18th edition

VOLUME 1

CECIL TEXTBOOK OF MEDICINE

Edited by

JAMES B. WYNGAARDEN, M.D.

Director, National Institutes of Health,
Bethesda, Maryland

LLOYD H. SMITH, Jr., M.D.

Professor of Medicine and Associate Dean,
University of California, San Francisco, School of Medicine,
San Francisco, California

1988

W. B. SAUNDERS COMPANY

Harcourt Brace Jovanovich, Inc.

Philadelphia/London/Toronto/Montreal/Sydney/Tokyo

W. B. SAUNDERS COMPANY
Harcourt Brace Jovanovich, Inc.

West Washington Square
Philadelphia, PA 19105

Library of Congress Cataloging-in-Publication Data

Textbook of medicine.

Published simultaneously as 1 v. and as a 2 v. set.

Includes bibliographies and index.

1. Internal medicine. I. Cecil, Russell L. (Russell La Fayette), 1881–1965. II. Wyngaarden, James B., 1924– . III. Smith, Lloyd H., 1924– . IV. Title: Cecil textbook of medicine. [DNLM: 1. Medicine. WB 100 T354]

RC46.T35 1988 616 86–27980

ISBN 0–7216–1848–0 (single v.)
ISBN 0–7216–1851–0 (set)
ISBN 0–7216–1849–9 (v. 1)
ISBN 0–7216–1850–2 (v. 2)

Acquisition Editor: John Dyson

Designer: Lorraine B. Kilmer

Production Manager: Frank Polizzano

Manuscript Editor: Donna Walker

Indexer: Nancy Guenther

CECIL TEXTBOOK OF MEDICINE

ISBN 0–7216–1848–0 Single Volume
ISBN 0–7216–1849–9 Volume 1
ISBN 0–7216–1850–2 Volume 2
ISBN 0–7216–1851–0 Set

Last digit is the print number: 9 8 7 6 5 4 3 2 1

DOSAGE NOTICE

Every effort has been made by the authors, the editors, and the publisher of this book to ensure that dosage recommendations are precise and in agreement with the standards of practice accepted at the time of publication.

However, dosage schedules are changed from time to time in the light of accumulating clinical experience and continuing laboratory studies. This is most likely to occur in the case of recently introduced products.

We urge, therefore, that you check the package information data for the manufacturer's recommended dosage to be certain that changes have not been made in the recommended dose or in the contraindications for administration. In addition, there are some quite serious situations in which drug therapy must be individualized and expert judgment advises the use of a higher dosage or administration by a different route than is included in the manufacturer's recommendations. Throughout the text examples of such instances are indicated by a footnote.

THE EDITORS

PREFACE

Medicine is forever mutable. Although certain general principles remain, medical science moves on. Changes in medical practice follow—not in continuous flow, it is true, but nevertheless in rapid sequence. The pace has quickened as we approach the last decade of the twentieth century. New technologies have revolutionized molecular genetics, neurobiology, immunology, cell biology, and structural biology; the application of these disciplines to all branches of the traditional biomedical sciences proceeds apace. The structure of DNA was elucidated only a generation ago. Now it can be confidently predicted that the whole human genome of approximately three billion nucleotide base pairs (the information equivalent to a thousand large telephone books) will be sequenced within the next decade. The language of the new biology has already permeated medicine. Beyond these contributions from the biological sciences, new applications of the physical and mathematical sciences, especially in diagnostic imaging (CT, MRI, PET, sonography) and in the use of the computer, have radically altered medical practice. In such a climate of change medical competence itself is mutable. It must be constantly renewed or else it will erode.

In order to reflect the best in medical practice, a major textbook of medicine must also be constantly renewed. In that spirit this edition of the *Cecil Textbook of Medicine* has been thoroughly revised, the 18th such revision in a span of more than 60 years. Approximately one third of the book is "new" in that different authors have been selected, in this way assuring that their chapters have been completely recast. All other chapters have been revised and updated by their current authors, carefully chosen authorities in their respective subjects. A revised *Cecil* must reflect the problems of the day. As an example, nowhere is this more apparent than in its attention to the acquired immunodeficiency syndrome (AIDS), the most dramatic medical epidemic of our time. In the 17th edition of *Cecil*, this new and baffling syndrome was described in a single chapter of two pages in the section on Diseases of the Immune System. In this current edition are new chapters on "Retroviruses That Cause Human Disease" (R. C. Gallo), "Acquired Immunodeficiency Syndrome" (J. E. Groopman), "AIDS Dementia and Human Immunodeficiency Virus Brain Infection" (R. W. Price), "Cryptosporidiosis" (R. Soave), and "Giardiasis" (D. P. Stevens), as well as expanded descriptions of other disorders that accompany AIDS—Kaposi's sarcoma, pneumocystosis, *Mycobacterium avium-intracellulare* infections, etc. Examples of other chapters reflecting areas of medical progress include "Natriuretic Factors" (P. Needleman) and the expanded treatment of "Slow Virus Infections of the Nervous System." Lyme disease has been transferred from being listed as a form of infectious arthritis and now receives more extensive discussion as a systemic disorder in the section on Spirochetal Diseases. New chapters have been added on "Clinical Decision Making" (S. G. Pauker), "Control of Unintended Injuries and Those Due to Violence" (S. B. Hulley), and "The Health of the Physician" (L. H. Clever). All of these and many other changes throughout the 18th edition, including updated and annotated references, are designed to maintain the traditional theme of *Cecil* as providing "authoritative clinical guidance and a reasoned, scientific basis for the pursuit of medicine."

In this 18th edition the reader will note a major change in format, the first use of color in *Cecil* (other than that of color plates to illustrate specific entities). The introduction of this single additional color is designed to add clarity to headings and figures throughout the book. This innovation is part of a continuing program to make the book more attractive and easier to use.

Cecil not only stands alone; it is also the senior member of an extended family. Four current books are linked to the *Cecil Textbook of Medicine* by design, format, and editorial responsibility. *Cecil Essentials of Medicine* (edited by T. E. Andreoli, C. C. J. Carpenter, F. Plum, and L. H. Smith, Jr.) offers a more abbreviated description of the realm of internal medicine. Designed primarily for the medical student, for whom the authoritative compendium of *Cecil* may sometimes seem formidable, it does not attempt to be complete. Nevertheless it serves as a useful entry guide into the study of medicine. *Review of General Internal Medicine* (edited by the editors of *Cecil*) has appeared in a 4th edition in parallel with this 18th edition of *Cecil*. As before, its 1200 questions and answers are designed to be of general educational benefit as well as to reinforce the value of *Cecil* as a reference text. *Pathophysiology: The Biological Principles of Disease* (edited by L. H. Smith, Jr., and S. O. Thier) gives a more extensive description of the scientific basis of medical practice than can be contained within a book such as *Cecil*, which must devote most of its attention to the practicalities of clinical description, diagnosis, prognosis, and therapy. *Medical Microbiology and Infectious Diseases* (edited by the late A. I. Braude) gives a more extensive description of the world's experience with the infectious and parasitic diseases.

Editing a major textbook is a complex task, as one attempts to balance content, format, style, integration, and innovation. The editors have been privileged to work with an admirable group of colleagues in this shared responsibility. Fred Plum has continued in his role as Editor for Neurologic and Behavioral Diseases. We welcome Thomas W. Smith as our new Consulting Editor for Cardiovascular Diseases. He joins a seasoned team of fellow Consulting Editors: Thomas E. Andreoli (Renal Diseases), Charles C. J. Carpenter (Infectious Diseases), Robert J. Lefkowitz (Therapeutics), John F. Murray (Respiratory Diseases), David G. Nathan (Hematologic and Hematopoietic Diseases), William E. Paul (Immunology), and Marvin H. Sleisenger (Diseases of the Digestive System). The Consulting Editors continually review their respective sections of this complex book and bring us their ideas and expertise concerning modifications. Our special gratitude is extended to the 325 contributors who have written the 543 chapters that collectively comprise this 18th edition. The ultimate value and authenticity of *Cecil* lies not with the editors but with the scholarship and experience that these individual physicians and scientists have brought to this joint enterprise.

"Language is the armoury of the human mind; and at once contains the trophies of its past, and the weapons of its future conquests." The weaponry of language, in Coleridge's image above, does not always come fully burnished in submitted manuscripts. As in the 17th edition, we have been most fortunate to work with seasoned editorial assistants in Bethesda (Margaret Quinlan) and in San Francisco (Judith Serrell), without whose dedication and skill this large project could not have been completed. At W. B. Saunders Company, Lorraine Kilmer, Donna Walker, and Frank Polizzano carried out with experienced professionalism the intricate task of formatting, editing, and assembling the book, made more complex this time by the use of color. The overall editor at the W. B. Saunders Company for this 18th edition of *Cecil* was John Dyson, who has been an invaluable guide, colleague, and good friend. We are deeply indebted to him for his extensive contributions in bringing to completion this 18th edition of a venerable book.

JAMES B. WYNGAARDEN, M.D.
LLOYD H. SMITH, JR., M.D.

CONTRIBUTORS

FRANCOIS M. ABBOUD, M.D.

Professor of Internal Medicine and of Physiology and Biophysics, University of Iowa College of Medicine. Head, Department of Internal Medicine, University of Iowa Hospitals and Clinics, Iowa City, Iowa.

Shock

DAVID H. ALPERS, M.D.

Professor of Medicine and Chief, Division of Gastroenterology, Washington University School of Medicine. Physician, Barnes Hospital; Consultant, Jewish Hospital of St. Louis, St. Louis, Missouri.

Principles of Nutritional Support: Enteral Nutritional Therapy

DAVID F. ALTMAN, M.D.

Associate Clinical Professor of Medicine and Associate Dean, University of California, San Francisco, School of Medicine. Attending Physician and Director, Gastroenterology Clinic, University of California Medical Center, San Francisco, California.

Food Poisoning; Diseases of the Rectum and Anus

WILLIAM J. C. AMEND, Jr., M.D.

Clinical Professor of Medicine and Surgery, University of California, San Francisco, School of Medicine. Attending Physician, Moffitt Hospital, San Francisco, California.

Renal Transplantation

W. FRENCH ANDERSON, M.D.

Chairman, Department of Medicine and Physiology, National Institutes of Health Graduate Program; Adjunct Professor, Graduate Genetics Program, George Washington University, Washington, D.C. Attending and Admitting Physician, Clinical Center, National Institutes of Health, Bethesda, Maryland.

Expectations from Recombinant DNA Research

THOMAS E. ANDREOLI, M.D.

Edward Randall, III Professor and Chairman, Department of Internal Medicine, University of Texas Medical School at Houston. Chief of Medicine, Hermann Hospital; Consultant, M. D. Anderson Hospital, Houston Texas.

Approach to the Patient with Renal Disease; Disorders of Fluid Volume, Electrolytes, and Acid-Base Balance; The Posterior Pituitary

VINCENT T. ANDRIOLE, M.D.

Professor of Internal Medicine and Chief, Infectious Disease Section, Yale University School of Medicine. Attending Physician, Yale-New Haven Hospital, New Haven, Connecticut.

Urinary Tract Infections and Pyelonephritis

CLAUDE D. ARNAUD, M.D.

Professor of Medicine and Physiology, University of California, San Francisco, School of Medicine. Chief, Endocrine Unit, Veterans Administration Medical Center, San Francisco, California.

Mineral and Bone Homeostasis; The Parathyroid Glands, Hypercalcemia, and Hypocalcemia; The Ultimobranchial Cells and Calcitonin

BERNARD M. BABIOR, M.D., Ph.D.

Member, Department of Basic and Clinical Research, Scripps Clinic and Research Foundation. Staff Physician, Division of Hematology-Oncology, Cecil H. and Ida M. Green Hospital of Scripps Clinic, La Jolla, California.

Function of Neutrophils and Mononuclear Phagocytes; Disorders of Neutrophil Function

GEORGE M. BAER, D.V.M.

Chief, Rabies Laboratory, Viral and Rickettsial Zoonoses Branch, Centers for Disease Control, Atlanta, Georgia.

Rabies

GROVER C. BAGBY, Jr., M.D.

Professor of Medicine and Head, Division of Hematology and Medical Oncology, Oregon Health Sciences Center School of Medicine. Acting Chief, Section of Hematology-Oncology, Veterans Administration Medical Center, Portland, Oregon.

Leukopenia; Leukocytosis and Leukemoid Reactions

ROBERT W. BALOH, M.D.

Professor of Neurology, University of California, Los Angeles, UCLA School of Medicine. Staff Physician, UCLA Medical Center and UCLA Neuropsychiatric Institute, Los Angeles, California.

The Special Senses

H. J. M. BARNETT, M.D.

Professor of Neurology, University of Western Ontario. Staff Physician, Clinical Neurological Sciences, University Hospital; The Verschoyle P. Cronyn Scientific Director and Chief Executive Officer of the John P. Robarts Research Institute, London, Ontario, Canada.

Introduction to Cerebrovascular Diseases; Cerebral Ischemia and Infarction; Spontaneous Intracranial Hemorrhage

ROBERT B. BARON, M.D.

Assistant Clinical Professor of Medicine, University of California, San Francisco, School of Medicine. Director of Screening and Acute Care, University of California, San Francisco, Hospitals and Clinics, San Francisco, California.

Protein-Calorie Undernutrition

DAVID W. BARRY, M.D.

Adjunct Professor of Medicine, Duke University School of Medicine. Vice-President of Research, Wellcome Research Laboratories, Burroughs Wellcome Company. Staff Physician, University Hospital, Durham, North Carolina.

Antiviral Therapy

WILLIAM H. BARRY, M.D.

Nora Eccles Harrison Professor of Cardiology, University of Utah School of Medicine. Attending Cardiologist, University of Utah Hospital, Salt Lake City, Utah.

Cardiac Catheterization and Angiography

JOHN G. BARTLETT, M.D.

Professor of Medicine, Johns Hopkins University School of Medicine. Chief, Division of Infectious Diseases, Johns Hopkins Hospital, Baltimore, Maryland.

Lung Abscess; Clostridial Myonecrosis and Other Clostridial Diseases; Pseudomembranous Colitis; Botulism; Tetanus

MICHAEL BARZA, M.D.

Professor of Medicine, Tufts University School of Medicine. Attending Physician, Department of Medicine, Division of Geographic Medicine and Infectious Diseases, New England Medical Center, Boston, Massachusetts.

Diseases Caused by Pseudomonads; Listeriosis; Erysipeloid

DAVID A. BASS, M.D., D.Phil.

Professor of Medicine, Division of Infectious Diseases and Immunology, Bowman Gray School of Medicine of Wake Forest University. Attending Physician in Infectious Diseases, North Carolina Baptist Hospital, Winston-Salem, North Carolina.

Eosinophilic Syndromes

STEPHEN G. BAUM, M.D.

Professor of Medicine, Mount Sinai School of Medicine of the City University of New York. Director, Department of Medicine, Beth Israel Medical Center; Associate Chairman, Department of Medicine, Mount Sinai Hospital, New York, New York.

Mycoplasmal Infections; Adenovirus Diseases

JOHN D. BAXTER, M.D.

Professor of Medicine and of Biochemistry and Biophysics, University of California, San Francisco, School of Medicine. Director, Metabolic Research Unit, and Chief, Section of Endocrinology, Moffitt Hospital, San Francisco, California.

Principles of Endocrinology; Disorders of the Adrenal Cortex

WILLIAM S. BECK, M.D.

Professor of Medicine and Tutor in Biochemical Sciences, Harvard Medical School. Physician and Director, Hematology Research Laboratory, Massachusetts General Hospital, Boston, Massachusetts.

Megaloblastic Anemias

CHARLES E. BECKER, M.D.

Professor of Medicine, University of California, San Francisco, School of Medicine. Head, Division of Occupational Medicine and Toxicology, San Francisco General Hospital, San Francisco, California.

Principles of Occupational Medicine

DONALD P. BECKER, M.D.

Professor of Surgery/Neurosurgery, University of California, Los Angeles, UCLA School of Medicine. Chief, Neurosurgical Service, UCLA Medical Center, Los Angeles, California.

Injuries to the Head and Spine

MICHAEL D. BENDER, M.D.

Associate Clinical Professor of Medicine, University of California, San Francisco, School of Medicine. Chief of Medicine and Director of Medical Education, Peninsula Hospital and Medical Center, Burlingame, California.

Diseases of the Peritoneum; Diseases of the Mesentery and Omentum

PAUL E. BENDHEIM, M.D.

Attending Neurologist and Head, Laboratory of Degenerative Neurologic Diseases, Department of Pathological Neurobiology, New York State Institute for Basic Research, Staten Island, New York.

Creutzfeldt-Jakob Disease

J. CLAUDE BENNETT, M.D.

Chairman and Professor, Department of Medicine, University of Alabama at Birmingham. Physician-in-Chief, University of Alabama Hospitals, Birmingham, Alabama.

Rheumatoid Arthritis

PAUL D. BERK, M.D.

Albert A. and Vera G. List Professor of Medicine and Chief, Division of Hematology, Mount Sinai School of Medicine of the City University of New York. Attending Physician, Mount Sinai Hospital and Bronx Veterans Administration Medical Center, New York, New York.

Erythrocytosis and Polycythemia; Myeloproliferative Disorders

J. THOMAS BIGGER, Jr., M.D.

Professor of Medicine and of Pharmacology, Columbia University College of Physicians and Surgeons. Attending Physician, Presbyterian Hospital in the City of New York; Director, Arrhythmia Control Unit, Columbia-Presbyterian Medical Center, New York, New York.

Cardiac Arrhythmias

DANIEL D. BIKLE, M.D., Ph.D.

Associate Professor of Medicine, University of California, San Francisco, School of Medicine. Co-Director, Special Diagnostic and Treatment Unit, Veterans Administration Medical Center; Attending Endocrinologist, University of California, San Francisco, Hospitals and Clinics, San Francisco, California.

Vitamin D; Osteomalacia and Rickets

J. MICHAEL BISHOP, M.D.

Professor of Medicine and Director, The G. W. Hooper Foundation, University of California, San Francisco, School of Medicine, San Francisco, California.

Oncogenes

ALAN L. BISNO, M.D.

Professor, Department of Medicine, Division of Infectious Diseases, University of Tennessee College of Medicine. Attending Physician, Memphis Regional Medical Center and University of Tennessee Medical Center; Consulting Physician, Baptist Memorial Hospital, Memphis, Tennessee.

Rheumatic Fever

D. MONTGOMERY BISSELL, M.D.

Professor of Medicine, University of California, San Francisco, School of Medicine. Attending Physician, University of California, San Francisco, Hospitals and San Francisco General Hospital Medical Center, San Francisco, California.

Porphyria

DANIEL S. BLUMENTHAL, M.D., M.P.H.

Professor and Chairman, Department of Community Health and Preventive Medicine, Morehouse School of Medicine. Attending Physician, Hughes Spalding Medical Center, Atlanta, Georgia.

Intestinal Nematodes; Angiostrongyliasis

GILES G. BOLE, M.D.

Professor of Internal Medicine, Associate Dean for Clinical Affairs, and Senior Associate Dean, University of Michigan Medical School. Attending Physician, University of Michigan Hospitals; Consultant, Ann Arbor Veterans Administration Hospital, Ann Arbor, Michigan.

Diseases Associated with Arthritis; Miscellaneous Forms of Arthritis; Nonarticular Rheumatism; Synovial Tumors

THOMAS D. BOYER, M.D.

Associate Professor of Medicine, University of California, San Francisco, School of Medicine. Chief of Gastroenterology, Veterans Administration Medical Center, San Francisco, California.

Cirrhosis of the Liver; Major Sequelae of Cirrhosis

PHILIP S. BRACHMAN, M.D.

Professor, Master of Public Health Program, Department of Community Health, Emory University School of Medicine, Atlanta, Georgia.

Anthrax

JEROME S. BRODY, M.D.

Professor of Medicine and Director of Pulmonary Center, Boston University School of Medicine. Staff Physician, University Hospital and Boston City Hospital, Boston, Massachusetts.

Diseases of the Pleura, Mediastinum, Diaphragm, and Chest Wall

PHILIP A. BRUNELL, M.D.

Professor of Pediatrics, The University of Texas Medical School at San Antonio. Attending Physician, Medical Center Hospital and Santa Rosa Medical Center, San Antonio, Texas.

Varicella

JOHN D. BRUNZELL, M.D.

Professor of Medicine, University of Washington School of Medicine. Attending Physician, University Hospital, Seattle, Washington.

The Hyperlipoproteinemias

REBECCA H. BUCKLEY, M.D.

J. Buren Sidbury Professor of Pediatrics and Professor of Immunology, Duke University School of Medicine. Chief, Division of Allergy and Immunology, Department of Pediatrics, Duke University Medical Center, Durham, North Carolina.

Primary Immunodeficiency Diseases

WARD E. BULLOCK, M.D.

Arthur Russell Morgan Professor of Medicine and Director, Division of Infectious Diseases, University of Cincinnati College of Medicine, Cincinnati, Ohio.

Leprosy

PAUL A. BUNN, Jr., M.D.

Professor of Medicine and Head, Division of Medical Oncology, University of Colorado School of Medicine. Head, Division of Medical Oncology, University Hospital, Denver, Colorado.

Paraneoplastic Syndromes; Tumor Markers

DAVID M. BURNS, M.D.

Associate Professor of Medicine, University of California, San Diego, School of Medicine, La Jolla. Medical Director, Department of Respiratory Therapy, Division of Pulmonary and Critical Care Medicine, University of California Medical Center, San Diego, California.

Tobacco and Health

THOMAS BUTLER, M.D.

Associate Professor of Medicine, Case Western Reserve University School of Medicine. Attending Physician, University Hospitals of Cleveland, Cleveland, Ohio.

Typhoid Fever; Shigellosis; Yersinia Infections; Nonsyphilitic Treponematoses; Relapsing Fever

JOEL N. BUXBAUM, M.D.

Professor of Medicine, New York University School of Medicine. Chief, Rheumatology Section, Veterans Administration Medical Center; Attending Physician, Bellevue Hospital, New York, New York.

The Amyloid Diseases

PETER H. BYERS, M.D.

Professor, Departments of Pathology and Medicine (Medical Genetics), University of Washington School of Medicine, Seattle, Washington.

The Marfan Syndrome; The Ehlers-Danlos Syndrome

ANDREI CALIN, M.D.

Consultant Rheumatologist, Royal National Hospital for Rheumatic Diseases, Bath, Ireland.

The Spondyloarthropathies

CHARLES C. J. CARPENTER, M.D.

Professor of Medicine, Brown University Program in Medicine. Physician-in-Chief, Miriam Hospital, Providence, Rhode Island.

Introduction to Microbial Diseases

JOHN P. CELLO, M.D.

Associate Professor of Medicine, University of California, San Francisco, School of Medicine. Chief of Gastroenterology, San Francisco General Hospital Medical Center, San Francisco, California.

Carcinoma of the Pancreas

BRUCE A. CHABNER, M.D.

Director, Division of Cancer Treatment, National Cancer Institute, National Institutes of Health, Bethesda, Maryland.

Principles of Cancer Therapy

ROBERT M. CHANOCK, M.D.

Chief, Laboratory of Infectious Diseases, National Institute of Allergy and Infectious Diseases, National Institutes of Health, Bethesda, Maryland.

Respiratory Syncytial Virus; Parainfluenza Viral Diseases

BAYARD CLARKSON, M.D.

Professor of Medicine, Cornell University Medical College. Chief, Hematology/Lymphoma Service, Department of Medicine, Memorial Hospital for Cancer and Allied Diseases, New York, New York.

The Chronic Leukemias

LINDA HAWES CLEVER, M.D.

Clinical Professor of Medicine, University of California, San Francisco, School of Medicine. Chairman, Department of Occupational Health, Presbyterian Hospital of Pacific Presbyterian Medical Center, San Francisco, California.

The Health of the Physician

RAY E. CLOUSE, M.D.

Assistant Professor of Medicine, Washington University School of Medicine. Assistant Physician, Barnes Hospital, St. Louis, Missouri.

Parenteral Nutrition

CHARLES G. COCHRANE, M.D.

Adjunct Professor of Pathology, University of California, San Diego, School of Medicine. Member, Department of Immunology, Research Institute of Scripps Clinic, La Jolla, California.

Immune Complex Diseases

MARTIN G. COGAN, M.D.

Associate Professor of Medicine and Associate Staff Member, Cardiovascular Research Institute, University of California, San Francisco, School of Medicine. Attending Physician and Medical Director, Acute Hemodialysis Unit, Moffitt-Long Hospitals, San Francisco, California.

Specific Renal Tubular Disorders

ALAN S. COHEN, M.D.

Conrad Wesselhoeft Professor of Medicine, Boston University School of Medicine. Chief of Medicine and Director, Thorndike Memorial Laboratory, Boston City Hospital, Boston, Massachusetts.

Specialized Diagnostic Procedures in the Rheumatic Diseases

JORDAN J. COHEN, M.D.

Professor and Associate Chairman of Medicine, University of Chicago Pritzker School of Medicine. Chairman of Medicine, Michael Reese Hospital and Medical Center, Chicago, Illinois.

Vascular Disorders of the Kidney

LAWRENCE S. COHEN, M.D.

The Ebenezer K. Hunt Professor of Medicine, Yale University School of Medicine. Attending Physician, Yale-New Haven Hospital, New Haven, Connecticut.

Diseases of the Aorta

WILLIAM G. COUSER, M.D.

Professor of Medicine, University of Washington School of Medicine. Head, Division of Nephrology, University Hospital, Seattle, Washington.

Glomerular Disorders

JAMES D. CRAPO, M.D.

Professor of Medicine, Duke University School of Medicine. Chief, Division of Allergy, Critical Care and Respiratory Medicine, Duke University Medical Center, Durham, North Carolina.

Physical, Chemical, and Aspiration Injuries of the Lung

PHILIP E. CRYER, M.D.

Professor of Medicine and Director, Metabolism Division, Washington University School of Medicine. Physician, Barnes Hospital, St. Louis, Missouri.

The Adrenal Medulla and The Sympathetic Nervous System; The Carcinoid Syndrome

RONALD G. CRYSTAL, M.D.

Chief, Pulmonary Branch, National Heart, Lung and Blood Institute, National Institutes of Health, Bethesda, Maryland.

Interstitial Lung Disease

ANTONIO R. DAMASIO, M.D.

Professor and Head of Neurology, University of Iowa College of Medicine. Attending Neurologist, University of Iowa Hospitals and Clinics, Iowa City, Iowa.

Regional Diagnosis of Cerebral Disorders; Focal Disturbances of Higher Functions

RONALD P. DANIELE, M.D.

Professor of Medicine and Pathology, University of Pennsylvania School of Medicine. Attending Physician and Director of the Interstitial Lung Disease Program, Hospital of the University of Pennsylvania, Philadelphia, Pennsylvania.

Asthma

MICHAEL DECK, M.B., B.S.

Professor of Clinical Radiology, Cornell University Medical College. Attending Radiologist, Chief of Neuroradiology, and Vice-Chairman, Department of Radiology, New York Hospital, New York, New York.

Radiologic Imaging of the Neurologic Patient

ANDREW DEISS, M.D.

Associate Professor of Medicine, University of Utah School of Medicine. Associate Chief of Staff for Research and Development, Veterans Administration Medical Center, Salt Lake City, Utah.

Wilson's Disease

VINCENT W. DENNIS, M.D.

Professor of Medicine, Duke University School of Medicine. Chief, Division of Nephrology, Duke University Medical Center, Durham, North Carolina.

Investigations of Renal Function

IVAN DIAMOND, M.D., Ph.D.

Director, Ernest Gallo Clinic and Research Center; Vice- Chairman and Professor, Department of Neurology, and Professor of Pediatrics and Pharmacology, University of California, San Francisco, School of Medicine. Attending Neurologist, University of California, San Francisco, Hospitals, San Francisco General Hospital Medical Center, and Veterans Administration Medical Center, San Francisco, California.

Nutritional Disorders of the Nervous System

CHARLES A. DINARELLO, M.D.

Professor of Medicine and Pediatrics, Tufts University School of Medicine. Physician, New England Medical Center Hospital, Boston, Massachusetts.

Pathogenesis of Fever; The Acute Phase Response

RAPHAEL DOLIN, M.D.

Professor of Medicine, University of Rochester School of Medicine and Dentistry. Head, Infectious Diseases Unit, University of Rochester Medical Center and Strong Memorial Hospital, Rochester, New York.

Enteroviral Diseases

R. GORDON DOUGLAS, Jr., M.D.

E. Hugh Luckey Distinguished Professor in Medicine and Chairman, Department of Medicine, Cornell University Medical College. Physician-in-Chief, New York Hospital, New York, New York.

Immunization; Introduction to Viral Diseases; Influenza; Herpes Simplex Virus Infections

DOUGLAS A. DROSSMAN, M.D.

Associate Professor of Medicine and Psychiatry, University of North Carolina at Chapel Hill School of Medicine. Attending Physician, North Carolina Memorial Hospital, Chapel Hill, North Carolina.

The Eating Disorders

DAVID J. DRUTZ, M.D.

Adjunct Professor of Medicine, University of Pennsylvania School of Medicine. Vice-President, Biological Sciences, Smith Kline & French Laboratories, Philadelphia, Pennsylvania.

Actinomycosis; Nocardiosis; The Mycoses

DAVID T. DURACK, M.B., D.Phil.

Professor of Medicine, Microbiology and Immunology, Duke University School of Medicine. Chief, Division of Infectious Diseases, Duke University Medical Center, Durham, North Carolina.

Pneumococcal Pneumonia; Infective Endocarditis

THEODORE C. EICKHOFF, M.D.

Professor of Medicine, University of Colorado School of Medicine. Director of Internal Medicine, Presbyterian-Saint Luke's Medical Center, Denver, Colorado.

Bartonellosis; Trench Fever; Q Fever; Colorado Tick Fever

RONALD J. ELIN, M.D., Ph.D.

Clinical Professor of Pathology, Uniformed Services University of the Health Sciences School of Medicine. Chief, Clinical Chemistry Service and Clinical Pathology Department, Clinical Center, National Institutes of Health, Bethesda, Maryland.

Reference Intervals and Laboratory Values of Clinical Importance

EDWARD A. EMMETT, M.B., M.S.

Professor and Director, Division of Occupational Medicine, Johns Hopkins Medical Institutions. Staff Physician, Johns Hopkins Hospital; Consulting Physician, Wyman Park Medical Center, Baltimore, Maryland.

Occupational Diseases of the Skin

ANDREW G. ENGEL, M.D.

William L. McKnight-3M Professor of Neuroscience, Mayo Medical School. Attending Physician, St. Mary's Hospital and Rochester Methodist Hospital, Rochester, Minnesota.

Diseases of Muscle and Neuromuscular Junction

JEROME ENGEL, Jr., M.D., Ph.D.

Professor of Neurology and Anatomy, University of California, Los Angeles, UCLA School of Medicine. Attending Neurologist and Chief of Clinical Neurophysiology Laboratories, UCLA Center for Health Sciences and UCLA Neuropsychiatric Institute, Los Angeles, California.

The Epilepsies

STANLEY FAHN, M.D.

H. Houston Merritt Professor of Neurology, Columbia University College of Physicians and Surgeons. Attending Neurologist, Neurological Institute of New York and Presbyterian Hospital in the City of New York, New York, New York.

The Extrapyramidal Disorders

DOUGLAS V. FALLER, Ph.D., M.D.

Assistant Professor, Harvard Medical School. Assistant Physician, Dana Farber Cancer Institute; Assistant in Medicine, Children's Hospital, Boston, Massachusetts.

Diseases of the Spleen

BARRY L. FANBURG, M.D.

Professor of Medicine, Tufts University School of Medicine. Chief of Pulmonary Division, Department of Medicine, New England Medical Center, Boston, Massachusetts.

Sarcoidosis

ANTHONY S. FAUCI, M.D.

Director, National Institute of Allergy and Infectious Diseases, National Institutes of Health, Bethesda, Maryland.

Glucocorticosteroid Therapy

DOUGLAS T. FEARON, M.D.

Professor of Medicine and of Molecular Biology and Genetics, Johns Hopkins University School of Medicine. Director, Division of Molecular and Clinical Rheumatology, Johns Hopkins Hospital, Baltimore, Maryland.

Complement

MARK FELDMAN, M.D.

Professor, Department of Internal Medicine, University of Texas Health Science Center at Dallas. Associate Chief of Staff for Research and Development, Veterans Administration Medical Center, Dallas, Texas.

Peptic Ulcer: Complications

PHILIP J. FIALKOW, M.D.

Professor and Chairman, Department of Medicine, University of Washington School of Medicine. Physician-in-Chief, University Hospital; Attending Physician, Harborview Medical Center, Seattle, Washington.

Clonal Development and Stem Cell Origin of Proliferative Disorders

DANIEL B. FISHBEIN, M.D.

Medical Epidemiologist, Viral and Rickettsial Zoonoses Branch, Centers for Disease Control, Atlanta, Georgia.

Rabies

ALFRED P. FISHMAN, M.D.

William Maul Measey Professor of Medicine, University of Pennsylvania School of Medicine. Attending Physician, Hospital of the University of Pennsylvania, Philadelphia, Pennsylvania.

Pulmonary Hypertension

GARRETT A. FITZGERALD, M.D.

Professor of Medicine and of Pharmacology, Vanderbilt University School of Medicine. Attending Physician, Department of Medicine and S.C.O.R. in Hypertension, Vanderbilt University Medical Center, Nashville, Tennessee.

Prostaglandins and Related Compounds

KATHLEEN M. FOLEY, M.D.

Associate Professor of Neurology and Pharmacology, Cornell University Medical College. Associate Attending Neurologist and Chief, Pain Service, Memorial Sloan-Kettering Cancer Center, New York, New York.

Pain and Its Management

BERNARD G. FORGET, M.D.

Professor of Medicine and Human Genetics; Chief of Hematology Section, Department of Medicine, Yale University School of Medicine. Attending Physician, Yale-New Haven Hospital, New Haven, Connecticut.

Sickle Cell Anemia and Associated Hemoglobinopathies

DAVID W. FRASER, M.D.

President, Swarthmore College, Swarthmore, Pennsylvania. Adjunct Professor of Medicine, University of Pennsylvania School of Medicine, Philadelphia, Pennsylvania.

Legionellosis

F. CLARKE FRASER, Ph.D., M.D.

Professor of Clinical Genetics, Departments of Biology and Pediatrics and the McGill Centre for Human Genetics, McGill University Faculty of Medicine. Medical Geneticist, Montreal Children's Hospital, Montreal, Quebec, Canada.

Genetic Counseling

JOSEPH F. FRAUMENI, Jr., M.D.

Associate Director for Epidemiology and Biostatistics, National Cancer Institute, National Institutes of Health. Adjunct Professor of Epidemiology, Department of Preventive Medicine and Biometrics, Uniformed Services University of the Health Sciences School of Medicine, Bethesda, Maryland.

Epidemiology of Cancer

WILLIAM T. FRIEDEWALD, M.D.

Associate Director for Disease Prevention, National Institutes of Health, Bethesda, Maryland.

Epidemiology of Cardiovascular Disease

GARY D. FRIEDMAN, M.D., M.S.

Assistant Director for Epidemiology and Biostatistics, Division of Research, Kaiser Permanente Medical Care Program, Oakland, California. Associate Clinical Professor of Medicine and of Family and Community Medicine, University of California, San Francisco, School of Medicine, San Francisco; Lecturer in Epidemiology, School of Public Health, University of California, Berkeley, California.

The Preventive Health Examination

JAMES F. FRIES, M.D.

Associate Professor of Medicine, Stanford University School of Medicine, Stanford, California.

Approach to the Patient with Musculoskeletal Disease

LAWRENCE A. FROHMAN, M.D.

Professor of Medicine, University of Cincinnati College of Medicine. Director, Division of Endocrinology and Metabolism, and Director, General Clinical Research Center, University of Cincinnati Medical Center, Cincinnati, Ohio.

Neuroendocrine Regulation and Its Disorders; The Anterior Pituitary

PATRICIA A. GABOW, M.D.

Associate Professor of Medicine, University of Colorado School of Medicine. Director, Medical Services, Denver General Hospital, Denver, Colorado.

Cystic Disease of the Kidney

ROBERT C. GALLO, M.D.

Chief, Laboratory of Tumor Cell Biology, National Cancer Institute, National Institutes of Health, Bethesda, Maryland.

Retroviruses That Cause Human Disease

JEFFREY A. GELFAND, M.D.

Associate Professor, Division of Geographic Medicine and Infectious Diseases, Department of Medicine, Tufts University School of Medicine. Physician, New England Medical Center Hospital, Boston, Massachusetts.

Advice to Travelers

JOHN W. GITTINGER, Jr., M.D.

Professor of Surgery and Neurology and Chairman, Division of Ophthalmology, University of Massachusetts Medical School. Chief of Ophthalmology, University of Massachusetts Medical Center, Worcester, Massachusetts.

Eye Diseases

JOHN H. GLICK, M.D.

Professor of Medicine, University of Pennsylvania School of Medicine; Director, University of Pennsylvania Cancer Center. Attending Physician, Hospital of the University of Pennsylvania, Philadelphia, Pennsylvania.

Hodgkin's Disease

SHERWOOD L. GORBACH, M.D.

Professor of Medicine and Community Health, Tufts University School of Medicine. Attending Physician, New England Medical Center Hospital, Boston, Massachusetts.

Diseases Caused by Non–Spore-Forming Anaerobic Bacteria

JARED J. GRANTHAM, M.D.

Professor of Medicine and Director, Nephrology Division, University of Kansas College of Health Sciences and Hospital School of Medicine, Kansas City, Kansas.

Acute Renal Failure

BRUCE M. GREENE, M.D.

Associate Professor of Medicine, Case Western Reserve University School of Medicine. Associate Chief, Division of Geographic Medicine, University Hospitals of Cleveland, Cleveland, Ohio.

Onchocerciasis

JOSEPH C. GREENFIELD, M.D.

James B. Duke Professor and Chairman, Department of Medicine, Duke University School of Medicine. Chief, Division of Cardiology, Duke University Medical Center, Durham, North Carolina.

Electrocardiography

JAMES H. GRENDELL, M.D.

Assistant Professor of Medicine and Physiology, University of California, San Francisco, School of Medicine. Attending Physician, San Francisco General Hospital Medical Center, San Francisco, California.

Vascular Diseases of the Intestine

JEROME E. GROOPMAN, M.D.

Associate Professor of Medicine, Harvard Medical School. Attending Physician and Chief of Hematology/Oncology, Department of Medicine, New England Deaconess Hospital, Boston, Massachusetts.

Langerhans Cell Granulomatosis; The Acquired Immunodeficiency Syndrome

CARL GRUNFELD, M.D., Ph.D.

Associate Professor of Medicine, University of California, San Francisco, School of Medicine. Co-Director, Special Diagnostic and Treatment Unit, Veterans Administration Medical Center, San Francisco, California.

Pancreatic Islet Cell Tumors

RICHARD L. GUERRANT, M.D.

Professor of Medicine and Head, Division of Geographic Medicine, University of Virginia School of Medicine. Attending Physician, University of Virginia Hospital, Charlottesville, Virginia.

Campylobacter Enteritis; Enteric Escherichia coli *Infections*

JOHN L. HAMERTON, D.Sc.

Professor of Human Genetics and Pediatrics, University of Manitoba Faculty of Medicine. Scientific Staff, Health Sciences Centre and St. Boniface General Hospital, Winnipeg, Manitoba, Canada.

Chromosomes and Their Disorders

DONALD H. HARTER, M.D.

Benjamin and Virginia T. Boshes Professor of Neurology, Northwestern University Medical School. Attending Neurologist, Northwestern Memorial Hospital, Chicago, Illinois.

Parameningeal Infections

WILLIAM L. HASKELL, Ph.D.

Associate Professor of Medicine, Stanford University School of Medicine, Stanford, California.

Exercise and Health

BARTON F. HAYNES, M.D.

Professor of Medicine and Chief, Division of Rheumatology and Immunology, Duke University School of Medicine, Durham, North Carolina.

Wegener's Granulomatosis and Midline Granuloma

JOHN P. HAYSLETT, M.D.

Professor of Medicine and Chief, Section of Nephrology, Yale University School of Medicine. Attending Physician, Yale-New Haven Hospital, New Haven, Connecticut.

Renal Disease in Pregnancy

LOUIS A. HEALEY, M.D.

Clinical Professor of Medicine, University of Washington School of Medicine. Attending Physician, Virginia Mason Hospital, Seattle, Washington.

Polymyalgia Rheumatica and Giant Cell Arteritis

BERNADINE P. HEALY, M.D.

Chairman, Research Institute, Cleveland Clinic Foundation, Cleveland, Ohio.

Miscellaneous Conditions of the Heart: Tumor, Trauma, and Systemic Disease

DONALD A. HENDERSON, M.D., M.P.H.

Dean and Professor of Epidemiology and International Health, Johns Hopkins School of Hygiene and Public Health, Baltimore, Maryland.

Variola and Vaccinia

ERIK L. HEWLETT, M.D.

Professor of Medicine and Pharmacology and Head, Division of Clinical Pharmacology, University of Virginia School of Medicine. Attending Physician, University of Virginia Hospital, Charlottesville, Virginia.

Diphtheria

J. ALLAN HOBSON, M.D.

Professor of Psychiatry, Harvard Medical School. Principal Psychiatrist, Massachusetts Mental Health Center, Boston, Massachusetts.

Sleep and Its Disorders

EDWARD W. HOLMES, M.D.

Professor of Medicine and Associate Professor of Biochemistry, Duke University School of Medicine. Chief of Metabolism, Endocrinology, and Genetics, Department of Medicine, Duke University Hospital, Durham, North Carolina.

Disorders of Purine Metabolism

LEWIS B. HOLMES, M.D.

Associate Professor of Pediatrics, Harvard Medical School. Pediatrician and Chief, Embryology-Teratology Unit, Massachusetts General Hospital, Boston, Massachusetts.

Congenital Malformations

PHILIP C. HOPEWELL, M.D.

Professor of Medicine, University of California, San Francisco, School of Medicine. Associate Chief of Medical Service, San Francisco General Hospital Medical Center, San Francisco, California.

Critical Care Medicine

DONALD R. HOPKINS, M.D., M.P.H.

Deputy Director, Centers for Disease Control, Atlanta, Georgia.

Dracunculiasis

RICHARD B. HORNICK, M.D.

Professor of Medicine, University of Rochester School of Medicine and Dentistry. Attending Physician, Strong Memorial Hospital, Rochester, New York.

Salmonella Infections Other Than Typhoid Fever; Tularemia; Introduction to Rickettsial Diseases; The Typhus Group; Rocky Mountain Spotted Fever; Other Tick-Borne Rickettsioses; Rickettsialpox; Scrub Typhus

DONALD W. HOSKINS, M.D.

Clinical Associate Professor of Medicine, Divisions of International Medicine and Digestive Diseases, Department of Medicine, Cornell University Medical College. Vice-President of Medical Affairs and Attending Physician in Medicine, Doctors Hospital; Associate Attending Physician, New York Hospital, New York, New York.

Trichinellosis

DAVID S. HOWELL, M.D.

Professor of Medicine and Director of Arthritis Division, Department of Medicine, University of Miami School of Medicine; Medical Investigator, Veterans Administration Medical Center. Attending Physician, James M. Jackson Memorial Hospital, Miami, Florida.

Osteoarthritis; The Painful Shoulder; The Painful Back

R. RODNEY HOWELL, M.D.

David R. Park Professor and Chairman, Department of Pediatrics, University of Texas Health Science Center at Houston. Pediatrician-in-Chief, University Children's Hospital at Hermann; Consultant in Pediatrics, M. D. Anderson Hospital and Tumor Institute; Consultant in Pediatrics, Shriners Hospital for Crippled Children, Houston, Texas.

The Glycogen Storage Diseases; Pentosuria; Essential Fructosuria and Hereditary Fructose Intolerance

STEPHEN B. HULLEY, M.D., M.P.H.

Professor of Epidemiology, Medicine and Health Policy, University of California, San Francisco, School of Medicine. Director, Clinical Epidemiology Program, San Francisco General Hospital Medical Center, San Francisco, California.

Principles of Preventive Medicine; Control of Unintended Injuries and Those Due to Violence

JULIANNE IMPERATO-McGINLEY, M.D.

Associate Professor of Internal Medicine, Cornell University Medical College. Associate Attending Physician, New York Hospital, New York, New York.

Disorders of Sexual Differentiation

WALDEMAR G. JOHANSON, Jr., M.D.

Professor and Chairman, Department of Internal Medicine, University of Texas Medical School at Galveston. Full-time Active Staff Physician, University of Texas Medical Branch Hospitals, Galveston, Texas.

Introduction to Pneumonia; Pneumonia Caused by Aerobic Gram-Negative Bacilli; Recurrent Aspiration Pneumonia

KENNETH P. JOHNSON, M.D.

Professor and Chairman, Department of Neurology, University of Maryland School of Medicine. Attending Neurologist, University of Maryland Hospital, Kernan Hospital for Crippled Children, and Mercy Hospital; Staff Neurologist, Veterans Administration Medical Center, Baltimore, Maryland.

Syphilitic Infections of the Central Nervous System

ALBERT R. JONSEN, Ph.D.

Professor of Ethics in Medicine and Chief, Division of Medical Ethics, Department of Medicine, University of California, San Francisco, School of Medicine, San Francisco, California.

Ethics in the Practice of Medicine

JOHN P. KANE, M.D., Ph.D.

Professor of Medicine and of Biochemistry and Biophysics, University of California, San Francisco, School of Medicine. Attending Physician, University of California Hospitals, San Francisco, California.

The Judicious Diet

ALBERT Z. KAPIKIAN, M.D.

Head, Epidemiology Section, Laboratory of Infectious Diseases, National Institute of Allergy and Infectious Diseases, National Institutes of Health, Bethesda, Maryland.

The Common Cold; Viral Gastroenteritis

MANUEL E. KAPLAN, M.D.

Professor of Medicine, University of Minnesota Medical School. Chief of Hematology/Oncology, Veterans Administration Medical Center, Minneapolis, Minnesota.

Hemolytic Disorders: Introduction; Acquired Hemolytic Disorders

SAMUEL KAPLAN, M.D.

Professor of Pediatrics and of Medicine, University of Cincinnati College of Medicine. Director, Division of Cardiology, Children's Hospital Medical Center, Cincinnati, Ohio.

Congenital Heart Disease

SAMUEL L. KATZ, M.D.

Wilbert Cornell Davison Professor and Chairman, Department of Pediatrics, Duke University School of Medicine, Durham, North Carolina.

Whooping Cough; Measles; Rubella

ALAN S. KEITT, M.D.

Associate Professor of Pathology and Medicine, University of Florida College of Medicine. Director, Hematology Laboratories, Shands Teaching Hospital, Gainesville, Florida.

Introduction to the Anemias; Anemia Due to Bone Marrow Failure

ELLIOTT KIEFF, M.D., Ph.D.

Block Professor of Medicine and Molecular Genetics, University of Chicago Division of Biological Sciences Pritzker School of Medicine. Chief, Section on Infectious Diseases, University of Chicago Hospital, Chicago, Illinois.

Infectious Mononucleosis: Epstein-Barr Virus Infection

BENJAMIN KISSIN, M.D.

Professor Emeritus in Psychiatry, State University of New York Health Sciences Center at Brooklyn, Brooklyn, New York.

Alcohol Abuse and Alcohol-Related Illnesses

SAULO KLAHR, M.D.

Joseph Friedman Professor of Renal Disease and Director, Renal Division, Washington University School of Medicine. Physician, Barnes Hospital; Staff Physician and Consultant in Nephrology, Jewish Hospital of St. Louis, St. Louis, Missouri.

Structure and Function of the Kidneys

JAMES P. KNOCHEL, M.D.

Vice-Chairman and Professor of Internal Medicine, University of Texas Health Science Center at Dallas. Chief, Medical Service, Veterans Administration Medical Center; Senior Attending Physician, Parkland Memorial Hospital, Dallas, Texas.

Disorders Due to Heat and Cold

JUHA P. KOKKO, M.D., Ph.D.

Professor and Chairman, Department of Medicine, Emory University School of Medicine. Chief of Medicine, Emory University Hospital and Grady Memorial Hospital, Atlanta, Georgia.

Chronic Renal Failure

EDWIN H. KOLODNY, M.D.

Professor of Neurology, Harvard Medical School, Boston. Associate Neurologist, Massachusetts General Hospital, Boston; Consultant in Neurology, McLean Hospital, Belmont, Massachusetts.

Gaucher's Disease; Niemann-Pick Disease

HERMES A. KONTOS, M.D., Ph.D.

Professor of Medicine; Chairman, Division of Cardiology; and Vice-Chairman, Department of Medicine, Virginia Commonwealth University Medical College of Virginia School of Medicine, Richmond, Virginia.

Vascular Diseases of the Limbs

STEPHEN M. KRANE, M.D.

Professor of Medicine, Harvard Medical School. Chief of Arthritis Unit, Massachusetts General Hospital, Boston, Massachusetts.

Connective Tissue Structure and Function

RICHARD M. KRAUSE, M.D.

Dean and Robert W. Woodruff Professor of Medicine, Emory University School of Medicine, Atlanta, Georgia.

Streptococcal Diseases

GUENTER J. KREJS, M.D.

Professor and Chairman, Department of Medicine, Karl-Franzens-Universitat, Graz, Austria.

Diarrhea

WILLIAM L. KRINSKY, M.D., Ph.D.

Associate Professor of Epidemiology, Section of Medical Entomology, Yale University School of Medicine, New Haven, Connecticut.

Arthropods and Leeches

DONALD J. KROGSTAD, M.D.

Associate Professor of Medicine and Pathology, Washington University School of Medicine. Co-Director, Microbiology and Serology Laboratories, Barnes Hospital; Assistant Physician, Barnes Hospital and Jewish Hospital of St. Louis, St. Louis, Missouri.

Amebiasis

JAMES P. KUSHNER, M.D.

Professor of Medicine and Chief, Division of Hematology- Oncology, University of Utah School of Medicine. Attending Physician, University of Utah Hospital and Veterans Administration Medical Center, Salt Lake City, Utah.

Normochromic Normocytic Anemias; Hypochromic Anemias

SYLVIA A LACK, M.D.

Director, Chronic Pain Program, Gaylord Hospital, Wallingford. Attending Physician, Gaylord Hospital, Wallingford; World War II Memorial Hospital, Meriden; and Veterans Administration Medical Center, Newington; Consultant in Hospice Care, St. Mary's Hospital, Waterbury, Connecticut.

Care of Dying Patients and Their Families

DAVID J. LANG, M.D.

Professor of Pediatrics, University of Southern California School of Medicine, Los Angeles. Pediatrician-in-Chief and Director of Infectious Diseases, Children's Hospital of Orange County, Orange, California.

Cytomegalovirus Infection

P. REED LARSEN, M.D.

Professor of Medicine, Harvard Medical School. Senior Physician and Director, Thyroid Unit, Brigham and Women's Hospital; Investigator, Howard Hughes Medical Institute, Boston, Massachusetts.

The Thyroid

JOHN LASZLO, M.D.

Professor of Medicine (on leave), Duke University School of Medicine, Durham, North Carolina. Vice-President for Research, American Cancer Society, New York, New York.

Oncology: Introduction

ROBERT B. LAYZER, M.D.

Professor of Neurology, University of California, San Francisco, School of Medicine. Attending Neurologist, University of California, San Francisco, Hospitals and Clinics, San Francisco, California.

Degenerative Diseases of the Nervous System

GERALD M. LAZARUS, M.D.

Milton B. Hartzell Professor and Chairman, Department of Dermatology, University of Pennsylvania School of Medicine, Philadelphia, Pennsylvania.

Panniculitis and Disorders of the Subcutaneous Fat

ROBERT J. LEFKOWITZ, M.D.

James B. Duke Professor of Medicine, Duke University School of Medicine, Durham, North Carolina.

Pharmacologic Principles Related to the Autonomic Nervous System

E. CARWILE LeROY, M.D.

Professor of Medicine, Medical University of South Carolina College of Medicine. Attending Physician, Medical University Hospital, Charleston Memorial Hospital, and Veterans Administration Medical Center, Charleston, South Carolina.

Systemic Sclerosis

BERNARD LEVIN, M.D.

Professor of Medicine, University of Texas Health Science Center at Houston. Attending Physician, M. D. Anderson Hospital and Tumor Institute, Houston, Texas.

Ulcerative Colitis

MICHAEL D. LEVITT, M.D.

Professor of Medicine, University of Minnesota Medical School. Attending Gastroenterologist and Associate Chief of Staff for Research, Veterans Administration Medical Center, Minneapolis, Minnesota.

Pancreatitis

BRIAN J. LEWIS, M.D.

Clinical Professor of Medicine, University of California, San Francisco, School of Medicine. Attending Physician, Cancer Research Institute, University of California, San Francisco, Hospitals and Clinics, San Francisco, California.

Breast Cancer

ROBERT A. LEWIS, M.D.

Senior Vice-President and Director of Basic Research, Syntex Research, Palo Alto. Clinical Associate Professor of Medicine, Stanford University School of Medicine, Stanford, California.

Mastocytosis

LAWRENCE M. LICHTENSTEIN, M.D.

Professor of Medicine, Johns Hopkins University School of Medicine. Staff Physician, Good Samaritan Hospital, Baltimore, Maryland.

Anaphylaxis; Insect Sting Allergy

IRIS F. LITT, M.D.

Associate Professor, Department of Pediatrics, Stanford University School of Medicine. Director, Division of Adolescent Medicine, Stanford University Hospital and Children's Hospital at Stanford, Stanford, California.

Adolescent Medicine

JOHN N. LOEB, M.D.

Professor of Medicine, Columbia University College of Physicians and Surgeons. Attending Physician, Presbyterian Hospital in the City of New York, New York, New York.

Polyglandular Disorders

D. LYNN LORIAUX, M.D., Ph.D.

Clinical Director, National Institute of Child Health and Human Development, National Institutes of Health, Bethesda, Maryland.

Hirsutism

DONALD B. LOURIA, M.D.

Professor and Chairman, Department of Preventive Medicine and Community Health, University of Medicine and Dentistry of New Jersey–New Jersey Medical School, Newark, New Jersey.

Trace Metal Poisoning

ROBERT G. LUKE, M.B., Ch.B.

Professor of Medicine, University of Alabama School of Medicine. Director of Nephrology Division, University of Alabama Hospitals, Birmingham, Alabama.

Dialysis

SAMUEL E. LUX, M.D.

Professor of Pediatrics, Harvard Medical School. Chief, Division of Hematology-Oncology, Children's Hospital, Boston, Massachusetts.

Hereditary Defects in the Membrane or Metabolism of the Red Cell

ADEL A. F. MAHMOUD, M.D., Ph.D.

Professor of Medicine and of Molecular Biology and Microbiology, Case Western Reserve University School of Medicine. Attending Physician, University Hospitals of Cleveland, Cleveland, Ohio.

Introduction to Protozoan and Helminthic Diseases; Schistosomiasis

STEPHEN E. MALAWISTA, M.D.

Professor of Medicine and Chief, Section of Rheumatology, Department of Internal Medicine, Yale University School of Medicine. Attending Physician, Yale-New Haven Hospital, New Haven, and Veterans Administration Medical Center, West Haven, Connecticut.

Lyme Disease; Infectious Arthritis

PETER F. MALET, M.D.

Assistant Professor of Medicine, University of Pennsylvania School of Medicine. Attending Physician, Gastrointestinal Section, Department of Medicine, Hospital of the University of Pennsylvania and Veterans Administration Medical Center, Philadelphia, Pennsylvania.

Diseases of the Gallbladder and Bile Ducts

HENRY J. MANKIN, M.D.

Edith M. Ashley Professor of Orthopaedics, Harvard Medical School. Chief of Orthopaedic Service, Massachusetts General Hospital, Boston, Massachusetts.

Bone Tumors

AARON J. MARCUS, M.D.

Professor of Medicine, Cornell University Medical College. Chief, Hematology-Oncology, and Attending Physician, Veterans Administration Medical Center; Attending Physician, New York Hospital, New York, New York.

Hemorrhagic Disorders: Abnormalities of Platelet and Vascular Function

ANDREW M. MARGILETH, M.D.

Professor of Pediatrics, Uniformed Services University of the Health Sciences School of Medicine, Bethesda. Consultant in Pediatrics, Walter Reed Army Medical Center, Washington, D.C.; Bethesda Naval Hospital, Bethesda; and Malcolm Grow U.S. Air Force Medical Center, Camp Springs, Maryland.

Cat Scratch Disease

ALEXANDER R. MARGULIS, M.D.

Professor and Chairman, Department of Radiology, University of California, San Francisco, School of Medicine. Chief of Radiology, University of California, San Francisco, Hospitals and Clinics, San Francisco, California.

Overview of Imaging Techniques and Projection for the Future

HENRY MASUR, M.D.

Professor of Clinical Medicine, George Washington University School of Medicine and Health Sciences, Washington, D.C. Deputy Chief, Critical Care Medicine Department, Clinical Center, National Institutes of Health, Bethesda, Maryland.

Toxoplasmosis; Pneumocystosis

ALVIN M. MATSUMOTO, M.D.

Assistant Professor of Medicine, University of Washington School of Medicine. Attending Physician, Division of Gerontology and Geriatric Medicine, Geriatric Research, Education, and Clinical Center, Veterans Administration Medical Center, Seattle, Washington.

The Testis

RICHARD A. MATTHAY, M.D.

Professor of Medicine and Associate Director, Pulmonary Section, Department of Internal Medicine, Yale University School of Medicine. Associate Director, Winchester Chest Clinic; Co- Director, Medical Intensive Care Unit; and Attending Pulmonologist, Yale-New Haven Hospital, New Haven, Connecticut.

Chronic Airways Diseases; Abnormalities of Lung Aeration

J. BRUCE McCLAIN, M.D.

Associate Professor of Medicine, Uniformed Services University of the Health Sciences School of Medicine, Bethesda, Maryland. Chief, Infectious Disease Service, Walter Reed Army Medical Center, Washington, D.C.

Rat-Bite Fevers; Leptospirosis

T. DWIGHT McKINNEY, M.D.

Professor of Medicine, University of Texas Health Science Center at San Antonio. Attending Physician, Medical Center Hospital and Audie L. Murphy Memorial Veterans Hospital, San Antonio, Texas.

Tubulointerstitial Diseases and Toxic Nephropathies

IRENE MEISSNER, M.D.

Assistant Professor of Neurology, University of Western Ontario. Staff Physician, Clinical Neurological Sciences, University Hospital, London, Ontario, Canada.

Introduction to Cerebrovascular Diseases

RONALD P. MESSNER, M.D.

Professor of Medicine and Director, Section of Rheumatology, University of Minnesota. Attending Physician, University of Minnesota Hospital and Clinics, Veterans Administration Medical Center, and Hennepin County Medical Center, Minneapolis, Minnesota.

Polymyositis

LOUIS H. MILLER, M.D.

Head, Malaria Section, Laboratory of Parasitic Diseases, National Institute of Allergy and Infectious Diseases, National Institutes of Health, Bethesda, Maryland.

Malaria

THOMAS P. MONATH, M.D.

Director, Division of Vector-Borne Viral Diseases, Center for Infectious Diseases, Centers for Disease Control, Public Health Service, Department of Health and Human Services, Ft. Collins, Colorado.

Arthropod-Borne Viral Encephalitides

WILLIAM L. MORGAN, M.D.

Professor of Medicine, University of Rochester School of Medicine and Dentistry. Associate Chairman, Department of Medicine, Strong Memorial Hospital, Rochester, New York.

Clinical Approach to the Patient

DEANE F. MOSHER, M.D.

Professor of Medicine and Physiological Chemistry and Head, Section of Hematology, University of Wisconsin Medical School, Madison, Wisconsin.

Disorders of Blood Coagulation

ARNO G. MOTULSKY, M.D., D.Sc.

Professor of Medicine and Genetics, University of Washington School of Medicine. Attending Physician, University Hospital and Providence Medical Center, Seattle, Washington.

Hemochromatosis; Hereditary Syndromes Involving Multiple Organ Systems

S. HARVEY MUDD, M.D.

Chief, Section on Alkaloid Biosynthesis, Laboratory of General and Comparative Biochemistry, National Institute of Mental Health, Bethesda, Maryland.

Homocystinuria

MAURICE A. MUFSON, M.D.

Professor of Microbiology and Chairman, Department of Medicine, Marshall University School of Medicine. Associate Chief of Staff for Research, Veterans Administration Medical Center; Staff Physician, Cabell Huntington Hospital and St. Mary's Hospital, Huntington, West Virginia.

Viral Pharyngitis, Laryngitis, Croup, and Bronchitis

JOHN F. MURRAY, M.D.

Professor of Medicine, University of California, San Francisco, School of Medicine. Chief of the Chest Service, San Francisco General Hospital Medical Center, San Francisco, California.

Respiratory Diseases: Introduction; Respiratory Structure and Function; Respiratory Failure

BRYAN D. MYERS, M.B.

Professor of Medicine, Stanford University School of Medicine. Acting Chief, Division of Nephrology, Stanford University Hospital, Stanford, California.

Diabetes and the Kidney

DAVID G. NATHAN, M.D.

Robert G. Stranahan Professor of Pediatrics, Harvard Medical School. Physician-in-Chief, Children's Hospital, Boston, Massachusetts.

Introduction to Hematologic Diseases

PHILIP NEEDLEMAN, Ph.D.

Professor and Head, Department of Pharmacology, Washington University School of Medicine, St. Louis, Missouri.

Natriuretic Factors

FRANKLIN A. NEVA, M.D.

Chief, Laboratory of Parasitic Diseases; Member, Section on Clinical Parasitology, Laboratory of Clinical Investigation, National Institute of Allergy and Infectious Diseases, National Institutes of Health, Bethesda, Maryland.

American Trypanosomiasis; Leishmaniasis

CHRISTOPHER J. L. NEWTH, M.B.

Associate Professor of Pediatrics, University of Southern California School of Medicine. Director, Pediatric Intensive Care, Children's Hospital of Los Angeles, Los Angeles, California.

Bronchiectasis; Cystic Fibrosis

ARTHUR W. NIENHUIS, M.D.

Deputy Clinical Director and Chief, Clinical Hematology Branch, National Heart, Lung and Blood Institute, National Institutes of Health, Bethesda, Maryland.

Hemoglobin Synthesis; The Thalassemias

ALAN S. NIES, M.D.

Professor of Medicine and Pharmacology, University of Colorado School of Medicine. Attending Physician, University Hospital, Denver, Colorado.

Principles of Drug Therapy; Interactions Between Drugs; Adverse Reactions to Drugs

CHARLES P. O'BRIEN, M.D., Ph.D.

Professor of Psychiatry, University of Pennsylvania School of Medicine. Chief, Psychiatry Service, Veterans Administration Medical Center, Philadelphia, Pennsylvania.

Drug Abuse and Dependence

ROBERT K. OCKNER, M.D.

Professor of Medicine and Director of Liver Center, University of California, San Francisco, School of Medicine. Chief of Gastroenterology, Moffitt-Long Hospitals, San Francisco, California.

Clinical Approach to Liver Disease; Hepatic Metabolism in Liver Disease; Laboratory Tests in Liver Disease; Approaches to the Diagnosis of Jaundice; Acute Viral Hepatitis; Toxic and Drug- Induced Liver Disease; Chronic Hepatitis

WILLIAM D. ODELL, M.D., Ph.D.

Chairman, Department of Internal Medicine, and Professor of Medicine and Physiology, University of Utah School of Medicine, Salt Lake City, Utah.

Endocrine Manifestations of Tumors: "Ectopic" Hormone Production

JERROLD M. OLEFSKY, M.D.

Professor of Medicine, University of California, San Diego, School of Medicine. Staff, Medical Research Services, Veterans Administration Medical Center, La Jolla, California.

Diabetes Mellitus

SUZANNE OPARIL, M.D.

Professor of Medicine and Associate Professor of Physiology and Biophysics, University of Alabama School of Medicine. Attending Cardiologist, University Hospital, Birmingham, Alabama.

Arterial Hypertension

ERIC A. OTTESEN, M.D.

Staff Physician, Clinical Center, National Institutes of Health, Bethesda, Maryland, and Children's Hospital National Medical Center, Washington, D.C.

Filariasis

CHARLES Y. C. PAK, M.D.

Professor of Internal Medicine, University of Texas Health Science Center at Dallas, Dallas, Texas.

Renal Calculi

FRANK PARKER, M.D.

Professor and Chairman, Department of Dermatology, Oregon Health Sciences University School of Medicine. Staff Physician, Oregon Health Sciences University Teaching Hospital and Veterans Administration Medical Center, Portland, Oregon.

Cutaneous Manifestations of Internal Malignancy; Skin Diseases

STEPHEN G. PAUKER, M.D.

Professor of Medicine and Chief, Division of Medical Information Sciences, Department of Medicine, Tufts University School of Medicine. Chief, Division of Clinical Decision Making, Department of Medicine, New England Medical Center, Boston, Massachusetts.

Clinical Decision Making

WILLIAM E. PAUL, M.D.

Chief, Laboratory of Immunology, National Institute of Allergy and Infectious Diseases, National Institutes of Health, Bethesda, Maryland.

The Immune System: Introduction

HERBERT A. PERKINS, M.D.

Clinical Professor of Medicine, University of California, San Francisco, School of Medicine. Scientific Director, Irwin Memorial Blood Bank, San Francisco, California.

Blood Transfusion

JOSEPH K. PERLOFF, M.D.

Streisand/American Heart Association Professor of Medicine and Pediatrics, University of California, Los Angeles, UCLA School of Medicine, Los Angeles, California.

Diseases of the Myocardium

WALTER L. PETERSON, M.D.

Associate Professor of Medicine, University of Texas Health Science Center at Dallas. Chief, Gastroenterology Section, Veterans Administration Medical Center, Dallas, Texas.

Peptic Ulcer: Medical Therapy; Gastrointestinal Hemorrhage

SIDNEY PHILLIPS, M.D.

Professor of Medicine, Mayo Medical School. Director, Gastroenterology Unit, and Consultant in Gastroenterology, Mayo Clinic, Rochester, Minnesota.

Disorders of Gastrointestinal Motility

THEODORE L. PHILLIPS, M.D.

Professor and Chairman, Department of Radiation Oncology, University of California, San Francisco, School of Medicine. Consulting Physician, University of California, San Francisco, Hospitals and Clinics, Veterans Administration Medical Center, and Mt. Zion Hospital and Medical Center, San Francisco, California.

Radiation Injury

NATHANIEL F. PIERCE, M.D.

Professor of Medicine, Johns Hopkins University School of Medicine; Professor of International Health, Johns Hopkins University School of Hygiene and Public Health, Baltimore, Maryland. Research Coordinator, Global Diarrhoeal Diseases Control Programme, World Health Organization, Geneva, Switzerland.

Cholera

F. XAVIER PI-SUNYER, M.D.

Professor of Clinical Medicine, Columbia University College of Physicians and Surgeons. Director, Division of Endocrinology and Metabolism, and Associate Director, Obesity Research Center, St. Luke's-Roosevelt Hospital Center, New York, New York.

Obesity

FRED PLUM, M.D.

Anne Parrish Titzell Professor and Chairman, Department of Neurology, Cornell University Medical College. Neurologist-in- Chief, New York Hospital–Cornell Medical Center, New York, New York.

Approach to the Neurologic Patient; Disorders of Consciousness and Arousal; The Dementias; Autonomic Disorders and Their Management; Disorders of Motor Function

CHARLES E. POPE II, M.D.

Professor of Medicine, University of Washington School of Medicine. Chief of Gastroenterology, Veterans Administration Medical Center, Seattle, Washington.

Diseases of the Esophagus

RICHARD L. POPP, M.D.

Professor of Medicine and Associate Chairman, Department of Medicine, Stanford University School of Medicine, Stanford, California.

Echocardiography

CAROL S. PORTLOCK, M.D.

Associate Professor of Medicine, Yale University School of Medicine. Staff Physician, Yale-New Haven Hospital, New Haven, Connecticut.

Introduction to Neoplasms of the Immune System; The Non- Hodgkin's Lymphomas; Burkitt's Lymphoma

JEROME B. POSNER, M.D.

Professor of Neurology, Cornell University Medical College. Attending Neurologist and Chairman, Department of Neurology, Memorial Sloan-Kettering Cancer Center, New York, New York.

Pain and Its Management; Nonmetastatic Effects of Cancer on the Nervous System; Disorders of Consciousness and Arousal; Episodic Loss of Motor Function; Disorders of Sensation; Mechanical Lesions of the Spine and Related Structures

RICHARD W. PRICE, M.D.

Associate Professor of Neurology, Cornell University Medical College. Associate Attending Neurologist, Memorial Hospital and New York Hospital; Associate Member, Memorial Sloan-Kettering Cancer Center, New York, New York.

Introduction to Viral Infections of the Nervous System; Acute Viral Meningitis and Encephalitis; Herpes Virus Infections of the Nervous System; Poliomyelitis; Slow Virus Infections of the Nervous System

BASIL A. PRUITT, Jr., M.D.

Professor of Surgery, Uniformed Services University of the Health Sciences, Bethesda, Maryland. Commander and Director, U.S. Army Institute of Surgical Research, Fort Sam Houston, Texas.

Electric Injury

CHARLES PUTMAN, M.D.

Dean and Vice-Provost for Research and Development, Duke University School of Medicine. Professor of Medicine and Radiology, Duke University Medical Center, Durham, North Carolina.

Radiography of the Heart

THOMAS C. QUINN, M.D.

Senior Investigator, National Institute of Allergy and Infectious Diseases, National Institutes of Health; Associate Professor of Medicine, Johns Hopkins University School of Medicine. Attending Physician, Clinical Center, National Institutes of Health, Bethesda, and Johns Hopkins Hospital, Baltimore, Maryland.

African Trypanosomiasis

CHARLES E. RACKLEY, M.D.

Anton and Margaret Fuisz Professor of Medicine and Chairman, Department of Medicine, Georgetown University School of Medicine. Physician-in-Chief, Department of Medicine, Georgetown University Hospital, Washington, D.C.

Valvular Heart Disease

SAMUEL RAPOPORT, M.D., Ph.D.

Assistant Professor of Neurology, Cornell University Medical College. Assistant Attending Neurologist, New York Hospital, New York, New York.

Neurologic Diagnostic Procedures

ROBERT W. REBAR, M.D.

Professor, Department of Obstetrics and Gynecology, and Head, Section of Reproductive Endocrinology and Infertility, Northwestern University Medical School. Attending Physician, Northwestern Memorial Hospital, Chicago, Illinois.

The Ovaries

FLOYD C. RECTOR, Jr., M.D.

Professor of Medicine and Physiology, University of California, San Francisco, School of Medicine. Staff Physician, University of California Hospitals and Clinics, San Francisco, California.

Obstructive Nephropathy

CHARLES E. REED, M.D.

Professor of Medicine, Mayo Medical School. Consultant in Internal Medicine and Allergic Diseases, Mayo Clinic and Foundation, Rochester, Minnesota.

Drug Allergy

SEYMOUR REICHLIN, M.D., Ph.D.

Professor of Medicine, Tufts University School of Medicine. Chief, Endocrine Division, New England Medical Center, Boston, Massachusetts.

The Pineal

CHARLES T. RICHARDSON, M.D.

Bertha M. and Cecil D. Patterson Professor of Medicine, University of Texas Health Science Center at Dallas. Chief of Staff, Veterans Administration Medical Center, Dallas, Texas.

Gastritis; Peptic Ulcer: Pathogenesis; Zollinger-Ellison Syndrome

RONALD F. RIEDER, M.D.

Professor of Medicine and Director of Hematology, State University of New York Health Science Center at Brooklyn. Attending Physician, Kings County Hospital Center, Brooklyn, New York.

Unstable Hemoglobins; Abnormal Hemoglobins with Altered Oxygen Affinity; Methemoglobinemia and Sulfhemoglobinemia

B. LAWRENCE RIGGS, M.D.

Professor of Medicine, Mayo Medical School. Consultant, Division of Endocrinology and Metabolism, Mayo Clinic and Foundation, Rochester, Minnesota.

Osteoporosis

RICHARD S. RIVLIN, M.D.

Professor of Medicine, Cornell University Medical College. Chief, Nutrition Service, Memorial Sloan-Kettering Cancer Center, and Chief, Nutrition Division, New York Hospital–Cornell Medical Center, New York, New York.

Disorders of Vitamin Metabolism

WILLIAM O. ROBERTSON, M.D.

Professor of Pediatrics, University of Washington School of Medicine. Medical Director, Seattle Poison Center and Washington Poison Network, Children's Orthopedic and Medical Center, Seattle, Washington.

Common Poisonings

RICHARD K. ROOT, M.D.

Professor and Chairman of Medicine, University of California, San Francisco, School of Medicine. Physician-in-Chief, Department of Medicine, University of California, San Francisco, Hospitals and Clinics, San Francisco, California.

The Compromised Host

IRWIN H. ROSENBERG, M.D.

Professor of Medicine, Physiology, and Nutrition, Tufts University School of Medicine. Physician, Tufts–New England Medical Center, Boston, Massachusetts.

Inflammatory Bowel Diseases: Introduction; Crohn's Disease

JOHN ROSS, Jr., M.D.

Professor of Medicine and Head, Division of Cardiology, Department of Medicine, University of California, San Diego, School of Medicine, La Jolla. Attending Physician, University of California Medical Center, San Diego, California.

Cardiac Function and Circulatory Control

RUSSELL ROSS, Ph.D.

Professor of Pathology and Adjunct Professor of Biochemistry, University of Washington School of Medicine, Seattle, Washington.

Atherosclerosis

DAVID A. ROTTENBERG, M.D.

Associate Professor of Neurology, Cornell University Medical College. Associate Attending Neurologist, New York Hospital and Memorial Hospital, New York, New York.

Disorders of Intracranial Pressure

DAVID W. ROWE, M.D.

Associate Professor of Pediatrics, University of Connecticut School of Medicine. Staff Physician, John Dempsey Hospital, University of Connecticut Health Center, Farmington, Connecticut.

Osteogenesis Imperfecta

JOHN W. ROWE, M.D.

Associate Professor of Medicine, Harvard Medical School. Chief of Gerontology, Beth Israel and Brigham and Women's Hospitals, Boston; Director, Geriatric Research Education Clinical Center, Veterans Administration Medical Center, West Roxbury, Massachusetts.

Aging and Geriatric Medicine

ROBERT M. RUSSELL, M.D.

Associate Professor, Tufts University School of Medicine. Attending Gastroenterologist, Tufts–New England Medical Center; Associate Director, USDA Human Nutrition Research Center, Boston, Massachusetts.

Nutrient Requirements; Nutritional Assessment

DAVID C. SABISTON, Jr., M.D.

James B. Duke Professor and Chairman, Department of Surgery, Duke University School of Medicine. Chief of Staff, Duke University Hospital, Durham, North Carolina.

Surgical Treatment of Coronary Artery Disease

R. BRADLEY SACK, M.D., Sc.D.

Professor of International Health, Johns Hopkins University School of Hygiene and Public Health. Staff Physician, Johns Hopkins Hospital and Francis Scott Key Medical Center, Baltimore, Maryland.

The Diarrhea of Travelers

ROBERT A. SALATA, M.D.

Assistant Professor of Medicine, Case Western Reserve University School of Medicine. Attending Physician and Director of the Travelers Clinic, University Hospitals, Cleveland, Ohio.

Brucellosis

SYDNEY E. SALMON, M.D.

Professor of Internal Medicine, University of Arizona College of Medicine. Chairman, Cancer Activities Committee, University Hospital, Tucson, Arizona.

Plasma Cell Disorders

JOHN SALVAGGIO, M.D.

Henderson Professor and Chairman, Department of Medicine, Tulane University School of Medicine. Senior Physician, Charity Hospital at New Orleans; Active Staff, Tulane University Hospital; Consulting Physician, Veterans Administration Medical Center, New Orleans, Louisiana.

Allergic Rhinitis

JAY P. SANFORD, M.D.

Professor of Medicine and Dean, F. Edward Hebert School of Medicine, and President, Uniformed Services University of the Health Sciences. Attending Physician, Walter Reed Army Medical Center and Naval Hospital, Bethesda, Maryland.

Snake Bites

BRUCE F. SCHARSCHMIDT, M.D.

Professor of Medicine, University of California, San Francisco, School of Medicine. Attending Physician, University of California, San Francisco, Hospitals and Clinics and Moffitt- Long Hospitals, San Francisco, California.

Bilirubin Metabolism and Hyperbilirubinemia; Parasitic, Bacterial, Fungal, and Granulomatous Liver Disease; Inherited, Infiltrative, and Metabolic

Disorders Involving the Liver; Acute and Chronic Hepatic Failure and Hepatic Transplantation; Hepatic Tumors

HERBERT H. SCHAUMBURG, M.D.

Professor and Chairman, Unified Department of Neurology, Albert Einstein College of Medicine of Yeshiva University. Attending Neurologist, Bronx Municipal Hospital Center and Montefiore Medical Center, Bronx, New York.

Diseases of the Peripheral Nervous System

ALAN N. SCHECHTER, M.D.

Professor of Biology, Johns Hopkins University, Baltimore; Professorial Lecturer in Biochemistry, George Washington University, Washington, D.C. Chief, Laboratory of Chemical Biology, National Institute of Diabetes and Digestive and Kidney Diseases, National Institutes of Health, Bethesda, Maryland.

Hemoglobin Structure and Function

LAWRENCE R. SCHILLER, M.D.

Clinical Assistant Professor of Internal Medicine, University of Texas Health Science Center at Dallas. Director of Gastrointestinal Research and Associate Attending Physician, Baylor University Medical Center, Dallas, Texas.

Peptic Ulcer: Epidemiology, Clinical Manifestations, and Diagnosis

H. RALPH SCHUMACHER, Jr., M.D.

Professor of Medicine, University of Pennsylvania School of Medicine. Director, Rheumatology-Immunology Center, Veterans Administration Medical Center; Attending Rheumatologist, Hospital of the University of Pennsylvania, Philadelphia, Pennsylvania.

Calcium Crystal Deposition Arthropathies; Relapsing Polychondritis; Multifocal Fibrosclerosis

BENJAMIN D. SCHWARTZ, M.D., Ph.D.

Professor of Internal Medicine, Washington University School of Medicine; Investigator, Howard Hughes Medical Institute. Associate Physician, Barnes Hospital and Jewish Hospital of St. Louis, St. Louis, Missouri.

The Major Histocompatibility Complex and Disease Susceptibility

CHARLES H. SCOGGIN, M.D.

Senior Scientist and Vice-President, Eleanor Roosevelt Institute for Cancer Research; Professor of Medicine, University of Colorado School of Medicine. Staff Physician, University Hospital, Denver, Colorado.

Pulmonary Neoplasms

CHARLES R. SCRIVER, M.D.C.M.

Professor, Departments of Biology and Pediatrics and Center for Human Genetics, McGill University Faculty of Medicine. Physician and Director, Division of Medical Genetics, Montreal Children's Hospital, Montreal, Quebec, Canada.

Hyperaminoaciduria

S. K. K. SEAH, M.D., Ph.D.

Associate Professor of Medicine, McGill University Faculty of Medicine. Attending Physician, Montreal General Hospital; Consulting Physician, Montreal Chinese Hospital, Montreal, Quebec, Canada.

Hermaphroditic Flukes

STANTON SEGAL, M.D.

Professor of Pediatrics and Internal Medicine, University of Pennsylvania School of Medicine. Senior Physician and Director, Division of Biochemical Development and Molecular Diseases, Children's Hospital of Philadelphia; Attending Physician, Hospital of the University of Pennsylvania, Philadelphia, Pennsylvania.

Galactosemia

ROBERT M. SENIOR, M.D.

Professor of Medicine, Washington University School of Medicine. Director, Respiratory and Critical Care Division, Jewish Hospital of St. Louis, St. Louis, Missouri.

Pulmonary Embolism; Fat Embolism Syndrome

F. JOHN SERVICE, M.D., Ph.D.

Professor of Medicine, Mayo Medical School. Consultant in Endocrinology and Metabolism, Mayo Clinic, Rochester, Minnesota.

Hypoglycemic Disorders

RALPH SHABETAI, M.D.

Professor of Medicine and Associate Director of Cardiology, University of California, San Diego, School of Medicine. Chief of Cardiology, Veterans Administration Medical Center, La Jolla, California.

Diseases of the Pericardium

WILLIAM R. SHAPIRO, M.D.

Professor of Neurology, Cornell University Medical College. Attending Neurologist, Memorial Sloan-Kettering Cancer Center and New York Hospital, New York, New York.

Intracranial Tumors

JOHN N. SHEAGREN, M.D.

Professor of Internal Medicine and Associate Dean, University of Michigan Medical School. Chief of Staff, Veterans Administration Medical Center, Ann Arbor, Michigan.

Shock Syndromes Related to Sepsis; Staphylococcal Infections

DEAN SHEPPARD, M.D.

Associate Professor of Medicine, University of California, San Francisco, School of Medicine. Director, Lung Biology Center, San Francisco General Hospital, San Francisco, California.

Occupation Pulmonary Disorders

ROBERT E. SHOPE, M.D.

Professor of Epidemiology, Yale University School of Medicine, New Haven, Connecticut.

Introduction to Arthropod-Borne Viral Diseases; Viral Hemorrhagic Fevers

DONALD H. SILBERBERG, M.D.

Professor and Chairman, Department of Neurology, University of Pennsylvania School of Medicine. Chairman of Neurology, Hospital of the University of Pennsylvania, Philadelphia, Pennsylvania.

The Demyelinating Diseases

SOL SILVERMAN, Jr., M.D., D.D.S.

Professor and Chairman, Division of Oral Medicine, University of California, San Francisco, School of Dentistry. Attending Dentist, Moffitt-Long Hospitals, San Francisco, California.

Oral Medicine

FREDERICK R. SINGER, M.D.

Professor of Medicine, University of Southern California School of Medicine. Associate Program Director, General Clinical Research Center, Los Angeles County/University of Southern California Medical Center, Los Angeles, California.

Paget's Disease of Bone

EDUARDO SLATOPOLSKY, M.D.

Professor of Medicine, Washington University School of Medicine. Director, Chromalloy American Kidney Center; Physician, Barnes Hospital; Consulting Physician, Jewish Hospital of St. Louis, St. Louis, Missouri.

Renal Osteodystrophy

MARVIN H. SLEISENGER, M.D.

Professor and Vice-Chairman, Department of Medicine, University of California, San Francisco, School of Medicine. Chief of Medical Service, Veterans Administration Medical Center; Attending Physician, Moffitt-Long Hospitals, San Francisco, California.

Gastrointestinal Diseases: Introduction; Miscellaneous Inflammatory Diseases of the Intestine

WILLIAM S. SLY, M.D.

Chairman, E. A. Doisy Department of Biochemistry, St. Louis University School of Medicine. Consulting Geneticist, Cardinal Glennon Memorial Hospital for Children, St. Louis, Missouri.

The Mucopolysaccharidoses

LLOYD H. SMITH, Jr., M.D.

Professor of Medicine and Associate Dean, University of California, San Francisco, School of Medicine, San Francisco, California.

Medicine as an Art; Primary Hyperoxaluria; The Hyperphenylalaninemias; Histidinemia; The Hyperprolinemias and Hydroxyprolinemia; Disease of the Urea Cycle; Branched-Chain Aminoaciduria; Disorders of Pyrimidine Metabolism; Phosphorus Deficiency and Hypophosphatemia; Disorders of Magnesium Metabolism

THOMAS W. SMITH, M.D.

Professor of Medicine, Harvard Medical School and M.I.T. Division of Health Sciences and Technology. Chief, Cardiovascular Division, and Senior Physician, Brigham and Women's Hospital; Consultant in Medicine, Massachusetts General Hospital; Consultant in Cardiology, Children's Hospital and Dana Farber Cancer Institute, Boston, Massachusetts.

Approach to the Patient with Cardiovascular Disease; Heart Failure

RALPH SNYDERMAN, M.D.

Adjunct Professor of Medicine, Duke University School of Medicine, and University of California, San Francisco, School of Medicine. Attending Physician, Duke University Hospital, Durham, North Carolina.

Mechanisms of Inflammation and Tissue Destruction in the Rheumatic Diseases; Behcet's Disease

ROSEMARY SOAVE, M.D.

Assistant Professor of Medicine and Public Health, Cornell University Medical College. Assistant Attending Physician, Department of Medicine, New York Hospital–Cornell Medical Center, New York, New York.

Cryptosporidiosis

ROGER D. SOLOWAY, M.D.

Professor of Medicine, University of Pennsylvania School of Medicine. Associate Chief, Gastrointestinal Section, Hospital of the University of Pennsylvania, Philadelphia, Pennsylvania.

Diseases of the Gallbladder and Bile Ducts

NICHOLAS A. SOTER, M.D.

Professor of Dermatology, New York University School of Medicine. Attending Physician, University Hospital, Bellevue Hospital Center, and Manhattan Veterans Administration Hospital, New York, New York.

Urticaria and Angioedema

P. FREDERICK SPARLING, M.D.

Professor of Medicine and Professor and Chairman of Microbiology and Immunology, University of North Carolina at Chapel Hill School of Medicine. Attending Physician in Infectious Diseases, North Carolina Memorial Hospital, Chapel Hill, North Carolina.

Sexually Transmitted Diseases

WALTER E. STAMM, M.D.

Professor of Medicine, University of Washington School of Medicine. Head, Infectious Disease Division, Harborview Medical Center, Seattle, Washington.

Disease Caused by Chlamydiae

ALFRED D. STEINBERG, M.D.

Medical Director, U.S. Public Health Service; Chief, Cellular Immunology Section, Arthritis and Rheumatism Branch, National Institute of Arthritis and Metabolic Diseases, National Institutes of Health. Attending Physician, Clinical Center, National Institutes of Health, Bethesda, Maryland.

Systemic Lupus Erythematosus

DAVID P. STEVENS, M.D.

Associate Clinical Professor of Medicine, Case Western Reserve University School of Medicine. Assistant Physician, University Hospitals, Cleveland, Ohio.

Giardiasis; Other Protozoan Diseases

LYNNE WARNER STEVENSON, M.D.

Assistant Professor of Medicine, University of California, Los Angeles, UCLA School of Medicine, Los Angeles, California.

Diseases of the Myocardium

DANIEL P. STITES, M.D.

Professor and Vice-Chairman, Department of Laboratory Medicine, University of California, San Francisco, School of Medicine. Attending Physician, University of California, San Francisco, Hospitals and Clinics, San Francisco, California.

Diseases of the Thymus

RAINER STORB, M.D.

Professor of Medicine, University of Washington School of Medicine. Member, Fred Hutchinson Cancer Research Center, Seattle, Washington.

Bone Marrow Transplantation

GORDON J. STREWLER, M.D.

Associate Professor of Medicine, University of California, San Francisco, School of Medicine. Clinical Investigator, Veterans Administration Medical Center, San Francisco, California.

Osteonecrosis, Osteosclerosis, and Other Disorders of Bone

WADI N. SUKI, M.D.

Professor of Medicine and of Physiology and Molecular Biophysics, Baylor College of Medicine. Chief, Renal Section, and Senior Attending Physician, Methodist Hospital, Houston, Texas.

Hereditary Chronic Nephropathies

MORTON N. SWARTZ, M.D.

Professor of Medicine, Harvard Medical School. Chief, Infectious Diseases Unit, Massachusetts General Hospital, Boston, Massachusetts.

Bacterial Meningitis; Meningococcal Disease; Infections Caused by Hemophilus Species; Babesiosis

NORMAN TALAL, M.D.

Professor of Medicine and Microbiology, University of Texas Health Science Center at San Antonio. Chief, Section of Clinical Immunology, Audie L. Murphy Memorial Veterans Hospital, San Antonio, Texas.

Sjögren's Syndrome

CLIFFORD TASMAN-JONES, B.Sc., M.B., Ch.B.

Associate Professor of Gastroenterology and Human Nutrition, University of Aukland Medical School. Senior Consultant Physician, Aukland Hospital Board, Aukland, New Zealand.

Disturbances of Trace Mineral Metabolism

ROBERT B. TESH, M.D., M.S.

Associate Professor of Epidemiology, Department of Epidemiology and Public Health, Yale University School of Medicine, New Haven, Connecticut.

Dengue; West Nile Fever; Phlebotomus Fever; Rift Valley Fever; Fevers Caused by Alphaviruses

RICHARD C. THIRLBY, M.D.

Assistant Professor of Surgery, University of Texas Health Science Center at Dallas. Assistant Chief of Surgery, Veterans Administration Medical Center; Attending Surgeon, Parkland Memorial Hospital, Dallas, Texas.

Peptic Ulcer: Surgical Therapy

LEWIS THOMAS, M.D.

Professor, State University of New York at Stony Brook; Professor Emeritus, Memorial Sloan-Kettering Cancer Center, New York, New York.

Medicine as a Very Old Profession

GEORGE TOLIS, M.D., M.Sc.

Auxiliary Professor of Medicine, McGill University Faculty of Medicine, Montreal, Quebec, Canada; Professor of Medicine, University of Crete Medical School. Director, Division of Endocrinology and Metabolism, Hippokrateion Hospital, Athens, Greece.

Nonmalignant Diseases of the Breast

PHILLIP P. TOSKES, M.D.

Professor of Medicine, University of Florida College of Medicine. Director, Division of Gastroenterology, Hepatology and Nutrition, J. Hillis Miller Health Center, Gainesville, Florida.

Malabsorption

GARY J. TUCKER, M.D.

Professor and Chairman, Psychiatry and Behavioral Sciences, University of Washington School of Medicine, Seattle, Washington.

Psychiatric Disorders in Medical Practice

J. BLAKE TYRRELL, M.D.

Clinical Professor of Medicine, University of California, San Francisco, School of Medicine, San Francisco, California.

Disorders of the Adrenal Cortex

JOUNI UITTO, M.D., Ph.D.

Professor of Dermatology, Biochemistry, and Molecular Biology and Chairman, Department of Dermatology, Jefferson Medical College of Thomas Jefferson University. Staff Physician, Thomas Jefferson University Hospital, Philadelphia, Pennsylvania.

Pseudoxanthoma Elasticum

JACK A. VENNES, M.D.

Professor of Medicine, University of Minnesota Medical School, Minneapolis. Staff, University of Minnesota Hospitals and Clinics and Veterans Administration Medical Center, Minneapolis; Consulting Staff, Hennepin County Medical Center, Minneapolis, and St. Paul-Ramsey Medical Center, St. Paul, Minnesota.

Gastrointestinal Endoscopy

FRANCIS WALDVOGEL, M.D.

Professor of Medicine, University of Geneva. Physician-in- Chief, Clinique Medical Therapeutique, University Hospital of Geneva, Geneva, Switzerland.

Osteomyelitis

SUSAN D. WALL, M.D.

Assistant Professor, University of California, San Francisco, School of Medicine. Chief, Abdominal Imaging, Veterans Administration Medical Center, San Francisco, California.

Diagnostic Imaging Procedures in Gastroenterology

PATRICK C. WALSH, M.D.

David Hall McConnell Professor and Director, Department of Urology, Johns Hopkins University School of Medicine. Urologist-in-Chief, James Buchanan Brady Urological Institute, Johns Hopkins Hospital, Baltimore, Maryland.

Diseases of the Prostate

STANLEY J. WATSON, Ph.D., M.D.

Associate Professor of Psychiatry and Associate Director of the Mental Health Research Institute, University of Michigan Medical School, Ann Arbor, Michigan.

The Endorphin Family of Opioid Peptides

HOWARD J. WEINSTEIN, M.D.

Associate Professor of Pediatrics, Harvard Medical School. Associate Physician, Dana Farber Cancer Institute and Children's Hospital, Boston, Massachusetts.

The Acute Leukemias

RICHARD P. WENZEL, M.D., M.Sc.

Professor of Medicine and Preventive Medicine and Director, Division of Clinical Epidemiology, Department of Internal Medicine, University of Iowa College of Medicine. Director, Hospital Epidemiology Program, University of Iowa Hospitals and Clinics, Iowa City, Iowa.

Prevention and Treatment of Hospital-Acquired Infections

CATHERINE M. WILFERT, M.D.

Professor of Pediatrics and Microbiology, Duke University School of Medicine. Staff Physician, Duke University Hospital, Durham, North Carolina.

Foot and Mouth Disease; Mumps

JAMES T. WILLERSON, M.D.

Professor of Medicine and Director, Cardiology Division, University of Texas Health Science Center at Dallas. Chief of Cardiology, Parkland Memorial Hospital, Dallas, Texas.

Sudden Cardiac Death; Angina Pectoris; Acute Myocardial Infarction

RICHARD D. WILLIAMS, M.D.

Professor and Chairman, Department of Urology, University of Iowa College of Medicine. Head of Urology, University of Iowa Hospital; Chief of Urology Section, Veterans Administration Medical Center, Iowa City, Iowa.

Anomalies of the Urinary Tract; Tumors of the Kidney, Ureter, and Bladder

T. FRANKLIN WILLIAMS, M.D.

Director, National Institute on Aging, National Institutes of Health, Bethesda, Maryland.

Management of Common Problems in the Elderly

JOHN WILLIAMSON, B.Sc., M.B., B.S.

Visiting Anaesthetist, Townsville General and Mater Hospitals; Consultant in Diving Medicine, Townsville General Hospital, Townsville, North Queensland, Australia.

Venomous and Poisonous Marine Animals

SIDNEY J. WINAWER, M.D.

Professor of Clinical Medicine, Cornell University Medical College. Attending Physician and Chief, Gastroenterology Service, Memorial Sloan-Kettering Cancer Center, New York, New York.

Neoplasms of the Stomach; Neoplasms of the Large and Small Intestine

MARTIN S. WOLFE, M.D.

Clinical Professor of Medicine, George Washington University School of Medicine and Health Sciences; Clinical Associate Professor of Medicine, Georgetown University School of Medicine. Attending Physician, George Washington University Hospital and Georgetown University Hospital, Washington, D.C.

The Cestodes

SHELDON M. WOLFF, M.D.

Endicott Professor and Chairman, Department of Medicine, Tufts University School of Medicine. Physician-in-Chief, New England Medical Center Hospital, Boston, Massachusetts.

The Febrile Patient; The Vasculitic Syndromes; Polyarteritis Nodosa Group

EMANUEL WOLINSKY, M.D.

Professor of Medicine and Pathology, Case Western Reserve University School of Medicine. Head, Division of Microbiology, Department of Pathology, Cleveland Metropolitan General Hospital, Cleveland, Ohio.

Tuberculosis; Other Mycobacterioses

JERRY WOLINSKY, M.D.

Professor of Neurology, University of Texas Health Science Center at Houston. Attending Neurologist, Hermann Hospital, Houston, Texas.

Subacute Sclerosing Panencephalitis; Neurologic Disorders Associated with Altered Immunity or Unexplained Host-Parasite Alterations

DANIEL G. WRIGHT, M.D.

Associate Professor of Medicine, Uniformed Services University of the Health Sciences; Adjunct Associate Professor of Medicine, George Washington University School of Medicine and Health Sciences. Chief, Department of Hematology, Walter Reed Army Institute of Research, Walter Reed Army Medical Center, Washington, D.C.

Familial Mediterranean Fever

JAMES B. WYNGAARDEN, M.D.

Director, National Institutes of Health, Bethesda, Maryland.

Medicine as a Science; Medicine as a Public Service; The Use and Interpretation of Laboratory-Derived Data; Human Heredity; Inborn Errors of Metabolism; Metabolic Diseases: Introduction; Fabry's Disease; Alcaptonuria; Gout; Acatalasia

LOWELL S. YOUNG, M.D.

Clinical Professor of Medicine, University of California, San Francisco, School of Medicine. Director, Kuzell Institute for Arthritis and Infectious Diseases; Chief, Division of Infectious Diseases, Pacific Presbyterian Medical Center, San Francisco, California.

Antimicrobial Therapy

BARRY L. ZARET, M.D.

Robert W. Berliner Professor of Medicine, Professor of Diagnostic Radiology, and Chief of Cardiology, Yale University School of Medicine. Chief of Cardiology, Yale-New Haven Hospital, New Haven, Connecticut.

Nuclear Cardiology

ELIZABETH J. ZIEGLER, M.D.

Professor of Medicine, University of California, San Diego, School of Medicine, La Jolla. Attending Physician, University of California, San Diego, Medical Center, San Diego, California.

Extraintestinal Infections Caused by Enteric Bacteria

CONTENTS

(Detailed table of contents begins on the following page)

CONTENTS

PART VIII CRITICAL CARE MEDICINE

PART IX RENAL DISEASES

PART X GASTROINTESTINAL DISEASES

PART XI DISEASES OF THE LIVER, GALLBLADDER, AND BILE DUCTS

PART XII HEMATOLOGIC DISEASES

PART XIII ONCOLOGY

PART XIV METABOLIC DISEASES

PART XV NUTRITIONAL DISEASES

PART XVI ENDOCRINE AND REPRODUCTIVE DISEASES

PART XVII DISEASES OF BONE AND BONE MINERAL METABOLISM

PART XVIII INFECTIOUS DISEASES

Section 1 Introduction

Section 2 Bacterial Diseases

Pneumonia

COLOR PLATES

PLATE 1 DIABETES MELLITUS

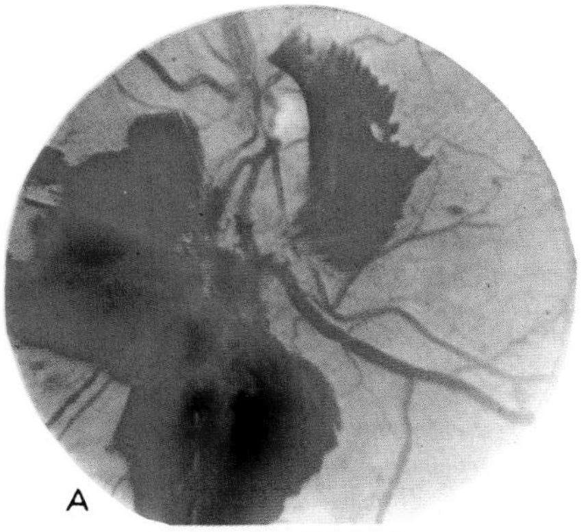

A

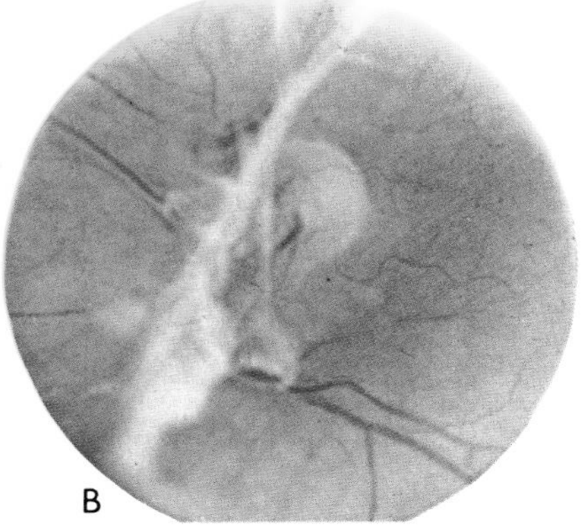

B

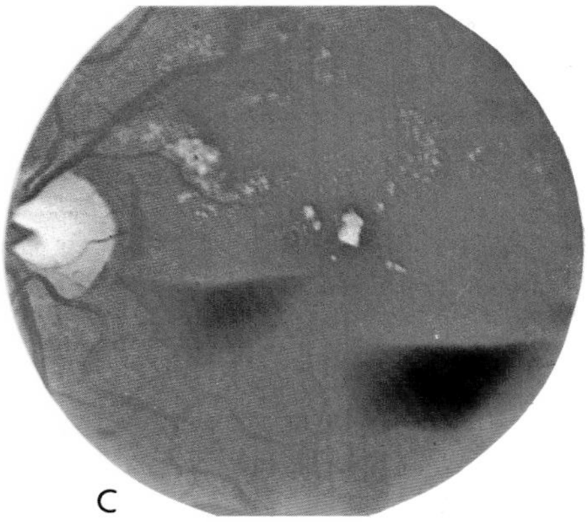

C

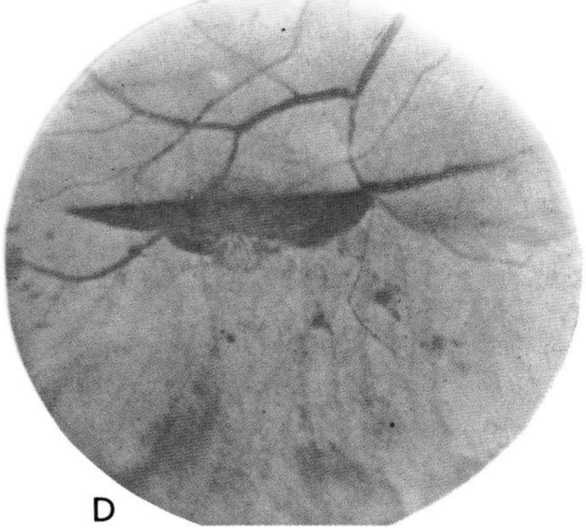

D

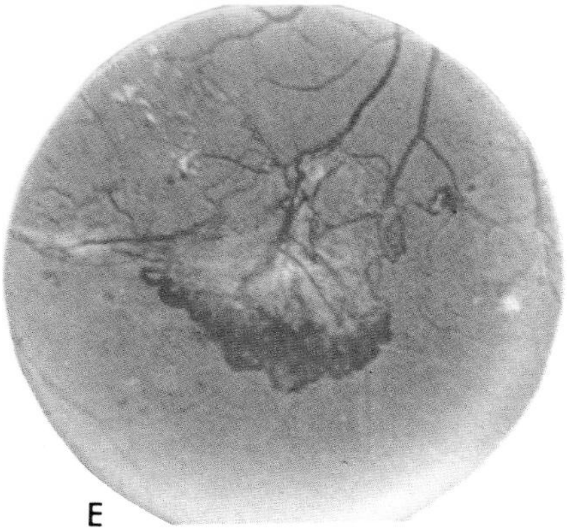

E

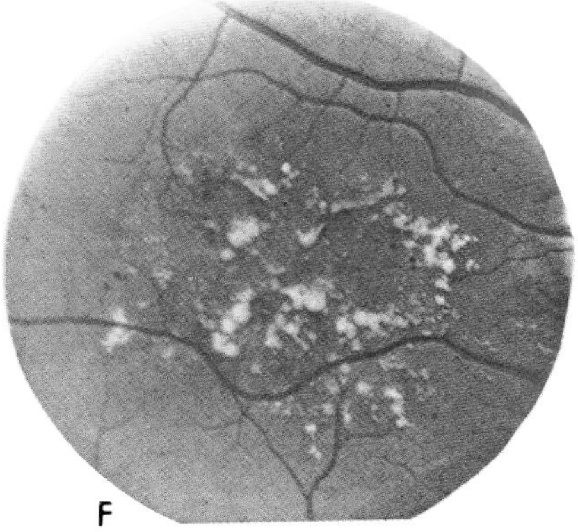

F

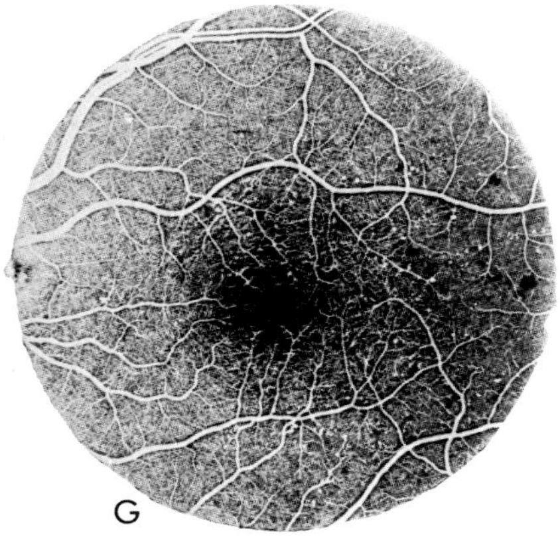

G

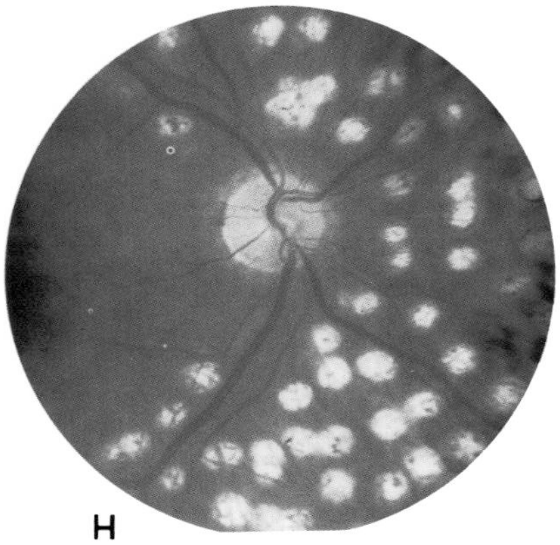

H

A, Vitreous and preretinal hemorrhage from the disc area secondary to disc neovascularization.

B, Fibrous band resulting from going into a quiescent stage of retinopathy one year after slide *A* was taken. Patient maintained quiescent stage for eight years until he died a cardiac death.

C, Preretinal hemorrhages in region of macula which also has exudates and superficial hemorrhages. Note boat-shaped dependency type of hemorrhage.

D, Preretinal hemorrhage at site of frond of neovascularization. Note the new vessel fan underneath the boat-shaped preretinal hemorrhage. It is these new vessels which rupture spontaneously or with minimal stress.

E, Extensive fan of new vessels with fibrous network elevated forward into vitreous. Feeding vessels come from multiple arteries and veins at the retinal level, the entire process being analogous to an angioma.

F, Characteristic waxy exudates in macular zone accounting for decrease in vision, apparently due to incompetent capillaries and leaking from central areas of rings of waxy exudates where the red blotches are noted.

G, Fluorescein angiography in a diabetic, showing some very fine microaneurysms and some tiny areas of capillary closure but with good parafoveal network of vessels and 20/20 vision. These are early changes of diabetic retinopathy probably not seen on ophthalmoscopy. (Courtesy of Dr. L. Aiello.)

H, Photograph of retina following laser therapy, showing circumscribed areas of destruction and fibrous replacement. (Courtesy of Dr. M. B. Landers, III.)

PLATE 2 HEMATOLOGIC DISEASES

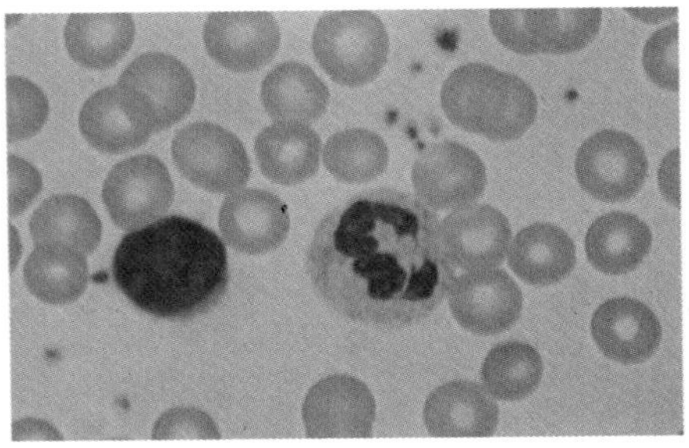

A, Normal peripheral blood smear showing an adult lymphocyte at the left, a mature segmented poly in the center, scattered platelets in the background, and normal appearing red blood cells. Note the normal central one-third pallor of the red cells (× 1200).

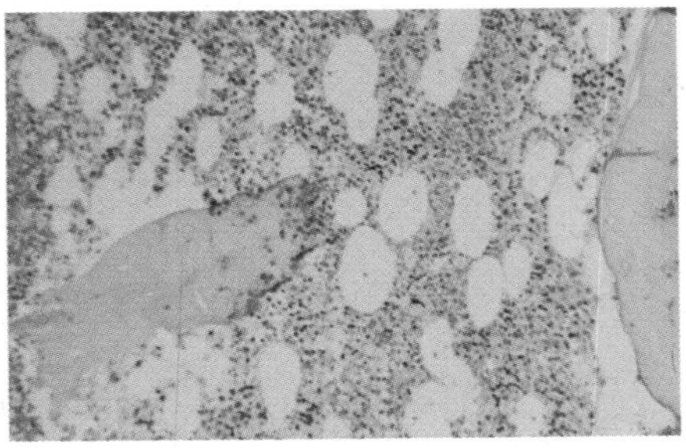

B, Normal bone marrow biopsy, low power. Note the normal fat content, about 50 per cent of the marrow. Normal hematopoietic cells are seen, including scattered megakaryocytes (× 100).

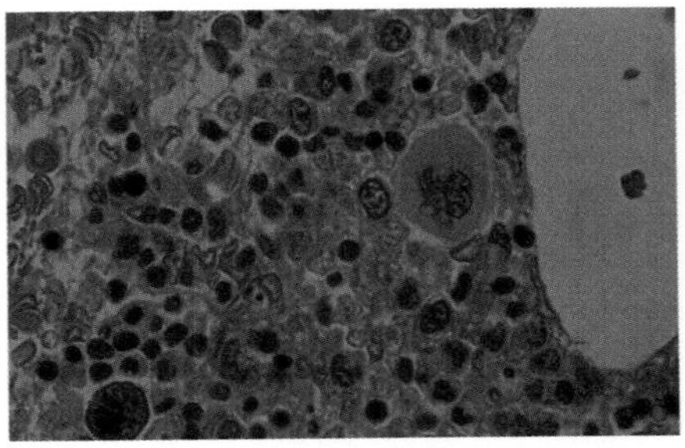

C, Normal bone marrow biopsy, high power. Note the detail of the background megakaryocytes, as well as scattered myeloid and erythroid cells in a ratio of approximately 3:1 (× 1000).

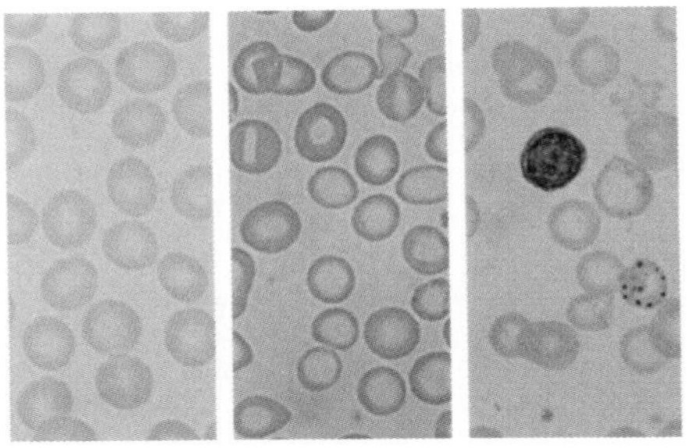

D, Peripheral blood smear showing normal red blood cells (left panel) compared with hypochromic cells of iron deficiency (central panel) or chronic lead poisoning (right panel). In the right panel note the prominent basophilic stippling. The cells are hypochromic as well as macrocytic (× 1200).

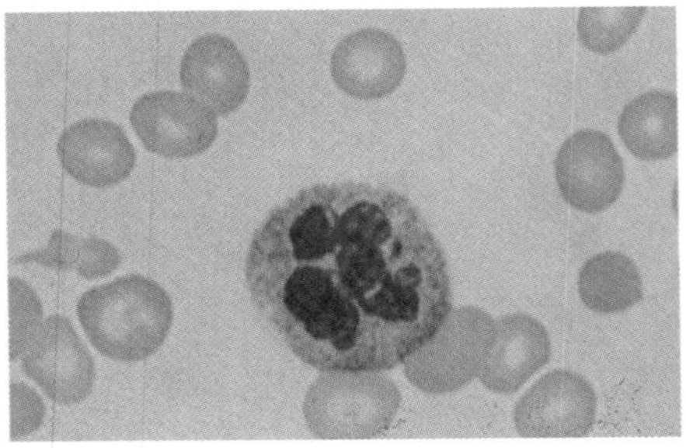

E, Peripheral blood smear showing a gigantic poly (macrocytic hypersegmented poly) in a patient with pernicious anemia. A few macrocytic red cells are noted, along with mild poikilocytes (× 1200).

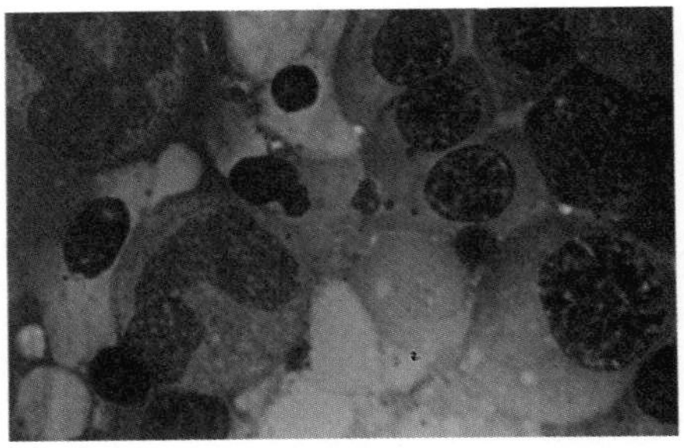

F, Marrow showing megaloblastic findings. Note the megaloblastic erythroid cells, characterized by maturation arrest. Nuclei have open chromatin while the cytoplasm shows early normal hemoglobinization. Several giant metamyelocytes are noted as well.

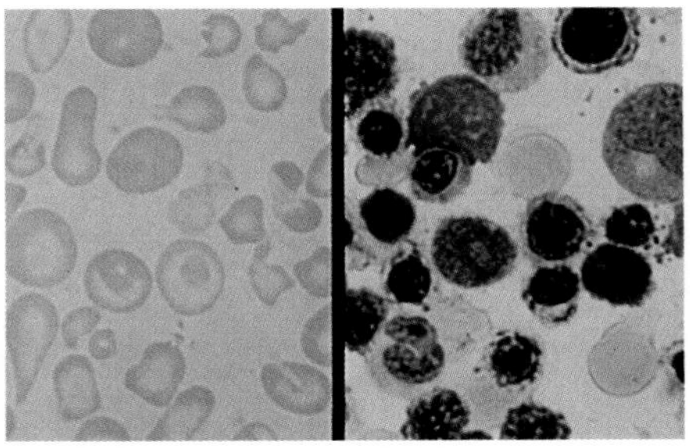

G, Thalassemia major showing marked anisocytosis, poikilocytosis, hypochromia, and target cell formation in the peripheral blood (left panel) and striking erythroid hyperplasia in the right panel, from the bone marrow (× 1200).

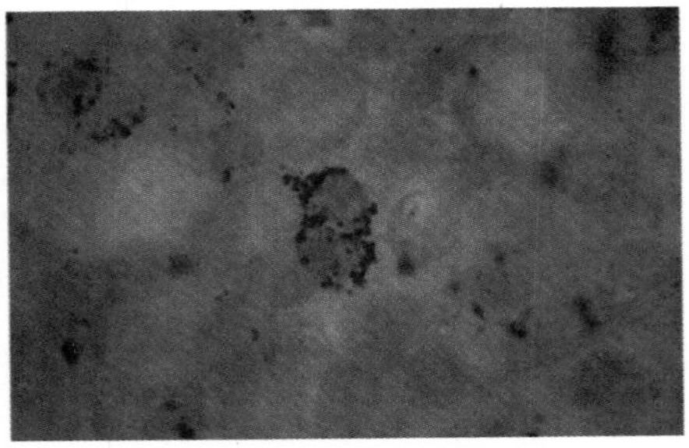

H, Bone marrow smear showing classic ringed sideroblasts. The normoblasts show clumps of iron (hemosiderin) surrounding the nucleus, resulting in a "ring." Physiologically, no more than two or three dots of iron are normally present. Prussian blue stain (× 1200).

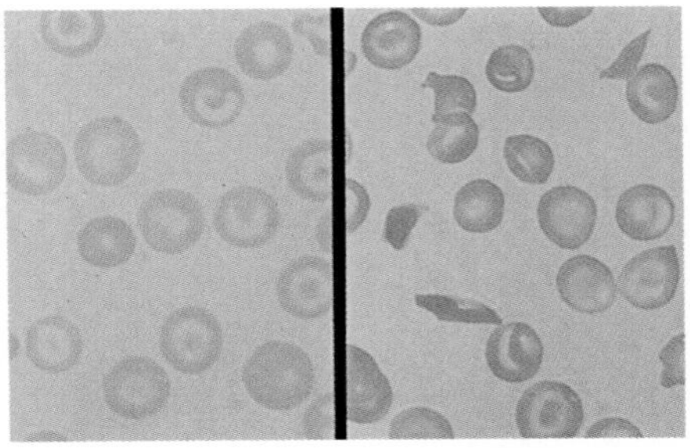

I, Peripheral blood smears from hemoglobin C trait (CA) (left panel) showing target cells and a few spherocytes, and hemoglobin S-C disease (right panel) showing sickled cells as well as target cells and other deformed red cells (x 1200).

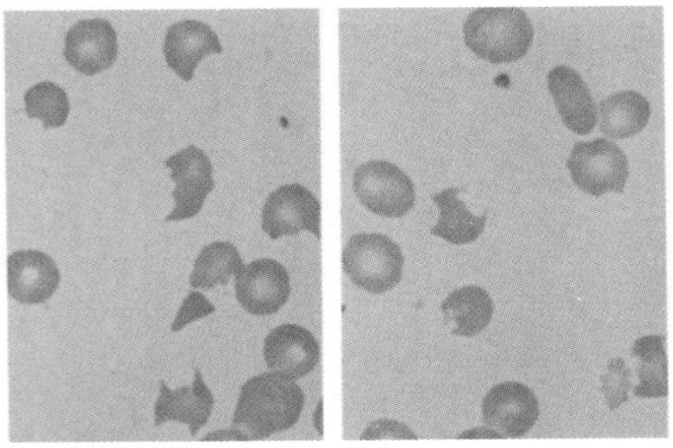

J, Peripheral blood smear from a patient with the hemolytic-uremic syndrome, showing striking schistocytes, also called helmet cells. Note the ragged and deformed red cells caused by rapid intravascular hemolysis due to physical factors (× 1200).

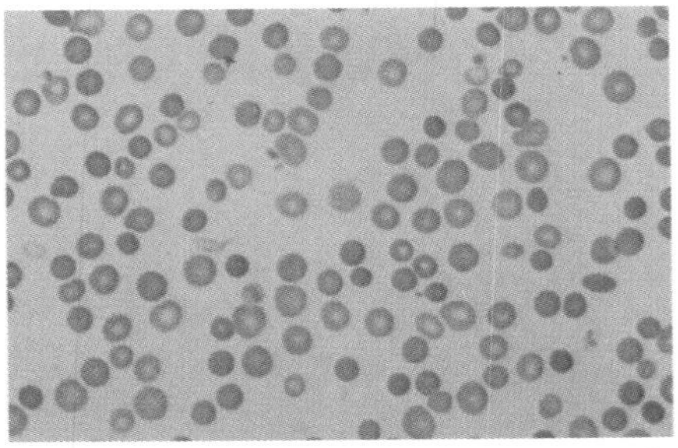

K, Peripheral blood smear from a patient with hereditary spherocytosis showing numerous spherocytes characterized by small size and dense hemoglobin stain. Scattered normal size red cells are also noted, along with occasional larger erythrocytes representing young cells (reticulocytes) (× 400).

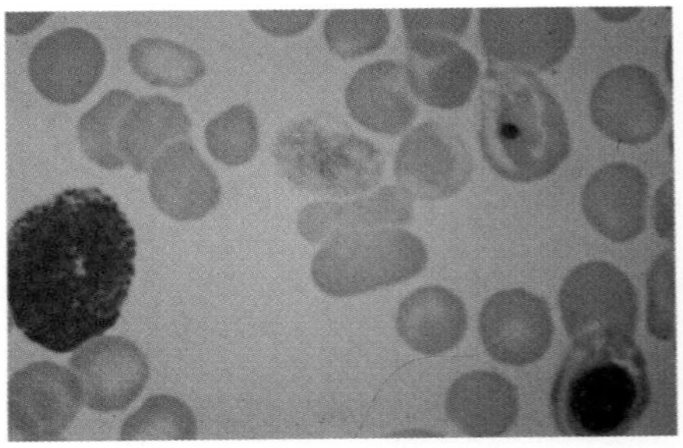

L, Peripheral blood smear showing a Howell-Jolly body in the erythrocyte in the right upper area of the slide. The round, dense granule represents nuclear DNA. At the lower right is a nucleated red cell. A giant platelet is present in the middle of the slide and a basophil is noted in the lower left corner. The patient had an underlying myeloproliferative disorder with a recent splenectomy (× 1200).

PLATE 3 HEMATOLOGIC DISEASES

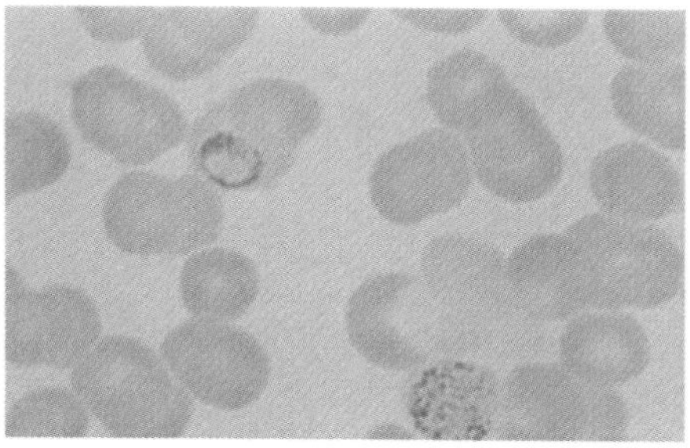

A, Peripheral blood showing malaria parasites within two red blood cells. Note the ringed form in the upper red cell and the numerous parasites in the lower red cell (× 1200).

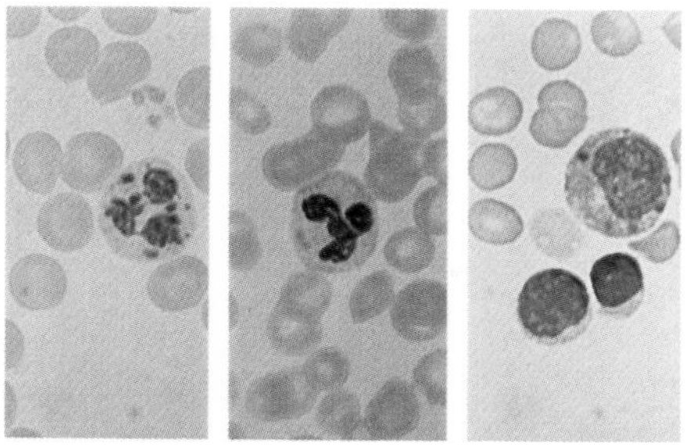

B, Leukocyte inclusions. *Left,* Giant basophilic granules in the Chediak-Higashi anomaly. *Center,* Basophilic inclusions (Döhle's bodies) within immature granulocytes. *Right,* Myelocyte with basophilic granules in Chediak-Higashi syndrome (× 1200).

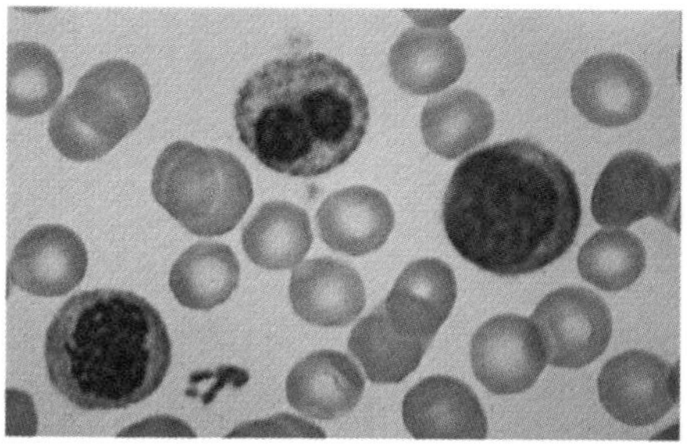

C, Pelger-Huët cells in the peripheral blood of a patient with chronic myeloid leukemia. Note the mature neutrophil in the center with an unsegmented adult poly in the lower left corner. A myeloblast is seen in the right of the slide (× 1200).

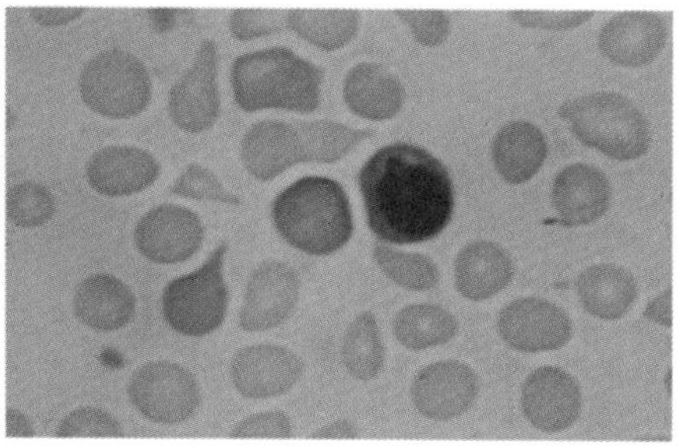

D, Peripheral blood smear showing leukoerythoblastic features, from a patient with myeloid metaplasia. Note the large nucleated red cell along with numerous tear drop–shaped red cells. Polychromatophilia is also present. Not seen in this slide are immature myeloid cells (× 1200).

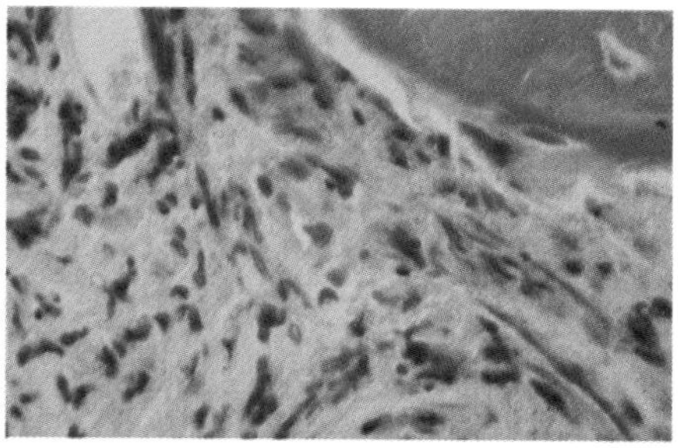

E, Myelofibrosis. Bone marrow biopsy showing intense fibrous tissue and primitive marrow reticulum cells replacing normal bone marrow elements (× 1000).

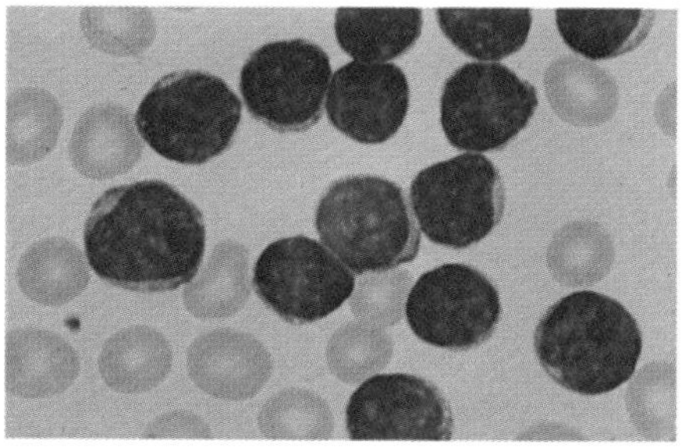

F, Chronic lymphocytic leukemia. Peripheral blood smear showing a majority of small mature-appearing lymphocytes, characterized by clumped nuclear chromatin and a rim of cytoplasm (× 1200).

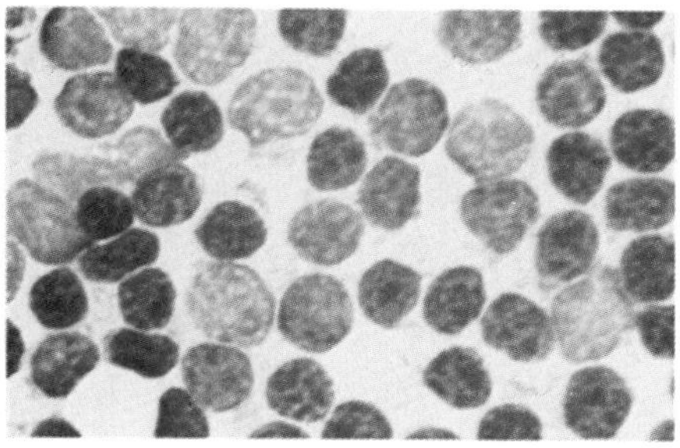

G, Bone marrow. Chronic lymphocytic leukemia showing dense infiltration by small mature-appearing lymphocytes with clumped chromatin and scanty cytoplasm (× 1200).

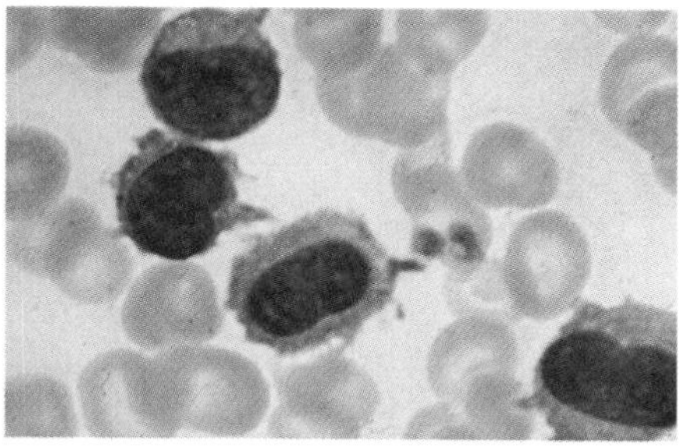

H, Hairy cell leukemia. Peripheral blood showing medium sized lymphoid cells with cytoplasmic strands or "hairs." Nuclei are somewhat immature (light staining) and indented in some of the cells. Indistinct nuclei are evident (× 1200).

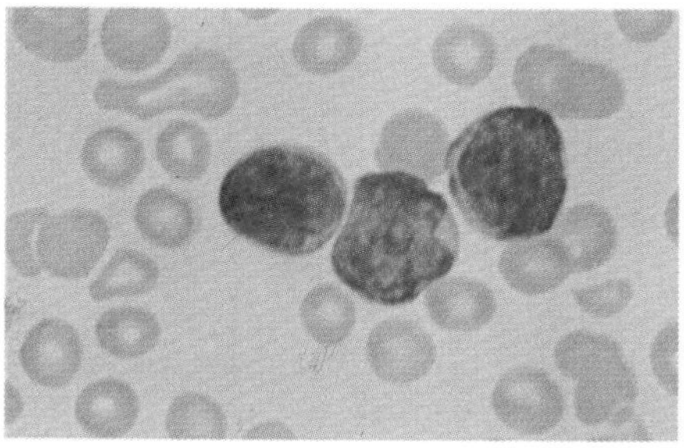

I, Acute lymphocytic leukemia. Peripheral blood showing three lymphoblasts, characterized by small size, immature light staining chromatin pattern, indistinct nuclei, and scanty cytoplasm (× 1200).

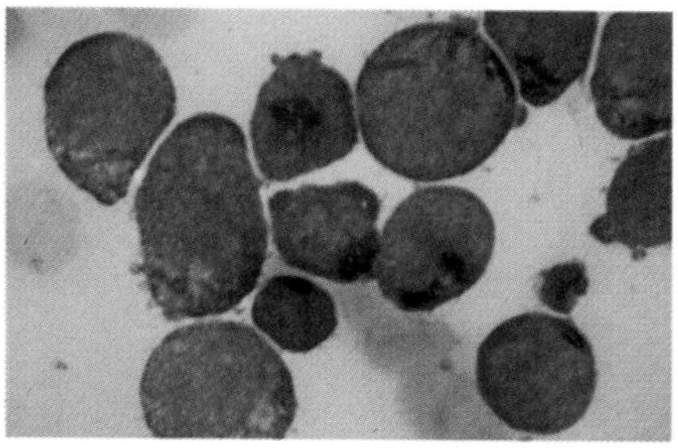

J, Acute myelogenous leukemia. Peroxidase stain showing marked positive activity in the majority of blasts, including the presence of Auer rods (× 1200).

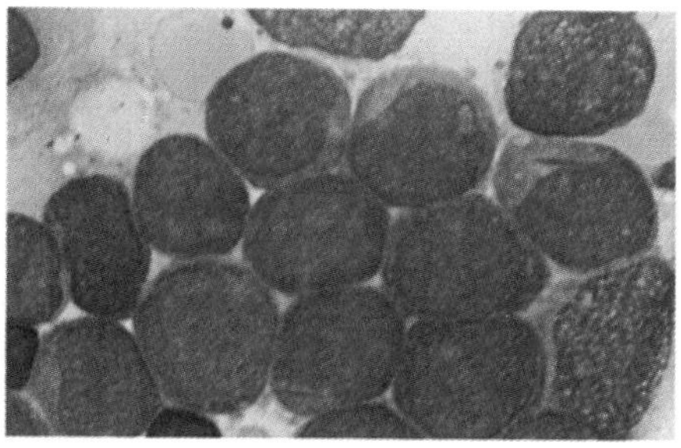

K, Acute myelogenous leukemia. Bone marrow, Giemsa stained, showing myeloblasts, some with prominent Auer rods (× 1200).

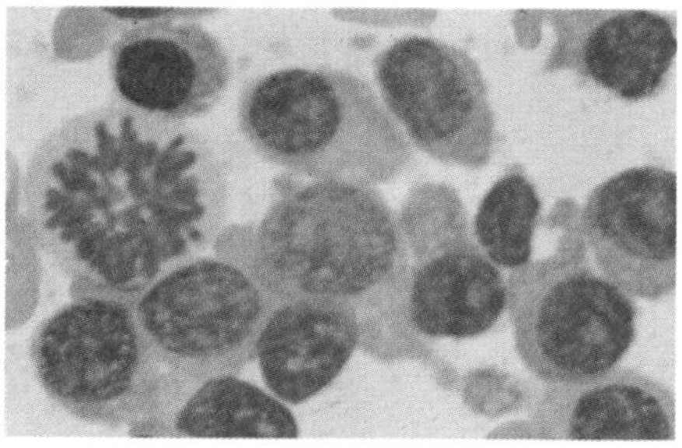

L, Multiple myeloma. Marrow shows a clump of immature plasma cells with eccentric nucleus, prominent nucleoli, and deep blue cytoplasm. A mitosis is present (× 1200).

PLATE 4 LYME DISEASE

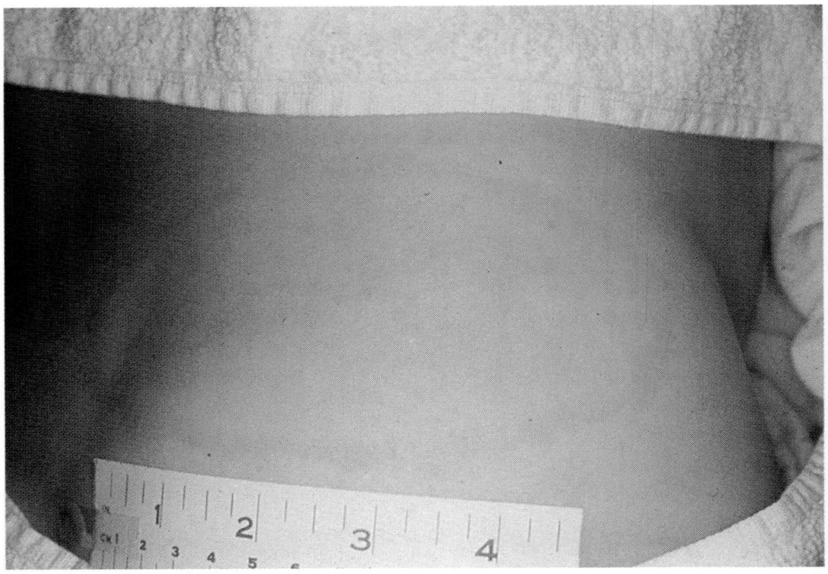

A

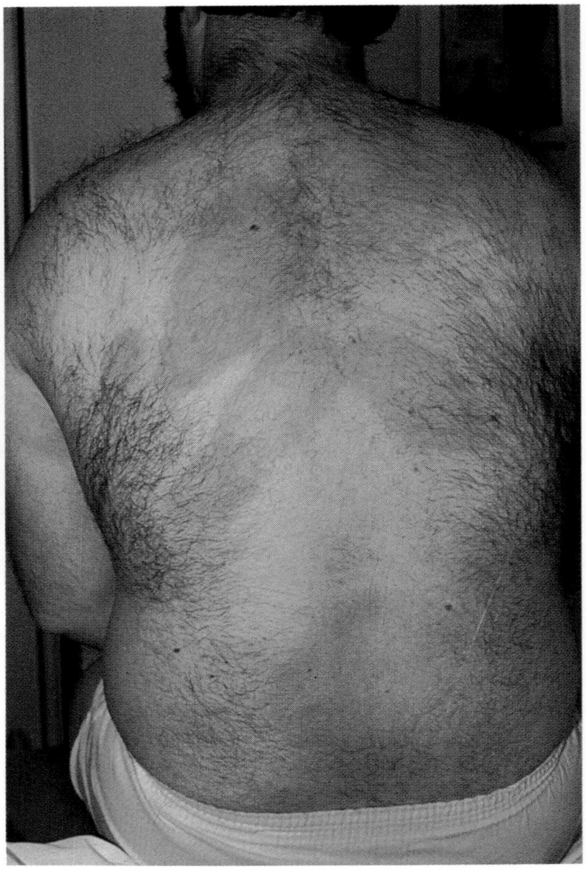

B

Major dermatologic manifestations of Lyme disease.
A, Erythema chronicum migrans (ECM). In a 17-day-old lesion, an expanding red margin surrounds an area of central clearing. ECM is the clinical hallmark of Lyme disease.
B, Four days after onset of ECM, this patient has developed secondary annular lesions; some of their borders have merged. (From Steere AC, Bartenhagen NH, Craft JE, et al.: The early clinical manifestations of Lyme disease. Ann Intern Med 99:76–82, 1983.)

PLATE 5. *See figure on the opposite page.*

A to *D* show various erythrocyte forms of falciparum or vivax malaria (× 1500).

A, "Ring forms" of *Plasmodium falciparum.* Note the delicate rings and an erythrocyte containing two organisms.

B, Trophozoite of *Plasmodium vivax.* The red cell is enlarged, Schüffner's dots are seen, and the parasite is large and ameboid.

C, Schizont of *Plasmodium vivax* with at least 18 merozoite nuclei.

D, Gametocyte of *Plasmodium falciparum.* The crescent or banana shape is characteristic.

E, Trypanosoma rhodesiense in the peripheral blood. It has a nucleus, posterior kinetoplast, undulating membrane, and flagellum (× 1500).

F, Spleen smear showing a cell filled with *Leishmania donovani.* The rod-shaped kinetoplast and large round nucleus appear as two adjacent red dots.

G, Methenamine silver nitrate stain of clump of *Pneumocystis* cysts. They appear as black circles against the blue background (× 800).

H, Stool sample observed by light microscopy, showing a motile *Entamoeba histolytica* moving in a straight line across the field. The ameba contains lucent vacuoles and shows a pseudopod directed to the upper right (× 500).

(*A, C, D,* and *F* are photographs taken by T. C. Jones from the Cornell Parasitology teaching slides; *B* is from the collection of H. Zaiman, originally photographed by M. Wittner; *E* and *G* were provided by R. B. Roberts; *H* is a photograph of fresh material provided by T. C. Jones.)

PLATE 5 PROTOZOAN DISEASES

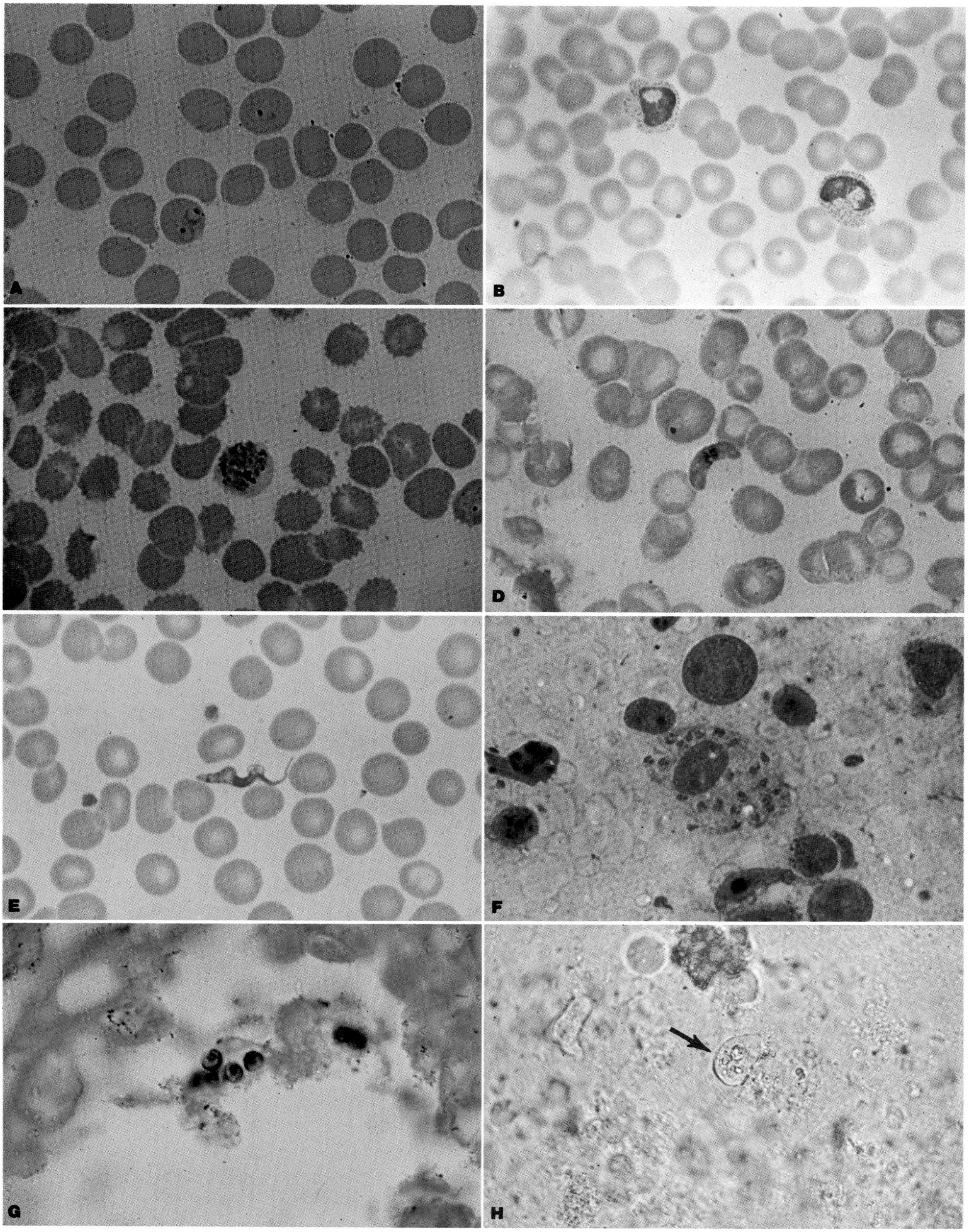

See legend on the opposite page.

PLATE 6 SKIN DISEASES

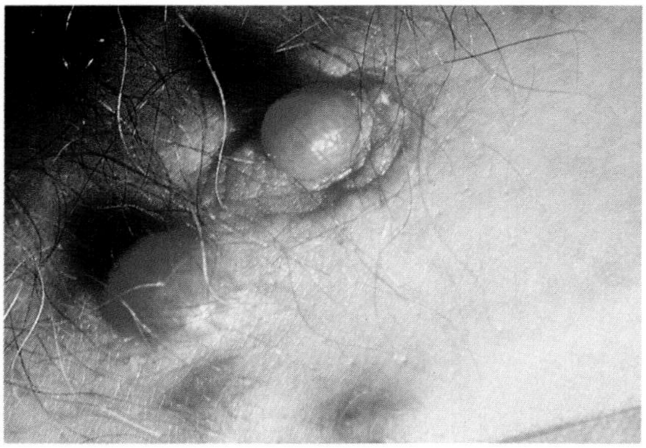

A, Skin metastases. Firm, hard, red nodules.

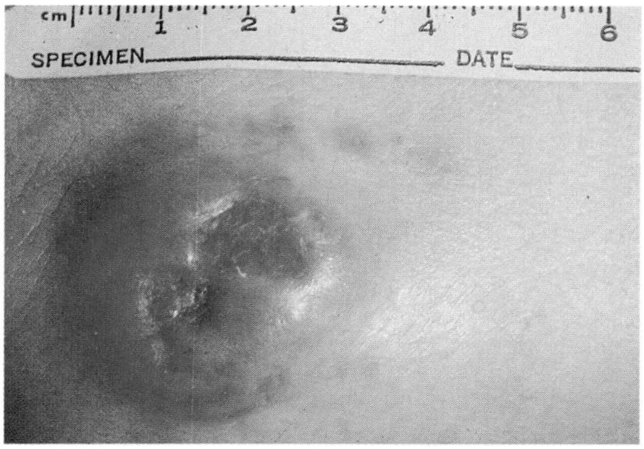

B, Mycosis fungoides, tumor stage.

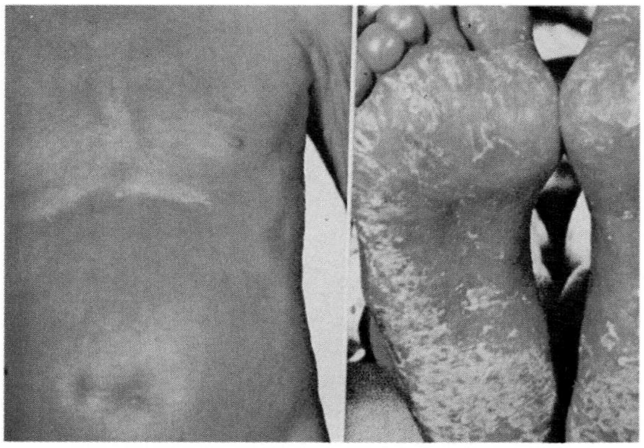

C, Sezary syndrome, exfoliative dermatitis stage.

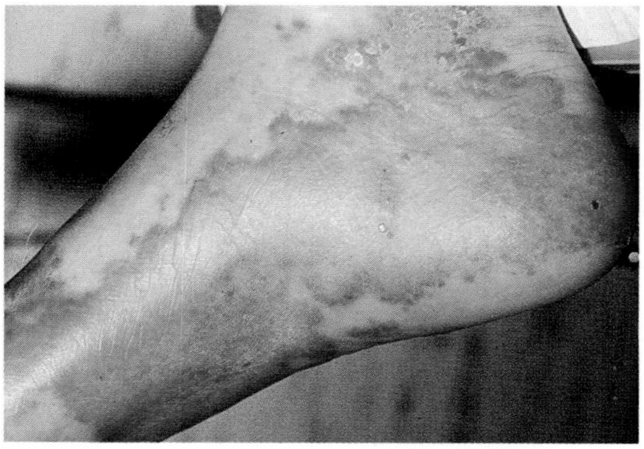

D, Classic Kaposi's sarcoma.

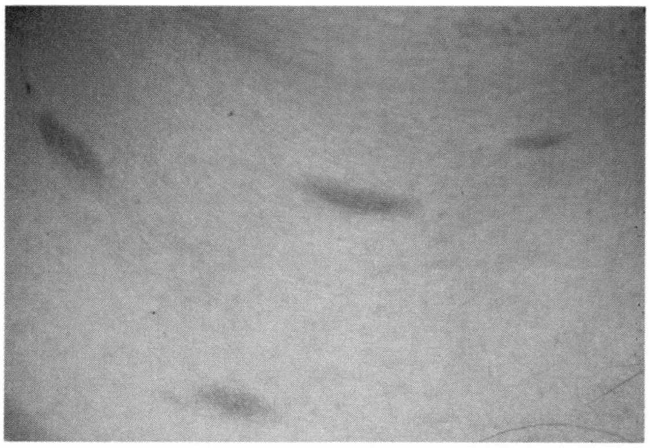

E, Kaposi's sarcoma in AIDS. Red-brown macules, papules, and nodules characteristically appear over the upper body.

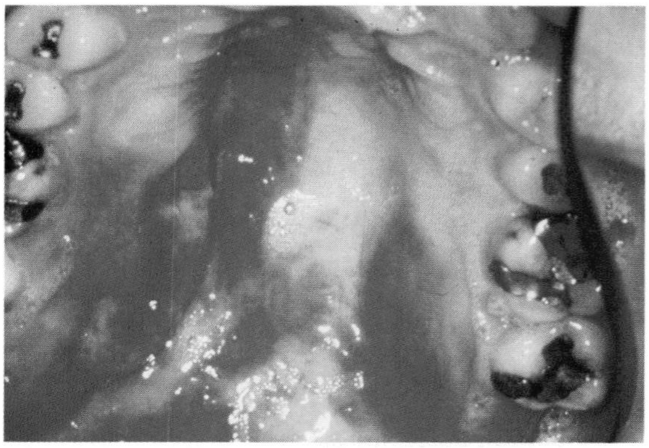

F, Kaposi's sarcoma in AIDS. Involvement of the oral mucosa.

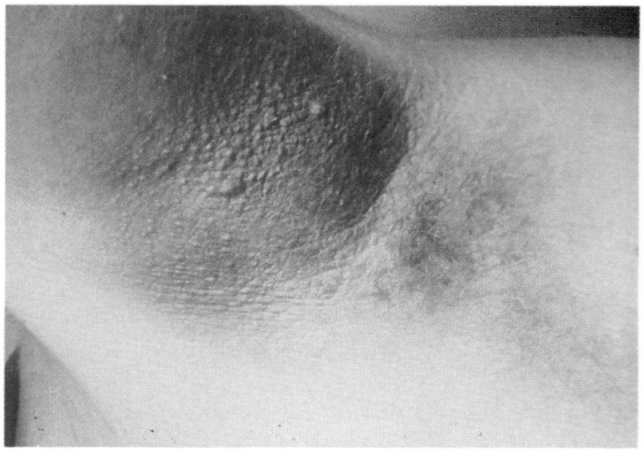

G, Acanthosis nigricans. Axillary lesion.

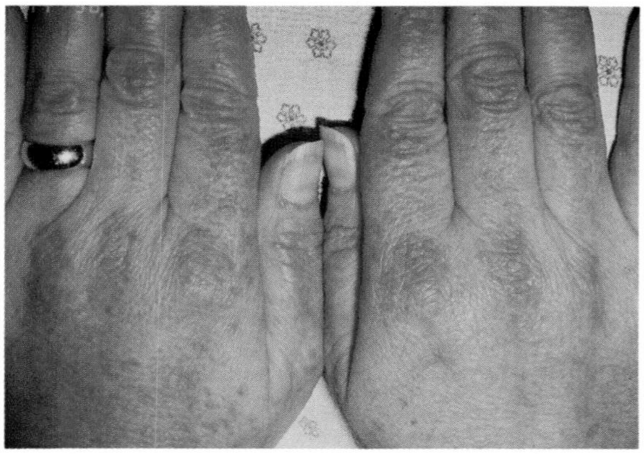

H, Dermatomyositis. Gottron's papules over the knuckles.

PLATE 7 EYE DISEASES

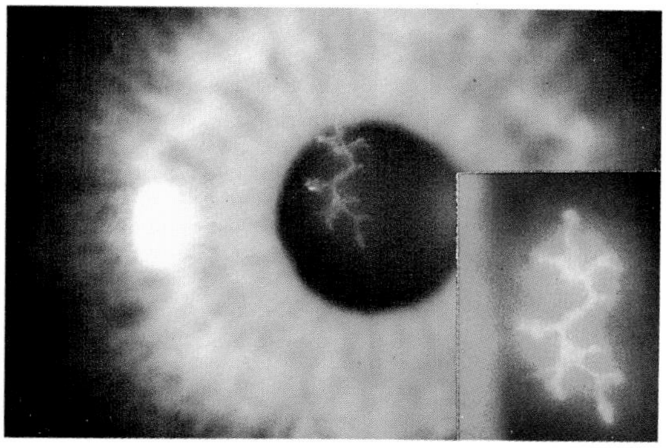

A, Herpesvirus hominis corneal epithelial dendrite in diffuse light and (inset) in light passed through a cobalt blue filter after fluorescein staining.

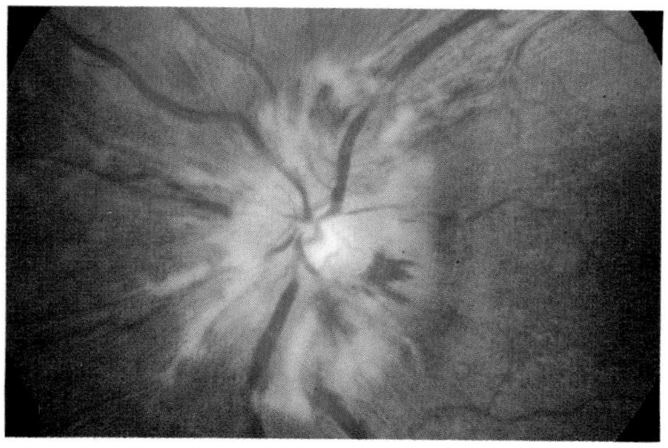

B, Papilledema in a young person. Note disc swelling, hemorrhages, and exudates with preservation of the physiologic cup.

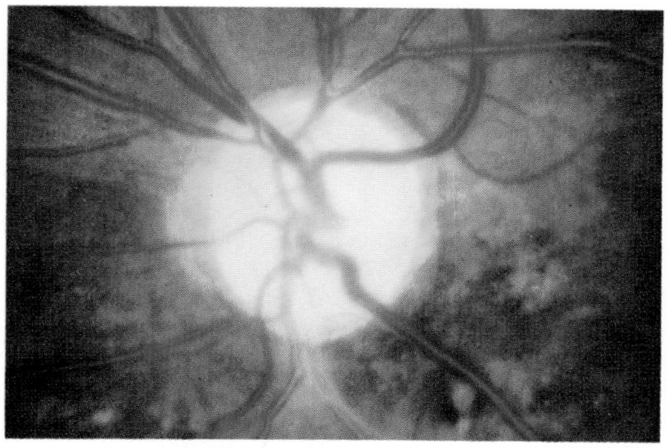

C, Primary optic atrophy in a young black man. The disc is pale, but there is no cupping or gliosis. The glial tissue seen over an inferior arteriole is a normal variant.

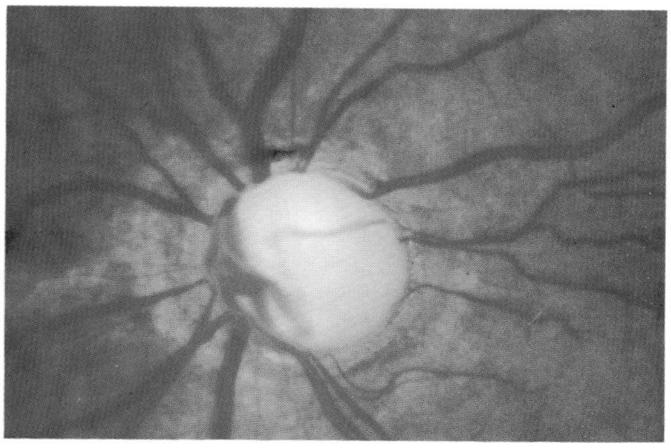

D, Advanced glaucomatous optic atrophy. Vessels curve over the edge of the almost complete cup and disappear into its depths.

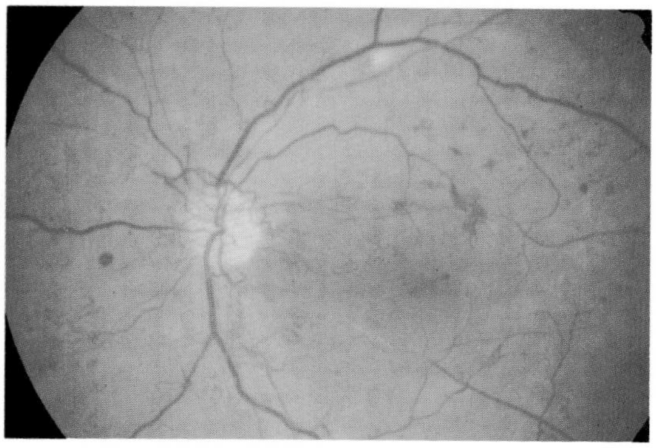

E, Proliferative diabetic retinopathy. Dot and blot hemorrhages appear diffusely, with neovascularization forming at the disc and along the major vascular arcades.

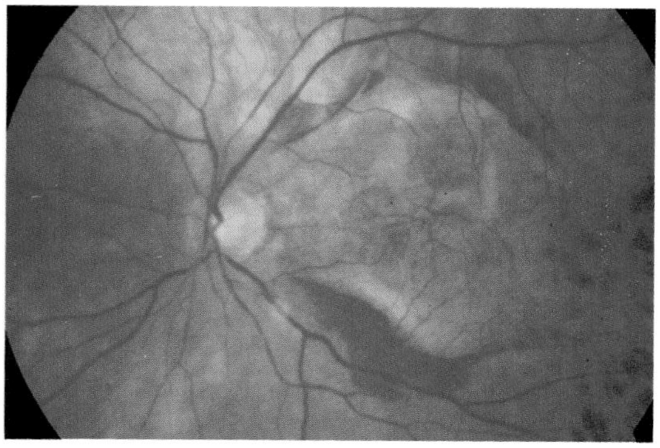

F, Age-related macular degeneration. A neovascular net lies in the macula with surrounding hemorrhage.

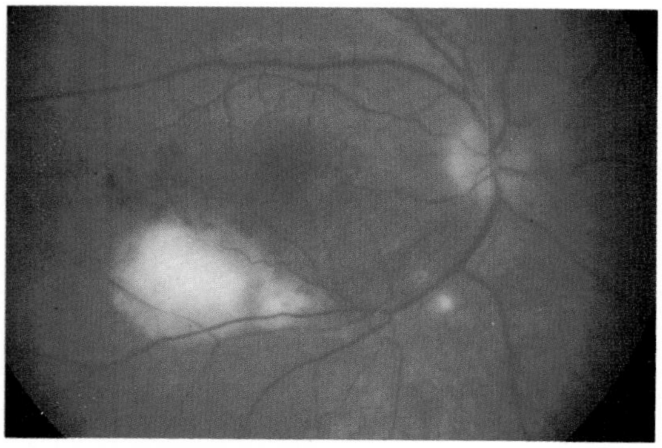

G, Cytomegalovirus retinitis. Hemorrhage and retinal necrosis lie along the inferotemporal vascular arcade.

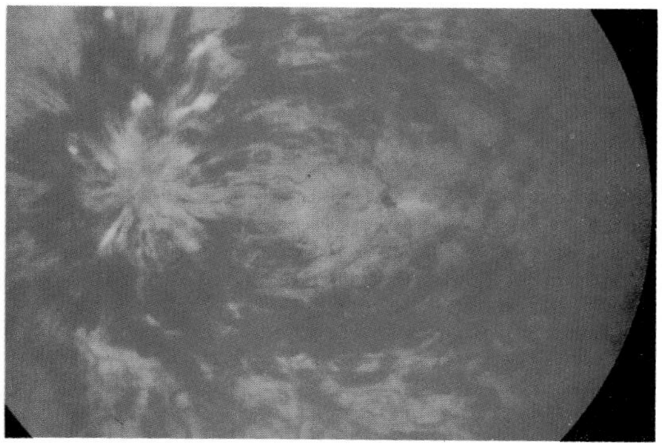

H, Central retinal vein occlusion. Note disc swelling and diffuse hemorrhages.

Photographs taken by Mr. Harry Kachadoorian, C.R.A., University of Massachusetts Medical School, Worcester, Massachusetts

PLATE 8 DISORDERS OF VITAMIN METABOLISM

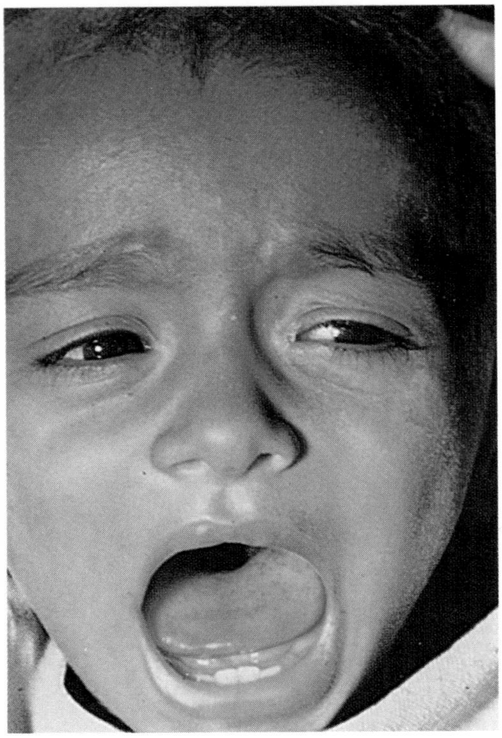

A

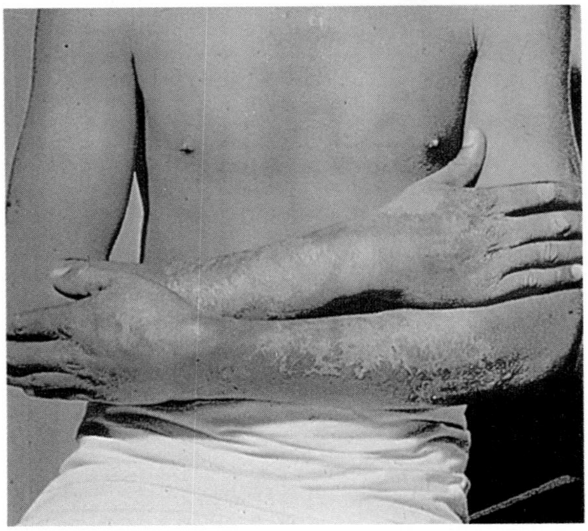

B

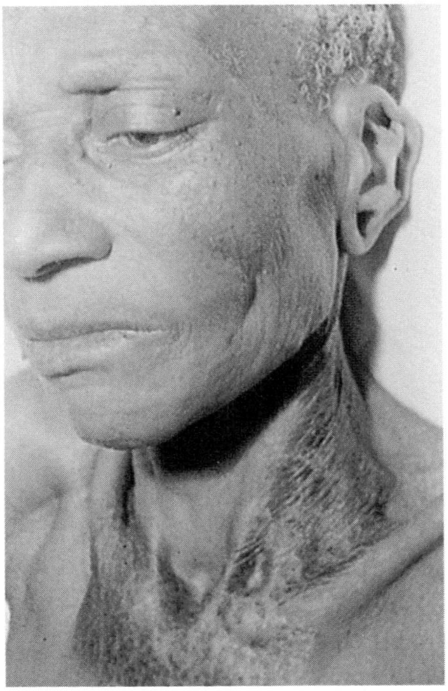

C

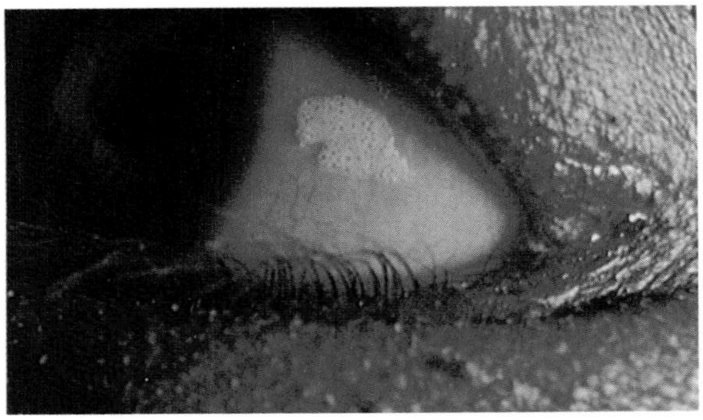

D

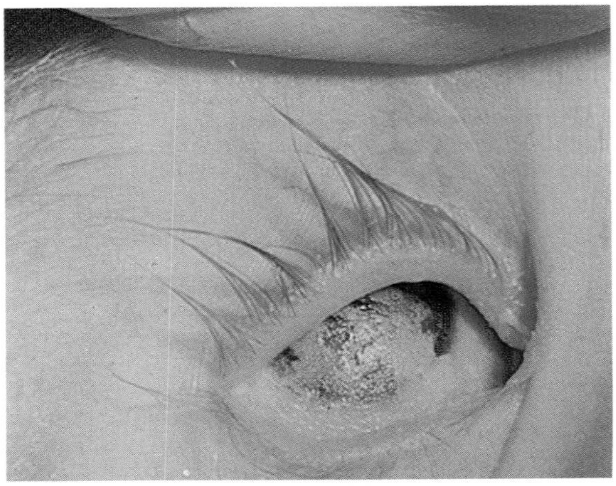

E

A, Magenta tongue, an abnormality commonly observed in patients with riboflavin deficiency, but probably not completely specific for deficiency of this vitamin. The tongue is purplish red and painful.

B, Early pellagra affecting the arms, resulting from dietary deficiency of niacin. The dermatitis begins with erythema, progresses to blebs and bullae, and in later stages becomes rough, cracked, and brittle, as shown here. Lesions are most prominent in sun-exposed skin but are not necessarily restricted to these areas.

C, Casal's necklace, a broad collar over the neck, is a classic manifestation of pellagra. Skin changes are similar to those shown in *B.*

D, A large, diffuse, foamy Bitot's spot, observed in the conjunctiva of a patient with vitamin A deficiency.

E, Advanced Bitot's spot involving cornea and conjunctiva, producing marked impairment of vision.

PART I

MEDICINE AS A LEARNED AND HUMANE PROFESSION

The *Cecil Textbook of Medicine* is addressed to medical students, residents, fellows, and practitioners of all ages. It deals with the body of knowledge of human disease. In contrast, these introductory essays are presented mainly for those now entering the profession, for students deserve a broader perspective of medicine than is offered by its subject matter alone.

1 MEDICINE AS AN ART

Lloyd H. Smith, Jr.

What is medicine? "Medicine is not a science but a learned profession, deeply rooted in a number of sciences and charged with the obligation to apply them for man's benefit." In this eloquent statement from an earlier edition of this book, Walsh McDermott defined medicine as a human activity undertaken for the benefit of others whether in the area of public health, "statistical compassion," or in the care of the individual patient.

Medicine can also be defined in other terms. It is a mutable body of knowledge, skills, and traditions applicable to the preservation of health, the cure of disease, and the amelioration of suffering. The boundaries of medicine blend into psychology, sociology, economics, and even into cultural heritage. Disease may be encoded in the genome; disease may also be encoded by the deprivations of poverty and ignorance. Medicine must therefore be concerned not only with an abnormal molecule but also with an abnormal childhood. As such it is open ended in a way that is both humbling and exhilarating to those who pursue it as a career.

Medicine is continually changing. The honored verities of one generation become the shopworn shibboleths of the next. Much of what we now so confidently espouse, including that compressed within this edition, will amuse our successors as being remarkably bizarre in its naiveté. Medical competence is based on the continuing pursuit of ever changing concepts. It must be renewed as the substance of medicine itself is transformed.

The practice of medicine is far more than the application of scientific principles to a particular biologic aberration. Its focus is on the patient whose welfare is its continuing purpose. That purpose of medicine is self evident in theory, but more difficult to sustain under the pressures of medical practice. For example, it is tragically easy for the patient to become merely the repository in which a disease or a syndrome has chosen to manifest its particular silhouette. During the training years every physician has subconsciously participated in what might be termed the personification of disease. A case of meningitis is admitted through the emergency room; a pheochromocytoma will be discussed at Grand Rounds. It is perhaps inevitable that a disease becomes symbolically an entity to the physician who must become familiar with all of its manifestations and guises. In the art of medicine the physician must be the advocate of the patient as well as the adversary of disease. It is the patient who is personified rather than the disease.

THE PATIENT. The description of a patient is simply that of a fellow human being in need of help. The patient comes seeking help because of a problem relating to his or her health. This subjective judgment carries with it disquieting concerns, although these may be unexpressed. Anxiety is present even in the most stoical of patients; this fact must never be forgotten or disregarded by the physician. The patient's anxiety may be specific—for example, in a fear of cancer with all that implies in the public mind concerning pain, degradation, and inexorable death. More often the anxiety is amorphous: fear of loss of independence or employment; fear of failure to meet obligations to one's family or to retain the regard of a loved one; or fear of an inability to maintain a life of dignity and significance. In the rush to crystallize a chief complaint and present illness the physician too often brushes aside these considerations.

The patient presents to the physician on alien and unfamiliar ground—in the structured and artificial setting of an office, a clinic, or a hospital bed. This form of health care of the individual, as opposed to health care in the aggregate, is often described by the unfelicitous phrase "the personal encounter system." Unfortunately it often seems distressingly like confrontation to the patient, who comes after all for comfort, not for encounter. Each human being is unique within a life that is enormously complex—in heredity, early experiences, cultural and psychologic environment, education, opportunities, successes, failures, fantasies, emotional commitments, motivations, and in the adjustments and compromises that serve to cripple or to mature. Living, therefore, is the ultimate personal encounter system. With an extensive and diverse experience the patient comes to the physician with "a problem." A chief complaint is requested. Defenses must be lowered and the emotions that spill out may be distressing. The patient's response must be selective and brief; as a result it is not infrequently distorted, perhaps even misleading.

What does the patient want when coming to see a physician? There are certain common hopes and expectations. Patients want to be listened to, so that their fears and concerns can be fully expressed and the burden shared. They want physicians to be interested in them as fellow human beings in a compassionate but nonjudgmental fashion. They expect professional competence incorporating the best in medical science and technology. They want to be reasonably informed as to the probable cause of their concerns and what the future is likely to hold. They want not to be abandoned. To each patient these desires and expectations vary in relative importance. It is notable that not all patients expect to be cured. These expectations will be further discussed in the light of how the physician should endeavor to meet them.

TRADITIONAL EXPECTATIONS OF PATIENTS. *Patients want to be listened to and understood.* This has been well expressed by Wilfred Trotter, a great English neurosurgeon:

". . . As long as medicine is an art, its chief and characteristic instrument must be human faculty. We come therefore to the very practical question of what aspects of human faculty it is necessary for the good doctor to cultivate. . . . The first to be named must always be the power of attention, of giving one's whole mind to the patient without the interposition of oneself. It sounds simple but only the very greatest doctors ever fully attain it. It is an active process and not either mere resigned listening or even politely waiting until you can interrupt. Disease often tells its secrets in a casual parenthesis. . . ."

Eventually the medical record must be organized in a logical and consistent fashion. But a history rarely unfolds that way. Patients do not divulge their fears in neat paragraphs or in direct responses to a cascade of queries. It is important to let patients tell their own stories. The manner of formulation and expression of symptoms and anxieties may be as informative as the medical data transmitted. The good physician is an attentive listener, with an ear for Trotter's "casual parenthesis."

Patients want physicians to be interested in them as fellow human beings. This interest cannot be that of the unusual "case" of the carcinoid syndrome or of hairy cell leukemia; the center of interest must be the patient as a person. It is difficult for the physician to feign such an interest, for patients are very perceptive, especially during the vulnerability that illness induces. In the practice of medicine the physician will encounter all of the virtues and vices to which mankind is heir. The physician need not be morally neutral in personal judgments, but these must be stringently excluded from professional activities. The response of the physician to human frailty and fallibility should be that of compassion rather than cynicism, of interest in the infinite variety of human experience rather than of repulsion from its aberrations.

Patients expect professional competence in medical science and technology. The physician must be a scholar both to attain professional competence and to sustain it during times of revolutionary changes in science and technology. All of the other attributes of the good physician will be of little avail in the absence of sound scholarship. Compassion is no substitute for knowing what should be done. The education of the physician and the role of the physician as a scientist will be discussed more fully below.

Patients want to be kept reasonably informed. The physician must listen to and communicate with the patient. Time must be set aside for this. Failure to do so is a serious error, for silence is a form of communication that is usually adverse. The physician should voluntarily answer questions of concern to the patient. The physician must also inform the patient concerning the illness and what it implies. A number of books have been developed to assist in patient education and are often quite effective in translating medical terminology into lay terms. Furthermore, clubs for mutual support and education have been formed by patients who share their common experiences with such chronic disabilities as ileostomies or amputations. Admirable and important as these are, they do not obviate the need for patients to learn from their own physicians about their particular illnesses and what they may mean in and for their future lives. This need extends beyond the legal confines of informed consent, which is now an important issue in medical practice.

Patients want not to be abandoned. Death comes to everyone. There are finite limits to what can be accomplished by medical science and technology in the alleviation of suffering and the prolongation of life. This fact is well known to both patients and physicians. When that limit is reached, the physician often feels powerless and even guilty that no more can be done. As a consequence there is a tendency to withdraw attention and direct it elsewhere. Nothing could be a greater mistake. It is at the margins of medical science that the role of the physician is enhanced. It is here that the art of medicine comes to the forefront in the care of the patient, whether it be by emotional support, relief of pain, small adjustments in medicines or diet, daily conversation and examination, or other methods to show that the patient is still someone of dignity and worth in whom interest has not been lost and for whom hope has not been abandoned. And when no more can be done for the patient it is time to care for the family. It is this caring role rather than the curing role of the physician that is so well described in Ch. 4 by Lewis Thomas. At this stage, as Walsh McDermott has written, "it is up to each of us to follow to the fullest measure the charge laid down long ago for the physician to become himself the treatment."

THE PHYSICIAN. The physician has both chosen and been chosen to enter an arduous and demanding profession, the origins of which stretch back to antiquity. Part priest, part shaman, part mystic, part alchemist, the physician of the past reflected the beliefs and expectations of the time and met a perceived need of fellow men. The history of medicine is part of the heritage of every physician and reflects the cultural history of each society.

The physician enters a profession with established values and traditions of ethical conduct and responsibilities. But each physician, as each patient, is unique. The physician is not a disembodied instrument that can be passively shaped by the profession, but rather a human being with innate strengths and weaknesses that must be recognized in order to meet the expectations of patients and of the profession, not least of which are those standards established for oneself. The qualities of the ideal physician are easy to state but difficult to attain: compassion, sincere interest in one's fellow man, knowledge of human nature, tact, equanimity, sustained scholarship, curiosity, and high ethical standards. Physical and mental vigor might be added to those traits, for the life of the physician is not for the languid or the disengaged. No one has been endowed with or ever fully achieves excellence in all of these qualities. One must first know oneself and judge how one can most closely approach those ideals in one's professional life.

THE EDUCATION OF THE PHYSICIAN. Barriers are encountered at the very beginning in the initial selection for medical school as many seek entry for few positions. Undergraduate education is sometimes distorted and breadth of personal experience curtailed in a grim and often distasteful race for competitive acceptance. This inadvertent feedback inhibition not infrequently results from erroneous conceptions of what may or may not impress admission committees of medical schools. Nevertheless, the phenomenon remains as a concern to all who are interested in the future of our profession. Admission committees of medical schools too often exercise allosteric control over the higher education of those destined to enter our profession.

The Basic Science Years. In the standard curriculum of medical school in the United States two years are largely devoted to the sciences basic to medicine and two years to clinical training. Fortunately there are a number of interesting variations on this thematic progression which diminish its rigidity and permit the student to re-explore basic science after an introductory clinical experience.

In the United States students usually arrive at medical school after an intensive four-year experience at a college or a university. They anticipate a scholarly atmosphere of a graduate school which will prepare them to enter the practice of a profession for which they hold idealistic expectations. Instead they are immediately assailed with a formidable array of "basic sciences" linked to the structure and function of the human organ systems. New facts constitute not so much an intellectual feast as an engorgement. Each discipline is attended by devotees who are passionately persuaded of the seminal role of their segment of science in the future of the profession. This commitment is translated into the basic academic commodity, curricular time, in which these cluttered wares are exhibited. Awed by the dimensionless task, students struggle with uneven success to assimilate and survive, conscious always that their receptor mechanisms are overloaded and of a continuing sense of high output failure. They look forward in hope that subsequent years will reward their endurance in the more congenial atmosphere of the clinic.

This is patently a caricature, as all will recognize. It can be said, as Mark Twain said of Wagner's music, "it is not as bad as it sounds." The quality of basic science in medical schools is often superb; the substance of modern science has a certain grandeur; many faculty members are gifted in imparting a sense of intellectual adventure to their students; finally, many students now arrive at medical school with a mature understanding of one or more of the fundamental disciplines of biology. Nevertheless this caricature contains elements of truth as seen from the perspective of medical students. The central question is not whether basic science is necessary for medical research, since few would deny its importance there, but whether it is relevant in the education of every physician to the degree to which it is currently emphasized. In the real world of patient care, public health, and medical economics, should the student have to struggle with the intricacies of post-transcriptional modifications of messenger RNA, or is this merely a rite of passage prescribed by a science-obsessed faculty? This is a reasonable question and calls for a response other than a simple reference to flexnerian orthodoxy.

A knowledge of the scientific underpinnings of medicine is clearly necessary in order to marshal the basic information required to understand a patient's illness and to be able to reason logically about the problems of diagnosis and therapy. If there were any doubt on that point, it would be quickly dispelled by random perusal of this book. Much of the basic science which seems abstruse and irrelevant today will find its way into clinical practice in the not too distant future. Medical research is only one step removed from patient care.

Beyond the assimilation of scientific information, there is an even more important consideration. Many of you will have most of your professional experience in the twenty-first century. The changes in medical science and technology will be enormous and largely unpredictable. Only the scientific method will remain unaltered as an invaluable instrument with which fallible man can acquire new knowledge and, equally important, debride that which proves fallacious. It is imperative that students learn the scientific method as part of their education if they are to participate critically and effectively in a changing profession. How can this be done? Perhaps the best method is to participate personally, even for a relatively brief period of time, in a research project so that learning comes from first hand experience. If that does not prove practical, one can pursue some scientific topic in depth and write a critical analysis of it. It is important to learn one area of inquiry in great detail, even though it may have to be a limited area, in order to penetrate to its frontier. It is only there that science can be understood as a process rather than as a repository.

The Clinical Years. In his perceptive essay "On Becoming a Clinician," in an earlier edition of this textbook, Paul B. Beeson described many of the disquieting stresses to which the student is subjected on entry into the clinical years. Every medical student will benefit from reading those thoughts from one of America's most distinguished physicians. Most students enter the clinical years with a sense of relief, but it is relief linked with anxieties. Some of these anxieties cluster around the following questions:

How can I cope with the uncertainties of clinical medicine?

What are the boundaries of clinical medicine? How much and what am I supposed to learn?

How will I function in my interactions with patients?

How will I measure up to the expectations of my colleagues?

How will I be able to maintain my own identity as an individual in a profession that so obsessively dominates my time and energy?

Other questions could be formulated. Each student possesses a unique idiotype of anxieties that cannot be purged by platitudes. Each will arrive at personal answers, or more likely at personal accommodations, through experience.

THE UNCERTAINTY PRINCIPLE OF CLINICAL MEDICINE. There is an "uncertainty principle" in medicine as there is in physics. The practice of medicine is inexact and will remain so. If it were not, it would be a science or a technology rather than an art. The measuring instrument is personal and unique. Subjective mensuration defies precision. Who can quantify nausea or the severity of pain? Symptoms may be forgotten, suppressed, or amplified when filtered through the grid of personality. Available data are often indirect, incomplete, or even contradictory. Patients respond in varying fashions to treatment across the range from simple reassurance (which is rarely simple) to surgical or pharmaceutical interventions. Clinical medicine is often based on experience and judgment—which are largely euphemisms for a knowledge of probabilities.

The process of formulating a diagnosis or selecting a therapy is not as arbitrary as it first seems. There are rational means for narrowing the range of diagnostic possibilities: a precise description of symptoms; an accurate and thorough characterization of physical findings; selective laboratory studies to evaluate the functions of organ systems; a synthesis of information to define syndromic patterns; a marshaling of information on etiology and pathogenesis. All of this requires attention to detail, consistency of work habits, and good intellect.

Hypotheses are formed and algorithms branch away from various entry points as new data are obtained which support or fail to support a working diagnosis. This process of clinical reasoning is often best displayed in the Clinicopathologic Conference (CPC). In the absence of certainty, best guesses must be utilized and in making informed guesses, generally dignified as judgments, the clinician actually relies upon subliminal statistics.

Medical decisions based on probabilities are necessary but also perilous. Even the most astute physician will occasionally be wrong. The wise physician will often recognize that a decision is erroneous and discard or modify the hypothesis on which it is based. The best decision may be approached only by successive approximations. Action may have to be taken despite lack of confirmation of a hypothesis (working diagnosis). Chester M. Jones, a noted clinical teacher, used to say: "If you cannot make a diagnosis, make a decision." Despite the remarkable contributions of science and technology, clinical medicine is frequently inexactitude in action. The student entering the clinical years will quickly realize the dangers to the welfare of the patient of dogmatism in clinical practice. The ambiguities and errors that you will encounter in your own experience and observe in the work of others should be an antidote to arrogance. Some errors are inevitable and should not humiliate you, but they should teach humility.

CLINICAL MEDICINE AS A DISCIPLINE WITHOUT BOUNDARIES. The basic sciences are demanding but, as taught in medical schools, they have reasonably defined margins. It is true that these margins are somewhat artificial, since the disciplines of modern biology merge almost imperceptibly into one another. Nevertheless, the educational responsibilities of the medical student can often be designated within the subject material of a lecture course, syllabus, and textbook. Not so in clinical medicine. The student emerges into an open-ended system of bewildering complexity in which science is blurred by sociology; psychology interacts with economics; and traditions and ethical concepts are buffeted by new imperatives. Within this complicated system, the practice of clinical medicine goes forward. The student does not encounter a theoretical discipline to be observed and analyzed in tranquility, but is abruptly thrown into the structured workings of the second largest industry in the United States where the health and even the survival of many people are at stake on a daily basis.

Based on previous educational experiences, students often ask, "How much am I expected to learn in this course?" No one can supply a satisfactory answer. The student stands on the threshold of a learning experience in clinical medicine that will extend over the remainder of an active career as a physician. Learning must have that stretch if the student is to meet the responsibilities of a physician. The course is merely a contrived entry point into that longitudinal experience. More advanced faculty members, medical residents, or even senior students in other rotations in medicine seem remarkably well informed. Yet no single individual has a balanced knowledge in all aspects of medicine. The specialist will often be adept only within a defined subset of medicine, and even the generalist will be uneven in many areas of information. Within this confusing and sometimes overwhelming setting the student must become an independent scholar in medicine—independent in the sense that never again will others outline or circumscribe the subject material.

Most students adapt themselves remarkably quickly to the changed environment of clinical medicine. The new language of the hospital, including its acronymic barbarisms (SOB, PERLA, COPD, etc.), no longer jar the ear, and the concepts of pathophysiology being applied at the bedside awaken latent memories. The student learns that there are habits of thought and clusters of associations so that the physician does not laboriously go back to first principles to meet each new clinical problem. These thought patterns are efficient and useful if they do not gel into medicine by reflex and aphorism. The student learns by listening, participating, observing, arguing, reading, and reflecting. As earlier generations of students have discovered, the intensity of the experience and the special chemistry of confronting the clinical problem of a specific patient serve to fix the information received in one's memory with a vividness far beyond that obtained from even the most brilliant lecture.

Beyond the required participation in clinical rotations, how should the student approach the study of medicine? It would be presumptuous to give a doctrinaire answer. Medical students have usually been seasoned by five or six years of higher education before they begin the study of clinical medicine and during those years have developed their own best methods of learning. In approaching internal medicine, in contrast perhaps to some more circumscribed specialties, it will usually prove most valuable to study in depth the specific problems presented by one's own patients rather than beginning with a systematic approach to cover all of the discipline. In this way one can exploit the intense immediacy of those experiences which, supplemented by conferences, rounds, seminars, conversations, and all of the other ways of learning on the fly, will usually converge to give a broad familiarity with the subject. A share in the responsibility of caring for a patient is a powerful stimulus to learning.

What is the role of the *Cecil Textbook of Medicine* in the learning process? This book attempts to provide the student or the physician with succinct but authoritative summaries about diseases or groups of diseases. Essays written by more than 250 acknowledged experts in their respective fields represent collectively a systematic approach to internal medicine. The chapters are designed to give a basic, lucid, and up-to-date consensus concerning the state of the art in our understanding of specific diseases, but they cannot be all inclusive. Many of the topics discussed within a few pages have received more extended treatment elsewhere as separate monographs. Each of the subspecialty areas (cardiology, gastroenterology, endocrinology, etc.) is the subject of textbooks similar in size to this one. The student should therefore cultivate the habit of consulting at least some of the carefully selected references that extend the information supplied in this basic text.

In general it is also wise for students to begin reading medical journals early in their study of clinical medicine. In this way a start can be made toward the regular study of current medical literature and also the foundations of one's own medical library can be laid. Each student may have a personal preference. The most frequently read medical journal by students and practitioners is the *New England Journal of Medicine*. It is particularly useful for the student with its CPC, surveys of medical progress, editorial comments on current topics, original articles, and lively correspondence. In this manner the student establishes an early acquaintance with the frontiers of medicine and with its issues, uncertainties, and controversies.

THE STUDENT AND THE PATIENT. One of the student's earliest concerns on entering clinical medicine is how to interact with patients and how to assume the traditional role of a physician. The student is concerned that personal insecurities will impair effective communication with patients in whose care he or she is now called upon to participate. Rarely does this turn out in practice to be a serious problem. The expectations of most patients in the physician-patient interaction, discussed above, are realistic ones. Patients are usually aware of the progression of assigned responsibilities in the student-house staff-faculty team and do not expect omniscience or authoritarianism from the student. Not infrequently the patient forms a special attachment to the student, especially if the student has been perceptive enough to listen in the sense described above by Wilfred Trotter. If the student respects the personal dignity of the patient as a fellow human being, and listens in a sensitive manner, the patient responds with gratitude and returns that respect. Even when patients are initially perceived as hostile or belligerent, the student must maintain equanimity and try to understand the sources of these reactions. Do not allow yourself to be drawn into the flippant cynicism that sometimes passes for sophistication in the subculture of student and house staff training. Francis Peabody's sentient summary is still most apt, "for the secret of the care of the patient is in caring for the patient."

STUDENTS AND THEIR COLLEAGUES. Beginning in the clinical years the relationships of students with their colleagues in medicine undergo a subtle change. No longer are they merely the passive recipients of data and concepts supplied by the faculty through lectures, conferences, syllabi, or laboratories. They are participating with graduated responsibilities in the practice of medicine. A point in the medical history or a question asked by the student may prove decisive in arriving at the solution of a clinical problem. Frequently the most effective teachers of students are the house staff or more advanced students. Students will find many residents to be splendid teachers who not only make them feel at home on the service but also take the extra time to include them in all of the discussions. On most teaching services there is a certain amount of badinage or gamesmanship which enlivens interactions. If this is recognized as such, and not taken too seriously, it can serve to enhance rather than demean the learning experience. As a student you must not hesitate to ask questions or bring up new points of view and must not be intimidated by your current position in this shifting hierarchy. Even the chief medical resident faced similar qualms only a few years ago. But above all, remember that it is the patient's welfare, and not your own ego, that is paramount.

THE PHYSICIAN AS A NONPHYSICIAN. Beginning in the basic science years but exacerbated in the clinical years, students often become concerned about the level of commitment demanded of them. How much of a life that is finite in time and energy must be devoted to medicine? What is the boundary between dedication and obsession? After all one does not really become a physician; one remains a human being who has acquired certain knowledge and skills that allow one to function as a physician during specific periods of time. What should those times be? How and when does one shift roles from being a physician to being a "nonphysician"? This is, of course, a generic question that is as applicable to science, art, business, or any other human activity as it is to medicine.

The student will not readily find an all-embracing answer to this question. Each student will most likely evolve a personal answer and it will be an operational one representing the integral of microcompromises and adjustments made throughout one's subsequent career. The "complete physician," narrowly construed, would be a very poor physician if he were merely an observer rather than a participant in the pageantry of his time. Physicians owe it to themselves, to their families, to society, and to their patients not to become simply skilled but detached automatons. On the other hand, the practice of medicine is not a job but a profession that cannot be sealed off into convenient hours for earning one's living. To attempt to do so smacks of dilettantism. Between these extremes one must decide for oneself where the compromises will be made along the varying border between personal and professional life. Tensions will remain, but properly channeled they can be creative and rewarding.

2 MEDICINE AS A SCIENCE

James B. Wyngaarden

The practice of medicine rests firmly upon a foundation of biologic and behavioral sciences, which in turn trace their evolution to chemistry, physics, mathematics, psychology, anthropology, and epidemiology. During college and medical school years, the physician acquires both an extensive knowledge base in science and a comfortable familiarity with the ways of science. But scientific knowledge is not static. It undergoes continuous remodeling as new discoveries are made and erroneous interpretations are discarded. As a consequence, preservation of professional competence throughout a working lifetime is a daunting challenge. It requires a continuing growth of knowledge, a critical assessment of new hypotheses and scientific advances, and a selective incorporation of the most useful of these into one's own practice.

Advances in biologic science and accompanying technologic developments underlie most of the medical progress of the past half century, which has so remarkably advanced the ability of the physician to intervene in illness. Much of this progress has been in fundamental or "basic" science, conducted in the pursuit of understanding for its own sake. Significant progress has also resulted from research conducted by physician-scientists with a specified clinical goal in mind—for example, the elucidation of a disease mechanism or the critical evaluation of a therapeutic practice. Advances in medicine also continue to occur through serendipity or by astute clinical observations concerning patients or groups of patients and their illnesses. Nevertheless, the only rational approach to finding new methods for prevention or treatment is based on scientific explanations of the causes and mechanisms of disease.

Some years ago, Comroe and Dripps* traced the origins of ten major clinical innovations in cardiovascular and pulmonary medicine in an effort to identify the antecedents of these advances. Over 60 per cent of the enabling discoveries were in the category of basic science; over 40 per cent were the result of research carried out without any particular clinical application in mind. These observations are probably representative of medical progress in general.

The ability to control infections with antibiotics, hypertension with antihypertensive agents, and inflammatory reactions with glucocorticoids represents remarkable advances that have contributed to a lengthening of life expectancy. But the agenda is far from being fulfilled. The major health care problems of our time lie in the continued existence of diseases for which we can as yet do little. Even if the best of contemporary medicine were universally available, cancer would continue to kill, rheumatoid arthritis would continue to cripple, and schizophrenia would continue to render insane. We have no definitive answers for these diseases and for many more the descriptions of which constitute the substance of this book—or else we have what Lewis Thomas has called a "halfway technology," measures capable of modifying and ameliorating illness but not of prevention or cure. Medicine as a science is incomplete. It will remain so, for science itself is by its nature incomplete.

The present bioscientific character of medical practice is a relatively recent development. Throughout most of recorded history, medicine was anything but scientific, being dominated by empiricism and shackled by dogma. Diagnoses were inexact, causes of diseases poorly understood, and therapies frivolous and haphazard. Interventions by physicians consisted of bleeding, purging, cupping, administration of infusions of every known plant and of solutions of every known metal, and prescription of every possible diet—with no scientific foundation for these practices. Nor could there be such a foundation, for the scientific base did not yet exist.

Harbingers of change emerged slowly in the early nineteenth century, as new principles of physics and chemistry were applied to medicine. Physiologists stressed functions of organs and tissues. Its exemplars, especially Claude Bernard (1813–1878), emphasized the experimental method in establishing biologic knowledge and the necessity of basing medical practice in such knowledge. Pathologists, led by Virchow (1821–1902), stressed the critical study of normal and abnormal tissues and the correlation of features of disease with precise anatomic observations. Bacteriologists, with Pasteur (1822–1895) and Koch (1843–1910) in the vanguard, began to identify the microorganisms and to implicate specific organisms in specific diseases—the anthrax bacillus in anthrax, the tubercle bacillus in consumption, the pneumococcus in lobar pneumonia, the streptococcus in puerperal fever. The groundwork for future therapies was being laid by these great Western European scientists, but there was relatively little that physicians could do about most illnesses at the time. Their major contributions were diagnostic, prognostic, and supportive. By correct diagnosis they could advise concerning outcome. By common-sense supportive measures they could provide comfort and maximize opportunities for recovery. But interventions were as likely as not to make things worse. The first edition of Osler's *Textbook of Medicine* in 1892 was revolutionary for its skepticism and its therapeutic nihilism, as this outstanding physician and teacher condemned the majority of nostrums and remedies as useless, even harmful.

Slowly, specific therapies—insulin for diabetes, liver extract for pernicious anemia—or specific immunizations—diphtheria antitoxin, pneumococcic antisera—appeared. But it was not until the decade of 1935 to 1945 that the entry of sulfonamides and penicillin into clinical medicine made curable a large number of previously lethal and untreatable diseases. It is customary to date the beginnings of modern medicine from these relatively recent events.

The language of contemporary biologic science has become

*Comroe JH, Dripps RD: The top ten clinical advances in cardiovascular-pulmonary medicine and surgery between 1945 and 1975: How they came about. Bethesda, Md., Public Inquiries and Reports Branch, National Heart, Lung, and Blood Institute, National Institutes of Health, 1977.

increasingly biochemical. The compositions of organs, tissues, cells, organelles, and membranes have been defined. The biosynthesis and catabolism of hundreds of compounds have been elucidated. The regulation of body processes has been described at progressively finer levels and in chemical language. Many pharmacologic agents are now understood in terms of specific loci and mechanisms of action. The expansion of new knowledge continues at a pace that is bewildering to all but experts in a given field. Current advances are particularly rapid in immunology, molecular and cellular biology, peptide research, and structural biology. A beginning has been made in explaining human behavior in mechanistic terms, as more and more chemical mediators and pharmacologic modifiers are discovered.

We are in a molecular age of basic biologic science. The molecular influence pervades all the traditional disciplines underlying clinical medicine. Approximately 200 inborn errors are now understood in terms of specific missing or abnormal enzymes or other proteins. There are more than 240 known abnormal human hemoglobins, and for each of these the precise structural defect in the DNA of the mutant gene can be defined. Membrane, cytoplasmic, and nuclear receptors for hormones and drugs are exploding upon us, and old as well as new diseases are being defined in terms of receptor abnormalities—for example, type II hypercholesterolemia and nephrogenic diabetes insipidus. Recognition of opiate receptors has led to the discovery of endogenous peptides (endorphins) with analgesic activity. Their localization gives promise of further understanding of the limbic system, affective states, and addictions. The number and function of neurotransmitters has greatly increased, and these and other advances in neuroscience portend exciting developments in understanding how the brain works. DNA sequencing techniques and restriction endonucleases now permit precise identification of the exact structural alteration of the gene in an increasing number of hereditary diseases. The complete sequencing of the human genome is now technically possible; about 0.2 per cent of it has already been done. Gene therapy—both pharmacologic modification of specific gene action and physical replacement of damaged genetic segments—is now possible in experimental systems.

Much of the recent fundamental information in science has been obtained by the process of reductionism—the exploring of details, and the details of details, until all the smallest bits of the structure, or the smallest parts of the mechanism, are exposed to scrutiny. The scientists responsible for our evolving understanding of biologic systems know that the reductionist approach must often precede reconstitutive endeavors. Scientific progress rests on myriads of small observations, tedious measurements, and the findings of investigators asking humble, answerable questions. Instead of reaching for the whole truth, the scientist examines small, defined, and clearly separable phenomena. The pattern of science is a stepwise extension of what came before, with an occasional quantum leap forward through great discovery.

The examples of advances in medical science mentioned above have been largely drawn from the areas of ultrastructure, biochemistry, and molecular biology. In biology these disciplines have arbitrary and porous boundaries: physiology, pharmacology, neurosciences, cell biology, molecular biology, biochemistry, immunology, biophysics—all are in a phase of confluence, and the common language is chemistry. Medicine is not only a branch of applied biology, however. It also subsumes many aspects of psychology, sociology, anthropology, and economics. These disciplines, too long neglected or denigrated as "soft science," are now increasingly recognized as germane to medicine as a discipline and the practice of medicine as a profession.

Critics of the bioscientific strategy of medicine have claimed that the great advances that have dramatically reduced mortality rates consist in the improvement of the environment, the correction of malnutrition, and the control of infectious diseases through immunizations and antimicrobial agents, and that the relevant medical breakthroughs largely occurred before the prodigious expansion of federal support of biomedical science begun in the early 1950's. They contend that the enormous expenditures that have made the United States pre-eminent in biomedical research have produced too little in the way of medical advance to justify their continuation and have instead fostered the development of an extremely costly technology that has had only a minimal effect upon mortality statistics. They propose that the bioscientific strategy of medicine should be replaced by an ecologic strategy for health.

These critics ignore several important realities: (1) A bioscientific strategy for medicine and an ecologic strategy for health are not mutually exclusive, and examples of contributions of both strategies are readily at hand. (2) Major advances have occurred since 1950 that have revolutionized the outlook in individual diseases or disease groups—for example, in Hodgkin's disease, acute lymphocytic leukemia of children, Parkinson's disease, and Wilson's disease. (3) Advances based on the bioscientific strategy have reduced as well as increased health care costs. (4) Such advances have rested in most instances on a deeper and clearer understanding of underlying disease mechanisms. (5) The elucidation of a disease mechanism and the devising of rational therapy usually depend upon the application of basic scientific knowledge to a clinical problem—for instance, the definition of pathways of purine synthesis led to the development of a xanthine oxidase inhibitor (allopurinol) for the control of hyperuricemia and hyperuricaciduria.

The list of human diseases for which there are as yet no definitive measures for prevention or cure is still formidable. Fresh insights into the nature of these diseases are needed. These insights can come only from continued basic research. But the expansion of the knowledge bank of the past quarter century justifies great optimism for the eventual control and cure of major diseases and the possible elimination of premature death from illness.

The practice of medicine is both a science and an art. A skilled physician must have extensive medical knowledge, which is the bedrock of technical competence. In addition, he or she must have judgment, tact, decisiveness, restraint, compassion, interest, time, and other personal qualities of caring and dedication. The science and the art of medicine must remain intimately linked if physicians are to be maximally effective. The student studies the science of medicine first, masters it early, and returns to it frequently. The physician acquires the art of medicine—the skillful application of medical knowledge and judgment in the optimal care of the patient—more gradually and with experience.

THE PHYSICIAN AS A SCIENTIST. Since medicine is derived from a number of sciences relevant to the health of individuals or of groups, physicians must be trained as scientists to utilize these complex disciplines effectively.

To be a scientist, the physician must have more than rote scientific knowledge or even fluency in its particular jargon. Physicians must be conversant with the processes of scientific inquiry—how data are obtained and evaluated; how hypotheses are framed, modified, or discarded; the uses and limitations of inductive reasoning. In short, they must understand science as an intellectual instrument that has been slowly perfected over centuries. Only in this way can they remain attentive to medical progress as a critical and independent participant. Otherwise they will be in danger of being the passive purveyor of medical fashions. Both the spirit and rigor of science are necesary for the physician to become and remain a scholar in medicine. Medical practice itself contains many of the elements of scientific inquiry in the pursuit and evaluation of data (history, physical examination, laboratory studies) and in framing a hypothesis (tentative clinical diagnosis).

As a scientist the physician is the beneficiary of both the fruits of scientific research and of the mental discipline of the scientific method. To a greater or lesser degree the physician also has the opportunity to contribute personally to medical progress. Most medical research is now carried out by teams of participating investigators in elaborately equipped laboratories that utilize the advanced instrumentation and technology of modern science. There is still scope, however, for scientific contributions made by inquiring physicians based on their own experiences in patient care. Much of medical progress has derived from this kind of curiosity in the past. In addition, this form of clinical research, on whatever modest scale it may be engaged in, adds excitement and zest to professional life. As Thomas Hobbes has written: "Desire to know why, and how, curiosity, which is a lust of the mind, that by a perseverance of delight in the continued and indefatigable generation of knowledge, exceedeth the short vehemence of any carnal pleasure."

THE PHYSICIAN AS A HUMANIST. Since the physician deals with fellow human beings in need of help, the patient and the public have every reason to assume that the physician is a humane and caring person as well as a competent practitioner. Yet a crisis of confidence appears to have beset modern medicine.* As the technology and complexity of medicine have increased, medical care has become more institutionalized and its delivery depersonalized. This is a particular risk when many different expert consultants or technologists are called upon to participate each in some segment of a given patient's workup and care. There is a widely held view that the increasingly complex science and technology of medicine are responsible for a decline of compassion in medicine, as though there were something inherently contradictory between science and humanity, between technology and compassion. There is, of course, no reason that scientific knowledge and compassion should be in conflict. Science and technology underlie most of the advances of medicine that enable contemporary physicians to render more effective medical care than their professional forebears were able to offer. Glick even views computed tomography as a technologic advance of extraordinary compassion. Its use has spared patients many more difficult, painful, and dangerous procedures and has permitted definitive diagnoses to be made earlier. Physicians cannot be made more compassionate by downgrading science any more than students can be made more humanistic by study of the humanities. If there is a decline in compassion among physicians, its causes must lie elsewhere. Glick suggests that "the fundamental problems lie for the most part outside the medical establishment, within society as a whole. The physician is largely a reflection of society. . . . Basic human character traits are well developed by the time a student enters medical school." He suggests that the prime examples of humane medicine are to be found in persons in whom service to humanity ranks as a higher priority than personal gratification. That characteristic is a reaffirmation of Hippocrates and of Osler and of every other truly great physician. Its expression is enhanced whenever good science and complex technology are applied for the benefit of the patient by a caring physician or any other personnel who participate in the delivery of medical services to people.

*Glick SM: Humanistic medicine in a modern age. N Engl J Med 304:1036, 1981.

3 MEDICINE AS A PUBLIC SERVICE

James B. Wyngaarden

Medicine is a serving profession, one that exists not for its own sake but for the benefit of others. "The responsibilities of medicine are threefold: to generate scientific knowledge and to teach it to others; to use the knowledge for the health of an individual or a whole community; and to judge the moral and ethical propriety of each medical act that directly affects another human being" (McDermott).

We have already discussed the generation of scientific knowledge and the way in which scientific advances continually modify and extend the practice of medicine. In the application of an increasingly technologic medicine, new and sometimes discomfiting issues arise. This chapter will briefly introduce selected issues in the practice of medicine faced by the physician as a member of modern society.

PATTERNS OF MEDICAL PRACTICE. Practitioners who apply medical knowledge for the benefit of patients are of two sorts: those who deal personally with individual patients and those who deal with people as groups. We call the latter activity *community medicine,* which is a component of public health. In community medicine, group membership is usually determined by geographic location or census tract. The members of such a community are not self-selected on the basis of perception of disease; rather, they are identified as members of the community on the basis of other common characteristics, usually location. At any one time a community will comprise many more people who are healthy than who are ill. Important functions of community medicine are the provision of appropriate health services for its members, the continuous surveillance of the population for discovery of individuals in need of care, and the creation of entry points for those so identified. These are large social challenges, as yet imperfectly attained. Marked unevenness in access to and in utilization of physician services remains a problem in most countries. In the United States these problems have been ameliorated but by no means solved by Medicare and Medicaid programs for financing of hospital and physician services. Important though these topics are, they are beyond the scope of this book, which is principally oriented toward the care of the individual patient. By and large the constituency described in this book consists of self-selected patients who consult a physician because of *dis-ease,* i.e., concern about their personal health.

Physicians who render personal medical care do so in a variety of practice patterns, ranging from solo practices to partnerships, to multispecialty groups, to full-time situations in an organized clinic or a medical school faculty, to Health Maintenance Organizations (HMO's) or Independent Practice Associations (IPA's). The traditional doctor-patient relationship, in which the patient identifies a specific physician as his or her own personal doctor, may exist within any of these practice patterns. Many patients want a personal physician who knows them, who is available for first contact and continuing care, and who offers a portal of entry to specialists for those conditions warranting referral. This type of practice, termed "primary care," characterizes activities of general practitioners, family physicians, and general internists, as well as of many pediatricians and obstetricians. Often their services are complemented by nurse-clinicians or physician associates. Physicians who see patients in referral for common conditions that do not require high technology, and who characteristically see them in an office or community hospital setting, are said to be offering "secondary care." Those who manage patients with complex illnesses requiring high technology, or the use of powerful, high-risk drugs or procedures, or specialized knowledge of limited availability, are said to be rendering "tertiary care." University hospitals and many large urban referral hospitals frequently function as "tertiary care centers." But categories of activities are not always clearly separable. Community hospitals and subspecialists often practice a mixture of primary and secondary care medicine. Large teaching hospitals generally offer a full spectrum of services—primary care in their clinics, secondary care as a community referral center, tertiary care for patients who have complex medical problems or who are critically ill.

The provision of continuing comprehensive care has traditionally required a high order of accessibility on the part of the primary care physician. In the following essay, Dr. Thomas eloquently describes the repetitive interruptions of sleep that characterized the nights of his general practitioner father. In recent decades physicians have sought relief from the overwhelming physical and emotional drain of continuous availability with its potentially excessive cost to personal and family life. Solo practitioners arrange to cross-cover each other, partners arrange on-call schedules, and metropolitan physicians often refer nocturnal and weekend patients to emergency rooms. In some group practices, individual doctor-patient relationships have been supplanted by a team approach. These changes in professional mores reflect evolving attitudes on the extent to which compassionate behavior in the practice of medicine should be allowed to dominate a physician's time and personal life. In times past availability was one of the few valuable services an individual physician could offer patients. When no one in the profession had many answers to illness, and treatment consisted largely of evaluation, prognosis, and emotional support, the reassuring presence of the physician constituted in itself the fulfillment of the Hippocratic Oath. As the science and technology of medicine have expanded, no one doctor can any longer be expert in all areas, and the care of the patient, when something is seriously wrong, necessarily becomes a collective effort. The personal interest of each physician continues to be essential, so that there may be a series of satisfying doctor-patient relationships. However, the patient usually wants one doctor as his or her personal advocate, regardless of the extent of sharing of medical responsibility.

THE PATIENT AS A CONSUMER. Some of the traditional and universal expectations of patients have been discussed in the initial essay, "Medicine as an Art." The general trend toward greater consumer awareness has created many new patient expectations. Patients now understand a great deal more about the human body and its disorders than they did a generation ago. As a consequence they expect more detailed information from the physician. Teaching about science and health in grade schools and high schools has improved greatly. Newspapers, magazines, and television regularly inform the public of advances in medicine. Many communities offer health seminars to the general public. Home medical encyclopedias are widely available. The individual has been admonished to take personal responsibility for his or her own health through weight control, dietary discretion, limitation of intakes of saturated fats and of salt, regular exercise, moderation in or abstinence from smoking and drinking, attention to the purity of water and of air, and appropriate diversions from work. These measures are widely accepted as contributing to physical and mental health. For those with chronic illnesses there are primers prepared by voluntary health agencies or the United States Public Health Service. In many instances there are clubs to join, organized about a diagnosis (e.g., lupus erythematosus clubs) or a procedure (e.g., laryngectomy clubs). One can send a coupon and urine sample to test for diabetes or have one's blood pressure checked at the supermarket. Ethnic groups at increased risk for certain diseases can avail themselves of screening programs for sickle cell disease or Tay-Sachs carrier status. Such measures and others have publicized medical progress and have kindled high expectations for imminent "breakthroughs." Such anticipations are often fanned by an overly exuberant press. All of these factors combine to place increased demands upon the physician to inform in greater detail and to anticipate increasingly sophisticated inquiries from patients and relatives.

The public is also well aware that substantial tax dollars have been spent on medical research and on the production of more physicians since World War II. They have come to view excellent medical care and access to it as birthrights. For the majority of Americans these birthrights have been achieved, but important segments of our society and of many societies throughout the world are still excluded from optimal medical care by poverty, location, or both. For many of those with access to care, the costs have become a preoccupation. The percentage of the American gross national product spent on medical care has risen substantially for two decades and is now about 11 to 12 per cent. In part this reflects the extension of medical care to individuals for whom it was only marginally available in the past. In larger part this reflects the costs of progress in medicine. Drugs are now available to treat conditions that in times past could only be observed. New technologies in medicine permit diagnostic and therapeutic procedures scarcely dreamed of a decade or two ago. The rising costs of medical care are particularly pronounced in circumstances in which partial solutions are much more expensive than the ultimate cure is likely to be. The classic example is poliomyelitis. Current examples include the expensive technology of renal dialysis and transplantation for chronic kidney failure and of coronary bypass surgery and heart transplantation for coronary artery disease. Doctors control many of the expenditures in medical care and therefore must share in the serious concerns about its escalating costs. They decide on hospitalization, order diagnostic studies, prescribe the drugs patients take, or recommend surgery. Control of costs of medical care is a lively topic in the public arena.

The advancing technology of medicine has enabled more and more interventions in the natural course of disease. An increasing number of parts of the body can be replaced by transplanted organs or mechanical substitutes. The term "invasive procedure" has become commonplace in our lexicon. The potential of such procedures for diagnostic information or therapeutic achievement is awesome. Benefits of scientific medicine can now be proffered to patients thought beyond help only several years ago. When all goes well, one is exhilarated by the wonder of the success. But high-risk procedures in high-risk patients cannot always go well. There are unanticipated complexities of disease, adverse biologic responses, genetic differences, flaws of judgment, variations in physicians' skills, mechanical failures. Often the doctor or the hospital or the pharmaceutical company is held responsible, sometimes for events beyond anyone's control.

DEFENSIVE MEDICINE. High-technology medicine has carried with it a lowering of the threshold for litigation on the part of patients when something does go wrong. Some physicians respond by the practice of "defensive medicine." This has at least three components. The first is informed consent. In concept this is unassailable. The patient clearly has the right to have anything that is proposed fully explained in advance, and the right to give or withhold consent. Three or four decades ago informed consent was largely limited to anesthesia and operating permits. Today, informed consent often involves written descriptions of procedures that include explicit accounts of every conceivable misfortune that has ever followed a given diagnostic test, drug therapy, or surgical procedure. Many persons appreciate such candor, but some become frightened and forego needed tests or therapy. Many patients sign forms based on discussions they do not really understand. In such instances the practice clearly is not achieving its intended goals.

Defensive medicine also may extend the medical workup that a prudent physician will perform in a given circumstance. When clinical concern results in an appropriate history, physical examination, and laboratory study, the patient is clearly the beneficiary. But when studies of marginal value are ordered or excessive consultations are requested, solely because of fear of potential litigation, the costs of medical care are driven upward to no good end. Yet physicians are often on the horns of a dilemma, often forced by the perception of their own best interests to exceed what is in the patient's best interest. Experienced physicians who are secure in their knowledge and competence will rely less on extensive studies and wide-ranging consultations than will more apprehensive or tentative doctors.

Defensive medicine also mandates the keeping of more thorough records. In case of challenge to adequacy or competence of care, the written record is the physician's defense. The record should contain all relevant data pertaining to the patient. It should also contain all important data pertaining to the doctor's opinions or conclusions, decisions, prescriptions, actions, and communications. The evolution of thoughts and responses should be clearly discernible from the record. If such entries are recorded at appropriately frequent intervals, an effective reconstruction of events is possible, should the need arise. These are, of course, all benchmarks of good medical practice. But the growing necessity for increasingly detailed documentation has its cost in time. When added to other items of escalating paper work in medical practice, this translates into reduced professional productivity. If defensive medicine benefits the patient, the additional costs may be justified, but in terms of the aforementioned responses the cost-benefit ratio is at present unknown.

PUBLIC ACCOUNTABILITY. The privilege of practicing medicine is increasingly coupled with accountability in the exercise of this stewardship. Private accountability has always been implied in the doctor-patient relationship. The entry of substantial public money into the field of medical care has also brought with it new forms of public accountability and regulation of medical practice.

A profound change is currently under way in the manner in which the private sector is being paid by the federal government for care of elderly and medically indigent patients; the principle of cost reimbursement has been superseded by one of prospective payment. Hospitals are now compensated according to predetermined allowances based on average days of stay and average ancillary charges for each of several hundred diagnosis-related groups into which patients are placed. In addition, peer review organizations have been given considerable power to regulate the system and insure adherence to guidelines concerning admission, early discharge, readmission, or interhospital transfer. Expenses in excess of reimbursement allowances are absorbed by the hospital; savings are banked by the hospital. Funds for graduate medical education have been reduced.

The revisions of federal programs have the dual objective of assuring quality medical care and controlling the rate of growth of the costs of our health care system. Early indications are that hospitals and physicians are making the required adjustments to new conditions, but long-term impacts will not be known for some additional years.

In the final analysis, quality of care depends upon the ability and wisdom of the physician; the adequacy of facilities and equipment; access to safe and effective therapeutic agents; the quality of professional education and training; personal standards of performance, integrity, and dedication; and a resolute self-discipline. The ultimate contract is between the patient and the doctor, and this relationship must be based on mutual trust and mutual respect. Third party participation must not be allowed to supplant that venerable tradition.

4 MEDICINE AS A VERY OLD PROFESSION

Lewis Thomas

I first heard the term "medical ethics" in my childhood, a long time ago. Then, it referred to a small set of unambiguous, nonphilosophical matters worried over only by doctors and their families and related exclusively to money. Doctors who advertised, overcharged their patients, surreptitiously took over the care of patients already being looked after by another doctor, or split fees with other doctors were unethical and that was what the word meant. Doctors who performed abortions were not unethical, they were immoral or criminal, or both. Human experimentation was not unethical because there was no such activity, or perhaps it is better to say that it was not realized, even by practicing doctors, that experiments were performed on patients in the normal course of medical practice.

This was a time ago and medicine has changed a great deal, more than is remembered by most people, changed so much that even those old enough to have lived though the whole period have difficulty in recognizing the connections between the old enterprise and the new one. For, in a certain sense, it is like that: it is as though we gave up altogether one kind of profession called medicine and then took up another one. A long look backward is needed to see the change.

I am just old enough to take that sort of view, first-hand, having been born into a doctor's family during the last decades of the profession's former existence as an applied art, then growing up in a household sustained by that endeavor, then being trained as a doctor at the very turning point when it began to change into something like a science, and finally pursuing a career in the profession which was the result of that evolution. In those years it was easier to shift from one field to another, perhaps because the requirements for deep expertise were less demanding in the absence of so many detailed facts to comprehend. Thus, I had a close professional look at several disciplines along the way: pediatrics, internal medicine, pathology, infectious disease, immunology, and administration. All of these have changed so much in recent years that I cannot imagine people climbing over departmental walls and specialty boards so easily. On the other hand, I do envision a time ahead when the clinical sciences will come to share the same ground in their base of knowledge. Before long, a post-M.D. period of training in internal medicine and molecular genetics might serve to prepare a young graduate for almost any discipline, in the kind of medicine that lies somewhere ahead.

My father began the practice of medicine in 1905. He was a busy and successful general practitioner for most of his life, switching to become a self-trained and self-certified surgeon in his latter years, as was the custom at that time. During all his years in general practice he possessed only small bits of science, used solely for the purpose of diagnosis, and almost no science at all for therapy. What he did, for treating disease, was to "look after" people. This was all he, or anyone else, knew how to do, and it had little to do with technology.

Indeed, if it became known in the small town I grew up in that a doctor had become locally famous for his technical capacity to treat this or that disease, the question of medical ethics was automatically raised by the local establishment. Claims for being able to treat disease were almost, not quite but almost, grounds for being charged with quackery, and usually the charge was warranted. In those days quackery abounded.

Not to say that treatments for illness were not used by doctors, but these were more like gestures of reassurance, sometimes like incantations or amulets. Prescriptions were written in Latin of great complexity for numberless compounds, most of them green and bitter-tasting but without any known biologic properties, issued for all kinds of complaints, but neither my father nor other doctors of this time had any real faith in them. The best that could be said for the treatments was that they did no harm, which, by the way, was considerably more than could be said for the medicine of his father's time, or his grandfather's. I don't recall ever hearing about a suit for malpractice during my father's professional lifetime. The question simply didn't arise. Nobody could possibly have been damaged by the therapy available, even less by omitting it.

The doctors of his generation were mostly passive, and the things they did in their practices were mostly watching and waiting. They had been educated at the end of the first great revolution in medicine, and a large part of their education emerged out of the destruction and abandonment of masses of misinformation which preceding generations of physicians had taken for granted.

For a great many centuries, the technology of therapeutic medicine had been based on something rather like pure guesswork, and anybody's theory stood a good chance of being incorporated into dogma for the generations to follow. It was taken for granted that medicine, to be effective, had to be a strenuous, perilous sort of enterprise, and if things like these were not done the most ordinary kinds of illness would surely end fatally. There was no disease for which a treatment was not recommended. It is sometimes complained by today's medical students that the mountains of reductionist facts to be learned and set in memory are more than the mind can cope with, but the students just before my father's generation had a lot more to complain about. Looking through any textbook of medicine or pediatrics in the last years of the nineteenth century must have caused the learner's heart to sink. Every other page is filled with bizarre, esoteric pieces of therapy, each one to be performed exactly as laid out and learned (since none of them made any intrinsic sense) by rote. Poliomyelitis had to be treated by injections of strychnine, the application of leeches over the spine, the administration by mouth of extracts of belladonna and ergot, potassium iodide, huge doses of mercurial purgatives, faradic stimulation of the muscles, bleeding, and cupping. Meningitis required all these things, plus the spreading of cantharides ointment over the head and spine, strong enough to produce large blisters. Since all patients were treated more or less alike, there were almost no controlled investigations, and chance observations were quickly turned from anecdotes to tradition. Even so esteemed and skilled a pediatrician as Abraham Jacobi wrote in his famous 1896 textbook, concerning erysipelas, "The recovery of a young man observed with such symptoms lately I attribute solely to the large quantities of brandy administered."

Bleeding had been the sovereign therapy throughout the century before my father's entry into practice. The conventional treatment for tuberculosis and rheumatic fever was the removal each day of about a pint of blood, or enough to cause blanching, weakness, faintness, and a palpable weakening of the pulse: early *shock,* in short, facilitated even more by calomel and antimony in doses arranged to produce violent diarrhea and vomiting. George Washington, by the way, is reported to have been treated for a peritonsillar abscess by the removal of 82 ounces of blood in his last, fatal illness. The point of all this was the doctrine, passed down through the centuries from Galen, that disease—any disease—was caused by the congestion of blood in one organ or another.

Protests against this kind of medicine had been raised as early as the 1830's, and a few observant physicians, here and abroad, took a careful look at what doctors were doing in the treatment of typhoid fever and delirium tremens and realized that they were doing a lot more harm than good. It very slowly dawned on the profession that a great many patients with various illnesses were capable of getting well all by themselves, without any treatment, and that many of the treatments then popular were probably making matters worse, but it took long decades before this kind of medicine was given up. At the same time, a genuine scientific activity, equivalent to the natural history of that day, got underway. Reliable classifications of human disease were constructed, based on careful clinical observations and correlated with the discoveries being made in the emerging field of pathology. Slowly but surely, during the latter part of the nineteenth century, the natural history of disease came to dominate medical education, and the art of making an accurate diagnosis and forecasting the likely outcome of every illness became the highest skill and the indispensable craft of the practicing physician.

This is what the doctors of my father's generation were trained to do. At the same time, largely under the influence of Sir William Osler, they were trained to be skeptical about treating disease. There were a few things they could do, but only a few. Malaria could be treated with quinine, digitalis was used with skill for heart failure, and morphine was the great standby—the most respected of all the drugs in the pharmacopoeia—for pain.

By the time I arrived in medical school in the mid-1930's there had been a few genuine advances, but still only a few: liver extract for pernicious anemia, insulin for diabetes, the early vitamins, immunization against diphtheria and tetanus, antiserum for pneumococcal pneumonia, not much else. I was taught at Harvard Medical School, as my father had been taught at Columbia, that treating disease would be the least of my future responsibilities. The doctor's job was to recognize the nature of disease with precision, so that he could explain to the patient, and to the patient's family, what was happening to him and how it was most likely to turn out.

This task, the explaining of illness, was the most important part of what was then called the art of medicine. It still is. Indeed, it has been a central duty of medicine, justifying all those millennia of the profession's existence, dating all the way back to our origins in shamanism. When you think about it, the first thing a sick person wants to know—and the sicker he is the more urgently he wants to know it—is "What's gone wrong?" And, in the same breath, "What happens next?" "Am I going to live?"

The quality of medicine's answers to these questions, and therefore the very usefulness of the doctor, were always matters of doubt until the great medical reform of the late nineteenth century. By the time of Osler, and in the decades that followed, science became the basis for explanation, and the answers became correspondingly more reliable.

It is easy to see why the mere act of explaining was so important, once you realize what being ill was like in the era before the discovery of antibiotics and the nearly successful conquest of infectious disease. Living was a considerably more chancy enterprise then. If you developed typhoid fever, which was still a common illness in the early years of my father's practice, you knew you were in for two months of constant high fever, deep malaise and debilitation, and the risk at any time of hemorrhage or perforation of the intestine.

You had about one chance in four of dying. If it was lobar pneumonia, which was the most common serious infection when I was a medical student, you had the prospect of dying or recovering spectacularly on your own within a shorter period—two weeks or so. The greatest danger of all, feared by everyone, was tuberculosis. People worried then about TB as they worry now about cancer, but for better reasons; people of all ages died from tuberculosis, and there was nothing at all to be done about it. Rheumatic fever, the cause of rheumatic heart disease, was the first thing to worry about whenever a young child developed a sore throat, and if you didn't worry about this you had to worry about poliomyelitis. The chief cause of insanity, filling the state hospitals of that time, was syphilis of the brain.

It was an enormous relief to be told that you or your family had none of these things the matter, and this was the function of a good doctor. But there was, of course, a lot more to the practice of medicine than simply explaining things.

When I was starting out as an intern, swept off my feet by the new demands for science in treating infectious disease, I used to wonder what my father did to keep so busy in his practice back in the days when there were no sulfonamides, no penicillin, no way of treating anything. Throughout my childhood, the telephone rang all day and all night in our house, and I remember waking up most nights at the sound of my father heaving out of bed and off in the family car on house calls, carrying along his black doctor's bag which contained almost nothing of any real value. There was nothing exceptional about his practice; this is what life was like for all the doctors in town when I was growing up. And yet, there was very little that he could do. He was, by the way, fully aware of this himself, as were his colleagues; he used to complain sometimes that most of the time he felt helpless; he was never really convinced that anything he did made a real difference to the outcome of an illness, in any of his patients, in all his life in medicine.

There is a mystery here, and it is an aspect of medicine that has been forgotten by too many people, doctors and patients alike. Once the nature of the illness had been identified for what it was, and the news conveyed to the patient, several other things happened. First of all, the doctor took on the responsibility for the outcome, for better or worse. And, perhaps most important of all, he stood by. Standing by was, getting down to brass tacks, what the doctor did: he might not have anything much in that black bag, and no magical potions to serve up, and certainly nothing that he could put into or get out of a computer, but he did have his presence, and that made a difference. Sir William Osler used to teach that it could make all the difference in the world: if the doctor understood what was occurring in his patient, and made that understanding available, and made himself available at the same time as a source of hope and strength, these acts of professional skill could turn the tide. I believe these things, even though I do not understand them.

I have one other piece of reminiscence about the medicine of 50 years ago, which has some bearing on the general problem of the future of medicine and medical science. It is this: 50 years ago, just before the profession underwent its transformation and the art began to incorporate science and technology, no one had the ghost of an idea that anything was about to happen. It was taken for granted by my generation that the medicine we were being taught in the year 1935 was precisely the medicine that would be with us for the rest of our lives. We expected nothing to change. If anyone had tried to tell us that the power to control bacterial infections was just around the corner, or that open-heart surgery or kidney transplants would be possible within two decades, or that some kinds of cancer would be cured by chemotherapy, or that there would soon be within reach a comprehensive biochemical explanation, in the most reductionist detail, for genetics and genetically determined diseases, we would have reacted in blank disbelief. We had no reason to believe that medicine would ever change. We knew that subacute bacterial endocarditis and tuberculous meningitis were always fatal; we regarded schizophrenia as a totally unapproachable and insoluble problem; we believed that mental retardation was an act of nature for which we would never have an explanation, much less a treatment. All this has, of course, changed. Tuberculosis has vanished as a threat to the life of young children. There are so many new clues to the underlying mechanism of neoplasia that it is now a problem to make the right choice of a research line to pursue; senile dementia is out in the open, recognized now as one of the great challenges to medical science in our time.

And so forth. What this recollection tells me is that we should keep our minds wide open to the future. It is going to be different, whatever we think today. And, since change is inevitable, we should be spending more of our thought and energy making sure that the air is right for changes that seem to be in the right direction. This means, from my point of view, which I acknowledge as being self-interested and wholly prejudiced, more science.

We cannot go back to the old days in medicine. We should never allow ourselves to forget the healing property of a physician's presence and we should hang on to this mysterious gift even though we cannot explain it, but we cannot return to the era when that was all there was in medicine. We are nowhere near yet to where we should be; we are beset all around by the imperfections in our profession; we do a lot of things the wrong way and neglect doing essential things we could be doing better; even so, there is no prospect for changing medicine for the better in the years ahead except through science, more and profounder science.

But when people in my position say things like this we are well advised to add a cautionary footnote or two. We are always at risk of sounding like making too many promises, and speaking out of hubris, and we are not as candid as we ought to be about the extent of our ignorance. We are not about to change the world, nor are we in possession of a level of scientific understanding so powerful as to frighten people with what we might do next. We are, I'd say, *pretty* good at using science in medicine, but, thus far, only pretty good.

I wish there were some formal courses in medical school on Medical Ignorance; textbooks as well, although they would have to be very heavy volumes. We have a long way to go.

It is easy, these days, to look ahead. Medicine is being transformed before our eyes, and the power of our technologies for diagnosis and treatment is increasing with every month's new journal.

But I do not foresee any real change in the fundamental responsibility of doctors. Whatever they may gain in the way of technology in the decades ahead, I hope that they will be bound by the same deeply personal obligation to serve their patients. I hope my profession will never lose the memory of this obligation, for it is all we have in the way of historical continuity, the only real link to our professional ancestors.

I remember a short story from real life which illustrates an aspect of the responsibility of doctoring which does not find emphasis in many textbooks of medicine. Some years back I was invited to give a lecture on antibiotics at the annual meeting of a county medical society in a remote part of Mississippi. The audience was almost entirely made up of general practitioners, real country doctors. For the president of the society, a man in his 40's, this meeting was the major event of the year and one of the major occasions in his professional life; he was to be inducted formally into the office of president and had his speech prepared and ready. Just as the meeting began he was handed a note and left the auditorium to take a telephone call. That was the last I saw of him until three hours later, when he came back looking tired and worn out. I knew that he was deeply disappointed to have missed what should have been his own professional triumph, and I asked him what had happened. It was a call from a family of an elderly patient of his who had just died, he said. He felt that he ought to be there, to help the family, and to be useful. He simply had to be there, he said.

This was about 30 years ago, but I've never been able to forget that doctor and his example of good doctoring that evening. It's not quite the same thing as open-heart surgery or curing meningitis, but if I were looking around for a role model for today's medical students to look at very closely, I'd pick that country doctor in the backwoods countryside of Mississippi, if I could find him.

5 ETHICS IN THE PRACTICE OF MEDICINE

Albert R. Jonsen

"The responsibilities of medicine are threefold: to generate scientific knowledge and to teach it to others; to use the knowledge for the health of an individual or a whole community; and to judge the moral and ethical propriety of each medical act that directly affects another human being." With these words, Dr. Walsh McDermott opened his chapter, Medicine in Modern Society, in earlier editions of this textbook. Textbooks of medicine communicate the knowledge that constitutes the science of medicine and explain its application in the art of medicine. The third responsibility, "to judge the moral and ethical propriety of each medical act," is not expounded in the textbooks. Yet no one enters the profession of medicine without becoming vividly aware of its ethical tradition. The science and the art are imparted to students along with implicit ethical imperatives: to seek the patient's benefit, to avoid harm, to be respectful and compassionate, to preserve confidences, and to maintain competence. Medical students see these values embodied in their best professors, although as Louis Lasagna has said, students "may quickly absorb the moral atmosphere around them without questioning it." Physicians praise these values in their best colleagues, past and present. Some physicians fail to honor this ethical tradition; social and financial influences exert counterforces against it. Still, the ideals are clear and their vitality in the behavior of many individual physicians is remarkable.

The current revival of interest in medical ethics was not stimulated by a plague of immorality among physicians. It has not arisen because there is general disdain of, or disagreement about, the general principles of medical ethics. Rather, it has been fostered by a growing awareness on the part of physicians and the public that these general principles often seem inadequate to new situations. In some instances, widely publicized events have dramatized this inadequacy: the "God Committee," which selected patients "of social worth" in the early days of chronic hemodialysis; the Karen Ann Quinlan case; the Willowbrook hepatitis studies. In addition, interested scholars from medicine, philosophy, theology, sociology, and the law have attempted to analyze critically the general principles and to discern how they apply to the contemporary science and practice of medicine. In this way, a new discipline has arisen, sometimes called "bioethics."

Although the issues discussed in this new discipline are compelling, the discussions are necessarily general and abstract. The physician, however, must make decisions about the care of patients; often, those decisions will have ethical implications. The general and abstract must become particular and concrete. It is not enough to have a sincere attitude about, for example, discontinuing life-support systems. It is not sufficient to read a moving essay on allowing the dying "to die in dignity." Attitudes and information must be transformed into choices and practice. When the occasion arises, the ethical problems in the care of a patient must be assessed as skillfully as the patient's medical problem.

Every physician is familiar with the method of organizing clinical information: presenting symptoms and signs, history, physical exam, laboratory data. The competent physician evaluates these elements in seeking a diagnosis and selecting a treatment. A parallel method for reaching an ethical decision can be formulated. In almost any sort of clinical-ethical problem—be it withdrawing treatment, obtaining informed consent, preserving a confidence, or allocating a scarce resource—the facts and values necessary for a careful assessment can be displayed and evaluated under four headings: (1) indications for medical intervention, (2) patient's preferences, (3) patient's quality of life, and (4) external factors. This chapter will briefly explain how these four topics can be helpful in reaching an ethical decision. Thoughtful review of the relevant facts and values can put order into what is often a very confused consideration. Orderly consideration may not, of course, always reach the most suitable conclusion, but it should help avoid the two extremes that often distort clinical-ethical decisions: rash and precipitate action or paralyzing indecision. Both extremes can lead to tragedy for the physician, the patient, the family, and the institution.

INDICATIONS FOR MEDICAL INTERVENTION. Patients approach physicians with the hope of receiving the benefit of improved health or care in illness. The habitual activity of a physician is to gather information from and about the patient and to evaluate it with a view to determining whether or not medical intervention can benefit the patient. Clinical judgment, in which informed and careful estimates are made of the probable benefits and risks of each step in diagnosis and therapy, reflects the primary ethical responsibility of the physician. The most ancient rule of medical ethics is the Hippocratic dictum, "As to diseases, make a habit of two things—to help, or at least to do no harm." This duty manifests the "principle of beneficence," which ethicists designate as one of the fundamental ethical principles. They define it as "the duty to help others further their important and legitimate interests. . . ."

In most encounters between physician and patient, fulfillment of this duty is ethically unproblematic (although it may be medically difficult). Patients can inform the physician of the legitimate interests they wish furthered: they wish their health restored, their pain and symptoms relieved, their disabilities alleviated, their fears allayed. Physicians often respond with actions which have as their goal some specific benefit corresponding to those interests: elimination of meningococci by administration of penicillin G, control of blood pressure of 180/115 by an antihypertensive agent, prevention of the symptoms of celiac sprue by a gluten-restricted diet, and so forth. The interests of the patient and the response of physician center on benefits which reflect the goals of medical intervention: (1) restoration of health, (2) relief of symptoms, (3) restoration of function or maintenance of impaired function, (4) saving endangered life, and (5) supporting the patient by counseling and education. While all of these goals are seldom fully attained, they are the objectives which define the benefits of medicine.

At times, however, it might be asked whether one or another of these benefits is, in truth, a "benefit" for a particular patient. This question may occur to physician or to family in circumstances in which the patient is no longer able to declare his or her own interests. Typical clinical situations in which this sort of problem appears are as follows:

Case 1. A 38-year-old man with AIDS suffers a second episode of *Pneumocystis carinii* pneumonia. He is admitted to the ICU in respiratory failure, becomes hypotensive, acidotic, and septic. He is mentally incompetent. Should he be intubated?

Case 2. A 69-year-old woman has multiple sclerosis, diagnosed 30 years ago. She is now paraplegic and has begun to experience mood disturbance and to show signs of intellectual deterioration. She is brought to the hospital for treatment of pneumonia. Should she be treated?

In these cases, the first important ethical consideration is also the important clinical consideration: what objectives can be achieved by medical intervention? The answer must not be sought in the expected immediate results of some specific clinical intervention, but in those fundamental goals of medicine noted above.

The first formulation of the ethical question must be a realistic assessment of what might be accomplished by intervention (both in terms of the nature of the accomplishment and the probability of its occurrence). In Case 1, the only goal likely to be accomplished is a short prolongation of organic life. This, in and of itself, is not a proper goal of medicine. It is highly questionable that the physician has a duty to sustain and prolong human life when no prospect for any other human function is in view. The duty to prolong life in this sense has no roots in the history of medical ethics; it is an "artifact" of modern intensive care techniques. The physician's ethical obligation to initiate or continue treatment arises from the real probability that treatment will produce genuine benefit to the patient.

In Case 2, several of the goals of medicine can be achieved. Despite the woman's ultimate prognosis, she can be restored to her previous condition and helped in a number of ways. In terms of medical indications, she should be treated. However, her own preferences and the future quality of her life are added considerations. These are treated under the next two headings.

THE PREFERENCES OF THE PATIENT. If benefiting the patient means furthering that person's best interests, the patient's preferences, in general, should determine what constitutes benefit and harm. Individuals are usually the best advocates for their own interests. Recent critics of medicine accuse physicians of "paternalism," of assuming, because of their dominance over patients, the right to judge what is in that person's interest. Certainly, the history of medicine reveals an ethic colored by paternalism. The Hippocratic Oath states, "I will use treatment to help the sick, according to my ability and judgment." The patient's "ability and judgment" are not mentioned. In the past, "compassionate deception" was recommended "for the patient's good." Informed consent is a modern notion. Contemporary medical ethics, in the opinion of some of its proponents, consists almost entirely of the debate over paternalism and autonomy.

Autonomy, the personal liberty to make one's own choices and plan one's own life, is one of the central concepts of ethics. All of us value it highly in our own lives. An ethicist has written, "To respect autonomous agents is to recognize with due appreciation their own considered value judgments and outlooks even when it is believed that their judgments are mistaken."

In the practice of modern physicians, paternalism and autonomy are seldom in stark contrast. Physicians may be deficient in communicating information; often patients' preferences are not elicited or are disregarded. However, most modern physicians consider themselves advisors and, when important questions arise about diagnosis, prognosis, and therapy, they will inform patients of their options and respect their preferences. The practice of informed consent is growing and the practice of deception waning. Still, there are situations in which serious ethical questions about autonomy must be asked. Two, in particular, occur from time to time in clinical practice: the refusal of recommended treatment believed by the physician to be critical for the patient's well-being, and the decision to treat or not to treat mentally incompetent patients.

Case 3. A 46-year-old woman has all of the indications for coronary angiography. She is known to the physician as timid and fearful. In the office, she is extremely nervous. Her physician fears she may refuse angiography if told the risks. Should she be told?

Case 4. A 54-year-old man, brought to the emergency room, has signs and symptoms strongly indicative of myocardial infarction. He is alert and oriented. He refuses hospitalization and insists on returning home. Should he be restrained?

The physician's anticipation that the patient may refuse recommendations (Case 3) does not justify deception, even though disclosure should be careful and sympathetic. Grounds for this anticipation may be weak. Should the patient suffer an adverse experience about which she was not informed, trust in the physician would be shaken. Deception fails to respect the patient. It undermines confidence in the profession. Should the informed patient actually refuse an intervention, efforts can be made to ascertain the motive and, if it is fear or misunderstanding, to deal with these. Actual refusal by an alert and competent person (Case 4) should be respected once the physician has made serious efforts to assure understanding and to ascertain competence. Similarly, if the woman with multiple sclerosis (Case 2) had no mental deficit, her refusal of treatment for acute disease should be respected.

Autonomy implies competence. Competence consists of the ability to deliberate about information and to draw conclusions: the conclusions need not be "true" or "sensible" or "correct." Clinical evidence of disorientation, confusion, psychosis, or even "peculiar judgments" when metabolic disturbance is suspected can cast doubt on competence. In the absence of clinical evidence of incompetence, it should not be presumed.

Case 5. A 32-year-old man known to his physician as a Jehovah's Witness has been treated for four years for peptic ulcer. He arrives at the hospital bleeding severely and refuses blood. He is lethargic and somewhat disoriented.

Case 6. A 19-year-old college student comes to the infirmary complaining of severe headache, malaise, and stiff neck. She has a fever of 39.4° C, and her pupils are contracted. Spinal fluid shows gram-positive diplococci. She refuses antibiotics but offers no reason.

In Case 4, the refusal of the patient with myocardial infarction to be hospitalized, no solid evidence of incompetence exists. The refusal of hospitalization possibly arises from denial, a common human psychologic mechanism rather than a mark of incompetence. The decision may be foolish and its consequences tragic. But the physician, after attempts at explanation and persuasion, does not bear responsibility for that patient's autonomous choice. Case 5 reveals a patient who is not, at that moment, competent. However, his history verifies long commitment to a doctrine, the consequences of which, it can be presumed, he accepts. His refusal should be respected. The "reasonableness" of that doctrine, in the eyes of others, is irrelevant. Case 6 shows a person who, while appearing oriented, might be presumed incompetent. She has a high fever; she offers no reason for refusal, and the consequences of refusal are certain and serious.

Most ethicists acknowledge that if a person truly is incapable of deciding rationally and freely, a form of limited paternalism is ethical. It involves making judgments in a person's best interest *temporarily*—until such persons are again capable of doing so for themselves. Thus, restraining a person in the hospital whose insistence on leaving appears to arise from a metabolically altered mental state could be justified, but only until the condition clears. However, such paternalism is justified only when there is solid evidence to suspect lack of competence. Vague affirmations, such as "It's his sickness talking," or "She is too emotional to make the right decision," hardly meet this standard. In general, the ethical principle of respect for autonomy requires a physician to formulate a judgment about the best interest of the patient, to offer that judgment to the patient for consideration, and to abide by the patient's considered decision. When the patient lacks ability to express such a decision, the physician should formulate a judgment based upon the best available evidence of that person's preferences: from past experience with the patient, from family and friends, from written directives, and so forth.

QUALITY OF LIFE. The phrase "quality of life" is used when people make judgments about the goodness or satisfaction of the life they are living, or about some part of it. It is a very subjective judgment: one arthritic patient might say, "My life is pretty poor quality. I've a lot of pain and not much mobility."; another might say, "I've got a lot of pain and not much mobility, but I have good quality life, since I can still read and listen to my music." At times it may be quite vague, as when one reads in a chemotherapy research consent form, "This treatment is intended to improve your quality of life; however, any treatment may decrease your quality of life." Doctors and patients alike are interested in life of high quality. In their dealings with each other, that interest dictates efforts to alleviate pain and symptoms, to stop the ravages of disease, and to allay fear and anxiety. Individuals are the best judges of the quality of their own lives. In recent years, however, the phrase has taken on a rather special meaning in medical discussions.

Those discussions often take place about a patient who is severely ill and whose only prospects are a life of pain or extreme limitation. At times, the patient's limitations may not be the result of a current acute illness, but of some other disorder, such as congenital retardation. Again, the patient's life might be one of deprivation or degradation. Still again, the patient may exist in a persistent vegetative state. In such cases, when acute medical intervention is needed, the question may be asked, "Is a life of such quality worth saving?"

The problems raised by this question are extremely complex. In general, several points should be made about the use of "quality of life" as a factor in clinical decisions. First, reports by the person who is living the life should be distinguished from the observations of other parties: the former have a higher claim to validity than the latter.

Second, all quality of life judgments are value judgments. Some of these value judgments can be amply supported by reference to certain manifest facts, such as the perception that someone is in great pain or is depressed. Other value judgments are less dependent on facts and more on personal or social predilections or prejudices, such as disdain for persons of low intelligence, the unproductive, and the unsuccessful.

In clinical decisions, the former sort of value judgments legitimately carry considerable weight; the latter, in general, should not be influential (often such "moralistic" attitudes are implicit and have to be uncovered). There are two reasons for this: medicine has long attempted to eliminate moralistic judgments from clinical decisions and to care for suffering persons simply because they are suffering. Reliance on any such criteria starts one down the slippery slope: the terminally ill are judged worthless, then the mentally ill, then the chronically ill, and so forth. The tragic consequences of this reasoning have marred medicine's history in this century. The less dramatic, but still tragic consequences for patients of certain social and economic status or of certain "unacceptable" life styles have been frequently documented. Quality of life is, then, an extraordinarily subtle notion. Its meaning in clinical decisions must be carefully scrutinized and cautiously applied.

EXTERNAL FACTORS. The three previous themes bear on the well-being, the preferences, and the qualities of the patient as an individual. In addition to these, it is sometimes necessary to consider factors external to the patient. These are the effects created in others' lives or in society by decisions made about the patient. Some of these are burdens: costs incurred by families, institutions, or society; hardships imposed upon relatives; dangers posed to other parties. Some are benefits: relief from hardships, protection of others, teaching and research potential associated with treatment. How are these external factors to be weighed in clinical decisions?

Certain external factors have long been branded as unethical: a physician prolonging useless treatment for profit alone; a family allowing a relative to die for the sake of inheritance. Others have been closely scrutinized and their role in ethical decisions carefully delineated: the use of patients for research purposes, the revealing of confidences for the benefit of others. The general rules are clear in these instances (although their application is often unclear). Except in very special circumstances, patients can be used for research only with their express consent, and, should the research procedure increase their risks, there should be some expectation of compensatory benefit to the patient. Confidences obtained in the course of care must be maintained unless there is well-founded anticipation that, because of lack of that information, notable harm is very likely to come to another party.

The influence of cost of care on clinical decisions is currently being debated. The import of this external factor on clinical decisions must be viewed even more cautiously than quality of life considerations. In principle, it is safe to say that only when patient preferences are unclear or unknown, when likelihood of benefit is low, and when the quality of the expected outcome is poor, the costs of continued care, for the family and for society, may become a legitimate consideration in deciding to forego life-sustaining treatment.

At the level of policy rather than of clinical decision, there may be determinations whether certain classes of patients should receive certain treatments, e.g., persons over or under a given age will not receive chronic hemodialysis; whether certain modalities of treatment will be developed and made available, e.g., a totally implantable artificial heart; whether a preventive modality should be developed in preference to a high-technology therapy. These policies should be designed not only in view of efficiency but also in view of the imperatives of distributive justice, the fair distribution of burdens and benefits throughout a society.

In general, policy determinations should not dictate clinical decisions about particular patients. Policy determinations should be made at that level where authority is properly situated, where public scrutiny can take place, and where information is available. External factors, while important, deserve the lowest priority in ethical decisions about patient care. Only when the objectives of honoring the patient's wishes and providing a benefit to the patient cannot be reasonably met should these factors be considered as important and decisive. Obviously, in any particular case, there will be discussion about the nature of these objectives and the probability of their attainment.

CONCLUSIONS. Ethical positions are neither entirely a matter of private preference nor a matter of general principles.

They are a mixture of preferences, principles, and facts. The mixture is often confused. Since it is the responsibility of the competent practitioner "to judge the moral and ethical propriety of medical acts," the confusion should be dispelled as much as possible. In each difficult case, the ethical perplexity should be clearly stated, the facts carefully discerned, personal prejudices exposed, and the relevant principles thoughtfully examined. This chapter has suggested a method for organizing these elements in view of a clinical decision. However, a method alone will not resolve the problems. Content, in the form of appreciation of ethical values and understanding of ethical principles, must be inserted into the method. Some reading should be done in the now voluminous and valuable literature in medical ethics. Consultation with persons familiar with these issues should be sought. Frank conversation with all involved—the patient, the family, house officers, and nurses—should be promoted. In this way, the practitioner will deserve to be called not only competent but also responsible.

Ad Hoc Committee on Medical Ethics, American College of Physicians: American College of Physicians Ethics Manual. Part I: History of medical ethics, the physician and the patient, the physician's relationship to other physicians, the physician and society. Ann Intern Med 101:129, 1984.

Ad Hoc Committee on Medical Ethics, American College of Physicians: American College of Physicians Ethics Manual. Part II: Research, other ethical issues. Recommended reading. Ann Intern Med 101:263, 2984.

Beauchamp TL, Childress JF: Principles of Biomedical Ethics. 2nd ed, New York, Oxford University Press, 1983. *An excellent systematic treatment, more philosophical than practical, of the basic principles which should underlie medical practice and health care.*

Beauchamp TL, Walters L (eds.): Contemporary Issues in Bioethics. 2nd ed. Encino, CA, Dickenson Publishing, 1982. *A comprehensive anthology of philosophical background and current problems.*

Jonsen AR, Siegler M, Winslade W: Clinical Ethics: A Practical Approach to Ethical Decisions in Clinical Medicine. 2nd ed. New York, Macmillan, 1986. *A practical guide to frequent ethical problems posed to the practitioner; explains the four considerations of medical indications, patient preferences, quality of life, and external factors.*

Reich W (ed.): Encyclopedia of Bioethics. New York, The Free Press-Macmillan, 1978. *An invaluable reference work of comprehensive, concise entries on most of the issues of biomedical ethics.*

Siegler M: Recommended reading in medical ethics. Ann Intern Med 101:268, 1984. *A selection of articles from medical literature on the major ethical problems encountered by the practitioner of internal medicine.*

Walters L (ed.): Bibliography of Bioethics. The Kennedy Institute of Ethics. Washington, DC, Georgetown University, annual. *A comprehensive compilation of citations of English language literature in medical ethics. Issued annually and available as Bioethicsline, a computerized information system of the National Library of Medicine.*

SUMMARY

These introductory essays have been both discursive and eclectic. Medicine is almost boundless in scope as we move toward the last decade of the twentieth century. Although much has changed, there is much that has remained the same in its traditions and common purposes. Eight centuries ago Moses ben Maimon (Maimonides) prayed:

"Grant me an opportunity to improve and extend my training, since there is no limit to knowledge. Help me to correct and supplement my educational defects as the scope of science and its horizon widen day by day. Give me the courage to realize my daily mistakes so that tomorrow I shall be able to see and understand in a better light what I could not comprehend in the dim light of yesterday."

The *Cecil Textbook of Medicine* has been dedicated to furnishing "a better light" for more than half a century. It is a privilege to be associated with this 18th edition of a book that has become an institution in medical education.

JAMES B. WYNGAARDEN AND LLOYD H. SMITH, JR.

PART II

HUMAN GROWTH, DEVELOPMENT, AND AGING

6 ADOLESCENT MEDICINE

Iris F. Litt

The teenager is a psychosocially and physically unique individual, and this uniqueness has important implications for health and health care. In addition to the age-specific features of this period of life, there are significant differences among adolescents, based upon their rates of pubertal development as well as their developmental stages within adolescence. The view of the adolescent from the physical standpoint reveals the importance of stage of pubertal development, rather than chronologic age, as an organizing principle, owing to the wide variability in timing of pubertal events. From a psychosocial perspective, early adolescents, middle adolescents, and late adolescents have many psychosocial and cognitive characteristics shared with others in their own age groups. There is a growing tendency to combine these vantage points and recognize the areas of interaction between pubertal and psychosocial development.

PSYCHOSOCIAL DEVELOPMENT

During adolescence, certain tasks must be mastered if the child is going to evolve into a successful adult in our society. These include the "tasks of adolescence": the process of separation from the protective milieu of the family and, with it, development of independence; incorporation of the physical and emotional effects of pubertal hormonal changes into one's self-concept; development of a clear sexual identity and a sense of sexual adequacy; educational and vocational decision making; and achievement of the capacity for intimacy. Accomplishing these goals may, in actuality, take a lifetime, but the physician caring for adolescents may encounter opportunities to assist in the psychosocial development of the adolescent.

The physician may foster development of independence by encouraging the adolescent to make his or her own appointments, by promising confidentiality when appropriate, by handing the prescription directly to the adolescent patient, rather than to the parent, and so on. Encouraging the parent of a chronically ill adolescent to assign household chores, to provide an allowance, and to allow going to friends' houses for "overnights" may prevent infantilization at the time when adolescents must be allowed to experience their emerging maturity. Failure to do so often results in "acting-out" behavior. One consequence of the stereotype of adolescents as rebellious patients is that physicians may expect them to be noncompliant with prescribed medication. When this stereotype is examined, however, it is found that the incidence of noncompliance is no different among adolescents than among adult patients, in the range of 40 to 50 per cent. The factors associated with noncompliance among adolescents are, however, different. Self-concept is the single most important predictor of compliance: The teenager who has a positive self-image is likely to follow the physician's advice. Moreover, the risk of noncompliance is great with any medication that affects appearance adversely, such as a systemic corticosteroid. The patient's satisfaction, a valid predictor of compliance for adult patients, is also important for the adolescent patient, but, here again, its determinants are different. The satisfied adolescent patient is the one whose privacy is respected, who is afforded the courtesy of confidentiality, and who is informed about the reasons for laboratory testing. Self-concept is also related to the risk of pregnancy during adolescence. Poor self-concept may place the young adolescent girl at increased risk of an exploitative relationship or cause her to lack the confidence to set limits within a sexual relationship. Low self-concept is also associated with poor compliance with oral contraceptives.

Among the many causes of poor self-concept is the timing of pubertal maturation. For males, maturing earlier than the peer group appears to be an advantage, associated with popularity and athletic prowess, whereas a late-maturing male is predisposed to poorer educational performance and lower self-image. For girls, the effects vary with the environmental context; for example, early maturers who remain in a kindergarten-through-eighth grade school exhibit no apparent ill effect from being out of synchrony with their peer group, whereas those early maturers who move to a junior high school have a higher incidence of poor self-image, have a lower grade-point average, and date more. Timing of pubertal development may also influence selection of sports involvement. Early maturing females tend to have more adipose tissue, are more buoyant, and therefore may be channeled into swimming. The late-maturing girl, on the other hand, with her shorter upper to lower body ratio and leaner body may be more likely to become a ballet dancer or runner. An increase in body fat accompanies normal pubertal development in females, who often have difficulty reconciling it with our society's idealized female form of a skinny fashion model. Their dissatisfaction may result in dieting and the risk of nutritional deficiencies. This puberty-associated dieting may be the forerunner of anorexia nervosa in the predisposed individual (see Ch. 13).

The physician may assist the adolescent's development of a healthy sense of sexual identity and adequacy by offering reassurance about the normality of secondary sex characteristics and genitalia during the course of a routine physical examination. This is particularly important when gynecomastia is observed, as this common phenomenon often causes concern to the adolescent male, who is unlikely to have the courage to inquire about it. The female adolescent with asymmetry of her breasts or one who has not gotten pregnant despite having had unprotected intercourse, or the male teenager who has never impregnated his sexual partner, all may be questioning their sexual adequacy and normality. Even more problematic is the male adolescent who has a renal or urologic condition. The separation of reproductive from excretory function and structure may not be known or apparent to the apprehensive patient, though this is often assumed by his physician. A useful method for allaying such fear may be concrete explanations about anatomy and pathogenesis of the condition, prefaced by a comment like the following: "Some other boys who have had this operation have been worried that it may interfere with their ability to have sex. I don't know if you have had this worry, but I want to reassure you that it will not."

COGNITIVE DEVELOPMENT

The issues of counseling and confidentiality in the context of health care delivery to adolescents are complicated by the developmental differences in cognition among them. Piaget classified children and adolescents on the basis of discrete stages of cognitive development (Table 6–1). According to this schema, most early adolescents would be considered to be at the stage of concrete operational thinking, whereas the middle and late adolescent would be more likely to have progressed to the highest stage of development, that of formal operations. This stage is distinguished by the ability to generate hypotheses that may be tested without their actual enactment. Moreover, the person in the stage of formal operations can think abstractly, entertain multiple contingencies simultaneously, and is able to generalize from one situation to another and to consider potential behavioral consequences logically without actually having to experience them. Piaget's static, categoric approach to cognitive development has been challenged. Newer research in the field stresses "trends" in development. For example, the thinking of the younger individual would now be regarded as being more "empirico-deductive" than that of the older adolescent, who is viewed as being more "hypothetico-deductive." Whatever the system used to evaluate cognition, it is important for the physician working with the adolescent patient to be able to assess his or her capacity for understanding the information conveyed and to be able to use it in a manner conducive to improving health status. For example, the adolescent female who is not able to think abstractly may have difficulty adhering to a regimen of oral contraceptives designed to prevent pregnancy. Similarly, truly informed consent to participate in a research project may not be obtainable from an adolescent subject unable to consider hypothetic consequences of his or her decision to participate or not.

PUBERTAL DEVELOPMENT

The Endocrinology of Puberty

The signal that initiates puberty remains elusive but it is known that just prior to puberty there is decreasing sensitivity of the hypothalamus and pituitary to circulating estrogen and testosterone and to the restraining influence of the hypothalamic arcuate neuron gonadotropin-releasing hormone. The latter secretion is a pulsatile secretion and is associated with sleep. The onset of puberty is marked by increased secretion of luteinizing hormone (LH) by the pituitary during sleep in a pulsatile fashion. The amplitude and frequency of LH pulses increase as puberty progresses. In late puberty, the adult pattern of approximately 12 pulses, evenly distributed over the course of a 24-hour period, is reached. There is a sex difference in gonadotropin secretion during puberty: A dramatic increase in LH levels occurs during early puberty in boys and later in girls. Follicle-stimulating hormone (FSH), on the other hand, rises gradually throughout puberty in boys and manifests an early rise in girls. The effect of the gonadotropin rise in boys is to stimulate testicular production of testosterone. In females, the gonadotropin rise (predominantly involving FSH) stimulates the ovary to produce estradiol, with serum levels rising incrementally as puberty progresses. Cyclic fluctuations in estradiol levels are noted around the time of menarche. Estrone, derived from conversion of estradiol and adrenal androstenedione, reaches its peak at sex maturity rating (SMR) 2 in girls. In boys, both estrone and estradiol (derived from conversion of adrenal and testicular testosterone and androstenedione) contribute to the frequent occurrence (in 30 to 50 per cent) of gynecomastia during SMR 2 and 3. Circulating sex hormones exert a constant or tonic negative feedback upon the hypothalamus in both sexes. The female experiences, additionally, a cyclic positive feedback loop by which increasing levels of circulating estrogens in the follicular phase cause a surge in LH. Sex hormone binding globulin levels fall in males during puberty. As only unbound sex hormones are physiologically active, this results in levels of free testosterone that are more than twice the female level. Prolactin secretion by the pituitary is augmented by estrogen, resulting in higher levels in females than males, peaking between SMR 2 and 3. Prolactin response to thyrotropin-releasing hormone (TRH) stimulation, however, peaks at SMR 4 to 5.

TABLE 6–1. PIAGET'S ERAS AND STAGES OF LOGICAL AND COGNITIVE DEVELOPMENT

Era I	(ages 0–2): The era of sensorimotor intelligence
Era II	(ages 2–5): Symbolic, intuitive, or prelogical thought
Era III	(ages 6–10): Concrete operational thought
Era IV	(age 11–adulthood): Formal operational thought

Growth Hormone and Somatomedin-C

Growth hormone is also produced in a pulsatile fashion, during sleep stages 3 and 4 in early puberty. Somatomedins are responsible for the anabolic activity of growth hormone. Somatomedin-C (IGF-1) levels are age dependent and rise in conjunction with advancing development of secondary sex characteristics during puberty. Accordingly, their levels correlate better with stage of sexual maturation than chronologic age.

Physical Growth During Puberty

During puberty, a growth spurt is experienced by every organ system in the body, with the exception of the central nervous system, which remains stable in size, and the lymphoid system, which undergoes involution. The most noticeable changes produced by the pubertal growth spurt are in height, weight, and the secondary sex characteristics.

The pubertal height spurt occurs during midpuberty (SMR 3 to 4) in most individuals, with its peak occurring at an average age of 12 years in girls and 14 years in boys. During this height spurt, males gain 10.3 ± 1.54 cm per year and females gain 9.0 ± 1.03 cm per year. The growth velocity is greater the earlier it occurs. There is an orderly pattern of linear growth, beginning with the foot, followed within six months by the lower leg and then the thigh. Growth of the upper extremity and of the trunk occurs after that of the lower extremity. The later onset of the growth spurt in males than females results in a longer period of prepubertal growth and, hence, longer legs in the former. Assessment of height during puberty should be undertaken using a height velocity curve, which records increments in height per year (Fig. 6–1).

Approximately four months after the peak of leg-length acceleration, there is an increase in the biacromial and biiliac diameters, the former of greater magnitude in males and the latter in females, resulting in characteristic sex differences in adult physiques. At about the same time, the cranial bones

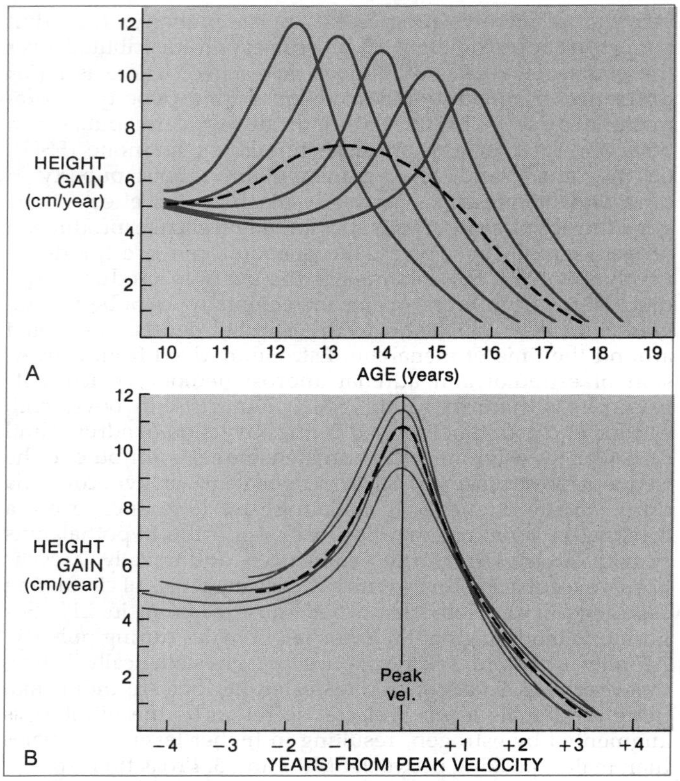

FIGURE 6–1. The relation between individual and mean velocities during the adolescent spurt. *A*, The individual height velocity curves of five boys of the Harpenden Growth Study (solid lines) with the mean curve (dashed) constructed by averaging their values at each age. *B*, The same curves all plotted according to their peak height velocity. (Adapted from Tanner JM: Fetus Into Man. Cambridge, MA, Harvard University Press, 1978, p 12.)

undergo a growth spurt, particularly the jaw, which becomes more prominent, especially in boys. Elongation of the pharynx causes lowering of the hyoid bone. Dentition is another reflection of pubertal development. The cuspids (canines) and first molars of the primary dentition are shed by early adolescence, at which time the permanent cuspids and the first and second premolars erupt in their place. The timing of appearance of the second permanent molar correlates well with that of menarche. The third molars, "wisdom teeth," erupt during late adolescence.

Bone age can be determined from a roentgenogram of the hand, which is compared with standards in an atlas. During puberty, there is close correlation between bone age and stage of sexual maturation (SMR—see below).

Although both sexes experience a weight spurt during puberty, its origin is different in males and females. In males, it is due to increase in muscle mass, and in females, to fat tissue. Eight per cent of body composition is about average fat content in both sexes throughout childhood. At puberty, males experience a loss in fat tissue, whereas it begins to increase in the female and reaches approximately 22 per cent when pubertal growth is complete (SMR 5).

Secondary Sex Characteristics

Estrogen and testosterone have a profound effect on a variety of tissues and organs during puberty. These effects are collectively referred to as secondary sex characteristics. These include voice change, body and facial hair in males, breast development in females, and axillary and pubic hair in both sexes. Of these changes, those that are most consistent in pattern and timing are pubic hair in both sexes and breast development in females. Accordingly, these traits have formed the basis for categorization of the stages of pubertal development, generally referred to as sex maturity ratings (SMR's).

Stages of Pubertal Development (SMR's): Breast

SMR 1: Childlike. No breast development.
SMR 2: Appearance of a breast bud.
Increase in diameter of the areola. Average age is 11.2 ± 1.6 years.
SMR 3. Enlargement of the breast. Average age is 12.15 ± 1.09 years.
SMR 4. The areola and papilla enlarge to form a mound above the underlying breast tissue. Average age is 13.11 ± 1.15 years.
SMR 5. Adult configuration with areola and underlying breast tissue in same plane. Average age is 14.5 ± 1.6 years.

Stages of Pubertal Development (SMR's): Pubic Hair

SMR 1: Childlike. No pubic hair.
SMR 2: Hair is fine, long, silky, and lightly pigmented. Distributed in the midline, along the separation of the labia majora in females and the base of the phallus in males. Average age is 11.9 ± 1.5 years in females and 12.3 ± 0.8 years in males.
SMR 3: Hair is darker and coarser and begins to curl. It extends upward and laterally. Average age is 12.7 ± 0.5 years in females and 13.9 ± 1.04 years in males.
SMR 4: Adult texture and distributed to cover the mons pubis. Average age is 13.4 ± 1.2 in females and 14.36 ± 1.08 years in males.
SMR 5: Adult texture. Distributed beyond the mons to the medial aspect of the thighs. Average age is 14.6 ± 1.1 years in females and 15.3 ± 0.8 years in males.

Stages of Pubertal Development (SMR's): Male Genitalia

SMR 1: Childlike. Testes average 2 ml in volume.
SMR 2: Scrotal skin begins to redden and thin. Scrotum narrows proximally, testes enlarge, and left testis lowers. Penis begins to lengthen. Mean age is 11.64 ± 1.07 years.
SMR 3: Testes continue to enlarge. Growth of corpora cavernosa penis contributes to widening, as well as lengthening, of penis. Mean age is 12.85 ± 1.04 years.
SMR 4: Further enlargement of testes and penis. Scrotum darkens. The glans becomes prominent. Average age is 13.7 ± 1.02 years.
SMR 5: Testes have reached adult size of approximately 25 ml and weight of 20 gm. Full reproductive capability by this stage. Average age is 15.1 ± 1.1 years.

"Primary" Sex Characteristics

The sine qua non of puberty is attainment of reproductive function. To this end, there is considerable growth of the reproductive organs. As indicated above, this process in the male commences with enlargement of the testes as a result of the growth in size of their seminiferous tubules and the number of Leydig's and Sertoli's cells. The epididymis, seminal vesicles, and prostate enlarge as well. The capacity for ejaculation is achieved approximately one year after testicular growth begins, coincident with appearance of pubic hair (SMR 2). For most, the first ejaculatory episode occurs in the context of masturbation, followed about one year later by nocturnal emissions. The median age for appearance of sperm in the first morning urine sample is 13.5 to 14.5 years. The timing of spermarche is unrelated to other manifestations of puberty, occurring at any SMR from 1 to 5 and antedating the peak height velocity. Although complete reproductive capability is not reached until SMR 5, it is possible for impregnation to occur much earlier. Accordingly, anticipatory guidance about pregnancy prevention should commence during early to middle adolescence for males.

Increasing levels of estrogen during pubertal development lead to endometrial thickening, enlargement of the corpus, and increase in cellular content of actomyosin, creatine phosphokinase (CPK), and adenosine triphosphate (ATP), presumably in preparation for menses and childbirth. Menarche occurs at a mean age of 13.3 ± 1.3 years, although its timing corresponds better with developmental than chronologic age.

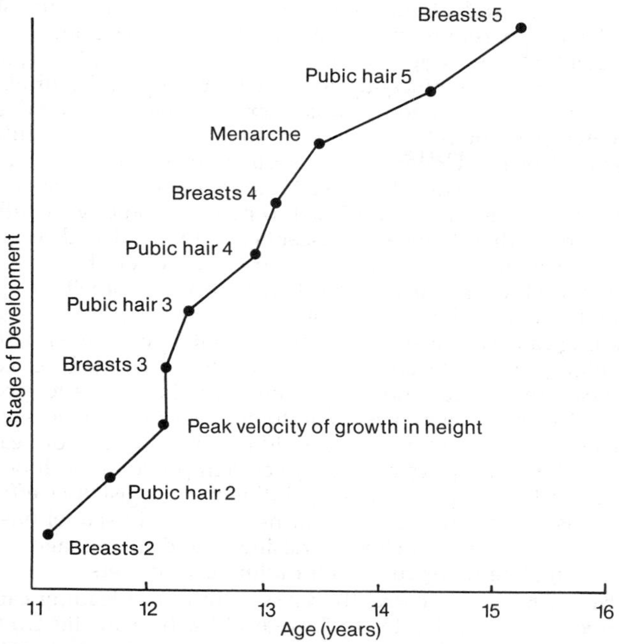

FIGURE 6–2. Sequence of breast and pubic hair development in adolescent girls.

Ten per cent of girls have menarche at SMR 2, 20 per cent at SMR 3, 60 per cent at SMR 4, and the remaining 10 per cent at SMR 5. In addition, there is close concordance between menarche and the peak of the weight velocity curve, which follows by approximately six months the peak of the height velocity curve. The inter-relationships of timing of pubertal events are shown in Figures 6–2 and 6–3. These inter-relationships are useful in the clinical assessment of the young adolescent who is concerned about her failure to begin to menstruate. Regardless of her chronologic age, she should be further evaluated if she is more than one year older than her mother or siblings at the time they experienced menarche, if she is at SMR 5, or if her bone age is 14.5 years or greater. In addition, failure to begin pubertal development by the age of 11 years should be cause for concern. Menarche occurs earlier

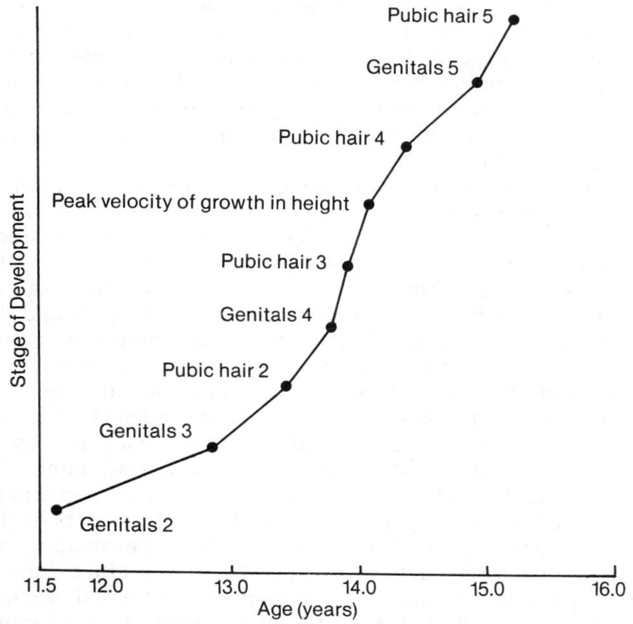

FIGURE 6–3. Sequence of genital and pubic hair development in adolescent boys.

in the obese than the lean adolescent female. Moreover, weight loss of as little as 10 per cent of body weight may result in cessation of menstruation, as can vigorous athletic training with or without weight loss. Full reproductive capability is typically reached within a year following menarche, but some adolescents ovulate regularly from the time of menarche, underscoring the need for timely education about pregnancy risk.

HEALTH PROBLEMS OF ADOLESCENTS

The image of adolescents as healthy and therefore not in need of health care has been fostered by a number of factors. Among them is the fact that this age group contributes only 11 per cent of office visits to physicians, the majority for gynecologic or obstetric care or acute injuries. However, data from the National Health Examination Survey of 1966 to 1970 reveal that 20 per cent of presumably healthy 12- to 17-year-olds have previously undiagnosed health problems, the majority of which are related to the rapid growth and maturation that characterize puberty.

Health Problems Related to Puberty

Skeletal System. The marked osseous growth during puberty renders the skeletal system vulnerable at this time. For example, Osgood-Schlatter disease or slipped capital femoral epiphysis and idiopathic scoliosis occur primarily during puberty. Certain neoplasms of osseous origin, such as osteogenic sarcoma, have their peak incidence at this time. Functional problems such as pitcher's elbow or "shin splints" are manifestations of adolescents' propensity for overinvolvement in athletic activities, and fractures are common sequelae of adolescent risk-taking behavior and resultant accidents.

Endocrine System. Failure to achieve puberty at the appropriate time is often the symptom that leads to diagnosis of endocrinopathies, such as pituitary insufficiency, during adolescence. Conversely, syndromes of precocious puberty or exaggerated adrenarche (e.g., hirsutism and acne) may result in discovery at this time of disorders of excess production of hormones (e.g., adrenal hyperplasia or hypothalamic or ovarian tumor). Euthyroid goiter is a common condition of adolescent females and is often the first sign of Hashimoto's thyroiditis.

Gynecologic. Gynecologic problems are common during this age period. They may be the result of previously undiagnosed congenital abnormalities, endocrinopathies, or exposure to oncogenic agents in utero, or they may be acquired as a result of adolescent sexual experimentation.

Primary dysmenorrhea is almost exclusively an adolescent medical problem. One third of adolescent females suffer from severe, incapacitating dysmenorrhea. It is the leading cause of short-term school absence among female teenagers, yet is easily preventable. Intervention is based on suppressing production of prostaglandins $F_{2\alpha}$ and E_2, which are produced in excess by the endometrium of patients with dysmenorrhea. Alternatively, inhibiting ovulation, and thereby the corpus luteum's production of progesterone, which primes the myometrium to the effects of the prostaglandins, will be effective. The first is accomplished through the use of cyclo-oxygenase inhibitors; the second goal is obtained with oral contraceptives. Failure to respond to these approaches should prompt laparoscopy to diagnose possible endometriosis.

Menometrorrhagia also presents special issues when it occurs in this age group. The differential diagnosis can be approached by separating those conditions that are painful from those that are painless (Table 6–2). The most common cause of menometrorrhagia in the adolescent is so-called dysfunctional uterine bleeding. This condition results from the anovulatory cycles following menarche in which estrogen is unopposed by progesterone, causing buildup of proliferative endometrium and its subsequent shedding. Management

TABLE 6–2. DIFFERENTIAL DIAGNOSIS OF MENOMETRORRHAGIA

Painless	Painful
Systematic	Trauma
Coagulopathy	Threatened abortion
Congenital	Salpingitis
von Willebrand disease	Intrauterine device
Acquired	
Aspirin sensitivity	
Aplastic anemia	
Anticoagulant treatment	
Neoplasm-bone marrow infiltration	
Idiopathic thrombocytopenia	
Endocrine	
Hypothyroidism	
Oral contraceptives—used improperly	
Local	
Gynecologic	
Dysfunctional uterine bleeding	
Neoplasm	

From Litt IF: Menstrual problems during adolescence. Pediatr Rev 4:203, 1983.

of menometrorrhagia in the adolescent includes reassurance (the young patient who develops this problem with her first menstrual period, in particular, will be extremely frightened), cardiovascular support if blood loss has been excessive, and appropriate diagnostic tests (remembering that results of certain of these tests may be altered by the administration of estrogens). Treatment with a combination of high-dose estrogen (for hemostasis) and progestin (to oppose endogenous estrogen effect), as may be found in Enovid (mestranol and norethynodrel), is effective except in cases of pregnancy, trauma, or infection.

Another menstrually associated condition of particular importance in adolescents is toxic shock syndrome (see Ch. 271). Forty-two per cent of cases reported during its peak years of 1980 to 1982 were in this age group.

A number of other gynecologic conditions of adolescents result from sexual experimentation. The reported incidence of sexual intercourse among American girls between 13 and 19 years of age increases from 10 to 50 per cent and with it an increase in sexually transmitted diseases and pregnancy.

Pregnancy during adolescence continues to be a major problem in the United States, which is distinguished by having the highest rate of any of the developed countries. Close to one-half million 15- to 19-year-olds become pregnant yearly. In addition, over the past two decades, there has been nearly a 200 per cent rise in the rate of out-of-wedlock births in this age group, as well as an increase in the number of unmarried adolescents who elect to keep their babies, rather than place them for adoption. Among those under the age of 15 years, the pregnancy rate continues to rise, with 30,000 births last year. In addition to the psychosocial sequelae of adolescent births (such as adverse educational, vocational, economic, and marital outcomes), those who become pregnant under the age of 15 years are generally at increased risk for obstetric and perinatal complications such as toxemia, postpartum hemorrhage, postpartum infection, and small-for-gestational age and stillborn infants.

Sexually Transmitted Disease (STD). Adolescents have the highest rate of sexually transmitted disease of any age group. The most common of the STDs are gonorrhea and chlamydial infection. Physicians should routinely test for the possible presence of other STDs when one is discovered, treat with the shortest effective methods, including parenteral antibiotics when feasible, and extend confidentiality to contacts.

Violence

Accidents, homicides, and suicides together are responsible for 70 per cent of adolescent deaths. Anticipatory guidance, prevention, and identification and referral of the youngster at risk are therefore important roles for the physician.

Accidents. Although athletic injuries and accidental drowning contribute significantly to their morbidity and mortality, the greatest toll among adolescents is taken by accidents involving motor vehicles. Sixteen- to 19-year-olds constitute 8 per cent of the United States population, yet account for 17 per cent of vehicular fatalities. Passengers in cars driven by adolescents account for 63 per cent of automotive deaths. More male than female adolescents are involved as drivers in fatal accidents, and most of these occur between the hours of 8 P.M. and 4 A.M. Aside from failure to use seatbelts in cars and to wear helmets on motorcycles, alcohol abuse is the leading cause of most motor vehicular fatalities. Lowering the drinking age to 18 years has been associated with a 5 per cent increase in fatal automotive accidents. Talking with adolescent patients about their use of automotive safety devices and alcohol use prior to driving should be a routine part of health care. Moreover, physicians may act to improve the well-being of their teenaged patients by influencing legislative efforts such as those directed at requiring seatbelts in school buses, use of motorcycle helmets, raising the drinking age, and imposing late-night curfews for adolescent drivers.

Suicide. Suicide currently ranks as the third leading cause of death among the 15- to 19-year-old cohort in the United States. Completed suicides are more likely to occur in males, whereas female adolescents are more likely to make uncompleted attempts. Sex differences also exist regarding the method used in the attempt; males are more likely to use violent methods, such as shooting, hanging, or wrist slashing, whereas females are more prone to ingestion of drugs. Chronically ill adolescents are at high risk for suicide, and their own medication may be ingested in the suicide attempt. Alternatively, the medication is often that of the parent with whom the teenager is in conflict. Assessment of the seriousness of the adolescent's suicide attempt becomes crucial to planning following such an act. The physician may be surprised to learn that the youngster who ingested a bottle of antibiotics was actually expecting to die as a result or, conversely, that the one who took a bottle of acetaminophen resulting in admission to the intensive care unit had erroneously thought the substance harmless and was only trying to get some attention from his or her parents. The adolescent who fails in an initial suicide attempt is at increased risk for a subsequent serious one, if the crisis has not been adequately addressed in the interim. Simply attending to the pharmacologic or surgical sequelae of the attempt does little to resolve the underlying conflict. Short-term hospitalization is often effective in providing a secure setting for the teenager and impressing parents with the need to seek help for the contributing problems.

Identification of the adolescent at risk for suicide prior to an attempt presents an even greater challenge to the physician. Mood swings from deep despair to the heights of elation are not uncommon during adolescence, but persistence of the depressed mood should be regarded as a potential sign of trouble. According to Puig-Antich, depression should be considered persistent if it lasts for at least three consecutive hours for three or more periods each week. Expressions of hopelessness and helplessness are also serious signs of depression. Disturbance of eating or sleeping may or may not be found in the depressed adolescent. A family history of depression is a useful predictor of seriousness. Some depressed adolescents may, alternatively, appear perpetually euphoric and may engage in socially self-destructive behavior such as drug use or sexual promiscuity. In evaluating the adolescent suspected of depression, it may be useful to inquire about plans for the future. When none are expressed or when the response is "what does it matter, I won't be here much longer," serious depression is obvious. When there is a suggestion of depression, the physician should not hesitate to inquire if the teenager has ever felt so sad that death was viewed as preferable. If answered in the affirmative, the existence of a suicide plan should be sought and such a patient should be immediately evaluated by a psychiatrist. Such questioning will not prompt suicidal thoughts in a youngster who has not already had them and will be greeted with relief by the one who has.

Substance Abuse

Experimentation with drugs serves a variety of purposes for adolescents in our society. It may symbolize attainment of adult maturity or rejection of parental values, facilitate peer acceptance, reduce stress, and, for some, provide an opportunity to explore the limits of new cognitive abilities through hallucinogenic effects. Intervention strategies for preventing or stopping drug use by adolescents must consider these various developmentally adaptive implications. Since more than 90 per cent of adolescents have experimented with either alcohol or marijuana by the time of high school graduation, the focus of the physician's involvement should be on the functional and physical implications of use rather than on the simple ascertainment of use or non-use.

Overall use of illicit drugs by high school seniors has decreased from a peak of 39 per cent in 1979 to 32 per cent in 1983 (Johnston et al.). Decline of marijuana use to 5.5 per cent is largely responsible for this finding. Declines have also been recorded for use of amphetamine, methaqualone, LSD (lysergic acid diethylamide), barbiturates, tranquilizers, and phencyclidine. Heroin and inhalant use has decreased markedly from their mid 1970's peaks to 1 per cent and 4 per cent, respectively. By contrast, however, cocaine use has doubled and smokeless tobacco is now used by approximately 20 per cent of male adolescents. Other sex differences include the increase in smoking by adolescent females and their 45 per cent lifetime incidence of use of diet pills. Alcohol is the most widely abused substance by this age group, with 93 per cent reporting use at some time and 5.5 per cent citing daily use. The time of greatest risk for initiation of cigarette smoking and alcohol and marijuana use is prior to the age of 20 years. Follow-up studies of adolescent "problem" drinkers demonstrated that one half of the males and one quarter of the females continued to have drinking problems as young adults.

Pubertal growth and development may be adversely affected by the use of drugs during this period of life. That the incidence of menstrual dysfunction resulting from drugs is higher in adolescents than adult women suggests greater vulnerability of the hypothalamic-pituitary-ovarian axis in the young. Heroin appears to block release of gonadotropin-releasing hormone. Amphetamines interfere with stage 4 sleep and may thus impair secretion of gonadotropins in early puberty. Induction of smooth endoplasmic reticulum of the liver by a variety of abused substances, such as opiates, barbiturates and tobacco smoke, has the potential for accelerating metabolism of hormones important for pubertal development, such as estrogens.

Regular use of any drug will eventually diminish the youngster's ability to function appropriately in school, to hold a job, or to operate a motor vehicle. An "amotivational" syndrome has been described in chronic marijuana users who lose interest in age-appropriate behavior.

The "infectious disease" model of prevention has little relevance to the problem of adolescent drug or alcohol abuse, nor are "scare" techniques effective. A more realistic approach is one that anticipates that most adolescents will experiment with some drug at some point and is designed to delay that event as long as possible, to limit the extent of use, and to prevent its use in conjunction with operating a motor vehicle. Presentation of factual information about medical complications of drug use by health professionals appears to have some positive impact. Strategies that enable young adolescents to resist peer pressure to smoke, by the use of trained peer counselors using role-playing techniques, have significantly reduced the onset of smoking in a number of studies.

GROWTH AND DEVELOPMENT

Gross RT, Duke PM: Effects of early versus late physical maturation on adolescent behavior. In Levine MD, Carey WB, Crocker AC, et al. (eds.): Developmental-Behavioral Pediatrics. Philadelphia, W. B. Saunders Company, 1983. *Pubertal development and psychosocial adjustment affect each other. Their interrelationships are well described in this review article.*

Grumbach MM: The neuroendocrinology of puberty. In Krieger DT, Hughes JC (eds.): Neuroendocrinology. Sunderland, Mass., Sinauer Associates, 1980. *The intricacies of neuroendocrine pathways and developmental interrelationship are presented in an easily understood manner.*

Kagan J, Coles R (eds.): Twelve to Sixteen: Early Adolescence. New York, W. W. Norton and Company, 1972. *A series of papers on various psychosocial aspects of adolescent development.*

Litt IF: Adolescent health care. In Green M, Haggerty RJ (eds.): Ambulatory Pediatrics. Edition 3. Philadelphia, W. B. Saunders Company, 1984. *Useful information and suggestions for approaching and screening adolescents in an ambulatory setting.*

Litt IF: Menstrual problems during adolescence. Pediatr Rev 4:203, 1983. *A review of special issues in care of adolescents with menstrual disorders.*

Litt IF, Martin JA: Development of sexuality and its problems. In Levine MD, Carey WB, Crocker AC, et al. (eds.): Developmental-Behavioral Pediatrics. Philadelphia, W. B. Saunders Company, 1983. *Development of sexuality begins at birth and is influenced by a variety of social, psychological and physical factors thereafter. This article reviews the process.*

Marshall WA, Tanner JM: Puberty. In Davis JA, Dobbing J (eds.): Scientific Foundations of Pediatrics. Edition 2. Baltimore, University Park Press, 1974. *A concise, current review of the physiology and endocrinology of puberty with excellent charts and tables.*

Zacharias L, Wurtman RJ: Age at menarche. N Engl J Med 280:868–875, 1969. *The multifactorial influences on menarcheal timing are chronicled.*

DEPRESSION (SUICIDE)

Beck AT, Beck R, Kovacs M: Classification of suicidal behaviors: Quantifying intent and medical lethality. Am J Psychiatry 132:285, 1975. *Useful in the assessment of seriousness of a suicidal attempt in patients of any age.*

Mattsson A: Adolescent depression and suicide. In Friedman SB, Hoekelman RA (eds.): Behavioral Pediatrics. New York, McGraw-Hill Book Company, 1980. *Useful categorization of manifestations of depression in the adolescent.*

Pugh-Antich J, Rabinovich H: Major child and adolescent psychiatric disorders. In Levine MD, Carey WB, Crocker AC, et al. (eds.): Developmental-Behavioral Pediatrics. Philadelphia, W. B. Saunders Company, 1983. *A summary of the psychobiology of adolescent behavioral disorders and their management.*

SUBSTANCE ABUSE

Alan Guttmacher Institute: Teenage Pregnancy: The Problem That Hasn't Gone Away. New York, Alan Guttmacher Institute, 1981. *Summary of statistics relating to adolescent sexual activity, pregnancy, abortion and contraceptive use.*

Jessor R, Jessor SL: Adolescence to young adulthood: A twelve-year prospective study of problem behavior and psychosocial development. In Mednick S, Hornway M (eds.): Longitudinal Research in the United States. New York, Praeger, 1984. *A comprehensive prospective assessment of early psychosocial predictors of drug use during adolescence as well as its implications for adult behavior.*

Johnston LD, O'Malley PM, Bachman JG: Highlights from Drugs and American High School Students, 1975–1983. U. S. Dept. of Health and Human Services, Public Health Service, Alcohol, Drug Abuse and Mental Health Administration, 1984. *A longitudinal study of trends in adolescent drug use.*

Kandel DB, Logan JA: Patterns of drug use from adolescence to young adulthood: 1) Periods of risk for initiation, continued use, and discontinuation. Am J Public Health 74:660, 1984.

7 AGING AND GERIATRIC MEDICINE

John W. Rowe

THE DEMOGRAPHIC IMPERATIVE

The Longevity Revolution

Over the next several decades, the practice of medicine in North America will be increasingly influenced by the health care needs of our rapidly enlarging elderly population. The portion of our population over age 65 years has grown from 4 per cent in 1900 to its current level of 11.6 per cent. As

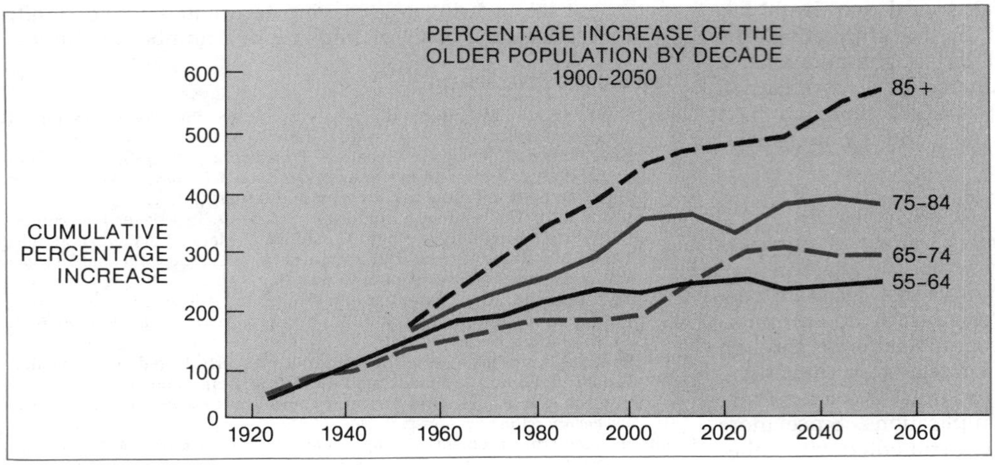

FIGURE 7–1. Past and projected increases in the elderly by decade. (Source: Bureau of the Census, Current Population Reports, Service P-25, No. P52, 1984.)

members of the post World War II "baby boom" age, projections call for a steady rise in the number of elderly in the United States from 25.5 million in 1980 to 64 million in 2030, when one of every five Americans will be 65 years or older. These changes reflect decreased death rates not only in youth and middle age but also in old age: Life expectancy at age 65 has risen from 11.9 years in 1900 to 16.4 years in 1980.

A second demographic shift of major importance is hidden within the general increase in the number of older persons. The elderly population itself is aging rapidly (Fig. 7–1). The longevity revolution has even affected the very old, as the past three decades have brought a 26 per cent reduction in mortality rates in individuals over age 80 in the United States. During the 1980's, it is estimated that the 65- to 69-year-old age group will increase by 13.6 per cent, whereas those 75 to 79 years will increase by 28.8 per cent and those over the age of 85 years will increase by a dramatic 52.4 per cent!

Coupling Longevity with Health

These remarkable improvements in lifespan have focused attention on improving health span and maintaining functional ability in old age. The general health status of older persons is substantially better than is often assumed. Objective health data show a pattern in which vigorous old age predominates. Dependency and institutionalization are the exception rather than the rule, since only 5 per cent of America's elderly reside in nursing homes at any one time. Most community-dwelling older Americans are cognitively intact and fully independent in their activities of daily living.

However, as individuals age they accumulate disabilities and diseases, and doctor visits increase. A substantial portion of community-dwelling elderly report major activity limitations due to chronic conditions. These functional impairments are clearly age related. The proportion of elderly that requires assistance with basic activities increases from approximately 5 per cent at ages 65 to 74 to nearly 12 per cent at ages 75 to 84 to approximately 35 per cent above the age of 85 (Fig. 7–2). Even if one maintains functional independence into old age, the risk of prolonged frailty is still high. For independent persons between the ages of 65 and 70 years, about 60 per cent of the remaining years will be characterized by independence; this proportion falls to 40 per cent at age 85.

Compression of Morbidity

The now familiar mortality curve for a modern aging population (Fig. 7–3*C*) has beneath it two additional clinically relevant curves, one describing the effect of age on the portion of the population in good health (i.e., morbidity curve, Fig. 7–3*A*) and another describing the transition of diseased aging individuals from the asymptomatic to the symptomatic or functionally impaired state (disability curve, Fig. 7–3*B*).

A major health policy issue relates to the relationship between future changes in morbidity and disability in an aging population. The question is whether we will see a prolongation of dependency (i.e., widening of gap between curves of Fig. 7–3*B* and *C*) or whether active life expectancy will increase (i.e., compression of morbidity), as health promotion and disease prevention strategies become increasingly effective and curve 7–3*B* shifts rightward toward the mortality curve. The initial claim that as mortality declines, morbidity will also decline, has recently been challenged by studies suggesting that the increased lifespan of the oldest old is not accompanied by decreased morbidity and may actually result in more dramatic increases in the need for health care services, unless our understanding of disease in old age, and our capacity to treat it, improve substantially.

BIOLOGIC THEORIES OF AGING

Theories Relating to Alterations in Proteins

Error in Protein Synthesis

This theory holds that age-associated impairments in cellular function result from an accumulation of errors in protein

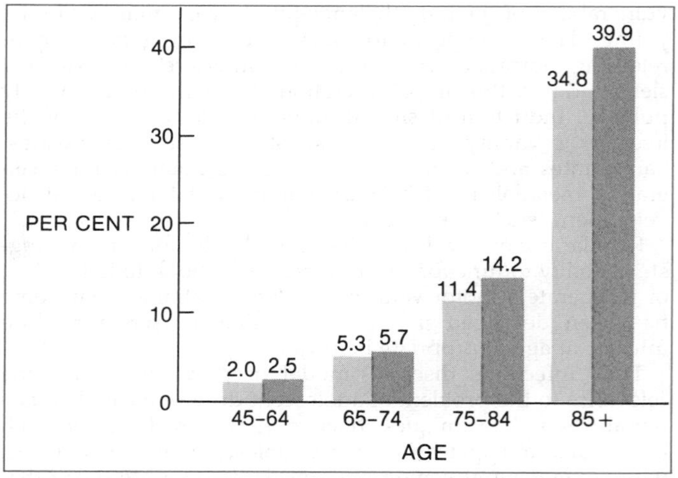

FIGURE 7–2. Percentages of adults, by age group, requiring assistance in basic activities (walking, bathing, dressing, using the toilet, transferring from bed to chair, eating, going outside) and in home-management activities (shopping, chores, meals, handling money) because of chronic disease. Colored bars denote basic activities and gray bars home-management activities.

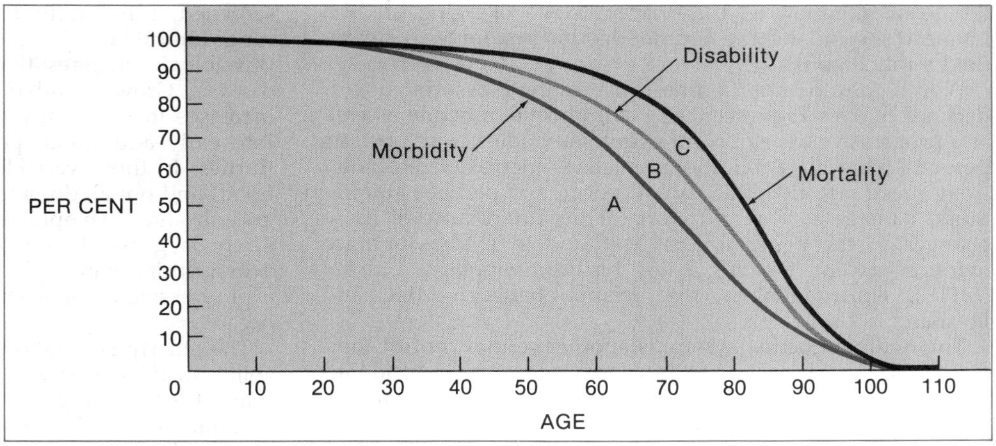

FIGURE 7–3. Mortality (observed), morbidity (hypothetical), and disability (hypothetical) survival curves for females in the United States in 1980.

synthesis. It is reasoned that random errors in DNA, transcription, or translation accumulate with aging to a level that markedly impairs cell function. Substantial basic research in aging over the past two decades has shown that both transcription and translation maintain their fidelity with advancing age and that aging is characterized by a remarkable constancy of the composition of a variety of physiologically important proteins. Specific findings inconsistent with the error catastrophe theory include the facts that aged fibroblasts cultures infected with viruses do not have a decreased virus yield, that newly synthesized enzymes from tissues in the aged are found to contain no synthetic errors, that experimentally induced errors fail to produce an error catastrophe, and that there is no increase in the infidelity of tRNA's with age and no age-related differences in the accuracy of poly(U)-directed protein synthesis. Thus, the error theory is considered by many to be disproven.

Post-translational Modifications (Cross-Linkage Theory)

This theory is based on findings that although transcription and translation are intact with age, *altered* proteins accumulate with advancing age. Thus, post-translational modifications may be important in mediating age-related losses in cell and organ function. A number of physiologically critical enzymes have been shown to undergo post-translational modifications with age, though these changes are by no means universal. One important post-translational modification—glycosylation—appears to be important in age-related development of increasing opacification in crystalline lens protein and eventual development of cataracts. Another modification, increased cross-linking, is central to the major aging modifications in collagen and might have direct clinical consequences for arteriosclerosis and other diseases. Cross-links should not be considered important only in extracellular tissues, since an age-related increase in cross-links has also been shown to occur in DNA. There are a number of criticisms of this theory, including the lack of evidence for varied rates of post-translational change in the same class of molecules in different species despite the remarkable diversity in species specificity of lifespan. Although it is unlikely that post-translational modifications are central to all aging-related biologic decrements, there is general agreement that they may play an important role in the emergence of some clinical consequences of aging.

Altered Protein Turnover

Another aspect of protein chemistry that has attracted substantial gerontologic attention is alteration with age in the *rate* of protein biosynthesis. Although there appears to be no mis-synthesis of proteins with age, many proteins are *produced more slowly* in aged cells than their younger counterparts. Delays have been identified in all of the four major stages of protein synthesis, including amino acylation of tRNA, initiation, elongation, and termination.

In addition, lysosomal pathways for *elimination* of proteins are substantially altered with age, with some proteins being degraded more quickly than in younger cells and others more slowly. Future experiments involving recombinant DNA techniques to correct modifications in these lysosomal pathways may permit evaluation of the impact of these changes on cell aging.

DNA Damage and Repair Theory

The intact fidelity of protein synthesis with age does not exclude major age-related alterations in DNA, since a substantial portion of DNA is responsible for regulatory rather than synthetic activities. The DNA damage and repair theory focuses on the facts that, throughout life, DNA is constantly damaged and that age-related impairments in the repair mechanisms might be expected to be associated with progressive declines in cellular function. Although modifications in DNA repair capacity with age have been identified, these have generally not been well correlated with lifespan, suggesting either that DNA repair defects are not important in aging or that, to date, investigations have not focused on the critical repair mechanisms.

Free Radical Theory

Free radicals are highly reactive atoms or molecules bearing an unpaired electron, which can cause random damage to structural proteins, enzymes, informational macromolecules, and DNA. In mammals the most important source of free radicals is the reduction of oxygen, with subsequent development of hydrogen peroxide. The free radical theory holds that advancing age is associated with an accumulation of low-level free radical damage, which leads to the physiologic and clinical consequences associated with aging. Normal defense mechanisms against free radical damage include a number of endogenous antioxidants, including selenium-containing glutathione peroxidase, superoxide dismutase, DNA repair mechanisms, and alpha-tocopherol. Preliminary support for this theory rests in studies that indicate that animals whose oxygen consumption is high in proportion to their size have shorter lifespans and that administration of antioxidants results in modest increases in life expectancy. Within primates, the levels of the cellular antioxidant superoxide dismutase correlate well with lifespan. In addition, in lower forms of life, mutations leading to defects in production of free radical quenching enzymes are associated with shorter lifespan.

Organ System Theory (Pacemaker Theory)

This theory holds that certain organs or organ systems decline with advancing age and their loss of function drives the systemic aging process. The organs that have attracted the most attention as the "pacemakers" of aging are the immune system and the neuroendocrine system, particularly the hypothalamus.

With regard to immunosenescence, aging is associated with declines of over 75 per cent in T lymphocyte function as well as a progressive development of autoantibodies, with obvious potential clinical ramifications, such as increased morbidity from infections, increased risk of cancer, and perhaps autoimmune damage as well. Support for the importance of these changes in the aging process is found in studies of mice identical except for the major histocompatibility complex (MHC), which show a close relation between MHC and lifespan.

The neuroendocrine system is another central control complex in which marked age-related changes have been identified and that has been targeted as a possible aging pacemaker. Sympathetic nervous system responsiveness is increased with age, and it has been postulated that this increase might be responsible for a number of age-related changes, such as hypertension, impaired carbohydrate tolerance, and altered sleep architecture. Investigators have also sought to identify the presence of a "death hormone," a substance that is produced in increasing amounts with advancing age and that might regulate the aging process, or perhaps a "Methuselah hormone," which is present in decreasing amounts with advanced age. To date, no firm data are available to support the presence of such substances.

These theories focusing on individual organ systems as major regulators of systemic aging suffer from the weaknesses that not all organisms known to age have well-developed immune or neuroendocrine systems and that such theories would fail to explain the origin of the changes in the pacemaker system itself.

GENETIC ASPECTS OF AGING

Despite the apparent lack of evolutionary value to increases in lifespan beyond the reproductive years, gerontologists have long been attracted to the notion that just as growth and development are clearly regulated by a systematic turning on and off of various genes, so aging might represent a process in which systematic modifications in gene expression result in age-related physiologic and pathologic changes. Several of the theories of aging discussed above are linked by the likelihood that the basic mechanisms of aging—whether they be decreases in the production of antioxidants, impairments in DNA structure or repair, or age-related modifications of protein disposal systems or T lymphocyte function—may all have a genetic basis.

Substantial information exists that supports the view that genetic factors are important to the aging process. There is a remarkable species specificity to lifespan. Within an individual species, the life expectancy of identical twins is more similar than that of nonidentical twins, which in turn is more similar than that of siblings. On a more basic level, recent studies in *Caenorhabditis elegans*, a nematode, have identified mutant varieties with lifespans that exceed normal lifespans by 50 per cent. In some of these strains, the lifespan extension appears to be due to a single gene change. These findings suggest that more intensive genetic approaches are promising avenues for future research in aging.

CLINICAL IMPACT OF THE AGING PROCESS

Distinction Between Successful and Usual Aging

A thorough understanding of age-related physiologic changes that occur in humans, in the absence of disease, is critical to diagnosis and management of disease in old age. These physiologic changes influence the presentation of disease, its response to treatment, and the complications that ensue. Cross-sectional and longitudinal studies in carefully screened, community-dwelling groups across the adult age range indicate that increasing age is accompanied by inevitable physiologic changes that are separate from the effects of disease. Growth and development, characterized by rapid increases in many physiologic functions, generally continue into early adulthood, peaking in the late twenties or early thirties. In those variables that change with age after adulthood, and not all do, a linear decline begins at the end of the growth and development phase and continues into old age. There is generally no pleasant plateau during the middle years, during which physiologic function is stable, but rather a progressive age-related reduction in the function of many organs.

The elderly population is characterized by substantial variability in the severity of age-related physiologic changes, as rates of organ aging vary substantially among healthy elderly individuals. Physiologically, it seems that as individuals become older, they become less like each other. This may be due, in part, to lifestyle differences that confound the effects of aging. For instance, although maximal oxygen consumption has repeatedly been shown to decline with age, studies also indicate that oxygen consumption increases in response to exercise training in older persons, with older master athletes achieving levels higher than those seen in normal young adults. As greater attention is paid to the potential beneficial effects of exercise, diet, smoking cessation, moderation in alcohol intake, and so forth, we may encounter increasing numbers of robust elders who demonstrate *successful aging*, i.e., not only lack of disease, but also physiologic performance only moderately below that of healthy young adults. However, the fact remains that most older adults exhibit another syndrome, that of usual aging, in which the effects of aging per se are mixed with adverse effects of confounding environmental, dietary, or lifestyle factors. Most data in the literature on the physiology of aging exclude diseased individuals and provide a description of usual aging.

Distinction Between Aging and Disease

Since age has an important influence on numerous physiologic variables, and since detection of disease depends upon the determination that an individual is different from what would be expected by virtue of his age, it is important to establish age-adjusted criteria for clinically relevant variables to facilitate differentiation of the physiologic consequences of usual aging from those of concomitant diseases. Such criteria have been in wide clinical use for many years for several clinically important functions. For example, spirometric measures of pulmonary function are commonly expressed as "per cent of expected" for age and body size. Similarly, the validity of an exercise tolerance test as a suitable stress for detection of ischemic heart disease is judged on the basis of age-adjusted achievements of maximum heart rates. Standardized criteria are also available for age-related changes in glomerular filtration rate (GFR) and oral glucose tolerance, although variability of these functions is great among the elderly and individual determinations are required to guide diagnosis or therapy. If measurement of GFR is not available, application of age-related standards of renal function is facilitated by the fact that the age-related decline in creatinine clearance (approximately 10 ml per minute per decade) is balanced by a similar reduction in endogenous creatinine production. Thus, serum creatinine levels remain unchanged in spite of substantially lower GFR's in older patients. Familiarity with age changes in renal function and the hepatic oxidizing system is of particular importance in guiding drug therapy in the elderly (see below).

Interaction of Aging and Disease

There is a wide spectrum of interaction between aging processes and diseases, ranging from a lack of interaction at one extreme to age changes that have direct adverse clinical sequelae. Several specific clinically relevant points along this continuum can be identified.

Physiologic Variables that Do Not Change with Age

Perhaps the most important phenomenon seen in the aged, from a clinical standpoint, is no age-related change at all. Too frequently, clinicians attribute a disability or abnormal physical or laboratory finding to "old age," when the actual cause may be a specific disease process. Often there is no influence of age on the specific variable being evaluated. For example, old patients with low hematocrit values may be incorrectly characterized as having "anemia of old age" and be assured that no diagnostic evaluation or treatment is warranted. Data from several sources clearly indicate that in healthy, community-dwelling elders, there is no age-related change in hematocrit. Thus, a low hematocrit level in an elderly individual cannot be ascribed to normal aging and requires prompt investigation and treatment. Other common clinical measures not strongly influenced by age include fasting blood glucose level, serum electrolyte concentrations, blood pH and carbon dioxide content, and numerous hormone levels, including those of insulin, cortisol, thyroxine, and parathyroid hormone.

Impaired Homeostasis in the Elderly

This category encompasses age-related reductions in the function of numerous organs that place the elderly person at special risk of increased morbidity from coincident pathologic changes in those organs. Although usual age-related declines in physiologic function are not so severe as to result in impairments in function under basal circumstances, these declines are of sufficient magnitude to reduce physiologic reserve and thus to move old individuals closer to the clinical threshold for the emergence of symptoms. Declines in basal immune, renal, and pulmonary function and the declines in glucose tolerance and cardiac function during physiologic stress all place the elderly at risk for earlier emergence or greater severity of clinical disease. This fact can be illustrated with several clinically relevant examples:

1. Aging is associated with significant progressive reductions in the dopamine content of the substantia nigra. These decreases may interact with pathophysiologic changes to account for the increasing prevalence of Parkinson's disease in late life and are also consistent with the well-recognized enhanced susceptibility of older individuals to extrapyramidal side effects of neuroleptic agents.

2. Age-related reductions in pulmonary function are so substantial that healthy individuals in the ninth decade of life frequently have only one half of the pulmonary function of their 30-year-old counterparts. Thus, acute bacterial pneumonias of equal initial severity are much more likely to induce a serious clinical manifestation in the elderly. In addition, the marked decline in immune function with age will also be expressed as an impaired capacity to respond to the infecting agent and a subsequent worsening of the clinical picture.

3. Since usual renal function in older persons may be as much as 40 per cent less than in healthy younger adults, the loss of one kidney due to ureteral obstruction, vascular occlusion, or trauma is more likely to result in a clinically significant reduction in overall renal function in an old patient than in a healthy younger individual.

4. The mortality associated with severe burns increases dramatically with advancing age throughout adulthood (Fig. 7–4). This effect, which reflects the multiple parallel reductions in physiologic function during middle age and early senescence, is apparent well before diseases become highly prevalent and exemplifies the impaired homeostasis associated with the physiologic changes with age.

Altered Presentation of Disease in the Elderly

Age-related alterations in disease presentation have long been recognized as being of major importance to the practice of geriatric medicine. Many diseases occurring in both young and old adults have manifestly different clinical presentations and natural histories, depending upon the age of the individual. These disorders should not be regarded as being either more or less severe in the elderly, but just different. One example is hyperthyroidism. Young individuals often present with agitation, anxiety, an elevated heart rate and blood pressure, hyperactive deep tendon reflexes, complaints of weight loss and irritability, hyperkinesis, and a palpable goiter. In the older person with thyroid hormone levels equally elevated, irritability and hyperkinesis are infrequent and goiter is rare. In addition, deep tendon reflexes may be normal or even hypoactive, and the older patient may present a deactivated clinical picture ("apathetic thyrotoxicosis"). Physicians not familiar with presentation of thyroid hormone excess in the elderly may miss the diagnosis early on, thus permitting the adverse sequelae to persist.

Another disorder that is revealed differently in different

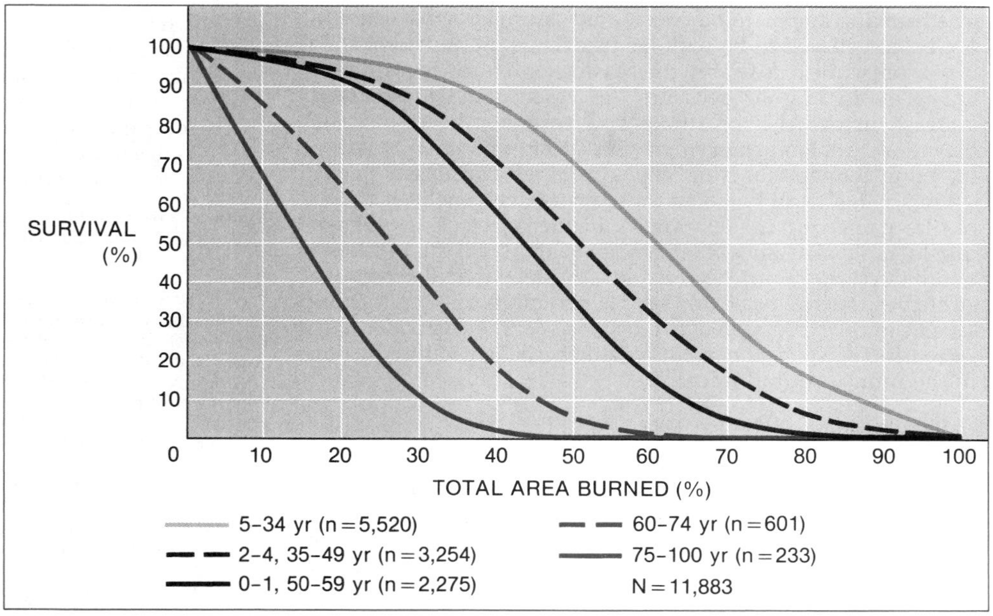

FIGURE 7–4. Survival of patients as a function of the total percentage of body surface burned and age.

age groups is uncontrolled diabetes mellitus. In children and young adults, uncontrolled diabetes is generally manifested as diabetic ketoacidosis. By contrast, the elderly with uncontrolled diabetes will frequently present with hyperosmolar nonketotic coma, with blood glucose levels markedly higher than in ketoacidosis and a relative or absolute lack of circulating ketones. Thus, the elderly may present with obtundation or in coma secondary to markedly high blood osmolality, whereas younger individuals are more likely to present with severe metabolic acidosis, polyuria, or volume depletion or any combination. The physiologic mechanisms underlying these major effects of age on presentation of common diseases remain unexplained.

HEALTH PROMOTION AND DISEASE PREVENTION IN THE ELDERLY

Not many years ago, it would have seemed paradoxical to discuss health promotion and disease prevention for the elderly. Recently, however, this has become an important theme in geriatrics in view of both the remarkable increases in longevity and the awareness that the physiologic and pathophysiologic changes associated with advancing age may be much more reversible than was previously appreciated. This *plasticity* of the aging process is reflected in findings that moderate exercise (30 minutes three times weekly) retards age-related loss of bone mineral content in elderly women, including individuals in their ninth decade of life living in long-term care facilities. Similarly, even though elderly smokers have a much higher risk of cardiac mortality than nonsmokers, quitting smoking late in life is associated with a rapid and sustained reduction in mortality from coronary disease. Clearly, one should not assume that risk factors are necessarily cumulative in their impact or that little is to be gained by altering long-term habits or treating longstanding disorders in the elderly.

A note of caution is required concerning health promotion and disease prevention strategies in the elderly population. Attempts to improve the quality of old age require an understanding of the risk factors for common diseases in the elderly and the efficacy of strategies to decrease the risk of morbidity. Simplistic generalizations of findings in young and middle-aged groups to the elderly are fraught with difficulty. The elderly clearly represent a select group of survivors with physiologic alterations that may influence pathophysiologic processes.

Another aspect of prevention in the care of the elderly is recognition that physiologic or pathologic changes so common in advancing age as to be considered "normal aging" should not be considered to be without risk. Thus, although systolic blood pressure increases with advancing age, it is also clear that rises in systolic pressure are associated with marked increase in the risk of stroke and coronary heart disease. Elevations in blood sugar represent another potentially harmful aging change that is usually considered harmless.

Finally, it should be noted that remarkable beneficial effects can be gained by modest delays in the onset of age-related disorders. For instance, the increase with age in the incidence of hip fracture among the very old is so steep that if preventive strategies, such as calcium supplementation or exercise, delayed clinical expression of osteoporosis for five years, without increasing lifespan, the result would be a 50 per cent reduction in the number of hip fractures.

MEDICATION USE IN OLDER PERSONS

Numerous studies have documented that old people have more trouble with medications than do the adult population in general. The aged use an excessive proportion of the prescription and over-the-counter drugs consumed in the United States. Athough the elderly represent less than 12 per cent of our population, they purchase 25 per cent of the drugs sold in America. This excess consumption of medications is accompanied, not surprisingly, by higher rates of side effects. Of equal importance is that when older people consume the same drugs with the same frequency as the young, toxicity is still more frequent and severe in the elderly. Often, standards for the use of current therapeutic agents were developed in young adults, and simplistic application of these guidelines to the elderly is often hazardous. Rates of adverse drug reaction rise steadily after age 50, and patients over 60 years old are twice as likely to suffer an adverse drug reaction as younger patients. Those over 80 years have a one in four risk of drug intoxication, twice the rate seen in patients under 50 years. Hospital stays are prolonged for all patients with adverse reactions, but older patients remain hospitalized the longest.

This increased toxicity of medication use in the elderly has three components: special vulnerability due to the physiologic effects of aging (drug-age interaction); modification of drug effects by multiple diseases often present in frail elders (drug-disease interaction); and the interactions of a given pharmacologic agent with the other medications, over the counter or prescribed, that the individual is taking (drug-drug interaction).

With regard to drug-age interactions, the changes with aging that occur in hepatic drug oxidation systems and in renal function have their major clinical impact on alterations in the pharmacokinetics of many medications. Several very commonly used medications such as digitalis and aminoglycoside antibiotics are excreted primarily via renal mechanisms and thus have prolonged half-lives in many elderly compared with younger adults, necessitating an adjustment in treatment schedules. These pharmacokinetic considerations are frequently compounded by parallel changes in pharmacodynamics, inasmuch as the tissues of elderly individuals, especially the central nervous system, become more sensitive to some agents with advancing age. Older persons are more sensitive than younger adults to the sedative effects of benzodiazepines and to the analgesic effects of narcotics. The combination of alterations in pharmacokinetics and pharmacodynamics is often further influenced by changes in body composition in the elderly. The average old individual has more fat and less lean body mass per kilogram of body weight than the younger adult. Thus, the volumes of distributions of many agents, such as diazepam, will be altered in the elderly. Similarly, circulating levels of serum albumin fall moderately with age and influence free circulating levels of medications that are highly protein bound, such as phenytoin.

Drug-disease interactions are particularly common in the elderly. It is not uncommon to have five or six major diagnoses exist in as many organ systems of a frail elderly patient. The resulting frequent worsening of one illness by treatment of another leads to disproportionately longer hospital stays and increased frequency of complications. Drug-drug interactions are clearly more common in the elderly in view of the polypharmacy noted above.

Andres R, Bierman EL, Hazzard WR: Principles of Geriatric Medicine. New York, McGraw-Hill Book Company, 1985. *A detailed comprehensive textbook of geriatrics.*

Finch CE, Schneider EL: Handbook of the Biology of Aging. Edition 2. New York, Van Nostrand–Reinhold, 1985. *An encyclopedic reference text, very detailed and well referenced, covering all aspects of aging from plants and nematodes through detailed system-by-system discussions of human aging.*

Greenblatt DJ, Seller EM, Shader RI: Drug therapy: Drug disposition in old age. N Engl J Med 306:1081, 1982. *A useful review of the principles of geriatric pharmacology.*

Hayflick L: Theories of biological aging. *In* Andres R, Bierman EL, Hazzard WR (eds.): Principles of Geriatric Medicine. New York, McGraw-Hill Book Company, 1985, pp. 9–22. *This chapter provides a detailed review of the major current biologic theories of aging, with a good historical review and balanced perspectives of the evidence for and against each theory.*

Katz S, Branch LG, Branson MH, et al.: Active life expectancy. N Engl J Med 309:1218, 1983. *This important paper coined the phrase "active life expectancy" and provides information on the functional capacity of the elderly.*

Rowe JW: Clinical research in aging: Strategies and directions. N Engl J Med

297:1332, 1977. *An overview of the perils, pitfalls and opportunities for clinical gerontologic research.*

Rowe JW: Health care of the elderly. N Engl J Med 312:827, 1985. *A detailed, heavily referenced review of the physiologic changes with age and their clinical influence, with additional updates on several geriatric diseases, including dementia, incontinence, and osteoporosis.*

Rowe JW, Besdine RW: Health and Disease in Old Age. Boston, Little, Brown and Company, 1982. *A concise practical textbook of geriatric medicine for students and practitioners. Emphasis on both normal aging and age-related diseases.*

Salzman C: Clinical Geriatric Psychopharmacology. New York, McGraw-Hill, 1984. *A very concise, practical clinical guide to use of psychotropic medications in the elderly with numerous references and instructive clinical vignettes.*

Schneider EL, Brody JA: Aging, natural death, and the compression of morbidity—another view. N Engl J Med 309:854, 1983. *A detailed update of evidence for and against the compression of morbidity hypothesis.*

8 MANAGEMENT OF COMMON PROBLEMS IN THE ELDERLY

T. Franklin Williams

A physician must approach the care of elderly persons with an informed, comprehensive, balanced perspective about aging itself and about the diseases and disabilities that commonly occur in older people. The previous section has described the physiologic changes that normally occur with aging. From the clinical perspective it is important to keep in mind that most older people are in reasonably good health and, despite some decline in maximum functional ability, can still function well at all ordinary activities. There are many persons in their eighties and nineties who can and do carry on all usual living activities, take long walks, are intellectually sharp with good memories, continue to be sexually active, and most of the time are symptom free. Thus when someone, no matter how old, comes to a physician with a complaint of discomfort or dysfunction, the complaint should not be dismissed as being simply "old age," but should be investigated and treated appropriately.

At the same time, a physician must understand that with increasing age people do accumulate chronic diseases and disabilities. Over the age of 65, 80 per cent have one or more chronic conditions; among the most common are some form of arthritis (present in 40 per cent in national surveys), hearing impairment (30 per cent), and chronic cardiac conditions (20 per cent). One in five persons over the age of 75 may be expected to have diabetes. In those 75 or older, four or more identifiable chronic problems are commonly present.

In addition to recognizing and treating the acute and chronic *diseases* that occur, the physician must give attention to the functional losses, the *disabilities* that are present, and attempt to reverse or minimize them no matter what can or cannot be done about underlying chronic diseases. The ultimate goal of care for elderly persons should be to restore or maintain as much function as possible—to help the patient to maintain as much independence of living, as much of a preferred lifestyle, as possible. Such a rehabilitative approach is an essential part of the therapy.

In those elderly patients who have some irreversible functional losses and thus need regular assistance, an additional part of the plan for care must be identification of who will provide the needed help and where. The extent and quality of family support and the potentials for community or institutional support services must be determined and worked into the overall, ongoing therapeutic program.

SPECIAL FEATURES OF THE WORKUP OF ELDERLY PATIENTS

HISTORY TAKING. Special attention should be given to the history of other (chronic) conditions in addition to the immediate chief complaint and to obtaining additional historical information from close relatives and previous records. An older person, like any patient consulting a physician, is most interested in having the immediate problem addressed and may tend to downplay past history and other chronic but less troubling conditions. It is the interaction of multiple diseases, the necessity to deal simultaneously with these multiple problems, that is one of the distinguishing characteristics of geriatric medicine. A closely related necessity is to obtain complete information on all drugs the patient is taking, both prescribed and over-the-counter medications. The numbers and variety are often astounding, and unfavorable drug interactions commonly contribute to the patient's discomfort and dysfunctions. A good technique is to have the patient (or responsible family member) bring in all the medications the patient is taking, for review, on each office visit.

Certain common functional problems should be explicitly inquired about: any history of falling; any episodes of urinary incontinence; any disturbances in sleep; and any difficulties with vision, hearing, or sexual function.

One must keep in mind the atypical presentations of common acute problems: pneumonia presenting as confusion, acute myocardial infarction as sudden weakness, or an acute abdomen as refusal to eat.

It is a good practice whenever possible to talk with one or more close family members to obtain their observations on the patient's functional status, mood, and daily routines, including intake of food and medicines. Such additional information is absolutely essential if there is evidence of dementia or depression in the patient—in such circumstances the patient may give quite a misleading story. If the patient is living alone (as a third or more of older women are), then it will be desirable or even necessary to have the benefit of observations from a home visit by the physician or by a visiting nurse or social worker.

Any person who has lived 70 years or more will almost always have had previous medical or surgical care, in or out of hospital, and may well have seen several specialists. It should be routine practice, when taking on the care of such a patient (as primary physician or consultant), to obtain summaries or copies of all previous records, including results of all diagnostic tests. Such information should help both in managing current problems and in reducing the extent of further diagnostic tests that are needed. In particularly complex or unclear situations, there should be direct discussion with physicians who have previously seen the patient.

PHYSICAL EXAMINATION. As part of a regular complete physical examination of an older patient, certain features should receive special attention, depending in part on clues from the history. These include evaluation of mobility, of mental status, and of mood. The ability of the patient to move around adequately and the degree of stability in balance and gait can be appraised to a degree from simple observation of the patient as he or she arrives. But because of the commonness of gait and balance disturbances in old people, and in particular if there is any history of falls or near-falls, these characteristics should be explicitly evaluated. The patient should be observed taking a prescribed walk down the corridor, turning and returning. Does each foot carry through a full swing with each step? Is there any limp? Is there any tendency to lean or fall to one side? Is the pace at a usual speed? One should perform the Romberg test and test the patient's ability to maintain balance when purposely given a moderate shove. One should also check for orthostatic hypotension and for any evidence of arrhythmia.

In assessing mental status, it is a good practice to use a standard, short mental status examination as a screening test for any degree of mental impairment and as a benchmark for comparisons on future occasions. Katzman (1986) recommends one of three such tests. Evidence of any degree of mental inadequacy should lead to a thorough investigation of the extent and possible causes of dementia (see below).

Also, in light of the often unrecognized occurrence of depression in older persons, the physician should specifically assess mood. Here, too, short, standardized screening tests are useful—for example, the test developed by Brink et al. (1982).

In light of the frequency of poor eating practices by older persons, particularly those living alone, special attention should be given to any indications of poor nutrition—weight loss, anemia, vitamin deficiency. A careful oral examination is important. Also in light of the frequency of functionally limiting problems, hearing and vision should be adequately tested; joint mobility and muscular strength should be thoroughly evaluated; and the possibility of peripheral neuropathy should be considered.

ASSESSMENT OF FUNCTIONAL STATUS. All aspects of daily functioning should be evaluated by history and physical examinations. Loss of ability to carry out such functions makes the older person dependent on others, at home or in institutional care. These functional characteristics include the usual activities of daily living (ADL): feeding oneself, bathing, dressing, toileting, ambulation, and continence. In addition, the person, particularly if living alone, may need to be able to carry out the "instrumental" activities of daily living (IADL), i.e., those activities necessary for maintenance of the immediate environment: obtaining food, cooking, laundering, housecleaning, transportation, use of telephone, managing medications.

ADDITIONAL DIAGNOSTIC TESTS. The same general principles for choosing diagnostic tests for younger patients should apply in the workup of older patients: The aim is to obtain any information that will help in clarifying the cause of disease or the functional loss, *if* this information will likely lead to effective therapy. The special circumstances that arise more often in older than in younger patients are those in which, because of the other chronic complicating problems, the best judgment may be not to proceed with any form of treatment that may be risky or unpleasant and offers only minimal chance for improvement. Such judgments should be weighed in consultation with the patient and close family before diagnostic procedures are embarked on: If the treatment plans will not be changed by the outcome of the procedure, then it should not be done.

However, because of the tendency, referred to earlier, to dismiss treatable problems of elderly patients as being simply the concomitants of old age, it is important to identify any potentially reversible condition and to use relevant diagnostic aids. An adequate use of diagnostic tests is especially indicated in the common, functionally disabling conditions faced by older people. These are discussed below.

ASSESSMENT OF FAMILY AND COMMUNITY SUPPORTS. A final essential element in the workup of a frail, elderly person, i.e., a patient who may face the necessity of ongoing help with daily activities, is the collection of information about the home environment, the family relationships, the degree of supporting services potentially available, the degree of "burn-out" or exhaustion that may have already occurred, and the availability of home care services and institutional services in the community. A visiting nurse or social worker can be very helpful in obtaining some of these services and in helping to integrate them into an overall plan.

DIAGNOSIS AND MANAGEMENT OF MAJOR COMMON PROBLEMS OF ELDERLY PATIENTS

EPISODES OF ACUTE ILLNESS. Older people with diminished reserves and chronic diseases are more prone to injuries, acute infections (especially respiratory), and other acute illnesses than are younger people, and are also more likely to decompensate at such times. It is a common observation that an old person, previously mentally competent at home, may become quite confused on admission to the strange environment of a hospital under the stresses of an acute illness. Careful attention must be given to every aspect of the patient's status, looking for the appearance of heart failure, overt diabetes, delirium, or increased risk of falling. Drug regimens should be kept simple and the possibility of deleterious effects of overdosage or drug interactions should be continuously reviewed.

Recovery from an acute illness will also take longer than in a younger person, and there is real risk that the previous functional level may not be regained. As early as possible in an episode of acute illness the older patient should be helped to be up and about, to keep joints supple and muscular strength as intact as possible, to retain or regain urinary continence through use of regular toilet facilities, to dress and feed oneself, and engage in social exchanges in usual ways, i.e., out of bed and dressed. The patient should remain in familiar home surroundings or return there as quickly as possible. Convalescent and rehabilitative efforts should be continued as long as any progress is being made.

DEMENTIA. The loss of mental competence is one of the most common and most distressing of functional disabilities in older persons, affecting about 5 per cent of those over age 65 and 20 per cent of those over age 80. We now know that dementia is *not* a feature of normal aging but instead is due to one or another of several disease processes. The most common form of dementia in old people is that of the Alzheimer's type, accounting for 50 per cent or more of cases. This is a (usually) progressive dementia associated with considerable cerebral atrophy and characteristic pathologic changes in selected regions of the brain, with neurofibrillary tangles within neurons and degenerating plaques at end-plates. These damaged neurons are producing far less of the neurotransmitter acetylcholine (and possibly other neurotransmitters also) than normal. With the accumulating evidence that the deficiency in this neurotransmitter is the cause of the failure in mental function, various research efforts are in progress to find ways to achieve more production of acetylcholine (for example, through providing substrate) or to delay its destruction or prolong its effectiveness. Thus far, results are inconclusive.

Other causes of dementia in the elderly include damage from multiple small infarcts or one or more larger infarcts secondary to cerebrovascular disease, metabolic or endocrine disorders such as hypothyroidism and vitamin B_{12} deficiency, brain tumors, brain injury (such as late dementia in professional boxers, which has the same pathologic changes as Alzheimer's disease), Korsakoff's dementia of chronic alcoholism, and the condition known as normal-pressure hydrocephalus. Most importantly, severe depression can present as dementia, reversible with successful treatment of the depression. Indeed, a number of the possible causes are potentially reversible or treatable. Thus it is essential, when confronted by an older person with any signs of dementia, to conduct a thorough differential diagnostic evaluation. This should include comprehensive mental testing to define the extent of the dementia, specific tests for all of the treatable causes, and in most instances, a computed tomographic (CT) scan that can usually identify or exclude infarcts and tumors and can help diagnose normal-pressure hydrocephalus. The finding of cerebral atrophy alone on the CT scan would be consistent with, but not diagnostic of, dementia of Alzheimer's type, inasmuch as a significant degree of atrophy occurs in the normal aging process without loss of mental function.

The physician should be sensitive to the alarm older patients and family members may have at the least sign of any aberration in mentation and should be able to reassure them that "benign forgetfulness" is a common trait at all ages. Benign forgetfulness characteristically is the inability to recall a name or some specific element of a prior experience, when one thinks one should be able to do so. The person can recall many related features of the person or episode and knows precisely what element or name is not being recalled. Usually recall of that element will occur later, unexpectedly. In contrast, a person with progressive dementia will have no recollection of the entire episode, as if it never happened, or can make only feeble, ineffective efforts to reconstruct the identity of the forgotten subject.

If the final diagnosis is dementia of the Alzheimer's type or one of the other irreversible dementias, the physician, nurses, and social workers must treat the family as well as the patient and help them to make the best of a distressing situation. The long-established daily activities of the patient in familiar surroundings should be maintained as much as possible, with avoidance of surprises or new and different decisions to be made. Family members should be helped to understand the disease and also the fact that the patient will likely not understand what is going on. They should be helped to accept the services of home support personnel to assist in the care of the patient—housekeeper, personal care aide, home health aide, or nurse—as needed to help prevent "burn-out" on their part; to accept respite care for the patient (temporary full-time care given in the home or a temporary nursing home admission) so that the family members may get away for a vacation or a special occasion; and to accept permanent nursing home care for the patient if this becomes best for everyone. They should be informed of support groups like the Alzheimer's Disease and Related Dementias Association (ADRDA), chapters of which now exist in most larger communities, and should be put in touch with social agencies and legal resources if necessary to help in making various legal and financial arrangements. The physician's involvement in all of these aspects may seem to some to be peripheral to the practice of medicine but in fact is central to the physician's primary goals of maintaining the health and functioning of the patient and the patient's family to the maximum extent possible. In working with problems like these the physician needs the close participation of well-informed nurses and social workers who can take the lead in management of many aspects.

The physician should keep in mind (and the family should be reminded) that any sudden worsening of dementia is not consistent with Alzheimer's disease and is likely a sign of some complicating acute illness.

DEPRESSION. Depressive reactions of varying degrees of severity are more common in elderly persons than has been recognized and warrant more attention in diagnosis and treatment. As a person lives into later years, losses are inevitable—death of family members and friends, usually "loss" of job through retirement, usually less income, often loss of some degree of health, less vigor, possibly loss of familiar home environment through moving. Some degree of grief and reactive depression is to be expected in response to such losses, but emotionally healthy older persons will work through such grief and return to their usual level of mood, outlook, and activity. Persistence of depressive symptoms may represent activation of a longer-standing depressed state or appearance of a new disorder.

If depression is suspected, it should be thoroughly evaluated with psychiatric consultation and perhaps treated by therapeutic trials of antidepressant drugs. In severe instances not responsive to drugs, electroshock therapy has been found to be successful in many elderly patients. The use of psychostimulants (methylphenidate, dextroamphetamine) in very introverted patients may be useful as a first, temporary step, preparatory to antidepressant drugs or electroshock therapy.

FALLS. Falling is common as people become older, occurring as often as once a year or more in half of those over age 75. In addition to the accompanying risk of injury—with up to 5 per cent of falls there may be fracture of the hip or arm—one or more falls may lead to such a fear of further falling that an older person will severely limit mobility and activities. Falls are often also a harbinger of other diseases or disabilities; one study in the United Kingdom has reported twice the overall mortality from various causes in the year following a first fall in older people, compared with age- and sex-matched persons who did not fall.

A number of risk factors contribute to the likelihood of falling, and it is typically the multiplicity of such risk factors in the same person that makes falling highly likely, rather than any one of them. These include diminished distant vision, deafness, disturbances in balance, abnormal gait, weakness in the lower extremities, decreased mental status, orthostatic hypotension, depression, and effects of drugs on alertness. All such factors should be searched for and as many as possible corrected as a part of regular preventive care and especially at the time of any fall.

Environmental hazards also contribute to the risk. A home visit by at least one of the professionals should include observation and recommendations for correcting such environmental hazards as poor lighting, rugs that can slide, objects blocking usual walkways, lack of nonslipping strips and handgrips in bathtubs, and lack of handrails on stairs.

A person who has fallen should be thoroughly examined for subtle signs of injury or fracture and for any underlying or associated disease condition, including a new febrile illness, painless myocardial infarction, and stroke. If any such risk factor is present and not fully correctable, the patient should be taught to use a walking aid such as a cane or walker.

URINARY INCONTINENCE. Lack of control of urination is far more common than generally recognized; some studies suggest that up to 50 per cent of older women have this problem. It has been referred to as the "closet disease" of old age because of the high frequency of denial of its presence—out of embarrassment or the mistaken view that nothing can be done about it. Older persons living alone may become oblivious to its presence, unaware of the odors that are obvious to visitors. Frequent urinary incontinence, particularly night-time incontinence, by a person living with family is a major cause of caregiver exhaustion and the precipitating reason for their seeking institutional care. Within long-term care institutions, urinary incontinence in a resident means that such a person must be cared for at a skilled nursing or high-intensity intermediate level of care, even if otherwise the person might manage well in a minimal care setting.

For all of these reasons it is important for the physician, in evaluating any older patient, to determine (from patient, family, or visiting nurse) whether the patient has any problem with urinary incontinence and, if so, to conduct a thorough diagnostic workup and, based on the findings, to undertake appropriate treatment. In most instances the problem can be eliminated or controlled.

A good first step in evaluating reported or suspected urinary incontinence is to arrange to have an "incontinence diary" kept by the patient or caregiver—a daily record for several days of just when episodes of incontinence occur, roughly how much urine is spilled, the circumstances—while up and about or in bed or while on the way to the bathroom but "didn't quite make it"—and whether the patient is aware of the episode. In some instances simply keeping such a diary leads a previously careless person to achieve satisfactory control. The diary provides information on the magnitude of the problem and clues to possible causes.

Further workup of the incontinence should proceed from simple to more complex tests, as needed. Urinalysis and culture may indicate a urinary tract infection that, if eliminated, will result in restoration of continence. Observing whether there is any urinary spillage with coughing or straining in the upright position (after adequate hydration) may point to stress incontinence Catheterization after the patient has attempted to void completely can provide evidence for an obstructed or atonic bladder and overflow incontinence.

The most common cause of urinary incontinence in older people is instability of the detrusor system of the bladder—the loss of normal neurologic inhibiting influences as the bladder fills. The detrusor muscle, if uninhibited, will begin to contract spontaneously when filling has reached relatively small volumes, 150 ml or less, and the patient will find it difficult or impossible to suppress the tendency to void. Unequivocal diagnosis of this condition requires cystometric studies and such should be done when needed; some physicians who are thoroughly familiar with the differential diagnosis of incontinence may choose to use first a trial of therapy for the presumptive diagnosis of instability, once other causes such as those referred to above have been eliminated.

In persons with stress incontinence or detrusor instability, the use of biofeedback and other training exercises has been found to help a number of patients to control this problem. Assuring quick access to a toilet, such as use of a bedside toilet at night, can help a person with detrusor instability reach the toilet in time. If stress incontinence in women is associated with major anatomic changes, e.g., severe uterine prolapse, or when prostatic obstruction in men is the apparent cause, surgical intervention may be indicated.

Drugs with anticholinergic effects are successful in decreasing detrusor instability in some patients; their use is often limited by undesirable anticholinergic effects in other organ systems, such as dry mouth and disturbances in gastrointestinal function. At least theoretically, anticholinergic drugs could worsen dementia of the Alzheimer's type (see above). Efforts have been made to identify drugs of this type whose effects are mainly on the bladder. Oxybutynin has smooth muscle–relaxing as well as anticholinergic effects, and imipramine has at least theoretically useful sympathomimetic and anticholinergic actions.

When overflow incontinence is secondary to a distended, atonic bladder (as with diabetic neuropathy), cholinergic drugs may be helpful.

Even if none of the above approaches is effective, acceptable management of the incontinence may be achieved through use of special waterproof pants with absorbent liners, the use of special absorbent pads on the bed, specially fitted collecting devices in women, and in selected patients the use of intermittent straight catheterization. The use of chronic indwelling catheters is rarely indicated.

PRESSURE ULCERS AND CONTRACTURES. These are unfortunate and for the most part preventable common complications of chronic illness in frail older people. Even a few hours of total immobility, as after a stroke or in the recovery period following surgery, will likely result in pressure damage to the skin and subcutaneous tissues; as little as a day or two of immobility in a joint may lead to contracture formation. Once these problems develop, correcting them is a long, tedious, and expensive process.

Preventive measures for any patient at risk of developing pressure (decubitus) ulcers or contractures should include regular, frequent passive or active movement of joints and turning, assiduous skin care, careful attention to avoiding potential damage from wrinkled bed clothes, and care in lifting, not pulling, a patient while changing his or her position. A patient should be sitting in a chair and also walking as much as possible; while sitting he or she should shift weight at least every 15 to 20 minutes.

Once pressure ulcers have developed, even greater attention should be paid to the preventive practices just described. The ulcer should be kept clean, with scrubbing and soaking three to four times a day; mild antiseptic cleansing solutions such as half-strength povidone are better than stronger agents, which may cause further tissue damage. A good practice is to leave wet-to-dry gauze dressings on the wound. Surgical debridement of any necrotic tissue should be done.

As important as local care of the wound is attention to adequate general nutrition and to the treatment of any systemic disease that may cause a general catabolic response. With good wound care in a patient who is adequately nourished and otherwise well or recovering, ulcers will heal rapidly; the presence of chronic infection elsewhere, or poor nutrition, can thwart the effectiveness of even the best wound care. With large ulcers, once the wound surface is thoroughly healthy, skin grafting may be indicated.

Minor degrees of contractures can often be corrected with regular, frequent, careful stretching exercises, following a regimen established for the patient by a physical therapist. More severe and unresponsive contractures may require surgical correction. Such a step can be valuable and justified if it helps to restore mobility and independence or significantly eases nursing care burdens.

DECISIONS ABOUT LONG-TERM CARE. Elderly persons who acquire chronic, irreversible functional losses must have appropriate ongoing supportive services: The goal should be to substitute help only to the extent necessary, thus preserving the maximum possible degree of independence for the patient.

Often the need for decisions arises at a time of crisis: Already borderline functional capabilities of the older person may have further deteriorated owing to a new condition, e.g., injury, stroke, and so on, or the caregiving spouse or child may become ill or unable to continue the previous extent of care. The physician, in collaboration with other professionals (e.g., visiting nurse, social worker) and the patient and family, must weigh the relative merits and feasibility of maintaining the patient at home with support services or arranging care in a nursing home or intermediate care facility. Most older people strongly prefer to continue living in their familiar home settings, and most families desire to help the patient to stay there. Through thoughtful use of various supportive services—meals on wheels, housekeeper, personal care or home health aides, day programs—it is possible to maintain many such patients at home whose care needs would have equally well justified nursing home admission. The cost of the external supporting services in such instances may be only 50 to 60 per cent as much as the nursing home alternative; the family clearly makes up the difference through their own provision of personal care, meals, and so forth.

These features are discussed here because with the continually growing numbers of very elderly persons in our society there will be major increases in the pressures on our long-term care systems, and physicians will continue to be involved at the critical points of decision making where careful efforts to help stabilize and maintain many patients at home will be most important. Comprehensive geriatric evaluation services are becoming available, as ambulatory or inpatient units, in many settings. They have been shown to be valuable for consultative help at these critical points in the lives of many older people and their families.

CARE OF TERMINALLY ILL ELDERLY PERSONS. "Aging" and "dying" are so often thought of as almost synonymous that the problems of how to approach terminal care and how far to go in heroic or extraordinarily expensive diagnosis and treatment are considered by many to be issues that primarily appear in the care of the aged. The actual picture is somewhat different. Almost all of the circumstances in which inevitable death can be predicted in a fairly short time occur in patients with advanced cancer, at any age. For elderly patients with terminal cancer the same principles of care apply as for younger patients: When patient, family, and the responsible physician have agreed that no further efforts at curative therapy are warranted, the primary goal should be comfort care, avoiding heroics.

Similar decisions can be made in instances in which an older person has had such irreversible loss of mental function that he or she has little, if any, remaining apparent contact with surroundings and communication with others, especially family or nursing personnel. If those who are closest to the patient agree on the hopelessness of further curative or extraordinary treatment, including their view that this is also what the patient would say for himself or herself (or perhaps did say earlier, verbally or in writing, such as in a "living will"), then comfort care should be the practice. In fact, despite frequently expressed views that physicians order too much heroic, expensive care for elderly patients in hopeless situations, one study has found evidence for this in only 10 per cent of instances in two hospitals (and in most of those it was the family that insisted on such efforts); in 90 per cent of the cases everyone involved agreed that putting primary emphasis on comfort care had been appropriately accomplished.

What is comfort care? The precise details will vary with the condition of each individual patient. Overall, the physician should be concerned to see that pain is relieved, that whatever may give the patient enjoyable days (and nights) is done (preferred foods, cleanliness, comfortable positioning, visits by family or friends, outings), and that no diagnostic or treatment efforts are undertaken that may be unpleasant or painful or that will not contribute to comfort. These guidelines do not eliminate all ambiguity: For example, what should the physician decide when confronted with a new infection such as pneumonia in a patient in whom comfort care is the primary goal? If no treatment is given, the patient will likely have several days of very uncomfortable respiratory distress and may or may not survive. Comfort care in this instance would probably include respiratory therapy to help clear the airway and use of an oral antibiotic, avoiding painful injections or intravenous therapy.

Blazer DG: Depression in Late Life. St. Louis, C. V. Mosby, 1982. *A thorough and practically useful presentation of this topic, including information on incidence and prevalence, diagnosis and differential diagnosis, and effective modes of therapy.*

Brink TL, Yesavage TF, Lum O, et al: Screening tests for geriatric depression. Clin Gerontol 1:37, 1982. *A validated, useful screening test for depression in older people.*

Katzman R: Alzheimer's disease (medical progress). N Engl J Med 314:964, 1986. *An excellent summary of current knowledge of pathophysiology, possible causes, diagnosis, and management of this condition, including references to useful screening tests for dementia.*

Radebaugh TS, Hadley E, Suzman R (eds.): Symposium on falls in the elderly: Biological and behavioral aspects. Clin Geriatr Med 1, No. 3, August, 1985. *This NIH symposium covers the many inter-related risk factors contributing to this major cause of disability among older people.*

Resnick HM, Yalla SV: Current concepts: Management of urinary incontinence in the elderly. N Engl J Med 313:800, 1985. *A good summary of our current understanding of this condition and successful approaches to management.*

Rubenstein LZ, Campbell LJ, Kane RL (eds.): Geriatric assessment. Clin Geriatr Med (in press). *With increasing recognition of the value of comprehensive geriatric assessment, this volume provides up-to-date information on when, where, how, and by whom such assessment may best be done.*

9 CARE OF DYING PATIENTS AND THEIR FAMILIES

Sylvia A. Lack

Dying patients need to maintain their self-esteem as their dependency on others increases. Physical distress erodes self-confidence and undermines the ability to make decisions and to give as well as to receive. Good symptom control frees the patient to work on existential and practical matters. Many, regardless of intellectual capability or social class, struggle to answer such questions as the following: "What has been the meaning of my life?" "Am I prepared for death and the life after?" Indeed, faced squarely with the fact of death, physicians are forced to consider such questions for themselves. The resultant unease may be a reason for the subtle withdrawal perceived by many patients.

THE PHYSICIAN AND DEATH

It is natural for a physician to feel unhappy when a patient recognizably deteriorates. One way of responding is to work compulsively against the disease until the patient dies. This is clearly beneficial when there is realistic expectation that the disease can be arrested. This chapter does not focus on the management of such patients, but on care for those *dying* with cancer and other chronic, degenerative illness. When death is inevitable, it is counterproductive to continue fruitless efforts to cure, especially when they only add to the patient's discomfort.

At the end of life the physician's two principal functions of curing disease and relieving suffering can become increasingly incompatible. For those in whom prognostic indicators show little or no prospect of rehabilitation, the caring physician has to shift gears and concentrate on the patient's immediate well-being. This requires an enlarged perspective, including awareness of the needs of the family and the possibilities of home care. Care of the dying, although analytic, is relaxed, with emphasis on listening and availability. Such care must be the best that skilled nursing and medicine can provide, ideally embodying the organizational characteristics found in the hospice movement (Table 9–1). It keeps abreast of developments while at the same time avoiding ineffective therapy.

AVOIDING INAPPROPRIATE TREATMENT

In the dying patient with irreversible underlying disease, the aim of treatment is to make remaining life comfortable and as meaningful and dignified as possible. It is no longer to preserve life at all costs. When cure is no longer possible, disease control and palliation should be considered. When disease escapes control, the emphasis moves to symptom relief and comfort as ends in themselves. What may be appropriate treatment when disease is reversible may be ineffective—and thus poor medical care—in the dying. Cardiac resuscitation, artificial ventilation, intravenous fluids, nasogastric tubes, and antibiotics are all primarily measures for use in acute or acute-on-chronic illness. They assist toward recovery of health or an enjoyable, stable state. Their use in the dying or severely, permanently brain damaged is justified only when specifically directed to providing comfort. The question is not, "to treat or not to treat," but to care enough to select the most appropriate treatment in light of the patient's biologic potential.

No particular type of treatment is in itself inappropriate for any category of patient. Instead, the therapeutic aim should be kept clearly in mind when treatment is employed. Terminal hemorrhage does not mandate blood transfusion, but rather sedation and constant companionship. Terminal pneumonia—if symptomatic—may be treated with antitussives and antipyretics. If these fail to control symptoms, antibiotics may be indicated, but the clinical setting must dictate the choice.

TABLE 9–1. CHARACTERISTICS OF A HOSPICE PROGRAM

1. Coordinated home care—inpatient beds with sufficient administrative autonomy and flexibility to provide intensive personal care.
2. Patient/family regarded as the unit of care.
3. Physician-directed services.
4. Provision of care by an interdisciplinary team.
5. An emphasis on control of symptoms (physical, sociologic, psychologic, spiritual).
6. Services available on a 24-hour-a-day/7-day-a-week/on-call basis, with emphasis on medical and nursing skills—including at-home availability.
7. Utilization of volunteers as an integral part of the interdisciplinary team.
8. Bereavement follow-up.
9. Structured staff support and communications systems.
10. Patient/family acceptance on the basis of health needs, not ability to pay.

COMMUNICATION

The value of good communication cannot be overemphasized. Technical, scientific, and clinical competence is not enough. Those who advocate a conspiracy of silence often convey by action and expression the message they are trying to avoid. It is impossible not to communicate. At a time of increasing uncertainty, the message a patient needs to receive is "You are safe." Only part of this can be said in words:

"One of us will always be available."

"I will be back as often as it takes to get this pain under control."

"Whatever happens, I am going to do all I can to help."

Most of this fundamental communication is nonverbal, transmitted by demonstration and behavior. Normal courtesies are maintained—the handshake, level eye-to-eye contact, a seat taken if at all possible. Greetings include the patient's name and often in this day of fragmented care, a reintroduction of oneself, with a reminder of one's role. Others within hearing range are acknowledged—the neighboring patient and others accompanying the familiar physician.

Once trust is established, a patient will often indicate with a question or statement that he is ready to hear more.

"I don't think I can take this much longer, doctor."

"The wife hopes I'll be home by Christmas? . . . "

"I want to stop chemotherapy; it's not doing me any good."

Total candor is not the only alternative to evasion. No one wants to hear harsh and brutal truths, but almost everyone wants to know what is going on. Words and concepts can be tailored to individual culture, beliefs, fears, frustrations, strengths, and courage. The physician's responsibility is to foster clarity and honesty, but not to force an unwilling patient into realities beyond his capacity to cope psychologically.

SYMPTOM CONTROL

Pain can be a major symptom in the terminal stages of many illnesses, especially cancer. Patients with a diagnosis of cancer frequently wait in a misery of apprehension for pain to start. Since, however, about 50 per cent of cancer patients never develop severe pain, this must be emphasized to such persons. Furthermore, for those who do have severe pain, much can be done to alleviate it, so that optimism and determination are justified. A valid base of trust can be maintained in the area of pain management, despite inability to control the disease process itself. The first mild pain should be taken seriously and controlled. This establishes confidence that the physician does have skills to prevent discomfort. This confidence will be a powerful ally if pain becomes troublesome later in the illness.

The goal of effective control is a pain-free patient with normal affect. The very sick patient may doze when external stimuli are minimal but is able to rouse and be alert to friends, family, and surroundings without drug-induced stupor or euphoria. A normal mental state can be sustained through a three-faceted approach as follows:

1. Identification of the primary cause and exacerbating factors.
2. Maintenance of *continuous* pain relief.
3. Ease of administration.

Narcotics for Selected Terminal Pain

Pharmacologic control of terminal pain is not usually a matter of exotic new techniques, but the correct use of drugs already known. The aim of treatment is to manage pain so that it will not return. Breakthrough or recurring pain erodes confidence while generating anxiety and fear. Constant pain control is achieved through adequate analgesia given at regular, well-timed intervals. This method uses smaller drug doses, minimizes side effects, and allows the dose to be increased as the disease progresses.

In mild pain aspirin or acetaminophen is used; for moderate pain codeine or dextropropoxyphene is effective; for severe pain morphine is the drug of choice. Useful alternatives are hydromorphone and oxycodone. Twycross and Lack (1986) have shown that there is no clinically observable difference between morphine and heroin when given orally in individually optimized doses at regular intervals (Table 9–2).

Meperidine has a two- to three-hour duration of action—rather short for continuous control. Narcotics with longer action are methadone and levorphanol, but these drugs may accumulate in the body, as their half-lives are much longer than their durations of action. In particular, levorphanol

TABLE 9–2. STRONG NARCOTIC ANALGESICS: APPROXIMATE ORAL EQUIVALENTS TO MORPHINE SULFATE

Analgesic	Proprietary Name	Potency Ratio with Morphine Sulfate[1]		Duration of Action (Hours)[2]
Pethidine/meperidine	Demerol	1/8	*1/12*[3]	2–3
Dipipanone*	in Diconal	1/2	*1/3*	3–5
Papaveretum	Omnopon, Pantopon	2/3	*1/2*	3–5
Oxycodone†[4]	in Percodan, Percocet; Tylox (capsule); Oxycodyne syrup	1	*2/3*	3–5
Dextromoramide*	Palfium	2[5]	*1.5*	2–4
Methadone	Physeptone, Dolophine	3–4[6]	*2–3*	6–8
Levorphanol	Dromoran, Levo-dromoran	5	*3*	4–6
Phenazocine*	Narphen	5	*3*	4–6
Hydromorphone†	Dilaudid	6	*4*	3–4

*Not available in the United States.
†Not available in Britain.
[1] *Multiply* dose of stated drug by the potency ratio to determine the equivalent dose of morphine sulfate.
[2] Dependent to a certain extent on dose, often longer lasting in very elderly and those with considerable liver dysfunction.
[3] Column of figures in italics refers to approximate potency ratio with *diamorphine* (heroin).
[4] Oxycodone is available in Britain only as oxycodone pectinate suppositories (q.v.).
[5] Dextromoramide—single 5-mg dose is equivalent to 15 mg of morphine (diamorphine, 10 mg) in terms of *peak* effect but is generally shorter acting; overall potency rate adjusted accordingly.
[6] Methadone—single 5-mg dose is equivalent to 7.5 mg of morphine (diamorphine, 5 mg). It has a prolonged plasma half-life, which leads to accumulation when given repeatedly. This means it is several times more potent when given regularly.
(From Twycross RG, Lack SA: Symptom Control and Control of Alimentary Symptoms in Far Advanced Cancer. Edinburgh, Churchill Livingstone, 1986. With permission.)

accumulation in the older patient manifests clinically by the onset of confusion and restlessness several days after starting regular administration.

Narcotics are used when non-narcotics, used correctly, fail to control pain. Some pains are not narcotic responsive. Other methods are sought for tension headache, postherpetic neuralgia, dysesthesia, gastric distention, and muscle spasm. The severity and type of pain guide the choice of analgesic, not the estimate of life expectancy.

Hospice workers have not found narcotic dependence or tolerance to be a practical problem. Addiction, in the popular sense, is rare in patients with no history of drug abuse, despite the widespread use of narcotics for pain control. Drug dependence as defined by the World Health Organization has two components: psychic and physical. Psychic dependence, an overpowering drive to take a drug, occurs in pain patients most commonly after the use of "p.r.n." injections in inadequate dosage. Each request becomes a reminder of the dependence on drugs and the person who administers them. It is preventable by the use of oral narcotics and regular administration. This frees the patient both from the ritual of injections and from continually asking for relief from the presence or threat of pain. With regular analgesia, the self-perpetuating spiral of pain, dependence, and misery is never started. Physical dependence is of little relevance in the patient with limited life expectancy and does not prevent gradual narcotic reduction if the disease goes into remission.

Tolerance is not a problem if the narcotic is precisely adjusted to the degree of pain the patient is experiencing. Patients remain pain free on the same dose for many weeks or months. With the exception of the first few days, when the pain is being brought under control, the total daily dose does not fluctuate unless disease progression increases nociceptive stimuli. The detailed management of cancer pain, both terminal and otherwise, is addressed in Ch. 27.

Unwanted effects should receive prompt management. Constipation is so common that a regular narcotic is never prescribed without concomitant attention to the bowels. Stool softeners, peristaltic agents, and small bowel flushers counteract the antiperistaltic narcotic effect. Nausea and vomiting, which are also initiation side effects and are not universal, can be prevented by the use of a piperazine phenothiazine or haloperidol. Persistent sedation is often due to factors other than the morphine.

Other Factors in Symptom Control

Insomnia is treated resolutely. Night nurses carry a special responsibility for emotional comfort, for discomfort is often worse at night when the patient is alone with his or her pain and fear. The cumulative effect of many sleepless, pain-filled nights is a substantial lowering of the pain threshold.

The therapeutic environment (Table 9–3) is important: light, flowers, art, and, most significantly, caring people.

Physical discomfort looms large in the lives of dying patients, and medicine for the dying must be concerned with smooth sheets, back rubs, relieving constipation, and getting up at night. A person lying in a wet bed is not interested in reassuring words. Patients and families can cope with many emotional crises if they are cared for with common sense and professional skills.

TABLE 9–3. SOME INGREDIENTS OF A THERAPEUTIC ENVIRONMENT FOR THE DYING

Freedom for pets and children to visit
Open visiting at all hours of the day and night
Provision for overnight stays for the family
Arrangements for patient and friends to eat together
Provision of edible food at any time
Nursing and other staffing patterns allowing for interdisciplinary conferences
Mobility for even the bedridden patient to facilitate trips outside and attendance at parties, religious services, concerts, and the like

There is never a time when "nothing more can be done." Remedies for all the common problems in terminal disease can be compiled. A problem-oriented approach treats each symptom on its own merit. Thus the patient becomes not Mr. Doe with incurable cancer, but Mr. Doe—the man with severe pain for which we can do a great deal. This enables the physician, as part of the team, to approach the patient with an optimistic, realistic attitude. Effective teamwork mandates that the health team gather regularly in conference to work out a coordinated approach.

Inclusion of the family in planning fosters an atmosphere of cooperation and support. If their questions are not answered speedily and satisfactorily, they may stop following their physician's advice and abandon the entire carefully constructed regimen. The attending physician, nurses, and home health aide must also understand the therapy. A visitor's doubts may undermine the positive advantages created by confidence. For the patient, underlying mechanisms are explained in simple terms: "Your shortness of breath is partly due to the illness and partly due to fluid at the base of the right lung. There is some degree of 'waterlogging' throughout the body, particularly in the lungs, and you are slightly anemic—people with your sort of illness often are. I cannot get rid of the underlying tumor—you know that—but this is what we are going to do about the extra fluid. . . ."

The fact that you, the doctor, understand why he or she, the patient, is having trouble is reassuring. No longer is this condition shrouded in mystery. The doctor understands. Treatment options are discussed with the patient, and, if possible, an immediate course of action is decided upon together. Few things are more demeaning to a person's self-esteem than to be disregarded in discussions concerning treatment. The dying have a right to be treated for what they usually are: sane, sensible adults. While it is wise not to promise too much, it is important to reassure the patient that the doctor is going to stand by and do all possible to ensure comfort.

Confidence is crucial to successful symptom management. The patient may resist a drug regimen because of a lifelong habit of never giving in or resorting to drugs. Other reasons for resistance may be fear of constipation, addiction, nightmares, and confusion. Once identified through sensitive inquiry, these fears can be dealt with by discussion, education, and control of unwanted effects. In addition to pressing symptoms such as pain, vomiting, and dyspnea, patients may experience a variety of other discomforts. These include dry mouth, altered taste, anorexia, constipation, frequency, pruritus, cough, and insomnia. Because patients tend to be reluctant to bother their doctor about such symptoms, physicians should inquire about them from time to time.

Bedside assessment precedes treatment. Treatment for the same symptom may vary considerably from patient to patient. In the dying, symptoms are caused by multiple factors, some treatable and some not. Best results are obtained by aggressively dealing with the treatable elements. Instead of attempting *immediately* to relieve the symptom completely, the physician can wear down the problem a little at a time. It is surprising how much can be achieved with determination and persistence. Comprehensive treatment is not limited to the use of drugs. Thus, pruritus is relieved in the majority without resorting to antihistaminic drugs. Application of emollient cream to dry, itching skin several times a day and elimination of soap are frequently sufficient.

Clearly defined medical leadership is vital. Frequent contact with specialist colleagues and readiness to consult with others will assist the physician in the search for symptom relief, but the patient should be discouraged from attending a succession of outpatient clinics.

DYING AT HOME

Although home care is not for all, it is a cost-effective alternative that has historic tradition and has proved to be a well-received option in contemporary communities. Physician availability, information about community resources, 24-hour coverage, and education of family members are crucial issues when keeping someone home to die.

Every family must have a sense of security in order to carry on. Most need professional reassurance, and the home visits of a trusted physician are a great boost to morale. Much discomfort can be assessed and alleviated at the bedside, but not over the phone. In some states, an at-home pronouncement visit is necessary to avoid legal complications. Bereavement counseling can then begin when the death certificate is put aside and the physician inquires:

"Tell me about the last few hours, how have you managed?"

Reassuring the family that "you did well" will help them to overcome feelings of helplessness and guilt.

Change comes quickly in terminal illness and can be planned for by discussion and practical measures, such as a supply of parenteral essentials kept in the home. Common crises include refusal of medication, impaction, disorientation, new pain, and the onset of incontinence or of coma. Poor preparation precipitates premature inpatient admission. Even the best laid plans may prove inadequate, but families often manage if someone who knows the patient is available at any time of the day or night.

Medication regimens should be kept simple to understand and easy to administer, even at the expense of pharmacologic purity. An impossibly complex schedule will not be followed. Short-acting narcotics such as meperidine are rarely satisfactory at home. Similarly, a two-hourly medication regimen is impossible to maintain for long.

THE LAST TWENTY-FOUR HOURS

Careful assessment is still necessary if the patient is to be kept comfortable. Temporary relief from a painful bedsore can be obtained by the application of a local anesthetic gel, which might not be used when life expectancy is longer. A distended bladder can be relieved by catheterization. The sound of rattling secretions can often be diminished by positioning and scopolamine. Pain will not be troublesome at the very end if control has previously been good. There is no final crescendo of pain. Analgesic requirements may decrease. Patients may, however, experience pain even when drowsy. In addition, they may be physically dependent on narcotics. Withdrawal restlessness may mar their peace if narcotics are stopped. For these reasons it is advisable to continue analgesia by suppository or injection when the patient cannot swallow. At one hospice 60 per cent of patients are able to swallow until a few hours before death and need no change in drug administration. Another 25 per cent require one or two narcotic suppositories; only 15 per cent need an injection. Only one fourth of the original daily dose is needed to prevent withdrawal symptoms, so rigid adherence to the previous schedule is not necessary. Morphine every six to eight hours will usually suffice.

Both staff and relatives are informed that, at this late stage, any injection may be the last. This information may allay in *advance* any lingering fears about "killing the patient":

"She might die just five minutes after you give her the four o'clock injection. How will you feel if that happens? You understand that it would be just a coincidence because she is going to die very soon anyway? We are using injections only to keep her out of pain."

The advent of the modern hospice has done much to raise expectations in both the public and health care professions. We must be wary of replacing one caricature by another—the old image of death as negative and despairing with the new image that "death is beautiful." It does not help to underestimate the problems. Good terminal care is hard work. The very highest standards may be achieved on paper, but this is a futile exercise unless every aspect is tailored to the vagaries of the individual patient and family.

Health and Public Policy Committee, American College of Physicians: Drug therapy for severe, chronic pain in terminal illness. Ann Intern Med 99:870, 1983. *A position paper authoritatively endorsing six principles elaborated by the modern hospice movement over the past 20 years.*

Hinton J: Talking with people about to die. Br Med J 3:25, 1974. *Sixty dying patients comment on their discussions with doctors and nurses, and give their opinions of what degree of truth is desirable.The assumed principle is that the views of dying people count.*

Lack SA: Hospice—a concept of care in the final stage of life. Conn Med 43:367, 1979. *Describes hospice as a specialized health care delivery system, emphasizing the essential administrative characteristics of a program organized to meet the needs of the dying and their families.*

Lasagna L: Heroin: A medical me too. N Engl J Med 304:1539, 1981. *A succinct rationale, with good references, emphasizing why improved terminal pain control in the United States does not require the legalization of heroin.*

Saunders C: Hospice care. Am J Med 65:726, 1978. *The founder traces the origins of the modern hospice movement, correcting some misconceptions in the popular press and defining the position of good terminal management within the mainstream of medicine.*

Twycross RW, Lack SA: Symptom Control and Control of Alimentary Symptoms in Far Advanced Cancer. Edinburgh, Churchill Livingstone, 1986. *More extensive elaboration and detailed discussion of the analytic methods of pain relief and symptom control mentioned in this chapter.*

PART III

PERSONAL HEALTH CARE AND PREVENTIVE MEDICINE

10 PRINCIPLES OF PREVENTIVE MEDICINE

Stephen B. Hulley

In the early part of this century the efforts of preventive medicine were focused on the predominant cause of illness and death at the time, infectious disease. In western countries, governmental provisions to control the spread of disease with modern water and sewage systems complemented the success of the medical profession in putting into practice the developing science of immunization. These programs combined with improved nutrition, better medical care, and other factors to make death from infectious disease an uncommon event (Table 10–1). This remarkable accomplishment has now brought life expectancy to unprecedented levels and has left, as the major causes of death and disability, the noninfectious and chronic diseases. A new set of strategies has evolved to prevent the chief causes of mortality today: coronary heart disease, cancer, stroke, and injury.

Preventive medicine is based on epidemiologic studies that have identified risk factors for these conditions. Many of these risk factors are aspects of individually chosen lifestyles: cigarette smoking (the most important single cause of preventable death) and eating, drinking, and exercising habits. This has changed the nature of the therapeutic relationship. The patient must take on the larger responsibility of making the necessary lifestyle changes, and the physician must now add the role of health counselor to his list of clinical duties.

RISK MODIFICATION

The process of guiding lifestyle change *begins* with serving as a model. A physician who has healthy habits and provides an appropriate environment (prohibiting smoking in the waiting room, for example) has set the stage for successful intervention. The *second step* is to identify the individual characteristics of the patient, testing for the presence of risk factors and exploring motivations for changing, and for not changing, unhealthy habits. The *third step* is to provide a clear message about the scientific facts on the relationship between risk factors and disease, specifying, for example, the nature and extent of the adverse health consequences of cigarettes.

The *fourth step* is to formulate and apply recommendations for change. Behavior modification, an approach to health education with origins in the conditioned response research of Pavlov and Skinner, has five components: (1) involving the patient as a partner in choosing attainable objectives and in making a firm commitment (a written contract may be helpful); (2) adjusting the environment to promote the desired behavior (by not keeping unhealthy food in the home, for example); (3) negatively reinforcing undesired behavior (through criticism or aversive techniques); (4) positively reinforcing desired behavior (through praise or rewards); and (5) involving the family and other social supports. Many clinics include staff with special skills in behavioral medicine, but even in the absence of formal training, physicians can accomplish a great deal just by addressing and lending importance to these activities. In addition to serving as health counselors themselves, physicians can guide the patient's access to other resources for lifestyle changes by providing pamphlets (obtained free from organizations like the American Heart Association) and by referral to appropriate books, support groups, and health professionals.

Whatever the intervention approach, the *fifth step* is a sustained effort to follow up on the risk factor levels. Habits are difficult to change, and health counselors need to have the tenacity and imagination to try a variety of approaches over the years. This does not mean harassing an unwilling or unsuccessful patient. The best health counselors are sensitive to the preferences of their patients and make wise decisions about when to promote recommendations for change and when to leave the patient alone.

TABLE 10–1. ANNUAL MORTALITY RATES AND YEARS OF LIFE LOST PREMATURELY IN THE UNITED STATES IN 1900 AND IN 1980

Causes of Death*	1900 Annual Mortality (rate/100,000)	1980 Annual Mortality (rate/100,000)	Years of Potential Life Lost Before Age 65 by Persons Dying in 1980
Diseases of the heart	137	336	1,636,000
Malignant neoplasms	64	184	1,804,000
Cerebrovascular disease	107	75	280,000
Injuries	83	69	4,487,000
All others	1330	214	2,199,000
Total	1721	878	10,406,000

*The causes of death are the four most common in 1980. The statistics, which are not age adjusted, are subject to the usual inaccuracies of death certificate attribution. The top three causes of death in 1900 were pneumonia and influenza (202/100,000), tuberculosis (194/100,000), and diarrhea and enteritis (143/100,000).

TABLE 10–2. FIFTEEN AREAS OF ENDEAVOR FOR PREVENTIVE MEDICINE ESTABLISHED BY THE U.S. DEPT. OF HEALTH AND HUMAN SERVICES IN 1979

Topics that Are Covered in Chapters of this Section
Smoking and health
Injury prevention
Control of stress and violent behavior
Nutrition
Physical fitness and exercise
Misuse of alcohol and drugs
Immunization
Topics that Are Addressed Elsewhere in this Book
High blood pressure control
Sexually transmitted diseases
Toxic agent control
Occupational safety and health
Surveillance and control of infectious diseases
Topics that Are the Concern of Other Specialties
Family planning
Pregnancy and infant health
Fluoridation and dental health

IMPLICATIONS OF CHRONIC DISEASE PREVENTION

If the entire population were fully successful in the lifestyle changes proposed in this second wave of preventive medicine efforts in the twentieth century, the chief causes of premature death in western countries might become far less common. In addition to further extending life expectancy, the potential reward of fully effective lifestyle intervention is the possibility that most people could live their full lifespan without major illness or disability.

Speculation of this sort is based, in part, on the remarkable decline in mortality observed in the United States over the past 15 years. The chief component of the decline is coronary heart disease, which has decreased more rapidly in the United States than in any other nation (2 per cent per year). It seems reasonable to attribute this, in part, to the changes in lifestyle that are occurring in this country: the substantial decline in the national prevalence of smoking and of inadequately treated hypertension, the decrease in the mean serum cholesterol level, and the movement in the population to become more physically fit.

The extent and thrust of preventive medicine today have been established by formal health goals in 15 areas of endeavor, created in 1979 by the U.S. Department of Health and Human Services (Table 10–2). For each of these topics, there are specific objectives for the nation to achieve by 1990 that address health status, risk factor levels, public and professional awareness, provision of health services, and mechanisms for evaluation. This section of *Cecil Textbook of Medicine* addresses the 7 of the 15 topics that are part of personal health care.

SUMMARY

The emergence of chronic and noninfectious disease as the predominant cause of death and disability in western nations has been accompanied by a growing importance of lifestyle factors as causal agents in health and disease. Among these, cigarette smoking is the single most important modifiable health hazard; excessive use of alcohol, sedentary lifestyle, and improper diet are also important. The clinician's role in preventive medicine still begins with immunization and treatment of such medical conditions as hypertension, but it now extends to health counseling: examining a patient's risk factors, educating the patient, listening to preferences for changing (or not changing) lifestyle, implementing the appropriate behavioral interventions, and following up on the progress of these personal health care strategies over the years.

Freis JR: Aging, natural death, and the compression of morbidity. N Engl J Med 303:130, 1980. *Speculation on the potential ability of lifestyle intervention to postpone chronic disease beyond the normal lifespan of 85 years. See also the response—another viewpoint—in* N Engl J Med 309:854, 1983.

Levy RI: Declining mortality in coronary heart disease. Arteriosclerosis 1:312, 1981. *Analysis of secular trends in heart disease; the United States has the most rapid decline of any nation.*

Martin AR, Coates TJ: A clinician's guide to helping patients change. West J Med. In press (1987). *Practical guidelines in helping patients modify their risks.*

Mason JO, Tolsma DD: Personal health promotion. West J Med 141:772, 1984. *Review of history of lifestyle intervention programs and extent of the current problem.*

Public Health Service, U.S. Dept of Health and Human Services: The 1990 Objectives for the Nation: A mid course review. 1986. *Update on progress in achieving the 1990 objectives.*

U.S. Dept. of Health, Education and Welfare: Healthy People: The Surgeon General's Report on Health Promotion and Disease Prevention. DHEW Publication No. 79–55071, 1979. *Summary of trends in illness and death rates from 1900 to the 1970's.*

U.S. Dept. of Health and Human Services: Promoting Health—Preventing Disease: Objectives for the Nation. DHHS, 1980. *Specific objectives for health promotion and protection in 15 topics, to be achieved by 1990.*

11 TOBACCO AND HEALTH

David M. Burns

Cigarette smoking is the largest preventable public health problem currently existing in the United States. An estimated 300,000 deaths per year, one sixth of the total mortality in the United States, occur prematurely secondary to the smoking habits of the American population.

Tobacco use, both oral and smoking, was introduced to European settlers by the American Indian, and tobacco was one of the main cash crops in revolutionary America. However, the invention of a cigarette-making machine in the 1880's and, around the turn of the century, of matches that could be carried safely resulted in a marked shift in tobacco consumption from predominantly pipes, cigars, and chewing tobacco to predominantly cigarettes. Per capita cigarette consumption in the United States increased from 54 in 1900 to a peak of 4336 in 1963. This dramatic switch to cigarette use was followed some 20 to 25 years later by an equally dramatic rise in deaths from lung cancer. The risks associated with tobacco smoking appear to be closely related to the amount of smoke inhaled. Smokers who have used only pipes or cigars tend not to inhale, and therefore the majority of the health risks are correlated with cigarette consumption (Table 11–1).

In the early part of the century, cigarette smoking was

TABLE 11–1. INCREASED RISKS FOR CIGARETTE SMOKERS

Cardiovascular Disease
Coronary artery disease
Peripheral vascular disease
Aortic aneurysm
Stroke (at younger ages)
Cancer
Lung
Larynx, oral cavity, esophagus
Bladder, kidney
Pancreas
Lung Disorders
Cancer (as noted above)
Chronic bronchitis with airflow obstruction
Emphysema
Complications of Pregnancy
Infants—small for gestational age, higher perinatal mortality
Maternal complications—placenta previa, abruptio placentae
Gastrointestinal Complications
Peptic ulcer
Esophageal reflux
Other
Osteoporotic fractures
Altered drug metabolism

largely a male phenomenon, but in the late 1930's and early 1940's women began to smoke in large numbers. Currently, smoking habits in young adults are similar for the two sexes. The prevalence of cigarette smoking is declining in both men and women in the United States population. In contrast, a major new marketing effort for smokeless tobacco has led to a dramatic resurgence of snuff use, particularly among adolescent males.

CIGARETTE SMOKE

Tobacco smoke is a complex mixture of some 4000 individual constituents. The smoke is a combination of pyrolysis and distillation products distributed between a particulate phase and a gas phase. Tar is the total particulate matter of the smoke once the water vapor and nicotine have been removed and contains the bulk of the carcinogenic effect of whole smoke. The gas phase of the smoke has a number of irritating and ciliotoxic agents, as well as high levels of carbon monoxide (1 to 5 per cent).

FACTORS DETERMINING RISK

The risks due to cigarette smoking are not evenly spread across the smoking population; they vary with differences in individual smoking habits and the presence of other risk factors. For each of the major diseases associated with smoking, the risk increases with the "dose" of smoke to which an individual has been exposed. The risk increases with increasing number of cigarettes smoked per day, depth of inhalation, and duration of the smoking habit. The risk also increases with the younger age at which regular smoking is begun. The risks due to adolescent and preadolescent smoking may be magnified by a vulnerability of the cardiovascular and respiratory systems during growth and maturation.

A given dose of smoke exposure may interact with other personal characteristics or environmental exposures to magnify the risk of disease greatly. Thus, the risks incurred by cigarette smoking in someone with elevated blood pressure or high levels of asbestos exposure are much larger than the risks for smokers without those characteristics. In addition, the presence of smoking-induced disease in one organ system (e.g., chronic obstructive lung disease) may alter the ability to treat or survive a second disease process (e.g., lung cancer).

CARDIOVASCULAR DISEASE

Cigarette smokers have almost twice the risk of nonsmokers of developing a myocardial infarction or dying of coronary heart disease. This relative risk of heart disease is even greater at younger ages, when the incidence of disease would otherwise be very low. The relative risks for sudden death from coronary disease, peripheral vascular disease, and aneurysm of the aorta are even higher. In contrast, cigarette smokers have only a slightly greater risk of developing angina pectoris, and an increased risk of stroke is demonstrable only in smokers at younger ages.

The magnitude of the risk of coronary heart disease associated with cigarette smoking is equivalent to the risks associated with elevated blood pressure or elevated serum cholesterol. The per cent of the population with smoking as a risk factor is substantially larger than the percentage with either elevated blood pressure or elevated serum cholesterol. As a result, *smoking ranks as the largest avoidable cause of coronary heart disease in the American population.*

Cigarette smoking acts as an independent risk factor for coronary heart disease; that is, its effect is not explained by levels of other risk factors. However, when more than one risk factor is present, smoking interacts with the other major risk factors to increase the risk synergistically (Fig. 11–1). The presence of smoking, or of either of the other risk factors, increases the risk by 31 per 1000, compared with the risk of someone with none of the risk factors. The presence of a

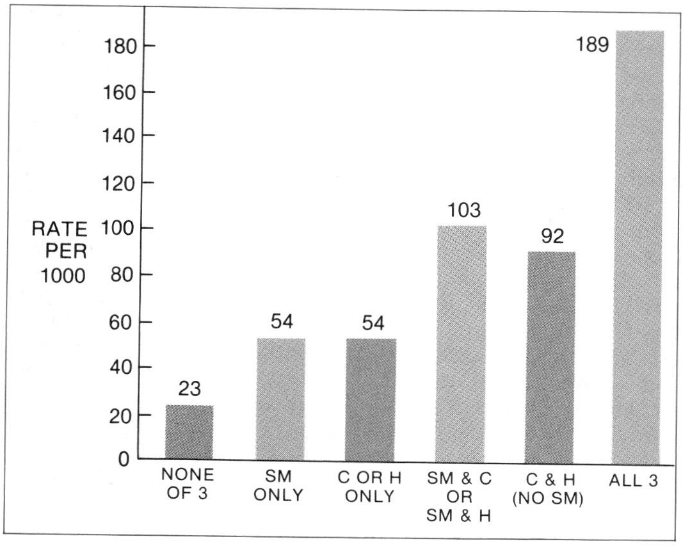

FIGURE 11–1. Major risk factor combinations, 10-year incidence of first major coronary events, men age 30 to 59 at entry, Pooling Project. Risk factor status at entry: Definitions of the three major risk factors and their symbols are hypercholesterolemia (C) = $\geq$ 250 mg/dl; elevated blood pressure (H) = diastolic pressure $\geq$ 90 mm Hg; cigarette smoking (SM) = any current use of cigarettes at entry.

second risk factor in someone who smokes results in an increase in risk of 49 per 1000 over the risk when only one risk factor is present, and the addition of a third risk factor increases the risk by 86 per 1000. The actual risk that exists is always greater than the sum of the risks measured independently, suggesting that when multiple risk factors are present they interact to create more disease. This interaction may occur by accelerating the development of atherosclerosis, or it may occur by increasing the likelihood or severity of a myocardial infarction for any given level of atherosclerosis.

Smokers have more atherosclerosis than nonsmokers, particularly in the aorta. Smoking a cigarette results in an increase in heart rate and blood pressure, necessitating a greater myocardial oxygen delivery, while the carbon monoxide in the smoke increases the blood's carboxyhemoglobin level, thus decreasing its oxygen-carrying capacity. Cigarette smoking also increases platelet adhesiveness and lowers the threshold for ventricular fibrillation and may thereby play a role in the acute events surrounding some thrombotic myocardial infarctions.

Cigarette smoking has a more profound effect on the peripheral vascular bed than on the coronary or cerebral vessels. Over 90 per cent of patients with atherosclerotic peripheral vascular disease are cigarette smokers. The cessation of cigarette smoking is a critical therapeutic intervention in these patients; and in those who fail to quit, there is a higher incidence of amputation, and surgical therapy is dramatically less successful.

The risk of coronary heart disease due to smoking is present at all ages beyond 30, but smoking is responsible for a greater proportion of coronary deaths in younger age groups than in older age groups. This risk declines dramatically with the cessation of cigarette smoking. By five years after the last cigarette, the risk in those who had smoked less than one pack per day approximates the risk in lifelong nonsmokers. For those who had smoked more than one pack per day, a small residual risk of coronary heart disease may persist.

CANCER

Lung cancer is the largest cause of death from cancer in men and women (Ch. 70). *Approximately 85 per cent of mortality due to lung cancer is causally attributed to cigarette smoking and is therefore potentially preventable.* No other single agent has been examined in as much detail, is more firmly established as a causal agent, or is responsible for more cancer deaths than cigarette smoking.

Cigarette smokers are ten times more likely to develop lung cancer than nonsmokers. This risk is proportional to the number of cigarettes smoked per day, increasing to 20 to 25 times the risk of the nonsmoker in those who smoke two or more packs of cigarettes per day. The risk is also increased in those who inhale more deeply or began smoking at a younger age. Lung cancer death rates begin to increase rapidly after age 35 (Fig. 11–2). Cigarette smoking causes all of the major types of lung cancer, including squamous cell, adenocarcinoma, oat cell, and large-cell carcinoma. Asbestos exposure and uranium mining interact synergistically with cigarette smoking to increase the risk of lung cancer dramatically.

The relative risks of developing *laryngeal cancer* for the cigarette smoker closely track those of lung cancer, but the total number of cases is smaller and the survival better. Cigarette smokers are five times more likely to develop *cancer of the oral cavity and esophagus,* and there appears to be a synergistic interaction between cigarette smoking and alcohol consumption for cancer of the larynx, oral cavity, and esophagus. Cigarette smoking is also a major contributing factor in *cancers of the bladder, kidney, and pancreas,* and an association between cigarette smoking and *gastric and cervical cancers* has been noted. The use of chewing tobacco or snuff can cause cancers of the cheek or gum. Overall, tobacco consumption is responsible for approximately 30 per cent of the total United States cancer mortality.

Cigarette smoking induces changes in the respiratory epithelium that progress from hyperplasia to dysplasia and even to carcinoma in situ. Tobacco smoke contains a variety of tumorigenic agents, including several that can act as complete carcinogens. In addition, tumor initiators, promoters, and cocarcinogens have been identified in smoke. The impact of these tumorigenic agents may be magnified by the ciliotoxic agents in the smoke that interfere with the normal clearance mechanisms of the lung and result in a prolonged retention of the carcinogenic agents in the lung.

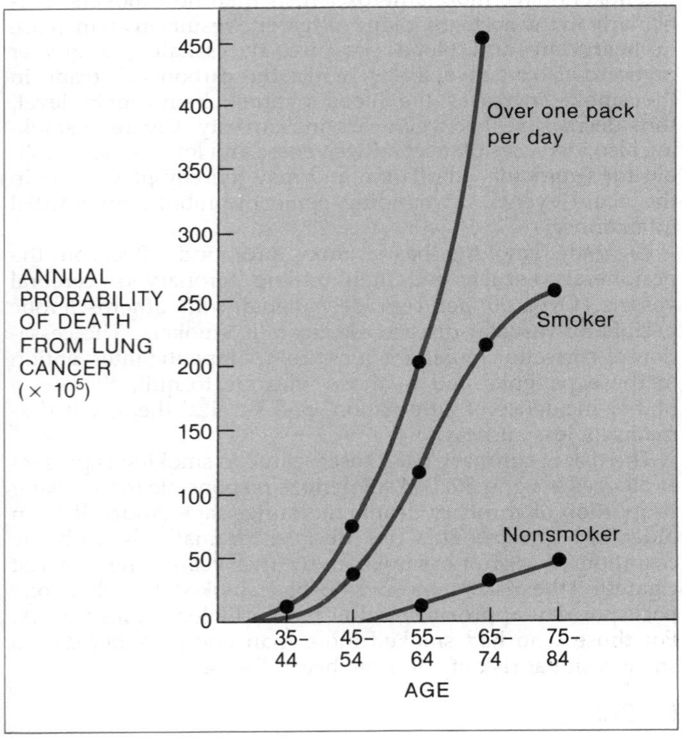

FIGURE 11–2. Annual death rate from lung cancer in nonsmokers, smokers in general, and those who smoke more than one pack per day.

Cessation of cigarette smoking results in a lessening of the risk of cancer in comparison with the risk to the continuing smoker. The risk for light smokers approximates the risk of the nonsmoker by 10 to 15 years after cessation. Heavy smokers have a residual two- to threefold increased risk that is proportional to their lifetime exposure to smoke.

CHRONIC OBSTRUCTIVE PULMONARY DISEASE (COPD)

Cigarette-induced lung injury is characterized by three overlapping syndromes: cough and mucus hypersecretion, bronchitis with airflow obstruction, and emphysema (see Ch. 61). By age 60 most cigarette smokers have changes in the airways and some degree of pathologic emphysema, but only the minority have symptomatic ventilatory limitation. An increased prevalence of cough can be demonstrated in cigarette smokers by the early teens, and abnormalities in the small airways are present in many smokers by early adulthood. However, it is not clear that either of these changes predicts those who will eventually go on to develop symptomatic chronic airflow limitation.

The cigarette smoking habit is the major predictor in a population for the development of COPD. The prevalence of COPD and risk of death from COPD increase with the number of cigarettes smoked per day and the depth of inhalation, as does the prevalence of chronic cough and sputum production, rate of decline in the measurements of expiratory airflow, and degree of anatomic emphysema.

In contrast to nonsmokers, the majority of cigarette smokers examined at autopsy have some degree of emphysema and hypertrophic changes of the respiratory epithelium. However, only a minority of cigarette smokers manifest clinically significant airflow obstruction. Those who develop chronic airflow obstruction may be a subset of the smoking population identifiable by a rapidly declining FEV_1 early in the course of disease. In any event, it is rare for symptomatic chronic airflow obstruction to develop in anyone who maintained normal measures of expiratory airflow through age 45.

Cessation of cigarette smoking is of some benefit at all preterminal stages of ventilatory impairment. Changes in the small airways and early declines of FEF_{25-75} may reverse within one year of cessation. Cough and sputum production also lessen, and the annual rate of decline in measures of expiratory airflow moderates and approximates the rate of decline in nonsmokers. These changes are probably related to reversal of the chronic inflammatory changes in the large and small airways and the recovery of ciliary function, as there is no evidence that the emphysematous process is reversible.

Lungs of smokers contain increased numbers of alveolar macrophages and polymorphonuclear leukocytes, probably drawn there as part of the inflammatory response to the irritants in the smoke. These cells produce elastase, which is capable of degrading the structural elements of the lung, resulting in a loss of elastic recoil. This destructive process is normally limited by blood-borne antiproteases. However, cigarette smoke contains a number of oxidants that destroy the function of these protective proteins, and the result is an imbalance in the protease-antiprotease system favoring degradation and rupture of alveolar walls.

RISKS FOR WOMEN

There is essentially no protective effect of being female for the risks of developing cancer or chronic lung disease. Much of the premenopausal difference in cardiovascular risk enjoyed by women disappears in those who smoke.

In addition to the risks defined for men, women also incur additional risks related to pregnancy and use of oral contraceptives. Infants of smoking mothers are small for their gestational age in weight, length, and head circumference, and they experience a higher perinatal mortality, particularly if other determinants of a high-risk pregnancy are present. The smoking mothers are also at greater risk for the maternal complications of pregnancy, especially placenta previa and abruptio placentae.

Women who smoke and use oral contraceptives are at dramatically increased risk of cardiovascular disease. They are over 30 times more likely to develop a myocardial infarction, and about 20 times more likely to have a subarachnoid hemorrhage, than their nonsmoking peers who do not use oral contraceptives.

INVOLUNTARY SMOKING

Environmental tobacco smoke contains most of the toxic and carcinogenic compounds identified in mainstream smoke; and therefore the question is not whether these agents can cause disease, but rather whether the dose and mode of exposure experienced in involuntary smoking carry a measurable risk. Absorption of smoke constituents from the environment has been documented in both infants and adults, and a number of epidemiologic studies have demonstrated health effects in humans.

Involuntary smoking can cause lung cancer in nonsmokers. The risk is small in comparison to active smoking but is large in comparison to other carcinogenic exposures experienced by the general population. From 500 to 5000 lung cancers per year have been estimated to result from involuntary smoking.

The majority of nonsmokers express annoyance and experience eye and respiratory tract irritation on exposure to smoke. Individuals with pre-existing disease may become more symptomatic on exposure to smoke, particularly those with allergies, and possibly those with chronic heart and lung disease.

Infants of smoking parents have a higher incidence of bronchitis and pneumonia in the first year of life, and the children of smoking mothers experience a developmental lag in lung growth.

CIGARETTES WITH LOW TAR AND NICOTINE

The machine-measured yield of tar and nicotine for the average cigarette smoked by the American population has been steadily declining. Unfortunately this decline in tar yield has not been matched by a proportional drop in the disease risks of smoking these cigarettes. Smokers of lower yield cigarettes have a slightly lower risk of lung cancer than smokers of the high-yield cigarette, but this benefit disappears if they increase the number of cigarettes they smoke per day. There is also a lower prevalence of cough and phlegm, but probably no major impact on the risk of developing cardiovascular disease or chronic airflow obstruction. There are two major reasons why the decline in machine-measured tar and nicotine yield has not been accompanied by a concomitant reduction in biologic effect: (1) Many smokers may compensate for the decline in yield by increasing the number of cigarettes smoked per day, or by inhaling more deeply, thereby negating any possible reduction in smoke exposure "dose." (2) The machine-measured yield may not correspond to the yield when the cigarette is actually smoked. This is particularly true for the very low-yield cigarettes that have vents or channels designed into the filter so that the machine draws very little smoke through the filter. These vents can be occluded by the smoker, or the volume of the puff increased, with a resultant dramatic rise in the yield. For these cigarettes, the measured tar and nicotine yields have almost no relation to either actual yield or biologic potency.

An additional concern is the wide variety of flavoring and other additives that have been used to compensate for the decline in tobacco content. These additives are considered trade secrets and may be added to the cigarette without informing the public of their presence and without any review for toxic effects. These additives represent a major gap in the understanding of the disease risks associated with smoking the modern cigarette.

PEPTIC ULCER DISEASE

Cigarette smokers have a greater incidence of gastric and duodenal ulcers and delayed healing of these ulcers. Smoking also relaxes the esophageal sphincter and may contribute to esophageal reflux.

DRUG METABOLISM AND DIAGNOSTIC TESTS

Several of the constituents of tobacco smoke are capable of inducing hepatic microsomal systems, which then alter the metabolism of other drugs. Theophylline, phenacetin, antipyrine, caffeine, and imipramine are metabolized more rapidly by smokers, and adjustment in the dosage may be required with cessation. Smokers have lower blood levels of vitamins C and B_{12}. Hematocrit and hemoglobin levels, as well as carboxyhemoglobin levels, are elevated in smokers; and smoking is one cause of an elevated red cell volume. Smokers also have small alterations in the other diagnostic tests, including a higher leukocyte count, but these differences are not usually clinically significant for an individual patient.

PIPE AND CIGAR SMOKING

Pipe and cigar smokers who have never smoked cigarettes have a lower risk of cardiovascular disease, lung cancer, and chronic airflow obstruction than do cigarette smokers. They have similar risks of cancer of the upper respiratory tract. These differences are due to the tendency of pipe and cigar smokers not to inhale the more irritating smoke of these forms of tobacco. Cigarette smokers who switch to pipes and cigars do tend to inhale, however, and so it is not clear that switching to a pipe or cigars results in a lowering of the risks for the cigarette smoker.

SMOKELESS TOBACCO USE

The re-emergence of oral snuff use among male adolescents in the last several years has generated substantial public health concern. Smokeless tobacco use can cause cancer of the cheek and gum and gingival recession. It may also increase the risk of other oral cancers, and regular use of snuff can lead to nicotine addiction.

SMOKING BEHAVIOR AND CESSATION

The initiation of regular cigarette smoking occurs almost exclusively during adolescence and early adulthood. The availability of cigarettes and a variety of peer pressures and needs to model adult behavior lead to developing regular smoking behavior, particularly in those adolescents with limited social and academic success. The maintenance of smoking behavior in the adult is conditioned by other factors. The cigarette is used for nonverbal communication, for accentuation of positive feelings, for the reduction of negative feelings, and for coping with stress. An individual may use cigarettes sometimes for stimulation and sometimes for sedation. The result is a pattern of use that builds the cigarette into the way the smoker learns to deal with the world, and the cessation of smoking requires the smoker to give up a major coping mechanism.

Cigarette smoking fulfills all the criteria for an addiction, including a defined withdrawal syndrome. Nicotine almost certainly plays a role in the addictive process, but nicotine alone will not reverse the withdrawal syndrome. Nicotine probably provides a transient pharmacologic stimulus around which the human organism builds a series of psychologic or psychopharmacologic reflexes. These reflexes can be designed to meet the specific needs of an individual, thereby personalizing the cigarette habit. The psychologic and sociologic utility of the smoking behavior may vary qualitatively and quantitatively from individual to individual, and therefore it is not surprising that no single cessation technique will work for all individuals.

The physician can play an important role in cessation. Most smokers say that they would attempt to quit if told to do so by a physician; and, when told, up to one third will actually try to quit.

Successful intervention by the physician to alter smoking behavior requires the acceptance of smoking as a medical problem necessitating both treatment and follow-up. The initial intervention by the physician should consist of the following: asking about the patient's smoking status, reviewing the benefits of quitting, making a firm recommendation to quit, and negotiating an actual quitting date with the patient. Assistance in quitting should be provided through referral to local cessation programs or through provision of self-help materials. Prescription of nicotine gum increases the chances of successful cessation when used in conjunction with some other behavior intervention. Follow-up visits or phone calls also improve the success of cessation attempts, and follow-ups should be scheduled at two weeks after the quit date. Smokers should be encouraged to try to quit "cold turkey" rather than tapering down. A variety of rapid smoking techniques (rapidly smoking several cigarettes to produce adverse symptoms) have been shown to improve cessation rates. Effective intervention by the physician can be delivered in 3 to 5 minutes with 1 to 2 follow-up contacts.

A variety of organizations provide cessation assistance, both in groups and with individual or self-help programs, and these organizations can be located in the telephone directory or by contacting the local heart, lung, or cancer societies.

American Heart Association: Report of the ad hoc committee on cigarette smoking and cardiovascular diseases. Circulation 57:404A, 1978. *A report of the combined experience of the major coronary heart disease incidence studies relating the presence of risk factors to risk of coronary heart disease.*

Fielding JE: Smoking: Health effects and control. N Engl J Med 313:491, 555, 1985. *An overall review of smoking issues.*

Health and Public Policy Committee, American College of Physicians: Methods for stopping cigarette smoking. Ann Intern Med 105:281, 1986. *A review of smoking cessation methods.*

U.S. Dept. of Health and Human Services: The Health Consequences of Smoking: The Changing Cigarette. DHHS Publication No. (PHS) 81–50156, 1981. *A detailed discussion of what is known about low-yield cigarettes and the problems associated with them.*

U.S. Dept. of Health and Human Services: The Health Consequences of Smoking: Cancer. DHHS Publication No. (PHS) 82–50179, 1982. *A review of the evidence on smoking and cancer from the perspective of causality.*

U.S. Dept. of Health and Human Services: The Health Consequences of Smoking: Cardiovascular Disease. DHHS Publication No. (PHS) 84–50204, 1983. *A review of the evidence on smoking and cardiovascular disease.*

U.S. Dept. of Health and Human Services: The Health Consequences of Smoking: Chronic Obstructive Lung Disease. DHHS Publication No. (PHS) 84–50205, 1984. *A review of the evidence on smoking and lung disease.*

U.S. Dept. of Health and Human Services: The Health Consequences of Smoking: Involuntary Smoking. DHHS Publication (CDC) 87-8398, 1986. *A review of the evidence of involuntary smoking.*

U.S. Dept. of Health and Human Services: The Health Consequences of Using Smokeless Tobacco. DHHS Publication No. (PHS) 86–2874, 1986. *A review of the health effects of using snuff.*

12 CONTROL OF UNINTENDED INJURIES AND THOSE DUE TO VIOLENCE

Stephen B. Hulley

Deaths from injury are the fourth most common cause of death in the United States; they number more than 150,000 each year and are the leading cause of death for young and middle-aged people in the age range 1 to 45. The problem is even larger if *nonfatal* injuries, some of which cause permanent disability, are considered: There are several hundred injury-related emergency room visits for every death from injury. One third of all deaths from injury are due to motor vehicles, one third result from other forms of unintended injury (falls are the most common, followed by drowning, fires, and poisoning), and the remaining third are due to violence (homicide and suicide).

Each of these causes of death and disability has risk factors that identify high-risk groups and that are susceptible to physician-mediated efforts to prevent occurrence or recurrence. Yet until recently, injury control has been largely ignored by the medical and public health establishment; it is the sleeping giant of preventive medicine.

THE EPIDEMIOLOGY OF UNINTENDED INJURIES

Motor vehicle fatalities decreased by one third in the 1970's after automobile safety regulations and the 55 mile per hour national speed limit were instituted, but most of the benefit has since been lost as average speeds have returned to higher levels and smaller cars (which have a twofold higher crash fatality rate) have become more prevalent. Deaths due to motor vehicles rise to alarmingly high levels among young adults, particularly males (Fig. 12–1). The impact of this is brought home by the current projection that 1.4 per cent of all 15-year-old boys in the United States will die of an injury before age 25. The most important modifiable risk factors are excessive alcohol intake, which plays a role in half of all fatal crashes, and the failure to observe speed limits and use seatbelts.

Half of all deaths from unintended injury are unrelated to traffic. Falls are the commonest cause (27 per cent of the 49,048 such deaths in 1980), followed by drowning (15 per cent), fire (12 per cent), poisoning (6 per cent), adverse effects of medical care (5 per cent), unintended firearm use (4 per cent), aspiration of food (4 per cent), airplane crashes (3 per cent), machinery accidents (3 per cent), aspiration other than food (3 per cent), electric current (2 per cent), and other less common causes. These deaths tend to have a common pattern of risk factors, including male sex, old age, low income, and alcohol intake.

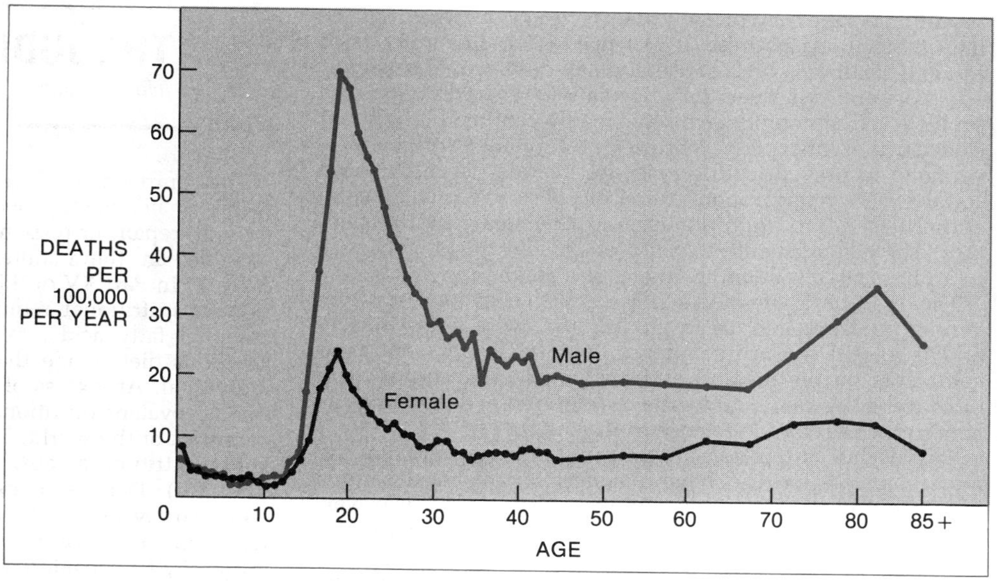

FIGURE 12–1. Age-specific death rates of motor vehicle occupants in the United States in 1976. The very high rates in 16- to 30-year-old males are a major component of the premature loss of life in this country. (From Haddon W, Baker SP: Injury control. In Clark D, MacMahon B [eds.]: Preventive and Community Medicine. Boston, Little Brown & Co, 1981, pp 109–140.)

Implications for Medical Practice

Injury prevention has assumed an important role in the practice of medicine only in the field of pediatrics. Perhaps it has not received more attention in internal medicine because the term "accident" connotes an event that has occurred by chance and is therefore unavoidable. This is far from the case; there are many lifestyle risk factors for injuries that are suitable for intervention with various behavioral techniques. (For this reason, the term "unintended injury" is now preferred over "accident," and the term "motor vehicle crash" over "motor vehicle accident.") The potential for preventing premature death and disability is substantial, and injury prevention advice could become as important in the general practice of medicine as the more familiar interventions on risk factors for cardiovascular disease and cancer.

Advice on preventing *motor vehicle injuries* begins with widely known precepts such as observing the speed limit and using a diagonal-lap or other well-designed seatbelt. From the medical viewpoint, patients should be warned when drugs that impair performance are prescribed, especially those like diazepam that may interact with alcohol. But the most important concern is alcohol itself. The knowledge that a particular patient drinks heavily should prompt a clinician to point out the danger to that individual and to others. Intervention can include counseling on ways to alter alcohol habits and on the use of other drivers, alternative forms of transportation, or different locations for drinking. The alarming motor vehicle crash rate among teenagers can be approached by counseling parents on the rules that they can establish for when and how their teenage children may drive (e.g., curfews for use of the family car). Society plays an important role in these areas—for example, in setting the penalties for drunken driving and for the minimum age for licensing—and physicians can be an important force behind social legislation of this sort.

Injuries due to *falls* in the elderly can be prevented by designing an environment that makes falls less likely (e.g., by providing handrails and night lights and by removing loose rugs) and that reduces the extent of injury should a fall occur (e.g., through avoiding sharp corners and selecting a home without stairs). The clinician should undertake regular tests and appropriate correction of problems with vision and should identify and treat diseases that impair mobility and balance, advising against heavy alcohol use and avoiding drugs that contribute to these problems. Hip fracture has received less attention than it deserves (there are more than 200,000 each year, involving one of every three women who reach extreme old age, and half of these die or are permanently disabled). White women are at the greatest risk and should receive treatment to retard osteoporosis (Ch. 250). This may include postmenopausal estrogens for some and should always include advice about calcium intake (1000 to 1500 mg per day in the diet or as calcium carbonate supplements), about not smoking (cigarettes are a risk factor for hip fracture), and about being physically active.

Many of the other causes of unintentional injury can be controlled by discussing the role of excess alcohol and other specific risk factors with patients. *Drowning*, for example, can be made less likely by placing barriers between small children and all bodies of water and by instruction in water safety rules. Injury due to *fires* can be reduced by counseling on the dangers of smoking (cigarettes are the commonest cause of fire-related deaths) and on the value of smoke detectors and fire extinguishers.

THE EPIDEMIOLOGY OF INJURY DUE TO VIOLENCE

The homicide rate in the United States has doubled in recent years and now exceeds 20,000 per year. One third of all homicides are between family members, and another third involve people who know each other. In the United States, more than half of all homicides are carried out with handguns. Countries like England, Sweden, and Japan that have strict handgun ownership laws have handgun homicide rates that are 100-fold lower; these countries also have lower overall rates of homicide. It is difficult to estimate the rates of nonfatal injury due to violence (assault, wife beating, rape, and child abuse), but each is undoubtedly far more common than homicide. Suicide rates have increased slightly in recent years, particularly in young men. Almost all forms of violent injury are more common in the male sex and in the socioeconomically disadvantaged, and all are commonly associated with excessive alcohol intake.

Implications for Medical Practice

The medical profession's role in dealing with the death and disability that result from violent behavior begins at an individual level. One focus is on preventing the occurrence (primary prevention) or recurrence (secondary prevention) of violent episodes, and the other is on providing medical, psychiatric, and social service care for the victims. Victims of assault and rape may present themselves for treatment of the injury, but those involved in violence within the family, such as wife beating, child abuse, or self-destructive behavior, often do not volunteer the information. The existence of a problem can sometimes be discovered by gentle probing about clues such as unexplained bruises or depressed affect. Interventions to prevent future episodes include psychiatric and social service referral, notification of police and public health authorities (when appropriate), and counseling by the clinician. The management of such problems is a major challenge to a physician's wisdom, courage, and skill.

The medical profession's most effective avenue for preventing violence may be in guiding the evolution of society and its rules. Doctors are important opinion leaders, and their comments on the medical and epidemiologic facts can help mold public opinion and legislation directed at such things as handgun control and violence in the media.

Approaches of this sort are probably the only way that the medical profession can have an effect on the most serious injury control issue of our age: the prevention of nuclear war. In addition to their general civic responsibility to express their views on this problem, some physicians regard it as a professional responsibility to educate community leaders and acquaintances on medical realities such as the false security of civil defense plans that would be inoperable in the event of a nuclear attack.

SUMMARY

Injuries are the most important cause of premature death and disability in western countries. One third of all deaths from injury are due to motor vehicle crashes, one third to other unintended causes (especially falls), and one third to intentional violence. Interventions designed to prevent each of these sources of injury are a useful and neglected focus for preventive medicine.

Physicians can play a major role in counseling individual patients about lifestyle factors that prevent motor vehicle crash injuries (e.g., avoiding alcohol in excess, using seatbelts, and setting curfews for teenage drivers) and about those that prevent other forms of unintended injuries (e.g., avoiding alcohol in excess and various medical and environmental strategies to prevent falls and osteoporosis). Physicians need to take a greater role in the primary and secondary prevention of injury due to violence. In addition, medical professionals can contribute to the emergence of societal measures dealing with hazards to health that range from drunken driving to nuclear war.

Baker SP, O'Neill B, Karpf RS: The Injury Fact Book. Lexington, Mass., D. C. Heath & Company, 1984. *A fascinating and readable book that comprehensively describes the epidemiology of injury: who is especially at risk and what are the potentially modifiable risk factors.*

Cassel C, McCally M, Abraham H: Nuclear Weapons and Nuclear War: A Source Book for Health Professionals. New York, Praeger Publishers, 1984. *Reports on the medical, biologic, psychologic, and ethical implications by many of the major medical writers on this topic.*

Institute of Medicine: Injury in America. Washington, D. C., National Academy Press, 1985. *The research agenda in the area of injury prevention and control.*

Perry BC: Falls among the elderly: A review of the methods and conclusions of epidemiologic studies. J Am Geriatr Soc 30:367, 1982. *Risk factors and prevention of falls in the elderly.*

Riggs BL, Melton LJ: Involutional osteoporosis. N Engl J Med 314:1676, 1986. *Good review of strategies for preventing osteoporosis.*

Robertson LS: Injuries: Causes, Control Strategies and Public Policy. Lexington, Mass., D. C. Heath & Company, 1983. *Thoughtful discussion of injury control strategies and policy implications.*

Trunkey DD: Trauma. Sci Am 249:28, 1983. *A surgeon's perspective on the epidemiology, prevention, and treatment of injuries.*

13 THE JUDICIOUS DIET

John P. Kane

The composition of an individual's diet and its relationship to his or her energy needs and to special requirements for growth, repair, or response to stress are among the important variables in the maintenance of health or the advent of disease. In Part XV of this book, there is an extensive discussion of nutritional requirements for calories, amino acids, essential fatty acids, minerals, and vitamins. Obviously, a judicious diet is one that meets these requirements for the individual. An excess of calories leads to obesity, one of the most prevalent nutritional disorders found in the developed countries of the world. This is discussed in detail in Ch. 216. Undernutrition can also produce serious impairment of health (Ch. 214). Deficits or excesses of other nutrients lead to a wide variety of specific disorders. In this chapter, however, we shall be concerned with variables within what would ordinarily be considered an adequate diet but that may influence the susceptibility of the individual to four major classes of disease: atherosclerosis, hypertension, cancer, and urolithiasis.

In few areas relevant to health is there so much misinformation and faddism as in the prevailing public arena concerning diets. Billions of dollars are spent in this major national industry to promote an astonishing variety of nostrums and dietary aberrations alleged to maintain holistic health, vitality, and attractiveness, or to reverse the process of disease. By and large, these programs are ingenious but harmless instruments to defraud the credulous. In some cases, however, they either produce harmful dietary abnormalities or delay the patient's seeking effective medical care. Physicians need to be informed about the dimensions of this cultism in order to be able to advise their patients and to participate effectively in the development of controlling public policy.

DIET AND ARTERIOSCLEROSIS

Lipids, primarily free and esterified cholesterol, constitute a major part of atherosclerotic plaques. In current models of atherogenesis, lipids enter the artery wall via plasma lipoproteins. These lipoproteins include low density lipoproteins (LDL), intermediate density lipoproteins (IDL), and, perhaps to a lesser extent, very low density lipoproteins (VLDL). More extensive descriptions of these lipoproteins and of their metabolism are given in Ch. 183. Elevated levels of LDL and IDL are strongly associated epidemiologically with accelerated atherogenesis. For instance, the risk of coronary heart disease in the United States, where the average level of serum cholesterol in an adult male is approximately 230 mg per deciliter, is several-fold higher than in rural Japan, where the average is about 160 mg per deciliter. The atherogenicity of VLDL appears to depend in part on qualitative properties of these lipoproteins. The finding of impaired acceptance of cholesteryl esters by VLDL of hypertriglyceridemic patients with arteriosclerosis suggests that the atherogenic effect may be exerted primarily via impaired retrieval of cholesterol from peripheral sites. An inverse relationship between plasma levels of high density lipoprotein (HDL) cholesterol and risk of coronary heart disease has been noted in a number of epidemiologic surveys, suggesting that total HDL levels may reflect the efficiency of mechanisms involved in the centripetal (retrieval) pathways of cholesterol transport.

The risk of coronary heart disease has been shown to correlate with levels of cholesterol in plasma as low as 180 mg per deciliter. The majority of individuals in industrialized western nations would therefore be expected to benefit from reduction of levels of serum cholesterol, reflecting primarily changes in the content of LDL in plasma. The results of several intervention studies tend to support this contention. Increasing the levels of HDL in plasma in order to increase the mobilization and retrieval of cholesterol might be equally attractive, but no studies of the effect of such an intervention on heart disease have yet appeared.

A single pattern of dietary modification is appropriate for individuals with nearly all types of primary hyperlipidemia (excepting only primary chylomicronemia), as well as for those individuals in the population at large who have less striking elevations of levels of atherogenic lipoproteins. The elements of this "universal" diet will be considered individually.

1. *Reduce body weight to the ideal.* This manipulation primarily induces a marked reduction in elevated VLDL levels. It also effects some reduction in LDL cholesterol levels and may increase HDL cholesterol levels slightly. Maintenance of ideal body weight is the most effective means of forestalling the appearance of type II diabetes, itself a risk factor for atherosclerosis.

2. *Decrease the intake of saturated fat.* This change effects a potent and uniform lowering of LDL cholesterol. The typical American diet contains approximately 40 per cent or more of calories as fat (15 per cent saturated fat). Levels of 30 per cent of calories as fat (8 per cent saturated fat) can be achieved easily, and 20 per cent (5 per cent saturated) is attainable with major modifications of food selection. To achieve the 30 per cent level of dietary fat, fat-rich meats, dairy products, and items such as certain baked goods must be restricted. To achieve the 20 per cent level, major substitution of vegetable protein sources for meats must be made.

When the intake of saturated fats is decreased, there are several possible sources of replacement calories: polyunsaturated fats, monounsaturated fats, or carbohydrates. Major substitution with polyunsaturated fat may result in lower levels of HDL cholesterol and of the principal HDL protein, apolipoprotein A-I. Furthermore, polyunsaturated fatty acids are susceptible to hydroperoxidation, which could lead to generation of free radical chains and perhaps to carcinogenesis. Monounsaturated fats, abundant in certain vegetable oils such as olive oil, do not increase LDL levels and do not hydroperoxidize readily. HDL cholesterol levels are somewhat higher with use of monounsaturates than with diets that are low in total fat. Major substitution of carbohydrate for fat is associated with modest elevations of plasma triglyceride levels in the short term, but these levels return to normal after a period of several months. Strict vegetarians tend to have lower levels of both LDL and HDL than individuals on a typical American diet, but the changes in LDL levels are of much greater magnitude. Furthermore, potentially important differences in composition of HDL are seen, with an increased ratio of phospholipid to cholesterol.

Recently, attention has been drawn to certain features of omega-3 fatty acids, principally eicosapentaenoic and docosahexaenoic acids, contained in marine fish oils. These fatty acids appear to have a unique ability to reduce elevated levels of VLDL and chylomicrons in plasma at doses of 15 to 20 grams per day. Plasma levels of LDL may be decreased modestly in individuals with normal or moderately elevated levels of plasma cholesterol, accompanied by some decrease in HDL cholesterol levels. The marked decreases in plasma triglycerides that occur are due at least in part to inhibition of VLDL secretion. Omega-3 fatty acids moderately reduce formation of thromboxane B_2 in platelets, inhibiting their aggregation and adhesion, an effect that may account in part for the low incidence of arteriosclerotic heart disease in populations for whom temperate and subarctic marine fish are a major food source.

Overall, a major reduction of saturated fat should be made from levels found in Western diets, and carbohydrate should be used in large part to provide the requisite caloric replacement. Small amounts of polyunsaturated fats from plant sources should be used to provide essential fatty acids. The use of fish oils might be considered if hypertriglyceridemia is present.

3. *Decrease the intake of cholesterol.* Reduction of dietary saturated fats automatically eliminates much cholesterol; however, rich sources such as organ meats and egg yolks should be restricted specifically. The effect of restriction of cholesterol on LDL levels varies widely among individuals. This variation appears to reflect two factors: (a) There is an approximately four-fold difference among individuals in the fraction of dietary cholesterol that is absorbed. (b) There are differences in the degree to which dietary cholesterol is capable of suppressing endogenous cholesterogenesis. Lacking metabolic ward studies on a given patient, it must be presumed that reduction of dietary cholesterol is likely to be of benefit. The typical American diet provides 500 mg or more of cholesterol per day, but an intake of 250 to 300 mg per day is relatively easily achieved, and intakes of 100 mg per day can be achieved with more rigorous mixed diets. Strict vegetarian diets contain no cholesterol.

4. *Restrict alcohol.* Alcohol should be limited in all cases to maintain ideal body weight. VLDL secretion is increased dramatically by even limited use of alcohol. Therefore, alcohol should always be restricted in the diet of individuals with elevated serum triglycerides. Increased alcohol intake may be associated with elevated levels of HDL cholesterol, but it is not yet clear whether this change represents subspecies of HDL that participate in centripetal cholesterol transport. No categorical presumption of beneficial effects of alcohol on HDL can yet be made.

5. *Other factors.* Increased dietary fiber appears to have marginal effect on serum lipoprotein levels, though certain sources of fiber, such as oat or wheat bran, appear to reduce LDL levels slightly. In addition, saponins in foodstuffs such as oats may decrease absorption of cholesterol. The ingestion of lecithin, which is widely suggested by health food advocates, also lacks significant effect, as do a number of vitamins and minerals that have been similarly recommended.

Individuals following this judicious dietary regimen usually show reductions of 10 to 15 per cent of plasma cholesterol levels on the basis of reduction of saturated fats. An additional reduction of up to 10 per cent may be achieved by restriction of cholesterol. Based on large epidemiologic studies, it can be roughly estimated that at least a twofold reduction in risk of coronary disease would be expected in the American population if such modifications of lipid levels were uniformly achieved.

DIET AND HYPERTENSION

Essential hypertension has been assumed to result from a constitutional inability to excrete sodium chloride efficiently, because of which calcium ions accumulate in arteriolar smooth muscle cells, increasing their tonicity. Indeed, evidence from cross-transplantation studies in animals and from human renal transplants lends credence to the existence of such a mechanism. Cross-cultural studies also have shown, in the aggregate, convincing positive correlation between blood pressure and intake of salt. More recently, patient populations with essential hypertension have been found to be heterogeneous with respect to renin levels, plasma calcium concentrations, response to individual antihypertensive drugs, and sensitivity to dietary salt. Normotensive individuals and perhaps half of American patients with hypertension do not show a pressor response to increased dietary salt. Thus, justification for the prescription of reduced salt intake appears to be limited to individuals with salt-sensitive hypertension and members of their kindreds. Most Americans consume 10 to 20 grams of salt per day; an intake of 4 grams is a more reasonable goal for individuals in such kindreds. It has been reported, without convincing evidence, that increasing calcium intake can reduce blood pressure. If true, this effect would probably be restricted to a subset of patients. Furthermore, indiscriminate increase in calcium intake could result in augmentation of urinary calcium excretion in individuals with absorptive hypercalciuria (Ch. 90). Thus, no basis yet exists for the general recommendation of increased calcium intake for the prevention of hypertension.

DIET AND CANCER

The consumption of certain major food components is epidemiologically correlated with an increased incidence of some types of cancer. Although the mechanisms of these associations are still largely unknown, a judicious diet at this time involves changes that would be expected to minimize these risks. A number of components that occur in foods naturally or are formed or added during processing are recognized as mutagens in bacterial test systems (Ames test) or as carcinogens or promoters of carcinogenesis in tests in whole animals. Prudence would dictate elimination of these compounds from human consumption to whatever extent is practicable, because definitive studies demonstrating specific risks of these agents in humans may emerge only slowly.

DIETARY FAT. An increased incidence of cancer of the breast, colon, and prostate is epidemiologically related to a high consumption of total fat. Enhancement of chemical carcinogenesis by dietary fat has also been demonstrated in several animal models. Total fat intake correlates best with carcinogenesis at high levels, but polyunsaturated fats appear to be most important at lower levels of intake. Polyunsaturated fats are substrates for hydroperoxidative reactions initiating free radical chains, and therefore they probably should not constitute a major component of the diet. Reduction of total fat intake, with an increased content of complex carbohydrates, is completely compatible with the "prudent" diet for prevention of arteriosclerotic heart disease. In fact, in multination comparisons coronary heart disease and cancer of the breast show a strong correlation.

FIBER. Carcinogens formed in the bowel may play a major role in development of carcinoma of the colon. It has been suggested that increased fiber in the diet, which would decrease the duration of contact of carcinogens with the mucosa, might reduce the risk of cancer. Only minimal epidemiologic support for this view has been forthcoming, and with the possible exception of pentosans from wheat, fiber has not been proven effective in animal models.

ALCOHOL. Alcohol consumption has been found to correlate with risk of carcinoma of the mouth, pharynx, and esophagus. It also appears to be teratogenic in humans and causes congenital malformations, mental dysfunction, and growth retardation in infants born to alcohol-abusing mothers. Alcohol metabolism produces acetaldehyde, which is both mutagenic and carcinogenic, in addition to other mutagenic and carcinogenic compounds.

RELATIONSHIP OF CANCER RISK TO LOW LEVELS OF CHOLESTEROL IN PLASMA. An increased risk of cancer has been associated epidemiologically with very low levels of serum cholesterol. Such an association when present is always weak and tends to be present only in the lowest range of cholesterol levels. Further, in nearly 20 prospective population studies, half have shown no such correlation, especially in those in which sufficient time elapsed between measurement of serum lipids and detection of cancer to minimize the number of pre-existing cancer cases. Furthermore, the risk of colon and rectal cancer is positively correlated with serum cholesterol levels. The correlation of higher levels of cholesterol in plasma with risk of coronary disease is very strong. Thus it appears that dietary modifications directed at lowering the risk of coronary disease should not be abandoned on the premise that a significant increase in the risk of cancer would ensue.

FOOD PREPARATION AND PRESERVATION. Exposure of meats to high temperatures, as in charcoal broiling, may be of importance in oncogenesis because of the formation of compounds with very high carcinogenic potential. In addition to benzo(a)pyrene, several mutagenic pyrolysates formed from amino acids are recognized. Considerable evidence both from epidemiology and from animal studies has linked components of wood smoke in smoked foods to carcinoma of the gastrointestinal tract. Nitrites, used as preservatives in meats, react with a number of natural amines and even certain medications to form nitrosamines, which are mutagenic. This reaction is favored by low pH; hence it proceeds readily in the stomach. Mutagenesis by nitrosamines is readily demonstrated, and clinical observations tend to link nitrites with carcinogenesis of the stomach and esophagus, at least. Vitamin C inhibits the formation of nitrosamines in vitro. Increased intake of this vitamin by the public may account in part for decreases in the incidence of gastric carcinoma observed in recent years. At the present state of our knowledge, restriction of nitrites and nitrosamines in the diet would appear reasonable. This is complicated by the presence of large amounts of nitrates, which can be reduced to nitrites, in certain vegetables that have been overfertilized by growers. The average American ingests about 75 mg of nitrate, 0.8 mg nitrite, and 1 μg of preformed nitrosamines daily.

NATURALLY OCCURRING CARCINOGENS AND MUTAGENS. Several species of *Aspergillus* molds produce aflatoxins, which are among the most potent natural carcinogens. These agents are carcinogenic in a number of animals, chiefly causing carcinoma of the liver. Induction of tumors of colon, lung, and kidney has also been observed. Aflatoxins have been linked strongly to hepatocellular carcinoma in humans in Africa and Asia, probably acting in concert with hepatitis B virus. Aflatoxins have been found chiefly in peanuts, apple products, and grains stored under moist conditions. Efforts to reduce the intake of these agents center on proper storage of foods. Emerging awareness of other naturally occurring mutagens and carcinogens may be expected to lead to an evaluation of their importance in human carcinogenesis. Among these agents are allyl isothiocyanate and the flavonoids quercetin and kaempferol found in many plant sources; hydrazine derivatives found in many mushrooms; safrol of sassafras; the methyl xanthines of coffee, tea, and cocoa; and phorbol esters and pyrrolizidine alkaloids found in herbal teas.

NATURAL INHIBITORS OF CARCINOGENESIS. Some naturally occurring compounds appear to inhibit carcinogenesis by certain agents. Tocopherols, which interrupt free radical chains, are capable of reducing the carcinogenicity of doxorubicin (Adriamycin) and daunomycin and are protective against oxygen radical damage to tissues. Certain indoles found in cruciferous vegetables (broccoli, cabbage, cauliflower, etc.) inhibit the carcinogenicity of benzo(a)pyrene, and substituted isothiocyanates found in these plants inhibit the carcinogenesis induced by polycyclic aromatic hydrocarbons. Higher intakes of retinol and beta-carotene have been correlated with reduced risk of cancer in several studies. This effect should be considered unproven, however, until further evidence is brought forth. Selenium, a cofactor in the reduction of hydroperoxides, also may confer resistance to free radical–mediated carcinogenesis.

DIET AND UROLITHIASIS

Certain general measures that should reduce the risk of urolithiasis are applicable to the general population (also see Ch. 90). Sufficient intake of water to ensure a daily urine volume of 2 to 3 liters is a most important preventive measure and is useful in all forms of urolithiasis. Restriction of dietary purine intake is also desirable because uricosuria can enhance the crystallization of calcium oxalate as well as uric acid stones. Restriction of the intake of red meats, recommended for reduction of saturated fat intake, also tends to reduce the "acid ash" residue of urine, diminishing the urinary excretion of calcium.

Moderate restriction of oxalate intake would appear reasonable in the general population in view of the prevalence of oxalate stones. More stringently reduced intake should be advised for individuals who have had one or more oxalate stones, because the incidence of recurrence tends to be high. The oxalate content is particularly high in rhubarb, spinach, chard, beets, citrus pulp, pecans, peanuts, sweet potatoes, and a number of berries and fruits. Reliable new methods for the determination of oxalate in foods have now led to the availability of lists of oxalate-rich foods for use by the patient. Because calcium in the intestine inhibits the absorption of oxalate, moderate intake of calcium, distributed throughout the day, is probably indicated in the prevention of oxalate urolithiasis. Citrate appears to inhibit the crystallization of calcium with oxalate. Some patients with calcium oxalate urolithiasis have low levels of citrate in urine. Regular intake of citrate-rich, pulp-free fruit juices appears to be a reasonable intervention. In general, restriction of dietary calcium should be limited to patients with hypercalciuria.

SUMMARY

Epidemiologic and experimental data are sufficient to support the following recommendations for dietary modifications among the general populace. Caloric intake should be adjusted to achieve and maintain ideal body weight. Fat intake should be reduced to 30 per cent of total calories (8 per cent as saturated fat) or less, and cholesterol intake to 150 mg, or less, per day. Even moderate use of alcohol should be avoided in individuals with hypertriglyceridemia. Complex carbohydrates should be used to make up the caloric deficits resulting from these changes. Individuals with a predisposition to hypertension should limit salt intake to 4 grams per day. Prudence would also suggest reasonable limitation of charcoal-broiled and smoked foods and foods rich in nitrites or nitrates.

Ames BN: Dietary carcinogens and anticarcinogens: Oxygen radicals and degenerative diseases. Science 221:1256, 1983. *A comprehensive review of mutagens and carcinogens in the diet.*

Ames BN: Food constituents as a source of mutagens, carcinogens, and anticarcinogens. In Knudsen I (ed.): Genetic Toxicology of the Diet. New York, Alan R. Liss, Inc, 1986, pp 3–32. *A discussion of mechanisms by which food constituents can promote or retard the formation of tumors.*

Committee on Diet, Nutrition, and Cancer. Assembly of Life Sciences, National Research Council: Diet, Nutrition and Cancer. National Academic Press, 1982. *A comprehensive evaluation of the roles of dietary components and additives in carcinogenesis.*

Connor WE, Connor SL: The dietary prevention and treatment of coronary heart disease. In Connor WE, Bristow JD (eds.): Coronary Heart Disease: Prevention, Complications, and Treatment. Philadelphia, J. B. Lippincott, 1985, pp 43–64. *A review of principles and practical measures in modification of plasma lipoprotein levels by diet.*

Havel RJ: Dietary regulation of plasma lipoprotein metabolism in humans. Prog Biochem Pharmacol 19:110, 1983. *A discussion of mechanisms underlying dietary effects on lipoproteins.*

MacGregor GA: Sodium is more important than calcium in essential hypertension. Hypertension 7:628, 1985. *A discussion putting forth arguments for the role of salt in hypertension.*

Menkes MS, Comstock GW, Vuilleumier JP, et al.: Serum beta-carotene, vitamins A and E, selenium, and the risk of lung cancer. N Engl J Med 315:1250, 1986. *Epidemiologic evidence relating beta-carotene and vitamin E to a reduced risk of lung cancer.*

Törnberg SA, Holm L-E, Carstensen JM, et al.: Risks of cancer of the colon and rectum in relation to serum cholesterol and beta-lipoprotein. N Engl J Med 315:1629, 1986. *A clinical study demonstrating a positive correlation of serum cholesterol level and risk of cancer in the lower bowel and rectum.*

Willett WC, Stampfer MJ, Colditz GA, et al.: Dietary fat and the risk of breast cancer. N Engl J Med 316:22, 1987. *An important study that confirms high dietary fat as a risk factor, with a useful bibliography of 37 references.*

14 EXERCISE AND HEALTH

William L. Haskell

The biologic and psychologic benefits ascribed to exercise are extremely diverse and vary substantially with regard to scientific documentation of a causal relationship. Some of these benefits have been definitively established and are achievable by anyone who exercises appropriately. Other benefits, frequently promoted by exercise advocates, usually do not occur, and at times inappropriate advice has been given that has placed patients at undue risk for exercise-caused morbidity or mortality. As with many other areas of health promotion, enthusiasm to help others by encouraging them to exercise can easily outstrip the scientific basis for such actions. While the idea that exercise might promote health is not new, many of the details regarding specific health benefits and exercise requirements are still much debated and under investigation.

EXERCISE AND PHYSICAL WORKING CAPACITY

The most effective method of achieving an increase in physical working capacity or "physical fitness" is through a systematic increase in habitual exercise (exercise training). This increase in capacity is an adaptative response by the body to the stress placed on various tissues and biologic functions by the increased metabolic or physical demands of the exercise. If the appropriate type of exercise is performed at the proper intensity, duration, and frequency, sedentary individuals of all ages will achieve significant improvements in physical working capacity. After training, they will be able to exercise at a greater intensity and for a longer duration than before. Also, at the same submaximal exercise intensity they will experience less fatigue. This increase in functional capacity is due to enhanced metabolic capacity of skeletal muscle, increased capacity for substrate and oxygen delivery to the muscle, and changes in autonomic nervous system regulation during exercise.

Increases in physical working capacity often are equated inappropriately with improvements in health status or disease prevention. This is an important and often difficult distinction to make: that while a very high level of physical fitness usually requires good health, an improvement in fitness does not ensure an increase in resistance to disease or a reduction in clinical manifestations. For example, patients with disorders such as emphysema, diabetes, or hypertension can significantly increase their working capacity through exercise without necessarily changing the severity of their disease or their medical prognosis. Becoming more physically fit and improving health status are interrelated but not synonymous.

HEALTH BENEFITS OF EXERCISE

Most of the health-related benefits of exercise appear to result from the increase in metabolism required to provide the energy needed for skeletal muscle contraction. This increase in demand for energy triggers a number of adaptations designed to enhance the efficiency and capacity of the skeletal muscle to perform work and minimize fatigue. Adaptations also occur in those systems that support the increased energy requirements of skeletal muscle, including the nervous, endocrine, cardiovascular, respiratory, and skeletal systems.

CORONARY HEART DISEASE. The area of greatest scientific inquiry regarding the health benefits of exercise has been its potential role in the prevention of coronary heart disease (CHD). In 1952 J. H. Morris and colleagues published data demonstrating that the conductors on double-decker buses in London developed fewer manifestations of CHD than did the less active bus drivers. Since then it has been repeatedly, but not exclusively, demonstrated that men and women who select more active jobs or leisure-time pursuits tend to experience fewer fatal and nonfatal CHD events. While these studies do not demonstrate a cause and effect relationship, the direction of the association is positive and quite consistent, the magnitude of the differences in CHD events is clinically meaningful, and the amount of exercise performed during leisure time associated with lower CHD risk is well within the capacity of most clinically healthy adults. As of yet no randomized trial of adequate design has been performed to determine if an increase in exercise by sedentary adults free of clinically evident CHD on entry into the study would significantly reduce future CHD events.

The six controlled clinical trials so far conducted to evaluate the effects of exercise training on recurrent cardiac events in patients following myocardial infarction have yielded statistically negative results. In three of these six studies, the exercise group tended to have fewer events ($0.05 < p < 0.10$), and in all of the studies the adherence to exercise training was sufficiently poor to raise questions regarding their adequacy as a test of the exercise hypothesis. Thus, no definitive evidence exists to substantiate that an *increase in exercise* will reduce either the primary or the secondary occurrence of CHD clinical events.

There are several mechanisms by which exercise could act to reduce CHD risk. Exercise might maintain or increase oxygen supply to the myocardium by decreasing the progression of atherosclerosis, increasing coronary collateralization, or enlarging the diameter of proximal coronary arteries. Only preliminary evidence has been published documenting that any of these changes occur in humans. Several studies have demonstrated potentially beneficial blood clotting-fibrinolysis activity and altered plasma lipoprotein profiles following training. These changes might improve the coronary blood flow in some individuals.

In contrast to very little evidence for any exercise-induced increase in myocardial oxygen supply, there is unequivocal evidence that endurance exercise training decreases myocardial oxygen demand. This decrease in demand is achieved primarily by a decrease in heart rate at rest and decreases in heart rate and systolic blood pressure during submaximal exercise. These changes are most likely produced by a modification in central nervous system regulation of cardiovascular function (decreased sympathetic and increased parasympathetic drive) and an increase in blood volume, with little, if any, change occurring in intrinsic myocardial function.

CARBOHYDRATE METABOLISM. A potentially important and often unrecognized health benefit of exercise is its effect on carbohydrate metabolism. During large-muscle, dynamic exercise of moderate intensity, the glycogen stored in skeletal muscle is used for the production of energy and becomes partially depleted. For the next 24 to 72 hours this glycogen is replaced by the uptake of glucose from the blood. In addition to this acute effect of increased glucose removal, there also is a more chronic training effect that increases the sensitivity of insulin receptors in skeletal muscle and adipose tissue and thus the rate of glucose removal at any given level of plasma insulin. This "insulin-sparing" effect of endurance exercise training probably decreases long-term insulin production and may reduce the risk of insulin deficiency developing with increasing age.

OSTEOPOROSIS. The bone mineral loss that occurs with aging is accelerated by inactivity, especially bed rest. While exercise will not prevent all of this loss, it appears to provide some benefit. For example, in a survey of 59 postmenopausal women, level of habitual activity was one of the major determinants of bone mass as measured by computerized tomography scanning. In the more active women, arm and leg bone mass was greater after accounting for the effects of age, body weight, and calcium intake. Also, when 18 elderly women exercised 3 times per week for 30 minutes each session, an increase in bone mineral content was observed (2.3 per cent), while 12 women who remained sedentary during this time showed a decrease of 3.3 per cent ($p < 0.005$). These experiences support the use of exercise requiring the movement of body weight against gravity as part of a comprehensive program of osteoporosis prevention.

WEIGHT CONTROL. More physically active individuals tend to weigh less than their sedentary counterparts and at any given body weight have a greater muscle mass. Even though calorie consumption frequently goes up when sedentary people substantially increase their exercise, they usually experience some adipose tissue loss. In addition to the increase in calories expended during the exercise, there is some evidence that *resting metabolic rate* is increased for an extended period after exericse. *Basal metabolic rate* at any given body weight may also increase. For these reasons, exercise, along with proper nutrition, can improve health status by contributing to the maintenance of optimal body composition.

PSYCHOLOGIC STATUS. Many physically active people state that the major health benefit that keeps them exercising is their improved psychologic status. They report less anxiety and depression, more self-confidence, and an increased ability to cope with at-home and job-related stress. How frequently such benefits will occur when sedentary people take up exercise is not known, nor is there any understanding of how to design an exercise program to maximize the positive psychologic effects. Whether or not a biologic basis, rather than just a "situational basis," exists for improvements in psychologic status has not been established. Proposed explanations for a biologic basis are the decrease in circulating catecholamines produced by exercise training and the acute increase in beta-endorphins that occurs during and following vigorous exercise. Regardless of the mechanism, consideration should be given to getting sedentary people up and away from chronic stress-producing environments and having them participate in an exercise of their choice.

OTHER DISORDERS. There are a number of other situations in which patients with an established disease tend to show some clinical improvement if they exercise properly, but there is no good evidence that exercise prevents these disorders. Diseases included in this category are chronic obstructive lung disease (emphysema and bronchitis), mild or labile hypertension, and intermittent claudication. There are no data supporting the notion that exercise prevents any infectious disease. More active people have a greater morbidity and mortality from accidents than would be the case if they remained sedentary!

A Comment on Safety

When recommending exercise for health promotion, one does battle with the proverbial two-edged sword. Inappropriate exercise literally can pose dangers to limbs and life. The most commonly encountered problem is that of musculoskeletal discomfort or injury due to trauma or overuse. Of more severe consequence, but much less frequent, is the precipitation of a major cardiac event, usually ventricular fibrillation. However, the likelihood is remote that exercise will cause a cardiac arrest in individuals without underlying cardiac disease.

There are many other health risks of exercise, but these usually are limited to individuals with established disease (e.g., diabetes, asthma, or renal failure) or occur with very extended or competitive exercise. The most important of these risks is the development of severe heat injury (Ch. 541). The total prevention of these injuries cannot be achieved if adults are to increase their exercise, but the risks can be reduced by proper medical evaluation, individualized exercise recommendations, and improved public education.

MEDICAL EVALUATION

Guidelines vary regarding the type of medical evaluation recommended prior to initiating a health-oriented exercise program. Advice depends on the specific exercise plan to be undertaken, as well as the person's age and clinical status. For sedentary people who plan to undertake a low-level program such as walking, no special medical examination is recommended unless they currently are under treatment for cardiopulmonary, metabolic, or musculoskeletal disorders. Such patients should be evaluated by a physician prior to an increase in exercise. For persons under age 40 who are free of clinically evident cardiopulmonary, metabolic, or musculoskeletal disorders, no special medical evaluation is considered necessary if they also are free of major cardiopulmonary disease risk factors (hypertension, hypercholesterolemia, or cigarette smoking). For persons under age 40 with disease or increased cardiopulmonary risk, and for all people over age 40, it is recommended that they have a medical examination prior to beginning vigorous exercise. Although recommended, but not required, for clinically healthy persons, an electrocardiographic and blood pressure–monitored exercise tolerance test should be included in the medical evaluation of patients with cardiopulmonary, metabolic, or musculoskeletal disorders. Such tests should be symptom limited and monitored by a physician.

IMPLICATIONS FOR MEDICAL PRACTICE

The *type* of exercise that provides the greatest health benefits and permits the greatest increase in energy expenditure with the least fatigue consists of performing rhythmic contractions of large muscles to move the body over a distance or against gravity. Such exercise frequently is referred to as being endurance or "aerobic," since, if it is performed at an intensity that is moderate relative to the person's capacity, most of the resynthesis of high-energy compounds in the muscle is performed in the presence of oxygen. Included in this type of exercise is walking, hiking, jogging or running, cycling, cross-country skiing, swimming, active games and sports, selected calisthenics, and vigorous at-home or on-the-job chores. While very specific activities may be required when training for athletic competition, for health purposes any exercise of this type seems to be of benefit if performed frequently enough at the proper intensity (Table 14–1).

The exercise-induced changes that contribute to health are achieved when the exercise *intensity* is somewhat greater than that usually performed by the individual. This increase intensity or overload causes adaptations that allow the metabolic needs of the muscles during exercise to be more readily met. While exercise intensities that are even slightly greater than that usually performed will produce changes, the usual recommendation is that exercise for optimizing health should be performed at 50 to 75 per cent of the individual's oxygen transport (aerobic) capacity or at 60 to 85 per cent of maximum achievable heart rate during exercise. Using these guidelines, exercise training heart rates for individuals 30 years of age would range from 114 to 162 beats per minute, whereas at age 60 the range would be from 86 to 137 beats per minute. For most people this recommendation produces a substantial intensity overload, since they usually do not exercise at more than about 40 per cent of their aerobic capacity during everyday activities.

The exercise *duration* to be recommended will depend on the person's health or fitness goals and exercise capacity as well as on the type of exercise being performed. One interpretation of the data available on exercise and health is that

TABLE 14–1. THE EXERCISE PRESCRIPTION

Type of Exercise
Primarily aerobic
Stretching for flexibility
Resistance exercise for muscle tone
Intensity
Moderate relative to capacity (50%–75%)
Target heart rate = 60%–85% MHR
Maximum heart rate (MHR) = 220 − age
Duration
25–45 minutes per session
Target of 300 kilocalories per session
Frequency
Daily if intensity <65% MHR and duration <30 minutes
Every other day if intensity >65% and duration >30 minutes
Session
Warmup, 3 to 5 minutes
Conditioning, 15 to 40 minutes
Cool-down, 2 to 5 minutes
Progression
Use exercise log
Keep pulse in target range
Evaluate every 2–4 weeks or each visit
Warning Signs
Severe musculoskeletal pain
Claudication
Chest pressure/pain, discomfort
Unusual shortness of breath
Dizziness, nausea, vomiting

people who do even a little bit of exercise on a regular basis are better off than those who do almost nothing. A reasonable goal seems to be an energy expenditure over usual activities of approximately 300 kilocalories per session with a *frequency* of at least every other day. Most clinically healthy adults have the capacity to expend from 400 to 700 kilocalories per hour while performing activity of moderate intensity; thus they can expend 300 kilocalories in 25 to 45 minutes. Activities meeting this goal include walking or jogging 4 kilometers, cycling or swimming for 30 minutes, or playing several sets of singles tennis lasting for 45 minutes. While lower intensity exercise such as walking or gardening will not produce a large increase in exercise capacity, if performed for longer periods or more frequently, it seems to provide many of the health benefits derived from more vigorous exercise (e.g., facilitates weight control, bone mineral retention, etc.).

SUMMARY

Inactivity does not appear to be the sole cause of any major disease, but a physically active lifestyle improves general health status and retards many of the functional impairments that frequently occur with aging. Success in initiating and maintaining an exercise program is most likely to occur when it is individually designed and takes into account the person's goals, interests, skills, and exercise opportunities, as well as exercise capacity. Instructions should be given to set aside a time for exercise and to fill it with a variety of activities, rather than selecting a single activity as the sole basis for increasing exercise for health purposes. The exercise plan should be convenient to perform, fit within the general lifestyle of the individual, and be considered fun or at least enjoyable. Success at exercise is increased when the individual has acquired the *knowledge* of what is to be done and why, the *confidence* that success can be achieved, and the *patience* to wait for the benefits to accrue.

American College of Sports Medicine: Guidelines for Graded Exercise Testing and Exercise Prescription. 3rd ed. Philadelphia, Lea & Febiger, 1986. *Comprehensive guidelines for the exercise testing and training of healthy persons and patients.*

Paffenbarger RS, Hyde RT, Weng AL, et al: Physical activity, all-cause mortality, and longevity of college alumni. N Engl J Med 314:605, 1986. *Report of major study supporting the relationship between sedentary habits and increased mortality from chronic diseases, especially ischemic heart disease.*

Siscovick DS, Weiss NS, Fletcher RH, et al: The incidence of primary cardiac arrest during vigorous exercise. N Engl J Med 311:874, 1984. *Important conceptual study presenting data on both cardiovascular risk and benefits of vigorous exercise in the general population.*

Vranic M, Lavina H, Lickley A, et al: Exercise and stress in diabetes mellitus. In Davidson JK (ed.): Clinical Diabetes Mellitus: A Problem Oriented Approach. New York, Thieme, 1986, pp 172–205. *Review of exercise effects on glucose metabolism and insulin production and uptake in response to exercise by healthy persons and diabetic patients.*

15 ALCOHOL ABUSE AND ALCOHOL-RELATED ILLNESSES

Benjamin Kissin

About 90 million Americans drink alcoholic beverages in one form or another, some occasionally, some moderately but regularly ("social drinkers"), and some heavily ("heavy drinkers"). About 10 million Americans drink enough to cause difficulties in their personal and/or social adjustment ("problem drinkers"). Of these, about 6 million drink sufficiently, over a long time period, to produce the stigmata of alcohol dependence ("alcoholism").

The medical syndromes associated with alcohol abuse fall generally under four major categories: (1) acute alcohol intoxication, (2) alcohol dependence or "alcoholism," (3) acute alcohol withdrawal syndromes, and (4) medical complications. Alcohol abuse, like the abuse of any other psychoactive drug, is the consequence of the action of a specific pharmacologic agent in a specific individual. The specific clinical syndromes of alcohol abuse derive directly from the pharmacologic effects of ethyl alcohol (ethanol) on body tissues and secondarily from the adaptive responses of the body to excessive exposure to alcohol (tolerance and physical dependence). Alcohol-related illnesses are mainly nutritional in origin and are discussed principally, along with specific organ systems as well, in Chapters 217 and 467.

PHARMACOLOGY OF ETHANOL

ABSORPTION AND METABOLISM. Ethanol is usually ingested in a concentration of 5 per cent (beer), 12 per cent (wine), 20 per cent (reinforced wines), or 43 per cent (86 proof whiskey). The distinctive flavor of different alcoholic beverages is a function of the contained congeners (e.g., higher alcohols, aldehydes), as may also be some complications of heavy drinking (e.g., hangovers). However, the major effects of drinking are due to the content of ethanol itself. Ethanol is rapidly absorbed from the stomach and intestines into the bloodstream, thus accounting for its quick pharmacologic action. It is also rapidly metabolized so that a moderate dose will usually clear from the blood in about one hour. Its absorption and metabolic breakdown make ethanol a fast-acting but short-lasting drug.

Ethanol diffuses rapidly into all aqueous compartments of the body (extracellular and intracellular), so that the blood concentrations of ethanol directly reflect concentrations of the chemical throughout the body. About 10 per cent of the ethanol in the body is directly eliminated by diffusion through the kidneys or lungs, and concentrations in alveolar air and urine can be utilized to estimate blood concentrations. The rest is metabolized in the liver. The rate-limiting element in this sequence is hepatic alcohol dehydrogenase, which, in a 70-kg man, can metabolize about 9.0 grams of ethanol (about three fourths of an ounce of whiskey) per hour. This results in a decrease in the blood level of approximately 15 mg per deciliter per hour. Ingestion of ethanol at a greater rate produces cumulatively rising blood levels.

The conversion of nicotinamide-adenine dinucleotide (NAD) to NADH during the oxidation of ethanol shifts the redox equilibrium and causes metabolic disturbances such as hyperlipidemia and hyperuricemia. Since alcohol dehydrogenase is located almost entirely in the liver, neutral fat deposition (fatty degeneration) occurs in the liver of about 90 per cent of alcoholics.

Alcohol dehydrogenase occurs in various isoenzyme forms, which metabolize ethanol at different rates. Orientals and American Indians tend to have increased hepatic levels of an atypical isoenzyme that metabolizes alcohol unusually rapidly and produces high levels of acetaldehyde. This is thought to produce the characteristic "Oriental flush," a reaction that occurs in about 80 per cent of genetically Mongoloid individuals.

NEUROPHARMACOLOGY. Ethanol is a powerful depressant of the central nervous system with pharmacologic effects similar to those of ether and chloroform. Ethanol is miscible with fats and rapidly enters cell membranes. It is thought that the neuropharmacologic action of ethanol is exercised through neuronal cell membrane effects (1) upon the activation of calcium ion (Ca^{++}), (2) upon the action of the Na^+ K^+ ATPase pump, or (3) more directly, through the production of increased fluidity.

Because parts of the brain respond differently to ethanol, its behavioral effects may differ from its neuropharmacologic ones; e.g., the depressant effects of ethanol upon inhibitory control centers may release excitatory behavior. Alcohol tends to depress the brain from above downward, first affecting the cortex, then the limbic system and cerebellum, next the reticular formation, and finally the lower brain stem.

In low doses, alcohol acts both as a stimulant (disinhibitor) and as a relaxant; it is widely used for these effects. The drug is also a euphoriant; perhaps the majority of alcoholics drink mainly for this effect. In larger doses, alcohol is a rapidly acting and potent anxiolytic-analgesic and is frequently taken by agitated individuals to obtain relief.

ACUTE ALCOHOL INTOXICATION

Acute alcohol intoxication occurs infrequently in social drinkers, more frequently in heavy drinkers, and most frequently in problem drinkers and alcoholics. The pattern of aberrant responsiveness is a function of the blood alcohol level (BAL) and of pre-existing tolerance. Alcoholics have a high level of behavioral and physiologic tolerance to ethanol so that they may require blood alcohol levels almost 100 mg per deciliter higher than social drinkers to show comparable impairment. Some alcoholics function adequately with a BAL of 250 mg per deciliter, a concentration at which social drinkers become stuporous (Table 15–1).

Acute alcohol intoxication occurs in two stages. In nontolerant individuals, a BAL of about 100 to 200 mg per deciliter will result in disinhibition and hyperexcitability; with a BAL of above 250 mg per deciliter, stupor and coma usually ensue. Although these two syndromes are part of a continuum, there

TABLE 15–1. BLOOD ALCOHOL LEVELS AND SYMPTOMS

Level (mg/dl)	Sporadic Drinkers	Chronic Drinkers
50 (party level)	Congenial euphoria	No observable effect
75	Gregarious or garrulous	Often no effect
100	Incoordinated Legally intoxicated	Minimal signs
125–150	Unrestrained behavior Episodic dyscontrol	Pleasurable euphoria or beginning incoordination
200–250	Alertness lost → lethargic	Effort required to maintain emotional and motor control
300–350	Stupor to coma	Drowsy and slow
>500	Some will die	Coma

is a sufficient change in symptoms at about the level of 200 to 250 mg per deciliter (depending on individual tolerance) to warrant their separate description.

EXCITATORY STAGE. The social use of alcoholic beverages usually produces a BAL of about 50 mg per deciliter, with a sense of relaxation and of well-being. At levels of 75 mg per deciliter, most individuals tend to feel more relaxed and sociable; a few become garrulous or hostile. At about 100 mg per deciliter, signs of ataxia begin. Coordination and judgment may be impaired at the same time that self-assurance increases. At this level, driving may be hazardous; most state laws define "driving while intoxicated" at a BAL of 100 mg per deciliter or higher.

At BAL's of about 125 to 150 mg per deciliter, behavioral changes occur that usually reflect the underlying personality. Some individuals continue to become more congenial, sociable, and disinhibited; some become hostile and aggressive; and some turn inward and become silent and depressed. Increasing BAL's usually continue to be associated with increasing personality-specific responsivities until the more narcotic effects of ethanol begin to manifest themselves at or about the 200 to 250 mg per deciliter level.

In susceptible persons alcohol may precipitate great agitation and acts of violence. To treat this condition one should give intramuscular benzodiazepines in cautiously increasing doses in order to avoid cumulative narcosis with the alcohol (see below). Individuals who show marked depressive reactions while under the influence of alcohol should be given verbal support until the effects wear off.

DEPRESSANT STAGE. When the BAL rises higher than about 200 to 250 mg per deciliter in nontolerant individuals, and to more than about 300 to 350 mg per deciliter in problem drinkers, the individual passes into a depressant syndrome. This condition requires immediate medical care. BAL's must be taken and evaluated; a single BAL of 300 mg per deciliter should not be interpreted as contravening treatment, since a reservoir of unabsorbed alcohol may be present in the stomach and small intestine. Gastric lavage should be undertaken to reduce this reservoir and to prevent vomiting and pulmonary aspiration. Vital systems must be maintained, with the administration of oxygen, intravenous fluids, and, rarely, ventilatory and circulatory support. Antidotes are ineffective.

HANGOVERS. Ethanol is strongly toxic to both brain and stomach, and its alcohol and aldehyde congeners are even more so, explaining the high incidence of postintoxication malaise, headache, giddiness, tremor, and nausea. These symptoms are generally self limited and respond readily to antacids and aspirin. More serious symptoms occur in more persistent but not yet fully alcoholic drinkers, in whom the so-called "hangover" may actually be an early withdrawal syndrome.

ALCOHOLISM (Alcohol Dependence)

Alcoholism is a drug-dependence syndrome resulting from the prolonged excessive use of ethanol. It is characterized by (1) a "high-risk" individual, (2) the development of self-perpetuating mechanisms producing addiction, (3) a more or less typical clinical course, and (4) specific complications and sequelae. The progressive clinical course is marked by repeated episodes of intoxication followed generally by characteristic withdrawal symptoms.

PREDISPOSING FACTORS. Predisposing factors that contribute to susceptibility to alcoholism may be biologic, psychologic, or social.

Studies of adoptees raised by nonalcoholic foster parents indicate a strong *genetic component* in alcoholics. Upon reaching adulthood, the children of alcoholic biologic parents have a four-fold greater incidence of alcoholism than those of nonalcoholic parents, even where no differences in alcohol consumption exist in the adopting families.

Psychopathology is found more frequently in alcoholics as a group than in nonalcoholics, although it is uncertain which is cause and which effect. The proven occurrence of significant brain damage as a result of prolonged alcoholism lends some weight to the latter argument. Nevertheless, some alcoholics show a characteristic psychologic immaturity, and the reportedly 8 to 10 per cent incidence of major psychoses among alcoholics is significantly higher than the 1 to 2 per cent in the general population. Agitated schizophrenics and manic-depressives not infrequently use alcohol as a means of self-medication. On the other hand, many alcoholics show no evidence of psychologic disturbance prior to the onset of their alcoholism.

Social influences can be the dominant influence in determining the level of drinking. Such factors include sex, ethnicity, religion, nationality, socioeconomic status, occupational subculture, family patterns, and peer pressure. In general, the level of psychopathology in a drug abuser is generally inversely proportional to the acceptability of that form of drug abuse in that individual's subculture. Thus, women alcoholics tend to show more psychopathology than do men, Jewish alcoholics more than Irish, and middle-class heroin addicts more than ghetto addicts.

THE ADDICTIVE CYCLE. Alcoholism (alcohol dependence, alcohol addiction) is the end result of a series of interacting processes that initiate and then perpetuate heavy drinking. The ingestion of alcohol provides temporary gratification of a need for euphoria or temporary relief from some psychologic or physical tension. However, chronic ethanol ingestion induces psychologic and physiologic processes that increase the desire for more alcohol; the substance that satisfies the need paradoxically increases the need.

The sequence in the elaboration of the addictive cycle in alcoholism is (1) primary psychologic dependence, (2) tolerance, (3) physical dependence, and (4) secondary psychologic dependence.

Psychologic Dependence. The first self-perpetuating mechanism is *primary psychologic dependence*. This reflects behavioral conditioning: An action and experience rewarded, either by pleasure or by the relief of pain and discomfort, will be reinforced by every similar succeeding action and experience. Primary psychologic dependence is the cornerstone of the dependency syndrome to all three classes of psychoactive drugs—the depressants, the stimulants, and the hallucinogens. Secondary psychologic dependence develops with the onset of physical dependence and is characterized by the need to drink to prevent withdrawal symptoms.

The combination of these two types of psychologic dependence is translated clinically into the subjective symptoms of *craving*, symptoms manifested as a continuous preoccupation with thoughts of drinking and with an overwhelming desire for alcohol. Craving is especially strong when reinforced by external stimuli such as a bottle of liquor. With long-term abstinence, there is a decline in the manifestations of both types of psychologic dependence, with craving tapering off to a low level after about six months of abstinence and more or less disappearing after about two years. However, craving can be reactivated thereafter by exposure to a strongly stimulating situation, e.g., the bar or tavern previously frequented.

Tolerance. With the continued ingestion of large doses of alcohol, metabolic changes result in an increased tolerance to ethanol. This is manifested clinically as a decreased responsivity to a given dose of alcohol or as the need to ingest a larger dose in order to obtain a desired effect. Tolerance occurs at three physiologic levels.

1. *Metabolic tolerance* results from the increased efficiency of hepatic enzymes breaking down ethanol to its metabolic end-products.
2. *Physiologic or intracellular tolerance* accounts for the major

increase in tolerance to ethanol, reflected in the behavioral and physiologic resistance to high doses of alcohol. The mechanisms of physiologic tolerance are thought to involve intracellular metabolic changes in the central nervous system and may be similar to those for barbiturates and other sedatives but are different from those for the opiates. Thus, individuals tolerant to ethanol show cross-tolerance to barbiturates and vice versa. Also, withdrawal symptoms from either drug can be relieved by administration of the other.

3. *Behavioral tolerance* is considered to be an overall learning response that enables the person to maintain behavioral function while under the influence of ethanol.

Physical Dependence. The same cellular changes that result in physiologic tolerance presumably are responsible for physical dependence. Neurons develop increased excitability to compensate for the depressant effects of chronic alcohol intake. If ethanol levels then drop sharply, a marked increase occurs in central nervous system irritability. The presence of physical dependence on ethanol is expressed by the phenomena of withdrawal.

When a high level of physical dependence develops in alcoholics, withdrawal symptoms become persistent because of the constant rise and fall of the BAL. The alcoholic finds that he is comfortable only while his BAL is rising; a falling BAL is accompanied by distressing withdrawal symptoms. Since quick and effective relief is obtained by alcohol ingestion, withdrawal symptoms become important factors in maintaining drinking behavior. During particularly heavy drinking bouts, severe withdrawal symptoms result whenever the physically dependent alcoholic seeks to stop drinking; this sequence leads to a compulsive pattern of drinking known clinically as *loss of control or inability to abstain.*

CLINICAL COURSE. Problem drinking and alcoholism are progressive syndromes characterized in most instances by repeated episodes of intoxication (in some problem drinkers and in some alcoholics, titration of drinking may conceal such episodes). With the development of physical dependence, the tempo of drinking tends to accelerate, and there is increased evidence of physical, psychologic, and social impairment. Besides developing multiple physical ailments, affected individuals tend to become careless in personal appearance, indifferent to family and social responsibilities, and inadequate at work. The addition of these stresses to already overburdened physiologic and psychologic resources tends further to increase drinking behavior.

An early sign of developing alcoholism is *blackouts*. These are episodes of temporary amnesia occurring during periods of intensive drinking. The amnesia is usually for periods of hours to a day or so, but with prolonged drinking may last up to a week. The syndrome is a characteristic anesthetic effect of alcohol on the brain; it is a precursor to the more chronic forms of brain damage secondary to chronic alcohol abuse.

The acute alcohol withdrawal syndrome occurs episodically after prolonged periods (two to three weeks) of extremely heavy drinking (a fifth of hard liquor daily or its equivalent). It is precipitated either by the cessation of drinking or by a sharp decrease in intake. Many individuals enter treatment for alcoholism after being hospitalized for acute alcohol withdrawal. After a week or so, many of these patients continue to show a low-grade withdrawal syndrome characterized by tremulousness, agitation, and insomnia. This constellation, labeled the *protracted abstinence syndrome*, may persist, to a greater or lesser degree, for up to six months. During this period, the individual is particularly susceptible to the effects of alcohol, since the entire addictive cycle is readily reactivated. Hence it is important with patients hospitalized during acute alcohol withdrawal to be certain that they are adequately detoxified before discharge.

TREATMENT OF ALCOHOL ABUSE. The major goal is to help the patient achieve and maintain total abstinence. The suggestion that treated problem drinkers sometimes may return safely to social drinking has no demonstrated merit and should be discounted. The achievement of abstinence is difficult enough without the interference produced by the reinforcing effects of even small amounts of alcohol. Rehabilitation requires a reconstruction of physical, psychologic, and social adjustment, to help overcome the long-term dependence upon alcohol. Nor is this a short-term affair. The perpetuating mechanisms of the addictive cycle remain very active during the first six months of abstinence and moderately active for the first two or three years of sobriety. The individual in therapy should be encouraged to undertake treatment for at least a two-year period, during which time the necessary physical, psychologic, and social adjustments can occur.

The three most effective treatment modalities for problem drinking and alcoholism are *disulfiram* (Antabuse), *psychotherapy* or counseling, and *Alcoholics Anonymous*. Disulfiram is a slowly excreted, long-acting medication that inhibits the action of acetaldehyde dehydrogenase. Because it is slowly metabolized and slowly excreted, once appropriate blood levels are established by a priming regimen (500 mg daily for one week), each single daily dose of 250 mg will maintain adequate blood levels for the next three or four days. Alcohol in any form is converted by alcohol dehydrogenase to acetaldehyde, but its further degradation is blocked by the action of disulfiram on acetaldehyde dehydrogenase. The piling up in the blood of acetaldehyde, a highly toxic substance, produces prostrating nausea, vomiting, diffuse flushing, and a shocklike reaction. The emergency treatment for the Antabuse-alcohol reaction consists of intravenous fluids and antihistamines. Most alcoholics who have experienced this reaction are careful not to repeat it, and many achieve and maintain abstinence with this drug.

Psychotherapy or the counseling of individuals who are abusing alcohol is directed (1) toward achieving abstinence and (2) toward accomplishing the changes in psychologic and social adjustment necessary to maintain it. Alcoholics Anonymous (AA), an association of ex-alcoholics, provides the companionship of those who have been able to overcome alcohol addiction; it also offers the strong social support and acceptance that alcoholics so often lack and so desperately need. The greatest chance for success in treating an alcoholic lies with continued supportive counseling by the physician plus the patient's participation in AA.

ACUTE ALCOHOL WITHDRAWAL SYNDROMES

Physically dependent alcoholics who go on a lengthy bout of heavy drinking for a period of one or more weeks will, upon reduction or cessation of alcohol intake, develop *acute alcohol withdrawal syndrome* characterized by cortical (behavioral) and beta-adrenergic (autonomic) hyperexcitability. Either pattern may predominate.

DELIRIUM TREMENS. *Delirium tremens* (DT's) represents the most severe type of acute alcohol withdrawal, with marked symptoms of cortical and brain stem hyperexcitability.

The patient in DT's represents an acute medical emergency, since the untreated mortality rate is about 15 per cent, largely from complications such as pneumonia or acute hepatitis. Affected patients are characteristically disoriented, agitated, hallucinating, tremulous, and perspiring. The pulse and respirations are rapid, blood pressure may be high or low, and body temperature is usually elevated. There may be severe muscle cramps because of an associated acute myopathy or generalized paresthesias because of a diffuse polyneuropathy. Nausea and vomiting often signify acute gastritis that induced the reduced alcohol intake and precipitated the acute episode.

The course of fully developed DT's usually follows upon alcohol withdrawal or decline by about three to five days, often after a preceding period of increasing restlessness, tremor, and behavioral agitation. A certain percentage follows upon withdrawal seizures. In untreated or inadequately treated cases, confusion and disorientation may last for several weeks. With adequate treatment, most severe symptoms clear within ten days; lesser ones may last for up to six months.

The specific treatment of delirium tremens involves the substitution of a long-acting drug that is cross tolerant for alcohol. Benzodiazepines are the agents of choice for inducing sedation. Treatment for moderately severe cases consists of diazepam, 25 to 50 mg orally four times daily for the first several days, with gradually tapering doses thereafter. In patients with more severe cases, particularly in those with convulsions, diazepam, 5 to 10 mg intravenously, should be used every one to two hours until the condition is stabilized. Fluids, electrolytes, and thiamine, 100 mg, should be given parenterally. A careful search should be made to detect and treat infection. Good nursing care is essential to provide the necessary physical and psychologic support (Table 15–2).

WITHDRAWAL CONVULSIONS. In *withdrawal convulsions* (*"rum fits"*) generalized convulsions occur usually singly but sometimes in short runs or even as status epilepticus following a decline in the BAL. Seizures usually occur in the period of 12 to 48 hours after cessation of drinking. Various causative mechanisms have been suggested for withdrawal seizures, including chronic hypocapnia or hypomagnesemia, but none stand as proved. The attacks usually are without focal features, and consistently focal signs deserve further investigation. Otherwise, computed tomographic (CT) scans of the brain are negative, as are interictal electroencephalographic (EEG) recordings. Treatment consists of stopping the acute convulsions with intravenous diazepam, plus giving a single dose of phenytoin (Dilantin) (see Ch. 493) to prevent immediately recurring seizures. Signs of impending delirium tremens emerge postictally in perhaps one third of cases. "Rum fits" occur only on withdrawal from alcohol; prophylactic, chronic treatment with anticonvulsants is useless.

IMPENDING DELIRIUM TREMENS. The most common clinical manifestation of the acute alcohol withdrawal syndrome is *impending delirium tremens*. Mild-to-moderate symptoms of withdrawal are evident, mainly those associated with beta-adrenergic brain stem discharge. Mild agitation, vasomotor changes, tremors, and insomnia sometimes respond to the alpha-adrenergic drug clonidine, an active antagonist to beta-adrenergic discharge. However, treatment with cross-tolerant benzodiazepines is both more specific and more effective. A mild case may be controlled with 10 to 20 mg of diazepam given orally four times daily for several days. Moderate cases will require up to 20 to 30 mg of the same drug four times daily for a few days, with gradual tapering off over a period of seven to ten days.

ACUTE ALCOHOLIC HALLUCINOSIS. In *acute alcoholic hallucinosis*, auditory hallucinations dominate the clinical picture as opposed to the more common visual hallucinations seen in delirium tremens. In addition, there is characteristically less agitation and tremulousness. Consequently, the clinical picture looks more like that of an acute schizophrenic episode than like that of alcohol withdrawal, and differential diagnosis may be difficult. However, a history of prolonged heavy drinking, followed by a sudden decrease or cessation, reveals the diagnosis. Treatment is the same as for delirium tremens. Recovery may require weeks to a month or more.

ALCOHOL-RELATED ILLNESSES

Medical conditions secondary to prolonged alcohol abuse fall generally into two categories: (1) nutritional diseases caused by dietary insufficiency and (2) diseases caused by the direct toxic effects of ethanol. Because alcoholic beverages provide 7 calories per gram of ethanol, an individual consuming a fifth of 86 proof liquor daily will derive about 2500 calories from alcohol alone. Under such conditions, most alcoholics consume little other food. Since liquor contains no vitamins, minerals, amino acids, or other essential nutritional elements, alcoholics often show marked nutritional deficiencies. Superimposed on this metabolic insufficiency, the direct toxic effect of ethanol produces further damage. Although the diseases secondary to alcohol abuse are generally categorized as either nutritional or toxic, both effects are probably involved in most cases.

Alcohol-related illnesses can involve all organ systems in the body. Table 15–3 indicates alcohol-related illnesses that are due predominantly to the direct toxic effects of prolonged alcohol ingestion and those that are more probably secondary to malnutrition. The effects may be difficult to separate, since most alcoholics are both heavy drinkers and malnourished.

TABLE 15–2. TREATMENT OF SEVERE TREMULOUSNESS OR DELIRIUM TREMENS

1. Attempt control by reassurance and observation.
2. Treat systemic problems promptly.
3. Treat uncontrollable agitation: Control with diazepam, 10 mg IV given slowly, followed by 5–10 mg IV, slowly every 15 minutes to induce calmness. Once calm, maintain with diazepam, 5–10 mg IV every 1–4 hours.
4. Continuously supply and balance electrolytes and vitamins, especially thiamine.

TABLE 15–3. ALCOHOL-RELATED ILLNESSES DUE TO TOXIC AND NUTRITIONAL EFFECTS OF ETHANOL

Organ	Syndromes Due to Toxic Effects	Syndromes Due to Nutritional Effects
Brain	Alcoholic dementia (cortical atrophy)	Wernicke-Korsakoff syndrome (Ch. 467) Cerebellar degeneration Central pontine myelinosis (secondary to electrolyte changes during therapy)
Nerves		Peripheral polyneuropathy (Ch. 305) (thiamine deficiency)
Heart	Alcoholic cardiomyopathy (Ch. 53) Arrhythmia	Beriberi heart disease (thiamine deficiency)
Blood	Leukopenia, anemia, thrombocytopenia	Macrocytic hyperchromic anemia (Ch. 136) (folic acid deficiency)
Gastrointestinal tract	Acute and chronic gastritis (Ch. 99) Acute and chronic pancreatitis (Ch. 108) Carcinoma of the head and neck and of the esophagus	Malabsorption syndrome (Ch. 136) (folic acid deficiency)
Liver	Fatty degeneration Acute hepatitis Laennec's cirrhosis	Laennec's cirrhosis (Ch. 126 to 128)
Metabolic	Hyperlipidemia (Ch. 183) Hyperuricemia (exacerbation of gout)	
Endocrine	Male sexual impairment Increased fetal risk (fetal alcohol syndrome)	
Immune system	Increased susceptibility to infection	
Electrolyte disturbances	Hypocalcemia Hypomagnesemia Hypophosphatemia Acute water intoxication Alcoholic hyperosmolality Alcoholic ketosis	

PROGNOSIS

Prognosis in alcoholism is related to the stage and severity of the disease process. Morbidity and mortality can be divided into two major categories: that directly associated with alcohol abuse and that associated with alcohol-related illness.

PROGNOSIS IN THE ALCOHOLISM SYNDROME. Perhaps the most serious consequences of the alcoholism syndrome are deaths related to alcoholic behavior. It has been estimated that 50 per cent of highway fatalities are caused by drunken driving, with half of the victims alcoholic. Twenty-five per cent of suicides have a history of prolonged alcoholism. In deaths due to drug overdose, alcohol is the associated agent most commonly found. The combined mortality rates of these three behavioral aberrations, together with those associated with alcohol-related medical illnesses, make alcoholism and its behavioral and medical complications the fourth most common cause of death in the United States after heart disease, strokes, and cancer.

Facts belie the generally negative public opinion about the prognosis of alcoholics. In most industrial alcoholism treatment programs where workers are socially stable and (because of the risk to jobs and pensions) well motivated, recovery rates run at the 70 to 80 per cent level. This remarkably high "cure" rate is probably accounted for mainly by early detection when most of the patients are still problem drinkers and have not yet developed the physical and social stigmata of advanced alcoholism. Once the latter develop, success rates seldom exceed 40 to 50 per cent. Early identification and intervention remain the most important steps in the treatment of alcoholism.

PROGNOSIS OF ALCOHOL-RELATED MEDICAL ILLNESSES. The prognosis for specific alcohol-related medical illnesses varies with the nature of the illness and with its severity. Practically no alcohol-related medical illness can be cured if the patient continues to abuse alcohol. The major component of the treatment of alcohol-associated medical illness is the treatment of the underlying alcoholism.

Harper C, Kril J: Brain atrophy in chronic alcoholic patients: A quantitative pathological study. J Neurol Neurosurg Psychiatry 48:211, 1985. *Evidence for common occurrence of cortical and brain stem atrophy in chronic alcoholics.*

Helzer JE, Robins LN, Taylor JK, et al.: The extent of long term moderate drinking among alcoholics discharged from medical and psychiatric treatment facilities. N Engl J Med 312:1678, 1985. *A conclusive demonstration that chronic alcoholics cannot successfully revert to moderate social drinking.*

Kissin B: Medical management of the alcoholic patient. In Kissin B, Begleiter H (eds.): The Biology of Alcoholism. Vol. 5. New York, Plenum Press, 1977. *Description of the role of the family physician in the diagnosis and treatment of alcoholism.*

Mendelson JH, Mello NK: Biologic concomitants of alcoholism. N Engl J Med 301:912, 1979. *A medical progress article reviewing studies dealing with the mechanistic aspects of genetics, metabolism, consequences, behavior, and speculated causes of alcohol addiction.*

Sellers EM, Kalant H: Alcohol intoxication and withdrawal. N Engl J Med 294:757, 1976. *An excellent didactic article dealing with all aspects of acute treatment.*

Thompson WL, John AD, Maddrey WL, et al.: Diazepam and paraldehyde for treatment of severe delirium tremens. A controlled trial. Ann Intern Med 82:175, 1975. *Establishes the clear superiority of diazepam for acute treatment and outlines a clear and effective plan for management.*

16 DRUG ABUSE AND DEPENDENCE

Charles P. O'Brien

Drug abuse is currently a significant problem at every level of our society. It is likely that the average physician will encounter many patients exhibiting behavioral or medical complications of licit or illicit drug use, but the relationship of the symptoms to drugs often goes unrecognized. Early diagnosis, which is critical for effective treatment, is difficult because, at an early stage, patients rarely fit the addict stereotype.

Clinicians have been mainly concerned with *tolerance* and *physical dependence*. *Tolerance* is the result of a homeostatic process in which the body adapts to the repeated effects of a drug. This adaptation tends to compensate for the pharmacologic effects, with the result that higher doses are required to achieve an effect. With daily dosing, tolerance increases and a state of *physical dependence* can occur. *Physical dependence* is indicated by the presence of a rebound known as a *withdrawal syndrome* that follows interruption of dosing. Withdrawal phenomena tend to be opposite to the effects of the drugs themselves. Thus a drug that produces sedation leads to hyper-reflexia and irritability during withdrawal, and a stimulant withdrawal is followed by weakness and depression.

Behavioral effects are the pivotal diagnostic criteria, however, not simply tolerance and physical dependence. Moreover, with some drugs, *intermittent use* that does not cause tolerance or a withdrawal syndrome may produce behavioral or social consequences that urgently require treatment. *Drug abuse* is therefore defined as a maladaptive pattern of use of any substance that persists despite social, psychologic, or medical consequences. This pattern of use may be intermittent and does not meet the criteria for dependence. *Drug dependence* is a behavioral syndrome that involves compulsive drug taking, neglect of constructive activities, and adverse social effects and *may* include pharmacologic tolerance and physical dependence.

RECOGNITION. Since early diagnosis is so important, the physician should have a high index of suspicion for including drug abuse in the differential diagnosis of any patient. The abuse pattern that presents the most difficulty is that of a successful middle-class adult whose substance abuse is detected incidental to a routine physical examination or during treatment of an unrelated disorder. Invariably, such patients will deny that drug or alcohol abuse is a problem. Physicians must be aware that denial of problems and minimizing of the drug or alcohol use are fundamental aspects of the syndrome. These patients usually will not admit to a problem until it becomes so severe that there is no alternative, by which time, treatment is much more difficult.

The diagnosis of drug abuse or dependence is basically a clinical deduction. The physician should use all of the available information, including the patient's history, information from relatives or the employer, physical examination, and laboratory tests. Blood or urine tests showing the presence of drugs or their metabolites can be useful but also can be misleading. The toxicologic tests, when properly done and confirmed, indicate use within a varying period of time, depending on the drug and its dose. Such tests do not disclose pattern of use or the presence of dependence. Metabolites of some drugs, such as marijuana, remain in the urine for at least several days following a single dose. Thus the tests require interpretation and integration with other clinical information.

Clues discovered on the physical examination include the presence of scars from numerous intravenous injections ("tracks") or the presence of edematous arms and veins that are difficult to find. Chronic sinusitis or a scarred and perhaps perforated nasal septum suggests "snorting" of cocaine, a powerful vasoconstrictor. Frequent injuries due to falls or auto accidents are seen in sedative abusers as well as alcoholics. Infections such as abscesses, hepatitis, respiratory infections, and endocarditis are well-known risks of drug abuse. The most devastating disease associated with drug abuse is the acquired immune deficiency syndrome (AIDS). In the late 1980's, intravenous drug users have become a major reservoir for the AIDS virus (Ch. 346).

Physicians must also be alert to the signs of drug abuse in

order to avoid unwittingly prescribing medications that will perpetuate the dependence. Patients taking sleeping medications, pain medications, or antianxiety agents on a chronic basis may visit several physicians in order to obtain a larger drug supply. Others will deliberately feign illness, particularly pain syndromes. Some will have read textbooks and recite classic descriptions of acute renal calculus, migraine headache, or pancreatitis. Physicians should be particularly wary of patients who ask for a specific medication or who claim to have an "allergy" to nonnarcotic pain medication.

Jaffe J: Drug addiction and drug abuse. In Gilman AG, Goodman LS, Rall TR, et al (eds.): The Pharmacological Basis of Therapeutics. Edition 7. New York, Macmillan, 1985, pp 532–581. *Thorough discussion of pharmacologic and clinical aspects of drug abuse.*

Senay, EC: Substance Abuse Disorders in Clinical Practice. Boston, John Wright, 1983. *Very practical and concise guide to diagnosis and treatment of drug dependence.*

SEDATIVES

Examples of sedatives include the following:

1. Ethanol
2. Barbiturates
3. Meprobamate (Miltown)
4. Glutethimide (Doriden)
5. Diazepam (Valium)
6. Lorazepam (Ativan)
7. Alprazolam (Xanax)
8. Flurazepam (Dalmane)
9. Triazolam (Halcion)

These drugs are central nervous system depressants, and all are capable of producing abuse, tolerance, and physical dependence. Their withdrawal syndromes are generally similar, although the sedatives come from different chemical categories (e.g., alcohol, barbiturate, benzodiazepine). Their effects are additive, and they are often used in combination. This aspect is particularly important in considering interactions with alcohol (Ch. 15) and in treating patients who are dependent on multiple sedatives with different durations of action.

Patterns of Abuse

There are two basic patterns of sedative drug abuse other than that with alcohol: One is produced inadvertently by taking prescription sedatives without proper concern for their potential to produce dependence, and the second involves deliberate use of sedatives to obtain a "high."

PRESCRIPTION SEDATIVES. The problem of improper use of prescription sedatives is a concern to all physicians because these drugs are among the most widely prescribed of all drugs throughout the world. They have legitimate medical uses in the short-term treatment of insomnia, anxiety, and seizure disorders. The chronic use of medication for insomnia, however, often leads to problems because insomnia is merely a symptom. It may signal the presence of an underlying illness, or it may simply require a change in activity patterns, but chronic use of sedatives simply adds a new problem. After daily use for several weeks, tolerance develops, and sleep difficulties may return, often in a modified form. The patient may have become dependent, however, on the daily ingestion of the sedative. If the drug is stopped, a rebound occurs, with the appearance of symptoms worse than those experienced prior to treatment. All sedatives are not equal in their tendency to produce this iatrogenic insomnia. Long-acting benzodiazepines, for example, are unlikely to produce rebound effects at usual doses. Other liabilities are associated with their use, however, such as "hangover" effects, which produce subtle neuropsychologic deficits and may mimic dementia in older persons. On balance, insomnia should not be treated with drugs except for brief periods of time.

Another pattern associated with the prescription of sedatives is that found in the treatment of anxiety. Benzodiazepines (e.g., diazepam, alprazolam) are the most effective medications available for the treatment of anxiety, and they produce relatively less sedation than older medications used for this purpose, such as meprobamate or phenobarbital. Symptoms of anxiety are widespread such that about 15 per cent of all Americans receive a prescription for one of these drugs in a single year. Approximately 6 per cent of the population take benzodiazepines chronically, and this leads to *tolerance* and *physical dependence*. This does not imply *abuse* because the patient may be taking the benzodiazepine for a legitimate anxiety disorder. It does mean, however, that since the patient perceives less sedation, there may be a tendency to increase the dose. It also implies that the patient should be warned about withdrawal symptoms if the drug is terminated abruptly. Occasionally, a patient who allows his prescription to run out is brought to an emergency room because of benzodiazepine withdrawal seizures. Some of these patients are mislabeled as "addicts," even though they have never used more of the antianxiety medication than was ordered. Others, however, become deliberate abusers of sedatives after beginning treatment for anxiety under a doctor's orders and may purposely increase their dose while obtaining medication from several different physicians. Benzodiazepines in general have a relatively low abuse potential, and such cases of deliberate abuse are rare.

DELIBERATE SEDATIVE ABUSE. Sedatives are used at parties by groups of abusers, usually adolescents and young adults, to obtain a "high." The "high" appears to be a form of disinhibition or release and depends partially on the setting in which the drug is taken. As with alcohol, increasing the dose produces depression and eventual loss of consciousness. A dangerous aspect of sedative abuse is that tolerance to the sought-after subjective effects rapidly develops, but tolerance to the depressant effects on the brain stem remains low. As the experienced user increases the dose to obtain a "high," he or she may unexpectedly reach the dose that depresses vital functions and threatens survival.

The most popular deliberately abused sedative over the past 10 to 15 years has been methaqualone (Quaalude), reputed to be an aphrodisiac. Although methaqualone probably does not enhance sexual performance, the drug was so widely abused that the manufacturer withdrew it. Counterfeit versions of methaqualone continue to be available "on the street" in some areas.

Certain benzodiazepines are popular sedatives for abuse and are available for purchase through illicit channels. Diazepam has been popular among abusers, and, more recently, alprazolam has been used by the drug subculture. Although benzodiazepines in general are not preferred drugs of abuse, those with more rapid onset, such as diazepam and alprazolam, may be sought.

Abstinence Syndrome

The withdrawal syndrome following sedative dependence is similar to alcohol withdrawal. Among the sedatives, the syndrome differs in onset, duration, and severity, depending on the dose and duration of action of the drug used and the duration of daily use. The long-acting benzodiazepines, such as diazepam, may have a withdrawal syndrome whose onset is delayed for several days following the termination of the drug. At doses within the therapeutic range, withdrawal symptoms may consist of only mild irritability, complaints of peculiar sensations, diaphoresis, and sleep disturbance accompanied by rebound increases in rapid eye movement (REM) sleep. The symptoms may be similar to the anxiety symptoms for which the drug was initially prescribed. At higher doses, the sedative withdrawal syndrome is more severe and can be life threatening. Major abnormalities include paroxysmal electroencephalographic (EEG) changes, generalized seizures, or a toxic psychosis similar to delirium tremens. During withdrawal from somewhat less, but still high, doses of benzodiazepines (the equivalent of 100 mg of diazepam per day), myoclonic jerking movements without loss of consciousness may be seen. Restlessness, anxiety, tremulousness, and weakness occur, and these are often accompanied by orthostatic hypotension, nausea, cramps, and vomiting. Irritability, anxiety, depressive symptoms, and neuropsychologic deficits may persist for weeks or months.

Treatment

The acute withdrawal syndrome should be considered a serious medical illness usually requiring inpatient treatment. Close monitoring for cardiac arrhythmias or seizures is necessary. Several detoxification techniques are available, each requiring the substitution of a prescribed sedative with cross-tolerance for the drug on which the patient is dependent. The physician should not simply accept the history, but rather determine the level of dependence by giving a test dose of a known sedative, such as diazepam or pentobarbital. If the patient shows no evidence of slurred speech or sedation after a test dose of 20 to 40 mg of diazepam, a higher level of dependence is indicated, and the daily sedative dose should be adjusted accordingly. Gradual detoxification using diazepam can be accomplished over 1 to 3 weeks, although in some treatment centers where diazepam is the object of much drug-seeking behavior and manipulation by patients, phenobarbital is preferred. Patients dependent on both a short-acting sedative, such as alcohol, and a long-acting drug, such as diazepam, should be watched for a biphasic withdrawal. The alcohol withdrawal peaks and subsides during the first week, but the diazepam withdrawal may not be evident until early in the second week. Patients dependent on both an opioid, such as heroin, and a sedative should be maintained on a low dose of methadone until the sedative withdrawal is completed. After detoxification, the patient must be put in a treatment program to prevent recurrence, as described at the end of this chapter.

Hallstrom C, Lader M: Benzodiazepine withdrawal phenomena. Int Pharmacopsychiatry 16:235, 1981. *Description of subtle symptoms of benzodiazepine withdrawal.*

O'Brien CP, Woody GE: Sedative hypnotic and anti-anxiety agents. In Frances AJ, Hales R (eds.): American Psychiatric Association Annual Review, Vol 5. Washington, APA Press, 1986, pp 186–199. *Review of diagnosis, treatment, and prevention of sedative abuse.*

STIMULANTS

Examples of stimulants include the following:

1. Cocaine
2. Dextroamphetamine
3. Methamphetamine
4. Methylphenidate (Ritalin)
5. Phenmetrazine (Preludin)
6. Diethylpropion (Tepanil)

Patterns of Abuse

Cocaine has suddenly become the major drug of abuse in the United States, excluding alcohol, and the problem continues to grow. The enormous profits available to drug dealers have spawned a huge supply system so that despite increased federal efforts, cocaine supplies have increased so rapidly that the price has declined. Not only is cocaine available to a wider audience, especially children, but also its users have developed clever new and efficient ways to administer the drug, increasing its potency and dangerousness.

Until recently, cocaine hydrochloride was available as a white powder through illicit channels in an adulterated form and at a cost so high that only the affluent could afford to use it regularly. The typical mode of administration was "snorting," which consists of application of the powder to the nasal mucous membranes. Intravenous injection of an aqueous solution was also used, resulting in a more rapid onset and greater likelihood of seizures. However, inhalation of the "free base" alkaloidal form of cocaine has been found to be the most convenient and efficient system for delivering the drug to the brain. A technique for converting the hydrochloride salt into cocaine "free base" using alkalinization and extraction with ether or other organic solvents while heating has become well known because of the devastating fires that sometimes result. During the mid 1980's, this solvent technique has been replaced by a mass-produced solid form of "free base" called "crack." Crack is produced by sodium bicarbonate extraction of cocaine hydrochloride, and the agent can be sold in small, yellow-white lumps for as little as $5 to $10 per dose. When heated in a small pipe, the cocaine vapor can be inhaled, producing a brief and very intense "high." This drug is clearly the *most addicting substance* yet encountered by clinicians. Dependence can be produced very rapidly, perhaps in days and certainly in weeks. Users may administer the drug continuously for several days without eating or sleeping. The widespread availability of "crack", its cheap price, and its proneness to produce dependence have led to problems in all strata of society.

The sought-after effect of cocaine is an intense "high" or euphoria, which is often described in sexual terms but is claimed to be "better than sex." The euphoria may last only a few minutes, depending on the dose and mode of administration. The after-effect is one of depression and craving for more cocaine. During a period of regular cocaine use, the person becomes irritable and suspicious. High doses may result in persecutory delusions or hallucinations, but these are more common with longer acting stimulants such as amphetamines. Families and friends of chronic cocaine users often note personality changes not observed by the users themselves. Alcohol, sedatives, opioids, and marijuana are often taken concurrently to combat the anxiety and irritability experienced by those using cocaine regularly. Users deprived of cocaine experience intense craving, depression, apathy, fatigue, and sleepiness.

Amphetamines have a longer duration of action than cocaine, but many of the effects are similar. These drugs have been used by physicians for a variety of conditions, including weight reduction, narcolepsy, and attention deficit disorder. Amphetamines have not been shown to be of value in weight reduction programs, and their use for all purposes has been curtailed by legal restrictions. Because they produce effects that are mostly pleasant, patients have a tendency to increase the dose of all stimulants and to take them longer than the prescribing physician intended. Tolerance develops rapidly to the stimulant effects of amphetamines, but with higher doses, toxic effects are common. These effects can resemble acute paranoid schizophrenia with delusions and hallucinations. Cessation of amphetamines produces a withdrawal syndrome similar to that after cocaine use and with depressive symptoms that may continue for several months.

The milder stimulants, such as methylphenidate and phenmetrazine, rarely are associated with abuse problems, but they should be prescribed only when specifically indicated and with awareness of their abuse potential.

Pharmacology

Cocaine acts at dopaminergic and other aminergic synapses by blocking reuptake of the neurotransmitter and presumably resulting in enhanced synaptic activity. Systemic effects of cocaine and amphetamine include increased cardiac contraction, increased blood pressure and heart rate, dilated pupils, constriction of peripheral blood vessels, rise in body temperature, relaxation of the bronchial musculature, and increases in central venous pressure, pulmonary arterial pressure, and renal blood flow. Cocaine is an effective topical local anesthetic and vasoconstrictor of mucous membranes. Low doses of stimulants increase alertness and physical and cognitive ability. Stimulants do reduce appetite, but significant tolerance to this effect develops. When stimulants are discontinued, a rebound increase in weight often leaves the person heavier than before the drug was taken.

Heavy users report acute tolerance to the euphorigenic effects of cocaine when the drug is used repeatedly at a single occasion. However, a day or two later, a "high" can again be obtained at approximately the same dose as previously. Tolerance to the respiratory and cardiac stimulatory effects of cocaine does occur. Although abrupt cessation of stimulant use produces a distinct withdrawal syndrome as described above, it is generally limited to *behavioral* evidence of brain dysfunction rather than marked by the development of physical signs. During the excessive periods of sleep seen during withdrawal, the EEG shows increase in the proportion of REM sleep and nightmares may occur. Rarely, withdrawal has been marked by headaches, profuse sweating, muscle cramps, disorientation, and confusion.

Adverse Effects

The most common adverse effect of cocaine use is loss of control, so that a severe dependence syndrome occurs with neglect of all constructive activities. *Acute cocaine toxicity* is dose related and is characterized by sympathomimetic effects, including tachycardia, hypertension, hyperthermia, and arrhythmias, and is followed by seizures, brain stem depression, and cardiorespiratory collapse. Stroke, coma, intracranial vasculitis, myocardial infarction, and sudden death have each been occasionally observed following cocaine binges. At lower doses the acute toxic effects may be marked by a brief period of paranoid behavior with hallucinations. *Acute amphetamine toxicity* is also characterized by excessive sympathomimetic stimulation and more commonly produces grossly paranoid behavior mimicking acute paranoid schizophrenia. There may be stereotyped compulsive behavior, tactile hallucinations consisting of "bugs" crawling under the skin, and visual or auditory hallucinations.

Chronic use of intranasal cocaine commonly causes ulceration or perforation of the nasal septum. Chronic users are typically debilitated and subject to infections as a result of neglect of hygiene, lack of sleep, and poor nutrition. There is evidence of dopamine cell damage in the brains of animals treated chronically with stimulants. This raises the possibility of an increased risk for later development of Parkinson's disease. There are also clinical reports of increased schizophrenic disorders in chronic stimulant users. Chronic cocaine use among pregnant women results in a high incidence of premature, low birth weight, and neurologically abnormal infants.

Treatment

Treatment of the anxiety reactions and irritability produced by cocaine or amphetamines can be accomplished with benzodiazepines. Acute psychotic reactions may require haloperidol if amphetamines are involved, but reactions produced by cocaine are usually self limiting. Withdrawal from stimulant dependence requires a supportive environment and protection from the supply of cocaine. Intense cravings for cocaine are the most prominent of the withdrawal symptoms, and these have been attributed to a state of dopamine depletion in the brain. To reverse these effects, the dopamine receptor agonist bromocriptine has been used experimentally to ease the acute withdrawal. The most difficult aspect of treatment is the prevention of relapse when the patient returns to his or her normal environment and is confronted with opportunities to re-establish the habit. This aspect of treatment is discussed at the end of this chapter.

Ellinwood EH: Amphetamines/anorectics. In Dupont RL, Goldstein A, O'Donnell J (eds.): Handbook on Drug Abuse. National Institute on Drug Abuse, U. S. Government Printing Office, 1979, pp 221–231. *Review of clinical and pharmacologic aspects of stimulant abuse.*

Washton A, Gold MS: Chronic cocaine abuse: Evidence for adverse effects on health and function. Psychiatr Ann 14:733, 1984. *Clear evidence of adverse consequences of chronic cocaine use.*

OPIOIDS

Examples of opioids include the following:

Agonists

1. Morphine
2. Methadone
3. Meperidine (Demerol)
4. Oxycodone (Percodan)
5. Propoxyphene (Darvon)
6. Heroin
7. Hydromorphone (Dilaudid)
8. Fentanyl (Sublimaze)
9. Codeine

Mixed agonist-antagonists

1. Pentazocine (Talwin)
2. Nalbuphine (Nubain)
3. Buprenorphine (Buprenex)
4. Butorphanol (Stadol)

Antagonists

1. Naloxone (Narcan)
2. Naltrexone (Trexan)

Opiates are derivatives of the opium poppy plant, which contains more than 20 alkaloids. Heroin, morphine, and codeine are examples of commonly used *opiates*. Synthetic drugs that act via opiate receptors in the body are called *opioids*. The body also produces peptides that act at these receptors as neurohormones or neurotransmitters and are called *endogenous opioids*.

Patterns of Abuse

Opioid abuse has been a problem in the United States for well over 100 years. The patterns have changed considerably since the turn of the century, when most of the opium-dependent persons were either Civil War veterans or users of patent medicines. At the current time, there are two abuse patterns in this country. The smaller group by far involves patients initially treated by a physician for a legitimate pain problem with opioid drugs. The pain may become chronic, and the dose is increased, usually at the patient's demand. The treatment may have begun with something mild, such as propoxyphene or pentazocine, but it tends to progress to the more potent opioids, such as oxycodone or hydromorphone. Prescriptions may be refilled excessively, and patients may visit more than one physician for medication or may frequent emergency rooms. Such individuals will vehemently deny being addicts; they are just seeking relief of pain. On closer examination, however, they usually turn out to have symptoms of anxiety or depression that are temporarily relieved by opioids.

The second pattern is that of intentional misuse of opioids for their euphoria-producing ability. Intermittent heroin use, primarily among males in the inner city, typically begins during adolescence, and dependence ensues within a year or two of first use. Development in all areas—educational, social, occupational, and even psychosexual—is curtailed by use of heroin. It is not known how many people begin experimenting with heroin and stop using it. Those who continue to use heroin develop tolerance to its euphorigenic effects, continue to increase the dose, and soon find that they must use the drug daily to avoid withdrawal even while chasing that elusive first "high."

Older users tend to introduce younger ones to heroin and to techniques of crime required to support the "habit." Street heroin available in the United States tends to be diluted many times so that there may be an average of only 4 to 10 mg of heroin in a typical 100-mg bag. Furthermore, the heroin on the street at any given time may be more or less potent, depending on the supply and the pressure from law enforcement agencies. Most street heroin users have relatively mild degrees of physical dependence in terms of number of milligrams of heroin or its equivalent in morphine or methadone per day. Heroin-dependent persons, although they insist that they are seeking a "high," actually fear withdrawal and will go to great lengths to obtain sufficient drug to inject themselves one to three times per day.

Some heroin users discover that prescription medications are more reliable than street drugs because the latter have no quality control. Hydromorphone is a very potent opioid that cannot be distinguished from heroin even by experienced users under double-blind conditions. Addicts may visit physicians or emergency rooms and feign pain to obtain opioids. Occasionally, unscrupulous physicians may simply sell prescriptions for whatever the addict requests. A few addicts have had prescription pads printed with their own name and a false Drug Enforcement Agency (DEA) number in an effort to trick pharmacists. Some of the prescription drugs prized on the street are not even the more potent ones. For example, a major problem in some large cities has been pentazocine abuse. The pattern is to obtain tablets of this mixed agonist-antagonist designed for oral use, dissolve the tablets in water under heat, mix them with another drug, such as an antihistamine (tripelennamine), and inject the mixture. Some addicts claim that they prefer the "high" obtained this way to that obtained from heroin. The manufacturer of pentazocine has recently begun supplying the tablets combined with naloxone, an opioid antagonist that is effective parenterally but not orally. Thus if the pentazocine tablets are taken intravenously, the naloxone will counteract the opioid effects, thus frustrating the abuser. Another weak opiate that is abused in combination is codeine. Mixed with glutethimide, a sedative, it is favored by a number of drug abusers.

In recent years, heroin dependence has spread from the inner city to the middle class. The same supply system that distributes cocaine and marijuana also makes heroin available. Some educated and employed persons seeking a "thrill" prefer the effects of heroin. Others learn to use heroin to combat some of the unpleasant anxiety and irritability produced by chronic cocaine use.

Pharmacology

Opioids act at specific receptors that are widely distributed throughout the body in virtually all major organ systems. Since these receptors are heavily represented in the endocrine, cardiovascular, gastrointestinal, and nervous systems, the effects of opioids are many and varied. The potency of individual drugs appears to depend on receptor affinity as well as metabolism. Heroin, for example, is diacetylmorphine, which has high lipid solubility and enters the brain rapidly. It is hydrolyzed to morphine, which is the form active at opiate receptors. Other opioids have similar systemic effects but reach brain receptors less rapidly. The mixed agonist-antagonist drugs, such as pentazocine, butorphanol, and nalbuphine, appear to act as agonists at kappa opiate receptors, but they also act as antagonists at mu (morphine) receptors. Thus, pentazocine can relieve pain on its own but, if given to someone already receiving morphine, will displace the morphine and precipitate withdrawal symptoms. Pure antagonists, such as naloxone and naltrexone, have no opiate-like effects, but they can reverse overdose and precipitate withdrawal if given *after* an opioid and can prevent opiate effects if given *before* the opioid.

After heroin injection, traces of morphine can be found in the urine for about 12 to 48 hours, depending on the dose and the laboratory detection technique. Quinine, a common adulterant of street heroin, persists longer, but it is also found in legal substances such as tonic water. Parenteral injections of morphine or methadone have equal analgesic effects and persist for four to six hours, whereas heroin is three times as potent, and meperidine and codeine are one tenth as potent as morphine. Codeine, meperidine, and methadone remain active when taken orally, and the duration of action of methadone is extended considerably when taken orally. For prevention of withdrawal in dependent persons, methadone remains active for 24 to 30 hours, far longer than its analgesic effect.

Opioids appear to produce analgesia, at least in part, by activation of an endogenous pain control system mediated via opiate receptors. Inhibition of pain sensation occurs at the spinal level as well as within the brain. Opioids are much more effective for clinical pain with anxiety than for experimental pain in research subjects. Opioids produce a reduction in anxiety, some sedation, and a feeling of well-being or euphoria. This effect seems important to their clinical usefulness and to their abuse potential as well. It is this euphoria that is sought by street addicts and that probably leads some medical patients to abuse prescribed opioids.

Tolerance to the euphoric effects of opioids develops rapidly, resulting in a tendency for users to increase their dose, if possible. Only partial tolerance develops to other effects, such as pupillary constriction, inhibition of gastrointestinal contractions, and suppression of anterior pituitary function.

Adverse Effects

Acute opioid overdose occurs when a user inadvertently injects a much higher dose than expected. This also can occur when a previously tolerant person returns to opioid use after a long interval, so that most of his or her tolerance has been lost. Many of the "overdoses" found with street heroin are now thought to have been due to a reaction to some of the adulterants rather than to the opiate. Acute reactions to adulterants, including quinine, allergic reactions, and synergistic interactions among several drugs used simultaneously may produce the *acute heroin reaction*. The syndrome is marked clinically by the rapid development of cyanosis, pulmonary edema, respiratory distress, and altered levels of consciousness progressing to coma. Increased intracranial pressure and occasionally seizures can develop. Fever to 40°C may occur initially and persist for 48 hours in association with leukocytosis. The pupils are usually pinpoint, although dilated, nonreactive pupils may occur with hypoxia or use of multiple drugs. The pathologic picture includes pulmonary congestion and edema and frequently cerebral edema.

Opioids themselves are surprisingly nontoxic even when used in substantial daily doses for many years. There is partial tolerance to their pharmacologic effects on the endocrine system. Thus females on methadone initially are amenorrheic, but the cycle usually returns in 6 to 12 months. Cortisol, luteinizing hormone, and testosterone levels are depressed while the patient is on methadone. Sexual response may be delayed; sperm count and ejaculate volume are reduced. Since street heroin users tend to have frequent periods of partial withdrawal, their endocrine systems are in turmoil. In contrast, a level dose of methadone induces some order, and the effects are reversible when the opioid is terminated. Chronic constipation may persist throughout opioid use.

The major adverse effects of opioid use come from the adulterants found in street drugs and the nonsterile practices typically followed by users. Skin abscesses, cellulitis, and thrombophlebitis are the most frequent complications. Pentazocine injection causes chronic ulcers and sclerosis of muscle in the areas of injection. Septicemia and bacterial endocarditis with involvement of either or both sides of the heart are seen. *Staphylococcus aureus* is frequently the causative agent in right-sided endocarditis. Peripheral and pulmonary embolic phenomena occur.

Viral hepatitis has long been common among intravenous drug abusers owing to the practice of sharing needles during an injection session. In recent years, this illness has been overshadowed by the appearance of AIDS. In 1986, 50 to 60 per cent of patients in methadone programs in some large cities tested positive for HIV antibodies, and it has been suggested that this group is particularly susceptible to the infection because the drugs suppress host resistance. Most of those being treated for AIDS had not previously received treatment for their drug abuse. AIDS not only is becoming a major cause of death among intravenous drug abusers but also threatens the general population because the abusers constitute a major reservoir for the virus.

Among applicants for drug abuse treatment, 75 to 80 per cent of heroin users have significantly abnormal liver function tests. These findings may be related to persistent chronic hepatitis, but alcohol, malnutrition, allergic phenomena, and the toxic effects of adulterants may contribute. Pulmonary complications include pneumonia, abscess, infarct, and tuberculosis. Disseminated extrapulmonary tuberculosis has been reported. Angiothrombotic pulmonary hypertension and granulomatosis result from the intravenous injection of foreign bodies, including talc or cotton. Other complications include nephropathy, local arterial occlusion, phlebitis, mycotic aneurysms, and necrotizing angiitis.

Neurologic complications of street heroin use include transverse myelitis, acute inflammatory polyneuropathy, peripheral nerve lesions, toxic amblyopia secondary to quinine, and muscle disorders, including acute rhabdomyolysis with myoglobinuria and a fibrosing chronic myopathy. Septic states may lead to bacterial meningitis and brain, subdural, and epidural abscesses. Tetanus may result from dirty needles.

Pregnant addicts suffer a high incidence of toxemia and premature deliveries. About 50 per cent of their newborns require treatment of withdrawal symptoms.

Treatment

There are more distinctly different kinds of treatment available for dependence on opioid drugs than for any other type of drug dependence. As with other drugs, the prevention of relapse to drug-seeking behavior is the most difficult aspect, as described later. The treatment of *acute overdose* is effective and straightforward. In any emergency situation in which opioid overdose is suspected, naloxone should be administered, preferably intravenously. The patient will have constricted pupils, and a dose of 0.4 mg of naloxone should cause an increase in pupil size, respiratory rate, and alertness within several minutes. Repeated doses may be necessary if the patient does not respond within several minutes to the first dose. An absent response to naloxone excludes the diagnosis of opioid overdose.

There is virtually no risk in giving naloxone, but the potential benefits mean that it should be tried even in doubtful cases. There are, however, two pitfalls that should be mentioned. One is that not only will naloxone reverse the overdose, but also it will go beyond mere reversal and actually precipitate *withdrawal* symptoms in opioid-dependent persons. To avoid this, the dose of naloxone should be titrated according to the level of consciousness and respiratory rate. The second is that the overdose may recur as the naloxone is metabolized. Naloxone should be titrated via an intravenous drip or repeated every 2 to 3 hours with careful monitoring of vital signs for at least 24 hours.

The opioid withdrawal syndrome varies in severity and duration, depending on the specific drug, dose, and duration of use. The typical heroin-dependent person notes the onset of withdrawal six to ten hours after the last injection. Feelings of drug craving, anxiety, restlessness, irritability, sweating, rhinorrhea, and yawning develop early. These are followed by dilated pupils, sneezing, piloerection, anorexia, nausea, vomiting, diarrhea, abdominal cramps, bone pains, myalgias, tremors, sleep disturbance, and, very rarely, convulsions or cardiovascular collapse. Untreated, these symptoms peak at 36 to 48 hours and gradually subside over 5 to 10 days. Withdrawal is generally not life threatening, and it has been compared with a severe case of the "flu." There is also a protracted abstinence syndrome consisting of mild symptoms of anxiety, sleep disturbance, and autonomic nervous system instability, which may persist for six months after acute withdrawal. Longer acting opioids, such as methadone, produce an abstinence syndrome that develops more slowly and with less intensity but that persists much longer.

Medically assisted withdrawal is usually accomplished using methadone, beginning with a test dose of 20 mg. If 20 mg has no appreciable effect on the signs and symptoms within one hour, an additional 20 mg can be given. The methadone can be gradually reduced over seven to ten days. An alternative is clonidine, an $alpha_2$-adrenergic agonist/partial agonist, which produces complex central effects that result in reduced central adrenergic outflow. Developed for the treatment of hypertension, clonidine has also been found to reduce many of the signs of autonomic dysfunction during opioid withdrawal. Thus clonidine can be useful in situations in which methadone is not available. Beginning with low doses of 0.1 to 0.2 mg to minimize the possibility of postural hypotension, clonidine can be increased to 1 to 1.5 mg daily in divided doses over four to ten days and then tapered over the next five days.

CANNABIS (Marijuana and Hashish)

Cannabis is not a single drug, but rather a complex preparation containing many biologically active chemicals. Δ-9-Tetrahydrocannabinol (Δ-9-THC) accounts for most of the pharmacologic effects of the complex.

Patterns of Abuse

Cannabis has been used in many societies as a form of folk medicine and for relaxation, but throughout the 1970's, its use increased explosively in the United States. In 1979, more than 50 million Americans reported using the drug at least once, and 9 per cent of high school seniors reported daily use. In the 1980's, the popularity of this drug has declined somewhat, but it is still in widespread use. The vast majority of users smoke marijuana cigarettes or hashish pipes in groups in which the ritual of preparation and sharing is part of the social interaction. Others demonstrate a compulsive pattern of daily use, with lives dominated by the acquisition and use of cannabis.

Pharmacology

Cannabis preparations are three to four times more potent when smoked than when taken orally. After inhalation, effects begin within three minutes, they peak within one hour, and the subject reports feeling "normal" within three hours. There is evidence, however, that psychomotor effects, such as impairment on eye tracking and vigilance tasks, may be evident for up to 11 hours after a single dose.

The acute physiologic effects of cannabis are dose related and include an increase in heart rate, conjunctival vascular congestion, decreased intraocular pressure, bronchodilation, increased airway conductance, and peripheral vasodilation. Dryness of mouth, fine tremors, ataxia, nystagmus, nausea, and vomiting have been noted. Sleep patterns are altered, and orthostatic hypotension occurs infrequently.

Psychoactive effects depend on the dose, route of administration, personality and experience of the user, and the environment in which the drug is used. Enhanced perceptions of colors, sounds, and tastes have been reported. Time seems to pass slowly, and the ability to learn new facts is impaired. There is often some drowsiness and inattentiveness, which may account for some of the poor performance on driving simulators. *Motor vehicular driving performance is definitely impaired by cannabis*, and this may persist for several hours after the period of obvious intoxication. Tolerance and physical dependence have been experimentally demonstrated with regular cannabis use. This is not relevant to the occasional user, but daily heavy users show clinical evidence of withdrawal when deprived of access to cannabis.

Cannabis contains chemicals with unusually high lipid solubility and thus a high affinity for brain tissue. Metabolites persist for several weeks, although their biologic significance is unknown. Urine tests for marijuana can remain positive for more than a week after a dose and even longer in chronic users. Positive urine tests have also been experimentally demonstrated in subjects who simply sat in a small room for several hours where marijuana was being smoked.

Cannabis derivatives have been investigated for their therapeutic potential in several illnesses. The antiemetic effect has been useful to some patients in reducing the nausea produced by cancer chemotherapy. The accompanying psychologic effects have so far limited its usefulness. Glaucoma, convulsive seizures, asthma, and muscle spasticity are other conditions in which a cannabis or a synthetic analogue may eventually prove useful.

Adverse Effects

Most clinicians believe that regular cannabis use by adolescents impairs maturation and often results in poor social and scholastic adjustment. Although there is no way to experimentally demonstrate causality, cannabis use is associated with poor academic performance. Occasional users have fewer problems, but acute panic, paranoid reactions, and frightening distortions of body image are sometimes experienced. Rarely, these reactions are severe enough to require emergency room treatment. Such reactions seem to be more common with higher doses and with oral administration than with smoking, which is easier to titrate. Patients with a history of schizophrenia may be particularly sensitive to adverse consequences of cannabis and should be warned to avoid it.

The cardiac stimulatory effects of cannabis may pose a threat to patients with cardiovascular disease. Chronic smoking of cannabis produces inflammatory changes in the bronchi and sinusitis. Cannabis is carcinogenic experimentally, but clinical studies are confounded by the concurrent use of tobacco by virtually all regular cannabis smokers.

Treatment

The acute anxiety reactions produced by cannabis are seldom severe enough to warrant medical attention. Treatment should be supportive and reassuring, with frequent reminders of the drug-induced nature of the symptoms. Benzodiazepines may be indicated in more severely agitated states. For the chronic heavy user, treatment is much more difficult. Such patients typically insist that treatment is not necessary and they feel no need to stop using cannabis on a daily basis. Meanwhile, they are failing in school or employment. Psychotherapy is unlikely to be of value unless the cannabis consumption can be interrupted. Hospitalization or entrance into a therapeutic community may be indicated, if the patient can be so persuaded. Medication is usually not required to treat withdrawal, and the drug-free patient clears mentally over several weeks. Psychotherapy is often necessary in addition to removing the cannabis.

Marijuana and Health: Report of a Study by a Committee of the Institute of Medicine: Division of Health Sciences Policy. Washington, D.C., National Academy Press, 1982. *Critical review of the published reports of marijuana effects on organ systems and behavior.*

PSYCHEDELICS

Psychedelic drugs include the following:

1. Lysergic acid diethylamide (LSD)
2. Dimethyltryptamine (DMT)
3. Phencyclidine (PCP)
4. Mescaline
5. Psilocybin
6. 5-Methoxy-3,4-methylene dioxyamphetamine (MDMA; "ecstasy")

Many drugs at some dose will produce hallucinations, but the drugs classified here reliably produce distortions in perception or in thinking as a primary effect, even at low dose. This category represents several chemical classes and different mechanisms of action. Phencyclidine, in particular, differs from the others in that it produces, in addition to hallucinations, analgesia and amphetamine-like stimulation.

Patterns of Abuse

Hallucinogenic drugs are among the oldest known psychoactive drugs, having long served as adjuncts to religious practices in some societies. During the 1960's they became well known on college campuses, where they were used in an effort to "gain insight" or experiment in expanding the potential of the mind. Physicians in emergency rooms were frequently called upon to treat young people suffering from "bad trips" or adverse reactions to these sessions. One of the problems with the use of illicit supplies of these drugs is their gross mislabeling. Chemical analysis of samples obtained from street purchases shows that phencyclidine ("angel dust," PCP) and by-products of phencyclidine are often the active ingredient in LSD or psilocybin purchases. Thus users often get unexpected and severe effects. Phencyclidine is available only from clandestine laboratories—hence its purity varies widely. The by-products produced during phencyclidine synthesis may cause severe toxic symptoms.

The use of psychedelics declined in the later 1970's and early 1980's, but the use of PCP has recently shown an upsurge. The typical pattern of psychedelic drug use involves intermittent rather than daily use. Recently, there has been great interest in MDMA, known as "ecstasy." This drug has been reported to facilitate insight and maturation and thus enhance the effects of psychotherapy. A few therapists have supported this notion and encouraged their patients to use MDMA. The drug has never been studied in any organized clinical trial, however, and thus there is no evidence to support these claims. Similar claims were made for LSD in the past, and serious attempts failed to demonstrate scientifically a beneficial effect. Both MDMA and the closely related MDA have been shown to be toxic to serotonergic nerve cells.

Pharmacology

LSD is the most potent psychedelic drug known. The usual illicit street dose is around 200 μg, but doses as low as 20 μg produce psychologic effects in susceptible individuals. Central sympathomimetic stimulation occurs within 20 minutes of oral ingestion and is characterized by mydriasis, hyperthermia, tachycardia, elevated blood pressure, piloerection, increased alertness, and facilitation of monosynaptic reflexes. Nausea and vomiting occasionally occur.

Psychoactive effects of LSD develop within one to two hours. These vary with the subject, dose, setting, expectation, and mood. Perceptions are heightened and may become overwhelming. Afterimages are prolonged and may overlap with ongoing perceptions. There may be a sense of unusual clarity, and one's thoughts may assume extraordinary importance. Time seems to pass slowly, and body distortions are commonly perceived. True hallucinations, usually visual, may occur in susceptible individuals. Mood is highly variable and labile and may range from expansive reactions characterized by euphoria and self-confidence to a constricted reaction marked by depression and panic.

The syndrome begins to clear after 10 to 12 hours, but fatigue and tension may persist for an additional 24 hours. The duration of action of mescaline is about 12 hours and that of psilocybin is 4 to 6 hours. Tolerance develops within three to four days to repeated daily doses of LSD, but recovery is rapid and weekly use of the same dose is possible.

Phencyclidine comes in various forms (powder, liquid, capsule, and tablet) and often is taken inadvertently when the user is expecting something else. It produces a prompt stimulant effect similar to that with amphetamine and usually a feeling of euphoria. Ataxia, slurred speech, nystagmus, and feelings of numbness are common. At higher doses, frightening and bizarre visual hallucinations can arise. There may be hostile or aggressive behavior and amnesia for the episode. With still higher doses, catatonia and coma occur, with the patient's eyes open and the pupils partially dilated. Heart rate and blood pressure are elevated. Tolerance to the stimulant effects occurs, and mild withdrawal symptoms have been observed in daily users.

Adverse Effects

The acute reactions such as panic or psychosis ("bad trip") are the most common complications of psychedelic use. With LSD, these vary in intensity and occasionally have led to suicide or self-injury. Phencyclidine is more likely to produce a severe reaction that results in suicide, often by drowning. Assaults and murders have been attributed to the effects of phencyclidine, and aggressive behavior can occur during the psychotic episode.

Prolonged psychotic episodes sometimes occur after psychedelic use. It is not known whether these can occur only in individuals who have pre-existing tendencies toward psychosis. Many clinicians believe that chronic use or high doses of psychedelics, especially phencyclidine, can produce prolonged psychosis even in healthy individuals.

Overdose resulting in death can occur with phencyclidine. The syndrome can progress rapidly from aggressive psychotic behavior to coma with elevated blood pressure, dilated pupils, muscular rigidity, arrhythmias, and seizures.

Another adverse effect of psychedelic use is known as "flashbacks." These are a brief reappearance of the hallucinations or distortions experienced during the acute ingestion, recurring days or weeks after the last psychedelic dose. "Flashbacks" appear to be more common with heavy use, and they eventually disappear without treatment.

Treatment

The use of medication in an emergency situation with a patient suffering from an unknown drug reaction can be dangerous owing to progression of the street drug effect with further absorption from the gut and to possible drug interactions with any prescribed medications. Thus treatment of acute panic reactions is best accomplished, when possible, by a supportive environment, observation, and reassurance. In severely agitated patients, intramuscularly administered lorazepam or haloperidol can be used. Prolonged psychosis requires hospitalization and treatment with neuroleptics.

Treatment of phencyclidine overdose may require support of vital signs. Gastric lavage with activated charcoal may prevent further absorption of the drug. To enhance the excretion of phencyclidine, acidification of the urine may be accomplished acutely by intravenously administered ammonium chloride, 75 mg per kilogram per day in four divided doses, or ascorbic acid, 500 mg every four hours, with repeated monitoring of blood pH, blood gases, blood urea nitrogen (BUN), blood ammonia, and electrolytes. If symptoms are mild, cranberry juice and 1 or 2 grams of ascorbic acid given orally four times per day may be sufficient.

Anticholinergic Compounds

Effects in some ways similar to those of psychedelic drugs may be produced by ingestion of the alkaloids *atropine, hyoscyamine, and scopolamine* in their natural forms. These are found in "herbal teas" and a variety of proprietary medications, and several deaths from their use have occurred. Excessive use of *antihistaminic* compounds with anticholinergic effects also occurs. Psychoactive effects are those of an acute toxic delirium with confusion, visual or tactile hallucinations, and amnesia for the episode. Symptoms of the potent peripheral effects of the intoxication include dilated pupils, tachycardia, dry mouth, flushing, and hyperthermia. Treatment is symptomatic and consists of protecting the patient from self-injury, providing fluids, and reducing the fever. Administration of cholinesterase inhibitors and lorazepam intramuscularly may be indicated in severe cases. Phenothiazines are contraindicated because of their anticholinergic effects. Anticholinergic drugs are sometimes sold as hallucinogenics, thus creating a potentially dangerous additive interaction if a phenothiazine is administered in the emergency room to treat a "bad trip."

INHALANTS

Examples of inhalants include the following:

1. Toluene (airplane glue)
2. Gasoline
3. Amyl nitrite
4. Kerosene
5. Carbon tetrachloride
6. Nitrous oxide

Chemicals that are volatile at room temperatures and that produce perceptible changes in brain function when inhaled have been popular among certain groups as a means of producing altered states of consciousness. There are characteristic patterns for each chemical.

Organic solvents, such as toluene, are typically used by children beginning at about age 12. During the 1970's, 10 to 12 per cent of high school seniors reported having tried some inhalant as a drug at least once. The material is usually placed in a plastic bag, and the vapors are inhaled. Dizziness and intoxication are described after several minutes of inhalation. Inhalant abuse also involves the use of aerosol sprays containing fluorocarbon propellents. Prolonged exposure or daily use may result in toxic effects on several organ systems, including cardiac arrhythmias, bone marrow depression, cerebral degeneration, and damage to liver, kidney, and peripheral nerves. Death has occasionally been attributed to inhalant abuse, probably via the mechanism of cardiac arrhythmias, especially accompanying exercise or associated with upper airway obstruction.

Amyl nitrite is a yellowish, volatile, inflammable liquid with a fruity odor. It produces dilation of smooth muscle and has been used in the past for treatment of angina. In recent years, amyl nitrite has been used to enhance orgasm, particularly by male homosexuals. It is sold in the form of room deodorizers and can produce a feeling of "rush," flushing, and dizziness. Adverse effects include palpitations, postural hypotension, and headache progressing to loss of consciousness.

Nitrous oxide, alone or in combination with oxygen, and *halothane* are sometimes used as intoxicants by medical personnel. Compulsive use and chronic toxicity have not been reported, but there are obvious acute dangers of the unauthorized use of such potent agents.

Treatment

Since the effects of solvents are brief, specific acute treatments are generally not indicated. When inhalant use is chronic or associated with other psychiatric diagnoses, specific psychiatric treatment and measures to prevent relapse are indicated.

Lewis JD, Moritz D, Mellis LP: Long term toluene abuse. Am J Psychiatry 138:368, 1981. *Case reports and review of the literature.*

Sharp CW, Brehem ML: Review of Inhalants: From Euphoria to Dysfunction. NIDA Research Monograph Series No. 15, National Institute on Drug Abuse, Rockville, Md. 20857. *Good review of clinical and toxicologic aspects of the spectrum of inhalant problems.*

NICOTINE

The medical consequences of the smoking of tobacco products are covered in many chapters of this book because the effects are so widespread. As the dangers of smoking have become so well known, it has become more apparent that the smoking of cigarettes can produce a very powerful dependence on nicotine. Cessation of smoking may be very difficult even in patients who strongly desire to remain abstinent (Ch. 11).

ILLICIT SYNTHETIC DRUGS (Designer Drugs)

The so-called designer drugs are produced in clandestine laboratories, and they vary in their composition and purity. Fentanyl analogues have been produced that have extremely potent opioid actions and have resulted in overdose deaths. Other attempts at synthesis of opioids have resulted in toxic compounds. A recent example is MPTP, a toxic by-product of botched attempts to synthesize a meperidine (Demerol) analogue, which produces an irreversible Parkinson's syndrome (Ch. 468). Other chemicals recently found in street samples are phenethylamines, which are analogues of amphetamine and various analogues of phencyclidine. In evaluating the drug history of any patient, the physician must remember that those who purchase drugs on the street have no way of knowing what they actually take.

TREATMENT OF DRUG DEPENDENCE

The treatment of drug dependence involves four stages (Table 16–1): acknowledgment, detoxification, pharmacotherapy, and psychiatry.

ACKNOWLEDGMENT OF THE PROBLEM. Rarely does a patient in the early and most treatable phase of drug dependence spontaneously volunteer for treatment. Friends or relatives who observe the signs of a drug problem must confront the patient. Often the family physician is in a good position to notice the problem early and convince the patient to enter treatment. Confrontation is best accomplished when several concerned people approach the patient together in a firm but supportive way. When confronted with evidence of a drug problem, most persons will continue to deny its existence, making persistence necessary.

DETOXIFICATION. The pharmacologic aspects of detoxification were covered in the discussions of specific drug categories. In some cases, hospitalization is mandatory, particularly when there is a large degree of physical dependence. If, however, the drug taking can be interrupted while the individual remains an outpatient, this can be far less expensive and just as effective. "Treatment programs" that advertise a 30-day inpatient treatment of drug dependence are misleading, because the heart of effective treatment is the continued therapy, usually lasting months or years, designed to prevent relapse after the patient returns to work or school. Frequently, the patient has so much cognitive impairment during the detoxification period that he or she retains little of therapy or education provided during this first phase.

PHARMACOTHERAPY. This mode of therapy has been discussed under specific drug categories. For the most part, this involves treatment of specific psychiatric disorders, such as affective disorders or psychosis commonly associated with a particular form of drug dependence. It must be remembered that patients who have abused one drug will have a strong likelihood of abusing a prescribed psychoactive drug. For this reason, antianxiety agents or sedatives should rarely, if ever, be prescribed in the rehabilitation of drug-dependent persons.

Certain pharmacotherapies are directed at the drug-seeking behavior rather than an associated psychiatric disorder. The use of disulfiram (Antabuse) in the treatment of alcoholics is discussed in Ch. 15. Opioid-dependent patients, who have repeatedly relapsed after detoxification, can be transferred from use of illicit drugs to methadone maintenance. The patient can then be maintained on a steady dose of methadone as a substitute for his or her opioid drug of choice. The advantage is that the patient is stabilized owing to the long duration of action of methadone and, if properly managed, experiences no "highs" or "lows." Patients are able to function well on methadone and perform complex tasks competently, including, for those physicians who require this treatment, the practice of medicine. The methadone enables the patient to participate in a rehabilitation program, including psychotherapy. Methadone may involve several years of maintenance and must be used only in authorized programs in which staff have received specialized training.

Naltrexone (Trexan) is a new drug that is a relatively long-acting opioid antagonist. Before receiving this medication, patients must first be thoroughly detoxified, or the naltrexone will precipitate withdrawal. Since naltrexone blocks opiate receptors, the effects of impulsive opioid use are prevented while naltrexone is in the body. This new treatment has been successful in conjunction with a comprehensive rehabilitation program, including a wide range of psychotherapies. The problem is that naltrexone must be taken at least two or three times per week to protect against relapse and it requires strong motivation on the part of the patient to remain opioid free.

PSYCHOTHERAPY. Psychotherapy is generally similar across all classes of drugs. It should be started as early as possible in the treatment program, but it is of little value when the patient is still intoxicated or confused. This treatment is, however, completely compatible with pharmacotherapy, such as psychoactive medication, methadone, naltrexone, disulfiram, or nicotine chewing gum. Such psychotherapy is broadly defined and involves counseling regarding job hunting or legal problems, family therapy, group therapy, individual therapy, all types of behavioral treatments, and self-help programs such as Narcotics Anonymous. The purpose of these treatments is to teach the patient

TABLE 16–1. TREATMENT OF DRUG DEPENDENCE

	Confrontation	Detoxification	Pharmacotherapy	Psychotherapy
Sedatives	S	Diazepam or phenobarbital	Antidepressants as needed	S
Stimulants	I	Not usually needed	Antidepressants or neuroleptics	I
Opioids	M	Methadone or clonidine	Methadone, naltrexone, or antidepressants	M
Cannabis	I	None	Antidepressants as needed	I
Psychedelics	L	None	Neuroleptics as needed	L
Inhalants	A	None	None	A
Nicotine	R	Nicotine gum	None	R

alternate behaviors to drug ingestion and to enable him or her to deal more effectively with problems of living. The general physician often can convince patients to join a specialized treatment program and can collaborate in the medical aspects of the treatment. Severe forms of drug dependence, however, are best managed by a treatment team specially trained in this area of medicine.

Childress AR, McLellan AT, O'Brien CP: Behavioral therapies for substance abuse. Int J Addict 20:947, 1985. *Comprehensive review of behavioral therapies for dependence disorders.*

Woody GE, Luborsky L, McLellan AT, et al: Psychotherapy for opiate addiction: Does it help? Arch Gen Psychiatry 40:639, 1983. *Largest controlled study of psychotherapy in addiction found definite benefits for psychotherapy, and the benefits were greatest for those with significant coexisting psychiatric disorders.*

17 IMMUNIZATION

R. Gordon Douglas, Jr.

Childhood immunizations continue to receive major emphasis as methods of controlling infectious diseases. A standard recommendation for such immunizations is presented in Table 17–1. Detailed immunization recommendations for the common childhood diseases are best secured from two standard references: the current issue of the Red Book of the American Academy of Pediatrics and the Collective Immunization Recommendations by the Advisory Committee on Immunization Practices of the United States Public Health Service.

It is also important to maintain immunizations begun in childhood and to utilize those immunizations primarily intended for adults. The internist must ensure that routine immunizations such as diphtheria-tetanus and influenza are up to date and that adequate records are maintained. He also must recognize special situations that require less commonly used products or booster doses of common immunizing agents.

Both active and passive immunizing agents are available (Tables 17–2 and 17–3). Active immunization, which is most often carried out in anticipation of exposure to a disease, is achieved by using one of the following as immunogens: inactivated virus or viral protein, live attenuated virus, bacterial protein, or bacterial polysaccharides. Live attenuated virus vaccines are associated with greater and more durable immunity than inactivated viral vaccines, but this is achieved at the expense of greater inherent risks. Bacterial proteins and polysaccharides are effective immunogens, but their protective effect is not lifelong.

Passive immunization, which is used for individuals who have recently been or may soon be exposed to a disease, is achieved by using immune globulin (IG), a preparation of pooled human immune globulins that contain specified amounts of antibody against diphtheria, measles, one type of poliovirus, hepatitis A, and hepatitis B. Specific immune globulin preparations are also available, e.g., those against varicella zoster, tetanus, rabies, or hepatitis B. They are obtained from donor pools preselected for high antibody content. Human immune globulins are not associated with a risk of transmitting hepatitis A and B. They are much less likely to evoke hypersensitivity reactions than are immune globulins derived from animals. When using animal-derived antitoxins, intradermal testing for hypersensitivity should always precede their administration.

The physician must consider the risks and benefits to an individual patient when administering a vaccine or immune globulin. With regard to risks, certain general principles must be kept in mind. Hypersensitivity to any vaccine component is a contraindication to use of that vaccine. This is of most concern with vaccines grown in eggs, such as measles, mumps, and influenza vaccine. This risk may be assessed by history of ability to eat eggs without adverse effects. Although acute hypersensitivity reactions may also be a theoretic problem with vaccines grown in cell cultures, such reactions are very rare. Hypersensitivity to antibiotics (e.g., neomycin) contained in vaccines is another possible risk. However, penicillin is not used in the manufacture of any vaccine, and information concerning specific components of a vaccine is available in the package insert. Persons with acute febrile illness should not be vaccinated until they recover to avoid additive toxicity and possible diminished response.

Patients with altered immunity or household contacts of such persons should not be given live attenuated virus vaccines because of the risk of disseminated disease. In addition, live attenuated virus vaccines should not be given to pregnant women, except in rare circumstances, because of theoretic risk to the fetus.

Persons receiving live attenuated vaccines should not receive immune globulin or hyperimmune globulin simultaneously, since passively acquired antibody can interfere with the response to such vaccines. Children under 12 months of age should not be given measles, mumps, or rubella vaccines because of possible interference with antibody response by maternal antibody. Several vaccines can be given together without loss of efficacy. For example, influenza and pneumococcal vaccines may be given simultaneously (in different sites), and trivalent oral polio vaccine may be given with combined measles-mumps-rubella vaccine without alteration of antibody responses. Patients receiving intermittent immunosuppressive drugs should be given inactivated vaccines between courses of therapy to maximize antibody responses.

TETANUS. Tetanus toxoid is highly effective and provides long-lasting protection. Antitoxins persist at protective levels, for ten years or more in individuals who have received a full-immunizing series. There are four preparations; tetanus toxoid absorbed (T), tetanus and diphtheria toxoids adsorbed (for adult use) (Td), diphtheria and tetanus toxoids and pertussis vaccine (DTP), and diphtheria and tetanus toxoids adsorbed (for pediatric use) (DT). The aluminum phosphate adsorbed

TABLE 17–1. RECOMMENDED SCHEDULE FOR ACTIVE IMMUNIZATION OF NORMAL INFANTS AND CHILDREN*

Recommended Age†	Vaccines‡	Comments
2 mo	DPT-1, OPV-1	Can be given earlier in areas of high endemicity
4 mo	DPT-2, OPV-2	6-wk to 2-mo interval desired between OPV doses to avoid interference
6 mo	DPT-3	An additional dose of OPV at this time is optional in areas with a high risk of polio exposure
15 mo§	MMR, DPT-4, OPV-3	Completion of primary series of DPT and OPV
25 mo§	*Hemophilus* B polysaccharide vaccine	Can be given at 18-23 mo for children in groups who are thought to be at increased risk of disease, e.g., day-care center attendees
4–6 yr**	DPT-5, OPV-4	Preferably at or before school entry
14–16 yr	Td	Repeat every 10 yr throughout life

*From Immunization Practices Advisory Committee, Centers for Disease Control: New recommended schedule for active immunization of normal infants and children. MMWR 35:578, 1986.

†These recommended ages should not be construed as absolute; 2 mo can be 6 to 10 weeks, for example.

‡DPT = diphtheria and tetanus toxoids and pertussis vaccine. OPV = oral, attenuated poliovirus vaccine containing poliovirus types 1, 2, and 3. MMR = live measles, mumps, and rubella viruses in a combined vaccine. Td = Adult tetanus toxoid and diphtheria toxoid in combination, which contains the same dose of tetanus toxoid as DTP or DT and a reduced dose of diphtheria toxoid.

§Simultaneous administration of MMR, DTP, and OPV may be given.

**Up to the seventh birthday.

TABLE 17–2. COMMONLY USED ACTIVE IMMUNIZING AGENTS IN ADULTS

Disease	Type of Material	Preparation	Dosage Schedule*	Other Uses, Comments
Routine use for all adults:				
Tetanus	Bacterial toxoid	Tetanus toxoid combined with diphtheria toxoid, adult type (Td); tetanus toxoid (T)	IM at least every 10 yr	Management of wounds
Diphtheria	Bacterial toxoid	Diphtheria toxoid combined with tetanus toxoid, adult type (Td)	IM at least every 10 yr	Management of contacts of cases of diphtheria
Use in selected populations:				
1. *Elderly persons and persons with chronic disease*				
Influenza	Inactivated virus	Influenza virus vaccines, trivalent	SC annually	Annual immunization of high-risk individuals: persons with chronic heart or lung disease or other chronic diseases, nursing home residents, age > 65 yr; medical personnel
Pneumococcal disease	Bacterial polysaccharide	Pneumococcal polysaccharide vaccine	SC once	Immunization of high-risk persons over 2 yr of age
2. *Postexposure prophylaxis of animal bites*				
Rabies	Inactivated virus	Human diploid cell rabies vaccine (HDCV)	Five 1-ml doses	Pre-exposure prophylaxis only in special situations
3. *Adolescents and young adults*				
Rubella	Live attenuated virus	Rubella virus vaccine, live	SC once	Adolescent and adult females who are unimmunized or who have no serum antibodies; hospital workers
Measles	Live attenuated virus	Measles live vaccine	SC once	Adolescents and young adults who have not had measles and have no serum antibodies to measles or have not received previous live virus vaccine; postexposure protection.
Mumps	Live attenuated virus	Mumps virus vaccine, live	SC once	Prepubertal and adolescent males who have not had mumps or mumps vaccine
4. *Special groups*				
Hepatitis B	Inactivated virus	Hepatitis B vaccine	Three doses	Persons at high risk of exposure to hepatitis B; health care workers, hemodialysis patient, users of illicit injectable drugs; and other travelers
Poliomyelitis	Live attenuated virus	Poliovirus vaccine, live oral, trivalent (oral polio vaccine, OPV) Poliomyelitis vaccine (inactivated polio vaccine, IPV)	Three doses Three doses	Not for routine use; IPV for primary immunization of special groups of adults; OPV for boosters in special situations; need for routine booster not established

*IM = Intramuscularly; SC = subcutaneously.

preparations induce more persistent antitoxin titers than fluid forms. DTP and DT are used only for primary immunization and boosters in infants and young children. For all persons over seven years of age, Td is the immunizing preparation of choice because of the increasing frequency of reactions with age to the full dose of diphtheria toxoid contained in DT. T is available for those allergic to diphtheria toxoid. For immunization of individuals not immunized as infants, a series of three doses of Td should be given intramuscularly, the second dose four to eight weeks after the first, and the third, six months to one year after the second. A single booster immunization of Td is recommended for adults every ten years.

Tetanus Prophylaxis in Wound Management. For a clean minor wound, Td is recommended only if the history of tetanus immunization is uncertain, if fewer than three doses had previously been administered, or if it is more than ten years since the last dose. For all other wounds, Td is indicated unless the patient has received three or more doses of toxoid within five years. In addition, for those with such wounds and incomplete or uncertain vaccine status, 250 units of tetanus immune globulin (TIG) should be considered with Td in separate syringes and at separate sites. Adsorbed Td is preferred over fluid toxoid for administration with TIG because of delayed absorption of the toxoid.

DIPHTHERIA. Diphtheria immunizations significantly decrease the occurrence and severity of clinical disease. Protective levels of antibody persist for at least ten years following a primary series or booster doses of diphtheria toxoid. Diphtheria toxoid is combined with tetanus toxoid and pertussis vaccine (DTP) for use in infants and young children, or with tetanus toxoid (Td), adult type, for use in persons over seven years of age. The diphtheria component in the latter material is only 10 to 25 per cent of that in DTP. A separate diphtheria toxoid is not available in the United States. The primary and booster immunization schedules described for tetanus provide adequate protection against diphtheria.

Diphtheria Immunization for Case Contacts. All asymptomatic, unimmunized close contacts of patients with diphtheria should receive either benzathine penicillin or erythromycin as well as diphtheria toxoid. Since the risk of diphtheria is low in those receiving chemoprophylaxis, diphtheria antitoxin should not be administered. Antitoxin, which is of equine origin, may be useful in therapy of diphtheria. Immediate hypersensitivity reactions occur in 7 per cent and serum sickness in 5 per cent.

INFLUENZA. Influenza epidemics can be expected almost every winter. Immunization efforts are aimed at protecting those at greatest risk of serious illness or death. At highest risk are those with chronic heart or lung disease and residents of nursing homes and other chronic care facilities. At high risk are persons with other underlying conditions, such as asthma, malignancy, and immunosuppressive disorders, those over 65 years of age, and children on chronic aspirin therapy. More than 10,000 deaths have occurred in 18 winters between 1957 and 1986, and on several occasions the number has exceeded 40,000.

Influenza vaccines are composed of highly purified inactivated virus. Whole virion (whole virus) and subvirion (split

TABLE 17–3. PASSIVE IMMUNIZATIONS FOR ADULTS

Disease	Name of Material	Comments and Use
Tetanus	Tetanus immune globulin human (TIG)	Management of tetanus-prone wounds
Diphtheria	Diphtheria antitoxin, equine	Treatment of established disease, high frequency of reactions to serum of nonhuman origin
Rabies	Rabies immunoglobulin, human (RIG)	Postexposure prophylaxis of animal bites
Rubella	Immune globulin, human (IG)	May modify or suppress symptoms but does not prevent infection or viremia
Measles	Immune globulin, human (IG)	Prevention or modification of disease in contacts; not for control of epidemics
Hepatitis A	Immune globulin, human (IG)	Protection of household contacts; control of epidemics; pre-exposure prophylaxis for travelers
Hepatitis B	Immune globulin, human (IG) Hepatitis B immune globulin, human (HBIG)	HBIG for needle stick or mucous membrane contact with HBsAG-positive persons; HBIG for infants born to mothers with HBsAg-positive hepatitis; IG for all other contacts
Herpes zoster/Varicella	Varicella zoster immune globulin (VZIG)	Persons under 15 years of age with underlying disease who have not had varicella and who are exposed to varicella
Erythroblastosis fetalis	Rh immune globulin (RhIG)	Rh-negative women who give birth to Rh-positive infants or who abort
Hypogamma-globulinemia	Immune globulin intravenous	Maintenance therapy
Idiopathic thrombocyto-penic purpura	Immune globulin intravenous	Therapy of acute episodes
Botulism	Monovalent E antitoxin, equine Bivalent A and B antitoxin, equine Trivalent A, B, and E antitoxin, equine	Treatment of botulism trivalent is preferred; most effective is type E
Snakebite	Antivenin, equine (North American coral snake antivenin) Antivenin, equine, Crotalidae, polyvalent	Specific for North American coral snake, *Micrurus fulvius* Effective for viper and pit viper, including rattlesnakes, copperheads, moccasins
Spider bite	Antivenin, equine	Specific for black widow spider, *Latrodectus mactans*, and other members of the genus

virus) preparations are available. In children, split virus vaccines have been associated with fewer side effects than whole virus vaccines, but in adults the vaccines are comparable. Each year vaccine composition is changed to reflect the most recent serotypes circulating in the United States and worldwide. The vaccine is almost always a trivalent vaccine containing two influenza A virus strains, as well as an influenza B virus strain. The protective efficacy against both influenza A and influenza B is about 70 per cent.

A small percentage of subjects will have local reactions consisting of redness and induration, which last 1 to 2 days. Fever and other systemic symptoms occur in only 1 to 2 per cent of subjects, begin 6 to 12 hours after vaccination, and persist for 1 to 2 days. Immediate reactions are extremely rare. In addition to vaccinating those in the highest risk and high-risk categories, persons such as health care workers and family members capable of nosocomial transmission of influenza to high-risk persons should be vaccinated.

PNEUMOCOCCAL DISEASES. Pneumococcal pneumonia, meningitis, otitis media, and bacteremia occur with increased frequency in persons with sickle cell anemia, anatomic or functional asplenia, agammaglobulinemia, multiple myeloma, renal failure, cirrhosis and alcoholism, or basal skull fractures with cerebrospinal rhinorrhea. Persons with diabetes mellitus or chronic cardiorespiratory, hepatic, or renal disease and persons of increased age may also be at increased risk. Vaccine is intended for individuals who are at high risk.

A 23-valent polysaccharide vaccine containing types (Danish) 1, 2, 3, 4, 5, 6B, 7F, 8, 9N, 9V, 10A, 11A, 12F, 14, 15B, 17F, 18C, 19F, 19A, 20, 22F, 23F, 33F is available. These types have been shown to cause 90 per cent of bacteremic pneumococcal disease in the United States. Antibody responses in healthy persons over two years of age are excellent, and the vaccine has been shown to prevent pneumococcal disease. The duration of immunity is unknown. Mild local side effects occur in 50 per cent of subjects. Booster doses should not be given. Influenza and pneumococcal vaccine can be administered in different sites simultaneously without impairment of immune response or enhancement of side effects.

RABIES. ***Postexposure Prophylaxis.*** Postexposure rabies immunization should always include both passively administered antibody and vaccine, except for persons who have previously been immunized with rabies vaccine and have a documented adequate rabies antibody titer.

Rabies vaccine (human diploid) (HDCV) is an inactivated vaccine prepared from rabies virus growth in human diploid cell cultures. Rabies immune globulin, human (RIG) is antirabies gamma globulin concentrated from plasma of hyperimmunized human donors; it contains 150 international units (IU) per milliliter.

Following exposure to animals known or suspected to be rabid, five 1-ml doses of HDCV are given intramuscularly. The first dose is given as soon as possible after exposure, and additional doses are given on days 3, 7, 14, and 28 after the first dose.

At the time of the bite and concurrent wtih vaccine, RIG is administered only once at the beginning of antirabies prophylaxis to provide antibodies until the patient responds to vaccination. The dose is 20 IU per kilogram. If possible, up to half the dose of RIG should be thoroughly infiltrated in the area around the wound, and the rest should be administered intramuscularly.

Pre-exposure Immunization. Vaccine may be offered to persons in high-risk groups such as veterinarians, animal handlers, and laboratory workers. For pre-exposure immunization, three 1-ml injections of HDCV are given intramuscularly, one on each of days 0, 7, and 21 or 28. Booster doses should be given every two years for persons with continuing risk of exposure.

Adverse reactions to HDCV include local pain, erythema, swelling, and itching in about 25 per cent of patients, and mild systemic reactions such as headache, nausea, abdominal pain, muscle aches, and dizziness in about 20 per cent. Rare neurologic reactions have been reported; however, causal relationship has not been established.

RUBELLA. All persons should be immune to rubella. Evidence of immunity includes documented proof of having received vaccine or laboratory studies showing immunity, but not a clinical history of disease. All others should be vaccinated, particularly women of childbearing age and susceptible hospital workers, who, if infected, might transmit rubella to pregnant patients. Because of the theoretic risk to the fetus, females of childbearing age should receive vaccine only if they are not pregnant and must understand that they should not become pregnant for three months after vaccination. If a woman who has no immunity to rubella is pregnant, vaccine should be administered in the immediate postpartum period prior to discharge from the hospital. Administration of anti-Rho(D) immune globulin or other blood products is not a contraindication to rubella vaccination. Vaccinating susceptible children whose mothers or other household contacts are pregnant does not present a risk. Vaccination after exposure may not prevent illness, but it is not harmful.

Live attenuated rubella virus vaccine is prepared in human diploid cell cultures. It is available as a monovalent vaccine or in combination with measles (MR) or measles and mumps (MMR) vaccines. A single dose of vaccine induces antibodies in more than 95 per cent of susceptible persons, and vaccine-induced immunity is protective against clinical illness from natural exposure. Although the duration of immunity is not known, it is expected to be long term.

Rash and fever are occasional side effects. Arthralgia and transient arthritis, usually involving the small peripheral joints, may occur in up to 40 per cent of subjects. They generally begin two to ten weeks after vaccination, persist for one to three days, and rarely recur. Allergic reactions have not been associated with this vaccine, and it may be safely administered to persons with allergies to eggs, ducks, and feathers.

MEASLES. All adolescents and adults who have not had measles confirmed by a physician, who do not have laboratory evidence of measles immunity, or who have not been adequately immunized with live measles vaccine when 12 or more months of age should receive vaccine. Persons born prior to 1957 are likely to have been infected naturally and need not be vaccinated. Those vaccinated from 1963 to 1967 may have received inactivated vaccine and should be revaccinated. Persons who received live attenuated vaccine during that period, however, are considered adequately protected. Although established immunity is preferable, live measles vaccine, given within 72 hours of measles exposure, may provide protection.

Live attenuated measles virus vaccine, prepared in chick embryo cell cultures, is available as a monovalent vaccine or in combination with rubella (MR), mumps (MM), or mumps and rubella (MMR). Antibodies that are protective against measles develop in 95 per cent or more of vaccinees. The duration of protective effect, although unknown, appears to be long.

About 5 to 15 per cent of vaccinees will develop fever, beginning about the sixth day after vaccination and lasting up to five days. Transient rashes have been reported rarely. Encephalitis has been reported approximately once for every one million doses administered. No allergic reactions have been associated with the vaccine even among persons with allergies to eggs, chickens, and feathers. Measles vaccine is inactivated by heat and light; it should be stored at 2 to 8°C and protected from light to avoid vaccine failure.

Immune globulin (IG) has been shown to be effective in preventing or modifying measles in a susceptible person exposed less than six days previously. The dose is 0.25 ml per kilogram of body weight. Live measles vaccine can be given after three months. Although effective in individuals, IG should not be used instead of live measles virus vaccine to control epidemics.

MUMPS. Although mumps is generally self-limited, it may be moderately debilitating; and complications involving the central nervous system, including deafness, occur rarely. Orchitis may occur in up to 20 per cent of clinical mumps cases in postpubertal males, but sterility is rare. Susceptible adolescents and adults should be vaccinated against mumps unless otherwise contraindicated. Susceptibility can be determined by documentation of disease by a physician or laboratory or by documented immunization with live mumps vaccine when the subject was 12 months or more of age. Mumps vaccine is not recommended for persons born prior to 1957, because they are likely to have been infected naturally and generally may be considered immune. Live attenuated mumps virus vaccine, prepared in chick embryo cell cultures, induces antibodies in over 90 per cent of recipients. The duration of immunity is unknown but is probably long lasting. Side effects are very rare and include allergic reactions, rash, and pruritus. No deaths have been reported.

HEPATITIS. Hepatitis B vaccine consists of purified inactivated hepatitis B surface antigen (HBsAg) particles obtained from chronic carriers or HBsAg made by genetically engineered yeast. Most data are available with the older vaccine. It is indicated for persons at high risk of exposure to hepatitis B, such as health care workers exposed to blood or blood products, hemodialysis patients, homosexual males, users of illicit injectable drugs, recipients of certain blood products, certain institutionalized individuals, household or sexual contacts of chronic carriers of HBsAg, and some international travelers. Vaccine is administered intramuscularly in three 20-μg doses at time 0, month 1, and month 6. Vaccine must be given in the deltoid; antibody responses are lower when the vaccine is given in the buttocks. Immunosuppressed and hemodialysis patients should receive 40-μg doses. Doses are one half of this value with the new recombinant vaccine. Efficacy is 80 to 95 per cent up to two years after vaccination. Local reactions and low-grade fever are mild and infrequent. There is no evidence of association with subsequent development of acquired immunodeficiency syndrome (AIDS). There are no contraindications, and there is no risk to those who are carriers or already immune.

Immune globulin (IG) offers effective protection against the clinical manifestations of hepatitis A. When exposure has occurred, 0.02 ml per kilogram of IG is given intramuscularly to persons with close personal contact who have not had hepatitis A. Usually, this means household or day care, but not school, hospital, office, or factory contacts. However, when outbreaks occur that are related to a school or institution, IG may be used to protect contacts. It should be given as early as possible after exposure but may be given up to two weeks thereafter, and protection will be achieved in approximately 80 to 90 per cent of the contacts. It is also useful for pre-exposure prophylaxis for travelers.

For hepatitis B, two preparations are available: IG and hepatitis B immunoglobulin (HBIG). IG produced since 1977 contains anti–hepatitis B antibodies. It may reduce the clinical severity of hepatitis B infection when infection is contracted by the percutaneous or oral route with a small viral inoculum. HBIG is prepared from donor pools preselected for high titer of antibody to hepatitis B (titer >1:100,000). It is recommended for acute exposure following a needle contact or a mucous membrane contact with HBsAg-positive blood. The dose is 0.06 ml per kilogram administered as soon as possible but within 24 hours, and a second dose is administered 25 to 30 days after the first. If HBIG is not available, IG may be given in the same dosage schedule. The first dose (20 μg) of a three-dose vaccine regimen should also be given. For infants born to mothers who are antigen (HBsAG) positive, 0.5 ml, together with hepatitis B vaccine (10 μg), given within 12 hours is recommended. Second and third doses of vaccine should be given at month 1 and month 6. Women at high risk should be screened prenatally for HBsAG. HBIG does not prevent maternal transmission. HBIG may also be used for those with sexual contact with HBsAG-positive persons.

POLIOMYELITIS. The risk of paralytic poliomyelitis is very small in the United States today, but it is important to maintain immunity of the population to prevent further outbreaks.

Routine primary vaccination of adults in the United States is not necessary. Most adults are already immune by virtue of wild-type poliovirus infection or prior vaccination. Vaccine is recommended in the following adults: laboratory workers handling specimens that may contain polioviruses, health care workers who are in close contact with patients who may be excreting polioviruses, and members of communities or specific population groups with disease caused by wild polioviruses. There are no data to substantiate a harmful effect of vaccine on the fetus, but it is advisable to avoid vaccination during pregnancy if possible. Immunocompromised patients, or household contacts of such patients, should not be given vaccine because of their substantially increased risk of vaccine-associated disease. Inactivated vaccine is safe in such patients, although development of protective immune response does not always occur.

Two types of poliovirus vaccines are currently licensed in the United States: oral polio vaccine (OPV) and inactivated polio vaccine (IPV). Both contain all three poliovirus types. The effectiveness of these vaccines is attested to by the dramatic decline in poliomyelitis since their introduction. For primary immunization of normal adults and young children, OPV is preferred because it induces intestinal immunity, is simple to administer, is well accepted by patients, and results in immunization of some contacts. For children it is usually given beginning at two months of age—an exception to the rule that maternal antibody interferes with development of protective antibody following live attenuated virus vaccines.

For adults who were not previously vaccinated, IPV may be considered because the risk of vaccine-associated paralysis following OPV is slightly higher in adults than in children, although it is exceedingly low in both groups. Three doses of IPV should be given at intervals of 1 to 2 months, and a fourth dose at 6 to 12 months after the third. For those who previously received only one or two doses of vaccine, the remaining required doses of either vaccine, regardless of interval, should be given. For those who have had a complete course, a booster dose of OPV may be given for high-risk individuals, but the need for such doses has not been established. Nonimmune parents of infants who are given OPV need not be vaccinated, but there is an exceedingly small risk of OPV-associated paralysis. Therefore, some physicians may wish to give these adults two doses of IPV one month apart or the full series before children receive OPV. If immediate protection is needed, OPV is recommended. IPV has not been associated with serious side effects in the past 20 years.

MENINGOCOCCAL DISEASE. Vaccines against *Neisseria meningitidis* serogroups A, C, Y, and W135 are now available in the United States. Routine vaccination against meningococcal disease is not recommended. The vaccines are reserved to control outbreaks of meningococcal disease caused by one of these serotypes. In the event of an epidemic caused by these serogroups, the population at risk should be identified by some reasonable boundary, and all residents or those at highest risk should be vaccinated. Vaccination should also be considered an adjunct to antibiotic chemoprophylaxis for household contacts of persons with meningococcal disease caused by these serogroups.

Four vaccines are available: monovalent A, monovalent C, bivalent A and C, and multivalent A, C, Y, and W135 combined. They are chemically defined antigens consisting of purified bacterial capsular polysaccharides, each inducing specific serogroup immunity. They have been shown to induce protective antibodies in more than 95 per cent of susceptible persons. A single dose of vaccine is sufficient. Local reactions to the vaccine are infrequent and mild, and serious side effects have not been reported.

***HAEMOPHILUS INFLUENZAE* TYPE B DISEASE.** *H. influenza* type B is the most common cause of bacterial meningitis in the United States, occurring mostly among children less than five years of age. In addition, other serious infections occur with this pathogen: epiglottitis, sepsis, cellulitis, septic arthritis, osteomyelitis, pericarditis, and pneumonia. Recently, a vaccine composed of the purified capsular polysaccharide of *H. influenzae* type B has been licensed. Over 90 per cent of children more than two years of age develop protective levels (0.15 μg per milliliter) of antibody in response to this vaccine.

It is recommended for all children at 24 months of age. For those at high risk, vaccination at 19 months may be considered. At present, insufficient data are available to recommend routine use in older children and adults at high risk of *H. influenzae* type disease.

Mild local reactions lasting less than 24 hours have occurred in up to 50 per cent and systemic or febrile reactions in fewer than 1 per cent. It may be given simultaneously with DTP.

TYPHOID. Routine administration of typhoid vaccine is no longer recommended for persons in the United States. Selective immunization is indicated for persons with intimate exposure to a documented typhoid carrier such as would occur with continued household contact. There is no reason to use typhoid vaccine for persons in areas of natural disaster such as floods or in rural summer camps. The adult dosage is 0.5 ml subcutaneously on two occasions, separated by four or more weeks.

TUBERCULOSIS. An attenuated strain of *Mycobacterium bovis*, bacille Calmette Guérin (BCG), may be protective against infection with *Mycobacterium tuberculosis.* It is not recommended for general use in this country. It is reserved for uninfected persons living in unavoidable contact with an uncontrolled infected person, or for groups with excessive rates of new infection that cannot be controlled by other measures. Excessive rates have been defined as more than 30 cases per 10,000 population.

OTHER DISEASES FOR WHICH ACTIVE IMMUNIZATIONS ARE AVAILABLE. A number of other vaccines licensed in the United States are used only for laboratory or field personnel working with the infectious agent or for other persons with unusual occupational exposure. These include cholera vaccine, smallpox vaccine, plague vaccine, anthrax vaccine, and Rocky Mountain spotted fever vaccine. Live virus vaccines for control of adenovirus types 4, 7, and 21 are available for military but not civilian use. Adenovirus vaccines are not attenuated, but rather produce immunity without disease when introduced into the gastrointestinal tract instead of the respiratory tract, the natural portal of entry.

VARICELLA. Varicella zoster immune globulin (VZIG) is prepared from pooled plasma containing high titers of antibody to varicella virus and is intended primarily for susceptible, immunodeficient children after significant exposure to chickenpox or zoster. VZIG is effective in preventing or modifying varicella infection in immunodeficient patients if administered within 96 hours after exposure. Because of the short supply of VZIG, it is distributed through regional blood centers, and its use is restricted to persons with one of the following illnesses or conditions: leukemia or lymphoma, congenital or acquired immunodeficiency, immunosuppressive treatment, or newborns of mothers who had onset of chickenpox less than five days before delivery or within 48 hours after delivery. In addition, exposure to chickenpox or varicella must have been via household contact, playmate contact, hospital contact, or contact between mother and newborn. The recipient should have a negative or unknown prior history of chickenpox and, for most purposes, be less than 15 years of age, since few patients 15 years of age or more are at risk of infection. The recommended dosage of VZIG is one vial for each 10 kg (22 lb) of body weight, up to a maximum of five vials. Thus, it would be advisable to screen immunodeficient children with a negative or unknown history of chickenpox for antibody to varicella zoster virus when first seen or first hospitalized, to avoid unnecessary administration of VZIG.

ERYTHROBLASTOSIS FETALIS. Rh immune globulin (RhIG) is effective in preventing erythroblastosis fetalis. RhIG is prepared from donors with high Rh antibody titer. It is recommended for Rh-negative women who give birth to Rh-positive infants or who undergo abortion. A single dose should be given within 72 hours after exposure, be it for delivery or abortion. Immunosuppression is transient, and RhIG may be required for Rh-negative women after each birth or abortion.

IMMUNE DEFICIENCY STATES. Intravenous immune globulin offers several advantages over intramuscular preparations: Therapeutic plasma levels can be achieved immediately, and dosage is not limited by muscle mass or bleeding tendencies. Such preparations contain antibodies to most common bacterial and viral pathogens.

Intravenous immune globulin has been shown to be useful in immunodeficiency states and in idiopathic thrombocytopenic purpura (ITP). For prophylaxis in immunodeficiency states, the usual dose is 100 to 200 mg per kilogram monthly. In patients with ITP, a dose of 400 mg per kilogram daily for five days is usual.

BOTULISM. Several preparations of equine antitoxin for passive immunization against *Clostridium botulinum* toxin are available; trivalent containing A, B, and E antitoxins; bivalent A and B; and monovalent E antitoxins. Although the effectiveness of these preparations in treatment is not well established, their use is recommended. The trivalent antitoxin is preferred because of its broader coverage and higher content of antibody. It is available from the Centers for Disease Control. One to three vials of this antiserum should be given intramuscularly as early as possible when botulism is suspected. Twenty per cent of patients will have untoward reactions. Testing for hypersensitivity should always precede its use.

SNAKEBITE. Specific antivenin is effective in neutralizing the systemic effects of snakebite. Two preparations are available: One is polyvalent for snakes of the Crotalidae family, including rattlesnakes, copperheads, moccasins, pit vipers, and vipers; the second is specific for coral snake, *Micrurus fulvius*, bites.

SPIDER BITES. A specific antivenin is highly effective for treatment of systemic effects following bites by the black widow spider, *Latrodectus mactans*, and other members of the genus. The dose is one vial (2.5 ml) intramuscularly.

Hollinger FB, Troisi CL, Pepe PE: Anti-HBs responses to vaccination with a human hepatitis B vaccine made by recombinant DNA technology in yeast. J Infect Dis 153:156, 1986. *Report of duration and magnitude of the antibody responses to new recombinant hepatitis.*

Immunization Practices Advisory Committee, Centers for Disease Control: General recommendations on immunization. Ann Intern Med 98:615, 1983. *Definitions, principles, and routine childhood immunization schedules.*

Immunization Practices Advisory Committee, Centers for Disease Control: Diphtheria, tetanus, and pertussis, guidelines for vaccine prophylaxis and other preventive measures. Recommendation of the Immunization Practices Advisory Committee. Ann Intern Med 103:896, 1985. *Good review of disease and preventive measures.*

Immunization Practices Advisory Committee, Centers for Disease Control: Recommendations for protection against viral hepatitis. Morbidity and Mortality Weekly Report 34:313, 1985. *Summary of nomenclature, risks, vaccine usage, and IG and HBIG usage in hepatitis A, B, non A–non B, and delta.*

Immunization Practices Advisory Committee, Centers for Disease Control: Prevention and control of influenza. Morbidity and Mortality Weekly Report 35:317, 1986. *Presents new strategy for prevention and control of influenza: prioritization of patients.*

Immunization Practices Advisory Committee, Centers for Disease Control: New recommended schedule for active immunization of normal infants and children. Morbidity and Mortality Weekly Report, 35:577, 1986.

18 THE PREVENTIVE HEALTH EXAMINATION

Gary D. Friedman

The primary purpose of preventive health examinations is to maintain or improve health. The rationale is that early detection of disease or of high risk of subsequent disease can lead to treatment or remedial measures that will prevent or postpone morbidity, disability, or mortality.

An "annual physical" for asymptomatic adults was once accepted as good medical practice. In recent years periodic health examinations have become controversial: (1) The costs of a thorough medical history, physical examination, and standard laboratory tests would be enormous if these procedures were annually and universally applied. (2) Many elements of traditional checkups have not been shown to benefit asymptomatic persons. On the other hand, certain simple examination procedures and screening tests can prolong life and prevent disability.

ROUTINE TESTS AND PROCEDURES OF PROVEN OR PROBABLE VALUE IN PREVENTIVE CARE FOR ADULTS. A test is suitable for routine use if it can detect a serious and relatively common disease at an early stage, or at a predisease high-risk stage, when treatment or intervention would be more effective. Furthermore, the test should be relatively economical in terms of both money and professional time. Although controversy continues about some, a few tests or procedures meet these criteria; a few others are of probable value but less universally accepted (Table 18–1).

Routine chest radiographs can now be justified only in settings where tuberculosis is common; they have not proved to be effective in reducing mortality from lung cancer. Although still controversial because of poor sensitivity and specificity, a tonometry test for glaucoma may also be of net benefit. Doubts about tests of probable value revolve primarily around the benefits of treatment compared with the harm of labeling (e.g., mild asymptomatic diabetes mellitus), the high relative frequency and high cost of evaluating false-positive results (e.g., occult blood in the stool), and the low yield of significant disease in the asymptomatic patient (e.g., palpating the abdomen).

ADDITIONAL BENEFITS OF PREVENTIVE HEALTH APPRAISALS. Detecting disease or abnormalities is not the only benefit of the preventive health examination. Negative findings are also of value in the reassurance they provide to the patient, especially if the patient has received what he or she perceives to be a thorough examination. In contemplating cuts in the content of routine checkups, physicians and health care planners must weigh the immediate economic gains against the possible decrease in this reassurance if patients perceive the examinations to be abbreviated or cursory.

A lengthy and thorough examination when a patient is first seen permits collection of baseline data that may be useful when symptoms develop later. For example, an electrocardio-

TABLE 18–1. THE PREVENTIVE HEALTH EXAMINATION

Of Accepted Value	Of Probable Value
Medical History of:	
1. Smoking, particularly cigarettes	1. Postmenopausal uterine bleeding
2. Drinking alcohol to excess	2. Immunization status
3. Failure to wear seatbelts	3. Use of nonmedicinal drugs other than alcohol
	4. Lack of regular physical activity
Physical Examination:	
1. Assessment of obesity	1. Search for cancers or precancerous lesions of the skin, mouth and pharynx, thyroid, abdomen, testes, uterus, prostate, and lymph nodes
2. Measurement of blood pressure	
3. Search for cancer or precancerous lesions of the breast and rectum	
Laboratory or Diagnostic Studies:	
1. Mammography in women at least 50 years of age	1. Hemoglobin or hematocrit
	2. Test of stool for occult blood
2. Sigmoidoscopy for cancer or polyps	3. Baseline electrocardiogram
	4. Blood glucose
3. Papanicolaou test for cervical cancer	5. Tuberculin skin test (in high-risk groups)
4. Serum cholesterol concentration	
5. Serologic test for latent syphilis and a cervical culture for gonorrhea (in individuals at high risk for venereal disease)	

gram, recorded when the patient is young and healthy, provides a useful benchmark for evaluating electrocardiograms taken later if chest pain or arrhythmia occurs. Also, the additional time spent in obtaining a medical and social history, examining the patient, and discussing the patient's concerns helps to establish a good doctor-patient relationship. Further, certain valuable information can be obtained during a thorough first examination and need not be sought routinely again. A good example is rheumatic heart disease detected by history and cardiac auscultation.

MULTIPHASIC AND SELECTIVE SCREENING. Screening tests aimed at early disease detection are sometimes offered singly, as in special programs to detect tuberculosis, diabetes mellitus, or breast cancer. Clearly it is more economical and efficient to test for several diseases at a single visit than for single diseases at several visits. Multiphasic screening provides several tests comparatively economically at one patient visit and can be used as part of a periodic health examination. Components of health screening or health examinations may be used for some patients and not others, depending on previous findings, risk characteristics, past medical history, or current symptoms of the patient. For example, once a baseline electrocardiogram has been taken, it need not be repeated at each succeeding health examination unless it initially revealed an abnormality or unless cardiovascular symptoms or indicators of high risk occur. This use of screening tests is known as selective or discriminate screening.

FREQUENCY OF EXAMINATIONS. It is not clear how frequently preventive health examinations, either basic or thorough, should be performed. The physician must strike a balance between excessive costs and low yield of too frequent examinations, and the chance that an important and controllable condition will develop and become irreversible if examinations are not provided often enough. Several sets of recommendations have been made recently based on available evidence and "prudent" judgment (see references). A common theme is that the incidence of most disabling and fatal diseases increases with age. Thus, basic examinations containing essential tests such as blood pressure measurement and breast palpation should increase in frequency from once in several years in the patient's twenties to annually in the fifties or sixties and older. As age advances it is advisable to observe the patient for losses in hearing, vision, and mental functioning as well. Even if losses are irreversible, knowledge of these limitations will aid in advising the patient and his or her family. Clearly, in our present state of knowledge, clinical judgment must play an important role both in deciding on the frequency of examinations and in selecting examination components for individual patients based on their age, sex, past medical history, and current risk status.

A health examination is of little value without appropriate follow-up, including treatment of early disease if indicated and counseling to encourage favorable changes in risk factors and a healthier lifestyle.

American Cancer Society: Report on the cancer-related health checkup. CA 30:194, 1980. *This is a critical evaluation of methods of early detection of cancer.*

Breslow L, Somers AR: The lifetime health-monitoring program: A practical approach to preventive medicine. N Engl J Med 296:601, 1977. *This review of health examinations contains recommendations that emphasize a changing approach for different age groups and the need for cost-effective preventive measures.*

Canadian Task Force on the Periodic Health Examination (Spitzer W, chairman): The periodic health examination. Can Med Assoc J 121:1193, 1979; 130:1276, 1984; 134:721, 1986. *This is a summary of a thorough review of various components of preventive health examinations and preventive care. The need for a selective rather than a routine approach is emphasized.*

Council on Scientific Affairs, Division of Scientific Activities, American Medical Association: Medical evaluation of healthy persons. JAMA 249: 1626, 1983. *This is a brief compilation of recommendations concerning health examinations at all ages, reviewed in the context of current and previous positions of the American Medical Association.*

Frame PS: A critical review of adult health maintenance. J Fam Pract 22:341, 417, 511; 23:29, 1986. *This is a recently updated and very readable review of major elements of the adult health examination with specific recommendations.*

Medical Practice Committee, American College of Physicians: Periodic health examination: A guide for designing individualized preventive health care in the asymptomatic patient. Ann Intern Med 95:729, 1981. *This review of periodic health examinations provides a diagrammatic summary of recommendations that are viewed as minimal preventive measures to be applied to apparently well asymptomatic individuals at low medical risk.*

19 THE HEALTH OF THE PHYSICIAN

Linda Hawes Clever

Physicians are a curious lot. On the one hand, they have decreased major health risks by not smoking. On the other hand, they usually avoid having immunizations for rubella and hepatitis B, illnesses that can be devastating both to them and to their patients. The purpose of this chapter is to review available data about the lives, deaths, and personal health practices of physicians and to make recommendations about health maintenance activities for physicians.

PHYSICIANS' WORK

Physicians work harder than most people. They work 15 hours per week longer than other professionals; take less vacation time (four weeks per year versus eight weeks per year for most other professionals); and work more years than the general population and therefore have a shorter retirement (3.1 years versus 7.8 years). They also have unique responsibilities and duties.

Demands of Practice

Physicians cite special pressures generated by patients and patients' families. These include unwarranted but firmly held expectations of cure, relief, or certainty. Physicians are disturbed by inflicting pain during diagnostic tests, coping with their own minor or grievous errors, and dealing with dying patients. Physicians feel angry or guilty about work with "difficult" patients or being unable to answer questions. They dislike medical politics, paperwork, and committee work. Public policy changes spawn concerns about preserving the quality of patient care, competition from other physicians and health practitioners, independence, the funding of both research and graduate medical education, and income maintenance. Professional liability casts a long shadow, with a 10 per cent increase per year in medical malpractice suits. The world changes rapidly; morale wavers.

Family and Lifestyle Tensions and Pleasures

It has been said that physicians have one of the few socially acceptable reasons for abandoning a family. The rigors of being "on call" (albeit occurring less frequently now as more physicians enter group and hospital- or institution-based practice) can interfere with family plans. Laser-focus on professional responsibilities leads to muddled values, constricted relationships, and stunted personal growth. Taxing schedules can clash with parenting and squelch creativity. Even reading for pleasure, attending church, and exercise may be squeezed out by the time or priority crunch.

Fairness requires comments on the "other" side. Although continuation of high prestige and income may be uncertain and pressures mount, there are numerous intrinsic pleasures in the medical profession. Making precision diagnoses, teaching, counseling, providing support and motivation, and, indeed, ameliorating suffering, treating disease, and saving lives are noted by physicians to be particularly satisfying. Developing personal relationships with patients and their families and earning a good living have appeal. Working with people during existential crises and dealing with the most private aspects of their lives and bodies provide staggering yet exhilarating experiences.

PHYSICIANS' HEALTH

Overall Mortality

Unfortunately, data about health status of physicians are scattered and rarely provide comparisons with other professionals. It is possible to infer, however, that despite the complexities and challenges of physicians' work and lives, *they are at least as healthy as the general population in most respects.*

Age-specific death rates for physicians are less than those for the white male population in the United States. On the whole, (1) the age-related mortality of male physicians has had a 61 per cent decline since 1929; (2) male physicians had 25 per cent less mortality and female physicians had 16 per cent less mortality than the white United States population compared by age and sex (Goodman study). Firm conclusions about the relative longevity of specialists and nonspecialists await further studies.

Disease-Specific Mortality

TOBACCO-RELATED ILLNESS. About one third of Americans smoke; fewer than 10 per cent of physicians smoke; and fewer than 5 per cent of physicians under 30 years of age smoke. Cigarette smoking is a grave health hazard (Ch. 11). Since physicians have usually smoked less than the general public and smoke far less now, it is not surprising that *smoking-related mortality among physicians is plummeting.* Deaths from lung cancer in male physicians in California halved between 1950 to 1959 and 1970 to 1979; other smoking-related diseases had striking declines (bronchitis, chronic obstructive pulmonary disease, and cancers of the esophagus and mouth). Although the incidence of fatal arteriosclerotic cardiovascular disease among physicians *was* higher than in the general population, it is now lower.

SUICIDES. On the darker side, *early death from suicide* appears to be excessive among physicians. Numbers are impressive for the general population: Suicides account for about 18 deaths per 100,000 in males and about 5 deaths per 100,000 in females. These figures combine to make suicide the eighth commonest cause of death in this country. Despite numerous methodologic problems, some generalizations about suicide by physicians are warranted. Male physicians probably commit suicide twice as often as the United States white male population. Female physicians take their own lives at a rate slightly more than triple that of white American women who are not physicians. Differences in suicide rates by specialty have not been verified because of inadequate sample size, although there is a suggestion of an increased incidence among psychiatrists. Professionals in other health sciences such as dentistry and pharmacy have substantially higher suicide rates than physicians. Similar results have been found in England and Wales. Overall, however, data are marred by incorrect reporting or under-reporting, small numbers, and inadequate comparison groups by age, sex, and profession. Speculations to explain existing data are plentiful. It is not surprising that physicians may have the same sorts of characteristics that drive others to suicide. These include a variety of family-related markers such as (1) death of a close relative during childhood or thereafter, (2) being single, and (3) excessive or incomplete integration into a family unit. Depression is an extremely important element (see Ch. 462). Other psychiatric diagnoses such as severe personality disorder or psychosis may also be causative. A history of a prior suicide attempt serves as a warning of high suicide risk. Financial problems, poor health, and substance abuse often contribute as well. Special problems that may incline physicians toward suicide include professional isolation, the tensions of training or practice, unrealistic expectations, rifts in relationships, the exhaustion and emotional burdens of patient care, and pre-existing psychiatric vulnerability.

Morbidity

The age-specific death rate of physicians is lower than that of other Americans, but it could be even better if several factors were not in effect. For example, most physicians *do not have their own doctor* who can provide health promotion and surveillance. Fortunately, from the standpoint of risk management, two thirds of physicians in their fifties and above have routine health examinations. Self-treatment, curbstone consultations, and delays because of embarrassment about professional courtesy can impede diagnosis and treatment. Denial may slow care. A pathologic extension of denial is the "physician invulnerability syndrome," which is characterized by the conviction that the personal and family problems, the aggravations, and the diseases that affect others cannot or will not affect the physician. Fear plays an important part in this "syndrome."

Substance Abuse

There is considerable reason for concern about the incidence of alcohol and drug abuse among physicians. Reliable, recent statistics are scarce, however. Past studies have suggested that alcoholism among physicians is at least double that of the general population (see Ch. 15). Current literature supports parity. Drug abuse may be somewhat more prevalent among physicians than other Americans. Regardless of population comparisons, of course, *substance abuse is a deadly problem for physicians, their families, and their patients.* Damage to patients resulting from confusion, inattention, poor judgment, unavailability, or psychomotor deficits often occurs before the physician seeks, or is forced, into care. A substantial majority of physicians in impaired physician rehabilitation programs are under treatment for drug and/or alcohol abuse alone. Automobile and private plane accidents are associated with intoxication, as are family dissolution and substance abuse in children of abusers (see Ch. 16). Although denial seems to play a major role at the inception of addiction ("I won't get hooked; *I'm* not susceptible"), and denial makes therapy more challenging, physicians seem to have a better prognosis, with treatment, than other middle-class substance abusers.

PERSONAL HEALTH PRACTICES OF PHYSICIANS

Many health promotion efforts for adults target smoking cessation, good nutrition, exercise, and moderation of alcohol intake. Immunization for adults is also receiving attention. Seatbelt use has been touted by national agencies, the media, and various professional groups and societies. The exceptional record of physicians in smoking avoidance has already been described, but other health habits seem to be less exemplary. For example, although most physicians report that they are careful about dietary fat, calories, and/or salt, 29 to 58 per cent acknowledge that they are overweight. Thirty-seven to 73 per cent of physicians do not engage in weekly vigorous exercise; indeed, gardening is a favorite recreation. Although moderation in frequency and volume of alcohol consumption is the norm, 13 to 24 per cent of physicians drink daily, and 20 per cent have at least two drinks when they do drink. Up to 10 per cent of physicians may be problem drinkers.

Immunization

By and large, physicians have an abysmal record of immunization for diseases that can affect them or that they can transmit. For example, between only 10 and 31 per cent of rubella antibody–negative physicians who work with children, pregnant women, and other patients receive rubella vaccine. At least 84 per cent of physicians are susceptible to hepatitis B (and, therefore, delta hepatitis), but very few house officers or attending physicians receive hepatitis B vaccine. The incidence of immunization of physicians for tetanus/diphtheria, polio, and influenza is unknown. Since health risks and costs are low, results are favorable, and the professional liability of not being vaccinated is high, wise physicians get vaccinated.

Seatbelt Use

Seatbelt use by physicians is the least well-documented good health habit. In one study, physicians did use seatbelts more often than did attorneys. One might extrapolate from other factors that correlate with seatbelt use (such as educational level, regular visits to a dentist, and nonsmoking) that physicians buckle up more often than others. Such a practice would be felicitous, since (1) many physicians drive hundreds of miles per week; (2) each American has a one in three chance of being disabled by an automobile injury during his or her lifetime; (3) always using a seatbelt can reduce the risk of serious injury or death by greater than one half.

Effects of Good Health Habits by the Physician on Others

Good health practices not only improve the health and lives of physicians themselves but also can affect others as well. As implied above, moderation of alcohol use and eschewing of drug use by physicians can prevent direct harm to patients. Vaccination of physicians can prevent transmission of infectious diseases. Smoking cessation by physicians can even decrease injury to others by reducing side-stream smoke. Of great importance is the observation that *physicians' personal health habits help determine advice that they give to patients.* Physicians with good health habits (regarding smoking, weight, exercise, and alcohol) are likely to counsel primary prevention; physicians with poor health habits are unlikely to provide any health promotion advice, nor do they even counsel tertiary prevention.

TABLE 19–1. SUGGESTIONS TO PHYSICIANS ABOUT GOOD HEALTH

Do:
1. Get help when you need it. Don't deny; don't delay.
2. Fasten your seatbelt—always.
3. Get antibody screening and appropriate vaccination for hepatitis B, tetanus/diphtheria, influenza, rubella, pneumonia, polio, and measles.
4. Practice moderation in diet and alcohol intake.
5. Exercise regularly and sensibly.
6. Engage fully in the pageantry of living in activities with your family, friends, and community.
7. Cultivate your creativity; be interested, not just interesting, and use your sense of humor.
8. Start planning for your retirement 25 to 30 years before your goal.
   a. Feel free to relish your profession, and if you don't, consider important changes.
   b. Get reputable, professional help with financial planning.

Do not:
1. Smoke.
2. Use nonprescribed drugs.
3. Ignore your family and friends in the frenzy of serving others or meeting their demands.
4. Short-circuit your own needs for personal and intellectual growth.
5. Be only a physician—be a person.

RECOMMENDATIONS

Basically, physicians, in concert with their own physician and family, need to analyze their own health and health behavior (Table 19–1). They need to assess pain and pleasure, risks and benefits. If change is necessary or desirable, a plan needs to be developed. Barriers need to be removed, incentives and rewards incorporated, and progress documented and celebrated.

Clever LH, Arsham GM: Physicians' own health—some advice for the advisors. West J Med 141:846, 1984. *This review article covers a broad spectrum of morbidity and mortality statistics and personal health habits of physicians. It also makes specific recommendations for good health in physicians.*

Goodman LJ: The longevity and mortality of American physicians, 1969–1973. Milbank Mem Fund Q 53:353, 1975. *This paper is a classic because of its statistical methods and breadth and depth of coverage. Sex, age, geography, and medical specialty are analyzed.*

McAuliffe WE, Rohman M, Santangelo S, et al.: Psychoactive drug use among practicing physicians and medical students. N Engl J Med 315:805, 1986. *This well-referenced research paper shows that physicians' use of psychoactive drugs is not too different from that of other professionals. High drug use by younger physicians and poor education of most physicians about drugs and alcohol are a call to action to avoid expanding physician impairment, however.*

Linn LS, Yager J, Cope D, et al.: Health habits and coping behaviors among practicing physicians. West J Med 144:484, 1986. *This thorough and refreshing paper explores the complex, arcane interactions of physicians' health habits and emotional health. It can be a cornerstone of further research and understanding of physicians' behavior.*

Roy A: Suicide in doctors. Psychiatry Clin North Am 8:377, 1985. *Its important topic, incisive commentary, and 44 references make this short paper especially useful.*

PART IV

PRINCIPLES OF DIAGNOSIS AND MANAGEMENT

20 CLINICAL APPROACH TO THE PATIENT

William L. Morgan, Jr.

The scientific basis of medical practice is well established, but only recently has the time-honored *art of medicine* come under scientific scrutiny. Medical educators are now beginning to understand how a physician relates to a patient and are introducing new ways to teach noncognitive skills. Data-gathering skills of interviewing and physical examination can be taught with standardized patients or a videotape. Strategies to select and interpret laboratory tests make the diagnosis of disease more scientific. Problem-oriented records have improved the organization and display of medical information. Understanding the role of a physician enables one to adapt such innovations to medical practice. What follows is a description of the abilities needed by a physician to care for a patient.

A task force of the American Board of Internal Medicine studied clinical competence in internal medicine by analyzing the components of the medical encounter (Tables 20–1 and 20–2). Knowledge, skills, and attitudes are the abilities required of a physician caring for a patient. The major tasks involved in solving a medical problem include data gathering, diagnosis, and patient care.

ABILITIES REQUIRED OF A PHYSICIAN

Noncognitive Abilities

Appropriate attitudes, habits, and interpersonal skills are important abilities needed to develop a positive physician-patient relationship. Without effective attitudes and interpersonal skills, and despite keen intellect and medical knowledge, a physician can fail in relating to and caring for a patient. The physician who is motivated primarily by concern for the patient's welfare is more likely to provide the conditions for an effective relationship. The essence of this relationship has never been better stated than in Peabody's classic 1927 article: "One of the essential qualities of the clinician is interest in humanity, for the secret of the care of the patient is caring for the patient."

ATTITUDES AND HABITS. Humanistic qualities, the assumption of responsibility, and continuing scholarship are among the major expectations of a physician. Humanistic qualities include integrity, respect, and compassion for the patient. Moral and ethical values are also essential components of clinical competence. Despite patients' psychological handicaps and failure to comply with treatment, the effective physician is sympathetic and nonjudgmental.

The assumption of full responsibility for the care of a patient is a fundamental requirement of the competent physician. This responsibility includes continuing care despite personal inconvenience and emotional demands of the patient. The physician is committed to doing what is best for the patient, and, when necessary, seeks the help of others.

Continuing scholarship is also an essential requirement of an effective physician. Rapid advances in medical sciences, and the resulting diagnostic and therapeutic innovations, make obsolete yesterday's method of medical practice. Each individual learns to recognize deficiencies in knowledge and adopts a plan to keep up with new information. This plan includes reading journals and texts, attending courses and hospital teaching rounds, and undertaking self-study programs. Continuing scholarship requires self-discipline to set aside personal time on a regular basis. An effective way to learn is to pursue knowledge about the disease at the time one sees a patient with a specific illness.

INTERPERSONAL SKILLS. Being able to relate to the patient, to family members, and to others caring for the patient is of particular importance. The ability to communicate well is the basis for effective interpersonal relationships. This communication includes encouraging the patient to share symptoms and personal concerns. One should be aware of nonverbal messages that convey significant information about emotional problems. The physician also has the obligation to transmit information to the patient about the illness itself and about its prognosis and treatment. Competence means communicating well despite intellectual, socioeconomic, and language barriers.

It is a responsibility of the physician to talk with family members, while at the same time respecting patient confiden-

TABLE 20–1. ABILITIES REQUIRED OF A PHYSICIAN

- Noncognitive abilities
  - Attitudes and habits
  - Interpersonal skills
  - Motor and technical skills
- Intellectual abilities
  - Knowledge
  - Organization
  - Synthesis
  - Clinical judgment

Modified from American Board of Internal Medicine: Clinical competence in internal medicine. Ann Intern Med 90:403, 1979.

TABLE 20–2. TASKS REQUIRED OF A PHYSICIAN

- Data gathering
  - Medical history
  - Physical examination
  - Diagnostic studies
- Diagnosis or problem definition
- Medical care

Modified from American Board of Internal Medicine: Clinical competence in internal medicine. Ann Intern Med 90:403, 1979.

tiality. Knowing with whom to talk and how much to say requires considerable skill. The competent physician also communicates effectively with others caring for the patient. This interpersonal skill includes the ability to present the patient's problem orally and to transmit information through written orders and the written record.

MOTOR AND TECHNICAL SKILLS. Manual skills are necessary in gathering information from the patient as well as in applying specific treatment. Being able to do a well-ordered and accurate physical examination requires effective motor skills. Diagnostic procedures such as biopsies, sampling of body fluids, or endoscopy also depend on motor and technical skills. Examples of treatment involving these skills include performing minor surgery and using machines for life support. Learning new techniques and continuing to practice them are major requirements for maintaining technical competence.

Intellectual Abilities

Disease is a scientific, impersonal term. *Illness* is personalized and refers to disease in a specific patient. Intellectual skills are directed to the understanding, diagnosis, and theoretical management of disease. Noncognitive abilities deal more with the individual. In approaching a medical problem, the physician begins with relevant medical knowledge and synthesizes the information into an integrated concept. Clinical judgment is used to resolve the problem.

To apply medical knowledge to a patient problem, the physician draws on pertinent medical facts from memory, from clinical experience, and from other sources such as journals, textbooks, and experts. An understanding of pathophysiology helps in anticipating the expected course of the disease. Information derived from the patient, together with medical knowledge, is organized into a logical sequence. Synthesis of organized medical knowledge involves integration of medical facts into practical concepts, which are altered as the patient's condition changes or when new information becomes available. Organization and synthesis of information are important in all tasks of a physician, including data gathering, diagnosis, and planning for study and treatment. The highest level of cognitive ability is clinical judgment, where intellectual skills are called upon to solve problems. The physician makes clinical decisions by discriminating between alternative courses of action. Clinical judgment is used to decide what is of greatest benefit to the patient with the least risk and cost.

TASKS REQUIRED OF A PHYSICIAN

When a patient comes for help, the physician follows a logical series of steps, which are called clinical tasks. The physician first obtains the medical history, does a physical examination, and conducts laboratory studies. Based on this information, an initial diagnosis is made upon which definitive medical care is based.

Data Gathering

MEDICAL HISTORY. The most powerful diagnostic tool of the physician is the interview. By this means, one learns the chronological events and the symptoms of the patient's illness. Diagnostic hypotheses are generated and tested as the patient's history unfolds, resulting in the formulation of the most likely diagnoses at the completion of the interview. These hypotheses are extended, confirmed, or refuted by the subsequent physical examination and diagnostic studies.

The interview has considerable importance beyond "history taking" or the gathering of medical facts. It is the principal means of initiating and developing a relationship with the patient. The interview is a shared experience with goals for both participants. For the patient, the goal is alleviation of distress and restoration of health. The patient must be satisfied that the person rendering medical care is not only professionally competent but is also interested in him as an individual. For the physician, the primary objective is to obtain the information needed to understand the illness and to initiate appropriate treatment. This objective is accomplished by demonstrating concern for the patient and by being willing to listen to his personal as well as medical problems. The overt demonstration of concern by the physician will help to build the physician-patient relationship and secure the patient's cooperation.

The most important component of the medical history is the patient's present illness. Here, the interviewer develops a detailed and sequential reconstruction of the symptoms and events contributing to the current illness. The social history is also of considerable importance. The inquiry with interest and empathy into the personal events of the patient's life, while affording the patient time to relate these events, helps to establish a strong physician-patient relationship. Knowledge of the patient's personal circumstances and relationships to others leads to better understanding of his problems and ways of coping with them. More effective planning for the future care of the patient takes place when the limitations imposed on the current life situation are known.

When pursuing information in the interview, the physician begins with open-ended or nondirective questions and concludes with specific questions. Such an approach allows the patient time to respond and to elaborate on his problems. Failure to take time to listen may be interpreted by the patient as a lack of interest on the part of the interviewer and can result in a perfunctory and noninformative interview. To initiate the interview with a series of specific questions may also inhibit the full development of the history. Encouraging the patient to speak freely as the interview proceeds is important, since only the patient can describe what he has been experiencing. On the other hand, the patient does not necessarily understand what the interviewer needs to learn from him. The physician therefore actively pursues the interview in order to develop organization and content. The patient soon learns that events must be dated, sequences established, and symptoms precisely described. Dates and times serve to anchor the history in such a way that relationships between symptoms and events are more clearly understood. Knowledge of disease and clinical syndromes enables the physician to anticipate symptoms the patient does not mention. It is often necessary to intervene in order to clarify terms the patient uses, including medical or quasi-medical terms. Some patients, when asked to tell of their own illnesses, may omit their symptoms altogether and persist in describing only what other doctors said and did. It should be made clear that the interviewer is more interested in learning about the patient's specific symptoms and not the interpretation of those symptoms.

In conducting an effective interview, the physician adapts to the personality of the patient and to limitations imposed by illness. Patients who are especially talkative or who wander from the subject need to be guided back to the pertinent issues. Patients with poverty of associations are encouraged to elaborate on their problems. When an interview becomes primarily a question and answer session, it is likely that the patient is unable to go into detail because of illness or that the interviewer is using poor technique and is therefore missing valuable historical information. In a seriously ill patient, one gives priority to those aspects of the history that appear more relevant to the immediate situation. Other patients, because of the type of disease, may be handicapped in relating their stories. When the interview is limited because of the patient's illness, information is derived from other sources such as family, friends, and previous hospital records. A subsequent interview of the patient at a more opportune time is often valuable.

The appearance and responses of the patient during the

interview are diagnostically helpful. The physical examination begins the moment the patient is seen. One studies the patient's appearance, his emotional state, and his physical and mental limitations. Not only is close attention paid to the overt meaning of what is said, but the interviewer is also alert to nonverbal cues. The physician's own feeling of being uncomfortable, uneasy, or unhappy often reflects the attitude of the patient.

The interview, a powerful diagnostic tool, goes far beyond collecting the facts of illness. Through knowledge and experience, the physician delineates subtle symptoms and interrelationships that are often unrecognized by the patient. A skillful interviewer will uncover personal feelings and circumstances underlying the illness. An interview conducted with sensitivity and concern will help to build a strong relationship between the patient and physician.

PHYSICAL EXAMINATION. A general screening examination is conducted following the interview. This examination is influenced by diagnostic hypotheses developed during the interview which direct the physician to do a more detailed study in the area of suspected abnormality.

Consideration for the patient continues during the physical examination. Privacy is provided for dressing and undressing, and the examination is done with appropriate draping. Both the physician and the patient need to be in a comfortable position throughout the examination in order to apply techniques properly. In certain parts of the examination, the physician tells the patient how to cooperate and forewarns him of any uncomfortable impending maneuver. In general, the examination is done in silence except for necessary instructions to the patient. Talking hinders the physician from concentrating fully on possible underlying abnormalities. The examination is carried out with meticulous care, gentleness, and sensitive attention. One avoids comments or facial expressions that can be misinterpreted by the patient as indicating concern or puzzlement. The physician is also alert to signs of patient fatigue or discomfort.

There are two major principles underlying an efficient physical examination. First, the examination is done by regions; second, there is a well-organized order of examination. To be efficient, one approaches regions sequentially, for example, the head, the neck, the posterior thorax and lungs, the anterior thorax and lungs, and the heart. This type of regional approach also takes into account the comfort of the patient by eliminating the need for frequent shifts in position. One begins with a general survey of each region and then focuses on component parts. If no abnormality is found, the examination is brief but comprehensive. If an abnormality is present, it is studied meticulously, using special maneuvers if necessary. One takes advantage of the symmetry of the human body by comparing one side with the other. In this way, subtle changes are recognized. Small differences in the lung examination, for example, are better detected by cross-comparing symmetrical areas of each lung than by examining each lung individually. Following a prescribed order of examination by regions does not imply a lack of flexibility. The examination varies with the condition of the patient and the type of problem present. Evidence of disease in one area alerts the physician to possible related abnormalities in other areas. If the initial physical examination has not been entirely satisfactory, one does not hesitate to return at a later time to recheck findings when circumstances for reexamination may be more favorable.

Observation is an often neglected technique of great importance. Studying the patient and his surroundings yields helpful diagnostic information. By noting what is on the bedside table, for example, one gains insight into the patient's interests and habits and the support of family and friends. Specifically, one looks for reading materials, cigarettes, and the presence of cards or gifts. When beginning to examine each region, the physician pauses to observe. For example, an enlarged thyroid gland will readily be seen when a patient extends his neck slightly and swallows; asymmetry of respiratory motion will be more easily observed from the foot of the bed with the patient on his back; and holding an end of a tongue blade lightly at the cardiac apex will magnify the visible impulse of a left ventricular gallop.

The physician learns to do a comprehensive screening examination. Depending on the condition of the patient, the examination will need to be adapted to special circumstances. The patient may be bed-bound and so ill that the examiner requires assistance with positioning. In an acute emergency where an abbreviated physical examination is carried out with deliberate speed, one simultaneously does a brief interview, obtains laboratory work, and initiates treatment. If the patient has a neurologic problem, a complete neurologic examination is done. Regardless of the problem and the condition of the patient, the physician is considerate, systematic, and logical in approach. One keeps in mind diagnostic possibilities, looks for unsuspected disease, and interrelates abnormal findings that may explain the patient's illness.

DIAGNOSTIC STUDIES. Laboratory tests and diagnostic procedures are obtained following the interview and physical examination. A few initial screening tests are usually done to detect unsuspected common entities, such as anemia, diabetes, or chronic renal disease. Studies are discriminatingly chosen to confirm one's impression and are not used in a routine or excessive way to search for unexpected diagnoses. After considering each of the patient's problems, the physician decides which studies are needed, both to confirm the diagnostic impression and to rule in or out other possibilities. If the prevalence of a problem is low and no effective treatment is available, few diagnostic tests are indicated. Laboratory tests and diagnostic procedures are of value not only to help make the diagnosis, but also to assess the severity, course, and prognosis of the disease and to follow the effect of therapy.

When choosing diagnostic studies, the physician begins with those that yield the most comprehensive information and carry the least risk for the patient. The diagnosis frequently becomes apparent with simple tests; more expensive or potentially hazardous studies may not be required. Laboratory tests are often overemphasized. These tests have limitations in accuracy, and there may be errors and misinterpretation of results. The physician's own clinical findings and judgment take precedence in the interpretation of laboratory data.

Potentially hazardous diagnostic or therapeutic procedures require competence on the part of those doing them. Plans for procedures are discussed with the patient, including possible risks. Time is taken to alleviate patient concern and to interpret the results. In carrying out diagnostic studies and treatment, consultant assistance is often required. The physician in charge of the patient takes into account the expert advice of consultants but continues to supervise overall care and makes the ultimate decisions.

Recent research into clinical decision making has been helpful in creating a better understanding of the selection and interpretation of diagnostic tests and procedures. Knowledge of the sensitivity and specificity of diagnostic studies leads to their more rational selection. *Sensitivity* is the probability that a test will be positive when the disease is present. *Specificity* is the probability that the test will be negative when the disease is not present. For example, to exclude the possibility of lupus erythematosus, one chooses a sensitive test such as the antinuclear antibody test. The more specific double-stranded DNA antibody test is ordered to confirm the diagnosis.

Diagnosis or Problem Definition

The physician uses the scientific method in clinical problem solving, as does the investigator in conducting an experiment.

Clinical information is analyzed to develop working hypotheses that are confirmed or refuted by obtaining further information. Problem solving begins at the time the physician initiates the interview. The symptoms and course of the illness lead to the formulation of several diagnostic hypotheses. These diagnostic possibilities direct further questioning of the patient in order to determine which hypothesis best fits the illness. Hypotheses are repeatedly generated and tested during the interview. As the physician completes the interview and physical examination, one or two possibilities usually become more likely and others less likely. With further information, an attempt is made to explain the patient's presenting illness with a single preliminary diagnosis. This goal is often attainable in young patients but seldom in older ones, in whom multiple diagnoses are usually required. One takes into account the likelihood of the disease process in making a preliminary diagnosis. The most common diseases are considered first, particularly those diseases for which specific treatment is available.

Cognitive or intellectual skills are used in formulating a diagnosis. A physician continually refers to knowledge of medical facts and pathophysiology in analyzing information pertaining to the patient's illness. This analysis consists of collecting information and synthesizing it into integrated concepts compatible with known diseases. Abnormal findings are localized anatomically and are interpreted in terms of their structure and function. Clinical judgment is used to weigh the diagnostic possibilities by assigning values to the data in order to arrive at the most likely conclusion. The experienced clinician is able to apply these intellectual processes rapidly and continually while interviewing the patient.

The written record is used to clarify the physician's diagnostic thinking. When there are several diagnostic possibilities explaining the symptoms and events of the present illness, a differential diagnosis is carried out. For each diagnosis considered, the physician weighs information favoring that possibility against information that makes the diagnosis unlikely. Consideration of alternative possibilities in the differential diagnosis is helpful in directing the physician to select diagnostic studies that confirm or exclude each possible diagnosis. In addition to indicating the most likely diagnosis that explains the present illness, the physician lists in descending order of importance all other active problems affecting the patient. This list includes not only specific diseases, but also such problems as the recent loss of a spouse or exposure to environmental toxins. The physician considers all possible factors in the patient's illness, including psychological stresses and underlying conditions that may alter resistance. The functional impact of the illness in terms of its severity and the degree of resulting disability is also taken into account.

Clinical decisions are influenced by policies determined by tradition, by the medical literature, and by the practice of colleagues. These policies may be based on simplistic or even erroneous reasoning. Greater attention needs to be paid to clinical policies that have been shown to be valid. Ongoing investigation of diagnostic reasoning will eventually lead to better understanding of the ways clinicians solve medical problems. The diagnostic thinking of physicians as they interview standardized patients has been studied, and decision analysis has contributed logic theory to problem solving, including the use of probability and decision trees.

Medical Care

The term *medical care* is used rather than the more authoritative *patient management,* because it expresses personal concern and responsibility for all of the patient's problems. In caring for a patient, physician attitudes of integrity, respect, and compassion are particularly important, as is the ability to communicate effectively. In addition, the intellectual skills of the physician are necessary attributes. Up-to-date medical knowledge of pharmacological principles and advances in technology are required. Clinical judgment is used in prescribing drugs, in selecting therapeutic procedures, and in implementing consultant opinions. Knowing when *not* to treat is as important as knowing when to treat. New drugs and procedures are ordered with caution. A full understanding of their potential complications is necessary to be sure that negative side effects do not outweigh possible advantages. To be fully effective, the physician needs the requisite knowledge and skills to treat acute life-threatening illness as well as the supportive staying power to care for the chronically ill patient. One learns to care for patients in a variety of environments: in the office, in the emergency room, in the hospital, by telephone, or when the patient is housebound or in a nursing home.

The care of the patient involves far more than prescribing drugs and completing therapeutic procedures. Attention is paid to the preventive aspects of disease, to the patient's psychological problems, and to conflicts arising from home or place of work. Immunization for infectious disease and advice to avoid smoking and excessive drinking are obvious examples of preventive measures. The patient may need to alter his way of living, if job stress plays a role. Psychiatric or family counseling may help when there are major psychological problems.

Good communication with the patient is required in order to educate him about his illness, its management, and its prevention. A better informed patient will be more motivated to comply with treatment. The ability to communicate well is also needed when dealing with responsible family members and with others caring for the patient. Diabetes mellitus is an excellent example of an illness that requires education and the help of others. The patient needs to understand the disease in order to know why diet is important, why blood sugar levels are high, and why insulin is used. He learns the potential complications and how to prevent them. Nurses help the patient learn to test glucose levels and to use an insulin syringe; dietitians teach a diabetic diet.

In providing excellent care, the competent physician knows how frequently a patient should be seen and how extensive an evaluation is necessary. These decisions require good clinical judgment and a rationale for each action. It is important for the physician to instruct the patient how to obtain medical care at all times, particularly in an acute emergency or when the physician is not available. Above all, the physician demonstrates a continuing personal interest in the patient, is the patient's advocate, and assumes responsibility for all of his health care needs.

THE MEDICAL RECORD

The primary purpose of the medical record is to document the medical experience of the patient. This information is used by those concerned with the patient's current and future care. Legally, it is a public document available to other physicians and to health care providers, to the court by subpoena, and to insurance companies. The medical record varies in format and detail, depending on whether the patient is seen in an ambulatory setting or in the emergency room or is admitted to the hospital.

A major contribution to the organization of the medical record has been the introduction of the problem-oriented method. Of particular importance are the problem list and the problem-oriented progress notes. The medical record of the patient may be organized by combining the traditional format of the history and physical examination with the identification of active problems. If there is a single major problem that is not clearly defined, a formulation is written. The physician gives the reasons for the diagnosis and weighs evidence for and against other diagnostic possibilities. When there are several active problems, these are discussed separately, each with a diagnostic and therapeutic plan.

The problem list is particularly useful when following an

ambulatory patient who has chronic illness and multiple problems. A list of active and inactive problems serves as an index to the record. In this way, problems are summarized and can be quickly reviewed. Problem-oriented progress notes help to organize ongoing clinical information. During the course of an illness, they enable one to easily follow individual problems through the record.

Establishment of the scientific basis of the art of medicine will lead to future clarification of each step of the medical encounter between the patient and physician. The expert clinician's resolution of a problem is not easily understood. Research defining the abilities and tasks of a physician will help to eliminate the dichotomy between the art and science of medicine.

American Board of Internal Medicine: Clinical competence in internal medicine. Ann Intern Med 90:402, 1979. *The major components of the medical encounter are analyzed, which include the abilities required of an internist, the tasks performed to solve a medical problem, the medical illness, and the patient.*

Eddy DM: Clinical policies and the quality of clinical practice. N Engl J Med 307:343, 1982. *A description is given of some of the sources of errors and biases in clinical policy making, with suggested ways to improve the quality of clinical policies.*

Elstein AS, Shulman LS, Sprafka SA: Medical Problem Solving. An Analysis of Clinical Reasoning. Cambridge, Mass., Harvard University Press, 1978. *A detailed, yet readable textbook gives the results of five years of research on medical problem solving and decision making based on the performance of selected internists and students in a variety of experimental situations.*

Griner PF, Panzer RJ, Greenland P: Clinical Diagnosis and the Laboratory. Logical Strategies for Common Medical Problems. Chicago, Year Book Medical Publishers, 1986. *This book provides a review of the scientific approach to selecting and interpreting diagnostic tests and procedures. Preferred diagnostic strategies are given for specific commonly considered clinical problems in adult medicine.*

Kassirer JP, Gorry GA: Clinical problem solving. A behavioral analysis. Ann Intern Med 89:245, 1978. *Tape-recorded interviews of simulated patients by experienced clinicians are studied to determine how hypothesis generation is used in clinical problem solving.*

Morgan WL, Engel GL: The Clinical Approach to the Patient. Philadelphia, W. B. Saunders Company, 1969. *This is a step-by-step guide to interviewing the patient, organizing the physical examination, and handling clinical information, with particular emphasis on how to relate to the patient.*

Weinstein MC, Fineberg HV: Clinical Decision Analysis. Philadelphia, W. B. Saunders Company, 1980. *A detailed quantitative analysis is given of clinical decision making, which includes the use of decision trees and probabilities and the assigning of values to possible outcomes.*

21 CLINICAL DECISION MAKING

Stephen G. Pauker

The primary role of the physician is to make decisions—about what tests to order, about what test results mean, about what drugs to administer, about whether or not to perform surgery. Virtually all medical decisions are made beneath a cloak of uncertainty—about diagnosis, about the effectiveness of therapeutic alternatives, about prognosis. Classic medical education has rarely included a formal approach to decision making in an uncertain world, despite its central position in medical practice. Over the past two decades, normative prescriptive techniques, borrowed from the military and business worlds, have been applied increasingly to medicine.

The benefits of these approaches rest on their explicit nature, on their unyielding requirements for information, and on the ability to ask "What if?" What if this disease were more likely? What if surgery were more effective but also engendered a higher risk? What if the patient is an octogenarian? What if the optimal time for diagnostic testing had passed and the test's sensitivity were therefore diminished? Of course, these approaches also carry significant cost: They are unfamiliar to most physicians, sometimes require extra effort, and always require the decision maker to confront uncertainty and to be explicit about his or her assumptions and data base.

Clinical decision analyses are often confused with clinical algorithms or flow charts, which have gained increasing popularity as media for representing and communicating management strategies. The latter are compact schemata for summarizing a set of rules of "if-then" statements that can lead the clinician down an established management pathway. It would be possible, for example, to translate many of the management strategies in this book into flow charts. Unfortunately, algorithms do not provide a process for creating such rules; they are most often the implicit product of singular or communal experience, although algorithms are sometimes annotated to describe the rationale that underlies them. Indeed, some investigators have used the decision analytic techniques described in this chapter to help formulate algorithms.

THE INTERPRETATION OF DATA

In making a diagnosis, the physician moves continually between two tasks: data gathering and data interpretation. The former task involves identifying potential data elements and deciding which elements to select. The latter task involves modifying a set of hypotheses based on new data elements; those new elements might be drawn from the patient's history, from the physical examination, from laboratory tests, or from the patient's response to diagnostic or therapeutic maneuvers. In each case, however, the new data might suggest new diagnostic hypotheses and almost always will modify the clinician's strength of belief in existing hypotheses. Those beliefs can be most conveniently represented as *probabilities*, the likelihood of each diagnosis on a scale from 0 to 1, which can be manipulated by several basic rules:

1. The probability of a diagnosis being false ($P_{no\ dis}$) equals $(1 - P_{dis})$ where P_{dis} is the probability of the diagnosis.
2. The list of alternative diagnoses must be exhaustive, and the probabilities must sum to 1.0 (thus, one often includes a category "other" in the list of diagnoses).
3. The various hypotheses must be mutually exclusive (thus, if one hypothesis is that diseases a and b coexist, then the explicit hypothesis "diseases a and b" must be included).
4. Among these mutually exclusive diagnoses, the probability that the patient has at least one of several diagnoses equals the sum of their probabilities [thus, $P_{a\ or\ b}$ equals $(P_a + P_b)$].
5. If events are independent, then their joint probability equals the product of the probabilities (thus, $P_{a\ and\ b}$ equals $P_a \times P_b$).
6. If events are dependent, then their joint probability equals the product of the probability of the first (P_a) and the conditional probability of the second, given the first ($P_{b/a}$).

Bayes' Rule

In this context, data are interpreted using Bayes' rule, a relation among probabilities that allows the clinician to modify his or her level of belief in each hypothesis based on incremental data. The technique begins with the probability of each disease before knowledge of the incremental finding. These probabilities are called the *prior probabilities* and are often estimated by the prevalence of each disease. Next, for each disease the *conditional probability* of the incremental finding ($P_{finding/dis_i}$) is specified. Although these probabilities can be combined using the equation for Bayes' rule

$$P_{dis_i/finding} = \frac{P_{dis_i} \times P_{finding/dis_i}}{\sum_{i=1}^{n} P_{dis_i} \times P_{finding/dis_i}}$$

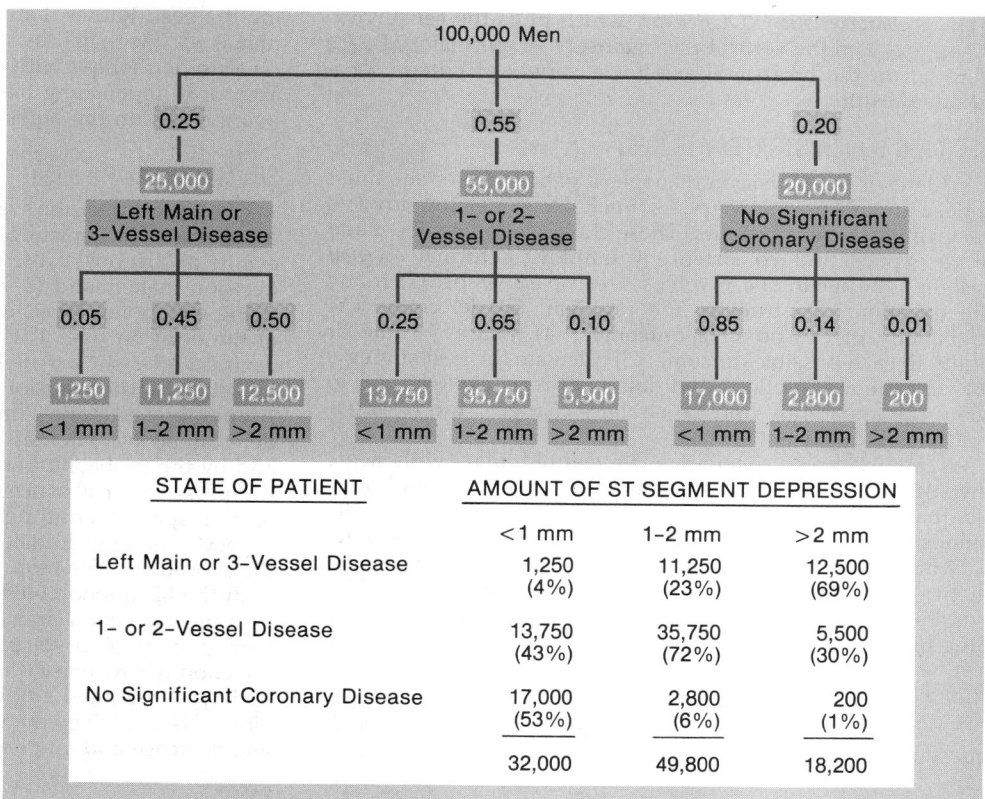

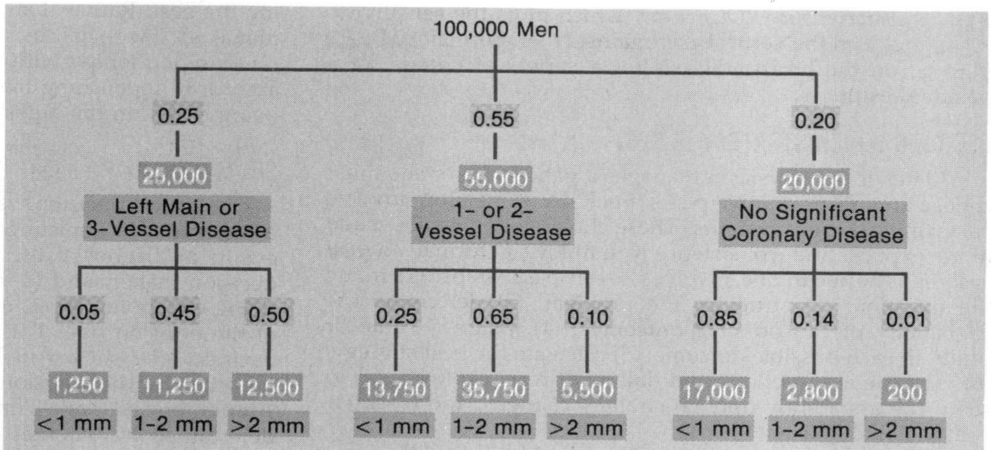

STATE OF PATIENT	AMOUNT OF ST SEGMENT DEPRESSION		
	<1 mm	1-2 mm	>2 mm
Left Main or 3-Vessel Disease	1,250 (4%)	11,250 (23%)	12,500 (69%)
1- or 2-Vessel Disease	13,750 (43%)	35,750 (72%)	5,500 (30%)
No Significant Coronary Disease	17,000 (53%)	2,800 (6%)	200 (1%)
	32,000	49,800	18,200

FIGURE 21–1. Cohort flow model of Bayes' rule used to interpret an exercise tolerance test in a 50-year old man with typical angina. Consider a cohort of 100,000 such men: 25 per cent have left main or 3-vessel disease, 55 per cent have 1- or 2-vessel disease, and 20 per cent are free of significant coronary disease. If the conditional probabilities of < 1 mm, 1–2 mm, and > 2 mm of ST depression are as shown and determine how many men from each diagnostic subgroup will have each finding, then of the 1250 + 13,750 + 17,000 (or 32,000) men with < 1 mm of ST depression, 17,000, or 53 per cent, will have no significant coronary disease, 43 per cent will have 1- or 2-vessel disease, and 4 per cent will have left main or 3-vessel disease.

it is almost always easier to use the tabular form of the technique (Table 21–1) or the cohort flow form (Fig. 21–1).

In the simplest case, the physician considers a single disease and interprets a diagnostic test, which is either positive or negative. In that situation, the probability of a positive test in a patient who has the disease, $P_{positive\ test/dis}$, is called the *sensitivity* of the test, and the probability of a negative test in a patient who does not have the disease, $P_{negative\ test/no\ dis}$, is called *specificity* of the test. The examples in Table 21–1 and Figure 21–1 demonstrate common settings in which implicit test interpretation is fraught with error: (1) In the setting of a low prior probability of disease, a positive finding often does not suggest a very high probability of disease unless the test is extremely specific; and (2) in the setting of a high prior probability of disease, a negative finding often does not suggest a very low probability of disease unless the test is extremely sensitive. Especially in those situations, it would be important to interpret the finding in an explicit and formal manner, using probabilities as described here.

When interpreting several findings, the calculated posterior or revised probabilities based on the first finding become the prior probabilities for interpreting the next finding in a sequential application of Bayes' rule. In such circumstances, the several findings may not be conditionally independent of one another. For example, in the diagnostic evaluation of a patient suspected of having a pulmonary embolism, the chest radiograph and the lung scan are not conditionally independent: In the setting of a normal chest film, a perfusion scan with a segmental defect is far more suggestive of pulmonary embolism than the same scan result in a patient with the radiologic findings of chronic pulmonary disease. In such situations, the probability of the finding must be conditioned on both disease and on the other dependent findings ($P_{finding/dis\ and\ other\ findings}$).

Many findings are innately continuous in nature, e.g., a serum creatine kinase level, the size of the liver, and the size of the left atrium. For a given finding to be positive or negative, one must first establish a *criterion* for defining a positive result. Furthermore, to determine the conditional probabilities of a given finding, one needs a separate *gold standard* to define the presence or absence of each disease. Changing either the gold standard or the test criterion will change the conditional probabilities of the findings. For example, if a positive exercise tolerance test is defined as one with ≥ 1 mm ST depression, then the sensitivity for the diagnosis of coronary disease would be 81 per cent and the specificity would be 85 per cent (see data in Fig. 21–1). On the other hand, if a positive result were defined as > 2 mm ST depression, then the sensitivity would be only 23 per cent but the specificity would be 99 per cent. In general, a more strict criterion (e.g., > 2 mm compared with ≥ 1 mm of ST depression) increases specificity and decreases sensitivity; a more lax criterion increases sensitivity and decreases specificity. The relations among sensitivity, specificity, and the definition of a positive finding are summarized by a *receiver*

TABLE 21–1. USING BAYES' RULE TO INTERPRET A SPUTUM CYTOLOGIC STUDY DEMONSTRATING ATYPICAL CELLS IN A NONSMOKER WITH A PULMONARY NODULE

A Diagnosis	B Prior Probability	C Conditional Probability of Observed Test Result	D Product (Col B times Col C)	E Revised or Posterior Probability (Col E/Sum)
Cancer	0.01	0.40	0.004	0.04
No Cancer	0.99	0.10	0.099	0.96
		Sum =	0.103	

Step 1: List diagnoses in Column A.
Step 2: List prior probabilities in Column B.
Step 3: List conditional probabilities of finding in Column C.
Step 4: Multiply Columns B and C and place products in Column D.
Step 5: Divide each entry in Column D by sum of Column D and place quotients in Column E.

operator characteristic (ROC) curve, which plots the sensitivity, $P_{\text{positive result/dis}}$, on the vertical axis against (1 − specificity), $P_{\text{positive result/no dis}}$, on the horizontal axis for a variety of criteria for a positive result.

DECIDING WHICH STRATEGY IS BEST

Whenever the physician manages a patient, he or she must choose among alternative plans. Such decisions often involve balancing risks and benefits. These choices often can be made more explicit and consistent by employing formal *decision analysis*. The technique involves seven basic steps: (1) frame the question; (2) structure the problem; (3) determine the probability of the possible outcomes; (4) assign a value or utility to each possible outcome; (5) calculate the best strategy; (6) vary the assumptions and data over reasonable ranges to see if the apparently optimal strategy changes; and (7) interpret the analysis.

As an example, consider a 54-year-old man with acute myelogenous leukemia complicating longstanding lymphoma. The patient is immunosuppressed by chemotherapy and develops a persistent fever, pulmonary infiltrates, and respiratory distress without clear etiology and despite empiric treatment with antibiotics and antituberculosis drugs. The possibilities of empiric therapy with amphotericin and open lung biopsy are raised.

Framing the Question

Formal decision analysis is designed to answer specific questions by evaluating well-specified alternatives and choosing the best. Rather than asking "How should this patient be managed," we shall ask which of three alternatives is best: (1) empiric therapy with amphotericin, (2) conservative therapy, or (3) open lung biopsy with the amphotericin decision being based on the biopsy results.

Structuring the Problem

The typical decision tree contains three basic elements: (1) decision nodes depicting choices, (2) chance nodes depicting events or diagnostic alternatives not under the control of the decision maker, and (3) outcome or terminal nodes summarizing events not explicitly occurring within the time horizon of the decision tree. This problem can be represented by the decision tree shown in Figure 21–2. The three choices are depicted by the decision node at the left. In both the "No Amphotericin" and "Amphotericin" strategies, prognosis is determined by whether or not a fungal infection is present and by the probability of short-term survival, conditioned on the presence or absence of fungal infection and on whether or not specific antifungal therapy is given. In the "Lung Biopsy" strategy, initially there is a chance of dying during the procedure. The biopsy may be either positive or negative, with the likelihood being determined by the prior probability of fungal infection and the sensitivity and specificity of the biopsy. If the biopsy is positive, then the probability of fungal infection will increase (the revised probability being calculated by Bayes' rule) and amphotericin will be administered. If the biopsy is negative, then the probability of fungal infection will decrease and amphotericin will be withheld.

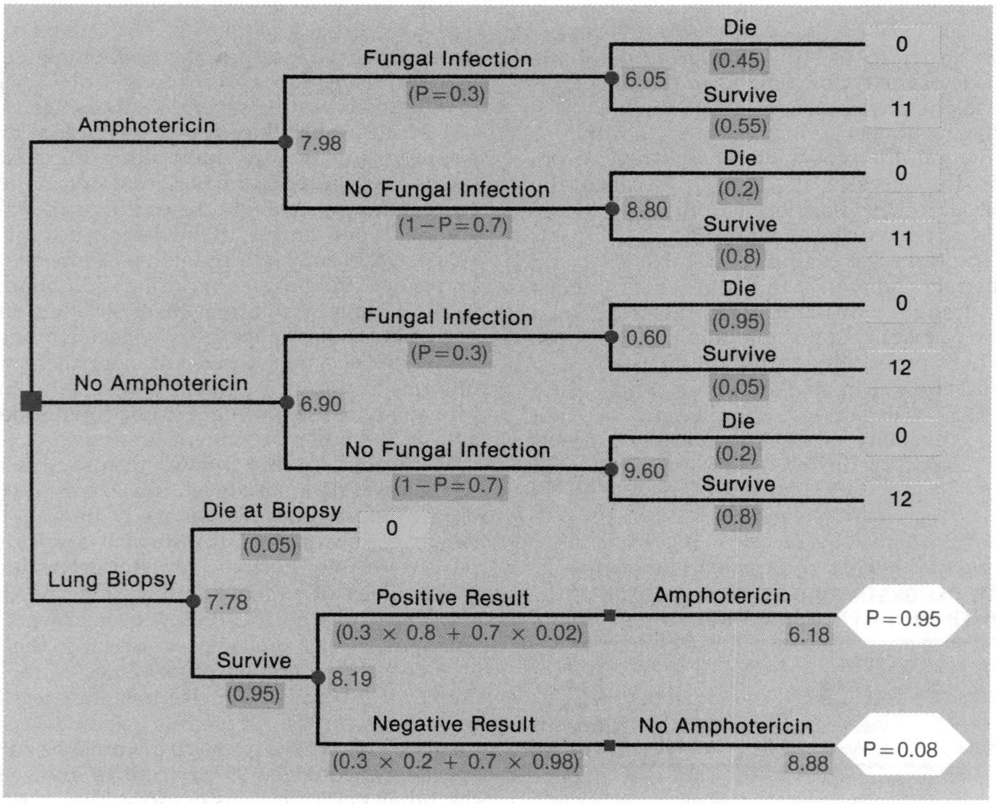

FIGURE 21–2. Decision tree depicting management choices in an immunosuppressed man with fever and pulmonary infiltrates. Decision nodes appear as squares. Chance nodes appear as circles. Outcome or terminal nodes appear as rectangles that contain the assigned utilities (in this case as quality-adjusted months of survival). Probabilities are shown shaded red on each branch of each chance node. The hexagons at the end of the "Lung Biopsy" strategy represent the use of the "No Amphotericin" and "Amphotericin" subtrees (which are used in the first two branches of the main decision node) with the probability of fungal infection being modified to 0.95 and 0.08 after a positive and negative biopsy, respectively, by the application of Bayes' rule. Calculated expected utilities are shown solid red within ovals. The sensitivity of the biopsy is taken as 0.8; the specificity is taken as 0.98. P = Probability of fungal infection.

Determining the Probabilities

In a decision tree, probabilities describe the present state of the patient (e.g., whether or not fungal disease is present) and the patient's prognosis. In both cases, these estimates can be based on the literature or on expert opinion. In either case, the physician uses descriptions of the past experience of other similar patients to predict the current and future state of the patient at hand.

In this case, we estimated the probability of fungal infection to be 30 per cent; we estimated the chance of dying from untreated fungal infection to be 95 per cent and the chance of dying from treated fungal infection to be 45 per cent. If fungal disease is not present, we estimated that the probability of death during this hospitalization to be 20 per cent. We estimated that, in this setting, lung biopsy would be associated with a 5 per cent mortality, a sensitivity of 80 per cent in diagnosing fungal infection, and a specificity of 98 per cent.

Assigning Utilities

The relative value of each possible outcome is summarized on a single consistent scale by a utility. Such scales can be arbitrary (e.g., 0 being the worst outcome and 100 being the best) or can describe the outcomes in identifiable units (e.g., five-year survival, years of life, years of disease-free survival, or even dollars spent). One useful metric can be *quality-adjusted life expectancy*, in which average survival is depreciated by long- and short-term morbidities. If such a metric is used, it is sometimes possible for the patient or the patient's family to contribute to the decision by expressing their attitudes about quality of life.

In this case, we shall use average survival modified by the short-term morbidity of amphotericin therapy. We estimated that survival would be 18 months if the patient achieves a remission of his leukemia but only 3 months if he does not. Because we assumed the chance of remission to be 60 per cent, the average survival for this man, if he survived the acute event, would be 60 per cent × 18 plus 40 per cent × 3, or 12 months. Although many physicians are very conservative in using amphotericin, the literature suggests that death and permanent renal failure are extremely rare complications of that drug; most side effects involve short-term toxicity. We assumed that the average duration of amphotericin therapy would be 2 months and that short-term morbidity would, on average, diminish quality of life during that period to half of what it otherwise would have been. Thus, we subtracted 1 month from the life expectancy to account for this morbidity, yielding a quality-adjusted survival of 11 months if amphotericin is administered. We assigned a utility of 0 to death during this acute illness.

Calculating the Expected Utility

In evaluating a tree, the decision maker follows two basic rules: (1) When facing a choice, select the option with the highest utility or expected utility; (2) when evaluating a chance event, the expected utility is the weighted average of the utilities of its outcomes, with the weights being the respective probability of each outcome. In applying these rules, the decision maker begins at the distal outcome nodes of the tree and sequentially calculates the average or expected utility of each node, moving toward the proximal decision node.

In this case, consider first the top branch of the decision node, the "Amphotericin" strategy. The highest distal chance node describes the short-term consequences of a fungal infection treated with specific antifungal therapy. There is a 0.45 probability of dying (utility 0) and 0.55 probability of surviving (utility 11 quality-adjusted months). Thus, the average or expected utility of this chance node is 0.45 × 0 plus 0.55 × 11, or 6.05 quality-adjusted months. Similarly, the expected utility of amphotericin in the absence of a fungal infection (the second distal chance node) is 0.2 × 0 plus 0.8 × 11, or 8.8 quality-adjusted months. The expected utility of the "Amphotericin" strategy is the weighted average of these two expected utilities: 0.3 × 6.05 plus 0.7 × 8.8, or 7.98 quality-adjusted months. In a similar fashion, we calculated the expected utility of "No Amphotericin" to be 6.9 quality-adjusted months.

Next we consider the lowest branch of the main decision node: the "Lung Biopsy" strategy. As depicted at the end of the "Positive" result branch, the expected utility is calculated using the "Amphotericin" subtree, with the probability of fungal infection being increased to 0.95. In that case, the expected utility is 0.95 × 6.05 plus 0.05 × 8.8, or 6.18 quality-adjusted months. Similarly, the expected utility of the "Negative" result branch is calculated with the "No Amphotericin" subtree, with the probability of fungal infection being decreased to 0.08, yielding 0.08 × 0.6 plus 0.92 × 9.6, or 8.88 quality-adjusted months. The weighted average of these expected utilities depends on the probability of a positive result (0.3 × 0.8 plus 0.7 × 0.02, or 0.25). The expected utility of the entire strategy is a weighted average of this result (8.19 quality-adjusted months) and the 5 per cent chance of a procedure-related death (utility 0), providing an expected utility of 7.78 quality-adjusted months.

Performing Sensitivity Analyses

Having calculated the expected utility in the baseline case, we next examine various central assumptions to determine whether reasonable variations in those assumed values will change the conclusions. Such sensitivity analyses initially examine variables one at a time, usually beginning with the "softest" data. Such analyses are often called *one-way sensitivity analyses* (see Fig. 21–3).

Typically, one strategy will be best for all values of the variable below a certain cutoff, and another strategy will be best for all values above that cutoff. The value at which the strategies have equal expected utility is called the *threshold* value for that variable. In addition to finding relevant threshold values, it is often important to examine the magnitude of the differences in expected values of the various strategies. If those differences are very small and potentially clinically insignificant, then the decision may well be a *close call*, and

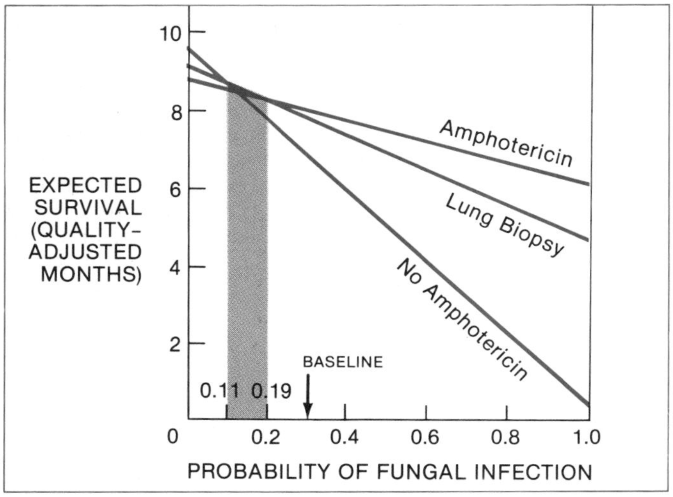

FIGURE 21–3. One-way sensitivity analysis of the effect of changing the probability of fungal infection in the decision tree shown in Figure 21–2. If the probability of fungal infection is zero, then the "No Amphotericin" strategy is best. If the probability of fungal infection is 100 per cent, then empiric amphotericin therapy is best. Lung biopsy is the optimal strategy in the narrow region between the two thresholds (vertical color bar) at 0.11 and 0.19. The baseline value of 0.3 is shown by the arrow.

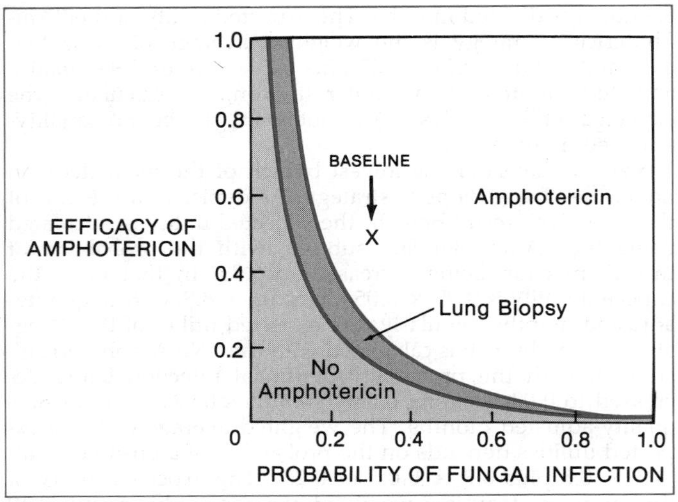

FIGURE 21–4. Two-way sensitivity analysis of the relation between the probability of fungal infection (horizontal axis) and the efficacy of amphotericin (vertical axis). Each combination of values corresponds to a unique point on the graph. All combinations falling in the lighter shaded area correspond to settings in which "no amphotericin" is the best strategy. All combinations falling in the darker shaded area correspond to settings in which "lung biopsy" is best. The baseline values correspond to the bold X, which lies within the settings in which amphotericin is best.

there may be relatively little to gain or lose in selecting one management plan over another. With sufficient time and energy or with adequate computational support, the clinician also can examine the effect of simultaneous changes in two or more variables. Such multiway sensitivity analyses are often summarized by decision diagrams that specify the best strategy for each combination of values (see Fig. 21–4).

In this case, the softest piece of data is the likelihood that this patient has a fungal infection. The one-way sensitivity analysis of this variable is summarized in Figure 21–3. Another central variable is the effectiveness of amphotericin in enhancing survival in an immunosuppressed patient known to have fungal disease. We define the *efficacy* of therapy to be $1 - (P_{die/Ampho}/P_{die/No\ Ampho})$. Thus, the probability of dying despite appropriate therapy equals the probability of dying without therapy times (1 − efficacy). If efficacy were 0, then $P_{die/Ampho}$ would equal $P_{die/No\ Ampho}$; if efficacy were 100 per cent, then $P_{die/Ampho}$ would be 0. The baseline value is 0.53, and the threshold value for this variable is 0.28. If the efficacy exceeds that threshold, then empiric amphotericin should be given. If the efficacy is below 0.15, then amphotericin therapy should be withheld. If the efficacy falls between these thresholds, then lung biopsy is the best strategy. Clearly, if the efficacy of therapy is changed, then the threshold probability of fungal disease will also change and vice versa. This two-way sensitivity analysis is summarized in Figure 21–4.

Interpreting the Analysis

Although there may well be a temptation to perform clinical decision analyses just to determine the best management strategy, the analyst would do the patient a disservice by stopping at that point. Every analytic model is merely an approximation of the underlying medical dilemma. The careful analyst must explore the model to discover its limitations. Only then can the clinician have reasonable confidence in its conclusions. One of the central benefits of a clinical decision analysis should be a better understanding of the clinical problem and a delineation of the settings in which the planned strategy is proper.

In this analysis, we see that empiric therapy with amphotericin is appropriate for any patient who has at least a moderate likelihood (over 20 per cent) of fungal infection. Therapy based on the results of lung biopsy is best only for the narrow wedge of patients falling in the darker shaded region of Figure 21–4. This region would be broadened if lung biopsy had a lower complication rate but would still be limited by the imperfect sensitivity of the test: Some patients with potentially treatable fungal infections would be denied therapy if their biopsy yielded falsely negative results. The major driving force is the surprisingly benign characteristics of amphotericin. Although patients receiving the drug have significant short-term morbidity, very few develop permanent renal insufficiency and even fewer die.

COST-BENEFIT AND COST-EFFECTIVENESS ANALYSIS

The practice of medicine in a world of limited resources sometimes leads the physicians to consider not only what is "best" for the patient but also the resources that such medical care will use. In such contexts, cost-benefit and cost-effectiveness analyses can be used to establish policies. Because those policies may affect the way he or she practices medicine, the physician should understand some of the underlying principles. The basic logic of such analyses is quite similar to that described above; the difference lies in the utility scales that measure the relative worth of the potential outcomes. When resources and societal issues are considered, outcomes are often measured by their economic impact. Economists argue that the magnitude of a cost depends on, among other things, *when* that cost is incurred. Money saved or spent immediately is worth more than money saved or spent in the future. This principle is called the *discounting* of future benefits and costs: Future costs and benefits are diminished by a fixed proportion for each year into the future when such cost and benefits occur. When several different utilities are considered (e.g., survival and economic costs), some analysts argue that all utility scales should be discounted at the same rate; other analysts argue that discounting should be restricted to monetary factors. When considering the economics of medical care, we should be careful to distinguish actual *costs* from *charges*, which may be quite distorted by particular billing practices or insurance plans. We also should consider *indirect costs* (e.g., heating and cleaning in the hospital and even malpractice insurance) and *induced costs* (e.g., the diagnostic evaluation of patients with falsely positive screening test results and even the medical care for treating cancer that develops years later in a patient who is "saved" from tuberculous pneumonia).

In a *cost-benefit analysis*, economic impact is the only utility scale used: All benefits are measured in those terms. Thus, if a strategy increases survival, that benefit is translated into its monetary equivalent: Each year of life saved would be associated with a societal worth, perhaps based on economic productivity. If the benefits minus the costs of a given strategy are positive, the program contributes in the net to society. Presumably, the bigger the difference, the larger the contribution. If the costs of a strategy exceed its benefits, the program should not necessarily be rejected. Society might well wish to underwrite such a program. For example, extending the life of a disabled, elderly nursing home resident might not provide net economic benefit to society, but our ethical values argue strongly against withdrawing care from such individuals.

Because the economic value of life and improved quality of life are difficult to quantify, we often turn to *cost-effectiveness analyses*, in which two separate utility measures are analyzed simultaneously, e.g., monetary costs and years of life saved. The results are expressed as the *ratio* of cost to benefits. That ratio does not measure the overall worth of a single strategy; rather, it is used to compare strategies. Often the strategy that engenders greater resource costs is also the strategy that provides the greater effectiveness. Thus, one usually examines the ratio of the difference in costs to the difference in effectiveness (the *marginal cost-effectiveness ratio*), which might be expressed as additional dollars spent per additional year of life saved or even as additional dollars spent per additional cancer detected. Such analyses rarely tell the decision maker in an absolute sense which strategy is best: They provide only a measure of cost per unit of gain. Some external standard, perhaps established by society, must be applied to decide how much money is too much to spend to gain a year of life. Such analyses can also help when we must choose among alternate uses for a fixed amount of resource, i.e., a budget. When we have only another $100,000 to spend, should we "buy" one heart transplant, five coronary bypass operations, or a year of therapy for 1000 hypertensive men? These are difficult decisions, but physicians must now contribute to the discussion, hopefully in a logical, explicit, and useful way.

Diamond GA, Forrester JS: Analysis of probability as an aid in the clinical diagnosis of coronary-artery disease. N Engl J Med 300:1350, 1979. *Provides data and techniques for the interpretation of exercise testing in the context of various clinical presentations of coronary disease.*

Gottlieb JE, Pauker SG: Whether or not to administer amphotericin B to an immunosuppressed patient with hematologic malignancy and undiagnosed fever. Med Decision Making 1:75, 1981. *The detailed clinical decision analysis that forms the basis for the amphotericin decision model.*

Griner PF, Mayesski RJ, Mushlin AI, et al: Selection and interpretation of diagnostic tests and procedures. Ann Intern Med 94:553, 1981. *Primer on Bayes' rule with many examples.*

Kassirer JP: The principles of clinical decision making: An introduction to decision analysis. Yale J Biol 49:149, 1976. *Conversational introduction to building decision trees for professional football and medicine.*

Kassirer JP, Moskowitz AJ, Lau J, et al.: Decision analysis: A progress report. Ann Intern Med, February, 1987. *Review of the literature and classification of techniques and clinical questions.*

Lusted LB: Introduction To Medical Decision Making. Springfield, Ill., Charles C Thomas, 1968. *One of the first monographs suggesting how probability theory could be applied to medicine.*

McNeil BJ, Keeler E, Adelstein SJ: Primer on certain elements of medical decision making. N Engl J Med 293:211, 1975. *General introduction to Bayes' rule, ROC analysis, and information theory.*

Pauker SG, Kassirer JP: Medical progress: Decision analysis. N Engl J Med, January, 1987. *A tutorial about new techniques.*

Plante DA, Kassirer JP, Zarin DA, et al.: A clinical decision consultation service. Am J Med 80:1169, 1986. *Description of experience using clinical decision analysis in the care of individual patients.*

Raiffa H: Decision Analysis: Introductory Lectures on Choices Under Uncertainty. Reading, Mass., Addison-Wesley, 1968. *The classic introduction to decision theory for business students.*

Weinstein MC, Fineberg HV, Elstein AS, et al.: Clinical Decision Analysis. Philadelphia, W.B. Saunders Company, 1980. *Overall introduction replete with examples.*

22 THE USE AND INTERPRETATION OF LABORATORY-DERIVED DATA

James B. Wyngaarden

The basic workup of a patient begins with the acquisition of information. The experienced clinician will acquire a discerning and sensitive history and perform a thorough physical examination and such laboratory tests as may be necessary to evaluate the general health of the patient, to arrive at a specific diagnosis, to assess the functional status of involved organs, or to provide a basis for monitoring effectiveness of therapy.

Until two decades ago only a few laboratory tests were performed routinely in the workup of a patient. When screening was practiced, the panel of tests was usually limited to hemoglobin (or hematocrit) determination, blood cell counts, urinalysis, stool examination for occult blood, and perhaps a chest x-ray and an electrocardiogram, particularly in adults. Additional tests were ordered only when suggested by the clinical assessment. In this setting an attending physician could evaluate the reasoning process that led a physician in training to order a serum calcium determination or a serum alkaline phosphatase assay. The ordering of laboratory procedures was a consequence of the intellectual discipline of constructing a logical differential diagnosis or of the need to monitor the progress of a patient, e.g., one in diabetic ketoacidosis. Thus it was a vital component of the educational process itself.

In 1966 Thiers published a provocative study comparing the results of a screening battery of 11 tests run by an automated multichannel analyzer with those of tests specifically ordered on the same patients by physicians as part of the admission workup. The screening battery detected twice as many abnormal test results as were uncovered by selective ordering. The most common findings were elevated glucose or uric acid concentrations. Ensuing developments were rapid. Ingenious automated analyzers brought an increasing number and variety of tests within the reach of all practitioners. The cost of such a screening battery fell rapidly until soon one could obtain 12 to 18 test results for no more than the cost of 3 or 4 selected tests run manually a decade earlier.

The inclusion of a panel of chemical tests or enzyme assays of blood (or urine) became a routine component of a basic medical workup. For more than a decade, medical students and resident physicians have been brought up with a dependency upon such screening batteries of chemical measurements. Only a few hospitals resisted the temptation to institute such screening procedures and continued the traditional practice of letting the intellectual evaluation of the patient determine the indications for further laboratory procedures. The pendulum has now begun to swing back, as the limited utility of large panel testing has become more generally recognized. Only a small number of "screening tests" (history, physical examination, stool guaiac test, and blood pressure measurement) have actually been shown to improve the health outcome of asymptomatic outpatients. Admission screening tests, such as a "Chem 12," complete blood count, or sedimentation rate, have a relatively low yield: Fewer than 1 per cent lead to a "new" diagnosis. In fact, fewer than 10 per cent of Chem 12 data are ever used clinically, and as few as 40 per cent of "abnormal" results initiate a follow-up. Furthermore, unnecessary hospitalization has occurred when one laboratory test result of a screening panel was "abnormal" by chance on a statistical basis alone. Whenever 20 procedures are done, whose "normal" range is defined as the central 95 per cent segment, one test result will, on the average, fall outside this range on the basis of chance alone. Statistically, 40 per cent of all Chem 12 panels performed on healthy individuals will result in one "abnormal" result. Repetition of tests showing such aberrant results contributes to the high cost of medical care, but only rarely to the detection of significant dysfunction or disease. As a consequence of this additional experience, some of the larger teaching hospitals have discontinued screening panels. This movement has been accelerated by the exclusion of routine screening procedures from the list of reimbursable expenditures by some third-party payers of medical services.

In order to utilize the results of laboratory tests intelligently (and economically), the physician must be able to evaluate the validity of the test result, understand principles of variation and distribution of values, and integrate the data received from the laboratory with the information acquired from the patient. If the test result deviates from values found in a healthy control population, is the difference trivial, or is it indicative of important dysfunction? Should the test be repeated? How often need a particular measurement be followed up? What additional tests or studies are indicated on the basis of these leads?

The more information the physician has, the more effective the physician should be in caring for the patient. To ensure that this is the result requires knowledge of science and medicine, clinical judgment, and a profound respect for the limitations of the laboratory. One of the best ways of acquiring the constructively critical attitude so essential to the proper evaluation of laboratory data is to work in a laboratory for a while. There is a paradox in the present pattern of medical education: At a time of increasing reliance upon an expanding array of laboratory tests in the practice of medicine, learning experiences in the laboratory have largely been eliminated from the medical curriculum!

SOME LIMITATIONS OF THE LABORATORY

CRITERIA FOR EVALUATION OF LABORATORY METHODS. A trustworthy laboratory test must pass critical evaluations of analytic specificity, sensitivity, accuracy, and precision.

Specificity refers to the detection of the substance in question and no other. It is doubtful that any test is absolutely specific for the substance being measured. There is always some other substance around that is capable of reacting. In biochemical analyses this limitation is most serious in tests dependent upon color development, less in the case of assays dependent upon degradation of the analyte by purified enzymes, and perhaps least in such procedures as atomic absorption spectroscopy.

Sensitivity refers to the ability of the test to detect the substance in question at the required concentrations, namely, those at which the compound exists in body fluids.

Accuracy refers to the quantitative detection of the correct amount of the substance being measured. This property rests upon both specificity and sensitivity. A test may be accurate in the absence of certain interfering drugs, and only in a certain range of values. It may fail this criterion under other conditions.

Precision embodies *repeatability*, the obtaining of the same result on samples analyzed in replicated fashion, and *reproducibility*, representing quality control over time.

THE "LAW OF ERRORS." Early in the nineteenth century, the German mathematician and physicist, Johann C. F. Gauss, introduced the "law of errors." This law states that in repeated measurements of the *same* object or substance, the random component on the errors will be distributed about the mean as a frequency function. This distribution, which is bell shaped, is often called "normal" or "gaussian." Note that the law applies to repeated measurements of the same item. Its extension to a population of those items is justifiable only under certain circumstances, for not all distributions are bell shaped, and not all bell-shaped distributions are gaussian. The matter of distributions will be discussed further below, when we consider the topic of "normal range" of a biologic variable.

SOURCES OF VARIANCE

These include some factors under the control of the clinician, such as the dietary preparation of the patient and the techniques of collection and handling of samples. Reduction of variance to an acceptable minimum requires compulsive attention to every detail of the process.

LABORATORY ERRORS. There is imprecision in every measurement. In tests run by hand, pipetting, timing, reading, and recording errors occur. They are more frequent when technicians are overworked or fatigued. It is common to find greater scatter of results of replicate tests at the end of the day than at the beginning. Technician fatigue can be largely eliminated by automation, but there will always remain the technical limitations of machines and the human error in the preparation of reagents, in the standardization of instruments, and in the copying of test results. The last is not totally avoided by the computer print-out, as even typewriters make misteaks. Quality control varies widely from laboratory to laboratory. Split samples submitted to different laboratories may show surprising disparities in results.

DRUG INTERFERENCE. According to Osler, humans are distinguished from all other members of the animal kingdom by their desire to take drugs. Since many patients do not regard proprietary pain remedies or vitamins as drugs, the physician may obtain a negative drug history unless questions are appropriately phrased. Drugs have great potential for interference with laboratory tests. High-resolution chromatography of urine yields about 300 peaks of ultraviolet-absorbing materials. Two hundred and fifty of these disappear if the "normal subject" abstains from salicylates and vitamins for a few days. Salicylates, vitamins, and many other drugs or their metabolites also produce chromogens that interfere with certain analytic methods employed in automated tests, particularly of the urine.

DISTRIBUTIONS OF VALUES

There is widespread belief among medical students and graduate physicians that if the sample of test results from a healthy population is large enough, the distribution will be "normal" (gaussian); that on this assumption one may justifiably determine a mean value ($\bar{x}$) and its standard deviation (s); that the value, $\bar{x} \pm 2s$, will include the central 95 per cent of all measurements; that this segment of the distribution is the "normal range"; and that values that fall outside this range are by definition "abnormal." These beliefs are erroneous in many instances. The experimental fact is that for about one half of the methods of clinical chemistry, the distribution is smooth, unimodal, and skewed and that $\bar{x} \pm 2s$ does not cut off the desired central 95 per cent. For example, among the distributions of serum calcium, inorganic phosphorus, magnesium, alkaline phosphatase, total proteins, albumin, uric acid, and blood urea, only that of albumin is gaussian. All others are skewed, leptokurtic, or both. In such situations, the value $\pm$ 2s will cut off many more measurements in one tail of the distribution than the other. The uncritical application of principles of normal distributions in situations in which variables are not normally distributed sometimes leads to values of $\bar{x} - 2s$ that are negative, surely a biologic absurdity.

We should discard the notion that the distribution of values in healthy persons is generally gaussian and should avoid estimating the mean and standard deviation for distributions that are nongaussian (see Fig. 22–1).

One can avoid the question of gaussian distribution by use of *nonparametric* methods for estimating the reference range, that is, methods that do not involve any a priori assumption regarding the parental distribution shape except that it is

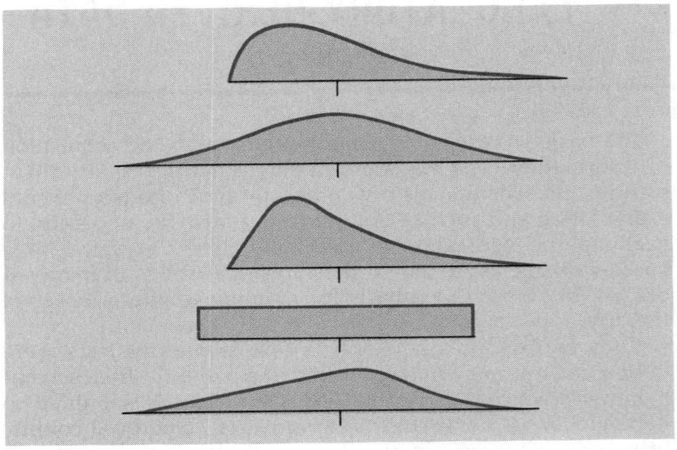

FIGURE 22–1. Five distributions with the same mean and standard deviation ($\bar{x}$ = 4, s = 2.83). From top to bottom: X_4^2, normal, lognormal, rectangular, and mixture of two normals. (From Elveback LR: Mayo Clinic Proc 47:93, 1972, with permission.)

continuous. Two nonparametric methods of normal range estimation are the method of *percentile estimates* with associated nonparametric confidence intervals and the method of non-parametric *tolerance intervals*, which include a specified proportion of the population with a specified probability.

Physicians are familiar with the percentile method of expressing interindividual variation through the use of pediatric growth charts of height and weight. The method avoids the arbitrary distinction of normal and abnormal. It also removes the aura of precision of the standard deviation. The percentile method appropriately fits the real world of nongaussian distributions.

From every laboratory test for which a good normal-value study has been done, the laboratory can report not only the result but also the percentile corresponding to that result and appropriate to the age and sex of the patient under study. With this information the clinician can appreciate just how common or how unusual the test result is. The percentile method is superior to an arbitrary definition of a normal range, such as $\bar{x} \pm 2s$, even in those few cases in which a distribution is gaussian, for it indicates for each test result the relationship of that result to the healthy population. The percentile method is also superior to the definition of the normal range as the range of all observed values in a healthy sample population, for the latter method seriously underestimates any selected segment, e.g., the central 95 per cent, in small samples, and overestimates it in large samples.

The percentile method does not systematically over- or underestimate any selected range, regardless of sample size. If one wishes to cut off the lowest and highest 2.5 per cent, or 5 per cent, one simply orders all values and finds the value that cuts off the desired percentage of observations at either tail of the distribution. Obvious outlier values are discarded. The complete percentile range is readily defined. No assumptions are required about distribution shape except that it is continuous. From the size of the healthy population represented in the distribution, the confidence limits of a given percentile may be ascertained, with known probability, by reference to standard tables. The method should appeal particularly to clinicians who utilize local norms, which are often based on small samples.

THE "NORMAL RANGE." From this discussion, it is clear that "normal range" is an arbitrary and potentially misleading term. By whatever method it is defined, the normal range will exclude observations of the parental distribution of healthy subjects and will very likely include some values of other distributions. What the clinician desires are cut-off points at either end of a distribution that include nearly all values of healthy individuals in the central segment, and very few values of other distributions, i.e., that the numbers of false-positive and false-negative values are both minimized. Ingrained habits will probably lead us to select the central 95 per cent of the parental distribution as "clinical limits," even though there is no magic in this number. Some clinical investigators advocate use of the central 90 per cent.

The term "normal range" has come in for substantial criticism. The connotation of a sharp demarcation between normal and abnormal values is unfortunate and usually erroneous. A value may fall outside the range, $\bar{x} \pm 2s$, or the central 95 per cent segment, on the basis of chance alone. The present consensus is that laboratory results should be interpreted in relationship to "reference intervals" rather than normal ranges. In most instances the quoted reference intervals for a given laboratory test result are the same as the previously published normal ranges, but the term emphasizes the manner in which such intervals are determined, and avoids an assumption of normality or abnormality of the test result. The newer terminology requires the laboratory to describe what it is using as a reference population to generate the interval values.

Influence of Age. The distributions of values of many plasma constituents vary with age in the apparently healthy population. For example, plasma cholesterol concentrations in men, 90 per cent limits, are 216 mg per deciliter in the 20- to 29-year age group and 258 mg per deciliter in the over 50-year age group (Table 22–1).

TABLE 22–1. PLASMA CHOLESTEROL CONCENTRATIONS ASSOCIATED WITH INCREASED RISK OF CARDIOVASCULAR DISEASE*

Age, yr	Total Cholesterol,* mg/dL		LDL† Cholesterol,* mg/dL		HDL† Cholesterol,‡ mg/dL (Increased Risk)
	Moderate Risk	*High Risk*	*Moderate Risk*	*High Risk*	
Men					
0–14	173	190	106	120	38
15–19	165	183	109	123	30
20–29	194	216	128	148	30
30–39	218	244	149	171	29
40–49	231	254	160	180	29
≥50	230	258	166	188	29
Women					
0–14	174	170	113	126	36
15–19	173	195	115	135	35
20–29	184	208	127	148	35
30–39	202	220	143	163	35
40–49	223	246	155	177	34
≥50	252	281	170	195	36

*Values are adopted from the 75th percentile (moderate-risk) and 90th percentile (high-risk) values obtained by the Lipid Research Clinics.

†LDL indicates low-density lipoproteins; HDL, high-density lipoproteins.

‡The HDL cholesterol values for the lower fifth percentile were taken from the Lipid Research Clinics.

Reprinted from Hoeg JM, Gregg RE, Brewer HB Jr: An approach to the management of hyperlipoproteinemia. JAMA 255:512, 1986. Copyright 1986, American Medical Association.

Influence of Sex. Distributions in men may differ from those in women. For example, in women, cholesterol values analogous to those cited above for men are 208 and 281 mg per deciliter, respectively. Plasma urate concentration values, mean and 90 per cent limits, are 4.9 (2.7 to 7.2) mg per deciliter in men and 4.0 (2.5 to 6.3) mg per deciliter in premenopausal women. Mean serum calcium values in normal men decline 0.0068 mg per deciliter per year from age 20 to age 80. Those of women show no regression against age. This is an important point in the diagnosis of hyperparathyroidism, which is chiefly a disease of the older age group.

Other Influences. These include weight (creatinine values), diet (triglycerides), drugs (diuretics), environment (altitude—hemoglobin), lifestyle (vegetarian diet), habits (alcohol), and the analytic methods themselves.

BIOLOGIC REFERENCE INTERVALS. In a few instances, sufficient data are available to set reference intervals on the basis of risk assessments. For example, Table 22–1 shows reference intervals for total, LDL, and HDL cholesterol in plasma selected on the basis of moderate and high risk, as determined by epidemiologic studies.

Another example concerns urate concentration values. An electrolyte solution with the sodium concentration of plasma is saturated with urate at 6.4 to 6.8 mg per deciliter. In addition, proteins of plasma bind urate equivalent to about 4 per cent of the amount in solution. Values above 7.0 (perhaps 7.2) mg per deciliter represent supersaturation and are associated with increased risk of renal stone and clinical gout. The magnitude of the risk factor increases as urate concentration values rise above 7.0 mg per deciliter. The 95 per cent limits of serum urate values in "healthy" male New Zealand Maoris are 4 to 10 mg per deciliter, and 10 per cent of adult males develop gout. Surely values of serum urate above 7.0 mg per deciliter in this male population cannot be considered "normal," even though they fall within the reference interval as selected by the usual criteria.

DISCONTINUOUS DISTRIBUTIONS. Some traits may be distributed bimodally or trimodally. Such relationships are most likely in families in which there is a monogenetic disease characterized by a chemical abnormality. For example, measurements of galactose-1-phosphate uridyltransferase activity in the families of patients with transferase deficiency galactosemia are distributed trimodally. The effects of two and of one mutant allele are clearly distinguishable from the normal and from each other. Assay values in the three modes are zero, 7.5 to 13.5 units, and 19.5 to 32 units. The intermediate enzyme assay values are found in subjects who are presumed heterozygotes by pedigree analysis. It is common to hear the term "heterozygote value" applied to an enzyme activity value approximately one half of normal. This practice is justifiable only when assay data are combined with pedigree data, for there may be other reasons for a reduced enzyme assay value that have nothing to do with genetics.

An apparently continuous distribution with marked skewing may at times be dissected into two or even three distribution modes by appropriate clinical and pedigree studies. For example, the distribution of plasma cholesterol concentrations in familial hypercholesterolemia displays marked overlap between subjects who are clinically normal and those who are heterozygotes by pedigree analysis. Similarly, there is considerable overlap between heterozygotes and abnormal homozygotes. Only a complete family pedigree permits adequate definition of the range of values in each distribution mode.

THE PHYSICIAN AND THE LABORATORY TEST RESULT

The tables at the end of this book contain values that define the reference intervals for a large number of substances commonly measured in clinical medicine. They represent the best data currently available, but are subject to all the uncertainties discussed above. In some instances more selective data of an age- and sex-matched control population will need to be consulted by the physician.

Clinical judgment will always be required in the interpretation of laboratory data. For example, a blood urea nitrogen (BUN) concentration of 22 mg per deciliter is not a normal value for a patient on a very low protein diet. Also, electrolyte values of sodium at 145 mEq per liter, potassium at 3.5 mEq per liter, chloride at 98 mEq per liter, and CO_2 at 30 mEq per liter may indicate metabolic alkalosis even though all individual values fall within published reference intervals.

Laboratory tests are critical to the diagnosis of disease and management of patients. The physician must know the limits of reliability and usefulness of each test result in the clinical setting of the individual patient. This is particularly true when all deviant test results have returned to normal but the patient is not improving. It is especially when laboratory data provide little or no help that the patient needs a doctor.

Dales LG, Friedman GD, Collen MF: Evaluating periodic multiphasic health checkups: A controlled trial. J Chronic Dis 32:385, 1979. *Only a limited number of screening tests (history or physical examination, stool test for occult blood, and blood pressure) actually improve health outcome of asymptomatic outpatients.*

Dixon RH, Laszlo J: Utilization of clinical chemistry services by medical house staff. Arch Intern Med 134:1064, 1974. *Less than 10 per cent of data obtained from a panel of 12 tests were used clinically.*

Elveback LR, Guillier CL, Keating FR: Health, normality, and the ghost of Gauss. JAMA 211:69, 1970. *Of eight distributions evaluated, only that of serum albumin was "normal" or gaussian.*

Hoeg JM, Gregg RE, Brewer HB, Jr: An approach to the management of hyperlipoproteinemia. JAMA 255:512, 1986. *One of the best examples relating reference intervals to epidemiologic risk factors.*

Keating FR, Jones JD, Elveback LR, et al.: The relation of age and sex to distribution of values in healthy adults of serum calcium, inorganic phosphorus, magnesium, alkaline phosphatase, total proteins, albumin, and blood urea. J Lab Clin Med 73:825, 1969. *A study of the age- and sex-dependency of several constituents of serum. The downward trend to serum calcium values with age in men is particularly noteworthy.*

Korvin CC, Pearce RH, Stanley J: Admissions screening: Clinical benefits. Ann Intern Med 83:197, 1975. *Admission screening tests have a relatively low benefit. Fewer than 1 per cent lead to new diagnoses of significance to the patient.*

Mainland, D: Remarks on clinical "norms." Clin Chem 17:267, 1971. *An excellent article explaining the use of nonparametric methods for establishing reference intervals.*

Parkerson GR, Eisenson HJ: Association of patient and physician characteristics with follow-up of abnormal laboratory results. J Fam Pract 11:943, 1980. *As few as 40 per cent of abnormal results initiate clinical follow-up.*

23 OVERVIEW OF IMAGING TECHNIQUES AND PROJECTION FOR THE FUTURE

Alexander R. Margulis

HISTORICAL PERSPECTIVE

Radiology has undergone tremendous changes in the post–World War II decades. Progress in technologic developments related to medical imaging has been continuously accelerating, making diagnostic radiology one of the most exciting areas of diagnostic medicine during the last few years. Diagnostic imaging has been and continues to be the direct beneficiary of some of the areas of technology that are most heavily subsidized by governments and industry. Space exploration provided miniaturization of imaging equipment components. Extremely high-resolution television techniques used for space exploration and photographing of the earth's surface and advances in computers and techniques of storage of information have contributed to the development of digital radiography, highly advanced x-ray computed tomography (CT) machines, positron emission tomography, and magnetic resonance imaging. These modalities, although expensive, are eventually cost effective because they significantly reduce invasiveness and permit the performance of many procedures on an outpatient basis. Because of this they have found ready acceptance and have rapidly proliferated, not only in the United States, but throughout the Western world and Japan.

PRESENT STATUS OF RADIOLOGIC IMAGING

Conventional Radiography

The term "conventional radiography" is a misnomer today. Equipment that was considered advanced in the early 1970's is today hopelessly obsolete. Although there have been no breakthroughs in x-ray tube design, the generators and controls have been computerized; the television cameras are smaller and more reliable; and the equipment as a whole has grown more functional and often multipurpose. The highly specialized, extremely expensive rooms used in the past for angiography only are changing, particularly in small hospitals, into rooms that can be used for many different procedures, including digital subtraction fluoroscopy (Fig. 23–1). Even conventional darkrooms are being replaced by daylight developing facilities, which save space, time, and personnel. These trends of saving space, time, and personnel will become even more evident in the future as departments of radiology will have to become smaller and more intensively active and will have to serve inpatients and outpatients with the same equipment over longer hours each day.

As computers improve and the capacity to store data increases, the present halide film will be replaced by laser discs or other similar devices that will significantly reduce the size of filing areas and permit rapid and reliable access to images projected on television monitors. Hard copies will be instantly available in multiple formats similar to x-ray computed tomography.

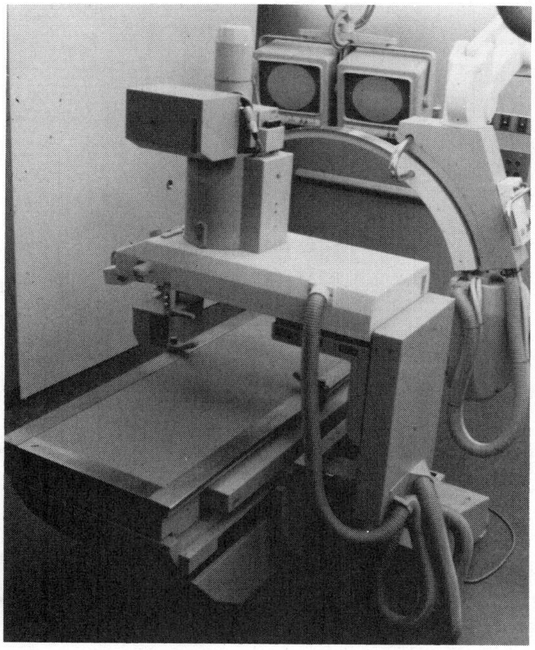

FIGURE 23–1. Photograph of a bi-plane fluoroscopic and radiographic multipurpose room with digital fluoroscopy. Multiple types of procedures are performed in this room: interventional, angiography, biliary procedures (including gallstone removal), gastrointestinal examinations, myelography, etc. Machines of this type, although expensive, are cost efficient because they are in constant use.

As videotaping improves and better resolution is obtained, fluoroscopic information will be recorded on tape and diagnostic frames will be recorded on multiformatted hard copy as the only record. This will result in reduced radiation exposure and eventually in cost saving.

Digital Radiography and Fluoroscopy

Digital subtraction fluoroscopy did not fulfill all the expectations that greeted it when it was introduced at the end of the 1970's. It was expected then that all arteriography would be performed intravenously, noninvasively, with images showing excellent detail. This has not occurred, and angiography still requires that large amounts of iodine-containing contrast media be injected intravenously through catheters advanced into large veins. Even then, owing to breathing or involuntary motion, blurring detracts from the quality of the images. At this time intra-arterial injections of small amounts of contrast medium appear to be the best method for performing digital subtraction angiography (Fig. 23–2). Further improvements in digital subtraction fluoroscopy will probably occur, and eventually it can be expected that most arteriography will be performed with some modification of digital radiography. This is also being facilitated by the continual decrease in price of the equipment.

Computed Tomography

Computed tomography has become an indispensable diagnostic tool in a modern hospital as well as in sophisticated outpatient centers throughout the United States, Canada, most of Western Europe, and particularly Japan. For the last ten years there has been a steady improvement in the quality of images. The speed of scanning, which indirectly also results in better spatial resolution, has come down to 1 second for conventional CT scanners and is in the 50 msec range for the cine CT scanner, an advanced scanner with no moving parts. Computed tomography is today considered to be an excellent method for the examination of the brain (Fig. 23–3) and spine. It is still the modality of choice for the examination of the mediastinum and chest, as well as the abdomen. It is a tomographic examination in the axial plane, but it also allows redisplay of images in any plane (Fig. 23–4). CT numbers accurately reflect the average density of small tissue volume elements and can be used to identify various tissues, fluids, and lesions. Computed tomography is of great advantage in showing tumors, abscesses, ruptures of organs, and accumulation of fluid, with high accuracy. Since the introduction of magnetic resonance imaging, CT has remained the examination of choice for organs in the peritoneal cavity and the alimentary tube, with magnetic resonance imaging rapidly replacing it in most other areas.

Ultrasonography

Diagnostic ultrasonography, or ultrasound, uses a pulse echo device to record reflected waves of a sound beam in two dimensions. The resolution of sonographic images is inferior

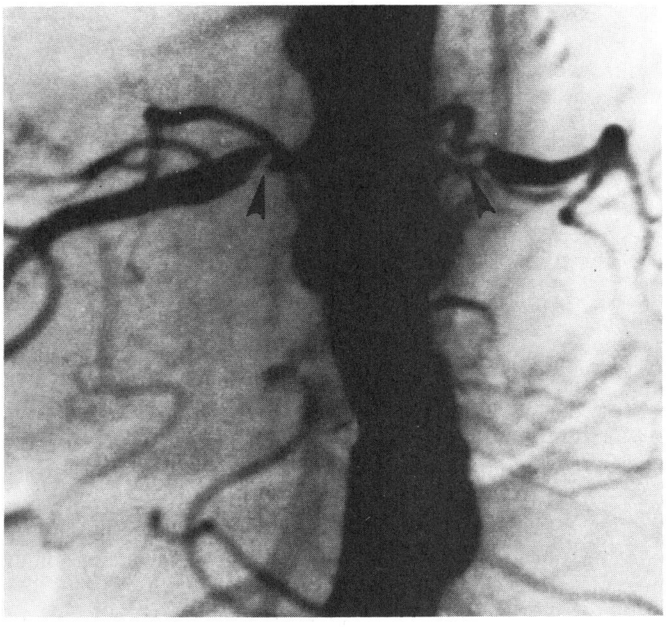

FIGURE 23–2. Intra-arterial digital subtraction aortogram showing bilateral renal artery stenoses (*arrowheads*).

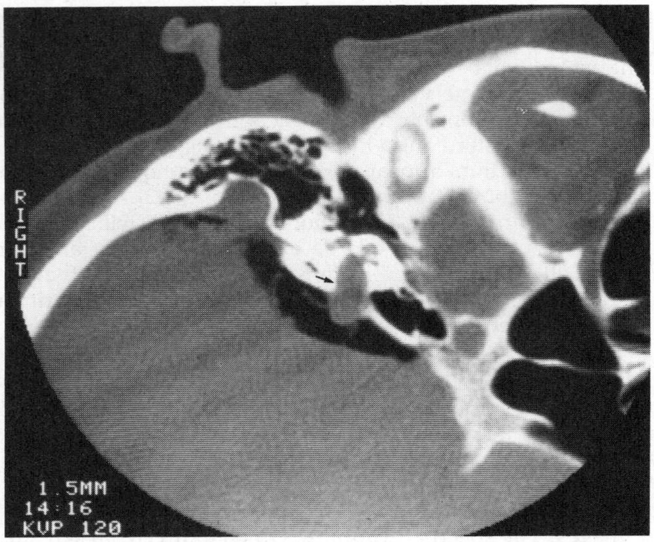

FIGURE 23–3. High resolution axial view computed tomogram showing an acoustic neuroma widening the internal acoustic meatus. The lesion itself (*arrow*) is seen with outstanding detail.

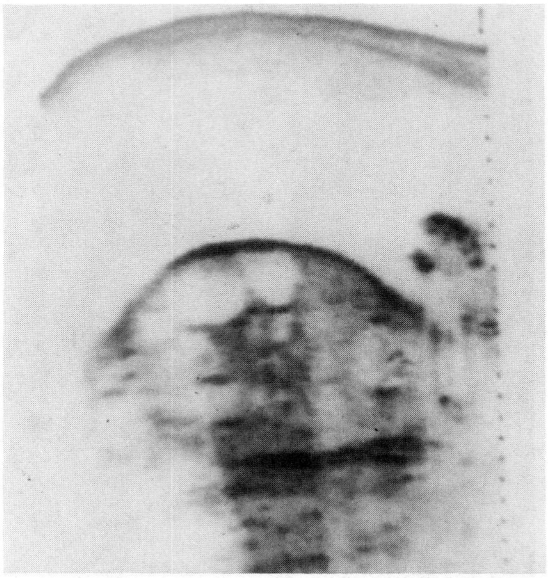

FIGURE 23–5. Multiple dilated loops of small bowel are demonstrated by ultrasound in this fetus with jejunal atresia.

to the image obtained from computed tomography or magnetic resonance. The great advantages of this modality, however, are (1) it is relatively inexpensive, (2) it is rapid, (3) it can produce images in real time, (4) it can obtain images in any plane without revision of format, (5) because of its speed it is ideal for directing certain interventional procedures, and (6) no biologic hazards have been demonstrated within the diagnostic range. It does not depend on ionizing radiation. The disadvantages of the method are that (1) it is highly dependent on operator skill, (2) its spatial resolution and resolving power lag behind those of computed tomography and magnetic resonance imaging, and (3) no good contrast media are available at present. In the diagnostic range, ultrasound is of no use in examining the lungs, the brain through the intact skull of an adult, the spine, or areas where there is a great deal of gas. Ultrasound images, however, exceed the quality of CT in asthenic or cachectic individuals. It is currently the method of choice in examining the female pelvis, particularly in obstetrics. An entire field of intrauterine diagnosis of fetal abnormalities by ultrasound has developed, leading also to surgical intrauterine interventions, again guided by ultrasound (Fig. 23–5). Ultrasonography is also of great use in diagnosis of abnormalities of the neonatal brain through the intact skull and in the intraoperative diagnosis of brain abnormalities through open skull flaps.

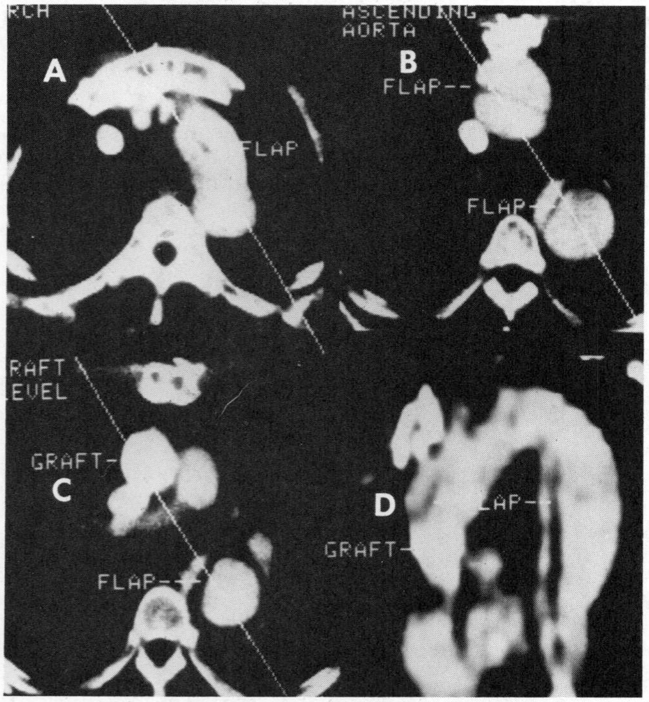

FIGURE 23–4. Dissecting aneurysm of the descending thoracic aorta demonstrated with exquisite detail on dynamic computed tomography reformatted along a plane shown by the dotted line on three axial tomograms at different levels and demonstrated in this illustration under A, B, and C. The flap is seen as a vertical dark line on the reformatted image (D). The Teflon graft was introduced a short time before this examination.

Magnetic Resonance Imaging

Magnetic resonance imaging (MRI) is a new imaging modality that has been derived from chemical magnetic resonance. For imaging, hydrogen protons give the best images. The strength of the signal will indicate the amount of hydrogen modified by tissue relaxation parameters, T1 and T2. T1, also known as the spin lattice parameter, is dependent on the interaction of other nuclei with hydrogen. T2 depends on the influence of protons on each other. It is also referred to as the spin-spin parameter. The intensity of the signal is also affected by the proton bulk motion effect, which results from the fact that is takes approximately 50 msec for the signal emanating from protons to register. If the protons move through the plane of imaging at a faster rate, the signal will not be recorded. This permits evaluation of speed of flow through blood vessels and visualization of patent blood vessels without contrast media. In addition, the image on MRI is influenced by the technique of acquisition of data. These techniques are so numerous that it is possible to individualize them for given tissue abnormalities and anatomic areas. By applying the right sequence, a great deal of information about the nature of normal and abnormal tissues can be obtained. Magnetic resonance imaging has several characteristics that are advantages when compared with other imaging modalities. Besides giving information about tissue chemistry and metabolic and biochemical data, MRI offers superb resolving power. This is due to contrast resolution that is considerably

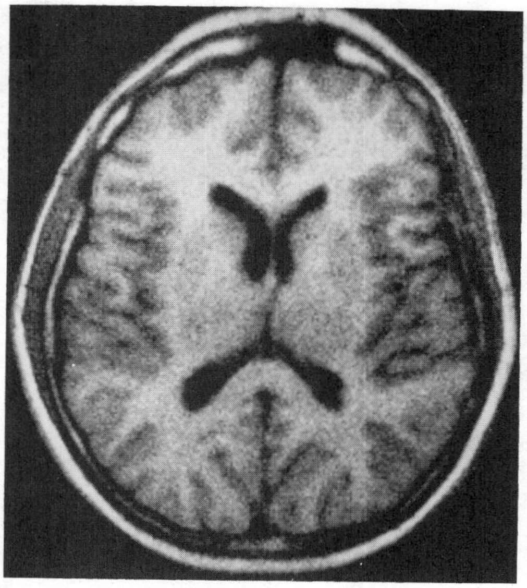

FIGURE 23–6. Axial section through the normal brain with MRI. Notice the excellent demonstration of the ventricles and gray and white matter.

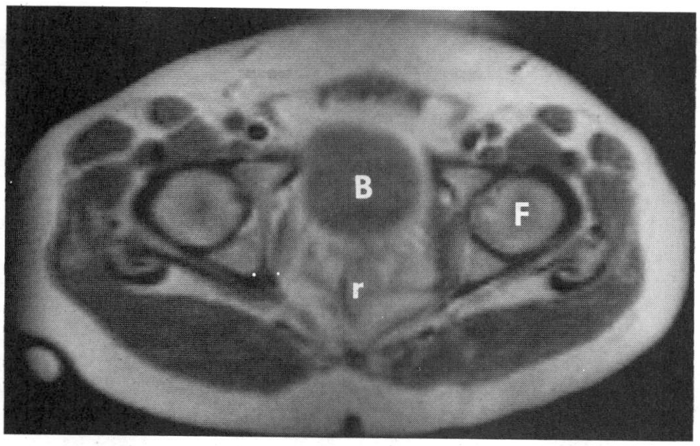

FIGURE 23–8. Axial MRI section through the pelvis of a male. B, Urinary bladder; r, rectum; F, femoral head.

better than that of CT, with spatial resolution becoming comparable to CT. Furthermore, MRI can provide tomographic sections in any desired plane. By exciting section after section while the remagnetization occurs in the original section, multiple simultaneous sections can be obtained in a relatively short time.

Magnetic resonance imaging is already superior to any other imaging modality in the examination of the brain (Figs. 23–6 and 23–7), spinal cord, cancellous bone, the male and female pelvic organs, and the urinary bladder (Figs. 23–8 and 23–9). With the use of surface or specially designed small coils, it is the best method for the examination of large joints (Fig. 23–10). It will probably shortly replace arthrography of the knee, hip, shoulder, and temporomandibular joint. Magnetic resonance imaging has been very successful in the examination of the spine, particularly with the use of surface coils. With respiratory and electrocardiographic (ECG) gating, it is providing diagnostic images of the heart (Fig. 23–11) and mediastinum of quality unsurpassed by other modalities. It is as valuable in the examination of the liver, particularly in the search for metastases, hepatocellular carcinomas, and hemangiomas. It has advantages over other techniques in the examination of the kidneys. Magnetic resonance imaging does not show calcifications. Magnetic resonance imaging is currently of no value in the examination of the small bowel and its mesentery and has only limited applications in the examination of the pancreas. It is promising in the staging of tumors of the rectum and esophagus. Further drawbacks are relatively slow scanning (in minutes), the expense of the equipment and siting, the large amounts of space necessary for the facility, and the danger of loose metallic objects flying into the machine. Other disadvantages are the inability to examine patients with pacemakers, large metallic prostheses, prosthetic heart valves made with magnetic materials, or freshly introduced vascular magnetic clips or to study patients who are in need of continuous observation and require life-support systems. The drawback of slow scanning by MRI will soon be eliminated by the development of rapid scanning sequences (in seconds), which use different pulses, resulting in reduced flip angles of protons, and imaginative handling of data by the computer.

Magnetic resonance imaging is highly sensitive in detecting disease, but its sensitivity is not matched by specificity. The

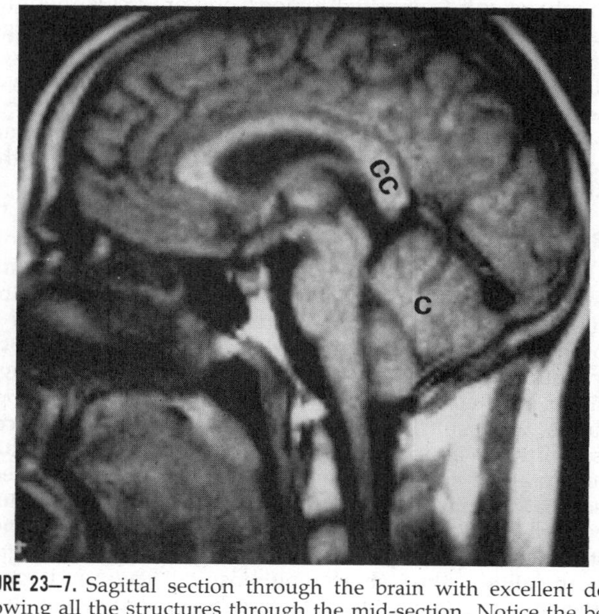

FIGURE 23–7. Sagittal section through the brain with excellent detail showing all the structures through the mid-section. Notice the beautiful demonstration of the gyri, corpus callosum (cc), and cerebellum (c).

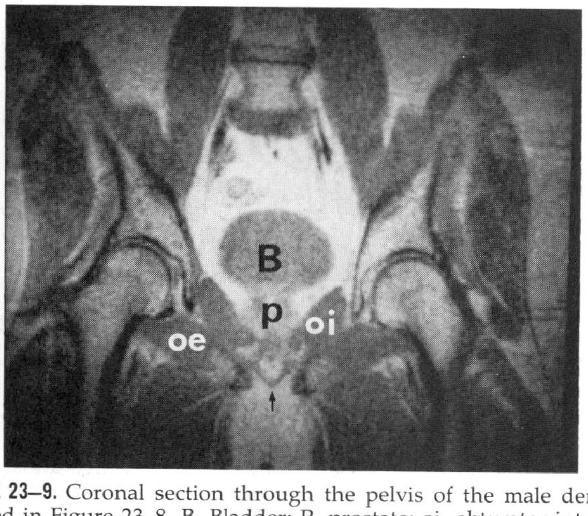

FIGURE 23–9. Coronal section through the pelvis of the male demonstrated in Figure 23–8. B, Bladder; P, prostate; oi, obturator internus muscle; oe, obturator externus muscle; arrow, bulbus spongiosus.

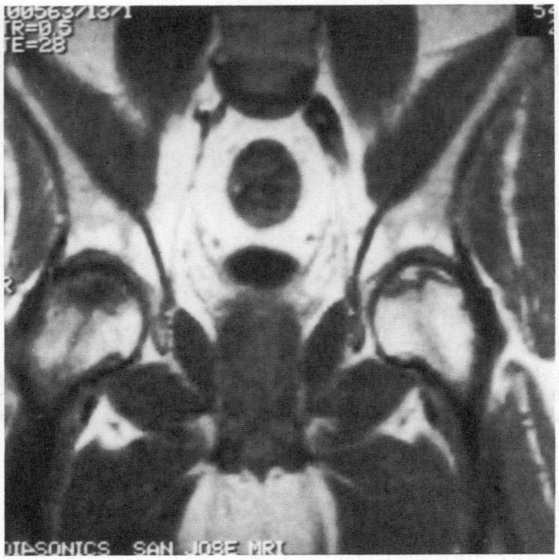

FIGURE 23–10. MRI of bilateral osteonecrosis of the femoral heads. The changes are more advanced on the right.

latter will be improved with the development of paramagnetic contrast media and localized tissue spectroscopy using spectra of multiple elements: ^{31}P, H, ^{19}F, ^{23}Na, ^{15}N, and so on.

The Algorithmic Approach

With many different radiologic modalities, the physician is often in a dilemma as to which examination is indicated and, if several are to be requested, in what order they should be performed. The algorithmic approach offers a logical sequence in which one examination follows the previous one, depending on its results, in order to provide a definitive diagnosis. This approach relies very much on the equipment available as well as on the skills of the operators. It is often linked with local experience and sometimes is tinged with prejudice. The best approach for selecting the proper procedures results from a continuing dialogue between the clinician and radiologist in which the two familiarize each other with the newest developments and experiences. A typical example of an algorithm is in the evaluation of jaundice (Ch. 120). When chemical

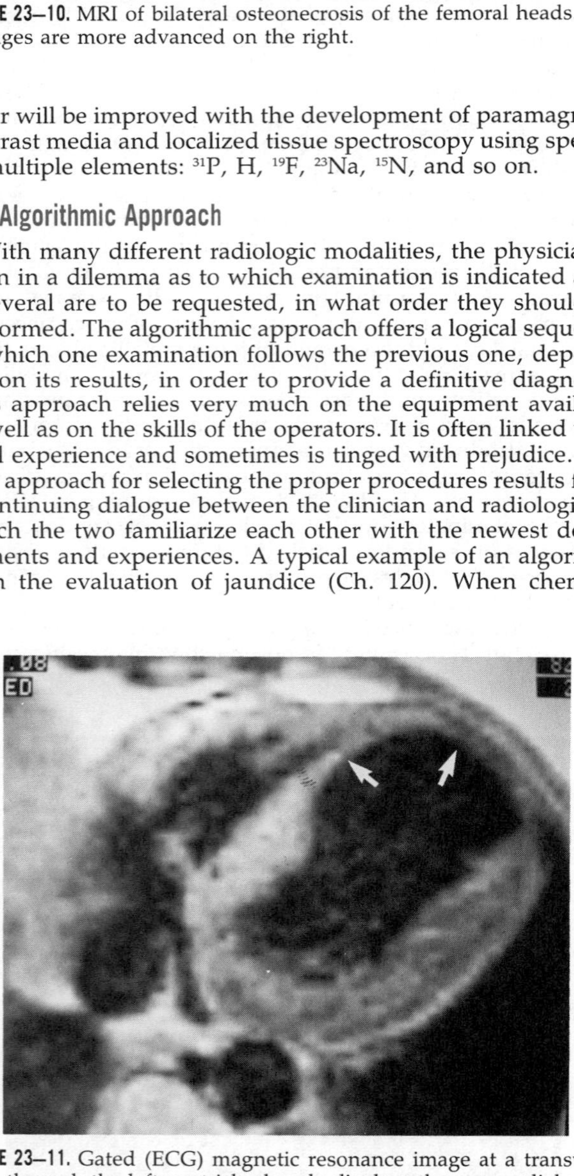

FIGURE 23–11. Gated (ECG) magnetic resonance image at a transverse level through the left ventricle sharply displays the myocardial walls. In this patient with a prior anteroseptal myocardial infarction, the image shows severe thinning of the anterior septum and anterior wall of the left ventricle (*arrows*).

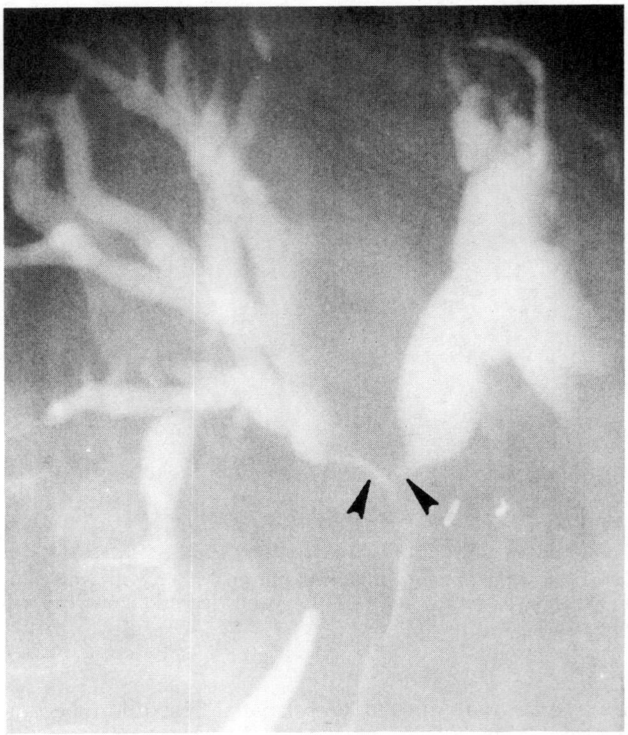

FIGURE 23–12. Percutaneous transhepatic cholangiogram demonstrates high-grade obstructing lesion of the proximal common hepatic duct involving the ductal bifurcation (*arrowheads*). Biopsy demonstrated cholangiocarcinoma.

tests indicate that the jaundice is most likely due to obstruction, the next procedure is ultrasonography (if that capability exists locally) to determine the width of the biliary tree. If the ducts are dilated, and depending on whether the history suggests tumor or stone, either endoscopic retrograde cholangiography (ERC) or percutaneous transhepatic cholangiography is performed. If a stone is found to be obstructing, sphincterotomy is performed by ERC, and if a tumor is seen, either percutaneous transhepatic cholangiography or ERC is performed (Fig. 23–12) with the introduction of drainage through a stent. Computed tomography or MRI is then done for staging of the tumor in order to determine whether surgery is indicated and, if so, whether it is likely to be curative or palliative. For curative surgery, decompression is often valuable. For palliation, an internal stent introduced percutaneously may be all that is necessary. Magnetic resonance imaging has greatly changed many of the previous algorithms as the method is used with increasing frequency.

Financial Considerations

The cost of radiologic equipment has soared; in most hospitals modern imaging equipment has overwhelmed equipment budgets. The sophistication and expense of the equipment necessitate an organized referral system to prevent duplication of equipment and to allow utilization of imaging systems to their best advantage. Noninvasive imaging procedures can result in shorter hospital stays, in avoidance of hospitalization altogether, and in almost complete elimination of exploratory surgery. When surgery is necessary, precise preoperative diagnosis shortens the procedure and reduces the number of complications. Properly utilized and properly distributed imaging systems can enhance outpatient diagnostic capabilities, thus shortening hospital stays and greatly reducing the number of acute care hospitals needed. Interventional radiologic procedures are relatively less invasive than surgical procedures. Their advances have already served in avoiding or shortening hospitalizations and significantly reducing the number of complications and expense of open surgery. The elimination of hospital beds resulting from all these procedures should eventually lead to enormous cost savings.

FUTURE DEVELOPMENTS IN IMAGING

With the continuous advances in the development of computers and television systems, combining increased versatility and decreased cost, diagnostic imaging can expect to make progress in several new directions. It can be expected that the departments of radiology of the future will become totally computerized, integrating into the hospital's general computer system. This means that images themselves as well as reports will be instantly available on television monitors on wards along with laboratory information and information from medical records and pathologic studies. These systems will be expensive but at the same time will be cost effective, saving on personnel, communication, and duration of hospital stay of the patient. Computers will also help to store data correlating clinical information and allowing the most efficient and most rational algorithmic approaches for reaching the correct diagnosis. Computers will therefore help physicians, surgeons, and radiologists to reach the correct, least invasive, and most time-saving sequence of diagnostic studies. Similarly, artificial intelligence based on clinical experience and previous imaging results will also help in selection of the proper techniques, sequences, and planes of imaging for magnetic resonance. This again will result not only in improving clinical results but also in making the use of equipment more cost effective and less traumatic for patients.

These remarkable advances in imaging will increasingly attract the interest and collaboration of other physicians (such as internists, neurologists, ophthalmologists, obstetricians, neurosurgeons, and surgeons) with the radiologist in the field of diagnostic imaging in order to optimize progress through the exchange of experience and ideas. Localized tissue magnetic resonance spectroscopy will provide further advances not only in making imaging yield morphologic information but also in making it possible to follow metabolic processes and specifically identify diseases.

HISTORICAL AND GENERAL REFERENCES

Grigg ERN: The Train of the Invisible Light. Springfield, Ill., Charles C Thomas, 1965. *An extensive, well-illustrated review of the development of roentgenology from its earliest days.*

DIGITAL RADIOGRAPHY AND FLUOROSCOPY

Enzmann DR, Djang WT, Riederer SJ, et al: Digital subtraction angiography: Current status and use of intra-arterial injection. Radiology 146:669, 1983. *A clever technical review of two approaches to digital angiography.*

Foley WD, Milde MW: Intra-arterial digital subtraction angiography. Radiol Clin of North Am 23:293, 1985. *A clear, objective view of the subject.*

Riederer SJ, Kruger RA: Intravenous digital subtraction: A summary of recent developments. Radiology 147:633, 1983. *An extensive summary of multiple approaches with the advantages and disadvantages of each.*

COMPUTED TOMOGRAPHY

Boyd DP: Computerized-transmission tomography of the heart using scanning electron beams. In Higgins CA (ed.): CTT of the Heart: Experimental Evaluation and Clinical Application. Mt. Kisco, N.Y., Futura Publishing Company, 1983. *The author describes an original approach to the generation of a scanning x-ray beam that permits the achievement of cine computed tomography.*

Lee JKT, Sagel SS, Stanley RJ (eds.): Computed Body Tomography. New York, Raven Press, 1982. *A well-illustrated, modern, complete textbook on computed tomography of the body. Particularly good sections on kidney and liver.*

Moss AA, Gamsu G, Genant HK (eds.): Computed Tomography of the Body. Philadelphia, W.B. Saunders Company, 1983. *A large, complete, up-to-date textbook. Particularly good sections on the mediastinum, the digestive tract, and the spine.*

ULTRASONOGRAPHY

Callen PW (ed.): Ultrasonography in Obstetrics and Gynecology. Philadelphia, W.B. Saunders Company, 1983. *A well-illustrated and organized textbook on modern ultrasound applications in the field of obstetrics and gynecology.*

Sarti DA, Sample WF (eds.): Diagnostic Ultrasound. Text and Cases. Boston, G.K. Hall & Company, 1980. *Still the best-illustrated book on ultrasonography, with exquisite illustrations.*

MAGNETIC RESONANCE

Budinger TF, Margulis AR (eds.): Medical Magnetic Resonance Imaging and Spectroscopy: A Primer. Berkeley CA, Society of Magnetic Resonance in Medicine, 1986.

James TL, Margulis AR (eds.): Biomedical Magnetic Resonance. San Francisco, Radiology Research and Education Foundation, 1984.

Margulis AR, Fisher MR: Present clinical status of magnetic resonance imaging. Magnet Res Med 2:309, 1985.

Pykett IL: NMR imaging in medicine. Sci Am 246:78, 1982. *An imaginative, clear, and well-illustrated explanation of the physics and techniques of NMR.*

ECONOMIC DATA AND BENEFITS

Margulis AR, Shea WJ, Jr: Advances in Imaging Technology and Their Impact on Medicine. Mackenzie Davidson Memorial Lecture, April 1986. Forty-fourth Annual Congress of the British Institute of Radiology, Bristol, April 1986.

Newton DR, Witz S, Norman D, et al: Economic impact of CT scanning on the evaluation of pituitary adenomas. Am J Neurol Radiol 4:57, 1983. *A carefully designed study showing the economic benefits of computed tomography in one selected condition where controls were available.*

Norman D, Ulloa N, Brant-Zawadzki M, et al: Intraarterial digital subtraction imaging cost considerations. Radiology 156:33, 1985. *Irrational handling of new technology.*

24 PRINCIPLES OF DRUG THERAPY

Alan S. Nies

Because all patients respond differently to drugs, individualization of drug dosages is required so that therapy will be effective and nontoxic. A basic tenet of clinical pharmacology is that a closer relationship exists between the concentration of drug in the blood and the drug's effect than between drug dose and effect. The relationship between drug concentration and effect has fostered the study of the factors influencing drug movement in the body, a science called pharmacokinetics (Fig. 24–1). Rational drug therapy requires a basic understanding of pharmacokinetic principles that can be applied to patient care. In this way the amount of drug delivered to the target tissue can be controlled within a definable and safe range.

ABSORPTION. When a dose of drug is administered, it must first be absorbed into the systemic circulation to produce its effects. The simplest case is that of the drug's being given intravenously, in which absorption is obviously complete and immediate. For all other routes of administration, there will be a delay in the drug's reaching the circulation, and the absorption may be incomplete. Drug absorption is the only part of the pharmacokinetic process that can be influenced by the physician and the pharmaceutical industry. Most drugs are absorbed by passive diffusion into the circulation from their site of administration. Since the process of diffusion is dependent upon the concentration of drug contacting the absorbing surface, the rate of absorption can be influenced by affecting the rate of dissolution of the dosage form. Depot intramuscular preparations of some drugs (e.g., penicillin, progesterone) slowly release the active drug into tissue fluids, from which it can be absorbed into the circulation. In this way, drug levels in the blood can be maintained by a continuous absorption process for many hours or many days even though the drug is rapidly eliminated from the body. A similar technique can be used for oral drug administration. Long-acting oral preparations can be formulated for drugs with rapid elimination by producing a dosage form that slowly releases the active drug from a matrix. The duration of sustained absorption from an oral preparation, however, is

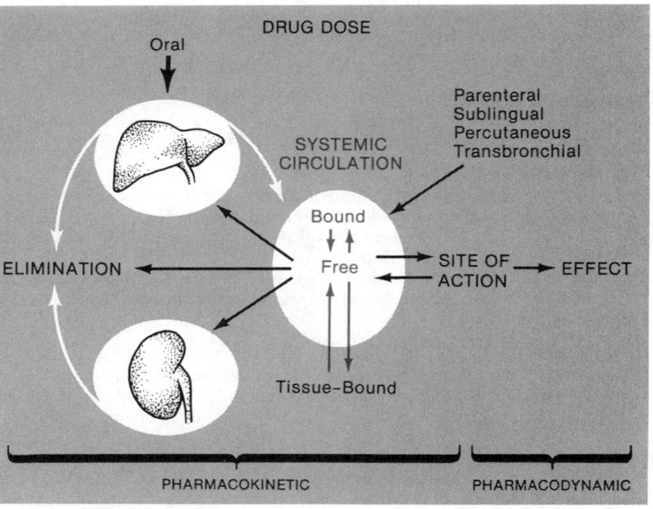

FIGURE 24–1. Drug movement in the body. The variation in effects following a given dose is related to pharmacokinetic and pharmacodynamic factors. The systemic circulation can be sampled to determine the pharmacokinetics.

limited by the gastrointestinal transit time. Drugs that are slowly dissolved and slowly absorbed may be affected by alterations in gut transit time more so than drugs that are rapidly and completely absorbed. An increase in gut motility will lead to a decrease in the extent of absorption of slowly absorbed drugs (such as digoxin), whereas a decrease in motility may actually increase the extent of absorption.

Depending on the drug, absorption can occur from sites other than the gastrointestinal tract, subcutaneous tissue, or muscle. Some lipid-soluble drugs can be absorbed from the skin or through the oral or bronchial mucous membranes. Nitroglycerin can be absorbed percutaneously, buccally, and sublingually. When given as a sublingual tablet or sprayed into the mouth, nitroglycerin is rapidly absorbed into the systemic circulation and produces a transient effect. When applied to the skin, nitroglycerin has a slow but sustained absorption lasting several hours for the ointment or 24 hours with a sustained release patch. The transdermal route also can be used for scopolamine, estradiol, and clonidine. However, most drugs cannot be absorbed well from the skin or oral mucous membrane because of the limited surface utilized for absorption and the solubility characteristics of the drug. Occasionally, percutaneous absorption is an unwanted side effect of drugs (e.g., steroids) applied to the skin to produce topical effects.

The sublingual, transbronchial, and percutaneous routes of absorption have the advantage of delivering the drug directly into the systemic circulation. By contrast, when absorbed by the intestine, the drug enters the portal circulation and is presented to the liver, where a portion of the drug can be eliminated before reaching the systemic circulation (Fig. 24–1). Thus, nitroglycerin can be absorbed readily from the intestine but is rapidly destroyed by the liver so that only a fraction of the orally administered dose reaches the circulation. A similar situation exists for propranolol, in which over half of an orally administered dose is removed by the liver. Hepatic removal during absorption of the drug from the gut is called "first pass" or "presystemic" elimination and, along with poor absorption from the intestine, accounts for the need to give larger oral than parenteral doses of some drugs to achieve equivalent pharmacologic effects. "Oral bioavailability" is the quantitative expression relating the amount of drug reaching the systemic circulation after oral administration to the amount after intravenous administration. Oral bioavailability ranges from 0 per cent (no drug reaches the systemic circulation) to 100 per cent (all of the ingested dose reaches the systemic circulation). For some drugs, such as lidocaine and morphine, the oral bioavailability is sufficiently low to preclude oral administration. Formulation of oral preparations can affect bioavailability. There are well-documented examples of differences in bioavailability for different brands of the same drug. In addition, sustained-release preparations often show greater interpatient variability in bioavailability than standard formulations of the same drug. For all calculations utilizing the oral dosage, the dosage must be corrected for less than complete bioavailability.

DISTRIBUTION. Once absorbed into the systemic circulation, the drug must distribute throughout the body. If the drug is rapidly administered intravenously, it is first delivered to the well-perfused tissues and only more slowly distributed to less well-perfused tissues. By measuring drug concentrations in plasma at various times after a drug is administered, a curve can be described from which distribution and elimination can be quantified. For example, if 100 mg of lidocaine is given as an intravenous bolus to an adult, the curve in Figure 24–2 results. This curve of lidocaine concentration versus time can be separated into an early distribution phase, during which the drug rapidly disappears from the circulation, and a later elimination phase, during which the drug in the blood is in equilibrium with drug in the tissues and is more gradually eliminated from the body (Fig. 24–2). The effects of most drugs are related to the plasma concentration during the elimination phase. However, whether the plasma concentration of the drug during the distribution phase is predictive of drug effects depends on the particular drug. For a drug such as lidocaine that quickly reaches its sites of action, the initial concentrations shortly after a bolus of drug can produce therapeutic antiarrhythmic effects and toxic effects on the heart or brain. On the other hand, digoxin is an example of a drug that requires time to equilibrate or be transported to its receptors. When given intravenously, digoxin does not produce maximal effects for four to eight hours, during which time the blood levels are falling as the drug equilibrates with tissues. After the equilibration period of eight hours, digoxin concentrations fall more slowly, and only then does the digoxin concentration correlate with the drug's effects.

Apparent Volume of Distribution. The relationship between the amount of drug in the body and the concentration of drug in the plasma is defined as the "apparent volume of distribution" (V_D) of the drug:

$$V_D = \frac{\text{amount of drug in the body}}{\text{concentration of drug in plasma}}$$

The V_D is the "apparent" volume needed to contain the entire amount of drug if the drug were everywhere at the same concentration as in the plasma. The apparent volume of distribution of a drug during the elimination phase can be determined from a graph of the plasma drug concentration versus time by extrapolating the elimination phase back to zero time, giving the C_{P_0} (plasma concentration at time 0), an estimate of the concentration of drug in the plasma that would have been achieved by the intravenous dose of drug if the drug had been distributed throughout the tissues instantaneously. Thus:

$$V_D = \frac{\text{IV dose}}{C_{P_0}}$$

In Figure 24–2, the C_{P_0} for lidocaine is 0.84 mg per liter following a 100-mg dose. The V_D for lidocaine, therefore, is 100 mg ÷ 0.84 mg per liter = 119 liters. The V_D for several drugs are shown in Tables 24–1 and 24–2.

The apparent volume of distribution frequently does not correspond to any given body fluid compartment. For many

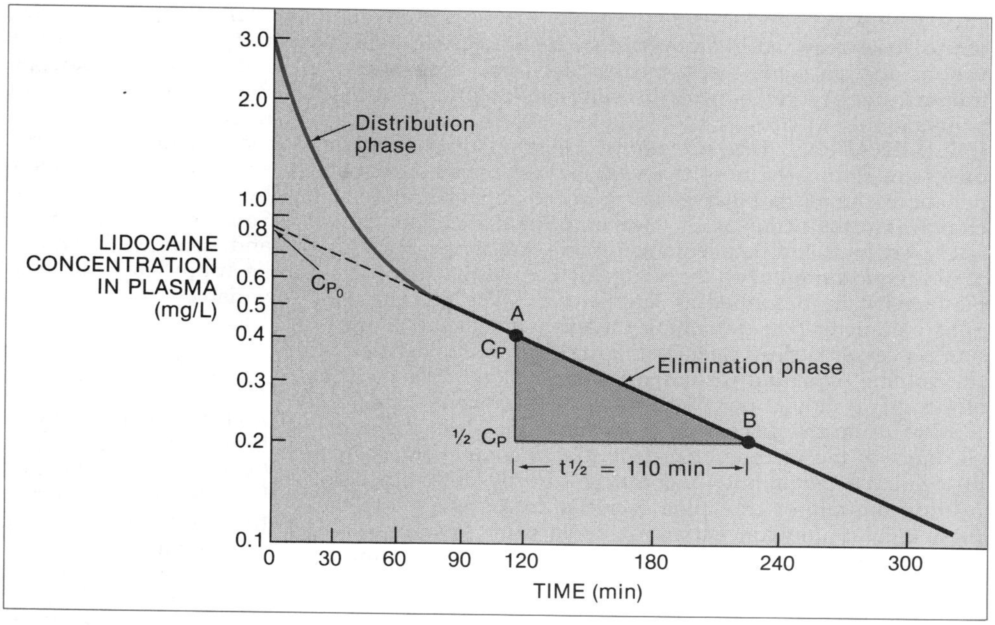

FIGURE 24–2. Lidocaine concentrations on a log scale plotted against time in minutes following a 100 mg bolus given intravenously to a 70-kg person. The C_{P_0} is the concentration of lidocaine in plasma that would be achieved if the dose was distributed instantaneously to the tissues. C_P at point A is twice the concentration of lidocaine at point B. The time between point A and point B is the half-life (t½).

drugs the V_D is larger than the entire body. For example, digoxin has a V_D of 7 liters per kilogram or about 500 liters in a 70-kg person. When a 0.5-mg dose of digoxin is administered intravenously, it distributes in this "apparent volume" of 500 liters to give a plasma concentration of 1 μg per liter or 1 ng per milliliter. A large apparent volume of distribution is merely an expression of the fact that most of the drug in the body is not in the plasma but is bound to the tissues at a greater concentration than in the plasma. For phenytoin and ethanol the V_D is 0.6 liter per kilogram. Although this figure approximates the value for total body water, it need not be the case that these drugs are distributed only in body water. The V_D is an empirically determined constant that allows one to relate the plasma concentration to the amount of drug in the body and should not be given a physiologic interpretation relating to real body volumes.

LOADING DOSES. One use of the apparent volume of distribution is to calculate the loading dose required to achieve a desired plasma drug concentration. From Figure 24–2 the apparent volume of distribution of lidocaine is 119 liters in a 70-kg person or 1.7 liters per kilogram. In order to establish rapidly a therapeutic plasma lidocaine concentration of 2 mg per liter, a loading dose of 238 mg (desired concentration × V_D) must be given. After the distribution phase, the loading dose (238 mg) will be contained in an apparent volume of 119 liters, resulting in a plasma concentration of 2 mg per liter. However, because lidocaine and many other drugs can produce toxic effects during the distribution phase, the entire loading dose should not be given in a single bolus; to do so would produce lidocaine concentrations during the distribution phase that would be potentially toxic. The initial high concentrations after a loading dose can be avoided by giving the desired amount of drug in divided doses or as an infusion rather than a bolus. In addition, the loading of drug into the body can be stopped if early signs of drug toxicity occur. If the drug can be given orally, a loading dose may be given that could cause toxicity if given intravenously. Because of the gradual absorption from the intestine, the drug has time to distribute to the tissues during the absorption process, and the very high peak drug concentrations that result from an intravenous bolus do not occur. As an example, the V_D of phenytoin is 0.6 liter per kilogram or 40 liters in a 70-kg adult. To achieve a low therapeutic plasma concentration of 10 mg per liter requires a loading dose of 400 mg. Since phenytoin has an oral bioavailability of 80 to 85 per cent, an oral loading dose of 500 mg will deliver 400 mg to the systemic circulation. The 500 mg of phenytoin can be given safely as a single oral dose even though the 400-mg loading dose given as a bolus intravenously could cause a cardiac arrest. If a patient has an inadequate plasma level, a loading dose can be used to achieve a therapeutic level rapidly. A patient with a phenytoin level of 5 mg per liter can be given a 400-mg phenytoin load (or 500 mg orally) to increase his level by 10 mg per liter to 15 mg per liter.

The estimates of all pharmacokinetic parameters, including the apparent volume of distribution, are derived from an

TABLE 24–1. PHARMACOKINETIC PARAMETERS FOR SOME COMMONLY USED DRUGS

	Cl_r* (ml/min)	Cl_{nr}† (ml/min)	Per Cent‡ Nonrenal	V_D (liter/kg)	t½ (hours)	Per Cent** Bound
Aminoglycosides	70	3	5	0.3	2–3	<10
Digitoxin	0	3	100	0.6	165	97
Digoxin§	110	40	30	7	36	25
Disopyramide	60	40	40	0.8	6	20–70
Lidocaine	60	800	95	1.7	1.7	70
Lithium	30	0	0	0.6	15	0
Penicillin G	350	35	10	0.2	0.5	65
Phenobarbital	1.5	4	70	0.6	86	50
Procainamide	330	120	30	1.6	3	65
Quinidine	100	200	65	2.5	7	75
Theophylline¶	0	55	100	0.5	7	55

*Cl_r = renal clearance for an adult with a creatinine clearance of 100 ml per minute.

†Cl_{nr} = nonrenal clearance for an adult.

‡Per cent nonrenal is the nonrenal clearance as a percentage of the total clearance.

§The oral bioavailability of digoxin is 65 per cent from the tablet and 95 per cent from the capsule.

¶Aminophylline is 85 per cent theophylline.

**Per cent bound to plasma proteins.

TABLE 24–2. DRUGS SHOWING DOSE-DEPENDENT KINETICS

	Maximal Metabolic Rate	Volume of Distribution
Salicylate	4000 mg/day	0.2–0.6 liter/kg*
Ethanol	8000 mg/hour	0.6 liter/kg
Phenytoin†	700 mg/day‡	0.6 liter/kg

*The volume of distribution of salicylate increases with increasing dose.

†The oral bioavailability of phenytoin is 80 per cent.

‡Some individuals have a lower maximal metabolic rate.

"average" patient and are therefore only first approximations of the doses required in an individual patient. Clinical observations and in some cases, measured plasma drug concentrations give information to the clinician for proper dosage adjustments.

ELIMINATION. ***Drug Clearance.*** Once in the circulation, drugs are eliminated from the body by two major processes: hepatic metabolism–biliary excretion and renal filtration-secretion into the urine. With a few important exceptions, the rates of hepatic and renal elimination are directly proportional to the concentration of the drug in the plasma, a process mathematically described as "first order." The pharmacokinetic parameter best describing the efficiency of the elimination processes is drug clearance. Drug clearance is defined as the volume of a fluid (usually plasma or blood) from which all drug is removed per unit of time. Clearance is a familiar term to clinicians discussing renal function. Thus creatinine clearance is the volume of plasma that is completely cleared of creatinine per minute and can be directly determined by relating the rate of creatinine excretion into the urine to the plasma creatinine concentration. Renal drug clearances can be determined in the same way by dividing renal excretory rate of the drug by the plasma drug concentration. Hepatic drug clearance is, by analogy to renal clearance, the volume of blood or plasma entirely cleared of drug by the liver and is therefore the rate of removal of drug by the liver divided by the concentration of drug in blood or plasma. Total body drug clearance (Cl) is the sum of all the individual organ clearances, which consists of renal (Cl_r) and nonrenal (Cl_{nr}) clearances. Total drug clearance is the rate of drug elimination by all processes ($\dot{R}$) divided by the plasma concentration (C_p):

$$Cl = \frac{\dot{R}}{C_p}$$

The clearance of drug by the liver and kidney can be influenced by the blood flow to the clearing organ, the binding of drug to the plasma proteins, and the activity of the processes responsible for drug removal, such as hepatic enzyme activity, glomerular filtration rate, and renal secretory processes. In physiologic terms, drug clearance by an organ is the product of organ blood flow (Q) and the fraction of the drug in the blood extracted on a single passage through the organ (E): $Cl = QE$. The extraction ratio, E, is calculated by dividing the arteriovenous difference in drug concentration ($C_a - C_v$) by the arterial drug concentration (C_a):

$$E = \frac{C_a - C_v}{C_a}$$

Clearance is *independent* of the distribution of drugs in the body (i.e., the V_D), since the eliminating organs "see" and can remove only the drug present in the blood.

Drug Half-Life. Both the clearance and the distribution of drug in the body influence the amount of time necessary to eliminate drug from the body. The proportion of the apparent volume of distribution cleared of drug per unit of time is a constant called the "first order elimination rate constant," or k_e:

$$k_e = \frac{Cl}{V_D}$$

This constant describes the exponential disappearance of drug from the plasma with time during the elimination phase. When plotted on semi-log graph paper, as in Figure 24–2, the exponential elimination phase is a straight line with a slope of k_e. A conceptually more useful term describing the time required to eliminate drug is the drug's elimination half-life ($t\frac{1}{2}$), which is the time required to reduce the plasma concentration of drug (and hence the body load of drug) to half the initial concentration. For drugs with first order elimination, the $t\frac{1}{2}$ is independent of drug concentration. The $t\frac{1}{2}$ is frequently determined graphically as in Figure 24–2, and mathematically the half-life is the natural logarithm of 2 (indicating a reduction of drug concentration by half) divided by the elimination rate constant: $t\frac{1}{2} = \ln 2/k_e = 0.693/k_e$. Since the elimination rate constant is related to both clearance and volume of distribution as independent variables, it can be appreciated that half-life must also be related to these two variables:

$$t\tfrac{1}{2} = \frac{0.693\ V_D}{Cl}$$

As the apparent volume of distribution increases, the half-life is prolonged for any given drug clearance, since a greater "volume" must be cleared of drug; as clearance increases, half-life shortens for any given V_D. A change in half-life frequently is used as an index of a change in efficiency of drug elimination, but this is true only when the apparent volume of distribution is unchanged. Hepatic, renal, and cardiovascular disease not only can decrease drug clearance but also can alter the apparent volume of distribution. Half-life, being affected by both V_D and Cl, may be affected to a greater or lesser extent than drug clearance, and therefore $t\frac{1}{2}$ may not indicate the degree of abnormality in drug elimination. For example, patients with congestive heart failure have a 50 per cent reduction in the clearance of lidocaine and may, in addition, have a similarly contracted volume of distribution of the drug. Since both Cl and V_D can be reduced by a similar magnitude, the half-life may be unchanged and not give any clue to the abnormal lidocaine clearance and the need for reduced infusion rates to avoid toxicity. (See "Maintenance Doses" below for discussion of the relationship of clearance to steady-state blood concentration.)

For exponential or first order drug elimination, an infinite time is required to eliminate drug entirely from the body. Only half the drug is eliminated in the first half-life, half the remaining drug eliminated in the second half-life, and so forth. Thus, by starting with an effective blood level, which we shall call 100 per cent, 50 per cent will be present after one half-life, 25 per cent after two half-lives, 12.5 per cent after three half-lives, 6.25 per cent after four half-lives, and 3.125 per cent after five half-lives, as shown in Figure 24–3 for lidocaine. For practical purposes, most drugs can be considered to be eliminated completely when less than 10 per cent of the effective concentration remains in the body, requiring three to four half-lives. For lidocaine (Fig. 24–3) this time is about six hours.

DRUG ACCUMULATION. When drug is given as a sustained infusion or in repeated doses, drug accumulates in the body until a steady state is achieved, at which time the amount of drug being administered is equal to the amount of drug eliminated so that body stores and plasma levels remain constant. The time course of drug accumulation, like the time course of elimination, is determined by the drug's elimination half-life, these processes being mirror images of each other (Fig. 24–3). Thus, accumulation to half the ultimate steady state occurs in one half-life, 75 per cent in two half-lives, 87.5 per cent in three half-lives, and 93.75 per cent in four half-lives. For practical purposes, the steady state is considered achieved when 90 per cent of the ultimate accumulation occurs, requiring three to four half-lives. For drugs with short half-lives, accumulation occurs rapidly and loading doses to achieve immediate therapeutic concentrations may not be necessary. For drugs with long half-lives, accumulation occurs slowly and loading doses are frequently required to achieve a therapeutic effect prior to waiting for full accumulation to occur. Regardless of whether a loading dose is given, the

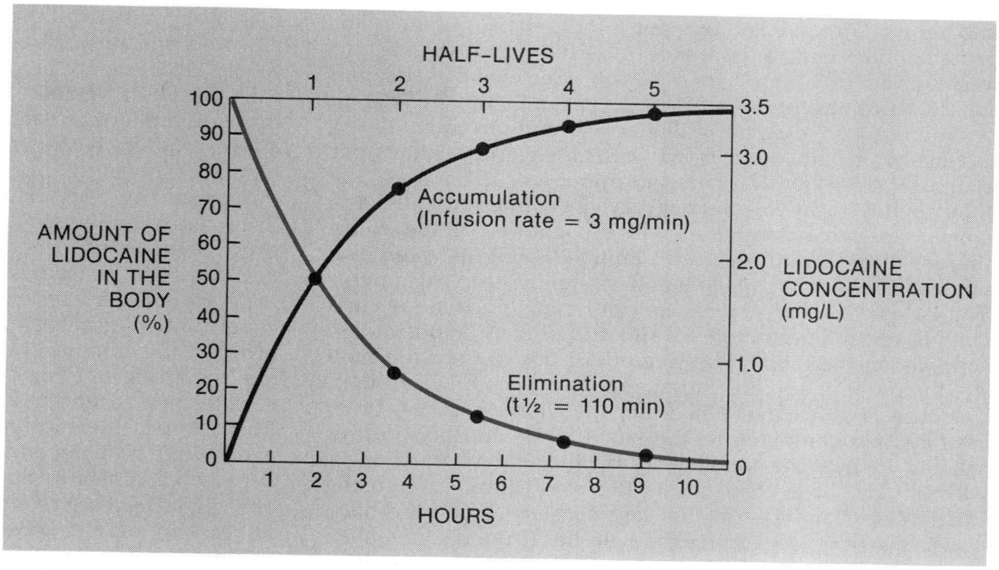

FIGURE 24–3. The accumulation of lidocaine during an infusion of 3 mg per minute and the elimination of lidocaine after the drug is discontinued. Time is indicated in hours and in half-lives and concentration in milligrams per liter. The amount of lidocaine in the body is the percentage remaining after discontinuation of the drug (elimination curve—color) or the percentage of the ultimate steady-state value achieved by the chronic infusion (accumulation curve). The two curves are mirror images of each other.

ultimate steady-state concentration achieved depends only on the maintenance dose and drug clearance. The loading dose only allows one to hasten the approach to a therapeutic concentration of drug. Figure 24–3 shows the accumulation of lidocaine to a steady state during a constant intravenous infusion of 3 mg per minute. The ultimate steady-state plasma level is approached with a half-life of 110 minutes. A loading dose would be required to achieve therapeutic concentrations more quickly.

When a drug is given intermittently, such as procainamide, illustrated in Figure 24–4, the average concentration approaches steady state with the same time course as during a constant infusion. The more frequently doses are given, the smaller the differences between peak and trough plasma concentrations, and the closer the intermittent dosing approximates an intravenous infusion.

Whenever the drug doses or infusion rates are changed, a new steady state will be achieved. The approach to the new steady state also is dependent on the half-life so that three to four half-lives will be required before the plasma concentrations and body stores of drug are at 90 per cent of the new steady state. Therefore, the effects of a dosage adjustment will not be immediate and will not be fully expressed for a time that is dependent on the drug's half-life.

MAINTENANCE DOSES. Steady state is achieved when the rate of drug administration equals the rate of drug elimination. The rate of drug administration is either the infusion rate (I) or the dose per unit time (D/t), and the rate of drug elimination is the product of drug clearance (Cl) and the drug concentration (C_p). Therefore, during a steady-state infusion, $I = ClC_p$, and during intermittent dosing, $D/t = ClC_p$. Note that the steady-state concentrations are independent of the distribution of the drug and are solely dependent on drug clearance and the rate of drug administration. The equations for steady state can be used to calculate the infusion rate or the intermittent dose required to achieve a desired plasma concentration, and, conversely, the plasma concentration at steady state produced by a known infusion rate can be used to calculate drug clearance. With the value for V_D (Table 24–1), half-life can also be calculated from the steady-state data as $0.693\ V_D/Cl$. For example, in an adult without heart failure or liver disease, the clearance of lidocaine is about 860 ml per minute (Table 24–1). In order to maintain a therapeutic concentration of 3.5 μg per milliliter, an infusion rate of 3 mg per minute must be given: $I = ClC_p = 860$ ml per minute × 3.5 μg per milliliter = 3000 μg per minute = 3 mg per minute. This is the steady-state value illustrated in Figure 24–3. The half-life for lidocaine in this patient is 0.693 (1.7 liters per

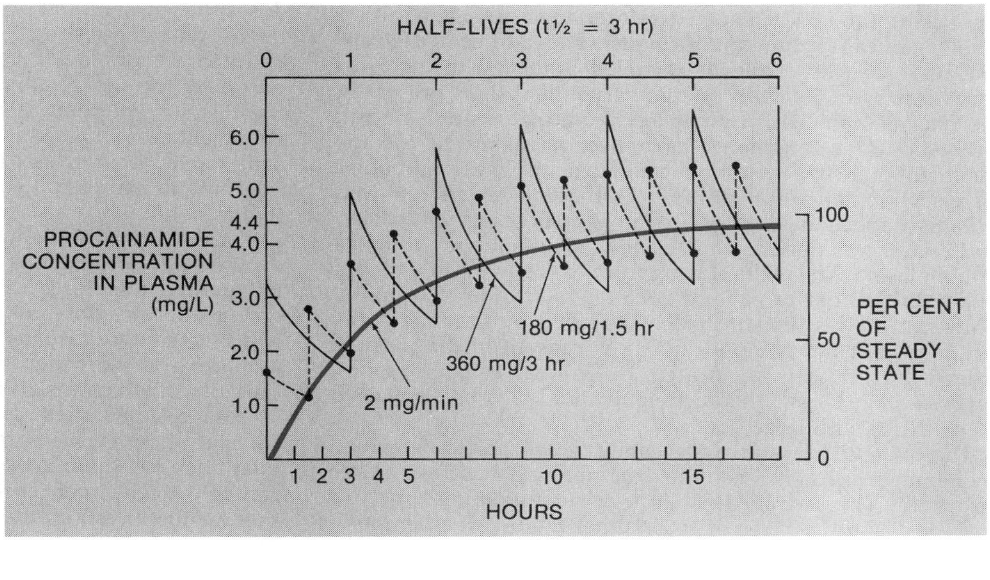

FIGURE 24–4. The accumulation to steady state of procainamide given as an infusion of 2 mg per minute (smooth curve) or intermittent doses of 180 mg per one and one half hours (dashed line) or 360 mg per three hours (solid line). Regardless of the method of administration, the accumulation follows the same time course and requires three to four half-lives to reach 90 per cent of steady state.

kilogram × 70 kg)/0.86 liters per minute = 96 minutes. For procainamide with a clearance of 450 ml per minute, an infusion rate of 2 mg per minute will achieve and maintain a steady-state concentration of 4.4 μg per milliliter: I = 450 ml per minute × 4.4 μg per milliliter = 2 mg per minute. The half-life of procainamide in this patient is 0.693 (1.6 liters per kilogram × 70 kg)/0.45 liters per minute = 172 minutes, or about 3 hours. If procainamide is given intermittently, the same average concentration will be achieved if the entire amount of drug infused over 3 hours (360 mg) is given as a single dose every 3 hours or half that amount every 90 minutes (Fig. 24–4). Obviously, drug concentrations fluctuate when a drug is given intermittently, and the degree of fluctuation depends on the interval between drug doses, the drug half-life, the route of administration, and the speed of absorption. If a dose is given every half-life, the fluctuation will be at most 100 per cent, that is, the blood levels and body stores will fall to half the initial level by the end of the dosage interval. The dose then boosts the blood level back to the initial value. The dose in this case consists of half the body stores, which is lost during the half-life. If the drug is given more often than the half-life, the fluctuations will be less, with the ultimate example being an infusion in which there is no fluctuation. In each case, the drug lost during a dosage interval is replaced by the dose to maintain the steady state. Usually drugs are given at least every half-life to avoid extreme fluctuations of blood levels. Only if very high concentrations are nontoxic or continuously effective plasma levels are not required can a drug be given much less frequently than one half-life. When a dose is given orally, absorption from the gut occurs gradually, and therefore peak concentrations are lower and fluctuations in plasma levels are less than if the same dose were administered as an intravenous bolus. In fact, with sustained-release oral formulations, absorption can be sustained over most of the dosage interval, resulting in minimal fluctuations in plasma levels.

DRUG REMOVAL FOLLOWING OVERDOSE. The principles described above can be used to predict the efficacy of hemodialysis or hemoperfusion in removing drug following an overdose. To be a valuable addition to the therapy of overdose, the drug removal process must make a substantial contribution to overall clearance of the drug and the amount of drug removed must be a significant portion of the body load. Consider the case of a digoxin overdose in an adult producing a plasma digoxin level of 8 ng per milliliter. The body load of digoxin is $V_D \times C_p$ or 500 liters × 8 μg per liter = 4 mg. At a clearance of 100 ml per minute with the hemoperfusion apparatus, the rate of drug removal with a C_p of 8 ng per milliliter is $Cl \times C_p$ = 100 ml per minute × 8 ng per milliliter = 800 ng per minute = 48 μg per hour, or only 1 per cent of the body load. Therefore, hemoperfusion cannot be of significant value in reducing the body stores of digoxin. The reason so little drug is removed is related to digoxin's very large V_D of 500 liters so that very little drug is present in the plasma from which it can be cleared. Recently, digoxin antibodies (Fab fragment) have become available for the treatment of life-threatening digoxin toxicity. These antibodies have such a high affinity for digoxin that the drug is removed from tissue sites, including those areas responsible for toxicity, and becomes trapped as an inactive digoxin-antibody complex in the plasma. This shift of drug from tissue to plasma results in a reduction of the V_D for digoxin by a factor of 10 or more. Thus not only is digoxin toxicity reduced by binding to the antibody, but much more digoxin is present in the plasma, from which it can be cleared by normal renal excretory processes. In theory this technique could also be applied to other drugs with large V_D.

The other circumstance that limits the benefit to be gained by hemoperfusion is when the drug normally has a very large clearance. The clearance of the tricyclic antidepressants, for instance, is in the range of 1000 ml per minute. If a hemoperfusion apparatus could clear the drug at 100 ml per minute, it would add only 10 per cent to the normal clearance and would therefore not be of substantial value.

DOSE-DEPENDENT PHARMACOKINETICS. For a few drugs, the pharmacokinetics do not follow the rules outlined above, and such drugs are said to have dose-dependent, nonlinear, or saturation kinetics (Table 24–2). For these drugs the amount of drug eliminated is not directly related to the drug concentration (first order), but as the concentration of drug is increased, the relative amount of drug eliminated decreases (i.e., clearance decreases) until a maximal rate of drug metabolism is achieved that is independent of drug concentration, at which point drug elimination is termed zero order. If the amount of drug administered exceeds the maximal metabolic rate for drug elimination, the drug will accumulate indefinitely and very high blood levels will result. Phenytoin is the most important example of a therapeutic agent with dose-dependent kinetics. With phenytoin, clearance is not constant but decreases at increasing dose so that any given increase in dose will result in a disproportionate increase in plasma concentration, and therefore dosage adjustments must be made cautiously. A dose of 300 mg of phenytoin daily may give a plasma level of 8 μg per milliliter, and a dose of 400 mg per day a plasma level of 25 μg per milliliter. Since all patients differ in their ability to eliminate phenytoin, proper dosage adjustments are difficult to predict for an individual patient. In practice, plasma concentration measurements (see below) must be used to establish a proper maintenance dose. High-dose salicylate therapy also behaves in a dose-dependent manner, as does ethanol. However, ethanol is eliminated by zero order kinetics at all doses, and therefore its elimination is much more predictable than that of phenytoin and salicylate, for which the elimination changes from first order to zero order over the therapeutic range.

USE OF PLASMA DRUG CONCENTRATION TO GUIDE THERAPY. The principles outlined above allow the clinician to choose a loading and maintenance dose based on the desired plasma concentration to achieve therapeutic effects and minimize the risk of toxicity. The underlying premise is that following distribution of a dose, the concentration of drug in plasma is in equilibrium with drug at the site of action and therefore is a direct reflection of the drug at the target site (Fig. 24–1).

However, the published pharmacokinetic data on which initial dosage recommendations are based are averages for a population and usually need modification for the individual patient. Dosage adjustment is best accomplished when the therapeutic effects of the drug are readily quantifiable. Thus, antihypertensive drugs can be given in a dose sufficient to lower blood pressure, and oral anticoagulants can be given in doses that prolong the prothrombin time into the therapeutic range. With these drugs the desired effect is the appropriate endpoint, and plasma concentrations of the drug are not necessary for dosage adjustment. For many drugs, however, the desired endpoint is difficult to assess clinically, either because there is no readily quantifiable measurement to assess drug effect or because the disease being treated has an intermittent expression so that the clinician cannot be certain that a therapeutic effect has been achieved. Two good examples are epilepsy and sporadic cardiac arrhythmias, in which drug dosage adjustments are difficult to make with precision. Frequently, therefore, patients with sporadic arrhythmias or epilepsy receive doses of drugs based on the average patient, and if these doses are ineffective or toxic, the drug is deemed a failure and the patient is "resistant" or "intolerant" to the therapy, in which case other drugs are tried.

Dosage adjustment can be aided by using the plasma concentration in cases in which there are no other easily quantifiable endpoints by which the drug's therapeutic effects can be gauged. In order for the plasma concentration to have therapeutic meaning, the drug in plasma must be in equilib-

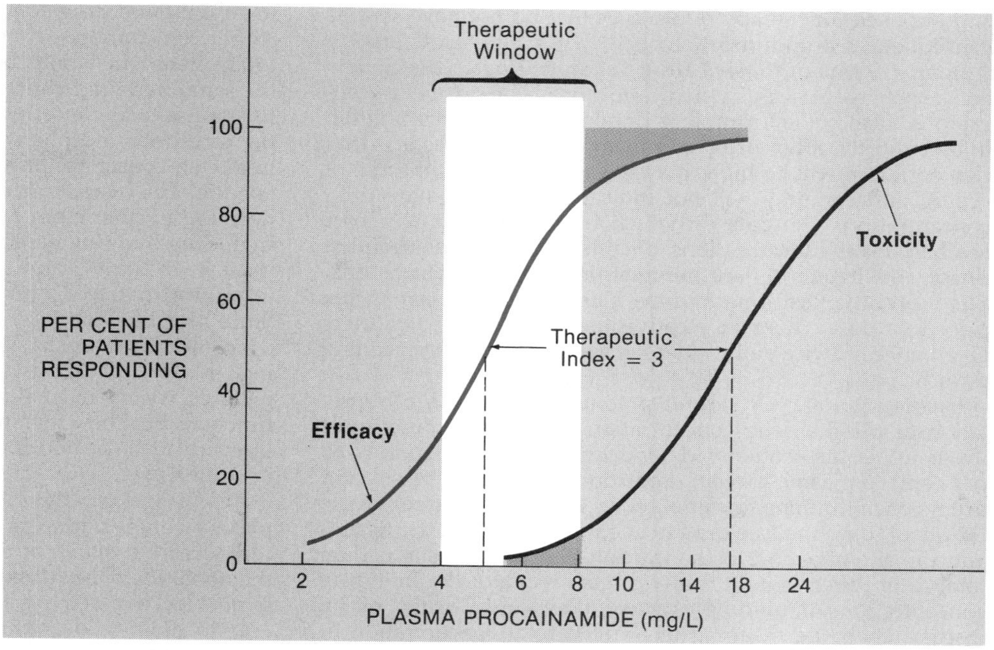

FIGURE 24–5. Population dose-response curves for the antiarrhythmic and acute toxic effects of procainamide. The therapeutic window is the range encompassing most of the therapeutic dose-effect curve and includes less than 10 per cent of the toxic dose-effect curve. The toxic dose divided by the therapeutic dose is the therapeutic index, here shown for 50 per cent of the population. Individual patients may lie anywhere on these curves.

rium with drug at the site of action and the effects must be reversible. If a drug has irreversible effects, such as the effect of aspirin to inhibit platelet aggregation, the plasma level will not correlate with effect. Fortunately, such situations are uncommon.

The sources of variation in drug effects can be divided into pharmacokinetic and pharmacodynamic factors. Those factors that alter the plasma drug concentration resulting from a given dose are the pharmacokinetic variables—absorption, distribution, and clearance. Those factors that alter the response to a given plasma level are the pharmacodynamic variables. If the pharmacodynamic variation among patients is very large, then plasma drug concentrations will not be a helpful guide for therapy. Fortunately, pharmacokinetic factors account for the major variation in response among patients for many drugs, and this variability can be managed with the use of plasma drug level monitoring.

Therapeutic Window. For plasma levels to be a useful guide to therapy, the range of drug concentrations required for optimal therapeutic effects with minimal toxicity must be established. This range is called the "therapeutic window" and is determined experimentally for each drug in a group of patients who are carefully observed for desired and toxic drug effects (Fig. 24–5). The width of the therapeutic window relates to the steepness of the concentration-effect curve and is an index of the pharmacodynamic variability in the population being treated. For procainamide, illustrated in Figure 24–5, the therapeutic window is 4 to 8 mg per liter. The separation between the therapeutic and toxic concentration-effect curves is an index of the toxicity of the drug frequently referred to as the "therapeutic index," which is the toxic dose divided by therapeutic dose. For procainamide the therapeutic index is ~3. With all drugs there is overlap between the therapeutic and toxic ranges. In addition, since the therapeutic window is based on a population of patients, one cannot be certain of the optimal drug concentration for a given patient. Although most patients will achieve a therapeutic effect within the therapeutic range, a few patients require concentrations below or above the range. Similarly, toxicity begins to occur in some patients within the therapeutic window, but the incidence of side effects increases sharply as the therapeutic range is exceeded. Therefore, the plasma concentration cannot be an infallible guide to safe and effective therapy, since it controls only the pharmacokinetic variability and not the pharmacodynamic variability. It is undoubtedly better, however, than the use of a standard dose that allows for no variability.

Table 24–3 lists some drugs for which therapeutic windows have been established. These drugs have several common characteristics: First, their pharmacologic effects are not readily quantifiable; second, they are used for therapy of serious or life-threatening illness so that therapeutic inefficacy cannot be tolerated; and third, their toxicity is serious, and the therapeutic index is small. Therapeutic windows are not required for drugs that have a very large therapeutic index

TABLE 24–3. THERAPEUTIC WINDOWS

Drug	Therapeutic Range
Cardiovascular Drugs:	
Digitoxin	10–25 μg/liter
Digoxin	0.8–2 μg/liter
Disopyramide	2–6 mg/liter
Flecainide	0.2–1 mg/liter
Lidocaine	1.5–5 mg/liter
Mexiletine	0.5–2 mg/liter
Procainamide	4–8 mg/liter
Quinidine	2–6 mg/liter
Theophylline	8–20 mg/liter
Tocainide	4–12 mg/liter
Antiseizure Drugs:	
Carbamazepine	6–12 mg/liter
Ethosuximide	40–80 mg/liter
Phenobarbital	15–30 mg/liter
Phenytoin	10–20 mg/liter
Valproic acid	50–100 mg/liter
Antibiotics:*	
Amikacin‡	20–40 mg/liter
Carbenicillin	100–300 mg/liter
Gentamicin‡	5–10 mg/liter
Penicillin G†	1–25 mg/liter
Tobramycin‡	5–10 mg/liter
Others:	
Lithium	0.5–1.5 mEq/liter
Nortriptyline	50–150 μg/liter
Salicylate	<300 mg/liter

*Actual concentration required related to minimal inhibitory concentration for infecting bacterium.
†1 mg of penicillin = 1.6 × 10^6 units.
‡Peak levels.

and are used for therapy of diseases that do not have serious consequences if undertreated.

Interpretation of Plasma Drug Concentrations. TIMING. Several problems exist in interpretation of plasma drug concentrations. If the blood sample is drawn during the distribution phase shortly after drug administration, the plasma drug concentration will be high, may not reflect drug at the site of action, and certainly will not indicate the steady-state drug concentration. The data on which the therapeutic windows are based are concentrations obtained after the distribution phase and frequently are minimal or trough concentrations. Therefore, the best time to draw blood for drug assay is just prior to a dose, during a steady-state infusion, or, for drugs given once or twice daily, at least eight hours after a preceding dose.

PROTEIN BINDING. A second potential problem in interpretation of plasma drug concentration is abnormal binding of drugs to plasma proteins. Many drugs are highly bound (>80 per cent) to plasma protein, and routine assays of plasma for drug concentrations include total (bound plus free) drug. However, only the free drug is in equilibrium with the tissues and the site of action. If the fraction bound is constant, then total drug concentration is an accurate index of the free drug concentration. If binding is altered by other drugs or by disease, then the meaning of a given total concentration of drug will be changed, since a greater proportion of the drug will be unbound. Both liver and kidney disease can alter the protein binding of some drugs (phenytoin, digitoxin, clofibrate, diazoxide, some sulfonamides, valproic acid, and salicylic acid) either by changing the quantity of protein (decreased albumin in liver disease and nephrotic syndrome) or by competition for binding between the drug and endogenous compounds that accumulate in patients with uremia or jaundice. In addition, one drug may compete with another for binding to plasma proteins. Measurement of unbound drug may be required for proper interpretation of the plasma concentration in these circumstances, since if more drug is unbound, the effects or toxicity of any given total plasma concentration will be increased. Unfortunately, most clinical laboratories are not capable of measuring unbound drug concentrations.

Decreased plasma protein binding can also change the kinetics of drug disposition. The volume of distribution will increase because less drug remains in the plasma as the increased free fraction distributes to the tissues. Whether changes in clearance occur with changes in plasma protein binding depends on whether the clearing organ can strip drug from the protein, in which case clearance will not change, since in this circumstance it does not depend on the free drug fraction. However, for many drugs the clearance is restricted to free drug, in which case drug clearance will increase as binding to plasma proteins decreases, since a larger fraction of the total is available for elimination. With these drugs, however, the clearance of *free* drug is unchanged. An unchanged clearance of free drug means that the average plasma free drug concentration will be unchanged at steady state, although protein binding is decreased. However, the total drug concentration will decrease because of the increased drug clearance. Since free drug concentration is not changed and free drug determines the effects of most drugs, the daily dose of drug need not be changed. The best-studied example is that of phenytoin, which is normally >90 per cent bound to plasma albumin. In patients with uremia, phenytoin binding can decrease to 70 per cent so that the unbound fraction increases from 10 to 30 per cent. As a consequence of the increase in free fraction, the apparent volume of distribution of phenytoin increases and clearance increases. The plasma concentration of total phenytoin falls as a result of the increased clearance, but the average free concentration at steady state is unchanged. A therapeutic phenytoin level with 90 per cent protein binding is 10 to 20 mg per liter, corresponding to an unbound drug concentration of 1 to 2 mg per liter. With 30 per cent unbound, the corresponding therapeutic level of total phenytoin would be 3.3 to 6.7 mg per liter to achieve the same free drug concentration. Obviously, if the goal were to attain a total concentration of 10 to 20 mg per liter with 30 per cent unbound phenytoin, toxicity would result, since the free drug concentration would be threefold higher than therapeutic. The overall pharmacokinetic change resulting from a decrease in phenytoin binding is an unchanged clearance of free drug, an increased clearance of total drug, a lesser increase in the V_D, and a consequent decrease in the half-life to approximately 8 hours from the normal 18 to 24 hours. Since the half-life is shortened but the average free drug concentration is unchanged by the change in phenytoin binding, the total daily dose of phenytoin should be the same in patients with renal failure as in patients with normal renal function, but the drug should be given every 8 hours instead of every 12 to 24 hours to avoid unwanted large fluctuations in drug level.

ACTIVE METABOLITES. A third pitfall in interpretation of the plasma concentration of some drugs is the presence of unmeasured but active or toxic drug metabolites. Propranolol is metabolized to 4-hydroxypropranolol, which has beta-adrenergic–blocking activity. Procainamide is metabolized to *N*-acetylprocainamide, which has antiarrhythmic activity. The importance of active metabolites depends on their intrinsic activity and toxicity and the extent to which they accumulate relative to the parent compound. In situations in which a metabolite accounts for a significant portion of the drug's activity or toxicity, the metabolite must be measured along with the parent drug for proper interpretation.

PHARMACODYNAMIC CHANGES. A final factor altering the interpretation of plasma levels is a physiologic or pathologic change that alters the response to a given plasma concentration. For instance, a change in serum potassium, magnesium, or calcium concentration will alter the toxic concentration-effect relationship for digoxin such that concentrations not usually associated with adverse effects may now be toxic. The development of tolerance to a drug will also distort the relationship of plasma concentration to effect. Tolerance can be defined as a reduction in response to a given concentration of drug at the site of action and has been described for drugs of abuse, particularly opiates. However, with the recent emphasis on drug delivery systems capable of producing constant blood levels of therapeutic drugs over many hours or days, the possibility of tolerance to the beneficial effects of these drugs is worrisome. The tolerance reported with the chronic use of beta-adrenergic agonists for asthma and heart failure may be due to a reduction in the density of beta-adrenergic receptors during chronic agonist stimulation (see Ch. 26). More recently, tolerance to the therapeutic effects of nitroglycerin has been described with the 24-hour transdermal delivery systems.

These alterations in pharmacodynamics of the drug response emphasize the fact that plasma drug concentrations must be interpreted with other clinical and laboratory data that may influence the response to the drug.

ALTERATIONS OF DRUG DOSES IN DISEASE STATES. ***Renal Disease.*** A decrease in renal function will result in a decreased renal clearance of drugs. Whether a dosage adjustment is required depends on the toxicity of the drug and the importance of renal clearance for drug elimination. If the drug has significant toxicity and the kidney accounts for most of the drug's elimination, then dosage adjustments must be made in patients with renal disease to avoid toxicity. On the other hand, if the drug is nontoxic, dosage adjustment is less critical even if the drug accumulates in patients with renal failure. For instance, penicillin is cleared >90 per cent by the kidneys, but because it is relatively nontoxic, dosage adjustments are not required for low-dose therapy (600,000 to 1,200,000 units per day). However, if massive doses of penicillin are required, then dosage adjustments must be made to avoid penicillin toxicity.

Fortunately, renal drug clearance is closely correlated with the clearance of creatinine even for those drugs that are eliminated by tubular secretion. For this reason, an adjustment of the average drug dose can be calculated from the creatinine clearance. The process is simple: The calculated renal drug clearance is reduced by the same proportion as the reduction from 100 ml per minute in the measured creatinine clearance or the creatinine clearance calculated by the formula:

$$\text{creatinine clearance} = \frac{(140 - \text{age}) \times \text{weight (kg)}}{72 \times \text{serum creatinine (mg/dl)}}$$

for males, with the creatinine clearance for females being 85 per cent of that for males. If the drug is cleared by nonrenal (usually hepatic) mechanisms as well as by renal mechanisms, only the renal clearance (Cl_r) is adjusted; the nonrenal clearance (Cl_{nr}) remains normal. Assuming that the same average plasma concentration (C_p) is desired in patients with renal failure, the dose is adjusted in direct proportion to the change in total clearance, since $Cl \times C_p$ = dose/time. Renal and nonrenal clearances for some drugs are listed in Table 24–1. Consider as an example of this approach the alteration of digoxin dosage in renal failure. The average renal clearance of digoxin is 110 ml per minute at a creatinine clearance of 100 ml per minute; the nonrenal clearance is 40 ml per minute. If the measured creatinine clearance is 50 ml per minute, or half normal, then the renal clearance of digoxin is reduced by a similar fraction; thus, Cl_r (digoxin) = 55 ml per minute in this patient. If the nonrenal clearance is assumed to be unchanged, the total digoxin clearance is $Cl_{nr} + Cl_r = 40 + 55 = 95$ ml per minute in the patient with a creatinine clearance of 50 ml per minute, versus a total digoxin clearance of $40 + 110 = 150$ ml per minute in a patient with normal renal function. The total digoxin clearance is therefore reduced by the fraction $\frac{95}{150}$ and the dose should be adjusted using the same fraction. If the average dose is 0.25 mg per day, this would be decreased to $\frac{95}{150} \times 0.25$ mg $= 0.16$ mg per day. These calculations can give only a first approximation of the appropriate dose for an individual patient, since they are based on the average dose for the average patient. In practice, a dose conveniently close to the calculated dose is administered to the patient, and the patient's response and/or plasma drug concentrations are monitored. With the information provided by either the plasma drug concentrations or clinical observations, the dosage can be adjusted.

If the desired plasma concentration is known, one can calculate the dosage directly from the drug clearance, since dose/t = $Cl \times C_p$. For example, an average procainamide concentration of 5 μg per milliliter is desired in a patient with a creatinine clearance of 50 ml per minute. The total procainamide clearance is $\frac{50}{100} \times 330\ (Cl_r) + 120\ (Cl_{nr}) = 285$ ml per minute. An infusion of 1.4 mg per minute ($Cl \times C_p$) or a dose of 250 mg every three hours will achieve and maintain the desired plasma concentration.

Although drug clearance is the best way to calculate doses for drugs, clearance data are not available for many drugs. For a few drugs, published nomograms are available to guide dosage. It would be preferable, both from a practical and from an intellectual standpoint, to be able to use a more generally applicable method to calculate proper dosage. Two such methods are outlined in the next two paragraphs.

For many drugs, the elimination rate constant (k_e) is known. If the apparent volume of distribution is unchanged in renal disease, then the k_e and Cl are proportional ($k_e = Cl/V_D$) and the change in k_e can be used to adjust the dose in a manner entirely analogous to the use of changes in clearance to adjust dose. Like clearance values, the elimination rate constant can be expressed as the sum of the rate constants for the separate eliminating organs; thus $k_e = k_{renal} + k_{nonrenal}$. Values for k_r and k_{nr} are listed in Table 24–4. To use these values to adjust dosage in renal insufficiency, the procedure is exactly the same as with the clearance calculations used above. Thus, k_e for amikacin in a patient with normal renal function is 0.31, which is made up of $k_r = 0.3$ and a $k_{nr} = 0.01$. The dose alteration in a patient with a creatinine clearance of 25 ml per minute is calculated as follows: The k_r for the patient is 25/100 $\times$ 0.3 = 0.08. The k_e therefore is $k_r + k_{nr} = 0.08 + 0.01 = 0.09$ versus the normal k_e of 0.31. The dose of amikacin must therefore be reduced to $\frac{0.09}{0.31}$ or 30 per cent of the usual dose per unit time. As can be readily appreciated, the dose of amikacin is reduced almost in proportion to the reduction in creatinine clearance, since the nonrenal elimination is negligible until creatinine clearance is reduced to very low values (i.e., <15 ml per minute). Several other drugs are like amikacin in this regard and are in Group A in Table 24–4. For all these drugs, dosage adjustment can be made by multiplying the usual dose by the fraction of the creatinine clearance remaining in the patient. When the patient has essentially no renal function, then the small k_{nr} may be used to calculate doses as illustrated above. For drugs that have nonrenal elimination that is a substantial fraction (e.g., 20 to 50 per cent) of the total elimination, the dosage reduction in renal insufficiency will be less than the reduction in creatinine clearance and can be calculated as illustrated above. These drugs are in Group B. If the nonrenal elimination is greater than 50 per cent of the k_e, then the dosage usually does not need to be adjusted for changes in renal function. In all cases, the calculations adjust only the average dose, and blood level determinations are required to make final dosage adjustments. This is particularly true if nonrenal elimination may also be reduced, as in liver or cardiac disease.

A final method for estimating the average dose in patients with renal failure is to use the per cent nonrenal elimination determined in normal individuals. These values are listed in Tables 24–1 and 24–4 and are frequently available for drugs even if clearances or elimination rate constants are not. This method uses the nomogram in Figure 24–6, in which creatinine clearance is plotted against the drug clearance as a per cent of normal. The black lines intersecting the black ordinate are for drugs that have a nonrenal elimination of from 0 to 50 per cent in a normal individual. The nomogram is used by drawing a perpendicular line to the creatinine clearance until it intersects the black line corresponding to the drug of interest. The per cent drug clearance can then be read directly from the red ordinate, and the dosage adjusted accordingly. For instance, consider the amikacin example calculated above. Since the per cent nonrenal elimination in a normal individual is ~5 per cent, the clearance values for amikacin fall on the line intersecting the ordinate at 5 per cent in Figure 24–6. The drug clearance as a percentage of normal for a creatinine clearance of 25 ml per minute is ~30 per cent (as indicated by the dotted line), and the dose of this drug in the patient with a creatinine clearance of 25 ml therefore must be 30 per cent normal.

The reduction in dose per unit time can be applied to patient care by giving either the reduced dose at the usual interval or the same dose at a longer interval. By both methods the average plasma level will be the same, but the fluctuations in plasma concentration will be less when the reduced dose is given at the usual intervals.

Loading doses for most drugs used in patients with renal failure need not be adjusted for creatinine clearance because V_D is usually close to normal. However, since the t½ of

TABLE 24–4. THE RENAL ELIMINATION RATE CONSTANTS (k_r), NONRENAL ELIMINATION RATE CONSTANTS (k_{nr}), AND PER CENT NONRENAL ELIMINATION IN A NORMAL INDIVIDUAL FOR SELECTED DRUGS

	k_r (per hour)	k_{nr} (per hour)	Per Cent Nonrenal
Group A (>80% renal)			
Acyclovir	0.2	0.02	10
Amantidine	0.05	0.005	10
Amikacin	0.3	0.01	5
Amoxicillin	0.6	0.1	10
Ampicillin	0.5	0.06	10
Atenolol	0.10	0.005	5
Bretylium	0.07	0.01	15
Carbenicillin	0.5	0.05	10
Cefamandole	0.84	0.04	5
Cefazolin	0.3	0.02	5
Cefoxitin	1.0	0.05	5
Cephalexin	0.7	0.03	5
Cephalothin	1.4	0.03	5
Cephradine	0.5	0.05	10
Colistin	0.3	0.02	10
Flucytosine	0.24	0.01	5
Gentamicin	0.3	0.02	5
Kanamycin	0.3	0.01	5
Methicillin	1.2	0.15	10
Methotrexate	0.07	0.007	10
Moxalactam	0.3	0.02	5
Oxypurinol*	0.03	0.003	10
Penicillin G	1.3	0.1	10
Polymyxin B	0.13	0.02	10
Streptomycin	0.24	0.01	5
Tetracycline	0.07	0.01	10
Ticarcillin	0.6	0.06	10
Tobramycin	0.3	0.01	5
Vancomycin	0.12	0.003	5
Group B (50–80% renal)			
Cefotaxime	0.6	0.28	30
Cephapirin	0.9	0.3	25
Cimetidine	0.27	0.09	25
Dicloxacillin	0.6	0.6	50
Erythromycin	0.30	0.15	35
Ethambutol	0.09	0.09	50
Isoniazid (slow acetylators)	0.12	0.12	50
Lincomycin	0.1	0.06	40
Nadolol	0.03	0.01	25
Nafcillin	0.7	0.5	40
Oxacillin	1.1	0.35	25
Oxytetracycline	0.065	0.015	20
Ranitidine	0.25	0.08	25
Trimethoprim	0.03	0.03	50
Group C (<50% renal)			
Amphotericin B	0.01	0.02	70
Chloramphenicol	0.02	0.3	80
Clindamycin	0	0.25	100
Doxycycline	0.005	0.03	80
Flecainide	0.013	0.03	70
Isoniazid (fast acetylators)	0.1	0.4	80
Mexiletine	0.006	0.06	90
Minocycline	0	0.06	100
Rifampin	0	0.25	100
Sulfamethoxazole	0.01	0.06	85
Tocainide	0.02	0.03	60

*Oxypurinol is the major active metabolite of allopurinol.

renally cleared drugs is prolonged in these patients, drug accumulation during initiation of therapy with maintenance doses will be slower. Because of the slower accumulation, a loading dose may be required in patients with renal failure in order to achieve a therapeutic blood concentration rapidly, whereas patients with normal renal function may not need a loading dose for the same drug. Digoxin, for example, with a half-life of 1.5 days in a patient with normal renal function will accumulate to 90 per cent of steady-state levels in 5 days (3 to 4 half-lives), and many patients need not be loaded, since this accumulation is sufficiently rapid to produce the desired therapeutic effects. On the other hand, in a patient without renal function, digoxin half-life increases to five days. If the anephric patient is begun on the appropriately reduced maintenance dose of digoxin, accumulation to the same steady-state level will take more than 15 days to occur. In this case, a loading dose may be desired to achieve a more rapid effect without waiting for drug accumulation. However, whether or not a loading dose is given, the ultimate steady-state drug concentration will be the same and, as always, depends only on drug dose and drug clearance.

Patients with end-stage renal disease are usually supported with hemodialysis. Dialysis can remove some therapeutic drugs from the circulation and necessitate supplemental dosing to maintain a therapeutic effect. The most important characteristics of the drug that determine the ability of dialysis to remove a significant amount of drug from the body are the V_D, drug binding to plasma proteins, and the nonrenal clearance of the drug. Of these, V_D is the most important parameter, and only if it is less than 1 liter per kilogram can significant amounts of drug be removed by dialysis. Dialysis is also more effective in drug removal if the drug is not highly bound to plasma proteins and is normally cleared primarily by the kidneys. Since clearance of drugs by hemodialysis is limited to a maximum of ~100 ml per minute, drugs that have a relatively small extrarenal clearance (< 400 ml per minute) may have a significant increment in their removal rate during hemodialysis even if they are not normally cleared by the kidney. For instance, aminoglycosides have a small V_D, low binding to plasma protein, and mostly renal clearance and are therefore removed to a significant extent by hemodialysis. Theophylline, although not normally cleared by the kidneys, has a relatively small V_D, a nonrenal clearance of 55 ml per minute, and moderate protein binding and therefore may be sufficiently removed during a three to six hour hemodialysis session to require a modest supplemental dosage. For most drugs that require supplemental therapy after hemodialysis to maintain a therapeutic effect, blood level determinations are available as a guide.

Some drugs form metabolites that are active or toxic and are eliminated by the kidneys. In patients with renal insufficiency, these metabolites may accumulate and produce effects. As an example, procainamide is in part excreted unchanged and in part metabolized to *N*-acetylprocainamide, which has antiarrhythmic effects and can produce toxicity. The metabolite may achieve concentrations in renal failure that are manyfold higher than the parent drug and can contribute to the antiarrhythmic effects and toxicity of procainamide. Since the concentration of metabolites is not routinely measured by drug assay laboratories, the plasma concentration of parent drug can be misleading. Drugs with renally excreted active or toxic metabolites include (in addition to procainamide) meperidine, propoxyphene, allopurinol, acetohexamide, clofibrate, nitrofurantoin, and nitroprusside. If alternative drugs are available for the treatment of patients with renal insufficiency, it is probably best to avoid these drugs when active or toxic metabolites may accumulate.

Hepatic Disease. Although many drugs are biotransformed by the liver, no quantitative predictor of the degree of abnormality in drug metabolism is available for patients with liver disease. Severe liver disease can result in a decreased metabolic capacity for a large number of drugs. If the indices of the liver's capacity to form proteins (serum albumin level and prothrombin time) are abnormal, then it is probable that drug metabolism will also be abnormal, and the doses of those drugs that are metabolized by the liver should be reduced. Acute liver disease has an inconstant and unpredictable effect on drug metabolism, but, in general, drug metabolism is not as abnormal as with chronic liver disease.

With chronic liver disease, portacaval anastomoses may develop. Not only will this decrease the blood flow to the liver with consequent reduction in clearance of some drugs,

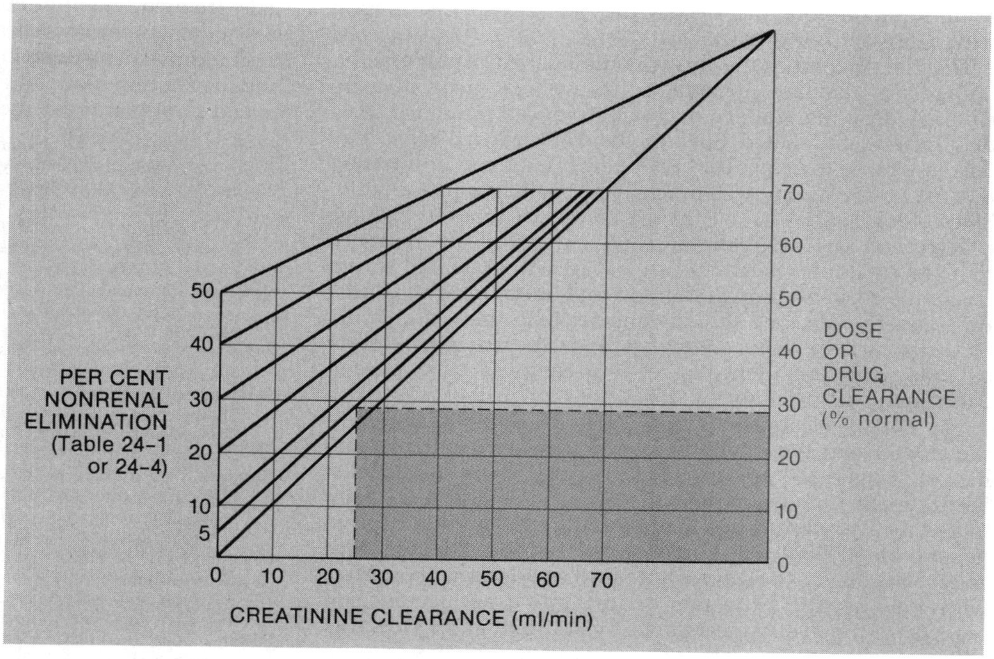

FIGURE 24–6. Nomogram for calculation of drug doses in patients with renal disease. The dose of any drug in a patient with renal disease (as a per cent of normal) is determined by connecting a line from the measured or calculated creatinine clearance to the black line that corresponds to the per cent nonrenal elimination for the drug of interest (from Table 24–1 or 24–4). The point of intersection is then extended to the red axis, where the dose per unit time is read directly. The dotted line indicates that in a patient with a creatinine clearance of 25 ml per minute the dose of amikacin, which normally has 5 per cent nonrenal elimination, must be reduced to approximately 30 per cent of normal.

but the portacaval shunting can allow drug absorbed by the gut to pass directly into the systemic circulation and bypass the liver, thereby avoiding the "first pass" or "presystemic" elimination. For those drugs that are largely extracted from the blood by the liver (e.g., propranolol, metoprolol, lidocaine), portacaval shunting will allow a much greater fraction of an orally administered dose to reach the systemic circulation.

Hemodynamic Disorders. Pharmacokinetics can be affected in several ways by disorders of the circulation. Hypotension and poor cardiac output reduce renal blood flow, glomerular filtration rate, and hepatic blood flow. As with primary renal disease, the impairment in renal drug excretion may be estimated by the change in creatinine clearance and dosage adjustments made accordingly. The effects of reduced hepatic blood flow on drug metabolism are highly dependent on the drug. For drugs that are essentially completely cleared from the blood on a single passage through the liver, i.e., when the extraction from blood is close to 100 per cent, a reduction in liver blood flow will reduce hepatic drug clearance proportionately. On the other hand, many drugs that are metabolized are extracted poorly by the liver, and for these drugs a reduction in liver blood flow has relatively little influence on their hepatic clearance. A complicating factor is that circulatory abnormalities also can result in hepatic congestion or tissue hypoxia that can impair hepatocellular function, so that drug metabolism may be reduced during hypotensive states independent of the effects of blood flow on drug delivery to the liver. Therefore, it is difficult to predict the proper dosage of hepatic metabolized drugs in individual patients with circulatory abnormalities. Certainly a drug such as lidocaine that has a very high hepatic clearance will be cleared less well in congestive heart failure or shock, and the maintenance infusion rates must be reduced by about half in these situations to avoid toxicity.

The distribution of some drugs is also affected by hemodynamic changes. For several drugs with large distribution volumes (lidocaine, quinidine, and procainamide), the apparent volume of distribution is decreased in heart failure and shock, and loading doses should also be reduced to avoid toxic plasma concentrations. However, for theophylline, a drug with a relatively small volume of distribution, the apparent volume of distribution is not changed by heart failure. Since data are not available for most drugs, we advise a conservative approach to loading and maintenance doses of toxic drugs in the setting of congestive heart failure or shock, with careful monitoring of the clinical status and plasma levels to guide further dosage adjustments.

USE OF DRUGS IN THE ELDERLY. Elderly persons (over 65 years) comprise 11 to 12 per cent of the United States population, but about 30 per cent of all prescriptions are written for this group of patients. In addition to prescription drugs, 70 per cent of elderly patients regularly use over-the-counter medications, primarily analgesics, compared with only 10 per cent of the general adult population. As an individual ages, changes occur that may affect drug kinetics and drug action. These age-related changes accentuate the normal interindividual variation in drug effects, thus making the elderly the most diverse segment of the adult population in terms of their drug responses. Because of the changes that occur with aging and the large numbers of drugs used in this population, the elderly are also highly susceptible to drug interactions.

The pharmacokinetic changes that may occur in the elderly are related to changes in body composition as well as to changes in function of pharmacokinetically important organs. The changes in gastrointestinal function that occur with aging are a decrease in gastric acid secretion, a decrease in mucosal absorptive surface of the small bowel by about 30 per cent, and a decrease in splanchnic blood flow by about 40 per cent. In spite of these changes, very few studies have shown much effect of aging on drug absorption. This is probably because most drugs are well absorbed and do not require very much of the small bowel for their absorption.

The distribution of drugs may change markedly with aging, probably because lean body mass and total body water decrease as the percentage of total body fat increases. In addition, the plasma concentration of albumin decreases, probably as a result of decreased albumin production by the liver, and this may affect those drugs that are bound to plasma albumin. Alpha$_1$-acid glycoprotein, the major plasma protein that binds basic drugs, is not diminished with aging. Because of the changes in body composition, water-soluble drugs that are not bound to plasma proteins may have a reduced apparent volume of distribution. However, for lipid-soluble drugs, such as many psychotropic agents, the volume of distribution relative to body weight may be increased, probably because of the increased percentage of body weight as fat. For water-soluble, albumin-bound drugs, the changes in distribution with aging are not predictable.

The clearance of many drugs is diminished in the elderly. Both drugs that are metabolized as well as those that are eliminated by the kidneys may have reduced clearance. Cardiac output and blood flow to the kidneys and liver may decrease by 30 to 40 per cent with aging. Glomerular filtration rate may be reduced by as much as 50 per cent in the elderly. Since older persons have a decreased muscle mass, they have a decreased rate of creatinine production. For this reason a reduced creatinine clearance can coexist with a normal serum creatinine concentration as defined for young, healthy adults. As a general rule, one should consider that renal elimination of drugs will be reduced by up to 50 per cent in elderly patients without evidence of renal disease and make dosage adjustments accordingly.

The hepatic clearance of drugs may also be diminished in the elderly, but the interindividual variability in the metabolism of drugs is so large as to preclude any useful predictions. Both hepatic blood flow and the intrinsic ability of the liver to metabolize some drugs may be reduced. The reduction in hepatic blood flow will influence the hepatic elimination of drugs with high extraction ratios, such as lidocaine. For drugs with low hepatic extraction ratios, the drug-metabolizing capacity of the liver appears to be most important. Drugs that are metabolized by the hepatic mixed function oxidase system are more likely to be affected by aging than those drugs that are metabolized by conjugation reactions.

Elimination half-life of many drugs is increased with aging. This is a combination of the effect of changes in the apparent volume of distribution and of changes in metabolic or renal clearance. Frequently, elimination half-life can be prolonged even without changes in drug clearance. This is true with diazepam, which has an increased apparent volume of distribution with no change in metabolic clearance, and this combination of changes produces a prolonged elimination half-life.

The age-related changes that occur with target-organ responsiveness are as important as the changes in pharmacokinetics. There is an increased sensitivity to a variety of drugs. The antianxiety agents and sedative hypnotic agents produce greater degrees of depression of central nervous system function in the elderly than in the young even at the same plasma levels. The hypotensive side effects of many psychotropic drugs are greater in the elderly because of reduced functioning of baroreceptor reflexes. Hemorrhage with anticoagulants is more common in the elderly even with good control of the clotting parameters. These changes in pharmacodynamics require the use of smaller doses of drugs in the elderly, even if the kinetics of the drug are not altered.

The following general principles derive from studies of drugs in the elderly: (1) Drugs that are eliminated by the kidneys will very likely have a reduced clearance, and the doses required to achieve the same blood concentration may be 50 per cent of those required in a young population. (2) Drugs that are eliminated by the liver may be less affected, but for parenterally given drugs such as lidocaine that have high hepatic clearances, the reduction in liver blood flow would be expected to decrease the clearance of the drug. In addition, some individuals may have a reduction in hepatic drug metabolism, and enzyme induction may not occur as readily in the elderly. (3) The sensitivity of target organs to drugs is increased for central nervous system depressants and probably for other drugs as well. Thus, the elderly constitute a population in whom drug use is likely to be marred by enhanced toxicity, and physician awareness of the possibility of altered drug disposition or effects is mandatory. It is a population in which drugs should be used in the lowest effective doses and only in individuals in whom they are absolutely necessary. That this is not commonly done is indicated by the numbers of drugs taken by elderly individuals, frequently without well-defined endpoints or even well-defined therapeutic indications. Frequent reviews of the patient's drug history, including over-the-counter medications, and discontinuation of those drugs that are not necessary would greatly improve medical care for the elderly population.

Benet LZ, Sheiner LB: Design and optimization of dosage regimens: Pharmacokinetic data. In Gilman AG, Goodman LS, Gilman A (eds.): The Pharmacological Basis of Therapeutics. Edition 7. New York, Macmillan, 1985, pp 1663–1733. *This series of tables lists the pharmacokinetic parameters of over 150 drugs with references to the literature. This represents the most concise and complete listing currently available and is the source for some of the data in Table 24–4.*

Bjornsson TD: Nomogram for drug dosage adjustment in patients with renal failure. Clin Pharmacokin 11:164, 1986. *This review of drug elimination in renal disease uses an approach to dosage adjustment similar to the nomogram in this chapter. There is an extensive compilation of over 130 drugs that can be used as a reference for those drugs not in Table 24–1 or Table 24–4.*

Chennavasin P, Brater DC: Nomograms for drug use in renal disease. Clin Pharmacokin 6:193, 1981. *This is a critical review of a variety of published nomograms for determination of creatinine clearance from serum creatinine and for drug dosing in patients with renal disease.*

Gerber JG: Drug usage in the elderly. In Schrier RW (ed.): Clinical Internal Medicine in the Aged. Philadelphia, W.B. Saunders Company, 1982, pp 51–65. *This chapter is an excellent summary of pharmacokinetic principles applied to the elderly patient. The 49 references serve as an entry to the recent literature.*

Reidenberg M: The binding of drugs to plasma proteins and the interpretation of measurements of plasma concentrations of drugs in patients with poor renal function. Am J Med 62:466, 1977. *This review discusses the problems that arise when drug binding to plasma protein is altered by renal disease.*

Wilkinson GR, Shand DG: A physiological approach to hepatic drug clearance. Clin Pharmacol Ther 18:377, 1975. *This article discusses hepatic drug clearance in relation to blood flow, enzyme activity, and plasma protein binding. The concepts are valuable for physiologically oriented individuals.*

25 INTERACTIONS BETWEEN DRUGS

Alan S. Nies

Good medical practice frequently demands treatment with multiple drugs for a single disease in an attempt to maximize therapeutic effects and minimize side effects. When one is treating multiple diseases, the number of coadministered drugs increases, as does the possibility of undesirable interactions occurring between the drugs. Entire textbooks have been written in an attempt to list all of the possible drug interactions. It is obviously impossible for a clinician to remember such lists, and frequently the *clinically important* drug interactions are lost in the midst of large listings of interactions that are based on undocumented case reports, animal experimentation, or theory.

Not all drug interactions that occur are clinically important or even clinically recognized. The reasons for this include the fact that (1) many drugs have such large therapeutic indices that toxicity does not result when there are moderate increases in drug concentration, and thus changes in concentration due to a drug interaction may not be perceived; (2) the disease being treated may not be serious so that a change of drug concentration to less than therapeutic levels may not be easily recognized; (3) many drugs are given without well-defined therapeutic endpoints, making the drug effect difficult to assess, and therefore changes in drug effect will not be recognized; (4) there is a large intersubject variability due to genetic, environmental, and disease factors that may obscure many drug interactions. These comments are not to imply that drug interactions are not important. Drug interactions will be important if the drug has easily recognizable toxicity and a low therapeutic index such that small increases in amount of drug in the body produce significant toxicity. Second, drug interactions will be recognized and important if the diseases that are being controlled with the drug are serious or potentially fatal when undertreated. Third, drug interactions will be recognized if the therapeutic endpoints for the drug are clearly defined or if drug levels are used to maximize therapy for a given drug. Thus major interactions have been reported with anticoagulants and oral hypoglycemics, both of which have easily recognizable toxicity with low therapeutic indices. Drug interactions are reported with antiseizure medication and antiarrhythmic drugs; not only do these drugs have recognized toxicity, but also the diseases being treated become clinically manifest if the amount of drug is inadequate. Drug interactions have also been recognized with cardiac glycosides when blood levels are used to maximize efficacy in some patients.

Clinically important drug interactions are related to either (1) changes in the amount of drug or active metabolite available at the site of action, the so-called pharmacokinetic drug interactions, or (2) changes in drug effect without a change in pharmacokinetics, the pharmacodynamic drug interactions. These latter interactions may result from interactions at a receptor site, from independent actions of two drugs either adding to or counteracting the effects of each other, or from one drug altering the cellular milieu, thus changing the effects of another drug.

PHARMACOKINETIC DRUG INTERACTIONS

These interactions involve the processes of absorption, distribution, renal elimination, and metabolism such that there is a change in the amount of a drug (or an active metabolite) at the site of action. These are the best understood and generally most important drug interactions in clinical medicine. They can be subdivided into those that result in a decreased amount of drug at the site of action and hence a decrease in effect and those that have an increased amount of drug at the site of action and hence an increased effect.

Interactions Resulting in Less Drug Available at the Site of Action

DECREASED ABSORPTION. Since drug absorption generally occurs across the gastrointestinal mucosa by passive diffusion, one drug would not be expected to compete with another for absorption. However, drugs may physically interact in the lumen of the gastrointestinal tract so as to cause decreased absorption. Cholestyramine and colestipol, resins used to bind bile acids and to lower serum cholesterol, can also bind a number of drugs if they are simultaneously present in the gastrointestinal lumen. Thus cholestyramine can diminish the absorption of thyroxin, cardiac glycosides, warfarin, and corticosteroids. It is highly likely that other drugs will also bind to the steroid-binding resins, so that one is advised to view concurrent therapy of these resins with other drugs with caution.

Tetracyclines are potent chelating agents that form insoluble complexes with metal ions such as magnesium, calcium, and aluminum, commonly found in antacids, as well as with iron, with the result that the absorption of tetracycline is reduced. Sucralfate used for peptic ulcer disease has been reported to reduce the absorption of warfarin. Kaolin used to halt diarrhea will effectively inhibit the absorption of some drugs such as lincomycin and digoxin. In addition, drug products may contain "inert" substances that can interact with other drugs. For instance, para-aminosalicylic acid (PAS) contains bentonite (a kaolin-like substance), which can hamper the absorption of coadministered rifampin.

If a drug is susceptible to degradation at acid pH, anything that delays emptying of the stomach, such as a drug with anticholinergic properties, can result in more degradation of the coadministered acid-sensitive drug, e.g., penicillin G or L-dopa, and thus a decrease in the amount of drug absorbed. Conversely, a drug that speeds gastric emptying, such as metoclopramide, can increase the absorption of acid-unstable drugs. With most other drugs only the time course of absorption is changed so that drug absorption is faster if gastric emptying is enhanced or is slower if gastric emptying is delayed, but the total amount of drug absorbed is unchanged. Whether a change in rate of absorption results in any important clinical effects depends on whether rapid absorption is necessary for drug effect, in which case drug effect will be diminished. Usually, if total absorption is unchanged, then there will not be an important interaction, particularly during chronic administration of drugs.

The pH of the gastrointestinal fluid has little predictable effect on drug absorption. Almost all drugs are absorbed to the greatest extent in the small intestine rather than in the stomach. The classic teaching that acidic drugs, such as aspirin, are best absorbed in the stomach at acid pH because less drug is ionized is untrue. Actually, aspirin is more rapidly absorbed from an alkaline medium, since dissolution is enhanced.

ALTERED DISTRIBUTION. Some drugs reach their site of action via active transport. In this case, drugs can compete with each other for the transport mechanism, and thus one drug can impair the ability of another to reach its site of action. In order to produce blockade of adrenergic activity, the antihypertensive drugs guanethidine, guanadrel, and bethanidine must be actively transported by an amine transport system into adrenergic neurons. This transport system can be interfered with by tricyclic antidepressants, high doses of phenothiazines, and some sympathomimetic amines. Thus coadministration of guanethidine with one of these other compounds will effectively block the antihypertensive effects of guanethidine. This is an undesirable interaction with guanethidine; however, with the antiarrhythmic drug bretylium, sympathetic blockade produces orthostatic hypotension as an unwanted side effect. Bretylium also gains access to adrenergic neurons via the same amine transport system used by guanethidine. Therapeutic advantage can be taken of a drug interaction that blocks access of bretylium to its antiadrenergic site of action. Thus tricyclic antidepressants or ephedrine will reverse bretylium's sympathetic blocking effects but will not affect the direct antiarrhythmic effects of bretylium.

ENHANCED METABOLISM. Several drugs can increase the ability of the liver to metabolize other drugs. Phenobarbital, other barbiturates, phenytoin, rifampin, glutethimide, griseofulvin, ethanol, phenylbutazone, chronic smoking, certain chlorinated hydrocarbons such as lindane and DDT, carbamazepine, and primidone have all been associated with induction of hepatic microsomal, drug-metabolizing enzymes. The amount of enzyme induction that occurs appears to be under genetic control and so not all individuals experience quantitatively similar effects when taking an inducing agent.

Induction of hepatic metabolizing enzymes can affect many drugs. The effects are greatest when the drugs are given orally, because all of the drug must perforce pass through the liver prior to reaching the systemic circulation. Therefore, even for drugs that have a systemic clearance that is largely dependent upon hepatic blood flow, the amount of drug that escapes metabolism on the first pass will be influenced by enzyme-inducing drugs. Some examples of drugs that can have their metabolism induced are oral anticoagulants, quinidine, digitoxin, corticosteroids, low-dose contraceptives, some beta-adrenergic blockers, mexiletine, and theophylline. The induction of corticosteroid metabolism has produced some interesting effects, including (1) inappropriate interpretation of low-dose dexamethasone suppression tests in which the enhanced metabolism of dexamethasone produced by enzyme induction resulted in too low a dexamethasone concentration to inhibit normal steroidogenesis; (2) exacerbation of steroid-dependent asthma; and (3) rejection of a renal transplant by individuals who required steroids and received an enzyme-inducing agent.

Frequently the most critical time comes when the inducing agent is discontinued. At this time the drug-metabolizing activity gradually decreases, and drug toxicity can occur if dosage adjustments are not made of other coadministered drugs. This phenomenon has been described most frequently with induction of warfarin metabolism and resultant warfarin toxicity when the inducting agent is discontinued.

Interactions Resulting in More Drug Available at the Site of Action

ENHANCED ABSORPTION. In general, absorption is not a common process in which drugs can interact to enhance efficacy. One exception is with acid-unstable drugs and enhanced gastric emptying mentioned above. Another potential interaction is with relatively poorly absorbed drugs, such as digoxin, with which absorption occurs throughout the gastrointestinal tract. With such a drug a decrease in intestinal motility could enhance the degree of absorption by prolonging contact with the absorbing mucosa.

ALTERED DISTRIBUTION. Many drugs are bound to plasma proteins, and drug so bound is not available for action at receptors or for distribution throughout the body. In addition, for many compounds only the free drug is available for metabolism or excretion. The drug bound to plasma protein, therefore, acts as an inactive reservoir of drug in the blood. Since drugs can compete with each other for binding to plasma proteins, a potential for interactions exists. Pure plasma protein–binding interactions, however, rarely are clinically significant. The one probable exception to this is the displacement of albumin-bound bilirubin by sulfonamides or salicylates, thus allowing the bilirubin to distribute into the tissues and cause kernicterus in jaundiced infants. With drug/drug interactions, however, when a drug is displaced from plasma protein binding, it will very rapidly distribute into the apparent volume of distribution so that the increase in free drug concentration in the plasma is always considerably less than suggested by experiments in vitro. The larger the apparent volume of distribution, the less of an impact a displacement from protein binding will have. Following the immediate displacement and redistribution of the drug, the free fraction generally is readily available for metabolism or excretion, and the clearance processes in the body will reduce the free drug concentration to that which existed prior to the protein binding interaction (Fig. 25–1). Therefore the effect of such an interaction will be small, transient, and frequently not recognized clinically. The relationship of free drug to total drug, however, will be changed by such drug interactions, and therefore the interpretation of plasma drug assays that measure total drug in blood may have to be altered (see Ch. 24). Some drugs will interact with other drugs by more than one mechanism, and so interactions at protein-binding sites can coexist with interactions at a metabolic site. These dual drug interactions can be clinically important. However, it is not the displacement from protein binding that makes these interactions clinically important but rather the alteration of metabolism that does so. These dual drug interactions include interactions of phenylbutazone and sulfinpyrazone with warfarin and sulfaphenazole with tolbutamide.

Displacement of drugs from tissue-binding sites has only recently been recognized as a situation for drug interactions. Such an interaction would decrease the apparent volume of distribution of the drug and increase the plasma drug concentration. However, if the dose, plasma drug binding, and drug clearance are not altered, the plasma levels will be only transiently elevated, since steady-state plasma concentrations are independent of the apparent volume of distribution. Thus an interaction resulting in only a displacement from tissue stores would not be easily detected. However, as with displacement interactions from plasma protein, drugs can interact at multiple sites. Thus quinidine will displace digoxin from tissue-binding sites, but the persistent elevation in digoxin plasma concentration that results from the interaction is due to quinidine's ability to reduce the clearance of digoxin.

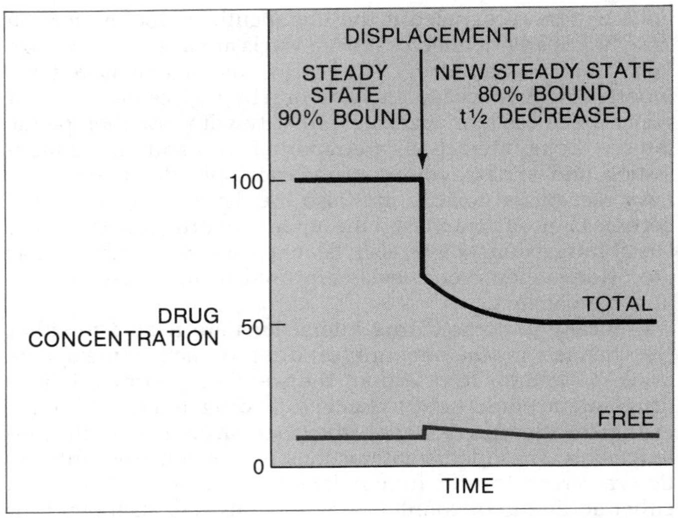

FIGURE 25–1. The effects of altered plasma drug binding on total and free plasma concentrations of the drug. The drug is assumed to be bound 90 per cent to albumin, not bound to tissues, and to have a V_D of 8.5 L. At the arrow an agent is given that displaces the drug from albumin such that binding is reduced to 80 per cent. The expected changes are an immediate increase in free drug concentration by only 40 per cent, with a fall of total concentration to 70 per cent of the initial value. Since the free drug clearance is not altered by this interaction, a new steady state will be achieved with the same free drug concentration and a reduction of total concentration to 50 per cent. For drugs with larger volumes of distribution, i.e., more tissue binding, the immediate increase of free concentration will be even less than in this example, but the ultimate steady-state condition of unchanged free drug concentration and a halving of the concentration of total drug will be the same. (Adapted from Shand et al.: In Handbook of Experimental Pharmacology. Vol 28, No 3, pp 272–314, 1975.)

DECREASED METABOLISM. Inhibition of drug metabolism can have a profound effect on drug disposition, resulting in drug toxicity. Inhibition of the metabolism of one drug by another occurs rapidly, and the enhanced effect or toxicity therefore often occurs shortly after the interaction takes place. Some drugs seem to be rather specific for inhibiting the metabolism of other individual drugs. However, there are a few drugs that can inhibit the metabolism of many drugs. The most commonly used such drug is cimetidine, which can inhibit the metabolism of theophylline, warfarin, diazepam, phenytoin, lidocaine, chlordiazepoxide, propranolol, carbamazepine, digitoxin, imipramine, quinidine, and probably others. The recently approved antiarrhythmic drug amiodarone also appears to be a potent inhibitor of the metabolism of many other drugs, including warfarin, phenytoin, and quinidine. Other important interactions resulting from decreased metabolism are listed in Table 25–1. As with other interactions resulting in an increased amount of drug at the sites of action, the most important examples are drugs that have a low therapeutic index and easily recognized, serious toxicity. The interaction of phenylbutazone or sulfinpyrazone and warfarin is a good example of an important interaction with a complex mechanism. Warfarin exists as R and S stereoisomers, with the S isomer being five times more potent an anticoagulant than the R isomer. Since phenylbutazone and sulfinpyrazone displace warfarin from plasma albumin, the normal occurrence would be for warfarin clearance to be increased by the interaction as more free drug becomes available for metabolism. In fact, this is true for R warfarin, but the metabolism of the more potent S warfarin is inhibited so that unbound S warfarin accumulates, although the total warfarin levels are unchanged or even decreased. It is the increased concentration of unbound S warfarin that results in enhanced anticoagulation.

TABLE 25–1. INHIBITION OF DRUG METABOLISM

Metabolism of	Inhibited by
Phenytoin	Isoniazid (in slow acetylators), chloramphenicol, cimetidine, clofibrate, phenylbutazone, disulfiram, sulfaphenazole, dicoumarol, amiodarone
Tolbutamide	Chloramphenicol, phenylbutazone, clofibrate, sulfaphenazole, dicoumarol
Warfarin	Phenylbutazone, alcohol, disulfiram, allopurinol, cimetidine, disopyramide, sulfinpyrazone, trimethoprim-sulfamethoxazole, metronidazole, amiodarone
Azathioprine, 6-mercaptopurine	Allopurinol
Catecholamines, tyramine	Monoamine oxidase inhibitors
Theophylline	Cimetidine, erythromycin, troleandomycin
Phenobarbital	Valproic acid

In addition to inhibition of hepatic drug metabolism via mixed function oxidase, inhibition of metabolism at other enzyme sites can be important. Thus monoamine oxidase inhibitors can inhibit the metabolism of catecholamines and tyramine at multiple sites, allowing for build-up of these substances and the so-called "cheese reaction" due to enhanced catecholamine release with the ingestion of tyramine-containing foods. Allopurinol inhibits xanthine oxidase, which can be important for the metabolism of azathioprine and 6-mercaptopurine as well as for production of uric acid. If allopurinol is given, much less azathioprine or 6-mercaptopurine is needed for equivalent effects. As discussed above, ethanol can induce hepatic microsomal drug-metabolizing enzymes. However, if ethanol is present, it can also act as an inhibitor of drug metabolism. Thus drugs given to an individual who is intoxicated may have an enhanced effect, whereas drugs given to an individual who has been drinking chronically but is no longer intoxicated may have diminished effect.

DIMINISHED RENAL EXCRETION. Some important drug interactions occur when active transport of one drug across the renal tubule is interfered with by another drug. Most of the reported interactions occur at the acid transport site. Thus probenecid is given to decrease penicillin clearance and thereby increase penicillin blood levels. Phenylbutazone can inhibit the renal clearance of hydroxyhexamide, an active metabolite of acetohexamide, and thereby increase its hypoglycemic effect. Salicylates, phenylbutazone, and probenecid can inhibit the renal elimination of methotrexate and enhance its effect. Drugs can also interact at the renal tubular site for active transport of bases, which is the probable mechanism whereby cimetidine and amiodarone reduce the renal clearance of procainamide.

Quinidine can inhibit the elimination of digoxin into the urine. The exact tubular site at which this interaction occurs is not known, but it is a significant interaction resulting in increased digoxin blood levels and effects. Verapamil and amiodarone also interact with digoxin by inhibiting renal excretion.

Decreased renal excretion of lithium occurs when proximal tubular reabsorption is enhanced. Since lithium and sodium are handled similarly in the proximal tubule, anything that results in more proximal tubular sodium reabsorption will also affect lithium in the same way. Thus dietary salt restriction, salt depletion due to diarrhea, and diuretics acting at more distal segments of the nephron can reduce renal lithium excretion, requiring a reduction in lithium dose. Indomethacin also reduces lithium clearance, probably by enhancing proximal tubular reabsorption of the ion.

PHARMACODYNAMIC DRUG INTERACTIONS

There are numerous examples of drugs interacting with each other at receptor sites or having additive effects by acting at separate sites on cells. Thus vitamin K can inhibit the effects of warfarin. Propranolol can interact with epinephrine by blocking the beta-adrenergic receptors and thus allowing the alpha-adrenergic effects of epinephrine to be unopposed, which can result in severe hypertension. Clonidine has been shown to have its antihypertensive effects in humans inhibited by tricyclic antidepressants. The mechanism for this is not entirely worked out but might be an interaction at an alpha-adrenergic receptor in the brain.

Examples of drugs producing additive effects are also common, such as the negative cardiac inotropic effects of disopyramide adding to the negative inotropic effects of beta-adrenergic blockers, producing heart failure. Two drugs that may affect the eighth cranial nerve, such as ethacrynic acid and aminoglycosides, may produce additional ototoxicity if given together. Drugs that affect neuromuscular function such as curare will have an enhanced effect if given with aminoglycosides, lincomycin, clindamycin, quinidine, or quinine, which also affect neuromuscular function.

One drug may alter the normal homeostatic mechanisms, resulting in a change in the internal milieu and thereby enhancing or diminishing the effect of another drug. The best-studied example of this type of interaction is the effect of diuretics to produce hypokalemia, which enhances the toxicity of cardiac glycosides.

Some drug interactions have not been well characterized, although the interaction is clearly significant. This is true for the interaction of warfarin with clofibrate. Clofibrate has a marked effect to increase the efficacy of warfarin, but there do not appear to be sufficient pharmacokinetic changes to account for this effect even though clofibrate may displace warfarin from plasma protein.

When viewed in perspective, drug interactions are only one of many factors that can alter the response of patients to drugs. Clinicians must be aware of the serious interactions and have well-defined therapeutic goals so that altered amounts or effects of drugs will become evident. The only way to accomplish this is to individualize therapy using effects or plasma drug levels when appropriate. This is particularly important for drugs with low therapeutic indices or during treatment of serious illnesses. Care must be used when a drug regimen is changed in any major way. If an interaction is appreciated, dosage adjustments can be made, and the two drugs often can be used together effectively. Drug interactions are an accepted fact of modern medical practice and should not be ignored, nor should they be overly feared.

Gerber MJ, Tejwani GA, Gerber N, et al.: Drug interactions with cimetidine: An update. Pharmacol Ther 27:353, 1985. *Cimetidine is the most commonly used drug that inhibits the metabolism and/or renal excretion of other drugs. This article reviews the increasing number of drug interactions reported with cimetidine.*

Hansten PD: Drug Interactions. 5th ed. Philadelphia, Lea and Febiger, 1985. *This frequently revised text is a useful compilation of known drug interactions. The interactions listed are referenced, and a estimate of probable clinical significance of the interaction is given.*

McElnay JC, D'Arcy PF: Protein binding displacement interactions and their clinical importance. Drugs 25:495, 1983. *This is a current review that emphasizes the fact that pure binding displacement interactions are unlikely to be of clinical significance.*

Serlin MJ, Breckenridge AM: Drug interactions with warfarin. Drugs 25:610, 1983. *Warfarin is a good model drug to study drug interactions, since its effects are easily measured, and hemorrhage is a readily detectable adverse effect. The several mechanisms of drug interactions affecting warfarin are reviewed with the relevant literature cited.*

Shand DG, Mitchell JR, Oates JA: Pharmacokinetic drug interactions. In Gillette JR, Mitchell JR (eds.): Handbook of Experimental Pharmacology, Vol 28, No 3. Concepts in Biochemical Pharmacology. New York, Springer-Verlag, 1975, pp 272–314. *This is a thorough review of pharmacokinetic mechanisms whereby drugs can interact. It is not a complete listing of potential drug interactions, although many illustrative examples for the various mechanisms are given.*

26 ADVERSE REACTIONS TO DRUGS

Alan S. Nies

Although difficult to quantify, there is little doubt that adverse reactions to drugs constitute an inevitable consequence of modern therapeutics. No drug is devoid of the potential to do harm, and benefit versus risk decisions are made with every decision to start drug therapy. Most ill patients require multiple drugs, and this increases the risk not only of adverse drug reactions but of drug interactions as well. Frequently it is difficult to be certain that an adverse effect is due to an individual drug because of the confounding effects of the underlying disease and the use of multiple drugs.

Studies to determine the incidence of adverse reactions are derived largely from medical services at academic hospitals. The Boston Collaborative Drug Surveillance Program found a 5 per cent incidence of adverse drug reactions, most of which were minor and self limited. Other studies have estimated a higher incidence, particularly in very ill or elderly patients. In a recent study of complications on a medical ward, adverse drug effects were the largest contributor to iatrogenic events, accounting for 42 per cent of all such occurrences. About 18 per cent of patients admitted to the hospital had an adverse drug effect, and 19 per cent of these were life threatening or resulted in serious disability. Drugs implicated in such studies include digitalis, theophylline, nitrates, lidocaine, and other antiarrhythmics, anticoagulants, benzodiazepines, antihypertensives, and antibiotics.

The recent studies do not indicate that the incidence of adverse drug reactions is decreasing. On the contrary, the risk may be increasing as the number of potent drugs available increases. The studies assessing the incidence of drug problems in an academic medical center cannot be generalized to other therapeutic situations such as outpatient clinics, office practices, or community hospitals. Since one of the major determinants of a drug reaction is how ill the patient is and how many drugs he is receiving, it is likely that adverse drug reactions occur much less commonly in situations outside the large general hospital. Also, it is impossible with present data to make a quantitative statement of risk versus benefit of medical therapy. It is clear that adverse reactions cannot be completely prevented even under the best of circumstances. Nonetheless, it is reasonable to continue investigation into ways to assess the risk and to reduce both the incidence and severity of these adverse reactions.

MECHANISMS OF ADVERSE DRUG REACTIONS

Unwanted effects of drugs are due to (1) exaggerated responses to the known desired or unwanted pharmacologic effects of the drug; (2) immunologic reactions to the drug or its metabolites; and (3) toxic effects of a drug or its metabolite. "Idiosyncratic" effects may be due to any of these mechanisms. The extension of the normal pharmacology accounts for most adverse drug effects. However, since these effects are predictable, they often may be avoided or treated by careful dosage adjustment without necessarily discontinuing drug treatment. The immunologically mediated and toxic adverse effects of drugs are less predictable and may be so severe as to require discontinuation of the offending drug. These latter effects are the least well understood, but mechanisms of some of the toxic drug effects have been discovered. Many reactions initially labeled immunologic may be due to other mechanisms. With time the mechanisms of the "idiosyncratic" drug reactions will be determined so that such reactions may be anticipated or avoided. All organ systems can be affected by drugs, and drug-induced disease should be a consideration in the differential diagnosis of most syndromes that present to an internist.

EXAGGERATED RESPONSES TO DRUGS

Excessive drug effects result from altered pharmacokinetics or altered target-organ response, as discussed in the previous chapters. Thus adverse drug effects are more common in the elderly, in patients with abnormal renal or hepatic function, and in patients receiving other drugs that may result in pharmacokinetic or pharmacodynamic interactions.

An example of a disease exaggerating the unwanted effects of a normally innocuous drug is the reduction in glomerular filtration rate produced by nonsteroidal anti-inflammatory drugs in patients who have activation of their sympathetic nervous system and/or increased plasma renin activity as a result of hepatic, renal, or cardiovascular disease. This adverse effect is a consequence of the same pharmacologic action responsible for the salutary effects of the drug, namely, inhibition of cyclo-oxygenase activity with a reduction in prostaglandin synthesis.

In addition, patients may have genetic abnormalities that make them susceptible to one or another effects of a drug. These genetic differences may be quantitative deviations from the norm or qualitative abnormalities. An example of such quantitative differences is the variability in hepatic drug oxidation that is described by a unimodal frequency distribution. Twin studies have indicated that genetic differences account for much of the variation between individuals in the metabolism of phenytoin, phenylbutazone, warfarin, ethanol, nortriptyline, and salicylate. In addition, several drug metabolic processes are controlled by genes at a single locus, such as slow acetylation of isoniazid, some sulfonamides, and procainamide; deficient parahydroxylation of phenytoin; deficient hydroxylation of debrisoquin; deficient hydroxylation of mephenytoin; deficient *N*-glucosidation of amobarbital; and deficient hydrolysis of succinylcholine. The excessive drug effects resulting from the genetically determined slow metabolic processes reflect increased drug available at the site of action.

In addition to these quantitative differences in drug metabolism, there are genetic abnormalities that result in qualitatively different responses to drugs. These reactions are due to known properties of the drug that are usually not important but become markedly exaggerated owing to the genetic defect. Thus individuals with a deficiency of the enzyme activity of glucose-6-phosphate dehydrogenase (G6PD) are unable to cope with the oxidative stress produced by some drugs, and hemolysis results. Drugs having this effect include primaquine, aspirin, sulfonamides, nitrofurantoin, sulfones, vitamin K, probenecid, quinidine, and quinine. In a similar manner, genetic deficiency of methemoglobin reductase results in inability to maintain hemoglobin in the ferrous form, resulting in methemoglobinemia upon exposure to some oxidizing drugs such as sulfones, sulfonamides, and nitrites. Likewise certain abnormal hemoglobins may be unstable and result in drug-induced hemolysis or methemoglobinemia. Frequently patients with these "pharmacogenetic" syndromes are unaware that there is any abnormality until they are challenged with a drug that produces the adverse effect.

TOXIC AND IMMUNOLOGIC REACTIONS

Adverse drug reactions in these categories are often lumped together because it is frequently difficult to be certain of the etiology of an individual reaction (Table 26–1). Some reactions that previously were considered to be immunologic have been shown to be toxic.

Toxic reactions include direct effects of a drug on a target organ, such as the nephrotoxicity and ototoxicity produced

TABLE 26–1. "ALLERGIC" DRUG REACTIONS

Type of Reaction	Example (not inclusive)
Definite Immunologically Mediated Syndromes	
1. Immediate hypersensitivity (IgE-mediated) reactions	Penicillin-induced anaphylaxis Insulin-induced wheal and flare
2. Cytotoxic reactions	Drug-induced destruction of formed elements in the blood: Penicillin-induced hemolytic anemia Quinidine- or quinine-induced thrombocytopenia Phenylbutazone-induced granulocytopenia
3. Immune complex–induced vasculitis	Serum sickness–like reactions to penicillin, sulfonamides, and other drugs presenting as fever, rash, palpable purpura, arthralgia, and/or lymphadenopathy
4. Delayed hypersensitivity reactions	Contact dermatitis from topically applied drugs
Possible Immunologically Mediated Syndromes but with Unknown Mechanism	
1. Skin rashes of various types	Many drugs and a variety of skin eruptions
2. Stevens-Johnson syndrome	Sulfonamides, penicillins, phenytoin, phenylbutazone
3. Fever	Antibiotics, quinidine, methyldopa, allopurinol, procainamide
4. Pneumonitis	Loeffler's syndrome
5. Lupus erythematosus–like	Procainamide, hydralazine, isoniazid
6. Hepatic dysfunction	Chlorpromazine-induced cholestasis ? Methyldopa-induced hepatitis
7. Renal dysfunction	Interstitial nephritis from methicillin, furosemide, allopurinol
8. Lymphadenopathy	Phenytoin, sulfonamides

by aminoglycosides. In other cases drugs are metabolized to reactive intermediates that can covalently bind to cellular components, often near the site of metabolism, and produce toxicity. This mechanism is well established for the hepatotoxicity produced by overdoses of acetaminophen. During therapeutic use of acetaminophen the small amount of reactive metabolite formed by oxidative metabolism is rapidly detoxified by interacting with reduced glutathione. With overdose, however, the glutathione is depleted, and the reactive metabolite attacks hepatic macromolecules, resulting in liver damage. Other sulfhydryl-containing compounds such as *N*-acetylcysteine or cysteamine can protect the liver by reducing the amount of toxic metabolite that remains unreacted with a sulfhydryl-containing compound. Other drugs may produce liver disease by somewhat similar mechanisms. Isoniazid-induced hepatitis may result from acetylation to acetylisoniazid that can be hydrolyzed to acetylhydrazine, which can be oxidized to a reactive metabolite. One might expect from this theory that individuals who rapidly acetylate isoniazid would be more susceptible to the hepatotoxicity. However, recent data indicate that the opposite may be true. This apparent discrepancy may be related to observations that rapid acetylators not only form acetylisoniazid rapidly but also quickly convert this metabolite to diacetylisoniazid, which is nontoxic. Slow acetylators, on the other hand, form acetylisoniazid gradually but are much less able to convert it to diacetylisoniazid. Consequently, more of the acetylisoniazid is available for hydrolysis to acetylhydrazine and subsequent oxidation to the reactive metabolite. However, there remains considerable controversy regarding the relevance of this theory to the clinical hepatitis that results from isoniazid, and it is clear that other factors, such as the patient's age, are also important.

Hepatocellular damage, such as that produced by methyldopa or halothane, is frequently considered to be immunologically produced. However, it is entirely possible that reactive metabolites could be important for these as well as a variety of other drugs that produce hepatotoxicity on occasion.

Immunologic reactions to drugs account for 5 to 10 per cent of all adverse drug reactions and probably result from the drug or a reactive metabolite combining with a protein to form an antigenic drug-protein complex that stimulates the immune response. Without such a reaction, most drugs, which have a molecular weight less than 1000, would not be able to elicit an immunologic response. The typical immunologic reaction requires a latent period of 10 to 20 days for stimulation of the production of antibodies and activated immune effector cells that cause the allergic reaction. After the initial exposure, however, the allergic reaction will occur with a much shorter or no latent period after re-exposure to the drug. Drug hypersensitivity can produce mediator release, initiate cell lysis, activate the complement system, or activate cellular hypersensitivity reactions.

The most dramatic allergic reaction is anaphylaxis, or IgE-mediated hypersensitivity. Penicillin is the most common drug to produce anaphylaxis, but many other drugs or diagnostic agents (such as Bromsulphalein) can produce this life-threatening reaction. A history of penicillin allergy increases the risk of this reaction occurring, but most (75 per cent) of the 100 to 300 patients dying of penicillin-induced anaphylaxis each year have no history of penicillin allergy. Oral penicillin seems to have a lower incidence of reactions than parenteral penicillin.

Skin testing with penicilloyl polylysine, penicillin G, and penicilloic acid can identify patients at risk for anaphylaxis. Skin tests should be used if there is a history of penicillin allergy and penicillin therapy is considered mandatory. Some day it may be common to skin test all patients who are to receive penicillin, but this is not current practice.

Cytotoxic allergic reactions occur when the drug binds to the surface of a cell and is then attacked by antibody. Penicillin-induced hemolytic anemia is of this type. Immune complexes of drug and antibody may become adsorbed to the cell membrane, resulting in complement-mediated cytotoxicity. Thrombocytopenia and hemolytic anemia due to quinine or quinidine are examples of immune complex–mediated cytotoxicity. Methyldopa-induced Coombs' positivity that occurs in up to 20 per cent of patients on therapy for over six months is of unknown etiology but results in antibodies directed at the Rh loci of the red cell. However, the continued presence of the drug is not necessary for the immune reaction to continue, and the Coombs' positivity only gradually resolves upon discontinuation of the drug.

Circulating immune complexes of drug and antibody can produce serum sickness (see Ch. 420, 431), a vasculitic syndrome produced by deposition of immune complexes. Penicillin, sulfonamides, thiouracil, cholecystographic dyes, phenytoin, and other drugs can cause serum sickness.

Drug-induced lupus syndromes as caused by procainamide, hydralazine, and isoniazid may be associated with circulating immune complexes. In this case the drug or a reactive metabolite may interact with nuclear material to allow formation of antinuclear antibodies. The drug-induced systemic lupus erythematosus (SLE) (see Ch. 436) differs from spontaneous lupus by being uncommon in blacks and by only rarely causing nephritis. The acetylator phenotype also is important in drug-induced lupus. Hydralazine-induced lupus is very uncommon in fast acetylators. Procainamide-induced lupus occurs with smaller doses of drugs and at an earlier time after starting the drug in slow acetylators, although fast acetylators are also at risk.

In addition to the immune phenomena outlined above, many other syndromes are attributed to drug allergy. These include a variety of skin rashes, drug fever, pulmonary reactions, hepatocellular or cholestatic reactions, interstitial nephritis, and lymphadenopathy. For most of these reactions, the exact immune mechanism is unknown. One interesting syndrome that is sometimes classified as immune but may involve other mechanisms as well is that of aspirin sensitivity. In some patients this syndrome resembles IgE-mediated allergy with rhinitis, sinusitis, nasal polyps, and asthma. However, other cyclo-oxygenase inhibitors, such as indomethacin and meclofenamate, also produce asthma in many of these patients, suggesting a possible etiologic role for an arachidonic acid metabolite, such as a leukotriene, rather than an immunologic mechanism. It seems likely that several syndromes of aspirin sensitivity exist.

Some adverse drug reactions mimic anaphylactic reactions but are not immune mediated. Such reactions are due to direct release of mediators by drugs and are called anaphylactoid reactions. Reactions to radiocontrast dyes are of this type. The risk of re-exposure to the dye is unpredictable and skin testing is of no value. If re-exposure is absolutely necessary, pretreatment with steroids and antihistamines is the current practice.

RECOGNITION AND IDENTIFICATION

Adverse drug effects must first be suspected to be recognized. In some situations, the adverse effect mimics the illness being treated (for instance, arrhythmias caused by antiarrhythmic drugs or antibiotic-induced fever). In other instances, the reaction is more obviously drug induced, as is the case with characteristic skin rashes or anticoagulant-induced bleeding. The first confirmation of an adverse reaction is its disappearance with drug withdrawal. In some cases it may be warranted to readminister the putative offending drug cautiously if it is likely that the drug will be required again for therapy. In the case of serious allergic or toxic reactions, however, this may be too dangerous. Tests in vitro are occasionally helpful for drug-induced thrombocytopenia or hemolytic anemia but are not useful for most drug reactions. Skin testing is of value with penicillin, insulin, and horse serum.

Adverse reactions will continue to occur as long as potent drugs are available. Most of the reactions are predictable. The unexpected toxic and immunologic reactions remain a problem that continues to stimulate discussions as to how to detect rare adverse effects. During the process of drug development, reactions occurring less often than 1 per 1000 patients will not be detected. In addition, drugs are developed by testing in patients who have well-defined diseases, are not on many other drugs, are not pregnant, and are usually neither in the pediatric nor the geriatric populations. After approval, however, all patient populations may be exposed to the drug. Therefore, the adverse effects of a new drug frequently are not discovered until after marketing. Different systems exist for early detection of drug reactions after marketing. A major mechanism is an early warning that results from anecdotal reports by practicing physicians to pharmaceutical companies, drug regulatory agencies, or most commonly as letters published in general medical journals. Following the first alerts, a verification mechanism is required. It is in this area that much remains to be learned. Postmarketing surveillance of patients taking drugs will not be effective for uncommon drug reactions unless sample sizes of more than 100,000 patients are followed. Surveys of patients with certain diseases to determine the incidence of use of the drug suspected to have caused the illness (case-control study) may be a more efficient way to detect drug-induced illness for rare adverse effects. However, the alert practitioner has been and will continue to be the primary individual who makes the initial important observation that often provides the first clue to an unsuspected adverse drug reaction.

Davies DM (ed.): Textbook of Adverse Drug Reactions. Oxford, Oxford University Press, 1977. *This well-referenced book is organized by specific syndromes, with a discussion of the drugs that may cause the syndrome. General problems of detecting and verifying adverse reactions are also discussed.*

Faich GA: Adverse-drug–reaction monitoring. N Engl J Med 314:1589, 1986. *This is a review of the adverse-reaction monitoring program at the FDA and indicates that spontaneous reporting of drug reactions by physicians is critical to providing early warnings of previously unsuspected drug risks.*

Jick H: Adverse drug reactions: The magnitude of the problem. J Allergy Clin Immunol 74:555, 1984. *This report from the Boston Collaborative Drug Surveillance Program is the leading article in a symposium on allergic drug reactions.*

Mitchell JR, Jollow DJ: Metabolic activation of drugs to toxic substances. Gastroenterology 68:392, 1975. *This is a review of adverse drug reactions that result from metabolism of drugs to reactive metabolites that covalently bind to tissue macromolecules.*

Patterson R, Anderson J: Allergic reactions to drugs and biologic agents. JAMA 248:2637, 1982. *Part of the "primer on allergic and immunologic diseases," this short review outlines the mechanisms of immunologic reactions to drugs. The authors provide relevant references and distinguish between allergic reactions for which the immune mechanisms are established and those that are only conjectured to be immunologically mediated.*

Steel K, Gertman PM, Crescenzi C, et al.: Iatrogenic illness on a general medical service at a university hospital. N Engl J Med 304:638, 1981. *This study of a medical service indicates an 18 per cent incidence of iatrogenic illness, of which 42 per cent were drug related.*

27 PAIN AND ITS MANAGEMENT

Kathleen M. Foley and Jerome B. Posner

INTRODUCTION

Pain is the most common symptom for which patients seek medical assistance. To manage pain, the physician must understand its nature—the relationship between its medical, psychologic, and social aspects—and must establish a relationship of mutual trust with the patient. The physician's therapeutic task is twofold: to discover and treat the cause of the pain and to treat the pain itself, whether or not the underlying cause is treatable. Advances in knowledge of the physiology, pharmacology, and psychology of pain perception have led to improved care of patients with both acute and chronic pain (see also Ch. 466), but a lack of generally agreed-upon definitions and classification of pain has hampered communication among physicians. To provide a more common ground for the evaluation and treatment of patients with pain, the International Association for the Study of Pain (IASP) has proposed a working definition: Pain is "an unpleasant sensory and emotional experience associated with either actual or potential tissue damage, or described in terms of such damage." The IASP has also developed a taxonomy of pain syndromes that serves as a universal classification of pain syndromes (see references).

TYPES OF PAIN

Clinically, pain can be classified *temporally* as acute or chronic, *physiologically* as somatic, visceral, or deafferentation, and *etiologically* as medical or psychogenic.

TEMPORAL CHARACTERISTICS. Patients with severe *acute pain* can usually give a clear description of its location, character, and timing. Furthermore, objective signs, particularly of autonomic nervous system hyperactivity, with tachycardia, hypertension, diaphoresis, mydriasis, and pallor are present. The pain is usually self-limited (e.g., postoperative pain, acute traumatic pain). The patient's ability to tolerate acute pain is influenced by the setting of the pain, its duration, and its psychologic significance. Treatment of both the cause of acute pain and the pain itself is usually possible. Pain lasting longer than three months' duration is usually considered *chronic*. In patients with chronic pain, the localization, character, and timing of the pain are often more vague, and because the autonomic nervous system adapts, signs of autonomic hyperactivity disappear. Significant changes occur in the psychologic, social, and functional status of patients with chronic pain, often requiring a multidisciplinary approach to treatment, including pharmacologic, behavioral, and rehabilitative therapeutic approaches.

PHYSIOLOGIC CHARACTERISTICS. *Somatic pain* results from activation of peripheral receptors and somatic efferent nerves, without injury to the peripheral nerves or central nervous system. The pain can be either sharp or dull but is typically well localized and intermittent. *Visceral pain* results from activation of visceral nociceptive receptors and visceral efferent nerves and is characterized as a deep aching, cramping sensation, often referred to cutaneous sites. *Deafferentation or causalgic pain* results from direct injury to peripheral receptors, nerves, or central nervous system. It is typically burning and dysesthetic and often occurs in an area of sensory loss (e.g., postherpetic neuralgia). The autonomic nervous system plays a significant modulatory role in all three types of pain but is most prominent in visceral and deafferentation pain. The somatic and visceral types of pain are readily managed with a wide variety of nonopioid or opioid analgesics, anesthetic blocks, and neurosurgical approaches. In contrast, deafferentation pain responds minimally to nonopioid and opioid analgesics and to anesthetic and neurosurgical procedures.

ETIOLOGIC CHARACTERISTICS. Patients with chronic pain can generally be classified into one of three major etiologic groups, allowing for some overlap. The first group includes patients with chronic pain associated with *structural disease*. Such pain occurs, for example, with rheumatoid arthritis, metastatic cancer, and sickle cell anemia and is usually characterized by prolonged episodes of pain alternating with pain-free intervals or by unremitting pain waxing and waning in severity. Successful treatment of the pain is closely allied with treatment of the disease, but in certain instances treatment of the pain is the only therapeutic goal, e.g., the dying cancer patient with pain. Psychologic factors may play an important role in exacerbating or relieving pain, but analgesic drug therapy is the mainstay of therapy while attempting to treat the underlying disease.

The second group comprises patients who suffer from *psychophysiologic disorders* causing pain. In these patients, structural disease such as a herniated disc or torn ligaments may once have been present but psychologic factors have caused chronic physiologic alterations, such as muscle spasm, which produce pain long after the underlying defect has healed. Typically, such patients are physically inactive and spend much of their time thinking and talking about their pain, often leading to social and emotional isolation. Patients are more impaired by their "chronic illness behavior" than by a defined pathologic condition. They usually respond poorly to analgesic drugs and often suffer from iatrogenic complications, such as adverse drug reactions and ineffective surgical procedures. They use health care resources excessively. Successful treatment can be expected only through a structured rehabilitation program designed to modify pain behaviors and not through medical intervention designed to correct pathologic conditions. Multidisciplinary pain clinics that diagnose and treat intractable pain exist in many centers and should be utilized to evaluate and treat such patients.

Patients of the third group complain of pain that appears to have neither a structural nor a physiologic basis. These patients probably suffer from *somatic delusions*. Such patients usually have serious psychiatric disorders, and the history of the pain is so vague and bizarre and its distribution so unanatomic as to suggest the diagnosis. These patients respond only to psychiatric therapy.

ASSESSMENT OF PAIN

No objective tests (except observing patient behavior) assess the severity of pain or even its presence. Therefore, the physician must accept the patient's report, taking into consideration his or her age, cultural background, environment, and psychologic circumstances known to alter reaction to pain.

A thorough history, general physical examination, and careful neurologic examination are imperative in any patient complaining of pain. The description of the nature and distribution of the pain may be so characteristic (e.g., trigeminal neuralgia or tabetic lightning pains) that it allows no other diagnosis. Inquiry should be made concerning (1) the temporal pattern of pain, (2) its distribution, (3) exacerbating factors, and (4) relieving factors. For example, headache beginning early in the morning before arising suggests increased intracranial pressure, whereas headache occurring late in the day is more suggestive of tension. Back pain and sciatica made worse by sitting or walking suggest disc disease, whereas back pain and sciatica that are worse while the person is in bed indicate intraspinal tumor. Back pain and sciatica exacerbated by cough or sneeze suggest intraspinal disease, whereas similar pain not exacerbated by cough or sneeze is indicative of disease in the pelvis. Pain in the back or legs exacerbated by straight-leg raising suggests disease of the nervous system, whereas a similar pain exacerbated by rotating the hips suggests pelvic or hip disease. All pain is relieved to some extent by distraction and a pleasurable environment and is exacerbated by anxiety or psychologic stress.

A careful psychiatric history, looking particularly for signs and symptoms of depression, should be elicited from all patients. The distinction between pain and suffering should be made by both the physician and the patient. Specifically, physicians should inquire about the degree to which pain has interfered with the patient's activities, whether he or she is having difficulty sleeping, and whether there is a change in appetite or bowel habits. Early morning awakening, anorexia, and constipation are somatic manifestations of depression and may either be caused by chronic pain or exacerbate the effects of the pain.

A general physical examination must be performed. Both the physical and the laboratory examination should begin with the assumption that the site of pathologic change is at the site of pain. The painful areas should be examined for swelling and redness as well as for any obvious deformity. (The pain of herpes zoster usually precedes the rash, and occasionally on examination one may note the faintest reddening of the skin in a dermatomal distribution.) The areas reported as painful should be palpated, the temperature estimated, and points of tenderness sought. (If the site of pain is in a soft tissue, bone, or joint, it should be tender to palpation as well as spontaneously painful.) Joints should be taken through a full range of motion, and the effect of movement on the pain assessed. Nerve trunks going to the extremities should be palpated and stretched by movement of that member (e.g., straight-leg raising: abduction and extension of the arm). Inflamed and compressed nerve roots and nerve plexuses are more painful when stretched. A careful neurologic examination must also be performed. If there are neurologic abnormalities (e.g., weakness, sensory loss, and reflex changes) in the painful part, one can infer that nervous system disease is responsible for the pain. However, the absence of neurologic abnormalities on first examination does not guarantee that the nervous system is free of disease, because the process may simply not have advanced beyond the stage of selectively involving pain pathways. For example, a Pancoast's tumor may cause shoulder and arm pain before other signs of neural involvement, such as Horner's syndrome or motor or sensory loss, appear.

Finally, laboratory examinations are performed. If the site

of disease appears to be in bones or joints, radiographs, computed tomography (CT) scans, or radioisotope scans may localize it. First attention should be paid to the local site of pain, but the physician should be familiar with the common referred patterns of pain (e.g., hip disease commonly causes knee pain, cardiac pain is frequently referred to the ulnar aspect of the arm and forearm, the pain of renal colic may be felt primarily in the groin and testicle, and pain resulting from disease of the throat may be referred to the ear).

Referred pain is pain perceived at a site remote from the source of the disturbance. Usually, referred pain is perceived as cutaneous and is evoked by disease of deep structures innervated by the same dermatome. Referred pain may be associated with cutaneous hyperalgesia and even relieved by procaine injection into the area of referral. When pain is referred to the same dermatome or myotome that innervates the diseased structure (e.g., pain down the medial aspect of the arm [T1-T2] produced by myocardial infarction or angina pectoris), it is often helpful in diagnosis. However, pain is sometimes referred a great distance from the primary site to segments not similarly innervated, and in such cases the mechanism is perplexing (e.g., anginal pain referred to the jaw). Various theories, such as division of the same nerve into deep and superficial branches, release of chemical mediators into the nervous system, and convergence of cutaneous and visceral nerves into a common synaptic pool at the spinal cord, all explain the dermatomal referral of pain but fail to explain pain at remote sites.

MANAGEMENT OF PAIN

Recent advances in pain research provide a scientific rationale that has improved treatment. These include better and more effective use of standard drug therapy (non-narcotic, narcotic, and adjuvant analgesic drugs), the development of new drugs and the use of novel routes of drug administration, more selective anesthetic and neurosurgical approaches, and the integration of behavioral approaches to pain control.

General Principles (Table 27–1)

1. Pain is best managed by treating the underlying disorder (e.g., steroids for giant cell arteritis relieve headache and jaw or temporalis muscle pain promptly; radiation therapy for bone pain caused by cancer is often helpful), but in many patients the pain is chronic and the physician is able neither to treat the underlying disturbances nor to offer specific therapy for that type of pain.

2. Pain should be treated early and promptly. The persistence of untreated pain results in significant psychologic morbidity, most commonly anxiety and depression with a sense of loss of control and hopelessness. Early treatment that provides prompt and continuous pain relief is crucial to prevent further compromise of the patient's emotional resources.

3. Multiple therapeutic approaches, often delivered simultaneously, should be utilized because different treatment modalities may be additive or synergistic when used together rather than separately. For example, combinations of narcotic and non-narcotic analgesics provide greater analgesia than either alone. Nonpharmacologic methods, such as relaxation techniques and cognitive coping skills, coupled with physical therapy and vocational rehabilitation, can often help in selected patients with chronic pain, especially when added to judicious drug therapy.

4. Narcotic drugs should be used with discrimination, but they should not be withheld if alternative therapy is ineffective. Long-term use of narcotics produces tolerance and physical dependence. Tolerance is the term used to describe increasing dose requirements to maintain analgesia. *Physical dependence* means that the signs and symptoms of withdrawal will appear if the narcotic drug is abruptly discontinued. These effects should not be confused with psychologic dependence or "*addiction*," which implies both a craving for the drug for effects other than analgesia and drug abuse behavior. The percentage of patients who actually become psychologically dependent on narcotics when they are given to treat medical illness is unknown, but recent data suggest that psychologic dependence is unusual in patients treated for pain when the pain is later relieved by other means.

5. Psychologic factors play a major role in chronic pain and must be carefully assessed. However, no patient should be diagnosed as having "psychogenic" pain until an exhaustive examination has ruled out structural disease. Depression should be identified and treated, and since the tricyclic antidepressants have analgesic properties as well, they are useful adjuvant analgesic drugs, particularly in patients with neuropathic pain.

6. Placebo effects are important. A positive analgesic response from intramuscular saline indicates only that the patient is a placebo responder. It does not suggest that the pain is unreal or less severe than reported by the patient. Misuse of placebo creates distrust between the patient and the physician and interferes with adequate pain assessment and management. In most clinical studies, up to one third of patients report relief of pain when given a placebo.

TABLE 27–1. GUIDELINES FOR THE USE OF ANALGESICS IN PAIN MANAGEMENT

1. Tailor drugs to nature and severity of pain
2. Know the pharmacology of the drug prescribed
   a. Know the duration of the analgesic effect
   b. Know the pharmacokinetic properties of the drug (duration of action and half-life)
   c. Know the equianalgesic doses for the drug and its route of administration (Table 27–2)
3. Adjust the route of administration to the patient's needs using oral, rectal, subcutaneous, intramuscular, intravenous, epidural, and intrathecal routes
4. Administer the analgesic on a regular basis after initial titration of the dose
5. Use drug combinations to provide additive analgesia and reduce side effects, e.g., nonsteroidal anti-inflammatory drugs, antihistamine (hydroxyzine), amphetamine (dextroamphetamine)
6. Avoid drug combinations that increase sedation without enhancing analgesia, e.g., benzodiazepine (diazepam) and phenothiazine
7. For narcotics, anticipate and treat side effects
   a. Sedation
   b. Respiratory depression
   c. Nausea and vomiting
   d. Constipation
   e. Multifocal myoclonus and seizures
8. When using narcotics, watch for the development of tolerance
   a. Switch to an alternate narcotic analgesic
   b. Start with one half of the equianalgesic dose and titrate to pain relief
   c. Use adjuvant analgesics and anesthetic and neurosurgical approaches
9. Prevent acute withdrawal
   a. Taper drugs slowly
   b. Use diluted doses of naloxone (0.4 mg in 10 ml of saline) to reverse narcotic-induced respiratory depression in the physically dependent patient and administer cautiously
10. Do not use placebos to assess pain

Drug Therapy

Analgesic drugs can be divided into three groups: Group I—the non-narcotic analgesics, such as aspirin and acetaminophen and the nonsteroidal anti-inflammatory drugs (NSAID's), act peripherally, probably on pain receptors; Group II—the narcotic agonist and antagonist drugs activate opiate receptors in the central and peripheral nervous systems; and Group III—the adjuvant analgesic drugs are designed for management of symptoms other than pain but produce relief in certain pain states (carbamazepine for trigeminal neuralgia) or potentiate narcotic analgesics. These three groups represent the mainstay of therapy for patients with acute and chronic pain. Effective use of these drugs requires

TABLE 27–2. NON-NARCOTIC ANALGESIC DRUGS

Drug	Indications	Equianalgesic Dose	Starting Dose (mg), Range/24 hr	Comments
Aspirin	Often used in combination with narcotics	650	650	Contraindicated in hepatic and renal dysfunction; avoid during pregnancy, in hemolytic disorders, and in combination with steroids
Acetaminophen	Like aspirin	650	650	Like aspirin
Ibuprofen	Higher analgesic potential than aspirin	ND	200–400	Like aspirin
Fenoprofen	Like ibuprofen	ND	200–400	Like aspirin
Diflunisal	Longer duration of action than ibuprofen; higher analgesic potential than aspirin	ND	500–1000	Like aspirin
Naproxen	Like diflunisal	ND	250–500	Like aspirin

ND = not documented.

an understanding of their pharmacologic characteristics and selection of a particular drug and dose geared to the needs of the individual patient.

NON-NARCOTIC ANALGESICS (Table 27–2). Aspirin, acetaminophen, and the nonsteroidal anti-inflammatory drugs are the first-line agents for the management of mild-to-moderate pain, and in patients with severe pain these drugs potentiate the effects of narcotic analgesics. Non-narcotic analgesics have a ceiling effect, and their long-term use is limited by gastrointestinal and hematologic side effects. The choice and use of these drugs must be individualized, with the patient receiving maximal levels of one drug before another is tried. If pain control is ineffective or the non-narcotic agents poorly tolerated, the use of narcotic analgesics is indicated. In general, the use of narcotics is limited to acute structural or chronic, irreversible structural pain, as in cancer.

NARCOTIC ANALGESICS (Table 27–3). The narcotic analgesics vary in potency, efficacy, and adverse effects. They are classified as agonist or antagonist drugs depending on their ability to bind to the opiate receptors and produce analgesia. The narcotic *agonist* drugs, such as morphine, bind to specific opiate receptors, resulting in analgesia. These

TABLE 27–3. NARCOTIC ANALGESIC DRUGS

Class	Drug	Indications	Equianalgesic Dose (mg)*	Starting Dose (mg) Range/24 hr	Comments
Morphine-like agonist, mild to moderate pain	Codeine	Often used in combination with non-narcotic analgesics	32–65	32–65	Impaired ventilation; bronchial asthma; intracranial pressure
	Oxycodone	Shorter acting; in combination with non-narcotic analgesics, limiting dose escalation	5	5–10	Like codeine
	Meperidine	Shorter acting; biotransformed to normeperidine; toxic metabolite	50	50–100	Normeperidine accumulates with repetitive dosing, causing CNS excitation; not for patients with renal dysfunction or receiving monoamine oxidase inhibitors
	Proproxyphene hydrochloride (Darvon)	Used in combination with non-narcotic analgesics; long half-life; biotransformed to potentially toxic metabolite (norpropoxyphene)	65–130	65–130	Propoxyphene and metabolite accumulate with repetitive dosing; overdose complicated by convulsions
Mixed-agonist antagonist	Pentazocine	In combination with non-narcotics, in combination with naloxone to discourage parenteral abuse	50	50–100	May cause psychotomimetic effects, may precipitate withdrawal in narcotic-dependent patients
Morphine-like agonists, moderate to severe pain	Morphine	Lower doses for aged patients; those with impaired ventilation; bronchial asthma; increased intracranial pressure; liver failure	10–60	30–60	Standard of comparison for narcotic-type analgesics
	Hydromorphone (Dilaudid)	Like morphine	1.5–8.0	4–8	Slightly shorter acting high-potency IM dosage form available for tolerant patients
	Methadone (Dolphine)	Like morphine; may accumulate with repetitive dosing, causing excessive sedation	10–20	10–20	Good oral potency; long plasma half-life
	Levorphanol (Levo-Dromoran)	Like methadone	2–4	2–4	Like methadone
	Oxymorphone (Numorphan)	Like morphine IM	1	See "Comments"	Not available orally
	Meperidine (Demerol)	Normeperidine (toxic metabolite) accumulates with repetitive dosing, causing CNS excitation; not for patients with impaired renal function or those receiving monoamine oxidase inhibitors	75–300	Not recommended	Slightly shorter acting; used orally for less severe pain
	Codeine	Like morphine	130–180	See "Comments"	Used orally for less severe pain

*Dose given intramuscularly or by mouth.
IM = intramuscular; CNS = central nervous system.

TABLE 27–4. ADJUVANT ANALGESIC DRUGS

Class	Drug	Indications	Starting Dose (mg), Range/24 hr	Comments
Anticonvulsants	Phenytoin (Dilantin)	Neuropathic pain, acute lancinating type (tic)	100, 100–300	Start with low doses; titrate slowly
	Carbamazepine (Tegretol)	Acute lancinating type (tic)	100, 200–800	Useful in paroxysmal nerve pain
Antidepressants	Amitriptyline, Imipramine	Deafferentation pain, e.g., postherpetic neuralgia	10, 10–150	Start at low dose and titrate slowly; has analgesic properties
Amphetamine	Dextroamphetamine	Somatic and visceral pain, e.g., postoperative	2.5, 10	Additive analgesia in combination with narcotics; reduces sedative effects
Antihistamine	Hydroxyzine	Somatic and visceral pain	25, 100	Additive analgesia in combination with narcotics; antiemetic, antianxiety properties
Phenothiazine	Methotrimeprazine (Levoprome)	Somatic and visceral pain; useful in narcotic-tolerant patients with GI obstruction and pain	10 (IM), 10–40 (IM)	Has antianxiety and antiemetic effects; available only in IM preparation
Steroids	Prednisone	Somatic and deafferentation pain, e.g., inflammatory pain, reflex sympathetic dystrophy	5, 5–60	Anti-inflammatory, antiemetic, analgesic effects
	Dexamethasone		0.5, 0.5–16	

IM = intramuscular; GI = gastrointestinal.

agents are commonly used in the management of chronic pain of structural cause, such as cancer pain. The narcotic *antagonist* drugs block the effect of morphine at its receptor. Included in this category is a group of drugs with analgesic properties referred to as the mixed agonist-antagonist drugs. These drugs are often used in acute postoperative pain management but are of limited use in chronic pain management for several reasons: They produce psychotomimetic effects with increasing doses; only pentazocine is available in oral form and only in combinations with naloxone, aspirin, or acetaminophen; they precipitate withdrawal in narcotic-dependent patients. Effective use of narcotic analgesics requires balancing of the desirable effect of pain relief with the undesirable side effects of nausea, vomiting, mental clouding, sedation, tolerance, and physical dependence. These undesirable effects impose a practical limit on the dose one can give a particular patient.

Much of the difficulty encountered with the clinical use of narcotics arises from individual variation, consisting of differences in response of specific patients to the same drug dose. Thus, although Tables 27–2 to 27–4 can serve as reference points, individualization of drug treatment is the cardinal rule of management. Drugs should be given in sufficient amounts and at time intervals close enough to achieve adequate pain relief. "Weak" narcotics, such as codeine, propoxyphene, and oxycodone, are selected to treat moderate pain. If the pain remains unrelieved, the "strong" narcotic analgesics, such as morphine, hydromorphone, levorphanol and methadone, should be employed. To ensure adequate dosing schedules, one must know the clinical pharmacology of the narcotic analgesics, including their duration of analgesic effect, their half-lives, and the equianalgesic doses for both oral and parenteral routes of administration. For example, the plasma half-lives of the narcotics vary widely and do not correlate with their analgesic time courses. Both methadone, with a half-life of 15 to 30 hours, and levorphanol, with a half-life of 12 to 16 hours, produce analgesia for only 4 to 6 hours. With repeated doses, these drugs accumulate in plasma and can result in excessive sedation and respiratory depression. It is necessary to adjust the dose and schedule, considering both the patient's degree of pain relief and the plasma half-life of the drug when it is introduced.

Knowledge of the equianalgesic doses when a switch is made from one medication to another or from one route of administration to another prevents undermedication. However, cross-tolerance is not complete, and patients tolerant to the analgesic effects of one narcotic can often be given another to provide better analgesia. The usual rule is to begin with one half of the calculated equianalgesic dose of the new drug and increase as required.

Medication should be administered on a regular basis, with the interval between doses based on the duration of the analgesic effect. The pharmacologic objective is to maintain the plasma level of the drug above the "minimal effective concentration for pain relief." The time required to reach steady state after repeated administration depends on the half-life of the drug; full assessment of the analgesic efficacy of a drug regimen may take 24 hours for a drug such as morphine or up to 5 to 7 days for methadone.

Combinations of drugs enable the physician to improve pain relief without escalation of the narcotic dose. Several combinations have been proven effective, including a narcotic plus a non-narcotic (aspirin, acetaminophen, or ibuprofen), a narcotic plus an amphetamine (dextroamphetamine, 10 mg) or a narcotic plus an antihistamine (100 mg of hydroxyzine given intramuscularly). Other drugs such as diazepam and chlorpromazine do not provide additive analgesia and may produce additive sedative effects.

Oral administration of drugs is the most practical route, but the choice must be made according to the needs of the patient. Several alternate methods of drug administration have been developed to maximize pharmacologic effects and minimize the undesirable effects associated with standard methods. The approaches that are most useful in the management of acute or chronic pain with chronic medical illness include slow-release morphine preparations effective for 8 to 12 hours, enabling a full night's rest; continuous subcutaneous and intravenous infusions for patients who are unable to tolerate oral analgesics because of gastrointestinal obstruction or malabsorption and in whom repeated parenteral dosing is difficult because of limited muscle mass or a bleeding diathesis; and epidural and intrathecal narcotic administration via temporary catheters or implanted pumps. This last approach minimizes the distribution of drugs to receptors in the brain stem and cerebral hemispheres, avoids the side effects of systemic administration, and is effective in selected patients with cancer pain who are unable to tolerate the excessive sedation or mental clouding associated with an oral or parenteral route.

Side Effects of Narcotics. Side effects of the narcotic analgesics should be anticipated and treated. *Sedation and drowsiness* vary with the drug dose and may occur after either single or repeated administration. Reducing the individual dose and prescribing it more frequently, switching to a drug with a short plasma half-life (hydromorphone), using an amphetamine (dextroamphetamine, 2 to 5 mg) in combination with the narcotic twice daily, and discontinuing all other sedative drugs are useful approaches to counteract the sedative effects.

Respiratory depression is the most serious adverse effect, but tolerance develops rapidly, allowing prolonged use of narcotics for chronic pain. If respiratory depression occurs, it can be reversed by administering the specific narcotic antagonist naloxone in a dose of 0.4 mg per milliliter. In patients receiving narcotics for prolonged periods who develop respiratory depression, diluted doses of naloxone (0.4 mg in 10 ml of saline) should be infused slowly to reverse the respiratory depression but prevent precipitation of severe withdrawal symptoms. The occurrence of *nausea and vomiting* with one drug does not mean that all narcotics will produce similar symptoms. Changing to an alternate narcotic or using an antiemetic in combination commonly obviates this effect. Tolerance rapidly develops to the emetic effect of narcotics so that after a few days antiemetics often are unnecessary. *Constipation* should be prevented by the provision of a regular bowel regimen, including cathartics, stool softeners, and careful attention to diet. *Multifocal myoclonus* may occur with toxic doses of any narcotic. The most common offender is meperidine because of the accumulation of the active metabolite normeperidine, which can cause seizures. Since the half-life of normeperidine is 16 hours, it may take several days for toxic side effects to clear. Patients should be switched to morphine to control their pain and managed symptomatically for seizures.

Tolerance is common when patients receive narcotic analgesics chronically for pain. The earliest sign is a decrease in the duration of effective analgesia. Increasing the frequency of drug administration of the dose provides improved pain relief. There is no limit to tolerance, and the dose of drug should not be the major concern of the prescribing physician. Adjuvant drugs and anesthetic and neurosurgical methods sometimes help to manage pain in the tolerant patient. These guidelines notwithstanding, the management of pain with narcotic analgesics is difficult and requires meticulous attention by the physician.

ADJUVANT ANALGESICS (Table 27–4). The adjuvant analgesics include several different categories of drugs, including anticonvulsants, phenothiazines, tricyclic antidepressants, antihistamines, amphetamines, and steroids (see Table 27–4). Carbamazepine and phenytoin are useful in the management of patients with some neuropathic pain syndromes, e.g., trigeminal neuralgia. The mechanism of action is through suppression of the spontaneous neuronal firing that commonly occurs with nerve injury. For both drugs, the minimal effective concentration for analgesia is unknown.

Certain phenothiazines have potent analgesic effects. Methotrimeprazine (Levoprome) has an analgesic potential close to that of morphine (15 mg given intramuscularly is equivalent to 10 mg of morphine given intramuscularly). This drug helps manage severe pain in patients tolerant to narcotic analgesics. The tricyclic antidepressants both enhance the analgesic effects of morphine and have independent analgesic properties. Doses of 10 to 75 mg administered orally are used to treat postherpetic neuralgia. The analgesic effects of these drugs occur independently of their antidepressant properties. The antihistamine hydroxyzine and the amphetamine dextroamphetamine are also sometimes helpful adjuvants. Steroids produce analgesia in patients with acute inflammatory diseases and in patients with tumor infiltration of bone or nerve or both.

Alternate Methods of Pain Control

A variety of nonpharmacologic therapeutic approaches can be used alone or in combination with the analgesic drugs. These include physical therapy, trigger point injections, transcutaneous nerve stimulation, and certain behavioral approaches, all of which should be familiar to general physicians. Technically demanding anesthetic and neurosurgical approaches require consultation with pain experts. Certain guidelines apply to these procedures:

1. Evaluate thoroughly the nature of the pain and the prognosis of the patient's primary disease. Neurolytic nerve blocks and neuroablative and neurostimulatory surgical procedures often yield only temporary relief in patients with chronic pain and are not useful for deafferentation pain. In contrast, patients with cancer pain of somatic origin who are not expected to live for more than several months are excellent candidates for such procedures.
2. Nondestructive procedures, such as transcutaneous electrical stimulation or temporary blocks with local anesthetics, should be tried first.
3. Start with the least destructive procedure. For example, try continuous epidural local anesthetics to manage perineal pain before initiating an intrathecal neurolytic block.
4. Evaluate patients psychologically. If psychologic factors play a major role in the pain, such procedures will not help and will often exacerbate the condition.
5. Inform the patient fully of the potential risks and benefits of the planned procedure.

PHYSICAL THERAPY. Chronic pain is commonly associated with reduced physical activity and splinting or immobilization of the injured body part. A graded exercise program with appropriate use of splints and braces and reactivation of the injured part plays a pivotal role in re-establishing the functional status of the patient. Local rubbing and transcutaneous electrical stimulation for "counterirritation" may help to mobilize the patient with a localized pain. Trigger point injections with either saline or a local anesthetic provide dramatic relief of painful muscle spasm.

BEHAVIORAL THERAPY. Behavioral approaches that often improve the patient's coping mechanism include breathing exercises to increase relaxation, coping strategies to integrate pain symptoms into a functioning lifestyle, and improving control over psychologic factors of anxiety, fear, and demoralization associated with chronic pain.

ANESTHETIC PROCEDURES (Table 27–5). Local anesthetics and injectable neurolytic agents are sometimes useful in managing both acute and chronic pain that occupies a well-defined anatomic site. Sympathetic blocks, for example, often predict the relief that can be expected from sympathectomy in treating causalgia due to peripheral sensory nerve damage. Blocking nerves with short- or long-acting anesthetics determines in a reversible manner whether semipermanent nerve blocks will be effective and what side effects they might have. In some patients, particularly when muscle spasm plays a major role in pain production, repeated temporary blocks produce long-lasting relief of pain. If an anesthetic nerve block has been effective temporarily and then begins to lose its efficacy, neurolytic agents, such as phenol, alcohol, and freezing (cryoanesthesia), can be used to destroy nerve structures. The principal pathologic effect produced by these neurolytic agents is demyelination with secondary nerve degeneration. Because peripheral nerves and roots have overlapping sensory functions, multiple nerves and roots must be blocked to yield adequate pain control. Since such blocks may paralyze as well as anesthetize, they have a limited role in extremity pain and are most useful to treat thoracic and

TABLE 27–5. TYPES OF ANESTHETIC PROCEDURES COMMONLY USED IN CHRONIC PAIN

I. Nerve Blocks	
Peripheral	Pain in discrete dermatomes in chest and abdomen
Epidural	Unilateral lumbar or sacral pain Midline perineal pain Bilateral lumbosacral pain
Intrathecal	Midline perineal pain Bilateral lumbosacral pain
Autonomic	
Stellate ganglion	Reflex sympathetic dystrophy, e.g., frozen shoulder Arm pain
Lumbar sympathetic	Reflex sympathetic dystrophy Lumbosacral plexopathy Vascular insufficiency of the lower extremity
Celiac plexus	Midabdominal pain
II. Continuous Epidural Infusion with Local Anesthetic	Unilateral and bilateral lumbosacral pain Midline perineal pain
III. Chemical Hypophysectomy	Diffuse bone pain
IV. Inhalation Therapy	Generalized pain Incident pain
V. Trigger Point Injection	Focal muscle pain

abdominal pain or perineal and sacral pain in patients with cancer.

Neurolytic agents can be injected into the epidural or intrathecal space as well as into peripheral nerves or roots. However, the limitations of motor weakness and autonomic dysfunction make this technique suitable for only a limited number of patients. Neurolytic blocks find their best use in the management of well-defined localized pain caused by cancer. Their role in managing pain of nonmalignant origin is controversial because they work for only a limited period of time. There is a real risk of adding morbidity without providing pain relief, and they are not effective in managing deafferentation pain.

Blocks of the cervical (stellate ganglion) and lumbar sympathetic chains are most useful in managing limb pain associated with vascular or peripheral nerve injury, as occurs in diabetic peripheral vascular disease and reflex sympathetic dystrophy. Celiac plexus block is the procedure of choice to manage visceral pain from pancreatic carcinoma.

Intermittent or continuous epidural infusions of local anesthetics are useful for temporary relief of chronic pain involving the lumbosacral plexus and sacrum. This approach is most useful to treat an acute exacerbation of chronic cancer pain. The technique does not result in cross-tolerance with opiate analgesia, and it can be appropriately titrated to provide anesthesia without interruption of motor or autonomic function.

Two other anesthetic approaches used to manage diffuse pain include chemical hypophysectomy and intermittent inhalation therapy with nitrous oxide. Chemical hypophysectomy involves the injection of alcohol into the sella turcica under radiologic control. It is used to control pain in patients with widespread bony metastases. Pain relief is reported in 35 to 75 per cent of patients, and many patients experience pain relief independent of whether the pituitary ablation causes tumor regression. Nitrous oxide is used to manage chronic pain in the dying patient, particularly acute incident pain or procedure-related pain. It is administered in oxygen through a non-rebreathing face mask with concentrations ranging from 25 to 75 per cent.

NEUROSURGICAL PROCEDURES (Table 27–6). Pharmacologic procedures requiring neurosurgery include placement of intraventricular, epidural, or intrathecal catheters and implanted reservoirs or pumps to infuse agents used to manage selected patients with pain and cancer in whom systemic drugs are either ineffective or associated with excessive side effects. These approaches are not useful in managing non–cancer-related chronic pain problems.

Neurostimulatory procedures are performed by implanting electrodes in or on the desired portion of the nervous system and leading the electrodes to an implanted conductive receiver attached to an external transmitter. The technique allows the patient to control the timing and intensity of the stimulation. Electrical stimulation of the dorsal columns of cervical or thoracic spinal cord sometimes controls bilateral deafferentation pain. Unfortunately, tolerance to the analgesic effect alters long-term usefulness of this procedure. Electrodes are usually placed in the epidural space over the dorsal column rather than directly on the spinal cord, thus reducing the risk of cord damage. Electrical stimulation of the periventricular gray matter of the brain stem also has been used for chronic deafferentation pain, especially if dorsal column stimulation or neurolytic blocks fail. Stimulation is delivered for no longer than 20 to 25 minutes at a time, three or four times a day. Tolerance develops more rapidly with increased use of the stimulator. Both animal studies and observations on human beings indicate that periventricular stimulation is associated with total body analgesia but without a decrease in sensory or motor function. This procedure is still experimental and is available in only a few specialized centers.

Medial thalamic stimulation is used to manage chronic but unilateral intractable pain. Electrodes are placed stereotactically in medial thalamus contralateral to the pain. Stimulation results in localized analgesia. This procedure is used to manage the thalamic pain syndrome, phantom limb pain, and peripheral nerve injury pain, particularly when pain involves the head or neck. About 50 per cent of patients with localized deafferentation pain respond to thalamic stimulation.

In addition to neurostimulatory procedures, portions of the nervous system from peripheral nerves to the cerebral cortex can be lesioned to relieve pain. The most commonly used procedures are dorsal root entry zone lesions and cordotomy. Other procedures have had only limited success and are marked by significant neurologic morbidity. Dorsal root entry zone (DREZ) lesions interrupt the sensory nerve roots as they enter the dorsal horn of the spinal cord. An electrode is introduced for a distance of 2 to 3 mm into the medial sulcus on the dorsal surface of the spinal cord, and a radiofrequency lesion is made. This procedure is most useful in managing

TABLE 27–6. NEUROABLATIVE, NEUROSTIMULATORY, AND NEUROPHARMACOLOGIC PROCEDURES

Site	Neurostimulatory	Neuroablative	Neuropharmacologic
Peripheral nerve	Transcutaneous and percutaneous electrical nerve stimulation	Neurectomy	Local anesthetics
Nerve root		Rhizotomy	Local anesthetics Neurolytic agents*
Spinal cord	Dorsal column stimulation	Dorsal root entry zone lesions Cordotomy Myelotomy	Epidural and intrathecal opiates*
Brain stem	Periaqueductal stimulation	Mesencephalic tractotomy	Intraventricular opiates*
Thalamus	Thalamic stimulation	Thalamotomy	
Cortex		Cingulumotomy Frontal lobotomy	
Pituitary		Trans-sphenoidal hypophysectomy*	Chemical hypophysectomy*

*Procedures restricted for the treatment of chronic cancer-related pain.

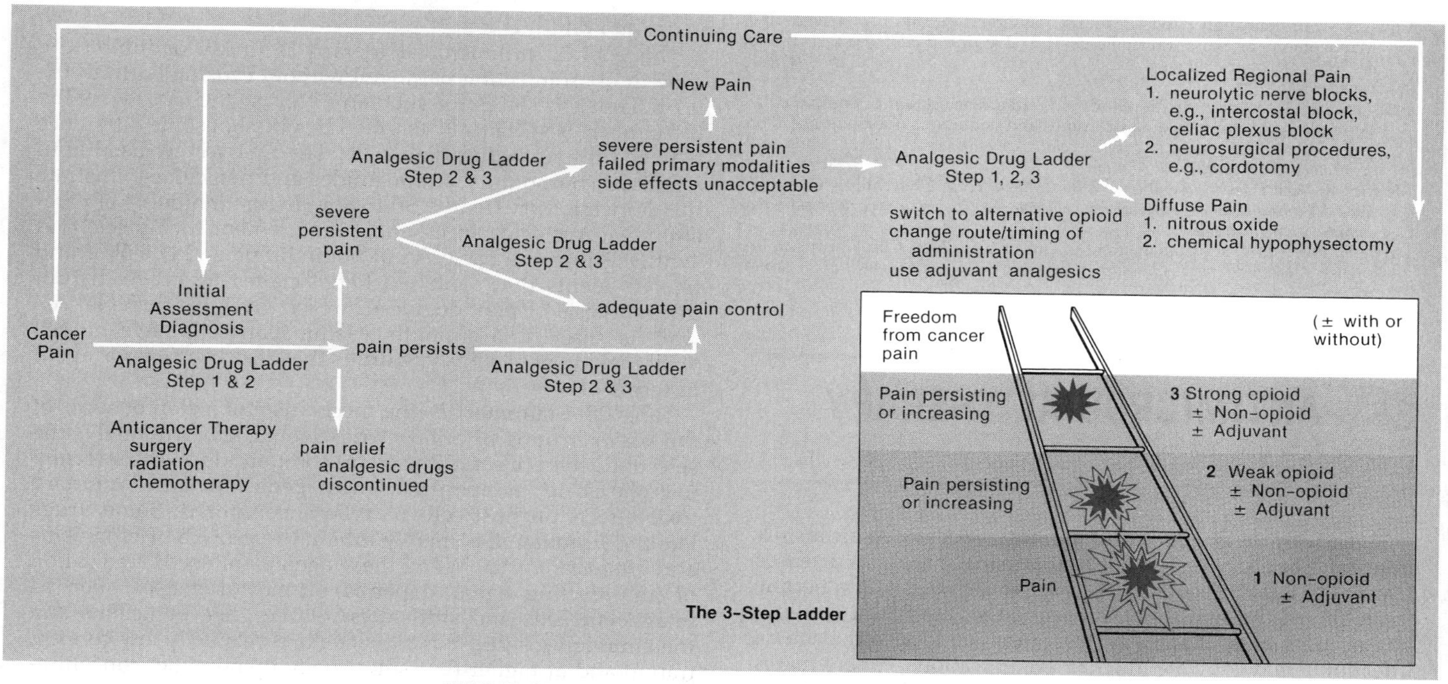

FIGURE 27–1. Algorithm for the management of cancer pain.

the continuous pain of peripheral nerve injury (e.g., postherpetic neuralgia, avulsions of the brachial or lumbar plexus). It is effective in 50 to 75 per cent of patients so treated. Postoperative complications occur in 20 per cent of patients and consist of ipsilateral clumsiness and weakness, usually transient, of the arm or leg. Cordotomy is the most useful neurosurgical procedure for relief of chronic somatic pain and the most commonly used procedure for the management of patients with localized cancer pain. Cordotomy can be performed as a percutaneous stereotactic radiofrequency procedure or as an open surgical ablation. Because the spinothalamic tract is selectively interrupted, only pain and temperature sensation are lost (on the contralateral side of the body). Cutaneous sensation and motor power remain intact, although some ipsilateral weakness or ataxia occurs transiently in about 20 per cent of patients. Cordotomy is most useful to manage unilateral pain below the neck. Initial pain relief occurs in 90 per cent of patients. This figure drops to 50 per cent at six months and about 40 per cent at the end of one year. One to 2 per cent of postcordotomy patients develop burning dysesthesias (anesthesia dolorosa), which are often as distressing as the original pain. Because of both the limited duration of its effectiveness and the risk of producing deafferentation pain, cordotomy is not indicated for management of chronic nonmalignant pain. Bilateral cordotomy can be performed to manage midline or perineal pain associated with cancer. If performed in the cervical area, bilateral cordotomy risks producing sleep-induced apnea (Ondine's curse). The second risk of bilateral cordotomy is bladder dysfunction. With unilateral cordotomy, 7 to 10 per cent of patients develop mirror pain on the opposite side of the body even when the original pain is relieved. Mirror pain can occur in the absence of a definable lesion in the affected area, and its pathogenesis is unknown. Other neuroablative procedures are rarely used.

Management of Cancer Pain

Figure 27–1 provides an algorithm for the management of cancer pain. It attempts to integrate assessment techniques, drug therapy, and anesthetic, neurosurgical, and behavioral approaches and stresses continuity of care. Treatment of cancer pain must begin with a careful diagnostic assessment that addresses not only the medical nature of pain but also its psychologic and social components. At the time of assessment, a plan is developed to treat both the cancer, if possible, and the pain itself. If the anticancer treatment is effective, pain relief usually occurs, and the drugs used for analgesia can be discontinued without difficulty. Pain relief begins with analgesic drugs. Incorporated in Figure 27–1 is the World Health Organization's Cancer Pain Relief Program. It proposes an analgesic drug ladder moving from nonopioid drugs alone or in combination with adjuvant drugs through weak opioids to strong opioids. If pain relief is achieved with this program, no further therapy is necessary. In patients with severe, persistent pain not responsive to analgesic drugs or in whom the side effects of the drugs are not tolerated, physicians should first try switching to alternate analgesics or changing the route or timing of drug administration. For example, intrathecal opioids are indicated for relief of pain in patients in whom systemic analgesics produce confusion or excessive sedation.

If the pain is unresponsive to analgesic drugs and is localized (e.g., intercostal pain from tumor infiltration of the chest wall), neurolytic blocks are indicated. If the pain is unilateral and below the waist, cordotomy should be considered. For more diffuse pain unresponsive to analgesics, neurostimulatory procedures, including nitrous oxide inhalation and chemical hypophysectomy, may be considered. Behavioral approaches, which include relaxation techniques, breathing exercises, and cognitive control of pain, serve as adjuvants and should be integrated into the management of patients with chronic pain.

As the algorithm indicates, whatever the techniques of pain management used in patients with cancer, the physician is responsible for delivering continuing care, constantly reassessing both the diagnosis and the treatment to achieve optimum relief of pain and suffering for both patient and family.

Cousins M, Bridenbaugh P (eds.): Neural blockade. In Clinical Anesthesia and Management of Pain. Philadelphia, J.B. Lippincott Co, 1980. *This text describes the commonly used anesthetic procedures in acute and chronic pain management.*

International Association for the Study of Pain: Classification of chronic pain, descriptions of chronic pain syndromes and definitions of pain terms. Pain [Suppl] 3:S1–S225, 1986. *This useful volume contains descriptions of chronic pain syndromes and definitions of pain terms.*

Melzack R, Wall P (eds.): Textbook of Pain. New York, Churchill Livingstone, 1984. *A compendium of the anatomy, physiology, and pharmacology of pain and common pain syndromes.*

Payne R, Foley KM: The management of cancer pain. Med Clin North Am (in press). *A detailed review of the current approach to pain management in the cancer patient.*

28 ANTIMICROBIAL THERAPY

Lowell S. Young

The advent of antimicrobial therapy represented an historic milestone in the cure and control of many infectious diseases. Invariably fatal infections, like bacterial endocarditis, became treatable for the first time. Subsequently, abundant evidence has accumulated that early treatment of localized bacterial infections may obviate further complications. The greatest progress during the modern era of antimicrobial therapy has been in the treatment of acute bacterial infections, although a few chronic diseases such as tuberculosis have become well controlled. New developments offer promise in controlling viral diseases and parasitic infections that are a major burden on much of mankind. There have been some modest developments in the antifungal area as well. Nonetheless, the initial enthusiasm that greeted the introduction of new agents with antibacterial activity has been tempered by a more sobering perspective. Antimicrobial agents are not always innocuous to the host, and their widespread usage appears to have fostered increasing drug resistance throughout the world. The growing complexities of antimicrobial therapy appear to be related to the rapid proliferation of agents of several classes, increasing drug resistance, and a greater recognition of interactions between pharmacologic agents.

SOME DEFINITIONS

The terms *antibiotic, antimicrobic,* and *chemotherapeutic agent* have often been used interchangeably to designate defined chemical substances that possess activity against specific microorganisms. Indeed, the earliest definition of an antibiotic was a substance produced in nature by living microbes that inhibited the growth of other microbial organisms at low concentrations. Viewed in this light, antibiotics seem to be a product of evolution and may confer a selective advantage to the producer in a specific ecosystem. Technically, antibiotics differ from chemotherapeutic agents in that the latter represent the products of chemical synthesis, such as the sulfonamide dyes that were subsequently found to have antibacterial activity. Antibiotics in common use, such as penicillins and aminoglycosides, are derived from natural products but from a functional point of view may be considered interchangeable with chemotherapeutic agents. As the development of new antibacterial agents has proliferated, restrictive technical terms have become outdated. For instance, new penicillins, cephalosporins, and aminoglycosides contain synthetic or semisynthetic modifications of existing structures that confer potent new biologic activity. The term *antimicrobic* has been proposed to describe all substances with antimicrobial activity whether of natural or synthetic origin, but its acceptance has been variable.

GENERAL PRINCIPLES

The goal of antimicrobial therapy is to kill or inhibit the growth of an infecting pathogen without causing harm to the host. Thus, the basis for such an effect is *selectivity*, whereby the parasite is specifically targeted by virtue of some difference between it and mammalian cells. The first widely used antimicrobial compounds, sulfonamides and penicillins, illustrate this principle very clearly. Sulfonamides are inhibitors of para-aminobenzoic acid, an essential requirement for nucleic acid synthesis in many bacteria but not in humans. Penicillins and related agents that contain a beta-lactam ring act to disrupt the synthesis of peptidoglycan, which gives the bacterial cell wall its shape and strength. Mammalian cells have no cell wall, making penicillin-type drugs the ideal antibacterial agent in terms of selectivity.

Table 28–1 summarizes the mechanism of action of some of the major groups of antibacterial agents. Unfortunately, the selective action of some important compounds on the infecting microbe is not as specific as with penicillin, and important toxic effects on host cells may be encountered. Some drugs like the sulfonamides merely inhibit the growth of organisms and are *bacteriostatic*. When these agents are used, eradication of an infecting agent depends on host defenses such as phagocytic cells and antibodies. Others, like penicillins and the aminoglycosides, inhibit bacteria at relatively low concentration and at higher (but still usually therapeutic) concentrations can kill them; these are *bactericidal* agents. These designations of a bacteriostatic or bactericidal agent may vary depending on the type of organism: Penicillin G is usually bactericidal for gram-positive cocci but is only static against the enterococcus (*Streptococcus faecalis*), while chloramphenicol is usually bacteriostatic even at very high concentrations but can be bactericidal against *Hemophilus influenzae*. Spectrum refers to range of microorganisms affected by a particular agent, which varies from relatively narrow for low doses of penicillin G to quite broad for large doses of the new cephalosporins. Breadth of spectrum is not necessarily related to mechanism of action.

The interaction between a microbe and therapeutic agent can be complex, and many important variables affect outcome. Intrinsic virulence differs considerably between infecting agents so that the progression of infection ranges from a very indolent tempo to a fulminating course. Host factors influence selection of bactericidal versus bacteriostatic agents and the breadth of spectrum of therapy. The site of infection influences dose and duration of treatment. The proliferation of therapeutic choices compels the physician to obtain in-depth knowledge of any agent prescribed. Treatment can be guided by laboratory studies, but therapeutic choices must be based on knowledge of antimicrobial spectrum, mode of action, pharmacology, toxicity, and all major factors that affect drug activity.

IDENTIFICATION OF THE INFECTING AGENT

It is highly desirable to have the infecting agent identified prior to initiation of treatment, but in most circumstances culture confirmation and tests in vitro of antimicrobial susceptibility will not be available for at least a day. Clinical decision making is usually based on a perception of probabilities and on simple tests, the most important of which is the Gram stain. Even the latter is not necessary in the case of exudative pharyngitis, because the only treatable bacterial causes of the syndrome are hemolytic streptococci and now, rarely, *Corynebacterium diphtheriae*. Other isolates can usually be ignored and therapy with a penicillin initiated. When only a single infecting organism seems likely, therapy with a narrow-spectrum agent is preferable.

TABLE 28–1. MECHANISM OF ACTION OF ANTIMICROBIAL AGENTS

Agent	Site of Action	Effect	Cidal	Static
Penicillins, Cephalosporins	Cell wall	Inhibit cross-linking of peptidoglycan resulting in spheroplast formation	+	Occasionally
Vancomycin	Cell wall	Block transfer of pentapeptide from cytoplasm to cell membrane	+	Occasionally
Polymyxin B, Colistin	Cytoplasmic membrane	Bind phospholipid and disrupt membrane	+	
Aminoglycosides	Ribosome	Bind to 30S ribosomal subunit, thereby inhibiting attachment of messenger RNA; also affect transfer RNA	+	
Tetracyclines	Ribosome	Bind to 30S subunit and inhibit binding of transfer RNA		+
Chloramphenicol	Ribosome	Bind to 50S subunit and inhibit messenger RNA translation	Occasionally	+
Erythromycin, Clindamycin	Ribosome	Inhibit messenger RNA translation	Occasionally	+
Rifampin	Nucleic acid synthesis	Impaired RNA formation by inhibiting DNA-dependent RNA-polymerase	+	Occasionally
Metronidazole	Nucleic acid synthesis	Damages nucleic acid structure	+	
Quinolones	Nucleic acid synthesis	Inhibit DNA gyrase	+	
Sulfonamides	Nucleic acid synthesis	Competitive inhibition of para-amino benzoic acid, thereby blocking formation of thymidine and purines		+

In reality, many infectious processes initially begin as mixed infections: The aspiration of secretions into the lung usually results in the deposition of many types of oral microbes that can lead to pneumonia or lung abscess, or the perforation of an abdominal viscus leads to release of millions of aerobic and anaerobic bacteria into the abdominal cavity. What may survive to be cultured in respiratory secretions or from abdominal drainage may well be the hardiest of bacteria, and not necessarily all of those that were associated with initial infectious morbidity. Not all mixed infectious processes require treatment with broad-spectrum therapy, but the presence of multiple pathogens might explain clinical failure when a mixed infection is being treated and only one component of that infection is being affected by a particular drug regimen.

Initiation of antibiotic therapy prior to obtaining appropriate cultures is perhaps the leading explanation for the failure to document infecting pathogens. On the other hand, the Gram stain or immunofluorescent staining of secretions can identify the cause of infection after treatment is started. Irrespective of when it is done, the Gram stain can provide valuable semiquantitative information about predominant pathogens and can help the clinician decide whether a subsequent culture result can actually be relied upon. For instance, the validity of a sample of respiratory secretions is greatly enhanced by the detection of phagocytic cells such as neutrophils or alveolar macrophages. In contrast, the presence of squamous epithelial cells should be the basis for rejecting the validity of expectorated sputum, since they reflect oropharyngeal contamination. With regard to quantitative evaluation of a potentially infected body fluid, isolation of greater than 10^5 organisms per milliliter has been accepted as establishing the validity of a urine culture result. However, microscopic examination of uncentrifuged urine may still yield an approximate idea of the degree of infection (any organism seen corresponds with 10^5 bacteria per milliliter), as well as the nature of the infection that is taking place in the urinary tract. Isolation of organisms in pure culture from blood or normally sterile body fluids (like spinal fluid) is an unambiguous laboratory result that establishes an infectious etiology. Occasionally, some bloodstream infections are polymicrobial. Some blood culture isolates may be rejected as contaminants. The latter are usually skin flora like corynebacteria or *Staphylococcus epidermidis*. However, repeated isolation of such organisms from blood culture in association with signs of infection calls for careful clinical assessment. *Staphylococcus epidermidis* and corynebacteria can be valid pathogens in immunosuppressed subjects and patients with prosthetic devices.

SUSCEPTIBILITY, RESISTANCE, AND ANTIBACTERIAL SPECTRA

Appropriate antimicrobial therapy is based on the results of laboratory tests and validated by the clinical effect of treatment. Test results and treatment are not always consistent: Patients who have excellent or intact host defenses may recover from infection irrespective of whether the antibiotic they receive has an effect on the infecting agent. Some important pathogens like Salmonella species are very susceptible in vitro to cephalosporin antibiotics, but clinical efficacy has been poor. Nevertheless, in a serious deep-seated or bloodstream infection, laboratory tests do provide an invaluable guide to the selection or adjustment of therapy. Usually a microbe is considered susceptible to an antibacterial agent if it can be inhibited or killed by a concentration of the drug that is realistically achievable at the site of the infection. The levels of drug that must be achieved in the host will vary depending on the site of infection and could be limited by toxic side effects. A common practice is to set the range of susceptibility at or above realistically achievable blood levels, but there are some notable exceptions. For instance, some agents like nalidixic acid or nitrofurantoin are rapidly excreted in the urine, and only very low blood levels are achieved. Low doses of drugs that are effective for some infections are totally inadequate for deep-seated infections. The best example is the relatively low dose of benzyl penicillin G that is required to cure pneumococcal pneumonia, sometimes less than 100,000 units of penicillin per day, which contrasts with the dose of approximately 20 million units per day that may be necessary to treat pneumococcal endocarditis or meningitis. With aminoglycosides the levels for effective therapy of bloodstream infections have been projected to be in the range of 4 to 6 μg per milliliter of gentamicin or tobramycin, and such concentrations are usually accepted as the upper boundary for susceptibility in vitro. However, it is clear that the peak levels of aminoglycosides like gentamicin and tobramycin are sustained for less than an hour. Nonetheless, that time period seems sufficient to achieve rapid killing of many bacterial strains.

Many methods have been introduced to determine the susceptibility of bacteria to antimicrobials in vitro. They have been best standardized for rapidly growing organisms. The most common involve measuring inhibition of growth in a broth medium or the measurement of growth inhibition around an antibiotic-impregnated disk placed on the surface of agar containing the test strain (disk diffusion test). By varying drug concentrations in a series of test tubes or wells, the broth dilution test yields quantitative data on the drug concentration required to inhibit the organism, the minimum inhibitory concentration, or MIC (usually expressed in micrograms per milliliter). Subcultures of broth media make it possible to determine the concentration of drug that kills the test strain—the minimum bactericidal concentration, or MBC. In the disk diffusion test only growth inhibition can be determined, but the diameter of the zone of inhibition usually correlates inversely with the MIC. The two methods give generally similar results (with the disk test being perhaps somewhat easier to perform) and for most infections susceptibility results based on inhibitory measurements are satisfactory. In treating endocarditis, meningitis, and septicemias occurring in immunocompromised hosts, MBC data on infecting isolates are desirable. Bactericidal activity appears to be a requisite for cure of enterococcal endocarditis, as penicillin G or ampicillin inhibits but does not kill this group of organisms. The phenomenon of "tolerance" has also been observed: a wide discrepancy, 32-fold or more, between MIC and MBC. Some investigators believe that strains of staphylococci isolated from endocarditis or osteomyelitis that prove to be tolerant to penicillins or vancomycin should be treated with the addition of gentamicin or rifampin, but this policy remains controversial.

Table 28–2 summarizes the susceptibilities of clinically important gram-positive and gram-negative bacteria in vitro and indicates agents of choice and alternative therapies. The darkened squares (resistant or not indicated) may include drug-pathogen combinations for which clinical evidence fails to support an effect in vitro. Susceptibility testing in vitro is needed because no one agent is predictably effective against all categories of bacteria and because of the increasing incidence and changes in patterns of resistance. There are a few exceptions to this dogma, such as the uniform susceptibility of Group A streptococci to penicillin. On the other hand, relative resistance (intermediate susceptibility) of pneumococci to penicillin G may be increasing, and it is advisable to test blood and cerebrospinal fluid (CSF) isolates.

Antimicrobial resistance may be absolute, in which case increasing the concentration of the agent has no effect, and relative, in which case it may be overcome by dose augmentation. The basis and mechanisms of resistance have become complex, and the simplest approach is to consider (a) the genetic basis for resistance and (b) the actual mechanisms involved. Chromosomal alterations or mutations were the first basis for resistance recognized. These occurred at a relatively predictable rate. Subsequently, a much more common genetic basis has emerged: Plasmids or extrachromosomal DNA elements include R-factors or genetic elements that encode for synthesis of enzymes that functionally inactivate or modify antibiotics. The rapid spread of resistance in some hospital and community settings has been related to acquisition of plasmids by the process of conjugation among gram-negative bacilli and transduction by phages among gram-positive cocci. The mechanisms of resistance are summarized in Table 28–3. The most familiar are the beta-lactamases that hydrolyze to varying degrees agents possessing the beta-lactam ring (penicillins, cephalosporins, monobactams). A great variety of these have been described, occurring in both cocci and bacilli and of both a constitutive and an inducible nature. The latter poses real problems in laboratory diagnosis, as organisms that are initially thought to be susceptible (like Enterobacter species) may harbor inducible enzymes. Beta-lactamases may be of either chromosomal or plasmid origin and are usually responsible for high level resistance that cannot be overcome by dosage escalation. Inactivation can destroy the usefulness of drugs outside the beta-lactam class. A growing number of R-factor–encoded enzymes have been identified that can modify aminoglycosides by the addition of an adenyl, acetyl, or phosphorylating group to hydroxyl or amino groups on the drug structure. These additions create a sterically altered molecule with ablated or reduced antibacterial activity. Conversely, the design of innovative new antimicrobial agents that prove invulnerable to inactivating enzymes involves further modifications of antibiotic structures that can block the access of inactivating enzymes to target sites. In this sense, the development of new aminoglycosides is analogous to the substitutions that protect the beta-lactam ring from hydrolysis and yield the antistaphylococcal penicillins.

One of the most worrisome mechanisms of resistance involves the ability of bacteria to exclude antimicrobial agents from the cell. Aminoglycosides are actively transported into bacteria, but high-level, multiresistant strains seem to be impermeable to all aminoglycosides. These appear to arise from chromosomal mutation and are selected by aminoglycoside use. The active transport system for aminoglycosides is oxygen dependent. This probably explains the lack of effect of aminoglycosides on anaerobic bacteria, since anaerobic conditions impair the activation of the transport system.

Another type of enzymatic resistance is illustrated by organisms that have acquired a plasmid-encoded "bypass" enzyme that subverts the metabolic block of the sulfonamides.

To have an effect, antibiotics that resist hydrolysis or modification must enter the bacterial cell and reach their target site. Target site alteration explains sudden high-level streptomycin resistance (30S ribosomal subunit) or erythromycin resistance (50S ribosomal subunit). The basis for these changes appears to be chromosomal mutations. A similar basis is postulated for alterations in penicillin-binding proteins, which can result in both low- and high-level resistance.

The indiscriminate use of antimicrobial agents generally favors the emergence of resistance. Antibiotics are not mutagens and do not "create" resistant bacteria. Rather, usage selects for strains that are resistant by virtue of chromosomal mutations or spread of plasmids among the bacterial population. Emergence of resistance during treatment is common with some gram-negative rods such as Serratia and Pseudomonas. This phenomenon must be distinguished from superinfection, whereby a new and usually resistant pathogen becomes a secondary invader. Superinfection may be a consequence of prolonged high-dose therapy and may be avoided by use of narrow-spectrum agents in doses that are not excessive.

PHARMACOLOGIC FACTORS

Laboratory conditions for testing antibacterial agents may differ strikingly from conditions in vivo. In clinical situations the rates of growth of bacteria may be slow, thus affecting the rapidity with which cell wall–active drugs can work. More important, blood and tissue concentrations fluctuate with frequency and method of dosing, and the concentration of drug at the active site of infection may differ from that in body fluids that are more easily sampled. The distribution of agents even within the same class can vary considerably, as they may be metabolized, inactivated, and eliminated by different pathways. Such factors have a crucial effect on the size of doses, the interval between dosing, and possible drug toxicity. Also, the properties of the infecting agent may affect dosing. After exposure of bacteria to an antibiotic, a certain proportion of the population is killed or inhibited and there may be a significant lag time before multiplication of bacteria resumes after the drug concentration falls. This time interval for regrowth has been called the "postantibiotic effect." For different organisms and with different antibiotics, there may be varying postantibiotic effects. Thus, intermittent dosing of agents may be quite feasible if there is rapid killing and a long postantibiotic effect. Some of the more recalcitrant organisms like Pseudomonas regrow rapidly after exposure to antipseudomonal penicillins, and there is very little postantibiotic effect. This argues for more frequent or even continuous dosing, but for the great majority of clinical situations the

TABLE 28–2. SUSCEPTIBILITIES OF CERTAIN BACTERIA TO SELECTED ANTIBIOTICS

Group	Organism	SULFONAMIDES	TRIMETHOPRIM/SULFAMETHOXAZOLE	PENICILLIN G/AMPICILLIN	METHICILLIN/NAFCILLIN/OXACILLIN	CARBENICILLIN/TICARCILLIN	AZLOCILLIN/MEZLOCILLIN/PIPERACILLIN	CEPHALOTHIN/CEPHAPIRIN/CEFAZOLIN	CEFUROXIME/CEFAMANDOLE	CEFOXITIN	CEFOTAXIME/CEFTIZOXIME/MOXALACTAM	CEFTAZIDIME/CEFOPERAZONE/CEFSULODIN	GENTAMICIN/TOBRAMYCIN/SISOMICIN	AMIKACIN/NETILMICIN	POLYMIXIN B/COLISTIN	ERYTHROMYCIN	CLINDAMYCIN	TETRACYCLINES	CHLORAMPHENICOL	VANCOMYCIN	RIFAMPIN	ISONIAZID	NALIDIXIC ACID	METRONIDAZOLE
GRAM POSITIVE	Cl. difficile																			1				2
	Cl. perfringens			1	3	3	3	3	3	3	3					2			2	3				2
	Listeria			1		3	3	3	3	3	3					2	3	3	2	3				
	Corynebacterium diphtheriae			1		3	3									1	3	2			2			
	Corynebacteria, other																			1	②			
	Nocardia	1	1	2		3	3	3			3					3		3	3		3			
	Streptococcus			1		3	3	3	3	3	3					2				2				
	Str. faecalis			①		3	3						①			3			3	2				
	Staph. aureus (pen. sens.)			1	3	3	3	3	3	3	3	3				2	3		3	3	3			
	(pen. resis.)				1			2	2	2	3	3	3	3		3	3		3	2	3			
	(meth. resis.)																			1	②			
	M. tuberculosis												3	3							①	①		
GRAM NEGATIVE	Treponema pallidum			1		3	3	3	3							2		2						
	E. coli		3			3	3		3	2	1		1	2	3									
	Klebsiella sp.		2					2	2	2	1		1	1	3									
	Enterobacter		2								3		2	1	3									
	Serratia		2								1		2	1										
	Proteus mirabilis		3	1		3	3	3	3	3	3	3	1	1										
	Providencia												2	1										
	Salmonella		2	1		3	3												1					
	Shigella		1	2																			3	
	Vibrio		2	2														1	3					
	P. aeruginosa					②	1					1	1	1	3									
	Pseudomonas, other																							
	Acinetobacter												2	1										
	Campylobacter															1	3	2	2					
	Legionella		3													1		3			2			
	Hemophilus		2						3		1								1					
	N. gonorrhoeae			1					3	2	2													
	N. meningitidis			1		3	3				3					2			2		3			
	Bacteroides					3	3			2							1		1					1
	Brucella		1															1			②			
	Yersinia		2															1	2					
	Rickettsia																	1	1					

KEY:
- 1 Agent(s) of choice
- 2 Alternative agent
- 3 Usually susceptible
- ☐ (white box) Variably susceptible
- ▒ (shaded box) Resistant or not indicated
- ◯ Use in combination

TABLE 28–3. MECHANISMS OF ANTIBACTERIAL RESISTANCE

Antimicrobial Agent	Mechanisms	Representative Organisms
Beta-lactams (penicillins, cephalosporins, carbapenems, monobactams)	Destruction by beta-lactamase	*Staphylococcus aureus* Enterobacteriaceae *Pseudomonas aeruginosa* *Hemophilus influenzae*
	Alteration of penicillin-binding proteins	*Neisseria gonorrhoeae* *Streptococcus pneumoniae* *Staphylococcus aureus*
	Cell wall impermeability	Enterobacter species *Pseudomonas aeruginosa*
Aminoglycosides	Enzymatic modification by N-acetylation, O-phosphorylation, or N-adenylation	*Staphylococcus aureus* Enterobacteriaceae *Pseudomonas aeruginosa* *Streptococcus faecalis*
	Membrane transport O_2 dependent	Anaerobes
	Cell wall impermeability	*Pseudomonas aeruginosa* Serratia species *Streptococcus faecalis*
	Altered 30S ribosome (streptomycin)	Enterobacteriaceae
Chloramphenicol	O-acetylation	*Staphylococcus aureus*
	Cell wall impermeability	Enterobacteriaceae *Pseudomonas aeruginosa*
Erythromycin, clindamycin	Alteration of 23S RNA	*Staphylococcus aureus*
Quinolones	Altered DNA gyrase	Enterobacteriaceae
	Cell wall impermeability	*Pseudomonas aeruginosa*
Tetracyclines	Decreased permeation plus enhanced removal	Enterobacteriaceae
Sulfonamides	Altered dihydrofolate synthetase	*Staphylococcus aureus* Enterobacteriaceae *Neisseria gonorrhoeae*
Trimethoprim	Altered dihydrofolate synthetase	Enterobacteriaceae
	Cell wall impermeability	*Pseudomonas aeruginosa*
	Alternate enzymatic pathway	Enterococci

latter has proved impractical and clinical superiority of continuous dosing has not been established.

Table 28–4 summarizes the recommended doses and some pharmacologic data on most of the commonly used agents. Tissue penetration is linked to serum protein binding. The quantity of drug that diffuses into a site of infection is related to the "peak" or maximum serum concentration of free or unbound drug and the duration that the maximum level is maintained. On the other hand, therapeutic outcome does not always correlate with protein-binding affinity, probably because protein binding is usually easily reversible. Lipid solubility of an antibiotic is another factor affecting tissue penetration and influences the ability of an agent to pass through membranes by nonionic diffusion. Penetration of drug into the spinal fluid is related not only to the drug itself but also to the degree of inflammation in the meninges. Lipid-soluble agents such as chloramphenicol, isoniazid, rifampin, sulfonamides, and metronidazole penetrate spinal fluid well. Aminoglycosides, amphotericin B, and polymyxins do not penetrate well even in the face of inflammation. Penicillins and vancomycin generally penetrate CSF when inflammation is present. Most antibiotics commonly used are excreted primarily through the kidney, but notable exceptions include erythromycin and chloramphenicol. Thus, it may be possible to treat infections of the urinary tract with doses smaller than are required for serious systemic disease, because high urine levels are achieved with most agents. Urine and bile regularly contain higher concentrations of antibiotics than does serum. Penicillins and tetracyclines are concentrated in bile, but aminoglycosides enter bile less well, particularly when liver disease or obstruction is present. Drugs like tetracyclines and clindamycin diffuse readily into bone and have been used successfully in osteomyelitis. Agents that enter prostate tissue well include sulfonamides, trimethoprim, erythromycin, and doxycycline. Some drugs may fail because of pharmacokinetic properties. For instance, amoxicillin is so well absorbed in the small intestine that effective therapeutic levels are usually not achieved in the colon, thereby limiting use for Shigella infections.

Factors besides drug levels per se may limit drug activity. Purulent secretions and high concentrations of calcium and magnesium ions antagonize aminoglycoside activity. Erythromycin and aminoglycosides have markedly diminished activity in acidic environments. Cephalosporins like cephalothin can be metabolized to relatively inactive derivatives, but metabolites of cefotaxime are still quite active.

There is evidence that a high ratio of bactericidal activity in serum (e.g., serum diluted 1:8 or greater possessing a killing effect) against infecting strains is associated with therapeutic success. Such activity may merely reflect the serum concentration required to achieve effective therapy at a site of infection. It should not be assumed that a given dose corrected for weight or body surface area will reliably produce the same levels in all patients. With agents like aminoglycosides that are potentially toxic, therapeutic monitoring is clearly indicated during serious systemic infection. For example, gentamicin peak (postinfusion) levels should exceed 4 μg per milliliter and trough (or "valley") levels should be less than 2 μg per milliliter. Route of administration is important, since orally administered drugs may be poorly absorbed in serious systemic infections. For patients who are in shock, intramuscular or subcutaneous injections should clearly be avoided and all medications should be given intravenously.

MODIFICATION OF DRUG DOSES IN RENAL AND HEPATIC FAILURE

Since the majority of antibiotics are excreted via the kidney, dosage adjustment must be considered in moderate-to-severe renal failure. Many studies have related serum creatinine level or creatinine clearance to degree of dosage modification, and useful nomograms have been derived that may aid in the calculation of dosage. Table 28–4 indicates the agents affected by renal failure and dialysis. Many of these guidelines have been derived by study of patients who are in the "steady state," i.e., patients in renal failure who are on dialysis programs but who may not be infected. Thus, they may not manifest the hemodynamic instability that is often present in patients with serious systemic infection. In unstable patients, there is no substitute for accurate assays of serum or plasma drug concentrations as a guide to appropriate dosing. While dosage modification is indicated in patients with serious renal failure, the initial doses should probably be the same. The

TABLE 28–4. DOSAGE, PHARMACOLOGIC FACTORS, AND ADJUSTMENT IN RENAL AND HEPATIC FAILURE

Class/Agent	Dose *Systemic Infection*	*Oral*	Protein Binding (%)	Normal Serum Half-Life (Hrs)	Dose Adjustment *Hepatic Failure*	Dose Adjustment *Renal Failure*	Serum Levels Affected by Dialysis
Aminoglycosides							
Amikacin	5–7 mg/kg/q8	—	0	2–3	No	Major	Yes
Gentamicin	1.7 mg/kg/q8	—	0	2–3	No	Major	Yes
Netilmicin	1.7 mg/kg/q8	—	0	2–3	No	Major	Yes
Tobramycin	1.7 mg/kg/q8	—	0	2–3	No	Major	Yes
Antifungal Agents							
Amphotericin B	0.7–1 mg/kg/d	—	90	24	No	No	No
Flucytosine	40 mg/kg/q6	Yes	10	3	No	Major	Yes
Ketoconazole	6 mg/kg/d	Yes	98	8	Avoid	No	No
Miconazole	5 mg/kg/q6–8	—	92	2.2	Avoid	No	No
Antituberculous Agents							
Ethambutol	15 mg/kg/d	Yes	10	1.5	No	Major	Yes
Isoniazid	5 mg/kg/d	Yes	10	3	Yes	Minor	Yes
Rifampin	10 mg/kg/d	Yes	70	3	Yes	Minor	No
Cephalosporins							
Cefaclor	7 mg/kg/q6	Yes	20	1	No	Yes	Yes
Cefamandole	30 mg/kg/q6	—	70	1	No	Yes	Yes
Cefazolin	15 mg/kg/q6	—	80	2	No	Major	Yes
Cefotetan	30 mg/kg/q12	—	85	3	No	Major	Yes
Cefoxitin	30 mg/kg/q6	—	70	0.7	No	Yes	Yes
Cephalothin	30 mg/kg/q6	—	70	0.7	Minor	Yes	Yes
Cephalexin	7 mg/kg/q6	Yes	15	1	No	Yes	Yes
Cefoperazone	30 mg/kg/q8–12	—	90	2	Some	Minor	Yes
Cefotaxime	30 mg/kg/q6	—	50	1.2	Some	Minor	Yes
Cefsulodin†	30 mg/kg/q6–8	—	20	1.6	No	Major	Yes
Ceftizoxime	30 mg/kg/q6–8	—	50	1.3	No	Minor	Yes
Ceftriaxone	30 mg/kg/q12–24	—	90	8	No	Yes	Yes
Ceftazidime	30 mg/kg/q8	—	60	2	No	Major	Yes
Moxalactam	30 mg/kg/q8–12	—	50	2	No	Major	Yes
Penicillins							
Amoxicillin	7 mg/kg/q6	Yes	20	1	No	Yes	Yes
Ampicillin	30 mg/kg/q6	Yes	20	1	No	Yes	Yes
Azlocillin	50 mg/kg/q6	—	50	1	Minor	Major	Yes
Carbenicillin	70 mg/kg/q4	—	50	1	Minor	Major	Yes
Cloxacillin	7 mg/kg/q6	Yes	95	0.5	Minor	Minor	Yes
Dicloxacillin	7 mg/kg/q6	Yes	97	0.5	Minor	Minor	No
Methicillin	30 mg/kg/q4–6	—	30	0.5	No	Minor	No
Mezlocillin	50 mg/kg/q6	—	50	1	No	Major	Yes
Nafcillin	30 mg/kg/q4–6	—	90	0.5	Yes	Minor	No
Oxacillin	30 mg/kg/q4–6	—	90	0.5	Yes	Minor	Yes
Penicillin G	0.3–4 million U q4–6h	Yes	60	0.5	No	Yes	Yes
Penicillin V	7 mg/kg/q6	Yes	80	1	No	Minor	Yes
Piperacillin	40 mg/kg/q6	—	50	1	Minor	Major	Yes
Ticarcillin	40 mg/kg/4–6	—	50	1	Minor	Major	Yes
Quinolones							
Ciprofloxacin	10 mg/kg/q12	Yes	30	3	No	Major	Yes
Nalidixic acid	15 mg/kg/q6	Yes	90	1.5	No	Avoid	No
Norfloxacin	6 mg/kg/q12	Yes	15	3	No	Major	Yes
Tetracycline							
Chlortetracycline	7 mg/kg/q6	Yes	50	5	Avoid	Avoid	No
Demeclocycline	7 mg/kg/q12	Yes	50	10	Avoid	Avoid	Yes
Doxycycline	1.5 mg/kg/q12–24	Yes	90	15–20	No	No	No
Minocycline	3 mg/kg/q12–24	Yes	90	15	Avoid	Avoid	No
Oxytetracycline	7 mg/kg/q6–12	Yes	35	8	Avoid	Avoid	No
Tetracycline HCl	7 mg/kg/q6	Yes	50	7	Avoid	Avoid	No
Sulfonamides							
Sulfadiazine	15 mg/kg/q6	Yes	50	3	Avoid	Major	Yes
Sulfamethoxazole	12 mg/kg/q8	Yes	50	6	Avoid	Major	Yes
Trimethoprim (used with above)	2.3 mg/kg/q8–12	Yes	60	10	No	Major	Yes
Sulfisoxazole	15 mg/kg/q6	Yes	50	6	Avoid	Major	Yes
Other Agents							
Aztreonam	30 mg/kg/q8	—	60	2.0	No	Major	Yes
Chloramphenicol	7–15 mg/kg/q6	Yes	30	1.5	Some	Minor	Yes
Clindamycin	7 mg/kg/q6	Yes	90	2.5	Some	Minor	No
Colistin	2 mg/kg/q12	—	0	5	No	Avoid	No
Erythromycin	7 mg/kg/q6	Yes	20	1.5	Some	No	No
Imipenem	7.5 mg/kg/q6	—	15	1	No	Avoid	Yes
Metronidazole	15 mg/kg/q6	Yes	20	8	No	No	Yes
Nitrofurantoin	1 mg/kg/q6	Yes	60	0.3	No	Avoid	No
Polymyxin B	1.5 U/kg/q12	—	0	5	No	Avoid	No
Spectinomycin	30 mg/kg	—	0	2	No	Avoid	No
Vancomycin	7 mg/kg/q6	Yes*	10	6	No	No	No

*Not systemically absorbed.
†Investigational drug in the United States.

timing of the second dose should probably be based on levels anticipated from nomograms, but peak levels after the end of the second dose and third dose should be monitored in order to calculate the next doses. Increased trough concentrations may help to warn of incipient toxicity. As a general principle, many pharmacologic agents are given every three to four half-lives. In renal failure these half-lives are prolonged many-fold. One strategy is to prolong the interval between maintenance doses, which can result in fairly high "peak" or postinfusion levels and rather prolonged (and occasionally subtherapeutic) troughs. Another strategy is to give more frequent doses but to decrease the size of maintenance doses. Subtherapeutic levels may be avoided by the latter tactic, but the approach could be more nephrotoxic (as in the case of aminoglycoside agents). Dialyzable agents are similarly cleared by peritoneal or extracorporeal hemodialysis. Following dialysis a dose approximately two thirds to three quarters of a maintenance dose should be given, depending upon the degree of removal of the antibiotic by dialysis and the timing of the previous maintenance dose.

Several important antibiotics are metabolized in the liver and are partially excreted in the bile. Agents primarily metabolized by the liver include the sulfonamides, chloramphenicol, and tetracycline. There is usually little reason to alter the dose of penicillin, cephalosporins, and aminoglycosides in patients with liver disease. Even with erythromycin, ethambutol, and clindamycin, there is little evidence that dosage reduction is necessary except in severe hepatic failure. For instance, clindamycin should probably be reduced to half-normal doses after two to three days of treatment. Chloramphenicol total dosage should be restricted to 1.5 to 2.0 grams per day (adult) and erythromycin should be reduced to perhaps one half the normal dose after two or three days of treatment. Drugs to be avoided in hepatic failure include sulfonamides and tetracyclines.

COMBINATION ANTIMICROBIAL THERAPY

Use of combinations of antibacterial agents is exceedingly common. The rationale for their use may be summarized as follows: (1) Prior to the identification of pathogens infecting critically ill subjects, combinations offer a broader, more comprehensive antibacterial spectrum than a single agent. (2) Use of a drug combination may eradicate an infection that cannot be cured by a single agent, such as the effect of penicillin on enterococci. Addition of an aminoglycoside or a potentiating agent such as rifampin may result in bactericidal activity at a deep-seated focus of infection, as in endocarditis. (3) Combinations are indicated in the treatment of mixed infections, since not all of the pathogens may be susceptible to a single agent. (4) Combinations may decrease the opportunity for emergence of resistance. This has been best documented in tuberculosis. (5) Combinations may interact additively or synergistically against infecting organisms. As a result, there may be an enhancement of antibacterial activity and/or enhanced rate of killing. The latter may lead to more rapid clearing of infection with reduction in duration of therapy. Combinations may permit the use of a lower dosage of one or more components of the regimen, particularly the more toxic component, thereby avoiding undesirable side effects. More rapid killing or greater potency in vivo may be more directly beneficial in patients with impaired host defenses. Some clinical studies suggest an improved clinical response not only when drugs used to treat endocarditis interact synergistically but in sepsis occurring in immunocompromised patients.

The converse of synergism is antagonism between antimicrobial agents. This is best described for combinations of bactericidal plus bacteriostatic agents. Penicillin-type drugs require cell growth to exert their lethal effect. When penicillins are combined with static drugs like tetracycline, only growth inhibition may result. Clinical studies in humans indicate poorer results in treatment of pneumococcal meningitis with penicillin plus tetracycline than with penicillin alone.

Empiric therapy is presumptive or "blind" therapy where clinical severity of likely infection dictates that treatment be started. It is not necessarily combination therapy, as some single agents can still be quite effective. Intelligent choices in the absence of microbiologic information can be made based on the clinical syndrome and the likely infecting pathogen. Epidemiologic factors as well as host factors enter into the decision. The setting in which the patient develops infection or a prior exposure or travel history can be of considerable value. Pneumonias contracted outside of the hospital are usually due to streptococci (and pneumococci) and penicillin-sensitive anaerobes. An "atypical" or diffuse pattern raises the likelihood that community-acquired pneumonia will be better treated with erythromycin than penicillin. Infections that occur in the nosocomial setting or in markedly neutropenic patients should always be initially treated with therapy directed against gram-negative bacilli.

Table 28–5 summarizes recommendations for initial empiric therapy by clinical syndrome.

SPECIFIC ANTIMICROBIAL AGENTS

Table 28–2 summarizes recommended choices of antimicrobial agents for specific infecting agents. The organisms are

TABLE 28–5. INITIAL EMPIRIC THERAPY FOR SERIOUS INFECTION

Syndrome	Qualifying Factors	Recommended Treatment
Septicemia	Immunocompromised Host	
	Neutrophil Count >500 μl	Cephalosporin (cefazolin) + aminoglycoside (gentamicin, tobramycin)
	Neutrophil Count <500 μl	Piperacillin or ceftazidime + aminoglycoside (amikacin, tobramycin)
	Normal Host	
	Urinary source	Ampicillin + gentamicin or third-generation cephalosporin
	Biliary source	Ampicillin + gentamicin or third-generation cephalosporin
	Abdominal or pelvic source	Aminoglycoside + clindamycin or cefoxitin, or broad-spectrum penicillin
	No source	Oxacillin + gentamicin
	Neonate	
	<48 hrs old	Ampicillin + either cefotaxime or ceftriaxone
	>48 hrs old	Ampicillin + oxacillin + aminoglycoside
Meningitis	<6 years	Ampicillin + cefotaxime or ceftriaxone
	>6 years	Ampicillin or penicillin G
Brain Abscess		Penicillin G + cefotaxime or ceftriaxone + metronidazole
Pneumonia	Community acquired	Ampicillin or penicillin G ± erythromycin
	Postinfluenzal	Antistaphylococcal penicillin or cephalosporin
	Postaspiration	Ampicillin or clindamycin
	Nosocomial	Azlocillin or piperacillin + aminoglycoside, or third-generation cephalosporin + aminoglycoside

divided into gram-positive and gram-negative isolates, and antimicrobial agents that are similar are grouped together. Clearly, such a table oversimplifies the appropriate choices for various agents. In some situations, there is no clear-cut agent of first choice, and any member of a class may be appropriate. Differences in pharmacology, cost, and side effects might lead to a selection of one agent in preference to another. There is an increasing divergence in antibacterial spectrum among the newer beta-lactam agents, such as the antipseudomonal penicillins and the third-generation cephalosporins. Among the aminoglycosides, anticipated efficacy may be expressed as follows: While gentamicin and tobramycin remain the most widely prescribed, gram-negative bacilli that are resistant to these agents are more likely to be inhibited by netilmicin and amikacin.

Few oral agents are listed in Table 28–2, but it may be inferred that any of the oral antistaphylococcal agents such as cloxacillin or dicloxacillin could be used to treat mild infections due to penicillinase-producing staphylococci. The spectrum of oral cephalosporins such as cephalexin or cephradine mimics that of cephalothin or cefazolin. In the case of Group A hemolytic streptococci, it would not be necessary to test for susceptibility of these organisms against penicillin G and related penicillins in vitro, since all would be expected to be susceptible. It would, however, be highly desirable if one were to use a penicillin against the Klebsiella species to test that penicillin for susceptibility in vitro; it should probably not be presumed that antibiotics such as piperacillin or mezlocillin will be effective in vitro and in vivo without specific testing. Some agents should always be used in combination to treat serious bloodstream or systemic infections, such as antituberculous therapy (isoniazid plus at least one other agent) or enterococcal sepsis with or without endocarditis (the combination of either a penicillin or a vancomycin with an aminoglycoside). Older agents of the aminoglycoside class such as streptomycin or kanamycin are no longer widely used because their activity is more comprehensively covered by newer drugs (gentamicin and amikacin). The exception to this might be in the conventional therapy of *Mycobacterium tuberculosis,* for which streptomycin is still indicated.

Sulfonamides and Sulfa-Containing Combinations

Sulfonamides were the first chemotherapeutic agents to be introduced into wide clinical use. They are bacteriostatic and previously were quite active against many gram-positive and gram-negative organisms. They are, however, no longer among the first choices for serious systemic infections, the exception being *Nocardia asteroides* infections. Sulfonamides remain effective therapy for coliform organisms causing community-acquired urinary tract infections, but they are unreliable against hospital-acquired microorganisms. More commonly used to treat a wide variety of more serious bacterial infections is the fixed combination (1:5) of trimethoprim and sulfamethoxazole. Synergism in vitro against many enteric bacteria can be demonstrated with this combination, yet trimethoprim is a highly active agent itself. A major argument in favor of continued use of the fixed combination is that it may reduce the likelihood of the development of resistance to one component in the pair. Trimethoprim/sulfamethoxazole is usually active against enteric bacteria and *H. influenzae* (including most penicillinase-producing strains), and it has been effective in parasitic infections such as *Pneumocystis carinii* pneumonia. The diffusion of trimethoprim into prostate fluid makes it a useful agent in prostatic infections. Central nervous system penetration is good. The oral preparation is well absorbed, although a parenteral form is available for patients in whom gastrointestinal absorption may be erratic. Occasional side effects include neutropenia and all of the dermal and systemic hypersensitivity reactions that have been well associated with sulfonamides.

Penicillin G and Related Agents

The primary spectrum of penicillin G (benzyl penicillin) is gram-positive, with such organisms as *Streptococcus pyogenes, Streptococcus pneumoniae,* and *Streptococcus viridans* remaining exquisitely susceptible. Procaine penicillin is readily administered intramuscularly, and because of slow absorption, dosing of 600,000 units every 12 hours remains effective therapy for pneumococcal pneumonia. Benzathine penicillin is a long-acting (two to three weeks) agent that is slowly released after intramuscular injection and provides therapeutic levels for streptococcal pharyngitis and some forms of syphilis and prophylactic effect against acute rheumatic fever. For oral use in mild respiratory infections, phenoxymethyl penicillin (V) is acid stable and preferable to penicillin G. In large doses penicillin G is still effective against *Neisseria meningitidis,* most *N. gonorrhoeae,* and anaerobic organisms including Clostridium species, but usually not against strains of *Bacteroides fragilis.* Against enterococci, penicillin G or ampicillin should be used in combination with an aminoglycoside such as streptomycin or gentamicin. Ampicillin may be preferable in the treatment of Salmonella, central nervous system infections due to Hemophilus strains, and *Listeria monocytogenes.* When used in large doses, penicillin G or ampicillin is effective against a few gram-negative organisms, most notably *Proteus mirabilis* (but not other Proteus species). Penicillin G and related penicillins should not be used against the great majority of coagulase-producing staphylococci, most of which now produce beta-lactamases.

Antistaphylococcal Penicillins

The antistaphylococcal penicillins are beta-lactamase–stable and relatively narrow in spectrum. Parenteral preparations include methicillin, nafcillin, and oxacillin. There is little choice among this category of agents in terms of antistaphylococcal activity. There may be some differences in side effects, with methicillin possibly associated with more hypersensitivity nephritis and oxacillin with a greater incidence of abnormal serum elevations of hepatic enzymes. When used in appropriate doses, the central nervous system penetration is probably adequate to treat meningitis. The oral antistaphylococcal agents should not be used to treat serious infections, but mild or moderately severe infections may respond to dicloxacillin or cloxacillin. Combination of antistaphylococcal penicillins with an aminoglycoside or rifampin has been recommended for refractory staphylococcal infections or when the isolates demonstrate tolerance. *Staphylococcus epidermidis* may produce beta-lactamase like most coagulase-positive *Staphylococcus aureus.* However, serious infections like prosthetic valve endocarditis are better treated with vancomycin plus rifampin or an aminoglycoside.

Broad-Spectrum Penicillins and Related Compounds

Although ampicillin and amoxicillin are technically classified as broad-spectrum penicillins, the extended spectrum really only includes *Escherichia coli, H. influenzae,* Salmonella, and Shigella species. Even then, amoxicillin should not be used orally for Shigella infections because excellent absorption from the upper gastrointestinal tract results in subtherapeutic levels in the lower gut. Other penicillins like carbenicillin, ticarcillin, mezlocillin, azlocillin, or piperacillin are notable for their activity against *Pseudomonas aeruginosa,* most Proteus species, and anaerobic pathogens such as *Bacteroides fragilis.* On a weight basis, carbenicillin and ticarcillin have relatively weak antipseudomonal activity and so must be used in considerably larger doses than most penicillins, in the range of 18 to 30 grams a day for adults (200 to 400 mg per kilogram). The large sodium load given with such doses may aggravate congestive failure and cause electrolyte abnormalities. While these antipseudomonal penicillins are important agents for serious infections, emergence of resistance and variable stability to beta-lactamases has led to the tendency to combine these agents with an aminoglycoside. They are quite active against the coccal organisms that ampicillin usually inhibits, but none of these agents should be used against coagulase-positive staphylococci. The combination of a beta-lactamase inhibitor (clavulanate) with amoxicillin or ticarcillin confers stability to staphylococcal penicillinase and broadens coverage of some gram-negative bacilli. Other potential uses of extended-spectrum penicillins include treatment of infection caused by Acinetobacter species, Listeria, and a variety of anaerobes. Like the antistaphylococcal penicillins, their half-life is relatively short, but protein binding is low. Thus, frequent dosing at four- to six-hour intervals is usually necessary. Newer antipseudomonal penicillins such as mezlocillin, azlocillin, or piperacillin are augmented in their antipseudomonal activity, in the case of the latter two approximately six- to eight-fold by weight in comparison to carbenicillin when organisms are tested at low inoculum concentrations. On the other hand, the tendency has been to use smaller doses of these more potent penicillins in order to avoid the side effects associated with large doses of carbenicillin. The result is that no clear-cut clinical differences have been found between these agents when they are used in combination with aminoglycosides. Some of these newer penicillins, such as mezlocillin and piperacillin, have variable activity against Klebsiella species and must be tested prior to use.

Newer compounds that possess a beta-lactam nucleus (and thus are related to the penicillins) include (1) imipenem, an agent with very broad activity against gram-positive and gram-negative bacteria; and (2) monobactams, such as aztreonam or carumonam.* These latter compounds are entirely devoid of activity against gram-positive bacteria, but, like the third-generation cephalosporins, they are potent agents for treatment of gram-negative bacillary infections.

Cephalosporins

Cephalosporins are structurally related to penicillins, yet there are major differences in activity between these agents in vitro and in vivo. The first cephalosporins, such as cephalothin, cephaloridine, and cefazolin, were effective against penicillinase-producing staphylococci as well as pneumococci and streptococci (except enterococci). Additionally, they offered good activity against several important gram-negative pathogens such as *E. coli*, Klebsiella, and *Proteus mirabilis*. Despite activity in vitro, they are not effective against Salmonella and Shigella and do not penetrate the blood-brain barrier. The enormous popularity of these agents appears related to a low incidence of side effects, fairly broad coverage against community-acquired respiratory and urinary tract pathogens, and the availability of both oral and parenteral dosing. Nevertheless, these compounds have not been considered the agents of choice for any serious systemic infections. They have been successfully used to treat patients with a history of mild penicillin-type reactions, such as rash, but not urticaria or anaphylaxis. With the development of newer cephalosporins the principal advantages of these older compounds (often referred to as "the first generation") have been in the prophylactic surgical usage and relatively greater activity against penicillinase-producing *Staphylococcus aureus*.

The so-called "second-generation" cephalosporins offer a few improvements over cephalothin and cefazolin. Cefoxitin is a compound with fairly consistent activity against *B. fragilis*. Cefamandole and cefuroxime lack the anaerobic spectrum of cefoxitin but have modestly improved activity against some gram-negative organisms not inhibited by the first generation, such as *H. influenzae* and Enterobacter species. Oral agents include cefaclor, which has greater activity against penicillinase-producing *H. influenzae* than cephalexin.

*Investigational drug in the United States.

The newest cephalosporins (often referred to as "third generation"), or structurally related compounds such as moxalactam, a 1-oxy-beta-lactam, have markedly enhanced activity against enteric bacteria as well as variable coverage of *P. aeruginosa*. These compounds are stable against the beta-lactamases of *H. influenzae* and *N. gonorrhoeae* and cross the blood-brain barrier in sufficient concentrations to offer effective therapy for gram-negative meningitis (with perhaps the exception of *P. aeruginosa* infection). Among the agents shown to be effective in gram-negative central nervous system infections are cefotaxime, moxalactam, ceftazidime, and ceftriaxone. Several of these agents have a much longer half-life than first-generation cephalosporins, permitting dosing intervals of 8 to 12 hours. In the case of one agent, ceftriaxone, once-a-day dosing has been possible in some infections because of an eight-hour half-life. The antipseudomonal activity of these compounds is variable; nonetheless, newer antipseudomonal cephalosporins like cefsulodin* and ceftazidime represent some of the most potent antipseudomonal agents introduced into clinical practice, and these compounds appear to be significantly safer than aminoglycosides. Table 28–6 summarizes the relative properties of these agents, as well as selected comments. As a general rule, the increased activity against gram-negative pathogens is also coupled with relatively diminished activity against gram-positive cocci. While the gram-positive, particularly antistaphylococcal, coverage of these agents may be satisfactory for initial therapy, serious staphylococcal disease as well as pneumococcal infection is better and certainly more economically treated with older beta-lactam agents (e.g., oxacillin, penicillin G, respectively). These agents are also not without serious untoward effects, including the triggering of disulfiram reactions, inhibition of platelet adhesiveness, and hypoprothrombinemia. In many patients with community-acquired and mild to moderately severe nosocomial infections, third-generation cephalosporins offer the potential of effective single-agent therapy. The results in immunocompromised hosts suggest that these compounds may still be more efficacious when combined with aminoglycosides.

Chloramphenicol

Chloramphenicol is an oral or parenterally administered drug whose spectrum makes it useful for a wide variety of bacterial and rickettsial infections. The antibacterial spectrum includes gram-positive organisms such as streptococci and staphylococci, but the agent has not been considered to be one of the more potent antistaphylococcal compounds. It is usually bacteriostatic except against *H. influenzae*, against which it is bactericidal. Many enteric organisms are inhibited by chloramphenicol, but Pseudomonas strains are usually resistant. Important therapeutic uses include typhoid fever, central nervous system infections, anaerobic infections, intraocular infections, and serious rickettsial infections. Against *B. fragilis*, it remains one of the most useful agents. On the other hand, chloramphenicol has been associated with severe hematologic toxicity. In the great majority of individuals receiving courses in excess of one week of chloramphenicol, there is a dose-dependent inhibition of erythropoiesis. Some patients, estimated at 1 in 50,000, have developed irreversible aplastic anemia following oral or parenteral dosing. While it remains a highly effective agent in selected situations, there are now a number of very reasonable alternatives to chloramphenicol. The unpredictability of the hematologic toxicity should lead physicians to reserve this agent for serious infections in which there are major indications for avoiding alternative drugs.

*Investigational drug in the United States.

TABLE 28–6. THIRD-GENERATION CEPHALOSPORINS AND RELATED COMPOUNDS

Agent	Protein Binding (%)	Peak Serum Levels (μg/ml) After 1 gm I.V.	Half-Life (Hours)	Comments
Aztreonam*	60	50	2	No activity vs. gram-positive organisms
Cefmenoxime*	77	40	1	Weak antipseudomonal activity
Cefoperazone	90	125	2.1	Primary excretion is biliary with little dose adjustment in renal failure
Cefotaxime	38	40	1.1	Good CNS penetration but weak antipseudomonal activity
Cefsulodin*	30	65	1.5	Primarily antipseudomonal activity, not much else
Ceftazidime	20	70	1.9	Potent antipseudomonal activity
Ceftizoxime	30	75	1.4	Potent gram-negative activity except for Pseudomonas
Ceftriaxone	85	140	8.0	Very long half-life, good CNS penetration, but poor antipseudomonal activity
Imipenem	15	50	0.9	Broad gram-positive and gram-negative activity
Moxalactam	50	60	2.3	Good anaerobe coverage but associated with coagulopathy.

*Investigational drug in the United States.
CNS = central nervous system.

The Tetracyclines

Tetracyclines inhibit a wide range of gram-positive and gram-negative bacteria as well as Mycoplasma species, but they are not agents of choice for any serious bacterial infections. Their activity against gram-positive organisms is static, and the results do not appear to approach those obtained with bactericidal agents. Gram-negative coverage includes *E. coli* and Klebsiella species, but there are major gaps in their spectrum, including Pseudomonas, Serratia species, and other serious nosocomial pathogens. Tetracycline may be useful in urinary tract infections, rickettsial infections, mycoplasmal infections, and the prophylaxis or treatment of traveler's diarrhea (caused by toxigenic *E. coli*). Older preparations such as chlortetracycline or oxytetracycline have been supplanted by tetracycline HCl, minocycline, or doxycycline. The last-named two preparations have certain pharmacologic advantages, including less frequent dosing, and doxycycline may be used in renal failure.

Erythromycin

This is the most commonly available member of the class of macrolide antibiotics. Traditionally, erythromycin has been regarded as an agent of second choice for streptococcal and staphylococcal infections, to be used in those patients with history of serious penicillin allergy. In this regard, erythromycin remains a useful agent, but its primary appeal in recent years has been its clinical efficacy against several important new causes of infection such as Mycoplasma, Legionella, Chlamydia, and Campylobacter species. Against all of these pathogens, erythromycin can be considered the agent of choice. In serious respiratory infections, erythromycin should be administered parenterally, but this use is associated with high incidence of phlebitis. The compound is one of the safest of all antimicrobials, but mild gastrointestinal disturbances are common. Several oral preparations are available, but none seems clinically superior.

Clindamycin and Lincomycin

Clindamycin and lincomycin mimic some of the spectrum of erythromycin. Their major advantage over erythromycin is greater activity against anaerobes, particularly *B. fragilis.* Nonetheless, the antianaerobic spectrum of these compounds is not complete. In the treatment of intra-abdominal infections these agents are usually combined with aminoglycosides for gram-negative coverage. A major problem with clindamycin therapy has been antibiotic-associated diarrhea and pseudomembranous colitis. The incidence and severity of this complication vary, and the problem is not always associated with clindamycin. The development of gastrointestinal symptoms on treatment should be a warning to discontinue use of these agents.

Metronidazole

Metronidazole has long been used for the therapy of trichomoniasis, amebiasis, and giardiasis. Subsequently, it has been found to be a highly effective and bactericidal agent against many anaerobic pathogens, including *B. fragilis.* It is available in both oral and parenteral forms and must be considered the therapy of choice for *B. fragilis* infections involving deep-seated foci such as heart valves and the central nervous system. Many infections involving anaerobes are mixed processes that also involve aerobic organisms. Because it is almost exclusively active against anaerobic pathogens, metronidazole is usually combined with other antimicrobials. The drug must be metabolized to its active form. Its excellent distribution, rapid bactericidal activity, and penetration in "closed spaces" are appealing characteristics, but it also has the potential of inducing disulfiram reactions and potentiating the effects of warfarin (Coumadin). There is concern about metronidazole's carcinogenicity in animals and mutagenicity in bacteria. These effects have not been demonstrated in humans, but it seems wise to restrict this agent to use in severe infections.

Rifampin

Rifampin is a semisynthetic derivative of rifamycin B and has been used principally for the therapy of tuberculosis. It is one of the most potent and effective antituberculous agents available, with a spectrum that includes both *M. tuberculosis* and atypical organisms. It has been found to be very active against the wide variety of gram-positive and gram-negative organisms, including staphylococci (both coagulase-positive and coagulase-negative) and Legionella species. The compound is one of the few that has been effective in terminating meningococcal carrier state, and it inhibits methicillin-resistant staphylococci. The principal drawback to the use of rifampin is that almost all microorganisms have the ability to develop resistance rapidly. Therefore, even in tuberculosis this drug must be combined with another active agent. It seems useful as an adjunct to other antibacterial agents, such as in combination with antistaphylococcal penicillins to treat "tolerant" strains in endocarditis and meningitis. It inhibits methicillin-resistant staphylococci but is best used with vancomycin. Another potential advantage has been excellent penetration into phagocytic cells. A disadvantage, however, is its potent ability to induce enzymes that decrease the half-life of a number of other pharmacologic agents, including steroids, sulfonylureas, and digitoxin.

Vancomycin

Initially developed during an intense search for agents active against coagulase-producing staphylococci, this agent developed a reputation for efficacy as well as toxicity to the eighth cranial nerve and to renal function. More modern preparations of vancomycin do not appear to be strongly associated with these side effects. Indeed, the compound has been used effectively to treat serious infections in patients with renal failure because it is not significantly excreted by the kidneys; prolonged bactericidal activity results from widely spaced doses. The spectrum includes not only *Staphylococcus aureus*, but also *Staphylococcus epidermidis*, *Staphylococcus faecalis* (enterococci), and Corynebacteria species. Vancomycin has not been considered an agent of primary choice for *Staphylococcus aureus* but is an effective alternative in the penicillin-allergic patient. In prosthetic valve endocarditis caused by *Staphylococcus epidermidis*, it is often considered the agent of choice in combination with rifampin or gentamicin or both.

Aminoglycosides

Aminoglycosides are rapidly bactericidal against most of the clinically important gram-negative bacilli, including enteric bacteria and *P. aeruginosa*. Most isolates of *Staphylococcus aureus* are also inhibited by aminoglycosides. The initial compounds of this series, like streptomycin, were also shown to be effective against *M. tuberculosis*, and in combination with a penicillin, either streptomycin or gentamicin offers the best available therapy for deep-seated enterococcal infections. Older agents like streptomycin, neomycin, and kanamycin are considerably less useful today because they appear to be relatively more toxic or have been supplanted by agents with greater activity against *P. aeruginosa*. The contemporary aminoglycosides include gentamicin, tobramycin, netilmicin, and amikacin. The last two compounds offer some advantages in that they are stable to inactivation by some of the plasmid-encoded enzymes that acetylate, adenylate, or phosphorylate the older agents. Thus, amikacin or netilmicin may be preferred to treat infections caused by gentamicin- or tobramycin-resistant strains, but susceptibility testing in vitro is necessary because some isolates may be resistant to all agents within this class. Rapid bactericidal effect and good distribution except for the central nervous system make these highly desirable compounds for the treatment of serious systemic gram-negative infections. Unfortunately, aminoglycosides are toxic to renal function, can cause eighth cranial nerve (both cochlear and vestibular function) and renal damage, and occasionally manifest curare-like effects. Pharmacologically, there is a narrow range between the therapeutic levels achievable by dosing every 8 to 12 hours and levels that are associated with toxicity. Aminoglycoside therapy should be closely monitored by frequent blood level determinations in treating serious infections, when large doses are used for prolonged courses. These agents are either additive or often synergistic with beta-lactam compounds against pathogens such as *P. aeruginosa*, Serratia species, and other gram-negative rods. For immunocompromised hosts, aminoglycosides remain an important component of therapy, usually as part of a combination with a beta-lactam agent. Aminoglycosides do not penetrate well into the central nervous system or bone and are not absorbed via the oral route. They are perhaps overused as topical agents and in that setting the rapid emergence of resistance has been documented. For prophylaxis in colonic surgery, older aminoglycosides like neomycin or kanamycin may suffice in regimens that transiently suppress the growth of aerobic bowel flora.

Spectinomycin also belongs to the aminoglycoside class and is used exclusively for the treatment of gonorrhea when penicillin-type agents have failed. Such antigonococcal activity is shared by other members of the class.

Polymyxin, Colistin (Polymyxin E)

Polymyxin B and colistin (polymyxin E) are closely related cationic polypeptide detergents that bind to the lipoproteins of many gram-negative outer cell membranes. They are rapidly bactericidal in vitro, particularly against *P. aeruginosa* and enteric rods except Proteus species and Serratia. These agents are without effect against gram-positive organisms. Resistance has rarely emerged on therapy. Because of poor clinical results and nephrotoxic potential, the use of these compounds has decreased markedly. Lack of clinical efficacy could be due to properties of poor diffusion and rapid binding to tissues.

Quinolones

The quinolone group of agents includes older compounds like nalidixic acid and newer, more active agents such as ciprofloxacin,* norfloxacin, and ofloxacin.* Nalidixic acid has few modern uses and may be regarded as a urinary antiseptic for suppression of chronic infection. The newer quinolones have very broad activity against both gram-positive and gram-negative organisms (including Mycoplasma and Legionella) and can be administered orally. Their use is best defined for urinary tract infection and, depending on pharmacology, for respiratory and bone infection. Quinolone therapy for serious systemic infections requires additional study.

Urinary Antiseptics

Mandelamine, nitrofurantoin, and nalidixic acid are agents that are effective only in urinary tract infections, and usually as suppressive therapy in chronic infections. Resistance to some of these compounds may emerge rapidly. They may be useful in situations where the goal is suppression rather than a cure because of unremediable anatomic abnormalities. Gastrointestinal side effects have been commonly associated with each of these preparations. Additionally, the optimum antibacterial effect of mandelamine is at urine pH of less than 5.0, so that additional acidification of the urine with acidic substances is required for efficacy.

DURATION OF THERAPY

There are no easy formulas for determining duration of therapy, although a practical guide is treating for two to four days after defervescence and resolution of signs of infection. The site of infection, host factors, the nature and antimicrobial susceptibility of infecting organisms, the severity of infections, and the response to treatment should be taken into consideration. For bloodstream infections not accompanied by endocarditis or bone involvement, 10 to 14 days is a usual course of treatment. Most respiratory infections are adequately treated in the same interval. Uncomplicated meningitis caused by the meningococcus or pneumococcus is probably adequately treated by seven to ten days of high-dose parenteral penicillin G. Endocarditis, deep-seated bone infections, and infections involving prostheses require a minimum four- to six-week course of treatment but in some cases more. It is important to remember that signs of inflammation, particularly pulmonary infiltration, may persist long after infecting organisms are killed or contained by host defenses, and delayed resolution of lung infiltrates is not uncommon. On the other hand, deep-seated infections like endocarditis and osteomyelitis may have to be treated for periods long after subsidence of signs of infection. Thus, the decision to continue or stop treatment at the end of an appropriate interval must be based on the thorough clinical examination and careful reasoning. Patients with impaired host defenses may require longer therapy than those individuals who are basically healthy. A single dose of an effective antimicrobial agent may be adequate to cure lower urinary tract infection involving the bladder, but a much longer duration, on the order of several weeks, is required to ensure therapeutic success in treatment of intrarenal infection.

---

*Investigational agents.

FAILURE TO RESPOND TO TREATMENT

One of the most important clinical dilemmas is the persistence of fever and other manifestations of infection after a course of costly and potentially toxic therapy has been started. At the same time that every component in antimicrobial therapy is being reassessed, an alternative explanation for fever, pain, and inflammation must also be sought. For instance, tumors or hypersensitivity reactions can incite febrile reactions. Usually, an interval of two to five days is necessary in order to judge the efficacy of treatment. At that point, the following are indicated: (1) Assessing the accuracy of the diagnosis of infection; (2) determining if the drug selection is appropriate, and particularly if the dose and mode of administration are responsible for the lack of success of therapy; and (3) searching for (a) presence of anatomic abnormalities, (b) foreign body, (c) undrained abscess, (d) infarction of tissue, (e) development of superinfection, (f) emergence of resistance, or (g) presence of a simultaneous infectious process that is not being treated by antibacterial therapy. If these are unrevealing, a noninfectious origin of fever or drug reaction should be considered.

In the severely immunosuppressed host, fever and signs of infection may persist despite appropriate therapy. In these patients clinical failure of drug treatment is more realistically regarded as host failure; if any improvement is possible in this difficult situation, it usually correlates with improvement in underlying disease or the immunologic status of the host. If an infection is documented and responds poorly to initially prescribed treatment, then a change to an alternate regimen is indicated. If signs and symptoms progress or new complications appear in spite of seemingly appropriate treatment, a change in therapy is indicated as well as a search for superinfection or an undiagnosed process such as a viral or fungal infection. One of the greatest clinical dilemmas is presented by the patient in whom drug fever or a hypersensitivity reaction is suspected but in whom discontinuing treatment could be dangerous. In such individuals, it is usually prudent to give alternative medication rather than stop antibacterial therapy.

ANTIBIOTIC TOXICITY AND UNTOWARD REACTIONS

A large proportion of drug reactions is related to antimicrobial agents. As many as 10 per cent of patients receiving penicillins and sulfonamides experience some type of toxic or hypersensitivity reaction. These reactions can be fatal, as in the anaphylaxis associated with penicillin or the aplastic anemia due to chloramphenicol. Table 28–7 summarizes some of the major untoward reactions to antibiotics. The majority of toxic reactions are, however, short lived and reversible. Nephrotoxicity secondary to aminoglycosides may be averted by careful therapeutic drug monitoring. A commonly recognized complication of antibiotic therapy is diarrhea and/or pseudomembranous colitis. This is due to bowel overgrowth by *C. difficile*, which elaborates an exotoxin that is responsible for symptoms. Discontinuation of antibiotic therapy will usually lead to resolution of treatment, but some patients require vancomycin or metronidazole.

Besides anaphylaxis, other hypersensitivity reactions include fever, hemolytic anemia, serum sickness, and a wide variety of dermal reactions that include rash and exfoliation. When serious infection is being treated, mild hypersensitivity reactions may be suppressed by a variety of symptomatic medications. Manifestations of hypersensitivity such as rash may fade despite continued treatment, as is common with ampicillin. The decision to continue therapy in the face of such reactions must be based on severity of infection and the lack of reasonable alternatives. Another issue of great clinical importance that is not fully resolved is the potential cross-reactivity between penicillins and cephalosporins. However, the great majority of patients who have only rash following exposure to penicillin, ampicillin, or related penicillins can be safely treated with cephalosporin compounds. The immediate hypersensitivity-type reactions such as anaphylaxis, wheezing, and urticaria should be carefully noted. Patients with a history of immediate reactions to penicillin should not be rechallenged with cephalosporins unless they have life-threatening infections and can be observed under close medical supervision.

MAJOR ANTIBIOTIC DRUG INTERACTIONS

An increasing number of interactions have been reported between antimicrobials, or antimicrobials and other pharmacologic agents that seriously ill patients may be receiving. Some of these are summarized in Table 28–8. Some noteworthy examples include the induction of hepatic enzymes by rifampin, which may hasten the metabolism of other anti-

TABLE 28–7. UNTOWARD EFFECTS OF SOME ANTIMICROBIAL AGENTS

Target	Agent	Mechanism	Manifestation
Endocrine	Ketoconazole	Altered steroid synthesis	Gynecomastia
	Sulfonamides	Block iodine uptake	Goiter
Gastrointestinal	All agents, esp. ampicillin, clindamycin	(1) Altered bowel flora	Diarrhea
		(2) Exotoxin of *Clostridium difficile*	Pseudomembranous colitis
	Isoniazid, rifampin, tetracyclines	Hepatocellular necrosis	Hepatitis
	Neomycin	Villous damage	Malabsorption
Hematologic	Chloramphenicol	(1) Protein synthesis inhibition	Reversible anemia, leukopenia
		(2) Idiosyncratic	Aplastic anemia
	Carbenicillin, others	Inhibition of platelet aggregation	Bleeding
	Moxalactam	Impaired prothrombin synthesis	Bleeding
	Penicillins, many others	Impaired leukopoiesis, thrombopoiesis	Neutropenia, thrombocytopenia
	Sulfonamides	G-6-PD deficiency	Hemolytic anemia
Kidney	Aminoglycosides, polymyxins	Tubular damage	Renal failure
	Amphotericin	Tubular damage	Hypokalemia, renal failure
	Carbenicillin	Na-K exchange	Hypokalemia
	Penicillins	Interstitial nephritis	Renal failure
	Sulfonamides	Tubular crystallization	Renal failure
Nervous System	Aminoglycosides	(1)Damage to hair cells of Corti	Deafness
		(2) Vestibular damage	Vertigo
		(3) Neuromuscular blockade	Respiratory arrest
	Isoniazid	Pyridoxine antagonism	Neuropathy
	Penicillins, cephalosporins	Cortical irritation	Seizures
	Polymyxins	Neuromuscular blockade	Respiratory arrest
Pulmonary	Nitrofurantoin	Interstitial inflammation	Fibrosis
Skin	Tetracyclines	Bind to dermal structures	Photosensitivity
	Penicillins, sulfonamides, tetracyclines, others	Allergic reactions	Rash, serum sickness, erythema multiforme

TABLE 28–8. IMPORTANT ANTIBIOTIC DRUG INTERACTIONS

Antimicrobial Agent	Interacting Drug	Result
Amphotericin B	Curariform drugs	Increased curare-like effect
Aminoglycosides	Neuromuscular blockers (i.e., tubocurarine, pancuronium)	Additive blockade
	Diuretics: ethacrynic acid, furosemide	Increased ototoxicity
	Antibiotics: amphotericin B	Increased nephrotoxicity
	Carbenicillin/ticarcillin (other penicillins)	Inactivation, resulting in reduced activity
Ampicillin/Amoxicillin	Allopurinol	Rash
Cephalosporins (cefamandole, cefoperazone, moxalactam)	Alcohol	Disulfiram reaction
Chloramphenicol	Warfarin	Decreased warfarin metabolism and inhibition of vitamin K–producing gut bacteria, thus increasing prothrombin time
	Phenytoin	Decreased phenytoin metabolism levels
	Oral hypoglycemic agents	Increased hypoglycemia
Isoniazid	Warfarin, phenytoin	Increased risk of toxicity by decreased drug metabolism
	Disulfiram	Psychosis
	Rifampin, para-aminosalicylic acid	Additive hepatotoxicity
	Oral contraceptives	Decreased contraceptive effect
Metronidazole	Alcohol	Disulfiram-like reaction (nausea)
	Disulfiram	Psychosis
Nalidixic Acid	Warfarin	Increased prothrombin time
Polymyxins	Curariform drugs	Increased curare-like effect
Quinolones	Theophylline	Increase quinolone blood levels
Rifampin	Warfarin, phenytoin	Decreased warfarin, phenytoin effect
	Isoniazid	Additive hepatotoxicity
	Methadone	Withdrawal symptoms
	Oral contraceptives	Decreased contraceptive effect
	Steroids	Decreased steroid effect
Sulfonamides	Procaine	Decreased sulfonamide effect
	Hypoglycemic agents	Hypoglycemia
	Warfarin, phenytoin	Displace drugs from protein-binding sites causing increased warfarin and phenytoin effects
Tetracyclines	Antacids, oral iron	Decreased tetracycline absorption

biotics or drugs. An unexplored area of drug interactions is that which may involve more than two agents. Penicillins like ampicillin or carbenicillin gradually inactivate aminoglycosides like gentamicin in renal failure, when a long half-life for both types of drugs provides opportunity for complexing between the two classes of agents. While this effect is not apparent when patients have normal renal function, the net effect in patients in renal failure is effectively to lower the levels of circulating aminoglycosides and penicillin.

USE OF TOPICAL ANTIBIOTICS

Topical antibiotics or antiseptics have been commonly applied to burns and open wounds, and they are often incorporated into irrigants. A few studies suggest that topical agents can suppress bacteria in burn wounds and reduce sepsis originating from this source. Some topical antiseptics, such as those that contain iodine, are probably too toxic to inflamed tissues and their local application should be discouraged. Topically applied antibiotics can provide only surface suppression of microbial flora. They also provide ample opportunity for development of resistance, since large numbers of organisms may be present on injured skin. Antibiotics in irrigants may be irritating, may be absorbed in large quantities so as to cause increased toxicity, and may offer little advantage over irrigation per se.

Bennett WM, Aronoff GR, Morrison G, et al.: Drug prescribing in renal failure: Dosing guidelines for adults. Am J Kidney Dis 3:155, 1983. *A highly practical guide to antibiotic dose reduction in renal failure.*

Garrod LP, Lambert MP, O'Grady F: Antibiotics and Chemotherapy. London, Churchill-Livingstone, 1981. *Succinct text oriented to microbiologists, but with much information useful to clinicians.*

McGowan JR Jr: Antimicrobial resistance in hospital organisms and its relationship to antibiotic use. Rev Infect Dis 5:1033, 1983. *An important subject exhaustively reviewed.*

Medical Letter: Choice of antimicrobial drugs. Med Lett Drugs Ther 26:19, 1984. *A somewhat conservative but practical compendium of "drugs of choice" and alternative agents for most pathogens.*

Neu HC: Relation of structural properties of beta-lactam antibiotics to antibacterial activity. Am J Med 79(Suppl 2A):2, 1985.

Siegenthaler WE, Bonetti A, Luthy R: Aminoglycoside antibiotics in infectious diseases. Am J Med 80(Suppl 6B):2, 1986. *Succinct summary of this group of agents, which remain important in modern antimicrobial chemotherapy.*

Young LS: Empirical antimicrobial therapy in the neutropenic host. N Engl J Med 315:580, 1986. *Summarizes, with relevant references, the debate over the merits of combination antimicrobial therapy versus the use of a single agent for empiric treatment of immunocompromised hosts.*

29 ANTIVIRAL THERAPY

David. W. Barry

Advances in our knowledge of basic virologic replicative mechanisms have led to the discovery of a number of new antiviral agents within the past decade. This chapter reviews clinical experience with these agents and examines the criteria to be considered before any new therapy is established as safe and effective. Only those agents that have withstood the tests of time and scientific scrutiny will be described.

Some antiviral agents have been available for over 20 years. Certain fundamental principles of viral infections prevent direct extrapolation from knowledge gained from antibacterial therapy. Viruses are obligate intracellular parasites and must divert normal host cell metabolism into providing the constituents for the reproduction of new viral particles. Thus the effectiveness of any antiviral drug will depend not only on its ability to penetrate mammalian cell membranes but also on its capacity to inhibit viral-directed metabolic functions and viral replication. In addition, in some instances, viral deoxyribonucleic acid (DNA) or viral ribonucleic acid (RNA)–directed cDNA may be integrated into the human genome, where it cannot be attacked by any known agent or process. Limited success has been achieved with agents that appear to inhibit viral replication from this genomic template. Furthermore, host immune function has a greater influence on the outcome of viral than bacterial infections in humans. Finally, the influence of intracellular metabolism and replication has slowed, complicated, or prevented the establishment of the relationship between the sensitivity of the virus to a drug in vitro, achievable serum levels of the agent, and its ability to cure an infection.

Evaluation of the effectiveness of antiviral agents is difficult because a number of virus infections are self-limited or mild, with virus replication often well past its peak by the time the physician is consulted. Therapeutic intervention will therefore usually occur simultaneously with the rising tide of the body's own defenses, and a "placebo effect" is prominent in mild and self-limited illnesses. Even in the case of acquired immunodeficiency syndrome (AIDS) or chronic hepatitis B infection, the clinical course is so variable that, as with milder infections, any study on the effectiveness of an antiviral that is not double blind and placebo controlled must be regarded with skepticism.

CHEMOTHERAPEUTIC AGENTS

Herpesvirus Infections

The earliest examples of successful antiviral chemotherapy have been the treatment of superficial infections of the eye caused by herpesviruses. Details of therapy may be found in the ophthalmologic literature, and only certain pharmacologic aspects of the treatment of these viral infections will be discussed here. The majority of the agents found to be effective in the treatment of herpetic keratitis interfere with viral DNA synthesis. Some, such as trifluorothymidine, idoxuridine, and cytosine arabinoside, are relatively toxic when given systemically because they also interfere with DNA replication in rapidly dividing host cells such as myelocytes and lymphocytes. However, when they are given topically in the eye, only minimal amounts are absorbed. Others, such as adenine arabinoside, acyclovir, and interferon, have much more limited toxicity even when given systemically. The final selection of an antiherpes keratitis agent will thus depend on such factors as local tolerance, allergic reactions, observed or potential drug resistance, rapidity of healing, depth of corneal ulceration, and the cost of the drug.

IDOXURIDINE. The first effective antiherpes drug to be developed was idoxuridine, also known as 5-iodo-2′-deoxyuridine or IUDR. It is an analogue of deoxythymidine and is chemically related to trifluorothymidine, which will be discussed later. The action of IUDR results in part from its inhibition of thymidine kinase but more significantly from its inappropriate incorporation into viral or host cell DNA and its formation of false base pairs with guanine rather than adenine. When given in the usual regimen of one drop of a 0.1 per cent aqueous solution in the affected eye every hour, IUDR will cure 75 to 90 per cent of patients with the milder or "dendritic" form of herpes keratitis. A 0.5 per cent ointment is also available. Unfortunately, IUDR cures a lower percentage (40 to 50 per cent) of patients with the more severe "geographic" ulcers. It appears to be relatively ineffective in patients who have deeper disease involving the corneal stroma or the uveal tract. Some patients are intolerant of or allergic to the drug and develop bothersome edema and erythema of the periorbital tissue. Resistance to the drug in vivo and in vitro develops fairly rapidly. As with all other antiherpes agents, IUDR does not eradicate "latent" virus when the organism is in a metabolically inactive state and when herpes nucleic acid may be integrated with host cell DNA. Thus, recrudescent infections are common (approximately 50 per cent will recur within two years) and add credence to the pessimism concerning complete cure of herpes infections.

Comparable success has not been obtained in systemic use of IUDR. For a number of years IUDR was used to treat herpes encephalitis but critically controlled studies showed that it was not effective. Accordingly, IUDR should not be used for this purpose; in addition, systemic toxicity predisposes the patient to serious superinfection and bleeding. Its use topically, even combined with dimethylsulfoxide, in the treatment of various cutaneous herpes and zoster infections has produced unimpressive results.

ADENINE ARABINOSIDE. Another nucleoside analogue that has been shown to be effective in the treatment of herpetic keratitis is adenine arabinoside, also known as vidarabine, ara-A, or Vira-A. It is phosphorylated intracellularly, and the triphosphate noncompetitively inhibits viral DNA polymerase more efficiently than host cellular DNA polymerase. The 3 per cent ophthalmic ointment applied every three hours has been associated with cure rates of keratitis higher than with IUDR. Like IUDR, it is ineffective against stromal and uveal tract disease. It is also the first drug shown to have some activity in herpes simplex encephalitis, lowering the mortality rate from 70 per cent to approximately 30 to 40 per cent. Some survivors were left with severe and permanent neurologic residua, and its effectiveness was obvious only in those patients who were not stuporous or comatose when therapy was initiated. Its use in this illness has been supplanted by acyclovir (see below). Multicenter studies have demonstrated that intravenous ara-A can also significantly reduce the high mortality rate in disseminated neonatal herpes simplex infections if administered early. As with herpes encephalitis, some survivors are left with significant sequelae. Intravenous ara-A has also been shown to produce some clinical improvements, including the prevention of visceral complications, in immunocompromised patients with cutaneous herpes zoster, although the overall clinical improvement was not dramatic. To produce these benefits, the drug must be given within 72 hours of infections, and conflicting data exist showing that the clinical benefit is seen only in younger (<35 years of age) or older (>38 years of age) individuals.

Treatment of other viral infections has met with varying success. Ara-A has some beneficial influence on the biochemical markers of chronic active hepatitis, but the degree and permanence of these changes are more impressive when it is given with prolonged courses of interferon, although toxicity is increased. It does not appear to be effective in preventing or curing cytomegalovirus pneumonia.

Ara-A also has a number of significant disadvantages, the first of which is its relative insolubility. Often an adult's daily dose (10 to 15 mg per kilogram intravenously) must be given in 2 or more liters of fluid—a potential hazard in patients with encephalitis, who often have significantly elevated intracranial pressure. In addition, the drug is rapidly deaminated to the relatively ineffective hypoxanthine arabinoside. Because of its insolubility and almost immediate deamination, the drug must be given as a continuous infusion over 12 to 24 hours, a cumbersome dosing schedule to maintain. Maximal levels of less than one fourth to one third of the inhibitory dose in vitro for most herpesviruses are achieved in the serum, an observation that must not necessarily engender newer concepts of intracellular micropharmacokinetics in order to explain the apparent clinical activity of the drug. The phosphorylated analogue (ara-AMP) is considerably more soluble, but clinical trials showed it to be ineffective in herpes encephalitis, possibly because it must be dephosphorylated before it can enter infected cells. At high doses, ara-A suppresses the bone marrow, although considerably less than cytosine arabinoside. Higher dosage regimens have been associated with tremors, hyperexcitability, and seizures. These reactions are more common in patients with compromised renal or hepatic function and is likely the result of higher blood and tissue levels. Like IUDR, it is not effective when applied topically to oral or genital herpetic lesions.

TRIFLURIDINE. Trifluridine, also known as trifluorothymidine, TFT, or Viroptic, is, like IUDR, an analogue of deoxythymidine. It is suitable only for topical use in the treatment of herpetic keratitis (one drop of a 1 per cent solution every two hours). When given intravenously, TFT induces significant bone marrow suppression, but applied topically in the eye, it produces only minimal adverse reactions, primarily mild stinging and burning in a low percentage of patients. Its major advantage is a higher cure rate than that for IUDR, and possibly ara-A, in herpetic keratitis. It is significantly better than IUDR for both dendritic and geographic ulcers and has also proved effective in those cases clinically or virologically resistant to either IUDR or ara-A. The drug has also shown some promise in certain adenovirus infections of the eye. It is not effective when applied topically to cutaneous lesions such as those of herpes genitalis or herpes labialis.

ACYCLOVIR. The next effective antiherpes agent to be developed was the acyclic nucleoside 9-(2-hydroxyethoxymethyl) guanine, also known as acyclovir, acycloguanosine, or Zovirax. It is similar in structure to guanosine but only half the ribose ring is present, yielding an "acyclic" structure. Its wide therapeutic index is based upon its selectivity as a substrate for virus-specified thymidine kinase. Normal host cell thymidine kinase does not effectively utilize acyclovir as a substrate. Herpesvirus-specified thymidine kinase converts acyclovir to its monophosphate, which is then transformed by cellular enzymes to di- and triphosphates. The triphosphate is both an inhibitor of and a substrate for herpesvirus-specified DNA polymerase. Because it does not contain a 3′ carbon, its incorporation into viral DNA selectively stops virus replication. The cellular α-DNA polymerase in infected cells is also inhibited by the triphosphate, but only at concentrations several-fold higher than those that inhibit the viral-specified DNA polymerase. Since acyclovir is preferentially taken up and converted to its active form by herpesvirus-infected cells, it has a low toxic potential for normal, uninfected cells.

Experiments in vitro have shown acyclovir to be effective against herpes simplex types I and II, varicella-zoster virus, and Epstein-Barr virus, but less potent against cytomegalovirus. Intravenous regimens of 5 to 10 mg per kilogram every eight hours produce peak serum levels of 4 to 15 μg per milliliter. If the solubility of the drug in renal tubular fluid (2.5 mg per milliliter at 37°C) is exceeded, through rapid infusion, poor hydration, or coexistent renal failure, tubular obstruction can occur and lead to usually reversible renal failure. The drug penetrates into the cerebrospinal fluid moderately well (~50 per cent of serum levels) and the inhibitory concentrations for herpes simplex, varicella-zoster, and Epstein-Barr viruses range from ~0.01 to 2 μg per milliliter. Intravenous acyclovir has been shown to be effective in the treatment of mucocutaneous herpes infections and in varicella-zoster infections in normal as well as immunocompromised patients. It is more effective than ara-A in the treatment of herpes encephalitis and as effective as ara-A in herpes neonatalis. Although there are suggestions of efficacy in acute and chronic mononucleosis, additional studies are required to define its therapeutic index in these illnesses. It does not appear to be effective in cytomegalovirus infections. Acyclovir has limited absorption from the gastrointestinal tract (15 per cent), yet a regimen of 200 to 400* mg every four hours has been shown to ameliorate genital herpes infections. Most striking is the fact that 200 mg taken orally two to five times per day effectively prevents the appearance of recurrent genital lesions. Like IUDR, ara-A, and TFT, it is very effective when applied topically to the lesions of herpes keratitis.

DHPG. The agent 9-1(1,3-dihydroxy-2-propoxymethyl) guanine (DHPG)† is a very close analogue of acyclovir and has shown great usefulness in the treatment of cytomegalovirus (CMV) infections. The presence of a 3′ carbon allows it to be phosphorylated very efficiently, by metabolic processes yet to be identified, in CMV-infected cells. Most CMV isolates are inhibited in vitro by levels of 1 to 5 μg per milliliter. It is also active against herpes simplex virus and varicella-zoster virus, but its use in these infections is limited because it has significantly greater toxicity than acyclovir in these infections. Although it produces severe and usually irreversible damage to spermatogenic tissue in animals and men, careful dose titration has permitted successful treatment of CMV retinitis and gastroenteritis, primarily in AIDS patients. Retinal lesions from CMV usually recur shortly after DHPG has been discontinued, often necessitating persistent treatment for as long as the patient remains severely immunocompromised. It is the only drug known to eliminate CMV from the pneumonic lesions of bone marrow transplant recipients. Unfortunately, this has not been associated with an improved clinical outcome.

*Exceeds manufacturer's recommended dosage.
†Investigational agent.

Poxviruses

METHISAZONE. One of the earliest chemotherapeutic agents to demonstrate anti-DNA virus activity was 1-methylisatin-3-thiosemicarbazone, also known as thiosemicarbazone, methisazone, or Marboran.* In the early 1960's it was found to have a wide antiviral spectrum in vitro, most impressively against variola, the virus that caused smallpox. Several prophylactic studies conducted during that decade showed a reduction in secondary attack rates among household contacts of smallpox cases. Methisazone did not significantly decrease the mortality rate in those who did develop the disease, nor was it effective in acute smallpox infections.

With the worldwide eradication of smallpox over the past two decades, this drug has seen little use. Nevertheless, methisazone is probably effective in treating complications of smallpox vaccination such as vaccinia gangrenosa, vaccinia necrosum, and generalized vaccinia, particularly when used in conjunction with vaccinia immune globulin. Smallpox vaccination has virtually disappeared, except in the military, and thus little use for this drug is expected in the future.

Influenza

AMANTADINE. One of the most significant advances in anti-RNA virus therapy was the development of amantadine, also known as Symmetrel. A drug with an odd, birdcage-like structure, it was first found to have antiviral activity in the early 1960's. In tissue culture, influenza A viruses, but not influenza B viruses, are inhibited by amantadine. Drug resistance can be induced fairly readily in vitro, although the clinical significance of this observation has yet to be established. The gene determining resistance has been linked with that governing the matrix protein. Amantadine appears to inhibit either viral penetration or viral uncoating within the cell by as yet undefined mechanisms. The concentration required to inhibit 50 per cent of the virus in tissue culture (ID_{50}) ranges between 0.1 and 6 μg per milliliter; the ID_{100} is often closer to 25 μg per milliliter. After a single oral dose of 2.5 to 4.0 mg per kilogram (roughly equivalent to the usual adult dose of 200 mg per day) peak serum levels of 0.3 to 0.5 μg per milliliter are attained. Significant concentration (10- to 60-fold) occurs in both mouse and human lung tissue. Amantadine has a very long half-life (20 to 24 hours) and two to three days are required before a steady state is reached. Eventually 90 to 99 per cent is excreted unchanged in the urine, and thus very significant dose reductions must be made in patients with compromised renal function.

Amantadine taken prophylactically provides protection rates against influenza infection in the range of 70 to 90 per cent (similar to that observed following the inoculation of influenza vaccines). At the usual therapeutic and prophylactic

*Experimental drug available from Burroughs Wellcome Company.

dose of 100 mg twice a day, amantadine will induce adverse reactions in 10 per cent or more of recipients. These reactions are generally more frequent and more severe in older individuals, who need most to be protected from influenza. Fortunately, these reactions are generally not severe and consist most often of mild agitation, confusion, mental depression, and insomnia. Adverse reactions are more common or more prominent when the patient is also taking antihistamines, but those of amantadine alone are not greater than those of antihistamines alone. Overdosages associated with blood levels above 1.5 μg per milliliter have led to severe central nervous system reactions, including coma and convulsions.

Amantadine also appears to be active against influenza when given orally. This efficacy, however, is more difficult to define, and the difference in the rates of significant clinical improvement between drug- and placebo-treated groups is often marginal. Sophisticated tests, such as those measuring frequency-dependent compliance, have shown that the duration of the diminished pulmonary function that occurs for a number of weeks after influenza may be markedly shortened by the use of amantadine during acute illness. Whether amantadine is effective in the treatment of primary influenza pneumonia has not been established. An analogue, rimantadine, which has been used in some European countries and has been studied in the United States, is reported to have a better therapeutic toxic ratio than amantadine.

Respiratory Syncytial Virus

RIBAVIRIN. Convincing and consistent results of double-blind, placebo-controlled studies of ribavirin (1-β-D-ribofuranosyl-1,2,4,-triazole-3-carboxamide), also known as Virazole, have become available. This analogue of guanosine or inosine appears to inhibit inosine monophosphate dehydrogenase and thus interferes with the de novo synthesis of guanine nucleotides necessary for viral replication. Ribavirin is converted by cellular enzymes to ribavirin triphosphate (RTP). RTP also inhibits GTP-dependent capping of the 5′ end of viral mRNA's. It is active against a broad spectrum of RNA and DNA viruses in vitro, although precise levels of sensitivity are dependent on the cell substrate employed in the assays. When given in doses of 333 mg every eight hours for ten days, ribavirin is effective in the treatment of Lassa fever. Although clinical studies of ribavirin in herpes and influenza infections have yielded inconclusive or mixed results, the use of continuous or semicontinuous aerosolized ribavirin (20 mg per milliliter in water) for a minimum of three days ameliorated the course of respiratory syncytial virus infection in children. Few adverse reactions were noted, although oral dosages* of 600 to 1200 mg per day for 5 to 14 days have been associated with reversible depressions in red cell counts and elevations of bilirubin. This anemia appears to be caused in part by the accumulation of RTP within erythrocytes, which cannot efficiently cleave the phosphate moieties and allow exit of the molecule from the cell. The half-life of ribavirin in erythrocytes is therefore much prolonged (approximately 40 days), and erythrocytes heavily ladened with RTP have a significantly shortened survival. Higher doses of ribavirin are also directly marrow suppressive. Loading doses of 1200 mg t.i.d., followed within a few days by a regimen of 300 mg b.i.d., yield serum levels of 6 to 15 μmol (and cerebrospinal fluid levels of 7 to 11 μmol). Hemolytic anemia is said not to occur if serum levels of ribavirin are kept below 20 μmol, although several patients required transfusions when this regimen was used over an eight-week period. Ribavirin is also mutagenic, tumorigenic, and teratogenic, and thus additional experience must be gained before a precise therapeutic index can be determined, particularly in infections requiring higher or more prolonged dosing regimens.

*Oral use not recommended by the manufacturer. Approved for aerosol administration only.

Human Immunodeficiency Virus

AZIDOTHYMIDINE. This compound is also known as AZT, zidovudine, Retrovir, Compound S, and BW509U. It is identical to thymidine with the exception that an azido (N_3) group has been substituted for a hydroxyl group in the 3′ position of the sugar moiety. AZT is monophosphorylated by cellular thymidine kinase, then di- and triphosphorylated by other as-yet-unidentified cellular enzymes. The triphosphate form inhibits retroviral reverse transcriptase at concentrations 100-fold less than those required to inhibit cellular DNA polymerase. Because of the azido in the 3′ position, it is also a DNA chain terminator. Many aerobic gram-negative bacteria and most animal and human retroviruses are inhibited by low concentrations (<0.5 μg/ml) of AZT, and animal studies have shown positive therapeutic and prophylactic effects in these infections.

Clinical studies in humans have shown that the drug is well absorbed (60 to 70 per cent) following oral administration, has a half-life of approximately one hour, has low (30 per cent) serum binding, is excreted primarily in the inactive glucuronidated form, and penetrates well into the CNS, with CSF concentrations averaging about 50 per cent of simultaneous serum concentrations. A double-blind, placebo-controlled study showed that AZT could ameliorate most of the clinical and immunologic manifestations of severe HIV infections, including the incidence of opportunistic infections and deaths, over a six-month observation period. The dosage used in the study was 250 mg by mouth every four hours, but a number of patients required dose reduction because of marrow suppression. AZT causes a macrocytic anemia secondary to inhibition of DNA replication in red and white cell precursors. The severity of the anemia is directly proportional to the degree of pre-existing impairment in the patient's marrow reserve. AZT also caused a moderate incidence of nausea and headaches in these patients.

Additional studies are required to determine the full therapeutic profile of this drug. Such studies would include its use in milder manifestations of HIV infection as well as its use with other agents, such as acyclovir (with which it is synergistic in vitro), interferon, colony stimulating factor, and other immunostimulants.

BIOLOGIC AGENTS

INTERFERON. The most prominent and perhaps the most promising biologic agent used for the therapy of virus infections is interferon. This protein has a molecular weight of approximately 20,000. It is a natural compound produced by many types of cells, particularly lymphocytes, in all vertebrate and possibly invertebrate species, but its activity is fairly species specific. In tissue culture, it is effective against a wide variety of viruses if the cells have been treated with interferon before virus is added to the medium. The mechanism of action of interferon is still being elucidated, but it appears to act by interfering with translation functions once the virus has entered the cell. Interferon has an extremely high specific activity of approximately 1 billion units per milligram of protein (1 unit of interferon = the amount required to reduce viral plaques in tissue culture by 50 per cent). It is produced by infecting human lymphocytes, lymphoblasts, or fibroblasts with a virus or exposing them to a chemical inducer. The cells respond by releasing interferon into the medium, and the material is then purified by a number of complex chemical steps. Alternatively, the gene for interferon production can be inserted in bacteria, allowing for large-scale and efficient production of this complex protein.

Unfortunately, the early promise of interferon in the potential treatment of a host of viral infections has been eclipsed by its toxicity or the appearance of chemical antivirals with a better therapeutic index. It is effective in the topical treatment of herpes keratitis, but numerous other effective agents are available, although it may somewhat enhance their effectiveness. Sprayed intranasally, interferon partially attenuates the symptoms of experimental rhinovirus infections, but bothersome nasal congestion and bleeding associated with a dense submucosal accumulation of lymphocytes preclude its clinical use to prevent upper respiratory viral infections. High-dose interferon (up to 5.1×10^5 units per kilogram) is effective in limiting the severity and progression of both herpes zoster and varicella infections in immunocompromised patients, but the common adverse reactions of fever, lassitude, prostration, and myalgias render it clearly less useful than other agents, such as acyclovir. Parenteral interferon can lower or ablate the serum markers of chronic hepatitis B infection, but the permanence and clinical significance of these changes will remain unclear until additional long-term studies are completed.

The most impressive activity of interferon is in the treatment of infection caused by human papillomaviruses. These agents cause juvenile laryngeal papillomas, which can cause severe and debilitating illness in children, and they also cause genital warts (condyloma acuminatum). Daily doses of 1 to 5 million units per square meter of body surface area induce significant lesion reduction or disappearance in the majority of patients. Additional studies will determine the duration of permanence of these remissions. Some of the more common adverse reactions diminish with long-term therapy, but less common ones, such as hypotension and hepatic and cardiac damage, can be severe. Therefore, only patients with the most severe forms of papillomavirus infections are suitable candidates for long-term interferon therapy.

IMMUNE GLOBULINS. Purified globulins have been used as "postexposure prophylaxis" for viral illness for a number of years. Such "prophylaxis" is in reality treatment of the viral infection before it is clinically manifest. Since antibodies cannot enter cells, they are effective only when the virus is circulating in the blood or when the newly formed viruses are spreading through interstitial fluid rather than via direct cell-to-cell contact. Antibodies may also exert their effect by attaching to a cell that has a viral antigen expressed on its surface, allowing complement and/or lymphocytes to destroy the infected cell. Serum prepared from patients convalescing from the illness to be treated, or serum selected to contain high titers of antibody to the virus to be treated, usually produces the best clinical results. The dosage to be given is often expressed in terms of volume (milliliters per kilogram). This is somewhat misleading, because the appropriate dose will be a factor not only of the volume of the serum preparation but also of the concentration of antibody within it. In some instances, this has been standardized.

Human globulin has been shown to be effective in several clinical situations. These include measles, rabies, and hepatitis A and B. Discussion and schedules of globulin therapy are provided under the individual topics. As newer chemical antivirals become available, the importance of these biologics that do not affect replicating viruses will wane.

Barry DW, Blum MR: Antiviral drugs: Acyclovir. In Turner P, Shand DG (eds.): Recent Advances in Clinical Pharmacology. New York, Churchill Livingstone, 1983, pp 57–80. *A review of preclinical and clinical studies of acyclovir.*

Bauer DJ: The Specific Treatment of Virus Diseases. Lancaster, United Kingdom, MTP Press Ltd., 1977. *This book contains an excellent review of the principles of antiviral chemotherapy. Excellent analysis of clinical data relating to methisazone.*

Bean B, Braun C, Balfour HH: Acyclovir therapy for acute herpes zoster. Lancet 2:118, 1982. *Intravenous acyclovir was effective in these normal patients, but crystalluria can occur if infusions are given too rapidly.*

Bryson YJ, Dillon M, Lovett M, et al.: Treatment of first episode of genital herpes simplex virus infection with oral acyclovir. N Engl J Med 308:916, 1983. *This double-blind, placebo-controlled study demonstrated good efficacy with minimal side effects.*

Collaborative DHPG Treatment Study Group: Treatment of serious cytomegalovirus infections with 9-(1,3-dihydroxy-2-propoxymethyl) guanine in patients with AIDS and other immunodeficiencies. N Engl J Med 314:801, 1986. *Those with retinitis did well. Those with pneumonia did poorly.*

Evans AS (ed.): Viral Infections of Humans. New York, Plenum Medical Book Company, 1976. *The most complete text on the epidemiology, pathophysiology, diagnosis, and therapy of viral infections.*

Fields BF (ed.): Virology. New York, Raven Press, 1985. *This impressive tome covers all aspects of virology, including recent data on the pathophysiology of virus infections as well as chemotherapeutic inhibition of replicative processes.*

Galasso, GJ, Merigan TC, Buchanan RA (eds.): Antiviral Agents and Viral Diseases of Man. 2nd ed. New York, Raven Press, 1984. *This book reflects the status of antiviral chemotherapy in 1984.*

Goepfert H, Sessions RG, Gutterman JU, et al.: Leukocyte interferon in patients with juvenile laryngeal papillomatosis. Ann Otol Rhinol Laryngol 91:431, 1982. *Clear demonstration of the activity of interferon in this viral-induced "proliferative" disease.*

Hall CB, McBride JT, Gala CL, et al.: Ribavirin treatment of respiratory syncytial viral infection in infants with underlying cardiopulmonary disease. JAMA 254:3047, 1985.

Heidelberger C, King DH: Trifluorothymidine. Pharmacol Ther 6:427, 1979. *Excellent review of this drug by its originator.*

Hirsch MS, Swartz MN: Antiviral agents. N Engl J Med 302:903, 949, 1980. *This concise review contains up-to-date information on antivirals, particularly acyclovir and interferon.*

McCormick JB, King IJ, Webb PA, et al.: Lassa fever: Effective therapy with ribavirin. N Engl J Med 314:20, 1986.. *Clear reduction in mortality if therapy begun within the first week of illness.*

Oxford JS, Drasar FA, Williams JD: Chemotherapy of Herpes Simplex Virus Infections. New York, Academic Press, 1977. *This book thoroughly examines drugs affecting double-stranded DNA virus replication.*

Whitley RJ, Alford CA, Hirsch MS, et al.: Vidarabine versus acyclovir therapy in herpes simplex encephalitis. N Engl J Med 314:144, 1986. *This study showed the superiority of acyclovir in decreasing death rate as well as incidence of neurologic sequelae.*

Whitley RJ, Nahmias AJ, Soong SJ, et al.: Vidarabine therapy of neonatal herpes simplex virus infections. Pediatrics 66:495, 1980. *Demonstration of the activity of ara-A in neonatal herpes.*

Whitley RJ, Soong SJ, Dolin R, et al.: Early vidarabine therapy to control the complications of herpes zoster in immunosuppressed patients. N Engl J Med 307:971, 1982. *This article contains the results of a multicenter, double-blind study, which showed the effectiveness of ara-A in herpes zoster.*

Yarchoan R, et al.: Administration of 3′-azido-3′-deoxythymidine, an inhibitor of HTLV-III/LAV replication, to patients with AIDS or AIDS-related complex. Lancet 1:575, 1986.

30 GLUCOCORTICOSTEROID THERAPY

Anthony S. Fauci

In 1949, Hench and coworkers reported marked clinical improvement in patients with rheumatoid arthritis treated with cortisone. During the next 30 years glucocorticosteroids became a major factor in the successful chemotherapy of a wide range of diseases, particularly those in which inflammation or immunologically mediated phenomena played a prominent role. However, these agents have proved a mixed blessing, for glucocorticosteroid therapy is also marked by a high incidence of deleterious and often devastating side effects. Perhaps as much as with any therapeutic agents, the use of corticosteroids requires an appreciation of the toxic as well as the beneficial effects of these drugs, since the one is almost invariably associated with the other. An understanding of the mechanisms of action as well as of the advantages and disadvantages of different glucocorticosteroids, and their treatment regimens, is essential for the physician to exercise appropriate clinical judgment in their use.

BIOCHEMISTRY AND PHARMACOLOGY. Cortisol (hydrocortisone) is synthesized endogenously from cholesterol via pregnenolone and progesterone. Approximately 95 per cent of the endogenous cortisol in the circulation is bound to plasma proteins, particularly to a specific corticosteroid-binding globulin (CBG or transcortin); a lesser amount is bound to albumin. Cortisol is rapidly removed from the circulation with a plasma half-life of approximately 90 minutes. Cortisol is rapidly metabolized in a number of tissues, especially the liver. Less than 2 per cent of the cortisol produced is excreted in the urine unchanged. The active moiety of cortisol is the

11-betahydroxyl group. Exogenously administered compounds such as cortisone and prednisone, which are 11-keto compounds, lack glucocorticosteroid activity until they are converted in vivo into the corresponding 11-betahydroxyl compounds cortisol and prednisolone. This reaction occurs chiefly in the liver. Patients with serious impairment of liver function should be given prednisolone instead of prednisone in order to ensure availability of the active compound.

There are a number of synthetic analogues of cortisol in clinical use today. These differ in their plasma half-life, relative anti-inflammatory potency, and salt-retaining potency (Table 30–1). Among them, cortisone and cortisol have the highest sodium-retaining potency. For this reason, these agents are rarely the steroids of choice in situations requiring long-term administration, except as replacement therapy in adrenal insufficiency. Certain cortisol analogues such as dexamethasone are much less susceptible than cortisol to metabolic degradation. Thus, their plasma half-lives are longer, contributing to their greater relative anti-inflammatory potency.

MECHANISMS OF GLUCOCORTICOSTEROID ACTION. Most, if not all, of the cellular and tissue responses to glucocorticosteroids are initiated via the common denominator of an intracellular glucocorticosteroid receptor, which is present in virtually every mammalian tissue. Exogenously administered glucocorticosteroids are thought to penetrate the cell membrane and bind with high affinity, but reversibly, to this receptor. The hormone-receptor complex then migrates to the cell nucleus and binds to nuclear protein. The association of the steroid-receptor complex with nuclear DNA modulates gene expression. Specific mRNA's then code for proteins that are thought to be responsible for the expression of the glucocorticosteroid effect. The predominant protein induced by glucocorticoids is lipocortin, which is a potent inhibitor of phospholipase A_2. Certain cases of resistance to steroid therapy have been associated with receptor defects, particularly in the refractoriness of some patients with acute lymphoblastic leukemia to glucocorticosteroid therapy.

The effects of glucocorticosteroids subsequent to receptor binding, are complex. Glucocorticosteroids are most often administered for their anti-inflammatory and immunosuppressive effects (the use of these agents as tumoricidal drugs in various chemotherapeutic protocols is discussed in Ch. 176). They are also occasionally administered to stabilize the cardiovascular system, as in hypotensive states arising from sepsis or other causes of cardiovascular collapse. Their efficacy in these latter situations is controversial. Proposed mechanisms of their efficacy in shock include a vasoconstrictive effect on the capillary bed either directly or via potentiation of the action of alpha-adrenergic agents, an increase in cardiac contractility and cardiac output, maintenance of capillary wall integrity, and prevention of tissue breakdown.

Another clinical use of glucocorticosteroids is in the treatment of brain edema, particularly that resulting from brain tumors. The precise mechanisms by which steroids work in this setting are unclear. In situations in which vascular permeability is altered, steroids may act by maintaining vascular integrity, as also postulated in shock. In situations in which brain edema occurs in the presence of an apparently intact vasculature, the mechanisms of steroid effect are even more speculative. However, in these situations the effects are probably related, at least in part, to a decrease in the accumulation of sodium in the tissue edema.

Glucocorticosteroids are also administered therapeutically to ameliorate certain types of hypercalcemia, such as that associated with sarcoidosis and certain neoplasms. The therapeutic effect is related to an increase in renal excretion of calcium and a decrease in calcium absorption from the gastrointestinal tract.

The mechanisms whereby glucocorticosteroid administration results in anti-inflammatory and immunosuppressive effects are also complex. Glucocorticosteroids cause a rapid (four to six hours after administration) but transient lymphocytopenia and monocytopenia, not by lysis and destruction of cells, as in certain animal models, but by a redistribution of cells out of the circulation into other lymphoid compartments, which renders the cells less accessible to sites of inflammation and immune reactivity. In steroid-induced lymphocytopenia, thymus-derived (T) lymphocytes are more markedly depleted than bone marrow-derived (B) lymphocytes; similarly, within the T lymphocyte population, certain subsets of cells are more markedly affected than others. This has potential clinical relevance, since certain immunologically mediated diseases express abnormalities predominantly of specific subpopulations of cells. On the other hand, steroid administration results in a neutrophilia by mobilizing neutrophils from the bone marrow reserve, prolonging the circulating half-life of these cells, and blocking the free migration of these cells out of the circulation into inflammatory and other extravascular sites. One mechanism of this blockage of cell migration is interference with the initial adherence of neutrophils to the microvasculature endothelium. In addition, steroids may block the interaction of various chemotactic factors with neutrophils. Glucocorticosteroid administration also causes a profound eosinopenia. Although the mechanisms of this effect are unknown, the eosinophils are thought to be redistributed out of the circulation similarly to lymphocytes following steroid administration. Furthermore, in vivo and in vitro, glucocorticosteroids interfere with chemotaxis of eosinophils.

Besides affecting the movement and circulatory kinetics of inflammatory and immunologically competent cells, glucocorticosteroids can also have direct effects on their functional capabilities. These include effects of cell activation, proliferation, and differentiation; generation and release of cell products; levels of mediators of inflammation and immune reactions, as well as the response of certain cell types to such mediators; phagocytosis; antigen processing; cytotoxic effector functions; and several others. Various cell types may be selectively sensitive or resistant to the effects of steroids on one or another functional capability. Steroid sensitivity of different cell types also may vary, depending on the stage of activation of the cell. The direct effect of glucocorticosteroids on the functional capability of a cell usually requires higher sustained concentrations of hormone than does their effect on the traffic of the cell.

Of the two major circulating phagocytic cells in humans, the monocyte is much more sensitive to direct suppression of its functional capabilities by steroids than the neutrophil. This has clinically relevant implications, since the monocyte is one of the focal cells in the formation of granulomas, which are quite sensitive to the suppressive effects of glucocorticosteroids. Granulomatous *hypersensitivity* diseases are generally responsive to steroid therapy, whereas infectious diseases such as tuberculosis and certain fungal diseases that are characterized by granulomatous reactions are prone to exacerbation and relapse during high-dose glucocorticosteroid therapy.

TABLE 30–1. COMPARISON OF COMMONLY USED GLUCOCORTICOSTEROID PREPARATIONS

Compound	Equivalent Potency (mg)	Sodium-Retaining Potency	Plasma Half-Life (minutes)
Cortisone	25	2+	30
Hydrocortisone (cortisol)	20	2+	90
Prednisone	5	1+	60
Prednisolone	5	1+	200
Methylprednisolone	4	0	180
Triamcinolone	4	0	300
Dexamethasone	0.75	0	200

Although many antibody and immune complex–mediated diseases are treated with glucocorticosteroids, the antibody-forming cells (B lymphocytes and plasma cells) are relatively resistant to the suppressive effects of these agents. Extremely high doses of drug are required to suppress antibody production by B cells and their progeny. The beneficial effects of steroids in antibody and immune complex–mediated diseases are most likely through indirect effects on the inflammatory response subsequent to the binding of antibody or deposition of immune complexes. At least one of the mechanisms of therapeutic efficacy of glucocorticosteroids in certain of the autoimmune hemolytic anemias and other cytopenias is blockage of the clearance of antibody-coated cells by the reticuloendothelial system.

Glucocorticosteroids are used extensively and beneficially in the treatment of asthma and immediate hypersensitivity allergic conditions. The precise mechanisms responsible are not well understood. Although glucocorticosteroids cause a circulating eosinopenia, the precise role of the eosinophil in allergic and asthmatic reactions is unclear. Glucocorticosteroids have very little effect on serum IgE levels or on the early-phase components of immediate hypersensitivity (Type I) immunologic reactions, although they do alter the late-phase components. In certain systems, glucocorticosteroids induce an increase in intracellular cyclic adenosine monophosphate (cAMP), which in turn is associated with a decrease in release of certain mediators of inflammation. Corticosteroids also decrease the biosynthesis of prostaglandins and leukotrienes, most likely by inducing the synthesis of lipocortin, which inhibits the activity of membrane phospholipase A_2, thus decreasing the availability of arachidonic acid for subsequent conversion by the cyclo-oxygenase and lipoxygenase pathways. Although corticosteroids do not protect animals against histamine-induced shock, several days of steroid treatment can decrease the histamine content of certain tissues. Furthermore, corticosteroids inhibit IgE-mediated release of histamine from human basophils after prolonged incubations. Finally, glucocorticosteroids suppress the expression of lymphocyte surface receptors for the Fc portion of IgE as well as the glycosylation of IgE-binding factors.

TREATMENT OF DISEASE STATES WITH GLUCOCORTICOSTEROIDS. Diverse disease states, with widely differing causes and pathophysiologic mechanisms, have been treated effectively with corticosteroids. These include disorders requiring merely physiologic or replacement doses of the hormone, such as adrenal insufficiency, as well as diseases of suspected or proven inflammatory and/or immunologic mediation, which require pharmacologic doses of drug. These diseases include the connective tissue disorders, particularly systemic lupus erythematosus, rheumatoid arthritis, acute rheumatic fever, dermatomyositis and polymyositis, and mixed connective tissue disease; several of the vasculitides; the idiopathic nephrotic syndrome; severe asthma; various hypersensitivity and allergic states; prophylaxis and treatment of organ transplant rejection; noninfectious granulomatous diseases such as sarcoidosis; autoimmune hemolytic anemia and the immunologically mediated cytopenias; a wide range of dermatologic and ophthalmologic conditions; and several others. Corticosteroids have proven effective in the amelioration of brain edema but have been inconsistent in septic shock and as adjunctive therapy to antibiotics in infections such as tuberculous meningitis.

From the standpoint of the physician, the critical issue is usually not whether the steroid will have a beneficial effect, but the choice of the most appropriate therapeutic regimen in a given patient at a specific phase of a particular disease.

DESIGN OF GLUCOCORTICOSTEROID THERAPEUTIC REGIMENS. The number of possibilities for different steroid regimens is enormous. To facilitate the proper choice, certain fundamental issues must be addressed. The first and most obvious is whether the disease is serious enough to warrant glucocorticosteroid therapy. A closely related question is whether the disease necessitates long-term administration of the drug for a reasonable therapeutic effect to be realized. For example, in mild asthma that is relatively well controlled on bronchodilators, or rheumatoid arthritis that is well managed on nonsteroidal anti-inflammatory agents, there is little question that administration of glucocorticosteroids would ameliorate symptoms even more. However, the required long-term use of even low doses of steroids militates strongly against their use in such situations. On the other hand, one would not hesitate to administer even massive doses (1 gram of methylprednisolone per dose) for limited periods of time in disorders such as status asthmaticus and acute organ transplant rejection. In clinical situations in which it is generally agreed that glucocorticosteroid therapy will be necessary for more than a brief time, other issues must be addressed by the physician. These include consideration of patient disposition to known toxic side effects of steroid therapy such as diabetes mellitus, peptic ulcer, psychiatric difficulties, osteoporosis (older individuals), exacerbations of underlying infections such as tuberculosis, and other potential hazards. If this is the case, alternative therapeutic regimens or modification of the steroid regimen (alternate-day therapy as opposed to daily therapy) to lessen the incidence of such side effects must be considered.

Local Versus Systemic Therapy. In some clinical situations, local glucocorticosteroid therapy that delivers high concentrations of drug directly to the involved site is much preferable to systemic administration of drug. Typical examples are certain dermatologic conditions such as contact dermatitis, in which steroid-containing creams and ointments can be applied directly. However, if a large enough area is exposed to the steroid for a sufficient amount of time, absorption can be great enough to result in systemic effects. Other examples of local administration include topical conjunctival administration of corticosteroids for a variety of ocular conditions as well as steroid enemas for ulcerative proctitis. The latter situation is especially prone to systemic absorption of drug, since denuded mucous membrane is exposed to the hormone.

One of the most important advances in the development of glucocorticosteroid agents has been inhaled aerosol steroids used in the treatment of bronchial asthma. In patients with steroid-dependent asthma, inhalants such as beclomethasone sprayed into the airways via the mouth in doses of two inhalations (100 μg) three to four times per day have allowed a reduction of systemic steroid dosage—and in some individuals, discontinuation of systemic steroid therapy—while controlling symptoms in large numbers of patients. Nasal instillation of aerosol steroids has also proved effective in certain cases of allergic rhinitis.

Type of Agent Employed. Although relatively few glucocorticosteroid preparations are used by clinicians, several factors must be considered in the choice of a steroid agent. A steroid preparation that possesses little or no mineralocorticoid activity is generally preferred in order to avoid the sodium-retaining side effects. Among the commonly used preparations, cortisol (hydrocortisone) has the greatest degree of mineralocorticoid activity. One of the major uses of this agent is in replacement therapy for adrenal insufficiency. Most normal adults secrete about 20 mg of endogenous cortisol per day, and so adults with nearly complete adrenal insufficiency (Addison's disease) require approximately 20 mg of hydrocortisone per day in a single or divided dose. The mineralocorticoid effect is desirable in this situation. In fact, an additional mineralocorticoid (usually fludrocortisone, 0.1 mg per day) is generally administered to the addisonian patient. Hydrocortisone is also indicated in stress situations such as severe trauma and extensive surgical procedures in patients who are or have recently been receiving glucocorticosteroid therapy and may be relatively addisonian (see below).

Among the commonly employed glucocorticosteroids, dexamethasone and methylprednisolone have the least sodium-retaining properties, while prednisone and prednisolone exhibit a slight to moderate degree, significantly less than hydrocortisone (Table 30–1).

Ever since the development of synthetic glucocorticosteroids, great effort has been made to develop agents that are potent and long acting but relatively nontoxic. Unfortunately, as a general rule, there is a correlation between duration of plasma half-life, potency, and toxic side effects. For example, dexamethasone is longer acting, more potent, and associated with greater deleterious side effects than the more commonly used prednisone. From a strictly anti-inflammatory or immunosuppressive standpoint, it would be desirable to administer a high dose of a long-acting agent at frequent intervals for an extended period of time in order to induce and maintain disease remission. However, the toxic side effects of such a regimen render it unacceptable except under the most extraordinary circumstances. In situations such as in the chronic connective tissue diseases, it is more appropriate to employ a short-acting agent such as prednisone in a single dose in the morning or on alternate days. Shorter acting agents are essential for the construction of long-term regimens that closely mimic the normal diurnal cortisol cycle. What then is the indication for a potent long-acting agent such as dexamethasone? Although there are no absolute indications, dexamethasone is generally considered to be the steroid of choice in clinical situations in which sustained high levels of potent glucocorticosteroids are desirable for limited periods of time, as in brain edema.

Dose and Dose Interval of Glucocorticosteroid Administration. BURST OR INTERMITTENT THERAPY. Examples of common, relatively minor ailments for which "burst" or intermittent administration of glucocorticosteroids is employed are poison ivy and poison oak dermatitis. Patients are generally given 60 mg of prednisone for two to three days, followed by rapid tapering of drug by 10-mg decrements over several days until complete discontinuation of therapy. On this regimen, there is little danger of complications. There are other situations that call for short periods of "massive" doses of glucocorticosteroid. Some of the most common are treatment of acute organ transplant rejection and of septic shock. The efficacy of such regimens is clearly documented for organ transplant rejection, in which methylprednisolone is given in doses of several grams per day for a limited time (usually three to five days), followed by conversion to more standard regimens of 60 to 100 mg of prednisone, which is then tapered according to the individual clinical situation. Methylprednisolone is generally employed for the burst therapy because of its relatively low sodium-retaining activity and high potency. Such brief courses of massive-dose steroid therapy have also been used in some cases of acute deterioration in certain connective tissue diseases, particularly systemic lupus erythematosus with active nephritis. The efficacy of such an approach is not certain at this time.

DAILY GLUCOCORTICOSTEROID THERAPY. The most commonly employed regimen for inflammatory and immunologically mediated diseases is the administration of prednisone on a daily basis either as a single dose in the morning or in divided doses over the day. A given dose of a relatively short-acting agent such as prednisone is more potent in its anti-inflammatory and immunosuppressive properties when administered in daily divided doses. Divided dose therapy is also attended by a greater incidence of complications, particularly suppression of the hypothalamic-pituitary-adrenal (HPA) axis. Administration of the same total amount of drug in a single dose on alternate days provides less anti-inflammatory and immunosuppressive effect but also produces significantly fewer toxic side effects. Ideally, a short-acting agent should be administered in a manner that closely mimics the normal diurnal cortisol cycle—namely, peak levels of cortisol early in the morning (6 to 8 A.M.), with tapering off by mid to late afternoon so that the low levels late at night release the pituitary gland from feedback inhibition and permit secretion of adrenocorticotropic hormone (ACTH). The therapeutic aim is to deliver the hormone in a bolus without interrupting the normal feedback mechanisms and thus without disrupting the normal pattern of steroid levels. Persistence of supraphysiologic or pharmacologic levels of hormone late in the day likely accounts for the toxic "tissue" effects and surely accounts for the suppression of the normal HPA cycle seen with divided dose administration of glucocorticosteroids.

Virtually all therapeutically effective regimens of daily divided dose glucocorticosteroid will have some of these effects. Even single daily doses as low as 15 to 20 mg per day of prednisone will cause both toxic tissue effects and HPA axis suppression. Because of its longer plasma half-life, a single dose of dexamethasone will likely have the same deleterious side effects as an equivalent anti-inflammatory dose of prednisone given in divided doses over the day. Since most of the complications of glucocorticosteroid therapy are dose, dose interval, and time related, one should administer the smallest possible dose in the least toxic dose interval over the shortest period of time sufficient to control disease activity. It is inappropriate to initiate steroid therapy in a patient with a flagrantly active inflammatory disease by administering a low dose of a short-acting drug (prednisone) in a single daily dose or on alternate days in order to avoid toxic side effects. It is just as inappropriate to allow a patient whose disease has been put into remission by high doses of divided daily prednisone to remain on that regimen for an inordinate period of time.

Since the diseases that are treated with glucocorticosteroids are heterogeneous and of varying severity, it is difficult to set strict rules for drug administration. However, there can be general and flexible guidelines. For example, if a patient presents with an inflammatory or hypersensitivity disease that is quite active, one should initiate therapy with prednisone at a dose of at least 1 mg per kilogram per day in up to three divided doses. Although this is a potentially toxic regimen if administered over an extended period of time, it may be essential in order to induce a remission of disease. A less aggressive therapeutic regimen may fail while still subjecting the patient to side effects. Once remission has been attained, attempts should be made to taper to the least toxic regimen, with the ultimate goal of completely discontinuing the drug if possible. A common mistake is to leave the patient on the regimen that induced remission while the toxic side effects go unnoticed for some time. Once clinical remission is induced, the divided daily dose can gradually be consolidated into a single daily dose of the same total amount. If remission is maintained, the daily dose can gradually be tapered while monitoring closely for symptoms of disease exacerbation, adrenal insufficiency, or withdrawal (see below). Tapering is continued to the lowest possible dosage that can maintain remission or until the drug is discontinued. Adjunctive therapy with, e.g., nonsteroidal anti-inflammatory drugs for connective tissue diseases, or disodium cromoglycate in asthma, often facilitates the tapering schedule. The advantage of converting from daily divided doses to a single daily dose is that the normal diurnal cortisol cycle can be closely mimicked, which will better acclimate the body to the ultimate discontinuation of therapy. One of the most effective regimens for a smooth tapering of glucocorticosteroid therapy is to convert from a daily divided dose to a single daily dose to an alternate-day administration and ultimately to complete discontinuation (see below).

ALTERNATE-DAY GLUCOCORTICOSTEROID THERAPY. Many inflammatory diseases can be maintained in clinical remission by alternate-day glucocorticosteroid therapy. The rationale is to deliver at regular intervals (every 48 hours) a dose of a short-acting steroid that will maintain the suppression of disease activity while avoiding the toxic side effects associated with single daily dose or divided daily dose regimens. The drug is administered in a single dose in the morning at a time when the normal endogenous cortisol level is at its peak, with maximal feedback suppression of ACTH secretion already occurring. By evening, the administered drug is no longer present in the circulation and the HPA axis will secrete ACTH, which in turn will stimulate the secretion of endogenous cortisol the following morning, when the patient will not be receiving exogenous hormone. In this way, the normal endogenous cortisol levels will maintain the patient's homeostatic function on the "off" day of exogenous steroid. The following day the drug is again administered, and the pharmacologic effect is apparently sufficient to maintain the disease in clinical remission.

It may be necessary to initiate exogenous hormone therapy on a daily basis or even in divided doses to induce remission of an active inflammatory process. However, once the process is adequately suppressed, doses of steroid as widely spaced as 48 hours may be adequate to maintain the disease in remission.

The logistics of conversion from a daily to an alternate-day steroid regimen are difficult. Two common pitfalls are attempting to accomplish the conversion too rapidly and failing to give a sufficient amount of drug on the "on" day. On the basis of the plasma half-life of prednisone, the highest practical single dose that one could administer on an alternate-day basis without suppressing the cortisol cycle on the "off" day is 120 mg. In actual practice, however, 80 to 100 mg is probably maximal. Clearly, a short-acting agent must be used, since administration of a long-acting agent such as dexamethasone on alternate days is intrinsically contradictory. Thus, if a patient is receiving 60 mg of prednisone per day, the daily dose is gradually tapered to 40 or 50 mg per day. At this point, the dose on the ultimate "on" day is immediately doubled to 80 or 100 mg. The dose on the ultimate "off" day is gradually tapered by 5- to 10-mg decrements over several cycles until it reaches 20 mg, and then by 2.5-mg decrements until the patient is receiving no drug that day. The rapidity with which the dosage is tapered on the "off" day varies considerably among patients and depends on the underlying disease and the tolerance of the patient to the tapering process. The judicious use of nonsteroidal anti-inflammatory agents during the tapering process can often prove most helpful. Once the patient has reached a true alternate-day regimen, the dose on the "on" day is maintained for variable periods of time, depending upon individual patient factors, and then it, too, can be tapered to the lowest possible dose required to maintain remission, which may be complete discontinuation of therapy. Although not every patient who requires glucocorticosteroids will be maintained on an alternate-day regimen, such a regimen should be attempted when possible.

ACTH VERSUS GLUCOCORTICOSTEROIDS. There is no convincing evidence that ACTH is superior to glucocorticosteroids in the treatment of any disease. Furthermore, glucocorticosteroids are preferable to ACTH for a number of reasons. ACTH must be injected, whereas glucocorticosteroids can be administered orally. The ACTH effect depends on the stimulation of release of variable amounts of cortisol from the adrenal gland, whereas the dose of administered glucocorticosteroid can be precisely controlled. In addition, ACTH stimulates other hormones, such as androgens and mineralocorticoids, which may have undesirable side effects. Also, administration of ACTH may result in hyperpigmentation.

APPROACH TO HPA AXIS SUPPRESSION. One of the most disputed topics in glucocorticosteroid therapy is the duration of steroid administration that will result in HPA axis suppression. A closely related topic is the duration of HPA axis suppression following cessation of steroid therapy. It is virtually impossible to identify the shortest period of therapy or the smallest dose at which clinically significant suppression of the HPA axis will occur. The most conservative estimates will be given here.

Patients who have received the equivalent of 30 mg of prednisone per day for more than a week should be considered to have sustained suppression of the HPA axis. This may be asymptomatic except under conditions of severe stress. In patients who have been exposed to high doses of glucocorticosteroids daily over a prolonged period of time, as much as 12 months may be required following cessation of therapy before normal hormonal response to stress returns. If patients who are suspected of HPA axis suppression are to be subjected to severe stress such as a major surgical procedure, they should receive parenteral hydrocortisone in doses of 100 mg every four to six hours during surgery and for several days thereafter, depending on the recovery period.

It is possible to determine the integrity of the HPA axis in a patient who has recently received glucocorticosteroid therapy. The standard test is to administer 50 units of ACTH as a constant intravenous infusion over six to eight hours and measure the resulting rise in plasma cortisol. Alternatively, synthetic ACTH (beta 1-24 ACTH) can be given as a rapid intravenous infusion (250 μg), with measurement of plasma cortisol at 30 minutes and one hour after injection. In patients with normal adrenal glands, plasma cortisol levels should rise to at least 30 μg per milliliter.

Once glucocorticosteroid therapy has been withdrawn, recovery from suppression of the HPA axis is a gradual process, the rate of which varies considerably among patients. There are no proven manipulations to hasten this process. Hypothalamic-pituitary function returns before adrenocortical function. The use of ACTH has not been proved to hasten recovery of HPA function. Conversion to alternate-day steroid therapy prior to withdrawal generally leads to a less symptomatic recovery, but it does not hasten the process. Suppression of the HPA axis can be associated with a diverse array of symptoms.

WITHDRAWAL SYNDROMES. Withdrawal from glucocorticosteroid therapy may result in both subjective and objective manifestations of adrenal suppression. Features of withdrawal may include lethargy, weakness, anorexia, nausea, fever, arthralgia, orthostatic hypotension with syncope, hypoglycemia, weight loss, and desquamation of the skin. The entire symptom complex may relate to HPA axis suppression, for which replacement therapy is indicated. However, exacerbation of certain underlying diseases may manifest similar symptoms. It is essential for the physician to monitor the patient closely, with appropriate diagnostic measures aimed at determining disease activity as well as integrity of the HPA axis. If the patient manifests HPA axis suppression, reinstitution of glucocorticosteroid therapy with more gradual withdrawal is indicated.

A number of patients may manifest a physical or psychologic dependence on glucocorticosteroids and yet have neither exacerbation of underlying disease nor suppression of normal HPA function. If the dependence is psychologic, appropriate counseling and encouragement are indicated. However, physical dependence may exist in the face of normal HPA function, since the tissues may have been acclimated to high levels of glucocorticosteroids for such a period of time that, despite "normal" levels of cortisol, the patient experiences symptoms of steroid deprivation. Under these circumstances, reinstitution of physiologic doses of a short-acting drug such as prednisone, followed by a more protracted tapering period, may be indicated. Finally, certain patients may manifest biochemical evidence of HPA axis suppression without evidence of exacerbation of underlying disease and without symptoms.

COMPLICATIONS OF GLUCOCORTICOSTEROID THERAPY. The major limiting factor in the use of glucocorticosteroid therapy is the wide array of deleterious side effects that may occur. The frequency and severity of glucocortico-

TABLE 30–2. COMPLICATIONS OF GLUCOCORTICOSTEROID THERAPY

Central nervous system	Endocrinologic
Pseudotumor cerebri	Suppression of HPA axis
Psychiatric disorders	Growth failure
Musculoskeletal	Secondary amenorrhea
Osteoporosis with spontaneous fractures	Metabolic
Aseptic necrosis of bone	Hyperglycemia and unmasking of genetic predisposition to diabetes mellitus
Myopathy	Nonketotic hyperosmolar states
Ocular	Hyperlipidemia
Glaucoma	Alterations of fat distribution (typical cushingoid appearance)
Cataracts	Fatty infiltration of the liver
Gastrointestinal	Drug interactions (decreased anticoagulant effect of ethyl biscoumacetate)
Peptic ulceration	Fibroblast inhibition
Intestinal perforation	Inhibition of wound healing
Pancreatitis	Subcutaneous tissue atrophy (striae, purpura, ecchymosis)
Cardiovascular and fluid balance	Suppression of host defenses
Hypertension	Immunosuppression, anergy
Sodium and fluid retention	Effects on phagocyte kinetics and function
Hypokalemic alkalosis	Increased incidence of infections
Hypersensitivity reactions	
Urticaria	
Anaphylaxis	

steroid-related complications are directly related to the dose, duration, and schedule of therapy. Although all the complications listed in Table 30–2 have been amply documented, the direct cause-effect relationship between drug administration and complications has not been equally convincing for each of the complications. For example, there is a high incidence of spontaneous peptic ulcer in certain diseases that are treated with glucocorticosteroids, particularly rheumatoid arthritis. In addition, other gastrointestinal irritants such as the nonsteroidal anti-inflammatory agents are often administered concomitantly with the steroid. In the absence of adequately controlled studies, it is difficult to determine whether glucocorticosteroids increase the incidence of peptic ulceration. Also, daily administration of steroid is associated with an increase in infectious disease complications. Several diseases that are treated with steroids, such as lymphoid malignancies and systemic lupus erythematosus, have defects of host defense. These act synergistically with the steroid-induced compromise of host defenses to result in an increased incidence of opportunistic infections. On the other hand, patients with asthma who are treated with steroids do not seem to have an increased incidence of infections. This may be related to the otherwise normal host defenses of these patients as well as to the low doses of steroid usually employed. By contrast, osteoporosis and cataracts are commonly and directly related to glucocorticosteroid therapy.

Questions often arise about the effects of steroid therapy on delayed cutaneous hypersensitivity responses. This effect is variable and dose related. Generally, patients receiving less than 80 mg of prednisone on alternate days have intact delayed cutaneous hypersensitivity. By contrast, patients receiving daily steroid will generally become anergic if the dose is 15 mg of prednisone or greater, with the onset of anergy usually within days after initiation of therapy. Following cessation of therapy, if all other factors involved in delayed hypersensitivity are intact, responses generally return within ten days to two weeks.

Glucocorticosteroids are not considered to increase teratogenic risk among newborns of mothers who receive steroids during pregnancy. However, such infants should be monitored for adrenal insufficiency during the neonatal period. Also, since glucocorticosteroids are excreted in breast milk, inhibition of endogenous steroid production as well as growth suppression can occur in infants who are breast fed by mothers receiving the hormone.

Baxter JD, Rousseau GG: Glucocorticoid Hormone Action. New York, Springer-Verlag, 1979. *An excellent book with comprehensive and sophisticated coverage of basic mechanisms of glucocorticoid action. One of the outstanding works on steroid hormone action, with contributions by recognized leaders in the field.*

Dixon RB, Christy NP: On the various forms of corticosteroid withdrawal syndrome. Am J Med 68:224, 1980. *An excellent, lucidly written discussion of corticosteroid withdrawal syndromes, with use of case presentations as example.*

Fauci AS: Alternate-day corticosteroid therapy. Am J Med 64:729, 1978. *Concise editorial discussion on usefulness and limitations of alternate-day glucocorticosteroid therapy.*

Fauci AS, Dale DC, Balow JE: Glucocorticosteroid therapy: Mechanisms of action and clinical considerations. Ann Intern Med 84:304, 1976. *An extensive review of mechanisms of action of glucocorticosteroids as they relate to therapeutic efficacy in the treatment of inflammatory and immunologically mediated diseases. Practical outlines of the design and modification of therapeutic regimens.*

Kehrl JH, Fauci AS: The clinical use of glucocorticoids. Ann Allergy 50:2, 1983. *An updated review article on the theoretic and practical aspects of the use of corticosteroids in clinical medicine.*

Thorn GW: Clinical considerations in the use of corticosteroids. N Engl J Med 274:775, 1966. *This superb article remains the classic treatise on the rational use of corticosteroid therapy.*

Udelsman R, Ramp J, Gallucci WT, et al.: Adaptation during surgical stress. A reevaluation of the role of glucocorticoids. J Clin Invest 77:1377, 1986. *An updated article establishing that the permissive actions of physiologic glucocorticoid replacement are both necessary and sufficient to tolerate surgical stress.*

Zora JA, Zimmerman D, Carey TL, et al.: Hypothalamic-pituitary-adrenal axis suppression after short-term, high-dose glucocorticoid therapy in children. *This updated study firmly establishes that short-term, high-dose glucocorticoid therapy produces only transient suppression of the hypothalamic-pituitary-adrenal axis.*

31 PHARMACOLOGIC PRINCIPLES RELATED TO THE AUTONOMIC NERVOUS SYSTEM

Robert J. Lefkowitz

ORGANIZATION AND PHYSIOLOGY OF THE AUTONOMIC NERVOUS SYSTEM

The autonomic nervous system regulates the functions of smooth muscle, the heart, and glands. It is composed of two major divisions, termed sympathetic and parasympathetic, which are anatomically, physiologically, and biochemically quite distinct. Activation of the sympathetic system leads to the classic "flight or fight" responses of tachycardia, increased force of cardiac contraction, vasoconstriction, mydriasis, bronchodilation, and hyperglycemia. Parasympathetic nervous activity results in a situation better exemplified by "an old man sleeping after dinner," with slow heart rate, noisy respirations (caused by bronchial constriction), meiosis, and saliva running out of the corner of his mouth. Auscultation of the abdomen would reveal loud bowel sounds.

Anatomically, the *sympathetic nervous system* is composed of pathways that originate from neurons with cell bodies in the "thoracolumbar" segments of the spinal cord. These preganglionic neurons synapse in the sympathetic ganglia with postganglionic neurons, which in turn innervate end-organs, including vascular, gastrointestinal, and genitourinary smooth muscle and the heart.

By contrast, the *parasympathetic pathways* originate from neurons that have their cell bodies in the "craniosacral" portions of the neuraxis, including the midbrain, the medulla, and the sacral portions of the spinal cord. Preganglionic fibers synapse in peripheral ganglia that are in general closer to innervated organs than is the case with the sympathetic system.

Communication between neurons in the autonomic nervous system, and between neurons and effector cells, is mediated by chemicals called neurotransmitters. Acetylcholine encodes communication between preganglionic and postganglionic neurons in both the sympathetic and parasympathetic nervous systems. Norepinephrine is generally the neurotransmitter at sympathetic postganglionic nerve endings, whereas acetylcholine is the transmitter at parasympathetic postganglionic nerve endings.

The *adrenal medulla* is anatomically and functionally analogous to the sympathetic ganglia. Its chromaffin cells are innervated by typical preganglionic fibers. The major product of the adrenal medulla is epinephrine, which is secreted into the bloodstream. Epinephrine has many of the same biologic activities as the sympathetic neurotransmitter norepinephrine. Because of the strong analogies and the concerted physiologic functioning of the sympathetic system and the adrenal medulla in situations such as stress or fright, these two components are often considered a unified "sympathoadrenal system."

NEUROTRANSMITTERS. A great deal is known about the biochemical basis of neurotransmission as mediated by norepinephrine in the sympathetic and acetylcholine in the parasympathetic system. Several discrete processes have been identified and elucidated. These include the mechanisms of (1) biosynthesis of transmitter in nerves, (2) storage of transmitter within granules in sympathetic and parasympathetic nerve endings, (3) release of transmitter at synapses, (4) interaction of transmitter with receptors on effector cells, and (5) termination of transmitter activity by reuptake and/or metabolizing processes.

There is a great diversity of physiologic autonomic effects and, because so much is known about neurotransmitter function, therapeutic interventions that modify autonomic function are among the most rational and important at the physician's disposal. For both the sympathetic and parasympathetic nervous system an understanding of the basic organization and physiology permits predictions of not only therapeutic but also adverse effects of a wide variety of drugs. The purpose of this chapter is to delineate the general principles underlying pharmacologic approaches that modify autonomic nervous system function. Although examples are provided, the reader is referred to other chapters for details of dosage, administration, and specific indications of individual drugs in disease states.

Each of the processes described above, including biosynthesis, uptake and storage in granules, release, receptor binding, and degradation of neurotransmitters, is susceptible to pharmacologic manipulation. A much wider variety of therapeutic interventions is possible in the sympathetic system than in the parasympathetic system, and these are summarized in Figure 31–1.

For the parasympathetic system the major clinical interventions involve drugs that act as agonists or antagonists at postsynaptic muscarinic receptors. Agents are also available that, by inhibiting the destruction of acetylcholine, lead to cholinergic agonist effects at postsynaptic receptors (cholinesterase inhibitors). Botulinum toxin appears to cause neuromuscular blockade by blocking release of acetylcholine from cholinergic nerves.

ADRENERGIC AND CHOLINERGIC RECEPTORS

Of the therapeutic interventions indicated in Figure 31–1, the most important relate to drugs that stimulate or block the postsynaptic receptors for adrenergic and cholinergic neurotransmitters. The concept that there are specific receptor molecules that mediate the effects of hormones has been popular throughout most of this century. This hypothesis has gained additional support over the past decade from radioligand binding studies, which have permitted the direct identification of these sites in cells with radioactively labeled drugs. Some of these receptors have been purified, and their genes have been cloned, leading to elucidation of their complete primary amino acid sequences.

Any discussion about receptors depends on certain essential pharmacologic concepts. Adrenergic receptors are the cellular sites at which catecholamines or related drugs are initially bound. The binding of drugs with adrenergic receptors induces changes in the receptors, which then lead to a series of events in the cell, resulting in the characteristic physiologic effects of the drug. Thus adrenergic receptors are recognition sites on the plasma membrane that transduce the interaction of catecholamines with the cell into a physiologic response. Agonist drugs are those capable of inducing a response. A "full" agonist causes a maximal response, whereas a "partial" agonist causes a qualitatively similar response of lesser magnitude. An "antagonist" is a drug that interacts with the receptor but elicits no response on its own. However, by occupying the receptor an antagonist may reduce the effect of an agonist. The "intrinsic activity" of a drug is a measure of its maximal effect. The intrinsic activities of full agonists are defined to be 1.0, whereas those of antagonists are 0. Partial agonists have intrinsic activities greater than 0 but less than 1.

The interaction of a drug with a receptor involves the notion of affinity or potency. Affinity is a measure of the avidity or tightness with which a drug combines with a receptor. The greater the affinity of a drug for a receptor, the lower the concentration of the drug necessary to occupy any specified fraction of the receptors. The affinity of a drug is unrelated to its intrinsic activity. Thus some drugs may have very great affinity for a receptor but virtually no intrinsic activity, e.g., potent antagonists.

ALPHA- AND BETA-ADRENERGIC RECEPTORS. Modern concepts concerning adrenergic receptors, the sites of action of epinephrine and norepinephrine, have their origin in the work of Raymond Ahlquist in 1948. He suggested that there were two main classes of adrenergic receptors, which he termed alpha and beta. This demarcation was based on the relative potencies of several agonist drugs for stimulation of physiologic responses in several tissues. The two major patterns observed were epinephrine>norepinephrine>>isoproterenol (alpha) and isoproterenol>epinephrine>norepinephrine (beta). He suggested that two distinct types of adrenergic receptors (alpha and beta) mediated responses displaying distinct potency series. Virtually all adrenergic responses fell into one or the other category. Table 31–1 lists some typical alpha and beta receptor–mediated adrenergic responses.

Although alpha- and beta-adrenergic receptors were originally defined by their agonist potency series, highly specific antagonists were subsequently developed, such as propranolol for the beta-adrenergic receptors and phentolamine for the alpha receptors. Refinements in the classification of adrenergic receptors have occurred over the past three decades with the realization that there are subtypes of both alpha- and beta-adrenergic receptors. For the beta-adrenergic receptors these were originally distinguished based on relative potencies of epinephrine and norepinephrine. Thus at beta$_1$-adrenergic receptors, such as those mediating positive inotropic effects in the heart, epinephrine and norepinephrine are of similar potency. By contrast, at beta$_2$-adrenergic receptors, such as those found in vascular and bronchial smooth muscle, epinephrine is much more potent than norepinephrine.

Beta$_1$- and beta$_2$-adrenergic receptors both appear to function by mediating stimulation of the plasma membrane-bound enzyme adenylate cyclase. The cyclic adenosine monophosphate (cAMP) generated in response to such stimulation leads to phosphorylation of key target proteins by cAMP-dependent protein kinases. Alteration in the functioning of such proteins as a result of phosphorylation presumably then leads to the

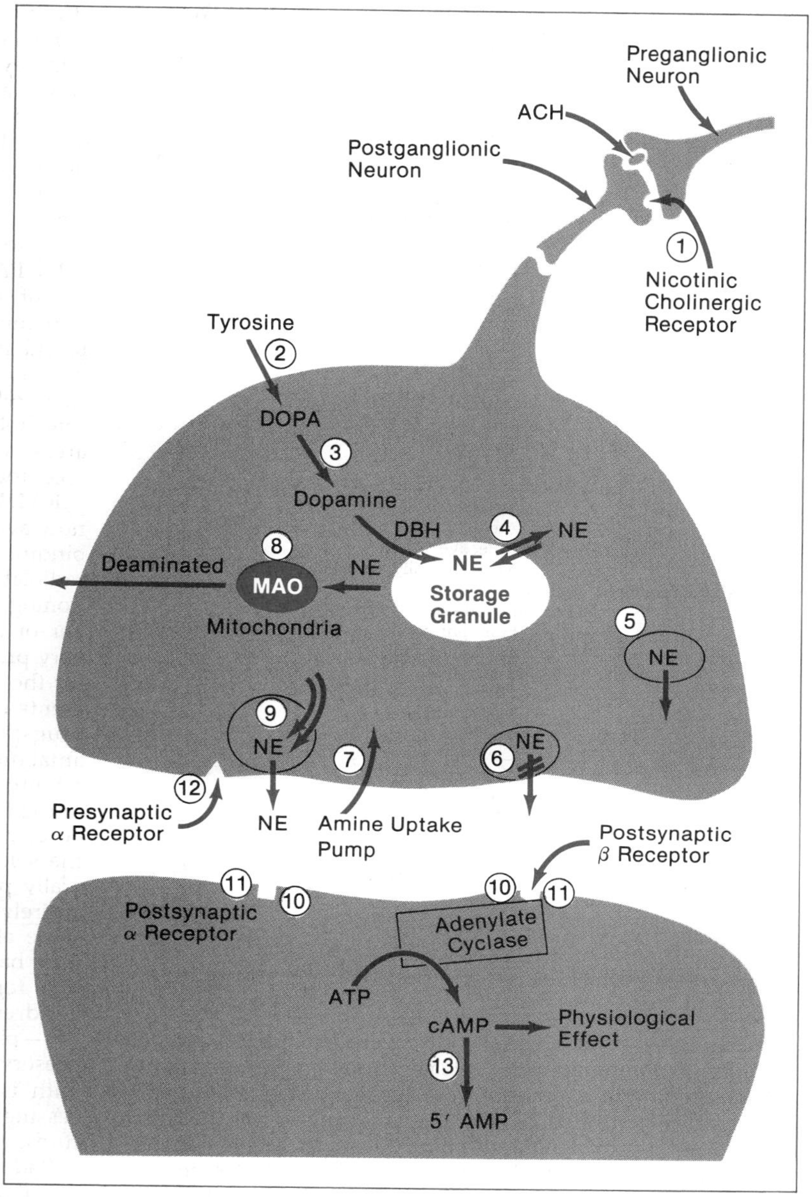

FIGURE 31–1. Therapeutic interventions in the peripheral adrenergic nervous system. Abbreviations: ACH = acetylcholine; DBH = dopamine beta hydroxylase; DOPA = dihydroxyphenylalanine; NE = norepinephrine; MAO = monoamine oxidase. (1) Competitive antagonism of nicotinic cholinergic receptors on postganglionic neuron in autonomic ganglia, e.g., trimethaphan. (2) Inhibition of transmitter (norepinephrine) synthesis, e.g., alpha methyl-p-tyrosine. (3) Drugs that enter the normal biosynthetic pathway and are transformed into "false neurotransmitters," e.g., alpha-methyldopa→→alpha-methylnorepinephrine. (4) Drugs that prevent the storage of transmitter in granules by inhibiting transport across storage granule membrane, e.g., reserpine. (5) Drugs that deplete transmitter from granules by displacement, e.g., guanethidine. (6) Drugs that inhibit the release of norepinephrine, e.g., bretylium. (7) Drugs that deplete neuronal norepinephrine by blocking the amine transport system of the neuronal membrane, e.g., cocaine or imipramine. Another major mechanism for the termination of norepinephrine action is by metabolism by catechol-o-methyl transferase. (8) Inhibition of metabolic destruction of transmitter, e.g., monoamine oxidase inhibitors. Relation of enzyme inhibition to therapeutic effects not clear, e.g., pargyline. (9) Indirectly acting agonists that displace norepinephrine from storage granules, e.g., tyramine, amphetamine (solely indirect), ephedrine, and metaraminol (also have direct actions). (10) Blockade of postsynaptic alpha receptors (e.g., phentolamine, phenoxybenzamine, prazosin) or beta receptors (propranolol). (11) Agonists that occupy postsynaptic receptors and mimic the effect of the neurotransmitter, e.g., isoproterenol (beta), phenylephrine (alpha). (12) Presynaptic alpha-adrenergic receptors. Although agonists and antagonists that specifically act through these receptors are not in general use, some adverse effects of other drugs, e.g., tachycardia after phentolamine administration, may be due to occupancy of these receptors. (13) Inhibition of breakdown of cyclic AMP by phosphodiesterase, e.g., aminophylline.

characteristic physiologic or pharmacologic effects of beta-adrenergic drugs.

A number of agonist and antagonist drugs showing preferential selectivity (affinity) for $beta_1$- or $beta_2$-adrenergic receptors are known, and some of these are summarized in Table 31–2. Many drugs show no preference for one or the other receptor subtype. The clinical use of these drugs is

TABLE 31–1. SOME EXAMPLES OF ADRENERGIC RECEPTOR–MEDIATED RESPONSES

$Beta_1$-adrenergic receptors	
	Heart—positive inotropism
	Adipose tissue—lipolysis
$Beta_2$-adrenergic receptors	
	Vascular smooth muscle—relaxation
	Bronchial smooth muscle—relaxation
$Alpha_1$-adrenergic receptors	
	Vascular smooth muscle—contraction
$Alpha_2$-adrenergic receptors	
	Platelets—aggregation
	Presynaptic nerve terminal—inhibition of norepinephrine release
	Postsynaptic—vascular smooth muscle contraction, some vascular beds

discussed below. The beta-adrenergic receptor subtypes in various tissues are listed in Table 31–2.

Alpha-adrenergic receptor subtypes are even more distinct than the beta receptor subtypes, differing not only in pharmacologic specificity but also in biochemical mechanism of action. $Alpha_1$ or typical "postsynaptic" alpha receptors are found, for example, in vascular smooth muscle, where they mediate the vasoconstrictor effect of sympathetic nerve stimulation. Pharmacologically, such $alpha_1$ receptors are characterized by their very high affinity for certain alpha antagonists such as prazosin and phenoxybenzamine. Typical alpha-adrenergic agonists such as phenylephrine and methoxamine stimulate these $alpha_1$ receptors quite effectively. Although the molecular mechanisms mediating $alpha_1$-adrenergic receptor effects are not clearly understood at present, a distinct signaling system appears to be involved. This leads to the hydrolysis of polyphosphoinositides to two second messengers, inositol trisphosphate and diacylglycerol. Inositol trisphosphate leads to the release of intracellular calcium from intracellular stores, whereas diacylglycerol activates the ubiquitous enzyme protein kinase C.

A second major subclass of alpha-adrenergic receptors,

TABLE 31–2. EXAMPLES OF SOME DRUGS THAT INTERACT WITH ADRENERGIC RECEPTORS

A. Beta-adrenergic agonists		
	Not receptor subtype selective ($beta_1$ and $beta_2$)	
		Isoproterenol
		Epinephrine
	Relatively $beta_1$-adrenergic selective	
		Norepinephrine
		Dobutamine
	Relatively $beta_2$-adrenergic selective	
		Metaproterenol
		Isoetharine
		Salbutamol
		Terbutaline
B. Beta-adrenergic antagonists		
	Not receptor subtype selective ($beta_1$ and $beta_2$)	
		Propranolol
		Alprenolol
		Timolol
		Pindolol
		Oxprenolol
		Nadolol
	Relatively $beta_1$ selective	
		Metoprolol
		Atenolol
	Relatively $beta_2$ selective	
		None clinically available
C. Alpha-adrenergic agonists		
	Not receptor subtype selective ($alpha_1$ and $alpha_2$)	
		Epinephrine
		Norepinephrine
	Relatively $alpha_1$ selective	
		Phenylephrine
		Methoxamine
	Relatively $alpha_2$ selective	
		Clonidine
		Guanabenz
		Guanfacine
D. Alpha-adrenergic antagonists		
	Not receptor subtype selective ($alpha_1$ and $alpha_2$)	
		Phentolamine
		Some ergot alkaloids
	$Alpha_1$ selective	
		Prazosin
	$Alpha_2$ selective	
		None clinically available

termed $alpha_2$, was originally discovered to play a role in regulating norepinephrine release from nerve terminals. While norepinephrine release from adrenergic nerve terminals is primarily controlled by the rate of firing of the neuron, norepinephrine in an autoinhibitory fashion acts to reduce the amount of norepinephrine released. This effect seems to be mediated by alpha-adrenergic receptors (since it is blocked by classic alpha-adrenergic antagonists) that have distinct pharmacologic characteristics and are possibly located on presynaptic sites on the nerve ending itself. Stimulation of these receptors by norepinephrine in the synaptic cleft serves to reduce the amount of norepinephrine released by subsequent nerve impulses.

In recent years alpha-adrenergic receptors with pharmacologic properties virtually identical to the "presynaptic" receptors described above have been found in a variety of "postsynaptic" locations, e.g., the platelet. In addition, $alpha_2$-adrenergic receptors play a distinct role in mediating effects on smooth muscle contraction in some vascular beds. Because $alpha_2$-adrenergic receptors may be found in both pre- and postsynaptic locations, it seems preferable to use the designations $alpha_1$ and $alpha_2$ rather than the earlier terminology of "presynaptic" and "postsynaptic" alpha receptors. Physiologic effects of $alpha_1$ and $alpha_2$ receptor stimulation are summarized in Table 31–1.

A variety of drugs demonstrate selective affinity for $alpha_2$ receptors. Among agonists the most notable examples are clonidine and related drugs. Yohimbine, a plant alkaloid antagonist, also is somewhat selective for $alpha_2$ receptors. The classic alpha-adrenergic antagonists phentolamine and the ergot alkaloids are not selective and possess comparable affinity for $alpha_1$ and $alpha_2$ receptors. Subtype selectivity of some alpha-adrenergic drugs is listed in Table 31–2.

In several model systems such as the platelet, stimulation of $alpha_2$-adrenergic receptors inhibits the enzyme adenylate cyclase. The resultant reduction in cellular cAMP levels mediates the alpha-adrenergic effect in question—in this case, platelet aggregation. It is not yet known whether adenylate cyclase inhibition is the common biochemical basis of all $alpha_2$-adrenergic effects. $Alpha_1$-adrenergic effects do not seem to involve modification of adenylate cyclase activity.

DOPAMINE RECEPTORS. Catecholamines are also capable of interacting with a third class of receptors termed dopamine receptors. Peripheral dopaminergic receptors are found in the renal and mesenteric vasculature, where they mediate vasodilation. These receptors are characterized by their relatively higher affinity for dopamine than for other catecholamines. Dopamine receptors are also found in certain areas of the brain, such as the corpus striatum. Dopaminergic receptors will not be considered further in this chapter.

RADIOLIGAND BINDING STUDIES. Direct methods are now available to measure adrenergic receptors by radioligand binding techniques. These techniques involve the use of radiolabeled drugs to tag the receptors in whole-cell or cell-homogenate preparations. Such studies have provided a number of insights of clinical relevance. These methods permit very precise and direct measurement of the affinities of drugs for the various adrenergic receptor subtypes. Such measurements indicate that even for presumably "subtype" selective drugs, the "selectivity" is only relative. Thus a $beta_1$ selective antagonist such as metoprolol has only 10- to 50-fold higher affinity for $beta_1$ receptors in the heart than for $beta_2$ receptors in the lung. As the dose of such a compound is raised, it will occupy increasing numbers of $beta_2$ as well as $beta_1$ receptors; the selectivity therefore is not absolute. Thus, it is not generally possible to block the $beta_1$ receptors in the heart and entirely spare the $beta_2$ receptors in the lung. By contrast, some $alpha_1$ receptor selective antagonists such as prazosin may have as much as 10,000-fold higher affinity for $alpha_1$ than for $alpha_2$ receptors.

Adrenergic receptor subtypes are distinct molecular entities—proteins—the pharmacologic properties of which are preserved even through extensive purification. In analogy with isoenzymes, they may represent "isoreceptors," possessing relatively subtle differences in their molecular structures.

Radioligand binding studies have also documented the wide distribution of binding sites throughout the central nervous system that have properties identical to the $beta_1$ and $beta_2$ and $alpha_1$ and $alpha_2$ receptor binding sites present in the peripheral nervous system. In most cases the physiologic role of these "central" adrenergic receptors is not known. It is, however, clear that $alpha_2$-adrenergic receptors in the vasomotor center act to decrease sympathetic outflow and hence sympathetic tone. This is possibly a major site of action of clonidine, an antihypertensive $alpha_2$ agonist.

PHYSIOLOGIC REGULATION OF RECEPTORS. Adrenergic receptors are subject to a wide variety of modulating influences that regulate their numbers and binding properties. For example, chronic exposure of beta receptors to high concentrations of agonists leads to a decrease in the number of beta-adrenergic receptors and a decrease in their efficiency for stimulating adenylate cyclase. The result is a decrease in beta-adrenergic responsiveness often termed *desensitization*. Similar findings have been documented for certain alpha-adrenergic receptors. This may explain the decreased responsiveness of asthmatics to chronically administered beta-agonist bronchodilators. Antagonists do not cause such desensitization effects. Indeed, hypersensitization may occur when receptors are chronically occupied by antagonists. Under such circumstances the number of receptors on cells may increase with the potential for supersensitivity when the antagonist drug is discontinued. (See below for discussion of "propranolol withdrawal syndrome.")

In certain animal models the number of beta receptors may be increased in hyperthyroidism. This provides one possible mechanism for the salutary effect of propranolol in relieving the hyperadrenergic symptoms of hyperthyroidism.

ACETYLCHOLINE RECEPTORS. Most of the principles discussed in relation to receptors for the sympathetic nervous system also apply to receptors for the parasympathetic system. Receptors for acetylcholine appear to be of two major types defined in terms of affinities for interaction with a variety of selective antagonists. The cholinergic receptors present on autonomic effector cells are of one major type termed "muscarinic" cholinergic receptors. These receptors are blocked by muscarinic antagonists such as atropine and stimulated not only by cholinergic agonists such as carbachol but also by drugs that prolong the effect of acetylcholine by blocking its hydrolysis.

The second major type of receptor for acetylcholine is termed "nicotinic" and mediates the effects of the neurotransmitter in autonomic ganglia (sympathetic and parasympathetic) as well as at neuromuscular junctions. The cholinergic receptors of the autonomic ganglion are blocked by antagonists such as hexamethonium or trimethaphan. These nicotinic receptors can be distinguished from the nicotinic receptors of skeletal muscle, which are selectively blocked by antagonists such as decamethonium. Thus there are in effect two subtypes of nicotinic receptors. These are sometimes referred to as N_1 (autonomic ganglia) and N_2 (neuromuscular junction).

The various types of cholinergic receptors have also been studied by ligand binding techniques. The different types of receptors appear to be distinct biochemical entities subject to regulation by excessive stimulation (tolerance or desensitization) as well as other factors.

Nicotinic receptors appear to function by regulating Na^+ conductance and consequent depolarization. By contrast, muscarinic cholinergic receptors may function by inhibiting adenylate cyclase in analogy with the alpha$_2$-adrenergic receptors that inhibit adenylate cyclase in the platelet.

SYMPATHOMIMETIC AMINES

In addition to the various amines that act directly on adrenergic receptors, there are several drugs that appear to act indirectly by causing the release of endogenous catecholamines from nerve terminals. Their pharmacologic effects are therefore similar to those of norepinephrine or epinephrine, i.e., they cause beta-adrenergic stimulation of the heart and alpha-adrenergic mediated vasoconstriction. These drugs include metaraminol, mephentermine, and ephedrine. Since these drugs work by causing secretion of endogenous transmitter, their prolonged use is associated with tachyphylaxis resulting from depletion of transmitter stores.

The most important therapeutic effects of epinephrine and norepinephrine are due to their actions on the heart and smooth muscle. Isoproterenol, epinephrine, and norepinephrine all have strong positive inotropic and chronotropic effects caused by interaction with cardiac beta receptors. In addition, epinephrine and norepinephrine generally have a vasoconstrictor effect (vascular alpha receptors), whereas isoproterenol is a strong and selective vasodilator by virtue of its interaction with vascular beta$_2$ receptors but not with vasoconstrictor alpha receptors. Since epinephrine can also combine with the beta$_2$ receptors, it may also cause vasodilation under certain circumstances. These catecholamines, as well as several related agents such as dopamine and dobutamine, may be used to stabilize the circulation in some forms of shock (see Ch. 44 for details).

Beta-adrenergic sympathomimetic amines may also be used to increase cardiac rate and improve atrioventricular conduction in patients with heart block. Alpha agonists such as metaraminol may be used to elevate blood pressure transiently to revert paroxysmal atrial tachycardia to normal sinus rhythm by provoking a reflex vagal discharge that may slow the heart rate. Their use in such circumstances should always be by slow intravenous infusion with careful monitoring of blood pressure.

Adrenergic agonists used in the treatment of hypertension include clonidine and guanabenz, which are relatively selective alpha agonists that appear to have primarily a central nervous system site of action. Rapid discontinuation of antihypertensive treatment with clonidine has occasionally been reported to be associated with marked rebound hypertension. This syndrome may be associated with transient elevations in catecholamine release, and hence alpha-adrenergic antagonists may be of use in its treatment.

A major application of beta-adrenergic agonists is in the treatment of asthma. Epinephrine by injection and isoproterenol by inhalation have long been used to achieve bronchodilation by stimulation of beta$_2$-adrenergic receptors. In recent years a number of beta$_2$ selective agonists have been developed. These include isoetharine, terbutaline, salbutamol, and metaproterenol. These agents have the advantage of causing somewhat less beta$_1$-adrenergic receptor stimulation and hence have less tendency to cause tachycardia for any given level of beta$_2$ stimulation (bronchodilation).

Adverse side effects are often a predictable consequence of the interaction of adrenergic agonists with adrenergic receptors of similar specificity in organs other than those in which specific therapeutic effects are sought. Some examples include tachycardia with bronchodilators and ectopic rhythms after inotropic or vasopressor agents.

ADRENERGIC ANTAGONISTS

BETA-ADRENERGIC BLOCKERS. Beta-adrenergic antagonists are among the most widely used drugs in the practice of medicine. As with adrenergic agonists, both therapeutic and adverse effects of beta-adrenergic antagonists are readily understood in terms of their competitive occupancy of beta-adrenergic receptors. Propranolol is the prototypic example of a beta antagonist. Propranolol and a number of related compounds also possess a direct "membrane stabilizing," "local anesthetic, or quinidine-like" effect, which gives them additional utility in the treatment of certain arrhythmias. These direct membrane effects can be dissociated from beta-blocking properties by the fact that the receptor blocking effects reside largely in the (–) stereoisomer, whereas the membrane effects are present equally in both the (+) and (–) stereoisomers. These membrane effects also appear to require somewhat higher blood concentrations.

Some, but not all, beta blockers also possess intrinsic sympathomimetic properties; i.e., they have intrinsic activities greater than 0. This means they are weak "partial agonists." Several of the earliest beta-adrenergic antagonists such as dichlorisoproterenol possessed such activity to an extent that markedly limited their therapeutic utility. Propranolol does not possess intrinsic sympathomimetic effects; it is a pure antagonist. Of the commonly used beta blockers, only pindolol and acebutolol have significant intrinsic sympathomimetic effects.

Propranolol is readily absorbed from the gastrointestinal tract, but much of the compound is immediately extracted from the portal circulation by the liver. There is marked patient-to-patient variability in hepatic metabolism, which leads to great differences in plasma drug concentrations at any given dose. An important metabolite of propranolol, 4-OH propranolol, is very active biologically, although it has a shorter half-life. Most of the propranolol in the circulation is bound to plasma proteins.

In normal persons the half-life of propranolol is quite short. The usual dosage range is 40 to 320 mg per day, with great variations observed in the dose required for optimal effects.

Propranolol has generally been administered orally four times daily because of its short half-life. However, especially in the treatment of hypertension, twice-a-day dosage is adequate. In contrast to the hepatic metabolism and short plasma half-life of propranolol and metoprolol is the renal excretion of atenolol and nadolol in largely unchanged form. As a result, these drugs are eliminated from the plasma much more slowly, which may permit once-a-day dosage.

It is believed that abrupt withdrawal of propranolol may be followed in some patients by a transient period of "supersensitivity" to catecholamines. This is especially important in patients with ischemic coronary artery disease. This phenomenon has been called the "propranolol withdrawal syndrome" and may be manifested by arrhythmias, angina, and myocardial infarction. The existence of such a syndrome and the possible basis for such supersensitivity is controversial. Experimental work in animals and humans indicates that propranolol therapy may be associated with an increase in beta receptor number in certain tissues. Many physicians prefer to taper the dosage of propranolol rather than to stop it abruptly, especially in patients with coronary artery disease.

Propranolol has equal affinity for $beta_1$- and $beta_2$-adrenergic receptors. The same is true of timolol, alprenolol,* oxprenolol,* and pindolol. In recent years several antagonists have been developed that have relative selectivity for the $beta_1$ receptors in the heart. The first of these, practolol, led to a variety of ocular, dermatologic, and other adverse effects that precluded its use in humans. More recently several other agents such as metoprolol, atenolol, and tolamolol* have become available and seem to possess some $beta_1$ selectivity. The indications for and clinical pharmacology of metoprolol are similar to those of propranolol. The potential advantage of such agents is the decreased tendency to provoke bronchospasm in susceptible subjects compared with propranolol (see below). Table 31–3 compares the important properties of several of the beta-adrenergic receptor-blocking drugs.

There are several major indications for the use of beta-adrenergic antagonist agents. In general, all of the agents have similar activities regardless of selectivity or partial agonism.

Angina. The salutary effect appears to be due primarily to a reduction of myocardial oxygen consumption as a consequence of decreased pulse rate, myocardial contractility, and, in hypertensive patients, blood pressure. Propranolol is one of the mainstays of medical therapy in many patients, and its effects may be additive with those of nitrates.

Hypertension. Beta blockers have become a very important part of antihypertensive therapeutic programs. They are used either as first-line monotherapy or often added as a second drug to a diuretic. Despite their proven efficacy, the mode of action of the drugs remains uncertain and may be related to decreased cardiac output, decreased renin release, central nervous system mechanisms, or other effects. These drugs are particularly effective in combination with a peripheral vasodilator such as hydralazine, since the reflex and possibly deleterious cardiac stimulation evoked by the vasodilator is blocked by the beta antagonist. Another positive feature of propranolol as an antihypertensive drug is that it is generally well tolerated, which is important when chronic therapy and patient compliance are required, as in hypertension.

*Investigational drug for this purpose.

Arrhythmias. Antiarrhythmic effects of beta blockers are the result of both beta receptor blockade and quinidine-like effects. The drug is most useful in situations in which ectopic rhythms caused by excess catecholamines (e.g., pheochromocytoma) or digitalis are involved. (See also "Hyperthyroidism," below.) In emergency situations propranolol can be administered intravenously in doses that are a small fraction of the usual oral dose.

Hyperthyroidism. Certain manifestations of hyperthyroidism such as hyperdynamic circulation, palpitations, and tremors mimic a "hyper–beta-adrenergic" state and may reflect alterations in the beta receptors themselves. These symptomatic manifestations are often dramatically improved by beta-adrenergic antagonists. A particular indication is in the circumstance of "thyroid storm" with difficult-to-control metabolic (e.g., hyperthermia) and cardiovascular (e.g., paroxysmal atrial fibrillation with rapid ventricular response) complications. Digitalis may be particularly ineffective in treating the rapid ventricular response to atrial arrhythmias in such patients, and beta blockers are often uniquely useful. This is one circumstance in which propranolol administration in the presence of congestive heart failure is not contraindicated, since it may reverse the underlying cause (very rapid arrhythmia).

Other Uses. Beta antagonists have also been found useful in circumstances in which ventricular outflow is compromised by hypertrophy and transient increases in cardiac contractility such as hypertrophic cardiomyopathy and tetralogy of Fallot. In addition, propranolol is used for prophylaxis of migraine.

Also, some beta blockers are used after myocardial infarction, since they have been shown to decrease the incidence of both reinfarction and sudden death.

Several other uses, such as benign familial tremor, are promising but currently still under investigation. The beta blocker timolol is used topically for the treatment of open-angle glaucoma.

Beta blockers are also used in the symptomatic treatment of certain of the manifestations of pheochromocytoma. However, they should never be used in the absence of concomitant alpha-adrenergic blockade, since marked hypertension may result.

Side Effects. The adverse effects of beta blockers, like their therapeutic actions, are largely consequences of their competitive occupancy of beta-adrenergic receptors. These include depression of cardiac contractility resulting from loss of normal sympathetic support with precipitation of previously latent or incipient congestive heart failure; worsening or precipitation of high degrees of heart block; and bronchoconstriction caused by blockade of bronchial $beta_2$-adrenergic receptors in susceptible individuals. When bronchoconstric-

TABLE 31–3. PROPERTIES OF SOME BETA-ADRENERGIC RECEPTOR–BLOCKING DRUGS

Drug	Relative Potency (Propranolol = 1)	Relative $Beta_1$ Selectivity	Intrinsic Sympathomimetic Activity	Membrane-Stabilizing Activity	Plasma Half-Life (hrs)
Acebutolol	0.3	+	+	0	3–4
Atenolol	1	+	0	0	6–9
Metoprolol	1	+	0	0	3–4
Nadolol	1	0	0	0	14–24
Pindolol	6	0	+ + +	+	3–4
Propranolol	1	0	0	+ +	3.5–6
Timolol	6	0	0	0	3–4

tion occurs, the usual beta-agonist bronchodilators may be ineffective owing to the very high affinity of propranolol for beta-adrenergic receptors. In such circumstances, drugs such as aminophylline, which dilate airway smooth muscle without the need for beta receptor interactions, are particularly useful.

In diabetics requiring insulin, propranolol may, in rare cases, cause or worsen hypoglycemia by interfering with beta-adrenergic–mediated hyperglycemic counter-regulatory mechanisms. It may also mask those symptoms of hypoglycemia that are mediated by beta-adrenergic stimulation, such as tachycardia or pupillary dilation. The presence of incipient congestive heart failure, heart block or impaired cardiac conduction, history of bronchoconstriction, or brittle diabetes may represent contraindications to the use of beta-adrenergic antagonists.

Other reported adverse effects with beta blockers include lethargy, depression, lightheadedness, and mild diarrhea.

ALPHA-ADRENERGIC ANTAGONISTS. Alpha-adrenergic blockers are used much less frequently than are the beta antagonists. Until recently the two most commonly employed agents have been phentolamine and phenoxybenzamine. Phentolamine is a classic rapidly reversible (i.e., "competitive") antagonist, whereas phenoxybenzamine is an irreversible ("noncompetitive") alpha-adrenergic antagonist. Thus, after occupancy of alpha receptors by phenoxybenzamine, a stable covalent bond forms between the drug and some portion of the receptor by an alkylation mechanism. This may lead to a very prolonged duration of action.

The major indication for these two drugs is in patients with known or suspected pheochromocytoma. As described in Ch. 242, phentolamine may be used in diagnosing pheochromocytoma, in which its injection leads to a marked drop in blood pressure. This potentially hazardous maneuver is only rarely indicated. Both phenoxybenzamine and phentolamine are used to prevent the hypertension of pheochromocytoma, for which they represent highly specific therapy. They are particularly useful in the perioperative period, when large fluctuations of serum catecholamines may occur (Ch. 242). Other than in patients with pheochromocytoma, non–subtype selective alpha antagonists such as phentolamine do not appear particularly useful in the treatment of hypertension.

Adverse effects of alpha antagonists such as phentolamine include nasal stuffiness, orthostatic hypotension, tachycardia, positive inotropic effects, and worsening angina. These effects may be explained, at least in part, by the observation that phentolamine is very potent not only at postsynaptic vascular alpha$_1$ receptors, which mediate smooth muscle contraction, but also at presynaptic alpha$_2$ receptors. Blockade by phentolamine of the alpha$_2$ receptor–mediated autoinhibitory effect of endogenous norepinephrine leads to increased release of norepinephrine in the heart. This increased concentration of norepinephrine causes enhanced stimulation of beta-adrenergic receptors, resulting in positive inotropic and chronotropic effects.

Prazosin is a highly selective alpha$_1$ antagonist that is useful in the treatment of hypertension. It exerts its major antihypertensive effect by reversible blockade of postsynaptic alpha$_1$ receptors. Prazosin is the most potent alpha$_1$-blocking drug currently available. In marked contrast to phentolamine, prazosin is an extremely weak antagonist of alpha$_2$ receptors both in physiologic studies and in direct radioligand binding experiments. This may explain why prazosin is apparently more effective as an antihypertensive agent than non–subtype selective alpha-adrenergic blocking drugs such as phentolamine. The very weak affinity of prazosin for alpha$_2$ receptors presumably accounts not only for its relatively better antihypertensive effect but also in part for the absence of certain adverse effects that are characteristically seen with non–subtype selective alpha blockers (see above). First, tachycardia is uncommon with prazosin. Since it is so weak in blocking alpha$_2$ receptors, enhanced norepinephrine release would not be expected. Second, since enhanced "norepinephrine overflow" from sympathetic nerves does not occur with prazosin, beta-adrenergic stimulation of renin secretion is absent and plasma renin concentrations do not generally rise with prazosin as they do with other alpha-adrenergic antagonists. Also, prazosin would not be expected to block the alpha$_2$ receptors, which are conjectured to inhibit renin release.

Another use of prazosin is in the management of patients with severe and intractable congestive heart failure. The beneficial hemodynamic changes are due to a combination of decreased mean arterial pressure (decreased "afterload") and decreased venous tone leading to decreased venous return (decreased "preload") (see Ch. 43).

In addition to the agents discussed above, a number of other drugs not normally thought of as "alpha blockers" have significant alpha-adrenergic antagonist potency. In particular, phenothiazines such as chlorpromazine and butyrophenones such as haloperidol are relatively potent alpha blockers. This may explain why hypotension is encountered with these drugs.

CHOLINERGIC DRUGS

ANTAGONISTS. Postganglionic parasympathetic cholinergic receptors are of one major type termed muscarinic. The major clinical muscarinic antagonist is atropine, one of the oldest drugs in medicine. Scopolamine is a closely related alkaloid.

Atropine blocks the effects of the parasympathetic nervous system on smooth muscle, cardiac muscle, and various glandular cells. Because atropine blocks the cardiac actions of the vagus nerve it increases the rate of firing of the sinoatrial node and facilitates conduction through the atrioventricular node. Accordingly atropine can be used in the treatment of atrioventricular block or sinus bradycardia, as for example in the setting of myocardial infarction or after digitalis excess. The drug is generally used intravenously or subcutaneously in such circumstances.

Atropine and less purified preparations of belladonna alkaloids also reduce gastrointestinal motility and gastric secretion and may be useful in symptomatic treatment of peptic ulcer disease.

As with the adrenergic antagonists, adverse effects of atropine are largely extensions of the therapeutic effects of receptor blockade. These include dry mouth, urinary retention, constipation, and blurred vision. Large doses may cause hallucinations, marked agitation, dilated pupils, and dry skin. In cases of severe atropine poisoning anticholinesterases such as physostigmine are quite effective (see below).

CHOLINERGIC AGONISTS. The actions of administered acetylcholine-like drugs are due to their interaction with both muscarinic receptors (parasympathetic effectors) and nicotinic receptors (autonomic ganglia). Because of its rapid inactivation by acetylcholinesterase, acetylcholine itself is not effective systemically. Several synthetic esters of choline are more resistant to hydrolysis and are therefore of greater therapeutic utility. Methacholine (acetyl-beta-methylcholine) and bethanechol have purely muscarinic effects, whereas carbamylcholine is both nicotinic and muscarinic. Such drugs have limited therapeutic applications. They are used occasionally, for example, in cases of postoperative urinary retention.

ANTICHOLINESTERASES. Inhibition of cholinesterases by inhibitors that bind reversibly to the active site of the enzyme leads to a competitive decrease in the rate of hydrolysis of acetylcholine, thus raising the concentration of the neurotransmitter at nicotinic and muscarinic receptors. Several such drugs are physostigmine, a naturally occurring alkaloid, and the synthetic agents neostigmine, pyridostigmine, and edrophonium. These agents may be used for their nicotinic actions in the treatment of myasthenia gravis (see Ch. 518). Because edrophonium is so short acting, it may be used intravenously to help determine if myasthenia gravis is actually present (marked improvement in symptoms) but is not used therapeutically in this disease. These drugs may also be used for their muscarinic actions to treat paralytic ileus or postoperative urinary retention.

Another application is in the treatment of paroxysmal atrial tachycardia, either alone or in conjunction with carotid sinus massage to stimulate the vagal fibers to the heart. Edrophonium is generally used for this purpose.

Several organophosphorous agents such as diisopropyl fluorophosphate (DFP) and parathion are used in insecticides and are potent *irreversible* inhibitors of cholinesterases. They appear to act by phosphorylation of the active site of the enzyme. Cases of poisoning result from absorption of the agent through the skin or gastrointestinal tract or by inhalation. Symptoms may have a subtle onset with signs of excess cholinergic stimulation, i.e., salivation, hyperhidrosis, pupillary constriction and muscle twitching, and nausea. A relatively specific antidote, pralidoxime, reactivates the enzyme by removing the phosphate group. Atropine is generally used acutely to relieve symptoms.

GANGLIONIC BLOCKERS

Ganglionic blockers competitively antagonize the nicotinic effect of acetylcholine in the autonomic ganglia. They have limited therapeutic applications at present. Because tonic sympathetic nerve outflow to vasculature is reduced after ganglionic blockade, these agents reduce blood pressure. Examples are hexamethonium* and trimethaphan. They are potent drugs and when administered by slow intravenous infusion can be used to titrate the blood pressure in hypertensive emergencies and aortic dissection. As expected, they have a variety of severe side effects that limit their therapeutic utility. These include postural hypotension, ileus, urinary retention, and, at high infusion rates, respiratory arrest.

Frishman WH: Beta-adrenoceptor antagonists: New drugs and new indications. N Engl J Med 305:500, 1981. *A detailed review of the pharmacodynamics and pharmacokinetics of all the commonly available beta blockers.*

Lefkowitz RJ, Caron MG, Stiles GL: Mechanisms of membrane receptor regulation: Biochemical, physiological and clinical insights derived from studies of the adrenergic receptors. N Engl J Med 310:1570, 1984. *An overview of physiologic and pathophysiologic factors found to regulate adrenergic receptor binding sites.*

Yusuf S, Peto R, Lewis J, et al.: Beta blockade during and after myocardial infarction: An overview of the randomized trials. Prog Cardiovasc Dis 27:335, 1985. *The basis for the use of beta-adrenergic receptor blockers to reduce post–myocardial infarction morbidity and mortality.*

*Investigational drug for this purpose.

32 COMMON POISONINGS

William O. Robertson

DEFINITION. Man's chemical environment was recognized as a threat to health long before the birth of Christ. Well-documented outbreaks of occupational mercury and lead "poisonings" had been recorded and preventive measures implemented by 200 B.C. The Middle Ages saw arsenic poisoning employed as a political weapon. More recent times have seen increasing recognition of industrial toxins, "accidental poisoning" in childhood, purposeful overdoses in adults, adverse reactions to drugs, and environmental hazards for us all. The common theme is entrance of an exogenous chemical into an organism and subsequent disruption of its metabolism. The term "poison" has undergone quantitative redefinition so that now such ubiquitous substances as table salt and drinking water are firmly established as being "poisonous." Finally, the host-organism itself has contributed to a better comprehension of the word "poison," as genetic variability has been recognized to determine the impact of a given molecule in such hereditary disorders as phenylketonuria, glucose-6-phosphate dehydrogenase deficiency, and others. As man's understanding of life has expanded, the connotation of poisoning has undergone substantial evolution.

ETIOLOGY. Approximately 1.2 million chemical entities had been identified and coded by 1950; the number had risen to more than 4.3 million by 1976. By 1987, the number will exceed 10 million. Although not all of these compounds have been marketed, many new organic compounds have appeared in the home and the workplace. For example, available formulations of pesticides have increased fifty-fold over the past 30 years. Moreover, manufacturing processes have released additional compounds (e.g., dioxins) into the workplace or the environment with capabilities of serving as poisons.

New chemical techniques have permitted prompt and complete identification of poisonings and have uncovered the causes of such diverse entities as Minamata disease (teratogenesis consequent to methyl mercury), an outbreak of ascending paralysis affecting more than 4000 with more than 400 deaths in Iraq (also caused by methyl mercury), the "gray syndrome" in premature infants (caused by chloramphenicol), mesotheliomas induced by asbestos, and an epidemic of angiosarcoma of the liver among industrial workers (caused by vinyl chloride). Nevertheless, many unknowns remain and justify careful prospective monitoring of industry, of the home, and of the environment.

INCIDENCE. Over the past 25 years progressively more reliable data have been gathered about deaths from poisonings, the leading agents, and the number of such deaths attributable to each among children less than five years old and among the overall population (Table 32–1). Although concerns for infants and toddlers prompted the creation of our nation's Poison Center Network, deaths from poisoning among that group have plummeted over the past 30 years; these children were, fortunately, greatly under-represented in 1984, accounting for only 2.2 per cent of poisoning deaths despite the fact that their "accidental ingestions" account for 61 per cent of the 900,513 human exposures summarized by the National Data Collection System of the American Association of Poison Control Centers. Among adults precise data

TABLE 32–1. DEATHS DUE TO ACCIDENTAL POISONING IN THE UNITED STATES, 1982

	All Ages	Under 5 Years	5–44 Years	45+ Years
Total: Solids and Liquids	3474	67	2295	1112
Medications	2862	41	2000	821
Analgesics, antipyretics	1171	16	835	282
Opiates	559	2	501	56
Sedatives, hypnotics	141	0	99	52
Psychotropic drugs	265	7	171	87
Other central nervous system (CNS) drugs	216	1	188	27
Other drugs	1375	24	865	486
Nondrugs	612	26	295	291
Alcohol	412	0	199	213
Paints, solvents, and cleaning agents	84	8	50	26
Pesticides	29	5	12	12
Corrosives, caustics	27	5	4	18
Foods, plants	7	0	4	3
Others	53	8	26	19
Gases and vapors	1259	37	707	515
Carbon monoxide	1022	21	584	417

Data from National Safety Council: Accident Facts. Chicago, National Center for Health Statistics, 1985.

are more difficult to retrieve. Incomplete data attest that a minimum of 12,000 deaths occur annually as a result of suicide by poisoning.

EPIDEMIOLOGY. There are significant differences in the epidemiology of poisonings among children under five years of age compared with the remainder of the population. With adults, occupational and industrial exposures, suicide gestures or attempts, and homicides depend upon host factors and environmental settings as well as involved chemicals. In contrast, among children under five, host and environmental factors are less variable. In the United States, occurrences peak at 24 to 32 months of age, and more male than female children are involved; poisonings happen most frequently between 11 A.M. and 12 noon or between 5 and 6 P.M. and in places of easiest exposure—the kitchen, the bedroom, and the bathroom. In addition, illness in the family or "life stress situations" increase the likelihood of accidental ingestion.

PREVENTION. Avoiding exposure to the toxin is the ultimate precaution; among adults, a variety of approaches have been employed—some with obvious effectiveness, others without. For example, the use of mercury in the felting process of hats has been outlawed since 1941; that source of mercury poisoning has disappeared in the hatting industry. Beryllium has been excluded from fluorescent light bulbs, and that source of exposure no longer exists. Similarly, where arsenic has been eliminated from pesticidal preparations and where naphthylamine has been eliminated from the rubber industry, human illness has been avoided. Some of these steps have resulted from legislative processes; others are the result of voluntary activity on the part of industry or an aware public.

Among children some approaches have also proved effective; others are without much evidence of success. For example, efforts directed at altering toddlers' exploratory behaviors in family settings have not proved effective. In contrast, the use of safety caps on medicine bottles had important consequences. For the ten-year period between 1959 and 1969, almost 100 deaths occurred annually from accidental salicylate poisoning in children under five; in 1978, only 12 such deaths were reported. Several variables have been cited as definitely contributory: (1) the manufacturers' voluntary reduction of the number of tablets as well as of the amount of aspirin per bottle; (2) the introduction of a favorable flavor to the "baby aspirin" as an attractive alternative to larger tablets; (3) programs of professional and public education; (4) the appearance of acetaminophen as a rival to aspirin, with its subsequent capture of 30 per cent of the analgesic-antipyretic market, and more recently, their replacement by still newer nonsteroidal anti-inflammatory drugs (NSAID's); and (5) the mandated use of safety caps or child-resistant containers. All have had an impact, but current professional opinion holds that safety caps have contributed approximately 60 per cent of the variance. As safety caps have subsequently been applied to other prescription products and dangerous household items such as petroleum distillates and caustics, their impact has been felt there also. Unfortunately, safety caps may have a negative effect among the geriatric population, among whom as many as 50 per cent cite them as contributing to their lack of compliance in taking prescribed medications.

Since 1953, more than 500 poison centers have been established across the country to provide professionals and patients with ingredient information, toxic potentials, and treatment alternatives. Initially, the FDA's National Clearinghouse of Poison Control Centers was intended to serve as the coordinating unit; it also provided technical information to centers. In recent years, several microfiche systems—particularly "Poisondex" (Micromedex, Denver)—have been developed to catalogue product information and to outline management approaches; they are capable of storing information on more than 300,000 products in a limited space and in an easily retrievable manner. Moreover, such microfiche systems avoid filing errors and permit updating of information on a quarterly basis. With recent advances in computer technology—e.g., hard disk drives, laser processing, and so forth—these data systems are now available on self-contained personal computer packages.

Over the years the American Association of Poison Control Centers has served to produce educational material aimed at preventing poisoning, to establish standards for the operation of poison centers, to conduct self-assessment examinations for those staffing poison centers, and to implement a nationwide program aimed at regionalizing the poison center network. More recently, the American Academy of Clinical Toxicology and the American Board of Medical Toxicology have been developed to serve as the specialty society and certifying body, respectively, to further the academic and professional goals of physicians involved in such programs.

DIAGNOSIS. The diagnosis of an accidental (or a purposeful) poisoning can be made only if considered; this is true for either the adult or child with unexplained signs or symptoms. Once the possibility of poisoning is entertained, a careful search is made for a possible container and its label or for a solid medication form and its drug-identifying imprint; next, the toxic potential of the substance can be verified from existing information or by contacting the nearest poison center. Often the presenting clinical signs and symptoms are so characteristic as to permit diagnosis—i.e., the hyperventilation (following vomiting) of acute salicylism, the extrapyramidal manifestations of phenothiazine reactions. Sometimes diagnostic confirmation can be established by the patient's response to a specific antidote, e.g., naloxone. On other occasions, analysis of specimens of body fluids—blood, urine, vomit, gastric contents, or stool—is necessary for diagnosis. As a generalization, "routine toxic screens" have proved to be of relatively little value in the child and are decried by many experts as inaccurate, confusing, and not helpful in the adult. Where the history or the environment provides a lead to the potential toxins, modern technology is proving increasingly useful. In the absence of such leads, helpful results are admittedly scarce.

Particularly helpful to toxicologists have been the Consumer Product Act of 1970 and the Commission Coordinating Safety Packaging Regulations, which have promulgated adequate labeling of hazardous substances across the country. *The label on the container is the single most useful information in accidental poisonings.* In the absence of a label, generic information about ingredients of household, industrial, and pharmaceutical products is available from a poison center or from a particularly useful textbook: Clinical Toxicology of Commercial Products. The information on the prescription bottle, on the package insert, or from the imprint of the solid medication form (such imprints exist on virtually all tablets and capsules) is equally important and ought to be diligently pursued.

Once the ingested poison has been identified, the problem remains to determine its potential for harm in the particular patient. That potential depends upon the amount and form ingested, the toxicity of the agent, the time lapse involved, and a variety of host factors. The amount ingested can sometimes be estimated by observers or by determining the amount of material remaining in the container. The toxicity of a particular poison can be assessed by reference to known data on human experiences, to animal LD50's, and to derivative "minimal lethal doses." One must be particularly cautious about overinterpreting LD50's or animal studies; in many instances the results are not transferable to the human. A toxicity rating has proved useful in estimating the degree of risk to the patient (Table 32–2).

In recent years, toxicologic analysis of body fluids has assumed an increasingly significant role in the diagnosis and management of poisoning, but it remains a relatively small one. Technical developments perfecting chemical analysis by mass spectrophotometry, gas-liquid chromatography, and

TABLE 32–2. TOXICITY RATING*

Rating	Probable Lethal Dose *mg/kg*	Probable Lethal Dose *For 70-kg Man*
6—Super toxic	<5	A taste <7 drops
5—Extremely toxic	5–50	7 drops to 1 tsp
4—Very toxic	50–500	1 tsp to 1 oz
3—Moderately toxic	500 mg–5 grams	1 oz to 1 pint
2—Slightly toxic	5–15 grams	1 pint to 1 quart
1—Practically nontoxic	>15 grams	>1 quart

*From Gosselin RE, Hodge HC, Smith RP: Clinical Toxicity of Commercial Products. 5th ed. Baltimore, Williams & Wilkins Company, 1984.

spin resonance now allow toxic screening for a variety of poisons from minuscule amounts of body fluids. Commercial laboratories as well as a number of hospital, public health, and university laboratories provide qualitative and quantitative analyses for sedatives, narcotics, psychotropics, heavy metals, pesticides, and other compounds, all of which enable a speedy and accurate diagnosis. Nevertheless, such determination (e.g., specifying the type and amount of barbiturate in the blood) often does not alter management of the patient. Thus, in instances of barbiturate overdose, measurements of blood gases and pH prove more effective in coping with the clinical problem than does the quantitative determination of barbiturate level. Notable exceptions occur when specific quantification is critical in deciding on therapy—e.g., the use of acetaminophen blood levels and the Matthews-Rumack nomogram in deciding on the use of its antidote (*N*-acetylcysteine) before clinical signs or symptoms of illness appear, or the use of the serum salicylate concentration and the Done nomogram in determining the need for therapy in acute salicylate ingestion; and the value of the serum iron concentration along with clinical signs and symptoms in contemplating chelation therapy with desferrioxamine for iron poisoning. So too, identifying the presence of methyl alcohol or ethylene glycol can be critical in therapeutic management. Regardless of these several exceptions, the point remains that historical and clinical features plus the routinely available laboratory tests are usually paramount. Assisting the physician are a number of texts listed at the end of this chapter.

TREATMENT. Even before the ingested (or inhaled) substance has been identified and its toxic potential determined, first aid measures and supportive care ought to be initiated. Subsequent efforts are directed toward (1) preventing absorption of the substance; (2) curtailing its conversion in the body to its active form or hastening its conversion to an inactive one; (3) neutralizing or counteracting its clinical effect; and (4) enhancing its excretion from the body. In the majority of instances instituting measures to enable the patient to tolerate the temporary impact of the toxin and then to recuperate on his or her own remains the most effective course of action and often prevents subsequent poisonings as a result of overzealous treatment.

Supportive Measures. Prompt attention to supportive measures before a crisis has arisen, is, in fact, usually the single most critical element in managing the overdosed patient. The airway must be maintained, ventilation assured, cardiac output sustained, peripheral vascular collapse avoided, convulsions controlled, and hypertension and increased intracranial pressure lowered. Physical and chemical options ought to be carefully reviewed in advance of the patient's arrival if possible. Life support mechanisms can tide the patient over a period of compromised function as a result of anesthesia, an accidental overdose, or the purposeful induction of "barbiturate coma." But those measures must be carefully planned, carried out by skilled personnel, and monitored in detail if optimal benefit is to be achieved.

Prevention of Absorption. This is best accomplished in the conscious child or adult by *induction of emesis* as opposed to gastric lavage. Although gastric lavage has a tradition in emergency medicine, its yield of ingested material falls short of the returns by emesis. Moreover, despite improved emergency transport systems, there are significant time delays in delivering the patient to a health care facility where lavage can be undertaken. During that time, significant absorption takes place. By contrast, efforts to induce vomiting can be initiated in the home—particularly if syrup of ipecac is available there. If not, it is readily obtained from local pharmacies, 24-hour corner groceries, emergency vehicles, and neighbors. One should administer 15 ml to a child or 15 to 30 ml to an adult together with 200 to 300 ml of any fluids—water, soft drinks, milk, or juices—and wait 10 to 15 minutes with an appropriate receptacle for vomiting to occur. If no vomiting ensues in 20 minutes, one should repeat the initial dose of syrup of ipecac and administer more fluids. If no syrup of ipecac is available, one should try gagging the patient but should be prepared for failure; one should then encourage the patient to drink 30 to 45 ml of liquid dishwashing detergents (anionic or nonionic but *not* cationic detergents) together with 240 ml of fluid. If the patient has already arrived in the emergency room, apomorphine can be used. It proves effective in four to five minutes but results in a drowsy patient despite use of naloxone. In all circumstances one should avoid table salt as an emetic agent; its use can compound the problem with acute hypernatremia. One should always avoid emesis in the comatose or convulsing patient or in the patient who has ingested a caustic. Syrup of ipecac proves effective in acute phenothiazine ingestions, but not in the face of chronic overdose; any form of emesis is maximally effective in the first one to one and a half hours after ingestion; seldom is it useful after two to three hours' delay.

Gastric lavage, using a large-bore tube and 1000 to 3000 ml of half-strength saline as the rinse, together with terminal instillation of activated charcoal, is the only option for the unconscious patient. In patients over two years of age, concomitant use of a cuffed endotracheal tube is indicated to avoid aspiration. Despite the fact that most toxins are absorbed rapidly and thus escape delayed evacuation efforts, on occasion substantial portions of ingested agents have been recovered, especially in suicidal patients who have consumed poisons that delay gastric emptying, slow intestinal motility, or depress overall body function. In those instances attempts at evacuation are recommended, but cannot be expected to be effective in more than one of five patients.

Activated charcoal can be used to complement either of the measures discussed above, but not with syrup of ipecac until after emesis has occurred. The large surface area of charcoal permits significant adsorption of the toxin, precluding its absorption from the gut. Given by mouth or via nasogastric tube in amounts of 5 to 15 times the amount of the ingested toxin, activated charcoal has diminished absorption by as much as 50 per cent with significant therapeutic benefits. Recent pharmacologic research supports the contention that absorption may be prevented by early intervention with charcoal, but equally importantly, finds that excretion of those compounds that are recycled via the gastrointestinal tract can be significantly increased by repetitive oral instillation of activated charcoal.

Cathartics, laxatives, enemas, and *colonic irrigations* are "heroic" measures devoid of evidence of effectiveness; in fact, cathartics can increase the rate of absorption of some barbiturates.

Inhibition of metabolism of a potential toxin to its active form or conversion to an inactive form is an option and, when feasible, may prove beneficial. For example, methyl alcohol becomes active only after it is converted to formaldehyde and formic acid; administering ethyl alcohol to the patient takes advantage of substrate competition (it is favored over methyl alcohol by the enzymatic processes involved), permitting significant reduction in the rate of metabolism of methyl alcohol and resulting in diminished formation of formaldehyde and formic acid, which in turn can be more easily scavenged by existent metabolic processes.

In other instances, enhancement of enzymatic activity may *activate* a toxin. For example, pretreatment of the pregnant woman and fetal liver with phenobarbital will enhance conjugation of bilirubin, but such pretreatment augments the conversion of carbon tetrachloride to its deleterious metabolite.

Chelating agents also limit the entry of certain toxins into metabolic pathways and augment excretion of the inactivited material. This approach has been particularly useful in poisonings by heavy metals—treatment of arsenic, mercury, and lead with dimercaprol (BAL), D-penicillamine, and edetate (EDTA), respectively. Similarly, desferrioxamine is useful in both acute and chronic iron poisoning.

Specific antidotes to counteract the effects of specific toxins are limited to a few compounds, but when one exists its usefulness is great. Paramount is the example of naloxone, an opiate derivative, which, when administered in adequate amounts (often *considerably more* than the recommended 0.4 mg) to a patient with heroin overdose, results in patient's sitting up and talking within 20 seconds! Administered to the nonoverdosed patient, naloxone is devoid of any action, thus constituting a unique example of an antagonist drug without any agonist effects. Most other antidotes have agonist as well as antagonist effects. Common examples of such antidotes include atropine for organophosphate and carbamate insecticide poisoning, methylene blue for methemoglobinemia, nitrites plus thiosulfate for cyanide ingestion, *N*-acetylcysteine for acetaminophen overdoses, and diphenhydramine for phenothiazine-induced extrapyramidal reactions. In addition, recent advances in immunology have resulted in the use of portions of antibodies ("Fab" fragments) to "neutralize" the clinical effects of overwhelming digoxin poisonings. Introduced as Digibind, this antidote is still limited in its availability; the nearest Poison Center should be contacted for available details. Moreover, monoclonal antibodies to various toxins are being developed for possible clinical use—either via injection into the patient or by being affixed to perfusion columns.

Enhancing elimination of a toxin can be accomplished by several mechanisms. For example, in carbon monoxide poisoning, use of 100 per cent oxygen by ventilatory mask has both theoretic and practical benefit. In instances of phencyclidine ingestion, continuous gastric lavage, taking advantage of "ion trapping" of the recycled phencyclidine via the gastric mucosa, is reported to be effective. Ion trapping is also employed in acute salicylate poisoning via alkalinization of the urine. In the kidney tubule, free salicylate molecules ionize in the presence of an alkaline medium and are not resorbed, thus being "captured" in the urine and excreted into the bladder. In contrast, amphetamine (a weak base) is captured in the kidney tubule by acidifying the urine with ascorbic acid or ammonium chloride. In general, forced osmotic diuresis, particularly chemical diuresis with common diuretics (e.g., furosemide), is of little or no benefit in enhancing the excretory processes.

By contrast, *dialysis* and *hemoperfusion* have proved to be effective therapeutic tools, although not as effective as had been initially believed. For example, a decade ago many patients with barbiturate overdose were subjected to extracorporeal or peritoneal dialysis; today, less than 1 in 300 such patients is so treated. If renal shutdown has occurred, as in mercury poisoning, dialysis will prove lifesaving, although it is unlikely to augment excretion of the mercury molecule. Exceptions do exist, as in dialysis for ethylene glycol overdoses. Hemoperfusion and lipid dialysis both serve as effective mechanisms in eliminating specific offending substances from the body, e.g., ethchlorvynol. To be effective, a significant proportion of the total body toxin must be present in the blood and must not be tightly bound to serum protein. For many compounds, such as digoxins, tricyclic antidepressants, and phenothiazines, these conditions are not met, and dialysis and hemoperfusion do little to reduce the total body burden of toxin. Knowledge of the "apparent volume of distribution" of a compound permits prediction of the usefulness of dialysis or hemoperfusion (see Ch. 80.1).

Occasionally, still other techniques, such as *exchange transfusions* in boric acid or iron poisoning, may be useful. So-called gut lavage, a virtually continuous through-and-through rinse of the bowel via instillation of large amounts of physiologic fluids into the intestine through a nasogastric tube, has been reported effective in paraquat overdoses when no alternatives exist. Careful consideration of the metabolic pathways of the involved substance combined with empiric evidence of previous outcomes serves as the best guide for management.

Treatment of Specific Common Poisonings. In addition to the general principles of treatment discussed above, a few common poisonings warrant specific mention.

Aspirin (salicylate) poisoning formerly accounted for 20 per cent of ingestions among children under five years of age; today, it is responsible for only 1 to 2 per cent. However, it remains a concern for all age groups—particularly because of its widespread use as a potential suicidal agent among the elderly. Acute ingestions in excess of 100 mg per kilogram of body weight deserve induction of emesis; aspirin leads to rapid metabolic acidosis in children under four years of age and to initial respiratory alkalosis in the adult. Both groups vomit; this permits early detection and helps in differentiation from acetaminophen ingestion. Alkalinizing the urine proves remarkably effective with the single acute ingestion; one should consult the Done nomogram for prognosis. The administration of intravenous $NaHCO_3$ (3 mEq per kilogram of body weight) to young children usually proves effective in raising urine pH above 7.0. A later second or third dose of approximately one half of that amount may be necessary to sustain alkalinization of the urine and thereby promote ionization and reduce reabsorption of salicylate. The use of acetazolamide to alkalinize the urine should be avoided; its mechanism of action also accelerates transport of salicylate into the central nervous system (CNS). Urinary elimination of the salicylate moiety removes the cause of the acidosis—a far more effective approach to therapy than treatment of the systemic acidosis itself. In the adult, initial blood pH may be elevated; nonetheless, it is the urine pH that is critical to monitor. In general, additional potassium administration is necessary only for the chronically intoxicated patient or later in the course of acute intoxications in adults. Occasionally dialysis may be warranted, but ordinarily general supportive measures prove sufficient. Chronic overdoses are far less responsive to any specific interventions, but supportive treatment can be crucial.

Acetaminophen has captured 30 per cent of today's analgesic-antipyretic market; liquid formulations are being augmented by solid preparation forms, some of which are in "extra strength" dosages. In Britain, acetaminophen has been a particularly popular suicidal substance; management is often complicated by the fact that no significant symptoms may appear until after irreversible liver damage has occurred. If recognized early—preferably less than 12 hours and certainly less than 24 hours after ingestion—determination of the serum level and comparison of it against standards on the Matthews-Rumack nomogram permit an appropriate decision about the possible use of an antidote, either *N*-acetylcysteine or methionine (both sulfhydryl donors). Both appear to enter into metabolic pathways via glutathione mechanisms and to preclude the formation of an epoxide derivative of acetaminophen that binds covalently to liver macromolecules, resulting in liver cell destruction. An intravenous preparation of the antidote is available that is strongly favored and widely used in Britain; it ought to be available in the United States soon. Currently, only an oral form is available in the United States, and its use presents difficulties because of associated emesis.

Of special note is the apparent diminished susceptibility to toxicity in the preadolescent compared with the adult.

Significant overdoses of *anticholinergic substances* in various forms (e.g., tricyclic antidepressants, atropine, antihistamines, phenothiazines, jimson weed) produce fever, flushing, widely dilated pupils, and CNS signs and symptoms varying from somnolence and coma to delirium and seizures. Each of these specific drugs may also produce additional specific symptoms by other mechanisms—e.g., diphenhydramine hydrochloride (Benadryl) occasionally results in extrapyramidal reactions; tricyclic antidepressants cause cardiac arrhythmias. For this class of drugs, physostigmine is available both as a diagnostic agent and as a therapeutic substance; because administration of physostigmine may itself induce seizures in 15 to 20 per cent of treated patients, its use has declined significantly. The dose is 0.5 mg administered slowly intravenously for the child under five and 1 to 2 mg for the adult, repeated as often as necessary to control seizures. Today, however, most centers rely on diazepam treatment instead. In all instances atropine should be immediately available during physostigmine infusion, and Valium also ought to be available should a convulsion occur. Tricyclic antidepressant overdoses are now numerically the most serious of prescription medicine hazards. These are best approached by using diazepam (Valium) or phenobarbital to control seizures, by maintaining a blood pH above 7.45 to prevent tachyarrhythmias either by administering $NaHCO_3$ or by controlled ventilation in the obtunded patient, and by use of conventional cardiac drugs should arrhythmias ensue.

Acute petroleum distillates (hydrocarbons) cause their most significant damage as a function of their initial action on the lungs via aspiration; such aspiration occurs at the time of ingestion or inhalation. Both in laboratory animals and in humans, large amounts of various petroleum distillates have been consumed and retained without development of any signs or symptoms save for odoriferous eructations ("smelly burps") and diarrhea. As a general rule, neither lavage nor induction of emesis is indicated in such ingestions unless some additional toxin (e.g., parathion) has been dissolved in the hydrocarbon. When such is the case, induction of emesis has supplanted gastric lavage as the treatment of choice. When pulmonary aspiration has occurred, supportive measures are introduced; antibiotics and steroids are widely used but without much evidence of effectiveness.

Carbon monoxide (see Ch. 537) ranks high as a contributor to common poisonings, suicides, and accidental deaths. The mechanism of action involves acute interruption of both oxygen transport and oxygen metabolism, with a rapid cessation of life functions. Prompt recognition of exposure and removal of the patient from the contaminated environment are essential. Hastening of excretion of carbon monoxide by administration of oxygen and consideration of hyperbaric oxygen treatment are currently the hallmarks of management.

Caustic compounds, including acids and alkalis, appear to exert their toxic effects largely via alterations of pH and their consequences on the gastrointestinal tract. Experimental evidence suggests that the damage done by alkalis is complete within 30 seconds after exposure; that done by acids may be somewhat slower to appear. Current recommendations of management are avoidance of major efforts to empty the gastrointestinal tract, neutralization of the offending compound by the administration of a protein-containing substance (such as milk), and careful assessment of the esophagus for the possibility of acute burns. This last point frequently necessitates esophagoscopy because the presence or absence of burns in the mouth proves nonpredictive of the status of the esophagus. In addition to concerns about the acute situation—managed by dilatation, steroids, and antibiotics—much interest now focuses on follow-up for 20 to 40 years because of a significantly increased risk of carcinoma of the esophagus.

Cyanide has gained its deserved reputation for toxicity by its ability to inhibit oxygen utilization at the level of the cell via cytochrome oxidase inhibition; severe metabolic acidosis can occur almost instantaneously. Most exposures are occupational; occasional exposures are the result of homicidal efforts, particularly associated with capsule tampering, and rare consequences are found subsequent to *l*-mandelonitrile-β-glucuronic acid (Laetrile) administration or nitroprusside overdose. As soon as cyanide poisoning is suspected, administration of nitrite—via a 3 per cent solution intravenously or amyl nitrite inhalation—is crucial. It converts hemoglobin to methemoglobin, which selectively binds cyanide. This is followed by administration of sodium thiosulfate to convert cyanide to the less toxic thiocyanate. Recent experience in Europe suggests the use of dicobalt edetate may be even more effective—but avoidance is the goal.

Drugs of abuse haunt the profession, the emergency room, and our society. Were the offending agent easily identified with certainty—e.g., heroin—the immediate remedy would be obvious—naloxone. Such instances are almost nonexistent; more than 90 per cent of what is bought and sold "on the street" is not what it has been represented to be. Even imprinted capsules have been counterfeited in efforts to "con" the buyer. In other instances the basic ingredient has been "cut" with an inert substance or "laced" with some other psychoactive substance. Enormous geographic variations seem to exist across the country, with phencyclidine ("angel dust," PCP) being particularly popular in Los Angeles and Detroit, Ritalin in Seattle, and heroin and cocaine ("crack") in New York.

The laboratory may be helpful in instances of opiate overdose but is of virtually no value for lysergic acid diethylamide (LSD) or PCP (see Ch. 466). As a consequence, symptomatic management predominates; the unconscious or convulsing adult may routinely be approached as a potential heroin addict, an alcoholic, or a hypoglycemic individual; the hyperactive, "spacey" patient prompts consideration of PCP, LSD, and related sympathomimetic agents (amphetamine, phenylpropanolamine, etc), as well as recreational cocaine or psychosocial decompensation. Supportive measures may include monitoring, restraints, sedatives (diazepam is "customary"). succinylcholine, hydration, and ventilatory and cardiac measures. As a generalization, the acute management proves far more successful than treatment of the underlying problem, but efforts ought to be directed at the latter, as it provides the only true solution to the basic problem.

Ethyl alcohol (see Ch. 467) is mentioned here to stress its ubiquity and the epidemiologic point that it is remarkably prevalent as a cause of admission to hospital for children, with both purposeful and accidental ingestions, as well as a cause of birth defects among newborns. Also, ethyl alcohol augments the potential toxicity of a number of other compounds, such as diazepam.

Halogenated hydrocarbons (including chlorinated insecticides such as chlorophenothane, or DDT) serve as a source of a myriad of occupational, industrial, and pharmacologic exposures. Almost invariably lipid soluble, most are readily absorbable by the gastrointestinal tract, the respiratory epithelium, or the skin. Fortunately, most are metabolically rather stable compounds within the human organism; thus reproduction of still more hazardous metabolites is minimized. Nonetheless, many of the compounds gain access to fat storage deposits or neural tissue and cause both central and peripheral nervous system symptoms. For some (e.g., 2,3,7,8-tetrachlorodibenzodioxin, or dioxin) there are concerns about long-term toxicity and teratogenicity. Treatment modes include elimination of subsequent exposures, attempts to retrieve unabsorbed quantities from the gastrointestinal tract, and general supportive measures in response to symptoms.

Iron salts ($FeSO_4$, Fe gluconate) represent a hazard confined almost exclusively to children who "accidentally" consume prenatal tablets. To date, virtually no cases of acute poisoning have been reported in adults. While initial reports of a 50 per cent mortality rate were greatly inflated (instead it hovers at approximately 1 per cent), iron poisoning typifies the problem of the "unsuspected toxin" about which parents, parent surrogates, and physicians may be uninformed. When ingestions are known to exceed 50 to 60 mg per kilogram or when serum levels (taken three to six hours after ingestion) exceed 400 to 500 μg per deciliter, observation and chelation with desferrioxamine ought to be seriously considered, particularly if clinical symptoms such as upper abdominal pain, nausea, and vomiting are present. Management of the acute ingestion calls for prompt gastric emptying and instillation of a 5 per cent solution of sodium bicarbonate into the stomach in an attempt to minimize absorption of the resultant ferrous carbonate compound. More serious overdoses have prompted heroic measures, including surgical extirpation of ingested tablets and attempts at exchange transfusion. To date, studies have documented no serious consequences from ingestion of iron as a component of children's chewable vitamin preparations.

Methanol and *ethylene glycol* present significant problems of metabolic acidosis in clinically poisoned patients. Diagnosis is often considered following discovery of an unexplained anion gap. These compounds both depend upon alcohol dehydrogenase for their metabolism. The current approach to therapy takes advantage of this situation and provides ethanol (5 to 10 grams per hour intravenously) as a competitive inhibitor of toxin metabolism—thus slowing the formation of toxic metabolites, formaldehyde, and formic acid from methanol, or glycoaldehyde and glycolic, glyoxylic, and oxalic acids from ethylene glycol, to rates of formation permitting these products to be disposed of by ordinary metabolic or excretory pathways. By contrast, for large overdoses hemodialysis may be required to eliminate the offending toxin.

Organophosphate and carbamate insecticides can both prove exquisitely toxic in minute amounts. The mechanism of action involves inhibition of acetylcholine metabolism via cessation of cholinesterase function. Prompt recognition of symptoms secondary to acute exposure can prove lifesaving. Detecting symptoms secondary to chronic exposure (e.g., peripheral neuropathy) can serve to eliminate much patient distress and employee unhappiness. In general, acute distress is ushered in via excessive secretions in the upper airway, with respiratory distress, diffuse muscular weakness, nausea, vomiting, and collapse. Treatment requires prompt and repeated administration of large amounts of atropine for both types of poisoning. Pralidoxime (2PAM) is also strongly recommended to assist in the rejuvenation of cholinesterase levels. Introduced in large measure as a "safer" replacement for DDT these compounds have been responsible for large numbers of acute poisonings but, as far as can be determined, are yet to be implicated in carcinogenicity, teratogenicity, or chronic liver disease.

Paraquat (and its associated congeners) is a particularly popular and effective herbicide. While controversy rages about the consequences of environment exposures, no controversy exists on the issue of acute, purposeful overdoses; they are devastating. Paraquat is a harsh gastrointestinal irritant that also inhibits renal function; its most destructive impact is on the respiratory tract, where it inhibits superoxide dismutase and kills via "oxygen toxicity." Current approaches to therapy favor such dramatic efforts as "gut lavage," with some suggestion that hemoperfusion might be warranted. However, overdoses are likely to be lethal.

Theophylline and its congeners have been recognized as inducing seizures, cardiac arrhythmias, and occasional deaths in overdose situations. More recently, "therapeutic misadventures" have been recognized; inadvertent overdoses, alterations of theophylline metabolism by viral infections and nutritional variations, and the tendency to use theophylline in large quantities for relatively minor illnesses all increase the likelihood of such occurrences. Beta blockers can be used in managing the clinical symptoms of overdose—particularly the associated anxiety and tachycardia—but should not be used in asthmatic individuals. Children seem more resistant to the serious side effects than do adults, but occasionally both groups may have to be considered for hemoperfusion. Peritoneal and extracorporeal hemodialysis have both been reported to be ineffective.

Although ingestions of *plants and plant elements* constitute the single most frequent reason for telephoning poison centers, the overall problem is best put in perspective by Fraser's analysis of Britain's most recent 20-year experience with poisonings:

> Plants are the most overrated poisons of childhood. In earlier decades there were occasional deaths, most caused by the umbelliferae (particularly hemlock water dropwort) and the solanaceae (various nightshades). From 1958 to 1977 there were three deaths, and in one the role of the ingestion in the child's demise is doubtful. The others were caused by hemlock and by *Amanita phalloides* (death cup), both in children aged five and nine. Laburnum is frequently cited as the most toxic and commonly fatal poisonous plant in both children and adults, but there appears to be no report this century of childhood poisoning death. One adult death in unusual circumstances has been recorded.

CONCLUSION. Chemical hazards have always been a way of life. Today their numbers continue to escalate. But modern technology permits both identification and quantification of minuscule amounts of some toxins—uncovering, for example, tamperings with cyanides. As a consequence, the physician is well advised to add possible poisoning to the differential diagnosis for any unexplained collection of signs or symptoms in a patient of any age. Moreover, unless the physician is confident of the timeliness and completeness of his or her understanding about a specific item, additional consultation is strongly advised.

Arena J, Drew RH: Poisoning: Chemistry, Symptoms and Treatment. 5th ed. Springfield, Ill., Charles C Thomas, 1986. *Derived from years of experience and leadership in the poisoning field, this book is well organized, carefully edited, and readable, with a remarkable collection of cases and common sense.*

Dreisbach RH, Robertson WO: Handbook of Poisoning. 12th ed. Los Altos, Calif., Lange Publishing Company, 1987. *This pocket-sized book is both comprehensive and concise. Up-to-date and always helpful to review for omissions in one's approach, it proves particularly valuable to the primary care physician.*

Goldfrank LR, Flomenbaum N, Lewin N, et al.: Toxicologic Emergencies. 3rd ed. Norwalk, CT, Appleton-Century-Crofts, 1986. *Probably the most clinically relevant and readable of all the texts available, it summarizes a remarkable amount of experience in readily retrievable form—and in a format aimed at anticipating the reader's needs.*

Gosselin RE, Hodge HC, Smith RP: Clinical Toxicology of Commercial Products. 5th ed. Baltimore, Williams & Wilkins Company, 1984. *Long established as the "bible" of the field, this compendium provides a concise overview of poisoning issues, as well as a thorough and well-edited clinical description of approximately 50 generic poisonings. It has a comprehensive listing of trade-name entities and generic items in household and commercial product fields. Authoritative the world over.*

Haddad LM, Winchester JF: Clinical Management of Poisoning and Drug Overdose. Philadelphia, W. B. Saunders Company, 1983. *A recent book with contributions chiefly by American experts, this is currently the most comprehensive text for the recognition and clinical management of poisoning.*

Klaassen CD, Amdur MD, Doull J: Toxicology: The Basic Science of Poisons. 3rd ed. New York, Macmillan, 1986. *This text constitutes the "compleat" basic science approach for the toxicologist. With 42 contributors and critical editing, the final product covers the field from salt to water to radiation.*

Proudfoot A.: Diagnosis and Management of Poisoning. Oxford, Blackwell Scientific Publications, 1982. *Stemming from the extensive experience of Edinburgh's Regional Poison Center, this clinically oriented manual ought to prove of special benefit to physicians seeking instantaneous updates on management concepts.*

Journals: Virtually any clinical journal may prove the source of a fascinating case report or a valuable review in the field of poisoning. Lancet, JAMA, N Engl J Med, and the traditional medical and pediatric specialty journals are particularly valuable resources. In the more limited field of clinical toxicology the following are of note: (1) Veterinary and Human Toxicology: The official journal of the American Association of Poison Control Centers and the American Academy of Clinical Toxicology, always updating the clinical field. (2) The American Journal of Emergency Medicine, published by W. B. Saunders Company. (3) Clinical Toxicology: A blend of industrial, environmental, and accidental cases appears here, together with results of bench research. (4) Emergency Medicine: A controlled circulation journal particularly noted for "The Toxic Emergency," a monthly contribution of Donald Kunkel. (5) Medical Toxicology: Newly published, focuses on definitive reviews and is worldwide in perspective.

PART V
PRINCIPLES OF HUMAN GENETICS

33 HUMAN HEREDITY

James B. Wyngaarden

The appreciation of genetic factors as arbiters of human disease is a relatively recent development in medical history. Scattered references to inheritance of biologic characteristics may be found in the records of several millenia, including the frequently cited Talmudic exemption from circumcision of males born into families of bleeders, but discernible patterns of hereditary transmission were recognized first in the eighteenth and nineteenth centuries. In the 1750's Maupertuis described the autosomal dominant inheritance of polydactyly. The essential features of X-linked inheritance of hemophilia were described in the early 1800's by several writers and the pattern formally outlined by Nasse in 1820. The pattern of inheritance now recognized as autosomal recessive was described by Adams in 1814, and the biologic consequences of consanguinity first reported by Bemiss in 1857. In 1876, Galton introduced the twin method of separating effects of heredity from those of environment; later he initiated quantitative studies of polygenic inheritance.

Genetics as an experimental science owes its origins to Gregor Mendel and his cross-breeding of garden peas, tall and short, yellow seed and green seed, round seed and wrinkled seed. From these studies Mendel derived concepts of dominant and recessive traits, hereditary factors (which we now call *genes*), alternative factors (*alleles*), true breeding plants with two identical factors (*homozygotes*), and nontrue breeding plants with alternative factors (*heterozygotes*). His experiments led to the formulation of laws of *unit inheritance* (that "factors" retain their identity from generation to generation and do not blend in the hybrid), of *segregation* (that two members [alleles] of a single pair of factors [genes] are never found in the same gamete but always segregate), and of *independent assortment* (that members of different pairs of genes [nonalleles] assort to gametes independent of one another). These laws, formulated in 1865, had almost no immediate impact on biologic thought, but they are now cornerstones of genetics. They were rediscovered about 1900 by several workers independently and first applied to human disease by Sir Archibald Garrod in his concept of "inborn errors of metabolism" in 1908.

In 1944 Avery and his associates at the Rockefeller Institute established that the hereditary information in the transforming principle of pneumococci resided in its deoxyribonucleic acid (DNA). From that date onward DNA has been considered the basic material of the gene. In 1953 Watson and Crick proposed a molecular model for the structure of DNA, consisting of two polynucleotide strands twisted together in a double helix with the purine and pyrimidine bases facing inward and attached to each other, binding the two chains. This model offered a rational structure for replication of DNA and for storage of hereditary information within sequences of purine and pyrimidine bases. This structure has since been established by x-ray crystallography. The genetic code, namely the precise triplet sequences of purine and pyrimidine bases in the structural gene that specify the individual amino acids of a polypeptide chain, was discovered by Nirenberg in 1961.

The amount of DNA in each human cell is sufficient to code for approximately 1 millon polypeptides of average length. Estimates of the number of structural genes in humans range from 50,000 to 100,000; large amounts of DNA constitute noncoding sequences whose function is as yet obscure. Only a small number of structural genes has been identified. In the most recent update of his catalogue of *Mendelian Inheritance in Man*, McKusick lists phenotypic variations or diseases of 1906 established genetic loci, thus implying that at least that many genes have undergone mutation so as to cause human disease or polymorphism. In humans, hereditary information is distributed in 23 pairs of chromosomes—22 pairs of autosomes and one pair of sex chromosomes (X+Y, male; X+X, female)—plus the impaired "mitochondrial chromosome" (see below).

Genetics is concerned with the study of hereditary variations. Most of these variations are not harmful; indeed, they confer a distinct biologic advantage by enabling the species to adapt to changing environments. When variations are extreme and impair the health, fitness, or reproductive capacity of the individual, we consider them diseases. These extreme variations are of three principal types: (1) chromosomal aberrations, (2) single-gene differences that exhibit mendelian patterns of inheritance, and (3) polygenic disorders, in which two or more, often multiple, genes each contribute to the characteristic in question. Examples of the first two categories are relatively easy to recognize. They are discussed in Ch. 34 and Ch. 36. Many genetic diseases are dependent upon environmental factors for their expression, e.g., phenylalanine ingestion in phenylketonuria or milk ingestion in galactosemia. Other hereditary diseases are kept in abeyance by specific environmental factors: Scurvy is an inborn error of metabolism (absence of the hepatic enzyme that converts L-gulonolactone to L-ascorbic acid in man, monkey, and guinea pig) kept in remission by vitamin C; metabolic cretinism is foiled in its expression by the administration of thyroid hormone. The greatest difficulty in sorting out the relative importance of genetic and environmental influences is encountered with common diseases. In disorders such as rheumatoid arthritis, essential hypertension, and coronary artery disease, genetic influences are important but hard to identify in specific biochemical terms. In most polygenic disorders, genetic factors are multiple and still beyond definition.

The pace of genetic advance across the full spectrum of molecular biology to human heredity is currently very rapid. The revolution in biology of the past three decades is increasingly molding medical science and practice. New insights into the genetic control of the immune response (see Ch. 425) are explaining disease susceptibilities and facilitating organ and tissue transplantation. Susceptibility to cancer is being explained by the interplay between oncogenes, antioncogenes and environmental exposures (see Ch. 169). As additional genetic mechanisms are disclosed, they will illuminate more and more human diseases and from time to time suggest new avenues of therapy.

THE FAMILY HISTORY. A careful family history is indispensable in the assessment and understanding of hereditary disease. The interviewer should ascertain whether anyone in the family has had a condition similar to that of the patient, and whether this condition or any other "runs in the family." Particularly in the case of rare disorders one should inquire whether the parents are related, and, if this is not known, whether they or their families came from the same village or community and whether their forebears may have intermarried. Since some disorders are more common in certain ethnic groups than in others, the ethnic origin of the parents should also be elicited.

The rarer the recessive disorder in a specific population, the greater is the likelihood of parental consanguinity. Tay-Sachs disease is relatively rare in non-Jews, in whom the gene frequency is low, but a high proportion of non-Jewish parents of Tay-Sachs children are consanguineous. By contrast, Tay-Sachs disease is relatively common in Jews of eastern European origin, in whom the gene frequency is relatively high. In parents of Jewish children with Tay-Sachs disease in the United States the frequency of consanguinity is only slightly higher than in the general population.

Certain ethnic backgrounds increase the likelihood of certain diagnostic possibilities while decreasing that of others. Thalassemia is chiefly a disorder of people of the Mediterranean region and of Southeast Asia, familial Mediterranean fever is a disorder of Armenians and Sephardic Jews, acatalasia is a disease of Japanese and Koreans, and gout is very common among the Maori. By contrast, cystic fibrosis is rare in blacks, phenylketonuria is uncommon in Jews, and sickle cell anemia does not occur in Caucasians.

PEDIGREE ANALYSIS. The chief method of study of an inherited disease in humans is the observation of its pattern of distribution in kindreds, i.e., of its pedigree pattern. The construction of a pedigree pattern begins with the individual first detected, who is referred to as the proband, index case, or propositus (female = proposita). The pedigree pattern allows one to judge whether the distribution conforms to mendelian principles of segregation and assortment and thus represents single-factor inheritance. Patterns that do not conform to mendelian principles may represent polygenic traits in which a number of genes each contributes a minor effect. Valid pedigrees depend on accurate and extensive information about the kindred. This information is likely to be more reliable when based on observer detection than when based on memory.

MONOGENIC DISORDERS. Disorders caused by single mutant genes show one of four simple (mendelian) patterns of inheritance: (1) autosomal dominant, (2) autosomal recessive, (3) X-linked dominant, or (4) X-linked recessive. Dominant traits are those expressed in the heterozygote (as well as in the homozygote or hemizygote). Recessive traits are those expressed in the homozygotes (or hemizygotes) but silent in the heterozygote. The terms *dominant* and *recessive* refer to the phenotypic expression of the trait, not to the expression of the gene. Thus it is incorrect to speak of a dominant or recessive gene. A gene is either expressed or not expressed. Whether the trait is considered dominant or recessive often depends upon the level of observation. Sickle cell anemia is a recessive trait, i.e., it requires a double dose of the abnormal gene for expression at the clinical level. Nevertheless, the sickle gene is expressed in single dose as well, giving rise to carriers with SA hemoglobin. Recessive traits are *codominant* when viewed biochemically at the level of the gene product.

With few exceptions, each of the approximately 1900 mendelian diseases is rare. The overall population frequency of monogenic disorders is about 10 per 1000 live births, comprising about 7 per 1000 dominants, about 2.5 per 1000 recessives, and about 0.4 per 1000 X-linked conditions (see Table 33–1).

TABLE 33–1. PREVALENCE OF SELECTED MONOGENIC DISORDERS AMONG LIVEBORN INFANTS*

Disorder	Estimated Prevalence
Autosomal Dominant	
Familial hypercholesterolemia	1 in 500
Polycystic kidney disease	1 in 1250
Huntington's disease	1 in 2500
Hereditary spherocytosis	1 in 5000
Marfan's syndrome	1 in 20,000
Autosomal Recessive	
Sickle cell anemia	1 in 625 (U.S. blacks)
Cystic fibrosis	1 in 2000 (Caucasians)
Tay-Sachs disease	1 in 3000 (U.S. Jews)
Cystinuria	1 in 7000
Phenylketonuria	1 in 12,000
Mucopolysaccharidoses (all types)	1 in 25,000
Glycogen storage disease (all types)	1 in 50,000
Galactosemia	1 in 57,000
Homocystinuria	1 in 200,000
X-linked	
Duchenne muscular dystrophy	1 in 7000
Hemophilia	1 in 10,000

*Data assembled from Galjaard, Carter, and Motulsky.

If a particular disease shows a mendelian pattern of inheritance, its pathogenesis, no matter how complex, must be due to a single abnormal protein molecule. For example, in sickle cell disease, such seemingly unrelated disturbances as hemolytic anemia, painful crises, nephropathy, vascular occlusions, and *Salmonella* osteomyelitis are all physiologic consequences of a single missense mutation, resulting in a single amino acid substitution in the β-globin chain. When two or more phenotypic characters are controlled by a single gene, that gene is said to have *pleiotropic* effects.

AUTOSOMAL DOMINANT TRAITS. Autosomal genes are those genes situated on chromosomes other than the X or Y. When there are two alleles, A and a, at a locus, three possible genotypes exist: AA, Aa, and aa. Genotypes AA and aa are *homozygotes*; Aa is a *heterozygote*.

Dominant traits are fully manifest in the presence of a gene in the heterozygous state, i.e., when only one abnormal gene (*mutant allele*) is present and the corresponding partner allele on the homologous chromosome is normal. Figure 33–1 shows

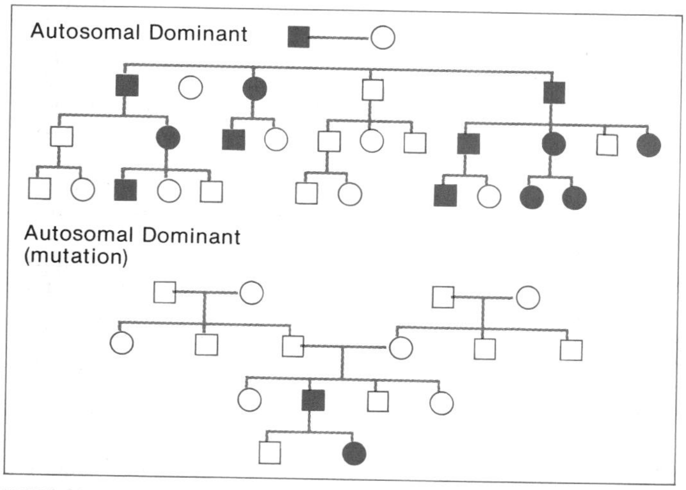

FIGURE 33–1. Pedigrees of autosomal dominant traits. In the lower pedigree the normal parents of the affected individual suggest the possibility of a new mutation. Solid symbols indicate those affected. (For details see text.)

a typical pedigree of transmission of an autosomal dominant trait. The following features are characteristic: (1) Each affected individual has an affected parent (unless the condition arose by a new mutation in a germ cell that formed the individual); (2) an affected individual will bear, on average, an equal number of affected and unaffected offspring; (3) males and females will be affected in equal numbers; (4) each sex can transmit the trait to male and female offspring (i.e., male-to-male transmission is possible); (5) normal children of an affected individual will have only normal offspring; and (6) when the trait does not impair viability or reproductive capacity, there will be *vertical* transmission of the trait through successive generations.

Most autosomal dominant disorders show two additional characteristics that are not seen in recessive disorders: (1) marked variability in severity, or *expressivity*, and (2) delayed age of onset. Dominant traits in humans often exert only mild effects. Occasionally the expression of the abnormal gene is so weak that a generation appears to be skipped because the carrier of the abnormal gene is clinically normal. When this is the case, the trait is said to be *nonpenetrant*. When a gene of a dominant trait exists in the homozygous state, the effect may be very severe, perhaps lethal. Examples are common in animals in which experimental matings can be constructed, but rare in humans, because matings of two affected heterozygotes are exceptional. One example is homozygous familial hypercholesterolemia. Others possibly include achondroplasia and Osler-Weber-Rendu syndrome. Delayed age of onset is seen in Huntington's disease and adult polycystic kidney disease. These disorders do not become manifest clinically until adult life, even though the mutant gene has been present since conception.

In every autosomal dominant disease some affected persons owe their disorder to a new mutation rather than to an inherited allele. Since a reasonable estimate of the frequency of mutation is of the order of 5×10^{-6} mutations per gene per generation, and since a dominant trait requires a mutation in only one of the parental gametes, one would expect that about 1 in 100,000 newborn persons would possess a new mutation at any given genetic locus. Many mutations will be silent or will involve a recessive function and not be manifest in a single gene dose. However, others will cause a defective gene product that gives rise to a dominant trait.

The percentage of patients with dominant disorders that represents a new mutation is inversely proportional to the effect of the disease upon *biologic fitness*, i.e., survival to adult life, and reproductive capacity. If a dominant mutation produces early death or absolute infertility, genetic transmission is impossible, and all cases represent new mutations. In tuberous sclerosis, the severe mental retardation reduces biologic fitness to about 20 per cent of normal, and the proportion of cases due to new mutations is about 80 per cent. In dominant conditions such as familial hypercholesterolemia, in which there is no reduction in biologic fitness, virtually all cases have a family pedigree showing classic vertical transmission

New mutations appear to be more frequent in the germ cells of fathers of relatively advanced age. Both Marfan's syndrome and achondroplastic dwarfism display such "paternal age effect." Fathers of sporadic cases of both conditions are an average of five to seven years older than the general population of fathers or than fathers who transmit these syndromes because of an inherited mutation. Diagnosis of a new mutation must exclude low expressivity of the trait in the carrier parent and also mistaken paternity.

The molecular basis of most of the more than 900 autosomal dominant disorders is obscure. Because in a dominant disorder expression of the mutation in only 50 per cent of the gene product may be sufficient to cause disease, the mutations are likely to involve two classes of proteins: (1) those that regulate complex metabolic pathways, such as membrane receptors as in familial hypercholesterolemia, and (2) key nonenzymic or structural proteins, such as hemoglobin or collagen, or a membrane protein as in hereditary spherocytosis.

In contrast to recessive disorders, in which an enzyme deficiency is the rule, defective enzymes are only rarely found in dominant disorders. Deficiencies of *Cl-esterase inhibitor* in hereditary angioedema and of *uroporphyrinogen-1 synthetase* in acute intermittent porphyria are exceptions to this general rule.

AUTOSOMAL RECESSIVE DISORDERS. Autosomal recessive conditions are clinically apparent only in the homozygous state, i.e., when both alleles at a particular genetic locus are mutant alleles. Figure 33–2 shows a typical pedigree of an autosomal recessive trait. The following features are characteristic: (1) The parents are clinically normal; (2) only siblings are affected; (3) males and females are affected in equal proportions; (4) if an affected individual marries a homozygous normal person, none of the children will be affected but all will be heterozygous carriers; (5) if an affected individual marries a heterozygous carrier, one half of the children will be affected, and the pedigree pattern will superficially suggest a dominant trait; (6) if two individuals who are homozygous for the same mutant gene marry, all of their children will be affected; (7) if both parents are heterozygous at the same genetic locus, one fourth of their children will be homozygous affected, one fourth will be homozygous normal, and one half will be heterozygous carriers of the same mutant gene; and (8) the less frequent the mutant gene is in the population, the greater is the likelihood that the affected individual is the product of consanguine parents.

In actual practice, unless the kinship is very large, the ratio of affected to unaffected sibs is frequently greater than one in four. Inclusion of probands in the enumeration loads the results in favor of the trait. In a sibship of 100 or even 10 the loading factor is not pronounced. However, in all ascertainable one-child sibships the involvement is 100 per cent, in two-child sibships it is 67 per cent (when the fundamental probability is 50 per cent), in three-child sibships it is 57 per cent, and so on. In small sibships a correction must be made for *bias of ascertainment*. The simplest method is to exclude the proband from the calculation and to determine the proportion of affected children among the remaining sibs.

In most autosomal recessive conditions the clinical presentation tends to be more uniform than in dominant diseases, and the onset is often early in life. Recessive disorders are commonly diagnosed in childhood. Approximately 800 well-established recessive traits have been recognized in humans, and in over 250 of these the mutant enzyme or other protein has been identified.

A *completely* recessive disease is one in which the heterozygote is clinically normal. When some features of the disease are detectable in the heterozygote, the disease is sometimes said to show *intermediate inheritance*, or to be *incompletely recessive* or *incompletely dominant*. The ambiguity of these terms

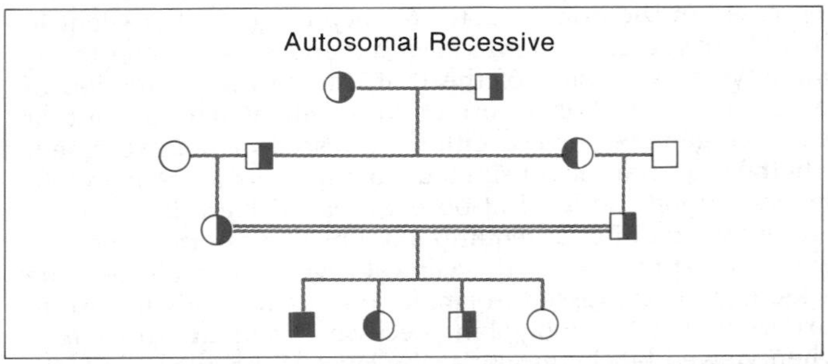

FIGURE 33–2. Pedigree of autosomal recessive trait. Note that both parents are heterozygous. One sib is affected, two are carriers, and one is normal. Double line (═══) indicates that parents are related by descent (first cousins).

from classic genetic studies of phenotypes is further emphasized by results of different methods of detection of gene effects. In many instances of completely recessive inheritance, refined biochemical observations enable the recognition of the trait in the clinically normal heterozygote. An example is Tay-Sachs disease, in which clinically normal parents and some sibs can be shown to be heterozygotes by assay of hexosaminidase A in leukocytes. Because of its importance in genetic counseling the detection of healthy heterozygous carriers of genes that in the homozygous state cause overt disease is one of the most significant aspects of medical genetics. Since by definition a dominant trait is one that is detectable in the heterozygous state, Tay-Sachs disease (and many others) is recessive when the clinical phenotype is considered and dominant when the biochemical phenotype is determined.

In pure form a recessive disease requires the inheritance of identical mutant genes from both parents. When the mutant genes are rare, the likelihood that any two unrelated parents are carriers for the same defect is small. Inheritance of two different mutant genes derived from the same locus gives rise to *heteroallelic compounds*. Individuals with Hb SC disease are genetic compounds who have inherited a different abnormal β-globin gene from each parent. Genetic compounds are also known in cystinuria, phenylketonuria, certain of the mucopolysaccharidoses, "homozygous" familial hypercholesterolemia, and several other disorders.

If the parents of a child with a recessive disorder have a common ancestor who carried a mutant gene, then the likelihood that two of the descendants would each have inherited the gene becomes relatively great. The less frequent the gene, the stronger is the likelihood that an affected individual has resulted from a consanguine mating. First cousins share, on the average, one eighth of their genes. When two first cousins marry, an offspring has, on the average, one sixteenth of the loci homozygous for a gene derived from a common ancestor. In general, offspring of first-cousin mating are slightly more likely to have congenital malformations, as well as mental defects and metabolic diseases, than are children born to unrelated parents.

Increased frequency of consanguinity will not be observed if the recessive disease is common. Sickle cell anemia, phenylketonuria, cystic fibrosis, and Tay-Sachs disease are examples in which the carrier (heterozygote) state is frequent in certain populations and in which consanguinity is usually not present in the parents. Increase in consanguinity would also not be expected in dominant or X-linked traits or genetic compounds.

A high percentage of recessive disorders involves abnormalities of enzyme proteins. In most reactions the normal maximal enzyme activity is greatly in excess of catalytic requirements; i.e., the concentration of a substrate is usually maintained at a point well below saturation for the enzyme that metabolizes it. Hence a reduction to 50 per cent of normal activity in a heterozygote does not impair the health of the carrier, whereas a total or near total deficiency may result in a serious inborn error of metabolism. These conditions are discussed in Ch. 34.

X-LINKED INHERITANCE. Diseases or traits that result from genes located on the X chromosome are termed X-linked. Since the female has two X chromosomes, she may be either heterozygous or homozygous for the mutant gene, and the trait may exhibit recessive or dominant expression. The male has only one X chromosome and therefore is *hemizygous* for X-linked traits. Males can be expected to express X-linked traits regardless of their recessive or dominant behavior in the female. Thus, the terms X-linked dominant or X-linked recessive refer only to expression of the trait in females.

Since males transmit their X chromosome only to daughters, an important feature of X-linked inheritance is the absence of male-to-male transmission. Affected males transmit the trait to all of their daughters and none of their sons.

Since the female carries two X chromosomes in each cell, it might be expected that the concentrations of proteins determined by genes on the X chromosome would be twice that of males who carry only one X chromosome per cell. This is not the case, and the explanation is provided by the process of X-inactivation first proposed by Mary Lyon, and often termed the *Lyon hypothesis*. In all adult female cells only one of the X chromosomes is genetically active. Early in differentiation one of the X chromosomes becomes inactive and forms the *Barr body*. Inactivation is random so that for each cell there is an equal probability that the paternally or maternally derived X chromosome will be inactivated. Once one of the two X chromosomes is inactivated, the same X chromosome remains inactive throughout all subsequent cell divisions. Thus, on the average one half of the cells of a female will express the X chromosome of her father, and one half of her mother: In this respect the normal female is a mosaic. If one of the X chromosomes carries a mutant gene, the probability is that the mutant phenotype will be expressed in one half of her cells. However, this statistical probability may be disturbed in at least two ways: (1) Since inactivation of one of the X chromosomes occurs early in development and is random, some females may by chance have many more cells that carry an active X chromosome derived from one parent than from the other; and (2) if one of the X chromosomes carries a mutant gene that confers a metabolic disadvantage upon cells with that mutation, these cells may survive less frequently during development, and the female offspring may have cells that carry predominantly or exclusively the active X chromosome without the mutation.

Over 120 loci have been identified on the human X chromosome, and many have been mapped to specific regions on the long or the short arm of the chromosome.

X-Linked Dominant Traits. This mode of inheritance (Fig. 33–3) is uncommon. Its characteristic features are as follows: (1) Females are affected about twice as often as males, (2) heterozygous females will transmit the trait to both sexes with a frequency of 50 per cent, (3) hemizygous affected males will transmit the trait to all of their daughters and none of their sons, and (4) the expression is more variable and generally less severe in heterozygous females than in hemizygous affected males. Examples of X-linked dominant inheritance include the Xg(a^+) blood group, vitamin D-resistant (hypophosphatemic) rickets, and pseudohypoparathyroidism.

Some rare X-linked dominant disorders occur only in the heterozygous female, because the condition is lethal in the hemizygous affected male. Additional characteristics of this form of inheritance are as follows: (1) An affected mother will transmit the trait to one half of her daughters (heterozygotes), and (2) an increased frequency of abortions occurs in affected women, the abortions representing affected male fetuses. Examples of disorders that appear to fit this mode of inheritance include incontinentia pigmenti, focal dermal hypoplasia, orofaciodigital syndrome, and hyperammonemia caused by ornithine transcarbamylase deficiency.

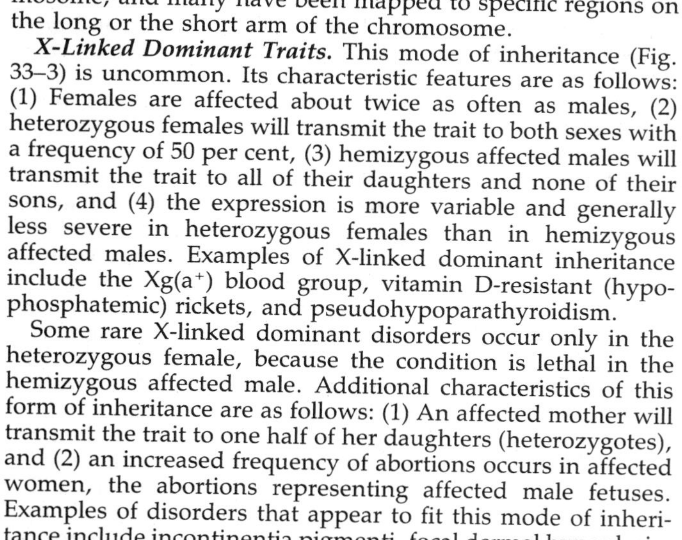

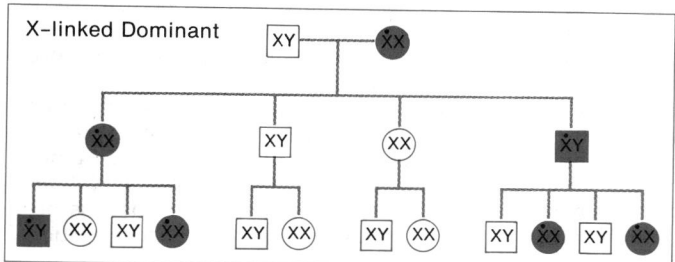

FIGURE 33–3. Pedigree of dominant X-linked trait. The X chromosome bearing the abnormal gene is designated by a small dot.

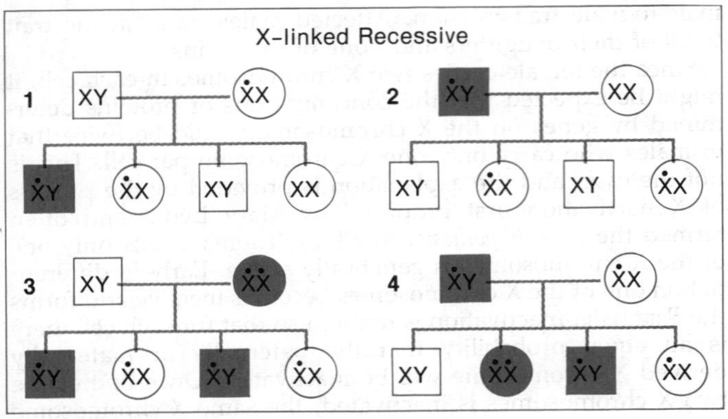

FIGURE 33–4. Pedigrees of X-linked recessive trait. The X chromosome bearing the abnormal gene is designated by a small dot. Affected individuals are indicated by solid squares (males) and circles (females). Pedigree 1 is commonly observed; pedigree 4 is rare.

X-Linked Recessive Traits. This mode of inheritance (Fig. 33–4) is relatively common. Its characteristic features are as follows: (1) The disorder is fully expressed only in the hemizygous affected male. (2) Heterozygous females are usually normal; occasionally they may exhibit mild features of the disorder; rarely they may be almost as severely affected as the hemizygous affected male (this variability is attributed to the probability that a disproportionate percentage of *normal* X chromosomes of the heterozygous female may have been inactivated early in development [see "Lyon hypothesis," above]). (3) On average, a heterozygous female will transmit the trait to one half of her sons (hemizygous affected), but the other half will be normal. (4) On average, one half of daughters of a heterozygous female will be carriers and one half will be normal. (5) All daughters of an affected male married to a normal female will be carriers, and no sons of such a union will be affected (no father-to-son transmission). (6) In the rare event of the union of an affected male and a heterozygous female, one half of daughters will be homozygous affected and one half will be heterozygous carriers; one half of sons will be hemizygous affected (maternal inheritance) and one half will be normal. Thus in this situation, one half of all offspring will be affected. (7) If the trait is rare, parents and relatives will be normal except for male relatives in the female line; e.g., on average, one half of maternal uncles will be affected. This "uncle and nephew" pattern gives rise to an *oblique* pedigree pattern, in contrast to the vertical pattern of autosomal dominant conditions and the horizontal pattern of autosomal recessive conditions.

Examples of X-linked recessive conditions include hemophilia A, Duchenne form of muscular dystrophy, the Lesch-Nyhan syndrome, glucose-6-phosphate dehydrogenase deficiency, and Fabry's disease. In several of these, e.g., Duchenne muscular dystrophy and Fabry's disease, heterozygous females may exhibit mild or even moderately severe forms of the disease. Color blindness is also an X-linked inherited trait, but it is sufficiently frequent (occurring in about 8 per cent of Caucasian males) that the occurrence of homozygous color-blind females is not rare.

It is important to distinguish between X-linked inheritance and *sex-influenced autosomal dominant inheritance*. Baldness and hemochromatosis are examples of autosomal dominant traits that are sex influenced. Heterozygous females express the gene for baldness only when a source of testosterone becomes available (e.g., a masculinizing tumor of the ovary). Heterozygous females rarely develop clinical hemochromatosis because menstruation and pregnancy mitigate the accumulation of iron.

Y-LINKED INHERITANCE. A gene on the Y chromosome will be transmitted through the father to all of his sons and none of his daughters. The only genes currently known to be located on the Y chromosome are those that determine "maleness" and an antigen that influences graft rejection.

POLYGENIC INHERITANCE. Most phenotypic traits are determined by the collaboration of many genes at different loci rather than by single gene effects. Polygenic inheritance is suggested for traits that show continuous variation in the form of a normal distribution curve. Height and intelligence are examples of polygenic traits in which the extremes of the distribution are not necessarily considered abnormal. Parents and offspring, and on average siblings also, have 50 per cent of their genes in common. Second-degree relatives share on average one fourth of all genes $(\frac{1}{2})^2$, and third-degree relatives (cousins) share one eighth $(\frac{1}{2})^3$. Thus as the degree of relation becomes more distant, the probability of inheriting the same combination of genes is reduced, and the degree of resemblance is likely to be less.

Many of the common chronic diseases of adults (such as essential hypertension, diabetes mellitus, hyperuricemia, hypercholesterolemia, coronary artery disease, and schizophrenia) and the common birth defects of children (such as cleft palate and lip and congenital heart disease) that tend to run in families fit best into the category of *multifactorial genetic disease*. This category should be suspected when the pedigree of a disease does not support inheritance in a simple dominant or recessive manner. In multifactorial genetic disease there is both a polygenic component and an environmental component of causative factors. In the population at large there are *risk* genes present in low frequency. If in any one individual there is a particularly large number of risk genes, the latent disorder becomes overt. When an individual inherits just the right combination of risk genes, he or she passes beyond a "risk threshold" at which environmental factors may determine the expression and severity of disease (Fig. 33–5). In order for another family member to develop the same disease, that individual would have to inherit the same or nearly similar combination of genes. The likelihood of such an occurrence is clearly greater in first-degree than in more distant relatives. The chances of any relative's inheriting the right combination of risk genes also decrease as the number of genes required for the expression of a given trait increases. Elegant and complex mathematical models have been advanced for polygenic-multifactorial disease, but these should not obscure the fact that each of the risk genes must express itself, like any other gene, by way of a specific biochemical product. Eventually the vague concept of genetic susceptibility of polygenic inheritance must yield to the basic premise that genes control the synthesis of specific proteins with specific functions.

The hypothesis of polygenic components in the inheritance of multifactorial disease has been given a potential mechanistic basis by the demonstration that as many as 28 per cent of all gene loci may contain polymorphic alleles that vary among

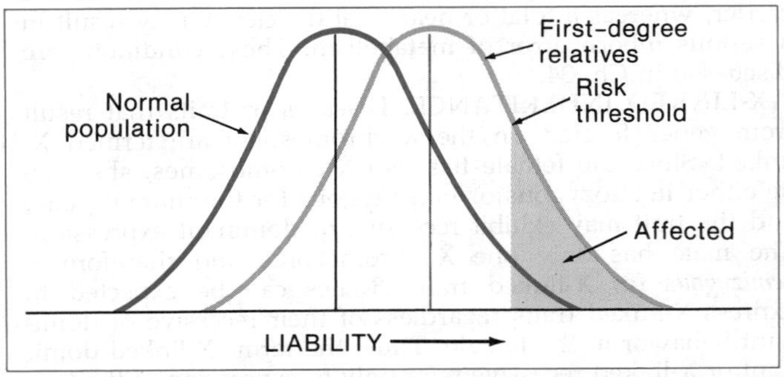

FIGURE 33–5. Diseases that conform to a polygenic multifactorial model of inheritance lead to an increased prevalence of disease among the relatives of affected individuals. This increased prevalence is most evident among first-degree relatives.

individuals. Such a large degree of variation in normal genes provides basis for variation in genetic predisposition with which other genetic or environmental factors can interact. To date genetic loci most prominently associated with disease susceptibility are those composing the major histocompatibility (MHC) locus or human leukocyte antigen (HLA) system. The HLA system consists of four distinct but closely linked, highly polymorphic loci situated on the short arm of chromosome 6. These loci as ordered on the chromosome are HLA-A, HLA-C, HLA-B, and HLA-D/DR. The A, B, C, and DR loci are defined serologically; the D locus controls lymphocyte (LD) antigens detectable by the mixed lymphocyte reaction (MLR). The D and DR (D-related) loci are closely linked but may not produce identical antigens. The products of these genes are proteins that are found on the surface of body cells and that enable an individual's immune system to distinguish its own cells (self) from those of someone else (nonself). Each HLA locus in the population consists of multiple alleles, each of which produces an immunologically distinct protein. HLA-A has at least 20 alleles, HLA-B has at least 42, C has at least 8, D has at least 12, and DR has at least 10 identified thus far. The inheritance of certain alleles predisposes to the development of certain diseases, in some instances when the individual is exposed to a particular environmental challenge. For example, the frequency of B27 allele in the white population is approximately 8 per cent. In patients with ankylosing spondylitis the frequency of B27 is over 90 per cent. In Australian aborigines and black Africans the B27 antigen is virtually absent and the frequency of ankylosing spondylitis is sharply reduced. A Caucasian with the B27 antigen is approximately 120 times more likely to develop ankylosing spondylitis than one who does not posses the antigen; the increased liability among Japanese with the B27 antigen is 300 times. Reiter's syndrome may follow an infection of the bowel or urinary tract with *Shigella*, *Salmonella*, or *Yersinia* organisms. No less than 20 per cent of B27-positive individuals with *Shigella* infections will develop Reiter's syndrome. Other disease associations of the HLA system are discussed in Ch. 425.

Multifactorial or polygenic inheritance must not be confused with *genetic heterogeneity*. Hypercholesterolemia and hyperuricemia behave as multifactorial traits when viewed at the population level. At the family level, however, it is sometimes possible to identify a single locus that is mainly responsible for the disease in that family. Examples include familial hypercholesterolemia, an autosomal dominant trait present in about 5 per cent of subjects with premature myocardial infarctions, which in single-gene dosage produces atherosclerosis in the absence of any extraordinary environmental factor; or hypoxanthine-guanine phosphoribosyltransferase deficiency, an X-linked recessive trait present in about 0.5 per cent of subjects with gout, which in the hemizygous state produces marked purine overproduction without any relationship to obesity or alcohol consumption.

MITOCHONDRIAL INHERITANCE. Each mitochondrion contains several circular chromosomes that code for certain ribosomal and transfer ribonucleic acids (RNA's) and for 13 polypeptides involved in oxidative phosphorylation, the chief function of the mitochondrion. The mitochondrial code differs from that of nuclear DNA and that of any contemporary prokaryote; it is similar to that of bacteria. Mitochondrial inheritance is exclusively matrilineal. Lebar's optic atrophy and certain myopathies associated with "ragged-red fiber" disease are thought to involve mitochondrial inheritance.

GENE FREQUENCY. The distribution of a mutant gene in the general population may be calculated on the basis of the Hardy-Weinberg equation. If the frequency of a particular gene A is p, then that of its alternative allele is $(1 - p) = q$. There will be three genotypes in the population: Those who are homozygous AA, those who are heterozygous Aa, and those who are homozygous aa. In a randomly mating population the frequencies of these genotypes will be in the proportion p^2(AA), 2pg(Aa), and q^2(aa). An important consequence of this distribution is that irrespective of the initial frequency of the genes A and a in the population, the proportion of the three genotypes will tend to remain constant in succeeding generations, provided that there is no difference in biologic fitness of any of the genotypes. If there is unequal viability or fertility among the three genotypes, or if mating is not random, the frequency calculations require considerable correction, and in small populations major changes in gene frequency can occur on the basis of chance alone.

If the frequency of a recessive disease in a particular population is known, the frequency of heterozygous carriers and of the abnormal gene can be calculated. Thus for a recessively inherited disease aa (q^2) with a frequency of 1 per 10,000 (e.g., albinism), the frequency of the gene a (q) will be 1 per 100, and that of heterozygous carriers will be $2 \times p \times q = 2 \times 99/100 \times 1/100 =$ approximately 1 in 50. Thus, in this particular example there will be 200 clinically unaffected carriers of the abnormal gene for every affected individual. Table 33–1 lists the frequency of several inherited diseases. Cystic fibrosis, a recessively inherited disease, has a prevalence in the white population of about 1 per 2500 (q^2); thus the frequency of the gene (q) is 1 in 50 and of heterozygous carriers is approximately 1 in 25, or 4 per cent of the white population. A similar calculation with respect to sickle cell anemia among United States blacks ($q^2 = 1/625$) yields a frequency of heterozygous carriers of 1 in 12.5, or 8 per cent of the United States black population.

The frequency of most genes in the population is relatively stable. When a gene is rare and severely disadvantageous, the rate of its introduction into a population by spontaneous mutation is balanced by the rate of elimination of the disadvantageous gene by natural selection. The frequency of the disadvantageous gene, however, can be stabilized at a high level if the heterozygotes are slightly favored (increased biologic fitness) and leave a greater number of progeny than either homozygote. When a rare form of a species is present at a frequency that cannot be maintained by recurrent mutation alone, a *balanced polymorphism* is said to exist. Usually this means that the rarer of two allelic forms occurs with a frequency of at least 1 per cent of the population. When this is found, *heterozygote advantage* should be suspected. An example of such a balanced polymorphism is the increased resistance of individuals heterozygous for the sickle cell trait to falciparum malaria. Although persons with sickle cell disease (homozygotes, SS hemoglobin) often die before they can reproduce, and thus remove the sickle cell gene from the population, the prevalence of heterozygotes (SA hemoglobin) may nevertheless reach 40 per cent in certain West African populations. Death from falciparum malaria is much less frequent in carriers of the sickle cell trait than in noncarriers, and thus the heterozygote does have an advantage. Whether the extraordinary frequency of heterozygotes for the sickle gene in West Africa is due entirely to differential mortality or in part to differential fertility is uncertain, but this example suffices to illustrate that the effects of genes can be assessed only in relation to a particular environment. In most instances, however, a distinct advantage for the heterozygote of a polymorphic trait (of which there are many; see Ch. 34) cannot be demonstrated, and the possibility exists that certain polymorphic traits are genetically neutral.

The term *genetic load* has been used to describe the total genetic disability of a population. It comprises both a *mutational load*, based on recurrent mutation of a normal gene to a lethal or sublethal gene, and a *segregational load*, resulting from segregation of the harmful gene from advantaged heterozygotes, as in the example of sickle cell heterozygotes discussed above. Each individual has been estimated to have three to eight genes, which, if homozygous instead of heterozygous, would be lethal. The relative contribution of the segregational and mutational loads to the total genetic load is uncertain.

THE HUMAN GENE MAP. Over 1780 autosomal loci are known, on the basis mainly of characteristic patterns of inheritance of alternative forms of a particular trait. Some chromosomal mapping information is available for over 30 per cent of these loci. In addition, over 120 loci have been assigned to the X chromosome, and about an equal number are suspected but unproved.

Assignment of a locus to a specific chromosome is based on a variety of methods: (1) study of linkage of traits in large families with multiple alleles at two loci; (2) co-segregation of specific proteins and single chromosomes in clones from somatic cell hybrids; (3) DNA-RNA in situ hybridization; (4) deductions from amino acid sequences of proteins; (5) deletion mapping or gene dosage effects; (6) induction of microscopically detectable chromosomal change by adenovirus; (7) DNA/cDNA molecular hybridization in solution or "Cot analysis" of somatic cell hybrids containing a small number of human chromosomes; (8) DNA restriction endonuclease techniques; and (9) chromosomal aberrations.

About 68 per cent of gene assignments have been made on the basis of somatic cell hybridization studies (method 2, above), about 22 per cent on the basis of linkage of traits in families (method 1), and about 20 per cent from in situ hybridization studies (methods 3 and 7). (Many foci have been mapped by two or more methods.)

Some interesting observations have emerged. Structural genes for enzymes that catalyze sequential steps in a metabolic pathway are as a rule not located on the same chromosome. Thus, whereas in bacteria the enzymes for sequential metabolic steps are often determined by linked genes, thus assuring coordinate regulation of activity, the situation in humans is quite different. This finding accords with the lack of evidence for coordinate regulation of enzyme activity, or for an operon-like organization of structural genes, in eukaryotic cells. Even the subunits of polymeric proteins may be coded by genes on different chromosomes. The genes for the α chains of hemoglobin are on chromosome 16, whereas that for the β chain is on chromosome 11. Lactate dehydrogenase is an example of an enzymic protein that is constituted by subunits coded by genes on different chromosomes: LDH-A by a gene on chromosome 11, LDH-B by one on chromosome 12.

When the location of a gene is known, physicians can use the concept of gene linkage to predict which individual in a given family will be affected by a given trait. For example, the locus for the gene specifying the Rh blood group factor and the locus for the gene producing one form of the dominant trait, hereditary elliptocytosis, occur in close proximity on chromosome 1. Thus, if a subject with hereditary elliptocytosis transmits the anomaly to an offspring, the offspring will usually inherit the allele that is present at the Rh locus on the chromosome. If the Rh allele on this chromosome happens to be a rare one in the population (such as r′), one can assume that whichever offspring inherits the r′ allele at the Rh locus will also inherit the abnormal allele at the elliptocytosis locus.

Carter CO: Monogenic disorders. J Med Genet 14:316, 1977. *An estimate of birth frequencies of selected genetic conditions.*

Cavalli-Sforza LL, Bodmer WF: The Genetics of Human Populations. 2nd ed. San Francisco, W. H. Freeman and Company, 1978. *An authoritative textbook of human genetics.*

Galjaard H: Genetic Metabolic Diseases. Early Diagnosis and Prenatal Analysis. Amsterdam, Elsevier/North Holland Biomedical Press, 1980. *An 850-page book on hereditary disorders, about one third of which is devoted to methods and results of prenatal diagnosis.*

McKusick VA: The anatomy of the human genome. Am J Med 69:267, 1980. *An excellent discussion of the basis and significance of the assignment of more than 350 genes to specific chromosomes, with a catalogue of assignments up to mid 1980.*

McKusick VA: Human Genetics. 2nd ed. Englewood Cliffs, N.J., Prentice-Hall, 1969. *An excellent introductory survey of human genetics.*

McKusick VA: Mendelian Inheritance in Man. 7th ed. Baltimore, Johns Hopkins University Press, 1986. *A catalogue of autosomal dominant, autosomal recessive, and X-linked phenotypes, with brief descriptions and literature references for each.*

Motulsky AG: Frequency of sickling disorders in U.S. blacks. N Engl J Med 288:31, 1973. *Gives estimated prevalence of all sickling disorders in the population (HB SS disease, Hb SC disease, and Hb S-β thalassemia).*

Vogel F, Motulsky AG: Human Genetics: Problems and Approaches. 2nd ed. Berlin, Springer-Verlag, 1986. *A superb and up-to-date treatment of human genetics.*

34 INBORN ERRORS OF METABOLISM

James B. Wyngaarden

The inspired concept of inborn errors of metabolism, developed by Archibald Garrod in the first decade of this century, marks the birth of biochemical genetics. Garrod's studies of alcaptonuria, pentosuria, albinism, and cystinuria led to the proposal of a new category of diseases in which a block in a metabolic pathway arises from an inherited deficiency of a specific enzyme. This concept was proved in 1948 when Gibson found a deficiency of NADH-dependent methemoglobin reductase in recessive methemoglobinemia. This was soon followed by the discovery in 1952 by Cori and Cori of a deficiency of glucose-6-phosphatase in von Gierke's disease, in 1953 by Jervis of phenylalanine hydroxylase deficiency in phenylketonuria, and in 1956 by LaDu of homogentisic acid oxidase deficiency in alcaptonuria as originally predicted by Garrod. By 1987 deficiencies of over 215 different enzymes have been associated with hereditary disease. Of even greater importance in the history of genetics was the remarkable insight in Garrod's hypothesis that the primary action of a gene is to control the synthesis of a specific enzyme. Decades later Beadle (1945) independently proposed the one gene–one enzyme hypothesis anticipated by Garrod.

In 1949 Pauling, Itano, and associates observed that sickle cell hemoglobin exhibited abnormal electrophoretic behavior and introduced the concept of *molecular disease,* in which a structural alteration in a macromolecule accounted for a specific functional change that was responsible for a disease state. In 1953 Ingram demonstrated the substitution of a single amino acid residue in the β-chain of sickle cell hemoglobin, confirming the concept of molecular disease and initiating an ever-lengthening series of findings of structural alterations in macromolecules that result from gene mutations. For a time "missing" enzyme diseases and hemoglobinopathies were thought to represent distinct categories of disease, perhaps representing defects of control and structural genes, respectively. More sensitive techniques have disclosed low levels of residual activity of the deficient enzyme in many inborn errors of metabolism. In some cases the mutation has affected a critical portion of the enzyme, radically reducing its catalytic activity; in others the mutation has rendered the enzyme highly unstable. In the case of erythrocytes that lack a nucleus and cannot continue to synthesize new protein, enzyme lability results in low enzyme activity values in the older cells. In several instances amino acid sequence studies of enzymes have disclosed single amino acid substitutions analogous to the defect in sickle hemoglobin. Thus many inborn errors of metabolism are molecular diseases in which the *primary* defect lies in the genetic specification of the protein.

Although most of the well-defined inborn errors of metabolism are inherited as recessive conditions, in principle any human phenotype showing mendelian genetics must be based on a specific variant or missing protein. Thus not only autosomal and X-linked recessive but also autosomal and X-linked dominant conditions may be expressed through abnormal proteins. Examples in which a mutant protein has been identified include autosomal recessive, alcaptonuria (homogentisic acid oxidase); X-linked recessive, Lesch-Nyhan syndrome (hypoxanthine–guanine phosphoribosyltransferase); autosomal dominant, acute intermittent porphyria (uroporphyrinogen I synthetase). No example of an X-linked dominant condition in which the mutant protein has been identified can be cited as yet. In one condition of this category, vitamin D–resistant (hypophosphatemic) rickets, a defect in phosphate transport is suspected but the membrane carrier has not been identified. The concept of inborn errors of metabolism has broadened considerably since first propounded by Garrod. A reasonable definition would include any condition of clinical significance that shows a mendelian mode of inheritance, but in practice the term is restricted to conditions that have recognizable biochemical manifestations.

A mutant protein that cannot be detected by functional assay may nevertheless retain immunologic reactivity. However, in some instances no protein can be detected by functional or immunologic means. In the terminology of microbial genetics, the former class of mutants is frequently called CRM(+) ("krim" positive) and the latter CRM(−). The presence of CRM(+) material suggests that the genetic defect is due to a mis-sense mutation with a consequent amino acid substitution that destroys the activity but not the antigenicity of the mutant enzyme. In most cases in which mutant enzymes have been studied, cross-reactive material has been detected. However, in the Lesch-Nyhan syndrome only 1 CRM(+) mutant has been found among 14 studied. At the pseudocholinesterase locus, 17 CRM(+) mutants and 18 CRM(−) mutants have been recognized. A CRM(−) reaction does not prove that no protein is present; the protein may be so altered that both enzyme function and immunologic reactivity have been lost.

Mutation does not necessarily result in loss of enzyme activity. Several examples of increased activity are known. The best examples are three types of phosphoribosylpyrophosphate synthetase overactivity associated with purine overproduction and gout. In one there is a 2.5-fold increase in enzyme activity per molecule; in another, excessive activity is a reflection of diminished affinity for normal intracellular nucleotide inhibitors; in a third, the overactivity results from an increased affinity for ribose 5-phosphate, a substrate of the reaction. All of these changes reflect alterations of enzyme structure. Some of the clinical conditions in which an abnormality of a specific protein has been observed are listed in Tables 34–1 and 34–2. Others include deficiencies of peptide hormones, abnormalities of binding proteins (receptor diseases) and of epidermal proteins, and defects in transmembrane transport (e.g., cystinuria). Chromosome mapping data exist for many inborn errors. Some examples are given in Table 34–3.

ETIOLOGY. The etiology of an inborn error of metabolism is a mutant gene. If the amino acid sequence of the mutant protein is known, it is possible to deduce the nature of the mutation from the genetic code. The human variant of glucose-6-phosphate dehydrogenase, G6PD Hektoen, differs from normal G6PD in a single amino acid substitution, HIS →TYR. This substitution corresponds to a mutation from GTA(or G) to ATA(or G) in a codon in the structural gene for G6PD. Most of the amino acid sequence information of human mutant proteins has been obtained from studies of red blood cell proteins, such as hemoglobin and G6PD. At least four types of mutations can be discerned by this approach: deletions, duplications, mis-sense mutations, and frame-shift mutations.

Another type of mutation, the non-sense mutation, has also been demonstrated in humans, using DNA restriction enzyme analysis and DNA sequencing techniques. The partial nucleotide sequence of β-globin mRNA isolated from a unique patient with homozygous β°-thalassemia disclosed a replacement of an adenine by a uracil in the codon for position 17. This changed the RNA codon from AAG to AUG, a termination codon. As a result a nonfunctional partial β-chain, only 16 amino acids long, was synthesized. Hb McKees-Rock represents another example of mutation of an amino acid codon to a terminator codon, but in this case the β-globin is shortened by only two amino acids and is functional.

DNA cloning techniques permit direct study of the altered DNA sequence in many human mutations, even those that involve genes that code for quantitatively minor proteins, such as most enzymes. These recent developments are discussed in Ch. 35.

PATHOGENESIS OF GENETIC DISEASE. The consequence of a mutation will depend on the function normally served by the product of the gene. Mutations in genes for rRNA or tRNA would very likely affect protein synthesis generally and might be incompatible with life. No such mutations have been identified in mammalian systems, although they are known in bacteria.

Defects involving nonenzymic proteins undoubtedly account for a large number of genetic diseases, but relatively few have been defined biochemically. The hemoglobinopathies are an exception. Over 580 hemoglobin variants are now known. A few additional examples exist. In one of these, the ZZ variant of α-1-antitrypsin deficiency, two amino acid substitutions (mis-sense mutations) in α-1-antitrypsin lead to the production of a modified protein that is not susceptible to normal post-translational processing. As a consequence carbohydrate residues are not added to the protein in the normal manner, and the defective glycoprotein accumulates in liver cells, possibly because the altered molecule cannot be secreted. Other examples in which a specific mutant protein has been identified, although the precise molecular alteration has not yet been defined, include the abnormal plasma membrane receptor in familial hypercholesterolemia, the abnormal cytoplasmic androgen receptor in the complete form of testicular feminization, an abnormal insulin in familial hyperproinsulinemia, and an abnormal protein called dynein in the microtubules of cilia in Kartagener's syndrome.

The largest number of known inborn errors of metabolism involves deficiencies of enzymes that catalyze discrete steps in biosynthetic or catabolic sequences. The consequences of metabolic blocks depend upon the function of the affected sequence and the properties of the affected substrates. In some conditions the disease is manifested by the inability to form a specific product, as in the failure of melanin production in one form of albinism. In others, accumulation of the precursor of a blocked reaction results in toxicity or in a storage disease. In phenylketonuria the block in phenylalanine hydroxylase results in accumulation of phenylalanine and overproduction of toxic phenylketone products. Deficiencies of various catabolic enzymes explain the progressive tissue accumulations in the mucopolysaccharidoses and sphingolipidoses. In some enzyme deficiencies, disease results from failure to modify another protein. For example, in some types of Ehlers-Danlos syndrome collagen polypeptide synthesis is normal but enzymes essential in cross-linking are deficient, with the result that fragile collagen is produced.

Polymorphism. Many proteins exist in two or more forms in the population. These multiple forms are the result of multiple genes (*alleles*) at the same genetic locus. If the most common allele at a given locus accounts for fewer than 99 per cent of the alleles in the population, *polymorphism* is said to occur. By definition, when polymorphism exists at a genetic locus, at least 2 per cent of the population must be heterozygous at that locus. Table 34–4 lists selected proteins for which polymorphism has been demonstrated electrophoretically. Many of these genetically determined variations in protein structure are unassociated with clinical disease.

Polymorphism appears to be very common. As many as 28 per cent of genetic loci coding for enzyme and other proteins of erythrocytes and serum show multiple alleles in the population, but this figure may be as low as 2 per cent of loci of

TABLE 34–1. DISORDERS IN WHICH DEFICIENT ACTIVITY OF A SPECIFIC ENZYME HAS BEEN DEMONSTRATED IN HUMAN BEINGS*

Condition	Enzyme with Deficient Activity
Acatalasia	Catalase
Acid phosphatase deficiency	Acid phosphatase
Acyl CoA dehydrogenase deficiency	Acyl CoA decarboxylase
Adrenal hyperplasia I	20,22 Desmolase
Adrenal hyperplasia II	3-β-Hydroxysteroid dehydrogenase
Adrenal hyperplasia III	Steroid cytochrome P450-21-hydroxylase
Adrenal hyperplasia IV	11-β-Hydroxylase
Adrenal hyperplasia V	17-α-Hydroxylase
Albinism	Tyrosinase
Alcaptonuria	Homogentisic acid oxidase
Aldosterone deficiency I	18-Hydroxylase (corticosterone methyl oxidase I)
Aldosterone deficiency II	18-OH-Dehydrogenase
Alpha-methylacetoaceticaciduria	β-Ketothiolase
Anemia, megaloblastic	Dihydrofolate reductase
Apnea, drug-induced	Pseudocholinesterase
Argininemia	Arginase
Argininosuccinic aciduria	Argininosuccinate lyase
Aspartylglycosaminuria	Special hydrolase (AADG-ase)
Ataxia, intermittent	Pyruvate decarboxylase
Carnosinemia	Carnosinase
Cerebrotendinous xanthomatosis	Mitochondrial 26-hydroxylase
Cholesteryl ester deficiency (Norum-Gjone disease)	Lecithin cholesterol acyltransferase (LCAT)
Citrullinemia	Argininosuccinate synthetase
Coproporphyria	Coproporphyrinogen III oxidase
Crigler-Najjar syndrome	Glucuronyl transferase
Cystathioninuria	γ-Cystathionase
2,8-Dihydroxyadenine nephrolithiasis	Adenine phosphoribosyl transferase
Disaccharide intolerance I	Invertase
Disaccharide intolerance II	Invertase, maltase
Disaccharide intolerance III	Lactase
Ehlers-Danlos syndrome, type VI	Collagen lysyl hydroxylase
Ehlers-Danlos syndrome, type VII	Procollagen peptidase
Ehlers-Danlos syndrome, type IX	Lysyloxidase
Ethanolaminosis	Ethanolamine kinase
Fabry's disease	α-Galactosidase A
Farber's lipogranulomatosis	Ceramidase
Formiminotransferase deficiency	Formiminotransferase
Fructose intolerance	Fructose-1-phosphate aldolase "B"
Fructose-1,6-diphosphatase deficiency	Fructose-1,6-diphosphatase
Fructosuria	Hepatic fructokinase
Fucosidosis	α-L-Fucosidase
Galactokinase deficiency	Galactokinase
Galactose epimerase deficiency	Galactose epimerase
Galactosemia	Galactose-1-phosphate uridyl transferase
Gangliosidosis, G_{M1}, type I or infantile	β-Galactosidase A,B
Gangliosidosis, G_{M1}, type II or juvenile	β-Galactosidase A,B
Gangliosidosis, G_{M2} (Tay-Sachs disease)	β-Hexosaminidase A
Gangliosidosis, G_{M2}, juvenile	β-Hexosaminidase A
Gangliosidosis, G_{M2}, adult	β-Hexosaminidase A
Gangliosidosis, G_{M2} (Sandhoff's disease)	β-Hexosaminidase B
Gangliosidosis, G_{M3}	UDP-N-acetyl-galactosaminyl transferase
Gaucher's disease	Acid β-glucosidase
G6PD deficiency (favism, primaquine sensitivity, etc.)	Glucose-6-phosphate dehydrogenase
Glutaric aciduria I	Glutaryl-CoA dehydrogenase
Glutaric aciduria II	Acyl-CoA dehydrogenase
Glutathionemia	γ-Glutamyl transferase
Glycogen storage disease Ia	Glucose-6-phosphatase
Glycogen storage disease Ib	Glucose-6-phosphate translocase
Glycogen storage disease II	α-1,4-Glucosidase
Glycogen storage disease III	Amylo-1, 6-glucosidase
Glycogen storage disease IV	Amylo-(1,4 to 1,6)-transglucosidase
Glycogen storage disease V	Muscle phosphorylase
Glycogen storage disease VI	Liver phosphorylase
Glycogen storage disease VII	Muscle phosphofructokinase
Glycogen storage disease VIII	Liver phosphorylase kinase
Gout, primary	Hypoxanthine-guanine phosphoribosyl transferase
Gout, primary	PP-ribose-P synthetase (increased)
Granulomatous disease, X-linked	NADPH oxidase ?
Gynecomastia, familial	Aromatase (elevated)
Hemolytic anemia	Adenosine triphosphatase
Hemolytic anemia	Adenylate kinase
Hemolytic anemia	Aldolase A
Hemolytic anemia	Diphosphoglycerate mutase
Hemolytic anemia	γ-Glutamylcysteine synthetase

Condition	Enzyme with Deficient Activity
Hemolytic anemia	Glucose-6-phosphate dehydrogenase
Hemolytic anemia	Glucose phosphate isomerase
Hemolytic anemia	Glutathione peroxidase
Hemolytic anemia	Glutathione reductase
Hemolytic anemia	Glutathione synthetase
Hemolytic anemia	Hexokinase
Hemolytic anemia	Phosphoglycerate kinase
Hemolytic anemia	Pyrimidine 5′-nucleotidase
Hemolytic anemia	Pyruvate kinase
Hemolytic anemia	Triosephosphate isomerase
Histidinemia	Histidine:ammonia lyase
HMG-CoA lyase deficiency	3-Hydroxy-3-methylglutarate-CoA lyase
Homocystinuria I	Cystathionine beta-synthase
Homocystinuria II	*N*(5,10)-Methylenetetrahydrofolate reductase
4-Hydroxybutyricaciduria	Succinic semialdehyde dehydrogenase
Hydroxyprolinemia	Hydroxyproline oxidase
Hyperalaninemia	β-Alanine-α-ketoglutarate aminotransferase
Hyperammonemia I	Ornithine transcarbamylase
Hyperammonemia II	Carbamyl phosphate synthetase
Hyperammonemia III	*N*-Acetylglutamate synthetase
Hyperglycerolemia	ATP:glycerol phosphotransferase
Hyperglycinemia, ketotic I	Propionyl CoA carboxylase, α subunit
Hyperglycinemia, ketotic II	Propionyl CoA carboxylase, β subunit
Hyperglycinemia, nonketotic form	Glycine formiminotransferase
Hyperlysinemia	Lysine-α-ketoglutarate reductase
Hyperprolinemia I	Proline oxidase
Hyperprolinemia II	δ-1-Pyrroline-5-carboxylate dehydrogenase
Hypoglycemia	Glycogen synthase
Hypophosphatasia	Alkaline phosphatase
Ichthyosis, X-linked	Steroid sulfatase
Immunodeficiency disease	Adenosine deaminase
Immunodeficiency disease	Purine nucleoside phosphorylase
Immunodeficiency disease	Uridine monophosphate kinase
Intestinal lactase deficiency (adult)	Lactase
Isovaleric acidemia	Isovaleryl CoA dehydrogenase
Ketoacidosis, infantile	Succinyl CoA:3-ketoacid CoA-transferase
Krabbe's disease	Galactocerebroside β-galactosidase
Lactic acidosis, congenital	Dihydrolipoyl dehydrogenase
Lactosyl ceramidosis	Neutral β-galactosidase
Leigh's necrotizing encephalomyelopathy	Pyruvate carboxylase
Lesch-Nyhan syndrome	Hypoxanthine-guanine phosphoribosyl transferase
Lipase deficiency, congenital	Lipase (pancreatic)
Lipoprotein lipase deficiency (type I hyperlipoproteinemia)	Lipoprotein lipase
Lysine intolerance	L-Lysine:NAD-oxidoreductase
Male pseudohermaphroditism	Testicular 17,20-desmolase
Male pseudohermaphroditism	Testicular 17-ketosteroid dehydrogenase
Male pseudohermaphroditism	Steroid 5α-reductase
Mannosidosis	α-Acid-mannosidase
Maple sugar urine disease	Branched-chain keto acid decarboxylase
Metachromatic leukodystrophy I	Arylsulfase A (cerebroside sulfatase)
Methemoglobinemia	NAD-methemoglobin reductase
Methionine adenosyl transferase deficiency (hypermethioninemia)	Methionine adenosyl transferase
β-Methyl crotonyl glycinuria I	β-Methyl crotonyl-CoA carboxylase
Methylmalonic aciduria I (vitamin B_{12}-unresponsive)	Methylmalonic CoA mutase
Methylmalonic aciduria II (vitamin B_{12}-responsive)	5′-Deoxyadenosyl transferase
Mitochondrial myopathy	NADH-CoA reductase
Mucolipidoses II and III	*N*-Acetylglucosamine-1-phosphotransferase
Mucolipidosis IV	Ganglioside neuramindase
Mucopolysaccharidosis IH (Hurler's)	α-L-Iduronidase
Mucopolysaccharidosis IS (Scheie's)	α-L-Iduronidase
Mucopolysaccharidosis II (Hunter's)	Sulfo-iduronidase sulfatase
Mucopolysaccharidosis IIIA (Sanfilippo's)	Heparan sulfate sulfatase
Mucopolysaccharidosis IIIB (Sanfilippo's)	*N*-Acetyl-α-D-glucosaminidase
Mucopolysaccharidosis IIIC	Acetyl-CoA:alpha glucosaminide *N*-transferase
Mucopolysaccharidosis IIID	*N*-Acetyltransglucosamine-6-sulfate sulfatase

TABLE 34–1. DISORDERS IN WHICH DEFICIENT ACTIVITY OF A SPECIFIC ENZYME HAS BEEN DEMONSTRATED IN HUMAN BEINGS* *Continued*

Condition	Enzyme with Deficient Activity
Mucopolysaccharidosis IVA (Morquio's)	Galactosamine-6-sulfate sulfatase
Mucopolysaccharidosis IVB	β-Galactosidase
Mucopolysaccharidosis VI (Maroteaux-Lamy)	Arylsulfatase B
Mucopolysaccharidosis VII	β-Glucuronidase
Multiple carboxylase deficiency, late-onset	Biotinase
Multiple carboxylase deficiency (several forms)	Holocarboxylase synthetase
Myeloperoxidase deficiency with disseminated candidiasis	Myeloperoxidase
Myopathy	Myoadenylate deaminase
Myopathy, lipid	Carnitine palmitoyl transferase I or II
Niemann-Pick disease, A and B	Sphingomyelinase
Niemann-Pick disease, C	Cholesterol esterification defect
Ornithinemia with gyrate atrophy	Ornithine ketoacid aminotransferase
Orotic aciduria I	Orotate phosphoribonyl transferase and orotidine-5′ phosphate decarboxylase
Orotic aciduria II	Orotidylic decarboxylase
Oxalosis I (glycolic aciduria)	Alanine: glyoxylate aminotransferase
Oxalosis II (glyceric aciduria)	D-Glyceric dehydrogenase
5-Oxoprolinuria (pyroglutamic aciduria)	Glutathione synthetase
Pentosuria	L-Xylulose reductase
Phenylketonuria I	Phenylalanine hydroxylase
Phenylketonuria II	Dihydropteridine reductase
Phenylketonuria III	Dihydrobiopterin synthetase
Porphyria, acute hepatic	Porphobilinogen synthetase
Porphyria, acute intermittent	Uroporphyrinogen I synthetase
Porphyria, congenital erythropoietic	Uroporphyrinogen III cosynthase
Porphyria cutanea tarda	Uroporphyrinogen decarboxylase
Porphyria variegata	Protoporphyrinogen oxidase
Prolidase deficiency	Prolidase
Protoporphyria	Heme synthetase (ferrochelatase)
Pulmonary emphysema, or cirrhosis	α-1-Antitrypsin
Pyridoxine-dependent infantile convulsions	Glutamic acid decarboxylase
Pyrimidinemia	Dihydropyrimidine dehydrogenase
Pyruvate carboxylase deficiency	Pyruvate carboxylase
Refsum's disease	Phytanic acid α-oxidase
Renal tubular acidosis with deafness	Carbonic anhydrase B
Rickets, vitamin D dependent	25-Hydroxycholecalciferol 1-hydroxylase
Saccharopinuria	Saccharopine dehydrogenase
Sarcosinemia	Sarcosine dehydrogenase complex
Sialidosis	α-Neuraminidase
Sulfite oxidase deficiency	Sulfite oxidase
Sulfite oxidase and xanthine dehydrogenase deficiency	Molybdenum cofactor
Thyroid hormonogenesis, detect in, II	Iodide peroxidase
Thyroid hormonogenesis, defect in, IV	Iodotyrosine dehalogenase (deiodinase)
Trimethylaminuria	Trimethylamine oxidase
Trypsinogen deficiency	Trypsinogen
Tyrosinemia I	Para-hydroxyphenylpyruvate oxidase
Tyrosinemia II (Richner-Hanhart syndrome)	Tyrosine transaminase
Urocanase deficiency	Urocanase
Valinemia	Valine transaminase
Wernicke-Korsakoff syndrome	Transketolase
Wolman's disease	Acid lipase
Xanthinuria	Xanthine oxidase
Xanthurenic aciduria	Kynureninase
Xeroderma pigmentosum	Ultraviolet-specific endonuclease
Xylosidase deficiency	Xylosidase

*Based upon McKusick VA: Mendelian Inheritance in Man. 7th ed. Baltimore, Johns Hopkins University Press, 1986, pp xxxi–xxxvi, with modifications.

the more abundant proteins of the cell. An average individual is demonstrably heterozygous at 7 per cent of loci. Since only about one third of base changes alter the charge of a protein, each individual may actually be heterozygous at as many as 20 per cent of loci.

At most genetic loci (e.g., the gene for β-globin) one standard allele accounts for the vast majority of alleles in the population, and alternative alleles are rare. At other loci, no single allele occurs with sufficient frequency to be designated as standard or normal. The α-chain of haptoglobin, a plasma protein, represents one such extreme example of genetic polymorphism. In this instance all polymorphic forms of haptoglobin appear to function equally in hemoglobin binding. Polymorphisms represent conspicuous examples of human biochemical diversity.

TABLE 34–2. SOME DISORDERS IN WHICH A DEFICIENCY OF A PLASMA PROTEIN HAS BEEN DEMONSTRATED IN HUMAN BEINGS

Condition	Plasma Protein
Afibrinogenemia	Fibrinogen
Agammaglobulinemia, X-linked	IgA, IgG
Agammaglobulinemia, selective IgA	IgA
Agammaglobulinemia, selective IgG	IgG
Analbuminemia	Albumin
Atransferrinemia	Transferrin
Complement deficiency states, selective C1q, C1r, C1s, C2, C3, C4, C5, C6, C7, C8	C1q, C1r, C1s, C2, C3, C4, C5, C6, C7, C8
Factor VII deficiency	Factor VII
Factor X (Stuart factor) deficiency	Factor X
Fibrin-stabilizing factor deficiency	Factor XIII
Hageman trait	Factor XII
Hemophilia A	Factor VIII
Hemophilia B	Factor IX
Hereditary angioedema	C1-inhibitor
Hypoprothrombinemia	Factor II
Parahemophilia	Factor V
PTA deficiency	Factor XI

PTA = plasma thromboplastin antecedent.

Genetic Heterogeneity. When two or more mutations produce identical or closely similar clinical syndromes, *genetic heterogeneity* is said to exist. In some instances the mutations may be at different loci (*nonallelic* genes), whereas in others they may occur in different portions of the same locus (*allelic* genes). Hemophilia can be caused by a mutation at either of two distinct loci on the X chromosome, one leading to a deficiency of factor VIII (classic hemophilia) and the other to a deficiency of factor IX (Christmas disease). By contrast, the multiple variants of G6PD, over 315 as of 1986, represent different structural gene mutations at a single locus. A striking example of both allelic and nonallelic heterogeneity is hereditary methemoglobinemia, which can be produced by at least ten different mutations at three distinct loci: two at the locus for the α-chain of hemoglobin, three at the locus for the β-chain, and at least five at the locus for NADH methemoglobin reductase.

In view of the multiple alleles that occur at virtually all genetic loci, persons who appear to be homozygous for a genetic trait may actually have inherited different abnormal alleles from each parent. Such individuals are said to be *genetic compounds*. The clinical syndrome in a genetic compound may be intermediate in severity and manifestations between the syndromes produced by homozygosity for either allele. A classic example is hemoglobin SC disease, which results when an offspring inherits a Hb S gene ($\beta\text{-}6^{glu \rightarrow val}$) from one parent and a Hb C gene ($\beta\text{-}6^{glu \rightarrow lys}$) from the other. Another is the mucopolysaccharide storage disease resulting from inheritance of one gene for Hurler's disease (severe) and one for Scheie's disease (mild). In both these examples the severity is intermediate between the diseases associated with the respective homozygous states. Table 34–5 lists selected inherited diseases for which genetic compounds have been demonstrated.

TABLE 34–3. METABOLIC DISEASES THAT HAVE BEEN MAPPED TO SPECIFIC AUTOSOMES*

Disease	Chromosome†
Disorders of carbohydrate metabolism	
Glycogen storage disease, Type II (Pompe's disease)	17
Galactosemia	9p
Galactokinase deficiency	17q
Galactose-4-epimerase deficiency	1p
Disorders of amino acid metabolism	
Classic phenylketonuria (phenylalanine hydroxylase deficiency)	1p
Atypical phenylketonuria (dihydropteridine reductase deficiency)	4
Argininosuccinic aciduria	7
Citrullinemia	9
Transcobalamin II deficiency	9q
Tetrahydrofolate methyltransferase deficiency	1
Disorders of lipoprotein and lipid metabolism	
Familial lecithin:cholesterol acyltransferase deficiency	16q
Disorders of lysosomal enzymes	
Mucopolysaccharidosis, Type VI (Maroteaux-Lamy syndrome)	5
Mucopolysaccharidosis, Type VII (β-glucuronidase deficiency)	7
Fucosidosis	1p
Mannosidosis	19
Wolman's disease and cholesteryl ester storage disease	10
Lysosomal acid phosphatase deficiency	11p
Metachromatic leukodystrophy	22q
Sandhoff's disease	5q
Tay-Sachs disease	15q
Generalized gangliosidosis	3
Disorders of steroid metabolism	
Adrenogenital syndrome (steroid 21-hydroxylase deficiency)	6p
Disorders of purine and pyrimidine metabolism	
Adenine phosphoribosyltransferase deficiency	16
Adenosine deaminase deficiency	20q
Nucleoside phosphorylase deficiency	14q
Disorders of metal metabolism	
Hemochromatosis	6p
Disorders of the blood and blood-forming tissues	
Glucosephosphate isomerase deficiency	19
Hexokinase deficiency	10
Triosephosphate isomerase deficiency	12p
Elliptocytosis	1p
Sickle cell anemia and all other β-chain variants	11p
Hemoglobin Constant Spring and all other α-chain variants	16p
α-Thalassemias	16p
β-Thalassemias	11p
Disorders of immune and other defense systems	
C2 deficiency	6p
C3 deficiency	19p
C4 deficiency	6p

*Modified from McKusick VA: Am J Med 69:267, 1980.
†These numbers indicate the chromosome that carries the particular locus. The chromosome arm is indicated when known: p = short arm; q = long arm.

TREATMENT OF INBORN ERRORS OF METABOLISM. Treatment of the patient with an inherited disorder depends upon accurate diagnosis and an understanding of the pathophysiology of the disease, including an appreciation of the interaction of genetic and environmental factors. Well-known examples are phenylketonuria, which predisposes to toxic reactions to dietary phenylalanine, and G6PD deficiency, which predisposes to hemolysis following ingestion of fava beans, during the course of acute viral hepatitis and infectious mononucleosis, or after administration of certain drugs, including aspirin and phenacetin. In such instances control of environmental factors may mitigate or neutralize the effect of the genetic change.

The balance of this chapter will be devoted to a discussion of forms of treatment of value in specific hereditary disorders.

Dietary Restriction of Substrate. Dietary restriction will often reduce the excessive substrate that accumulates behind a metabolic block. A general reduction in protein intake will prevent brain damage in disorders of the urea cycle associated with ammonia intoxication, including argininosuccinicaciduria and citrullinemia. A diet low in phenylalanine is effective in preventing growth and mental retardation in phenylketonuria, if started soon after birth. A fructose-free diet controls the symptoms of hereditary fructose intolerance resulting from deficiency of fructose-1-phosphate aldolase. Similarly, a diet that is virtually galactose free will avert brain damage and cataract formation in children with galactokinase or galactose-1-phosphate uridyl transferase deficiency.

Replacement of the Deficient End-Product. A metabolic block may also result in a critical shortage in the product of the reaction or later products of the sequence. Replacement may alleviate the deficiency state. Goiter resulting from a block in thyroxine production can be treated and cretinism prevented by replacement of thyroid hormone. In the adrenogenital syndromes, corticosteroid administration supplies the missing hormone, corrects the disordered steroidal secretory pattern, and leads to remission of the clinical manifestations. In orotic aciduria, administration of uridine supplies the pyrimidines needed for hematopoietic functions and corrects the macrocytic anemia, and also suppresses orotic acid synthesis and urolithiasis.

TABLE 34–4. SOME PLASMA PROTEINS AND CELLULAR ENZYMES THAT EXHIBIT ELECTROPHORETICALLY DETECTABLE POLYMORPHISMS*

Protein	Locus Name
Plasma proteins	
Haptoglobin (α-chain)	Hp α
Transferrin	Tf
Vitamin-D binding protein	Gc (for group-specific component)
Ceruloplasmin	Cp
α-1-Antitrypsin	Pi (for protease inhibitor)
α-1-Acid glycoprotein	Oro (for orosomucoid)
β-2-Glycoprotein I	—
Properdin factor B	Bf
Complement	
Second component	C2
Third component	C3
Fourth component	C4
Sixth component	C6
Enzymes	
Pancreatic amylase	AMY_2
Cholinesterase	E_2
Red blood cell enzyme	
Acid phosphatase 1	ACP_1
Adenosine deaminase	ADA
Adenylate kinase	AK_1
Carbonic anhydrase 2	CA_2
Diaphorase (NADPH-dependent)	DIA_2
Esterase D	ESD
Galactose-1-uridyltransferase	GALT
Glucose-6-phosphate dehydrogenase	Gd
Glutamic pyruvic transaminase	GPT
Glutathione peroxidase	GPX
Glutathione reductase	GSR
Glyoxalase I	GLO
Peptidase A	PEPA
Peptidase C	PEPC
Peptidase D	PEPD
Phosphoglucomutase 1	PGM_1
Phosphoglucomutase 2	PGM_2
Phosphogluconate dehydrogenase	PGD
Uridine monophosphate kinase	UMPK
White blood cell enzymes	
Aconitase (soluble)	$ACON_S$
Cytidine deaminase	CDA
α-L-Fucosidase	αFUC
α-Glucosidase	αGLUC
Glutamic-oxaloacetic transaminase (mitochondrial)	GOT_M
Hexokinase 3	HK_3
Malic enzyme (mitochondrial)	ME_M
Phosphoglucomutase 3	PGM_3

*From Giblett ER: Ann Rev Genet 11:13, 1977.

TABLE 34–5. INHERITED METABOLIC DISEASES FOR WHICH GENETIC COMPOUNDS HAVE BEEN DEMONSTRATED*

α-1-Antitrypsin deficiency
Cystinosis
Cystinuria
"Homozygous" familial hypercholesterolemia (LDL receptor-internalization defect)
Galactosemia (galactose-1-phosphate uridyltransferase deficiency)
Gaucher's disease (glucocerebrosidase deficiency)
Glucosephosphate isomerase deficiency
Hemoglobin α-chain variants
Hemoglobin β-chain variants
Hurler-Scheie syndrome (α-L-iduronidase deficiency)
Iminoglycinuria
Metachromatic leukodystrophy (cerebroside sulfatase deficiency)
Hereditary methemoglobinemia (NADH dehydrogenase deficiency)
Phenylketonuria (phenylalanine hydroxylase deficiency)
Pseudocholinesterase deficiency
Pyruvate kinase deficiency

*Modified from McKusick VA: Am J Hum Genet 25:446, 1973.
LDL = low density lipoprotein; NADH = reduced form of nicotinamide adenine dinucleotide.

Depletion of Storage Substances. In some hereditary disorders the clinical consequences result from accumulation of stored materials in the tissues, and removal of the excess material may ameliorate the effects of the genetic lesion. Removal of stored copper in Wilson's disease by penicillamine and of excess iron in hemochromatosis by frequent phlebotomy illustrates this approach. Use of uricosuric agents to deplete the body of uric acid in tophaceous gout and of cholestyramine to reduce serum cholesterol levels in familial hypercholesterolemia are additional examples.

Use of Metabolic Inhibitors. When a toxic metabolite accumulates because of a metabolic error, it may be possible to control its production by use of an appropriate metabolic inhibitor. Allopurinol inhibits xanthine oxidase and controls uric acid production in gout and 2,8-dioxyadenine production and renal stone formation in patients with homozygous adenine phosphoribosyltransferase deficiency. Clofibrate, which inhibits synthesis or release of glyceride from the liver, reduces blood lipid levels to normal in type III hyperlipoproteinemia.

Amplification of Enzyme Activity. Many enzyme proteins require cofactors for biologic activity. In some inborn errors the mutation affects the ability of the apoenzyme to combine with its cofactor. In other genetic disorders there is a metabolic defect in the conversion of a precursor vitamin to its active cofactor form. In both situations administration of the appropriate cofactor may increase the catalytic activity of the apoenzyme. Pyridoxine (vitamin B_6) is a cofactor for cystathionine synthetase. In more than one half of patients with homocystinuria caused by deficient synthetase activity, administration of large doses of pyridoxine partially overcomes the block in homocysteine metabolism. Similarly the ketoacidosis of some patients with methylmalonicaciduria is corrected by treatment with pharmacologic doses of vitamin B_{12}, and the clinical and hematologic abnormalities of patients with hereditary dihydrofolate reductase deficiency are corrected by administration of small doses of 5-formyltetrahydrofolate, which bypasses the metabolic block (replacement of deficient end-product).

Phenobarbital and certain other drugs increase production of smooth endoplasmic reticulum and of certain of its enzymes, including NADPH-cytochrome C reductase, cytochrome P-450, and several drug-hydroxylating enzymes. Administration of phenobarbital to patients with unconjugated hyperbilirubinemia in a variant of the Crigler-Najjar syndrome or with Gilbert's syndrome may reduce plasma bilirubin levels following induction of hepatic glucuronyltransferase.

Replacement of Mutant Protein. Direct replacement of the missing protein is an attractive approach to the treatment of recessively inherited diseases. Greater success has been achieved in deficiencies of nonenzymic than of enzymic proteins. Examples include replacement of gamma globulin in agammaglobulinemia, of albumin in analbuminemia, and of factor VIII in hemophilia. In each of these cases, the deficient gene product is a plasma protein. The metabolic and immunologic defects of patients with adenosine deaminase deficiency are transiently corrected by infusion of irradiated erythrocytes containing normal levels of adenosine deaminase.

Much less success has attended efforts to replace missing enzymes that normally function within cells. Enzyme infusions have been attempted in the mucopolysaccharidoses, Gaucher's disease, Tay-Sachs disease, and Pompe's disease, but therapeutic benefits are unproved. The lysosomal storage diseases are perhaps the best candidates for treatment by administration of exogenous enzyme, for cells have highly specific mechanisms for taking up exogenous proteins and delivering them to lysosomes. However, the exogenous protein must bind to a specific recognition site on the plasma membrane of the target cell so that it can be selectively internalized. Enzymes have been coupled covalently to other molecules for which tissues contain receptors, on the theory that in this manner the enzyme might be conveyed to the lysosomes along with the primary ligand. This type of experimental work holds promise for the future.

Modifying the Mutant Protein. Many proteins can be modified by the addition of subgroups. For example, sickle cell hemoglobin can be carbamylated by cyanate at the valine in position 1 of the β-chain, which then blocks the hydrophobic bonding of the normal val-1 to the mutant val-6 of β-globin of Hb S, thereby preventing sickling in vitro. Severe toxic reactions, such as peripheral neuropathy, sharply limit the clinical usefulness of cyanate therapy in patients with sickle cell disease. Nevertheless, this approach holds promise for the future.

Organ Transplantation. Allotransplantation of the organ in which the deficient enzyme is normally synthesized has been attempted in a variety of inherited diseases. The greatest experience has involved renal transplantation, which has been performed in Alport's syndrome, renal amyloidosis, cystinosis, Fabry's disease, Gaucher's disease, oxalosis, and some other conditions. The results in most instances have paralleled those of renal transplantation for other forms of end-stage renal disease. There has been no evidence of reactivation of the renal lesion in patients with Alport's syndrome, or of development of cystinosis or Fabry's disease in the transplanted kidneys. Amyloidosis has recurred in the graft on rare occasions. By contrast severe recurrent oxalosis has developed in a number of transplanted kidneys, and end-stage renal failure resulting from oxalosis is not now considered an indication for renal transplantation. Patients with Fabry's disease have developed measurable levels of the missing enzyme, ceramide trihexosidase, in plasma following renal transplantation, and there have been a few long-term survivals. Nevertheless, renal transplantation in patients with inborn errors of metabolism should be limited to replacement of failed kidneys. Results do not warrant use of renal transplantation primarily for enzyme replacement.

Transplantation of allogenic marrow has successfully corrected a number of immunodeficiency states, including lymphopenic hypogammaglobulinemia (Swiss type), Wiskott-Aldrich syndrome, and severe combined immunodeficiency disease.

Liver transplantation has been successful in cases of hepatic failure from Wilson's disease, α-1-antitrypsin deficiency, and homozygous familial hypercholesterolemia. Heart transplantation has been employed in many cases of hereditary cardiomyopathy.

Surgical removals also play a role in certain hereditary disorders. Examples include splenectomy in hereditary spherocytosis and colectomy in preventing neoplastic transformation in polyposis of the colon. Also, surgery offers a quick and permanent cure for polydactyly as well as for certain other dominantly inherited defects.

Genetic Engineering. The use of recombinant DNA technology in the diagnosis and treatment of inborn errors is discussed in Ch. 35.

Giblett ER: Genetic polymorphisms in human blood. Ann Rev Genet 11:13, 1977. *A review of polymorphic protein in blood, including alloantigens of red and white blood cells and plasma proteins, and electrophoretic variants of plasma and cellular components.*

McKusick VA: Phenotypic diversity of human diseases resulting from allelic series. Am J Hum Genet 25:446, 1973. *An analytical review of different disorders that can result from series of mutations involving the same gene.*

Stanbury JB, Wyngaarden JB, Fredrickson DS, et al. (eds.): The Metabolic Basis of Inherited Disease. 5th ed. New York, McGraw-Hill Book Company, 1983. *Authoritative discussions of all inborn errors of metabolism for which there is a substantial body of metabolic or biochemical information.*

35 EXPECTATIONS FROM RECOMBINANT DNA RESEARCH

W. French Anderson

Over the past dozen years, a revolution has occurred in DNA research, variously referred to as recombinant DNA technology, genetic engineering, molecular cloning, gene splicing, or biotechnology. The new DNA research is beginning to make a major impact on clinical medicine in four major areas: (1) understanding of the molecular basis of human (particularly genetic) diseases, (2) prenatal diagnosis, (3) production of human biologic products, and (4) gene therapy. Categories 1 to 3 are already a reality, whereas human gene therapy is fast approaching that status.

THE MOLECULAR BASIS OF HUMAN DISEASES

Although the human diseases studied by recombinant DNA techniques at present are the genetic diseases, the power of this technology is beginning to be felt in many other areas of human physiology and pathophysiology. All living processes are ultimately controlled by genes. Therefore, as genes are "cloned" (i.e., isolated) and as their products (which can be obtained in large amounts once the gene is cloned; see below) are studied both in vitro and in vivo, more is learned about the reactions that the genes govern. The result is that the normal physiology of a process becomes better understood. An example is the regulation of the hematopoietic system. As the genes for various growth factors and cytokines are obtained and their products made available for study (e.g., granulocyte-macrophage colony-stimulating factor, [GM-CSF], erythropoietin, interleukin-2 [Il-2], and so forth), a much clearer understanding is emerging on how proliferation and differentiation are controlled in the bone marrow. Another example is the immune system, in which the genes for the various cell surface receptors (e.g., Il-2 receptor, T-cell receptor, and so on) are being cloned and analyzed.

It is the genetic diseases, however, that have primarily benefited from the recombinant DNA revolution. Most studied are the thalassemias and hemoglobinopathies (see Ch. 142, 143). A decade ago the genetics of beta-thalassemia was extremely confusing. There were various clinical classifications to account for the range of severity seen. It was assumed that there must be different genotypes and that many patients were probably genetic compounds. Now, most of the genotypes that can produce beta-thalassemia have been sequenced, and the mechanisms underlying the various beta-zero and beta-plus thalassemias have been elucidated (see Ch. 142). Not only has this information led to a better comprehension of the thalassemia syndromes, but also it has made prenatal diagnosis and genetic counseling much more accurate. Similar progress in the understanding of a number of other genetic diseases is under way.

PRENATAL DIAGNOSIS

Prenatal diagnosis can be used for the detection of a number of genetic diseases; see, for example, the discussion in the chapter on sickle cell anemia (Ch. 143). Recombinant DNA technology has greatly expanded the accuracy, range, and safety of this procedure. Previously, it was necessary to obtain the gene product in sufficient amounts to be detectable by biochemical methods. For example, in the prenatal diagnosis of beta-thalassemia, fetal blood would be sampled at around 18 weeks of gestation (either by fetoscopy or placental aspiration), with a 5 per cent fetal mortality rate. Globin chains would then be fractionated. Analysis of fetal DNA, on the other hand, can be carried out on a small number of amniotic cells (with a fetal mortality rate of only 0.3 per cent) or from chorionic villi (with a fetal loss of 4 per cent but with the distinct advantage of making a diagnosis as early as 9 to 10 weeks of gestation).

There are a number of techniques that can be used to analyze fetal DNA for single-gene disorders. First is the straightforward method of restriction endonuclease mapping. A restriction enzyme cuts DNA at a specific short (4- to 6-nucleotide) sequence. If a genetic disorder alters the sequence recognized by a restriction enzyme, digestion of the fetal DNA with that enzyme provides an immediate diagnosis. Unfortunately, there are only a few situations in which this technique is applicable (e.g., sickle cell anemia). A second procedure is to make a linkage analysis with a restriction fragment length polymorphism (known as RFLP) (see Ch. 34). This approach will become increasingly valuable as sufficient RFLP's are located to make a roadmap of the entire human genome. Finally, a procedure that promises to be extremely valuable is the use of oligonucleotide probes that are specific for individual mutations. In theory, every genetic disease could be detected directly by hybridizing a normal and "mutant" oligonucleotide probe to a sample of fetal DNA.

It is clear that the new technology will revolutionize prenatal diagnosis. What is uncertain is how long it will take to transfer these sophisticated procedures from research laboratories to routine clinical use.

HUMAN BIOLOGICS PRODUCED BY BIOTECHNOLOGY

Genetic engineering is currently being used by biotechnology companies to produce large quantities of previously unavailable human biologics (usually peptides or proteins). What products are being made? Why these products? How are they being made? How good are they?

The first human proteins produced by the new technology are now being evaluated in clinical trials: Insulin, growth hormone (GH), and α and β interferon have been licensed by the United States Food and Drug Administration (FDA); gamma interferon, interleukin-2 (Il-2), and tumor necrosis factor (TNF) are under study. In each case, they were chosen because of the importance of the protein in treating specific human disease states (either established: insulin, GH; or postulated), the commercial market expected for the compound, and the ability to apply recombinant DNA techniques to synthesize large quantities of the human protein in bacteria (or in yeast or other cells) inexpensively.

The Technology

A gene is a sequence of nucleotides in DNA that code for a product. In order to get a bacterium (the most common biologic "factory" in use at present) to produce a human protein, it is necessary to obtain a DNA copy of the protein—in other words, to obtain a piece of double-stranded DNA that carries the precise sequence of nucleotides that code for the protein. This DNA is then inserted into a bacterial plasmid—a circle of naturally occurring nonchromosomal DNA that replicates freely in the cytoplasm of a bacterium. Any gene (bacterial, plant, animal, or human) that is inserted into the plasmid with the correct control signals can, in theory, be transcribed and translated into protein within the bacterium. The synthesized protein can then be purified from the bacterial cells.

There are a number of ways to acquire a human gene suitable for engineered protein production in bacteria. One procedure is to sequence a portion of the human protein of interest and then, by using the genetic code, determine the DNA sequence that would give the known amino acid sequence. Then a segment of DNA one and one half to several dozen nucleotides long is chemically synthesized (longer DNA molecules are very difficult to synthesize and purify) that will be exactly complementary to a portion of the expected sequence of the messenger RNA (mRNA). "Exactly complementary" means that the DNA "probe" will have T (thymine) where the mRNA has an A (adenine), a C (cytosine) where the mRNA has a G (guanine), and so forth. This DNA probe can be tagged with radioactivity and then be used to find (by hybridization) the desired mRNA in extracts of the appropriate human cells. The mRNA is isolated, purified, and shown to be capable of being translated in vitro to give the predicted human protein. This mRNA is then transcribed into full-length complementary (or copy) DNA, called cDNA, by the enzyme reverse transcriptase. The resulting DNA is an exact code of the mRNA for the human protein. It can now be made double stranded (by the action of other enzymes) and inserted into a bacterial plasmid along with the appropriate control signals.

Several requirements must be met in order to obtain large quantities of human proteins in bacteria. The human gene must be attached within the plasmid to a bacterial control signal that will be switched on at a high level. Several such "promoter" regions are used, including those from the lactose operon, from the bacteriophage lambda, and so on. Second, other regulatory signals (for example, a binding site so that the transcribed RNA will attach to and be translated by ribosomes) must be present adjacent to the human gene. Third, any hard-to-handle portion of DNA (for example, nucleotides producing a leader sequence of amino acids or an intervening sequence) should be removed, since bacteria are not equipped to carry out many of the post-transcriptional and post-translational modifications that eukaryotic cells can perform. Fourth, the human protein must be protected from proteinases within the bacterium.

How good are these biologically engineered human proteins? They should be perfectly acceptable for administration to patients. In most cases, they should be pure and contain no infectious contaminants or animal antigenic material. However, unless purified extensively, they might contain clinically relevant amounts of bacterial antigenic substances. In addition, since some products isolated directly from the body have a number of biologic compounds bound to them, the clinical effect of a "pure" engineered product (e.g., albumin) might be somewhat different from that of the natural product.

The Next Products

What human biologics are now under development? Those being prepared for human trials fall into four broad categories; vaccines, blood components, neurohormones, and diagnostics.

VACCINES. The first recombinant DNA vaccine approved by the FDA (July 1986) for clinical use was that for hepatitis B. Specific vaccines for influenza and malaria are in clinical trials. Potential vaccines for a number of other diseases are currently in preparation, e.g., leprosy, tuberculosis, typhoid, acquired immunodeficiency syndrome (AIDS), and so forth. This new generation of vaccines should be superior to those in use today. A precise portion of the antigenic surface of a virus or a parasite can be selected and the DNA complement to this moiety prepared. Since a bacterial control signal will transcribe any sequence of DNA attached to it, the DNA coding for just the antigenic site desired can be inserted into bacteria for large-scale production of material. Or the DNA could be inserted into, for example, vaccinia in order to take advantage of a well-characterized vaccination agent. It appears to be possible to prepare highly specific vaccines by this approach.

BLOOD COMPONENTS. Several different types of blood components are being prepared for clinical trials.

Clotting Factors. The genes for factor VIII, von Willebrand's factor, and factor IX have been obtained. Human protein C has also been cloned.

Albumin. The great demand for albumin as a plasma expander has resulted in a major effort to produce human albumin in bacteria. The advantages of engineered albumin (besides increased availability and decreased cost) should be that there will be no risk of hepatitis, AIDS, or other infectious contamination.

Thrombolytic Agents. Blood clots are a major cause of death and disabling diseases in the United States. Consequently, readily available clot-specific thrombolytic agents would be clinically useful. Biotechnology is being employed to isolate the genes for, and to engineer the production of, tissue-type and urokinase-type plasminogen activators. These proteins should be superior to the currently available agents, urokinase and streptokinase. Considerable progress has been made toward bringing tissue plasminogen activators to market.

Biologic Response Modifiers. Besides the family of interferons, Il-2, and TNF, which are under active clinical investigation, other cytokines (Il-1, GM-CSF, human granulocyte CSF, and so forth) are undergoing engineered production. Considerable effort is under way to identify other factors, particularly a molecule that would stimulate the earliest pluripotent stem cell. Major advances in clinical manipulation of the immune system are expected when the genes of the major histocompatibility complex and the immunoglobulin gene families are more fully understood.

NEUROHORMONES. This complex group includes a large number of hormones, various neuropeptides, and the neurotransmitters with their receptors. Insulin and growth hormone are already being tested clinically; peptides from the pro-opiomelanocortin family should be available shortly.

DIAGNOSTICS. Since viruses consist of sequences of DNA or RNA with a coat, diagnostic techniques that would rapidly and accurately identify the presence of specific viruses in body tissues or fluids by using DNA probes are being developed.

OTHER AREAS. Finally, two other areas need to be mentioned. A further understanding of oncogenes and their role in cancer should lead to the development of drugs or antibodies that could be used to inhibit specific steps in the pathway leading from a normal to a malignant cell. Second, the tremendous potential of recombinant DNA research to produce useful new agricultural plants and improved farm animals should have a large effect on the food supply of the world.

GENE THERAPY

By gene therapy is meant the insertion of a normal gene into the appropriate cells of a patient in such a way that the exogenous gene produces a product that will cure, or at least ameliorate, the genetic defect. For some genetic conditions (specifically those caused by a single gene mutation that produces a defective product that can be isolated), gene therapy should be a beneficial therapeutic procedure in the future.

The Technology of Gene Therapy

It is now possible by the use of recombinant DNA technology to isolate specific normal genes from the DNA of human tissue. A gene can be isolated if it can be recognized, and it can be recognized if the protein product that it makes can be isolated. The defective product in many genetic diseases is a protein (e.g., an enzyme in many of the inborn errors of metabolism; beta-globin in sickle cell anemia or Cooley's anemia). In a manner similar to that described above in the section on human biologics, a DNA probe can be synthesized. With this probe it is possible to locate the gene in human DNA, isolate (i.e., clone) it, and purify it. Any gene can be cloned once a probe for the gene exists.

The cloned gene can be inserted into cells in any one of a number of ways. The three most commonly used techniques are (1) microinjecting directly into a cell's nucleus, (2) forming a calcium phosphate precipitate of the DNA and then incubating tissue culture cells with this precipitate, and (3) inserting the gene into a nonpathogenic virus and infecting cells with this recombinant virus. All three procedures have been used successfully to insert cloned genes into cells growing in tissue culture. By far, the most efficient procedure at present is the use of retrovirus-based vectors carrying exogenous genes.

Vectors derived from retroviruses possess several advantages as a gene delivery system. First, up to 100 per cent of cells can be infected and can express the integrated viral (and exogenous) genes. Second, as many cells as desired can be infected simultaneously. Third, under appropriate conditions, the DNA can integrate as a single copy at a single, albeit random, site. Finally, the infection and long-term harboring of a retroviral vector usually does not harm cells. Several retroviral vector systems have been developed; those projected for human use are constructed from the Moloney murine leukemia virus. Evidence obtained from studies with experimental animals and in tissue culture indicates that retroviruses can be used as a reasonably efficient delivery system.

The next question is, what target cell to use? At present, the only human tissue that can be used effectively for gene transfer is bone marrow. No other cells (except, perhaps, skin cells) can be extracted from the body, grown in culture to allow insertion of exogenous genes, and then successfully reimplanted into the patient from whom the tissue was taken. In the future, as more is learned about how to package the DNA and to make it tissue specific, the intravenous route would be the simplest and most desirable. However, attempting to give a foreign gene by injection directly into the bloodstream is not advisable with our present state of knowledge, since the procedure would be enormously inefficient and there would be little control over the DNA's fate.

Studies are considerably more advanced with bone marrow than skin cells as a recipient tissue for gene transfer. Bone marrow consists of a heterogeneous population of cells, most of which are committed to differentiate into red blood cells, white blood cells, platelets, and so on. Only a small proportion (0.1 to 0.5 per cent) of nucleated bone marrow cells are stem cells (that is, blood-forming cells that have not yet differentiated into specific cell types and that divide as needed to maintain the marrow population). In gene therapy, it would be these stem cells that would be the primary target.

Initial Disease Candidate for Gene Therapy

For many years, clinical investigators thought that the human genetic diseases most likely to be the initial ones successfully treated by gene therapy would be the hemoglobin abnormalities (specifically, beta-thalassemia) because these disorders are the most obvious ones carried by blood cells, and bone marrow is the easiest tissue to manipulate outside the body. Regulation of globin synthesis, however, is unusually complicated. Not only are the embryonic, fetal, and adult globin chains carefully regulated during development, but also the subunits of the hemoglobin molecule are coded by genes on two different chromosomes. To understand the regulatory signals that control such a complicated system and to develop means for obtaining controlled expression of an exogenous (i.e., inserted by gene therapy) beta-globin gene will take considerably more research effort. It now appears that the most likely gene to be used in the first experiments on human gene therapy is adenosine deaminase (ADA), the absence of which results in severe combined immunodeficiency disease (in which children have a greatly weakened resistance to infection and cannot survive the usual childhood diseases).

ADA deficiency has a number of features that make it an ideal initial candidate.

1. The disease can be cured by infusion of normal bone marrow cells from a histocompatible donor. Selective replication of the normal marrow cells appears to take place. This observation offers hope that defective bone marrow can be removed from a patient, the normal ADA gene inserted into a number of cells through gene therapy, and the treated marrow reimplanted into the patient, where it may have a selective growth advantage. If selective growth occurs, elimination of the patient's own marrow would not be necessary. If, however, corrected marrow cells have no growth advantage over endogenous (i.e., the patient's own untreated) cells, then partial or complete marrow destruction (either by irradiation or by other means) may be required in order to allow the corrected marrow cells an environment favorable for expansion. The latter situation (which will probably be necessary in most other genetic diseases) would require much greater confidence that the gene therapy procedure would work before a clinical trial should be undertaken.
2. Experience with mismatched bone marrow transplantation has demonstrated poor results for ADA deficiency. There is not a good alternative therapy for patients without a matched donor.
3. The entire pathophysiology of the disease appears to be confined to the lymphoid population of the marrow. Therefore, successful treatment of these cells should be curative.
4. Regulation of the inserted gene does not need to be precise, since individuals with levels of 5 to 5000 per cent of normal ADA activity are relatively symptom free.

Ethics

The ethics of gene therapy in humans has been discussed for many years. Essentially all observers have stated that they believe that it would be ethical to insert genetic material into a human being for the sole purpose of medically correcting a severe genetic disorder in that patient—in other words, somatic cell gene therapy. Attempts to correct a patient's reproductive cells (i.e., germ line gene therapy) or to alter or improve a "normal" person by gene manipulation (i.e., enhancement or eugenic genetic engineering) are controversial areas. However, somatic cell gene therapy for a patient suffering a serious genetic disorder would be ethically acceptable if carried out under the same strict criteria that cover other new experimental medical procedures. The techniques now being developed by clinical investigators for human application are for somatic cell, not germ line, gene therapy.

What criteria should be satisfied prior to the time that somatic cell gene therapy is tested in a clinical trial? Three general requirements are that it should be shown in animal studies that (1) the new gene can be put into the correct target cells and will remain there long enough to be effective; (2) the new gene will be expressed in the cells at an appropriate level; and (3) the new gene will not harm the cell or, by extension, the animal. These criteria are very similar to those required prior to the use of any new drug, therapeutic procedure, or surgical operation. The requirements simply state that the new treatment should get to the area of disease, correct it, and do more good than harm.

Although retroviruses have many advantages for gene transfer, they also have disadvantages, which lead to questions about safety. One problem is that they can rearrange their own structure, as well as exchange sequences with other retroviruses. There is a built-in safety feature with the mouse retroviral vectors now in use, however; these mouse structures have a very different sequence from known primate retroviruses, and there appears to be little or no homology between the two. Therefore, it should be possible, with continuing research, to build a safe retroviral vector.

Even with a "safe" vector, however, the problem of insertional mutagenesis remains. Since a retroviral vector incorporates into the genome randomly, it may inactivate an important gene or, worse, activate an oncogene. It is uncertain how great a danger this problem poses. As with any new clinical protocol, the total expected benefit for the patient must be weighed against potential risks. Ultimately, local institutional review boards and the National Institutes of Health, the latter through its Working Group on Human Gene Therapy, must decide if a given protocol is ready for human application.

Present Capabilities

What is the present capability for transferring a functional gene into an intact animal in a manner that has potential clinical application? Encouraging results have been obtained in mice as well as in nonhuman primates and sheep.

Several laboratories have successfully carried out a bone marrow transplantation (BMT)/gene transfer protocol in mice. A neomycin resistance gene (carried by a retroviral vector) has been transferred into murine bone marrow cells, followed by the reinsertion of the treated marrow cells into lethally irradiated mice. After several months, the fully reconstituted animals were shown still to carry a functioning neomycin resistance gene in their bone marrow and peripheral blood cells. Analysis demonstrated that, in some animals, all the blood cell lineages contained the active gene.

It has been more difficult to obtain expression of a human gene in vivo in mice. However, when a retroviral vector was built in which the human ADA gene was regulated by a primate (SV40) promoter, excellent expression of the human gene could be obtained in primate cells in culture. T and B cells isolated from patients with ADA deficiency were shown to produce normal human ADA after insertion of the ADA gene. When a protocol similar to the mouse BMT/gene transfer procedure was carried out in nonhuman primates using the primate-promoted ADA vector, several monkeys were found to carry and express the human ADA gene in a small number of their blood cells several months after treatment. These results offer encouragement that retroviral vectors may soon be sufficiently developed to be used in a clinical trial of gene therapy.

There are some genetic diseases that might be most optimally treated in utero rather than waiting until after birth, when some irreversible damage may already have occurred. Recent experiments in fetal sheep suggest that, at least in this animal model, a gene can be inserted into fetal blood cells that have been removed and then reinfused during midpregnancy. The gene (in this case, the neomycin resistance gene previously studied in mice) is active and continues to function for at least several months after the birth of the lamb. Thus, in utero gene therapy is a theoretic possibility.

What still needs to be done? First, the efficiency of the BMT/gene transfer should be improved. Although positive selective pressure may take place in patients with ADA deficiency, there is no assurance that the inserted ADA gene will be adequately expressed in stem cells as well as in mature T and B cells. Therefore, the more efficient the gene transfer procedure is, the higher is the likelihood that the patient will be helped. Second, the procedure should be shown to be reproducible. Only a few animals have been studied up to this point. Third, the safety of the procedure should be verified. Do the animals develop a viremia? Is there any indication that the vector has spread from the bone marrow to other cells (including germ cells)? Are there any signs of a malignancy or other pathologic condition?

Overview

It now appears that effective delivery-expression systems are becoming available that will allow reasonable attempts at somatic cell gene therapy. The first clinical trials will probably be carried out within the next couple of years. The initial protocols will be based on treatment of bone marrow cells with retroviral vectors carrying a normal gene. Patients severely debilitated by having no normal copies of the gene that produces the enzyme ADA are the most likely first candidates for gene therapy.

Gene therapy is a procedure with enormous potential. It should, in the future, provide a cure for hereditary diseases caused by a single gene defect. It is even possible that the germ line might be corrected so that the children of a patient will also be free from disease. This would be, indeed, a powerful therapeutic tool. But some claims made about the potential of genetic engineering in humans are highly unlikely. Patients with multigenic diseases, in which the genes as well as the intracellular products involved are unknown, will not be candidates for gene therapy for a long time to come, if ever. Likewise, characteristics such as personality and intelligence are probably outside the realm of this technique's potential. Only traits produced by identifiable single genes can be approached by genetic engineering. Of course, if, as now seems the case, some very widespread pathologic conditions (namely, lipid deposition in vessels to produce atherosclerosis) are influenced by identifiable individual genes, then gene therapy might have a far wider application than currently visualized.

The power to cure a genetic defect is an awesome one. But the goal of biomedical research is, and has always been, to alleviate human suffering. Gene therapy, with proper safeguards imposed by society, is a logical part of that effort.

Anderson WF: Prospects for human gene therapy. Science 226:401, 1984. *This review summarizes the medical, technical, and ethical issues involved in human gene therapy.*

Parkman R: The application of bone marrow transplantation to the treatment of genetic diseases. Science 232:1373, 1986. *This recent review places gene therapy in the context of present-day treatment of genetic disorders, particularly bone marrow transplantation.*

Walters L: The ethics of human gene therapy. Nature 320:225, 1986. *This commentary surveys the social issues related to gene therapy.*

Weatherall DJ: The New Genetics and Clinical Practice. 2nd ed. 2. Oxford, Oxford University Press, 1985. *This well-written, easy-to-follow, small volume describes the clinical implications of recombinant DNA technology.*

36 CHROMOSOMES AND THEIR DISORDERS

John L. Hamerton

Cytogenetics is the study of the chromosomes and their behavior as it relates to transmission of the genetic material from parent to offspring. Errors in chromosome behavior and structure are the cause of a wide range of clinical syndromes.

Humans have 46 chromosomes, which consist of 22 pairs

of homologous chromosomes (identical in regard to morphology and constituent gene loci) and one pair of sex chromosomes (X and Y), one partner of each pair being derived from the mother and one from the father. The genes are arranged along the chromosomes in linear order, each gene having a precise position or *locus*. Genes that have their loci on the same chromosome are said to be *linked*, or more precisely, to be *syntenic*. Alternate forms of a gene that occupy the same locus are called *alleles*. Any one chromosome bears only a single allele at a given locus, although in the population as a whole there may be multiple alleles, any one of which can occupy that specific locus.

CELL DIVISION

The number of chromosomes found in somatic cells is constant and is termed the diploid (2n) number. Each gamete, however, has only half the *diploid* number and is said to be *haploid* (n). In order to maintain this regularity two types of cell division occur: *mitosis*, which is the cell division occurring in somatic tissues during growth and repair, and *meiosis*, which is the specialized form of cell division occurring during the formation of the gametes.

MITOSIS. The function of mitosis is the distribution and maintenance of the continuity of the genetic material in every cell of the body. This process consists of a number of different phases, which results in an equal distribution of the chromosomes to the two daughter cells. The cell cycle has four stages: mitosis or M, G_1, S, and G_2. The G_1 phase follows mitosis, during which RNA and protein synthesis occurs. S is the period during which DNA replication takes place and the DNA content of the cell doubles, and G_2 is the period during which energy requirements for cell division are built up and any repair of errors in DNA synthesis takes place.

MEIOSIS (Fig. 36–1). This process occurs only during the formation of the gametes and results in four daughter cells, each with the haploid number of chromosomes. In males each primary spermatocyte forms four functional spermatids that develop into sperm, while in females each oocyte forms only one ovum, the remaining products of meiosis being nunfunctional polar bodies.

The first division of meiosis consists of an extremely long and complex *prophase* during which DNA replication occurs. This is divided into a number of stages during which crossing over and reassortment of genetic material occur. Initially the chromosomes are apparently single threads that begin to shorten and thicken. This is followed by the commencement of pairing of homologous chromosomes (*synapsis*). After pairing is completed, the chromosomes continue to shorten and are now known as *bivalents*, which are held together only at specific points (*chiasmata*). At this stage of prophase each homologous chromosome can be seen to be visibly doubled (two chromatids) so that each bivalent, which continues to shorten and thicken, consists of four chromatids.

The end of prophase is marked by the disappearance of the nuclear membrane and the formation of a spindle, heralding entry into *metaphase* of the first meiotic division. The bivalents are arranged on the equatorial plate of the spindle as a result of a series of complex chromosome movements. The homologous centromeres are undivided at this point and lie opposite each other on the equatorial plate (co-orientation). As soon as this process is complete, the paired homologues separate and move to opposite poles (*anaphase*). The cell then proceeds to the second meiotic division.This is essentially a mitotic

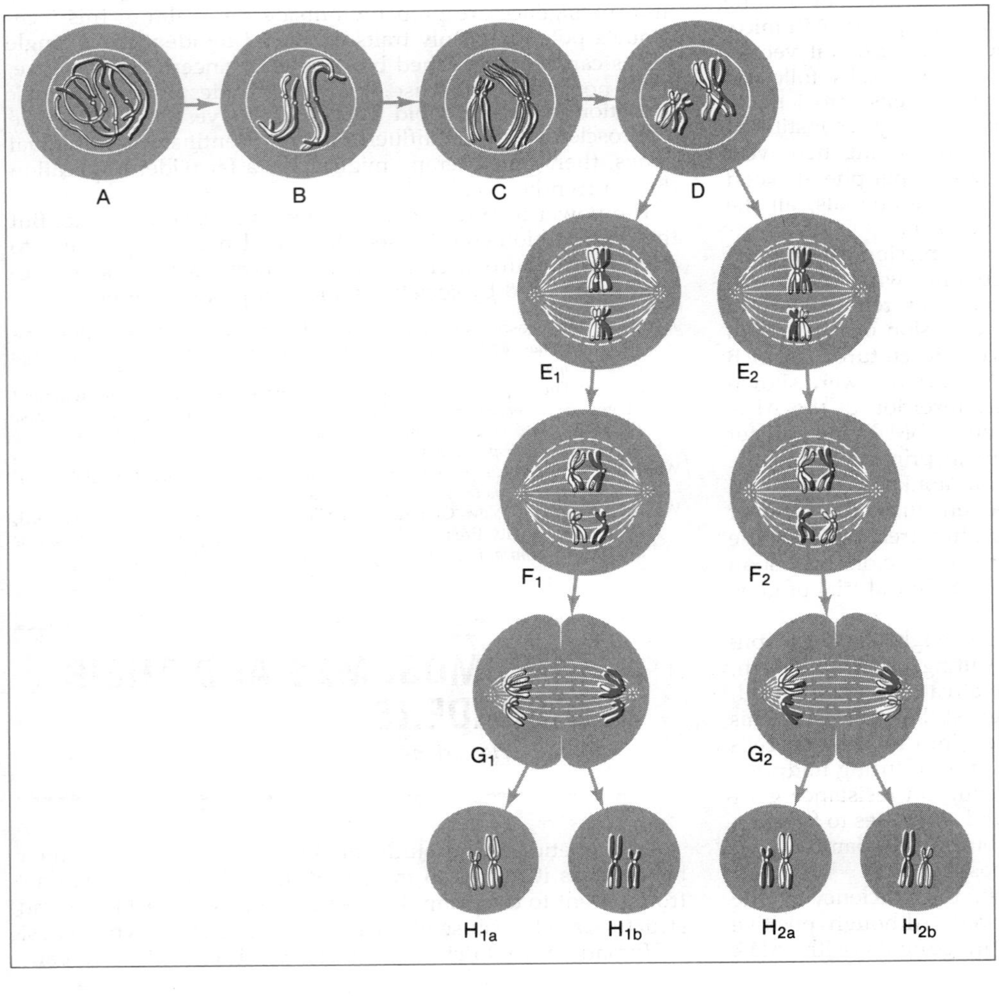

FIGURE 36–1. The stages of the first division of meiosis. Paternal and maternal chromosomes are shown in red and white, respectively. A to D, Stages of prophase. E to G, Metaphase 1 to anaphase 1. H1 to H2, Daughter cells with haploid number of chromosomes prior to entering the second division of meiosis. Note the chromosome exchanges that have taken place.

division in which the chromosomes have already doubled so that there is no need for DNA synthesis. In addition, the genetic material has undergone exchange at meiosis I so that the sister chromatids are not genetically identical.

The major consequences of meiosis are threefold: (1) the halving of the chromosome number; (2) the co-orientation of the bivalents on the metaphase plate, which ensures the regular distribution of the chromosomes to the daughter cells; and (3) the independent assortment of genetic material that results both from genetic crossing over and from the random assortment of the maternal and paternal homologues to the two daughter cells in meiosis I.

Two processes are fundamental to meiosis: chromosome pairing, which results in formation of the bivalents, and chiasma formation. Chiasmata have two main functions: They are the points on the chromosomes at which genetic crossing over takes place, and they serve to maintain bivalent association throughout the prophase and metaphase. Meiosis thus ensures genetic variability as a result of random segregation of the parental homologous chromosomes and the exchange of genetic material by crossing over between nonsister chromatids.

METHODS FOR THE PREPARATION OF CHROMOSOMES

Since nondividing chromosomes cannot be analyzed, dividing cells are required for chromosome analysis. The cell type most commonly used is the mitogenically stimulated peripheral blood lymphocyte. Skin fibroblasts, bone marrow cells, amniotic fluid cells, and chorion villus cells are also used for special tests. Dividing cells are accumulated at metaphase. Colcemid added to the culture medium toward the end of the culture period is most commonly used to accomplish this. The cells are then subjected to hypotonic treatment, followed by fixation and spreading on microscope slides. The slides are then stained.

Staining techniques may result in either a nonbanded or a banded appearance of the chromosomes. Most laboratories today use one of several banding techniques, since this results in a great deal of additional information.These methods provide a means for the precise identification of an extra or missing chromosome and the precise localization of breakpoints in chromosome rearrangements (Fig. 36–2).

Recent developments have resulted in the expansion of the number of visible bands from between 200 and 300 to between 1000 and 2000. This allows the recognition of small deletions and duplications. Most laboratories today work with chromosomes in which between 400 and 800 bands can be recognized.

HUMAN CHROMOSOME NOMENCLATURE

The 46 human chromosomes consist of three types designated by the position of the centromere or primary constriction. These are metacentric, submetacentric, and acrocentric, depending upon whether the position of the centromere is median, submedian, or terminal. Now that each individual chromosome pair can be recognized, the chromosomes are numbered from 1 to 22 in descending order of length. In the female the two sex chromosomes, designated X chromosomes, are identical, while in the male the two sex chromosomes, designated X and Y, are morphologically different.

Chromosome Variants

This term refers to consistent minor chromosome changes often involving the short arms of the acrocentric chromosomes, the long arm of the Y chromosome, or the constitutive heterochromatin near the centromere of chromosomes 1, 9, and 16. These have little obvious clinical significance but may be useful as genetic markers. They occur much more frequently in the population than do major chromosome abnormalities, and they often segregate in families in a mendelian manner. Recent studies suggest that about 70 per cent of newborn infants carry one or more variant chromosomes.

Nomenclature

The nomenclature used to describe the chromosomes, chromosome bands, chromosome variants, and chromosome rearrangements is given in detail in ISCN (1985). A shorthand notation is used to describe the chromosome complement of an individual. In this notation the number of chromosomes

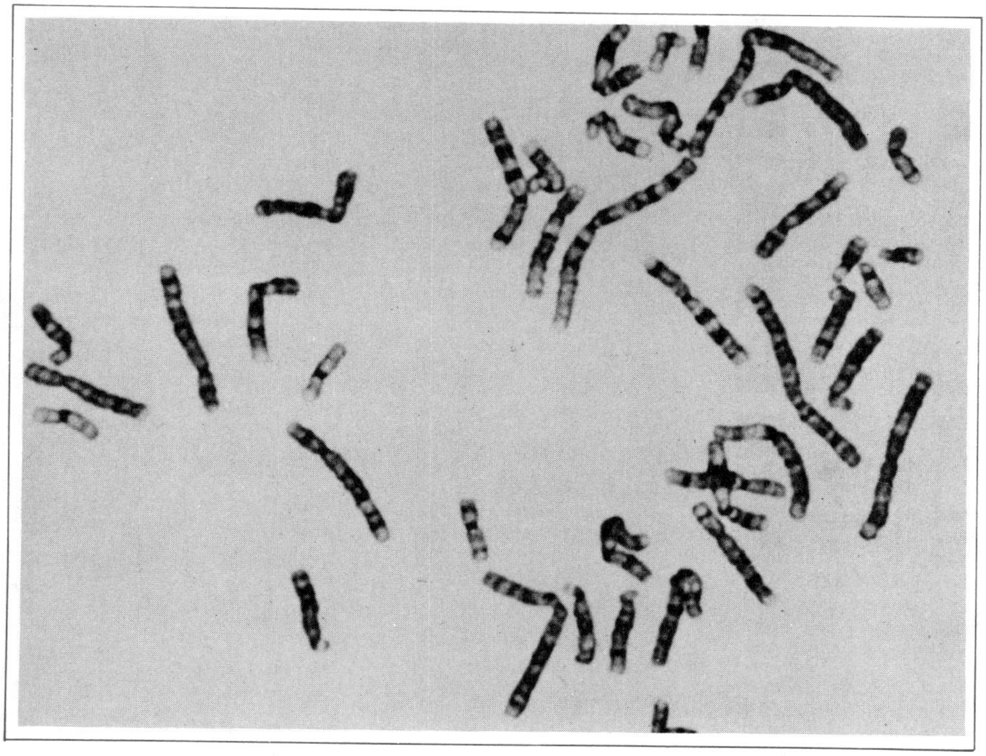

FIGURE 36–2. Human chromosomes at mitotic metaphase. G-banding, approximately 550 band stage. (Courtesy of Dr. H. S. Wang.)

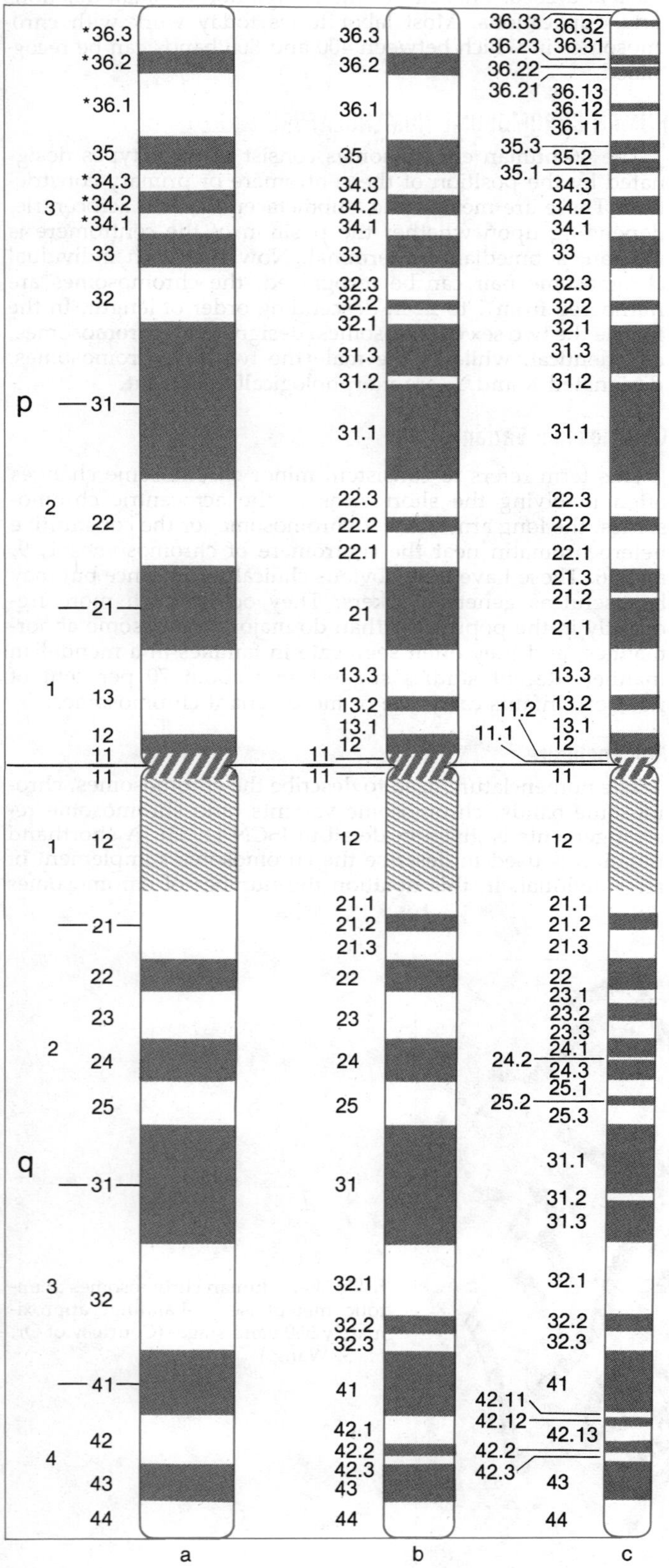

FIGURE 36–3. Human chromosome 1. Idiogram showing chromosome bands at different resolutions. *a*, Approximately 400 bands; *b*, 550 bands; *c*, 850 bands. The band nomenclature and subdivision are according to the internationally agreed system (ISCN 1985).

is specified first, followed by the listing of the sex chromosomes. Thus a normal female karyotype is designated 46,XX and a normal male karyotype 46,XY. Any deviations from a normal karyotype are written after the sex chromosomes. An individual autosome is referred to by its number, its short arm by the letter "p," and its long arm by the letter "q." A "+" or "−" sign written after the p or q indicates an increase (+) or decrease (−) in the length of the arm. When written before a designated chromosome the sign indicates that the chromosome is extra (+) or missing (−).

Examples: 46,XY,18q− describes a male with 46 chromosomes, including one chromosome 18 whose long arm is diminished in length.

47,XX,+21 describes a female with 47 chromosomes, including an extra chromosome 21 in addition to the 46 chromosomes of the normal karyotype.

A diagrammatic representation of the human chromosome 1 showing differing degrees of chromosome banding is given in Figure 36–3.

CHROMOSOME ABNORMALITIES

Chromosome abnormalities can be divided into two classes: abnormalities of number and of structure.

Abnormalities of Chromosome Number. These arise from nondisjunction, that is, from *the failure of two homologous chromosomes in the first division of meiosis or of two sister chromatids in mitosis or the second division of meiosis to pass to opposite poles of the cell* (Fig. 36–4). Nondisjunction results in cells with abnormal chromosome numbers. If these cells are gametes, fertilization will result in a zygote with an abnormal chromosome number. If nondisjunction occurs during an early cleavage division of a zygote, then a chromosome mosaic may result. This is an individual with two or more cell lines differing in chromosome complement. Table 36–1 gives examples of chromosome abnormalities resulting from nondisjunction.

TABLE 36–1. EXAMPLES OF CHROMOSOME ABNORMALITIES DUE TO NONDISJUNCTION IN HUMANS

Sex Chromosomes	Autosomes†
47,XXY (Klinefelter's syndrome) *46,XY/47,XXY	21-trisomy (47,XX or XY, +21)
47,XYY	13-trisomy (47,XX or XY, +13)
47,XXX	18-trisomy (47,XX or XY, +18)
45,X (Turner's syndrome) *45,X/46,XX (ovarian dysgenesis)	21-monosomy (45,XX or XY, −21)

*Examples of chromosome mosaics due to nondisjunction or chromosome loss during an early cleavage division.

†In describing a chromosome abnormality the words "trisomy" and "monosomy" refer simply to an additional or missing chromosome.

Abnormalities of Chromosome Structure. These result from chromosome breakage and reunion. When a chromosome breaks it can rejoin in its old form (restitution) or it can rejoin with another broken chromosome (reunion). Reunion leads to a structural rearrangement that can be *balanced* or *unbalanced*. If it is balanced the amount of genetic material is presumed to be identical to that found in a normal cell, and there is a simple rearrangement of the distribution of this material. Types of balanced rearrangements include the balanced reciprocal translocation, robertsonian translocations, and inversions. Balanced chromosome rearrangements do not usually lead to any clinical change. If the rearrangement is unbalanced this indicates loss or gain of chromosome material.

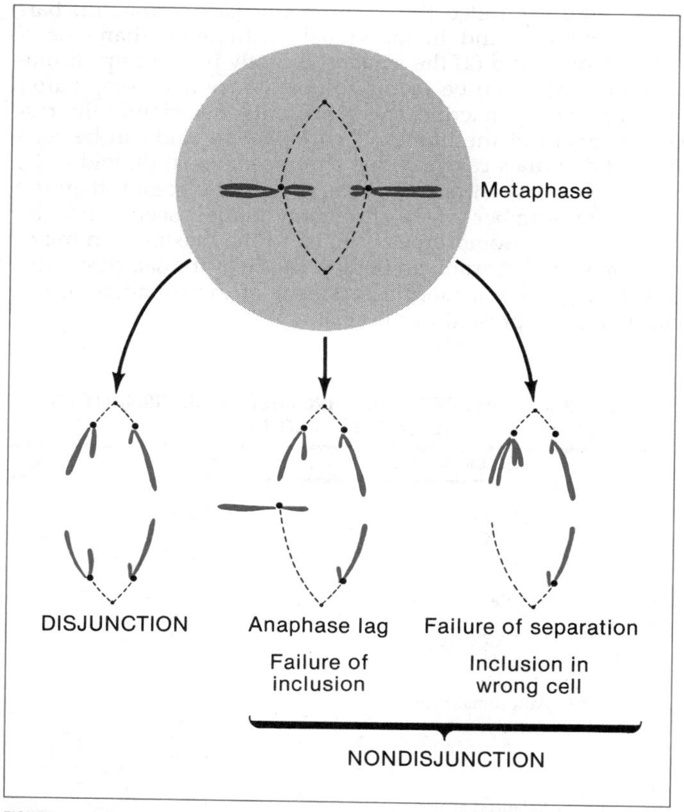

FIGURE 36–4. Diagram illustrating chromosome disjunction and two types of nondisjunction—anaphase lagging and failure of separation. (From Hamerton JL: Human Cytogenetics, Vol 1. New York, Academic Press, 1971.)

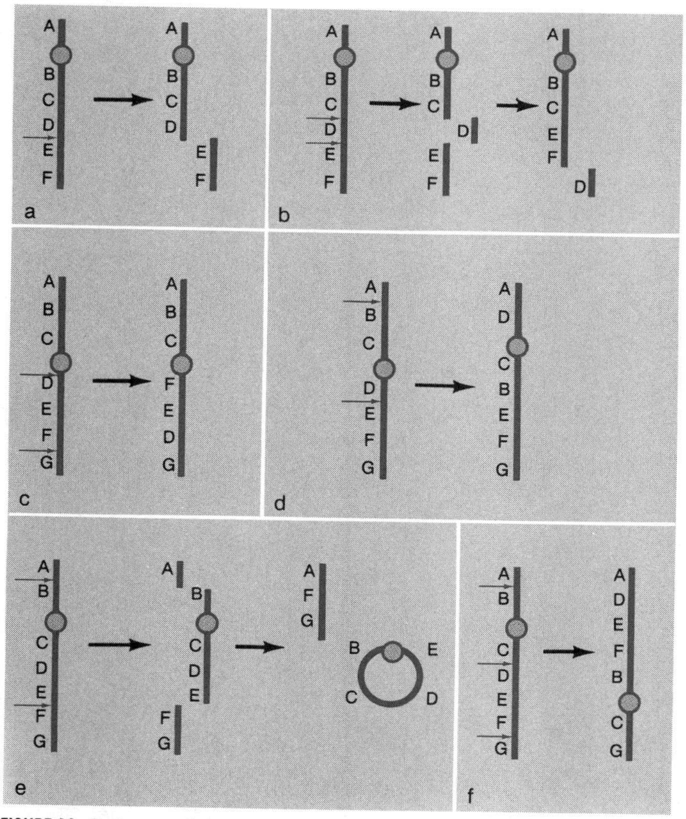

FIGURE 36–5. Types of chromosome rearrangement: *a*, terminal deletion; *b*, interstitial deletion; *c*, paracentric inversion; *d*, pericentric inversion; *e*, ring chromosome; *f*, segmental shift. (From Hamerton JL: Human Cytogenetics, Vol 1. New York, Academic Press, 1971.)

Loss includes a deficiency or a deletion. Gain includes a duplication. Such unbalanced rearrangements will usually result in changes in the clinical phenotype.

CHROMOSOME DELETION. Deletion is the loss of a chromosome segment following chromosome breakage. Deletions may be terminal or interstitial or result in ring chromosomes (Fig. 36–5*A*, *B*, and *E*).

INVERSIONS (Fig. 36–5*C* and *D*). These result from two chromosome breaks and inversion of the intervening segment and can be detected only by chromosome banding studies that show a changed banding sequence. Inversions result in disturbances in chromosome pairing and in the formation of unbalanced as well as balanced gametes.

BALANCED RECIPROCAL TRANSLOCATION (Fig. 36–6). This results from exchange of chromosome segments between nonhomologous chromosomes. An individual carrying such a rearrangement will have a higher frequency of abnormal gametes as the result of a disturbance in chromosome pairing at meiosis. Such individuals will themselves have a balanced chromosome complement and be clinically normal, but they may have a high risk of having congenitally malformed children and/or spontaneous abortions. Normal children may also be born, and such persons require careful genetic counseling.

ROBERTSONIAN TRANSLOCATION. This is a specific type of unequal reciprocal translocation that occurs between acrocentric chromosomes, resulting in the formation of a new metacentric chromosome from two acrocentric chromosomes. Such rearrangements may be important in the transmission of Down's syndrome when one of the chromosomes involved is chromosome 21, the other usually being chromosome 14.

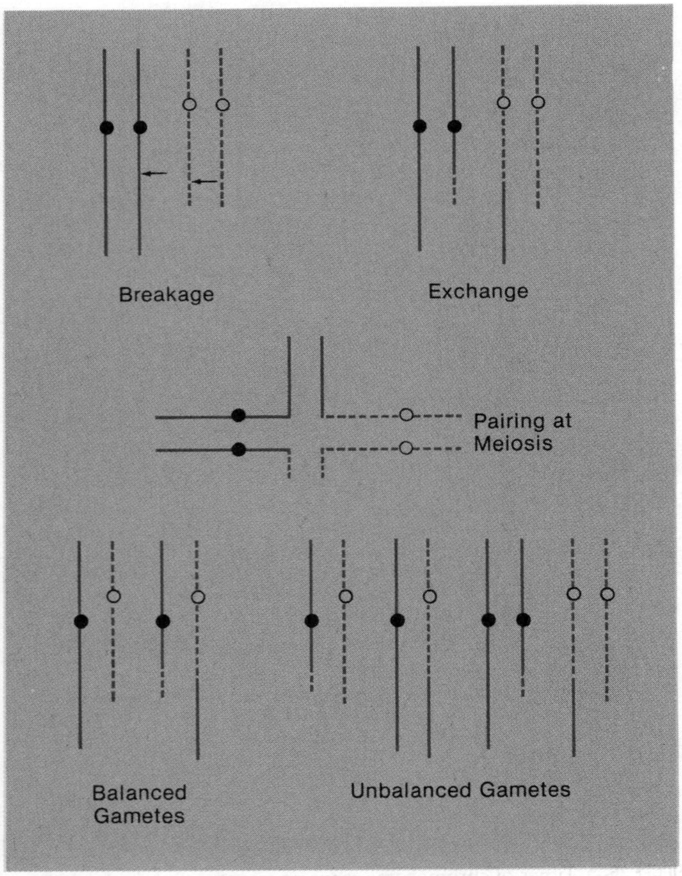

FIGURE 36–6. Consequences of reciprocal translocation. Note both balanced and unbalanced gametes are possible as a result of segregation of the exchanged chromosomes.

POPULATION CYTOGENETICS

Chromosome abnormalities form a significant component of the deleterious genetic load carried by the human population. About 6 per 1000 newborn babies have a major chromosome abnormality that may result in some degree of morbidity or mortality at some time during life. The frequency of the different types of chromosome abnormalities found when large numbers of newborn infants are screened is shown in Table 36–2.

Chromosome abnormalities found among infants at birth are, however, only a very small proportion of the total load of chromosome abnormalities seen at conception. The majority of these are lethal or sublethal and are lost during gestation as either very early abortions or failure of implantation (monosomies, and so on), or as recognized abortions and perinatal deaths. This group includes most trisomies, triploids (3n), and tetraploids (4n). A significant proportion of infants dying in the perinatal and neonatal periods have been shown to have a major chromosome abnormality. About 50 per cent of all embryos and fetuses spontaneously aborted have a chromosome abnormality, and about 6 per cent of stillborn infants and those dying in the perinatal period have abnormal chromosomes.

In addition to the large amount of data on newborn babies and spontaneous abortions, there are now data on large numbers of mothers who have received amniocentesis because of a maternal age of 35 and over. A recent study of over 50,000 amniocenteses shows that, overall, about 2 per cent of the fetuses in midtrimester pregnancies in mothers aged 35 and above have a chromosome abnormality.

SEX CHROMATIN

There are two types of sex cromatin that can be seen in somatic cells: (1) the interphase chromocenter, which represents the genetically inactivated and condensed X chromosome, which is called the X chromatin (sex chromatin, Barr body) and is found in individuals with more than one X chromosome; and (2) the smaller, brightly fluorescing chromocenter, which can be seen by fluorescence microscopy after staining with quinacrine; this represents the brightly fluorescent segment of the human Y chromosome and can be seen in all individuals carrying this chromosome. In diploid cells, the number of X chromosomes is always one greater than the maximum number of X chromatin bodies seen, and the number of Y chromosomes is equal to the maximum number of fluorescent Y chromatin bodies. Study of the sex chromatin can thus provide a rapid assessment of the numbers of sex chromosomes present in the cells.

TABLE 36–2. FREQUENCY OF CHROMOSOME ABNORMALITIES AMONG LIVE BIRTHS*

Sex Chromosomes	Frequency
Male	
47,XYY	1:1022
47,XXY	1:1022
Other	1:1277
Female	
45,X	1:9586
47,XXX	1:958
Other	1:2739
Autosomal trisomics	
+D	1:18984
+E	1:8136
+G	1:802
Balanced structural	1:517
Unbalanced structural	1:1675
Total	1:167

*Based on 54,952 babies: 35,779 males, 19,173 females.

TABLE 36–3. COMMON SEX CHROMOSOME ABNORMALITIES

Chromosome Complement	Eponym	X Chromatin	Frequency (live birth)	Phenotype
Males				
47,XXY	Klinefelter's syndrome	Positive	1:1000	Often tall, eunuchoid males with hypogonadism, feminine distribution of hair, gynecomastia, testicular atrophy after puberty with hyalinized tubules, Leydig cell hyperplasia, often low IQ. May have psychosocial difficulties (see Ch. 235).
47,XYY	—	Negative	1:1000	Often no phenotype abnormalities; usually tall to very tall. May have psychosocial problems.
Females				
45,X and other variants of the X chromosome and mosaics	Turner's syndrome or ovarian dysgenesis	Negative or positive	1:10,000	These patients have ovarian dysgenesis with webbing of neck, short stature (< 153 cm). Often congenital heart disease, skeletal defects, and renal anomalies. This is Turner's syndrome. Other patients may have ovarian dysgenesis without webbing of the neck and with much less frequent somatic anomalies. Invariably they are of short stature (< 153 cm) (see Ch. 237).
47,XXX	None	Double	1:1000	This is extremely variable. Often no phenotypic abnormalities but may be mentally retarded or may have psychosocial problems. Often fertile although may be infertile.

Late-replicating X chromosomes can be identified by autoradiography using tritiated thymidine or by the incorporation of 5-bromodeoxyuridine (BUDR) into DNA in place of thymidine, followed by staining with a dye that differentiates between BUDR and thymidine (the Hoechst-BUDR technique). It is now known that the condensed, late-replicating X chromosomes are genetically inactivated. This inactivation is a random process that may affect either the maternal or the paternal X chromosome at random, occurs early in embryogenesis, and remains fixed for a given cell lineage (Lyon's hypothesis).

The clinical significance of this phenomenon is best demonstrated in females heterozygous for a gene carried by the X chromosome. Such females will have two types of somatic cells in their bodies, one in which the normal allele is inactivated and the other in which the abnormal allele is inactivated. Thus studies on clones of cells (colonies of cells derived from a single progenitor) may allow differentiation between the active and inactive X chromosome and the identification of carrier females. Examples of diseases in which carrier detection has been based on this phenomenon include the Lesch-Nyhan syndrome, Fabry's disease, testicular feminization syndrome, and mucopolysaccharidosis type II (Hunter's syndrome).

Clinical Cytogenetics

Sex Chromosomes

The major features of a few common sex chromosome abnormalities are summarized in Table 36–3. Other sex chromosome abnormalities include the rare females with four or five X chromosomes, as well as males with multiple X and Y chromosomes. Such individuals are usually mentally retarded and may have somatic anomalies. Individuals with various degrees of chromosome mosaicism have also been reported, most frequently as variants in Klinefelter's syndrome or Turner's syndrome.

Autosomes

The clinical features of the three best known autosomal trisomies are listed in Table 36–4.

Other autosomal trisomies in fetuses surviving to term include trisomies 8, 9, and 22. All other autosomes have been reported as trisomic among spontaneous abortions. The advent of banding techniques has greatly widened the scope of chromosome pathology, and numerous examples of chromosome imbalance resulting from deletion or duplication of chromosome material have been reported. Such chromosome imbalance results in dysmorphic features and often developmental and mental retardation.

INDICATIONS FOR CHROMOSOME STUDY

Chromosome abnormalities result in a significant amount of clinical pathology, and chromosome studies should be initiated to rule out this etiologic factor in a patient when a recognizable chromosome syndrome is suspected; in patients with two or more unexplained major congenital malformations involving different systems possibly combined with the presence of minor malformations; and in patients with unexplained developmental or mental retardation. Certain cases of abnormal sexual development, leukemia, and certain solid

TABLE 36–4. THREE BEST-KNOWN AUTOSOMAL TRISOMIES

Chromosome Complement	Eponym	Frequency (live birth)	Phenotype
21-Trisomy (47,XX, +21 47,XY, +21)	Down's syndrome Mongolism	1:700	Typical facial appearance, epicanthic folds, oblique palpebral fissures, broad bridge of the nose, protruding tongue, open mouth, square-shaped ears, flattened facial profile. Invariable mental retardation, muscular hypotonia, and often congenital heart disease (Fig. 36–7).
18-Trisomy (47,XX, +18 47,XY, +18)	Edwards' syndrome	1:8000	Full-term infants of low birth weight with severe mental and motor retardation. Usually have a prominent occiput and frequently occurring facial abnormalities, including micrognathia, a Grecian nose, low-set and malformed ears, cleft lip and palate. Flexion deformities of fingers are often severe. Mental retardation is often severe. They are sublethal, and survival for more than a few months is rare.
13-Trisomy (47,XX, +13) 47,XY, +13	Patau's syndrome	1:20,000	Usually low birth weight infants of full-term gestation with a typical facial appearance, including a broad nose, hypertelorism, microphthalmia, anophthalmia, often with coloboma, and micrognathia. They are usually microcephalic, ears are low-set and malformed, and there is a large broad and bulbous nose. There are often flexion deformities and frequent polydactyly and syndactyly. Survival is usually very short.

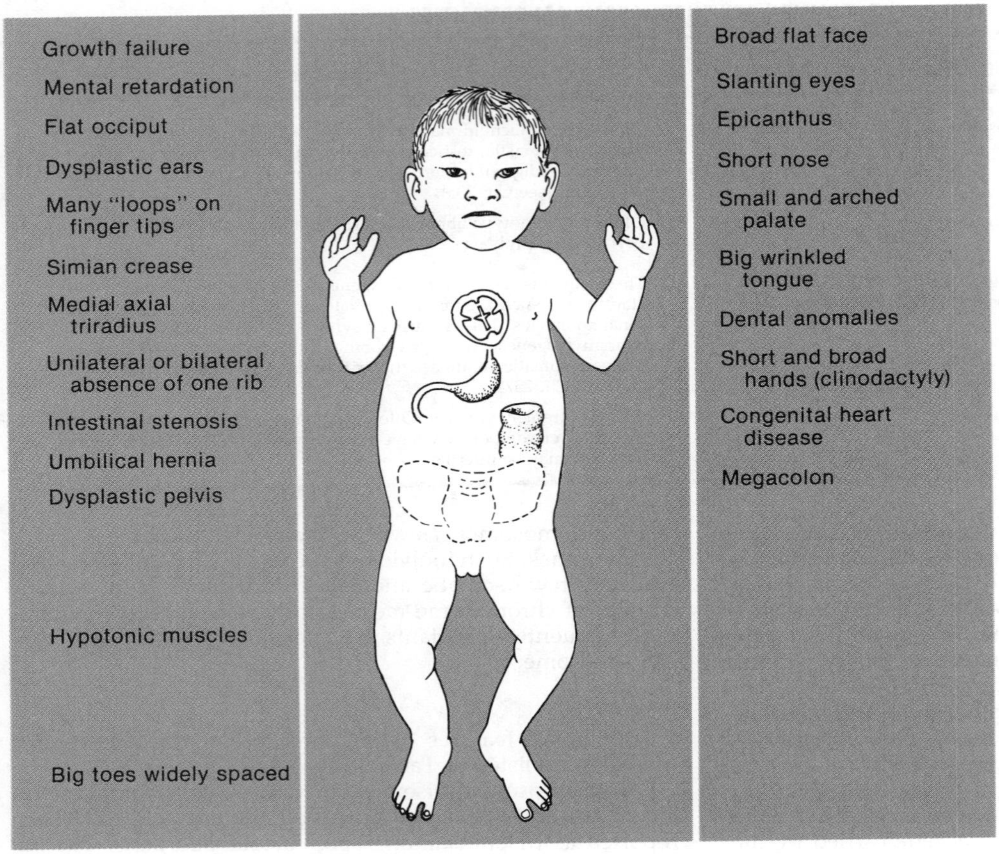

FIGURE 36–7. Clinical findings in trisomy 21. (From Vogel F, Motulsky AG: Human Genetics: Problems and Approaches. Berlin, Springer-Verlag, 1986.)

tumors associated with congenital malformations and known to be associated with specific chromosome abnormalities (aniridia, Wilms' tumor, retinoblastoma) require chromosome studies. Chromosome banding is mandatory to identify the chromosome involved as well as to rule out possible structural changes not detectable by other means.

Chromosome Breakage Syndromes

Three diseases are commonly associated with unrepaired chromosome breaks. These are Fanconi's anemia (FA), ataxia-telangiectasia (AT), and Bloom's syndrome (BS). These are so characterized because in addition to their typical clinical features they share the propensity to chromosome breakage that can be seen in cultured cells and that commonly occurs with several times the frequency observed in normal individuals. Each of these diseases is inherited as an autosomal recessive condition. Two of these conditions are associated with congenital malformations (BS and FA), and all three have an increased frequency of malignancy. This may be the consequence of alterations in DNA repair process.

Sister chromatids can be differentially stained by a modification of the Hoechst-BUDR technique. This permits the identification of exchanges between sister chromatids. Such sister chromatid exchanges (SCE) occur with an increased frequency in BS and in normal individuals may be increased as the result of exposure to chromosome-damaging agents.

Heritable Fragile Sites

Chromosome breakage is usually random; however, some individuals may exhibit breakage or a nonstaining chromosome region (chromosome gap) at a specific site in a significant proportion of metaphases. In many cases such sites may be induced by the use of folate-deficient culture medium, although a few sites are folate insensitive. These specific sites, known as fragile sites, may represent alterations in the DNA and are often heritable. While most fragile sites are not associated with disease or other clinical problems, the fragile site at Xq28 is known to be associated with one common form of X-linked mental retardation among males.

PRENATAL DIAGNOSIS

The diagnosis of chromosome abnormalities at midtrimester gestation is now a routine procedure for certain pregnancies. It involves the aspiration of a small sample of amniotic fluid (amniocentesis), culturing of the fetal cells contained in the fluid, and determination of the karyotype of these cells and thus of the fetus. The major indications for the use of this technique for the detection of chromosome abnormalities are: (1) Maternal age—usually offered to all mothers over the age of 35 at the time of delivery; (2) presence of a parental chromosome abnormality—if one parent is a balanced translocation carrier and particularly if the translocation was detected as the result of the previous birth of a clinically abnormal infant; (3) previous trisomy—those cases in which the mother has previously had a trisomic infant or possibly in which she is known to have had a previous instance of spontaneous abortion in which the abortus was karyotyped and shown to be trisomic; and (4) abnormal levels (high or low) of alpha-fetoprotein.

The safety and reliability of amniocentesis as a diagnostic technique have now been well established by numerous studies, and it is generally accepted that amniocentesis increases the risk of miscarriage by between 0.5 and 1 per cent above the inherent risk for that individual without intervention. Other risks of the test, including fetal and maternal morbidity, are negligible. In competent hands the test has been shown to have a near 100 per cent reliability for the detection of chromosome abnormalities.

Recently, direct transcervical aspiration of chorionic villi (chorionic villus sampling, or CVS) has been used for prenatal diagnosis, and several randomized, controlled trials of CVS compared with genetic amniocentesis (GA) are in progress in different countries. These trials will determine whether CVS is as safe, accurate, and reliable as GA. If it is found to be an acceptable alternative, then the diagnosis of chromosome abnormalities may be moved from the second to the first trimester of pregnancy.

DeGrouchy J, Turleau C: Clinical Atlas of Human Chromosomes. 2nd ed. New York, John Wiley & Sons, 1984. *A review of chromosomal syndromes with numerous illustrations and references.*

Hamerton JL: Population cytogenetics: A perspective. In Adonolfi M, Baron P, Giarnelli F, et al. (eds): Pediatric Research: A Genetic Approach. London, Heineman Medical Books, 1982. *Deals with frequency of chromosome abnormalities in populations.*

ISCN: An International System of Human Cytogenetic Nomenclature. Birth Defects Original Article Series 21:1–116. New York, March of Dimes, 1985. *The basic handbook of nomenclature rules for human chromosomes including high-resolution banding.*

Vogel F, Motulsky AG: Human Genetics: Problems and Approaches. 2nd ed. Berlin, Springer-Verlag, 1986. *A detailed treatise on human genetics from both a basic and a clinical viewpoint. Numerous references. Chapter 2 deals extensively with human cytogenetics.*

Yunis JJ: The chromosomal basis of human neoplasia. Science 221:227, 1983. *A review of our current knowledge about chromosome abnormalities and gene mapping in relation to human tumors.*

37 CONGENITAL MALFORMATIONS

Lewis B. Holmes

INCIDENCE

Two per cent of newborn infants have serious malformations, most of which are compatible with survival. Many additional malformations, such as genitourinary, vertebral, and heart defects, are identified during childhood and the teenage years. Many adults with congenital malformations are unaware of the significance of these problems for their health or the potential significance for their unborn children.

ETIOLOGIES

The recognized causes of malformations include genetic abnormalities, environmental factors, and the combined effects of mutant genes and environmental factors, i.e., multifactorial inheritance (Table 37–1). Multifactorial inheritance is the most common of these etiologies. However, at least 40 per cent of all malformations cannot be explained. One example of a cause that is neither environmental nor genetic is a vascular abnormality. Occlusion of blood vessels during development has been postulated to cause intestinal atresia and hydranencephaly; absence of vessels and abnormal persistence of vessels have been observed in absence of the radius and absence of the tibia.

A few hereditary malformations have been shown to be due to biochemical abnormalities, such as a deficiency of 5α-reductase in individuals with pseudovaginal perineoscrotal hypospadias, an autosomal recessive disorder characterized by ambiguous genitals. An abnormal alpha-2 chain in type I collagen has been identified in skin fibroblasts from a woman with type I osteogenesis imperfecta, a skeletal dysplasia inherited as an autosomal dominant trait (see Ch. 201).

In multifactorial inheritance, clinical studies of human and laboratory examples have shown that several genes (including major genes) are involved, as well as environmental factors such as maternal influences, uterine factors, the season of the year, and socioeconomic class. Most individuals with a malformation attributed to multifactorial inheritance are the only affected members of their families. However, affected individuals have an increased risk of having affected sibs or affected children. The recurrence risk is usually between 1 and 10 per cent, which is 10 to 40 times greater than the incidence of the malformation in the general population.

About 0.6 per cent of newborn infants have a major chromosome abnormality, but many do not survive to the adult years. Down's syndrome results from the most common trisomy, and survival of most affected newborns to the adult years is now expected. In trisomy 21, the associated chromosome abnormality in 95 per cent of the cases, the extra chromosome comes from the mother 75 per cent of the time. Since women over age 35 now are having a smaller portion of all pregnancies, 80 per cent of the infants with Down's syndrome are being born to women of less than 35 years.

Common sex chromosome abnormalities, such as 47,XYY and 47,XXX, are usually not associated with any congenital malformations. Boys with 47,XXY (Klinefelter's syndrome) may have abnormal physical features that are evident in the teenage years. Girls with the 45,X (Turner's) syndrome are usually recognized in infancy because of associated lymphedema, webbed neck, heart defects, and short stature or in the teenage years because of failure of puberty to occur spontaneously.

CLINICAL RELEVANCE

The following examples illustrate the potential significance of a malformation to the affected adult and his or her children.

Relevance to the Health of the Affected Person

CONGENITAL ABSENCE OF ONE KIDNEY. About 1 in 700 infants has unilateral renal agenesis. Most affected individuals are asymptomatic. However, they have an increased risk of structural malformations of the ureter, such as ureteropelvic junction stricture, and associated infections, hypertension, and so forth. The affected female may have a bicornuate uterus or absence of the half of the uterus on the same side as the renal aplasia. Affected males may have absence of the vas deferens on the same side. Parents with unilateral renal

TABLE 37–1. RECOGNIZED ETIOLOGIES OF MALFORMATIONS PRESENT IN ADULTS

	Examples
1. Genetic abnormalities	
a. Single mutant gene	
i. Autosomal dominant trait	Polycystic kidney disease, adult type Polysyndactyly
ii. Autosomal recessive trait	Mohr's syndrome (oro-facial-digital syndrome, type II)
iii. X-linked dominant trait	Telecanthus-hypospadias (BBB) syndrome
iv. X-linked recessive trait	Metacarpal 4-5 fusion
b. Chromosome abnormalities	
i. Trisomy of autosomes	Down's syndrome
ii. Interstitial deletion	Aniridia-Wilms' tumor
iii. Sex chromosome abnormalities	45,X (Turner's syndrome); 47,XXY (Klinefelter's syndrome)
2. Environmental factors	
a. Uterine factors	Amniotic band syndrome
b. Intrauterine infection	Congenital rubella syndrome
c. Drugs	Fetal hydantoin syndrome
3. Genetic plus environmental factors (multifactorial inheritance)	Heart defects Cleft lip and/or palate Hypospadias Pyloric stenosis Hirschsprung's disease

agenesis have an increased risk of having infants with either the same malformation or bilateral renal agenesis, which is fatal.

BRACHYDACTYLY, TYPE E. Owing to premature closure of epiphyses, persons with this autosomal dominant disorder have short hands and feet with a variable pattern of shortening of the first, fourth, and fifth metacarpals and metatarsals and distal phalanges of the thumb and great toe. They also have a mild-to-moderate degree of shortness of stature. Severe hypertension is often a problem in the affected teenager and young adult. This cause of the hypertension has not been determined.

BRANCHIO-OTO-RENAL SYNDROME. The person with this autosomal dominant disorder has a pattern of malformations that includes malformed ears, preauricular tags, preauricular sinus, and branchial cleft sinus. The mildly affected adult is often not diagnosed until a more severely affected child is born. The affected adult may have significant hearing loss or renal hypoplasia.

KLIPPEL-FEIL SYNDROME. The person with fusion or hemivertebrae of one or more cervical vertebrae usually has a short neck, limited rotation of the head, a low hairline, and a webbed neck. Common associated problems include hearing loss, heart defects, Sprengel's deformity, and genitourinary anomalies, such as aplasia of mullerian structures.

POLYCYSTIC KIDNEY DISEASE. The affected individual with the adult form has an increased risk of having cerebral aneurysms and pancreatic cysts. Prenatal diagnosis using DNA probes is now possible.

Relevance to Increased Risk of Having Affected Children

MULTIFACTORIAL INHERITANCE. The adult with one of the common malformations attributed to this process has an increased risk of having an affected child. For malformations that show an altered sex ratio, the sex of the affected parent is important in determining the risk of having an affected child (Table 37–2). In general, the parent of the less frequently affected sex has a greater risk of having affected children. For example, *intestinal aganglionosis* (Hirschsprung's disease) is much more common in males than females, but the affected female has a much greater risk of having affected children (Table 37–2).

With early surgical closure and better treatment of the associated hydrocephalus and urinary tract infections, males and females with *spina bifida* (myelomeningocele) are surviving to adult years and often have normal intelligence. Both affected males and females may be fertile. The affected adult has an increased risk of about 3 per cent that each child will have a neural tube defect.

HYPERTELORISM. The mother who has a broad bridge of the nose and hypertelorism* has an increased risk of having severely malformed sons. For example, the female who carries the X-linked gene for the telecanthus-hypospadias (BBB) syndrome will show only hypertelorism, but sons who inherit this gene have a severe malformation syndrome that may include hypertelorism, broad nasal bridge, cleft lip and palate, heart defects, imperforate anus, hypospadias, and mental deficiency. Mothers with the autosomal dominant disorder known as the Opitz-Frias (or G) syndrome also have hypertelorism and a broad bridge of the nose. Their affected sons and daughters have at birth aspiration due to a laryngotracheoesophageal cleft, stridor, and associated malformations such as cleft lip, heart defects, hypospadias (males), and imperforate anus. Unfortunately, the physical feature of broad nasal bridge and hypertelorism is nonspecific and the risk for the woman with no affected children cannot be determined.

MENTAL RETARDATION. There are many causes of mental retardation. The mildly retarded woman without striking physical abnormalities may be a carrier of significant and relatively common genetic abnormalities that give her an increased risk of having severely affected sons. Two examples are the fragile-X syndrome and the Coffin-Lowry syndrome. The fragile-X syndrome is a common cause of mental retardation, mild facial abnormalities, and sometimes macroorchidism in males. The affected female may show mosaicism for the marker X chromosome, an abnormality of the distal portion of the long arm of the X chromosome that can be identified in cytogenetic studies only if special media and processing are used. The woman who has the X-linked gene for the Coffin-Lowry syndrome shows only mild mental retardation, short stature, short and hyperextensible hands, and tufted distal phalanges. The affected male is much more severely affected, with severe mental deficiency, short stature, stiff joints, coarse facial features, pectus carinatum, and large, soft hands.

*Hypertelorism can be determined most precisely from an anteroposterior radiograph that shows an increased bony interorbital distance.

TABLE 37–2. RISK OF AFFECTED CHILDREN FOR PARENT WITH MALFORMATION ATTRIBUTED TO MULTIFACTORIAL INHERITANCE

Malformation	Risk of Affected Child (per cent)	Prevalence of Condition in General Population (per cent)
1. Intestinal aganglionosis (Hirschsprung's disease)	2.0	0.02
2. Hypospadias	6.0	0.8
3. Club foot	1.4	0.13
4. Congenital hip dislocation	4.3	0.8
5. Ventricular septal defect	4.0	0.2
6. Pyloric stenosis	4 (affected father) 13 (affected mother)	
7. Cleft palate	6.2	0.3
8. Spina bifida (meningomyelocele)	3.0	0.14

PRENATAL DIAGNOSIS

The techniques used most often for diagnosing malformations in the fetus are cell culture of amniocytes removed at 16 to 18 weeks of gestation, assay for alpha-fetoprotein (AFP) in the amniotic fluid and maternal serum, and ultrasound imaging. Early amniocentesis is now offered at 12 to 14 weeks of pregnancy at some medical centers. Parents who have previously had a child with trisomy 21 have a 1 per cent risk of recurrence regardless of the mother's age. To rule out this possibility amniocentesis for chromosome analysis is offered. For the woman who has previously had a child with anencephaly or spina bifida, prenatal diagnosis includes amniocentesis to measure the level of AFP and ultrasound imaging for hydrocephalus, the cranial defect in anencephaly, and the spinal defect in meningomyelocele. If the level of AFP is elevated, a neural tube defect is confirmed by an increase in the level of acetylcholinesterase in the amniotic fluid. Both the amniocytes removed at amniocentesis and the chorionic villi removed transcervically at 9 to 11 weeks of gestation can be used to identify chromosome abnormalities, hemoglobinopathies, and metabolic disorders in the fetus. Limb malformations, such as absent radius, ectrodactyly, hydrocephalus, and bilateral renal agenesis, can be investigated with ultrasound imaging. However, the accuracy of this method of prenatal diagnosis is not known.

Prenatal screening for neural tube defects is now available as an option in prenatal care. Serum AFP is measured in the mother at 16 to 18 weeks of pregnancy. The pregnant woman with an elevated serum level of AFP on two occasions should have prenatal studies, including amniocentesis for AFP and acetylcholinesterase and ultrasound imaging. Errors in diagnosis result from incorrect gestational age and alterations in the range of normal values in obese women and in women with diabetes mellitus. Elevations in AFP also occur in twin pregnancies, intrauterine death, and other malformations such as esophageal atresia, omphalocele, and hereditary nephrosis. A skin-covered neural tube defect, such as a lumbar meningocele, will be missed in prenatal screening with serum AFP. In general, prenatal AFP screening is most effective if carried out by individuals who are experienced in identifying the causes of false-positive and false-negative values and who educate the parents initially about the steps involved and the benefits and accuracy of the testing.

FETAL SURGERY

Catheters have been introduced to relieve malformations that cause obstruction of the flow of urine or of cerebrospinal fluid. This approach is experimental. One major problem is to identify an abnormality early enough to permit intervention before the fetus has suffered irreversible damage, such as the lung hypoplasia that is a cause of death in infants with oligohydramnios from urinary tract obstruction. Another problem is that the fetus in whom only hydrocephalus or urinary tract obstruction is visible by ultrasound may have multiple malformations that will be apparent only after birth.

PREVENTION OF MALFORMATION

Pregnant women with several different medical diseases or exposures have an increased risk of having children with birth defects. If the patient is informed of this risk before conception or soon after conception, these risks can be either lessened or eliminated. These efforts at prevention require special efforts in education, as most women receive routine prenatal care too late to benefit from counseling. Specific opportunities in prevention include the following:

CHRONIC ALCOHOLISM. Exposure of the fetus to high maternal levels of alcohol causes growth retardation before and after birth, microcephaly, brain malformations, mental deficiency, a characteristic pattern of craniofacial features, and at times other malformations, such as vertebral anomalies and spina bifida (fetal alcohol syndrome). The lower the level of exposure, the less the risk of damage to the fetus. If the pregnant woman decreases her alcohol consumption at any time in pregnancy, it is beneficial to the fetus, although a decrease before or soon after conception is the most beneficial.

DIABETES MELLITUS. The woman with insulin-dependent diabetes mellitus is two to three times more likely to have a child with serious malformations than the nondiabetic woman. The malformations include spina bifida, anencephaly, heart defects, vertebral and genitourinary malformations, and multiple malformations. The risk of having a malformed infant correlates inversely with the quality of control of her disease, glucose metabolism in particular, very early in pregnancy. The lower the level of glycosylated hemoglobin before or soon after conception, the lower her risk of having a malformed child.

MATERNAL PHENYLKETONURIA (PKU). Children with PKU identified at birth through neonatal screening for metabolic diseases will have normal development and intelligence if the dietary treatment (low phenylalanine, low protein) is begun soon after birth. The diet is usually discontinued in the early school years. However, successfully treated females with PKU who are no longer on the diet have a risk of over 90 per cent that any pregnancy will either end in a spontaneous abortion or result in a child with microcephaly and mental deficiency, and often heart defects as well. The risk of damage to the fetus correlates with the blood level of phenylalanine in the mother. If the woman with PKU resumes the low-phenylalanine diet before conception she has her best chance of having a normal child. If the diet is resumed in the first trimester, as soon as she knows she is pregnant, the child is less severely damaged than if no dietary treatment is used during pregnancy. Unfortunately, many young women with PKU are not aware of their risk of having children with serious birth defects.

Bergsma D (ed.): Birth Defects Compendium. 2nd ed. New York, Alan R. Liss, Inc., 1979. *An up-to-date, brief summary on all common birth defects.*

Briggs GG, Freeman RK, Yaffe SJ: Drugs in Pregnancy and Lactation. 2nd ed. Baltimore, Williams & Wilkins Company. *A summary of current information on the potential teratogenic effect of many common exposures.*

Jacobs PA, Glover TW, Mayer M, et al.: X-Linked mental retardation: A study of 7 families. Am J Med Genet 7:471, 1980. *A thorough study of this very common hereditary cause of mental deficiency in affected males and carrier females.*

Lenke RR, Levy HL: Maternal phenylketonuria and hyperphenylalaninemia. N Engl J Med 303:1202, 1980. *The results of an international survey of the teratogenic effect of PKU in the pregnant woman and the attempts at prevention.*

Reeders ST, Zerres K, Gal A, et al.: Prenatal diagnosis of autosomal dominant polycystic kidney disease with a DNA probe. Lancet 2:6, 1986. *The report of this new development.*

Report of the U.K. Collaborative Study on Alpha-Fetoprotein in Relation to Neural-tube Defects. Amniotic-fluid alpha-fetoprotein measurement in antenatal diagnosis of anencephaly and open spina bifida in early pregnancy. Lancet 2:651, 1979. *A summary of the findings in the U.K. Collaborative Study of using maternal AFP screening to detect fetuses with spina bifida and anencephaly.*

Smith DW: Recognizable Patterns of Human Malformation. 3rd ed. Philadelphia, W.B. Saunders Company, 1982. *A thorough tabulation of recognized malformation syndromes.*

Temtamy SA, McKusick VA: The Genetics of Hand Malformations. New York, Alan R. Liss, Inc., 1978. *The best source of information on malformations of the hands, arms, and legs.*

38 GENETIC COUNSELING

F. Clarke Fraser

Genetic counseling is the process whereby patients and their families are helped to deal with a problem created by the occurrence, or potential occurrence, of a disorder in the family that they think may have a genetic basis. The need for genetic counseling starts with one or more questions. "My child is born with Nevererdofit syndrome. What caused it? Will it happen again? Should we stop having children?" "My grandfather has developed Huntington's disease. Might I get it?" "I have fallen in love with my cousin. Would our children all be malformed or mentally retarded?" "I volunteered for a screening program and they say I have the gene for Tay-Sachs disease. What harm will it do?" "I am 35 years old and I read that I should have a test that will make sure my baby will be normal. Should I?"

In many cases the genetic principles underlying the answers to such questions are simple and should be in the repertoire of every physician. Some cases require more sophisticated calculations or special tests and can be referred to a genetic counselor. The answers may depend not only on genetic principles but also on complex social and ethical issues that will require several interviews and perhaps the effort of both the family physician and the genetic counselor to resolve.

DIAGNOSIS

The first step in the counseling process is to confirm, or establish, the diagnosis (Fig. 38–1). This may already have been done, or it may require special tests (karyotype, carrier detection tests, and so forth). Do not ignore the family history, which may sometimes be an aid to diagnosis. Genetic heterogeneity (see Ch. 34) may confound the issue and require special tests to be done on the patient or family members. In

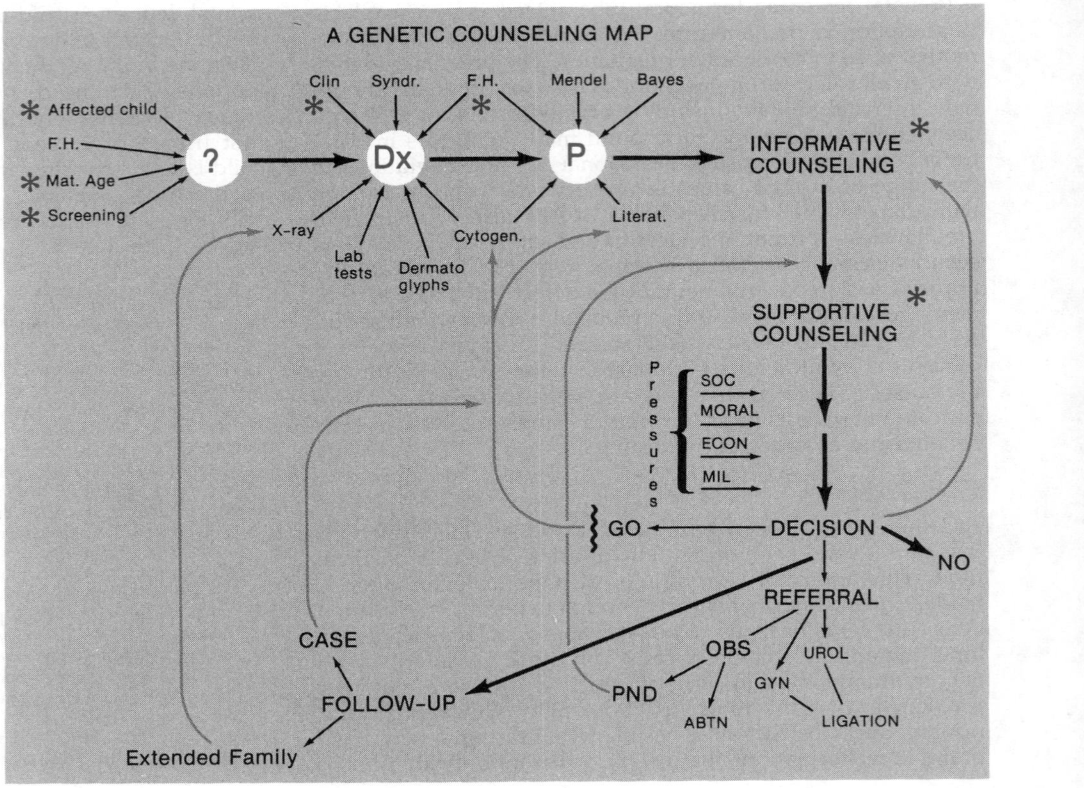

FIGURE 38–1. Map of the genetic counseling process. It begins with a question, raised by the advent of a child with a ? genetic disorder, other aspect of the family history, etc. There must be a diagnosis (Dx), which may depend on information from clinicians, syndromologists, x-ray studies, laboratory tests, dermatoglyphics, cytogenetics, and the family history (FH). To answer the question usually requires estimating a probability (P), using information from the family history, cytogenetics, the literature, the mendelian principles, and Bayesian calculations. Following informative and supportive counseling (often influenced by social, moral, economic, and family pressures) the counselee may reach a decision either to refrain from reproduction or to go ahead. Both of these may require appropriate referral. If the "GO" decision results in a recurrence, further counseling may be required. Follow-up of the counselee and the extended family may result in reentry into the process. Asterisks indicate where the physician can play an important role. (Reprinted with permission from Nora JJ, Fraser FC: Medical Genetics: Principles and Practice. 2nd ed. Philadelphia, Lea and Febiger, 1981.)

some cases, a specific diagnosis cannot be reached and the counseling must be done on an "either-or" basis—an unsatisfactory situation, but informed uncertainty is better than erroneous certainty.

ESTABLISHING "P"

The next step is to derive the probability, P, of the event that concerns the counselee, usually a risk of recurrence. Prerequisite to this is a carefully taken *family history*, which will serve not only as the basis for calculating P but also as a screening procedure that may pick up additional warning signals relevant to the counselee (this function applies also to the routine family history taken as part of the workup of any patient). A near relative with a neural tube defect may make the counselee eligible for prenatal diagnosis even though the condition for which she was referred does not. A sib or parent with non–insulin-dependent diabetes mellitus puts the counselee at increased risk for this disease; this raises the question of early detection tests and preventive measures. The same applies to most common, familial disorders, including hypertension, early coronary disease, the common neoplasms, and the common psychoses.

If the disease is known to have a *mendelian basis*, P can often be calculated on the basis of the known mode of inheritance (see Ch. 33). In some cases bayesian algebra can be used to improve the precision of the estimate by using additional family information. For instance, if a man's parent has Huntington's disease, which has a variable age of onset, the man had a 50 per cent chance of inheriting the gene at conception, but the longer he lives, free of the disease, the more likely it is that he did not inherit the gene. Similarly, for a woman who had a 50 per cent chance of inheriting the gene for hemophilia from her mother, the chance that she did inherit it diminishes with each unaffected son she bears. The precise probability can be calculated for the specific family situation. If the calculations tax the mathematical abilities of the physician, a genetic counselor can be consulted.

The rapid advances in mapping the human genome (Ch. 35) and particularly the use of DNA markers (RFLP's) are making it possible, in an increasing number of diseases, to identify carriers of mutant genes either before onset of the disease (e.g., Huntington's chorea) or prenatally (e.g., hemoglobinopathies, cystic fibrosis of the pancreas).

Diseases that do not fit the mendelian rules of family segregation often fit the expectations for *multifactorial inheritance*, particularly if they are known to be common (1 in 1000 or so) and familial. For these conditions the risk increases with the genetic proximity to an affected relative and with the number of affected relatives. Empiric estimates of average risks are available for counselees of varying degrees of relationship to the affected individual, and these can be modified upward or downward, according to the numbers of affected and unaffected relatives, by formulae based on the assumption of multifactorial inheritance.

Empiric estimates of risk must also be used for *chromosomal disorders*. We know the frequencies of liveborn trisomics at various maternal ages (see Ch. 36) and the probability of a recurrence after having had one.

Estimating risks for carriers of balanced chromosomal rearrangements is more difficult. One can derive the theoretic ratios of balanced to unbalanced offspring, but actual segregations are usually not random, and the question of whether theoretically possible unbalanced products will be viable or nonviable complicates the issue. Both segregation ratios and viability will vary with the length and position of the rearranged segments, and it is difficult to obtain enough data for any one rearrangement to derive segregation ratios. The genetic counselor can use a combination of general principles and empiric knowledge to obtain an estimate of the risk but must recognize the uncertainties involved.

Finally, there is the uncomfortably large group of disorders, particularly those involving mental retardation and dysmorphic features, for which the risk of recurrence is unknown. It may be as high as 1 in 4, for an as yet unrecognized autosomal recessive syndrome, or less than 1 per cent for an unrecognized environmental teratogen. Since unrecognized autosomal recessive syndromes will, one hopes, be in the minority (unless these is parental consanguinity), the risk in such cases will average out as low.

INFORMATIVE COUNSELING

Once P has been established as precisely as possible, we pass on to the stage of "informative counseling"—imparting the prognosis, probability of recurrence, and reproductive options to the counselee or counselees.

The processes by which families reach their reproductive decisions are complex, variable, and not well understood. Odds seem more easily appreciated than percentages, and the term "chances" does not have the opprobrious overtones of "risks." A statement such as, "if 20 couples who have had a baby like John each have another baby, on the average one of them would be like John and 19 would not," is easier to understand and less threatening than "the risk of your next baby's being affected is 5 per cent." Make sure they understand that the odds are the same for each child, and that (when the odds are one to three, for example), if they have one affected child, it does not mean that the next three will be normal.

Imparting the information may be relatively simple if the risk is so low as to be reassuring, and the nature of the disorder is well known to the counselees, who may have first-hand experience with it, or if the risk and burden are so high that no further reproduction is contemplated. It is in the intermediate group, who must decide on various reproductive options, often complicated by a host of social, ethical, economic, and family pressures, that genetic counseling may be most helpful.

SUPPORTIVE COUNSELING

This process involves helping the family to choose, among the various options, the one that is best for their own particular set of circumstances. Obviously, informative and supportive counseling go on together and are separated only for didactic purposes.

Who should do the counseling may depend on the local scene. If the physician knows the family best and the genetics is simple, the physician may be the most suitable counselor. If the genetics and the reproductive options are complex, the genetic counselor may be the appropriate resource. Often the two can work together in helping the family to reach an informed and responsible decision.

Parents often tend to ignore the numerical risk and focus on the burden; they may work toward a decision by trying out, in their imagination, various scenarios and selecting the "least-lose" option that they could live with. The risk of recurrence may, in this process, be incorporated into the burden. The "1" in the odds may loom large even if the denominator is quite big, particularly if the counselee is a pessimist. "No matter how big the *n* is in the 1 in *n* odds, the 1 never goes away."

The process of deciding may take some time, and the counselees may need several sessions with a counselor, as new issues or questions come up. Throughout this time, the counselor acts as both a source of information and a sounding board, trying to steer an understanding and supportive course between paternalistic directiveness ("with that high a risk, you shouldn't have children") and Olympian detachment ("It's your decision; don't ask me to make it for you.").

REFERRAL

Having reached a decision, the counselee or counselees may require referral—for tubal ligation (fallopian or vas deferens), artificial insemination, prenatal diagnosis, or care during the next pregnancy.

PRENATAL DIAGNOSIS

Prenatal diagnosis has changed the face of genetic counseling, since, for a growing number of conditions, it can change odds to certainty. It behooves the physician to know what categories of disorder are eligible, and although he or she cannot be expected to keep up with the latest additions to the list, it is at least possible to establish rapport with a clinical genetics center where this information can be found.

Techniques used in prenatal diagnosis include visualization by ultrasound examination or, less frequently, x-ray. Ultrasound will detect structural malformations such as anencephaly and overt spina bifida, renal agenesis, polycystic kidney disease, and exomphalos. As techniques improve, the array of detectable defects increases, and it is now possible to detect a remarkable number of disorders, including cleft lip, cleft palate, various heart malformations, microphthalmia, and some types of short-limb dwarfism. Fetoscopy permits direct examination, blood sampling, and even skin or muscle biopsy, although the risk of miscarriage may be as high as 5 per cent, even in experienced hands.

Amniotic fluid can be obtained by amniocentesis at 12 to 14 weeks of gestation, with a risk of fetal damage or induced miscarriage that seems well below 1 per cent in experienced hands. The cells can be cultured for karyotyping or biochemical studies. The fluid can be examined for alpha-fetoprotein, hormones (adrenogenital syndrome), intestinal enzymes (imperforate anus), or other appropriate chemicals. Techniques for chorionic biopsy are now becoming available that will allow examination of cells with the same genotype as the fetus as early as 8 to 10 weeks of gestation, permitting earlier diagnosis and, if necessary, termination of pregnancy. This along with the increasing array of conditions that can be diagnosed prenatally, will exacerbate the problems, both ethical and practical, involved in deciding what conditions and what circumstances justify the procedure. Genetic counselors tend to be nondirective, assuming that the parents (presumably well informed and conscientious) are in the best position to balance the burden of caring for an affected child against that of the guilt and suffering of a midtrimester abortion. They tend to draw the line, however, at prenatal diagnosis for nonpathologic conditions, and in particular the determination of sex for reasons of social preference.

The physician's main responsibility would seem to be to ensure that prospective parents at risk are aware that prenatal diagnosis is possible. The desire to practice good preventive medicine may be reinforced by the risk of litigation in cases in which parents have a child affected by some serious condition for which prenatal diagnosis is available and were not told about it. The main indications to be kept in mind are the following:

1. Maternal age: in most centers 35 or more at the expected time of birth.
2. Neural tube defect in a previous child, in the counselee, or in a first-degree relative. The risk of recurrence in a child or sib ranges from 1.5 to 10 per cent, depending on the frequency in the general population, and the risk for a nephew or niece is close to 1 per cent. Neural tube defects in this context include spina bifida occulta if there are multiple vertebral defects or spinal dysraphism. The advisability of maternal serum screening for neural tube defects by alpha-fetoprotein determination is a complex question, which must be answered for each population, depending on the frequency of neural tube defects and the availability of adequate laboratory, amniocentesis, and genetic counseling resources.
3. Chromosomal rearrangement in a parent. Couples who have had two or more spontaneous abortions deserve karyotyping, as about 1 in 20 will be found to carry a balanced chromosome rearrangement.

4. Sex determination, when the mother is at risk for being a carrier of an X-linked disorder not amenable to prenatal diagnosis.

5. A growing list of inborn errors of metabolism and other mendelian disorders, including the hemoglobinopathies. The dramatic advances in molecular genetics are rapidly expanding the number of such conditions (see Ch. 34 and 35).

6. Structural anomalies detectable by ultrasound, x-radiography, or, possibly, fetoscopy.

In most centers the number of positive diagnoses is about 2 per cent of the total number of cases, and the main benefit is to relieve anxiety and to allow couples who would otherwise refrain from having children, because of their high risk, to go ahead, without fear of the disorder in question.

FOLLOW-UP

The final stage in the genetic counseling process is the follow-up. As with any patient, follow-up is advisable to keep track of the results. The content of the informative counseling should be summarized in a letter, and a telephone call or note a few months later will establish whether the information has been understood, whether new questions have arisen, or whether new circumstances have changed the odds.

It may also be necessary to follow up the extended family. Often the discovery that a couple is at risk for a genetic disorder means that other family members are at risk, particularly in the case of autosomal dominant and X-linked disorders.

In diseases for which treatment is available, such as Wilson's disease or multiple polyposis of the colon, early detection in high-risk relatives is vitally important. Often, it may be possible to test individuals known by pedigree analysis to be at risk for carrier status. The hemoglobinopathies, glucose-6-phosphate dehydrogenase (G6PD) deficiency, Duchenne muscular dystrophy (creatine kinase levels), hemophilia (factor VIII clotting versus antigenic activity), and Tay-Sachs disease are examples. Cystic fibrosis will soon be on the list.

Good preventive medicine requires that these relatives be informed of their risks. This may require some ingenuity to avoid breaches of confidence. Sometimes a key family member will take on the role of genetic advocate, or an approach through the family doctor may solve the problem. One way or another, one strives to avoid the tragedy of an affected child, born to parents whose family history placed them at increased risk, and who bitterly demand, "Why didn't somebody tell me?"

Bergsma D: Birth Defects Compendium. 2nd ed. New York, Alan R. Liss, 1979. *A useful compilation of descriptive and etiologic data on dysmorphic syndromes and other birth defects.*

Brock DJH: Early diagnosis of fetal defects. Cur Rev Obstet Gynaecol 2:165, 1982. *A review of prenatal diagnosis.*

Capron AM, Lappé M, Murray RF (eds): Genetic counselling: Facts, values, and norms. Birth Defects 20:1, 1979. *A multiauthored volume on the concepts, psychology, ethics, and legal issues in genetic counseling.*

Fraser FC: Taking the family history. Am J Med Genet 34:585, 1963. *A discussion of family history-taking at various levels from routine office to research.*

Fraser FC, Nora JJ: Genetics of Man. Philadelphia, Lea and Febiger, 1986. *A textbook oriented toward medical students.*

Lippman-Hand A, Fraser FC: Genetic counseling—the postcounseling period. II. Making reproductive choices. Am J Med Genet 4:73, 1979. *The third in a series of articles on the psychodynamics of genetic counselees.*

McKusick V: Mendelian Inheritance in Man. 7th ed. Baltimore, The Johns Hopkins University Press, 1986. *An exhaustive catalogue of disorders showing mendelian inheritance.*

PART VI
CARDIOVASCULAR DISEASES

39 APPROACH TO THE PATIENT WITH CARDIOVASCULAR DISEASE

Thomas W. Smith

Common to the care of all patients with cardiovascular disease is a data base on which sound diagnostic and therapeutic decisions can be made. This chapter outlines an approach to cardiovascular data collection that emphasizes general principles and strategies and is intended to complement the more specific consideration of disease entities in the chapters that follow. One of the endlessly fascinating aspects of medicine is that each patient presents to the physician a unique story of his or her past history and present illness. Textbook descriptions of disease therefore convey at best a set of findings that the author regards as typical but that never quite fit in detail the findings present in any one individual patient. Hence, an open mind is essential during the evaluation of each patient so that diagnostic possibilities are not overlooked or prematurely discarded.

A dazzling array of diagnostic tests is now available for the evaluation of patients with evident or suspected cardiovascular disease. Sensitivity and specificity are known, or can be estimated, for each method under a given set of clinical circumstances. Redundancy must be avoided to achieve a favorable cost:benefit ratio (e.g., radionuclide ventriculography will often yield information regarding ventricular function that can be obtained from a two-dimensional echocardiogram, and both methods may be superfluous if the patient undergoes left ventriculography as part of a cardiac catheterization procedure). The emerging discipline of decision analysis (see Ch. 21) should help in formulating strategies in the development of an adequate cardiovascular data base.

Although accurate diagnosis is a key element in patient care, prognosis is also vitally important to the patient and often to the physician, who must formulate a program of treatment. Information over and above that needed to establish a diagnosis is typically required to allow an accurate prediction of outcome. This exercise in probability statistics is challenging and deserves careful attention as an essential component of the comprehensive care of the patient.

COMPONENTS OF THE CARDIOVASCULAR WORKUP

The three essential components of the clinical data base are the history, physical examination, and laboratory studies. Although this sequence of data acquisition will typically be followed, the value of returning to the bedside (often repeatedly) to refine the assessment of historical information and physical findings as the workup progresses cannot be overstated.

History

The cardinal symptoms of cardiovascular disease are listed in Table 39–1. *Dyspnea* and the related items in the first line are discussed in detail in Ch. 43. Historical information is particularly important in distinguishing among heart failure, pulmonary disease (including pulmonary emboli), metabolic disturbances producing acidosis, and anxiety as factors causing dyspnea. The nature of onset and duration of symptoms, relation to position, and precipitating and alleviating factors all provide important clues to the underlying pathophysiologic process.

Fatigue and *weakness* are common to many physical and emotional disease states and are nonspecific; nevertheless, it is important to record quantitative information in the history (e.g., flights of stairs or distance on level ground that the patient can manage) for current and future reference. *Cough*, initially dry and irritative, is a common early manifestation of elevated left-heart filling (and hence pulmonary venous) pressures. *Hemoptysis* should be characterized in regard to color and nature of admixture of blood and sputum to help distinguish between pulmonary (e.g., bronchitis, pulmonary infarction) and cardiac causes (e.g., pulmonary edema, hemorrhage from loss of bronchial vein integrity, as in mitral stenosis). *Cyanosis* is discussed in Ch. 43.

Chest pain should be characterized in terms of location, quality, course of onset and offset, duration, and precipitating and alleviating factors. Pain due to ischemic heart disease is considered in Ch. 51.1. Pericardial pain is more likely to be left sided, sharp in character, and related to breathing and position. Pleuritic pain also tends to be localized and sharp and is related to breathing or coughing. Chest wall pain is often long lasting and associated with tenderness to pressure applied at the trigger area.

Palpitation refers to an awareness of the heart beat, usually occurring in response to a change in cardiac rhythm or rate or by increased contractile force. It is a common anxiety-related symptom in patients without heart disease. Awareness of irregularity of the heart beat is more closely correlated with cardiac rhythm disturbances. *Dizziness* and *syncope* are frequent manifestations of cardiac arrhythmias and demand careful evaluation, often with 24-hour electrocardiographic (ECG) monitoring. These symptoms also occur as a consequence of orthostatic hypotension due to reduced blood volume, vasodilator drugs, or autonomic dysfunction. Obstruction to venous return from any cause will also predispose

TABLE 39–1. CARDINAL SYMPTOMS OF CARDIOVASCULAR DISEASE

Dyspnea, orthopnea, paroxysmal nocturnal dyspnea, wheezing
Fatigue, weakness
Cough, hemoptysis
Cyanosis
Chest pain
Palpitations, dizziness, syncope
Edema
Pain in extremities with exertion (claudication)

to these symptoms. *Claudication* refers to pain or an uncomfortable sensation of tiredness, usually in calf and/or thigh muscles, that occurs in response to exertion and is relieved by rest. This common symptom of peripheral arterial insufficiency is further discussed in Ch. 57.

Edema refers to swelling, usually of a dependent part of the body, due to retention of excess fluid. It is typically maximal in the feet at the end of the day and resolves, at least partially, by morning. Local factors such as deep venous disease predispose to unilateral edema. Patients confined to bed usually accumulate fluid in the sacral area.

The Physical Examination

Five elements constitute the cardiovascular physical examination. These are

1. Physical appearance
2. Venous pressure and pulse contours
3. Arterial pressure and pulse contours
4. Movement of the heart
5. Auscultation

PHYSICAL APPEARANCE. This is important in assessing the nature and severity of heart disease and also in providing clues to systemic diseases that affect the heart. Important cardiac problems are frequently encountered in patients with Marfan's syndrome, Turner's syndrome, Down's syndrome, the pickwickian syndrome, scleroderma, and thyroid disease, all of which are often recognizable on the basis of careful inspection of the patient's appearance. The funduscopic examination yields important information with regard to hypertension, diabetes mellitus, and sometimes infective endocarditis (Roth's spots). Cheyne-Stokes respirations are often seen in patients with advanced heart failure. Sometimes a highly specific cardiac diagnosis can be made on the basis of the physical appearance, such as the association of atrial septal defect with the bony abnormalities of the upper extremity which constitute the Holt-Oram syndrome. Cyanosis and clubbing of the fingertips indicate right-to-left shunting in patients with congenital heart disease.

VENOUS PRESSURE AND PULSE. Both external and internal jugular veins require careful inspection: external for estimation of mean right atrial pressure and internal for wave form as well as pressure. Figure 39–1 illustrates the typical features of the normal jugular venous pulse and indicates the terminology applied to the various aspects of this wave form. The A wave reflects right atrial contraction and occurs immediately prior to the carotid arterial pulse and first heart sound. The X descent occurs with right atrial relaxation and continues with early right ventricular contraction. The C wave, often superimposed on the beginning of the A wave, coincides with the carotid pulse itself. The V wave in the normal jugular venous pulse represents passive right atrial filling behind a closed and competent tricuspid valve. The Y descent reflects sudden termination of the V wave with right ventricular relaxation and opening of the tricuspid valve. The X descent is normally the more evident of the two declining phases of the jugular venous pulse. These phenomena are best noted with the patient so positioned that the top of the venous column can be observed throughout the cardiac cycle. Estimation of the central venous pressure is accomplished by estimating its height in centimeters above the sternal angle of Louis, adding 5 cm to allow for the normal relation of the right atrium to the external chest wall. Normal venous pressure varies from 5 to 10 cm of H_2O. The A wave tends to be accentuated in disease states characterized by reduced right ventricular compliance, tricuspid stenosis, or rhythm disturbances in which the atrium contracts against a closed tricuspid valve ("cannon" A waves). Tricuspid insufficiency produces systolic or regurgitant waves that obliterate the normal jugular venous V waves. Abnormalities associated with pericardial disease are discussed in Ch. 54.

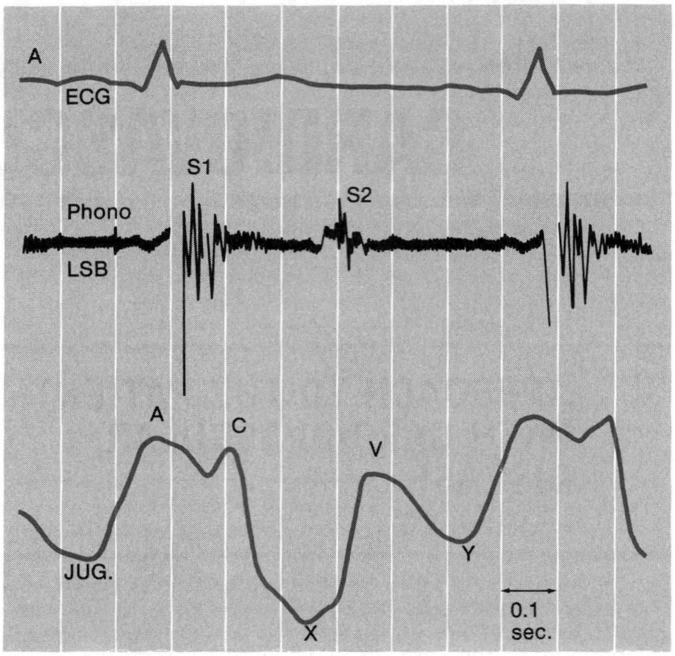

FIGURE 39–1. Normal jugular venous pulse.

ARTERIAL PRESSURE AND PULSE. Examination of the arterial pulse yields critically important information regarding the cardiovascular system. Arterial pressure should always be measured in both arms because of the unexpected discrepancies that are encountered in disease states or that are occasionally due to congenital anomalies. Use of a cuff of appropriate size is essential, and the arterial blood pressure should be recorded in both supine and standing position to assess volume status and the adequacy of reflex vasoconstrictor responses. Pulsus paradoxus refers to a decrease in systolic blood pressure of greater than 10 mm Hg on inspiration and is a typical feature of pericardial tamponade.

The carotid arteries provide the most direct reflection of cardiac activity because of their central location in proximity to the left ventricle and aorta. The amplitude of the carotid pulse is typically increased under circumstances associated with higher cardiac output, including fever, anemia, hyperthyroidism, and arteriovenous fistulas. The regularity (or lack thereof) indicates disturbances of rhythm or hemodynamics as in pulsus alternans. The wave form of the arterial pulse yields clues regarding runoff from the aorta, as in aortic insufficiency or arteriovenous fistula; a bisferiens quality is often present in aortic insufficiency and should be distinguished from the spike-and-dome contour encountered in patients with hypertrophic cardiomyopathy with obstruction (i.e., hypertrophic subaortic stenosis). The volume of the carotid pulse is typically reduced in heart failure and in mitral or aortic stenosis. Peripheral arterial pulses other than the carotid pulses should be felt and compared, with particular attention to a pulse delay at the femoral artery as a manifestation of coarctation of the aorta. Patients with claudication should have their lower extremity pulses examined both at rest and with exercise, since the latter maneuver will often accentuate asymmetries.

MOVEMENT OF THE HEART. Observation, palpation, and percussion are the traditional means for physical examination of cardiac movements. Inspection of the precordium will reveal asymmetries that serve as clues to chronic cardiac hypertrophy, particularly in congenital disease. The partial left lateral decubitus position is optimal for observation as well as palpation of the left ventricle in most patients. Diffuse left parasternal cardiac movement is often best appreciated with the heel of the palm, whereas higher frequency events (S_1, ejection clicks, S_2, opening snap, and thrills) are best felt with firm pressure and the tactile use of the fingertips. Precordial movements should be described at the apex, left parasternal area, and the right and left second intercostal spaces. The normal tapping impulse of the left ventricular apex is replaced by a more diffuse and sometimes dyskinetic impulse in patients with cardiac enlargement from a variety of causes. Displacement of the left ventricle is typically downward and to the left with cardiomegaly. Systolic overload with concentric hypertrophy increases the duration of the apex impulse and can be distinguished from the hyperdynamic impulse accompanying volume overload lesions, such as mitral or aortic insufficiency. Right ventricular enlargement produces a left parasternal systolic lift that is occasionally mimicked by the anterior motion of the heart with systolic expansion of the left atrium in the presence of severe mitral insufficiency. Pulmonary hypertension may be accompanied by a palpable pulmonary artery segment in the second left interspace and by a palpable pulmonic component of the second sound (P_2). Prominent third or fourth heart sounds can often be palpated as well as heard.

Thus, with the data gleaned from physical appearance, the venous and arterial pulse characteristics, and cardiac motion properties, the experienced clinician is armed with substantial information about cardiac anatomy and physiology before employing the stethoscope.

AUSCULTATION. Satisfactory cardiac auscultation requires a stethoscope that fits the ears snugly but comfortably and has the shortest tubing consistent with convenient use. The examination should be carried out in a quiet area, which sometimes requires moving the patient to a more suitable place when ambient noise levels are excessive. A systematic approach, as in all facets of physical examination, is important. Apart from the most obvious and dramatic auscultatory events, one generally hears only what one listens for. Beginning at the apex, the timing and nature of the first and second heart sounds are determined. Separable components of these events should be carefully noted. If the first sound has more that one component, S_4, asynchronous closure of mitral and tricuspid valves, and ejection clicks must be distinguished. Higher frequency transient systolic and diastolic sounds are listed in Table 39–2 and should be listened for explicitly. Murmurs should be identified and characterized, using the diaphragm to distinguish high-frequency events and the bell for lower frequency sounds. The examination should include listening with the patient sitting and leaning forward, supine, and in the left lateral decubitus position. Standing, exercising, isometric handgrip, and the Valsalva maneuver will be important in specific circumstances, as outlined in the chapters that follow.

The plethora of sophisticated laboratory examinations now available should refine, rather than render obsolete, physical diagnostic skills. Every opportunity should be taken to review physical findings with the additional insights provided by noninvasive and invasive laboratory studies.

TABLE 39–2. SYSTOLIC AND DIASTOLIC SOUNDS

Systolic
- Early
  - Ejection sounds (aortic, pulmonary)
  - Systolic ejection clicks (mitral apparatus)
  - Opening click of aortic valve mechanical prosthesis
- Mid to late
  - Mitral valve clicks (prolapse)

Diastolic
- Early
  - Opening snaps
  - Early third sound of pericardial constriction or mitral regurgitation
  - Opening click of mitral valve mechanical prosthesis
  - "Tumor plop" of atrial myxoma
- Mid
  - Third heart sound or gallop (S_3)
  - Summation gallop (S_3 + S_4)
- Late (presystolic)
  - Fourth heart sound (S_4)

Laboratory Studies

Laboratory studies of patients with cardiovascular disease run the gamut from routine examinations (chest radiograph, electrocardiogram) that should be performed on virtually every patient being evaluated to highly sophisticated techniques that would be appropriate for specific individual subsets of patients. Remarkable progress in the past decade in noninvasive techniques now permits adequate evaluation of many patients without need for cardiac catheterization. Nevertheless, catheterization and angiography are essential components of the cardiovascular workup in most patients with advanced valvular or coronary artery disease.

ELECTROCARDIOGRAM. The standard 12-lead electrocardiogram remains a cornerstone of the clinical cardiologic evaluation. Although vectorcardiography and other more sophisticated approaches have their proponents, the standard 12-lead ECG remains a highly cost-effective screening test. It is reviewed in detail in Ch. 42.4. Detailed clinicopathologic correlations accumulated over two generations provide a wealth of background information. The most important applications are in assessment of cardiac arrhythmias, in which analysis of the P wave and the QRS complex, and their temporal relation to each other, forms the basis for the definition and clinical diagnosis of cardiac rhythm disturbances. Existence and location of myocardial ischemia and infarction represent other important components of the information inherent in the ECG. Right and left ventricular hypertrophy patterns, as well as right and left atrial abnormalities, are well described. Characteristic electrocardiographic findings are frequently important in the assessment of congenital heart disease.

The 12-lead electrocardiogram augmented with a standard exercise protocol is important in the assessment of ischemic heart disease (see Ch. 51.1). Both establishment of coronary artery obstructive disease and useful prognostic information are available from this study. Risk stratification in patients who have had myocardial infarctions is heavily dependent upon the exercise ECG. The predictive accuracy of the exercise ECG examination for coronary artery disease in specific patient subsets is well defined. It is important not only to classify ST-segment depression but also to assess duration of exercise, maximum heart rate achieved, time of onset of ST-segment depression, and time of resolution. A decrease in blood pressure during exercise correlates closely with advanced three-vessel or left main coronary artery obstructive disease. As in all such examinations, the diagnostic and predictive accuracy is dependent on the population of patients studied, and false-positive exercise ECG results are relatively commonly encountered in women, especially from populations with a low predicted incidence of obstructive coronary artery disease.

Assessment of symptoms of palpitations, dizziness, and syncope now rests heavily on the 24-hour (Holter) ECG. This approach is essential in the evaluation of cardiac arrhythmias and of response to antiarrhythmic drug regimens. Recent technical advances permit the assessment of transient ST-segment and T-wave changes reflecting myocardial ischemia, findings of particular value in the assessment of patients with variable threshold or "silent" ischemia.

CHEST RADIOGRAPH. This is a component of virtually every cardiovascular evaluation. Important findings are reviewed in Ch. 42.1. Chest radiography always supplements, rather than replaces, physical examination, since both approaches yield complementary information. Current practice usually limits the radiographic examination to the posteroanterior and lateral views. Echocardiography yields more accurate and specific information regarding individual chamber sizes. Evidence of calcification of cardiac structures should be sought on the chest radiograph, although fluoroscopic examination is generally more sensitive for this purpose.

ECHOCARDIOGRAPHY. This noninvasive technique uses high-frequency sound waves that reflect from cardiac structures, permitting the imaging of cardiac anatomy and motion. The technique is considered in detail in Ch. 42.3. Two-dimensional echocardiography has largely replaced the conventional M-mode display, although the latter provides superior quantitative details regarding wall thickness and chamber dimensions. This examination is now standard in the assessment of ventricular function and valvular abnormalities.

The Doppler method has rapidly gained acceptance and yields important additional information on intracardiac blood flow, shunts, and valvular stenosis and regurgitation. In selected patients, echocardiographic information, together with full clinical assessment, will permit valvular surgery without prior cardiac catheterization. Echocardiography is diagnostic in cases of left atrial myxoma, mitral valve prolapse, and hypertrophic cardiomyopathy. It is frequently useful for visualization of vegetations on heart valves in patients with infective endocarditis. Pericardial fluid and tamponade are routinely assessed by echocardiography, which is also useful in guiding pericardiocentesis.

RADIONUCLIDE STUDIES. These tests involve injection of radioisotopes into the circulation with detection by special instrumentation. One of the most useful of these techniques is radionuclide ventriculography, also referred to as gated blood pool scanning. Technetium 99m (^{99m}Tc) bound to albumin stays in the blood pool and permits imaging of the size and contractile function of cardiac chambers. Special applications include detection of intracardiac shunts by "first pass" methods. Most commonly, the technique is used to assess left and right ventricular function by measurement of end-systolic and end-diastolic dimensions, permitting evaluation of regional wall motion and the derivation of values for right and left ventricular ejection fractions.

Scanning with radioactive thallium (^{201}Tl) permits assessment of myocardial perfusion. The radioisotope is injected at maximum exercise and localizes in cardiac muscle as a function of coronary flow; areas of diminished myocardial perfusion are visualized as "cold" spots on the myocardial image. Viable but ischemic myocardium subsequently fills in with more homogeneous ^{201}Tl distribution, whereas previous infarction produces a persistent cold spot.

Scanning with ^{99m}Tc pyrophosphate is used to visualize areas of myocardial necrosis and is useful in evaluation of patients with suspected myocardial infarction when other studies are equivocal. These techniques are discussed in detail in Ch. 42.4.

CLINICAL APPLICATION. The safety of noninvasive techniques tempts the clinician to overutilize them, since no physical harm is likely to result and some incremental information is often obtained. Cost-effectiveness considerations must be kept in mind, however, and the use of these tests must be orchestrated so that the essential clinical decisions can be made without unnecessary cost and inconvenience to the patient. In particular, noninvasive test information will often be superfluous if the patient is destined to undergo complete evaluation by cardiac catheterization and angiography.

CARDIAC CATHETERIZATION. This invasive approach provides information on intracardiac and vascular pressures and flows. Gradients across stenotic valves and great vessels can be measured and systemic and pulmonary blood flows quantified. Contrast agents can be injected selectively to define the anatomy of cardiac chambers, coronary vessels, and pulmonary and peripheral vessels. The technique of cardiac catheterization and angiography is considered in detail in Ch. 42.5. This diagnostic approach will usually be employed when a cardiac surgical procedure is under consideration.

Other applications of cardiac catheterization include electrophysiologic studies with pacing and mapping procedures to evoke and localize the source of cardiac rhythm disturbances. Endomyocardial biopsy is now a standard technique for the assessment of transplant rejection, unexplained cardiomyopathy, suspected myocarditis, suspected infiltrative diseases such as cardiac amyloidosis, or doxorubicin cardiotoxicity.

Cardiac catheterization procedures form the basis for therapeutic interventions, including percutaneous transluminal coronary angioplasty, or ablative procedures, such as those under development for the management of patients with Wolff-Parkinson-White syndrome refractory to drug therapy.

Although cardiac catheterization involves substantial expense and a small but finite risk of morbidity and mortality, this approach remains indispensable in the assessment of a wide array of cardiac problems that remain unsolved after complete noninvasive assessment. A frequent problem is the adult patient with a chest pain syndrome consistent with angina pectoris but with a negative or equivocal exercise electrocardiogram. Such patients may be severely disabled by these symptoms and attendant anxiety. Even though coronary artery surgery may not loom as a likely therapeutic approach, coronary arteriography can be of substantial value, especially when normal coronary anatomy is found, directing the diagnostic evaluation in more productive directions and restoring a previously incapacitated patient to full activity.

ELEMENTS OF A COMPLETE CARDIOVASCULAR DIAGNOSIS

Coordinated use of the history, physical examination, and laboratory studies will permit a full diagnosis to be established in nearly all patients, including the following five elements:

1. Etiology of the cardiovascular problem
2. Anatomic abnormalities, including quantification to the extent possible
3. Physiologic status, including pressures, flows, and relevant gradients
4. Functional capacity (see Table 39–3)
5. Prognosis

Diagnostic Strategies

The most appropriate approach to a patient with suspected cardiovascular disease will depend on the age and clinical presentation of the patient. A systolic ejection murmur at the base in a healthy teenager with an otherwise normal clinical evaluation, including ECG and chest radiograph, should ordinarily constitute adequate grounds for reassurance and avoidance of more elaborate studies. In an elderly patient with a systolic ejection murmur at the base, slow-rising carotid arterial pulses, and symptoms suggesting possible aortic stenosis, however, the chest radiograph, electrocardiogram, and echocardiogram with Doppler study will be necessary, at a minimum, to determine whether further and more aggressive evaluation is warranted.

Since prevention is a highly desirable goal in cardiovascular medicine, certain diagnostic tests may be warranted in individual patients even in the absence of specific symptoms. In addition to careful history and physical examination, serum cholesterol measurements will be appropriate in many patients, especially those with a family history of coronary artery disease, to assess risk and to guide therapeutic intervention. Use of exercise electrocardiography in sedentary, middle-aged individuals who are contemplating an exercise program remains controversial; many physicians would advocate this procedure, especially if the patient has risk factors for coronary artery disease.

TABLE 39–3. A COMPARISON OF THREE METHODS OF ASSESSING CARDIOVASCULAR DISABILITY

Class	New York Heart Association Functional Classification	Canadian Cardiovascular Society Functional Classification	Specific Activity Scale
I	Patients with cardiac disease but without resulting limitations of physical activity. Ordinary physical activity does not cause undue fatigue, palpitation, dyspnea, or anginal pain.	Ordinary physical activity, such as walking and climbing stairs, does not cause angina. Angina with strenuous or rapid or prolonged exertion at work or recreation.	Patients can perform to completion any activity requiring ≥ 7 metabolic equivalents, e.g., can carry 24 lb up eight steps; carry objects that weight 80 lb; do outdoor work (shovel snow, spade soil); do recreational activities (skiing, basketball, squash, handball, jog/walk 5 mph).
II	Patients with cardiac disease resulting in slight limitation of physical activity. They are comfortable at rest. Ordinary physical activity results in fatigue, palpitation, dyspnea, or anginal pain.	Slight limitation of ordinary activity. Walking or climbing stairs rapidly, walking uphill, walking or stair climbing after meals, in cold, in wind, or when under emotional stress, or only during the few hours after awakening. Walking more than two blocks on the level and climbing more than one flight of ordinary stairs at a normal pace and in normal conditions.	Patient can perform to completion any activitiy requiring ≥ 5 metabolic equivalents but cannot and does not perform to completion activities requiring ≥ 7 metabolic equivalents, e.g., have sexual intercourse without stopping, garden, rake, weed, roller skate, dance fox trot, walk at 4 mph on level ground.
III	Patients with cardiac disease resulting in marked limitation of physical activity. They are comfortable at rest. Less than ordinary physical activity causes fatigue, palpitation, dyspnea, or anginal pain.	Marked limitation of ordinary physical activity. Walking one to two blocks on the level and climbing more than one flight in normal conditions.	Patient can perform to completion any activity requiring ≥ 2 metabolic equivalents but cannot and does not perform to completion any activities requiring ≥ 5 metabolic equivalents, e.g., shower without stopping, strip and make bed, clean windows, walk 2.5 mph, bowl, play golf, dress without stopping.
IV	Patient with cardiac disease resulting in inability to carry on any physical activity without discomfort. Symptoms of cardiac insufficiency or of the anginal syndrome may be present even at rest. If any physical activity is undertaken, discomfort is increased.	Inability to carry on any physical activity without discomfort—anginal syndrome *may be* present at rest.	Patient cannot or does not perform to completion activities requiring ≥ 2 metabolic equivalents. *Cannot* carry out activities listed above (Specific Activity Scale, Class III).

Reproduced by permission of the American Heart Association, Inc., from Goldman L, et al: Comparative reproducibility and validity of systems for assessing cardiovascular functional class: Advantages of a new specific activity scale. Circulation 64:1227, 1981.

There is no simple formula for defining the data base that is adequate for clearance of patients for noncardiac surgery. A simple, informal stress test of walking up one or more flights of stairs to observe the presence or absence of dyspnea or chest discomfort will often obviate the need for more expensive and elaborate formal exercise testing. When extensive procedures such as peripheral vascular surgery or abdominal aortic aneurysm resection are contemplated in older patients with known or suspected coronary artery disease, aggressive diagnostic work-up, sometimes including cardiac catheterization and coronary arteriography, may be necessary because of limitations imposed by vascular disease on exercise electrocardiography or other approaches to assessment of cardiac reserve requiring exercise stress.

Perloff JK: Physical Examination of the Heart and Circulation. Philadelphia, W. B. Saunders Company, 1982. *A pocket-sized compendium of up-to-date information, well illustrated and referenced.*

40 EPIDEMIOLOGY OF CARDIOVASCULAR DISEASE

William T. Friedewald

Cardiovascular diseases have been the major health problem and the leading cause of death in the United States for several decades. The various statistics defining the magnitude of the problem are staggering. Estimates suggest that over 60 million people have some form of cardiovascular disease. In 1985, 981,000 people died of cardiovascular diseases, which accounted for 47.3 per cent of all deaths. This problem also ranks as the leading reason for social security disability, limitation in physical activity, and hospital bed use, accounting for 46 million bed days in 1984. In 1982 it was estimated that cardiovascular diseases carried a direct health expenditure cost of $48 billion and additional indirect costs of $54 billion.

COMPONENTS OF CARDIOVASCULAR DISEASE

Cardiovascular disease is a general diagnostic category consisting of several separate diseases. One component, congenital heart disease, occurs at a rate of approximately 7 per 1000 live births, leading in 1983 to 6100 deaths, 3500 of which occurred before the age of one year. Another component, rheumatic heart disease, has had a dramatic 90 per cent decline over the last 40 years in the age-adjusted death rate (Table 40–1). Although 1.6 million people still have the disease, with approximately 6100 deaths in 1985, it has become a minor contributor to the overall cardiovascular disease problem. Coronary heart disease and cerebrovascular disease continue to be the major components of cardiovascular disease. Each year an estimated 1.25 million heart attacks occur (of which 800,000 are first attacks), leading to 534,000 deaths in 1985. Ten per cent of men and 3.3 per cent of women aged 45 to 64 years have overt coronary heart disease, and over the age of 65, these percentages increase to 13.4 in men and 9.4 in women. Cerebrovascular disease is found in 1.7 per cent of men (1.4 per cent of women) between the ages of 45 and 64 and 5.6 per cent of men (5.8 per cent of women) aged 65 and older, with 152,000 deaths due to this cause in 1985.

CARDIOVASCULAR DISEASE MORTALITY

These diseases have not always been the major health problem of the United States. In 1900 the five leading causes of death were (1) pneumonia and influenza combined, (2) tuberculosis, (3) diarrhea, enteritis, and ulceration of the intestines, (4) diseases of the heart, and (5) intracranial lesions of vascular origin. These categories all had rates greater than 100 per 100,000 population. By 1940, only two disease categories still had rates greater than 100 per 100,000: diseases of the heart and cancer and other malignant tumors. The infectious diseases had, to a large extent, been controlled, and

TABLE 40–1. AGE-ADJUSTED DEATH RATES* FOR MAJOR CARDIOVASCULAR DISEASES AND ALL OTHER CAUSES OF DEATH COMBINED IN THE UNITED STATES, 1905 TO 1985

			Cardiovascular Diseases			
Year	All Causes	All Causes Except Cardiovascular Diseases	Total	*Coronary Heart Disease*	*Cerebrovascular Diseases*	*Rheumatic Heart Disease*
1905	1673.5	1315.9	357.6	NA	134.4	NA
1915	1443.4	1072.6	370.8	NA	123.3	NA
1925	1299.9	920.5	379.4	NA	114.2	NA
1935	1165.8	777.9	387.9	NA	94.4	NA
1945	947.4	556.9	390.5	NA	85.4	18.4
1955	764.6	368.5	396.1	200.0	83.0	11.2
1960	760.9	367.4	393.5	214.6	79.7	9.6
1965	739.0	364.8	374.2	215.8	72.7	7.4
1970	714.3	368.0	346.3	200.4†	66.3	6.3
1975	630.4	337.0	293.4	170.1†	53.7	4.8
1980	585.8	325.4	260.4	149.8	40.8	2.6
1985	545.3‡	316.6	228.7	127.3	33.1	1.8

*Rate per 100,000 population age adjusted to the United States population, 1940.
†Comparability ratio applied to convert rate to level comparable to rates for 1980 and 1985.
‡Estimated.
NA = not available.

their mortality rates have continued to fall to the present. The "epidemic" of cardiovascular disease, especially coronary heart disease had begun. By 1963, the mortality rate from coronary heart disease reached a peak; there has been a progressive and steady decline since then (Fig. 40–1). Despite the continued magnitude of the coronary heart disease problem, the focus recently has been on this dramatic reversal. Not only is the percentage of decline large, but also the impact on the total number of deaths in the United States is large and has led to an increase in life expectancy. In fact, the recent rate of improvement in life expectancy compares with that seen in the 1940's, when tuberculosis and other infectious diseases were being controlled. In 1983 a 45-year-old person could, on the average, expect to live 3.3 years longer than would have been expected in 1963. Estimates suggest that 45 per cent of this declining total mortality rate is due to the decline in coronary heart disease. The decline in death due to cerebrovascular disease, though even more impressive with a 63 per cent decrease since 1950, has been less of a contributing factor because it is less prevalent.

Declines in coronary heart disease mortality have been greater in younger adults, but there has been a remarkable uniformity among blacks and whites and among men and women. Despite some early doubts when the reversal in rates was beginning, this decline in coronary mortality is real and not artifactual. It cannot be explained by (1) problems in trend measurement, such as a shift in classifying deaths as due to some other disease, (2) the waning of periodic respiratory epidemics that can contribute to the death of many patients with coronary heart disease, or (3) the depletion of the pool due to other causes of death in people expected to be susceptible to coronary heart disease. In addition, the decline has been too steep and long lasting to be reasonably explained by a simple random, temporary downturn. Determining precisely when the true decline began is complicated by these factors, but the increasing rate most likely changed to a decline beginning in the mid 1960's, perhaps somewhat earlier in women.

Data from other countries during the same period offer a perspective on understanding the United States rates. The multinational data in Figure 40–2 are for coronary heart disease death rates averaged over the four ten-year age groups for men 35 to 74 years of age. These data are not comparable to the age-adjusted rates in the table, but they still offer an important perspective for comparing the changes over time. During the period 1969 to 1978, among the 27 countries compared, the United States had the largest decrease in its coronary heart disease mortality rate and moved from second to eighth in rank. During this period, four other countries (Australia, New Zealand, Canada, and Israel) also had significant declines, whereas several others (e.g., Scotland and Northern Ireland) had increases despite having had initially high rates. Although the large absolute difference in rates by country in any given year might suggest that the genetic

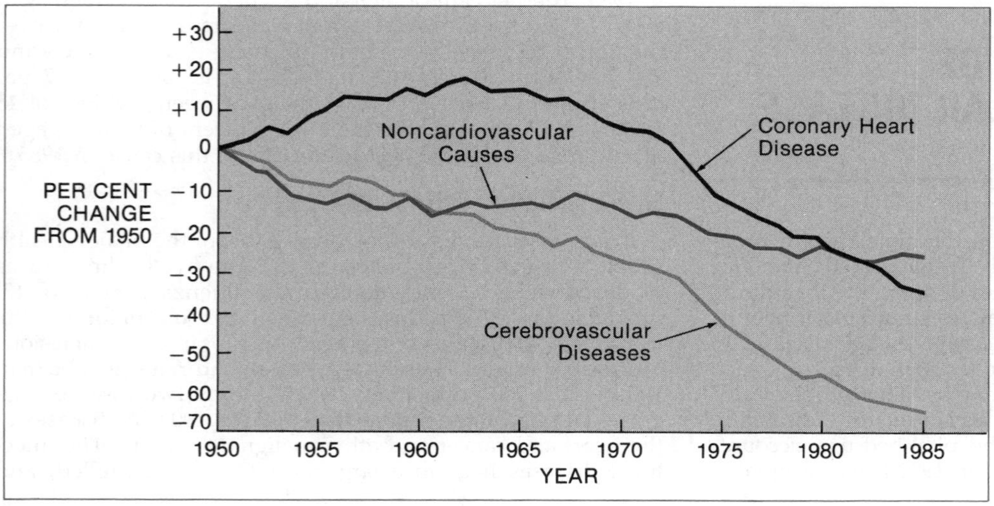

FIGURE 40–1. Per cent change in age-adjusted death rates for coronary heart disease, cerebrovascular diseases, and noncardiovascular causes of death in the United States, 1950 to 1985. (Source: Vital Statistics of the United States, National Center for Health Statistics.)

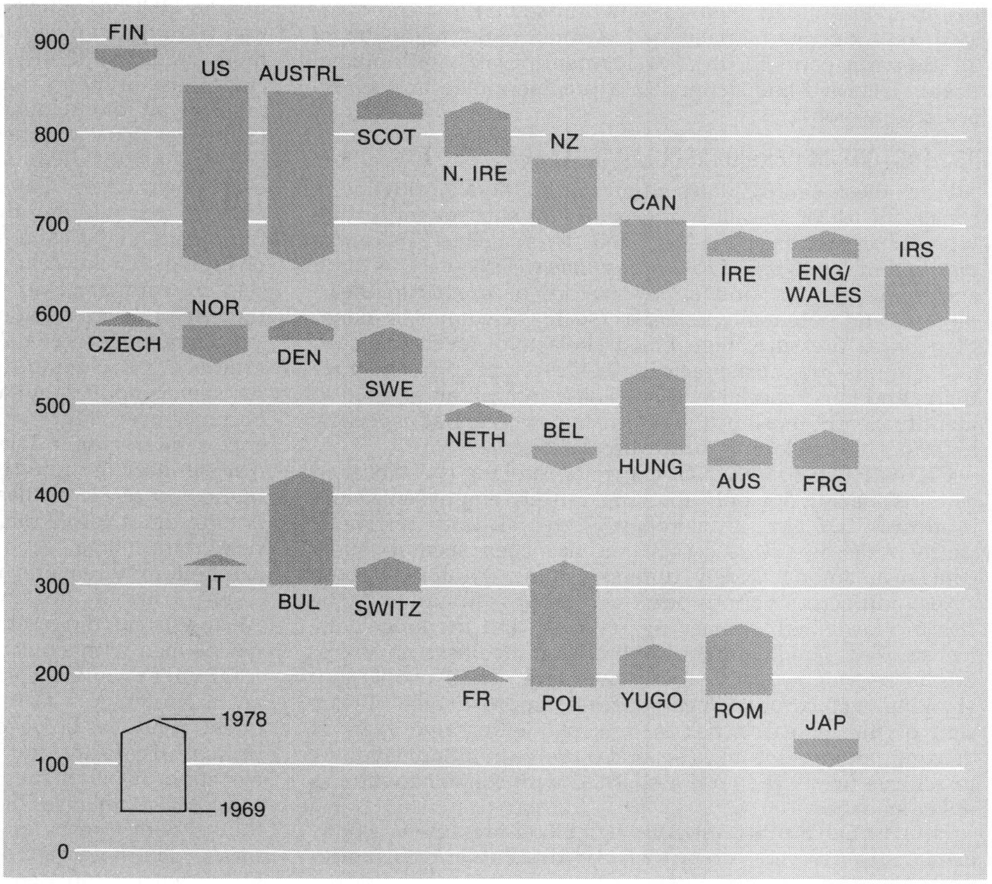

FIGURE 40–2. Coronary heart disease mortality rates per 100,000 population for men ages 35 to 74 by country (1969 to 1978). (Source: World Health Organization, World Health Statistics Annual, 1970 . . . 1981.)

differences among the populations account for this range, the large changes within a country over time demonstrate that regardless of genetic factors, the disease process can be significantly modified. Identification of the factors specifically responsible for these changes has proved to be difficult. Although the relative contributions of prevention efforts versus improved treatment modalities or improved general health measures have not been distinguishable, all most likely have contributed.

ATHEROSCLEROSIS AND CARDIOVASCULAR DISEASE

The major pathologic process leading to disease of the heart and blood vessels is atherosclerosis, with hypertension either a contributing or a primary problem. Atherosclerosis in its most malignant and rare form begins in early childhood and becomes rapidly manifest as clinical coronary heart disease or sudden death in adolescence. The more common and highly prevalent form begins to develop in adolescence and slowly progresses over several decades, gradually occluding the arterial lumen and eventually manifesting clinically as a stroke, angina pectoris, claudication, myocardial infarction, or, most devastatingly, as sudden death. Although the factors that may lead to an acute clinical event, such as arterial spasm, acute thrombosis, or embolism, are not completely understood, the underlying, if not immediate, problem is predominantly atherosclerosis.

Laboratory and clinical research efforts continue in the search for the underlying cause or causes of atherosclerosis, examining those factors that may initiate the process as well as those that may cause the milder, highly prevalent, presumed early forms of the disease (i.e., fatty streaks on the arterial surface) to progress in many individuals to the more serious, complicated, and obstructing form of the disease. Other research efforts are concentrating on the later, but still preclinical, stages of the process, searching for improved and more quantitative diagnostic techniques. Meanwhile, epidemiologic research efforts have made and continue to make major contributions to both prevention and treatment approaches to the cardiovascular disease problem through identification of personal and environmental characteristics that markedly increase an individual's probability of developing specific cardiovascular diseases.

RESEARCH IN CARDIOVASCULAR DISEASE

The research approach that has been repeatedly used in several large observational studies of cardiovascular disease is exemplified by the Framingham Heart Study, begun in 1948 in a relatively small town in Massachusetts. A sample (5209 men and women aged 30 to 62) of the total population agreed to be part of this study, undergoing thorough examinations every two years, with intense follow-up for the development of both fatal and nonfatal diseases. This population has remained under close scrutiny continuously since originally recruited and examined over the two-year period from 1948 to 1950. Similar studies have been performed in other groups in the United States, as well as around the world. In Tecumseh, Michigan, 8624 men and women, in Evans County, Georgia, 3102 men and women, in Albany, New York, 1913 male civil servants, and in Chicago, Illinois, 1264 male gas company employees and 1983 male employees of the Western Electric Company were recruited and observed over several years. The critical elements of these studies have been the (1) inclusion of relatively large numbers of people to allow for important and sufficiently powerful subsample analyses, (2) enrollment of participants by methods that would make them reasonably representative of the total population from which they were recruited, (3) careful determination of all the variables (such as height, blood pressure, smoking and dietary histories, and blood chemical determinations) in a standardized, reproducible manner, and (4) meticulous follow-up of all the participants for the development of fatal and nonfatal events recorded and defined in a predetermined and standardized fashion.

RISK FACTORS IN CARDIOVASCULAR DISEASE

From these United States studies and others worldwide, a consistent list of so-called risk factors for subsequent cardiovascular disease has been identified. These risk factors can be grouped into two broad categories: *unmodifiable* (such as older age, male gender, and family history of premature heart disease) and potentially *modifiable* (such as cigarette smoking, high blood pressure, high blood cholesterol level, diabetes, and the less prognostic factors of overweight, physical inactivity, and psychosocial factors). These factors can be used to identify clearly those in the population who are at especially high risk of developing cardiovascular disease.

CIGARETTE SMOKING. Cigarette smoking is established as a risk factor not only for lung cancer, emphysema, and bronchitis but also for coronary, cerebral, and peripheral vascular disease. This association has been seen in many countries, among widely different ethnic groups, in both sexes, and across various adult age groups. In addition, the risk increases with heavier cigarette use and the longer one has smoked. Equally important has been the observation that this increased risk falls rapidly over time when people quit smoking. For coronary heart disease, approximately 40 per cent of the increased risk is removed within five years of quitting, although it takes several more years of nonsmoking to achieve finally the level associated with someone who has never smoked.

HIGH BLOOD PRESSURE. High blood pressure is a powerful risk factor for cerebrovascular disease, as well as for coronary heart disease and the atherosclerotic process directly. An estimated 58 million people have high blood pressure, defined as a level equal to or greater than 140 mm Hg systolic or 90 mm Hg diastolic or as being on a regimen of antihypertensive medications. An important result of the epidemiologic studies was the observation that the relationship between blood pressure and cardiovascular risk was not only a positive one (a higher blood pressure resulted in a higher disease rate) but also a smooth one (there was no sharp breakpoint in the curve such that below a certain blood pressure level the risk remained constant or became nonexistent). Thus, the lower the blood pressure, within reasonable physiologic limits, the lower the level of risk. These observations prompted several important intervention trials, which have now clearly established the value of aggressively treating elevated blood pressure.

BLOOD CHOLESTEROL LEVELS. A clear and positive relationship between blood cholesterol levels and subsequent coronary heart disease has repeatedly been demonstrated. Later information refined the nature of this association but did not weaken it. Cholesterol in the plasma is transported by the lipoproteins. The cholesterol level associated with the low density lipoprotein (LDL) fraction was seen to be positively correlated with coronary heart disease, whereas the cholesterol associated with the high density lipoprotein (HDL) was negatively correlated (the higher the level, the lower the risk). These initial observations have been verified in several different populations and were shown to be independent of each other, as well as of other known risk factors. As with blood pressure and cardiovascular disease risk, for both LDL cholesterol and HDL cholesterol, the curve is smooth (in the populations studied, there was no breakpoint in the curve observed). The evidence regarding HDL, though more recent than that for LDL, supports a powerful role for HDL in coronary heart disease risk and may explain some of the difference in risk between men and women, with women having average levels of HDL higher than men. The ratio of LDL to HDL, an efficient method of combining the information from the two separate measures, has been shown to be more predictive than either measure alone. The appropriate clinical use of the mix of LDL, HDL, and/or LDL:HDL values must await more information and experience. Information from over 350,000 American men screened for eligibility in the Multiple Risk Factor Intervention Trial demonstrated that even down to and below levels of total blood cholesterol of 182 mg per deciliter the risk continues to fall off. Recent intervention studies in hypercholesterolemic men have demonstrated that lowering blood cholesterol levels lowers subsequent coronary heart disease morbidity and mortality and the rate of progression of coronary atherosclerosis.

Each of these three risk factors alone can be used to separate groups of people into those at high or low risk. But as these risk factors occur simultaneously in individuals, the risk range becomes even larger (Fig. 40–3). Based on the Multiple Risk Factor Intervention Trial screenee data, the coronary heart disease mortality rate (1.6/1000 screenees) for nonsmokers in the lowest tertile of diastolic blood pressure, and cholesterol is nine times lower than the rate (14.6/1000) for the highest risk group, using only these three variables. As can be seen, age uniformly remains one of the most powerful factors at all levels of risk, as does male gender, with women realizing a 10- to 20-year differential before attaining the same level of risk as men with similar risk factors.

OBESITY. Initial epidemiologic data identified obesity as an important risk factor for coronary heart disease. Subsequent analyses, however, suggested that obesity was not a primary risk factor, but rather that it acted indirectly through elevation of blood pressure and of blood cholesterol levels. More recent analyses of the data from the Framingham Heart Study, with longer follow-up of people in the cohort, have once again suggested that obesity is indeed a primary risk factor that acts independently of these other factors. Clinically, the resolution of this issue of primary versus secondary causation is somewhat irrelevant. Weight reduction should lower the risk of coronary heart disease, whether it acts through a lowered blood pressure and/or cholesterol level or as a lowered risk factor itself.

DIABETES. Diabetes is a powerful and independent risk factor for cardiovascular disease, which remains the major cause of death in diabetic persons. An important remaining issue is whether an elevated blood glucose level is responsible for the observed higher rate of cardiovascular disease and, if it is, whether lowering or, preferably, normalizing the glucose level will lower the risk. Regardless of the answers, for the present the important observation is that diabetic individuals are at higher risk of cardiovascular disease, and thus careful attention should be paid not just to the blood glucose level and its control, but also to the other risk factors that may coexist in a given patient and additionally elevate the risk.

PHYSICAL INACTIVITY. An association between a less active lifestyle and increased risk of coronary heart disease has been shown in multiple longitudinal and cross-sectional studies in such diverse groups as London transit workers, United States longshoremen, and United States college graduates. However, studies establishing a clear cause-and-effect relationship have not been forthcoming. One of the major problems in the randomized studies investigating this question has been adherence to the prescibed exercise regimen. Another problem is that as people begin an exercise program, other factors change as well. Overweight people tend to lose weight; HDL cholesterol levels rise; the diet tends to change; and those individuals who are cigarette smokers frequently stop smoking. Although these covarying factors make the scientific evaluation of physical exercise as an isolated risk factor difficult, they tend to favor the recommendation of a prudent exercise program because of the multiple healthful consequences of such activity.

Other risk factors for cardiovascular disease have been

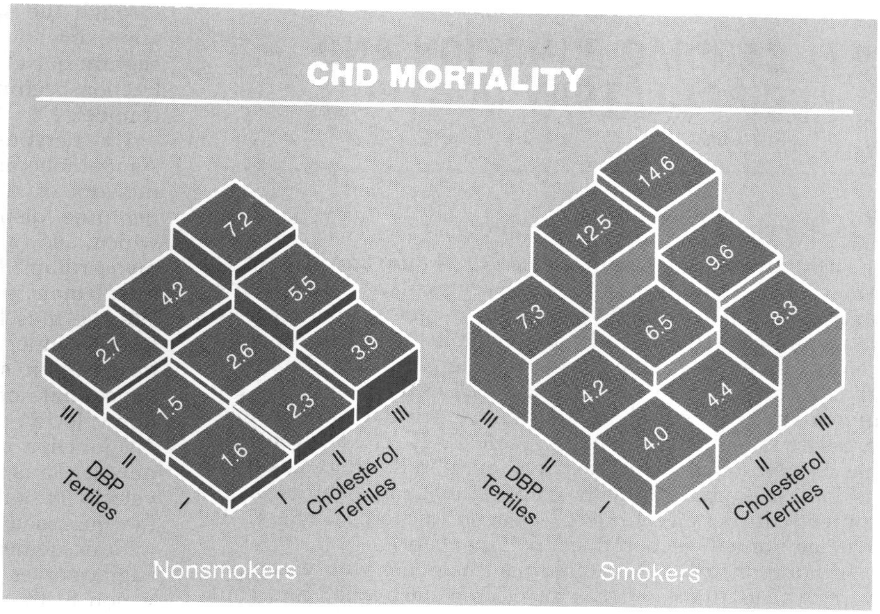

FIGURE 40–3. Age-adjusted CHD mortality rates/1000 screenees for the Multiple Risk Factor Intervention Trial among smokers and non-smokers for cholesterol tertiles (I = ≤ 196, II = 197–228, III = ≥ 229) and diastolic blood pressure (DBF) tertiles (I = ≤ 79, II = 80–87, III = ≥ 88).

identified in single or multiple studies, but further information is needed to establish them as independent, important prognostic factors.

RISK FACTORS AFTER MYOCARDIAL INFARCTION. After surviving a myocardial infarction, the primary risk factors become those related to the infarct itself and the damage to myocardial tissue. As part of the Coronary Drug Project clinical trial, 2789 post–myocardial infarction patients were given usual medical care and observed over a period of five years. The most powerful factors increasing risk in this group were persistent resting electrocardiographic abnormalities (namely ST segment depression and ventricular conduction defects), use of diuretics, a higher (and therefore more activity-restrictive) New York Heart Association functional classification, and a higher heart rate. Although the traditional risk factors, such as cigarette smoking and elevated blood cholesterol levels and blood pressure, remained prognostic, they were weaker factors overshadowed now by primary damage to the myocardium. In addition, with sudden death as the initial clinical presentation of cardiovascular disease in approximately one quarter of patients, it is obviously important to establish effective prevention modalities before the onset of clinical disease. Much current myocardial infarction research is focusing on therapeutic approaches that seek to minimize the extent of myocardial damage or even prevent the development of the infarct entirely. Nonetheless, the greatest potential for continuing and accelerating the decline in cardiovascular disease rates rests with prevention or treatment of the factors that lead to clinical presentation of disease and more profoundly of the factors that lead to or accelerate the atherosclerotic process.

CHANGES IN RISK FACTORS. Significant changes have occurred nationally in the major modifiable risk factors. In 1965, 52 per cent of men aged 20 or greater were cigarette smokers. In 1983 that figure had dropped to 35 per cent (age adjusted). For women the change has been modest, falling from 34 per cent in 1965 to 30 per cent in 1983. From 1965 to 1983, consumption of tobacco fell from 11.5 to 6.6 pounds per capita. In 1971 and 1972 only 16.5 per cent of people with high blood pressure (defined as a level equal to or greater than 160 mm Hg systolic or 95 mm Hg diastolic or as being on a regimen of antihypertensive medication) were effectively controlled. By the late 1970's, this figure had increased to 34 per cent. During this same period, visits to a physician for high blood pressure increased by 35 per cent. In addition, salt sales fell from 2.2 pounds per capita in 1972 to 1.4 in 1985. Average blood cholesterol levels in men fell from 217 mg per deciliter in the period between 1960 and 1966 to 211 in the late 1970's. Annual per capita consumption of several foods changed over the 20-year period from 1964 to 1984. Vegetable fat and oil consumption rose from 32.5 to 48.1 pounds, whereas that of animal fats and oils fell from 18.3 to 13.5 pounds; butter use fell from 6.9 to 5.0 pounds, and the number of eggs eaten fell from 322 to 264 per person per year. These impressive changes clearly demonstrate that the United States public can and will modify lifestyle behavior and suggest that additional gains in the prevention of the cardiovascular diseases can be made.

Food Consumption, Prices and Expenditures, 1964–1984. Economic Research Service, U.S. Department of Agriculture. Statistical Bulletin No. 736, December 1985. *A collection of tables on the food system, marketing, nutrition, and demand for food in the United States.*

Goldman L, Cook EF: The decline in ischemic heart disease mortality rates: An analysis of the comparative effects of medical interventions and changes in lifestyle. Ann Intern Med 101:825, 1984. *An interesting attempt at quantification of the relative contribution of lifestyle and treatment factors on the decline in coronary heart disease mortality.*

Gordon T, Garcia-Palmieri MR, Kagan A, et al.: Differences in coronary heart disease in Framingham, Honolulu and Puerto Rico. J Chronic Dis 27:329, 1974. *A valuable comparison of the relationship between risk factors and subsequent coronary heart disease in three geographically and ethnically diverse populations.*

Grundy SM, Ad Hoc Committee to Design a Dietary Treatment of Hyperlipoproteinemia: Recommendations for the Treatment of Hyperlipidemia in Adults: A Joint Statement of the Nutrition Committee and the Council on Atherosclerosis of the American Heart Association. Arteriosclerosis 4:445A, 1984. *A succinct review of the hyperlipidemias and hyperlipoproteinemias with treatment recommendations and 265 references.*

Health, United States, 1985. U.S. Department of Health and Human Services, Public Health Service, National Center for Health Statistics. DHHS Publication No. (PHS) 85–1232, December 1985. *A frequently updated report presenting national data on morbidity and mortality, health delivery costs, and prevention programs with detailed tables.*

The Joint National Committee on Detection, Evaluation, and Treatment of High Blood Pressure: The 1984 Report of the Joint National Committee on Detection, Evaluation, and Treatment of High Blood Pressure. Arch Intern Med 144:1045, 1984. *A succinct and authoritative review of the major clinical issues involving high blood pressure with a list of key references.*

Kaplan NM, Stamler J: Prevention of Coronary Heart Disease: Practical Management of the Risk Factors. Philadelphia, W.B. Saunders Company, 1983. *A concise, informative, and readable summary of the current information on the risk factors for coronary heart disease.*

Proceedings of the Conference on the Decline in Coronary Heart Disease Mortality. U.S. Department of Health, Education, and Welfare, Public Health Service. DHEW Publication No. (NIH) 79–1610, 1979. *A careful review of the issues bearing on the decline with a useful appendix.*

World Health Statistics Annual 1970–1985. World Health Organization. *International vital statistics and population data in tabular form by country.*

41 CARDIAC FUNCTION AND CIRCULATORY CONTROL

John Ross, Jr.

FUNCTIONAL ANATOMY OF THE HEART

The right ventricle is thin walled (3 to 4 mm) and somewhat irregular in shape, with the interventricular septum being largely formed by the left ventricle. The right ventricle is more compliant than the left, the upper limit of normal for right ventricular end-diastolic pressure being 6 mm Hg (Table 41–1). The left ventricle has a thicker wall (8 to 9 mm), and the upper limit of normal for the left ventricular end-diastolic pressure is higher (12 mm Hg, Table 41–1). The left ventricle has an ellipsoidal shape, shortens more in its short axis than its long axis, and normally empties about two thirds of its contents during ejection (see "ejection fraction," Table 41–1, average normal ejection fraction 65 per cent).

In addition to its four muscular chambers with accompanying valves, the heart has an electrical activation and conduction system, an autonomic neural supply, and a coronary circulation. The three main coronary arteries divide into lesser branches and eventually send small, penetrating vessels directly into the myocardium to supply a very dense capillary network. During coronary vasodilation, approximately one capillary per muscle cell provides a rich blood supply to the heavily working myocardium.

The electrical subsystem includes the sinoatrial (SA) node, comprising special pacemaker cells with continuous phase 4 depolarization, and the atrioventricular (AV) node, which exhibits delayed or decremental conduction, allowing atrial depolarization to precede ventricular depolarization by approximately 140 msec and atrial contraction thereby to serve as a "booster pump" for filling the ventricles. From the AV junction (or node) the electrical impulse rapidly spreads through the specialized His-Purkinje conduction system in approximately 40 msec to reach the ventricles, which contract slightly out of phase (left before right), left ventricular contraction beginning about 50 msec after the onset of the QRS complex.

The nervous subsystem supplying the heart consists of sympathetic and parasympathetic divisions. There is a rich network of sympathetic nerve terminals containing norepinephrine distributed throughout the atria and ventricles, which allows reflex regulation of the contractility of the myocardium. The beta-adrenergic receptors on the myocardial sarcolemma also permit circulating catecholamines to stimulate the muscle during stress. The sympathetic nerves also heavily innervate the SA node and AV junction, where increases in sympathetic tone increase the heart rate (enhanced rate of phase 4 depolarization) and improve conduction velocity, thereby decreasing conduction time through the AV junction and improving synchronicity of the ventricular muscle. Thus, enhanced strength of contraction and increased velocity of both muscle contraction and relaxation accompany the increased heart rate during sympathetic stimulation, as with excitement or exercise. Parasympathetic fibers from the vagus nerves containing acetylcholine provide heavy innervation to the right and left atria, the SA node, and the AV junction, but there are few parasympathetic nerve terminals in the ventricles or the conduction system below the AV junction. Activation of the parasympathetic system has a slowing effect on the SA node (reduced rate of phase 4 polarization) and slows conduction through the AV junction, providing reciprocal neural control with the sympathetic nervous system. The contractility of atrial muscle is depressed by parasympathetic stimulation, but there is minimal effect on the ventricles because of their sparse innervation by this branch of the autonomic nervous system.

Unlike skeletal muscle, cardiac muscle can regulate its contractility, or inotropic state. The force of cardiac muscle contraction, as well as its velocity is normally regulated in large part by the amount of free calcium (Ca^{++}) that is released by the action potential. Events associated with arrival of the action potential at the myocyte trigger release of calcium from the sarcoplasmic reticulum; calcium then binds to a subunit of troponin on the actin filament, causing a conformational change that uncovers the active site and allows a tension-generating bond to occur between actin and myosin. More calcium allows more sites to bind. *Between* contractions, the sarcoplasmic reticulum (together with subsarcolemmal binding sites) rapidly and actively sequesters calcium, so that the level at the myofilaments falls below that required for the actin-myosin interaction. Calcium enters the cell during phase 2 of the action potential and is extruded against an electrical and chemical gradient by an ATP-driven sarcolemmal calcium pump and by a 3:1 sodium for calcium exchange mechanism across the sarcolemma, which is driven mainly by the sodium gradient generated by the sodium/potassium ATPase membrane pump. Myocardial contractility is normally increased by catecholamines, which stimulate the beta receptors and augment intracellular cyclic adenosine monophosphate (AMP), which leads to increased calcium influx during the action potential. Increasing extracellular calcium also augments myocardial contractility.

A variety of mechanisms stimulate myocardial contractility in the failing heart. Digitalis, by inhibiting membrane sodium/potassium ATPase, causes an increase of intracellular sodium, which decreases the sodium gradient, thereby leading to increased intracellular calcium and enhanced contractility. Beta-adrenergic agonist drugs such as dobutamine are used to treat the acutely failing heart as well. Some newer positive inotropic agents (e.g., amrinone and milrinone) act largely by inhibiting phosphodiesterase, leading to increased intracellular cyclic AMP, and other new drugs are under study that may directly affect calcium influx during the action

TABLE 41–1. PRESSURES AND VOLUMES IN THE NORMAL HEART

Pressures
- Left sided
  1. Left atrial pressure (normal mean pressure ≤ 12 mm Hg)
  2. Left ventricular pressure
     a. Peak systolic pressure (same as aorta)
     b. Maximum dP/dt (1200–3500 mm Hg/sec)
     c. Left ventricular end-diastolic pressure (normal ≤ 12 mm Hg)
  3. Aorta
     a. Systolic pressure (wide normal range, usually 100–150 mm Hg in adults)
     b. Diastolic pressure (wide normal range, usually 60–90 mm Hg in adults)
- Right sided
  1. Right atrial pressure (normal mean pressure ≤ 6 mm Hg)
  2. Right ventricular pressure
     a. Peak systolic pressure (normal 15–30 mm Hg)
     b. Right ventricular end-diastolic pressure (normal ≤ 6 mm Hg)
  3. Pulmonary artery
     a. Systolic pressure (normal 15–30 mm Hg)
     b. Diastolic pressure (normal 4–12 mm Hg)

Volumes
- Left sided (at rest)
  1. Left ventricular end-diastolic volume (normal 70–100 ml/m^2)
  2. Left ventricular end-systolic volume (normal 25–35 ml/m^2)
  3. Stroke volume (wide normal range, usually 40–70 ml/m^2)
  4. Ejection fraction (stroke volume divided by end-diastolic volume [normal 0.55–0.80])

Time-related measurements
  1. Heart rate (wide normal range, usually 60–100 beats/minute)
  2. Cardiac index (2.5–4.2 liters/min/m^2)

Resistances
  1. Systemic vascular resistance (770–1500 dynes sec cm^{-5})
  2. Pulmonary vascular resistance (20–120 dynes sec cm^{-5})

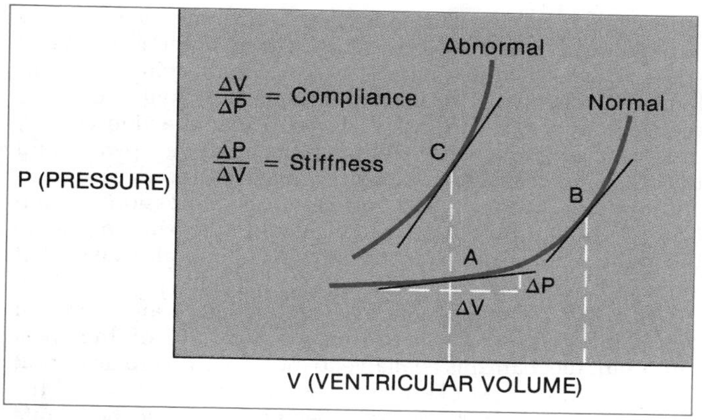

FIGURE 41–1. Diastolic pressure-volume curves of left ventricle under normal conditions and in the presence of severe ventricular hypertrophy (abnormal). Note the nearly exponential shape of the curves. The stiffness at any point on the normal curve ($\Delta P/\Delta V$) is shown by a tangent. Notice that ventricular stiffness increases (tangent A to tangent B) with ventricular filling to a larger ventricular volume. The stiffness of two ventricular chambers can be compared at a common volume, and comparison of the stiffness of the normal with that of the abnormal (hypertrophied) ventricle shows that the latter is markedly increased (tangent A versus tangent C). Compliance is the inverse slope ($\Delta V/\Delta P$) of the curve, and therefore the abnormal ventricle has a markedly reduced compliance. (Adapted from West JB (ed): Best & Taylor's Physiological Basis of Medical Practice. 11th ed. Baltimore, Williams & Wilkins Co., 1985).

potential or increase the sensitivity of the myofilaments to calcium.

DIASTOLIC PROPERTIES OF THE HEART. A major feature of cardiac muscle is its intrinsic stiffness while at rest. Unlike skeletal muscle, which, when isolated from its bony supports, can be overstretched easily, cardiac muscle at first stretches readily but then, when stretched further while in the relaxed state, it reaches an elastic limit, giving a much steeper relation between length and resting tension at long muscle lengths than in skeletal muscle. Thus, there is intrinsic stiffness within the walls of the ventricles, particularly the left ventricle, which tends to prevent overdistension with sudden changes in the venous return to the heart.

This property of heart muscle results in a nearly exponential relation between cardiac volume and pressure wherein small changes in volume produce large pressure changes as the ventricle is further filled beyond the upper limit of normal for left ventricular end-diastolic pressure (Fig. 41–1). Thus, the slope of this relation or chamber stiffness ($\Delta P/\Delta V$) increases as the ventricle is filled, and compliance ($\Delta V/\Delta P$) falls. Of course, when an abnormal chamber, such as a hypertrophied left ventricle, is compared with a normal chamber at the same cardiac volume, the entire diastolic pressure-volume relationship is shifted upward and steepened (Fig. 41–1), and the abnormal chamber is said to be stiffer or less compliant than normal. Even in chronically dilated hearts (as in the normal heart), it does not appear possible to stretch sarcomere lengths much beyond 2.2 μm, so that the heart never appears to operate on a descending limb of the sarcomere length-tension relation.

Although emphasis is often placed on a description of the systolic function of the heart, a greater appreciation of the importance of the diastolic properties of the heart has developed in recent years. A thick, hypertrophied ventricle with decreased compliance causes increased resistance to filling. This frequently leads to atrial dilation and hypertrophy in order to maintain the atrial contribution to ventricular filling. The importance of this contribution is apparent in patients with severe hypertrophy caused, for example, by aortic stenosis or hypertrophic obstructive cardiomyopathy. Loss of an appropriately timed atrial contraction (as with atrial fibrillation) often results in marked exacerbation of the left-heart failure. In these patients, during sinus rhythm the left ventricular end-diastolic pressure is markedly elevated owing to a large A wave, whereas mean diastolic pressure, which is reflected back through the pulmonary veins into the lungs, is maintained at a lower level. When atrial contraction and the A wave "kick" are lost, however, there is an increase in mean left atrial and pulmonary venous pressures in an attempt to maintain the same level of end-diastolic pressure and cardiac output. This frequently leads to disabling dyspnea.

CARDIAC CONTRACTION AND ITS REGULATION

DETERMINANTS OF CARDIAC PERFORMANCE. There are four major determinants of the performance of both ventricles; the discussion will be focused primarily on the left ventricle, however.

1. Preload
2. Afterload
3. Contractility
4. Heart rate

The Preload. This refers to the loading condition on the heart at the end of diastole, which is primarily set by the venous return to the heart. In isolated heart muscle, it is defined as the force stretching the resting muscle to a given length prior to contraction. In the intact heart, it is less easily defined. Estimates of preload include measurements of the ventricular end-diastolic volume or the end-diastolic pressure (although the two are not linearly related, Fig. 41–1), and in acutely ill patients, it may be convenient to measure the ventricular "filling pressure" (the mean right or left atrial pressure, or the pulmonary artery wedge pressure) as an index of the preload. Within limits, as the preload increases, there is an increase in cardiac performance manifested by an increase in systolic pressure development or the volume of blood ejected. This represents the ascending limb of the familiar Frank-Starling relationship.

This overall relationship is often referred to as a ventricular function curve (Fig. 41–2). Some measure of cardiac performance, such as the stroke volume or stroke work (stroke volume × arterial pressure) is plotted as a function of some measure

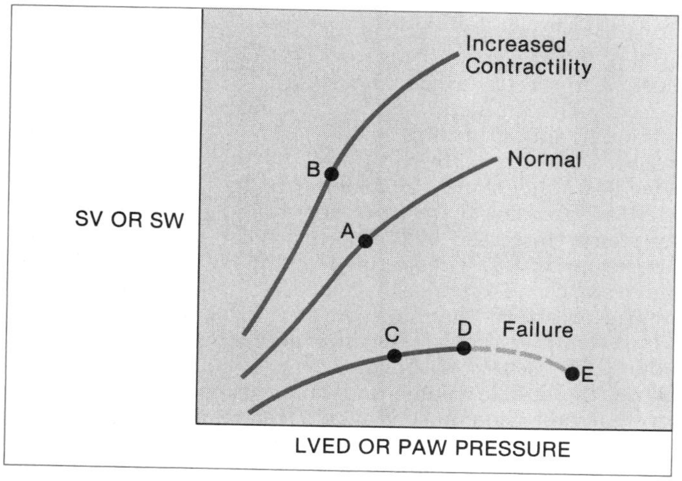

FIGURE 41–2. Left ventricular function curves relating the left ventricular filling pressure to ventricular performance expressed as stroke volume (SV) or stroke work (SW). The filling pressure can be expressed as either the left ventricular end-diastolic (LVED) pressure or the pulmonary artery wedge (PAW) pressure. Curves indicate normal, increased, or depressed ventricular contractility. Points A and B show the effects of a positive inotropic drug, which increases ventricular performance while reducing the filling pressure. See text for further discussion.

of the preload, such as the filling pressure or the end-diastolic pressure. The concept of the ventricular function curve is important, since it allows an objective assessment of the contractility of the ventricles. For example, the normal ventricle has a steep function curve, relatively small changes in end-diastolic pressure producing large changes in performance, whereas the failing ventricle has a downwardly displaced and flattened curve (Fig. 41–2). Such curves can permit a comparison between subjective signs or symptoms and objective measurements. Since the failing left ventricle operates near the peak of its ventricular function curve, the combination of a high filling pressure and low cardiac output (Fig. 41–2, point *D*) explains the clinical picture of dyspnea and fatigue (see Ch. 43).

An important distinction must be made between the right atrial pressure, which represents the filling pressure of the right ventricle and can be estimated from the jugular veins, and the left atrial pressure, which is the filling pressure of the left ventricle. The mean left atrial pressure can be assessed from the mean pulmonary artery (or "capillary") wedge pressure, often measured by a flow-directed balloon catheter. In manipulating the volume status of the acutely ill patient, except in cases of isolated right ventricular failure, it is preferable to measure the left ventricular filling pressure, because the failing left ventricle usually has a more important role in determining arterial pressure and the forward cardiac output.

The Afterload. Afterload refers to the load against which the ventricle must contract when it ejects blood. In isolated heart muscle, it can be accurately defined as the load (or force) resisting shortening after the muscle is stimulated to contract. In the intact heart, afterload is often estimated as the systolic arterial pressure. A better measure of the afterload is the systolic wall stress, which can be related to the systolic pressure, heart size, and wall thickness through the simplified Laplace relation:

$$\sigma = \frac{PR}{2h}$$

in which σ = wall stress or force/cross-sectional area, P = intraventricular pressure, R = radius of chamber (radius of curvature of the wall), and h = wall thickness.

The effect of afterload on performance is relatively straightforward. As arterial pressure is increased, the stroke volume tends to fall because the ventricle has greater difficulty in ejecting blood against a higher load. Such an effect is seen most clearly in experimental preparations when the preload is held constant (and cannot compensate for changes in afterload), and an inverse relation between the afterload (or systolic ventricular pressure) and the stroke volume is observed. In the intact circulation, changes in preload and afterload are closely related. For example, as the arterial pressure is increased in the normal heart, the left ventricle has greater difficulty in ejecting blood, which results in larger end-systolic and end-diastolic volumes, and the increasing preload then tends to restore the stroke volume.

If systemic vascular resistance and arterial pressure are reduced by use of a vasodilator drug in a patient with heart failure, the stroke volume and cardiac output will increase. Severe hypotension must be avoided, since it will compromise coronary blood flow and therefore reduce cardiac performance. The principle of afterload reduction has become one of the most important concepts in the therapy of both acute and chronic heart failure.

Contractility. The inotropic state, or contractility, refers to the vigor of contraction of heart muscle and is best defined in isolated heart muscle as an increased velocity and extent of shortening when the loading conditions (preload and afterload) do not change. Contractility is altered under normal conditions primarily by reflex release of norepinephrine from adrenergic nerve terminals in the myocardium, as well as by adrenal release of catecholamines during various forms of stress. Drugs such as digitalis increase contractility, whereas hypoxia, ischemia, acidosis, and certain antiarrhythmic agents reduce contractility. In terms of ventricular function curves, drugs that increase contractility shift the curve upward and to the left, increasing stroke volume or stroke work at a given end-diastolic pressure (Fig. 41–2). With depression of contractility, the ventricular function curve shifts down and to the right, with a reduction in stroke volume at a given left ventricular end-diastolic pressure (Fig. 41–2).

Heart Rate. The frequency of contraction is an important determinant of cardiac performance and one of the most important mechanisms available to increase the cardiac output (cardiac output = stroke volume × heart rate), provided the venous return is increased (see below). Increased heart rate has a modest positive inotropic effect, increasing the velocity and extent of shortening while reducing the duration of contraction. During the response to moderate exercise, when the venous return increases, a higher heart rate is mainly responsible for the change in cardiac output, since the increase in stroke volume is relatively small.

The level of the heart rate may be an important indicator of the cardiovascular status of an individual patient. For example, in a patient with acute failure who has a sinus tachycardia of 140 beats per minute, the marked reduction in stroke volume is compensated for by the tachycardia in order to maintain an acceptable cardiac output. Other factors that can raise the resting heart rate must also be considered, including fever, anemia, thyrotoxicosis, and anxiety.

ASSESSMENT OF CARDIAC PERFORMANCE. Quantitative indices of cardiac performance can be measured in the cardiac catheterization laboratory or in critical care units. For reference, normal pressures, cardiac volumes, cardiac output, and vascular resistance are listed in Table 41–1. Volume measurements are normalized to allow interpatient comparison by dividing by the body surface area (square meters), obtained from a standard table based on height and weight. The maximum value of the first derivative of left ventricular pressure during isovolumetric systole (dP/dt) is sometimes used as a measure of contractility. One very useful index of ventricular function is the ejection fraction, which is the stroke volume divided by the end-diastolic volume. A normal ejection fraction of the left ventricle is 0.55 or greater, and in severe heart failure the ejection fraction may be reduced to less than 0.20.

As discussed above, *ventricular function curves* (Fig. 41–2) are often employed to demonstrate changes in inotropic state, whereas changes in preload move the ventricle up and down on a *single* curve. Experimentally, they are produced by progressive infusions of fluid, whereas in the clinical setting often only two points on a curve are available, before and after an intervention.

When two ventricular function curves are compared, they generally are compared at the same level of mean arterial pressure, since, as discussed above, the stroke volume of the ventricle is changed by altered afterload. Hence, decreased afterload would shift the relation between stroke volume and filling pressure upward, and increased afterload would shift the relation downward. In heart failure, such an effect caused by increased blood pressure is sometimes represented as an apparent "descending limb" of function. In such a setting, the preload reserve is exhausted and increased arterial pressure will result in movement from point *D* to *E* (Fig. 41–2), whereas lowering the afterload would move the ventricle from *E* to *D*, improving stroke volume and cardiac performance.

Venous return and cardiac output curves can be used to represent cardiocirculatory responses under experimental conditions, and although venous return curves cannot be performed in humans, they allow insight into the highly important role of the venous return. The heart behaves as a demand pump, ejecting whatever blood is returned to it under normal conditions, and only in heart failure or when filling is impaired (as in constrictive pericarditis) does the heart itself become the limiting factor for cardiac output. Therefore, the return of blood to the heart (the venous return), which is regulated by a number of mechanical, neural, and humoral factors, through its influence on preload is a key determinant of cardiac performance under normal conditions.

In A.C. Guyton's analysis, cardiac function is represented by a cardiac output curve that intersects a venous return curve at any given-state condition (Fig. 41–3). Noncardiac factors that influence the venous return include the volume of blood in the vascular bed (transfusion shifts the venous return curve upward, whereas bleeding shifts it downward). The position of the venous return curve is also affected by neurohumoral factors, increased sympathetic tone shifting the venous return curve upward and to the right and vice versa; venoconstriction produced by increased sympathetic tone also displaces blood from the peripheral circulation toward the central (cardiopulmonary) circulation, whereas decreased tone to the veins causes pooling of blood in the peripheral circulation. With this framework, changes in *both* cardiac performance and peripheral circulatory regulation (venous return) can be represented as they influence the cardiac output. Positive inotropic interventions, decreased afterload, and other factors shift the cardiac output curve upward, and opposite effects, including heart failure, shift it downward (Fig. 41–3).

The importance of venous return can be illustrated by the response to electrical cardiac pacing to increase the heart rate, a response in which myocardial contractility is increased. Since no significant effects on the peripheral circulation occur, no change in the cardiac output is observed. This response occurs because the normal heart operates near the flat portion of the normal venous return curve (near the point of venous

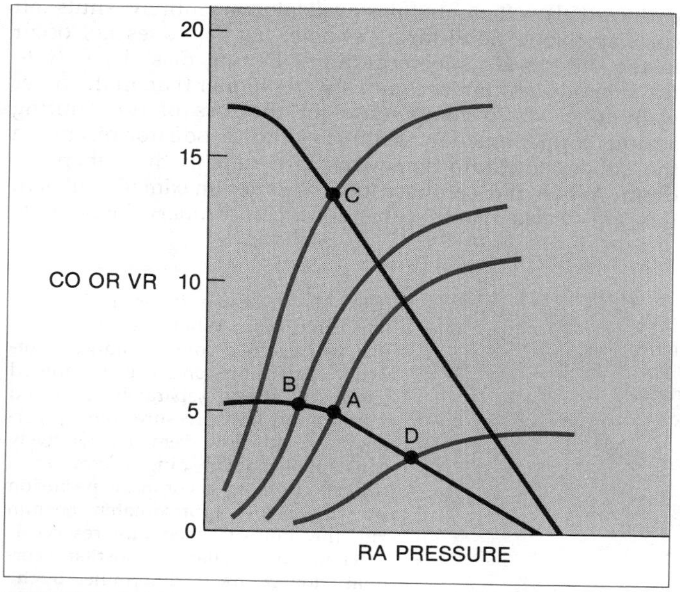

FIGURE 41–3. Relationship between the filling pressure of the heart, expressed as the right atrial (RA) pressure, and either cardiac output (CO) or venous return (VR). Venous return curves are represented as an inverse relation between the cardiac output or venous return and the right atrial pressure; the lower curve represents normal conditions and the upper curve shows the effect of marked sympathetic stimulation during exercise. The series of cardiac output curves shows a positive relation between right atrial pressure and cardiac function. Any steady-state condition is represented by the intersection of these two curves. Shown are normal conditions (A), electrical pacing of the heart (B), severe exercise (C), and heart failure (D). See text for further discussion.

collapse), and therefore even though the cardiac output curve is shifted upward, the venous return curve is unchanged, and there can be no alteration of the cardiac output (Fig. 41–3, point *A* to *B*). The response to exercise using this diagram is discussed subsequently under integrated responses.

REGULATION OF MYOCARDIAL OXYGEN CONSUMPTION

The heart is almost entirely supplied with energy from ATP and creatine phosphate produced by aerobic metabolism, and for practical purposes, the total energy expenditure of the normal heart can be equated with its oxygen consumption. The myocardial oxygen consumption ($M\dot{V}O_2$) of the left ventricle can be determined using the Fick principle as the product of its coronary blood flow and the arteriovenous oxygen difference, calculated using blood samples from an artery and from the coronary sinus. Since the heart is a continuously active organ, its oxygen consumption is high relative to other organs, and the $M\dot{V}O_2$ of the normal human left ventricle at rest is approximately 6 to 8 ml per minute per 100 grams.

The determinants of the $M\dot{V}O_2$ of the heart (most of which is used by the left ventricle) consist of the basal oxygen consumption, which supplies energy for cell maintenance processes including the calcium and sodium pumps, protein synthesis, and so on. The remainder of the oxygen expenditure is controlled by the type of activity that the heart is called upon to perform. The determinants of $M\dot{V}O_2$ are

1. Basal oxygen requirements
2. Systolic pressure (or wall stress)
3. Heart rate
4. Myocardial contractility (inotropic state)
5. Wall shortening against a load (related to cardiac work)

Systolic pressure, heart rate, and *contractility* are the major determinants of $M\dot{V}O_2$, whereas shortening of the wall utilizes relatively less oxygen. There is a nearly linear relation between systolic pressure development by the left ventricle and $M\dot{V}O_2$, and with the Laplace equation, this relation can also be expressed as systolic wall stress versus $M\dot{V}O_2$. Thus, as systolic pressure doubles, the $M\dot{V}O_2$ of the left ventricle approximately doubles. There is also a nearly linear relationship between heart rate and the $M\dot{V}O_2$ and, again, an approximate doubling of the $M\dot{V}O_2$ occurs as the heart rate increases twofold. If the heart rate and systolic pressure are held constant and a positive inotropic agent is administered, a rather marked increase in $M\dot{V}O_2$ can be demonstrated, associated with a pronounced increase in the velocity of shortening and some increase in the extent of myocardial fiber shortening. It is possible that this extra energy expenditure is related, at least in part, to increased oxygen use by the calcium sequestration mechanism of the sarcoplasmic reticulum. Decreased contractility of the myocardium has been shown to cause a reduction of $M\dot{V}O_2$.

The oxygen cost of myocardial fiber shortening against a load is relatively low. This is exemplified by experiments in which the systolic arterial pressure was elevated while the cardiac output and heart rate were held constant, and a marked stimulation of $M\dot{V}O_2$ was produced, whereas if the cardiac output was increased over a wide range while the arterial pressure and heart rate were constant, only small changes in $M\dot{V}O_2$ occurred. These findings indicate a high oxygen cost of "pressure work" and a relatively low oxygen cost of "volume work." The importance of heart rate and systolic pressure has resulted in the use of simplified indices of $M\dot{V}O_2$, such as the heart rate × blood pressure (the "double product"). In clinical studies, this provides a means of estimating the effect of an antianginal drug (such as a beta blocker) on cardiac oxygen requirements during exercise.

The fact that myocardial energy expenditure, expressed as $M\dot{V}O_2$, is closely linked to mechanical cardiac performance carries important implications in various disease states. For example, in valvular heart disease, chronic mitral regurgitation places a large volume overload on the heart due to the low impedance backward leak into the left atrium. In this condition, the systolic left ventricular pressure is not elevated, and since the left ventricle is performing extra "volume work," the $M\dot{V}O_2$ of the left ventricle is not significantly increased. Therefore, in the absence of coronary artery disease, oxygen supply-demand imbalance and angina pectoris are rarely seen in chronic mitral regurgitation. In contrast, in patients with aortic stenosis, the high left ventricular systolic pressures with elevated $M\dot{V}O_2$ of the entire chamber can lead to reduction of coronary vasodilator reserve. Therefore, subendocardial ischemia with angina pectoris is quite common in aortic stenosis, particularly during exercise or when left ventricular failure is beginning to occur, even in the absence of coronary artery disease. Of course, in chronic coronary artery disease, during exercise virtually all of the major determinants of $M\dot{V}O_2$ are augmented, and in the presence of a stenosed coronary artery with impaired vasodilator reserve, coronary blood flow cannot keep pace with enhanced oxygen demands, and regional myocardial ischemia with angina pectoris occurs (see Ch. 51.1).

REGULATION OF CORONARY BLOOD FLOW

In keeping with the high energy requirements of the normal myocardium, coronary blood flow is relatively high, averaging 60 to 90 ml per minute per 100 grams in the normal human left ventricle when an individual is at rest. Extraction of oxygen by the heart is the highest of any organ, so that little additional oxygen extraction can occur during stress. This means that changes in oxygen demand of the heart are met chiefly by alterations in oxygen supply through changes in coronary blood flow, reflected by a nearly linear positive relation between the $M\dot{V}O_2$ and the coronary blood flow. Although cardiac metabolism is the main determinant of coronary blood flow, several additional factors can be of importance:

1. $M\dot{V}O_2$
2. Coronary perfusion pressure
3. Systolic compression
4. Alpha-adrenergic tone to the coronary arteries (or exogenous vasoconstrictors)
5. Vasodilators (epinephrine, exogenous vasodilator substances)

Since the $M\dot{V}O_2$ is influence by each of the major determinants of cardiac performance, coronary blood flow is altered in the appropriate direction. There is evidence that release of the ATP metabolite adenosine, a potent coronary vasodilator, is involved in some of the responses of the coronary blood flow to altered cardiac performance and metabolism, although a number of other stimuli to vasodilation (such as decreased PO_2, decreased pH, and increased K^+ during enhanced metabolic activity) may also be important.

Under normal conditions, the mean coronary perfusion pressure is not a major determinant of coronary blood flow, except as it affects the systolic arterial pressure and therefore the $M\dot{V}O_2$. Of course, on a moment-to-moment basis, the phasic pattern of coronary blood flow to the left ventricle shows a slow fall during diastole as the aortic pressure falls, as well as a sharp drop during systole as the squeezing action of the left ventricular wall compresses the intramural vessels and shuts down coronary blood flow, particularly to the subendocardial layers. However, the mean flow has been shown to be independent of the mean coronary perfusion pressure within certain limits, a phenomenon termed "autoregulation." Studies in which the coronary arteries are perfused *separately* from the aorta show that between mean coronary perfusion pressures of about 60 mm Hg and 150 mm Hg coronary blood flow is maintained constant, provided that the $M\dot{V}O_2$ of the heart does not change (Fig. 41–4). When the coronary perfusion pressure drops below 60 mm Hg, the coronary bed reaches the limit of autoregulation and tends to become fully dilated; at that point, perfusion pressure becomes the major determinant of coronary blood flow, and flow will drop as pressure falls below that value with an exponential relation between pressure and flow typical of a passive blood vessel (Fig. 41–4). Obviously, in coronary artery disease the coronary perfusion pressure can become extremely important, since the perfusion pressure beyond an area of stenosis may be relatively low.

Systolic compression of coronary vessels in the inner (subendocardial) left ventricular wall almost entirely shuts off coronary blood flow during systole, but this does not occur in the outer wall (subepicardium). During diastole, flow to the subendocardium becomes slightly higher than in the outer wall, in order to compensate for the loss of flow during systole, a phenomenon that makes the vasodilator reserve in the subendocardium somewhat *less* than in the subepicardium. When the coronary bed becomes maximally dilated, this effect also makes subendocardial coronary blood flow

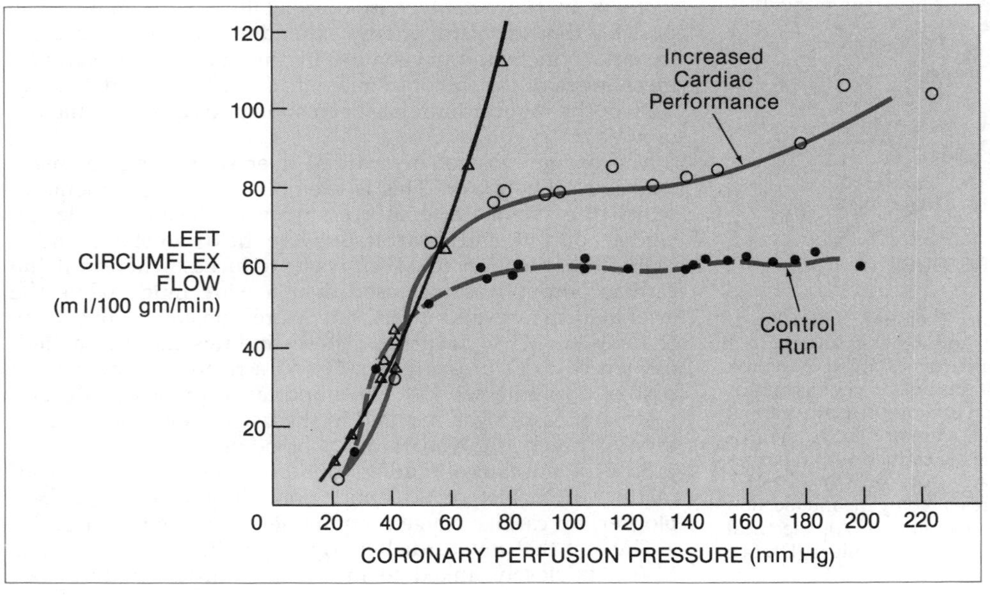

FIGURE 41–4. Autoregulation in the coronary circulation. When the left ventricular work is held constant and the coronary perfusion pressure is altered (coronary artery separately perfused from a controlled pressure source), coronary blood flow remains relatively constant over a wide range (*closed circles*, control run). At a coronary perfusion pressure below approximately 60 mm Hg, the limit of vasodilator reserve is reached, autoregulation is lost, and coronary flow is directly determined by the coronary perfusion pressure. The pressure-flow relation then falls on a curve of maximum vasodilation (passive pressure-flow curve of a distensible blood vessel, *open triangles*). Coronary blood flow is regulated at a higher level when cardiac performance and hence $M\dot{V}O_2$ are increased (*open circles*, increased cardiac performance). (Adapted from West JB (ed): Best and Taylor's Physiological Basis of Medical Practice. 11th ed. Baltimore, Williams & Wilkins Co., 1985).

highly dependent upon the time available for diastolic perfusion. For example, if heart rate increases under such circumstances, systolic time per minute is increased at the expense of diastolic time, and coronary flow will fall. This can occur in coronary artery disease, when, during exercise, the heart rate increases and coronary blood flow consequentially falls beyond an area of coronary stenosis (decreased oxygen supply), in the face of increased oxygen demands. Beta-adrenergic blockade is often used to treat angina pectoris in this setting (Ch. 51.1).

Alpha-adrenergic constrictor influences on the coronary vascular bed have been demonstrated. Although such an effect is of relatively minor significance under normal conditions, under certain circumstances of reflex activation it can be of great significance. There is recent evidence that under conditions of exercise-induced ischemia, alpha-adrenergic coronary vasoconstrictor tone exists and can be reduced by vasodilators or by alpha-adrenergic blockade.

A variety of substances can relax the smooth muscle of coronary arteries, including nitroglycerin and calcium channel blockers, and these are used to treat angina due to coronary artery spasm, as well as exercise-induced angina pectoris. Certain prostaglandins and agents such as vasopressin and ergonovine are coronary vasoconstrictors.

REGULATION OF THE PERIPHERAL CIRCULATION

The heart pumps blood sequentially through the pulmonary and systemic circulations. Throughout the circulation, the small arterioles provide the main site for vascular resistance regulation. The normal distribution of peripheral blood flow at rest is shown in Figure 41–5. There is a wide variability in cardiac output distribution and in oxygen extraction by various organs; for example, the kidneys have a high blood flow (20 per cent of the cardiac output) and a low oxygen extraction, whereas the coronary circulation has a lower flow but a much higher oxygen extraction (Fig. 41–5). The large conduit arteries have a high velocity of blood flow (aorta = 31 cm per second), whereas in the capillaries, the enormous total cross-sectional area results in marked slowing of blood flow (0.05 cm per second), allowing exchange of metabolites. The veins contain 75 to 80 per cent of the total blood volume in the circulation and serve a capacitance function, i.e., as a blood volume reservoir.

The general organization of the systemic circulation is such that the arterial bed serves as a pressure reservoir from which the circulations to the various organs operate in parallel (Fig. 41–5). Thus, each organ takes the blood supply that it requires by regulating its *local* vascular resistance primarily on the basis of metabolic needs (autoregulation, as discussed earlier for the coronary circulation), whereas the *total* peripheral vascular resistance (TPVR) is primarily controlled by cardiovascular reflexes and maintains the pressure in the arteries. Thus, the blood pressure, which equals the product of the cardiac output and the TPVR (blood pressure = cardiac output × TPVR), is protected by the reflexes. For example, during exercise the vascular resistance in exercising skeletal muscles decreases markedly, and despite the increase in cardiac output, the blood pressure might fall were it not for a reflex increase in vascular resistance in nonexercising muscles and certain other areas.

REFLEX NEURAL CONTROL. The autonomic nervous system and certain neurohumoral factors maintain circulatory homeostasis through regulation of the heart rate, myocardial contractility, vascular tone in the arterioles and small veins, and the blood volume (discussed in a subsequent section).

The high-pressure baroreceptors, which sense stretch in the walls of arteries, are located in the carotid sinuses and aortic

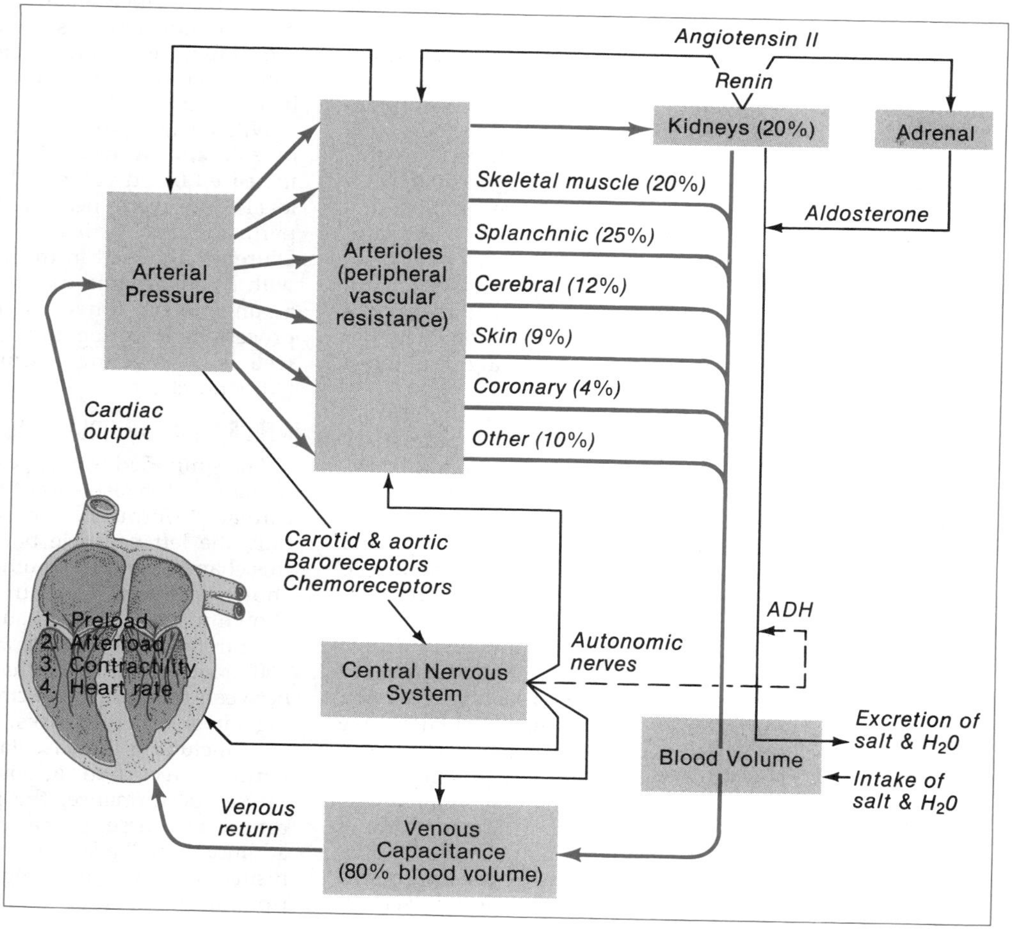

FIGURE 41–5. Schematic representation of the circulatory system. See text for details.

arch. They increase their afferent impulse traffic when the blood pressure rises, and vice versa, and these nerve impulses pass through the cardiovascular regulatory centers in the medulla, which alter the relative magnitude of efferent vagal and sympathetic impulses. For example, as arterial pressure is increased, the enhanced impulse traffic stimulates the vagus to slow the heart rate and simultaneously inhibits the cardioaccelerator center. Simultaneously, the vasoconstrictor center is also inhibited, reducing sympathetic tone to the peripheral arterioles and also lowering venous tone. Thus, the reduced peripheral vascular resistance and venous return, together with the slowed heart rate, lower the increased blood pressure toward its previous level. With a decrease in blood pressure, as with moderate bleeding, this reflex arc would reduce vagal tone and enhance sympathetic tone, both of which would cause the heart rate to increase, which, together with increased myocardial contractility and venous tone, would increase the cardiac output, whereas increased arteriolar tone would enhance peripheral vascular resistance. All of these factors would rapidly restore the lowered blood pressure toward its previous level. With a significant drop in blood pressure, reflex release of catecholamines from the adrenal glands also occurs.

Reflex control of the heart and circulation is also under the influence of higher brain centers, as when marked emotional stress activates the sympathetic nervous system. Such central stimulation, as well as reflex activation of the sympathetic nervous system via receptors in the exercising skeletal muscle, produce the marked sympathetic stimulation of exercise. At rest, there appears to be little sympathetic tone affecting heart rate or myocardial contractility, and the heart rate is primarily under the control of parasympathetic influences.

Chemoreceptors lying in the carotid bodies near the carotid bifurcation and in the aortic arch respond to changes in pH, Pco_2, and Po_2. When ventilation is controlled experimentally, reduced oxygen tension, increased carbon dioxide tension, or lowered pH stimulates the chemoreceptors and leads to an elevation of the systemic arterial pressure and bradycardia. Marked hypotension can also make the brain stem itself ischemic and result in severe peripheral vasoconstriction mediated through the sympathetic nerves, and under such circumstances, the chemoreceptors may contribute to this vasoconstriction. However, the major normal physiologic effect of the chemoreceptors is the control of respiration, hypoxemia producing hyperpnea, which, in turn, stimulates low-pressure stretch receptors in the lungs to cause peripheral vasodilation. Thus, even though under unphysiologic conditions when respiration is held constant the major effect of stimulating the chemoreceptors is vasoconstriction, whether or not this response has a role in regulating the intact circulation is unclear.

Low-pressure baroreceptors (stretch receptors) are also located in the heart, particularly in the atria and the pulmonary veins, with fewer in the ventricles. Increased stretch of the atrial receptors can induce tachycardia (the Bainbridge reflex). More marked stretch of these low-pressure receptors produces a depressor reflex, with withdrawal of sympathetic tone and a fall in peripheral vascular resistance, which contributes to high-pressure baroreceptor regulation of the blood pressure. It has been considered that syncope in some patients with aortic stenosis and high intracardiac pressure may be due to activation of these intracardiac receptors. Increased stretch of the low-pressure receptors also causes renal vasodilation through reduction of sympathetic tone, whereas hemorrhage causes renal vasoconstriction, and it may be that the primary role of these low-pressure receptors is in regulating blood volume.

REGULATION OF BLOOD VOLUME. The magnitude of blood volume is an important factor affecting cardiovascular function, and it is important in long-term regulation of the blood pressure. Some of the factors involved in the maintenance of extracellular fluid and blood volume are listed on the right-hand side of Figure 41–5. Loss of fluid volume occurs primarily through the kidneys, whereas sweating, respiratory, and gastrointestinal losses are less important (except during extreme conditions). Since approximately 20 per cent of the resting cardiac output passes through the kidneys, they provide an ideal location for regulating sodium and water balance. In addition, the hypothalamic osmoreceptors that regulate thirst and antidiuretic hormone (ADH) secretion are of great importance. Since these subjects are discussed in detail in Ch. 77, only selected cardiovascular factors are mentioned here.

An increase in blood volume, as might occur by increased intake of salt and water, would increase the cardiac output. This, in turn, would tend to raise arterial pressure and renal perfusion and thus augment urine output, which would then decrease blood volume back toward normal. Atrial receptors sensitive to stretch are responsible for vasodilating reflexes to the kidneys, as mentioned, and atrial receptors also reflexly stimulate the central nervous system to diminish the secretion of ADH. These factors would tend to increase the output of urine and sodium excretion. A decrease in effective blood volume would have opposite effects.

An additional highly important control mechanism for the regulation of arterial pressure and blood volume is the renin-angiotensin system (see Ch. 47). Reduction in renal perfusion (reduced pressure and flow) is sensed by the juxtaglomerular apparatus, which releases renin, whereas increased effective blood volume shuts off the stimulus for renin release. (This response forms the basis for alterations in sodium intake and volume as provocative tests for altering renin levels.) Renin enzymatically promotes the formation of angiotensin I from a precursor in the bloodstream, which is then converted to angiotensin II by the converting enzyme. Angiotensin II is a powerful vasoconstrictor, but this may not be its most important effect, since small subpressor doses of angiotensin II increase aldosterone secretion. Aldosterone, in turn, acts on the kidney to promote retention of salt and water, thereby counteracting the original stimulus of decreased effective blood volume.

With congestive heart failure, there is increased retention of salt and water, which leads to edema formation and increased blood volume. There may be increased aldosterone levels in severe heart failure secondary to reduced renal perfusion and activation of the renin-angiotensin system. Diuretics are used in this setting, and in severe heart failure with hyponatremia that is unresponsive to diuretics, use of an angiotensin-converting enzyme inhibitor may reverse this process by lowering angiotensin II and aldosterone levels, as well as by lowering vascular resistance and afterload on the left ventricle.

INTEGRATED CARDIOVASCULAR RESPONSES

The simplified overview of the circulatory system illustrated in Figure 41–5 also shows the four factors directly influencing cardiac performance. These factors affect performance of not only the left ventricle but also the right ventricle, although this chamber and the pulmonary circulation are not separately shown in Figure 41–5. In addition, a number of factors not shown in this diagram, such as the prostaglandins and atrial natriuretic factor, also can affect overall circulatory function.

It is important to emphasize the significance of interactions between the peripheral circulation and the heart in considering integrated responses. Certain peripheral circulatory factors, including the vascular resistance and the venous capacitance, affect two important mechanical determinants of cardiac performance, the preload and the afterload. Venous return, of course, primarily determines the cardiac output. In addition, feedback control by neurohumoral reflex mechanisms simultaneously regulates both the heart and the peripheral circulation.

CHANGES IN VENOUS RETURN. Changing from the supine or sitting to a standing position causes venous blood to pool in the distensible veins of the abdomen and lower extremities, leading to an immediate drop in the venous return and cardiac output and in the blood pressure. However, prompt action of cardiovascular reflexes via the baroreceptor mechanism causes an increase in vascular resistance, tending to restore the blood pressure toward normal, and further stimulates restoration of the cardiac output by sympathetic reflexes, which enhance the heart rate and the contractility of the myocardium. A more marked stimulus, the Valsalva maneuver, which is useful in the physical diagnosis of heart murmurs, causes a marked decrease in the venous return to the heart because of the abrupt elevation of intrathoracic pressure, and after 15 to 20 seconds, the associated drop in blood pressure produces reflex tachycardia and increased myocardial contractility. During this phase of the maneuver, cardiac murmurs associated with blood flow across a narrowed valve, such as that of aortic stenosis, diminish in intensity because of the reduced cardiac output, whereas the murmur associated with hypertrophic cardiomyopathy increases owing to the reduced heart size and increased contractility.

Vasodilator drugs that have a considerable venodilating effect, such as nitroglycerin and nitroprusside, can have different effects on the cardiac output in the normal circulation and in congestive heart failure. Thus, in the normal circulation the cardiac output falls with nitroprusside, since the venous return curve is shifted downward as blood volume is displaced from the central circulation and pooled in the peripheral veins (decreased effective blood volume), whereas during cardiac failure, the associated unloading of the left ventricle by the arteriolar-dilating action of this drug releases blood from the central circulation, which counterbalances the drug's venodilator effect; therefore, the venous return curve is not shifted downward, and the marked shift upward of the cardiac output curve owing to reduced afterload results in an increased cardiac output (Fig. 41–3, D to A).

It is also important to note that certain chronic cardiac conditions can limit the venous return to the heart because of impaired cardiac filling. These include chronic constrictive pericarditis and restrictive cardiomyopathy.

CHANGES IN HEART RATE. The lack of effect on cardiac output of changing heart rate by electrical pacing over a wide range has been previously discussed (see Fig. 41–5). But the usual increases in heart rate that occur as a component of cardiocirculatory reflex responses are ordinarily accompanied by increased myocardial contractility, venoconstriction, and an increased cardiac output. Below a certain level of heart rate, as in complete heart block with a ventricular rate of 40 beats per minute, the resting cardiac output may not be maintained, since the stroke volume is maximal (preload reserve fully utilized) and the ventricular output becomes rate limited. In addition, with marked resting tachycardia (approaching 200 beats per minute or more), as in paroxysmal atrial or ventricular arrhythmias, the available diastolic filling time is shortened because of the increased number of contractions per minute, and inadequate ventricular filling leads to a fall in the cardiac output. The loss of an appropriately timed atrial contraction in some dysrhythmias may further contribute to inadequate cardiac filling.

EXERCISE. Many mechanisms can come into play to cause the increased cardiac output that accompanies normal exercise. In individuals with some degree of physical training, the heart rate is lowered both at rest and with exercise, and during low levels of exercise, increased stroke volume, combined with a mild increase in heart rate, augments the cardiac output. With marked exercise, as sympathetic stimulation and circulating catecholamine levels increase, the increased venous return causes further utilization of the Frank-Starling mechanism, and the stroke volume is further enhanced as increased myocardial contractility augments the ejection fraction. However, the most important cardiac mechanism allowing a very high cardiac output during intense exercise in such individuals is augmented heart rate, which may reach 180 beats per minute or higher. Increased myocardial contractility combines with decreased total peripheral vascular resistance (caused by marked vasodilation in the exercising muscles) to shift the cardiac output curve upward (Fig. 41–5).

In addition, increased sympathetic tone shifts the venous return curve upward, and it is steepened by decreased venous and arteriolar resistance (Fig. 41–5). Therefore, the intersection of the venous return and cardiac output curves occurs at a markedly increased cardiac output, with only a mild elevation of the right atrial pressure (Fig. 41–5, point C). Thus, *both* peripheral and circulatory adaptations are involved in the exercise response.

Braunwald E (ed.): Heart Disease: A Textbook of Cardiovascular Medicine. 2nd ed. Philadelphia, W.B. Saunders Company, 1984, pp 409–466. *Up-to-date review of cardiac performance from the cellular level to the intact heart. Also includes the pathophysiology of heart failure.*

Guyton AC: Circulation Physiology: Cardiac Output and Its Regulation. Philadelphia, W.B. Saunders Company, 1963. *Classic text on the importance of venous return and the relationship between venous return and cardiac output.*

Ross J Jr: Cardiac function and myocardial contractility: A perspective. J Am Coll Cardiol 1:52, 1983. *Current concepts concerning left ventricular function under normal and abnormal loading conditions, including heart failure and valvular heart disease.*

West JB (ed.): Best and Taylor's Physiological Basis of Medical Practice. 11th ed. Baltimore, Williams & Wilkins Company, 1985, pp 207–262. *Basic physiology text that assumes little advanced knowledge. Pathophysiologic examples are concerned with cardiac function, circulatory control, myocardial oxygen consumption, and coronary circulation.*

42 SPECIALIZED DIAGNOSTIC PROCEDURES

42.1 Radiography of the Heart

Charles E. Putman

The standard posteroanterior (PA) and lateral chest radiographs are the most frequently used imaging procedures in evaluating the heart. The examination is simple to perform and requires relatively inexpensive equipment and very little technical expertise. The advantages of chest radiographs in the evaluation of the cardiac patient are as follows: (1) an experienced observer may detect significant abnormalities not available by other noninvasive methods; (2) recognized abnormalities may be followed, and response to therapy can be documented; and (3) results are easily reproducible, and the radiograph provides a reliable comparative index to changing pathology or alteration of normal cardiovascular function.

TECHNIQUE

There is considerable variation in the configuration of the normal cardiac silhouette. The two most important factors influencing cardiac size and shape are (1) thoracic cavity dimensions and symmetry of the musculoskeletal structure and (2) intrathoracic pulmonary pressure. As the diaphragm descends during normal inspiration, the heart will become smaller and more vertical and conversely during expiration the heart will be larger and more transverse. If the radiograph is exposed during a Valsalva maneuver, there will be a decrease in heart size because of decreased venous return secondary to increased intrathoracic pressure. Variation of technical factors from one examination to another may be responsible for misinterpretation of cardiac dimensions.

INTERPRETATION

To evaluate the cardiovascular status adequately, a systematic approach to reading the standard PA and lateral radiographs is necessary (Figs. 42–1 and 42–2). In addition to evaluating the heart, one should study the great vessels, the pulmonary vascularity, the pleura, the bones, the abdominal viscera, and the extrathoracic structures that may provide useful clues to diagnosis. It is necessary to know which chambers and vascular structures contribute to the cardiac boundaries in the two standard views (Figs. 42–1 to 42–4). When there is suggestive evidence of heart disease, two additional views, the right and left anterior oblique views, may be obtained (Figs. 42–5 and 42–6). These four radiographs are called "the cardiac series" and are usually obtained following the swallowing of barium sulfate to outline and distend the esophagus. Encroachment on the esophageal column by enlarged or displaced cardiac chambers can then be more easily ascertained and the appropriate differential diagnosis facilitated. The value of these views in defining specific cardiac pathology is illustrated in Figures 42–7 to 42–10.

HEART SIZE. Cardiac enlargement is the single most important observation in the suspect cardiac patient, and yet it can be a difficult assessment from the chest radiograph. Various measurements of heart size have been suggested, but the most reliable is a nomogram published by Ungerleider and Gubner. A series of tables indicates predicted normal transverse cardiac diameter for adults of various heights and weights. In actual practice, these tables are rarely used, and instead the cardiothoracic ratio is employed. This measurement is determined by dividing the maximal transverse diameter of the heart by the maximal transverse diameter of the thorax on the PA radiograph. The normal cardiothoracic ratio averages 0.45, but values up to 0.55 may be seen in normal subjects with a greater than average stroke volume. Measurements from the chest radiographs (Figs. 42–1 and 42–2), like other measurements in medicine, are only statistically reliable when applied to subgroups and are therefore less consistent for a given individual. Radiographic cardiac measurements are most meaningful when they can be compared with measurements from previous radiographs of similar quality and technique. Solitary chamber enlargement without cardiomegaly is usually better delineated by the electrocardiogram or echocardiogram than by the radiograph.

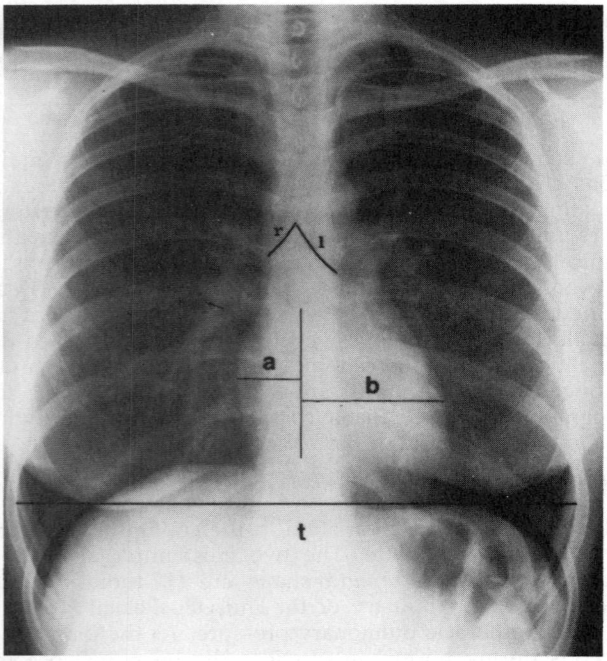

FIGURE 42–1. Normal PA view: a = Transverse diameter of the heart to the right of the midline; b = transverse diameter of the heart to the left of the midline; t = transverse diameter of the thorax; l = lower margin of the left stem bronchus; r = lower margin of the right stem bronchus. The measurements of the right descending pulmonary artery (*arrow*) are 10 to 15 mm for males and 9 to 14 mm for females. The maximal normal angle between the two bronchi is 75 degrees for adults in deep inspiration. The cardiothoracic ratio = a + b/t.

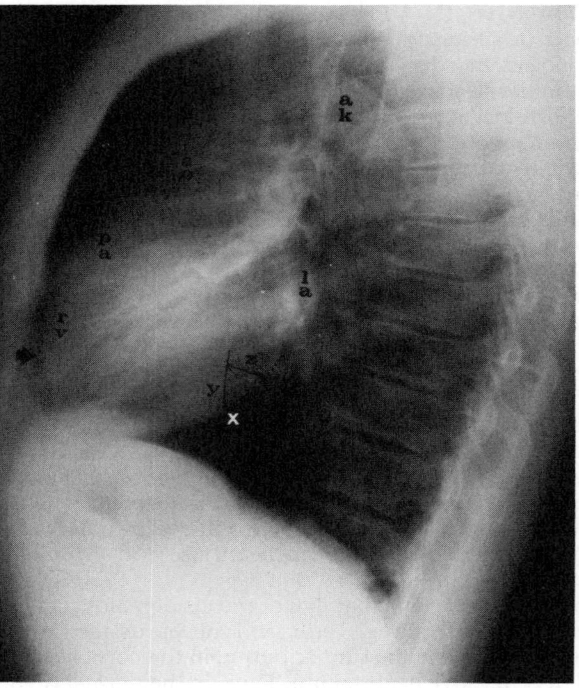

FIGURE 42–2. Normal lateral view. x = The crossing point between the inferior vena cava and the posterior border of the left ventricle; y = distance from point x, 2 cm cephalad along the inferior vena cava; z = posterior dimension of the left ventricle (according to Hoffman and Rigler), which should be smaller than 1.8 cm. Other abbreviations are as in Figure 42–3. Arrow points to the removal position of the subpericardial fat line (very close to the sternum).

PULMONARY VESSELS. Following the determination of cardiac size and chamber predominance, an evaluation of the pulmonary vessels allows for a more precise differential diagnosis. There are four basic patterns of abnormal pulmonary circulation identified by the standard radiograph. Certain groups of diseases may be identified on the basis of (1) decreased flow, (2) increased flow, (3) increased pulmonary resistance, or (4) pulmonary venous hypertension. Each has a specific radiographic pattern that allows for discrimination.

With *decreased pulmonary flow* (e.g., tetralogy of Fallot) there is a decrease in size of the central and peripheral vessels. *Increased pulmonary flow* is indicative of high output states (e.g., hyperthyroidism) or more commonly of left-to-right shunts (e.g., atrial septal defect). With small shunts, no abnormality may be detected by the standard radiograph. Larger shunts cause enlargement and tortuosity of the central and peripheral vessels (Fig. 42–7). Increased pulmonary resistance or *pulmonary arterial hypertension* is identified by dilatation of the central vessels and narrowing or attenuation of the peripheral vessels. *Pulmonary venous hypertension* is a more common hemodynamic state and is usually due to mitral stenosis or left ventricular failure. In upright humans 60 to 70 per cent of the blood flow normally goes to the lower portion of the chest. This can be appreciated on the standard PA radiograph by visualizing larger vessels at the lung bases than in the upper zones of the lung. Pulmonary venous hypertension produced by increased resistance distal to the pulmonary capillaries causes distention and recruitment of upper lobe vessels because of diversion of blood from the constricted

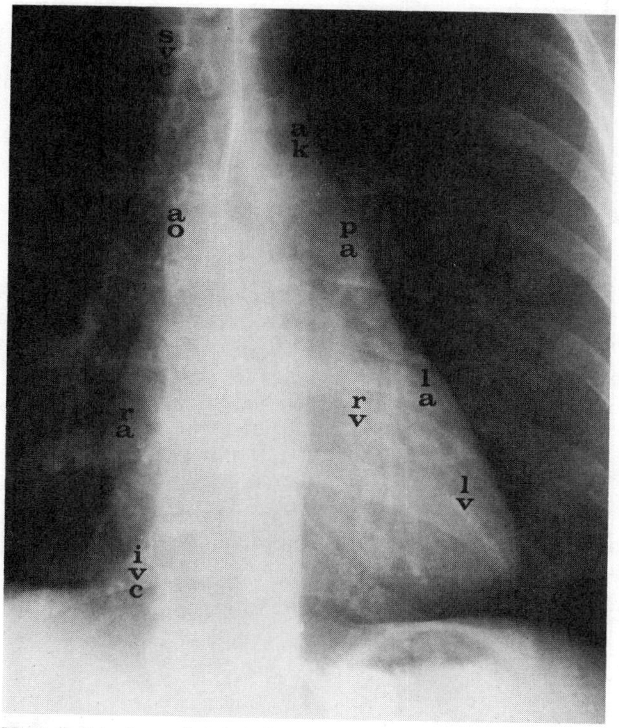

FIGURE 42–3. PA view of the chest with barium in the esophagus. The major border-forming cardiovascular structures are marked as follows: ak = aortic knob (the arch joining the transverse and descending portions of the thoracic aorta); pa = pulmonary artery (the pulmonary trunk); la = left atrium; lv = left ventricle; rv = right ventricle (left lateral border); ivc = inferior vena cava; ra = right atrium; ao = ascending aorta; svc = superior vena cava.

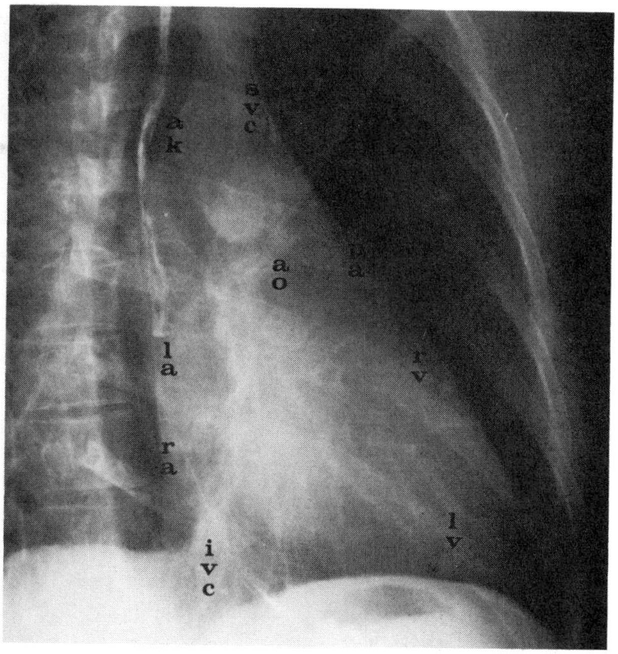

FIGURE 42–5. Forty-five degree right anterior oblique (RAO) view with barium in the esophagus. Abbreviations are as in Figure 42–3.

lower zones. Radiographically, this produces an equalization of vascular caliber between the upper and lower lobes. As left atrial pressure increases, upper lobe vessels become larger than lower lobe vessels (Fig. 42–11*A*). The ability of the radiograph to detect these subtle changes in left atrial pressure is an adequate indication to obtain chest radiographs periodically in patients who are prone to heart failure, e.g., the hypertensive patient.

HEART FAILURE. Other radiologic signs of incipient congestive heart failure may not be so obvious. When the pulmonary venous pressure exceeds 20 mm Hg, fluid will begin to accumulate in the interstitium of the lung. Radiographically, this is detected by the appearance of Kerley's B lines (edema of interlobular septa), which are thin horizontal reticular lines seen most often in the costophrenic angles (Fig. 42–11*B*). Also, the hilar structures may be indistinct and the peripheral vessel margins hazy. As the pulmonary venous pressure exceeds 30 mm Hg, alveolar edema and pleural effusion appear—classic radiographic signs of congestive heart failure.

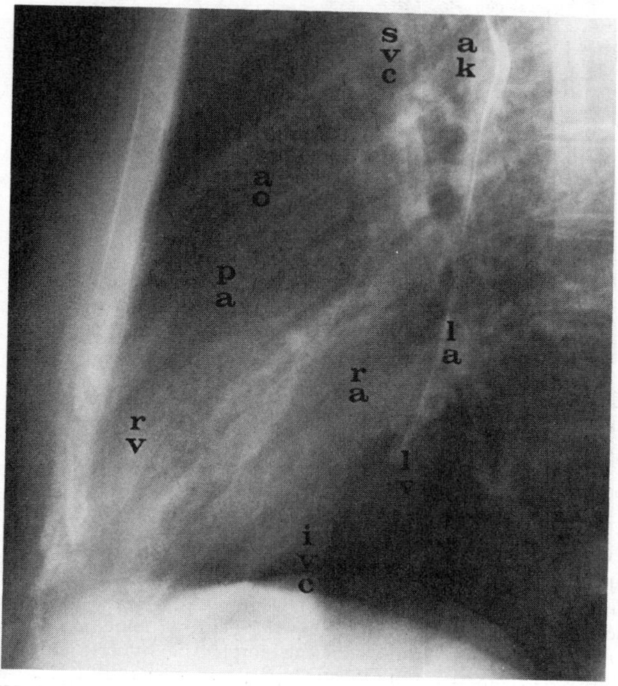

FIGURE 42–4. Left lateral view of the chest with barium in the esophagus. Abbreviations are as in Figure 42–3.

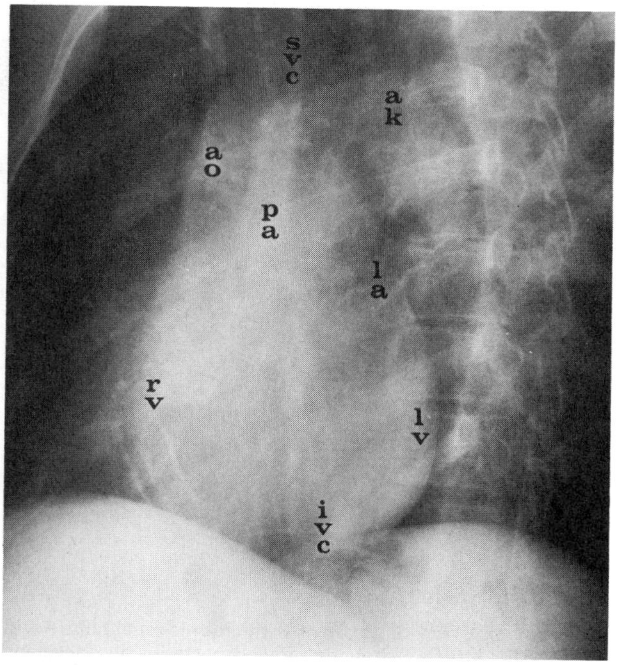

FIGURE 42–6. Sixty degree left anterior oblique (LAO) view without barium in the esophagus. Abbreviations are as in Figure 42–3.

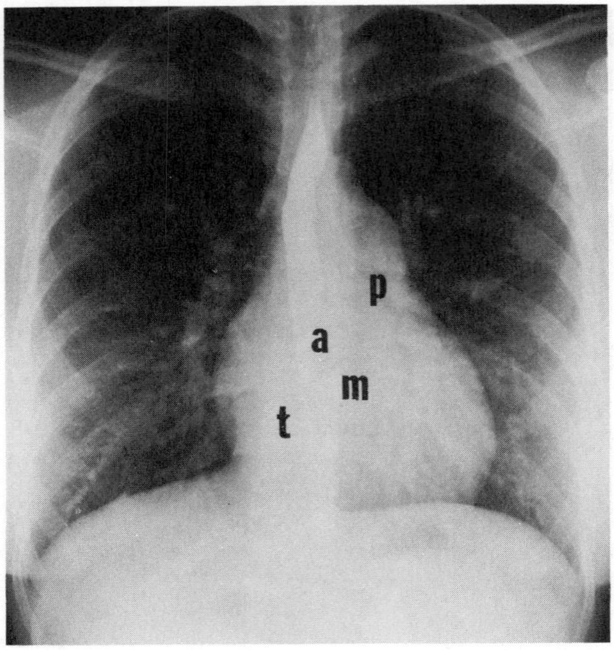

FIGURE 42–7. PA view of a patient with secundum atrial septal defect showing bilateral increase in pulmonary vascularity, right-sided cardiomegaly, marked dilatation of the pulmonary trunk, and an inconspicuous aortic knob. There is no deviation of the barium-filled esophagus or double density to suggest left atrial enlargement. The four cardiac valve positions are marked as follows: a = aortic valve; m = mitral valve; p = pulmonic valve; t = tricuspid valve.

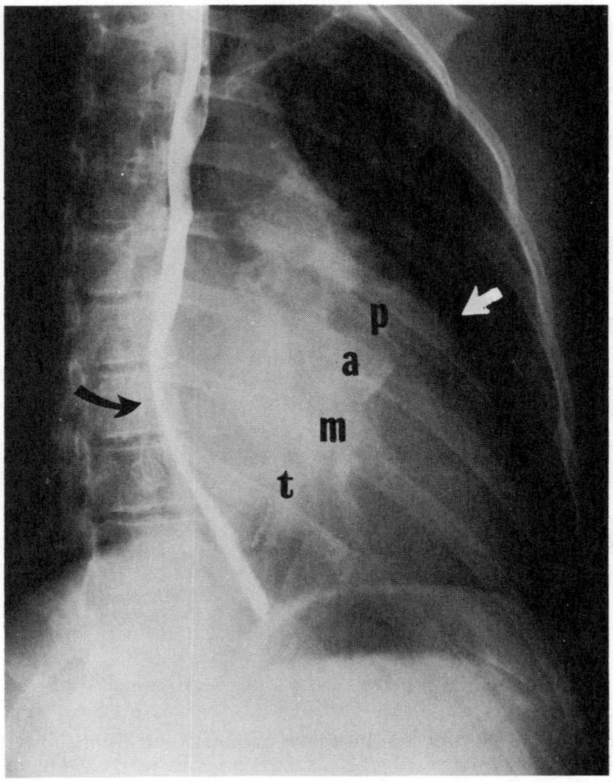

FIGURE 42–9. RAO view of a patient with mitral stenosis. Note that the barium-filled esophagus is deviated posteriorly by the enlarged left atrium (*curved arrow*). The right ventricular enlargement presents as an anterior bulge along the upper cardiac border (*straight arrow*). The four cardiac valve positions in this view are designated as in Figure 42–7.

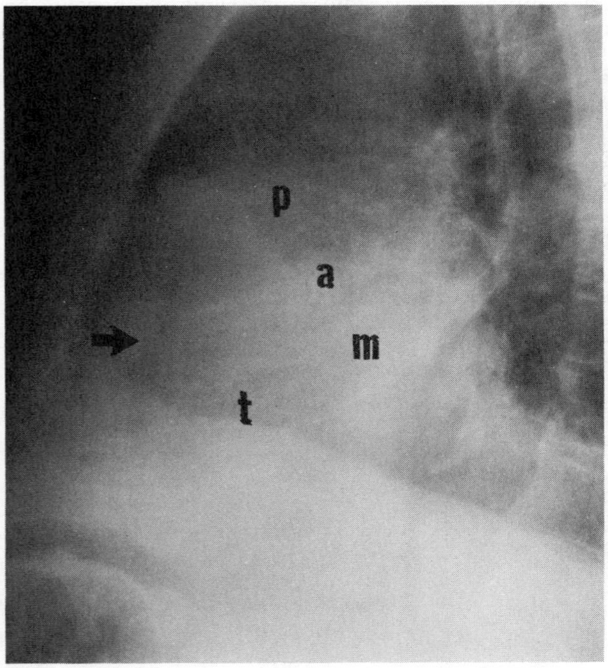

FIGURE 42–8. Lateral view of a patient with chronic renal failure with a large pericardial effusion showing marked posterior displacement of the subepicardial fat line (*arrow*). The four valve positions are marked in the same manner as in the PA view (Fig. 42–7).

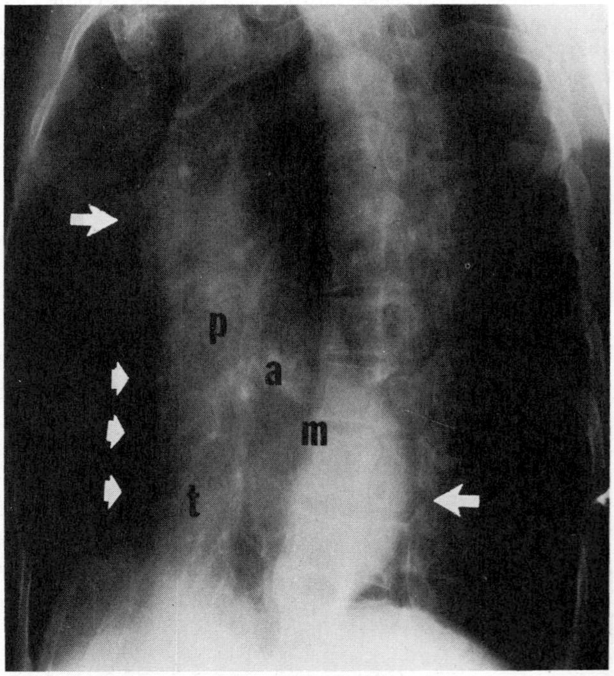

FIGURE 42–10. LAO view of a patient with aortic valve stenosis. The four valve positions are labeled as in Figure 42–7. Heavy aortic valve calcification is visible (a). The upper long arrow points to the post-stenotic dilatation of the ascending aorta. The hypertrophied left ventricle is marked by the lower long arrow posteriorly. The three short arrows point to the left anterior cardiac border formed by the normal right ventricle.

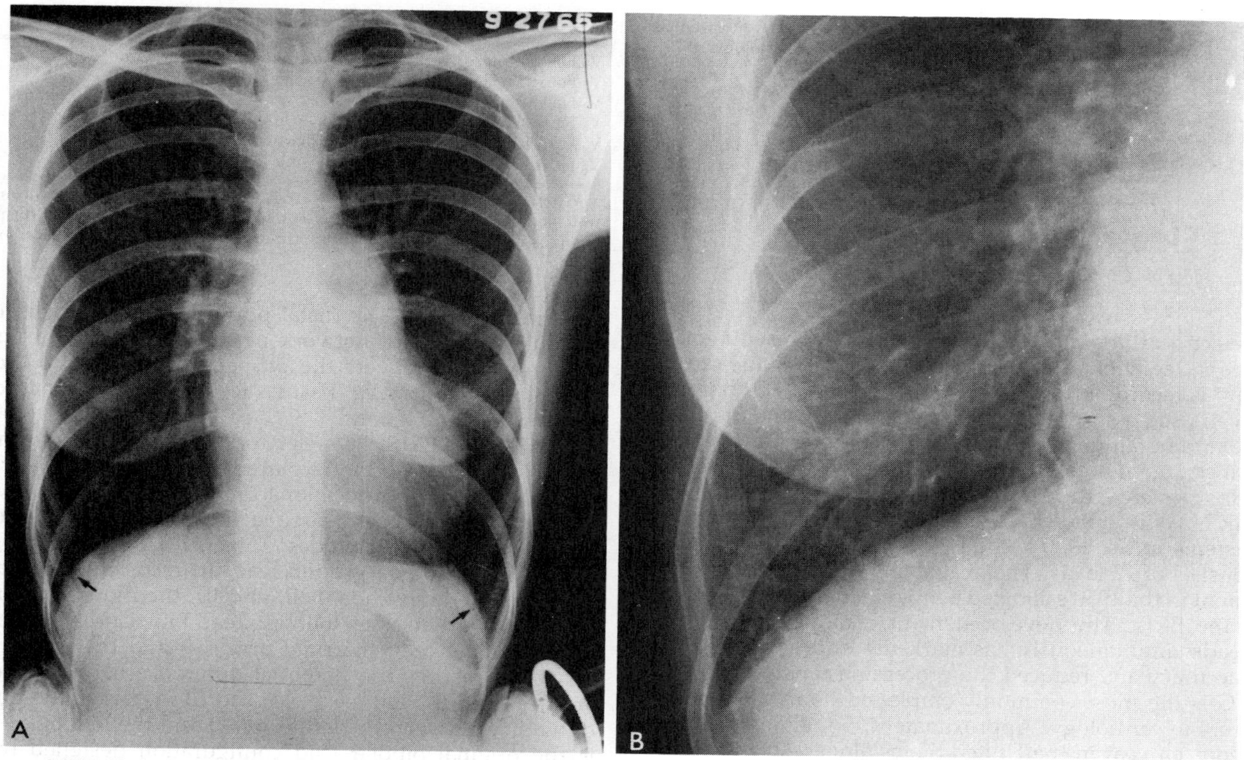

FIGURE 42–11. Patients with severe mitral stenosis. *A*, PA view shows striking redistribution of pulmonary blood flow. Note dilatation of upper and central vessels and constriction of lower and peripheral vessels. Arrows indicate Kerley's B lines in both costophrenic sulci. *B*, Magnified view of the right lower lung zone, showing multiple distinct Kerley's B lines.

PERICARDIAL EFFUSION. A large heart does not always imply heart failure but may be indicative of pericardial effusion. A rapidly enlarging cardiac silhouette without evidence of pulmonary venous congestion strongly suggests pericardial fluid accumulation, especially if of the "water-bottle" configuration. A more definitive radiographic sign of pericardial effusion is the inward displacement of the subepicardial fat line (Fig. 42–8; compare with Fig. 42–2).

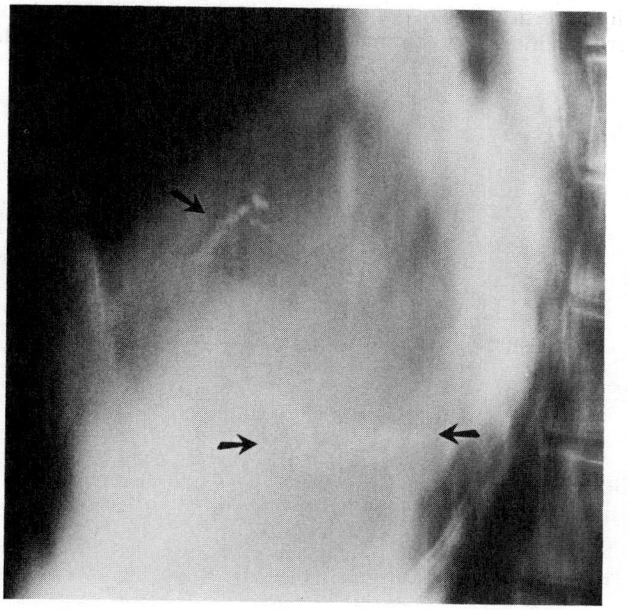

FIGURE 42–12. Lateral tomogram of a patient with severe calcific mitral stenosis. The heavily calcified mitral valve is indicated by the two opposing arrows. The upper arrow points to a heavily calcified anterior descending coronary artery.

FLUOROSCOPY. Fluoroscopy, the technique for visualizing the body structures in real time using a continuous x-ray beam and projecting the image on a recording device such as a television monitor, is a technique commonly applied to evaluate dynamic function of various organ systems. Occasionally it may clarify questionable abnormalities depicted on the standard two- or four-view radiographs of the heart. Pulsation and calcification are better evaluated by fluoroscopy than by static films. Pericardial calcification is curvilinear and is usually seen in the anterior portion of the cardiac shadow. Valvular calcifications are usually seen as multiple dense opacities in the respective valve regions (Figs. 42–10 and 42–12). Myocardial calcification, following myocardial infarction, is linear in distribution and usually occurs at the cardiac apex. Fluoroscopy can reveal faint calcifications in the coronary vessels (Fig. 42–12), which always signify atherosclerosis.

Decrease in cardiac pulsations is suggestive of pericardial effusions, constrictive pericarditis, cardiomyopathy, or generalized cardiac failure. Localized decrease in cardiac motion may be seen in myocardial infarction, and paradoxical movement may be indicative of a ventricular aneurysm. However, regional myocardial contraction abnormalities may not be reliably demonstrated by fluoroscopy. Echocardiography has become the method of choice in this context. Increased cardiac motion on fluoroscopy may indicate hyperthyroidism, hypertension, anemia, or aortic insufficiency.

An accurate assessment of the standard radiograph in the evaluation of the suspect or known cardiac patient will depend on an understanding of normal anatomy and physiology, and an appreciation of the reliability and limitations of the radiographic image. Accurate and skillful radiographic interpretation requires a thorough knowledge of the clinical history and physical findings, as well as of radiographic signs.

Chen JT: The plain radiograph in the diagnosis of cardiovascular disease. Radiol Clin North Am 21(4):609–623, 1983. *This article is the most comprehensive review of the conventional radiograph in evaluation of the cardiovascular system. The bibliography accompanying this paper is current and thorough.*

Colley RN, Capp MP, Lester RG, et al.: Plain Film Diagnosis of Cardiovascular Disease. Syllabus Set 14, Copyright American College of Radiology, 1979. *This is an excellent syllabus and self-evaluation text encompassing all aspects of the interpretation of conventional radiographs. A broad spectrum of cardiac cases is presented, always emphasizing the correlation of the radiographic abnormalities with pertinent clinical, laboratory, and electrocardiographic data.*

42.2 Electrocardiography

Joseph C. Greenfield, Jr.

The electrocardiogram (ECG) is a graphic representation of the electrical activity generated by the heart during the cardiac cycle and is recorded from the body surface. In 1903, Wilhelm Einthoven used a string galvanometer to record the first EKG (Elektrokardiogramm, Ger.) Shortly thereafter, a clinically useful instrument was manufactured by the Cambridge Scientific Instrument Company. Following the pioneering work of Frank N. Wilson and his associates in the development of lead systems in the 1930's, the ECG became standardized. It now consists of 12 leads. The availability of the direct-writing instrument in the 1950's allowed a rapid increase in the routine use of the ECG. The development of recorders that obtain three leads simultaneously has markedly improved the diagnostic accuracy and reduced the processing time. At present, the ECG is the most commonly employed noninvasive diagnostic tool in cardiology. Approximately 75 million ECG's are recorded each year in the United States alone.

ELECTROPHYSIOLOGY. Cardiac muscle may be conveniently divided into specialized conducting tissue and nonspecialized myocardial tissue. While all myocardial cells possess the potential for electrical activity, the rate and pattern of depolarization and subsequent repolarization differ markedly in different regions of the heart. Some cells of the specialized conducting tissue possess the potential for spontaneous depolarization, a process termed automaticity.

The electrical activity of all myocardial cells is made possible by the presence of ionic gradients maintained across the membranes of individual cells. The concentration of intracellular potassium is approximately 30 times greater than its extracellular concentration, and it is the diffusion of this ion out of the cell that results in a resting transmembrane potential of approximately −90 mV in the fully repolarized state. The extracellular sodium concentration is approximately 15 times greater than its intracellular concentration, and the rapid influx of this ion into the cells results in the usual process of rapid cellular depolarization. When cells are partially depolarized to less than −55 mV, however, the sodium channels in the cell membrane are no longer operative, and a slower depolarization process may occur that predominantly involves calcium ions.

Myocardial activation normally begins with the spontaneous calcium-dependent depolarization of cells within the sinoatrial (SA) node located at the junction of the right atrium and superior vena cava. The impulse then propagates in a wavelike fashion through the atrial myocardium to the atrioventricular (AV) node located in the lower portion of the interatrial septum. Conduction through the AV node primarily involves the calcium-dependent process of depolarization and is delayed owing to membrane properties of nodal cells. The membrane properties in the proximal and distal segments of the AV node vary such that conduction in the proximal segment is slow and may occur with decrement, whereas conduction in the distal segment is more rapid.

The impulse is rapidly transmitted through the bundle of His, which then bifurcates into the narrow right bundle branch (RBB) and the fibers that become the left bundle branch (LBB). The LBB divides further into two main collections of fibers forming the anterior (superior) and posterior (inferior) fascicles. The distal portion of the specialized conducting system is a network of smaller fibers, the Purkinje system, which delivers the propagated impulse to the nonspecialized ventricular tissue, resulting in a synchronized myocardial contraction.

TABLE 42–1. POSITION OF CHEST LEADS

V_1	Fourth intercostal space (ICS) at the right sternal border
V_2	Fourth ICS at the left sternal border
V_3	Halfway between V_2 and V_4
V_4	Fifth ICS at the left midclavicular line
V_5	Fifth ICS at the left anterior axillary line
V_6	Fifth ICS at the left midaxillary line

When several sequential ECG's are to be obtained, e.g., in the coronary care unit, it is important to mark the location of the chest electrodes to minimize changes in the waveform resulting from variation in electrode placement.

LEAD SYSTEMS. Five electrodes are used in the standard ECG lead system. One is placed on each of the four limbs and one at different locations on the anterior chest wall (in instruments that record three leads simultaneously, there are six separate chest electrodes; Table 42–1). The right leg electrode functions as a ground lead. In recording the standard frontal plane limb leads, I, II, and III, the right arm, left arm, and left leg are used as follows: Lead I measures the potential difference between the right arm (−) and the left arm (+). Lead II measures the potential difference between the right arm (−) and the left leg (+). Lead III measures the potential difference between the left arm (−) and the left leg (+). This is the original bipolar lead configuration designed by Einthoven. The other three frontal plane leads, aV_R, aV_L, and aV_F, are constructed using a modified central terminal of Wilson, which augments the voltage output, hence the prefix aV. The exploring electrode, placed on the right arm (aV_R), left arm (aV_L), and left leg (aV_F), functions as a positive unipolar lead. The relationship among the six frontal plane leads is shown in Figure 42–13. The six chest leads also function as positive unipolar leads, using the central terminal as the reference point. The ECG leads are displayed in sequence, beginning with lead I, II, and III, followed by aV_R, aV_L, and aV_F, and then the chest leads from V_1 through V_6. A normal ECG recorded in this manner is illustrated in Figure 42–14.

The ECG is recorded on a paper chart, using a standard paper speed of 25 mm per second. The paper is marked with a light vertical line every millimeter (0.04 second) and a heavy vertical line every 5 mm (0.20 second). The paper also has

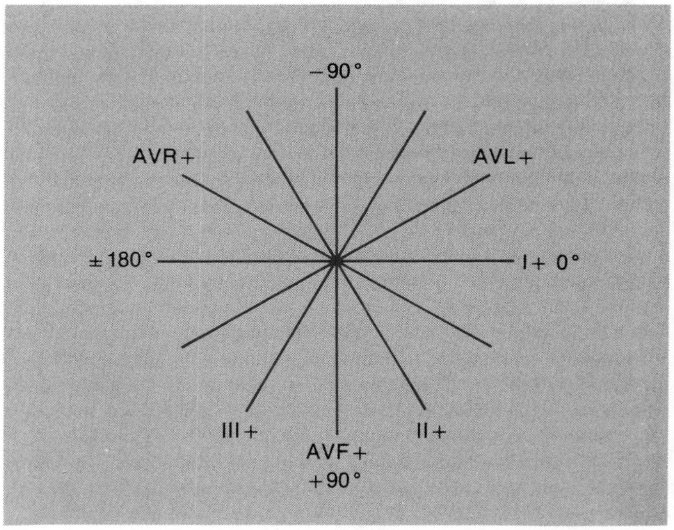

FIGURE 42–13. The limb leads are used to form a hexaxial reference system for the frontal plane. The axis of each lead is separated by approximately 30 degrees from the axes of the two adjacent leads.

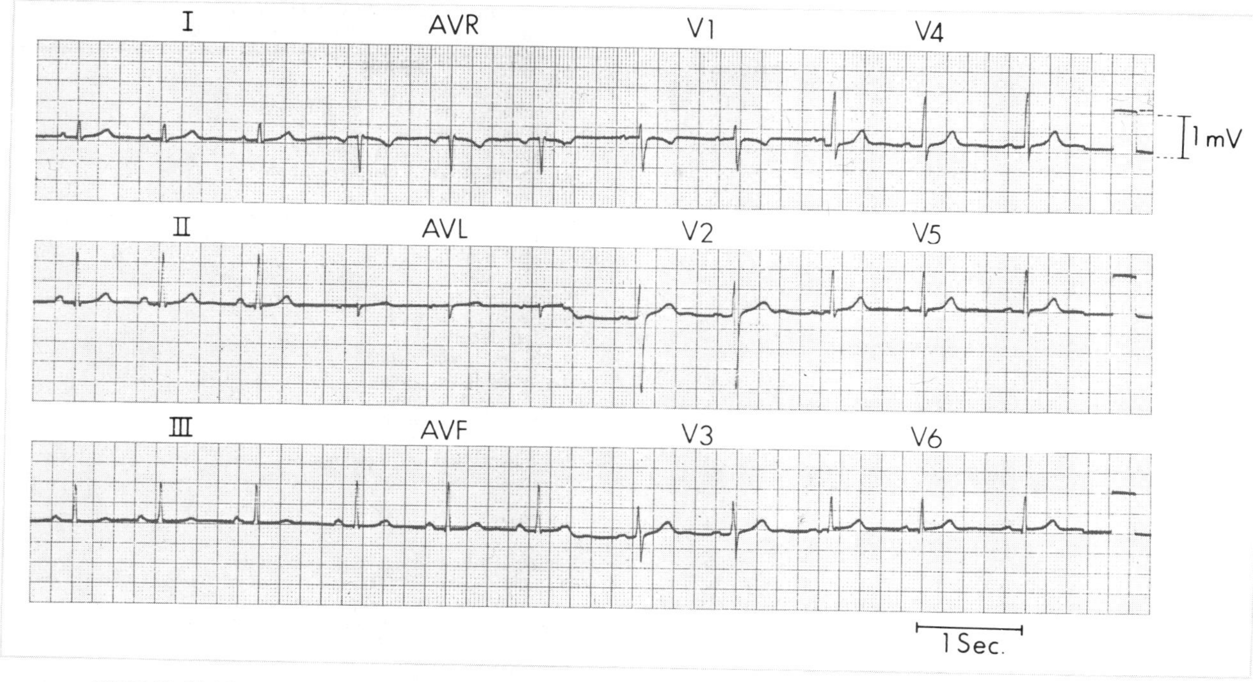

FIGURE 42–14. Normal electrocardiogram; the three leads in each column or lead set are recorded simultaneously.

horizontal lines separated by 1 mm and a dark horizontal line every 5 mm. Vertical deflection is calibrated in terms of voltage so that 10 mm equals 1.0 mV.

WAVEFORMS. The waveforms and intervals of the ECG are shown in Figure 42–15. The P wave is the electrical activity recorded during atrial depolarization and, in the normal ECG, precedes ventricular depolarization. The QRS complex occurs during ventricular depolarization. The Q wave is the initial downward deflection, the R wave is the initial upward deflection, and the S wave is the second downward deflection. A second upward deflection or a third downward deflection is defined as R′ or S′, respectively. A Q, R, and S may not be present in each lead; e.g., if the entire lead is negative, it is termed a QS wave. The time from the onset of the P wave to the beginning of ventricular depolarization is the PR interval; normally the range is 0.12 to 0.20 second. The QRS duration is normally less than 0.10 second. The T wave is inscribed during the period of ventricular repolarization. The electrical activity during atrial repolarization is usually masked by the QRS complex. The interval from the end of ventricular depolarization to the beginning of the T wave is termed the ST segment. The interval from the onset of ventricular depolarization to the end of the T wave is the QT interval. This interval is a function of rate. A small deflection following the T wave is the U wave; the precise origin of this waveform is unknown.

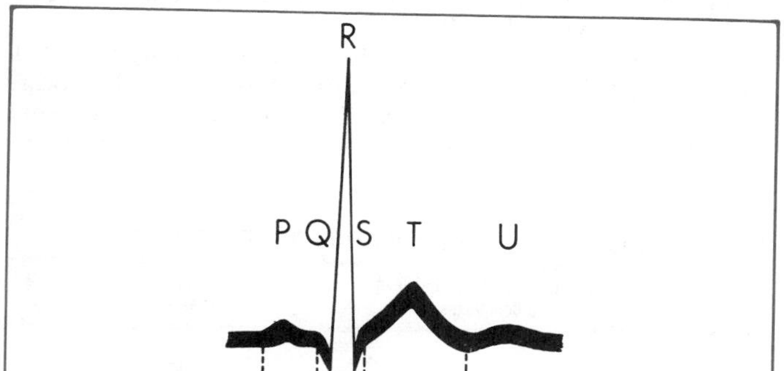

FIGURE 42–15. The ECG waveforms and intervals (horizontal bars) are illustrated. For description, see text.

LEARNING ELECTROCARDIOGRAPHY. There are two general approaches to learning electrocardiography: (1) the pattern recognition method and (2) the spatial vector approach. In the former, the student memorizes the multiple normal and abnormal waveforms for each lead and gains the necessary expertise through experience in interpreting a large number of ECG's with clinical correlation. This technique is used by all experienced electrocardiographers, and illustrations of this approach are provided in the legends of Figures 42–18 to 42–22. In the spatial vector approach, popularized by R. P. Grant, the waveform is reduced to a vector representing the magnitude and direction of the mean electrical forces of P, QRS, and T. Using this technique, the student can quickly learn to define the normal ECG and the major abnormalities. This approach is based on the fact that the magnitude of a wave in any lead is a function of the relationship between the electrical axis of the heart and that lead (Fig. 42–16). From the hexaxial reference system of the six frontal plane leads illustrated in Figure 42–13, the spatial vector approach can be used to obtain the mean frontal plane axis for the normal electrocardiogram (Fig. 42–14). The QRS complex is upright (positive) in lead I; thus the mean axis must be between +90 degrees and −90 degrees—i.e., on the positive side of a line perpendicular to lead I. Since the QRS complex is also positive in leads II and III, the axis must be between +30 and +90 degrees. Since the mean QRS complex is slightly negative in lead aV_L, the mean QRS vector is approximately +70 degrees. A similar determination then can be made for P and T waves. In the frontal plane, the mean P vector should be between 0 and +80 degrees, and the mean QRS and T vectors should lie between −30 and +90 degrees. A mean QRS vector more negative than −30 degrees is considered left-axis deviation and more positive than +90 degrees is defined as right-axis deviation. The angle between the mean QRS and T vectors in the frontal plane should be less than 80 degrees. Application of the spatial vector tech-

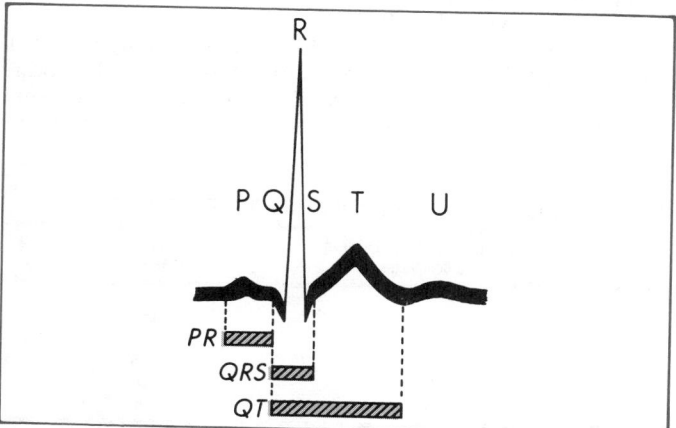

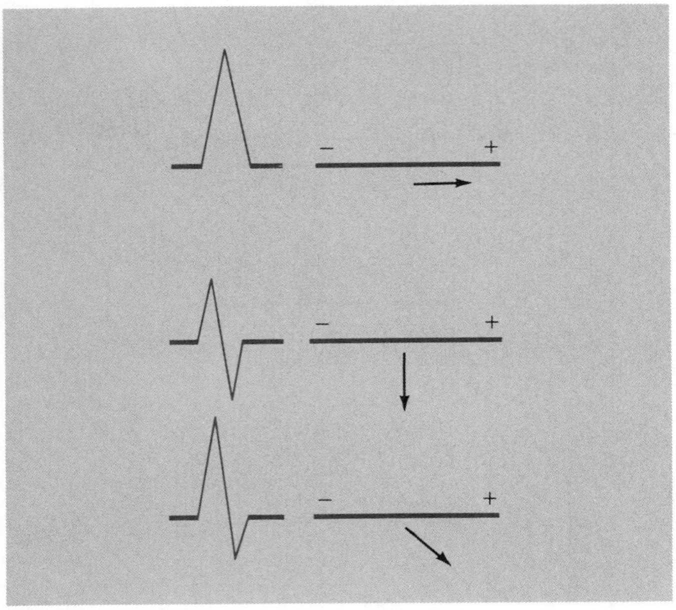

FIGURE 42–16. Determination of the relationship between the mean electrical axis of a wave and the waveform in a given lead. The top row depicts an entirely positive waveform; thus, the axis is parallel to the lead. In the second row the waveform is biphasic and the summation of the positive and negative parts is zero. In this instance, the mean electrical axis of the wave is perpendicular to the lead. (Note that the arrow could be drawn in the opposite direction and still be perpendicular to the lead.) In the third row, a biphasic waveform is shown in which the majority of the area is positive. The mean electrical axis is roughly at a 45-degree angle to the lead.

TABLE 42–2. DIAGNOSTIC CATEGORIES IN WHICH AN ECG IS USEFUL

Arrhythmias	+ +
Electronic pacemaker function	+ +
Intraventricular conduction disturbances	+ +
Chamber enlargement	
Left and right atrial enlargement	+
Left and right ventricular hypertrophy	+
Myocardial infarction	
Old	+
Acute	+
Myocardial ischemia	+
Pericardial disease	
Pericarditis	±
Pericardial tamponade	±
Electrolyte disturbances	
Hypo- and hyperkalemia	+
Hypo- and hypercalcemia	+
Miscellaneous disorders	
Congenital heart disease	±
Muscular dystrophy	±
Emphysema and/or cor pulmonale	±
Pulmonary emboli	±
Hypothermia	±
Myxedema	±
Drug effects	
Antidysrhythmic drugs (e.g., quinidine)	±
Digitalis	±
Antineoplastic agents (e.g., doxorubicin)	±
Phenothiazine derivatives (e.g., chlorpromazine)	±
Antidepressant drugs (e.g., amitriptyline)	±
Antiparasitic compounds (e.g., emetine)	±

The symbols indicate the necessity for ECG to establish diagnosis:
+ + ECG is essential for diagnosis.
+ ECG is important for diagnosis.
± ECG may be useful for diagnosis.

nique to the transverse plane is somewhat more difficult, since the six precordial leads do not define a precise reference system. An estimate of the vector can be obtained by noting when the waveforms make their transition from a negative to a positive deflection. In a normal ECG, the QRS transition is between V_2 and V_5, and the T wave makes its transition before the QRS. The next step is to determine the direction of the initial 0.04 second vector of the QRS. It is this portion of the QRS that defines the presence of myocardial infarction. The initial 0.04 second vector should lie between 0 and +90 degrees in the frontal plane; outside this range it suggests myocardial infarction (see Fig. 42–19). The direction of the terminal 0.04 second vector is used to aid in the diagnosis of ventricular conduction abnormalities (see Fig. 42–21).

APPROACH TO INTERPRETING AN ECG. The diagnostic categories in which an ECG may be useful are outlined in Table 42–2. In interpreting an ECG, it is important to develop a routine so that each aspect of the recording is carefully analyzed. Since the waveforms of the ECG are influenced to a certain extent by the age and body habitus of the patient, this information should be available to the electrocardiographer. The following eight sequential steps are necessary for proper ECG interpretation.

1. *Quality of the ECG recording.* This includes proper standardization (Fig. 42–17), lead placement (Fig. 42–18), and identification of significant artifact. The student must learn to evaluate the quality of the recording and not interpret an inadequately recorded ECG. Serious misdiagnosis can result if the quality of the ECG is ignored.

2. *Measurements.* The heart rate can be estimated adequately by employing the method outlined in Table 42–3. The amplitude, duration, and intervals of the various waveforms are usually measured in the standard frontal plane limb leads. Abnormality of the QRS duration, PR interval, and QT interval also is determined in these leads. Proper measurement of the waveforms is enhanced by simultaneous recording of three leads, since the inter-relationships between the waveforms can be easily seen. The QT interval must be corrected for heart rate. The corrected QT interval (QT_c) is given by Bazet's formula:

$$QT_c = \frac{QT}{\sqrt{\text{RR interval (seconds)}}}$$

and should be between 0.33 and 0.47 second.

3. *Determination of rhythm.*

4. *Examination of P wave.* Determine if atrial enlargement (see Fig. 42–20) or intra-atrial block is present.

5. *Examination of QRS.* Determine if myocardial infarction (Fig. 42–19), ventricular hypertrophy (Fig. 42–20), or ventricular conduction defect (Fig. 42–21) is present.

6. *Examination of ST segment.* Determine if subendocardial (Fig. 42–22) or epicardial (Fig. 42–19) injury is present; abnormal displacement of the ST segment is defined by convention as injury. The ST segment is shortened in hypercalcemia and prolonged in hypocalcemia.

7. *Examination of T wave.* Defining the significance of T wave abnormalities is the most difficult aspect of electrocardiography. In general, marked T wave abnormalities that occur either without other ECG abnormalities or with myo-

TABLE 42–3. DETERMINATION OF HEART RATE

Interval in Large Boxes Between Two Complexes	Heart Rate (beats/min)
1	300
2	150
3	100
4	75
5	60
6	50

The ECG recording paper is marked vertically by light lines; every fifth line is heavily marked. The time increment separating two heavy lines (one large box) is 0.20 second. To determine the rate rapidly, note the interval between two complexes and estimate the rate from this table.

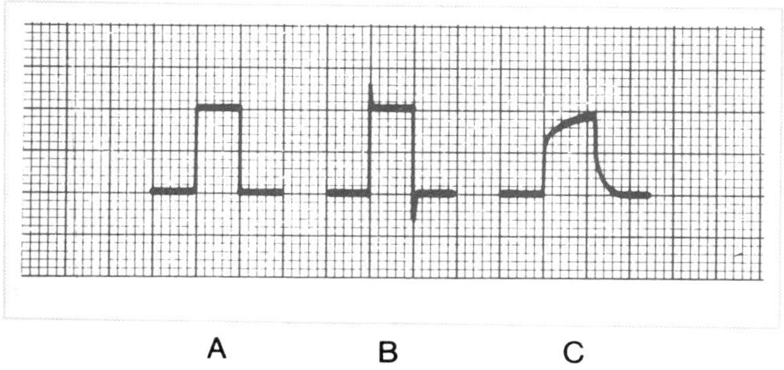

FIGURE 42–17. In *A*, a correct standardization having a true square wave response is illustrated. *B* represents a standardization obtained from an instrument in which the response is underdamped; the amplitude of the waves will be spuriously enhanced. In *C*, the recorder is overdamped, resulting in both a spuriously decreased amplitude and an increased width of the waveform.

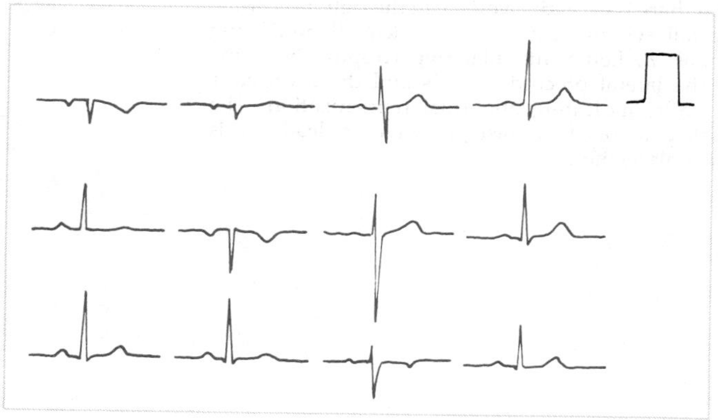

FIGURE 42–18. Two examples of incorrect lead placement from the same patient illustrated in Figure 42–14. Both the left and right arm leads and chest leads V1, 2, 3 are reversed. Reversal of the arm lead results in a mirror image recording of lead I and is easily recognized, since the P wave is negative. If missed, a spurious diagnosis of lateral wall infarction may be made. Reversal of the right precordial leads may result in an incorrect diagnosis of either right ventricular hypertrophy or posterior wall infarction.

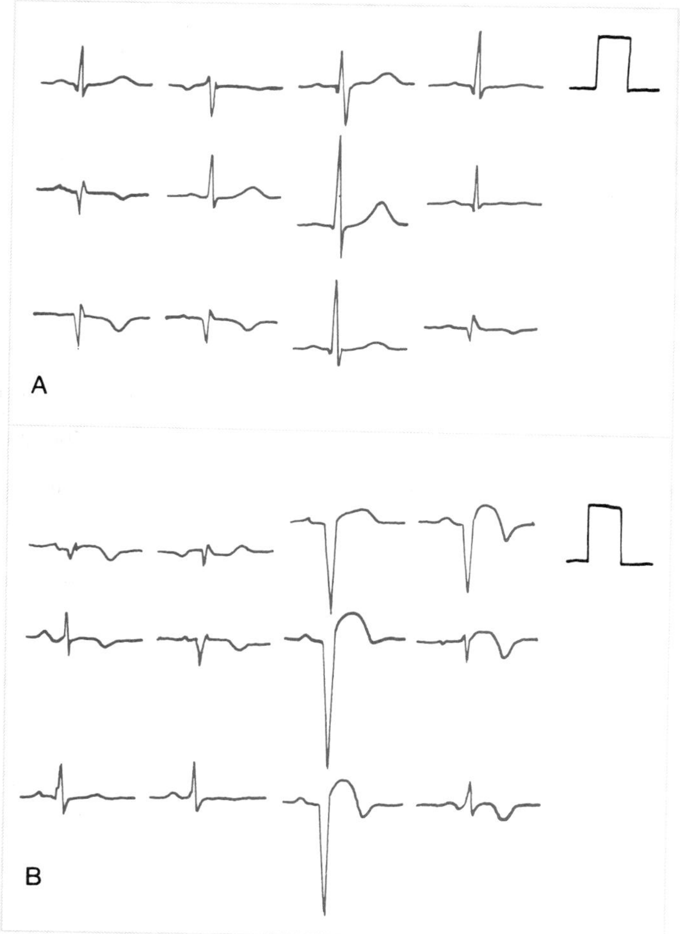

FIGURE 42–19. The ECG lead sets are recorded in the same sequence as in Figure 42–14. *A*, Inferior and posterior infarction. Note the abnormal superiorly and anteriorly directed initial forces, i.e., significant Q waves in leads II, III, and AVF, and a broad R wave in V1. Note the concomitant negative T waves in the same frontal plane leads (inferior ischemia). *B*, Anterolateral myocardial infarction. The initial forces are posterior and to the right, i.e., extensive Q waves in leads I, AVL, and V1 through V4. Also note the concomitant ST segment elevation (epicardial injury) and T wave inversion (anterior ischemia) in the precordial leads, indicating that the myocardial infarction is probably acute.

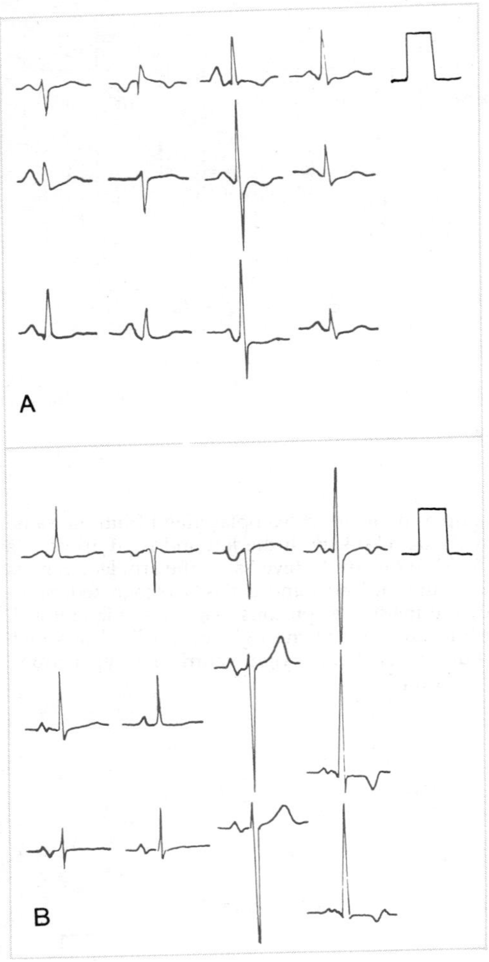

FIGURE 42–20. *A*, Right ventricular hypertrophy. The mean frontal plane axis is to the right, and there is excessive voltage in the right precordial leads. Also note the tall symmetrical P wave in lead II, indicating right atrial enlargement. *B*, Left ventricular hypertrophy. Note the excessive voltage in the lateral precordial leads and the inverted T waves in the same leads, indicating abnormal repolarization. The wide (greater than 0.12 second) biphasic P wave in lead V1 is indicative of left atrial enlargement.

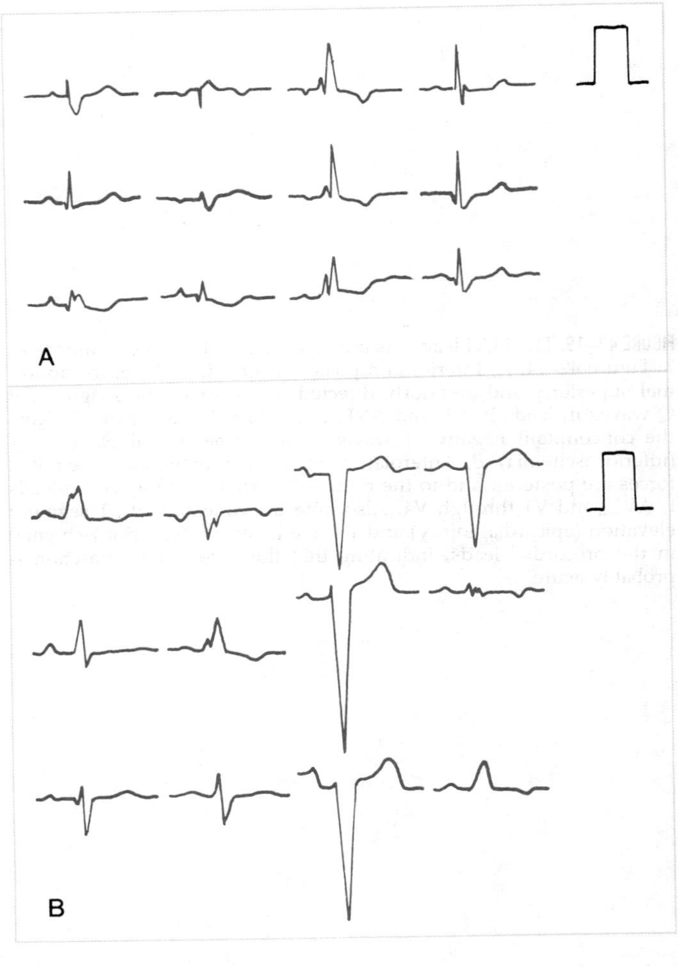

FIGURE 42–21. *A*, Right bundle branch block. The QRS duration is greater than 0.12 second, and the axis of the terminal 0.04 second of the QRS is to the right and anterior. *B*, Left bundle branch block. The QRS duration is greater than 0.12 second, and the terminal 0.04 second of the QRS is to the left and posterior. Note the secondary T wave changes in leads I and V6.

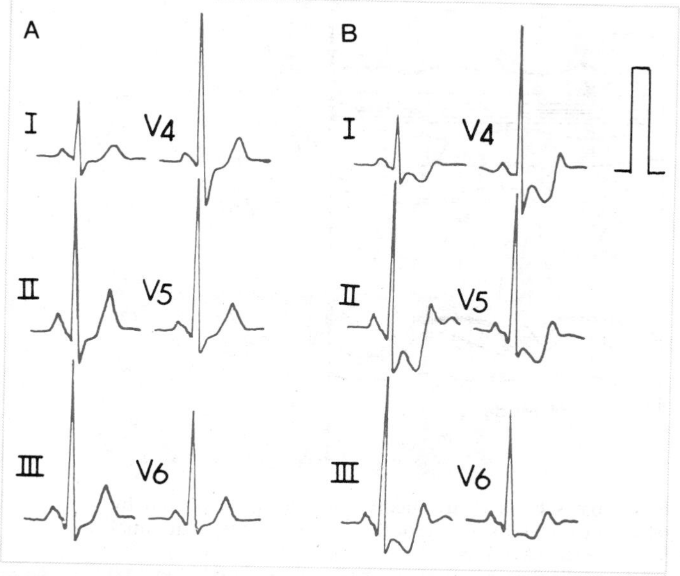

FIGURE 42–22. Recording obtained (*A*) prior to and (*B*) during an exercise test. Note the depression and downward sloping of the S-T segment wave during exercise. This is a typical pattern of subendocardial injury.

cardial infarction are defined as ischemic or primary T wave changes (Fig. 42–19). T wave abnormalities that occur with conduction defects or ventricular hypertrophy are spoken of as secondary. Abnormal T waves are seen in hypertrophy (Fig. 42–20). The T waves also are important in the diagnosis of drug effects and electrolyte abnormalities.

8. *Comparison with patient's previous ECG's.* It is extremely important to compare a new tracing with a previous electrocardiogram for two reasons: (1) although the ECG may still be within the normal range, significant changes may have occurred since the previous record; and (2) a comparison allows the electrocardiographer to date specific abnormalities and may have important therapeutic implications.

COMPUTER INTERPRETATION OF THE ECG. The development of algorithms to process and interpret ECG's has progressed to the point that, at present, there are several acceptable programs available for routine clinical use. Although these programs are helpful in decreasing processing time, they must be viewed as an assist device to the electrocardiographer and not as a replacement.

OTHER RECORDING TECHNIQUES. Several of the other ECG recording techniques and their uses are described in Table 42–4.

The vectorcardiogram (VCG) is used to obtain a true orthogonal lead system (XYZ leads) so that the cardiac dipole is in the center of the chest. The most commonly employed lead system was devised by E. Frank. It is time consuming to record a VCG properly, and for this reason the VCG has not been generally accepted in clinical medicine. The VCG is primarily beneficial in teaching electrocardiography and in

TABLE 42–4. DIAGNOSTIC USES OF OTHER ECG RECORDING TECHNIQUES

Vectorcardiograms: old myocardial infarction, ventricular hypertrophy, ventricular conduction abnormalities
Body surface mapping: precise definition of instantaneous depolarization and repolarization—primarily experimental at present
Exercise electrocardiography: transient subendocardial or transmural injury
Ambulatory monitoring: arrhythmias, transient subendocardial injury
Transtelephone monitoring: arrhythmias, pacemaker function
His bundle recordings: arrhythmias and conduction defects
Esophageal leads: arrhythmias

enhancing the diagnosis of myocardial infarction, conduction defects, and ventricular hypertrophy.

A further refinement of this approach is body surface mapping, in which multiple precordial leads are obtained and a computer is utilized to generate a continuous body surface map of the change in electrical potential during depolarization and repolarization. These techniques are still in the experimental stage, but ultimately may prove to be important in obtaining the maximal information available from the electrical activation of the heart.

The ECG stress test is a widely used physiologic technique designed to assess the ability of the coronary circulation to deliver oxygen at a rate commensurate with the metabolic needs of the myocardium. Because myocardial metabolism is almost entirely aerobic, an inadequate increase in coronary flow quickly results in ischemia of the inner layers of the heart. The concomitant ST segment changes have been empirically defined as subendocardial injury. The characteristic ST segment response is a flat (square wave) or downward-sloping ST segment of 0.1 mV or greater measured 0.08 second after the end of the QRS complex (Fig. 42–22).

Chou TC, Helm RA: Clinical Vectorcardiography. 2nd ed. New York, Grune & Stratton, 1974. *Complete coverage of vectorcardiography.*

Lipman BS, Massie E, Kleiger RE: Clinical Scalar Electrocardiography. 6th ed. Chicago, Year Book Medical Publishers, 1973. *Excellent general text covering all phases of electrocardiography.*

Marriott HJL: Practical Electrocardiography. 7th ed. Baltimore, Williams & Wilkins, 1983. *A comprehensive description of electrocardiography.*

42.3 Echocardiography

Richard L. Popp

PULSED REFLECTED ULTRASOUND

Echocardiography includes a family of diagnostic procedures that use ultrahigh-frequency sound waves to record the structure of the heart, and the blood flow velocities within the heart, throughout the cardiac cycle. Sound frequencies in the range of 1 to 10 million cycles per second, or megaHertz (MHz), are transmitted from a piezoelectric crystal along a carefully defined path within the thorax. A transducer is placed on the chest wall, and a short burst of ultrasound is transmitted through the chest and into the underlying cardiac structures. The transducer then acts as a sound receiver until the next pulse. At each interface of materials with differing acoustic impedance, part of the sound is reflected or refracted and the remaining sound energy is further transmitted for subsequent acoustic reflection. The acoustic reflecting interfaces oriented perpendicular to the path of sound travel produce reflected sound that is received by the transducer on the chest wall as an "echo" of the transmitted sound. The location of each reflecting surface relative to the transducer can be calculated from the known velocity of sound in tissue and the elapsed time between sound transmission and reception of the echo. This series of depth readings is displayed on an oscilloscope for each pulse of sound, as shown in Figure 42–23. The strength of each echo is indicated by the brightness of the signal on the display device. Blood within the heart chambers usually gives signals of low amplitude that are not displayed. This "brightness-modulated" (B-mode) record of the reflecting interfaces is the building block for both two-dimensional (2D) and time-motion (M-mode) echocardiography.

One thousand pulses per second are created with typical instruments used clinically. A high sampling rate facilitates tracking motion of cardiac structures, yet there is usually enough time for the sound to return from even the most distant reflectors before the next pulse. Sequentially directing

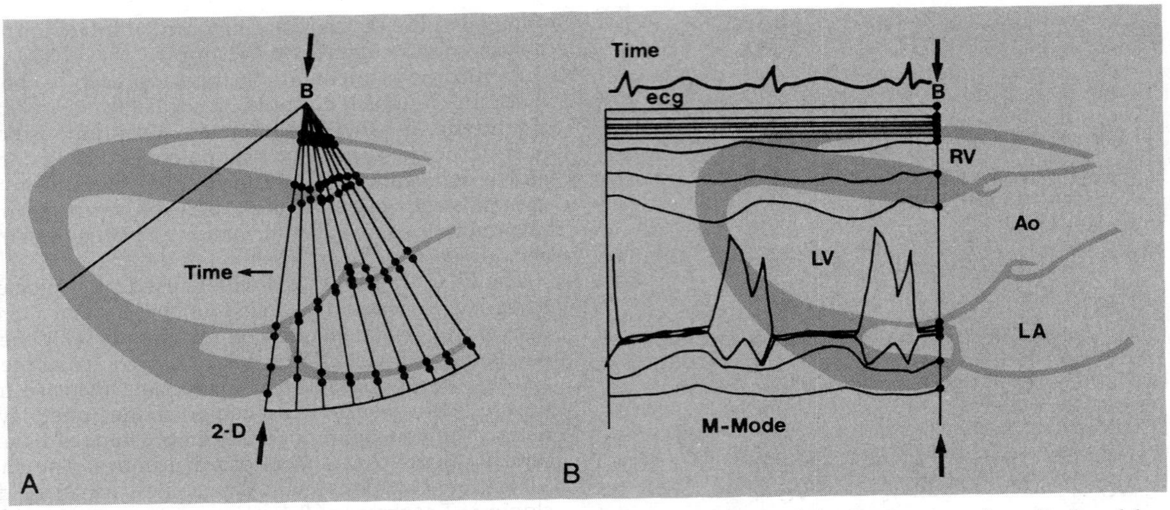

FIGURE 42–23. *A*, A schematic two-dimensional (2-D) image of a cross-section of the heart oriented as displayed by echocardiography. The sound transducer is located on the anterior chest wall to the left of the sternum, at B. Sequential sound pulses and the returning echoes from reflecting interfaces are displayed as individual lines (*large arrows*), with dots of light defining the loci of reflectors. B = brightness-modulated display. Many such lines, accumulated over 1/60 to 1/15 second, make up a single 2-D image. *B*, A schematic time-motion (M-mode) echocardiogram produced by tracing out the location of structures moving during the cardiac cycle under a stationary sound transducer. As in *A*, the transducer on the chest wall creates a B-mode (B, *arrows*) display of sequential pulses and traces the motion pattern of each echo-producing interface. The M- and W-shaped patterns represent the anterior and posterior mitral valve leaflets, respectively. Ao = Aorta; ecg = electrocardiogram; LA = left atrium; LV = left ventricle; RV = right ventricle. (Modified from Popp RL, Rubenson DS, Tucker CR, et al: Echocardiography: M-mode and two-dimensional methods. Ann Intern Med 93:844, 1980.)

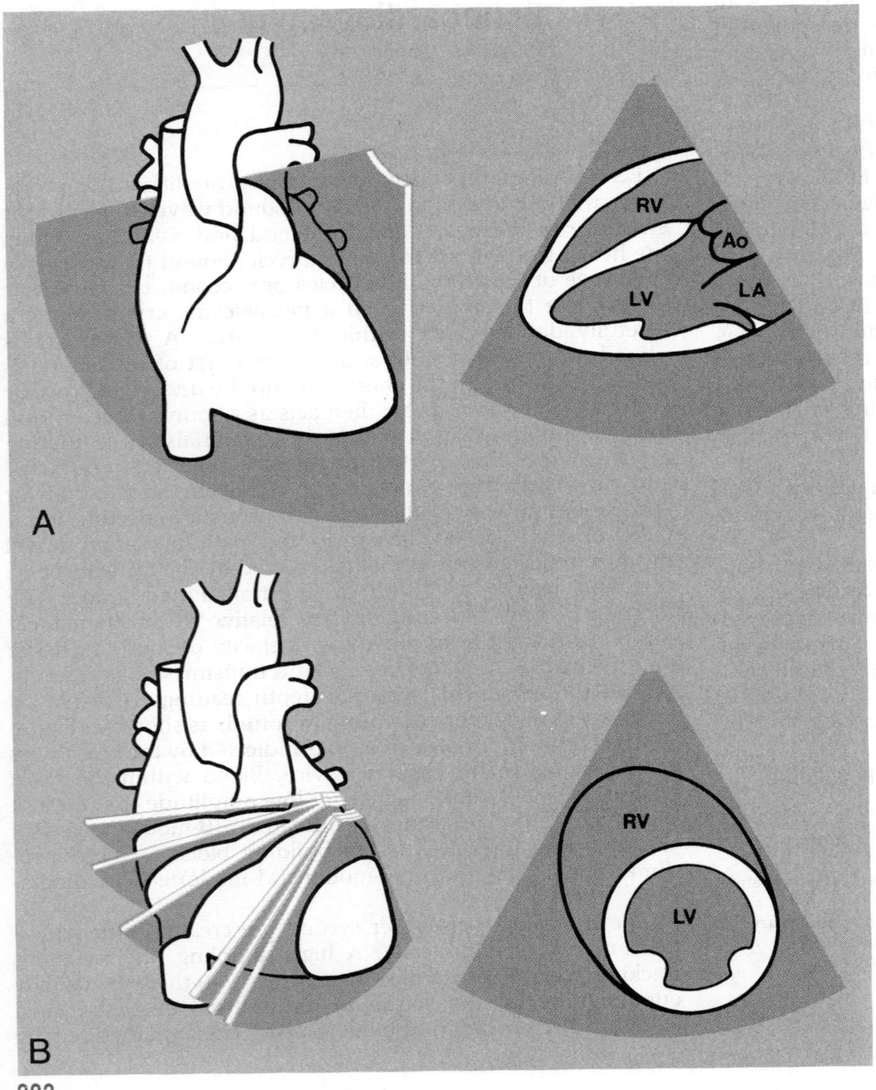

FIGURE 42–24. Schematic illustration of some standard 2-D imaging planes used for clinical cardiac studies. *A*, Parasternal transducer position, with the imaging plane oriented parallel to the long axis of the left ventricle (LV) and intersecting a portion of the right ventricular outflow tract (RV), aortic root (Ao), and left atrium (LA). *B*, Transducer position as in *A*, but the imaging planes (six illustrated) are oriented parallel to the left ventricular short axis.

Illustration continued on opposite page

the sound beam along a given path, usually a pie-shaped sector of a circular plane, for each successive pulse produces a two-dimensional map of the structures underlying the transducer, called a two-dimensional (2D) echocardiogram (Fig. 42–23). Clinical instruments sweep the sound beam through an arc of 60 to 90 degrees, by electronic or mechanical means, to create an imaging plane for visualizing a cross-section of the heart. Thus each 2D ultrasonic image is made up of multiple individual lines of sound reflection information. Depending on the basic pulse repetition rate, the time required for a single sound pulse to travel round trip through the thorax, and the number of such pulses per 2D image, 15 to 60 individual 2D image frames per second are available for interpretation. The images usually are presented on a digital scan converter that interpolates data between the scan lines and gives the impression of watching the heart in motion. The standardized examination provides multiple 2D cross-sectional planes through all parts of the heart using specific transducer locations, as shown in Figure 42–24. The dynamic three-dimensional structure of the heart can be understood by mentally assembling these multiple slices. An electrocardiogram is included as a reference signal in these studies.

A single direction of the sound beam, within the 2D image, may be selected for special attention and very high sampling rate. In this case, a given sound beam direction is repeatedly sampled, and the motion along the path of the sound beam is displayed with respect to time. The usual display is on an oscilloscope or strip chart recorder and is called a time-motion, T-M, or M-mode echocardiogram (right panel, Fig. 42–23). This method of recording is especially useful for identifying precise timing of motion of cardiac structures, such as valves, with respect to the electrocardiogram, phonocardiogram, or Doppler echocardiogram (to be described below). Historically, the M-mode echocardiogram was the first to be used.

Normal or abnormal patterns of cardiac chamber size and connection, wall thickness, wall motion, valve structure, and valve motion all are well assessed by echocardiographic study (Figs. 42–25 and 42–26). It is the method of choice for visualizing many abnormal structures, such as vegetations of infective endocarditis, intracardiac tumors, mural thrombi, and pericardial fluid.

During acute and chronic ventricular ischemia and acute infarction, the echocardiographic images accurately show the extent of myocardial thinning and segmental akinesis or dyskinesis. Exercise-induced segmental abnormalities may be observed as well. The acute complications of myocardial infarction that may be detected by imaging and Doppler echocardiography include pericardial effusion with or without cardiac tamponade, flail mitral leaflet (ruptured papillary muscle), acute mitral regurgitation of papillary muscle dysfunction, acute ventricular septal defect, myocardial rupture with pseudoaneurysm formation, infarct expansion producing true aneurysm, and right ventricular infarction.

Echocardiographic imaging also may be performed "invasively," as when transesophageal transducers are used or during thoracotomy with direct application of the transducer to the epicardium. These approaches produce superb images owing both to lack of sound scattering in the thorax and to the feasibility of using very high-frequency (5 to 10 MHz) ultrasound, which has high physical resolution but poor soft tissue penetration. Intravenous injections of many fluids, such as physiologic saline solution, contain myriad microbubbles of gas, which may be visualized by echocardiography as they travel through the right side of the heart. The gas does not

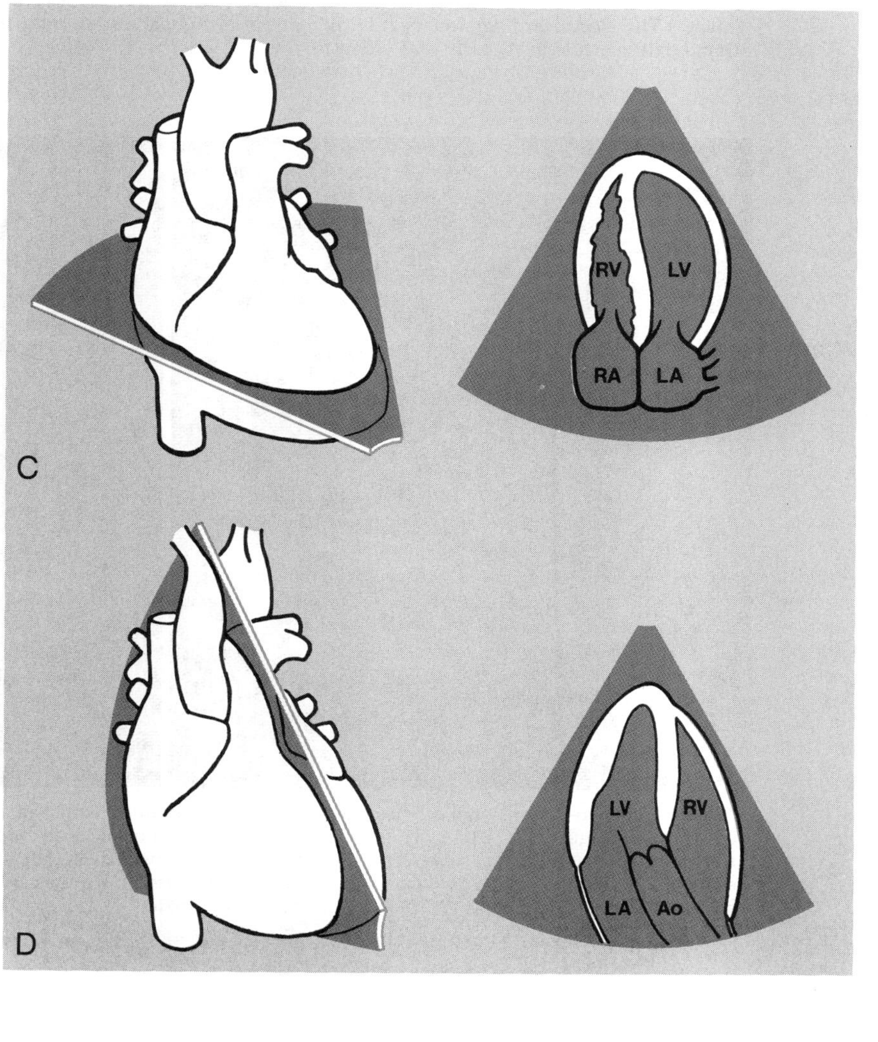

FIGURE 42–24 *Continued C,* Apical transducer position, with the imaging plane oriented to show the four main chambers of the heart (4-chamber view). The 2-D image is displayed relative to the transducer so that the cardiac apex is shown near the transducer. RA = right atrium. *D,* Transducer position as in C, but the imaging plane is oriented parallel to the left ventricular long axis, as in panel *A.* (Redrawn from Popp RL, Fowles RE, Coltart DJ, et al.: Cardiac anatomy viewed systematically with two-dimensional echocardiography. Chest 75:579, 1979.)

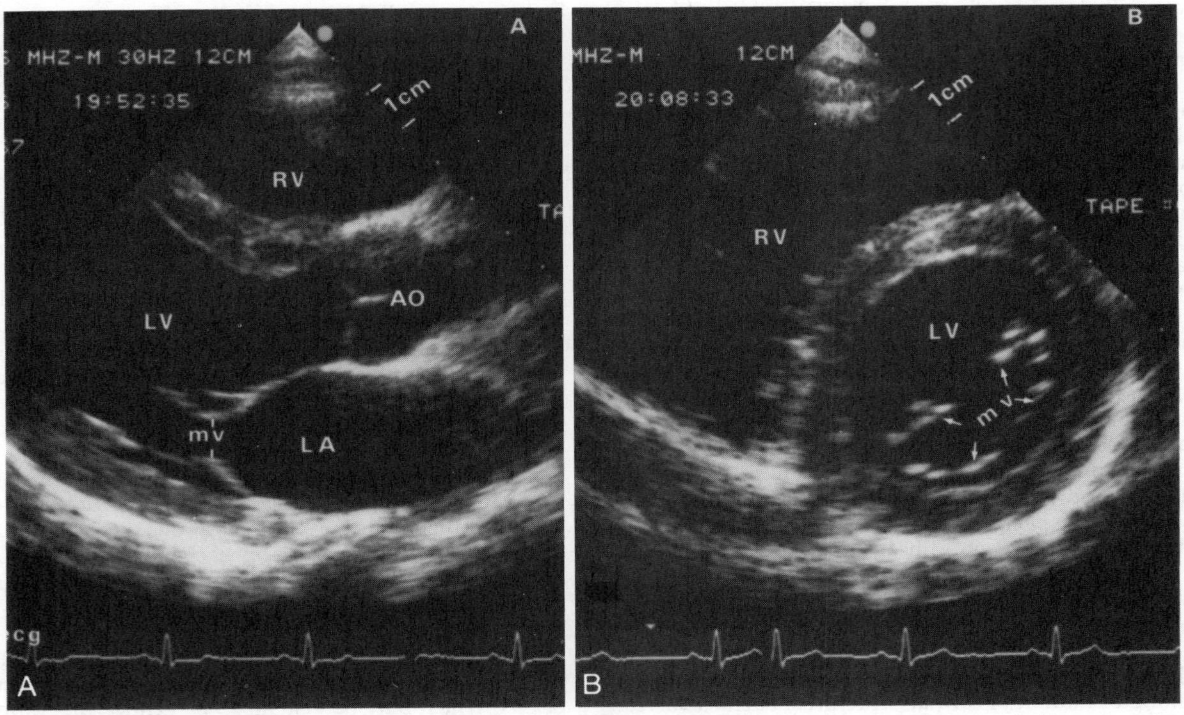

FIGURE 42–25. Two-dimensional echocardiographic images of a normal heart. Panels *A* and *B* were obtained with transducer positions and imaging plane orientations as shown in Figure 42–24*A* and *B*, respectively. Abbreviations as in Figure 42–24. mv = Mitral valve leaflets. (Note depth calibration scale at 1-cm intervals along right margin of each image.) The electrocardiograms (ecg) at the bottom of the panels are interrupted to indicate the timing of each image frame (late diastole in *A*, early diastole in *B*).

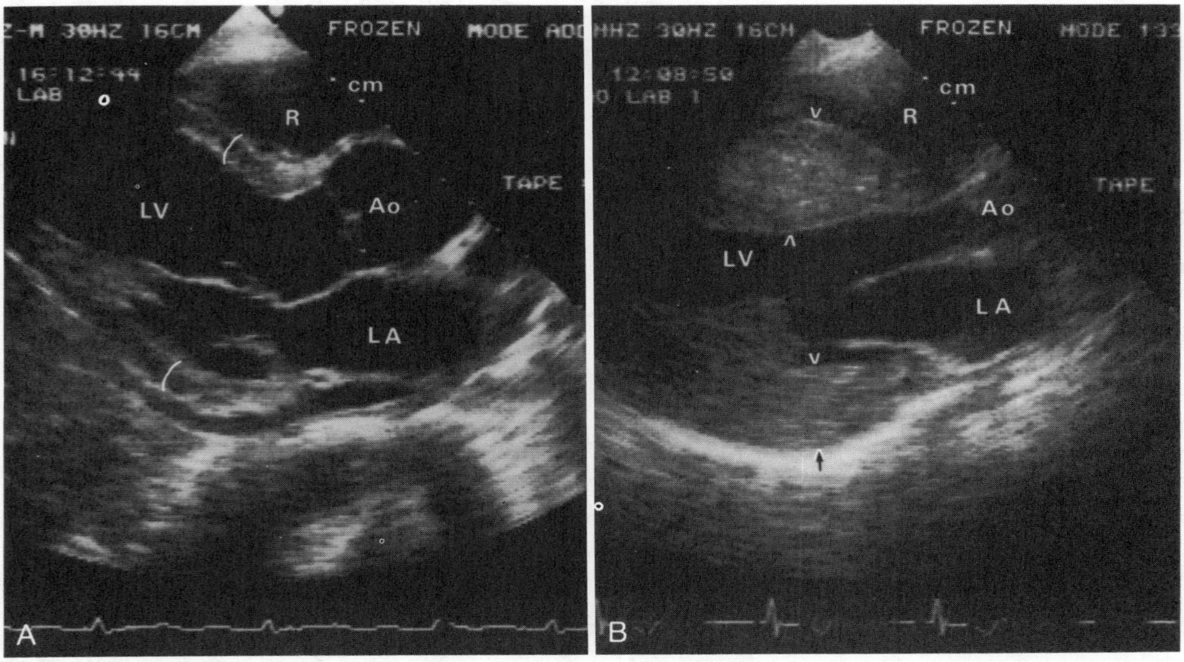

FIGURE 42–26. Two-dimensional echocardiographic images obtained with transducer position and image plane orientation as shown in Figure 42–24*A*. *A*, The left ventricle (LV) has normal wall thickness (white brackets). A relatively echo-free space posterior to the lower bracket, and extending toward the left atrium (LA), represents a small pericardial effusion. *B*, The LV cavity is small and the walls (*arrowheads*) are massively thickened in a patient with concentric hypertrophic cardiomyopathy. Ao = Aorta; cm = centimeter scale; R = right ventricle.

pass through the pulmonary capillary bed, so if microbubble echoes are seen immediately in the left side of the heart, one may assume an intracardiac shunt is present, and a delayed appearance implies an intrapulmonary shunt. Direct intra-aortic or intracoronary injection of various contrast agents has been used in attempts to visualize coronary perfusion areas of the left ventricle and experimentally to assess washout rates with altered coronary flow.

DOPPLER ULTRASOUND

Sound energy is transmitted as a series of compression-rarefaction waves with a given periodicity or wave frequency. Sound reflected from stationary surfaces has the same basic frequency as the transmitted sound, as shown in Figure 42–27. However, if the reflector or reflectors are moving relative to the direction of sound transmissions, the sequential interaction of the compression-rarefaction waves with the reflector results in a change in the frequency of the sound, as shown in Figure 42–27. This frequency shift is the Doppler effect, and it enables calculation of the velocity of the reflector if one knows the originally transmitted frequency, the received frequency, the speed of sound in the medium (soft tissues), and the angle between the sound beam and the direction of the moving reflectors. The moving column of blood, with its cells and fluctuations in spatial distribution of cells, is the source of the Doppler frequency shift measured by echocardiography. An indicator of the beam direction undergoing Doppler frequency analysis is superimposed on the 2D image to help orientation and facilitate placing the beam in the general direction of flow. Fortunately, the change in frequency obtained with clinical instruments is in the audible range, so one may optimally match the direction of the sound beam with the direction of the blood flow by adjusting the transducer while listening to the signal. A beam-to-flow angle of zero degrees is desirable, since the calculated velocity is a function of the cosine of this angle ($\cos 0° = 1$), but an angle of up to 20 degrees produces underestimation of velocities of up to only 6 per cent.

Blood flow toward or away from the transducer produces an increase or decrease in sound frequency, respectively, so both the velocity and the direction of the blood are measurable. These signals are usually displayed with velocites calculated from received Doppler shifted frequencies plotted versus time. The velocity spectrum is arranged above or below a baseline to convey information on flow direction, as shown in Figures 42–28 and 42–29.

Pulsed wave (PW) Doppler echocardiography is performed with pulses of ultrasound as described above, and frequency analysis is possible for sound returning from any given distance from the transducer. Thus, a signal received during systole from the left atrium and indicating high-velocity flow directed into the atrium from the ventricle signifies mitral regurgitation. This technique has proved especially valuable in locating intracardiac shunts, such as atrial or ventricular septal defects (Fig. 42–28) and patent ductus arteriosus. Since the product of the mean flow velocity (centimeters per second) and cross-sectional flow area (square centimeters) is volumetric flow (cubic centimeters per second), flow within the pulmonary artery or left ventricular outflow tract, or across the tricuspid or mitral valves, can be estimated. Comparison of flows across the pulmonary artery and aorta give an estimate of shunt flow across the septal defects, for example. Measurement of cardiac output by this method is useful clinically; however, the procedure is technically demanding.

PW methods provide spatial resolution but have limited velocity resolution because of the physical-mathematical constraints of sampling periodically. This trade-off is the opposite of that with continuous wave (CW) Doppler echocardiography, which uses one transducer to transmit, and another to receive, reflected sound continuously. CW Doppler methods have no spatial resolution within the path of the beam but can display frequency shifts corresponding to very high flow velocities. A major series of applications of Doppler echocardiography derives from the relationship of measured velocities to corresponding drops in pressure within the heart or vascular system. A cardiac valve stenosis presents an obstacle to flowing blood, which results in an increased velocity through the area of obstruction. This convective acceleration is the major factor producing a drop in pressure (ΔP, or pressure gradient) across the stenosis. The pressure difference can be accurately estimated instantaneously by CW Doppler echocardiography from the maximum flow velocity (V) achieved ($\Delta P = 4V^2$), as first shown by Holen and coworkers (1976). The ability to obtain intracardiac and intravascular pressure information noninvasively has been a significant advance in the capabilities of echocardiography. Many patients with aortic or mitral stenosis or both now have adequate preoperative hemodynamic assessment on the basis of clinical features and echocardiography only. The method for calculating instantaneous and mean pressure drops across a stenotic aortic valve is shown in Figure 42–29.

The pressure drop across a stenotic valve is dependent on both the valve area and the blood volume crossing the valve per unit of time. Aortic valve area is accurately estimated by applying the Gorlin formula (see Ch. 42.5) using Doppler ultrasound–derived values for ejection time, stroke volume, and pressure gradient. Alternatively, one may calculate the flow per beat (see above) from the mean flow velocity and

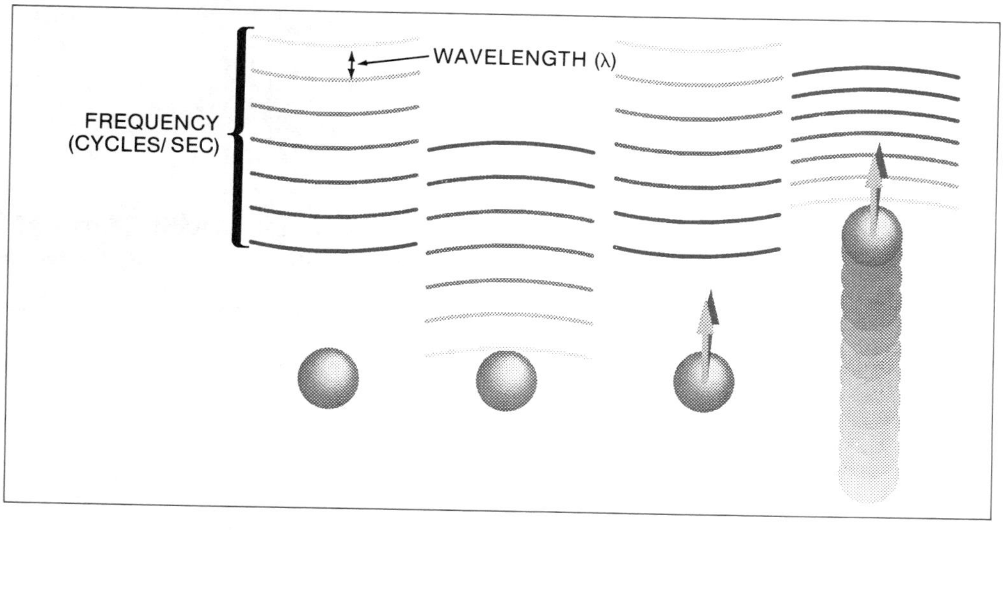

FIGURE 42–27. Schematic diagram of the Doppler principle as applied in echocardiography. From left to right: Sound waves of a given frequency (cycles/sec) and wave length (λ) are transmitted into the chest. Sound reflected from a stationary target has the same frequency as that transmitted. Sound directed toward a moving target will interact with the reflector and alter the frequency of the returning sound by a factor related to the speed of the moving target, the original sound frequency, and the angle of interception of the two.

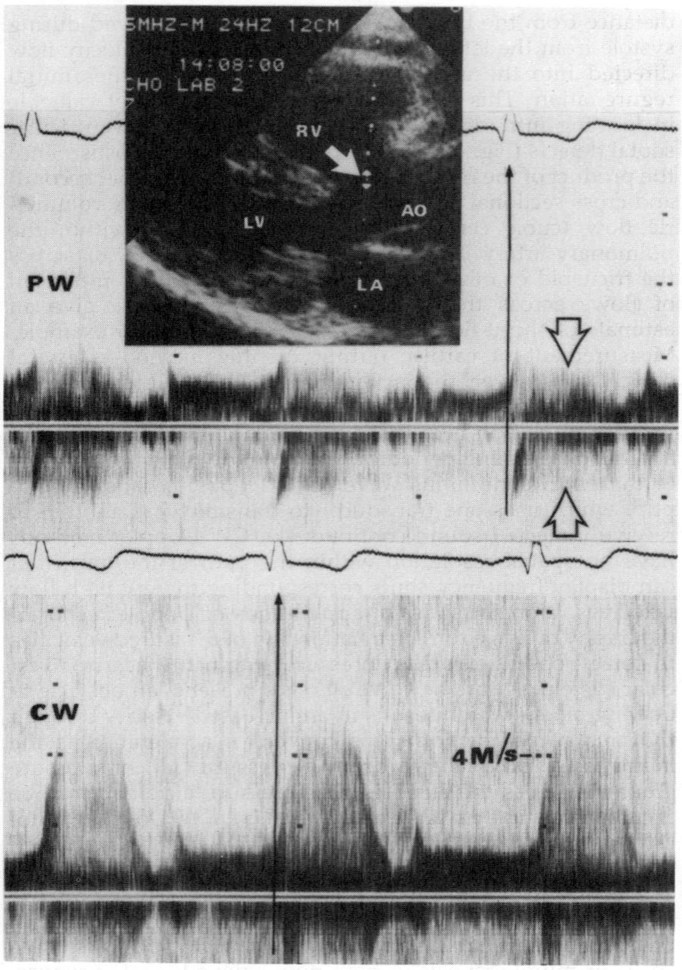

FIGURE 42–28. Methods of displaying a Doppler echocardiographic study in a patient with ventricular septal defect. The black panel above is a 2-D image taken with transducer position and image plane orientation as in Figure 42–24A. The white arrow points to the sample volume indicator for pulsed-wave (PW) Doppler ultrasound analysis. This illustration is from a patient with a large defect of the septum between the right ventricle (RV) and left ventricle (LV). The white panels below are spectral displays of the Doppler ultrasound signals in a patient with a small ventricular septal defect. The PW record indicates a frequency shift (*open arrows*) from the area of the sample volume (above), which occurs in systole after the onset of the electrocardiographic QRS (*long arrow*). The continuous-wave (CW) record indicates high-velocity (>4 M/s) flow somewhere along the dotted line shown above. The systolic pressure difference between the right and left ventricles can be calculated from the CW signal as shown in Figure 42–29. The location of the signal origin is defined by PW, while the CW signal defines high-flow velocity quantitatively but is ambiguous regarding signal locus. Other abbreviations as in Figure 42–23.

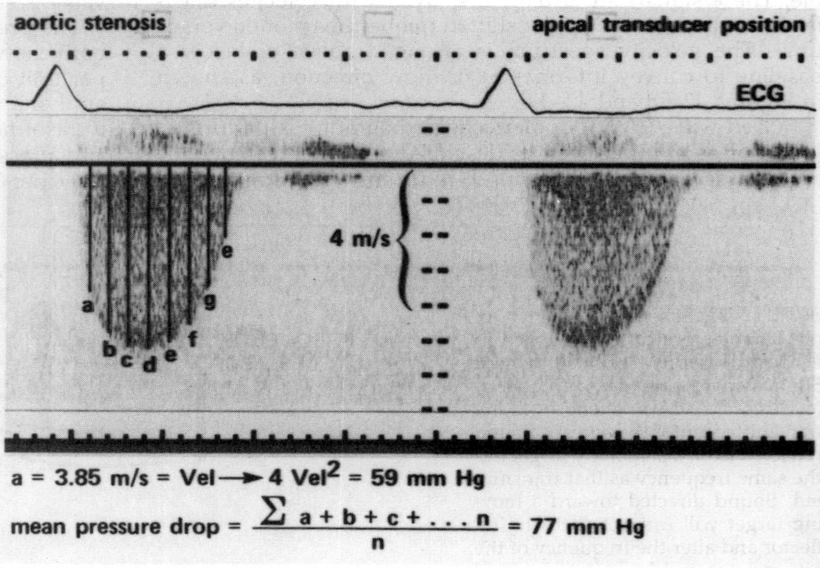

FIGURE 42–29. Continuous-wave Doppler ultrasound recording of aortic outflow velocities from a patient with aortic stenosis. The transducer is at the apex, so flow toward the aorta is registered below the baseline in this spectral display of velocity (M/s) vs. time. The systolic signal occurs after each QRS of the electrocardiogram (ECG). Instantaneous (vertical lines a through e) maximum velocities (Vel) are assumed to occur in the most narrow part of the stenosis and to correspond to instantaneous pressure drops across the stenosis. The formulae for calculating the instantaneous and mean pressure drops in mm Hg are given below. n = Number of samples.

$$a = 3.85 \text{ m/s} = \text{Vel} \longrightarrow 4\,\text{Vel}^2 = 59 \text{ mm Hg}$$

$$\text{mean pressure drop} = \frac{\sum a + b + c + \ldots n}{n} = 77 \text{ mm Hg}$$

cross-sectional area of the left ventricular outflow tract immediately below the stenotic valve and assume this same flow is represented by the product of the mean flow velocity within, and the cross-sectional area of, the stenotic valve. The outflow tract flow velocity, outflow tract area, and aortic valve flow velocity are obtainable, permitting calculation of the aortic valve area. This method is reliable even when aortic regurgitation is present. It is fortuitous that the time required for the pressure drop across the mitral valve to reach one half of the maximum level is directly related to the valve area at virtually all clinically relevant flows. Thus mitral valve area may be accurately calculated from data developed by Holen and colleagues (1977) without the necessity for measuring stroke volume.

Recording the velocity of blood flowing across a narrow orifice between any two chambers or cardiovascular loci permits calculation of the absolute pressure level in one chamber if the pressure in the other chamber is known. For example, the systolic pressure difference between the right ventricle and right atrium can be calculated from the velocities recorded from tricuspid regurgitant flow. The sum of jugular venous or right atrial pressure and the atrioventricular pressure difference is the right ventricular systolic pressure. The prevalence of tricuspid regurgitation detectable by Doppler echocardiography sufficient to perform this calculation ranges from over 90 per cent (in normal subjects) to 80 per cent (in patients with cardiomyopathy and pulmonary hypertension). This concept is useful in assessing ventricular pressures in ventricular septal defect and is under investigation for several conditions. Quantitating the pressure gradient across prosthetic valves and assessing the central or perivalvular origin of regurgitant prosthesis leaks noninvasively are major advances because the alternative of catheter placement to get similar information may require trans-septal catheterization of the left side of the heart or direct left ventricular puncture.

Advancing microprocessor technology for high-speed processing of ultrasonic echoes has permitted superposition of flow direction and velocity information, obtained from Doppler frequency shift analysis throughout the imaging field, upon the 2D image itself. The velocity data are coded in color and shade for direction and velocity, respectively, and are presented as a color velocity map within the cardiac chambers of the 2D image at frame rates of 12 to 30 per second. This flow velocity tomographic image is similar to angiographic projectional images in that it gives the appearance of blood moving normally or abnormally across the valves and within the chambers. Clinical instruments generally provide standard 2D, M-mode, PW, and CW Doppler audio and spectral displays as well as the color flow velocity images.

Echocardiography has some advantages over competing imaging technologies. These include no risk from ionizing radiation, portability of equipment, noninvasive imaging, high imaging rate, no requirement for contrast injection, and generally low cost for the study. Its disadvantages include poor-quality images in 5 to 20 per cent of various patient groups and lack of complete quantitative data from most clinical laboratories.

Feigenbaum H: Echocardiography. 3rd ed. Philadelphia, Lea & Febiger, 1986. *This encyclopedic text is useful for the neophyte as well as the advanced student. Its strength in discussion of M-mode and 2D methods is not quite matched in areas discussing Doppler ultrasound.*

Hatle L, Angelsen B: Doppler Ultrasound in Cardiology. 2nd ed. Philadelphia, Lea & Febiger, 1985. *The most authoritative text on this subject. The chapters on the physics of blood flow and Doppler analysis are excellent. The comprehensive illustrations of pathologic and normal flow velocity patterns are superb. Much of the information included is not published elsewhere.*

Holen J, Aaslid R, Landmark K, et al.: Determination of pressure gradient in mitral stenosis with a non-invasive ultrasound Doppler technique. Acta Med Scand 199:455, 1976. *The classic work describing the clinical use of the relationship between maximum blood velocity detected by Doppler ultrasound and pressure gradient calculated from the velocity.*

Holen J, Aaslid R, Landmark K, et al.: Determination of effective orifice area in mitral stenosis from non-invasive ultrasound Doppler data and mitral flow rate. Acta Med Scand 201:83, 1977. *Original description of the pressure half-time method for estimation of mitral orifice area using Doppler ultrasound.*

Popp RL, Macovski A: Ultrasonic diagnostic instruments. Science 210:268, 1980. *A more detailed discussion of the instrumentation for producing ultrasonic images than given in this chapter.*

42.4 NUCLEAR CARDIOLOGY

Barry L. Zaret

Nuclear cardiology is based upon the ability of externally placed instruments to detect, define, and quantify radiation emanating from cardiac structures following injection of a radioisotope. The utility of nuclear procedure for defining pathophysiologic, prognostic, and diagnostic phenomena in cardiac patients has been established. The procedures can be safely repeated and are suitable for both imaging and biodistribution studies. Changes in cardiac function, cardiac blood volume, myocardial perfusion, and metabolism can be evaluated routinely.

CARDIAC PERFORMANCE

At present, a major clinical application of nuclear cardiology is in the assessment of global and regional cardiac performance. This is achieved with radionuclides that remain within the intravascular space during the period of study. Computer technology is critical for appropriate measurement. Cardiac performance can be assessed in two general ways: during the first pass of the isotope through the central circulation or following its equilibration in the cardiac blood pool. First-pass radionuclide angiocardiography is completed within 30 seconds following intravenous injection of a technetium-99m compound. There is temporal and anatomic segregation of the radioactive bolus during its first transit through the central circulation. Thus it is possible to make concomitant measurements of right and left ventricular function without concern that radioactivity present in one ventricle is interfering with the analysis of the other. Analysis of time-activity curves generated from the respective ventricular regions allows determination of ventricular ejection fraction (Fig. 42–30). Count rates emanating from a cardiac chamber are proportional to the volume of the chamber. In addition to analysis of ejection fraction, rates of ventricular filling and emptying, and ventricular volumes, quantitative and qualitative assessments of regional wall motion can be made from the same data (Fig. 42–31).

The alternative and more widely used approach to assessing cardiac performance involves complete equilibration of the radionuclide within the intravascular space. Physiologic signals are introduced that convert the conventional static imaging procedure into a dynamic assessment of cardiac function. To obtain this goal, technetium-99m is bound to the patient's own erythrocytes. The technetium-99m label remains evenly distributed throughout the intravascular blood volume for several hours. With the use of the electrocardiogram, nuclear data are segregated according to the time of their occurrence within the cardiac cycle. The R wave peak corresponds to maximal (end-diastolic) radioactivity. Data are summed over several hundred cardiac cycles, and composite data are quantified and displayed as sequential 10- to 50-msec points, which together define a representative cardiac cycle. The ventricular volume curve derived from these data is suitable for direct measurement of ejection fraction, rates of filling and ejection, and ventricular volumes. The data also may be displayed as a series of images that, when projected in cinematic format, provide a direct visual assessment of the regional contraction patterns of the heart (Fig. 42–32). Newly developed computer techniques now make it possible also to quantify regional motion accurately.

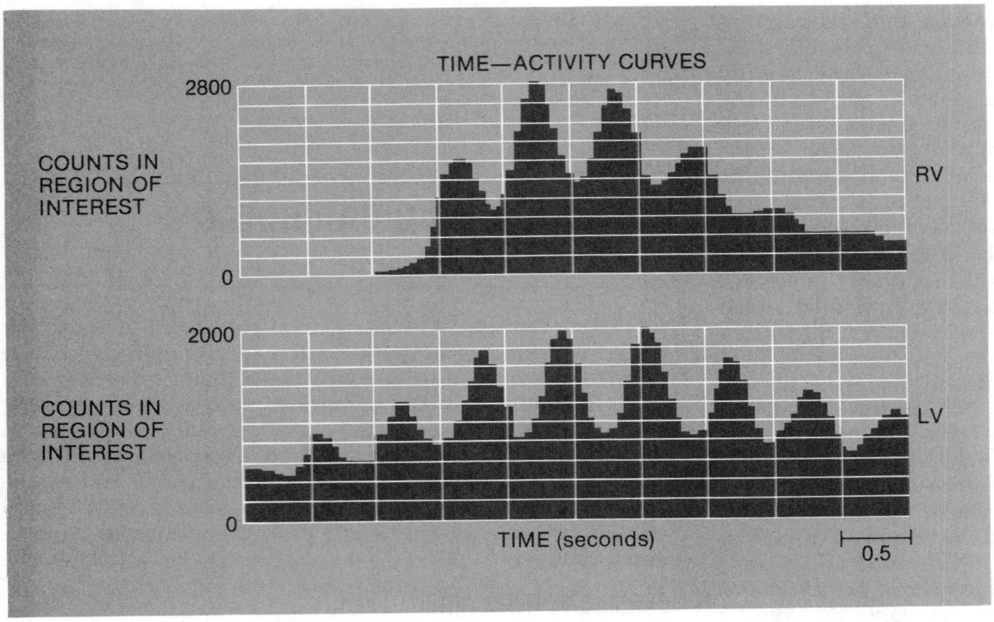

FIGURE 42–30. Right ventricular (RV) and left ventricular (LV) time-activity curves obtained at 20 frames per second with the computerized multicrystal scintillation camera. Analysis of these time-activity curves allows determination of ventricular ejection fraction. (Redrawn from Berger HJ, et al.: Semin Nucl Med 9:275, 1979.)

Both first-pass and equilibrium techniques can be employed to study cardiac performance under conditions of rest and exercise. Data may be accumulated during supine, semisupine, or upright bicycle exercise. Often critical data concerning cardiovascular status emerge only when the patient is evaluated during stress. The normal response to exercise involves an augmentation in the pump function of both ventricles. Normal ventricular reserve generally is defined as an increase in ejection fraction of each ventricle of at least 5 per cent (in absolute ejection fraction units) and the presence of normal regional wall motion. Abnormal exercise ventricular reserve may be encountered in a variety of pathophysiologic conditions involving coronary artery disease and intrinsic myocardial, valvular, and congenital heart disease.

The study of cardiac performance employing nuclear techniques has been particularly useful in patients with coronary artery disease. The ejection fraction is the single best clinical indicator of global ventricular pump performance. This index is of major prognostic importance in patients with coronary artery disease, either immediately following myocardial infarction or in the chronic stable phase of disease. Analysis of the ventricular ejection fraction is based upon radioactivity counts taken over the entire cardiac cycle. It is not dependent upon geometric assumptions concerning ventricular shape or ventricular volume. In coronary artery disease, particularly following myocardial infarction, asymmetric contraction patterns are common. In these ischemic ventricles, cavitary shapes frequently cannot be approximated by idealized geometric models. Consequently, in coronary artery disease, ejection fraction is measured most accurately by the nuclear approach. Using portable equipment, it is possible to study cardiac performance at the bedside of the acutely ill in coronary and intensive care units. Such studies have demonstrated substantial abnormalities in the functioning of the ischemic left ventricle during the acute phase of myocardial infarction. Abnormalities of both left and right ventricles can be identified. Right ventricular infarction occurring in the course of inferior wall infarction has been identified and further defined. The important negative prognostic impact of functional left ventricular aneurysm formation during acute anterior infarction has been defined. Assessment of regional and global function also is an important means of evaluating the effect of thrombolytic therapy for acute infarction.

Abnormalities of ventricular performance are found in approximately 85 per cent of patients with coronary artery disease studied during exercise stress. Myocardial ischemia is reflected in abnormal ventricular reserve. Abnormal responses of the ejection fraction may be encountered in a variety of conditions, but the development of new regional abnormalities of wall motion is quite specific for coronary artery disease. Abnormal exercise performance has important prognostic implications, particularly following infarction.

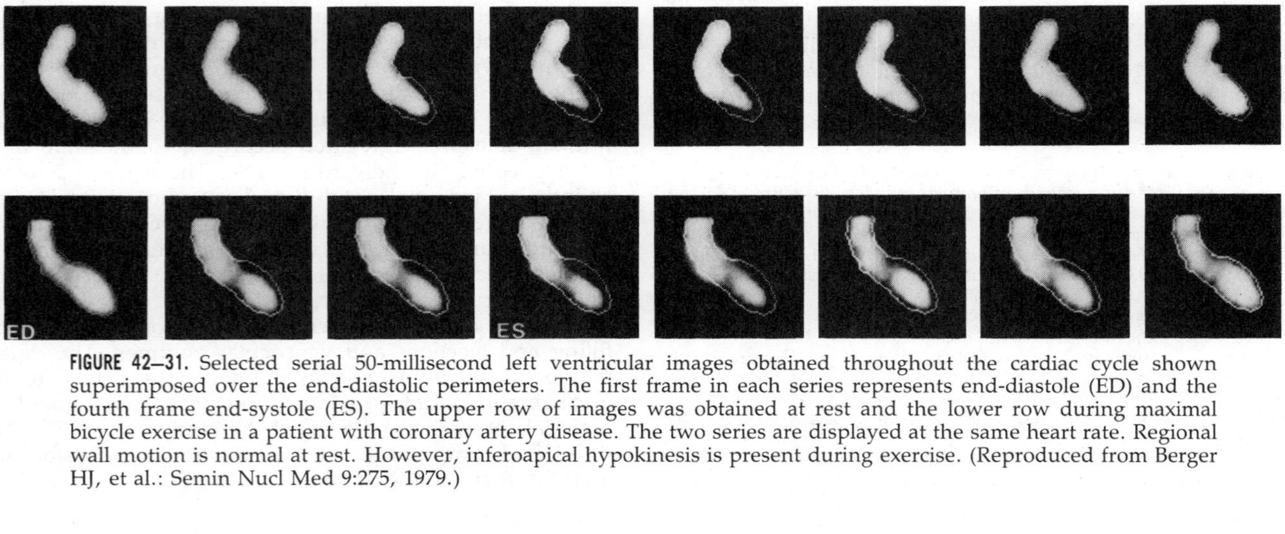

FIGURE 42–31. Selected serial 50-millisecond left ventricular images obtained throughout the cardiac cycle shown superimposed over the end-diastolic perimeters. The first frame in each series represents end-diastole (ED) and the fourth frame end-systole (ES). The upper row of images was obtained at rest and the lower row during maximal bicycle exercise in a patient with coronary artery disease. The two series are displayed at the same heart rate. Regional wall motion is normal at rest. However, inferoapical hypokinesis is present during exercise. (Reproduced from Berger HJ, et al.: Semin Nucl Med 9:275, 1979.)

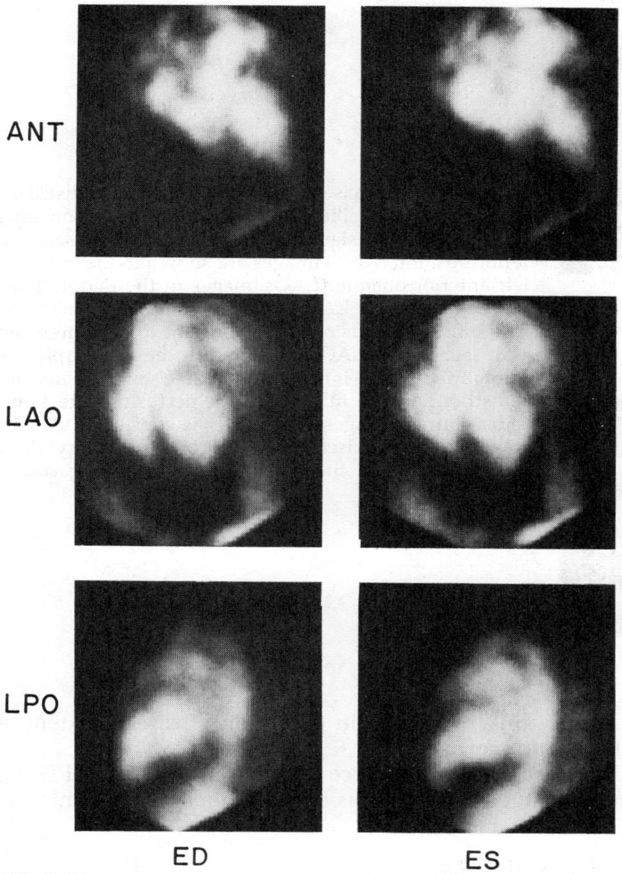

FIGURE 42–32. Gated cardiac blood pool studies obtained in the anterior (ANT), 45-degree left anterior oblique (LAO), and left posterior oblique (LPO) positions. End-diastolic images (ED) are shown on the left and end-systolic (ES) on the right. Note that radioactivity is present throughout the entire cardiac blood pool. A large anteroapical left ventricular aneurysm is appreciated in all three positions. Note that in the LAO position image the left ventricle is the posterior cardiac structure and the right ventricle the anterior structure. These are separated by the interventricular septum, which is displayed as an area devoid of radioactivity. (Reproduced from Berger HJ, et al.: Radiol Clin North Am 18:441, 1980.)

Radionuclide assessment of ventricular performance may also be employed in the evaluation of patients with valvular disease at rest or exercise. Resting measurement of cardiac function provides important preoperative prognostic data and may also be of value in defining the physiologic significance of valvular lesions such as mitral regurgitation. For example, normal left ventricular function in a patient with severe mitral regurgitation would imply a primary valvular problem, whereas severe ventricular dysfunction would suggest secondary mitral regurgitation resulting from diffuse myocardial disease. Assessment of performance under hemodynamic stress may help define the advent of irreversible damage in valvular heart disease. This is particularly important in aortic regurgitation, in which irremediable change in left ventricular function is frequently present by the time valve surgery is considered.

Assessment of ventricular performance is critical to the understanding and treatment of congestive heart failure. Knowledge of the degree of impairment in ventricular performance has prognostic and therapeutic relevance. In addition, an important group of patients with primary diastolic dysfunction (normal systolic function and impaired measures of diastolic filling) has been defined. Such patients require other than conventional therapy for heart failure.

Radionuclide studies also have been employed in the evaluation of myocardial function in patients with lung disease in which the major hemodynamic burden falls on the right ventricle. Right ventricular performance can probably be evaluated best with the first-pass technique. Abnormalities in right ventricular performance have been noted at rest and during exercise in patients with chronic obstructive pulmonary disease and have been related to the degree of impairment in ventilatory performance. Pharmacologic interventions may modify abnormal right ventricular performance.

These techniques also have been utilized for long-term studies assessing cardiac therapy. A prototype example has been the application of first-pass radionuclide angiocardiography for the serial assessment of ventricular function in patients receiving the antineoplastic agent doxorubicin. Use of this agent has been limited by the frequent development of a drug-induced cardiomyopathy. Serial measurement of cardiac ejection fraction during the course of therapy has led to a set of guidelines of dosage and schedule that help avert cardiotoxicity.

In addition, left-to-right shunts can be detected and quantified during performance of the first-pass radionuclide angiocardiogram. With this technique, a time-activity curve is generated from a region in the lung field. In the presence of a shunt, early recirculation is detected. The curve can be deconvoluted so that the major components can be quantified and the pulmonic-systemic blood flow ratios determined.

MYOCARDIAL PERFUSION IMAGING

Myocardial perfusion imaging utilizes radionuclides that traverse the myocardial capillary system and enter the myocardial cell. The radionuclide currently employed for these studies is thallium-201. This tracer is considered a potassium analogue, since its distribution generally mirrors that of intracellular potassium. Thallium-201 is produced in the cyclotron and has a physical half-life of approximately 72 hours. After intravenous injection it is rapidly extracted and distributed within the myocardium according to regional myocardial blood flow and regional cellular viability. Recently, a new group of technetium-99m perfusion tracers has been developed. These compounds are now being investigated actively; in the future, they may replace thallium.

At rest, the normal myocardial perfusion image demonstrates homogeneous uptake in the left ventricular wall with a central area of decreased activity corresponding to the left ventricular cavity. In approximately 20 per cent of normal persons, there is a region of decreased uptake at the cardiac apex corresponding to a normal relative thinning of this portion of the left ventricle. Abnormal image patterns will demonstrate a zone of decreased myocardial perfusion as a region of relatively decreased radionuclide uptake. Images are obtained in multiple positions. This is necessary to confirm the presence of a defect and define its location. The normal right ventricle is not visualized at rest because of its smaller mass compared with that of the left ventricle.

In the resting state, abnormalities usually represent either acute or remote myocardial infarction. However, studies have also demonstrated perfusion defects at rest in patients with unstable angina or coronary spasm (either spontaneous or induced by ergonovine maleate) or, rarely, in patients with severe obstructive coronary disease in the absence of clinical evidence of acute ischemia. Defects are noted with high sensitivity during the early hours of acute myocardial infarction. Within the first six hours, virtually all infarcts may be identified. After 24 hours, sensitivity falls to 80 to 90 per cent.

In most patients with coronary artery disease without previous infarction, myocardial perfusion patterns appear normal at rest. This is to be expected, since from a pathophysiologic standpoint coronary blood flow is relatively uniform at rest, even in the presence of severe coronary obstruc-

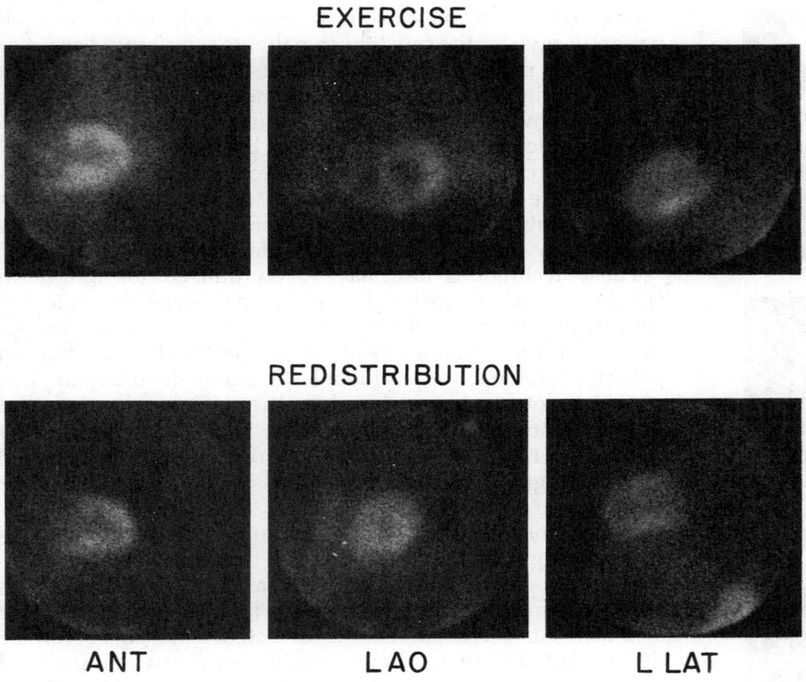

FIGURE 42–33. Exercise (upper panels) and redistribution (lower panels) thallium-201 myocardial perfusion images in a patient with significant coronary artery disease. Anterior position (ANT) images are shown in the left panels, left anterior oblique (LAO) images in the middle panels, and left lateral (L LAT) images in the right panels. Note a significant perfusion defect present in the anteroseptal wall seen in the LAO image and in the anteroapical wall seen in the L LAT image during exercise, with substantial redistribution and filling in of the perfusion defect on the redistribution images. This study is consistent with transient myocardial ischemia and coronary artery disease involving at least the left anterior descending coronary artery.

tion. The major physiologic abnormality in coronary disease is diminished coronary vascular reserve. Therefore, to detect perfusion abnormalities in coronary disease it is necessary to study patients under conditions of increased myocardial blood flow. Most work has employed exercise as an appropriate stress. Thallium 201 is injected at peak exercise, and imaging is begun within ten minutes after injection. Since thallium is rapidly extracted by myocardium, it can be injected during the period of maximal heterogeneity of regional myocardial blood flow, and its distribution will reflect this heterogeneity. Comparison of images obtained immediately following exercise with those obtained following a redistribution phase two to four hours after exercise allows definition of transiently ischemic zones (Fig. 42–33). Defects present on exercise but not at redistribution are most consistent with transient ischemia; defects that are unchanged are most consistent with previous infarction and scar; and defects that are present at redistribution but are markedly increased during exercise are most consistent with transient ischemia superimposed upon the scar. The overall sensitivity of this technique for detecting significant ischemic disease is approximately 80 per cent. The specificity of the technique is excellent. This technique is of greatest value diagnostically in patients with equivocal exercise electrocardiograms, abnormal baseline electrocardiograms, or suspected false-positive or false-negative conventional exercise tests. Both imaging with the patient at rest and exercise/redistribution studies have been of value in evaluating thrombolysis and reperfusion. Exercise studies also have been of value in assessing prognosis following infarction and in evaluating patients after coronary angioplasty.

An alternative means of stress perfusion imaging involves use of the coronary vasodilator, dipyridamole. Thallium myocardial distributions following dipyridamole provide data comparable to those noted with exercise. However, with pharmacologic stress, evaluation is based upon differences in flow without implying ischemia, whereas with exercise, evaluation is based upon heterogeneity of flow, generally associated with ischemia.

Thallium planar imaging is becoming increasingly quantitative. Computer techniques now provide objective definition of the presence and extent of defects as well as quantification of regional tracer washout kinetics. Kinetic analysis has added a new dimension to diagnostic and functional assessment, with particular relevance in definition of disease extent and efficacy of reperfusion.

Single photon emission computed tomography (SPECT) of thallium studies currently is under evaluation. Its clinical role awaits further definition.

INFARCT-AVID IMAGING

An additional radionuclide approach involves definition of acute myocardial infarction and regions of acute myocardial necrosis. This is performed with "infarct-avid" radiotracers, which bind selectively to regions of acute infarction. The current agent for this procedure is technetium-99m stannous pyrophosphate, although recent research suggests that radiolabeled antimyosin antibody also may be employed. With this technique, acute infarcts are visualized as regions of increased radionuclide uptake. The mechanism of abnormal pyrophosphate accumulation appears to be related to regional calcium deposition, as well as binding to denatured proteins. Pyrophosphate uptake also is dependent upon sufficient residual blood flow to allow entry of the radioactive tracer.

The infarct zone can be visualized within 24 to 48 hours of the onset of infarction. Maximal visualization generally occurs from 48 to 72 hours after the infarct. Images usually are not positive within the first 24 hours unless thrombolysis has occurred. Images generally are no longer positive seven to ten days after the infarct. From the standpoint of diagnosis, pyrophosphate imaging appears to be a sensitive means of detecting acute myocardial infarction as well as extension of the infarct. Sensitivity is less in patients with nontransmural compared with transmural infarction. Pyrophosphate infarct imaging is most valuable in patients presenting several days after infarction when other studies are equivocal or nondiagnostic.

POSITRON TOMOGRAPHY

This technique involves imaging and quantification of the intracardiac distribution of positron-emitting radionuclides. By virtue of the types of radionuclides available and the instrumentation employed, this technique has provided new insight into metabolism and coronary flow. Since carbon-11 is a positron emitter, a variety of biologically active compounds can be radiolabeled and used for imaging. These include fatty acids, receptor ligands, and neurotransmitters. Although still primarily research in nature, these studies offer great potential for ultimate clinical application. Because of the cost involved and general need for an on-site cyclotron, this technique currently remains experimental and localized to only a few centers.

In addition to positron studies, additional metabolic studies have been obtained using conventional imaging. Studies to date have focused on radioiodinated fatty acids and their analogues.

Berman DS, Garcia EV, Maddahi J, et al.: Thallium-201 myocardial perfusion scintigraphy. In Freeman LM (ed.): Freeman and Johnson's Clinical Radionuclide Imaging. New York, Grune & Stratton, 1984, pp 479–536. *A detailed clinical and technologic explication of myocardial perfusion imaging.*

Pohost GM, Higgins CB, Morganroth J, et al. (eds.): New Concepts in Cardiac Imaging: 1986. Chicago, Year Book Medical Publishers, 1986. *This book contains detailed chapters on perfusion imaging, equilibrium blood pool studies, and positron emission tomographic studies. The contrasting efficacy of other imaging approaches is also outlined in other chapters in this volume.*

Zaret BL, Berger HJ: Techniques of nuclear cardiology. In Hurst JW (ed.): The Heart. 6th ed. New York, McGraw-Hill Book Company, 1986, pp 1809–1858. *A comprehensive review of current clinically relevant aspects of nuclear cardiology with 255 individual references cited.*

42.5 Cardiac Catheterization and Angiography

William H. Barry

Cardiac catheterization provides a unique, comprehensive, and quantitative assessment of cardiac structure and function. As facilities have become more widely available and the risks have decreased, there has been a progressive tendency to employ catheterization in the diagnosis and management of patients with heart disease. With the development of additional techniques such as bedside hemodynamic monitoring, intracardiac electrophysiologic testing, endomyocardial biopsy, and percutaneous transluminal coronary angioplasty, it is increasingly important for the internist to understand the indications, capabilities, and risks of cardiac catheterization.

INDICATIONS FOR CARDIAC CATHETERIZATION AND ANGIOGRAPHY

In general, cardiac catheterization and angiography are performed when the history, physical examination, and noninvasive studies have provided insufficient information to allow a definitive decision about diagnosis or treatment. The accuracy of noninvasive evaluation has increased remarkably recently, because of the greatly improved sensitivity and specificity of two-dimensional echocardiography combined with Doppler procedures, radionuclide ventriculography, thallium 201 myocardial perfusion scintigraphy, and fast computed atrial tomographic (CAT) and magnetic resonance imaging (MRI) scanners. Therefore, cardiac catheterization is performed most frequently to quantify the severity of disease present and to determine whether the patient is a candidate for surgical intervention. In Table 42–5 are shown the diagnoses of a typical series of patients referred for cardiac catheterization. As can be seen, the vast majority of patients undergoing this procedure have coronary artery disease, with patients having valvular disease a distant second. In Table 42–6 are listed the usual indications for cardiac catheterization and coronary angiography in patients with coronary artery disease or valvular heart disease.

TECHNIQUES AND THEIR HAZARDS

ARTERIAL AND VENOUS ACCESS. Two basic approaches are used for insertion of catheters into arteries and veins. The first involves incision of the skin overlying the vessel, dissection of the vessel free of surrounding tissue, and incision of the vessel with direct insertion of the catheter. This method is usually reserved for the brachial artery or antecubital vein. The advantage of this technique is that one has direct access to the vessels, so that they may either be tied off (vein) or repaired (brachial artery) after completion of the catheterization procedure. This procedure decreases the likelihood of hematoma formation. The disadvantages of the technique are that an incision is required in the skin, increasing the patient's discomfort in the postcatheterization period, and that there is a significant (2 to 3 per cent) incidence of thrombosis of the brachial artery. For these reasons, and because it requires a longer time to perform, this technique is less commonly employed than the percutaneous method. However, it may be preferred in patients with severe atherosclerotic disease of the aorta or iliofemoral arteries.

In the Seldinger technique, an artery or vein is punctured percutaneously with a needle, and a thin, flexible guide wire is then inserted through the needle into the vessel and advanced up the vessel. The needle is withdrawn over the wire, and then a catheter may be inserted directly over the wire, or a short arterial or venous sheath may be inserted, using a dilator, over the wire and into the vessel to provide access. The percutaneous technique is employed most frequently for the femoral artery and vein, the axillary artery, or the subclavian or internal jugular vein. This technique is relatively simple, and no sutures are required. The disadvantage is that one does not have direct control of the vessels after withdrawal of the catheters or sheaths, and control of postcatheterization bleeding may be more difficult than with the direct-approach. Patients must therefore be relatively immobile at least four to six hours. At present, the percutaneous femoral approach in which the femoral artery and femoral vein are punctured is most commonly utilized for cardiac catheterization.

Because of potential hemostasis problems after the procedure, elective cardiac catheterization is usually not performed if the prothrombin time is greater than 18 seconds. To decrease the risk of thrombosis during the catheterization procedure, heparin is frequently used for catheterization of the left side of the heart. The anticoagulant effect of heparin is usually reversed with protamine at the termination of the procedure, before the final withdrawal of the sheath or catheter. The main risks of arterial or venous puncture and subsequent catheter manipulation are thrombosis of the vessel, hemorrhage, cerebrovascular accident, and myocardial infarction induced by clot from the tip of the catheter or dislodgment of atherosclerotic material. Table 42–7 summarizes the incidence of complications during cardiac catheterization and coronary angiography. Catheterization of the left side of the heart generally carries a much higher risk than catheterization of the right side of the heart because of the ability of the lung vascular bed to filter out thrombi. Angiography carries a higher risk than simple pressure measurements of the left side of the heart because of the additional catheter manipu-

TABLE 42–5. DIAGNOSES OF 562 PATIENTS CONSECUTIVELY STUDIED

Coronary Artery Disease (CAD)	Valvular Disease	CAD and Valvular Disease	Cardiomyopathy	Normal Persons	Congenital Heart Disease	Miscellaneous
62.6%	16.7%	6.0%	5.9%	6.4%	1.4%	0.9%

Adapted from Barry WH, et al.: Cathet Cardiovasc Diagn 8:401, 1979.

TABLE 42–6. POSSIBLE INDICATIONS FOR CARDIAC CATHETERIZATION AND ANGIOGRAPHY

Suspected Coronary Artery Disease

1. Angina, especially if:
   - unstable
   - refractory to treatment
   - strongly positive treadmill ECG
   - young person with positive family history
2. After acute myocardial infarction, if:
   - angina
   - positive treadmill result
3. In selected patients suspected to have "silent" ischemia
   - occupational hazards
   - strong family history of infarction/sudden death
4. Patients with ischemic cardiomyopathy and congestive heart failure (CHF)
5. In patients with high risk (age, diabetes, lipid disorder) prior to major noncardiac surgery; in patients at risk for coronary artery disease in whom cardiac surgery is planned.

Suspected Valvular Disease

1. Aortic stenosis
   - angina
   - syncope
   - CHF
2. Aortic regurgitation
   - CHF
   - angina
   - progressive cardiac enlargement
3. Mitral stenosis*
   - CHF refractory to digitalis and diuretics
   - Recurrent emboli with atrial fibrillation
4. Mitral regurgitation
   - CHF
   - Progressive cardiac enlargement

Additional Miscellaneous Indicators

Congenital heart disease
Pericardial disease
Other: Percutaneous transluminal coronary angioplasty
Electrophysiologic study
Biopsy
Hemodynamic monitoring

*Operation may be performed without catheterization if diagnosis is certain.

TABLE 42–7. COMPLICATIONS OF CARDIAC CATHETERIZATION AND ANGIOGRAPHY*

Complication	Incidence (%)
Death	0.14
Myocardial infarction	0.07
Cardiovascular accident	0.07
Arrhythmia	0.56
Vascular complications	0.57
Other	0.41
TOTAL	1.82

*Data on 53,581 patients.
Adapted from Kennedy JW: Complications associated with cardiac catheterization and angiography. Cathet Cardiovasc Diagn 8:5, 1982.

lation, selective placement of the catheters within the coronary arteries, and use of angiographic contrast solution, especially in patients with more severe cardiac diseases.

PRESSURE MEASUREMENTS. Measurement of intracardiac pressure is an essential part of the cardiac catheterization procedure. Pressures are measured by attaching the end of the fluid-filled catheter to an external pressure transducer. The pressure waveform transmitted through the fluid-filled catheter deforms a pressure-sensitive diaphragm in the transducer, which changes the resistance of an electrical circuit and allows recording of the pressure waveform as voltage signals. Phasic pressure waveforms up to 12 Hz may be recorded with this technique (Fig. 42–34). During routine catheterization of the right and left sides of the heart, all the pressures within the heart are measured, with the usual exception of the left atrial pressure. The pulmonary capillary "wedge" position, in which a segment of the pulmonary arterial tree is occluded either with the catheter tip or with a small balloon attached to the end of a catheter (a flow-directed Swan-Ganz type of catheter), gives a pressure that resembles closely the true left atrial pressure (Fig. 42–34). Normally, the diastolic pressure of the pulmonary artery is very close to the mean wedge pressure. However, in patients with tachycardia or with increased pulmonary vascular resistance, pulmonary artery end-diastolic pressure may be significantly higher than the mean wedge pressure. The normal values for intracardiac pressures are given in Ch. 41.

In addition to the average pressures, the shape and magnitude of the waveforms frequently contain diagnostic information. For example, in mitral regurgitation there is a large v wave in the left atrial or pulmonary artery wedge pressure recording (Fig. 42–35). A large v wave in the right atrial pressure tracing indicates tricuspid insufficiency. Simultaneous pressures are usually measured in the pulmonary wedge position and left ventricle to quantitate mitral valve function. A pressure gradient in diastole between the pulmonary wedge pressure and left ventricular diastolic pressure is seen, for example, in mitral stenosis (Fig. 42–36). Left ventricular and aortic pressures are measured simultaneously to assess aortic valve function.

Comparison of pressures in different chambers can be very useful. In patients with pericardial constriction, there is equalization of the right atrial and the pulmonary artery wedge pressures, and the mean right atrial pressure is greater than one third of the right ventricular systolic pressure. Measure-

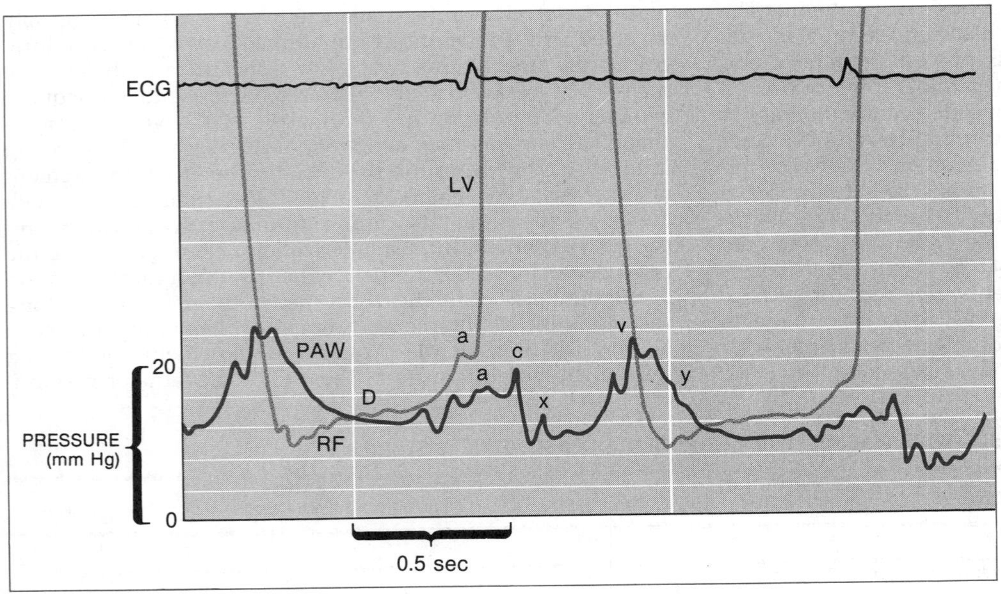

FIGURE 42–34. Simultaneous pulmonary artery wedge (PAW) pressure and left ventricular pressure (LV) in a normal patient. RF = Rapid LV filling; D = diastasis of LV filling; a = atrial contraction pressure wave. Note the delay of the PAW pressure relative to LV pressure.

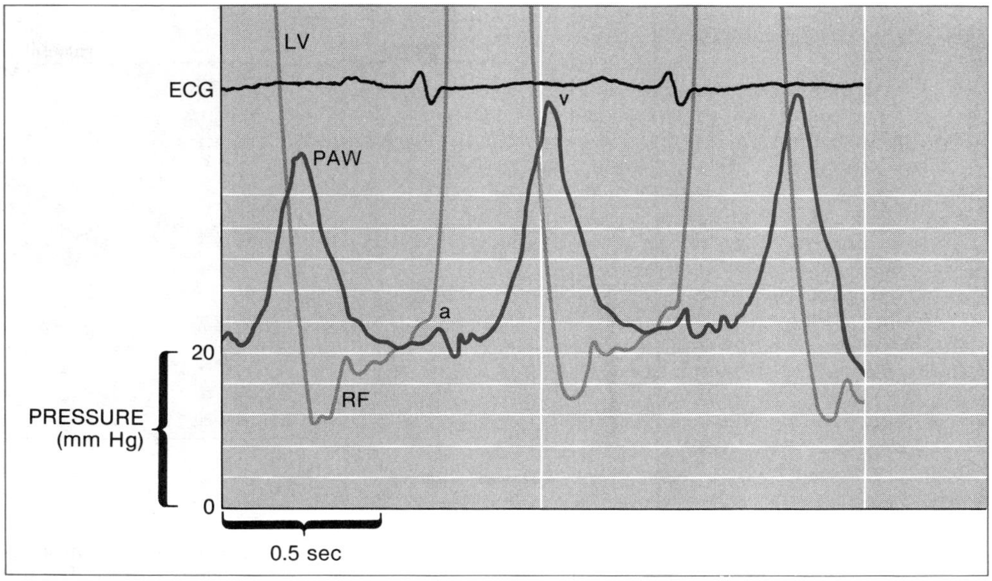

FIGURE 42–35. Simultaneous PAW and LV pressures in a patient with severe mitral regurgitation. Note large v wave, with rapid y descent.

ment of intracardiac pressures during exercise or pacing stress may also provide useful information. For example, patients with mitral stenosis or mitral insufficiency may have relatively normal resting pressures but abnormally high pulmonary artery wedge pressures with exercise. Patients with coronary artery disease may have normal left ventricular diastolic pressures at rest, which elevate markedly during the stress of pacing tachycardia owing to ischemic left ventricular dysfunction.

MEASUREMENT OF CARDIAC BLOOD FLOW. Another important part of cardiac catheterization is measurement of cardiac output. In the Fick method, oxygen consumption is measured by collecting all expired air over a three-minute period into a bag and determining the oxygen content in the expired air. This allows determination of oxygen consumption in milliliters per minute. Collection of samples from the pulmonary artery (mixed venous sample) and a systemic artery allows determination of the arteriovenous (A-V) oxygen difference. If the value for hemoglobin concentration in the blood is known, this allows calculation of the milliliters of blood that had to flow through the lungs to acquire the amount of oxygen consumed. (See bottom of page.)

Cardiac output may be normalized by dividing by body surface area (m^2) and expressed as cardiac index. The determined cardiac output by the Fick technique is most accurate when the cardiac output is low and thus the A-V oxygen content difference is large. In patients with intracardiac shunts, correction for the shunt must be made. This occurs most commonly in adult patients with atrial septal defects or ventricular septal defects with a left-to-right shunt. The pulmonary artery saturation in these conditions is elevated relative to the true mixed venous saturation, which is most closely approximated by the superior vena cava saturation. Standard methods for quantification of left-to-right and right-to-left intracardiac shunts exist.

Another method commonly used for measurement of cardiac output is dye dilution, in which indocyanine green dye is injected in a peripheral vein, with continuous sampling of the dye concentration from a peripheral artery. The cardiac output is calculated as $\frac{i}{c \times t}$, where i is the quantity of indicator injected, c is the average arterial concentration of the indicator during its first pass, and t is the total duration of the dye concentration curve in the arterial blood. The product of c and t is easily measured as the area under the first-pass curve determined by planimetry. The error of the dye dilution indicator curve is greatest in patients with extremely low outputs or with mitral or aortic regurgitation. The dye curve is also distorted by the presence of intracardiac shunts and in fact may be used in certain circumstances to diagnose the presence and direction of an intracardiac shunt. The indicator dye curve output is most accurate in patients with high cardiac output and a narrow A-V oxygen difference.

The thermodilution method is another dilution indicator method; in this case, the indicator is not dye, but cold saline injected into the right atrium. Temperature changes are detected with a thermistor in the pulmonary artery. The advantages of the thermodilution method are that it is relatively unaffected by mitral and aortic regurgitation and that it may be repeated frequently to measure serial outputs. It is influenced by respiration, by the presence of shunts that increase pulmonary flow, and by the presence of tricuspid regurgitation. At the presence time, the Fick method is most commonly employed in the cardiac catheterization laboratory, and the thermodilution method is most commonly utilized in intensive care unit settings where patients are being monitored with catheters in the right side of the heart.

From measurements of cardiac output and pressure gradients across vascular beds, the systemic and pulmonary vascular resistances may be calculated. Elevations in systemic vascular resistance are important in patients with chronic congestive heart failure and may identify those patients who will respond favorably to vasodilator therapy. Pulmonary vascular resistance is frequently elevated in patients with severe left ventricular failure and elevated wedge pressures, in patients with mitral valve disease, in patients with left-to-right shunts, and always in patients with primary pulmonary hypertension. Measurement of changes in pulmonary and

$$\text{Cardiac output (liters/min)} = \frac{\text{oxygen consumption (ml } O_2\text{/min)}}{\text{A-V } O_2 \text{ difference (ml } O_2\text{/liter blood)}}$$

$$\text{A-V } O_2 \text{ difference (ml } O_2\text{/liter blood)} = 13.9 \times \text{hemoglobin (gm/dl)} \times (\%\text{ sat A} - \%\text{ sat V})$$

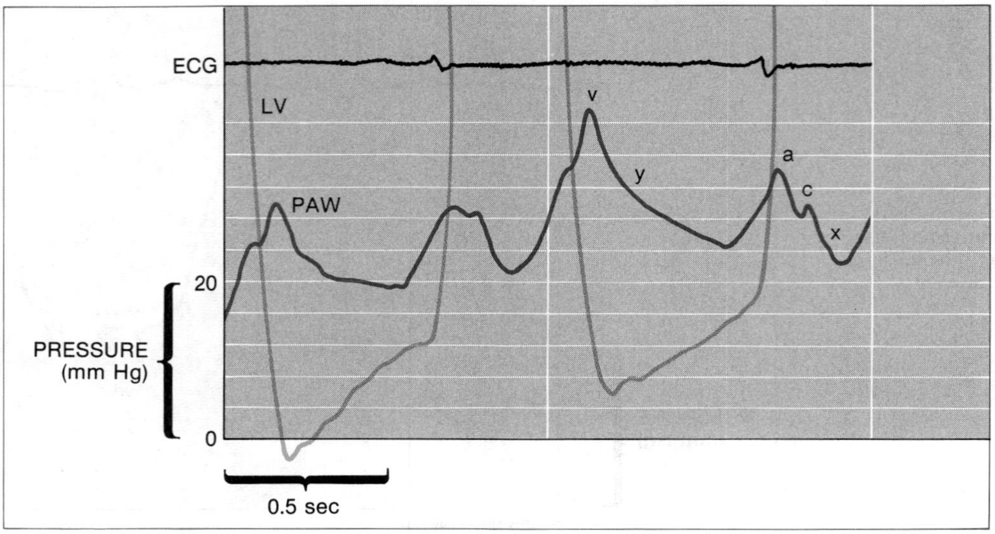

FIGURE 42–36. Simultaneous PAW and LV pressures in a patient with mitral stenosis. Notice slow y descent, and the large gradient throughout diastole between PAW and LV diastolic pressures. The actual mitral valve area (M.V.A.) may be estimated as:

$$\text{M.V.A.} = \frac{\text{diastolic mitral flow (ml/sec)}}{38\sqrt{\text{diastolic pressure gradient}}}$$

Thus, for a given M.V.A., the pressure gradient across the valve goes up as the *square* of mitral valve flow. This explains why the PAW pressure rises so markedly with increased cardiac output and hence increased mitral valve flow. Increased heart rate shortens diastolic time, and hence increases the mitral valve flow rate per unit of diastolic time at any given cardiac output.

systemic vascular resistances and in cardiac outputs and pressures before and after administration of vasodilator drugs may be helpful in guiding treatment of patients with specific disorders and is frequently employed, in the catheterization laboratory setting.

Measurement of pressure gradients across the aortic, mitral, tricuspid, or pulmonic valve allows estimation of valve area utilizing the Gorlin formula (see Fig. 42–36). The calculated valve area may differ significantly from the true value, particularly in situations of very low cardiac output or valvular insufficiency. Nevertheless, this measurement is often useful in guiding surgical interventions.

ANGIOGRAPHY. During routine cardiac catheterization, left ventriculography and coronary angiography are commonly performed. In left ventriculography, contrast material is injected into the left ventricular chamber and cineangiographic filming is performed at 30 to 60 frames per second. Ejection fraction is determined as the fraction of end-diastolic ventricular volume ejected each systole. In patients with mitral or aortic regurgitation, the angiographic regurgitant volume can be estimated by comparing the angiographic stroke volume and the forward stroke volume determined by the Fick method. However, because of frequent inaccuracies in absolute volume measurements by angiographic methods, the degree of regurgitation is usually graded on a simple 1+ to 4+ scale. In patients with coronary artery disease, segmental contraction abnormalities are frequently present, and these may be quantified by a variety of regional indices of left ventricular performance.

Adverse effects of left ventriculography include a negative inotropic effect due to calcium binding by the contrast agent and an intravascular volume–expanding effect due to hyperosmolality of the contrast material. The myocardial depressant effects of contrast agents are usually not a problem unless left ventricular function is severely compromised. In these patients, the risks of left ventriculography may be reduced by using nonionic, non–calcium-binding contrast agents or by use of digital image enhancement techniques that permit use of a small volume of contrast material, or both.

Injection of dye into the aortic root allows assessment of the degree of aortic insufficiency, and right ventricular contrast injection allows assessment of the tricuspid valve. Pulmonary angiography may be performed to assess the pulmonary vasculature and to detect presence of pulmonary emboli.

Coronary cineangiography is performed by injecting a contrast agent selectively into the right or left main coronary ostia and filming at 30 frames per second. The degree of coronary artery obstruction in multiple views is assessed by measuring the percentage of narrowing of the artery at the site or sites of obstruction or by determining the percentage of area of stenosis by video densitometric measurements. The presence and location of collateral vessels to partially or totally occluded coronary segments are also determined. In patients with no or only minor coronary artery narrowings, but with a suggestive history of chest pain, ergonovine may be infused intravenously to precipitate coronary artery spasm, which then can be documented angiographically.

Insertion of a catheter into the coronary tree may precipitate coronary occlusion by provoking spasm, by dislodging thrombus, or by dissecting the arterial wall. With current techniques, however, these complications are rare (see Table 42–6). Recent developments (nonionic contrast material, smaller high-flow catheters, and digital coronary angiographic image enhancement techniques) can be expected to decrease further the risk of this procedure.

Barry WH, Grossman W: Cardiac catheterization. In Braunwald E. (ed.): Heart Disease. Philadelphia, W.B. Saunders Company, 1984.

Cowley MJ. Vetrovec GW, Di Sciascio G, et al.: Coronary angioplasty of multiple vessels: Short term outcome and long term results. Circulation 73:1314, 1985. *Representative report of current success rate and complications.*

Grossman W: Cardiac Catheterization and Angiography. Philadelphia, Lea & Febiger, 1980. *Excellent comprehensive text on catheterization and angiography.*

Kennedy JW: Complications associated with cardiac catheterization and angiography. Cathet Cardiovasc Diagn 8:5, 1982. *Excellent description of type and incidence of complications.*

Rahimtoola SH, Zipes DP: Consensus statement of the state of the art of electrophysiological testing in the diagnosis and treatment of patients with cardiac arrhythmias. Circulation, April 1987. *Summary of current status of invasive electrophysiologic testing.*

43 HEART FAILURE

Thomas W. Smith

The heart generates the motive force to satisfy the metabolic needs of tissues by delivery of blood containing oxygen and nutrients. The minute-to-minute adjustments in the distribution of the cardiac output according to physiologic priorities (e.g., muscular exercise, heat loss, and digestion) require a complex regulatory system that must also serve to protect vital organs such as the heart and brain when cardiac output is compromised.

The normal or failing heart, in terms of its structure and function, may be examined as a pump, as a muscle, or as a component of the circulatory system. This chapter will address aspects of heart failure common to the various disease entities discussed in subsequent chapters.

GENERAL ASPECTS

The term *heart failure* is generally used as a synonym for myocardial failure, emphasizing the impaired performance of the heart as a muscle and as a pump. It also provides a rationale for medical treatment. Subsequent chapters deal with syndromes in which the cause of circulatory compromise lies elsewhere, such as in abnormalities of the heart valves or pericardium or inappropriate heart rates.

Imbalance between circulatory demands and cardiac response sets the stage for the syndrome of heart failure. Volume overload is generally tolerated better than pressure overload. Aortic or mitral insufficiency produces *volume* overload that may be tolerated for years without overt heart failure; *pressure* overload from aortic stenosis, in contrast, usually results in much earlier onset of heart failure. Gradually developing overloads are accommodated better than acute overloads. Thus, gradually developing chronic mitral regurgitation is often present for years without signs of failure, whereas acute mitral regurgitation from a ruptured chorda tendinea can precipitate life-threatening pulmonary edema.

The myocardium adapts quite differently to volume and pressure loads. Volume overloads typically produce dilation followed by hypertrophy; pressure overloads characteristically elicit concentric hypertrophy until late in the natural history when dilation supervenes. Primary myocardial disease usually results in both dilation and hypertrophy.

Precipitating stresses (see Table 43–2) often tip the balance of the compromised heart toward decompensation and constitute important items for therapeutic attention.

CLINICAL CATEGORIES OF HEART FAILURE

Types of heart failure are often categorized according to five features: duration (acute or chronic), initiating mechanisms, the ventricle primarily affected, the clinical syndrome, and the underlying physiologic derangements.

Acute Versus Chronic Heart Failure

The clinical manifestations of heart failure often begin insidiously and progress gradually into a chronic state. Alternatively, onset may be abrupt, as after myocardial infarction.

Compensatory mechanisms in both acute and chronic heart failure include increased systemic vascular resistance and redistribution of blood flow. However, these adaptive mechanisms in acute and chronic heart failure differ quantitatively and sometimes also in direction. For example, *acute* distention of the left atrium generally promotes a sodium-poor diuresis, whereas *chronic* distention of the left atrium elicits salt and water retention.

Initiating Mechanisms

Each initiating mechanism has its own distinctive characteristics. For example, the symptoms and signs that evolve in rheumatic heart disease differ from those of hypertensive heart disease, whereas both have a different natural history from that of cor pulmonale. Even a single etiology, arteriosclerosis, may have distinctly different consequences, depending on the size and location of affected vessels: Progressive narrowing and gradual occlusion of distal branches of the coronary arteries may be so covert that shortness of breath and fatigue may be misinterpreted as the general physical decline of advancing age. In contrast, abrupt closure of a major coronary artery may result in myocardial necrosis followed by an acute low output state or by progressive chronic heart failure.

Left Versus Right Heart Failure

One ventricle bears the brunt of many disease processes and fails before the other. Because of the prevalence of cardiac disorders that overload or damage the left ventricle, heart failure most often begins with that ventricle. Breathlessness is the most common presenting symptom and is a direct consequence of elevated left ventricular filling pressure and pulmonary congestion. When the right ventricle fails, systemic venous congestion and peripheral edema predominate. Left ventricular failure is the most common cause of right ventricular failure, and breathlessness may improve as right ventricular output falls and pulmonary congestion diminishes.

The mechanism by which left ventricular failure causes the right ventricle to fail is not clear. Pulmonary hypertension secondary to left ventricular failure may contribute, but the degree of pulmonary hypertension is often insufficient to constitute a formidable burden on the right ventricle. Interdependence of the two ventricles, with failure of shared muscle in the ventricular septum, may also contribute. How often right ventricular failure causes left ventricular failure is still a matter of debate, complicated by the high frequency of independent and unrelated left ventricular disease in elderly patients with right ventricular failure.

The combination of left and right ventricular (biventricular) failure, with elevated filling pressures of both ventricles causing pulmonary and systemic venous hypertension, is known as "congestive heart failure." This term implies reduced effort tolerance, breathlessness, distended neck veins, hepatic engorgement, and peripheral edema.

Backward Versus Forward Heart Failure

"Backward failure" refers to elevated cardiac filling pressures and attributes to the consequent venous congestion a critical role in the evolution of the syndrome of heart failure. "Forward failure" refers to decreased cardiac output and inadequate perfusion of organs. This distinction has limited clinical usefulness and has largely been replaced by more specific consideration of ventricular filling pressures and cardiac output.

High Versus Low Output Failure

The separation into "high" and "low" output failure distinguishes certain clinical manifestations, rather than causes, of myocardial failure. It serves: (1) to distinguish a type of myocardial failure ("high output failure") in which the circulation remains brisk and the extremities tend to remain warm despite elevated venous pressures and a lower cardiac output than existed prior to the onset of heart failure; (2) to emphasize that the cardiac output and the circulatory adjustments during heart failure are conditioned by the state that existed prior to heart failure; and (3) to relate etiology to typical clinical features of heart failure. In regard to this last point, the more common causes—arteriosclerosis, hypertension, myocardial disease, valvular disease, and pericardial disease—tend to produce low output states; other, less common causes, including hyperthyroidism, Paget's disease of bone, anemia, beriberi, and arteriovenous fistula, tend to be associated with high output states. The essence of cardiac failure, however, remains the inability of the heart to increase its output appropriately in relation to demand.

Congestive Failure Versus Congested State

Elevated volume of the circulation, with preserved ventricular function, characterizes the "congested state." It is commonly encountered in intensive care facilities, where vigorous volume infusions are often used to combat systemic hypotension. It is encountered on a chronic basis in severe anemia and chronic renal insufficiency and less often in Paget's disease or beriberi. In these situations, venous hypertension results from expanded intravascular volume, rather than from impaired myocardial contractile state.

In time, myocardial failure may supervene but may then be difficult to detect on clinical grounds alone, because the hyperkinetic circulation tends to persist and the congestion may be only modestly increased. Cardiac catheterization, however, discloses an inadequate increase in cardiac output for the increment in oxygen uptake during exercise. Identification of the transition from a "congested state" to "congestive heart failure" is of greater theoretic than practical importance, since correction of inciting factors and administration of diuretics are effective in both situations.

SUBCELLULAR BASIS FOR CONTRACTION

Cardiac contraction is initiated by depolarization of the sarcolemmal membrane, which activates slow calcium channels that undergo a transient increase in calcium permeability. The resulting calcium influx triggers the release of a much larger amount of calcium from the sarcoplasmic reticulum with consequent sarcomere shortening; the sarcoplasmic reticulum then resequesters calcium to turn off myofilament interaction, permitting myocardial relaxation.

Contractile force in heart muscle is generated by interactions among contractile proteins in repeating units (sarcomeres) that compose the individual muscle fibers (myofibrils). Within each sarcomere, the contractile proteins are arranged in thick filaments consisting of myosin and thin filaments consisting of actin and the modulator proteins troponin and tropomyosin. Interaction of calcium with one of three proteins composing troponin initiates the contractile process by removing a troponin-tropomyosin–induced inhibition of thick and thin filament interaction.

Changes in the length of heart muscle during contraction and relaxation are explained by the sliding filament hypothesis. During contraction, the thin actin filaments are propelled past the myosin thick filaments by force generated by ATP-dependent movement of cross-bridges consisting of the head portion of the myosin molecule. As the muscle shortens, the cross-bridges disengage and then engage other sites with a ratchet-like action. Depending on the number of cross-bridges that interact at a given time, different tensions will be developed. Uptake of cytosolic calcium by the sarcoplasmic reticulum allows cross-bridge disengagement and relaxation to occur. Abundant mitochondria generate energy for the contractile machinery by oxidative phosphorylation fueled by free fatty acids and, to a lesser extent, glucose.

For the sarcomere, as for the whole heart (see Preload, below), the tension developed during contraction is directly related to its end-diastolic length. Stretching to permit optimal thick and thin filament overlap increases the ability of individual contractile elements to develop force. There are still many uncertainties regarding molecular details of the contractile process, and much is still to be learned about cardiac "success" as an essential background against which to examine basic mechanisms in cardiac "failure."

PATHOPHYSIOLOGIC INTERPLAY

Because of their location, structure, and function, the heart and lungs operate as a functional unit. The continuity of the muscle that surrounds the ventricular chambers, the shared ventricular septum, and the encasing pericardium ensure coordinate function, yet each ventricle functions as a separate muscular pump with its own atrial booster pump. In the normal heart, at least 50 per cent of the ventricular end-diastolic volume is ejected with each beat. Although many properties of ejection are inherent in the architecture and physiology of cardiac muscle, adaptability to changing metabolic needs is provided by a superimposed set of neurohumoral adjustments that modulate cardiac contractility.

Each ventricle has its own capacity to withstand and repair the stresses imposed by normal and abnormal function. The two ventricles also have different designs in keeping with their different physiologic functions. Before birth, both ventricles bear similar pressure loads. After birth, the right ventricular work load decreases as pulmonary arterial pressure falls, and the durability of right ventricular performance thus tends to exceed that of the left ventricle. These prospects are enhanced by the greater prevalence of diseases that compromise the left side of the heart and its blood supply.

ASSESSMENT OF CARDIAC PERFORMANCE

In terms of its performance, the heart may be assessed as a pump, as a muscle, or as a component of the circulatory system. Hemodynamic pressure and flow measurements characterize its behavior as a pump. Principles of muscle mechanics are used to describe its behavior as a muscle. Its adequacy as a component of the circulatory system is reflected in the consequences of reduced cardiac output, redistribution of blood flow, organ hypoperfusion, and pulmonary or systemic venous congestion.

Heart as a Pump: Hemodynamics

By the time overt heart failure is apparent, a variety of mechanisms operate to compensate for its diminished performance. Despite an inappropriately low cardiac output, the blood pressure at rest tends to remain normal or even increases.

CARDIAC OUTPUT. In response to peripheral demands, a complex set of control mechanisms modulates heart rate and the extent of stretch and shortening of myocardial fibers and, hence, the stroke volume and the cardiac output (stroke volume times heart rate). Three principal variables determine the stroke volume (Table 43–1): preload, afterload (resistance to ventricular emptying during systole), and the contractile state of the heart. For practical purposes, three of the principal determinants of cardiac output—preload, afterload, and heart rate—are readily measured. Contractile (inotropic) state remains difficult to assess in quantitative terms. Ejection fraction is commonly used as an index (albeit impure) of contractile state, and the maximum rate of pressure rise during the isovolumetic phase of systole (dP/dt) is a useful measure.

Relationships among these determinants vary with the state of the heart and circulation. Thus when contractility is impaired, stroke output and cardiac output tend to be maintained by ventricular dilation (Frank-Starling mechanism), limiting the value of cardiac output as a measure of inotropic state to experimental circumstances in which preload, afterload, and heart rate can be held constant.

Indicator-dilution techniques are useful for the bedside determination of cardiac output. In resting adults, the normal range is between 2.5 and 3.6 liters per minute per square meter of body surface area. Decreased cardiac output at rest occurs only in advanced stages of cardiac impairment. A

TABLE 43–1. TERMS USED TO DESCRIBE DETERMINANTS OF CARDIAC PERFORMANCE

Term	Relation to Cardiac Function
Afterload	Resistance that the ventricle must overcome during systole in order to eject the stroke volume. The two major determinants are aortic impedance (see below) and left ventricular volume.
Energetics	Generally determined as myocardial oxygen consumption. For any contractile state, the wall tension developed and maintained during contraction represents the major mechanical determinant of oxygen consumption. An increase in myocardial wall tension occurs in heart failure as filling pressure increases and the ventricle dilates, thereby increasing the energy cost of contraction (see Fig. 43–3).
Impedance (during ejection)	Instantaneous relationship between rate of change in aortic pressure and aortic blood flow. The aortic input impedance reflects the forces external to the heart that impose a load on the left ventricle, including stiffness of aortic wall. Determined primarily, but not exclusively, by total peripheral vascular resistance to runoff from the arterial tree. Normal peripheral resistance is approximately 1500 dynes • sec/cm^{-5} or 15 peripheral resistance units (also known as Wood's units).
Inotropic state	A measure of contractility.
Preload	Rigorously, stretch of myocardial fibers at end-diastole; commonly used as a synonym for venous return to the heart or end-diastolic volume.

blunted cardiac output response to exercise occurs much earlier. Supine exercise in normal subjects should increase the cardiac output by at least 600 ml per minute for each 100-ml increment in oxygen consumption; lower values indicate reduced cardiac performance. In heart failure the arteriovenous oxygen difference is abnormally wide, resulting chiefly from the low oxygen content of venous blood returning to the heart. Oxygenation of blood in the lungs remains nearly normal until pulmonary vascular congestion becomes sufficiently severe to create ventilation-perfusion mismatch with effective shunting, or abnormal diffusion barriers to oxygen transport.

During exercise, cardiac output normally increases as a linear function of oxygen consumption, although for any level of exercise the cardiac output tends to be lower in the upright position. Increases in cardiac output in the upright posture are accomplished principally by increases in heart rate rather than in stroke volume. In heart failure, cardiac output is particularly dependent on heart rate, both at rest and during exercise.

VENTRICULAR END-DIASTOLIC PRESSURE AND VOLUME (PRELOAD). Impaired systolic ventricular emptying leads to an increase in the end-systolic residual volume of blood in the ventricle, predisposing to an increase in end-diastolic volume. Since this is inconvenient to measure or monitor, ventricular end-diastolic pressure is customarily followed for clinical purposes on the premise that a change in pressure is effected by a change in ventricular volume. Exceptions occur, however, including structural changes in the myocardium (fibrosis, edema, and hypertrophy) and pericardial constriction that cause disproportionate rises in end-diastolic pressure relative to volume. Acute ischemia also produces transient reduction in left ventricular compliance. Conversely, in some states of chronic volume overload, compliance increases so that increased volumes are accommodated at end-diastole with relatively modest pressure increases.

A left ventricular end-diastolic pressure greater than 12 to 15 mm Hg is abnormal. The corresponding upper limit for the right ventricle is 6 to 10 mm Hg. It is straightforward to estimate the right ventricular end-diastolic pressure by measuring the central venous pressure. In the absence of mitral obstruction or increased pulmonary vascular resistance, pulmonary arterial diastolic pressure approximates left ventricular end-diastolic pressure. Pulmonary capillary wedge pressure or diastolic pressure measured with a Swan-Ganz catheter is widely used in intensive care settings to monitor left ventricular filling pressures.

To summarize, the performance of heart muscle depends on two essential components: fiber length (Frank-Starling mechanism) and inherent contractility (inotropic state). The normal heart autoregulates to maintain cardiac output. The variables involved are preload, afterload, contractility, and heart rate. With chronic overloading, the heart undergoes dilation, hypertrophy, or both.

PRELOAD. According to the Frank-Starling mechanism, an increase in end-diastolic volume (preload) results in more forceful contraction with enhancement of ventricular emptying and stroke volume. A unique ventricular function curve exists for each state of contractility (Fig. 43–1). The curve for a failing ventricle is shifted downward and flattened such that stroke volumes are reduced despite abnormally high end-diastolic volumes or pressures. The elevated filling pressures are responsible for congestion and edema in the venous beds leading to the failing ventricle.

In the normal heart, the Frank-Starling mechanism serves to match the stroke outputs of the two ventricles. In heart failure, this mechanism plays the additional role of helping to support the cardiac output.

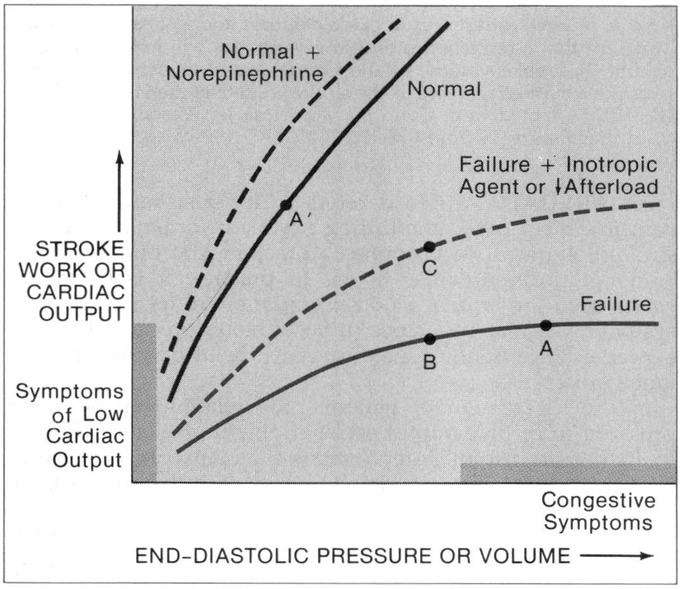

FIGURE 43–1. Schematic diagram demonstrating the relationship between ventricular end-diastolic pressure or volume and cardiac index in a normal and a failing heart. The normal left ventricle increases its stroke output as preload (often measured clinically as pulmonary capillary wedge pressure) increases, moving up the ascending limb of the curve until reserve is exhausted. In heart failure, the ventricular function curve is displaced downward and to the right. An increase in contractility, as after administration of norepinephrine or digitalis, displaces the curve to the left; i.e., a larger stroke output is accomplished at any given filling pressure. A and A′ represent the operating points at rest of a hypothetical patient with heart failure and of a normal person, respectively. Reduction of physical activity allows the failing heart to meet the demands of the metabolizing tissues. Treatment of heart failure by a reduction in preload (e.g., with a diuretic or a vasodilator acting predominantly on the venous bed) causes a shift from point A to B on the same ventricular function curve. Administration of a positive inotropic agent or a vasodilator producing afterload reduction will shift the curve as shown, resulting in improvement of the circulatory state in the direction shown by a shift from point A to C.

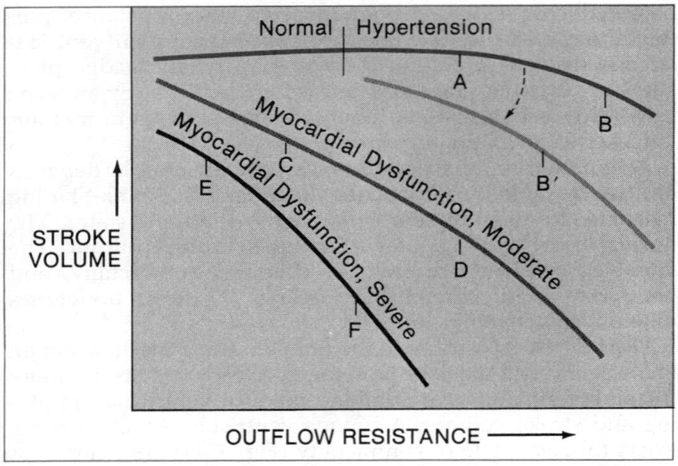

FIGURE 43–2. Relation of left ventricular stroke volume to systemic outflow resistance in normal and diseased hearts. A family of curves may be described, depending on the severity of the myocardial disease. If cardiac function is normal, a rise in resistance results in hypertension, since cardiac output remains fairly constant. Heart failure in a hypertensive patient could be shown by a move to either point B, a high resistance with normal function, or point B′, which represents a shift to a slightly depressed ventricular function curve. When myocardial dysfunction is more severe, as shown by the lower two curves, blood pressure is no longer directly determined by resistance, since stroke volume and resistance are inversely related. Consequently, arterial pressure may be similar at points E and F despite marked differences in cardiac output and resistance. It is also apparent that a reduction in outflow resistance will not affect significantly the stroke volume of the normal ventricle. However, it can produce a marked increase in the stroke volume of the failing ventricle (F →E). (Adapted from Cohn JN, Franciosa JA: Vasodilator therapy of cardiac failure. N Engl J Med 297:27, 1977.)

AFTERLOAD. Afterload refers to the resistance that the ventricle must overcome during systole in order to eject the stroke volume. It incorporates all factors that oppose shortening of the ventricular fibers. In practice, it is estimated either from the arterial blood pressure or from calculation of systemic vascular resistance (ratio of blood pressure to flow, expressed in units of dynes • sec/cm^{-5} or in peripheral resistance units).

In the assessment of patients, the relationship of blood pressure to cardiac output and peripheral resistance (P/Flow = R) is quite useful. Interventions that cause an increase in cardiac output without changing systemic blood pressure must cause vasodilation, thereby decreasing peripheral vascular resistance or afterload. Improved emptying of the left ventricle is usually accompanied by a decrease in its filling pressure (pulmonary wedge or diastolic pressure).

If preload and contractility remain constant, increasing afterload in the normal heart tends to decrease both the extent and the speed of contraction to a minor extent. Reduction in afterload has the opposite effects. Within broad physiologic limits, the normal ventricle maintains a relatively constant stroke volume as afterload is increased (Fig. 43–2). The impaired ventricle responds quite differently, with progressive diminution in its ability to eject blood against a given afterload as the severity of myocardial dysfunction advances. Figure 43–2 illustrates the rationale for afterload reduction in the management of heart failure.

CONTRACTILITY (INOTROPIC STATE). Modulation of sympathetic nervous activity provides the major component of short-term adjustment of contractile state in the normal heart and also mediates increases in heart rate and venous tone. Unlike the Frank-Starling mechanism, the increase in force and velocity of contraction is accomplished without any increase in fiber length (end-diastolic volume). Contractility does not limit the output of the normal heart. By contrast, the failing heart is limited in its myocardial performance, as indicated by displacement of the ventricular function curve, which is shown in Figure 43–1.

An objective index of myocardial contractility that could be measured independent of myocardial fiber length would be useful (1) to assess the effects on the myocardium of interventions such as the administration of digitalis or other inotropic agents; (2) to determine serial changes in inotropic state in an individual during the evolution of heart failure and in response to treatment; and (3) to compare the inotropic state in different individuals. However, distinction between the effects of loading conditions and intrinsic contractility is difficult because of the strong influence of loading on hemodynamic measurements. Changes in preload or afterload can modify ventricular performance greatly without affecting intrinsic inotropic state. Since conventional hemodynamic measurements do not take heart size into account, comparisons of contractility in hearts of different size are difficult to interpret.

Ejection Fraction. This term denotes the fraction of the right or left ventricular end-diastolic volume ejected per beat. It is useful as an integrative measure of contractility and is determined by contrast ventriculography, by gated radionuclide imaging, or by echocardiography. The normal left ventricular ejection fraction ranges from 0.56 to 0.78. A reduced ejection fraction in a patient with normal valves and a dilated ventricle strongly suggests decreased contractility, particularly in the absence of increased afterload. Abnormalities of regional myocardial function are often evident in the pattern of ventricular contraction demonstrated by these techniques.

Other Techniques. Simultaneous graphic recording of the electrocardiogram, phonocardiogram, and carotid arterial pulse contour provides another noninvasive means of assessing cardiac function. This approach does not readily distinguish between inotropic state and other determinants of cardiac performance, and interpretation is greatly complicated by disturbances in conduction or the presence of valvular disease. Accurate measurement of dP/dt can be accomplished at cardiac catheterization and provides a measure of contractile state less subject to the influence of loading conditions than most other approaches.

CHRONIC COMPENSATORY MECHANISMS. In chronic heart failure compensatory mechanisms include tachycardia, increased contractility due to sympathetic nervous activity, dilation, and hypertrophy. The increase in sympathetic activity is a mixed blessing, since it tends to increase systemic vascular resistance in addition to its salutary effects on cardiac output by increasing the heart rate and inotropic state.

Heart Rate. Chronic tachycardia characterizes decompensated heart failure. The increase in rate stems in part from cardiac reflexes stimulated by distention of structures at the venoatrial junctions (Bainbridge reflex). Tachycardia is, in terms of energy, an expensive way to support the cardiac output, and it is possible to precipitate heart failure by inducing sustained tachycardia.

Dilation. Progressive ventricular dilation typically occurs with the transition from compensation to overt failure. Dilation may serve as a useful compensatory mechanism for a time via the Frank-Starling relationship, but with progressive disease it ultimately becomes inadequate to maintain stroke output or does so only at the cost of markedly elevated filling pressures.

Mechanisms contributing to the inability of the dilated heart to maintain adequate function include (1) ultrastructural changes with slippage of sarcomeres during progressive dilation; as a result, they are not stretched to generate optimal contractility; and (2) increased wall tension (law of Laplace, Fig. 43–3) resulting in increased myocardial oxygen consumption; a corollary is that in contrast to the normal heart, in which the wall tension decreases in the course of systole, wall tension tends to remain high in the dilated heart. Thus chronic

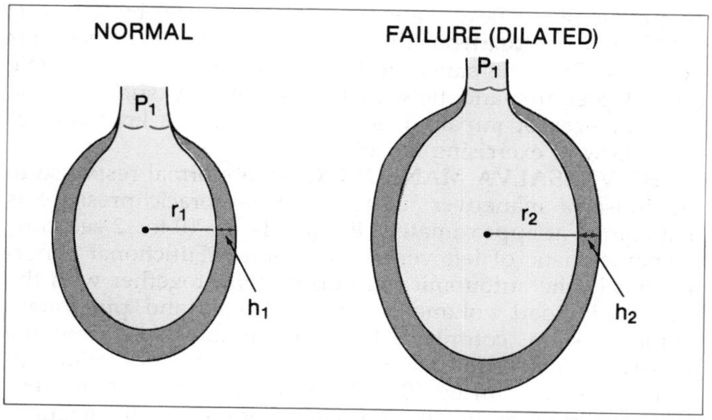

FIGURE 43–3. Laplace relationship applied to the dilated heart. The tension developed in the wall of the heart during systole (T) is a directional force that is proportional to the product of the mean pressure that the wall is supporting (P) and the mean radius (r). Dilation of the heart ($r_2 > r_1$) at the same pressure ($p_1 = p_2$) increases wall tension ($T_2 > T_1$). Should the wall become thinner during dilatation, the wall stress would increase as the cross-sectional area of myocardium (h) decreased (equation 2). The use of wall force (equation 3), which is proportional to the pressure and volume of the chamber, eliminates considerations of chamber size and shape and of the thickness of the myocardial wall.

Wall tension = Force per circumferential length of myocardium

$$= \frac{P \cdot \pi r^2}{2\pi r} \quad (1)$$

$$= \frac{P \cdot r}{2}$$

Wall stress = Force per cross-sectional area of myocardium

$$= \frac{P \cdot \pi r^2}{2\pi r h} \quad (2)$$

$$= \frac{P \cdot r}{2h}$$

Wall force = Pressure · cross-sectional area of chamber

$$= P \cdot r^2 \quad (3)$$

dilation has important limitations as a compensatory mechanism in cardiac failure.

Hypertrophy. Sustained abnormal pressure or volume loads lead to an increase in ventricular mass. This involves increased protein synthesis and perhaps decreased degradation in response to mechanical overload or dilation. The stimulus for hypertrophy appears to involve an increase in wall stress and possibly in the energy requirements of a chronically dilated heart with elevated filling pressures.

The hypertrophy pattern depends on the nature of the load. Chronic volume overloading leads to increased total mass as the chamber size enlarges, but wall thickness changes little ("eccentric" hypertrophy). By contrast, chronic exposure to increased pressure (e.g., systemic hypertension or aortic stenosis) leads to a "concentric" hypertrophy pattern in which end-diastolic volume remains unchanged but wall thickness increases.

Abnormal electrical conduction patterns can interfere with the normal, smoothly coordinated contraction pattern of the normal heart, as can myocyte loss with focal or diffuse fibrosis. Ischemic myocardial damage may lead to hypertrophy and remodeling of residual muscle because the geometry of the abnormal ventricle causes it to operate at a mechanical disadvantage and also because normal muscle must work, and expend energy, in moving and stretching adjacent damaged muscle or scar.

In early or mild hypertrophy, muscle mass and capillary vessels increase proportionately, preserving the nutritive and contractile properties of the myocardium. With progressive hypertrophy, additional sarcomeres are laid down, wall thickness increases, and ventricular wall stress tends to be maintained at a normal level despite increased cavity pressure, as indicated in equation 2, Figure 43–3. This process ultimately exacts a price, however, since increased wall thickness often leads to increased wall stiffness (reduced compliance), thus necessitating a disproportionate rise in filling pressure to maintain adequate end-diastolic ventricular volume. This leads to elevated pulmonary or systemic venous pressures, which contribute to symptoms of dyspnea or peripheral edema. In addition, beyond a certain point, coronary flow reserve diminishes and contractile function declines. Thus, once unremitting hypertrophy begins, the myocardium has embarked on the road to overt failure.

Despite the depressed contractile state associated with later stages of hypertrophy, circulatory function is maintained for a time by the combination of increased muscle mass, dilation, and augmented sympathetic drive. With continuing loss of myocardial contractility, or loss of muscle cells (e.g., from ischemic or inflammatory processes), circulatory compensation can no longer be maintained. The typical clinical and hemodynamic manifestations of congestive heart failure then emerge as cardiac output fails to meet demands and filling pressures increase.

Heart as a Muscle

Consideration of the ventricular performance of the failing heart usually centers on the contraction phase. Events during diastole, however, influence ventricular compliance and hence filling pressures, as well as the subsequent contraction and the energy supply for contraction and relaxation.

RELAXATION AND DISTENSIBILITY. Diastolic filling of the ventricle depends on the time available (a function of heart rate), the timing and properties of atrial systole, and the diastolic properties of the ventricle. Relaxation of cardiac muscle is an energy-requiring process (see above) that is quite vulnerable to adenosine triphosphate (ATP) depletion caused by ischemia. Although heart failure per se does not necessarily impair ventricular relaxation, associated processes of hypertrophy, fibrosis, and ischemia may reduce chamber distensibility and further increase filling pressures. This problem can be particularly severe in hypertrophic cardiomyopathy and in diseases such as amyloidosis that markedly reduce left ventricular diastolic compliance.

ENERGETICS. The heart depends on aerobic metabolism for its supply of energy, the bulk of which is spent to support contraction. The major determinants of oxygen consumption of the heart include the interrelated components of rate, ventricular pressure, volume, work, wall tension, and contractile state. The time integral of systolic tension relates closely to myocardial oxygen consumption, whereas fiber shortening has a minor effect on myocardial oxygen consumption.

The cellular and biochemical basis for heart failure remains unsettled. It is generally agreed that there are no consistent defects in energy metabolism or in protein synthesis and turnover. Current investigation is centered on excitation-contraction coupling and mechanisms that control calcium homeostasis.

Compensatory mechanisms in advanced heart failure tend to increase myocardial oxygen requirements by several mechanisms, including increased preload due to salt and water retention and enhanced sympathetic drive with consequently increased afterload, contractility, and heart rate. Increased preload and afterload are also the result of activation of the renin-angiotensin-aldosterone system.

Heart as Component of the Circulatory System

With loss of cardiac reserve and onset of overt heart failure, peripheral mechanisms are called upon to sustain blood pressure and cardiac output.

VENOUS HYPERTENSION. As the ejection fraction falls and the ventricle fails to empty properly during systole, the volume of unexpelled blood increases with an accompanying increase in diastolic pressure in the ventricles and in the atrium and proximal veins. Other elements that contribute to the venous hypertension include (1) increased tone in venous capacitance vessels; (2) blood volume expansion as a consequence of renal sodium and water retention; and, on occasion, (3) incompetence of mitral or tricuspid valves with regurgitation of blood from ventricle to atrium as the valve becomes incompetent from intrinsic valvular disease, papillary muscle dysfunction, ventricular dilation, or inadequate closure during an arrhythmia.

PERIPHERAL MECHANISMS TO SUSTAIN BLOOD PRESSURE AND CARDIAC OUTPUT. To sustain and distribute the cardiac output, and to maintain systemic arterial pressure, important peripheral mechanisms are activated.

In the normal circulation, the cardiac output doubles in response to a four- or fivefold increase in total body oxygen consumption. When functional impairment is such that the cardiac output cannot keep pace with peripheral demands, blood flow is redistributed to defend vital areas such as the brain and heart. The autonomic nervous system participates in this modulation of the circulation and contributes also to activation of mechanisms that mediate the retention of sodium and water.

Peripheral vasoconstriction and tachycardia characterize the common forms of heart failure. However, despite a generalized increase in sympathetic nervous activity, norepinephrine stores in the heart muscle are depleted because of its enhanced turnover rate. Pharmacologic agents such as reserpine or guanethidine, which further deplete cardiac catecholamine stores, aggravate heart failure, as do beta-adrenergic antagonists such as propranolol.

The contribution of the parasympathetic nervous system to the control of heart rate and baroreceptor activity is impaired in heart failure, but therapeutic consequences of these phenomena are not yet clear.

Peripheral Vasoconstriction. Peripheral arteriolar and venous constriction, mediated in large part by increased sympathetic nervous activity, is an important compensatory mechanism in heart failure that has both positive and negative consequences, as noted earlier. The second regulatory system that contributes to elevated peripheral vascular resistance is the renin-angiotensin system (see Ch. 47). The extent to which accumulation of sodium and water in the arteriolar wall contributes to increased arteriolar resistance is as yet unclear.

Venoconstriction augments venous return by facilitating the return of blood to the central veins, increasing central venous pressure and hence preload. The principal determinant of elevated filling pressures, however, is the inability of the failing ventricle to eject the venous return.

Redistribution. Maintenance of oxygen and substrate delivery to brain and myocardium during states of limited cardiac output requires diversion of flow from skin, kidneys, splanchnic viscera, and skeletal muscle. This redistribution of blood flow initially occurs during activity or stress as cardiac output fails to increase sufficiently to meet the increment in metabolism; in severe heart failure, redistribution operates also at rest. The redistribution of blood flow to essential beds depends on the balance among sympathetic innervation, renin-angiotensin system activity, and local metabolism. The vasculature of skin, kidney, splanchnic beds, and skeletal muscle is richly innervated. Furthermore, these tissues have relatively low metabolic rates, permitting sympathetic nervous and angiotensin II–mediated vasoconstriction to override local vasodilator effects of metabolites. By contrast, the circulations to brain and myocardium are less subject to alpha-adrenergically mediated vasoconstrictor influences because these organs, with their high oxygen consumption, produce metabolic dilator substances that offset increased sympathetic tone.

Under normal physiologic circumstances, exercise with the attendant need for heat dissipation induces an increase in cutaneous blood flow. Patients in heart failure, by contrast, fail to increase cutaneous flow despite this increased need for heat loss. Thus the patient in heart failure preserves systemic arterial pressure and flow to vital organs by suffering the consequences of impaired heat loss as well as limitation of blood flow to exercising muscle groups.

THE VALSALVA MANEUVER. An abnormal response to the Valsalva maneuver, in which intrathoracic pressure is maintained at approximately 40 mm Hg for 10 to 12 seconds, is characteristic of left ventricular failure. Functional abnormalities in the autonomic nervous system, together with the expanded blood volume in the left heart and pulmonary venous system, contribute to an abnormal response to the Valsalva maneuver in patients with left ventricular failure. In normal subjects during 10 to 12 seconds of increase in intrathoracic pressure to 40 mm Hg, there is a characteristic decrease in blood pressure and pulse pressure and increase in heart rate; at cessation of straining, the blood pressure, pulse pressure, and bradycardia tend to overshoot. By contrast, in the presence of left ventricular failure there is a "square wave" response of blood pressure. Blood pressure increases at the onset of straining, stays elevated throughout the maneuver, and decreases abruptly to baseline after the maneuver with no overshoot; there is little, if any, change in pulse pressure, and tachycardia is absent. The blunting of reflex changes results from the absence of stroke output or arterial pulse pressure changes during the phase of reduced venous return, and hence no reflex changes are elicited.

SALT AND WATER RETENTION. As overt heart failure develops, there is typically a decrease in renal blood flow and glomerular filtration rate, with an associated redistribution of renal blood flow. These changes contribute to the sodium and water retention that characterizes heart failure, but the nature and extent of the response differ according to the severity of heart failure, as discussed subsequently under diuretics. Hemodynamic abnormalities are undoubtedly involved in activating the renin-angiotensin-aldosterone system both via direct effects on the kidney and via indirect effects stemming from activation of mechanoreceptors in the distended left atrium. Recognition of the role of hyperaldosteronism in the genesis of sodium and water retention has resulted in the development of aldosterone antagonists as useful adjuncts in the therapy of heart failure.

Sweat and saliva are sodium poor in patients with decompensated heart failure. Antidiuretic hormone (arginine vasopressin) levels tend to be elevated in heart failure and may contribute to elevated systemic vascular resistance, but probably are not important in salt or water retention.

An increase of about 10 to 20 per cent in circulating blood volume contributes to maintenance of cardiac output and perfusion of vital organs in moderate-to-severe heart failure, augmenting ventricular end-diastolic volume and thereby tending to improve ventricular performance. The resulting elevation of filling pressure, however, promotes edema formation by raising venous and capillary pressures proximal to the failing ventricle. By the time the circulating blood volume has increased by 20 per cent, the extravascular fluid volume may well have increased by a factor of two.

Exercise Testing

On the premise that the circulatory function of the heart has failed when it can no longer provide sufficient oxygen and nutrients to satisfy metabolic needs, graded treadmill or bicycle exercise testing has been used investigatively to determine maximum total body oxygen uptake (aerobic capacity). The endpoint of fatigue generally coincides with the point at which aerobic metabolism can no longer meet tissue demands and lactate production begins (anaerobic threshold). This approach has also been used to assess quantitatively the effects of therapeutic interventions for the treatment of heart failure.

CLINICAL MANIFESTATIONS OF HEART FAILURE

The signs and symptoms of heart failure depend on which ventricle has failed and the severity and duration of failure. The clinical picture in left ventricular failure is dominated by *symptoms* of pulmonary congestion and edema. By contrast, right ventricular failure is dominated by *signs* of systemic venous congestion and peripheral edema. Weakness, fatigue, and effort intolerance are common to right or left ventricular failure as well as biventricular failure.

Left Ventricular Failure

The symptom of breathlessness predominates in the patients with left ventricular failure and varies with position and activity. Noteworthy physical signs are most evident in the heart, the lungs, or respiratory control mechanisms.

DYSPNEA. Dyspnea (breathlessness) during limited exertion is typically the earliest symptom of left heart failure and is usually associated with an increased rate of breathing (tachypnea). Although many details of the physiologic basis for the sensation of dyspnea remain unclear, some aspects of the etiology of respiratory symptoms from pulmonary congestion deserve consideration. Since the bronchial capillaries drain for the most part via the pulmonary veins, congestion tends to develop in alveolar and bronchial vascular networks simultaneously. Interstitial edema surrounding pulmonary capillaries appears to stimulate juxtacapillary receptors known as J-receptors, which in turn elicits a reflexly mediated pattern of rapid and shallow breathing. At the same time, bronchial congestion stimulates mucus production, and the distended bronchial capillaries may rupture, with resulting cough and hemoptysis. Bronchial mucosal edema causes increased resistance in small airways, producing wheezing and respiratory distress known as cardiac asthma. The increased work of moving fluid-laden, noncompliant lungs must be accomplished in the face of decreased blood flow to respiratory muscles and also increased diffusion barriers to oxygen exchange across the alveolar-capillary interface, contributing to respiratory muscle fatigue and the sensation of dyspnea.

In any event, the symptom of dyspnea in left heart failure clearly relates to the increase in blood volume and interstitial fluid content of the lungs at the expense of air. Ventilation increases, and the awareness of dyspnea becomes more severe as minute ventilation approaches the maximal ventilatory capacity.

ORTHOPNEA. Dyspnea that occurs soon after lying flat (and is relieved by sitting up) is known as orthopnea. The pathophysiologic basis for orthopnea is the increase in venous return from the lower extremities and splanchnic bed to the lungs in the recumbent position, together with the reabsorption of peripheral edema that accumulates during the day. Orthopnea is a relatively reliable marker for left ventricular failure, whereas the dyspnea associated with chronic lung disease or musculoskeletal disorders is not typically aggravated by lying flat. Patients usually learn to avoid dyspnea of this sort by sleeping with the head and thorax on two or more pillows. In advanced heart failure, orthopnea may be so severe as to cause the patient to sleep upright in a chair. An orthopneic cough has the same significance as orthopnea and is presumably the consequence of venous congestion and edema, as discussed previously. Patients with left heart failure may also complain of precordial distress in the supine position that is difficult to distinguish from symptoms caused by myocardial ischemia.

NOCTURIA. In early heart failure, limitation of renal blood flow with upright activity during the day gives way to more normal renal perfusion and diuresis while supine at night. This causes nocturia, a common early symptom of incipient heart failure.

PAROXYSMAL NOCTURNAL DYSPNEA. Severe respiratory distress may arouse the patient from sleep. Relief is urgently sought by sitting up and often by finding an open window. Such episodes are caused by marked exacerbations of pulmonary vascular congestion and edema during supine sleep. Blunting of the respiratory center response to sensory input from the lungs during sleep, together with increased venous return, allows pulmonary venous congestion and edema to accumulate and trigger the alarming episode of breathlessness.

ACUTE PULMONARY EDEMA. In an episode of acute left ventricular failure, pulmonary venous and capillary pressure can increase abruptly to levels exceeding plasma oncotic pressure, with consequent rapid accumulation of edema fluid in the interstitial spaces and alveoli. Interstitial pulmonary edema leads to an increase in respiratory rate (see foregoing discussion) and tends to produce alveolar hyperventilation and respiratory alkalosis. However, when free fluid enters the alveoli and bronchioles, respiratory acidosis may occur owing to an intolerable increase in the work of breathing. Hypoxemia also occurs commonly because of imbalances between alveolar ventilation and alveolar blood flow (ventilation-perfusion mismatch or "shunting").

Symptoms of pulmonary edema may begin with a nonproductive cough, with wheezing, or with frank dyspnea. Apart from tachypnea and possibly evidence of underlying heart disease on physical examination, few physical signs may be present initially. Later, as free fluid accumulates in distal airways, rales become audible at the lung bases and extend upward accompanied by rhonchi as the episode progresses. In severe acute pulmonary edema, the patient is typically pale, sweating, cyanotic, gasping for breath, and sometimes producing pink or blood-tinged frothy sputum.

HEMOPTYSIS. Rust-colored sputum containing heart failure cells (alveolar macrophages containing hemosiderin) sometimes occurs in severe chronic left heart failure and is seen with particular frequency in patients with advanced mitral stenosis. Frankly bloody sputum should suggest the possibility of pulmonary infarction, but expectoration of substantial quantities of blood can also occur as a consequence of rupture of engorged bronchial capillaries in patients with severe chronic left heart failure, including that caused by uncorrected mitral stenosis.

CHEYNE-STOKES RESPIRATION. Advanced heart failure may be accompanied by periodic breathing with alternate periods of apnea and hyperventilation. Due to slowing of the circulation time from lungs to brain, the arterial P_{O_2} reaches its peak and the arterial P_{CO_2} its nadir during apnea. At this time alveolar gas tensions are exactly opposite. During hyperpnea the alveolar P_{O_2} reaches its peak and the alveolar P_{CO_2} its nadir. Thus, changes in arterial blood gases are responsible for the cyclic ventilation, which in turn causes the changes in alveolar gas tensions. As would be expected from this delay of the normal negative feedback loop, the longer the circulation time, the longer are the cycles of hyperventilation and apnea. The neurologic changes of advanced age predispose to Cheyne-Stokes breathing, as does cerebrovascular disease.

Physical and Laboratory Signs of Left Heart Failure

The patient with decompensated left heart failure is generally tachypneic, pale, dusky, and sweaty. The handshake is cold because of peripheral vasoconstriction, and tachycardia is present. The pulse pressure is usually narrow, often with a modest increase in diastolic pressure. The neck veins are not distended if the left ventricle alone has failed.

THE HEART. Cardiac enlargement is often evident with inspection, percussion, and palpation of the apical impulse and is confirmed by radiographic examination, although this finding is more typical of valvular or primary myocardial disease than of ischemic heart disease. With increased left heart filling pressure pulmonary venous pressure increases and the pulmonary arterial pressure must also increase. The pulmonic component of the second heart sound (P_2) therefore tends to increase in intensity. In the presence of left ventricular dilation, papillary muscle dysfunction, or both, the mitral valve leaflets may fail to appose properly, resulting in mitral incompetence.

Gallop Rhythm. The presence of a protodiastolic third heart sound (S_3 gallop) in an adult with heart disease usually signifies the presence of heart failure. The timing of the normal first and second sounds and the abnormal third sound, in conjunction with an increased heart rate, results in the characteristic cadence of the gallop rhythm. The third heart sound occurs in early diastole coincident with rapid ventricular filling. The S_3 gallop appears to be produced by vibrations of the ventricular walls as the rapidly inflowing blood is abruptly arrested. A third heart sound is a normal finding in children and in young adults.

Presystolic gallop rhythms result from the atrial contribution to ventricular filling. The atrial or S_4 gallop is characteristic of decreased ventricular compliance and typically results from left ventricular hypertrophy or ischemia rather than from myocardial dysfunction or failure. When a patient with an audible fourth heart sound develops overt heart failure, a third sound may appear, causing a quadruple rhythm. If the heart rate is sufficiently rapid or the PR interval is prolonged, S_3 and S_4 may merge, producing a summation gallop. The presence of a summation gallop has the same clinical implication as other protodiastolic (S_3) gallop rhythms.

Pulsus Alternans. The presence of alternating strong and weak beats (the fundamental rhythm remaining regular) usually signifies advanced heart failure. Pulsus alternans can be detected by palpation or by sphygmomanometry and often follows an atrial or ventricular premature beat for several cycles. Mechanical alternans of this sort is only rarely associated with electrical alternans. Pulsus alternans has been attributed to a severe disturbance of excitation-contraction coupling, the detailed pathophysiology of which is unclear.

THE LUNGS. The sequence of pulmonary findings with advancing left heart failure has been described in the foregoing section on acute pulmonary edema.

THE ELECTROCARDIOGRAM. Electrocardiographic abnormalities result from underlying cardiac disease, therapeutic agents (e.g., digitalis), or both and yield little information regarding the functional status of the heart.

RADIOLOGIC ASPECTS. The chest radiograph is usually quite helpful in the diagnosis and assessment of left ventricular failure (see Ch. 42.1). The cardiac silhouette is typically, but not invariably, enlarged and may assume telltale configurations that are determined by the underlying disease process. In contrast to normal, the pulmonary vasculature is prominent in the upper lung zones, reflecting pulmonary venous hypertension and redistribution of blood flow because of encroachment upon the lower lung vessels by edema and possibly fibrosis. Enlarged hilar shadows and prominent septal lines, particularly near the costophrenic angles (Kerley's B lines), are typical findings. Alveolar edema results in a generalized clouding of the lung fields but can occur in focal or patchy distributions that are difficult to distinguish from pneumonia. Pleural effusions sometimes occur in predominantly left-sided heart failure but are more characteristic of biventricular failure. Interstitial and alveolar edema may lessen or disappear with onset of right ventricular failure. A widened superior vena cava shadow suggests right ventricular failure and systemic venous congestion.

PULMONARY FUNCTION TESTS. The course of left ventricular failure, including the response to treatment, can be followed by consecutive determinations of vital capacity, although this practice has been largely supplanted by other approaches in recent years. With interstitial pulmonary edema, expiratory flow rates at low lung volumes are reduced and distal airways tend to close prematurely during expiration, trapping gas within the lungs and disturbing the normal relation of ventilation to perfusion. This produces a widening of the alveolar-arterial P_{O_2} difference and a decrease in arterial P_{O_2} due to venous admixture. Arterial oxygen saturation is typically nearly normal, however, unless intrinsic lung disease is present. The arteriovenous oxygen content difference increases with decreasing cardiac outputs as tissue extraction of oxygen becomes more complete. Systemic arterial P_{CO_2} remains normal or low unless ventilation is compromised in the course of pulmonary edema. Endotracheal intubation and assisted ventilation may be indicated if progressive carbon dioxide retention is documented by serial blood gas measurements.

Right Ventricular and Biventricular Failure

CLINICAL MANIFESTATIONS. Isolated right ventricular failure is uncommon in adults and is usually a consequence of cor pulmonale secondary to intrinsic lung disease or, on occasion, chronic volume overload from a congenital atrial septal defect. Right ventricular failure is encountered most often as a complication of left ventricular failure. In the presence of elevated right heart filling pressures, neck veins are distended and fill from below. Hepatic enlargement and tenderness to gentle palpation result from passive congestion, and compression causes further distention of the neck veins (hepatojugular reflux). In the presence of biventricular failure, signs of right ventricular failure may dominate, but the presence of dyspnea and rales should suggest additional left ventricular failure. Accompanying low cardiac output results in signs of increased sympathetic nervous activity and of organ hypoperfusion. It should be remembered that a critically lowered cardiac output from any cause sufficient to produce metabolic acidosis will occasion hyperventilation in defense of acid-base balance, and this must be distinguished from the tachypnea of left heart failure.

Advanced right-sided or biventricular failure may be associated with anorexia, weight loss, and malnutrition ("cardiac cachexia"). Digitalis excess, high doses of diuretics, and electrolyte disturbances often contribute to the genesis of this manifestation of end-stage heart failure.

Cyanosis. Cyanosis is caused by 5 or more grams per 100 ml of unoxygenated hemoglobin in the subpapillary venous plexus of the skin. This occurs in right heart failure because the congested venules contain blood from which considerable oxygen has been extracted because of the slow flow. This is typically accompanied by relatively normal arterial P_{O_2} values unless intrinsic lung disease or intracardiac shunting is present. Cyanosis is usually absent in left heart failure unless caused by a complication (e.g., pneumonia) or by pulmonary edema.

Abnormal Heart and Lungs. Although dyspnea accompanying left ventricular failure may be partially relieved by onset of right ventricular failure, some dyspnea usually persists, together with tachypnea and basal rales. Tricuspid valvular insufficiency commonly accompanies severe right ventricular dilation and failure and contributes to systemic venous engorgement. The murmur of tricuspid insufficiency is distinguished from that of mitral insufficiency by its location (lower left border of sternum), by its tendency to increase during inspiration, and by associated physical signs, such as hepatic pulsation and systolic waves in the jugular venous pulse. Doppler echocardiography greatly assists in the assessment of this problem. Pleural effusion, often unilateral, is more common in right-sided or biventricular than in isolated left ventricular failure.

Systemic Venous Congestion. Elevation of systemic venous pressure is a sine qua non of right heart failure. Responsible mechanisms include (1) the inability of the failing ventricle to eject the venous return without abnormally high filling pressures, causing (2) an increase in the volume of blood in the large systemic veins; and (3) increased venomotor tone resulting from increased sympathetic nervous system activity.

Increased systemic venous pressure is responsible for the hepatomegaly, occasional splenomegaly, and peripheral edema that characterize decompensated right ventricular failure. Usually less apparent are the associated congestion and edema of the gastrointestinal tract.

Pressure in the jugular venous system, a useful index of right atrial pressure, may be estimated from the height of the column of blood distending the cervical veins. The cervical veins are normally flat in the upright posture in the absence of raised intrathoracic pressure, whereas in right heart failure they are prominent and distended. The wave form of venous pulsation is usually best appreciated from inspection of the right internal jugular vein, adjusting the angle of the patient's upper body to bring out the top of the venous pressure column. Tricuspid insufficiency distorts the normal venous pulse by producing a systolic or C-V wave that has no counterpart in the normal jugular venous pulse. Occasionally, compression over the liver is necessary to display the increased blood volume in the venous system, but the examiner must avoid being misled by venous distention from involuntary expiration against a closed glottis (Valsalva's maneuver).

Liver. The liver is typically enlarged and tender in right heart failure. If the onset is acute, right upper quadrant pain may result from constraint of the swollen liver by its tight capsule. Splenomegaly is uncommon except in prolonged passive congestion of the liver, and pain or tenderness of the spleen should raise the question of superimposed systemic embolization and splenic infarction.

Early congestion of the liver may cause modest increases in the concentrations of hepatic enzymes such as alkaline phosphatase in serum, and increases in serum bilirubin may occur. Hyperbilirubinemia from this cause usually consists of a combination of conjugated and unconjugated bilirubin. Frank jaundice is uncommon unless hepatic congestion is associated with longstanding pulmonary congestion or pulmonary infarction.

Hypoglycemia may occur if cardiac output is severely compromised and hepatic congestion is marked and protracted. This is attributed to depletion of liver glycogen stores and increased formation of lactic acid from glucose induced by hypoxia.

Repeated and prolonged episodes of right heart failure with reduced hepatic blood flow and elevated venous pressures can cause atrophy and centrilobular necrosis of liver cells and can lead to extensive fibrosis ("cardiac cirrhosis") that is difficult to distinguish from posthepatitic cirrhosis. Hepatic failure with precoma or coma is a rare, preterminal complication of this sequence of events.

Extracellular Fluid Compartments. The fluid compartments of the body are normally maintained constant by neurohormonally mediated interplay among intake (governed by thirst and appetite), exchanges of fluid and electrolytes (governed by passive and active transport mechanisms), and excretion (regulated primarily by the kidneys). In heart failure, excessive retention of sodium and water by the kidneys results in an isosmotic expansion of extracellular fluid, including the circulating blood volume. In mild heart failure, retention of sodium and water may serve to expand the blood volume to sustain venous return and the forward output of the failing heart through the Frank-Starling mechanism. However, retention of salt and water only exacerbates pulmonary and systemic congestion and edema when the myocardium can no longer respond positively to increased filling pressure and volumes.

The distribution of excess extracellular ("third space") fluid varies among patients. Under the influence of gravity, edema accumulates in the feet and ankles of ambulatory patients but shifts to the sacral region in the bedridden patient. Localization occurs in areas of low tissue pressure, such as the back of the ankle. Colloid osmotic pressure and the integrity of the lymphatic system also influence extracellular fluid distribution.

Peripheral Edema. Dependent edema developing over the course of the day and subsiding by morning is a characteristic feature of right heart failure. It is a direct consequence of elevated systemic venous pressure and is typically preceded by a gain in weight. Persistent edema is accompanied relatively frequently by complications such as low-grade cellulitis, and the combination of edema and sluggish venous flow predisposes to deep venous thrombosis and pulmonary embolism.

Pleural Effusion. The infrequency of hydrothorax in isolated right ventricular failure dictates that the association of pleural effusion and cor pulmonale should lead one to search for another cause, such as pulmonary infarction. It is, however, common in biventricular failure. Hydrothorax results from impaired removal of isotonic fluid from the pleural space because of elevated venous pressures in both the pulmonary and the systemic circulations, compromising transcapillary exchange of water at the pleural surface and also impeding lymphatic drainage. Hydrothorax contributes to dyspnea reflexly, probably by stimuli from lungs and chest wall, as well as by displacing ventilated lung tissue from the relatively fixed volume of the thoracic space. Pulmonary embolism and infarction may contribute to pleural effusion in two ways: by transit of fluid from the infarcted area of the lung and to the pleural space or by aggravation of heart failure.

Ascites. The presence of free fluid in the abdominal cavity is a late manifestation of right heart failure, usually associated with systemic venous hypertension, peripheral edema, and hydrothorax. It is commonly encountered in the setting of tricuspid valve disease or chronic constrictive pericarditis. Elevated pressures in portal and hepatic veins and in the systemic veins draining the peritoneum contribute to the formation of ascites, but renal retention of sodium and water is a prerequisite. It may contribute to anorexia and can cause abdominal discomfort or pain in patients with severe right ventricular failure.

Pericardial Effusion. Patients with chronic heart failure commonly have increased amounts of fluid in the pericardial sac that can be demonstrated echocardiographically. Only rarely, however, does it accumulate to an extent that produces further hemodynamic compromise (tamponade).

Anasarca. Advanced and protracted right ventricular failure without adequate treatment can cause edema fluid to accumulate throughout the body, most conspicuously in subcutaneous tissues as well as abdominal and thoracic cavities. Face and arms are typically spared until the preterminal stages of failure. This clinical picture occurs rarely in the present era of potent diuretics.

Gastrointestinal Tract. Systemic venous hypertension leads to edema of the bowel wall. These changes interfere with absorption of drugs or foods only when heart failure is severe, but reduced bioavailability of furosemide and perhaps other drugs can occur under these circumstances. In severe congestive heart failure, anorexia, nausea, and vomiting may occur from reflex, central, local, or drug-induced causes. Protein-losing enteropathy can occur in the setting of severe right heart failure.

Brain. Nonspecific complaints, including headache and insomnia, are common in heart failure and are usually attributable to some diminution of cerebral blood flow and triggering mechanisms such as dyspnea that contribute to insomnia. Neurologic or behavioral aberrations are more frequent when the burdens of a limited cardiac output are superimposed on antecedent neurologic disease (e.g., cerebrovascular disease or prior stroke) or on personality disorder. Irritability, restlessness, and limited attention span are associated with severe congestive heart failure. Stupor and coma supervene when cardiac output is critically reduced.

Kidney. Oliguria occurs with decompensation in isolated right or left heart failure but is more prominent in the latter or in biventricular failure. The urine is sodium poor but has a relatively high specific gravity (1.020 to 1.030). Prerenal azotemia is common, particularly in the presence of intrinsic renal disease or after vigorous diuresis. Azotemia with high urine specific gravity is characteristic of heart failure (and dehydration) and stands in contrast to the low specific gravity expected with renal insufficiency due to intrinsic renal disease. Blood urea nitrogen is typically elevated out of proportion to serum creatinine. Proteinuria is common but does not usually exceed 1 gram per day.

Other Manifestations. In chronic severe congestive heart failure, weakness and gradual loss of tissue mass are frequent concomitants and may progress to cachexia. At this late stage, the patient is usually suffering from anorexia and often gastrointestinal symptoms and electrolyte disturbances as well. Although organ hypoperfusion and congestion play an important part in this syndrome, the physician must maintain vigilance to avoid additional contributions from overvigorous use of digitalis and diuretics.

Anxiety. This is a common feature of cardiac disease by the time the heart fails. Manifestations of anxiety may be difficult to distinguish from symptoms of the underlying cardiac disorder because of the nonspecific nature of complaints such as breathlessness. Symptoms related to hyperventilation as well as palpitations may contribute to the patient's anxiety by reinforcing the impression that organic heart disease is present. The physician must proceed with the separate assessment of organic and psychosomatic aspects of the disease process, recognizing that a careful history and physical examination, together with judicious use of noninvasive diagnostic methods, will usually establish the extent to which organic heart disease is responsible for the patient's symptoms.

CLINICAL MANAGEMENT OF HEART FAILURE

General Approaches

The management of congestive heart failure includes three general types of approaches. The first is removal of the underlying cause. This is the first priority in all cases and includes measures such as surgical correction of valvular lesions or congenital malformation. It also includes medical treatment of hypertension or infective endocarditis when present.

The second approach consists of removal of precipitating causes of heart failure. Frequently the initial development or exacerbation of heart failure is related not to worsening of the underlying cardiac condition but rather to a superimposed stress. Typical factors that can precipitate overt congestive heart failure, apart from changes in the status of the heart itself, are listed in Table 43–2.

TABLE 43–2. PRECIPITATING OR EXACERBATING FACTORS IN CONGESTIVE HEART FAILURE

Increased demand:
- Anemia
- Fever
- Infection
- Fluid overload
- Increased dietary salt intake
- High environmental temperature
- Renal failure
- Hepatic failure
- Thyrotoxicosis
- Arteriovenous (A-V) shunt (Paget's disease of bone)
- Respiratory insufficiency
- Emotional stress
- Pregnancy
- Obesity

Arrhythmias
Pulmonary embolism
Ethanol ingestion
Thiamin deficiency
Uncontrolled hypertension
Poor compliance with therapeutic regimen
Drugs
- Beta-adrenergic blockers
- Antiarrhythmic drugs (e.g., disopyramide)
- Salt-retaining drugs
  - Steroids
  - Nonsteroidal anti-inflammatory agents

The third set of measures, treatment of clinical manifestations of heart failure, will occupy the remainder of this chapter. This approach may in turn be divided into three categories, as summarized in Table 43–3:

1. Measures to improve the contractile performance of the heart.
2. Measures to reduce cardiac work.
3. Measures to control excessive retention of salt and water.

As listed in Table 43–3, several therapeutic entities are available in each category. Cardiac glycosides and sympathomimetic agents constitute the principal drugs that enhance the pumping performance of the failing heart. In addition, placement of a pacemaker may improve pumping performance either by supporting a more appropriate heart rate or by restoring atrial augmentation of ventricular filling if synchronous atrioventricular contraction can be achieved (see Ch. 45).

Reduction of the work load of the failing heart can be accomplished by physical and emotional rest, by appropriate treatment of obesity, and by vasodilator therapy. Under specific circumstances, assisted circulation with the intra-aortic balloon pump can usefully contribute to this goal.

Finally, control of the excessive retention of salt and water is approached by instituting a low-sodium diet and the use of diuretic drugs. Under some circumstances, mechanical removal of fluid will be of value.

These measures are customarily applied in a stepwise fashion, as outlined in detail in Table 43–4.

Strategy of Heart Failure Management

The many etiologies and degrees of severity of heart failure demand an individualized approach to each patient. Nevertheless, certain general principles apply to the management of various subsets of patients. It is usually not appropriate to institute specific therapeutic measures until symptoms of overt heart failure occur—that is, until the patient makes the transition from functional class I to class II. The first approach in all instances will include judicious limitation of activity, advising the patient to avoid physical exertion that produces undue dyspnea or exhaustion. The degree of restriction should be tailored to the severity of heart failure. It is important not to limit activity so severely that skeletal muscle deconditioning, rather than the underlying cardiac problem,

TABLE 43–3. MEASURES IN THE MANAGEMENT OF CONGESTIVE HEART FAILURE

A. Improve pump performance of the failing ventricle
   1. Cardiac glycosides (digoxin)
   2. Sympathomimetic drugs (dopamine, dobutamine)
   3. Other positive inotropic drugs (amrinone)
   4. Pacemaker for bradycardia or loss of atrioventricular synchrony

B. Reduction of cardiac work load
   1. Rest (physical and emotional)
   2. Correction of obesity
   3. Vasodilator drugs
   4. Assisted circulation (e.g., intra-aortic balloon counterpulsation)

C. Control salt and water retention
   1. Limit dietary sodium intake
   2. Diuretics
   3. Mechanical removal of fluid
      a. Thoracentesis
      b. Paracentesis
      c. Dialysis
      d. Phlebotomy

TABLE 43–4. STEPS IN THE MANAGEMENT OF CHRONIC CONGESTIVE HEART FAILURE

	Functional Class		
Steps	*II*	*III*	*IV*
A	*Restrict physical activity:* Limit competitive sports and heavy labor	Reduce work schedule; rest periods during day	Limit to house and finally to bed and chair
B	*Dietary sodium restriction:* Eliminate salt shaker and heavily salted foods	Eliminate salt in cooking and at table (Na intake ~ 1.2 to 1.8 grams)	As in III, plus low-sodium foods (Na intake <1 gram)
C	*Diuretics:* Thiazide or low-dose loop diuretic	Loop diuretic (progressive doses); consider adding distally acting (K-sparing) diuretic	Loop diuretic with distally acting (K-sparing) and/or thiazide diuretic
D	*Digitalis glycosides:* Conventional maintenance doses →	→	Dose to maintain serum level in 1.5 ng/ml range
E		*Vasodilators:* Hydralazine and isosorbide dinitrate *or* captopril	Intravenous nitroprusside
F			*Other inotropic drugs (intravenous):* Dopamine, dobutamine, amrinone
G			*Consider cardiac transplantation* *Thoracentesis, paracentesis* *Dialysis* *Assisted circulation (e.g., intra-aortic balloon pump)*

becomes the limiting factor in the patient's activity. Physical activity should, however, be markedly restricted in the setting of acute decompensation of chronic heart failure, a situation in which hospitalization will generally be advisable.

Diuretics or cardiac glycosides may be added in early class II, with the choice of one or both based on the balance between risk and expected benefit. In many cases, modest doses of digoxin and a mild diuretic such as thiazide will restore the patient to an essentially asymptomatic state. Dietary sodium restriction may be limited to avoidance of heavily salted foods and the use of the salt shaker at the table. Special low-sodium foods are expensive and can be so unpalatable as to impair nutrition.

When symptoms persist or evolve on the simple regimen outlined above, intensification of the diuretic regimen is usually the next step. Depending upon the etiology of the heart failure, vasodilators may be instituted in late class II or class III failure. Problems such as mitral regurgitation will be particularly amenable to successful treatment with vasodilators, as discussed below.

As the severity of heart failure advances, increased restriction of physical activity is usually necessary, and patients will often require rest periods during the day as class III symptoms evolve. When patients remain symptomatic during ordinary activity on a program that includes digitalis, loop diuretics, and vasodilators, hospitalization is often advisable to search for precipitating causes and to consider the possibility of more aggressive approaches. In patients who have progressed to functional class IV, hospitalization will usually be advisable and the use of intravenous sympathomimetic agents can be considered, as well as optimization of the vasodilator, diuretic, and cardiac glycoside regimens. In younger patients who meet appropriate criteria, cardiac transplantation should also be considered at this time.

During episodes of decompensation, the hazards of deep venous thrombosis and pulmonary embolism must be guarded against, and the use of minidose heparin (see Ch. 57) is a relatively safe and effective approach during hospitalization. At these times, emotional as well as physical rest is important, and anxiety-provoking situations should be carefully avoided. Marked anxiety or insomnia may be treated with benzodiazepines such as diazepam or the shorter-acting agent triazolam.

DIET. Rigid salt restriction can usually be avoided until diuretics are no longer capable of controlling the accumulation of salt and water. Water intake will, in general, not require specific restriction unless dilutional hyponatremia supervenes.

OXYGEN. Patients with hypoxia, and certainly those with pulmonary edema, will benefit from oxygen inhalation, conveniently given by nasal prongs at 4 to 6 liters per minute. In general, supplemental oxygen is worthwhile whenever the arterial oxygen saturation falls below 90 per cent. This will be a particularly effective way of reducing right ventricular afterload, since oxygen is a potent pulmonary arteriolar vasodilator.

PHYSICAL REMOVAL OF FLUID. The availability of potent diuretics limits the need for thoracentesis or paracentesis, but these procedures may be important diagnostically when the accumulation of fluid in serous cavities is not readily explained on the basis of heart failure alone. Pulmonary embolism, for example, is a relatively common cause of pleural effusion, and a diagnostic thoracentesis will often provide critically important information leading to this diagnosis. Drainage of pleural or ascitic fluid should be carried out slowly, at a rate of not more than about 1500 ml per hour, and the total quantity of fluid removed on any single occasion should not exceed about 1500 ml because of the risk of fluid shifts from the vascular to the extravascular compartment, with consequently inadequate ventricular filling pressures. Particular caution is required in patients (such as those with aortic stenosis or hypertrophic cardiomyopathy) who have reduced ventricular compliance and require high ventricular filling pressures to maintain adequate stroke volume.

Acute Pulmonary Edema

Acute pulmonary edema is a medical emergency in which the immediate therapeutic goals are to (1) improve oxygenation; (2) reduce venous return (preload); (3) reduce anxiety; and (4) treat causal and precipitating factors. Placement of flow-directed pulmonary artery (Swan-Ganz) and arterial lines for monitoring of pressures and arterial blood gases will often be advisable. The patient is placed in a trunk-up, legs-down posture and given humidified 100 per cent oxygen, by positive pressure mask if possible. Vital signs are monitored frequently, and an intravenous cannula is inserted for secure intravenous access. Arterial blood gas, blood urea nitrogen (BUN) or creatinine, electrolyte, and complete blood count measurements are obtained at once. An electrocardiogram and chest radiograph (taken with a portable machine if necessary) should also be obtained, and electrical conversion of supraventricular or ventricular tachyarrhythmias should be considered if present and if not due to digitalis excess.

Morphine given intravenously (2 to 10 mg, repeated every 10 to 15 minutes) will reduce venous return and allay anxiety; naloxone should be available in case of respiratory depression. Nitroglycerin given sublingually or possibly intravenously will further reduce venous return; nitroprusside given intravenously may be used if the blood pressure is adequately maintained and afterload reduction is desirable. Furosemide should be given intravenously in a 20- to 40-mg dose and repeated in increasing doses as necessary to achieve a diuresis. Aminophylline, 250 to 500 mg given slowly intravenously (5.6 mg per kilogram), will be useful to relieve bronchospasm and promote diuresis but can exacerbate sinus or ectopic tachycardias.

If severe respiratory distress persists, tourniquets applied to three of four extremities and rotated every 15 to 20 minutes may be of value. If respiratory acidosis (pH of 7.10 or less) or severe hypoxemia (Po_2<50 mm Hg) persists, endotracheal intubation and controlled positive pressure ventilation should usually be instituted. Phlebotomy or hemodialysis deserves consideration in refractory cases. Digitalis has a secondary role in this clinical setting, except occasionally in the management of supraventricular tachyarrhythmias. Superimposed hypotension and low cardiac output states are considered in Ch. 44. Concurrently, vigorous attention should be directed to the identification and management of precipitating factors (Table 43–2).

Digitalis Glycosides

Cardiac glycosides have been used in the management of heart failure for more than 200 years and remain the only drugs currently available for long-term ambulatory use that have a positive inotropic effect. The unusually narrow therapeutic-toxic ratio of cardiac glycosides renders them particularly difficult to use, and the clinician should have a detailed understanding of the actions and pharmacokinetics of one drug of this class, such as digoxin. Because digoxin has supplanted almost entirely the use of other cardiac glycosides in the United States, the discussion will focus on this agent.

BASIC MECHANISM OF CARDIAC GLYCOSIDE ACTION. A consensus exists that the sequence of events leading to the positive inotropic effect of digitalis on both normal and failing cardiac muscle is as summarized in Figure 43–4. The digitalis glycosides bind to the extracellular facing aspect of NaK-ATPase, the enzyme constituting the "sodium pump" that moves sodium and potassium across cell membranes against their respective concentration gradients. The complete amino acid sequences of the alpha and beta subunits of the enzyme are known. When a cardiac glycoside binds to the alpha subunit, that individual sodium pump unit is completely inhibited. When a fraction of NaK-ATPase sites on a cardiac myocyte are occupied, intracellular sodium concentration tends to rise. Through the mechanism of sodium-calcium exchange, this leads in turn to augmentation of the intracellular calcium content. Since calcium constitutes the trigger that leads to the contractile event, the increase of intracellular calcium stores (up to a point) enhances the contractile state of both normal and failing myocardium.

The electrophysiologic toxicity commonly observed with excessive doses of digitalis is probably due to the same fundamental mechanism of sodium pump inhibition. At higher doses and myocardial concentrations of the drug, impairment of sodium and potassium transport leads to characteristic disturbances of impulse formation and conduction, as discussed below. It is likely that intracellular calcium overload contributes to the cardiotoxicity of the digitalis glycosides, at least under the circumstances that have been studied experimentally.

ELECTROPHYSIOLOGIC EFFECTS. Table 43–5 summarizes the major electrophysiologic effects of digitalis on the heart. Most of the antiarrhythmic effects of digitalis are the results of its actions at the level of the atria and atrioventricular junction. These effects are largely mediated by increased vagal tone, rather than by direct effects of cardiac glycosides, although the latter can be documented at the upper end of the dose range. Of particular importance in the management of supraventricular tachyarrhythmias is the tendency of digitalis to lengthen the refractory period and to slow conduction in the atrioventricular node. At toxic doses and blood levels, digitalis enhances sympathetic nerve traffic to the heart, thus increasing the propensity to ectopic impulse formation at atrial, atrioventricular junctional, and ventricular levels.

HEMODYNAMIC EFFECTS. The positive inotropic action is a direct effect of digitalis on cardiac myocytes in isolated muscle as well as the intact heart. Endogenous norepinephrine stores are not necessary to permit expression of this effect. A useful way to appreciate the effect of digitalis on the intact circulation is by consideration of the ventricular function curves shown in Figure 43–1. In contrast to diuretics, which

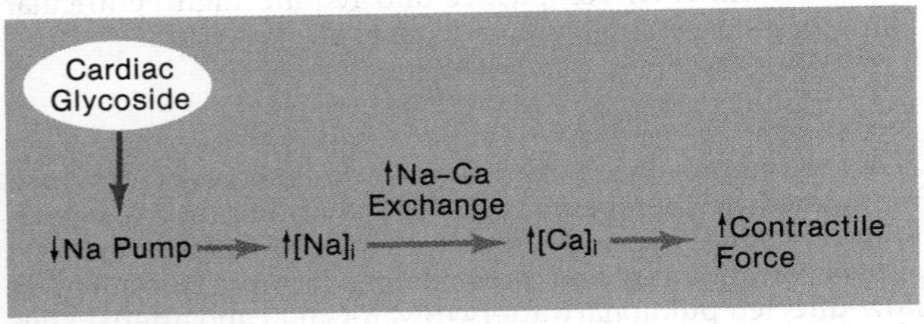

FIGURE 43–4. Schematic representation of the mechanism of inotropic action of cardiac glycosides. Binding of digitalis to NaK-ATPase inhibits this enzyme and hence the active outward transport of Na^+ across the myocardial cell membrane. Na^+ pump inhibition leads to increased intracellular Na^+ ($[Na]_i$) content and activity, which in turn alters Na-Ca exchange with consequent increase in Ca influx, decrease of Ca efflux, or both. The resulting increase in intracellular Ca ($[Ca]_i$) is presumed to mediate the observed increase in myocardial contractile force.

TABLE 43–5. EFFECTS OF DIGITALIS ON CARDIAC ELECTROPHYSIOLOGY

Property	Effect
Pacemaker Automaticity	
S-A node	→ ↓ (↑, after atropine or toxic doses)
Purkinje fibers	↑
Excitability	
Atrium	→*
Ventricle	variable*
Purkinje fibers	↑*
Membrane Responsiveness	
Atrium	variable* (↓, after atropine)
Ventricle	↓ (toxic doses)
Purkinje fibers	↓ (toxic doses)
Conduction Velocity	
Atrium, ventricle	↑ (slight)*
A-V node	↓
Purkinje fibers	↓
Effective Refractory Period	
Atrium	↓ (↑, after atropine)
Ventricle	↓
A-V node	↑
Purkinje fibers	↑*

Key: The arrows indicate the direction, not the magnitude, of the changes indicated: ↑, increased; ↓, decreased; →, no significant change.

*Decreased with high or toxic doses of digitalis.

From Moe GK, Farah AE: Digitalis and allied cardiac glycosides. In Goodman LS, Gilman A (eds.): The Pharmacological Basis of Therapeutics. 5th ed. New York, The Macmillan Company, 1975, p 661.

reduce preload and shift the circulatory state to the left along a given ventricular function curve, a positive inotropic agent will shift the entire curve upward and to the left toward the normal curve. Since contractility does not limit cardiac output in the normal circulation, digitalis would not be expected to change output in normal subjects. This is the case. As soon as the contractile state becomes limiting, however, digitalis will increase cardiac output and lower filling pressures of both the right and the left ventricles. Thus, cardiac glycosides are of clinical value in patients with congestive heart failure in the presence or absence of supraventricular tachyarrhythmias such as atrial fibrillation or atrial flutter. Although opinion is less uniform regarding patients in sinus rhythm, recent studies have documented benefit in the majority of patients who have dilated, failing ventricles with poor systolic function. These patients must be carefully distinguished from those with relatively noncompliant ventricles and elevated filling pressures, but normal ejection fractions at rest, who are unlikely to benefit. Thus, patients who are most likely to benefit are those having cardiomegaly with impaired systolic contraction, often accompanied by S_3 gallops. There is no convincing evidence of desensitization or tolerance to the cardiac effects of digitalis, and the positive inotropic effects are sustained over periods of months and years in patients with congestive heart failure.

To summarize, as pathologic processes, such as ischemia, volume or pressure loads, or primary myocardial disease, lead to reduced contractility, compensatory mechanisms emerge. Elevated end-diastolic pressure and volume will augment ventricular performance through the Frank-Starling mechanism. Sympathetic tone will tend to increase, thus enhancing contractile state, and the process of ventricular hypertrophy will generate additional contractile elements. Each of these mechanisms, however, exacts a price. Excessive elevation of filling pressures results in pulmonary or peripheral edema. Excessive sympathetic tone results in tachycardia and inappropriately increased peripheral vascular resistance as well as increased myocardial oxygen consumption. With the progression of underlying cardiac disease, the compensatory mechanisms will ultimately fail, or the consequences of these mechanisms will become limiting (for example, with emergence of pulmonary edema). Administration of cardiac glycosides under these circumstances will enhance myocardial contractility, decreasing the dependence of the circulation on compensatory mechanisms and providing improved cardiac reserve. Improved ventricular function will yield a higher cardiac output at any given ventricular filling pressure. With the alternative therapeutic modalities now available, there is little virtue in giving cardiac glycosides to the point of toxicity. Rather, conventional doses (see below) resulting in serum digoxin concentrations not exceeding 1.5 to 1.7 ng per milliliter appear to yield the best risk-benefit ratio.

PHARMACOKINETICS, BIOAVAILABILITY, AND DOSAGE CONSIDERATIONS. Summarized in Table 43–6 are the important pharmacokinetic variables and dosage ranges for cardiac glycosides in current clinical use. The values cited are averages, and individual variation is to be expected.

Digoxin. This is the most widely used preparation in the United States, particularly in hospitalized patients. Its virtues include flexibility of route of administration and intermediate duration of action. Digoxin is excreted exponentially (i.e., first-order kinetics) with a half-life of about 36 hours in young, healthy, normal subjects. In older patients with cardiac disease but without nitrogen retention, a half-life of 48 hours represents a more appropriate first approximation. Such patients will excrete approximately one third of body stores daily, for the most part in unchanged form, although about 10 per cent of patients excrete substantial quantities of the inactive metabolite dihydrodigoxin, which arises through bacterial biotransformation in the gut lumen. The excretion of digoxin by the kidney is directly proportional to glomerular filtration rate (and hence creatinine clearance) and is relatively independent of the rate of urine flow in patients with intact renal function. Clearance may decrease somewhat in patients with prerenal azotemia. There is also evidence for some secretion of the drug at the renal tubular level.

Therapy can be instituted in patients without urgent indications by starting the daily maintenance dose without a loading dose. This results in stable plateau concentrations of the drug in four to five excretory half-lives, or about one week. In patients with severe renal impairment, the half-life of the drug is prolonged to as much as four to five days, and steady-state levels are reached on a daily maintenance regimen only after three to four weeks.

Digoxin is extensively bound to tissues (large volume of distribution), and the drug is consequently not effectively

TABLE 43–6. PHARMACOLOGY OF CARDIAC GLYCOSIDES

Agent	Gastrointestinal Absorption	Onset of Action* (minutes)	Peak Effect (hours)	Average Half-Life†	Principal Metabolic Route (Excretory Pathway)	Average Digitalizing Dose		Usual Daily Oral Maintenance Dose ‖
						Oral‡	*Intravenous§*	
Ouabain	Unreliable	5–10	½–2	21 hours	Renal; some gastrointestinal excretion	—	0.30–0.50 mg	—
Deslanoside	Unreliable	10–30	1–2	33 hours	Renal	—	0.80 mg	—
Digoxin	55%–75%¶ (Lanoxicaps 90%–100%)	15–30	1½–5	36–48 hours	Renal; some gastrointestinal excretion	1.25–1.50 mg	0.75–1.00 mg	0.25–0.50 mg††
Digitoxin	90%–100%	25–120	4–12	4–6 days	Hepatic#; renal excretion of metabolites	0.70–1.20 mg	1.00 mg	0.10 mg
Digitalis leaf	About 40%	—	—	4–6 days	Similar to digitoxin	0.80–1.20 g	—	0.10 g
Lanatoside C	10%–40%	—	—	Similar to digoxin	Renal	10 mg	—	0.5–1.5 mg
Gitalin**		—	—	4–6 days	Similar to digitoxin	6 mg	—	0.25–1.25 mg
Acetyldigitoxin	About 70%	20–30	8–10	Similar to digitoxin	Similar to digitoxin	2.0–3.0 mg	1.4–1.6 mg	0.1–0.2 mg

Modified from Smith TW: Drug Therapy: Digitalis glycosides. N Engl J Med 288:719, 1973.

*For intravenous dose.

†For normal subjects (prolonged by renal impairment with digoxin, ouabain, and deslanoside and probably by severe hepatic disease with digitoxin and digitalis leaf).

‡Divided doses over 12 to 24 hours at intervals of 6 to 8 hours.

§Given in increments for initial subcomplete digitalization, to be supplemented by further small increments as necessary.

‖ Average for adult patients without renal or hepatic impairment; varies widely among individual patients and requires close medical supervision.

¶For tablet form of administration (may be less in malabsorption syndromes and in formulations with poor bioavailability).

#Enterohepatic cycle exists.

**Gitalin is a mixture of cardiac glycosides, the principal one of which is digitoxin.

††Approximately 20 per cent lower maintenance doses are required if gel solution in capsules (Lanoxicaps) is used.

removed from the body by hemodialysis. Lean body mass should be used for purposes of dosage calculation. Infants and children absorb and excrete digoxin much as do adults, although secretion at the renal tubular level may be somewhat more important in prepubertal patients.

An important interaction between digoxin and quinidine has been described, leading to a substantial increase in steady-state serum digoxin levels (averaging about twofold) when conventional quinidine doses are added to a maintenance digoxin regimen. Increases in the serum digoxin level are also observed when verapamil or amiodarone are given concurrently.

Bioavailability of digoxin in the standard tablet formulation is 55 to 75 per cent. The higher estimate is usually used in converting oral to intravenous doses. A recently marketed preparation in which digoxin is dissolved in an encapsulated gel gives higher bioavailability, requiring a slight adjustment in the standard maintenance doses, as noted in Table 43–6. Previously marketed preparations with poor bioavailability properties are no longer available in the United States, thanks to appropriate controls imposed by regulatory agencies.

The maintenance digoxin dose required to replace daily losses will vary from about 37 per cent of the body content in patients with normal renal function to 14 per cent in patients with essentially no renal function. The latter figure is an average, however, and some patients will require substantially more or less than the maintenance dose that would be predicted by the 14 per cent figure. A useful approximation of daily per cent of loss of digoxin from the body is given by the following expression:

$$\text{Per cent daily loss} = 14 + \frac{C_{Cr} \text{ in ml/min}}{5}$$

Useful nomograms have been developed for loading and maintenance doses of digoxin, but it is important that these be used only as first approximations and that the patient be followed closely until a stable steady state is reached. Adjustments subsequently will be required with changes in renal function, related either to intrinsic renal disease or to altered renal perfusion due to cardiac disease.

Digitoxin. This cardiac glycoside is the least polar and the most slowly excreted of the cardiac glycosides in common use. It is the principal constituent of the whole leaf of the digitalis plant. Gastrointestinal absorption of digitoxin is virtually complete. The drug binds avidly to serum albumin, and only about 3 per cent of the drug circulates in the free, pharmacologically active state at conventional doses and serum levels. It thus differs substantially from digoxin, which is only about 23 per cent bound to plasma proteins at usual doses. Because of the high degree of serum protein binding, renal clearance of digitoxin is minimal and the drug is metabolized to a variety of poorly defined derivatives, presumably in the liver. Some enterohepatic cycling occurs in the case of digitoxin but is not important for digoxin. The half-time for digitoxin excretion averages about five to six days and is not appreciably affected by altered renal function.

Standard pharmacology texts give details of pharmacokinetics of other glycosides such as deslanoside and ouabain, which are rarely used at present in the United States.

DIGITALIS USE IN CONGESTIVE HEART FAILURE. The therapeutic use of digitalis in patients with normal sinus rhythm is complicated by the lack of any easily measurable therapeutic endpoint, such as that provided by the ventricular rate in patients with atrial fibrillation. Digitalis is of value in patients with symptoms and signs of heart failure due to ischemic cardiomyopathy, valvular disease, hypertensive heart disease, many types of congenital heart disease, and dilated cardiomyopathies and in some patients with cor pulmonale and overt right ventricular failure. The drug is of no demonstrated benefit in isolated mitral stenosis with normal sinus rhythm unless right ventricular failure is present. Similarly, little benefit can be expected in patients with pericardial tamponade or constrictive pericarditis. The latter disease states are all characterized by mechanical limitations to cardiac function, rather than by impairment of myocardial contractility. In hypertrophic cardiomyopathy with an obstructive element, digitalis may in fact be deleterious if left ventricular contractility increases and produces greater outflow obstruction. As noted previously, patients with symptoms of dyspnea on exertion due to high diastolic filling pressure from decreased ventricular compliance, but with well-preserved ejection fractions, are unlikely to benefit from digitalis if sinus rhythm is present.

The prophylactic use of digitalis in patients with diminished cardiac reserve who are expected to undergo a major stress such as surgery remains controversial. Many clinicians prefer to withhold digitalis until a specific indication arises.

The use of digitalis in the management of supraventricular rhythm disturbances is considered in Ch. 45. The drug is potentially dangerous in patients with Wolff-Parkinson-White syndrome.

INDIVIDUAL SENSITIVITY TO DIGITALIS. Table 43–7 lists factors that influence the sensitivity of individual patients to digitalis. These are factors intrinsic to the patient, rather than factors that influence *apparent* sensitivity, such as alterations in drug bioavailability or in the excretion pattern of the drug.

Electrolyte and Acid-Base Disturbances. Potassium depletion increases the likelihood that patients will develop digitalis toxicity. Hypokalemia has a primary arrhythmogenic effect of its own and also tends to increase cellular binding of digitalis glycosides. Potassium depletion must be guarded against carefully in patients on potassium-wasting diuretics. Magnesium depletion also predisposes to digitalis toxicity and is a common concomitant of diuretic therapy. Elevated serum calcium levels may enhance ventricular automaticity and may also predispose to digitalis toxicity.

Acid-base disturbances appear to exert their effects largely through shifts in serum potassium concentration, and the acid-base disturbances per se usually have little effect within the range commonly encountered clinically.

Drug Interactions. Several drugs, including cholestyramine, colestipol, and neomycin, decrease absorption of orally administered digoxin, as do nonabsorbable antacids and Kaopectate. Quinidine, verapamil, and amiodarone all increase steady-state serum digoxin levels.

Type and Severity of Underlying Heart Disease. The most important factor influencing individual digitalis sensitivity is the type and severity of underlying heart disease. Otherwise healthy subjects are remarkably tolerant of large doses of digitalis, and toxicity typically manifests itself as disturbances of atrioventricular conduction rather than life-threatening tachyarrhythmias. In patients with advanced heart failure or severe focal ischemia, however, the therapeutic ratio of digi-

TABLE 43–7. FACTORS INFLUENCING INDIVIDUAL SENSITIVITY TO DIGITALIS

Type and severity of underlying cardiac disease
Serum electrolyte derangement
Hypokalemia or hyperkalemia
Hypomagnesemia
Hypercalcemia
Hyponatremia
Acid-base imbalance
Concomitant drug administration
Anesthetics
Catecholamines and sympathomimetics
Antiarrhythmic agents
Thyroid status
Renal function
Autonomic nervous system tone
Respiratory disease

talis is remarkably low, and these patients may experience potentially life-threatening toxicity at doses and serum levels no more than twice the optimal amount.

Digitalis and Coronary Artery Disease. The effects of digitalis on myocardial oxygen consumption, and therefore its use in patients with ischemic heart disease, depend primarily on the prior state of the ventricle. In the normal-size ventricle, the enhanced contractile state may modestly increase oxygen consumption. If failure and ventricular dilation are present, however, digitalis administration will tend to reduce cardiac dimensions and thereby reduce wall tension (Laplace's relation) such that myocardial oxygen consumption may not increase or may even be reduced. It is important, therefore, to assess carefully the state of ventricular function prior to instituting digitalis therapy in patients with ischemic disease.

The role of digitalis therapy after acute myocardial infarction remains controversial. Other measures are generally preferable in the management of mild congestive heart failure in this setting. When symptoms and signs of overt left ventricular failure persist despite optimal use of diuretics, digitalis may be added at about 75 per cent of the usual loading dose. The loading dose should be given over a period of 18 to 24 hours with close monitoring of cardiac rhythm. It is customary to use digoxin in the presence of atrial fibrillation, which is typically a manifestation of heart failure in patients with acute myocardial infarction.

Some evidence suggests that patients may experience excess mortality when maintained on digitalis in the long-term following acute myocardial infarction, but most studies indicate that the mortality trends are accounted for by baseline variables such as greater severity of heart failure, rather than a deleterious effect of conventional doses of digoxin.

Advanced Age. It is unlikely that advanced age per se has an independent adverse effect on digitalis tolerance, but the reduced renal and pulmonary functions that attend advanced age require appropriate consideration.

Renal Failure. Factors influencing digitalis absorption and elimination, as well as rapid shifts in electrolytes with hemodialysis, predispose to digitalis toxicity. It is wise to leave an extra margin of safety in digitalis doses in managing these patients.

Thyroid Disease. Hyperthyroidism tends to reduce the response of patients to digitalis, whereas hypothyroidism increases the likelihood of digitalis toxicity. The failure of a patient with atrial fibrillation to respond to standard doses of digoxin with appropriate slowing of the heart rate should raise the question of occult thyrotoxicosis.

Pulmonary Disease. It is generally agreed that patients with chronic pulmonary disease, and especially with acute respiratory insufficiency, experience an increased frequency of digitalis intoxication. This may be related both to the underlying lung disease and hypoxia and to the sympathomimetic drugs that these patients often receive. It should be assumed that patients with a variety of pulmonary diseases may be sensitive to the arrhythmogenic effects of conventional doses and serum levels of cardiac glycosides.

SERUM DIGITALIS CONCENTRATIONS. Assay of serum digoxin concentration is routinely performed in most clinical laboratories, usually with the radioimmunoassay technique. There is a relatively constant ratio of serum or plasma to myocardial digoxin concentration, and thus the clinical effect of digoxin is directly related to the serum level. Nevertheless, there is considerable overlap in serum levels between patients with and without evidence of toxicity. Thus, serum concentration data must always be interpreted in the overall clinical context. Mean serum digoxin concentrations in groups of patients without evidence of toxicity, and with an expected therapeutic effect, average 1.4 ng per milliliter. Doubling the digoxin dose in a patient on a steady-state regimen can be expected to double the serum concentration when a new steady state is reached.

Serum digitoxin concentrations average about tenfold higher than those of digoxin because of the binding of digitoxin to serum proteins.

The upper limit of the "therapeutic" range for digoxin is usually taken as about 2.0 ng per milliliter, but patients with supraventricular tachyarrhythmias, including atrial fibrillation and atrial flutter, may require appreciably higher levels to gain adequate control of the ventricular response and may tolerate these higher levels with no evidence of toxicity. Conversely, unusually sensitive patients may experience toxicity at serum levels as low as 1.0 ng per milliliter. It is not necessary to monitor serum digoxin levels routinely in patients who are doing well on standard maintenance doses of the drug. Serum levels may be of use, however, in the assessment of unexpected responses to therapy, including lack of the expected therapeutic response (Is the patient taking the drug?) or in situations in which digitalis toxicity is suspected (for example, multifocal ventricular premature beats in a patient with overt congestive heart failure who is taking digoxin).

DIGITALIS TOXICITY. At the cellular level, exposure to excessive levels of cardiac glycosides causes increased automaticity and decreased conduction. These abnormalities are reflected in a broad array of rhythm disturbances that are often difficult to distinguish from those caused by underlying heart disease.

Sinus Node and Atrium. Slowing of the sinus rate in patients with congestive heart failure is largely mediated by improved cardiac function and withdrawal of elevated sympathetic tone. Sinus rate is not a very useful indicator of digitalis effect, since it will tend to remain rapid in the presence of fever, infection, anemia, thyrotoxicosis, or a variety of other conditions that predispose to sinus tachycardia. At high toxic doses, digitalis can cause direct depression of sinus node automaticity, or more likely sinoatrial exit block, which will produce bradyarrhythmias.

Atrioventricular Node. The effective refractory period of the atrioventricular (AV) node is prolonged by digitalis, chiefly through increased vagal activity. In addition, the conduction velocity through the AV junction is reduced. As digoxin doses are increased, first-degree block (PR interval $>$ 0.20 second) may appear, followed by second-degree AV block of the Mobitz type I or Wenckebach variety (see Ch. 45). With still higher doses, complete AV dissociation and third-degree block can occur. A typical manifestation of digitalis toxicity in the presence of atrial fibrillation is AV dissociation, often accompanied by increased automaticity of pacemakers in the AV junction. This causes regularization of a previously irregular ventricular rate.

His-Purkinje System. Digitalis-induced increase in the automaticity of cells in the His-Purkinje system is a relatively common manifestation of digitalis excess and is responsible for rhythm disturbances, including ventricular premature beats, ventricular bigeminy, and ventricular tachycardia. Table 43–8 shows the approximate relative incidence of rhythm disturbances most commonly produced by digitalis.

Clinical Manifestations of Digitalis Toxicity. GASTROINTESTINAL SYMPTOMS. Anorexia, nausea, and vomiting are common consequences of digitalis toxicity. Unfortunately, these are present prior to the onset of rhythm disturbances in only about 50 per cent of cases.

NEUROLOGIC SYMPTOMS. Headache, fatigue, malaise, disorientation, confusion, delirium, and seizures can occur, and visual symptoms, including disturbances of color vision, are well known. In fact, the gastrointestinal symptoms actually arise from the effects of digitalis on the chemoreceptor trigger zone in the medulla rather than as a result of direct irritation of the gastrointestinal system.

MASSIVE CARDIAC GLYCOSIDE OVERDOSE. Suicidal or accidental digitalis overdose can produce the entire array of typical cardiac arrhythmias, including refractory ventricular fibrilla-

TABLE 43–8. RELATIVE INCIDENCE OF CARDIAC ARRHYTHMIAS ATTRIBUTED TO DIGITALIS TOXICITY IN 14 STUDIES (926 PATIENTS)

Rhythm Disturbance	Number of Arrhythmias	Per Cent of Patients with This Arrhythmia
Ventricular ectopic rhythms	567	62
AV block	314	34
1°	91	
3°	82	
Atrial arrhythmias	248	27
Sinoatrial arrhythmias	106	11
AV dissociation	92	10
AV junctional rhythms	138	15

AV = atrioventricular.
Data from Fisch C, Stone JM: Recognition and treatment of digitalis toxicity. *In* Fisch C, Surawicz B (eds): Digitalis. New York, Grune & Stratton, 1969, pp 162–173, with permission.

tion. In addition, hyperkalemia is sometimes encountered owing to interference with sodium and potassium transport across cell membranes throughout the body. This must be taken into account in considering the use of potassium supplements in cases in which massive toxicity may occur.

Treatment of Digitalis Intoxication. The most important element of successful treatment is early recognition that a cardiac rhythm disturbance is due to digitalis toxicity. For many of the most common manifestations, such as occasional ventricular premature beats, first-degree AV block, or atrial fibrillation with a slow ventricular response, temporary withdrawal of the drug with electrocardiographic monitoring (if indicated) until the arrhythmia has disappeared will constitute adequate management. The maintenance dose should then be adjusted to prevent recurrence. Arrhythmias that impair cardiac function because of rates that are too rapid or too slow, or those that suggest the possibility of progression to more malignant arrhythmias, require more aggressive management. Ventricular tachycardia due to digitalis toxicity requires immediate vigorous treatment. Bradyarrhythmias, including sinus bradycardia, sinoatrial arrest, or exit block, and atrioventricular block of second or third degree can sometimes be treated effectively with atropine, 0.5 to 1.0 mg given intravenously. Pervenous electrical pacing should be instituted if atropine is not rapidly effective.

POTASSIUM. Potassium repletion is useful in the treatment of ectopic tachyarrhythmias when hypokalemia is present or when the serum potassium level is in the low normal range. Potassium must be given with caution in other circumstances because of the risks of hyperkalemia, particularly in the presence of renal impairment or of conduction disturbances.

PHENYTOIN AND LIDOCAINE. These are the most useful drugs in the treatment of ectopic rhythm disturbances caused by digitalis. They tend to have minimal adverse effect on sinoatrial or AV conduction. Phenytoin* is given in a dose of 100 mg by slow intravenous infusion, repeated every five minutes until onset of toxicity or control of the arrhythmia, followed by an oral maintenance dose of 400 to 600 mg per day if control of the rhythm disturbance is achieved. Lidocaine is given intravenously in 100-mg bolus doses every three to five minutes, followed by a maintenance intravenous infusion of 15 to 20 μg per kilogram of body weight per minute, as required to maintain control of the rhythm disturbance and to avoid neurologic signs and symptoms.

PROPRANOLOL. Beta blockade has been useful in the treatment of some arrhythmias caused by digitalis excess but tends to decrease conduction as well as myocardial contractility and therefore is not widely used in this setting.

QUINIDINE AND PROCAINAMIDE. These drugs carry a risk of depression of sinoatrial and atrioventricular node function and can also depress myocardial contractility. Other agents are usually preferable for use in digitalis toxicity.

*This use is not listed in the manufacturer's directive.

DIRECT CURRENT (DC) COUNTERSHOCK (also see Ch. 45). This is generally inadvisable in the presence of digitalis intoxication because it may evoke severe arrhythmias in this setting. However, it must occasionally be used when other methods have been ineffective in the presence of a life-threatening arrhythmia. Risk is decreased when lower energy levels are employed, and careful titration of dose is essential. In general, ventricular tachycardia will convert easily at an energy level of 25 watt-seconds or less. Cardioversion is generally a benign procedure in patients without digitalis-induced rhythm disturbances.

STEROID-BINDING RESINS, HEMODIALYSIS, AND HEMOPERFUSION. These techniques have not been demonstrated to be effective in the management of advanced digitalis intoxication and are not recommended. Hemodialysis may be of value in controlling the serum potassium level in patients with refractory hyperkalemia.

DIGOXIN-SPECIFIC ANTIBODIES. Purified Fab fragments of digoxin-specific antibodies have recently been released for treatment of advanced digitalis toxicity of sufficient severity to be potentially life threatening. More than 400 patients have now been treated, with a high degree of efficacy and with no major adverse side effects. This approach is recommended for patients in whom conventional measures are not rapidly effective.

Diuretics

Salt and water retention with consequent expansion of the intravascular and interstitial compartments is a sine qua non of chronic congestive heart failure and accounts for many of the common signs and symptoms. Elimination of excess salt and water is an essential goal in management of heart failure.

Two stages characterize diuretic use: first, the elimination of accumulated excess fluid; and second, maintenance of optimal "dry" weight. Care of patients in the hospital typically focuses on elimination of excess fluid, which is facilitated by the controlled salt intake and limited activity of hospitalized patients. Maintenance of optimal fluid balance out of hospital requires adjustments in the context of the individual patient's diet and activity. A sound approach is the use of the mildest diuretic program that is consistent with maintenance of appropriate fluid balance and a salt intake that promotes a nutritious diet. Severe sodium restriction is usually unnecessary except in very severe congestive heart failure. Overly rigorous restriction of sodium intake, together with use of potent diuretics, is a well-known formula for impaired renal function, oliguria, and prerenal azotemia, particularly in the elderly.

CONTROL OF SODIUM BALANCE. The key role of diuretics in management of heart failure relates to the central role of the kidney as a target of many of the neurohumoral and hemodynamic changes that occur in heart failure. Reduced cardiac output causes activation of the renin-angiotensin system in the kidney, with consequent reduction in renal blood flow and increased glomerular filtration fraction, leading to increased resorption of salt and water by the proximal tubule. Elevated plasma angiotensin II levels contribute to increased systemic vascular resistance and increase aldosterone release from the adrenal. Increased renal sympathetic nerve activity also tends to reduce renal blood flow and to release renin from the macula densa, as well as directly augmenting sodium resorption along other segments of the nephron. Intrarenal blood flow redistribution contributes to the formation of relatively concentrated urine. Plasma vasopressin levels are frequently elevated in patients with heart failure, causing further limitation of free water clearance. Together with the increase in thirst of patients with advanced heart failure, this leads to a hyponatremic state that is a particularly ominous prognostic sign in heart failure.

Diuretics intervene in the pathophysiology of heart failure by reducing the reabsorption of sodium and its accompanying

TABLE 43–9. PROPERTIES OF DIURETIC DRUGS

Diuretic	Brand Name	Principal Site and Mechanism of Action	Effects on Urinary Electrolytes	Effects on Blood Electrolytes and Acid-Base Balance	Extrarenal Effects	Usual Dosage*	Drug Interactions
Thiazides and Related Compounds							
Chlorothiazide	Diuril	*Distal tubule:*	$\uparrow Na^+$	$\downarrow Na^+$, particularly in elderly patients	$\uparrow$ Glucose	500–1000 mg, IV or p.o.	Efficacy reduced by prostaglandin inhibitors
Hydrochlorothiazide	Hydrodiuril	Enhance NaCl	$\uparrow Cl^-$	$\downarrow Cl$, $\uparrow HCO_3^-$—	$\uparrow$ LDL/triglycerides	25–100 mg/day	
Trichlormethiazide	Metahydrin	reabsorption and	$\uparrow K^+$	mild metabolic	(may be dose	2–8 mg/day	Reduces renal clearance of
Chlorthalidone	Hygroton	$\downarrow Ca^{++}$ excretion	$\uparrow H^+$	alkalosis	related)	25–100 mg/day	lithium
				$\uparrow$ Uric acid			
Metolazone	Zaroxolyn		$\uparrow Mg^{++}$ $\downarrow Ca^{++}$	$\uparrow Ca^{++}$		5–10 mg/day	Synergistic effects on NaCl and K^+ excretion with loop diuretics
Indapamide	Lozol	Smooth muscle vasodilator *Proximal tubule:*			Extrarenal effects less marked with indapamide	2.5–5 mg/day	
Acetazolamide	Diamox	Carbonic anhydrase inhibitor	$\uparrow Na^+$, $\uparrow K^+$ $\uparrow HCO_3^-$	Metabolic acidosis	$\uparrow$ Ventilatory drive $\downarrow$ Intraocular pressure	250–500 mg/day	May be useful in alkalemia due to other diuretics
Osmotic Diuretics							
Mannitol	Osmitrol	*Proximal tubule* (primarily)	$\uparrow Na^+$, $\uparrow Cl^-$	$\uparrow$ Extracellular volume transiently	$\downarrow$ Intracranial pressure	50–200 grams/day, IV	May enhance loop diuretic effectiveness by maintaining GFR
Glycerol	Glyrol		$\uparrow H_2O$		$\downarrow$ Intraocular pressure	1–1.5 grams/kg, p.o.	
Loop Diuretics							
Furosemide	Lasix	*Thick ascending limb of loop of Henle:* Inhibition of Na/K/Cl cotransport	$\uparrow\uparrow Na^+$	Hypochloremic alkalosis ($\uparrow HCO_3^-$)	Acute: $\uparrow$ Venous capacitance	20–600 mg/day, p.o. or IV	Tubular secretion delayed by competing organic acids (renal failure) and some drugs
Bumetanide	Bumex		$\uparrow\uparrow Cl^-$		$\uparrow$ Systemic vascular resistance	0.5–40.0 mg/day	
Piretanide†			$\uparrow K^+$ $\uparrow H^+$ $\uparrow Mg^{++}$,Ca^{++}	$\downarrow K^+$, $\downarrow Na^+$, $\downarrow Cl^-$ $\uparrow$ Uric acid (less than thiazide)	Chronic: $\downarrow$ Cardiac preload	6–20 mg/day	Effectiveness reduced by prostaglandin inhibitors
Ethacrynic Acid	Edecrin	$\uparrow$ Renin, AII; $\uparrow$ PG's			Ototoxicity	50–150 mg/day	
Indacrinone				Uricosuric potency depends upon ratio of $\pm$enantiomers in final drug			Additive ototoxicity with aminoglycosides Excessive hypotension may occur in patients treated chronically with diuretics and begun on ACE inhibitors
Potassium-Sparing Diuretics							
Spironolactone	Aldactone	*Aldosterone antagonist*	$\uparrow K^+$ $\uparrow Na^+$ $\uparrow Cl^-$ $\uparrow HCO_3^-$	$\uparrow K^+$, particularly in patients with $\downarrow$ GFR; metabolic acidosis	Gynecomastia Antiandrogen effects	25–200 mg/day	Useful adjunct to therapy with K^+-wasting diuretics
Canrenone							
Triamterene	Dyrenium	*Inhibit Na^+/H^+ exchanger:*				100–300 mg/day	Triamterene with indomethacin may cause abrupt $\downarrow$ GFR
Amiloride	Midamor	Primary effect is in distal nephron				5–10 mg/day	Triamterene may cause renal calculi

*Route of administration is p.o. except as noted.
†Investigational drug.
AII = Angiotensin II; PG = prostaglandin; GFR = glomerular filtration rate; LDL = low density lipoproteins; ACE = angiotensin-converting enzyme inhibitor.

anions, as well as water, by the renal tubule. The four major classes of diuretics in current clinical use are summarized in Table 43–9. Each of these agents affects renal tubular function in a distinct way, and each tends to produce a characteristic set of abnormalities in electrolyte patterns, fluid balance, and acid-base homeostasis. The more potent the diuretic, the greater the potential risk for severe and sometimes life-threatening disturbances of electrolyte and acid-base balance.

THIAZIDES. Because of their effectiveness by oral administration, their predictable effects, and their relative freedom from toxicity, thiazide diuretics are very commonly used in the management of heart failure. The thiazide diuretics include several agents with chemical and pharmacologic similarities. The prototype is chlorothiazide. Chlorthalidone and metolazone are heterocyclic compounds that share the basic benzothiadiazine nucleus. All of these drugs inhibit sodium chloride reabsorption in the distal tubule. This effect is not dependent upon the weak carbonic anhydrase inhibitory activities common to most of these drugs. By inhibiting sodium chloride transport in the distal tubule, dilution of tubular fluid is prevented and delivery of solute and water to the hydrogen- and potassium-secreting sites in the collecting duct is enhanced. Calcium reabsorption is also promoted by the thiazides, probably by enhancement of calcium entry into epithelial cells of the distal tubule and perhaps by mild volume depletion as well.

The thiazides are useful in the initial management of mild-to-moderate congestive heart failure. Their utility is limited, however, by avid solute reabsorption in the more proximal nephron segments. Thiazides are largely ineffective when the glomerular filtration rate is less than 30 ml per minute. They are often useful in the treatment of refractory edema in combination with loop diuretics, as discussed subsequently.

Potentially troublesome side effects include potassium depletion, hyperuricemia, glucose intolerance, and plasma lipid elevations, as discussed below. Care must be taken to avoid gastric and small bowel irritation from the potassium chloride supplements that are often required in conjunction with thiazide diuretics.

CARBONIC ANHYDRASE INHIBITORS. Related to the thiazides are the carbonic anhydrase inhibitors, of which acetazolamide is the only agent currently available. This drug results in urinary sodium and bicarbonate losses until the plasma bicarbonate level falls to the point at which renal tubular bicarbonate reabsorption (both proximal and distal) exceeds the filtered load of bicarbonate. Thus, these agents tend to have a transient effect. The sodium and potassium loss accompanying bicarbonate excretion is moderate, but acetazolamide may be of value in patients with high serum bicarbonate levels, as may occur in cor pulmonale or metabolic alkalosis. The presence of metabolic acidosis, e.g., from renal failure or hepatic failure, constitutes a contraindication to its use.

LOOP DIURETICS. These agents are the most potent diuretics in common clinical use and are capable of inducing a natriuresis of up to 20 per cent of the filtered load of sodium for limited periods. They are of particular value in three situations: in acute pulmonary edema, used intravenously; in severe or refractory heart failure; or when renal function is impaired. Ethacrynic acid is chemically different from furosemide and its analogues but appears to share a similar set of pharmacologic properties. These diuretics act to inhibit the Na/K/2 Cl transport system that is responsible for solute reabsorption in the thick ascending limb of the loop of Henle. Each of these drugs is secreted into the tubular lumen by the organic acid secretory pathway, and their effects may therefore be delayed or decreased by exogenous (e.g., probenecid) or endogenous (organic anion accumulation in uremia) competitive inhibitors of the transporter.

Gastrointestinal absorption of furosemide, the most commonly used of the loop diuretics, is variable, with an average bioavailability of 60 per cent. This is substantially diminished when the drug is given with meals. Congestive heart failure appears to decrease absorption of both furosemide and bumetanide. The nonsteroidal anti-inflammatory drugs, including aspirin, tend to blunt the natriuretic response to all of the loop diuretics.

The loop diuretics in general produce systemic hemodynamic changes that precede and are presumably unrelated to the degree and extent of diuresis they induce. Acute administration of furosemide causes a rapid increase in venous capacitance, with a consequent decline in cardiac filling pressures. This effect is accompanied by an increase in plasma renin activity that can produce an appreciable rise in systemic vascular resistance. These effects on the peripheral vasculature tend to plateau in the lower dose range at about a 20-mg intravenous dose of furosemide. Although the loop diuretics are potent inhibitors or Na/K/2 Cl cotransport, this process is not clinically important outside the kidney, except in the cochlea, where it is thought to account for the eighth nerve toxicity that is seen with loop diuretics, particularly ethacrynic acid. The ototoxicity of loop diuretics is synergistic with that of aminoglycoside antibiotics.

Bumetanide and piretanide tend to have higher bioavailability and greater potency than furosemide and may be slightly less ototoxic. Other differences among these closely related compounds appear to be small and probably clinically unimportant.

An important advantage of the loop diuretics is their rapid onset of action, with a diuretic response typically appearing within a few minutes of intravenous administration.

ORGANOMERCURIAL DIURETICS. With the availability of potent oral diuretics, these agents are no longer part of the contemporary management of heart failure.

POTASSIUM-SPARING DIURETICS. Two groups of drugs fall into this class: (1) the aldosterone antagonists; and (2) the direct inhibitors of sodium permeability in the collecting duct. The aldosterone antagonist most frequently used is spironolactone, although canrenoate and canrenone have essentially identical effects. The aldosterone antagonists compete with the native hormone for cytoplasmic receptors in responsive cells, ultimately reducing sodium reabsorption. Therapeutic efficacy of these agents is limited when used alone, but they are often useful in combination with other potent diuretics.

Amiloride and triamterene are structurally related compounds that inhibit sodium uptake in collecting duct epithelial cells by blocking sodium-hydrogen exchange. A principal effect of these drugs is to reduce renal potassium secretion, which may be useful in concert with the action of potassium-wasting compounds such as the thiazides and loop diuretics, but which may lead to clinically important hyperkalemia, particularly in patients with renal failure. The potassium-sparing diuretics tend to cause a mild metabolic acidosis. In patients with chronic obstructive pulmonary disease, these agents may be preferred to diuretics that enhance renal hydrogen losses and secondarily reduce ventilatory drive. Apart from causing hyperkalemia, these drugs are relatively benign. Spironolactone can cause troublesome gynecomastia.

OSMOTIC DIURETICS. These agents are rarely of use in the management of heart failure, but it should be remembered that radiographic contrast dyes are filtered by the glomerulus and act as osmotic diuretics, increasing urinary loss of salt and water. This volume-contracting effect can be important in fragile patients, such as those with severe aortic stenosis. An important characteristic of osmotic diuresis is its ability to maintain urine flow even at very low glomerular filtration rates, as occur in hypotension or dehydration.

COMBINED DIURETIC REGIMENS. Combined use of diuretics in patients with heart failure is usually considered for two main reasons: to avoid electrolyte disturbances that occur with the isolated use of a powerful agent such as a loop diuretic, especially in chronic therapy; and to augment salt and water excretion in the face of refractory edema. A third possible indication is the avoidance of ototoxicity from large doses of loop diuretics.

Combined use of potassium-sparing diuretics with a more proximally acting agent such as a thiazide or a loop diuretic constitutes a common practice. The potassium-sparing diuretics limit potassium and hydrogen loss induced by diuretics that act more proximally.

The combination of a loop diuretic with a thiazide often results in a synergistic augmentation of salt and water excretion. This combination of agents is capable of producing marked intravascular volume depletion and electrolyte disturbances. Potassium wasting can be severe, and serum potassium levels require close monitoring. In general, this combination of diuretics should be initiated in a hospital setting, with careful regulation of the regimen on an outpatient basis with weight measurements taken daily and frequent checks of serum electrolyte and creatinine levels.

COMPLICATIONS OF DIURETIC THERAPY. Problems complicating diuretic therapy include intravascular volume depletion and hypotension from overly vigorous diuresis; hyponatremia, often due to prolonged diuretic therapy with inadequate sodium intake and often with excessive water intake; hypokalemia from the use of thiazides or loop diuretics, or both, with inadequate potassium supplementation, predisposing to digitalis intoxication; hyperkalemia from potassium-sparing diuretic administration and potassium supplements; metabolic alkalosis with or without potassium depletion; hyperuricemia secondary to thiazide or loop diuretic administration; magnesium depletion, often occurring in parallel with potassium losses; and increased serum low density lipoproteins and triglyceride levels in patients receiving thiazides.

As a final comment, many patients treated for congestive heart failure spend a period of weeks developing the excessive fluid accumulation that characterizes this disease state; there is little virtue and much potential harm in attempting to correct this problem in an unduly short period of time. In general, in the absence of acute pulmonary edema, a reasonable goal (even in the era of DRG's) is about 1 kg of fluid loss per day.

Vasodilators

Cardiac function has a strong dependence on the resistance and capacitance properties of the peripheral vascular bed. Thus, vasodilator therapy in heart failure is designed to reduce the preload or afterload, or both, of a failing ventricle by relaxing vascular smooth muscle in the periphery. This approach to the management of heart failure improves survival in patients with continuing symptoms of heart failure who are taking digitalis and diuretics. This approach is an addition to, rather than a substitute for, use of cardiac glycosides and diuretics.

PRINCIPLES OF VASODILATOR THERAPY. As summarized in Figure 43–2, the normal ventricle is able to respond to increased afterload with an increase in the force of contraction such that there is little, if any, change in stroke volume until extreme elevations in afterload are encountered. As the ventricle fails, the relationship between afterload and stroke volume shifts downward and to the left so that a relatively modest change in outflow resistance causes a substantial alteration in stroke volume. This constitutes both a pathophysiologic problem and a therapeutic opportunity. The opportunity follows from the uniform increase in peripheral vascular resistance observed in untreated patients with decompensated congestive heart failure. Activation of the sympathetic nervous system and of the renin-angiotensin system accounts for most of the increase in peripheral resistance. These responses of the peripheral vascular system to a perceived decrease in cardiac output have survival value under conditions of hemorrhage or dehydration by redirecting the cardiac output to essential beds, including the brain and coronary circulation. Since congestive heart failure was presumably not an evolutionary pressure, it is not surprising that these primitive mechanisms for the defense of blood flow to vital organs prove maladaptive in the patient with chronic congestive heart failure.

As illustrated in Figure 43–1, the failing heart responds to a reduction in afterload by shifting its ventricular function curve toward normal, although the inotropic state remains unchanged. An attractive feature of afterload reduction is the ability to increase cardiac output without increasing preload or myocardial oxygen consumption.

VASODILATOR AGENTS. In the following discussion, primary consideration is given to vasodilator therapy for left ventricular failure, although the failing right ventrical will also benefit from reduced pulmonary vascular resistance. The most potent afterload-reducing agent in the pulmonary circulation is oxygen; there is, as yet, no drug that reliably exerts a preferential afterload-reducing effect in the pulmonary circulation.

The action of vasodilator drugs is described in terms of effects on the venous bed (preload) or the arteriolar bed (afterload). Table 43–10 summarizes data on the vasodilators in current clinical use in the management of heart failure.

Venous Dilators. These reduce the vascular smooth muscle tone in the systemic venous bed, increasing its capacitance and shifting blood volume from the arterial to the venous side of the circulation. Thus, patients with pulmonary vascular congestion and edema due to high left heart filling pressures will obtain symptomatic relief, limited only by the necessity to maintain a level of preload that results in an adequate forward cardiac output. The most selective agents for this purpose are the nitrates, including nitroglycerin and the longer-acting orally administered compounds, such as isosorbide dinitrate. Many investigators believe that much or most of the clinical benefit of vasodilator use derives from the venous dilator component. In chronic congestive heart failure,

TABLE 43–10. MAJOR VASODILATOR DRUGS*

Drug	Mechanism of Action	Venous Dilating Effect (Preload Reduction)	Arteriolar Dilating Effect (Afterload Reduction)	Usual Dosage	Comments
Nitroglycerin	Direct	+ + +	+	10–100 μg/min, IV 5–20 mg, transdermal 0.4 mg, s.l.	Tolerance may be a problem with sustained continuous use. May be used sublingually to control acute increases in left atrial pressure.
Isosorbide dinitrate	Direct	+ + +	+	5–20 mg q. 2 hr, s.l. 10–60 mg q. 4 hr, p.o.	Improved survival shown in chronic CHF when used with hydralazine.
Nitroprusside	Direct	+ + +	+ + +	5–150 μg/kg/min IV; usual dose, 50–75 μg/kg/min	Used IV only. Drug is light sensitive. Hazard of thiocyanate or cyanide toxicity with prolonged high doses.
Hydralazine	Direct	0	+ + +	10–75 mg q. 6 hr p.o.	Sustained benefit in heart failure not shown when used as sole vasodilator.
Phenoxybenzamine	Alpha-adrenergic blockade (nonselective)	+ +	+ +	10–20 mg q. 8 hr p.o.	Current use is limited.
Phentolamine	Alpha-adrenergic blockade (nonselective)	+ +	+ +	5 mg q. 4–6 hr IV	Current use is limited.
Prazosin	Alpha-adrenergic blockade ($alpha_1$ selective)	+ + +	+ +	1–5 mg q. 6 hr p.o.	Extra caution required with initial doses. Tolerance requires dosage adjustments.
Trimazosin†	Alpha-adrenergic blockade and undetermined mechanism	+ + +	+ +	50–450 mg b.i.d., p.o.	Investigational use only.
Captopril	Angiotensin converting enzyme inhibitor	+ + +	+ +	6.25–25.0 mg q. 6–8 hr, p.o.	Approved by F.D.A. for use in chronic CHF. Acute renal failure can occur with initial doses; initiate use with extra caution. Avoid potassium-sparing diuretics.
Nifedipine	Calcium channel blockade	+	+ +	10–30 mg q. 6 hr, p.o. 10–40 mg q. 6 hr, p.o.	Negative inotropic effect may be unmasked in severe CHF.

*All of these agents may cause severe hypotension, and special caution is required with initial use, particularly in patients with severe congestive heart failure. Heart rate changes with all agents listed are usually minor unless a hypotensive response elicits reflex tachycardia; prazosin can cause bradycardia with initial use.

†Investigational drug.

CHF = congestive heart failure; F.D.A. = Food and Drug Administration.

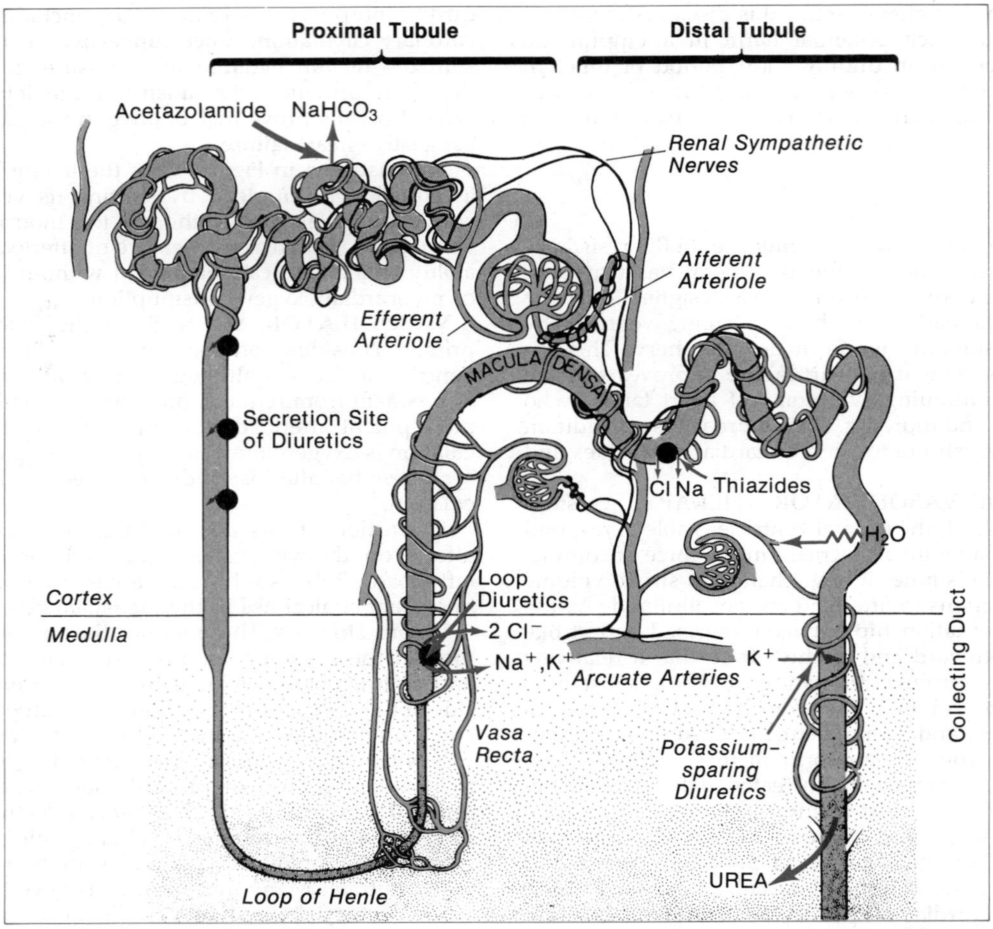

FIGURE 43–5. Sites of diuretic action in the mammalian nephron. Fluid resorption across the proximal tubule accounts for approximately two thirds of the resorption of filtered sodium and H_2O. Neuronal, hormonal, and hemodynamic factors, both extrinsic and intrinsic to the kidney, affect the volume and content of urine formation by altering the rate of formation of glomerular filtrate, thereby altering the balance of Starling forces between the proximal tubule and postglomerular peritubular capillaries. Agents that alter the rate of formation of glomerular filtrate, such as angiotensin-converting enzyme inhibitors, may enhance the delivery of solute and water to more distal segments of the nephron that are sensitive to diuretics. Nonsteroidal anti-inflammatory drugs may diminish the glomerular filtration rate, thus reducing the flow of urine to distal diuretic-sensitive portions of the nephron. A reduction in systemic blood pressure, or in renal artery pressure distal to the stenotic arterial lesion, below that necessary for formation of glomerular filtrate will render the kidney refractory to any diuretic. With the exception of the osmotic diuretics that are freely filtered at the glomerulus, most diuretics reach their site of action along the nephron after being secreted into the tubular lumen by the organic anion secretory transport system of the straight proximal tubule (pars recta).

About one third of the glomerular filtrate arrives at the descending limb of Henle's loop; no active transport of solute occurs here, although the tubular epithelium is highly permeable to water, which leaves the nephron for the increasingly hyperosmotic medullary interstitium. Most of the solute transport responsible for maintaining the hypertonicity of the medullary interstitium occurs in the water-impermeable thick ascending limb of Henle's loop. Here, a NaK cotransport system in the luminal membrane is coupled to the uptake of two chloride ions, a process dependent upon the electrochemical driving force for sodium generated by the NaK-ATPase on the basolateral membrane of these cells. This Na/K/2 Cl cotransport system on the luminal membrane of the tubular cells is the site of action for the loop diuretics (furosemide, bumetanide, and ethacrynic acid). Inhibition of cation transport by loop diuretics prevents the normal generation of the hypertonic medullary interstitium, thus reducing the osmotic gradient for free water clearance of ADH-sensitive tubular cells in the collecting duct, and also delivers large amounts of solute and water to the distal nephron, thus overwhelming distal Na^+ and Cl^- resorption sites.

The thick ascending limb approaches its own glomerulus as it reenters the cortex and passes between the afferent and efferent arterioles to form the juxtaglomerular apparatus (JGA), the tubular contribution to which is termed the macula densa. Loop diuretics may directly stimulate the release of renin by the JGA, an action that may contribute to the extrarenal vascular effects of these drugs. The distal convoluted tubule begins beyond the macula densa. Na^+ and Cl^-, as well as other ions (e.g., Ca^{++}) are resorbed in this segment. The thiazide diuretics and related drugs inhibit NaCl resorption in this segment, although the mechanism is unknown; they also enhance Ca^{++} resorption by tubular cells in this segment. Salt resorption by this distal, water-impermeable portion of the nephron allows the formation of a dilute urine, hence the term "cortical diluting segment." Thiazide-induced inhibition of NaCl resorption in this segment therefore may lead to hyponatremia, particularly when accompanied by elevated ADH levels and increased thirst.

The cortical collecting duct actively resorbs NaCl via an aldosterone-sensitive mechanism. This leads to increased net resorption of Na^+ into cells and hence to a lumen negative potential difference that favors the secretion of K^+ and H^+ ions. This is why increased Na^+ concentrations and high flow rates in the cortical collecting duct, as after loop or thiazide diuretic administration, leads to enhanced passive K^+ secretion. Anti-aldosterone drugs, such as spironolactone, competitively inhibit aldosterone's binding to its receptor, thereby limiting Na^+ permeability by the apical membrane and reducing K^+ secretion.

As illustrated, the blood supply to each nephron is derived from several sources. The afferent arteriole that enters the glomerulus is richly innervated with sympathetic nerve endings, particularly as it enters the glomerulus at its vascular pole within the juxtaglomerular apparatus. Increased sympathetic discharge to the kidney results in increased net NaCl resorption even in the absence of changes in glomerular hemodynamics. Elevated efferent sympathetic activity, as is often seen in decompensated congestive heart failure, would be expected to result in avid retention of solute due to reduced renal perfusion, increased renin release, and enhanced tubular resorption of solute. Dopamine is a potent renal vasodilator and may directly affect tubular epithelia to reduce NaCl resorption, thus acting as a natriuretic agent. Exogenously administered dopamine, particularly when infused at rates of 5 μg per kilogram per minute, may be a useful adjunct to diuretic therapy in selected patients with advanced CHF.

administration of agents that preferentially dilate the arteriolar bed without a preload-reducing component, such as minoxidil and hydralazine, fail to show sustained benefit.

Arteriolar Dilators. These reduce left ventricular afterload and tend to redistribute blood flow among organ beds in ways that are, unfortunately, not always predictable. The improvement in blood flow to exercising skeletal muscle is relatively limited. Nevertheless, the forward stroke output of the left ventricle is delivered with a lower wall tension, such that myocardial oxygen consumption is favorably affected. The most selective agent routinely used in obtaining an afterload-reducing effect is hydralazine.

The balanced vasodilators exert an effect on both preload and afterload through a generalized relaxing effect on vascular smooth muscle. The prototype short-acting agent of this kind is nitroprusside. This agent has found widespread application in the management of acute heart failure states, including acute pulmonary edema. Used with care, it can also improve the circulatory state of patients with combined hypotension and low forward output, provided that adequate arterial pressure can be maintained by the use of volume loading or inotropic drugs or both. The tendency of nitroprusside to reduce systemic arterial pressure is offset to a considerable extent by the increased stroke output. The unloading effect of nitroprusside is most helpful when the left ventricular filling pressures are maintained in the vicinity of 15 mm Hg, which may require administration of intravenous fluids. An important advantage of nitroprusside in intensive care unit settings is its short duration of action, permitting minute-to-minute titration of the circulatory state.

A regimen frequently employed to obtain a balanced vasodilator effect is hydralazine and nitrates, often given as the long-acting oral preparation isosorbide dinitrate. In an important multicenter study (Cohn, 1986), the protocol randomly assigned patients who were symptomatic while taking digitalis and diuretics to hydralazine with isosorbide dinitrate, to prazosin, or to placebo. The group treated with hydralazine and nitrates showed a 38 per cent mean reduction in mortality during the initial year of treatment, and the improved survival was sustained to the three-year point. The prazosin-treated group showed no significant difference from the placebo group.

The angiotensin-converting enzyme inhibitor captopril is now available as a balanced vasodilator for the management of patients with advanced heart failure. Multicenter trials have demonstrated sustained improvement in symptoms and exercise tolerance, although a study designed to examine the issue of survival has not yet been completed. Many clinicians find that captopril provides a relatively simple and controllable approach to vasodilator therapy, and it is the vasodilator of choice in many centers. Special care is required in administering initial doses of captopril, which can produce severe hypotension and renal failure. In general, the initial dose should not exceed 6.25 mg, and institution of therapy for patients with advanced heart failure is best carried out in the hospital.

Only about one half of patients who appear to be reasonable candidates for vasodilator use in advanced heart failure can tolerate the drugs initially, and only half of that group (or 25 per cent of the total) still show demonstrable benefit at the end of three months. Although these figures may be improved by careful selection of patients and judicious use of available agents, the fact remains that many patients with advanced heart failure are unable to tolerate vasodilators, chiefly because of postural hypotension.

Refractory Heart Failure

Therapeutic advances have left in their wake a subset of patients with marked impairment of ventricular function (often with left ventricular ejection fractions in the 10 to 20 per cent range) who survive but are severely symptomatic on maximal tolerated doses of digitalis, diuretics, and vasodilators. Those aged 50 years or less who meet additional relevant criteria (including preserved function of other organ systems, no elevation of pulmonary vascular resistance, no glucose intolerance, no active infection) may deserve consideration of heart transplantation after detailed explanation of the potential risks and benefits of this procedure. This procedure now has relatively widespread application since the advent of cyclosporine for immunosuppression, and more than 50 centers in the United States now have active programs. Survival exceeds 50 per cent at 5 years in larger series, compared with an expected mortality well in excess of 50 per cent at 12 months in patients treated by conventional means, and functional recovery is often gratifying.

Treatment of acute decompensation using intravenous beta-adrenergic or dopaminergic agonists, or both, is covered in Ch. 44. Longer-term use of orally active adrenergic drugs has proved disappointing because of rapid development of tolerance and cannot be recommended. Intermittent use of intravenous dobutamine for ambulatory patients with severe heart failure is under investigation, as are several phosphodiesterase inhibitor drugs, including amrinone, milrinone,* and enoximone,* that have both vasodilator and positive inotropic properties related to enhancement of cyclic adenosine monophosphate levels in vascular smooth muscle and myocardium. Although symptoms are improved in some patients treated with these investigational agents, evidence of improved survival is lacking. The artificial heart has been developed sufficiently for placement in several patients, but results to date have been disappointing because of unsolved thromboembolic problems.

*Investigational drug.

ACKNOWLEDGMENT: The author is indebted to Alfred P. Fishman, M.D., the author of this chapter in the seventeenth edition, for his valuable advice regarding the structure and content of the sections of this chapter dealing with general aspects, categories, pathophysiology, and clinical findings in heart failure. Ralph A. Kelly, M.D., has made major contributions to the coverage of diuretics, including Figure 43–5.

Berger BE, Warnock DG: Clinical uses and mechanisms of action of diuretic agents. In Brenner BM, Rector FC (eds.): The Kidney. Philadelphia, W. B. Saunders Company, 1986, pp 433–455. *A compact summary of clinically relevant information as stated in the title.*

Braunwald E, Mock MB, Watson JT (eds.): Congestive Heart Failure. New York, Grune & Stratton, 1982. *A series of informative monographs covering all aspects of heart failure, originally presented at an NIH-sponsored conference intended to summarize the current state of the art.*

Captopril Multicenter Research Group: A placebo-controlled trial of captopril in refractory congestive heart failure. J Am Coll Cardiol 2:755, 1983. *A well-designed controlled trial demonstrating improved clinical state and effort tolerance among 92 patients with heart failure refractory to digitalis and diuretics randomized to additional treatment with placebo or the angiotensin-converting enzyme inhibitor captopril, which was subsequently approved by the United States Food and Drug Administration for the indication of congestive heart failure.*

Cohn JN, et al.: Effect of vasodilator therapy on mortality in chronic congestive heart failure: Results of a VA cooperative study. N Engl J Med 314:1547, 1986. *Random assignment of 642 men with heart failure on digitalis and diuretics (which were continued) to additional placebo, prazosin, or hydralazine and isosorbide dinitrate. At a mean follow-up of 2.3 years, this study showed improved survival (risk reduction of 34 percent) among patients treated with hydralazine and nitrates. Mortality in the prazosin-treated group was indistinguishable from that in the group receiving placebo. Overall mortality, as expected, was high (36 to 47 per cent at three years). Additional useful references on vasodilator therapy in heart failure are cited.*

Colucci WS, Wright RF, Braunwald E: New positive inotropic agents in the treatment of congestive heart failure: Mechanisms of action and recent clinical developments. N Engl J Med 314:290, 349, 1986. *This two-part review article covers the stated subjects well, with a clinical emphasis.*

New Concepts in the Mechanisms and Treatment of Congestive Heart Failure. Am J Cardiol 55:1A, 1985. *This symposium, chaired by J. N. Cohn, includes up-to-date discussions of current problems in the study of heart failure. Epidemiology is well summarized by W. McF. Smith.*

Smith TW (ed.): Digitalis Glycosides. Orlando, Fla., Grune & Stratton, 1986. *This 348-page book summarizes available information on all aspects of the basic and clinical pharmacology, clinical use, and toxicity problems related to the cardiac glycosides.*

Smith TW, Braunwald E: The management of heart failure. In Braunwald E (ed.): Heart Diseases. 3rd ed. Philadelphia, W. B. Saunders Company, 1987. *A detailed consideration of general and specific aspects of congestive heart failure management with 562 references.*

44 SHOCK

*François M. Abboud**

Shock is a complex clinical syndrome that demands vigilant medical attention, careful hemodynamic monitoring, and thorough understanding of the basic principles of circulatory control and of the pharmacology of cardiac and vasoactive drugs. This chapter covers the basic principles of *circulatory control* as they relate to the shock syndrome, the *cellular mechanisms* involved in the pathogenesis of shock, and the *therapy* of shock.

DEFINITION. Shock, regardless of cause, is a failure of the circulatory system to maintain cellular perfusion and function. This results in cellular membrane dysfunction, abnormal cellular metabolism, and eventually cellular death.

CAUSES. Table 44–1 lists the most common clinical situations associated with decreased cardiac output, hypotension, decreased tissue perfusion, capillary endothelial injury, and cellular damage.

CLINICAL PICTURE. The classic clinical presentation is one of a patient who is hypotensive (with a systolic blood pressure of 90 mm Hg or less); has a tachycardia with a thready pulse; is hyperventilating; has cold, clammy, cyanotic skin; and has a dulled sensorium ranging from agitation to stupor or coma. The patient is frequently oliguric, with a urinary output of less than 20 ml per hour.

This clinical picture is not always present, and the recognition of the subtle or early presentation of shock may be crucial. For example, a patient may have a "normal" blood pressure (i.e., 110/70), but this may actually represent "relative hypotension" if the patient has a history of hypertension. Early shock may be indicated only by unexplained agitation or tachycardia in the absence of cardiovascular collapse. Some patients with septic shock may initially present with warm hyperperfused extremities (so-called warm shock) due to abnormal peripheral vasodilatation.

Frequently, the clinical findings follow a progressive pattern as shock evolves from the early compensated phase to the advanced stages (Table 44–2). In addition, the signs and symptoms of the underlying precipitating disease are present, e.g., severe pain of acute myocardial infarction or dissecting aneurysm, visible bleeding, burn, peritonitis, sepsis, or trauma.

PATHOPHYSIOLOGY AND STAGES OF SHOCK. The basic elements in the pathogenesis of shock are portrayed in Figure 44–1.

Stage I: Compensated. Hypotension may be caused either by a fall in cardiac output or by vasodilatation. The fall in cardiac output and hypotension trigger compensatory mechanisms, which restore arterial pressure and blood flow to the more vital organs such as brain and heart. Symptoms and signs are minimal, and appropriate intervention is most effective.

Stage II: Decompensated. In this stage, the compensatory mechanisms to maintain perfusion of vital organs are insufficient. Evidence of decreased cerebral perfusion may be apparent from the mental state of the patient; decreased renal perfusion may reduce urinary output, and patients with coronary artery disease may experience myocardial ischemia. The external appearance of the patient also reflects excessive sympathetic discharge, with cyanosis, coldness, and clamminess of the skin. The majority of patients are recognized in this phase, and rapid aggressive intervention to restore cardiac output and perfusion of the tissues may reverse the shock syndrome.

Stage III: Irreversible. Excessive and prolonged reduction of tissue perfusion leads to significant alterations in cellular membrane function, aggregation of blood corpuscles, and "sludging" in the capillaries. The vasoconstriction that has taken place in the less vital organs in order to maintain blood pressure is now excessive and has reduced flow to such an extent that cellular damage occurs.

Arterial pressure continues to fall progressively to a critical level at which the perfusion of vital organs is reduced. Critical impairment of renal perfusion leads to acute tubular necrosis. Ischemia of the gastrointestinal tract leads to necrotic damage

*The author acknowledges the assistance of David W. Ferguson in the revision of this chapter.

TABLE 44–1. CAUSES OF SHOCK AND INITIATING MECHANISMS

I. **Decreased intravascular volume**
   A. Acute hemorrhage (e.g., gastrointestinal bleeding, retroperitoneal bleeding, ruptured aortic aneurysm, hemoptysis, hemothorax, trauma)
   B. Excessive fluid loss
      1. Vomiting (intestinal or pyloric obstruction)
      2. Severe diarrhea, sweating, and dehydration
      3. Excessive urine (e.g., diabetes mellitus, diabetes insipidus, excessive diuretics, diuretic phase of acute renal failure)
      4. Peritonitis, pancreatitis, splanchnic ischemia, intestinal obstruction, and gangrene
      5. Trauma and extensive muscle injury
      6. Burns
   C. Vasodilatation (relative hypovolemia)
      1. Neurogenic: drug induced (e.g., anesthesia, ganglionic and adrenergic blockers, overdoses such as barbiturates, poisons); nervous system damage (e.g., spinal cord injury, cerebral vascular accident, severe dysautonomia)
      2. Metabolic, toxic, or humoral vasodilatation: septicemia (gram-negative endotoxemia or gram-positive bacteremia); acute adrenal insufficiency, anaphylactic reaction

II. **Cardiac**
   A. Acute myocardial infarction
   B. Myocarditis, myocardial depression (hypoxia, acidosis, septic shock, myocardial depressant factors [MDF], drugs, hypoglycemia), severe low-output failure
   C. Acute valvular insufficiency, myocardial rupture, septal perforation
   D. Arrhythmias: severe bradycardia, tachycardia, and fibrillation
   E. Mechanical compression or obstruction
      1. Pericardial effusion or tamponade
      2. Positive pressure ventilation, tension pneumothorax
      3. Pulmonary embolism
      4. Ball-valve thrombus or atrial myxoma

III. **Microcirculatory endothelial injury and aggregation of corpuscles**
   A. Anaphylaxis
   B. Disseminated intravascular coagulation
   C. Burns, septic shock, trauma

IV. **Cellular membrane injury**
   A. Septic shock
   B. Anaphylaxis
   C. Ischemia, prolonged hypoxia, pancreatitis, tissue injury

TABLE 44–2. CLINICAL FINDINGS AT VARIOUS STAGES OF SHOCK

Stages	I Compensated*	II Decompensated	III Irreversible
Arterial blood pressure	N or ↓	↓	↓ ↓
Heart rate	↑	↑ ↑	↑ ↑ → ↓ ↓
Pulse pressure	↓	↓ ↓	↓ ↓
Cardiac output	↓	↓ ↓	↓ ↓ ↓
Respiratory rate	N	↑	↑ ↑ → ↓ ↓
Mental status	Anxiety	Obtunded	Coma
Urinary output	N or ↓	↓ ↓	Anuria
Skin	Cool	Mottled	Cold, cyanotic

*N = no change. A high cardiac output and warm skin may be present in septic shock.

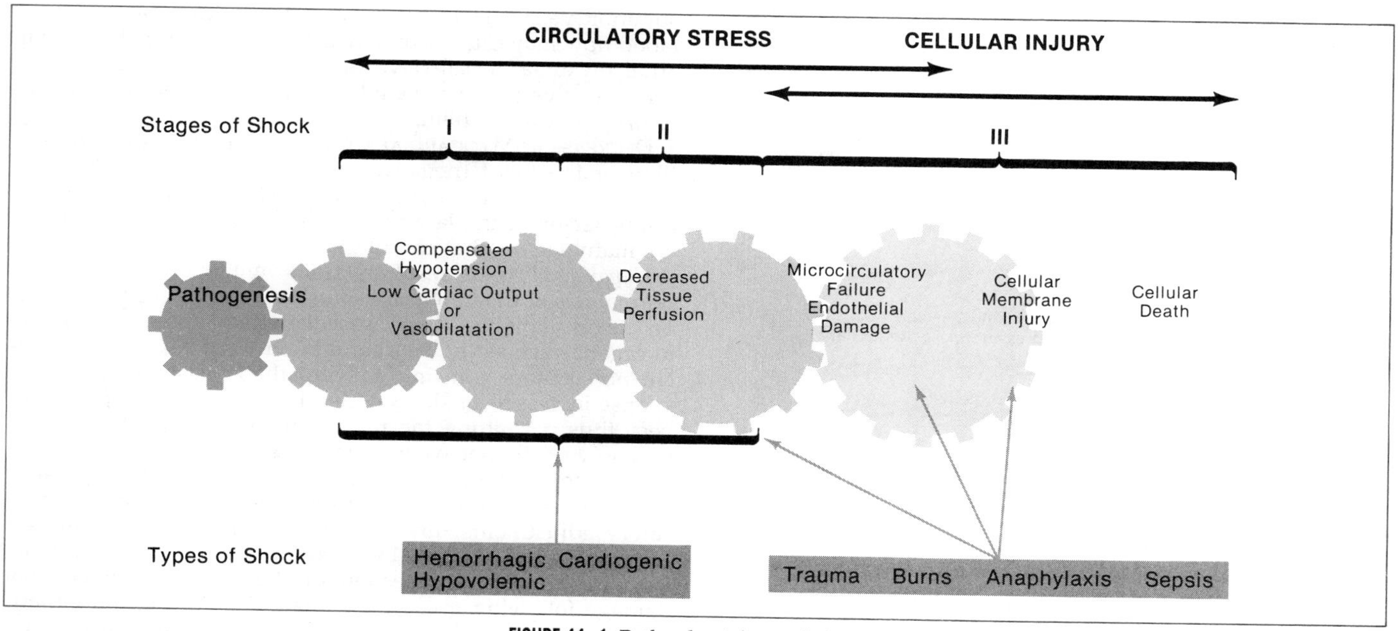

FIGURE 44–1. Pathophysiology of shock.

of the mucosa and absorption into the circulation of bacteria and toxic bacterial products that have detrimental effects on other organs and may lead to generalized endothelial damage with disseminated intravascular coagulation. Bacterial toxins react with neutrophils and cause the release of vasodilator polypeptides that contribute to the fall in arterial pressure. The severe acidosis resulting from anaerobic metabolism also contributes to vasodilatation. The decreased perfusion pressure of the coronary vessels, particularly in patients with coronary disease, results in reduction of myocardial perfusion, which in turn decreases myocardial contractility and creates a vicious cycle as the decreased contractility causes further decrements in arterial blood pressure. Hypoxia impairs reflex neurogenic circulatory adjustments that help in maintaining arterial pressure. Damage to the capillary endothelium leads to loss of fluid and protein through the capillaries, with exacerbation of hypovolemia and hypotension. Damage to cellular membranes from ischemia leads to leakage of lysosomal enzymes and intracellular ions, to progressive reduction in high energy phosphate reserves, and to cellular destruction.

CIRCULATORY CONTROL IN SHOCK

Major Determinants of Tissue Perfusion

The major determinants of hemodynamics and tissue perfusion are listed in Table 44–3. Perfusion of any organ depends upon systemic arterial pressure (which is the driving force for blood to flow through all organs), the resistance offered by the vasculature of that organ, and the patency of nutritional capillaries. Systemic arterial pressure is in turn determined by cardiac output and the resistance of the total vascular tree. Vascular resistance is predominantly a function of the radius or caliber of blood vessels. Vascular caliber is influenced by neurogenic, humoral, and myogenic factors that regulate the tone of vascular smooth muscle. Thus blood flow to any one organ depends on cardiac function and on vascular muscle tone and caliber in all the arterial tree as well as in the organ itself. The determinant of exchange of substrates and metabolites with the tissues is the microcirculation. A patent nutritional capillary network is the critical interface between the circulation and the cell.

This discussion deals with cardiac, vascular, and microcirculatory factors.

CARDIAC FACTORS. Cardiac output is the product of heart rate and stroke volume. A rate of 70 beats per minute and a stroke volume of 70 ml per beat give a cardiac output of approximately 5 liters per minute, an amount more than sufficient to deliver 250 ml of oxygen per minute to all the tissues. This consumption of oxygen reflects metabolic needs at rest. A drop in cardiac output below 2 liters per minute per square meter is an indication of severe shock.

Heart Rate. Tachycardia usually increases cardiac output, but a marked increase in heart rate may limit cardiac diastolic filling time and result in a low cardiac output and arterial blood pressure. For example, ventricular tachycardia or rapid atrial fibrillation in a patient with recent myocardial infarction causes a reduction in cardiac output and arterial pressure that, if uncorrected, could result in cardiogenic shock. Immediate treatment to restore heart rate is essential. In considering the treatment of tachycardia in shock, one has to be cautious in avoiding treatment of a "compensatory tachycardia" often seen in patients with fever, anemia, sepsis, hemorrhage, or severe hypovolemia. Tachycardia is often an appropriate reflex circulatory adjustment to maintain cardiac output.

Extreme bradycardia may also cause a low output and hypotension. Sinus bradycardia and atrioventricular block are often seen immediately following myocardial infarction and should be reversed if they contribute to hypotension.

Stroke Volume. A decrease in stroke volume may be caused by (1) a decrease in cardiac filling, (2) a decrease in myocardial contractility, or (3) an increased afterload (Fig. 44–2).

DECREASE IN CARDIAC FILLING PRESSURE. The amount of blood filling the ventricles at the end of diastole is the "preload," and it regulates the subsequent contraction and stroke volume (Starling's law of the heart). Although there are many factors that determine preload, such as the rate and duration of filling, ventricular compliance, and venous tone, a most important determinant is total blood volume. Reduction in blood volume may be either absolute or relative to the capacity of the vascular tree. Absolute reductions in blood volume are apparent when blood or fluids are lost, causing a hypovolemic state leading to hypovolemic shock. This is seen in hemorrhage (either external or internal bleeding), excessive vomiting, diarrhea, burns, renal loss of fluids such as in diabetes mellitus or diabetes insipidus, excessive diuresis, and exces-

TABLE 44–3. MAJOR DETERMINANTS OF HEMODYNAMICS AND TISSUE PERFUSION

I. Systemic arterial pressure
A. Total vascular resistance
1. Total arteriolar resistance, vascular muscle tone
a. Tissue metabolism
b. Neurohumoral factors, toxins
2. Viscosity of blood
B. Cardiac output
1. Heart rate
2. Stroke volume
a. Cardiac filling pressure (preload)
i. Venous (vascular) tone
ii. Blood volume (total and central)
Capillary hydrostatic pressure: post-precapillary resistance
Capillary permeability
Oncotic pressure, plasma proteins
iii. Posture
iv. Atrial contraction
v. Diastolic filling time (heart rate)
vi. Mechanical obstruction (e.g., pericardial tamponade, pulmonary embolus)
b. Myocardial contractility
i. Arterial blood pH, Po_2
ii. Myocardial O_2 supply:
Increase supply:
↑ Diastolic arterial pressure (norepinephrine, dopamine)
Capillary diffusion
Coronary dilatation (nitroglycerin, dopamine, metabolites)
Decrease supply:
↓ Diastolic arterial pressure (isoproterenol, vasodilators)
Coronary artery disease, myocardial infarction
Hypoxia, anemia
iii. Myocardial O_2 demand
Increase demand:
↑ Cardiac size (pulmonary wedge pressure)
↑ Afterload (systolic arterial pressure, impedance)
↑ Contractility (norepinephrine, dopamine, isoproterenol) and heart rate
Decrease demand:
↓ Cardiac size
{ Digitalis, ↑ ejection fraction
{ Venodilatation (nitroprusside, nitroglycerin, phentolamine)
{ Diuretics
↓ Afterload, impedance (vasodilators)
↓ Contractility and heart rate
iv. Humoral factors
Catecholamines
Myocardial depressant factors
v. Drugs
Increase norepinephrine, dopamine, isoproterenol, digitalis
Decrease propranolol, anesthetics
c. Afterload
i. Arterial blood pressure, vascular impedance
ii. End-diastolic cardiac wall tension
iii. Severe aortic stenosis
II. Organ vascular resistance
A. Occlusive arterial disease
B. Local arteriolar resistance
C. Local venular resistance
D. Viscosity of blood
III. Patency of nutritional capillaries
A. Precapillary sphincter tone
B. Intracapillary aggregation of corpuscles
C. Capillary endothelial integrity

sive perspiration without fluid replacement. Internal losses of fluid occur in peritonitis, pancreatitis, intestinal obstruction with extravasation of fluid, splanchnic ischemia with bowel necrosis and gangrene, fractures with extensive muscle trauma, hemothorax, and hemoperitoneum.

Relative decreases in blood volume occur when there is loss of vascular tone because of the administration of anesthetics or ganglion blockers, after spinal cord injury, and in patients with neuropathy or autonomic insufficiency. Pooling of blood thus results in a decrease in cardiac filling pressure. Compression of the heart may also prevent its filling, as is seen during pericardial tamponade, in tension pneumothorax, or in the superior vena caval syndrome. Mechanical obstruction to blood flow may cause hypotension and shock in patients with atrial myxoma, a ball-valve thrombus, or pulmonary embolism. Positive pressure ventilation may also decrease venous return and cardiac filling.

DECREASE IN MYOCARDIAL CONTRACTILITY. Reduced contractility of the heart (negative inotropic effect) is the primary cause of shock after myocardial infarction, and it is a complicating factor in the late phases of shock of any type. There are many factors that contribute to it.

Hypoxia. Hypoxia resulting from ventilation-perfusion abnormalities of the lung occurs in shock and has several effects on the circulation. A direct, vascular effect causes vasodilation in organs such as the heart and brain. Hypoxia also activates chemoreceptors, causing a sympathetic vasoconstrictor response in vessels of skeletal muscle, skin, and the splanchnic bed, thus permitting the redistribution of blood to the vital organs with higher oxygen demand. When the central nervous system is hypoxic and ischemic, a significant sympathetic discharge also takes place. Despite these and other compensatory adjustments, myocardial performance is impaired in the presence of decreased arterial Po_2. The severity of arterial hypoxia is often a reflection of the extent of myocardial damage following myocardial infarction. It is an important, potentially reversible cause of depression of myocardial contractility.

Acidosis. Acidosis results from anaerobic metabolism with release of lactate, from decreased renal perfusion with accumulation of organic acids, and possibly from hypoventilation of certain pulmonary segments, leading to respiratory acidosis. Acidosis reduces myocardial contractility and the vasoconstrictor response to various neurohumoral factors.

Myocardial Ischemia and Perfusion Pressure. Myocardial performance depends on perfusion of the ischemic myocardium, which is determined to a great extent by the level of arterial diastolic pressure. The fall in arterial pressure during hemorrhagic or hypovolemic shock in patients with coronary artery disease may cause myocardial ischemia. Restoration of arterial pressure is critical to preservation of myocardial function. In the presence of coronary artery disease, resistance to flow is due largely to structural changes in the vessel wall, and vasomotor tone is minimal because of excessive accumulation of vasodilator metabolites downstream from the site of coronary narrowing. Thus arterial pressure becomes the determinant of perfusion of the ischemic segment through collateral vessels or across a narrowing or a plaque.

Increased Myocardial Oxygen Demand Relative to Supply. Although oxygen supply to the ischemic myocardium is in-

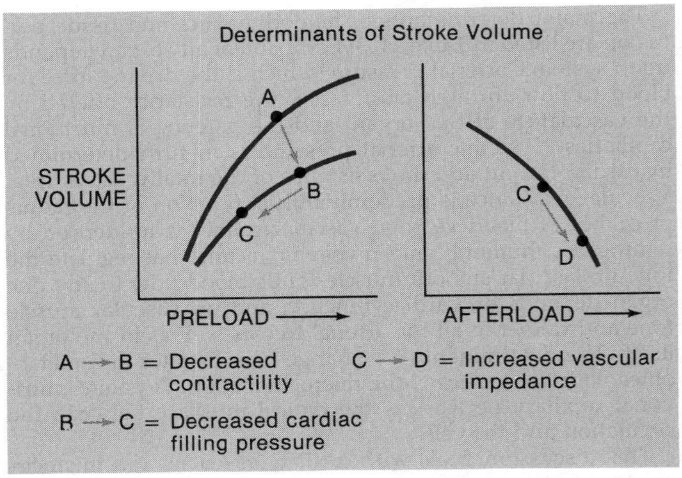

FIGURE 44–2. Determinants of stroke volume.

creased by increasing arterial pressure, hypertension is detrimental, as it increases myocardial work and oxygen demand. Conversely, hypotension decreases myocardial work and oxygen needs, but it also reduces myocardial perfusion as mentioned above. Judicious restoration of arterial pressure is necessary.

Increased cardiac size is associated with increased myocardial wall tension, which causes greater myocardial oxygen consumption. Drugs such as isoproterenol may increase myocardial oxygen demand out of proportion to the associated increase in coronary flow.

Other Factors that Depress Contractility. Drugs such as the barbiturates may depress cardiac output by a direct effect on the myocardium. More frequently, myocardial depression occurs from suppression of the adrenergic drive with propranolol, ganglion-blocking drugs, catecholamine depleters such as reserpine or guanethidine, or high spinal anesthetics, or with such conditions as spinal cord injury or an intracranial lesion involving the medullary centers. These interventions not only depress myocardial contraction but also decrease peripheral vascular tone.

Myocardial depressant factors may be released from damaged cells in various organs during shock from burns, pancreatitis, septicemia, or hemorrhage, and add an element of myocardial depression. Oxygen free radicals generated during ischemia and reperfusion may cause significant myocardial depression.

INCREASE IN AFTERLOAD. To eject the stroke volume the ventricle has to generate enough force to oppose the end-diastolic wall tension, the arterial pressure, and the vascular impedance. In severe heart failure with high ventricular end-diastolic pressure, cardiomegaly, and very low cardiac output, a vasodilator agent that decreases afterload by reducing vascular impedance and cardiac size may increase stroke volume.

VASCULAR FACTORS. These determine the resistance to blood flow and transcapillary exchange. Resistance to flow of blood is determined by the viscosity of blood and by the length and the cross-sectional area of the vessels. The cross-sectional area is the most important component, because the calculated resistance is inversely proportional to the fourth power of the radius of the vessels. The radius is in turn determined by the tone of vascular smooth muscle in the wall of the vessels. Vascular smooth muscle tone is modulated by neurogenic influences mediated primarily through the sympathoadrenal system and by circulating humoral and local metabolic factors.

Neurogenic Control. Sympathoadrenal discharge to the circulatory system is regulated by medullary neurons in the vasomotor center. Activity of these neurons is modulated by afferent neural impulses originating in various receptors located in strategic areas around the body. Important among these receptors are arterial and cardiac baroreceptors, chemoreceptors, somatic receptors in skeletal muscle, and thermal receptors. Activities originating in various parts of the central nervous system (cerebellum, fastigial and vestibular nuclei, and hypothalamus) also impinge upon the vasomotor center to modulate its output. Activation of cardiac sensory receptors, particularly those in the left ventricle, during volume expansion and stretch of the myocardium, inhibits sympathoadrenal activity. Conversely, reduction in the stretch of these ventricular receptors during hypovolemia and hemorrhage release the sympathoadrenal efferent activity to cause reflex tachycardia and vasoconstriction, to restore arterial blood pressure, and to release renin. The arterial baroreceptors, activated by a rise in blood pressure, suppress sympathoadrenal tone; conversely, during hypotension they increase sympathoadrenal drive and restore arterial pressure.

Severe hypoxia, often associated with shock from any cause, activates the chemoreceptor reflex and causes an increase in sympathoadrenal drive. The reduction of central or cardiopulmonary blood volume and arterial pressure during hemorrhage activates the cardiopulmonary reflex and the arterial baroreceptor reflex simultaneously, and the two reflexes are synergistic with respect to the final sympathetic efferent activity. Similarly, the combined activation of the arterial baroreceptor reflex by hypotension and the chemoreceptor reflex by hypoxia results in a significant synergistic effect on the ventilatory response as well as the circulatory sympathetic drive.

Conversely, there may be situations in which reflex responses have competing effects. This may occur, for example, when cardiac receptors are activated following acute myocardial infarction by the dyskinetic bulge of the left ventricle, while the arterial baroreceptors are inactivated because of hypotension. In the experimental preparation the inhibitory influence of the bulging left ventricular wall on the sympathetic outflow predominates and overrides the arterial baroreflex, preventing vasoconstriction and thus causing a decrease in the afterload of the damaged left ventricle. Teleologically, this effect may be beneficial, as it will tend to decrease left ventricular work following its acute insult.

There have been few studies of the effects of endotoxin on neurocirculatory reflexes. An increase in baroreceptor activity for any level of arterial blood pressure has been reported in endotoxemia, a situation that would tend to inhibit sympathoadrenal tone, and might explain in part the decreased vascular resistance often seen in septic shock.

Humoral Factors. The release of hormones such as renin, vasopressin, steroids, prostaglandins, and kinins is partly mediated through the sympathoadrenal system and cardiovascular mechanoreceptors and partly through direct and indirect cellular effects of toxins, ischemia, and antigens in various organs. These hormones have direct cardiovascular and renal effects and indirect effects on central or peripheral adrenergic transmission.

RENIN-ANGIOTENSIN. A fall in arterial blood pressure or an increase in sympathoadrenal sympathetic discharge to the kidney causes the release of renin. The resulting formation of angiotensin causes peripheral vasoconstriction, maintains arterial pressure, stimulates the release of aldosterone to retain sodium and water, and has an intrarenal effect on tubular sodium reabsorption that also permits greater sodium and water retention and preserves blood volume during hypotensive states.

VASOPRESSIN. This important water-retaining and constrictor hormone is released from the posterior pituitary primarily in response to increases in osmolality and may also play a role in the circulatory control in shock. Its release is reduced by stretch of the left atrial receptors during hypervolemia or by stretch of the arterial baroreceptor during hypertension; conversely, during hemorrhage and systemic hypotension, or when patients are on cardiopulmonary bypass, the blood levels of vasopressin increase significantly. Thirst and the release of vasopressin may be induced by a central nervous system action of angiotensin.

KININS. A variety of potent vasodilator polypeptides is formed by the action of certain proteolytic enzymes on plasma protein precursors. Bradykinin serves as the prototype for this class of endogenous peptides. Their major physiologic role may be the local regulation of blood flow and function of such organs as the salivary gland, pancreas, and kidney. In pathophysiologic states, kinins are believed to play a part in the hyperemia associated with inflammation and as vasodilators in hypotension produced by anaphylactic reactions. Renal kinins may cause diuresis and natriuresis.

SEROTONIN AND HISTAMINE. Serotonin released from platelets and histamine released from mast cells during anaphylaxis or during complement activation in shock may play an important role in regulating local vascular tone and capillary permeability.

PROSTACYCLIN AND THROMBOXANE A_2. Prostaglandins may be released in various organs during ischemia and may contribute to the reactive hyperemia and vasodilatation. The prostaglandin endoperoxides formed in platelets and in blood vessels are pivotal in the synthesis of two potent substances with opposing effects on the formation of thrombi. Prostacyclin, a powerful vasodilator and inhibitor of platelet aggregation, is synthesized in the vascular wall, mostly in the endothelial layer, from endoperoxides. In the platelets, however, endoperoxides are converted to thromboxane A_2, which causes vasoconstriction and platelet aggregation. In shock, damage to endothelial cells may inhibit synthesis of prostacyclin; in addition, platelets may release thromboxane A_2, causing intravascular platelet aggregation, clumping, and vasoconstriction.

ENDORPHINS. β-Endorphin and adrenocorticotropin are stored in the pituitary gland and secreted concomitantly under stress. β-Endorphins may contribute directly or indirectly to myocardial depression in shock. Studies in endotoxin *(E. coli)* shock and hemorrhagic shock in animals indicate that the specific opiate antagonist, naloxone, rapidly reverses the hypotension primarily through a positive inotropic effect on the heart. Naloxone has minimal cardiovascular effects in the absence of shock. The beneficial effect of synthetic steroids in experimental shock may be caused by suppression of β-endorphins. It is difficult, however, to demonstrate a convincing beneficial effect of either naloxone or steroids on humans in shock.

Local Autoregulatory Adjustment of Blood Vessels. Blood vessels have an intrinsic ability to regulate vascular tone and thereby maintain blood flow over a wide range of perfusion pressures. This property is referred to as the autoregulatory capacity for blood flow and is independent of systemic neurogenic influences or humoral factors. Different vascular beds vary with respect to their ability to maintain blood flow. The cerebral, coronary, and renal circulations are most potent. Thus during a fall in arterial pressure, vasodilatation of the cerebral, coronary, and renal vasculatures maintains blood flow and oxygen delivery to the brain and heart as well as sodium and water balance. Although a myogenic response intrinsic to the smooth muscle may explain the phenomenon, accumulation of tissue metabolites following a transient period of ischemia may also cause vasodilatation and restore blood flow. The specific mediator of metabolic vasodilatation is not known, but it is likely that a combination of changes in oxygen, carbon dioxide, and hydrogen ions and other cations, in osmolality, in the amount of adenosine compounds, and in Krebs cycle intermediates and other metabolites released in the immediate environment of blood vessels contributes to adjustments in vascular tone.

MICROCIRCULATION AND TRANSCAPILLARY EXCHANGE. Perhaps the most critical aspect of the pathogenesis of shock takes place at the level of the microcirculation. Delivery of a significant amount of blood to an organ does not guarantee that all the segments of that organ and all capillaries are perfused appropriately.

Intraorgan Blood Flow Distribution. Adequate tissue perfusion depends on blood flow through vascular channels in which diffusion between the blood and tissues can occur. These are referred to as nutritional capillaries, as contrasted with nonnutritional vessels that do not permit capillary exchange. The latter are also referred to as arteriovenous shunts, although there may be little anatomic evidence for the existence of such shunts. An example of the importance of the intraorgan redistribution of blood flow is observed in myocardial infarction, in which an increase in coronary blood flow may not increase perfusion to the infarcted segment. Under some circumstances a coronary vasodilator might redistribute flow away from ischemic into nonischemic regions.

Similarly, intraorgan blood flow distribution may be critical in the kidney. Acute tubular necrosis associated with shock may reflect a reduction in glomerular filtration in the outer cortex because of a localized increase in vascular resistance in this region and a selective reduction in blood flow. Interventions that alter total renal blood flow can produce significant redistribution of flow within the kidney; for example, renal vasoconstriction following adrenergic discharge tends to shunt blood away from the outer cortex, whereas renal vasodilators such as furosemide shunt blood toward the outer cortical nephrons.

Pre- and Postcapillary Resistance. The *precapillary sphincters* regulate the patency of nutritional or "exchange" capillaries. The tone of those spincters may be modulated by neurohumoral factors that contribute to the circulatory adjustments in shock. The metabolic products at the local tissue level are important determinants of the patency of these sphincters, which regulate the total capillary surface area and in turn determine the intravascular-extracellular fluid and solute exchange. The capillary hydrostatic force driving fluid out of the capillaries into the extracellular space is dependent on the ratio of post- to precapillary resistances. In hypovolemic or hemorrhagic shock, the fall in arterial pressure causes activation of the sympathoadrenal system, constriction of precapillary resistance vessels, and a fall in capillary hydrostatic pressure, facilitating movement of fluids from the extracellular into the intravascular space. This partially restores intravascular volume. Hematocrit and viscosity of blood and plasma oncotic pressure fall. The decline in plasma oncotic pressure may be partially corrected by rapid synthesis of new proteins. However, with persistent hypotension and ischemia, the vasoconstrictor response of precapillary resistance vessels becomes less pronounced because of tissue acidosis while resistance of *postcapillary* vessels (venules) increases. This creates a situation in which more fluid is lost from the vascular to the interstitial space. Thus, *venular resistance* and the reactivity of venules to the various vasoactive agents involved in shock become important. Venules may even be *relatively* more reactive than precapillary resistance vessels to catecholamines, which activate constrictor alpha receptors. This differential effect in favor of postcapillary vasoconstriction also further increases hydrostatic pressure and intravascular fluid loss. One might consider the administration of a venodilating drug in late stages of shock, in which failure of the microcirculation is a predominant factor.

Capillary Permeability and Oncotic Pressure. Colloidal osmotic pressure is a major determinant of intravascular volume. Albumin (molecular weight 69,000) is the main osmotically active protein in plasma. The balance between colloidal osmotic pressure and capillary hydrostatic pressure determines the balance between intravascular and extracellular fluid spaces. A significant degree of hypovolemia and hemoconcentration may take place either because of excessive capillary hydrostatic pressure from an increase in the ratio of post- to precapillary resistance or because of a reduction in plasma protein and consequently reduction of plasma oncotic pressure. Reduction of plasma protein occurs as a result of increased capillary permeability and loss of plasma protein from the intravascular to the extracellular space. The balance between oncotic and hydrostatic pressures is also an important determinant of the level of pulmonary edema and is critical in the management of the shock lung syndrome. Plasma oncotic pressure should be restored through careful selection of the type of fluid to be used in volume replacement. Fluids containing crystalloids may be undesirable, as these further decrease the oncotic pressure. Administration of blood or colloids may be more appropriate to reduce pulmonary edema if pulmonary venous (or wedge) pressure is low. If there is increased vascular permeability in the lung because of damage to pulmonary capillaries, only a fall in hydrostatic pressure reduces pulmonary interstitial fluid. Positive end-expiratory pressure or an increase in oncotic pressure does not help.

Shock resulting from increased vascular permeability, as in anaphylactic shock or snake venom poisoning, is characterized by a dramatic reduction of plasma volume. Hematocrit rises sharply and oncotic pressure drops. This increase in capillary permeability may be partly related to release of histamine, metabolites, or humoral factors that alter endothelial permeability.

Intravascular Hemagglutination and "Blood Sludging." Erythrocytes, leukocytes, and platelets undergo agglutination to a variable degree in association with the shock syndromes in thermal burn, sepsis, trauma, and perhaps even hemorrhage. These aggregates may cause obstruction of capillaries as well as arterioles. The precipitating events are numerous. They may include platelet aggregation by catecholamines; damage to endothelial lining of small blood vessels and capillaries with subsequent fibrin deposition and accumulation of microthrombi; hypoxia increasing the rigidity of red cells; oxygen free radicals generated by endothelial cells or neutrophils; and release of vasoactive peptides and anaphylatoxins as a result of complement activation. These may cause additional damage to endothelial cells and increase the tone of precapillary sphincters, leading to further reduction in tissue perfusion and cellular injury.

Disseminated intravascular coagulation is a syndrome often seen in shock, particularly from gram-negative septicemia. The syndrome causes renal cortical necrosis, generalized ischemic damage of multiple organs, consumption of coagulation factors, and bleeding, and may also contribute to the pathogenesis of shock lung.

Shock Lung. Pathologic studies of the lungs in patients dying from shock may reveal marked capillary dilatation, pulmonary edema, alveolar hemorrhages, massive pulmonary vascular congestion and hyaline membrane formation, atelectasis, superimposed bronchial pneumonia, and, if the patient survives for weeks or months after the initial injury, pulmonary fibrosis. Shock affects the lung by producing endothelial damage in the vast capillary bed or precapillary arterioles. Microaggregates of platelets, polymorphonuclear leukocytes, and red cells block capillaries, destroy capillary endothelial cells by releasing hydrolytic enzymes and/or superoxide radicals, and eventually cause the increased capillary permeability that is responsible for the pulmonary interstitial edema seen in shock. The trigger for aggregation of neutrophils in the lung is not clear. Complement is a likely candidate; C5a produced with the activation of complement may cause white cells to aggregate in the lung. One must also keep in mind the role of lymphatic drainage. Lymph flow is greatly increased in the very early stages of shock, and patients dying in hemorrhagic shock may have a widely distended pulmonary lymphatic system filled with proteinaceous material.

The decrease in pulmonary blood flow may also interfere with production of surfactant. Lack of surfactant reduces the patency of alveoli and perpetuates leakage of fluid across pulmonary arterioles. Pulmonary venular constriction in response to tissue hypoxia may also contribute to pulmonary capillary congestion. It is also possible that with cerebral ischemia and hypoxia, neurogenic influences on the lung may cause a differential increase in venular resistance and increase capillary hydrostatic pressure and permeability. During *Pseudomonas* infusions in animals, there may be a direct effect of the endotoxin on capillary permeability, although sometimes a delayed response suggests an immune reaction with release of serotonin, contributing to pulmonary edema. Regardless of its cause, the damage to pulmonary capillary endothelium in shock perpetuates both the resistance to blood flow and systemic hypoxia and accelerates cellular death.

CELLULAR AND BIOCHEMICAL FACTORS IN SHOCK

OXYGEN-HEMOGLOBIN (Hb) AFFINITY. Arterial blood with normal hemoglobin and oxygen saturation of 90 per cent at a Po_2 of 100 mm Hg carries close to 20 ml of oxygen per deciliter to the tissues. The mixed venous blood has an oxygen saturation of 75 per cent at a Po_2 of 40 mm Hg and contains 15 ml of oxygen per deciliter. The normal arteriovenous oxygen difference is 5 ml per deciliter. The extraction of oxygen from Hb by the tissues is not complete and depends to a large extent on the affinity of oxygen to Hb, i.e., the shape of the oxygen-Hb dissociation curve. Hydrogen ions (Bohr effect), carbon dioxide, and 2,3-diphosphoglyceric acid (2,3-DPG) cause greater dissociation of oxygen from Hb because of their preferential affinity for reduced hemoglobin. The concentration of 2,3-DPG in red cells results from a side reaction of glycolysis and increases during anemia, hypoxia, and acidosis. A drop in hemoglobin, hypoxia, and acidosis may thus be partly compensated for by a shift of the oxygen dissociation curve to the right, favoring greater delivery of oxygen to the tissues at the same Po_2. This compensatory mechanism, in addition to the increase in cardiac output, provides for better oxygenation as extraction of oxygen from the oxygen reserve in venous blood increases. In certain tissues, however, such as the myocardium, extraction of oxygen at rest is already large, and any additional oxygen demand or a decrease in oxygen-Hb dissociation such as in alkalosis requires greater delivery of oxygen, i.e., higher coronary blood flow.

In shock, the pH, carbon dioxide, and 2,3-DPG levels are changing, and one cannot calculate oxygen extraction from values of Po_2 because the shape of the oxygen dissociation curve cannot be predicted accurately. It is preferable to measure oxygen content or saturation of venous and arterial blood; if saturation is lower than predicted from values of Po_2, one can deduce that there is a shift of the dissociation curve to the right, and vice versa. Overzealous correction of acidosis with bicarbonate may, through the Bohr effect on Hb affinity for oxygen, actually reduce oxygen delivery to the tissues. Hypophosphatemia reported during hyperalimentation may decrease 2,3-DPG and oxygen delivery.

CELLULAR STRUCTURE AND FUNCTION IN SHOCK. Survival of aerobic cells depends on availability of substrates and oxygen to the mitochondria, which provide most of the high-energy phosphate needs of the cell and utilize most of the available oxygen in the process. During oxidative phosphorylation, 36 moles of adenosine triphosphate (ATP) are produced per mole of glucose, whereas in the anaerobic state, glycolysis provides only 2 ATP molecules during the breakdown of 1 glucose molecule. Synthesis of ATP from adenosine diphosphate (ADP) is associated with the most active state of respiration in mitochondria (state 3 respiration) and is determined by cell energy demands. In addition to oxidative phosphorylation and ATP synthesis, mitochondria bind and accumulate calcium. This function determines calcium availability for other intracellular organelles and thereby regulates biochemical processes of contractile events, as in cardiac or vascular muscle.

Two processes may lead to cellular death. One is a marked inhibition of the electron transport system caused by severe ischemia or anoxia or by administration of cyanide or actinomycin A. This process leads to depletion of ATP, and the electron microscopic appearance of cells undergoing that type of death does not show any calcium phosphate accumulation in the mitochondria, presumably because of inhibition of the energy-dependent calcium transport mechanism. The other type of cell death is initiated by an injury to the cell membrane caused by activation of complement, or by antigen-antibody reaction, or by administration of certain polyenes, such as amphotericin B, or certain bacterial or microbiologic products, such as phospholipases or antitoxin. This type of cellular membrane damage is generally characterized by the precipitation of calcium phosphate in mitochondria, presumably because active processes requiring ATP are preserved until late stages and calcium can be transported into mitochondria.

Several structural changes take place in cellular membranes in shock. The earliest manifestation consists of swelling of the cell associated with an increase in intracellular sodium and clumping of nuclear chromatin, followed by dilation of the endoplasmic reticulum. In this phase the cell membrane is unstable, and "blebs" may appear at the surface. The mitochondria will then begin to swell, and electron-dense clumps of flocculent material will appear within them. As the swelling of the mitochondria continues, Ca^{++} may or may not accumulate in them, depending on the type of cellular damage. The process of cell death becomes irreversible, lysosomes begin to disappear, and finally the cell is converted to a mass of debris, with large inclusions resembling myelin.

One can relate the sequence of structural changes in the cellular membranes to specific biochemical changes. Initially there is probably an increase in cellular permeability for sodium and water causing cellular swelling, followed by increased sodium-potassium ATPase activity in an attempt to drive sodium out of the cell. Increased membrane ATPase activity might eventually lead to depletion of ATP and cyclic adenosine monophosphate (AMP), the latter leading to alteration of cellular responses to insulin, glucagon, catecholamines, and other hormones. For example, the effect of insulin on glucose uptake in muscle of animals that have been subjected to hemorrhagic shock is reduced. The unresponsiveness to insulin in peripheral tissues may be one of the reasons for hyperglycemia following injury or in shock. There is also a decrease in ATP, particularly in liver in early shock and in most other organs in late shock. It is difficult to determine the critical level of ATP necessary for cellular function, but it is believed that as long as there is ADP and oxygen, and substrate is provided, ATP generation can be resumed within minutes if mitochondrial structure is preserved. The organs that are most seriously affected in shock include, in descending order, the liver, kidneys, muscle, and lung.

MITOCHONDRIAL FUNCTION. Hypoxia may reduce the rate of ATP synthesis by mitochondria, but it does not cause significant damage to mitochondrial membrane functions unless it is severe, sustained, or associated with ischemia, which also reduces the availability of other substrates. In fact, adaptation to hypoxia appears to take place such that when mitochondria are isolated from animal tissues after the animals have been exposed to brief periods of hypoxia (at a PO_2 of 30 to 40 mm Hg), their capacity to respire and synthesize ATP in vitro is enhanced. In contrast to hypoxia, hemorrhagic and endotoxin shock reduce calcium transport by mitochondrial membranes, particularly in organs that become ischemic; state 3 respiratory activity and ATP synthesis and mitochondrial ATPase activity are inhibited, and finally mitochondrial damage ensues. The mechanism by which ischemia and endotoxins induce mitochondrial damage is not known. Whether such mitochondrial changes are direct effects of deprivation of vital substrates or are secondary to release of lysosomal enzymes, changes in intracellular pH, or other changes in cellular ionic environment with accumulation of metabolites is not apparent.

Glucocorticoids may exert a protective effect on mitochondrial function in endotoxemia in rats. Very large doses of glucocorticoids completely protect the mitochondria when rats are given a lethal dose (LD) 60 of endotoxin. The protective effect is not apparent, however, when an LD 90 is given. One may summarize the mitochondrial effects by saying that hypoxia by itself triggers some adaptive mechanisms that tend to increase respiratory activity if oxygen and ADP become available. In contrast, ischemia and endotoxemia can induce significant mitochondrial damage that heralds cellular death.

THE LYSOSOMAL THEORY. Lysosomes are cytoplasmic granules that contain a variety of potent hydrolytic enzymes bound in a latent form. These enzymes are capable of hydrolyzing a wide variety of both natural and synthetic substances and can digest all intra- and extracellular macromolecules if they are released from their membranes. When released from the organelles, either inside or outside the cell, as a consequence of certain forms of cellular injury, they may contribute to the pathogenesis or the propagation and perpetuation of shock. They are most active at an acid pH, which would make them potentially more destructive in the setting of hypoxia and shock.

Numerous morphologic and biochemical observations implicate the lysosomal enzymes in the perpetuation of shock, but at this time the evidence for their primary involvement is not convincing. In organs such as liver, spleen, and intestine, the lysosomes enlarge and lose their granules during the early phases of shock. This is associated with a decrease in the total activity of lysosomal hydrolases in tissues and a corresponding increase in activity in the soluble fraction of the tissue homogenate. This indicates a loss of lysosomal membrane integrity in vivo. The lysosomes obtained from animals in shock demonstrate an enhanced release of enzymes in vitro. A reduction in lysosomal membrane integrity has also been observed in animals after administration of endotoxin. In several animal studies the levels of hydrolases found in blood, lymph, or serum seem to correlate with severity of shock.

The appearance of a *myocardial depressant factor* or factors (MDF) in shock, although still controversial, may be an indirect manifestation of the effect of lysosomal enzymes. In experimentally induced pancreatitis and in a variety of other shock states, plasma MDF activity closely parallels lysosomal hydrolases in the plasma. It has been suggested that pancreatic ischemia associated with shock results in the release of lysosomal and other enzymes within the pancreas. These enzymes act on an endogenous substrate to yield a peptide with low molecular weight and MDF activity, which is then released into the circulation. The resulting myocardial depression maintains the state of low cardiac output and sustains shock.

Another indication of the involvement of MDF has been the reproducibility of the shock syndrome with infusion of lysosomal hydrolases in animals. These animals demonstrate the hypotension, circulatory collapse, and pathologic changes in the tissues that are seen in other experimental forms of shock.

Other suggestive evidence of the involvement of MDF has been the responsiveness of certain animals in shock to large amounts of corticosteroids. In vitro, corticosteroids stabilize the lysosomal membranes and prevent their lysis. Treatment with steroids suppresses circulating serum levels of lysosomal hydrolases in a variety of shock states.

Endotoxemia is associated with increased levels of serum hydrolases, but in vitro the endotoxins do not increase the lysis of lysosomes. It has been suggested that endotoxins may cause the formation of a lysosomal releasing factor, LRF, through activation of the alternative as well as the classic complement pathways. Activation of complement in fresh human serum has been found to generate a factor (LRF) that stimulates human polymorphonuclear leukocytes to release their lysosomal enzymes. This factor has many of the properties of human C5a.

COMPLEMENT ACTIVATION IN SHOCK. The complement system consists of a series of discrete plasma proteins that are present as inactive precursors until they are activated by highly specific biochemical reactions (see Ch. 418). Activation of the complement system results in the cleavage of several low molecular weight vasoactive peptides from the complement molecules. These peptides in turn have a wide variety of significant biologic effects. For example, during the activation of C2, a cleavage product occurs that has kinin-like activity, which then can significantly influence capillary permeability. Two other activation peptides, C3a and C5a, release histamine from mast cells, have chemotactic activity, and constrict vascular smooth muscle. Another fragment, C3b, acts as an opsonin and facilitates phagocytosis. Polymorphonuclear leukocytes may be attracted chemotactically through activation of esterases on their surface and may release their lysosomal enzymes if the concentration of the complement reaction product C5a is large enough. Platelets may have an increase in their procoagulant activity, and endothelial cells may contract. In addition to the direct and indirect effects of the fragments of activated complement on cells, their aggregation as decamolecular complexes on the surface of the cell membranes causes cellular destruction. The expressions of all these effects are increased capillary permeability; increased leukocyte accumulation and infiltration; release of lysosomal enzymes; and activation of intravascular coagulation factors. Clinically, these result in such entities as glomerulitis, necrotizing vasculitis, the Shwartzman reaction, thrombocytopenia, and other manifestations of microcirculatory collapse and intravascular plugging seen in prolonged shock and in endotoxemia.

Although the side effects of complement activation in shock are detrimental, leading to cellular death, the fundamental biologic activities of the complement components are beneficial in enhancing phagocytosis and mediating the inflammatory response to local infection or irritation, in the vital neutralizing of viruses, and, finally, in modulating the immune response.

OXYGEN FREE RADICALS. Oxygen free radicals generated during ischemic reperfusion of myocardium may contribute significantly to myocardial depression and injury. They include superoxide anion, hydrogen peroxide, and hydroxyl radicals, which are produced in vascular endothelium and neutrophils by the degradation of membrane phospholipids and the subsequent metabolism of arachidonic acid or by the conversion of xanthine dehydrogenase to xanthine oxidase and subsequent oxidation of hypoxanthine.

The unpaired electron in these radicals may react with any cellular component, but particularly with unsaturated fatty acids and sulfhydryl amino acids, and cause cellular damage. The scavengers of oxygen radicals, such as superoxide dismutase and catalase, and the competitive antagonist of xanthine oxidase, allopurinol, have proved protective against myocardial injury in different animal models. The clinical documentation of the relative importance of these factors and the effectiveness of their elimination awaits further experimentation in humans.

TREATMENT OF SHOCK

GENERAL PRINCIPLES. There are five main goals in the management of the patient in shock: (1) rapid recognition of the shock state, (2) correction of the initiating insult (e.g., pericardiocentesis, defibrillation, hemostasis, antibiotics), (3) correction of the secondary consequences of the shock state (e.g., hypovolemia, acidosis, hypoxemia, disseminated intravascular coagulation), (4) maintenance of the function of vital organs (e.g., cardiac output, arterial pressure, urinary output), and (5) identification and correction of aggravating factors. All five goals are approached simultaneously. The prognosis of a patient in shock is determined in part by the etiology of the shock state (e.g., hypovolemic traumatic shock in a young, healthy adult carries a mortality of less than 20 per cent in many centers, while cardiogenic shock due to massive anterior infarct carries a mortality of more than 70 per cent even in the most aggressive medical center). Prognosis is also affected by the duration of shock and consequent secondary organ dysfunction and by the speed of recognition and appropriateness of medical intervention.

A key element in the therapy of a patient in shock is hemodynamic monitoring.

PATIENT MONITORING. Management of the patient in shock requires accurate and serial measurements of heart rate and rhythm, respiratory rate and adequacy of gas exchange, systemic blood pressure and cardiac filling pressures, cardiac output and tissue perfusion indices, and end-organ function (mental status, urine output, liver function, etc.).

1. *The electrocardiogram* permits serial assessment of cardiac rate and rhythm and promptly detects serious arrhythmias such as premature ventricular beats, ventricular tachycardia or fibrillation, third-degree heart block, serious sinus bradycardia, and atrial arrhythmias. In addition, serial 12-lead ECG's may allow an indirect assessment of the severity of myocardial ischemia.

2. *Arterial blood gases and pH.* These should also be monitored routinely. Correction of acidosis and hypoxia is essential in management of early phases of shock.

3. *Central venous and Swan-Ganz catheters.* The monitoring of central venous pressure provides an index of the status of absolute and relative blood volume and of the need for fluid replacement. The catheter should be inserted through the antecubital or external jugular vein; only if the physician is experienced should it be introduced through the subclavian or internal jugular vein. Central venous pressure obtained with the catheter advanced to the superior vena cava is normally between 5 and 8 mm Hg, but it should be elevated to 10 mm Hg if one is to expect an adequate cardiac output in patients in shock. Central venous pressure reflects the filling pressure of the right ventricle and hence is an adequate indicator of cardiac filling pressure *only* in patients who have no underlying cardiac or pulmonary disease and are not on a mechanical ventilator. The central venous pressure is probably adequate only for the initial management of young adults suffering from traumatic hypovolemic shock. In the patient with known or suspected cardiac or pulmonary disease, or in whom management includes the use of positive pressure ventilation, state of the art management requires the use of a Swan-Ganz catheter to measure pulmonary capillary wedge pressure as an indicator of left ventricular filling pressure. In addition, the Swan-Ganz catheter allows serial assessment of cardiac output and provides a route for oximetric studies.

The filling pressure of the left ventricle can be estimated from measurement of the "pulmonary capillary wedge" pressure with a Swan-Ganz balloon-tip catheter. A triple-lumen thermodilution catheter is introduced intravenously with or without fluoroscopy but with electrocardiographic monitoring. Its tip is advanced to the pulmonary artery; the balloon is inflated with air, and it can be floated to a wedge position in one of the pulmonary arteries. The recorded pressure downstream from the inflated balloon is the "pulmonary capillary wedge" pressure, and the appearance of the left atrial pressure wave form on the oscilloscope confirms the position of the catheter tip. The wedge pressure reflects left ventricular end-diastolic pressure, but a discrepancy between the two may occur if there is severe mitral stenosis or left atrial tumors. If for some reason one is unable to get the wedge pressure, the pulmonary artery diastolic pressure may be a useful index of the wedge pressure.

The Swan-Ganz catheter has been modified to include an extra lumen that allows measurement of right atrial pressure simultaneously with the wedge pressure. Another modification includes a temperature sensor device at the tip that allows detection of changes in temperature following injection of cold dextrose in the right atrium, and the temperature dilution curve obtained with the temperature sensor provides an estimate of cardiac output. Further modifications of the Swan-Ganz catheter allow the continuous monitoring of intracardiac electrocardiogram and of oxygen saturation in blood and introduction of a pacing wire through a right ventricular port.

The Swan-Ganz catheter is expensive, and complications such as arrhythmias, sepsis, or pulmonary infarction may accompany its use. Nevertheless, it is a very important tool for monitoring patients in shock and for providing important data for judicious administration of fluids and sympathomimetic amines. The catheter should probably be removed within 72 hours after its insertion to avoid sepsis or pulmonary infarction and should not be left continuously in the "wedged" position. The normal wedge pressure is 12 mm Hg, but it often needs to be raised to 15 or 20 mm Hg in shock in order to maintain adequate organ perfusion unless there is pulmonary edema.

A discrepancy between right atrial and left atrial pressures may occur in patients with acute myocardial infarction, sepsis, or trauma when a high left atrial or pulmonary capillary wedge pressure may be accompanied by a low right atrial pressure, and under those circumstances monitoring right atrial pressure alone may lead to excessive administration of fluids. Conversely, patients with pulmonary disease, pulmonary embolism, pulmonary hypertension, and right ventricular infarction have relatively high levels of right atrial pressure compared with the pulmonary capillary wedge pressure, and avoidance of fluids under those circumstances may deprive the patient of important therapy. In addition to providing information on pressure, the triple-lumen Swan-Ganz catheter provides proximal and distal ports for sampling of right atrial and pulmonary arterial blood for oximetry to rule out a left-to-right intracardiac shunt. The sampling of "mixed venous" (pulmonary arterial) and systemic arterial blood to measure the oxygen content allows the estimation of cardiac output, since output equals oxygen consumption divided by arteriovenous oxygen difference. The use of a thermodilution catheter permits serial direct measurements of cardiac output by the thermodilution technique. At least three consecutive samples of thermodilution curves with less than 10 per cent variance should be averaged.

4. *Urinary catheter*. This allows the routine hourly measurement of urinary output. A decline in urinary output to less than 20 ml per hour is an indication of inadequacy of arterial pressure and renal perfusion. It is a sensitive index of progress of the shock syndrome and reflects the effectiveness of management. The most frequent cause of oliguria in shock is hypovolemia. Fluid deficits are often underestimated, particularly in the presence of sepsis. If oliguria persists despite adequate administration of fluid and elevated wedge pressure, diuretic therapy may be necessary to avoid acute renal tubular necrosis, which complicates prolonged hypotension.

5. *Arterial catheterization for arterial pressure monitoring*. Patients with severe or persistent hypotension and shock in whom it is difficult to measure blood pressure with the sphygmomanometer are candidates for intra-arterial pressure monitoring. There is often a discrepancy between intra-arterial pressure measurements and cuff pressure. There may be a low or even no recordable arterial pressure by the cuff technique when intra-arterial pressure by cannulation is normal or even at times slightly elevated. This discrepancy may result from severe peripheral vasoconstriction and low output and pulse pressure. Since the sphygmomanometric measurement of arterial pressure in shock may be erroneously low, it is advisable to palpate the femoral artery in the groin to get a better index of the strength of the pulse pressure and to introduce an arterial cannula for monitoring arterial pressure before administering vasopressors or resorting to counterpulsation. An arterial cannula also allows the frequent determination of blood gases and pH. The radial, brachial, or femoral arteries may be cannulated. The radial artery is the preferred site for cannulation with the lowest complication rate. Brachial or femoral arterial cannulation is preferred in patients who are severely hypotensive, who are on large doses of vasoactive drugs, who are markedly vasoconstricted, and in whom the radial artery is difficult to palpate.

6. *Cardiac output*. Measurement of cardiac output by thermal or dye dilution techniques is used for management of selected patients or for evaluation of new therapeutic regimens. The mixed venous blood oxygen content may be used as an index of total body perfusion. Within certain limitations, one can estimate the effectiveness of total body perfusion and delivery of oxygen to tissues by monitoring oxygen content of mixed venous or pulmonary arterial blood. The assumptions are that total body oxygen consumption is constant or does not change drastically and that arterial oxygen content is high and does not vary significantly. An arteriovenous oxygen difference of 6 ml per deciliter or more indicates poor tissue perfusion.

MANAGEMENT. ***General Measures.*** Management consists of primary therapy, directed at the underlying insult, and secondary therapy, directed at consequences of the shock state. Patients in shock may be in pain and frightened. They should be reassured and put in a horizontal position with legs slightly elevated, unless this position is uncomfortable or causes shortness of breath. In that case, they should be allowed to be in the most comfortable position. Pain should be relieved with morphine sulfate intravenously, preferably in small repeated doses of 2 to 5 mg; if side effects occur, such as hypotension, cold clammy skin, bradycardia, nausea, and vomiting, atropine may provide some relief. Another analgesic, meperidine, 50 to 100 mg, may be given intravenously. Intravenous fluid and monitoring of various functions should begin promptly to guide further therapy. Oxygen, norepinephrine, or dopamine may be initiated while the cause of shock is determined. Reversible factors that decrease cardiac output and cause hypotension should be corrected promptly (i.e., tension pneumothorax, marked acidosis or alkalosis, cardiac tamponade).

Correction of Hypovolemia. Hypovolemia may occur in any type of shock whether or not it is associated with external signs of blood or fluid loss. If there is no evidence of actual fluid or blood loss, there may be a significant shift of fluid from the intravascular to extracellular space because of increased capillary permeability and endothelial damage. This may occur in any vascular bed, but more specifically in the splanchnic and the pulmonary vasculature. In any shock syndrome associated with decreased tissue perfusion, fluid may also shift intracellularly because of changes in cellular membrane permeability and increased intracellular sodium and water. Fluid replacement is essential for restoration of cardiac output. Without an adequate filling pressure, there will not be an adequate cardiac output. The administration of potent cardiotonic drugs in the presence of hypovolemia and low cardiac filling pressure may be ineffective and may potentially aggravate the clinical condition rather than improve it. On the other hand, these drugs increase cardiac output significantly if left ventricular end-diastolic pressure and volume are adequate.

If the patient has cardiogenic shock or if there are signs of pulmonary congestion or edema, one should insert a Swan-Ganz balloon catheter into the pulmonary artery or pulmonary arterial wedge position for measurements of pulmonary artery diastolic pressure or pulmonary capillary wedge pressure. If pulmonary artery diastolic or pulmonary artery wedge pressure is less than 15 mm Hg, one should give 100 ml of Ringer's lactate, saline, or dextran every 10 to 15 minutes. If perfusion improves and wedge pressure remains less than 15 mm Hg, one should continue infusion at the same rate, trying to achieve a pressure between 15 and 20 mm Hg. If perfusion of tissues is unchanged or worse, if wedge pressure increases above 20 mm Hg, or if there are signs of pulmonary congestion, one should stop volume expansion. Improvement in tissue perfusion is evaluated by examining the degree of cyanosis, clamminess of the skin, level of arterial blood pressure, and urinary output, as well as the sensorium and alertness of the patient, blood gases, and pH.

If a Swan-Ganz catheter is not available or if pulmonary artery diastolic pressure or wedge pressure cannot be obtained, insertion of a central venous catheter is a helpful guide for administration of fluids. If central venous pressure is less than 10 mm Hg, one should expand volume until arterial pressure and tissue perfusion return to satisfactory levels, central venous pressure is between 10 and 15 mm Hg, or pulmonary congestion develops. Central venous or pulmonary capillary wedge pressures should be measured with careful reference to a constant point marked on the chest at the level of the right atrium or the phlebostatic axis. Patients who are on respirators or are receiving positive pressure assistance or positive pressure ventilation will have an abnormally elevated pressure. Under those circumstances, the filling pressure should be recorded at the time the respirator is transiently disconnected.

Treatment for hemorrhagic hypotension is with blood replacement, but while waiting for typing and cross-matching, the patient should be given saline or Ringer's lactate. The effects of these fluids are transient, because the crystalloids will rapidly leave the intravascular space. A more effective treatment might include colloids that stay longer in the circulation and increase oncotic pressure. This is particularly important when patients have manifestations of the shock lung syndrome, when extensive endothelial damage and interstitial edema are suspected, or when patients are chronically ill or malnourished and have hypoalbuminemia. Under those circumstances, dextran or mannitol, albumin, or plasma would expand blood volume. The excretion of dextran or mannitol by the kidney will increase oncotic pressure in Bowman's capsule and create a favorable hydrostatic-oncotic pressure gradient across the glomerulus, facilitating filtration even at low arterial pressure. If arterial pressure is not rapidly restored or oliguria persists despite administration of diuretics such as furosemide in conjunction with fluid replacement, then there might be danger of overexpansion of plasma volume and accentuation of pulmonary edema.

Development of pulmonary edema is closely correlated with the gradient between plasma oncotic and pulmonary artery wedge pressure, which reflects the capillary hydrostatic pressure in the lung. Plasma oncotic pressure of normal adults is approximately 25 mm Hg whereas pulmonary wedge pressure is 10 to 12 mm Hg. Capillary filtration takes place normally in the lung despite a low hydrostatic and a relatively high oncotic pressure, because of the equally high interstitial oncotic pressure in the lung. Plasma oncotic pressure may fluctuate. After 12 hours of bed rest, for example, it declines markedly. If oncotic pressure remains significantly higher (>8 mm Hg) than pulmonary capillary hydrostatic pressure, the risk of pulmonary edema is negligible; but if oncotic pressure is only 1 to 3 mm Hg higher than pulmonary wedge pressure, the patient is at high risk for pulmonary edema.

Types of Fluid. Isotonic saline solution contains 140 mEq of sodium and 140 mEq of chloride, whereas Ringer's lactate solution has 130 mEq of sodium, 4 mEq of potassium, 108 mEq of chloride, and 28 mEq of lactate. Lactate and acetate are converted to bicarbonate and maintain the alkalinity of the blood. When large volumes of fluid are administered, isotonic saline causes a dilution acidosis, which can be avoided if Ringer's lactate is used.

Human serum albumin comes in two concentrations, 5 grams per deciliter, which is the usual dose used, or 25 grams per deciliter salt-poor albumin. The 25 grams per deciliter solution is necessary only in the presence of severe hypoalbuminemia. An alternative is purified plasma protein, which is free of hepatitis virus contamination but has some contamination with vasoactive substances such as prekallikrein activator, causing the Food and Drug Administration to express concern about its use. Both albumin and purified plasma protein are expensive. They cost between $70 and $300 per 500 ml and represent a significant strain on blood donor programs. They should not be used indiscriminately.

There are two types of dextran: dextran 40 with 40,000 molecular weight and dextran 70 with approximately 70,000 molecular weight. Dextran 70 comes in a 6 per cent solution, and dextran 40 comes in a 10 per cent solution. Dextran 70 maintains vascular volume for up to 24 hours. While dextran 40 volume expansion lasts only a few hours owing to rapid renal clearance, the effective volume expansion is nearly twice as great as that of an equal volume of infused 5 per cent albumin or dextran 70. Dextran solutions cost one third to one half as much as albumin. If given in amounts exceeding 1 liter, they may cause serious side effects, including platelet dysfunction and abnormalities in bleeding and coagulation, the nature of which are not clearly defined, and occasional anaphylactoid reactions. Approximately 5 per cent of patients receiving dextran have had such reactions, but very few of these are fatal. It should probably be avoided in patients with hypofibrinogenemia and bleeding dyscrasias.

With dextran 40 there is an incidence of acute renal failure, presumably because the rapid filtration of the low molecular weight dextran into the urine is accompanied by maximal reabsorption of the filtered salt and water, leading to a high intratubular concentration with an increase in intratubular viscosity and possibly physical occlusion of the renal tubule by dextran precipitates. This does not seem to occur with dextran 70 because it is filtered at a much slower rate owing to its molecular size.

Another colloid is hydroxyethyl starch or hetastarch, which maintains volume expansion almost twice as long as dextran 40 and has fewer side effects. It interferes minimally with coagulation, it has a very mild anaphylactoid effect, and its cost is one third that of albumin. New synthetic oxygen-carrying compounds are currently under investigation for use in the setting of acute hemorrhagic shock.

CORRECTION OF HYPOXIA. Oxygenation of the patient and interpretation of serial blood gases require the use of high-flow oxygen delivery systems, where the delivery system supplies the entire inspired gas mixture. The currently used high-flow systems include intubation with mechanical ventilation or T-tube devices, or tight-fitting face masks making use of the Venturi principle. These systems deliver a fixed inspired oxygen concentration ($F_{I_{O_2}}$), allow careful titration of oxygen as a drug, and permit the calculation of alveolar-arterial oxygen gradients that require a constant $F_{I_{O_2}}$. Low-flow systems (such as nasal prongs or simple face masks) do *not* deliver the entire inspired gas mixture, and hence the $F_{I_{O_2}}$ varies with the rate and depth of ventilation. While more comfortable, these low-flow systems are much less accurate.

Adequacy of the airway should be assessed in any patient in shock. If the patient is obtunded and cannot protect his or her airway, intubation with a cuffed endotracheal tube is essential. Occasionally the use of positive pressure respirators to improve gas exchange is necessary. Positive pressure ventilation may simultaneously decrease the venous return by increasing intrathoracic pressure and thereby perpetuate and aggravate a low-output state. Also, 100 per cent oxygen by mask may lead to toxic changes in the lung if continued more than a few hours. Thus when a respirator is required, the preferred approach is to select an $F_{I_{O_2}}$ of 50 per cent and to increase the $F_{I_{O_2}}$ and employ positive pressure only if needed to achieve a P_{O_2} of about 70 mm Hg.

CORRECTION OF ACIDOSIS. If arterial blood pH is less than 7.3 and respiratory acidosis has been ruled out, it is advisable to give 1 ampule of sodium bicarbonate intravenously (50 mEq per 50 ml). If the arterial blood pH is less than 7.2, 2 ampules may be administered and values repeated for further therapy in 15 to 30 minutes. Overcorrection of acidosis to alkalosis may decrease oxygen delivery to tissues by shifting the oxyhemoglobin dissociation curve to the left. Serial assessment of arterial blood gases permits careful titration of $NaHCO_3$. There is a risk of pulmonary edema with large volumes of $NaHCO_3$.

TREATMENT OF ARRHYTHMIAS. Arrhythmias, particularly after myocardial infarction, may limit cardiac output and perpetuate shock.

Sustained ventricular tachycardia may be treated first with intravenous lidocaine in a bolus of 1.5 to 2.0 mg per kilogram; if there is associated hypotension or any evidence of hemodynamic deterioration, synchronized electrical countershock should be used immediately. Ventricular fibrillation should be treated immediately with countershock. If the first or second shock is unsuccessful, the patient must receive closed chest massage, mouth-to-mouth respiration, and possibly intravenous sodium bicarbonate before again attempting electrocardioversion. In patients who fail to respond to adequate doses of lidocaine and have recurrent refractory ventricular fibrillation or tachycardia, bretylium tosylate in a bolus dose of 5 mg per kilogram of body weight is the next preferred agent.

Accelerated idioventricular rhythm is seen frequently in patients with myocardial infarction, particularly in those with diaphragmatic infarction. The rate is slightly faster than sinus rhythm, and a period of sinus bradycardia seems to favor the development of this arrhythmia. This is usually a benign rhythm and does not require therapy unless it degenerates into rapid ventricular tachycardia.

Supraventricular arrhythmias (atrial tachycardias, flutter, fibrillation, or junctional rhythms) should generally be treated pharmacologically with calcium channel blockers (e.g., verapamil), beta blockers (e.g., propranolol), or digitalis glycosides. But if the rhythm persists or there is an associated hypotension or hemodynamic deterioration, synchronized countershock therapy should be utilized. Sinus bradycardia, if severe (less than 40 beats per minute), can contribute to hypotension. It is commonly associated with inferior infarction, and, if accompanied by frequent premature ventricular beats, restoration of a more rapid sinus rhythm can eliminate them. Atropine is most effective intravenously in incremental doses of 0.4 mg to 2 or 3 mg. If bradycardia persists and hypotension or other signs of hypoperfusion are evident, electrical pacing should be instituted.

Conduction disturbances such as atrioventricular block carry a variable prognosis. The conduction disturbance that occurs with inferior infarction has a better prognosis than that associated with anterior infarction. It generally occurs early, is associated with sinus bradycardia, and may be caused by a temporary reflex increase in vagal tone to the conduction system or by atrioventricular nodal ischemia with only localized necrosis of this discrete structure. In anterior wall infarction heart block is related to ischemic damage of the three fascicles of the conduction system, which results from a more extensive degree of necrosis and is associated with higher mortality. Patients with inferior infarction benefit from temporary electrical pacing if they do not respond to atropine, whereas those with anteroseptal infarction generally require a permanent pacemaker, and the correction of the electrical disturbance may not alter their prognosis.

Treatment of Sepsis. Both gram-negative and gram-positive organisms have been associated with septic shock (see Ch. 259). In gram-negative septicemia, *E. coli* is the predominant organism, and infections with *Klebsiella-Aerobacter* (enterobacter) groups are not uncommon; endotoxin is an important factor in the pathogenesis of this syndrome. Gram-positive infections without endotoxemia, such as in pneumococcal pneumonia, *Staphylococcus aureus* infections, or streptococcal bacteremia, may cause shock. Chronic alcoholism is a common associated illness among these patients. The toxic shock syndrome, a complication of *S. aureus* infection most commonly associated with tampon usage in women, is discussed in Ch. 271.

The characteristic hemodynamic abnormality in septic shock (whether gram-positive or gram-negative) is a marked decrease in peripheral vascular resistance; cardiac output may be increased, normal, or decreased. In contrast, in cardiogenic shock cardiac output is low and peripheral resistance is normal, increased, or occasionally decreased, and in hypovolemic shock cardiac output is low and peripheral resistance is increased. The treatment of septic shock includes the aggressive treatment of the infection with antibiotics and drainage of any abscesses. Although cardiac output may be normal or high, it may be insufficient to meet metabolic needs of the tissues. An absolute or relative decrease in intravascular volume requires fluid administration. Crystalloids or colloids are given to restore and raise central venous pressure to levels of 10 to 15 mm Hg or pulmonary wedge pressure to 20 mm Hg. In these patients who have marked peripheral vasodilation in the face of arterial hypotension, a potent peripheral vasoconstricting agent such as norepinephrine may be the agent of choice if correction of intravascular volume fails to provide adequate arterial blood pressure.

Use of Steroids. The use of steroids in shock remains controversial. If used, they are given early and in large doses. Their potential beneficial effect appears to be related primarily to their action on cellular membranes. Steroids interact with biomembranes and probably become incorporated within their bilayer structures. A stabilizing effect on biomembranes has been demonstrated in vitro in studies of lysosomes isolated from animals treated with these agents. These lysosomes acquire a resistance to lysis in vitro. Apparently this beneficial action of corticosteroids is not related to their glucocorticoid properties. For example, testosterone is another potent membrane-stabilizing agent. The reason for the continued question concerning the effectiveness of corticosteroids is that the consequences of membrane stabilization by corticosteroids in vivo are not really known. Experimental studies in animals subjected to septic, endotoxin, or hemorrhagic shock indicate improved survival with administration of corticosteroids. In shock, considerable damage to the microcirculation may be attributed to membrane interactions between platelets, polymorphonuclear leukocytes, and endothelium. Activation by the bacteria of the alternative complement pathway with the release of various peptides may favor platelet aggregation with endothelium and leukocytes, clot formation, and obstruction of the microcirculation. Corticosteroids may prevent these membrane interactions in vivo. Steroids may also prevent the pituitary release of β-endorphins, which may cause myocardial depression. Animals pretreated with cortisone or naloxone (β-endorphin antagonist) exhibit an impressive resistance to endotoxin-mediated shock. Use of corticosteroids in doses of 30 mg per kilogram of methylprednisolone as early as possible in patients with septicemia and hypotension may be justifiable (but see also Ch. 30). The extension of the use of corticosteroids to patients with cardiogenic shock is unwise. There is evidence that malignant arrhythmias develop after the administration of corticosteroids to such patients, and the incidence of ventricular aneurysms may be increased.

It is claimed that corticosteroids have significant cardiovascular effects with possible alpha receptor blocking activities, but pharmacologic studies indicate that the steroids have little, if any, significant direct cardiovascular action; they may augment the action of catecholamines, but they do not block alpha receptors.

Sympathomimetic Amines. These drugs are used to increase cardiac output through their cardiotonic effect and to redistribute blood flow to vital organs by their selective vasoconstricting action; by virtue of these two effects, they raise arterial pressure and allow perfusion of ischemic regions, particularly in the myocardium, through collateral vessels. There are two potential problems with their use. If arterial pressure is elevated significantly, the hypertension may be detrimental, as it increases myocardial work and oxygen demand. Thus judicious elevation of arterial pressure to levels between 110 and 120 mm Hg systolic pressure would be reasonable. One cannot predict the optimal arterial pressure necessary to perfuse the coronaries in any particular patient because one does not know the severity of coronary disease and its extent, or the extent of myocardial reserve that would allow the heart to cope with a slight increase in afterload induced by the rising arterial pressure. Nevertheless, hypotension, particularly following myocardial infarction, should be corrected and arterial pressure maintained. The second potential problem with these drugs is their vasoconstricting effect; however, some vasoconstriction can be beneficial if it occurs in nonvital organs and if it is associated with increased cardiac output. This combination of effects raises arterial pressure and improves perfusion of vital organs. Therefore the proper use of sympathomimetic amines in shock requires a thorough knowledge of their cardiovascular effects. Their action depends upon their affinity for various types of adrenergic receptors (see Ch. 31).

ADRENERGIC RECEPTORS. The adrenergic receptors may be classified as alpha or beta receptors with respect to their cardiovascular action. The alpha receptors are predominantly in blood vessels and mediate vasoconstriction. The beta receptors are present in the blood vessels as well as the myocardium. Activation of the beta-1 receptors in myocardium causes an increase in myocardial contractility and in heart rate, whereas activation of beta-2 receptors in blood vessels causes vasodilation. The same catecholamine may activate both alpha and beta receptors, depending on dose and the organ in which it is acting (Table 44–4). The sympathomimetic amines that are available clinically include norepinephrine, epinephrine, dopamine, isoproterenol, phenylephrine, and dobutamine. The relative actions and potencies of these agents are summarized in Tables 44–5 and 44–6.

NOREPINEPHRINE. Norepinephrine increases myocardial contractility by activating beta-1 receptors and thus may increase cardiac output. In blood vessels it activates primarily alpha, or vasoconstricting, receptors. The magnitude of its effect on alpha receptors varies from one organ to another. It is a very potent vasoconstrictor in skin, muscle, and splanchnic beds, whereas in the coronary vessels it activates the beta-2 receptors as well as the alpha receptors; and because there is a paucity of alpha receptors in the coronary vessels in contrast to other vascular beds, the drug causes vasodilatation of the coronaries.

It offers several distinct advantages in the treatment of shock. It increases cardiac output and redistributes blood flow away from the extremities and toward the heart and brain and increases arterial pressure, which in turn increases coronary flow to ischemic myocardium. It should be administered intravenously through an indwelling catheter to avoid the risk of extravasation, which results in necrosis of subcutaneous tissues. Two ampules of Levophed (4 mg base per ampule) may be dissolved in 500 ml glucose and water and an infusion started at a very low rate to determine the smallest dose necessary to maintain arterial pressure between 100 and 120 mm Hg, which should provide adequate perfusion to the heart, brain, and kidney (unless the patient was hypertensive or has extensive arteriosclerotic disease). A dose of 4 μg per minute may occasionally be adequate; however, many patients require up to 40 μg per minute; and in general if such doses are necessary to maintain pressure, prognosis is poor. The average dose is between 10 and 15 μg per minute. If hypoxia, hypovolemia, and acidosis have been corrected, the lack of response to norepinephrine is probably an indication of significant myocardial damage. Norepinephrine may be the preferred agent in the management of profound hypotensive septic shock.

TABLE 44–4. ADRENERGIC RECEPTORS

Receptor Type	Site	Action
Beta-1	Mycocardium Sinoatrial node Atrioventricular	↑ Atrial and ventricular contraction ↑ Heart rate ↑ Atrioventricular conduction
Beta-2	Arterioles Lung	Vasodilation Bronchial dilation
Alpha	Arterioles Venules Veins	Vasoconstriction

TABLE 44–5. RELATIVE ADRENERGIC POTENCIES

Amine	Alpha (Vascular)	Beta-1 (Cardiac)	Beta-2 (Vascular)
Norephinephrine	+ + + +	+ + +	+
Epinephrine	+ + +	+ + + +	+ +
Dopamine	+ +	+ + + +	+ +
Isoproterenol	0	+ + + +	+ + + +
Phenylephrine	+ + + +	0	0
Dobutamine	+	+ + + +	+ +

DOPAMINE. This is a naturally occurring precursor of norepinephrine. Its cardiovascular effect depends on its dose and the type of receptor that it activates. When given in low doses, less than 3 μg per kilogram per minute, it has a vasodilator action in the renal, mesenteric, cerebral, and coronary vessels because of activation of dopaminergic (DA) receptors. DA-1 postsynaptic receptors mediate vasodilatation and DA-2 presynaptic receptors prevent the release of endogenous norepinephrine. In doses of 3 to 10 μg per kilogram per minute, it increases myocardial contractility and cardiac output through the activation of beta-1 receptors. In larger doses of more than 20 μg per kilogram per minute, it causes vasoconstriction through activation of alpha-adrenergic receptors of arteries and veins in most vascular beds. Thus this drug may redistribute blood flow away from the extremities and toward the kidney, gut, heart, and brain; however, it may be necessary to give large doses to maintain arterial pressure and coronary blood flow, particularly following myocardial infarction; these large doses tend to oppose the beneficial vasodilator effects in some vascular beds. Dopamine may cause nausea and vomiting and increased cardiac irritability in some patients.

EPINEPHRINE. Epinephrine activates myocardial beta-1 receptors and vasoconstrictor alpha receptors in most vessels except in skeletal muscle and coronary vessels, where it activates beta-2 receptors when administered in low doses. It increases cardiac output but redistributes flow away from the kidney and splanchnic circulations toward skeletal muscle. Given in a dose range from 2 to 30 μg per minute intravenously, its effect on the redistribution flow is not optimal, and its effect on arterial pressure is only modest because of its vasodilator effect in skeletal muscle.

ISOPROTERENOL. Isoproterenol is a synthetic sympathomimetic amine that activates primarily vascular beta-2 receptors, causing vasodilatation, and myocardial beta-1 receptors, increasing cardiac output. The magnitude of the vasodilator effect of isoproterenol varies in different vascular beds, depending on the density of beta-2 receptors and the affinity of the drug for them. The major vasodilator action of isoproterenol is in skeletal muscle beds.

This drug is not recommended in either cardiogenic or septic shock. In cardiogenic shock, isoproterenol significantly increases myocardial oxygen requirement, and, despite the increase in coronary flow, the ischemic region of the myocardium may be hypoperfused as indicated by increased lactate production. Its use should be limited to the treatment of atropine-resistant complete heart block in an attempt to maintain an idioventricular rhythm and hemodynamic stability until more definitive therapy with pacing can be carried out.

TABLE 44–6. RELATIVE INITIAL HEMODYNAMIC EFFECTS

Amine	Heart Rate	Arterial Pressure	Cardiac Output	Systemic Resistance
Norepinephrine	↑	↑ ↑	↑ →	↑ ↑
Epinephrine	↑	↑	↑	↑ →
Dopamine	↑	↑	↑	↑ →
Isoproterenol	↑	↓ →	↑ ↑	↓
Phenylephrine	→	↑	→ ↓	↑ ↑
Dobutamine	→	→	↑	→

Isoproterenol may prevent the recurrence of ventricular tachycardia associated with the long QT syndrome and presenting as *"torsades de pointes."* The usual dose of isoproterenol is 2 to 20 μg per minute.

DOBUTAMINE. Dobutamine is a synthetic sympathomimetic amine that has predominant beta-1 activity. In contrast to dopamine, dobutamine has much less alpha-vasoconstricting activity but equal positive inotropic effects. Thus, in equal inotropic doses, dobutamine tends to lower the pulmonary capillary wedge pressure while dopamine tends to increase it. Dobutamine is also reported to have a lower incidence of cardiac arrhythmias. In experimental models of canine infarction, the administration of dobutamine results in significantly smaller infarcts compared with dopamine, possibly owing to the intracardiac release of norepinephrine produced by dopamine. Thus, especially in the setting of acute myocardial infarction with low output but no significant hypotension, dobutamine may be a preferred agent over dopamine for improvement in the cardiac output.

One can summarize the use of sympathomimetic amines by saying that the goal is to attain an arterial pressure adequate to perfuse the kidney, the ischemic myocardial segment, and the brain without overloading the left ventricle. The drug used should redistribute blood flow toward the more vital organs and away from skin and muscle for the optimal utilization of the limited cardiac output in shock. Finally, the drug should also have an inotropic action, and drugs such as methoxamine and phenylephrine, which cause arterial vasoconstriction only by activating alpha receptors without stimulating the heart, should be avoided. With these goals in mind, norepinephrine, dopamine, and dobutamine should be chosen in the management of shock.

Vasodilator Therapy in Shock. The beneficial effects of vasodilator therapy are (1) to decrease myocardial oxygen demands by decreasing preload or cardiac filling pressure and cardiac size and decreasing afterload by decreasing arterial pressure and arterial impedance, and (2) to dilate microcirculatory vessels.

The effectiveness of vasodilators (nitroprusside, nitroglycerin, phentolamine, or hydralazine) is impressive in the acutely failing heart following myocardial infarction without shock and with an elevated left ventricular end-diastolic pressure or capillary wedge pressure over 20 to 25 mm Hg; but the presence of *hypotension* should be a contraindication to the use of this therapy alone. Under these circumstances one may have to use a vasodilator drug along with norepinephrine or dopamine.

REDUCTION IN PRELOAD. One can reduce oxygen demand of the myocardium by decreasing cardiac volume in patients who have a high filling pressure. Reduction in cardiac size decreases myocardial wall tension, which is a major determinant of myocardial oxygen requirements. It may be achieved by administration of diuretics or venodilator drugs, which reduce filling pressure by pooling blood in the peripheral veins. The goal of "venodilator therapy" is to decrease preload and cardiac size and not to decrease arterial blood pressure. This effect is desirable as long as cardiac filling pressure does not drop excessively, causing a drop in cardiac output. In some patients with severe pulmonary congestion and high cardiac filling pressure with systemic arterial hypotension, it may be necessary to combine vasodilator therapy with another drug that will cause selective arteriolar vasoconstriction in certain organs and will increase peripheral vascular resistance and raise and maintain arterial pressure, such as dopamine or norepinephrine.

REDUCTION IN AFTERLOAD. This is a beneficial effect of the vasodilators, because it will decrease the arterial impedance against which the left ventricle ejects its blood; thus cardiac output improves. This is desirable as long as it is not associated with a significant reduction in systemic arterial diastolic pressure, particularly in patients who are normotensive or have borderline hypotension. The dose of vasodilator drug must be adjusted so that it will not cause a significant reduction in diastolic arterial pressure. Any drop in arterial pressure by more than 10 mm Hg should be avoided, and the diastolic pressure should certainly not be allowed to decrease below 65 mm Hg. Reduction in afterload is ideal in patients with chronic severe congestive failure with high filling pressure, pulmonary congestion, and low cardiac output, but without a significant reduction in arterial pressure. Patients with cardiomyopathy but without coronary artery disease may be the best candidates for this therapy.

Neither a vasodilator alone nor propranolol, which also reduces myocardial oxygen demand, has a place in the management of cardiogenic hypotension following myocardial infarction. The elimination of the cardiotonic effect of the normal sympathetic drive by propranolol may significantly impair cardiac output and precipitate failure. If the patient has continuing pain and *a normal or elevated blood pressure,* despite administration of narcotics, morphine or meperidine, and nitroglycerin, administration of propranolol might then be considered.

MICROCIRCULATORY VASOCONSTRICTION AND ALPHA RECEPTOR BLOCKERS. In some patients, despite prolonged administration of dopamine or norepinephrine, tissue perfusion is not improved. The reason may be that myocardial infarction or cellular damage is extensive. It is also possible that constriction of microcirculatory vessels may be preventing perfusion of exchange capillaries. The alpha receptor blocker phentolamine has a specific effect on vasoconstricting alpha receptors and does not block beta receptors in the myocardium. Thus the cardiotonic effect of sympathomimetic amines is not prevented, yet vasoconstricting effects at the microcirculatory level are antagonized. Phentolamine has a greater inhibitory effect on alpha receptors in venules and veins than in arterioles, and its dilator action may therefore be greater in veins than in arterioles. This effect calls for a note of caution, because rapid relaxation of large veins may abruptly lower cardiac filling pressure if the patient is hypovolemic. For this reason, it is essential to ascertain that the patient has received adequate amounts of fluid before giving phentolamine.

NITROPRUSSIDE. This is a very effective vasodilator drug that causes relaxation of veins to decrease preload and some relaxation of arterioles to decrease arterial impedance. It may be started intravenously at a dose of 16 μg per minute and increased to 200 μg per minute with constant monitoring of arterial and cardiac filling pressures. Occasionally larger doses have been necessary. Prolonged administration may lead to thiocyanate toxicity.

NITROGLYCERIN. This is also a very effective vasodilator with predominant effects on the venous system and lesser effects on arteriolar resistance vessels. When given as an intravenous infusion of 15 to 100 μg per minute, it reduces preload and is useful in congestive heart failure complicating acute myocardial infarction, particularly when the wedge pressure is high and the arterial pressure is normal. Intravenous nitroglycerin may also cause coronary vasodilatation and improve subendocardial flow.

In cardiogenic shock with arterial hypotension and an elevated pulmonary artery wedge pressure, the combination of intravenous nitroglycerin and dopamine may be appropriate.

Other vasodilator drugs, such as hydralazine, which primarily exert an action on the arterioles, would not be very effective in reducing cardiac size and myocardial oxygen demand, and may be detrimental in causing a significant reduction in arterial blood pressure.

DIGITALIS. It is advisable not to use digitalis in patients in cardiogenic shock due to acute myocardial infarction even if there is evidence of pulmonary congestion and an elevated pulmonary artery wedge pressure. In the setting of acute myocardial infarction it may increase myocardial irritability.

In addition, the renal excretion of digoxin may be impaired because of decreased renal perfusion and arterial blood pressure.

Mechanical Ventricular Assistance and Surgical Treatment in Cardiogenic Shock. Intra-aortic balloon counterpulsation may be beneficial in cardiogenic shock. The balloon is introduced into the aorta at the end of a catheter inserted through the femoral artery via surgical cutdown or percutaneously via the Seldinger technique. It is inflated during early diastole and is collapsed during systole. This sequence decreases afterload during ejection and increases coronary perfusion pressure and coronary flow during diastole. Improvement of the hemodynamic status has been observed, but because a large number of patients with myocardial infarction and shock have extensive coronary artery disease, the long-term survival is still disappointing. Balloon counterpulsation appears to be of greatest potential benefit in support of patients who have seriously compromised hemodynamics after myocardial infarction, are refractory to medical management, and are candidates for a surgical procedure. This mechanical assistance sustains the hemodynamics during cardiac catheterization and coronary arteriography in preparation for surgery. Emergency revascularization surgery or infarctectomy, which has been carried out in some centers, has not been uniformly encouraging. Two complications of myocardial infarction require surgical intervention and carry a reasonable prognosis; these are ruptured papillary muscle and interventricular septal perforation. In both, there is decreased ejection from the left ventricle and a fall in arterial pressure. Attempts to increase systemic arterial pressure with drugs exaggerate the regurgitation or the left-to-right shunt. In these circumstances, selective lowering of arterial systolic pressure with intra-aortic balloon counterpulsation is ideal, as it will facilitate ejection and reduce mitral regurgitation or left-to-right shunt. A significant reduction in afterload and vasodilatation may also be achieved with drugs such as nitroprusside or nitroglycerin, but the associated fall in diastolic pressure may extend the myocardial ischemia. Surgical management, as soon as it is feasible and safe, should be the course to pursue. Severe papillary muscle dysfunction or papillary muscle rupture (the posterior more frequently than the anterior) may cause significant left ventricular failure, and the surgical replacement of the mitral valve has been satisfactory, particularly in patients with good myocardial function. Patients with a perforation of the ventricular septum have congestive failure in association with the sudden appearance of a pansystolic murmur, often accompanied by a thrill. Clinically, it is often impossible to differentiate this condition from a ruptured papillary muscle. The demonstration of a left-to-right shunt by cardiac catheterization or radionuclide angiography confirms the diagnosis. Rupture of the septum should be treated surgically, preferably six to eight weeks after infarction, so that the margins of the defect can have sufficient scar tissue to permit surgical closure with relative ease.

Abboud FM, et al.: Reflex control of the peripheral circulation. Prog Cardiovasc Dis 18:371, 1976; and Abboud FM, Thames MD: Interaction of cardiovascular reflexes in circulatory control. In Shepherd J, Abboud F (eds.): Handbook of Physiology. Bethesda, Md., American Physiological Society, 1984, pp 675–753. *These are reviews of factors that regulate peripheral vascular resistance (neural, humoral, local, and metabolic). The characteristic behavior of different vascular beds and various vascular segments is described. The role of cardiac sensory receptors, arterial baroreceptors, and chemoreceptors in the reflex control of the circulation is also described. Circulatory adjustments to various stressful conditions, including hypotension, acute myocardial infarction, and hypoxia, in animals and in humans are discussed.*

Berne R: The coronary circulation. In The Handbook of Physiology, Section 2: The Cardiovascular System. Bethesda, Md., American Physiological Society, 1979, pp 873–952. *This is a thorough review of the factors that regulate coronary blood flow, with emphasis on the potential metabolic determinants and interplay between local metabolic control and neurogenic control.*

Chaudry IH: Cellular mechanisms in shock and ischemia and their correction. Am J Physiol (Regulatory Integrative Comparative Physiology 14) 245:R117, 1983. *This is a review that deals specifically with cellular and subcellular alterations in shock. The potential mechanisms responsible for mitochondrial abnormalities, for alterations in cellular nucleotide levels, for the reduction in transmembrane potential, and for the increase in sodium-potassium ATPase activity are discussed. The depression of the reticuloendothelial system phagocytic activity and the release of lysosomal enzymes are also mentioned. The therapeutic attempts to restore cellular integrity by providing specific substrates are reviewed briefly, with emphasis on the proven effectiveness of ATP $MgCl_2$ as an adjunct therapy in restoring cellular function and improving survival rates in experimental shock.*

Goldberg LI: Dopamine—clinical uses of an endogenous catecholamine. N Engl J Med 291:707, 1974; and Goldberg LI, Rajfer SI: Dopamine receptors: Applications in clinical cardiology. Circulation 72:245, 1985. *These are reviews of the cardiovascular and renal actions of dopamine, of its hemodynamic effects in humans, and of its effectiveness in the treatment of shock. The action of dopamine is contrasted with that of other sympathomimetic amines. A regimen for its use in shock and its adverse effects are described.*

Goldfarb RD, Glenn TM: Regulation of lysosomal membrane stabilization via cyclic nucleotides and prostaglandins—the effects of steroid and indomethacin, pp 147–166. *The authors review data that suggest a significant change in the integrity of myocardial lysosomes during myocardial ischemia and propose that intramyocardial lysosome stability can be positively correlated with myocardial cyclic AMP/cyclic guanosine monophosphate (GMP) ratio. Furthermore, intramyocardial cyclic AMP concentration was negatively correlated with prostaglandin A and E concentrations. In that study, indomethacin treatment decreased myocardial prostaglandin A and E concentration approximately 60 per cent following coronary arterial ligation. One might conclude that myocardial infarction induces synthesis and release of prostaglandins, which, in turn, induce alterations in intramyocardial cyclic nucleotide ratio such that release of lysosomal enzymes is promoted. In a section of the monograph entitled* Therapeutics of Shock and Trauma *(pp 199–322), several authors review different approaches considered at the experimental stage. These include the use of dibutyryl cyclic AMP; a comparison of methylprednisolone and hydrocortisone in the treatment of shock patients (double-blind study suggesting that methylprednisolone may have a more beneficial effect); the use of calcium channel blockers in the treatment of shock, particularly after myocardial infarction, which may have a direct cellular effect that could be beneficial independently of changes in perfusion; the use of the antiproteolytic enzyme aprotinin in endotoxin shock, which preserves the phagocytic function of the reticuloendothelial system (aprotinin antagonizes serine endopeptidases and thus prevents the conversion of prekallikrein to kallikrein and consequently the conversion of kininogen to kinin) and protects the integrity of the capillaries and prevents aggregation of leukocytes in endotoxin shock.*

Lefer AM, Schumer W (eds.): Molecular and Cellular Aspects of Shock and Trauma. New York, Alan R. Liss Inc, 1983. *This volume represents the proceedings of a USA-Japan Binational Conference on this topic held in June, 1982. New concepts in cellular and metabolic aspects of shock and their therapeutic implications were reviewed. Following are brief comments on some of the article.*

Lefer AM: Pharmacologic and surgical modulation of myocardial depressant factor (MDF) formation and action during shock, pp 111–123. *This is a review of the chemical properties and the formation as well as the pathophysiology of MDF. There are no specific antagonists to MDF, and the author reviews the means of prevention of its formation and some of the pharmacologic approaches to counteracting its action.*

The Cell in Shock. Proceedings of a Symposium on Recent Research Developments and Current Clinical Practice in Shock. The Upjohn Company, April, 1976. *Several important concepts are reviewed. For example:* Baue AE: Mitochondrial function in shock, pp 11–15. *This article reviews Dr. Baue's research on the cellular events that may take place during shock and ischemia. A sequence of cellular membrane damage, mitochondrial dysfunction, and lysosomal breakdown is discussed.* Trump BF: The role of cellular membrane systems in shock, pp 16–19. *This is a detailed analysis of the sequential structural changes that occurs in cells in shock correlated with biochemical changes.* Goldstein IM: Lysosomes and their relation to the cell in shock, pp 30–34. *The potential role of lysosomal enzymes in cellular destruction in endotoxin shock is reviewed. The mechanisms of lysosomal enzyme release from human leukocytes, microtubule assembly, and membrane fusion induced by a component of complement are reviewed. A lysosomal releasing factor, or LRF, sharing many of the components of human C5a, appears to stimulate human polymorphonuclear leukocytes to release lysosomal enzymes selectively.* Müller-Eberhard HJ: The significance of complement activity in shock, pp 35–38. *This is a brief review of the complement system, its activation, and its role in the release of vasoactive peptide, which may contribute to the syndrome of shock.*

The Organ in Shock. Proceedings of the Second Symposium on Recent Research Developments and Current Clinical Practice in Shock. The Upjohn Company, April, 1977. *The following are brief comments on some of the articles:* Mela LM: Oxygen's role in health and shock, pp 8–15. *Dr. Mela reviews the membrane alterations induced by ischemic cell injury that are characteristically different in each organ, reflecting the particular organ's most delicately balanced plasma membrane functions. The author emphasizes that hypoxia alone does not induce inhibition in mitochondrial activity, whereas ischemia does.* Ayres, SM: The shock lung, pp 24–31. *The role of lymphatics, capillary permeability, and arteriovenous shunts in the pathogenesis of the shock lung syndrome is reviewed, and the structural and functional changes in the lungs are discussed.* Mueller HS: The heart and oxygen transport, pp 38–49. *This is a review of the treatment of coronary shock in patients with acute myocardial infarction. A careful survey of the hemodynamic changes and of survival in response to various catecholamines, and intra-aortic balloon counterpulsation, is described. Emphasis is placed on the early recognition and aggressive management of patients with incipient ventricular failure to improve survival rate. Caution regarding the use of vasodilators in patients who have low systolic blood pressure is expressed, and potential use of intra-aortic balloon counterpulsation coupled with an aggressive work-up and surgical approach to severe cardiogenic shock unresponsive to medical management is discussed.*

Werns SW, Shea MJ, Lucchesi BR: Free radicals and myocardial injury: Pharmacologic implications. Circulation 74:1, 1986. *The authors review the growing evidence that oxygen free radicals generated during ischemia and reperfusion may contribute significantly to myocardial depression and injury. The mechanisms for generation of these oxygen free radicals and their removal by therapeutic interventions are discussed. The potential clinical implications are important in view of the more aggressive management of acute myocardial infarction with thrombolytic therapy and the frequently noted post-reperfusion myocardial depression and arrhythmias.*

Ziegler EJ, McCutchan JA, Fierer J, et al.: Treatment of gram-negative bacteremia and shock with human antiserum to a mutant *Escherichia coli.* N Engl J Med 307:1225, 1982. *This is a randomized controlled trial of human J5 antiserum in patients with gram-negative bacteremia and shock. The antiserum was prepared by vaccinating healthy men with heat-killed* E. coli *J5 mutant, which lacks lipopolysaccharide-oligosaccharide side chains so that the core (which is nearly identical to that of most other gram-negative bacteria) is exposed for antibody formation. The antiserum reduced death substantially.*

45 CARDIAC ARRHYTHMIAS

J. Thomas Bigger, Jr.

Optimal management of cardiac arrhythmias requires knowledge of their (1) mechanism, etiology, and natural history and (2) effect on the hemodynamic state. Before selecting therapy, the physician should thoroughly assess the patient's physical, psychologic, and biochemical state. The chosen treatment, whether drugs, devices, or surgery, must be monitored closely for its initial and continued effectiveness and for adverse effects. In this chapter we will discuss mechanisms, electrocardiographic (ECG) recognition, and management of cardiac arrhythmias.

ANATOMIC CONSIDERATIONS

Normal Specialized Impulse-Generating and Conducting System

SINUS NODE. The sinus node is situated on the right anterolateral margin of the junction between the superior vena cava and the right atrium. The node surrounds a large central artery arising from the right (55 per cent) or left circumflex coronary artery (45 per cent). Two types of special muscle fibers are found in the node: P (pacemaker) and T (transitional) cells. P cells are small (diameter of 5 to 10 microns) ovoid or stellate cells that have a low density of mitochondria, sarcoplasmic reticulum, and myofibrils, suggesting a lack of contractile function. P cells occur in tight clusters and attach only to other P cells or T cells; intercellular attachments are sparse, correlating with the slow conduction found in the sinus node.

T cells are intermediate in size, structure, and cellular organization between P cells and ordinary atrial myocardium. T cells may attach either to P cells or to working myocardial cells. Perinodal T cells surround the sinus node and presumably serve both to organize impulses leaving the node and to hinder access of premature ectopic atrial impulses.

INTERNODAL TRACTS. Three internodal tracts connecting the sinus node to the atrioventricular (AV) node have been described: anterior, middle, and posterior. The *anterior internodal tract* also connects to the left atrium via the interatrial bundle of Bachmann. The three internodal tracts are widely separated in the interatrial septum but converge above and behind the AV node.

Internodal tracts contain working atrial cells interspersed with large cells that resemble ventricular Purkinje cells. Because internodal pathways are difficult to trace by serial microscopic sections, some doubt their presence or functional significance. Internodal tracts continue to function in high extracellular K^+ concentrations, a property that has been used to demonstrate their functional continuity and preferential internodal conductivity.

ATRIOVENTRICULAR NODE. The AV node lies beneath the endocardium of the right atrium near the septal leaflet of the tricuspid valve and immediately anterior to the ostium of the coronary sinus. The AV node artery usually arises from the right coronary artery. In the central portion of the AV node, the myocytes form tangled swirls with ample interconnections. Ultrastructurally, cells in the mid AV node resemble the sinus node T cells. Toward the distal end of the AV node, myocytes palisade into linear arrays as they form the bundle of His.

The region between the ostium of the coronary sinus and the posterior margin of the AV node is richly supplied by cholinergic ganglia. Retronodal chemoreceptors may trigger vagal reflexes during ischemia of the posterior wall of the heart. These reflexes can produce marked bradycardia, peripheral vasodilatation, nausea, sweating, and salivation.

THE HIS-PURKINJE SYSTEM. The AV bundle (bundle of His) is a thick, cable-like structure, about 15 mm in length, that emerges from the anterior, inferior border of the AV node (Fig. 45–1). The bundle of His penetrates the central fibrous body and courses to the crest of the muscular interventricular septum, where it divides into left and right bundle branches. The His bundle is the only normal route for AV conduction. Damage to the AV bundle can cause AV conduction delay or block. The His bundle is generously supplied with arterial blood from the anterior and posterior descending coronary arteries; therefore, extensive coronary disease is required to produce ischemic damage.

The left bundle branch is a broad sheet of fibers that cascade under the noncoronary cusp of the aortic valve and down the left side of the interventricular septum. The left bundle branch connects first with myocardium in the septum and near the papillary muscles, causing early activation of these regions.

The right bundle branch emerges from the bundle of His and courses down the right side of the interventricular septum to make its first connections with ventricular myocardium near the base of the anterior papillary muscle. From here, the peripheral branches of the right bundle spread up the interventricular septum and the free wall of the right ventricle.

The terminal Purkinje fibers form extensive interconnected lacy networks on the endocardial surface of both ventricles. In human hearts, no cells of the Purkinje type can be identified in the outer two thirds of the ventricular walls. Purkinje cells are large—15 to 30 mm in diameter and 20 to 100 mm in length. The nucleus is round and centrally located in the cell, and Purkinje fibers contain fewer myofibrils and mitochondria than working ventricular muscle. External to the sarcolemmal basement membrane is a thick surface coat of negatively charged glycoproteins that function in Ca^{++} binding and exchange. Intercalated discs are well developed in Purkinje fibers and provide low-resistance pathways for current flow and for diffusion of K^+.

Function of the Specialized Impulse-Generating and Conducting System

The normal heart beat begins in the sinus node and spreads slowly through the perinodal fibers to reach specialized atrial tracts and ordinary atrial muscle (Fig. 45–1). The specialized atrial tracts transmit the cardiac impulse rapidly from the sinus node to the AV node and to the left atrium. The cardiac impulse slows dramatically in the AV node, accounting for most of the PR interval in the ECG. Conduction accelerates tremendously in the His bundle, and excitation of the bundle branches and peripheral Purkinje fibers occurs with blazing speed. The great mass of ordinary ventricular muscle is activated almost simultaneously over much of its endocardial surface. Then, activation spreads from endocardium to epicardium to complete cardiac excitation.

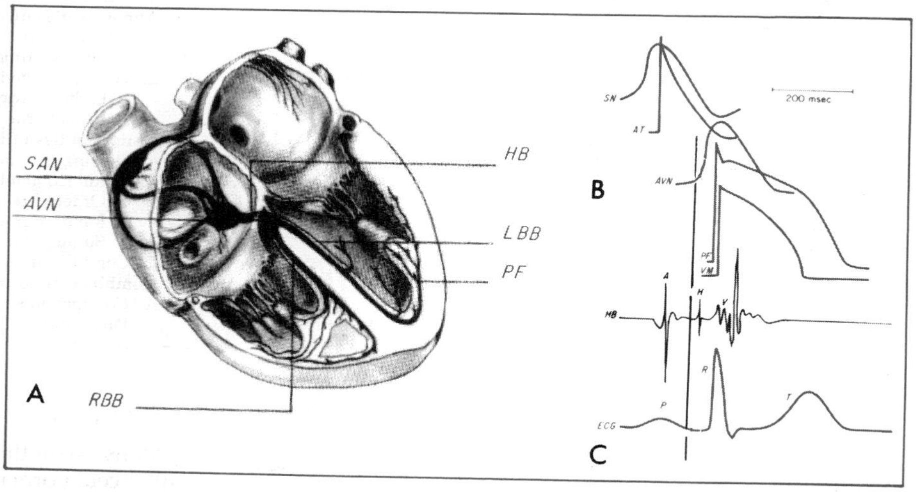

FIGURE 45–1. The anatomy and characteristic action potentials of the specialized impulse-generating and conducting system of the heart. *A*, A diagram of the conduction system of the heart. SAN = Sinoatrial node; AVN = atrioventricular node; HB = bundle of His; RBB = right bundle branch; LBB = left bundle branch; PF = Purkinje fiber. *B*, Typical action potentials from the sinus node (SN), atrium (AT), atrioventricular node (AVN), Purkinje fiber (PF), and ventricular muscle (VM). *C*, Relationship of deflections in the His bundle (HB) electrogram to depolarization of the sites shown in *B* and to the electrocardiographic deflections. Depolarization of the lower atrial septum (A), bundle of His (H), and ventricular septum (V) is recorded in the bipolar His bundle electrogram. The H deflection partitions the P-R interval into two subintervals: the A-H interval, representing atrioventricular nodal conduction, and the H-V interval, which measures conduction to the His-Purkinje system. (From Braunwald E.: Heart Disease: A Textbook of Cardiovascular Medicine. Philadelphia, W. B. Saunders Company, 1980.)

BRIEF REVIEW OF CARDIAC CELLULAR ELECTROPHYSIOLOGY

Resting Potentials

The sarcolemma of cardiac cells is a hydrophobic phospholipid bilayer. Protein molecules cross the entire width of the membrane, provide hydrophilic channels, and permit hydrated cations or anions to cross the sarcolemma. Ion-selective channels and energy-dependent ion pumping establish transmembrane gradients of Na^+ and K^+ that determine the resting voltage difference of about −80 to −90 mV across the sarcolemma, the *resting transmembrane voltage* (Vm).

Action Potentials

When cardiac cells activate, a complex sequence of voltage changes occurs as a function of time and membrane ionic currents. Figure 45–2 diagrams the four phases of a Purkinje fiber *action potential*. Sinus and AV nodal cells have a slowly rising phase 0 and lack distinct phases 1, 2, and 3 (Fig. 45–1). Many cells hold a steady level of transmembrane voltage during phase 4, whereas automatic fibers in the sinus node and His-Purkinje spontaneously depolarize during this period and can initiate impulses that propagate to the rest of the heart.

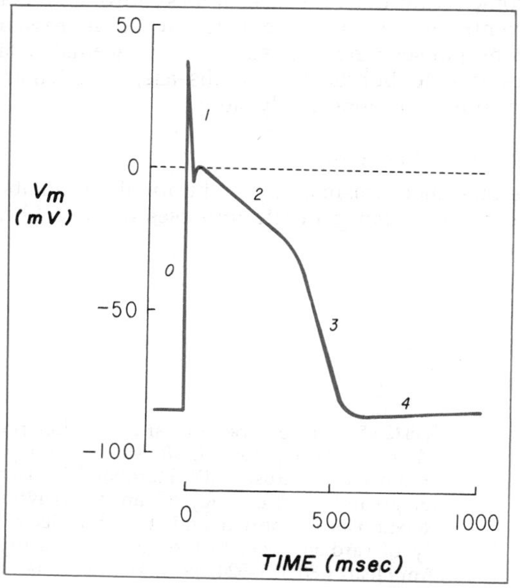

FIGURE 45–2. The cardiac action potential of a Purkinje fiber has five distinct phases: rapid depolarization (0), early repolarization (1), the plateau (2), rapid repolarization (3), and diastole (4). (From Braunwald E.: Heart Disease: A Textbook of Cardiovascular Medicine. Philadelphia, W. B. Saunders Company, 1980.)

The ionic basis for cardiac action potentials is still a subject of debate and active study.

Overdrive Suppression

In the normal heart, P cells in the sinus node depolarize and overdrive subsidiary pacemaker cells in the atrial specialized tracts, coronary sinus region, or His-Purkinje system. The faster subsidiary pacemakers are overdriven, the more Na^+ enters the cell per unit of time. As the $[Na]_i$ increases, the activity of the Na^+/K^+ exchange pump becomes more electrogenic, i.e., the ratio of the Na^+ out to K^+ in will increase, hyperpolarizing the cell and counteracting pacemaker activity. If the dominant pacemaker stops, there will be a pause in rhythm. However, as the $[Na]_i$ is pumped out, outward pump current will decline until spontaneous depolarization resumes. As the pump current declines, firing rate in the subsidiary pacemaker will increase gradually, producing the well-known "warmup" behavior.

Fast and Slow Responses

Cardiac action potentials are classified as *fast* or *slow* responses (see Table 45–1). The *fast response* (Fig. 45–3) is generated by intense inward [Na]; has a large, fast-rising phase 0; propagates rapidly; and has a large safety factor for conduction. Working myocardial cells in the atria, ventricles, and Purkinje fibers have fast responses. The *slow response* has a slowly rising phase 0, propagates slowly, and has a low safety factor for conduction (Fig. 45–3). Cells in the sinus node, pectinate muscles, AV node, and AV rings have slow responses. Depolarization in slow-response fibers is due to slow inward current (i_{si}) carried by Ca^{++} and, to a lesser extent, Na^+ ions.

Refractoriness

The concept of refractoriness is used to explain the pathogenesis of many arrhythmias and the mechanism of action of antiarrhythmic drugs. The effective refractory period, the minimum interval between two propagating responses, is

TABLE 45–1. COMPARISON OF SLOW AND FAST ACTION POTENTIALS

Electrophysiologic Characteristics	Slow Potential	Fast Potential
Resting potential	Low (−40 to −70mV)	High (−75 to −90mV)
Action potential amplitude	40 to 80 mV	90 to 120 mV
Phase 0 $\dot{V}$ max	1 to 10 V/sec	200 to 800 V/sec
Overshoot	0 to 15 mV	10 to 30 mV
Conduction velocity	0.01 to 0.1 meter/sec	0.5 to 3.0 meter/sec
Stimulus-dependent action potential amplitude	Yes	No
Threshold voltage	−50 to −30 mV	−75 to −65 mV
Depolarizing current carried by	Ca^{++} (Na^+)	Na^+
Ionic current activates	Slow (0.5 msec)	Fast (10 to 20 msec)
Ionic current inactivates	Slow (0.5 msec)	Fast (50 to 100 msec)
Channel blocked by	Mn^{++}, La^{+++}, verapamil, diltiazem, nifedipine	Tetrodotoxin, class 1 antiarrhythmics

closely linked to action potential duration in fast-response fibers because recovery from inactivation in the Na^+ channel closely parallels repolarization. However, in sinus and AV nodal cells (slow responses), refractoriness can outlast full repolarization so that the effective refractory period is much longer than the action potential duration.

Responsiveness and Conduction

The term *membrane responsiveness* describes the response of a cardiac fiber to a stimulus. Changes in the maximum rate of depolarization during phase 0 ($\dot{V}$max) provide an index of changes in availability of the Na^+ current. In cardiac Purkinje fibers and other fast-response fibers, $\dot{V}$max is strongly dependent on Vm at the instant of excitation; as soon as the fiber is fully repolarized, it is fully responsive. In slow-response fibers, responsiveness does not return until well after repolarization is complete. There is a considerable safety factor for conduction in fast-response fibers; $\dot{V}$max must be reduced to less than one half of normal before conduction velocity decreases. The safety factor is much lower in slow-response fibers so that premature impulses are likely to experience substantial conduction delay or block.

MECHANISMS OF CARDIAC ARRHYTHMIAS

An arrhythmia is an abnormality of rate, regularity, or site of origin of the cardiac impulse or a disturbance in conduction that causes an abnormal sequence of activation. Arrhythmias may arise because of alterations in impulse generation, impulse conduction, or both (Table 45–2).

TABLE 45–2. MECHANISMS RESPONSIBLE FOR CARDIAC ARRHYTHMIAS

I. Abnormalities of impulse generation
- A. Alterations of normal automaticity
- B. Abnormal automaticity
- C. Triggered activity
  1. Early afterdepolarizations
  2. Late afterdepolarizations

II. Abnormalities of impulse conduction
- A. Slowing of conduction and block
- B. Unidirectional block and re-entry
  1. Ordered re-entry
  2. Random re-entry
  3. Summation and inhibition
- C. Conduction block, electrotonus, and reflection

III. Combined abnormalities of impulse generation and conduction
- A. Conduction showed by phase 4 depolarization
- B. Parasystole

Arrhythmias Due to Abnormalities of Impulse Generation

Many arrhythmias arise because of either depressed or enhanced normal automaticity. Abnormal automaticity and triggered activity also are important mechanisms for arrhythmogenesis.

ALTERED NORMAL AUTOMATICITY. Only a few cardiac cell types develop normal automaticity: sinus node, internodal tracts, fibers near the ostium of the coronary sinus, distal AV node, and the His-Purkinje system.

Sinus Node. The rate of firing in the sinus node can be altered by autonomic activity or intrinsic disease. Increased vagal activity can slow or stop sinus node pacemakers by increasing membrane K^+ conductance of P cells. Increased sympathetic traffic to the sinus node causes sinus tachycardia.

Purkinje Fibers. Augmented automaticity due to increased sympathetic nerve activity in the His-Purkinje system is a common cause of human arrhythmias. Atrioventricular junctional pacemakers can fire faster than a normal sinus node because of selective traffic on sympathetic nerves, local release of catecholamines, or enhanced responsiveness of beta-adrenergic receptors. In addition, vagal and autonomic activity can increase together; the vagus slows sinus rate and AV conduction, whereas sympathetic traffic increases the firing rate in the His-Purkinje system.

In diseased hearts, automaticity in the His-Purkinje system may become reduced. In the sick sinus syndrome, it is typical for the ventricular escape pacemakers to be depressed, producing long pauses when the sinus node pacemaker fails. In AV block due to bundle branch disease, ventricular pacemakers also may be abnormally slow.

Abnormal Impulse Generation

Numerous mechanisms, e.g., abnormal automaticity or triggered activity, can generate impulses even in fibers that

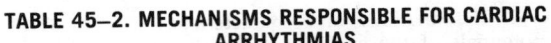

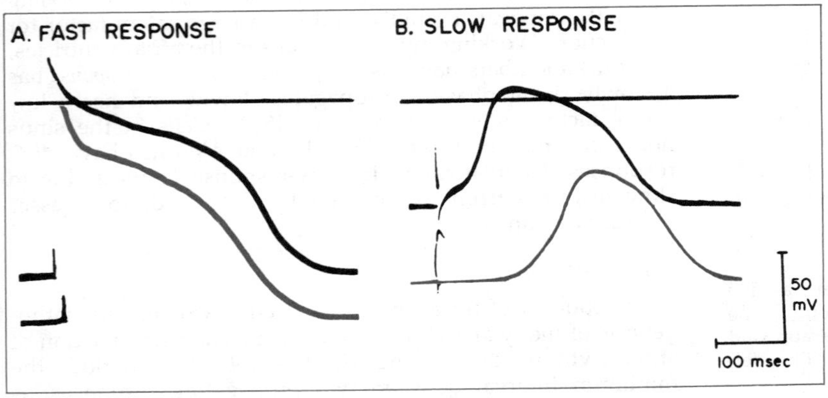

FIGURE 45–3. Two types of cardiac action potentials: (*A*) fast action potential, (*B*) slow action potential. (From Wit AL, Rosen MR, Hoffman BF: Electrophysiology and pharmacology of cardiac arrhythmias. II. Relationship of normal and abnormal electrical activity of cardiac fibers to the genesis of arrhythmias. Am Heart J 88:515–524, 1974. With permission of the publisher.)

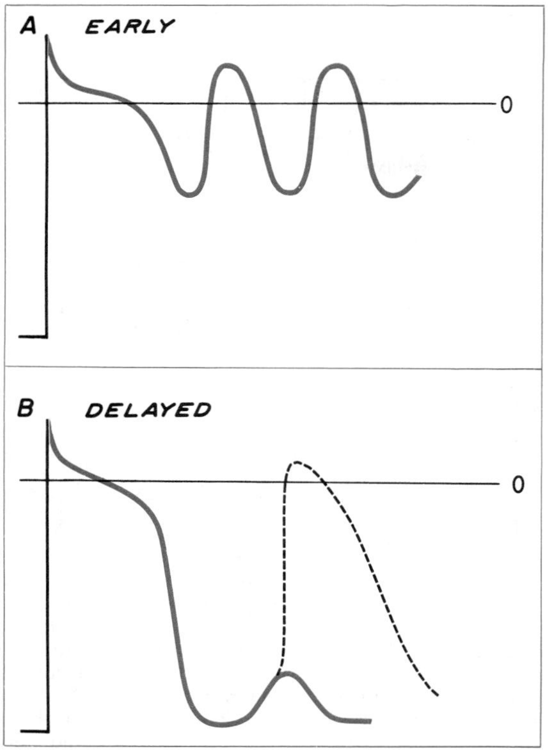

FIGURE 45–4. After-depolarizations and triggered activity. *A*, Early after-depolarization. Repolarization of the Purkinje fiber is interrupted by two secondary depolarizations, which can activate adjacent fibers and cause arrhythmias, e.g., torsades de pointes. *B*, Delayed after-depolarizations. After full repolarization, the Purkinje fiber depolarizes. If the after-depolarization reaches threshold voltage, a propagating response can occur. (From Bigger JT: Electrophysiology for the clinician. Euro Heart J 5(Suppl B):1–9, 1984.)

are incapable of normal automaticity, e.g., ordinary atrial or ventricular muscle cells.

ABNORMAL AUTOMATICITY. Abnormal automaticity refers to spontaneous diastolic depolarization in depolarized cells. Purkinje fibers, atrial cells, and ventricular cells can show spontaneous diastolic depolarization and repetitive automatic firing when their resting Vm is reduced to −60 mV or below. Abnormal automaticity is seen in Purkinje fibers depolarized by acute myocardial infarction. Abnormal automaticity and repetitive firing can be evoked in normal atrial or ventricular cells by applying depolarizing current. Abnormal automaticity is not readily suppressed by overdrive pacing.

TRIGGERED ACTIVITY. Repetitive firing in heart muscle can be caused by triggered activity. Triggered activity is *not* a form of automaticity but is capable of producing a sustained tachyarrhythmia. Two primary mechanisms can initiate triggered activity: early afterdepolarizations and delayed afterdepolarizations (Fig. 45–4).

Early Afterdepolarizations. Early afterdepolarizations are secondary depolarizations that occur before repolarization is complete, often from the action potential plateau (Fig. 45–4). Experimentally, early afterdepolarizations have been produced in cardiac Purkinje fibers by stretching or crushing, hypoxia, cooling, low $[K]_o$, high $[Ca]_o$, catecholamines, and chemicals and drugs (such as veratrine, aconitine, quinidine, sotalol, or *N*-acetylprocainamide). Torsades de pointes (see below) in humans is thought to be the counterpart of triggered activity due to early afterdepolarizations.

Delayed Afterdepolarizations. A delayed afterdepolarization is a secondary depolarization occurring after full repolarization has been achieved but is dependent on a prior action potential (Fig. 45–4). Delayed afterdepolarizations can reach threshold and cause a single premature depolarization or trigger a series of impulses. Delayed afterdepolarizations can be induced easily by digitalis in the His-Purkinje system and with more difficulty in specialized atrial or ordinary ventricular cells. Some of the digitalis-induced ventricular tachycardias in humans have characteristics that resemble triggered activity produced by digitalis in isolated tissue preparations. In the atria, coronary sinus, and mitral valve, delayed afterdepolarizations and triggered activity can be caused by catecholamines.

Arrhythmias Caused by Abnormalities of Impulse Conduction

Re-entry seems to be a common cause of cardiac arrhythmias in humans, particularly paroxysmal supraventricular tachycardia and constantly coupled ventricular premature depolarizations. Re-entrant arrhythmias usually are started by an initiating premature depolarization, i.e., are self-sustained but are not self-initiated. To start re-entry, one-way conduction block must occur and there must be an anatomic or functional "barrier" that forms a circuit (Fig. 45–5). In addition, the path length of the re-entrant circuit must be greater than the wavelength of the cardiac impulse (wavelength = conduction velocity × refractory period). For re-entry to occur, conduction must be very slow, refractoriness very short, or both. Re-entry has been demonstrated in anatomic loops (e.g., rings of Purkinje fibers) and around anatomic obstacles (e.g., scars). Re-entry occurring in unbranched bundles or sheets of cardiac muscle has been given specialized names, e.g., reflection or leading circle re-entry.

Re-entry can be subdivided into random and ordered forms. In random re-entry, the cardiac impulse conducts over circuits that change their location and size as a function of time, e.g., atrial and ventricular fibrillation. In ordered re-entry, the circuit for re-entrant activity is relatively constant.

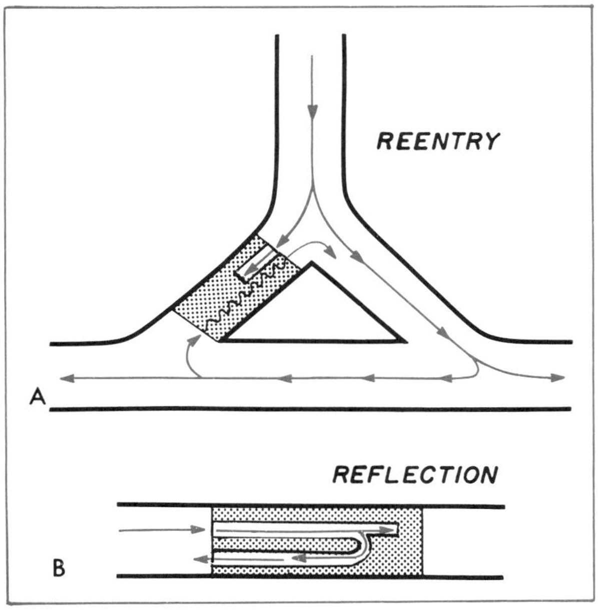

FIGURE 45–5. Two models of re-entry according to Schmitt and Erlanger. *A*, Diagram showing a loop of cardiac fibers that could represent either a terminal branch of a Purkinje fiber ending on ventricular muscle or a loop of the Purkinje syncytium. In this case, one-way block and slow conduction permit re-entry. *B*, A linear strand of cardiac muscle showing a depolarized zone in a portion of its cross section. One-way block occurs in the depolarized zone, permitting the propagating impulse to reflect back in the direction from which it came. (From Braunwald E.: Heart Disease: A Textbook of Cardiovascular Medicine. Philadelphia, W. B. Saunders Company, 1980.)

LEADING EDGE RE-ENTRY. Re-entrant excitation can be initiated in vitro by premature stimulation in small, thin pieces of normal atrium that contain no anatomic obstacles of loops of tissue. Conduction is slowed because activation occurs when the tissue is partially refractory. Block occurs in some regions because of local differences in refractory periods. The pathway for re-entrant activity can stabilize and be sustained.

Cranefield PF: The Conduction of the Cardiac Impulse. Mount Kisco, NY, Futura Publishing Company, 1975. *A monograph that reviews the concepts of fast and slow action potentials and their role in the genesis of re-entrant cardiac arrhythmias.*

Fozzard HA, Haber E, Jennings RB, et al. (eds.): The Heart and Cardiovascular System: Scientific Foundations. New York, Raven Press, 1986. *The section on cardiac electrophysiology and arrhythmias contains detailed reviews of current knowledge and thought on the electrophysiology of the heart, the genesis of cardiac arrhythmias, and the epidemiology of human arrhythmias. Other sections contain excellent reviews of the embryology, anatomy, and pathology of the heart. Profusely illustrated and exhaustively referenced.*

Hackel DB: Anatomy and pathology of the cardiac conducting system. In Edwards JE, Lev M, Abell MA (eds.): The Heart. Baltimore, Williams & Wilkins Company, 1974, pp 232–247. *A concise description of the normal anatomy and pathology of the conduction system.*

Noble D: The Initiation of the Heartbeat. London, Oxford University Press, 1979. *An account of cardiac electrophysiology for medical students and clinicians who are unfamiliar with electronics and mathematics. The most difficult concepts of cardiac excitation are explained clearly and concisely. Selective references to the classic papers on electrophysiology.*

DIAGNOSTIC APPROACHES TO CARDIAC ARRHYTHMIAS

The history, physical examination, 12-lead electrocardiogram, 24-hour continuous electrocardiographic recordings, exercise tests, intermittent electrocardiographic recorders, and clinical electrophysiologic studies are the primary tools used in the diagnosis of cardiac arrhythmias. Decisions about treatment may require other laboratory studies to define better the etiology of heart disease, other aspects of the functional status of the heart, e.g., left ventricular function or perfusion, or function of other organ systems.

History and Physical Examination

The primary purposes of the history are (1) to formulate a hypothesis about the presence and type of arrhythmia; (2) to detect factors that trigger the onset of the arrhythmia or intensify arrhythmic symptoms; (3) to establish the frequency and pattern of occurrence of the arrhythmia; and (4) to establish the functional consequences of the arrhythmia.

The physical examination provides information about the presence and type of heart disease and the degree of functional impairment caused by heart disease. The physical examination in conjunction with the ECG can aid in the differential diagnosis of arrhythmias. A regular tachycardia, 150 per minute, with a wide QRS complex is compatible with many arrhythmias and the physical examination during tachycardia can provide the key to the diagnosis.

Electrocardiography

The ECG is the most important test to obtain for arrhythmia diagnosis. A long, continuous recording of a lead with clear-cut P waves should be made. Usually, a systematic analysis of the rhythm strip with the aid of calipers permits a definitive diagnosis. The rate and the regularity of PP and RR intervals, the constancy of the PR interval, and the ratio of atrial to ventricular complexes should be noted. Even when every P wave and QRS complex is identified, the ECG pattern may be compatible with more than one diagnosis. Ladder diagrams are helpful for displaying the possibilities in an unequivocal manner (Fig. 45–6).

Carotid Sinus Pressure

Taking ECG rhythm strips during carotid sinus pressure is a valuable bedside maneuver for diagnosis of cardiac arrhythmias. Carotid massage activates a reflex arc that increases the

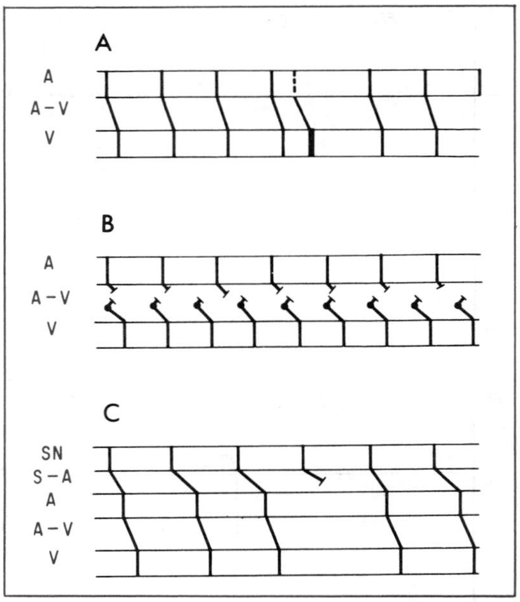

FIGURE 45–6. Ladder diagrams of cardiac rhythm. A = Atrium; A-V = atrioventricular junction (the A-V node and His-Purkinje system); V = ventricle; SN = sinus node; S-A = sinoatrial junction. *A*, Sinus rhythm with atrial premature depolarization (APD). Atrioventricular conduction of the APD is slower than for sinus impulses because the atrioventricular node is partially refractory. The broad line in the ventricular tier indicates aberrant ventricular conduction of the APD, which occurs because the premature impulse arrives during the relative refractory period of the His-Purkinje system. *B*, Atrioventricular junctional rhythm. The A-V junctional automatic rhythm captures the ventricles but shows retrograde block. The sinus node controls the atria, but the sinus impulse finds the A-V node refractory and is blocked; i.e., there is interference between the sinus and junctional rhythm. *C*, Type I (Wenckebach) sinoatrial block. The sinus impulse travels through the perinodal junctional tissues with increasing delay until block finally occurs. (From Braunwald E.: Heart Disease: A Textbook of Cardiovascular Medicine. Philadelphia, W. B. Saunders Company, 1980.)

vagal traffic to the heart. The most important use of carotid sinus pressure is to aid in the analysis of rapid, regular tachycardia when P waves are not clearly apparent. The responses of various arrhythmias to carotid sinus massage are listed in Table 45–3.

Carotid sinus pressure carries significant risks, particularly in older patients, i.e., syncope, convulsions, stroke, prolonged asystole, or ventricular tachyarrhythmias. In patients with digitalis toxicity, carotid sinus pressure may provoke malignant ventricular arrhythmias.

Special Procedures to Detect Atrial Activation

All of the P waves must be identified to make rhythm analysis reliable. P waves can be detected using special lead placement, e.g., the Lewis lead, esophageal electrograms, or transvenous bipolar catheter electrodes.

Ambulatory Electrocardiographic Recording

In 1961, Holter described the technique of ambulatory ECG recording. A light, portable tape recorder makes continuous 24-hour ECG recordings while the patient performs his or her usual daily activities and records activities and symptoms in a diary. The primary uses of ambulatory ECG recordings in individual patients are listed in Table 45–4.

INTERMITTENT RECORDERS. When symptoms occur only occasionally, intermittent recorders permit monitoring lasting from a few days to many weeks, even though the ECG recordings are brief (seconds to minutes). The recorders may be attached to the patients continuously or intermittently.

TABLE 45–3. EFFECT OF CAROTID SINUS PRESSURE ON TACHYARRHYTHMIAS

Arrhythmia	Response to Carotid Sinus Pressure
Sinus tachycardia	1. Gradual slowing during massage, gradual speeding after massage
Paroxysmal supraventricular tachycardia (AV nodal)	1. No effect or 2. Abrupt conversion to sinus rhythm or 3. Slight slowing
Paroxysmal supraventricular tachycardia (anomalous AV connection)	1. No effect or 2. Abrupt conversion to sinus rhythm or 3. Slight slowing
Nonparoxysmal supraventricular tachycardia	1. No effect or 2. Atrioventricular block, slowed ventricular rate or 3. Gradual slowing of ventricular rate (rare)
Atrial flutter	1. Atrioventricular block, slowed ventricular rate or 2. No effect or 3. Atrial fibrillation
Atrial fibrillation	1. Atrioventricular block, slowed ventricular rate or 2. No effect
Ventricular tachycardia	1. No effect or 2. Atrioventricular dissociation

AV = atrioventricular.

Hard-Wired Recorders. Intermittent recorders of the "hard-wired" type are continuously attached to the patient by electrodes and cables. Patients activate these recorders by pressing a switch. Some units have 40 to 100 seconds of electronic memory and sample the ECG continuously, replacing old data with new. When activated, 30 to 60 seconds of ECG prior to patient activation are recorded. Data are retrieved from "hard-wired" systems either by direct playback or by telephonic transmission.

Intermittently Attached Recorders and Telephonic Transmission. These devices are typically about the size and shape of a radiopaging unit. The patient applies ECG leads when symptoms occur. Units with memory can store one to three ECG samples for subsequent telephone transmission. Commercial services provide immediate evaluation of the ECG transmission. Transmissions are acted on in accordance with the instructions of the patient's physician.

TABLE 45–4. INDICATIONS FOR LONG-TERM CONTINUOUS ECG RECORDINGS

I. Detect and quantify arrhythmias or conduction defects in patients with symptoms (e.g., syncope or other central nervous system symptoms, palpitations, or angina pectoris)

II. Quantification of arrhythmias, conduction defects, or ischemia in patients with predisposing conditions
- A. Sick sinus syndrome
- B. Pre-excitation syndromes
- C. AV conduction defects
- D. Pacemaker malfunction
- E. Mitral valve prolapse
- F. Long QT syndrome
- G. Post myocardial infarction
- H. Angina pectoris
- I. Hypertrophic or dilated cardiomyopathy
- J. Heart failure

III. Evaluate activity
- A. For potential to cause arrhythmias or conduction defects
- B. To evaluate ischemia during activity

IV. Evaluate therapy
- A. Antiarrhythmic drug treatment
- B. Fad diets
- C. Drugs with adverse cardiac effects
- D. Pacemakers
- E. Automatic implantable cardioverter defibrillator
- F. Surgery
  1. Ischemia or arrhythmias after coronary artery bypass graft surgery
  2. Pre-excitation after division of anomalous AV connection
  3. AV conduction after surgical division or catheter ablation of the His bundle

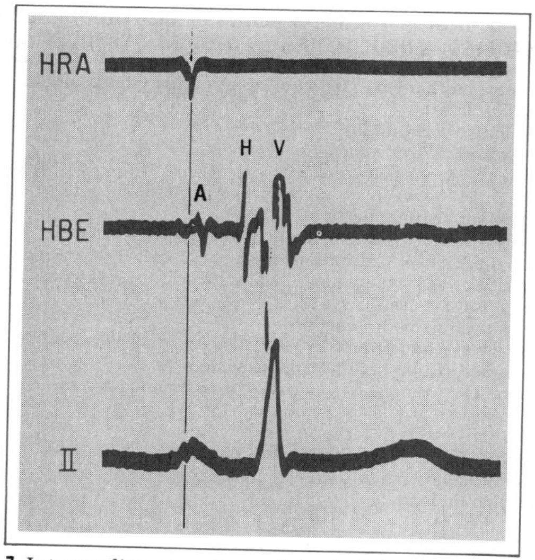

FIGURE 45–7. Intracardiac recordings. A high right atrial bipolar electrogram (HRA), His bundle bipolar electrogram (HBE), and tracing from lead II of the electrocardiogram. A = Atrial depolarization; H = depolarization of the His bundle; V = depolarization of the upper ventricular septum. The P-A interval represents intra-atrial conduction time (upper to lower atrium); A-H represents atrioventricular nodal conduction; and H-V represents the His-Purkinje conduction time. The thin vertical line correlates the onset of atrial activation in the three recordings. (From Braunwald E.: Heart Disease: A Textbook of Cardiovascular Medicine. Philadelphia, W. B. Saunders Company, 1980.)

Intracardiac Recording and Stimulation (Endocardial Electrical Stimulation)

Over the past 20 years, intracardiac recording and stimulation have developed as a diagnostic and therapeutic tool for the management of human cardiac arrhythmias. Local electrical activity can be recorded from the portions of the heart that are electrically silent on the body surface ECG, e.g., sinus node, His bundle, right bundle branch, left bundle branch, and selected sites in the right or left ventricle. The sequence and time of activation of atria and ventricles can be mapped and AV conduction can be partitioned into AV nodal and His-Purkinje components (see Fig. 45–7). Recordings from selected sites are used with pacing and programmed stimulation sequences to evaluate automaticity, conduction, refractoriness, and the causes of arrhythmias in intact humans. These techniques not only have enhanced our understanding of arrhythmias and conduction defects but also have improved our ability to select and evaluate therapy. Some of the major clinical uses of electrophysiologic studies are listed in Table 45–5.

Bigger JT Jr, Reiffel JA, Coromilas J: Ambulatory electrocardiography. In Platia EV (ed.): Nonpharmacologic Management of Cardiac Arrhythmias. Philadelphia, J. B. Lippincott Company, 1986, pp 36–61. *A comprehensive review of the technology, indications, and clinical uses of ambulatory electrocardiography. Liberally illustrated and referenced.*

Horowitz LN, Josephson ME, Kastor JA: Intracardiac electrophysiologic studies as a method for the optimization of drug therapy in chronic ventricular arrhythmias. Prog Cardiovasc Dis 23:81, 1980. *Gives the details of electrophysiologic methods for evaluating drug therapy of malignant ventricular arrhythmias.*

Josephson ME, Seides SF: Clinical Cardiac Electrophysiology: Techniques and Interpretations. Philadelphia, Lea & Febiger, 1979. *A detailed description of the techniques of clinical electrophysiology and the interpretation of the findings. Intended for the internist and clinical cardiologist without an extensive background in cardiac electrophysiology.*

Morganroth J: Ambulatory Holter electrocardiography: Choice of technologies and clinical uses. Ann Intern Med 102:73, 1985. *A concise review of the current status of ambulatory electrocardiography.*

TABLE 45–5. INDICATIONS FOR CLINICAL ELECTROPHYSIOLOGICAL STUDIES—ENDOCARDIAL ELECTRICAL STIMULATION

I. To evaluate mechanism, site, and extent of arrhythmia and/or conduction defect
- A. Sick sinus syndrome
- B. Pre-excitation syndrome
- C. Supraventricular tachycardia
- D. Distinguish between supraventricular arrhythmias with aberration and ventricular arrhythmia
- E. Type I AV block with bundle branch block
- F. Type II AV block with normal QRS
- G. Bifascicular block occurring in acute myocardial infarction

II. To search for a cause for syncope
- A. Evaluate sinus node function
- B. Evaluate AV node function
- C. Evaluate function of His-Purkinje system
- D. Evaluate functional characteristics of anomalous AV connections
- E. Provoke arrhythmias
  1. Supraventricular tachycardia
  2. Atrial flutter or fibrillation
  3. Ventricular tachycardia

III. To evaluate therapy
- A. Drug therapy
  1. Prevent inducible arrhythmias
  2. Measure conduction and refractoriness in anomalous AV connections
  3. Evaluate adverse effects
     a. Sinus node function
     b. AV node function
     c. His-Purkinje system
     d. Effect on device function
- B. Surgical therapy
  1. Preoperative endocardial catheter mapping
     a. Location of anomalous AV connections
     b. Location of VT circuit
     c. Need for concomitant pacemaker implantation
  2. Postoperative evaluation
     a. Presence of anomalous AV connections
     b. Arrhythmia inducible
- C. AICD therapy
  1. Preoperative evaluation
     a. Determine that VT or VF is inducible
     b. Determine that VT or VF is drug resistant
     c. Determine need for concomitant pacemaker implantation
  2. Intraoperative evaluation
     a. Determine quality of right or left ventricular sensing electrograms
     b. Determine quality of patch electrograms for the probability density function
     c. Determine defibrillation thresholds
     d. Induce clinical arrhythmia to test sensing and termination of ventricular arrhythmias by the AICD
  3. Postoperative evaluation
     a. Induce VT or VF to test the performance of the AICD
     b. Acquaint the patient with the symptoms during AICD discharge
- D. Pacemaker therapy
  1. Evaluate condition for suitability for pacemaker therapy
     a. Supraventricular tachycardia—reciprocation in the AV node
     b. Supraventricular tachycardia—reciprocation in anomalous AV connections
  2. Determine the information needed to select pacemaker type and parameters

IV. To apply ablation therapy
- A. Posterior septal anomalous AV connections
- B. AV node
- C. Ventricular tachycardia

AICD = automatic implantable cardioverter defibrillator; VT = ventricular tachycardia; VF = ventricular fibrillation.

SPECIFIC CARDIAC ARRHYTHMIAS

Clinically, cardiac arrhythmias are classified by their presumed site of origin, i.e., atrial, AV junctional, or ventricular, and as premature complexes, bradycardia, or tachycardia. It would be desirable to use the precise mechanism to classify cardiac arrhythmias, but this is impossible because we do not know the precise mechanism of many arrhythmias. For some arrhythmias, e.g., the ventricular arrhythmias, prognostic significance can be assigned with reasonable precision. When this is the case, a prognostic classification is useful for guiding decisions about management. In this section, we will use a classification based on the site of origin and rate as the framework in which to discuss the definition, pathophysiology, electrocardiographic diagnosis, significance, and management of each arrhythmia. The emergency and chronic treatments of cardiac arrhythmias are outlined in Tables 45–6 and 45–7.

ATRIAL ARRHYTHMIAS

Sinus Rhythm

ECG DIAGNOSIS. Sinus rhythm is recognized in the ECG by a normal atrial rate and P wave vector, i.e., an upright P wave in leads III and aV_F. The PR interval is normal in classic sinus rhythm. In adults, sinus rates below 60 or 50 per minute are called sinus bradycardia and those above 100 per minute, sinus tachycardia. Heart rate changes synchronized with breathing are called sinus arrhythmia and are caused by changes in autonomic nervous activity. Sinus arrhythmia is more pronounced in children and young adults than the elderly. Marked sinus arrhythmia can be difficult to distinguish from sinoatrial block or ectopic atrial rhythms.

CLINICAL FEATURES. Resting heart rate in sinus rhythm varies with age: from 130 to 160 per minute in infants to 50 to 100 per minute in adults. Sex, temperature, emotion, effort, and neurohumoral factors also influence sinus rate. The maximum heart rate during exercise varies from almost 200 per minute in healthy young persons to less than 140 per minute in the elderly. Many drugs increase or decrease the sinus rate, usually by interacting with autonomic mechanisms.

MANAGEMENT. Sinus bradycardia is treated only when symptomatic. When acute and symptomatic sinus bradycardia is due to increased vagus nerve activity, heart rate can be increased by intravenous (IV) atropine injection. Rarely, IV isoproterenol infusion may be needed. Chronic symptomatic sinus bradycardia is an indication for an electronic pacemaker. Treatment of sinus tachycardia is based on the cause, usually non-cardiac.

Atrial Premature Depolarizations

Atrial premature depolarizations (APD's) arise in the atria outside the sinus node. Atrial premature depolarizations occur in normal and diseased hearts. In heart disease, APD's herald sustained arrhythmias such as atrial flutter, atrial fibrillation, or paroxysmal supraventricular tachycardia.

ECG DIAGNOSIS. Atrial premature depolarizations typically have premature P waves, abnormal P wave morphology, and a prolonged PR interval. Early APD's can be difficult to see because the P wave is superimposed on the T wave. In addition, APD's can block the AV node discharge to produce pauses that can be misinterpreted as a sinus pause or sinoatrial block. Usually, APD's reset the sinus node so that the sum of the pre- and post-extrasystolic PP intervals is less than two sinus cycles (see Fig. 45–8). If sinus reset does not occur because the APD occurs late or the perinodal refractory period is long, a compensatory pause will occur. An APD can conduct aberrantly, causing the QRS complex to be wide and bizarre like a ventricular premature depolarization (see Fig. 45–9). Aberrant conduction occurs when APD's activate one of the bundle branches, usually the right, during its relative refractory period. Left bundle branch block aberrancy implies an abnormality in the left bundle branch (see Fig. 45–9).

MANAGEMENT. The objectives of treating APD's are to control symptoms or prevent sustained symptomatic arrhythmias. In patients with normal hearts, treatment should be focused on general hygienic measures; rest and reducing the use of tobacco, alcohol, or caffeine often reduce the frequency of APD's. In some patients with intermittent, sustained atrial arrhythmias, APD's should be treated with digitalis or class I, II, or IV antiarrhythmic drugs to prevent sustained arrhythmias.

TABLE 45–6. EMERGENCY TREATMENT OF CARDIAC ARRHYTHMIAS

Arrhythmia	Usual First Treatment	Other Effective Treatments	Comments
Atrial fibrillation	Digitalis	Cardioversion; propranolol; acebutolol; verapamil	If hypotensive due to rapid ventricular rate, cardiovert. Avoid propranolol or verapamil in patients with heart failure or hypotension. Avoid digitalis or verapamil in Wolff-Parkinson-White syndrome.
Atrial flutter	Cardioversion	Digitalis; verapamil; propranolol; acebutolol; rapid atrial pacing	Very large doses of digitalis, e.g., 4–6 mg, often are required to achieve AV block in atrial flutter.
Paroxysmal supraventricular tachycardia (AV nodal)	Vagal maneuvers; verapamil	Digitalis; propranolol; acebutolol; procainamide	Do not treat wide QRS complex tachycardia with verapamil unless the diagnosis of PSVT is certain. Use cardioversion for PSVT with hypotension.
Paroxysmal supraventricular tachycardia (anomalous AV connection)	Vagal maneuvers; verapamil	Cardioversion	If the RP interval suggests anomalous AV connection, an electrophysiologic study should be considered.
Sick sinus syndrome	Pacemaker	Digitalis; pacemaker plus class I antiarrhythmic drug	Digitalis usually improves atrial tachyarrhythmias without aggravating sinus bradycardia or AV block.
Nonparoxysmal AV junctional tachycardia	Stop digitalis	Potassium; observation	If the arrhythmia is caused by digitalis toxicity and serum K^+ is low, digitalis should be stopped and potassium should be given.
Sustained ventricular tachycardia	Cardioversion	Lidocaine; procainamide	If ventricular tachycardia is well tolerated, intravenous lidocaine or procainamide can be tried.
Ventricular fibrillation	Cardioversion		Lidocaine or bretylium tosylate or propranolol may be helpful when ventricular fibrillation recurs several times immediately after cardioversion.
Digitalis toxic atrial tachycardia with block or ventricular tachycardia	Lidocaine; phenytoin	Potassium	Avoid cardioversion or bretylium tosylate, which may precipitate ventricular fibrillation.
Digitalis toxic asystole or AV block	Pacemaker	Fab fragments of digoxin-specific antibodies; dialysis	If associated with malignant hyperkalemia, these rhythms are always fatal unless treated promptly with Fab fragments of digoxin-specific antibodies.

PSVT = paroxysmal supraventricular tachycardia.

TABLE 45–7. CHRONIC TREATMENT OF CARDIAC ARRHYTHMIAS

Arrhythmia	Usual First Treatment	Other Effective Treatments	Comments
Atrial fibrillation	Digitalis	Class I antiarrhythmic drug and digitalis; digitalis and propranolol; digitalis and verapamil	Class I antiarrhythmic drugs are used to maintain sinus rhythm; propranolol, acebutolol, or verapamil is used as an adjunct to control ventricular rate in atrial fibrillation
Atrial flutter	Class I antiarrhythmic drug	Digitalis; propranolol; verapamil	—
Paroxysmal supraventricular tachycardia (AV nodal)	Digitalis	Class IC antiarrhythmic drug; propranolol	—
Paroxysmal supraventricular tachycardia (anomalous AV connection)	Class IC antiarrhythmic drug	Class IA antiarrhythmic drug	Surgical ablation is preferable if patient also has atrial fibrillation with rapid ventricular response, if the anomalous AV connection has a short refractory period, or if the patient is noncompliant or has adverse effects from drugs.
Sick sinus syndrome	Pacemaker	Pacemaker and digitalis; pacemaker and class I antiarrhythmic drug	With the arrhythmias effectively treated, prognosis is determined by the severity of associated heart disease
High-grade AV block	Pacemaker		No drugs are needed.
Symptomatic ventricular premature depolarizations	Class I antiarrhythmic drug	Beta blocker	For benign and potentially malignant ventricular arrhythmias, class IC drugs are the most effective and usually have the lowest incidence of adverse effects. When heart failure is present, disopyramide and flecainide are relatively contraindicated.
Symptomatic unsustained ventricular tachycardia	Class I antiarrhythmic drug	Beta blocker	Class IC drugs are the most effective and usually have the lowest incidence of adverse effects. When heart failure is present, disopyramide and flecainide are relatively contraindicated.
Sustained ventricular tachycardia	Class I antiarrhythmic drug	Class III antiarrhythmic drug	Treatment must be guided by a method with proven high predictive accuracy, e.g., endocardial electrical stimulation. A common sequence of drugs is class IA → class IA + class IB → class IC → class III. If drugs fail or cannot be evaluated, an implantable cardioverter defibrillator usually is the best treatment. In selected cases, surgical excision of the arrhythmogenic tissue is the best choice.

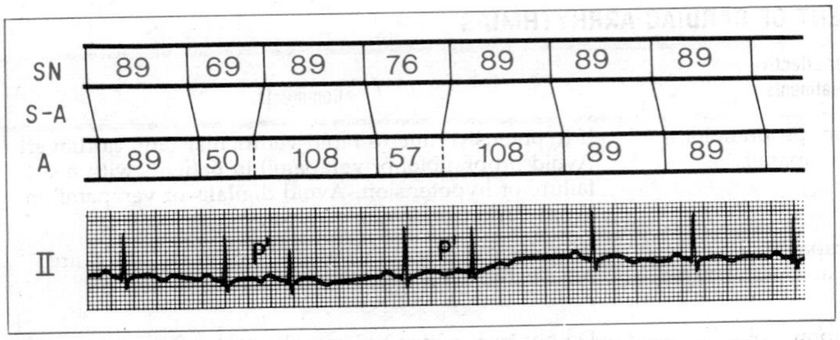

FIGURE 45–8. Atrial premature depolarization (APD). The ladder diagram correlates with the events in the lead II electrocardiographic strip below. SN = Sinus node; S-A = junctional tissues between sinus node and atrium; A = atrium. The time intervals in the ladder diagram are given in msec × 10^{-1} (e.g., 89 represents 890 msec). The third and fifth P waves are APD's (P′). These P′ waves are premature and inverted. The P′-R interval is prolonged, and QRS duration is normal. The APD's capture the sinus node and reset it; therefore, the pause following APD's is less than compensatory. (From Braunwald E.: Heart Disease: A Textbook of Cardiovascular Medicine. Philadelphia, W. B. Saunders Company, 1980.)

Paroxysmal Supraventricular Tachycardia

ECG DIAGNOSIS. Typically, paroxysmal supraventricular tachycardia (PSVT), also known as paroxysmal atrial or nodal tachycardia and reciprocating AV nodal tachycardia, has the following electrocardiographic features: a regular, rapid rate of 150 to 230 per minute; QRS complex duration less than 100 msec; and an abnormal P wave in a fixed relationship to each QRS. The P wave often is superimposed on the T wave or the QRS complex. Paroxysmal supraventricular tachycardia starts abruptly, usually started by an atrial or ventricular premature depolarization. Often, the atrial rate in PSVT will be about 180 per minute. The rate of PSVT is often faster in infants and children, in the Wolff-Parkinson-White (WPW) syndrome, and in thyrotoxicosis. The rate of PSVT is likely to be slower when AV node disease or certain drugs are present. The RR intervals in typical PSVT are extremely regular except for the first or last few cycles of an episode. Carotid sinus massage either has no effect on PSVT or terminates it. In the presence of AV nodal disease or drugs that depress nodal conduction, e.g., digitalis or verapamil, fixed 2:1 AV block or AV Wenckebach can occur during PSVT.

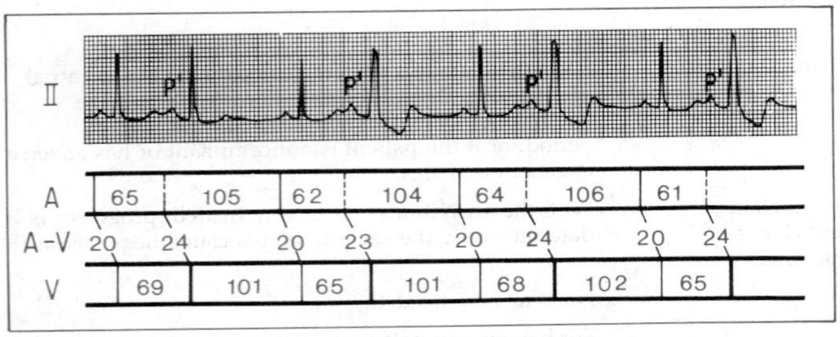

FIGURE 45–9. Atrial premature depolarizations (APD's) with aberrant conduction. The ladder diagram depicts the events in the lead II electrocardiographic strip above. A = Atrium; A-V = atrioventricular node and His-Purkinje system; V = ventricle. Time intervals are in msec × 10^{-1} (65 represents 650 msec). APD's are represented by dashed lines in the atrial tier; the wide QRS complexes are represented by a wide bar in the ventricular tier. APD's occur in a bigeminal pattern. The even (ectopic) P waves (P′) are premature and have configurations slightly different from the odd P waves. Although the P-P′ interval is relatively long (>600 msec), the P′-R interval is also prolonged, and the QRS complex following each P′ is aberrant (left bundle branch block configuration)—a pattern of aberration suggesting bundle branch disease. Note that the QRS complex after the longest P-P′ interval (second QRS) is least aberrant. (From Braunwald E.: Heart Disease: A Textbook of Cardiovascular Medicine. Philadelphia, W. B. Saunders Company, 1980.)

The QRS complexes may be wide owing either to a pre-existing wide QRS or to aberrant conduction of the rapid atrial rhythm, resembling ventricular tachycardia. If atrioventricular dissociation can be documented, the rhythm originates in the subatrial location and is not PSVT. His bundle electrography can differentiate between PSVT and ventricular tachycardia (Fig. 45–10).

The mechanism of PSVT is often AV nodal re-entry initiated by an APD. In the WPW syndrome, the PSVT is re-entrant, using the anomalous AV connection in the retrograde direction and the AV node in the antegrade direction (see Fig. 45–11).

Nonparoxysmal atrial tachycardia probably is due to ectopic automaticity or triggered activity in the atrium. Atrial tachycardia with AV block suggests digitalis toxicity, particularly if the atrial rate is slow.

CLINICAL FEATURES. PSVT occurs in normal as well as diseased hearts. Attacks of PSVT begin abruptly, cause palpitations, and may also end abruptly after a period of time. The patient may learn maneuvers that are likely to stop the tachycardia, e.g., cough, Valsalva's maneuver, or facial immersion. The hemodynamic effects of PSVT vary tremendously and depend on rate and underlying mechanical reserve of the heart. When the rate of PSVT is rapid, e.g., 180 to 220 per minute, systemic arterial pressure usually falls and diastolic filling pressures rise in both ventricles, even in persons without heart disease. Prolonged and rapid supraventricular tachycardia is likely to cause marked salt and water retention.

MANAGEMENT. Either vagal maneuvers (e.g., Valsalva's maneuver or carotid sinus massage) or verapamil is effective in about 90 per cent of the episodes. When PSVT causes hypotension or heart failure, DC cardioversion should be used. For prevention of recurrences of PSVT due to AV nodal re-entry, digitalis usually is tried first. If digitalis fails, potent class I antiarrhythmic drugs (see below, Specific Antiarrhythmic Drugs, and Tables 45–9 to 45–11) are quite effective. Surgical interruption (see Table 45–16) of the anomalous AV conduction pathway may be preferred to drugs in the WPW syndrome with recurrent symptomatic tachyarrhythmias.

Atrial Flutter

ECG DIAGNOSIS. Typically, atrial flutter has the following electrocardiographic features: a rapid atrial rate, 250 to 350 per minute; a narrow QRS complex; and a ventricular rate of about 150 per minute, i.e., 2:1 AV conduction ratio (see Fig. 45–12). In atrial flutter, the baseline of the ECG has a characteristic sawtooth or undulating appearance best seen in leads II, III, and aV_F. An AV conduction ratio greater than 2:1 suggests AV node disease or drug effect. Rarely, atrial flutter will conduct to the ventricles with a 1:1 ratio, resulting in a ventricular rate of about 300 per minute and hemodynamic collapse. The QRS complex usually is normal during atrial flutter but may be wide owing to pre-existing bundle branch block.

CLINICAL FEATURES. Atrial flutter usually signifies either intrinsic heart disease or adverse extrinsic influences on the heart. Atrial flutter is associated with scarred atria due to rheumatic heart disease, coronary heart disease, or primary myocardial disease. In addition, atrial flutter is associated with atrial enlargement, e.g., in interatrial septal defect, mitral or tricuspid stenosis or regurgitation, or chronic ventricular failure. Atrial flutter occurs in toxic or metabolic conditions that affect the heart, e.g., thyrotoxicosis, alcoholism, or beriberi, or when the pericardium is inflamed or infiltrated, e.g., with pneumonia or bronchogenic carcinoma. In all these conditions, atrial flutter is much less common than atrial fibrillation. Atrial flutter tends to be unstable, either reverting to sinus rhythm or converting to atrial fibrillation. Probably because the atria contract vigorously in atrial flutter, systemic emboli are less common than during atrial fibrillation.

MANAGEMENT. The best choice for the acute treatment

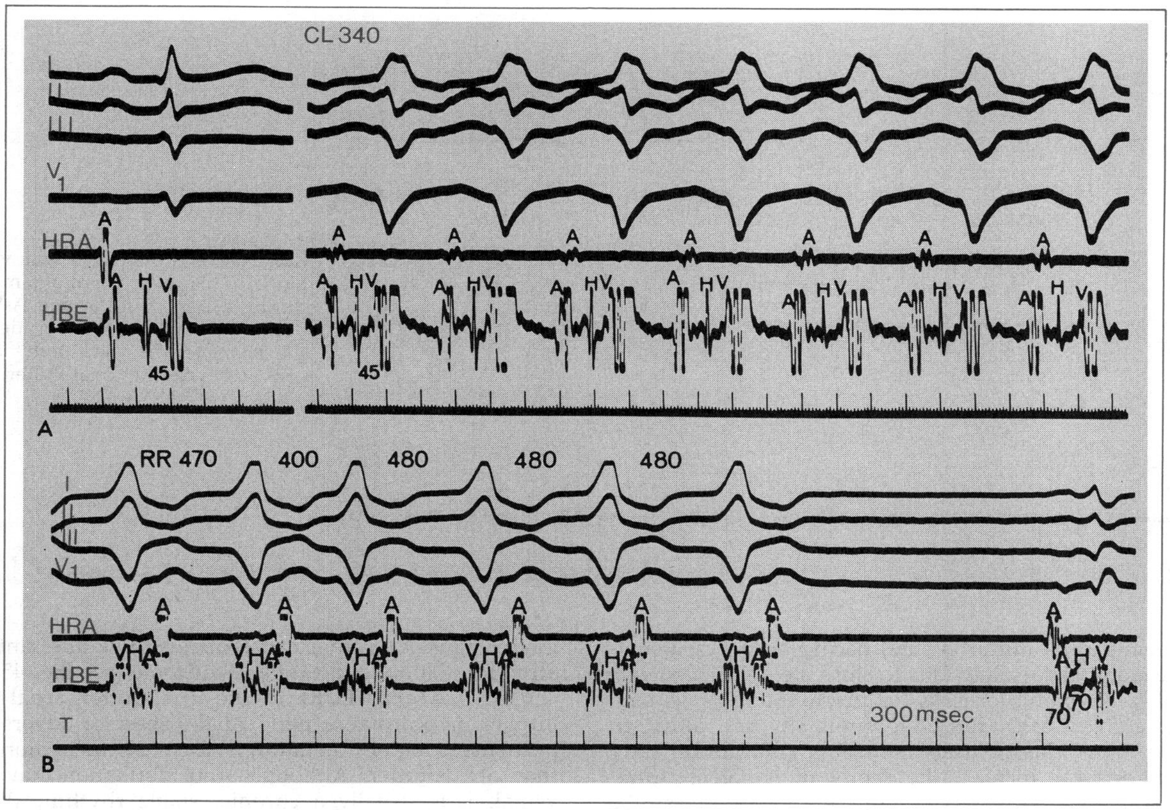

FIGURE 45–10. His bundle recording in regular tachycardia with a wide QRS complex. *A*, Supraventricular tachycardia. The left panel is a record taken during sinus rhythm; the QRS is normal. The right panel is a record taken during tachycardia; a left bundle branch block pattern is present. The normal H-V interval in the His bundle electrogram (HBE) indicates that the rhythm is supraventricular tachycardia with aberrant conduction. *B*, Ventricular tachycardia. The last six depolarizations of a tachycardia and the first of sinus rhythm are shown. A left bundle branch block pattern is present during the tachycardia. In the His bundle electrogram, the ventricles depolarize (V) before the bundle of His (H), indicating that the rhythm is ventricular tachycardia. Ventriculoatrial conduction shows a stable 1:1 pattern. (From Caracta AR, Damato AN: Significance of His bundle electrocardiography. In Fowler NO (ed.): Cardiac Diagnosis and Treatment. 2nd ed. New York, Harper and Row, 1976, pp 979–1008.)

FIGURE 45–11. Mechanism of supraventricular tachycardia utilizing an accessory pathway. The upper panel demonstrates an electrocardiogram recorded in a patient with Wolff-Parkinson-White syndrome during straight atrial pacing and the introduction of a premature atrial beat. The first five beats are preceded by a stimulus artifact (S); a short P-R interval and a wide QRS complex indicate the presence of pre-excitation. Following the introduction of a premature beat, a narrow QRS tachycardia is initiated. The events underlying this supraventricular tachycardia are diagrammatically shown in the lower panels. During sinus rhythm (A), fusion is present owing to conduction over the A-V node (AVN) and the accessory pathway (AP). In B, an atrial premature depolarization blocks the accessory pathway and conducts with delay over the A-V node, thus dissociating the activity of the normal and accessory pathways. In C, the impulse conducting through the ventricle travels retrograde over the accessory pathway and re-enters the atrium, establishing a tachycardia. D demonstrates schematically the re-entry circuit underlying supraventricular tachycardia resulting from re-entry confined to the A-V node.

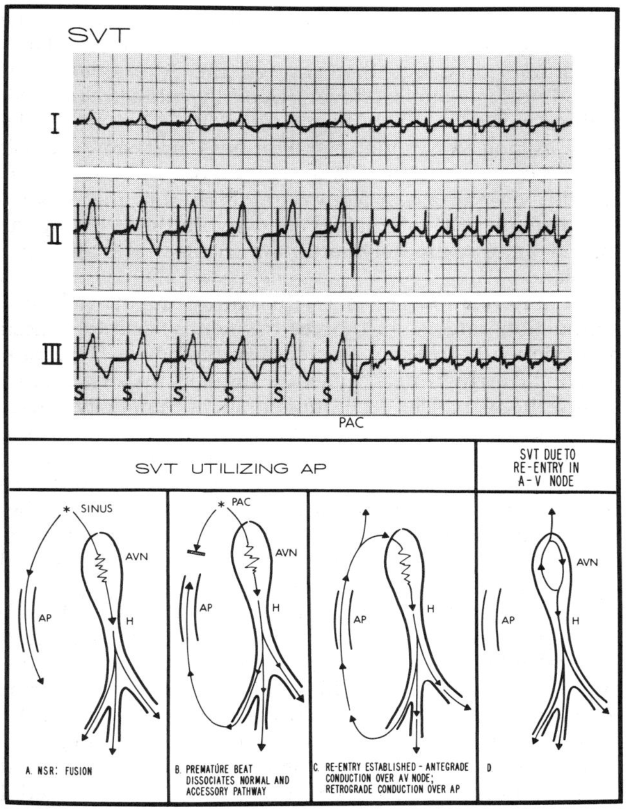

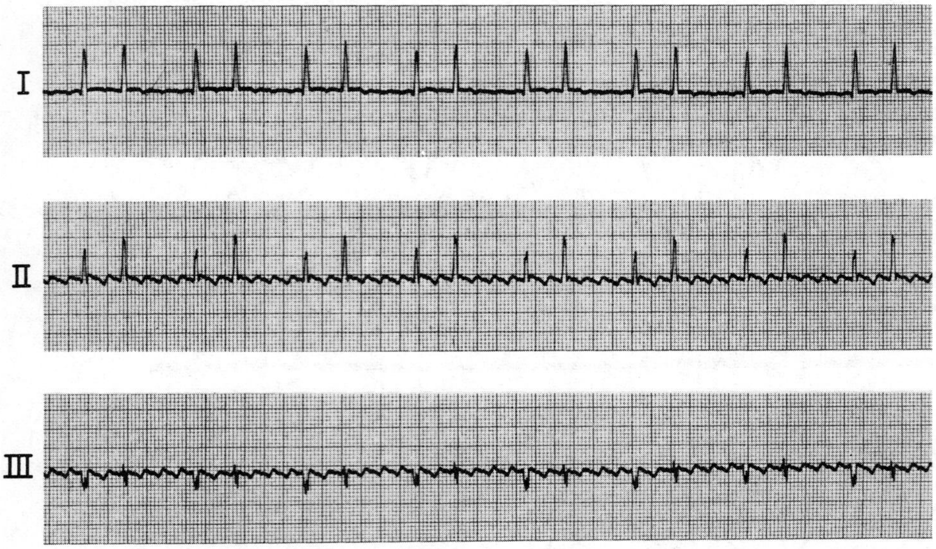

FIGURE 45–12. Atrial flutter with varying A-V block. This electrocardiogram, recorded during a period of varying A-V block induced by a vagal maneuver, demonstrates the characteristic "sawtooth" appearance of P waves during atrial flutter.

of symptomatic atrial flutter is atrial pacing or DC cardioversion because digitalis usually fails to slow the ventricular rate and digitalis, verapamil, or class I antiarrhythmic drugs usually fail to convert atrial flutter to sinus rhythm, although quinidine or other class I drugs may slow atrial flutter rates dramatically and can increase the degree of AV block. Intravenously administered verapamil or beta blockers can be useful temporizing measures to control heart rate while arrangements are made for DC cardioversion. A class I antiarrhythmic drug with or without digitalis is the usual treatment to prevent recurrence of atrial flutter.

Atrial Fibrillation

ECG DIAGNOSIS. Atrial fibrillation has the following features: absence of P waves; irregular atrial activity at a rate of 350 to 600 per minute; and rapid, irregularly irregular ventricular depolarization (150 to 200 per minute). The cardinal feature is the presence of fibrillatory waves best seen in ECG leads II, III, aV_F, or V_1 and at slow ventricular rates. Conditions or drugs that shorten the AV nodal refractory period, e.g., exercise, fever, hyperthyroidism, or catecholamines will increase the ventricular rate. Conversely, factors that prolong AV nodal refractoriness will slow ventricular rate. Because atrial fibrillation is so common, this diagnosis should be entertained for any rapid rhythm that has irregularly irregular RR intervals. Patients with the WPW syndrome may develop extremely rapid ventricular rates during atrial fibrillation.

Atrial fibrillation coexists with many other arrhythmias and conduction defects. Two occur frequently, and their management depends critically on a correct diagnosis. The first is AV junctional arrhythmias caused by digitalis toxicity. As digitalis slows the ventricle, AV junctional automaticity increases. First, junctional escape complexes will terminate long RR intervals, or the ventricular rate will become regular at a slow rate. Then, the junctional focus accelerates to produce nonparoxysmal AV junctional tachycardia. The second is aberrant conduction of supraventricular impulses that must be distinguished from ventricular premature depolarizations (VPD's). The duration of refractoriness in the His-Purkinje system is directly proportional to the preceding RR interval. In atrial fibrillation, aberrant conduction is likely when a short RR interval follows a long one, the Ashman phenomenon (see Fig. 45–13). Aberrant conduction usually produces a triphasic (RSR') right bundle branch block configuration in lead V_1 and normal initial forces. Ventricular premature depolarizations usually have a mono- or biphasic QRS pattern in lead V_1, have abnormal initial QRS forces, and are followed by a longer pause. Another cause of repetitive aberrant QRS's in atrial fibrillation is the WPW syndrome (see Fig. 45–14).

CLINICAL FEATURES. Like atrial flutter, atrial fibrillation implies myocardial or pericardial disease or adverse extrinsic influences. Atrial fibrillation is about 20 times more common than atrial flutter. Although atrial fibrillation may be paroxysmal, it is usually a chronic, stable rhythm. When atrial fibrillation occurs abruptly in patients with serious heart disease, the consequences may be dramatic, e.g., disconcerting palpitations, pulmonary edema, or angina pectoris. If the ventricular rate is well controlled with digitalis, atrial fibrillation may cause little hemodynamic impairment and is compatible with decades of uneventful survival. As with atrial flutter, atrial fibrillation occurs in many etiologic forms of heart disease. Chronic atrial inflammation and lack of effective atrial contraction promote left atrial thrombi and increased risk for systemic emboli. Atrial fibrillation may occur as an isolated arrhythmia in patients without heart disease or any other systemic illness. This condition has been called "lone atrial fibrillation."

MANAGEMENT. The objective of treating acute atrial fibrillation is to slow the rate. For symptomatic hypotension, immediate cardioversion is indicated. Usually, rate is controlled with IV digoxin (see Table 45–11). Verapamil or beta-blocking drugs are useful adjuncts for achieving rate control but can aggravate heart failure or cause hypotension. Digitalis and verapamil are best avoided in patients with the WPW syndrome because they can increase the ventricular rate and trigger ventricular fibrillation.

Multifocal Atrial Tachycardia

ECG DIAGNOSIS. The ECG features of multifocal atrial tachycardia are frequent APD's, often occurring in runs that

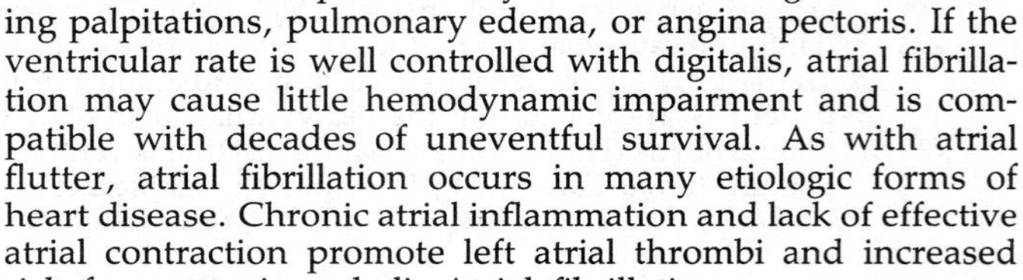

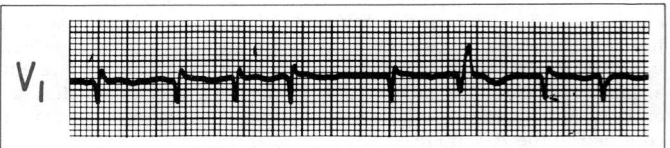

FIGURE 45–13. Aberrant conduction in atrial fibrillation (the Ashman phenomenon). The sixth QRS complex has a right bundle branch appearance. Note that this complex ends a long R-R–short R-R sequence and that its initial forces are similar to those of the other QRS complexes. These features suggest aberrant conduction of a superventricular impulse. (From Braunwald E.: Heart Disease: A Textbook of Cardiovascular Medicine. Philadelphia, W. B. Saunders Company, 1980.)

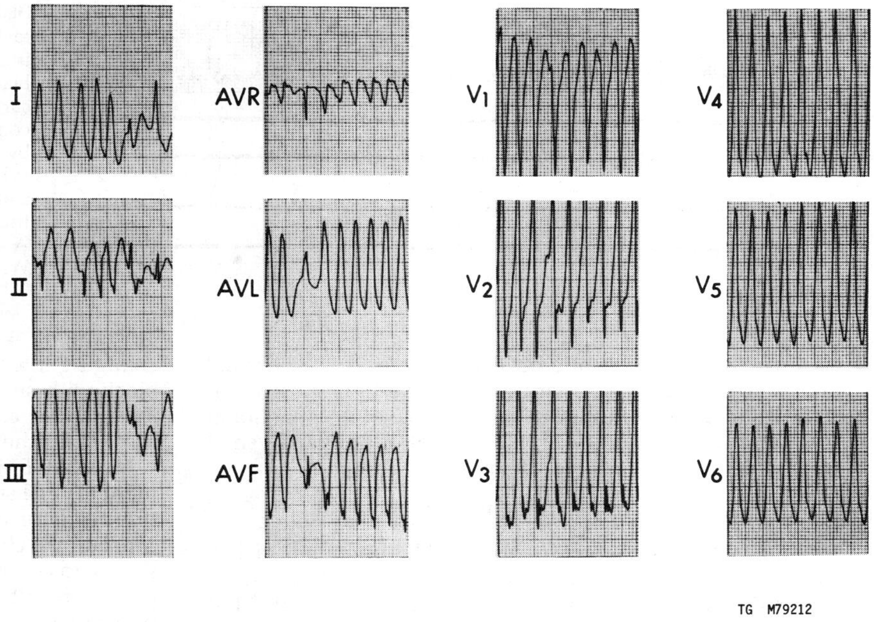

FIGURE 45–14. Atrial fibrillation in the Wolff-Parkinson-White syndrome. The electrocardiogram demonstrates the irregularly irregular response associated with anomalous-appearing QRS complexes resulting from atrial fibrillation with rapid conduction over the accessory pathway to the ventricle.

have dramatically different P wave morphology and marked variability in PP interval.

CLINICAL FEATURES. This rhythm occurs in patients with decompensated or overtreated chronic obstructive pulmonary disease. These patients often have severe derangement of arterial blood gases and electrolytes and are being treated aggressively with theophylline or catecholamines or both.

MANAGEMENT. Multifocal atrial tachycardia is resistant to digitalis therapy. Therapy is directed at improving ventilation and eradicating infection to improve arterial blood gases. The dose of bronchodilators may need to be reduced as well. Verapamil can be used to control the arrhythmia while the other medications are adjusted.

Sinoatrial Block

ECG DIAGNOSIS. Impulses generated in the sinus node may conduct slowly or block in the junction between the sinus node and atrium. First-degree sinoatrial (SA) block, i.e., a delay in conduction from sinus node to the atrium, cannot be recognized in the standard ECG but can be identified by electrophysiologic studies. Second-degree SA block can be diagnosed electrocardiographically. Type I second-degree SA block is recognized by Wenckebach periodicity of the PP intervals (see Fig. 45–15). In type II second-degree SA block, the PP interval suddenly lengthens to a value almost precisely twice that of the usual PP interval. Third-degree SA block causes atrial arrest.

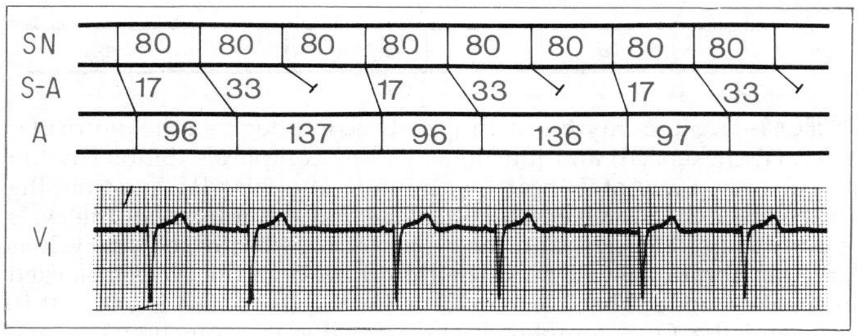

FIGURE 45–15. Second-degree sinoatrial block, type I (Wenckebach). The ECG shows periodicity of the P waves and QRS complex. The PR is constant. This pattern is consistent with a constant sinus node rate of 75 per minute (sinus cycle length = 800 msec) with 3:2 sinoatrial shock. The sinoatrial conduction times are assumed. (From Braunwald E.: Heart Disease: A Textbook of Cardiovascular Medicine. Philadelphia, W. B. Saunders Company, 1980.)

CLINICAL FEATURES. Sinoatrial block indicates intrinsic sinus node disease, electrolyte disturbance, or an adverse drug effect, most often digitalis. Class I antiarrhythmic drugs also cause SA block in patients with pre-existing sinus node dysfunction.

Sick Sinus Syndrome. The sick sinus syndrome is characterized by intrinsic inadequacy of sinus node pacemaking or conduction failure between the sinus node and the rest of the atrium, or both. In the bradycardia-tachycardia syndrome, recurrent supraventricular tachyarrhythmias alternate with sinus bradycardia or subatrial bradyarrhythmias or both. Conduction disturbances are common in the atria, AV node, bundle branches, and ventricles, but ventricular ectopic activity is rare.

Symptoms in sick sinus syndrome may be intermittent, varied, and difficult to correlate with ECG changes. Syncope, dizziness, and palpitations are common, probably because these symptoms are used for case finding and diagnosis. Congestive heart failure or angina can be aggravated. Cerebral thromboembolism is common in the bradycardia-tachycardia syndrome. Treatment of atrial fibrillation in the sick sinus syndrome can cause severe bradycardia. A temporary ventricular pacemaker should be used when attempting to convert atrial fibrillation with slow ventricular rate.

MANAGEMENT. Persistent, symptomatic sinus bradycardia is an indication for pacemaker therapy. Digitalis can be used to control the atrial tachyarrhythmias and, contrary to expectation, usually does not aggravate coexistent bradyarrhythmias. After pacemaker implantation, class I antiarrhythmic drugs can be used to control tachyarrhythmias. Symptoms can be improved with pacemaker therapy in the bradycardia-tachycardia syndrome, but cerebral thromboembolism continues. The prognosis of effectively treated sick sinus syndrome is determined by the associated heart disease.

ATRIOVENTRICULAR JUNCTIONAL ARRHYTHMIAS

Atrioventricular Junctional Premature Depolarizations

ECG DIAGNOSIS. Atrioventricular junctional premature depolarizations are much less common than either atrial or ventricular premature depolarizations. Typical ECG features are an abnormally premature or absent P wave and a premature QRS complex with a normal configuration. The position of the premature P wave (P′) is critical to the diagnosis.

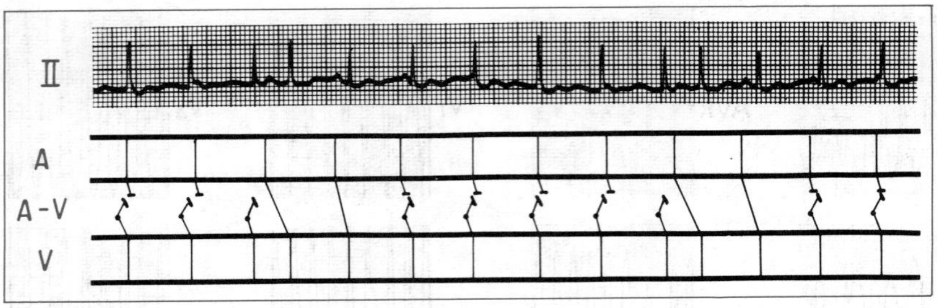

FIGURE 45–16. Nonparoxysmal atrioventricular junctional tachycardia with atrial capture of the ventricles. Two independent rhythms coexist: sinus tachycardia at 107 beats per minute and atrioventricular junctional tachycardia at 115 beats per minute. Sinus rhythm always controls the atria. The ventricles are usually controlled by the A-V junctional focus, because its rate is faster. When time relationships are appropriate, atrial depolarizations propagate through the A-V junction and capture the ventricles. (From Braunwald E.: Heart Disease: A Textbook of Cardiovascular Medicine. Philadelphia, W. B. Saunders Company, 1980.)

The P′ may occur 0.10 second or less before or during or 0.20 second or less after the premature QRS. The P′ is inverted in leads II, III, and aV_F. The clinical significance of AV junctional premature depolarizations is similar to that of nonparoxysmal AV junctional tachycardia (see below).

Nonparoxysmal Atrioventricular Junctional Tachycardia

ECG DIAGNOSIS. Nonparoxysmal AV junctional tachycardia is caused by enhanced automaticity in the AV junction. The junctional focus depolarizes at a rate between 70 and 130 per minute (see Fig. 45–16). The QRS complex usually is normal or slightly aberrant. If the AV junctional focus captures the atria, the retrograde P may be positioned 0.10 second or less in front of the QRS, simultaneous with the QRS, or 0.20 second or less after the QRS. This arrhythmia often is associated with AV nodal conduction impairment and AV dissociation. The atrial rhythm may intermittently capture the junctional focus and ventricle (see Fig. 45–16).

CLINICAL FEATURES. Nonparoxysmal AV junctional tachycardia has great significance because it is associated specifically with acute inferior myocardial infarction, digitalis toxicity, acute carditis (e.g., viral myocarditis or acute rheumatic fever), or surgical trauma.

MANAGEMENT. Treatment should be focused on the underlying condition, e.g., myocarditis or digitalis toxicity. In acute inferior myocardial infarction, and after open heart surgery, nonparoxysmal AV junctional tachycardia is usually transient and requires no therapy. In digitalis toxicity, this arrhythmia should prompt intensive management of toxicity.

Atrioventricular Block

ECG DIAGNOSIS. Atrioventricular block is classified as first, second, and third degree. First-degree AV block, i.e., a prolonged PR interval, is caused by conduction delay in the AV node. Second-degree AV block is subdivided into type I (AV nodal) and type II (His-Purkinje). Type I second-degree AV block has characteristic Wenckebach periodicity, i.e., the PR interval prolongs with each cycle until a P wave fails to conduct to the ventricles (see Fig. 45–17). The longest RR interval is less than twice the shortest RR interval. Type II second-degree AV block is recognized by the sudden failure of a P wave to conduct to the ventricles without previous lengthening of the PR interval. Type II AV block nearly always occurs in patients with bundle branch disease, and the site of block is distal to the AV node.

In third-degree AV block, sinus or some other atrial rhythm controls the atria, whereas the ventricles are controlled by an independent AV junctional or ventricular pacemaker. The QRS usually is prolonged, and the ventricular rate is between 35 and 50 per minute.

CLINICAL FEATURES. First-degree AV block produces no symptoms but may cause the first heart sound to be soft because the AV valves almost close before ventricular contraction. Second-degree AV block usually causes no symptoms unless the ventricular rate becomes very slow. It may be possible to discern second-degree AV block by characteristic pulse intervals, intermittent, prominent "A" waves, and changing intensity of the first heart sound. In complete heart block with sinus rhythm, the pulse is slow, full, and regular; intermittent cannon "A" waves occur in the jugular venous pulse; and the first heart sound varies in intensity.

MANAGEMENT. First-degree AV block requires no treatment. Type I second-degree AV block usually resolves without the need for a temporary pacemaker. When type I block is caused by a chronic AV junctional disease, block can progress slowly to complete AV block. Type II second-degree AV block usually results from chronic bundle branch disease and often progresses to complete heart block. Chronic, symptomatic second- or third-degree AV block should be treated with an implanted pacemaker.

VENTRICULAR ARRHYTHMIAS

Ventricular Premature Depolarizations (VPD's)

ECG DIAGNOSIS. The QRS is premature, wide, and often bizarre in appearance; the ST segment and T wave are opposite in direction to the QRS complex; and no premature P wave precedes the premature QRS complex (see Fig. 45–18). As the impulse leaves its ectopic site of origin, it activates the ventricle in an abnormal sequence, accounting for the striking QRS-T changes. Typically, the VPD is followed by a fully compensatory pause, i.e., the RV interval, and the VR interval is equal to two RR intervals in sinus rhythm (see Fig. 45–18). Ventricular premature depolarizations may be *interpolated* between two successive sinus complexes. "Concealed" retrograde conduction of the interpolated VPD into the AV node causes the PR interval of the subsequent sinus complex to prolong. Certain patterns of VPD's have special names. When every other QRS is a VPD, the pattern is termed *bigeminy;* a

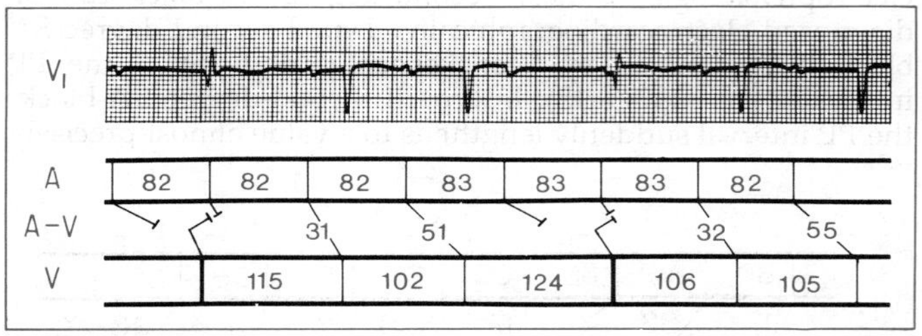

FIGURE 45–17. Sinus rhythm with type I second-degree atrioventricular block (Wenckebach) and junctional escape complexes. Sinus rhythm is regular at a rate of 73 beats per minute. The third P wave from the left begins a 3:2 Wenckebach cycle. The first P-R interval of the cycle is quite long (0.31 sec), and the P-R increment in the second cycle is large (an additional 0.20 sec). The third P wave of the cycle is blocked in the A-V node. The P-R interval following the pause is short (0.10 sec), and the QRS complex is aberrant; this is a junctional escape complex. The tracing demonstrates both impaired conduction and enhanced automaticity in the A-V junction. Type I A-V block nearly always occurs in the A-V node, and A-V junctional escape complexes are presumed to arise in the bundle of His or the most proximal portions of the bundle branches. (From Braunwald E.: Heart Disease: A Textbook of Cardiovascular Medicine. Philadelphia, W. B. Saunders Company, 1980.)

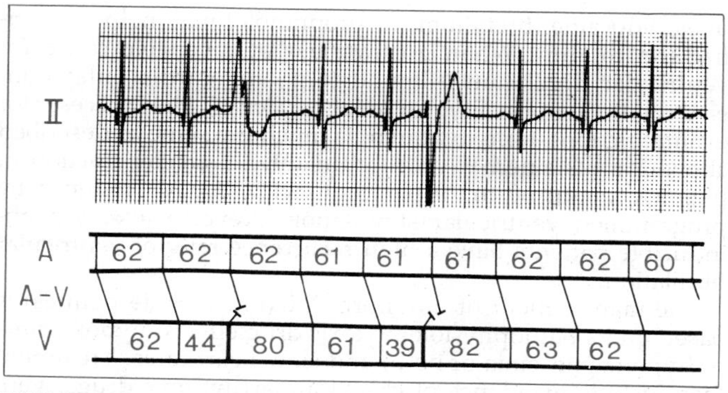

FIGURE 45–18. Multiformed ventricular premature depolarizations. The third and sixth QRS complexes are VPD's with strikingly different configurations. Also, the coupling interval of the two VPD's differs by 50 msec. Such a difference in configuration may be due either to a different site of origin or to a difference in the sequence of ventricular activation from the same site of origin. (From Braunwald E.: Heart Disease: A Textbook of Cardiovascular Medicine. Philadelphia, W. B. Saunders Company, 1980.)

VPD every third QRS is termed *trigeminy*; and two successive VPD's are termed a *pair* or a *couplet*.

CLINICAL FEATURES. Infrequent VPD's are commonly found even in young persons, and VPD frequency increases with age. Although sporadic VPD's in persons with normal hearts do not seem to affect outcome adversely, VPD's confer significant risk of subsequent cardiac death in persons with heart disease. When VPD's are caused by drug toxicity, e.g., digitalis, quinidine, or tricyclic antidepressants, lethal rhythm disturbances may ensue unless the drug is discontinued. A strong association exists between myocardial infarct size and the frequency of VPD's in acute myocardial infarction, and a weak association exists between poor left ventricular function and frequency of VPD's during recovery.

MANAGEMENT. The most important issue in the treatment of VPD's is the selection of patients for treatment. In general, only symptomatic VPD's need treatment, and class IC or class II antiarrhythmic drugs (see Table 45–9) are the first choices for treatment of benign and potentially malignant ventricular arrhythmias. Intravenously administered lidocaine or procainamide is usually used to treat VPD's occurring immediately after myocardial infarction or cardiac surgery.

Ventricular Tachycardia

ECG DIAGNOSIS. The most prevalent definition of ventricular tachycardia (VT) is three or more VPD's in succession at a rate of 100 per min or greater. Ventricular tachycardia may be unsustained, i.e., last less than 15 to 30 seconds, or sustained (see Fig. 45–19). In a tachycardia with wide QRS complexes, two findings strongly suggest VT: *ventricular captures* and *fusion complexes*. Sinus impulses may capture the ventricle during VT, producing either a normal QRS (ventricular capture) or a QRS intermediate in contour between normal and the QRS of ventricular tachycardia (fusion complex). Sustained VT can be difficult to distinguish from supraventricular arrhythmias with a wide QRS complex. A His bundle recording can easily distinguish between these two possibilities (Fig. 45–10).

CLINICAL FEATURES. Unsustained VT nearly always occurs in patients with heart disease, most often in those with coronary heart disease. After myocardial infarction, about 10 per cent of patients have VT detected by a single 24-hour continuous ECG recording. Patients with class III or IV heart failure have a 40 to 50 per cent prevalence of VT in a 24-hour ECG. Most episodes of VT in either setting are brief, i.e., three to five consecutive VPD's, and asymptomatic yet increase the risk of dying two- to fourfold. Sustained VT is rare and has a poor prognosis. As with other tachyarrhythmias, the severity of symptoms in sustained VT is related primarily to the rate of the tachycardia and left ventricular function. Sustained VT is prone to deteriorate into ventricular fibrillation (Fig. 45–19).

MANAGEMENT. The management of symptomatic, unsustained VT is the same as that described above for VPD's. Sustained VT in chronic heart disease is treated acutely with IV lidocaine or procainamide, if the patient is hemodynamically stable, or by DC cardioversion, if unstable (Fig. 45–19). Baseline studies should include 48 hours of continuous ECG recording, exercise testing, and endocardial electrical stimulation. The drug-dose finding and long-term management of these patients should be guided by rigorous methods with high predictive accuracy. The standard method is endocardial electrical stimulation. A programmatic noninvasive approach using 24-hour continuous ECG recordings and exercise tests also can be used. The usual sequence for drug testing is class IA (e.g., quinidine or procainamide), IA plus IB (e.g., quinidine and mexiletine), IC (e.g., encainide or flecainide), and finally III (amiodarone). If an effective drug is not found, an implantable defibrillator is usually the best treatment. In selected cases, surgery is the best choice.

Accelerated Idioventricular Rhythm

ECG DIAGNOSIS. Accelerated idioventricular rhythm (AIVR) is defined as three or more consecutive QRS complexes of ventricular origin with a rate between 50 and 100 per minute (see Fig. 45–20). Fusion QRS complexes often begin or end an episode of AIVR.

CLINICAL FEATURES. Accelerated idioventricular rhythm occurs in about 30 per cent of patients during the course of either inferior or anterior acute myocardial infarction. Accelerated idioventricular rhythm frequently follows coronary reperfusion. This rhythm is usually asymptomatic and therefore needs no treatment. The incidence of ventricular fibrillation and hospital mortality is not increased in patients who have AIVR.

Ventricular Parasystole

ECG DIAGNOSIS. Ventricular parasystole is an automatic rhythm in the His-Purkinje system that competes with sinus

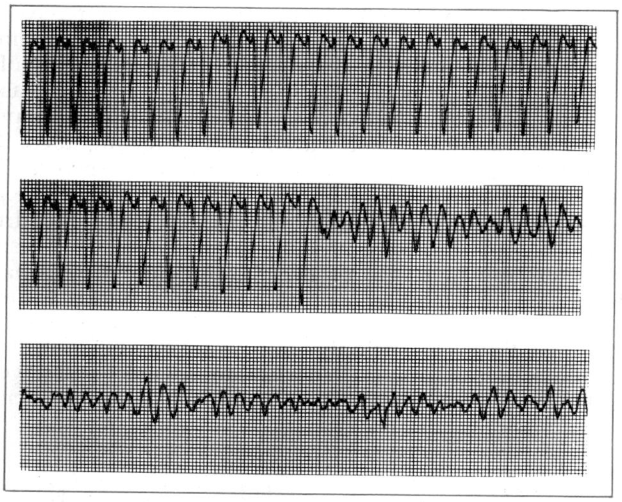

FIGURE 45–19. Ventricular tachycardia and ventricular fibrillation. Three continuous strips from lead V4 of a Holter electrocardiograph. The top strip shows ventricular tachycardia at 214 cycles per minute—an unusually rapid rate for ventricular tachycardia. Ventricular fibrillation begins in the middle strip and continues on the bottom strip. Note the irregularity in amplitude and period of deflections recorded during ventricular fibrillation. (From Braunwald E.: Heart Disease: A Textbook of Cardiovascular Medicine. Philadelphia, W. B. Saunders Company, 1980.)

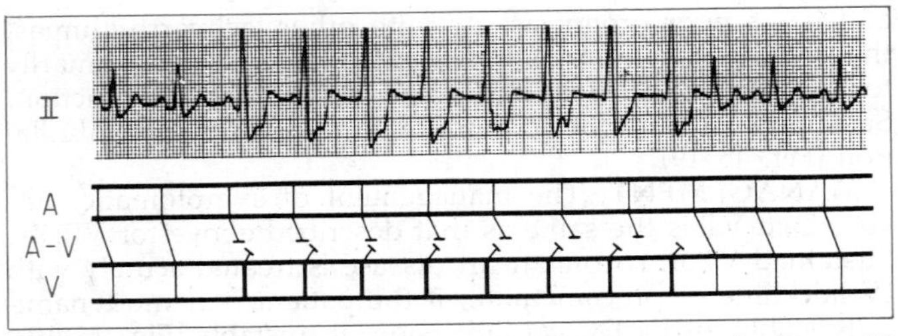

FIGURE 45–20. Accelerated idioventricular rhythm. Sinus rhythm at 88 cycles per minute is interrupted by a rhythm with wide QRS complexes at 95 cycles per minute. Note that the P-R interval progressively shortens at the onset of the ventricular rhythm and that sinus rhythm continues unperturbed by the ventricular rhythm (atrioventricular dissociation). After eight QRS complexes of ventricular rhythm, sinus rhythm resumes. (From Braunwald E.: Heart Disease: A Textbook of Cardiovascular Medicine. Philadelphia, W. B. Saunders Company, 1980.)

rhythm. Parasystole has two cardinal features: variable coupling of VPD's and a common denominator for interectopic intervals. Entrance block removes the parasystolic focus from the suppressant influence of the sinus impulses, permitting a stable automatic rhythm to emerge; the ectopic focus will activate the ventricle every time it fires unless the ventricle is refractory (Fig. 45–20).

CLINICAL FEATURES. Parasystole often is resistant to antiarrhythmic drug therapy, and untreated patients seem to have a good prognosis.

Ventricular Flutter and Fibrillation

ECG DIAGNOSIS. The electrocardiographic diagnosis of ventricular flutter is made when the ventricular tachyarrhythmia has large sinusoidal or zigzag QRS's and the rate is between 240 and 280 per minute. Multiform VT, or torsades de pointes, is recognized by the periodic twisting of the points of the QRS complexes (see Fig. 45–21). Ventricular fibrillation is recognized in the ECG by the absence of QRS complexes and T waves and the presence of low-amplitude baseline undulations that are variable in both amplitude and periodicity (see Fig. 45–19).

CLINICAL FEATURES. Ventricular flutter is rarely recorded, because it is unstable and tends to convert to sinus rhythm or, more often, to ventricular fibrillation. Ventricular flutter or fibrillation is catastrophic. Cardiac pumping ceases instantly, the patient loses consciousness, and, if cardiopulmonary resuscitation is not started within a few minutes, the patient will die. Identifiable causes are acute myocardial ischemia or infarction; marked electrolyte disturbances, e.g., hypokalemia; marked hypothermia; electrocution; and drug toxicity. Most victims of ventricular fibrillation who are resuscitated do *not* have one of these conditions but do have advanced coronary atherosclerosis and poor ventricular function.

MANAGEMENT. The only effective treatment for ventricular fibrillation is prompt defibrillation. In most cases, ventricular fibrillation will not recur after defibrillation. When it does, lidocaine, bretylium, or propranolol may help to stabilize the rhythm. When no transient or reversible cause for ventricular fibrillation is found (e.g., myocardial infarction, electrolyte abnormality, or drug toxicity), the process for evaluating long-term treatment is much the same as described above for sustained VT. Unfortunately, a smaller fraction of patients, about 60 to 70 per cent, will have VT induced by programmed ventricular stimulation. Nevertheless, the uninducible patients have a high recurrence rate for ventricular fibrillation.

The management of multiform VT (torsades de pointes) is based on its pathophysiology: toxic drug effects, hypokalemia or hypomagnesemia or both, and slow heart rates. Treatment may include avoidance of class I antiarrhythmic drugs, ventricular pacing, reducing the level of the culprit drug, repletion of electrolytes, and catecholamine or magnesium sulfate infusion.

PROGNOSTIC CLASSIFICATION OF VENTRICULAR ARRHYTHMIAS. Table 45–8 outlines the classification of ventricular arrhythmias as determined by the presence of heart disease, left ventricular function, and arrhythmia characteristics. Prognosis is an important basis for deciding whom to treat and how to sequence the treatment choices.

Bigger JT Jr, Reiffel JA: Sick sinus syndrome. Ann Rev Med 30:91, 1979. *A comprehensive review of the human sinus node dysfunction. Liberally referenced.*

Marriott HJL: Practical Electrocardiography. Baltimore, Williams & Wilkins Company, 1983. *A textbook designed to emphasize the simplicities of the ECG, provide only those concepts that make everyday ECG interpretation more intelligible, and provide illustrations and discussion of all-important ECG patterns. Excellent for learning or reviewing the ECG patterns of arrhythmias.*

Zipes DP: Specific Arrhythmias: Diagnosis and treatment. In Braunwald E (ed.): Heart Disease: A Textbook of Cardiovascular Medicine. Philadelphia, W. B. Saunders Company, 1984, pp 683–743. *Detailed description of the clinical features, electrocardiographic recognition, and treatment of cardiac arrhythmias. Contains 48 figures and 375 references.*

ANTIARRHYTHMIC DRUGS

Classification of Antiarrhythmic Drugs

Antiarrhythmic drugs have been classified according to their mechanisms of action into four classes (see Table 45–9). One could think of digitalis as having class V drug action, i.e., a strong cholinergic action that can repolarize stretched or damaged atrial cells and thereby speed conduction. Digitalis glycosides slow conduction in the AV node, tending to abolish re-entrant rhythms that use that structure.

Use-Dependent Block of Ionic Channels—An Antiarrhythmic Action

Many antiarrhythmic drugs act on ionic channels in the sarcolemma. Class I antiarrhythmic drugs block the Na^+ channel so that ionic conductance falls to zero until the drug dissociates from the channel. Most class I drugs bind to open or inactivated channels; drug-associated channels have slow or incomplete reactivation. Drug binding and Na^+ channel blockade increase with rate, producing *use-dependent block.* If the association and dissociation of drug from the Na^+ channel both are rapid, use-dependent block will attain a steady state after a few action potentials, and if the interval between action potentials is reasonably long, little block will persist at the

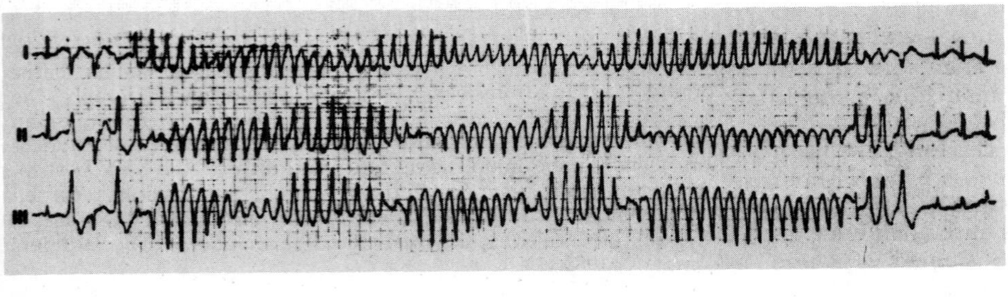

FIGURE 45–21. Torsades de pointes. Sinus rhythm associated with a long Q-T interval is present at the beginning and at the end of this rhythm strip. Sinus rhythm is interrupted by a rapid wide QRS tachycardia. Note that during the tachycardia, the direction of the points of the QRS complex appears to revolve around an imaginary isolelectric line. (From Krikler DM, Curry DVL: Br Heart J 38:118, 1976. With permission of the British Heart Journal and authors.)

TABLE 45–8. PROGNOSTIC CLASSIFICATION OF VENTRICULAR ARRHYTHMIAS

	Benign	Potentially Malignant	Malignant
Risk for sudden death	Very low	Moderate	High
Clinical presentation	Palpitations; detected by routine examination	Palpitations; detected by routine examination or screening	Palpitations; syncope; cardiac arrest
Heart disease	Usually absent	Present	Present
Cardiac scarring and/or hypertrophy	Absent	Present	Present
VPD frequency	Low to moderate	Moderate to high	Moderate to high
Paired VPD and/or unsustained ventricular tachycardia	Absent	Common	Common
Sustained ventricular tachycardia	Absent	Absent	Present
Hemodynamic effects of arrhythmia	Absent	Absent; mild	Moderate; severe

VPD = ventricular premature depolarization.
The characteristics listed in this table are typical and do not represent the full range of observations. For example, benign ventricular arrhythmias can be frequent and, occasionally, repetitive.

time of the next action potential upstroke. If dissociation is slow, use-dependent block will require many action potentials to develop fully, and a significant degree of block will remain at the time of each action potential upstroke.

SPECIFIC ANTIARRHYTHMIC DRUGS

This section gives a brief summary of the pharmacology and indications for each antiarrhythmic drug. This information is supplemented by information given in tables; Table 45–10 gives pharmacokinetic data for the drugs, and Table 45–11 gives information on dosing and on contraindications, precautions, and adverse effects.

Class IB Antiarrhythmic Drugs

LIDOCAINE. Lidocaine is a local anesthetic used frequently, since the early 1960's, for the intravenous treatment of ventricular arrhythmias in the intensive care unit setting because of two major advantages: It reaches a steady state rapidly after starting or changing the dose, and it lacks significant adverse hemodynamic effects.

Pharmacology. Lidocaine prevents re-entrant rhythms, decreases automaticity in Purkinje fibers, and increases the ventricular fibrillation threshold. Lidocaine has an intense depressant action on depolarized tissues, but almost none on normal cardiac cells. The drug has a negligible effect on the ECG. Lidocaine shortens the effective refractory period (ERP) of the His-Purkinje system. It has no significant effect on the autonomic nervous system.

Indications. Lidocaine is used only for ventricular arrhythmias, particularly those caused by acute myocardial infarction, open heart surgery, and digitalis intoxication. Lidocaine is relatively ineffective for ventricular arrhythmias in chronic coronary heart disease or cardiomyopathy.

Pharmacokinetics. Lidocaine is administered intravenously and, rarely, intramuscularly. Plasma lidocaine concentration dynamically follows the hepatic blood flow. About 70 per cent of lidocaine in the plasma is bound to alpha$_1$-acid glycoprotein, an acute phase reactant. At a given total plasma concentration, the free concentration will fall as the alpha$_1$-acid glycoprotein increases in the first few days after infarction or surgery.

TABLE 45–9. CLASSIFICATION OF ANTIARRHYTHMIC DRUGS ACCORDING TO THEIR MECHANISM OF ACTION

Class / Action	Drugs
I. Sodium channel blockade	
A. Minimal phase 0 depression Slow conduction 0 to 1+ Shorten repolarization	Lidocaine; mexiletine; tocainide
B. Moderate phase 0 depression Slow conduction 2+ Prolong repolarization	Quinidine; procainamide; disopyramide
C. Marked phase 0 depression Slow conduction 4+ Little effect on repolarization	Encainide; flecainide
II. Beta-adrenergic blockade	Propranolol; acebutolol
III. Prolong repolarization	Amiodarone; bretylium; sotalol
IV. Calcium channel blockade	Diltiazem; verapamil

MEXILETINE. Mexiletine is a new orally active local anesthetic that is similar to lidocaine chemically and electrophysiologically.

Pharmacology. Mexiletine has an antiautomatic effect on Purkinje fibers and depresses phase 0 of fast action potentials more than lidocaine. It shortens the action potential duration and refractoriness of Purkinje fibers and ventricular muscle cells. Mexiletine has little effect on the ECG.

Indications. Like lidocaine, this drug is not indicated for atrial arrhythmias, and its efficacy is less than the class IA or class IC antiarrhythmic drugs for ventricular arrhythmias. In chronic coronary heart disease or cardiomyopathy, the drug is about 60 per cent effective in controlling unsustained ventricular arrhythmias.

PHENYTOIN. Phenytoin* is an anticonvulsant drug that is electrophysiologically very similar to lidocaine and has no significant effect on the ECG. Phenytoin has complex central autonomic actions that decrease efferent traffic on cardiac sympathetic nerves in digitalis toxicity. Phenytoin has no peripheral cholinergic or beta-adrenergic–blocking activity.

Indications. Phenytoin is used to treat paroxysmal atrial flutter or fibrillation, supraventricular arrhythmias, and ventricular arrhythmias caused by digitalis but is ineffective for the common atrial arrhythmias, e.g., atrial flutter, atrial fibrillation, and PSVT. Phenytoin is effective against ventricular arrhythmias after acute myocardial infarction or open heart surgery, but lidocaine is easier to use. Plasma concentrations above 10 μg per milliliter are effective for reducing ventricular arrhythmias in the year after myocardial infarction. Phenytoin, like other class I antiarrhythmic drugs, is relatively ineffective against recurrent, drug-resistant VT in patients with chronic coronary heart disease.

Pharmacokinetics. The enzymes that metabolize phenytoin can saturate at antiarrhythmic plasma concentrations, causing plasma concentration to rise sharply to toxic levels. Phenytoin should not be infused because its alkaline pH causes severe phlebitis.

TOCAINIDE. Tocainide is an orally effective analogue of lidocaine that has cardiac electrophysiologic effects almost identical to those of lidocaine and has almost no effects on the ECG. In addition, it is well tolerated hemodynamically.

Indications. Tocainide is indicated for the oral treatment of ventricular arrhythmias. The drug is similar to mexiletine in its efficacy, i.e., it controls about 60 per cent of the chronic unsustained ventricular arrhythmias. There is about a 70 per cent concordance between the responses to IV lidocaine and oral tocainide.

*This use of phenytoin is not listed in the manufacturer's directive.

Text continued on page 270

TABLE 45–10. PHARMACOKINETIC PROPERTIES OF ANTIARRHYTHMIC DRUGS

Drug	Volume of Distribution (liters/kg)	Half-time of Elimination (hr)	Bioavailability (%)	Major Route of Elimination	Protein Binding (%)	Effective Plasma Concentration (μg/ml)
Digoxin	10.0	24–72	50–80	Kidney	25	>0.0008
Lidocaine	1.0	1–3	—	Liver	70	1.5–5
Mexiletine	9.5	8–14	80–90	Liver	60	0.7–2.0
Phenytoin	0.7	18–30	60–80	Liver	90	8–20
Tocainide	3.0	10–14	80–90	Kidney; liver	10	6–15
Disopyramide	0.8	7–9	75–90	Kidney	Dose dependent	2–5
Procainamide	2.0	3–6	75–85	Kidney; liver	15	4–20
Quinidine	2.5	5–9	70–80	Liver	90	2–6
Encainide	4.0	1–3	20–40	Liver	80	—
Flecainide	10.0	13–30	>90	Kidney; liver	40	0.2–1.0
Acebutolol	1.2	2–4	35–45	Kidney; liver	25	—
Propranolol	4.0	3–6	20–50	Liver	>90	0.04–0.9
Amiodarone	60.0	500–1000	30–40	Liver	>95	0.5–2.5
Bretylium	6.0	8–12	20–30	Kidney	5	—
Diltiazem	5.5	2–6	40–50	Liver	75	0.5–2.0
Verapamil	4.0	4–10	10–35	Liver	90	0.1–0.2

TABLE 45–11. DOSING AND ADVERSE EFFECTS OF ANTIARRHYTHMIC DRUGS

	Usual IV Dose		Usual Oral Dose				
	Loading	*Maintenance*	*Loading*	*Maintenance*	Contraindications	Precautions	Adverse Effects
Digoxin							
Tablets 0.125, 0.25, 0.5 mg	—	—	0.5–1.00 mg p.o., followed by 0.125–0.375 mg p.o. in 6–8 hr	0.125–0.375 mg p.o. once a day	Hypersensitivity to the drug	Reduce dose in renal insufficiency; hypokalemia, hypomagnesemia, and hypercalcemia predispose to digitalis toxicity; may accelerate the ventricular response to atrial flutter or fibrillation in Wolff-Parkinson-White syndrome; may worsen outflow obstruction in HOCM; serum digoxin concentration increased by quinidine and verapamil; absorption may be increased by some antibiotics; use cautiously with beta blockers or calcium channel antagonists in atrial fibrillation	Ventricular arrhythmias, including ventricular tachycardia; accelerated junctional rhythms; atrial tachycardia with AV block; AV dissociation; progression of AV block Anorexia; nausea, vomiting; visual disturbances; weakness
Lanoxicaps capsules 0.05, 0.1, 0.2 mg	—	—	—	0.1–0.3 mg p.o. once a day			
IV 2-ml ampule, 0.25 mg/ml	0.5–1.00 mg IV, followed by 0.125–0.375 mg IV in 6–8 hr	—	—	—			
Pediatric preparation 1-ml ampule, 0.1 mg/ml	0.015–0.030 mg/kg IV, followed by 0.005–0.010 mg/kg/day (age dependent)	—	—	—			
Lidocaine							
IV	50–100 mg IV over 2–5 min; may repeat 50 mg after 5 min	10–40 μg/kg/min	—	—	Known hypersensitivity to local anesthetics of the amide type; patients with Stokes-Adams syndrome or with severe degrees of sinoatrial, AV, or intraventricular block in the absence of a pacemaker	Accumulation in heart failure, in hepatic or renal insufficiency, or after prolonged infusions; reduce dosage in children and elderly patients; safety in malignant hyperthermia not established; cimetidine and propranolol increase plasma lidocaine concentration	Bradycardia, hypotension, and cardiovascular collapse Drowsiness; confusion; dizziness; respiratory depression and arrest; vomiting; visual disturbances; convulsions; twitching; unconsciousness; allergic reactions secondary to lidocaine sensitivity
IM	300 mg IM	—	—	—			

TABLE 45–11. DOSING AND ADVERSE EFFECTS OF ANTIARRHYTHMIC DRUGS *Continued*

	Usual IV Dose		Usual Oral Dose				
	Loading	*Maintenance*	*Loading*	*Maintenance*	Contraindications	Precautions	Adverse Effects
Mexiletine Capsules 150, 200, 250 mg	—	—	400 mg p.o.	200–400 mg p.o. q. 8 hr	Cardiogenic shock; pre-existing second- or third-degree AV block in the absence of a pacemaker	Patients with first-degree AV block, sinus node dysfunction, intraventricular conduction abnormalities, hypotension, heart failure, liver disease; may worsen arrhythmias; mexiletine levels increased by cimetidine; use cautiously in patients with a history of seizures, hypotension, heart failure, or liver disease	GI distress; lightheadedness; tremor; coordination difficulties; diplopia; paresthesia; confusion
Phenytoin* Tablets 100 mg	—	—	Day 1, 400 mg Day 2, 300 mg Day 3, 300 mg (1000 mg total)	100 mg p.o. t.i.d.; 200 mg p.o. b.i.d.	History of hypersensitivity to hydantoin products; sinus bradycardia, sinoatrial block, second- or third-degree AV block; Stokes-Adams syndrome	Use cautiously in presence of hypotension and myocardial depression; may worsen arrhythmias; discontinue if skin rash develops; may cause hypoglycemia; multiple drug interactions; may be associated with congenital malformations	Hypotension and bradycardia with rapid IV injection Nystagmus, ataxia, slurred speech; Stevens-Johnson syndrome; sensory neuropathy; lymphadenopathy; pancytopenia; megaloblastic anemia; gingival hyperplasia; hyperglycemia; hypocalcemia
Extended capsules 100 mg	—	—	—	300 mg or 400 mg p.o. q. day			
IV 2-ml ampules, 50 mg/ml 5-ml ampules, 50 mg/ml	100 mg IV q. 5 min to a maximum of 1000 mg	—	—	—			
Tocainide Tablets 400, 600 mg	—	—	—	400–800 mg p.o. q. 8 hr	Hypersensitivity to this drug or to local anesthetics of the amide type; second- or third-degree AV block in the absence of a pacemaker	May cause blood dyscrasias, pulmonary fibrosis, pneumonitis; may aggravate heart failure or worsen ventricular arrhythmias; may accelerate the ventricular response in atrial fibrillation; accumulates in severe renal or hepatic insufficiency	Nausea, vomiting; light-headedness; dizziness; tremor; diplopia; paresthesia; confusion; *agranulocytosis;* thrombocytopenia; hypoplastic anemia
Disopyramide Capsules 100, 150 mg	—	—	300 mg p.o.	100–200 mg p.o. q. 6 hr	Cardiogenic shock; pre-existing second- or third-degree AV block in the absence of a pacemaker; congenital QT prolongation; known hypersensitivity to the drug	*Use cautiously with left ventricular dysfunction,* sick sinus syndrome, bundle branch block, or AV block; prior digitalization suggested for atrial flutter or fibrillation to prevent increase in ventricular rate; may precipitate myasthenia crisis, glaucoma, or urinary retention; may cause hypoglycemia; serum level may be lowered by phenytoin	*Heart failure;* worsening of arrhythmias; AV block; hypotension; may cause significant prolongation of QRS and QT intervals *Urinary retention;* dry mouth; constipation; blurred vision; impotence; cholestatic jaundice; fever; thrombocytopenia; granulocytopenia; gynecomastia
Norpace CR (controlled release) 100, 150 mg	—	—	—	200–400 mg p.o. q. 12 hr			
Procainamide HCl Tablets, capsules 250, 375, 500 mg	—	—	1 gm p.o.	500–1250 mg p.o. q. 3–4 hr	Second- or third-degree AV block unless a pacemaker is present; torsades de pointes; lupus-like syndrome; hypersensitivity to the drug	Reduce dosage in renal insufficiency; may accelerate the ventricular response in atrial fibrillation or atrial flutter; may exacerbate myasthenia gravis	Hypotension; worsening of ventricular arrhythmias; myocardial depression; AV block
Procainamide SR (sustained release) 250, 500, 750, 1000 mg	—	—	—	1000–3000 mg p.o. q. 6–8 hr			

*This use of phenytoin is not listed in the manufacturer's directive.

TABLE 45–11. DOSING AND ADVERSE EFFECTS OF ANTIARRHYTHMIC DRUGS ***Continued***

	Usual IV Dose		Usual Oral Dose				
	Loading	*Maintenance*	*Loading*	*Maintenance*	**Contraindications**	**Precautions**	**Adverse Effects**
Procainamide HCl for IV use	100 mg injected q. 5 min IV for 7–10 doses or 20 mg/min infusion IV for 40–60 min	20–80 μg/kg/min	—	—			*Lupus-like syndrome;* GI distress; *agranulocytosis;* hemolytic anemia; fever; thrombocytopenia; rash; myalgia; hallucinations, psychosis
Quinidine sulfate							
Tablets 100, 200, 300 mg	—	—	—	200–500 mg p.o. q.i.d.	Hypersensitivity to quinidine; complete AV block; complete bundle branch block or other severe intraventricular conduction defects exhibiting marked QRS widening; myasthenia gravis; arrhythmias due to digitalis toxicity	May accelerate the ventricular response to atrial flutter or atrial fibrillation; *concurrent use with digoxin will increase plasma digoxin levels;* drugs that increase hepatic drug-metabolizing enzymes decrease the plasma concentration of quinidine; may worsen heart failure; test dose recommended because of idiosyncratic response; may require change in oral anticoagulant dose	Hypotension; worsening of ventricular arrhythmias; asystole; may increase AV or bundle branch block; may cause significant prolongation of QRS and QT intervals; *syncope; torsades de pointes* *Diarrhea;* nausea; *thrombocytopenia;* hemolytic anemia; granulocytopenia; fever; visual disturbances; hypersensitivity reaction; cinchonism; rash
Quinidine Extentabs (sustained release) 300 mg	—	—	—	300–600 mg p.o. q. 8–12 hr			
Quinidine gluconate 330 mg (200-mg quinidine base)	—	—	—	330–660 mg p. o. q. 8 hr			
Quinidine polygalacturonate 275 mg (200-mg quinidine base)	—	—	—				
Encainide*							
Tablets 25, 35, 50 mg	—	—	—	25–50 mg p.o. t.i.d.	Second- or third-degree AV block or right bundle branch block with associated hemiblock unless a pacemaker is in place; cardiogenic shock; known hypersensitivity	May worsen sinus node dysfunction; increases pacing thresholds; may suppress ventricular escape rhythms; reduce dose with renal insufficiency; cimetidine increases encainide serum concentration	*New or worsened ventricular tachycardia or ventricular fibrillation;* second- or third-degree AV block Dizziness, vertigo; visual disturbances; headache; leg cramps
Flecainide							
Tablets 100 mg	—	—	—	100–200 mg p.o. b.i.d.	Second- or third-degree AV block or right bundle branch block with associated hemiblock unless a pacemaker is in place; cardiogenic shock; known hypersensitivity to the drug	May worsen sinus node dysfunction; increases pacing thresholds; may suppress ventricular escape rhythms; avoid concurrent administration of disopyramide or verapamil	*New or worsened ventricular tachycardia or ventricular fibrillation* in patients with sustained ventricular arrhythmias; *heart failure;* second- or third-degree AV block Dizziness; *visual disturbances;* dyspnea; hepatic dysfunction; blood dyscrasias
Acebutolol							
Capsules 200, 400 mg	—	—	—	200–600 mg p.o. q. 12 hr	Severe sinus bradycardia; second- and third-degree AV block; overt cardiac failure; cardiogenic shock	Exacerbation of angina may occur or myocardial infarction may occur following abrupt withdrawal; may mask symptoms of hypoglycemia or hyperthyroidism; cautious use in renal insufficiency or with concurrent alpha-adrenergic or catecholamine-depleting drugs	Congestive heart failure; bradycardia; hypotension; increase in AV block Fatigue; headache; dizziness; arterial insufficiency; bronchospasm; impotence

*Investigational drug.

TABLE 45–11. DOSING AND ADVERSE EFFECTS OF ANTIARRHYTHMIC DRUGS *Continued*

	Usual IV Dose		Usual Oral Dose				
	Loading	*Maintenance*	*Loading*	*Maintenance*	Contraindications	Precautions	Adverse Effects
Propranolol							
Tablets 10, 20, 40, 60, 80, 90 mg	—	—	—	10–160 mg p.o. q. 6 hr*	Cardiogenic shock; sinus bradycardia; second- or third-degree AV block; asthma; congestive heart failure	Exacerbation of angina may occur or myocardial infarction may occur following abrupt withdrawal; may mask symptoms of hypoglycemia or hyperthyroidism; may cause severe sinus bradycardia following termination of tachycardia; may worsen hypertension in pheochromocytoma unless used with an alpha-adrenergic–blocking drug	Congestive heart failure; bradycardia; increase in degree of AV block; hypotension Bronchospasm; arterial insufficiency; Raynaud's phenomenon; mental depression; sleep disturbances; weakness; impotence; disorientation; memory loss; blood dyscrasias
Inderal LA capsules 80, 120, 160 mg	—	—	—	One daily*			
IV 1-mg ampule	1–3 mg, at rate ≤ 1 mg/min	—	—	—			
Amiodarone							
Tablets 200 mg	—	—	800–1600 mg per day for 1–3 weeks; 600–800 mg per day for 4 weeks	400 mg per day	Severe sinus node dysfunction; marked sinus bradycardia; second- or third-degree AV block; history of syncope due to bradycardia unless a pacemaker is in place	Raises serum digoxin concentration; potentiates the effect of oral anticoagulants; increases levels of quinidine, procainamide, phenytoin; may potentiate bradycardia or AV block when used with beta blockers or calcium antagonists; may worsen arrhythmias	Sinus bradycardia *Pulmonary fibrosis;* interstitial pneumonitis; corneal microdeposits; photosensitivity; blue-gray pigmentation; hypo- and hyperthyroidism; *hepatic injury;* nausea, vomiting; anorexia; constipation; tremor; malaise; gait disturbance; *peripheral myopathy or neuropathy*
Bretylium tosylate							
IV 50 mg/ml	5–10 mg per kg IV	1 mg/min infusion or 5–10 mg/kg IV q. 6 hr	—	—	—	*Severe hypotension may occur in patients with fixed cardiac output;* may aggravate digitalis toxicity; reduce dosage in renal insufficiency	*Hypotension, especially postural hypotension;* transient hypertension and increased frequency of ventricular arrhythmias Nausea and vomiting, usually with rapid IV infusion; increased sensitivity to catecholamines
IM	5–10 mg per kg IM	—	—	—	—		
Diltiazem							
Tablets 30, 60 mg	—	—	—	30–90 mg p.o. q. 6–8 hr	Sick sinus syndrome; second- or third-degree AV block in absence of a ventricular pacemaker; systolic BP < 90 mm Hg	Cautious use in renal or hepatic insufficiency; additive effects on AV conduction when used with digitalis or beta blockers	Bradycardia; hypotension; AV block Edema; headache; nausea; dizziness; rash; abnormal hepatic enzymes
Verapamil							
Tablets 80, 120 mg	—	—	—	80–160 mg p.o. q. 6–8 hr	*Severe left ventricular dysfunction; hypotension or cardiogenic shock;* sick sinus syndrome (except with a pacemaker); second- or third-degree AV block; concurrent intravenous beta blockers and intravenous verapamil; known hypersensitivity to verapamil	Reduce oral dose with hepatic dysfunction; avoid use with disopyramide; use cautiously with renal insufficiency, beta blockers, quinidine, or severe HOCM; will raise serum digoxin level; *may accelerate ventricular response in atrial flutter or fibrillation in the presence of an accessory AV connection;* may potentiate activity of neuromuscular blocking agents	Hypotension; AV block; heart failure; bradycardia; asystole (with IV use); *severe hypotension or ventricular fibrillation when given IV to patients with ventricular tachycardia* Peripheral edema; headache; elevation of liver function test values; constipation
IV formulation 5 mg vials 10-mg vials	5–10 mg IV over 2–5 min; after 30 min, 10 mg IV if needed	—	—	—			

*Dose and interval depend on indication.
IV = intravenous; HOCM = hypertrophic obstructive cardiomyopathy; GI = gastrointestinal.

Class IA Antiarrhythmic Drugs

DISOPYRAMIDE. Disopyramide suppresses normal automaticity in Purkinje fibers and depresses phase 0 of the action potential and conduction in the atria and ventricles. Disopyramide may be somewhat more potent than quinidine in increasing atrial or ventricular refractoriness but seems less potent in the His-Purkinje system. Therapeutic concentrations cause little change in heart rate or PR or QT intervals and increase the QRS duration by about 25 per cent. It increases the ERP in the atrium and ventricle, but not in the AV node or His-Purkinje system. Disopyramide has a prominent anticholinergic action that counteracts its direct effects on the sinus and AV nodes.

Indications. Disopyramide is indicated for the oral treatment of symptomatic, unsustained ventricular arrhythmias. It also will terminate attacks of PSVT and will decrease the frequency of recurrences. It is about as effective as quinidine for preventing recurrence of atrial fibrillation after cardioversion. Disopyramide prolongs the refractory period of anomalous AV connections and can control arrhythmias in the WPW syndrome.

PROCAINAMIDE. Procainamide has been used since the 1950's for treatment of atrial and ventricular arrhythmias. The cardiac electrophysiologic effects of procainamide are similar to those of disopyramide and quinidine. It suppresses automaticity in cardiac Purkinje fibers, slows the phase 0 depolarization in fibers with fast action potentials, and delays repolarization and increases refractoriness in the atrium, His-Purkinje system, and ventricle. Procainamide produces a small increase in the PR and QT intervals in the ECG and produces a 20 to 30 per cent increase in the QRS duration at therapeutic plasma concentrations. In addition, procainamide increases slightly the ERP of the atrium, has little effect on the refractoriness of the AV node, and prolongs the conduction time and refractoriness of the His-Purkinje system slightly in humans. Procainamide has no significant anticholinergic or alpha-adrenergic–blocking properties.

Indications. Procainamide is indicated for the treatment of atrial fibrillation, atrial flutter, PSVT, premature ventricular depolarizations, and ventricular tachycardia. It can suppress digitalis-induced toxic ventricular arrhythmias, but lidocaine or phenytoin is a better choice.

Pharmacokinetics. Procainamide is biotransformed in the liver to *N*-acetylprocainamide (NAPA). In the steady state, the plasma NAPA concentrations can equal or exceed those of the parent drug. NAPA is qualitatively different electrophysiologically from procainamide; it has a weak effect on phase 0 depolarization and a pronounced effect on action potential duration and refractoriness, a class III action. NAPA is eliminated by the kidney and can accumulate to toxic levels when renal or congestive heart failure is present.

QUINIDINE. Quinidine, an alkaloid derived from the bark of the cinchona tree, has been used for the treatment of atrial and ventricular arrhythmias since the 1920's.

Pharmacology. Quinidine has powerful direct effects on most types of cardiac cells and has significant anticholinergic and alpha-adrenergic–blocking activity. Quinidine has little effect on the automaticity of normal sinus nodes but can markedly depress abnormal sinus nodes. It substantially decreases automaticity of normal cardiac Purkinje fibers but has little effect on abnormal automaticity. Quinidine increases atrial and ventricular pacing and fibrillation thresholds; depresses phase 0 of atrial, ventricular, and Purkinje cells; and delays repolarization and increases the ERP of atrial, ventricular, and Purkinje cells. In humans, quinidine causes a small increase in heart rate and in the PR, QRS, and QT intervals in the ECG and usually prolongs the HV interval slightly.

Indications. Quinidine is indicated for the chronic treatment of atrial flutter or fibrillation, PSVT, and symptomatic ventricular arrhythmias. For symptomatic benign or potentially malignant ventricular arrhythmias, the quinidine dose is titrated until symptoms are controlled and unsustained VT is 90 or more per cent suppressed. Quinidine is selected for malignant arrhythmias if it renders them uninducible by programmed ventricular stimulation or if it abolishes unsustained VT from Holter recordings.

Class IC Antiarrhythmic Drugs

ENCAINIDE. Encainide is a class IC antiarrhythmic drug that became available for use in the United States in 1987. Encainide has little effect on the normal sinus node but can depress abnormal sinus nodes. It decreases spontaneous phase 4 depolarization in Purkinje fibers and markedly depresses phase 0 in fast-response cardiac cells. Encainide slows conduction substantially and shortens the ERP in the atrium, the ventricle, and the His-Purkinje system. In humans, chronic oral encainide prolongs the refractory periods on the atrium, ventricle, and anomalous AV connections. It increases the AH and HV intervals and the PR, QRS, and QT intervals in the ECG. The increase in QRS duration is greater than that caused by class IA drugs. Encainide has two active metabolites, *O*-demethylencainide (ODE) and 3-methoxy-*O*-demethylencainide (MODE). The metabolites have more potent electrophysiologic effects and longer elimination half-times than encainide. Encainide is notable for minimal myocardial depression in patients with poor left ventricular function.

Indications. At the present time, encainide is indicated only for the treatment of symptomatic ventricular arrhythmias. However, it has been shown to be extremely effective against PSVT in the WPW syndrome, and it is being investigated for its effectiveness against atrial flutter and fibrillation and AV nodal re-entrant tachycardia.

FLECAINIDE. Flecainide is a new class IC antiarrhythmic drug that has little effect on the normal sinus node but can depress abnormal sinus nodes. It decreases spontaneous phase 4 depolarization in Purkinje fibers and markedly depresses depolarization in fast-response cardiac cells. The drug slows conduction substantially in the atrium, the ventricle, and the His-Purkinje system. Flecainide shortens repolarization in the atrium, the ventricle, and the His-Purkinje system. In humans, flecainide prolongs the refractory periods of the atrium, ventricle, and anomalous AV connections. It increases the AH and HV intervals and the PR and QRS intervals in the ECG. The increase in QRS duration is much greater than that seen with class IA drugs. Flecainide can aggravate left ventricular dysfunction.

Indications. Flecainide is indicated for symptomatic, unsustained VT and frequent VPD's and for life-threatening arrhythmias, such as sustained VT. Flecainide is not currently indicated for atrial arrhythmias, but early studies suggest that, like encainide, it will have an important role in the future.

Class II Antiarrhythmic Drugs

PROPRANOLOL. Propranolol was the first beta blocker approved in the United States and has been on the market more than 20 years. Of the many beta-adrenergic–blocking drugs now approved for use, only acebutolol, propranolol, timolol, and esmolol are approved for the treatment of arrhythmias, and only propranolol, timolol, and metoprolol are indicated to reduce cardiovascular mortality after myocardial infarction. There are many significant differences among the beta-adrenergic–blocking agents in terms of cardioselectivity, intrinsic sympathomimetic action, electrophysiologic effects, and pharmacokinetics.

Pharmacology. Beta blockers decrease automaticity in the sinus node and His-Purkinje systems when it is enhanced by sympathetic influences but have little effect when catecholamines are absent. Propranolol has little effect on phase 0 depolarization of cardiac fibers at low concentrations. At high concentrations, i.e., 1000 to 3000 ng per milliliter, phase 0 depolarization is depressed. Propranolol shortens, whereas other beta blockers can prolong, action potential duration in atrial, ventricular, and particularly His-Purkinje cells; these effects are unrelated to beta-blocking activity. In humans, propranolol and other beta blockers increase the ERP of the AV node, a major antiarrhythmic effect but have little effect on atrial or ventricular refractoriness.

Indications. Propranolol is indicated for supraventricular arrhythmias, particularly those induced by catecholamines or those associated with the WPW syndrome or thyrotoxicosis; for symptomatic APD's; and for control of the ventricular rate in atrial flutter or fibrillation. It is also indicated for ventricular arrhythmias caused by catecholamines. Propranolol or another beta blocker is often chosen for the treatment of symptomatic but benign VPD's.

Class III Antiarrhythmic Drugs

AMIODARONE. Amiodarone is a benzofuran derivative, 37 per cent iodine by weight, originally developed as a smooth muscle relaxant and coronary vasodilator to treat angina pectoris. In 1986, amiodarone was approved by the United States Food and Drug Administration (FDA) as a last-resort treatment for malignant ventricular arrhythmias. There have been no controlled studies of its efficacy.

Pharmacology. Amiodarone substantially prolongs action potential duration and ERP in atrium, ventricle, and Purkinje fibers (a class III action). Amiodarone slows sinus rate by a direct effect. Under laboratory conditions, amiodarone can have a substantial class I effect. In humans, amiodarone slows the sinus rate, and it increases the PR and QT intervals in the ECG, with less effect on the QRS. In addition, it increases the atrial, AV nodal, and ventricular refractory periods and prolongs the HV intervals.

Indications. Amiodarone is indicated only for treatment of recurrent ventricular fibrillation or recurrent, hemodynamically unstable, sustained VT that has not responded to documented adequate doses of other antiarrhythmic drugs or when alternative agents cannot be tolerated. Treatment must be assessed by a method with high predictive accuracy. Endocardial electrical stimulation is the method of choice. About 20 per cent of patients with inducible VT can be rendered uninducible, and these patients do very well. In another 40 to 50 per cent, the VT rate slows enough to prevent significant symptoms during sustained VT. In this group, recurrences of VT are not reduced much but usually are not fatal. Patients who have inducible symptomatic, sustained VT after being loaded with amiodarone should be considered for some alternate treatment. Because of the serious nature of the arrhythmias for which amiodarone is indicated and the unpredictable time course of effect, amiodarone should be started in a monitored hospital setting.

BRETYLIUM TOSYLATE. Bretylium is a postganglionic adrenergic neuron blocker approved for intramuscular or intravenous use as an antiarrhythmic drug.

Pharmacology. Bretylium causes marked lengthening of the action potential duration and ERP of ventricular muscle and Purkinje fibers (class III action). It is selectively taken up in peripheral adrenergic nerves and causes the acute release of norepinephrine; later, it produces chemical sympathectomy, preventing the norepinephrine release during nerve action potentials. Bretylium has no significant effect on phase 0 depolarization or conduction (i.e., it has no class I action), but it does increase the ventricular fibrillation threshold. Bretylium does not depress myocardial performance but can cause severe postural hypotension by interfering with the efferent limb of the baroreceptor reflex arc.

Indications. Bretylium is indicated for the therapy and prophylaxis of ventricular fibrillation and for the treatment of life-threatening ventricular arrhythmias, e.g., sustained VT, that have failed to respond to first-line antiarrhythmic drugs, e.g., lidocaine. Use of bretylium should be restricted to intensive care units. Ventricular fibrillation usually responds within minutes, whereas the full effect on unsustained VT and VPD's takes hours.

Class IV Antiarrhythmic Drugs

VERAPAMIL. Verapamil is a papaverine derivative long used as a coronary vasodilator. Later, its calcium channel–blocking properties were discovered, and in 1981 it was approved for treatment of angina pectoris and supraventricular arrhythmias.

Pharmacology. Verapamil slows spontaneous firing in isolated sinus node preparations; the effect is less marked in vivo because of reflex sympathetic nervous activity by peripheral vasodilation. Verapamil decreases normal automaticity in Purkinje fibers and abolishes delayed afterdepolarizations and triggered activity in experimental digitalis toxicity. It prolongs refractoriness and conduction in the AV node by blocking Ca^{++} channels. This action accounts for the ability of verapamil to terminate and prevent PSVT. Verapamil can abolish experimental VT due to slow potentials. In addition, it can delay ischemic injury and prevent arrhythmogenic electrophysiologic effects caused by transient ischemia. Verapamil also has alpha-adrenergic–blocking properties. In humans, verapamil slows the heart rate and increases the PR interval without any change in the QRS and QTc.

Indications. Intravenous verapamil is indicated for a rapid conversion of PSVT to sinus rhythm (see Table 45–11). The quick effectiveness of verapamil has made it a drug of first choice in emergency rooms and offices. Verapamil should not be given to patients with wide QRS tachycardias until the rhythm is *proven* to be PSVT.

Verapamil can provide temporary control of rapid ventricular rate in atrial fibrillation. A 5- to 10-mg IV dose of verapamil will slow the ventricular rate about 20 per cent for 15 to 30 minutes while a more permanent treatment is being established. Verapamil can be used orally to prevent PSVT or help to control the ventricular rate in atrial flutter or fibrillation.

Bigger JT Jr, Hoffman BF: Antiarrhythmic Drugs. In Gilman AG, Goodman LS, Rall TW, et al. (eds.): The Pharmacological Basis of Therapeutics. 7th ed. New York, The Macmillan Company, 1985, pp 748–783. *A concise summary of the pharmacology and clinical use of antiarrhythmic drugs. Selectively referenced.*

Siddoway LA, Roden DM, Woosley RL: Clinical pharmacology of old and new antiarrhythmic drugs. Cardiovasc Clin 15:199, 1985. *A discussion of the pharmacodynamics, pharmacokinetics, drug interactions, and clinical use of antiarrhythmic drugs. Extensively referenced.*

ELECTRICAL DEVICES IN THE MANAGEMENT OF CARDIAC ARRHYTHMIAS

Temporary or permanent cardiac pacemakers and DC cardioversion or external defibrillation are well-established forms of electrical therapy. In 1985, an automatic implantable cardioverter defibrillator was approved by the FDA.

Cardiac Pacemakers

Permanent pacemakers were first implanted in the 1960's, and over the ensuing 25 years, the pacemaker industry has matured, providing highly sophisticated and diverse products for the management of bradyarrhythmias, and, to a lesser extent, tachyarrhythmias. About 100,000 pulse generators are implanted each year in the United States, about one half of the world's pacemaker implants. There are approximately 500,000 patients with pacemakers living in the United States.

INDICATIONS FOR CARDIAC PACING. The joint report of the American College of Cardiology and American Heart Association grouped pacemaker use into three classes: I, definitely indicated; II, possibly indicated; and III, not indicated (see Table 45–12). Pacing is indicated for bradycardia

TABLE 45–12. DEFINITE INDICATIONS FOR IMPLANTED PACEMAKER

A. Complete heart block, permanent or intermittent, with any one of the following complications:
   1. Symptomatic bradycardia
   2. Congestive heart failure
   3. Conditions that require treatment with drugs that suppress ventricular escape rhythms
   4. Asystole ≥ 3 seconds or ventricular rate <40 per minute
   5. Mental confusion that clears with pacing

B. Patients with complete heart block or advanced second-degree AV block that persists after myocardial infarction

C. Chronic bi- or trifascicular block with intermittent complete heart block or type II second-degree AV block associated with symptomatic bradycardia

D. Sinus node dysfunction with documented symptomatic bradycardia

E. Hypersensitive carotid sinus syndrome with recurrent syncope and asystole >3 seconds provoked by minimal carotid sinus pressure

F. Symptomatic supraventricular tachycardia that does not respond to medical treatment

with complete heart block or advanced second-degree AV block with symptoms such as transient dizziness, light-headedness, near syncope or syncope, marked exercise intolerance, or congestive heart failure. Asymptomatic conditions that are definite indications are permanent high-grade AV block after myocardial infarction or surgical repair of congenital heart disease, or complete heart block with a ventricular rate of less than 40 per minute.

LEAD PLACEMENT. More than 90 per cent of permanent pacing leads are placed via cephalic, subclavian, or external jugular veins. Most transvenous leads are stainless steel, multifilament, helical coil wires insulated with polyurethane or silicone rubber. These leads are small, steerable, and fracture resistant. Leads are anchored by tines or a screw-in arrangement at their tips. Both unipolar and bipolar electrodes are commonly used. For simple ventricular pacing, one lead is placed in the right ventricular apex. For dual chamber pacing, a second lead is placed in the right atrium.

PULSE GENERATORS. Modern pacemaker generators weigh 40 to 50 gm, are powered by lithium batteries that last seven to 10 years, and have circuitry for sensing intracardiac electrograms. Pacemakers can be interrogated to evaluate the pulse generator or reprogrammed to meet changing requirements. Multiprogrammability provides flexibility in obtaining diagnostic information and individualizing the pacemaker prescription.

MODES OF CARDIAC PACING. Pacemaker modes are expressed in the three- or five-letter notation proposed by the Inter-Society Commission for Heart Disease Resources. Table 45–13 shows the first three letter codes. The three letters indicate the chamber paced, the chamber sensed, and the response to sensing. The fourth and fifth positions describe programmable and antitachycardia features and are used less frequently.

SELECTION OF THE PACEMAKER MODE. Selection of the appropriate pacemaker has become more complex as options have become more diverse. Table 45–14 summarizes common selections, considering the atrial rhythm and status of AV and VA conduction.

Rate-Responsive Pacing. Many patients who would benefit from heart rate increase during exercise have relative contraindications for DDD pacing (see footnote, Table 45–14), e.g., inadequate sinus node function of atrial fibrillation. Rate-responsive pacing can be provided by sensing activity with a piezoelectric accelerometer mounted in the pulse generator case. Heart rate can be increased by as much as 90 per minute, i.e., from 60 at rest to 150 during exercise. Cardiac output and the patient's ability to perform daily activities also increase.

COMPLICATIONS. Transvenous implants are associated with cardiac perforation, arrhythmias, infection, thrombosis, emboli, and lead pipe fracture or displacement. Thoracotomy carries the risk of general anesthesia, bleeding, infection, postoperative respiratory compromise, and late threshold increases. With either route of implantation, the pulse generator may erode through the skin. Pacemakers can be inhibited by intense magnetic fields such as large telephone transformers, microwave devices, diathermy, cautery, antitheft devices, and certain types of motors, e.g., electric razors. Unipolar pacemakers may be inhibited by local myopotentials.

The "pacemaker syndrome" was first defined as light-headedness or syncope related to long cycles of AV asynchrony that occurred during VOO or VVI pacing. The definition also includes (1) episodic weakness or syncope associated with alternating AV synchrony and asynchrony; (2) inadequate cardiac output associated with continued absence of AV synchrony or with fixed asynchrony (persistent VA conduction); and (3) the patient's awareness of beat-to-beat variation in vascular pulsation.

PACEMAKER FOLLOW-UP. Implanted pacing devices require careful follow-up. Regular transtelephonic monitoring permits early detection of battery depletion. At the present time, the principal problem in pacemaker follow-up is the

TABLE 45–13. CODE FOR PACEMAKER MODES

Chamber Paced	Chamber Sensed	Mode of Response
V = Ventricle	V = Ventricle	I = Inhibited
A = Atrium	A = Atrium	T = Triggered
D = Double (atrium and ventricle)	D = Double (atrium and ventricle)	D = Double (atrium triggered and ventricle inhibited)
	O = None	R = Reserve
		O = None

TABLE 45–14. INDICATIONS FOR PACING MODES

	Atrial Rhythm		
AV Conduction	*Normal*	*Bradycardia*	*Bradycardia-Tachycardia*
Normal	None indicated	AAI	AAI
AV block; normal VA conduction time	VDD, DDD	DDD, DVI	DVI, VVI
AV block; prolonged VA conduction time	DVI	DVI	DVI

AAI: Fixed-rate atrial pacing occurs unless inhibited by sensed atrial depolarizations. This mode can be used for patients with symptomatic sinus node dysfunction and normal AV conduction.

VDD: Ventricular pulses are delivered when atrial depolarization is sensed and inhibited when ventricular depolarization is sensed. The VDD mode is used when adequate atrial rates and sensing are present, along with high-grade AV block and normal VA conduction. VDD pacing provides atrial augmentation of ventricular filling and avoids the pacemaker syndrome but is contraindicated for patients with supraventricular tachyarrhythmias.

DVI: Both chambers are paced at a preselected rate and AV interval. Pacing is inhibited by ventricular, but not atrial, activity. The DVI mode is used when synchronous AV contraction is needed in patients with symptomatic atrial bradycardia. The pacing rate does not increase during exercise. DVI pacing is contraindicated in patients who have supraventricular tachyarrhythmias.

DDD: Both atria and ventricles are paced and sensed. The atrial or ventricular pacemaker pulses are inhibited when either atrial or ventricular premature activity is detected. When atrial activity is sensed, a ventricular pulse is provided. This mode of pacing provides synchronous AV contraction over a wide range of heart rates. DDD pacemakers are adaptive: totally inhibited in sinus rhythm with normal AV conduction; AAI pacing during sinus bradycardia with normal AV conduction; VDD pacing during sinus rhythm with impaired AV conduction; DVI pacing during sinus bradycardia with impaired AV conduction. DDD pacemakers are contraindicated in patients with persistent or frequently occurring atrial tachyarrhythmias and those with long VA conduction times who can develop pacemaker-mediated reciprocating tachycardia.

VVI: This mode can be used for any symptomatic bradyarrhythmia. The VVI mode is contraindicated in patients who have had the pacemaker syndrome (see text), those with congestive heart failure, or in those who need rate-responsive pacing.

diversity of pacemaker models and methods for interrogating pacemaker function.

DC Cardioversion

DC cardioversion was introduced in 1962 and has become a mainstay in the management of cardiac arrhythmias. Cardioversion depolarizes all or most of the heart, interrupts reentrant circuits, and terminates arrhythmias. It is effective for atrial fibrillation, atrial flutter, PSVT, ventricular tachycardia, or ventricular fibrillation. Drug-resistant arrhythmias, e.g., atrial flutter, may respond readily to DC cardioversion. Because of its speed, cardioversion is preferable to drug therapy for arrhythmias that adversely affect hemodynamics, such as rapid atrial arrhythmias, sustained ventricular tachycardia, or ventricular fibrillation. Elective cardioversion is indicated for atrial fibrillation of recent onset (< 6 months) to control symptoms and hemodynamic abnormalities and to lower the risk of systemic embolism.

LIMITATIONS AND CONTRAINDICATIONS. Chronic atrial fibrillation, i.e., that greater than 6 to 12 months in duration, is so likely to recur after cardioversion that digitalis therapy may be preferred. Contributing causes, e.g., hyperthyroidism, pericardial inflammation, pulmonary thromboembolism, chronic obstructive pulmonary disease, or alcohol abuse, should be controlled before cardioversion; otherwise, atrial fibrillation is likely to recur. Sinus rhythm is difficult to maintain after cardioversion of atrial fibrillation in patients with heart failure or large left atria (> 45 mm in diameter by echocardiography). In the bradycardia-tachycardia syndrome, cardioversion often produces inadequate rhythms and atrial fibrillation usually resumes within a few hours. Cardioversion is contraindicated for arrhythmias caused by digitalis intoxication because it can precipitate ventricular fibrillation.

ANTICOAGULATION. Despite the lack of controlled evaluation, most patients who have been fibrillating for more than three weeks are treated with anticoagulants before cardioversion, particularly those with (1) a history of embolization, (2) a prosthetic mitral valve, (3) an enlarged left atrium, or (4) congestive heart failure. The prothrombin time is kept at 2.5 times the normal value with warfarin for about three weeks before and a week after cardioversion.

RESULTS. The immediate results of cardioversion are excellent (Table 45–15). The main long-term problem is reversion to atrial fibrillation. Class I antiarrhythmic drugs decrease the chance of recurrence of atrial fibrillation one year after cardioversion from about 75 to 50 per cent.

COMPLICATIONS. Few complications attend technically excellent cardioversion. Occasionally, transient SA or AV block or ventricular arrhythmias occur immediately after DC shock, especially when digitalis dosage is excessive. In the sick sinus syndrome, the sinus may fail to resume control of cardiac rhythm after cardioversion. Atropine, isoproterenol, and/or external pacing usually will maintain the patient until a temporary transvenous pacemaker can be inserted. Occasionally, worsening heart failure or frank pulmonary edema occurs within a few hours after cardioversion. The cause of this syndrome is unknown. Elevation of myocardial creatine kinase after DC cardioversion is rare.

TABLE 45–15. ENERGY FOR CARDIOVERSION/DEFIBRILLATION

Arrhythmia	Recommended Initial Energy* (joules)	Comments
Atrial flutter	50	100% conversion; most will convert with about 25 joules.
Atrial fibrillation	200	85–95% conversion; a few patients may require 300–400 joule DC shocks to cardiovert.
Paroxysmal supraventricular tachycardia	100	100% conversion
Ventricular tachycardia	50	90–95% conversion; 80% will convert with <10 joules, but a few need 100 joules or more.
Ventricular fibrillation	300–400	90–95% defibrillation; many will convert at 200 joules or below, but time is of the essence in successful defibrillation.

*An energy level with a high probability of converting the arrhythmia

Automatic Implantable Cardioverter Defibrillator

The first automatic implantable defibrillator (AID), a device that responded only to ventricular fibrillation, was implanted in 1980. The first automatic implantable cardioverter defibrillator (AICD) was implanted in 1982. This unit detects and cardioverts ventricular tachycardia as well as providing defibrillation.

INDICATIONS. The AICD is recommended for patients who have had a documented episode of life-threatening ventricular tachyarrhythmia or cardiac arrest not associated with the acute phase of myocardial infarction. In addition, patients should have inducible ventricular tachycardia or ventricular fibrillation unsuitable for drug or surgical therapy.

IMPLANTATION. The electrode systems are implanted via a thoracotomy. The 292-gram power unit is implanted subcutaneously in an abdominal pocket. During implantation, defibrillation thresholds and detection of ventricular tachycardia/fibrillation are tested extensively to ensure proper function. The AICD usually lasts 18 to 24 months or 100 discharges.

The device monitors the ECG continuously. When ventricular tachycardia of fibrillation is detected and verified, the AICD charges its capacitors and delivers a 20- to 30-joule pulse.

FOLLOW-UP. The AICD is a complex device that requires careful follow-up. Potential problems with the device include (1) depletion of the battery, (2) lead breakage or migration, (3) inappropriate discharges, (4) infection, and (5) skin erosion. After implantation, a magnet test should be performed every two months to evaluate the device and reform the capacitors.

Between 1980 and the end of 1986, more than 1000 AID or AICD units were implanted. Follow-up reveals a one-year cardiovascular mortality of about 10 per cent and a sudden death rate of about 2 per cent. Although the device is complex and expensive, it is highly effective for selected patients with malignant ventricular arrhythmias.

DeSilva RA, Graboys TB, Podrid PJ, et al.: Cardioversion and defibrillation. Am Heart J 100:881, 1980. *A thorough review of the history, theory, and practice of cardioversion and defibrillation.*

Echt DS, Armstrong K, Schmidt P, et al.: Clinical experience, complications, and survival in 70 patients with the automatic implantable cardioverter/defibrillator. Circulation 71:289, 1985. *A description of a large experience with the implantable defibrillator. Provides an excellent perspective on the current use of the device.*

Frye RL, Collins JJ, DeSanctis RW, et al.: Guidelines for permanent cardiac pacemaker implantation, May 1984. J Am Coll Cardiol 4:434, 1984. *A report of a task force to review cardiac pacing. The report defines current indications for cardiac pacing and makes recommendations about the selection of devices for treatment of specific clinical problems. This report is used as a standard by the medical profession, regulatory agencies, and reimbursement sources.*

Mirowski M: The automatic implantable cardioverter-defibrillator: An overview. J Am Coll Cardiol 6:461, 1985. *A review of the concepts, evolution, clinical use, and follow-up of the automatic implantable cardioverter defibrillator by the originator of the device.*

Parsonnet V, Bernstein AD: Pacing in perspective: Concepts and controversies. Circulation 73:1087, 1986. *A perspective on cardiac pacing. Provides a concise view of the history, development, current practice, and future directions in cardiac pacing.*

TABLE 45–16. SURGERY FOR CARDIAC ARRHYTHMIAS

Arrhythmia	Operative Approach
Atrial fibrillation	Ablation of AV node and implantation of a pacemaker; left atrial exclusion (highly experimental)
Ectopic atrial focus	Excision of the focus after accurate mapping
PSVT (Pre-excitation)	Surgical division of anomalous AV connection
PSVT (AV nodal)	Partial catheter ablation of AV node; division of His bundle and implantation of pacemaker
Ventricular tachycardia (coronary heart disease)	Endocardial resection guided by mapping
Ventricular tachycardia (arrhythmogenic right ventricular dysplasia)	Simple ventriculotomy; isolation of arrhythmic site
Ventricular tachycardia (after repair of tetralogy of Fallot)	Resection of infundibulectomy scar
Multiform ventricular tachycardia (long QT syndrome)	Left stellate ganglionectomy

PSVT = paroxysmal supraventricular tachycardia.

SURGICAL TREATMENT OF CARDIAC ARRHYTHMIAS

The objective of arrhythmia surgery (Table 45–16) may be (1) to remove the arrhythmic focus, (2) to interrupt a re-entrant pathway, or (3) to prevent the ventricles from responding to supraventricular tachyarrhythmias. For surgery to be seriously considered, the arrhythmia must pose significant risk to life or interfere substantially with the quality of life.

Supraventricular Arrhythmias

INTERRUPTION OF THE BUNDLE OF HIS. Atrial flutter and fibrillation can be palliated by interruption of the His bundle and implantation of a ventricular pacemaker when drug therapy cannot control ventricular rate. The need for such surgery has diminished with the advent of beta-adrenergic blockers, verapamil, and catheter ablation.

Catheter Ablation. Recently, a catheter technique for His bundle ablation has been found to be safe and effective. With the use of fluoroscopy, a multielectrode catheter is placed so as to record the bundle of His depolarization. Then, one or more large energy shocks are delivered to the electrode (cathode) that records the largest His bundle depolarization. Shocks can be repeated until AV conduction is interrupted.

REMOVAL OF AUTOMATIC FOCI. Automatic or tiny re-entrant ectopic foci can be excised or ablated. The key to removal or ablation is accurate localization by epicardial and/or endocardial activation mapping.

INTERRUPTION OF RE-ENTRANT PATHWAYS. Surgery is very effective for paroxysmal supraventricular tachycardia (PSVT) that uses an anomalous AV connection as an essential portion of the circuit or for atrial fibrillation with rapid ventricular response in the Wolff-Parkinson-White syndrome. Preoperative electrophysiologic studies delineate the mechanism of PSVT, the site of the accessory AV connection, and the route of cardiac excitation during PSVT. During operation, the anomalous AV connection or connections are located precisely using cardiac stimulation and epicardial or endocardial mapping during sinus rhythm, ventricular pacing, and PSVT. Traditionally, division of anomalous AV connections is done on cardiopulmonary bypass with the atrium open. More recently, dissection and cryoablation have been used successfully without cardiopulmonary bypass. Centers with major programs obtain cure rates of greater than 85 per cent with surgical mortalities of less than 1 per cent. These results usually make surgery a better choice than drug treatment.

Sustained Ventricular Tachycardia

VENTRICULAR ANEURYSMS. The largest surgical experience has been gathered in patients with recurrent, sustained ventricular tachycardia (VT) and coronary heart disease; most of these patients have left ventricular aneurysms, two- or three-vessel disease, and severely impaired left ventricular function. The rate of VT tends to be slow and easily induced and can be mapped during electrophysiologic studies. Accurate preoperative endocardial maps are critical because adequate maps are often impossible to obtain at surgery. At surgery, the arrhythmogenic tissue is removed or ablated with a cryoprobe. Map-guided excision, isolation, or cryoablation is about 80 per cent effective in controlling sustained VT during one to three years of follow-up. However, the perioperative mortality is about 15 to 20 per cent, primarily because of advanced coronary disease and severity of left ventricular dysfunction.

ARRHYTHMOGENIC RIGHT VENTRICULAR DYSPLASIA. Patients who have VT due to right ventricular arrhythmogenic dysplasia usually can be cured by an incision across the dysplastic area that shows the latest activation in sinus rhythm and earliest activation during VT. Small areas of dysplasia can be excised, and large areas can be isolated if simple incision is not feasible.

TETRALOGY OF FALLOT. Ventricular tachycardia occurs rarely in patients who have had total repair of tetralogy of Fallot. Epicardial excitation mapping at surgery shows that VT arises in the right ventricular infundibular scar and scar resection effects a cure.

LONG QT SYNDROME. Patients with the congenital form of the long QT syndrome can have recurrent attacks of malignant, multiform VT of the torsades de pointes type. These rhythms are associated with cardiac arrest and sudden cardiac death. Unequal sympathetic nerve traffic to the heart is part of the explanation for the heterogeneous electrophysiologic condition of the ventricles. Excision of the left stellate ganglion markedly reduces the mortality rate in high-risk patients with the congenital long QT syndrome.

Cox JL, Gallagher JJ, Cain MM: Experience with 118 consecutive patients undergoing operation for the Wolff-Parkinson-White syndrome. J Thorac Cardiovasc Surg 90:490, 1985. *A review of a large, successful experience with surgery for anomalous AV connections.*

Cox JL: The status of surgery for cardiac arrhythmias. Circulation 71:413, 1985. *A perspective on surgery for both supraventricular and ventricular arrhythmias.*

Klein GJ, Guiraudon GM: Surgical therapy of cardiac arrhythmias. Cardiol Clin 1:323, 1983. *A summary of present and future concepts that form the basis for surgical treatment of cardiac arrhythmias.*

46 SUDDEN CARDIAC DEATH

James T. Willerson

DEFINITION AND FREQUENCY. The definition of *sudden cardiac death* used in this chapter is the sudden cessation of effective cardiac contraction resulting from ventricular tachycardia-fibrillation or asystole. Sudden cardiac death claims approximately 1200 lives daily in the United States. It is the leading cause of death among men between the ages of 20 and 60, and approximately 25 per cent of patients dying suddenly have had no previously recognized symptoms of heart disease. Sudden cardiac death among women is approximately one fourth as frequent as among men.

ETIOLOGY AND PATHOGENESIS. Important data regarding the individual who suffers sudden cardiac death come from the Seattle Heart Watch study. During a six-year period of 1710 episodes of ventricular fibrillation, there were 346 long-term survivors. Cobb has shown that most instances of sudden cardiac death are not related to identifiable acute myocardial infarcts, which were detected by electrocardiography in only 19 per cent of patients hospitalized after resuscitation from ventricular fibrillation. Nevertheless, the majority of individuals resuscitated have extensive coronary artery disease, including 75 per cent with multivessel involvement. Patients experiencing cardiac arrest without concomitant acute myocardial infarcts have a considerably higher incidence of recurrent sudden death in the next two years than do those with acute infarcts. The annual recurrence rate is approximately 30 per cent for those within acute infarcts.

It seems likely that the most critical etiologic factor is electrophysiologic instability related to chronic ischemic heart disease, cellular damage associated with cardiomyopathy, or chronic severe valvular heart disease. Since the frequency of recurrence of sudden death is high in those with chronic ischemic heart disease without acute infarcts, it is important to protect such patients with antiarrhythmic agents and, when appropriate, also with coronary artery revascularization and/or an internal cardiac defibrillator, or "antitachycardiac" pacemaker.

Most patients experiencing sudden death have chronic ischemic heart disease or chronic myocardial scarring and ventricular dysfunction. However, sudden death from ventricular arrhythmias occurs in some individuals with mitral valve prolapse, in some with left ventricular outflow obstruction, including valvular aortic stenosis and asymmetric septal hypertrophy, and in some with hereditary prolongation of the QT interval with or without associated deafness. Sudden death also occurs in individuals with various cardiomyopathies, in those with chronic valvular insufficiency and myocardial dilatation and/or hypertrophy, in those with cardiac tamponade, in some young athletes while they are exercising, and in an occasional individual suddenly aroused or frightened by an external event. Sudden death from a ventricular arrhythmia may also occur in the Wolff-Parkinson-White syndrome; in those with advanced atrioventricular block without pacemakers, or with diffuse conduction system disease ("sick sinus syndrome"); and in severe electrolyte alterations, including hypokalemia, hyperkalemia, and hypercalcemia. Drug overdose, particularly with cardiac glycosides, may also be a cause for sudden cardiac death. Additional causes for sudden death or death within a few hours that do not initially involve the heart include intracerebral or subarachnoid hemorrhage, pulmonary emboli, severe drug overdose, hypoxia associated with chronic obstructive lung disease or lung injury, dissecting aortic aneurysms, and rupture of an aortic aneurysm.

In order to reduce the frequency and risk of sudden death in susceptible individuals, at least two additional developments are needed: (1) better means to identify those at risk and (2) better understanding of mechanisms involved in ventricular tachycardia or fibrillation in susceptible patients. Although most patients who experience sudden death have heart disease, the risk factors for atherosclerosis do not singly or in combination identify a subset of patients prone to sudden death. The mechanism of sudden death is ordinarily ventricular fibrillation.

IDENTIFICATION OF HIGH-RISK PATIENTS. In patients with acute infarction, certain types of ventricular premature beats are considered precursors of ventricular fibrillation. In coronary care units, more than seven ventricular premature beats per minute, multiform ventricular premature beats, ventricular premature beats occurring on or close to the apex of the T wave, and runs of two or more ventricular premature beats are considered potential harbingers of ventricular tachycardia or fibrillation. These "malignant ventricular premature beats" are ordinarily suppressed by pharmacologic agents such as lidocaine. However, some patients with acute myocardial infarcts have ventricular tachycardia or fibrillation without precursor ventricular arrhythmias. Moreover, there is a relationship between recurrent ventricular tachycardia or fibrillation and the overall size of myocardial infarcts, such that patients with large infarcts may have recurrent ventricular (and supraventricular) arrhythmias.

In patients with chronic ischemic heart disease, only advanced grades or complex ventricular premature beats and the presence of important ventricular dysfunction predict sudden cardiac death. The frequency of sudden death and of ventricular premature complexes increases with age. In addition, the frequency of ventricular premature beats increases in relationship to the extent of ventricular damage from earlier myocardial infarcts. Ventricular ectopic activity is often more frequent and complex in patients with multivessel coronary artery disease than in those with only single-vessel involvement. Therefore, a knowledge of the extent of coronary disease and of ventricular dysfunction may be useful in predicting the risk of sudden death. Specifically, patients with a left ventricular ejection fraction of 40 per cent or less and (1) frequent ventricular premature beats ($\geq$ 8 per hour) and/or (2) complex ventricular premature beats have a several-fold increased risk of sudden death in the initial six months after myocardial infarction. An increased risk has also been claimed for patients demonstrating repetitive ventricular beating following ventricular stimulation. Dynamic myocardial scintigraphic characterization of ventricular function at rest and during submaximal exercise in patients with acute infarction before hospital discharge may identify those most at risk for future coronary events. Increasing in popularity are techniques that determine the efficacy of a particular antiarrhythmic regimen prior to hospital discharge in patients at risk, including electrophysiologic studies in a cardiac catheterization laboratory, which test individual vulnerability for sustained ventricular arrhythmias while the patient is on and off selected antiarrhythmic agents. This approach is important because merely administering an antiarrhythmic agent to a patient with the hope of preventing sudden death is often not successful. Schaffer and Cobb (1975) reported that 73 per cent of 64 patients with recurrent ventricular fibrillation were receiving antiarrhythmic therapy at the time of sudden death. This information emphasizes the need to select and optimize antiarrhythmic therapy for the individual patient. It is also important to realize that antiarrhythmic agents, particularly quinidine and procainamide (Pronestyl), given in normal doses to the patient with a prolonged QT interval, may cause life-threatening ventricular arrhythmias, including a ventricular tachycardia known as *torsade de pointes.* In addition, each of the available antiarrhythmic agents has a certain incidence of causing ventricular ectopic beats ("proarrhythmic effect") even when given at normal doses.

PREVENTION OF SUDDEN DEATH. Beta blockers without intrinsic sympathomimetic activity have been shown to reduce mortality from cardiac events in selected patients in the months to years after myocardial infarction. Left stellate ganglionectomy may also reduce the risk of sudden deaths in patients with hereditary prolongation of the QT interval and recurrent ventricular tachycardia and/or fibrillation. However, it is critically important that we develop an improved understanding of mechanisms that initiate and sustain life-threatening ventricular arrhythmias in patients in diverse clinical settings. Unanswered questions include the following: Do platelet aggregation and subsequent thromboxane A_2 and/or serotonin release play a role in leading to sudden death in patients with coronary artery disease but without identifiable acute myocardial infarction? Are the important ventricular arrhythmias that develop with acute myocardial ischemia related primarily to re-entrant mechanisms or to increased ventricular automaticity resulting in part from variations in regional concentrations of potassium or catecholamines, from alterations in autonomic nervous system activity, from alterations in adrenergic receptor numbers or affinity, or from local accumulation of phospholipid degradation products? It is important to determine why some individuals with chronic congestive heart failure and others with chronic cardiomegaly and ventricular dysfunction are at risk of sudden death from ventricular arrhythmias. It is not clear at present whether increased triglyceride uptake and the inability of injured myocardial cells to metabolize long-chain fatty acids contribute to the ventricular arrhythmias of ischemic heart disease. Specific myocardial cellular mechanisms associated with increased risk of ventricular arrhythmias need to be elucidated, as does the role of psychologic stress in the initiation of ventricular arrhythmias in humans.

Extensive efforts are being made to develop more effective means of correcting recurrent and life-threatening ventricular arrhythmias. New antiarrhythmic agents are being developed and tested but still unavailable is one or more agents with (1) marked efficacy against ventricular and supraventricular arrhythmias, (2) few or no important side effects, and (3) the need for relatively infrequent administration, i.e., once per day. Amiodarone has proved to be useful in the control of recurrent ventricular tachycardia when other antiarrhythmic agents have failed, but there is a relatively high risk of important side effects, including pneumonitis and pulmonary fibrosis, in patients treated with this agent. Surgical resection of ventricular sites of ectopic impulse formation has been successfully utilized following epicardial and endocardial "activation mapping" in the treatment of patients with sustained ventricular tachycardia. Surgical revascularization has been successful in reducing mortality from ventricular dysrhythmias in selected patients with extensive coronary artery stenoses. Mirowski has developed an implantable automatic defibrillator capable of identifying and then spontaneously discharging and converting ventricular tachycardia-fibrillation to sinus rhythm. This device is useful in allowing prompt conversion of life-threatening ventricular arrhythmias when adequate control is not provided by antiarrhythmic agents and the patient is clearly at risk for sudden death. Implantable, programmable pacemakers capable of sensing and correcting ventricular tachyarrhythmias by rapid and brief pacing have also been developed and are alternative methods for treating high-risk patients.

Bigger JT Jr., Fleiss JL, Kleiger R, et al.: The relationships among ventricular arrhythmias, left ventricular dysfunction, and mortality in the 2 years after myocardial infarction. Circulation 69:250, 1984. *A thorough review of these relationships.*

Cobb LA, Baun RS, Alvarez H III, et al.: Resuscitation from out-of-hospital ventricular fibrillation: 4 year follow-up. Circulation 51, 52(Suppl III):III, 1975. *A follow-up of patients following resuscitation from sudden death.*

Doyle JT, Kannel WB, McNamara RM, et al.: Factors related to the suddenness of death from coronary disease: Combined Albany-Framingham Studies. Am J Cardiol 37:1073, 1976. *An epidemiologic study of factors involved in sudden death.*

Hoffman BF, Dangman KH: The role of antiarrhythmic drugs in sudden cardiac death. J Am Coll Cardiol 8:104A, 1986. *A thorough description of the relative advantages and disadvantages of antiarrhythmic agents.*

Horowitz LN, Harken AH, Kastor JA, et al.: Ventricular resection guided by epicardial and endocardial mapping for treatment of recurrent ventricular tachycardia. N Engl J Med 302:589, 1980. *Aggressive but effective surgical techniques for abolishing ventricular rhythm disturbances are described.*

Kannel WB, Doyle JT, McNamara PM, et al.: Precursors of sudden coronary death: Factors related to incidence of sudden death. Circulation 51:606, 1975. *A review of risk factors related to sudden death.*

Lown B: Sudden cardiac death: The major challenge confronting contemporary cardiology. Am J Cardiol 43:313, 1979. *A thorough review of this subject.*

Mirowski M, Reid PR, Mower MM, et al.: Termination of malignant ventricular arrhythmias in man with an implanted defibrillator. N Engl J Med 303:322, 1980. *The development of an implantable defibrillator is described.*

Mukharji J, Rude RE, Poole K, et al.: Risk factors for sudden death after acute myocardial infarction: Two-year follow-up. Am J Cardiol 54:31, 1984. *Patients with recent myocardial infarction and left ventricular ejection fractions < 40 per cent and > 8 ventricular beats per hour are at increased risk of sudden death.*

Willerson JT: Prevention and control of ventricular arrhythmias (editorial). N Engl J Med 303:332, 1980. *A review of the prevention and control of sudden death.*

47 ARTERIAL HYPERTENSION

Suzanne Oparil

DEFINITION

Arterial hypertension is defined as elevated arterial blood pressure (BP). Since BP in the general population falls on a gaussian curve of normal distribution, it is not possible to define with precision the limits of "normal" BP. In addition, the BP of a given individual varies widely over time, depending on many variables, including sympathetic activity, posture, state of hydration, and skeletal muscle tone. Accordingly, any definition of hypertension must be arbitrary. The Joint National Committee on Detection, Evaluation and Treatment of High Blood Pressure recommends the scheme shown in Table 47–1 for the diagnosis of hypertension in patients aged 18 years or older. The diagnosis of hypertension in adults is made when the average of two or more diastolic BP measurements on at least two subsequent visits is 90 mm Hg or higher or when the average of multiple systolic BP readings on two or more subsequent visits is consistently greater than 140 mm Hg (Table 47–2). The patient should be clearly informed that a single elevated reading does not constitute a diagnosis of hypertension but is a sign that further observation is required (Table 47–3).

Essential, or primary, hypertension is arterial hypertension of unknown cause. Over 95 per cent of all cases of arterial hypertension are in this category.

Secondary hypertension is arterial hypertension of known cause. Fewer than 5 per cent of all cases of systemic hypertension are in this category. The importance of identifying patients with secondary hypertension is that they sometimes may be cured by surgery or can be easily controlled by specific medical treatment. Thus the morbidity and mortality of potentially ineffective empiric medical therapy can be avoided and the cumulative cost of medical treatment reduced. The most common causes of secondary hypertension are summarized in Table 47–4.

Benign hypertension is a descriptive term for uncomplicated hypertension, usually of long duration and mild-to-moderate severity. Benign hypertension may be primary or secondary.

Malignant hypertension is the syndrome of markedly elevated BP (diastolic BP usually > 140 mm Hg) associated with papilledema. Accelerated hypertension is the syndrome of markedly elevated BP associated with hemorrhages and exu-

TABLE 47–1. CLASSIFICATION OF BP

Range (mm Hg)	Category*
Diastolic	
< 85	Normal BP
85–89	High normal BP
90–104	Mild hypertension
105–114	Moderate hypertension
≥ 115	Severe hypertension
Systolic, when diastolic BP is < 90	
< 140	Normal BP
140–159	Borderline isolated systolic hypertension
≥ 160	Isolated systolic hypertension

*A classification of borderline isolated systolic hypertension (systolic BP, 140 to 159 mm Hg) or isolated systolic hypertension (systolic BP, > 160 mm Hg) takes precedence over a classification of high normal BP (diastolic BP, 85 to 89 mm Hg) when both occur in the same person. A classification of high normal BP (diastolic BP, 85 to 89 mm Hg) takes precedence over a classification of normal BP (systolic BP, < 140 mm Hg) when both occur in the same person.

Reprinted with permission from The 1984 Report of the Joint National Committee on Detection, Evaluation, and Treatment of High Blood Pressure. Arch Intern Med 144:1045, 1984.

TABLE 47–2. FOLLOW-UP CRITERIA FOR FIRST-OCCASION MEASUREMENT

Range (mm Hg)	Recommended Follow-Up*
Diastolic	
< 85	Recheck within 2 yr
85–89	Recheck within 1 yr
90–104	Confirm promptly (not to exceed 2 mo)
105–114	Evaluate or refer promptly to source of care (not to exceed 2 wk)
≥ 115	Evaluate or refer immediately to a source of care
Systolic, when diastolic BP is < 90	
< 40	Recheck within 2 yr
140–199	Confirm promptly (not to exceed 2 mo)
≥ 200	Evaluate or refer promptly to source of care (not to exceed 2 wk)

*If recommendations for follow-up of diastolic and systolic BP's are different for those aged 18 years or older, the shorter recommended time period supersedes and a referral supersedes a recheck recommendation.

Reprinted with permission from The 1984 Report of the Joint National Committee on Detection, Evaluation, and Treatment of High Blood Pressure. Arch Intern Med 144:1045, 1984.

dates (grade 3 Kimmelstiel-Wilson [K-W] retinopathy). If untreated, accelerated hypertension presumably progresses to a malignant phase. Both the accelerated and the malignant types of hypertension are associated with widespread degenerative changes in the walls of resistance vessels. They are usually characterized by extreme BP elevations, sudden onset, a fulminant course, and evidence of severe, generalized vascular damage, including grade 3 or 4 K-W retinopathy, hypertensive encephalopathy, hematuria, and renal dysfunction. Malignant hypertension is usually fatal unless treated promptly and vigorously. If BP can be controlled, prognosis depends on the state of renal function.

Complicated hypertension is the descriptive term for arterial hypertension of any etiology in which there is evidence of cardiovascular damage related to the BP elevation. Hypertensive complications commonly include stroke, congestive heart failure, renal failure, myocardial infarction, and arterial aneurysm.

Labile hypertension, sometimes referred to as prehypertension or the hyperkinetic heart syndrome, is a descriptive term for intermittent hypertension in which some BP measurements are elevated and some are normal in the untreated patient. Patients with labile hypertension tend to maintain pressures that are above average for the general population and are at greater risk of cardiovascular morbidity and mortality than the general population. As a group, these patients manifest increased cardiac output, more rapid heart rate, and higher left ventricular ejection rate than either the normotensive population or the population of patients with stable hypertension. The proportion of such patients who go on to develop sustained hypertension and secondary vascular damage varies from 10 to 70 per cent in published series.

TABLE 47–3. FOLLOW-UP CRITERIA FOR SECOND-OCCASION MEASUREMENT

Range (mm Hg)	Recommended Follow-Up*
Diastolic	
< 85	Recheck within 2 yr†
85–89	Recheck within 1 yr
≥ 90	Evaluate or refer promptly to a source of care
Systolic, when diastolic BP is < 90	
< 140	Recheck within 1 yr
≥ 140	Evaluate or refer promptly to a source of care

*If recommendations for follow-up of diastolic and systolic BP's are different for those aged 18 or older, the shorter recommended time period supersedes and a referral supersedes a recheck recommendation.

†Rechecking within one year is recommended for persons at increased risk of progressing to higher BP's, including family history of hypertension or cardiovascular event, weight gain or obesity, black race, use of an oral contraceptive, and excessive ethanol consumption.

Reprinted with permission from The 1984 Report of the Joint National Committee on Detection, Evaluation, and Treatment of High Blood Pressure. Arch Intern Med 144:1045, 1984.

TABLE 47–4. CAUSES OF SECONDARY HYPERTENSION

Systolic and diastolic hypertension
- Renal vascular disease
- Renal parenchymal disease
- Renin-secreting tumors
- Syndromes of mineralocorticoid excess
  - Primary aldosteronism
  - Overproduction of 11-deoxycorticosterone (DOC), 18-OH DOC, and other mineralocorticoids without accompanying defects in steroid synthesis
  - Congenital adrenal hyperplasia
  - Ingestion of licorice of carbenoxolone
- Pheochromocytoma
- Oral contraceptives
- Pregnancy
- Coarctation of the aorta
- Cushing's syndrome
- Hyperparathyroidism
- Acromegaly
- Increased intracranial pressure
- Open heart surgery

Isolated systolic hypertension
- Aging
- Decreased peripheral vascular resistance
  - Arteriovenous shunts
  - Paget's disease of bone
  - Beriberi
- Increased cardiac output
  - Anemia
  - Thyrotoxicosis
  - Aortic valvular insufficiency

ETIOLOGY

Pathophysiologic factors that have been implicated in the genesis of essential hypertension include increased sympathetic nervous system activity, overproduction of an unidentified sodium-retaining hormone, chronic high sodium intake, increased or "inappropriate" renin secretion, deficiencies of various vasodilatory substances such as prostaglandins, congenital abnormalities of the resistance vessels, and unknown genetic factors. It is likely that essential hypertension represents a collection of diseases or syndromes with distinct pathophysiologic features. The most common etiologies of secondary hypertension are summarized in Table 47–4. The neurohumoral and circulatory abnormalities that are responsible for these forms of hypertension are discussed below.

INCIDENCE AND PREVALENCE

More than 60 million persons in the United States have hypertension. The prevalence of hypertension is higher among blacks than whites, and it increases with age in all groups (Fig. 47–1). The reason for the increased prevalence of hypertension among blacks is unclear, but it has been variously attributed to heredity, greater salt intake, and greater environmental stress. The rise in BP over time in a population is related to both aging and the level of BP: The higher the BP, the greater the rate of change in pressure over time. Hypertension is more common in men than in women up to approximately age 50; after that time, hypertension is more common in women (Fig. 47–1). The reason for the increased prevalence of hypertension in postmenopausal women is unknown.

PATHOGENESIS

Essential Hypertension

HEMODYNAMICS. Elevation of BP results from any disturbance of the circulation that increases cardiac output or

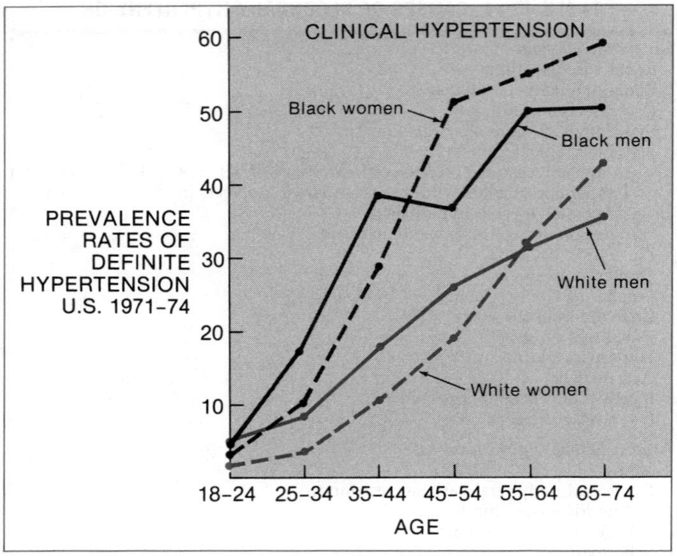

FIGURE 47–1. The prevalence of hypertension in the United States defined as a systolic blood pressure of at least 160 mm Hg or a diastolic blood pressure of at least 95 mm Hg. (From Health and Nutrition Examination Survey, 1971–1974. Source: Advance Data, Vital and Health Statistics of the National Center for Health Statistics, No. 1, October 18, 1976.)

total peripheral resistance, or both. Increases in total peripheral resistance elevate both systolic and diastolic pressures. Cardiac output is elevated early in the course of essential hypertension. Patients with hypertension of recent onset show a pattern of increased cardiac output, tachycardia, increased dp/dt, and venoconstriction, with normal or even low peripheral vascular resistance at rest. In contrast, patients with longstanding established hypertension usually have a slightly decreased cardiac output and increased peripheral vascular resistance. Thus, increased cardiac output plays a role in the initiation of essential hypertension, and elevated peripheral resistance is more important in its maintenance. Longitudinal studies of untreated hypertensive patients have documented a fall in cardiac output, due mainly to a decrease in stroke volume, and an increase in total peripheral resistance over time.

The elevation in cardiac output seen in persons with labile hypertension has been related to increased sympathetic nervous system function with enhanced venoconstrictor tone and a resultant redistribution of blood volume from the periphery to the cardiopulmonary segments (central redistribution of blood volume). Central blood volume, the volume of blood in the heart and lungs, is generally normal or increased in the presence of decreased total blood volume in these patients. Further, forearm venous distensibility is diminished in untreated patients with essential hypertension, indicating that venoconstrictor tone is increased.

AUTONOMIC FUNCTION. The autonomic nervous system is involved in both the initiation and the maintenance of elevated arterial pressure in essential hypertension. In patients with early hypertension, both parasympathetic and sympathetic control mechanisms are abnormal. The tachycardia, increased cardiac output, increased dp/dt, and venoconstriction characteristic of these patients are due to a combination of diminished resting parasympathetic inhibition and enhanced sympathetic stimulation. These patients have elevated plasma renin and norepinephrine levels and enhanced vascular responses to stress as a consequence of their increased sympathetic activity. The concentration of norepinephrine in cerebrospinal fluid from patients with essential hypertension is higher than in healthy normal volunteers, suggesting that noradrenergic pathways in the central nervous system are hyperactive in persons with essential hypertension.

Patients with essential hypertension have an exaggerated pressor response to stress and an exaggerated depressor response to relaxation. Blood pressure falls during sleep, meditation, and other states of relaxation and rises during isometric exercise and the stress of mental arithmetic in these patients to a greater extent than in normotensive control subjects. The impressive fall in BP that is frequently seen when a hypertensive patient is removed from the home environment and brought into the hospital suggests that environmental stress exacerbates hypertension. The increased prevalence of hypertension in urban populations compared with rural groups and the occurrence of age-related rises in BP in societies with changing value systems but not in those with a stable social structure provide evidence for a psychogenic contribution to essential hypertension. Stress presumably mediates its pressor effect through the sympathetic nervous system.

HUMORAL CONTROL OF PRESSURE AND VOLUME. ***Renin-Angiotensin System.*** Renin is a proteolytic enzyme that is synthesized, stored, and secreted mainly in the kidney, but also in brain and blood vessel walls. Renin cleaves its glycoprotein substrate, angiotensinogen, to produce angiotensin I (Fig. 47–2). Angiotensin I is a decapeptide prohormone that is activated by conversion to the octapeptide angiotensin II via angiotensin-converting enzyme. Angiotensin II is a potent vasoconstrictor and stimulator of aldosterone synthesis and secretion. It also has pressor and dipsogenic effects through actions on the central nervous system and on facilitation of norepinephrine release from sympathetic nerve terminals. Angiotensins I and II are destroyed in peripheral capillary beds by a number of enzymes, the angiotensinases.

Kallikrein-Kinin System. The kallikrein-kinin system is involved in the maintenance of BP by control of regional blood flow and water and electrolyte excretion. Kinins are potent vasodilator and natriuretic peptides released from inactive precursors, the kininogens, by the kininogenases, a group of serine proteases that includes the plasma and glandular kallikreins. The kinins are rapidly inactivated in the circulation, suggesting that, rather than producing systemic vasodilatation, their physiologic role is to maintain regional blood flow and, in the case of the kidney, to influence sodium excretion. One of the kinin-inactivating enzymes, kininase II, also catalyzes the conversion of angiotensin I to II (Fig. 47–2). Thus, the same enzyme generates a vasoconstrictor peptide (angiotensin II) and hydrolyzes a vasodilator/natriuretic peptide (bradykinin). Kallikrein in the luminal plasma membrane of the distal tubule catalyzes the formation of kinins that effect a natriuresis by (1) inhibiting sodium transport in the distal nephron, (2) causing renal vasodilatation, and (3) altering the osmotic gradient of the renal medulla.

The kallikrein-kinin system also alters renal blood flow and sodium handling indirectly by effects on the renin-angiotensin-aldosterone system and on renal prostaglandins (Fig. 47–3). Kallikrein stimulates renin release and activates inactive renin. Further, kinins stimulate the synthesis of vasodilator prostaglandins, probably by activation of phospholipase A_2 and increased release of arachidonic acid. Part of the vasodilator effect of the kinins is mediated through the release of prostaglandins. Conversely, angiotensin, aldosterone, and prostaglandins, as well as arginine vasopressin (AVP), can stimulate the release of renal kallikrein and perhaps the intrarenal formation of kinins.

Both reductions and elevations in urinary kallikrein excretion have been described in patients with various forms of hypertension. Whether these abnormalities in kallikrein excretion are etiologically related to the hypertension is uncertain.

Prostaglandins. Prostaglandins (PG) in kidney and blood vessel walls participate in BP regulation through both their

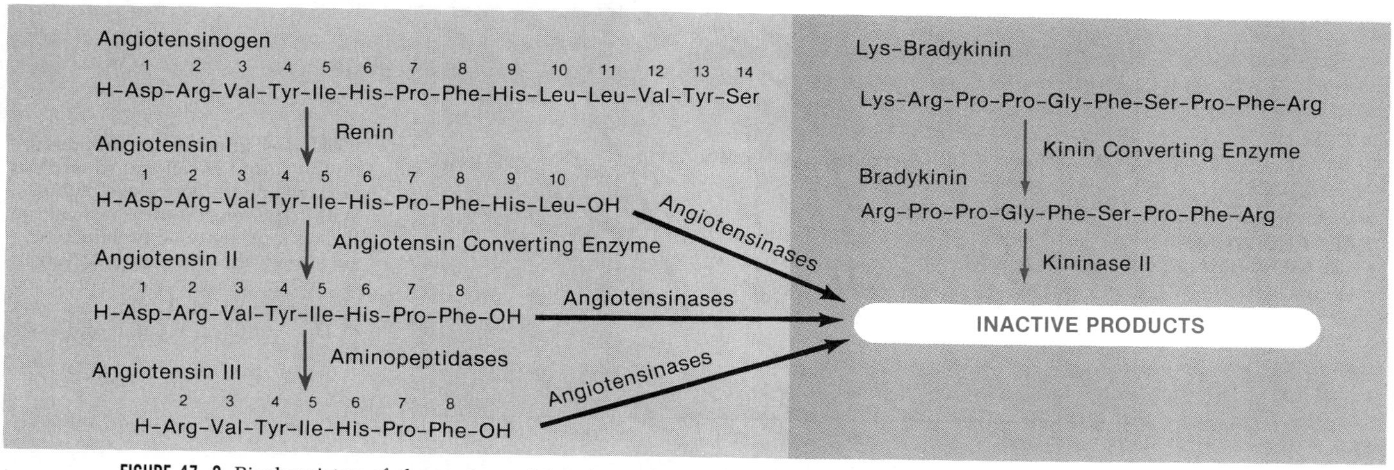

FIGURE 47–2. Biochemistry of the renin-angiotensin system and its interaction (via converting enzyme or kininase II) with the kallikrein-kinin system.

intrinsic effects and their interactions with other vasoregulatory systems. Prostaglandins stimulate the kallikrein-kinin and renin-angiotensin systems, and prostaglandin production is stimulated by both bradykinin and angiotensin II (Fig. 47–3). The antihypertensive effects of the prostaglandins predominate over their pressor effects, since intravenous administration of their precursor, arachidonic acid, generally lowers BP, whereas indomethacin, which inhibits prostaglandin production, tends to exacerbate hypertension.

Prostaglandins oppose the vasoconstrictor effects of a number of humoral agents. Prostaglandins E_2 and I_2 decrease the release of norepinephrine during sympathetic nerve stimulation and reduce the vasoconstrictor effect of infused norepinephrine. Further, prostaglandins whose synthesis is stimulated by angiotensin II attenuate the vasoconstrictor effects of angiotensin II.

Prostaglandins, principally PGE, which are found in high concentrations in the renal medulla, act as local vasodilators and powerful natriuretic agents. It has been proposed that the prostaglandins operate in concert with the kallikrein-kinin system to maintain renal blood flow and facilitate natriuresis, thus opposing those factors that elevate BP through intrarenal mechanisms.

Prostaglandin metabolism may be altered in patients with essential hypertension. Urinary excretion of PGE_2 is often depressed in essential hypertension but not in hypertension secondary to aldosterone excess or renovascular disease, suggesting that reduction of renal PGE_2 synthesis in essential hypertension may be a primary abnormality rather than a secondary response to the elevated BP. These data, coupled with the observation that renal kallikrein-kinin activity is often reduced in essential hypertension, are consistent with the interpretation that these local renal hormones regulate systemic BP and vascular resistance through control of renal blood flow and sodium excretion.

Arginine Vasopressin. Arginine vasopressin (AVP), the mammalian antidiuretic hormone, has pressor effects that are mediated by direct actions on vascular smooth muscle and by indirect actions on the brain, including resetting of the baroreceptor. Levels of AVP in plasma and urine are elevated in patients with renovascular hypertension and in a subset of patients with essential hypertension. Whether AVP plays an etiologic role in the hypertension or represents a marker of other neurohumoral abnormalities remains to be determined.

Atrial Natriuretic Peptides. Mammalian atria synthesize, store, and release into the circulation peptides with potent diuretic, natriuretic, and vasorelaxant properties. The atrial natriuretic peptides inhibit the action of endogenous vasoconstrictors and reduce aldosterone synthesis. These properties suggest that the atrial natriuretic peptides may be physiologic regulators of sodium, volume, and pressure homeostasis or may play a role in the pathogenesis of hypertension, or both. Plasma levels of atrial natriuretic peptide in patients with untreated essential hypertension are two- to eightfold greater than those in control normotensive subjects. The mechanism by which circulating atrial natriuretic peptide levels are elevated in hypertensive subjects likely involves a combination of increased left atrial stretch secondary to systemic hypertension and increased right atrial stretch secondary to volume expansion.

RENAL SODIUM HANDLING. Hemodynamic, neural, and humoral factors all participate in the control of volume

Figure 47–3. A schematic representation of the interactions of the renal kallikrein-kinin, renin-angiotensin, and prostaglandin systems. Solid lines represent stimulation or conversion, and dotted lines inactivation or inhibition. LBK = Lysyl-bradykinin; BK = bradykinin; ACE = angiotensin-converting enzyme. (From Smith MC, Dunn MJ: Renal kallikrein, kinins and prostaglandins in hypertension. In Brenner BM, Stein JH (eds): Contemporary Issues in Nephrology. Vol. 8. New York, Churchill Livingstone, Inc., 1981, by permission.)

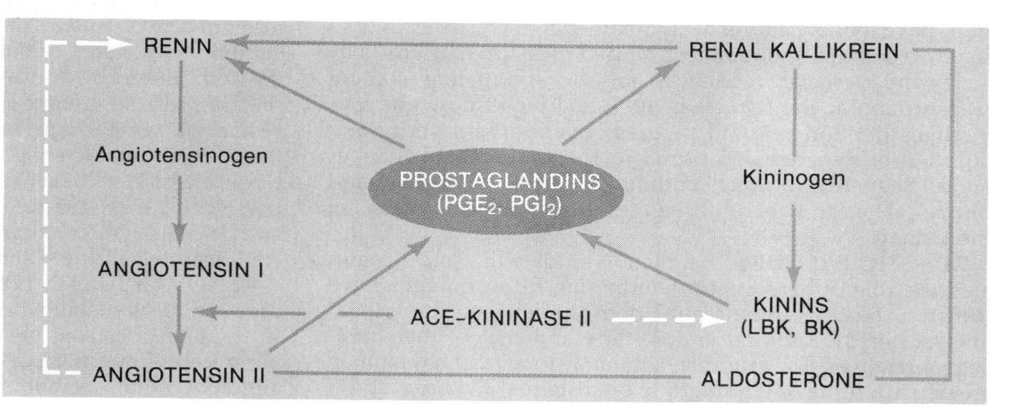

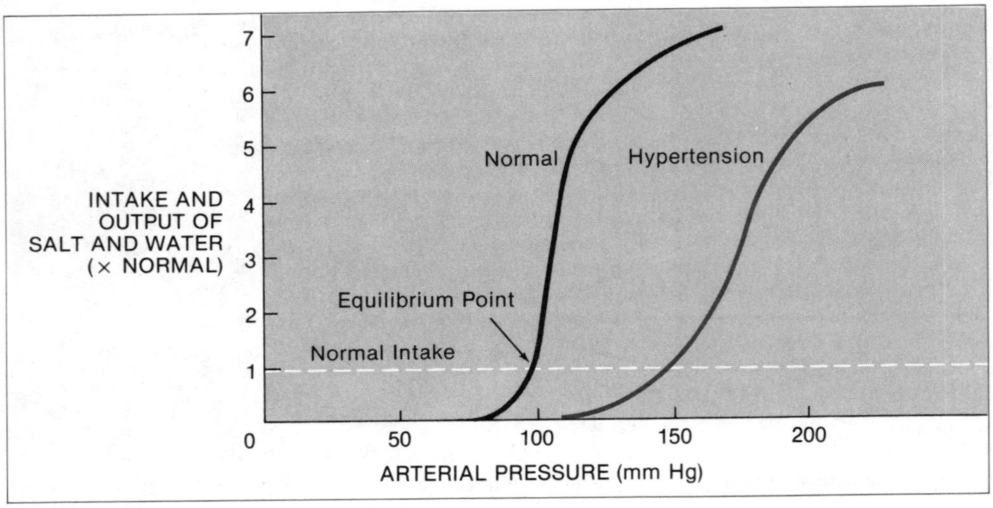

FIGURE 47–4. Effect of arterial pressure on the output of salt and water from normal and hypertensive kidneys. With hypertension there is a shift to the right of the renal function curve such that the pressure natriuresis occurs at a higher level of blood pressure. (Adapted from the work of Dr. Arthur C. Guyton and associates.)

and pressure homeostasis by regulating renal sodium handling. The normal kidney plays an important role in maintaining intravascular volume and arterial BP. It responds to increments in perfusion pressure by increasing sodium and water excretion, thus reducing intravascular volume and restoring arterial pressure to normal levels (Fig. 47–4). Normally, sodium intake and output are balanced at a mean perfusion pressure of 100 mm Hg. An alteration in this relationship, such that higher perfusion pressures are needed to produce a natriuresis, would facilitate the development and maintenance of hypertension. A variety of neurohumoral factors, intrinsic and extrinsic to the kidney, can influence the relationship between perfusion pressure and sodium excretion. Intrinsic factors include angiotensin II, prostaglandins, and kinins; extrinsic factors include circulating catecholamines, AVP, aldosterone, and sympathetic nervous activity. In addition, a kidney subjected to elevated pressure over time develops structural changes that limit its ability to excrete sodium and water in response to increases in pressure.

A defect in the excretion of salt and water may be central to the pathogenesis of many, if not all, forms of hypertension. Animal models provide evidence that changes in the renal circulation due to increased sympathetic nervous system activity favor salt and water retention and the genesis of hypertension. Renal denervation delays the development of hypertension in these models. Renal abnormalities have also been demonstrated in patients with essential hypertension. In patients with established uncomplicated essential hypertension, renal blood flow tends to be reduced in the presence of a normal or slightly reduced glomerular filtration rate. Alterations in renal blood flow and tubular function in uncomplicated essential hypertension usually result from reversible arteriolar vasoconstriction rather than from fixed structural changes. Many patients with established essential hypertension have enhanced renal sympathetic tone, which could facilitate sodium retention and blunt a pressure natriuresis by increasing vascular resistance and by stimulating sodium reabsorption at the tubular level. Renal blood flow and glomerular filtration rate fall progressively as the severity and duration of hypertension increase. These functional changes are consequences of longstanding elevations in pressure and can be related to structural changes in resistance of vessels of the kidney.

GENETIC FACTORS. Population studies that have examined the role of heredity in determining BP in humans have shown a direct quantitative relationship between the arterial pressure of the subjects under study and that of their first-degree relatives. For example, a monozygotic twin has a much greater risk of having borderline or sustained hypertension if his or her twin has either condition. To date, no specific set of BP-regulating genes has been identified, nor have genetic markers that permit early detection of individuals at risk for developing hypertension been characterized.

Hypertensive Crisis

Approximately 1 per cent of hypertensive patients enter an accelerated phase characterized by severe hypertension and necrotizing arteriolitis, leading to progressive end-organ damage that may be irreversible if the hypertension is untreated. Hypertensive crisis is a medical emergency; left untreated, the five-year mortality rate is 100 per cent. This syndrome can result from essential hypertension or from hypertension secondary to any cause, except coarctation of the aorta, and is particularly common in patients with renovascular hypertension. The triggering mechanism for the development of arteriolar lesions has been related to the absolute level or rate of rise of arterial pressure, the presence of disseminated intravascular clotting in association with microangiopathic hemolytic anemia, or activation of the renin-angiotensin system. Whatever the initiating mechanism, the syndrome is perpetuated by deposition of fibrin in arteriolar walls, which in turn leads to retinopathy, renal damage, and increased renin release.

Secondary Hypertension

ORAL CONTRACEPTIVE–INDUCED HYPERTENSION. Approximately 5 per cent of women who use oral contraceptives experience the new onset of hypertension, which resolves with withdrawal of oral contraceptive therapy. Mechanisms by which oral contraceptives may precipitate hypertension in a genetically susceptible host include stimulation of angiotensinogen synthesis with secondary increases in renin activity and angiotensin II generation, increased renal sodium and water retention, increased cardiac output, increased adrenocorticotropic hormone (ACTH) synthesis and release with secondary overproduction of aldosterone, and enhanced sympathetic nervous system activity. It is likely that genetic characteristics, such as family history of hypertension and black race, as well as environmental characteristics, such as pre-existing and occult renal disease, obesity, and middle age (> 40 years), increase susceptibility to oral contraceptive–induced hypertension.

RENOVASCULAR HYPERTENSION. Renovascular disease produces sustained elevation of circulating renin activity. In the face of a fixed obstruction to perfusion, the intrarenal baroreceptor and perhaps the macula densa are stimulated to augment renin secretion. Angiotensin and aldosterone are increased secondarily, resulting in sodium and water retention, but because of a block in the feedback loop proximal to the intrarenal baroreceptors, renin production cannot be turned off. In renovascular hypertension, renin levels are elevated primarily and aldosterone levels secondarily. Elevated circulating angiotensin II and aldosterone levels are primarily responsible for BP elevation early in the course of renovascular hypertension, and increased sodium and water retention and enhanced sympathetic nervous system activity play dominant roles in the maintenance of hypertension in the chronic phase of the syndrome. Deficiencies of antihypertensive factors, such as prostaglandins and renomedullary neutral lipid, may also contribute to the pathogenesis of this form of hypertension.

Any lesion that obstructs either large or small renal arteries can cause renovascular hypertension. The most common and clinically important of these are intrinsic lesions of the large vessels, because they can be physically removed and the hypertension either cured or ameliorated. Atherosclerotic disease is found in two thirds of patients with renovascular hypertension; fibrous or fibromuscular disease, in one third. Patients with atherosclerotic renal artery lesions tend to be older and to have higher systolic BP measurements and more frequent extrarenal arterial disease than patients with essential hypertension and are more likely to develop target-organ damage. Patients with fibromuscular disease tend to be younger and predominantly female and are less likely to develop cardiovascular complications. Prognosis is generally worse in atherosclerotic disease than in fibromuscular disease.

PRIMARY ALDOSTERONISM. Primary aldosteronism is the most common of the syndromes of mineralocorticoid excess. Despite its low prevalence in hypertensive populations (< 1 per cent), the syndrome has received much attention because it can be easily suspected by the finding of depressed serum potassium levels and can frequently be cured by surgery.

Primary aldosteronism is a syndrome of hypertension associated with hypokalemia, suppressed plasma renin activity, and increased aldosterone production in which the other abnormalities result from the relatively autonomous secretion of aldosterone. Autonomous production of aldosterone is associated with excessive salt and water retention, which leads to an increase in effective blood volume and suppression of renin release. Since mineralocorticoid production is not angiotensin dependent, the feedback loop is interrupted, and excessive mineralocorticoid production continues. Renin is therefore suppressed, and the level of aldosterone is elevated. Hypokalemia is a direct consequence of the effects of aldosterone on the renal tubule, but the pathogenesis of the hypertension remains poorly understood. Increases in plasma volume have been described but are inconstant findings. Hemodynamic studies suggest that increased peripheral resistance is important in maintaining the hypertension.

PHEOCHROMOCYTOMA. Pheochromocytoma is a rare but important cause of surgically curable hypertension. Although it accounts for less than 0.5 per cent of all cases of hypertension, diagnosis is critical because pheochromocytomas may be malignant, the hypertension may be severe and refractory to conventional antihypertensive treatment, and patients with unrecognized pheochromocytoma are subject to hypertensive crises during anesthesia and angiography and following administration of drugs such as guanethidine and the ganglion blockers.

Pheochromocytoma is a tumor of neural crest origin that produces sustained or paroxysmal hypertension by releasing catecholamines, usually a combination of norepinephrine and epinephrine, into the circulation. Ninety per cent of pheochromocytomas are located in the adrenal medulla, and 10 per cent of these are bilateral. The remaining 10 per cent are scattered in the distribution of autonomic tissue. Fifteen per cent of all pheochromocytomas are malignant. These are generally slow growing and resistant to radiation therapy. They usually metastasize to lymph nodes, liver, lung, and bone. Malignant pheochromocytomas and their metastases may or may not be functional. Pheochromocytomas are common in patients with neurocutaneous syndromes such as von Recklinghausen's disease and in families with the syndromes of multiple endocrine adenomatosis. Patients with pheochromocytoma have an increased incidence of neuroectodermal tumors, including brain tumors.

DIAGNOSIS

Initial Evaluation

The initial evaluation of the hypertensive patient is designed to establish the diagnosis of arterial hypertension, grade its severity, determine the need for treatment, and assess the likelihood of a secondary cause for the hypertension. The Joint National Committee on Detection, Evaluation, and Treatment of High Blood Pressure has published guidelines for the detection, follow-up, and stepped-care therapy of hypertensive patients.

BLOOD PRESSURE MEASUREMENT. The accurate and reproducible measurement of BP by the cuff technique is the most critical part of the diagnostic evaluation. On the initial visit, the BP should be taken after the patient has been seated comfortably for at least five minutes with his or her arm bared. Constriction of the upper arm by a rolled sleeve should be avoided, as it distorts the BP measurement. Two or three measurements should be taken at each visit, and at least two minutes should be allowed between readings. Proper cuff size is critical to accurate BP measurement. The width should be about two thirds the width of the arm (15 cm in most adults), and, more important, the bladder cuff should be long enough to circle the arm. Falsely elevated readings can be obtained when the bladder is too short, and the error is magnified if the cuff is also too narrow. Mercury manometers are preferred, but aneroid manometers can be used if they are standardized frequently against a mercury manometer.

To obtain an accurate systolic pressure, the cuff should be inflated rapidly to at least 30 mm Hg above the systolic pressure, as determined by palpation of the radial artery. This inflation is necessary to avoid underestimating the pressure because of the auscultatory gap, an unexplained disappearance of Korotkoff's sounds for some interval between systole and diastole. The systolic reading is taken as the level of pressure at which clear Korotkoff's sounds are heard with each heart beat. The diastolic reading is taken at the level both when sounds become muffled (Korotkoff phase IV) and when sounds disappear (phase V). Both readings should be recorded. It is not known whether the level of muffling or of disappearance is a more accurate reflection of the intra-arterial diastolic pressure, so selection of one over the other as the clinical measurement of diastolic pressure is a matter of convenience and reproducibility.

The use of home BP recordings by either the patient or another person in the household or the use of 24-hour ambulatory BP recordings, or both, is useful, particularly in monitoring patients with labile hypertension, anxious patients whose BP readings tend to be falsely elevated in the doctor's office, and patients whose doses of antihypertensive medications need to be adjusted frequently. Home recordings should be taken at various times of day, in various positions, and during periods of stress and relaxation in order to assess the effects of diurnal variations in hormones, posture, and emotional state of BP. Standard sphygmomanometers and stethoscopes are appropriate for this purpose; most automated indirect BP measuring devices are inaccurate and should not be used. The patient's skill at BP measurement should be tested at frequent intervals by a professional.

Selection of Patients for Evaluation for Secondary Hypertension

Once a diagnosis of stable hypertension has been established, the need for antihypertensive treatment should be assessed, and, where indicated, diagnostic evaluation for secondary causes of hypertension should be undertaken. In view of the rarity of secondary causes of hypertension and the high cost and risk of elaborate diagnostic studies, the routine pretreatment workup should be limited to defining the severity of the hypertension and to identifying its complications and associated cardiovascular risk factors. All of the secondary causes combined account for less than 5 per cent of the adult hypertensive population, but since some patients with secondary hypertension are potentially curable, diagnostic evaluation is warranted in selected patients. These include the following:

1. Those in whom routine history, physical examination, or routine laboratory data suggest a specific secondary cause.
2. Those who are younger than 30 years of age, since they have the greatest prevalence of correctable secondary hypertension.
3. Those in whom drug therapy is inadequate or unsatisfactory.
4. Those whose BP has suddenly worsened.

MEDICAL HISTORY. A careful, complete history should be obtained and a physical examination should be performed in all hypertensive patients before therapy is started. The medical history should include any previous history of hypertension, including prior and current antihypertensive treatment; a history of factors regarded as predisposing to hypertension, including excessive salt intake, the use of oral contraceptives or other estrogen preparations, stressful occupation, and a family history of hypertension and its complications; evidence of hypertensive complications, including congestive heart failure, coronary artery disease, renal dysfunction, and stroke; and a history of other cardiovascular risk factors, including diabetes, obesity, cigarette smoking, and lipid abnormalities. A history of weakness, muscle cramps, and polyuria suggests hypokalemia and the possibility of hyperaldosteronism; a history of headaches, palpitations, or hyperhidrosis suggests pheochromocytoma.

PHYSICAL EXAMINATION. The physical examination should include two or more BP measurements, at least one of which is obtained in the standing position; funduscopic examination for hypertensive retinopathy; careful examination of the cardiovascular system for evidence of congestive heart failure, cardiomegaly, myocardial dysfunction, and peripheral vascular disease; examination of the abdomen for bruits; auscultation over all scars for evidence of arteriovenous fistulas; and a careful neurologic examination for the stigmas of stroke.

LABORATORY EVALUATION. Pretreatment laboratory tests can be restricted to those generally performed as part of a routine medical checkup; hematocrit, urinalysis, creatinine or blood urea nitrogen levels, serum potassium levels, chest film, and electrocardiogram. Other tests, which can be obtained as part of most automated blood chemistry batteries, such as the blood glucose, serum cholesterol, and serum uric acid levels, are helpful in assessing other cardiovascular risk factors and can be used as a baseline for monitoring the effects of antihypertensive treatment. Serial electrocardiograms and echocardiograms may be useful in assessing the effects of hypertension and antihypertensive treatment on the heart.

Hypertensive Crisis

Patients with accelerated hypertension usually present with hypertension encephalopathy, rapidly progressive renal insufficiency, or acute left ventricular failure. Hypertensive encephalopathy is characterized by the rapid onset of confusion, headache, visual disturbances, seizures, and, in severe cases, somnolence and even coma. Increased intracranial pressure with papilledema occurs, presumably resulting from failure of autoregulation of cerebral blood flow with breakthrough vasodilatation and secondary extravasation of intravascular contents. Death from a cerebrovascular accident frequently occurs if the hypertension is untreated, but the encephalopathy usually clears rapidly following successful antihypertensive treatment. Renal damage secondary to necrotizing arteriolitis results in proteinuria, hematuria, and azotemia. Assuming that the blood pressure can be controlled, the presence of renal damage at the time of diagnosis has prognostic significance. The five-year survival of treated patients with grade IV retinopathy and azotemia is 23 per cent and that of nonazotemic patients, 64 per cent.

Evaluation of Patients for Secondary Causes of Hypertension

ORAL CONTRACEPTIVE–INDUCED HYPERTENSION. The diagnosis of oral contraceptive–induced hypertension can be made by documenting the onset of hypertension de novo during contraceptive therapy and the resolution of the hypertension upon drug withdrawal. This form of hypertension usually begins during the first year of oral contraceptive administration.

Oral contraceptive–induced hypertension can, in part, be prevented by avoiding use of these agents in women who are at high risk. Evidence of thromboembolic disease or chronic hypertension of any cause is an absolute contraindication to use of oral contraceptives. A family history of hypertension and a personal history of pre-existing or occult renal disease or of pregnancy complicated by hypertension are relative contraindications to oral contraceptive use. Women over 35 years of age, particularly if obese, should be cautioned about the increased risk of developing hypertension while ingesting oral contraceptives. Such patients should be followed closely: BP measurement and a funduscopic examination should be performed and an interval history obtained on several occasions during the first year of treatment and at yearly intervals thereafter.

RENOVASCULAR HYPERTENSION. Patients most likely to have renovascular hypertension include those with hypertension of abrupt onset, especially in the young or in those in late middle age; those with malignant hypertension or sudden acceleration of benign hypertension; and those who have failed to respond to medical therapy. Generally, these patients have moderately severe to severe fixed diastolic hypertension. The presence of an upper abdominal bruit, particularly one that is systolic-diastolic or continuous in timing, is high pitched, and radiates laterally from the midepigastrium, is strongly suggestive of functionally significant renal artery stenosis. Such bruits have been described in one half to two thirds of patients with surgically proved renovascular hypertension. Because of the cost of the diagnostic evaluation for renovascular hypertension, diagnostic study should be reserved for patients with one or more of the characteristics discussed above.

Screening tests, including the rapid-sequence or hypertensive intravenous pyelogram (IVP), abdominal ultrasonography, and pharmacologic screening with a converting enzyme inhibitor, have some role in the preliminary evaluation of patients for renovascular hypertension, particularly in those in whom the index of suspicion for the syndrome is low. The lack of specificity of these screening procedures limits their usefulness, however, so that, in patients in whom the index of suspicion of renovascular hypertension is high, it is reasonable to move directly to definitive diagnostic testing, which generally requires hospitalization.

Definitive diagnosis of functionally significant renal artery stenosis is made by a combination of *selective renal angiography*

TABLE 47–5. ANTIHYPERTENSIVE AGENTS THAT INHIBIT RENIN RELEASE

Agent	Trade Name
Beta-adrenergic–blocking agents	
Propranolol	(Inderal)
Metoprolol	(Lopressor)
Nadolol	(Corgard)
Atenolol	(Tenormin)
Timolol	(Blocadren)
Acebutolol	(Sectral)
Combined alpha- and beta-adrenergic–blocking agent	
Labetalol	(Normodyne)
Sympatholytic agents	
Alpha-methyldopa	(Aldomet)
Clonidine	(Catapres)
Guanabenz	(Wytensin)
Reserpine	(Serpasil)
Guanethidine	(Ismelin)
Ganglion-blocking agent	
Trimethaphan camsylate	(Arfonad)

and differential renal vein renin measurement. Renal angiography is needed to define the anatomy of the stenotic renal artery in order to plan the approach to revascularization. Documentation of the functional significance of an anatomic lesion requires demonstration of increased renin production by the involved kidney. When renin activity in the venous effluent from the involved kidney is 1.5 or more times that of the uninvolved side and when the uninvolved side can be shown not to produce renin, the probability of improvement in BP after renal revascularization is approximately 90 per cent. Stimulation of renin release with provocative maneuvers—such as tilting, salt deprivation, or administration of vasodilators, diuretics, or converting enzyme inhibitors—has been shown to enhance selectively renin release from the affected kidney. Converting enzyme inhibitors increase the renal vein renin ratio in patients with hypertension secondary to unilateral renal artery stenosis by two mechanisms: lowering BP and blocking feedback inhibition of renin release by angiotensin II. A convenient regimen is administration of 25 mg of captopril p.o. two to four hours before the procedure. The diagnosis of surgically remediable renal artery stenosis can be missed when renal vein sampling is performed in the unstimulated state or when renin-suppressing antihypertensive drugs (Table 47–5) are not discontinued prior to study. False-positive lateralization secondary to excess stimulation of renin release has not been reported.

PRIMARY ALDOSTERONISM. The diagnosis of primary aldosteronism should be considered in patients with refractory hypertension, particularly those with spontaneous or diuretic-induced hypokalemia. A normal plasma potassium value on screening does not rule out the diagnosis of primary aldosteronism. Many (7 to 38 per cent) patients with primary aldosteronism have intermittently normal plasma potassium values, particularly if dietary sodium is restricted or potassium supplementation is given. In a recent prospective study of 80 patients with primary aldosteronism, all of whom were referred for evaluation because of spontaneous hypokalemia, diuretic-induced hypokalemia, and/or refractory hypertension, only 73 per cent had spontaneous hypokalemia (serum potassium level < 3.5 mEq per liter on a normal sodium intake) and only 86 per cent had provoked hypokalemia (serum potassium level < 3.5 mEq per liter on a high sodium intake for three days) (Table 47–6). More than one half of patients in this series developed moderately severe hypokalemia (serum potassium level < 3.0 mEq per liter) while on usual diuretic therapy. Thus, although reliance on serum potassium measurements in screening would cause the diagnosis of primary aldosteronism to be missed in about one fourth of patients, hypokalemia does provide an important clue to the presence of primary aldosteronism. Approximately 50 per cent of hypertensive patients with unprovoked hypokalemia have primary aldosteronism, whereas less than 0.5 per cent of those with normal plasma potassium levels have the syndrome. When hypokalemia is observed, the concomitant measurement of urinary potassium excretion when the patient is not taking diuretics is valuable in distinguishing primary aldosteronism from other causes. Inappropriate potassium wastage (> 40 mEq per 24 hours) is seen in primary aldosteronism with hypokalemia, but not in hypokalemia of other causes.

The best single test for identifying patients with primary aldosteronism is the measurement of aldosterone excretion after three days of salt loading (Table 47–6). Under these conditions, most patients with primary aldosteronism have aldosterone excretion rates of greater than 14.0 μg per 24 hours. There is little or no overlap with the range of values obtained in normal subjects or in patients with essential hypertension. Measurements of plasma renin activity and plasma and urinary aldosterone levels obtained under uncontrolled dietary conditions are not useful in screening for primary aldosteronism, and plasma renin measurements made under conditions of stimulation (sodium restriction, diuretic administration, and upright posture) are inadequate to rule out the diagnosis of primary aldosteronism.

Adenoma Versus Hyperplasia. Once a presumptive diagnosis of aldosterone excess is made, additional procedures are needed to differentiate between adrenal adenoma—or, rarely, carcinoma—and bilateral adrenal hyperplasia as sources for the hormone. A solitary adrenal cortical adenoma is the cause of primary aldosteronism in 60 to 85 per cent of cases; bilateral adrenal cortical hyperplasia is the cause in the remaining 15 to 40 per cent. Aldosterone-producing adenoma is generally associated with more severe hypertension, more extreme aldosterone elevation and renin suppression, and more marked electrolyte imbalance than hyperplasia. The distinction is important in guiding therapy, as patients with adrenal adenomas can have their hyperaldosteronism and

TABLE 47–6. SENSITIVITY AND SPECIFICITY OF VARIOUS SCREENING TESTS FOR PRIMARY ALDOSTERONISM[a]

Test	Standard	Sensitivity (no. of patients)	Specificity (no. of patients)
Serum potassium[b]	Spontaneous (< 3.5 mEq/liter)	0.73 (58/80)	0.94 (66/70)
Serum potassium[c]	Provoked (< 3.5 mEq/liter)	0.86 (70/80)	0.96 (67/70)
Plasma renin activity[d]	Suppressed (< 2.0 ng/ml/hr)	0.64 (51/80)	0.83 (58/70)
Aldosterone excretion rate [c]	Nonsuppressible (> 4 μg/24 hr)	0.96 (77/80)	0.93 (65/70)
Plasma aldosterone concentration[c]	Nonsuppressible (> 22 ng/dl)	0.72 (31/43)	0.91 (31/34)

[a]Sensitivity = percentage of subjects with disease who have positive results. Specificity = percentage of subjects without disease who have negative results. Standards for aldosterone excretion rate and plasma aldosterone concentration represent the upper 95 per cent range of values obtained in subjects with essential hypertension.

[b]Normal sodium intake for three to five days.

[c]High sodium intake for three days.

[d]Low sodium intake for four days.

Reprinted with permission from Bravo EL, Tarazi RC, Dustan HP, et al.: The changing clinical spectrum of primary aldosteronism. Am J Med 74:641–651, 1983.

hypertension cured by unilateral adrenalectomy, whereas those with bilateral hyperplasia often remain hypertensive even after both adrenal glands are removed.

Several techniques are available for localizing aldosterone-producing adenomas. Computed tomography (CT) scanning can resolve adrenal tumors that are more than 1.0 cm in diameter and has a localizing accuracy of 75 per cent for aldosteronomas. In patients with suspected bilateral adrenal cortical hyperplasia, the CT scan reveals either bilateral adrenal enlargement or normal-appearing glands. Computed tomographic scans have largely replaced ^{125}I-19-iodocholesterol scintiscans in the diagnostic evaluation of patients with primary aldosteronism. Computed tomographic scanning offers several practical advantages over radioisotope studies, including immediate availability of results, lower absorbed radiation doses, greater convenience for the patient, and greater availability to the physician. Direct adrenal vein sampling by percutaneous catheterization, with measurement of adrenal venous aldosterone levels, is the most accurate (90 per cent accuracy in experienced hands). Elevated values with a less than twofold difference between sides suggest bilateral hyperplasia; aldosterone-producing adenomas generally result in a more than tenfold difference between sides. Adrenal venography, although accurate in localizing adrenal tumors, is no longer in general use because of the high incidence (5 to 10 per cent) of retroperitoneal and intra-adrenal hemorrhage.

In summary, when biochemical findings suggest the presence of an aldosterone-producing adenoma, an adrenal CT scan should be performed and can be considered diagnostic if an adrenal mass is clearly identified. If the results of the CT scan are inconclusive, adrenal venous sampling for aldosterone is indicated.

PHEOCHROMOCYTOMA. The most common signs and symptoms of pheochromocytoma include unusually labile hypertension; symptomatic paroxysms of hypertension and tachycardia characterized by "spells" with headache, palpitations, sweating, pallor, and hypertension; accelerated hypertension, hypertension refractory to conventional therapy; hypermetabolism and weight loss; abnormal carbohydrate metabolism; and pressor responses to induction of anesthesia or antihypertensive treatment. Most patients with pheochromocytoma are symptomatic, so it is legitimate to use symptoms and physical signs in screening patients for the tumor. Biochemical tests need to be performed only in patients who have clinical evidence of the disorder.

Diagnosis of pheochromocytoma requires the demonstration of increased concentrations of catecholamines or their metabolites, or both, in plasma or urine and the localization of a tumor via CT scanning, radionuclide techniques, or angiography. Measurements of 24-hour urinary excretion of VMA (3-methoxy-4-hydroxymandelic acid) and of metanephrine and normetanephrine are the most commonly used screening tests for pheochromocytoma because of their low cost, simplicity, and general availability. Assay of plasma catecholamines offers advantages over measurement of urinary catecholamines or metabolites, or both, in that it eliminates the unreliability inherent in 24-hour urine collections and artifacts secondary to interference from drugs and angiographic contrast media. Measurement of plasma catecholamines is more reliable than 24-hour assessment of urinary metanephrines or VMA, or both, in screening for pheochromocytoma as long as appropriate precautions are taken in obtaining plasma samples. Patients must be resting and the stress of venipuncture avoided by insertion of an indwelling catheter 20 to 30 minutes before sampling. Plasma catecholamine levels are usually enormously elevated in patients with pheochromocytoma compared with controls with essential hypertension (Fig. 47–5). In contrast, urinary metanephrine and VMA values in patients with pheochromocytoma show substantial overlap with the range of values obtained in patients with essential hypertension.

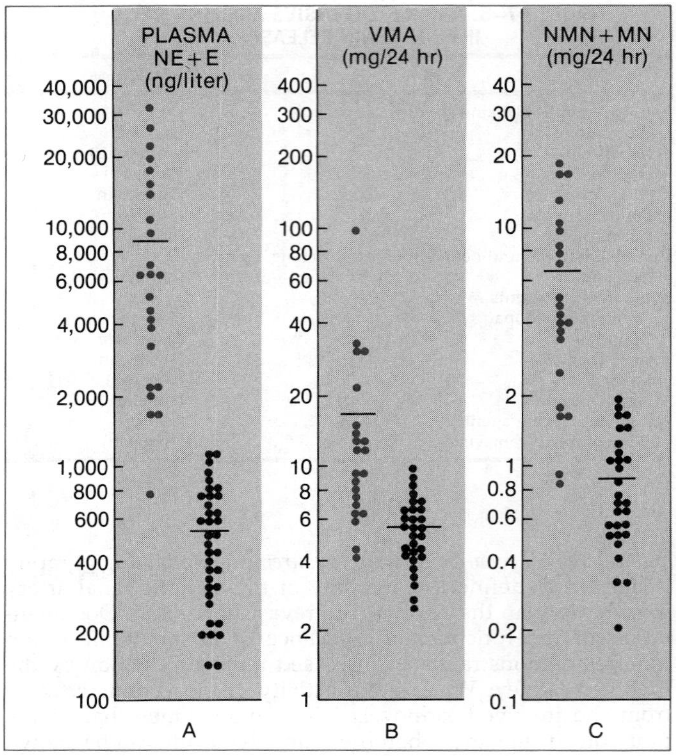

FIGURE 47–5. *A,* Plasma norepinephrine (NE) and epinephrine (E) measured at rest in patients with (*red circles*) and without (*black circles*) evidence of pheochromocytoma. All but 1 of the 23 patients with pheochromocytoma had plasma catecholamine values greater than the highest value in patients without pheochromocytoma. *B* and *C,* Twenty-four hour urinary vanillylmandelic acid (VMA) and total metanephrines (NMN + MN) collected on the same day as blood drawing for the determination of plasma catecholamines in patients depicted in *A.* (Reprinted, with modifications, from Bravo EL, et al.: Circulating and urinary catecholamines in pheochromocytoma. N Engl J Med 301:684,1979.)

The sensitivity and specificity of plasma catecholamine assays in the diagnosis of pheochromocytoma can be enhanced by repeating the assays after administration of clonidine or pentolinium. In normal subjects or patients with essential hypertension, stimulation of central alpha-adrenergic receptors with clonidine or administration of a ganglion blocker suppresses plasma norepinephrine by blunting central sympathetic outflow. These agents have no effect on plasma norepinephrine levels in patients with pheochromocytoma, in whom circulating norepinephrine levels depend on autonomous release from the tumor. Interestingly, both groups show similar reductions in BP and heart rate, measured with the patient supine, after administration of these agents, suggesting that catecholamines secreted by the tumor are not responsible for the maintenance of hypertension in patients with pheochromocytoma. The clonidine and phentolamine suppression tests are useful adjunctive procedures to rule out pheochromocytoma in hypertensive patients with suggestive symptoms and borderline resting catecholamine values. Caution must be employed in the use of the clonidine suppression test in patients who are being maintained on antihypertensive treatment, as serious hypotensive reactions have been reported in that group.

Once a presumptive diagnosis of pheochromocytoma has been made by demonstrating elevations in plasma catecholamine levels or by a positive clonidine or phentolamine suppression test, localization studies are indicated. In most cases the tumor can be localized by adrenal CT scanning. For the 10 per cent of pheochromocytomas that are smaller than the resolving power of the CT scan (1.0 cm in diameter) or are located outside the adrenal glands, other means of localization are required. The guanethidine analogue ^{131}I-metaiodobenzylguanide(^{131}I-MIBG) is useful in imaging pheochromocytomas that are undetectable by CT scan. False-negative results have been reported with both CT and ^{131}I-MIBG scans. In such cases, selective arteriography or differential venous catheterization with measurement of regional plasma catecholamines, or both, may help in localizing the tumor. These procedures are associated with appreciable risk to the patient, so they are indicated only if the scans are negative.

TREATMENT

General Considerations

The goal of antihypertensive therapy is to reduce excess cardiovascular morbidity and mortality due to hypertension. In any given patient, the decision to initiate therapy is governed by the extent of the BP elevation and the presence or absence of cardiovascular complications or additional cardiovascular risk factors, or both. Antihypertensive treatment is indicated in patients with diastolic BP measurements of 95 mm Hg or higher and in those with lesser elevations (90 to 94 mm Hg) who are at high risk of developing cardiovascular morbidity or mortality. The high-risk group includes patients with target-organ damage, diabetes mellitus, and/or other major risk factors for coronary artery disease. The initial goal of therapy is to lower diastolic BP to levels less than 90 mm Hg with minimal adverse effects. A reasonable further goal is the lowest diastolic BP consistent with safety and tolerance. An effort should be made to correct other cardiovascular risk factors in all hypertensive patients.

In patients with moderate-to-severe hypertension, even partial BP reduction has been shown to decrease cardiovascular morbidity. Therefore, in these patients, a more limited therapeutic goal may be accepted if side effects are intolerable at doses necessary to achieve normal BP. For patients with diastolic BP readings in the range of 90 to 94 mm Hg who are otherwise at low risk, an initial trial of nonpharmacologic therapy with careful BP monitoring should be carried out. If the diastolic BP remains higher than 90 mm Hg despite nonpharmacologic therapy, use of antihypertensive drugs should be considered, although controlled clinical trials have not demonstrated a clear benefit from effective antihypertensive treatment in this subset of patients.

Antihypertensive treatment is probably indicated in isolated systolic hypertension, since pharmacologic therapy has recently been shown to be well tolerated and effective in lowering BP in this group. Patients with systolic pressures greater than 160 mm Hg are generally considered to deserve treatment. The efficacy of such treatment in reducing cardiovascular morbidity and mortality has yet to be demonstrated, however.

Nonpharmacologic Therapy

Modifications in diet and lifestyle are generally more difficult to achieve than the administration of antihypertensive medication, so they should be considered adjuncts to drug therapy in hypertension. However, since the behavioral modifications useful in hypertensive persons are not costly and are generally beneficial in promoting good health, their gradual introduction should be attempted in all hypertensive patients. Institution of such measures in patients already on antihypertensive treatment may obviate the need for medical therapy or reduce the dosage requirements for adequate control.

Dietary sodium restriction is the most efficacious of all nonmedical measures in the treatment of hypertension. Moderate restriction of salt intake (to 4 to 6 grams per day) lowers BP and potentiates the antihypertensive effect of diuretics in hypertensive subjects. Conversely, a high sodium intake (15 to 20 grams per day) may overcome the antihypertensive effect of diuretics. An additional benefit of moderate sodium restriction is protection from diuretic-induced hypokalemia: In the sodium-restricted subject, less sodium is delivered to the distal exchange site and kaliuresis is minimized. Moderate sodium restriction can be effected by the simple and tolerable measures of not adding salt to food during preparation or at the table, avoiding dairy products, and avoiding processed foods to which salt is added as the preservative. Salt substitutes in which sodium is replaced with potassium are useful in hypertensive patients who do not have renal dysfunction. This form of dietary therapy should be attempted in all hypertensive subjects and may enhance the ease of control with conventional antihypertensive therapy.

Restriction of caloric intake in order to control obesity produces substantial decrements in BP, even if ideal body weight is not achieved. There appears to be a causal relationship between obesity and hypertension, and obesity may be a risk factor for coronary artery disease, independent of hypertension. In addition, obesity is an important marker for susceptibility to hypertension in the young: Body weight and weight gain are associated with the development of hypertension in children. Since caloric and sodium restriction and a reduction in saturated fats and cholesterol can easily be combined, a dietary approach to the treatment or prevention of hypertension and atherosclerotic disease has great appeal. Weight reduction should be an integral part of therapy for all obese persons (> 115 per cent of ideal weight) with hypertension. The practical problem with such an approach is widespread nonadherence to weight reduction regimens.

Dietary calcium supplementation lowers BP in some patients with essential hypertension. The mechanism of this effect is uncertain but has been related to calcium-induced natriuresis. The magnitude of this effect and the risk/benefit ratio of adding calcium to the diet are currently under investigation. Until more complete data are available, it is premature to advocate dietary calcium supplementation as a general therapeutic measure in hypertensive patients.

Reduction of alcohol consumption may be useful in the management of hypertension, since ingestion of more than 2 ounces of alcohol per day is associated with an increased prevalence of hypertension. *Coffee* has not been found to have such a deleterious effect. *Cigarette smoking* can elevate BP, but when a hypertensive patient stops smoking, BP does not usually change appreciably. The failure of smoking cessation to lower BP has been attributed to concomitant weight gain.

Relaxation techniques and other methods designed to minimize psychogenic stress have been explored in the treatment of hypertension. The theoretic basis for this approach is the observation that excess mental stress may raise the BP in humans, presumably via activation of the sympathetic nervous system. Reports on the antihypertensive efficacy of techniques of behavior modification, such as yoga, biofeedback, and meditation, have been mixed. Various relaxation and biofeedback therapies or combinations of such treatments may produce modest BP reduction in selected groups outside the laboratory for as long as one year. However, controlled studies with longer periods of follow-up are needed before these techniques can be recommended for widespread application in the treatment or prevention of hypertension. Other means of reducing stress, such as enforced vacations or job changes and the use of sedatives and tranquilizers, have not been systematically evaluated.

The role of exercise in the prevention and treatment of hypertension has not been adequately assessed. Studies in small groups of hypertensive patients have shown that BP is lowered significantly (mean of 14/10 mm Hg) after physical training. The numbers of patients studied and the duration of follow-up in these studies are inadequate to determine whether the beneficial effects of exercise are reproducible and sustained. The potential benefits of exercise include a relaxation effect and weight loss.

Pharmacologic Therapy

Ideally, therapy should be tailored to correct the specific disturbance responsible for initiating or maintaining elevated BP. Patients in whom hypertension is associated with elevated or suppressed plasma renin activity, increased cardiac output, increased effective intravascular volume, or enhanced sympathetic tone may be candidates for individualized therapy aimed at the specific abnormality. In practice, however, detailed characterization of hormone patterns and hemodynamics in most patients with essential hypertension is not feasible and adds little to the efficacy of drug therapy.

The empiric selection of antihypertensive medication is directed toward a variety of goals. Treatment should be inexpensive, long acting, effective over the long term, and associated with minimal side effects. It should control systolic and diastolic hypertension whether the patient is supine or upright, without impairing postural regulation of BP. Expensive and complicated drug regimens are frequently associated with poor compliance and treatment failure, particularly when they disturb sexual function, mood, or alertness.

In recent years, considerable attention has been devoted to improving compliance with antihypertensive regimens. Improved education of the patient, with direct involvement of patients in their own care by having them measure and record their own BP, has been shown to improve control. Instituting treatment early in the course of the disease, when BP measurements are minimally elevated and target-organ damage has not developed, helps to ensure compliance because simpler, less costly drug regimens with fewer associated adverse effects can be used. Other new approaches, such as simplifying diagnostic evaluations to minimize cost and inconvenience to the patient and using ancillary personnel in routine management and education of the patient, are beneficial in improving adherence of the patient to antihypertensive therapy.

Appropriate utilization of currently available drugs will permit adequate control of BP in most (80 to 90 per cent) patients. The guiding principle of antihypertensive treatment in ambulatory patients is to control BP using the simplest regimen possible (fewest drugs in the lowest doses administered over the most convenient dosage schedule). This is usually implemented by a stepped-care program, in which therapy is started with a small dose of a single drug and the dose of that drug is increased until either the BP is controlled or the maximal therapeutic dose is achieved. Additional drugs are then added, one at a time, in increasing doses until the BP is controlled. An example of such a stepped-care regimen is given in Figure 47–6. Alternative regimens can be used as required, based on the patient's experience and preferences. In patients who present with moderately severe to severe hypertension, it may be desirable to initiate treatment with more than one agent, because it can be predicted that a single agent will not be adequate to control the BP. It is generally advisable to see the patient once every one to two weeks while the BP is being titrated downward and once every three to four months once the BP is controlled. This interval is thought to be necessary to reinforce the need for compliance, to assess the patient for side effects of the medication, and to titrate the dosage of antihypertensive drugs. Recommended dose ranges for individual drugs are listed with each agent in Tables 47–7 and 47–8.

TABLE 47–7. DIURETICS

Generic Name	Trade Name (manufacturer)	Adult Dosage (mg/day)	Duration (hr)	Dispensing Unit (mg)
Benzothiadiazine Diuretics				
Thiazides				
Chlorothiazide	Diuril (MSD)*	250–500	6–12	250, 500
Hydrochlorothiazide	Esidrix (CIBA)	25–50	12–18	25
	HydroDIURIL (MSD)			50
	Oretic (Abbott)			
Bendroflumethiazide	Naturetin (Squibb)	5–20	18–36	2.5, 5.0, 10
Benzthiazide	Aquatag (Tutag)	25–50	12–18	50
	Diucen (Central)			
	Edemex (Savage)			
	Exna (Robins)			
	Lemazide (Lemmon)			
Cyclothiazide	Anhydron (Lilly)	1–2	18–24	2
Hydroflumethiazide	Saluron (Bristol)	25–50	18–24	50
Methyclothiazide	Aquatensen (Wallace)	2.5–10.0	24–48	5.0, 2.5
	Enduron (Abbott)			
Polythiazide	Renese (Pfizer)	2–4	24–48	1, 2, 4
Trichlormethiazide	Methahydrin (Merrell Dow)	2–4	24–48	2
	Naqua (Schering)			4
Indapamide	Lozol (USV Pharmaceutical)	2.5–5.0	18–24	2.5
Phthalimidines				
Chlorthalidone	Hygroton (USV Pharmaceutical)	25–50	24–72	25, 50, 100
	Chlorthalidone (Parke-Davis)			25, 50
	Thalitone (Boehringer Ingelheim)			
Metolazone	Zaroxolyn (Pennwalt)	2.5–5.0	12–24	2.5, 5.0, 10.0
	Diulo (Searle)			2.5, 5.0, 10.0
Quinazolines				
Quinethazone	Hydromox (Lederle)	50–100	18–24	50
Loop Diuretics				
Furosemide	Lasix (Hoechst-Roussel)	20–1,000	3–6	20, 40, 80
Ethacrynic acid	Edecrin (MSD)	50–400	3–6	25, 50
Bumetanide	Bumex (Roche)	0.5–2.0	1–4	0.5, 1.0
Potassium-sparing Diuretics				
Spironolactone	Aldactone (Searle)	50–100	3–6	25, 50, 100
	Spironolactone (Parke-Davis)			25
Triamterene	Dyrenium (SKF)*	50–100	3–6	50, 10
Amiloride	Midamor (MSD)	5–10	24	5

*MSD = Merck Sharp & Dohme; SKF = Smith Kline & French.

TABLE 47–8. ANTIHYPERTENSIVE DRUGS IN AMBULATORY TREATMENT OF HYPERTENSION

Generic Name	Trade Name (manufacturer)	Adult Maintenance Dose (mg/day)	Frequency of Administration (times/day)	Duration of Action (hr)
Sympatholytic Agents				
Centrally acting alpha-adrenergic agents				
Methyldopa	Aldomet (MSD)†	250–2000	2	6–12
Clonidine	Catapres (Boehringer Ingelheim)	0.2–0.8	2	6–12
Guanabenz	Wytensin (Wyeth)	8–64	2	8–12
Reserpine and rauwolfia alkaloids	Serpasil (CIBA)	0.1–0.25	1	24
Beta-adrenergic–blocking agents				
Propranolol	Inderal (Ayerst)	40–640	2	6–12
Metoprolol	Lopressor (CIBA)	100–450	2	12
Atenolol	Tenormin (ICI)	50–100	1	24
Nadolol	Corgard (Squibb)	40–320	1	24
Timolol	Blocadren (MSD)	20–60	2	6–12
Pindolol	Visken (Sandoz)	10–60	2	6–12
Acebutolol	Sectral (Wyeth)	400–1200	1 or 2	12–24
Alpha-adrenergic–blocking agent				
Prazosin	Minipress (Pfizer)	2–20	2 or 3	3–6
Mixed alpha- and beta-adrenergic–blocking agent				
Labetalol	Normodyne (Schering), Trandate (Glaxo)	200–800	2	3–6
Ganglion-blocking agent				
Mecamylamine	Inversine (MSD)	25	2	12–24
Peripherally acting sympatholytic agent				
Guanethidine	Ismelin (CIBA)	10–300	1	24
Direct Vasodilators				
Hydralazine	Apresoline (CIBA)	20–300	2 or 3	6
Minoxidil	Loniten (Upjohn)	5–100	1 or 2	up to 72
Converting Enzyme Inhibitors				
Captopril	Capoten (Squibb)	75–450	3	4–8
Enalapril	Vasotec (MSD)	5–40	1 or 2	12–24
Calcium Channel–Blocking Agents*				
Nifedipine	Procardia (Pfizer)	30–120	3 or 4	6–8
Diltiazem	Cardizem (Marion)	90–240	3 or 4	6–8
Verapamil	Isoptin (Knoll), Calan (Searle)	240–480	3 or 4	6–8

*These agents have not been approved by the Food and Drug Administration (FDA) for the treatment of hypertension.
†MSD = Merck Sharp & Dohme.

STEP 1. Agents that should be considered as initial therapy include thiazide diuretics, beta-adrenergic blockers, and converting enzyme inhibitors (Fig. 47–6). Any of these agents given as monotherapy will control BP in the majority of patients with mild to moderate hypertension with a minimum of adverse effects.

Thiazide diuretics have been used as initial therapy in all of the major clinical trials of antihypertensive treatment. Advantages of these agents include efficacy in almost all classes of hypertensive patients, low cost, convenient dosing schedules, and potentiation of other antihypertensive drugs. Disadvantages include induction of electrolyte imbalance (hypokalemia and hypomagnesemia) with associated ventricular ectopic activity; hypercholesterolemia and hypertriglyceridemia, which enhance the tendency to develop atherosclerosis; hyperglycemia; and hyperuricemia, which may precipitate gout (Table 47–9). Despite these disadvantages, diuretics are the preferred step 1 agent in volume-dependent forms of hypertension, in blacks, and in older patients.

The beta-adrenergic blockers are preferred step 1 agents in patients with a hyperdynamic circulatory state (indicative of increased sympathetic activity) and in patients with coronary artery disease, as they have proved useful in heart attack prevention. Disadvantages of beta blocker therapy include exacerbations in obstructive pulmonary disease, asthma, and peripheral vascular insufficiency; fatigue; sexual dysfunction; bradycardia; and hypertriglyceridemia and reductions in high density lipoprotein (HDL) cholesterol.

The converting enzyme inhibitors may prove to be advantageous as step 1 agents in patients with renin-dependent hypertension. When given as monotherapy to unselected patients with essential hypertension, captopril restores BP to normal in approximately 50 per cent of cases; the remainder require addition of a diuretic or of a diuretic and beta-adrenergic blocker to achieve satisfactory BP control. Superior results may be obtained with the newer, more potent converting enzyme inhibitors, such as enalapril and lisinopril.* Advantages of converting enzyme inhibitors as step 1 therapy include paucity of subjective adverse effects and an absence of metabolic effects. Disadvantages include high cost and the lack of efficacy in patients whose hypertension is not renin dependent, including blacks and those with volume-dependent forms of hypertension.

STEP 2. Patients whose BP is not controlled with a step 1 drug require the addition of a second agent. Figure 47–6 summarizes therapeutic options frequently used at step 2. Step 2 agents should be added in small doses initially; then the dose should be increased until BP is controlled, the patient experiences adverse effects of the treatment, or the maximal dose is reached.

STEP 3. If step 2 therapy is inadequate in controlling BP, a third agent should be added. Figure 47–6 summarizes therapeutic options frequently used at step 3.

STEP 4. If the third step of therapy is ineffective, an additional agent that has a different mechanism of action should be added. Figure 47–6 summarizes therapeutic options frequently used at step 4.

Once BP is controlled on a stable dosage of antihypertensive drugs, fixed-dose combination tablets may be substituted in order to simplify the patient's regimen and reduce medication costs. Use of fixed-dose combination tablets provides the convenience of taking several drugs in a single tablet but has several disadvantages. The durations of action of the various components are frequently different, and the dosages may

*Investigational agent.

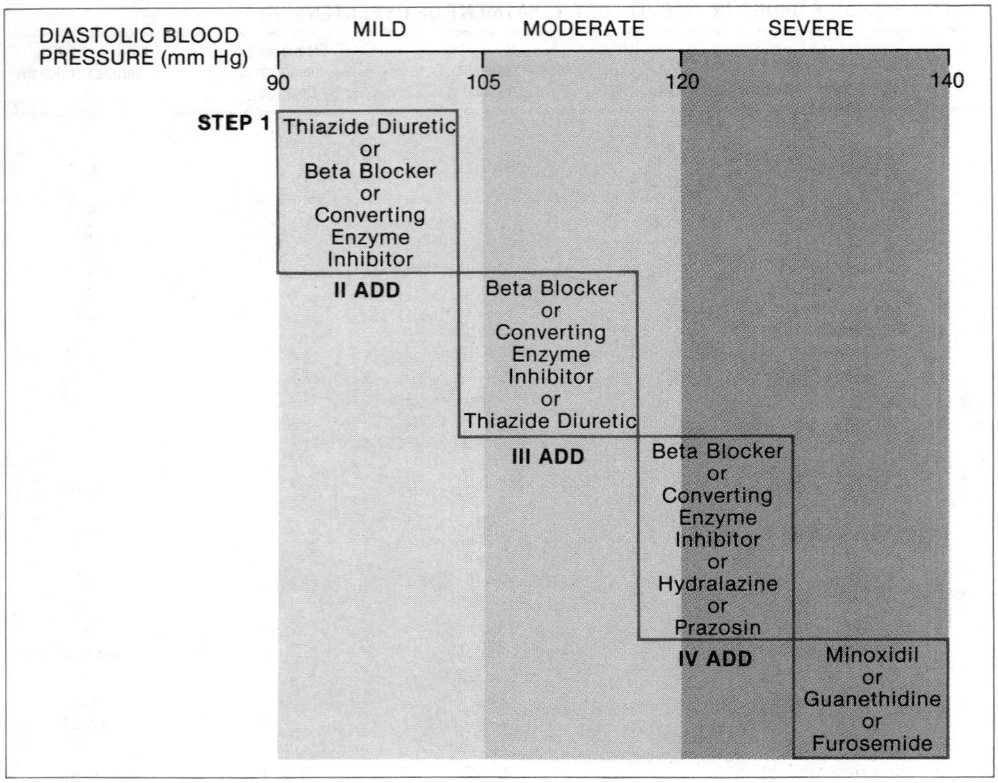

FIGURE 47–6. General antihypertensive ("stepped care") regimen.

not be appropriate for the patient's needs. The fixed-dose ratio precludes the adjustment of doses of constituent drugs to suit requirements of the individual patient.

"Step-down" therapy, or reduction of drug dosages, may be attempted in patients whose BP has been controlled for longer than one year. Administration of the lowest maintenance dose of therapy consistent with adequate BP control has the advantages of minimizing cost and adverse effects of treatment. Downward titration of doses or withdrawal of antihypertensive medications should be carried out only under careful medical supervision.

Systolic Hypertension in the Elderly

Elderly patients with rigid aortas have decreased baroreceptor responsiveness and are highly susceptible to postural hypotension when antihypertensive treatment is started. This susceptibility can be minimized by beginning with very small doses of drug and increasing dosage slowly. It has been recommended that diuretic treatment begin with half the usual starting dose, since small volume losses may give rise to large falls in pressure. Vasodilators, in small doses, are favored as second agents rather than sympatholytic drugs because the latter frequently cause central nervous system depression and may exacerbate postural hypotension.

Hypertensive Crisis

The goal of treatment in hypertensive crisis is to lower the BP as rapidly as possible to levels adequate to arrest progressive end-organ damage without causing hypoperfusion. Table 47–10 lists the antihypertensive drugs most commonly used in the management of hypertensive crisis, with recommended doses and common adverse effects. Intravenous furosemide should be administered along with these agents to assist in controlling BP and to prevent complicating fluid retention. The drug of choice in hypertensive crisis is sodium nitroprusside because it is almost always effective, has a very rapid onset of action, and has an antihypertensive effect that can be regulated precisely if monitoring facilities are available.

Secondary Hypertension

ORAL CONTRACEPTIVE–INDUCED HYPERTENSION. All patients who become hypertensive while on oral contraceptive treatment should have the drug withdrawn immediately. A treatment algorithm for such patients is outlined in Figure 47–7.

RENOVASCULAR HYPERTENSION. In general, the approach to patients with renovascular hypertension is to attempt revascularization with percutaneous transluminal angioplasty at the time of diagnosis in those with anatomically favorable lesions. If angioplasty is initially unsuccessful in dilating a lesion, or if restenosis occurs, the procedure can be repeated. If repeat angioplasty is unsuccessful, surgical revascularization should be attempted in patients with favorable lesions who can tolerate the procedure, particularly those whose BP is controlled even with medical treatment or whose renal function is deteriorating. In patients with anatomically unfavorable lesions, those who are not surgical candidates, and those whose BP can be controlled on antihypertensive drugs, medical treatment is indicated. Reliance on medical treatment is greater in patients over 50 years of age who have atherosclerotic renal artery disease and overt extrarenal vascular disease than in younger patients with fibromuscular disease. The relative efficacy of medical, percutaneous angioplastic, and surgical treatment of renovascular hypertension has never been rigorously evaluated in a randomized, controlled prospective study, so it is difficult to make firm recommendations about which therapeutic modality should be chosen for a given patient with this syndrome.

Percutaneous Transluminal Angioplasty. Dilatation of the renal artery is technically successful in 60 to 70 per cent of patients with atherosclerotic disease and 90 per cent of those with fibromuscular disease. Complete occlusion of the renal artery and bilateral renal artery stenosis have been successfully treated with transluminal angioplasty, as have the fibrotic, scarred lesions of renal transplant arterial stenosis and stenosis at the site of previous renal arterial repair. In contrast, atherosclerotic lesions located at the ostium of the renal artery

TABLE 47–9. ADVERSE DRUG EFFECTS

Drugs	Side Effects	Precautions and Special Considerations
	*Diuretics**	
Thiazides and related sulfonamides	Hypokalemia, hyperuricemia, glucose intolerance, hypercholesterolemia, hypertriglyceridemia, and sexual dysfunction	May be ineffective in renal failure; hypokalemia increases digitalis toxicity; and hyperuricemia may precipitate acute gout
Loop diuretics	Same as for thiazides	Effective in chronic renal failure; cautions regarding hypokalemia and hyperuricemia same as above; and hyponatremia may be found, especially in the elderly
Potassium-sparing agents		Danger of hyperkalemia in patients with renal failure
Amiloride hydrochloride	Hyperkalemia	—
Spironolactone	Sexual dysfunction	—
Triamterene	Gynecomastia, mastodynia, and sexual dysfunction	—
	—	
	Adrenergic Antagonists	
Beta-adrenergic blockers†	Bradycardia, fatigue, insomnia, bizarre dreams, sexual dysfunction, hypertriglyceridemia, decreased high-density lipoprotein cholesterol	Should not be used in patients with asthma, chronic obstructive pulmonary disease, congestive heart failure, heart block (greater than first degree), and sick sinus syndrome; use with caution in patients with diabetes and peripheral vascular disease
Central-acting adrenergic inhibitors	Drowsiness, dry mouth, fatigue, and sexual dysfunction	—
Clonidine	—	Rebound hypertension may occur with abrupt discontinuance
Guanabenz	—	Same as for clonidine
Methyldopa	—	May cause liver damage and positive direct Coombs' test
Peripheral-acting adrenergic inhibitors		—
Guanadrel sulfate	Sexual dysfunction and nasal congestion	
	Orthostatic-hypotension and diarrhea	Use cautiously in elderly patients because of orthostatic hypotension
Guanethidine monosulfate	Same as for guanadrel	Same as for guanadrel
Rauwolfia alkaloids	Lethargy	Contraindicated in patients with a history of mental depression; use with caution in patients with a history of peptic ulcer
Reserpine	Same as for rauwolfia alkaloids	Same as for rauwolfia alkaloids
$Alpha_1$-adrenergic blocker		
Prazosin hydrochloride	"First-dose" syncope, orthostatic hypotension, weakness, and palpitations	Use cautiously in elderly patients because of orthostatic hypotension
Combined alpha and beta-adrenergic blockers		
Labetalol hydrochloride‡	Asthma, nausea, fatigue, dizziness, and headache	Contraindicated in cardiac failure, chronic obstructive pulmonary disease, sick sinus syndrome, and heart block (greater than first degree); use with caution in patients with diabetes
	Vasodilators	
Vasodilators	Headache, tachycardia, and fluid retention	May precipitate angina in patients with coronary heart disease
Hydralazine hydrochloride	Positive antinuclear antibody (without other changes)	Lupus syndrome may occur (rare at recommended doses)
Minoxidil	Hypertrichosis, ascites (rare)	May cause or aggravate pleural and pericardial effusions
	Angiotensin-Converting Enzyme Inhibitors	
Angiotensin-converting enzyme inhibitors	Rash and dysgeusia (rare)	Can cause reversible acute renal failure in patients with bilateral renal arterial stenosis; neutropenia may occur in patients with autoimmune collagen disorders; and proteinuria may occur (rare at recommended doses)
	Calcium Channel–Blocking Agents§	
Calcium channel–blocking agents	Headache, hypotension, and dizziness	—
Diltiazem hydrochloride	Nausea	Use with caution in patients with congestive heart failure or heart block
Nifedipine	—	—
Verapamil hydrochloride	Flushing, edema, and constipation	Same as for diltiazem

*See Table 47–7 for a list of these drugs.
†Sudden withdrawal of these drugs may be hazardous in patients with heart disease.
‡This drug has not been approved by the Food and Drug Administration (FDA).
§These agents have not been approved by the FDA for the treatment of hypertension.
Modified from The 1984 Report of the Joint National Committee on Detection, Evaluation, and Treatment of High Blood Pressure. Arch Intern Med 144:1045, 1984.

TABLE 47–10. ANTIHYPERTENSIVE DRUGS FOR PARENTERAL ADMINISTRATION IN MANAGEMENT OF HYPERTENSIVE CRISIS

Drugs	Dosage: Intramuscular (mg*)	Dosage: Intravenous: Single Dose (mg*)	Dosage: Intravenous: Continuous Infusion (μg/kg/min)*	Onset of Action	Adverse Effects
Direct Vasodilators					
Sodium nitroprusside (Nipride)†	—	—	0.5–10	Instantaneous	Nausea, vomiting, muscle twitching, apprehension, sweating, thiocyanate intoxication
Diazoxide (Hyperstat)	—	50–100 at 5 to 10-min intervals until satisfactory BP response is achieved	Rarely used	3–5 min	Tachycardia, palpitations, flushing, headache, nausea, vomiting, aggravation of angina or congestive heart failure or both, hyperglycemia, hyperuricemia, hypotension
Hydralazine (Apresoline)	10–40 at 30-min intervals until satisfactory BP response is achieved	10–20‡ at 30-min intervals until satisfactory BP response is achieved	Rarely used	Intramuscularly, 30 min; intravenously, 5–10 min	Tachycardia, palpitations, flushing, headache, vomiting, aggravation of angina or congestive heart failure or both
Sympathetic Blocking Drugs					
Ganglion-blocking agents					
Trimethaphan camsylate (Arfonad)	—	—	4–90	5–10 min	Urinary retention, paralytic ileus, paralysis of pupillary reflex and accommodation of eye, dry mouth, orthostatic hypotension
Central nervous system–active agents					
Methyldopate hydrochloride (Aldomet ester)	—	250–500§; may be repeated at 6-hr intervals	—	2–3 hr	Drowsiness
Alpha-receptor–blocking agents					
Phentolamine (Regitine)†	5–15	5–15 (rapid injection essential)	—	Instantaneous	Tachycardia, flushing
Labetalol	—	50 (over a 1-min period)	3 to a total dose of 200 mg in malignant hypertension; 300 mg in pheochromocytoma	Instantaneous	Postural dizziness with or without postural hypotension; paradoxical pressor responses have been reported; nausea, vomiting, scalp tingling, burning in throat and groin

*Start with the smallest dose shown. Subsequent doses and intervals of administration should be adjusted according to the blood pressure response.

†Start infusion slowly and adjust rate according to response to BP. Constant surveillance is mandatory. Concentration of solution can be adjusted according to patient's fluid requirements.

‡The total dose should be contained in a volume of at least 20 ml, and the solution should be administered from a 20- or 50-ml syringe. Blood pressure should be monitored continuously while the injection is being made. Rate of injection should not exceed 0.5 ml per minute. To avoid hypotension, the injection should be stopped frequently when the BP is falling.

§Diluted up to 100 ml and injected during a 30- to 60-minute period.

Modified from The 1984 Report of the Joint National Committee on Detection, Evaluation, and Treatment of High Blood Pressure. Arch Intern Med 144:1045, 1984.

respond poorly to balloon dilatation, and angioplasty should not be attempted in patients with such lesions.

Complications of percutaneous transluminal angioplasty, including occlusion of the renal artery secondary to intimal dissection or thrombosis, renal artery perforation, retroperitoneal bleeding, and balloon rupture, are uncommon. Many of these complications require emergency surgery, however, so renal angioplasty should be done only with the backup of a vascular surgeon. Hypotension immediately after angioplasty can be a problem, particularly in patients who have had severe hypertension or who have been maintained on large doses of antihypertensive drugs up to the time of angioplasty. Special attention should be given to keeping these patients well hydrated.

Long-term results of transluminal dilatation for renal artery stenosis, as assessed by vessel patency and effect on BP, are promising. Approximately 85 per cent of patients with technically successful angioplasties show sustained improvement in BP control. Life-table analysis gives a cumulative success rate of 81 per cent for a three-year period: The cure rate (diastolic BP < 90 mm Hg with no medication) is 20 per cent; the improvement rate (diastolic BP < 100 mm Hg with decreased medication) is 65 per cent. Cure rates and improvement rates in fibromuscular disease are greater than in atherosclerotic disease.

In summary, percutaneous transluminal dilatation of the renal artery offers advantages over renovascular surgery that include lower cost, morbidity, and mortality; greater ease of documenting results by recording pressures across the stenosis before and after dilatation; and ease of repetition if restenosis occurs. Disadvantages include technical failure in 10 to 20 per cent of cases due to inability to pass through the stenosis or inability to dilate the artery when very firm lesions or ostial lesions are present.

Renovascular Surgery. In most published series, the overall surgical cure rate of patients with hypertension secondary to unilateral renal artery stenosis is 40 to 50 per cent; the improvement rate is approximately 50 per cent, and the failure rate is 10 per cent. Results in patients with fibromuscular disease are better than in those with arteriosclerotic disease, and morbidity and mortality rates are lower in the former group. Results in unilateral disease are better than in bilateral disease. Preoperative duration of hypertension is also an important predictor of the outcome of renovascular surgery. Approximately 80 per cent of patients who have had hypertension for less than five years before surgery, but only 25 per cent of those who have had hypertension for more than five years, show a favorable BP response. Recently, improved results (1 to 2 per cent mortality and low morbidity rates) in renovascular surgery have been attributed to sophisticated

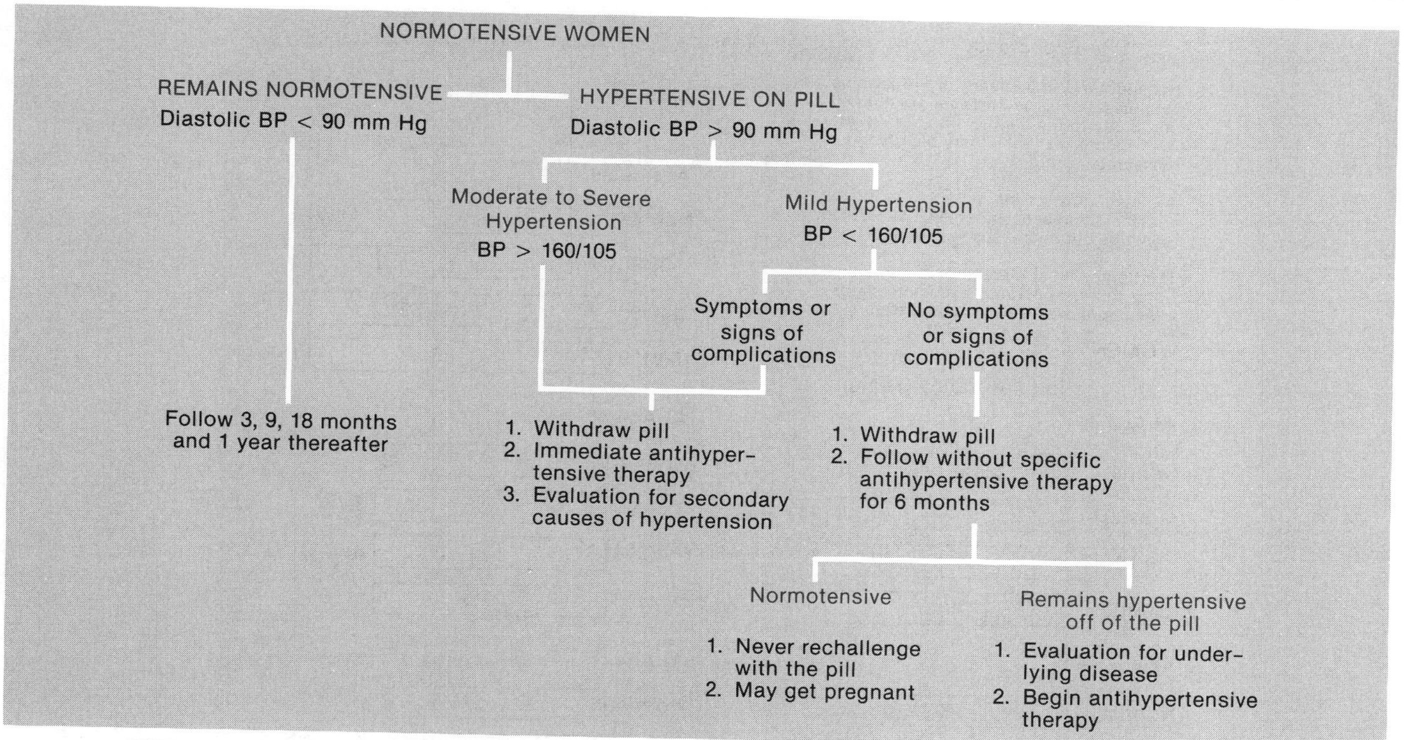

FIGURE 47–7. Diagnosis and management of oral contraceptive pill hypertension. (Reprinted with permission from The Journal of Reproductive Medicine 15:205, 1975.)

preoperative screening, preoperative correction of coexisting coronary or cerebrovascular disease, and employment of methods of revascularization, such as hepatorenal, splenorenal, or ileorenal bypass or autotransplantation, that obviate operation on a severely diseased aorta.

In summary, the noninvasive nature, low cost, and low morbidity of percutaneous renal angioplasty make it the procedure of choice in the initial approach to patients with renovascular hypertension and disease confined to the renal artery. Renovascular surgery should be reserved for those patients who are not candidates for angioplasty or for those whose artery cannot be successfully dilated because of the particular lesions present.

Medical Treatment. Converting enzyme inhibitors administered alone or in combination with a diuretic are effective in controlling BP while sparing renal function and maintaining negative sodium balance in patients with renovascular hypertension secondary to unilateral renal artery stenosis. These regimens are simple and well tolerated and represent the medical treatment of choice in most patients with renovascular hypertension. Converting enzyme inhibitors induce acute, reversible renal failure in a subset of patients with renovascular hypertension: those with bilateral renal artery stenosis or renal artery stenosis in a solitary kidney, whether native or allograft, or those with unilateral renal artery stenosis and severe parenchymal disease in the contralateral kidney. This form of reversible renal insufficiency is a consequence of impairment in the autoregulation of glomerular filtration secondary to blockade of the intrarenal renin-angiotensin system in the presence of reduced renal artery perfusion pressure. This explanation assumes that there is (1) enhanced intrarenal angiotensin II production under conditions of impaired renal perfusion and (2) a preferential constrictor effect of angiotensin II on the efferent arteriole, causing enhanced postglomerular vascular tone, thus maintaining an effective filtration pressure and glomerular filtration rate. Autoregulation of glomerular filtration rate, which is dependent on an intact intrarenal renin-angiotensin system, is lost when a converting enzyme inhibitor is administered.

Careful monitoring of renal size and function is mandatory in patients who are undergoing medical treatment for renovascular hypertension even if BP control is satisfactory. Deterioration of renal function and loss of renal mass can occur rapidly in patients with atherosclerotic disease who are treated medically. Progressive loss of renal mass, presumably related to parenchymal ischemia due to progression of the renal artery lesion, is common in medically treated patients with renovascular hypertension and does not appear to be related to BP control. Significant reduction in renal length is the most sensitive index of loss of renal mass. Serial (every three to six months) estimates of renal size, as by intravenous pyelography (IVP) or ultrasonography, are important in the follow-up of patients who are being treated medically for renovascular hypertension.

PRIMARY ALDOSTERONISM. The treatment of choice for hypertension secondary to an aldosterone-producing adenoma is unilateral adrenalectomy. In 70 to 80 per cent of cases, surgery restores both blood pressure and electrolytes to normal levels. Administration of spironolactone in doses of 200 to 400 mg per day for four to eight weeks can be used to predict the response to surgery: If spironolactone restores the BP to normal, a good surgical result can be expected; but if BP is unaffected by spironolactone, surgery is not likely to be successful.

Occasionally, the syndrome of primary aldosteronism is caused by adrenal carcinoma. The treatment of choice in this case is surgery, particularly if there is no evidence of metastasis. Alternatively, pharmacologic therapy—including aldosterone antagonists (spironolactone) and inhibitors of steroid biosynthesis, such as aminoglutethimide (Cytadren or trilostane) or the adrenolytic agent *o,p*′-DDD—can be used.

In patients with bilateral adrenal hyperplasia, remission of hypertension after bilateral total adrenalectomy occurs in only 18 to 35 per cent of cases. Chronic spironolactone administra-

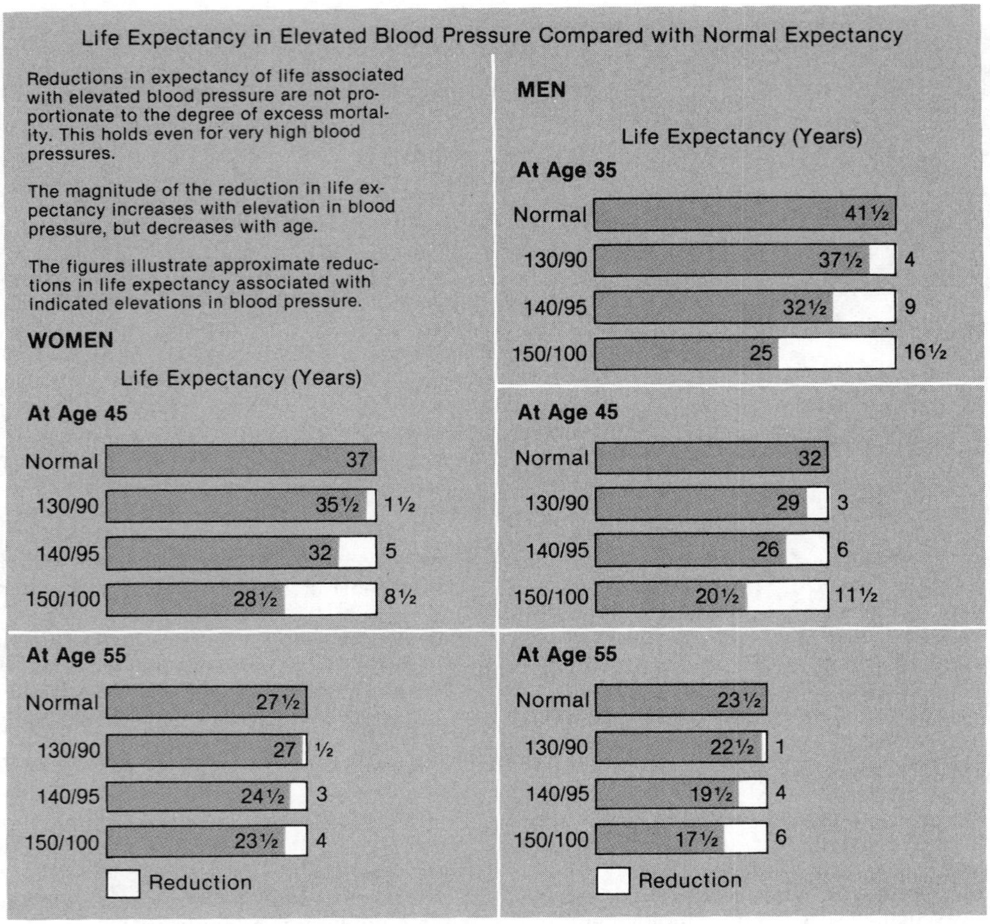

FIGURE 47–8. Life expectancy table. Normal means 120/80 mm Hg or less. (From Metropolitan Life Insurance Company: Blood Pressure: Insurance Experience and Its Implications, New York, Metropolitan Life Insurance Co., 1961.)

tion in doses greater than 200 mg per day is effective in controlling hypertension in these patients. The adverse effects of the drug, including nausea, vomiting, gynecomastia, impotence, hirsutism, and intermenstrual bleeding, limit its chronic use. In patients who are intolerant of spironolactone, amiloride may be an appropriate substitute.

PHEOCHROMOCYTOMA. Treatment of pheochromocytoma is surgical unless the tumor is metastatic or the patient is inoperable for other reasons. Patients should be prepared with alpha-adrenergic–blocking agents (phenoxybenzamine, prazosin, or labetalol) for one to two weeks before surgery to block the pressor effects of circulating norepinephrine and expand intravascular volume.

If surgery cannot be performed, patients can be managed medically with alpha-and beta-adrenergic blockers or the new combined alpha- and beta-adrenergic antagonist labetalol. Alpha-methylparatyrosine (Demser) inhibits tyrosine hydroxylase, the rate-limiting enzyme in catecholamine biosynthesis, thus reducing catecholamine production by the tumor and secondarily lowering BP. The many adverse effects of alpha-methylparatyrosine, including sedation, diarrhea, galactorrhea, anxiety, tremulousness, and crystalluria, limit its clinical usefulness.

PROGNOSIS

The excess mortality associated wiith hypertension is related mainly to cardiovascular disease and cerebral hemorrhage. Natural history studies in the era prior to the development of antihypertensive therapy showed that the mean age of onset of hypertension was the early 30's and the mean survival was 20 years. Thus life expectancy in hypertensive subjects was shortened by 15 to 20 years on the average. Survival was shorter for men (20 per cent surviving for 20 years) than for women (50 per cent surviving for 20 years) (Fig. 47–8). Further, subjects with hypertension of early onset and with more severe hypertension had shorter life expectancies. The prognosis for women was thought to be better because of their lower incidence of coronary artery disease and accelerated hypertension. Despite the variable rate of progression of hypertensive vascular disease, the average hypertensive pa-

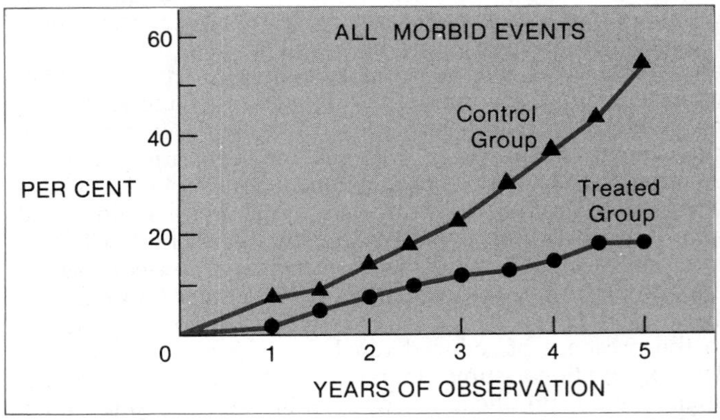

FIGURE 47–9. Life-table analysis, comparing the percentage of incidence of cardiovascular complications over a five-year period in controls versus treated patients with initial diastolic blood pressure between 90 and 114 mm Hg. (From Freis ED: VA Cooperative Study: JAMA 213:1143, 1970. Copyright 1970, American Medical Association.)

tient was free of symptoms and vascular complications for most of the duration of the syndrome.

The cardiovascular complications of hypertension include stroke secondary to cerebral hemorrhage or thrombosis, coronary artery disease with associated angina pectoris and acute myocardial infarction, left ventricular hypertrophy, congestive heart failure, aortic dissection, renal insufficiency, and peripheral vascular disease with intermittent claudication.

Controlled studies have demonstrated that effective antihypertensive treatment reduces the incidence of cardiovascular complications. In the Veterans Administration Cooperative Study, a randomized, double-blind prospective clinical trial in 523 male patients whose initial diastolic pressures ranged from 90 to 129 mm Hg, treatment with a combination of hydrochlorothiazide, reserpine, and hydralazine caused a sharp reduction in the incidence of stroke, congestive heart failure, accelerated hypertension, and renal failure. Although antihypertensive treatment did not significantly reduce the incidence of myocardial infarction or sudden death, there was a trend suggesting fewer fatal myocardial infarctions in treated subjects. Life-table analysis of these results indicates that over a five-year period the risk of developing a serious cardiovascular complication was reduced from 55 to 18 per cent by treatment (Fig. 47–9). The reduction in cardiovascular morbidity was related to the level of diastolic BP that was attained with treatment: Partial control of BP resulted in partial reductions in cardiovascular morbidity and mortality.

More recently, controlled trials in patients with mild hypertension (diastolic BP of 90 to 104 mm Hg) have uniformly shown that control of BP with antihypertensive drugs protects against stroke, left ventricular hypertrophy, congestive heart failure, and progression to more severe hypertension. Two studies, the Hypertension Detection and Follow-up Program (HDFP) and the Australian National Trial, demonstrated a benefit of antihypertensive therapy in reducing fatal and nonfatal coronary events. By contrast, a clear benefit from effective antihypertensive treatment has not been demonstrated in the subset of patients with a diastolic BP of 90 to 94 mm Hg. For that reason and because of concerns about the toxicity of antihypertensive agents, pharmacologic treatment of patients with mild hypertension is not always recommended.

Bravo EL, Tarazi RC, Gifford RW, et al.: Circulating and urinary catecholamines in pheochromocytoma: Diagnostic and pathophysiologic implications. N Engl J Med 301:682, 1979. *Comparison of the value of measuring plasma catecholamines versus urinary excretion of catecholamine metabolites in the diagnosis of pheochromocytoma. Plasma catecholamine measurement is a much more sensitive and specific diagnostic procedure than the measurement of urinary catecholamine metabolites.*

Bravo EL, Tarazi RC, Dustan HP, et al.: The changing clinical spectrum of primary aldosteronism. Am J Med 74:641, 1983. *A prospective study of 80 patients with primary aldosteronism (70 with adenoma and 10 with hyperplasia) that demonstrated that (1) measurements of serum potassium concentration and plasma renin activity are inadequate screening tests; (2) excessive aldosterone production measured as urinary aldosterone excretion rate after three days of salt loading is highly sensitive and specific for identifying patients with primary aldosteronism; and (3) the most accurate localizing procedure for adrenal adenoma is selective adrenal venous sampling for plasma aldosterone concentration.*

Genest J, Koiw E, Kuchel O: Hypertension. 2nd ed. New York, McGraw-Hill, 1983. *A comprehensive textbook that covers all aspects of the pathophysiology of systemic hypertension in animals and in humans.*

Hypertension Detection and Follow-up Program Cooperative Group: The effect of treatment on mortality in "mild" hypertension. N Engl J Med 307:976, 1983. *Evidence of significantly reduced five-year mortality in patients with mild hypertension and no evidence of end-organ damage treated with stepped care in special clinics compared with those treated according to usual community standards. These findings were interpreted as supporting a recommendation that in patients with mild hypertension, treatment should be considered early, before end-organ damage occurs.*

Kaplan NM: Clinical Hypertension. 4th ed. Baltimore, Williams & Wilkins Company, 1986. *A comprehensive textbook that covers the pathogenesis, diagnosis, and treatment of all forms of clinical hypertension.*

The 1984 Report of the Joint National Committee on Detection, Evaluation, and Treatment of High Blood Pressure. Arch Intern Med 144:1045, 1984. *Detailed recommendations for the diagnosis and pharmacologic and nonpharmacologic treatment of systemic hypertension.*

Oparil S, Haber E: The renin-angiotensin system. N Engl J Med 291:389, 1974. *A detailed and authoritative review of the biochemistry and physiology of the renin-angiotensin system.*

Oparil S, Katholi RE: Humoral control of the circulation. In Garfein OB (ed.): Cardiovascular Physiology: A Review. New York, Academic Press (in press). *A review of the hormonal and neural mechanisms that control normal cardiovascular homeostasis. It provides a useful basis for understanding the perturbations that occur in systemic hypertension.*

Veterans Administration Cooperative Study Group on Antihypertensive Agents: Effects of treatment on morbidity in hypertension: I. Results in patients with diastolic blood pressures averaging 115 through 129 mm Hg. JAMA 202:1028, 1967. *Demonstration that male hypertensive patients with diastolic blood pressure averaging 115 mm Hg or above represent a high-risk group in which hypertensive therapy exerts a significant beneficial effect.*

Veterans Administration Cooperative Study Group on Antihypertensive Agents: Effects of treatment on morbidity in hypertension: II. Results in patients with diastolic blood pressure averaging 90 through 114 mm Hg. JAMA 213:1143, 1970. *Demonstration that treatment of male patients with mildly elevated blood pressure is more effective in preventing congestive heart failure and stroke than in preventing the complications of coronary artery disease and that the degree of benefit of treatment is related to the level of prerandomization blood pressure.*

48 PULMONARY HYPERTENSION

Alfred P. Fishman

The pulmonary circulation is a highly distensible, low-resistance vascular bed interposed between the systemic veins and the systemic arteries. Its major function is gas exchange with ambient air. It differs from the circulation to other organs in that it is perfused by the entire output of the right ventricle (the cardiac output) and from the systemic circulation in that it lacks elaborate mechanisms for regulating blood pressure. Because of its large capacity, its great distensibility, and its low resistance, the pulmonary circulation is not prone to become hypertensive. When pulmonary hypertension does occur, it is usually secondary to cardiac or pulmonary disease. Only on rare occasion is "primary" or "unexplained" pulmonary hypertension encountered. Nonetheless, although uncommon, "primary" pulmonary hypertension is of considerable theoretic interest for the understanding of the clinical picture, natural history, and management of uncomplicated pulmonary hypertension.

The normal pulmonary hemodynamics of adults residing at sea level and at altitude are indicated in Table 48–1. Because of the passive nature of the pulmonary vascular bed, the pulmonary arterial pressure—particularly in hypertensive states—must be assessed with respect to the pulmonary blood flow (cardiac output). For a cardiac output of 5 to 6 liters per minute, the normal pulmonary arterial pressure at sea level is about 20 mm Hg systolic and 12 mm Hg diastolic, with a mean of about 15 mm Hg; the same level of blood flow is asssociated with higher pressures at altitude. Pulmonary arterial pressures also tend to increase somewhat with age.

Pulmonary hypertension is a colloquialism for pulmonary *arterial* hypertension. Unless otherwise stipulated, the term refers to *chronic* pulmonary hypertension. Acute pulmonary hypertension occurs most often clinically as a result of pulmonary embolism or the adult respiratory distress syndrome. This chapter will be confined to the chronic states.

Criteria for pulmonary hypertension depend on the altitude: In the resting individual at sea level, a *mean* pulmonary arterial pressure greater than 19 to 20 mm Hg establishes the diagnosis; the corresponding limit at altitude is higher—at about 15,000 feet, a *mean* pulmonary arterial pressure greater than 25 mm Hg signifies pulmonary hypertension. Pulmonary hypertension is important only if it imposes a heavy burden on the right ventricle. Thus mild pulmonary hypertension is clinically insignificant because it can be well tolerated by the right ventricle for a lifetime. However, mild pulmonary hy-

TABLE 48–1. REPRESENTATIVE VALUES AT REST FOR THE NORMAL PULMONARY CIRCULATION AT SEA LEVEL AND AT ALTITUDE

	Sea Level	14,900 ft
Pulmonary arterial pressure (mm Hg, systolic/diastolic, mean)	20/12, 15	38/14, 25
Cardiac output (liters/min)	6.0	6.0
Cardiac index (liters min/m², body surface area)	3.1	3.1
Left atrial pressure (mm Hg)	5.0	5.0
Pulmonary vascular resistance (R units*)	0.1†	0.2

*R units express calculated resistance in terms of $\frac{\text{mm Hg}}{\text{ml/sec.}}$. To convert to C.G.S. units (dynes · sec · cm^{-5}), the value in R units is multiplied by 1328.

†Based on the data in this table, at sea level, $R = \frac{15 - 5}{6000/60} = 0.1$ R units.

pertension at rest generally signifies higher levels during exercise or upon exposure to a pulmonary vasoconstricting stimulus, e.g., hypoxia. Not infrequently, pulmonary hypertension remains subclinical until an explanation is sought for unanticipated right ventricular failure. This is so because the normal right ventricle can handle comfortably a moderate afterload; e.g., it can generate systolic pressures of about 50 mm Hg. It can also cope with heavier work loads if allowed time to hypertrophy. However, when inordinate loads are imposed, e.g., pulmonary arterial pressures approximating systemic arterial pressures, it is destined to fail. Moreover, at high levels, hazards other than ventricular failure often supervene, including a propensity to syncope, precordial pain, and sudden death.

Pulmonary *venous* hypertension is a different entity with respect to etiology, pathogenesis, clinical manifestations, and management. It is said to exist when pulmonary venous or left atrial pressure exceeds 12 mm Hg; this limit applies to altitude as well as to sea level. In the normal pulmonary circulation an acute increase in pulmonary venous pressure to the range of 20 to 30 mm Hg increases the risk of pulmonary edema. The same levels are less threatening when sustained chronically, as in mitral valve disease, presumably by thickening of the walls of the fluid-exchanging vessels in the lungs. However, in these individuals, a further increment in venous pressure—as by exercise or infusions—topples them into pulmonary edema.

THE NORMAL PULMONARY CIRCULATION

Structure

In the normal adult, the small muscular arteries and arterioles constitute the "resistance" vessels. In the adult at sea level, these vessels are thin-walled and sparsely equipped with muscle; in the fetus and in the native resident at altitude, the muscle is thicker and more extensive. In contrast to the pulmonary circulation, the normal bronchial circulation is minute but capable of undergoing remarkable proliferation in congenital heart disease and in pulmonary disorders involving local suppuration and fibrosis.

Hemodynamics

Because of the low resistance and high distensibility of the pulmonary vascular bed and the pulsatile nature of pulmonary blood pressure, the large pulmonary blood flow is accomplished by only a small drop in mean pressure between the pulmonary artery and the left atrium (Table 48–1). The mean pressure difference is ordinarily about 5 to 10 mm Hg.

Calculated pulmonary vascular resistance has become a popular tool for assessing the state of the normal and abnormal pulmonary circulation and for detecting pulmonary vasoconstriction or vasodilation. Unfortunately, interpretation in terms of vasomotor activity can be clouded by passive changes that occur when pulmonary vascular blood pressures, or flow, or both are changing. For example, exercise normally elicits a passive decrease in resistance due to distention of open vessels and recruitment of vessels that were previously closed. Also, clinical short-cuts, such as the substitution of pulmonary arterial pressure for the pressure drop between pulmonary artery and left atrium, deprive the calculation of any physiologic meaning, although it may still suffice in pulmonary hypertensive states as an empiric tool. Finally, since the calculation involves a ratio, interpretation in terms of clinical significance can become highly subjective. For example, a decrease in calculated pulmonary resistance involving a drop in pulmonary arterial pressure in conjunction with an increase in cardiac output (while heart rate and left atrial and systemic blood pressures remain unchanged) would seem preferable for the welfare and favorable prognosis of a patient to the same decrease in resistance brought about by an increase in cardiac output, an unchanged pulmonary arterial pressure, and tachycardia.

A large increase in cardiac output, i.e., three times that at rest, increases pulmonary arterial pressure in the normal lung by only a few millimeters of mercury. But after restriction of the pulmonary vascular bed by disease or surgery, lesser increments in pulmonary blood flow elicit more striking increases in pulmonary arterial pressure.

The role of increase in the pulmonary blood volume is much more subtle and less susceptible to measurement. The normal pulmonary blood volume is about 500 ml, approximately 100 ml of which is in the pulmonary capillaries. Expansion of the pulmonary blood volume limits the distensibility of the pulmonary circulation and decreases the capability for avoiding sizable increments in pulmonary arterial pressure by recruiting new vessels. The pulmonary blood volume expands as cardiac output increases and during systemic vasoconstriction.

Although autonomic nerves supply the pulmonary vascular tree, they are far less effective in mediating vasoconstriction or vasodilation than are local stimuli. Indeed, hypoxia acting within the lungs is the most powerful mechanism for eliciting pulmonary vasoconstriction, particularly if reinforced by a concomitant acidosis. The mechanism by which hypoxia exerts its local pressor effect is unknown. Hypercapnia also exerts a pressor effect, presumably by way of the local acidosis that it generates.

CLINICAL MANIFESTATIONS

As indicated above, most cases of pulmonary hypertension are secondary (Table 48–2). As a rule, in these pulmonary hypertensive states, the clinical picture is dominated by the signs and symptoms of the underlying disease, which also shapes the natural history, prognosis, and response to treatment. The clinical entity of "primary pulmonary hypertension," in which the heart and lungs are not etiologically related to the pulmonary hypertension, is described subsequently.

SECONDARY PULMONARY HYPERTENSION

As causes of secondary pulmonary hypertension, heart or lung diseases dominate in numbers. Less impressive in number but of great clinical importance because of the potential for prevention and cure on the one hand and catastrophe on the other is pulmonary thromboembolic disease. Heart disease exerts its effects by increasing pulmonary blood flow or pulmonary venous pressure. In contrast, lung disease and thromboembolic disease cause pulmonary hypertension by increasing resistance to blood flow, albeit by different mechanisms.

TABLE 48–2. CLASSIFICATION OF CHRONIC PULMONARY (ARTERIAL) HYPERTENSION

I. **Secondary**
  A. Cardiac Disease
    1. Acquired disorders of the left side of the heart causing pulmonary venous hypertension
      Left ventricular failure
      Mitral valve disease
      Left atrial myxoma
      Decrease in left ventricular compliance
    2. Congenital heart disease
      Pre-tricuspid
      Post-tricuspid
  B. Occlusive Pulmonary Vascular Disease
  C. Respiratory Disorders
    1. Interstitial fibrosis
    2. Obstructive airways disease
    3. Combined fibrosis, emphysema, and chronic bronchitis
    4. Alveolar hypoventilation despite normal lungs
    5. Adult respiratory distress syndrome
    6. Multiple systemic diseases
II. **Primary**

Cardiac Disease

Acquired disorders of the left side of the heart and certain types of congenital heart disease often lead to pulmonary hypertension.

ACQUIRED DISORDERS OF THE LEFT SIDE OF THE HEART. Left ventricular failure is the outstanding cause of pulmonary hypertension. It is also the most common cause of right ventricular failure. Rarely is the level of pulmonary hypertension sufficient to account for the right ventricular failure. The discrepancy is usually attributed to concomitant failure of the muscle in the ventricular septum.

Myocardial disorders and lesions of the mitral and aortic valves are the most common left ventricular disorders leading to pulmonary hypertension. Occasional instances also occur of constrictive pericarditis, which compromises primarily the compliance of the left ventricle, thereby increasing its end-diastolic pressure. All first raise pulmonary venous pressure, which, in turn, evokes an increase in pulmonary arterial pressure that is necessary to maintain antegrade flow. How this automatic adjustment is accomplished is unclear. But, in time, three types of morphologic changes appear: (1) occlusive intimal and medial changes in pulmonary *precapillary* vessels as well as in pulmonary venules and veins; (2) perivascular interstitial edema, which not only contributes directly to the increase in resistance to blood flow but also stimulates perivascular fibrosis; under the influence of gravity, the vascular and perivascular changes are most marked in the dependent portions of the lungs; and (3) occlusion of small pulmonary vessels by emboli or thrombi; especially in states of slowed systemic blood flow, emboli are much more apt to arise from thrombi in the veins of the extremities than from the right side of the heart. Depending on the reversibility of the vascular and perivascular lesions, surgical relief of the pulmonary venous hypertension, as by mitral valve commissurotomy or replacement, generally reduces the pulmonary arterial pressure.

CONGENITAL HEART DISEASE. At term, pulmonary arterial pressure approximates aortic pressure and is generally about 70/40, with a mean of 50 mm Hg. After birth, the combination of closure of the ductus arteriosus and pulmonary vasodilation causes pulmonary arterial pressure to fall rapidly to about one half of systemic levels. Thereafter, a gradual drop usually brings pulmonary arterial pressures to normal adult values in one to four weeks.

Congenital defects that produce left to right shunting of blood within the heart or between the great vessels are commonly associated with pulmonary arterial hypertension. But acute left to right shunts per se do not produce appreciable pulmonary hypertension in normal lungs unless flow is massive, i.e., at least three times greater than normal. Therefore, even though the increase in pulmonary blood flow produced by the left to right shunt is often the cardinal initiating element in this type of pulmonary hypertension, important contributing factors are the degree of arterial hypoxemia and the duration of the hemodynamic abnormalities. The interplay of these mechanisms leads to occlusive pulmonary vascular changes that, depending on the congenital defect, preferentially damage pulmonary vascular intima or media and inflict different degrees of pulmonary vascular injury. Not infrequently, as the hemodynamic abnormalities persist, the anatomic changes in the pulmonary resistance vessels take over as the dominant mechanism in sustaining the pulmonary hypertension and in determining its reversibility.

It was noted above that the pulmonary vascular lesions in pulmonary arterial hypertension are somewhat variable. However, sustained increases in pulmonary arterial pressure and arterial hypoxemia are generally associated with medial hypertrophy, whereas large pulmonary blood flows usually elicit intimal proliferation. Once pulmonary hypertension becomes chronic, distinctions between pressure and flow effects on the vascular wall tend to blur. In addition, as the pulmonary hypertension approaches systemic levels, various consequences of necrotizing arteritis supervene, including plexiform and angiomatoid lesions. Congenital defects in which pulmonary hypertension persist from birth also seem to interfere with the normal involution of the pulmonary resistance vessels so that the characteristic thin-walled resistance vessels of the normal adult lung fail to evolve. To complicate matters further, atherosclerotic lesions in the pulmonary hypertensive circulation and local thrombi or emboli add a final hypertensive element to the occlusive pulmonary vascular processes.

Important differences exist with respect to the natural history of pulmonary hypertension caused by "pre-tricuspid" congenital defects (e.g., secundum atrial septal defect) on the one hand and "post-tricuspid" congenital defects (e.g., ventricular septal defect) on the other. These are described elsewhere in this volume.

Occlusive Pulmonary Vascular Disease

The causes of secondary pulmonary hypertension due to occlusive vascular disease vary with geography. In the United States and Europe, extensive obliteration of the pulmonary arterial tree by pulmonary emboli is a common cause. In other parts of the world, other etiologies predominate. Thus, in Egypt, where schistosomiasis is endemic, pulmonary vascular disease caused by mechanical obstruction and hypersensitivity reactions is not uncommon. Elsewhere, filariasis is considered to be an important cause of pulmonary hypertension. In the United States, sickle-cell disease, the most common cause of pulmonary vascular thrombosis, rarely causes pulmonary hypertension. Several types of cancer, notably choriocarcinoma, can embolize the pulmonary circulation after the tumor has invaded the liver or the inferior vena cava.

Another important, but less common, cause of obliterative pulmonary vascular disease is the connective tissue disorders, such as systemic lupus erythematosus. Although it is generally held on morphologic grounds that connective tissue disorders of the lungs favor large, rather than small, vessels, recent improvements in the sensitivity and diversity of serologic testing for autoimmune disorders have lent credence to the proposition that connective tissue disorders may affect the small pulmonary vessels more often than previously believed.

The common denominator in pulmonary hypertension due to chronic obliterative pulmonary vascular disease is amputation and occlusion of large segments of the pulmonary circulation, abetted by pulmonary vasoconstriction largely attributable to systemic arterial hypoxemia. Early in the course of embolic pulmonary vascular disease, systemic arterial hypoxemia is mild and contributes little of the pulmonary arterial hypertension. Preterminally, however, as the right ventricle fails, the role of the "anatomic venous admixture," or "shunt," increases considerably as the oxygen content of blood returning to the lung decreases because of the slowed circulation and greater oxygen extraction in peripheral tissues.

In patients who have chronic pulmonary hypertension secondary to pulmonary emboli, two different types of pathogenetic sequences can usually be identified: (1) *clinically detectable* thromboembolic disease originating in systemic veins that is either progressive, overlooked, or neglected, and (2) a syndrome of "multiple pulmonary emboli" that is covert and mimics primary pulmonary hypertension in its clinical expression and natural history. In the latter type, precapillary vessels throughout the lung are partially or totally occluded by organized clots. Since the lesions are microscopic, only lung biopsy or autopsy can distinguish multiple pulmonary emboli from primary pulmonary hypertension. Although the possibility exists that the multiple pulmonary "emboli" are in reality multiple pulmonary thrombi secondary to widespread endothelial damage, by the time the nature of the disorder is recognized, scarring has occurred and the practical implications for management are no different from those of primary pulmonary hypertension.

Usually management involves antithrombotic therapy, occasionally supplemented by surgical elimination of the veins from which the emboli originate. Much less amenable to medical or surgical interventions are the covert multiple pulmonary emboli, in which the source and occurrence of pulmonary emboli are inapparent during life.

Tachypnea is a hallmark of pulmonary emboli. It persists during sleep and is generally associated with tachycardia. This pattern of rapid, shallow breathing is indistinguishable from that arising from stiffened lungs of any cause, e.g., interstitial pulmonary edema. And, by analogy with pulmonary interstitial edema, vagal afferent impulses arising from juxtacapillary (J) receptors and irritant receptors are generally believed to be responsible. The result of the rapid, shallow breathing is alveolar and dead space hyperventilation that, in turn, decreases the P_{CO_2} in arterial blood and alveolar gas and widens the alveolar-arterial difference in P_{O_2}. Indeed, the combination of arterial hypoxemia, hypocapnia, and a widened alveolar-arterial gradient for P_{O_2} suggests pulmonary emboli.

Since there is no obstructive disease of the airways to cloud the clinical picture, right ventricular enlargement secondary to pulmonary hypertension is manifested in pure form (see Primary Pulmonary Hypertension).

The "gold standard" for detecting pulmonary emboli is selective, high-resolution pulmonary angiography. However, even this paragon is not perfect, especially in detecting multiple pulmonary emboli of minute vessels. More expedient, but far less certain, are lung scans that have great consistency when normal in excluding pulmonary emboli and, when abnormal, in pinpointing areas of the lungs to be explored by selective angiography. By the time the characteristic chest radiograph of pulmonary hypertension has evolved, angiography and lung scans are rarely of much help in distinguishing healed multiple pulmonary emboli from primary pulmonary hypertension. But, on occasion, they do settle the issue by disclosing one or more organized clots in the pulmonary arterial tree. Right-sided heart catheterization is often done to determine the level of the pulmonary arterial hypertension, to confirm that pulmonary wedge pressures are normal, to assess the state of right ventricular performance, and to test the efficacy of pulmonary vasodilator agents.

Once pulmonary hypertension has been established in the patient with thromboembolic disease, it is generally irreversible. Therefore, preventive measures, directed at the source of emboli, hold more promise than treatment. The medical and surgical approaches to thromboembolic disease are described elsewhere in this volume.

As symptomatic measures, oxygen-enriched inspired mixtures are often helpful in relieving breathlessness, in enhancing cerebration, in relieving arterial hypoxemia, and, thereby, in decreasing the level of pulmonary hypertension. However, unless arterial hypoxemia is marked, the drop in pulmonary arterial pressure during oxygen breathing is rarely striking, and it is usually unclear whether the slight relief in pulmonary arterial pressure is due to a decrease in cardiac output or to pulmonary vasodilation. Almost invariably, once the diagnosis is entertained or established, anticoagulation is initiated even if a search for the sources of emboli proves fruitless. The investigation and treatment are rarely more than gestures, because the pulmonary disease is usually too far advanced for impressive improvement to occur or for the downhill course of the disease to be arrested. Pulmonary vasodilators have not proved to be a reliable form of therapy.

Other forms of secondary obliterative pulmonary vascular disease are usually equally difficult to manage unless a reversible component can be identified, as in a connective tissue disorder that responds to steroids. The lessons learned from pulmonary embolic disease are the importance of prevention and early intervention to control or eliminate the systemic venous (rarely cardiac) source of clots to the lungs.

Respiratory Disorders

Respiratory disorders elicit pulmonary hypertension in different ways: widespread interstitial fibrosis and/or inflammation in the vicinity of the minute pulmonary vessels, by encroaching upon vascular lumens, thereby limiting their distensibility and amputating peripheral segments of the pulmonary vascular tree; obstructive airways disease by causing arterial hypoxemia; conglomerate fibrosis, emphysema, and chronic bronchitis by a combination—in varying proportions—of distorting, encasing, and occluding large segments of the pulmonary vascular tree and promoting vasoconstriction of the pulmonary resistance vessels by inducing alveolar hypoxia and arterial hypoxemia.

INTERSTITIAL FIBROSIS. Familiar examples of this category are sarcoidosis, asbestosis, and radiation fibrosis. Lymphangitic spread of carcinoma within the lungs can produce the same functional effect.

The clinical picture is generally dominated by dyspnea and tachypnea; cough is rarely a prominent feature. The chest radiograph is particularly diagnostic in disclosing a widespread pattern that is consistent with either interstitial fibrosis or infiltration, or both. Corticosteroids are usually the main hope in therapy, often in conjunction with enriched oxygen mixtures. Oxygen therapy holds little promise for relieving pulmonary hypertension unless appreciable arterial hypoxemia is present at rest.

OBSTRUCTIVE AIRWAYS DISEASE. Chronic bronchitis and emphysema ("chronic obstructive lung disease, or COPD") is the most common cause of pulmonary hypertension and cor pulmonale. Even though chronic bronchitis and emphysema generally coexist, it is the chronic bronchitis that is predominantly responsible for the alveolar hypoxia and the low P_{O_2}, high P_{CO_2}, and resultant low pH that lead to pulmonary hypertension. Emphysema per se probably does predispose to pulmonary hypertension by amputating segments of the pulmonary vascular bed. But emphysema does not cause pulmonary hypertension, even when rarefaction of the lungs is extensive, because ventilation-perfusion relationships are not severely deranged as in chronic bronchitis. Cystic fibrosis provides another illustration of the importance of chronic obstructive airways disease in evoking pulmonary hypertension. Here, as in chronic bronchitis, the basic mechanism is persistent alveolar hypoxia, arterial hypoxemia, and, to a lesser extent, respiratory acidosis resulting from ventilation-perfusion abnormalities.

The indiscriminate use of "COPD" to designate the spectrum of obstructive airways disease, without distinguishing between predominant bronchitis and predominant emphysema, tends to promote ambiguity with respect to perceptions of the natural history of this group of diseases. In essence, pulmonary hypertension (often leading to cor pulmonale) is encountered in two different settings: episodically in the "pink puffer" during an acute respiratory infection and chronically in the "blue bloater," with periodic exacerbations during an acute respiratory infection. In the "blue bloater" the course of the pulmonary hypertension is inexorably progressive. It is noteworthy that in the patient first seen during a bout of respiratory failure, clinical distinction between a "pink puffer" and a "blue bloater" is often impossible. However, after recovery from the acute episode, distinction is usually quite simple.

One of the cardinal signs of pulmonary hypertension is right ventricular enlargement. However, recognition of right ventricular enlargement may be difficult in obstructive airways disease because of hyperinflation and cardiac rotation. Right ventricular failure often is accompanied by striking cyanosis, unexplained drowsiness or inappropriate behavior, distended neck veins, warm hands, suffused conjunctivas, hepatomegaly, and edema of the extremities. Right ventricular gallops (S_3 and S_4) are generally present, and the murmur of tricuspid insufficiency can often be elicited. Not only is the liver generally displaced downward by the low diaphragm, but it is also enlarged and tender to gentle pressure over the abdomen. Hepatomegaly is invariably associated with distended neck veins and often with peripheral edema. Once suspicion is raised that the clinical picture of right ventricular failure stems from ventilation-perfusion abnormalities, an arterial blood sample will confirm that the P_{O_2} is low (P_{O_2} < 40 to 50 torr), the P_{CO_2} is high (P_{CO_2} > 50 torr), and respiratory acidosis is present. Such arterial blood gas tensions are rare in left ventricular failure unless the patient is in frank pulmonary edema. The chest radiograph is often more helpful in detecting right ventricular enlargement retrospectively than during right ventricular failure.

Electrocardiographic evidence of right ventricular enlargement is also often equivocal in patients with bronchitis and emphysema because of rotation and displacement of the heart, widened distances between electrodes and the cardiac surface, and the predominance of dilation over hypertrophy in the cardiac enlargement. Indeed, if right ventricular enlargement is apparent, it can be assumed that the degree of cardiomegaly is severe.

Because of these limitations, it is not surprising that standard electrocardiographic criteria for right ventricular enlargement apply in about only one third of patients with chronic bronchitis and emphysema who have right ventricular hypertrophy at autopsy. Consecutive changes in the electrocardiogram are often more useful than a single electrocardiogram in detecting right ventricular overload due to pulmonary hypertension. As the arterial P_{O_2} drops to distinctly subnormal levels (e.g., below 60 to 70 torr while awake), T waves tend to become inverted, biphasic, or flat in the right, precordial leads (V_1 to V_3), the mean electrical axis of the QRS shifts 30 degrees or more to the right of the patient's usual axis, ST segments become depressed in leads II, III, and aVF, and right bundle branch block (incomplete or complete) often appears. These changes tend to reverse as arterial oxygenation improves.

In the patient with bronchitis and/or emphysema in whom pulmonary hypertension has been elicited or aggravated by a bout of bronchitis or pneumonia, the goal of therapy is to maintain tolerable levels of arterial oxygenation while waiting for the upper respiratory infection to subside. If the pulmonary hypertension is acute, modest enrichment of inspired air with oxygen, as by 28 per cent oxygen delivered by a Venturi mask, generally suffices to relieve arterial hypoxemia and to restore pulmonary arterial pressures toward normal. Considerable improvement may also be accomplished even in the individual who has chronic pulmonary hypertension by sustained (virtually continuous) breathing of oxygen-enriched air that restores arterial P_{O_2} to nearly normal values.

Once the right ventricle has failed, cardiotonic agents must be used cautiously beause of the threat of arrhythmias posed by arterial hypoxemia and respiratory acidosis. Moreover, after adequate oxygenation has been achieved, the need for digitalis and diuretics often decreases, since the hemodynamic burden on the right ventricle (i.e., the pulmonary arterial hypertension) decreases. Even though each episode of acute hypoxia and acidosis seems to elicit about the same increment in pulmonary arterial pressure, each bout of pulmonary hypertension appears to leave behind a slightly higher level of pulmonary hypertension after recovery.

Arterial blood gas composition is the therapeutic compass to the control of pulmonary hypertension in obstructive airways disease. The degree of hypoxia is usually underestimated by conventional practice for blood sampling, since hypoxemia is regularly more marked during sleep than during waking hours. In managing ambulatory patients, serial determinations of the hematocrit may serve as a practical clue to the occurrence of covert arterial hypoxemia. However, once right ventricular failure has set in, there is no substitute for determining arterial P_{O_2} and P_{CO_2} as a guide to therapy. Ensuring the return of arterial oxygenation toward normal is much more vital than is the administration of cardiotonic measures. When respiratory infection has triggered the episode of pulmonary hypertension, a vital strategy for achieving a lasting improvement in arterial oxygenation is the administration of an appropriate antibiotic. While awaiting the salutary effects of antibiotic therapy, attention is paid to hydration, to postural drainage, and to adequate alveolar ventilation. The management of respiratory acidosis is described elsewhere in this volume.

Phlebotomy was once popular as an ancillary measure because of the prospect that increased blood viscosity contributes importantly to the pulmonary hypertension. This practice has fallen into disuse. Polycythemia is rarely severe enough to be a serious problem in cor pulmonale that is associated with bronchitis and emphysema.

Vasodilators have recently been tried in various types of secondary pulmonary hypertension, including that due to obstructive airways disease. The agents tried are the same as those outlined for primary pulmonary hypertension and their efficacy is far less impressive or predictable. To date, the most reliable approach to pulmonary vasodilation in obstructive arterial hypoxemia is enriching inspired air with oxygen.

CONGLOMERATE FIBROSIS, EMPHYSEMA, AND CHRONIC BRONCHITIS. Pulmonary hypertension is uncommon in uncomplicated silicosis or tuberculosis. By contrast, in patients in whom smouldering, long-standing tuberculosis or conglomerate, massive fibrosis has shrunk and distorted the lungs, pulmonary hypertension is virtually the rule. The likelihood of pulmonary hypertension (and cor pulmonale) is enhanced by chronic pleurisy, fibrothorax, or excisional surgery, which exert their effects by a combination of anatomic restriction of the vascular bed and disturbances in gas exchange. Of all of these derangements, the disturbances in gas exchange are most susceptible to relief. Although these combinations are generally complicated, the principles of management are those outlined above for obstructive airways disease. Unfortunately, therapeutic triumphs are uncommon, because of the fixed anatomic changes.

ALVEOLAR HYPOVENTILATION IN PATIENTS WITH NORMAL LUNGS. In those individuals who develop net alveolar hypoventilation even though their lungs are normal, as in those with ventilation-perfusion abnormalities, the common pathogenetic denominators are alveolar hypoxia and arterial hypoxemia, often reinforced by respiratory acidosis. The global alveolar hypoventilation in individuals with normal lungs generally originates in either an inadequate ventilatory drive in subtle upper airways obstruction, as in the sleep apnea syndromes, or in an ineffective chest bellows. Among the disorders associated with global alveolar hypoventilation are residual paralyses of respiratory muscles, unresponsive respiratory "centers," kyphoscoliosis, and extreme obesity. The corresponding clinical syndromes are considered elsewhere in this volume.

The clinical manifestations are detemined by the etiology and pathogenesis; the occurrence of pulmonary hypertension depends on the development of alveolar hypoxia sufficient to evoke arterial hypoxemia. Early in the disorder, when arterial hypoxemia (and hypercapnia) is minimial, cyanosis may appear only during exercise, as the ventilation fails to keep pace with the increased metabolic demand. Alternatively, as in the sleep apnea syndromes, arterial hypoxemia and hypercapnia may become appreciable only during sleep. Regardless of the underlying cause, an upper respiratory infection often topples the subject into acute respiratory failure and severe pulmonary hypertension.

For the patient in combined respiratory and cardiac (right ventricular) failure, the highest priority is to improve oxygenation. Success with this strategy results in a decrease in pulmonary arterial pressures, thereby relieving the overburdened right ventricle. Recently, potent but short-acting pulmonary vasodilators, such as prostacyclin, have been advocated for urgent relief of right ventricular overload. But, in this category of patients, pharmacologic therapy is rarely needed because of the efficiency of the oxygen therapy in promoting pulmonary vasodilation.

ADULT RESPIRATORY DISTRESS SYNDROME. In this disorder, pulmonary hypertension is quite common, occasionally in conjunction with pulmonary venous hypertension secondary to fluid overload but more often as a consequence of mechanical influences exerted by pulmonary edema and atelectasis operating in conjunction with respiratory acidosis. This concomitant disorder requires no special treatment, since it follows the course of the illness, decreasing spontaneously as the patient recovers.

MULTIPLE SYSTEM DISEASES. Pulmonary hypertension is occasionally caused by the pulmonary arterial lesions of connective tissue diseases, notably lupus erythematosus, scleroderma, and dermatomyositis. However, the most common cause of pulmonary hypertension in systemic disorders is sarcoidosis, not only because this disorder is more prevalent than the connective tissue disorders but also because of the proclivity of the parenchymal lesions for the vicinity of the small pulmonary arteries and arterioles.

PRIMARY (UNEXPLAINED) PULMONARY HYPERTENSION

Definition

Primary pulmonary hypertension is a synonym for "unexplained" pulmonary arterial hypertension. It is also a diagnosis of exclusion. As a rule, pulmonary veno-occlusive disease (see below) is not included under the rubric of primary pulmonary hypertension because, although unexplained in etiology, its pathologic features and pathogenetic mechanisms are different and usually quite distinctive.

The clinical diagnosis of primary pulmonary hypertension rests on three different types of evidence: (1) clinical, radiographic, and electrocardiographic manifestations of pulmonary hypertension; (2) demonstration by right-heart catheterization of the typical hemodynamic constellation of abnormally high pulmonary arterial pressures and pulmonary vascular resistance in association with a normal pulmonary wedge pressure and a nearly normal cardiac output; and (3) inability to attribute the pulmonary hypertension to a disorder of the heart, lungs, or systemic circulation.

With respect to corroborating the clinical diagnosis, the pathologist is most helpful in proving that the cause of the pulmonary hypertension is as obscure after death as it was during life. Unfortunately, the idea of a pathognomonic vascular lesion—notably the "plexiform" lesion—has not been rewarding on three accounts: (1) Primary pulmonary hypertension seems to be the final common pathway for multiple unknown etiologies; (2) the vascular lesions have been shown by biopsy and at autopsy to be quite heterogeneous; and (3) plexiform lesions probably represent a healed pulmonary arteritis and are diagnostic of one type of primary pulmonary hypertension if other causes of plexiform lesions can be excluded.

GENERAL FEATURES. Primary pulmonary hypertension is an uncommon disorder and, at autopsy, is responsible for about 1 per cent of all causes of cor pulmonale. A total of about 1000 cases have been reported.

After puberty, females predominate, most strikingly between 10 and 40 years of age. Before puberty, no sex difference is discernible. Consequently, the paradigmatic patient with primary pulmonary hypertension is a young woman in the prime of life without discernible cause for symptoms. This fact is sometimes useful in the clinical differentiation between primary pulmonary hypertension and pulmonary thromboembolic disease, which, unless preceded by a predisposing disease, trauma, or intervention, favors men, particularly in their later years.

Until recently, virtually all reports of primary pulmonary hypertension dealt with sporadic cases. About 25 families have now been identified in which the disease seems to be hereditary. The question has been raised whether detailed histories would demonstrate that some sporadic cases are actually familial.

Over the years, evidence has accumulated that primary pulmonary hypertension may be the end result of diverse etiologies, ranging from incomplete involution of the fetal circulation to autoimmunity, diet, and drugs (Table 48–3). The diversity of potential causes complicates management. In addition, they confuse descriptions of natural history. Thus, although the paradigm cited above indicates death within two to three years, several instances now exist of much longer life spans. Moreover, occasional instances are known of regression of the disease, most notably during the subsidence of the epidemic of primary pulmonary hypertension associated with the ingestion of the anorectic agent Aminorex in Europe between 1967 and 1970.

Pathology

The seat of the disease is the small pulmonary arteries (between 40 and 100 μ in diameter). The obliterative lesions are diverse, affecting one or more layers of the small muscular arteries and arterioles. In some instances, medial hypertrophy predominates; in others, combinations of inflammation and fibrosis coexist. The "classic" picture of concentric intimal fibrosis, necrotizing arteritis, and plexiform lesions encountered in the Aminorex epidemic is far from the rule. Pathologists can usually distinguish with confidence the obliterated vessels of primary pulmonary hypertension from those of multiple pulmonary emboli. An important basis for this distinction is the *concentric* pattern of the fibroelastosis that obliterates the vascular lumens in primary pulmonary hypertension and the *eccentric* fibroelastosis that follows organization of venous clots after pulmonary embolization. But these differences are not absolute.

Pathophysiology

The hemodynamic hallmarks of primary pulmonary hypertension studies at rest are well known: a high pulmonary arterial pressure in association with a nearly normal cardiac output and a normal left atrial (pulmonary wedge) pressure.

TABLE 48–3. SUGGESTED ETIOLOGIES FOR PRIMARY PULMONARY HYPERTENSION

Etiology	Comment
Autoimmune mechanisms	Especially in young women, associated with Raynaud's phenomenon and collagen diseases, such as disseminated lupus erythematosus, rheumatoid arthritis, progressive systemic sclerosis, polyarteritis nodosa, and dermatomyositis.
Persistence of fetal pulmonary vascular bed	A distinct syndrome in neonatal life that is questionably related to the adult syndrome.
Dietary pulmonary hypertension	Suggested by an outbreak of primary pulmonary hypertension related to an anorectic agent, Aminorex. Only 2% of those who ingested the drug developed pulmonary hypertension, suggesting individual predisposition. Pulmonary hypertension (with different vascular lesions) also produced experimentally by ingesting seeds of leguminous plant *Crotalaria spectabilis*.
Sustained vasoconstriction	A classic suggestion which is difficult to accept as initiating mechanism; more likely a contributing factor.
Combined portal and pulmonary hypertension	Common denominator suggested by occurrence of pulmonary hypertension in some patients with hepatic cirrhosis. Also related to mechanism of dietary pulmonary hypertension.
Multiple pulmonary emboli	Once considered to be the major cause of primary pulmonary hypertension. May still be difficult to distinguish on clinical grounds but can almost always be distinguished morphologically.
Familial pulmonary hypertension	Although familial instances do occur, and individual susceptibility has been demonstrated in some instances, the connecting links between inherited defect or predisposition and clinical disease are unclear.

As a result of this constellation, calculated pulmonary vascular resistance is high, generally leading to the logical conclusion that the resistance vessels, i.e., the small muscular arteries and arterioles, are the predominant sites of vascular obstruction. During exercise, as cardiac output increases, pulmonary arterial pressures increase; the increments in pressure in the pulmonary hypertensive circuit are generally much more striking than in the normotensive pulmonary circulation.

Most protocols using pulmonary vasodilators currently center on the response to rest and exercise. Several clinical and hemodynamic changes are sought as desirable endpoints:

1. Improvement in exercise tolerance. This increase in physical capacity is usually accompanied by an increase in cardiac output and presumably improved distribution of blood flow to peripheral organs and tissues.
2. A decrease in the level of pulmonary arterial hypertension, both at rest and during exercise.
3. A decrease in calculated pulmonary vascular resistance. Although this goal is often attained in acute experiments, its clinical value is doubtful unless an increase in cardiac output (with minimal increase in heart rate) occurs in conjunction with a decrease in pulmonary arterial pressure.
4. Agents that relax pulmonary vessels also usually cause vasodilation if they gain access to the systemic circulation, thereby unloading the left ventricle and calling into play the systemic baroreceptors. As a result, pulmonary blood volume and pressure may fall even though systemic arterial pressures remain virtually unchanged.

It remains to be learned if pulmonary vasodilation will promote long-term survival, even though there now seems to be little doubt that an increase in cardiac output, and the accompanying redistribution of systemic blood flow, can provide symptomatic relief.

Clinical Picture

In its early stages, the disease is difficult to recognize. In the sporadic case, the first clue is often an abnormal chest radiograph or electrocardiograph indicative of right ventricular hypertrophy. But these are late manifestations: By the time that these changes appear, pulmonary hypertension is moderate to severe and generally longstanding. Initial complaints, particularly easy fatigability and chest discomfort, are often dismissed except during the course of an epidemic, as that associated with Aminorex, or in familial pulmonary hypertension. Direct determination of pulmonary circulatory pressures by cardiac catheterization is currently the only way to prove the diagnosis.

When the disease is advanced, dyspnea, particularly during exercise, is common. Many patients are tachypneic and complain of nondescript chest pain as well as breathlessness. Other common symptoms are weakness, fatigue, and effort syncope. In time, right-sided heart failure develops. On rare occasion, an enlarged pulmonary artery causes hoarseness because of compression of the left recurrent laryngeal nerve.

Patients with severe pulmonary hypertension seem prone to sudden death. Thus, death has occurred unexpectedly during normal activities, cardiac catheterization, and surgical procedures, and after the administration of barbiturates or anesthetic agents. The mechanisms for sudden death are not clear.

On physical examination, the jugular venous pulse usually shows a prominent "a" wave. Right ventricular hypertrophy causes a cardiac thrust along the left sternal border, and a distinct impulse is palpable over the region of the main pulmonary artery. The pulmonic component of the second sound is markedly accentuated, the second heart sound is narrowly split, and an ejection click is heard in the pulmonic area. Often a fourth heart sound emanating from the hypertrophied right ventricle is heard at the lower left sternal border. In some patients an ejection murmur is audible at the pulmonic area; as pulmonary arterial pressures approximate systemic arterial levels, the murmur of pulmonary valvular insufficiency often appears.

Right ventricular failure is accompanied by jugular venous distention and a gallop (S_3); inspiration intensifies the gallop. The liver becomes enlarged and tender and a hepatojugular reflux can be elicited; in time dilation of the failing right ventricle leads to tricuspid insufficiency manifested by a holosystolic murmur, best heard in the fourth interspace to the left of the sternum, which increases in intensity during inspiration. The liver develops expansile pulsations synchronous with the heart beat. Hydrothorax and ascites are uncommon even in the face of hepatomegaly and peripheral edema.

In the early stage, the chest radiograph is generally normal. Later it shows cardiac enlargement in association with enlargement of the pulmonary trunk while the peripheral pulmonary arterial branches are attenuated; the lung fields appear oligemic. Although fullness of the central pulmonary arterial trunks and peripheral "pruning" are distinctive, appearances vary somewhat from patient to patient in accord with the level and pace of the pulmonary hypertension and the age of the patient. The electrocardiogram almost always shows some evidence of right ventricular enlargement and usually of right atrial enlargement. Radiographic evidence of right ventricular enlargement usually becomes overt only late in the course of the pulmonary hypertension.

Lung scans and angiography help to exclude multiple pulmonary emboli. Rarely do these procedures prove to be more enlightening than the standard chest radiograph.

The results of cardiac catheterization are consistent with diffuse obliterative disease of the pulmonary arterial tree: Pulmonary arterial hypertension is associated with a normal pulmonary wedge pressure and a normal, or nearly normal, cardiac output (see Pathophysiology). Cardiac catheterization is most valuable in excluding known causes of pulmonary arterial hypertension and in screening the response of the pulmonary circulation to vasodilator agents.

Diagnosis

The diagnosis of primary pulmonary hypertension rests on two pillars: (1) the detection of pulmonary hypertension, and (2) exclusion of known causes of high pulmonary arterial pressure. The history is of utmost importance. Before categorizing pulmonary hypertension as "primary" or "unexplained," due regard must be paid to the predilection of primary pulmonary hypertension for young women, its occasional familial occurrence, associated signs and symptoms of connective tissue disorders (e.g, Raynaud's phenomenon), and, above all, the likelihood of pulmonary thromboembolism. Pulmonary function tests are useful in excluding diffuse pulmonary disorders, paricularly interstitial fibrosis and granuloma. The value of cardiac catheterization in eliminating acquired or congenital heart disease has been indicated above. But even after these procedures, distinction is often not possible, particularly between primary pulmonary hypertension and pulmonary arterial hypertension secondary to multiple pulmonary emboli. Theoretically, this distinction is of great importance because of the possibility of intervening therapeutically in thromboembolic disease by using anticoagulants, inferior vena caval or common femoral vein ligation, or even pulmonary embolectomy. Unfortunately, by the time pulmonary hypertension is recognized, the anatomic lesions are generally so far advanced that the likelihood of arresting or reversing the obliterative pulmonary vascular disease in either disorder is exceedingly slim.

Treatment

GENERAL FEATURES. The aim of treatment in primary pulmonary hypertension is to decrease pulmonary arterial pressure, preferably in conjunction with an increase in cardiac output. By this combination, the afterload on the right ventricle will decrease and organ blood flow will improve. In recent years, attempts have been made to identify pulmonary vasodilators that, by decreasing pulmonary vascular resistance, will provide symptomatic relief and prolong life.

To aid in pursuing this goal, the National Heart, Lung, and Blood Institute has established a national registry by which experiences with the disease and with the use of pharmacologic agents can be shared. To date, about 200 patients have satisfied the criteria for inclusion in the registry. Although the data have not yet been analyzed in detail, enough information is already on hand to underscore the difficulties in evaluating therapy: (1) The natural history of primary pulmonary hypertension is inconsistent, probably in keeping with the diverse etiologies that can elicit pulmonary hypertension. (2) Instances are being reported of long-term survival without vasodilator therapy. (3) Unless documented by morphologic studies, i.e., lung biopsy or autopsy, secondary pulmonary hypertension—notably multiple pulmonary emboli and less often vasculitis—can masquerade clinically as primary pulmonary hypertension. (4) All vasodilators, except those destroyed during a single pulmonary circulation (currently acetylcholine and prostacyclin), cannot be administered so that they act solely on the pulmonary circulation; as a corollary, all run the risk of troublesome side effects on the heart and systemic circulation. (5) For both acute and chronic administration, optimal therapeutic doses are difficult to establish. (6) Criteria for efficacy in acute studies are inconsistent; many rely almost entirely on a drop in calculated pulmonary vascular resistance even though pulmonary arterial pressure usually remains unchanged and the work of the right ventricle increases. (7) Symptomatic improvement after the acute administration of a presumed pulmonary vasodilator is most closely related to an increase in cardiac output. (8) The acute response to a pulmonary vasodilator is not a reliable predictor of the chronic response. Because of these reservations, optimism for the use of pulmonary vasodilators in primary pulmonary hypertension remains cautious. The ideal would still be prevention (as in thromboembolic disease) or treatment according to etiology (e.g., corticosteroids for interstitial granulomas due to sarcoidosis).

Despite these general caveats and uncertainties, pulmonary vasodilator therapy continues to be tried in the hope that individual patients will respond. The pulmonary vasodilators currently in use are summarized in Table 48–4. Not shown are acetylcholine and prostacyclin, both of which have been used to assess the potential for pulmonary vasodilation. Although promising as agents for testing and for acute reduction of right ventricular overloading, neither is as yet available for chronic administration. Nor is oxygen listed, since it is only apt to cause pulmonary vasodilation if arterial hypoxemia coexists with pulmonary hypertension.

DIRECTLY ACTING DRUGS. Two agents in this category are currently in wide use to test acutely for responsiveness: nitroprusside and hydralazine.

Nitroprusside. Nitroprusside elicits vasodilation in both arteries and veins. It is ideal for acute testing, but cannot be administered chronically. Sublingual nitroglycerin has been tried for chronic administration of a nitrate. However, its effectiveness as a chronic pulmonary vasodilator has not been documented. Instead, when nitroprusside given intravenously does produce pulmonary vasodilation, oral therapy with long-acting nitrates is usually begun, using a combination of isosorbide dinitrate, which primarily causes venodilatation, and hydralazine, an alpha-adrenergic blocker, which acts primarily on the arterial resistance vessels (arterioles). The effectiveness of the isosorbide in this combination is conjectural.

Hydralazine. This agent is currently very much in vogue. It exerts its vasodilator effect predominantly on vascular smooth muscle, much more on arterioles than on veins. It also increases cardiac output, both by a positive inotropic effect and by tachycardia; the latter seems to originate centrally as well as peripherally in response to the drop in systemic arterial pressure that the drug produces. When used in the treatment of systemic hypertension, the incidence of side effects is high but many can be avoided, or eliminated, by concurrent administration of a beta-adrenergic antagonist, e.g., propranolol. Although experience with this agent in treating primary pulmonary hypertension is limited, enthusiasm is high.

Side effects have not been reported despite its high potential for evoking circulatory upsets. Noteworthy is the observation that during chronic hydralazine therapy, pulmonary arterial pressure remains high even though pulmonary vascular resistance drops, both at rest and during exercise, and even though the patients feel better and can do more. The basis for the sustained pulmonary hypertension is the concomitant increase in cardiac output. Unexplained is the increase in oxygen consumption during hydralazine therapy, possibly related to cutaneous vasodilatation and heat loss, a property that hydralazine shares with other cutaneous vasodilators.

DRUGS ACTING ON ADRENERGIC RECEPTORS. Two agents in this broad category are still quite popular: isoproterenol and phentolamine.

Isoproterenol. Isoproterenol is a powerful sympathomimetic amine that acts on beta receptors everywhere, leaving alpha receptors virtually unaffected. Its predominant effects are on the heart and the smooth muscle of vessels and bronchi. Intravenous administration raises the cardiac output because of the chronotropic and inotropic effects of the drug coupled with the increase in venous return effected by peripheral vasodilation. Sublingual or oral administration is unreliable. Its effectiveness as a pulmonary vasodilator has been remarkably unpredictable and inconsistent.

Phentolamine. Phentolamine (Regitine) in doses of 100 to 200 mg per day acts primarily on vascular smooth muscle to

TABLE 48–4. SOME VASODILATOR DRUGS CURRENTLY USED IN THE MANAGEMENT OF PRIMARY PULMONARY HYPERTENSION*

	Mechanism of Action	Acute Testing	Usual Maintenance Therapy	Major Side Effects; Comments
Nitroprusside	Directly on vascular smooth muscle; relaxes both systemic arteries and veins.	10 μg/min IV, increasing by 10 μg/min every 4 min until systemic systolic < 95 torr or PA† systolic > 10 torr over control (max 60 μg/min).	Hydralazine 10 mg every 6 h, increasing up to 50 mg every 6 h, + isosorbide dinitrate 10 mg every 6 h, increasing up to 50 mg every 6 h.	Systemic vasodilation and hypotension, cyanide toxicity at high concentrations. Half-life of a few minutes.
Hydralazine	Directly on vascular smooth muscle, presumably via prostacyclin production; greater dilator effect on arterioles than on veins; myocardial stimulant.	10 mg IV repeated once after 10 min. Resting hemodynamics followed by exercise 20 min later.	Hydralazine, start with 10 mg every 6 h, increase to 50–75 mg every 6 h.	Flushing, nasal congestion, conjunctivitis, CNS† stimulation, drug fever, muscle cramps. Lupus-like syndrome at doses of 200–400 mg/day. Side effects lessened by gradual increase in dosage. Surprisingly few side effects reported as yet in treating primary pulmonary hypertension.
Isoproterenol	Beta-adrenergic agonist; relaxes vascular smooth muscle when tone is high; increases venous return to heart; positive inotropic and chronotropic effects.	1 μg/min IV and increasing by 1 μg/min until heart rate > 120/min or PA systolic > 10 torr over control, up to maximum dose of 5 μg/min.	Isoproterenol (sublingual) 10 mg every 4 h, increasing up to 20 mg every 3 h. Terbutaline 5 mg tid.	Palpitation, tachycardia, flushing, cardiac arrhythmias exceedingly common.
Phentolamine	Alpha-adrenergic blocker; dilates both systemic arterioles and large veins; positive inotropic effect.	0.5 mg/min IV to a maximum of 10 mg.	Phentolamine 25 mg every 6 h, increasing to 50 mg every 3 h while awake. Phenoxybenzamine 10 mg daily, increasing by 10 mg every 4 days to a maximum of 40 mg daily. Prazosin 2 mg tid, increasing up to 5 mg tid.	Tachycardia, cardiac arrhythmias, angina, gastrointestinal stimulation.
Nifedipine§	Interferes with calcium fluxes in vascular smooth muscle.	10 mg sublingually repeated once after 15 min. Exercise 15 min later.	Nifedipine 50 mg bid.	Systemic vasodilation and hypotension; flushing, rhythm disturbances; dysesthesias, peripheral edema; currently the most popular vasodilator agent for empiric trial (without hemodynamic testing).

*Based on a table developed by a working group as part of suggested protocols for use by centers for primary pulmonary hypertension, recently established by the National Heart, Lung, and Blood Institute. Members of this working group were Drs. Edward H. Bergofsky (chairman), Michael Beaven, Alfred P. Fishman, Michael Heymann, John T. Reeves, Lynne M. Reid, and Marvin A. Sackner. (Reprinted with permission from Fishman AP [ed.]: Update: Pulmonary Diseases and Disorders. New York, McGraw-Hill Book Company, 1982.)

†PA = pulmonary arterial; CNS = central nervous system.

‡Some clinics prefer the calcium channel blocker diltiazem, up to 30 mg 3 times daily, for oral maintenance therapy.

§This use of nefedipine is not listed in the manufacturer's directive.

cause vasodilation; this direct effect is supplemented by a modest degree of blockade of sympathetic nervous activity and of antagonism to circulating catecholamines; higher doses elicit the full picture of alpha-adrenergic blockade, including marked gastrointestinal side effects. Its use has not been uniformly successful.

Quinazoline Derivatives. Prazosin also acts predominantly as an alpha-adrenergic blocking agent on vascular smooth muscle. It resembles nitroprusside in its effects on the systemic arterial and venous circulations. However, it has been reported to become increasingly ineffective during prolonged administration.

DRUGS THAT BLOCK CALCIUM TRANSPORT. The designation *calcium blocker* or *calcium antagonist* refers to a heterogeneous group of agents of different structural, pharmacologic, and electrophysiologic properties. The agents currently receiving the most clinical attention as potential pulmonary vasodilators are nifedipine and diltiazem. Of the two, nifedipine is the more popular. Verapamil, once used extensively, has fallen into disuse, largely because of its undesirable negative inotropic effect.

Nifedipine.* Nifedipine is a synthetic agent that is unrelated to other vasoactive or cardiotonic drugs. It is a potent, long-acting systemic vasodilator that has grown increasingly popular for the treatment of coronary vasospasm. No myocardial depressant effects have been demonstrated, nor does it seem to possess antiarrhythmic properties. In an experimental model of pulmonary hypertension in the dog, it was judged more effective than either verapamil or diltiazem. It is now the agent of choice for empiric therapy when hemodynamic trials of the various pulmonary vasodilators are not feasible as a preliminary.

OTHER AGENTS. Diazoxide has proved during the past few years to have too many untoward side effects to warrant the risk of using it, particularly because more manageable agents, like nifedipine, are available. Captopril has also proved disappointing, and its use has fallen off.

Arachidonic Acid Metabolites. Enthusiasm is currently high about the effectiveness of prostacyclin (PGI_2) in evoking pulmonary vasodilation in patients with primary pulmonary hypertension. This agent seems to have several attractive features: (1) It is a powerful relaxant of increased pulmonary vascular tone, i.e., it is a potent vasodilator; (2) it reduces pulmonary vascular resistance in a dose-dependent way so that dosage can be titrated to achieve maximal pulmonary vasodilation without undue systemic side effects, e.g., headache, nausea, flushing, and vomiting; (3) adverse effects stop when the infusion stops; and (4) it seems to indicate whether

*This use is not listed in the manufacturer's directive.

there is a vasoconstrictive element to the pulmonary hypertension that other pulmonary vasodilators might affect.

Among its disadvantages are (1) it is an investigational drug only available in a form fit for intravenous use, and (2) in some patients, it is ineffective or even increases pulmonary vascular resistance. Until the agent becomes widely available for clinical trials, this promising drug cannot be fully assessed.

HEART-LUNG TRANSPLANTATION. Many patients with primary pulmonary hypertension are unresponsive to pulmonary vasodilator therapy. Young individuals threatened by syncope and incapacitated by right ventricular failure are candidates for heart-lung transplantation. A few patients with primary pulmonary hypertension seem to have undergone this procedure successfully. However, organs for transplant are in short supply. In a few patients with primary pulmonary hypertension, continued infusion of prostacyclin for two months to two years has helped to tide over candidates for transplantation.

Prognosis

The diagnosis of primary pulmonary hypertension carries with it a poor prognosis. Although death usually occurs within a few years after the onset of symptoms, instances of long-term survival do occur. Exceptions to the rule of a short and fatal course were also reported in the Aminorex epidemic in patients in whom the drug was stopped. At present, there is no specific treatment for primary pulmonary hypertension. Pulmonary vasodilators have, in some patients, improved exercise tolerance and the quality of life but have not yet been shown to prolong life. Neither anticoagulants nor corticosteroids have been of value. The cause of death is generally right ventricular failure. In some patients, sudden death terminates the illness.

PULMONARY VENO-OCCLUSIVE DISEASE

In a few patients with unexplained pulmonary arterial hypertension the disease appears to originate in progressive obstruction of pulmonary veins. Characteristically, anatomic lesions in the pulmonary veins predominate, but pulmonary arteries and arterioles are also involved. The etiology is unknown, but the obstructive venous lesions seem attributable to thrombosis after local injury, possibly secondary to a viral infection.

When the pulmonary hypertension is suspected to originate distal to the pulmonary capillary bed, mitral valve disease or myocardial dysfunction, or even left atrial myxoma, has the greater likelihood of being the cause than does primary pulmonary venous obstruction. More esoteric etiologies for the pulmonary venous hypertension to be excluded are congenital atresia of pulmonary veins and coexistent phlebitis of systemic and pulmonary veins.

Predominantly children and young adults are affected, but the age range has been from infancy to 48 years. There seems to be no sex difference. Although hints exist of possibly related familial cardiac disorders, the patients are too few to do more than raise suspicion of a familial or common environmental cause.

Clinical suspicion of this disorder generally arises when a patient with congested and edematous lungs, consistent with occult mitral valvular disease or left ventricular failure, proves to have a normal mitral valve and left ventricle. However, this stereotype is not always encountered and some patients have carried the diagnosis of primary pulmonary arterial hypertension until autopsy disclosed the characteristic pulmonary venous lesions.

The cardinal signs are dyspnea and fatigue or exertion in conjunction with evidence of pulmonary hypertension, particularly radiologic evidence of postcapillary pulmonary hypertension without evidence of an increase in left atrial pressure. Pleural effusions are common. Cyanosis, syncope, hemoptysis, and finger clubbing have been inconsistent findings.

Cardiac catheterization discloses a high pulmonary arterial pressure, often with a normal pulmonary wedge pressure. The low wedge pressure has been attributed to discontinuities and channels of high resistance between the pulmonary capillaries and the pulmonary and bronchial venous channels so that wedging interrupts all sources of flow distal to the area blocked by the catheter. A few lung biopsies have been done during life.

Both lungs are involved, but the venous lesions may be more marked in one region than in another. As a rule, the pulmonary arteries as well as the pulmonary veins are affected, but the lesions are different. Most striking are the morphologic changes in the pulmonary veins and venules, which are narrowed or occluded by fibrous tissue; up to 95 per cent of the veins and venules may be affected, but complete occlusion is uncommon. Bronchial veins and bronchopulmonary anastomoses share in the occlusive process. Hypertrophy in the walls of the pulmonary arteries may be also quite striking, whereas the pulmonary capillary bed is generally unaffected. Thrombi in the pulmonary arteries are common. The lungs show congestion, edema, and focal fibrosis, which may become extensive.

Management has been disappointing, since the lesions are generally irreversible. The usual duration after recognition ranges from a few weeks in infants to several years in adults, with seven the maximum.

Bjornsson J, Edwards WD: Primary pulmonary hypertension: A histopathologic study of 80 cases. Mayo Clin Proc 60:16, 1985. *Describes the histologic features that seem to form the morphologic substrate for the increase in pulmonary vascular resistance that characterizes primary pulmonary hypertension.*

Fishman AP: Pulmonary circulation. In Fishman AP, Fisher A (eds.): Handbook of Physiology: The Respiratory System, Vol I. Bethesda, Md., American Physiological Society, 1986, pp 93–165. *A comprehensive survey of the regulation of the pulmonary circulation, particularly useful as a background for considering pathogenesis of clinical pulmonary hypertension. Emphasis is placed on the concept of pulmonary vascular resistance, the interpretation of pulmonary wedge pressures, and the identification of pulmonary vasomotor activity.*

Fishman AP: Pulmonary thromboembolism: Pathophysiology and clinical features. In Fishman AP (ed.): Pulmonary Diseases and Disorders. New York, McGraw-Hill Book Company, 1980, pp 809–826. *A succinct account of pulmonary thromboembolic disease that calls special attention to the category of multiple pulmonary emboli.*

Fishman AP, Pietra GG: Primary pulmonary hypertension. Ann Rev Med 31:421, 1980. *A review of current understanding of primary pulmonary hypertension with special emphasisis on etiology. Comprehensive bibliography.*

Groves, BM, Rubin LJ, Frosolono MF, et al: A comparison of the acute hemodynamic effects of prostacyclin and hydralazine in primary pulmonary hypertension. Am Heart J 110:1200, 1985. *Interest in this comparison for those using pulmonary vasodilator agents lies in the hypothesis that hydralazine, which can be taken orally, exerts its effects by way of prostacyclin, for which no oral form is yet available.*

Higenbottam T, Wheeldon D, Wells F, et al: Long-term treatment of primary pulmonary hypertension with continuous intravenous epoprostenal (prostacyclin). Lancet 1:1046, 1984. *This paper describes the first of now seven patients, unmanageable by oral vasodilators, who were treated by continous infusion of prostacyclin for months up to two years. After one year of continuous self-administration of prostacyclin intravenously, the patient remained greatly improved.*

Reitz BA, Wallwork JL, Hunt SA, et al: Heart-lung transplantation: Successful therapy for patients with pulmonary vascular disease. N Engl J Med 306:557, 1982. *Initial successful experiences with heart-lung transplantation are described, including three patients with primary pulmonary hypertension.*

Rubin LJ, Peter RH: Oral hydralazine therapy for primary pulmonary hypertension. N Engl J Med 302:69, 1980. *Hydralazine taken orally (50 mg q 6 hours) by four patients increased cardiac output and exercise tolerance, leaving pulmonary arterial pressure unchanged; heart rate increased in all. Although calculated vascular resistance fell in each instance, the hemodynamic burden of the right ventricle was unchanged. Clinical improvement was probably related to increased cardiac output.*

Trell E: Benign, idiopathic pulmonary hypertension. Acta Med Scand 193:137, 1973. *Two cases of unusually long duration of idiopathic pulmonary hypertension (about 27 and 40 years, respectively) are presented and discussed with respect to others reported in the literature. No autopsy or biopsy findings.*

Voelkel N, Reeves JT: Primary pulmonary hypertension. In Moser KM (ed.): Pulmonary Vascular Diseases. New York, Marcel Dekker, 1979, pp 573–628. *Excellent clinical and physiologic review of current understanding of primary pulmonary hypertension against a background of a large personal experience with both this disorder and the pulmonary hypertension of high altitude.*

Wagenvoort CA, Wagenvoort N: Pathology of Pulmonary Hypertension. New York, John Wiley & Sons, 1977. *Splendid morphologic treatise on primary pulmonary hypertension based on years of collecting pathologic material, careful analysis, and intriguing extrapolations from morbid anatomy to etiology and clinical syndromes.*

Weir EK, Reeves JT: Pulmonary Hypertension. Mt. Kisco, NY, Futura Publishing Company, 1984. *A collection of papers that summarize the current understanding of pulmonary hypertension and its various subsets. Considerable emphasis on management.*

49 CONGENITAL HEART DISEASE

Samuel Kaplan

Congenital diseases of the heart occur in about 8 to 10 of 1000 live births. The spectrum of severity varies widely. One fourth to one third are symptomatic in the first year of life, frequently as neonates. In others, such as in patients with a functionally normal bicuspid aortic valve, the lesion may remain silent throughout life. With the development of palliative or radical surgical treatment, another large group has evolved that was treated during infancy or childhood and has reached adult life. Accordingly, adults with congenital heart disease fall into several groups: Some have anomalies with a natural history for long survival, others have had successful palliative or "curative" surgery in childhood, and still others have had lesions that were mild in childhood but have increased in severity in adult life (e.g., aortic stenosis).

Etiology

The cause is usually unknown in individual patients. The etiology of congenital heart disease is thought to be multifactorial, primarily due to an interaction between genetic predisposition and intrauterine environmental factors. It is estimated that congenital heart disease is associated with chromosomal abnormalities in 5 per cent of cases and with single mutant genes and environmental factors in 3 per cent each. Among *chromosomal abnormalities* the prevalence of congenital heart disease is about 50 per cent in trisomy 21 (Down's syndrome), 95 per cent in trisomy 18, 90 per cent in trisomy 13, and 35 per cent in Turner's (XO) syndrome. Among *single mutant gene* disorders (autosomal dominant or recessive or X-linked phenotypes), the more frequent syndromes in which the heart is involved are hypertrophic cardiomyopathy and the syndromes of Noonan and Holt-Oram. Numerous *environmental factors* have been implicated. Women who contract rubella during the first trimester of pregnancy may give birth to infants with pulmonic stenosis (especially pulmonary artery branch stenosis), persistent patent ductus arteriosus, and less often other defects. Other viruses have also been implicated, but the evidence that they produce congenital heart disease is not so strong. These include cytomegalovirus, coxsackievirus, and herpesvirus. Among drugs implicated in congenital heart disease are the anticonvulsants, especially phenytoin and trimethadione, and lithium salts (with an apparent predilection for atrioventricular valve disease, especially Ebstein's malformation of the tricuspid valve), progesterone, warfarin, and amphetamines. The offspring of diabetic women are at greater risk for a variety of congenital heart diseases. Patent ductus arteriosus is more frequent in children born at high altitudes. It is estimated that about one half of the offspring of alcoholic mothers have congenital heart disease, usually left to right shunts.

Counseling

Parents of children with congenital heart disease are concerned about the cause and about the possibility of recurrence in future pregnancies. This concern is greatest when the child is first born or the baby succumbs during the neonatal period. An explanation should be offered about the known causes of congenital heart disease and guilt feelings allayed. The prevalence of congenital heart disease in a second infant is 2 to 5 per cent. Although this figure is higher than in the general population, it is still quite low and parents should be supported if they decide to have another child. When congenital heart disease has recurred in two siblings, the prevalence is higher in a third pregnancy (estimated to be 20 to 25 per cent). Many women with congenital heart disease who had corrective surgery during childhood have reached childbearing age. The prevalence of congenital heart disease in their children ranges from 3 to 16 per cent. Recurrence risks are low in the offspring of fathers with congenital heart disease.

Circulatory Shunts

Pathophysiology

MAGNITUDE AND DIRECTION. Factors that determine the magnitude and direction of intra- and extracardiac shunts are the size of the defect, pressure differences between the cardiac chambers or vessels, and resistance to ejection produced by outflow obstruction, as well as the ratio of systemic to pulmonary vascular resistance. Since normal systemic vascular pressures and resistances greatly exceed those in the pulmonary circuit, flow across small defects (such as ventricular septal defects) is from left to right but is limited in magnitude by the small opening. When the defect is large and nonrestrictive, peak systolic pressures in the ventricles are virtually identical, so that the direction and magnitude of flow are regulated by outflow resistance. If systemic vascular resistance significantly exceeds that in the pulmonary circuit with large defects (in the absence of pulmonic stenosis), torrential left to right shunts are present. The magnitude of the shunt is decreased as pulmonary vascular resistance approaches that in the systemic circuit, and it is bidirectional or right to left with continued increase of pulmonary resistance. When severe pulmonic stenosis is present, resistance to right ventricular ejection virtually equalizes peak systolic pressures in both ventricles so that flow across ventricular defects is right to left or bidirectional. A major determinant of direction and magnitude of shunting at the atrial level is the diastolic distensibility of the ventricles. Flow, frequently torrential, is from left to right, since the thin-walled right ventricle is easily filled even though atrial pressures are equal and low.

PULMONARY HYPERTENSION. This complication (see Ch. 48), common in congenital heart disease, results from increased pulmonary blood flow and/or resistance. Torrential pulmonary blood flow (as in secundum atrial septal defects) can be accommodated by the pulmonary circulation without increase in pressure. Pulmonary hypertension develops frequently in the presence of large defects at the ventricular level or communications between the aorta and pulmonary arteries. In infants and small children with these defects, "hyperkinetic" pulmonary hypertension is present. This term refers to a vasoactive pulmonary bed that undergoes vasodilation in response to oxygen or tolazoline. These agents reduce the level of pulmonary arterial pressure by pulmonary vasodilation even though pulmonary blood flow increases. Hyperkinetic pulmonary hypertension is uncommon in adults but is seen in some with secundum atrial septal defects. Generally, pulmonary vascular disease is present in adults, so that pulmonary vascular resistance is greatly increased even when pulmonary blood flow is not excessive (see Eisenmenger's Syndrome below). The status of the pulmonary vascular bed determines the clinical picture, prognosis, and feasibility of surgical treatment of intra- and extracardiac shunts. The goal of management is to prevent the development of severe pulmonary vascular changes by surgical ablation of the shunt. This implies serial measurements of pulmonary and systemic pressures and resistances, especially in infants and toddlers with large ventricular or aortopulmonary defects.

Right to Left Shunts

PULMONARY BLOOD FLOW AND SYSTEMIC DESATURATION. Right to left shunts are characteristically associated with arterial oxygen desaturation. The degree of desaturation is determined by pulmonary blood flow and the magnitude of right to left shunt. When effective pulmonary blood flow is markedly reduced (as in tetralogy of Fallot), systemic venous blood is ejected preferentially through the ventricular septal defect into the left ventricle and aorta, so that arterial oxygen saturation is severely reduced and cyanosis is obvious. On the other hand, right to left shunts may be associated with markedly increased pulmonary blood flow (as in transposition of the great arteries). In this situation pulmonary venous blood is almost fully saturated so that systemic arterial saturation is only moderately decreased. Cyanosis is not as intense in the latter group of patients, but they suffer from volume loading and failure of the left ventricle.

ARTERIAL HYPOXEMIA. *Cyanosis*, a dusky purple color of the skin but especially the mucous membranes and nail beds, is due to reduced hemoglobin in the arterial blood from right to left shunts. Clinical cyanosis may not be evident until the arterial oxygen saturation is below 85 per cent (normal is 94 to 98 per cent). *Clubbing* of fingers and toes is common, especially when arterial hypoxemia is marked. This sign may appear in childhood (beyond the age of one year) and is progressive. When arterial oxygen saturation returns to normal (at rest and during exercise), as occurs after surgical correction, clubbing regresses and even severe forms disappear within two to three years after operation.

Polycythemia results from adaptation of the hemopoietic system to the anoxic stimulus. This compensatory mechanism increases arterial oxygen content. When the hematocrit exceeds 65 to 70 per cent, blood viscosity increases so that the patient is at risk for intravascular thrombosis. Thrombi may develop in any organ system but are more frequent in the cerebral circulation (generally in the dural sinuses and cerebral veins) and pulmonary arteries. Dehydration increases the risk of intravascular thrombosis. Headaches are common in severely polycythemic patients (see Eisenmenger's Syndrome, below). The combination of iron deficiency anemia and polycythemia is not well tolerated. There is greater risk for intravascular thrombosis, and iron therapy is required even though this results in a further elevation of hematocrit. Severely polycythemic patients have a delicate balance between intravascular thrombosis and bleeding from coagulation defects. The more frequent abnormalities associated with a bleeding diathesis are a combination of thrombocytopenia, accelerated fibrinolysis, hypofibrinogenemia, prolonged prothrombin time, and prolonged partial thromboplastin time.

BRAIN ABSCESS AND PARADOXICAL EMBOLUS. Brain abscess occurs in older children and adults. Predisposing factors include previous occlusive microcirculatory disease from thrombosis or emboli. Clinical recognition may be difficult because the onset is insidious, symptoms are vague, and fever is low grade. In others, the onset is more acute, with headache, seizures, and localized neurologic signs that are dependent on the size and site of the abscess and the presence of increased intracranial pressure. The diagnosis is established with computed axial tomography or magnetic resonance imaging or both. Treatment is with antibiotics, generally followed by surgical drainage. In patients with right to left shunts, venous blood bypasses the lungs so that emboli arising from systemic veins enter the systemic circulation directly to occlude an artery anywhere in the body, especially the brain. This complication is rare.

SHUNT LESIONS

Atrial Septal Defect

Atrial septal defects occur more frequently in females and are designated according to their site in the septum. The most common are in the region of the fossa ovalis (*ostium secundum defect*) and are among the most prevalent congenital cardiac anomalies in adults. A less frequent variety (*sinus venosus defect*) occupies the upper part of the atrial septum and is closely related to the entry of the superior vena cava. This structure receives one or more anomalously draining pulmonary veins, usually from the right lung. (The *ostium primum defect* is discussed under Endocardial Cushion Defect, below).

The principal factors that determine the magnitude of the left to right shunt are the size of the defect, the relative compliance of the cardiac chambers, and the vascular resistances in the pulmonary and systemic circulations. If the defect is moderate or large (>2 cm in diameter in an adult), the greater distensibility of the right atrium and ventricle and the low pulmonary vascular resistance allow an abundant left-to-right shunt. On the other hand, in infancy the relatively thick and less compliant right ventricle limits the magnitude of left to right shunts. Large defects with torrential left to right shunts produce right atrial and ventricular enlargement, which encroaches on the left-sided chambers. Pulmonary pressures and resistances are generally normal. In the unusual instances in which they are elevated, the pulmonary circulation remains vasoactive, so that pressures and resistances return to normal after surgical ablation of the shunt. Those with severe pulmonary vascular disease are described under Eisenmenger's Syndrome.

DIAGNOSIS. Although symptoms are trivial and physical signs subtle, the diagnosis is usually made during childhood. However, many escape detection in the first decade of life and are recognized in later years only because of effort dyspnea and fatigue. Superimposed coronary artery disease or systemic hypertension can cause the left ventricle to be less distensible, favoring the development or worsening of these symptoms because of a further increase in left to right shunt and right volume overload. In some instances the presence of the defect is first appreciated when pulmonary hypertension develops with persistence of a torrential left to right shunt. The advent of atrial arrhythmias, fibrillation, flutter, or paroxysms of supraventricular tachycardia is not well tolerated. These events increase in frequency beyond the fourth decade. Some patients with an uncomplicated atrial septal defect are recognized for the first time because of an abnormal "routine" chest roentgenogram.

In children failure to gain weight is common but by no means the rule. The characteristic physical appearance is that of a thin child with nearly normal height and a gracile habitus. Generally, adults have a normal physical appearance, but again some are thin and gracile. The jugular venous pulse shows "a" and "v" waves of equal heights because the atria are in free communication. Dominant "a" waves suggest the presence of pulmonary hypertension, and dominant "v" waves are associated with tricuspid regurgitation. Right ventricular volume overload results in an easily palpable left parasternal lift. The importance of this sign cannot be overemphasized, and in some the dilated pulmonary artery is palpated in the second left interspace. The soft ejection systolic murmur, seldom accompanied by a thrill, is best heard at the upper left sternal edge and is produced by increased blood flow into the pulmonary artery. A loud murmur is widely transmitted to the chest anteriorly and posteriorly, especially in slightly built patients. The murmur is preceded by an accentuated first heart sound and sometimes by a pulmonic ejection sound. The auscultatory hallmark is the easily audible, widely split second heart sound. This split is virtually fixed in all phases of respiration and during the Valsalva maneuver. When the defect is large, a mid-diastolic murmur is audible at the lower left sternal edge and is produced by extravagant flow across the tricuspid valve. An early diastolic murmur of pulmonary regurgitation may accompany pulmonary hypertension, but this is rare.

The *electrocardiogram* shows right axis deviation and right ventricular hypertrophy (generally rsR' in right precordial leads). This pattern is due to terminal depolarization of the hypertrophied right ventricular outflow tract. Less frequent findings include tall P waves (because of right atrial enlargement), complete right bundle branch block, a prolonged PR interval, and Wolff-Parkinson-White syndrome. Supraventricular arrhythmias may be detected in untreated adults or many years after surgical closure of the defect. These consist of atrial fibrillation or flutter, paroxysmal atrial tachycardia, and multiple premature atrial contractions. Left axis deviation usually denotes the presence of an ostium primum atrial defect but is seen occasionally in secundum defects. Another rare finding is a normal electrocardiogram.

The *chest roentgenogram* is often distinctive, especially in adults. Varying degrees of cardiac enlargement are due to dilatation of the right atrium and ventricle, which displaces the normal or relatively small left-sided chambers posteriorly. The large pulmonary trunk contrasts with the smaller aortic knob, which is especially notable on the posteroanterior view. The primary branches of the pulmonary artery are enlarged and the vascularity increased toward the periphery of both lung fields.

Echocardiography not only is diagnostic but also is useful in excluding other suspected anomalies. In uncomplicated secundum atrial defects the right ventricular end-diastolic dimension is increased and the ventricular septal motion is flat or paradoxical. Real-time two-dimensional echocardiograms define the location and size of the defect and also confirm the significant enlargement of the right atrium. The deformity of the ventricular septum resulting from right ventricular volume overload is recognized, and its encroachment into the left ventricular cavity is visualized. Flow disturbance across the interatrial septum can be detected by measurements based on the Doppler principle. The pulmonary and aortic flows can be estimated by two-dimensional echo and Doppler techniques, and the difference between these flows represents the shunt volume. *Mitral valve prolapse* may be associated with secundum atrial septal defects and in many instances the suspicion is raised by the echocardiogram. Since various criteria are used for the echo diagnosis of mitral valve prolapse, caution should be exercised in the diagnosis of combined atrial septal defect and mitral valve prolapse. It is probable that the association has been overestimated.

There is an ongoing debate about whether *cardiac catheterization* is indicated in all patients. Physical examination supplemented by the electrocardiogram and chest roentgenogram usually suggests the diagnosis. This can be confirmed by visualizing the site of the defect by echocardiography and estimating the pulmonary-systemic flow ratio. However, this view is not held universally and some prefer to confirm the shunt by demonstration of a step-up in oxygen concentration between the vena cava and the right atrium, to define the site of entry of pulmonary veins, and to measure the level of pulmonary arterial pressure and resistance. The study should be undertaken in the adult in whom pulmonary hypertension or coexisting coronary artery disease is suspected.

NATURAL HISTORY. The vast majority of secundum atrial septal defects are recognized and treated surgically during childhood or adolescence. Spontaneous closure does occur, but this is usually prior to the age of about three years. Although life expectancy is shortened, adult survival is the rule and some live to an advanced age. Pregnancy is usually well tolerated, especially in women who were asymptomatic prior to pregnancy.

COMPLICATIONS. After the age of 40 years complications are frequent, and most patients who survive beyond the age of 60 years show symptoms of effort dyspnea and fatigue. Death may be unrelated to the defect, but when a relationship exists cardiac failure is the most common cause. Heart failure may be due to right ventricular failure alone or may be intensified by a dilated tricuspid valve ring with resultant incompetence. The prevalence of atrial arrhythmias increases after the fourth decade and may precipitate heart failure, especially when the ventricular response is rapid in the presence of a large shunt. Coronary artery disease or systemic hypertension may result in a less distensible left ventricle, which favors an increase in left to right shunting. Pulmonary hypertension may be due to the high pulmonary blood flow or may progress to a state in which pulmonary and systemic vascular resistances are virtually identical and the shunt is abolished or reversed (see Eisenmenger's Syndrome). Infective endocarditis is rare in isolated lesions.

TREATMENT. Treatment is surgical ablation of the shunt, especially when the pulmonary systemic flow ratio exceeds 2:1. This is preferably accomplished between the ages of about three and four years, when the surgical risk is minimal. In these young patients the right ventricular dimension returns to normal. Surgical treatment in older children and adolescents usually improves the size of the right-sided chambers, but they may not return to normal. When the operation is performed in adults, patchy fibrosis of the chronically volume-loaded right ventricle persists, as does some degree of right ventricular dilatation. These residua may explain the blunted chronotropic response during exercise, with resultant decreased cardiac output and decreased working capacity. Nevertheless, patients in the fifth, sixth, or even seventh decade with high pulmonary blood flow and low resistance benefit from surgical repair, which can be done with a comparatively low risk. Defects in older patients can be closed surgically despite moderate pulmonary hypertension and cardiac failure, provided there is still a significant left to right shunt. Operation is contraindicated when pulmonary vascular resistance is greatly elevated so that the shunt is abolished or reversed. Late-onset arrhythmias occur in fewer than 5 per cent, 10 to 20 years after surgery. The commonest are atrial flutter, atrial fibrillation, paroxysmal supraventricular tachycardia, and frequent premature atrial contractions. Less frequent arrhythmias are sick sinus syndrome, junctional tachycardia, and complete heart block.

Lutembacher's Syndrome

This condition consists of a secundum atrial septal defect with acquired mitral stenosis. Obstruction to left ventricular inflow aggravates the left to right shunt across the atrial septum. Atrial fibrillation is common. A prominent jugular "a" wave is visible because left atrial pressure is transmitted to the right atrium and the systemic venous return. Physical findings resemble those described under secundum atrial septal defects. Auscultatory findings of mitral stenosis are present but may not be obvious. The echocardiogram is diagnostic in that signs of mitral stenosis are superimposed on right ventricular volume overload. Patients with this condition derive great symptomatic relief after intracardiac repair.

Endocardial Cushion Defect

The embryonic endocardial cushions contribute to the development of the mitral and tricuspid valves and to the growth and convergence of the atrial and ventricular septa. Maldevelopment during this stage of cardiac morphogenesis results in varying degrees of complex malformations involving the atrioventricular valves and the atrial and ventricular septa. The *ostium primum defect* is situated in the lower portion of the atrial septum overlying both the mitral and tricuspid valves. A cleft in the anterior leaflet to the mitral valve is usual, and the tricuspid valve is frequently thickened but otherwise normal. The ventricular septum is intact functionally. *Common atrioventricular canal* (complete endocardial cushion defect) consists of a common defect of both the intra-atrial and intraventricular septa with a single atrioventricular valve. This valve, common to both ventricles, has an anterior and posterior leaflet with a lateral leaflet in each ventricle. This anomaly is relatively common in patients with Down's syndrome. *Transitional forms* are intermediate between atrioventricular canal and ostium primum defects.

OSTIUM PRIMUM DEFECTS. Ostium primum defects may be associated with recurrent lower respiratory tract infections with or without congestive heart failure during infancy and early childhood. However, the majority are asymptomatic and are recognized because of the murmur of mitral incompetence. In others, the degree of mitral regurgitation is trivial. The physical signs resemble those of ostium secundum defects with superimposed mitral regurgitation. The electrocardiogram is distinctive in that there is a superior counterclockwise frontal plane axis (left axis deviation), varying degrees of right ventricular hypertrophy (rsR[1] is common), and sometimes voltage criteria for left ventricular hypertrophy because of mitral regurgitation. The chest radiograph simulates an ostium secundum atrial septal defect. The echocardiogram is also characteristic, showing enlargement of both right ventricle and right atrium, a low lying atrial septal defect, and a cleft in the anterior mitral leaflet. The mitral valve apparatus is displaced so that the anterior mitral leaflet encroaches upon the left ventricular outflow. Cardiac catheterization demonstrates the left to right atrial shunt, the level of pulmonary arterial pressure, and the degree of mitral valve incompetence. Left ventriculography shows the characteristic "goose-neck" deformity produced by the abnormal position of the mitral valve. Surgical treatment is advised during infancy or childhood with the purpose of obliterating the left to right shunt and alleviating mitral valve incompetence. In adult life, many years after surgery, atrial arrhythmias may occur as described under secundum atrial septal defect. In addition, a small number of patients have progressive mitral valve incompetence that may require mitral valve replacement.

COMPLETE ATRIOVENTRICULAR CANAL. Congestive cardiac failure, significant elevation of pulmonary artery pressures, and resistances and intercurrent pulmonary infections are common during infancy. At that time surgical treatment is undertaken to attempt to prevent progression of these complications. Without treatment, survival of these patients to adolescence and adult life is usually associated with the development of severe pulmonary vascular disease (see Eisenmenger's Syndrome, p 316) or congenital obstruction to right ventricular outflow, which limits pulmonary blood flow.

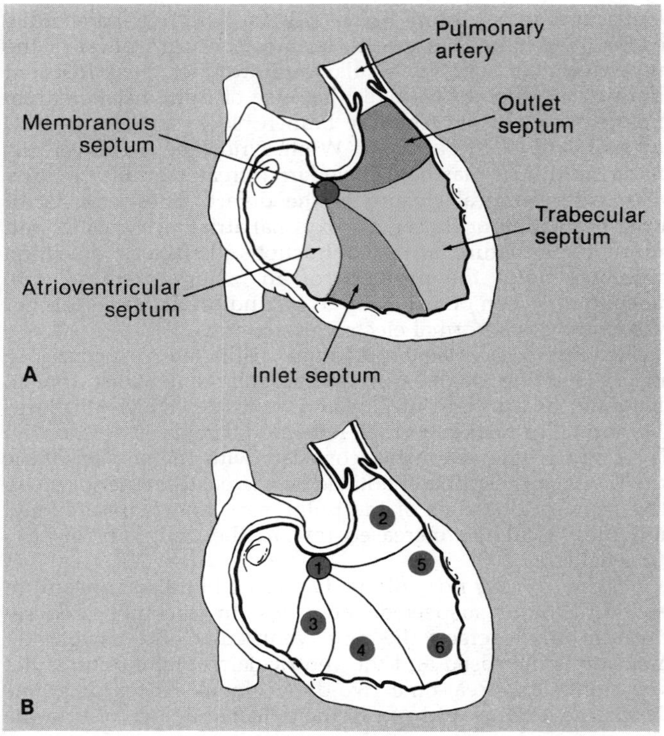

FIGURE 49–1. Diagrams of the right side of the ventricular septum. Anterior portions of the right ventricle and atrium have been removed, as has the tricuspid valve. *A*, Subdivisions of the ventricular septum. *B*, Locations of ventricular septal defects (VSD). 1. Perimembranous VSD (most common type). 2. Subpulmonic VSD (also known as infundibular, conal, or outlet VSD). 3. Atrioventricular canal VSD. 4, 5, and 6. Muscular VSD's in various parts of the septum; defects may be single or multiple. VSD's may extend to adjacent parts of the septum so that perimembranous VSD's may involve the inlet, trabecular, or outlet septum. The tricuspid valve may straddle the defect (rare in isolated VSD). Malalignment of the ventricular septum with override of a semilunar valve is unusual in isolated VSD and is more frequent with tetralogy of Fallot, double outlet ventricles, and truncus arteriosus and in some patients with transposition of the great arteries.

Ventricular Septal Defect

The commonest form of congenital heart disease is an isolated ventricular septal defect. Perimembranous defects are the most frequent (Fig. 49–1). The magnitude of the shunt depends on the size of the defect and status of the pulmonary vascular bed. A small defect limits the size of the left to right shunt so that cardiac chambers are normal in size and pulmonary arterial pressures and resistances remain within normal limits. Large defects are associated with a marked increase in pulmonary blood flow, as well as varying degrees of elevation of pulmonary arterial pressures and resistance. In these instances pulmonary vascular disease may be progressive, so that systemic and pulmonary vascular resistances are virtually equal (Eisenmenger's syndrome) (see Ch. 42.5).

SMALL VENTRICULAR SEPTAL DEFECTS. Spontaneous closure of the defect is frequent, especially in the first year of life, and is estimated to occur in more than one half of instances. If the defect does not close spontaneously within the first three years of life, it is likely that the clinical condition will remain unchanged. These patients are generally asymptomatic and have a normal heart size. A systolic thrill may be palpable at the lower left sternal edge and is accompanied by a harsh, loud pansystolic murmur that is widely distributed but loudest at the site of the thrill. The electrocardiogram and chest roentgenogram are normal. Generally these defects are too small to be visualized by two-dimensional echocardiograms, although turbulence is recorded in the right ventricle by the Doppler principle, especially in the outflow tract. It is now believed that spontaneous closure of a small ventricular septal defect may also occur in early adult life. This notion is based on the fact that congenital ventricular septal defects are seldom found in older adults. Sometimes the development of an ejection click heralds a course that in a few years is associated with complete disappearance of all abnormal auscultatory findings when the defect is completely closed. Uncomplicated small ventricular septal defects do not require surgical closure, and the only treatment is prophylaxis against infective endocarditis.

LARGE VENTRICULAR SEPTAL DEFECTS. Large defects with unrestricted flow from the left to the right ventricle and into the pulmonary vascular bed are common in early life and rare in adults. These defects are associated with increased pulmonary vascular pressure and resistance. Furthermore, volume loading of the left heart may lead to superimposed left ventricular failure. Symptoms are present during infancy, especially between the ages of two and six months, and are produced by congestive cardiac failure, poor physical development, and recurrent pulmonary infections. These infants may respond to anticongestive measures. If this improvement is maintained, especially beyond the age of one year, the defect frequently decreases in size, with continuing clinical improvement. However, in a significant number response to therapy is not maintained, physical development remains poor, and signs of pulmonary hypertension persist. In these instances surgical closure of the defect is indicated, since the mortality rate from surgery is acceptably low and soon after operation there is a growth spurt when heart failure and pulmonary hypertension regress.

Clinical improvement in some babies with a large ventricular septal defect may be due to the development of *acquired pulmonic stenosis*, which limits pulmonary blood flow. Generally, right ventricular outflow tract obstruction is due to infundibular hypertrophy and is progressive. During infancy or early childhood the clinical course changes in that signs of heart failure improve and heart size decreases because pulmonary blood flow is limited by the pulmonic stenosis. Right ventricular pressure rises to approximate that of the left ventricle, with resultant right to left shunting and cyanosis. The clinical picture resembles that of tetralogy of Fallot (see below).

VENTRICULAR SEPTAL DEFECT WITH AORTIC REGURGITATION. The ventricular septal defect is usually small or moderate in size and its presence is known from infancy. During childhood or adolescence aortic valve regurgitation occurs because of prolapse of the right or, at times, the noncoronary cusp. The clinical picture is extremely variable, from the asymptomatic child with a small left to right shunt and trivial aortic regurgitation to the symptomatic young adult with congestive cardiac failure, angina pectoris, massive cardiomegaly, and florid aortic regurgitation. The latter patient requires surgical closure of the defect and relief of aortic regurgitation; this generally requires aortic valve replacement. The asymptomatic patient with mild regurgitation needs to be observed closely. Some believe that closure of the ventricular defect will prevent further prolapse of the aortic valve. Others recommend simultaneous aortic valvuloplasty prior to the development of significant valvular regurgitation and left ventricular dysfunction.

VENTRICULAR SEPTAL DEFECT WITH LEFT VENTRICULAR–RIGHT ATRIAL SHUNT. The atrioventricular septum is divided by the insertions of the tricuspid valve and the mitral valve. The insertion of the tricupsid valve is below that of the mitral. Thus, this area is common to the right atrium and left ventricle, and a defect in this area allows shunting from the left ventricle directly into the right atrium. In others the defect is below the tricuspid valve and is associated with an abnormal tricuspid septal leaflet. The physical signs simulate those of an isolated small to moderate ventricular septal defect. If the shunt is above the tricuspid valve, cardiac catheterization demonstrates a left to right shunt at the atrial level that may be confused with an atrial septal defect; this issue is resolved by the fact that the physical signs are not compatible with an atrial septal defect and left ventriculography demonstrates direct opacification of the right atrium from the left ventricle. This condition should be treated surgically.

OTHER DEFECTS ASSOCIATED WITH VENTRICULAR SEPTAL DEFECTS. ***Patent Ductus Arteriosus.*** In some instances the murmurs of both lesions are audible, so that a continuous murmur is present at the upper left sternal edge and a holosystolic murmur is heard at the lower left sternal edge. However, in many patients the physical findings are dominated by either the ventricular defect or the patent ductus arteriosus. Echocardiography combined with the Doppler technique is helpful in the diagnosis, disclosing shunting at the ventricular level as well as a patent ductus arteriosus. Left ventriculography demonstrates the ventricular septal defect, and aortography is necessary to confirm the associated ductus arteriosus if this structure is not entered directly by the catheter from the pulmonary artery.

Secundum Atrial Septal Defect. In patients with a ventricular septal defect and an ostium secundum atrial septal defect, the clinical picture is usually dominated by the ventricular defect. This combination of defects is more likely to be present during infancy and may result in torrential pulmonary blood flow, pulmonary hypertension, and congestive heart failure. The defects are recognized by echocardiography and, if uncontrolled by medical measure, are both treated surgically during the same procedure.

Coarctation of the Aorta. Signs of coarctation of the aorta usually dominate, and sometimes the signs of ventricular septal defect are erroneously attributed to the collateral circulation associated with coarctation.

Communications Between the Aorta and Pulmonary Arteries

PATENT DUCTUS ARTERIOSUS. Persistent patency of the ductus arteriosus is more frequent in females, in premature babies, in infants born at high altitude, and in infants whose first trimester of intrauterine life is complicated by maternal rubella. The aortic end of the ductus is opposite the origin of the left subclavian artery, and the vessel enters the pulmonary artery, usually at its bifurcation.

The hemodynamic effects of a patent ductus arteriosus depend on the size of the communication, the length of the ductus, and the resistance relationships between the systemic and pulmonary circulations. Generally, the flow through the ductus is small to moderate so that pulmonary arterial pressures and resistances remain normal. These patients usually are asymptomatic, and the only abnormal physical sign is a typical continuous murmur. This murmur, sometimes accompanied by a thrill, is heard best at the upper left sternal edge, rises to a peak in late systole, continues without interruption through the second sound, and wanes during the course of diastole. Larger shunts with a significant aortic runoff result in a wide pulse pressure and a "waterhammer" or bounding arterial pulse. The left atrium and ventricle enlarge to accommodate the increased pulmonary blood flow, and this is recognized by a lateral and downward displacement of the apical impulse, which is lifting in character. The typical continuous murmur is still present, but in addition an apical mid-diastolic murmur may be audible because of increased flow across the mitral valve. When pulmonary arterial pressure and resistance rise to systemic levels, flow across the ductus is limited. In patients with pulmonary hypertension effort dyspnea is common, the wide pulse pressure disappears, and right ventricular enlargement is prominent. The auscultatory findings are dominated by those produced by pulmonary hypertension in that the typical continuous murmur disappears and is replaced by a short systolic murmur frequently preceded by an ejection click, a booming second heart sound due to loud pulmonic valve closure, and sometimes an early diastolic murmur of pulmonic valve incompetence. Occasionally the shunt through the ductus is reversed so that the descending aorta is perfused with desaturated pulmonary arterial blood. This results in cyanotic lower extremities with clubbing of the toes and normal color and shape of the fingers and fingernails.

The *electrocardiographic findings* are normal when the ductus is small. Moderate or large flows result in left ventricular hypertrophy. In the presence of severe pulmonary hypertension right ventricular hypertrophy dominates. The *chest roentgenogram* is normal if the flow is small. With larger flows the heart is enlarged because of left atrial and left ventricular prominence, the pulmonary arterial trunk and aorta are enlarged, and there is pulmonary plethora. With the development of severe pulmonary hypertension, heart size decreases, there is prominence of the right ventricle and especially the main pulmonary artery, and the size of the aorta may not be increased. In older patients the ductus may calcify. The *echocardiogram* defines and identifies the degree of chamber enlargement and visualizes the ductus. Evidence of continuous flow is recorded using the Doppler technique from the ductus arteriosus and the major pulmonary arteries.

Surgical correction is advisable by division of the ductus. In the adult with a large left to right shunt and normal pulmonary vascular resistance surgery is also advised. Extensive calcification of the ductus increases the surgical risk, but surgery should still be advised if the shunt is large. Occasionally, an adult is seen with a small, hemodynamically insignificant patent ductus. The decision of surgical treatment for these patients must take into account that they are at risk for infective endocarditis, but on the other hand they may remain asymptomatic and some may experience spontaneous closure of the defect. Thus individual judgment is required in these patients.

AORTIC-PULMONARY SEPTAL DEFECT. This rare anomaly consists of a communication between the ascending aorta and the pulmonary arterial trunk. The defect is generally large and associated with a torrential pulmonary blood flow and pulmonary hypertension. Congestive cardiac failure is common during infancy and childhood. In the absence of severe pulmonary hypertension the signs are dominated by a wide pulse pressure, cardiomegaly, a systolic murmur at the left and right upper sternal edges, and occasionally a continuous murmur. The electrocardiogram generally shows biventricular hypertrophy, although isolated left or right dominance may be present. Roentgenographic examination of the chest defines the degree of cardiomegaly and shows prominence of the pulmonary artery and ascending aorta, as well as pulmonary plethora. The echocardiogram is helpful in defining the presence of two semilunar valves (which excludes the diagnosis of truncus arteriosus) and shows a normal relationship of a large aorta and pulmonary artery. The diagnosis is confirmed by aortography. The hemodynamic effects are measured at the same time by cardiac catheterization. These defects usually require surgical correction.

TRUNCUS ARTERIOSUS. A single arterial trunk supplies the systemic, pulmonary, and coronary circulations. Both ventricles eject blood through a ventricular septal defect into the single trunk. The number of semilunar valve cusps varies from two to six, and in most patients pulmonary arteries arise from the ascending portion of the truncus proximal to the origin of the innominate artery. When the major source of pulmonary blood flow is from aortopulmonary collateral arteries, the condition is considered to be pulmonary atresia with ventricular septal defect (previously known as truncus arteriosus type IV or pseudotruncus arteriosus).

In the majority the pulmonary blood flow, pressure, and resistance are greatly increased, so that signs of heart failure appear in infancy. Cyanosis is minimal or absent. The heart is usually enlarged, the precordium is hyperdynamic, a systolic ejection murmur sometimes preceded by a click is audible along the left sternal edge, and the second heart sound is loud and generally single. Occasional patients survive infancy because of the development of severe pulmonary vascular disease, which limits pulmonary blood flow. The clinical picture in these patients simulates that of Eisenmenger's syndrome. Incompetence of the truncal valve or, less frequently, stenosis of this valve may complicate the picture at any age. The diagnosis is confirmed by cardiac catheterization and angiocardiography. Since rapid deterioration is frequent during infancy, surgical treatment is advised, at which time the ventricular septal defect is closed, the pulmonary arteries are detached from the truncus, and a conduit is inserted from the right ventricle to the pulmonary arteries.

Communication Shunts Between the Aortic Root and the Right Heart

CORONARY ARTERIAL FISTULA. A fistulous branch, most frequently from the right coronary artery, enters the right atrium or right ventricle and occasionally the pulmonary trunk. The right coronary artery becomes massively dilated. Although the volume of shunt from the coronary artery to the right heart is variable, it is usually small. The diagnosis is suspected when an atypically located continuous precordial murmur is heard. The electrocardiogram and chest roentgenogram are normal. Studies using the Doppler technique demonstrate the site of entry of the fistula: The diagnosis is confirmed with an aortic root injection of contrast material that demonstrates the large, tortuous right coronary artery and its site of entry into the right heart. Surgical treatment is advised.

CONGENITAL ANEURYSMS OF THE SINUSES OF VALSALVA. The usual aneurysm involves the right or noncoronary sinus, which begins as a blind pouch or diverticulum. The aneurysms may remain as unruptured diverticula but usually enter the right ventricle or right atrium. Patients with these aneurysms are generally asymptomatic and the left to right shunt is small. The diagnosis is suspected because of an atypically located continuous murmur and confirmed by injection of contrast material into the ascending aorta. Surgical treatment is advisable even in asymptomatic patients. Acute rupture of a large aneurysm in a previously healthy young adult produces a dramatic clinical picture. This is characterized by sudden onset of dyspnea, chest pain, brisk arterial pulses, and a loud continuous murmur. Cardiac failure with pulmonary edema supervenes rapidly. The electrocardiogram shows left or combined ventricular hypertrophy. The chest roentgenogram shows cardiomegaly with prominent vascular markings due to pulmonary arterial overcirculation and prominent pulmonary veins and signs of pulmonary edema. The diagnosis is confirmed by two-dimensional echocardiography and Doppler methods, supplemented by cardiac catheterization and aortography. Surgical correction is urgently indicated in acute rupture.

ANOMALOUS ORIGIN OF THE LEFT CORONARY ARTERY FROM THE PULMONARY TRUNK. The right coronary artery originates normally from the aorta, and the left coronary artery receives blood from intercoronary anastomoses so that blood flow in the left coronary artery drains *into* the pulmonary trunk. Thus left ventricular myocardial perfusion is significantly compromised. Generally symptoms are present within the first few months of life because of myocardial infarction, congestive cardiac failure, and mitral valve incompetence due to papillary muscle dysfunction. About 15 per cent of patients with this anomaly reach adult life because of exuberant intercoronary anastomoses, which may produce a continuous murmur. The electrocardiogram is important because signs of anterior and anterolateral myocardial infarction are present in a relatively young person. The chest roentgenogram shows cardiomegaly with dominance of the left ventricle. The origin of the left coronary artery from the aorta cannot be demonstrated by echocardiography. The diagnosis is confirmed by selective right coronary arteriography, which demonstrates the dilated right coronary artery, the intercoronary anastomoses, and opacification of the left coronary artery from these anastomoses as it enters the pulmonary artery. Reconstitution of normal coronary flow from the aorta to the left coronary artery is advised, although in many instances fibrosis of the left ventricle has resulted in permanent damage to ventricular function.

Pulmonary Arteriovenous Fistula

Fistulous communications between the pulmonary arteries and pulmonary veins may be multiple, small, and diffuse in both lungs or large and relatively localized. Hereditary hemorrhagic telangiectasia (Rendu-Osler-Weber syndrome) with angiomas of the buccal and nasal mucous membranes, gastrointestinal tract, and liver is present in about one half of patients or other members of their family. Desaturated pulmonary arterial blood flows through the fistula and enters the pulmonary vein without oxygenation. When total flow across the fistulous communications is significant, left atrial and left ventricular blood is desaturated, resulting in cyanosis and digital clubbing. Pulmonary arterial pressure remains normal because the flow across the fistula is at low pressure and resistance; cardiomegaly is unusual and heart failure uncommon. Hemoptysis may occur and is sometimes massive. Recurrent epistaxes and gastrointestinal bleeding are features of hereditary hemorrhagic telangiectasia. Transitory central nervous symptoms, including dizziness, vertigo, speech disturbances, visual aberrations, motor weakness, and convulsions, may result from paradoxical emboli, cerebral thromboses, or abscess. Findings on auscultation of the chest may be normal; in others soft systolic or continuous murmurs are audible anywhere in the chest. The electrocardiogram is usually normal. Roentgenographic examination of the chest shows the presence of large fistulas only. Selective pulmonary arteriography is diagnostic and visualizes the site, extent, and distribution of the fistulas. Large localized fistulous communications are treated surgically by lobectomy or wedge resection. Smaller communications may be obliterated by embolization; these emboli are introduced selectively through a strategically placed catheter in the branch of the pulmonary artery that feeds the fistula. Successful treatment is usually followed by disappearance of symptoms, although in some there is postoperative growth of small previously unrecognized fistulas and recurrence of symptoms.

OBSTRUCTIVE LESIONS WITH OR WITHOUT SHUNTS

Tetralogy of Fallot

The tetralogy of Fallot comprises a combination of four defects consisting of (1) right ventricular outflow tract obstruction (pulmonic stenosis), (2) ventricular septal defect, (3) overriding of the aorta above the ventricular defect, and (4) right ventricular hypertrophy. The pulmonic stenosis is usually a combination of obstruction at the valve as well as in the right ventricular outflow. The pulmonary arterial trunk may be short and smaller than normal, and there may be branch stenosis. The pulmonic valve is often bicuspid, may have a small ring, and occasionally is the only site of obstruction. Infundibular stenosis is produced by the anteriorly displaced hypoplastic infundibular (conal) septum. Occasionally, right ventricular outflow is completely obstructed (pulmonary atresia) and pulmonary blood flow is maintained by a patent ductus arteriosus and/or collateral flow via aortopulmonary collaterals. The ventricular septal defect is generally large, approximating the size of the aortic orifice; involves, but is not limited to, the membranous septum; and is related to the right and posterior aortic cusps. The ascending aorta is displaced anteriorly (dextraposed), and the aortic arch is to the right in about 20 per cent.

The severity of right ventricular outflow tract obstruction determines the hemodynamics and therefore the clinical picture. Severe obstruction is common, pulmonary blood flow is decreased, and blood is shunted from the right ventricle across the ventricular defect into the aorta. This right to left shunt results in systemic hypoxemia manifested as marked cyanosis, digital clubbing, and polycythemia. When obstruction to right ventricular outflow and a ventricular septal defect coexist without right to left shunting, the condition is known as acyanotic tetralogy of Fallot.

In severe cases, *cyanosis* is present from birth. In others, this finding develops in infancy, generally before the first birthday. The absence of cyanosis in the neonatal period is related to maintenance of pulmonary blood flow via a patent ductus arteriosis, which closes spontaneously in the first few months of life. Cyanosis increases in intensity progressively during the first years and is associated with poor physical development. *Dyspnea* with exertion is usual.

Hypoxic ("blue") spells occur primarily in infants with hypoxemia. These spells consist of a sudden onset of dyspnea, restlessness, increased cyanosis, gasping respirations, and syncope. They are associated with a further decrease of arterial Po_2 and a reduction of an already compromised pulmonary blood flow. These frightening episodes are treated by placing the child in a knee-chest position and by administering oxygen and intravenous bicarbonate if acidemia develops. The frequency and severity of these episodes can be reduced by oral propranolol. However, surgical treatment is generally indicated to increase pulmonary blood flow and thus relieve the hypoxemia.

Squatting is common in children with hypoxemia, who may assume this position to relieve dyspnea associated with exertion. Physical activity is usually resumed within a few minutes. Squatting decreases the magnitude of right to left shunt by increasing systemic vascular resistance and pulmonary blood flow. Adults seldom squat because they know the limitation of their exercise tolerance and discontinue physical activity before arterial Po_2 is significantly decreased.

Physical examination confirms the presence of delayed growth and development, cyanosis, and clubbing. Characteristically, the heart size is normal but the apical impulse is tapping owing to right ventricular hypertrophy. The systolic murmur, sometimes accompanied by a thrill, is produced by the right ventricular outflow tract obstruction. Auscultatory findings are variable; the systolic murmur, which is loudest at the upper left sternal edge but is widely transmitted, may be ejection in type or pansystolic. The murmur is less intense when the obstruction is severe. Aortic blood flow is increased, and this may result in an early ejection click. The second heart sound is single, produced by aortic valve closure, and pulmonic valve closure is generally inaudible. In rare instances a systolic and diastolic murmur may be audible in any part of the chest, anteriorly or posteriorly, and is produced by bronchial collateral flow to the lung or rarely by a patent ductus arteriosus. This auscultatory finding is frequent with pulmonary atresia.

Roentgenographically the heart size is normal, with a rounded, elevated cardiac apex likened to a wooden shoe (coeur en sabot). There is a concavity in the region of the main pulmonary artery, and the pulmonary vasculature is diminished. The aorta is large and arches to the right in 20 per cent. The *electrocardiogram* shows right axis deviation and right ventricular hypertrophy. Sometimes the P wave is tall and peaked. *Echocardiography* demonstrates the major intracardiac abnormalities. Echocardiographic examinations show the large ventricular septal defect, the degree of aortic override, and thick right ventricle; the right ventricular outflow tract obstruction may be visualized or inferred from Doppler turbulence in this area. The echocardiogram also helps to distinguish tetralogy of Fallot from other anomalies that may closely simulate this condition, namely, double outlet right ventricle with pulmonic stenosis, arterial transposition with pulmonic stenosis and ventricular septal defect, and a group of complex cardiac malformations consisting primarily of single ventricle and pulmonic stenosis.

These abnormalities are also excluded by *cardiac catheterization and angiocardiography*, and these tests are essential for surgical management. Cardiac catheterization confirms that the peak systolic pressures in both ventricles are virtually identical and that there is a significant gradient across the right ventricular outflow. The degree and direction of shunting at the ventricular level are also demonstrated. Arterial oxygen saturation is decreased and at rest is usually between 75 and 85 per cent. Selective right ventriculography identifies the site or sites of right ventricular outflow tract obstruction, the narrowed pulmonic valve ring, the presence of abnormalities of the pulmonary arterial trunk, and any stenoses of the pulmonary arterial branches (Fig. 49–2). In patients with pulmonary atresia, the anatomy of pulmonary blood flow is complex. Although there may not be filling of the main pulmonary artery, a central confluence of left and right intrapulmonary arteries may be present. Left ventriculogra-

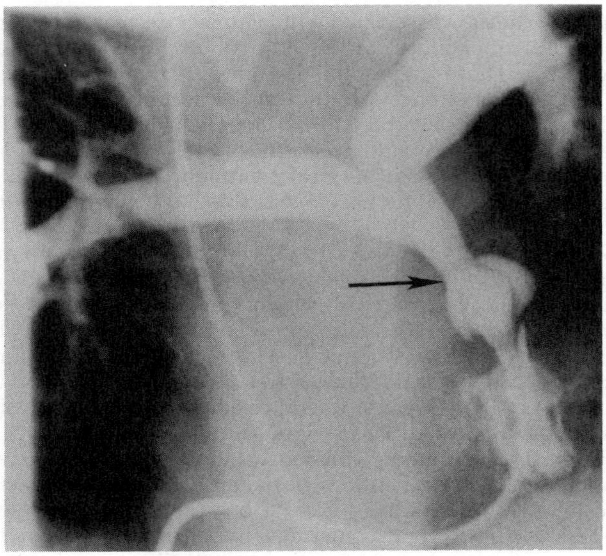

FIGURE 49–2. Cineangiograms in tetralogy of Fallot. Contrast injected in outflow of the right ventricle showing subvalvular obstruction, pulmonary valve stenosis with small annulus (*arrow*), and supravalvular stenosis with short pulmonary arterial trunk.

phy shows the position and size of the ventricular septal defect and the presence of an overriding aorta. In a few instances, a large coronary artery courses over the right ventricular outflow; preservation of this artery during surgical repair is essential. *Surgical treatment* is usually advised during infancy or childhood. The type of surgical procedure and its timing are still controversial. Infants with severe anoxemia in the first few months of life are frequently treated with a systemic to pulmonary arterial shunt to augment pulmonary arterial blood flow. Beyond the age of one to two years correction of the defect is advised, at which time any previous systemic to pulmonary shunt is taken down. Older children should have surgical correction of the anomaly because they are generally symptomatic. In all groups surgical correction is more difficult when there is severe deformity of the right ventricular outflow, including a small pulmonic valve ring. The surgical procedure consists of closure of the ventricular septal defect and relief of obstruction by infundibular resection and/or pulmonic valvotomy. Right ventricular outflow may need to be enlarged.

Ebstein's Anomaly of the Tricuspid Valve

This abnormality consists of an abnormal tricuspid valve that is displaced into the right ventricular cavity so that portions of the valve leaflet are attached to the right ventricular wall rather than to the atrioventricular ring. The portion of the right ventricle proximal to the tricuspid valve is thin, functions as an extension of the right atrium, and is known as "atrialized right ventricle." Leaflets of the tricuspid valve are generally redundant and frequently incompetent. The right atrium is large and an atrial septal defect or patent foramen ovale may be present. Increased right atrial pressure, as from tricuspid regurgitation, results in a right to left shunt across the atrial septum and cyanosis of varying degrees. Pulmonary blood flow is decreased.

Ebstein's anomaly in adults varies considerably in severity, so that many patients have active and productive lives, but survival beyond age 50 years is unusual. Symptoms vary in intensity, and with mild anomalies the only complaint is fatigue. Cardiac arrhythmias are frequent and generally supraventricular, the commonest being attacks of paroxysmal atrial tachycardia. The precordium is quiet to palpation. Auscultation reveals a systolic murmur, sometimes accompanied by a thrill over most of the anterior left chest, and third and fourth heart sounds are audible, resulting in triple or quadruple rhythms. A diastolic murmur is frequent, appears to be superficial, and may mimic a pericardial friction rub. Other auscultatory findings include multiple systolic ejection clicks and an opening snap of the tricuspid valve. The *electrocardiogram* shows right bundle branch block, tall and/or broad P waves, and a prolonged PR interval. Wolff-Parkinson-White syndrome (usually type B) is present in some. *Roentgenographic examination* shows a variable heart size; in extreme instances massive cardiomegaly is present because of great enlargement of the right atrium (Fig. 49–3). The outflow portion of the right ventricle is sometimes visible in the region usually occupied by the pulmonary artery in the posteroanterior view. The pulmonary vasculature is normal to decreased, and the aorta is small. The *echocardiogram* shows significant delay in tricuspid valve closure and an increased amplitude of motion of the tricuspid valve. The large right atrium and the displaced tricuspid valve can also be visualized. Surgical treatment should be advised in symptomatic patients, especially those with progressive cyanosis. Therapy consists of tricuspid valvuloplasty or valve replacement and ablation of the anomalous pathways between the atrium and ventricle in patients with Wolff-Parkinson-White syndrome and supraventricular tachycardia.

Tricuspid Atresia

In this condition there is no communication between the right atrium and right ventricle so that the entire systemic venous return enters the left heart through a defect in the intra-atrial septum. The left ventricle ejects blood into the normally related aorta and through a ventricular septal defect into the pulmonary arteries. If these vessels are transposed,

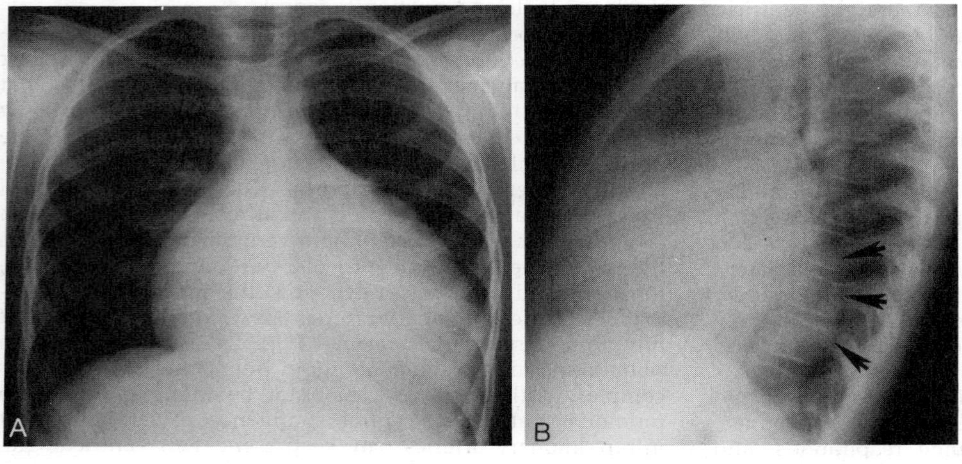

FIGURE 49–3. Chest roentgenograms in Ebstein's anomaly of the tricuspid valve. *A*, Posteroanterior view showing globular cardiac silhouette with narrow waist simulating pericardial effusion. *B*, Left anterior oblique view showing marked cardiomegaly due to massive right atrial enlargement, which extends posteriorly (*arrows*) and also encroaches on the anterior clear space.

the aorta arises from a hypoplastic right ventricle that fills from a ventricular septal defect. These patients have a marked increase in pulmonary blood flow and pressure so that heart failure and minimal cyanosis are common in infancy. Survival usually depends upon pulmonary arterial banding to limit pulmonary arterial flow. When the great arteries are normally related, the right ventricle can be minute and associated with marked pulmonic stenosis or atresia. In these patients pulmonary blood flow is derived from a patent ductus arteriosus or collateral bronchial flow. In other instances the left ventricle ejects its blood through a ventricular septal defect into a small right ventricle and then into the pulmonary artery.

Symptoms are usual during infancy and with decreased pulmonary blood flow consist of cyanosis, anoxemia, and poor physical development. Minimal cardiac enlargement is present, and the systolic ejection murmur along the left sternal edge is nonspecific. Left axis deviation with left ventricular hypertrophy is usual, and these *electrocardiographic findings* in the presence of cyanosis suggest the diagnosis. *Roentgenograms* of the chest show pulmonary undercirculation but are otherwise nonspecific. The *echocardiogram* confirms absence of the tricuspid valve, delineates the size of the small right ventricle, confirms the presence of a large left ventricle, and identifies the presence or absence of transposition of the great arteries. Most infants with decreased pulmonary blood flow require enlargement of the intra-atrial septal defect to ensure easy communication between the two atria as well as a systemic to pulmonary shunt. In later years more radical surgery is undertaken with anastomosis of the right atrium to the pulmonary artery and closure of the intra-atrial septal defect. This procedure effectively separates pulmonary and systemic blood flows, abolishes cyanosis, and improves exercise tolerance. A similar procedure is also used in patients who had pulmonary arterial banding during infancy.

Single Ventricle

Atrial blood empties through two separate atrioventricular valves or a common valve into a single ventricle from which the aorta and pulmonary artery arise. Associated cardiac abnormalities are present, but their nature varies considerably. The most frequent ones are transposition of the great arteries, pulmonic stenosis, and aortic origin from a rudimentary outlet chamber. The clinical picture depends on the nature of the associated anomalies. If pulmonic stenosis is severe, cyanosis and anoxemia dominate. In the absence of pulmonic stenosis pulmonary blood flow and vascular resistance are increased. The clinical picture is then dominated by congestive heart failure. Although these malformations are complex, surgical palliation is undertaken. In the presence of pulmonic stenosis the blood flow is increased with a systemic pulmonary shunt. On the other hand, high pulmonary blood flow is treated with a pulmonary arterial band. In later years, a surgical connection is established between the right atrium and pulmonary artery, and the atria are partitioned so that systemic venous return flows into the pulmonary artery and pulmonary venous return is ejected from the single ventricle into the aorta. When the aorta arises from a rudimentary chamber, systemic flow is dependent on an unobstructed communication between the single ventricle and the rudimentary chamber. This communication (the bulboventricular foramen) may narrow, resulting in a variable but often significant subaortic gradient. This complication may occur at any time, even postoperatively, and produces cardiomegaly and heart failure.

Inflow Obstruction to the Left Ventricle

Conditions of inflow obstruction are grouped together since they result in high pulmonary venous pressure with potential pulmonary edema. The lesions may occur anywhere from the insertion of the pulmonary veins into the left atrium to the area of the mitral valve. They are extremely rare abnormalities. *Pulmonary vein stenoses* at their site of entry into the left atrium are difficult to treat surgically or by balloon angioplasty. *Cor triatriatum* consists of a diaphragmatic partition of the left atrium. The upper portion receives the pulmonary veins, and the distal portion communicates with the mitral valve or through an atrial septal defect into the right atrium. The opening in the diaphragm is generally small so that symptoms are present in early life. The condition is surgically correctable by excision of the diaphragm and closure of associated atrial septal defects. *A supravalvular ring* above the mitral valve produces a similar clinical picture. *Congenital mitral stenosis* may be due to marked abnormality of the mitral valve apparatus, which includes fused, thickened mitral valve leaflets with short chordae, or the valve may have a parachute deformity in which the leaflets are also abnormal but the chordae converge and insert into a single papillary muscle.

Hypoplastic Left Heart Syndrome

Varying degrees of underdevelopment of the left side of the heart coexist, including marked underdevelopment of the left ventricle and atrium, and stenosis or atresia of the aortic and mitral orifices with hypoplasia of the ascending aorta. This complex malformation is a significant cause of cardiovascular death in the neonatal period. Attempts at surgical management have not been standardized.

OBSTRUCTIVE AND REGURGITANT LESIONS

Pulmonic Stenosis with Intact Ventricular Septum

Obstruction to right ventricular outflow can be valvular, subvalvular, supravalvular, or a combination of obstructions at these sites. Valvular obstruction, the most common variety, results from varying degrees of commissural fusion so that the deformed valve appears domelike. Dysplastic thick valve leaflets are less common and may accompany Noonan's syndrome (see Ch. 211). Subvalvular obstruction usually accompanies severe valvular stenosis, is due to infundibular hypertrophy, and occasionally is seen as an isolated abnormality with a normal pulmonic valve. Pulmonary arterial branch stenosis may be isolated or may occur at multiple sites and may be associated with supravalvular stenosis. These peripheral lesions are a feature of congenital rubella.

The hemodynamic consequences of valvular pulmonic stenosis are produced by the severity of obstruction. When the right ventricular outflow gradient is between 50 and 80 mm Hg the obstruction is considered to be moderate; pressures below and above that range are considered mild and severe, respectively. Pulmonary arterial pressure is normal or low. The arterial oxygen saturation is normal except when the obstruction is severe (sometimes with suprasystemic right ventricular pressure). Poor right ventricular compliance with or without an increase in right ventricular end-diastolic pressure increases right atrial pressure and may result in right to left shunting across the intra-atrial septum.

Symptoms are usually absent when the obstruction is mild or moderate, but when it is severe, effort dyspnea may be present. The physique is frequently normal, and some patients appear robust. When the stenosis is *mild*, the venous pressure is normal and the heart is not enlarged. A systolic murmur of varying intensity with midsystolic peaking is heard best at the upper left sternal edge and is preceded by a pulmonic ejection click. The second heart sound may be normal, but the pulmonic component is frequently delayed and of normal intensity. The electrocardiogram is normal or shows signs of minimal right ventricular hypertrophy. The chest *roentgenogram* shows prominence of the pulmonary arterial trunk because of poststenotic dilatation, but the heart size and pulmonary vasculature are normal. Echocardiography shows the domed stenotic valve. When pulmonic stenosis is *moderate*, the venous pressure may be normal or slightly elevated, with a prominent "a" wave in the jugular pulse. A right ventricular parasternal lift is palpable and may be accompanied by a systolic thrill at the upper left sternal edge. The systolic murmur, frequently preceded by an ejection sound, is accentuated in late systole. The second heart sound is split with a delayed and diminished pulmonic component. Electrocardiographic evidence of right ventricular hypertrophy is usual, sometimes with a prominent spiked P wave. The chest roentgenogram shows a normal or mildly enlarged heart, prominence of the pulmonary arterial trunk, and normal pulmonary vasculature. The abnormal valve is visualized by echocardiograms.

In *severe* pulmonic stenosis cyanosis may be present, owing to a small cardiac output or a right to left shunt across the intra-atrial septum. A large presystolic "a" wave is usual in the jugular venous pulse and the increased venous pressure may be transmitted to the liver, resulting in a presystolic pulsation. The heart is moderately or greatly enlarged, with a conspicuous parasternal right ventricular lift. The systolic ejection murmur is usually loud, frequently accompanied by a thrill, and audible maximally at the upper left sternal edge, but it may radiate widely over the entire precordium and into the neck and back. The murmur is accentuated in late systole, frequently encompasses the aortic component of the second heart sound, and may be preceded by an ejection sound. The pulmonic component of the second heart sound is either inaudible or soft and very late. The electrocardiogram shows gross right ventricular hypertrophy with tall P waves attributed to right atrial enlargement. The chest roentgenogram confirms the cardiac enlargement, prominence of the right ventricle and atrium, poststenotic dilatation of the pulmonary artery, and pulmonary vasculature that is either normal or decreased. The echocardiogram demonstrates systolic doming of the stenotic leaflets into the dilated pulmonary arterial trunk. In the presence of significant obstruction, the right ventricular wall is thick, the right atrium is enlarged, and the intra-atrial septum bows toward the left. The degree of obstruction is quantified with Doppler techniques by applying a modified Bernoulli equation using peak velocity of flow ($P = 4V^2$, where P = pressure gradient and v = peak flow velocity).

Cardiac catheterization demonstrates the pressure gradient across the pulmonic valve and determines the degree of severity. Selective right ventriculography visualizes the site and nature of the obstruction. During ventricular systole contrast material is seen as a jet through the domed stenotic valve. Subvalvular hypertrophy, which may intensify the obstruction, is also demonstrated by this method.

The clinical course of patients with mild obstruction is usually good, and progression of the disease is unusual, especially in adolescence and adult life. Many with moderate obstruction also do well, although their progress needs to be evaluated at regular intervals, especially during childhood. Progression of the obstruction is detected clinically by the change in character of the murmur, which becomes accentuated in late systole. Also, the width of the splitting of the second heart sound increases as the right ventricular pressure rises. These signs are associated with an increase in the severity of the electrocardiographic signs of the right ventricular hypertrophy.

Two options are now available for treatment of moderate to severe obstruction. These consist of surgical valvotomy or balloon valvuloplasty. There is a long experience with surgical treatment, and children with isolated pulmonic stenosis generally do well for many years after valvotomy. This is due to immediate decrease in right ventricular pressure after valvotomy. Pulmonic valve incompetence after surgery is usually mild, presents as a short early diastolic murmur, and is generally of no clinical significance. Recurrence of obstruction after surgery is extremely rare. The results of surgery in adults with severe obstruction may not be uniformly good. Right ventricular dysfunction may persist despite relief of the gradient, and this has been attributed to a poorly compliant right ventricle due to persistent hypertrophy and fibrosis. Pulmonic valvuloplasty for valvular stenosis is accomplished by a balloon catheter inserted percutaneously. Rapid inflation and deflation of the balloon placed across the valve annulus significantly increase the size of the valve orifice. When the valve is not dysplastic and greatly thickened, valvuloplasty is the treatment of choice in many institutions. Patients who have had this new form of treatment are at present being observed to determine whether the initial reduction of gradient is maintained over many years, and whether valvuloplasty produces significant pulmonic valve regurgitation.

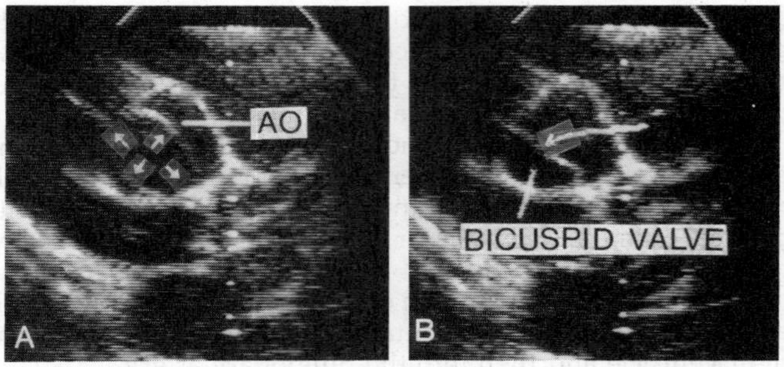

FIGURE 49–4. Short axis echocardiogram of bicuspid aortic valve. *A*, Open valve orifice during systole (*arrows*). *B*, Competent bicuspid valve during diastole. Arrow points to line of apposition of valve leaflets.

Bicuspid Aortic Valve

This condition is said to occur in about 2 per cent of the population. The valve consists of two commissures and two cusps, one of which is generally larger. The bicuspid aortic valve may have normal function so that there is no systolic gradient across the valve and during diastole the valve remains competent. This normal function may continue throughout life, and the bicuspid valve may be found only incidentally at necropsy. In others, abnormality of the aortic valve can be suspected during examination of teenagers or young adults. These findings relate to minor degrees of valvular obstruction and/or incompetence. The auscultatory findings consist of short, soft systolic murmurs heard at the upper right sternal edge. An early aortic ejection click, which precedes the murmur, excludes an innocent murmur. In others, the systolic murmur may be followed by a short, high-pitched early diastolic murmur of aortic incompetence. The diagnosis may be confirmed by echocardiography, which demonstrates only two aortic leaflets (Fig. 49–4).

The natural course of bicuspid aortic valves is variable. In some, the valve may function normally for many decades and produce no abnormal clinical signs. In others the valve leaflets become thickened, fibrotic, and calcified, so that clear signs of aortic stenosis of varying severity develop during early or midadult life. In others, there is eversion or prolapse of one of the aortic cusps, resulting in progressive aortic regurgitation that can become severe. A bicuspid aortic valve is particularly susceptible to infective endocarditis, which may convert a benign lesion into one associated with acute severe aortic regurgitation.

Congenital Valvular Aortic Stenosis

See Ch. 52 for a discussion of this lesion.

Subvalvular Aortic Stenosis (Discrete)

Obstruction to left ventricular outflow is produced by a fibrous membrane situated just below the aortic valve. The membrane is a collar-like structure extending from the intraventricular septum and involving the anterior mitral leaflet.

The high-velocity jet of blood flowing through the obstructed area during ventricular systole impinges on the aortic valve, which results in fibrous thickening and incompetence of the valve. The clinical picture simulates that of valvular aortic stenosis with important exceptions. An aortic ejection sound is usually absent, and the murmur occupies the whole of systole. This condition is frequently mistaken for a ventricular septal defect or mitral incompetence. Mild forms of obstruction may coexist with other lesions, especially a ventricular septal defect. This obstruction may be unrecognized at the time of surgical closure of the ventricular septal defect, and the obstruction may progress over the ensuing years. A useful differential sign is the presence of an early diastolic murmur of aortic valve incompetence, which is a common finding when the obstruction is moderate or severe. Laboratory findings simulate those described under valvular aortic stenosis. However, the echocardiogram is diagnostic in that the discrete membrane is visualized. Cardiac catheterization and angiocardiography are undertaken to measure the severity of obstruction and to outline the membrane by left ventriculography or aortography if the aortic valve is incompetent. Indications for surgery are liberalized, since continued damage to the aortic valve should be prevented. Excision of the membrane gives immediate good results, but complications include damage to the anterior mitral leaflet with resultant regurgitation or conduction abnormalities, including complete heart block from trauma to the intraventricular septum. Furthermore, there may be recurrence of obstruction from regrowth of the membrane.

A rarer form of subaortic stenosis is a long, narrow fibromuscular channel frequently associated with hypoplasia of the aortic ring. This disease is more frequent in childhood and is difficult to treat surgically because relief of obstruction may require enlargement of the aortic valve ring. In extreme cases a valve-bearing conduit is inserted between the left ventricle and the aorta.

Hypertrophic Cardiomyopathy

See Ch. 53.

Supravalvular Aortic Stenosis

The obstruction may be localized to a segmental hourglass-shaped narrowing immediately above the aortic sinuses. Beyond the area of obstruction the aorta may be normal in diameter or show varying degrees of tubular hypoplasia, frequently involving the ascending aorta but occasionally extending for a varying length along the course of the aorta, even to its bifurcation. Aortic valve leaflets may be thickened, with resultant mild aortic regurgitation. During systole the aortic valve leaflets may impinge upon the orifices of the coronary arteries so that coronary flow is impaired; this may be further aggravated by the coronary arteries themselves, which can be enlarged and tortuous but have a narrow lumen. Supravalvular aortic stenosis is frequently associated with the *Williams syndrome,* consisting of typical facies (broad, prominent forehead, flattened bridge of the nose, epicanthal folds, and long upper lip), mild mental retardation, and low-pitched voice; children with this syndrome are particularly friendly and converse easily. In the absence of the Williams syndrome, supravalvular aortic stenosis occurs sporadically and is sometimes familial. Pulmonary arterial branch stenosis may coexist. Carotid and brachial arterial pulses may be asymmetric, with more conspicuous pulses on the right side. This finding has been attributed to preferential flow into the innominate artery. Other components of the clinical picture simulate those described under valvular aortic stenosis. Echocardiography visualizes the ascending aorta, identifies the area of obstruction, and defines the degree of aortic hypoplasia. Cardiac catheterization and angiocardiography determine the severity of the obstruction, visualize the anatomy of the aorta and the obstruction, and demonstrate severity of pulmonary arterial branch stenosis, if present. Surgical treatment to relieve the obstruction is advised when the gradient is severe. However, surgical treatment is complicated, especially when the transverse and thoracic aortae are markedly hypoplastic.

Coarctation of the Aorta

Narrowing of the aortic lumen may occur at isolated or multiple sites in the aorta. By far the commonest site of discrete obstruction is just distal to the origin of the left subclavian artery. The lesion is more frequent in males and is also seen in patients with Turner's (XO) syndrome. Associated cardiac malformations are frequent, the commonest being a bicuspid aortic valve, congenital aortic stenosis with or without incompetence, ventricular septal defect, and lesions of the mitral valve with or without valvular regurgitation. Extensive collateralization usually develops, especially from branches of the subclavian, internal mammary, superior intercostal, and axillary arteries. These vessels join the intercostal arteries of the descending aorta and inferior epigastric branches of the femoral arteries, which allow channels for arterial blood to bypass the area of coarctation. These collateral vessels can become enormously enlarged and tortuous by early adult life.

Children and young adults are generally asymptomatic. However, hypertension may develop in the arteries above the coarctation and may be associated with epistaxis and throbbing headaches. Other symptoms include leg fatigue, complaints of cold extremities, and occasionally intermittent claudication. Beyond the second decade coarctation may be discovered by the finding of brachial arterial hypertension during routine physical examination. The methods of presentation in adults include infective endocarditis, usually involving the aortic valve, and rupture of the aorta or dissecting aneurysm may occur especially in the 20's and 30's. The site of rupture is either in the proximal aorta or in an aneurysm in the area of coarctation. Cerebral vascular disease with resultant cerebral hemorrhage or infarction may result from complications of hypertension or from the rupture of an aneurysm, usually of the circle of Willis. Hypertension and associated atherosclerosis of the coronary circulation may result in congestive cardiac failure, sometimes preceded by acute myocardial infarction. Pregnancy is usually well tolerated, especially if hypertension is controlled. However, the risk of aortic rupture is increased especially toward the end of the third trimester.

Classic signs of aortic coarctation are the disparity in pulsations and blood pressures of the arms and legs. The bounding pulses of the arms and carotid vessels contrast with the weak, delayed, or absent femoral and/or distal arterial pulses in the legs. Also, the blood pressure in the arms exceeds that in the legs. This applies especially to the systolic reading, and there is a further rise of systolic blood pressure in response to exercise. If the systolic arterial pressure in the right arm exceeds that of the left arm by more than 30 mm Hg, the left subclavian artery is involved in the coarctation. Collateral arterial circulation may be visible but is usually palpable, especially in the back, at the angles of the scapulae and in the axillae. Murmurs are variable in location, quality, and intensity. The usual is a precordial midsystolic murmur heard best at the left sternal edge, but it may be loudest in the back between the scapulae. Additional systolic or sometimes continuous murmurs are audible over the anterior or posterior chest and are produced by flow through the large, tortuous collateral arteries. The *electrocardiogram is* usually normal during childhood and adolescence. In adults, varying degrees of left ventricular hypertrophy are present. *Roentgenographic* examinations during childhood may not be striking. However, prominence of the left ventricle occurs thereafter and during adult life. The heart may be moderately enlarged. Notching of the inferior border of the ribs from collateral vessels is common. This may be unilateral if one of the subclavian arteries arises below the area of coarctation. Poststenotic dilatation of the descending aorta is usual and is demonstrated by a barium esophagram, and the prominent left subclavian artery produces a shadow in the left mediastinum. *Echocardiography* visualizes the area of coarctation, the large left subclavian artery, poststenotic dilatation of the descending aorta, and associated intracardiac anomalies, especially those of the aortic valve. These associated anomalies are confirmed by cardiac catheterization and selective left ventriculography and angiography. Coarctectomy is advised, preferably in early childhood between ages three and five years.

Pulmonic Valvular Regurgitation

Isolated congenital pulmonic valve regurgitation is rare and seldom produces symptoms; an early diastolic murmur at the upper left sternal edge is the only abnormal sign. However, pulmonic valvular regurgitation may accompany other conditions such as those associated with severe pulmonary hypertension or after surgical transection of the pulmonic valve ring for the treatment of severe obstruction of the right ventricular outflow.

Absence of Pulmonic Valve

Absence of the pulmonic valve is a congenital anomaly in which pulmonic valve leaflets are virtually absent. Although the lesion may be isolated it is usually associated with other defects, especially tetralogy of Fallot or isolated ventricular septal defect.

Vascular Rings and Other Aortic Arch Anomalies

The more common anomalies are double aortic arch, right aortic arch with left ligamentum arteriosum, origin of the right subclavian artery from the thoracic aorta distal to the left subclavian artery, anomalous origin of the innominate or left carotid arteries, and anomalous left pulmonary artery, which arises from the elongated pulmonary trunk and courses between the trachea and the esophagus. The clinical picture is extremely variable, and in many instances there are no symptoms. Tracheal compression, especially during infancy, produces respiratory distress with wheezing and a brassy cough. Dysphagia may occur in older patients. Surgery is advised in symptomatic patients to relieve the tracheal and esophageal compression.

THE TRANSPOSITIONS

Transposition of the Great Arteries

In this condition the aorta arises from the right ventricle and the pulmonary artery from the left ventricle. Systemic venous return is to the right atrium, and pulmonary venous return is to the left atrium. Systemic venous blood flows through the tricuspid valve into the right ventricle and is ejected into the aorta. Pulmonary venous blood flows from the left atrium through the mitral valve into the left ventricle and is ejected into the pulmonary artery. Thus, the circulations are parallel. Survival is dependent on mixture of blood through the foramen ovale, a ventricular septal defect, or patency of the ductus arteriosus. This condition is a common malformation that occurs predominantly in males, with symptoms in the neonatal period or soon thereafter.

ISOLATED "SIMPLE" TRANSPOSITION OF THE GREAT ARTERIES. In this malformation the ventricular septum is intact. Mixing of systemic and pulmonary blood occurs primarily from bidirectional shunting across the foramen ovale. This condition produces symptoms and signs of anoxemia in the neonate, is suspected in an otherwise normal neonate who is cyanotic and tachypneic, and is verified by echocardiography, which demonstrates the abnormal origin of the great arteries, as well as the fact that the aorta is usually anterior to the pulmonary artery. Emergency balloon atrial septostomy that ruptures the foramen ovale allows greater mixing at the atrial level and decompresses the left atrium. Generally, these babies do well for many months, until surgical treatment is undertaken, usually between the ages of 6 and 12 months. Currently, there is debate about the preferred method of surgical treatment. There has been greater experience with intra-atrial redirection of venous return so that systemic venous blood flows into the left ventricle and is ejected out the pulmonary artery; pulmonary venous return flows through the tricuspid valve and is pumped by the right ventricle into the aorta. Immediate results are excellent, but concern has been expressed about late onset of supraventricular arrhythmias (especially bradyarrhythmias and sick sinus syndrome) and about right ventricular failure and pulmonary edema, since this ventricle is ejecting blood into the aorta. Because of these concerns, the arterial switch operation was developed whereby the origins of the great arteries are transected and the pulmonary artery is connected to the stump of the vessel arising from the right ventricle and the aorta to the left ventricle with implantation of the coronary arteries into the new aorta.

TRANSPOSITION OF THE GREAT ARTERIES WITH VENTRICULAR SEPTAL DEFECT. When the septal defect is small, the clinical picture is similar to that of simple transposition, and many of these small defects close spontaneously. If the ventricular septal defect is large and nonrestrictive, significant mixing of blood occurs and symptoms are frequently delayed. The clinical picture is dominated by signs of congestive cardiac failure with minimal cyanosis. In the untreated state there is progressive pulmonary hypertension with severe pulmonary vascular disease. Treatment is required during infancy, and a number of options are available for surgical treatment. The greatest experience has been with a staged procedure. Pulmonary arterial banding is done during infancy to restrict pulmonary blood flow and prevent the onset of pulmonary vascular disease. In later years, usually during childhood, the second stage is undertaken, in which the pulmonary artery is debanded and transected, the ventricular septal defect is closed so that the left ventricle ejects blood into the aorta, and a conduit is placed from the right ventricle to the transected pulmonary artery *(Rastelli procedure)*. Another option consists of the arterial switch operation as described above.

TRANSPOSITION OF THE GREAT ARTERIES WITH PULMONIC STENOSIS. The importance of this condition is that it may closely simulate the clinical picture produced by tetralogy of Fallot. The condition generally requires an aortic pulmonary shunt during infancy to increase pulmonary blood flow and relieve the symptoms of anoxemia. In later years the Rastelli procedure is undertaken.

Double Outlet Right Ventricle

In this malformation both the pulmonary artery and the aorta arise from the right ventricle, and the only outlet from the left ventricle is a ventricular septal defect. The clinical picture simulates a large, uncomplicated ventricular septal defect with pulmonary hypertension. The echocardiogram is diagnostic in that there is discontinuity between the anterior mitral leaflet and the aorta, since the latter structure arises from the right ventricle. Uncontrollable heart failure and pulmonary hypertension are frequent during infancy so that pulmonary arterial banding is usually required. In later years, generally during childhood, the Rastelli operation is advised. Double outlet right ventricle may be complicated by pulmonic stenosis when the condition simulates that described under Tetralogy of Fallot.

Corrected Transposition (L Transposition of the Great Arteries)

This condition consists of *ventricular inversion* and transposition of the great arteries. Systemic venous blood enters a normal right atrium, flows through a mitral valve into the left ventricle, and is ejected into the pumonary artery. Pulmonary venous blood flows from the left atrium through a tricuspid valve into the right ventricle and is ejected into the aorta. If the condition is uncomplicated, blood flow and hemodynamics are normal. However, associated anomalies are usual, such as ventricular septal defect, pulmonic stenosis, left atrioventricular valve (tricuspid) anomalies, including an Ebstein-like malformation of this valve, and atrioventricular conduction abnormalities—frequently complete atrioventricular block. The clinical picture is dominated by the associated lesions. The chest roentgenogram may suggest the abnormal origin of the great arteries in that the ascending aorta occupies the upper left border of the cardiac silhouette in the posteroanterior view. Since ventricular inversion is present, the electrocardiogram may show absent q waves in leads I and V_6, initial q waves in III, aVF, and V_1, and prominent T waves in the right precordial leads. During surgical treatment the bundle of His may be injured because it is located abnormally, so that complete heart block may occur. In others, significant regurgitations via the Ebstein-like tricuspid valve requires valve replacement.

Anomalous Pulmonary Venous Connection

The anomalous pulmonary venous return may be partial or total. *Partial anomalous pulmonary venous return* simulates the clinical picture produced by a secundum atrial septal defect. In fact, one of these forms is the sinus venosus defect.

TOTAL ANOMALOUS PULMONARY VENOUS CONNECTION. The site of entry of the pulmonary veins may be supradiaphragmatic (into a left superior vena cava or vertical vein, coronary sinus, right superior vena cava, or right atrium) or infradiaphragmatic (portal vein, hepatic veins, or inferior vena cava). Thus, there is no connection between the pulmonary vein and the left atrium. Generally the pulmonary veins converge to form a single trunk, which then enters the systemic venous circulation. Varying degrees of pulmonary venous obstruction are present and depend on the length of the common pulmonary venous trunk before its entry into the systemic vein as well as localized areas of obstruction.

The clinical picture is variable. In some instances, especially those of infradiaphragmatic connection, pulmonary edema and cyanosis are present in the neonatal period or soon thereafter. When there is a large intra-atrial communication and obstruction to pulmonary venous return is moderate, symptoms occur in later infancy and the clinical picture is dominated by congestive cardiac failure. When pulmonary venous obstruction is absent and there is a large communication between the right and left atria, symptoms may be delayed until early childhood and very occasionally adolescence. The clinical picture of these patients simulates that produced by a large left to right shunt at the atrial level.

The *electrocardiogram* reflects the hemodynamic state so that symptomatic infants have marked right ventricular hypertrophy with prominent P waves. Chest *roentgenograms* in neonates with pulmonary venous obstruction are characterized by pulmonary edema with a normal heart size. In older infants the heart is large and pulmonary overcirculation evident. In older children with pulmonary venous connection to the left superior vena cava, the cardiac silhouette has the appearance of a snowman or figure 8. The supracardiac shadow is produced by marked dilatation of the left superior vena cava, innominate vein, and right superior vena cava. The *echocardiogram* shows signs of right volume overload, and sometimes a common venous trunk is visualized. *Cardiac catheterization* demonstrates the severity of pulmonary hypertension, and pulmonary arteriograms show return of contrast material to the pulmonary veins and their anomalous site of insertion into the systemic venous system. Surgical treatment is indicated when the common pulmonary venous trunk is anastomosed to the left atrium, the atrial septal defect closed, and the anomalous connection to the systemic venous system obliterated. Results of surgical treatment have been good, with greatest risk in symptomatic neonates.

CARDIAC MALPOSITION

Knowledge of the position of the heart as well as the location (situs) of abdominal viscera aids in defining the nature of these anomalies. Roentgenography of the abdomen helps identify abdominal situs by localizing the position of the stomach bubble and other abdominal structures, but many viscera cannot be visualized by this method alone. Generally, atrial and visceral situs are related; if the viscera are normally located, the atria have a normal position. In abdominal situs inversus, the left atrium is usually to the right and the right atrium to the left. Location of the atria is further and more accurately assessed by evaluation of the tracheobronchial air column on chest roentgenogram. A normal tracheobronchial tree with an epiarterial bronchus on the right indicates normal atrial situs, and this finding is independent of the position of the heart.

Dextrocardia

The heart is in the right chest, and the cardiac apex points to the right. Associated abdominal situs inversus (mirror-image dextrocardia) in adults is usually associated with a normally functioning heart. However, poorly motile cilia may result in sinusitis and bronchiectasis (Kartagener's syndrome). Dextrocardia may be discovered by physical examination when the heart sounds are more clear in the right chest or accidentally on a routine chest film. The electrocardiogram demonstrates the mirror image so that the P, QRS, and T are inverted in lead I; aV_R and aV_L are the reverse of normal, and the right precordial leads resemble those usually recorded from the left chest. *Isolated dextrocardia* with abdominal viscera in normal position (situs solitus) is invariably associated with various combinations of severe cardiac malformations, the commonest being ventricular inversion, single ventricle, pulmonic stenosis, abnormalities of the atrioventricular valves, and anomalies of systemic and pulmonary venous return.

Isolated Levocardia

Isolated levocardia is accompanied by varying degrees of anomalous position of abdominal viscera (heterotaxia) so that situs inversus is partial or complete. Severe cardiac malformations are usual, including various combinations of anomalies of systemic and pulmonary venous return, common atrioventricular canal, pulmonic stenosis or atresia, defects of the atrial and ventricular septa, and single ventricle.

Mesocardia

Mesocardia is the term used when the heart is centrally located in the chest or the cardiac silhouette on roentgenogram is toward the right chest. The cardiac anatomy is normal with normal relationships of the cardiac chambers, venous return, and origin of the great arteries. Cardiac malformations are usually absent.

Asplenia Syndrome

This condition is characterized by absence of the spleen, undefinable situs of the abdominal viscera (situs ambiguus), bilateral *right-sidedness*, and complex, severe cardiac malformations. Bilateral right-sidedness is identified by bilateral trilobed lungs with bilateral epiarterial bronchi. In the majority the liver is located centrally so that the liver edge is palpable across the entire upper abdomen. The stomach is located on the right in about half the patients, and varying degrees of malrotation of the small bowel are present. Both atria have the morphologic characteristics of the right atrium. Common cardiovascular anomalies include total anomalous pulmonary venous connection, transposition of the great arteries, pulmonic stenosis or atresia, complete atrioventricular canal, single ventricle, and dextrocardia. The condition is suspected in a deeply cyanotic male infant with dextrocardia and a centrally placed liver. Howell-Jolly and Heinz bodies in the peripheral red blood cells are suggestive of asplenia, but these findings are not conclusive. Infants with asplenia are susceptible to severe intercurrent infections so that continued antibiotic prophylaxis has been suggested as a preventive measure. Aortopulmonary shunts during infancy are indicated when severe anoxemia is present owing to pulmonic stenosis, and right atrial-pulmonary shunts (Fontan) are advised in later years.

Polysplenia Syndrome

The features of this condition are multiple splenic masses (two or more), ambiguous abdominal situs, and *bilateral left-sidedness;* while cardiovascular abnormalities are frequent, they are generally not as complex as in the asplenia syndrome. The lungs are bilobed and epiarterial bronchi are absent. The liver is frequently located centrally in the upper abdomen, and the stomach is right- or left-sided. Malrotation of the bowel is common. Both atria have the morphologic features of the left atrium. The hepatic segment of the inferior vena cava is frequently absent so that systemic venous return is by way of the azygos vein. The cardiac apex points to the left in the majority. Pulmonary venous return may be normal, arterial transposition is present in only a minority, and pulmonic stenosis is unusual. The cardiac malformations are generally associated with left to right shunts at atrial or ventricular levels.

THE ADULT WITH "UNCURED" CONGENITAL HEART DISEASE

Strategies of management of symptomatic patients with congenital heart disease have changed recently so that the majority are treated during infancy or early childhood. Many adolescents and adults now exist who have trivial lesions, have remained asymptomatic, and have lived a normal lifestyle. Other patients have anomalies that are silent until adult life. Palliative surgery may have been undertaken in another group who have remained relatively well and have now approached adult life. Another cohort of patients who may not have had surgical treatment during early life develop progressive pulmonary hypertension during childhood, and in adult life their lesions are associated with severe pulmonary vascular disease. This section discusses these groups of patients.

VENTRICULAR SEPTAL DEFECTS. A significant number of patients seen in pediatric cardiac clinics have trivial shunts across a small ventricular septal defect. They remain asymptomatic throughout the growing years, and as adults the only abnormal physical sign is a long, harsh systolic murmur, which may be accompanied by a thrill and is heard best at the lower left sternal edge. It is unusual to see such patients beyond the age of 40 years so that it has been assumed that many of these defects close spontaneously. While the defect remains, these patients are at risk to develop infective endocarditis and occasionally aortic regurgitation or discrete subaortic stenosis.

VALVULAR PULMONIC STENOSIS. Generally, asymptomatic children with mild pulmonic stenosis (resting peak right ventricular pressure less than one half of systolic systemic pressure) do not require surgical treatment. There is no consensus about the course of untreated mild to moderate pulmonic stenosis. The generally held belief, however, is that progressive increase in severity is unusual, especially if the patient is beyond the age of 12 years. This optimistic view also applies to those who had a valvotomy during childhood, which relieved the obstruction. Restriction of physical activity is not required, pregnancy is well tolerated, and, although infective endocarditis of the pulmonic valve is not common, prophylaxis is advisable at the time of risk for this complication.

CONGENITAL COMPLETE HEART BLOCK. Fetal echocardiography may be prompted by the recognition of intrauterine bradycardia, and this test unmasks the presence of complete atrioventricular (AV) block. This study is especially important during pregnancy of mothers with connective tissue disease, such as systemic lupus erythematosus, since the offspring are at greater risk for complete AV block. It is suggested that antinuclear antibodies of the IgG category cross the placenta and damage the fetal conduction system. This occurs in mothers whose disease is active but also when there are no overt clinical manifestations and only positive serologic evidence is present. In about 70 per cent of children with complete AV block the lesion is isolated, and the remainder have associated complex cardiac malformations, such as ventricular inversion or single ventricle. Familial complete AV block is well recognized. Adolescents and adults with isolated congenital complete AV block are usually asymptomatic, but it is not possible to predict episodes of syncope. The pulse rate is inappropriately slow for age. The large stroke volume and vasodilatation produce jerky pulses, systolic hypertension, and cardiomegaly. Cannon waves may be visible in the jugular venous pulse. The first heart sound varies in intensity and may be followed by a nonspecific systolic ejection murmur. The diagnosis is confirmed by the electrocardiogram, in which there is no constant relationship between the P waves and QRS complexes. Usually the QRS is of normal duration, which suggests that the site of the lesion is above the bundle of His. Marked ventricular slowing may be recorded by continuous, 24-hour electrocardiographic monitoring, especially during sleep. It is not known whether there is any relationship between the slow ventricular rates during sleep and the prognosis. Since patients with congenital complete AV block have been observed in late adult life, there is a generally held view that the prognosis is good. However, the lesion is not benign, in that complications may occur at any time and are not predictable. Syncope is an indication for implantation of a permanent pacemaker. Decisions about treatment in asymptomatic patients are more difficult. The demonstration of ventricular tachycardia or fibrillation during continuous electrocardiographic monitoring or graded exercise testing is an indication for pacemaker implantation. There remains a group of asymptomatic patients in whom treatment is not standardized, including those with premature ventricular contractions during and after exercise, extreme nocturnal bradycardia, and ventricular depolarization initiated from a focus low in the bundle of His.

EISENMENGER'S SYNDROME. This syndrome is associated with marked elevation of pulmonary vascular resistance with reversed or bidirectional shunt, which is intracardiac or between the aorta and pulmonary arteries. Thus, pulmonary vascular disease is the hallmark of this syndrome, and the site of the shunt is incidental. Medial hypertrophy of pulmonary arteries and arterioles is present and is associated with cellular, fibrotic, and fibroelastic intimal reactions, and in more severe forms plexiform lesions encroach into the lumen of the vessel. These changes in the pulmonary vascular bed are directly related to pulmonary arterial pressure. Extension of muscle into the peripheral arteries occurs when pulmonary hypertension is still associated with increased pulmonary blood flow. With progressive vascular disease, a reduction in the number of small arteries may precede obliterative pulmonary vascular disease.

Historically these patients are frequently symptomatic during infancy and early childhood because of congestive cardiac failure, poor physical development, and recurrent lower respiratory tract infections. As pulmonary vascular resistance rises, the left to right shunt decreases so that symptoms improve. These children may lead nearly normal lives, but their stamina is limited and mild exertional cyanosis is evident. In early adult life there is progressive anoxemia with intensification of cyanosis, digital clubbing may be extreme, and polycythemia increases. Progressive decrease in effort tolerance develops over many years, culminating in congestive cardiac failure in early or mid-adult life. Other symptoms include hemoptysis, angina pectoris attributed to right ventricular ischemia, syncope, and palpitations from premature atrial or ventricular contractions. Jugular venous pressure is increased, with a prominent "v" wave in the presence of complicating tricuspid valve regurgitation. Hepatomegaly and marked dependent edema with ascites are usual with heart failure. The heart size is increased to a variable extent, greatest when there are shunts at the atrial level and when there is complicating tricuspid and/or pulmonic valve incompetence. The precordium is active with a right ventricular heave along the left sternal edge. Pulmonary arterial pulsations and the second heart sound may be palpable at the upper left sternal edge. The systolic murmur varies in intensity and is frequently initiated by a pulmonic ejection click. The second heart sound is booming, single, or narrowly split in ventricular shunts, but wide, fixed splitting may be audible in isolated atrial shunts. Signs of pulmonary and/or tricuspid valve regurgitation are superimposed when there is dilatation of these valve rings secondary to pulmonary hypertension or right ventricular failure. The *electrocardiogram* shows marked right ventricular or biventricular hypertrophy with prominent P waves. Complete right bundle branch block may be present, especially when the shunt is at the atrial level. In others the electrocardiogram is influenced by the underlying anomaly (e.g., single ventricle, ventricular inversion, etc.). The *chest roentgenogram* confirms the degree of cardiomegaly. The pulmonary trunk is enlarged with prominence of the primary divisions, which diminish in caliber in the peripheral branches. The *echocardiogram* helps to identify the anatomy of the underlying intracardiac or extracardiac malformation. *Cardiac catheterization* is undertaken when the diagnosis cannot be established by clinical findings and noninvasive studies. One of the purposes of catheterization is to determine whether the pulmonary vascular bed is vasoactive, as indicated by a fall in pulmonary artery pressure and resistance during the breathing of 100 per cent oxygen. Another major indication is to exclude the presence of left ventricular inflow lesions, which result in elevation of pulmonary venous pressure and secondary pulmonary hypertension. Angiocardiography carries a small increased risk because the contrast medium may produce a fall in systemic vascular resistance and increased right to left shunting with a further fall in systemic arterial saturation.

Polycythemia may become extreme, and when the hematocrit exceeds 70 per cent excruciating headaches may occur. These are difficult to treat but do respond to repeated venesection. This treatment should not be undertaken lightly, since reduction of red cell count and blood volume is not tolerated. Heart rate and blood pressure are monitored during the procedure. Small aliquots of blood (± 30 ml) are removed and immediately replaced with a similar volume of fresh frozen plasma or human albumin. Repeated venesection results in iron deficiency anemia so that daily oral iron replacement is essential. The usual goal is to reduce the hematocrit to between 55 and 60 per cent. *Hemoptysis* occurs from rupture of pulmonary vessels or is due to pulmonary arterial thrombosis or embolism. This symptom is usually limited to adult life, blood loss is not excessive, and symptomatic treatment is all that is needed. However, hemoptysis can be life threatening if associated with hypotension, an increase in the degree of hypoxemia, and the development of acidemia. Long-term anticoagulation is not indicated. *Syncope and sudden death* cannot be predicted, but patients with Eisenmenger's syndrome between the ages of about 20 and 40 years are at risk. The mechanism is not clear but has been attributed to arrhythmias, probably ventricular tachyarrhythmias, which result in hypotension and an increase in right to left shunting. *Pregnancy* is not well tolerated and sudden death has been reported during the third trimester or in the postpartum period.

Treatment. Surgical treatment of the cardiac anomaly is contraindicated because these patients succumb to the effects of pulmonary vascular disease. Palliation has been successful in the presence of transposition of the great arteries, ventricular septal defect, and severe pulmonary vascular disease; the procedure involves redirection of the venous return (as described under Transposition of the Great Arteries), but the ventricular defect is not closed. The experience with transplantation of the heart and lungs is still small and follow-up is short, but this therapy is being watched with interest, since patients with progressive symptoms are at great risk of dying. Drugs have been used to attempt to manipulate pulmonary and systemic vascular resistance to reduce the right to left shunt; generally the results have been disappointing.

COMPLEX CARDIAC MALFORMATIONS. When pulmonic stenosis is an important part of the anomaly, surgical aortopulmonary shunting is undertaken during infancy or childhood to alleviate hypoxemia. In others with torrential pulmonary blood flow and pulmonary hypertension, pulmonary arterial banding is undertaken in infancy to prevent progressive pulmonary vascular disease. Many have now reached adolescence or adult life with normal or low pulmonary vascular resistance. These patients are candidates for operation using the Fontan principle (direct anastomosis of the right atrium to the pulmonary artery).

THE ADULT WITH SURGICALLY "CURED" CONGENITAL HEART DISEASE

Surgical treatment for extracardiac anomalies has been undertaken for four decades, and 30 years have elapsed since the introduction of surgical procedures for intracardiac congenital malformations. Immediate results after operation continue to be excellent, even dramatic, but it is now recognized that complications may develop many years after surgery.

INTRA-ATRIAL SURGERY. Many anomalies may be treated by an approach through the right atrium. These include atrial septal defects of all types, endocardial cushion defects, transposition of the great arteries, and total anomalous pulmonary venous connection. Frequently isolated ventricular septal defects are closed surgically transatrially and the defect (especially the more common perimembranous defect) is approached through the tricuspid valve and the shunt obliterated. Persistent *conduction disturbances* may occur immediately after operation or appear for the first time many years later. These consist of supraventricular arrhythmias (atrial flutter or fibrillation, paroxysmal supraventricular tachycardia, and junctional rhythm), sick sinus syndrome, or varying degrees of atrioventricular block. These rhythm disturbances occur even when there is complete anatomic correction of the abnormality. The treatment of these abnormalities in conduction is similar to the treatment of these arrhythmias of any cause. The *function of the right ventricle* and competence of the tricuspid valve have also been of concern especially in transposition of the great arteries.

INTRAVENTRICULAR SURGERY. Right ventriculotomy is the approach used in most patients who require intraventricular surgery. The more common lesions treated this way include some forms of ventricular septal defect, tetralogy of Fallot with or without pulmonary atresia, and various forms of transposition of the great arteries. Some of these complications may be reduced in future years, since earlier operation is being advised, especially in some patients with tetralogy of Fallot.

Conduction Disturbances. Permanent complete heart block from intraoperative trauma to the conduction system has decreased to a point where it is no longer a major problem soon after operation. *Bifascicular block* (left anterior hemiblock with complete right bundle branch block) may occur from intraoperative trauma to the bundle of His and its branches. These patients usually remain well for many years after operation, but the conduction abnormality may progress to complete AV block. Bifascicular block does not require treatment. *Sudden unexpected cardiac arrest* may occur many years after operation. While this catastrophe may occasionally occur from complete AV block, more frequent mechanisms are ventricular tachyarrhythmias and deterioration into ventricular fibrillation. The risk of ventricular tachycardia is higher in patients who have multiple unifocal or multifocal premature ventricular contractions at rest. Bursts of ventricular tachyarrhythmia may be recorded during 24-hour electrocardiographic recording or unmasked during or immediately after graded exercise testing. While these arrhythmias may occur in patients who have had adequate relief of right ventricular outflow tract obstruction and in whom the ventricular defect is closed, there appears to be greater risk when residual defects are present, such as severe pulmonic stenosis, persistent large shunts across the ventricular septum, and right ventricular aneurysms. Significant residual defects should be treated by reoperation, and the ventricular arrhythmia may be abolished by excision of arrhythmogenic right ventricular aneurysms. Medical treatment of the ventricular tachycardia is indicated and although there is a choice of many drugs, phenytoin (Dilantin) has been used with particular success.

Reconstruction of the Right Ventricular Outflow Tract. Treatment of extreme forms of tetralogy of Fallot, especially pulmonary atresia, and many forms of transposition of the great arteries with pulmonic stenosis or previous arterial banding, requires a prosthesis to establish continuity between the right ventricle and the pulmonary artery. During the last decade the most frequently used prosthesis consisted of a Dacron tube with an aortic valve bearing a porcine heterograft. The durability of this prosthesis is unpredictable, since recurrence of obstruction may occur anywhere along its length from narrowing of the anastomotic sites or from development of an exuberant neointima that encroaches on the lumen of the Dacron tube. Because of these complications, a human valve bearing aortic or pulmonary homografts is being used with greater frequency.

Congenital Aortic Stenosis. See above.

Valvular Pulmonic Stenosis. See above.

Coarctation of the Aorta. It is now common practice to advise surgical treatment of coarctation of the aorta in preschool years. One of the reasons for earlier operation is the notion that late-onset complications will be reduced. These complications in adult life have been related to recurrence of hypertension, progressive atherosclerosis, myocardial infarction, and cerebral vascular accidents. It is therefore advisable that patients who have had previous coarctation therapy be followed carefully so that treatment can be instituted, especially for hypertension, prior to the onset of some of these complications.

Adams FH, Emmanouilides GC: Moss' Heart Disease in Infants, Children and Adolescents. 3rd ed. Baltimore, Williams and Wilkins, 1983. *The standard comprehensive text on all aspects of congenital heart disease.*

Fontan F, Deville C, Quaegebeur J, et al.: Repair of tricuspid atresia in 100 patients. J Thorac Cardiovasc Surg 85:647, 1983. *Evolution of the principles for treatment of tricuspid atresia. These principles are also applicable to many complex cardiac malformations.*

Garson A, Nihill MR, McNamara DG, et al.: Status of the adult and adolescent after repair of tetralogy of Fallot. Circulation 59:1232, 1979. *Long-term results are evaluated with emphasis on complications in the adult.*

Giuliani ER, Fuster V, Brandenberg RO, et al.: Ebstein's anomaly. Mayo Clin Proc 54:163, 1979. *Clinical features and natural history are reviewed in a lucid manner.*

Goldberg SJ, Allen HD, Sahn DJ: Pediatric and Adolescent Echocardiography. 2nd ed. Chicago, Year Book Medical Publishers, 1980. *A comprehensive handbook describing the M-mode, two-dimensional, and Doppler features of congenital cardiac malformations.*

Kirklin JW, Barratt-Boyes BG: Cardiac Surgery. New York, John Wiley and Sons, 1986. *Comprehensive analyses of combined clinical experiences from two respected pioneers in all aspects of cardiac surgery, especially congenital heart disease.*

Krongrad E: Prognosis for patients with congenital heart disease and postoperative intraventricular conduction defects. Circulation 57:867, 1978. *A useful guide to mechanisms, prognosis and treatment.*

Liberthson RR, Boucher CA, Strauss HW, et al.: Right ventricular function in adult atrial septal defect. Am J Cardiol 57:56, 1981. *This preoperative and postoperative assessment has important clinical applications relative to the defects of preoperative right ventricular dysfunction and pulmonary hypertension on the expected result from operation.*

Meyer RA: Echocardiography. In Adams FH, Emmanouilides GC (eds.): Moss' Heart Disease in Infants, Children and Adolescents. 3rd ed. Baltimore, Williams and Wilkins, 1983, pp 58–82. *Up-to-date, concise, and well illustrated. Discusses anatomic features as well as cardiac performance.*

Perloff JK: The Clinical Recognition of Congenital Heart Disease. 3rd ed. Philadelphia, W.B. Saunders Company, 1986. *A book that focuses on the anatomic and physiologic derangements in congenital heart disease, setting the stage for an understanding of the history, physical signs, electrocardiogram, chest roentgenogram, and echocardiogram. All age groups are dealt with.*

Rabinovitch M: Pulmonary hypertension. In Adams FH, Emmanouilides GC (eds.): Moss' Heart Disease in Infants, Children and Adolescents. 3rd ed. Baltimore, Williams and Wilkins, 1983, pp 669–692. *Up-to-date information on quantitative structural analysis of the pulmonary vasculature bed in congenital heart disease.*

Roberts WC: Adult Congenital Heart Disease. Philadelphia, F.A. Davis Company, 1987. *The specific focus is on adults with congenital heart disease. Natural history and surgical treatment are considered.*

50 ATHEROSCLEROSIS

Russell Ross

Atherosclerosis is responsible for the majority of cases of myocardial and cerebral infarction and thus represents the principal cause of death in the United States and western Europe. Atherosclerosis is the descriptive term for thickened and hardened lesions of the medium and large muscular and elastic arteries. It is a lipid-rich lesion, in contrast with arteriosclerosis, which is the generic term used for thickened and stiffened arteries of all sizes. Other forms of arteriosclerosis include focal calcific arteriosclerosis (Mönckeberg's arteriosclerosis) and arteriolosclerosis, a disease of small vessels.

The lesions of atherosclerosis occur within the innermost layer of the artery, the intima, and are largely confined to this region of the vessel. The lesions are generally eccentric and, if they become sufficiently large, can occlude the artery and thus the vascular supply to a tissue or organ, resulting in ischemia or necrosis. If this occurs, it often leads to the characteristic clinical sequelae of myocardial infarction, cerebral infarction, gangrene of the extremities, or sudden cardiac death.

THE NORMAL ARTERY

The normal artery consists essentially of a tube lined on its luminal aspect by a continuous layer of endothelium and on its outer aspect by loose connective tissue containing fibroblasts and smooth muscle cells, which package an intermediate layer of pure smooth muscle cells that are bound together in such a manner that, by working with the elastic laminae and the collagen and proteoglycans that surround the cells, the smooth muscle cells contract and maintain the tonus of the artery wall as the blood flows through with each systole and diastole.

The lining cells of the artery, the endothelium, represent the interface with the cells of the blood. It is at this interface that different blood cell types can interact with the endothelium and, under appropriate circumstances, lead to the development of lesions of atherosclerosis. These cells are the platelet, the monocyte, and the lymphocyte. Their potential roles in atherogenesis will be discussed below.

THE LESIONS OF ATHEROSCLEROSIS

The two principal forms of atherosclerosis are the early lesion, or fatty streak, and the advanced lesion, or fibrous plaque, which can become an advanced complicated lesion.

The Fatty Streak

The fatty streak is the most common and ubiquitous lesion of atherosclerosis. It occurs at all ages and in Western society is present at birth in some infants and is common in young children. The lesions of atherosclerosis are confined principally to the intima. Initially, the fatty streak appears to contain a single cell type, a foam cell that consists of macrophages filled with lipids, principally in the form of cholesteryl esters. These macrophages are derived from blood-borne monocytes that are chemotactically attracted into the artery wall, where they develop into the foam cells. As the fatty streak enlarges, it does so by continuing attachment and migration of monocytes into the intima with their consequent development into macrophages. Subsequently, smooth muscle cells appear to migrate into the intima from the media and also begin to accumulate lipid and take on the appearance of foam cells. As the fatty streak becomes larger and more advanced, it contains varying numbers of smooth muscle cells mixed together with the predominant lipid-filled macrophages. Fatty streaks can be found in young individuals at the same anatomic sites that are later occupied by advanced lesions, as well as at sites where they may either regress and disappear or remain as fatty streaks throughout life.

The Fibrous Plaque

The fibrous plaque is also located in the intima and characteristically leads to the eccentric thickening of the artery that often results in occlusion of the lumen. The fibrous plaque is typically covered at its luminal aspect by a thickened cap of dense connective tissue containing a special form of flattened, pancake-shaped smooth muscle cell that has formed the dense collagenous matrix in which it is embedded. Beneath this cap, the lesion is highly cellular and contains large numbers of smooth muscle cells, some of which may be full of lipid droplets. It also contains numerous macrophages, many of which take the form of foam cells, together with variable numbers of T and B lymphocytes. These collections of cells usually overlie a deeper area of necrotic foam cells and debris. This necrotic area sometimes becomes calcified and often may contain cholesterol crystals. (Figure 50–1 details the cellular composition of a fibrous plaque.)

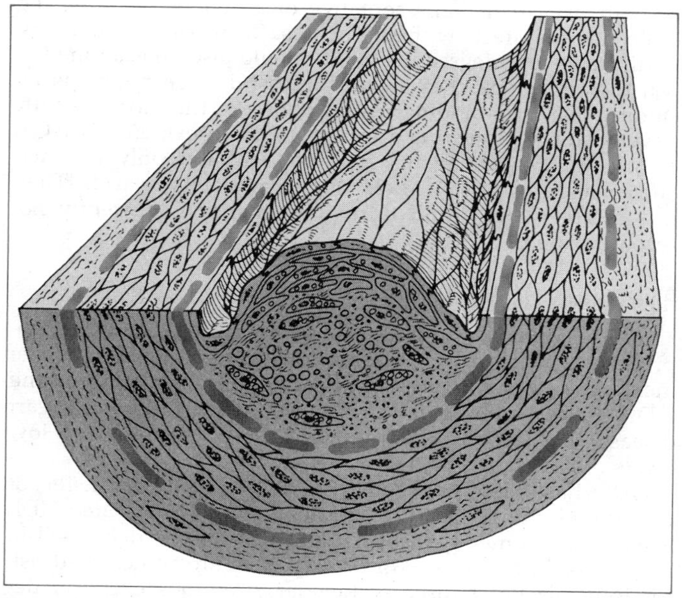

FIGURE 50–1. The *fibrous plaque,* which characteristically consists of numerous proliferated smooth muscle cells together with macrophages and variable numbers of lymphocytes. In this diagram, the fibrous plaque is covered by an intact endothelial monolayer and contains a fibrous cap of smooth muscle cells. These smooth muscle cells lie in a dense connective tissue matrix that covers a deeper collection of smooth muscle cells and macrophages, both of which may contain numerous lipid droplets and take the form of foam cells mixed together with variable numbers of lymphocytes. These collections of cells lie in a mixture of connective tissue matrix and free extracellular deposits of lipid. The fibrous plaque usually intrudes into the lumen owing to its proliferative nature. This diagram represents only in general terms the relative appearance of such a lesion.

The Complicated Lesion

The complicated lesion is a fibrous plaque that has undergone extensive degeneration and often calcification. It may contain ulcerations, cracks, and fissures, which serve as sites for platelet adherence, aggregation and thrombosis, and subsequent organization. When this occurs, thrombosis may result in sudden occlusion of the artery.

Morbid Anatomy of the Lesions

Fatty streaks are flat lesions that often appear as yellow discolorations on the surface of the artery but seldom intrude into the lumen and thus cause no clinical sequelae. The fibrous plaques and complicated lesions are raised lesions that are often pearly gray in appearance but may be discolored when associated with erythrocytes and thrombi.

Localization of the Lesions

The arteries most commonly involved with atherosclerosis are the aorta; the femoral, popliteal, and tibial arteries; the coronary arteries; the internal and external carotid arteries; and the cerebral arteries.

In the aorta, the abdominal portion is commonly involved with lesions of atherosclerosis at an earlier age, and, as in the thoracic aorta, lesions most commonly form around orifices of branches and bifurcations of the artery. There is a greater incidence of atherosclerotic lesions in the leg arteries, whereas they are relatively rare in the vessels of the upper limbs. Atherosclerosis of the smaller arteries, particularly those of the legs and the coronary arteries, is more common in cigarette smokers or in individuals who have glucose intolerance.

Coronary atherosclerosis is most prominent in the main stems of the coronary arteries, particularly in the segments closest to the ostia of the coronary vessel. The degree of luminal narrowing in the coronary arteries can be variable; however, atherosclerosis is generally present in the epicardial segment of the vessels, whereas the intramural coronary arteries are generally spared. Typically, after coronary bypass surgery, the perianastomotic site of the bypass is often (30 per cent of the time) involved in the development of a new lesion of atherosclerosis.

The carotid and cerebral arteries generally have a patchy distribution of the lesions of atherosclerosis, which often first appear at the base of the brain in the carotid, basilar, and vertebral arteries.

The pulmonary arteries are generally spared of lesions of atherosclerosis, except in association with pulmonary hypertension.

RISK FACTORS

The risk factor concept evolved from epidemiologic studies of the incidence of coronary artery disease conducted in the United States and in Europe. Prospective studies demonstrated a consistent association of characteristics observed in apparently healthy individuals with the subsequent incidence of coronary artery disease in the same individuals. These studies demonstrated an association between an increase in the concentration of plasma lipoproteins, principally low density lipoprotein (LDL) and thus plasma cholesterol (see Ch. 183), and the rate of occurrence of new events of coronary artery disease. Also observed was an increased incidence of the disease in relation to cigarette smoking, hypertension, clinical diabetes, age, male sex, obesity, stress and particular personality characteristics (denoted as type A), and genetic factors. Because of these associations, each of these characteristics was termed a risk factor for atherosclerosis (see Ch. 40). At least three independent predictors of risk for individuals within a population are valuable in anticipating increased incidence of atherosclerosis. These are hyperlipidemia, cigarette smoking, and hypertension.

Hyperlipidemia

There is a clear association between chronic hypercholesterolemia and increase in incidence of ischemic heart disease. The Framingham Study demonstrated this association, particularly in men between the ages of 20 and 40. When the plasma cholesterol levels are greater than 220 mg per deciliter, there is a marked increase in the relative incidence of myocardial infarction, which is most easily demonstrated in individuals with familial hypercholesterolemia. The range of normality is not entirely clear in defining cholesterol and triglyceride levels for a given population as they relate to increased risk of ischemic heart disease. However, in the United States, 220 mg per deciliter is considered to be the upper limit of normal for the plasma cholesterol level (although this is probably too high), which increases from birth through young adulthood until the age of approximately 50 in men and to somewhat older ages in women. Similarly, there is an age-related increase in plasma triglyceride levels. Triglyceride is associated with increases in very low density lipoproteins (VLDL), whereas elevation in plasma cholesterol level is generally associated with increase in LDL.

Abnormal accumulation of lipoproteins in the plasma can occur from overproduction, from deficient removal, or from a combination of these abnormalities. There are numerous forms of genetically derived hyperlipoproteinemias that are either monogenic or polygenic. Perhaps more common are forms of hyperlipoproteinemia that are secondary to other disease, such as diabetes, renal disease, alcoholism, hypothyroidism, and the dysglobulinemias, or to treatment with corticosteroids or estrogens (see Ch. 183).

HOMOZYGOUS FAMILIAL HYPERCHOLESTEROLEMIA. Patients with homozygous familial hypercholesterolemia (FH disease) represent one of the best demonstrations of the capacity of hypercholesterolemia to induce the cellular changes that lead to atherogenesis. Although FH disease is much rarer than the secondary hyperlipoproteinemias or other forms of genetic hyperlipidemia, we know a great deal about its course in humans and in an animal model, the Watanabe heritable hyperlipidemic rabbit, as well as diet-induced hypercholesterolemia in the nonhuman primate. In the case of genetic hyperlipidemia, the plasma cholesterol and LDL levels are inordinately high owing to faulty or missing LDL receptors. When LDL is bound to its normal receptor, it suppresses the activity of the rate-limiting enzyme for cholesterol synthesis, HMG-CoA-reductase. In individuals with FH disease, the liver and peripheral cells continue to synthesize large amounts of cholesterol because absent or faulty receptors fail to generate a feedback inhibitory signal and cholesterol synthesis goes on unabated. Under these conditions, plasma cholesterol levels reach 500 to 1000 mg per deciliter or higher, and rampant atherosclerosis develops, with advanced occlusive lesions. This can occur at very young ages, and myocardial infarcts have been described in young children with this disease.

TREATMENT OF HYPERCHOLESTEROLEMIA. The Lipid Research Clinic Trials have demonstrated that it is beneficial to lower plasma levels in patients with chronic elevations of LDL. These studies showed that the decrease in plasma cholesterol levels can be correlated with a reduction in the incidence of myocardial infarction and thus atherosclerosis. Premature ischemic heart disease is usually associated with hypercholesterolemia, particularly when levels of plasma cholesterol are greater than 260 mg per deciliter. When this occurs, the incidence of atherosclerotic disease can be as high as fivefold greater than for individuals with plasma cholesterol levels below 220 mg per deciliter.

Hypertriglyceridemia is usually associated with increases in VLDL in the plasma, which may be complicated by increases in cholesterol as well. Patients with increased VLDL levels who come from families with familial combined hyperlipidemia are at increased risk for atherosclerosis, whereas those with elevated VLDL levels from families with monogenic familial hypertriglyceridemia are not at increased risk. Increased VLDL levels can increase the risk of atherosclerosis if it accompanies other risk factors, such as diabetes mellitus or cigarette smoking.

It is important to examine all patients over the age of 20 for hyperlipidemia, particularly if they have a family history of premature ischemic heart disease. This is best done by measuring the concentrations of cholesterol and triglyceride in plasma after an overnight fast. Cholesterol levels above 250 mg per deciliter or triglyceride levels above 200 mg per deciliter, or both, are indicative of hyperlipidemia, requiring attention and therapy, the first step of which should be dietary intervention. Such patients should be brought to normal weight if this is excessive and maintained on a diet low in saturated fat and cholesterol. Those with hypertriglyceridemia should limit or eliminate intake of alcohol. In general, reduction of intake of calories, cholesterol, and saturated fat is the best approach to begin with in most patients. Severe hyperlipidemia with cholesterol levels in excess of 350 mg per deciliter or triglyceride levels in excess of 400 mg per deciliter, or both, is usually representative of a genetic disorder and often first manifests with xanthomas. Such patients' families, particularly first-degree relatives, should also be examined.

If dietary approaches are unsuccessful, then regimens including bile acid–binding resins or one of the more recently developed lipid-lowering drugs should be considered (see Ch. 183). Use of such agents is dependent not only on their efficaciousness, but on their long-term effects as well. Their use before puberty and during pregnancy is currently not recommended.

High Density Lipoprotein (HDL)

In epidemiologic studies, elevations of high density lipoprotein particles in the plasma are inversely related to the incidence of atherosclerosis and its sequelae. Elevation of the HDL cholesterol level is "protective" against ischemic heart disease; conversely, the individuals with abnormally low levels of HDL are at increased risk.

HDL has been postulated to participate in transfer of cholesterol out of cells. Women generally have elevated HDL levels prior to menopause. If their HDL level is decreased in association with diabetes or obesity, they are at increased risk for ischemic heart disease. Regular strenuous exercise, decreased cigarette smoking, and diet rich in some fish oils (eicosapentaenoic acid) are associated with increased HDL levels, although the basis for the increase is poorly understood.

Cigarette Smoking

Cigarette smoking is one of the most common risk factors associated with increased incidence of atherosclerosis, and when it is reduced or eliminated, the risk of developing the disease decreases. Stroke, myocardial infarction, and intermittent claudication are common in male cigarette smokers, who, together with female smokers, show an increased incidence of symptoms associated with atherosclerosis. In addition to atherosclerosis of the large coronary arteries, cigarette smokers characteristically have occlusive disease of the leg arteries. There is a mean increase of approximately 70 per cent in the death rate and a three- to fivefold increase in the risk of ischemic heart disease in males who smoke more than one pack of cigarettes per day, compared with nonsmokers.

Sudden death is frequently associated with cigarette smoking, and of particular importance is the observation that cessation of cigarette smoking leads within a year to reduction of the risk of the sequelae of atherosclerosis to levels of that of nonsmokers. The basis for atherosclerosis in cigarette smokers is not well understood.

Glucose Intolerance and Diabetes Mellitus

Both insulin-dependent and non–insulin-dependent diabetics show at least a twofold increase in the incidence of myocardial infarction, compared with nondiabetics. Younger diabetics have a marked increase in the risk of atherosclerosis and thus of ischemic heart disease, and diabetic women appear to be even more prone than diabetic men. Gangrene of the lower extremities is one of the principal sequelae of atherosclerosis in diabetics. It is not clear what factors are responsible for the increased incidence of atherosclerosis in diabetes.

Hypertension

Elevation in blood pressure is an important risk factor associated with increased incidence of atherosclerosis and is of particular importance since this is a factor that is easily diagnosed and highly treatable. The risk of atherosclerosis and its sequelae increases progressively with increase in blood pressure, and when the blood pressure exceeds 160 mm Hg systolic and 95 mm Hg diastolic in middle-aged men the risk is five times greater than in normotensive men with blood pressure of 140 mm Hg systolic and 90 mm Hg diastolic or less. The increase in diastolic pressure may be more important than that in systolic pressure in both hypertensive men and women. After the age of 50, hypertension may be more important as a risk factor in predicting increased incidence of atherosclerosis than hypercholesterolemia. Recent intervention studies of individuals with hypertension have demonstrated that a reduction of diastolic pressure levels below 105 mm Hg can significantly reduce the incidence of symptomatic cerebrovascular disease, ischemic heart disease, and congestive heart failure in men (see Ch. 47). When multiple risk factors are present, including hypertension, it is particularly important to treat the hypertension, since it is the most easily accessible and treatable aspect of this disease process.

Obesity

When body weight is greater than 20 per cent above the norm, there is an increased risk of ischemic heart disease. Obesity may particularly accelerate atherosclerosis in individuals below the age of 50. Obesity is generally associated with hypertriglyceridemia, hypercholesterolemia, glucose intolerance, and hypertension.

Physical Activity

There are many and conflicting studies related to the value of increased physical activity in reducing the incidence of ischemic heart disease. The Framingham Studies suggest that sedentary individuals are more susceptible to atherosclerosis and to sudden death than individuals who maintain an active lifestyle. It has been suggested that increased physical activity may elevate the level of high density lipoprotein. Appropriately supervised physical training can improve exercise performance in patients with angina due to ischemic heart disease.

Genetic Factors

Clearly, genetic factors are critical in atherosclerosis. The best example of this is the increased incidence of atherosclerosis in individuals with homozygous familial hypercholesterolemia and familial combined hyperlipidemia. Other risk factors, such as hypertension and diabetes mellitus, can also be inherited, and it is possible that protective factors, such as increased high density lipoprotein, may also be inherited, although the latter is not well understood. As a consequence, family history must be included in assessing the risk for a given individual.

THE PATHOGENESIS OF THE LESIONS OF ATHEROSCLEROSIS

The lesions of atherosclerosis as they occur in the intima of the artery essentially consist of three biologic entities. First and foremost of these is an increase in the number of intimal smooth muscle cells, together with an accumulation of macrophages and variable numbers of lymphocytes. The increased number of smooth muscle cells is responsible for the second entity, the formation of large amounts of connective tissue matrix containing collagen, elastic fibers, and proteoglycans. The third entity, lipid, accumulates within the smooth muscle cells and the macrophages and in many instances causes them to develop into foam cells. Lipid also accumulates within the surrounding connective tissue matrix. Thus the advanced lesions of atherosclerosis represent the culmination of a usually longstanding proliferative disease process in which it becomes important to understand the basis for the proliferation of smooth muscle, accumulation of macrophages, formation of new connective tissue, and accumulation of lipid.

The Response to Injury Hypothesis of Atherosclerosis

During the past decade, it has been possible to develop a hypothesis that takes into account most of what is known concerning risk factors, the biology of the artery wall, the cells involved, and the biologic processes that may result in the lesions of atherosclerosis.

The response to injury hypothesis of atherosclerosis suggests that some form of "injury" affects the lining endothelial cells. The injury may alter the functional characteristics of the endothelium, leaving the endothelium morphologically intact. Thus endothelial injury could alter the permeability of the endothelium, its nonthrombogenic character, its ability to form vasoactive substances and growth factors, and its capacity to regenerate. At the other extreme, endothelial injury may lead to endothelial cell-cell disjunction and endothelial retraction, exposing the underlying connective tissue or accumulated foam cells, such as macrophages, that form the first and ubiquitous lesion of atherosclerosis, the fatty streak.

In hypercholesterolemic animals, including nonhuman primates, swine, rabbits, and rats, the first change that occurs in the artery wall is a chemotactic attraction of circulating monocytes, which increasingly adhere to the surface of the endothelial cells in clusters located throughout the arterial tree. These adherent monocytes migrate on the surface of the endothelium, penetrate between endothelial junctions, localize subendothelially, accumulate lipid, and become intimal foam cells. The accumulation of these intimal monocytes that become converted to lipid-laden macrophages represents the initial lesion of atherosclerosis, the fatty streak. These fatty streaks expand by continued attraction and accumulation of monocytes in the artery. They also expand by migration of some smooth muscle cells from the underlying media into the intima, where they localize beneath the accumulated macrophages and also accumulate lipid.

With increasing time, level, and duration of hypercholesterolemia, a second series of changes occurs in the endothelial cells in which endothelial cell-cell junctions separate and endothelial cells retract, particularly at anatomic sites such as branches and bifurcations of the artery, where the flow characteristics of the blood may make the endothelium more susceptible to injury. If the endothelial cells retract and expose the underlying foam cells in the fatty streaks at the sites, then the exposed macrophages or connective tissue, or both, can be thrombogenic and induce platelets to adhere. Within one to two months, sites where mural thrombi have formed become loci of increased migration and proliferation of smooth muscle cells that accumulate and form large amounts of connective tissue matrix. Thus sites of platelet adherence and aggregation subsequently become sites of intimal smooth muscle proliferation.

At other anatomic sites, the endothelium may remain intact, but the fatty streak will expand by the continued attraction and accumulation of monocytes. Over a longer period of time, those areas that maintain an intact endothelial cover also appear capable of developing into a fibrous plaque.

Numerous investigations have attempted to determine what factors are responsible for the migration and proliferation of smooth muscle cells into the intima. Growth factors able to induce smooth muscle cell migration and proliferation can be formed and secreted by several cells. Of particular importance is the capacity of platelets to release growth factors and of activated macrophages to release the same as well as other types of growth factors. The growth factors that may play a critical role in atherogenesis include platelet-derived growth factor (PDGF), a potent growth factor for mesenchymal connective tissue cells such as fibroblasts and smooth muscle; fibroblast growth factor (FGF), an angiogenic agent; epidermal growth factor (EGF), an agent capable of stimulating the growth of epithelial cells; and transforming growth factor beta (TGF-beta), a factor that may act in an inhibitory fashion or, in other circumstances, synergistically with PDGF.

PDGF is a potent mitogen that, at nanogram and picogram levels, can induce cells such as those of smooth muscle to multiply and to form new connective tissue. Platelet-derived growth factor can be derived from platelets, from activated macrophages, and from appropriately stimulated or "injured" endothelial cells. Thus, if endothelial injury occurs, appropriate opportunities may be present for the release of mitogens

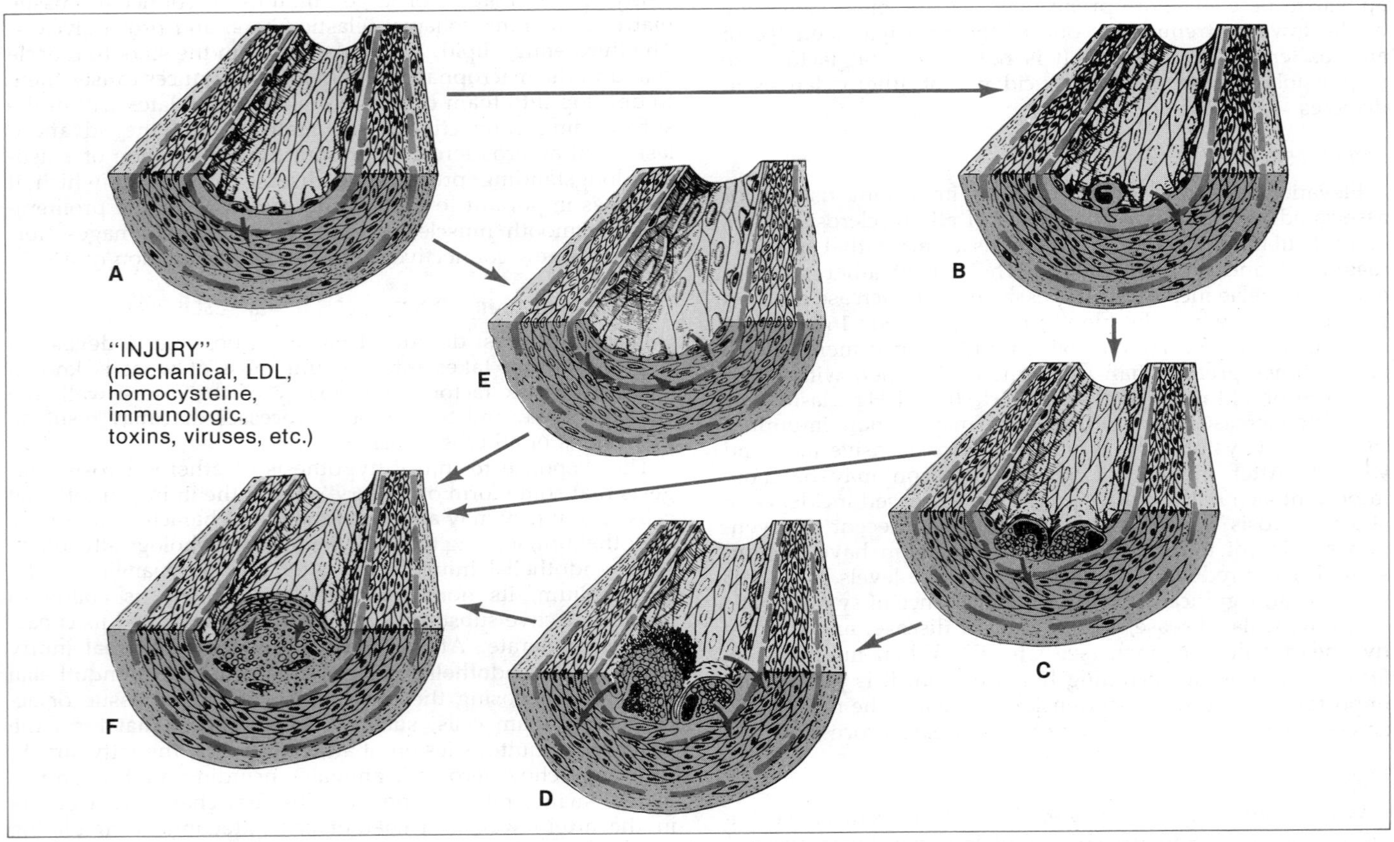

FIGURE 50–2. Endothelial injury: The response to injury hypothesis. Advanced intimal proliferative lesions of atherosclerosis may occur by at least two pathways. The pathway demonstrated by the clockwise (long) arrows to the right has been observed in experimentally induced hypercholesterolemia. Injury to the endothelium (*A*) may induce growth factor secretion (*short arrow*). Monocytes attach to endothelium (*B*), which may continue to secrete growth factors (*short arrow*). Subendothelial migration of monocytes (C) may lead to fatty streak formation and release of growth factors such as platelet-derived growth factor (PDGF) (*short arrow*). Fatty streaks may become directly converted to fibrous plaques (*long arrow* from *C* to *F*) through release of growth factors from macrophages or endothelial cells or both. Macrophages may also stimulate and or injure the overlying endothelium. In some cases, macrophages may lose their endothelial cover and platelet attachment may occur (*D*), providing three possible sources of growth factors—platelets, macrophages, and endothelium (*short arrows*). Some of the smooth muscle cells in the proliferative lesion itself (*F*) may form and secrete growth factors such as PDGF (*short arrows*).

An alternative pathway for development of advanced lesions of atherosclerosis is shown by the arrows from *A* to *E* to *F*. In this case, the endothelium may be injured but remained intact. Increased endothelial turnover may result in growth factor formation by endothelial cells (*A*). This may stimulate migration of smooth muscle cells from the media into the intima, accompanied by endogenous production of PDGF by smooth muscle as well as growth factor secretion from the "injured" endothelial cells (*E*). These interactions could then lead to fibrous plaque formation and further lesion progression (*F*). (Reproduced by permission from Ross R: The pathogenesis of atherosclerosis—an update. N Engl J Med 314:496, 1986.)

such as PDGF from all three cells. Such growth factor release may be related to increased incidence of atherogenesis in experimental animals. There is also some suggestion that smooth muscle cells, once they have been induced to proliferate in the artery wall, may in themselves be capable of expressing the gene for PDGF and of secreting this growth factor so that they may, in effect, stimulate themselves in an autocrine fashion to continue the proliferative response.

The response to injury hypothesis of atherogenesis suggests that the "injury" to the endothelium results in cellular changes that lead to a modified form of inflammation in which monocytes and lymphocytes enter the artery wall and the monocytes become macrophages that can secrete growth factors, act as scavenger cells, and accumulate lipid and become foam cells. The fatty streak then becomes converted into a smooth muscle proliferative lesion, or fibrous plaque, and probably does so by local release within the artery of growth factors derived from activated macrophages, injured endothelium, and/or platelets that may interact with the artery wall at sites where the protective cover of the endothelium may be altered. These changes are diagrammatically shown in Figure 50–2, which suggests how the lesions of atherosclerosis may form.

The response to injury hypothesis also offers an opportunity to consider means of preventing and intervening in the formation of the lesions of atherosclerosis. Clearly, alteration in lifestyle habits, including changes in dietary habits and alteration of risk factors associated with increased incidence of atherosclerosis, could be potentially important in preventing these cellular changes from occurring and possibly in inducing lesion regression.

Regression of Atherosclerosis

In experimental animals the fatty streak is clearly capable of regressing and disappearing entirely if hypercholesterolemic animals are placed on a normocholesterolemic regimen for a sufficient period of time. There is some evidence to suggest that fatty streaks can also regress in humans, based upon examination of individuals who decreased their dietary intake of lipids and atherogenic foods. Fibrous plaques, or complicated lesions in humans may also be partially reversible, based upon angiographic studies. It is not yet clear how far a lesion must progress before it becomes irreversible. Cessation of cigarette smoking is associated with decreased risk, and this in combination with treatment of hypertension, dietary intervention, treatment of diabetes mellitus, and removal, where possible, of other associated causes may be important in inducing regression of the lesions of atherosclerosis. More remains to be learned concerning this approach to reversing the disease process.

Prevention of atherosclerosis, rather than treatment, has to be the principal goal for all patients. In consideration of the association between hyperlipidemia and increased atherosclerosis, and with recognition of the decline in the death rate in the United States from premature ischemic heart disease, it becomes increasingly important to understand that early detection of risk and approaches toward change in dietary habits and in lifestyles are important in the prevention of atherosclerosis in individuals who may potentially be at increased risk. It is important to detect those who may be at increased risk on a familial basis, who may be hypertensive, who are cigarette smokers, or whose dietary habits could be altered with a resultant reduction in risk. Treatment of hypertension, as well as advice regarding diet, cigarette smoking, and exercise, can be valuable adjuncts to helping a patient deal with these problems. Pharmacologic treatment of hyperlipidemia should be limited to individuals at risk who do not respond adequately to dietary management. The long-term value of antiplatelet drugs and, potentially in the future, of drugs that may affect growth factor activity could be of importance in reducing the incidence of atherosclerosis and the long-term sequelae of this disease process.

Brown MS, Goldstein JL: How LDL receptors influence cholesterol and atherosclerosis. Sci Am 251:158, 1984. *A discussion of how LDL receptor interactions control cholesterol metabolism.*

Gordon T, Castelli WP, Hjortland MC, et al.: Diabetes, blood lipids, and the role of obesity in coronary heart disease risk for women. The Framingham Study. Ann Intern Med 87:393, 1977.

Gordon T, Castelli WP, Hjortland MC, et al.: High density lipoprotein as a protective factor against coronary heart disease. The Framingham Study. Am J Med 62:707, 1977. *These two papers represent epidemiologic studies that relate the role of several of the principal risk factors to atherosclerosis and indicate the potential protective effect of HDL in atherosclerosis.*

Report of the Working Group of Arteriosclerosis of the National Heart, Lung, and Blood Institute. Vol. 2. Department of Health, Education and Welfare (National Institutes of Health) Publication No. 82–2035. Washington, D.C., Government Printing Office, 1981. *This represents an overview of a large number of individuals who have examined both the epidemiology and the nature of the lesions of atherosclerosis.*

Ross R: The pathogenesis of atherosclerosis—an update. N Engl J Med 314:488, 1986.

Ross R, Glomset JA: The pathogenesis of atherosclerosis. N Engl J Med 295:369, 1976. *These two papers review the anatomic structure of the artery wall, lesions of atherosclerosis, and the potential roles of the cells in atherosclerosis. They provide a hypothesis for how atherogenesis may come about.*

Steinberg D: Lipoproteins and atherosclerosis: A look back and a look ahead. Arteriosclerosis 3:283, 1983. *A discussion of the role of lipoproteins and atherosclerosis that highlights many of the important questions.*

51 DISORDERS OF CORONARY ARTERIES

51.1 Angina Pectoris

James T. Willerson

Angina pectoris is the clinical term used to describe chest pain resulting from a relative oxygen deficiency in heart muscle. Angina occurs when oxygen demand exceeds oxygen supply. Most individuals with angina pectoris have underlying atherosclerotic coronary artery disease, but angina may also develop in some patients with ventricular hypertrophy, left ventricular outflow obstruction, severe aortic valvular regurgitation or stenosis, cardiomyopathy, or dilated ventricles in whom coronary artery stenoses are not present. The explanation for the development of angina in these circumstances is that under certain conditions even normal coronary arteries may not adequately supply hypertrophied, dilated, or failing heart muscle with oxygen. In some circumstances, a limited coronary vasodilator reserve may also explain angina pectoris, especially in some patients with left ventricular outflow obstruction (valvular aortic stenosis and idiopathic hypertrophic subaortic stenosis) or ventricular hypertrophy or both. Normal individuals do not develop angina, probably because the heart is protected from an important imbalance in oxygen delivery by other factors that limit physical activity, such as dyspnea and fatigue.

The predisposing pathologic alteration in coronary arteries ordinarily responsible for angina is atherosclerosis. Severe narrowing of the lumen of coronary arteries results in a decreased ability to deliver oxygen to areas supplied by the involved vessels. Consequently, under conditions of exercise, cold exposure, or emotional stress, or after eating, angina may develop. This is most easily understood by recalling that the primary determinants of oxygen demand in the heart are heart rate, contractile state, and wall tension. Emphasis upon relative oxygen demand makes it easier to understand why some individuals with valvular heart disease and associated ventricular hypertrophy develop angina even in the absence of coronary artery disease. Systolic pressure development is relatively costly in terms of oxygen utilization, and, together with ventricular hypertrophy and increased wall tension, is an important factor in the development of angina in patients with valvular aortic stenosis and without coronary artery stenoses. However, a limited coronary vasodilator reserve is also a factor. Development of angina in individuals with marked pulmonary hypertension may be the result of increased right ventricular pressure and hypertrophy.

Angina pectoris may also develop in individuals with severe volume overload of the ventricle, including those with aortic or mitral regurgitation. "Volume work" results in a smaller increase in oxygen demand than "pressure work" until important cardiac dilatation occurs. At this point, increased oxygen demand may not be met because of reduced diastolic coronary perfusion pressure. The presence of angina pectoris in patients with aortic regurgitation is often an ominous prognostic sign.

Angina may also occur because of extracardiac influences. In particular, severe anemia or carbon monoxide exposure limits the capacity of the blood to carry or release oxygen and may result in angina under conditions that the subject would otherwise tolerate well. Increases in systemic arterial pressure and consequent dilatation of the heart may result in angina pectoris. Increases in heart rate or contractile state, such as occur with hyperthyroidism, pheochromocytoma, or exogenous administration or endogenous release of catecholamines, may also result in angina pectoris.

Primary decreases in coronary blood flow and myocardial oxygen delivery, such as occur with progressive atherosclerosis, partial coronary artery thrombosis, coronary arterial spasm or transient platelet aggregation, may also lead to angina pectoris. Similarly, increases in coronary artery tone associated with platelet aggregation and the release of humoral mediators, such as thromboxane or serotonin or both, may interact with intrinsic narrowing in coronary luminal diameter to decrease coronary flow and oxygen delivery and result in angina. With primary decreases in coronary blood flow, there is no necessary association between symptoms and exertion, and the majority of the anginal episodes occur at rest. These patients usually have little change in heart rate or blood pressure prior to the onset of pain, or the pain occurs first and is followed only later by an increase in blood pressure or heart rate. Continuous electrocardiographic monitoring may document transient ST segment change with the onset of pain, either ST segment elevation indicating transmural ischemia or ST depression when subendocardial ischemia occurs. Alternatively, ST segment alterations may occur in the absence of chest pain, emphasizing the presence of *silent ischemia* in some patients with primary decreases in myocardial oxygen delivery and angina at rest.

PATHOPHYSIOLOGY. Angina occurs most commonly in circumstances in which regional myocardial oxygen demand exceeds oxygen availability. This occurs when myocardial oxygen demand is increased by (1) an increase in intramyocardial systolic tension resulting from increases in blood pressure, cold exposure, congestive heart failure, ventricular hypertrophy, or left ventricular outflow obstruction; increases in intramyocardial systolic tension are directly proportional to blood pressure and the radius of the ventricle (Laplace's rule); (2) an increase in heart rate, such as occurs with exercise or emotion; and (3) an increase in the contractile state of the myocardium, such as occurs during physical effort, with catecholamine administration, with fright, or with the use of certain pharmacologic interventions that increase inotropy and myocardial oxygen demand more than they increase myocardial oxygen delivery. Rest generally relieves angina that occurs with effort, emotion, or exercise. Nitroglycerin also relieves angina, typically within three to five minutes. The beneficial effect of nitroglycerin is related to its ability to dilate medium-sized penetrating coronary vessels and thus improve coronary blood flow and its distribution to the subendocardial ischemic region or regions and to its ability to dilate systemic veins so that venous return to the heart and ventricular end-diastolic volume are reduced, thereby reducing wall tension and oxygen demand.

CLINICAL DIAGNOSIS. Angina is typically described as a substernal or left precordial chest discomfort that is perceived as a "tightness" or "heaviness" ("like a weight on my chest") or as "a pressure." On occasion, the pain may radiate into the neck; it often radiates down the ulnar aspect of the left arm. It is typically produced by effort, exercise, emotion, or cold exposure or occurs after a large meal is eaten; it is relieved by rest or nitroglycerin. As mentioned earlier, it may also occur at rest as an expression of progressive atherosclerosis (more than 70 per cent luminal diameter narrowing), partial coronary artery thrombosis, coronary artery spasm, and/or platelet aggregation with the release of humoral mediators that increase coronary vascular resistance at sites of severe coronary arterial stenosis. Some patients do not describe their angina in typical terms but refer to it as "a hurt," "a little discomfort," or "a sharp pain." Others note the pain only in atypical locations, including the jaw, the teeth, the forearm, or the back. Some describe their angina as beginning in the epigastric region and radiating up into the chest. Finally, some patients have *silent* angina. Ten to 20 per cent of patients with both diabetes mellitus and coronary artery disease have silent angina, and in those with acute myocardial infarcts, 10 to 20 per cent are silent (painless) infarcts. Many patients after cardiac transplantation do not perceive angina even though coronary artery atherosclerosis occurs in the coronary arteries of the transplanted heart.

Left or right ventricular dysfunction may develop even with transient ischemic episodes. This may explain the dyspnea or orthopnea, paroxysmal nocturnal dyspnea, tachycardia, and alterations in blood pressure, including hypotension, that occur with some episodes of angina. Further, some patients develop transient murmurs of mitral or tricuspid regurgitation because of papillary muscle dysfunction occurring as a consequence of the ischemic process; acute mitral insufficiency may also contribute to the development of transient left ventricular failure during angina. Typically, left ventricular end-diastolic pressure rises during angina; this is a consequence of a reduction in ventricular compliance and, in some instances, possibly of incomplete relaxation of the ventricular muscle leading to increased left atrial and pulmonary venous pressures and the development of dyspnea, orthopnea, and pulmonary congestion during myocardial ischemia. Palpation of the precordium during an episode of angina may reveal a dyskinetic impulse. Auscultation may identify a third heart sound and rales or a murmur of mitral insufficiency. Occasionally, patients develop paradoxical splitting of their second heart sounds. The murmur of papillary muscle dysfunction reflects mild-to-moderate mitral regurgitation and is classically a mid to late systolic murmur, but it may be holosystolic.

Noncardiac problems may also cause chest pain, including peptic ulcer disease, pancreatitis, cholecystitis, esophageal reflux or spasm, and primary pulmonary abnormalities such as pneumonia, pulmonary embolism with infarction, atelectasis, and spontaneous pneumothorax. Other causes of chest pain that must be differentiated from angina pectoris are the pain of dissecting aortic aneurysm, musculoskeletal chest pain, and the pain that occurs with herpes zoster, which may develop before skin lesions occur.

CLINICAL CLASSIFICATION OF ANGINAL SYNDROMES. Table 51–1 lists the various coronary artery syndromes that should receive specific attention. Segregation of patients with coronary artery disease into the various anginal syndromes is useful diagnostically, therapeutically, and prognostically. Patients with stable angina usually have angina with effort or exercise or during other conditions in which myocardial oxygen demand is increased. This often occurs in a predictable manner and is usually relieved promptly by rest or nitroglycerin. However, some of these patients have angina

TABLE 51–1. ANGINAL SYNDROMES OF PATIENTS WITH CORONARY ARTERY DISEASE

Stable angina pectoris
Unstable angina pectoris (crescendo angina, angina at rest, and angina of recent onset)
Variant angina pectoris (Prinzmetal's angina)
Acute myocardial infarction

at variable levels of effort and, on occasion, also at rest, suggesting that intermittent increases in vascular smooth muscle tone and decreases in coronary blood flow contribute to the development of angina. Thus, in patients with stable angina, there may be a spectrum of pathophysiologic mechanisms responsible for angina leading to effort or emotion-related angina but also for angina occurring occasionally at lesser effort and even at rest.

Increasingly frequent angina with chest pain produced by less effort or provocation and occurring in a crescendo pattern is generally termed *unstable angina pectoris*. Patients with the initial development of angina at low levels of activity or at rest should probably be included in this category. Individuals with unstable angina pectoris often have pain at rest, and the pain may last for longer periods of time and be more difficult to relieve. Unstable angina should be considered a medical emergency and warrants hospitalization and evaluation of the patient for acute myocardial infarction.

Variant angina pectoris (Prinzmetal's angina) is defined as chest pain at rest in association with ST segment deviation (ordinarily ST segment elevation, but ST segment depression may also occur depending on the size of the coronary vessel in which spasm occurs) without preceding increase in heart rate or blood pressure. The mechanism of variant angina is coronary artery spasm shown by coronary arteriography often to involve large and medium-sized vessels with transmural myocardial blood flow distribution. As the chest pain disappears, the ST segment deviation resolves in association with relief of the coronary spasm. In most patients, many more episodes of ST segment deviation than of chest pain occur; therefore, continuous recording of multilead electrocardiograms is recommended for patients with this abnormality. In those circumstances in which the coronary artery spasm is prolonged, acute myocardial infarction, important ventricular arrhythmias, heart block, or death may occur.

Ten to 20 per cent of patients with Prinzmetal's angina have angiographically normal coronary arteries; this further emphasizes the role of spasm in the pathophysiology of variant angina. The most common arteriographic pattern is significant single-vessel stenosis involving the proximal portion of either the right or the left anterior descending coronary artery. However, any pattern of coronary artery disease may be seen. Although variant angina pectoris attributable to coronary spasm occurs as a specific syndrome, there is also speculation that spasm may be a factor in more patients with stable and unstable angina pectoris than previously realized and that it may contribute to the variable threshold angina found in some of these patients.

It is not clear which pathophysiologic factors are most important in the conversion of stable angina to the various anginal syndromes mentioned above. However, current interest centers on the role of platelet aggregability, hemorrhage into atherosclerotic plaques, increases in local vascular concentrations of thromboxane, serotonin, and histamine, and relative decreases in prostacyclin, tissue plasminogen-activating factor, and/or endothelial relaxing factor concentrations at the site of coronary arterial intimal injury or atherosclerotic plaque or both.

DIAGNOSTIC TESTS. An association of the chest pain with exercise, effort, and emotion and of relief with rest or nitroglycerin is presumptive evidence that the chest pain represents angina pectoris. In addition, certain diagnostic maneuvers, such as carotid sinus pressure or the Valsalva maneuver, may help to determine the etiology of chest pain. Both these maneuvers slow the heart rate and reduce the blood pressure as a consequence of increased vagal and reduced sympathetic tone.

One may also use certain tests to provoke angina. In particular, exercise testing on a bicycle or on a treadmill is often used for this purpose. The patient exercises at graded loads, starting from low and progressing to higher ones. Blood pressure and heart rate are monitored throughout, and multilead electrocardiograms (ECG) are obtained prior to, during, and toward the end of each exercise level (continuous multilead monitoring of the electrocardiogram is preferable). An exercise test result is positive if typical angina develops and/or if the test is associated with ST segment deviation of 1 mm or greater, flat or downsloping, 0.08 second after the ST junction. There are both false-positive and false-negative exercise test results, however. Particularly in women, false-positive results occur in up to 20 to 30 per cent of patients. False-positive results may also occur in patients with electrolyte abnormalities, in patients taking digitalis, and in those with ventricular hypertrophy, conduction abnormalities (including left or right bundle branch block), or ST-T wave abnormalities prior to the onset of exercise. In addition, in some patients with anatomically important coronary artery stenoses, diagnostic ECG changes do not occur with stress. The incidence of false-negative results with adequate exercise tests and multilead ECG analysis is at least 10 to 15 per cent. Additional hemodynamic and clinical variables monitored during the exercise testing are heart rate, systolic blood pressure, exercise work load achieved, and the development of frequent or complex ventricular ectopic beats. Angina that develops during exercise at a relatively low heart rate and blood pressure and/or at a low work load or a reduction in systolic blood pressure with exercise generally indicates more extensive and physiologically important coronary artery stenoses and a poorer prognosis with medical therapy. Prominent ST segment depression ($\geq$3 mm) developing at low or moderate exercise work loads often identifies more extensive coronary artery stenoses or a significant left main coronary artery stenosis or both. Frequent or complex ventricular ectopic beats occurring during exercise may subsequently be adequately suppressed by a beta blocker or a slow channel calcium antagonist.

Additions to the standard exercise ECG include the use of selected nuclear cardiology tests. One approach uses a myocardial perfusion agent such as thallium 201, which is injected at the peak of exercise. Myocardial scintigraphic images are obtained immediately thereafter. Regions of relative perfusion deficit observed during exercise that are normal at rest three to four hours later are generally indicative of physiologically significant coronary artery stenoses. When a maximal exercise effort is achieved, thallium 201 myocardial scintigraphy with tomographic imaging has a 90 per cent sensitivity and specificity in the noninvasive detection of anatomically important ($\geq$70 per cent luminal diameter narrowing) coronary artery stenoses.

An alternative approach is to label the patient's red blood cells in vivo with technetium 99m pertechnetate or to inject intravenously a radionuclide such as technetium-labeled albumin or technetium pertechnetate and obtain a radionuclide ventriculogram (RVG) at rest and at each level of exercise. With either approach, one may measure global and segmental ventricular performance at rest and at each exercise level and determine directly whether alterations in regional wall motion, ventricular volumes, or global ejection fraction occur. In individuals without important coronary artery stenoses or myocardial disease, ventricular ejection fraction increases with exercise, but in those with physiologically important coronary artery stenoses, and particularly those with multivessel disease, the ventricular ejection fraction usually decreases with exercise. Similarly, in the patient with physiologically important coronary artery stenoses, left ventricular end-systolic volumes increase rather than decrease, and segmental wall motion abnormalities may develop. With a maximal exercise effort, the sensitivity of RVG in detecting physiologically important multivessel or proximal coronary stenoses is approximately 90 per cent. However, the specificity is only approximately 50 per cent, since patients with myocardial and valvular heart disease may also demonstrate ventricular dysfunction at rest or with exercise or both.

CORONARY ARTERIOGRAPHY. Coronary arteriography is the most reliable diagnostic test currently available to detect anatomically important coronary atherosclerosis and to estimate the extent of such disease. Resting coronary blood flow is not decreased, but effort-related increases in coronary blood flow may be reduced by coronary artery luminal narrowing of 50 per cent or greater. Resting coronary blood flow may be reduced by luminal diameter narrowing of greater than 70 per cent. However, there are sometimes discrepancies between the apparent anatomic severity of a coronary artery stenosis and its physiologic significance; thus, exercise testing with or without the scintigraphic assessments may be important in evaluating the physiologic significance of apparently anatomic important coronary artery stenoses.

A subset of patients with angina has normal coronary arteriograms but objective evidence of myocardial ischemia by ECG criteria or by lactate production during rapid pacing or by both. This pattern occurs in some patients with ventricular hypertrophy or systemic arterial hypertension or both, and in others with no obvious underlying cardiovascular disease.

Indications for coronary arteriography in patients with angina vary. A widely accepted clinical indication is the presence of limiting angina in the patient on a good medical regimen. However, some practitioners also use coronary arteriography to evaluate young patients (those less than 40 years of age) who have had previous acute myocardial infarcts. Others use coronary arteriography and left ventricular catheterization to evaluate the cause of congestive heart failure in patients in whom the etiology is not clear. Radionuclide ventriculography and echocardiography with Doppler may also be used for this purpose, especially to characterize regional and global ventricular function, to exclude sizable ventricular aneurysms, to identify valvular regurgitation and to estimate its severity, and to detect intracardiac shunt lesions. Coronary arteriography may also be used to help resolve the etiology of undiagnosed chest pain that is limiting or frightening for the patient. In general, however, coronary arteriography is reserved for patients selected as potential candidates for coronary artery surgery or precutaneous transluminal coronary angioplasty (PTCA) because of symptomatic angina pectoris.

MANAGEMENT. The therapeutic approach to patients with angina pectoris can be medical or surgical. These alternatives are not mutually exclusive, since many patients continue to take long-acting nitrates, propranolol, a calcium antagonist, or combinations of these agents following coronary artery revascularization or PTCA. In addition, one does everything possible to correct underlying risk factors, such as smoking, systemic arterial hypertension, hypercholesterolemia, overweight, major stress, and emotional conflicts, and to encourage proper amounts of exercise, especially in younger individuals. Control of multiple risk factors, especially discontinuing smoking and reducing serum cholesterol concentrations, has a beneficial effect in reducing subsequent mortality risks; and in experimental animals with hypercholesterolemia and coronary artery stenoses, reductions in serum cholesterol may be associated with some regression of coronary artery plaques.

Patients with angina pectoris should be encouraged to carry nitroglycerin with them. Nitroglycerin (0.3 to 0.5 mg) should be taken sublingually when angina develops in order to prevent it from becoming severe; if one nitroglycerin tablet is ineffective, a second should be taken. In addition, the patient should sit or lie down in order to help relieve the pain. If the angina is not relieved by two or three nitroglycerin tablets and rest, the individual should go to the hospital for further evaluation, specifically concerning the possibility that he or she is having an acute myocardial infarct. Nitroglycerin may also be taken prophylactically prior to engaging in activities the individual knows will produce angina, i.e., before physical effort, sexual intercourse, or an emotional experience that cannot be avoided. Nitroglycerin tablets should be replaced every 6 to 12 months, since they deteriorate. One needs to be certain that important reductions in blood pressure or increases in heart rate do not occur following the administraton of nitroglycerin, because under these circumstances coronary flow to the vulnerable myocardium may actually decrease.

Long-acting nitrates may also be used. The effectiveness, proper dosage, and route of administration are subjects of controversy. However, isosorbide dinitrate may be taken sublingually or orally, and it exerts an effect similar to that of nitroglycerin for 40 to 60 minutes after its administration. Nitroglycerin ointment is also an effective long-acting agent in most patients. It is generally applied to a small area of the chest as a thin film. The nitrate preparations in common use today are described in Table 51–2. Over time, many individuals develop a tolerance to the hemodynamic effects from the nitrate preparations, such that the same dose of nitrate is much less effective or even ineffective. The cellular biochemical alterations responsible for tolerance to nitrates are not yet elucidated, but less frequent administration of a particular nitrate and mixing the nitrates so that one might rely on

TABLE 51–2. NITRATE PREPARATIONS USED IN THE TREATMENT OF ANGINA PECTORIS

Preparation	Dosage	Duration of Effect	Frequency of Administration
Sublingual nitroglycerin	0.3–0.5 mg	15–30 min	For individual episodes
Sublingual or chewable isosorbide dinitrate	2.5–10 mg	30 min to 1 hr	May be used instead of nitroglycerin
Oral isosorbide dinitrate (Isordil)	5–30 mg	2 hr	Every 2 to 3 hr while the patient is awake
Oral isosorbide dinitrate (Tembid), longer-acting preparation	40 mg	6–8 hr	Every 6–8 hr
Pentaerythritol tetranitrate (Peritrate)	10–40 mg	3–4 hr	Every 3–4 hr
Oral	80 mg	8–10 hr	Every 8–10 hr
Sustained-release oral nitroglycerin (Nitro-Bid)	2.5–6.5 mg	6 hr	Every 6 hr
Nitroglycerin ointment	Thin film on 1 to 2 inches over small area of anterior chest	4–6 hr	Every 4–6 hr
Nitroglycerin patches (sustained-release)	5–20 mg	More than 6 hr	Every 12–24 hr

Modified from Willerson JT, Hillis LD, Buja LM: Ischemic Heart Disease: Clinical and Pathophysiological Aspects. New York, Raven Press, 1982, p 189.

TABLE 51–3. BETA-ADRENERGIC ANTAGONISTS

Name	Beta-Blockade Potency Ratio (Propranolol—1.0)	Cardioselective*	Usual Therapeutic Dose Range (mg/day)	Elimination Half-life	Route of Excretion
Propranolol	1.0	0	80–480	3.5–6.0 hr	Urine
Timolol	6.0	0	5–40	4–5 hr	Urine
Oxprenolol†	0.5–1.0	0	40–360	2 hr	Urine
Sotalol†	0.3	0	80–480	5–13 hr	Urine
Metoprolol	1.0	+	100–800	3–4 hr	Urine
Pindolol	6.0	0	2.5–30.0	3.4 hr	Urine
Atenolol	1.0	+	100–400	6–9 hr	Approximately 40% of unchanged drug in urine
Alprenolol†	0.3	0	200–800	2–3 hr	Urine
Acebutolol	0.3	+	400–800	8 hr	Uncertain

*Seen only at low dosage.
†Investigational drug.
Reproduced with permission from Hillis LD, Firth BG, Willerson JT: Manual of Clinical Problems in Cardiology. 2nd ed. Boston, Little, Brown and Company, 1984, p 285.

nitroglycerin paste during the night hours and a long-acting nitrate, such as isosorbide dinitrate, during the day help to reduce the likelihood of tolerance.

The second major group of agents used to control angina comprises the beta-adrenergic–blocking drugs (Table 51–3). Beta-adrenergic blockers decrease heart rate and blood pressure responses to exercise and usually reduce the frequency of angina related to exercise or effort. They also decrease the inotropic response to exercise in normal hearts but may actually improve global and segmental left ventricular contractility for any particular exercise effort in patients with important coronary artery stenoses. The most common contraindications to the use of beta blockers are congestive heart failure, bradycardia, bronchospastic lung disease, and insulin-requiring diabetes. Second- or third-degree heart block is also a contraindication to the use of beta blockers. Relatively cardioselective beta blockers (such as metoprolol and alprenolol)* that exert their effects on heart rate and blood pressure rather than on bronchial dilatation are alternatives. However, at higher dosages, the relatively selective beta blockers exert a nonspecific beta-blocking effect.

The use of "slow channel" calcium antagonists, such as nifedipine, verapamil, or diltiazem, is gaining in popularity (Tables 51–4 and 51–5). These agents reduce calcium entry into myocardial and vascular smooth muscle cells. This effect results in a reduction in vascular contractility and vascular resistance. These agents are effective in treating patients with vasospastic angina (Prinzmetal's angina), but they are also useful in treating patients with stable angina pectoris. Some calcium antagonists decrease myocardial contractility and atrioventricular conduction (verapamil and diltiazem), so they must be used with caution in patients with congestive heart failure, bradycardia, or atrioventricular (AV) conduction blocks, but they do not augment bronchoconstriction and thus may be of particular benefit as an alternative to beta blockers for those with bronchospasm and chronic obstructive lung disease. Nifedipine decreases systemic vascular resistance, and therefore, clinically apparent reductions in cardiac contractility are usually not evident. Nifedipine does not decrease AV conduction. Thus, nifedipine is safer to administer to patients with bradycardia, heart failure, or AV conduction abnormalities. The effect of nifedipine in decreasing systemic vascular resistance is often associated with a reflex increase in heart rate that may preclude giving nifedipine (Procardia) to the patient with tachycardia.

*Investigational drug.

Many patients are given long-acting nitrates, beta blockers, and/or calcium antagonists concomitantly. Continuing angina at low levels of effort is generally considered an indication for coronary arteriography and, when appropriate, coronary artery revascularization or PTCA.

Carefully supervised and individually developed physical training and exercise programs are also appropriate for patients with stable angina. The major benefit of training appears to be to improve the hemodynamic response to exercise, including reducing heart rate and blood pressure changes for any given exercise effort. Exercise training may also improve skeletal muscle performance at any given blood flow, thus contributing to improved effort tolerance in patients with coronary artery disease. Whether exercise programs increase collateral coronary blood flow is controversial.

Pain relief occurs following complete bed rest in 90 per cent of patients with unstable angina. Patients who continue to have pain while at bed rest are given nitrates initially orally, sublingually, and/or topically. If angina at rest recurs or angina at low levels of effort persists, a slow channel calcium antagonist (nifedipine, verapamil, or diltiazem) should be administered. In the patient with a well-maintained blood pressure and heart rate who has continuing angina at rest or at a low level of effort and in whom coronary artery spasm (Prinzmetal's angina) is not believed to be the pathophysiologic mechanism, a beta blocker may be administered. In the patient believed to have coronary artery spasm, i.e., those having chest pain at rest with transient ST segment elevation during the episode of pain and without a preceding increase in heart rate or blood pressure, calcium antagonists should be used instead of a beta blocker. If angina at rest persists or recurs,

TABLE 51–4. PHARMACOLOGIC EFFECTS OF THE CALCIUM CHANNEL BLOCKERS

	Heart Rate		Conduction SA Node	Conduction AV Node	Myocardial Contractility	Peripheral Vasodilator	Cardiac Output	Coronary Blood Flow	Myocardial O_2 Demand
	Acute	*Chronic*							
Diltiazem	↓	↓	↓	↓	↓	↓	V	↑	↓
Nifedipine	↑	↑	—	↑	↓	↓↓	↑	↑↑	↓
Verapamil	↓	↓	↓	↓	↓↓	↓	V	↑	↓

↓ = decrease; ↑ = increase; — = no change; V = variable effect.
Modified from Packer M, Frishman WH: Calcium Channel Antagonists in Cardiovascular Disease. East Norwalk, CT, Appleton-Century-Crofts, 1984, p 13.

TABLE 51–5. CLINICAL USE OF CALCIUM CHANNEL BLOCKERS

	Dosage		Onset of Action		Therapeutic Plasma Concentration	Metabolism	Excretion
	Oral	*I.V.*	*Oral*	*I.V.*			
Diltiazem	30–90 mg q 6–8 hr	75–150 μg/kg (10–20 mg)	< 30 min	< 10 min	50–200 ng/ml	Deacetylation *N*-demethylation *O*-demethylation	60% fecal
Nifedipine	10–40 mg q 6–8 hr	5–15 μg/kg	< 20 min	< 5 min (3 min sl)	25–100 ng/ml	A hydroxycarboxylic acid and a lactone with no known activity	20–40% fecal 50–80% renal
Verapamil	80–120 mg q 6–12 hr	150 μg/kg (10–20 mg)	< 30	< 5 min	80–300 ng/ml	*N*-dealkylation *N*-demethylation Major hepatic first pass effect	15% fecal 70% renal

sl = sublingual.
Reproduced with permission from Packer M, Frishman WH: Calcium Channel Antagonists in Cardiovascular Disease. East Norwalk, CT, Appleton-Century-Crofts, 1984, p 8.

intravenous nitroglycerin is begun. In selected patients with angina at rest despite the therapy outlined above, intra-aortic balloon counterpulsation may be utilized. The equivalent of one to four aspirin per day has been shown to reduce the risk of death and myocardial infarction for up to two years after the development of unstable angina. If pain relief does not occur with bed rest and the use of appropriate drugs, the risk of subsequent myocardial infarction, sudden death, or important ventricular arrhythmias is increased.

Coronary arteriography is generally recommended in patients with unstable angina pectoris once the pain is controlled and a myocardial infarct is excluded. In the patient in whom angina at rest recurs despite a good medical regimen, cardiac catheterization and coronary arteriography become almost mandatory. This approach is recommended because 10 to 15 per cent of patients with this syndrome have significant (≥50 per cent stenosis) main left coronary artery disease; in these patients, coronary artery bypass surgery has been shown to prolong their lives. Approximately 10 per cent of patients with unstable angina have no angiographic evidence of significant coronary artery stenoses. Thus, in 25 per cent of these patients, the angiographic findings help to provide a therapeutic approach. In the remaining patients, identifying the location and extent of coronary artery disease is helpful prognostically, and in the patient with continuing angina at rest, the arteriographic findings allow the physician to consider coronary bypass surgery or angioplasty (PTCA).

Subsequently, in those patients in whom angina is controlled medically and in whom there are no coronary angiographic findings requiring revascularization, exercise testing is usually performed. Submaximal exercise tests are often obtained within four to ten days after the angina is controlled, followed several weeks later by a more vigorous exercise test. Patients with continuing angina or objective evidence of intermittent myocardial ischemia at low levels of activity despite a good medical regimen and those with significant three-vessel coronary artery stenoses and depressed left ventricular function (left ventricular ejection fraction, or LVEF <50 per cent) usually undergo coronary artery revascularization, either by coronary artery bypass grafting or by PTCA.

Variant angina is generally treated with nitrates or calcium antagonists or both, including nifedipine, verapamil, or diltiazem. Calcium antagonists appear to be particularly successful in reducing the frequency of episodes of coronary artery spasm. Direct coronary artery surgery and coronary angioplasty have not been as successful in these patients as in those with more typical angina pectoris, although these therapeutic approaches are used in patients with important underlying coronary artery stenoses in whom one cannot obtain symptomatic relief of the angina. One report (Bertrand, 1980) suggests that plexectomy coupled with coronary artery revascularization may be more successful than revascularization by itself.

DIRECT CORONARY ARTERY SURGERY. Large groups of patients now have undergone direct coronary artery surgery in the form of saphenous vein or internal mammary artery bypass grafting (see Ch. 51.3). These surgical procedures result in relief or reduction in the frequency of angina for months to years after the procedure in the majority of patients. For patients with significant left main coronary artery stenoses and/or three-vessel stenoses and impaired left ventricular function, improved survival has been documented following coronary artery revascularization. The best results from coronary artery surgery are obtained in (1) patients with "limiting angina" who are on a medical regimen and who have important proximal coronary artery narrowing but good distal vessels and (2) patients in whom the most important obstructing lesions can be bypassed completely with coronary revascularization. Recent evidence also suggests that the internal mammary artery graft represents the best surgical revascularization because of its durability and effectiveness.

Graft occlusion during the first year in most reported series varies from 10 to 12 per cent. Only a small additional percentage of grafts occlude during the second and third years. However, coronary artery surgery is a palliative procedure, and most patients redevelop angina months to years after the procedure. The most common reason for redevelopment of angina is progression of the intrinsic coronary artery disease. Incomplete revascularization may also be a cause for persistent angina or angina that develops soon after surgery. Graft occlusion and relatively inadequate revascularization with limited increases in coronary blood flow in grafted arteries subsequently are additional reasons for unfavorable results.

Grafted vessels may develop progressive atherosclerosis over time. This occurs most commonly in patients with hypercholesterolemia, in those with diabetes mellitus, and in those with important distal vascular disease such that coronary graft flow is reduced. Native coronary arteries proximal to the site of insertion of coronary artery bypass grafts may develop an accelerated pattern of atherosclerosis following coronary artery surgery. It is almost certainly beneficial to control serum cholesterol concentrations and correct all other risk factors as thoroughly as possible to provide the best opportunity for a prolonged period of coronary graft patency. The administration of aspirin preoperatively or within a few hours of the surgical procedure also appears to be useful in protecting the patency of the coronary artery bypass grafts.

There is a risk of perioperative myocardial infarction, but the frequency with which this occurs is controversial. If the electrocardiogram is used to document the frequency of perioperative infarction, estimates range from 1 to 10 per cent. However, if myocardial scintigraphic techniques are used, the incidence is approximately twice as high. This discrepancy probably reflects "non–Q wave" infarcts not detected by the electrocardiogram.

In addition to the subjective relief of angina that usually occurs for months to years following coronary artery revascularization, some patients also have objective improvement in ventricular function, both at rest and during exercise.

CORONARY ARTERY ANGIOPLASTY. Gruentzig introduced direct coronary artery dilatation with a balloon catheter (PTCA) for proximal coronary artery lesions. This procedure provides a means to increase luminal diameter in selected patients. Important complications occur relatively infrequently. Nevertheless, this procedure should be performed only with facilities available for subsequent direct coronary artery surgery, should that be necessary. Experienced surgeons have a success rate in carefully selected patients of greater than 80 per cent, with less than a 10 per cent risk of acute myocardial infarction or need for emergency coronary artery revascularization. The ideal coronary lesions for PTCA are those with moderately tight proximal stenoses over a short segment and without severe calcification or branch vessel involvement. Left main coronary lesions are not considered suitable for PTCA. Patients are generally pretreated with platelet-active agents (aspirin* and dipyridamole*) and a calcium antagonist in an attempt to reduce the risk of coronary artery spasm during and immediately following angioplasty. Approximately 30 per cent of patients develop restenosis of the dilated coronary artery in the initial six months following the procedure; thus, close follow-up with exercise testing and imaging assessments is important.

PROGNOSIS. There is extreme variance in symptoms and progression of coronary artery stenoses among patients. In some, angina may remain stable for many years. However, approximately 25 per cent of men and 12 per cent of women with angina can expect a myocardial infarct within 5 years. In the population over 55 years of age, the overall 5-year survival rate is 75 per cent for those with stable angina pectoris.

The prognosis of patients with chronic ischemic heart disease is related directly to the location and extent of physiologically important coronary artery stenoses and to left ventricular function. Patients with significant three-vessel coronary stenoses have an expected annual mortality of 6 to 8 per cent; if they also have had a previous myocardial infarction, the mortality rate is increased. On the other hand, patients with significant single-vessel coronary artery disease have an annual mortality rate on medical therapy of approximately 2 to 3 per cent. Patients with main left coronary artery disease equal to or greater than 70 per cent luminal diameter narrowing have a prognosis similar to those with severe three-vessel coronary disease. In fact, most patients with left main coronary artery disease have extensive additional coronary artery stenoses. Survival is also reduced in patients with left ventricular ejection fractions lower than 40 per cent and in those with frequent and complex ventricular ectopy and left ventricular dysfunction. As noted earlier, patients with significant multivessel coronary stenoses, impaired left ventricular function, and objective evidence of myocardial ischemia at relatively low work loads also have a reduced survival with medical therapy.

---

*Investigational uses.

Brensike JF, Levy RI, Kelsey SF, et al.: Effects of therapy with cholestyramine on progression of coronary arteriosclerosis: Results of the NHLBI Type II Coronary Intervention Study. Circulation 69:313, 1984. *A beneficial effect from lowering serum cholesterol values on progression of coronary arteriosclerosis is suggested by these data.*

Folts JD, Crowell EB, Rowe GG: Platelet aggregation in partially obstructed vessels and its elimination with aspirin. Circulation 54:365, 1976. *This study suggests that intermittent platelet aggregation can decrease coronary blood flow in narrowed canine coronary arteries.*

Hillis LD, Braunwald E: Myocardial ischemia. N Engl J Med 296:971, 1977. *A thorough review of myocardial ischemia.*

Hirsh PD, Hillis LD, Campbell WB, et al.: Release of prostaglandins and thromboxane into the coronary circulation in patients with ischemic heart disease. N Engl J Med 304:685, 1981. *Patients with unstable angina have increased transcardiac concentrations of thromboxane occurring in temporal association with unstable angina, thereby suggesting a possible role for platelet aggregation and the release of thromboxane in the pathophysiology of this syndrome.*

Johnson SM, Mauritson DR, Corbett JR, et al.: Double-blind, randomized, placebo-controlled comparison of propranolol and verapamil in the treatment of patients with stable angina pectoris. Am J Med 71:443, 1981. *In 18 patients with exertional angina, propranolol and verapamil were each effective.*

Kannel WB, Feinleib M: Natural history of angina pectoris in the Framingham Study: Prognosis and survival. Am J Cardiol 29:154, 1972. *Of 303 patients with angina followed long term, the mortality averaged about 5 per cent per year in men and 2 to 3 per cent per year in women.*

Maseri A, Severi S, DeNes M, et al.: "Variant" angina: One aspect of a continuous spectrum of vasospastic myocardial ischemia. Am J Cardiol 42:1019, 1978. *Vasospastic angina can occur in the presence of extremely variable degrees of coronary atherosclerosis and in any phase of ischemic heart disease.*

Roberts WC: The coronary arteries and left ventricle in clinically isolated angina pectoris: A necropsy analysis. Circulation 54:388, 1976. *Postmortem findings regarding coronary artery disease and ventriculographic abnormalities in patients with angina pectoris.*

Truett J, Cornfield J, Kannel WB: A multivariate analysis of the risk of coronary heart disease in Framingham. J Chronic Dis 20:511, 1967. *Detailed analysis of risk factors involved in the acquisition of coronary artery disease.*

Willerson JT, Hillis LD, Winniford M, et al.: Speculation regarding mechanisms responsible for acute ischemic heart disease syndromes. J Am Coll Cardiol 8:245, 1986. *Speculations regarding the etiologies for unstable angina and coronary artery spasm.*

51.2 Acute Myocardial Infarction

James T. Willerson

Myocardial infarction is the term used to describe irreversible cellular injury and necrosis occurring as a consequence of prolonged ischemia. Infarction may occur secondary to coronary occlusion, major reduction in blood flow to certain regions of heart muscle, or an insufficient increase in coronary blood flow relative to regional oxygen demand during periods of severe stress. In almost every instance, some degree of narrowing of coronary artery luminal diameter resulting from coronary atherosclerosis exists, but there are exceptions. Acute myocardial infarcts may also result from coronary artery dissection, coronary emboli, coronary artery spasm, vasculitis, anomalous origin of one of the coronary arteries from the pulmonary artery, and congenital coronary arteriovenous fistula.

The pathogenesis of coronary atherosclerosis is considered in detail in Ch. 50 and in brief in Ch. 51.1.

RISK FACTORS FOR CORONARY ARTERY DISEASE. Several epidemiologic studies have established that hyperlipidemia, especially hypercholesterolemia, constitutes a major risk factor predisposing to the development of premature atherosclerosis. Approximately one third of survivors of acute myocardial infarction at an age less than 60 years have some form of hyperlipidemia, defined as serum cholesterol and/or triglyceride levels above the ninety-fifth percentile for the control population. Other factors associated with an increased risk of development of coronary atherosclerotic disease include systemic arterial hypertension, smoking, lack of regular physical activity, and emotional stress. Risk factors are discussed more extensively in Ch. 40 and 50.

MECHANISMS OF ACUTE MYOCARDIAL INFARCTION. Acute myocardial infarction occurs primarily in patients with significant coronary artery disease (Fig. 51–1). In such patients, the primary determinants of vulnerability to acute myocardial infarction include (1) prolonged increases in myocardial oxygen demand under conditions in which increases in oxygen delivery cannot occur because of significant coronary artery disease (included are prolonged and marked increases in heart rate, contractility, and myocardial wall tension) or (2) primary decreases in oxygen delivery to the

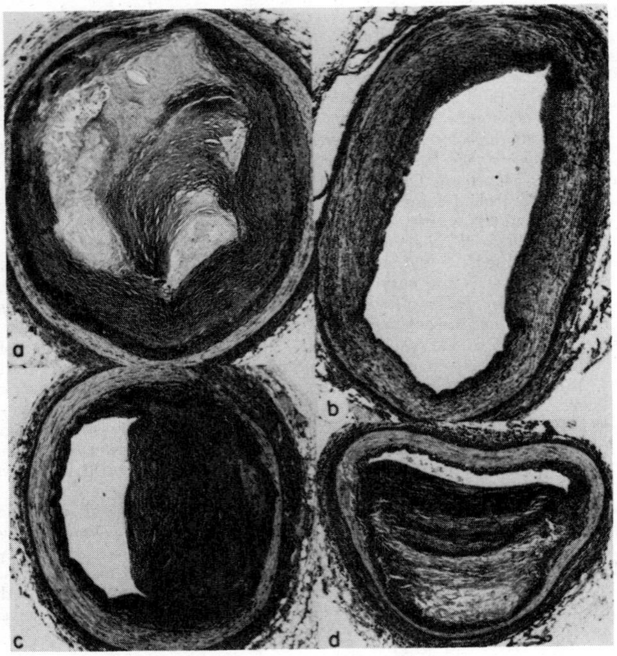

FIGURE 51–1. Sections of coronary arteries at sites of maximal narrowing in a 54-year-old woman who died suddenly at home. She had angina pectoris. *a*, Right coronary artery 3 cm from the aortic ostium. The lumen is more than 90 per cent obstructed. *b*, Left main coronary artery. *c*, Left circumflex coronary artery in the first 1 cm. *d*, Left anterior descending coronary artery 3 cm from the bifurcation of the left main coronary artery. These sections demonstrate the extent of coronary artery disease that may be present in an individual patient. (From Roberts WC: Circulation 48:1161, 1973. Reproduced by permission of The American Heart Association, Inc.)

myocardium. The latter may be caused by (1) coronary artery thrombosis, (2) coronary artery spasm, (3) hemorrhage into an atherosclerotic plaque, and (4) systemic arterial hypotension (coronary artery perfusion is dependent on mean and diastolic aortic blood pressure).

Several clinicopathologic studies of patients with fatal ischemic heart disease and clinical evaluations in patients with evolving acute myocardial infarcts have established that approximately 90 per cent of "Q wave infarcts" (usually transmural myocardial infarcts) are caused by proximal coronary artery occlusion by a thrombus. The coronary thrombosis generally occurs at a tight stenosis and often in association with hemorrhage into an ulcerated atherosclerotic plaque. In contrast, only about 30 per cent of "non–Q wave infarcts" (usually subendocardial myocardial infarcts) have an occlusive coronary thrombus in the infarct-related artery. Instead, most of these patients have significant multivessel coronary artery stenoses and a low-flow state, possibly associated with microthombosis due to platelet aggregation at sites of severe coronary artery stenosis.

In a clinicopathologic study of 100 episodes of acute ischemic heart disease, the incidence of acute coronary occlusion was 61 per cent (57 in situ thrombi, 2 thromboemboli, and 2 isolated plaque hemorrhages), including 90 per cent for transmural infarcts, 35 per cent for subendocardial infarcts, and 11 per cent for multifocal microinfarcts associated with clinical acute coronary insufficiency syndromes (Buja and Willerson). The incidence of plaque erosion or rupture with coronary thrombus formation was 68 per cent for infarcts of age three weeks or less but decreased to 20 per cent with older infarcts, probably because organization and healing made identification of these lesions more difficult. Other investigators, using serial section techniques, have described a higher incidence (usually over 90 per cent) of plaque erosion and rupture associated with major plaque hemorrhage and acute coronary artery thrombosis. Potential causative factors for plaque rupture include hemodynamic trauma, inflammatory or chemical injury to coronary artery endothelium and subendothelial tissue, increased intraplaque pressure resulting from infiltration of blood or other mechanisms, and coronary vasospasm. Factors to be considered in the development of coronary artery thrombosis are platelet aggregation; local increase of catecholamines; autonomic neural influences; and local alterations in fibrinolytic systems related to potential decreases in prostacyclin, tissue plasminogen-activating factor, and/or endothelial relaxing factor at sites of coronary artery stenosis and endothelial injury and to increases in thromboxane A_2 and serotonin released from aggregating platelets and/or infiltrating white blood cells at the same sites. Local increases in thromboxane A_2 and serotonin promote platelet aggregation and potentially are capable of altering coronary artery tone dynamically by increasing coronary vascular resistance, thereby decreasing coronary blood flow.

It also seems plausible that coronary artery thrombosis may develop without plaque disruption in severely stenotic coronary arteries. Experimental studies in canine models show increased coronary vascular resistance and reduced reflow in the necrotic or severely damaged subendocardium after 90 to 120 minutes of coronary artery occlusion. Coronary collateral flow may sometimes compensate for acute coronary thrombosis so that no important myocardial necrosis results. It seems likely that variations in the extent of generalized coronary atherosclerosis and of coronary collateral flow may influence the extent and location of acute infarction subsequent to acute coronary thrombosis.

Sudden cardiac death syndromes and acute myocardial infarction are usually separate entities with differing pathogenesis, since the majority of patients resuscitated from sudden death do not develop evidence of important myocardial infarction. Sudden cardiac death usually is caused by a primary ventricular arrhythmia, usually ventricular tachycardia or fibrillation, often produced by an acute ischemic event but not involving major coronary thrombosis, or it may be caused by ventricular ectopy occurring against a background of chronic coronary artery disease and ventricular scarring, but not necessarily triggered by acute myocardial ischemia.

RECOGNITION OF ACUTE MYOCARDIAL INFARCTS. ***History.*** The history is of the utmost importance in the recognition of acute myocardial infarction. Typically, the chest pain is severe and usually lasts until the patient receives analgesic medication from a physician. The pain is ordinarily described as being substernal or left precordial and as a "heaviness" or "tightness," or "like a weight on my chest," and is often associated with nausea and diaphoresis. The chest pain may radiate to the back, the neck, the jaw, or the left arm, particularly down its ulnar aspect. Occasionally, the pain may exist only in the back, the jaw, the left arm, or the neck. Chest pain in patients with acute myocardial infarcts generally lasts longer than 30 minutes and is typically the most severe pain an individual has experienced. Many patients have unstable angina pectoris for hours to days prior to their acute myocardial infarcts; by contrast, 10 to 20 per cent of patients have "silent," i.e., painless or relatively painless, infarcts. Painless infarction is noted with special frequency in diabetic patients and following cardiac transplantation.

Physical Examination. GENERAL. Patients with small myocardial infarcts, particularly non–Q wave infarcts, may not have detectable abnormalities on physical examination. At the other extreme, patients with more than 40 per cent irreversible cellular damage to the left ventricle often develop severe left ventricular failure with pulmonary edema and cardiogenic shock.

INSPECTION AND PALPATION. The findings depend on the extent of the myocardial damage. Most patients are in obvious discomfort. They are often diaphoretic, pale, and extremely anxious. Those with extensive damage develop a reduction in systemic arterial blood pressure ranging from mild to severe. Cardiogenic shock is defined as hypotension resulting from extensive myocardial damage with evidence of inadequate systemic perfusion, such as cool skin, mental confusion, and oliguria. Patients with extensive myocardial necrosis may also have an alternating force of their pulse (pulsus alternans). Most patients have frequent ventricular premature beats.

Patients with second- or third-degree atrioventricular block may have intermittent cannon A waves in their jugular venous pulse. Patients with atrial fibrillation lack an A wave and have an irregular pulse. Patients with right ventricular failure usually have an increased jugular venous pressure.

AUSCULTATION. Fourth heart sounds are almost invariably heard, and all the heart sounds are usually soft. When the mitral valve apparatus is damaged, a new murmur of mitral insufficiency may be audible. These murmurs have variable auscultatory characteristics and may occur in mid to late systole or be holosystolic. Acute mitral insufficiency occurs most commonly in patients with inferior, lateral, or subendocardial myocardial infarcts. Patients with inferior myocardial infarcts and structural damage to the tricuspid valve may develop tricuspid insufficiency. Rupture of the interventricular septum occurs most commonly in patients with acute anterior myocardial infarcts. Murmurs resulting from ventricular septal defects are located along the lower left sternal border and are holosystolic. They may radiate toward the cardiac apex. Acute interventricular septal defects are often associated with a systolic thrill along the left sternal border. The distinction between a holosystolic murmur caused by acute mitral insufficiency and a ruptured septum is not always clear on physical examination.

Third heart sounds may occur in patients with ventricular filling pressures of 15 mm Hg or greater (ventricular failure) or in those with at least moderately severe mitral insufficiency. The second heart sound is paradoxically split in some patients with left ventricular failure, in some with left bundle branch block, and in some during chest pain. The pulmonic closure sound is increased in intensity in patients with pulmonary hypertension resulting from left ventricular failure. Pericardial friction rubs are detected in less than 10 per cent of patients with acute myocardial infarcts. Patients with audible pericardial friction rubs are ordinarily those with the largest Q wave infarcts. If large pericardial effusions develop, heart sounds may be distant and the jugular venous pressure is elevated. Cardiac tamponade results in shock, pulsus paradoxus, distant heart sounds, and an elevated jugular venous pressure. Bibasilar or more extensive moist rales develop in patients with left ventricular failure. Pulmonary edema occurs with extensive myocardial infarction and in patients with myocardial ischemia superimposed on extensive myocardial infarction. Evidence of reduced peripheral perfusion accompanied by clear lungs and an elevated jugular venous pressure should raise the question of extensive right ventricular infarction in the patient with an inferior myocardial infarct.

Electrocardiographic Diagnosis. The electrocardiogram (ECG) provides an excellent means for recognition of acute Q wave myocardial infarction (Figs. 51–2 to 51–4). The characteristic sequence of ECG alterations with Q wave infarction is as follows: (1) the initial development of prominent, peaked T waves in the ECG leads, representing sites of epicardial injury; (2) the development of hyperacute ST segment elevation; and (3) the development of significant Q waves, i.e., of 0.04 second in duration, and/or loss of more than 30 per cent of the amplitude of the R wave (Fig. 51–2). The rate of evolution of these ECG changes is variable; they may occur in minutes or may be delayed for several hours. Some patients with acute myocardial infarcts have relatively normal electrocardiograms in the first few hours after the event. Problems in using the ECG to identify acute myocardial infarction are

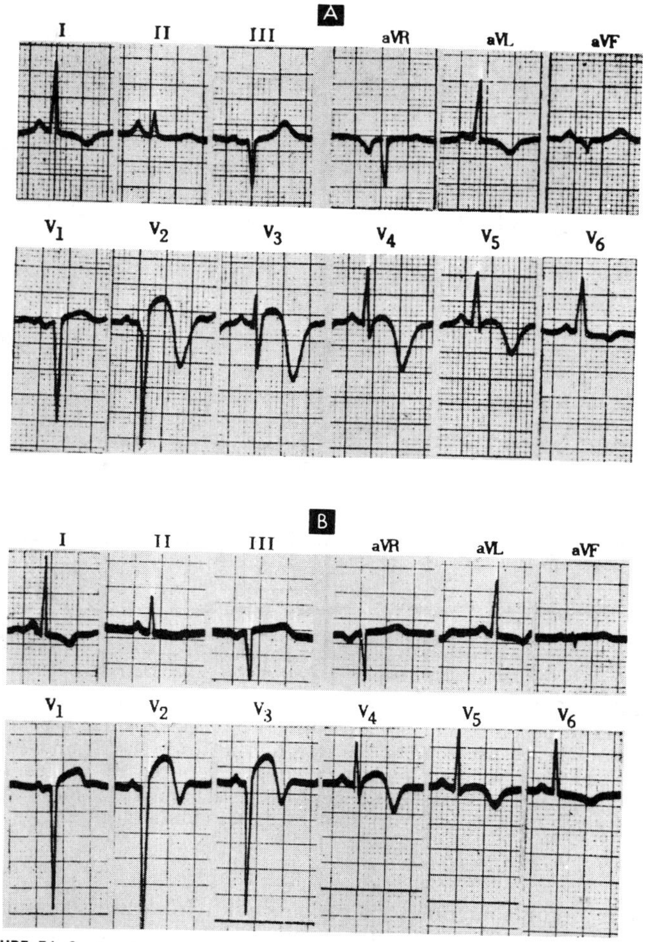

FIGURE 51–2. Acute anteroseptal myocardial infarction. Panel *A* was obtained on the day of hospitalization and demonstrates inverted T waves in V_2 through V_5 and a Q wave in V_2. Panel *B* was obtained three days later and shows further evolutionary changes compatible with an acute anteroseptal myocardial infarction. (Reproduced by permission from Lipman BS, Massie E, Kleiger RE: Clinical Scalar Electrocardiography. 6th ed. Chicago, Year Book Medical Publishers, 1979.)

as follows: (1) In patients with left bundle branch block, acute anterior myocardial infarcts are not recognized by the ECG; (2) in patients with previous Q wave infarction, recognition of new injury can be difficult; and (3) in individuals in whom rapid ECG evolution occurs, it may not be possible to differentiate old from new myocardial infarction. ST segment elevation may also occur (1) with normal early repolarization (Fig. 51–3); (2) with transient myocardial ischemia, as in Prinzmetal's angina or with ischemia in an area of previous myocardial damage; (3) in some individuals with chronic ventricular aneurysms; (4) transiently, following electrical cardioversion; (5) in the anterior precordial ECG leads in patients with left bundle branch block; (6) in patients with left ventricular hypertrophy; and (7) in some patients with hyperkalemia.

In contrast to the usefulness of the ECG in the recognition of Q wave myocardial infarcts, the ECG does not allow one to recognize acute non–Q wave myocardial infarction with certainty. The ECG demonstrates ST depression and T wave inversion with non–Q wave myocardial infarction; the only evolution is a return toward baseline. Unfortunately, subendocardial ischemia, ventricular hypertrophy, rapid heart rates, emotional influences, electrolyte alterations, and the use of certain medications, including cardiac glycosides, may produce the same ECG changes. Indeed, bizarre T wave altera-

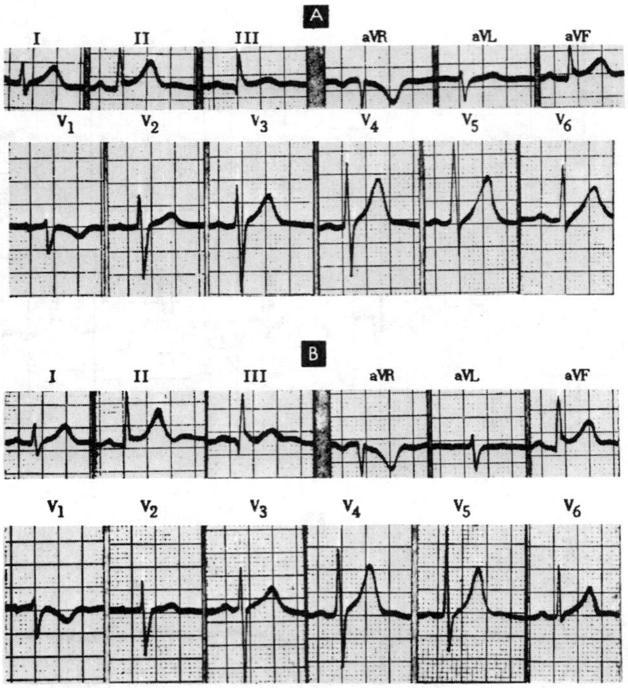

FIGURE 51–3. Normal early repolarization. The electrocardiograms obtained in panels *A* and *B* were taken two weeks apart in a patient without heart disease. The ST elevation in leads II, III, and AVF represent normal early repolarization. (Reproduced by permission from Lipman BS, Massie E, Kleiger RE: Clinical Scalar Electrocardiography. 6th ed. Chicago, Year Book Medical Publishers, 1979.)

tions occur sometimes in patients with intracranial hemorrhage. The only useful rule in the ECG recognition of non–Q wave myocardial infarction is that the deeper the ST segment depression and the longer it lasts, the more likely the presence of myocardial infarction.

Serum Enzyme Changes. Currently, the preferred enzymatic technique for detection of myocardial infarction is the measurement of creatine kinase (CK) and in particular the "myocardial specific" CK-MB isoenzyme measured by spectrophotometric, fluorometric, or radioimmunoassay technique. CK-MB increases in the sera of patients approximately 2 to 4 hours after acute myocardial infarction, peaks within 12 hours with small or reperfused infarcts and between 16 and 24 hours with large or non-reperfused infarcts, and often returns to normal within 24 to 36 hours after the event. Radioimmunoassay measurement of alterations in serum myoglobin concentration allows slightly earlier recognition of acute myocardial infarction, but at present there is no means to distinguish between myoglobin release from the heart and from the skeletal muscle when both are injured. Radioimmunoassay measurement of alterations in the serum concentration of the light chain of myosin may also allow a relatively early recognition of acute myocardial infarction. In the past, serial serum measurements of glutamic-oxaloacetic transaminase (SGOT), lactic dehydrogenase (LDH), or the LDH isoenzymes were used to recognize acute myocardial infarction.

Myocardial Scintigraphy. The use of radionuclide scintigraphic techniques to recognize acute myocardial infarction has gained in popularity (see Ch. 41.4). These techniques allow one to see the region or regions of acute myocardial infarction (infarct-avid imaging techniques) or to identify areas of severely decreased myocardial perfusion (cold spot imaging techniques). The prototype infarct-avid imaging agent is technetium 99m stannous pyrophosphate. This agent accumulates in irreversibly damaged myocardium one to five days after infarction; its sensitivity in the detection of acute infarction of 3 grams or larger is greater than 90 per cent when tomographic imaging is utilized. Thallium 201 is the perfusion imaging agent of choice at present. When used within 12 hours after acute infarction, its sensitivity is approximately 90 per cent. The extent of the initial ^{201}Tl defect and the volume of pyrophosphate uptake after acute myocardial infarction have prognostic significance; the larger the volume of pyrophosphate uptake or of the ^{201}Tl perfusion defect, the poorer the in-hospital prognosis. Finally, one may employ technetium-labelled red blood cells to evaluate the impact of acute myocardial infarction on regional and global ventricular function, using "dynamic myocardial scintigraphy." This technique allows one to measure or identify ventricular ejection fraction, ventricular volumes, regional wall motion, left-to-right shunts (i.e., ventricular septal defects), ventricular aneurysms, and valvular insufficiency, including mitral or tricuspid regurgitation.

DIFFERENTIAL DIAGNOSIS. The differential diagnosis of acute myocardial infarction theoretically includes every cause of chest pain, cardiac arrhythmia, and heart failure. Important diagnostic considerations are (1) unstable angina pectoris, (2) variant (Prinzmetal's) angina, and (3) dissecting aortic aneurysm. Less common as difficult diagnoses to exclude, but still sometimes important to differentiate, are (1) peptic ulcer disease, (2) pancreatitis, (3) cholecystitis, (4) pulmonary embolic disease, (5) spontaneous pneumothorax, (6) pericarditis, and (7) pneumonitis. Careful attention to the history and physical examination and the proper use of

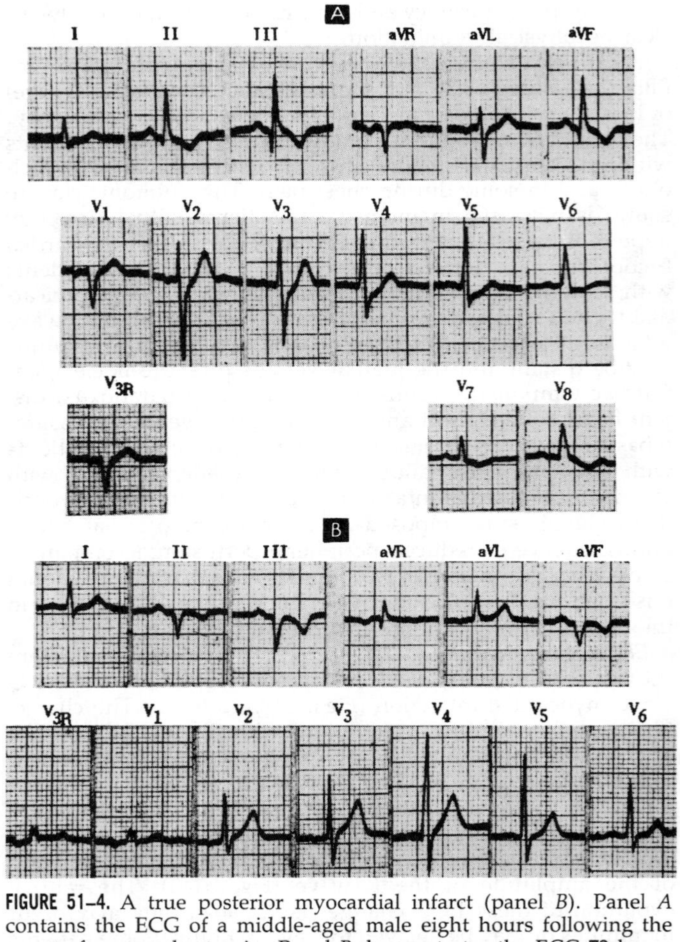

FIGURE 51–4. A true posterior myocardial infarct (panel *B*). Panel *A* contains the ECG of a middle-aged male eight hours following the onset of severe chest pain. Panel *B* demonstrates the ECG 72 hours later, at which time prominent R waves have developed in precordial leads V_1 and V_2. Panel *B* also demonstrates an acute inferior transmural myocardial infarct.

relevant blood tests, electrocardiograms, and myocardial scintigraphy usually allow one to make the proper diagnosis.

COMPLICATIONS OF ACUTE MYOCARDIAL INFARCTS. *Mechanical Complications.* Patients with cardiogenic shock as a consequence of extensive left ventricular damage occurring with acute myocardial infarction have a poor prognosis. Cardiac assistance devices such as intra-aortic balloon counterpulsation have reduced mortality slightly in patients with acute myocardial infarcts and cardiogenic shock, particularly when coupled with coronary artery revascularization or ventricular aneurysmectomy. However, the extent of myocardial damage is generally so severe that a majority of these patients still succumb.

An important complication of acute myocardial infarction is infarct extension or expansion. Approximately 10 per cent of patients extend their myocardial infarcts within the first five days. The incidence is slightly higher for those with anterior Q wave infarcts and those with subendocardial ischemia or non–Q wave infarction or both at hospital admission, and the consequences of infarct extension for patients in these groups are more serious. The incidence of infarct extension is approximately twice as high when assessed by laboratory methods as by clinical symptoms alone. Infarct expansion (dilatation of the infarct region secondary to stress-and-strain relationships) may be associated with worsening ventricular function and increased morbidity and mortality.

Other mechanical problems that may complicate acute myocardial infarction include papillary muscle dysfunction or rupture with consequent acute mitral regurgitation, and the development of a ventricular septal defect. Rupture of an entire papillary muscle is ordinarily fatal within minutes to hours owing to massive mitral regurgitation, which results in severe left ventricular failure and cardiogenic shock. Rupture of one head of a papillary muscle may be tolerated for longer periods of time, allowing clinical evaluation and occasionally surgical correction. Partial or complete rupture of a papillary muscle occurs in less than 5 per cent of patients with acute infarction. Dysfunction of a papillary muscle occurs more commonly when ischemia or infarction of the papillary muscle prevents proper coaptation of the mitral leaflets, causing mitral regurgitation. Patients with papillary muscle dysfunction generally have milder left ventricular failure and are responsive to medical intervention. Patients who develop acute mitral insufficiency usually do so within one to seven days after acute myocardial infarction.

Rupture of a portion of the ventricular septum is usually associated with a holosystolic murmur and systolic thrill along the left sternal border. Ventricular septal defects develop in about 1 per cent of patients with acute myocardial infarcts and often result in right and left ventricular failure. They may occur within hours or as late as 10 to 12 days following infarction. If ventricular failure is severe, one must consider emergency surgical correction even though surgical mortality rates are highest within the first month after myocardial infarction. Afterload reduction using intra-aortic balloon counterpulsation or pharmacologic means, or both, may benefit patients with ventricular septal defects or mitral regurgitation occurring acutely after myocardial infarction.

Ventricular aneurysms usually develop within hours of myocardial infarction and may enlarge over subsequent weeks or months. If sizable, they may result in congestive heart failure. They may also be associated with ventricular arrhythmias or with mural thrombosis and systemic embolization. Left ventricular endocardial thrombi can be demonstrated in at least 50 per cent of patients with ventricular aneurysms at autopsy.

Right ventricular infarction develops occasionally in patients with inferoposterior myocardial infarction. Occasionally, right ventricular involvement may be sufficient to cause systemic hypotension with low pulmonary capillary wedge and left ventricular filling pressures. Alternatively, extensive right ventricular infarction may simulate a large pericardial effusion and cardiac tamponade. Recognition is important, since proper therapy includes fluid administration, which is not usually employed in the hypotensive patient with a dominant left ventricular infarct. Right ventricular infarction may also lead to tricuspid valvular insufficiency secondary to papillary muscle dysfunction.

Arrhythmias and Heart Block. More than 90 per cent of patients develop ventricular premature beats in the first 72 hours after acute myocardial infarction. Ventricular premature beats can be suppressed by pharmacologic intervention in most patients. However, in those with large infarcts, they may be difficult to suppress, and death may occur because of medically refractory arrhythmias.

Various types of atrioventricular and intraventricular blocks (see Ch. 45) may occur as a consequence of acute myocardial infarction. First-degree heart block is common with acute inferior infarction, and as an isolated finding, it is not a cause for concern. Second-degree heart block of the Mobitz I type (Wenckebach block) also occurs following acute inferior infarction. It is usually transient, and even if it progresses to complete heart block, it is usually only temporary. Temporary pacemaker insertion is indicated only in patients with Mobitz I block who have slow ventricular rates resulting in syncope, congestive heart failure, angina pectoris, or ventricular arrhythmias. Mobitz II heart block occurs most often as a consequence of anterior myocardial infarction. The level of block is located below the atrioventricular junction within the ventricle. Mobitz II block should be treated with a pacemaker as soon as it is recognized. Permanent pacing is indicated in such patients at a later date.

Complete heart block may develop abruptly or follow either of the two forms of second-degree heart block described above. Complete heart block complicating acute anterior myocardial infarction is often permanent and usually requires permanent pacing. It often coexists with other signs of a large infarct, and the subsequent prognosis is poor. Complete heart block after inferior myocardial infarction is ordinarily only transient, and temporary ventricular pacing almost always suffices.

Acute left bundle branch block ordinarily develops as a consequence of a large anterior myocardial infarction. The risk of complete heart block in patients who develop left bundle branch block with acute infarction is approximately 40 per cent, and many physicians elect to insert a temporary pacemaker prophylactically. The acute development of right bundle branch block is not a reflection of infarct size and does not necessarily indicate a high risk of complete heart block. Bilateral bundle branch block (left-axis deviation and right bundle branch block, right-axis deviation and right bundle branch block, or first-degree atrioventricular block and left bundle branch block) that develops acutely after myocardial infarction indicates a large infarct and a relatively poor prognosis with a high risk of complete heart block. These patterns develop most commonly with anterior infarction, and temporary pace-makers should be inserted. Many patients who develop acute bilateral bundle branch block die as a consequence of a low-output state. Those patients who survive and have even transient atrioventricular block in the hospital should be paced permanently.

Other Complications. Other complications of acute myocardial infarction include (1) pericarditis, (2) pulmonary emboli, (3) lower extremity venous thrombosis, (4) systemic arterial embolization, (5) rupture of the heart, (6) Dressler's syndrome, and (7) the shoulder-hand syndrome. Pericarditis is evident clinically in 7 to 15 per cent of patients with acute infarcts. However, a higher percentage have transient pleuritic chest pain, which itself may indicate pericarditis. Pericarditis generally occurs with transmural infarcts of at least moderate size. Pericarditis may be recognized by auscultation of a pericardial friction rub, but the majority of patients with pericarditis in this setting do not have rubs. The pain of pericarditis must be distinguished from the pain of persistent angina. Anticoagulation should be avoided (if possible) in patients with pericarditis in order to minimize the risk of hemorrhagic pericardial effusion.

Pulmonary embolism is treated with heparinization followed by longer-term anticoagulation; lower extremity venous thrombosis is treated similarly. Systemic embolization is generally due to a mural thrombus developing in the damaged left ventricle, and when it occurs, anticoagulation is indicated. The visualization of a left ventricular thrombus in a patient soon after anterior myocardial infarction should also result in the administration of anticoagulants.

Rupture of the heart occurs one to ten days following infarction and is the cause of death in 2 to 15 per cent of fatal cases. Rupture is most common in patients with systemic arterial hypertension and following an initial anterior infarct. The classic clinical clue indicating myocardial rupture is "electromechanical dissociation," in which electrical activity persists without detectable blood pressure or pulse. When rupture occurs, death is ordinarily so rapid that surgical intervention is not possible. An occasional patient, however, may develop a slow leak of blood into the pericardial space, and clotting of blood may serve to compress and partially seal the tear in the heart. This may allow emergency pericardiocentesis and an attempt at surgical repair. Untreated survivors of a sealed-off rupture typically develop "false aneurysms" of the left ventricle; the "false aneurysms" have a high risk of rupture and should be repaired surgically.

Dressler's syndrome is characterized by pericarditis and pericardial effusion, pleural effusion, and often fever two weeks to nine months after myocardial infarction. The etiology of this syndrome is not clear. It is treated with aspirin or indomethacin. If these agents are unsuccessful, steroids usually relieve the chest pain, suppress the fever, and result in the ultimate disappearance of the effusions.

The shoulder-hand syndrome, of rare occurrence, consists of the development of pain and stiffness in the left shoulder or hand and vasomotor changes sometimes associated with muscle atrophy. Typically, it occurs several weeks to months after the infarct. It is believed that prolonged immobilization and bed rest used to treat patients with acute myocardial infarction in the past may have been responsible for the development of this problem.

ESTIMATION OF INFARCT SIZE. Accurate measurements of the extent of reversible and irreversible cellular damage are helpful. Such measurements should be relatively noninvasive, ideally should be applicable early in the patient's clinical course, should be capable of being repeated with reasonable frequency, should provide measurements of the extent of damage with various types of infarcts, and should be available generally. No perfect measurement of infarct size or of the extent of ischemic damage exists at present, but there are many promising developments. Included among these are (1) enzymatic indices of infarct size, including, most importantly, measurement of creatine kinase enzyme release from the heart; (2) electrocardiographic estimates of the extent of ischemic injury, including precordial electrocardiographic mapping to identify the extent of QRS alterations; (3) scintigraphic measurements of infarct size, including infarct-avid and cold spot techniques (see above); (4) dynamic myocardial scintigraphy to estimate abnormalities of global and segmental ventricular function, using either first-pass or equilibrium studies; and (5) two-dimensional echocardiography. Each of these techniques has its limitations, but each also provides important information concerning location or relative size of infarcts. For the scintigraphic measurements, it is necessary to use three-dimensional estimates of the extent of myocardial damage; tomographic cameras are available that provide three-dimensional estimates of infarct size and of the extent of perfusion defects and also allow estimates of global and regional ventricular function.

EVALUATION OF VENTRICULAR FUNCTION IN PATIENTS WITH MYOCARDIAL INFARCTS. Invasive and noninvasive techniques have been developed to allow more precise characterization of ventricular function in patients with reduced systemic arterial blood pressure and uncertain left ventricular functional status in order to assess the need for volume replacement, diuresis, or inotropic support. A flow-directed catheter, such as the Swan-Ganz catheter, allows measurement of left ventricular filling pressure without entering a systemic artery or the left ventricle. This balloon-tipped, flow-directed catheter may be placed in the pulmonary artery from a systemic vein. One positions the Swan-Ganz catheter in the pulmonary artery, either with the aid of fluoroscopy or with continuous pressure monitoring to identify the characteristic right atrial, right ventricular, and pulmonary artery pressures. Once the catheter is in the pulmonary artery, the balloon is partly inflated, allowing the measurement of pulmonary capillary wedge pressure. In the absence of mitral valve or pulmonary venous disease, the mean pulmonary capillary wedge pressure approximates the left ventricular end-diastolic or filling pressure. Measurements of left ventricular filling pressure with the Swan-Ganz catheter differentiate between hypotension because of hypovolemia and hypotension resulting from left ventricular failure. Cardiac output may also be measured. Patients with acute myocardial infarction and shock often benefit from an indwelling arterial cannula inserted to allow measurement of arterial pressure and moment-to-moment monitoring of pressure changes.

TREATMENT. Patients with proven or suspected acute myocardial infarction should be admitted to a coronary care unit, where their heart rate and rhythm are monitored continuously. In patients evaluated within the first three hours of the onset of symptoms with acute anterior Q wave myocardial infarcts, with new Q wave infarcts and previous myocardial infarction, or with new Q wave infarcts in a low-output state, thrombolytic therapy should probably be administered. Thrombolytic therapy (tissue plasminogen-activating factor, streptokinase, or urokinase) may be given intravenously or directly into the infarct-related coronary artery. When given intravenously four to five hours after the onset of symptoms suggestive of myocardial infarction, tissue plasminogen-activating factor appears superior to streptokinase in achieving thrombolysis. Successful thrombolytic therapy within the first one to two hours after the infarct appears to reduce infarct size, preserve segmental ventricular function, and reduce mortality in patients with anterior Q wave infarcts, in patients with previous infarcts, and in some patients in a low-output state. However, 20 to 30 per cent of patients develop rethrombosis of the infarct-related artery after successful thrombolytic therapy initially, despite the administration of heparin in the initial three to four days followed by warfarin or platelet-active agents (aspirin and dipyridamole) thereafter. Rethrombosis is most likely to occur in patients with the most severe, persistent residual coronary artery stenoses of the infarct-related artery.

Currently, it is not clear whether percutaneous transluminal coronary angioplasty (PTCA) should be used to dilate the infarct-related artery following thrombolytic therapy in an effort to reduce the risk of reocclusion. Future studies will probably identify a severity of residual coronary artery stenosis after thrombolytic therapy that would benefit from PTCA to prevent reocclusion of the infarct-related artery.

More than 90 per cent of patients with acute myocardial infarction have ventricular ectopy, which often requires pharmacologic suppression. Since many of the important complications of acute myocardial infarction occur in the first 96 hours after the event, it is advisable to keep patients in a coronary care unit for this period. Complete bed rest is recommended initially, followed by gradual mobilization of patients who are clinically stable. Emotional stimulation and strenuous physical effort are to be avoided. Chest pain during the initial 24 hours after the infarct is usually treated with narcotics, usually intravenous morphine or meperidine; thereafter, recurrent chest pain believed to represent angina is usually treated with nitrates, and a calcium antagonist, buffered aspirin, and/or beta blockers are used if angina persists. Recent data suggest that in-hospital infarct extension is reduced in patients with non–Q wave infarcts by the calcium antagonist diltiazem. Angina that recurs frequently at minimal activity despite nitrates, calcium antagonists, and/or beta blockers is often treated with a constant intravenous infusion of nitroglycerin. If this is unsuccessful, intra-aortic balloon counterpulsation may be used for temporary control of the angina. However, if this aggressive effort is required to control angina, one also prepares the patient for coronary arteriography, and if the coronary anatomy is suitable, PTCA or coronary artery revascularization is usually performed.

Two points of caution regarding persistent or recurrent angina at rest or at minimal effort in patients with acute myocardial infarction should be emphasized. One needs to determine that intermittent coronary spasm is not responsible for angina that occurs at rest. This determination may be accomplished by obtaining 24-hour multilead ECG monitoring, which allows identification of ST segment shifts (usually elevation) with and without anginal episodes. Such findings unassociated with preceding alterations in blood pressure or heart rate are presumptive evidence of coronary artery spasm or platelet aggregation or both at the site or sites of a severely narrowed coronary artery, causing further phasic reductions in coronary blood flow. Recurrent coronary spasm is treated with nitrates or calcium antagonists, or both, rather than with a beta blocker. Aspirin (one to four 300-mg tablets per 24 hours) may reduce the risk of reinfarction in patients with continuing angina at rest or at low levels of activity (unstable angina) after myocardial infarction. One also needs to be certain that recurrent chest pain after myocardial infarction is not due to pericarditis (which is usually treated with indomethacin or salicylates) or to some noncardiac problem such as atelectasis, pneumonia, pulmonary embolic disease, pancreatitis, peptic ulcer disease, or cholecystitis.

During the initial few hours after acute myocardial infarction, oxygen is usually administered by face mask or nasal cannula. Vital signs are checked frequently, chest pain is relieved with narcotics, and sedatives are provided as necessary. Reassurance that the chest pain will be relieved and that survival is likely is important. Specific complications of the acute myocardial infarction are recognized using the clinical criteria described earlier and the methods described in more detail later in this chapter. Anticoagulants are not administered uniformly to patients with acute myocardial infarction. Some physicians use low-dose heparin to prevent the post–myocardial infarction complications related to prolonged bed rest and restricted activity. Patients with documented left ventricular thrombi after infarction, those with embolic events, and those treated with thrombolytic therapy usually receive heparin for several days, followed by warfarin or platelet-active agents or both. Anticoagulants are relatively contraindicated in the very elderly, in patients with severe hypertension, bleeding diatheses, and peptic ulcer disease, and in those who develop pericarditis. Anticoagulants administered to patients with pericarditis complicating acute myocardial infarction may result in large hemorrhagic pericardial effusions and pericardial tamponade.

Smoking is prohibited in the coronary care unit; subsequently, one attempts to convince the patient to discontinue smoking altogether. The patient with an uncomplicated myocardial infarction is allowed to use a bedside commode, but those with shock, severe heart failure, or frequent and recurrent angina use a Foley catheter or bedpan. Stool softeners and laxatives are administered to prevent fecal impaction and to prevent the patient from straining to defecate.

Patients are allowed regular diets with the following exceptions: Extremes of hot or cold beverages are avoided in the first two or three days, salt restriction is provided for those with important heart failure, low-cholesterol diets are often used, and certain calorie and carbohydrate restrictions are provided for obese and diabetic patients, respectively. Diabetic patients receiving insulin are treated with regular insulin for the initial several days after their infarct.

Patients with uncomplicated myocardial infarction are usually discharged from the coronary care unit after three to four days to an "intermediate care" or "step down" unit. Such areas should be able to monitor heart rate and rhythm for several additional days. Most physicians begin a gradual rehabilitation program that encourages patients to be up in a chair several times a day beginning on approximately day 3 and to walk in their rooms and short distances outside their rooms by five to eight days after myocardial infarction. Patients with complications such as severe congestive heart failure, shock, important arrhythmias, or recurrent angina at rest or at low levels of effort remain in the coronary care unit until they are stable.

Some physicians recommend relatively early discharge from the hospital, even by seven or eight days after the event for patients with uncomplicated myocardial infarcts. Other physicians feel that 10 to 12 days in the hospital are indicated even for those with uncomplicated mycoardial infarcts. Patients with complicated myocardial infarctions remain in the hospital longer. Once at home, patients are gradually rehabilitated so that by four to six weeks they return to work and a more normal lifestyle. Resumption of sexual activity and mild exercise is allowed at approximately four weeks after myocardial infarction for asymptomatic patients. Angina that develops with minimal-to-moderate effort requires medical therapy with long-acting nitrates and, when appropriate, with a beta blocker or a calcium antagonist. Patients who continue to have symptoms at moderate or less effort while on good medical regimens should undergo coronary arteriography and should be considered for coronary artery revascularization. Patients, with their physicians' help, should also be encouraged to correct all risk factors, including overweight, hypercholesterolemia, cigarette smoking, and emotionally difficult circumstances. They should also be encouraged to get appropriate amounts of exercise in the future, but the exact type, duration, and level of effort should be guided by a physician. In addition, three recent studies have demonstrated that the beta-adrenergic antagonists timolol, metoprolol, and propranolol reduce mortality and the risk of reinfarction in selected patients with myocardial infarction when administered within a few hours to a few days after the myocardial infarction and continued for periods ranging from 90 days to 3 years. These beta blockers appear most protective in older patients, in those with larger and anterior infarcts, in patients with transient evidence of heart failure, and in patients with several previous infarcts. More work is needed to identify specific patients most likely to benefit from beta blocker therapy, but it appears that beta-adrenergic blockers have the potential to reduce mortality in patients with recent myocardial infarction considered to be at relatively higher risk for future coronary events. More recently, data have been provided to suggest that aspirin therapy (one 300-mg tablet) after infarction also reduces the risk of subsequent coronary events, especially in patients with well-preserved ventricular function, in patients following their initial myocardial infarction, and in patients with non–Q wave infarcts.

Protection of Ischemic Myocardium and Containment of Infarct Size. There has been considerable interest in the possibility that one may limit infarct size with pharmacologic or physiologic interventions that reduce myocardial oxygen demand, increase myocardial oxygen delivery (increase coronary blood flow), reduce inflammatory processes, reduce or retard lysosomal enzyme release, or alter metabolism or calcium influx in such a way as to prevent cell death. In experimental animals, pharmacologic interventions that increase coronary blood flow to the ischemically injured tissue (particularly the subendocardial region) have been effective in reducing the enzymatic, ECG, and morphologic indices of the size of experimentally induced myocardial infarction. Containment of infarct size depends on pharmacologic intervention within the first six hours after infarction. Beyond that time, some interventions are less successful or ineffective. In experimental animals, certain interventions may increase infarct size. This group includes those interventions that (1) increase myocardial oxygen demand, (2) divert coronary blood flow from the ischemic tissue, (3) reduce systemic arterial pressure and thereby coronary perfusion pressure, (4) alter myocardial metabolism in a detrimental manner, or (5) primarily decrease oxygen availability. In particular, the administration of isoproterenol or the development of hypotension, hypoglycemia, hypoxemia, and rapid heart rates results in an increase in infarct size in experimental animal models. Some of the interventions capable of limiting infarct size in experimental animal models are listed in Table 51–6.

Whether pharmacologic or physiologic interventions other than early thrombolytic therapy are capable of limiting infarct size in patients with acute myocardial infarction is at present unknown. In the future, continuing attention will probably be directed to determining the influence of thrombolytic therapy and selected pharmacologic interventions used together in reducing infarct size and preserving segmental and global left ventricular function.

PROGNOSIS. ***In Hospital.*** Most patients with acute myocardial infarction have an uncomplicated course. Some patients, however, develop life-threatening complications during the first one to two weeks, and others die (Table 51–7). In the early 1970s, 50 per cent or more of patients died prior to reaching the hospital; these deaths were due to ventricular arrhythmias that developed in the initial seconds or minutes following the onset of chest pain. Optimal emergency ambulance systems have achieved a 25 to 30 per cent reduction in the incidence of death prior to hospitalization in patients with acute myocardial infarction and sudden cardiac arrest syndromes.

TABLE 51–6. INTERVENTIONS CAPABLE OF LIMITING INFARCT SIZE IN EXPERIMENTAL ANIMAL MODELS

1. Interventions that reduce myocardial oxygen demand and myocardial work
   a. Beta blockers
   b. Calcium antagonists (nifedipine, verapamil, or diltiazem)
   c. Circulatory assistance (intra-aortic balloon counterpulsation)
2. Interventions that increase coronary blood flow to the damaged myocardium
   a. Nitrates (nitroglycerin)
   b. Calcium antagonists
   c. Hyperosmotic agents (hypertonic mannitol)*
   d. Hyaluronidase
   e. Corticosteroids
   f. Circulatory assistance
3. Agents that decrease inflammation, alter immunologic mechanisms, stabilize lysosomal membranes, and/or directly protect myocardial cells and sarcolemmal membranes
   a. Hyaluronidase
   b. Corticosteroids†
   c. Hypertonic agents (hypertonic mannitol)*
   d. Glucose, potassium, and insulin
   e. Cobra venom
   f. Calcium antagonists
   g. Phospholipase inhibitors
   h. Anti-inflammatory agents

*Effective for approximately one hour after experimental coronary occlusion when serum osmolality is increased by 30 to 40 mOsm.

†Given in modest dosage and only once or twice.

Table 51–7. POTENTIAL LIFE-THREATENING COMPLICATIONS OF ACUTE MYOCARDIAL INFARCTION

Ventricular arrhythmias (ventricular tachycardia, ventricular fibrillation, or asystole)
Extremely rapid atrial arrhythmias in association with extensive myocardial infarction (atrial flutter or atrial fibrillation)
Heart block (second- or third-degree types)
Marked bradycardia
Loss of atrial contribution to cardiac contraction (atrioventricular junctional rhythm)
Infarction ≧ 40 per cent of left ventricle
Extensive right ventricular infarction
Acute ventricular septal defects
Acute and severe mitral regurgitation
Severe pulmonary edema
Rupture of the heart
Systemic and/or pulmonary emboli

Overall mortality in patients with acute myocardial infarction who reach the hospital ranges from 3 to 30 per cent depending upon the population studied. In general, patients with anterior infarction have a higher mortality than patients with inferior infarction; this appears to be related to greater loss of left ventricular muscle with anterior infarcts.

Patients can be divided into groups with differing prognosis on the basis of initial hemodynamic measurements. Those without left ventricular failure and with a mean systolic arterial pressure of greater than 100 mm Hg, an average cardiac index greater than 2.5 liters per minute per square meter, and a normal pulmonary capillary wedge pressure (or pulmonary artery diastolic pressure) have relatively low mortality rates, i.e., approximately 3 to 12 per cent. Similarly, patients with left and right ventricular ejection fractions greater than 48 per cent have a relatively low in-hospital mortality risk. If death occurs in patients in these groups, it is generally from a ventricular arrhythmia, from later infarct extension, or from a mechanical complication such as myocardial, septal, or papillary muscle rupture. Patients with cardiogenic shock, including hypotension with systolic arterial pressures less than 90 mm Hg, with decreased peripheral perfusion without a reversible cause, with reduced cardiac index (less than 2.0 liters per minute per square meter), and with an increased pulmonary capillary wedge or pulmonary diastolic pressure (greater than 25 mm Hg) have a mortality of greater than 70 per cent. Those with clinical evidence of left ventricular failure and a normal or elevated systemic arterial pressure have an expected mortality rate of 5 to 30 per cent. Patients with left ventricular ejection fractions less than 40 per cent have substantially increased mortality risk in-hospital and following hospital discharge.

Following Hospital Discharge. Long-term mortality risks after recovery from an initial myocardial infarct are related to the presence of ventricular arrhythmias, the extent of myocardial damage, the presence or absence of additional myocardium at risk, and the age of the patient. Patients with left ventricular ejection fractions of 40 per cent and less are at increased risk for future coronary events and sudden deaths. Patients with eight or more ventricular premature beats per hour, coupled ventricular premature beats, and runs of ventricular tachycardia are also at increased risk of sudden death. Patients with both a left ventricular ejection fraction of 40 per cent or less and frequent or complex ventricular premature beats as defined above have an 11 times greater risk of sudden death in the ensuing six months than patients without these clinical characteristics. In addition, patients developing ST depression of 1 mm or greater or a reduction in their left ventricular ejection fraction or an increase in their left ventricular end-systolic volume at low levels of exercise prior to hospital discharge have an increased risk for new coronary events (new myocardial infarct, unstable angina, new or worsening heart failure, and sudden death) in the subsequent eight months. Similarly, patients developing reversible thallium 201 perfusion defects at low levels of exercise also are at increased risk for future coronary events. Finally, patients with previous anterior Q wave and non–Q wave infarcts also have an increased risk of subsequent myocardial infarction in the months following hospital discharge.

With regard to the patients described above, medical therapy should be developed as appropriate for the individual patient. However, when medical therapy does not prevent angina at rest, low-level exercise-induced angina, ECG changes, reductions in left ventricular ejection fractions, increases in left ventricular end-systolic volumes, or reversible perfusion defects, then cardiac catheterization with subsequent coronary revascularization should be considered.

Beta Blocker Heart Attack Study Group: The beta-blocker heart attack trial. JAMA 246:2073, 1981. *This study established the potential value of propranolol in reducing postinfarct mortality in patients.*

Buja LM, Willerson JT: Clinicopathologic correlates of acute ischemic heart disease syndromes. Am J Cardiol 47:343, 1981. *Detailed postmortem pathophysiologic correlates of anatomic and clinical relationships.*

Corbett J, Dehmer GJ, Lewis SE, et al.: The prognostic value of submaximal exercise testing with radionuclide ventriculography following acute myocardial infarction. Circulation 64:535, 1981. *This study demonstrates the prognostic value of submaximal exercise testing coupled with dynamic myocardial scintigraphy in predicting prognosis for patients after their myocardial infarcts. The scintigraphic data added substantially to the ability to predict future prognosis; measurements of alterations in ventricular function at rest and during exercise were more sensitive in predicting future prognosis than were ECG changes alone.*

Gibson RS, Watson DD, Craddock GB, et al.: Prediction of cardiac events after uncomplicated myocardial infarction: A prospective study comparing predischarge exercise thallium-201 scintigraphy and coronary angiography. Circulation 68:321, 1984. *Thallium 201 myocardial scintigraphy with submaximal exercise at hospital discharge following myocardial infarction may be used to identify patients at risk for future ischemic heart disease complications.*

Gruppo Italiano per lo Studio Della Streptochinasi Nell'infarto miocardico (GISSI): Effectiveness of intravenous thrombolytic treatment in acute myocardial infarction. Lancet 1:397, 1986.

Hjalmarson A, Herlitz J, Malek I, et al.: Effect on mortality of metoprolol in acute myocardial infarction. Lancet 2:823, 1981. *The beneficial influence of metoprolol on mortality risk in patients with recent myocardial infarction is demonstrated in this study.*

The I.S.A.M. Study Group: A prospective trial of intravenous streptokinase in acute myocardial infarction (I.S.A.M.): Mortality, morbidity, and infarct size at 21 days. N Engl J Med 314:1465, 1986. *This study provides data suggesting that intravenously administered streptokinase reduces infarct size when given to patients soon after myocardial infarction.*

Kennedy JW, Ritchie JL, Davis KB, et al.: Western Washington randomized trial of intracoronary streptokinase in acute myocardial infarction. N Engl J Med 309:1312, 1983. *Data suggest that mortality is reduced by successful thrombolytic therapy in patients with acute anterior Q wave infarcts.*

Maseri A., L'Abbate A, Baroldi G, et al.: Coronary vasospasm as a possible cause of myocardial infarction: A conclusion derived from the study of "preinfarction" angina. N Engl J Med 299:1271, 1978. *An interesting suggestion that coronary artery spasm may play a role in the pathogenesis of acute myocardial infarcts.*

Norwegian Multicenter Study Group: Timolol-induced reduction in mortality and reinfarction in patients surviving acute myocardial infarction. N Engl J Med 304:801, 1981. *This study provides evidence that timolol reduces the mortality risk and the likelihood of reinfarction when it is given chronically to patients after myocardial infarction.*

O'Neill W, Timmis G, Bourdillon P, et al.: A prospective, randomized clinical trial of intracoronary streptokinase versus coronary angioplasty for acute myocardial infarction. N Engl J Med 314:812, 1986. *Coronary angioplasty is an effective means of achieving thrombolysis acutely after myocardial infarction and also reduces the risk of postinfarction angina and protects regional ventricular function better than thrombolytic therapy alone.*

Rothkopf M, Boerner J, Stone M, et al.: Detection of myocardial infarction extension by CK-B radioimmunoassay. Circulation 59:268, 1979. *The frequency with which in-hospital extension of acute myocardial infarcts occurs is described in this study.*

The TIMI Study Group: Thrombolysis in myocardial infarction (TIMI Trial): Phase I findings. N Engl J Med 312:932, 1985. *Intravenously-administered tissue plasminogen-activating factor is superior to streptokinase in achieving thrombolysis when given approximately five hours after the event.*

Wackers FJ, Busemann S, Samson G, et al.: Value and limitations of thallium-201 scintigraphy in the acute phase of myocardial infarction. N Engl J Med 295:1, 1975. *A description of the advantages and limitations of a "cold spot" imaging technique, thallium-201 myocardial scintigraphy, in infarct recognition.*

Willerson JT, Parkey RW, Bonte FJ, et al.: Technetium stannous pyrophosphate myocardial scintigrams in patients with chest pain of varying etiology. Circulation 51:1046, 1975. *The applications and usefulness of an infarct-avid myocardial imaging technique, technetium 99m stannous pyrophosphate, in the recognition of acute myocardial infarcts are described.*

51.3 Surgical Treatment of Coronary Artery Disease

David C. Sabiston, Jr.

The development of coronary artery bypass grafts (CABG) has made a remarkable impact upon the management of ischemic heart disease. Each year some 800,000 patients in the United States survive an acute myocardial infarction, and approximately 175,000 undergo CABG. Complete relief of anginal pain is achieved in more than two thirds of patients following operation, and the life expectancy is increased in specific groups.

The *natural history* of coronary atherosclerosis is important in selecting therapy, since many factors are of prognostic significance. These include the number of coronary arteries involved, the severity of the lesions, the status of left ventricular function, and the presence of associated cardiac or systemic disorders. The prognosis of patients with angina is adversely affected by a familial history of coronary artery disease, cigarette smoking, hypertension, diabetes, and obesity.

SELECTION OF PATIENTS FOR SURGICAL THERAPY. Surgical management is usually indicated in patients with chronic stable angina in whom medical therapy has failed and in whom it is desirable to provide the highest likelihood of relief of myocardial ischemia. Moreover, CABG improves survival in those with left main coronary lesions as well as in patients with proximal left anterior descending (LAD) disease as a part of two-vessel disease and those with a positive exercise test for ischemia with two- or three-vessel disease (Table 51–8). Patients with left ventricular dysfunction also show improvement in wall motion following CABG. *Medical therapy* is better than or equal to surgical management in patients without evidence of myocardial ischemia and in those with one- or two-vessel disease without proximal LAD lesions, since long-term survival is not appreciably different.

In the selection of patients for CABG, noninvasive radionuclide angiocardiography is useful in assessment. This rapid, safe, and relatively simple technique makes possible an objective evaluation of ventricular function, including end-systolic and end-diastolic ventricular volumes, ejection fraction, cardiac output, and left ventricular wall motion. These parameters may be determined both at rest and during exercise. Patients with significant coronary artery disease may have essentially normal values at rest, but deterioration of cardiac function follows exercise. Thallium scans also quantify ventricular function and demonstrate abnormalities of wall motion. These techniques demonstrate the type, location, and extent of myocardial perfusion abnormalities and are often predictive of the role of CABG. Many now consider these techniques more reliable than exercise electrocardiography.

Coronary arteriography is essential in the selection of patients for CABG. Diseased vessels to be grafted should have a

TABLE 51–8. MEDICAL VERSUS SURGICAL MANAGEMENT OF PATIENTS WITH CHRONIC STABLE ANGINA

Surgical management better than medical therapy for
1. Relief of myocardial ischemia
2. Improving long-term survival in
   - Left main coronary artery disease
   - Three-vessel disease
   - Proximal left anterior descending disease (part of two-vessel disease)
   - Positive exercise test for ischemia in two- or three-vessel disease
3. Symptoms and pharmacologic therapy of ischemia
4. Left ventricular dysfunction due to myocardial ischemia

Adapted from Rahimtoola SH: A perspective on the three large multicenter randomized clinical trials of CABG for chronic stable angina. Circulation 72(Suppl V):123, 1985.

reasonable lumen (1.0 to 1.5 mm in diameter) and evidence of distal runoff indicative of a patent peripheral coronary bed. However, vessels that do not opacify distally may be found at operation to be patent. Both cardiac catheterization and noninvasive radionuclide arteriography provide helpful data for assessment of ventricular function. Certain features are apt to be associated with an increased surgical risk, including cardiomegaly, low ejection fraction (below 25 per cent), an increased left ventricular volume, large arteriovenous oxygen difference (greater than 6 volumes per cent), and an elevated left ventricular end-diastolic pressure. However, the presence of any one or a combination of these abnormalities does not necessarily represent a contraindication to operation or preclude a successful postoperative result.

Left ventricular *aneurysms* may follow myocardial infarction and are hazardous both for the paradoxical dilatation during systole, which makes the heart more inefficient, and as a source of systemic arterial emboli. These aneurysms may also be the site of electrical instability and may incite refractory dysrhythmias. Patients with aneurysms may also have coexisting valvular disease, which may further increase surgical risk.

Patients with *unstable angina* may be candidates for urgent CABG. Some patients can be managed by intensive pharmacologic therapy, but CABG may be preferable if the anginal pain is not rapidly controlled. Moreover, it has been shown in several series that patients with unstable angina initially treated by medical therapy ultimately require CABG. This fact became clear in the Coronary Artery Surgery Study (CASS), in which more than one third of patients ultimately required CABG. In a recent study of 100 consecutive patients with atypical angina on the coronary care unit, relief of anginal pain could not be obtained despite the use of intravenous nitroglycerin, propranolol, and nifedipine, and therefore CABG was performed. In this group, 52 had a myocardial infarction (6 hours to 30 days prior to operation) and 75 had serious disease as exhibited by either left main or three-vessel coronary disease or an ejection fraction less than 45 per cent. The operative mortality was only 4 per cent, and survival at one year was 90 per cent, showing that the procedure can be done in severely ill patients with superior results (Rankin, 1984).

Acute myocardial infarction may be associated with several complications requiring surgical therapy. An acquired ventricular septal defect (VSD) occurs in 1 to 2 per cent of patients with myocardial infarction, and the prognosis is poor, the survival being only 20 per cent at two months without operation. Surgical closure is indicated in nearly all patients, and it is preferable to allow healing of the infarct to permit the edges of the defect to become fibrotic and enable a better operative repair. Intractable cardiac failure may appear early and may require urgent operation. Multiple VSD's are present in approximately a third of these patients and should be carefully sought. The defects are generally closed with a plastic prosthesis, and CABG may be necessary to improve coronary blood flow. If early operation is mandatory, the results are less favorable than in patients able to survive for several weeks and undergo an elective procedure.

SURGICAL PROCEDURES. The techniques for CABG have progressively improved since the first use of a saphenous vein bypass graft for coronary disease in 1962 (Sabiston). Originally, most patients had autologous vein grafts, but the use of the internal mammary artery graft has dramatically increased in the past several years owing to improved long-term patency. It is preferable to use one or both internal mammary arteries in nearly all CABG procedures with venous grafts as necessary. It is important that the internal mammary artery be dissected with a sufficient pedicle of tissue to preserve the vasa vasorum and thus the blood supply of the arterial wall. Extracorporeal circulation is used with moderate *total body hypothermia,* and the temperature of the heart is further lowered by infusion of a potassium solution at 4°C to produce cardioplegia. To maintain a myocardial temperature of 10 to 15°C, cold saline or ice slush topically surrounds the heart. Intracoronary injection of potassium solution eliminates cardiac contraction and further reduces myocardial metabolism to a very low level. The motionless heart and bloodless operative field are ideal for performing the best coronary anastomoses. The use of very fine, monofilament sutures, often placed with the use of magnifying lenses, has been helpful in achieving long-term patency. Comparative data also show that *all* major coronary arteries with significant stenoses should be grafted. In addition, branches of the primary vessels are also frequently bypassed beyond significant stenoses. Approximately four grafts are currently inserted in the average patient.

The *surgical mortality* for CABG varies in accordance with the severity of the disease. The CASS randomized multicenter evaluation study sponsored by the National Institutes of Health (1975 to 1979) demonstrated a very low mortality in patients considered good risks. For those with Class I and Class II angina, who are less than 65 years of age, who do not have a history of congestive heart failure or previous CABG, and who have an ejection fraction greater than 35 per cent, the surgically treated group had an annual mortality for single-, double-, and triple-vessel disease of 0.8, 0.8, and 1.2 per cent, respectively, compared with an annual mortality in medically managed patients of 1.1, 0.6, and 1.2 per cent, respectively. In more recent series, the surgical mortality in patients undergoing CABG who do not have significant associated cardiac conditions is generally 1 per cent or less. In addition, attention must be given to the fact that medical therapy has also improved with greater utilization of agents such as nitrates, beta blockers, and calcium channel blockers.

POSTOPERATIVE MANAGEMENT. A number of postoperative problems may arise in patients following CABG and require prompt diagnosis and immediate therapy. Adequate oxygenation is essential, and ventilatory support should be assessed by blood gas P_{O_2}, P_{CO_2}, and pH. The cardiac output should be maintained at a normal level by continuous monitoring of central venous pressure, systemic arterial pressure, the electrocardiogam, and urinary output. Should the *low cardiac output syndrome* develop, dopamine, dobutamine, and other agents should be employed as necessary. In many patients, the pulmonary artery diastolic pressure, as well as left atrial pressure, should be continuously monitored through an indwelling catheter placed at operation. Cardiac dysrhythmias occur and may require the use of appropriate drugs, pacing, or electrical cardioversion. Temporary pacing wires should be placed at operation.

Certain special complications occur following CABG, such as perioperative myocardial infarction (2 to 5 per cent), and cause hypotension and cardiac conduction defects. Most postoperative infarctions are limited and only occasionally are associated with serious clinical symptoms. Cardiac dysrhythmias and pericarditis usually respond well to appropriate medication. A serious postoperative complication (about 1 per cent) is *mediastinitis,* which should be managed aggressively with open drainage and, in some instances, by placement of pedicle grafts.

RESULTS. In nearly all series, relief of pain is complete in approximately two thirds of patients following CABG, with pain in the remainder of patients being much improved. Early assessments at rest and at exercise show improvement of left ventricular function in the first week following CABG. Although CABG does not prevent subsequent myocardial infarction, if such occurs, the infarcts are smaller and have fewer untoward effects.

In all series following CABG, *graft patency* is critical to long-term prognosis. Approximately 85 per cent of patients have patent anastomoses at one year, with an attrition rate in the general range of 2 per cent annually. In one large series, the patency rate of saphenous vein grafts followed for five years or longer was 47 per cent, whereas that of the internal mammary artery grafts during the same period was 90 per cent (Lytle). Therefore, use of the internal mammary artery graft is indicated in nearly all patients.

The role of platelets and platelet inhibitors in the long-term patency of coronary grafts is of major significance, and long-term administration of aspirin and dipyridamole is clearly effective in reducing graft occlusion. Postoperatively, dipyridamole* should be given at a dose of 75 mg three times a day and aspirin* at a dosage of 325 mg three times a day orally and should be continued indefinitely.

Late graft changes include intimal fibrosis, which reduces luminal caliber or may produce complete obstruction. The graft may also thrombose, and this is generally the cause of early failure. In addition, technical difficulties at the site of the anastomosis, such as kinking, can produce obstruction. A distinctive *fibrous proliferation* also occurs. The basic atherosclerotic process may progress in the coronary arteries, and in one series followed one to four years postoperatively with repeat coronary arteriography, 55 per cent of the original lesions proximal to the graft progressed and 14 per cent of the ungrafted vessels showed progression (McLaughlin).

REOPERATION. Should the symptoms of angina pectoris reappear and coronary arteriography provide evidence that there is either occlusion of previous grafts or an increase in the severity of the original disease, consideration may be given to reoperation. Although the technical procedure is somewhat more difficult, favorable results can nevertheless be predicted in the majority of patients. In one series of 1000 consecutive patients undergoing reoperation, the surgical mortality declined from 5 per cent early in the series to 2 per cent. During the same time, the number of grafts placed at the second operation increased from 1.4 to 2.3 (Loop). The five-year actuarial survival for patients was 89 per cent and was affected by the extent of disease and preoperative level of ventricular performance.

PERCUTANEOUS TRANSLUMINAL CORONARY ANGIOPLASTY. Gruentzig introduced percutaneous transluminal coronary angioplasty (PTCA) in 1977, and it has since become an increasingly useful procedure for patients with coronary artery disease. During the past decade, this technique has assumed an important role in the management of both *chronic myocardial ischemia* and *acute myocardial infarction*, especially in association with the intracoronary administration of thrombolytic agents. Tissue plasminogen activator (TPA), which is a recombinant human tissue-type plasminogen activator and is associated with minimal toxic reactions, can be given with favorable results. Although originally PTCA was reserved for patients with early symptoms, single-vessel disease, short segmental stenoses, and favorable anatomy, on the basis of wider use, the indications have increased to include more severe disease and multiple lesions. Current estimates indicate that some 70,000 PTCA procedures are being done annually. Better guide wires, angioplastic catheters, larger balloons (3.5 mm), and greater experience have been responsible for this escalation and for an 80 to 90 per cent success rate. In approximately 5 per cent of patients, clinical deterioration occurs, with evidence of ischemia, angina, and ST segment changes. Appropriate intervention with pharmacologic agents, as well as further attempts to open stenotic lesions, is indicated, but emergency CABG may be necessary. If symptoms reappear several days to weeks later, such may be due to coronary arterial spasm and may be relieved by calcium channel–blocking agents. If symptoms continue, coronary arteriography should be repeated, with determination of whether a further angioplastic procedure is indicated or if CABG is needed. Following PTCA, patients should be given platelet-inhibiting drugs, including dipyridamole* and aspirin,* indefinitely.

*This use is not listed in the manufacturer's directive.

LONG-TERM SURVIVAL. The results of several randomized studies on the effect of CABG are available. The first convincing evidence that CABG improved longevity in patients with myocardial ischemia was the Veterans Administration Cooperative Study of patients with significant lesions of the *left main coronary artery*. The data showed that the survival of surgically treated patients at 3½ years was 88 per cent, whereas in those treated medically the survival was 65 per cent (Takaro). For patients with *three-vessel disease*, surgical management has generally been associated with increased survival, most impressively in the European Prospective Randomized Coronary Surgery Study. An eight-year follow-up in this series showed that patients managed surgically have an 89 per cent survival compared with 80 per cent for those managed medically. In the CASS Study, the survival at five years was 94 per cent in surgically managed patients compared with 82 per cent among those medically managed. The figures at the end of eight years were 92 per cent and 77 per cent, respectively (Rahimtoola).

*This use is not listed in the manufacturer's directive.

Austin EH, Odlham HN Jr, Sabiston DC Jr, et al.: Early assessment of rest and exercise following coronary artery surgery. Ann Thorac Surg 35:159, 1983. *In this study, significant improvement in left ventricular performance in patients following CABG was demonstrated at one week.*

Beller GA, Gibson RS, Watson DD: Radionuclide methods of identifying patients who may require coronary artery bypass surgery. Circulation 72 (Suppl V):V-9, 1985. *An excellent review of patient selection for CABG. The role of radionuclide technique in determining the type, location, and extent of coronary perfusion abnormalities as well as the status of myocardial performance in patients with angina pectoris.*

Chesbro JH, Clements IP, Fuster V, et al.: A platelet-inhibitor-drug trial in coronary-artery bypass operations: Benefit of perioperative dipyridamole and aspirin therapy on early postoperative vein-graft patency. N Engl J Med 307:73, 1982. *An excellent randomized study demonstrating the value of aspirin and dipyridamole maintaining long-term patency of coronary artery bypass grafts.*

Crean PA, Waters DD, Bosch X, et al.: Angiographic findings after myocardial infarction in patients with previous bypass surgery: Explantations for smaller infarcts in this group compared with control patients. Circulation 71:693, 1985. *A careful study of a series with myocardial infarction and CABG compared with controls. Those with CABG had smaller and less significant infarctions.*

Fuster V, Chesbro JH: Role of platelets and platelet inhibitors in aortocoronary artery vein-graft disease. Circulation 73:227, 1986. *Recent confirmatory evidence for use of platelet inhibitors to improve long-term graft patency.*

Gold HK, Fallon JT, Yasuda T, et al.: Coronary thrombolysis with recombinant human tissue-type plasminogen activator. Circulation 70:700, 1984. *The role of this relatively nontoxic and effective fibrinolysin is discussed.*

Jones RH, Floyd RD, Austin EH, et al.: The role of radionuclide angiocardiography in the preoperative prediction of pain relief and prolonged survival following coronary artery bypass grafting. Ann Surg 197:743, 1983. *An evaluation of the usefulness of radionuclide angiocardiography (RNA) in the selection and prognosis of patients with coronary artery disease. Calculations comparing the maximal increase in survival and complete pain relief, using multiple criteria known to provide prognostic information, showed that the* exercise response on RNA *is the single most important variable in selection of therapy.*

Loop FD, Lytle BW, Gill CC, et al.: Trends in selection and results of coronary artery reoperations. Ann Thorac Surg 36:380, 1983. *A large series of patients undergoing reoperation for myocardial revascularization are studied. Emphasis is placed upon the fact that the mortality is now relatively low, despite the technical difficulties encountered in some of these procedures. The results are quite favorable.*

Lytle BW, Loop FD, Cosgrove DM, et al.: Long-term (5 to 12 years) serial studies of internal mammary artery and saphenous vein coronary bypass grafts. J Thorac Cardiovasc Surg 89:248, 1985. *In this series of patients, the markedly improved patency rate of internal mammary grafts was clearly demonstrated compared with that of saphenous vein grafts.*

McLaughlin PR, Berman ND, Morton BC, et al.: Saphenous vein bypass grafting. Changes in native circulation and collaterals. Circulation 51–52(Suppl 1):66, 1975. *A carefully performed study of the continuing changes that occur in the coronary circulation after an initial diagnosis of stenotic atherosclerotic coronary disease. It emphasizes the need for continuing attention toward prevention of the basic process in addition to surgical therapy.*

Pryor DB, Harrell FE Jr, Lee KL, et al.: A study demonstrating the improving prognosis in medically treated patients with coronary artery disease. Am J Cardiol 52:444, 1983. *This study emphasizes that the mortality from coronary artery disease has decreased during the past decade and cannot be explained solely on the basis that less severe patients are being evaluated but is due at least in part to the decrease in mortality from coronary artery disease.*

Rackley CE: Advances in Critical Care Cardiology. Philadelphia, F. A. Davis Company, 1986. *An updated monograph of recent advances in the management of patients with acute cardiac problems. Appropriate diagnostic tests, together with a spectrum of medical therapy, transluminal coronary angioplasty, and CABG, are each thoroughly presented. There are notable discussions of the role and appropriate use of various cardiac pharmacologic agents, emergency procedures for myocardial ischemia, and the management of cardiac dysrhythmias.*

Rahimtoola SH: A perspective on the three large multicenter randomized clinical trials of CABG for chronic stable angina. Circulation 72(Suppl V):123, 1985. *A comparative review by an outstanding cardiologist of the three large and well-publicized multicenter clinical trials of CABG for chronic stable angina.*

Rankin JS, Newman GE, Muhlbaier LH, et al.: The effects of coronary revascularization on left ventricular function in ischemic heart disease. J Thorac Cardiovasc Surg 90:818, 1985. *A review of a series of patients with severe coronary artery disease and depressed myocardial function. CABG not only reverses exercise-induced ischemic ventricular dysfunction but can also have a similar effect on resting ventricular performance. Despite the fact that over 80 per cent of the patients in the study were New York Heart Association (NYHA) Stage IV, the mortality was 2.2 per cent.*

Rankin JS, Newman JR Jr, Califf RM, et al.: Clinical characteristics and current management of medically refractory unstable angina. Ann Surg 200:457, 1984. *A unique series of seriously ill patients, all on the coronary care unit, with refractory unstable angina who underwent CABG with excellent rate of survival.*

Sabiston DC Jr: The coronary circulation. The William F. Rienhoff, Jr. Lecture. Johns Hopkins Med J 134:314, 1974. *A review of the anatomic, physiologic, and pathologic aspects of the coronary circulation. The data presented are based upon experimental and clinical findings in the normal and pathologic coronary circulation and their relationships to surgical management. The first patient treated with a saphenous vein bypass graft for coronary artery disease in 1962 is described.*

Shearn DL, Brent BB: Coronary artery bypass surgery in patients with left ventricular dysfunction. Am J Med 80:405, 1986. *A study of a series of patients with poor left ventricular ejection fractions (less than 45 per cent) managed by CABG. Significant improvement in global left ventricular ejection fraction and regional left ventricular systolic function was demonstrated.*

Takaro T, Hultgren HN, Lipton MJ, et al.: Circulation 54(Suppl 3):107, 1976. *A randomized study showing definite superiority for long-term survival of surgical over medical therapy in patients with significant lesions of the left main coronary artery.*

Varnauskas E: Survival, myocardial infarction, and employment status in a prospective randomized study of coronary bypass surgery. Circulation 72(Suppl V):V, 1985. *A long-term report of the European Coronary Surgery Study Group indicating improved longevity in patients treated surgically as opposed to those managed medically. An eight-year result of survival is reported, together with five-year results on recurrent myocardial infarction and employment status of patients undergoing CABG compared with randomized controls.*

52 VALVULAR HEART DISEASE

Charles E. Rackley

The clinical manifestations of valvular heart disease result from either stenosis or incompetence of cardiac valves, or both. These mechanical disturbances lead to either pressure or volume overload on the affected chambers. The most frequently involved cardiac chamber in valvular heart disease is the left ventricle, which compensates for chronic volume or pressure overload with dilatation and hypertrophy. Myocardial oxygen requirements are related to the increased mechanical work and hypertrophy of the myocardium. In the advanced stage of valvular heart disease, myocardial decompensation, a reduction in cardiac output, and decreased coronary perfusion can impair oxygen delivery despite increased myocardial oxygen demands.

Although rheumatic heart disease remains prevalent in the temperate climates of the world, control of streptococcal infections in the United States has reduced the incidence of rheumatic fever and subsequent rheumatic heart disease. Today mitral valve prolapse is the most common valvular abnormality. A bicuspid aortic valve is the most common cause of aortic stenosis, but calcification of the degenerative aortic valve is recognized with increasing frequency in the aging adult.

Recognition of a heart murmur on physical examination is the usual means of initially diagnosing valvular heart disease. Thus, the clinical examination remains important for detection of valvular heart disease, recognition of cardiac deterioration, and assessment of follow-up status. The noninvasive technologies of electrocardiography, chest radiography, echocardiography, radionuclide angiography, and stress testing play an important role in assessing the impact of valvular heart disease on cardiac function and determining the timing of operative intervention. Cardiac catheterization continues to be important in the accurate measurement of gradients across stenotic valves, evaluation of left ventricular function, and recognition of concomitant coronary artery disease. In recent years advances in echocardiography have resulted in more accurate assessment of valvular orifice size, and catheterization is reserved to confirm impressions and to identify underlying coronary artery disease.

GENERAL APPROACH TO THE PATIENT WITH VALVULAR HEART DISEASE

History

The patient with valvular heart disease usually recalls a history of a heart murmur, and therefore the first recognition of the murmur may be helpful in establishing the etiology. Although cardiac murmurs are frequent in healthy, physicially active children and adolescents, congenital valvular etiologies are often recognized at birth. Detection of a heart murmur in early adulthood often suggests a rheumatic basis, whereas development of the murmur in later years is often due to the degenerative changes in valvular structure. In addition to ascertaining the earliest detection of the heart murmur, the physician should carefully assess the patient's physical activities and note the initial onset of dyspnea or fatigue. The physician's interpretation of the patient's symptoms dictates the appropriate timing of noninvasive and invasive cardiac studies as well as the decision for surgical correction.

Physical Examination

The physical examination of the patient with valvular heart disease should be performed in the standard manner. Particular attention should be paid to the vital signs. Fever should raise the possibility of infective endocarditis. Palpation of the peripheral pulse may indicate stenosis or incompetence of the aortic valve. The habitus can suggest Marfan's syndrome as well as other heritable disorders of connective tissue. Funduscopic examination can demonstrate subtleties in arterial pulsations in aortic incompetence or the characteristic hemorrhages or Roth's spots in infective endocarditis. Careful attention to the vessels in the neck can reveal abnormalities in venous pulsation reflecting right ventricular failure or tricuspid stenosis or incompetence. Carotid arteries reveal pulsatile abnormalities and transmitted bruits from the aortic valve.

Cardiac examination must include inspection, palpation, percussion, and auscultation. These maneuvers should be performed with the patient both in the sitting and in the recumbent positions. Auscultation at the apex, left sternal border, and pulmonic and aortic areas should be performed with the patient in the sitting, recumbent, and left lateral decubitus positions as well as after mild exercise. The remainder of the examination consists of documenting fluid retention, such as hepatic enlargement, ascites, and peripheral edema.

Laboratory Studies

Electrocardiogram

The electrocardiogram can provide information on atrial and ventricular enlargement. Left atrial enlargement is recognized by a prominent, prolonged, notched P wave in leads II, III, and aV_L, as well as in lead V_1. Left ventricular hypertrophy increases QRS voltage as well as ST-T wave abnormalities. Right ventricular hypertrophy produces right-axis deviation of the QRS complex as well as ST-T wave changes in leads V_1 and V_2. Atrial fibrillation often develops in the course of valvular heart disease from enlargement of the left atrium.

Chest Radiograph

Standard posteroanterior and lateral chest films provide information on heart size and chamber enlargement as well as evidence of pulmonary venous and arterial hypertension. Chest radiographs are useful in the follow-up of patients with valvular heart disease to detect changes in cardiac dimensions and alterations in pulmonary vascularity.

Echocardiography

Because of technical improvements, echocardiography has become a major noninvasive tool in the assessment of valvular heart disease. Valvular anatomy, pressure gradients, chamber dimensions, wall thickness, and ventricular function can be precisely assessed and quantitated using modern echocardiography. Valvular motion, calcification, orifice size, and the presence of infective endocarditis can all be determined with this technology.

Radionuclide Imaging

Radionuclide techniques can provide information on cardiac function, valvular incompetence, and the cardiac response to exercise. The imaging capability is particularly useful in evaluating the function of the right ventricle as well as tricuspid valve integrity. The response of the left ventricle to exercise is increasingly used to identify the earliest possible time for surgical correction of valvular abnormalities.

Exercise Testing

Standard exercise testing can be used to assess exercise capacity as well as document symptoms of dyspnea and fatigue. The test is useful in the initial and follow-up evaluations of patients with valvular heart disease to detect deterioration in cardiac performance.

Cardiac Catheterization

Cardiac catheterization remains a definitive procedure in the evaluation of valvular heart disease but, despite the improvements in techniques, is still limited by the number of times patients can tolerate this procedure. Objectives for cardiac catheterization are (1) to identify the underlying valve lesions, (2) to assess ventricular function, (3) to evaluate the anatomy of the coronary arteries, (4) to recognize any additional cardiac lesions, and (5) to assess the performance of prosthetic heart valves.

AORTIC STENOSIS

Etiology and Pathology

Aortic stenosis (Table 52–1) can result from a congenital abnormality, rheumatic fever, or degeneration with calcification in the aging patient. A bicuspid valve is the most common congenital abnormality, and invariably there is a raphe in one of the cusps that indicates failure of the commissure to develop. Rarely, a unicuspid valve can be present at birth. Although the bicuspid valve may not be initially stenotic, fibrosis and thickening lead to eventual reduction of the orifice size with calcification. Rheumatic fever produces scarring of the leaflet margins, and there is eventual fusion of the commissures with calcification. More than 50 per cent of adults with aortic stenosis will be found to have a bicuspid valve, but fibrosis and calcification may make it difficult to determine whether the valve is bicuspid or tricuspid. In the aging patient with degenerative aortic stenosis, calcium deposits usually develop in the sinuses and annulus, whereas the margins of the leaflets remain free.

In any of the conditions producing hemodynamic stenosis of the aortic valve, the systolic hypertension in the ventricular chamber is compensated by concentric hypertrophy of the myocardial wall. As myocardial failure develops from depression of the contractile state, dilatation of the ventricle will occur. Fibrosis of the myocardium also occurs. Myocardial oxygen consumption remains high owing to the elevation of systolic pressure within the left ventricle and the increase in left ventricular mass. Thus, significant aortic stenosis creates conditions in which high myocardial oxygen demands are inadequately supported by reduced oxygen supply, which leads to subendocardial ischemia. Eventually, with a decline in the inotropic state of the myocardium, the ventricle dilates and the ejection fraction is decreased below the normal range. Further elevation of the left ventricular end-diastolic pressure results in pulmonary venous hypertension The increased myocardial oxygen demands in aortic stenosis with the underperfused subendocardial myocardium can produce arrhythmias, chest pain, and even sudden death. In adults there may be coexistent coronary artery disease, which further contributes to myocardial ischemia.

Clinical Features

Chest pain, syncope, and heart failure are the characteristic symptoms of aortic stenosis, even though a gradient across the valve can exist for years before the patient develops symptoms. Children with a severe gradient can suddenly develop symptoms, whereas in adults the increase in mortality occurs later in the course of the disease.

The anginal chest discomfort is exertional and indistinguishable from that of ischemic heart disease. Approximately 50 per cent of patients with aortic stenosis who are above the age of 40 years will have underlying coronary artery disease whether exertional chest pain is present or not. Syncope can be an initial symptom of aortic stenosis and is probably related to the same mechanism as the chest pain, that is, critical reduction in myocardial oxygen supply with increased demands. Orthostatic syncope can result from the inability of the cardiac output to increase with abrupt assumption of the upright position, whereas exertional syncope is further aggravated by peripheral vasodilatation unaccompanied by an increase in cardiac output. Arrhythmias due to myocardial ischemia can also contribute to syncope and sudden death. When aortic stenosis is found at autopsy, approximately 15 per cent of the patients will have died suddenly without previous symptoms.

Heart failure in aortic stenosis generally reduces life expectancy to less than two years, whereas patients with syncope or angina may survive, on the average, two to five years. With calcification of the aortic valve, hemolytic anemia due to destruction of red cells can develop; furthermore, patients with aortic stenosis have an increased incidence of gastrointestinal bleeding resulting from angiodysplasia. Finally, patients with aortic stenosis are susceptible to infective endocarditis.

Physical Examination

In aortic stenosis, the typical physical findings include a delay in the upstroke of the peripheral pulse, a diamond-shaped crescendo-decrescendo systolic murmur, and hypertrophy of the left ventricle. The peripheral pulse is diminished in amplitude, delayed in upstroke, and prolonged owing to sustained ejection across the aortic valve (pulsus tardus et parvus). The changes in the peripheral pulse are caused by a reduction in the systolic pressure and a gradual decline in diastolic pressure. The harsh murmur is often transmitted to the carotid vessels, and a palpable thrill develops with a substantial gradient across the aortic valve.

Since the contour of the heart does not become enlarged with concentric hypertrophy, there may be no visible abnormalities on examination of the chest. However, the apical impulse of the pressure-overloaded ventricle may be sustained

TABLE 52–1. AORTIC STENOSIS

Etiology	Physiology	Symptoms	Physical Examination	Electrocardiogram	Chest	Echocardiogram	Catheterization	Medical Therapy	Surgical Therapy
Congenital Rheumatic Degenerative	LV* pressure overload LV hypertrophy Decreased LV compliance	Chest pain Syncope Heart failure	Delayed arterial pulse wave Aortic thrill Diamond-shaped aortic area, left sternal border and apex	LV hypertrophy	Normal cardiac size Poststenotic dilatation of ascending aorta	Anatomy of aortic valve/calcium Number of cusps LV wall thickness EchoDoppler estimate of valvular gradient Valvular area	Valvular gradient LV function Valvular area Coronary anatomy Mitral lesions	Endocarditis prophylaxis	Symptoms Gradient >50 mm Hg Valvular area <0.8 cm²

*LV = left ventricular.

even though localized. When the ventricle dilates owing to myocardial failure, there is lateral displacement of the impulse, which becomes more diffuse. Detection of palpable systolic vibrations over the primary aortic area, with the patient in the sitting position during full expiration, often correlates with a gradient across the aortic valve of more than 40 mm Hg. An atrial (S_4) gallop is usually audible, and an ejection click may be heard along the left sternal border. The aortic second sound becomes diminished, except in calcific stenosis of the elderly, in which the margins of the leaflets usually maintain their mobility. The diamond-shaped ejection murmur develops after the first sound, peaks in mid- and late systole, and disappears before the second heart sound. If an ejection click is present, the murmur develops immediately after the click and can sometimes be erroneously identified as a holosystolic murmur. The murmur is most intense over the aortic area and along the left sternal border, but in the elderly patient, the musical quality of the murmur can sometimes be loudest at the apex. The intensity in the apical area can be confusing and may make it difficult to distinguish this murmur from that of mitral regurgitation. A faint diastolic blow is often audible along the left sternal border, since the severely stenotic valve may have a mild degree of incompetence.

Laboratory Studies

Electrocardiogram

Left ventricular hypertrophy is the most common finding on the electrocardiogram, with an increase in QRS amplitude and ST-T changes of a strain pattern. Left-axis deviation can develop as well as conduction disturbances and left bundle branch block. As the left ventricle becomes noncompliant, there may be enlargement of the left atrium with a negative P wave in lead V_1. Because of myocardial fibrosis, Q waves can develop in the precordial leads, but these as well as the ST-T wave abnormalities are indistinguishable from underlying coronary artery disease.

Chest Radiograph

The heart size remains unchanged in the early phase of aortic stenosis, since hypertrophy does not increase the cardiothoracic ratio. There may be poststenotic dilatation and prominence of the ascending aorta. Calcification is often present but may require fluoroscopy for confirmation. Development of heart failure will enlarge the left ventricle and cause pulmonary congestion. Since a bicuspid aortic valve is sometimes associated with coarctation of the aorta, rib notching should always be sought on the chest film.

Echocardiogram

The echocardiogram can demonstrate thickening of the aortic leaflets, determine the number of leaflets, detect calcification of the valves, and reveal left ventricular wall thickness and function. Two-dimensional echocardiography can give an estimated size of the aortic orifice, and the Doppler technique can assess accurately the systolic pressure gradient across the valve. Thus, available echocardiographic techniques can provide accurate diagnosis and assessment of aortic stenosis (Fig. 52–1).

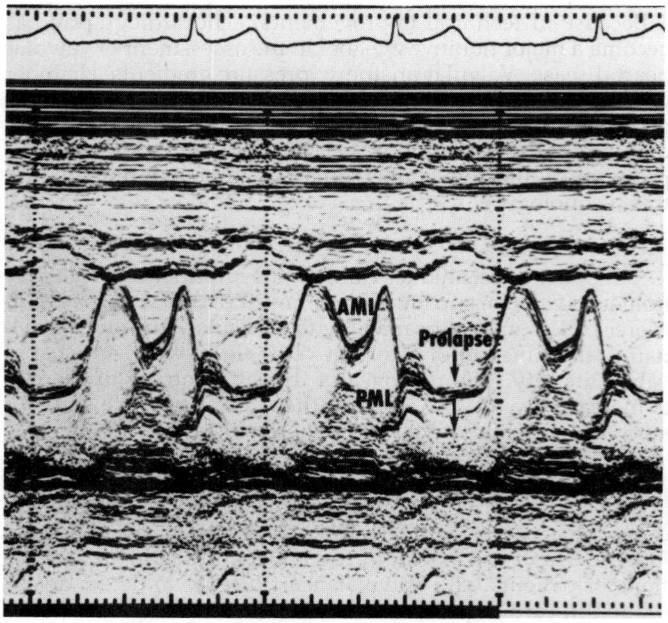

FIGURE 52–1. M-Mode echocardiogram of a patient with mitral valve prolapse. Note the systolic posterior motion of the anterior (AML) and posterior (PML) mitral valve leaflets.

Cardiac Catheterization

The pressure gradient across the aortic valve can be accurately measured with simultaneous measurements of left ventricular and aortic pressures. A decline in cardiac output will be associated with a reduced pressure gradient across the valve, and the valvular area will tend to be overestimated when the cardiac output is reduced and only the pressure gradient is analyzed.

The size of the normal aortic orifice is 2.5 to 3 cm², and mild stenosis develops when the orifice is reduced to 0.75 to 1.5 cm². Moderate stenosis is present when the valvular size is less than 0.75 cm² and severe stenosis when the valvular area is less than 0.5 cm². Surgery is usually advised when the aortic valve gradient is greater than 50 mm Hg or the valve area is less than 0.8 cm². Left ventricular angiography is helpful in determining the presence of mitral regurgitation. With the information available from echocardiography, cardiac catheterization may be primarily indicated for coronary arteriography, since 50 per cent of patients over the age of 40 years will have underlying coronary artery disease.

Differential Diagnosis

In children, valvular aortic stenosis has to be differentiated from congenital forms of both supra- and infravalvular lesions. In hypertrophic cardiomyopathy with obstruction, the systolic ejection murmur is similar to that of valvular aortic stenosis, but the peripheral pulse is hyperdynamic with a rapid upstroke and a double-notch or bisferious contour compared with the delayed upstroke observed in valvular stenosis. With rupture of the chordae or papillary muscle, acute mitral regurgitation may produce a harsh systolic murmur. This murmur can be transmitted to the left atrial wall and aorta, resulting in a palpable and audible "aortic" murmur. However, the murmur of acute mitral regurgitation transmitted into the aortic area is holosystolic rather than midsystolic. A systolic ejection murmur accompanies significant aortic regurgitation and is generally caused by turbulence of the large stroke volume across the aortic valve.

Medical Therapy

Prophylaxis with antibiotics is indicated for dental, genitourinary, and gastrointestinal procedures in the asymptomatic patient to reduce the likelihood of infective endocarditis. Prophylaxis should be routine throughout life in a patient with a stenotic or prosthetic valve. For dental and respiratory tract procedures, an adult should receive penicillin V, 2.0 gm orally one hour before, then 1.0 gm six hours later. For patients unable to take oral medications, 2 million units of aqueous penicillin G given intravenously (IV) or intramuscularly (IM) 30 to 60 minutes before a procedure and 1 million units 6 hours later may be substituted. For patients with prosthetic valves, ampicillin, 1.0 to 2.0 gm given IM or IV, plus gentamicin, 1.5 gm per kilogram given IM or IV, is recommended one-half hour before a procedure, followed by 1.0 gm of oral penicillin V six hours later. Alternatively, the parenteral regimen may be repeated once eight hours later. For patients allergic to penicillin, erythromycin, 1.0 gm, should be given orally one hour before the procedure, then 500 mg six hours later; or for parenteral administration, vancomycin, 1.0 gm, should be given IV slowly over one hour, starting one hour before, without a repeat dose. For genitourinary or gastrointestinal tract procedures, ampicillin, 2.0 gm given IM or IV, plus gentamicin, 1.5 mg per kilogram given IM or IV, is given one-half to one hour before a procedure, and a follow-up dose is administered eight hours later. For minor or repeated procedures, amoxicillin, 3.0 gm orally, is recommended one hour before a procedure and 1.5 gm six hours later. In children, appropriately reduced doses for each of these programs should be used.

If the patient with aortic stenosis develops a supraventricular tachycardia, digitalis and an antiarrhythmic drug may be necessary to slow the ventricular response. Development of chest pain warrants catheterization to evaluate underlying coronary artery disease, but the use of nitrates should be undertaken with great caution, since arterial pressure may fall and further reduce coronary blood flow. Since life expectancy is reduced when aortic stenosis becomes symptomatic, chest pain, syncope, or heart failure warrants appropriate studies and consideration for surgery.

Surgical Therapy

In children with aortic stenosis, surgery may be considered before the development of symptoms. If the pressure gradient is high, valvuloplasty can sometimes be performed before calcification has developed. The operative mortality for aortic valve replacement is 2 to 3 per cent and is less than 5 per cent if coronary bypass surgery is also performed. Even if heart failure has developed, surgery with prosthetic valve replacement can improve ventricular function. A mechanical valve will require long-term coagulation, but the porcine valve can be utilized in older patients or in those in whom anticoagulation is contraindicated. Currently, the porcine valve will usually last ten years or longer before deterioration in adults, but it is not recommended in children or adolescents. If indicated, coronary bypass surgery should also be performed at the time of valve replacement. The ten-year survival of combined aortic valve replacement and coronary revascularization approaches 55 per cent. Late cardiac events occur at a rate of approximately 6 per cent per year and include thromboembolic neurologic insults, myocardial infarction, congestive heart failure, endocarditis, bleeding, peripheral thromboembolism, and reoperation.

AORTIC REGURGITATION

Etiology and Pathology

Aortic regurgitation (Table 52–2) can be caused by disease conditions that render the aortic leaflets incompetent or affect the ascending aorta with dilatation of the annulus of the aortic valve. Rheumatic fever produces scarring and fibrosis of the valvular margins. Myxomatous degeneration of the aortic cusp can lead to incompetence. Hypertension, as well as arteriosclerosis, can be associated with scarring of the aortic valve and mild incompetence. Congenital lesions, such as bicuspid aortic valve, are predominantly stenotic, but scarring and calcification can result in associated incompetence as well. An aneurysm of the sinus of Valsalva may be associated with a ventricular septal defect as well as aortic regurgitation.

Conditions that affect the ascending aorta and produce valvular incompetence include syphilis, heritable disorders of connective tissue, arthritic diseases, and cystic medial necrosis of the aorta. In syphilis, the granulomatous process can result in calcification of the aorta, extreme dilatation, and ostial narrowing of the coronary arteries. Myxomatous degeneration of the aortic valve occurs in Marfan's syndrome. Ankylosing spondylitis, rheumatoid arthritis, and Reiter's syndrome are arthritic conditions that can cause aortic root dilatation and aortic cusp thickening. Cystic medial necrosis and aortic ectasia can produce extreme dilatation of the aorta with secondary aortic regurgitation. Aortic regurgitation can result from dissection of the aorta, perforation of the valve with infective endocarditis, rupture of a sinus of Valsalva, and mechanical complications of a prosthetic aortic valve.

Physiology

Aortic regurgitation imposes a volume overload on the left ventricle. Although the end-diastolic pressure may be normal or slightly elevated in the early phases, progressive regurgitation will elevate the end-diastolic pressure and dilate the chamber by slippage of myocardial fibers, sarcomere replication, and myocardial hypertrophy. These compensatory mechanisms support a large left ventricular stroke volume, which is often achieved with an ejection fraction above 50 per cent.

The systolic ejection of a large stroke volume into the high-impedance area of the systemic circulation increases the systolic pressure. Systolic wall stress or afterload can be maintained within the normal range by hypertrophy of the myocardium, but myocardial oxygen demand is significantly increased. A progressive decline in aortic diastolic pressure due to regurgitation of blood into the left ventricle can reduce coronary blood flow and thus create conditions for subendocardial ischemia in severe chronic aortic regurgitation.

The gradual volume overload of chronic aortic regurgitation can be tolerated for years before the inotropic state of the myocardium deteriorates. Eventually, the declining ejection fraction and inotropic state, along with limits to the dilatation hypertrophy mechanism, cause marked elevation of the left ventricular filling pressure with pulmonary venous capillary congestion.

Left ventricular hemodynamics in acute aortic regurgitation, compared with those in chronic aortic regurgitation, are immediately disturbed, since the regurgitant volume may be imposed on a normal end-diastolic volume. Under such circumstances, sudden incompetence of the aortic valve can severely elevate the left ventricular filling pressure, since the acute dilatation of the left ventricle is limited. With such rapid regurgitation through the aortic valve, the mitral valve may close prematurely, and the aortic diastolic murmur may persist beyond the diminished first heart sound.

TABLE 52–2. AORTIC REGURGITATION

Etiology	Physiology	Symptoms	Physical Examination	Electrocardiogram	Chest	Echocardiogram	Catheterization	Medical Therapy	Surgical Therapy
Chronic									
Rheumatic fever Connective tissue disorders Hypertension, atherosclerosis Syphilis Cystic medial necrosis Aortic ectasia Congenital heart disease	Chronic volume overload LV* dilatation LV hypertrophy	Fatigue Dyspnea Edema	Wide arterial pulse pressure Enlarged LV Diastolic aortic murmur Systolic ejection murmur Third sound Apical diastolic rumble	LV hypertrophy and strain	Enlarged LV Dilated aorta	Valvular anatomy Aortic root size Enlarged LV Mitral valve fluttering LV function	Contrast from aorta to LV LV function	Preload and after load reduction Diuretics Digitalis	LV systolic echo dimension >55 mm Ejection fraction <50%
Acute									
Endocarditis Aortic dissection Ruptured sinus of Valsalva Prosthetic valve	Acute LV diastolic pressure and volume overload	Pulmonary edema	Loud diastolic musical murmur Right and left sternal border radiation with thrill Soft S_1 and third sound Continuous murmur if rupture into right side of heart	LV strain	Pulmonary edema Normal heart size	Valvular anatomy Aortic size and intimal flap	Contrast from aorta to LV Aortic and intimal flap	Preload and afterload reduction	Urgent surgery

*LV = left ventricle or ventricular.

Clinical Course

Since the volume overload of aortic regurgitation is well tolerated, patients may remain asymptomatic for long periods of time. The patient may be aware of prominent precordial activity as well as exaggerated pulsation of the carotid arteries. Diffuse sweating patterns and vague abdominal discomfort are less frequent symptoms. The accelerated development of angina, heart failure, or sudden death within several years has been observed in patients with a pulse pressure greater than 140/40 mm Hg and left ventricular enlargement demonstrated on electrocardiography or chest radiograph. Dyspnea, orthopnea, and paroxysmal nocturnal dyspnea result from impaired left ventricular contractility in pulmonary venous hypertension. Although tachycardia may impair ventricular function, the shortened diastolic filling period can be beneficial in reducing the duration of the aortic regurgitation. Chest pain and syncope are infrequent symptoms. Chest pain is often associated with underlying coronary artery disease, and syncope is usually attended by arrhythmias.

With acute aortic regurgitation, pulmonary edema is often the presenting manifestation. Severe chest pain suggests aortic dissection when acute aortic incompetence develops.

Physical Examination

In aortic regurgitation, the physical findings reflect the large left ventricular stroke volume into the systemic circulation and the rapid diastolic run-off into the left ventricle. The peripheral pulse is characteristically bounding, and additional manifestations of the wide pulse pressure include head bobbing, pulsation of the retinal arterioles, bounding carotid pulse, pistol shot sounds over the femoral arteries, a to-and-fro murmur elicited from the femoral artery with slight compression of the stethoscope, and capillary pulsations in the nail beds. With connective tissue and arthritic diseases that produce aortic regurgitation, there may be characteristic changes in habitus, such as the musculoskeletal type in Marfan's syndrome and kyphosis of the thoracic spine in ankylosing spondylitis.

The precordium is hyperdynamic with a laterally displaced apical impulse. The auscultatory hallmark is the high-pitched, blowing, decrescendo diastolic murmur heard best along the left sternal border while the patient is in the sitting position during full expiration. As the regurgitation becomes more severe, a diastolic rumble or Austin Flint murmur due to vibration of the anterior leaflet of the mitral valve in the regurgitant jet may be audible at the apex. If the ascending aorta is dilated, the diastolic murmur may be heard along the right sternal border as well. With extreme left ventricular dilatation, mitral regurgitation can produce an apical systolic murmur, and heart failure is attended by a ventricular gallop at the apex.

With acute aortic regurgitation due to disruption of an aortic leaflet or dissection dilating the aortic annulus, the diastolic murmur may be harsh with palpable vibrations along the left sternal border. A perforated or prolapsed aortic leaflet, as well as the detached aortic intima from dissection, can generate prominent musical qualities in the diastolic murmur.

Laboratory Studies

Electrocardiogram

The electrocardiogram typically reveals left ventricular hypertrophy with increased QRS voltage amplitude and ST-T wave changes of the strain pattern. With acute aortic regurgitation, the hypertrophy may be absent, and the ST-T wave changes can indicate myocardial ischemia.

Chest Radiography

Significant cardiomegaly usually attends chronic aortic regurgitation, with the increase in size due to dilatation of the left ventricle. The ascending aorta is often prominent. Calcium in the aortic valve or annulus is best appreciated by fluoroscopy, but calcification of the ascending aorta caused by syphilis can be detected on the chest film. Left ventricular failure will be accompanied by pulmonary congestion and venous prominence.

Echocardiogram

Echocardiography has become the most useful noninvasive tool to recognize anatomic abnormalities of the aortic valve and to assess dimensions of the annulus and ascending aorta. The intensity of the regurgitant flow can be appreciated by the vibrations of the anterior mitral leaflet, and the echo-Doppler technique can estimate the severity of the regurgitation. Left ventricular chamber dimensions and wall thickness permit calculation of end-diastolic volume and hypertrophy. Finally, an end-systolic dimension of 55 mm has been proposed by several investigators to represent the limit of surgically reversible dilatation of the left ventricle so that aortic valve replacement should be performed before this chamber size is exceeded. Additional clinical experience has challenged the validity of the 55-mm systolic limit, since postoperative reduction in chamber size remains variable. Thus, echocardiographic studies of left ventricular dimensions and function are important in evaluation, follow-up, and timing for aortic valve replacement in aortic regurgitation.

Exercise Testing

Although exercise capacity can be measured and followed periodically in patients with aortic regurgitation, exercise testing is best clinically used in combination with radionuclide angiography. A reduction in exercise ejection fraction by 5 per cent or more is considered by some an indication for surgery even in the absence of symptoms.

Cardiac Catheterization

Cardiac catheterization can confirm the presence of aortic incompetence when contrast material injected into the aorta regurgitates into the left ventricle. The primary clinical indications for catheterization are to recognize coexisting lesions, such as mitral regurgitation, and to detect coronary artery disease. Dimensions of the aortic annulus and the ascending aorta will be useful for the choice of a prosthetic device in the operative procedure.

Differential Diagnosis

In the evaluation of a diastolic murmur along the left sternal border, aortic insufficiency is far more common than pulmonic insufficiency. The pulsatile characteristics of the peripheral circulation can be helpful in differentiating an aortic from a pulmonic origin of the diastolic murmur. In systemic hypertension, accentuated tambour qualities of the second heart sound can sometimes suggest mild aortic regurgitation, but the level of the diastolic blood pressure can be helpful in distinguishing incompetence from reverberations of the second sound. Any condition that causes aortic stenosis through immobility of the valve leaflets is often accompanied by some degree of aortic regurgitation.

Medical Therapy

Antibiotic prophylaxis is indicated for the prevention of endocarditis. When symptoms of heart failure develop, vasodilating agents such as hydralazine, prazocin, or nifedipine may be beneficial, but benefits are rarely maintained. Thus, the use of digitalis, diuretics, and afterload-reducing agents is primarily of short-term benefit in aortic regurgitation.

Surgical Therapy

A major clinical decision in aortic regurgitation is the timing of aortic valve replacement before irreversible dilatation of the left ventricle has developed. The echocardiographic dimensions and evidence of reduced left ventricular function are now being utilized to advise valve replacement before symptoms of heart failure have developed. Even after heart failure has developed, patients still improve clinically after aortic valve replacement. Valve replacement can be undertaken with a mortality of less than 3 to 5 per cent. The type of prosthetic valve will depend on the patient's age and the ability to be anticoagulated. In aortic dissection, there may also be replacement of the ascending aorta, since acute regurgitation requires intervention.

MITRAL STENOSIS

Etiology and Pathology

Rheumatic fever remains the predominant cause for mitral stenosis (Table 52–3). Calcification of the mitral valve annulus in the elderly patient can occasionally cause hemodynamic obstruction. Space-occupying lesions, such as left atrial myxoma, or thrombus formation can rarely obstruct the mitral valve. The characteristic pathologic change in rheumatic fever is fibrosis and scarring, particularly at the margins of the valve. This process can also extend into the chordae, with shortening and fusion. Eventually, fibrotic and destructive changes lead to calcification of the valve, and pulmonary hypertension with thickening of the pulmonary veins and capillaries, along with intimal and medial proliferation of the pulmonary arteries, occurs. With longstanding mitral stenosis and pulmonary hypertension, right ventricular hypertrophy and fibrosis develop.

Physiology

The hemodynamic abnormalities in mitral stenosis result from obstruction of diastolic blood flow into the left ventricle. The normal cross-sectional area of the mitral valve ranges from 4 to 6 cm^2, and turbulence of diastolic flow occurs when the valvular orifice is reduced below 2 cm^2. Increased demands for cardiac output, such as in exercise or fever, may be necessary to produce the diastolic murmur when the mitral valve orifice is reduced to 1.5 to 2 cm^2. In the second stage of progressive reduction in the mitral orifice size, a diastolic gradient develops between the left atrium and left ventricle under resting conditions when the valvular area is 1.5 to 1 cm^2. In the advanced stage, mitral orifice size is less than 1 cm^2, and left atrial and pulmonary hypertension becomes significant. The pulmonary capillary pressure often exceeds 20 to 25 mm Hg, and this leads to significant pulmonary arterial hypertension, pressure overload on the right ventricle, and compensatory hypertrophy of the right ventricle. Although the cardiac output can be maintained until the late stage of severe mitral stenosis, exercise will not produce a normal increase in cardiac output owing to impaired diastolic filling. Another hemodynamic complication in chronic mitral stenosis is atrial fibrillation due to left atrial enlargement. Atrial fibrillation and the increased ventricular response can aggravate hemodynamic abnormalities by reducing the diastolic filling period and leading to further elevation of pressure in the lungs.

Clinical Features

The average age at which rheumatic fever occurs is 10 to 12 years, and generally there is a 10-year period before the murmur of mitral stenosis can be detected. Mitral stenosis affects females more than males, and symptoms usually develop between the ages of 25 and 30 years. In temperate zones, mitral stenosis can accelerate in childhood, with severe hemodynamic impairment by the age of 10 to 12 years. Dyspnea is the most common symptom secondary to pulmonary venous hypertension and can be precipitated by any

TABLE 52–3. MITRAL STENOSIS

Etiology	Physiology	Symptoms	Physical Examination	Electrocardiogram	Chest	Echocardiogram	Catheterization	Medical Therapy	Surgical Therapy
Rheumatic Myxoma Calcification Congenital	Pressure overload LA* and pulmonary veins	Dyspnea Fatigue Palpitations Hemoptysis	Loud S_1 Opening snap Diastolic rumble Signs of pulmonary hypertension: RVH* $\uparrow P_2$ Diastolic blow	Broad, notched P wave in lead II	Enlarged LA Prominent pulmonary veins	Square wave of EF slope of mitral valve Estimation of gradient and orifice size	Elevated PA* wedge pressure and normal LV diastolic pressure	Dental prophylaxis Digitalis for atrial fibrillation Warfarin (Coumadin)	Symptoms Valvular area <1.0 cm^2

*LA = left atrium; RVH = right ventricular hypertrophy; PA = pulmonary arterial.

circumstance that increases cardiac output, such as exercise or febrile conditions. Paroxysmal atrial fibrillation can precipitate symptoms by increasing the ventricular rate. As the stenosis progresses, patients experience symptoms with minimal effort or at rest. With longstanding mitral stenosis and chronic pulmonary hypertension, the compensatory thickening of the pulmonary capillaries can protect the lungs from extravasation of fluid despite severe elevations of pulmonary pressure.

Systemic embolization resulting from underlying atrial fibrillation and left atrial thrombus development can also be a manifestation of mitral stenosis. Females can become symptomatic in the second trimester of pregnancy, when the blood volume increases significantly and elevates pulmonary pressures. As the blood volume diminishes late in the third trimester, the symptoms may slightly improve. With severe enlargement of the left atrium and infringement on the mainstem bronchus, persistent cough may develop. Hemoptysis can result from rupture of small vessels in the bronchi due to longstanding venous hypertension. Infective endocarditis can complicate mitral stenosis at any stage, but this generally occurs when mitral regurgitation is present as well.

Physical Examination

The classic physical findings of mitral stenosis are an accentuated first sound at the apex, an opening snap, and a diastolic rumble. If the condition is severe, the diminished peripheral pulse and blood pressure reflect a reduced left ventricular stroke volume. Patients may display typical "mitral facies" with florid congestion of the cheeks. The distended neck veins indicate right ventricular failure with secondary tricuspid regurgitation. If tricuspid stenosis coexists with mitral stenosis, a prominent *a* wave may be observed in the jugular vein.

Inspection of the precordium may reveal activity along the left sternal border, indicating right ventricular enlargement and pulmonary hypertension. On palpation, the accentuated first sound, the opening snap, and the diastolic rumble can sometimes be felt at the apex. With significant right ventricular dilatation, the left ventricular apical impulse may be displaced laterally, and the right cardiac border may be percussed to the right of the sternum. The opening snap can vary from 0.04 to 0.10 second after the second sound at the apex. The higher the left atrial pressure, the closer the opening snap to the second heart sound (S_2), and thus the S_2-OS interval indicates the severity of the mitral stenosis. The opening snap is a high-pitched sound and is heard best with the patient in the left lateral decubitus position. The opening snap can sometimes be appreciated at the base of the heart but must be differentiated from a split pulmonic second sound. The diastolic rumble at the apex is a low-pitched murmur following the opening snap. If sinus rhythm is present, there will be presystolic accentuation due to atrial contraction. Since the murmur of mitral stenosis may be faint in the early stages, to complete the physical examination, the patient should exercise by performing sit-ups or hopping on one foot to increase the heart rate. With the increased flow across the mitral valve, the diastolic rumble may be more easily detected.

The diastolic murmur of pulmonic insufficiency should be sought along the left sternal border, but this can be difficult to distinguish from aortic regurgitation. A widened systemic pulse pressure favors aortic versus pulmonic insufficiency with mitral stenosis. Rarely, tricuspid stenosis can simultaneously occur with the mitral stenosis. The murmur of tricuspid stenosis is heard along the lower left sternal border and is greatly accentuated with inspiration. Finally, some degree of mitral incompetence often accompanies mitral stenosis and will produce an apical systolic murmur of varying intensity.

Laboratory Studies

Electrocardiogram

The electrocardiographic changes of mitral stenosis include left atrial enlargement and right ventricular hypertrophy due to pulmonary hypertension. Characteristic notching and prolongation of the P wave are most prominent in leads II, III, and aV_F. The terminal portion of the P wave is usually negative in lead V_1. Right-axis deviation and an increased amplitude of the R wave in V_1 are evidence of right ventricular hypertrophy.

Chest Radiograph

Radiographic evidence of mitral stenosis includes left atrial enlargement, pulmonary venous hypertension, and right ventricular prominence. The enlarged left atrium produces a double contour along the right cardiac silhouette, as well as straightening of the left cardiac border due to the large left atrial appendage. This change produces elevation of the left mainstem bronchus. The pulmonary venous hypertension redistributes the blood flow to the apices of the lungs, with a reduction in blood volume of the lower lung. Pulmonary arterial hypertension renders the hilar arteries more prominent. Kerley's B lines due to fibrosis and lymphatic engorgement appear as transverse linear densities at the lung bases above the diaphragm.

Echocardiogram

The echocardiogram is the most accurate noninvasive technique for detection of mitral valve stenosis and is recognized by the characteristic square wave motion of the E to F slope of the valve during diastole. The concordant movement of anterior and posterior mitral valve leaflets is one of the cardinal echocardiographic findings in mitral stenosis. Calcification produces additional echoes from the stenotic valve. The two-dimensional echo can accurately measure the diastolic area of the mitral valve, and the echoDoppler technique can estimate the pressure gradient across the valve, as well as left atrial and left ventricular dimensions, and provide an assessment of left ventricular function. Thrombus or a myxoma in the left atrium will produce multiple echoes during diastolic filling.

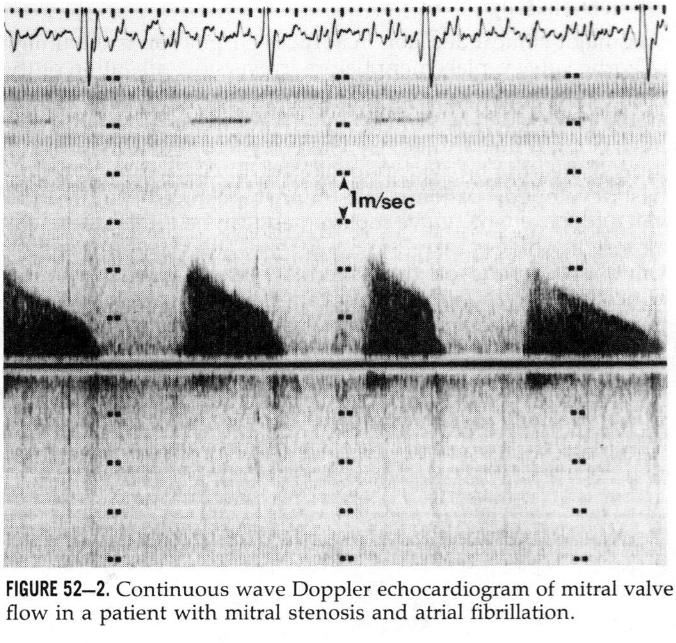

FIGURE 52–2. Continuous wave Doppler echocardiogram of mitral valve flow in a patient with mitral stenosis and atrial fibrillation.

Exercise Testing

Treadmill or bicycle exercise testing can establish aerobic capacity and the degree of exercise impairment. These observations can be useful in following the young patient with mitral stenosis during the early stages of the disease. The response of the heart rate to exertion and early symptoms of fatigue or dyspnea can be documented with an exercise test.

Cardiac Catheterization

Hemodynamic confirmation of mitral stenosis requires measurement of the diastolic pressure gradient across the mitral valve. Left atrial pressure can be obtained directly through trans-septal puncture or as reflected in the pulmonary capillary wedge pressure and recorded simultaneously with the left ventricular pressure. The Gorlin formula (see Ch. 42.5) permits calculation of the mitral orifice size based on the diastolic flow derived from the forward cardiac output and the simultaneous pressure gradient across the valve. The mitral valve gradient can vary from 5 to 25 mm Hg. In an individual without symptoms, mitral valve area can range from 1.5 to 2.0 cm^2. In those exhibiting symptoms with usual activity, valvular size may be 1.5 cm^2 or less, and patients with marked limitations usually have an orifice size less than 1.0 cm^2. Sometimes, a minimal mitral valve gradient is obtained under resting circumstances, but exercise can markedly increase pulmonary pressures to the level of heart failure. At the time of catheterization, associated valve lesions should be assessed, such as mitral regurgitation, aortic stenosis, and aortic regurgitation. If the patient is above 40 years of age, coronary arteriography should also be performed.

Differential Diagnosis

Several cardiac conditions can be confused with the symptoms and physical findings of mitral stenosis. A left atrial myxoma can produce dyspnea or syncope with an opening snap and a diastolic rumble. Primary pulmonary hypertension in young women can be associated with dyspnea and an accentuated pulmonic second sound, but other auscultatory findings are lacking. An atrial septal defect can mimic mitral stenosis with an accentuated first sound, opening snap, and diastolic rumble. However, the accentuated first sound is due to tricuspid valve closure, the opening snap is a split pulmonic second sound, and the diastolic rumble is created by flow across the tricuspid valve.

Medical Therapy

Medical therapy is directed at reducing the incidence of rheumatic fever, prophylaxis for infective endocarditis, control of atrial fibrillation with a rapid ventricular response, and anticoagulation for thromboembolic phenomena. The patient should continue on rheumatic fever prophylaxis until he or she is 30 years of age.

Since atrial fibrillation can aggravate and precipitate symptoms of pulmonary congestion, digitalis should be administered to control ventricular response. Anticoagulation on a chronic basis should be considered in all patients with mitral stenosis and atrial fibrillation. If the patient develops pulmonary edema with atrial fibrillation, cardioversion should be attempted. Ideally, the patient should be anticoagulated two weeks prior to elective cardioversion for atrial fibrillation. Quinidine should be started two days before the elective procedure, and if digitalis has been administered, this may be discontinued one day prior to the cardioversion. If cardioversion is successful, the patient should remain on long-term anticoagulation and quinidine therapy. For thromboembolic phenomena from the left atrium, anticoagulation is indicated. For acute embolism to the extremities or abdomen, surgical embolectomy may be beneficial.

Although considered experimental at present, valvuloplasty via catheter is being performed in selected patients with mitral stenosis, particularly in children or in young women desiring to become pregnant at a later date.

Surgical Therapy

The decision for surgery is based on the development of symptoms of pulmonary congestion during activity or at rest. In addition to pulmonary congestion, recurrent atrial fibrillation with aggravation of pulmonary congestion, thromboembolic phenomena, and hemoptysis can be indications for surgery. Mitral commissurotomy remains the procedure of choice with a pliable mitral valve without calcification on mitral regurgitation and carries an operative mortality of less than 1 per cent. This procedure should be considered particularly for the young female who has a desire for pregnancy. Sometimes commissurotomy can be performed before the development of significant symptoms. Patients may benefit for 5 to 20 years after commissurotomy, but if symptoms occur at a later time, mitral valve replacement may be required. Mitral valve replacement carries an operative mortality of 2 to 3 per cent. The type of mitral valve depends on the age of the patient as well as the circumstances for anticoagulation in a young female. The porcine valve can be inserted without the need for chronic anticoagulation but may require replacement after 10 years. If the valve is calcified or if the patient has had a previous commissurotomy, a prosthetic device is preferred. When there is a contraindication to anticoagulation, as in the aging patient, the porcine valve can be inserted.

Anticoagulation and antibiotic prophylaxis are required in patients with a prosthetic valve. Should atrial fibrillation persist with a rapid ventricular response, digitalis will still have to be administered. Long-term complications of prosthetic mitral valves, such as thrombus formation, infection, and mechanical dysfunction, are estimated to occur at a rate of 1 to 2 per cent per year. Thromboembolism occurs at a rate of 3 per cent per year with a mechanical mitral valve, whereas with the porcine valve, the incidence is 1 to 2 per cent per year.

MITRAL REGURGITATION

Etiology and Pathology

Mitral valve prolapse has now become the leading cause of mitral regurgitation (see next section), although rheumatic heart disease remains an important cause of mitral regurgitation (Table 52–4). Connective tissue disorders, coronary artery disease, annular calcification, and any condition producing left ventricular dilatation can create incompetence of the mitral valve. Several congenital cardiac conditions, such as partial atrioventricular (AV) canal, corrected transposition of the great arteries, and isolated cleft of the mitral valve seen with the ostium primum atrial septal defect, can be associated with mitral valve regurgitation.

Acute mitral regurgitation can result from sudden disruption of the normal function of the mitral valve apparatus. Ruptured mitral valve chordae from endocarditis, myxomatous degeneration of the valve, or trauma can produce sudden mitral regurgitation. Acute myocardial infarction can rupture the papillary muscle, and infective endocarditis can perforate the mitral valve leaflet or the chordae. Mechanical disturbances with a prosthetic mitral valve can lead to mitral incompetence.

Physiology

Incompetence of the mitral valve apparatus during systolic ejection permits regurgitation into the left atrium and pulmonary veins. The extent of the hemodynamic abnormalities imposed on the left ventricle and the left atrium is influenced by the chronic or acute nature of the valvular disturbance as well as the pre-existing functional state of the left ventricle. In chronic mitral regurgitation, a volume overload is imposed on the left ventricle, and the size of the regurgitant volume

TABLE 52–4. MITRAL REGURGITATION

Etiology	Physiology	Symptoms	Physical Examination	Electrocardiogram	Chest	Echocardiogram	Catheterization	Medical Therapy	Surgical Therapy
Chronic									
Prolapse Rheumatic Coronary artery disease Annular calcification Connective tissue disorder LV* dilatation Prosthetic valve	LV volume overload LV dilatation and hypertrophy LA* enlargement	Initially asymptomatic Fatigue Dyspnea	Holosystolic apical murmur Decreased S_1 Third sound	LV hypertrophy	Enlarged LV Enlarged LA	Enlarged LV and LA Mitral valve anatomy	Contrast from LV to LA LA v wave	Afterload reduction Diuretics Digitalis	Symptoms LV echo Diastolic dimension >60 mm†
Acute									
Ruptured chordae Ruptured papillary muscle Perforation of leaflet Prosthetic valve	Pressure overload LA and pulmonary veins No change in LV dimension	Acute pulmonary edema	Harsh holosystolic murmur radiating into back Third sound	No change Acute myocardial infarction	Normal LV and LA dimension Pulmonary edema	Abnormal mitral valve apparatus	Massive LA regurgitation Large v wave Normal-sized LA	Preload and afterload reduction	Surgery may be urgently required

*LV = left ventricle, ventricular; LA = left atrium atrial.
†Proposed.

will determine the increase in the end-diastolic volume. Systolic regurgitation into the left atrium produces a prominent v wave, which accentuates the normal filling of the left ventricle from the pulmonary venous inflow. With chronic mitral regurgitation, distensibility of the left atrium and pulmonary veins and increased compliant properties of the left ventricle permit rapid ventricular diastolic filling. As a result of the increased atrial and ventricular compliance, mean left atrial pressure and left ventricular end-diastolic pressure often remain within the normal range in chronic mitral regurgitation.

In *chronic mitral regurgitation,* the large total left ventricular stroke volume maintains the forward stroke volume despite the regurgitant volume into the left atrium. Total left ventricular output may reach six times the normal forward cardiac output. Left ventricular hypertrophy accompanies the increased left ventricular end-diastolic volume. Eventually, the contractile properties of the left ventricular myocardium decline, and the end-systolic volume is abnormally increased. The ejection fraction declines, even though the value may remain near the normal range in the early stage of left ventricular decompensation. An increase in the end-systolic volume elevates the pressure and wall stress values beyond those that can be attributed solely to changes in wall thickness or hypertrophy. This occurrence has been designated as a mismatch in afterload and preload. Even though the deterioration of the contractile state of the left ventricle may gradually elevate the left ventricular end-diastolic pressure, in rare instances the left atrium enlarges to such dimensions that ventricular end-diastolic and left atrial pressures remain normal, as encountered in the giant left atrium syndrome.

In coronary artery disease, mitral regurgitation results from abnormalities of posterior wall motion and papillary muscle function. Ischemia of the papillary muscle has been proposed as a mechanism, and disturbances in posterior wall motion are usually present with mitral regurgitation. When the residual scar after myocardial infarction exceeds 20 per cent of the total surface area of the ventricle, compensatory dilatation of the left ventricle is often attended by some degree of mitral regurgitation.

Severe dilatation of the left ventricle from either a primary volume overload or a secondary myocardial decompensation will eventually result in mitral regurgitation. Dilatation of the left ventricular chamber displaces the papillary muscles so that coaptation of the leaflets is impaired during systolic ejection. Conditions producing ventricular dilatation are further aggravated by depression of the contractile state, and the left ventricular hemodynamic abnormalities primarily reflect myocardial failure with an additional overload on the ventricle.

In *acute mitral regurgitation,* a sudden pressure overload is imposed on the left atrium and pulmonary veins from the left ventricular regurgitant volume. This pressure overload is intensified by the inability of the left atrium and left ventricle to dilate suddenly. The v wave in the left atrium may be as high as 60 to 70 mm Hg, resulting in acute pulmonary edema.

Clinical Features

When mitral regurgitation results from primary defects in the mitral apparatus, significant enlargement of the left ventricle develops, but the patient may remain symptom free with normal exercise tolerance. Since pulmonary venous hypertension and congestion are not features of mitral regurgitation in the early phase, fatigue due to reduced forward cardiac output is a more frequent symptom than dyspnea. Gradual impairment of the contractile state is attended by further enlargement of end-systolic and end-diastolic volumes and elevation of the left ventricular end-diastolic and left atrial pressures. Atrial fibrillation commonly develops when the left atrium enlarges and further aggravates heart failure.

In coronary artery disease, significant mitral regurgitation is usually accompanied by symptoms of impaired left ventricular function, such as dyspnea, fatigue, and orthopnea. This condition is sometimes designated as the ischemic cardiomyopathy syndrome. In acute syndromes of mitral regurgitation, pulmonary edema is often the initial presentation because of the suddenly imposed pressure and volume overload on the left atrium and pulmonary venous system.

Physical Examination

The typical physical finding of mitral regurgitation is the apical holosystolic murmur, but the intensity, variation during the ejection phase, and radiation over the precordium are influenced by the underlying mechanism. The peripheral pulse can sometimes be rapid in upstroke with a short duration because of the abbreviated systolic ejection time, since a large volume of blood is regurgitated into the left atrium. The precordium may reveal a diffusely hyperdynamic impulse, and the first heart sound at the apex is diminished. The characteristic holosystolic murmur radiates into the axilla and often to the left sternal border. A protodiastolic or ventricular gallop sound is frequently audible and may be followed by an early diastolic rumble due to the large inflow of blood from the left atrium. When mitral regurgitation is caused by left ventricular dilatation and depression of the contractile state, the systolic murmur may be mid-, late, or holosystolic. Under these circumstances, the systolic murmur is usually grade II/VI or less and is accompanied by a left ventricular (S_3) gallop sound.

In acute mitral regurgitation due to rupture of the mitral valve apparatus, the murmur is harsh, grade III or IV/VI, and accompanied by a palpable thrill at the apex.

Laboratory Studies

Electrocardiogram

In chronic mitral regurgitation, the electrocardiogram will show evidence of left ventricular dilatation and hypertrophy with increased QRS voltage and ST-T wave changes in the lateral precordial leads. Left atrial enlargement will produce a negative P wave in lead V_1, but atrial fibrillation often develops in the late stages. When coronary artery disease is the etiology of mitral regurgitation, there is often evidence of an inferior or posterior wall myocardial infarction.

Chest Radiograph

Left ventricular enlargement due to the volume overload can be appreciated from the standard chest film. Left atrial enlargement will cause a prominence along the right sternal border, but the pulmonary venous pattern may show no abnormalities until heart failure and venous congestion have developed.

Echocardiogram

The echocardiogram can define the anatomy of the mitral valve apparatus as well as left atrial and left ventricular chamber dimensions and function. Calcification of the valve leaflets and the annulus can be recognized. Depression of left ventricular ejection fraction and increases in end-diastolic and end-systolic dimensions are observed in secondary causes of mitral regurgitation with heart failure. With acute mitral regurgitation, a flail leaflet, ruptured chordae, or nidus of infection with infective endocarditis can sometimes be identified by the echocardiogram. The echoDoppler technique can assess the intensity of the regurgitant jet into the left atrium. Finally, left ventricular end-diastolic and end-systolic dimensions have been used to identify the optimal time for mitral valve replacement before significant and irreversible myocardial deterioration has taken place.

Exercise Testing

The standard exercise tests and radionuclide angiography can quantify functional capacity and document early deterioration in patients with mitral regurgitation.

Cardiac Catheterization

Left ventriculography confirms mitral regurgitation by demonstrating systolic regurgitation of contrast material into the left atrium. Although the magnitude of the regurgitation can be quantified, the mechanism is not always apparent from left ventriculography. Left ventricular end-diastolic and end-systolic dimensions can be utilized to calculate ejection fraction, left ventricular mass, wall stress, and regurgitant volume per beat into the left atrium. The difference between the angiographic left ventricular stroke volume—that is, the end-diastolic volume minus the end-systolic volume on left ventriculography—and the forward stroke volume, calculated from the Fick or thermodilution methods, yields the regurgitant stroke volume per beat across the mitral valve. Coronary artery disease and the wall motion abnormalities contributing to disturbance in mitral valve function can also be confirmed at catheterization. The prominent v wave of mitral regurgitation can be recorded in the left atrium or the pulmonary capillary wedge pressure tracing. In acute mitral regurgitation, dimensions of the left ventricle and left atrium may be normal, but the regurgitant v wave can rise to 60 to 70 mm Hg. Cardiac catheterization can also detect coexistent lesions in the aortic valve. Since the left ventricular ejection fraction may be misleading maintained in the normal range despite deterioration of the contractile state, additional assessment of the contractile state is important in all causes of mitral regurgitation. Calculation of end-systolic wall stress from pressure, volume, and wall thickness dimensions has proved useful in recognizing early deterioration of the contractile state in mitral regurgitation.

Differential Diagnosis

A holosystolic murmur identifies mitral regurgitation, even though the mechanism may not be apparent. Tricuspid regurgitation can cause a holosystolic murmur at the lower left sternal border, but inspiration accentuates the murmur more than in mitral regurgitation. If the murmur is not holosystolic, conditions such as aortic stenosis could be considered, along with papillary muscle dysfunction and mitral valve prolapse. In calcific aortic stenosis of the elderly patient, the murmur may sometimes be more prominent in the apex and may be confused with that of mitral regurgitation. A ventricular septal defect also causes a harsh holosystolic murmur at the lower left sternal border, but this generally radiates to the right of the sternum, compared with the axillary radiation of the murmur in mitral regurgitation.

Medical Therapy

In the early phase of mitral regurgitation without symptoms, only antibiotic prophylaxis is warranted. The same antibiotic program as described in the mitral stenosis should be administered to these patients. When atrial fibrillation develops, digitalis is indicated to slow the ventricular response. Afterload-reducing agents, such as nitrates and antihypertensive drugs, have been found useful in maintaining the forward stroke volume in mitral regurgitation. Once heart failure develops, diuretics and inotropic agents are required, but major consideration should be given to surgery.

Surgical Therapy

The operative mortality of mitral valve replacement in mitral regurgitation has remained higher than the 2 to 3 per cent in mitral stenosis and for the symptomatic patient may range from 5 to 10 per cent. In the past, surgery has been delayed until patients develop symptoms, but the advanced symptomatic stage and depressed left ventricular function contribute to high operative mortality rates. When the ejection fraction falls below 20 per cent, operative mortality for mitral valve replacement may be as high as 25 per cent. Therefore, surgery should be considered before the patient becomes extremely symptomatic. An echocardiographic diastolic dimension greater than 60 mm has been proposed as a predictor for mitral valve replacement. In the selection of the optimal prosthetic device, the patient's age, underlying condition, and circumstances for anticoagulation must be considered. The mechanical prosthetic valve in the mitral position is more likely to develop thrombotic material than in other locations, so anticoagulation must be maintained. Any contraindication to anticoagulation warrants consideration of a porcine valve. Thromboembolism in patients with mechanical valves who are on anticoagulation occurs at a rate of 3 per cent per year, and for preoperative functional classes I through III, there is a yearly mortality rate of 3 per cent over a ten-year follow-up period. With a porcine valve, the rate of thromboembolism is lower but may reach 1.5 per cent per year.

MITRAL VALVE PROLAPSE

Etiology and Pathology

Although an isolated systolic click has been regarded as benign for decades, echocardiography has identified prolapse of the mitral valve in as many as 5 per cent of the adult population. A variety of synonyms include the midsystolic click–late systolic murmur, click murmur syndrome, and Barlow's syndrome. Pathologic findings include myxomatous degeneration of the valve and redundancy of the valve leaflets. These changes can also involve the chordae as well as the mitral valve. Although the underlying mechanism is still incompletely understood, these changes in the mitral valve are seen with several connective tissue diseases, including Marfan's syndrome and osteogenesis imperfecta, and sometimes with coronary artery disease. The syndrome occurs most frequently in women in early adulthood and can also be found in families.

Physiology

The abnormalities of mitral valve prolapse can affect both anterior and posterior leaflets, but the posterior leaflet is most frequently involved. With the onset of ventricular systole, normal closure of the mitral valve takes place, but redundancy of the leaflets results in further upward motion of the valve into the left atrium. Sudden cessation of the valvular motion is thought to generate the click, and the lack of proper positioning of the two leaflets results in the systolic regurgitant murmur in mid- and late systole. Occasionally, both the anterior and posterior leaflets prolapse, and in extreme conditions, there can be extensive prolapse of both leaflets in the absence of a click or murmur. In a small number of patients, progressive degenerative changes in the valve or rupture of the chordae or both can produce severe mitral regurgitation.

Clinical Features

The majority of patients with mitral valve prolapse remain asymptomatic, but a spectrum of symptoms can be encountered. Symptoms include palpitations, fatigue, chest pain, orthostatic changes, and psychologic aberrations. Frequently, symptoms fail to correlate with the prominence of the physical findings and the extent of mitral regurgitation. Circulatory studies on changes in tilting, along with heart rate and blood pressure response changes, have lead to a diagnosis of dysautonomia in certain of these patients. In 10 to 15 per cent of affected individuals, palpitations may become frequent, and in a smaller number there may be progressive mitral regurgitation. Infective endocarditis occurs with a slightly higher incidence than in the normal population. Sudden deaths associated with this syndrome have been sporadically reported.

Physical Findings

Patients are often female, with a thin habitus and a narrow anteroposterior chest diameter. The principal findings are the early to midsystolic click and a mid- or late systolic murmur. The timing of the click as well as the characteristics of the murmur can vary widely. Often the murmur is crescendo and decrescendo, but it can be sustained in its frequency. The click or the murmur may be present alone, and not infrequently, both click and murmur are absent. The click and the murmur are influenced by the dimensions of the ventricle, and maneuvers that decrease ventricular filling, such as standing and the Valsalva maneuver, will result in movement of the click closer to the first sound, followed by early onset of the murmur. Conditions that increase filling of the ventricle, such as the squatting maneuver, can delay the onset of the click and the murmur.

Laboratory Studies

Electrocardiogram

The electrocardiogram may reveal a variety of T wave and ST segment changes, along with atrial or ventricular ectopic beats. Most commonly, the T wave is slightly inverted in the inferior and lateral precordial leads, and occasionally there is associated ST segment depression. Rarely, QT prolongation with deep coving of the T wave is seen in the precordial leads. Runs of premature beats, both from the atrium and the ventricle, can be recorded by Holter monitoring. Frequently, symptoms do not correlate with the frequency and occurrence of cardiac ectopic activity.

Chest Radiograph

The habitus is asthenic; the chest has a narrow anteroposterior diameter, and the cardiac silhouette is elongated.

Echocardiography

The echocardiogram is the diagnostic technique of choice for mitral valve prolapse. In one form, late systolic prolapse of the posterior leaflet resembles an inverted question mark. In the second form, there may be prolapse of the posterior leaflet throughout the systolic ejection phase with a hammock type of configuration. The echocardiographic findings of prolapse can be recognized in the absence of the click and the murmur. At other times, the click and murmur cannot be confirmed by echocardiographically evident prolapse of the leaflet. The standard for diagnosis of mitral valve prolapse is the two-dimensional echo, which can define the plane of the mitral annulus and demonstrate extension of the mitral valve leaflets beyond the annulus into the left atrium.

Exercise Testing

Stress testing can aggravate or precipitate cardiac irritability in these patients. Furthermore, the exercise test can document the patient's fatigue and musculoskeletal symptoms, which often are at variance with the echocardiographic findings.

Cardiac Catheterization

Although left ventriculography has been the standard invasive method for documenting redundancy and prolapse of the mitral leaflets, the precision of echocardiography has obviated the necessity of catheterization in the majority of patients with prolapse. Atypical chest discomfort sometimes requires coronary arteriography to exclude coronary artery disease. Wall motion abnormalities have been recognized on the ventriculogram, but these do not correlate with coexisting abnormalities in the coronary arteries. Prolapse of the tricus-

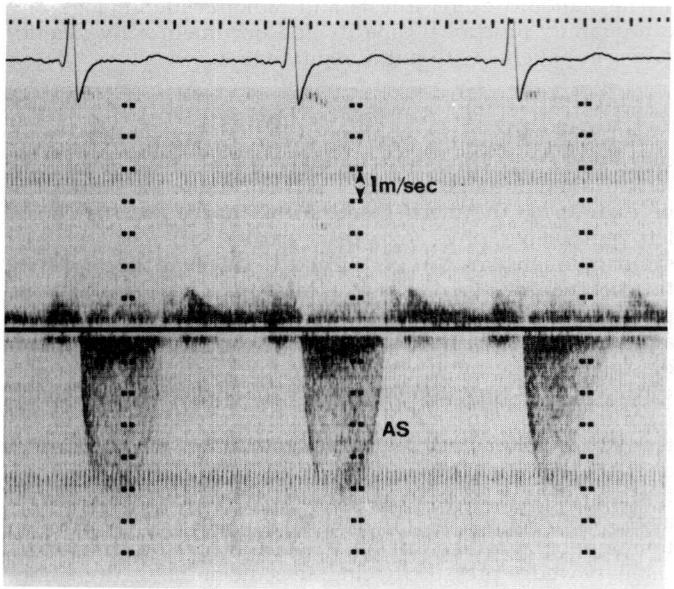

FIGURE 52–3. Continuous wave Doppler recording from the ascending aorta in a patient with severe aortic stenosis. The peak velocity is approximately 5 m/sec. Utilizing the modified Bernoulli equation, a peak instantaneous gradient across the aortic valve of 100 mm Hg can be calculated. Peak-to-peak gradient at catheterization was 80 mm Hg.

pid valve can also occur. With mitral valve prolapse in connective tissue disorders, there may be associated aortic regurgitation.

Differential Diagnosis

The mid- and late systolic murmur, as well as the crescendo-decrescendo qualities of mitral valve prolapse, can be similar to the murmur of regurgitation in papillary muscle dysfunction. In coronary artery disease or hypertrophic cardiomyopathy with obstruction, the crescendo-decrescendo murmur may be similar to that of mitral valve prolapse. However, the harsh intensity of the murmur is much louder with the hyperdynamic contraction of hypertrophic cardiomyopathy. Maneuvers that increase the murmur of mitral valve prolapse intensify the murmur of cardiomyopathy with obstruction even more. However, in the latter condition, the murmur is often holosystolic. If ventricular irritability is present, the intensity of the murmur of hypertrophic cardiomyopathy with obstruction will be much louder in the post-extrasystolic beat.

Treatment

The majority of patients with mitral valve prolapse require no treatment. Ventricular ectopy and symptoms of palpitations can be effectively managed with beta-blocking drugs. However, the fatigue in these patients can sometimes be aggravated with beta blockade. In patients with the prolonged QT interval or syncope, treatment with an antiarrhythmic is warranted. Infrequently, control of ectopy may be difficult despite the use of standard antiarrhythmic agents.

Infective endocarditis is a potential problem in these patients. Originally, all patients were advised to have antibiotic prophylaxis. Statistical studies now suggest that only those patients with an audible click and murmur should be treated with antibiotic prophylaxis. Patients with prolapse demonstrated on echocardiography without a click or murmur may be at no greater risk than the normal population. When mitral regurgitation becomes progressive with chamber enlargement or with ruptured chordae, mitral valve replacement may be necessary. Mitral valve reconstruction and mitral valve annuloplasty are preferred by some surgeons to total valve replacement. Fortunately, for the majority of patients, reassurance and conservative follow-up constitute the best treatment.

TRICUSPID STENOSIS

The most common cause of stenosis of the tricuspid valve remains rheumatic fever, but this condition is invariably associated with involvement of left-sided valves by the same rheumatic process. Rare conditions such as carcinoid tumor, endocardial fibroelastosis, and right atrial myxoma can create stenosis or obstruction of the tricuspid valve. Tricuspid stenosis causes right atrial hypertension and elevated systemic venous pressure. Stenosis of the tricuspid valve may serve as a protective mechanism for the pulmonary vascular bed in patients with mitral stenosis. Symptoms of tricuspid stenosis are dyspnea and fatigue, but the pulmonary manifestations of mitral stenosis can diminish with the development of significant stenosis of the tricuspid valve. Pulsations in the neck veins and peripheral edema develop.

Physical examination reveals a prominent, often giant, a wave in the neck veins caused by the vigorous atrial contraction against the stenotic valve. The diastolic murmur is heard best along the left lower sternal border and is presystolic if sinus rhythm is present or midsystolic with atrial fibrillation. The murmur increases prominently with inspiration, but an opening snap is barely heard. Since mitral stenosis is usually concurrent, the auscultatory maneuvers must specifically locate the tricuspid stenosis murmur. If tricuspid stenosis is the dominant hemodynamic lesion, pulmonary hypertension and right ventricular hypertrophy will not be detected on the physical examination.

The electrocardiographic finding is a tall, tented P wave in leads II, III, and aV_F with absence of right ventricular hypertrophy. The chest radiograph should reveal a large right atrium without prominence of the pulmonary arteries. The echoDoppler technique may detect and assess the gradient across the tricuspid valve. If cardiac catheterization is performed simultaneous catheters must be placed in the right atrium and the right ventricle for accurate detection of the pressure gradient. Respiratory variations will introduce inaccuracies in a pull-back tracing across the tricuspid valve. Treatment consists of antibiotic coverage. If surgery is performed for lesions in the left side of the heart, correction of the tricuspid lesion can also be undertaken.

TRICUSPID INSUFFICIENCY

Tricuspid insufficiency is, most commonly, secondary to right ventricular dilatation and hypertrophy. Tricuspid regurgitation can rarely result from infective endocarditis, trauma, prolapse, or congenital heart disease such as atrial septal defect or Ebstein's anomaly. Symptoms of tricuspid regurgitation are those of hepatic congestion or peripheral edema.

On physical examination, atrial fibrillation is commonly present and large cv waves can be detected in the jugular veins. The murmur is holosystolic along the left sternal border and increases with inspiration. The electrocardiogram often reveals atrial fibrillation without other significant features. The chest film will demonstrate a prominent right atrium and ventricle. The echocardiogram can document prolapse of the tricuspid leaflets as well as a nidus of infection or disruption of a chorda. Contrast-echo and echoDoppler techniques can accurately detect and assess the amount of tricuspid regurgitation. Therapy usually consists of treatment of conditions leading to right ventricular failure. Should surgery be performed for left-sided lesions, the tricuspid valve can be inspected. Often the leaflets are anatomically normal, and annuloplasty is indicated rather than valve replacement. If the tricuspid valve is replaced, along with insertion of mitral and aortic prostheses, mortality remains high at 20 per cent.

PULMONIC REGURGITATION

Regurgitation of the pulmonic valve is most invariably secondary to severe pulmonary hypertension, which can be caused by mitral stenosis, chronic lung disease, or pulmonary emboli. Inflammatory diseases and endocarditis can sometimes render the pulmonic valve incompetent, and previous surgery for congenital heart disease may create pulmonic regurgitation. The murmur (Graham Steell) is typically a high-pitched diastolic blow along the left sternal border similar to that in aortic regurgitation. No characteristic electrocardiographic changes are found, but the chest radiograph will often demonstrate a prominent pulmonary artery. The echoDoppler technique may detect turbulence in the pulmonary outflow tract. Cardiac catheterization is useful only to exclude aortic regurgitation as a cause of the diastolic murmur. Treatment consists of management of pulmonary hypertension with medical agents or occasionally with mitral valve surgery.

PULMONIC STENOSIS

Stenotic lesions of the pulmonic valve are almost always caused by congenital malformations (see Ch. 49). Rarely, hypertrophic cardiomyopathy can involve the right side of the heart with obstruction of the right ventricular outflow tract.

AORTIC VALVE DISEASE

Currie PJ, Seward JB, Reeder GS, et al.: Continuous wave Doppler echocardiographic assessment of severity of calcific aortic stenosis: A simultaneous

Doppler catheter correlative study in 100 adult patients. Circulation 71:1162, 1985. *A comparison of noninvasive and invasive estimates of aortic pressure gradients.*

Hoshino PK, Gaasch WH: When to intervene in chronic aortic regurgitation. Arch. Intern. Med 146:349, 1986. *A thorough review of noninvasive and invasive indications for the timing of aortic valve replacement in aortic regurgitation.*

Rackley CE, Edwards JE, Wallace RB, et al.: Aortic valve disease. In Hurst JW (ed.): The Heart. 6th ed. New York, McGraw-Hill Book Company, 1985, p 729.

Wood P: Aortic stenosis. Am J Cardiol 1:553, 1958. *A classic description of aortic stenosis.*

MITRAL VALVE DISEASE

Nishimura RA, McGoon MD, Shub C, et al.: Electrocardiographically documented mitral valve prolapse: Long term follow-up of 237 patients. N Engl J Med 313:1305, 1985. *A large clinical review with noninvasive criteria, for early mitral valve replacement.*

Rackley CE, Edwards JE, Karp RB: Mitral valve disease. In Hurst JW (ed.): The Heart. 6th ed. New York, McGraw-Hill Book Company, 1985, p. 754.

Rappaport E: Natural history of aortic and mitral valve disease. Am J Cardiol 36:221, 1975. *A ten-year follow-up of the stenotic and regurgitant lesions of the aortic and mitral valves.*

VALVE SURGERY

Cohn L, Allred E, Cohn L, et al: Early and late risk of mitral valve replacement. J Thorac Cardiovasc Surg 90:872, 1985. *A large review of the morbidity and mortality in porcine valve prostheses and prosthetic disc valves.*

Ivert TSA, Dismukes WE, Cobbs CG, et al.: Prosthetic valve endocarditis. Circulation 69:223, 1984. *An extensive review of a large series on prosthetic valve endocarditis.*

Magilligan DJ, Lewis JW, Tilley B, et al.: The porcine bioprosthetic valve twelve years later. J Thorac Cardiovasc Surg 89:499, 1985. *An extensive experience with the porcine prosthetic valve.*

53 DISEASES OF THE MYOCARDIUM

Joseph K. Perloff and Lynne Warner Stevenson

"Cardiomyopathy" means heart (cardio) muscle disease (myopathy). The term is appropriately applied to disorders characterized by *primary* involvement of ventricular myocardium. The cardiomyopathies are best classified according to their anatomic and pathophysiologic types as dilated, hypertrophic, or restrictive (Table 53–1, Fig. 53–1). In each category, the cause or causes may or may not be known.

DILATED CARDIOMYOPATHY

DEFINITION AND GENERAL DESCRIPTION OF FINDINGS. Dilated cardiomyopathy is characterized by an increase in left ventricular or biventricular internal dimensions without an appropriate increase in septal and free wall thicknesses. The essential physiologic impairment is in systolic function (depressed contractility).

Certain *general pathophysiologic principles* apply. Injured myocytes do not regenerate but are replaced by connective tissue. Hypertrophy of remaining cells does not adequately compensate for the loss of contractile elements. Ventricular volumes increase as ejection fractions fall, and the ventricles progressively dilate, especially the left. Stroke volume is initially maintained despite depressed ejection fraction, and compensatory tachycardia may help maintain cardiac output. This state of compensated systolic dysfunction is usually replaced by decompensated heart failure in which cardiac output is critically limited. The development of atrioventricular valve regurgitation adds to the hemodynamic burden and further depresses cardiac output. Hypervolemia and peripheral vasoconstriction contribute additionally to net ventricular overload.

TABLE 53–1. PATHOPHYSIOLOGIC CLASSIFICATION OF THE CARDIOMYOPATHIES

1. Dilated
2. Hypertrophic
   a. Asymmetric (eccentric)
   b. Symmetric (concentric)
3. Restrictive (nondilated, nonhypertrophic)
   a. Increased septal wall thickness
   b. Normal septal wall thickness

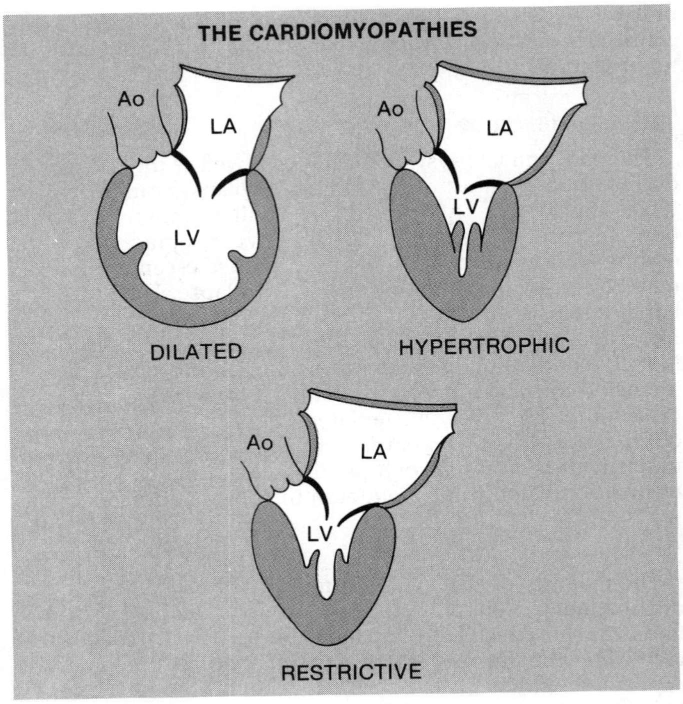

FIGURE 53–1. Schematic illustrations of dilated, hypertrophic, and restrictive cardiomyopathies. (Modified from Roberts WC, Ferrans VJ: Pathologic anatomy of the cardiomyopathies. Human Pathol 6:287, 1975. Reprinted with permission from W. B. Saunders Co.)

Two major threats confront the chronically afflicted patient, namely, progressive hemodynamic deterioration and sudden death. An insidious decrease in exercise tolerance is followed by frank exertional dyspnea, orthopnea, and paroxysmal nocturnal dyspnea. Both ventricles are usually involved, but the clinical manifestations of left ventricular failure generally predominate. The risk of sudden death is primarily the result of ventricular electrical instability—ventricular tachycardia or ventricular fibrillation. However, sudden death may also be due to systemic emboli from the left side of the heart or to pulmonary emboli.

On *physical examination*, the arterial pulse may be rapid (compensatory tachycardia) with a relatively small pulse pressure and pulsus alternans. The jugular venous pulse exhibits elevated A and V waves with preserved X and Y descents until the advent of tricuspid regurgitation, which increases the V wave and blunts the X descent. Precordial palpation identifies a displaced left ventricular impulse. Auscultation detects third and fourth heart sounds. Systolic murmurs originate from mitral and tricuspid regurgitation. Occasional patients have disproportionate right ventricular failure (peripheral edema, ascites, and painful hepatic congestion). An enlarged, tender liver exhibits an hepatic pulse that mirrors the jugular venous pulse.

The *electrocardiogram* may show nothing more than nonspecific ST-T wave abnormalities, but occasionally Q wave "infarct patterns" are present and are believed to reflect myonecrosis. Left bundle branch block is relatively frequent in chronic idiopathic dilated cardiomyopathy, but Chagas' disease is most commonly manifested by right bundle branch block.

The *chest roentgenogram* reveals varying degrees of cardiomegaly and pulmonary venous congestion. The increase in heart size principally reflects dilatation of the ventricles, although the atria are enlarged as well.

Two-dimensional echocardiography identifies increased internal dimensions of the ventricles at end-diastole, normal or reduced septal and free wall thicknesses, and depressed ventricular function. Although global hypokinesis is the rule, regional wall motion abnormalities occur and are believed to reflect zones of injury caused by a cardiotropic myonecrotic virus. Doppler echocardiography establishes the presence and degree of atrioventricular valve regurgitation. Technetium 99m radionuclide imaging sheds light on abnormal ventricular function and wall motion. The depressed response to exercise can be studied by technetium-99m scintigraphy and stress echocardiography. Magnetic resonance imaging provides refined morphologic information and, together with two-dimensional echocardiography, serves to identify left ventricular endocardial thrombi.

INCIDENCE. Over 10,000 deaths and 100,000 annual hospital admissions in the United States are attributed to dilated cardiomyopathy annually. Current estimates exceed 140 cases per million population per year, a threefold higher incidence than in 1970. The apparent increase probably reflects enhanced awareness and diagnostic accuracy.

ETIOLOGY, PATHOGENESIS, AND PATHOLOGY. The dilated cardiomyopathies are caused by primary myocardial injury that results in depressed systolic function and progressive ventricular dilatation. Table 53–2 lists most of the etiologic categories.

Myocardial inflammation—myocarditis—can be infectious or noninfectious. The majority of cases of dilated cardiomyopathy are believed to represent sequelae of myocarditis, generally infectious. Myocarditis, defined as inflammatory infiltrates and myocardial cell necrosis, is due to direct tissue invasion by the offending infectious agent, to an autoimmune process, or to toxins elaborated by an infectious organism. Every major type of infectious agent has been implicated as causative (Table 53–2), although with widely divergent incidence. In western Europe and the United States, infectious myocarditis is most commonly due to viruses, especially enteroviruses.

TABLE 53–2. ETIOLOGIC CLASSIFICATION OF THE DILATED CARDIOMYOPATHIES

- **I. Idiopathic**
- **II. Inflammatory**
  - A. Infectious
    1. Viral
    2. Bacterial
    3. Mycobacterial
    4. Parasitic
    5. Rickettsial
    6. Spirochetal
    7. Fungal
  - B. Noninfectious
    1. Autoimmune diseases
    2. Peripartum
    3. Hypersensitivity reactions
    4. Transplantation rejection
- **III. Toxic**
  - A. Ethyl alcohol
  - B. Chemotherapeutic agents
  - C. Elemental compounds
  - D. Catecholamines
- **IV. Metabolic**
  - A. Nutritional
  - B. Endocrinologic
  - C. Electrolyte abnormalities
- **V. Familial cardiomyopathy**
  - A. Neuromyopathic
    1. Progressive muscular dystrophy
    2. Myotonic muscular dystrophy
    3. Friedreich's ataxia
  - B. Hereditary dilated cardiomyopathy

The most convincingly documented cause of human myocarditis is coxsackievirus group B infection. Experimental murine coxsackievirus B3 infection results in an initial phase of active intramyocardial viral replication and cell necrosis during which physical exercise or immunosuppressive agents enhance replication of the virus and reinforce tissue injury. In the next phase, virus is not detectable in the myocardium. Instead, there is a population of thymus-derived lymphocytes apparently sensitized to myocytes. This phase of myocardial inflammation is believed to reflect immunologic virus-induced myocardial cellular injury caused by cytolytic thymus-derived T lymphocytes—immunopathic myonecrosis. Reduction of the offending lymphocyte population appears to coincide with a decrease in late myocyte injury. Infected animals may recover, die, or progress to a late third stage in which the dilated heart contains little or no inflammation but large areas of fibrosis.

The lymphocyte infiltration and myocyte necrosis of human viral myocarditis are found in the left and right ventricles and may be present in the atria as well. There is reason to believe that the left ventricle—the relatively high-pressure systemic chamber—responds more adversely to viral myocarditis than the less stressed right ventricle, which is a low-pressure, low-resistance pump.

Extensive lymphocytic infiltration and myocardial necrosis often occur in the absence of symptoms. It is likely, therefore, that many cases of primary myocarditis initially escape clinical detection. In the late phase of the natural history, active inflammatory cell infiltration is absent or nearly so. Chronic dilated cardiomyopathy is then characterized by the presence of areas of fibrosis interwoven among shrunken or hypertrophied myocytes. At this stage, the designation *idiopathic dilated cardiomyopathy* is commonly applied because thorough clinical evaluation fails to identify a specific cause in more than 80 per cent of patients so afflicted. Nevertheless, an association between myocardial inflammation initiated by cardiotropic viruses and the subsequent development of dilated cardiomyopathy is persuasive, as argued earlier.

In South America, up to 15 per cent of the rural population have primary myocardial injury due to infection by *Trypanosoma cruzi* (Chagas' disease). Chagas' cardiomyopathy is characterized by an acute tissue invasive phase followed by a chronic phase of extensive myocardial fibrosis believed to be the result of a lymphocyte- or an antibody-mediated autoimmune reaction. Chronic chagasic injury not only affects myocytes (with a peculiar propensity to cause apical left ventricular aneurysm) but also has a predilection for specialized tissues and for cardiac parasympathetic ganglia (denervation).

Noninfectious inflammation of the myocardium occurs with systemic diseases of connective tissues (autoimmune disorders), such as systemic lupus erythematosus. Of the *toxic agents* that directly injure ventricular myocardium, ethyl alcohol, or ethanol, is the commonest and has been implicated in at least 10 per cent of patients with dilated cardiomyopathy. The undesirable acute effects of ethyl alcohol on the myocardium are masked by the beneficial effects of peripheral vasodilatation and the positive inotropic response to released catecholamines, but ethanol in the autonomic blockaded heart causes a significant decrease in contractility. Both ethanol and acetaldehyde (its first metabolite) in sufficient concentrations can severely affect myocardial metabolism. Alcoholic cardiomyopathy is attributed to the toxicity of ethanol and acetaldehyde on the myocardial cell. In addition to the effects of ethyl alcohol and its metabolites, constituents of the brew may also depress contractility. Cobalt added to beer to stabilize foam is a case in point. In the beriberi heart disease of chronic alcoholics, high-output heart failure of thiamine deficiency is imposed upon the depressed myocardium of alcoholic cardiomyopathy. In addition, there is a positive epidemiologic association between excessive alcohol ingestion and systemic hypertension. An important clinical aspect of alcoholic cardiomyopathy is its reversibility, at least initially. However, pathologic studies late in the natural history reveal myocardial cell necrosis with replacement fibrosis.

A host of other toxic substances and drugs reportedly cause myocardial injury either as a result of excessive exposure or as idiosyncratic responses. Catecholamine excess may cause myonecrosis, and doxorubicin (Adriamycin) and other anthracycline chemotherapeutic agents are additional examples. The structural changes in response to anthracycline antitumor agents are dose related. Doxorubicin rarely results in acute heart failure and only occasionally produces acute arrhythmias and conduction disturbances. About 2 to 5 per cent of patients receiving 500 mg of the drug per square meter slowly develop overt heart failure, but over one half of patients have abnormal responses to exercise and exhibit histologic changes on endomyocardial biopsy. The microscopic pattern of doxorubicin-induced myocardial injury is characterized by the gradual appearance of vacuolar degeneration, myofibrillar loss, and juxtaposition of disrupted cells among normal cells.

The distinct clustering of *peripartum cardiomyopathy* in the last month of gestation and especially in the first three postpartal months supports the contention that the disorder is unique to pregnancy. Incidence has been estimated at from 1 in 3000 to 1 in 15,000 confinements. Myocardial inflammation is sufficiently frequent to warrant the designation "myocarditis," but the inflammation is not infectious. Despite diligent search, no role of cardiotropic viruses has been established. The peripartal myocardial injury is believed to result from an autoimmune reaction triggered by release of myocyte antigens from the late-term pregnant uterus.

Metabolic derangements that adversely affect systolic function and result in dilated cardiomyopathy include endocrinopathies, trace element deficiencies, and electrolyte abnormalities. In diabetes mellitus, systolic dysfunction with ventricular dilatation may be unrelated to large- or small-vessel coronary artery disease. Dilated heart failure in hyperthyroidism principally reflects pre-existing impairment of contractile reserve made clinically overt by the hypermetabolic state. An analogy is the high-output state of beriberi (vitamin B_1 deficiency) in chronic alcoholics. In classic Asian beriberi, however, dilated heart failure is due to thiamine deficiency per se in individuals without myocardial depression from other causes. Teenagers who excessively consume processed foods deficient in thiamine may suffer from heart failure provoked by heavy exercise. Although the principal initial physiologic effect of thiamine deficiency is on the peripheral circulation, persistent deficiency may lead to dilated cardiomyopathy. Abnormal regulation of carnitine, a cofactor in mitochondrial fatty acid metabolism, has also been associated with dilated heart failure.

A number of *electrolyte disorders* may aggravate pre-existing abnormalities of myocardial contractility. If the availability of calcium is inadequate, ejection fraction falls, as in patients receiving large transfusions of blood preserved with citrate, which chelates calcium, or in patients with hypoparathyroidism. Hypophosphatemia leads to inadequate stores of high-energy phosphate compounds, as in alcoholism, diabetes, and hyperalimentation. Magnesium, a cofactor for thiamine-dependent reactions and for sodium-potassium adenosine triphosphatase (ATPase), may be depleted by impaired gastrointestinal absorption or increased renal excretion(diuretics).

A number of heredofamilial *neuromyopathic disorders* are associated with dilated cardiomyopathy. Examples include X-linked, slowly progressive muscular dystrophy (Becker's dystrophy), certain patients in the late stages of Duchenne's dystrophy, Friedreich's ataxia, and the childhood form (but not the adult form) of myotonic muscular dystrophy.

DIAGNOSIS. Dilated cardiomyopathy should be suspected in relatively young patients who present with cardiac enlargement, congestive heart failure, systemic emboli, and ventricular arrhythmias. Chest pain indistinguishable from myocardial infarction (myonecrosis caused by the cardiotropic virus) sometimes accompanies acute myocarditis, but the mechanism of chest pain occasionally associated with chronic dilated cardiomyopathy is unclear. The diagnosis of dilated cardiomyopathy hinges on firm exclusion of pre-existing or coexisting heart disease. Cardiac catheterization has given way to noninvasive diagnostic procedures (see earlier) except for the exclusion of ischemic cardiomyopathy (coronary artery disease) in older patients, especially males.

If dilated cardiomyopathy presents sufficiently early in its course (persistent myocardial inflammation), throat and stool cultures and viral titers should be secured and serially compared. Up to 50 per cent of patients with clinical myocarditis have evidence of recent coxsackievirus B infection, especially types 1 to 5. Myocardial inflammation has been identified by gallium 67 scintigraphy, but more specifically by endomyocardial biopsy from the right ventricular septum. Biopsy positivity depends largely on when in the natural history the specimen is secured.

TREATMENT AND PROGNOSIS. Dilated cardiomyopathy confronts us with four major therapeutic concerns: the potential presence of ongoing myocardial injury, the hemodynamic state of the dilated heart, the threat of systemic emboli, and the risk of ventricular arrhythmias.

During the tissue-invasive stage of acute myocarditis, immunosuppressive agents provoke viral replication and are therefore proscribed. The majority of patients who present with active myocardial inflammation do so after the acute tissue-invasive stage. Attempts at pharmacologic suppression of persistent myocardial inflammation require documentation of the presence of inflammation. Although immunosuppression for biopsy-proven myocarditis in human subjects remains controversial, experience with cardiac transplant patients teaches us that immunosuppressive therapy can be lifesaving. Many patients with virally induced myocarditis improve during treatment with prednisone and azathioprine, and relapses have occurred after discontinuing immunosuppression. Whether or not immunosuppression is used, clinical status improves in up to one half of patients with biopsy-proven myocarditis. Not surprisingly, even patients who clinically improve usually have persistent abnormalities of ventricular systolic function. The grim prognosis of peripartum cardiomyopathy, coupled with evidence of noninfectious myocardial inflammation, argues for treatment with immunosuppressive agents, even though the relatively high incidence of spontaneous improvement is a confounding variable. If resolution occurs within six months after delivery, prognosis is good, although one half of such women have recurrences during subsequent pregnancies. Alcoholic cardiomyopathy often responds dramatically to abstention even after patients have become significantly symptomatic. Benefits previously attributed to strict bed rest in patients with dilated cardiomyopathy were largely the result of forced abstinence from ethyl alcohol. Continued ethanol consumption is associated with an inexorable deterioration and a three-year mortality of up to 80 per cent. Abstention should be undertaken in hospital so compliance can be assured, diet monitored, and arrhythmias controlled.

Doxorubicin (Adriamycin) cardiotoxicity is generally irreversible and is the cause of death in over 60 per cent of patients so afflicted. Careful monitoring during doxorubicin therapy minimizes the risk. Potential cardiomyopathy in response to doxorubicin can be identified by radionuclide angiography, two-dimensional echocardiography, or endomyocardial biopsy. Patients without additional cardiac risks are best studied after 450 mg per square meter of drug administration. Although a decline in ejection fraction at rest or with exercise arouses legitimate concern for myocyte damage, the frequency of false-positivity mandates that damage be confirmed by endomyocardial biopsy before therapy is withdrawn. Cardiotoxicity of doxorubicin is related not only to peak levels but also to cumulative dose. Toxicity is reduced by slow infusion rates.

In the treatment of the depressed hemodynamic state of dilated cardiomyopathy, digitalis glycosides have little to offer, and in fact toxicity is believed to be increased. Because the most disabling symptoms are due to circulatory congestion rather than to inadequate systemic perfusion, the establishment and maintenance of minimal ventricular filling pressures are critical to symptomatic control. Early in the natural history, this end can be achieved by empiric diuretic and vasodilator therapy adjusted according to symptomatic response. Should symptoms of circulatory congestion persist, especially in the face of relative systemic hypotension or declining renal function, hospitalization for insertion of a flotation catheter permits hemodynamic monitoring to seek a more effective regimen of diuretics and vasodilators.

The use of beta blockade in chronic dilated cardiomyopathy is seemingly contradictory and remains controversial. The theoretic benefit of reducing myocardial oxygen demand in the failing ventricle by beta-blocking agents has not been established by clinical trials. Some patients experience improvement in symptoms and ejection fraction, whereas in others serious decompensation ensues.

The risk of systemic emboli in dilated cardiomyopathy prompts use of long-term oral anticoagulants, which are obligatory if an endocardial thrombus announces itself as a systemic embolus or if a thrombus is found prior to embolization during noninvasive imaging. Systemic emboli arising from intracardiac thrombi occur in up to 30 per cent of patients with dilated cardiomyopathy, and pulmonary emboli are not uncommon.

The risk of ventricular arrhythmias is closely coupled with clinical and hemodynamic deterioration, but ventricular arrhythmias appear to be an independent variable in early mortality. Although patients with symptomatic ventricular tachycardia should be treated with antiarrhythmic agents, the value of such treatment for asymptomatic ventricular arrhythmias has not been established.

Prognosis of idiopathic dilated cardiomyopathy depends largely, but not exclusively, on the clinical and hemodynamic stages of the natural history at the time of presentation. Patients who are New York Association Class III or IV have a one-year mortality approaching 50 per cent and a five-year mortality of over 90 per cent. The lower the ejection fraction and cardiac index and the higher the left ventricular filling pressure, the higher the mortality. The above therapeutic recommendations may have dramatic impact on symptoms, but mortality remains high, although vasodilator therapy appears to reduce mortality in patients with mild symptoms. Hemodynamic failure and its complications account for only 50 to 70 per cent of mortality. Sudden death remains a major threat that is not convincingly reduced by antiarrhythmic agents, including amiodarone.

Cardiac transplantation has been performed in a total of more than 2500 patients, over one half of whom had primary dilated cardiomyopathy. The current one-year post-transplantation survival is 80 per cent, with a five-year survival of 60 per cent for patients on prednisone and cyclosporin immunosuppression. Limitation in donor availability restricts access to cardiac transplantation, and postoperative infection and rejection remain major causes of morbidity and mortality. Up to one third of candidates die before transplantation can be performed.

Dec GW, Palacios IF, Fallon JT, et al.: Active myocarditis in the spectrum of acute dilated cardiomyopathies: Clinical features, histologic correlates, and clinical outcome. N Engl J Med 312:885, 1985. *A series of 27 patients with dilated cardiomyopathy of recent onset in which biopsy-proven myocarditis and subsequent improvement were frequent, whether or not immunosuppressive drugs were given.*

Fowles RE, Mason JW: Role of cardiac biopsy in the diagnosis and management of cardiac disease. Prog Cardiovasc Dis 27:153, 1984. *This review includes a description of the biopsy procedure, the histology of many cardiomyopathies, and general indications for biopsy.*

Gillum RF: Idiopathic cardiomyopathy in the United States, 1970–1982. Am Heart J 111:752, 1986. *The discussion focuses on the difficulties in estimating the incidence of dilated cardiomyopathy and the apparent increase in incidence over the past ten years.*

Johnson RA, Palacios I: Dilated cardiomyopathies of the adult. N Engl J Med 307:1051, 1119, 1982. *An extensive review of the etiologies and diagnosis of dilated cardiomyopathies.*

Kantrowitz NE, Bristow MR: Cardiotoxicity of anti-tumor agents. Prog Cardiovasc Dis 27:195, 1984. *The review discusses the possible pathogenesis of cardiotoxicity and a strategy for monitoring cardiac injury.*

O'Connell JB, Costanzo-Nordin MR, Subramanian R, et al.: Peripartum cardiomyopathy: Clinical, hemodynamic, histologic, prognostic characteristics. J Am Coll Cardiol 8:52, 1986. *Characterization and prognosis of 14 patients who developed peripartum cardiomyopathy despite good general health and prenatal care. The relatively high incidence of myocarditis is documented and discussed.*

O'Connell JB, Henkin RE, Robinson JA, et al.: Gallium-67 imaging in patients with dilated cardiomyopathy and biopsy-proven myocarditis. Circulation 70:58, 1984. *Sixty-eight patients underwent gallium scans and endomyocardial biopsies. The study disclosed the sensitivity but lack of specificity of gallium imaging in diagnosing myocarditis.*

Perloff JK: Neurological disorders and heart disease. In Braunwald E (ed.): Heart Disease. 3rd ed. Philadelphia, W.B. Saunders Company, 1987. *A comprehensive review of the interplay between systemic neuromuscular disorders and cardiac involvement.*

Regan TJ: Alcoholic cardiomyopathy. Prog Cardiovasc Dis 27:141, 1984. *A comprehensive review of the pathogenesis, preclinical course, and prognosis of alcoholic cardiomyopathy.*

Reyes MP, Lerner AM: Coxsackie myocarditis—with special reference to acute and chronic effects. Prog Cardiovasc Dis 27:373, 1985. *A comprehensive review of the murine model of myocarditis and its relation to myocarditis in human subjects.*

THE HYPERTROPHIC CARDIOMYOPATHIES

DEFINITION. This category of disorders is represented grossly by asymmetric (eccentric) or symmetric (concentric) hypertrophy of the left ventricle in the absence of another cardiac or systemic disease capable of producing left ventricular hypertrophy (Table 53–1). In the asymmetric variety, the septum is disproportionately thick relative to the left ventricular free wall beneath the mitral annulus (Fig. 53–2). In the symmetric variety, the septum and left ventricular free wall are of equal thickness. Ventricular cavity size is normal or reduced in both types.

ETIOLOGY. Just over one half of patients with hypertrophic cardiomyopathy have clear evidence of genetic transmission, usually an autosomal dominant trait. Sporadic occurrences may represent new mutations, reduced penetrance in first-degree relatives, autosomal recessive transmission, or nongenetic occurrence. Biochemical determinants in the pathogenesis are not firmly established but have focused on two inter-related hypotheses—the proposed intrauterine links between myocyte development and norepinephrine stimulation and/or excess intracellular calcium.

PATHOLOGY. Genetic hypertrophic cardiomyopathy is characterized by two gross morphologic and two histologic features. The gross morphologic features are asymmetric septal hypertrophy and a catenoid ventricular septal configuration (Fig. 53–2). The most typical histologic feature—cellular disarray—is significantly more common (95 per cent of patients) and quantitatively considerably more extensive in hypertrophic cardiomyopathy than in other cardiac disorders or in normal subjects. In its proper clinical and pathologic context, extensive septal cellular disarray remains an important marker of genetic hypertrophic cardiomyopathy. The second histologic feature—thick-walled intramural coronary arteries with narrow lumens—occurs in more than three fourths of patients with genetic hypertrophic cardiomyopathy, especially in the ventricular septum. The pathogenetic and clinical significance of the thickened intramural coronary arteries is unresolved.

PHYSIOLOGY. Characterization of the physiologic derangements in genetic hypertrophic cardiomyopathy sets the stage for an understanding of the clinical manifestations, diagnosis, and treatment. The principal physiologic features include a hypercontractile left ventricular free wall (enhanced

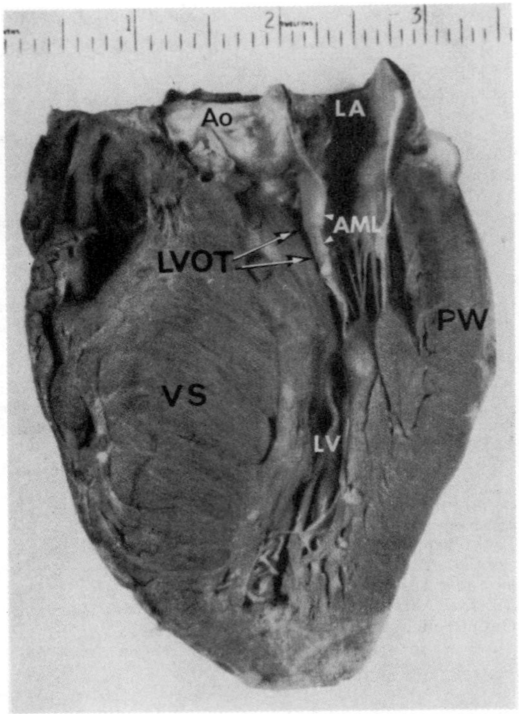

FIGURE 53–2. One of Teare's original cases of "asymmetrical hypertrophy of the heart." The ventricular septum (VS) is substantially thicker than the left ventricular posterior wall (PW). The cavity of the left ventricle (LV) is much reduced. The base of the ventricular septum bulges into the left ventricular outflow tract (LVOT) adjacent to the anterior mitral leaflet (AML). Ao = Aorta; LA = left atrium. (From Teare D: Asymmetrical hypertrophy of the heart in young adults. Br Heart J 20:1, 1958, with permission. Labels superimposed.)

systolic function), prolonged left ventricular isovolumetric relaxation (impaired diastolic function), hypocontractile ventricular septum, and left ventricular cavity obliteration. Normal ventricular contraction consists of an isovolumetric phase that occupies about 10 per cent of systole and an ejection phase with fiber shortening that occupies 80 to 90 per cent of systole. In genetic hypertrophic cardiomyopathy, a third phase is added. High-velocity ejection is completed in the first 60 to 80 per cent of systole, following which the cavity obliterates and the myocardium contracts isometrically. Thus, hypertrophic cardiomyopathy is characterized by enhanced systolic function, a prolonged and abnormally powerful isometric contraction phase followed by prolonged left ventricular isovolumetric relaxation (impaired diastolic function).

Classic genetic hypertrophic cardiomyopathy is accompanied by a singular physiologic feature that continues to generate lively interest and considerable controversy—the left ventricular to aortic dynamic pressure gradient (Fig. 53–3). Entrapment of the catheter tip during cavity obliteration spuriously elevates the recorded systolic pressure within the left ventricle. However, a true gradient has been ascribed to narrowing of the left ventricular outflow tract by the thick base of the ventricular septum, coupled with systolic anterior motion of the anterior mitral leaflet, which is usually accompanied by mitral regurgitation. Although the term "hypertrophic obstructive cardiomyopathy" is applied in this setting, it has been argued that neither the gradient nor systolic anterior motion of the anterior mitral leaflet is justifiably equated with the presence of true obstruction. The earlier term "idiopathic hypertrophic subaortic stenosis" has fallen out of use because hypertrophic cardiomyopathy is not necessarily so characterized, even though the disorder first came into prominence because of the systolic pressure difference across the subaortic portion of the left ventricular outflow tract.

The gradient is "dynamic," a term that calls attention to its lability and to its response to certain physical and pharmacologic interventions (Fig. 53–3). Interventions that reduce left ventricular internal dimensions (cavity size) intensify the gradient and vice versa. The gradient increases during the straining phase of Valsalva's maneuver; during prompt standing, especially from the squatting position; following the compensatory pause after a premature beat; and in response to isotonic exercise, tachycardia, digitalis, isoproterenol, amyl nitrite, and nitroglycerin. The gradient decreases during the overshoot phase of Valsalva's maneuver, during Muller's maneuver, upon squatting, in response to isometric exercise (handgrip), and in response to beta-adrenergic blockade or alpha-adrenergic stimulation. In patients with significant gradients, administration of inotropic drugs or volume-depleting diuretics can be accompanied by sudden and serious deterioration.

CLINICAL MANIFESTATIONS. The symptomatically overt disease typically becomes manifest in young adults (mid third decade), but it is not uncommon for patients to present after 60 years of age. In infants, the disorder announces itself

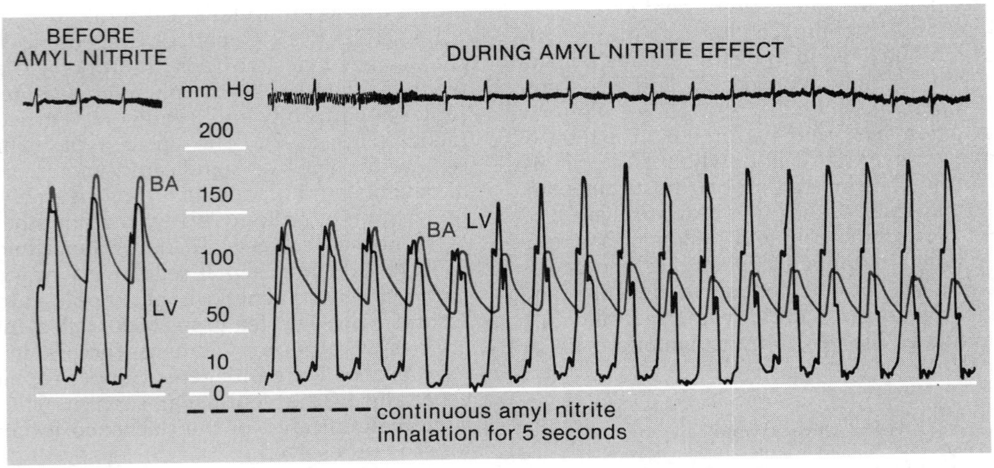

FIGURE 53–3. Tracings from a patient with asymmetric hypertrophic cardiomyopathy. The control tracing shows no outflow gradient. Amyl nitrite induced a peak LV-BA systolic gradient of 100 mm Hg. Observe the initial parallel fall in both left ventricular (LV) and brachial arterial (BA) pressures with subsequent divergence. (From Marcus FI, Perloff JK, De Leon AC: The use of amyl nitrite in the hemodynamic assessment of aortic valvular and muscular subaortic stenosis. Am Heart J 68:468, 1964, with permission.)

as a murmur and marked congestive failure, with the majority of afflicted babies dying before their first birthday. In adults, the clinical picture varies from incapacitating symptoms to asymptomatic relatives who exhibit few or no manifestations of illness except on echocardiography. It is dramatic but not uncommon for the disease to declare itself as syncope or sudden death in previously healthy young persons engaged in strenuous exertion. The commonest cluster of symptoms consists of dyspnea, fatigue, chest pain (similar to, if not identical with, angina pectoris), and syncope. The most prevalent symptom is dyspnea, which is intensified by exertion and which is a reflection of high end-diastolic and pulmonary venous pressures (left ventricular diastolic dysfunction). Symptoms are unrelated to the presence or degree of the left ventricular outflow gradient. Clinical deterioration is typically slow with two major exceptions—sudden death or the onset of atrial fibrillation. Loss of coordinated atrial contraction in the face of impaired left ventricular diastolic distensibility results in acute dyspnea (sudden increase in end-diastolic and pulmonary venous pressures).

In older subjects, chest pain coupled with electrocardiographic Q waves (see later) prompts a diagnosis of atherosclerotic coronary artery disease, which may coexist. However, symptoms resembling angina pectoris occur in relatively young patients without extramural coronary artery disease.

Cerebral symptoms vary from lightheadedness to frank syncope and are not strictly analogous to the cerebral symptoms in discrete aortic valve stenosis. Patients sometimes feel faint in the upright position (promptly corrected by lying down) or in response to physical exercise. Occasional patients report such a history for years without apparent clinical deterioration. Signs of cerebral hypoperfusion may in part reflect a fall in cardiac output due to physical interventions that decrease left ventricular cavity size and left ventricular filling. Arrhythmic syncope is ominous and heralds sudden death (see below).

The *physical examination* in asymptomatic patients without systolic gradients is unimpressive except for a relatively prominent left ventricular impulse and a fourth heart sound. The jugular venous pulse may exhibit a prominent A wave (increased force of right atrial contraction) that does not reflect pulmonary hypertension, but instead is a response to impaired distensibility of the right ventricular cavity caused by massive thickening of the ventricular septum. The increase in velocity of left ventricular ejection is reflected in the brisk rate of rise of the systemic arterial pulse while the blood pressure remains normal (small waterhammer pulse). Twin peaking results from a mid- to late-systolic trough, a feature better recorded than palpated. Precordial palpation sometimes detects a relatively uncommon but more characteristic *triple* apical impulse composed of double systolic movement coupled with presystolic distention. A systolic thrill may be present at the apex and toward the lower left sternal edge in patients with left ventricular outflow gradients, but the thrill corresponds more closely to mitral regurgitation than to the severity of the pressure gradient. Auscultation detects a prominent apical fourth heart sound, a normal first sound, and at the left base a second sound that is usually normally split, sometimes narrowly split or single, and occasionally paradoxically split. Despite the increased velocity of left ventricular ejection, aortic ejection sounds are sufficiently exceptional to call the diagnosis of hypertrophic cardiomyopathy into question. Systolic murmurs in patients with left ventricular outflow gradients represent combinations of midsystolic murmurs caused by increased velocity of ejection and a longer, if not holosystolic, apical murmur caused by mitral regurgitation. The murmur is typically loudest at the apex, with radiation into the axilla or to the left lower sternal edge, less prominently to the base, and seldom into the neck. The systolic murmur is important less because of its presence than because of the diagnostic significance of its response to physical and pharmacologic interventions (Table 53–3). Third heart sounds occur in the presence of mitral regurgitation and are occasionally followed by brief after-vibrations that create the auscultatory impression of a short mid-diastolic murmur. A high-frequency early diastolic murmur of aortic regurgitation makes the diagnosis of hypertrophic cardiomyopathy doubtful.

TABLE 53–3. EFFECTS OF BEDSIDE PHYSICAL INTERVENTIONS ON THE SYSTOLIC MURMUR OF ASYMMETRIC HYPERTROPHIC CARDIOMYOPATHY

Increased Intensity of Murmur
Dynamic exercise
Straining phase of Valsalva's maneuver
Prompt standing after squatting
Decreased Intensity of Murmur
Release (overshoot) phase of Valsalva's maneuver
Squatting
Isometric exercise (handgrip)

Normal *electrocardiograms* are confined to a minority of asymptomatic patients. The tracings are almost invariably abnormal in symptomatic patients with left ventricular outflow gradients. P wave morphology generally reflects a left atrial abnormality alone, but occasionally together with a right atrial configuration. The PR interval is often short but only rarely in conjunction with evidence of pre-excitation, even when the short PR interval is accompanied by initial force slurring reminiscent of delta waves. Atrial fibrillation, the commonest sustained supraventricular rhythm disturbance, is not associated with accelerated atrioventricular conduction.

Prominent Q waves occur in upwards of 50 per cent of cases. The Q waves tend to be abnormal because of their depth rather than their duration. The Q waves have been ascribed to abnormal electrophysiologic properties in areas of cellular disarray. Electrocardiographic evidence of left ventricular hypertrophy is common but not invariable and is reflected in the increased voltage and ST segment and T wave abnormalities. Giant T wave inversions in mid to left precordial leads imply *apical* hypertrophic cardiomyopathy.

In the *chest roentgenogram,* enlargement of the left atrium is relatively common, especially when mitral regurgitation coexists. Dilatation of the left atrium is most conspicuous when mitral regurgitation is accompanied by atrial fibrillation. Left ventricular size and contour range from normal to a prominent convex silhouette projecting to the left, inferior and posterior. The aortic root is typically inconspicuous, and calcification of aortic valve or mitral apparatus is absent.

The echocardiogram is the mainstay of the *laboratory diagnosis* of hypertrophic cardiomyopathy, providing virtually all necessary clinical diagnostic information. The cardinal echocardiographic features of genetic hypertrophic cardiomyopathy are disproportionate thickness of the ventricular septum with a septal/posterior left ventricular wall ratio of 1.5:1 or more, a small left ventricular cavity, and exaggerated contractility of the left ventricular free wall with a relatively hypocontractile ventricular septum. Two-dimensional echocardiography establishes the location and extent of disproportionate septal thickness and occasionally shows on real-time imaging a ground-glass appearance of the septum believed to be related to cellular disarray. Systolic anterior motion of the anterior mitral leaflet, an important feature of the echocardiogram in the presence of left ventricular outflow gradients, is almost invariably accompanied by mitral regurgitation established by Doppler interrogation. Doppler echocardiography is pivotal in establishing the patterns of left ventricular ejection and in characterizing the abnormal diastolic properties of the left ventricle (impaired relaxation).

Technetium 99m gated radionuclide ventriculography identifies the thickness of the ventricular septum, the relative motions of septum and free wall, and the left ventricular cavity size in diastole and systole. Magnetic resonance imaging, with its capability of recording in multiple planes, provides refined morphologic information.

Prior to noninvasive imaging (especially echocardiography), *cardiac catheterization* provided the standards for the clinical diagnosis of hypertrophic cardiomyopathy. The systemic arterial pulse pressure fails to increase in the beat ending the compensatory pause after a premature ventricular contraction. The significance of recorded differences in systolic pressure between left ventricular cavity and aortic root is still debated. The subaortic gradient, like the systolic murmur, is reinforced by pharmacologic interventions that reduce left ventricular cavity size (Table 53–3, Fig. 53–3), and the gradient, like the murmur, decreases in response to interventions that increase left ventricular cavity size. Left ventriculography reveals a relatively small, angulated chamber in diastole, with systolic cavity obliteration and mitral regurgitation. In older patients with chest pain, selective coronary angiography is necessary to resolve the issue of coexisting atherosclerotic artery disease.

An important variation on the foregoing theme is the excessive *concentric* hypertrophic cardiomyopathy occasionally found in mildly hypertensive elderly patients. Two-dimensional echocardiographic features include severe concentric left ventricular hypertrophy, reduced left ventricular cavity size, enhanced systolic emptying with cavity obliteration, and impaired diastolic function.

TREATMENT. Hypertrophic cardiomyopathy cannot be prevented, but echocardiographic identification of clinically occult disease in first-degree relatives is desirable and sets the stage for genetic counseling. Certain proscriptions are important, such as sudden, strenuous, or isometric exercise or the use of digitalis glycosides, beta-adrenergic stimulants, or nitrates, all of which reduce left ventricular cavity size and may significantly enhance symptoms. Prophylaxis for infective endocarditis is necessary when mitral regurgitation accompanies hypertrophic cardiomyopathy.

Treatment falls into two broad categories: first, relief of symptoms (especially dyspnea and chest pain); and second, control of arrhythmias. A prime pharmacologic objective is to improve abnormal left ventricular relaxation and to enhance diastolic filling. Beta-adrenergic blockade has been a keystone of medical therapy in this regard. The largest clinical experience has been with propranolol. Dyspnea and angina pectoris respond favorably, the latter more so than the former. Disappointing, however, is the long-term capability of propranolol in maintaining its beneficial effects. Only a minority of patients experience long-term improvement, and an increase in dosage is often accompanied by unacceptable side effects. Calcium channel blockers, especially verapamil, are important therapeutic alternatives. Nifedipine is less effective, and data on diltiazem are currently inadequate to provide a basis for judgment. Intravenous verapamil is capable of decreasing the left ventricular outflow gradient with maintenance of cardiac output. The mechanism of action is believed to be enhancement of left ventricular diastolic filling and a decrease in left ventricular systolic function in response to reduced myocardial uptake of calcium. Verapamil improves exercise capacity and relieves symptoms during short- and long-term therapy in patients who previously experienced inadequate symptomatic relief with beta receptor–blocking agents. The most serious adverse effects of verapamil are electrophysiologic, namely, atrioventricular dissociation, Wenckebach periods, or sinus arrest. Verapamil administration can also be accompanied by postural hypotension and pulmonary congestion, the latter generally requiring cessation of administration. Because of these adverse effects, the drug should be used with caution or not at all in patients with significant abnormalities of atrioventricular conduction or sinus node function or in patients with low systemic systolic blood pressure or clinical evidence of increased pulmonary venous pressure. Because the adverse electrophysiologic effects of verapamil are dose related, a reduction in dose sometimes permits continuation of the drug.

The foregoing therapeutic recommendations are also applicable to the mildly hypertensive elderly patient with symptomatic *concentric* hypertrophic cardiomyopathy (see earlier). In this setting, abnormal diastolic function and excessive systolic emptying are favorably influenced by beta antagonists and calcium channel blockers and are aggravated by conventional therapy with inotropic agents or vasodilators.

Antiarrhythmic therapy in genetic hypertrophic cardiomyopathy deals chiefly with atrial fibrillation or ventricular arrhythmias. Atrial fibrillation is properly regarded as a medical emergency and should be electrically cardioverted without delay (even before preconversion treatment with intravenous heparin) to circumvent the serious hemodynamic sequelae following loss of the atrial contribution to ventricular filling. Amiodarone (see below) is the most efficacious drug for maintaining sinus rhythm. Because of the relatively long interim between initial amiodarone administration and its sustained pharmacologic effect, heparin administration is advisable during that interval.

Ventricular arrhythmias are relatively common in hypertrophic cardiomyopathy and are represented by uniform or polymorphic premature ventricular beats occurring singly or repetitively. Because ventricular tachycardia and fibrillation are believed to be the chief causes of sudden death, antiarrhythmic suppression is pivotal. Treatment with conventional agents such as quinidine, disopyramide, or mexiletine has been disappointing, and propranolol-induced relief of angina pectoris and dyspnea has not been accompanied by a significant reduction in ventricular arrhythmias. The potentially malignant ventricular arrhythmias that prevail in genetic hypertrophic cardiomyopathy are essentially unknown in the hypertrophic cardiomyopathy of Friedreich's ataxia, whether asymmetric or concentric, and septal cellular disarray has not been found at necropsy in Friedreich's disease. Accordingly, the electrical instability inherent in cellular disarray may be the fundamental cause of ventricular arrhythmias in genetic hypertrophic cardiomyopathy. Amiodarone suppresses ventricular tachycardia in this setting, and long-term use of the drug may favorably influence the risk of sudden death.

Surgery is a therapeutic option in markedly symptomatic patients who do not respond satisfactorily to medical management. The most widely used operation is transaortic ventricular septal myotomy-myectomy, which consists of excising a portion of the hypertrophied septum. Surgery reduces or abolishes the left ventricular outflow gradient as well as the mitral regurgitation and appears to prevent progression of hypertrophy, although the operative risk is 5 to 10 per cent. Mitral valve replacement, a less desirable and seldom applied alternative, also eliminates the left ventricular outflow gradient and the mitral regurgitation. Because the symptoms in hypertrophic cardiomyopathy are not correlated with the presence or magnitude of the left ventricular outflow gradient, operation is believed to exert its beneficial effects for unestablished reasons that are apart from the reduction in gradient. Late postoperative progression to left ventricular dilatation and failure—dilated cardiomyopathy—is a serious and not exceptional sequel.

PROGNOSIS. Except for the infant with clinically overt hypertrophic cardiomyopathy in the first year of life, the natural history is usually characterized by slow progression. The most ominous threat is sudden death, which often occurs during exercise in persons who were previously clinically well. There is no necessary relationship between prognosis and the presence or degree of the left ventricular outflow gradient. Atrial fibrillation, however, is a poor prognostic eventuality accompanied by congestive heart failure and the risk of systemic embolization. Infective endocarditis is a complication related chiefly to the presence of mitral regurgitation. The transition of hypertrophic cardiomyopathy to dilated cardiomyopathy usually, but not necessarily, proceeds after septal myotomy-myectomy (see earlier). Less commonly, progressive left ventricular dilatation and failure occur as part of the natural history and have been ascribed to myocardial infarction with or without extramural atherosclerotic coronary artery disease.

In women of childbearing age, the prognosis accompanying pregnancy is good despite a number of undesirable hemodynamic variables during the course of gestation, labor, and delivery. The increases in cardiac output and left ventricular diastolic volume during pregnancy reduce the left ventricular outflow gradient, but the fall in systemic resistance counteracts this effect. Supine compression of the inferior vena cava by the gravid uterus impedes venous return, reduces left ventricular volume, and augments the left ventricular outflow gradient. Accordingly, pregnant patients with hypertrophic cardiomyopathy are advised to avoid the supine position toward term and during labor. A number of conflicting variables come into play during labor. Adrenergic stimulation associated with pain and stress, together with the Valsalva maneuver (bearing down), increases the left ventricular outflow gradient, but the rise in central blood volume during active uterine contraction has the opposite effect. The rapid decline in blood volume during the puerperium reduces left ventricular internal dimensions and intensifies the outflow gradient.

Criley JM, Siegel RJ: Has "obstruction" hindered our understanding of hypertrophic cardiomyopathy? Circulation 72:1148, 1985. *A concise, informative editorial summarizing the controversy regarding obstruction to left ventricular outflow in patients with asymmetric hypertrophic cardiomyopathy.*

Maron BJ, Merrill WH, Freier PA, et al.: Long-term clinical course and symptomatic status of patients after operation for hypertrophic subaortic stenosis. Circulation 57:1205, 1978. *Late results of operation were reviewed in 124 patients with hypertrophic cardiomyopathy. Surgical technique, operative risk, and short-term and long-term outcomes are reviewed.*

Maron BJ, Nichols PF, Pickle LW, et al.: Patterns of inheritance in hypertrophic cardiomyopathy: Assesment by M-mode and two-dimensional echocardiography. Am J Cardiol 53:1087, 1984. *This important paper focuses on the mode of inheritance of hypertrophic cardiomyopathy in 367 relatives from 70 families.*

Maron BJ, Roberts WC, Epstein SE: Sudden death in hypertrophic cardiomyopathy: A profile of 78 patients. Circulation 65:1388, 1982. *No morphologic or hemodynamic variable was characteristic of patients with hypertrophic cardiomyopathy and premature sudden death or cardiac arrest. The implication is an arrhythmogenic cause.*

McKenna WJ, Oakley CM, Krikler DM, et al.: Improved survival with amiodarone in patients with hypertrophic cardiomyopathy. Br Heart J 53:412, 1985. *The control of ventricular arrhythmias with amiodarone was associated with significantly improved survival, suggesting that the cause of sudden death is arrhythmogenic and that amiodarone may prevent death in patients with hypertrophic cardiomyopathy and ventricular tachycardia.*

Perloff JK: Pathogenesis of hypertrophic cardiomyopathy. In Goodwin JF (ed.): Heart Muscle Disease. Lancaster, England, MTP Press Ltd., 1985, pp 7–22. *Pathogenesis is dealt with in light of anatomic, physiologic, and clinical features of hypertrophic cardiomyopathy. The catecholamine hypothesis is elaborated.*

Rosing DR, Idanpaan-Heikkila U, Maron BJ, et al.: Use of calcium channel blocking drugs in hypertrophic cardiomyopathy. Am J Cardiol 55:185B, 1985. *An important long-term drug study dealing with 227 patients treated with verapamil. A policy regarding drug administration is recommended, and the beneficial and adverse effects are reviewed.*

Topol EJ, Traill TA, Fortuin NJ: Hypertensive hypertrophic cardiomyopathy of the elderly. N Engl J Med 312:277, 1985. *Excessive concentric left ventricular hypertrophic cardiomyopathy with reduced cavity size, enhanced systolic emptying, and impaired diastolic function was identified in elderly patients with mild systemic hypertension. Diagnostic and therapeutic implications are underscored.*

Wigle ED: Hypertrophic cardiomyopathy: A 1987 viewpoint. Circulation 75:311, 1987. *An editorial that takes the form of an excellent review of hypertrophic cardiomyopathy.*

THE RESTRICTIVE CARDIOMYOPATHIES

DEFINITION. Restrictive cardiomyopathies, the least common of the three major categories (Table 53–1), are characterized by a *primary* abnormality of *diastolic* ventricular function (impediment in filling) with normal or nearly normal systolic function (contraction). The term "restrictive cardiomyopathy" is not appropriately applied when the primary derangement is systolic function associated with variable degrees of diastolic impairment (late-stage dilated cardiomyopathy, for example). Nor is the term properly used to characterize the impaired diastolic function secondary to cardiac hypertrophy (hypertrophic cardiomyopathy, see above). In the restrictive cardiomyopathies, there is little or no increase in end-diastolic or end-systolic dimensions of either ventricle—hence the designation "nondilated, nonhypertrophic cardiomyopathy" or "congestive heart failure with normal systolic function." Restrictive cardiomyopathy functionally resembles constrictive pericarditis.

Myocardial stiffness refers to those effects that reflect changes in each unit of muscle, in contrast to *chamber stiffness,* which refers to changes in muscle mass rather than in unit of muscle. Chamber stiffness can be increased while myocardial stiffness is normal (left ventricular hypertrophy), whereas in restrictive cardiomyopathy, chamber stiffness is closely coupled to myocardial stiffness. Myocardial stiffness can be impaired for a host of reasons, many of which are shown in Table 53–4.

TABLE 53–4. ETIOLOGIES OF THE RESTRICTIVE CARDIOMYOPATHIES

- I. **Myocardial**
  - A. Infiltrative
    1. Amyloid
    2. Sarcoid
    3. Hemochromatosis
    4. Glycogen storage diseases
    5. Hurler's disease
    6. Fabry's disease
  - B. Noninfiltrative
    1. Idiopathic
    2. Radiation
    3. Scleroderma
- II. **Endomyocardial**
  - A. Endomyocardial fibrosis
  - B. Idiopathic hypereosinophilic syndrome

Infiltrative Restrictive Cardiomyopathies (Table 53–4)

AMYLOIDOSIS. Amyloid heart disease is the paradigm of the infiltrative cardiomyopathies. Classification of amyloidosis remains imprecise, although the hallmark of tissue injury in typical cardiac amyloidosis is replacement of normal contractile elements by interstitial deposits. The gross appearance of the heart in primary amyloidosis is occasionally normal, but the myocardium is characteristically firm, rubbery, and noncompliant, with ventricular cavities that are normal to small (Fig. 53–4). Histologically, insoluble fibrillar proteins are deposited in the interstitium of all four chambers. Primary amyloidosis also involves the pericardium and cardiac valves (especially atrioventricular) and infiltrates the sinus node in about 50 per cent of cases. Deposition of amyloid in the walls of intramural coronary arteries and arterioles is almost invariable and is held responsible for myocardial ischemia.

The pathophysiologic mechanisms of disturbed ventricular function and the clinical manifestations of cardiac amyloidosis are understood in light of certain morphologic details. *Interstitial* infiltration impairs diastolic function, leaving systolic function initially normal or nearly so. Systolic function is sometimes well preserved despite advanced amyloid deposition, although with progressive replacement of contractile elements, systolic function is reduced. Impaired ventricular distensibility results in elevated filling pressure and in a rise in pulmonary and systemic venous pressures analogous to constrictive pericarditis.

Biventricular circulatory congestion, the commonest overt clinical feature of cardiac amyloidosis, often presents as congestive heart failure of unknown cause. Right-sided congestion is typically dominant, with peripheral edema and occasionally ascites more evident than orthopnea and nocturnal dyspnea, which are usually absent or nearly so. Angina pectoris occurs in approximately one third of patients (amyloid

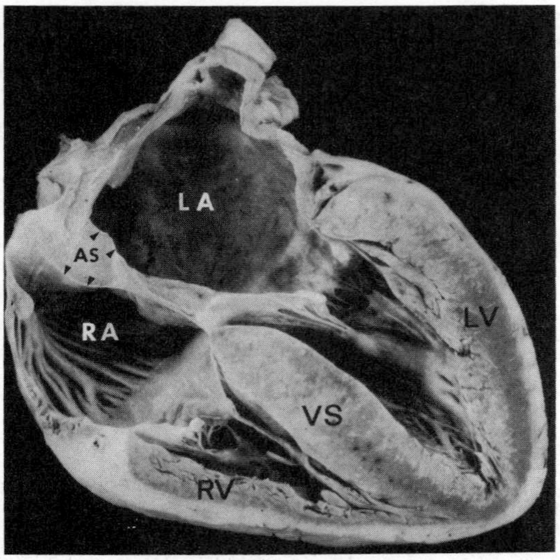

FIGURE 53–4. Pathologic specimen of a typical amyloid heart with thick, infiltrated ventricular septum (VS), left (LV) and right (RV) free walls, and atrial septum (AS). RA, LA = Right and left atria. (Courtesy of Dr. William Edwards, Mayo Clinic, Rochester, Minnesota.)

involvement of the coronary arteries; see above). Impaired atrioventricular conduction occurs in about 35 per cent of cases, with bundle branch block and atrial fibrillation less prevalent. Upwards of a third of patients experience orthostatic hypotension, lightheadedness, or syncope; sudden death is comparatively common.

Physical examination reveals peripheral edema without orthopnea or rales. The arterial pulse is normal or small. Pulsus alternans is usually absent because systolic function is relatively well preserved. The elevated jugular venous pulse is often visible only when the patient sits bolt upright, and it resembles the jugular pulse in constrictive pericarditis, including Kussmaul's sign. The left ventricular impulse is normal in location or only moderately displaced to the left, and its systolic movement is, as a rule, normal. Auscultation detects a soft first heart sound (PR interval prolongation), no murmur or soft systolic murmurs of atrioventricular valve regurgitation, and a third but not a fourth heart sound. Hepatomegaly is common, and ascites is occasionally present.

The electrocardiogram shows left atrial or right atrial P wave abnormalities and varying degrees of atrioventricular block. Abnormal infranodal conduction takes the form of left anterior fascicular block or isolated right or left bundle branch block. QRS voltage is characteristically low. Poor R wave progression or QS deformities in right precordial leads are believed to reflect myocardial replacement with amyloid.

In the chest roentgenogram, cardiac size and configuration are normal, including the atria, but in later stages, moderate cardiac enlargement reflects increased left ventricular internal dimensions. Radiologic signs of pulmonary venous congestion are almost invariable, and pleural effusions are common. Pericardial calcium is conspicuous by its absence.

Echocardiography, especially two-dimensional imaging, is the best means of identifying early cardiac amyloid infiltration and in gauging its subsequent progression. The early asymptomatic phase is manifested on echocardiography by a mild-to-moderate increase in left ventricular and/or right ventricular wall thicknesses. A useful and distinctive, but by no means invariable, feature of advanced cardiac amyloidosis is the granular sparkling appearance of the myocardium on two-dimensional real-time imaging. Avid myocardial pyrophosphate uptake is an important feature of advanced cardiac amyloidosis, and technetium-99m pyrophosphate myocardial scintigraphy is a safe, useful, and relatively specific diagnostic intervention in the proper clinical context. Endomyocardial biopsy remains the definitive means of identifying amyloid deposits in the heart, but the combination of circulatory congestion and a relatively small heart, together with the above features on electrocardiography, echocardiography, and technetium pyrophosphate myocardial scintigraphy, goes far in establishing the diagnosis without recourse to myocardial biopsy.

The treatment of cardiac amyloidosis is supportive, usually ineffective, and occasionally inadvertently harmful. Progression cannot be arrested, and regression of tissue deposits is unknown. Overzealous use of diuretics reduces left ventricular filling pressure and relieves symptoms of circulatory congestion, but at the expense of an obligatory and undesirable fall in cardiac output. Digitalis sensitivity should be underscored not only because of the proarrhythmic effects of the glycoside but also because of its effect on already depressed sinus node and atrioventricular (AV) node function. Also to be considered is the inability of the sinus node to act as an effective pacemaker following pharmacologic or electroconversion in patients with atrial fibrillation. A right ventricular endocardial pacemaker for high-degree heart block may be less than ideally effective because of amyloid deposits at the site of electrode implantation. Nitroglycerin for angina pectoris reinforces the orthostatic hypotension believed to be caused by amyloid infiltration of the autonomic nervous system or of the systemic resistance vessels.

SARCOIDOSIS. Primary cardiac involvement occurs when granulomas preferentially infiltrate the cephalad portion of the ventricular septum and the atrioventricular junction and His bundle. The left and right ventricular free walls, endocardium, pericardium, and rarely the cardiac valves or intramural coronary arteries may also be involved. Clinically overt myocardial infiltration occurs in about 5 per cent of patients with proven sarcoidosis, although myocardial granulomas are found in approximately 25 per cent of such patients at necropsy. Granulomatous myocardial infiltration is initially interstitial and is functionally reflected by impaired diastolic filling with normal or nearly normal systolic function. Injury of contractile elements with fibrous replacement subsequently results in impaired systolic function. Relevant to this discussion is the restrictive phase of sarcoid cardiomyopathy (increased ventricular filling pressure with pulmonary and systemic venous congestion), although pulmonary hypertension, high-degree heart block, and papillary muscle dysfunction are important features of the cardiac response to sarcoidosis. An elevated mean jugular venous pressure with tall but equal A and V waves and brisk X and Y descents is a feature of myocardial restriction and reflects biventricular restrictive cardiomyopathy or, less commonly, sarcoid involvement of the pericardium (effusion or constriction). On physical examination, a right ventricular impulse is inconspicuous or absent, and auscultation detects a prominent third heart sound due to rapid ventricular filling. The echocardiogram identifies impaired diastolic ventricular function without increased thicknesses of ventricular free walls and septum and initially with relatively well-preserved systolic function and comparatively little increase in ventricular end-diastolic dimensions. Echocardiography is useful in establishing myocardial restriction and in excluding a confounding pericardial effusion, but ultrasonic imaging is not sensitive in delineating functionally significant noncalcific pericardial constriction. Endomyocardial biopsy does not sample the most likely sites of cardiac involvement (see earlier). Perfusion imaging with thallium-201 is sometimes useful in detecting segmental defects of sarcoid infiltration of the myocardium. Increased myocardial uptakes of technetium-99m pyrophosphate and gallium have been reported in myocardial sarcoidosis.

Prognosis from the cardiac point of view reflects not only the restrictive cardiomyopathy but also the risks of ventricular arrhythmias, high-degree heart block, and pulmonary hypertension (see earlier). Steroid administration has been advocated for the treatment of patients with biopsy-proven myocardial sarcoidosis. Sarcoid granulomas in the heart are reportedly more responsive to steroids than granulomas in other organs, although the myocardial granulomas may be replaced by connective tissue, with aneurysmal thinning of the ventricular wall.

HEMOCHROMATOSIS. Iron is stored normally as ferritin in reticuloendothelial cells, but with the iron overload of hemochromatosis, the proportion of hemosiderin (an insoluble granular aggregate) to ferritin increases, and storage is chiefly in parenchymal cells, where it is potentially harmful. Impaired diastolic ventricular function (restrictive cardiomyopathy) reflects the presence of iron within myocardial cells prior to significant myocyte injury or fibrous replacement. During this stage, ventricular internal dimensions and systolic function are normal or nearly so despite increased thickness of the infiltrated ventricular septum and ventricular free walls. Myocyte disruption and replacement fibrosis subsequently result in impaired systolic function. Clinical manifestations depend upon where in this natural history a given patient falls. Progressive diastolic dysfunction with rising ventricular filling pressure is symptomatically expressed as effort dyspnea, right-sided failure may dominate the clinical picture. During the myocardial restrictive phase of hemochromatosis, the arterial pulse and blood pressure are normal, there is an increased mean jugular venous pressure with elevated A and V waves and brisk X and Y descents, a normal left ventricular impulse, and a prominent third heart sound. When systolic dysfunction supervenes, the physical signs resemble those of dilated cardiomyopathy (see earlier). In either case, hepatic enlargement may be due to the hemochromatosis per se and not to the passive congestion of restrictive cardiomyopathy.

The echocardiogram initially shows a nondilated, concentrically thick left ventricle with evidence of diastolic dysfunction but normal or nearly normal ejection fraction. Endomyocardial biopsy provides a tissue diagnosis and sheds light on the degree of iron deposition, on myocyte integrity, and on the presence and degree of myocardial fibrosis.

Heart failure need not be progressive but may respond to iron depletion therapy if initiated when cardiac muscle cells are viable and when there is relatively little myocardial fibrosis. The corollary to this observation is that prevention of myocardial fibrosis is achieved when early recognition of myocardial infiltration with iron is effectively treated by phlebotomy.

GLYCOGEN STORAGE DISEASE. Restrictive cardiomyopathy is commonest in type II (Pompe's disease), in which the glycogen within cardiac muscle cells is biochemically normal but present in excessive amounts. There is dramatic thickening of the ventricular septum and of right and left ventricular free walls with reduced cavity size and markedly impaired diastolic distensibility. Pompe's disease is always fatal, usually within the first two years of life. The electrocardiogram is unique, exhibiting a remarkable increase in QRS amplitude, together with a short PR interval. Two-dimensional echocardiography in clinical context is virtually diagnostic.

FABRY'S DISEASE. In this X-linked inborn error of metabolism, deficiency of the lysosomal enzyme α galactosidase leads to progressive deposition of glycosphingolipids in cardiac muscle, resulting in an increase in mass and myocardial restriction. The disease is relatively benign until the second or third decade, but cardiovascular involvement may lead to early death.

HURLER'S SYNDROME. This autosomal recessive disorder is the prototype of the mucopolysaccharidoses, which result from defects in the degradation of complex carbohydrates and mucopolysaccharides. Hurler's cells laden with mucopolysaccharide moities are found in the myocardial interstitium, together with interstitial fibrosis, imparting to the myocardium its characteristic firm consistency and resulting in reduced diastolic distensibility (restrictive cardiomyopathy). Approximately a third of deaths in Hurler's syndrome result from congestive heart failure, but it is difficult clinically to isolate the effects of myocardial involvement per se from the effects of infiltration of mitral and aortic valves and from the ischemic effects of infiltration of the coronary arteries and the sequelae of systemic hypertension. Survival into the early teens is exceptional.

Noninfiltrative Restrictive Cardiomyopathies

IDIOPATHIC RESTRICTIVE CARDIOMYOPATHY. This term applies the clinical and hemodynamic findings of restrictive heart disease in the absence of a morphologic cause. Ventricular cavity size is normal or nearly so, ventricular septal and wall thicknesses are increased little, if at all, and microscopic study, including histochemical stains, may show nothing more than mild interstitial fibrosis. Echocardiographic, hemodynamic, and angiographic evaluations disclose reduced diastolic distensibility, elevated filling pressures, and normal global systolic function. Relatively normal ventricular cavity size contrasts with marked biatrial dilatation in response to reduced ventricular compliance and atrioventricular valve regurgitation, especially tricuspid. Atrial fibrillation is not uncommon, and high-degree heart block often requires a permanent pacemaker. The chief differential diagnosis is noncalcific constrictive pericarditis. An abnormal jugular venous pulse, peripheral edema, and ascites reinforce that impression. At biventricular catheterization, slight but distinct differences in the filling characteristics of right and left ventricles favor restrictive cardiomyopathy, but the distinction is often imprecise. Magnetic resonance imaging is a diagnostic step forward in identifying the absence, presence, or degee of pericardial thickening and may distinguish idiopathic restrictive cardiomyopathy from noncalcific constrictive pericarditis. The clinical course may be protracted even in the presence of chronic atrial fibrillation and high-degree heart block, provided a permanent pacemaker is inserted. Inotropic agents such as digoxin are not beneficial in light of normal or nearly normal systolic ventricular function. Calcium antagonists (verapamil) or beta-adrenergic blockers have been recommended to improve diastolic distensibility and prolong diastolic filling time, but the efficacy of these drugs is unproven.

IRRADIATION RESTRICTIVE CARDIOMYOPATHY. Restrictive physiology develops disproportionately in the more exposed anterior right ventricle, which exhibits interstitial fibrosis. The differential diagnosis between irradiation restrictive cardiomyopathy and radiation injury to pericardium (thickening, effusion, and occasionally tamponade) is important.

SCLERODERMA HEART DISEASE. Insidious interstitial myocardial fibrosis may result, at least initially, in restrictive cardiomyopathy. Hemodynamically significant pericardial effusion is exceptional.

Endomyocardial Restrictive Disease (Table 53–4)

ENDOMYOCARDIAL FIBROSIS. This disorder accounts for 15 to 25 per cent of deaths due to heart disease in equatorial Africa and is encountered, but less often, in South America and Asia and more recently in western Europe and the United States. In the left ventricle, there is involvement of the posterior mitral leaflet with varying degrees of mitral regurgitation. Thrombi overlie the endocardial lesions. The outflow portion of the left ventricle and the anterior mitral leaflet are spared. In the right ventricle, there is dense endocardial fibrous thickening of the inflow tract and apex, with involvement of papillary muscles and chordae tendineae causing varying degrees of tricuspid regurgitation. The outflow tract of the right ventricle is uninvolved. Functional derangements consist of impaired diastolic filling and atrioventricular valve regurgitation with relatively well-preserved systolic function.

In the presence of intractable biventricular failure and atrioventricular valve regurgitation, surgical resection of the fibrous endocardium, together with valve replacement, is a therapeutic option.

THE IDIOPATHIC HYPEREOSINOPHILIC SYNDROME. In this disorder, signs and symptoms of organ involvement, especially heart and nervous system, are accompanied by persistent eosinophilia of 1500 eosinophils per cubic millimeter for at least six months or death before 6 months with lack of evidence of recognized causes of the eosinophilia despite meticulous evaluation. It has been persuasively argued that the idiopathic hypereosinophilic syndrome and endomyocardial fibrosis (see above) are the same disease at different stages of development. The capability of the eosinophil or its contents to cause tissue damage (the Gordon phenomenon) has been known for over 50 years and is held responsible for the primary damage to ventricular endocardium. Platelet thrombi form over the denuded endocardium with an evolution that ultimately results in pathologic findings indistinguishable from those described earlier in endomyocardial fibrosis. Rigorous treatment directed at lowering the eosinophil count (prednisone alone or with hydroxyurea) appears to alleviate clinical manifestations of myocardial restriction, stabilizing and perhaps reversing the cardiac disease and favorably influencing survival.

Cueto-Garcia L, Tajik AJ, Kyle RA, et al.: Serial echocardiographic observations in patients with primary systemic amyloidosis; Smith TJ, Kyle RA, Lie JT: Clinical significance of histopathologic patterns of cardiac amyloidosis. Mayo Clin Proc 59:547, 589, 1984. *Two comprehensive articles that deal with the pathology and serial echocardiographic diagnoses of cardiac amyloidosis.*

Dabestani A, Child JS, Henze E, et al.: Primary hemochromatosis: Anatomic and physiologic studies characteristic of the cardiac ventricles and their responses to phlebotomy. Am J Cardiol 54:153, 1984. *Clinically occult cardiac involvement was identified by echocardiography and equilibrium blood pool imaging. Therapeutic phlebotomy ameliorated or reversed the deleterious effects of cardiac iron deposition if initiated prior to irreversible connective tissue replacement.*

Fauci AS, Harley JB, Roberts WC, et al.: The hypereosinophilic syndrome. Ann Intern Med 97:78, 1982. *This comprehensive National Institutes of Health conference deals with clinical, pathophysiologic, and therapeutic considerations in the hypereosinophilic syndrome and with the relationship of the disorder to endomyocardial fibrosis.*

Siegel RJ, Shah PK, Fishbein MC: Idiopathic restrictive cardiomyopathy. Circulation 70:165, 1984. *This form of cardiomyopathy is characterized chiefly by elevated left and right ventricular filling pressures, normal global ventricular systolic function, and normal or nearly normal ventricular septal and wall thicknesses and internal dimensions in the absence of specific infiltrative disorders or of diseases of pericardium or coronary arteries.*

Silverman KJ, Hutchins GM, Bulkley BH: Cardiac sarcoid: A clinicopathologic study of 84 unselected patients with systemic sarcoidosis. Circulation 58:1204, 1978. *An extensive study of the pathology of sarcoid involvement of the heart with clinical correlations.*

Stewart JR, Fajardo LF: Radiation-induced heart disease: An update. Prog Cardiovasc Dis 27:173, 1984. *An informative review of the pathology, physiology, pathogenesis, diagnosis, treatment, and prevention of radiation-induced heart disease.*

54 DISEASES OF THE PERICARDIUM

Ralph Shabetai

Diseases of the pericardium typically present in one or more of three clinical forms: acute pericarditis, pericardial effusion, and pericardial constriction. Pericardial involvement may progress from inflammation to effusion and then constriction, or it may present as effusion or constriction without clinical evidence of preceding inflammation.

ETIOLOGY

The pericardium may be involved in a large number and variety of diseases. The most important are listed in Table 54–1. Pericardial disease may be asymptomatic, but may also cause dramatic symptoms and signs.

TABLE 54–1. MAJOR CAUSES OF PERICARDIAL DISEASE

1. Inflammation	
Virus	
Coxsackie (usually B)	(E)
Echo	(E)
Other	
Bacterial	
Pneumococcus	(E)
Staphylococcus	(E,C)
Meningococcus	(E,C)
Mycobacterium tuberculosis	(E,C)
Hemophilus influenzae	(C)
Other	
Fungus	
Histoplasma capsulatum	(E,C)
Other	
Other living organisms	
Parasites	(E)
Protozoa	(E)
Nonliving agents	
Trauma	(E,C)
Radiation	(E,C)
Chemical	
Chemotherapeutic agents	
2. Idiopathic	
(Many may be viral, but unproven)	(E,C)
3. Neoplastic	
Secondary to carcinoma of	
Lung	(E,C)
Breast	(E,C)
Other	
Lymphoma	(E)
Primary	
Mesothelioma	(E)
Other	
4. Metabolic	
Chronic renal disease	
Associated with dialysis	(E)
End-stage uremia	(E)
Myxedema	(E)
Chylopericardium	(E)
Hypoalbuminemia	(E)
5. Myocardial injury	
Myocardial infarction	
Acute	
Dressler's syndrome	(E)
Congestive heart failure	(E)
6. Trauma	(E,C)
Postpericardiotomy syndrome	(E)
Postoperative	(C)
7. Connective tissue disorders and hypersensitivity	
Acute rheumatoid fever	
Rheumatic arthritis	(C)
Systemic sclerosis	
Lupus erythematosus	
Drugs	
Procainamide	
Others	
8. Congenital	
Absence of left pericardium	
Partial	
Complete	
Cyst	
Other	

(E) = effusion common; (C) = constrictive pericarditis common.

The clinical syndromes of pericardial disease are listed in Table 54–2.

INFECTIONS WITH LIVING AGENTS. ***Virus Infection.*** Many viruses may cause pericarditis; the common offenders are listed in Table 54–1. The number of cases of idiopathic pericarditis that are caused by preceding viral infection is unknown.

Bacterial Infection. Bacterial pericarditis is still important, although the spectrum has altered. Pneumococcal pericarditis, once a frequent complication of pneumonia, is now rare, whereas infection by staphylococci, fungi, and exotic organisms is more common, especially in persons at either extreme

TABLE 54–2. CLINICAL SYNDROMES OF PERICARDIAL DISEASE

Dry, fibrinous pericarditis
Usually acute (R)
Lax pericardial effusion
Chronic effusive
Cardiac tamponade (R)
Constrictive pericarditis
Subacute
Chronic
Effusive-constrictive pericarditis

(R) = Relapse or recurrence common.

of age and in the immunologically compromised host. Meningococcal pericarditis may be a manifestation of either direct infection or hypersensitivity.

Tuberculosis. Tuberculous pericarditis is less common now that tuberculosis is better controlled and treated. Pulmonary tuberculosis may be present, but often pericardial effusion is an isolated manifestation. *Mycobacterium tuberculosis* can be recovered from only one third of effusions. Even pericardial biopsy findings are not uniformly positive. Commonly, the diagnosis is presumptive and based on circumstantial evidence, such as a positive skin test result or a history of recent contact.

Hemophilus influenzae infection is an important cause of constrictive pericarditis in children.

Fungal Infection. In an otherwise normal population fungal pericarditis is uncommon, but infection with *Histoplasma capsulatum* should be considered in patients who reside in the Ohio Valley. Similarly, coccidioidomycosis should be considered in patients who have been in the San Joaquin Valley of California.

PERICARDIAL INFLAMMATION CAUSED BY NONLIVING AGENTS. ***Trauma.*** Blunt and sharp trauma is an important cause of pericarditis and may lead to pericardial effusion with or without tamponade and ultimately to constrictive pericarditis. Common examples of acute trauma include gunshot and knife wounds. Impact against a steering wheel, explosions, and crushing are the major causes of blunt injuries.

Radiation. The pericardium may be exposed to considerable injury when radiotherapy is employed to treat neoplasia, for example, Hodgkin's disease and lung or breast neoplasms. The latent period between radiation and clinical pericardial disease may extend for many years.

PERICARDIAL DISEASE IN METABOLIC DISORDERS. ***Renal Disease.*** Pericardial disease continues to be one of the more frequent major complications of chronic dialysis and may cause cardiac tamponade. Fortunately, constrictive pericarditis is rare. The etiology is not understood: It may be a manifestation of end-stage renal disease, but the process of dialysis itself may be responsible in whole or in part.

Myxedema. Pericardial effusion may occur and accounts in part for apparent cardiomegaly on chest radiograph; it may also contribute to the low voltage and T wave inversion that, in addition to sinus bradycardia, characterize the electrocardiogram. Pericardial effusion may contain cholesterol crystals.

CHYLOPERICARDIUM. Chylopericardium, a pericardial collection of fluid bearing a large quantity of chyle may be idiopathic but often follows surgical or other trauma of the thoracic duct.

MYOCARDIAL INFARCTION. Acute dry, fibrinous pericarditis can be detected in about one third of patients with acute myocardial infarction. Autopsy evidence is more common. Acute pericarditis early in the course is often a contiguous inflammation over the infarction but may also represent reaction to myocardial injury. Rupture of an infarction, aneurysm, or pseudoaneurysm creates greater or lesser degrees of hemopericardium, the former usually ending fatally.

In some patients, pericarditis (often accompanied by effusion) occurs in the weeks or months following acute myocardial infarction. This syndrome (Dressler's) is thought to be a delayed autoimmune reaction and is often recurrent.

CONNECTIVE TISSUE DISORDERS. Pericardial reaction may occur in virtually all of these disorders. Acute pericarditis is a constituent of rheumatic pancarditis but does not progress to constriction. On the other hand, subacute constrictive pericarditis can occur in rheumatoid arthritis. Pericarditis is an important manifestation of lupus erythematosus, both spontaneous and induced by drugs such as procainamide, and can cause tamponade.

HEART FAILURE. In patients with fluid retention, small pericardial effusion may be seen by echocardiography.

CONGENITAL LESIONS AND CYSTS. Partial absence of the pericardium produces a striking abnormality on the chest radiograph. Pericardial cysts are more frequent. They are filled with clear fluid, and most often occupy the right cardiophrenic angle, although they may occupy atypical locations. They are benign and usually produce no symptoms.

ACUTE (FIBRINOUS) VIRAL OR IDIOPATHIC PERICARDITIS

SYMPTOMS. Findings are often preceded by generalized malaise and fever. The chief symptom is chest pain, which may be either sharp or crushing. Frequently, the pain is precordial but may shift to the left side, simulating pleurisy. Characteristically, the pain is relieved by sitting up and exacerbated by deep inspiration. Thus, pericardial pain has features that may suggest either myocardial ischemia or pleural inflammation. Referral of pain to the right trapezius ridge is a specific but uncommon sign of its pericardial origin.

CLINICAL FINDINGS. ***Pericardial Friction Rub: The Pathognomonic Sign of Pericardial Inflammation.*** Classifically, the rub has components accompanying atrial systole, ventricular systole, and ventricular diastole (see LMSB line, Fig. 54–1). Commonly, the rub is biphasic and must be distinguished from to-and-fro murmurs. When it is monophasic, it must be differentiated from systolic murmurs. It is typically superficial and scratchy, and although it may be widely distributed over the precordium, it is usually most apparent at the left sternal edge. Appreciation is enhanced by firm pressure with the diaphragm of the stethoscope. Changes in posture and the respiratory cycle may alter the intensity. Pericardial friction rubs are often transient and should be sought frequently when pericarditis is suspected. They must be distinguished not only from cardiac murmurs but also from mediastinal crunch due to air in the mediastinum, crepitations from surgical emphysema, and artifacts produced by movement of the skin against the stethoscope.

LABORATORY FINDINGS. ***Electrocardiogram.*** The typical findings of pericarditis are shown in Figure 54–2. ST segment elevation, although common, is not invariably present, depression of the ST segment being usual in leads aV_R and V_1. Depression of the PR segment, although highly specific, is less common than ST segment elevation.

On a single tracing and without clinical information, ST segment elevation cannot always be distinguished from the early repolarization normal variant or from the early stage of acute myocardial infarction. In the latter, evolution of the pattern in serial tracings is helpful. In acute pericarditis, the ST segment returns to baseline without inversion of the T wave (which may occur later if pericarditis becomes chronic), whereas in acute myocardial infarction, T wave inversion typically occurs before the ST segment becomes isoelectric.

Other Laboratory Findings. The erythrocyte sedimentation rate is elevated and there is variable leukocytosis. Viral titers may confirm the origin of the illness but are seldom performed in clinical practice. Gallium radioisotope scanning may display the epicardium, but this expensive test is required only in exceptional cases. Plasma levels of cardiac enzymes may be elevated, but this determination need not be made routinely.

DIAGNOSIS. The diagnosis can usually be made reliably from symptoms and signs. When any of the conditions listed

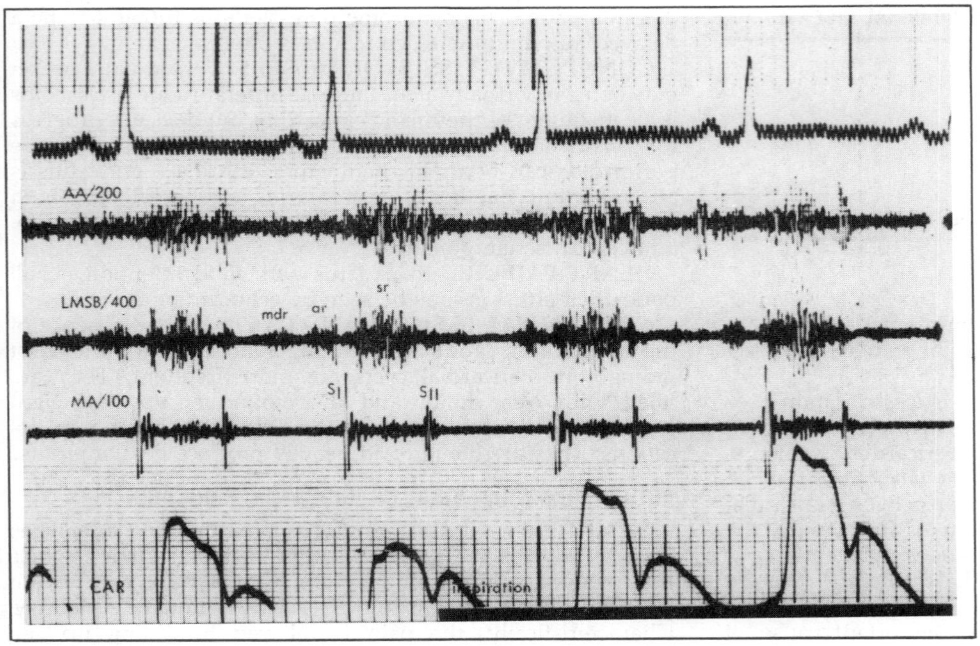

FIGURE 54–1. Phonocardiography of pericardial friction rub. AA = Aortic area; LMSB = left mid-sternal border; MA = mitral area. Note the three-component rub heard along the left mid-sternal border. Numbers refer to filter settings. (Reproduced by permission from Spodick DH: Am Heart J 81:114, 1971.)

in Table 54–1 is suspected, the symptoms and signs of pericarditis should be specifically sought and the diagnosis confirmed by electrocardiography. When the pain simulates that of pleurisy, pneumonia or pulmonary infarction must be considered. When it is retrosternal and crushing, myocardial infarction must be ruled out. On occasion, other major causes of chest discomfort, such as acute pulmonary embolism or dissection of the aorta, need to be considered.

CLINICAL COURSE, PROGNOSIS, AND MANAGEMENT. Commonly, this is a self-limiting disease. However, its natural history is seldom observed, as it usually responds rapidly to treatment with nonsteroidal anti-inflammatory agents such as indomethacin (25 to 50 mg three to four times a day) or ibuprofen. Even aspirin is often satisfactory. Resistant cases may require steroid treatment—for instance, prednisone, starting with 75 mg a day and rapidly tapering to the minimum dose that suppresses symptoms and signs.

Detectable pericardial effusion occurs in a small proportion of cases and may progress to cardiac tamponade. Similarly, acute pericarditis may rarely lead to chronic constrictive pericarditis.

Recurrent Pericarditis. Perhaps the most troublesome of all complications is frequent recurrence over a period of years. The patient is greatly disturbed by the frequent occurrence of disabling pain, and when steroidal agents must be used for resistant cases, their side effects may become significant.

PERICARDIAL EFFUSION

LAX PERICARDIAL EFFUSION. Pericardial effusions that do not raise intrapericardial pressure more than 3 or 4 mm Hg do not cause symptoms. The physical findings are variable and frequently do not provide valuable clinical clues. Pericardial effusion should be strongly suspected in the setting of acute pericarditis if the cardiopericardial silhouette is enlarged on the chest radiograph. A previous radiograph showing a normal-sized silhouette is particularly helpful. The diagnosis can be made with certainty by echocardiography (Fig. 54–3).

PERICARDIAL EFFUSION COMPLICATING ACUTE PERICARDITIS. When echocardiograms are performed routinely in acute pericarditis, effusion is found in a considerable proportion of cases. However, in clinical practice, echocardiography is not required if the heart size remains normal, there is no evidence of cardiac tamponade or myocarditis, and the findings subside within 48 to 72 hours after beginning treatment. Myocarditis should be suspected when depolarization changes, such as left or right bundle branch block, or conduction abnormalities develop and when a third heart sound is audible. In such cases, echocardiography is often

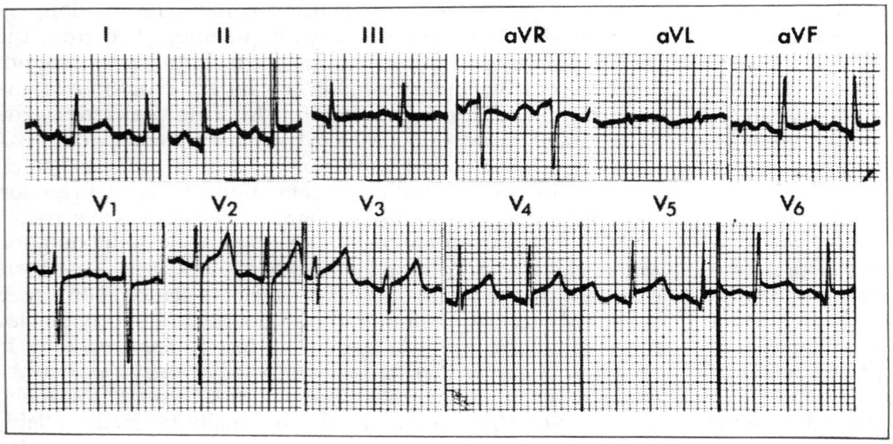

FIGURE 54–2. ECG from a case of acute pericarditis. Note the ST segment elevation in leads I, II, aVF and V_4 to V_6 and ST segment in leads aVR and V_1. (From Shabetai R: The Pericardium. New York, Grune & Stratton, 1980.)

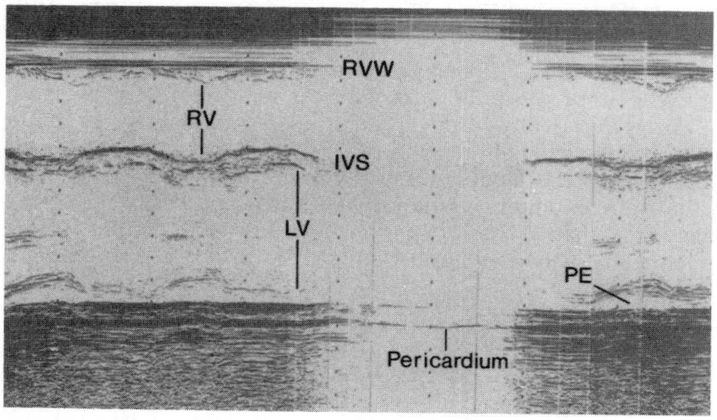

FIGURE 54–3. M = mode echocardiogram of moderate pericardial effusion. RVW = Right ventricular free wall; RV = cavity of right ventricle; IVS = interventricular septum; LV = left ventricular cavity; PE = pericardial effusion. The pericardial echo is identified in the middle of the photo, where other less echo-dense structures have been damped.

useful in distinguishing cardiac chamber enlargement from pericardial effusion.

ETIOLOGY OF PERICARDIAL EFFUSION. The causes of pericardial effusion are indicated in Table 54–1. Pericardial effusion must always be considered in patients who have or are likely to have one of these disorders, but especially when there is or has been evidence of acute pericarditis or when there is circulatory compromise. When the patient has a possible cause of cardiac tamponade or constrictive pericarditis, pericardial disease must be ruled out before attributing circulatory abnormalities to heart disease.

PERICARDIOCENTESIS. When the venous pressure is normal, systemic arterial hypotension is absent, and the etiology of pericardial effusion has been established with reasonable certainty, pericardiocentesis is seldom needed. On the other hand, if the clinician suspects or diagnoses purulent effusion, or cardiac tamponade that is not responding satisfactorily to medical treatment, removal of pericardial fluid via a needle or open drainage becomes necessary. In a smaller fraction of cases, pericardiocentesis is required to establish a tissue or bacteriologic diagnosis. In such instances, the relative merits of the less traumatic and less expensive pericardiocentesis, versus surgical drainage, must be weighed against local experience and preference and the relative importance of pericardial biopsy in establishing the diagnosis.

Lax pericardial effusions have minimal hemodynamic effects, but when large and chronic, as, for example, in idiopathic chronic effusive pericarditis, a number of clinicians recommend surgical drainage.

CARDIAC TAMPONADE

ETIOLOGY AND PATHOPHYSIOLOGY. Pericarditis of virtually any cause may be associated with pericardial effusion, and virtually any pericardial effusion can progress to cardiac tamponade. The important causes are indicated in Table 54–1. The pathophysiology is illustrated in Figure 54–4, taken from cardiac catheterization data from a patient with severe cardiac tamponade.

Normal pericardial pressure is subatmospheric (Fig. 54–4*F*) and approximates pleural pressure. When pericardial effusion rapidly accumulates, pericardial pressure rises abruptly because of the limited capacity of the parietal pericardium to stretch acutely (Fig. 54–4*D*). A few hundred milliliters accumulating rapidly can generate intrapericardial pressures in excess of 20 mm Hg, whereas a slowly developing effusion may assume gigantic proportions with only minimal elevation of intrapericardial pressure. In clinical practice, cases may be encountered anywhere between these two ends of the spectrum.

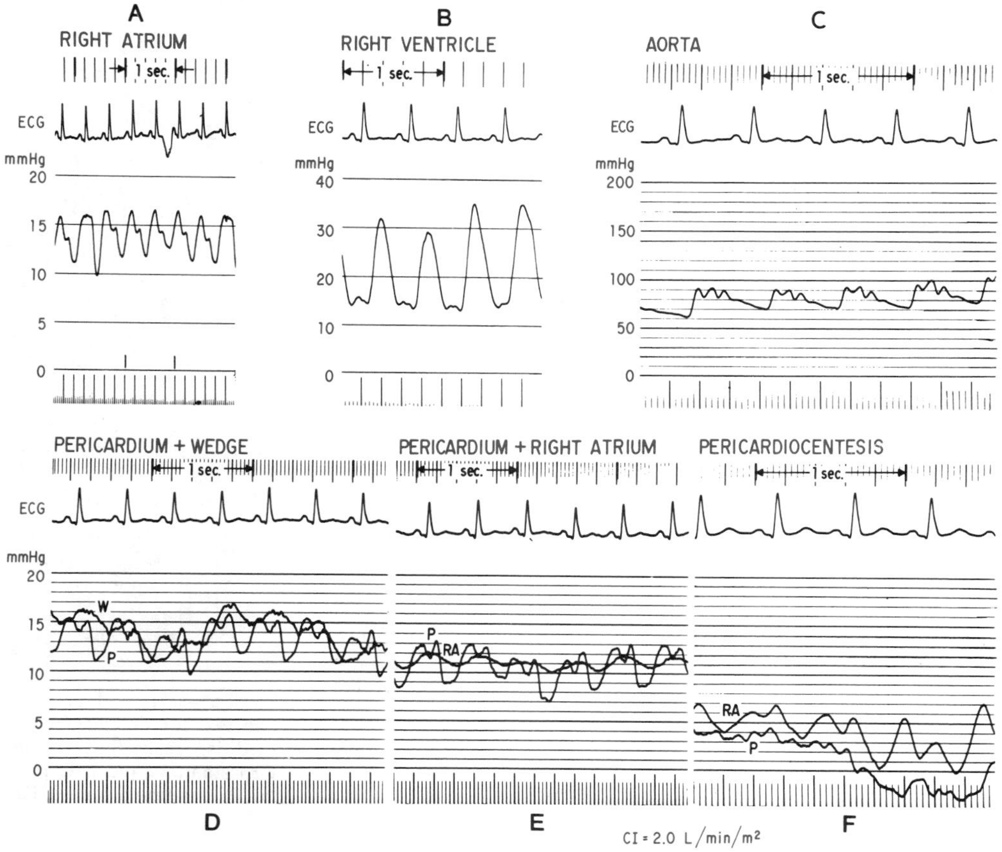

FIGURE 54–4. Hemodynamic data from a patient with cardiac tamponade. See text for discussion.

If effective circulation is to be maintained, systemic venous pressure must rise to equal intrapericardial pressure to maintain venous return. Figure 54–4*E* indicates equilibration of right atrial and pericardial pressure. Unless the pre-existing left ventricular diastolic pressure was higher than pericardial pressure during cardiac tamponade, this pressure also must rise to the same level to maintain filling of the left ventricle. Figure 54–4 *A* to *E* shows equally elevated pulmonary wedge, right atrial, right ventricular diastolic, and intrapericardial pressures. During inspiration the normal inspiratory drop of systemic venous pressure is maintained (Fig. 54–4*A*), but the normal systemic arterial systolic and pulse pressure drop is exaggerated during inspiration (Fig. 54–4*C*). The latter finding is termed pulsus paradoxus. Systemic arterial hypotension is absent (Fig. 54–4*C*) in mild-to-moderate cardiac tamponade. Surgical causes such as trauma or rupture of the heart or the aorta into the pericardium are usually associated with profound hypotension. In medical cases, cardiac output is often reduced to the range shown in Figure 54–4, but in surgical cases still lower cardiac outputs are often observed.

CLINICAL FINDINGS. The chief component in recognizing tamponade is thinking of it. Cardiac tamponade must be considered whenever evidence suggesting heart disease or heart failure develops in a patient who may reasonably be suspected of a disorder listed in Table 54–1. In extreme cases consciousness may be impaired, and arterial blood pressure may drop to shock levels. Frequently there is oliguria, because cardiac tamponade, and the resulting drop in cardiac output and blood pressure, is a powerful stimulus for sodium retention by the kidney. Pericardial pain may or may not be present; often there is a sensation of fullness of the chest and sometimes frank dyspnea.

Venous Pressure. Important evidence of cardiac tamponade includes abnormal jugular venous pulses. The venous pressure is elevated, usually considerably so, unless there is concomitant acute blood loss or severe dehydration. The right atrial (and therefore the jugular) pulse is monophasic, the normal inspiratory drop is maintained, and the predominant wave is the x descent, occurring when the ventricle ejects (Fig. 54–4*A*). The prominent x descent is detected as a sharp inward movement of the internal jugular pulse synchronous with the carotid pulse. The y descent is reduced or abolished because of the attenuated early diastolic dip of ventricular pressure (Fig. 54–4*B*).

Pulsus Paradoxus. Severe pulsus paradoxus may be detectable by palpation of any arterial pulse. When extreme, the pulse disappears during inspiration; when less extreme, it diminishes but can still be palpated. In the presence of severe hypotension, pulsus paradoxus may be difficult to detect, but then is usually more evident in large arteries. Pulsus paradoxus is quantified with a sphygmomanometer. As the cuff is deflated, pulsus paradoxus is estimated as the difference between pressure occurring when the first blood pressure sound can be heard only during expiration and that occurring when the sound is heard throughout the respiratory cycle. More accurate measurement requires direct monitoring of systemic arterial pressure. In clinical practice this intervention is necessary only when monitoring of arterial blood pressure is essential.

Friction Rub. In some cases of cardiac tamponade, a pericardial friction rub is present; otherwise, precordial examination tends not to be helpful.

LABORATORY FINDINGS. The echocardiogram is definitive. The chest radiograph usually shows cardiac enlargement, but in acute cases the volume of pericardial effusion may be too small to increase the cardiothoracic ratio. The electrocardiogram is often not helpful, but when pericardial effusion is large, especially in cardiac tamponade secondary to neoplasm, electrical alternans may occur. Alternation is usually confined to the QRS complex; more specific for pericardial effusion, but less common, is alternation of P, QRS, and T waves.

TREATMENT. Unless tamponade is mild or moderate and rapidly improves following medical treatment of the cause, prompt removal of pericardial fluid is mandatory. In acute cases only a small portion of the fluid need be removed, because of the steep pressure-volume curve of the pericardium. In experienced hands, pericardiocentesis has an acceptable risk. When experience is limited, tamponade is recurrent, or biopsy is needed, subxiphoid surgical drainage is preferred.

CONSTRICTIVE PERICARDITIS

DEFINITION AND ETIOLOGY. Constrictive pericarditis produces thickening, fibrosis, and often calcification of the pericardium with restriction of the diastolic filling of the ventricles. The most common causes are listed in Table 54–1. In the United States and western Europe, constrictive pericarditis most often is idiopathic, secondary to neoplasm or radiation, post-traumatic, or due to connective tissue disease. Tuberculosis and pyogenic infection are less common causes than they used to be. More subacute and fewer chronic cases are therefore seen, and heavy calcification of the pericardium is less frequent.

PATHOPHYSIOLOGY. The pathophysiology and hemodynamics are shown in Figure 54–5 from the study of a stock car driver with post-traumatic pericarditis. Panel A shows pressures recorded simultaneously from both ventricles. In early diastole there is a prominent dip of pressure, and in mid and late diastole the pressure forms a plateau. The two plateaus are elevated and equal. During early diastole, ventricular filling is faster than normal, signified by the early diastolic dip, at the end of which cardiac volume reaches the limit set by the rigid pericardium. The ventricular diastolic pressures are then elevated but do not rise through the remainder of diastole, signifying absence of further ventricular filling. Elevation of left ventricular diastolic pressure to approximately 20 mm Hg causes elevation of right ventricular systolic pressure.

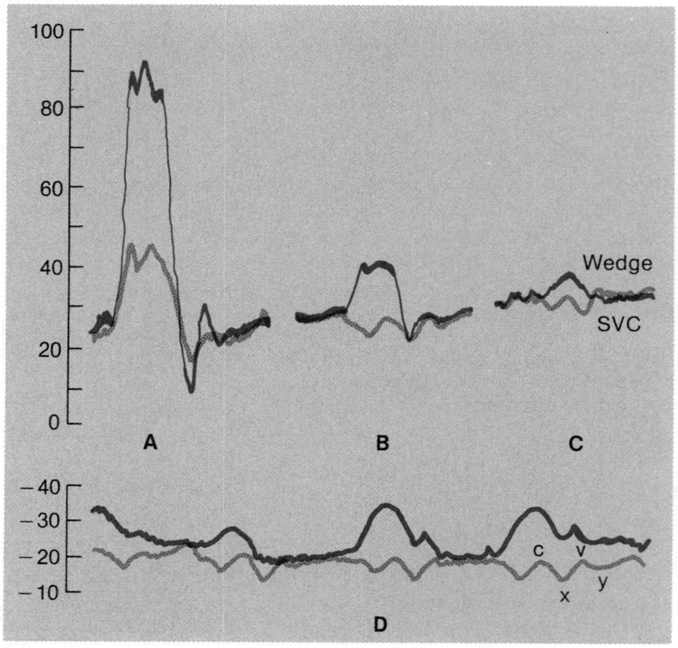

FIGURE 54–5. Hemodynamic data from a case of constrictive pericarditis. See text for details. (From Shabetai R: Profiles of constrictive pericarditis, restrictive cardiomyopathy and cardiac tamponade. In Grossman W [ed.]: Cardiac Catheterization and Angiography. 2nd ed. Philadelphia, Lea & Febiger, 1980.)

Panel B shows simultaneous pressure records from the right ventricle and right atrium. In contradistinction to cardiac tamponade, right atrial pressure is biphasic, showing a prominent x descent with ventricular ejection and prominent y descent coincident with the early diastolic dip of ventricular pressure. The y descent can be recognized at the bedside as a sharp inward movement of the jugular pulsation out of phase with the carotid pulse. Respiratory variation is absent. Panel C shows simultaneous pulmonary wedge and superior vena cava pressures, confirming equilibration of filling pressures on the two sides of the heart. Panel D shows pressures simultaneously recorded from the pulmonary artery and the pulmonary wedge position. In late diastole all cardiac pressures equilibrate around 20 mm Hg.

CLINICAL FINDINGS. Elevation of the filling pressure of the left side of the heart causes dyspnea and pulmonary congestion, which in severe cases is evident on the chest radiograph. Elevated filling pressure of the right side of the heart causes peripheral edema, hepatic enlargement, congestion, and dysfunction, and frequently ascites.

When ventricular filling is suddenly checked at the end of the early diastolic pressure dip, a loud third heart sound ("pericardial knock") is frequently audible. The apex beat may not be palpable, or there may be systolic retraction. Ascites is often prominent in relation to peripheral edema. The liver is usually enlarged and pulsatile. When present, palmar erythema, spider angiomas, and mild jaundice testify to severe, chronic hepatic congestion.

The abnormally small ventricular end-diastolic volume reduces stroke volume even when systolic function is well maintained, as it usually is.

LABORATORY FINDINGS. By chest radiography, the heart is normal in size to moderately enlarged. In chronic cases, particularly those associated with tuberculosis, calcification may be seen in the pericardium. The electrocardiogram usually shows T wave inversions and frequently a wide, notched P wave due to chronic elevation of left atrial pressure. In longstanding cases, atrial fibrillation often supervenes. Liver function test results are abnormal, and hypoalbuminemia may be compounded by protein-losing enteropathy.

Echocardiography. The echocardiogram is less helpful than in pericardial effusion. Sometimes increased thickness of the pericardium can be detected, especially if there is a small effusion. The cardiac walls move abruptly in early diastole and are stationary throughout middle and late diastole, corresponding with the hemodynamic alterations. Motion of the interventricular septum is often abnormal.

Other Imaging Techniques. The thickened pericardium is more adequately visualized by computerized tomography, which at present is the imaging technique of choice for chronic constrictive pericarditis. Magnetic resonance imaging promises to be as good or better.

DIAGNOSIS. Systemic venous congestion not explained by heart failure or other causes should suggest the possibility of constrictive pericarditis, especially when one of the etiologies listed in Table 54–1 is present or suspected. Although nonspecific systolic murmurs are common, murmurs of predominant valvular heart disease are absent.

When patients present with massive edema and liver dysfunction, the most common erroneous diagnosis is cirrhosis of the liver. This major error can be avoided by examination of the venous pressure in the neck. When the venous pressure is elevated, anasarca is generally due to cardiac or pericardial, not hepatic, causes.

Pericardial effusion may produce a large "water-bottle" heart on chest radiograph. Constrictive pericarditis may produce only minimal enlargement but may be detectable by calcification of this pericardium. Cardiac imaging shows normal systolic function and normal cardiac valves. The ventricles are often small and fill rapidly in early diastole but not at all for the remainder of diastole. This finding, together with increased thickness of the pericardium, establishes the diagnosis.

Restrictive cardiomyopathy is a disease of heart muscle (see Ch. 53) that mimics constrictive pericarditis. Characteristically, however, left ventricular diastolic pressure exceeds that on the right. In some cases, endomyocardial biopsy and occasionally exploratory thoracotomy are needed to establish the correct diagnosis.

TREATMENT. For the vast majority of patients, the treatment of choice is pericardiectomy. The patient may be prepared by modest diuresis. With modern techniques of cardiopulmonary bypass, especially in cases that are not too far advanced, the operation yields gratifying clinical improvement, full benefit may not be evident for about six months.

Engel PH: Echocardiographic findings in pericardial disease. *In* Fowler NO (ed.): The Pericardium in Health and Disease. Mt. Kisco, NY, Futura Publishing Company, 1985. *An up-to-date, well-written discussion.*

Klopfenstein HS, Schuchard G, Wann LS, et al.: The relative merits of pulsus paradoxus and right ventricular diastolic collapse in the early detection of cardiac tamponade. An experimental echocardiographic study. Circulation 71:829, 1985. *Describes the correlation between hemodynamics and echocardiographic abnormalities in cardiac tamponade.*

Shabetai R: The Pericardium. New York, Grune & Stratton, 1980. *A comprehensive monograph dealing with the normal pericardium and pericardial diseases.*

Shabetai R, Fowler NO, Fenton JC, et al.: Pulsus paradoxus. J Clin Invest 44:1882, 1965. *An experimental study of the mechanisms of pulsus paradoxus.*

Spodick DH: Pathogenesis and clinical correlations of the electrocardiographic abnormalities of pericardial disease. Cardiovasc Clin 8:201, 1977. *A well-illustrated and complete account of theory and clinical application.*

55 MISCELLANEOUS CONDITIONS OF THE HEART: TUMOR, TRAUMA, AND SYSTEMIC DISEASE

Bernadine P. Healy

CARDIAC TUMORS

Tumors of the heart and pericardium are uncommon, and as a cause of clinical cardiac disease they are especially rare. Consecutive autopsy studies suggest that primary tumors of the heart are seen in only 1 in 2000 postmortem examinations; tumors secondary to metastases are roughly 20 times more frequent than primary lesions. A number of factors have made cardiac tumors a more visible current medical problem. With improved medical diagnostic technology, we are more apt to recognize both primary and secondary cardiac tumors; and with better therapy, patients with metastatic neoplasms live longer, increasing the likelihood for the heart to develop secondary cancers.

In part because of their relative rarity as a cause of clinical heart disease, cardiac tumors often go unrecognized. A general awareness of the pathophysiology of the heart afflicted with tumor and the ways in which it so often mimics more common forms of heart disease is essential to diagnosis and recognition of options for therapeutic intervention.

Primary Tumors of the Heart

Primary tumors of the heart are almost always benign and are considerably less common than tumors secondary to metastatic disease. The myxoma, of endocardial origin, is overwhelmingly the most common and best known of the primary cardiac tumors. Less common is the rhabdomyoma, a benign congenital tumor of myocardium most often seen in children. The sarcoma is the predominant malignant form of primary heart tumor and includes a variety of types, such as rhabdomyosarcoma, angiosarcoma, and fibrosarcoma. Among these tumor types, the myxoma is of greatest clinical importance in terms of relative frequency, tendency to produce symptoms, and ease of diagnosis and therapy.

The cardiac myxoma has been recognized as a pathologic entity for several hundred years, occurring with an incidence of about 0.03 per cent at autopsy. Myxomas are typically solitary, smooth-surfaced, globular tumors, which vary in size from 1 to 8 cm (average 5 cm), and most are pedunculated. In about 90 per cent of cases they occur in the left atrium; most of the rest occur in the right atrium. They are attached to the interatrial septum in the region of the fossa ovalis. Clinical presentation is related to location of the tumor, as well as to the presence of a pedicle. Larger myxomas, generally over 3 cm in diameter, are more apt to be symptomatic. The presence of a pedicle, allowing the myxomas to move about in the cardiac chambers, also correlates with symptomatology.

Myxomas occur most frequently (75 per cent) in women and usually manifest with symptoms in persons between the ages of 35 and 60 years. Because myxomas are most commonly located in the left atrium, signs and symptoms of cardiac dysfunction are usually referable to left-sided cardiac disease. The most common clinical cardiac problem is congestive heart failure, present in roughly half of patients, and often the heart failure is paroxysmal and precipitated by positional change, such as lying down. Other signs include chest pain, murmurs of mitral stenosis or regurgitation or both, syncope, and arrhythmias (including atrial fibrillation, often paroxysmal in nature). Other, noncardiac manifestations of atrial myxomas include systemic or pulmonary embolism, fever, malaise, arthralgias, and hematologic abnormalities suggestive of chronic infection. With these clinical manifestations, it is not surprising that atrial myxomas often have been misdiagnosed as rheumatic mitral valve disease, infective endocarditis, fever of unknown origin, or connective tissue disease. Indeed, cardiac myxomas may be viewed as the "great simulators"; their correct clinical diagnosis is among the most challenging in internal medicine.

Some of the challenge and error in the clinical recognition of cardiac myxomas has been diminished by the advent of improved noninvasive techniques. Echocardiography, particularly two-dimensional study, readily identifies atrial tumors and has virtually eliminated the need for invasive contrast angiography. Radionuclide ventriculography (gated blood cardiac scan) will also identify a moving filling defect within the cardiac chambers and can be used in making the diagnosis of intracavitary tumor. Once the diagnosis of cardiac myxoma has been made, the only treatment is surgical excision. Undiagnosed atrial myxomas are often fatal, but when considered, are readily detected and, once detected, straightforwardly treated and virtually always cured.

Secondary Tumors of the Heart

The heart may be a target for secondary tumor invasion. Cancer has been reported to involve the heart in anywhere from 5 to 20 per cent of patients with metastatic malignant disease, with an apparent increase in reported involvement of the heart in recent years. Almost any type of primary neoplasm may involve the heart. Malignant melanomas are among the most common solid tumors that spread to the heart. Cardiac lesions occur in 40 to 50 per cent of patients with metastatic disease, and as a group, melanomas constitute approximately 3 per cent of all cardiac metastases. Leukemias frequently infiltrate the heart, with microscopic invasion evident in approximately half of patients. Other tumors that frequently metastasize to the heart include carcinomas of the lung, breast, and thyroid, the lymphomas, and the sarcomas, including Kaposi's sarcoma. Carcinomas of the lung and breast, because of their relative frequency among malignancies, together account for approximately 50 per cent of the secondary tumors of the heart.

What is most striking about cardiac invasion by metastatic tumor is that it is so often clinically silent, despite what may be extensive disease. The clinical manifestations of cardiac metastases are myriad and generally reflect the anatomic site of invasion. Congestive heart failure, cardiac arrhythmias, and signs of pericardial constriction are among the most common clinical manifestations of cardiac metastases. Myocardial ischemia and infarction may also result from coronary compression or invasion. Although most cardiac metastases are diagnosed post mortem, they may be clinically detected by a variety of means. When a malignant pericardial effusion is present, cytologic examination of pericardial fluid readily provides diagnosis. Identification of a mass in one or more cardiac chambers or of an irregularity in chamber contour or wall thickness may be accomplished by cross-sectional cardiac echocardiography, radionuclide ventriculography, or invasive contrast angiography. Pathologic examination is necessary, however, to identify tumor type. Unlike treatment for myxomas, surgery for primary or secondary malignancies of the heart is generally ineffective. The major role for cardiac surgery is to obtain tissue for pathologic diagnosis or to alleviate mechanical obstruction. Radiotherapy and chemotherapy are utilized, depending on tumor type.

CARDIAC DISEASE SECONDARY TO CANCER THERAPY. Cardiac disease or dysfunction may also occur as a consequence of chemotherapy and radiotherapy and may obscure even further the diagnosis of metastatic tumors of the heart. Many of the antineoplastic drugs, particularly doxorubicin (Adriamycin), produce a dose-dependent toxicity that leads to a dilated congestive cardiomyopathy. Doxorubicin causes a characteristic degeneration of the myocyte that can be detected by myocardial biopsy. Radiotherapy may also produce dose-dependent cardiac damage to all three layers of the heart. Pericarditis and pericardial effusions are most common, but fibrosis of the myocardium and of mural and valvular endocardium may occur. Prevention is the best therapy for radiation- and drug-induced cardiac damage, which is generally irreversible.

CARDIAC TRAUMA

Trauma is a major cause of morbidity and mortality in our society, and tragically it often affects those who are otherwise healthy. Cardiac trauma results from either a penetrating object or a nonpenetrating blunt assault on the thorax. Death may immediately occur as a result of asystole, ventricular fibrillation, or exsanguination. Those who survive long enough for transport to a hospital pose immediate diagnostic and therapeutic challenges.

Penetrating wounds of the heart are believed to be fatal in over 90 per cent of instances, with most patients never reaching medical attention. Stab and gunshot wounds may lacerate any portion of the heart. Pericardial laceration with cardiac tamponade or exsanguination is most common, usually in conjunction with rupture of some portion of the myocardium. Because of their anterior location, the right ventricle and pulmonary outflow tract are particularly susceptible. Valve lacerations leading to incompetence and coronary injuries leading to ischemia or infarction, or both, are of particular importance for survivors, who may be left with residual lesions.

The diagnosis of cardiac trauma in the setting of a penetrating wound of the thoracic cavity is not always straightforward. Patients usually present acutely with hypotension due either to cardiac tamponade or to hemorrhage. The diagnosis is assumed when profound hypotension is present in the setting of a penetrating mediastinal wound with or without an object in or near the cardiac silhouette. In this setting, emergency thoracotomy, preferably in an operating room, is virtually always necessary for both diagnosis and therapy. The wisdom of performing a diagnostic pericardiocentesis has been challenged, as false-negative readings may result from local clot formation. Pericardiocentesis may be necessary, however, to stabilize a patient with cardiac tamponade prior to emergency thoracotomy. Once the diagnosis of trauma has been made and cardiac surgical repair initiated, the survival rate may be as high as 70 per cent.

Nonpenetrating trauma to the chest cavity may also cause a similar range of cardiac injuries requiring emergency thoracotomy. Unlike penetrating wounds, however, physical evidence of trauma to the chest wall may be minimal or even absent, and the severity of chest wall trauma does not correlate with likelihood or extent of cardiac injury. Among the most common causes of cardiac trauma are steering wheel injuries to the sternum. Others include sports activities, industrial accidents, and personal assaults. The myocardium is the major site of injuries, which may range in severity from mild myocardial contusion to rupture of the ventricle or interventricular septum. Pericardial laceration, valve disruption, coronary artery thrombosis, or great vessel rupture, particularly of the ascending aorta, may also occur.

Diagnosis is difficult, since symptoms are often absent or misleading. Symptoms of chest pain similar to that associated with myocardial infarction are the most frequent. Cardiac arrhythmias and hypotension may also signal cardiac injury in the proper setting. Survivors of myocardial injury may develop false aneurysms with their usual complications. Early and late cardiac arrhythmias (atrial or ventricular) may be caused by myocardial contusions, and the electrocardiographic abnormalities may include those of myocardial infarction or acute pericarditis. Serum enzyme assays (creatine kinase, MB fraction) and echocardiography are helpful in making the diagnosis, and if coronary compromise is suggested, cardiac catheterization with coronary angiography would be appropriate. Treatment depends on the extent of cardiovascular compromise. Pain and arrhythmias alone are treated similarly to those of acute myocardial infarction, except that anticoagulants should be strictly avoided. Thoracotomy is necessary if there are signs of myocardial rupture or pericardial tamponade. Late complications, such as valvular or interventricular septal rupture or false aneurysms of the heart or aorta, require surgical correction.

CARDIAC MANIFESTATIONS OF SYSTEMIC DISEASE

The heart may be afflicted secondarily by a variety of systemic conditions and diseases. The most frequent cardiac manifestations of systemic disease are those common disorders that primarily involve the vascular system and produce cardiac dysfunction by virtue of increased volume or pressure load on the heart or interruption in blood flow to the myocardium. Systemic hypertension, whether essential, renal, or endocrine in cause, often leads to cardiac hypertrophy and heart failure. Atherosclerosis is a systemic vascular disease with the heart as a prime target. Less common are the anemias, which produce a volume load and at times hypoxic insult to the heart, leading to congestive heart failure. In addition to these widely recognized disorders, there are several systemic diseases that secondarily involve the heart in a distinctive fashion. Examples of these disorders include the connective tissue diseases (e.g., systemic lupus erythematosus [SLE], progressive systemic sclerosis and polyarteritis nodosa), endocrine-humoral disorders (thyroid disease, pheochromocytoma, and metastatic carcinoid), and systemic infiltrative disease (amyloidosis).

CONNECTIVE TISSUE DISEASES. Although the connective tissue diseases may affect the heart only secondarily, the cardiac disorder may dominate the clinical course. In systemic lupus erythematosus, the endocardium, myocardium, and pericardium all are potential targets. A fibrinous pericarditis is a common cardiac lesion and frequently produces clinical symptoms. Fibrofibrinous thrombotic lesions may develop on the surface of the cardiac valves (a condition termed Libman-Sacks endocarditis) and are usually clinically silent. On occasion this endocarditis may lead to significant mitral or aortic valve dysfunction. Myocarditis may occur but is an infrequent result of SLE. Coronary arteritis and thromboembolism may also develop, and in patients with corticosteroid-treated lupus, in particular, there may be accelerated coronary atherosclerosis.

Progressive systemic sclerosis (PSS) or scleroderma may produce cardiac dysfunction by means of its effect on the myocardium. Focal fibrosis and necrosis of myocardium may lead to a picture of dilated congestive cardiomyopathy. Morphologic and clinical evidence now suggests that the etiology of the myocardial disease in PSS is small vessel coronary spasm, causing ischemia, i.e., a Raynaud's phenomenon of the coronary arteries. Polyarteritis nodosa may cause a focal or a diffuse coronary arteritis, with formation of coronary thrombosis or aneurysm or both. The latter may lead to myocardial ischemia or infarction and, combined with systemic hypertension, to congestive heart failure. Cardiac manifestations of the connective tissue diseases are diagnosed and treated with the standard technology and methods used for valvular, myocardial, pericardial, or coronary disease. Therapy also includes the immunosuppressive drugs used for treatment of the systemic diseases.

ENDOCRINE-HUMORAL DISORDERS. Thyroid disease has long been known to target the heart. Thyroid hormone increases oxygen consumption and metabolic rate, has a direct inotropic and chronotropic effect on the heart, and has been shown to have a direct trophic effect on the myocardium, inducing a physiologic pattern of hypertrophy. The major clinical manifestation of thyroid hormone excess is a hyperkinetic heart and circulation. Other symptoms include a variety of arrhythmias (atrial fibrillation, in particular), and, with severe disease, congestive heart failure may develop. Although less common, hypothyroidism may produce an idiopathic dilated cardiomyopathy, but its etiology is obscure. More often, hypothyroidism causes bradycardia and pericardial effusions. The latter may contain cholesterol crystals, a finding believed to be characteristic of a myxedema-associated effusion. Identification of the basis for these cardiac disorders is confirmed by abnormal serum thyroxine levels. Thyroid hormone levels should be obtained routinely in patients with idiopathic atrial fibrillation and in those with heart failure of obscure etiology.

Pheochromocytomas, which are chromaffin cell tumors, produce norepinephrine and, to a varying degree, epinephrine, which may cause systemic hypertension as well as induce direct myocardial toxicity. Autopsy studies have shown focal myocardial contraction band necrosis and fibrosis in as many as 50 per cent of patients with this tumor. Similar lesions may be produced in experimental animals with catecholamine infusions and are believed to relate to norepinephrine-induced calcium overload. Although this tumor may cause cardiomyopathy, it is exceedingly rare.

CARDIAC AMYLOIDOSIS. This disorder may be primary but occurs most often secondary to systemic conditions, including multiple myeloma, systemic amyloidosis, familial Mediterranean fever, and aging. Amyloid may infiltrate myocardium and coronary arteries, and less often the cardiac valves, and typically causes increased myocardial mass and focal fibrosis. The latter leads to decreased myocardial compliance and ultimately congestive heart failure—a picture that may simulate hypertrophic or restrictive cardiomyopathy. Cardiac amyloid deposits may also affect the conduction system of the heart, causing a variety of arrhythmias. The diagnosis of cardiac amyloid is confirmed by myocardial biopsy. Therapy for the cardiac dysfunction of amyloidosis is the standard treatment for arrhythmias or heart failure or both. A proclivity to digitalis toxicity, possibly related to conduction system infiltration by amyloid, should be considered when treating heart failure in these patients.

Doherty NE, Siegel RJ: Cardiovascular manifestations of systemic lupus erythematosus. Am Heart J 110:1257, 1985. *A review article summarizing present information on the clinical and morphologic aspects of the heart in systemic lupus erythematosus.*

Follansbee WP, Curtiss EI, Medsger TA, et al.: Physiologic abnormalities of cardiac function in progressive systemic sclerosis with diffuse scleroderma. N Engl J Med 310:142, 1984. *Description of cardiac dysfunction in patients with PSS, showing by noninvasive techniques the relationship of circulatory disturbances to ventricular dysfunction.*

Frazee RC, Mucha P Jr, Farnell MB, et al.: Objective evaluation of blunt cardiac trauma. J Trauma 26:510, 1986. *A review of the cardiovascular consequences of blunt chest trauma, describing CK-MB elevations, arrhythmias, and ventricular dysfunction as assessed by echocardiography in a wide range of cardiac injuries.*

McDonnell PJ, Mann RB, Bulkley BH: Involvement of the heart by malignant lymphoma: A clinicopathologic study. Cancer 49:944, 1982. *A clinicopathologic study of the cardiovascular manifestations of lymphomatous involvement of the heart and a general review of the range of malignant tumors of the heart and how they cause cardiac dysfunction.*

Morkin E, Flink IL, Goldman S: Biochemical and physiologic effects of thyroid hormone on cardiac performance. Prog Cardiovasc Dis 25:435, 1983. *An in-depth and current review of the effect of thyroid hormone on the normal heart and its role in disease.*

Salcedo EE, Adams KV, Lever HM, et al.: Echocardiographic findings in 25 patients with left atrial myxoma. J Am Coll Cardiol 1:1162, 1983. *Describes the use of echocardiography to diagnose myxomas noninvasively.*

Schrader ML, Hochman JS, Bulkley BH: The heart in polyarteritis nodosa: A clinicopathologic study. Am Heart J 109:1353, 1985. *A clinicopathologic study of the heart in polyarteritis nodosa and a review of the literature.*

Skhvatsabaja LV: Secondary malignant lesions of the heart and pericardium in neoplastic disease. Oncology 43:103, 1986. *A review of clinical and laboratory data in 240 patients with metastatic tumors of the heart and pericardium, focusing on clinical symptoms and diagnosis.*

56 DISEASES OF THE AORTA

Lawrence S. Cohen

The aorta is vital to the proper functioning of every organ system in the body. The coronary arteries are the first arteries to arise from the aorta, followed by vessels of the head and central nervous system and then the gastrointestinal, renal, and genitourinary arteries. Disease in any segment of the aorta, therefore, can have profound consequences upon bodily function. The aorta is susceptible to four major disease processes: *aneurysm, dissection, arteriosclerotic occlusive disease,* and *aortitis*.

At its origin the aorta is approximately 3 cm in diameter. The ascending aorta is approximately 5 cm in length, coursing in a left-to-right direction in the same ejection axis as the left ventricle. The aortic arch is also approximately 5 cm in length and takes an upward, posterior, and leftward direction, terminating along the left border of the thoracic vertebrae. The aortic arch lies entirely within the superior mediastinum. The descending thoracic aorta is contained in the posterior mediastinum. It is a bit narrower than the ascending aorta and is approximately 20 cm in length. It runs to the diaphragm at the level of the twelfth thoracic vertebra and supplies the arteries to the spinal cord. The abdominal aorta is the continuation of the thoracic aorta, ending at the level of the fourth lumbar vertebra. The average length is 15 cm, with an average diameter of 2 cm at its origin and a slightly smaller diameter at its lower end.

ANEURYSM

Definition

An aneurysm is a widening of a vessel involving the stretching of fibrous tissue within the media of the vessel. A true aneurysm is a widening of the vessel, whereas a false aneurysm represents a localized rupture of the artery with sealing over by clot or adjacent structures. The natural history of aneurysms is to enlarge. Not only does the etiologic process tend to continue and progress but also the law of Laplace is a factor. As described by Laplace, the tension in the wall of a spherical chamber enclosing a fluid under pressure is related to this pressure under which the fluid is kept and the radius of curvature of the containing vessel. As the radius increases so does wall tension. Hence, enlargement of the vessel begets more enlargement.

It is convenient to classify aneurysms according to etiology, morphology, and location. Arteriosclerosis is the most common cause of aneurysms. Other causes are cystic medial necrosis, trauma, and infection, including syphilis. Rarer causes are rheumatic aortitis, Takayasu's syndrome, temporal arteritis, and relapsing polychondritis. Marfan's syndrome is characterized by cystic medial necrosis (Ch. 199). In some forms of Ehlers-Danlos syndrome, rupture of blood vessels, including the aorta, may occur. Aneurysms can be classified into three morphologic types: (1) fusiform, in which the aneurysm encompasses the entire circumference of the aorta and assumes a spindle shape; (2) saccular, in which only a portion of the circumference is involved and in which there is a neck and an asymmetric outpouching of the aneurysm; and (3) dissecting, in which an intimal tear permits a column of blood to dissect along the media of the vessel. This is often called a dissecting hematoma. Location is a further way to classify aneurysms. Aneurysms involve (1) the ascending aorta, including the sinuses of Valsalva; (2) the aortic arch; (3) the descending thoracic aorta, originating just distal to the left subclavian artery, and (4) the abdomen, most commonly distal to the renal arteries.

The most proximal portion of the ascending aorta comprises the sinuses of Valsalva. Aneurysms in this location are usually congenital in origin. Most involve either the right sinus or the right portion of the noncoronary sinus. Aneurysms of the sinus of Valsalva are often silent until they rupture into the right side of the heart, usually the right ventricle or right atrium. This event may occur spontaneously or may be a consequence of infective endocarditis. Other causes of aortic sinus aneurysm are Marfan's syndrome, syphilis, or infective endocarditis. Aneurysms of the ascending aorta may be arteriosclerotic, but cystic medial necrosis with or without other features of Marfan's syndrome is more common. Syphilis was once a common cause of ascending aortic aneurysm but has all but disappeared as an etiology. The more distal the aortic location of the aneurysm, the more likely it is to be arteriosclerotic.

Clinical Manifestations

Clinical manifestations of aneurysms of the thoracic aorta (other than rupture) are due to compression, distortion, or erosion of surrounding structures. Pain is the most common symptom. Pain in a gradually enlarging aneurysm is insidious and may be described as boring and deep. Increasing intensity of pain is an ominous sign and may presage impending rupture.

Aortic valve regurgitation may be associated with aneurysms of the ascending aorta. Distortion of the aortic annulus and separation of the aortic valve cusps accounts for the regurgitation. If regurgitation occurs rapidly, the clinical consequences can be dramatic, with the patient developing acute pulmonary edema. Many patients will develop a murmur of aortic regurgitation gradually and may be relatively asymptomatic. Aneurysms of the transverse aortic arch are less common than are aneurysms in other sites. The consequences of such aneurysms are often formidable, since the innominate and carotid arteries arise from the transverse aortic arch. In addition, the arch is contiguous with other vital structures such as the superior vena cava, pulmonary artery, trachea, bronchi, lung, and left recurrent laryngeal nerve. Symptoms may include dyspnea, stridor, hoarseness, hemoptysis, cough, or chest pain.

The most common site of an aneurysm of the thoracic aorta is between the origin of the left subclavian artery and the diaphragm. Arteriosclerosis is the most common cause, with age, hypertension, and probably smoking contributing as risk factors. One factor in the pathogenesis of aneurysms of the descending aorta may be the immobility of the aorta at this site and the unique stresses imposed on the aorta immediately distal to the left subclavian artery. Distortion of the architecture in this area may result in sufficient turbulence to cause elastic tissue degeneration, accelerated arteriosclerosis, and localized dilatation.

Pain from descending thoracic aortic aneurysm is often intrascapular but can vary considerably. Hoarseness may occur from stretching of the left recurrent laryngeal nerve. Hemoptysis may occur owing to leakage into the left lung. Thoracic aortic aneurysms, like those of the abdominal aorta, threaten life by potential rupture. They are rarely complicated by thrombosis or embolism. Thoracoabdominal aneurysms involve the celiac, superior mesenteric, and renal arteries. Fortunately, they are not common, for they represent a great challenge to the vascular surgeon. Although some are caused by cystic medial necrosis, most are of arteriosclerotic origin and occur in older men.

The most common form of aneurysm is the abdominal aortic aneurysm. The prevalence of this aneurysm at autopsy is in the 1 to 3 per cent range but is even more common in men over 60. Its frequency in men outnumbers that in women by 6:1. Almost all of these aneurysms are below the renal arteries. Most are of arteriosclerotic origin, but trauma, infection (including syphilis), and arteritis make up a small fraction. A fortunate feature of these aneurysms is their accessibility on physical examination. A mass that pulsates in all directions may well be an aneurysm, whereas a pulsation in one direction only is usually a transmitted pulsation through an overlying visceral mass. Rupture of an abdominal aneurysm is the greatest threat and may lead to a rapid demise because of shock and hypotension. Other less acute symptoms may also occur. Pain in the lower back is a sign of enlargement of the aneurysm and at times is a warning of impending rupture. Almost all abdominal aortic aneurysms are lined with clot or have ulcerated plaques. Embolization of atherothrombotic material may lead to a variety of symptoms, ranging from digital infarction to anuria from a shower of emboli to the kidneys.

The likelihood of rupture increases with increasing aortic aneurysm size. Sixty to 80 per cent of patients with lesions 7 cm or larger die of rupture, and 95 per cent of patients with lesions over 10 cm die of aneurysm rupture. The risk of rupture in aneurysms 5 cm or less is considerably lower. Given these data, general guidelines about surgical repair have emerged. Aneurysms associated with aortic thrombosis or distal embolic events should be repaired promptly. Aneurysms suspected of rupture or acute expansion should be treated surgically immediately. Although there are differences of opinion concerning when elective repair of asymptomatic aneurysms should be undertaken, once the aneurysm exceeds 5 cm in diameter, the prognosis on continued medical management becomes increasingly guarded.

Diagnosis

Palpation is usually the first step in diagnosing abdominal aneurysms. Ultrasound imaging is an excellent technique to confirm the diagnosis, as it is noninvasive, inexpensive, and accurate to within 2 to 3 mm of aneurysm size when compared with the findings at surgery. Computed tomographic (CT) scanning utilizing contrast material is equal in effectiveness to ultrasound in the detection and sizing of abdominal aortic aneurysms. Often lumbar spine x-ray films will clearly outline the walls of an abdominal aortic aneurysm if there is calcium in the walls. Aortography, either arterial or venous with digital subtraction, may not reflect the true size of the aneurysm; an extensive laminated clot may reduce the lumen.

Joyce JW: Aneurysmal disease. In Spittell JA Jr (ed.): Clinical Vascular Disease. Philadelphia, F. A. Davis Company, 1983, pp 89–101. *A concise summary of aneurysmal disease, including management guidelines for aneurysms in all aortic locations.*

Spittell JA Jr: Abdominal aortic aneurysms. Hosp Pract 21:105, 1986. *This is a short, well-illustrated practical management update. Modern diagnostic tools are discussed, and management strategies are reviewed.*

MARFAN'S SYNDROME

Patients with Marfan's syndrome (see Ch. 199) develop both aortic aneurysm and aortic dissection. Myxomatous degeneration of valve leaflets may also occur. The mitral valve cusps may be involved. The chordae tendineae may elongate or rupture, predisposing to mitral valve prolapse, or flail mitral valve with mitral regurgitation. Regurgitation at either the mitral or the tricuspid valve may be the most prominent finding in certain patients. However, the most commonly affected tissue is the aorta. The aorta enlarges, beginning with the sinuses of Valsalva. The enlargement most often extends to the innominate artery, although at times the entire aorta may be involved in what has been referred to as annuloaortic ectasia. Aortic dilation may begin as early as the fifth year of life or as late as the sixth decade.

Aortic regurgitation may occur secondary to participation of the aortic root in the development of an aortic aneurysm. Dissection of the aortic root may lead to acute aortic regurgitation. Dilation of the pulmonary artery is common.

Diagnosis

Dilation of the aortic root is easily measured by echocardiography. Two-dimensional echocardiography shows the classic flask-shaped dilation of the aorta extending from the aortic valve to the innominate artery (Fig. 56–1). Echocardiography may also be used to demonstrate the major complications of aortic root dilation, dissection of the aorta, and aortic regurgitation. The echocardiogram has also helped in defining the optimal time for operative intervention.

Therapy

It is now generally agreed, although not absolutely proven, that beta blockade may inhibit the pace of aortic dilation.

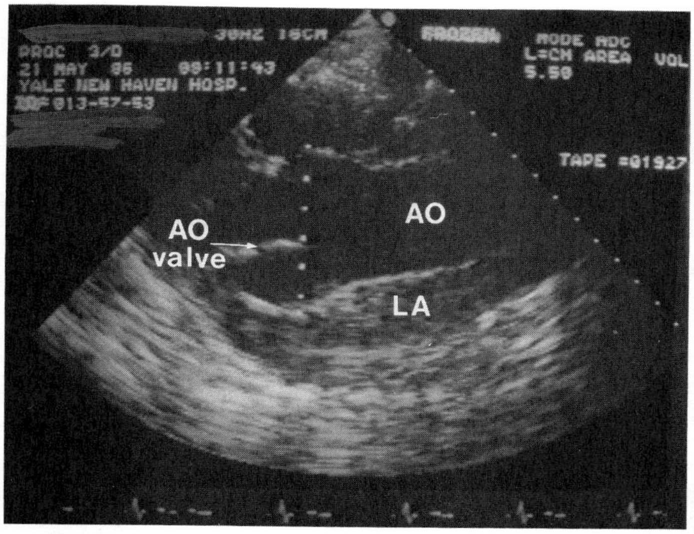

FIGURE 56–1. Echocardiogram, long axis parasternal view of a patient with Marfan's syndrome. The sinuses of Valsalva are flared and the aortic root is dilated.

Therefore, it is appropriate to obtain serial echocardiograms in patients thought to have Marfan's syndrome. When incipient dilation of the aorta is recognized, institution of a beta blocker may be warranted. By diminishing the velocity with which the left ventricle ejects blood, the forces on the weakened aortic wall may be lessened.

Complications of aneurysms in the ascending aorta account for more than 90 per cent of deaths from the Marfan's syndrome. The likelihood of both aortic dissection and aortic regurgitation increases as the size of the aortic root increases. Operation in the face of an acute dissection is fraught with considerable hazard. Therefore, prophylactic operation is recommended if the aortic root enlarges to 6 cm on echocardiography. The operation most commonly utilized for patients with the Marfan's syndrome is replacement of the ascending aortic aneurysm with a composite tube graft that includes a prosthetic valve at its proximal end. The coronaries are anastomosed to the sides of the tube graft. The aneurysm is wrapped around the tube graft to help establish hemostasis. The overall hospital mortality of the procedure is 2 per cent (Gott and colleagues). Although it may seem radical to recommend aortic replacement to a patient who may be asymptomatic, the adverse prognosis of the patient with Marfan's syndrome whose aorta dilates to greater than 6 cm in diameter probably warrants this recommendation.

Gott VL, Pyeritz RE, Magovern GJ Jr, et al.: Surgical treatment of aneurysms of the ascending aorta in the Marfan syndrome. N Engl J Med 314:1070, 1986. *The results of ascending aorta replacement with a composite graft in 50 consecutive patients with Marfan's syndrome are reported. Because of the unfavorable natural history of Marfan's syndrome, the authors recommend prophylactic repair when the aneurysm reaches a diameter of 6 cm.*

Halpern BL, Char F, Murdoch JL, et al.: A prospectus on the prevention of aortic rupture in the Marfan syndrome with data on survivorship without treatment. Johns Hopkins Med J 129:123, 1971. *This is one of the first articles to advocate the prophylactic use of beta blockers in patients with the Marfan's syndrome in order to prevent further dilation and dissecting aneurysm.*

DISSECTING ANEURYSM OF THE AORTA

The incidence of aortic dissections is not known exactly, but it is estimated that approximately 2000 acute cases occur in the United States each year.

Classification of aortic dissection is based upon duration and anatomic location of the dissection. Dissection is considered acute if it occurred within two weeks, and chronic if it occurred more than two weeks, prior to the institution of therapy.

Aortic dissection is more commonly classified by site of the intimal tear and extent of dissecting hematoma. In type I and type II dissections, the intimal tear is in the ascending aorta, usually within a few centimeters of the aortic valve. In type I aneurysms, the dissecting hematoma extends and involves at least the aortic arch and often the descending aorta as well. Type II aneurysms involve the ascending aorta only. Type III aneurysms are characterized by an intimal tear in the descending aorta, usually immediately distal to the left subclavian artery. The dissecting hematoma usually propagates distally but at times may extend in a retrograde manner to the aortic arch (Fig. 56–2).

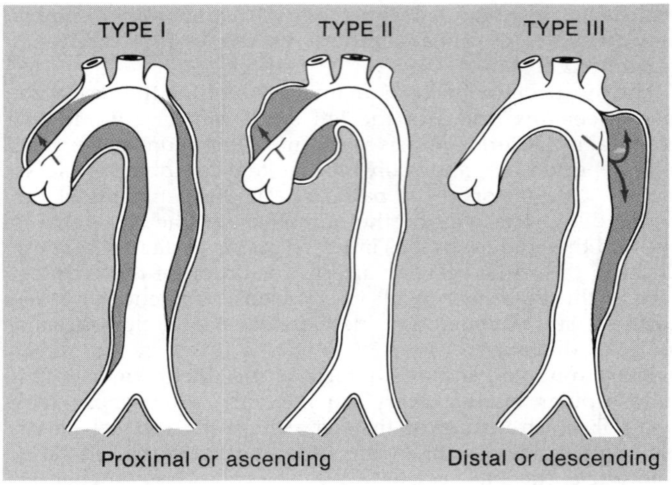

FIGURE 56–2. Classification of dissecting aneurysms of the aorta. (Modified from DeBakey.)

Etiology

The most consistent etiologic factor in aortic dissection is hypertension. Other conditions are associated with dissection in the absence of hypertension. Marfan's syndrome has been discussed. There is a peculiar association between pregnancy and dissection. It is postulated that hormonal changes during pregnancy may alter the composition of the aorta and make it more susceptible to rupture. Stresses and strains of labor may also be a factor.

Valvular aortic stenosis, particularly that due to a bicuspid valve, is associated with dissection. Turbulence established beyond the stenotic valve increases lateral forces, thereby enhancing the likelihood of an intimal tear and development of a dissection. The association between coarctation of the aorta and dissection is well known. The years of proximal aortic hypertension prior to repair of the coarctation may establish the conditions that ultimately lead to aortic dissection. In addition, there is a high incidence of bicuspid aortic valves in patients with coarctation of the aorta. Before the advent of antimicrobial agents, syphilitic aortitis was the most common cause of aortic dissection. It is now unusual. Trauma may be a cause of dissecting aneurysm. Other unusual etiologies are the Ehlers-Danlos syndrome and relapsing polychondritis.

Pathogenesis

Aortic dissection begins most frequently in an intimal tear in the ascending aorta a short distance above the aortic valve. The primary tear is often referred to as the *entry intimal tear*. The *re-entry* or *secondary tear* occurs more distally. The basic pathologic condition resides in the underlying media, the chief supporting layer of the aorta. Most tears are transverse or circumferential, reflecting the direction of the muscular fibers of the media.

The two key ingredients of aortic dissection are arterial hypertension and medial degeneration. In any given patient, one or the other of these abnormalities may be the more important. Many patients with Marfan's syndrome or the Ehlers-Danlos syndrome develop dissecting aneurysms without ever developing hypertension. Alternatively, individuals with longstanding hypertension may develop dissection without any apparent specific weakness of the aortic medial wall. Additional factors in the pathogenesis of aortic dissections are the anatomy and motion of the heart and great vessels themselves. The heart beats an average of 70 times per minute, over 80,000 times per day and over 35 million times per year. The heart is not absolutely fixed in place but is limited in its anterior-posterior movement by the sternum and vertebral column, respectively. Its motion is both side to side and twisting as it ejects blood into the ascending aorta. This produces a flexing stress in the ascending aorta and contributes to the frequency of ascending aortic dissections. The descending aorta becomes fixed distal to the left subclavian artery, accounting for the alternative predilection for dissection to occur at that site. Once an intimal tear occurs, the dissecting hematoma is propagated through the weakened medial wall. The forces that continue the propagation are the arterial pressure and the pulse wave properties (dp/dt) of left ventricular ejection. Some dissecting hematomas will rupture back into the aortic lumen at a distal site. Rupture may also occur externally into the pericardial or pleural space.

Clinical Manifestations

Pain is often excruciating and may occur primarily in the anterior chest. It may migrate to the back as the dissecting hematoma works it way down the aorta. Patients sometimes describe an accentuation of the pain with each heart beat suggesting the driving force of the pulse wave. Pain may occur in the neck, jaw, or teeth if the aortic arch is involved. Less common symptoms are syncope, stroke, paraplegia, or loss of pulses in any of the extremities. Rarely, a dissection may be clinically silent and be suggested only by an abnormal roentgenogram. If aortic regurgitation occurs owing to the dissection, patients may develop congestive heart failure. A diastolic murmur is usually present in these circumstances, although the duration of the murmur may be relatively short if the filling pressure in the left ventricle rises rapidly because of the acute nature of the regurgitation. Such murmurs may be heard commonly along the right sternal border.

The clinical presentation and physical findings in patients with aortic dissection are determined by the course taken by the dissecting hematoma. (1) Loss of any pulse can occur as the circulation to any major artery arising from the aorta may be compromised. (2) Aortic regurgitation may result from disruption of the supporting structures of the aortic valve. (3) Neurologic symptoms may occur if the head and neck vessels are compromised by the dissection. Paraplegia may occur owing to loss of blood supply to the spinal cord. A number of other physical findings may be seen in patients with aortic dissection. These include Horner's syndrome due to compression of the superior cervical ganglion, vocal cord paralysis and hoarseness due to pressure against the recurrent laryngeal nerve, superior vena cava syndrome, pulsating neck masses, dyspnea due to tracheal or bronchial compression, hemorrhagic pleural effusion, myocardial infarction if the hematoma dissects retrograde across a coronary ostium, and symptoms and signs of mesenteric infarction. Persistent fever has also been described.

Diagnosis

Time is often of utmost importance in management. Once the patient is stabilized, aortography should not be delayed. Routine laboratory tests do not generally add much to the diagnosis. Leukocytosis is a common but nonspecific finding.

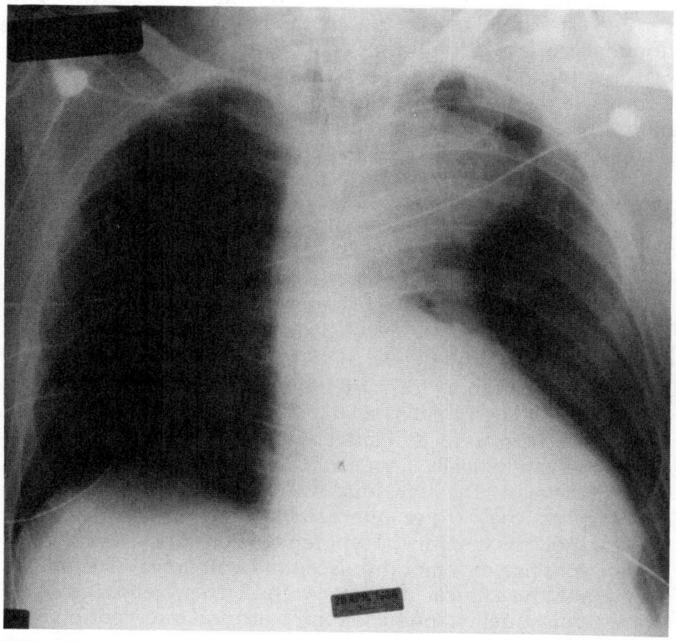

FIGURE 56–3. Chest roentgenogram of a patient with a dissecting aneurysm demonstrating marked enlargement of the aortic arch and descending aorta.

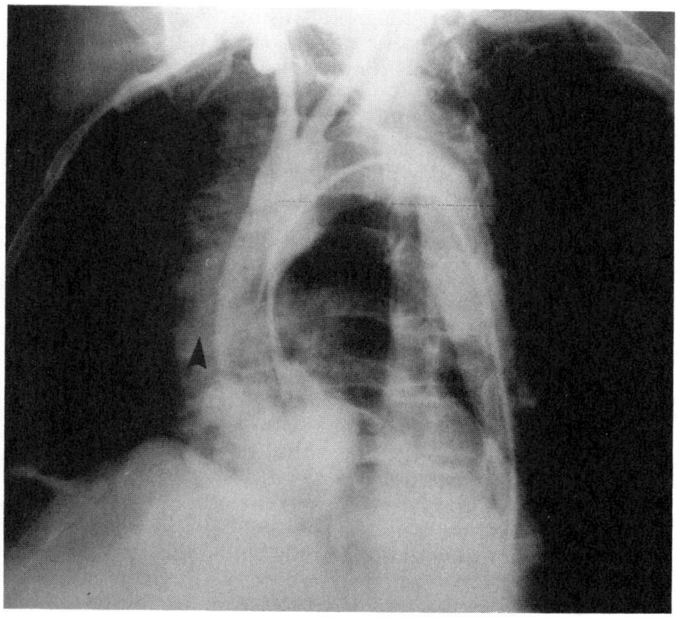

FIGURE 56–4. Aortic root angiogram in the left anterior oblique projection. The black arrowhead demonstrates the false lumen caused by the aortic dissection.

A chest roentgenogram may be normal but will often show widening of the aortic shadow (Fig. 56–3). Aortic angiography is the definitive procedure, yielding precise information necessary for proper management. The extent of the dissection, the entry and re-entry sites, the competence or degree of regurgitation of the aortic valve, and aortic branch vessel involvement can all be ascertained (Fig. 56–4).

The differential diagnosis of a patient with chest or back pain, pulmonary edema with a new murmur of aortic regurgitation, any acute neurologic syndrome, or sudden loss of pulse in an extremity should include aortic dissection.

Computed tomography with the use of contrast material is also highly accurate in demonstrating aortic dissection, although it is not always possible to perform this examination rapidly. Two-dimensional echocardiography does not necessitate the use of contrast agents or ionizing radiation and is easily performed. False-negative and false-positive diagnoses remain a problem with this procedure, but it is nevertheless useful (Fig. 56–5). Echocardiography can detect the presence

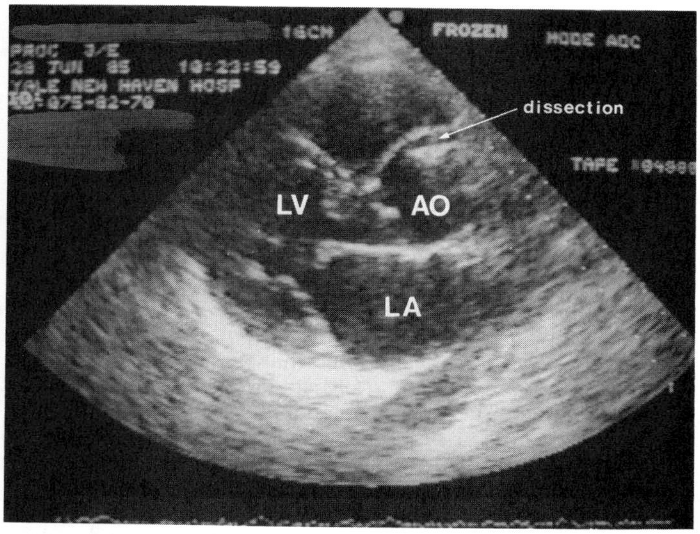

FIGURE 56–5. Echocardiogram, long axis parasternal view of a patient with dissecting aneurysm. The dissection arises in the proximal aortic root. LV = Left ventricle; AO = aortic root; LA = left atrium.

of aortic regurgitation. Magnetic resonance imaging is also capable of diagnosing aortic dissection and does not require the use of contrast agents for vascular imaging.

Prognosis

In untreated aortic dissection, the prognosis is poor. Approximately 20 per cent of patients die in 24 hours, 60 per cent in 2 weeks, and 90 per cent in 3 months. The principal cause of death is not the initial intimal tear but is related to the effects of propagation of the dissecting hematoma. Progressive aortic regurgitation may occur if the hematoma dissects in a retrograde direction. Rupture into the pericardial or pleural space is often a fatal complication.

Treatment

Prompt diagnosis and institution of therapy are critical to the success of treatment. Since the most important known factors in the propagation of the dissecting hematoma are hypertension and the rate of rise of the aortic pressure pulse (dp/dt), efforts must be undertaken to alter both of these. An intravenous drip of sodium nitroprusside is started, and the infusion is titrated to reduce the systolic blood pressure to 100 to 120 mm Hg. The infusion rate can usually be started at 1 μg per kilogram per minute. Simultaneously, propranolol should be given in intermittent intravenous boluses of 0.5 to 1.0 mg until the heart rate is in the range of 60 beats per minute. When possible, an intra-arterial line to measure blood pressure accurately and a central venous line or Swan-Ganz catheter should be utilized. Once the patient's blood pressure and other hemodynamic and clinical features are stable, aortography should be performed. Computed tomographic scanning or echocardiography may be of some diagnostic aid at this stage while awaiting aortography.

Operative intervention is usually indicated if the dissection involves the ascending aorta, as in Types I and II aneurysms. These aneurysms are unstable and pose the threat of retrograde dissection, rupture, severe aortic regurgitation, or fatal pericardial tamponade. This type of acute dissection can be corrected surgically with a mortality rate in the range of 20 per cent. Type III aneurysms that involve the distal or descending aorta can generally be treated medically. If the patient's condition stabilizes, drug therapy can be continued into the chronic phase. Surgical intervention for the patient with a Type III aneurysm is indicated if there is evidence of increasing size of the dissecting hematoma, impending rupture, inability to control pain, or bleeding into the pleural space.

The operative approach must be flexible and individualized. For patients with ascending aortic dissection and involvement of the annulus or root, it is often necessary to replace the entire aortic root and aortic valve with a composite conduit, which is attached proximally to the aortic annulus and distally to the aorta after obliteration of the false lumen. The coronary ostia are then reimplanted into the tubular graft. If the ascending aorta is involved but the sinuses of Valsalva are spared, operative repair consists of resection of the aneurysmal portion with replacement by a synthetic tubular graft. This same technique applies for descending aortic dissections. In all cases, the false lumen is obliterated. Management and follow-up of patients initially treated either surgically or medically is the same. Continued meticulous control of blood pressure and administration of beta blockers to control dp/dt are warranted. The systolic blood pressure should be kept below 130 mm Hg at rest and the heart rate below 72 beats per minute at rest.

Cooke JP, Safford RE: Progress in the diagnosis and management of aortic dissection. Mayo Clin Proc 61:147, 1986. *This is an excellent short article that concentrates on the available diagnostic studies in patients with aortic dissection.*

Eagle KA, Quertermous T, Kritzer GA, et al.: Spectrum of conditions initially suggesting acute aortic dissection but with negative aortograms. Am J Cardiol 57:322, 1986. *This study defines the differential diagnosis of aortic dissection, discusses the frequency of false-negative aortographic findings, and contrasts the clinical features of patients with and without dissection.*

Roberts WC: Aortic dissection: Anatomy, consequences, and causes. Am Heart J 101:195, 1981. *A well-illustrated review of aortic dissection with emphasis on pathologic findings.*

Slater EE, DeSanctis RW: The clinical recognition of dissecting aortic aneurysm. Am J Med 60:625, 1976. *The clinical, roentgenologic, and laboratory findings in 124 patients with dissecting aneurysm of the aorta are discussed. Patients with dissections of the proximal aorta were younger and had a higher incidence of Marfan's syndrome, cystic medial necrosis, anterior chest pain, pulse deficits, neurologic compromise, aortic regurgitation, and congestive heart failure. Back pain, hypertension, and atherosclerosis characterized patients with distal dissection.*

Wheat MW Jr: Acute dissecting aneurysms of the aorta: Diagnosis and treatment—1979. Am Heart J 99:373, 1980. *The author, a surgeon, presents arguments for vigorous medical therapy in order to control hypertension and rate of pressure development in the aorta.*

MISCELLANEOUS FORMS OF AORTITIS AND THE AORTIC ARCH SYNDROME

Arteritis

A number of inflammatory processes can involve the aortic arch and its major branches. Aortic arteritis, no matter what the etiology, may cause narrowing or occlusion of the major arch vessels. Blood supply to the areas supplied by the innominate artery, the left common carotid artery, and the left subclavian artery may be impaired. Symptoms may include transient ischemic attacks, syncope, disorders of vision or speech, claudication of the upper extremities or of the muscles of the jaw, decreased pulses in the neck and upper extremities, or symptoms of basilar artery insufficiency. As a group, these entities are called the aortic arch syndrome. They include aortitis due to syphilis, tuberculosis, giant cell arteritis, polyarteritis nodosa, Takayasu's syndrome, or dissecting aneurysm. Kawasaki's mucocutaneous lymph node syndrome may cause an aortitis, but the coronary arteries are the principal vessels involved. Giant cell arteritis may cause the aortic arch syndrome in addition to temporal and ophthalmic artery disease.

Takayasu's arteritis may be a more specific form of aortitis. Initially it was thought that the arteritic process was limited to the aortic arch and its branches. Subsequent studies have demonstrated that the arteritis is not confined to these areas. Three varieties are now recognized. In one type, the involvement is localized to the aortic arch and its branches. The second type involves the descending thoracic aorta and abdominal aorta without the arch. The third type contains features of both. There is a preponderance of females with "pulseless disease." Although early reports were more common in Japan, increasing numbers of patients are being recognized in the United States. The presence of hypertension with absent pulses in the upper extremities has caused this syndrome to be called reversed coarctation.

Lupi-Herrera E, Sanchez-Torres G, Marcushamer J, et al.: Takayasu's arteritis: Clinical study of 107 cases. Am Heart J 93:94, 1977. *A review of Takayasu's arteritis involving 107 patients. This entity is not limited to Asian patients. It is a nonspecific inflammatory process affecting the aorta and its main branches.*

TRAUMATIC AORTIC DISEASE

The most common form of trauma to the aorta is due to deceleration injuries, often seen in automobile accidents. Since the descending aorta is relatively immobile, deceleration injuries characteristically affect the portion of the aorta immediately distal to the left subclavian artery. Nonpenetrating aortic injury may cause internal bleeding with no external evidence of chest injury. Hypotension or shock, left hemothorax, absence of femoral pulses, and pale lower extremities round out the clinical picture. A chest roentgenogram may show mediastinal widening. Prompt surgical intervention may be life saving.

57 VASCULAR DISEASES OF THE LIMBS

Hermes A. Kontos

VASCULAR DISEASES OF THE LIMBS CAUSED BY ABNORMAL RESPONSES OF VASCULAR SMOOTH MUSCLE

Raynaud's Phenomenon and Disease

DEFINITION. Raynaud's phenomenon is a syndrome manifested by attacks of pallor and cyanosis of the digits in response to cold or to emotion. As the attack abates, these color changes are replaced by redness. When the disorder is primary, it is called Raynaud's disease, when it is secondary to another disease or cause, it is called Raynaud's phenomenon.

ETIOLOGY AND INCIDENCE. Raynaud's disease is the most common cause of Raynaud's phenomenon, accounting for 60 per cent of patients with this disorder. The cause of Raynaud's disease is unknown. Although it can begin at any age, it becomes clinically manifest most commonly between the ages of 20 and 40 years. Raynaud's disease is much more common in women than in men. Two theories have been advanced to explain its occurrence. Raynaud believed that it is caused by increased sympathetic nerve activity. However, measurements of the sympathetic nerve traffic in the median nerve failed to show differences between patients with Raynaud's disease and normal individuals. Lewis discovered that attacks of Raynaud's phenomenon could be induced after interruption of the sympathetic nerves. He concluded that the cause of the disorder was a fault in the arterial wall that rendered the vessels hyper-responsive to the vasoconstrictive effects of cold. He ascribed the vasospastic attacks to spasm of the digital arteries as a result of this hypersensitivity. Little is known about the defect in the vessel wall, which renders the vessel hypersensitive to cold. The circulation of the digits of patients with Raynaud's disease is not hypersensitive to infused norepinephrine. Also, determination of the arteriovenous concentration differences of norepinephrine and epinephrine across the hand showed that there was no excessive release of catecholamines from the hands of patients with Raynaud's disease. More recently, accelerated destruction of platelets and release of agents such as serotonin or thromboxane A_2 have been proposed as causing vasoconstriction in some patients with Raynaud's phenomenon. It is not known whether platelet destruction is the cause of spasm in such patients or a consequence of it.

In a recent study, 26 per cent of patients with the variant type of angina pectoris were found to have migraine, and 24 per cent were found to have Raynaud's phenomenon. This suggested that some patients with Raynaud's phenomenon may have a generalized defect that predisposes arteries in many regions to vasospasm. An association of Raynaud's phenomenon with idiopathic pulmonary hypertension has also been reported. This association may reflect a very high level of peripheral vascular tone secondary to the severe reduction in cardiac output.

Secondary Raynaud's phenomenon is observed frequently as a manifestation of the diseases listed in Table 57–1.

In the presence of arterial obstruction, vasoconstrictive stimuli that normally do not cause clinical manifestations result in more severe reduction in blood flow and may cause Raynaud's phenomenon.

Raynaud's phenomenon is very often associated with connective tissue diseases; it is particularly frequent in scleroderma. Almost all patients with scleroderma develop Raynaud's phenomenon at some time during the course of their illness. A distinctive syndrome consisting of calcinosis, Raynaud's phenomenon, abnormal esophageal motility, sclerodactyly, and telangiectasia (CREST syndrome) is recognized. Raynaud's phenomenon may be the presenting manifestation in connective tissue diseases and may precede the appearance of other manifestations by several years. The presence of abnormal nail fold capillaries in patients with Raynaud's phenomenon has predictive value for the future development of scleroderma. Structural changes in the vessel wall that limit flow and increase the sensitivity to vasoconstrictive influences appear to account for the frequent occurrence of Raynaud's phenomenon in these diseases. Vascular injury may also result from repetitive minor occupational trauma or from a severe exposure to cold, as in frostbite. Consequent hypersensitivity to cold causes Raynaud's phenomenon.

Neurogenic lesions cause Raynaud's phenomenon because of irritation of sympathetic nerves and consequent vasoconstriction. Intense or sustained vasoconstriction caused by drugs may also result in Raynaud's phenomenon, as in 3 to 6 per cent of patients taking beta-adrenergic receptor–blocking drugs. Propranolol is the main offender. These drugs block a beta-adrenegic vasodilative mechanism in the digits and may also enhance the vasoconstrictive effects of norepinephrine.

Intravascular aggregation or coagulation of blood elements may obstruct the vessels and cause ischemia and Raynaud's phenomenon.

PATHOPHYSIOLOGY. The pallor during the attack of Raynaud's phenomenon is explained by intense vasoconstriction or spasm of the digital arteries. This results in severe reduction in blood flow. In a later stage of the attack, the vasoconstriction becomes less severe, and the capillaries and veins are partially filled with blood whose hemoglobin becomes markedly deoxygenated. This accounts for the cyanosis. Upon rewarming, cyanosis is replaced by an intense red color associated with reactive hyperemia. Between attacks, blood flow to the digits is usually reduced, especially in patients who have trophic changes, but may be normal in some patients. In those patients without trophic changes, blood flow to the hand during maximum vasodilation is the same as in normal individuals, but it is severely reduced in those with trophic changes, a reflection of structural changes in the blood vessels.

TABLE 57–1. CAUSES OF SECONDARY RAYNAUD'S PHENOMENON

1. Occlusive arterial disease
   a. Arteriosclerosis obliterans
   b. Buerger's disease
   c. Arterial embolism
   d. Vasculitis
   e. Arterial thrombosis
2. Connective tissue diseases
   a. Scleroderma
   b. Rheumatoid arthritis
   c. Systemic lupus erythematosus
3. Vascular injury
   a. Repetitive minor occupational trauma, as in pneumatic hammer operators, pianists, or typists
   b. Frostbite
4. Neurogenic causes
   a. Thoracic outlet compression by cervical rib, by scalenus anticus muscle, or in hyperabduction syndrome
   b. Carpal tunnel syndrome
   c. Sympathetic causalgia
   d. Spinal cord diseases
5. Drugs or exposure to chemicals
   a. Ergotamine
   b. Ergotism
   c. Methysergide
   d. Polyvinyl chloride
   e. Beta-adrenergic receptor blockers
6. Intravascular coagulation or aggregation
   a. Cryoglobulinemia
   b. Cold agglutinins

PATHOLOGY. In the early stages of the disease, the digital blood vessels are histologically normal. In longstanding cases, the intima becomes thickened, and the media may be hypertrophied. In severe progressive cases, complete obstruction from thrombosis may occur, and gangrene of the tips of the digits may ensue.

CLINICAL MANIFESTATIONS. The onset of Raynaud's disease is usually gradual. The patient notices an occasional mild and short-lasting attack during winter. Over succeeding years, the severity and duration of the attacks may increase. A wide variation in severity is present. Most commonly, the attacks are provoked by exposure to cold. In some patients, attacks are also precipitated by emotion. The attacks may be terminated by rewarming, or they may abate spontaneously. Between attacks, in a warm environment, the patient is asymptomatic, and physical examination shows no abnormalities. Some patients, however, complain of chronically cold hands and feet, and they may have cold fingers with cyanosis on examination. In a typical attack of Raynaud's phenomenon, the digits become pale. Usually, all digits are affected symmetrically. The pallor is sharply demarcated at the level of the metacarpophalangeal joints, a reflection of spasm of the digital arteries. At a later stage during the attack, pallor is replaced by cyanosis. The patient may have feelings of coldness, numbness, and occasionally pain. Upon rewarming, the cyanosis is replaced by intense redness, and the patient may feel tingling or throbbing. Most commonly, only the hands are affected. Frequently, both hands and feet are affected. Rarely, the nose, cheeks, ears, and chin are affected also.

Atypical attacks are not infrequent. In these, the involvement of the digits may be asymmetric, with only one or two digits being affected. In some cases, only a portion of the digit is affected. In these instances, the most severely affected portion of the digit is the most distal one. Thus, one may see pallor of the fingertip or of the terminal phalanx of one digit. In other cases, more than one phalanx may be involved.

In severe, progressive cases, trophic changes may occur after a few years of involvement. The hair may disappear from the dorsal aspect of the digits. The nails grow more slowly and become brittle and deformed. The skin becomes atrophic, thin, and tight (sclerodactyly). Ulcerations may develop at the fingertips or around the nail bed. These heal slowly and may become infected. They are extremely painful, especially at night. When they heal, they leave characteristic small, pitted scars.

DIAGNOSIS. The diagnosis of Raynaud's phenomenon can usually be made on the basis of the history of vasospastic attacks in the digits, precipitated by cold and relieved by warming. In atypical cases or when the patient's description of the attack is not clear, provocation of an attack may be helpful. This may be done by immersing the hands in water at a temperature of 10 to 15°C. Whole-body exposure to cold is more successful in provoking attacks. A negative result does not exclude Raynaud's phenomenon.

In typical cases, Raynaud's phenomenon is easily distinguished from acrocyanosis, but when involvement is atypical, the differentiation may be more difficult. Distinguishing features include the following: The color changes in Raynaud's phenomenon are episodic, whereas in acrocyanosis they are sustained. Pallor is not a prominent feature of acrocyanosis. Cyanosis is the more typical color change, whereas in Raynaud's disease digital pallor is characteristic. In Raynaud's disease, only the digits are involved, whereas in acrocyanosis the color changes usually involve the whole hand or foot and sometimes even more proximal portions of the limbs. In Raynaud's disease the skin of the palms is usually dry, whereas in acrocyanosis it is wet and clammy with sweat. Finally, acrocyanosis rarely causes trophic changes and ulcerations.

Obstruction of major arteries from arteriosclerosis, angiitis, embolism, or thrombosis may lead to color changes in the digits that simulate Raynaud's phenomenon. The distinction is made by the demonstration of changes in arterial pulses and by the fact that the color changes in these disorders are likely to be confined to one limb rather than be symmetric. Arteriography, which demonstrates the arterial lesion, is helpful. However, secondary Raynaud's phenonenon may be superimposed upon any of these diseases. In Raynaud's phenomenon, Doppler velocity studies show patent arteries and sharply peaked blood flow velocity patterns in the digits. Arteriography shows normal major arteries and diffuse spasm of the digital arteries.

The distinction of Raynaud's disease from secondary Raynaud's phenomenon is based mainly on the exclusion of disorders known to cause secondary Raynaud's phenomenon. The exclusion of obstructive arterial disease is discussed above. Connective tissue disorders, particularly scleroderma, are excluded by the absence of arthralgias or arthritis, alterations of esophageal motility, and the absence of a pulmonary oxygen diffusion defect. The presence of a normal sedimentation rate and the absence of circulating autoantibodies, such as antinuclear antibodies, provide additional reassurance. A careful occupational history is necessary to exclude Raynaud's phenomenon secondary to minor repetitive trauma. A history of drug ingestion or exposure to chemicals is helpful in identifying drug-induced Raynaud's phenomenon. Neurologic disorders can be recognized by their somatic neurologic manifestations. Thoracic outlet compression syndromes can be excluded by the appropriate maneuvers. The presence of intravascular agglutination or coagulation of the blood elements may be suspected if, in the presence of cyanosis, the blood cannot be expelled from vessels by pressure, and when there are isolated areas of redness as the attack abates during rewarming. Confirmation is obtained by demonstrating the cold agglutinins or cryoglobulins in the patient's blood.

PROGNOSIS. The prognosis of patients with Raynaud's disease is good. There is no mortality associated with the disease and morbidity is low, it is generally limited to loss of portions of digits as a result of ulcerations. In approximately 50 per cent of patients with Raynaud's disease, the disorder improves and may disappear completely after several years. In only a fraction of 1 per cent of patients is amputation necessary. Approximately 15 per cent of patients with Raynaud's phenomenon eventually develop a connective tissue disorder, particularly scleroderma.

The prognosis in secondary Raynaud's phenomenon depends on the course of the primary disorder. In scleroderma, the prognosis is unsatisfactory, particularly when the disease has caused digital ulcerations.

TREATMENT. Management of patients with Raynaud's phenomenon must be tailored to the individual needs of the patient, taking into consideration the frequency and severity of the attacks (Table 57–2). All patients benefit from reassur-

TABLE 57–2. TREATMENT OF RAYNAUD'S PHENOMENON

Frequency and Severity of Vasospastic Attacks	Suggested Treatment
1. Rare or mild attacks	Protective measures, cessation of smoking, and no drug therapy
2. Frequent or severe attacks without trophic changes	Protective measures and calcium antagonists
3. Frequent attacks with trophic changes but no open ulcers	Protective measures plus calcium antagonists or oral reserpine plus liothyronine
4. Frequent attacks with active, painful ulcers	Intravenous PGE_1, intra-arterial reserpine followed by calcium antagonists; or reserpine plus liothyronine

TABLE 57–3. SOME DRUGS USEFUL IN THE TREATMENT OF RAYNAUD'S PHENOMENON

1. Calcium antagonists
   a. Nifedipine*
   b. Diltiazem*
2. Alpha-adrenergic receptor blockers
   a. Phenoxybenzamine*
   b. Tolazoline
   c. Prazosin*
3. Drugs that interfere with sympathetic nerve activity
   a. Reserpine*
   b. Guanethidine*
   c. Alpha-methyldopa*
4. Vasodilators
   a. PGE_1*
   b. PGE_2*
   c. PGI_2*
   d. Nitroglycerin (topical)*
5. Miscellaneous
   a. Liothyronine*

*Investigational drug for this purpose.

ance and protective measures against exposure to cold. The patients should limit the duration of exposure to cold to the greatest extent possible. They should wear heavy clothing, protecting not only the hands and feet but also the face and trunk, especially when there is a cold wind, this is important because exposure to cold of other portions of the body may reflexly induce vasoconstriction in the digits and precipitate Raynaud's phenomenon. When prolonged exposure to cold is unavoidable, the use of electrically powered or solid fuel–powered hand and foot warmers is advisable. These patients should be taught to recognize and terminate attacks by returning promptly to a warm environment, placing their hands in warm water, or using a warm-air hairblower to warm their hands rapidly. Smoking causes cutaneous vasoconstriction; therefore, tobacco smoking is contraindicated in Raynaud's phenomenon. The use of induced vasodilation by placing the hands in warm water (43°C) has been reported to raise skin temperature and minimize the severity of attacks of Raynaud's phenomenon. Biofeedback to teach patients to raise skin temperature voluntarily has been shown to limit the duration and frequency of vasospastic attacks, but its effect is nonspecific because it is also seen in control patients who received no such treatment and in those in whom biofeedback is used to teach relaxation.

The simple measures outlined above usually suffice for patients with infrequent or mild attacks. When Raynaud's phenomenon is more frequent or more severe, and especially when it has resulted in trophic changes or ulcerations, these measures need to be supplemented by drugs. The aim of drug therapy is to induce vascular smooth muscle relaxation, thereby relieving spasm, raising resting blood flow, and limiting the degree of ischemia during attacks. The drugs most frequently used in treating patients with Raynaud's phenomenon are shown in Table 57–3. For most patients, the drug of choice is a calcium antagonist. Nifedipine* has been found to be effective in several well-controlled, double-blind studies. The drug is administered at a dose of 10 to 20 mg three or four times daily. Diltiazem,* at a dose of 60 mg three or four times daily, may be substituted, if nifedipine is not well tolerated or if it causes side effects. In one study of very severely affected patients, verapamil was found not to be effective.

Reserpine* is the best-studied drug among the group that interferes with the function of the adrenergic nervous system. It is administered by mouth in doses of 0.1 to 0.5 mg daily. In cases in which ulcerations have developed, it may be given intra-arterially in a dose of 0.5 to 1 mg, dissolved in saline and administered into the brachial or radial artery by slow infusion over several minutes. The drugs in this group may

*Investigational drug for this purpose.

also be administered by means of tourniquet-controlled intravenous injection (Bier's block). The administration by the last two routes gives a much higher local concentration and largely avoids systemic side effects.

In controlled trials, nitroglycerin* ointment or topical prostaglandin E_2* (PGE_2) has been found effective in Raynaud's phenomenon. The topical application of these drugs is advantageous because their local relaxant action is not counteracted by reflex vasoconstriction, secondary to changes in blood pressure that may occur when they are given systemically.

Prostaglandin E_1* (PGE_1) or prostacyclin* (PGI_2) administered intravenously has a beneficial effect in patients with Raynaud's phenomenon. These drugs can be given by constant intravenous infusion in a dose of 6 to 10 ng per kilogram per minute for a few hours or up to three days. It is reported that the beneficial effect outlasts this therapy by several weeks.

A novel but effective way of inducing vasodilation in the digits is via the iatrogenic induction of hyperthyroidism by the administration of sodium liothyronine* (triiodothyronine), 75 μg daily. The resultant hypermetabolism elicits thermoregulatory reflex cutaneous vasodilation. The combination of triiodothyronine and reserpine has been found to be most effective.

Preganglionic sympathectomy to eliminate vasoconstrictor tone may have a beneficial immediate result, but the long-term results are disappointing. The duration of benefit is limited by regeneration of the nerves. If sympathectomy is contemplated, it is advisable to try sympathetic blockade with local anesthetics to verify a beneficial result. A recently devised technique that involves surgical stripping of the palmar and digital arteries to bring about a local sympathectomy may also be tried, but its results have not been fully evaluated.

Coffman JD, Davis WT: Vasospastic diseases: A review. Prog Cardiovasc Dis 18:123, 1975. *A comprehensive, well-referenced review of vasospastic diseases.*

Cohen RA, Coffman JD: β-Adrenergic vasodilator mechanism in the finger. Circ Res 49:1196, 1981. *Demonstration of a beta-adrenergic, humorally activated, vasodilative mechanism in the arteriovenous anastomoses of the human finger. Blockade of this mechanism may explain the occurrence of Raynaud's phenomenon in patients taking beta-adrenergic receptor–blocking drugs.*

Fagius J, Blumberg H: Sympathetic outflow to the hand in patients with Raynaud's phenomenon. Cardiovasc Res 19:249, 1985. *Demonstration that sympathetic nerve activity in patients with Raynaud's phenomenon under baseline conditions and during maneuvers that increase sympathetic nerve traffic does not differ from that in normal controls. The results do not support the theory that Raynaud's disease is caused by increased sympathetic nerve activity.*

Harper FE, Maricq HR, Turner RE, et al.: A prospective study of Raynaud's phenomenon and early connective tissue disease. Am J Med 72:883, 1982. *This study of capillaries of the nail fold shows that the presence of capillary abnormalities in patients with Raynaud's phenomenon may have predictive value for the future development of scleroderma.*

Kontos HA, Wasserman AJ: Effect of reserpine in Raynaud's phenomenon. Circulation 39:259, 1969. *An analysis of the effects of reserpine given intra-arterially and orally on hand blood flow in patients with Raynaud's disease. It also contains evidence against the hypothesis that defective catecholamine metabolism may account for Raynaud's disease. Beneficial results from oral administration of reserpine are also presented.*

Miller D, Waters DD, Warnica W, et al.: Is variant angina the coronary manifestation of a generalized vasospastic disorder? N Engl J Med 304:763, 1981. *Provocative study showing high incidence of migraine and Raynaud's phenomenon in patients with variant angina, suggesting the possibility that we may be dealing with a generalized vasospastic disorder.*

Smith CR, Rodeheffer RJ: Treatment of Raynaud's phenomenon with calcium channel blockers. Am J Med 78 (Suppl 2B): 39, 1985. *Concise consideration of the pathophysiology of Raynaud's phenomenon and review of available evidence concerning the effectiveness of treatment with calcium antagonists.*

Acrocyanosis

DEFINITION. Acrocyanosis is a rare disorder characterized by persistent cyanosis of the skin of the hands and, less commonly, of the feet associated with reduced skin temperature.

ETIOLOGY. Acrocyanosis is a primary disorder of unknown cause. It is much more common in women than in

*Investigational drug for this purpose.

men. The onset of the disease is usually in young adults or middle-aged persons. The high incidence of the disease among patients with psychiatric disorders is of unknown significance.

PATHOPHYSIOLOGY. The smaller precapillary vessels (arterioles) are abnormally constricted, causing reduction in blood flow and accounting for cyanosis and reduced skin temperature. The veins are secondarily dilated. Constriction of the arterioles occurs under normal environmental conditions and becomes more pronounced on exposure to cold because of increased sensitivity of these vessels to the effects of cold. An important feature of acrocyanosis is the reduced venous tone. No venous obstruction is present. These features can be demonstrated by elevating the involved limb and eliminating the blue color or intensifying the blue color by placing the limb in a dependent position and overfilling the veins.

CLINICAL MANIFESTATIONS. Patients with acrocyanosis have persistent blue discoloration of the hands. Less commonly, the feet are also involved. In some cases, the blue color extends to more proximal portions of the limbs. The skin is cold, and the palms are wet and clammy from sweat. No pallor is usually present. In some cases, there may be spots of pallor surrounded by confluent cyanosis. The blue color is intensified by exposure to cold, and it is converted into purplish or red color by exposure to heat. There are few accompanying symptoms. The patient has feelings of coldness and, occasionally, numbness. Ulcerations and other trophic changes are distinctly unusual. Patients with acrocyanosis seek medical advice either because they are frightened or because the cyanosis is cosmetically unappealing.

DIAGNOSIS. The distinction between acrocyanosis and Raynaud's phenomenon is discussed above in the section on Raynaud's phenomenon. Differentiation from cyanosis secondary to arterial obstruction can be made on the basis of normal pulses, by the bilateral and symmetric occurrence of acrocyanosis, and, if necessary, by the angiographic verification of absence of obstruction. The limitation of the cyanosis to the hands and feet, the improvement in a warm environment, and the absence of reduced arterial blood saturation distinguish acrocyanosis from generalized, systemic cyanosis.

TREATMENT. Since acrocyanosis is a benign disease, no drug therapy is usually required. Reassurance and protection from cold usually suffice. In some cases, cosmetic considerations or unusually severe symptoms may necessitate drug therapy. In these cases, the same drugs that are useful in Raynaud's phenomenon may be tried.

Lewis T, Landis EM: Observations upon the vascular mechanism in acrocyanosis. Heart 15:229, 1930. *Classic description of the clinical features of acrocyanosis. Evidence is presented showing that the disease is the result of an abnormal responsiveness of the smaller blood vessels.*

Livedo Reticularis

DEFINITION. Livedo reticularis is a reticular, bluish discoloration of the skin of the extremities that produces a lacy, irregular appearance outlining central areas of normal-appearing skin. The etiology is not known. The disorder usually begins in young individuals before age 20 to 30 years. It is equally common in men and women but more often symptomatic in women.

PATHOLOGY. Proliferative lesions of the arterioles of the skin with perivascular infiltration have been described. In some cases, there may be thrombosis of arterioles leading to cutaneous infarction and ulceration. Similar changes are seen in the veins.

PATHOPHYSIOLOGY. The mechanism of livedo reticularis is presumed to be similar to that of acrocyanosis, namely, constriction of arterioles followed by stasis and dilation of capillaries and veins. The latter are filled with desaturated blood. The reticular appearance of livedo reticularis reflects the anatomic arrangement of the affected vessels. It is believed that the bluish areas represent the arborizations of peripheral capillaries from central penetrating arterioles. Blood flow is faster in the central regions closer to the penetrating arteriole, whereas the more distant areas have lower flow, with consequent stasis and cyanosis.

CLINICAL MANIFESTATIONS. Patients seek medical attention for cosmetic reasons or because they are frightened by the bluish discoloration. The lower extremities are involved more often than the upper extremities. The patient usually has no symptoms. In some cases, there may be paresthesias or a feeling of coldness. The bluish discoloration becomes more intense on exposure to cold and may disappear in a warm environment. Ulcerations occur rarely; when they do, they appear in winter and heal in summer.

TREATMENT. In most cases no treatment is required. Protection from cold and abstinence from tobacco are useful. In severe cases, drugs useful in the treatment of Raynaud's phenomenon, such as nifedipine and reserpine, may be tried.

Feldaker M, Hines EA, Kierland RR: Livedo reticularis with ulcerations. Circulation 13:196, 1956. *Report of the clinical and pathologic features of 18 patients with livedo reticularis with ulcerations. A brief review of the earlier literature is included.*

Erythromelalgia (Erythermalgia)

DEFINITION. Erythromelalgia is a disorder manifested by episodes of erythema accompanied by increased skin temperature and by pain involving the feet and, less commonly, the hands. It may be primary or secondary to other disorders. These include obstructive arterial disease, polycythemia, and hypertension. There is no sex predilection, and the disease may occur at any age. It is occasionally hereditary.

PATHOPHYSIOLOGY. The symptoms of erythromelalgia are dependent on skin temperature. Rise in skin temperature above a certain level causes the manifestations. In each person this critical point is fairly constant. Vasodilation and consequent hyperemia are the usual causes of the rise in skin temperature. However, an increased blood flow is not essential, since once symptoms have been induced by heat, they may continue even though blood flow is reduced to zero with a cuff inflated above the systolic pressure levels. These features suggest that the cause of the disorder is abnormal sensitivity of the cutaneous pain fibers to heat or tension from the dilated blood vessels.

CLINICAL MANIFESTATIONS. The onset of the disease is gradual. With progression, the frequency and duration of the attacks become more pronounced. Eventually, symptoms may become almost continuous and cause total disability. During an attack the patient complains of burning pain, usually in the feet and, less commonly, in the hands. The pain is usually located in the balls of the feet and in the tips of the toes and in the corresponding parts of the hands. Pain is aggravated by dependency and ameliorated by elevation of the limbs. Exposure to heat aggravates the disorder, whereas cold provides relief. Trophic changes, ulcerations, and gangrene are rare.

DIAGNOSIS. Peripheral neuropathy may cause burning pain simulating erythromelalgia. The pain may be accompanied by cutaneous vasodilation. The detection of the associated sensory and motor manifestations of peripheral neuropathy should help distinguish this condition from erythromelalgia. Arteriosclerosis obliterans or thromboangiitis obliterans may also produce localized burning pain and redness. The alterations in the arterial pulses and the absence of high skin temperature distinguish these conditions from erythromelalgia. Vascular damage from prolonged exposure to cold, as after frostbite, may simulate erythromelalgia. In these cases, the condition is more persistent, and the history of cold exposure should help make the distinction possible.

TREATMENT. Avoidance of exposure to heat, particularly dry heat, prevents attacks of erythromelalgia. Elevation of the extremity and application of cold may terminate an attack. Aspirin, 0.5 gram orally, relieves the pain in many cases. The response is sometimes so striking that it is of diagnostic value. Vasoconstrictive agents, such as methysergide or epinephrine, or beta-adrenergic blocking agents, such as propranolol, have been reported to be effective in some patients. In secondary cases, treatment of the primary disorder may alleviate the attacks.

Babb RR, Alarcon-Segovia D, Fairbairn JF: Erythermalgia: Review of 51 cases. Circulation 29:136, 1964. *Description of the features of primary and secondary erythromelalgia based on a study of a large number of patients.*

Lewis T: Clinical observations and experiments relating to burning pain in the extremities, and to so-called "erythromelalgia" in particular. Clin Sci 1:175, 1933. *A classic paper with detailed clinical descriptions of the manifestations of erythromelalgia. The paper also presents clinical investigations pertinent to the pathogenesis of the disease.*

VASCULAR DISEASES OF THE LIMBS CAUSED BY DAMAGE FROM COLD

Immersion Foot (Trench Foot)

DEFINITION AND ETIOLOGY. Immersion foot is characterized by vascular damage resulting from prolonged exposure of the extremities to cold by wearing wet socks or wet footwear. Usually, the exposure is for several days at about 0°C. Dependency of limbs and immobility, as well as conditions that lead to general debility (lack of sleep and starvation), are contributory factors. The condition occurs primarily in soldiers at war.

Immersion foot has been described in survivors of shipwrecks, who were immobilized in crowded small craft for prolonged periods of time, and exposed to wetness and cold. Maceration of the skin with sea water and secondary infection also contribute.

PATHOPHYSIOLOGY. This condition results from vascular injury. The initial effect of cold is to cause vasoconstriction. Loss of heat is facilitated by moisture. The resultant ischemia causes tissue and vascular injury with increased endothelial permeability. There is extensive extravasation of protein and fluid. As a result, there may be increased hematocrit, sludging, and further aggravation of ischemia.

PATHOLOGY. Little is known about the earliest pathologic change in the blood vessels in immersion foot. Most of the available information has been obtained from advanced cases with extensive vascular injury and gangrene. In these cases, the small arteries exhibit periarterial fibrosis and thickening and may be occluded. The veins show perivenous fibrosis, inflammatory reaction, and hemorrhage. The nerves may also be affected. In cases of immersion foot at relatively high temperatures, hyperhydration of the plantar stratum corneum may be the only finding.

CLINICAL MANIFESTATIONS. Three successive stages, each with distinct clinical manifestations, are recognized. During exposure to the wet, cold environment, there is vasoconstriction. The involved extremity becomes pale and cool, and the patient has paresthesias and a feeling of coldness. A second hyperemic stage follows. Patients are observed most commonly during this stage, because this is when they seek attention. The involved extremity is red, hot, and edematous. There may be pain or paresthesias. The swelling may be aggravated by heat and by placing the limb in a dependent position. Subsequently, blebs appear, filled with serous or hemorrhagic fluid. Hemorrhages may occur into the skin and subcutaneous tissue. This stage may persist for several days. In severe cases, gangrene may supervene. The condition may be complicated by lymphangitis, cellulitis, and thrombophlebitis. Mild cases or those treated early may recover after this second hyperemic phase. In other cases, a third late vasospastic phase occurs in which there is increased sensitivity to cold and typical secondary Raynaud's phenomenon, with excessive sweating, pain, and paresthesias of the lower extremities. This phase may persist for years.

TREATMENT. If the patient is seen in the initial vasoconstrictive phase, bed rest with the extremity in the horizontal position and a warm environment are necessary. During the hyperemic phase, the extremity should be placed at heart level and kept cool to diminish edema. Local care to keep the foot dry and clean should be instituted to avoid infection. Control of pain may require analgesics or narcotics. Sympathectomy may be helpful in the hyperemic stage and also in preventing the late vasospastic phenomena.

Abramson DI, Lerner D, Shumacker HB, et al: Clinical picture and treatment of the later stage of trench foot. Am Heart J 32:52, 1946. *Clinical report based on the study of 633 patients with trench foot. Emphasis is placed on the late sequelae of the disorder.*

Frostbite

DEFINITION AND ETIOLOGY. Frostbite results from freezing of the tissues and consequent vascular injury. In most cases, frostbite occurs during prolonged exposure to temperatures below 0°C. Other environmental factors also play a role, such as high wind and humidity. Predisposing factors include vascular disease, inadequate clothing, lack of acclimatization, and general debility.

PATHOPHYSIOLOGY. Tissue damage results from cold-influenced vasoconstriction. Freezing causes water crystal formation in cells and dehydration. Endothelial damage with increased permeability to protein ensues, causes edema, and further contributes to stasis and eventual thrombosis.

PATHOLOGY. The vessels show endothelial swelling and vacuolization and proliferative changes. Subsequently, there are inflammatory reactions and atrophic changes in the skin.

CLINICAL MANIFESTATIONS. Initially, the patient notices a prickling sensation followed by numbness. The skin becomes bloodless and appears white and cold. This is followed by redness, swelling, and increased temperature. Blisters may form 24 to 48 hours after thawing. They are filled with either serous yellow or hemorrhagic fluid. There may be hemorrhages under the nail beds. Necrosis and gangrene may supervene. The subsequent course may be similar to that of sudden arterial occlusion, including ischemia and gangrene. Spontaneous amputation may require several weeks or months. After an attack of frostbite, the affected extremities may remain sensitive to cold for a period of time or permanently, and secondary Raynaud's phenomenon may occur.

TREATMENT. Frostbite should be treated with immediate rewarming. If frostbite affects deep tissues, rewarming should be done with water at 40 to 44°C. Muscular exercise of the involved limb and massage should be avoided, because they tend to increase edema and pain. If pain is severe, it should be treated with analgesics or narcotics. After the tissues have thawed, the exposed parts should remain at room temperatures. Vesicles should be left untouched, and the limb should be left exposed, without dressings. Antibiotic therapy should be used if infection is present. Sympathectomy has been reported to be beneficial in the initial stages as well as in preventing the delayed sequelae of frostbite.

Washburn B: Frostbite. N Engl J Med 266:974, 1962. *Comprehensive consideration of the clinical features, pathology, diagnosis, prevention, and treatment of frostbite.*

Chilblain (Pernio)

DEFINITION. Chilblain is an inflammatory condition of the skin of the extremities induced by cold and characterized by erythema, itching, and ulceration. The cause is unknown. It is more common in cold, damp climates, as in England, than in the United States. Women are affected more commonly than men. In most patients, the disease begins before the age of 20 years.

PATHOLOGY. In chronic cases, the lesions consist of angiitis with intimal proliferation, thickening of the arterial wall, and perivascular infiltration with lymphocytes and polymorphonuclear leukocytes. There may be necrosis of the adipose tissue and chronic inflammatory infiltrates in the subcutaneous tissue.

CLINICAL MANIFESTATIONS. Both acute and chronic forms of the disease are recognized. The typical patient is a young woman who, in the winter, notices bluish-red discoloration and edema of the skin of the lower limbs associated with burning and warmth. The lesions are persistent and are associated with itching. They generally last from 7 to 10 days and then clear up, sometimes leaving residual pigmentation of the skin. In severe cases, the lesions may become hemorrhagic, or blebs may appear. Infection may supervene.

With repeated exposure to cold, susceptible persons may develop chronic lesions. These are erythematous, ulcerative, and hemorrhagic lesions that begin as raised, red areas 0.5 to 1 cm in diameter. These lesions are then transformed into blebs and finally ulcerate. Healing occurs in the summer, leaving a permanently pigmented region.

DIAGNOSIS. Acute chilblain is distinguished from other forms of dermatitis by its characteristic distribution and by its relationship to cold. Chronic chilblain needs to be distinguished from erythema induration and erythema nodosum. Erythema induratum of Bazin is caused by *Mycobacterium tuberculosis.* If the infection is active, the differential diagnosis may be made by the microscopic demonstration or culture of bacteria. Erythema induratum affects the upper part of the legs more frequently than the lower part. The lesions are more nodular, deeper, and infiltrative. They are also more permanent, whereas those of chronic chilblain clear up in the summer. Erythema nodosum is a more acute process, and it is usually associated with a systemic reaction, consisting of fever, malaise, and arthralgias. There is no seasonal association.

TREATMENT. In mild cases, protection from cold, local application of anti-inflammatory ointments, avoidance of scratching, and cessation of smoking are usually sufficient. In more severe cases, drugs that have been found useful in the treatment of Raynaud's phenomenon, such as reserpine, may be effective.

Eskell J: Reserpine in the treatment of chilblains. Practitioner 189:792, 1962. *Report of a controlled clinical trial of reserpine in patients with chilblain showing excellent benefit.*

Lynn RB: Chilblains. Surg Gynecol Obstet 99:720, 1954. *Concise description of the clinical and pathologic features of chilblain.*

VASCULAR DISEASES OF THE LIMBS CAUSED BY ORGANIC ARTERIAL OBSTRUCTION

Arteriosclerosis Obliterans

DEFINITION. Arteriosclerosis obliterans consists of segmental arteriosclerotic narrowing or obstruction of the lumen in the arteries supplying the limbs.

ETIOLOGY AND INCIDENCE. The etiology of arteriosclerosis in general is discussed in another chapter (see Ch. 50).

Arteriosclerosis obliterans is the commonest cause of arterial obstructive disease of the extremities. The disease becomes clinically manifest usually between the ages of 50 and 70. It is unusual in individuals younger than 30 years of age. Men are affected more often than women. The lower limbs are involved much more frequently than the upper limbs. The most commonly affected vessel is the superficial femoral artery. The distal aorta and its bifurcation into the two iliac arteries and the popliteal artery are the next most frequent sites of involvement. The presence of diabetes mellitus influences arteriosclerosis obliterans in a number of important ways. In diabetics, arteriosclerosis obliterans is likely to be more progressive. This is reflected in a much higher incidence of intermittent claudication in diabetics. The disease affects arterial vessels of smaller caliber and more distally located vessels more frequently than in nondiabetics. The incidence of involvement of vessels below the knee with arteriosclerosis obliterans in diabetics is considerably higher than in nondiabetics.

PATHOLOGY. The lesions of arteriosclerosis obliterans are typical atheromatous plaques involving the intima of the arteries. As a rule, there is superimposed thrombus formation. The media of the vessels shows degenerative changes. Calcification of the media is frequent and may take the form of a ringlike arrangement, as in Monckeberg's sclerosis. Medial calcification is twice as frequent in diabetics as in nondiabetics. These arteriosclerotic lesions are segmental, and they are typically multiple. Weakening of the media may give rise to aneurysmal dilation of the involved artery. Such arteriosclerotic aneurysms are most common in the popliteal fossa or in the femoral artery below the inguinal ligament. They may be filled with thrombi.

PATHOPHYSIOLOGY. The arterial obstruction or narrowing causes reduction in blood flow during exercise or at rest. Clinical symptoms are caused by the consequent ischemia. The most important feature of the stenosis in determining ischemia is the cross-sectional area of the stenotic segment. Because the vascular bed of the extremities generally has a high resting vascular tone and, therefore, a large capacity for vasodilation, a moderate degree of stenosis can be compensated fully by downstream dilation. Stenoses that decrease the cross-sectional area of the vessel by less than 75 per cent do not usually affect resting blood flow. When the prevailing flow rates are high, as in exercise, decreases of 60 per cent or more in cross-sectional area are required before a reduction in flow occurs. Vasodilation in response to ischemia is the result of the action of local mechanisms. These include myogenic mechanisms related to reduction in intravascular pressure or metabolic mechanisms due to release of vasodilative metabolites from the ischemic tissues. These local mechanisms compete with neurogenic mechanisms that, when activated, cause vasoconstriction. Increased sympathetic activity, as from exposure to cold, may, therefore, induce ischemia in the presence of an arterial obstructing lesion.

The presence or absence of ischemia in the face of severe arterial stenosis or obstruction is frequently determined by the degree of development of collateral circulation. Some collateral vessels are present in the normal limb but are not used until obstruction takes place. They open up immediately after an acute arterial occlusion. Others take several weeks or months to become fully developed. Little is known about the responsiveness of collateral vessels. They are subject to neurogenic vasoconstriction from the action of adrenergic nerves. They dilate in response to increased blood pressure, resulting in improved collateral blood flow.

CLINICAL MANIFESTATIONS. The symptoms of arteriosclerosis obliterans are intermittent claudication, pain at rest, and trophic changes in the involved limb. Intermittent claudication denotes pain that develops in a limb on exercise and disappears when the patient rests. The pain is usually described as a cramp or a tightness or as severe fatigue of the exercising muscles. The amount of exercise necessary to induce the pain is usually constant for any given patient. The pain is usually bilateral. In some patients, the pain disappears by slowing the pace of walking without complete cessation of exercise. The location of the pain is distal to the arterial obstruction. The most frequently affected muscles are those of the calf, because of the high frequency with which the femoral artery is involved. The muscles of the lower part of the back, the buttocks, the thigh, and the foot may also be affected.

Pain at rest occurs when a pronounced reduction in resting blood flow is present. It is a sign of severe disease. The pain may be localized to one or more toes, or it may have a stocking-type distribution. The character of the pain is usually burning or gnawing. It is generally worse at night. It is improved by placing the limb in a dependent position and by cooling. There may be associated coldness and numbness, together with cyanosis or pallor of the extremity.

Examination discloses reduced or absent arterial pulses distal to the obstruction. There may be bruits audible over the aorta or its branches. These may be systolic, or they may be continuous. In advanced cases, examination may reveal signs of ischemia. The skin temperature may be abnormally low, or there may be pallor or cyanosis. Ischemic damage may cause persistent reddish or reddish-blue discoloration. There may be trophic changes, including a dry, scaly, and shiny skin. The hair may disappear, and the toenails may become brittle, ridged, and deformed. There may be ulcerations or gangrene. The ischemic ulcers are usually at pressure points and may be inflamed and painful.

Leriche's syndrome refers to isolated aortoiliac disease, which produces a fairly characteristic clinical picture. There is intermittent claudication of the low back, buttocks, and thigh or calf muscles. There is atrophy of the limbs and pallor of the skin of the feet and legs. Impotence may also be present. Arterial pulses in the legs are absent, they may be present but weak in the femoral arteries. Systolic bruits may be audible over the femoral arteries and lower abdomen.

Arteriosclerotic aneurysms may occur, and present as pulsatile, expansible masses in the popliteal fossa or in the femoral artery below the inguinal ligament. These may cause symptoms by pressure on adjacent structures, and, occasionally, by embolism of peripheral vessels or by hemorrhage into the tissues.

DIAGNOSIS. The diagnostic approach to the patient with arteriosclerosis obliterans should be directed at establishing the site of the arterial obstruction, its severity, the degree of ischemia, and the adequacy of the collateral circulation. Palpation of the arterial pulses and auscultation of bruits usually suffice to determine the presence and site of arterial obstruction. Trophic changes and alterations in skin color and temperature indicate ischemia. The latter, as well as the adequacy of the collateral circulation, can be further ascertained by determining the blood pressure at the ankle at rest and during exercise. Several tests may be helpful. With the patient in a warm environment, so that vasoconstrictor tone is low, the leg is raised to a 45-degree angle while the patient is supine. The color of the plantar surface of the foot is observed. Pallor during this test is indicative of severe arterial insufficiency. Venous and capillary filling times can be measured when the patient shifts from the recumbent to the sitting position. Ordinarily, delay in flushing by more than 20 to 30 seconds indicates inadequate collateral circulation. The systolic blood pressure in the dorsalis pedis or posterior tibial arteries can be determined with the use of a Doppler velocitometer at rest as well as during exercise. Ordinarily, this pressure should not be lower than 90 per cent of the level of systolic pressure in the brachial artery. In the presence of severe ischemia, pressures may fall to very low levels. As a rule, pressures less than 30 mm Hg indicate ischemia of sufficient severity to cause gangrene.

The confirmation of arterial obstruction is carried out by arteriography, which is essential to establish the exact anatomy of the arterial vessels and to determine the advisability of surgery.

Arterial embolism is usually distinguishable from arteriosclerosis obliterans because of the sudden onset of the ischemic manifestations and the usually unilateral involvement. Intermittent claudication may occur in severe anemia, in venous disease, and in muscle phosphorylase deficiency (McArdle's syndrome). These conditions are distinguished from arteriosclerosis obliterans by the presence of normal pulses. Ergotamine or methysergide toxicity may cause severe vasospasm, which may affect the large arteries and diminish pulses. The history of drug ingestion may help distinguish these from arteriosclerosis obliterans. In difficult cases, angiography shows the generalized vasospasm and absence of segmental obstructions. A number of conditions of nonvascular nature, such as arthritis and lumbar disc disorders, may cause pain in the limbs and may be confused with intermittent claudication. The presence of normal pulses and other manifestations of these diseases distinguishes them from arteriosclerotic obliterans. In diabetics, ulcerations may be present as a result of diabetic neuropathy. The cause of these ulcers may be difficult to ascertain in the presence of arteriosclerosis obliterans.

TREATMENT. Patients with arteriosclerosis obliterans without evidence of ischemia should be treated medically. Limitation of physical activity, avoidance of tobacco smoking (which causes vasoconstriction), and a regular exercise program are advisable. The treatment of hyperlipidemia, if present, may prevent development of new arteriosclerotic lesions. The control of diabetes, if present, is required. Patients should maintain the skin of the affected limbs clean, dry, and soft and protect it from cold and trauma. Infections and trauma should be attended to promptly. There is no evidence that vasodilative drugs are effective in the treatment of arteriosclerosis obliterans. In fact, they may be harmful under certain circumstances by lowering arterial blood pressure and reducing collateral blood flow or by diverting blood to proximal healthy areas, thereby reducing the perfusion pressure in the more distal portions of the limb. Pentoxifylline, 400 mg administered orally three times daily, has been shown in controlled trials to prolong the duration of exercise and the distance the patient is able to walk prior to the onset of claudication. The drug acts by increasing red cell membrane deformability, thereby reducing effective blood viscosity.

Surgical treatment is advisable when ischemia is present, or if intermittent claudication seriously interferes with the patient's activities. Surgery involves either endarterectomy of the stenotic artery or a bypass operation. Bypass can be performed with either a vein graft or synthetic material. Vein grafts are preferred because of the lower incidence of thrombosis. It is essential that the presence of patent vessels below the obstruction be ascertained before the grafting procedure is carried out. Axillofemoral or femorofemoral grafts for aortoiliac disease have been successful. The larger the size of the vessels grafted, the higher the rate of successful restoration of blood flow.

Percutaneous transluminal angioplasty offers an attractive alternative to surgery in the treatment of arteriosclerosis obliterans. It is simple, has low morbidity, and is less costly than surgery. In this technique, the segmental stenosis or obstruction is dilated by suddenly inflating a balloon introduced into the artery at the site of the lesion by percutaneous catheterization. High success rates and good long-term rates of patency of the dilated vessels have been reported. Angioplasty is more successful in larger vessels, when the stenotic segment is relatively short and when the vessel is not completely occluded.

If the anatomy of the disease makes surgery impossible and ischemic manifestations are present, bed rest is essential. The affected extremity should be kept in a slightly dependent position at 20 to 30 degrees below horizontal, and direct application of heat should be avoided. The limb is best kept warm by placing it under a cradle, under which the temperature is regulated below 38°C. Analgesics or narcotics may be required to control pain. Ulcers should be kept clean with warm saline soaks and debrided. Appropriate antibiotics should be used if infection is present. Intra-arterial administration of PGE_1* may be beneficial in patients with gangrene or ulceration in whom surgery is not possible. Amputation may be necessary to arrest advancing gangrene. The level of amputation is chosen by the presence of warm, viable tissue having normal color.

Long-term anticoagulants are of questionable value. Fibrin-

---

*Investigational drug for this purpose.

olytic therapy with intravenous streptokinase is reported to be helpful in a few patients with recent onset of the disease.

Preganglionic lumbar sympathectomy may be performed as an acute intervention to treat ischemic manifestations of arteriosclerosis obliterans. Before surgery, it must be demonstrated that the interruption of sympathetic nerves is likely to cause improvement in the circulation of the limb. This is done by inducing temporary sympathetic blockade with local anesthetics. This is essential, especially in diabetics in whom peripheral neuropathy may have already produced spontaneous sympathectomy. Sympathectomy does not influence the long-term prognosis of intermittent claudication.

PROGNOSIS. Arteriosclerosis obliterans in the absence of diabetes is a slowly progressive disease. No significant deterioration may be detected for several years. In the presence of diabetes, the disease tends to progress more rapidly, and the prognosis is less satisfactory. The location of obstructing lesions also influences the prognosis. When the lesions are in larger arteries, the probability of successful surgical intervention or percutaneous angioplasty is higher, and the prognosis is better. Frequently arteriosclerosis obliterans is only one of the manifestations of a generalized arteriosclerotic process. Mortality results from arteriosclerotic involvement of other vascular beds, such as the coronary or the cerebral circulation, with death from myocardial infarction or stroke.

Coffman JD: Intermittent claudication and rest pain. Physiologic concepts and therapeutic approaches. Prog Cardiovasc Dis 22:53, 1979. *A comprehensive, well-referenced consideration of the clinical features, diagnosis, and treatment of arteriosclerosis obliterans.*

Freiman DB, Spence R, Gatenby R, et al.: Transluminal angioplasty of the iliac and femoral arteries: Follow-up results with anticoagulation. Radiology 141:347, 1981. *Transluminal angioplasty for the treatment of obstructive disease of the iliac and femoral arteries. Excellent results are reported in 192 patients.*

Porter JM, Culter BS, Lee BY, et al.: Pentoxifylline efficacy in the treatment of intermittent claudication: Multicenter controlled double-blind trial with objective assessment of chronic occlusive arterial disease patients. Am Heart J 104:66, 1982. *A controlled trial of pentoxifylline in patients with intermittent claudication demonstrating objectively improved exercise tolerance.*

Schadt DC, Hines EA, Juergens JL, et al.: Chronic atherosclerotic occlusion of the femoral artery. JAMA 175:937, 1961. *A long-term follow-up study showing slow progression of arteriosclerosis obliterans.*

Thromboangiitis Obliterans (Buerger's Disease)

DEFINITION. Thromboangiitis obliterans is an obstructive arterial disease caused by segmental inflammatory and proliferative lesions of the medium and small arteries and veins of the limbs.

ETIOLOGY. The cause of thromboangiitis obliterans is unknown. Almost all patients with this disease are moderate or heavy smokers, particularly of cigarettes. Many show cutaneous hypersensitivity to intradermally injected tobacco products. There is a high prevalence of HLA-A9 and HLA-B5 antigens in affected persons. An autoimmune mechanism is suggested by a study of cellular and humoral immune responses of 39 patients with thromboangiitis obliterans. Lymphocytes from 77 per cent of these patients exhibited cellular sensitivity to human type I and type III collagen, both of which are constituents of the vascular wall. In addition, approximately 50 per cent had significant levels of anticollagen antibodies in their blood. By contrast, normal controls and patients with arteriosclerosis obliterans had considerably lower levels of cellular sensitivity to collagen and no circulating anticollagen antibodies.

INCIDENCE. Thromboangiitis obliterans is a disease mostly of young males. The disease begins most frequently between the ages of 20 and 40 years, and the ratio of men to women affected varies from 9:1 to as high as 75:1. There is a high prevalence of the disorder in Israel, the Orient, and in India as compared with the United States and Western Europe, suggesting the possibility of a genetic predisposition. The disease has been occasionally reported to occur in familial form.

PATHOLOGY. The disease affects small and medium-sized arteries and veins in segmental fashion. Acute lesions are manifested by proliferation of the intima and thrombosis. There is inflammatory infiltration with polymorphonuclear leukocytes, lymphocytes, and giant cells of all coats of the artery or vein, extending into the thrombus. The media remains intact. Calcium or cholesterol deposition does not occur. These lesions are distinguished from those of arteriosclerosis obliterans because of the more cellular thrombus, the preservation of the media, and the inflammatory infiltration of all coats of the vessel. Older lesions become less cellular, and eventually they may be transformed into a dense scar. Typically, in any one vessel, lesions of varying ages are seen.

CLINICAL MANIFESTATIONS. The typical patient with thromboangiitis obliterans is a young man who smokes cigarettes heavily, has manifestations of ischemia of the extremities, and has a history or evidence of superficial thrombophlebitis. Common presenting complaints are Raynaud's phenomenon with digital ulcerations or pain from ischemia. Pain in thromboangiitis obliterans may be of several types. The most frequent is pain at rest in one or more digits. This pain may be accompanied by manifestations of ischemia, such as color or temperature changes of the skin. This type of pain may be a forerunner of ulceration or gangrene. In the presence of these trophic lesions, there may be localized pain that is aching in character and more severe at night. Another type of pain may occur along the course of the inflamed blood vessels. Ischemic neuropathy may result and cause a paroxysmal, shocklike pain, which may follow the distribution of sensory nerves. Paresthesias may accompany this type of pain. Typical intermittent claudication occurs commonly in the lower extremities. It most often occurs in the arch of the foot because of involvement of the vessels of the leg and sparing of the femoral and iliac arteries. Some patients have intermittent claudication of the forearm or hand. Sensitivity to cold with paresthesias and the development of secondary Raynaud's phenomenon are common. Migratory superficial thrombophlebitis is manifested by the development of inflamed, tender, red segments of the superficial veins, which subside over a period of several weeks.

Physical examination discloses impaired arterial pulsations in the more distal portions of the limbs, such as the radial, ulnar, dorsalis pedis, and posterior tibial arteries. The more proximal arteries are normal, a finding that contrasts with arteriosclerosis obliterans. There may be cyanosis or pallor or persistent redness in the digits, and associated changes in temperature may be noted. Postural changes in color are also common. Gangrene or ulcerations of the digits may be present in both upper and lower extremities. Edema of the foot is common. Occasional patients have involvement of visceral arteries with stenosis or occlusion of mesenteric, coronary, cerebral, or renal arteries and manifestations of ischemia of these organs.

DIAGNOSIS. The diagnosis of thromboangiitis obliterans should be entertained when there is evidence of ischemia of the extremities from arterial occlusive disease in association with migratory superficial thrombophlebitis. The age and sex of the individual and the involvement of the upper extremities are additional helpful characteristics. Arteriography may be helpful in disclosing segmental multiple occlusions of the medium-sized and small arteries associated with collateral vessel visualization. The larger arteries are generally spared, a finding that also helps distinguish the disorder from arteriosclerosis obliterans. Final confirmation may be obtained only from biopsy material of an early lesion and histologic demonstration of the characteristic inflammatory and proliferative lesion of the disease.

PROGNOSIS. Thromboangiitis obliterans is not usually life threatening except in rare individuals in whom the visceral arteries are involved. The disease, however, results in disability and amputation of the extremities in a high percentage of cases. It is generally more rapidly progressive than arteriosclerosis obliterans, especially in individuals who refuse to stop smoking.

TREATMENT. Cessation of tobacco smoking is essential. Continuation of smoking results in a progressive course. If the patient stops smoking, new lesions do not develop or they develop more rarely. The approach to the patient with thromboangiitis obliterans is generally the same as that of patients with advanced arteriosclerosis obliterans. It consists of conservative measures, including protection from cold, local care in the event of ulceration or gangrene, and eventually amputation, if these lesions occur. Sympathectomy is tried frequently and may be effective, at least temporarily, if vasospasm is a prominent feature. Vasodilative drug therapy can be tried in cases of Raynaud's phenomenon with ulcerations, but its effectiveness is questionable.

Adar R, Papa MZ, Halpern Z, et al.: Cellular sensitivity to collagen in thromboangiitis obliterans. N Engl J Med 308:1113, 1983. *An important study showing high incidence of cellular sensitivity to collagen and the presence of circulating anticollagen antibodies in patients with thromboangiitis obliterans. The results have profound implications concerning the etiology of the disease and offer possible means of differentiating it from arteriosclerosis obliterans.*

McKusick VA, Harris WS, Ottesen OE, et al.: Buerger's disease: A distinct clinical and pathologic entity. JAMA 181:5, 1962. *A concise and thoughtful consideration of the clinical features, arteriographic findings, and histopathology of 30 cases with Buerger's disease.*

Sudden Arterial Occlusion

DEFINITION. Sudden arterial occlusion may result from obstruction of an artery of the extremity by embolism or by thrombosis in situ. The clinical manifestations are the result of the consequent ischemia.

ETIOLOGY. The major cause of sudden arterial occlusion is arterial embolism. The heart is the most frequent source of emboli in this syndrome. Emboli may arise from thrombi in the left atrium in the presence of atrial fibrillation or mitral valve disease, usually mitral stenosis. Emboli may also arise from mural thrombi from a myocardial infarction or in the presence of a cardiomyopathy. Septic emboli may arise from vegetations from the mitral or aortic valves in the presence of bacterial endocarditis. Less commonly, emboli may arise from an arteriosclerotic plaque in more proximal parts of the arterial tree or from aneurysms. In rare cases, the embolus may arise from the venous side and enter the arterial tree via a patent foramen ovale (paradoxical embolism). More rarely, the embolus consists of calcium fragments from a calcified valve leaflet, cholesterol crystals from an arteriosclerotic plaque, or foreign materials such as a bullet.

Sudden arterial thrombosis occurs in about 10 per cent of the cases of arteriosclerosis obliterans. The condition is rare in thromboangiitis obliterans or in polyarteritis nodosa. Acute arterial thrombosis may occur in conditions in which the coagulability of the blood is increased in the presence of normal vessels, such as in polycythemia vera or in cryoglobulinemia. Rarely, arterial thrombosis may occur in the presence of normal vessels in infections such as septicemia, pneumonia, peritonitis, tuberculosis, ulcerative colitis, and other debilitating diseases. Trauma from penetrating wounds, as from arterial puncture or catheterization, may cause arterial occlusion.

PATHOLOGY. The structure of emboli that arise from thrombi in the heart or from aneurysms is the same as that of the parent thrombi. Emboli lodge in an artery and obstruct the vessel. There may be extension of the thrombus distally by further clotting of the blood. The fate of the embolus varies. In some cases it may become organized and finally be recanalized, and in other cases it may become fragmented and the fragments may lodge in more distal vessels.

PATHOPHYSIOLOGY. The sudden arterial occlusion causes reduction of blood flow to the more distal portions of the limb and consequent ischemia. There have been suggestions that vasoactive agents released from the emboli, such as serotonin from platelets, may cause contraction of vascular smooth muscle in more distal portions of the vascular tree and result in vasospasm that further aggravates ischemia. The severity and extent of ischemia depend on the size of the vessel occluded and on the extent of collateral circulation. The larger the occluded vessel, the more likely it is that severe ischemia would result.

CLINICAL MANIFESTATIONS. Sudden arterial occlusion causes the abrupt onset of severe pain accompanied by manifestations of ischemia in about half the patients. In the remainder, the onset is gradual with either mild pain or numbness and paresthesias. Pain is present in about 75 per cent of the cases. There may be muscular weakness or outright paralysis. A saddle embolus of the aortic bifurcation causes abdominal pain, nausea, and vomiting and may result in a shocklike state.

Examination of the patient discloses diminished or absent pulses distal to the occlusion. Evidence of ischemia is present with low skin temperature and pallor or cyanosis or a combination of the two. If the occluded artery is superficial, the site of lodgment of the embolus may be identified as a tender region. The subsequent course depends on the adequacy of the collateral circulation. If this is adequate, gradual improvement occurs. Otherwise, gangrene supervenes.

DIAGNOSIS. The diagnosis of sudden arterial occlusion is usually relatively easy in the patient who has the acute onset of pain and ischemia of an extremity. If the cause is an embolus, its source may be evident. Rarely, patients with acute thrombophlebitis of the iliac and femoral veins may have feeble or absent arterial pulses and show manifestations resembling those of ischemia from an arterial embolus. In these cases, the demonstration of the feeble pulse and the presence of distended veins and pronounced edema help make the differentiation possible.

PROGNOSIS. The outcome of acute arterial obstruction depends on the size of the vessel affected, the age of the patient, the extent of the collateral circulation, and the timing of therapeutic intervention. When a large artery is occluded, the prognosis is poor without surgical treatment. In older patients with pre-existing arterial occlusive disease, the prognosis is poor because of obstruction of multiple vessels, including collateral vessels.

TREATMENT. The goal of therapeutic intervention is the removal or dissolution of the thrombus and re-establishment of patency of the occluded artery. This goal can be achieved by surgical embolectomy or by thrombolytic therapy. Urgent embolectomy is the preferred method of treatment when a large artery is occluded, such as with a saddle embolus of the bifurcation of the aorta. When smaller vessels are occluded and the thrombus is not easily accessible or when the patient's general condition does not permit surgical intervention, intravenous or intra-arterial streptokinase or urokinase may be given, if there are no contraindications for their use. Streptokinase is given intravenously as a bolus of 250,000 IU, followed by an infusion of 100,000 IU per hour. The infusion is continued for 72 hours. Intra-arterial administration can be used instead, in a dose of about one tenth of the intravenous dose; it can be coupled with angioplasty. Thrombolytic therapy is followed by conventional anticoagulants. The success rate of thrombolytic therapy is critically dependent on how early it is administered after the onset of symptoms. It is more effective for thrombotic lesions than embolic ones. Streptokinase or urokinase cannot be safely followed by surgery because of the danger of bleeding from the arteriotomy. The choice of therapy, therefore, must be carefully considered.

If neither therapeutic approach can be used, the patient should be treated conservatively. The patient should be placed at rest. The limb should be placed in a slightly dependent position under a cradle whose temperature is controlled at 30 to 35°C. Anticoagulation with heparin should be started as soon as possible to prevent extension of the thrombus and to prevent formation of additional emboli. If vasospasm is prominent, lumbar sympathectomy may be tried to reduce vasomotor tone and improve blood flow to the limb.

When a patient is treated by conservative medical measures, he or she should be followed closely for evidence of deterioration. If this occurs, immediate surgical intervention and embolectomy should be attempted. The results of embolectomy depend, to a large extent, on the timing of intervention. Therefore, surgery should not be delayed longer than a few hours. If therapy fails, gangrene may supervene, and amputation may become necessary.

Haimovici H: Peripheral arterial embolism. Angiology 1:20, 1950. *Detailed consideration of the clinical features of the arteries of the limbs based on study of 330 cases.*

Hargrove WC, Barker CF, Berkowitz HD, et al.: Treatment of acute peripheral arterial and graft thromboses with low-dose streptokinase. Surgery 92:981, 1982. *A report of good results from the use of intra-arterial streptokinase for the treatment of acute arterial thrombosis.*

Hinton RC, Kistler JP, Fallon JT, et al.: Influence of etiology of atrial fibrillation on incidence of systemic embolism. Am J Cardiol 40:509, 1977. *A study of the pathology of arterial embolism in 333 patients with atrial fibrillation. The paper emphasizes that the risk of embolism is independent of the cause of atrial fibrillation.*

VASCULAR DISEASES OF THE LIMBS CAUSED BY ABNORMAL COMMUNICATION BETWEEN ARTERIES AND VEINS

Arteriovenous Fistula

DEFINITION. Arteriovenous fistula is an abnormal direct communication between an artery and a vein.

ETIOLOGY. Arteriovenous fistulas in the limbs may be congenital or acquired. Congenital fistulas are usually multiple, acquired ones are usually single. The most common type is iatrogenic, created to carry out renal dialysis. Acquired arteriovenous fistulas may also result from trauma caused by penetrating wounds or surgical procedures.

PATHOPHYSIOLOGY. The low resistance of the direct communication between artery and vein results in a high arterial inflow into the vein, with a resultant increase in venous pressure. The elevated venous pressure causes engorgement of the vein and distention and may lead to the production of varicose veins. In the region of the fistula, blood flow is high, whereas more distal portions are deprived of capillary blood flow and may show ischemia and trophic changes.

Large fistulas cause a reduction in systemic vascular resistance and impose a burden on the heart because of the associated increase in cardiac output. Total blood volume may be increased. Left ventricular failure may eventually result.

PATHOLOGY. In the region of the fistula the veins become thickened, whereas the artery undergoes thinning and loss of elastic and muscular fibers in the media.

CLINICAL MANIFESTATIONS. The patient may be totally asymptomatic, and the discovery of the fistula may be accidental. In other cases, there may be pain in the location of the fistula, edema, varicosities, and asymmetry in the size of the limbs. In some cases, the presenting symptoms may be those of cardiac decompensation with dyspnea on exertion, palpitations, and orthopnea. Examination of the involved limb reveals tortuous, dilated, superficial veins and venous pulsation at the site of the fistula. The temperature of the skin may be high, and distal portions of the limb may show ischemic changes. A bruit or a thrill may be heard over the fistula during systole. At other times, a continuous bruit may be present. The extremity may be swollen, or the girth of the limb may be increased because of hypertrophy of the soft tissues. Temporary compression of the artery proximal to the fistula causes immediate increase in systemic vascular resistance and leads to reflex decrease in heart rate (Branham's sign), a change that may be helpful diagnostically.

DIAGNOSIS. When the fistula is superficial and large, the diagnosis can be made easily. If this is not possible from the physical examination, arteriography should be attempted for a definitive diagnosis. The oxygen saturation of the venous blood from the involved limb is higher than that of its contralateral part, and this comparison may be helpful in making the diagnosis.

TREATMENT. The treatment of choice is surgical intervention with closure of the fistula and re-establishment of the continuity of the involved artery and vein. If such restoration is not possible, ligation of the artery or vein or both may be necessary, but this may lead to arterial or venous insufficiency of the limb. In some cases, the fistula involves an anomalous artery. In this case, the ligation of the artery and the obstruction of the veins by the injection of sclerosing solutions may give a satisfactory result. It may not be practical to treat surgically patients with multiple fistulas. In these cases, conservative measures consisting of local care, relief of pain, and wearing elastic bandages may be helpful. If the fistula is inoperable and cardiac decompensation is present or threatened, amputation may be necessary.

Nickerson JL, Elkin DC, Warren JV: The effect of temporary occlusion of arteriovenous fistulas on heart rate, stroke volume, and cardiac output. J Clin Invest 30:215, 1951. *A classic study of the systemic hemodynamic effects of arteriovenous fistulas in a large number of patients.*

Rossi P, Carillo FJ, Alfidi RJ, et al.: Iatrogenic arteriovenous fistulas. Radiology 111:47, 1974. *A comprehensive review of 154 cases of iatrogenic arteriovenous fistulas. The paper provides a good review of the literature.*

Glomus Tumor (Glomangioma)

DEFINITION. Glomangioma, or glomus tumor, is a benign tumor of the glomus body.

PATHOLOGY. The glomus tumor is an encapsulated structure consisting of a hypertrophied arteriovenous anastomosis. The tumor varies in size from 0.5 to 2.5 cm in diameter. It can be found in various parts of the upper and lower extremities but is most frequently located in the nail beds.

CLINICAL MANIFESTATIONS. The most common symptom is severe burning pain in the location of the tumor. The pain may precede the appearance of the tumor. Pain may occur spontaneously, or it may be precipitated by exposure to heat or cold. Occasionally, the tumor is exquisitely sensitive to touch, and even the slightest pressure from contact with clothing may cause severe pain. Severe disability and atrophy of the limb from disuse may occur secondary to fear of pain. Examination of the involved area shows a reddish, purplish, or bluish mass that is sharply demarcated. At times, the tumor may not be easily visible or palpable. In this case, pressure with the head of a pin may help identify the location of the tumor. When it is located under the nail bed, the nail and the phalanx may be visibly deformed, thereby giving a clue to the location of the tumor.

TREATMENT. The glomus tumor is a benign tumor. Surgical excision results in complete relief without recurrence.

Cooke SAR: Misleading features in the clinical diagnosis of the peripheral glomus tumour. Br J Surg 58:602, 1971. *The clinical manifestations of glomus tumor are described based on the study of 24 cases.*

DISEASES OF THE VEINS OF THE LIMBS

Thrombophlebitis and Deep-Vein Thrombosis

DEFINITION. Thrombophlebitis refers to venous thrombosis with accompanying inflammation of the venous wall. For important practical reasons, superficial thrombophlebitis is distinguished from deep-vein thrombosis. Superficial thrombophlebitis does not cause embolic complications, but deep-vein thrombosis is a frequent cause of pulmonary embolism.

PATHOLOGY. Thrombi in veins consist mostly of red cells with a few platelets held together with fibrin. They propagate in the direction of the bloodstream by extension of the thrombotic process. They attach to the wall of the vein at one end, while the more proximal end floats freely into the lumen of the vessel. This is the portion that is commonly broken off and travels to the lungs. Varying degrees of inflammatory reaction of the venous wall may be present. Venous thrombosis may exist in the absence of inflammation, as is the case in some patients with malignancy. This is referred to as "phlebothrombosis." In most cases, however, inflammation and thrombosis coexist. The disorder may start as a pure thrombotic process, and inflammation usually occurs secondary to the presence of the thrombus.

INCIDENCE. Deep-vein thrombosis is a common disorder. It is more common in women than in men. All races seem to be affected equally, at least in civilized countries. The incidence of the disease increases with advancing age. The disease is very common in hospitalized patients. Approximately one third of the patients over age 40 who have undergone major surgery or have had an acute myocardial infarction develop deep-vein thrombosis. The incidence is even higher after certain operations such as repair of hip fractures or prostatectomy. Patients with thrombotic strokes have an equally high incidence of deep-vein thrombosis. This occurs almost exclusively in the paralyzed limb.

Superficial thrombophlebitis occurs most commonly in patients with varicose veins, possibly as a result of minor trauma. It is also frequent after pregnancy. A migratory type of superficial thrombophlebitis also occurs in patients with thromboangiitis obliterans.

PATHOGENESIS. Venous stasis, injury to the venous wall, and a hypercoagulable state are the three main factors that lead to venous thrombosis. In most cases, more than one of these factors are present, and their effect may be cumulative. The combination of venous stasis and changes in the clotting mechanism of the blood accounts for the increased incidence of deep-vein thrombosis in pregnancy and during administration of oral contraceptives. Venous stasis is the major factor in the development of venous thrombosis in patients with heart disease, in paralyzed patients, in patients undergoing major surgery, in those who have varicose veins, and in healthy individuals after long trips. Increased viscosity, leading to stasis, and alterations in the clotting factors of the blood account for the high incidence of polycythemia vera. Patients with familial deficiencies of certain anticlotting factors are susceptible to recurrent thrombophlebitis. These include deficiencies of antithrombin III, protein S, protein C, and heparin cofactor II. Injury to the venous wall may result from administration of certain vasoconstrictive or chemotherapeutic agents, or it may result from infectious agents. Patients with malignancies may have migrating thrombophlebitis, which has been attributed to low-grade activation of intravascular coagulation.

CLINICAL MANIFESTATIONS. The presence of superficial thrombophlebitis is usually easily ascertained by finding the inflamed vein. This may be apparent as a red, tender cord. By contrast, deep-vein thrombosis frequently causes few distinctive clinical features, about one half of patients with deep-vein thrombosis are asymptomatic. The first manifestation of deep-vein thrombosis may be the occurrence of pulmonary embolism. Pain in the region of the thrombosed veins at rest or only during exercise and edema distal to the obstructed veins are the usual symptoms of deep-vein thrombosis. Examination of the patient may disclose several helpful manifestations. Edema or pitting of the malleolar fossa may be present and may cause loss of the normal concavity of that portion of the leg. There may be a difference between the two legs in the circumference of the calf. A difference in maximal circumference in excess of 1.4 cm in men and 1.2 cm in women is highly suspicious. The temperature of the skin may be increased as a result of the inflammatory reaction, and palpation may disclose the thrombosed veins in the calf or in the popliteal fossa. There may be tenderness to palpation. Increased resistance or pain on voluntary dorsiflexion of the foot (Homans' sign) may be present. A useful sign is the presence of tenderness on inflation of a blood pressure cuff around the calf. Most normal individuals tolerate this without pain up to pressures of 160 to 180 mm Hg.

Thrombosis of the iliac and femoral veins usually presents with a characteristic clinical picture consisting of rapidly advancing swelling of the entire limb. The thrombosed vein may be tender if it extends below the inguinal ligament. Collateral distended veins may be present in the upper thigh. In some cases, secondary ischemia may occur as a result of the very high venous pressure that impedes arterial inflow. Cyanosis of the toes and even gangrene may occur under these circumstances.

Thrombosis of the subclavian vein may result in swelling of the upper extremity, and collateral veins may be present. In axillary thrombosis, a similar clinical picture occurs; the thrombosed vein may be felt in the axilla. A history of walking on crutches or sleeping in a sitting position on a bench with the arms behind the backrest may be helpful. Thrombosis of the superior vena cava causes increased venous pressure in the neck and face with distention of the neck veins in the upper part of the chest.

In septic thrombophlebitis, there may also be systemic manifestations of infection, such as fever, chills, and leukocytosis. In cases in which septic phlebitis begins from infected needles or catheters, an inflamed, tender cord may appear at the site of the venipuncture.

DIAGNOSIS. Ileofemoral thrombophlebitis is usually easily recognized by the rapid swelling of the entire limb, engorged collateral veins in the thigh, and signs of inflammation, such as increased skin temperature.

By contrast, in the majority of cases of deep-vein thrombosis involving the calf, popliteal area, and thigh, the clinical picture is not sufficiently distinctive to allow diagnosis with a high degree of confidence. Confirmation of the diagnosis must be provided by resorting to one or more of a number of diagnostic tests. The most commonly employed tests are the following:

X-ray Venography. Venography is one of the most accurate means of making the diagnosis of deep-vein thrombosis. The test involves the injection of a contrast medium into the venous system, which has been previously emptied of blood by gravity. The test relies on finding a filling defect or a sharp cutoff, indicating the presence of occluding thrombus in the vein. The test may result in inflammatory reaction followed by thrombosis in a few cases. It is sensitive and highly specific, for these reasons, venography is considered the "gold standard" in the diagnosis of deep-vein thrombosis.

Radionuclide Venography. This test is similar to x-ray venography except that instead of contrast medium, a radioisotope, such as ^{99m}Tc-macroaggregated albumin, is injected in a foot vein. External scanning detects venous obstruction and the presence of collateral circulation. In another variation of the technique, ^{99m}Tc-labeled red cells from the patient's own blood are injected intravenously, and a blood pool scan is obtained. The sensitivity and specificity of the technique are somewhat less than those of x-ray venography. The technique is probably better in detecting venous thrombosis in the thigh than in the calf.

Radioisotope-labeled Fibrinogen. This test consists of intravenous administration of fibrinogen labeled with ^{125}I and the subsequent incorporation of the radioactive material into the thrombus. The accumulation of radioactivity is detected by external counting. This test detects an active thrombophlebitis, it may be negative in cases in which the active process has stopped but thrombi exist in the veins. The reliability of the test depends on the location of the thrombus. It is of little use in detecting pelvic thrombi because of the high background due to the bladder and iliac arteries. It is most useful in detecting thrombosis of the calf. Another disadvantage is that it requires one or two days for a sufficient number of counts to build into the thrombosed vein for detection. This test is, therefore, most useful in longitudinal screening of high-risk populations.

Liquid Crystal Thermography. This test relies on the detection of small increases in skin temperature as a result of the venous inflammation. The test is easy to perform. It has high sensitivity but relatively low specificity. It can be a useful adjunct to ultrasonography or impedance plethysmography for monitoring patients at risk.

Ultrasonography. This test utilizes the Doppler principle to detect venous obstruction. Thus, during various maneuvers that alter venous flow, such as deep inspiration, Valsalva's maneuver, or leg compression, the ultrasonogram may detect the presence of obstructed veins. The disadvantages of the technique are that a high degree of stenosis is necessary for the test result to be abnormal and that it does not distinguish between occlusion from external pressure and occlusion by thrombus. Also, the result may be negative if an effective collateral circulation has developed. The test is most sensitive for thrombosis of the veins above the knee.

Impedance Plethysmography. This test detects alterations in blood volume of the extremities by detecting changes in the electrical impedance of the tissues. The test is carried out during respiratory maneuvers or during alterations in blood flow by occluding the limb with a pneumatic pressure cuff. Like ultrasonography, this test requires significant proximal obstruction for positive results. The reported sensitivity and specificity of the last two tests are high (over 90 per cent).

Choice of Tests. The choice of tests to be performed depends to a large extent on their availability. If all are available, it is preferable to use first ultrasonography and impedance plethysmography and resort to venography only if the results of these are inconclusive. The radioactive fibrinogen test and thermography should be reserved for screening of patients at high risk.

DIFFERENTIAL DIAGNOSIS. A number of conditions that cause localized pain or edema in the lower extremities may be confused with deep-vein thrombosis. A ruptured popliteal synovial membrane or cyst (Baker's cyst) may simulate most of the manifestations of venous thrombosis. The diagnosis can be suspected if there is a history or physical findings of arthritis of the knee joint. The diagnosis may be confirmed by an arthrogram revealing the entry of dye from the joint into the calf muscles. Rupture of the calf muscles may cause pain, tenderness, and edema and may simulate thrombophlebitis. The diagnosis can be made from the history of strenuous or unusual exercise, the presence of ecchymosis from extravasated blood, and the palpation of a hematoma. Sometimes the patient reports an audible snap during the activity when the pain first occurred. The differential diagnosis is important because anticoagulants are contraindicated in this condition. A severe muscle cramp may cause pain and swelling for a considerable period of time. Other manifestations of thrombophlebitis are, however, lacking in this situation. The pain of a lumbar disc may be localized in the calf. There are no other manifestations of venous thrombosis, however, and there may be neurologic findings to identify the cause of the pain. Lymphedema is recognized by its slower and gradual onset and the absence of signs of inflammation and of collateral veins. Finally, cellulitis may be confused with superficial thrombophlebitis.

COMPLICATIONS. Pulmonary embolism is a frequent and serious complication of deep-vein thrombosis. About 80 to 90 per cent of pulmonary emboli arise in the deep veins of the lower limbs. Although deep-vein thrombosis may begin frequently in the veins of the calf, it is only when the thrombosis extends above the knee that serious pulmonary embolism occurs.

About 5 per cent of patients with deep-vein thrombosis develop venous insufficiency with stasis dermatitis (postphlebitic syndrome). This is more likely to occur in those with more proximal venous obstruction. A rare complication of iliofemoral thrombophlebitis is venous claudication, in which the patient develops pain on exercise which is relieved by rest, as in arterial occlusive disease.

PROPHYLAXIS. Prophylactic therapy against deep-vein thrombosis should be attempted in high-risk patients (Table 57–4). The exact regimen used must take into consideration the risk of deep-vein thrombosis and consequent pulmonary embolism and the potential risk of hemorrhagic complications from the prophylactic therapy. Low-dose heparin is currently the most commonly used prophylactic technique. For surgical patients, this consists of administration of 5000 units of heparin subcutaneously 2 hours before surgery and then every 8 or 12 hours until the patient is ambulatory. This method is effective in reducing the incidence of deep-vein thrombosis and pulmonary embolism in patients subjected to a variety of surgical procedures. It is also effective in reducing the incidence of deep-vein thrombosis in patients following acute myocardial infarction, but it is not known whether there is also a reduction in the incidence of pulmonary embolism. Low-dose heparin has been shown to be ineffective in patients undergoing surgery for hip fracture and hip replacement, and its effectiveness has not been established in urologic procedures. Higher dose heparin adjusted to give an activated partial thromboplastin time (APTT) in the upper limits of the therapeutic range has been reported to be more effective than low-dose heparin. In addition, the administration of dihydroergotamine mesylate, 0.5 mg subcutaneously, together with low-dose heprin, is more effective in preventing deep-vein thrombosis than heparin alone in surgical patients. Warfarin and other similar drugs are also effective in protecting patients from thromboembolism during a variety of surgical techniques. Low molecular weight dextran given on the day of surgery and at suitable intervals thereafter has been reported in most cases to give favorable results. There is a risk of fluid overload, and, to a lesser extent, hemorrhagic complications. This method can be used in instances in which there is a high risk of bleeding from anticoagulants. Drugs that interfere with platelet aggregation, such as aspirin and other nonsteroidal anti-inflammatory agents, have not been

TABLE 57–4. PREVENTION OF VENOUS THROMBOEMBOLISM

Representative Patient Groups	1. Medical patients without predisposing factors on short bed rest 2. Young patients without predisposing factors undergoing brief (<1 hr) general surgical procedure	1. Medical patients with predisposing factors or on prolonged bed rest 2. Middle-aged or old patients without predisposing factors undergoing general surgical procedure longer than 1 hr	1. Patients with hip fracture 2. Patients undergoing extensive orthopedic or pelvic surgery 3. Middle-aged or old patients with predisposing factors or with previous venous thrombosis undergoing general surgical procedure longer than 1 hr
Approximate Incidence of Venous Thrombosis	5%	20–40%	50–70%
Approximate Incidence of Pulmonary Embolism	Almost zero	5%	10%
Suggested Prophylaxis	None	Low-dose heparin or intermittent pneumatic compression	Warfarin, low-dose heparin plus either intermittent pneumatic compression or dihydroergotamine; or higher dose heparin

shown convincingly to be effective as prophylactic agents. In patients in whom anticoagulation is contraindicated, such as patients with neurosurgical procedures, it is prudent to use conservative means of prophylaxis. These include early ambulation, elastic stockings, and external periodic calf compression. The external compression devices have been reported to be effective. There are no risks associated with their use; the only negative aspect is low patient acceptance during prolonged use, because they are uncomfortable or cumbersome.

TREATMENT. Antocoagulation is not necessary for the treatment of superficial thrombophlebitis. Local measures, sometimes coupled with administration of anti-inflammatory drugs, such as indomethacin, suffice to bring about healing and relief of symptoms.

Full anticoagulation is the preferred treatment for deep-vein thrombosis. Heparin is preferred for initiation of treatment because of its immediate action, whereas warfarin-type drugs may not become fully effective for a considerable period of time. Heparin inhibits coagulation by binding and activating antithrombin III, an inhibitor of activated factor X. Heparin is best administered by constant infusion. Initially a bolus of 5000 units is given intravenously, followed by constant infusion of 750 to 1000 units per hour. The dose is adjusted by monitoring the APTT so that a level about two times the normal control is achieved. APTT is checked four to six hours after the initial bolus and once a day thereafter. An alternative method is intermittent intravenous administration of 5,000 to 10,000 units every four to six hours. If no suitable veins are found, heparin may be administered subcutaneously in a dose of 15,000 to 30,000 units every 12 hours. After five days of heparin therapy, oral warfarin at a dose of 10 to 15 mg daily is given until the one-stage prothrombin time (PT) is one and one half to two times the normal level. Subsequently, a daily maintenance dose is administered to maintain the PT at the desired level. Warfarin brings about anticoagulation by decreasing the level of factors II, VII, IX, and X. Many drugs interact with warfarin. Some of them potentiate its action and others inhibit it. If the patient requires other drug therapy while on warfarin, each drug should be carefully screened for potential interaction. If bleeding occurs in the course of heparin therapy, its effect can be counteracted by administration of 1 mg of protamine per 100 units of heparin. If bleeding develops in the course of warfarin treatment, the patient should receive vitamin K_1 intramuscularly to reduce PT to the therapeutic range (0.25 to 1.0 mg usually suffices). If bleeding is serious, blood or fresh frozen plasma may be necessary.

Thrombolysis with fibrinolytic agents, such as streptokinase or urokinase, administered intravenously in patients with deep-vein thrombosis has been shown to achieve more complete dissolution of the thrombus and better preservation of the venous architecture than conventional anticoagulants. These drugs act by causing activation of plasminogen to plasmin, thereby causing dissolution of the thrombus. Steptokinase is administered intravenously as an initial bolus of 250,000 to 500,000 IU, followed by an infusion of 100,000 IU per hour for 24 to 72 hours. The effectiveness of the drug diminishes after the first 24 hours. Urokinase is less likely to cause anaphylactic reactions, but it is more expensive. It is given in a dose of 4400 IU per kilogram as a bolus, followed by an infusion of 4400 IU per kilogram per hour for the same duration as streptokinase. Thrombolytic therapy is the preferred method of treatment of patients with iliofemoral or subclavian-axillary vein thrombosis. In patients with more distal deep-vein thrombosis, the high effectiveness of heparin and its lower rate of hemorrhagic complictions render this the preferred method of treatment.

In patients in whom anticoagulation is contraindicated, simple measures—elevation of the extremity and local heat—should be used. When the risk of pulmonary embolism is low, as is the case of deep-vein thrombosis limited to the calf, these measures suffice. In patients with deep-vein thrombosis extending above the knee, in whom the risk of pulmonary embolism is high, implantation of an inferior vena caval filter or ligation of the inferior vena cava may also be considered. This form of therapy should also be used when anticoagulation needs to be terminated because of complications, when recurrent thromboembolism occurs in the presence of adequate anticoagulation, and when septic thromboembolic disease not controlled by antibiotics is present.

Bed rest should be continued until local signs of inflammation, including tenderness and edema, subside. After 7 to 15 days the patient is allowed to walk wearing elastic stockings. If no discomfort occurs, resumption of full activity is allowed one to two weeks later. Anticoagulation for three months is usually sufficient to prevent recurrence of deep-vein thrombosis.

Coon, WW: Epidemiology of venous thromboembolism. Ann Surg 186:149, 1977. *A detailed, well-referenced consideration of the epidemiology of venous thrombosis.*

Moser KM, Fedullo PF: Venous thromboembolism, three simple decisions (part 1). Chest 83:117, 1983. *A practical, well-reasoned approach to the prophylaxis and treatment for venous thrombosis is presented.*

Mudge M, Hughes LE: The long term sequelae of deep vein thrombosis. J Surg 65:692, 1978. *A report of long-term follow-up of patients who had evidence of venous thrombosis after surgery. The sequelae of venous thrombosis are described.*

The Multicenter Trial Committee: Dihydroergotamine-heparin prophylaxis of postoperative deep-vein thrombosis. JAMA 251:2960, 1984. *A multicenter investigation showing that the combination of dihydroergotamine and heparin is superior in preventing deep vein thrombosis in surgical patients to heparin or dihydroergotamine alone.*

Painter TD: Thrombophlebitis: Diagnostic techniques. Angiology 31:386, 1980. *Comprehensive consideration of the diagnostic techniques for venous thrombosis.*

Shafer KE, Jaffe AS: Thrombolytic therapy: Current and potential uses. Drug Ther 13:95, 1983. *A concise consideration of the uses of thrombolytic agents.*

Sharma GVRK, Cella G, Parisi AF, et al.: Thrombolytic therapy. N Engl J Med 306:1268, 1982. *Detailed consideration of the use of streptokinase and urokinase in vascular thrombosis.*

Wessler S, Gitel SN: Low-dose heparin: Is the risk worth the benefit? Am Heart J 98:94, 1979. *A review of the use of low-dose heparin for prophylaxis against venous thrombosis.*

Wessler S, Gitel SN: Warfarin: From bedside to bench. New Engl J Med 311:645, 1984. *A concise consideration of the mechanism of action and clinical uses of warfarin in thrombotic disease.*

Varicose Veins

DEFINITION. Varicose veins are prominent, abnormally distended, and tortuous veins.

INCIDENCE. Approximately 20 per cent of adults develop varicose veins. A familial history is present in 15 per cent of patients. They are more common in women than in men by a factor of 5 to 1. Most women date the onset of varicose veins from the time of pregnancy. The veins of the lower extremities are most frequently affected because of the effects of gravity on venous pressure.

ETIOLOGY. Congenitally absent or defective valves are a recognized cause of varicose veins in early life. Varicose veins may develop secondary to sustained elevations of venous pressure from obstruction of the veins. The cause of the obstruction may be thrombosis secondary to thrombophlebitis or external pressure, as is the case in pregnancy, ascites, and tumors. However, in most affected individuals, no clearly identifiable cause or precipitating factor can be found. The possibility of a genetically determined structural defect in the venous wall has been suggested. Individuals with varicose veins in the lower extremities have been found to have increased venous distensibility and reduced amounts of collagen and hexosamine in the wall of unaffected veins. In the face of such a generalized defect, a sustained elevation in venous pressure from the effects of gravity in the lower extremities or from other factors may lead to stretching of the walls and, finally, to incompetence of the valves and overdistention of the veins. An association of varicose veins with hemorrhoids and diverticulosis of the bowel suggests the possibility that increased intra-abdominal pressure during bowel movements may play a role in their pathogenesis.

CLINICAL MANIFESTATIONS. Most patients are asymptomatic, especially in the early stages of the disease. They may seek attention because the dilated, tortuous varicosities are cosmetically unappealing. In some cases, aching in the lower extremities and edema, especially after prolonged standing or exercise, may be present. The edema usually subsides overnight. When the communicating veins are incompetent, symptoms are more common. Prolonged venous insufficiency leads to the postphlebitic syndrome, with sustained edema, induration, and fibrosis. Eventually, trophic changes with brownish discoloration of the skin and ulceration may result. Ulcers usually occur above the medial malleolus. An incompetent communicating vein may be identified in the vicinity of the ulcer. The arterial pulses are normal, and no evidence of ischemia is present.

DIAGNOSIS. Clinical inspection suffices to make the diagnosis. The Trendelenburg test can identify the presence of defective valves and incompetent communicating veins. With the patient recumbent, the leg is elevated to empty the veins, and a tourniquet is then applied to occlude the superficial veins. The patient is instructed to resume the erect position, and the tourniquet is released. If the venous valves are incompetent, the veins immediately become distended as a result of the back flow. If two tourniquets are applied, the distention of the veins in the intervening portion of the limb identifies the presence of incompetent communicating veins. The patency of the deep venous system can be examined by venography. It is prudent to exclude other causes of edema, such as congestive heart failure and renal disease.

PROGNOSIS. The prognosis of uncomplicated superficial varicose veins is excellent. The postphlebitic syndrome, once established, is usually progressive and resistant to treatment.

TREATMENT. Simple measures usually suffice to treat uncomplicated varicose veins. These consist of frequent periods of rest with elevation of the limbs, external pressure with elastic stockings or bandages, and avoidance of obstruction of the veins by garments, such as girdles. In more severe or advanced cases, ligation and stripping of the saphenous veins or injection of sclerosing solutions may become necessary to prevent the postphlebitis syndrome. An injection/compression technique in which the sclerosing solution is injected into a vein emptied of blood, followed by compression by external pressure, is simple, cheap, and effective. It is widely used in Europe. When stasis ulcers are present, local care with warm, wet dressings is necessary. If infection is present, local and systemic antibiotics may be administered. If considerable fibrosis is present, it may be necessary to excise the entire area and carry out skin grafting to eliminate ulceration.

Beresford SSA, Chant ADB, Jones HO, et al.: Varicose veins: A comparison of surgery and injection/compression sclerotherapy Lancet 1:921, 1978. *A five-year follow-up comparing the effects of surgery and injection/compression sclerotherapy for varicose veins.*

Hobbs JT: The Treatment of Venous Disorders: A Comprehensive Review of Current Practice in the Management of Varicose Veins and Post-thrombotic Syndrome. Philadelphia, J. B. Lippincott Company, 1977. *A well-written, comprehensive consideration of the clinical features, diagnosis, and treatment of varicose veins and post-thrombotic syndromes.*

DISEASES OF THE LYMPHATIC VESSELS OF THE LIMBS

Lymphangitis

DEFINITION. Lymphangitis is an inflammation of the lymphatic vessels. It is usually of bacterial origin.

ETIOLOGY. In most cases the responsible infective agent is the hemolytic streptococcus or *Staphylococcus aureus*, coagulase-positive. The bacteria gain access to the lymphatics via local trauma or from ulcerations. In many instances no identifiable portal of entry can be found. Infection spreads from the lymphatics to the regional lymph nodes.

PATHOLOGY. Various stages of inflammation are found in the subcutaneous tissue and regional lymph nodes.

CLINICAL MANIFESTATIONS. The local manifestation of lymphangitis consists of a red streak that appears at the site of initial entry of the infective organism and extends to the regional lymph nodes. The latter are swollen and tender. There may be a surrounding area of cellulitis. Systemic accompaniments of infection may constitute the presenting manifestations.

DIAGNOSIS. The local manifestations of lymphangitis and the accompanying system reaction are usually sufficient to make the diagnosis. Leukocytosis with predominance of polymorphonuclear leukocytes may be present. Confirmation is obtained by culturing the organism from the portal of entry or from the subcutaneous tissues. Acute lymphangitis may be difficult to distinguish from a generalized cellulitis or from thrombophlebitis.

PROGNOSIS. With treatment the prognosis is good when one is dealing with an initial attack in an otherwise normal limb. In the case of recurrent attacks, lymphedema may develop and residual increase in the girth of the limb may occur.

TREATMENT. This consists of systemic administration of the appropriate antibiotics. In addition, surgical drainage of the focus of infection is important. Supportive measures, including rest and elevation of the infected limb and local warm, wet dressings, are also helpful. The use of elastic support hose may be necessary for a period of several weeks to prevent lymphedema. In recurrent cases, the causes of secondary lymphedema should be sought.

Schinger A, Martin WJ, Spittell JA: Acute lymphangitis and cellulitis. Minn Med 48:191, 1965. *Concise consideration of the clinical features, diagnosis, and treatment of lymphangitis.*

Lymphedema

DEFINITION. Lymphedema refers to edema from accumulation of lymph secondary to obstruction to its flow.

ETIOLOGY AND INCIDENCE. Lymphedema can be primary or secondary. The most frequent type of primary lymphedema is simple congenital lymphedema, which is not familial and is present at birth. A congenital familial form (Milroy's disease) is inherited as an autosomal dominant trait. Another hereditary form is associated with Noonan's syndrome in about 15 per cent of cases. Lymphedema praecox becomes manifest in puberty and is associated with congenital hypoplasia of the lymphatics. A late form may become manifest in middle age.

Primary lymphedema is more common in women. Most cases are manifest at birth or become apparent before age 40. A syndrome characterized by yellow nails, recurrent pleural effusion, and lymphedema is believed to be secondary to multiple lymphatic abnormalities in the areas involved. A familial syndrome consisting of recurrent intrahepatic cholestasis and lymphedema is probably due to defective hepatic lymphatic vessels as well as those in the extremity.

Secondary lymphedema results most commonly from trauma. It commonly results from surgical removal of lymph nodes and from fibrosis secondary to radiation following surgery for cancer. Lymphoma or metastatic carcinoma involving the lymph nodes may also cause obstruction to the flow of lymph and lymphedema. Filarial infection in the tropics is a cause of secondary lymphedema.

PATHOLOGY. In cases of congenital lymphedema there is absence or hypoplasia of the lymphatic vessels. In secondary lymphedema there are numerous small, irregular lymphatics, together with tortuous and sometimes greatly enlarged varicose lymphatic vessels.

CLINICAL MANIFESTATIONS. Typically, lymphedema begins gradually with an enlargement of the involved limb without other manifestations. The swollen extremity is soft and pitting. The edema subsides at night. With time, the skin becomes thickened and cannot be raised into a fold, and the edema becomes more persistent. The lower extremities are involved most often. In about half the patients the edema is unilateral. Superimposed lymphangitis and cellulitis may occur, and in longstanding cases lymphangiosarcoma may develop.

DIAGNOSIS. The diagnosis of lymphedema may be confirmed with a radioisotope lymphogram. ^{99m}Tc-labeled rhenium sulfur colloid or ^{99m}Tc-labeled antimony trisulfide colloid is injected in the web spaces of the foot. The ilioinguinal region is scanned 30 and 60 minutes later. In lymphedema, the uptake of isotope by the lymph nodes is reduced, whereas in edema due to venous obstruction it is greater than normal owing to increased lymph flow. The precise diagnosis of the type of lymphedema is made by lymphangiography. Contrast medium is injected directly into a lymphatic vessel in the foot, or a water-soluble contrast agent is injected intracutaneously and taken up by the lymphatics. By this technique, a distinction can be made between absence or hypoplasia of the lymphatic vessels on one hand, which characterizes congenital lymphedema, and the hyperplasia and numerous small lymphatics, which characterize secondary lymphedema, on the other.

PROGNOSIS. Primary lymphedema is usually a slowly progressive disorder, not easily amenable to treatment. The prognosis of secondary lymphedema depends on the cause. In cases in which it results from infection, it can be effectively managed by treatment with antibiotics.

TREATMENT. In primary lymphedema this is aimed at keeping the limb as free of edema as possible to prevent fibrosis and secondary infection. Frequent elevation of the limb, the use of elastic stockings, and the administration of diuretics may be useful. In cases not controlled by these simple measures, benzopyrones have been reported to be useful. These drugs break down protein by activating macrophages; hence, they reduce viscosity and facilitate the flow of lymph. Surgery may be tried in advanced cases to remove subcutaneous tissue and to induce new lymph vessel formation. Anastomosis of small lymphatic vessels with veins by microsurgery has been reported to give good results in some cases.

Allen EV, Ghormley RK: Lymphedema of the extremities: Etiology, classification and treatment; report of 300 cases. Ann Intern Med 9:516, 1935. *Comprehensive consideration of the clinical features of primary and secondary lymphedema in a large series of cases.*

Browse NL: The diagnosis and management of primary lymphedema. J Vasc Surg 3:181, 1986. *A concise account of the diagnosis and management of primary lymphedema.*

Browse NL, Stewart G: Lymphoedema: Pathophysiology and classification. J Cardiovasc Surg 26:91, 1985. *An up-to-date description of the pathophysiology and classification of lymphedema.*

Partsch H, Wenzel-Hora BI, Urbanek A: Differential diagnosis of lymphedema after indirect lymphography with iotasul. Lymphology 16:12, 1983. *Description of the usefulness of indirect lymphangiography using a water-soluble contrast medium for the differential diagnosis of lymphedema.*

Pillar NB: Lymphoedema, macrophages and benzopyrones. Lymphology 13:109, 1980. *Discussion of the role of macrophages in lymphedema. The effectiveness of benzopyrones in this disease is ascribed to activation of macrophages.*

PART VII
RESPIRATORY DISEASES

58 INTRODUCTION

John F. Murray

Respiration includes all the processes that contribute to O_2 uptake and CO_2 elimination. The lungs are the major organs of gas exchange, but the nose, oropharynx, extrapulmonary airways, brain, spinal cord, nerves, thoracic cage, respiratory muscles, lymph nodes and vessels, and cardiovascular system are also involved. Thus respiratory diseases, literally interpreted, include a large variety of abnormalities arising in all the different structures concerned with gas exchange. In general, a more limited definition applies, and respiratory diseases are considered to include disturbances of the air passages, lungs, pleura, chest wall, muscles of respiration, and mediastinum (excluding the heart, systemic vessels, and esophagus).

Acute respiratory diseases are probably the most common afflictions of humankind and are responsible for more absences from school and work than any other type of illness. Chronic respiratory diseases, particularly emphysema and bronchitis, are second only to cardiovascular diseases as causes of disability payments. Cancer of the lung kills more persons each year than any other kind of malignancy. Because of the remarkable incidence of these and other respiratory diseases, it is important that all physicians, not just internists and chest specialists, be well versed in the clinical manifestations and methods of diagnosis, treatment, and prevention of the most common disorders. The material concerned with respiratory diseases here and elsewhere in the book is intended as a primer of necessary knowledge with which to recognize and to treat the major respiratory diseases; additional information is available in the references cited at the end of each chapter.

Patients with respiratory disease often seek medical attention because they have at least one of three cardinal manifestations: *cough* (including its derivative hemoptysis), *chest pain*, and *dyspnea*. These are nonspecific and sometimes trivial abnormalities, but the frequency with which they are associated with serious underlying thoracic disease means that the complaints must always be considered carefully and often become the focus of diagnostic evaluations. Because of the clinical importance of cough, chest pain, and dyspnea, the mechanisms, special features, and diagnostic approach to each symptom are briefly reviewed in the following pages. Further information can be found under the headings of the specific diseases in which the sensations occur.

COUGH

Healthy persons seldom cough, their scant bronchial secretions, although constantly being produced, are imperceptibly carried up the tracheobronchial system by the action of cilia and, after reaching the pharynx, swallowed. Coughing is an essential defense mechanism that protects the airways from the adverse effects of inhaled noxious substances and also serves to clear them of retained secretions. Patients recognize that coughing indicates an abnormality, and this symptom is the second most common reason given for seeking medical advice.

MECHANISM. Coughing may be produced voluntarily, but more often it results from reflex stimulation. Extrathoracic cough receptors are located in the nose, oropharynx, larynx, and upper trachea. Intrathoracic rapidly adapting irritant receptors, which cause cough, are located in the epithelium of the lower trachea and large central bronchi, which are the air passages from which coughing is effective in clearing secretions or removing foreign material. Depending on which cough receptors are activated, afferent stimuli travel to the brain via the trigeminal, glossopharyngeal, superior laryngeal, or vagus nerves. Efferent pathways include the recurrent laryngeal nerves, to cause closure of the glottis, and the corticospinal tract and peripheral nerves, to cause contraction of the thoracic and abdominal musculature. The cough reflex begins with a deep breath followed by glottic closure, relaxation of the diaphragm, and contraction of the expiratory muscles. Collectively, these acts generate a positive pressure of 100 to 300 mm Hg within the thorax, which is suddenly released when the glottis opens. During cough, the *volume*-rate of flow out of the lungs (liters per second) is only slightly greater than or the same as it is during a forced expiratory maneuver, a fact that is not always appreciated. However, because the positive pressure in the pleural space is higher than the luminal pressure in the trachea and central bronchi, a pressure difference is created that causes the posterior membranous portion of the airway walls to fold inward and nearly to obliterate the lumen. By this means, the *linear* velocity of airflow through the narrowed channels (centimeters per second) is markedly increased, and a shearing force is created that dislodges secretions and particles from the mucosal surface.

PRODUCTIVE COUGH. The daily quantity of bronchial secretions produced by a normal person is not known, but it is sufficiently small to be removed by mucociliary action alone, and coughing and expectoration are not required. Secretions can accumulate in the tracheobronchial system in the presence of one or more of the following abnormalities: excessive production, altered physical properties, and deficient clearance. Thus, productive cough, which clears retained secretions from the airways, is an important defense mechanism and one of the hallmarks of acute and chronic inflammatory conditions of the lungs and airways. Patients who are unconscious, intubated, or for other reasons cannot cough must have their tracheobronchial secretions removed by suctioning to prevent the complications of atelectasis and/or bronchopulmonary infection.

NONPRODUCTIVE COUGH. In addition to the cough that serves an expectoration function, another type of cough—an irritative phenomenon—is encountered frequently. The stimulus may be mechanical, chemical, thermal, or inflammatory, including reactions from infection. There is increasing evidence that alteration of the surface epithelium of the major airways, into which the terminal filaments of irritant receptors are inserted, exposes the receptors more directly or somehow sensitizes them to the effects of stimulants; the cough reflex thus becomes hyper-reactive, and coughing occurs in response to ordinarily innocuous stimuli. When the causes of chronic cough are analyzed, asthma often heads the list. Indeed, chronic nonproductive cough, especially at night, may be the sole presenting complaint of patients who subsequently prove to have bronchial asthma.

COMPLICATIONS. Coughing seems to provoke more coughing. Paroxysms of coughing, as in pertussis, may terminate in vomiting, which seems to break the cycle. Paroxysmal attacks may also terminate in syncope. The mechanism of *cough syncope* is uncertain, but the effects of increased intrathoracic pressure on venous return, cardiac output, and blood flow to the brain are believed to play a role. At times, severe coughing attacks have continued to the point of utter exhaustion. The muscular force developed during coughing may be sufficient to cause occasional fractures of ribs *(cough fractures)* and even compression fractures of vertebral bodies.

DIAGNOSTIC APPROACH. It is difficult to generalize about a condition as common but as varied as coughing. Obviously, many episodes of coughing are innocent and transient. The essential first step in evaluating a patient complaining of cough is to obtain a thorough history with particular attention to the following aspects: (1) acute or chronic, (2) productive or nonproductive, (3) character, (4) time relationships, (5) type and quantity of sputum, and (6) associated features. A specific diagnosis of the cause of chronic intractable cough can be made by history alone in the majority (80 per cent) of patients.

An acute cough is usually associated with viral laryngotracheobronchitis but may signify other bronchopulmonary infections. Less commonly, acute episodes of coughing may be the chief manifestation of the inhalation of various immunologic or irritative substances. A chronic cough is the diagnostic hallmark of chronic bronchitis but also occurs in asthma, tuberculosis, bronchiectasis, and bronchogenic carcinoma. The frequency with which chronic bronchitis and bronchogenic carcinoma coexist, both being a complication of cigarette smoking, has led to the important axiom that *any change in the character or pattern of a chronic cough warrants immediate diagnostic evaluation, with special attention directed toward the detection of bronchogenic carcinoma.*

A productive cough usually implies an underlying inflammatory process, often infectious, whereas a nonproductive cough signifies a mechanical or other irritative stimulus. The character of the cough may be described as "brassy" from major airways involvement or "barking" or "croupy" from laryngeal disease. Paroxysmal coughing with "whoops" is characteristic of pertussis. A cough that occurs mainly at night may accompany congestive cardiac failure; one occurring at meals suggests esophagogastric disease, such as hiatal hernia or diverticulum; and the cough of severe bronchitis or bronchiectasis is often worse upon awakening because of pooling of secretions during sleep. Each of these patterns tends to recur repeatedly under similar circumstances.

A description of the secretions produced in association with cough is diagnostically useful. Foul-smelling sputum indicates anaerobic infection, as in lung abscess or necrotizing pneumonia. Abundant frothy saliva-like sputum is a well known but rare symptom of bronchoalveolar carcinoma. Pink foamy sputum, which is often voluminous, indicates pulmonary edema. In pneumococcal pneumonia, the classic rust-colored or "prune juice"–colored sputum may be observed. The chronic production of copious purulent sputum with intermittent blood streaking, especially on change of postures, is an important clue to bronchiectasis.

The associated features of coughing episodes are of considerable clinical importance: wheezing—a disorder with obstruction to airflow such as asthma; stridor—involvement of the pharynx–larynx–extrathoracic trachea; fever and chills—acute infection; weakness and weight loss—tuberculosis or other chronic infection or malignancy; and recurrent pneumonias—bronchiectasis, foreign body, or obstructing tumor. In view of the importance of cigarette smoking in the pathogenesis of cough, a careful smoking history is crucial to the evaluation of cough.

Physical examination may reveal signs of pulmonary involvement that provide clues to the specific diagnosis. Regardless of the presence or absence of physical findings, evaluation of significant cough entails roentgenographic examination of the chest. When indicated, simple pulmonary function tests will demonstrate abnormalities of airflow and/or lung volumes. In patients whose routine spirometric tests are normal, bronchial provocation studies are indicated. Appropriate studies of sputum, especially culture and cytology, are often the easiest and most direct way of establishing a diagnosis. Fiberoptic bronchoscopy or other special diagnostic tests are sometimes needed.

TREATMENT. The ideal treatment of cough is elimination of its underlying cause. This is possible in most kinds of bronchopulmonary infections by suitable antimicrobial treatment of the responsible microorganism. Cessation of cigarette smoking nearly always eliminates the cough of chronic bronchitis. Disabling, irritative nonproductive cough may be suppressed by an antitussive drug such as codeine, 15 mg every six hours. In contrast, productive cough should not be suppressed because retention of secretions impairs the distribution of inspired air, which worsens gas exchange, and promotes the development of atelectasis and secondary infection. Adequate hydration, not overhydration, is traditionally recommended, although its effect on pulmonary secretions is difficult to substantiate. Expectorants and ultrasonic aerosols have not been shown to be beneficial. When secretions are difficult to raise because of their physical properties and/or ineffective coughing, respiratory physical therapy with postural drainage and percussion may be helpful and a trial is warranted.

HEMOPTYSIS

Regardless of whether the sputum is grossly bloody or merely blood streaked, the expectoration of any blood whatsoever denotes hemoptysis. Patients with chronic bronchitis may produce faintly blood-tinged sputum from time to time, but apart from this exception every patient with hemoptysis deserves a thorough diagnostic workup. A substantial proportion of all patients who expectorate bloody sputum have a serious disease; approximate figures indicate bronchogenic carcinoma 20 to 30 per cent; bronchiectasis 20 to 30 per cent; bronchitis 10 to 20 per cent; and other inflammatory disorders, including tuberculosis, 10 to 20 per cent. Other conditions that may present with hemoptysis include pulmonary embolism, mitral stenosis, pulmonary arteriovenous fistula, and Goodpasture's syndrome. All series include an appreciable number (5 to 15 per cent) of undiagnosed cases despite complete investigation.

DIAGNOSTIC APPROACH. The amount of expectorated blood may vary widely, from slight streaking of sputum to massive exsanguinating hemorrhage. The patient may not be aware of the pulmonary origin of the bleeding and often states that the blood "welled up" in his or her throat. For this reason, patients with true hemoptysis may seek the services of an otolaryngologist. Although it is always wise to examine the nasopharynx thoroughly, it is rare that hemoptysis is due to lesions in the upper respiratory tract.

Bleeding of esophageal, gastric, or duodenal origin may be confused with bleeding from the respiratory tract. Hematemesis can usually be differentiated from hemoptysis by the presence of symptoms of gastrointestinal involvement such as nausea and vomiting, a history of peptic ulcer disease or alcoholism, or signs of cirrhosis. Prompt endoscopy will settle the issue in doubtful cases.

Historical and physical examinations may provide clues to the underlying cause of hemoptysis but are seldom diagnostic. Chest roentgenograms, which should be obtained in all patients complaining of hemoptysis, may reveal evidence of old or new inflammatory lesions, probable malignancies, or vascular abnormalities. At times, the underlying lesion may be obscured by the densities caused by the presence of blood itself. Once the bleeding has stopped, however, intra-alveolar blood usually clears within a week so that delayed roentgenographic examinations are often helpful. Routine laboratory evaluation should include a complete blood count and tests to exclude a coagulopathy. It is useful to collect and measure the quantity of blood coughed up.

Virtually every patient with significant hemoptysis should undergo bronchoscopy to determine the site of bleeding and its cause. If bleeding is brisk, the earlier this is done the better. Even if the cause cannot be ascertained during the initial examination, it is important to determine from which bronchus the blood is coming; this is absolutely necessary in patients bleeding massively who are being considered for surgery, but it is also extremely difficult because the tracheobronchial system contains so much blood that it is frequently impossible to identify a bleeding point. The fiberoptic bronchoscope is often used in patients with hemoptysis, but many experts prefer the rigid scope because its larger lumen permits easier aspiration of blood and, when necessary, control of bleeding by packing.

If surgical treatment is a consideration, the origin of the bleeding must be identified each time hemoptysis occurs. Even if a lesion is obvious on chest roentgenographic examination, the patient may be bleeding from an occult site. Similarly, even if a source of blood has been identified on a previous occasion, the blood may come from a different abnormality next time.

TREATMENT. Fortunately, intrapulmonary bleeding usually stops spontaneously. Until it does, the patient should be kept with the affected lung, from which the bleeding is occurring, in the dependent position; the airways should be kept free of blood—coughing may suffice but suction may be necessary; and strong sedatives, which abolish cough, should be avoided, but mild sedatives, to relieve anxiety, are often advisable. A thoracic surgeon should be notified about the problem, and an endotracheal tube and suction apparatus must be ready at the bedside. If massive bleeding suddenly occurs, the tube can be inserted blindly into the right main bronchus and the balloon inflated to separate the two lungs and keep the blood confined to one of them. If circumstances permit, it is even better to put a balloon catheter, under bronchoscopic guidance, into a lobar or segmental bronchus to isolate the blood to as small a region of lung as possible. Blood transfusions are given according to the usual clinical guidelines of quantity of blood lost, hematocrit, blood pressure, pulse rate, and urine output.

After the bleeding stops, the patient should be investigated as outlined to determine the cause of the hemorrhage as well as the extent and severity of the underlying disease(s). Then, in consultation with a thoracic surgeon, a rational decision can be made concerning the need for and likelihood of success of an operation. Ordinarily, localized lesions (e.g., bronchial adenoma or sequestration) are resected and generalized lesions (e.g., widespread bronchiectasis or multiple fistulas) are left alone. However, there is considerable clinical ground between these two extremes and each patient must be considered individually.

An even more difficult problem is the selection of patients with "massive" hemoptysis for emergency pulmonary resection, usually lobectomy but occasionally pneumonectomy. Part of the problem lies in defining what actually constitutes "life-threatening" hemorrhage. Emergency resection in the presence of bleeding from relatively localized, chronic conditions (e.g., broncholithiasis) produces good results; in contrast, in patients hemorrhaging from acute parenchymal infections (e.g., lung abscess), there is a high incidence of postoperative complications. Patients who bleed massively from bronchogenic carcinomas or extensive benign lesions that are nonresectable are particularly difficult; the method of bronchial or intercostal arterial catheterization and embolization with Gelfoam to occlude the bleeding site has been tried with some success in these patients.

CHEST PAIN

Various types of chest pain are extremely common. Chest pain is one of the most frequent symptoms that cause the sufferer to seek medical attention. Because there is no clear relationship between the intensity of the discomfort and the importance of its underlying cause, all complaints of chest pain must be considered carefully. Pain that is virtually diagnostic because of its typical pattern of onset, location, and relation to effort and to respiratory movements is found in pleurisy, intercostal neuritis, costochondral disease, and disorders of the chest wall. The location and character of pain from myocardial ischemia are also characteristic but may be simulated by the pain of acute and chronic pulmonary hypertension. Occasionally, chest pain is elusive and difficult to diagnose, but it must always be taken seriously. A *meticulous history* is essential in evaluating chest pain. From the patient's story alone, a differential diagnosis can be formulated that serves as the basis for subsequent examinations.

MECHANISM. The anatomy, physiology, and biochemistry of pain in the body are reviewed in Ch. 466. Chest pain is no different from other types in that receptors and afferent pathways transmit a stimulus to the central nervous system, where that stimulus is perceived as pain. However, the capacity of various intrathoracic structures to serve as a source of pain differs. The lung parenchyma and the visceral pleura covering it are insensitive to ordinarily painful stimuli. In contrast, pain often accompanies involvement of the parietal pleura, the major airways, the chest wall, the diaphragm, or the mediastinal structures, including the heart. The mechanism of pain in myocardial ischemia is unknown, but the actuating event is clearly an imbalance between myocardial oxygen supply and demand. The pain of pericarditis may be in part related to involvement of the adjacent pleura, thus accounting for the striking respiratory component of what is primarily a cardiac disease. Pain in the esophagus is provoked by stimulation of receptors from acid reflux or muscle spasm.

PLEURAL PAIN. Pleurisy, or acute inflammation of the pleural surfaces, usually causes chest pain that has several distinctive features. The pain is restricted in distribution rather than diffuse, is nearly always on one side or the other, and tends to be distributed along the intercostal nerve zones. Pain from diaphragmatic pleurisy is often referred to the shoulder and side of the neck. The most striking and important characteristic of pleural pain is its clear relationship to respiratory movements. The pain may be variously described as "achy," "sharp," "burning," or simply a "catch," but whatever its designation, it is typically worsened by taking a deep breath, and coughing or sneezing causes intense distress. Patients with pleurisy frequently also complain of dyspnea because the aggravation of their pain during inspiration makes them conscious of every breath. Movement of the trunk, including bending, stooping, or even turning in bed, increases pleural pain, and patients usually find and remain in the position in which movements of the affected region are most restricted.

The rapidity of development of pleural pain provides a clue to its cause. An immediate onset attends pulmonary embolism or spontaneous pneumothorax, a slower but still acute onset over a few hours, especially with fever and cough, accompanies pneumonia, finally, a gradual onset over days or even weeks, often associated with features of chronic illness such as weakness and weight loss, suggests tuberculosis or malignancy.

INTERCOSTAL NEURITIS. The distribution and superficial and knifelike quality of the pain of intercostal neuritis may resemble pleural pain and, sometimes, may even be mistaken for myocardial ischemia. Usually, the pain of intercostal neuritis is worsened by vigorous respiratory movements such as coughing, sneezing, and straining but, unlike pleurisy, not by ordinary breathing. A neuritic origin may be suggested by the presence of lancinating or electric shock sensations unrelated to movements, and hyperalgesia or anesthesia over the distribution of the affected intercostal nerve provides further confirmatory evidence.

COSTOCHONDRAL DISEASE. Pain localized to the costosternal cartilaginous junctions may be confused with other, more serious causes of chest pain. The discomfort is usually described as dull with a gnawing, aching quality; there is little if any relationship to respiratory or other movements, although the pain may be most noticeable when the patient is lying in bed at night. The diagnostic key lies in the fact that there is tenderness to palpation that is clearly localized to one or more of the costal cartilages. There may be redness, swelling, and enlargement of the costal bridges *(Tietze's syndrome)*, but the frequency of these is overemphasized. The most common sites of costosternal perichondritis are the second, third, and fourth cartilages, but any part of the large and complex cartilaginous shield along the central and lower portions of the anterior thoracic cage may be involved.

DISORDERS OF THE CHEST WALL. The system of joints, muscles, and fasciae involved in movements of the thoracic wall is complex. Because these structures are in constant motion throughout a person's life, it is surprising that "rheumatic" pains of the chest do not occur more frequently than they do. Fibrositis of the muscle-bone attachments may simultaneously involve the chest wall and other parts of the skeleton. Similarly, spondylitis of the thoracic spine may have its rib cage component, and many less definable skeletal disorders may produce discomfort in the chest. Localized pain in the thoracic cage may be related to unusually severe exercise or motion of the involved area. At times, the abnormality appears to be spontaneous, although even in these cases it is possible that pain was delayed in onset after either injury to the muscles of the chest wall or fractures of ribs during minor trauma or an unnoticed episode of coughing.

PULMONARY HYPERTENSION. The pain of pulmonary hypertension may simulate the pain of myocardial ischemia in its substernal location, its pattern of radiation, and its crushing or constricting quality. This type of pain may occur in patients with acute pulmonary hypertension from multiple and/or massive pulmonary emboli or in patients with chronic pulmonary hypertension from vasculitis or mitral stenosis. The mechanism of the pain is unknown, but it is believed to differ in the acute and chronic varieties. In the former it is related to sudden distention of the main pulmonary artery and stimulation of mechanoreceptors, and in the latter to an imbalance between the oxygen supplied to and utilized by the pressure-overloaded right ventricle. Although substernal pain related to the sudden onset of pulmonary hypertension is a well-recognized complication of pulmonary embolism, more commonly emboli cause pain in the lateral part of the chest that is typically pleuritic in character whether or not they produce pulmonary infarction.

MYOCARDIAL ISCHEMIA. Among the most important types of chest pain is that of myocardial ischemia, which is usually caused by coronary artery atherosclerosis (see Ch. 51). These attacks are provoked by an imbalance, which may be transient or permanent, between the supply of and demand for oxygen by the ventricular myocardium. Ischemic pain spans a continuum of severity from angina pectoris on the one hand to myocardial infarction on the other. Typical anginal pain is induced by exercise, heavy meals, and emotional upsets, the pain is usually described as a substernal "pressure," "constriction," or "squeezing" that, when intense, may radiate to the neck or down the ulnar aspect of one or both arms. Variant or Prinzmetal's anginal pain is similar in location and quality to typical angina pectoris but occurs in cycles at rest rather than during stressful episodes. Both typical and variant types of angina pectoris are relieved by coronary vasodilatory drugs such as nitroglycerin. Typical angina also decreases with rest or removing the inciting stress. In contrast, the pain of myocardial infarction, although similar in location and character to anginal pain, is usually of greater intensity and duration, is not alleviated by rest or by nitroglycerin, may require large doses of opiates, and is often accompanied by diaphoresis, nausea, hypotension, and arrhythmias. Although patients are often short of breath during attacks of myocardial ischemia, and myocardial infarction may induce severe pulmonary edema, the pain itself is neither related to breathing nor affected by respiratory movements.

OTHER SOURCES. Pericarditis causes pain that is usually pleuritic in nature but may be steady and substernal, typically, the pain is worse while the patient is recumbent or lying on the left side. Dissecting aneurysm of the aorta is associated with severe, unremitting anterior chest pain that often radiates through to the back or into the abdomen. A deep substernal pain may result from esophageal reflux or spasm or from spontaneous mediastinal emphysema. Finally, psychogenic disorders may be associated with various forms of chest pain, the most common of which is a substernal tightness or aching sensation that may last from 30 minutes to several days. The pain may vary somewhat in intensity from time to time, and the ancillary features of myocardial infarction and a respiratory component are absent.

DIAGNOSTIC APPROACH. The approach to the general problem of the diagnosis of chest pain varies according to how seriously ill the patient is when first seen. Patients with acute chest pain who are gravely ill, as evidenced by hypotension, intense dyspnea, profuse diaphoresis, agitation, and restlessness, are usually evaluated first in the emergency room. The chief diagnostic considerations in this common clinical complex are myocardial infarction, pulmonary embolism, and dissecting aneurysm, less likely possibilities are tension pneumothorax, pericardial tamponade, and ruptured esophagus. An initial tentative diagnosis can usually be made from the results of careful historical and physical examinations, supplemented by an electrocardiogram and chest roentgenograms. Except when the electrocardiogram reveals clear evidence of acute myocardial ischemia, definitive diagnosis depends on the results of later studies such as ventilation-perfusion lung scans, pulmonary angiography, aortography, serial enzyme determinations, and coronary artery catheterization.

Patients with less severe chest pain may present during an episode of pain or afterward. Again, a detailed history of the character and behavior of the pain provides the best guide for the selection of subsequent diagnostic studies. Most patients will require an electrocardiogram, ideally taken during an episode of pain, and chest roentgenograms; then, based on the results of these examinations, diagnostic evaluation proceeds as needed for the particular entities under consideration.

TREATMENT. The treatment of chest pain depends on its cause. Anginal pain responds to coronary artery vasodilator drugs, whereas myocardial infarction usually requires opiates, often in large doses. Pleural pain responds to analgesics, given as required. However, pleurisy in association with pneumonia may be alleviated by anti-inflammatory drugs such as indomethacin; in refractory cases, intercostal nerve block is needed. For costochondral and other types of chest wall pain, mild analgesia, reassurance, and time usually suffice; rapid relief can be obtained, when necessary, by injection of local anesthetic agents into the involved area.

DYSPNEA

When healthy persons undertake a steadily increasing amount of physical activity, they will eventually become aware of their breathing; the exercise required to provoke this sensation depends on their physical fitness. If they increase the level of activity even further, the awareness will increase as the sensation becomes progressively more unpleasant; if they stop exercising, the feeling will quickly disappear. The sensation experienced by normal subjects during physical exertion is aptly described as "shortness of breath" but not as dyspnea. The term dyspnea implies that the awareness is disproportionate to the stimulus and, moreover, that the sensation is abnormally uncomfortable. Many patients will describe their breathing discomfort as "breathlessness," but many others will complain only of "tightness," "choking," "inability to take a deep breath," "suffocating," and simply "can't get enough air." Thus dyspnea is difficult to define precisely and it is impossible to quantify. As with the evaluation of chest pain, a thorough history is required to explore all the vagaries of this elusive symptom.

MECHANISM. It is impossible to find a common mechanism for what appears to be the same or similar sensation of difficulty in breathing that may occur in respiratory, cardiac, erythropoietic, metabolic, and psychogenic disorders. Dyspnea in patients with respiratory diseases is believed to have a reflex origin and thus must begin with stimulation of receptors in one or more of the organs concerned with breathing. There are three types of intrapulmonary receptors (stretch, irritant, and C-fibers, which include the J- and probably other receptors), each of which has its afferent pathway to the central nervous system in the vagus nerve. There are also receptors in the muscles and tendons that participate in breathing, and chemoreceptors are situated in systemic arteries and the brain. The theory of "length-tension inappropriateness" postulates that misalignment of muscle spindles in the respiratory musculature serves as the genesis of dyspnea. Perhaps the best explanation is that dyspnea is the subjective perception of the intensity of the stimuli that are generated by *all* the receptors activated during or in association with the act of breathing.

PATTERNS. Dyspnea occurs with many underlying conditions and in several different patterns. Some of these are sufficiently characteristic to warrant separate designations. Episodes of breathlessness that wake patients from a sound sleep are called *paroxysmal nocturnal dyspnea;* these are most often observed in patients with chronic left ventricular failure but may also occur in patients with chronic pulmonary diseases because of pooling of secretions, gravity-induced decreases in lung volumes, or sleep-induced increases in airflow resistance. *Orthopnea,* or the onset or worsening of dyspnea on assuming the supine position, like paroxysmal nocturnal dyspnea, is found in patients with heart disease and occasionally in patients with chronic lung disease. The inability to assume the supine position (instant orthopnea) is particularly characteristic of the rare condition of paralysis of both hemidiaphragms. *Platypnea* denotes dyspnea that occurs in the upright position and *trepopnea* the even rarer form of dyspnea that develops in either the right or left lateral decubitus position. Both the terms *hyperpnea,* an increase in minute volume, and *hyperventilation,* an increase in alveolar ventilation in excess of carbon dioxide production, indicate that ventilation is increased above normal. However, neither term carries any implication about the presence or absence of dyspnea.

DIAGNOSTIC APPROACH. The differential diagnosis of the dyspneic patient begins with a careful history. In patients with chronic respiratory or cardiac disease, dyspnea initially develops only during physical activity, and the amount of exertion required to provoke the symptom relates in a general way to the severity of the underlying condition. Sudden episodes of dyspnea, unrelated to physical activity, typically occur with pulmonary embolism, spontaneous pneumothorax, and anxiety; the acute attacks in each of these disorders characteristically remit, but bouts of breathlessness may recur with varying severity.

The results of historical and physical examinations, routine blood tests, electrocardiography, and chest roentgenography nearly always indicate whether the dyspneic patient is suffering from a respiratory, cardiac, hematologic, renal, or hepatic abnormality. Special diagnostic studies are often then required to determine what specific kind of disease is present. Measurements of lung volumes, expiratory flow rates, and diffusing capacity, studies during exercise, and noninvasive tests of cardiac function are particularly valuable in three difficult clinical situations: (1) differentiating between dyspnea of cardiac and pulmonary origin and, if abnormalities of both systems coexist, as is often the case, estimating the severity of each; (2) identifying the presence of either pulmonary vascular obstructive disease or diffuse pulmonary infiltrative disorders in dyspneic patients whose routine studies, including chest roentgenograms, are normal; and (3) helping to establish, by ruling out significant cardiorespiratory abnormalities, that dyspnea in a given patient is psychogenic in origin (a diagnosis that is always tenuous).

TREATMENT. Unlike cough, for which there are effective antitussives, and pain, for which there are powerful analgesics, there is no category of medications for relief of dyspnea. Cure or alleviation of dyspnea depends on recognizing its origin and treating the basic abnormality. In acute reversible conditions, the dyspnea subsides along with improvement of its underlying cause. In chronic cardiac and pulmonary disorders, sufficient physical exertion will continue to provoke dyspnea, but even in these conditions rehabilitation programs can be used to enable patients to increase their physical activity up to the maximum of the limits imposed by their disease.

CONCLUSION

This introduction to the three most common and important symptoms of *all* diseases of the respiratory system is meant to supplement the material presented not only in the remainder of Part VII but also elsewhere in the book. Acute infections of the upper and lower respiratory tract caused by viruses, bacteria, fungi, protozoa, and helminths are discussed in Parts XVIII and XIX. Systemic diseases in which the lungs may be involved are also discussed elsewhere: Wegener's granulomatosis (Ch. 441), eosinophilic syndromes (Ch. 162), and the "collagen diseases" (Ch. 429 to 455). Various abnormalities of the pulmonary circulation, exclusive of pulmonary embolism, and pulmonary edema, an important disorder (not disease) of the lungs, are discussed chiefly in Part VI.

Adelman M, Haponik EF, Bleeker ER, et al.: Cryptogenic hemoptysis: Clinical features, bronchoscopic findings and natural history in 67 patients. Ann Intern Med 102:829, 1985. *Review of workup and outcome in patients with hemoptysis and no initial diagnosis; known causes discussed as well.*

Altose MD: Assessment and management of breathlessness. Chest 88(suppl):77S, 1985. *Brief but thorough discussion of current theories about the mechanisms of dyspnea.*

Schneider RR, Seckler SG: Evaluation of acute chest pain. Med Clin North Am 65:53, 1981. *Comprehensive description of pain arising from different organs within the thorax; 75 references.*

Stulbarg M: Evaluating and treating intractable cough. Medical Staff Conference, University of California, San Francisco. West J Med 143:223, 1985. *Excellent review of the pathophysiology, causes, diagnosis, and management of intractable cough; 49 references.*

59 RESPIRATORY STRUCTURE AND FUNCTION

John F. Murray

Respiration can be defined as "those processes concerned with gas exchange between an organism and its environment." This definition, which emphasizes that the chief function of the respiratory system is *gas exchange*, is sufficiently comprehensive to apply to all animals, ranging from simple one-celled protozoa to infinitely more complex mammals. In human beings, the basic processes leading to gas exchange, or the uptake of O_2 and the elimination of CO_2, are usually separated into four functional subdivisions:

1. *Ventilation*—the movement of air from outside to inside the body and the distribution of air within the tracheobronchial system to the gas exchange units of the lungs.
2. *Diffusion*—the movement of O_2 and CO_2 across the alveolar-capillary membrane between the gas in alveolar spaces and the blood in pulmonary capillaries.
3. *Perfusion*—the flow of mixed venous blood through the pulmonary arterial circulation, distribution of the blood to the capillaries of the gas exchange units, and removal of the blood from the lungs through pulmonary veins.
4. *Control of breathing*—the regulation of ventilation, usually in accordance with changing metabolic demands.

VENTILATION

Air moves from outside the body into the gas exchange units of the lungs because contraction of the muscles of respiration normally generates sufficient force to expand the lungs and chest wall and to overcome the resistance and inertia in the system. Accordingly, the volume of gas that reaches the individual gas exchange units is determined by the mechanical properties of the lung parenchyma, airways, and chest wall, and by the force provided by the muscles of respiration (or by a mechanical ventilator).

The amount of air that enters the lung with each breath is called the *tidal volume*. When the lungs are fully expanded, the amount of gas they contain is called the *total lung capacity*. The maximal volume of gas that a person can exhale from total lung capacity is called the *vital capacity*, and the amount of gas remaining in the lungs at the end of maximal expiration is called the *residual volume*. Another important static lung volume is the *functional residual capacity*, which is the volume of gas in the lungs at the end of a normal breath. The relationships among these different lung volumes, which vary in different disorders and which will be frequently referred to, are shown in Figure 59–1.

Static Properties

Both the lungs and chest wall are elastic structures. This means that they can be distended and, when the distending force is removed, they recoil back to their resting volumes. Although the lungs and chest wall are similar in this respect, they differ considerably in their respective resting volumes when there is no expanding force.

The elastic properties of isolated lungs are shown by the dashed line in Figure 59–1. The slope of the line, or the change in volume (ΔV) for a given change in pressure (ΔP), is known as the compliance of the lungs. This curve demonstrates that (1) the lungs collapse almost completely when there is no distending pressure, (2) the slope of the volume-pressure curve is relatively steep at low lung volumes (i.e., as the lungs are beginning to inflate, their compliance is high), and (3) at high lung volumes, the curve flattens (compliance decreases) so that little increase in volume results from a large increase in pressure. The elastic forces of the lungs originate within the tissues that are being stretched, particularly those containing elastin and collagen, and from the surface tension of the film of *surfactant* that lines the air-liquid interface of alveolar spaces. The static properties of the isolated chest wall (including the diaphragm and abdominal contents that must be displaced during breathing) are shown by the solid light red line in Figure 59–1. The chest wall is a compressible and distensible structure that contains an appreciable volume in its resting state. To decrease the volume of the thorax, a force must be applied to overcome the tendency of the chest wall to resist compression and recoil back to its resting position. Conversely, to increase the volume of the thorax, the applied force must overcome the elastic forces in the chest wall that also cause it to recoil back to its resting position.

It is useful conceptually to consider the behavior of the lungs and chest wall separately, but obviously they function together. Because their action is coupled by the pleural pressure that keeps each lung expanded against the chest wall, the lungs and chest wall ordinarily change their volumes by exactly the same amount. Thus the pressures required to change the volume of the respiratory system are obtained by simply adding the separate pressures necessary to inflate the

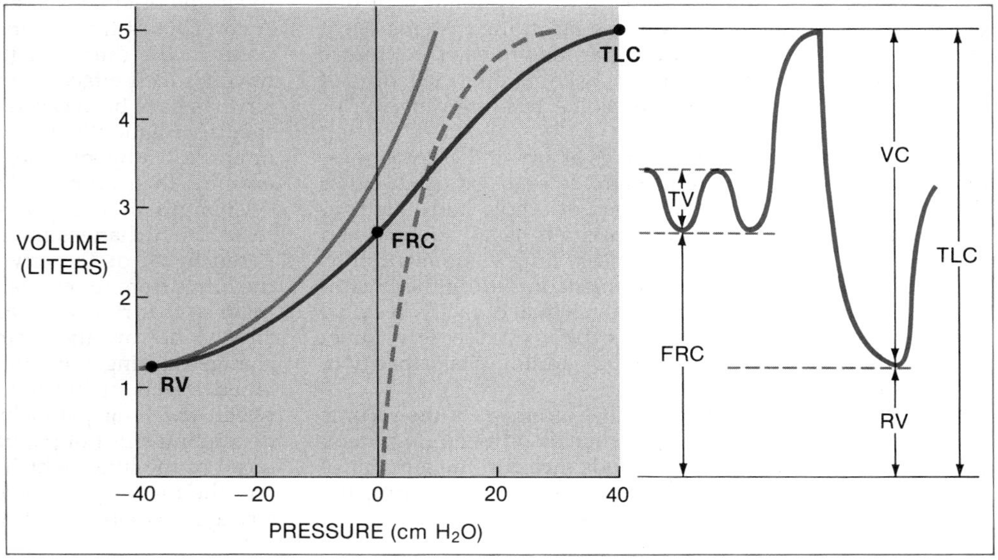

FIGURE 59–1. Schematic representation of the volume-pressure relationships of the chest wall (*solid light red line*), lungs (*dashed light red line*), and chest wall and lungs combined (*solid dark red line*). Total lung capacity (TLC) occurs when the lungs are fully expanded, and residual volume (RV) is the amount of gas remaining in the lungs at the end of a maximal expiration. Functional residual capacity (FRC) occurs at that volume at which the recoil pressures of the chest wall and lung are equal and opposite (i.e., the distending pressure = 0 cm H_2O). On the right is a spirometric tracing (volume-time) of the breathing maneuvers of the person whose pressure-volume curves are on the left. TV = Tidal volume; VC = vital capacity.

lungs and chest wall to a given volume. The solid line in Figure 59–1 indicates the pressure that must be produced by contraction of the respiratory muscles, or by a mechanical ventilator, to inflate or deflate both the lungs and chest wall. Figure 59–1 also shows that functional residual capacity is the volume at which the inward recoil force of the lungs is equal and opposite to the outward recoil force of the chest wall; in other words, functional residual capacity is that volume at which the net force of the respiratory system is zero.

During inspiration, the force developed by the contracting muscles of inspiration meets progressively increasing (inward) recoil forces from the combined expansion of the lungs and chest wall. Furthermore, because shortening muscle fibers generate progressively less force, inspiration finally ceases at that volume (total lung capacity) at which the weakening inspiratory muscle forces can no longer overcome the increasing forces required to expand the lungs and chest wall. Similarly, during expiration, the net force developed by the contracting muscles of expiration meets progressively increasing (outward) recoil forces from the chest wall. In children and young adults, expiration ceases at that volume (residual volume) at which the decreasing expiratory muscle forces can no longer overcome the increasing forces required to compress the chest wall. In older persons, residual volume is governed mainly by factors that regulate the caliber and patency of peripheral airways; thus even though the expiratory muscles are capable of further compression of the thorax, emptying is prevented by airway closure and trapping of gas in the lungs.

Vital capacity, or the volume between total lung capacity and residual volume, is determined by the factors that influence maximum inspiration and expiration, i.e., the balance of forces generated by the muscles of respiration and by the mechanical properties of the lungs and chest wall combined. Changes in these variables explain the characteristic changes in lung volumes that occur in patients with the respiratory disorders discussed in subsequent chapters.

Lung volumes also vary among healthy persons according to their age, sex, and physical structure (especially height). Because body build varies slightly from one ethnic group to another, it is important to have normal data that pertain to the population being studied. Measured volumes are usually expressed as both the observed value and the percentage of the predicted mean value for a normal subject of the same age, sex, and height. Measured values should not be considered abnormal unless they are clearly outside the range of values likely to be found in normal persons (100 per cent ± 20 per cent for vital capacity and 100 per cent ± 25 per cent for total lung capacity, residual volume, and functional residual capacity).

Vital capacity is easily measured with a spirometer or one of a variety of commercially available recording systems. Most spirometers can also be used to determine rates of expiratory airflow (see Dynamic Properties, below), but they do not measure total lung capacity, functional residual capacity, or residual volume.

To measure *all* the gas in the lungs at any of these volumes, one of two basically different methods must be used: either dilution or washout of an inert gas or whole body plethysmography. Functional residual capacity is usually determined because it is the normal end-expiratory lung volume and thus is an easy volume for subjects to maintain during the breathing test. After measuring functional residual capacity, residual volume is derived by subtracting expiratory reserve volume, and total lung capacity is obtained by adding vital capacity to the residual volume.

Gas dilution or washout involves measurement of the volume and concentration of an inert gas such as nitrogen (N_2), neon (Ne), or helium (He). These methods measure the amount of gas that communicates freely with the airways during the breathing maneuver; dilution or washout techniques do not detect gas trapped beyond closed (or very narrowed) airways and in poorly communicating regions, like bullae.

Body plethysmography involves placing the subject in the plethysmograph, a large airtight box resembling a telephone booth, and having him or her breathe through a mouthpiece in which a shutter can be closed to stop the flow of air. When the subject attempts to pant against the closed shutter, the volume of the thorax and gas in the lungs expands and contracts, which changes the pressure measured inside the mouthpiece. Movement of the thorax also changes the pressure in the box by compressing and expanding the gas surrounding the subject. From application of Boyle's law, which states that the pressure times the volume of a gas is constant if temperature remains the same, the volume of gas in the thorax can be calculated. The body plethysmograph measures all the gas present during the breathing maneuver, including that in freely communicating airspaces *and* any that may be trapped behind poorly communicating airways or in closed spaces (pneumothorax).

In normal subjects, measurements of functional residual capacity by dilution (or washout) and plethysmographic techniques are virtually identical. In contrast, in patients with airways obstruction or bullous disease, the communicating volume may be considerably less than the plethysmographic volume and the difference is a measure of the noncommunicating (sometimes called trapped) volume.

Dynamic Properties

To cause air to flow from outside the body into the gas exchange units, a muscular (or other mechanical) force must be exerted to overcome not only the elastic recoil properties of the lungs and chest wall but also their resistive and inertial properties. In contrast to distensibility, which is not affected by the rate of movement, the forces required to offset resistance and inertia are markedly influenced by the velocity of airflow. Except in a few patients (e.g., those with severe obesity), inertial forces are ordinarily small and usually ignored, thus only those factors affecting airways resistance need be considered in detail.

Resistance to airflow is affected chiefly by the caliber of the air passages. Although the diameter of each successive generation of airways decreases, the combined total cross-sectional area at any level increases steadily throughout the tracheobronchial tree from the main bronchi to the peripheral airways. This means that airways resistance progressively decreases and that most of the resistance of the human tracheobronchial tree resides in large airways: direct measurements reveal that between 50 and 80 per cent of total resistance to airflow originates in airways *greater than* 2 mm in diameter. A corollary of this observation is that substantial changes can occur in the caliber of the small peripheral airways without having much effect on total airways resistance. Hence, small airways have been called the lung's "quiet zone," and because they are frequently involved early in the evolution of clinically important lung disease, special tests have been devised to examine their functional behavior.

Changes in the cross-sectional area of airways can also result from changes in lung volume and diseases of the lung parenchyma or the airways themselves. During inflation of the lungs from functional residual capacity, airways are pulled open so that resistance to airflow decreases, during deflation, airways narrow and their resistance increases. Airway caliber changes during inflation and deflation because of the combined effects of the tethering action of the attachments between the lung parenchyma and small bronchioles and the distending effect of pleural pressure on larger airways. Elastic recoil of the lung, which governs the pull of the attachments and the magnitude of pleural pressure, affects the size of all airways. It follows that when elastic recoil is decreased, as in patients with emphysema, airways are narrowed and resistance is increased, this mechanism accounts for much of the airflow obstruction found in patients with emphysema.

Airway narrowing can also result from bronchospasm, edema of the mucosal lining, and secretions within the lumen. Also, changes in the viscosity and density of the inspired gas affect airways resistance, and gas mixtures of different densities are sometimes used to study the dynamic properties of the tracheobronchial system.

Resistance to airflow can be measured in a body plethysmograph; however, this procedure has limited clinical usefulness. Fortunately, the important dynamic properties of the respiratory system can be assessed by several readily available tests of airways function. The simplest and most widely used of these is the forced expiratory volume in one second (FEV_1), expressed as a ratio of the forced vital capacity (FVC), or FEV_1/FVC (Fig. 59–2). To perform the FVC maneuver, the subject inhales fully and then exhales as rapidly and completely as possible. In normal persons, the FVC equals the vital capacity from a slow or nonexpulsive maneuver, but in patients with airways obstruction, vigorous expiration may cause airways to narrow and close prematurely so that the FVC may be less than the vital capacity; the magnitude of the difference between the two values is an indication of the amount of air trapped behind compressed airways. The FEV_1/FVC decreases with age in normal persons after reaching adulthood and is usually higher in women than in men at all ages.

Additional measurements of airways behavior besides the FEV_1 can be obtained from the FVC maneuver (Fig. 59–2): several derivatives of time such as the $FEV_{0.5}$ and FEV_3 (the subscript denoting the number of seconds after beginning expiration at which the expired volume is measured), the maximal expiratory flow rate (MEFR or often $MEFR_{200-1200\ ml}$, indicating that the flow rate was measured between expired volumes of 200 and 1200 ml), and the maximal mid-expiratory flow rate (MMFR or often $MMFR_{25-75\%}$, indicating that the rate was measured between expired volumes of 25 and 75 per cent of the FVC). None of these has any particular advantage over the FEV_1 except that the MMFR is less dependent on the effort exerted by the subject than the other variables and reflects the flow properties of small as well as large airways.

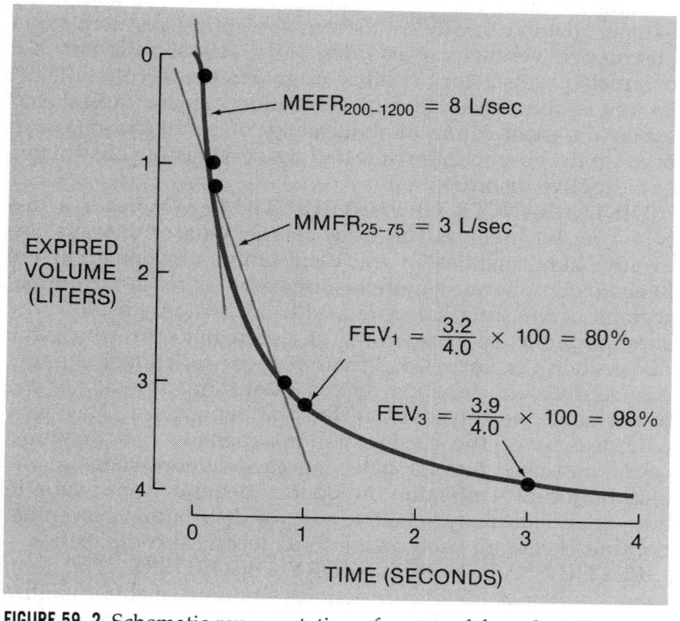

FIGURE 59–2. Schematic representation of a normal forced vital capacity (FVC) maneuver (expired volume against time, *heavy red line*) and the derivation of several variables commonly used to evaluate airways obstruction. $MEFR_{200-1200}$ = maximal expiratory flow rate, measured between expired volumes of 200 and 1200 ml, $MMER_{25-75}$ = maximal mid-expiratory flow rate, measured between 25 and 75 per cent of the total FVC, FEV_1 = forced expiratory volume in one second, expressed as percentage of total FVC, FEV_3 = forced expiratory volume in three seconds, expressed as percentage of total FVC.

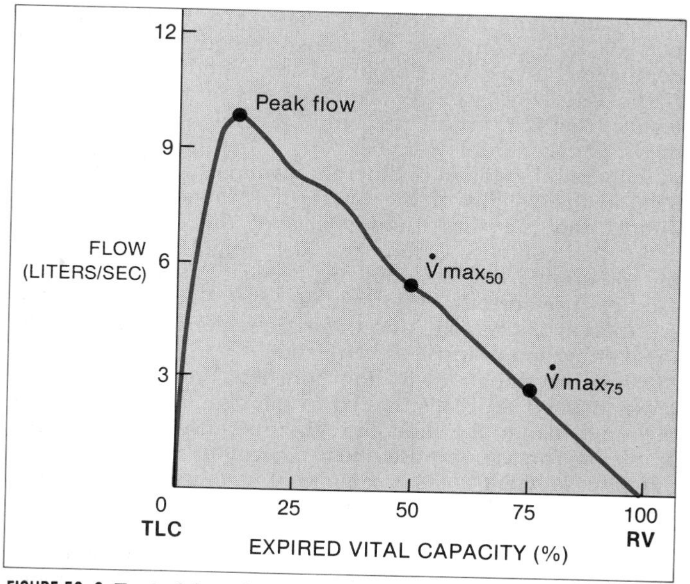

FIGURE 59–3. Typical forced expiratory flow-volume tracing of a normal adult man showing points of peak flow, maximal flow at 50 per cent expired vital capacity ($\dot{V}max_{50}$) and maximal flow at 75 per cent expired vital capacity ($\dot{V}max_{75}$). TLC = total lung capacity, RV = residual volume. (From Smith LH, Thier SO: Pathophysiology. The Biological Principles of Disease. Philadelphia, W. B. Saunders Company, 1981.)

Another way of examining the events during an FVC maneuver is by recording flow against volume instead of volume against time, which provides a maximal expiratory flow–volume curve (Fig. 59–3). From these records, maximal flow rates at any given fraction of the expired vital capacity, usually 50 per cent ($\dot{V}max_{50}$) or 75 per cent ($\dot{V}max_{75}$), can be determined and reported as the percentage of the predicted values for a subject of the same age, sex, and body size. The early portion of the maximal expiratory flow–volume curve, which includes peak flow, is determined by the effort exerted by the subject and is thus called the effort-*dependent* segment; the later portion is less influenced by effort and is called the effort-*independent* segment or that part of the curve during which expiratory airflow limitation occurs. Additional effort does not increase expiratory airflow (i.e., maximal velocity is limited), because "choke points" develop in those airways in which the velocity of airflow has increased to equal the speed at which pressures will propagate along the airways. Because events recorded in the effort-independent portion of the flow-volume curve require less cooperation and understanding by the subject, they are more reproducible than those in the effort-dependent portion.

Maximal expiratory flow-volume curves can also be recorded after a few breaths of 79 per cent He and 21 per cent O_2 (He-O_2) as well as after breathing room air (79 per cent N_2 and 21 per cent O_2). Although much has been learned about the behavior of the airways by comparing the curves obtained with the two gas mixtures, these tests have not proved as reliable as originally believed in detecting disease localized to peripheral (small) airways.

Distribution of Ventilation

During the movement of air from outside the body into the lungs during inhalation, the airstream is partitioned as it flows through the branching airways to the terminal respiratory units where gas exchange takes place. Even in healthy persons ventilation is not distributed uniformly, and marked derangements may develop in patients with lung disease.

The unevenness of ventilation found in normal subjects results from the vertical gradient of pleural pressure between the uppermost and lowermost parts of the lungs. The origins of the vertical gradient in different mammals are complex and include the weight of the lungs, their attachments at the hilum, and the shape and effects of the chest wall and abdominal contents, in humans, the weight of the lungs is the most important determinant. Because of the gradient in the pressure surrounding the lungs, alveoli are larger at the top than at the bottom, and there are regional differences in the distribution of inspired ventilation.

When breathing slowly from functional residual capacity, more inspired air is distributed to the dependent regions of the lungs than to the superior regions because the differences in pleural pressure cause the two regions to function on different segments of the same volume-pressure curve. Because the *change* in intrapleural pressure during quiet breathing is the same throughout the pleural space, the lower regions, which are operating on a steeper part of the curve and thus receive more volume for the same pressure change, inflate more than the upper regions. When inspiration continues to total lung capacity, alveoli at the top and bottom of the lungs inflate to nearly the same size because both regions are functioning on the flat portion of the volume-pressure curve even though the pleural pressure difference persists. When the rate of inspiratory airflow increases, as during exercise, the distribution of ventilation becomes more uniform than it is at rest.

During expiration, pleural pressure surrounding the most dependent portion of each lung becomes positive; this causes airways in that region to close. As expiration continues, airway closure progresses from the lowermost regions up the lungs, involving more and more airways. Regional differences in the distribution of ventilation can be examined by the test of closing volume (Fig. 59–4). After labeling alveolar gas by one of two methods (bolus or resident gas techniques), gas concentration measured at the mouth during the subsequent exhalation varies according to the sequence of regional emptying and occurs in four phases. Phase I reflects the composition of gas from the tracheobronchial system and contains none of the label; the concentration rapidly rises during Phase

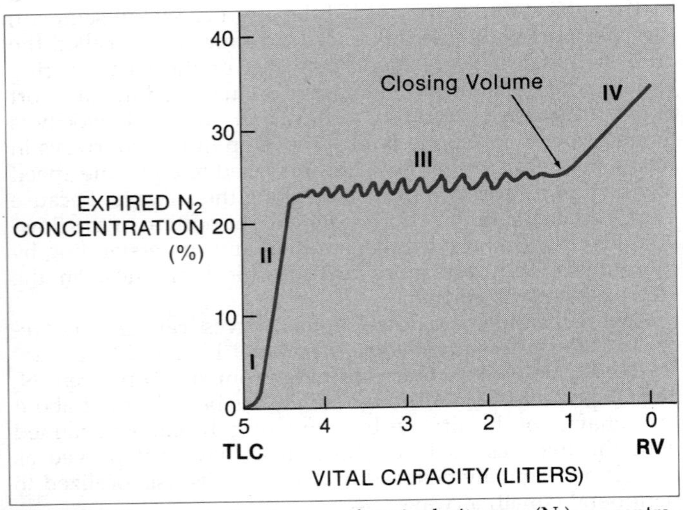

FIGURE 59–4. Representative tracing of expired nitrogen (N_2) concentration after taking a single breath of 100 per cent oxygen. An explanation of the four numbered phases (I, II, III, IV) is provided in the text. TLC = total lung capacity; RV = residual volume. (From Smith LH, Thier SO: Pathophysiology: The Biological Principles of Disease. Philadelphia, W. B. Saunders Company, 1981.)

II as alveoli containing the label begin to empty, a near-plateau is evident in Phase III as alveoli throughout the entire lung deflate; finally, the plateau terminates abruptly with a steep rise in concentration during Phase IV. Closing volume is the junction between Phases III and IV and is that volume at which airways in the dependent regions of the lung begin to close, accordingly, the rising concentration of the label in the subsequent expirate indicates the progressively increasing contributions from the preferentially labeled alveoli in the upper regions of the lung.

Because an increase in closing volume reflects premature closure or narrowing of airways, an increase in closing volume occurs in patients with lung disorders in which the caliber of peripheral airways is decreased from either decreased elastic recoil (e.g., in emphysema) or abnormalities of the airways themselves (e.g., in bronchitis or asthma). Furthermore, increases in closing volume have been detected in asymptomatic patients, usually smokers, and may be an early manifestation of lung disease. In addition, examination of the slope of Phase III is useful because it provides a sensitive measure of the adequacy of the distribution of ventilation. Well-ventilated units fill and empty more completely and rapidly than poorly ventilated units, this means that the concentration of the label will be lower in the better-ventilated regions that empty early during exhalation than in the poorly ventilated regions. Thus, the more uneven the distribution of ventilation within the lung, the steeper the slope of Phase III.

Other tests of the distribution of ventilation utilize the gamma ray–emitting properties of certain radioactive gases, chiefly ^{133}Xe, which are nontoxic and can be detected after inhalation in low concentrations by external counters. The distribution of ventilation can be assessed during a breath hold at end-inspiration after a single breath of ^{133}Xe or at intervals during its elimination by normal breathing after the lung has been labeled uniformly by rebreathing ^{133}Xe from a closed system.

Abnormalities of Ventilation

Lung diseases that cause abnormalities of ventilation are usually divided into two different categories: restrictive and obstructive ventilatory disorders. This classification is not completely satisfactory because it ignores the fact that disturbances of the distribution of ventilation are the earliest and by far the most common abnormality of ventilation and can occur in the absence of manifestations of coexisting obstructive or restrictive disorders.

DISTURBANCES OF DISTRIBUTION. Whenever a disease process involves the lung parenchyma or airways unevenly, abnormalities in the distribution of ventilation are likely to occur because more inspired gas will reach the normal regions of the lung compared with the regions distal to the sites of bronchial narrowing, or the regions in which the distensibility is impaired. Whether these functional changes can be detected depends on the extent and severity of the disease and the sensitivity of the test being used. The slope of Phase III of the closing volume maneuver is the most commonly used test for detecting early abnormalities in the distribution of ventilation. Frequency dependence of compliance is an extremely sensitive test for distribution of ventilation but is seldom used owing to its technical complexities.

RESTRICTIVE VENTILATORY DISORDERS. The term *restrictive ventilatory disorder* denotes a pattern of abnormalities in lung function. The word "restrictive" is employed to indicate a restriction of or limitation to the amount of gas within the lungs. Thus restrictive ventilatory disorders are characterized by reductions in lung volumes (Table 59–1). The hallmark of restriction is a decreased vital capacity, but because this change also occurs in obstructive ventilatory disorders, it is important to exclude the presence of airways obstruction (see Obstructive Ventilatory Disorders, below) or

TABLE 59–1. CHARACTERISTIC CHANGES IN LUNG VOLUMES AND TESTS OF AIRWAYS RESISTANCE IN PATIENTS WITH RESTRICTIVE AND OBSTRUCTIVE VENTILATORY DISORDERS*

Test	Restrictive	Obstructive
Vital capacity	Decreased	Decreased or normal
Residual volume	Decreased	Increased
Total lung capacity	Decreased	Normal or increased
RV/TLC	Normal or slightly increased	Markedly increased
FEV_1/FVC	Normal or increased	Decreased
MMFR	Normal or decreased	Decreased
Slope of phase III	Normal or increased	Increased

*Abbreviations: RV/TLC = residual volume to total lung capacity ratio; FEV_1/FVC = forced expiratory volume in one second to forced vital capacity ratio; MMFR = maximum mid-expiratory flow rate.

to demonstrate the presence of reductions in other lung volumes, particularly total lung capacity.

Many components of the lungs, chest wall, and respiratory control system determine the amount of gas that can be breathed into the lungs. Accordingly, restrictive ventilatory disorders can develop in diseases that (1) affect the chest wall or respiratory muscles (kyphoscoliosis, myasthenia gravis), (2) cause infiltrations in the lung parenchyma or airspaces (diffuse interstitial fibrosis, pulmonary edema), (3) involve the pleura (pleural thickening), (4) occupy space within the thorax (tumors, effusions, cardiac enlargement), and (5) occur after lung resection (pneumonectomy).

OBSTRUCTIVE VENTILATORY DISORDERS. The term *obstructive ventilatory disorder* denotes the constellation of abnormalities that result from limitation of expiratory airflow, regardless of its cause. Because the functional disturbances depend on the presence of increased airways resistance, obstructive ventilatory disorders are detected mainly by tests of the behavior of the respiratory system under dynamic conditions (Table 59–1). The FEV_1/FVC test is the most widely used, but tests of maximal flow-volume relationships are being used increasingly in the *early* diagnosis of airways obstruction, especially when the obstruction is situated in peripheral airways.

Obstructive ventilatory disorders are found in patients with asthma, bronchitis, emphysema, advanced bronchiectasis, or other diseases that cause narrowing of the tracheobronchial system. When the term "obstructive" was originally employed, it was not possible to differentiate among these various entities, so they were lumped together in the nonspecific category of chronic obstructive pulmonary disease. Now, however, it is possible by means of specialized tests of lung function to sort out the various diseases that cause airways obstruction, even when they coexist; the characteristic features of asthma, chronic bronchitis, and emphysema are described in subsequent chapters.

DIFFUSION

Diffusion can be defined as the movement of molecules from a region of higher to one of lower concentration; accordingly, diffusion tends to eliminate differences in concentration within the various regions accessible to the molecules. Diffusion is a passive process that results from the kinetic motion of the molecules, and no extra energy is required. In the lungs, O_2 moves by diffusion from alveolar gas into pulmonary capillary blood; similarly, in the peripheral tissues, O_2 moves by diffusion from capillary blood into neighboring cells. Carbon dioxide also moves by diffusion but usually in the direction opposite to that of O_2. Both O_2 and CO_2 undergo chemical reactions in the bloodstream at the start and finish of their journeys between the lungs and the peripheral tissues; O_2 reacts solely with hemoglobin, and CO_2 reacts in part with hemoglobin and in part to form bicarbonate.

Diffusing Capacity

The diffusing capacity of the lungs or any gas indicates the quantity of that gas that diffuses across the alveolar-capillary membrane per unit time in response to the difference in mean pressures of the gas within the alveolus and pulmonary capillary. Most inert gases (e.g., N_2) diffuse across the air-blood barrier so rapidly that the amount taken up by the lungs is not detectably limited by the diffusibility of the gas and the properties of the lungs and blood but is determined solely by the solubility of the gas and the volume of tissue and blood into which it can dissolve. This phenomenon enables use of highly soluble gases like acetylene, dimethyl ether, or nitrous oxide to measure lung tissue volume and pulmonary capillary blood flow.

The only two gases that can be used to measure the diffusing capacity of the lungs are O_2 and CO. Because of their unique ability to combine with hemoglobin, both have to diffuse across the alveolar-capillary membrane in large quantities to saturate the available hemoglobin at the gas pressure prevailing in the alveoli. Thus it may not be possible for complete equilibrium to occur before the hemoglobin-containing red blood cells leave the pulmonary capillaries and gas transfer ceases. Of the two gases, CO is much more widely used for the measurement of diffusing capacity than O_2 because of the ease and convenience of applying the various CO tests and because CO uptake is always diffusion limited. In contrast, O_2 uptake is not limited by diffusion (i.e., is not a test of diffusing capacity) in normal subjects except during heavy exercise or while breathing low concentrations of O_2.

Two general types of tests using CO are available that involve either a breath-holding maneuver (single-breath method) or continuous rebreathing (steady-state methods). These two methods yield systemically different results, largely because neither technique summarizes accurately the events taking place in the 100,000 gas exchange units of the lung, in each of which P_{CO} varies according to the ventilation and blood flow to the unit. Despite this shortcoming, measurements of pulmonary diffusing capacity have provided useful empiric information concerning the function of the lungs in healthy persons and patients with lung diseases.

The quantity of CO that will diffuse in a known period of time from alveolar gas into capillary blood and combine with hemoglobin in response to a given pressure difference between gas and blood depends on (1) the solubility and diffusibility of CO in each layer of the air-blood barrier, (2) the surface area and thickness of the barrier, and (3) the rate of the chemical reaction between CO and hemoglobin within red blood cells. Because the solubility and diffusibility of CO are physical characteristics that presumably do not change under ordinary circumstances, the two chief components of diffusing capacity are the area and thickness of the alveolar-capillary membrane available for diffusion (D_M) and the pulmonary capillary blood volume (Vc), both of which can be derived by performing several measurements of diffusing capacity (DL_{CO}) with the subject breathing gas mixtures of different concentrations of CO and O_2.

Normal values for CO-diffusing capacity depend chiefly on the person's lung volume and therefore closely correlate with body size, especially height. Approximately half the total resistance to diffusion of CO from alveolar gas to capillary blood resides in the membrane compartment and the other half in the chemical reaction that takes place in the pulmonary capillary blood volume. Accordingly, changes in the hemoglobin concentration have a calculable effect on total CO diffusion that should be taken into account when establishing the predicted "normal" value for a patient with anemia or polycythemia.

Diffusing capacity is normally higher in the supine than the erect posture because position changes the volume of blood in pulmonary capillaries, and at high compared with low lung volumes because inflation recruits alveolar-capillary surface. When blood flow to the lung increases, as in muscular exercise, capillary blood volume also increases owing to recruitment of previously nonperfused capillaries and dilatation of others; these phenomena account for the progressive increase in DL_{CO} during increasingly strenuous levels of exercise. Similarly, the elevated pulmonary arterial pressures encountered in persons who live at high altitudes also recruit capillaries, increase capillary blood volume, and cause an increase in "normal" DL_{CO}. For unexplained reasons (possibly genetic), natives of high altitudes have higher DL_{CO} values than sojourners fully acclimatized to the same altitude.

Abnormalities of CO-Diffusing Capacity

On the basis of the physiologic principles that govern the diffusion of CO, it can be inferred that DL_{CO} may increase or decrease in patients with various cardiopulmonary disorders that affect the membrane, the capillary blood volume, or both. When tests of diffusing capacity were first used to study patients with various forms of lung disease, it was assumed that abnormalities of gas transfer would result from thickening of the air-blood barrier by a pathologic process that lengthened the pathway for diffusion of gases; this concept led to the formulation of what became widely known as the *alveolar-capillary block syndrome*. The "block" meant that the distance CO molecules had to travel from gas to blood was increased and, in turn, that extra time was required for diffusion to reach equilibrium across the air-blood barrier. Now it is known that the importance of alveolar-capillary block has been greatly exaggerated because a decreased diffusing capacity is not a satisfactory cause for arterial hypoxia, especially in patients at rest; when a low PO_2 occurs, it is nearly always attributable to a ventilation-perfusion abnormality, or less often to a right-to-left shunt.

Pulmonary vascular disorders, such as pulmonary emboli and pulmonary vasculitis, that affect (directly or indirectly) the pulmonary capillary bed decrease DL by decreasing capillary blood volume. Similarly, DL_{CO} is reduced in patients with infiltrative disorders of the interalveolar septum that obliterate or destroy capillaries. This is the usual mechanism underlying reduction of DL_{CO} in patients with sarcoidosis, diffuse interstitial fibrosis, berylliosis, or collagen diseases of the lung.

Changes in the characteristics of the membrane account for a decreased DL_{CO} in patients with diseases in which some form of intra-alveolar filling process has occurred and the air-to-blood diffusion pathway is actually lengthened: pneumonia, pulmonary edema, alveolar proteinosis. A decrease in both membrane and blood volume components produces a low DL_{CO} in patients with disorders associated with removal or destruction of lung tissue, such as resectional surgery or emphysema.

An increase in DL_{CO} results occasionally from an increase in capillary blood volume secondary to hemodynamic changes in the pulmonary circulation: an increase in pulmonary arterial or left atrial pressures, as in congestive heart failure, or an increase in pulmonary blood flow, as in atrial septal defect. The DL_{CO} is sometimes increased in patients with bronchial asthma during an attack, but the cause of this change is not known.

PERFUSION

The pulmonary circulation delivers blood in a thin film to the gas exchange units so that O_2 uptake and CO_2 elimination can occur. The physiologic determinants of pulmonary blood flow are analogous to those of ventilation in that the total volumes of ventilation and blood flow must be adequate to meet metabolic needs, and the distribution of both must be such that proportionate amounts of inspired fresh air and incoming mixed venous blood are delivered to individual gas exchange units. Ventilatory volume is controlled by the factors that regulate breathing (see below), whereas the volume of blood flowing through the lungs is determined mainly by the extrapulmonary mechanisms that govern cardiac output.

Distribution of Pulmonary Blood Flow

Pulmonary blood flow is not distributed uniformly throughout the lungs but is normally greatest in the dependent regions where pulmonary arterial pressure is highest and, conversely, is least in the superior regions where pulmonary arterial pressure is lowest. In the upright subject under resting conditions, the apices of the lungs are barely perfused and considerably more blood flows, even allowing for differences in the amount of lung tissue, to the basilar regions. The presence of nonuniform blood flow, which is not matched by comparable changes in ventilation, leads to important differences between regions of the lung in their defense capabilities and efficiency of gas exchange.

Regional blood flow is also governed by local factors, the most important of which is vasoconstriction secondary to alveolar hypoxia. As a consequence, blood flow is redistributed away from poorly ventilated gas exchange units and the matching of ventilation and perfusion is preserved.

Distribution of pulmonary blood flow can readily be measured by injecting radioactive substances, such as ^{125}I-albumin aggregates or ^{133}Xe dissolved in saline, and then detecting their location in the lung with an external counter system. Abnormalities in the volume and distribution of pulmonary blood flow may result from diseases that involve the blood vessels themselves (emboli, vasculitis, emphysema), from compression of blood vessels (tumors, cysts), or from vasoconstriction of blood vessels (alveolar hypoxia secondary to local abnormality of ventilation).

Other Functions

The pulmonary circulation has important functions besides providing blood flow for continuous gas exchange: (1) it acts as a filter of virtually the entire venous drainage; (2) it supplies substrates for the nutrition and metabolic needs of the lung, including the synthesis of surfactant; (3) it serves as a reservoir of blood for the left ventricle; (4) it affects endocrine function by modifying the pharmacologic properties of a variety of circulating substances; and (5) it provides a large surface area for the absorption and filtration of liquids and solutes.

CONTROL OF BREATHING

The respiratory system must maintain gas exchange during periods of stress, such as exercise and other forms of increased metabolic needs. The O_2 consumption may increase more than ten-fold from rest to strenuous exercise; over this range, arterial PO_2 remains remarkably constant. The correspondence between the volume of ventilation and the demands for O_2 uptake and CO_2 elimination results from the responsiveness of three reasonably well-characterized receptor systems that interact to regulate breathing in normal persons and patients with a variety of disease states: (1) receptors in the airways and lung parenchyma, (2) peripheral chemoreceptors, and (3) central chemoreceptors. Nerve impulse traffic from these receptors is integrated and modulated in the medulla with impulses arising from higher centers in the brain. The medulla can be viewed as the main headquarters for initiating, processing, and relaying messages concerning breathing to other parts of the body via nervous pathways. Some of the resulting medullary neural activity may reach the cerebral cortex and evoke conscious perception of breathing (i.e., the symptom of dyspnea); other impulses may travel through efferent pathways in the autonomic nervous system to the lungs and other organs; still other impulses may descend in the spinal cord to be processed with afferent impulses from peripheral nerves at different cord segments before finally being transmitted to the muscles of respiration and other effectors.

Abnormalities of Control of Breathing

Variations, usually increases, in the rate and depth of breathing occur in patients with many common clinical disturbances such as fever, metabolic diseases, or psychiatric disorders. Several frequently used drugs (e.g., aspirin, antidepressants, and alcohol) also affect ventilation. *Hyperventilation* occurs when ventilation increases out of proportion to CO_2 production and arterial P_{CO_2} decreases; *hypoventilation* is the converse. *Hyperpnea* signifies an increase in the rate and depth of breathing, such as occurs during exercise, but carries no implication concerning arterial P_{CO_2} values. It should be emphasized that a decrease in the O_2 pressure (P_{O_2}) of arterial blood has several causes. In contrast, the pressure of CO_2 (P_{CO_2}) is governed simply by the relationship between CO_2 production ($\dot{V}_{CO_2}$) and CO_2 elimination by alveolar ventilation ($\dot{V}alv$):

$$P_{CO_2} = k\dot{V}_{CO_2}/\dot{V}alv$$

Because alveolar ventilation normally changes to keep pace wth CO_2 production, for practical purposes abnormal arterial P_{CO_2} values can always be interpreted as indicating hyper- or hypoventilation.

Abnormalities of the control of breathing can result from excitation of intrapulmonary receptors (pulmonary embolism, pneumonia, asthma), depression of peripheral chemoreceptors (natives of high altitudes, sedative drugs, severe chronic bronchitis), stimulation of peripheral chemoreceptors (drugs such as doxapram), depression of central chemoreceptors (sedative drugs, obesity, myxedema, neurologic disorders), and stimulation of central chemoreceptors (drugs such as aspirin, irritative neurologic lesions). Special tests of the ventilatory response to breathing gas mixtures with increased CO_2 or decreased O_2 and a test that determines the pressure developed during the first 0.1 second of breathing against a closed mouthpiece ($P_{0.1}$) help in defining the physiologic derangements among these disorders.

GAS EXCHANGE

The end-product of respiration is gas exchange, which in human beings consists of maintaining the values for P_{O_2} and P_{CO_2} in arterial blood within normal limits. As stated previously, respiration consists of ventilation, including the distribution of inspired air throughout the tracheobronchial system, diffusion, blood flow, including the distribution of mixed venous blood throughout pulmonary capilliaries, and the control of breathing. Each of these contributes in a unique way to gas exchange such that an impairment in one process cannot be compensated for by improvement in another.

Ambient air consists primarily of N_2 and O_2 with varying amounts of water vapor. As air is inhaled, it is warmed to body temperature and fully saturated with water vapor (P_{H_2O} 37° C = 47 mm Hg); the addition of water vapor has the effect of diluting the inspired mixture of N_2 and O_2 and reduces their respective pressures proportionately. During gas exchange in the alveoli, more O_2 is removed than CO_2 is added; this causes the volume of each respiratory unit to decrease slightly and raises the concentration and pressure of N_2 slightly. When ventilation and perfusion are each uniformly distributed to various units (Fig. 59–5), "ideal" conditions for gas exchange exist and there is no difference between the P_{O_2} values in (mean) alveolar gas and arterial blood. The alveolar-arterial P_{O_2} difference is an important measure of the uniformity of matching of ventilation and perfusion. The difference is derived from a direct measurement of the arterial P_{O_2}, which is subtracted from alveolar P_{O_2} ($P_{A_{O_2}}$) calculated according to the following equation:

$$P_{A_{O_2}} = P_{I_{O_2}} - P_{A_{CO_2}}\left[F_{I_{O_2}} + \frac{1 - F_{I_{O_2}}}{R}\right]$$

where $P_{I_{O_2}}$ = P_{O_2} of inspired gas, $P_{A_{CO_2}}$ = alveolar P_{CO_2} (usually assumed to equal arterial P_{CO_2}), $F_{I_{O_2}}$ = fractional concentration of O_2 in inspired gas, and R = respiratory exchange ratio (often assumed to equal 0.8).

However, gas exchange in healthy lungs is not perfect because there is a small (5 to 10 mm Hg) alveolar-arterial P_{O_2} difference, which occurs because of the normal presence of a slight nonuniformity in the distribution of ventilation with respect to perfusion and a small right-to-left shunt. It is also noteworthy that the sum of the pressures of the individual gases in mixed venous blood is less than the total atmospheric pressure. Because the tissues and spaces of the body are in approximate equilibrium with venous blood, these structures are also subatmospheric. The "suction" serves to keep the lung expanded against the chest wall and to cause the reabsorption of gas from tissue spaces (e.g., a pneumothorax).

Abnormal Gas Exchange

Measurements of arterial P_{O_2} and P_{CO_2} and calculations of the alveolar-arterial P_{O_2} difference are reliable guides to the overall adequacy of respiration. In determining whether or not an abnormalitiy is present, it must be remembered that normal values for P_{O_2}, but not P_{CO_2}, vary with age and that both P_{O_2} and P_{CO_2} are influenced by the altitude at which the subject is living. There are five physiologic mechanisms known to cause arterial hypoxia, defined as a decrease below normal of arterial P_{O_2}: (1) hypoventilation, (2) decreased diffusion, (3) ventilation-perfusion imbalance, (4) right-to-left shunting of blood, and (5) breathing air (or a gas mixture) with a low P_{O_2}. Except for a few uncommon clinical examples, such as breathing air with its P_{O_2} reduced by combustion of O_2 and addition of smoke or suffocation, item 5 can be ignored. Items 1 to 4 can be separated, at least for practical clinical purposes, by analyzing the values from a given blood specimen and a few easy tests.

HYPOVENTILATION. The simplest disturbance of gas exchange occurs when not enough fresh air is breathed into alveolar spaces to raise pulmonary capillary P_{O_2} to normal levels and to allow CO_2 to leave the bloodsteam. Although arterial P_{CO_2} may theoretically increase in patients with other disturbances of gas exchange (ventilation-perfusion abnormalities and right-to-left shunts), for clinical purposes an elevated value should be interpreted as indicating alveolar hypoventilation.

Pure hypoventilation is a relatively uncommon clinical event. When it is found, depression of the central nervous system resulting from anesthetic agents or other sedative drugs is the usual cause. More commonly, hypoventilation occurs in association with other disturbances of oxygenation. When these coexist, they can be recognized by the fact that the decrease in arterial P_{O_2} is more than can be accounted for by the increase in arterial P_{CO_2}.

IMPAIRED DIFFUSION. Decreased diffusion, from either loss of pulmonary capillaries or thickening of the air-blood barrier, does not usually cause important alveolar-arterial P_{O_2} differences *at rest*. Thus abnormalities of diffusion can be ignored in patients with arterial hypoxia whose blood specimens are obtained while they are resting. In contrast, impaired diffusion is one of the two major causes of severely worsening hypoxia during exercise (right-to-left shunting of blood is the other). Regardless of the cause of the diffusing impairment, under resting conditions there is sufficient time to allow gas transfer to reach equilibrium between gas and blood. However, during exercise, cardiac output and the velocity of blood flow through pulmonary capillaries increase; thus the time for gas transfer is reduced and alveolar-end-capillary P_{O_2} differences may occur.

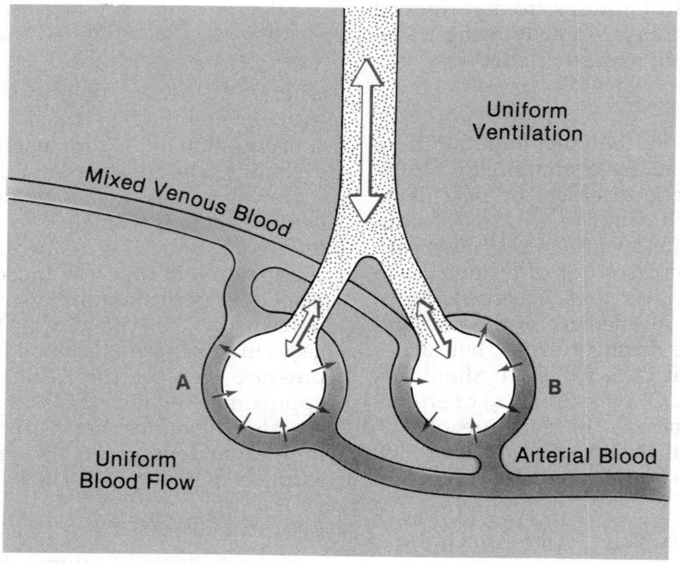

FIGURE 59–5. Schematic representation of gas exchange in an idealized two-compartment model of the lung in which there is uniform distribution of ventilation and blood flow. (Adapted from Comroe JH Jr, et al.: The Lung: Clinical Physiology and Pulmonary Function Tests. 2nd ed. Chicago, Year Book Medical Publishers, 1962. Reprinted by permission from the authors and Year Book Publisher, Inc.)

	A	*B*	*A + B*	*Units*
Alveolar ventilation	2.4	2.4	4.8	L/min
Pulmonary blood flow	3.0	3.0	6.0	L/min
Ventilation-perfusion ratio	0.8	0.8	0.8	
Mixed venous P_{O_2}	40	40	40	mm Hg
Mixed venous S_{O_2}	75	75	75	per cent
Mixed venous P_{CO_2}	46	46	46	mm Hg
Alveolar P_{O_2}	101	101	101	mm Hg
Arterial P_{O_2}	101	101	101	mm Hg
Arterial S_{O_2}	97.5	97.5	97.5	per cent
Arterial P_{CO_2}	40	40	40	mm Hg
Alveolar-arterial P_{O_2} difference	0	0	0	mm Hg

VENTILATION-PERFUSION MISMATCHING. Because the distributions of inspired air and pulmonary blood flow in normal lungs are neither uniform nor proportionate to each other, a slight ventilation-perfusion imbalance exists in healthy persons. Moreover, increased (above normal) mismatching of ventilation and perfusion is by far the most common cause of arterial hypoxia encountered clinically. Virtually all forms of lung disease are associated with a detectable ventilation-perfusion abnormality.

When a unit is underventilated relative to its perfusion (i.e., has a low ventilation-perfusion ratio), O_2 uptake by that unit must decrease so that the P_{O_2} of its end-capillary blood is lower than normal; P_{CO_2} tends to increase but cannot rise above the value in mixed venous blood (Fig. 59–5). Thus the process affects values for P_{O_2} more than P_{CO_2}. Furthermore, in those units that are overventilated owing to a redistribution of inspired air, the high ventilation-perfusion ratio causes P_{O_2} to increase and P_{CO_2} to decrease. But there is an important difference in the effects of these changes in pressures on the actual quantities (contents) of O_2 and CO_2 in the capillary blood leaving units with high ventilation-perfusion ratios. Given the shapes of the respective dissociation curves, O_2 content is not appreciably increased but CO_2 content is decreased. Thus increasing ventilation with respect to perfusion in some regions corrects the tendency to CO_2 retention that would otherwise exist but does not correct the hypoxia caused by low ventilation-perfusion relationships in other units. Another invariable consequence of a ventilation-perfusion abnormality is an increase in the alveolar-arterial P_{O_2} difference.

RIGHT-TO-LEFT SHUNTING. A small right-to-left shunt of blood is found in normal persons, and shunts of considerable magnitude may occur in patients with pulmonary disease. A right-to-left shunt may be visualized as a pathway(s) through which mixed venous blood flows from the right to the left side of the heart without having contacted functioning gas exchange units along the way. Thus there is a continuous admixture of venous blood that has flowed through the abnormal pathway with arterialized blood from normal pathways in the lungs. Arterial hypoxia and an increased alveolar-arterial P_{O_2} difference occur that vary in severity with the magnitude of the shunt and its O_2 content. Right-to-left shunts may occur through intracardiac communications in patients with congenital heart disease. In patients with lung disease, although shunts may be extremely large, they seldom occur through abnormal vascular channels such as pulmonary arteriovenous fistulas; instead, they are caused by blood perfusing normal vessels in regions of lung that are atelectatic or in which alveoli are filled with edema fluid, pus, or blood; in either case, because gas transfer is impossible, a shunt occurs.

The consequences of a right-to-left shunt are similar to those of a ventilation-perfusion imbalance owing to basic similarities between the two disturbances. A shunt can be viewed as an extreme ventilation-perfusion abnormality in which there is perfusion but *no* ventilation at all. It is impossible to differentiate between a ventilation-perfusion disturbance and a right-to-left shunt while the subject is breathing ambient air; therefore the effects of both are combined and designated as venous admixture or a "shunt-like" effect. The two causes of hypoxia can be separated by giving the patient 100 per cent O_2 to breathe and measuring arterial Po_2 after all the N_2 has been washed out of the lungs. When a ventilation-perfusion abnormality exists, the N_2 is replaced by O_2 and all the blood perfusing the lungs equilibrates at a high Po_2 (approximately 600 mm Hg); in this way 100 per cent O_2 is said to "correct" a ventilation-perfusion disturbance. In contrast, in the presence of a right-to-left shunt, the admixture of mixed venous blood continues despite breathing 100 per cent O_2 and arterial hypoxia persists. In fact, the alveolar-arterial Po_2 difference in patients with a right-to-left shunt is higher during breathing of 100 per cent O_2 compared with room air, whereas the opposite occurs in patients with ventilation-perfusion inequalities.

Significance of Arterial Blood Gas Values

The availability of accurate rapid analyzers for measuring Po_2, Pco_2, and pH has been one of the major clinical advances of the last 25 years. Virtually the entire therapeutic approach to patients with acute and chronic respiratory failure is dictated by the presence and magnitude of blood gas and pH abnormalities (see Ch. 72). Every physician should know the mechanisms of arterial hypoxia and how to differentiate them, because it is important clinically whether a patient's hypoxia results from hypoventilation, impaired diffusion, ventilation-perfusion mismatching, or right-to-left shunting. Evaluating the course and prognosis of the lung disease, determining the need for and outcome of therapy, and assessing disability, operability, and the limits of resection in patients considered for pulmonary surgery all depend to some extent on the findings of blood gas analysis. Thus all physicians who care for patients must become familiar with the technique of arterial puncture and must know how to interpret the results of blood gas analysis.

EXERCISE

Tests of pulmonary function are customarily performed with the subject seated at rest. The results of these studies provide useful information about the functional abnormalities that characterize common and important pulmonary diseases. Occasionally, the results of routine tests are perfectly normal in symptomatic patients, usually those with exertional dyspnea. In these circumstances, tests during exercise may reveal severe functional disturbances that lead to further evaluation and a diagnosis of either pulmonary vascular or parenchymal infiltrative diseases. Exercise tests are also essential to document the presence of and mechanisms underlying disability.

Cotes JE: Lung Function. 4th ed. Philadelphia, J. B. Lippincott Company, 1979. *Good textbook of pulmonary physiology.*

Hyatt RE: Expiratory flow limitations. J Appl Physiol 55:1, 1983. *Concise and understandable explanation of the wave-speed theory of expiratory flow limitation.*

Jones NL, Campbell EJM: Clinical Exercise Testing. Philadelphia, W. B. Saunders Company, 1982. *Comprehensive survey of and instructions for exercise testing.*

Murray JF: The Normal Lung: The Basis for Diagnosis and Treatment of Pulmonary Disease. 2nd ed. Philadelphia, W. B. Saunders Company, 1986. *Review of normal anatomy, pulmonary physiology, and structure-function correlations.*

Roussos C, Macklem PT (eds.): The Thorax, Parts A and B. New York, Marcel Dekker, Inc., 1983. *Extremely thorough, authoritative discussion of the interrelationships among the thorax, lungs, and respiratory muscles in health and disease.*

Torre-Bueno JR, Wagner PD, Saltzman HA, et al.: Diffusion limitation in normal humans during exercise at sea level and simulated altitude. J Appl Physiol 58:989, 1985. *Elegant study of the effects of diffusion limitation in normal persons.*

Wilson AF (ed.): Pulmonary Function Testing: Indications and Interpretations. Orlando, Fla., Grune & Stratton, 1985. *Good summary of pulmonary function testing; well referenced.*

60 ASTHMA

Ronald P. Daniele

DEFINITION AND PREVALENCE. Asthma is a disorder that is characterized by increased responsiveness of the trachea and bronchi to various stimuli, resulting in widespread narrowing of the airways. These changes are reversible either spontaneously or as a result of therapy. The currently accepted definition does not specify a cause or causes, identify unique clinical or pathologic features, or mention immunologic mechanisms. It does describe, however, the fundamental abnormality that is common to all asthmatic patients—reversible hyper-responsiveness of tracheobronchial smooth muscle.

Most asthmatic patients are diagnosed by a triad of episodic symptoms: wheezing, cough, and dyspnea. Characteristically, these signs and symptoms are highly variable in severity and duration. They may run the gamut from being completely absent for days, months, and even years to being protracted and unresponsive to outpatient therapy (status asthmaticus).

Asthma may afflict as many as 5 per cent of the population in the United States. In over half the cases it is diagnosed between ages 2 and 17 years, and in this group it is the leading cause of disease and disability. About one third of asthmatic patients are first diagnosed after 30 years of age.

CLASSIFICATION. Patients with asthma may be separated into two clinical groups, extrinsic and intrinsic (Table 60–1). Extrinsic asthma is characterized by childhood onset, seasonal variation, and a well-defined allergic history to a variety of inhaled allergens (atopy). The extrinsic form accounts for less than 10 per cent of all patients. Intrinsic asthma usually begins after the age of 30 and tends to be perennial and more severe; status asthmaticus is more common in this group. By definition, in intrinsic asthma an allergic etiology cannot be identified. More than 80 per cent of asthmatic patients have clinical features that are common to both groups, but for purposes of discussion each will be discussed separately.

PATHOLOGY. Most descriptions of the pathologic features of asthma come from patients dying in status asthmaticus. In these cases, the lungs are markedly distended and fail to collapse owing to the occlusion of most bronchi by thick, tenacious plugs of mucus, which often extend to the terminal bronchioles. Histopathologic hallmarks include bronchial smooth muscle hypertrophy, mucosal edema, thickening of the basement membrane, and inflammatory cells in submucosal tissue, particularly eosinophils. The lung parenchyma is

TABLE 60–1. CLASSIFICATION OF ASTHMATIC PATIENTS

Extrinsic*	Intrinsic*
Known external allergens	No known external allergens
Positive immediate skin tests	Negative skin tests
IgE raised in 50–60% of subjects	IgE normal or low
Onset usually in childhood or early adult life	Onset usually (but not invariably) in older adults
Intermittent asthma	More continuous asthma
Other allergies (hay fever and eczema) often present (54%)	Other allergies uncommon (7%)
Family history of multiple allergies (asthma, hay fever, eczema) common (50%)	Family history of multiple allergies less common (20%)

*Blood and sputum eosinophilia common in *both* groups.

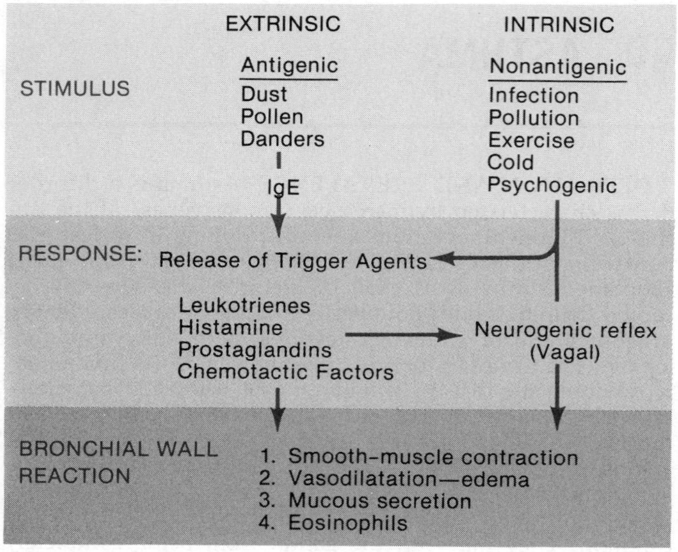

FIGURE 60–1. Dual pathways involved in the pathogenesis of bronchial constriction. (Adapted from Fishman AP [ed.]: Pulmonary Diseases and Disorders. New York, McGraw-Hill Book Company, 1980.)

remarkably spared with no evidence of fibrosis or destruction of the alveolar septa. Unexpectedly, similar abnormalities have been found in asthmatic patients dying from other causes who were presumably symptom free prior to death. The presence of mucous plugs in the small airways (less than 2 mm) of these patients may explain some of the persistent functional abnormalities (reduced midmaximum expiratory flow rate [MMF] and increased alveolar-arterial difference for Po_2) found even in asymptomatic patients.

PATHOPHYSIOLOGY OF EXTRINSIC ASTHMA. In extrinsic asthma, the sequence of events after sensitization leading to the pathologic features described above is shown in Figure 60–1. Inhaled allergens interact with specific IgE antibodies that are fixed to mast cells that line the tracheobronchial tree. Mast cells (and possibly basophils) that are sensitized with IgE are primed to respond to specific allergens when cell-bound IgE is bridged by divalent allergen. This membrane event signals mast cells to secrete a variety of mediators by two processes. First, preformed mediators contained in metachromatic granules of mast cells are released by a process of exocytosis. Important examples of preformed mediators include histamine, eosinophilic factors of anaphylaxis (ECF-A), and neutrophil chemotactic factor (NCF). In the second process, unstored mediators, such as slow-reacting substance of anaphylaxis (SRS-A) (now called the leukotrienes), platelet activating factors (PAF), and prostaglandins (PGD_2 and $PGF_{2\alpha}$), are synthesized and secreted by mast cells within minutes after antigen stimulation. Some of the properties and functional characteristics of these mediators are summarized in Table 60–2. For a more extensive discussion of mast cell structure and function, the reader is referred to Ch. 427.

Two advances have extended our knowledge of the role of mediators in asthma: the elucidation of the arachidonic acid metabolic pathways and the characterization and synthesis of SRS-A, which proved to be a group of compounds called leukotrienes. Leukotrienes, as well as prostaglandins, are synthesized from the 20-carbon unsaturated fatty acid, arachidonic acid (Fig. 60–2). Arachidonic acid is derived from cell membrane phospholipids by the action of phospholipases and may be converted by cyclo-oxygenase to prostaglandins and thromboxanes. A second pathway that is catalyzed by 5-lipoxygenase leads to the formation of 5-hydroperoxyeicosatetraenoic acids (5-HPETE) and then to an unstable intermediate, leukotriene A_4 (LTA_4). LTA_4 may then be converted to leukotriene B_4, a potent chemotactic factor for eosinophils and neutrophils. Alternatively, LTA_4 may be transformed by several cell types (mononuclear cells and basophils) into leukotriene C_4 by the enzymatic addition of glutathione (S-glutamylcysteinylglycine). Leukotriene C_4 may undergo further conversion to leukotriene D_4 (S-cysteinylglycine) by enzymatic removal of glutamine and then by removal of glycine to leukotriene E_4 (S-cysteine). SRS-A is composed of the cysteinyl-containing leukotrienes (LTC_4, LTD_4, and LTE_4), of which LTD_4 is the most potent bronchoconstrictor (Table 60–2). The leukotrienes are a thousand times more potent on a molar basis than histamine or $PGF_{2\alpha}$ and exert their effect predominantly in the small or distal airways. In asthmatic patients, allergens induce the release of leukotriene C_4, D_4, and E_4 from the lung tissue in amounts that correlate well with their capacity to induce bronchial contraction.

Secretion of primary mediators described in Table 60–2 apparently initiates the release of secondary mediators, such as serotonin, prostaglandins, and possibly kinins. Serotonin

TABLE 60–2. MEDIATORS IN THE ATOPIC INFLAMMATORY RESPONSE

Mediator	Molecular Characteristics	Source	Function
Histamine	Beta-imidazolylethylamine MW* = 111	Mast cells, basophils, preformed and stored in granules	Increases vascular permeability, bronchial smooth muscle contraction (H1 type) ↑ cyclic AMP in mast cells (H2 type) ↑ mucous secretion
Slow-reacting substance of anaphylaxis (SRS-A) Leukotrienes C_4 (LTC_4) LTD_4 LTE_4	Polyunsaturated substituted C-20 fatty acids MW ≃ 625 ≃ 500 ≃ 425	Mast cells eosinophils, mononuclears, lung cells? (not preformed)	Increases vascular permeability, bronchial smooth muscle contraction
Eosinophil chemotactic factors of anaphylaxis (ECF-A)	Tetrapeptides (Val/Ala-Gly-Ser-Glu), MW ≃ 360–390, and acid peptides	Mast cells, basophils, preformed and stored in granules	Attracts eosinophils
Neutrophil chemotactic factor (NCF)	Structure ? MW > 750,000	Mast cells, basophils, lung tissue, preformed and stored	Attracts neutrophils
Platelet-aggregating factors (PAF)	Phospholipids 1-0-alkyl-2-acetyl-sn-glyceryl-3-phosphorylcholine MW ≃ 520–550	Neutrophils, ? mast cells, basophils, other lung cells? (not preformed)	Aggregates platelets and release of other mediators (serotonin, PG)
Prostaglandins (PG)	Polyunsaturated C-20 fatty acids, MW ≃ 350	Mast cells, basophils, platelets, other lung cells? (not preformed)	↑ cyclic AMP PGE_1, PGE_2—dilate smooth muscle PGD_2, $PGF_{\alpha 2}$—contracts smooth muscle Release of PG probably stimulated by other mediators

*MW = molecular weight.

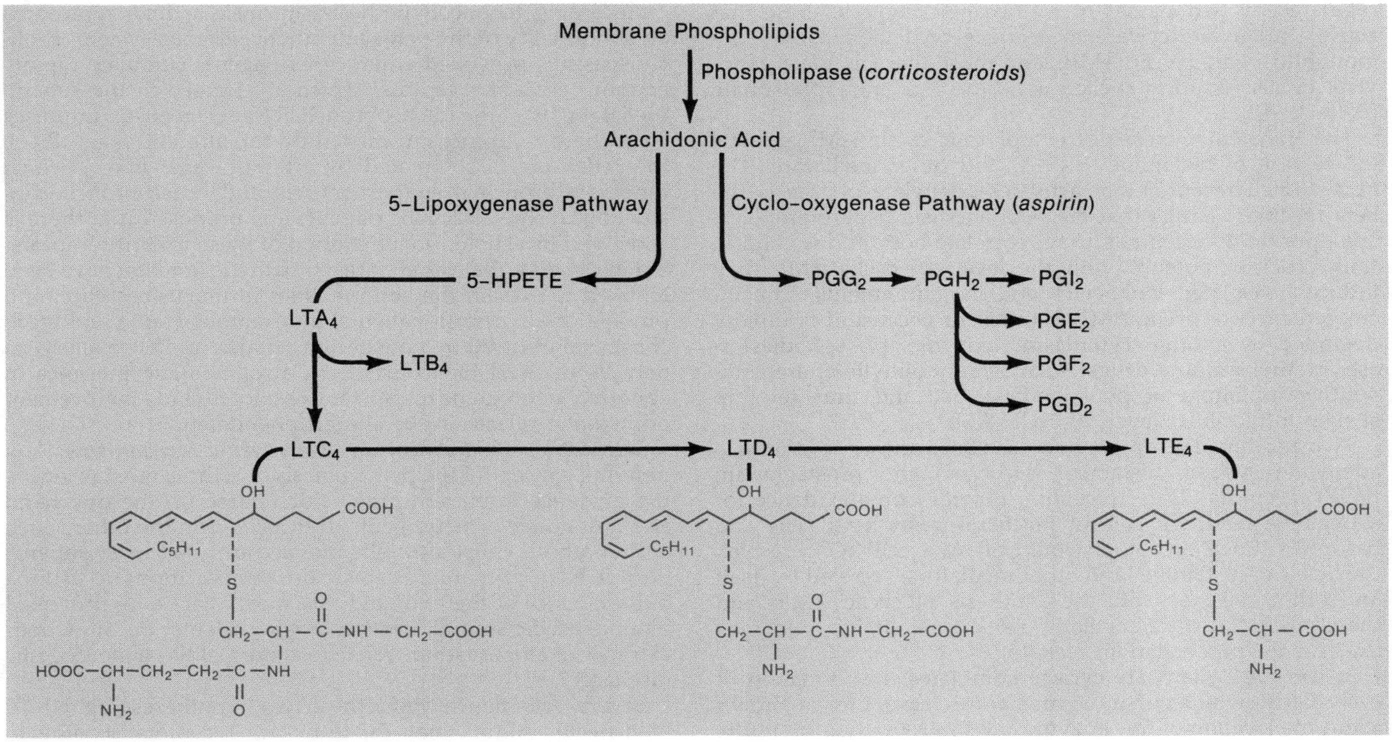

FIGURE 60–2. Arachidonic acid metabolic pathways. The figure depicts major prostaglandin (PG) products of the cyclooxygenase pathway. Also shown are the structural formulas of the three leukotrienes that constitute slow-reacting substance of anaphylaxis and that are generated through the lipoxygenase pathway. It is noteworthy that corticosteroids inhibit the phospholipases involved in synthesis of arachidonic acid. Aspirin inhibits the cyclooxygenase pathway. Not shown in the figure are thromboxanes that are derived from PGH_2.

constricts bronchial smooth muscle directly but may also induce bronchoconstriction by stimulating irritant receptors (see below). Prostaglandins of the E series (PGE_1 and PGE_2) are potent dilators of airways and blood vesesls. Although the lung is a major site for their production, the principal cell types involved are not defined.

The effects of these mediators may be viewed as two waves of an inflammatory response: The first is an immediate serous transudation caused by increased capillary permeability. The second occurs hours to days after antigen stimulation and involves the accumulation of inflammatory cells (*late-onset asthmatic response*).

In more than one half of asthmatic patients inhalation of specific allergens causes an immediate bronchoconstriction that resolves within minutes to hours and then recurs six to ten hours later. This *late-onset response* of the airways is thought to be associated with an accumulation of neutrophils, platelets, and eosinophils in the bronchial mucosa and submucosa. The reaction is initiated by mast cell (and basophil) degranulation and release of mediators, including leukotriene B_4, other eicosanoids, and eosinophil and neutrophil chemotactic factors. The arrival of neutrophils appears to elicit the infiltration of mononuclear cells in the submucosa, which may persist for several days. An appreciation of late-onset reactions is reshaping our thinking about asthma: It is not solely a syndrome of brief and reversible airways obstruction but also a disease involving a progressive, multistage inflammatory response. The identification of late-onset responses also has important therapeutic implications because they are poorly managed by standard bronchodilator therapy (beta$_2$ drugs and methylxanthines) (see below).

The eosinophil and neutrophil appear to play prominent roles in the late-onset reaction, especially in their capacity to inflict injury. Granular constituents derived from the eosinophil, particularly major basic protein, and the secretion of oxygen free radicals can injure bronchial epithelial cells, rendering the mucosa more permeable to allergens and possibly lowering the threshold of underlying irritant receptors.

Mast Cell Receptors—Intracellular Regulation. As shown in Figure 60–3, secretion by mast cells and basophils is

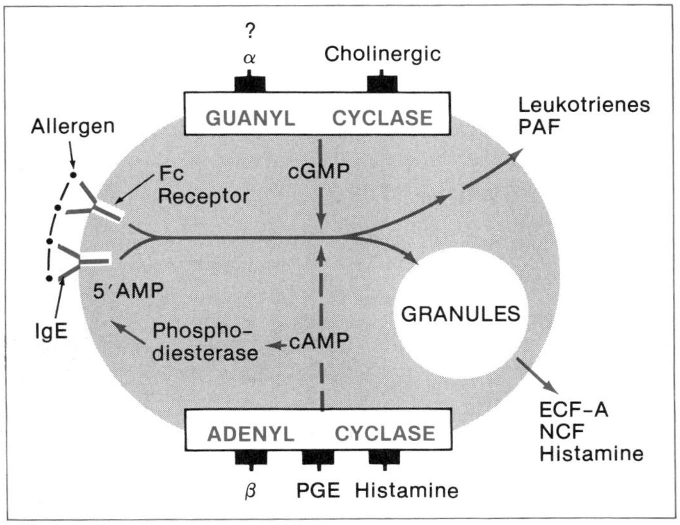

FIGURE 60–3. Membrane receptor interactions involving allergen-IgE and agonists that result in the stimulation of cyclic AMP or cyclic GMP and modulation of mediator release from mast cells and basophils. (From Fishman AP [ed.]: Pulmonary Diseases and Disorders. New York, McGraw-Hill Book Company, 1980.)

regulated by two classes of membrane receptors: those that activate adenylate cyclase to produce cyclic adenosine-3′,5′-monophosphate (cyclic AMP); and those that stimulate guanylate cyclase to form cyclic guanosine-3′,5′ monophosphate (cyclic GMP).

The transient increase of cytoplasmic cyclic AMP inhibits the release of histamine, SRS-A, and other mediators. The best-studied receptor that activates adenylate cyclase is the beta receptor. Drugs that are beta agonists (isoproterenol > epinephrine > norepinephrine) correlate both in dose and in rank order of potency with the levels of cyclic AMP they induce in isolated leukocytes and lung fragments. The increased level of cyclic AMP is transient because it is rapidly degraded by another cytoplasmic enzyme, phosphodiesterase. Methylxanthine drugs, such as aminophylline, are competitive inhibitors of phosphodiesterase and thus tend to sustain intracellular levels of cyclic AMP.

Two additional receptors have also been shown to stimulate adenylate cyclase: histamine (H_2 type) and prostaglandin (PGE) receptors. These receptors provide some evidence for a negative feedback control mechanism for mast cells and basophils. Such receptors would allow a cell to "perceive" the levels of histamine (and other mediators) secreted by itself and other cells, activate the synthesis of cyclic AMP, and thereby limit further mediator release. A similar role may exist for the prostaglandin receptor.

In contrast, guanylate cyclase stimulates the formation of cyclic GMP, which enhances mediator release. Less is known about the location of this enzyme and its associated receptors. However, a cholinergic receptor has been identified whereby acetylcholine stimulates the production of cyclic GMP.

According to a current hypothesis, the balance between the inhibitory (cyclic AMP) and excitatory (cyclic GMP) messenger molecules regulates mediator release. It has been proposed that asthma results from a partial blockade of beta receptor, leading to an imbalance of these regulatory molecules.

The elucidation of the mechanisms of mediator release in asthma has greatly extended our understanding of bronchospasm and provides a more rational basis for therapy. Nevertheless, most attacks of asthma are not precipitated by allergens.

INTRINSIC ASTHMA—PATHOPHYSIOLOGIC MECHANISMS. In intrinsic asthma, reversible airways obstruction is caused by a variety of stimuli that are nonantigenic and seemingly unrelated. Nonetheless, as shown in Figure 60–1, these stimuli lead to pathologic lesions similar to those seen in extrinsic asthma.

According to one hypothesis, intrinsic asthma represents an abnormality of the parasympathetic nervous system. Bronchospasm is provoked when certain agents stimulate rapidly adapting irritant receptors, which are located in the subepithelial region of the tracheobronchial tree (Fig. 60–4). Impulses from these receptors are carried by the afferent vagal fibers; the reflex arc is completed by efferent vagal fibers, which innervate bronchial smooth muscle and cause bronchoconstriction. In the asthmatic patient, it is proposed that there is a lowered threshold for stimulation of these irritant receptors. Similarly, disturbances in parasympathetic function have been invoked to explain the abnormalities in mucus secretion and production. In certain patients, for example, cough and bronchospasm induced by nonspecific irritants and even allergens may be relieved or abolished by atropine. The presence of abnormal neurogenic responses does not exclude involvement of mediator release in the allergic phenomenon.

Interaction of Mediator and Neurogenic Mechanisms. Any unifying concept of the pathogenesis of asthma must reconcile the evidence implicating mediator release on the one hand and autonomic or neurogenic dysfunction on the other. Such an hypothesis must also take into account that most patients do not have primarily extrinsic or intrinsic forms of asthma but a mixture of the two, and that most attacks are provoked by nonspecific stimuli, even in atopic patients. But how does extrinsic or atopic asthma relate to abnormalities in neurogenic discharge?

Several schemes may link these two hypotheses (Fig. 60–4). Nonspecific stimuli may excite irritant receptors, leading to bronchospasm by way of efferent vagal pathways. Allergen-antibody complexes may stimulate mast cells, releasing mediators that might have a direct action on smooth muscle as well as an indirect effect by stimulating irritant receptors and thereby producing bronchospasm. Alternatively, both nonspecific irritants and allergen-antibody interaction might stimulate mediator release from mast cells. Certain mediators, such as histamine and serotonin, are potent stimulants of irritant receptors. By such a scheme, stimuli may induce bronchospasm by direct action of mediators on smooth muscle or by indirect action that operates via neurogenic reflexes, or by both mechanisms.

The late-onset reactions may also be involved in the interaction between mediator release and neurogenic stimuli. An important feature of the late-onset response is an increase in airway hyper-reactivity. It is likely that the infiltration of the bronchial mucosa with inflammatory cells and continued release of mediators further stimulate irritant receptors. Late-

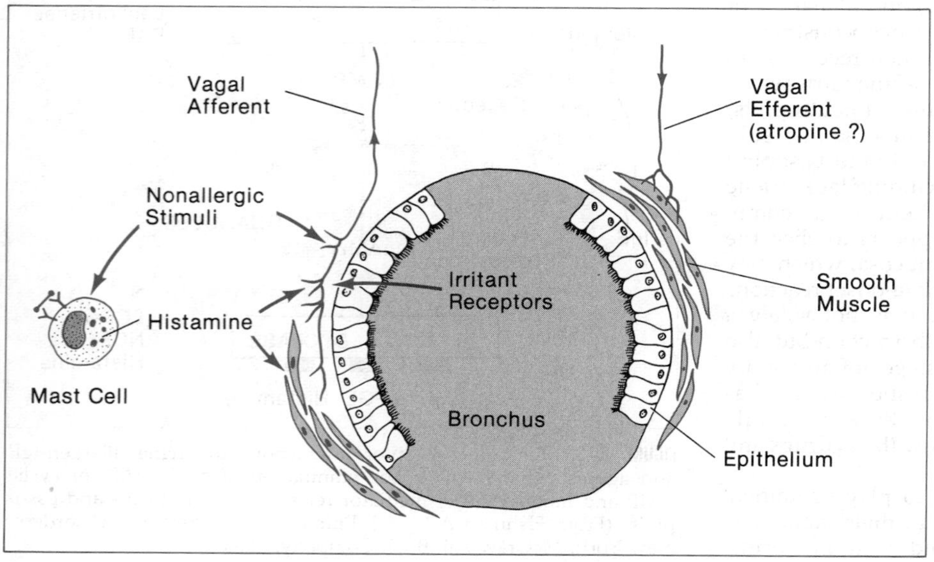

FIGURE 60–4. Possible interactions between mediators and neurogenic reflexes in the elicitation of bronchial smooth muscle contraction in asthma. Also indicated in the figure is one potential site of action for anticholinergic drugs in asthma.

onset reactions are caused not only by allergic stimuli but also by certain nonallergic provocative stimuli discussed below (e.g., viral infection and pollutants).

Nonallergic Provocative Stimuli. One of the most important nonspecific irritants is *respiratory tract infection*, particularly by viral agents. Both lower and upper respiratory infections may initiate or aggravate bronchospasm. This is not due to a hypersensitivity to the infecting agents, but is thought to result from the capacity of viral agents to lower the threshold for stimulation of irritant receptors.

Airborne pollutants may play a role in the pathogenesis of asthma. In "Tokyo-Yokohama asthma" and in "New Orleans asthma," a high density of air pollutants was found to have initiated or aggravated wheezing and dyspnea in asthmatic patients as well as in certain previously asymptomatic individuals who were later shown to have *hyperirritable* airways. Air pollutants (e.g., ozone) are thought to increase hyper-reactivity of bronchial smooth muscle by stimulating irritant receptors in the tracheobronchial tree.

A variety of *occupational dusts and fumes* may provoke asthmatic attacks in susceptible individuals. The onset of wheezing, cough, or dyspnea may be related to the working hours. More commonly, however, symptoms are not closely linked to occupation but may be delayed for several hours until after the patient has left the work place. Important diagnostic clues include a cyclic pattern in which symptom-free periods occur during weekends or vacations. Both allergic and irritant stimuli are thought to be involved in occupational asthma. A more extensive discussion of occupational asthma is contained in Ch. 536.

In some patients, *hyperpnea, laughing*, or *exercise* may also induce bronchoconstriction. Moreover, the inhalation of *cold air* may initiate or intensify bronchospasm. There are two hypotheses to explain how bronchospasm is induced by such diverse ventilatory maneuvers: One implicates mainly heat transfer from the respiratory tree; the other proposes that it is respiratory water loss, resulting in an increase in the osmolarity of the epithelial lining fluid. When all other variables are controlled, the major determinant is the volume of air that is to be warmed and humidified on inspiration. Heat and water loss occurs as the minute ventilation increases in response to exercise. This loss is independent of whether minute ventilation is voluntary or the result of exercise. Although it is unsettled regarding which mechanism is predominantly involved in exercise-induced asthma, both the inhalation of cold air and an increase in the osmolarity of lining fluid cause mediator release as well as stimulate vagal efferent pathways. Cromolyn or $beta_2$ drugs or both may blunt or prevent symptoms when given by inhalation prior to exercise. Measures that humidify and warm inhaled air, such as cold weather masks, are also helpful.

In about 10 per cent of asthmatic patients, a peculiar triad exists of *bronchospasm, nasal polyps*, and *sensitivity to aspirin*. Ingestion of aspirin, indomethacin, aminopyrine, or yellow food additives (e.g., tartrazine yellow) may induce severe bronchospasm, urticaria, and even hypotension. Interestingly, these patients are sensitive to acetylsalicylic acid but not to sodium salicylate. The reaction is not immunologic but appears related to an abnormality in prostaglandin metabolism, which is unmasked by these drugs. The arachidonic acid pathways may provide a clue to this abnormality (Fig. 60–2). In certain asthmatic patients, ingestion of aspirin or indomethacin, known inhibitors of cyclo-oxygenase, may divert arachidonic metabolism toward the lipoxygenase pathway and the production of spasmogenic leukotrienes.

Least understood are the *psychologic factors* that influence the asthmatic patient. It is thought that emotional stress influences bronchomotor tone, rendering it more susceptible to irritant and allergic stimuli.

Bronchospasm is usually induced by nonspecific stimuli that presumably involve nonimmunologic pathways. Allergic asthma also has a background of hyper-reactivity to nonspecific stimuli, and this abnormality may persist long after atopy disappears.

CLINICAL MANIFESTATIONS. In most patients, an asthma attack begins with a nonproductive cough and wheezing, usually followed by a tightness in the chest and dyspnea. In a minority of patients, cough may be the most conspicuous and even sole manifestation of the attack. Attacks frequently occur at night and during sleep. They usually do not last for more than several hours and resolve spontaneously or with therapy. The end of an attack is often heralded by a change to a productive cough with expectoration of mucous plugs and casts.

Physical findings of airway obstruction include prolonged expiration and wheezing in both phases of respiration. In more severe attacks, increasing dyspnea may be associated with a diminution of wheezing. This may lead to a silent chest, an especially serious finding that suggests impending respiratory failure. Severe attacks are also associated with lung hyperinflation, causing an increase in the anteroposterior diameter of the chest wall and the finding of hyper-resonance and low diaphragms on chest percussion. Important physical findings in gauging the severity of the attack are the patient's use of accessory respiratory muscles, sternocleidomastoid retractions, and the appearance of pulsus paradoxus. Cyanosis is a late and unreliable sign.

LABORATORY FINDINGS. A wet preparation of sputum of many asthmatic patients contains spiral casts (Curschmann's spirals), eosinophils, and Charcot-Leyden crystals. The presence of sputum and blood eosinophilia is suggestive of the diagnosis of asthma but does not distinguish between extrinsic and intrinsic types.

Arterial blood gases should be obtained only in patients experiencing severe asthmatic attacks or prolonged attacks that are unresponsive to bronchodilator therapy. Hypoxemia is invariably present during an acute attack and, when mild to moderately severe, is usually associated with a decrease in the arterial P_{CO_2} and an increase in arterial pH. Hypocapnia and respiratory alkalosis are due to increased alveolar ventilation. Respiration may be stimulated by increased chemical drive (when Pa_{O_2} is less than 60 torr), but neurogenic reflexes (irritant and stretch receptors are probably more important. Determination of arterial blood gases is important for two reasons. First, the degree of hypoxemia generally reflects the degree of mismatching of ventilation to perfusion ($\dot{V}/\dot{Q}$) and thus gives some objective measure of the severity of airways disease. Second, a *normal* or increased Pa_{CO_2} signals severe airway obstruction and impending respiratory failure.

Chest roentgenograms may demonstrate lung hyperinflation, usually without parenchymal infiltrates. However, in patients with severe disease, roentgenograms should be scrutinized for (1) infiltrates suggesting a respiratory infection; (2) atelectasis or collapse of a segment or lobe, implicating mucous plugging of a bronchus; and (3) the presence of pneumothorax or pneumomediastinum.

Pulmonary function tests are important in assessing the severity of an attack and the response to bronchodilator therapy and in providing objective information about the resolution of disease. Pulmonary function tests may also be used to define hyperirritable airways in an asymptomatic asthma patient by provoking increases in airway resistance with aerosolized doses of histamine or methacholine, which would have no effect in normal individuals. In addition, the degree of airway hyper-responsiveness, as measured by these challenge tests, may give a more precise assessment of the severity of asthma. Pulmonary function tests may also identify patients with exercise-induced asthma.

During the acute attack, airway narrowing decreases the forced expiratory volume in one second (FEV_1), the maximal midexpiratory flow rates (MMF), and the peak expiratory flow rates. When the FEV_1, is less than 25 per cent of predicted (e.g., <1.0 liter), it is often accompanied by other signs of severe disease (e.g., pulsus paradoxus). All lung volumes are affected in an acute attack. There is a decrease in vital capacity (VC), with large increases in residual volume (RV), functional residual capacity (FRC), and total lung capacity (TLC). The peak expiratory flow rate (PEFR) is a particularly useful measurement because it is easy to perform repeatedly and does not require the patient to do the entire forced expiratory maneuver. The devices available for such measurements are small and convenient and may be kept in the home so that patients can produce daily records of their airway function.

Signs and symptoms are not entirely reliable in assessing the severity of an asthma attack or the optimal response to therapy. For example, in patients whose symptoms remit and signs of wheezing disappear, FEV_1's may be 40 to 60 per cent of normal and residual volumes greater than 200 per cent of predicted. Moreover, in patients whose attack has resolved for weeks or months, maximal midexpiratory flow rates may remain abnormal. The latter test emphasizes that the peripheral airways (less than 2 mm in diameter) are "silent" zones where considerable airway disease and obstruction may exist without signs or symptoms. These considerations have important therapeutic and clinical implications because the tendency for asthmatic attacks to recur seems to depend on the degree of residual disease. Also, a subpopulation of patients may have disease that exists predominantly in peripheral airways.

During symptom-free periods, skin tests or specific serum IgE antibodies (RAST test) may be useful in demonstrating hypersensitivity to suspected allergens. The use of RAST avoids the risk of sensitization or anaphylaxis and the need to interrupt medication. When compared with skin testing, however, it does not improve on specificity or sensitivity. Moreover, a positive skin test does not necessarily mean that exposure to the same allergen will produce respiratory symptoms. Newer inhalational tests may be more precise in identifying offending agents, including those that are implicated in occupational asthma and late-onset asthmatic responses. Use of these tests should be restricted to atypical patients in whom usual approaches are insufficient to establish a causative role for inhaled antigens.

DIFFERENTIAL DIAGNOSIS. Recurrent bronchospasm may occur in other diseases such as congestive heart failure, pulmonary embolism, and chronic bronchitis (see Ch. 61). There is usually little difficulty in distinguishing bronchospasm of congestive heart failure, since it is associated with other signs of underlying cardiac dysfunction. Distinguishing features of recurrent pulmonary emboli include pleural pain and effusions, signs of venous disease in the lower extremities, and characteristic findings on radioisotope lung scans and arteriography. Episodic and reversible wheezing may occur in patients with chronic bronchitis. In these patients, however, a persistent and productive cough exists in a setting of hyperirritable airways. Bronchospasm usually responds to bronchodilator therapy.

TREATMENT. Management of the asthmatic patient may be divided into two phases: treatment of the acute episode and maintenance therapy. The major classes of drugs will be reviewed as a background for recommendations on their optimal use in the treatment of asthma.

Sympathomimetic Drugs. *Epinephrine* has direct beta-adrenergic action but also stimulates alpha receptors. Its usefulness is limited by its actions on the heart, its restrictive use by inhalational and parenteral administration, and its short duration of action. Epinephrine is used in the treatment of acute asthmatic attacks and for this purpose is usually given in adults subcutaneously (0.2 to 0.5 ml of a 1:1000 solution). Tolerance develops after repeated use.

Isoproterenol has a potent selective beta-adrenergic effect. It is not absorbed orally, it has a relatively short duration of action, and certain patients may become refractory to its effects. Isoproterenol is usually administered by inhalation.

There are two types of beta-adrenergic receptors: $Beta_1$ agonists are cardiac stimulants (e.g., tachycardia); $beta_2$ agonists relax bronchial smooth muscle and blood vessels. The potential for selective $beta_2$ activity has led to the generation of new beta agonists with reduced cardiac side effects. These include the resorcinols, such as *metaproterenol* and *terbutaline*. The advantages of these agents are rapid onset of action, the potential for oral administration, and longer duration of action. Both agents are available in the United States for parenteral, oral, and aerosol administration. Skeletal muscle tremors are the main side effect. Newer agents with similar advantages but apparently even greater $beta_2$ selectivity are now available in the United States (e.g., *albuterol*). The use of $beta_2$ agents will probably replace the use of older, less specific drugs such as ephedrine.

The administration of $beta_2$ drugs, such as albuterol, has a number of advantages when used by the inhalational compared with the oral route. These include a rapid onset of action, fewer systemic side effects (skeletal muscle tremors), and preservation of $beta_2$ selectivity. When given by mouth, $beta_2$ drugs have a longer duration of action but lose $beta_2$ selectivity.

Because at least one third of asthmatic patients use metered dose inhalers incorrectly, it is important for physicians to ascertain personally that their patients learn proper inhalational techniques to insure adequate delivery of the drug (e.g., $beta_2$ agonists, beclomethasone).

Methylxanthines. Methylxanthines were once thought to cause smooth muscle relaxation by their action on the cytoplasmic enzyme phosphodiesterase. At the therapeutic doses currently used, however, tissue concentrations result in little (about 10 per cent) inhibition of phosphodiesterase. Other possible mechanisms of action of the methylxanthines are the enhancement of diaphragmatic contractility and the blocking of adenosine receptors, which may also play a role in bronchoconstriction. The recommended therapeutic concentration of *theophylline* in plasma is between 10 and 20 μg per milliliter. Because of considerable variation in metabolism of the drug, maintenance doses may range between 500 and 5000* mg per day. Thus, when theophylline preparations are used alone, blood levels should be determined to establish the proper dosage. When levels exceed 20 μg per milliliter, anorexia, nausea and gastrointestinal upset, and central nervous system irritability may occur. Newer timed-release preparations show promise of achieving more stable blood levels, reducing side effects, and permitting twice-a-day administration. Patients with congestive heart failure and liver disease usually require lower maintenance dosages; smokers may require higher doses.

Corticosteroids. Why corticosteroids are so effective in the treatment of asthma remains unclear. They stabilize cellular lysosomal membranes, reduce cellular stores of histamine and SRS-A, and restore the responsiveness of leukocytes and airway smooth muscle to beta agonists. Interestingly, corticosteroids do not inhibit the release of mediators or influence their effect on target cells. Their main action may be to inhibit the late cellular inflammatory response. Nonetheless, steroids are important therapeutic agents in patients whose symptoms cannot be controlled with optimal combinations of bronchodilator therapy or whose disease becomes progressively severe and life threatening.

The onset of action, whether the drug is given intravenously or orally, occurs at about six hours. Thus, patients whose disease is severe enough to require intravenous steroids should continue to receive optimal doses of bronchodilator

*This dose exceeds manufacturer's maximum recommended dose.

therapy. Patients who require maintenance steroid therapy should receive a short-acting drug, such as *prednisone*, in a single morning dose, and the course of therapy should be as short as possible to reduce pituitary adrenal suppression. Because of reduced side effects, alternate-day administration is preferable, and the dose should be tapered as rapidly as possible. Patients receiving corticosteroid therapy should be monitored for complications such as ulcer disease, reactivation of tuberculosis, hypertension, diabetes, and cataracts.

Some synthetic steroids, such as *beclomethasone diproprionate*, can be delivered by inhalation. When doses are between 400 and 1200 μg (8 to 24 puffs daily),* there is minimal systemic absorption. Side effects include oropharyngeal candidiasis and exacerbation of rhinitis, nasal polyposis, and atopic dermatitis. Inhaled steroids are usually used to withdraw patients from long-term systemic steroids. In this situation, it is important to watch for signs of adrenal insufficiency. Inhaled steroids are used to prevent asthmatic symptoms; they should not be used to treat acute attacks because they can worsen symptoms.

The Cromones. *Disodium cromoglycate* is believed to reduce the release of chemical mediators by its action on the mast cell or basophil membrane. It is not a bronchodilator, and it does not have anti-inflammatory or antihistaminic effects. Thus, it is a prophylactic drug and is not to be used during an acute asthmatic attack. In fact, inhalation of the drug may initiate or aggravate bronchospasm. Metered dose inhalers (two puffs or 2 mg every four to six hours), which are now available in the United States, are easier to use and permit more effective delivery of cromolyn sodium than inhalation of the dry powder by turbo-inhaler (Spinhaler). Response or failure of response to cromolyn sodium is unpredictable. For example, not only patients with extrinsic asthma but also a significant number of patients with mixed or intrinsic asthma, particularly those with exercise-induced bronchospasm, may benefit from the drug. In patients who respond to the drug, it may be possible to reduce or eliminate the use of corticosteroids. Because of its low frequency of toxicity and side effects, a trial of therapy with cromolyn sodium should be carried out in patients with moderate-to-severe asthma in whom conventional bronchodilator therapy has been inadequate. Proper evaluation of the drug requires a four- to eight-week course of therapy.

Anticholinergic Agents. Atropine is one of the oldest treatments in asthma but has been all but abandoned because of its untoward side effects. Interest, however, has been rekindled in atropine-like drugs because of new insights into neurogenic mechanisms involving the vagal reflexes (Fig. 60–4) and the development of a congener of atropine (*ipratropium*), which is a nonabsorbable aerosol and remarkably free of side effects. Ipratropium may be useful as an adjunct to current therapy and of value to patients whose predominant symptom is chronic bronchitis or cough.

Calcium Antagonists. Another group of investigational drugs are the calcium antagonists. The translocation of calcium from the external medium or cell stores into the cytosol is a fundamental signal in the stimulation of mast cell and mucous gland secretion and smooth muscle contraction. With the aim of blocking this signal, calcium antagonists (*verapamil* and *nifedipine*) have been given by mouth or inhalation to asthmatic patients to alleviate bronchoconstriction. Some benefit has been achieved in patients with exercise-induced asthma, but the exact role of these agents in the management of asthma is unclear.

Management of the Acute Asthmatic Attack. There is no simple recipe for the management of the asthmatic patient. Each therapeutic program must be tailored to the patient. The following comments are meant to be general guidelines.

*This dose exceeds manufacturer's maximum recommended dose.

For patients with mild attacks, one drug may suffice. Therapy may begin with a theophylline preparation of a beta$_2$ sympathomimetic amine or both. Theophylline may be started at dosages (200 mg) that produce few or no side effects. If this is inadequate, the addition of a beta$_2$ sympathomimetic amine, preferably by inhalation (metered dose inhaler), may be effective with relatively low doses of theophylline. There is an additive effect when a beta-adrenergic agent is combined with theophylline. Thus, when used together, therapeutic doses and side effects of either agent may be reduced.

In the treatment of asthma, therapy should be guided by objective evidence (e.g., pulmonary function tests) rather than relying solely on the resolution of symptoms or signs. The measurement of FEV$_1$ or PEFR is appropriate and can be performed in the physician's office or at home (PEFR).

If asthma becomes progressively more severe or if the patient does not respond adequately to therapy after several hours of observation, then the patient should be hospitalized. Aminophylline may then be given by continuous intravenous infusion. The initial recommended dosage for adult patients is a loading dose of 5.6 mg per kilogram given over 15 to 30 minutes, followed by a continuous infusion of 0.9 mg per kilogram per hour for smokers, 0.6 mg per kilogram per hour for nonsmokers, and 0.3 mg per kilogram per hour for severely ill patients (e.g., congestive heart failure, pneumonia, and liver disease). Maintenance doses must also be reduced ($\simeq$ 0.3 mg per kilogram per hour) for patients taking certain drugs, such as cimetidine or triacetyloleandomycin, which interfere with hepatic microsomal enzymes. After 36 hours, theophylline levels should be measured. If patients have recently received theophylline, then the loading dose should be decreased (50 to 75 per cent) or eliminated to avoid toxic levels and a continuous infusion begun. Patients should also receive controlled oxygen therapy and physiotherapy to relieve bronchial secretions. Fluids are given by mouth or intravenous infusion to correct dehydration if present. Electrolyte imbalance, particularly hypokalemia, should be corrected. Tranquilizers and sedatives must be avoided.

If the patient remains unresponsive or the attack becomes more severe, then the patient must be hospitalized and treated with corticosteroids, with continuation of full dosages of bronchodilator therapy. The correct dosage for intravenous corticosteroids is unsettled. One regimen recommends 2 mg per kilogram of methylprednisolone sodium succinate initially, followed by 1 to 2 mg per kilogram every four to six hours. When clinical signs and objective evidence indicate that the patient is responding to therapy, usually after 48 to 72 hours, then steroids may be converted to oral preparations. Sixty mg of prednisone may be started as a single morning dose. If the patient continues to improve, it may be reduced by 5 mg every third or fourth day.

In some patients it may not be possible to withdraw steroids. In this situation, the following approaches may be tried: maintenance with the lowest possible dose given on alternate days, a trial of cromolyn therapy, or conversion to aerosolized steroids. It is important that the latter two agents should be started only after there has been an optimal therapeutic response for the acute attack.

Long-term Management. Maintenance therapy should be based on similar clinical and objective criteria as in treating the acute attack. For example, outpatient spirograms should be used routinely in following the patient. Also, the patient should be convinced as to the chronicity of the disease and dissuaded from adjusting or stopping medication when symptoms abate. Asthma should not be treated symptomatically.

It is also important to identify specific precipitating or triggering factors, including allergic and nonallergic stimuli. A thorough history may allow elimination of offending agents from the environment or occupation. Other underlying conditions such as chronic sinusitis should be carefully evaluated (e.g., sinus roentgenograms). The successful medical or surgical treatment of chronic sinusitis may have a dramatic impact on the treatment of asthma.

Immunotherapy with extracts of allergens may benefit certain allergic patients. This form of therapy, however, is just beginning to be established on firm scientific grounds.

Patients with late-onset asthmatic responses may not be adequately managed on maintenance bronchodilator therapy alone (beta$_2$ drugs and aminophylline). Beta$_2$ bronchodilators and theophylline are not effective in preventing or reversing the late-onset reactions. In contrast, corticosteroids inhibit as well as reverse the inflammatory response of the late-onset reaction. Cromolyn sodium is useful strictly because it is a prophylactic agent. Thus, the use of cromolyn sodium or steroids (by mouth or inhalation) or both may be necessary for successful long-term maintenance therapy of late-onset asthma. A trial of immunotherapy may also benefit this group of patients.

PROGNOSIS. There are about 9 million patients with asthma in the United States, and several thousand deaths per year are attributable to the disease. Statistics concerning the long-term prognosis of asthma are as variable as the disease. For example,the percentage of childhood asthma reported to persist until adult life varies from 26 to 78 per cent. Also, it is generally held, without good data, that adult asthma improves or disappears with age. Taken together, the evidence supports Osler's adage that "asthmatics pant their way into old age."

Anderson SD: Issues in exercise-induced asthma. J Allergy Clin Immunol 76:763, 1985. *A review of the pathophysiologic mechanisms involved in exercise-induced asthma. It contrasts the evidence implicating heat versus water loss as the primary stimuli for this phenomenon.*

Barnes NC, Costello JF: Mast-cell–derived mediators in asthma: Arachidonic acid metabolites. Postgrad Med 76:140, 148, 1984. *A clear and concise summary of a difficult subject dealing with arachidonic acid metabolic pathways. It describes how leukotrienes and prostaglandins are generated within the lung and their potential role in bronchoconstriction.*

Cherniack RM: Chronic and acute asthma: Key to successful management. Postgrad Med 75:87, 1984. *A practical review of management strategies for acute and chronic asthma.*

Kaliner MA: Hypotheses on the contribution of late-phase allergic responses to the understanding and treatment of allergic diseases. J Allergy Clin Immunol 75:311, 1985. *A current and concise review of the pathophysiologic events involved in the late-onset asthmatic reactions. It also discusses the clinical implications and the drugs that are efficacious in reversing or preventing late-onset reactions.*

McFadden ER Jr, Feldman NT: Asthma: Pathophysiology and clinical correlates. Med Clin North Am 61:1229, 1977. *A review that summarizes the correlations between manifestations and pulmonary function abnormalities.*

Morris HG: Mechanisms of action and therapeutic role of corticosteroids in asthma. J Allergy Clin Immunol 75:1, 1985. *A review of our current understanding of the mechanisms of action of corticosteroids in inhibiting the inflammatory response in asthma. It also identifies current indications, efficacy, and side effects of systemic and topical steroids that are used in the therapy of bronchial asthma. It contains an extensive bibliography.*

Nadel JA, Barnes PJ: Autonomic regulation of the airways. Ann Rev Med 35:451, 1984. *Reviews the sympathetic and parasympathetic innervation of the airways with particular reference to how they modulate smooth muscle tone and mucosal gland secretion. It also presents evidence implicating autonomic dysfunction in asthma.*

Sheppard D: Mechanisms of bronchoconstriction from nonimmunologic environmental stimuli. Chest 90:584, 1986. *A brief review that discusses the general mechanisms by which diverse inhaled agents cause bronchoconstriction by nonimmunologic mechanisms.*

Weinberger M, Hendeles L: Current concepts: Slow-release theophylline: Rationale and basis for product selection. N Engl J Med 308:760, 1983. *A review of the therapeutic strategies for theophylline. It also contains details on drug preparations and their doses.*

Woolcock AJ, Yan K, Salome CM, et al.: What determines the severity of asthma? Chest 87:209S, 1985. *A good discussion of epidemiologic and clinical factors that are considered to influence the severity of asthma.*

61 CHRONIC AIRWAYS DISEASES*

Richard A. Matthay

CHRONIC BRONCHITIS AND EMPHYSEMA

Chronic generalized airway disorders that are not the direct result of a "specific" bronchopulmonary disease are discussed in this chapter. Common to most of these diseases is chronic airways obstruction, caused most frequently by a diffuse involvement of peripheral (small) airways or, more rarely, by localized obstruction of central (large) airways. The designation *chronic obstructive pulmonary disease (COPD)* is an imperfect, although widely utilized, term, since it includes several specific disorders with different clinical manifestations, pathologic findings, therapy requirements, and prognoses.

Four *diffuse* airway disorders are examined in this chapter: simple chronic bronchitis, asthmatic bronchitis, chronic obstructive bronchitis, and emphysema. Some classifications include all of these entities in the broad term COPD. Moreover, various combinations of these disorders coexist; for instance, patients often have chronic obstructive bronchitis as well as emphysema. *Localized* airway obstruction, above and below the tracheal bifurcation, is discussed in a separate section of this chapter.

DEFINITIONS OF TERMS. Unfortunately, *chronic bronchitis* has been used variably to refer to a simple smoker's cough or, as in the British literature, to severe COPD. In this discussion, chronic bronchitis will be considered "simple," "obstructive," or "asthmatic" to reduce ambiguity. It is useful clinically to differentiate between the extremely common simple chronic bronchitis and the less common but often devastating form, chronic obstructive bronchitis. These two entities will therefore be described in separate sections.

Simple chronic bronchitis, a syndrome characterized primarily by a chronic productive cough, is the result of low-grade exposure to bronchial irritants in an individual without hyperreactive airways. This syndrome is associated with enhanced mucous secretion, reduced ciliary activity, and impaired resistance to bronchial infection. Simple chronic bronchitis is defined in clinical terms: (1) excessive production of mucus; (2) presence of symptoms, largely cough, on most days for at least three months annually during two or more successive years; and (3) exclusion of bronchiectasis, tuberculosis, or other causes of these symptoms. The term does not describe the underlying process, which may vary widely. The patient population ranges from those who are asymptomatic except for a morning "cigarette cough" productive of mucus in small amounts (*simple chronic bronchitis*) to patients with a severe disabling condition manifested by increased resistance to airflow, hypoxia, and often hypercapnia (*chronic obstructive bronchitis*). Chronic obstructive bronchitis, which develops in a relatively small proportion of individuals with simple chronic bronchitis, results in irreversible narrowing of air-

*Portions of this chapter were rewritten from the 17th edition of *Cecil Textbook of Medicine*, with permission from Benjamin Burrows.

TABLE 61–1. FEATURES OF THE EMPHYSEMATOUS AND BRONCHIAL TYPES OF COPD

	Emphysematous (Type A)	Bronchial (Type B)
Clinical features		
Dyspnea	Insidious onset, slowly progressive	Often noted first only during chest infections
Sputum	Usually scant and mucoid	Often copious and purulent
Weight loss	Often marked	Usually slight or absent
Chronic cor pulmonale with heart failure	Infrequent until terminal stages of the disease	Common
Chest examination	Quiet chest (except slight wheeze at end expiration), marked hyperinflation	Noisy chest, slight hyperinflation
Chest radiograph	Hyperlucent, overinflated lung; often regional attenuation of vessels	Often evidence of old inflammatory disease
Physiologic tests		
Total lung capacity	Increased	Normal or slightly decreased
Residual volume	Markedly increased	Moderately increased
Lung compliance, static	Increased	Near normal
Lung compliance, dynamic	Normal or slightly low	Very low
Lung recoil	Markedly reduced	Variable
Inspiratory airways resistance	Normal	Increased
Diffusing capacity	Markedly reduced	Variable
Arterial P_{O_2}	Slight reduction at rest; usually falls with exertion	Often very low at rest; variable change with exertion
Arterial P_{CO_2}	Usually normal or low	Often chronically elevated
Resting pulmonary artery pressure	Normal or slightly elevated at rest; increases with exertion	Often markedly elevated at rest
Cardiac output	Often low	Usually near normal

ways. Because the obstruction is in bronchioles and bronchi 2 mm or less in diameter, the term *small airways disease* has been used.

Exposure to bronchial irritants in individuals with hyper-reactive or "twitchy" airways can lead to bronchospasm (i.e., bronchial smooth muscle constriction), frequently accompanied by excessive mucous production and edema of bronchial walls. Recurrent episodes of symptomatic bronchospasm are called *asthma* (discussed in Ch. 60). The present discussion must consider bronchospasm, since a degree of reversible airways obstruction often accompanies other reactions to inhaled noxious agents. In fact, episodic airways obstruction is common in individuals with chronic bronchitis. This combination, called *asthmatic bronchitis,* may closely resemble classic asthma. The term *chronic asthmatic bronchitis* is applied in patients with persistent airways obstruction, a chronic productive cough, and a major problem of episodic bronchospasm.

Emphysema, another lung response to noxious stimuli, is characterized by abnormal, permanent enlargement of airspaces distal to the terminal bronchioles, accompanied by destruction of their walls, and without obvious fibrosis. The alterations of emphysema cause reduction in lung elastic recoil, which permits excessive airway collapse upon expiration and leads to irreversible airflow obstruction.

These definitions are not mutually exclusive; there is considerable crossover between the emphysematous (type A) and bronchial (type B) findings listed in Table 61–1. For example, most individuals with emphysema also have a chronic productive cough. It may be difficult to determine the relative importance of emphysema and chronic obstructive bronchitis, with obliteration of small airways. Accordingly, general terms such as *chronic obstructive pulmonary disease (COPD)* have been used to describe this clinical syndrome.

PATHOPHYSIOLOGY OF AIRWAYS OBSTRUCTION. Airways obstruction denotes slowing of forced expiration. As outlined in Ch. 59, the speed of forced expiration is determined primarily by three factors: intrinsic resistance of the airways, compressibility of the airways, and lung elastic recoil. Reduced maximum expiratory flow ($\dot{V}max$) results from high airways resistance, reduced lung recoil, and/or excessive airways collapsibility.

In general, a low FEV_1/FVC* ratio is indicative of airflow obstruction; the amount of reduction in FEV_1 itself establishes the severity of the obstruction (Fig. 61–1). Some prefer to use $FEF_{25-75\%}$, the average flow over the middle half of a forced expiration.

Actual $\dot{V}max$ values can be measured, commonly at 50 per cent or 75 per cent of the forced expired volume ($\dot{V}max_{50\%}$ or $\dot{V}max_{75\%}$, respectively*). $\dot{V}max_{75\%}$ has become popular in epidemiologic studies because it appears to be more sensitive than the FEV_1.

In clinical practice, FEV_1 is used more widely because it is easy to measure, is quite reproducible, has a relatively narrow normal range, and tends to reflect the clinical severity of disease.

A variety of physiologic abnormalities are associated with obstructive airways disorders (also discussed in Ch. 59). Increased venous admixture and hypoxemia develop owing to ventilation and perfusion mismatching. Unless there is an increase in overall ventilation, this mismatching also may lead to increased physiologic dead space and hypercapnia. Carbon dioxide retention is likely when airways obstruction is severe, respiratory muscle fatigue occurs, and the drive to breathe is depressed. Air trapping and an increase in residual volume develop because obstructed airways tend to close prematurely during a maximal exhalation. In emphysema, total lung capacity may be enhanced as well. The pulmonary diffusing capacity measurement is usually reduced in emphysema owing to loss of functioning alveolar capillary membrane surface area.

Because of the large total cross-sectional diameter of the small airways, marked alterations are required to produce discernible changes in the FEV_1 values. Several potentially more sensitive tests have been proposed to detect mild abnormalities of the small airways: closing volume, helium response of the maximal expiratory flow volume (MEFV) curve, and frequency dependence of compliance. These tests are specific for small airways abnormalities, but clinical application has not been established yet.

Burrows B: An overview of obstructive lung disease. Med Clin North Am 65:455, 1981. *This is the lead article of an 11-chapter symposium on obstructive lung diseases. The entire symposium is recommended reading and an excellent source of original references.*

Fishman AP: The spectrum of chronic obstructive disease of the airways. In

*FEV_1 = forced expiratory volume in one second; FVC = forced vital capacity; FEF = forced expiratory flow.

*Because use of these symbols has caused confusion, it has been suggested that $\dot{V}max_{50\%}$ and $\dot{V}max_{75\%}$ be expressed as $FEF_{50\%}$ and $FEF_{75\%}$, respectively. Moreover, $\dot{V}max_{75\%}$ as defined herein has sometimes been reported as $\dot{V}max_{25\%}$, the 25% referring to the portion of the FVC remaining when the flow measurement is made.

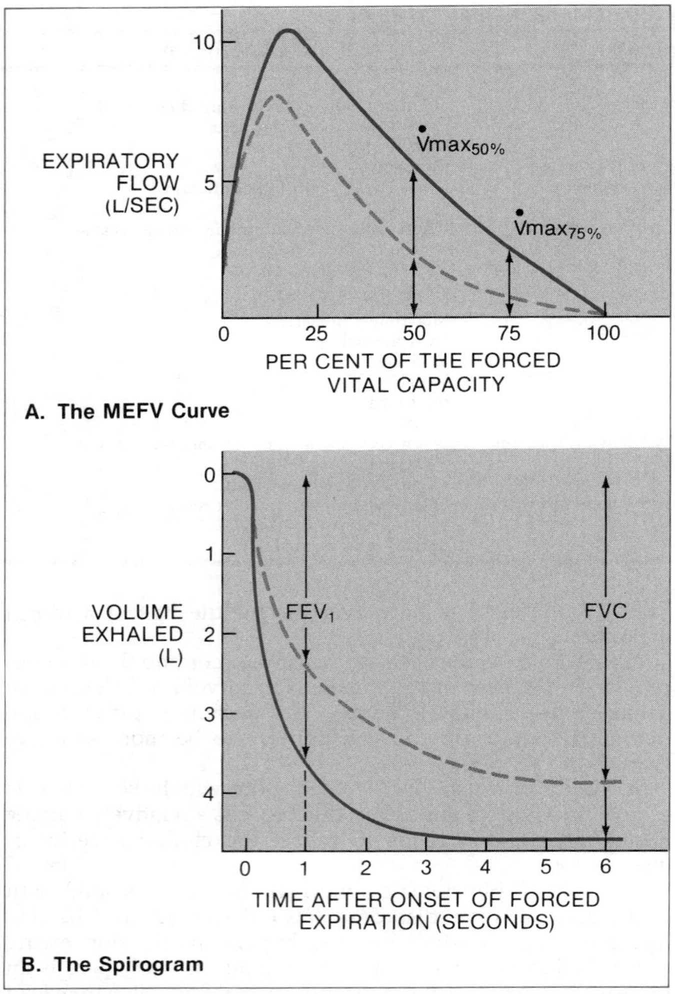

FIGURE 61–1. Solid lines are used to show a normal maximum expiratory flow-volume (MEFV) in *A* and a normal spirogram in *B*. Broken lines indicate typical curves for a patient with mild airways obstruction. Measurements of the forced vital capacity (FVC), the forced expiratory volume at one second (FEV_1), and forced flow rates at 50 per cent and 75 per cent of the FVC ($\dot{V}max_{50\%}$ and $\dot{V}max_{75\%}$) are depicted as vertical lines. (Adapted from Burrows B: Chronic airways disease. Cecil Textbook of Medicine. 17th ed.)

Fishman AP (ed.): Pulmonary Diseases and Disorders. New York, McGraw-Hill Book Company, 1980, p 458. *A concise, clearly written description of the different types of airways obstructive disorders and how they overlap.*

Snider GL, Kleinerman J, Thurlbeck WM, et al.: The definition of emphysema. Am Rev Respir Dis 132:182, 1985. *Up-to-date, succinct statement of the definition, anatomic subtypes, and clinical diagnosis of emphysema.*

Thurlbeck WM: The anatomical pathology of chronic airflow obstruction. Curr Pulmonol 4:1, 1982. *A good discussion of the pathologic conditions associated with airways obstruction.*

Simple Chronic Bronchitis and Asthmatic Bronchitis

PREVALENCE AND PATHOGENESIS. "Simple chronic bronchitis" refers to a productive cough that persists for at least three months of the year for two consecutive years. It affects 10 to 25 per cent of the adult population. Cough with sputum production is more common in men than in women and more common in persons over the age of 40 than in younger individuals. All forms of chronic bronchitis are strongly linked to cigarette smoking. Thus, a large proportion of cigarette smokers, particularly those over age 45, have simple chronic bronchitis. Some occupations involving dust (e.g., handling grain and mining) are associated with an abnormally high incidence of chronic bronchitis, even after statistics are corrected for smoking habits. Few individuals with simple chronic bronchitis consult a physician, and then the visit is usually prompted by acute or recurrent respiratory tract infections or wheezing in addition to chronic cough. *Chronic asthmatic bronchitis* tends to develop in elderly individuals, most commonly in smokers. Three direct effects of inhaling bronchial irritants cause chronic bronchitis: (1) stimulation of mucous secretion in the airways, (2) impaired mucous clearance due in part to interference with ciliary activity, and (3) lowered resistance to bronchopulmonary infection due to disturbed alveolar macrophage function. Cough develops owing to accumulation of secretions. As a result of bacterial colonization by organisms usually found in the nasopharynx, normally sterile bronchi now harbor organisms.

Although cigarette smoking is the most important of the identifiable causal factors, not all smokers develop mucus hypersecretion and no more than 15 to 20 per cent develop airflow obstruction. Little is known about the reasons for the variable susceptibility to hypersecretion and airflow obstruction in smokers or why reversible airways obstruction develops in many patients with chronic bronchitis. Retention of secretions may be a major factor in some instances. Immunologic factors and other mediators of bronchoconstriction may play a role, since some patients have subacute or chronic bronchospasm resembling classic asthma.

PATHOLOGY. Enlargement of mucous glands in the large airways, the most characteristic abnormality, is primarily due to increased numbers of their constituent cells (hyperplasia) rather than to enlargement of cells (hypertrophy). Retained bronchial secretions and variable degrees of inflammatory changes in the bronchial walls also are identified. Narrowing or obliteration of some small airways, increased mucus in these airways, and scattered centrilobular emphysema may be found, even though clinically significant obstruction is absent. Since asymptomatic smokers may have similar small airways and emphysematous changes, it is unclear whether these alterations are related to simple chronic bronchitis except through a common association with cigarette smoking.

CLINICAL MANIFESTATIONS. When the disease is mild, *cough* occurs on arising or usually after smoking the first cigarette of the day. The cough is productive of a small amount of mucoid sputum and occurs most regularly in the winter months. As the severity increases, the patient coughs throughout the day, symptoms are present throughout the year, sputum volume increases, and episodes of severe coughing develop. Near the end of a severe paroxysm of coughing, wheezing may occur, probably owing to cough-induced bronchospasm. Lying down may induce wheezing, which is probably caused by retained secretions, for cough often provides relief.

Symptoms associated with purulent sputum, suggesting overgrowth of bacteria, may reappear after a viral respiratory infection. *Haemophilus influenzae* and *Streptococcus pneumoniae* may be present, but sputum cultures usually show normal nasopharyngeal flora.

Bacterial organisms probably represent secondary pathogens rather than being the primary cause of these exacerbations of symptoms. During exacerbations, various degrees of bronchospasm also may develop, blurring the distinction between such episodes and asthma. Whereas *blood-streaked sputum* is noted occasionally, severe or repeated hemoptysis may indicate a more serious entity, such as pulmonary neoplasm.

The sputum may become chronically purulent as the disorder progresses, and the term *mucopurulent bronchitis* may be applied to this stage of the disease. Rarely, drug-resistant organisms (e.g., *Pseudomonas aeruginosa*) are identified on sputum cultures, especially if the patient has received multiple antibiotics.

In mild disease, physical examination may be normal. As the disease advances, variable coarse crackles, which may clear or change location with coughing, and scattered wheezes are heard. A forced expiratory maneuver often induces a wheeze or a paroxysm of coughing.

If reversible airway obstruction is present, the patient may resemble the typical asthmatic person, with wheezing and slowing of forced expiration as prominent features.

LABORATORY FINDINGS. The chest radiograph, blood counts, and differential smear are all normal in the uncomplicated case. Leukocytes and a mixed flora of organisms are noted on sputum examination. Although spirometry often shows some slowing of forced expiration, flow rates may be normal in simple bronchitis. Individuals with *chronic asthmatic bronchitis* may have severe airways obstruction even between acute attacks. During episodes of bronchospasm in patients with asthmatic bronchitis, functional abnormalities are more severe, and both blood and sputum eosinophilia may be present.

COURSE AND PROGNOSIS. In patients with simple chronic bronchitis, symptoms may fluctuate widely. Increased cigarette use, inclement weather, and acute respiratory infections all tend to enhance cough and sputum production. Cessation of smoking in mild cases usually leads to disappearance of symptoms. A slight reduction in ventilatory function is common in simple chronic bronchitis, but progressive respiratory insufficiency does not necessarily develop.

The long-term outcome of patients with asthmatic bronchitis has not been studied extensively. Some patients may become asymptomatic for years after an initial excellent response to therapy, whereas others require progressively more medication to control bronchospasm. Progress to irreversible airways obstruction occurs in at least a few patients despite good medical management.

DIFFERENTIAL DIAGNOSIS. A persistent, productive cough not attributable to an upper respiratory tract disorder, an allergic reaction of the airways, a specific endobronchial disease, or parenchymal lung disease justifies the diagnosis of chronic bronchitis. Exclusion of a parenchymal lesion requires a chest radiograph. Moreover, a careful upper airway examination should be done, and physical findings, such as a persistent, localized wheeze, must be sought to identify a localized airways disorder. Cystic fibrosis must be excluded in children and in young adults who have severe symptoms of chronic bronchitis (see Ch. 66). In addition, in individuals with one of the immotile cilia syndromes, symptoms of chronic bronchitis may be noted (see Ch. 65).

When there is no identifiable source of chronic bronchial irritation, the diagnosis of simple chronic bronchitis should be made with caution. Sputum and blood eosinophilia should be sought in a nonsmoking patient whose symptoms are associated with exposure to allergens or in a patient with episodes of combined wheezing and dyspnea. Asthmatic bronchitis, which may respond to bronchodilators or corticosteroids, is suggested by high eosinophil levels.

Bronchoscopy and even bronchography or a computed tomography (CT) scan may be indicated to rule out an endobronchial lesion or localized bronchiectasis in patients with severe or repeated hemoptysis or with physical findings suggesting localized disease. In the routine case, these procedures are not indicated.

Severe mucopurulent bronchitis may be difficult to distinguish from bronchiectasis. In fact, in persons with severe bronchitis, the bronchi may show mild, diffuse, cylindric dilatation. Saccular bronchiectasis is suggested by (1) repeated pneumonias in the same lung zone, (2) honeycombed areas on the chest radiograph, and (3) recurrent hemoptysis. Bronchography provides an accurate diagnosis, but this invasive procedure is usually indicated only if resection of the bronchiectatic area or areas is considered. Otherwise, there is little difference in therapy for mucopurulent bronchitis and bronchiectasis. Computed tomography of the chest has been used successfully to diagnose localized and diffuse bronchiectasis.

TREATMENT. Cigarettes and any other bronchial irritants should be removed initially, since this step alone may relieve the symptoms. If the symptoms persist after maximal effort to avoid provoking factors, the following measures are applied.

Antibiotic Therapy. Infection is considered present when the patient is producing a noneosinophilic purulent sputum. A seven- to ten-day course of tetracycline or ampicillin (1 gram daily in divided doses) or double-strength sulfamethoxazole-trimethoprim (one tablet twice daily) should be administered. Failure of this antibiotic therapy to clear the sputum warrants a sputum culture and sensitivity test. Successive doses of different antibiotics should be avoided, since this may lead to resistant flora. Therapeutic failure generally is due to inadequate drainage of the airways more often than to an improper choice of antibacterial drugs.

The antibiotic may have to be changed on the basis of drug susceptibility studies when resistant organisms are cultured from the sputum. (For severe purulent exacerbations, penicillin has proved to be inadequate therapy.)

Bronchodilators. The bronchodilator agents are the mainstays for managing bronchospasm associated with simple chronic bronchitis and for control of any reversible component of COPD. They are also useful in conjunction with bronchial hygiene therapy, described below. Both of the main classes of bronchodilators, the methylxanthines and the beta-adrenergic agonists, help to relieve bronchospasm and to prevent recurrent attacks. The inhaled route of administering beta-adrenergic drugs is usually more effective and rapid in relieving bronchospasm than the oral route. Patients must be carefully instructed, however, in the proper technique for utilizing inhalers. Inhaled atropine may exhibit a combined beneficial effect of reducing copious amounts of sputum and partially relieving bronchospasm in the person with severe bronchitis. The principles and details for therapeutic application of these agents are described in Ch. 60.

Corticosteroids. When significant airways obstruction persists or recurs in the patient with asthmatic bronchitis in spite of maximal therapy with bronchodilators, corticosteroids are indicated. If the patient is ambulatory, modest doses (e.g., 20 to 40 mg of prednisone per day) are administered for several days and then tapered to the lowest dose that will sustain improvement. Often, improvement is rapid, and the drug can be discontinued in seven to ten days. Thereafter, a short "burst" of corticosteroids is used to treat occasional relapses. In some patients, tapering corticosteroids leads to recurrence of symptoms. In these individuals, the dose should be maintained as low as possible to relieve bronchospasm and to prevent recurrent attacks. Alternate-day single-dose corticosteroids should be used if possible.

Once bronchospasm has been relieved and a maintenance dose of corticosteroid achieved, an inhaled, poorly absorbed preparation such as beclomethasone should be added. This medication is inhaled from a pressurized container, two to four puffs (100 to 200 μg) two to four times daily, depending upon the preparation. The inhaled agent may permit reduction in the maintenance dose of corticosteroid without recurrence of bronchospasm. When significant bronchospasm is present, inhaled corticosteroid agents should be avoided, since this medication may aggravate bronchoconstriction and fail to reach the distal airways. For some patients, premedication with an inhaled bronchodilator (e.g., a beta-adrenergic agent) may relieve airway irritation and permit successful use of inhaled corticosteroids. In general, inhaled corticosteroids replace 7.5 to 10 mg per day of oral prednisone.

After the addition of an inhaled agent, the dose of oral prednisone should be reduced slowly (over several months) to avoid adrenal insufficiency in a corticosteroid-dependent patient who has received months or years of systemic medication. In up to 30 per cent of patients, oropharyngeal candidiasis occurs owing to inhaled corticosteroids. This condition responds, however, to specific therapy and rarely requires discontinuation of the inhaled preparation. Nasal symptoms, previously controlled by oral prednisone, may recur, requiring reinstitution of oral agents.

Bronchial Hygiene. These measures are designed to clear retained bronchial secretions. Deep breathing followed by deliberate coughing is the most important maneuver. Sputum production may be more effective if the most involved lung regions are in the superior position (postural drainage) and chest percussion and vibration are applied.

Bronchial hygiene measures may be better tolerated and more effective if the patient is premedicated with an inhaled bronchodilator and then inhales a bland mist to loosen secretions. Although some patients are convinced of its efficacy, objective benefits of bland mist therapy have been difficult to establish. Because patients' reactions to this therapy vary, only measures that prove effective should be continued, since the full program is uncomfortable and time consuming.

To avoid inspissation of secretions, patients should be encouraged to keep well hydrated. Intravenous fluids may be required for acute exacerbations. Although the efficacy of expectorant medications has not been established, some authorities recommend 10 to 12 drops of a saturated solution of potassium iodide three times daily. This program is associated with a high rate of side effects, some severe; yet, it does seem effective in some patients. Cough syrups and lozenges have little effect on the viscosity of bronchial secretions, but they may relieve a "tickle" in the throats of many persons with bronchitis. Cough sedatives should be used only for acute episodes of a severe, nonproductive cough and are otherwise contraindicated.

Treatment of Severe Exacerbations. Severe exacerbations of asthmatic bronchitis can be life threatening, particularly when associated with severe airways obstruction. The approach to status asthmaticus outlined in Ch. 60 is appropriate, although the patient with asthmatic bronchitis may require more attention to bronchial hygiene measures to clear secretions than does the person with classic asthma.

Anthonisen NR, Manfreda J, Warren CPW, et al.: Antibiotic therapy in exacerbations of chronic obstructive pulmonary disease. Ann Intern Med 106:196, 1987. *Double-blind placebo controlled trial that reports significant benefit from antimicrobial therapy during exacerbations of chronic bronchitis.*

Burrows B: Irreversible airways obstruction and asthma. Pract Cardiol 8:69, 1982. *This article presents in more detail views concerning the overlap of reversible and irreversible airways obstructive diseases.*

Burrows B, Lebowitz MD, Barbee RA, et al.: Interactions of smoking and immunological factors in relationship to airways obstruction. Chest 84:657, 1983. *This paper presents evidence that chronic asthmatic bronchitis may result from an interaction of the irritant effects of smoking and immunologic factors.*

Iafrate RP, Massey KL, Hendeles L: Current concepts in clinical therapeutics: Asthma. Clin Pharmacol Ther 5:206, 1986. *A good review of the use of bronchodilators and corticosteroids in reversible airways diseases.*

IPPB Trial Group: Intermittent positive pressure breathing therapy of chronic obstructive pulmonary disease. Ann Intern Med 99:612, 1983. *This study establishes that there is no significant benefit in positive pressure breathing over other modalities of delivering bronchodilators.*

Sachs FL: Chronic bronchitis. In Pennington JE (ed.): Respiratory Infections: Diagnosis and Management. New York, Raven Press, 1983, p 113. *Comprehensive review of the etiologic role and need for therapy of respiratory infection during exacerbations of chronic bronchitis.*

Chronic Obstructive Bronchitis and Emphysema

PREVALENCE AND PATHOGENESIS. As a major cause of chronic disability in older individuals, chronic obstructive bronchitis and emphysema (COPD) rank only behind heart disease and schizophrenia in the United States. Chronic obstructive pulmonary disease is the fifth leading cause of death in the United States, and there has been a 22 per cent increase in the death rate from this condition over the past 20 years. Approximately 65,000 individuals die yearly from COPD in the United States, one half of the number dying annually from lung cancer.

Emphysema is common and increases with age. It is present at autopsy in approximately 65 per cent of adult men and 15 per cent of adult women. The prevalence of emphysema is strongly related to cigarette smoking.

Chronic obstructive pulmonary disease is usually diagnosed between ages 55 and 65. The greater incidence in men than in women most likely reflects the lower incidence of smoking in women in earlier decades. Recent trends, however, show that more teenage girls than boys are starting to smoke. Thus, in several decades COPD may be as common or more common in women.

Smoking. Patients with COPD have some combination of chronic obstructive bronchitis and pulmonary emphysema, both of which are closely associated with cigarette smoking. The chronic, progressive destruction of the alveolar structures characteristic of emphysema is thought to occur because of an imbalance between the proteases (proteolytic enzymes) and antiproteases in the lower respiratory tract. According to this concept, proteases, particularly neutrophil (PMN) elastase and possibly elastases in pulmonary alveolar macrophages (PAM's), work unimpeded to destroy alveolar structures and their elastin network. Cigarette smokers have increased numbers of PAM's, and PMN's are recruited into their lungs so that increased numbers of both cell types are recoverable on bronchoalveolar lavage. Recruitment of PMN's into the lungs may occur as a result of the elaboration of chemotactic factors by PAM's stimulated by cigarette smoke. Moreover, smoke components can cause elastase to be released by PMN's by inducing cytotoxic reactions and by stimulating secretion from viable cells. Macrophages exposed to cigarette smoke in vitro or in vivo increase secretion of an elastase-like enzyme. This potential for a greatly increased protease (primarily elastase) burden must be counteracted by the antiprotease defense system of the lungs.

The protease-antiprotease theory of the pathogenesis of emphysema has received further support from the recognition that patients with severe (homozygous phenotype) $alpha_1$-antitypsin deficiency have markedly reduced levels of serum $alpha_1$-antitrypsin and progressive panacinar emphysema. As might be expected, patients with severe $alpha_1$-antitrypsin deficiency have little or no $alpha_1$-antitrypsin in their lower respiratory tracts when studied by bronchoalveolar lavage. Nor do they have alternate antiprotease protection against neutrophil elastase.

Cigarette smokers without $alpha_1$-antitrypsin deficiency also show reduced elastase inhibitory capacity, compared with nonsmokers, because of inactivation of $alpha_1$–proteinase inhibitor ($alpha_1$-PI). Chemical oxidation of $alpha_1$-PI by material in cigarette smoke is postulated as a major cause of the observed decrease in elastase inhibitory capacity. Smoking may interfere with elastin repair mechanisms, as documented by studies both in vivo and in vitro.

Severe genetic deficiency of serum $alpha_1$-antitrypsin occurs in 0.5 to 2 per cent of patients with COPD. Typically, in such individuals, emphysema is likely to develop by age 40 in smokers and by age 60 in nonsmokers. Presumably, prolonged exposure to irritants, primarily cigarette smoke, further reduces lung antiprotease defenses and induces low-grade inflammation and destructive changes in the parenchyma of the lungs.

The protease-antiprotease hypothesis of the pathogenesis of emphysema does not readily explain all of the observations in experimental and human emphysema. For instance, experimental enzyme-induced emphysema is panacinar rather than centrilobular, the more common type in humans with chronic airflow obstruction. Moreover, it does not explain the predominant localization of centrilobular emphysema to the upper lung zones or of panacinar emphysema to the lung bases or of paraseptal emphysema to the regions beneath the pleura and adjacent to fibrous septa. There is a close relationship between slowing of forced exhalation and cigarette smoking. The average heavy smoker has a 40 to 45 ml per year decline in FEV_1, whereas the average nonsmoking adult shows a decline of only 20 to 25 ml per year. Nonsmokers with $alpha_1$-antitrypsin deficiency have approximately an 80 ml per year decline in FEV_1; cigarette smokers with this deficiency have approximately a 150 ml per year decline. When individuals with $alpha_1$-antitrypsin deficiency stop smoking, this excess rate of decline in FEV_1 ceases. Nevertheless, the average effect of cigarette smoking alone does not explain the more severe reduction in FEV_1 noted in patients with COPD. Moreover, why is it that only a minority of smokers develop clinically significant COPD? Some individuals may be particularly susceptible for various reasons: respiratory disorders in childhood, intercurrent respiratory infections, or genetic factors, for example.

Can COPD be detected early by screening lung function in young to middle-aged adults? Longitudinal studies are attempting to identify susceptible cigarette-smoking individuals with an excessive rate of decline in pulmonary function throughout adult life. The hypothesis is that the individual who will develop COPD later in life should be identifiable by age 40 because he or she will show at least a mild ventilatory abnormality by then. There is no direct evidence yet, however, that any physiologic test applied early in life identifies the individual who will develop disabling COPD.

$Alpha_1$-Antitrypsin Deficiency. A deficiency in serum antiproteolytic activity associated with a susceptibility to COPD has been noted in several families. The protease inhibitor, or "Pi," phenotype of the subject determines the serum's trypsin inhibitory capacity. Two M genes (Pi MM phenotype) are present in normal individuals. When only Z genes are present (Pi ZZ phenotype), serum $alpha_1$-antitrypsin levels are severely reduced (< 50 mg per deciliter), and the $alpha_1$-antitrypsin that is present in plasma is less effective in inhibiting neutrophil elastase than $alpha_1$-antitrypsin in individuals with the Pi MM phenotype. Deficiency of $alpha_1$-antitrypsin is transmitted as an autosomal recessive trait. This antiproteolytic deficiency, present in approximately 1:4000 of the population, is associated with hepatitis in infancy and the development of emphysema in the third, fourth, and fifth decades. Present in 3 to 5 per cent of the population, the heterozygous state (Pi MZ phenotype) is associated with a moderately reduced serum antiproteolytic activity, but no predilection for developing an excess of respiratory disorders. Several other Pi genes have been identified (of which S is the most common), but only the Z gene clearly leads to COPD. In Ch. 125, the hepatic manifestations of $alpha_1$-antitrypsin deficiency are discussed.

PATHOLOGY. Alveolar wall destruction with a nonuniform pattern of airspace enlargement is the basic abnormality in emphysema. The orderly appearance of the acinus and its components is disturbed and may be lost, as airspaces are fewer in number but enlarged. In centrilobular emphysema, the process is most severe in the central portion of the lobule, whereas in panacinar emphysema the defect occurs uniformly throughout the acinus. Both centrilobular and panacinar emphysema may be noted in the same lung. In severe centrilobular emphysema, the entire acinus ultimately may become involved. Centrilobular emphysema generally is the most common form of emphysema in patients with chronic airflow obstruction.

In large airways, inflammation is noted in and around air passages, with narrowing of the lumina, impaction of mucus, and obliterative changes. Small airways abnormalities usually are not obvious on cursory examination and require careful morphometric studies.

CLINICAL MANIFESTATIONS. Dyspnea is usually the predominant complaint, but some patients consult a physician initially because of cough, wheezing, recurrent respiratory infections, or, occasionally, weakness or weight loss. Patients may date the onset of chronic symptoms to an acute respiratory infection. In some, shortness of breath is present only during acute exacerbations.

A productive cough is usually present, associated with a thick or "sticky" sputum varying widely in quantity. Copious amounts of purulent sputum production, coupled with a severe cough, are noted by some patients.

The physical examination may be normal relatively early in the illness (FEV_1 >1.0 liter). Auscultation of the chest may reveal rhonchi, or the chest may be quiet, particularly in patients with extensive emphysema. Wheezing, which may be absent on quiet breathing, can often be heard on forced exhalation. As the disease progresses, marked hyperinflation with low diaphragms and a reduced area of cardiac dullness are common. After minimal exertion or even at rest, labored breathing, at times through pursed lips, may be noted. Patients tend to lean forward on their elbows when sitting, assuming a stooped posture, while using accessory muscles of respiration. Cyanosis and dependent edema may be noted.

Occasionally, patients first seek medical attention when signs of right heart failure due to cor pulmonale appear. In such cases, the FEV_1 is likely to be below 1 liter and the arterial P_{O_2} below 45 mm Hg. The pulmonary hypertension in these patients with COPD and cor pulmonale is most closely related to the severity of hypoxemia.

Table 61–1 shows features of relatively distinctive COPD clinical syndromes and their associated underlying pathologic conditions. These two clinical types of COPD, emphysematous (type A) and bronchial (type B), represent extremes of presentation; most individuals, if followed chronically, develop a mixture of findings from the type A and type B groups. Type A patients, described as "pink puffers," often hyperventilate, maintaining a normal or nearly normal arterial O_2 tension and CO_2 tensions. In contrast, type B patients, "blue bloaters," often have a low arterial O_2 tension, high CO_2 tension, cyanosis, and right-sided congestive heart failure. The "blue bloater" syndrome may also result from disordered breathing during sleep, a common problem in patients with COPD.

LABORATORY FINDINGS. The routine blood count and differential study are normal except for erythrocytosis in some COPD patients with hypoxemia. When eosinophilia is found, a reversible (asthmatic-bronchitic) component of the disease should be suspected.

Early in the disease, the chest radiograph may be normal; however, in severe emphysema, lung hyperinflation and an increased retrosternal airspace, with flattening of the diaphragms and regional attenuation of blood vessels, are usually noted. Frank bullae outlined by hairline margins are present in some cases. The chest radiograph should not be the sole basis for the diagnosis of COPD, for individuals with perfectly normal lung function may have radiographic findings typical of the disease. Chest CT can be used to determine the presence of emphysema and to quantify its severity with reasonable accuracy.

Persistent reduction in forced expiratory flow rates is the most typical finding in COPD. Two lung volume measurements, the residual volume and the residual volume/total lung capacity ratio, are elevated. Ventilation-perfusion mismatch and nonuniformity of ventilation are also typical findings, whereas arterial hypoxemia and physiologic shunting vary among patients. When the diffusing capacity is very depressed and the total lung capacity is clearly elevated, emphysema is likely to be extensive.

Ventilation and perfusion lung scans should be interpreted cautiously when pulmonary emboli are suspected. These scans reveal the uneven ventilation and perfusion typical of COPD. Areas of diminished perfusion may be mistaken for pulmonary emboli. Accordingly, when pulmonary embolism is suspected in a patient with COPD, a pulmonary angiogram is often required for definitive diagnosis.

The electrocardiogram tends to be normal, particularly early in the course of the disease. Later, the axis is shifted to the right, and there are early R waves in the precordial leads V_1 and V_2 and net negative electrical forces in leads V_5 and V_6. Especially during exacerbations, peaked P waves ("p pulmonale") are present. Unfortunately, these changes do not correlate well with pulmonary artery hypertension and cor pulmonale. The presence of R waves over the right precordium is the most reliable indication of cor pulmonale.

COURSE AND PROGNOSIS. Initially, there is a variable response to bronchodilator therapy, dependent upon the degree of bronchospasm. Thereafter, the disease progresses slowly, with an annual average decrement in FEV_1 of 50 to 75 ml. Because the variability in FEV_1 may be greater than the true annual decline, a follow-up of several years is required to determine the rate of loss of lung function. If the patient stops smoking, cough and sputum production may cease. However, most other symptoms progress gradually.

In terms of absolute FEV_1, patients are dyspneic upon moderate exertion when the value is 1.2 to 1.5 liters; they are forced to be relatively sedentary at 1.0 liter; and they are often invalids when the FEV_1 is 500 ml or less. As the FEV_1 drops below 1 liter, severe arterial hypoxemia, hypercapnia, and cor pulmonale often are evident.

Median survival varies considerably. Despite initially very low FEV_1 values, some individuals live 12 to 15 years. Generally, however, when the FEV_1 is more than 1.2 liters, patients survive about ten years; when the FEV_1 is 1.0 liter, survival is approximately five years; and when the FEV_1 is less than 700 ml, survival is about two years. Signs of a poor prognosis include a resting tachycardia, severe arterial hypoxemia or hypercapnia or both, and evidence of cor pulmonale. If a patient resides at altitudes higher than 3500 feet, longevity is reduced.

Increased cough and dyspnea are hallmarks of periodic worsening of the disease. Symptoms characteristically occur after an acute respiratory infection and may be accompanied by bronchospasm. Such exacerbations in patients with severe COPD may be life threatening and may lead to acute respiratory failure as well as right heart failure. The latter occurs secondary to pronounced increases in pulmonary artery pressure and pulmonary vascular resistance, which, in turn, are due primarily to hypoxic pulmonary vasoconstriction.

DIFFERENTIAL DIAGNOSIS. Three criteria are required to diagnose COPD: (1) The FEV_1 must be reduced, and this reduction must be proportionately more than any lowering in the FVC (i.e., both the FEV_1 per cent predicted and the FEV_1/FVC ratio must be depressed); (2) in spite of intensive, prolonged medical treatment, this slowing of forced expiration must persist; and (3) other bronchopulmonary disease that might explain the observed physiologic abnormalities must be excluded. Sufficient evidence for the last criterion generally includes absence of extensive parenchymal abnormalities on the chest radiograph and absence of any signs of upper airway obstruction, such as neck mass, stridor, or narrowing of the upper airway on chest radiograph. Irreversibility of the obstructive ventilatory defect may be more difficult to establish. This is discussed further in the treatment section.

Assessing the relative contribution of emphysema and intrinsic airway changes can also be difficult. Emphysema is usually severe when the diffusing capacity is very depressed and the chest radiograph shows hyperlucent lungs with attenuation of the vascular markings. In contrast, if the diffusing capacity is normal or nearly normal, extensive emphysema is unlikely. Esophageal balloon measurements, which are required to assess lung elastic recoil (the best guide to the severity of emphysema), are seldom justified as part of the clinical evaluation.

If there is a family history of emphysema or if an emphysema type of COPD develops at an early age, a homozygous $alpha_1$-antitrypsin deficiency should be considered. Suspicion is heightened when the patient is a nonsmoker or a woman or when the chest radiograph shows a bibasilar distribution of emphysematous changes. Laboratory confirmation is provided by almost complete absence of $alpha_1$-globulin, by a markedly reduced serum trypsin inhibitory capacity, and, most specifically, by demonstrating a pattern of a pure Z phenotype on crossed immunoelectrophoresis of the serum.

TREATMENT. The following are therapeutic goals in patients with COPD: (1) to relieve the portion of airway obstruction that is reversible; (2) to control cough and sputum production; (3) to eliminate and prevent airway infections; (4) to increase exercise tolerance to the maximum allowable at the individual's level of physiologic deficit; (5) to control remedial disease complications, such as arterial hypoxemia and cardiovascular problems; (6) to avoid smoking and other airway irritants, narcotics and sedatives, and noncritical surgery, all of which aggravate the disease; and (7) to relieve the anxiety and depression that are often present in the patient with COPD.

In spite of treatment, most patients with severe COPD show progressive ventilatory deterioration; yet, therapy should not be withheld. A comprehensive therapeutic program can reduce symptoms, decrease the frequency of hospital admissions, prevent premature death, and permit patients to lead a more active and satisfying life.

A formal rehabilitation program using a team approach is effective. Nevertheless, good results also can be obtained by a dedicated individual physician assisted, perhaps, by an office nurse who can help patients with physical therapy and bronchial hygiene measures.

Initial Treatment. During the initial visit, it is impossible to predict with certainty the degree of reversibility of airway obstruction in a patient with COPD. Therefore, all patients should be considered as having potentially reversible disease. Bronchodilators should be administered according to tolerance, as outlined in the therapy for asthmatic bronchitis and asthma. Smoking should be discontinued and other bronchial irritants avoided. As mentioned in the therapy for simple chronic bronchitis, bronchial hygiene measures and, when indicated by purulent mucous production, antibiotics should be used. Diuretics should be given when heart failure is present. In addition, the Pneumovax vaccine and yearly administration of the influenza vaccine are indicated.

The effects of this initial therapy both on symptoms and on pulmonary function test results should be determined and adjustments made in medication to minimize side effects. Apparently ineffective measures (e.g., postural drainage that leads to no symptom relief or sputum production) should be discontinued. Next, if further reversibility of the disease is considered possible, a three- to four-week trial of corticosteroids can be initiated. Several findings suggest that corticosteroids may help: (1) provide a more than 20 per cent improvement in FEV_1 after acute inhalation of a bronchodilator; (2) provide a similar increase in FEV_1 after several days or weeks of intensive bronchodilator therapy; (3) a history of acute attacks of wheezing not precipitated by exertion or of marked fluctuation in symptoms; (4) a noisy chest or wheeze upon auscultation; (5) sputum or blood eosinophilia; (6) provide any evidence of atopy, such as a history of hay fever, positive results in allergy skin tests, or an elevated level of serum IgE; (7) associated nasal polyps or vasomotor rhinitis; (8) a normal pulmonary diffusing capacity; or (9) provide normal chest film except for hyperinflation.

Generally, 20 to 40 mg of prednisone daily is given for three to four weeks, and spirometry tests are used to assess the efficacy of this medication. Other bronchodilators are continued at full doses. When improvement is noted, the corticosteroid dose should be tapered to the lowest maintenance dose possible, as outlined for asthmatic bronchitis. If there is no significant improvement in FEV_1 (e.g., > 20 per cent), corticosteroids should be tapered slowly and discontinued.

Maintenance Therapy. Frequently, objective improvement (i.e., increase in FEV_1) cannot be demonstrated with bronchodilator therapy. Yet, oral theophylline, combined with an inhaled beta-adrenergic agent, is recommended to prevent superimposed bronchospasm. In COPD, theophylline can (1) enhance respiratory muscle function, in both the fatigued and the nonfatigued state; (2) augment right and left ventricular systolic pump function while decreasing pulmonary artery pressures and pulmonary vascular resistance (potentially helpful in patients with cor pulmonale); and (3) in some patients, reduce dyspnea. The beta-adrenergic agents also improve biventricular systolic pump performance and decrease pulmonary vascular resistance. Whether any of these potentially salutary effects are additive or synergistic when oral theophylline is administered in conjunction with beta-adrenergic agents has not been established.

Aerosolized adrenergic agents also are used (1) to relieve acute attacks of dyspnea; (2) prior to exposure to known bronchial irritants, such as cold air; or (3) as a regular part of a bronchial hygiene program.

If a patient with COPD shows improvement in airflow rates (particularly FEV_1) with bronchodilators or adrenocortical hormones, these agents should be maintained as in asthmatic bronchitis. Those with a productive cough, retained secretions, or repeated episodes of bronchopulmonary infection should be treated with the same measures as described for simple chronic bronchitis. In addition, some other forms of treatment are uniquely applicable to patients with COPD.

Physical Therapy. Exercise has not been shown to improve lung function, but it may enhance cardiovascular fitness and train skeletal muscles to function more efficiently, thus increasing exercise tolerance. Accordingly, unless contraindicated by an underlying cardiac abnormality, progressively increasing exercise (usually walking) should be prescribed. In most cases, the program can be recommended directly by the physician, but if the patient is severely disabled, a trained physical therapist can initiate an appropriate exercise program. Arterial blood gas levels should be obtained at rest and exercise prior to instituting a vigorous exercise program, particularly if the FEV_1 is less than 1 liter. Supplemental oxygen should be used during exercise if the patient becomes severely hypoxemic.

Although breathing exercises probably do not alter the usual breathing pattern of patients with COPD, occasionally they are recommended to encourage diaphragmatic breathing. Perhaps it is more useful and more realistic to teach patients slow, deep breathing as a quicker, more effective method for relieving dyspnea rather than rapid, shallow "panic" breathing. Breath holding should be avoided during exertion. Many authorities now recommend inspiratory muscle training by breathing against a graded resistor, but mechanical devices, intermittent positive pressure breathing (IPPB) machines, and emphysema belts are of unproven value.

Oxygen Therapy. In some individuals with COPD, there are clear indications for home oxygen therapy. One indication is development of severe exertional hypoxemia ($Pa_{O_2} < 40$ mm Hg) in patients who respond to supplemental oxygen therapy with an increase in exercise tolerance. A second indication is found in patients with severe, persistent arterial hypoxemia at rest ($Pa_{O_2} < 55$ mm Hg) accompanied by secondary signs of hypoxemia after all other therapeutic measures have been exhausted and the patient has completely recovered from exacerbation of the disease. Both continuous oxygen therapy and that spanning 12 to 15 hours per day prolong survival, but continuous therapy (i.e., 10 to 24 hours per day) is associated with longer survival. To raise the Pa_{O_2} to the necessary 60 to 80 mm Hg usually requires 1 to 3 liters of oxygen per minute via nasal prongs.

Since patients may become habituated to this therapy and thus increase their invalidism, oxygen should not be prescribed solely for episodes of dyspnea.

Environmental Control. All patients with severe COPD should be cautioned to avoid high altitudes and should reside at altitudes below 4000 feet. Supplemental oxygen may be required for those with severe hypoxemia when they travel by air. A change in residence may be indicated in patients who live in areas with heavy air pollution.

Cold winter climates are avoided by some patients who find relief in either warm desert climates or warm, humid regions. No specific climate has been shown to alter the overall course of the disease. Accordingly, the economic and social hardships of a move should be weighed carefully against the potential symptomatic benefit provided by relocation to a more agreeable climate. Before moving, the patient should spend a trial period in the new climate to assess symptomatic benefit.

Treatment of Edema and Cor Pulmonale. Even in the absence of frank right-sided congestive heart failure, pedal edema is common and control is usually obtained with small doses of diuretics. Ankle edema associated with cor pulmonale is more difficult to control, but oxygen combined with diuretics often will suffice. Digitalis is useful for enhancing right ventricular function only if there is concomitant left heart failure; accordingly, digitalis should be reserved for combined right and left heart failure. Phlebotomy is not required in most oxygen-treated patients but may transiently relieve central nervous system symptoms, especially when the hematocrit is above 60 per cent.

Treatment of Hypercapnia. Chronic hypercapnia is common in late stages of COPD, but it requires no therapy. However, during exacerbations, blood gases must be monitored closely for severe respiratory acidosis, and all narcotics, sedatives, and tranquilizers should be avoided. In patients with stable chronic hypercapnia, mechanically assisted ventilation and respiratory stimulants are unnecessary.

Surgical Therapy. In the absence of significant emphysema (e.g., manifested by a moderate-to-severe reduction in diffusing capacity), bullectomy may benefit patients with large bullae compressing normal or nearly normal lung. Careful, detailed preoperative evaluation is required to select suitable operative candidates.

Supportive Measures. Careful, detailed education of the patient regarding the nature of the disease is essential. The significance of symptoms such as purulent sputum production, potential side effects of medication, and therapeutic goals should be explained. A prompt, prearranged treatment plan should be discussed with the patient for intercurrent exacerbations.

Above all, within the limits of respiratory impairment and within the constraints of therapy, these patients should be encouraged to live active lives with daily exercise. Some patients benefit from vocational rehabilitation and occupational therapy.

Replacement Therapy in Severe Alpha$_1$-Antitrypsin Deficiency Emphysema. Chronic, weekly replacement therapy with intravenous alpha$_1$-antitrypsin concentrate of normal plasma has been undertaken at the National Heart, Lung and Blood Institute in individuals with severe alpha$_1$-antitrypsin deficiency. Serum alpha$_1$-antitrypsin was elevated to levels likely required for effective antielastase protection of the lungs (average post-therapy level achieved, 130 mg per deciliter; average pretherapy level, 31 mg per deciliter). Alpha$_1$-antitrypsin levels after bronchoalveolar lavage increased in these individuals to about 60 per cent of normal, associated with an equivalent restoration of functional antineutrophil elastase activity. Moreover, the incidence of adverse reactions was limited to a transient postinfusion fever in less than 1 per cent of the patients.

Recently, recombinant DNA methodology has been used to produce alpha$_1$-antitrypsin. The future may bring widespread clinical application of this potentially less expensive material in patients with the Pi ZZ phenotype. When only mild airways disease is present, this therapy will re-establish the lung antineutrophil elastase defenses and protect the alveolar walls from elastolytic attack.

Treatment of Exacerbations. Antibiotics, increased bronchodilator medications, and even corticosteroids often are indicated for acute exacerbation. Immediate hospitalization is indicated for severe hypoxemia, increasing carbon dioxide tension, or congestive heart failure. Ch. 43 and 72 outline the management of decompensated cor pulmonale and acute respiratory failure, respectively, The same management utilized in patients with status asthmaticus is indicated in COPD patients with superimposed refractory bronchospasm.

Anthonisen NR: Hypoxemia and O_2 therapy. Am Rev Respir Dis 126:729, 1982. *A quality review of the British and American studies establishing that oxygen therapy prolongs life in patients with hypoxemic COPD.*

De Marco FJ Jr, Wynne JW, Block AJ, et al.: Oxygen desaturation during sleep as a determinant of the "blue and bloated" syndrome. Chest 79:621, 1981. *One of several papers by this group of investigators proposing that sleep-related breathing disorders are important in COPD patients.*

Higgins MW, Keller JB: Estimating your patient's risk of COPD. J Respir Dis 4:97, 1983. *This paper discusses the use of routine spirometric testing to detect subjects who are at high risk of developing clinically significant airways obstructive disease.*

Janoff A: Elastases and emphysema: Current assessment of the protease-antiprotease hypothesis. Am Rev Respir Dis 132:417, 1985. *Reviews ten years of progress in elucidating the pathogenesis of emphysema.*

Petty TL (ed.): Chronic Obstructive Pulmonary Disease. 2nd ed. New York, Marcel Dekker, 1985. *Comprehensive statement on all aspects of COPD.*

Snider GL (ed.): Emphysema. Clin Chest Med 4:327, 1983. *Quality monograph emphasizing the pathology and pathogenesis of emphysema.*

LOCALIZED AIRWAY OBSTRUCTION

Extrinsic compression of airways, intraluminal obstruction, and diseases of the airways themselves all can cause localized airway obstruction. Signs and symptoms depend upon location of the obstruction, whether it is partial or complete, variable or fixed. The discussion of localized lesions is divided into obstructions above and below the bifurcation of the trachea.

Obstruction Above the Tracheal Bifurcation

PARTIAL OBSTRUCTION. Stridor, frequently accompanied by inspiratory retraction of the intercostal spaces, is the principal finding in partial obstruction above the main (tracheal) carina. On both forced inspiration and forced expiration, airflow rates are reduced, and there may be a characteristic appearance to the MEFV curve. As shown in Figure 61–2, the site and nature of the obstruction determine the findings on spirometry. When the obstruction is severe, hypoxemia and hypercapnia may result owing to reduced overall ventilation.

Among the intrinsic airway diseases that can cause partial airway obstruction are (1) tonsil and adenoid enlargement, especially in young children; (2) stenosing lesions secondary to trauma; (3) neoplasms or granulomatous processes (e.g., sarcoidosis, fungi) involving the hypopharynx, larynx, vocal cords, or trachea; (4) bilateral paralysis of the vocal cords; (5) spasm or edema of the larynx; or (6) inflammation in several locations—the pharynx (e.g., peritonsillar abscess), the larynx (e.g., croup), or the trachea (e.g., diphtheria). An enlarged thyroid, a paratracheal neoplasm, or a mediastinal infection can cause extrinsic compression of the airway. An artificial airway, tracheostomy, or surgical repair is indicated when the primary cause of the obstruction cannot be eliminated.

COMPLETE OBSTRUCTION. Rapid asphyxiation results unless complete obstruction above the main carina is relieved promptly. There is a pathognomonic presentation with absent airflow at the mouth in spite of both inspiratory efforts and inspiratory retraction of the intercostal muscles. Aspiration of poorly chewed food (so-called "café coronary") is the most common cause of acute obstruction. If a sharp blow to the back fails to dislodge the obstructing material, forced pressure is applied to the epigastrium—the *Heimlich maneuver*.

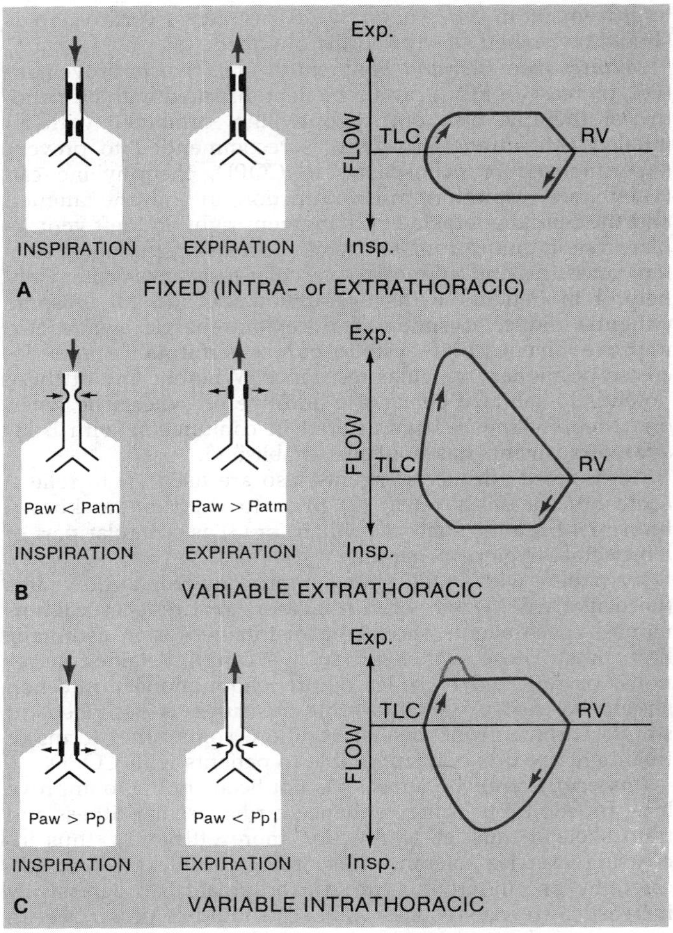

FIGURE 61–2. Airways obstruction above the carina may produce characteristic flow-volume abnormalities, depending on the type and site of obstruction. *A,* If the obstruction is fixed, both inspiratory and expiratory flows will be decreased whether the obstruction is intrathoracic or extrathoracic (for purposes of illustration, obstruction is shown in both locations). Note that this pattern is usually seen when the obstruction is at the level of the thoracic inlet. *B,* When a variable obstruction is extrathoracic in location, the airway narrows during inspiration when airway pressure (Paw) is less than atmospheric (Patm) and inspiratory flow is diminished. Expiratory flows are often limited but to a lesser extent. *C,* When a variable obstruction is intrathoracic in location, airway pressure is less than pleural pressure (Ppl) during expiration, and expiratory flow is diminished. Inspiratory flows are often limited but to a much lesser extent. (Reproduced with permission from Burrows B, et al.: Respiratory Disorders—A Pathophysiologic Approach. 2nd ed. Copyright 1983 by Year Book Medical Publishers, Inc., Chicago.)

When the glossopharyngeal structures fall back in some obese individuals, complete obstruction of the upper airway occurs. Local abnormalities in the hypopharynx may also cause complete upper airway obstruction, resulting in disordered breathing, especially during sleep. Frequent awakening, a troubled sleep, and somnolence are characteristic. This clinical picture, often confused with the pickwickian syndrome and other forms of sleep disorders, is discussed in Ch. 458.

Obstruction Below the Tracheal Bifurcation

PARTIAL OBSTRUCTION. A primary neoplasm, compressing or growing into an airway, is the most common cause of obstruction below the bifurcation of the trachea.

Other causes include aspiration of foreign bodies, acute or chronic inflammatory lesions of the bronchi, and compression of bronchi by enlarged hilar lymph nodes or mucous plugs. A localized expiratory wheeze over the site of obstruction and hyperinflation of the lung distally are characteristic. Spirometry may be normal or only mildly abnormal because airflow from the remaining lung is unimpaired; yet, other tests will show nonuniformity of ventilation. A ventilation lung scan may reveal an area of diminished airflow. Bronchoscopy usually provides a definitive diagnosis, and treatment is directed at the cause of obstruction.

Infection and perhaps an abscess may develop with partial bronchial obstruction because of impaired secretion clearance from the distal lung. Partial obstruction of the proximal bronchus should be suspected in patients with recurrent infections in the same lung zone, slow resolution of pneumonia, or a lung abscess.

COMPLETE OBSTRUCTION. "Obstructive atelectasis" is a condition due to absorption of air into the bloodstream from lung distal to a complete obstruction. This condition is discussed in Ch. 62 under Atelectasis. Complete occlusion of a bronchus and resultant obstructive atelectasis may develop with progression of any of the above-mentioned causes of partial obstruction.

Heimlich HJ: A life-saving maneuver to prevent food-choking. JAMA 234:398, 1975. *The original report on a new standard method to remove aspirated food from the airway.*

Loughlin GM, Taussig LM: Upper airway obstruction. Semin Respir Med 1:131, 1979. *This is an excellent review of upper airways obstructive disorders in infants and children.*

Miller RD: Obstructing lesions of the larynx and trachea: Clinical and pathophysiologic aspects. In Fishman AP (ed.): Pulmonary Diseases and Disorders. New York, McGraw-Hill Book Company, 1980, p 490. *An excellent review of the causes, consequences, and treatment of tracheolaryngeal obstruction.*

62 ABNORMALITIES OF LUNG AERATION*

Richard A. Matthay

LOCALIZED HYPOAERATION (ATELECTASIS)

Atelectasis, or reduced aeration of the lung, is present in many bronchopulmonary disorders and assumes a variety of forms. A total loss of ventilation to a lung region (i.e., with total airway collapse) leads to a shunt wherein blood traversing this region fails to participate in gas exchange and behaves as if it were moving directly from the right to the left side of the heart. Accordingly, total atelectasis causes an "absolute" shunt. In contrast to the "shuntlike" effect of increased venous admixture present in most bronchopulmonary diseases, inhalation of 100 per cent oxygen does not fully correct the "absolute shunt."

TYPES OF ATELECTASIS AND THEIR PATHOGENESIS. *Obstructive atelectasis* is a condition of alveolar collapse that develops within a few hours after obstruction of an airway distal to the tracheal bifurcation. The collapse develops because gas in the lung behind the obstruction is slowly absorbed into the bloodstream. If the lung is filled with oxygen-rich gas rather than ambient air, the alveoli collapse more rapidly. Nitrogen in ambient air is poorly soluble, whereas oxygen is rapidly absorbed into the bloodstream. As a result, high inspired oxygen tensions encourage the development of atelectasis behind obstructing mucous plugs.

Contraction atelectasis occurs when fibrotic changes in a local area of the lung increase its recoil. Contraction, or shrinkage, of the involved lung, rather than complete airlessness, results.

Patchy atelectasis develops throughout the lung owing to alveolar instability in adult and infant (newborn) respiratory distress syndromes.

A large pneumothorax, pleural effusion, or other space-occupying lesion in the thorax can increase intrapleural pressure, causing a portion of the lung to decrease in volume. This *compression atelectasis* is more appropriately called *relaxation atelectasis* because the atelectasis results from the tendency of the lung to recoil when the distending forces are relaxed. As small airways close in the affected region because of marked relaxation atelectasis, any air remaining distally is absorbed into the bloodstream.

Although its pathologic significance is unclear, *platelike atelectasis* may be visible on the chest radiograph. This condition is characterized by horizontal radiopaque streaks, usually in the lung bases. Commonly associated with poor lung aeration, these streaks are seen when the patient has been unable to breathe deeply for a sustained period or when the diaphragm is elevated, such as after intra-abdominal surgery.

CLINICAL MANIFESTATIONS. The chronicity and extent of the process determine the physiologic and clinical consequences of atelectasis. When the obstruction evolves slowly, typical of bronchial neoplasms, usually few or no symptoms develop and hypoxemia is minimal. In contrast, profound dyspnea and severe hypoxemia often develop after acute collapse of a large section of the lung. As blood-flow through the nonventilated lung diminishes over several hours, symptoms and hypoxemia lessen. The acute picture typically includes development of obstructive atelectasis due to aspiration of a foreign body or due to retention of secretions (which may develop in the postoperative period).

The type of atelectasis determines the physical findings. In obstructive or contraction atelectasis, the physical findings depend upon the amount of lung involved. In major atelectasis, the trachea and mediastinum shift to the affected side, the diaphragm is elevated, and the involved hemithorax is smaller and shows less respiratory motion than the unaffected side. Patchy atelectasis is associated with findings like those of the respiratory distress syndrome reviewed in Ch. 72. The underlying condition (e.g., pleural effusion, pneumothorax, space-occupying lesion) determines the findings in relaxation atelectasis. Platelike atelectasis is primarily a chest radiographic diagnosis without distinctive abnormalities on physical examination.

DIAGNOSIS, TREATMENT, AND OUTCOME. The chest radiograph confirms the presence of atelectasis. When obstructive atelectasis is suspected, bronchoscopy is required to establish the etiology; it may be possible to remove the occluding material through the bronchoscope. However, a bronchogenic neoplasm should always be considered when obstructive atelectasis is present and the patient is not severely ill.

Treatment is directed at the underlying disorder in nonobstructive forms of atelectasis.

When relaxation atelectasis is relieved (e.g., by insertion of a chest tube for a large pneumothorax), the lung usually returns to normal. However, obstructive atelectasis often is accompanied by secondary complications, such as infection, which lead to abscess formation, localized bronchiectasis, and fibrosis. Moreover, after prolonged collapse, the affected lung may fail to re-expand after the obstruction is removed. The *middle lobe syndrome* provides a typical sequence of events. In this syndrome, the middle lobe bronchus in the right lung usually has been compressed by large hilar lymph nodes in tuberculosis or other granulomatous lung diseases. Even after the lymph nodes finally decrease in size, the affected lung fails to expand fully, there are often bronchiectatic changes, and the lobe may be a site of recurrent or chronic infection. Although less common, the same sequence of events may

---

*Portions of this chapter were rewritten from the 17th edition of *Cecil Textbook of Medicine* with permission from Benjamin Burrows.

occur in other lung regions. The involved lung may have to be resected if recurrent pneumonia, chronic suppuration, or repeated episodes of hemoptysis develop.

LOCALIZED HYPERAERATION

BLEBS AND BULLAE. Blebs are small collections of gas that are entirely enclosed within the visceral pleura. The gas resides between the multiple leaves of the visceral pleura rather than within the lung itself. Blebs are the uncommon result of dissection of air from the lung interstitium into the lung septa and thence into and between the layers of visceral pleura. Blebs are not clinically important except on the rare occasions that they rupture and cause a spontaneous pneumothorax. Sometimes blebs are visible on the plain chest radiograph, particularly in the lung apex; they are more easily seen when there is a pneumothorax and partial collapse of normal surrounding lung.

Bullae are larger airspaces in the parenchyma of the lung (> than 1 cm in diameter) that are associated with destruction. A bulla denotes severe, localized emphysema causing the formation of a large airspace. Bullae may occur with several different types of emphysema and are common in patients with chronic obstructive bronchitis and emphysema. Individuals without any generalized obstructive airways disorder and without diffuse emphysema also may develop bullae.

Bullae are commonly located in the apices of the lungs and are often multiple. A lack of an endothelial lining distinguishes bullae from cysts. Moreover, on the chest radiograph, bullae have "hairline" (thin) margins and, unlike cysts, are usually irregularly shaped, are frequently trabeculated, and rarely contain fluid.

When they become large enough to compromise the function of the remaining normal lung and cause shortness of breath, bullae are clinically important. However, like blebs, when small, they are of little significance, unless they rupture and lead to a pneumothorax.

A difficult clinical problem may be to ascertain whether dyspnea is secondary to diffuse emphysema of the lungs or to bullae (observed on the chest radiograph). Surgery may be indicated in the latter case, but it is contraindicated in the former. Ventilation-perfusion radionuclide lung scans, computed tomography (CT) scans, and pulmonary angiograms may be necessary to make this distinction and to evaluate the state of the remaining lung. As a rule, unless there is associated generalized obstructive airways disease, bullae that occupy less than half a hemithorax are not associated with severe dyspnea and significant functional impairment. Moreover, unless there is diffuse disease, severe slowing of expiratory airflow is unusual, even with very large bullae. An ideal surgical candidate has moderate-to-severe dyspnea, bullae that fill most of a hemithorax, only mild slowing of flow rates on forced expiration, good perfusion of normal remaining lung on lung scan and pulmonary angiogram, and no evidence of significant emphysema (e.g., the diffusing capacity measurement is normal or only moderately reduced, and lung compliance studies are normal).

The diagnosis is usually made by the sound chest radiograph; however, on physical examination, a tympanitic percussion sound and reduced breath sounds may be noted over very large bullae. The radiolucency of a very large bulla of the chest film may be mistaken for a pneumothorax.

BRONCHOGENIC CYSTS. Bronchogenic cysts may occur in the mediastinum or within the lung parenchyma. These congenital malformations can be differentiated from bullae by their epithelial lining. On the chest radiograph, mediastinal cysts are seen as masses in the hilar, paraesophageal or paratracheal, and, most commonly, subcarinal region. In the parenchyma, these cysts are most commonly in the lower lobes and are usually filled with a proteinaceous material until they may become infected and communicate with the bronchial tree. They may have thin, even paper-thin, walls. During early development, acquired lung cysts often have relatively thick walls; later even those resulting from lung abscesses often have very thin walls that simulate bullae.

Large cysts may cause respiratory symptoms in young children, but adults with these large lesions are usually asymptomatic, and the chest radiographic abnormality tends to be an incidental finding. In the differential diagnosis, mediastinal cysts must be distinguished from other mediastinal masses. Lung cysts must be differentiated from acute lung abscesses, cavitated carcinomas, and cystic bronchiectasis. Frequently, thoracotomy and resection of the lesion are required to obtain a specific diagnosis, although chest CT combined with needle aspiration has been useful for diagnosis and drainage.

Only when they have a bronchial connection (communication) do bronchogenic cysts manifest as abnormalities in lung aeration. Although often partially filled with fluid, they may appear as airspaces when there is a bronchial communication. Infection in fluid-filled cysts is unusual and may require that they be removed surgically after a course of antibiotics. Cysts containing air often can be distinguished from bullae by their regular outline, lack of trabeculation, and the presence of a fluid level. Distinguishing bronchogenic cysts in the lung from thin-walled cavities secondary to granulomatous infections, prior abscesses, prior pulmonary infarcts, and squamous cell carcinomas may be more difficult.

BRONCHOPULMONARY SEQUESTRATION. In *bronchopulmonary sequestrations* of the intralobular type, cystic lesions may be identified. This sequestration is caused by abnormal budding in the tracheobronchial tree of the early embryo. The involved area is most often in the bases of the lungs posteriorly, and the affected lung region is nonfunctional. On the chest radiograph, involved areas are opaque.

Only when there is a bronchial communication do air-containing cysts develop, and in such situations secondary infection is the prime concern. These lesions are asymptomatic and are incidental chest radiographic findings unless infection develops. An aortogram that shows an abnormal vascular supply distinguishes a sequestration from a simple cyst. The arterial supply to some sequestrations arises at least partially from below the diaphragm. Surgical excision is the only treatment.

THE UNILATERAL HYPERLUCENT LUNG. Swyer-James or Macleod's syndrome, a rare disorder, is generally discovered on chest radiograph. Increased translucency of one hemithorax is noted owing to diminished vascular markings in the lung on that side. On the inspiration chest radiograph, the affected lung is usually not hyperinflated. However, air trapping has been described, and an expiration chest radiograph may show hyperinflation of the affected lung relative to the other uninvolved lung and shift of the mediastinum to the unaffected side. Extensive bronchitis and bronchiolitis are usually noted on biopsy. These abnormalities likely date from childhood. In fact, in some children the condition develops six months to five years after viral bronchiolitis, and there is a history of some such incidence in more than half of the patients. Dyspnea, a productive cough, and occasionally hemoptysis may occur.

At bronchoscopy, there is no obstruction of the main bronchi. But bronchography shows irregular dilatation of the bronchi to the fifth order, with failure to fill the peripheral airways, and an appearance characteristic of bronchiolar obliteration. Patency of the pulmonary artery on the angiogram differentiates Swyer-James syndrome from pulmonary artery stenosis or atresia. On the affected side, the lung scan shows reduced ventilation and perfusion. Pulmonary function test findings are variable and usually include some evidence of airways obstruction and an increase in residual volume, suggesting air trapping. Severe expiratory obstruction of airflow is uncommon.

Resection is not indicated, and treatment is limited usually to managing infection.

Allison RS, Chirnside AM: Pulmonary sequestration: A review of 12 cases. NZ Med J 596:381, 1983. *Well-written, complete coverage of the types, presentation, and management of pulmonary sequestration.*

Boushy SF, Kohen R, Billig DM, et al.: Bullous emphysema: Clinical, roentgenologic and physiologic study of 49 patients. Dis Chest 54:327, 1968. *A good description of the range of manifestations seen with pulmonary bullae.*

Hamilton CR Jr, Ballinger WF II, Cader G: The unilateral hyperlucent lung syndrome. Bull Johns Hopkins Hosp 123:222, 1968. *A good review of this unusual syndrome.*

Primrose WR: Spontaneous pneumothorax: A retrospective review of etiology, pathogenesis, and management. Scott Med J 29:15, 1984. *Succinct, up-to-date review of spontaneous pneumothorax.*

Proto AV, Tocino I: Radiographic manifestations of lobar collapse. Semin Roentgenol 15:117, 1980. *A comprehensive review of chest radiographic features of lobar collapse.*

Rodgers BM, Harman PK, Johnson AM: Bronchopulmonary foregut malformations—the spectrum of anomalies. Ann Surg 203:517, 1986. *A review of the various foregut malformations, including both bronchogenic cysts and sequestration, complete with ultrasound and CT images and a quality bibliography.*

Wagner RB, Johnston MR: Middle lobe syndrome. Ann Thorac Surg 35:679, 1983. *The etiology, pathophysiology, and therapy of this syndrome are up to date.*

63 INTERSTITIAL LUNG DISEASE

Ronald G. Crystal

General Description

The interstitial lung diseases (ILD) are a heterogeneous group of diffuse inflammatory disorders of the lower respiratory tract. The term "interstitial lung disease" refers to the fact that the interstitium of the alveolar walls is thickened, usually by fibrosis. While this is true, the ILD are also characterized by derangements of the epithelial and endothelial cells of the alveolar walls and, in many cases, of the small airways and/or blood vessels of the lung parenchyma.

There are many disorders associated with ILD. In some, the ILD is the only manifestation; in others it is a part of a systemic disorder. The natural history of many of the ILD is one of slowly progressive loss of the functional alveolar-capillary units, often eventuating in respiratory insufficiency and death. Because of their insidious nature and the nonspecificity of the accompanying symptoms, such as dyspnea on exertion or a nonproductive cough, the ILD may go undiagnosed and untreated until large numbers of alveolar-capillary units become scarred and irrevocably lost.

These disorders are inflammatory diseases; the bulk of the damage to the lung parenchyma is caused by activated inflammatory cells that have accumulated in the alveolar structures. The diagnosis, staging, and treatment of the ILD require defining the character and intensity of the inflammation in the lung and the derangements of the alveolar structures caused by the inflammation.

Anatomy

The lower respiratory tract is composed of alveoli, grapelike units branching off the terminal bronchioles, and the vascular network of pulmonary arterioles, capillaries, and venules that bring blood to and from the lung (Fig. 63–1). The walls of the alveoli are lined by a single layer of epithelial cells resting on a thin, continuous basement membrane. Ninety-five per cent of the alveolar surface is covered by type I epithelial cells, with the remainder by type II epithelial cells, the cell that produces the surfactant, material that prevents alveolar collapse. Underneath the epithelial basement membrane is the alveolar interstitium, a region containing fibroblasts and supporting connective tissue matrix composed of collagen, elastic fibers, proteoglycans, and various glycoproteins. The pulmonary capillaries form a branching network of tubes lined by a single layer of endothelial cells resting on their own basement membrane. The capillaries weave through the interstitium such that the capillary basement membrane often abuts the epithelial basement membrane beneath the type I epithelial cells. It is at these sites that air and blood are in closest approximation and where gas exchange takes place.

The normal alveolar wall is thin (5 to 10 μm wide) compared with the space occupied by air (200 to 300 μm). In the ILD, the walls are thickened severalfold and the space for air is correspondingly less. The derangements that accompany the thickening of the alveolar walls in the ILD can be conceptualized in two groups (Fig. 63–2). In the distortion form of derangement, typified by sarcoidosis and the early phases of hypersensitivity pneumonitis, the alveolar walls are deformed by the accumulation of inflammatory cells in the interstitium, altering the normal architecture. Because there is little injury to the normal structures, this form of derangement is often reversible if the process causing the distortion is eliminated.

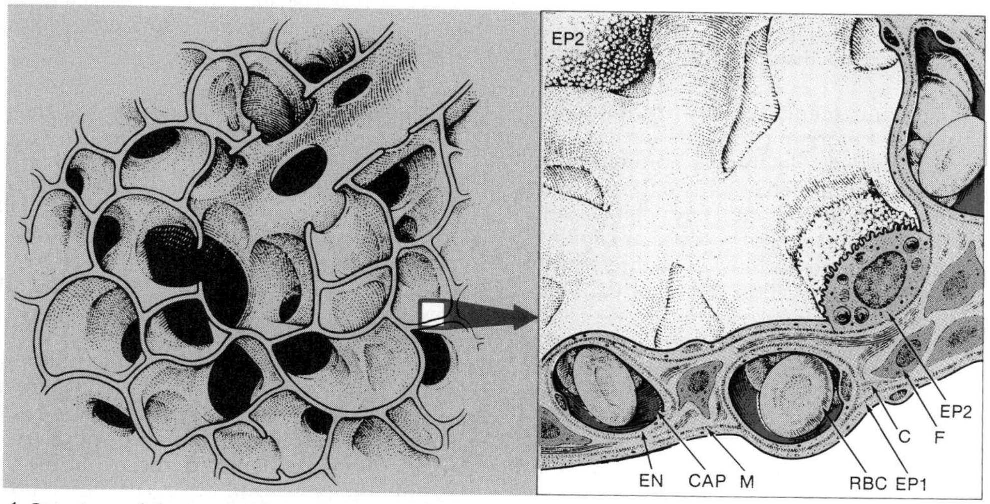

FIGURE 63–1. Structure of the normal lower respiratory tract. *Left*, Representation of a low-power view of the distal lung; the terminal bronchiole is shown but the pulmonary artery and vein are omitted. *Right*, Representation of a high-power view of an alveolus; the cut surface demonstrates the type I (EP1) and type II (EP2) epithelial cells, endothelial cells (EN), basement membranes (M), red blood cells (RBC) in the capillaries (CAP), fibroblasts (F), and connective tissue (C). Inflammatory cells are not shown. (Reprinted with permission from Crystal RG, Bitterman PB, Rennard SI, et al.: Interstitial lung diseases of unknown cause: Disorders characterized by chronic inflammation of the lower respiratory tract. N Engl J Med 310:154, 1984.)

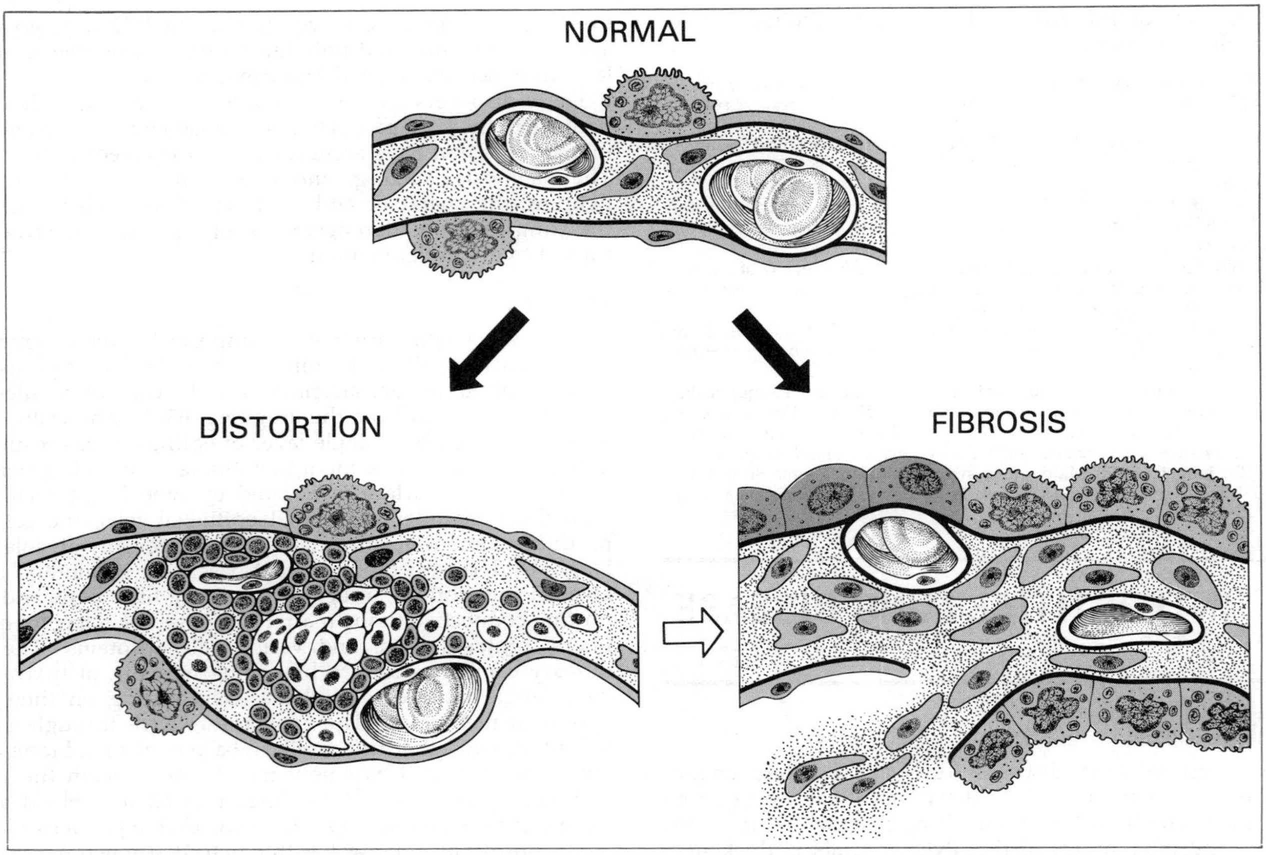

FIGURE 63–2. Typical forms of derangement of alveolar structures in the interstitial lung disorders. *Top*, Schematic of a cut surface of the normal alveolar wall. Shown are the type I and II epithelial cells, endothelial cells lining the capillaries, basement membranes, fibroblasts, and interstitial connective tissue. The few inflammatory cells normally present are not shown. *Lower left*, Schematic of a similar view of the alveolar wall deranged by the distortion caused by the accumulation of inflammatory cells. The example used is that of sarcoidosis, in which T lymphocytes, macrophages, and granulomas (massed accumulations of differentiated macrophages) distort the normal alveolar walls. *Lower right*, Schematic of a similar view of the alveolar wall deranged by fibrosis. The example used is that of idiopathic pulmonary fibrosis. In contrast to the distortion type of derangement, in which there is little damage and change in the lung parenchyma, in the fibrotic form of derangement the type I cells are injured, leaving denuded basement membrane. In some areas, the interstitial contents protrude into the airspace, causing intra-alveolar fibrosis. Note that some of the injured type I cells have been replaced by the type II cells and bronchiolar cells that have migrated down from the airways. Capillaries are injured; the basement membranes are thickened; there are expanded numbers of fibroblasts; and the density of connective tissue is increased. In the fibrotic type of derangement, there are also inflammatory cells distorting the alveolar wall (not shown), but this is overshadowed by the changes in normal parenchymal components. In some cases of the distortion type of derangement, there is sufficient damage to the parenchymal components that the derangements shift into a more fibrotic-type picture.

In the fibrosis form of derangement, typified by idiopathic pulmonary fibrosis and the inorganic dust disorders, the epithelial surface is often altered: Flat type I epithelial cells are lost, and the surface is repopulated with cuboidal cells derived from proliferating type II cells and bronchiolar cells migrating down from the terminal airways. Alveolar capillary endothelial cells are usually injured and lost. The interstitium is thickened with edema and proliferation of interstitial fibroblasts and accumulation of connective tissue products secreted by the fibroblasts, particularly collagen. The interstitium is scarred and fibrotic—hence the term "fibrotic lung disease" is also used to refer to these ILD. In the more aggressive forms of fibrosis-type derangements, there are breaks in the epithelial basement membrane through which the interstitial contents protrude; this often expands into intra-alveolar fibrotic masses called "intra-alveolar buds." As the fibrotic form of ILD progresses, the alveolar-capillary units become less distinguishable, and the lung parenchyma takes on the appearance of "end-stage lung" characterized by masses of fibrotic tissue interspaced with cystic areas representing the remnants of alveoli and dilated terminal bronchioles.

Epidemiology

The epidemiology for most of the ILD is not carefully defined, but it is estimated that in the United States their prevalence is approximately 20 to 40 per 100,000 of the population. Conventionally, the ILD are categorized as those of unknown and known etiology. Although there are more subcategories of ILD of known etiology than those of unknown etiology, in terms of total numbers of patients, more are of unknown etiology. The most common ILD of unknown etiology (Table 63–1) are idiopathic pulmonary fibrosis (IPF), chronic ILD associated with the collagen-vascular disorders, and sarcoidosis. Much less common are histiocytosis-X, Goodpasture's syndrome, chronic eosinophilic pneumonia, idiopathic pulmonary hemosiderosis, and the ILD associated with the pulmonary vasculitides. The other ILD of unknown etiology are very rare, with far fewer than 1000 cases of each reported in the world literature.

The ILD of known etiology are most commonly due to the inhalation of inorganic dusts, particularly crystalline silica, asbestos, and coal dust (Table 63–2), the hypersensitivity

TABLE 63–1. INTERSTITIAL LUNG DISEASES (ILD) OF UNKNOWN ETIOLOGY*

● Idiopathic Pulmonary Fibrosis (IPF)
● Sarcoidosis
● ILD Associated with the Collagen-Vascular Disorders
  Rheumatoid arthritis
  Progressive systemic sclerosis
  Systemic lupus erythematosus
  Polymyositis/dermatomyositis
  Sjögren's syndrome
  Mixed connective tissue disease
  Ankylosing spondylitis
Histiocytosis-X
Goodpasture's Syndrome
Idiopathic Pulmonary Hemosiderosis
Chronic Eosinophilic Pneumonia
Lymphocytic Infiltrative Disorders
  Immunoblastic lymphadenopathy
  Lymphocytic interstitial pneumonitis
  Pseudolymphoma
ILD Associated with Pulmonary Vasculitides
  Wegener's granulomatosis
  Lymphomatoid granulomatosis
  Churg-Strauss syndrome
  Systemic necrotizing vasculitides ("overlap" vasculitides)
  Hypersensitivity vasculitis
Inherited Disorders
  Familial idiopathic pulmonary fibrosis
  Neurofibromatosis
  Tuberous sclerosis
  Hermansky-Pudlak syndrome
  Niemann-Pick disease
  Gaucher's disease
ILD Associated with Pulmonary Airway Disease
  Bronchocentric granulomatosis
  Bronchopulmonary aspergillosis
Lymphangioleiomyomatosis
Alveolar Proteinosis
ILD Associated with Liver Disease
  Chronic active hepatitis
  Primary biliary cirrhosis
ILD Associated with Bowel Disease
  Whipple's disease
  Ulcerative colitis
  Crohn's disease
Weber-Christian Disease
Amyloidosis
Hypereosinophilic Syndrome
Pulmonary Veno-occlusive Disease
ILD Caused by Failure of Other Organs
  Chronic left ventricular failure
  Chronic left-to-right intracardiac shunt
  Chronic renal disease with uremia
Graft-versus-Host Disease
Recovery Phase of Adult Respiratory Distress Syndrome

*Disorders indicated with "●" are the most common ILD of unknown etiology.

pneumonitides (diseases caused by the repeated inhalation of organic dust—Table 63–3), and the drug-induced ILD (Table 63–4). Much less frequent are the ILD resulting from paraquat, radiation, the sequelae of known infectious agents, and the inhalation of gases, aerosols, chemical dusts, fumes, and vapors (Table 63–5). Occasionally, however, large populations develop ILD when exposed to a single agent at one time, such as occurred in Bhopal, India, in 1984 when methyl isocyanate was released into a crowded urban area.

Differential Diagnosis

The initial problem in assessing ILD is to differentiate it from other disorders that may also present with symptoms of respiratory deficiency and diffuse infiltrates on the chest radiograph (Table 63–6). In general, pulmonary edema, high-flow states, hemorrhage, and aspiration pneumonitis can be easily differentiated from the ILD by history and physical examination. The major problem is in ensuring that the patient does not have an infection or malignancy, diagnoses that require an appropriate evaluation of specimens from the lower respiratory tract for the presence of infectious agents or malignant cells, respectively. In some cases, such as HIV infection or filarial infestation, serologic studies are necessary.

The diagnosis of a specific ILD is made by a combination of historical, physical examination, blood, urine, roentgenographic, physiologic, scintigraphic, and bronchoscopic criteria. In addition, unless an agent of known etiology is apparent (e.g., long-term asbestos exposure), it is mandatory to evaluate the disease by morphologic means, usually by open lung biopsy. The only exception to this rule is when the ILD is in clear association with a systemic disorder (e.g., a collagen-vascular disease, Goodpasture's syndrome) in which the diagnosis can be made by evaluation of organs other than the lung.

Pathogenesis

The ILD are inflammatory disorders in which most of the derangements of the alveolar walls, including the fibrosis, are mediated by the accumulated inflammatory and immune effector cells. The inflammation, usually referred to as the "alveolitis" of the disease, not only involves the alveoli, but often involves the walls of small airways and sometimes the pulmonary blood vessels. The critical importance of the alveolitis is simply stated: Although dysfunction of the alveolar-capillary units causes the symptoms and impairment of the patient, it is the alveolitis that causes the derangements of the alveolar-capillary units, resulting in their dysfunction and eventual loss as gas-exchanging units (Fig. 63–3).

INITIATION OF THE ALVEOLITIS. Although it is not clear what initiates the inflammation in the ILD of unknown etiology, many of the processes that maintain the alveolitis are understood. For example, in idiopathic pulmonary fibrosis, alveolar macrophages, activated by immune complexes, release neutrophil-specific chemotactic factors that attract blood neutrophils to the lung. In contrast, in sarcoidosis, activated lung T lymphocytes release a monocyte-specific chemotactic factor that modulates the accumulation of blood monocytes in the alveolar structures.

For the disorders of known etiology, the causative agent most commonly activates the inflammatory cells that are normally present, which, in turn, propagate the alveolitis. Alternatively, the causative agent may directly injure the alveolar walls, and the resulting deranged tissue initiates the inflammation. For example, bleomycin, an antineoplastic drug, can injure lung parenchyma cells and by unknown mechanisms induce the formation of an alveolitis.

CHARACTER OF THE ALVEOLITIS. The inflammatory component of the ILD is defined by the number, type, and state of activation of the effector cells composing the alveolitis. The differences in the form and extent of the derangements

TABLE 63–2. INHALED INORGANIC DUSTS THAT CAUSE INTERSTITIAL LUNG DISEASE*,†

Silica (variants of SiO_2)
  ● Crystalline silica ("silicosis")
  Amorphous
Silicates
  ● Asbestos ("asbestosis")
  Talc (hydrated Mg silicates; "talcosis")
  Kaolin (china clay, hydrated aluminum silicate)
  Diatomaceous earth (Fuller's earth, aluminum silicate with Fe and Mg)
  Nepheline (hard rock containing mixed silicates)
  Aluminum silicates (sericite, sillimanite, zeolite)
  Portland cement
  Mica (principally K and Mg aluminum silicates)
Carbon (with or without crystalline silica)
  ● Coal dust ("coal worker's pneumoconiosis")
  Graphite ("carbon pneumoconiosis")
Metals
  Beryllium ("berylliosis")
  Aluminum ("aluminosis")
    Powdered aluminum ("aluminum lung")
    Bauxite (aluminum oxide; "Shaver's disease")
  Barium (powder of baryte or $BaSO_4$; "baritosis")
  Iron ("siderosis")
  Tin ("stannosis")
  Antimony (oxides and alloys)
  Mixed dusts
    Hematite (mixed dusts of iron oxide, silica and silicates; "siderosilicosis")
    Mixed dusts of silver and iron oxide ("argyrosiderosis")
  Hard metals
    Titanium oxide
    Tungsten, titanium, hafnium, niobium, cobalt, and vanadium carbides
    Cadmium
Rare earths (cerium, scandium, yttrium, lanthanum)
$CuSO_4$ neutralized with hydrated lime (Bordeaux mixture; "vineyard sprayer's lung")

*The most common inorganic dust–induced interstitial lung diseases are indicated with "●".

†Disorders given a specific name are indicated in quotes in parentheses; others are referred as "(name of the dust) pneumoconiosis."

TABLE 63–3. INHALED ORGANIC DUSTS THAT CAUSE INTERSTITIAL LUNG DISEASE*

Disorder	Causative Agent†
• Farmer's lung	*M. faeni, T. vulgaris, A. fumigatus, T. candidus*
• Humidifier lung, air conditioner lung	*T. vulgaris, T. candidus,* thermotolerant bacteria, protozoa, *Penicillium* species, *Naegleria gruberi*
• Bird breeder's disease‡	Avian proteins, feathers
Maple bark stripper's lung	*Cryptostroma corticale*
Cheese worker's lung	*A. clavatus, Penicillium caseii*
Malt worker's lung	*A. clavatus, A. fumigatus*
Sequoiosis	*Aureobasidium pullulans, Graphium* species
Paprika splitter's lung	*Mucor stolonifer*
Wheat weevil disease	*Sitophilus granarius*
Suberosis	*Penicillium frequentans*
Bagassosis	*T. sacchari*
Mushroom worker's lung	*M. faeni, T. vulgaris*
Pituitary snuff lung	Porcine and bovine proteins
Wood-pulp worker's disease	*Alternaria* species
Sauna-taker's disease	*Aureobasidium* species
Detergent worker's lung	*Bacillus subtilis*
Lycoperdonosis	*Lycoperdon bovista*
Rodent handler's disease	Serum and urine constituents
Dry rot disease	*Merulius lacrymans*
Wood-dust worker's lung	Unknown
Furrier's lung	Unknown
New Guinea lung	*Saccharomonospora irridis*
Coptic disease (mummy unwrapper's disease)	Antigens associated with mummy wrappings
"Summer type" disease	*Cryptococcus neoformans*
	§*Cephalosporium* species
	§*Streptomyces albus*
	§*Bacillus subtilis*

*The most common interstitial lung disorders caused by inhaled organic antigens are indicated with "•".

†M. = *Micropolyspora;* T. = *Thermoactinomyces;* A. = *Aspergillus.*

‡Includes pigeons, parakeets, budgerigars, turkeys, chickens, and ducks.

§Hypersensitivity pneumonitis has been described in association with these agents, in circumstances in which no common name has been given to the disorder.

to the lower respiratory tract in these disorders are defined by the sum of these characteristics.

In the normal lung there are approximately 80 inflammatory cells per alveolus. Most (greater than 80 per cent) are alveolar macrophages, phagocytic cells derived from blood monocytes. The remainder are lymphocytes, mostly T cells, but with a small number of B cells. Polymorphonuclear leukocytes are rare in the normal lung, although small numbers do accumulate with a long history of cigarette smoking. As a general rule, alveolar macrophages and T and B lymphocytes are not activated in the normal lung. Immunoglobulins are present in the normal lower respiratory tract (IgG > IgA >> IgM), as are most complement components. Macromolecules that defend against inflammatory injury, including antiproteases and antioxidants, are also present.

Active, untreated ILD are generally characterized by a marked increase in the number of inflammatory cells in the alveolar walls and on the alveolar epithelial surface. Commonly, this increase in numbers of effector cells is also characterized by a shift in their relative proportions. Different patterns of alveolitis are generally referred to by the cell types that are most abundant. For example, when the inflammation is dominated by neutrophils and macrophages it is referred to as a neutrophil-macrophage alveolitis. The alveolitis patterns most frequently observed in ILD are a macrophage-dominant alveolitis, a lymphocyte-macrophage alveolitis, and

TABLE 63–4. DRUGS THAT CAUSE INTERSTITIAL LUNG DISEASE

Antineoplastic Agents
- Azathioprine
- Bleomycin
- Cyclophosphamide
- Methotrexate
- Nitrosoureas
  - Carmustine (BCNU)
  - Lomustine (CCNU)
  - Semustine (methyl-CCNU)
  - Chlorozotocin (DCNU)
- Melphalan
- Busulfan
- Chlorambucil
- 6-Mercaptopurine
- 6-Thioguanine
- Mitomycin C
- Procarbazine
- Uracil mustard
- Zinostatin

Antibiotics
- Nitrofurantoin
- Penicillins
- Sulfonamides
- Erythromycin
- Tetracycline
- Isoniazid
- para-Aminosalicylic acid
- Niridazole

Cardiovascular Drugs
- Hydralazine
- Procainamide
- Beta blockers (propranolol, practolol, pindolol, acebutolol)
- Tocainide
- Amiodarone
- Reserpine

Central Nervous System Drugs
- Phenytoin
- Carbamazepine
- Chlorpromazine
- Imipramine
- Amitriptyline
- Methylphenidate
- Dantrolene
- Mephenesin

Ganglionic Blocking Agents
- Mecamylamine
- Hexamethonium
- Pentolinium

Anti-inflammatory Agents
- Gold salts
- Phenylbutazone
- Beclomethasone
- Naproxen

Oral Hypoglycemic Agents
- Chlorpropamide
- Tolbutamide
- Tolazamide

Miscellaneous
- Penicillamine
- Allopurinol
- Cromolyn sodium
- Hydrochlorothiazide
- Mineral oil
- Intravenous drugs containing particulate material
- Silicon used for tissue augmentation

TABLE 63–5. OTHER AGENTS KNOWN TO CAUSE INTERSTITIAL LUNG DISEASE

- Paraquat
- Radiation
- Sequela of Known Infectious Agents
  - Bacteria
  - *Mycoplasma*
  - Mycobacteria
  - *Legionella pneumophila*
  - Fungi
  - Parasites
  - Viruses
- Inhaled Agents Other Than Inorganic or Organic Dusts
  - Gases
    - Oxygen
    - Sulfur dioxide
    - Oxides of nitrogen
    - Methyl isocyanate
    - Chlorine gas
  - Aerosols
    - Aspiration pneumonia
    - Pyrethrum (a natural insecticide)
    - Fats
    - Toluene diisocyanate
    - Oils
  - Chemical dusts
    - Synthetic fibers (Orlon, polyesters, nylon, acrylic)
    - Bakelite
    - Vinyl chloride, polyvinyl chloride powder
  - Fumes
    - Oxides of Zn, Cu, Mn, Cd, Fe, Mg, Ni, Se, Sn, Sb, V, and brass
    - Diphenylmethane diisocyanate
    - Trimellitic anhydride
  - Vapors
    - Hydrocarbons
    - Mercury
    - Thermosetting resins

TABLE 63–6. DISORDERS INVOLVING THE LOWER RESPIRATORY TRACT THAT CAN BE CONFUSED WITH INTERSTITIAL LUNG DISEASE*

- Pulmonary Edema
- Neoplasms
  - • Leukemic infiltration
  - • Lymphoma
  - • Lymphangitic spread of carcinoma
  - Multiple metastases
  - Primary pulmonary malignancy
- Infections
  - • Viruses†
  - Fungi
  - Bacteria‡
  - • Mycobacteria
  - • Parasites§
  - • Mycoplasma
  - Psittacosis
  - Q fever
- Pulmonary Hemorrhage
- Aspiration

*Disorders frequently confused with the ILD are indicated with "•."

†Of the viruses known to involve the lung—influenza, cytomegalovirus (CMV), varicella zoster, and measles—HIV are most commonly confused with ILD.

‡Particularly *Legionella.*

§*Pneumocystis* and filarial disease are commonly mistaken for ILD.

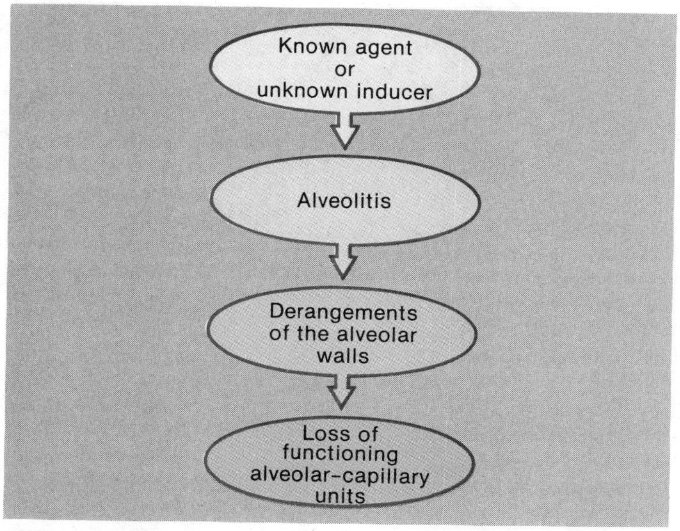

FIGURE 63–3. Pathogenesis of the interstitial lung diseases of unknown and known etiology. In both groups, the inflammation (alveolitis) is responsible for the bulk of the derangements of the alveolar walls. In some disorders, the deranged wall components may accelerate the alveolitis by recruiting additional inflammatory cells. In the disorders of known etiology, the causative agent may directly damage the alveolar structures, which, in turn, initiates and/or accelerates the alveolitis.

a neutrophil-macrophage alveolitis. Eosinophils play a role in the alveolitis of many ILD but rarely dominate it. Subcategories of the common alveolitis patterns have also been described. For example, the granulomatous lung disorders, sarcoidosis and berylliosis, are characterized by a T-helper cell macrophage alveolitis, while chronic hypersensitivity pneumonitis is usually characterized by a T-suppressor/cytotoxic cell macrophage alveolitis, sometimes including neutrophils.

In addition to the numbers and types of inflammatory cells present, the consequences of the alveolitis critically depend on the state of activation of these cells. The simple presence of the inflammatory cells in the alveolar structures distorts the alveolar walls but usually is not damaging. When activated, however, some inflammatory cells can injure the alveolar walls, particularly sensitive type I epithelial cells and capillary endothelial cells. If the alveolitis is self limiting, or if it is suppressed by therapy before the injury becomes too severe, the architecture of the lower respiratory tract can be re-established and normal lung function restored. If, however, the injury is extensive, with fibroblast proliferation and collagen deposition, the normal architecture of the affected alveolar-capillary units can never be fully re-established. Therapeutic success in treating ILD means suppression of the alveolitis and thus prevention of further loss of alveolar-capillary units.

DISTORTION AND FIBROSIS. Whether the derangements to the alveolar walls take the form of distortion and/or fibrosis is dictated by the characteristics of the alveolitis. Importantly, while the distortion type of derangement is usually reversible if the inflammation is suppressed, the consequences of the fibrosis form of derangement are commonly sufficient to prevent a return to the normal architecture.

Accumulation of sufficient numbers of any type of inflammatory cells results in some distortion of the tissue. However, this form of derangement is most important when the inflammation involves lymphocytes and macrophages, such as when there is an accumulation of activated T-helper lymphocytes that direct the formation of granuloma. Together, the T cells and masses of macrophages distort the normal architecture but usually do not cause permanent damage.

The fibrosis form of derangement is characterized by injury to parenchymal components, together with the accumulation of fibroblasts and their secreted connective tissue products. The neutrophil is the most damaging of all inflammatory cells by virtue of its highly reactive oxygen metabolites that are toxic to the parenchymal cells and its connective tissue-specific proteases that can damage the interstitial collagens and basement membranes. Injury to the epithelial basement membrane has profound consequences because the epithelial cells no longer have a surface upon which to migrate, making it impossible to reconstruct a normal alveolar surface. The eosinophil can also injure lung parenchymal cells and connective tissue, but on a per cell basis it is far less potent than the neutrophil. Activated human alveolar macrophages release toxic oxidants and thus can be cytotoxic to normal lung parenchymal cells. The macrophage also mediates the accumulation of fibroblasts and the connective tissue that characterizes the fibrosis type of derangement to the alveolar walls. The fundamental problem is the accumulation of fibroblasts in the alveolar walls. Since fibroblasts are major producers of collagen, the consequence of an increase in fibroblast numbers is an accumulation of collagen in the alveolar interstitium. As a result, the alveolar wall is thickened and scarred and has decreased compliance. The macrophage mediates the accumulation of fibroblasts by releasing exaggerated amounts of at least three mediators, platelet-derived growth factor, fibronectin, and alveolar macrophage-derived growth factor. Platelet-derived growth factor, a product of the *c-sis* oncogene, attracts fibroblasts and is a potent stimulus for fibroblasts to begin traversing the cell cycle. Fibronectin, a 440,000-dalton glycoprotein, attracts fibroblasts, attaches them to the extracellular matrix, and stimulates them to enter the cell cycle. The alveolar macrophage–derived growth factor, an 18,000-dalton protein, induces the fibronectin-primed fibroblasts to continue through the cell cycle and proliferate.

Clinical Features

HISTORY. Occasional patients are detected as having ILD because a routine chest radiograph is noted to be abnormal, but most come to medical attention because of symptoms related to the chest. All ILD are characterized by abnormalities in the transfer of oxygen from air to blood secondary to slowly progressive derangement of the lower respiratory tract. The initial symptoms are those of insufficient oxygen transfer, such as *fatigue* and *breathlessness with exertion.* These symptoms are often initially denied by the patient or are attributed to being "out of shape" or "overweight" or to a prior chest infection, usually a viral syndrome. As the disease progresses, the dyspnea becomes more apparent and eventually is felt at rest. In contrast to cardiac-induced dyspnea, paroxysmal nocturnal dyspnea and orthopnea are rare, as are platypnea and trepopnea. Nonproductive cough, pleuritic pain, and hemoptysis are less common presenting complaints. Early in the disease, chest pain is rare, although later, when pulmonary hypertension develops, substernal discomfort may be noted.

The history also plays an important role in the diagnosis of the type of interstitial disease. Since a large number of agents cause ILD, a careful exposure history is essential in order to determine not only the agents to which the patient has been exposed, but also the circumstances, intensity, and duration of exposure. Exposure to agents that cause ILD may be found in nonclassic situations. For example, silicosis has been described in workers involved in the manufacture of pencils, furniture, and tombstones; talcosis in the manufacture of rubber condoms; and hypersensitivity pneumonitis in office buildings where the offending organic antigen was located in the air conditioning system.

The lack of a history of exposure to a known agent that causes interstitial disease is very important to diagnosing the ILD of unknown etiology. For example, pulmonary sarcoidosis is very difficult to separate from berylliosis unless there is a negative history of beryllium exposure. Likewise, idiopathic pulmonary fibrosis is difficult to diagnose if an exposure history is unavailable or if there is a clear history of sufficient exposure to one or more agents that cause ILD. Some ILD of unknown etiology are associated with diseases that often involve other organs, such as the collagen-vascular disorders, primary biliary cirrhosis, and Wegener's granulomatosis, which may be suspected from the history.

PHYSICAL EXAMINATION. The chest expansion is typically reduced, reflecting the reduced total lung capacity of individuals with ILD. Most have fine, crackling inspiratory and expiratory rales, heard best at the posterior lung bases. These rales have a characteristic sound, described as "Velcro-like" (i.e., the sound of unwrapping a blood pressure cuff) or like the sound of rubbing hair together. Coarse rales, wheezing, and rhonchi are occasionally heard. As the disease progresses, these patients may be tachypneic at rest, but unlike emphysema victims, they do not use the accessory muscles of respiratory and do not assume the posture of placing their hands on their thighs to "fix" the upper body to assist in respiration.

Early in the disease, examination of the heart is normal. Later, an accentuated P_2 reflects mild pulmonary hypertension. Eventually, obvious evidence of pulmonary hypertension is noted, including a right ventricular heave. Patients with ILD rarely develop frank right-sided failure with liver enlargement and peripheral edema, presumably because they die from the complications of insufficient oxygen delivery before the right ventricle deteriorates.

Clubbing of the fingers and sometimes the toes is common in ILD, particularly in idiopathic pulmonary fibrosis and asbestosis. Cyanosis occurs, but usually very late in the disease. Other physical findings in ILD are those associated with problems with oxygen transport (e.g., left ventricular failure, central nervous system signs) and those characteristic of associated diseases (e.g., the rash of systemic lupus erythematosus, the skin changes of scleroderma).

LABORATORY STUDIES. No blood test is diagnostic for one ILD, and the intensity and character of the alveolitis are not reflected in the blood. The hemoglobin and hematocrit are usually normal despite associated hypoxemia, and the white blood cell count and differential usually bear no relationship to the alveolitis. In most ILD, the sedimentation rate is elevated.

A patient with suspected ILD should have routine blood screening tests for hematologic, liver, renal, and muscle abnormalities and collagen-vascular disorders. Other blood tests directed toward specific diseases may be ordered as the workup proceeds and specific disease is suspected. For example, serologic tests for antibodies against organic antigens are ordered only in the context of suspected hypersensitivity pneumonitis and anti–basement membrane antibodies only when there is suspected Goodpasture's syndrome.

Rheumatoid factor and antinuclear antibodies are occasionally present in low titer and do not necessarily indicate the presence of an underlying collagen-vascular disorder. Plasma immunoglobulins may be elevated, but this finding is usually nonspecific. Except in those circumstances in which the disease is systemic (e.g., sarcoidosis, a collagen-vascular disorder), other screening blood studies are generally normal.

The electrocardiogram (ECG) is usually normal in ILD except for evidence of pulmonary hypertension. As the loss of alveolar-capillary units progresses, the ECG demonstrates a pattern of right atrial and ventricular strain. The hypoxemia of ILD may exacerbate coexisting coronary heart disease, evoking arrhythmias and evidence of coronary insufficiency, particularly with exercise.

RADIOGRAPHIC STUDIES. The posteroanterior and lateral chest films play a major role in establishing the diagnosis of ILD, although 5 to 10 per cent of patients with biopsy-proven disease have a normal chest film. A ground-glass pattern may be seen early in the disease. More typically, the chest radiograph demonstrates a diffuse, finely nodular, reticular, or reticulonodular pattern usually more prominent at the bases (Fig. 63–4). As the disease evolves, the pattern becomes coarser, with cystic areas appearing and, finally, a honeycomb pattern. Initially the pulmonary arteries appear normal, but in the later stages of ILD evidence of pulmonary hypertension may be present.

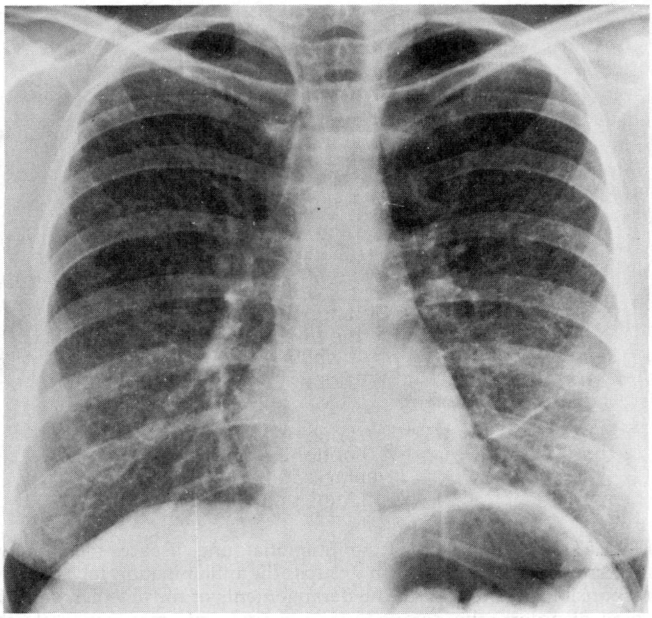

FIGURE 63–4. Chest radiograph of a patient with idiopathic pulmonary fibrosis, typical of the radiographic findings of many interstitial lung diseases. There is a diffuse reticulonodular infiltrate throughout the lung fields, most prominent at the bases. The heart and pleura are normal.

A definitive diagnosis of a specific ILD can never be made by the chest radiograph alone. However, certain radiographic patterns are characteristic of specific diseases or groups of diseases and thus are very helpful in establishing a diagnosis. For example, some ILD are also characterized by hilar and/or paratracheal lymph node enlargement, while others manifest pleural disease.

Except for rare circumstances, radiographic studies other than the routine chest film have little use in the evaluation of ILD. Oblique films, tomography, bronchography, and angiography are occasionally used to evaluate localized lesions on a background of ILD but usually are difficult to interpret. At present, computerized axial tomographic (CT) scans of the chest are not used in the evaluation of these patients except in the circumstance in which questionable pleural lesions are being evaluated.

PULMONARY FUNCTION TESTS. The classic physiologic alterations in ILD include reduced lung volumes (vital capacity, total lung capacity), reduced diffusing capacity, and a normal or supranormal ratio of forced expiratory volume in 1 second to forced vital capacity. In some ILD, sensitive tests such as flow-volume curves and maximum flow-static recoil curves can detect mild limitation of airflow. Measurement of static lung compliance demonstrates decreased lung volumes for a given transpulmonary pressure, and an increased maximal transpulmonary pressure, i.e., very high negative pressures (relative to the atmosphere), must be generated to open the fibrotic alveoli.

Arterial blood gases typically show mild hypoxemia; carbon dioxide retention is rare, even late in the course of the disease. Patients with ILD tend to hyperventilate and have a reduced P_{CO_2} and compensated respiratory alkalosis, mostly as a result of an increase in respiratory rate. The drive to hyperventilate is not due to hypoxemia or abnormalities in acid-base status but rather to the subjective sense of dyspnea or from an increased stimulation of the respiratory center from neural signals arising in the deranged lung parenchyma. With exercise, the arterial Po_2 drops, while the Pco_2 remains constant. The loss of alveolar-capillary bed in ILD and hence the limitation of cardiac output seriously impair oxygen delivery and thereby markedly limit the exercise tolerance of these patients. This leads to their propensity to suffer hypoxic damage to vital organs. The arterial pH is usually normal in ILD, but it can fall with exercise as a consequence of oxygen deprivation of muscles, which then resort to anaerobic metabolism.

At rest, the hypoxemia of ILD results from abnormal matching of pulmonary ventilation and perfusion. With exercise, however, an apparent "diffusion block" also contributes. It was originally thought that this resulted from a limited oxygen diffusion through the thickened alveolar walls, but it is now recognized to be due to red blood cells passing through the functioning pulmonary capillaries too rapidly to permit full saturation of hemoglobin. In rare instances, some of the hypoxemia of ILD results from shunts, either in the lung parenchyma or through a patent foramen ovale in the setting of pulmonary hypertension.

The loss of pulmonary capillary bed in ILD is associated with pulmonary hypertension, first with exercise only and later at rest. The pulmonary hypertension is thought to result from mechanical reasons (e.g., the loss of pulmonary capillary bed) and not from hypoxia-induced vasoconstriction or from local mediators. Right ventricular end-diastolic pressure rises late in the disease, but this rarely leads to frank right-sided failure.

SCINTIGRAPHIC STUDIES. Conventional ventilation and perfusion scans usually demonstrate diffuse abnormalities. The perfusion scans show multiple subsegmental areas of impaired perfusion. The normal, upright individual has limited blood flow to the upper lobes at rest. The perfusion scan in ILD, however, shows a redistribution of perfusion to the upper lobes resulting from the loss of pulmonary capillary bed and developing pulmonary hypertension. The ventilation scan shows multiple subsegmental areas of reduced ventilation. Comparison of the perfusion and ventilation scans demonstrates numerous areas of ventilation and perfusion mismatch. The presence of numerous perfusion defects limits the usefulness of these techniques in evaluation of patients with ILD with suspected pulmonary emboli. In such circumstances, pulmonary angiography is mandatory.

Gallium-67 scans are used to evaluate the alveolitis of ILD. Whereas the normal lung parenchyma takes up little gallium-67, ILD with an active alveolitis demonstrate positive gallium-67 lung scans with either a diffuse or a patchy pattern (Fig. 63–5). A high density of activated alveolar macrophages is thought to play a major role in the lung uptake of gallium-67 in these patients.

BRONCHOSCOPIC STUDIES. Most patients with suspected ILD are evaluated by fiberoptic bronchoscopy to rule out neoplastic or infectious disease. In selected patients (see below), transbronchial biopsy can be carried out at the same time.

The technique of bronchoalveolar lavage can be used to sample the inflammatory cells constituting the alveolitis. To accomplish this, the bronchoscope is wedged into a distal bronchus, and aliquots of sterile saline are used to recover the inflammatory cells and epithelial lining fluid of the lower respiratory tract. In normal individuals, 80 per cent or more of the recovered cells demonstrate alveolar macrophages, with the remainder being lymphocytes (almost all T lymphocytes). Polymorphonuclear leukocytes are normally very rare. In patients with ILD, the pattern of alveolitis is reflected by the cells recovered by lavage. For example, in pulmonary sarcoidosis, the proportions of T cells may be 30 to 60 per cent,

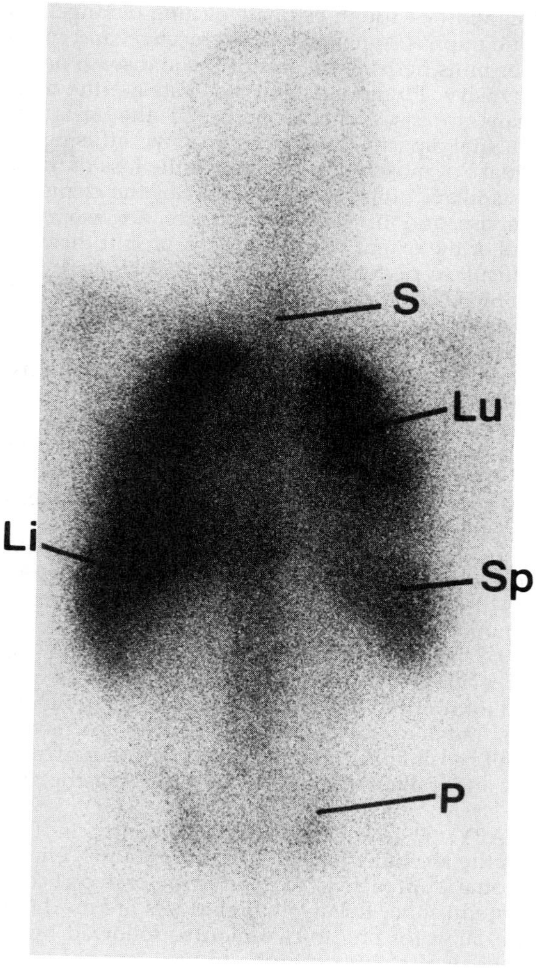

FIGURE 63–5. Gallium-67 scan of a patient with sarcoidosis. There is diffuse uptake of the isotope throughout the lung parenchyma (Lu). Structures that normally take up gallium-67 are also seen, including the spine (S), liver (Li), spleen (Sp), and pelvis (P).

while in idiopathic pulmonary fibrosis, the proportion of neutrophils is greater than 10 per cent. The diagnostic usefulness of bronchoalveolar lavage has not been established, but it can help to orient the clinician to the category of alveolitis that is present. Furthermore, because alveolar macrophages are phagocytic and ingest foreign materials present in the lung parenchyma, bronchoalveolar lavage can also be used to help diagnose specific agents that cause ILD, including inorganic dust diseases.

BIOPSY. The diagnosis of many ILD depends upon pathologic studies of lung parenchyma. The method of choice is the open lung biopsy, usually performed in the right middle lobe or lingula in an area of "average" disease as judged by the chest film. Transbronchial biopsy through the fiberoptic bronchoscope is useful for diagnosing sarcoidosis, but for most other ILD the samples are too small for a definitive diagnosis to be made.

Staging and Therapy

A patient with ILD should be evaluated to assess the contribution of the disease to his functional impairment. The activity of the disease process should be independently assessed. Once both are known, rational decisions can be made concerning prognosis and therapy.

ASSESSMENT OF IMPAIRMENT. The consequences of ILD are assessed by history, chest radiograph, and lung function testing. A careful history of the patient's sensation of breathlessness, combined with an estimate of exercise tolerance, allows a rough estimate of lung derangement. The chest radiograph is somewhat more objective, and comparison with prior films helps to determine if the disease has become more extensive. Pulmonary function tests are the most accurate means to assess impairment. Of the tests routinely available, vital capacity, total lung capacity, diffusing capacity, and arterial P_{O_2} most accurately gauge the loss of functioning alveolar-capillary units. Measurements of the changes in P_{O_2} with exercise and of static compliance are more sensitive indicators of the extent of the impairment, but these tests are more difficult to perform and are not widely available.

ASSESSMENT OF ACTIVITY. Alveolitis is confined to the lower respiratory tract, so that its character or extent is difficult to measure directly. Circulating immune complexes and angiotensin-converting enzyme have been suggested as measures of the alveolitis in idiopathic pulmonary fibrosis and sarcoidosis, respectively, but neither test is very sensitive or specific. Likewise, attempts to correlate the chest radiograph or lung function tests with morphologic evidence of the alveolitis have been disappointing, and thus neither can be used to accurately evaluate the alveolitis.

Open lung biopsy, bronchoalveolar lavage, and *gallium-67 scanning* are the best present methods to stage alveolitis. Open biopsy is the most accurate method but is very rarely performed more than once in the course of the disease. Bronchoalveolar lavage and gallium-67 scanning are both sensitive to and specific for the alveolitis, but neither has been fully validated for routine clinical use. At this time, bronchoalveolar lavage is most useful for evaluating the intensity of the neutrophil, eosinophil, and lymphocyte components of the alveolitis and gallium-67 scanning for the macrophage component.

THERAPY. The principal aim of therapy in ILD is to suppress the alveolitis. For the ILD of unknown etiology, the conventional approach is to treat with oral corticosteroids, usually prednisone. Relatively high doses are used (1 mg per kilogram daily) for one to two months followed by tapering doses over two to three months to maintenance levels (0.25 mg per kilogram daily), which are continued for varying periods of time. The corticosteroids are generally given once daily; it is not known if alternate-day regimens are equally effective. There has never been a large controlled trial of corticosteroids in any ILD, but some patients with ILD respond to corticosteroids in a fashion that cannot be explained by spontaneous remission. "Successful" therapy does not necessarily mean improvement in pulmonary function, chest radiograph, or subjective symptoms, since severely damaged alveoli are lost forever. In this context, successful suppression of the alveolitis usually means no further loss of alveoli. If improvement does occur, it likely results from suppression of the contribution of the inflammation itself to the derangements of the alveolar structures.

If the disease stabilizes, the corticosteroids are usually tapered. If the deterioration restarts after a period of quiescence, corticosteroids are often restarted, but their efficacy under these circumstances is limited. A variety of cytotoxic and other anti-inflammatory drugs have also been used in the treatment of the ILD of unknown etiology, but there has been no controlled series to demonstrate their efficacy.

For the ILD of known etiology, the initial treatment is to remove exposure to the causative agent. If the inflammation persists months after removal from the known agent, the patients are usually treated in a similar fashion to ILD of unknown etiology. The exception to this rule is in most of the pneumoconioses, for which no therapy is used.

In all ILD, attention should be given to prompt treatment of lung infections. Bronchodilators are sometimes used in mid to late course in these diseases to help mobilize secretions. Oxygen therapy, particularly with exercise, is often used as the patient reaches the late stage of ILD, but its efficacy in increasing the lifespan of these patients is unproven.

INTERSTITIAL LUNG DISEASES OF UNKNOWN ETIOLOGY

The ILD of unknown etiology represent the majority of all cases of ILD. Although of unknown etiology, each represents a specific entity with distinct features (Table 63–1). The best understood ILD of unknown etiology are idiopathic pulmonary fibrosis and sarcoidosis.

Idiopathic Pulmonary Fibrosis (IPF)

CLINICAL MANIFESTATIONS. IPF, the "classic" fibrotic lung disease, is characterized by a neutrophil-alveolar macrophage alveolitis and progressive scarring of alveolar-capillary units. In the past IPF was sometimes called the Hamman-Rich syndrome, but this designation is not generally used now. Typically, IPF presents in middle age, but all age groups can be affected. The sex distribution is equal. Patients present with dyspnea on exertion and/or a dry cough, often following a viral illness. Fever is rare. Physical examination demonstrates dry, bibasilar rales, often associated with clubbing of the fingers and sometimes of the toes. The chest radiograph typically shows a diffuse reticulonodular infiltrate most prominent at the bases without hilar or pleural abnormalities. Some patients have various "autoimmune" abnormalities that likely represent nonspecific epiphenomena. Circulating immune complexes are common. Pulmonary function tests are typical for ILD, with reduced volumes and diffusing capacity. Routine tests of airflow are normal, but sensitive tests reveal mild airflow limitation, an observation that correlates with morphologic evidence of narrowing of small airways. Patients with IPF have mild resting hypoxemia that drops significantly with physical activity. Typically, a resting P_{O_2} of 80 torr will fall to 50 torr with exercise equivalent to walking up one flight of stairs. Ventilation and perfusion studies reveal diffuse patchy abnormalities with mismatching of air and blood. The gallium-67 scan usually shows a diffuse uptake of isotope throughout the lung parenchyma, and bronchoalveolar lavage reveals an alveolitis pattern dominated by neutrophils and macrophages, with fewer numbers of lymphocytes and eosinophils. The epithelial lining fluid of the lower respiratory tract contains elevated levels of IgG, immune complexes, and neutrophil products, including collagenase and myeloperoxidase. Open lung biopsy shows a diffuse alveolitis that is patchy in its intensity. There is marked derangement of the alveolar walls with a fibrosis type pattern, including denudation of the epithelial basement membranes; replacement of the type I epithelial cells by type II epithelial cells and bronchiolar cells; loss of capillaries; and expansion of the interstitium with edema, increased fibroblast numbers, and masses of deranged collagen fibers. The epithelial basement membranes have holes through which the interstitial fibrosis extends into the airspaces.

The clinical course of IPF is characterized by progressive loss of alveolar-capillary units, with eventual respiratory failure and death an average of five years after the onset of symptoms. Occasional patients have a rapidly progressive course; others may live for ten or more years. IPF is associated with a higher than expected incidence of lung carcinoma, myocardial infarction, and pulmonary embolism.

DIFFERENTIAL DIAGNOSIS. Although the term "IPF" suggests that the diagnosis is one of exclusion, its features are so characteristic that the diagnosis is usually not difficult. Most confusion comes in separating ILD associated with the collagen-vascular disorders, which are systemic diseases, whereas IPF is compartmentalized to the lung. To exclude the ILD of known etiology that can mimic IPF, it is mandatory to take a careful history of past exposures to agents that can cause ILD. An open lung biopsy is necessary for diagnosis, but IPF cannot be diagnosed using morphologic criteria alone. While the biopsy features of IPF fit the morphologic categories of "usual interstitial pneumonitis (UIP)," "desquamative interstitial pneumonitis (DIP)," or, more commonly, a mixture of UIP and DIP, these features are not specific for IPF and can be found in other ILD of both known and unknown etiology.

PATHOGENESIS. IPF likely results from uncontrolled inflammatory processes that ensue after any of a variety of insults to the lower respiratory tract of susceptible individuals. There is likely an inherited susceptibility to this disease, but links to a specific genetic locus have not been made. The neutrophil-macrophage–dominated alveolitis, the first known manifestation of IPF, may be driven by immune complexes of unknown origin formed within the lower respiratory tract. The immune complexes are probably associated with enhanced lung B cell immunoglobin production, with at least some of the immunoglobulins directed against local self-antigens. These immune comlexes activate alveolar macrophages to release neutrophil-specific chemotactic factors that continuously recruit neutrophils to the alveolar structures. The neutrophils damage the alveolar walls by releasing toxic oxygen radicals and proteases. IPF macrophages spontaneously release exaggerated amounts of platelet-derived growth factor, fibronectin, and alveolar macrophage–derived growth factor and thus expand the numbers of fibroblasts, resulting in fibrosis of the alveolar walls.

STAGING AND THERAPY. The degree of lung damage in IPF is determined by history, chest radiograph, and pulmonary function testing. The intensity of the alveolitis of IPF can be gauged by gallium-67 scanning and bronchoalveolar lavage, with particular emphasis placed on the intensity of the neutrophil component of the alveolitis. Conventional therapy is use of corticosteroids, usually as lifelong therapy. Approximately 10 to 20 per cent of IPF patients improve with corticosteroids, particularly if the disease is detected early, before the alveolitis causes significant abnormalities. The second line of therapy is either the addition of massive doses of methylprednisolone sodium succinate (Solu-Medrol) (2 grams IV once weekly) or oral cyclophosphamide (1.5 mg per kilogram daily). Either approach helps suppress the alveolitis, but their long-term efficacy is unknown.

Sarcoidosis

Sarcoidosis (Ch. 69) is a multisystem granulomatous disease of unknown etiology characterized in affected organs by a T-helper lymphocyte–mononuclear phagocyte inflammatory process, noncaseating granulomata, and derangement of normal tissue architecture. While most organs can be affected by sarcoidosis, the lower respiratory tract is the site that most commonly causes morbidity and mortality. Pulmonary sarcoidosis is characterized by sharply circumscribed granulomata in the alveolar, bronchial, and vascular walls, composed of tightly packed cells derived from the mononuclear phagocyte system. In addition, the alveolar walls are deranged in a fashion similar to IPF, but much less so. Significant interstitial fibrosis occurs in 20 to 25 per cent of patients. Sarcoidosis is described in detail in Ch. 69 and will not be discussed further here.

ILD Associated with the Collagen-Vascular Disorders

All collagen-vascular disorders are associated with ILD. In most cases the collagen-vascular disorder is apparent before lung involvement is noted, but occasionally the ILD develops first and the other characteristic systemic signs and symptoms appear later. In either case, these disorders are frequently confused with IPF.

RHEUMATOID ARTHRITIS (Ch. 433). The ILD associated with rheumatoid arthritis include (1) an IPF-like disorder, (2) Caplan's syndrome (rheumatoid arthritis associated with coal worker's pneumoconiosis), (3) pulmonary parenchymal rheumatoid nodules, (4) pulmonary arteritis, and (5) apical fibrobullous disease. A few patients with rheumatoid arthritis have been described with dyspnea, severe irreversible airway obstruction with hyperinflation, and morphologic evidence of obliterative bronchiolitis. While some of this terminal airway disease may be related to penicillamine therapy, it may represent another manifestation of rheumatoid arthritis in the lung parenchyma.

The IPF-like disorder is by far the most common pulmonary manifestation of rheumatoid arthritis. Approximately 25 per cent of chest radiographs of patients with rheumatoid arthritis show interstitial changes, and the diffusing capacity is reduced in 50 per cent of all patients. In most cases the lung disease is much milder than IPF. The pathogenesis of the ILD is unknown but assumed to be the consequence of the same processes that affect the joints. The alveolitis is similar to IPF, but the neutrophil component is much less evident. There is no relationship between the extent of disease and the titer of the rheumatoid factor. Most cases of ILD associated with rheumatoid arthritis do not need to be treated. If treatment is instituted, guidelines similar to those for IPF are used. Gold salts, a common therapy for rheumatoid arthritis, can also induce ILD. There is no way to distinguish between gold salt– and rheumatoid arthritis–induced ILD, except that the gold-induced disease may reverse when the drug is discontinued.

PROGRESSIVE SYSTEMIC SCLEROSIS (PSS) (Ch. 527). The most common form of ILD associated with PSS is similar to IPF. The incidence of ILD among patients with PSS is very high; at autopsy, morphologic changes are found in 90 per cent and radiographic evidence of ILD is found in 30 to 40 per cent of patients. PSS patients with the CREST syndrome (calcinosis, Raynaud's phenomenon, esophageal involvement, sclerodactyly, and telangiectasia) rarely develop ILD. The ILD associated with PSS is generally indolent, but if it becomes symptomatic, the four-year survival rate is about 50 per cent. Although PSS is considered to be a connective tissue disorder with fibrosis as its main feature, patients with the ILD associated with PSS have an alveolitis, albeit milder than that of IPF. Gallium-67 scans are often positive. For most patients, the alveolitis is dominated by macrophages, but neutrophils and sometimes lymphocytes play a role. The ILD associated with PSS is associated with a higher than normal incidence of bronchogenic carcinoma, particularly bronchoalveolar cell carcinoma.

Occasional patients with PSS develop an ILD characterized by pulmonary hypertension with relatively less disease of the alveolar-capillary units. Morphologically, there is thickening of the pulmonary arteries with fibrosis and some inflammation. Many of these patients develop rapidly progressive respiratory failure.

The pathogenesis of the ILD associated with PSS is unknown. The therapeutic guidelines are unclear, although patients with progressive disease usually are treated in a similar fashion to those with IPF. Penicillamine has been suggested as an alternative therapy, but its efficacy is unproven.

SYSTEMIC LUPUS ERYTHEMATOSUS (SLE) (Ch. 436). The common manifestations of SLE in the lung include pleurisy with or without effusion, atelectasis, or acute pneumonitis. Less frequently, SLE manifests as uremic pulmonary edema, diaphragmatic dysfunction, parenchymal hemorrhage, or chronic ILD. Most cases of chronic ILD have pulmonary features similar to IPF, together with the systemic findings of SLE. Rarely, ILD associated with SLE can also present with a lymphocytic alveolitis similar to Sjögren's syndrome, a disorder similar to idiopathic pulmonary hemosiderosis, or a hypersensitivity vasculitis–like picture. Together, the incidence of acute and chronic pulmonary involvement in SLE is less than 20 per cent of all cases of SLE, and chronic ILD occurs in less than 5 per cent. Chronic ILD can appear insidiously or follow the acute pneumonitis of SLE, a severe illness characterized by fever, tachypnea, radiographic evidence of patchy or diffuse infiltrates, and hypoxemia. The pathogenesis of the ILD associated with SLE is thought to result from the deposition of circulating immune complexes in the alveolar walls. Therapy is usually with corticosteroids, but specific treatment guidelines have not been established. SLE can be associated with pulmonary infections, and this must be distinguished from ILD before corticosteroid therapy is started.

POLYMYOSITIS/DERMATOMYOSITIS (Ch. 443). The incidence of ILD in polymyositis/dermatomyositis is 5 to 10 per cent. Of all the collagen-vascular disorders, a higher proportion of patients who develop the ILD associated with polymyositis/dermatomyositis develop the ILD before the other systemic manifestations of the disease. The ILD is similar to IPF, but its pathogenesis is unclear. Patients are usually treated with corticosteroids, but methotrexate has been suggested as alternative therapy.

SJÖGREN'S SYNDROME (Ch. 438). Approximately 3 per cent of patients with Sjögren's syndrome develop ILD that manifests as either a mild IPF-like disease or, more commonly, a disorder with a lymphocyte-dominant alveolitis, similar to the lymphocytic infiltration of other organs in these patients. This lymphocytic form of ILD can be mild to severe and can undergo transformation to a lymphocytic malignancy, an event that is invariably fatal. Therapy of either ILD associated with Sjögren's syndrome is controversial; corticosteroids, immunosuppressive agents, and no therapy have all been advocated.

MIXED CONNECTIVE TISSUE DISEASE (Ch. 437). Up to 80 per cent of patients with this systemic disorder have ILD. The lung disease is usually IPF-like. Pulmonary hypertension is common and can occur without significant parenchymal involvement. Therapy is usually with corticosteroids with or without cytotoxic agents.

ANKYLOSING SPONDYLITIS (Ch. 434). Lung disease, manifested as chest wall restriction and upper lobe fibrobullous disease, occurs in about 1 per cent of patients with ankylosing spondylitis. Most patients are asymptomatic, but colonization with organisms such as *Aspergillus* or atypical mycobacteria is common, and hemoptysis and pneumothorax occur in the late stages of the disease. While HLA-B27 is strongly associated with ankylosing spondylitis, it is not common in those patients with the associated ILD. The morphology of the ILD is IPF-like, together with localized destruction of alveolar walls and bullae. There is no known therapy.

Histiocytosis-X

Histiocytosis-X (HX) (Ch. 161), also called "primary pulmonary histiocytosis" and "eosinophilic granuloma," is a fibrotic-destructive disorder of the lower respiratory tract associated with an intense mononuclear phagocyte–dominant alveolitis. HX is grouped with the other proliferative disorders of the mononuclear phagocyte system, such as Letterer-Siwe and Hand-Schüller-Christian disease. In adults, HX is primarily a lung disease, although bone, skin, and central nervous system manifestations do occur. At least 50 per cent of all patients have chronic symptoms, and the disease can be fatal. More than 1000 cases have been reported; most new patients are 20 to 40 years of age and there is an equal sex distribution. Almost all patients with HX have been cigarette smokers.

The patient with HX presents with a nonproductive cough, dyspnea on exertion, or chest pain. Spontaneous pneumothorax occurs in 10 per cent of cases; fever, weight loss, hemoptysis, and wheezing are occasionally noted. Bone involvement is present in a minority of patients. Posterior pituitary involvement with diabetes insipidus is unusual, as are skin lesions. Physical examination commonly reveals decreased breath sounds and rales. The chest radiograph shows upper and midzone small, irregular nodules superimposed on a delicate cystic pattern. The costophrenic angles are usually clear, and the pleura and hila are normal. Pulmonary function tests show a mixed restrictive-obstructive pattern with reduced lung volumes, reduced diffusing capacity, airflow limitation, and hypoxemia that worsens with exercise.

Definitive diagnosis is made by open lung biopsy. The disease is focal but poorly demarcated. There are sites of intense alveolitis dominated by alveolar macrophages and Langerhans cells. Gallium-67 scans are negative or only mildly positive. Bronchoalveolar lavage reveals a macrophage-dominant alveolitis and the Langerhans cells can be detected in lavage by ultrastructure and the T6 monoclonal antibody. The pathogenesis of this rare entity is discussed in Ch. 161. The lung disease in adults is considered untreatable.

Goodpasture's Syndrome

Goodpasture's syndrome (Ch. 81) is characterized by diffuse pulmonary hemorrhage, ILD, glomerulonephritis, and circulating antiglomerular basement membrane (anti-GBM) and anti–alveolar basement membrane (anti-ABM) antibodies. It is assumed that the anti-GBM and anti-ABM antibodies are identical and cross-react with identical components in the kidney and lung basement membranes. Goodpasture's syndrome can be mimicked by SLE, Wegener's granulomatosis, and the systemic necrotizing vasculitides. In the appropriate clinical setting, the diagnosis of Goodpasture's syndrome is straightforward but does require (1) demonstration of the circulating antibodies, (2) characteristic linear deposits of immunoglobulin along the glomerular basement membrane, and (3) demonstration that the antibodies (either those circulating or those eluted from the kidney) are specific. It is usually not necessary to obtain lung tissue to make the diagnosis, but the diagnosis can be confirmed by histologic and immunofluorescence study of lung tissue obtained by transbronchial biopsy.

Almost all of the anti–basement membrane antibodies in Goodpasture's syndrome are IgG, but IgA anti-GBM, and anti-ABM antibodies have been described in the setting of pulmonary hemorrhage and glomerulonephritis. The basement membrane antigen(s) against which the antibodies are directed is thought to be a portion of type IV (basement membrane) collagen that is somehow unmasked in the kidney and lung.

Goodpasture's syndrome occurs mostly in young men. In most cases, evidence of alveolar hemorrhage precedes the clinical evidence of renal disease. Hemoptysis occurs in almost all cases, tends to be recurrent, and occasionally is massive and life threatening. In such cases, death is from asphyxiation. Anemia is almost always present. The chest radiograph reveals interstitial and alveolar infiltrates. The patchy infiltrates due to the hemorrhage often clear, but the interstitial markings, reflecting chronic ILD, often remain. Histologic findings include alveolar hemorrhage, hemosiderin-laden macrophages, focal areas of alveolitis, and interstitial fibrosis. Linear deposits of IgG can be detected in the alveolar walls.

Spontaneous remissions of Goodpasture's syndrome can occur but are rare. Therapy generally consists of corticosteroids, cytotoxic agents, and plasmapheresis.

Idiopathic Pulmonary Hemosiderosis (IPH)

IPH is a rare disorder of unknown cause characterized by alveolar hemorrhage, iron deficiency anemia, transient parenchymal infiltrates on the chest radiograph, and ILD. The disease is most common in individuals less than 20 years of age, but adult cases are seen. The disease is occasionally found in families, but a genetic basis has not been proven. IPH is compartmentalized in the lung and must be distinguished from Goodpasture's syndrome, Wegener's granulomatosis, SLE, and the vasculitides.

The patient with IPH presents with repetitive acute episodes of dyspnea, cough with hemoptysis, and fever. Iron deficiency anemia is common. The chest radiographs associated with these acute episodes reveal transient infiltrates, a miliary pattern, or massive confluent shadows. On this background of intermittent episodes, a chronic ILD develops with increasing dyspnea, rales, clubbing, and pulmonary hypertension. While the childhood form of the disease is aggressive, with a mean survival of about three years, adult IPH tends to be more insidious. Lung function tests are typical for ILD, but the diffusing capacity may be falsely high owing to increased uptake of the carbon monoxide (used as the test gas) by free hemoglobin in the lung parenchyma. Hemosiderin-laden macrophages in sputum or lavage fluid suggest prior parenchymal hemorrhage. In the appropriate clinical setting, when there are no detectable anti-GBM antibodies, a definitive diagnosis of IPH can be made with an open lung biopsy revealing focal hemorrhage, a macrophage-dominant alveolitis with hemosiderin-positive macrophages, and typical findings of ILD. The pathogenesis of this disorder is unknown. Corticosteroids are generally used to treat the acute episodes and the chronic ILD, but there is no evidence regarding their efficacy.

Chronic Eosinophilic Pneumonia (CEP)

CEP is a chronic ILD characterized by cough, dyspnea, malaise, fever, night sweats, weight loss, variable degrees of blood eosinophilia, and a chest film revealing peripheral, nonsegmental, nonmigratory infiltrates. Hilar adenopathy rarely occurs. Asthma accompanies CEP in 50 to 60 per cent of cases. High proportions of eosinophils are sometimes recovered in sputum or by lavage. A very high sedimentation rate is common, and elevated levels of IgE during acute episodes have been described. The histologic findings of CEP include a diffuse alveolitis dominated by eosinophils and macrophages with fewer numbers of neutrophils and lymphocytes. Eosinophilic abscesses, multinucleated giant cells, angiitis of small pulmonary vessels, and interstitial fibrosis are common.

Although the stimulus to the accumulation of the eosinophils in the lung is unknown, the eosinophil can damage the cells and matrix of the alveolar walls through its release of toxic oxygen radicals, collagenase, and major basic protein, a highly charged polypeptide associated with the eosinophil granules.

An open lung biopsy is required to make a definitive diagnosis. However, because CEP usually responds dramatically to corticosteroids, a tentative diagnosis is often made on clinical grounds only without biopsy confirmation and corticosteroid therapy is instituted. In some patients, the disease is only partly suppressed by corticosteroids, and long-term treatment is required.

Lymphocytic Infiltrative Disorders

This is a group of rare, diffuse ILD characterized by infiltration of the alveolar structures by cells of the lymphocyte series. Most patients present with cough and dyspnea, occasionally with fever. All of the lymphocyte infiltrative disorders of lung can progress to frank lymphoma.

Immunoblastic lymphadenopathy (also called angioimmunoblastic lymphadenopathy) is a systemic disorder, usually of elderly individuals, characterized by generalized lymphadenopathy hepatosplenomegaly, and variable amounts of ILD. The disease has no known etiology, but associations with drugs have been reported, including antibiotics and phenytoin. A skin rash is observed in one third of cases; there may be a coexistent collagen-vascular disorder or hemolytic anemia. There are polyclonal increases in serum immunoglobulins. The alveolar structures exhibit a pleomorphic alveolitis representing all levels of lymphocyte differentiation. Diagnosis is usually made by lymph node biopsy. The disease can remit spontaneously, but patients die from progressive respiratory failure, infection, or malignancy. There is a variable response to therapy with corticosteroids and/or cytotoxic agents.

Lymphocytic interstitial pneumonitis is limited to the lung. The signs and symptoms are typical for an insidious, slowly progressive ILD. It is most common in women in their 40's, but it is observed in males and all age groups. The chest radiograph characteristically shows diffuse reticulonodular infiltrates. Most patients have dysproteinemias. Hyper- and hypogammaglobulinemia have been described, and an association with Sjögren's syndrome is common. The diagnosis is made by an open lung biopsy revealing diffuse parenchymal infiltration with mature lymphocytes, plasma cells, and immunoblasts. Granulomas are sometimes observed. Because the infiltrating cells may form germinal centers, the disease is sometimes called "pseudolymphoma." The prognosis of lymphocytic interstitial pneumonitis is variable, and some patients progress to end-stage lung disease or lymphoma. Treatment is with corticosteroids and/or immunosuppressive agents.

ILD Associated with Pulmonary Vasculitis

Many of the systemic vasculitides result in ILD as a consequence of a pulmonary vasculitis causing a secondary alveolitis and derangements of the alveolar structures.

Wegener's granulomatosis is a granulomatous vasculitis of the upper and lower respiratory tracts and glomerulonephritis (Ch. 441). There is a limited form of the disease without clinically apparent renal disease. All patients have pulmonary involvement, but only one third have symptoms related to the lungs. Airway involvement is common. The parenchymal lung disease can appear as discrete nodules and/or diffuse ILD; either can undergo necrosis and cavity formation. Hemoptysis, cough, sputum production, dyspnea, and pleuritic pain are common. Lung function tests reveal a mixed restrictive-obstructive pattern. Diagnosis is usually made by open lung biopsy. Untreated disease is usually fatal, but with cyclophosphamide therapy long-term survival is the rule.

Lymphomatoid granulomatosis is a systemic vasculitis involving the lung, skin, central nervous system, and kidneys. The lung is always affected, but involvement of other organs is variable. In the lung, the walls of the blood vessels are infiltrated with typical and atypical lymphocytes together with some granulomata, and there is associated ILD. A mild form of lymphomatoid granulomatosis has been described ("benign lymphocytic angiitis and granulomatosis"). The disease is most common in middle age. There are multiple, fleeting nodular densities on the chest film; occasionally there are diffuse infiltrates. Death is usually due to parenchymal destruction with sepsis and occasionally due to massive hemoptysis. The diagnosis is usually established by biopsy of the lung or skin. The lung disease often responds to corticosteroids and cyclophosphamide, but the central nervous system lesions do not. Lymphoma occurs in about 10 per cent of cases.

The *Churg-Strauss syndrome* ("allergic angiitis and granulomatosis") (Ch. 439) is a form of systemic necrotizing vasculitis that almost always involves the lung, unlike classic polyarteritis nodosa, which rarely does. The pulmonary manifestations, consisting of asthma and diffuse infiltrates, often precede systemic involvement by one or two years. An allergic history is common. An elevated sedimentation rate and total eosinophil count are common. The systemic vasculitis involves skin, heart, and gastrointestinal tract. Diagnosis is made by open lung biopsy, which shows a granulomatous vasculitis with eosinophilic infiltration, a secondary diffuse alveolitis, interstitial granulomata, and fibrosis. Treatment is the same as for the other pulmonary vasculitides.

"Hypersensitivity vasculitis" represents a heterogeneous group of vasculitides whose development is thought to be related to sensitization to antigens such as drugs or serum proteins. Skin involvement is most common; most cases do

not involve the lung. When they do there is a small-vessel polymorphonuclear leukocyte vasculitis with fibrinoid necrosis and secondary ILD. Diagnosis is usually made by skin biopsy, and the disorder is often self limiting. A similar disorder can occur in association with mixed cryoglobulinemia or Henoch-Schonlein purpura.

Inherited Disorders

There is a small group of rare ILD that are clearly inherited. Almost all are autosomal dominant disorders, although the autosomal recessive disorders Hermansky-Pudlak syndrome, Niemann-Pick disease, and Gaucher's disease may rarely be associated with interstitial lung disease.

FAMILIAL IDIOPATHIC PULMONARY FIBROSIS. This is a chronic, usually fatal autosomal dominant disorder identical to IPF. Symptoms usually begin in the fifth or sixth decade, but the disease can be manifested earlier. Some of the asymptomatic children of affected family members have evidence of a mild alveolitis yet with normal lung function, suggesting that the disease begins with an alveolitis.

NEUROFIBROMATOSIS (Ch. 477). Von Recklinghausen's disease is an autosomal dominant disorder characterized by pigmented skin lesions and neurofibromas of the peripheral and central nervous systems. In 10 to 20 per cent of adult cases there is a coexisting ILD and/or bullous lung disease. The ILD has histologic features similar to those of IPF, but it is not known whether it responds to similar therapies.

TUBEROUS SCLEROSIS (Ch. 477). This is a hamartomatous autosomal dominant disorder involving the central nervous system, skin, kidneys, eyes, bones, heart, and, in 1 per cent of patients, the lungs. Although the hamartomatous "tumors" are composed of various cell types in most affected organs, in the lung they are composed only of smooth muscle cells. The accumulation of smooth muscle cells in the alveolar interstitium causes ILD, together with parenchymal destruction. Unlike most ILD, there is little alveolitis. The chest radiograph shows diffuse infiltrates and honeycombing, and lung function tests show a mixed pattern with a dominant obstructive pattern. Pneumothorax is common. There is no known therapy.

ILD Associated with Pulmonary Airway Disease

This term refers to disorders in which the ILD is likely secondary to a primary airway disease. It is unclear if there are many such diseases or only one. The characteristic lesions are necrotic granulomata in the bronchial walls, with the bronchiolar lumens filled with palisading epithelioid cells, cellular debris, and polymorphonuclear leukocytes. There are usually a diffuse alveolitis and nongranulomatous fibrosis-type derangements of the alveolar walls. Approximately one third have asthma, blood eosinophilia, mucus plugging, fungal hyphae identifiable in the airways, and positive sputum cultures for *Aspergillus* organisms. These patients are usually referred to as having *"bronchopulmonary aspergillosis"* (see Ch. 376). It is unclear, however, whether the fungus is a primary cause of the disease or represents a secondary process.

The remaining two thirds of patients, referred to as having *"bronchocentric granulomatosis,"* do not have asthma, microscopic evidence of fungi, or blood eosinophilia. The disease can present in an insidious manner or as an acute febrile illness. The chest film usually shows nodular or mass lesions; diffuse infiltrates are seen in about 20 per cent of cases. Lung function tests demonstrate a mixed obstructive-restrictive pattern. Corticosteroids are usually the therapy of choice.

Lymphangioleiomyomatosis

This is a rare disease of women, usually of childbearing age, characterized by the proliferation of benign but atypical smooth muscle cells in walls of the lymphatics of the lower respiratory tract, pleura, mediastinum, and retroperitoneum. Although it is an ILD characterized by thickening and derangements of the alveolar walls, there is very little inflammation present. Eventual destruction of the alveolar walls is common. The clinical findings include dyspnea, recurrent unilateral or bilateral chylous pleural effusions, pneumothorax, hemoptysis, and occasionally peritoneal chylous effusions. The chest radiograph has a characteristic reticulonodular pattern on a background of diffuse cystic changes, similar to that seen in histiocytosis-X. Lung function tests reveal a mixed obstructive-restrictive pattern. An open lung biopsy is required to make the diagnosis. It has been theorized that the disease results from an abnormal response to estrogens, and thus oophorectomy, progesterone, and tamoxifen therapy have all been tried in these patients. There is no proven efficacy of such therapies, and the disease is almost always fatal, usually within 10 years of diagnosis.

Alveolar Proteinosis

In this disorder the alveoli are filled with a periodic acid-Schiff (PAS)–positive lipid and protein-rich granular material. There may be an accompanying mononuclear cell alveolitis and fibrosis-type derangements of the alveolar walls. Although of unknown etiology, alveolar proteinosis can be associated with silicosis, hematologic malignancies, bronchogenic cyst, and mycobacterial and fungal diseases of the lung. Why this material accumulates in the alveoli is unknown but is speculated to result from the breakdown of cells in the lower respiratory tract, from the overproduction of substances normally secreted into the alveolar spaces (e.g., surfactant), from increased transudation of plasma proteins, or from decreased alveolar clearance mechanisms.

The disease usually begins insidiously with dyspnea as the initial symptom. The chest radiograph has a characteristic diffuse, finely nodular alveolar filling pattern. Lung function tests show decreased lung volumes and diffusing capacity. There is usually hypoxemia secondary to pulmonary blood shunting by filled alveoli. Open lung biopsy is usually required for the diagnosis. However, in the appropriate clinical setting, bronchoalveolar lavage recovery of the typical material, together with transbronchial biopsy evidence of alveoli filled with PAS-positive material, is usually diagnostic. Alveolar proteinosis can be fatal but can also spontaneously resolve. The recommended therapy is massive whole lung lavage under general anesthesia. Corticosteroid therapy has no proven use and may lead to the development of opportunistic infections.

Miscellaneous Other ILD of Unknown Etiology

There are several ILD of unknown etiology that are reasonably well defined but so rare that there is little information available concerning their pathogenesis and no apparent guidelines relating to their staging and therapy. These are included by list in Table 63–1 but will not be discussed individually here.

INTERSTITIAL LUNG DISEASE OF KNOWN ETIOLOGY

Approximately 135 agents are known to cause ILD, but together they are responsible for only one third of all cases of ILD. In terms of numbers of patients that come to medical attention, the most important agents are crystalline silica, asbestos, coal dust, organic dusts of the *Micropolyspora* and *Thermoactinomyces* genera and those derived from avian proteins, some antineoplastic drugs, nitrofurantoin, and hyperoxia.

Inhaled Inorganic Dusts

ILD resulting from the chronic inhalation of an inorganic dust is called a "pneumoconiosis" (see Table 63–2). The most common are silicosis, asbestosis, and coal worker's pneumoconiosis. The common pneumoconioses are all characterized by fibrosis-type derangements of the lower respiratory tract.

There are several important principles relevant to understanding the pneumoconioses. (1) The dusts themselves cause little damage to the lung parenchyma; it is the inflammatory response to the dusts that causes the loss of functional alveolar-capillary units. (2) A number of defense mechanisms prevent such dusts from reaching the alveoli, and others remove most dusts that might reach the lower respiratory tract. Just because an individual has been exposed to an inorganic dust does not mean that the dust has necessarily caused ILD. (3) Abnormalities on a chest radiograph consistent with exposure to an inorganic dust do not prove that the individual has a functionally significant ILD. (4) These chronic disorders result from the inhalation of high concentrations of inorganic dusts over many years; i.e., history of a brief exposure sometime in the past is not sufficient evidence to implicate a particular dust. (5) No known therapy has proven efficacy for any pneumoconiosis; current "treatment" for all pneumoconiosis is permanent removal from inhalation of the causative agent. (6) Many individuals exposed to inorganic dusts also have a history of chronic cigarette smoking; this must be taken into account when evaluating these patients. (7) Physical evidence of the inorganic dust in the lung is useful but not critical in making the diagnosis of a common pneumoconiosis (silicosis, asbestosis, coal worker's pneumoconiosis) as long as the chronic exposure history is very clear and unambiguous. For the other inorganic dusts, however, biopsy evidence is required to make a definitive diagnosis. (8) While the miners and millers of these inorganic dusts represent the "classic" exposure situations, inorganic dust materials are widely used in manufacturing. A careful occupational history is required or the exposure history may be missed. *Coal worker's pneumoconiosis, silicosis, asbestosis,* and *berylliosis* are described in Ch. 536 on Occupational Lung Disease.

Inhaled Organic Dusts

The repeated inhalation of certain organic dusts (see also Ch. 536) causes a granulomatous ILD called *"hypersensitivity pneumonitis"* or *"extrinsic allergic alveolitis."* The term "hypersensitivity pneumonitis" is reserved for those ILD caused by organic dusts derived from living sources. A large number of organic dusts have been implicated (Table 63–3), but the most common are the thermophilic organisms of the *Micropolyspora* and *Thermoactinomyces* groups and those derived from avian proteins.

The nomenclature relating to hypersensitivity pneumonitis is confusing because the "name" of the disease usually refers to the situation of exposure (e.g., "maple bark stripper's disease," "humidifier lung") even though the organic dusts causing different "diseases" may be identical. For example, *Thermoactinomyces vulgaris* can cause "farmer's lung," "humidifier lung," and "mushroom worker's lung." The most common exposure situations are farmers exposed to moldy hay, individuals exposed to organic antigens growing in humidifiers and air conditioners, and bird breeders, particularly those raising pigeons. The other exposure situations are varied, and the list is ever expanding (Table 63–3).

Classically, four to six hours after inhalation of the antigen, a sensitized individual develops acute symptoms of hypersensitivity pneumonitis, including fever, cough, dyspnea, and malaise. The chest film at this time shows diffuse parenchymal infiltrates, and lung function tests demonstrate decreased lung volumes, decreased diffusing capacity, mild airflow limitation, and hypoxemia. If the individual is removed from the antigen exposure, there is gradual improvement in symptoms, the chest film, and lung function tests over a 24-hour period. If the exposures are few, there are few sequelae other than the acute episodes. However, in some individuals, for unknown reasons, repetitive exposure leads to a chronic ILD characterized by lymphocyte-macrophage alveolitis occasionally mixed with neutrophils. Initially, the derangements are of the distortion type, with lymphocytes and granulomata in the alveolar walls. Later, however, there are fibrotic changes, including intra-alveolar fibrosis. Rarely, the chronic form develops in an insidious manner without the acute episodes.

The diagnosis of hypersensitivity pneumonitis is made in the context of a history of exposure to a known causative antigen, the presence of ILD, the presence of antigen-specific antibodies in the blood, and an open lung biopsy demonstrating the characteristic morphology. The gallium-67 scan is usually positive, and bronchoalveolar lavage shows a lymphocyte-macrophage alveolitis, mixed with neutrophils when the exposure has been recent. When the history is typical, a biopsy is not necessary to make the diagnosis, but there must be a clear demonstration of the acute symptoms four to six hours after inhalation of the antigen.

The mechanisms by which sensitization to these organic dusts causes either the acute or chronic disease are unknown. T lymphocytes, the majority of which have suppressor/cytotoxic surface markers, are associated with the alveolitis. The T cells in the lung and blood are sensitized to the offending antigen. Besides the circulating antigen-specific immunoglobulins, there are increased levels of IgG and IgM in the lower respiratory tract. However, there is no evidence that the immunoglobulins play a role in the pathogenesis of the disease, and immune complexes have not been convincingly demonstrated in the lower respiratory tract. One of the confusing aspects of this disease is that, although many exposed individuals become sensitized to the organic antigen (as manifest by the presence of antigen-specific antibodies in the blood), only a very small proportion will develop either the acute or chronic symptoms of hypersensitivity pneumonitis.

The prognosis of chronic hypersensitivity pneumonitis is not clear. In those with farmer's lung, there is a 10 per cent mortality over six years, with an additional 30 per cent having significant functional impairment. Management of hypersensitivity pneumonitis is directed toward removing the patient from the source of antigen and suppressing the alveolitis, usually with corticosteroids.

Drug-Induced ILD

Drug-induced ILD are disorders in which the lower respiratory tract is structurally and/or functionally deranged as a result of a pharmacologic agent. The list of drugs reported to cause ILD is large (Table 63–4) and includes acute, subacute, and chronic ILD. Drug-induced ILD can be serious and sometimes fatal, but they are usually effectively treated simply by recognizing the disorder and discontinuing the responsible drug.

It is generally assumed that many of the drug-induced ILD are "hypersensitivity" reactions, but proof of an immune basis for these diseases is circumstantial at best. In many cases, it is thought that the drug injures the lung parenchyma in some fashion to initiate an alveolitis that propagates the injury.

Typically, the acute and subacute forms of drug-induced ILD present with respiratory decompensation following a prodrome of fever and cough. At this time there are usually increased heart and respiratory rates, dry rales, and, occasionally, cyanosis. The chest radiograph shows a patchy or diffuse reticulonodular infiltrate that can be confused with pulmonary edema. Pleural effusions are common. Blood studies often show eosinophilia and arterial hypoxemia and hypocarbia. Lung function tests are typical for ILD, and the gallium-67 scan is often positive. Open lung biopsy demonstrates parenchymal cell injury, edema of the alveolar wall, fibrin in the airspaces, and a patchy lymphocyte-macrophage alveolitis, sometimes mixed with neutrophils and/or eosinophils. In some cases, the course is rapidly downhill, requiring mechanical ventilation and oxygen administration. The disease is usually reversible if the drug is discontinued but can be fatal if this is not done early in the course.

One major area of confusion in conceptualizing and categorizing the drug-induced ILD disorders has resulted from the use of the term "pulmonary infiltration with eosinophilia (PIE) syndrome" to describe patients receiving drugs who develop an acute or subacute disorder characterized by blood eosinophilia and parenchymal infiltrates on the chest film. However, the PIE syndrome is far from diagnostic as a drug-induced ILD. Many nondrug-associated ILD of both known (e.g., acute beryllium-induced disease) and unknown etiology (e.g., IPF, sarcoidosis) can be associated with blood eosinophilia, and tropical pulmonary eosinophilia caused by filarial infestation presents in an identical manner. In addition, there is no evidence that the blood eosinophilia has any relevance to the pathogenesis of the disease in the lung. Thus, most clinicians have abandoned the concept of the "PIE syndrome" and simply think of these disorders as part of the spectrum of ILD in which the presence of blood eosinophilia is a helpful, but not definitive, clue to the diagnosis.

The chronic form of drug-induced ILD is much more insidious and difficult to associate with a drug as the etiologic agent. Fever is less common, and patients usually present with typical ILD. Occasionally there is blood eosinophilia. Because of the insidious nature of the chronic form of drug-induced ILD, many clinicians use lung function tests, particularly measuring the diffusing capacity, to follow patients on drugs commonly associated with the development of ILD. The gallium-67 scan is usually positive. Open lung biopsy usually shows a lymphocyte-macrophage alveolitis with mixed numbers of polymorphonuclear leukocytes. The derangements are fibrosis-type, often with intra-alveolar fibrosis. Unlike the acute and subacute forms of the drug-induced ILD, the chronic form often persists after the drug is discontinued. The reasons why this occurs are not clear, but it is likely that the injury to the parenchyma has been sufficient to establish a chronic alveolitis that propagates the disorder in the absence of the initial stimulus. In such cases, therapeutic strategies are directed toward suppressing the alveolitis, usually with corticosteroids.

ANTINEOPLASTIC AGENTS. *Bleomycin*-induced disease is common; up to 10 per cent of patients receiving bleomycin develop some ILD and 1 per cent die from the ILD. Toxicity from this agent occurs in both acute and chronic forms and is potentiated by concomitant therapy with oxygen or irradiation. *Busulfan* lung disease occurs in 2 to 3 per cent of those receiving the drug. The disease is chronic, usually takes at least one year of therapy before it appears, and usually does not respond to withdrawal of the drug or to corticosteroids. *Methotrexate*-induced ILD can appear in acute or chronic form. Leucovorin or corticosteroids are not protective, but recovery is common once the drug is stopped. There are increasing numbers of reports of ILD induced by the *nitrosoureas*. The incidence of toxicity is about 1 per cent and occurs two months to three years after initiation of therapy. *Procarbazine* causes an acute ILD with pleural effusions, peripheral eosinophilia, and an eosinophilic alveolitis. Although *cyclophosphamide* is used to treat many ILD of unknown etiology, it can rarely cause acute or chronic ILD. Several other antineoplastic agents are reported to cause ILD but very rarely.

ANTIBIOTICS. ILD induced by *nitrofurantoin* is a common adverse drug reaction, occurring in both acute and chronic forms. The acute form, five to ten times more frequent than the chronic form, occurs in sensitized individuals within one month of reinstituting treatment. The disease almost always clears when the drug is discontinued. The chronic disease occurs following 6 to 12 months of therapy. Approximately 60 per cent have positive antinuclear antibodies. The prognosis is good once the drug is stopped, but permanent loss of lung function is common, and approximately 10 per cent die from the disease. The ILD caused by other antibiotics are also mostly acute disorders and are very rare.

CARDIOVASCULAR DRUGS. *Hydralazine* and *procainamide* induce an acute ILD similar to that associated with systemic lupus erythematosus (SLE). In contrast to spontaneously occurring SLE, which is common in blacks and females, the ILD produced by both of these drugs occurs more commonly in whites and affects a significant number of males. Most affected individuals have serum antinuclear antibodies. The disease usually disappears when the drug is stopped. Other drugs that can cause a similar syndrome include isoniazid, phenytoin, and allopurinol. Increasingly, ILD has been observed in association with amiodarone, a useful antiarrhythmic agent. The ILD is usually dose dependent and self limiting but can be chronic even after the drug has been discontinued. The beta blockers can cause chronic ILD, but rarely. The disease is insidious and IPF-like but often associated with fibrosis elsewhere in the body.

OTHER DRUGS. *Gold salts* can induce ILD after one to six months of therapy and can be difficult to distinguish from the ILD associated with rheumatoid arthritis. The disease is thought to represent a hypersensitivity reaction. *Mineral oil*-induced ILD, sometimes called "lipoid pneumonia," results from the aspiration of mineral oil used as nose drops or ingested as a laxative. The open lung biopsy demonstrates a typical picture of lymphoid cells, lipid-laden macrophages, and fibrosis. With an appropriate history, however, the diagnosis can be made by recovering lipid-laden macrophages by bronchoalveolar lavage. The intravenous use of drugs meant for oral use can cause ILD by virtue of the presence of particulate material in the drugs, including talc, starch, maltose, or quinine. The disease is usually chronic and characterized by foreign-body granulomatous reactions affecting pulmonary capillaries.

Many other drugs are known to cause acute and/or chronic ILD, and the list is ever expanding. Because these disorders are all potentially curable if the drug is stopped, it is critical to have a high index of suspicion of drug-induced disease whenever confronted by a patient with ILD.

Other Agents Known to Cause ILD

Beyond inorganic dusts, organic dusts, and drugs, the most important known causes of ILD are paraquat, radiation, the sequelae of prior infectious processes, hyperoxia, and chronic aspiration pneumonia. The others are very rare and mostly represent anecdotal case reports (see Table 63–5).

PARAQUAT. Poisoning with the herbicide paraquat can occur with oral, parenteral, aerosol, or dermal exposure. Paraquat is available in granules, aerosols, and liquid concentrates; ingestion of the liquid either by accident or by suicidal intent is the most common means of paraquat poisoning. Paraquat is an extremely potent cause of parenchymal derangement and fibrosis and consequent respiratory insufficiency. As little as one teaspoon of the concentrate can be fatal. The disease is usually acute, but chronic cases have been described. In the acute cases, dyspnea, fever, fatigue, and gastrointestinal complaints follow one to five days after poisoning. Mouth, pharyngeal, and esophageal ulcerations are common following oral ingestion. Diffuse radiographic changes of ILD are quickly followed by rapidly progressive respiratory failure, usually requiring ventilatory support. Open lung biopsy reveals a neutrophil-macrophage alveolitis and alveolar wall derangements typical of ILD, but very severe. In addition to interstitial fibrosis, intra-alveolar fibrosis is common. In these acute cases, there is a rough correlation between plasma levels of paraquat and survival. If the plasma paraquat concentration eight hours after ingestion is greater than 1200 μg per liter, death is inevitable. In addition to these acute cases, intermittent low-dose skin exposure may be hazardous and lead to a chronic ILD.

Paraquat causes ILD by virtue of its propensity to be taken up by parenchymal cells of the lower respiratory tract, where it generates toxic oxygen radicals sufficient to damage the normal parenchymal components severely. There is a secondary alveolitis that further injures the parenchyma and mediates the development of fibrosis-type derangements. Treatment of paraquat poisoning is mostly supportive. Attempts should be made to remove the paraquat (gastric lavage with bentonite, Fuller's earth, or charcoal, followed by charcoal hemoperfusion). Since hyperoxia accelerates paraquat-induced injury, oxygen concentrations should be kept as low as possible. Antioxidant therapy (e.g., vitamin E) has been suggested, but its efficacy is unknown. In chronic cases, corticosteroids are usually used to suppress the alveolitis.

RADIATION. ILD resulting from thoracic irradiation is a common sequela of radiotherapy of breast, lung, or esophageal carcinoma and lymphoma and is potentiated by the concomitant use of antineoplastic drugs known to cause ILD. Radiation-induced lung disease is described in Ch. 539.

SEQUELA OF KNOWN INFECTIOUS AGENTS. All types of infections of the lower respiratory tract may occasionally result in significant injury and fibrosis. Usually, the ILD remains localized to the site of infection and does not progress after eradication of the infectious agent. A typical example is the localized upper lobe scars left by mycobacterial infection. ILD has been described following *Mycoplasma* infection as well as *Legionella* pneumonia, and there are scattered reports of viral infections causing a progressive ILD. Tropical pulmonary eosinophilia due to chronic microfilarial infestation is a subacute ILD (see Ch. 413.3) and can evolve into a chronic ILD.

INHALED AGENTS OTHER THAN INORGANIC OR ORGANIC DUSTS. These agents include gases, aerosols, chemical dusts, fumes, and vapors. Most are rare causes of ILD, and there is little information available concerning pathogenesis, clinical course, staging, or therapy. Most are acute disorders that reverse when the agent is removed unless significant injury to the parenchyma has occurred.

The most common gas causing ILD is *oxygen*. The inhalation of high concentrations of oxygen over several days often causes parenchymal lung damage, particularly in the setting of acute respiratory failure in the intensive care situation (see Ch. 72). Oxygen toxicity can also be chronic. In contrast, the inhalation of gases such as the oxides of nitrogen, chlorine gas, and sulfur dioxide almost always cause only acute injury; if the patient survives the initial insult and respiratory failure, there are rarely any sequelae. In contrast, many of the survivors of methyl isocyanate exposure develop chronic fibrosis-type ILD.

Aerosols are particles of liquid suspended in a gas. The most common examples of ILD due to aerosol inhalation are the acute and chronic ILD resulting from aspiration of gastric contents (see Ch. 537) and the aspiration of mineral oil. Exposure to aerosols of cooking oils, pyrethrum (a neutral insecticide used in commercial and household products), and toluene diisocyanate has also been implicated as a cause of ILD.

ILD due to the inhalation of chemical dusts such as synthetic fibers, bakelite, and vinyl chloride and polyvinyl chloride powder are probably hypersensitivity-type disorders similar to those associated with the repeated inhalation of organic dusts from living sources. Little is known about the clinical course of these disorders. ILD have also followed the inhalation of various fumes and vapors (Table 63–5).

Basset F, Ferrans VJ, Soler P, et al.: Intraluminal fibrosis in interstitial lung disorders. Am J Pathol 122:443, 1986. *Overview of the patterns of fibrosis in the interstitial lung disorders.*

Crystal RG, Bitterman PB, Rennard SI, et al.: Interstitial lung diseases of unknown cause: Disorders characterized by chronic inflammation of the lower respiratory tract. N Engl J Med 310:154, 235, 1984. *A useful review of the interstitial lung disorders of unknown etiology.*

Crystal RG, Ferrans VJ: Reactions of the interstitial space to injury. In Fishman AP: Pulmonary Diseases and Disorders. New York, McGraw-Hill (in press). *General concepts of the processes that derange the alveolar walls.*

Crystal RG, Gadek JE, Ferrans VJ, et al.: Interstitial lung disease: Current concepts of pathogenesis, staging, and therapy. Am J Med 70:542, 1981. *Overviews the current concepts of the pathogenesis of the interstitial lung disorders and emphasizes the current approaches to staging and therapy.*

Davis WB, Crystal RG: Chronic interstitial lung disease. In Simmons DH (ed.): Current Pulmonology, Vol V. New York, John Wiley and Sons, 1984, pp 347–473. *Reviews the recent observations in each of the interstitial lung disorders.*

Fanburg BL (ed.): Sarcoidosis and Other Granulomatous Diseases of the Lung. New York, Marcel Dekker, 1983. *A good general review of sarcoidosis.*

Keogh BA, Crystal RG: Alveolitis: The key to the interstitial lung disorders. Thorax 37:1, 1982. *Summarizes the importance of alveolitis in the interstitial disorders.*

Morgan WKC, Seaton A: Occupational Lung Diseases. 2nd ed. Philadelphia, W. B. Saunders Company, 1984. *Overall summary of the interstitial lung disorders resulting from the inhalation of inorganic dusts.*

Rom WN (ed.): Environmental and Occupational Medicine. Boston, Little, Brown and Company, 1983. *Well-referenced text detailing known environmental causes of interstitial lung disease.*

Schoenberger CI, Crystal RG: Drug induced lung disease. In Isselbacher KJ, Adams RD, Braunwald E, et al. (eds.): Harrison's Principles of Internal Medicine. Update IV, New York, McGraw-Hill Book Company, 1983, pp 49–74. *Details the pathogenesis and clinical findings in all of the drug-induced interstitial lung disorders.*

64 LUNG ABSCESS

John G. Bartlett

DEFINITION. Lung abscess literally means a collection of pus within a destroyed portion of the lung; thus there are numerous possible causes of such a lesion (Table 64–1). As used clinically, however, the term lung abscess refers to a pulmonary infection with parenchymal necrosis, generally caused by bacteria other than mycobacteria. Lung abscesses are usually solitary, but occasionally multiple discrete lesions are observed. Numerous small abscesses confined to a given region of the lung are sometimes referred to as "necrotizing pneumonia." Because they share a common pathogenesis, there is considerable overlap among aspiration pneumonia, lung abscess, and necrotizing pneumonia, and each of these may lead to and coexist with an empyema (a collection of pus within the pleural space).

ETIOLOGY. As indicated in Table 64–1, many different underlying processes can lead to the formation of a lung abscess. By far the most important are necrotizing pulmonary infections and, of these, anaerobic bacteria are responsible for

TABLE 64–1. CLASSIFICATION OF LUNG ABSCESS

I. Necrotizing infections
  A. Pyogenic bacteria (*Staphylococcus aureus, Klebsiella,* mixed anaerobes, *Nocardia asteroides*)
  B. Mycobacteria (*Mycobacterium tuberculosis, M. kansasii,* and *M. avium-intracellulare*)
  C. Fungi (*Coccidioides immitis, Histoplasma capsulatum*)
  D. Parasites (*Entamoeba histolytica, Paragonimus westermani*)

II. Cavitary infarction
  A. Bland embolism
  B. Septic embolism (*Staphylococcus aureus, Candida*)
  C. Vasculitis (Wegener's granulomatosis, periarteritis)

III. Cavitary malignancy
  A. Bronchogenic carcinoma
  B. Lymphoma
  C. Metastatic malignancies

IV. Other
  A. Infected cysts, bullae, or sequestration
  B. Necrotic conglomerate lesions (silicosis, coal miner's pneumoconiosis)

Adapted from Hirschmann JV, Murray JF: Pulmonary and lung abscess. In Petersdorf RG, et al. (eds.): Harrison's Principles of Internal Medicine. 10th ed. New York, McGraw-Hill Book Company, p 1532.

the majority. These organisms account for essentially all "putrid" lung abscesses and nearly all that have been classified as "nonspecific" or "primary." Most of these infections involve multiple bacterial species, which may include aerobic organisms. The dominant bacteria are *Fusobacterium nucleatum, Bacteroides melaninogenicus, B. intermedius*, peptostreptococcus, aerobic streptococci, and microaerophilic streptococci.

Pneumonia, particularly cases caused by *Staphylococcus aureus* and *Klebsiella pneumoniae,* may also be complicated by abscess formation. Less frequent but well-documented agents of lung abscess include *Streptococcus pyogenes* (group A beta-hemolytic streptococci), *S. pneumoniae* (especially type 3), *Streptococcus milleri, Hemophilus influenzae* (type B), *Pseudomonas aeruginosa, Pseudomonas pseudomallei* (melioidosis), *Actinomyces* (actinomycosis), *Legionella, Nocardia, Paragonimus westermani* (lung fluke), and *Entamoeba histolytica* (amebiasis). Enteric gram-negative bacilli other than *K. pneumoniae* may cause lung abscess, but this occurs almost exclusively in debilitated patients with severe associated medical-surgical conditions. Necrotizing alveolitis is a separate entity diagnosed by microscopic examination and usually caused by *Pseudomonas aeruginosa;* sometimes these microabscesses coalesce to form radiographically detectable cavities.

INCIDENCE AND PREVALENCE. The incidence of primary lung abscess has decreased substantially since the prechemotherapeutic era. Nevertheless, most large academic centers encounter 10 to 30 cases annually.

EPIDEMIOLOGY. Most lung abscesses, and nearly all involving anaerobic bacteria, involve the normal flora of the oropharynx. Abscesses involving *S. aureus* or gram-negative bacilli are more likely to be nosocomial in origin. Amebic lung abscess results from the direct extension of an hepatic abscess through the diaphragm into the lung. *Nocardia* causes lung abscess almost exclusively in immunocompromised hosts, especially in recipients of corticosteroids. Septic pulmonary emboli commonly lead to multiple solitary abscesses in noncontiguous sites and are usually caused by *S. aureus*, anaerobic bacteria, or *P. aeruginosa;* hematogenous abscesses are most often found in intravenous drug abusers with tricuspid valve endocarditis, patients with infected indwelling cannulas. Lung abscesses due to *Paragonimus westermani* and melioidosis are usually acquired in the Far East or Indonesia.

PATHOGENESIS. The formation of an anaerobic lung abscess nearly always involves two coexisting abnormalities: (1) periodontal sepsis such as gingivitis or pyorrhea, which provides the inoculum, and (2) aspiration, which provides access to the lung parenchyma. The usual causes for aspiration are those that compromise consciousness and the gag reflex, such as alcoholism, drug addiction, general anesthesia, seizure disorder, sedative use, or neurologic disorders. Other factors predisposing to aspiration include dysphagia resulting from esophageal disorders or neurologic deficits; disruption of the usual mechanical barriers as with nasogastric intubation, tracheostomy, or nasogastric feeding tubes; or pharyngeal anesthesia as seen with dental procedures or surgery involving the upper airway. Most healthy persons periodically aspirate small inocula from the upper airways, but these are readily cleared by the normal cough reflex and other pulmonary defense mechanisms without deleterious consequences. Patients who develop aspiration pneumonia and lung abscesses presumably do so because of the relatively large inocula of bacteria and failure of the usual protective mechanisms.

The initial lesion is pneumonitis, or "aspiration pneumonia," that typically involves dependent pulmonary segments, e.g., those favored by gravitational flow. The dependent pulmonary segments in patients who aspirate in the recumbent position are the superior segments of the lower lobes or posterior segments of the upper lobes. Aspiration in the upright or semi-upright position favors involvement of the basilar segments of the lower lobes. Patients who have a defined period of known or probable aspiration demonstrate with sequential radiographs that 7 to 14 days are usually required for the appearance of a typical air-fluid level on chest radiograph.

CLINICAL MANIFESTATIONS. Patients with anaerobic abscesses tend to have indolent symptomatology with medical complaints dating for two or more weeks before presentation. The usual symptoms are fever, malaise, cough, sputum production, and pleuritic pain. The frequent observation of weight loss and anemia provides testimony to the chronicity of the infection. There may be "chilliness," but frank rigors are rare and their presence suggests organisms other than anaerobes. The cough often becomes more productive at the time of cavitation, and it is at this time that the patient is most likely to note the onset of putrid sputum, which is considered diagnostic of anaerobic infection. Putrid sputum is found in 60 per cent of patients with a confirmed anaerobic etiology. Many patients will also note an unusually noxious taste to sputum. Most patients have a history of compromised consciousness or other risk factors for aspiration, and many have gingival crevice disease. Nevertheless, about 10 per cent of patients with anaerobic lung abscesses have no identifiable predisposing condition. Occasional patients with anaerobic lung abscesses are edentulous; the incidence of underlying bronchogenic neoplasms seems particularly high in this group. Patients with lung abscesses due to *S. aureus*, gram-negative bacilli, and amebae usually have a more fulminant course, with the precipitous onset of symptoms. Other features that may be noted in this group include chills, the lack of putrid discharge, and the absence of the usual associated findings. The physical findings in the early phases of disease are those of pneumonia, with or without a pleural effusion. At a later stage there may be amphoric or cavernous breath sounds, pleural effusions are common, and approximately 25 per cent of patients have an associated empyema.

DIAGNOSIS. The diagnosis of lung abscess is usually established with a chest radiograph showing a parenchymal infiltrate with a cavity containing an air-fluid level (Fig. 64–1). The differential diagnosis of this roentgenographic finding is included in Table 64–1. Certain roentgenographic features may provide clues to the presence of an infected cyst, bulla, or sequestration. Massive pulmonary fibrosis with necrosis from occupational exposure is usually distinctive. A loculated empyema with an air-fluid level may be differentiated from lung abscess with computerized tomography.

Studies for an etiologic agent are often hampered by the limitations of bacteriologic analysis of expectorated sputum. These specimens are useful in detecting mycobacteria, pathogenic fungi, and parasites, and they may be used for cytologic studies. However, routine aerobic cultures often give erroneous results, and they are not valid for meaningful anaerobic culture owing to the universal presence in oral secretions of anaerobes that contaminate the specimen during passage through the upper airways. Blood cultures are useful, primarily for patients with infections involving *S. aureus* or gram-negative bacilli, but most patients with anaerobic abscesses do not have bacteremia. Pleural fluid is a valuable culture source for both aerobic and anaerobic bacteria in any patient with an empyema, so that thoracentesis should be performed before treatment is begun. For most patients with anaerobic pulmonary infections restricted to the pulmonary parenchyma, the preferred specimen source is from a transtracheal aspiration or from a fiberoptic bronchoscopy utilizing a double-lumen catheter with a distal occluding plug combined with quantitative cultures. Each requires specimen collection prior to institution of antibiotic therapy. In most cases of anaerobic abscesses, the etiologic agents will not be defined and the therapeutic regimen will be selected empirically. Bronchoscopy, which used to be performed routinely in patients with lung abscesses, is now usually restricted to patients who fail to respond to antibiotic treatment or who

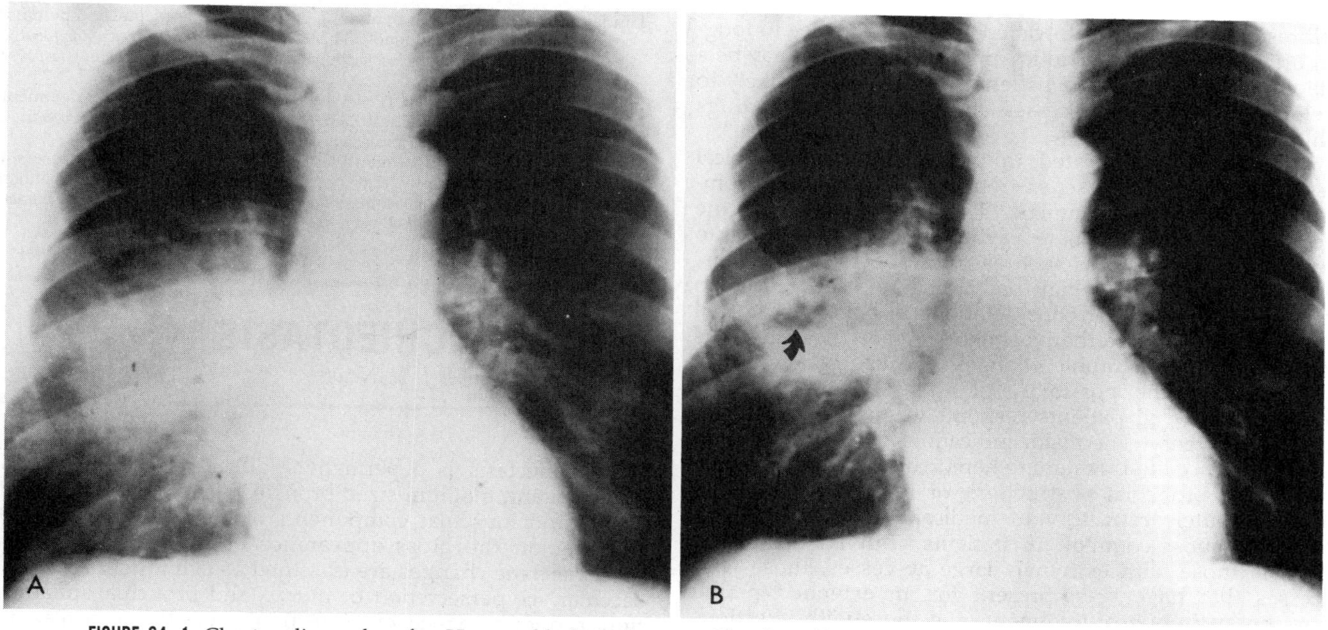

FIGURE 64–1. Chest radiographs of a 55-year-old alcoholic man. The first film (*A*) shows pneumonitis involving the superior segment of the right lower lobe, a common segment for aspiration pneumonia. The second radiograph (*B*), taken one week later, shows cavitation with an air-fluid level as indicated by the arrow. A transtracheal aspirate yielded *F. nucleatum*, *B. melaninogenicus*, and anaerobic streptococci. The final diagnosis was aspiration pneumonia with progression to lung abscess due to anaerobic bacteria.

have an atypical clinical presentation. Major concerns are a cavitating neoplasm, an obstructing tumor, or a foreign body.

TREATMENT. Obviously, treatment of lung abscess will depend on the underlying cause. For those due to infection, the most important facets of the treatment program are the administration of appropriate antibiotics and adequate drainage of any associated empyema. Physiotherapy with postural drainage should be utilized when possible; however, this must be done with considerable caution in patients with large lung abscesses because of the possibility of spillage of purulent contents with extensive involvement of other lobes.

The drugs of choice for the treatment of abscesses caused by aerobic pyogenic microorganisms, *M. tuberculosis*, fungi, and *Entamoeba histolytica* are reviewed in detail elsewhere in this volume. For aspiration-related lung abscess involving anaerobic bacteria, the three antimicrobial regimens recommended are penicillin, clindamycin, or penicillin plus metronidazole. Penicillin has traditionally been regarded as the favored drug on the basis of its long, well-established track record. There is considerable variation in the dosage recommendations, but most authorities recommend doses of 10 to 20 million units per day. This is continued until the patient is afebrile and clinically improved, at which time treatment is changed to intramuscular or oral penicillin using penicillin G, penicillin V, ampicillin, or amoxicillin in doses of 500 to 750 mg four times daily. Some authorities suggest an arbitrarily selected total duration of treatment of three to six weeks, whereas others continue treatment until the chest radiograph changes have cleared or there is only a small stable residual lesion. The latter criterion commonly requires two to four months or longer but may be necessary to prevent relapses.

Clindamycin is active against most penicillin-resistant anaerobes that are found in 20 to 25 per cent of cases, including many or most strains of *B. melaninogenicus*, *B. fragilis*, *B. ruminicola*, and *B. ureolyticum*. Some regard clindamycin as the preferred agent for all lung ascesses due to anaerobic bacteria; others advocate it only for patients who fail to respond to penicillin, have a contraindication to penicillin, or have a serious infection with a fulminant course. The usual regimen is 600 mg given intravenously every six to eight hours until the patient is afebrile and clinically improved, followed by 300 mg orally four times daily. An alternative regimen is penicillin G (above doses) combined with metronidazole (2 gm orally per day in two to four divided doses). Metronidazole is active against nearly all clinically important anaerobes, but penicillin must be added owing to the probable importance of aerobic and microaerophilic streptococci. The necessity to treat the aerobic components of mixed aerobic-anaerobic infections is controversial, but this is generally advocated for patients who are seriously ill or fail to respond to clindamycin. In selecting regimens for these mixed infections, it is important to note that most penicillins are equally effective against oral anaerobes. These include penicillin G, penicillin V, ampicillin, amoxicillin, carbenicillin, and piperacillin. However, antistaphylococcal penicillins, such as nafcillin or oxacillin, are considered inferior and unacceptable. Cephalosporins are considered nearly equivalent to penicillins in terms of in vitro activity, although the clinical experience is much more limited than it is with penicillin or clindamycin.

Patients with lung abscesses involving *S. aureus* should be treated with a penicillinase-resistant penicillin or a first-generation cephalosporin. Vancomycin is the preferred agent for methicillin-resistant strains of *S. aureus*. This agent or clindamycin may be used for patients with a contraindication to beta-lactam antibiotics. Penicillin G is the preferred agent for infections involving group A beta-hemolytic streptococcal infection. Antibiotic selection for infections involving gram-negative bacilli requires in vitro sensitivity data. This usually consists of an aminoglycoside combined with an expanded spectrum penicillin such as ticarcillin for *P. aeruginosa* or an aminoglycoside combined with a cephalosporin for *Enterobacteriaceae*. Sulfonamides are preferred agents for *Nocardia* infections.

The expected response to antimicrobial agents is subjective improvement with decreased fever within 3 to 7 days and elimination of fever within 7 to 14 days. The putrid odor of the sputum, when initially present, usually resolves in three to ten days. Radiographic response is delayed; in fact, there is often extension of the infiltrate and increased cavity size or new cavity formation during the first week. Chest radiographs should be followed at two- to three-week intervals with the expectation that infiltrates will clear and that there will be a small residual scar or a thin-walled cyst. Compliance to long-term oral regimens of antibiotics among outpatients may be a problem, particularly in the patient population most likely to develop primary lung abscesses and with expensive drugs such as clindamycin.

Bronchoscopy is indicated in patients with an atypical presentation and in those who fail to respond to recommended antimicrobial regimens. The major purpose of the procedure is to differentiate cavitating neoplasms and to detect underlying lesions, such as bronchogenic neoplasms, bronchostenosis, or a foreign body. It may also be used to facilitate drainage. Other considerations in patients who fail to respond include alternative infectious and noninfectious causes of roentgenographic changes, the use of alternative antibiotics, and the possibility of an empyema requiring drainage. Nearly all patients respond to antibiotics and do not require surgery. The major indications for surgery are an uncontrollable or life-threatening hemorrhage, a bronchogenic neoplasm, a bronchial obstruction, or a lung abscess that proves absolutely refractory to medical treatment. Medical failures are most common in patients with an obstructed bronchus, those with extremely large abscesses, those with abscesses that have been present for an extended period before the institution of treatment, and those with infections involving certain bacteria such as gram-negative bacilli. The usual surgical procedure is lobectomy. Patients with prohibitive operative risks may benefit from percutaneous drainage, but care must be taken to avoid contamination of the pleural space.

PROGNOSIS. The natural course of lung abscesses was best studied in the prechemotherapeutic era. Treatment at that time was nearly equally divided between conservative management using postural drainage and supportive care, and surgery. The mortality rate was about 33 per cent in both groups. An additional third of patients developed a chronic debilitating disease or suffered recurrent symptoms. The technique of resectional surgery was developed at about the time penicillin became available, and the relative merits of these two approaches as the primary therapeutic modality were widely debated. During the past two decades, however, the majority of patients have been treated with antibiotics alone, including those with "delayed closure" (i.e., the persistence of a cavity demonstrated by a chest radiograph at four to six weeks after the initiation of antibiotic therapy), because most of these cavities eventually resolve if the antibiotics are continued long enough. The mortality rate for aspiration-related lung abscess is currently reported at 5 to 6 per cent. Findings that herald a relatively poor prognosis include (1) large cavity size, particularly cavities greater than 6 cm in diameter, (2) prolonged symptoms prior to presentation, especially symptoms for over six weeks, (3) necrotizing pneumonia characterized by multiple small abscesses in contiguous segments, (4) patients who are elderly, debilitated, or immunologically compromised, (5) abscesses associated with bronchial obstruction, and (6) abscess due to aerobic bacteria, including *S. aureus* and gram-negative bacilli.

PREVENTION. The major preventive measures are factors used to reduce the incidence or magnitude of aspiration, appropriate care of periodontal disease, early treatment of pneumonia, and adequate courses of antimicrobials to prevent relapses.

Bartlett JG: Lung abscess. Johns Hopkins Med J 150:141, 1982. *The literature is reviewed, including a summary of bacteriologic studies, treatment guidelines, and prognosis.*

Bartlett JG, Gorbach SL, Tally FP, et al.: Bacteriology and treatment of primary lung abscess. Rev Respir Dis 109:510, 1974. *The authors report their experience with lung abscesses using transtracheal aspiration to define the infecting flora.*

Hagan JL, Hardy LD: Lung abscess revisited. A survey of 184 cases. Ann Surg 197:755, 1983. *Update on the surgical point of view concerning lung abscess; 11 per cent were operated on.*

Landay MJ, Christensen EE, Bynum LJ, et al.: Anaerobic pleural and pulmonary infections. Am J Roentgenol 134:233, 1980. *The authors review the roentgenographic features of anaerobic pleuropulmonary infections, including response to antibiotic treatment.*

Snow N, Lucas A, Horrigan TP: Utility of pneumonotomy in the treatment of cavitary lung disease. Chest 87:731, 1985. *A description of the procedure and results with percutaneous drainage.*

Stark DD, Federle MP, Goodman PC, et al.: Differentiating lung abscess and empyema: Radiography and computed tomography. Am J Roentgenol 141:163, 1983. *Nice demonstration that computed tomography is extremely useful in this important differential diagnosis.*

65 BRONCHIECTASIS

Christopher J. L. Newth

Bronchiectasis is a permanent dilatation of one or more proximal and medium-sized bronchi due to destruction of the elastic and muscular components of the bronchial wall. Depending on the gross appearance of the dilated segment, bronchiectatic changes are classified as cylindric, varicose, or saccular. Hypersecretion of mucus and bronchial inflammation secondary to recurrent infections cause the clinical expression of the disease.

PREVALENCE

Bronchiectasis was once a common disease, but effective vaccines for pertussis and measles and better antibiotics for tuberculosis and bacterial pneumonia have all but removed these conditions as precursors. Most new cases of this now rare disease have some predisposing genetic cause, with cystic fibrosis (Ch. 66) responsible for about half the cases. Sporadic events such as adenovirus infections still account for some bronchiectasis, as may congenital lesions (e.g., bronchomalacia), aspiration of gastric contents and foreign bodies, tumors, and external compression (by impairing mucociliary clearance and enhancing the chance of necrotizing infection of the bronchial wall).

PATHOLOGY

Bronchiectatic segments show dilated lumina filled with suppurative material and inflamed, often necrotic, mucosal surfaces. The infection extends into the bronchial wall, disrupting smooth muscle and elastic tissue. The ciliated columnar epithelium is replaced by nonciliated cuboidal cells or fibrous tissue, resulting in localized dilatation and eventually traction as a result of peribronchial scarring. *Cylindrical* (fusiform) bronchiectasis is mild bronchial dilatation with mucous plugging that is usually managed conservatively. *Varicose* bronchiectasis is a more advanced stage characterized by moderate dilatation and distortion of bronchi that resemble varicose veins. *Saccular* (cystic) bronchiectasis, which usually involves proximal (central) bronchi, is the most advanced form. The most common sites of involvement are the posterior basilar segments of the lower lobes, presumably because of the lack of gravitational drainage. The middle lobe of the right lung is also predisposed owing to angulation of the lobar bronchus at its takeoff; the presence of peribronchial lymph nodes at its origin, which may be involved in a number of pathologic processes; and the relative lack of collateral ventilation. Upper lobe bronchiectasis is most commonly secondary to tuberculosis or lung abscess.

CLINICAL MANIFESTATIONS

Bronchiectasis usually begins in childhood. In most cases, symptoms occur before the age of four years, and the majority are diagnosed within the first two decades of life.

The classic form of bronchiectasis is characterized by chronic cough with production of copious amounts of putrid sputum, fetid breath, emaciation, severe secondary bacterial pneumonias, repeated episodes of hemoptysis, cyanosis, digital clubbing, and reduced life expectancy. This presentation is now seldom seen, and bronchiectasis is more likely to be a manifestation of a systemic disorder than of a local pulmonary process. The most usual symptom now is a chronic productive cough that may be more distressful when the patient is recumbent owing to pooling of secretions. The amount and type of sputum produced vary markedly, but it is generally more voluminous and purulent during intercurrent infections. Frank hemoptysis is now uncommon, but blood-streaked sputum is present frequently. There are recurrent bouts of pneumonia, which usually involve the same pulmonary segment or lobe when the bronchiectasis is localized. Exertional dyspnea, clubbing, fatigue, and malaise may be noted in patients with extensive disease. The most characteristic finding on physical examination is persistent, moist, coarse rales over the area involved. If the disease is widespread, there may be generalized wheezing, evidence of air trapping, and progression to cor pulmonale, as in other forms of chronic obstructive pulmonary disease. *Sinusitis* is a frequent companion to diffuse bronchiectasis, but *secondary amyloidosis* and *metastatic abscesses* are now rare complications.

DIAGNOSIS

Bronchiectasis should be suspected in any patient with a chronic productive cough, particularly if there is intermittent blood streaking or increased purulence of the sputum. Knowledge of a precursor event or a genetic error that predisposes to bronchiectasis, or documentation of recurrent pneumonias (particularly those involving the same lobe or segment), should arouse suspicion further. The differential diagnosis for patients with chronic cough and sputum production includes foreign body aspiration, chronic bronchitis, tuberculosis, and chronic lung abscess.

The diagnosis of bronchiectasis depends on demonstrating the abnormal anatomy of the bronchial tree. This is usually accomplished radiologically. *Plain chest films* may be normal or may show only patchy infiltrates, bronchial crowding, or evidence of bronchial thickening, such as "tram tracks" and ring shadows. In advanced cases of saccular bronchiectasis, the diagnosis may be apparent from the presence of multiple cystic lesions with or without fluid levels. *Computed tomography* (CT) is an accurate screening device for bronchiectasis and is all that is required to confirm the diagnosis in most cases.

Bronchography is the definitive procedure with which to establish the diagnosis, determine the extent of involvement, and describe the distribution of lesions. However, because of its potential complications, it is indicated only in patients who are likely candidates for surgery. Bronchography should not be performed until exacerbations of cough, sputum production, and pulmonary infection have been thoroughly treated, since reversible changes that are similar to those of bronchiectasis may occur in the bronchi during this period.

Magnetic resonance imaging is sensitive for mucus impaction and peribronchial edema, but there is little experience with this technique in bronchiectasis.

Bronchoscopy does not establish the diagnosis of bronchiectasis but is useful for detecting conditions that cause obstruction and determining the source of bleeding and secretions.

Pulmonary function studies show a range of abnormalities depending on the extent and severity of disease. There is a correlation between the number of involved segments and the overall impairment of lung function. Regional ventilation-perfusion mismatch can be documented early by hypoxemia and radionuclide scan. In the later stages of diffuse bronchiectasis, the vital capacity is reduced, with marked airflow obstruction and airtrapping.

TABLE 65–1. DIAGNOSTIC FEATURES OF FAMILIAL BRONCHIECTASIS

Disorder	Clinical Findings	Laboratory Tests
Cystic fibrosis (Ch. 66)	Pancreatic insufficiency Mucoid *Pseudomonas* strain Obstructive azospermia Infertility	Sweat chloride
Immotile cilia syndrome	Infertility, sinusitis, otitis media +/− dextrocardia in Kartagener's syndrome	Electron microscopy of cilia Absent mucociliary clearance Immotility in living cells (nasal, sperm)
Alpha$_1$-antitrypsin deficiency	Emphysema, cirrhosis	Serum alpha$_1$-antitrypsin, Pi typing
IgG deficiency (Ch. 419)	Recurrent infections	Quantitative Ig IgG subclass
IgA deficiency (Ch. 419)	Autoimmune phenomena Atopy	Quantitative Ig
Williams-Campbell syndrome	Disease restricted to chest	Bronchographic expiratory collapse of proximal bronchi
Neutrophil deficiencies (Ch. 149)	Recurrent infections +/− thrombocytopenia +/− pancreatic disease	Blood smear Differential leukocyte count, NBT test*
Complement deficiencies (Ch. 418)	Recurrent infections	C3 levels, CH50 determination

*NBT = nitroblue tetrazolium dye.

Sputum culture often grows normal flora and, less commonly, *Streptococcus pneumoniae, Haemophilus influenzae,* and anaerobes. Patients with mucoid strains of *Pseudomonas aeruginosa* should be tested for cystic fibrosis. *Aspergillus* may grow in asthmatic patients with bronchiectasis secondary to bronchopulmonary aspergillosis.

Unless there has been an obvious predisposing event, all patients should be investigated for one of the familial causes of bronchiectasis (Table 65–1).

TREATMENT

The underlying anatomic defects are irreversible, so medical therapy is aggressively directed toward controlling symptoms and limiting or preventing progression of disease. Basic supportive measures include postural drainage to mobilize secretions, hydration, bronchodilators for patients with bronchospasm (and as an aid to ciliary clearance of mucus), discontinuation of smoking, and treatment of associated sinusitis. Expectorants are of questionable value. Antimicrobials are indicated for infectious exacerbations manifested by increased cough, blood streaking, and purulent sputum production. Progressive dyspnea, malaise, and weight loss may also indicate an infectious exacerbation. The choice of antibiotic should be guided by the results of sputum culture. However, these cultures often grow "normal flora," and in this circumstance ampicillin is appropriate for empiric use. Trimethoprim-sulfamethoxazole or tetracycline is usually adequate for those patients who have a contraindication to penicillins. A course of antibiotics may require from one to three weeks to achieve the desired therapeutic effect. Long-term courses and inhaled delivery of antibiotics have not been proved effective in the management of bronchiectasis with the sole exception of that occurring in cystic fibrosis. Oxygen should be used for hypoxia during an acute exacerbation and on a domiciliary basis for those with chronic respiratory insufficiency. Influenza vaccines should be administered annually.

Resectional surgery, once a mainstay of treatment, is now seldom indicated because (1) patients with mild symptoms usually respond well to medical therapy, (2) those with severe symptoms usually have extensive disease with many segments involved and limited pulmonary reserve, and (3) many patients with bronchiectasis frequently have a systemic disorder, and although their bronchiectasis may appear well localized initially, new sites of involvement develop later. The major indication for resectional surgery is localized disease that responds poorly to medical management, particularly in young patients with illness sufficient to impair their ability to live a normal life. Segmental resection or lobectomy in these patients may be curative. A now rare indication is massive hemoptysis from an aneurysmal vascular deformity in a bronchiectatic cavity. Embolization of bronchial arteries can be a successful (though usually only palliative) procedure in patients with significant hemoptysis who cannot tolerate pulmonary resection.

PROGNOSIS

Progression within involved segments is common, but extension to previously normal segments is unusual unless the underlying disease is a generalized process that predisposes the entire bronchial system (Table 65–1). As a general rule, patients with familial bronchiectasis have a tendency to improve during the second and third decades of life and may remain relatively stable with decreased pulmonary symptoms and good quality of life. There is, however, a reduced life expectancy.

Cochrane GM: Chronic bronchial sepsis and progressive lung damage. Br Med J 290:1026, 1985. *A concise review with 39 references, outlining current theory, research, and therapy.*

Davis PB, Hubbard VS, McCoy K, et al.: Familial bronchiectasis. J Pediatr 102:177, 1983. *A well-referenced review of the familial syndromes that lead to recurrent infections and bronchiectasis.*

Ellis DA, Thornley PE, Wightman AJ, et al.: Present outlook in bronchiectasis: Clinical and social study and review of factors influencing prognosis. Thorax 36:659, 1981.

Grenier P, Maurice F, Musset D, et al.: Bronchiectasis: Assessment by thin-section CT. Radiology 161:95, 1986. *A prospective study correlating CT with bronchography. The authors conclude that CT is a reliable, noninvasive method for detection and assessment of bronchiectasis.*

66 CYSTIC FIBROSIS

Christopher J. L. Newth

Cystic fibrosis (CF) is an autosomal recessive disease affecting both eccrine and exocrine gland function. Cystic fibrosis is characterized by elevated levels of sodium and chloride in sweat and by abnormally viscid secretions from mucous glands leading to chronic pulmonary disease in most and pancreatic insufficiency in 85 per cent, along with other manifestations (Table 66–1). It is the most common lethal genetic disease of the white population in the United States.

The abnormal gene (which is known to lie on chromosome 7) has a carrier rate of about 5 per cent in Caucasians, resulting in an incidence of CF of 1 per 1600 to 2000 births (compared with 1 per 17,000 in blacks and 1 per 100,000 in Asians). There is no test for heterozygotes for the CF gene, who are clinically normal. The disease is recognized in most patients prior to adolescence; rarely, the diagnosis may not be made until the third or fourth decade of life.

PATHOGENESIS

Obstruction and dilatation of glands and their ducts occur secondary to abnormal mucous clearance, which is presumed to be caused by the unknown basic biologic defect. However, no primary abnormalities of the mucoproteins secreted, of ciliary function, or of host defenses (including cell-mediated, humoral, and secretory immunity) have been demonstrated.

Although morphologically normal, the sweat glands in CF have defective tubular reabsorption of electrolytes or water or both, resulting in a striking increase in the levels of sodium and chloride in the sweat. Similar abnormalities have not been found in the secretions of other glands, with the exception of the submaxillary salivary glands.

CLINICAL MANIFESTATIONS

The major medical problems encountered in adolescents or young adults with CF are disorders of the tracheobronchial tree, the pancreas, and the gastrointestinal tract (Table 66–2). There are no abnormalities in the respiratory tract at birth; the earliest changes are hypertrophy of bronchial glands and metaplasia of goblet cells. Meconium ileus at birth, which occurs in about 10 to 15 per cent of CF patients, is the earliest common manifestation. The pulmonary problems increase and dominate the clinical picture as the patient gets older, whereas problems with malabsorption seem to decline.

Chronic pulmonary disease characterized by chest deformity, clubbing, and bronchiectasis is present in 97 per cent of adults with CF and is the major cause of morbidity and mortality. Pulmonary function tests show mixed obstructive and restrictive disease, with the obstructive element being dominant in most patients. The serial measurement of FEF 25–75 appears to be the most sensitive index of pulmonary decline. A sudden change, particularly in female adolescents, is a very serious

TABLE 66–1. CLINICAL MANIFESTATIONS OF CYSTIC FIBROSIS

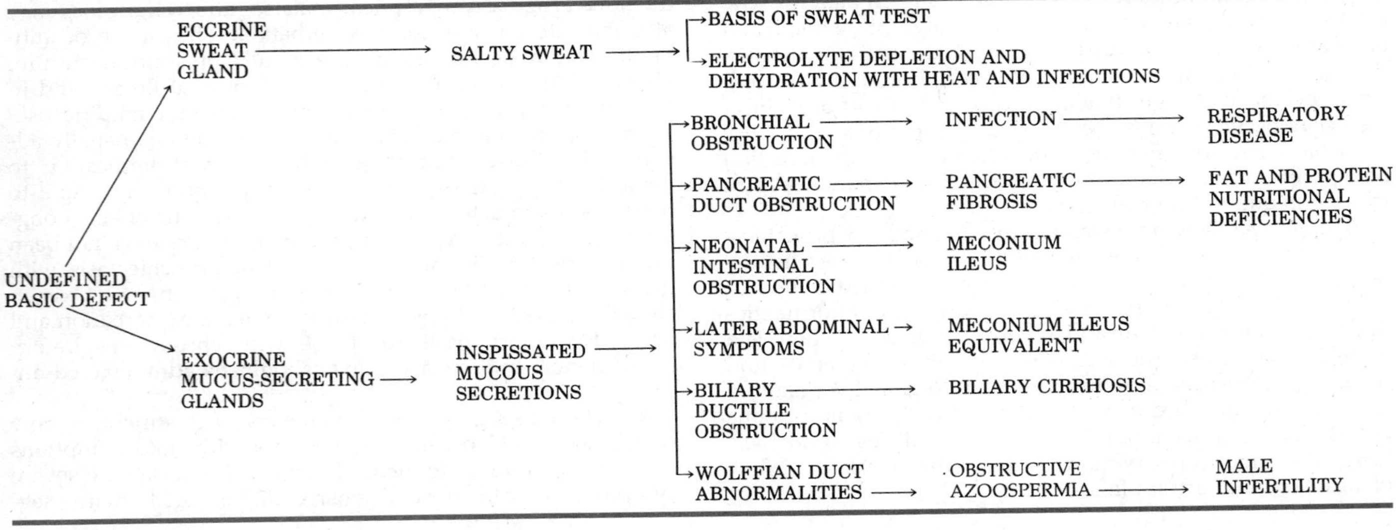

TABLE 66–2. CLINICAL MANIFESTATIONS OF CYSTIC FIBROSIS IN ADOLESCENTS AND ADULTS*

Clinical Feature	Percentage
Pulmonary disease	97
Hemoptysis	60
Pneumothorax	16
Nasal polyps	48
Cirrhosis	5
Heat prostration	5
Intestinal obstruction	21
Meconium ileus equivalent	24
Intussusception	5
Pancreatic insufficiency	95
Glucosuria	8

*Modified from di Sant'Agnese PA, Davis PB: Cystic fibrosis in adults. Am J Med 66:121, 1979.

sign. The respiratory disease is characterized by recurrent flareups of chronic bacterial bronchitis and bronchopneumonia, terminating in respiratory failure and death. The chronic bacterial infection is due primarily to mucoid strains of *Pseudomonas aeruginosa*. *Staphylococcus aureus*, which is present in about 50 per cent of adult patients, is rarely implicated in acute pulmonary complications. *Pseudomonas cepacia* occurs in the sputum of 5 to 10 per cent of patients with CF and is associated with a more rapid decline of pulmonary function. In adults with CF, minor hemoptysis occurs in 60 per cent, massive hemoptysis in 7 per cent, and pneumothorax in 16 per cent. Half of the adults with this disease have nasal polyps, but usually they are not obstructive. Over 70 per cent of patients die with cor pulmonale; the appearance of right ventricular failure usually means death within two years.

Pancreatic exocrine insufficiency occurs in 85 to 90 per cent of patients with CF. This results in deficient enzymatic hydrolysis of fats and proteins (Ch. 104). The salivary amylase allows normal carbohydrate metabolism. Malabsorption of fat may be associated with deficiencies in essential fatty acids such as linoleic acid and the fat-soluble vitamins (A, D, E, and K). Patients with residual pancreatic exocrine function tend to have better pulmonary function and probably a better prognosis. Pancreatic function may decline with age in those patients born without malabsorption.

Cystic fibrosis may also affect the small bowel, liver, bile ducts, and male reproductive organs. Intestinal obstruction secondary to meconium ileus may occur at birth. Later, distal small bowel obstruction, or "meconium ileus equivalent," occurs in about 20 per cent of older patients and is presumably related to inspissation of mucofeculent material. Patchy biliary cirrhosis may result in hepatic enlargement and rarely may progress to severe portal hypertension with varices. The incidence of cholelithiasis is increased owing to lithogenic bile rich in cholesterol. Diabetes mellitus occurs in about 10 per cent of adults, associated with decreased levels of insulin and glucagon secondary to pancreatic destruction The diabetes is relatively easy to control, and ketoacidosis is rare. Puberty, skeletal maturity, and the pubertal growth spurt are delayed in the majority of adolescents. Men are often infertile owing to reduced vasa deferentia function, and women, although able to conceive despite having an abnormal cervical mucus, frequently develop secondary amenorrhea as they deteriorate clinically. Pregnancies can be carried to term in most cases, with a 2.5 per cent risk of the infant's having CF.

DIAGNOSIS

Cystic fibrosis is diagnosed in nearly 80 per cent of patients in the first three years of life. The diagnosis should be suspected in any adolescent or young adult presenting with chronic bronchopulmonary disease and pancreatic insufficiency or obstructive azoospermia. For diagnosing CF, a quantitative pilocarpine iontophoresis sweat test should be performed in a laboratory with established expertise. At least 100 mg of sweat should be collected, and the results should be confirmed with a second test. Elevated sodium and chloride concentrations in sweat, exceeding 60 mEq per liter in children and 70 mEq per liter in adults, are diagnostic of CF.

Prenatal tests are available for the homozygous condition, but their reliability has not yet been established. In the first four to six weeks of life, when it is difficult to obtain sufficient sweat for testing, high serum concentrations of immunoreactive trypsin may prove to be diagnostic and can be used for routine newborn screening. Early detection of CF by such screening has not yet been shown to increase the long-term survival but does decrease morbidity in the first two years of life.

TREATMENT

An increasingly large number of patients with CF survive into adulthood, and an additional small number of patients with previously undiagnosed CF are identified in young adulthood. The major source of morbidity in later life is pulmonary disease. Vigorous pulmonary toilet is basic, and good bronchial clearance can be obtained with a combination of chest physical therapy, active coughing, and exercise. Patients should be encouraged to pursue any form of exercise within their capacity. About 50 per cent of adult patients have bronchial hyper-reactivity. Aerosols of bronchodilators in normal saline are sometimes partially effective. In occasional cases, airflow can be improved by oral corticosteroids without any evidence of worsening of the bronchopulmonary infection.

Antimicrobial agents are particularly important in the therapy of CF lung disease. Chronic antistaphylococcal therapy can be given orally for years without evidence of drug resistance or complications. Antipseudomonal agents are essential for acute exacerbations of bronchial infections and intermittent bouts of pneumonia. These infections generally remain localized in the lungs; bacteremia, empyema, and extrapulmonary spread are unusual. The initial treatment of *Pseudomonas aeruginosa* infection in adolescents and adults is most commonly a combination of intravenous tobramycin and ticarcillin. Subsequent modification should be based on the results of sputum cultures and in vitro sensitivity tests. Aerosolized antibiotics directed against *Pseudomonas aeruginosa* have been found efficacious in both acute and chronic bronchopulmonary exacerbations. When the bronchopulmonary exacerbation is due to *Pseudomonas cepacia*, the antimicrobial choice is usually extremely limited.

Most patients with pancreatic insufficiency can be maintained on a normal diet with supplemental pancreatic enzymes. The preferred agents are enteric-coated microsphere pancreatic enzyme preparations, such as Pancrease and Cotazym-S, given in doses of five to seven capsules per meal. The concomitant use of sodium bicarbonate or H_2-receptor antagonists (cimetidine, ranitidine) may also improve the fat and protein absorption, since the efficacy of pancreatic enzymes is markedly increased at higher intraluminal pH levels.

"Meconium ileus equivalent" can usually be treated with enemas or nasogastric suction. Surgery is necessary on rare occasions. The administration of increased amounts of pancreatic enzymes may reduce the frequency of this complication. The lithogenicity of the bile can be reversed with appropriate pancreatic enzyme replacement. No treatment is available for the hepatic or vas deferens abnormalities. Nocturnal oxygen therapy is being evaluated to determine if prevention of arterial oxygen desaturation during sleep decreases cardiopulmonary morbidity and prolongs survival. The psychosocial aspects of this disease are formidable, and, where possible, patients should be cared for by special units so that their manifold problems can be dealt with by staff experienced with their management.

PROGNOSIS

About half of the patients with CF in the United States live to be 20 years of age. In areas where patients are cared for by special units, such as those supported by the Cystic Fibrosis Foundation and National Institutes of Health (NIH), 50 per cent survive to at least 25 years of age, with males doing much better than females.

Factors associated with a better prognosis in CF are the male sex, maintenance of appropriate weight, single-system (gastrointestinal or pulmonary) involvement at presentation, and a normal chest radiograph within the first year of presentation. Preservation of pancreatic exocrine function is likely to be a good prognostic factor.

Beaudat A, Bowcock A, Buchwald M, et al.: Linkage of cystic fibrosis to two tightly linked DNA markers: Joint report from a collaborative study. Am J Hum Genet 39:681, 1986. *Two DNA markers (MET and D758) have been discovered which flank the CF locus on chromosome 7. The finding of these probes has implications for diagnosis as well as for final characterization of the CF gene itself.*

Di Sant'Agnese PA, David PB: Cystic fibrosis in adults. Am J Med 66:121, 1979. *An excellent review of the clinical aspects of CF as the disease is seen by the internist in the adolescent and adult patient.*

Estivill X, Farrall M, Scambler PJ, et al.: A candidate for the cystic fibrosis locus isolated by selection for methylation-free islands. Nature 326:840, 1987. *Description of a novel technique for honing in on the site of the abnormal gene responsible for cystic fibrosis.*

Kuzemko JA: Evolution of lung disease in cystic fibrosis. Lancet 1:448, 1983. *This article describes an interesting hypothesis that circulating pancreatic proteases may play a role in lung injury in CF, to be followed by superinfections with bacteria and/or viruses.*

Moss AJ: The cardiovascular system in cystic fibrosis. Pediatrics 70:728, 1982. *An extensive review, with 135 references, concerning the cardiovascular findings in CF, with special emphasis on the importance of cor pulmonale as a complication.*

Rodman HM, Doershuk CF, Roland JM: The interaction of two diseases: Diabetes mellitus and cystic fibrosis. Medicine 65:389, 1986. *The occurrence of diabetes mellitus in cystic fibrosis (approximately 15 per cent of CF patients over age 18) does not seem to affect the rate of progress of the disease.*

Spier S, Rivlin J, Hughes D, et al.: The effect of oxygen on sleep, blood gases, and ventilation in cystic fibrosis. Am Rev Respir Dis 129:712, 1984. *A study demonstrating the beneficial effect of nocturnal oxygen on sleep quality and on the arterial oxygen desaturation that occurs during REM sleep in CF. The hypoventilation that occurs in this sleep state was not made clinically worse.*

Wilcken B, Chalmers G: Reduced morbidity in patients with cystic fibrosis detected by neonatal screening. Lancet 2:1319, 1985. *An Australian study that documents the reduction in morbidity in the first two years of life in patients detected by neonatal immunoreactive trypsin screening by a dried blood spot method.*

67 PULMONARY EMBOLISM

Robert M. Senior

DEFINITION

Pulmonary embolism is the impaction of material into branches of the pulmonary arterial bed. Although they may completely prevent blood flow, most pulmonary emboli do not produce necrosis of lung parenchyma ("pulmonary infarction") because (1) a dual circulation (bronchial and pulmonary) supports lung parenchymal tissue, and (2) exchange of oxygen and carbon dioxide can occur directly between the tissue and alveolar gas. Most pulmonary emboli are blood clots ("thromboemboli"); much more rarely, neoplastic cells, fat droplets (Ch. 68), air bubbles, exogenous materials (such as talc and corn starch particles in intravenous drug abusers), or pieces of intravenous catheters and catheter introducers occlude pulmonary vessels. The ensuing discussion deals with pulmonary thromboembolism.

PATHOGENESIS

Pulmonary embolism is a complication of venous thrombosis: That is, emboli come from thrombi in peripheral veins, principally the deep veins of the lower extremities and pelvis (Ch. 57), and "travel" through the circulation to the pulmonary artery. In fact, in 70 per cent of patients with pulmonary thromboembolism, coexisting thrombi can be found in the deep veins of the thighs or pelvis. In the remaining cases, it is presumed that the emboli either come from other sites that escape detection or represent the entire thrombus that originated in the lower extremities. Thrombosis of superficial veins of the lower extremities does not lead to pulmonary thromboemboli, and thrombosis confined to deep veins in the leg distal to the popliteal vein infrequently leads to pulmonary thromboemboli. The renal veins can be a source of thromboemboli, particularly in patients with the nephrotic syndrome, but thromboemboli in nephrotic patients do not necessarily arise only from the renal veins. Pulmonary thromboemboli seldom originate in veins of the upper extremities, head or neck, but they may arise from mural thrombi in the right side of the heart. Venous thromboemboli may be trapped in the right atrium or ventricle, from which they embolize to the lungs intact or fragment in the heart and shower the lungs with emboli at one time or at different times.

Venous thrombosis can be attributed to one or more of the following: stasis of blood, increased tendency for blood to coagulate, and endothelial injury. Many clinical situations have been associated with risk of proximal deep venous thrombosis (Table 67–1), but, practically speaking, most are associated with decreased blood flow in lower extremity veins due to immobilization, elevated systemic venous pressure, extrinsic pressure on pelvic and lower extremity veins, intraluminal venous blockage from previous venous thrombosis, or decreased venous tone.

Pulmonary embolism occurs in 1 to 2 per cent of patients over age 40 following general surgery. The incidence is higher (5 to 10 per cent) with orthopedic surgery of the hip or knee. The risk associated with surgery is increased by advanced age, obesity, a lengthy operative period, underlying malignancy, pre-existent venous disease, prolonged bed rest after surgery, and postoperative infection. Venous stasis due to immobilization is probably a major reason for venous thrombosis associated with surgery, but other factors come into play: increased blood coagulability associated with release of tissue thromboplastin and exposure of subendothelium, postoperative decreased blood fibrinolytic activity, and vessel damage, particularly in surgery of the lower extremities or pelvis.

TABLE 67–1. CLINICAL RISK FACTORS FOR VENOUS THROMBOSIS AND PULMONARY THROMBOEMBOLISM

Common:
- Surgical and nonsurgical trauma, including burns
- Orthopedic injuries and procedures
- Age over 50
- Malignancy
- Immobilization (bed rest, stroke, prolonged travel, and so forth)
- Congestive heart failure
- Previous deep venous thrombosis
- Pregnancy, particularly in the puerperium and after cesarean section
- Estrogen therapy
- Obesity (?)

Uncommon:
- Acquired
  - Systemic lupus erythematosus
  - Inflammatory bowel disease
  - Nephrotic syndrome
  - Persistent thrombocytosis
  - Polycythemia vera
  - Paroxysmal nocturnal hemoglobinuria
- Inherited
  - Hemocystinuria
  - Antithrombin III deficiency
  - Protein C deficiency
  - Protein S deficiency
  - Dysfibrinogenemia

Cancers of the lung, breast, and abdominal viscera have a strong association with venous thromboembolism, and the thromboembolism may antedate clinical recognition of the malignancy. Factors released from tumors may increase blood coagulability, decrease fibrinolytic activity, and alter endothelial surfaces. Malignancies also predispose to deep venous thrombosis by leading to venous stasis through immobilization and surgical interventions. Prolonged bed rest from any cause and paralysis resulting from stroke are also associated with a high incidence of venous thrombosis. Pulmonary embolism is commonly found at autopsy in patients who die of congestive heart failure.

In pregnancy, multiple factors predispose to venous thrombosis: (1) venous stasis induced by compression on pelvic veins, increased intra-abdominal pressure, and hormonal relaxation of vascular smooth muscle; (2) altered blood rheologic properties; and (3) increased concentrations of factors in the coagulation cascade (fibrinogen, factors VII, VIII, IX, and XII), with concomitant reductions in antithrombin III and fibrinolytic activity. There may be an increased risk of thromboembolism during pregnancy, but there is clearly an increased risk in the puerperal period, particularly after cesarean section. Estrogen therapy has been associated with an increased incidence of venous thrombosis, and the risk appears related to the dose, but the precise degree of increased risk and the mechanisms involved are not certain. Multiple possibilities have been considered, including reduction in antithrombin III concentration, decreased plasminogen activator level, increased platelet aggregability, increased blood viscosity, and increased distensibility of peripheral veins leading to venous stasis.

When pulmonary embolism occurs without an obvious predisposing factor, hereditary conditions involving decreased antithrombotic proteins (antithrombin III, proteins C and S) or deficient plasminogen activators should be considered (Ch. 167).

INCIDENCE

Pulmonary embolism is a major cause of morbidity and death. The annual incidence in the United States has been estimated at approximately 600,000. About one third of the episodes are fatal, with nearly all of the fatalities either sudden (within one hour of onset) or undiagnosed during life. In approximately half of the people who die, there is serious underlying disease apart from venous thrombosis. Autopsy studies have reported pulmonary emboli as a major cause of death (10 to 20 per cent of all hospital deaths and 15 per cent of postoperative deaths). The incidence of fatal pulmonary embolism in hospitalized patients may be declining. In one medical center, autopsy-documented fatal pulmonary embolism fell from 9.3 per cent to 3.8 per cent over a recent ten-year period. Interestingly, during the same years, there was a concomitant increase, from 4 per cent to 12.3 per cent, in the percentage of adult patients given anticoagulant therapy.

PATHOPHYSIOLOGY

Pulmonary emboli produce respiratory and hemodynamic responses that reflect the extent of pulmonary vascular obstruction, the time elapsed since embolization, and the presence or absence of pre-existent heart or lung disease.

HYPERPNEA AND ALVEOLAR HYPERVENTILATION. Acute pulmonary embolism stimulates ventilation. The increase in minute ventilation, manifested clinically by increased respiratory rate, usually offsets the increased physiologic dead space produced by obstruction of the pulmonary vascular bed, so that the arterial Pco_2 ($Paco_2$) does not rise. On the contrary, the $Paco_2$ typically falls below 35 mm Hg, indicating that hyperpnea does not occur solely to preserve a normal $Paco_2$. Similarly, alveolar hyperventilation is not due to hypoxemia, as it occurs even when arterial oxygenation is normal, and it cannot be abolished with supplemental inspired oxygen. The stimulus for alveolar hyperventilation is unknown but presumably involves reflexes initiated from the pulmonary parenchyma in the area of the obstructed vessel. A reduction of $Paco_2$ below baseline may occur even among those with chronic hypercapnia. Although a lower than normal $Paco_2$ is usual, the $Paco_2$ rises in individuals who cannot increase their minute ventilation adequately to compensate for the increased physiologic dead space—for example, in those with neuromuscular disease, those receiving controlled mechanical ventilation, or those with severe pleuritic pain. The $Paco_2$ may also rise when there is massive embolization that confines pulmonary blood flow to a severely reduced portion of the pulmonary vascular bed.

HYPOXEMIA. A decrease in arterial oxygen tension (Pao_2) is common in acute pulmonary embolism. The mechanisms are complex. Ventilation-perfusion ($\dot{V}a/\dot{Q}$) inequality seems to be the predominant mechanism early in the course of pulmonary embolization, with intrapulmonary shunting the dominant cause after 48 hours. Regional bronchoconstriction, atelectasis, and pulmonary edema are postulated as the anatomic basis for these physiologic defects. If cardiac output fails to keep up with metabolic demands, as is common with massive pulmonary embolism, mixed venous oxygen saturation falls and accentuates the effects of abnormal $\dot{V}a/\dot{Q}$ and intrapulmonary shunting. If pulmonary hypertension develops and there is a patent foramen ovale, blood may be shunted from right to left within the heart, another factor causing arterial hypoxemia.

PULMONARY HYPERTENSION AND ACUTE COR PULMONALE. Pulmonary thromboembolism is the most common cause of acute pulmonary hypertension. The rise in pulmonary arterial pressure results primarily from mechanical blockage of the pulmonary vascular bed. Vasoconstrictive reflexes and mediators may also contribute. The rise in mean pulmonary arterial pressure tends to match the extent of blockage of the pulmonary arterial tree, but in patients without preexisting cardiac or pulmonary disease, mean pulmonary arterial pressure is usually below 20 mm Hg, unless pulmonary vascular obstruction exceeds 50 per cent. Pressures of 20 to 40 mm Hg occur only with 50 to 75 per cent obstruction. The pressure seldom goes above 40 mm Hg because the normal right ventricle is incapable of generating higher pressures. A mean pulmonary arterial pressure above 40 mm Hg indicates chronic right ventricular hypertrophy secondary to recurrent pulmonary emboli or other diseases. When a sudden and marked increase in pulmonary vascular resistance causes the mean pulmonary arterial pressure to approach 40 mm Hg, several events occur. Right ventricular diastolic pressure, right atrial pressure, and systemic venous pressure all increase. The cardiac index falls below 2.5 liters per minute per square meter, and systemic hypotension and other clinical signs of hemodynamic distress appear.

PATHOLOGY

Most episodes of acute pulmonary embolism involve multiple emboli. Both lungs are affected about two thirds of the time. Lower lobe vessels are involved more often than upper lobe vessels, and the right lung is affected more often than the left. Emboli in the main branches of the right or left pulmonary arteries are seen in only a small percentage of patients. A large embolus obstructing the main pulmonary artery or straddling the pulmonary artery bifurcation (so-called "saddle embolus") is uncommon even in fatal acute pulmonary embolism. When a thromboembolus is poorly organized, it is apt to fragment in passage through the heart and is thus more likely to impact in smaller vessels than are organized thromboemboli.

The likelihood that emboli will cause pulmonary infarction is determined by the size of the vessel involved, by the extent of obstruction, by the potential for delivery of bronchial arterial blood flow, and by the adequacy of ventilation to the lung tissue supplied by the blocked pulmonary artery. Occlusions of segmental arterial vessels or smaller branches are more likely to lead to infarction than are emboli lodged in larger vessels. Infarction is also more likely in the setting of elevated pulmonary capillary pressure from any cause—hence the frequency of infarction in patients with congestive heart failure—but otherwise healthy individuals can develop pulmonary infarcts. Histologically, pulmonary infarction is characterized by intra-alveolar hemorrhage and necrosis of alveolar walls, but little inflammation. Cavitation rarely develops without coexisting pulmonary infection or an infected thrombus, although it has recently been reported in the adult respiratory distress syndrome without associated infection.

CLINICAL MANIFESTATIONS

The clinical features of pulmonary embolism can be diverse and confusing and range from no symptoms to sudden death. Occasionally, the principal manifestations are fever, arrhythmias, or refractory congestive heart failure. Usually, however, the presentations are not obscure. Three clinical patterns predominate: (1) sudden dyspnea with no physical findings but tachypnea; (2) sudden pleuritic chest pain and dyspnea accompanied by findings consistent with pleural effusion and pulmonary consolidation; and (3) sudden apprehension, chest discomfort, and dyspnea, with findings of acute cor pulmonale (accentuated pulmonic closure sound in the second left interspace, right ventricular lift, jugular venous distention) and systemic hypotension. It is this last pattern that may culminate in death within a few minutes.

The type of pattern that develops depends upon the extent of pulmonary arterial tree blockage, whether there is pre-existing cardiopulmonary disease, and whether pulmonary infarction occurs. Severe disturbances in pulmonary and systemic hemodynamics seldom occur unless there is extensive vascular obstruction or pre-existent heart or lung disease. Pleuritic pain and signs of pulmonary consolidation and pleural effusion indicate that embolization involves one or more peripheral pulmonary arterial branches. Large discrepancies may exist between the severity of embolization and symptoms. Some patients with massive embolization may appear remarkably comfortable, whereas others with minimal embolization may show great distress.

The most common symptoms of pulmonary embolism are *dyspnea* and *chest pain*, each occurring in more than 80 per cent of patients (Table 67–2). *Tachypnea* is the most common sign. *Hemoptysis*, on the other hand, often considered typical, is not common. Its absence, therefore, is not evidence against pulmonary embolism. Similarly, deep venous thrombosis of the lower extremities is seldom clinically apparent.

TABLE 67–2. SYMPTOMS AND SIGNS IN 327 PATIENTS WITH PULMONARY EMBOLI

Symptoms*	Per Cent	Signs*	Per Cent
Chest pain	88	Respirations above 16/min	92
Pleuritic	74	Rales	58
Nonpleuritic	14	S_2P† increased	53
Dyspnea	84	Pulse above 100/min	44
Apprehension	59	Temperature above 37.8°C	43
Cough	53	Diaphoresis	36
Hemoptysis	30	Gallop	34
Sweats	27	Phlebitis	32
Syncope	13	Edema	24
		Murmur	23
		Cyanosis	19

*Apprehension, syncope, increased pulmonic component of the second heart sound, gallop, diaphoresis, murmur, and cyanosis occurred more often with massive emboli (angiographically at least two lobar arteries obstructed), whereas hemoptysis and pleuritic pain were more often present with submassive emboli.

†S_2P = intensity of the pulmonic component of the second heart sound.

(From Bell WR, Simon TL, DeMets DL: The clinical features of submassive and massive pulmonary emboli. Am J Med 62:355, 1977, with permission.)

DIAGNOSIS

Although the history and physical examination are the means by which the diagnosis of pulmonary embolism is suggested, a diagnosis that rests on clinical grounds alone is often incorrect. The differential diagnosis of pulmonary embolism can encompass many disorders, but principally those leading to acute shortness of breath, substernal or pleuritic chest pain, hemoptysis, and hemodynamic collapse. Thus, at times the possibility of pulmonary embolism must be distinguished from asthma, the hyperventilation syndrome, pneumothorax, pulmonary edema, a fractured rib, herpes zoster before the appearance of vesicles, pleurodynia, pleuritis due to collagen vascular diseases, pneumonia, empyema, bronchiectasis, bronchogenic carcinoma, acute myocardial infarction, pericarditis, dissecting aortic aneurysm, esophageal rupture, and upper abdominal processes such as acute cholecystitis. Several features point away from the diagnosis of pulmonary embolism: (1) the absence of a precipitating factor for deep venous thrombosis, (2) recurrent chest pain in the same location, (3) pleuritic chest pain of more than one week's duration that is increasing in severity, (4) pleuritic chest pain with negative findings on the chest radiograph, (5) hemoptyis of greater than 5 ml with negative findings on the chest radiograph, (6) pericardial friction rub, (7) purulent sputum, and (8) spiking fever in excess of 39°C lasting more than one week.

DIAGNOSTIC STUDIES. When pulmonary embolism is suspected, confirmation of the diagnosis depends upon establishing that there is intravascular obstruction to pulmonary arterial blood flow. The definitive means of making the diagnosis is by pulmonary arteriography; however, a high degree of certainty can also be achieved with ventilation-perfusion scanning. Other approaches to visualizing the pulmonary circulation (digital subtraction pulmonary arteriography) and novel methods of directly visualizing intrapulmonary blood clots (radioisotopically labeled platelets or monoclonal antibodies that recognize fibrin but not fibrinogen) are under development and may prove useful in the future.

Arterial blood gas measurements, the electrocardiogram, the chest radiograph, and thoracentesis may help in the evaluation of patients suspected of having pulmonary embolism, either by pointing toward or pointing away from diagnoses with which pulmonary embolism can be confused, but these studies lack specificity and therefore cannot be used in place of imaging the pulmonary circulation. Many efforts have been made to develop blood tests with specificity for the diagnosis of pulmonary embolism. None has been found useful.

Arterial Blood Gases. Typically in pulmonary embolism, there is a reduction in Pa_{O_2} and a concomitant reduction in Pa_{CO_2}. In patients with arteriographically proved acute pulmonary embolism who do not have previous cardiopulmonary disease, Pa_{O_2} values are less than 50 mm Hg in 13 per cent, 50 to 59 mm Hg in 19 per cent, between 60 and 80 mm Hg in 55 per cent, and greater than 80 mm Hg in 13 per cent. Even in those with a normal Pa_{O_2}, there is an increased alveolar-arterial oxygen difference, reflecting reduced efficiency of alveolar gas exchange. A Pa_{O_2} less than 50 mm Hg is confined to those with greater than 50 per cent occlusion of major pulmonary arterial branches; however, in individuals with underlying cardiopulmonary disease, less severe degrees of pulmonary vascular obstruction can be associated with severe hypoxemia. Arterial blood gas abnormalities have no specificity for pulmonary embolism (similar abnormalities occur in conditions with which pulmonary embolism is confused). Similarly, a normal Pa_{O_2} does not exclude pulmonary embolism.

Electrocardiogram. The main value of the electrocardiogram is to help exclude acute myocardial infarction. The most common finding in pulmonary embolism is sinus tachycardia. With emboli that provoke a substantial rise in pulmonary arterial and right-sided cardiac pressures, patterns of S_1, Q_3, T_3, inverted T waves in leads V_{1-3}, right ventricular strain, right-axis deviation, right bundle branch block, and atrial arrhythmias may occur. These changes, when they occur, are apt to be transient, lasting a few minutes or hours, disappearing as the pulmonary arterial pressure returns toward normal.

Chest Radiograph. A normal chest radiograph is uncommon in acute pulmonary embolism, but the usual radiographic findings are nonspecific: elevation of one of the hemidiaphragms with basilar atelectasis, infiltrates, and unilateral pleural effusion. Cardiac dilatation, dilatation of the main branches of the pulmonary artery, and zones of oligemia may occur with massive embolization. Besides lacking specificity, the chest radiograph shows a poor correlation with pulmonary arteriographic findings. Parenchymal densities tend to be in the lower lung fields, pleural based, and triangular and are commonly associated with pleural effusions. These densities usually represent extravasated blood rather than infarcted tissue. In summary, the principal value of the chest radiograph is to help exclude other possible diagnoses.

Thoracentesis. Pleural effusions, usually unilateral, are common with pulmonary embolism. The fluid is most often an exudate and is often hemorrhagic (but has a low hematocrit).

Ventilation-Perfusion Lung Scans. Isotopic scans of pulmonary perfusion ("$\dot{Q}$" scans) provide a sensitive, safe means of assessing regional pulmonary blood flow and therefore have proved of great value in the diagnosis of pulmonary embolism. They can be performed alone or in combination with isotopic scans of ventilation. The combination of scans ("$\dot{V}/\dot{Q}$ scans") increases the specificity of the $\dot{Q}$ scan. Ventilation-perfusion lung scanning has become the accepted means of initially assessing the patient suspected of pulmonary embolism. The strategy of using these scans is summarized in Figure 67–1.

A perfusion scan requires intravenous administration, with the patient supine, of technetium 99m–labeled particles of macroaggregated albumin or albumin microspheres, followed by scanning of the thorax with a gamma camera in six views (anterior, posterior, right and left lateral, and right and left posterior oblique). The particles, which are slightly larger in

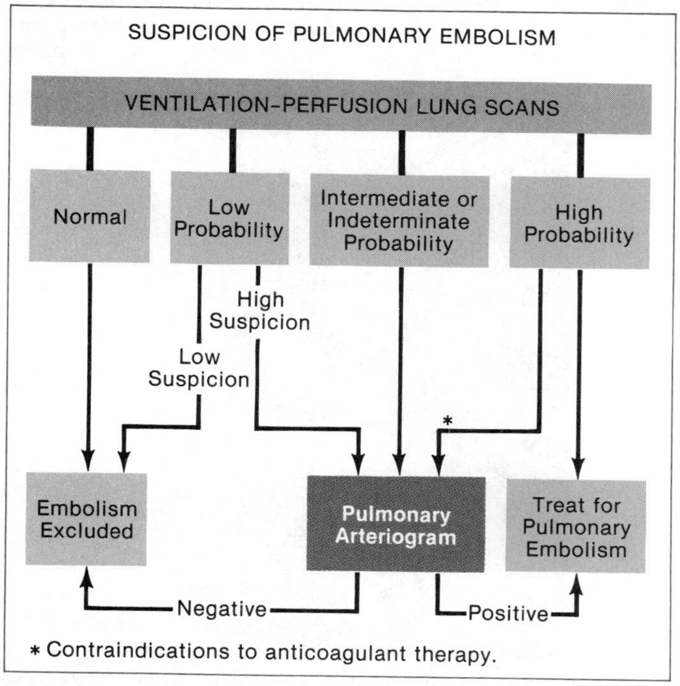

FIGURE 67–1. Ventilation-perfusion lung scanning in the evaluation of the patient suspected of having pulmonary embolism.

diameter than the cross-section of the precapillary vessels of the pulmonary circulation, are injected into a peripheral vein, flow through the peripheral and central venous circulation, the right side of the heart, and the main pulmonary arteries, and finally lodge in precapillary vessels, where they remain for hours and can be externally imaged. The standard dose of particles blocks less than 0.2 per cent of the pulmonary precapillary vessels in the normal pulmonary vascular bed. For a ventilation scan, the patient inhales and then rebreathes air containing a trace of radioactive gas, usually xenon^{133}. The procedure involves obtaining images on the initial breath, at equilibration (about five minutes later), and during the washout of the tracer, beginning when the patient is returned to breathing room air. Typically, the ventilation scan is done from only one view (posterior) and for technical reasons is best done before the perfusion scan. Besides xenon^{133}, two other isotopes are gaining usage for ventilation scanning: (1) krypton^{81m}, which has the advantage over xenon^{133} of enabling the scan to be obtained in the same views and at the same time as the perfusion scan, with minimal radiation exposure, and (2) technetium^{99m} diethylene triamine penta-acetate in aerosols, which is more convenient from the standpoint of stability of the preparation and ease of handling.

A normal perfusion scan eliminates the diagnosis of pulmonary embolism. A normal scan reveals a homogeneous distribution of isotopic activity with an image that conforms to the anatomic shape of the lungs. In the presence of a pulmonary embolus, the radiolabeled particles are prevented from reaching vessels distal to the embolus, and the scan shows one or more perfusion defects in the image. The sensitivity of the perfusion lung scan to pulmonary arterial obstruction is excellent, as obstruction of vessels 3 mm in diameter or more leads to defects. Perfusion defects may show some resolution within a few days, but substantial abnormalities commonly persist for several weeks and may be present even a year later.

Defects on perfusion lung scans are interpreted in conjunction with the chest radiograph. Defects that do not have a corresponding abnormality on the chest radiograph are scored by number and size for the probability of pulmonary embolism (Table 67–3). Single segment-sized defects and defects smaller than segments carry low probability (less than 10 per cent) for pulmonary embolism, whereas multiple defects that are segmental or larger carry a substantially higher probability for pulmonary embolism. Perfusion defects that have corresponding abnormalities on the chest radiograph are called indeterminate, although some evidence indicates that a perfusion defect can be assigned a probability of embolus score based upon its size relative to the radiographic abnormality.

TABLE 67–3. VENTILATION-PERFUSION LUNG SCANS: FREQUENCY OF EMBOLISM BY ARTERIOGRAPHY*

Interpretation	Scan Patterns	Frequency (%)
Normal	Normal perfusion	0
Low probability	Matching defects Small subsegmental defects with mismatch ($\dot{Q}$ defects smaller than chest roentgenogram abnormalities)	Less than 10
Intermediate probability	Single segmental defect with mismatch Multiple segmental defects with mismatch and match ($\dot{Q}$ defects same size as chest roentgenogram abnormalities)	20–30
High probability	Multiple segmental or lobar defects with mismatch ($\dot{Q}$ defects larger than chest roentgenogram abnormalities)	~90

*When perfusion scans are done without ventilation studies, the frequencies are lower.

(Adapted from Biello DR, Mattar AG, McKnight RC, et al.: Ventilation-perfusion studies in suspected pulmonary embolism. Am J Roentgenol 133:1033, 1979.)

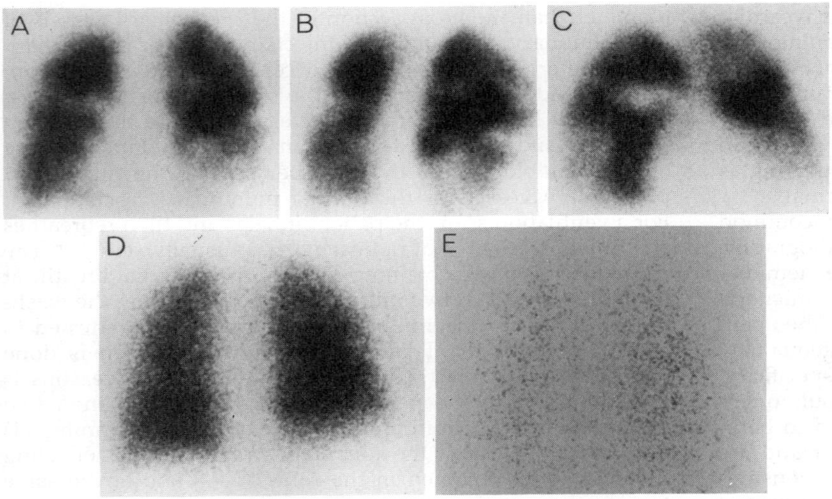

FIGURE 67–2. Selected views of ventilation-perfusion lung scans in a 60-year-old man who experienced sudden, severe shortness of breath 14 days after a suprapubic prostatectomy. The perfusion scans—(*A*) posterior, (*B*) right posterior oblique, and (*C*) left posterior oblique—show multiple segmental defects, whereas the ventilation scans are normal—(*D*) at equilibrium, (*E*) 1 minute of washout. This combination of scan findings indicates a high probability of pulmonary embolism and with the clinical setting is sufficient to make the diagnosis of pulmonary embolism. (Courtesy of Dr. Keith C. Fischer.)

The limitation of the perfusion scan is nonspecificity. Besides emboli, perfusion defects can be caused by lesions that compress pulmonary vessels, by increased pulmonary vascular resistance, by regional alveolar hypoxia, and by regional loss of pulmonary parenchyma, as in pulmonary emphysema. In practice, obstructive lung disease is the most common clinical condition causing perfusion defects that are not due to pulmonary embolism. Even in patients with known obstructive lung disease, perfusion scans are indicated when pulmonary embolism is suspected because they serve as a guide to selective angiography when the procedure is indicated.

Ventilation lung scans increase the specificity of perfusion scans for pulmonary emboli because pulmonary emboli do not usually disrupt regional ventilation as much as regional blood flow, unlike other causes of perfusion defects, especially obstructive lung disease. Ventilation scans may indicate the preservation of ventilation when there are perfusion defects ("$\dot{V}/\dot{Q}$ mismatches"), the loss of ventilation when there are perfusion defects ("$\dot{V}/\dot{Q}$ matches"), and delays of washin or washout indicative of obstructive lung disease. $\dot{V}/\dot{Q}$ mismatches establish a higher probability of pulmonary emboli than perfusion defects alone (Table 67–3). With some patterns of $\dot{V}/\dot{Q}$ mismatch, the diagnosis of pulmonary embolism can be made with virtual certainty (Fig. 67–2). Matched $\dot{V}/\dot{Q}$ defects are less likely to represent pulmonary embolism, but pulmonary embolism is not excluded. At large institutions, approximately 25 per cent of $\dot{V}/\dot{Q}$ studies are interpreted as being either normal or of high probability for pulmonary embolism.

Pulmonary Arteriography. *Pulmonary arteriography is the definitive test for the diagnosis of pulmonary embolism.* It involves insertion of a catheter into the pulmonary artery, usually by a percutaneous approach through one of the femoral veins. After the catheter is advanced at least as far as the right or left mainstem branch of the pulmonary artery, or more selectively into lobar or segmental branches, the contrast medium is injected and films are taken in rapid sequence. Radiographic images—supine, oblique, or lateral views—are examined for filling defects (Fig. 67–3) in branches of the pulmonary artery; these establish the diagnosis of pulmonary embolism. Abrupt terminations ("cut offs") of pulmonary arterial branches also point toward that diagnosis, although less definitely. The filling defects or cutoffs should be present in vessels of at least 2 to 3 mm in diameter. Other types of abnormalities, including delayed filling and diminished number of small vessels, are not diagnostic. Once a diagnosis of pulmonary embolism is made, the study is terminated. A negative study has rarely been proved wrong. Arteriography should be done promptly after the onset of symptoms, but it is doubtful that there will be major changes within a few days in most cases.

Pulmonary arteriography is indicated when scans are indeterminate or demonstrate an intermediate probability of pulmonary embolism. Arteriography is also warranted in the following circumstances: (1) when $\dot{V}/\dot{Q}$ scans suggest a high probability of pulmonary embolism but there are concerns about using anticoagulation therapy, (2) before using thrombolytic agents, (3) when there are clear-cut contraindications to anticoagulation therapy so that other forms of treatment will be needed, and (4) when there is an apparent failure of anticoagulation therapy and surgical treatment is being contemplated. When scans are interpreted as indicating a low probability of pulmonary embolism, a decision regarding arteriography should be guided by clinical suspicion. Thus, in patients in whom the possibility is high on the basis of clinical and laboratory tests, arteriography should be done. In approximately 10 per cent of these patients, an arteriogram will be positive. Clearly, therefore, a low probability $\dot{V}/\dot{Q}$ scan is not equivalent to an exclusion of pulmonary embolism. Indeed, some clinicians contend that pulmonary arteriography should be done routinely upon finding a low probability scan regardless of the strength of the clinical impression of pulmonary embolism. An approach to reduce the need for pulmonary arteriography has been to investigate the veins of the lower extremities using venography or noninvasive approaches such as impedance plethysmography or Doppler

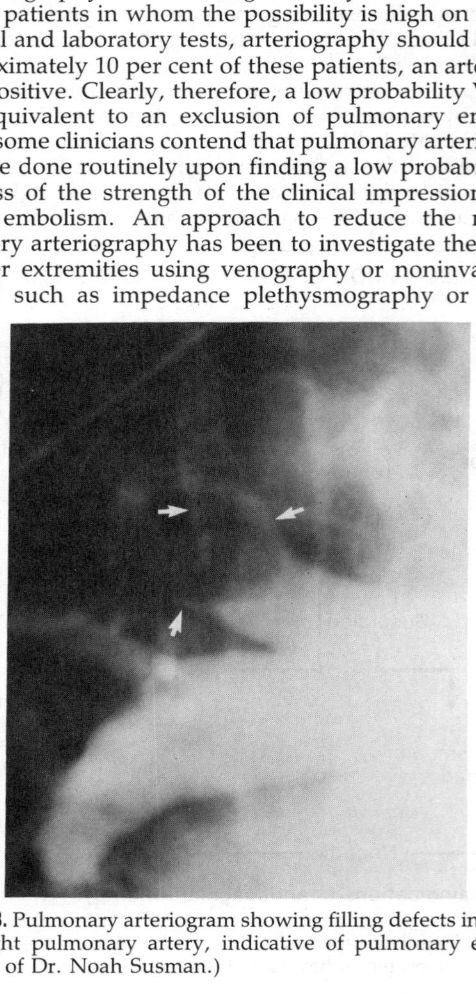

FIGURE 67–3. Pulmonary arteriogram showing filling defects in branches of the right pulmonary artery, indicative of pulmonary embolism. (Courtesy of Dr. Noah Susman.)

study. It is argued that a positive study of the extremity veins indicates the need for the same anticoagulant therapy necessary to treat pulmonary embolism and that a negative study of a lower extremity vein, along with a low-probability V̇/Q scan, excludes pulmonary embolism. While this concept has some merit, one must remember that in 30 per cent of patients with proven pulmonary emboli, studies of lower extremity veins are negative.

Many experts in this field believe that pulmonary arteriography is underutilized because physicians have concerns about the safety of the procedure. Pulmonary arteriography for the diagnosis of pulmonary embolism has proved very safe. In large series, the risk of a serious complication is 1 to 2 per cent and of death, about 0.25 per cent. The deaths have occurred almost exclusively in people with severe pulmonary hypertension who were given large amounts of contrast media.

THERAPY

Nearly all patients with acute pulmonary embolism who survive long enough to have the diagnosis confirmed will survive the acute episode. Accordingly, the primary goal of therapy is to prevent a recurrence that might be fatal. Additional goals are to reduce the morbidity of the acute episode and to prevent chronic pulmonary hypertension.

The overall therapeutic approach is summarized in Figure 67–4. The cornerstone of therapy is the use of anticoagulant drugs, since most patients with acute pulmonary embolism are hemodynamically stable and do not have a contraindication to anticoagulants. Patients who are treated with therapeutic doses of anticoagulants for an appropriate period seldom have a recurrence of pulmonary embolism, and fatal recurrences are rare indeed. Thrombolytic therapy accelerates restoration of pulmonary blood flow and normal pulmonary hemodynamics and therefore is the initial therapy for massive pulmonary embolism that has produced hemodynamic instability. When anticoagulants and thrombolytic agents are contraindicated or prove ineffective, therapy consists of interruption of the inferior vena cava, combined with pulmonary embolectomy in patients with hemodynamic instability.

Supportive measures can reduce the morbidity of the acute episode and on occasion are essential to tide the patient through a period of hemodynamic crisis. These include supplemental oxygen to correct hypoxemia, analgesics for pleuritic pain, and hemodynamic and ventilatory support.

ANTICOAGULANT THERAPY. Anticoagulant therapy prevents future embolization by preventing the formation of new deep venous thrombi and the propagation of residual thrombi in the deep venous system. During anticoagulant therapy, pulmonary emboli and residual deep venous thrombi either organize or undergo dissolution or both. Anticoagulation does not, however, hasten resolution of the thromboemboli within the lungs.

Table 67–4 presents a regimen for the use of anticoagulant agents. Heparin is the initial therapy because its effect is immediate. It may also be a more effective antithrombotic agent than warfarin. Heparin, an acidic glycosaminoglycan obtained from pig intestinal mucosa or beef lung, accelerates the inhibitory effect of antithrombin III upon the coagulation enzymes, thrombin, and Factors IXa, Xa, XIa, and XIIa. In patients who are suspected of having pulmonary embolism, an intravenous bolus of heparin (5000 units) should be given while diagnostic studies are under way, unless there is intracranial bleeding, intracranial lesions predisposed to bleed, or active internal bleeding, all of which are absolute contraindications to heparin.

Heparin is usually administered intravenously by continuous infusion. Intermittent intravenous injection and subcutaneous injection are alternative means of administration, but a higher incidence of bleeding complications may occur with intermittent injection, and it is difficult to establish the correct dose with the subcutaneous route. The risk of recurrent venous thromboembolism is low if the activated partial thromboplastin time is maintained 1.5 to 2 times the control (about 25 seconds beyond the control) at all times. Accordingly, this is the goal of therapy. The usual daily dose is 25,000 to 50,000 units. Heparin therapy should be monitored particularly closely during the first few days after the thromboembolic event, as the heparin requirements are greatest then.

The most common and most serious complication of heparin therapy is bleeding. The risk of bleeding may be more closely related to risk factors, such as trauma, recent surgery, recent invasive procedures, and the inhibition by heparin of platelet function, than to the absolute anticoagulant effect produced by the drug. Thrombocytopenia may also complicate therapy and cause bleeding. Approximately 10 per cent of patients exhibit platelet counts less than 100,000 per cubic millimeter

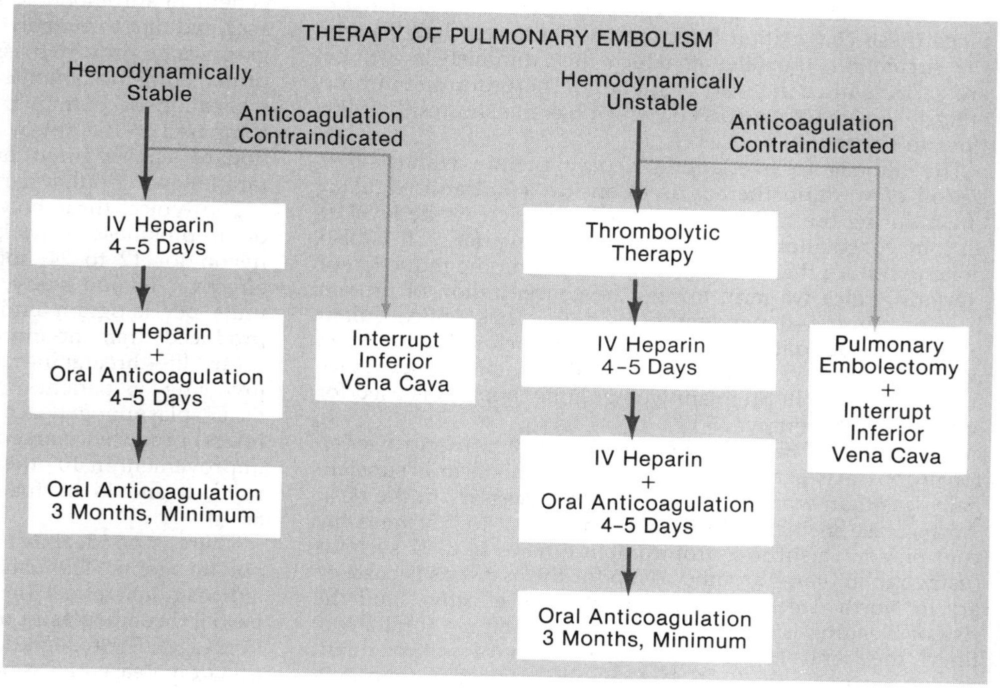

FIGURE 67–4. The therapy of pulmonary embolism.

TABLE 67–4. GUIDELINES FOR ANTICOAGULANT THERAPY WITH HEPARIN AND WARFARIN IN PULMONARY EMBOLISM

Embolism Suspected	Embolism Confirmed
Obtain baseline APTT,* PT,* and platelet count and give heparin bolus (5000–10,000 units) IV* Order diagnostic test: ventilation-perfusion lung scan or pulmonary arteriogram	Give loading dose of heparin (5000 units) and start constant IV infusion at approximately 1000 units/hr Monitor APTT at 4–6 hr and thereafter until the APTT is stabilized between 1.5 and 2.0 times control value Monitor platelet count while administering heparin Start warfarin by day 4 or 5 by instituting the estimated daily maintenance dose (usually 4–10 mg) After at least 7–10 days of heparin therapy and 4–5 days of joint therapy, stop heparin and check PT four hours later Maintain PT off heparin at 1.2 to 1.5 times control or pretreatment value (using rabbit brain thromboplastin) Maintain full-dose anticoagulation for at least 3 mo in patients without continuing risk factors, longer in other patients

*APTT = activated partial thromboplastin time; PT = one-stage prothrombin time (1.2 times control performed with rabbit brain thromboplastin is roughly equal to 2.0 times control with human brain thromboplastin); IV = intravenous.

(Adapted from Hyers TM, Hull RD, Weg JG: Antithrombotic therapy for venous thromboembolic disease. Chest 89:26S, 1986, with permission.)

during heparin therapy; there seems to be no correlation between this complication and the type of heparin used. The thrombocytopenia, which appears to have an immunologic basis, seldom occurs until after several days of therapy. A rare complication of heparin-induced thrombocytopenia is thrombosis, mainly of arteries. With long-term administration, heparin can cause accelerated osteoporosis.

After four to five days of heparin therapy, oral anticoagulation is begun with *warfarin*. Both agents are continued together for four to five days, after which the heparin is discontinued. Warfarin acts in the liver to inhibit the gamma-carboxylation of specific glutamic acid residues in several vitamin K–dependent coagulation cofactors: II, VII, IX, and X (Ch. 167). These gamma-carboxyglutamic acids are required for calcium binding and the expression of functional activity. Since these coagulation cofactors have different half-lives in the circulation, the rates at which they diminish in activity are variable after the start of therapy. The prothrombin time is most sensitive to factor VII, which has the shortest half-life (four to six hours).

The rationale for overlapping heparin therapy with the first period of warfarin therapy is to ensure a full anticoagulant effect during the time required for depression of the level of all four coagulation cofactors affected by warfarin. It is also done to reduce the risk of thrombosis during the induction of warfarin, since warfarin lowers the concentration of protein C, a vitamin K–dependent protein that has anticoagulant properties due to its capacity to degrade factors Va and VIIIa proteolytically. Warfarin is not used during pregnancy, since it is teratogenic. In pregnant women, only heparin is used for anticoagulant therapy.

The extent of the anticoagulant effect of warfarin needed for prophylaxis against venous thromboembolism is substantially less than what had been thought necessary in the past. An increase in the prothrombin time to 1.2 to 1.5 times the control, equivalent to a prothrombin time of 14 to 17 seconds (using rabbit brain thromboplastin for the assay, as is customary in North America), is sufficient to be effective, and the risk of bleeding is less than with therapy aiming for 1.5 to 2 times the control. The optimal duration of anticoagulant therapy is not known. It is generally advised to continue therapy for at least three months in all patients, to extend therapy as long as identifiable risk factors are resolving, and to give therapy indefinitely to patients in whom an increased risk for deep venous thrombosis is permanent.

THROMBOLYTIC THERAPY. Thrombolytic agents, by dissolving pulmonary emboli and thrombi in the deep venous system, can alleviate the hemodynamic disturbances caused by pulmonary emboli, eliminate the source of further emboli, and perhaps diminish postphlebitic complications in the lower extremities. Two thrombolytic agents, streptokinase and urokinase, have been used for a number of years. A third, tissue-type plasminogen activator (TPA), is currently in use in limited trials and should be generally available soon.

Streptokinase and *urokinase* convert circulating endogenous plasminogen to plasmin, a potent serine protease that dissolves fibrin. Urokinase cleaves plasminogen to plasmin directly, whereas streptokinase forms a complex with plasminogen, allowing expression of plasminogen's normally hidden active site, which then cleaves other plasminogen molecules to plasmin. At equivalent dosage, streptokinase is considerably cheaper than urokinase, but, unlike urokinase, it can produce febrile and allergic reactions. Plasmin formed by either agent lyses the fibrin clot in pulmonary emboli, but unfortunately it also cleaves other molecules in the circulation, including fibrinogen and factors V and VIII, and it leads to consumption of circulating plasmin inhibitors, in particular alpha 2-antiplasmin. Thus, besides solubilizing pulmonary emboli and deep venous thrombi, these agents can solubilize hemostatic plugs where they are important, such as at incisional sites, and can reduce hemostatic competence generally. *Tissue-type plasminogen activator*, which has been used widely in trials for acute coronary occlusion, has shown dramatic thrombolytic effects on pulmonary emboli in a small number of patients. It has the advantage of expressing little activity in the absence of fibrin.

These thrombolytic agents restore pulmonary arterial pressure and pulmonary perfusion toward normal faster than does heparin, but their use seems to result in no improvement in mortality or in pulmonary perfusion, compared with heparin, a few weeks after the acute episode. There is also no difference between thrombolytic agents and anticoagulants in the rate of recurrence of pulmonary embolism. Thrombolytic therapy appears to offer only an immediate short-term advantage over heparin, but studies do not exclude a life-saving benefit of thrombolytic therapy in some patients. It is now accepted that thrombolytic therapy should be given for angiographically proven massive pulmonary embolism that has produced hemodynamic instability. There may be better normalization of pulmonary capillary blood flow after a year compared to therapy with heparin only, but this is of questionable clinical importance, since pulmonary impairment is rare following pulmonary emboli in either case.

The typical thrombolytic regimen involves a loading dose of streptokinase or urokinase, followed by a continuous infusion for 12 to 24 hours, but other regimens may be as effective. In one study, a single bolus of urokinase, 15,000 units per kilogram into the right atrium over 10 minutes, produced dramatic improvements in 12 of 14 patients with acute, life-threatening pulmonary emboli. In another study involving 36 patients, short-term infusions of recombinant tissue plasminogen activator (50 to 90 mg over two to six hours) produced marked clot lysis in 24 patients and objective improvement in 10 others. Whatever thrombolytic regimen is used, it should be followed by anticoagulant therapy (Fig. 67–4).

There is no ideal test for monitoring patients given thrombolytic agents. The usual approach is to document either an anticoagulant effect (lengthening of the prothrombin time, partial thromboplastin time, or thrombin time) or evidence of fibrinogen/fibrin degradation (decreased fibrinogen concentration or increased titers of fibrin degradation products) or both.

Because these agents digest substrates besides fibrin in pulmonary emboli, proof that a thrombolytic agent has exerted some effect by these tests does not, however, prove an effect upon pulmonary emboli. Nor is it possible to use results from these tests to titrate the dose. On the other hand, clinical effectiveness is usually apparent from improvement in the patient's cardiopulmonary status.

Because thrombolytic agents may start or aggravate bleeding, they are absolutely contraindicated when there is active internal bleeding or within a few months of stroke, neurologic or ophthalmologic surgery, or head injury. They are relatively contraindicated within ten days of major surgical procedures or biopsies of internal organs or arteriographic studies, during pregnancy and the first ten days postpartum, and in a variety of medical states associated with increased risk of bleeding, such as severe hypertension. In the patient who is critically ill from pulmonary emboli, however, the danger of bleeding must be weighed against the potential benefits and the risks of alternate forms of therapy.

VENA CAVAL INTERRUPTION. The principal reasons for interruption of the inferior vena cava are (1) absolute contraindications to anticoagulant therapy (active internal bleeding and recent central nervous system lesions that are bleeding or are predisposed to bleed), (2) severe internal bleeding that develops during therapeutic anticoagulation, and (3) recurrent emboli despite adequate anticoagulation. Infrequently, vena caval interruption is necessary for septic embolism, after pulmonary embolectomy, or after massive embolization of such severity that further embolization might well be fatal. In the last-noted situation, anticoagulation therapy is used as well.

Like anticoagulation therapy, interruption of the vena cava is only preventive against future emboli. It does not promote resolution of emboli already in the lungs, and it does not alleviate the hemodynamic effects of emboli. In addition, it may not provide permanent protection against pulmonary embolism, since collateral veins bypassing the interruption can enlarge and provide other routes for thromboemboli to reach the lungs. Since most bleeding during anticoagulant therapy is not life threatening and can be controlled by reduction in anticoagulant dosage, a conservative approach is advised regarding the interruption of the vena cava. Similarly, recurrence of pulmonary embolism after anticoagulation therapy is begun should not be taken as an automatic indication for vena caval interruption. Unless massive embolism is documented angiographically, anticoagulation therapy should be continued, with maximal effort made to ensure an adequate anticoagulant effect at all times. As noted above, fatal pulmonary embolism is rare during therapeutic anticoagulation.

Methods of vena caval interruption include ligation or clipping, which must be done with the patient under general or spinal anesthesia, and the use of umbrellas or filters, which are inserted percutaneously through jugular or femoral veins with the patient under local anesthesia. Except in the case of septic embolism, percutaneous devices are preferred.

PULMONARY EMBOLECTOMY. Pulmonary embolectomy is rarely performed and is limited to patients with massive pulmonary emboli involving pulmonary arteries shown to be accessible on pulmonary angiography, with hypotension and end-organ (brain and kidney) dysfunction despite maximal medical support, and in whom there are contraindications to thrombolytic therapy or in whom thrombolytic therapy has proved ineffective. Few patients meet these conditions and survive long enough to have surgery. The surgical mortality for emergency pulmonary embolectomy is at least 25 per cent. In contrast, elective surgery for symptomatic, unresolved pulmonary emboli in large branches of the pulmonary artery has proved effective and reasonably safe. The procedure for chronic emboli, which amounts to an endarterectomy for removal of organized thromboemboli, can improve functional status, reduce pulmonary arterial pressure, and normalize pulmonary arterial perfusion and arterial oxygenation.

PROGNOSIS

The majority of deaths from pulmonary embolism occur either too quickly for therapy to be given or because the condition is not recognized. If pulmonary embolism goes untreated, survival is only 70 per cent, with death occurring as a result of recurrent thromboembolism within a few weeks of the first episode. In contrast, among those individuals in whom a diagnosis is made and therapy begun, 92 per cent survive and do so without sequelae. Among those few individuals who do not survive despite therapy, two thirds of the deaths are due to associated critical diseases. In those in whom death is due to pulmonary embolism, systemic hypotension is usually present at the onset of the episode, and pulmonary vascular obstruction is usually greater than 75 per cent. Even when hypotension and acute cor pulmonale are present at the onset of acute pulmonary embolism, however, it does not necessarily mean a fatal outcome. Clinical signs of massive embolization can subside quickly, presumably because vascular obstruction decreases as a result of fragmentation or remodeling of the emboli or because pulmonary vasoconstrictive reflexes and mediators dissipate. The presence of pulmonary infarction has no effect on survival.

In less than 1 per cent of those who survive acute pulmonary thromboembolization, the emboli persist and result in a chronic syndrome of exertional dyspnea, pulmonary hypertension, right ventricular enlargement, and right ventricular failure. Individuals presenting with this syndrome usually have a history that contains clues to recurrent episodes of pulmonary embolism and to conditions predisposing to venous thromboembolic disease.

PREVENTION

Several therapeutic regimens reduce the risk of deep venous thrombosis and by doing so reduce the risk of pulmonary thromboembolism. These regimens—which include early ambulation, low-dose subcutaneous heparin, low-dose warfarin, dextran, external pneumatic calf compression, and gradient elastic stockings—are easy to use, have minimal complications, and require essentially no laboratory monitoring. The most thoroughly proven regimen, low-dose subcutaneous heparin (5000 units twice daily), is effective for (1) general surgery patients with high-risk features (over age 40, obese, previous deep venous thrombosis or previous pulmonary embolism, current malignancy, and complex surgery), (2) patients undergoing urologic or gynecologic surgery (excluding procedures for gynecologic malignancies), and (3) patients with congestive heart failure and those recovering from acute myocardial infarction. Low-dose subcutaneous heparin is not effective for prophylaxis of deep venous thrombosis in patients with traumatic hip fracture. In that situation, low-dose warfarin or pneumatic compression should be used. Because there is some risk of bleeding with low-dose heparin, it should not be used in patients having intracranial or eye surgery or in those who have suffered spinal cord trauma. For these situations, pneumatic compression is a satisfactory, safe alternative. Prophylaxis for deep venous thrombosis should be given wider usage because it is the only way that a substantial reduction in fatal pulmonary embolism will be achieved.

Bounameaux H, Vermylen J, Collen D: Thrombolytic treatment with recombinant tissue-type plasminogen activator in a patient with massive pulmonary embolism. Ann Intern Med 103:64, 1985. *Describes dramatic resolution of life-threatening pulmonary embolism within a few hours after a bolus of tissue-type plasminogen activator delivered through a catheter placed in the right ventricle.*

Consensus Development Panel: NIH Consensus Development Conference Statement on the Prevention of Venous Thrombosis and Pulmonary Embolism. JAMA 256:744, 1986. *Summarizes current views about prophylactic therapy for deep venous thrombosis and concludes that such therapy is effective and should be used more widely.*

Dismuke SE, Wagner EH: Pulmonary embolism as a cause of death. JAMA 255:2039, 1986. *Reports a declining incidence of massive fatal pulmonary embolism in a university hospital between 1966 and 1980, coincident with an increased use of anticoagulants.*

Goldhaber SZ (ed.): Pulmonary Embolism and Deep Venous Thrombosis. Philadelphia, W. B. Saunders Company, 1985. *Detailed reviews of various aspects of pulmonary embolism.*

Goldhaber SZ, Markis JE, Meyerovitz MF, et al.: Acute pulmonary embolism treated with tissue plasminogen activator. Lancet 2:886, 1986. *Reports angiographic improvement in 34 of 36 patients, which was marked in 24, within six hours after receiving recombinant human tissue-type plasminogen activator intravenously.*

Heim CR, Des Prez RM: Pulmonary embolism: A review. Adv Intern Med 31:187, 1986. *Summarizes clinical aspects of pulmonary embolism.*

Hirsh J: Venous thromboembolism: Prevention, diagnosis and treatment. Chest 89:369S, 1986. *Articles on the management of pulmonary embolism.*

Huet Y, Lemaire F, Brun-Buisson C, et al.: Hypoxemia in acute pulmonary embolism. Chest 88:829, 1985. *Using the multiple inert gas technique to analyze alveolar gas exchange, this study shows that the mechanisms for hypoxemia in pulmonary embolism change during the course of the illness.*

Hyers TM (ed.): Symposium on pulmonary embolism and hypertension. Clin Chest Med 5:383, 1984. *Articles on various aspects of venous thromboembolism.*

Hyers TM, Hull RD, Weg JG: Antithrombotic therapy for venous thromboembolic disease. Chest 89:26S, 1986. *Describes how to use anticoagulants in the management of venous thrombosis and pulmonary embolism.*

Petitprez P, Simmoneau G, Cerrina J, et al.: Effects of a single bolus of urokinase in patients with life-threatening pulmonary emboli: A descriptive trial. Circulation 70:861, 1984. *Twelve of 14 patients with massive pulmonary embolism had rapid clinical improvement shortly after receiving one large dose of urokinase delivered in the right atrium over 10 minutes.*

Shafer KE, Santoro SA, Sobel BE, et al.: Monitoring activity of fibrinolytic agents: A therapeutic challenge. Am J Med 76:879, 1984. *Reviews the fibrinolytic system, mechanisms of fibrinolysis, and methods for monitoring therapy with fibrinolytic agents.*

68 FAT EMBOLISM SYNDROME

Robert M. Senior

DEFINITION

Fat embolism syndrome refers to the constellation of clinical manifestations that may develop when fat droplets impact in the pulmonary microvasculature and other microvascular beds, especially in the brain. The principal clinical features of fat embolism syndrome are respiratory failure, cerebral dysfunction, and petechiae.

CLINICAL SETTING

Fat embolism syndrome occurs almost exclusively as an early complication of traumatic fractures of the pelvis and of long bones, particularly the shaft of the femur. Delays in stabilization of fractures and periods of systemic hypoperfusion after trauma increase the risk of the syndrome. The syndrome develops in 2 to 25 per cent of persons with fresh long bone fractures, depending on criteria for the diagnosis and selection of patients at risk. In contrast, it rarely follows elective orthopedic surgery on long bones, even though fat droplets can be found routinely in the venous blood draining the operative sites. Other rare settings for fat embolism include massive soft tissue injury, severe burns, conditions associated with fatty liver, osteomyelitis and conditions causing bone infarcts such as sickle cell hemoglobinopathy, and prolonged corticosteroid therapy.

DIAGNOSIS

There are no laboratory tests that are diagnostic of fat embolism syndrome. Specifically, looking for the presence of fat droplets in the blood, urine, and sputum is not helpful in making the diagnosis, as droplets may not be present in patients who clearly have fat embolism syndrome but may be found after traumatic fractures in patients without evidence of the syndrome. The diagnosis is based on the presence of at least one of the following features within the first 72 hours after traumatic fracture: (1) otherwise unexplained dyspnea, tachypnea, arterial hypoxemia, and diffuse alveolar infiltrates on chest radiograph; (2) otherwise unexplained confusion or other signs of cerebral dysfunction, and (3) petechiae over the upper half of the body, including the axillae, conjunctivae, and oral mucosa. Further support for the diagnosis is provided by fluffy retinal exudates and hemorrhages and unexplained fever. The diagnosis is definite if all three criteria are present. The diagnosis is unlikely if the signs and symptoms first begin more than 72 hours after the injury. In this situation, pulmonary edema from massive fluid replacement, aspiration, sepsis, pneumonia, or venous thromboembolism is a more probable cause of respiratory distress.

PATHOGENESIS

The specific cellular mechanisms leading to fat embolism syndrome are not fully understood, but it is clear that the syndrome is not simply a consequence of mechanical obstruction of small vessels by fat droplets. An important aspect of the pathogenesis appears to be endothelial injury caused by fatty acids released from impacted fat droplets by lipoprotein lipase, with ensuing increased microvascular permeability and fluid leakage into interstitial spaces. Some data suggest that individuals who have had fat embolism syndrome after trauma have abnormalities of carbohydrate and lipid metabolism, increased capillary fragility, and abnormal neurohumoral responses to stress and are distinguishable by these characteristics from individuals with comparable trauma who did not develop fat embolism syndrome.

The fat droplets found in small vessels are from the trauma site. As the first microvascular bed encountered by fat droplets in the venous circulation, the lungs bear the brunt of fat embolization. Presumably, fat emboli in other organs, especially the brain, reach those sites by passing through the pulmonary microvasculature or through right-to-left shunts in the heart.

Although the effects of fatty acids upon endothelium appear to be important in the mechanism of lung injury, the pathogenesis of respiratory failure may be more complex in some cases. Other tissue components besides fat may be liberated from fracture sites, and these as well as the injured pulmonary endothelium may activate the clotting, complement, and contact systems. Thus, the pathogenesis of lung injury may be multifactorial, as in other forms of the adult respiratory distress syndrome, involving thrombosis, mediators of inflammation, and products of inflammatory cells.

Hypoxemia explains brain dysfunction in many cases, but not all. In some fatal cases, cerebral symptoms reflect direct brain injury, with many fat emboli and associated hemorrhage and necrosis. Moreover, patients with comparable hypoxemia from causes other than fat embolism syndrome seldom have brain dysfunction, and occasional patients with fat embolism syndrome have neurologic features that precede hypoxemia or are disproportionate to the degree of hypoxemia.

The reason for petechiae is not known, although in some patients there may be thrombocytopenia and disseminated intravascular coagulation. There is also no explanation for the striking localization of the petechiae to the pectoral regions and conjunctivae.

THERAPY

Management of fat embolism syndrome is supportive and usually consists primarily of ensuring good arterial oxygenation. Supplemental oxygen is given to maintain the arterial oxygen tension in the normal range, 75 to 90 mm Hg. If endotracheal intubation and ventilatory support are necessary, positive end-expiratory pressure may reduce the need for high concentrations of inspired oxygen. Restricting fluid intake and even giving diuretics, if systemic perfusion can be maintained, may minimize fluid accumulation in the lungs.

The role of corticosteroids is controversial; there is no clear-cut evidence that they are helpful.

In patients with acute long bone fractures, the risk of fat embolism syndrome is reduced by prompt surgical stabilization of the fractures and by correcting or preventing decreased systemic perfusion. In addition, administration of corticosteroids at a high dose for a short period (7.5 mg per kilogram of methylprednisolone intravenously at six-hour intervals for three days) seems to prevent development of the syndrome.

PROGNOSIS

The mortality from fat embolism syndrome is 10 per cent or less and thus is clearly much lower than the 50 per cent or greater mortality for most causes of the adult respiratory distress syndrome. Even severe respiratory failure seldom leads to death. In one report of 54 cases, there was not a single fatality from the syndrome, although severe hypoxemia was common during the acute stages.

Guenter CA, Braun TE: Fat embolism syndrome: A changing prognosis. Chest 79:143, 1981. *This study emphasizes that with modern respiratory care, death from post-traumatic fat embolism is unusual.*

Peltier LF: Fat embolism: An appraisal of the problem. Clin Ortho Rel Res 187:3, 1984. *Reviews clinical investigations of the source and composition of post-traumatic fat emboli and the pathogenesis of fat embolism syndrome.*

Rosen JM, Braman SS, Hasan FM, et al.: Nontraumatic fat embolization: A rare cause of new pulmonary infiltrates in an immunocompromised patient. Am Rev Resp Dis 134:805, 1986. *Describes fatal fat embolism syndrome in a patient with lymphoma who was receiving high-dose corticosteroid therapy.*

Schonfeld SA, Ployongsang Y, DiLisio R, et al.: Fat embolism prophylaxis with corticosteroids: A prospective study in high-risk patients. Ann Intern Med 99:438, 1983. *This study presents persuasive evidence for the efficacy of steroids in prevention of post-traumatic fat embolism syndrome.*

69 SARCOIDOSIS

Barry L. Fanburg

DEFINITION

Sarcoidosis, a multisystem granulomatous disease, begins most frequently in people between 20 and 40 years old. The etiology is unknown, but alterations in the immune system are clearly involved in its pathogenesis. Organ involvement is usually asymptomatic, and the disease most frequently regresses spontaneously, but it may progress to a more chronic state of fibrosis with severe functional impairment of various organs. No natural animal models of sarcoidosis have been discovered.

EPIDEMIOLOGY AND GENETICS

Sarcoidosis occurs with similar manifestations world wide, but its incidence differs strikingly, from 0.04 per 100,000 in Spain, for example, to 64 per 100,000 in Sweden. The reported numbers are susceptible to considerable error based upon procedures for evaluation, but large unexplained differences in prevalence clearly exist. The majority of cases occur during adulthood, but sarcoidosis is also present in the pediatric population.

The disease has been reported to be transmissible in experimental animals, but this work still has not been rigorously tested for confirmation. Sarcoidosis is not contagious in humans.

Familial occurrences have been reported in approximately 200 instances, but no specific patterns of parent-child or sibling relationships have emerged. Sarcoidosis has been reported in twins, with a preponderance of monozygotic over dizygotic twins. The disease seems not to be linked with specific human leukocyte antigen (HLA) types.

IMMUNOLOGY

A postulated schema for the immunopathology of sarcoidosis is presented in Figure 69–1. The macrophage most likely initiates the cellular response of sarcoidosis, possibly in response to some unknown presenting antigen. Various factors released by the macrophage, such as interleukin-1, cause accumulation and proliferation of helper T lymphocytes. Factors secreted by the lymphocytes attract and immobilize other inflammatory cells. In addition, B lymphocytes are stimulated to produce increased amounts of immunoglobulins, and fibroblasts are stimulated to proliferate.

As a result of these various immunologic interactions (1) inflammatory cells proliferate in the affected organ (forming the granuloma), (2) cutaneous delayed hypersensitivity responses to common antigens are depressed, and (3) immune globulins are synthesized and circulate in excess. In addition, circulating immune complexes may be present; high levels of serum antibodies to common environmental antigens such as *Mycoplasma pneumoniae* and various viruses frequently occur; antibody responses to immunization may be exaggerated; and circulating rheumatoid factor, antinuclear antibody, and autoantibodies to T lymphocytes may be present.

Intradermally injected extracts of homogenized tissue of involved organs from patients with sarcoidosis are capable of producing a delayed inflammatory reaction in patients with sarcoidosis. This antigen that causes the so-called *Kveim-Siltzbach reaction* has not been purified, and the basis for its response has not been defined. The reaction differs from a cutaneous delayed hypersensitivity reaction in that it takes four to six weeks to develop and then persists for several months.

CLINICAL PRESENTATION

Sarcoid lesions may develop in almost any organ system so that the clinical presentation is quite varied (Fig. 69–2). In fact, "silent" granulomas are frequently present in multiple organs. Most characteristically, the patient is asymptomatic, but the disease is detected by an abnormal chest radiograph, usually showing bilateral symmetric hilar adenopathy often associated with paratracheal adenopathy (Fig. 69–3) and/or reticulonodular parenchymal infiltrates. Patients with sarcoidosis may also present with hilar and paratracheal adenopathy in association with some combination of acute peripheral arthritis, uveitis, and erythema nodosum (the so-called acute sarcoidosis or Loeffgren's syndrome). Except for Loeffgren's syndrome, significant constitutional symptoms other than those of fatigue are unusual in sarcoidosis. When anorexia, weight loss, and fever are present, other diseases should be strongly considered.

Lungs

The lungs are the most frequently involved organ, and pulmonary symptoms, when present, include dyspnea on exertion, nonproductive cough, and wheezing. Dyspnea is usually caused by fibrotic or granulomatous pulmonary parenchymal disease, but it may also result from granulomatous obstruction of upper airways. Granulomas in the nose may cause nasal congestion and in the larynx may result in hoarseness. Hemoptysis is rare in sarcoidosis but may occur from an associated mycetoma in advanced cavitary sarcoidosis. Acute dyspnea secondary to a pneumothorax also occasionally develops in patients with more advanced fibrotic pulmonary disease. Pleural involvement has been reported but is unusual.

Skin

Erythema nodosum may be associated with sarcoidosis as a secondary vasculitic reaction. Sarcoid granulomas also occur directly in the skin to produce a variety of small, asymptomatic

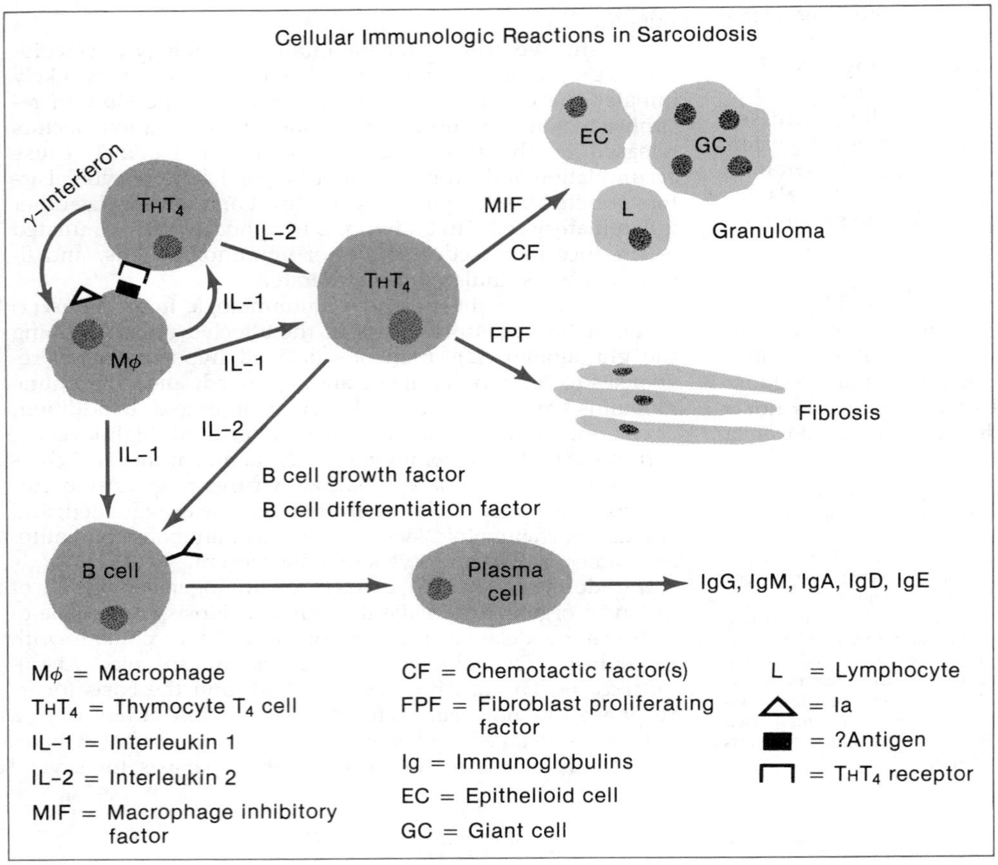

FIGURE 69–1. Immunologic abnormalities associated with sarcoidosis.

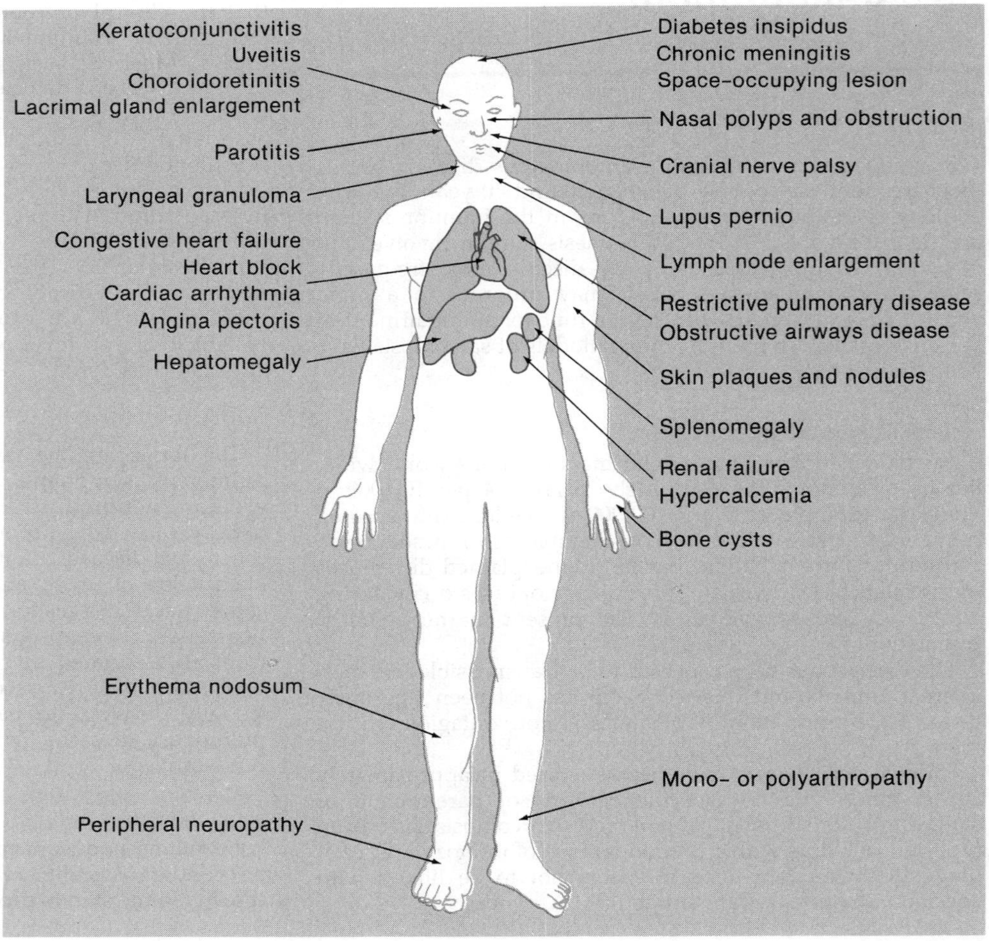

FIGURE 69–2. Organ abnormalities associated with sarcoidosis.

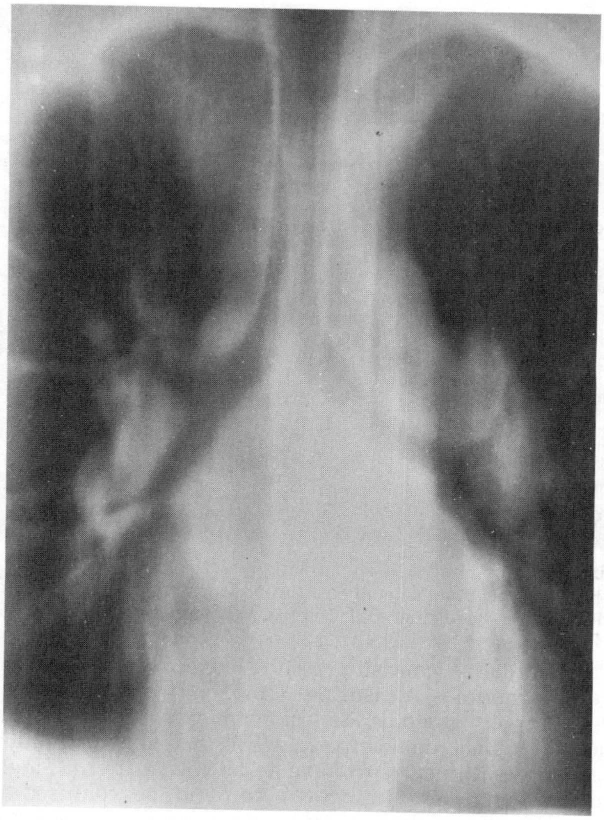

FIGURE 69–3. Tomogram of chest showing hilar and paratracheal adenopathy. (From Murray JF, Nadel J: Textbook of Respiratory Medicine. Philadelphia, WB Saunders Company, 1987.)

macular and papular lesions that are present either superficially or more deeply in the dermis. *Lupus pernio,* consisting of violaceous plaques over the nose, cheeks, and ears, is the most commonly described skin lesion. It may be disfiguring. Granulomas may also occur in scar tissue.

Eyes

Ophthalmologic lesions most commonly consist of inflammation of the uveal tract, but involvement of the conjunctiva, retina, and lacrimal glands may also occur. These lesions may produce nonspecific ocular symptoms of visual impairment and discomfort; chronic lesions may progress to blindness. Anterior uveitis in combination with parotitis and facial nerve palsy has been referred to as *Heerfordt's syndrome.*

Nervous System

Almost any portion of the neurologic system may be involved by sarcoidosis, and the diagnosis may prove difficult. The most common cranial nerve to be involved is the facial nerve, but any cranial nerve may be affected. Disease of the optic nerve may result in papilledema. Palsies of the ninth and tenth cranial nerves manifest as dysphagia, absent gag reflex, and vocal cord paralysis, and disease of the eighth cranial nerve occurs as deafness, tinnitus, and vertigo. Mono- or polyneuropathy of peripheral nerves causes sensory loss, paresthesias, or motor weakness. Meningitis produced by sarcoidosis is usually insidious in presentation and chronic in its course. Diabetes insipidus results from involvement of the hypothalamus or posterior pituitary gland. Granulomas of the brain may produce a space-occupying lesion and cause headaches, seizures, or focal symptoms. Rarely, personality changes have been observed, and the total constellation of findings resulting from multiple areas of involvement of the nervous system by sarcoidosis may bewilder the diagnostician.

Heart

Although cardiac granulomas are often present on autopsies of patients with sarcoidosis, symptomatic cardiac involvement is unusual. Granulomatous or fibrotic cardiac lesions resulting from sarcoidosis may cause congestive heart failure, heart block, arrhythmias (often ventricular), angina pectoris, ventricular aneurysm, recurrent pericardial effusion, or sudden death. Since these abnormalities may also be due to other causes, it may be difficult to prove a relationship to sarcoidosis. Cor pulmonale is an infrequent presentation, occurring usually in association with advanced pulmonary fibrosis, but there has been the rare report of pulmonary hypertension without severe restrictive lung disease.

Kidneys

Granulomas of the kidneys are usually infrequent and asymptomatic. When kidney failure occurs, other lesions such as pyelonephritis, nephrocalcinosis, and hyalinization of various kidney structures are present. The kidneys may be severely and irreversibly damaged by calcium nephropathy caused by altered calcium metabolism that produces hypercalcemia and hypercalciuria. Symptoms of kidney failure may be the predominant feature of sarcoidosis in these cases. Sarcoid lesions can enzymatically activate vitamin D precursors to 1,25-dihydroxycholecalciferol, thereby increasing intestinal absorption of calcium. The result may be hypercalcemia and hypercalciuria, with renal damage from nephrocalcinosis and recurrent nephrolithiasis.

Musculoskeletal System

Bones, joints, and muscles are frequently involved in sarcoidosis. Bone changes are found most commonly in chronic cases and are particularly common in blacks with chronic skin disease. The phalanges, metacarpals, and metatarsals are the bones most frequently involved. Osteoporosis, cystic or reticulated changes, and external manifestations of digital deformation and dystrophic nails may be present. Joints are usually spared destructive changes except in the vicinity of bone lesions.

Arthritic changes may also manifest acutely by mono- or polyarthralgias or arthritis of the larger joints, such as the ankles, knees, wrists, or elbows. The associated symptoms may be migratory and usually recede with no residual deformities. Although, like the liver, muscles frequently contain asymptomatic granulomas, acute myositis or chronic myopathy with associated muscular enzyme abnormalities are uncommon findings in sarcoidosis. Gout may complicate sarcoidosis, presumably owing to overproduction of purines in widespread granulomas.

Miscellaneous

Although diffuse granulomas may be present, clinical manifestations of liver, gastrointestinal, or pancreatic disease are very unusual. Similarly, clinical evidence for involvement of the endocrine and reproductive systems is rare. As noted earlier, posterior pituitary and hypothalamic involvement may result in diabetes insipidus. Hypopituitarism from anterior pituitary disease occurs very rarely and, when present, is associated with diabetes insipidus. Alteration in fertility by sarcoidosis has not been described. Peripheral lymph nodes, in contrast to hilar nodes, are seldom more than moderately enlarged and usually go unnoticed by the patient. Although the spleen is moderately enlarged in 5 to 10 per cent of patients, gross enlargement that causes discomfort and predisposes to rupture occurs rarely. Thrombocytopenia is occasionally present and may be associated with hypersplenism.

PHYSICAL FINDINGS

Physical findings in the chest in sarcoidosis are often normal despite radiographic abnormalities that may be extensive.

Fever is absent, except with Loeffgren's syndrome. Other physical findings usually relate to granulomatous or fibrotic involvement of a specific organ system. Skin lesions may be readily apparent or found only with careful examination. Subcutaneous or muscle nodules may be identified. Slit-lamp examination may be necessary to demonstrate ocular lesions. Lymph nodes are often palpable but usually only moderately enlarged. As noted above, hepatosplenomegaly may be present. Digits may be deformed by bone lesions, and the nails may be dystrophic in cases of chronic disease. Acute arthritic changes may be apparent, in particular in association with erythema nodosum, and must be differentiated from associated gout.

ROUTINE LABORATORY STUDIES

Routine laboratory evaluation may reveal lymphopenia, hyperglobulinemia, hypercalcemia, and/or hypercalciuria. The platelet count is rarely decreased. It is unusual for the sedimentation rate to be significantly elevated, except with Loeffgren's syndrome. Liver function tests may be moderately abnormal, and, in particular, alkaline phosphatase levels may be elevated. With complications of the disease, the expected but nonspecific changes in arterial blood gases and serum chemistries accompany respiratory or renal failure, respectively. Cerebrospinal fluid examination may show nonspecific pleocytosis and increased protein in meningitis caused by sarcoidosis.

DIFFERENTIAL DIAGNOSIS

The differential diagnosis of sarcoidosis depends largely upon the clinical presentation of the patient. With hilar lymphadenopathy, lymphoma is most frequently considered; with pulmonary parenchymal disease, a wide variety of diffuse interstitial diseases must be considered (Ch. 63). Tuberculosis and other granulomatous pulmonary infections must always be ruled out. Eosinophilic granuloma is another diagnostic possibility, particularly when diabetes insipidus is present. Exposure to beryllium may produce disease very similar to sarcoidosis. Pulmonary sarcoid nodules raise the possibilities of primary or metastatic tumor. Conglomerate lesions with hilar retraction or eggshell calcification of lymph nodes may be confused with silicosis. Hypercalcemia in sarcoidosis raises the question of a number of metabolic or malignant disorders, especially primary hyperparathyroidism (Ch. 247). Arthritis or arthralgia associated with sarcoidosis may be confused with acute rheumatic fever or gout. The isolated finding of granulomas on biopsy of various tissues raises the possibilities of foreign body reactions, fungal or tubercular infections, and malignancy associated with granulomatous reactions. Granulomas occurring only in the liver may result in confusion between granulomatous hepatitis and sarcoidosis. The presence of granulomas in the intestinal wall may suggest Crohn's disease. Finally, renal and hepatic impairment or cardiac abnormalities occurring in sarcoidosis may be caused by more common co-existing diseases rather than by sarcoidosis itself.

RADIOLOGIC EVALUATION

Radiologic evaluation of the chest is particularly useful in sarcoidosis, since the disease is so often asymptomatic and so often involves the thorax. Radiologic abnormalities that occur in sarcoidosis have been arbitrarily classified as follows: Grade 0—absence of abnormal radiographic findings; Grade 1—lymph node enlargement without pulmonary parenchymal abnormalities; Grade 2A—combination of lymph node and diffuse pulmonary parenchymal disease; Grade 2B—diffuse parenchymal disease without lymph node enlargement; and Grade 3—radiographic changes indicating more chronic disease with pulmonary fibrosis ("honeycombing" or hilar retraction). The most frequent parenchymal abnormality is reticulonodularity, consisting of fine linear densities and small, irregular nodules measuring 3 to 5 mm in diameter (Fig. 69–4). Large, conglomerate lesions may be present in association with hilar retraction (Fig. 69–5). Parenchymal infiltrates are at times "fluffy" and have an alveolar pattern. Single or multiple large nodules may occur and be confused with tumor. Small nodules may cause a miliary pattern suggestive of tuberculosis.

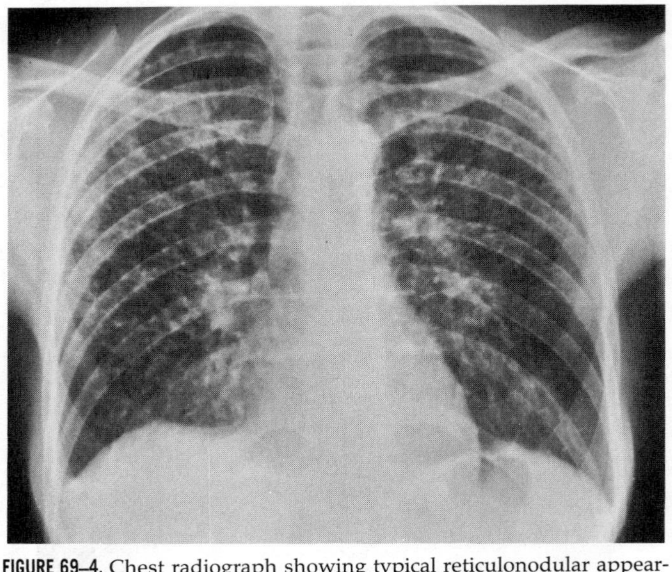

FIGURE 69–4. Chest radiograph showing typical reticulonodular appearance of parenchymal sarcoidosis. (From Murray JF, Nadel J: Textbook of Respiratory Medicine. Philadelphia, WB Saunders Company, 1987.)

A large variety of other changes may be present on the radiograph. Pleural effusion occurs rarely in sarcoidosis. Mediastinal or hilar lymph nodes may show eggshell calcification. In addition to bullous changes, true cavities may be present that, at times, contain mycetomas. Lobar atelectasis may be caused by intrabronchial granulomas, and postobstructive bronchiectasis may be present. In addition to the more common locations in the short tubular bones of the hands and feet, lytic or sclerotic bone lesions may occur in the ribs.

Computed tomographic (CT) scans can demonstrate lymphadenopathy more clearly and, in particular, can detect anterior mediastinal and subcarinal lymph nodes that have gone

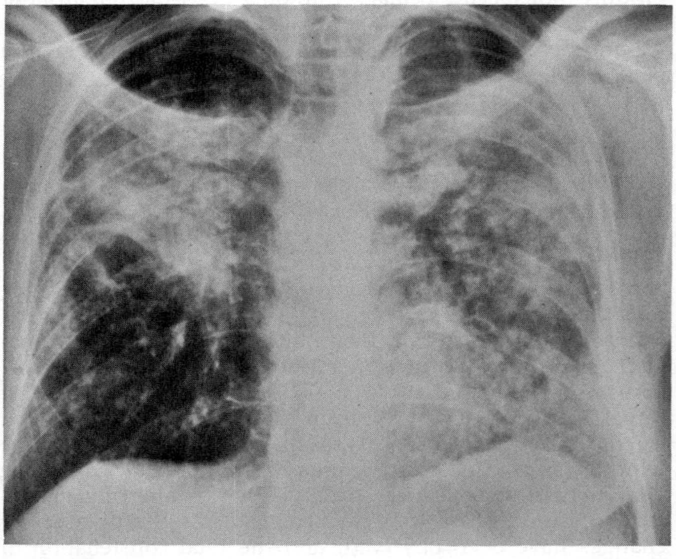

FIGURE 69–5. Chest radiograph showing large conglomerate lesions associated with hilar retraction. (From Murray JF, Nadel J: Textbook of Respiratory Medicine. Philadelphia, WB Saunders Company, 1987.)

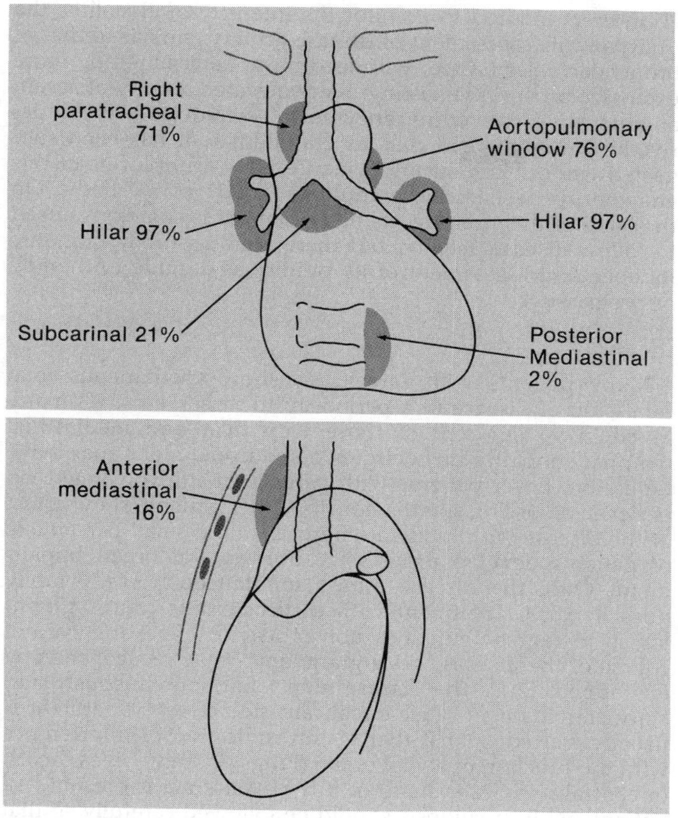

FIGURE 69–6. Schematic representation of CT detection of thoracic lymphadenopathy in sarcoidosis.

undetected on conventional films of the chest (Fig. 69–6). This examination, however, is needed in only a limited number of patients with sarcoidosis.

PHYSIOLOGIC CHANGES

The most common pulmonary physiologic changes occurring in sarcoidosis are decreases in vital capacity and diffusing capacity. Although useful in determining the extent of functional impairment at the onset and in following the course of the disease, physiologic changes do not correlate well with symptoms or radiologic abnormalities. At times pulmonary function studies are totally normal despite radiologic evidence of pulmonary disease. Conversely, functional abnormalities, especially of diffusing capacity, may be present when the lung parenchyma appears normal radiographically. Evidence of airway disease may also be present, and, at times, this is the predominant feature of sarcoidosis, causing confusion with asthma. An elevation in arterial P_{CO_2} is unusual, but moderate arterial hypoxemia may be present. As with other interstitial diseases, arterial hypoxemia often worsens with exercise.

APPROACH TO DIAGNOSIS

With a very typical presentation (i.e., bilateral symmetric hilar and paratracheal lymphadenopathy in an asymptomatic patient 20 to 40 years of age or in one with erythema nodosum, uveitis, and arthralgias), the clinical diagnosis of sarcoidosis can be made with a high degree of certainty by physicians familiar with this disease (Table 69–1). In all other cases in which the diagnosis is less clear, further support must be obtained by examination of biopsy material.

Diagnosis by Biopsy

Typical sarcoid granulomas consist of whorls of epithelioid cells surrounding multinucleated giant cells, which may or may not contain inclusion bodies (Fig. 69–7). Mononuclear

TABLE 69–1. FEATURES CONSIDERED IN THE DIAGNOSIS OF SARCOIDOSIS

Primary
1. Clinical and radiologic presentation
2. Biopsy material showing granuloma, but no mycobacterial, fungi, or refractile material

Secondary
1. Anergy to skin tests
2. Positive Kveim-Siltzbach reaction (infrequently performed)
3. Significant elevation of serum angiotensin I–converting enzyme with exclusion of other obvious diseases associated with elevation (i.e., Gaucher's disease, leprosy, and so on)

Current Research Modalities
1. Evaluation of cells obtained by bronchial lavage
2. Gallium-67 scanning

cells are present at the periphery of the granulomas, and various amounts of fibrosis and/or hyalinization are present throughout the tissue. True caseation does not occur. The histologic appearance, even when typical, is always nonspecific. To strengthen the diagnosis of sarcoidosis, infectious agents and foreign bodies must be excluded by special stains, cultures, and examination under polarized light.

What tissue should be examined by biopsy? In the absence of specific skin lesions, transbronchial biopsy of the lung is usually most specific, since rarely, if ever, will nonspecific granulomas be found (in contrast to liver or lymph nodes). Approximately 60 per cent of patients with sarcoidosis show granulomas on transbronchial lung biopsy even if their chest radiographs are normal; this number increases to 85 to 90 per cent when there is a parenchymal abnormality on chest radiograph. If the transbronchial biopsy yields negative findings but a high suspicion of sarcoidosis exists and there is obvious parenchymal disease on the chest radiograph, a repeat transbronchial biopsy may be justified. Other reasonable approaches at this juncture of evaluation include mediastinoscopy or, at times, open lung biopsy.

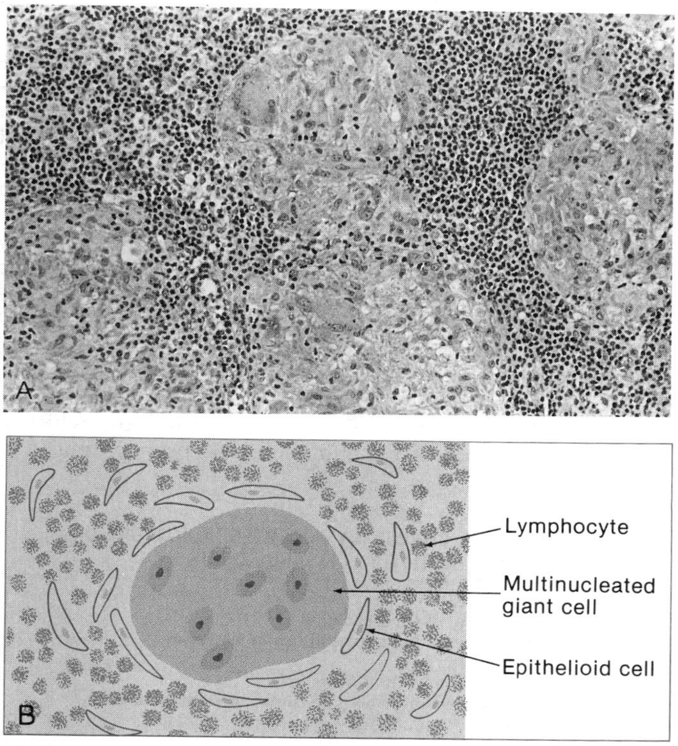

FIGURE 69–7. Typical histologic appearance of granuloma of sarcoidosis with accompanying schematic representation.

Blind conjunctival, lacrimal gland, or gingival biopsies are frequently not rewarding in the absence of overt disease at these locations. When these organs are involved, however, the yield is high. Biopsies of skin lesions are particularly useful, since they may show granuloma and, in association with other findings, may provide an easy diagnosis, if foreign body granuloma can be excluded. Biopsy of identifiable subcutaneous or muscle lesions also may be diagnostic. Biopsy of lesions of erythema nodosum shows a nonspecific panniculitis or vasculitis and therefore is not useful. Other localized lesions, such as those of the pharynx or larynx, require direct biopsy for diagnosis. Diagnosis by biopsy sometimes becomes problematic for neurologic disease caused by sarcoidosis when other tissues do not provide a positive diagnosis, since the involved tissue is often not easily accessible.

Other Available Tests

The Kveim-Siltzbach test lacks precision, and the required antigen is not readily available. It is therefore rarely used. Anergy to delayed hypersensitivity skin test antigens is a frequent finding but is obviously not diagnostic of sarcoidosis. Similarly, characterization of cells obtained by bronchial lavage and the use of gallium-67 scanning of the lungs are not in themselves diagnostic of sarcoidosis, although abnormalities consistent with that diagnosis may be found. For this reason, and because of cost and radiation exposure, these last two tests are not justified currently for diagnosis in clinical practice.

Serum angiotensin I–converting enzyme activity is often elevated in sarcoidosis, but a number of other diseases may be similarly associated with its increased activity (i.e., miliary tuberculosis, leprosy, Gaucher's disease). If these diseases can be readily excluded, measurement of this enzyme may be useful. This is the case when the primary diagnostic considerations are lymphoma and sarcoidosis, since angiotensin I–converting enzyme activity is not increased in lymphoma. Elevations of other proteolytic enzymes in serum, such as lysozyme and thermolysin-like metalloendopeptidase, have been evaluated but are not yet commonly used for diagnostic purposes.

ACTIVITY OF DISEASE

Sarcoidosis may remit spontaneously; the concept of "activity of disease" is therefore useful when considering therapeutic strategies (Table 69–2). "Activity of disease" is very difficult to define, since occult granulomatous lesions may exist throughout many tissues of the body. Clinical findings provide some indication of activity of disease, but often in a nonquantitative and imprecise way, especially when the patient is relatively asymptomatic. Radiologic and pulmonary function study changes also may be helpful in assessing "activity of disease." Bronchoalveolar lavage to measure the percentage of lymphocytes as a reflection of parenchymal inflammation has been advocated. A high percentage of lymphocytes has been referred to as high-intensity alveolitis, denoting a poorer prognosis, but this approach has not gained wide acceptance. Gallium-67 scanning of the lung, which is also thought to reflect inflammation, has been proposed as an indirect method to monitor the intensity of alveolitis; the utility of this assessment of disease activity, similar to that of bronchoalveolar lavage, will need to be determined by more extensive prospective testing. Since elevated activity of serum angiotensin I–converting enzyme in sarcoidosis may be derived from epithelioid cells or granulomas, it has been suggested without convincing evidence that serum levels of this enzyme may reflect the granuloma "load" of the body. On the basis of this premise, its measurement is sometimes used to follow disease activity, but there is no assuredly accurate independent assessment of its validity as a guide to therapy or prognosis.

TABLE 69–2. CURRENTLY ACCEPTED INDICATORS OF "ACTIVITY" OF SARCOIDOSIS

1. Clinical features
2. Worsening of symptoms
3. Worsening of pulmonary function tests/chest radiograph
4. Elevation of serum calcium level
5. Elevation of serum angiotensin I–converting enzyme level?
6. Gallium scanning positivity?
7. Evidence of alveolitis on bronchial lavage?

THERAPY

Many patients with sarcoidosis show spontaneous total remission of disease in a period up to three years. As many as 80 to 90 per cent of those with hilar and mediastinal lymphadenopathy or Loeffgren's syndrome alone may have remission; fewer patients with parenchymal involvement experience remission spontaneously. Other patients show arrest of the disease with moderate fibrosis, and a small percentage of patients develop progressive fibrosis and organ impairment. Once the disease remits spontaneously, only rarely does it recur. Treatment with corticosteroids causes granulomas to regress but does not appear to affect the natural course of the disease, since granulomas may recur if therapy is stopped. Since the disease may remit spontaneously and since steroids may cause significant side effects, treatment is usually started only if there is an indication of interference with the function of a vital organ (lungs, kidneys, eyes, heart, or central nervous system) or if hypercalcemia is present. All patients with sarcoidosis should be followed carefully so that therapy can be started as soon as deterioration of organ function has been detected.

Prednisone is usually the drug of choice for the treatment of sarcoidosis. The usual starting dose is 30 to 40 mg per day, but at times a schedule of 50 to 60 mg every other day is used for initial therapy. A response in terms of symptoms or radiologic findings should be seen within two to four weeks. The steroid dose should be tapered after several weeks, and the eventual maintenance dose should be the lowest one that is effective in maintaining the response that is being followed (see below). Often 10 to 15 mg of prednisone every other day, a dose that has a low risk of side effects, will suffice. Attempts to stop therapy may be tried after several months, but evidence of disease activity (symptoms, chest radiographic abnormalities, or worsening of pulmonary function) may recur, and prednisone may have to be restarted.

What are the best parameters to follow as indicators of disease activity? As noted earlier, measurements of disease activity are imprecise. Certainly, clinical symptoms should be assessed carefully, and chest radiographic and pulmonary function changes often give indication of disease activity. However, both radiographic abnormalities and pulmonary function changes correlate poorly with clinical parameters. Serum angiotensin I–converting enzyme levels are easily obtained and may provide clues to activity, but tests such as bronchial lavage and gallium-67 scanning are still largely experimental. Failure of response may indicate irreversible fibrosis, a situation in which steroid therapy causes more potential risk than benefit.

All of the usual side effects associated with steroid therapy may occur in patients treated for sarcoidosis (Ch. 30). The dose can usually be reduced sufficiently, however, so that infection with opportunistic organisms occurs rarely. Cosmetic problems of weight gain and fluid accumulation are often the most bothersome side effects. More difficult decisions about steroid therapy arise when there are associated disorders, such as diabetes mellitus, that may be exacerbated by these agents. Since tuberculin skin tests will become positive in patients with sarcoidosis who contract tuberculosis, appropriate prophylaxis or treatment should be given when the tuberculin skin test is positive or converts to positivity.

Topical steroids have been used for dermatologic and ophthalmologic lesions, and chloroquine and methotrexate have been used for sarcoidosis of the skin. Indomethacin and other nonsteroidal anti-inflammatory agents may be useful for arthritis occurring in Loeffgren's syndrome. Aerosolized steroids approved for use in the United States have not been effective for pulmonary sarcoidosis, but other aerosolized preparations are being tried in Europe. Sarcoidosis that manifests with bronchoconstriction does not respond well to conventional bronchodilator therapy other than steroids. It remains to be determined whether avoidance of sunlight will significantly influence calcium metabolism in sarcoidosis.

Bascom R, Johns CJ: The natural history and management of sarcoidosis. Adv Intern Med 31:213, 1986. *This is an excellent general review of this controversial area, with 138 references.*

Crystal RG, Roberts WC, Hunninghake GW, et al.: Pulmonary sarcoidosis: A disease characterized and perpetuated by activated lung T-lymphocytes. Ann Intern Med 94:73, 1981. *A good review of immunologic features in sarcoidosis.*

Delaney P: Neurologic manifestations in sarcoidosis, review of the literature with a report of 23 cases. Ann Intern Med 87:336, 1977.

Fanburg BL: Sarcoidosis and Other Granulomatous Diseases of the Lung. New York, Marcel Dekker, 1983. *A comprehensive textbook covering both clinical and experimental aspects of sarcoidosis.*

James DG, Williams WJ: Sarcoidosis and Other Granulomatous Disorders. Philadelphia, W. B. Saunders Company, 1985. *Another good monograph with an extensive review of all phases of sarcoidosis. Excellent clinical descriptions and comprehensive references.*

Roberts WC, McAllister HA Jr, Ferrans VJ: Sarcoidosis of the heart: A clinicopathologic study of 35 necropsy patients (Group I) and review of 78 previously described necropsy patients (Group II). Am J Med 63:86, 1977.

Rockoff SD, Ronatagi PK: Unusual manifestations of thoracic sarcoidosis. Am J Radiol 144:513, 1985. *A comprehensive coverage of radiologic features of sarcoidosis.*

Venet A, Hance AJ, Saltini C, et al.: Enhanced alveolar macrophage-mediated antigen-induced T-lymphocyte proliferation in sarcoidosis. J Clin Invest 75:293, 1985. *Further information about immunologic abnormalities in sarcoidosis.*

70 PULMONARY NEOPLASMS

Charles H. Scoggin

The lung can be involved in a variety of neoplasms (Table 70–1). Bronchogenic carcinoma accounts for over 90 per cent of all lung tumors. The major management questions of lung cancer are the following: Is the tumor resectable? Is the tumor small cell lung cancer? Other tumors may metastasize to the lung. Benign tumors of the lung are infrequent compared with malignant tumors.

BRONCHOGENIC CARCINOMA

Lung cancer, a primary neoplasm arising within the airways, is a frequent and important neoplasm. In the United States it is the leading fatal neoplasm of men and women. In 1985 approximately 135,000 cases of lung cancer were diagnosed in the United States, and approximately 110,000 people died of the cancer. The medical care of patients with lung cancer in the United States is estimated to cost more than $10 billion annually, approximately 1.5 per cent of the national health care expenditure. Lung cancer is strongly associated with the use of tobacco products, particularly with cigarettes. Although surgery or radiation therapy may lead to eradication of tumors in a small number of patients, the majority of people with lung cancer will have advanced disease at the time of diagnosis and will die of the disorder within one year of its detection. Determining the cell type and the stage of the disease is important in the clinical management of lung cancer, since these factors will affect treatment and prognosis. Four types of tumors account for 95 per cent of all lung malignancies: squamous cell (epidermoid), adenocarcinoma (including alveolar cell), large cell (also known as large cell anaplastic), and small cell lung cancer. Small cell lung cancer is distinguished from other types of lung cancer because it often shows a clinical response to chemotherapy.

TABLE 70–1. WORLD HEALTH ORGANIZATION CLASSIFICATION OF LUNG TUMORS

I. Epithelial tumors
  A. Benign
    1. Papillomas (squamous cell and "transitional")
    2. Adenomas (includes pleomorphic and monomorphic)
  B. Dysplasia, carcinoma in situ
  C. Malignant
    1. Squamous cell carcinoma (epidermoid carcinoma)
    2. Small cell carcinoma
    3. Adenocarcinoma (includes acinar, papillary, bronchiolar, alveolar, and solid with mucus formation)
    4. Large cell carcinoma (giant cell and clear cell)
    5. Adenosquamous carcinoma
    6. Carcinoid tumor
    7. Bronchial gland carcinomas (includes adenoid cystic and mucoepidermoid carcinoma)
    8. Others
II. Soft tissue tumors
III. Mesothelial tumors
  A. Benign mesothelioma
  B. Malignant mesothelioma
IV. Miscellaneous tumors
  A. Benign
  B. Malignant
    1. Carcinosarcoma
    2. Pulmonary blastoma
    3. Malignant melanoma
    4. Malignant lymphoma
    5. Others
V. Secondary tumors
VI. Unclassified tumors
VII. Tumor-like lesions
  A. Hamartoma
  B. Lymphoproliferative lesions
  C. Tumorlet
  D. Eosinophilic granuloma
  E. "Sclerosing hemangioma"
  F. Inflammatory pseudotumor
  G. Other

Incidence and Prevalence

No population group is exempt from lung cancer. Lung cancer is the leading cause of cancer-related death of men in 28 developed countries of the world. In 1986 lung cancer surpassed breast cancer as the leading cause of death from cancer in women in the United States. The worldwide incidence of lung cancer is anticipated to continue to increase owing to the spread of the use of cigarettes, particularly in the Third World.

Lung cancer as a major health problem is a phenomenon of the twentieth century. In 1912, only 374 cases of primary lung neoplasms had been reported in the world's medical literature. There is little doubt that the exposure to cigarette smoke and other carcinogens accounts for the rapid increase in the occurrence of lung cancer.

The exact incidence of each type of lung cancer is difficult to determine. Squamous cell carcinoma is thought to be the most frequent form of the tumor (30 to 35 per cent of all cases), followed by adenocarcinoma, large cell carcinoma, and small cell carcinoma. Adenocarcinoma may be the most frequent lung cancer of women currently, but there is evidence that small cell lung cancer may soon surpass it.

Lung cancer occurs principally between the ages of 45 and 75 years. All histologic types of lung cancer in men peak at approximately 70 to 74 years of age. In women adenocarcinoma peaks at an earlier age than in men (50 to 59 years).

Epidemiology

CIGARETTE SMOKING. About 80 to 90 per cent of all cases of lung cancer are caused by smoking cigarettes (see also Ch. 11 and 170). It is estimated that there are 50 million smokers in the United States. Cigarette smoking causes cancer in humans and experimental animals in a dose-dependent manner. Consumption of cigarettes is commonly quantitated as number of packs smoked per day and number of years smoked ("pack years"). A person who has smoked two packs per day for 20 years (40 pack years) has a 60- to 70-fold increased risk of developing lung cancer compared with a person who has never smoked. Because the duration of smoking is strongly associated with risk of lung cancer, the incidence and death rate from lung cancer are highest in the older age groups. Other factors that are important are depth of inhalation and tar and nicotine content of cigarettes.

Decreased smoking of cigarettes is associated epidemiologically with a declining incidence of lung cancer. A reduction in the prevalence of smoking among men in Sweden, Australia, Canada, and the United States has resulted in a reduction or slowing of deaths from lung cancer in men. A lag phase of about 20 years exists between an increase in cigarette smoking in a particular population and a rise in deaths from lung cancer. This lag is reflected in the current rise in deaths, from lung cancer among women of the United States, among whom there was an increase in cigarette consumption in the 1950's. A similar phenomenon is thought to account for increasing occurrence of lung cancer among Japanese men.

Passive inhalation of cigarette smoke may also be a risk factor for lung cancer. It is estimated that 4700 nonsmoking Americans died in 1985 from bronchogenic cancer due to passive smoking. Sidestream smoke has a higher concentration than mainstream smoke of carcinogens such as nitrosamines, naphthalene, and benzopyrene.

OCCUPATIONAL ASSOCIATIONS. Occupational exposures also increase the incidence of lung cancer: uranium (in miners), haloethers (such as dichloromethyl ether and chloromethyl methyl ether), arsenical fumes, isopropyl oil, nickel, metallic iron, iron oxide, and beryllium. Asbestos exposure in nonsmokers is associated with a four to fivefold increased incidence of lung cancer. Asbestos and radon gas probably act as cocarcinogens with cigarette smoke. Smoking increases the risk of bronchogenic cancer 80- to 90-fold in persons also exposed to asbestos. Radon gas exposure may also occur as an environmental pollutant in heavily insulated homes. As many as 12 per cent of homes in the United States may contain unhealthy levels of radon gas. Chronic inflammation of the lung, such as from interstitial fibrosis and areas of scarring, is associated with the occurrence of adenocarcinoma. Certain genetic determinants, such as levels of aryl hydrocarbon hydroxylase, may also be important.

Pathogenesis

CELL OF ORIGIN. The development of lung cancer is a multistep process. The pulmonary endodermal cell seem to be the common stem cell of origin of all lung cancer cell types. Because it demonstrates certain amine precursor uptake and decarboxylation (APUD) properties, small cell lung cancer has been hypothesized to arise from Kulchitsky's cell. There is no direct evidence to support this hypothesis, however.

CIGARETTE SMOKE. Cigarette smoke contains many carcinogens in both the gaseous and the particulate phases. Nitrosamines and other compounds are thought to be important in the gaseous phase. Carcinogens in the particulate phase include benzopyrene and related polycyclic aromatic hydrocarbons, nitrosonornicotine, polonium, and arsenic. Reduction in particulate factors correlates with decreased incidence of lung cancer. A 20 per cent reduction in risk of lung cancer has been associated with a 50 per cent reduction in tar delivery in cigarettes in the United States, Canada, and other countries.

CELLULAR CHANGES. In the natural history of bronchogenic cancer, bronchial epithelial cells first become cytologically abnormal. At this stage, they are not malignant nor are they invariably predictive of the eventual development of malignancy. The next step is carcinoma in situ, i.e., carcinomatous changes localized above the basement membrane and productive of no symptoms. The next change is epidermal invasion by tumor cells, followed by metastasis of the tumor. In situ tumors are indolent and slow growing. As malignancy progresses, so too does the rapidity of tumor spread.

CELLULAR EVENTS. Three aspects of the cellular events that attend the transformation of normal bronchial epithelial cells to malignant cells are important: (1) damage to cellular deoxyribonucleic acid (DNA); (2) alteration in cellular oncogene expression; and (3) tumor-derived factors that stimulate cellular division.

Cigarette smoke, ionizing radiation, and chemical carcinogens damage cellular DNA, in part through inducing chromosomal deletions and rearrangements and point mutations. The most widely recognized chromosomal abnormality seen in lung cancer is a deletion of genetic material in the 3p14 to 23 region in the malignant, but not the normal, cells of patients with small cell lung cancer. Activation of oncogenes appears to be a common event in bronchogenic carcinoma (Ch. 169). Expression of members of both the *ras* and the *myc* oncogene families has been found in lung tumor cells, in contrast to normal lung cells. Another important factor is the production of so-called autocrine growth factors by lung cancer cells. Cultured small cell lung cancer cells secrete growth factors into their media. This is thought to account for their decreased requirement for serum growth factors. One such factor is bombesin/gastrin–related peptide. These growth factors stimulate cell division constantly. They may be of future clinical importance in that monoclonal antibodies to bombesin/gastrin–related peptide inhibit tumor growth of cells in culture and in experimental animals.

Clinical Manifestations

SYMPTOMS OF LUNG CANCER (Table 70–2). Most patients with lung cancer have some symptoms that cause them to seek medical attention. A typical patient will present with pulmonary complaints such as cough, hemoptysis, and weight loss. Only 5 to 15 per cent of patients are asymptomatic when discovered to have bronchogenic carcinoma.

Some Characteristics of Specific Tumors. *Squamous cell, or epidermoid, carcinoma* usually begins as a central lesion that tends to invade locally. The patient often presents with symptoms referable to the airways, such as cough, dyspnea, or hemoptysis. It may also invade the chest wall, diaphragm, or mediastinum. Unlike other primary lung neoplasms, squamous cell tumors may cavitate.

Adenocarcinoma usually begins as a peripheral lesion. It is more aggressive than squamous cell carcinoma. Symptoms at the time of diagnosis often reflect invasion of lymph nodes, pleura, or the other lung or metastasis to other organs, such as the central nervous system or adrenal glands. *Bronchioloalveolar carcinoma,* a special subtype of adenocarcinoma, usually accounts for no more than 1 to 5 per cent of primary lung neoplasms. Bronchioloalveolar carcinoma often manifests as

TABLE 70–2. CLINICAL MANIFESTATIONS OF LUNG CARCINOMA

1. Due to primary lesions	
Cough	Wheezing
Dyspnea	Weight loss
Hemoptysis	Fever
Sputum	Pneumonia
2. Due to local extension	
Chest pain	Dysphagia
Hoarseness	Pericardial effusion
Superior vena cava syndrome	Pleural effusion
Pancoast's syndrome	Diaphragm paralysis
Horner's syndrome	
3. Extrapulmonary manifestations (see Table 171–1, p 1097)	

a solitary pulmonary nodule (approximately 60 per cent) but may also appear as a localized infiltrate or area of lobar consolidation mimicking infection. *Large cell carcinoma* usually manifests as a bulky peripheral mass.

Small cell lung cancer should be carefully distinguished from non–small cell lung cancer, from which it differs both in biologic features and in clinical manifestations (Table 70–3). Small cell lung cancer commonly begins as a central tumor, but 70 to 90 per cent of patients have disease outside the original hemithorax at the time of detection. Because of its propensity to metastasize and to produce paraneoplastic syndromes, small cell lung cancer is usually symptomatic for three months or less before diagnosis. In contrast, symptoms associated with squamous cell carcinoma appear, on the average, eight months before the diagnosis is made, and up to 25 per cent of patients with adenocarcinoma are asymptomatic at presentation. The severity of symptoms is also an important prognostic factor, particularly in small cell lung cancer. The more severe the tumor symptoms, the worse the prognosis.

Symptoms Referable to the Chest. Most patients with bronchogenic carcinomas present with symptoms referable to the chest, sometimes reflecting the area of lung involved. Central or endobronchial tumors can manifest as dyspnea, cough, hemoptysis, wheezing, or pneumonitis with fever and purulent sputum. Even small tumors may cause a disproportionately high degree of dyspnea. Hemoptysis, a common complaint, is more frequent in non–small cell lung cancer, since small cell lung cancer is often submucosal in location without ulceration into the airway itself. Peripheral tumors may manifest as chest pain due to pleural or chest wall involvement.

Spread to thoracic lymph nodes is common in lung cancer, especially in small cell lung cancer. Regional spread to hilar and mediastinal nodes may cause dysphagia due to esophageal compression, hoarseness because of recurrent laryngeal nerve compression, Horner's syndrome due to sympathetic nerve involvement, and elevation of the hemidiaphragm from phrenic nerve compression. Superior sulcus, or Pancoast's, tumor may involve the brachial plexus, resulting in a C7–T2 neuropathy with pain, numbness, and weakness of the arm.

Cardiac involvement is seen at autopsy in 20 to 25 per cent of patients with small cell lung cancer but less frequently in non–small cell lung cancer. Clinical findings of cardiac involvement are arrhythmias, cardiomegaly, and pericardial effusion with pericardial friction rub. Cardiac tamponade may occur.

Systemic Symptoms. Constitutional symptoms of anorexia, weight loss, and generalized weakness are common in lung cancer. Patients may also have fever without obvious infection.

Tumors that obstruct the superior vena cava cause the superior vena cava syndrome: swelling of the head and neck, breast enlargement, and prominence of the superficial veins of the thorax. Bronchogenic carcinoma, particularly small cell lung cancer, may demonstrate extrathoracic spread to other organ systems. Metastasis to the spinal cord causes spinal cord pain and symptoms of cord compression. Pain may precede weakness and sensory changes by days. Metastasis to the liver may cause pain, chemical dysfunction of the liver, and biliary obstruction. Metastasis to the bone may result in pain or bone marrow invasion.

Paraneoplastic Syndromes. Paraneoplastic syndromes are remote effects of tumor. They are described in detail in Ch. 173, 174, and 175, to which the reader is referred. They lead to metabolic and neuromuscular disturbances unrelated to the primary tumor, metastases, or treatment. Paraneoplastic syndromes may be the first sign of the tumor or of tumor recurrence. They do not necessarily indicate that a tumor has spread. Paraneoplastic syndromes often respond to treatment of the primary tumor. Osteoarthropathy associated with lung cancer is seen in up to 30 per cent of patients with lung cancer but is rare in patients with small cell lung cancer. Manifestations include digital clubbing and painful periosteal inflammation. Periosteal elevation usually involves the long bones. It may be confused with certain forms of arthritis, including rheumatoid arthritis. Endocrinologic manifestations are well recognized in bronchogenic carcinoma. Up to 10 per cent of epidermoid tumors secrete humoral factors resulting in hypercalcemia and hypophosphatemia. Metastasis to the adrenal glands may rarely result in adrenal insufficiency. Other endocrinologic manifestations, most common with small cell lung cancer, include Cushing's syndrome due to production of adrenocorticotropic hormone (ACTH), hyperpigmentation from production of melanocyte-stimulating hormone (MSH), and rarely the "somatostatinoma syndrome," which consists of vomiting, abdominal pain, diarrhea, mild diabetes, and cholelithiasis. Patients with lung cancer develop the syndrome of inappropriate antidiuretic hormone secretion (SIADH) in 10 to 15 per cent of cases (Ch. 173). Neuromyopathic manifestations of lung cancer are rare ($<$ 1 per cent) but may dominate the clinical picture when they occur (Ch. 174). Such manifestations include the Eaton-Lambert syndrome (seen in small cell lung cancer), polymyositis, subacute cerebellar degeneration, spinocerebellar degeneration, and peripheral neuropathies. Nonbacterial (marantic) endocarditis, migratory thrombophebitis (Trousseau's syndrome), and disseminated intravascular coagulation as complications of malignancy are described in Ch. 171.

PHYSICAL FINDINGS OF LUNG CANCER. Physical examination often does not reflect either the presence of lung cancer or the state of the disease. Digital clubbing may be found in up to 12 per cent of patients and gynecomastia in 5 to 7 per cent of patients (the latter most frequently associated with large cell anaplastic cancer). Acanthosis nigricans may be found with adenocarcinoma, and hyperpigmentation of the palms and soles may be seen with squamous cell carci-

TABLE 70–3. COMPARISON BETWEEN NON–SMALL CELL LUNG CANCER AND SMALL CELL LUNG CANCER

	Small Cell Lung Cancer	Non–Small Cell Lung Cancer
Cytopathology	Scant cytoplasm; indistinct nucleoli	Large amount of cytoplasm; prominent nucleoli
Cytogenetics	Deletion 3p14→23	No known specific chromosomal alteration
Biochemistry and Hormone Production	Multiple enzymes and hormones (neuron-specific enolase, creatinine kinase BB, L-dopa decarboxylase, ACTH, bombesin, ADH, somatostatin, MSH)	Ectopic hormone production rare; paraneoplastic syndromes less common than in small cell lung cancer
Clinical Presentation	Hemoptysis rare; most patients symptomatic at presentation; usually metastatic at presentation	Hemoptysis common, symptoms less frequent at time of presentation; dissemination at presentation less common than in small cell carcinoma
Treatment		
Surgery	Seldom, if ever, indicated	Primary hope for cure
Radiation	Limited role; palliation and perhaps prophylaxis of CNS metastasis	Palliation, possible cure
Chemotherapy	Main treatment (up to 80 per cent response)	Effect on survival undetermined

ACTH = adrenocorticotropic hormone; ADH = antidiuretic hormone; MSH = melanocyte-stimulating hormone; CNS = central nervous system.

noma (Ch. 175). Obstruction of the superior vena cava may cause superior vena cava syndrome. Examination of the head may disclose the presence of Horner's syndrome, i.e., a unilaterally constricted pupil, enophthalmos, narrowed palpebral fissure, and loss of sweating on the same side of the face. Endobronchial obstruction may result in a localized wheeze detected during physical examination of the chest. Lobar collapse may result in an area of decreased breath sounds and dullness to percussion. Decreased movement of a hemidiaphragm may occur as a consequence of phrenic nerve compression. Liver metastasis may cause hepatic enlargement or nodularity. Weakness, altered reflexes, and decreased sensation may be found in patients with tumors metastatic to the central nervous system.

Diagnosis of Bronchogenic Carcinoma

The diagnosis of lung cancer requires detecting the tumor, establishing its cell type, and defining the stage of the malignancy. Determining cell type is important because it guides the approach both to staging and to treatment.

THE CHEST RADIOGRAPH. The presence of lung cancer is usually suggested by abnormalities on the chest radiograph. The most frequent finding is a mass in the lung field. Lesions usually cannot be detected if they are < 5 to 6 mm. Tumors occur in the right lung more than in the left (3:2) and in the upper lobes more than in the lower lobes. Secondary manifestations seen on chest radiograph include lobar collapse, pleural effusion, pneumonitis, elevation of the hemidiaphragm, hilar and mediastinal adenopathy, and erosion of ribs or vertebrae due to metastases. Alveolar cell cancer can manifest as a localized infiltrate mimicking pneumonia.

HISTOLOGIC DIAGNOSIS. When lung cancer is suspected, the next step in evaluation after the chest radiograph should be that of obtaining tissue specimens for histologic examination. The diagnostic yield of sputum cytologic evaluation will depend upon the adequacy of the specimen, the expertise of the cytologist, the type of tumor, and the number of specimens examined (three to four specimens are considered adequate). Sputum cytologic study is more likely to be negative in patients with small cell lung cancer than in those with non–small cell lung cancer. A negative sputum study should never be regarded as conclusive evidence for absence of carcinoma.

Bronchoscopy is important both for determining if a tumor is present and for obtaining tissue for histologic diagnosis. The combination of bronchial brushing and forceps biopsy is positive 90 to 93 per cent of the time with tumors located in proximal airways. Bronchial washings are less successful (approximately 80 per cent positive). For lesions than are not proximal enough in the airways for direct visualization, transbronchial biopsy with fluoroscopic guidance may be utilized. Yield of histologic diagnosis is 25 per cent for tumors less than 2 cm in diameter and 65 per cent for larger lesions. Transbronchial needle aspiration can also be employed. Peripheral lesions can be aspirated using a transthoracic needle with guidance by multiplane fluoroscopy or chest computerized tomography (CT). Success rates as high as 95 per cent have been reported. Pneumothorax is the major complication. Contraindications to pulmonary biopsy include pulmonary hypertension, hypoxemia with carbon dioxide retention, and a bleeding diathesis.

If a diagnosis is not established by cytologic study of the sputum, bronchoscopy, or needle biopsy, thoracotomy may be necessary. The decision to undertake thoracotomy should be a reasoned one, weighing the importance to the patient of making the diagnosis against other factors such as age or other complicating illness.

In some circumstances, a histologic diagnosis can be made by biopsy of metastatic sites such as liver, lymph nodes, bone, or bone marrow. When the pleural space is involved with tumor, combined thoracentesis and pleural biopsy will provide a diagnostic yield of up to 90 per cent.

SCREENING STUDIES. Screening studies for early stages of lung cancer, using chest radiographs alone or in combination with sputum cytology, have been proposed for cigarette smokers who are 45 years of age or older. Early detection leads to higher resectability rate and longer survival from time of diagnosis (80 to 85 per cent five-year survival). Mass screening has not been shown to have an overall benefit, however, in decreasing mortality from lung cancer. Yearly sputum studies and chest radiographs may be reasonable in smokers over 45 years, particularly if they have been exposed to cocarcinogens such as asbestos or radon gas. Use of hematoporphyrin derivatives that accumulate in neoplastic tissue and are visible with fluorescent bronchoscopy is being explored as an adjunct to early diagnosis of lung cancer. Carcinoembryonic antigen (CEA), neural peptides, and neurogenic enzymes are not currently useful in detecting lung tumor, its metastases, or its recurrence.

Staging of Lung Cancer

Lung cancers are staged first for location (anatomic staging) and then for the patient's ability to withstand various treatments aimed at curing the tumor or increasing life expectancy (physiologic staging). Staging for non–small cell lung cancer differs from that for small cell lung cancer.

NON–SMALL CELL LUNG CANCER. For non–small cell lung cancer, the first and most important decision is whether or not the tumor is operable. Routine staging to exclude inoperable patients has increased survival of patients undergoing surgical resection of lung cancer. Table 70–4 lists a widely used tumor, node, and metastasis (TNM) system for classifying lung cancer.

Patients with stages I and II are considered candidates for surgical resection. Certain patients with stage III cancer may be candidates for surgery with postoperative irradiation of the mediastinum. Surgical resection of N2 disease is controversial. Detection of mediastinal lymph node involvement with cancer is best determined by mediastinoscopy for tumors in the right hemithorax. Tumor assessment of the left hemithorax requires an anterior exploration (Chamberlain procedure). Transbronchial and percutaneous needle aspiration is sometimes used to evaluate hilar lymph nodes. Size alone cannot be used to judge whether or not mediastinal lymph nodes are involved with metastatic cancer; however, enlarged nodes in the presence of known bronchogenic carcinoma argues strongly for metastatic disease. Computerized tomographic scanning of the chest is useful in excluding the presence of other tumors in the chest. In addition, scanning of the adrenal glands can be useful in determining if adrenal enlargement, possibly due to metastases, is present. Routine bone scan, CT scanning, liver scan, and bone radiographs are not recommended unless physical examination or history suggests that these organs are involved.

SMALL CELL LUNG CANCER. Small cell lung cancer has often metastasized at the time of diagnosis; the TNM system has not proved to be useful. Small cell lung cancer is defined as either limited or extensive (Table 70–5). Limited disease is confined to one hemithorax, with or without involvement of mediastinal lymph nodes. Spread of disease beyond this point is extensive. In addition, performance status is also an important prognostic factor. Survival correlates with degree of symptoms and functional impairment.

Treatment of Bronchogenic Carcinoma

NON–SMALL CELL LUNG CANCER. Both surgery and radiation therapy may benefit patients with non–small cell lung cancer, but chemotherapy remains experimental. Newer modalities such as laser bronchoscopy may lead to sympto-

TABLE 70–4. TNM CLASSIFICATION OF LUNG CANCER

Primary Tumor (T)

TX:	Tumor present as determined by presence of malignant cells in bronchopulmonary secretions, but not radiographically or bronchoscopically visible; no evidence of primary tumor
T0:	No evidence of primary tumor
T1S:	Carcinoma in situ
T1:	Tumor 3 cm or less surrounded by lung or visceral pleura, but without evidence of invasion proximal to lobar bronchus at bronchoscopy
T2:	Tumor more than 3 cm or tumor invading visceral pleura or associated with obstructive pneumonitis or atelectasis; involving less than entire lung; at broncoscopy, proximal extent of visible tumor must be within a lobar bronchus or at least 2.0 cm distal to carina
T3:	Tumor of any size with direct extension into chest wall, diaphragm, or mediastinal pleura or pericardium without involving heart, great vessels, trachea, esophagus, or vertebral body; also includes superior sulcus tumors and tumor in main bronchus within 2 cm of carina but not involving carina
T4:	Tumor of any size invading mediastinum or involving heart, great vessels, trachea, esophagus, vertebral body, or carina or presence of malignant pleural effusion.

Nodal Involvement

N0:	No demonstrable metastasis to regional lymph nodes
N1:	Metastasis to peribronchial or the ipsilateral, or both, hilar lymphnodes, including direct extension
N2:	Metastasis to ipsilateral mediastinal lymph nodes and subcarinal lymph nodes
N3:	Metastasis to contralateral mediastinal lymph nodes, contralateral hilar lymph nodes, ipsilateral or contralateral scalene or supraclavicular lymph nodes

Distant Metastasis (M)

M0:	No (known) distant metastasis
M1:	Distant metastasis present—specify site(s)

Stage Grouping

Occult carcinoma	TX	N0	M0
Stage 0	T1S	Carcinoma in situ	
Stage I	T1	N0	M0
	T2	N0	M0
Stage II	T1	N1	M0
	T2	N1	M0
Stage IIIa	T3	N0	M0
	T3	N1	M0
	T1–3	N2	M0
Stage IIIb	Any T	N3	M0
	T4	Any N	M0
Stage IV	Any T	Any N	M1

matic improvement by relieving endobronchial obstruction and may have a role in the treatment of carcinoma in situ.

Surgery. Surgical resectability of lung cancer is determined in large measure by the extent of lymph node metastasis. Patients with stage I and stage II non–small cell lung cancer (Table 70–4) should be treated with surgical resection aimed at cure. Patients with stage III disease characterized by ipsilateral intranodal mediastinal lymph node involvement may benefit from surgical resection of the primary and involved lymph nodes. Intranodal disease is defined as tumor completely confined within the capsule of the mediastinal lymph nodes. These patients should also receive postoperative mediastinal irradiation. Patients with superior sulcus tumors that have not metastasized to mediastinal lymph nodes or systemically should be treated with preoperative irradiation and en bloc resection. Irradiation is usually given as 3000 rads in ten treatments, followed in three to six weeks by surgical resection. En bloc surgical resection of tumors that have invaded the chest wall, but have not metastasized systemically or to the mediastinal lymph nodes may be of benefit. Surgical resection of both superior sulcus and chest wall tumors is associated with increased surgical mortality compared with other less extensive surgical resections of lung cancer.

TABLE 70–5. TWO-STAGE CLASSIFICATION FOR SMALL CELL LUNG CANCER

Limited Diseases (30%)
1. Primary tumor confined to hemithorax
2. Ipsilateral hilar lymph nodes
3. Ipsilateral and contralateral supraclavicular lymph nodes
4. Ipsilateral and contralateral mediastinal lymph nodes
5. Pleural effusion

Extensive Disease (70%): More advanced than limited
1. Metastasis in the contralateral lung
2. Distant metastasis (brain, bone, liver, etc.)

Limited resection of tumors yields results comparable to more extensive surgical procedures. In general, lobectomy is recommended. Even less extensive procedures, such as lobar segment and wedge resection, are usually reserved for patients with peripheral lesions or limited pulmonary function.

Approximately 40 per cent of patients with non–small cell lung cancer undergo thoracotomy, with an overall five-year survival from 10 to 35 per cent. At the time of thoracotomy, 75 per cent of patients undergo tumor resection with the aim at cure. The overall survival of patients resected for cure varies according to histopathologic type of tumor: squamous cell carcinoma, 37 per cent; adenocarcinoma, 27 per cent; large cell undifferentiated carcinoma, 27 per cent; and bronchoalveolar, 56 per cent. Stage of the tumor is also an important determinant of surgical survival: stage I, 54 per cent; stage II, 35 per cent; and stage III without systemic or mediastinal lymph node metastasis, 19 per cent.

Pulmonary function is another very important factor in the evaluation of patients for surgery. Forced vital capacity greater than 2 liters and a forced expiratory volume in the first second (FEV_1) of greater than 50 per cent of the forced vital capacity predict that a patient can tolerate the consequences of pneumonectomy. Radionuclide scanning has generally replaced differential spirometry as a method of assessing the lung to be resected for its contribution to overall respiration.

Elderly patients should not be excluded from consideration for resection of tumor. The most limiting factor of survival in this age group is not age, but the tumor. Bronchogenic carcinoma is a highly aggressive tumor in the elderly. Average life expectancy of patients with untreated tumor is eight months. This compares with an average life expectancy in the United States of 11.1 and 14.8 years, respectively, for men and women aged 70 years. Elderly patients carefully selected for surgery have a five-year survival of 35 to 42 per cent.

Radiation Therapy. Most non–small cell lung cancers are responsive to radiation treatment. Radiation therapy is indicated in patients with stage III disease without metastases or in stage I or stage II patients who refuse surgical treatment. A consistently small but reproducible group of patients with disease in the chest alone benefit from radiation treatment aimed at cure. Patients with operable lung cancer may have a five-year survival rate with radiation therapy alone of up to 21 per cent. Treatment is generally 5500 to 6000 rads by either split course or continuous fraction irradiation. Acute esophagitis is a common complication. Patients receiving irradiation of a lung for cure of cancer may develop radiation pneumonitis; therefore, patients must have pulmonary function equivalent to that necessary to tolerate pneumonectomy.

Most tumors will respond to irradiation by decreasing in size; however, treatment of patients with nonresectable non–small cell lung cancer with irradiation has been disappointing in prolonging survival.

Postoperative mediastinal irradiation is recommended in patients who have undergone resection and who have intranodal lymph node involvement, but preoperative and postoperative adjuvant radiotherapy for T2 and T3 tumors has not been shown to be beneficial and may even be detrimental. The single exception appears to be superior sulcus, or Pancoast's, tumor.

TREATMENT OF PATIENTS WITH DISSEMINATED NON–SMALL CELL LUNG CARCINOMA. Seventy per cent of patients with non–small cell lung cancer have unresectable disease at the time of diagnosis or thoracotomy. In such patients, irradiation and other forms of palliative treatment are very important.

Radiation. Irradiation effectively decreases tumor size to reduce endobronchial obstruction and to re-expand the atelectatic lung. Important intrathoracic complications may respond to irradiation: the superior vena cava syndrome, 80 to 90 per cent; hemoptysis, 84 per cent; cough 60 per cent; and atelectasis, 23 per cent. Radiation therapy may also palliate bone pain and cerebral metastases.

Chemotherapy. A response rate of 30 to 40 per cent in non–small cell lung cancer has been achieved with cisplatin regimens, especially in combination with etoposide (VP-16) and/or mitomycin-C. This should not be regarded as routine therapy. Substantive improvement in symptoms and survival remains to be proved. Potential benefit to the patient must be weighed against chemotherapy-induced side effects. The effectiveness of combined modalities such as chemotherapy plus radiotherapy or chemotherapy plus surgery is still unproved.

SMALL CELL LUNG CANCER. The median survival of untreated small cell lung cancer from the time of diagnosis is 2.8 months. Less than 1 per cent of untreated patients will survive five years. The treatments of choice for small cell lung cancer are chemotherapy and radiation. Surgical resection has little, if any, role, because at the time of detection the tumor has usually spread beyond the limits of surgical removal. For example, the mean survival with radiotherapy alone (284 days) is statistically greater than the mean survival with surgical treatment (199 days), although it remains very low.

Chemotherapy. Small cell lung cancer is highly responsive to chemotherapy. Moderately intensive therapy with three agents is usually given initially in an attempt to eradicate the tumor. The use of additional drugs beyond three is associated with a disproportionate increase in side effects compared with benefit. Examples of currently employed regimens are cyclophosphamide, methotrexate, and lomustine (CCNU); cyclophosphamide, doxorubicin, and vincristine; and cyclophosphamide, doxorubicin, and etoposide (VP-16). These regimens appear to be approximately equal in producing responses and long-term survival. Objective responses usually occur within 6 to 12 weeks after initiation of treatment. The effective length of treatment is yet to be established. Most protocols involve treatment for 12 months or less. Alternating non–cross-resistant combinations of drugs and using intensive therapy with autologous bone marrow transplantation have not been shown to increase survival. Combined modalities of irradiation and chemotherapy may be of use in limited disease, although this is yet to be conclusively proved.

Most chemotherapy regimens produce a greater than 80 per cent response rate in all patients. Complete response, defined as absence of any evidence of residual tumor, is seen in greater than 50 per cent of patients with limited disease and 20 per cent of patients with extensive disease. This results in a median survival of about 14 months in patients with limited disease and 7 months in patients with extensive disease. Twelve to 15 per cent patients with limited disease will survive 6 to 11 years.

Aggressive chemotherapy produces complications and symptoms in all patients. All experience anemia and leukopenia. Opportunistic infection is an important complication. Approximately 60 per cent of neutropenic patients experience febrile episodes. Herpes zoster occurs in 8 to 12 per cent of patients with small cell lung cancer treated with chemotherapy. Other complications include nausea, vomiting, alopecia, hemorrhagic cystitis, mucositis, electrolyte imbalance, possible cardiotoxicity, and peripheral neuropathy. A long-term complication of chemotherapy for small cell lung cancer is a secondary malignancy: leukemia, lymphoma, and other neoplasms. Risk appears to increase with intensity of drug dosage and the number of drugs utilized. Finally, patients successfully treated for small cell carcinoma are still at risk for non–small cell carcinoma.

Radiation Therapy. Radiation therapy is of proven benefit in controlling bone pain, spinal cord compression, superior vena cava syndrome, and bronchial obstruction. More than 90 per cent of patients have been reported to have palliation of symptoms due to brain metastases. The use of radiation therapy in combination with chemotherapy is controversial and should be reserved for experimental studies.

Prophylactic Cranial Irradiation. Although chemotherapy has increased the survival of patients with small cell lung cancer, this survival has been accompanied by an increased risk of relapse in the central nervous system. The cumulative risk of central nervous system metastases at two years may be as high as 80 per cent. This risk is reduced to about 3 to 12 per cent with the use of prophylactic cranial irradiation. Unfortunately, this decreased rate of brain metastasis is not associated with increased survival. Prophylactic cranial irradiation is generally reserved for patients who have achieved a complete response to chemotherapy, but even in these patients the benefit in terms of increased survival is slight. In all other patients cranial irradiation should be used when central nervous system metastases are diagnosed. Most patients who survive long term exhibit memory loss, confusion, ataxia, loss of vision, and dysphonia. This encephalopathy is probably a complication of cranial irradiation with a possible contribution by chemotherapy as well.

OTHER CONSIDERATIONS IN THE TREATMENT OF LUNG CANCER. *Bone Metastasis.* Metastasis of lung cancer to bone most frequently cause pain, but pathologic fracture may also occur. Bone involvement is best detected by bone scan, although large lesions will be visible radiographically. Pain can usually be palliated by radiation to the involved areas.

Hypercalcemia. Hypercalcemia is one of the most important complications of lung cancer. Serum calcium values in excess of 12 mg per deciliter are considered life threatening. Treatment is aimed at lowering the serum calcium level. Treatment of hypercalcemia is discussed in detail in Ch. 247.

Central Nervous System Metastasis. Metastases from lung cancer to the central nervous system usually cause symptoms in proportion to their size and location. Corticosteroids are effective in relieving acute symptoms of increased intracranial pressure in about 75 per cent of patients. Doses of 8 to 12 mg of dexamethasone should be acutely administered. Osmotic agents given to reduce intracranial pressure, such as a 20 per cent solution of mannitol intravenously, may be useful in treating cerebral herniation. Acute control of increased pressure should be followed by radiation therapy.

Pleural Effusion. Malignant pleural effusion frequently complicates bronchogenic carcinoma. It is exudative in nature. The diagnosis is made by cytologic examination of the fluid and by pleural biopsy. Effusions complicated by dyspnea or pain should be drained. If the fluid recurs, obliteration of the potential pleural space should be accomplished by introducing a sclerosing agent. This is best performed by insertion of a chest tube to drain the effusion completely, followed by the instillation of 1 gram of tetracycline dissolved in 100 ml of normal saline and 50 ml of 1 per cent Xylocaine into the chest through the tube. The tube should then be clamped and the patient turned into different positions to distribute the sclerosing fluid along the pleural surface. The tube is then allowed to drain until the amount of fluid over a 12- to 14-hour period is 100 ml or less. Malignant pleural effusions with pH less than 7.0 are associated with a very poor prognosis.

Weakness and Weight Loss. Weight loss, muscle weakness, and difficulty in eating are frequent and distressing manifestations of lung cancer. The pathophysiology of weight loss in lung cancer is poorly understood but can be partially explained by altered carbohydrate and protein metabolism and the release of toxic factors into the circulation. The use of aggressive nutritional support in lung cancer patients in whom traditional forms of treatment have been ineffective is of limited value and may even be adverse.

Cough and Dyspnea. Reversible causes of cough and dyspnea, such as bronchospasm, bronchitis, and pneumonitis, should be excluded. The mainstays of cough control are narcotic cough suppressants. Narcotics and tranquilizers used in low dosages may produce remarkable relief of severe dyspnea. When clearance of large airway secretions becomes difficult, patients may "rattle" when they breathe (so-called "death rattle"). This is particularly distressing to family members. In patients who are terminally ill, scopolamine, 0.4 to 0.6 mg subcutaneously every four hours as necessary, will tend to dry up secretions and relax the smooth muscle of the airways. It is preferred to atropine, since the former is a central nervous system depressant, in contrast to atropine, which is a stimulant.

Pain. The therapeutic goal of managing pain, the most common symptom of advanced lung cancer, should be not only its relief but also its prevention. Narcotics should be taken every four hours around the clock to prevent the patient from awakening with pain. There is no single optimal dosage schedule for narcotics. Most patients have their pain controlled with 30 mg of morphine, or its equivalent, given orally on a four-hour basis. Patients, families, and those caring for the patient should be counseled that tolerance and addiction do not present a real clinical problem in patients with advanced lung cancer. The most common adverse side effects of narcotic treatment are constipation and nausea, which must preferably be prevented, but treated aggressively if they appear.

Patients who have been treated for lung cancer with apparent success continue at risk for a second primary lung cancer, or "metachronous" tumor. Such tumors can be of identical or different histologic pattern from the first primary tumor. Metachronous tumors occur in 1 to 3 per cent of patients with lung cancer. Treatment is determined by the same factors that affect other primary lung tumors, however, the physiologic impact of treatment of the first primary cancer may limit surgical resection or radiation dosage.

Filderman AE, Shaw C, Matthay RA: Lung cancer part 1: Etiology, pathology, natural manifestations, and diagnostic techniques. Invest Radiol 21:80, 1986. *Particularly good for summarization of roentgenographic manifestations of primary pulmonary malignancies.*

Ginsberg RJ, Feld RJ (eds.): IV World Conference on Lung Cancer. Chest 89:314S, 1986. *Comprehensive summaries of epidemologic, diagnostic, and therapeutic aspects of lung cancer.*

Greco FA, Johnson DH, Hainsworth JD, et al.: Chemotherapy of small-cell lung cancer. Semin Oncol 12:31, 1985. *Summarizes current approaches to treatment of small cell lung cancer.*

Iannuzzi MJ, Scoggin CH: Small cell lung cancer: state of the art. Am Rev Respir Dis 134:593, 1986. *Focuses on clinical and investigational aspects of small cell lung cancer.*

Klastersky J, Sculier JP: Chemotherapy of non–small-cell lung cancer. Semin Oncol 12:38, 1985. *Specific discussion of issue of use of chemotherapy for treatment of non–small cell lung cancer. Contains information relevant to the decision on whether to offer treatment beyond surgery and radiotherapy.*

Marini N, McCormack P: Therapy of stage III (non-metastatic) lung cancer. Semin Oncol 10:95, 1983. *Reviews treatment of superior sulcus (Pancoast's) tumor.*

Peh SB Jr, Wernly JA, Aki BF: Lung cancer—current concepts and controversies. West J Med 145:52, 1986. *This medical progress article considers a variety of controversial methods and alternatives for management of patients with lung cancer, including classification, staging, radiotherapy, chemotherapy, and palliation.*

Risk NW: Selection of patients with non–small-cell lung carcinoma for surgical resection. West J Med 143:636, 1985. *Review of criteria for determining which patients should and should not receive consideration for surgical resection.*

Whang-Peng J, Bunn PA, Kao-Shan CS, et al.: A nonrandom chromosomal abnormality, del 3p(14–23), in human small cell lung cancer (SCLC). Cancer Genet Cytogenet 6:119, 1982. *Description of a chromosomal abnormality found in small cell lung cancer.*

Woolner LB, Fontana RS, Cortese DA, et al.: Roentgenographically occult lung cancer: Pathologic findings and frequency of multicentricity during a 10 year period. Mayo Clin Proc 54:453, 1984. *Details of the problem of occurrence of new primary tumor in patients treated for lung cancer.*

OTHER MALIGNANCIES OF THE LUNG

Carcinoid Tumors

These tumors, sometimes termed "bronchial adenomas," are in fact distinct entities with different clinical courses and histologic manifestations. Three types are recognized: bronchial carcinoids, cylindromas, and mucoepidermoid tumors. Tumors may manifest with endobronchial obstruction or hemoptysis. Carcinoid tumors, including bronchial carcinoids, are considered in Ch. 243.

Scheithauer BW, Carpenter PC, Block B, et al.: Ectopic secretion of a growth hormone–releasing factor: Report of a case of acromegaly with bronchial carcinoid tumor. Am J Med 76:605, 1984. *Reviews different extrapulmonary manifestations of bronchial carcinoid tumors.*

Primary Lymphoma of the Lung

Hodgkin's disease and non-Hodgkin's lymphoma are discussed in Ch. 158 and 160. Such lymphoma may arise in the lymph nodes of the chest or within the lung itself. Patients with tumor involving the lung may present with weight loss, fever, cough, or pleuritic chest pain. Pleural effusion may be an initial or complicating manifestation.

Non-Hodgkin's tumors arising within the parenchyma of the lung are often discrete masses with or without hilar and mediastinal lymph node enlargement. An intrathoracic Hodgkin's tumor mass may cavitate or compress the bronchial tree to cause atelectasis or postobstructive pneumonitis. A common differential diagnosis of hilar adenopathy is that between lymphoma and sarcoidosis (Ch. 69). Enlargement of anterior mediastinal lymph nodes suggests lymphoma, as this is an unusual region of lymphadenopathy in sarcoidosis.

Other lymphoproliferative disorders that involve the lung are pseudolymphoma and lymphocytic interstitial pneumonitis. Pseudolymphoma appears as a nodular lesion, whereas lymphocytic interstitial pneumonitis manifests as a diffuse infiltrate. The diagnosis is made by histologic examination of lung biopsy specimen. Distinguishing between benign disease and true pulmonary lymphoma may be difficult. Some patients who initially present with an apparently benign lymphoproliferative disorder later develop malignant lymphoma. The development of hilar or mediastinal lymphadenopathy suggests the presence of malignancy.

The diagnosis of lymphoproliferative disorders of the lung depends upon histologic examination of tissue obtained by bronchoscopy, transbronchial biopsy, mediastinoscopy, or thoracotomy.

The treatment of Hodgkin's and non-Hodgkin's lymphomas of the lung is by the use of radiation or chemotherapy as would be employed for nonpulmonary lymphoma (Ch. 158 and 160). Pseudolymphoma can be removed by surgical resection. No established treatment for lymphocytic interstitial pneumonitis exists, although chemotherapy has been attempted.

Colby TV, Carrington CB: Pulmonary lymphomas: Current concepts. Pathol Annu 14:884, 1983. *Presents criteria for and classification of pulmonary lymphoid lesions.*

Uncommon Primary Lung Malignancies

Cylindromas are the second most common tumors of the trachea and bronchi. (The most common tumors are bronchogenic carcinomas.) The tumors arise from the mucous glands of the bronchial epithelium. The most common symptoms are airway obstruction and cough. Men and women are equally affected, and the age of occurrence ranges from 30 to 65 years. The diagnosis is made by bronchoscopy and biopsy. Treatment is by surgical resection, although cure may be difficult owing to the tumor's propensity to metastasize.

Mucoepidermoid tumors also arise from the bronchial mucous glands and usually manifest in persons between the ages of

40 and 55. The diagnosis is made by the bronchoscopic finding of a polypoid endobronchial mass, followed by biopsy. Treatment is by surgical resection, with a better prognosis than with cylindroma. *Carcinosarcoma*, an unusual tumor, contains both malignant epithelial elements and sarcomatous changes. It may occur as a peripheral mass or as an endobronchial lesion. Treatment is by surgical resection. *Pulmonary blastomas*, which usually occur in the periphery of the lung, are thought to arise from mesoderm. Treatment is by surgical resection, but the prognosis is poor.

Primary sarcomas of the lung, which are very rare, include fibrosarcomas, leiomyosarcomas, hemangiopericytomas, and osteosarcomas. Treatment is by surgical resection. More recently, Kaposi's sarcoma has been recognized as a cause of pulmonary disease in patients with the acquired immunodeficiency syndrome (AIDS). It may be difficult to distinguish from infection. The diagnosis requires lung biopsy.

Olnibene FP, Steis RG, Macher AM, et al.: Kaposi's sarcoma causing pulmonary infiltrates and respiratory failure in the acquired immunodeficiency syndrome. Ann Intern Med 102:471, 1985. *Description of 66 patients with acquired immunodeficiency syndrome and 30 episodes of pulmonary Kaposi's sarcoma.*

Tumors Metastatic to the Lung

The lung may be involved from both hematogenous and lymphatic spread of carcinomas and sarcomas. Patients are often asymptomatic; however, metastatic lesions may cause dyspnea, cough, and chest pain. Diffuse hematogenous tumor spread may cause vascular obstruction manifested by corpulmonale with hilar enlargement and clear lung parenchyma.

The radiographic appearance of pulmonary metastases may give some clue to the primary tumor. Solitary nodules are usually associated with cancers from breast, colon, kidney, rectum, cervix, and melanoma. These tumors may also diffusely involve the lung, leading to multiple large nodules or micronodules. In addition, a micronodular pattern is also seen with tumors from the thyroid, trophoblastic tissue, or bone sarcomas. Large, well-defined pulmonary nodules, sometimes with associated hilar enlargement, occur with testicular germinal cell tumors.

Tumors that spread lymphatically include carcinomas from the stomach, pancreas, thyroid, larynx, and lung. These tumors may spread to lung lymphatics through hilar lymph nodes or from involvement of parenchymal lymphatics due to hematogenous metastases. Enlargement of lung lymphatics is radiographically visible as linear shadows similar to Kerley's lines.

Pleural involvement may appear as a pleural-based mass or as pleural effusion. Metastatic lesions, particularly synovial cell tumors and other bone tumors, may lead to pneumothorax. Certain metastatic lesions may cavitate: metastatic sarcomas, carcinomas of the colon, and epidermoid carcinomas of the head, neck, and the female reproductive system. Osteogenic sarcomas or chondrosarcomas display calcification in metastatic lesions.

The diagnosis of metastatic lesion is confirmed by histologic examination of tissue obtained by sputum cytology, fiberoptic bronchoscopy, or occasionally thoracotomy. Cytologic findings are positive in as many as 50 per cent of patients. Bronchoscopy and needle biopsy have similar success rates. Decisions on aggressiveness in seeking confirmation by tissue study of suspected metastatic lesions must be made thoughtfully. The risk to the patient must be weighed against the question of how the confirmation of metastasis will alter the management of the patient.

Treatment will usually be based upon management of the primary neoplasm. Certain metastatic lesions should be considered for surgical resection, especially those arising from osteogenic sarcomas. On occasion, resection of a solitary metastasis from other primary sources has been reported to be associated with increased survival, but usually without any controlled study. In considering surgical resection of a metastasis, the following criteria should be met: (1) absence of other metastatic lesions within the lung on CT, (2) no evidence of metastasis involving other organs, and (3) sufficient physiologic reserve to tolerate a more extensive resection if simple wedge resection is deemed inadequate. In general, this means that criteria used for determining tolerance of surgical resection of primary lung cancer should be applied when contemplating resection of metastatic lesions.

In summary, surgical resection of pulmonary metastasis should be considered when the primary tumor is under control, the patient is a good surgical risk, other approaches to treatment are unsatisfactory, and all of the tumor can be resected.

Beattie EJ: Surgical treatment of pulmonary metastases. Cancer 54:2729, 1984. *Brief review of metastatic lesions to the lung that may be appropriate for multiple surgical resections.*

Mountain CF, McMurtrey MJ, Hermes KE: Surgery for pulmonary metastasis: A 20-year experience. Ann Thorac Surg 38:323, 1984. *Report of results of the M.D. Anderson Hospital and Tumor Institute with surgical resection in 443 patients with various tumors metastatic to the lung.*

BENIGN NEOPLASMS OF THE LUNG

Benign neoplasms of the lung are uncommon. They may occur as solitary nodules within lung parenchyma or as endobronchial lesions. Symptoms are nonspecific and include cough, dyspnea, chest pain, and pneumonia.

HAMARTOMAS. Hamartomas, the most common benign tumors of the lung, are usually diagnosed in adults. The tumors consist of unorganized elements such as fat, fibrous tissue, epithelial tissue, cartilage, and calcification. Calcification leads to the "popcorn" radiographic appearance of the tumor. The majority of hamartomas occur as solitary nodules within lung parenchyma, but about 10 per cent are endobronchial. Hamartomas should be removed because of the potential complications of hemorrhage and bronchial obstruction resulting in atelectasis and pneumonia.

PAPILLOMAS. Papillomas, which arise form the trachea and bronchi, are most commonly found in children. They may be diffuse, leading to repeated pneumonias, bronchiectasis, atelectasis, and chronic infection. Because of diffuse involvement, management may be difficult and may require repeated bronchoscopy for attempt at removal of these tumors. Malignant changes may also occur.

Uncommon benign tumors of the lung include granular cell myoblastomas, lipomas, fibromas, leiomyomas, chondromas, and hemangiomas. They usually first appear as masses radiographically. Complications are similar to those of other benign neoplasms. Surgical removal is the usual treatment.

Arrignoni MG, Woolner LB, Bernatz PE, et al.: Benign tumors of the lung: A ten-year surgical experience. J Thorac Cardiovasc Surg 60:589, 1970. *Excellent review of 130 patients with benign tumors of the lung. Includes clinical, radiographic, and pathologic features.*

SOLITARY PULMONARY NODULE

A solitary pulmonary nodule is a single lesion, regardless of size, surrounded by lung parenchyma on at least two thirds of its circumference, not touching the hilum or mediastinum, and without associated atelectasis or pleural effusion. Important etiologies of solitary pulmonary nodules include neoplasia, infection, and collagen vascular disease. Because of wide varieties of cause and differing treatments, determining the etiology is very important (Table 70–6).

Etiology

Both benign and malignant tumors may manifest as a solitary pulmonary nodule. Approximately 40 per cent of solitary pulmonary nodules are malignant, and of these 85 to 90 per cent are bronchogenic carcinoma. Bronchogenic carcinomas that are detected as solitary nodules have a much more favorable prognosis (24 per cent five-year survival) than those with more complicated presentations (5 to 8 per cent

TABLE 70–6. ETIOLOGIES OF SOLITARY PULMONARY NODULES

1. Primary lung malignancies	
2. Metastatic malignancies to the lung	
3. Benign tumors or tumor-like conditions	
Hamartoma	Pseudolymphoma
Herniation of omentum	Herniation of liver
Hemangioma	
4. Pulmonary infections	
Fungal	Mycobacterial
Bacterial	Hydatid cyst
5. Foreign body pneumonitis	
Lipid pneumonia	Amyloidosis
Pneumoconiosis	Aspiration pneumonia
Talc granulomas	
6. Pulmonary vascular disorders	
Pulmonary infarct	Pulmonary hemosiderosis
Pulmonary hemorrhage	

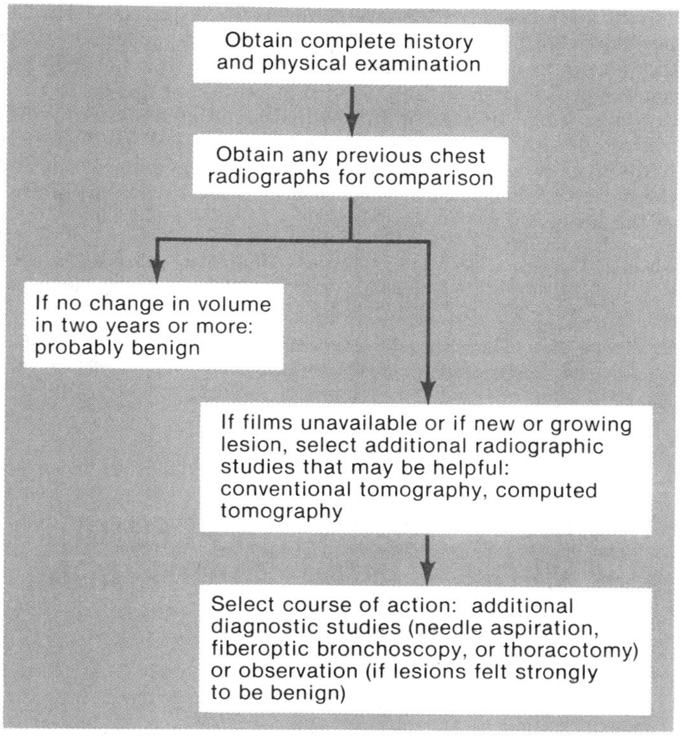

Obtain complete history and physical examination
Obtain any previous chest radiographs for comparison
If no change in volume in two years or more: probably benign
If films unavailable or if new or growing lesion, select additional radiographic studies that may be helpful: conventional tomography, computed tomography
Select course of action: additional diagnostic studies (needle aspiration, fiberoptic bronchoscopy, or thoracotomy) or observation (if lesions felt strongly to be benign)

FIGURE 70–1. Approach to the patient with a solitary pulmonary nodule.

five-year survival). Patients detected with solitary nodules at stage I of bronchogenic carcinoma have been reported to have almost a 50 per cent five-year survival. Most benign hamartomas appear as solitary pulmonary nodules. Three to 10 per cent of solitary pulmonary nodules are due to malignancies metastatic to the lung from other organs, especially from renal cell carcinoma, Wilm's tumor, Ewing's sarcoma, choriocarcinoma, bladder carcinoma, rhabdomyosarcoma, osteosarcoma, melanoma, and carcinomas of the breast, colon, testis, head, and neck.

The most common infection that presents as solitary nodules is that caused by *Coccidioides immitis*. Echinococcal cysts also may appear as a single nodule, as may the lesions of *Histoplasma capsulatum* and *Blastomyces dermatitidis*. Tuberculosis rarely manifests as a solitary pulmonary nodule.

Certain collagen vascular disorders may present as pulmonary nodules, especially rheumatoid arthritis and Wegener's granulomatosis. Although usually multiple lesions occur, occasionally only a single nodule may be seen. Unusual causes of solitary nodules are pulmonary infarcts and vascular malformations.

Evaluation

The sequence of the approach to a patient with a solitary pulmonary nodule is outlined in Figure 70–1. Evaluation of patients with solitary pulmonary nodules begins with a thorough history and physical examination. Travel to an area endemic for fungal disease such as coccidioidomycosis suggests, but does not prove, this etiology. Weight loss and other constitutional symptoms are consistent with malignancy, although early stages may be asymptomatic. Joint changes may suggest rheumatoid nodules. Age is also an important consideration. Primary lung cancer is uncommon in patients who have never smoked and who are below the age of 30 years. Patients over the age of 50 years with new solitary nodules, particularly if they have smoked, have an increased incidence of malignancy. Geography is also important. Fungal disease is a more common etiology in persons who reside or have recently visited the American Southwest, whereas malignancy is a more common cause of solitary nodules in individuals living in areas nonendemic for fungal infections such as coccidioidomycosis.

An important step in the evaluation of a solitary pulmonary nodule is a comparison of its radiographic appearance with that of a previous film. A lesion that has not enlarged in two or more years suggests a benign etiology. On the other hand, if the nodule is new or if there has been progressive enlargement, malignancy or infection is much more likely. Most malignant solitary nodules have a volume doubling time of 60 to 150 days with a mean of 120 days. In spherical lesions, an increase in diameter of 26 per cent equates to one doubling in volume. Calcification within the node is usually a sign of a benign lesion. Patterns of calcification seen with benign lesions are a dense central nidus of calcium, a concentric or laminated pattern, a diffuse pattern, or a clustered or "popcorn" pattern. Small amounts of calcium may be seen within 1 to 3 per cent of bronchogenic carcinomas or osteosarcomas metastatic to the lung. Computerized tomography has two important roles in evaluating solitary pulmonary nodules. First, imaging and densitometry can be helpful in detecting calcification. Tomograms of the lung may also serve this purpose. Second, other nodules not seen with standard anteroposterior and lateral chest radiographs may be detected on CT. The use of CT densitometry to identify malignancy by low density numbers remains experimental.

If a previous radiograph is not available, or if an enlarging lesion is suspected, the ultimate determination of etiology of a solitary nodule is dependent upon either culture confirmation of infection or histologic examination. A lesion can be considered benign only if a specific diagnosis is obtained. Sputum for tuberculosis should be obtained only if tuberculosis is highly suspected. Cytologic findings in sputum are positive in only 10 per cent or less of patients with endobronchially invisible bronchogenic carcinomas and 20 per cent of patients with malignancies metastatic to the lungs.

Once the etiology of a solitary nodule is ascertained, treatment will depend upon cause. When a lesion is not obviously benign, percutaneous transthoracic needle aspiration, fiberoptic bronchoscopy, or thoracotomy is indicated. Needle aspiration biopsy yields a specific diagnosis in 85 to 90 per cent of cases. It is helpful to establish a diagnosis of malignancy in patients in whom surgery is not contemplated but in whom a specific diagnosis will help guide management. Fiberoptic bronchoscopy with transbronchial biopsy and bronchial brushing has the advantage over needle aspiration because it is useful in staging lung cancer and has a lower complication rate. Success in obtaining a diagnosis is dependent upon the size of the nodule. Solitary pulmonary nodules less than 2 cm in size or within 2 cm of the hilum are difficult to diagnose with bronchoscopy. Thoracotomy is the most direct means of establishing a diagnosis. It also offers the best chance for cure of lung cancer. The possibility of small cell lung cancer is not necessarily a reason for avoiding thoracotomy. Surgical resection of small cell lung cancer presenting as a solitary pulmonary nodule may have a five-year survival comparable to that with other forms of nodular bronchogenic carcinoma treated with surgical resection (approximately 24 per cent). Indications for thoracotomy include suspicion that the lesion is malignant and resectable and the absence of major surgical risk factors. Contraindications are severe underlying lung disease or heart disease. Mediastinoscopy is indicated only if the chest radiograph shows mediastinal widening, if the solitary nodule is greater than 3 cm in diameter, or if the nodule is centrally located near the hilum of the lung.

Khouri, NF, Melziane MA, Zerhouni EA, et al.: The solitary pulmonary nodule: Assessment, diagnosis and management. Chest 91:128, 1987. *Practical review of clinical approach to solitary nodules, particularly in light of procedures other than thoracotomy.*

Stauffer JL: What to do when you detect a solitary pulmonary nodule. J Respir Dis 7:17, 1986. *Excellent summary of management of solitary pulmonary nodule based upon etiologic considerations and the yield of particular diagnostic approaches. Practical and rational.*

71 DISEASES OF THE PLEURA, MEDIASTINUM, DIAPHRAGM, AND CHEST WALL

Jerome S. Brody

THE PLEURA

ANATOMY AND PHYSIOLOGY. The pleura is composed of a single layer of mesothelial cells supported by a sparse network of connective tissue, vessels, and lymphatics. The parietal pleura covers the surface of the chest wall, diaphragm, and mediastinum, from which it separates with ease. It receives its blood supply from the systemic circulation and contains sensory nerve endings. The visceral pleura covers and adheres to the entire surface of both lungs. It receives its blood supply from the low-pressure pulmonary circulation and contains no sensory nerve fibers. Either pleural surface can be the site of a primary disease process; pleural disease, however, is most often an extension of, or a reflection of, disease that arises elsewhere.

The visceral and parietal pleural surfaces are separated by a potential space that is filled with 10 to 30 ml of fluid, which spreads out in a layer several angstroms thick. This serous fluid has a protein concentration of less than 2 grams per deciliter and a pH and glucose concentration similar to those of blood. The fluid in the pleural space turns over at a rate of 35 to 75 per cent per hour in a fashion dependent in part on Starling forces similar to those governing interstitial fluid exchange. Hydrostatic pressures are systemic in the parietal pleura (30 cm H_2O), pulmonary in the visceral pleura (10 cm H_2O), and subatmospheric in the pleural space itself (–5 cm H_2O at end expiration in normals). Colloid oncotic pressure results in pressure gradients of 25 cm H_2O from pleural space to each pleural surface. The net result of these forces is an inflow pressure gradient of 5 to 10 cm H_2O from parietal pleura to pleural space and an outflow pressure gradient of 5 to 10 cm H_2O from pleural space to visceral pleura. Augmenting this outflow pressure gradient are factors other than Starling forces such as pulmonary lymphatic flow, the relatively greater vascular bed in the visceral pleura, and the increased number of microvilli on visceral pleura mesothelial cells, all of which favor movement of fluid out of the pleural space.

The major forces involved in pleural fluid movement can help explain why fluid may accumulate in the pleural space. Excess hydrostatic forces or decreased oncotic pressures produce filtrates across intact capillary walls and result in protein-poor transudates. Breakdown of the normal formation-resorption mechanism because of damage to pleural capillaries (e.g., produced by inflammation) or blocking of lymphatics results in protein-rich exudates.

DIAGNOSTIC PROCEDURES. ***History and Physical Examination.*** Pleural pain and dyspnea are the symptoms most frequently associated with pleural disease, although considerable pleural disease can occur in the absence of symptoms. Pleural pain is usually unilateral, arising from irritation or inflammation of the parietal rather than visceral pleura. Because nerve fibers of the parietal pleura are derived from intercostal nerves, the pain may be referred to the abdomen, neck, or shoulder. Pleuritic pain is usually unilateral, sharp, and accentuated by deep breathing, coughing, or movement of the chest cage. The patient may find relief by splinting the area of involvement. Pleural pain often disappears once pleural effusion develops.

A collection of pleural fluid may produce respiratory dysfunction by compressing normal lung tissue and creating ventilation-perfusion mismatches, or by flattening the diaphragm and placing it at a mechanical disadvantage. These effects produce dyspnea in patients with otherwise normal lung function but may precipitate respiratory failure in patients with underlying lung disease.

The physical examination in pleural disease varies considerably, depending on the nature of the accompanying lung or systemic disease. Patients usually have rapid, shallow respirations, impaired chest wall motion (splinting), intercostal tenderness, and decreased breath sounds over the affected area. A pleural friction rub is the characteristic physical sign, but it is often entirely absent or audible for only 24 to 48 hours after the onset of the pain. Impaired percussion note, absent tactile fremitus, decreased or absent breath sounds, and E to A change of the spoken voice (egobronchophony) at the upper border of the fluid are frequent signs of pleural effusion.

Radiologic Examination. Up to 300 ml of pleural fluid may fail to be seen on the posteroanterior chest film. However, as little as 150 ml can be seen in a lateral decubitus film. Early signs of fluid accumulation include blunting and medial displacement of the normally sharp costophrenic angle and widening of the shadow between the gas-containing stomach and lower margin of the left lung. Larger volumes of fluid track up the pleural space, outlining the pleural fissures and producing a concave shadow with its highest margin along the pleural surface. Large amounts of pleural fluid may accumulate in the area between the lung base and diaphragm (subpulmonic effusion), producing the radiologic appearance of an elevated hemidiaphragm. In patients with small or subpulmonic effusions, bilateral decubitus roentgenograms will often reveal the presence of free pleural fluid and allow visualization of underlying lung tissue. Collections of pleural air and fluid (hydro-, pyo-, or hemopneumothorax) usually produce horizontal rather than concave areas of fluid. Loculated pockets of pleural fluid, pleural-based tumors, and parenchymal disease are often difficult to localize and define anatomically. Ultrasonic studies and computed tomography have provided more precise anatomic definition of pleural and contiguous parenchymal abnormalities.

Thoracentesis. Removal of pleural fluid serves both diagnostic and therapeutic functions. Diagnostic thoracentesis should be performed when the cause of the effusion is uncertain. Therapeutic thoracentesis should be performed when the effusion is producing symptoms or when infection is present within the pleural space. The patient is usually placed in a sitting position; the area of fluid is defined by physical examination; and, using sterile techniques, the fluid is removed. Diagnostic thoracentesis requires relatively small amounts of material, which may be obtained through a small-gauge needle. Therapeutic thoracentesis usually involves removing large amounts of fluid. However, no more than 1000 to 1500 ml of fluid should be removed at one time, since re-expansion pulmonary edema may occur as the fluid compressing the underlying lung is removed. Although pleural fluid can be classified as either transudative or exudative, the difference between transudate and exudate is relative and serves only to suggest likely categories of disease.

Transudates (Table 71–1) are defined by (1) a total protein content less than 3.0 grams per deciliter (or with a pleural fluid to serum protein ratio of less than 0.5) and (2) a lactic dehydrogenase (LDH) level of less than 200 units per milliliter (or a pleural to serum LDH level of less than 0.6). Such fluids usually have white blood cell counts less than 1000 per cubic millimeter. Transudates are usually seen in congestive heart failure or hypoalbuminemia, or with movement of peritoneal fluid into the pleural space.

Exudates (Table 71–2) exist if any one of the above criteria does not hold. They are most frequently produced by infection or malignancy. As there is overlap in these categories, white cell counts and differentials, acid-fast and Gram's stains, aerobic and anaerobic cultures, and cytologic analysis of fluid should be included in all studies of pleural fluid. A predominance of polymorphonuclear leukocytes is most compatible with bacterial infection, while a predominance of lymphocytes, particularly with a paucity of mesothelial cells, suggests tuberculosis. Lymphomas and lymphatic leukemias producing pleural disease also produce lymphocytic effusions. Pleural fluid eosinophilia is a nonspecific finding usually associated with effusions of long duration. Blood-tinged (serosanguineous) fluid may be produced by as few as 5000 red blood cells per cubic millimeter. Malignancy, trauma, and pulmonary infarction are the most frequent causes of bloody pleural effusion, although congestive heart failure and infection can produce serosanguineous effusions. Substantial amounts of pleural fluid with a high hematocrit (>10 per cent) nearly always indicate trauma, a neoplasm that has bled into the pleural space, or a vascular abnormality. A variety of special diagnostic studies can be performed on pleural fluid, and these studies will be mentioned under discussion of specific disease entities.

Pleural Biopsy. Needle biopsy of the pleura with a hook type needle (Cope or Abrams needle) is indicated in exudative effusions when the diagnosis is uncertain. Pleural biopsy provides a specific tissue diagnosis most frequently in tuberculosis and malignancy. Histologic examination with acid-fast stains and culture of pleural tissue add significantly to the diagnostic evaluation of tuberculous effusions. In each instance, pleural implants may be patchy so that diagnostic yield increases with repeat biopsies. Biopsy is usually reserved for those patients who have sufficient pleural fluid to separate safely visceral and parietal pleura. In patients with small or loculated effusions, localization of the fluid with ultrasound can increase the yield and safety of pleural biopsy.

Exploration of the Pleura. In 5 to 10 per cent of cases, a diagnosis cannot be established on the initial evaluation. In most instances, if one waits, either the effusion will not recur or its cause will become evident. The alternative approach, surgical exploration of the pleura, will usually provide the diagnosis. However, even in some of these patients the diagnosis will not be established. In most of these cases the effusion will not recur, although in 25 per cent the cause will prove to be a malignancy. An alternative to surgery is exploration of the pleura through a thoracoscope inserted percutaneously under general anesthesia. Experience with this approach has been limited in this country.

TABLE 71–1. CHARACTERISTICS OF PLEURAL FLUID TRANSUDATES

	Absolute Value	Pleural Fluid: Serum Ratio
Protein	<3.0 grams/dl	<0.5
Glucose	>60 mg/dl	1.0
WBC*	<1000	—
LDH*	<200 IU/liter	<0.6

*WBC = White blood cells; LDH = lactic dehydrogenase.

TABLE 71–2. EVALUATION OF PLEURAL FLUID EXUDATES

Test	Disease(s)
pH (<7.20)	Infection, malignancy, rheumatoid arthritis, esophageal rupture
Glucose (<60 mg/dl)	Infection, malignancy, rheumatoid arthritis
Amylase (>200 units/dl)	Pancreatic disease, malignancy, esophageal rupture
Rheumatoid factor, ANA,* LE* cells	Collagen vascular disease
Complement (decreased)	Lupus erythematosus, rheumatoid arthritis
Biopsy (+)	Malignancy, tuberculosis
RBC* (>5000/μl)	Pulmonary embolus, malignancy, trauma
Chylous effusion (triglycerides >110 mg/dl)	Trauma, malignancy

*ANA = Antinuclear antibodies; LE = lupus erythematosus; RBC = red blood cells.

PLEURAL INFLAMMATION AND EFFUSION. ***Pleural Transudates (Simple Hydrothorax).*** The most common cause of pleural transudates is congestive heart failure. Left ventricular failure increases hydrostatic pressure in visceral pleural vessels, thereby diminishing reabsorption. Right ventricular failure increases parietal pleural and central venous pressures, thereby increasing transudation and decreasing lymphatic reabsorption. Pleural effusions are often a manifestation of biventricular failure. Pleural effusion resulting from cardiac disease is most often bilateral and usually larger on the right side. If unilateral, right-sided effusions are most frequent. On rare occasions, effusions are localized within fissures, simulating lung masses that vanish as congestive heart failure regresses (phantom tumors). Chronic effusions from cardiac causes may increase their protein concentration such that the fluid may appear exudative. Hypoalbuminemia of any cause may produce transudative pleural effusions; these are usually bilateral and associated with fluid accumulation elsewhere in the body. Intra-abdominal disease may also produce large transudative hydrothoraces. Pleural effusions occur in 5 to 10 per cent of patients with cirrhosis of the liver. In these patients, ascites is usually evident, but massive effusions may appear with little or no demonstrable ascites. In this setting, peritoneal fluid appears to traverse the diaphragm either through lymphatics or through minor channels between muscle fibers in the diaphragm. The effusions are usually right sided but may be bilateral or left sided. A similar mechanism is thought to be responsible for all the pleural fluid that appears following peritoneal dialysis.

Tuberculosis. Localized tuberculosis of the pleura occurs in most patients with pulmonary tuberculosis but is usually clinically inapparent. Pleural tuberculosis may be the first manifestation of primary infection, producing a febrile illness with serous fluid and often no evidence of parenchymal disease. The effusion in this setting results from hypersensitivity to tubercular protein in pleural tubercles. The acute illness usually subsides, even if untreated, although a few such patients develop progressive primary tuberculosis. The purified protein derivative is usually positive, but skin test conversion may not yet have occurred. Patients with pleural manifestations of primary infection have a high risk of future disease, as two thirds develop clinically apparent tuberculosis within the succeeding five years. A second form of pleural tuberculosis occurs when parenchymal disease, usually reinfection tuberculosis, extends into the pleural space, producing a tuberculous empyema. Diagnosis in this case is relatively simple, since the patient will have a positive tuberculin skin test, evidence of parenchymal disease, and often positive sputum smears. Pleural fluid is exudative and usually reveals lymphocytosis; occasionally a predominance of polymorphonuclear leukocytes may be found initially. Acid-fast bacilli are rarely seen in pleural fluid, but histologic examination for granulomas and culture of material obtained at biopsy, together with culture of pleural fluid, yield the diagnosis in 80 to 90 per cent of cases. When uncertain, the pleural biopsy and purified protein derivative skin test should be repeated and the patient treated for tuberculosis until culture results are available. Treatment of all types of pleural tuberculosis is with standard antibiotic regimens (see Ch. 302), although tube drainage of tuberculous empyema may be necessary.

Pleural Effusions with Pneumonia. Inflammation of adjacent pleura occurs in most patients with pneumonia whatever the cause. The extent of pleural inflammation in bacterial pneumonia varies widely. There may be minor inflammation producing pleural pain with no clinically detectable fluid, exudative effusions containing inflammatory cells but no bacteria (parapneumonic or sympathetic effusion), or large collections of purulent fluid containing numerous bacteria (empyema). Antibiotics are usually sufficient for treating parapneumonic effusions, with thoracentesis being reserved for diagnosis or for relieving dyspnea.

Empyema tends to occur in bacterial diseases associated with tissue necrosis, e.g., infections with anaerobes, staphylococci, and gram-negative organisms. Gram's stains and aerobic and anaerobic cultures of pleural fluid are mandatory, although Gram's stains of sputum and the clinical picture are often the best initial means of identifying the infecting organism. Empyema fluid should be completely removed either by one to three thoracenteses, using a large-bore venous catheter, or by closed tube drainage. Appropriate systemic antibiotics are also required. Since bacteria are not always seen on Gram's stain, thick purulent fluid with more than 100,000 cells per cubic millimeter or fluid with pH values less than or equal to 7.20 should be treated as a presumptive empyema with drainage. In some instances, placement of the tube or catheter will require ultrasound or computed tomography to locate loculated effusions. Occasionally an empyema will be associated with air in the pleural space resulting from tissue necrosis, infection with a gas-forming organism, or communication of the bronchial tree with the pleural space (bronchopleural fistula). Tube drainage and adequate antibiotic coverage will result in closure of most such fistulas. Untreated, however, they can communicate with skin (bronchopleurocutaneous fistula) and require surgical therapy (open drainage with rib resection, decortication, myoplasty involving insertion of flaps of skin or intercostal muscles into the empyema space, or occasionally thoracoplasty). Surgery, however, should be postponed until prolonged drainage and antibiotic therapy have failed.

Pleural involvement by nonbacterial, nontuberculous infections is uncommon. Viral and mycoplasmal pneumonias rarely produce pleural symptoms. Fungal disease is also not characterized by pleural disease except in coccidioidomycosis, in which a hypersensitivity pleuritis over frank empyema can occur.

Pulmonary Embolus and Infarction. Pulmonary embolus frequently produces pleural disease, with more than half of patients having detectable effusions. These effusions are usually exudates, which often contain blood, although occasionally transudates may be found. Unless repeated embolization occurs, the effusion disappears with time and requires no treatment. Pulmonary embolus is discussed in detail in Ch. 67.

Hemothorax. Frank blood in the pleural space (pleural fluid hematocrit greater than 25 per cent of peripheral blood hematocrit) may be associated with either blunt or penetrating chest trauma, but may also result from spontaneous pneumothorax, hematologic disorders, and pleural malignancies. Left-sided hemothorax, particularly when associated with a widened superior mediastinum, may indicate dissection or rupture of the aorta. Pleural blood often does not clot and can be removed by thoracentesis. Small amounts of blood are readily reabsorbed via the lymphatics, but large collections should be removed by tube drainage. Persistent pleural bleeding requires surgical intervention.

Chylothorax. The leakage of thoracic duct lymph or chyle into the pleural space is most frequently due to *trauma* but may be due to *granulomatous disease* or to invasion of the thoracic duct by *tumor*. Lymphomas are most commonly implicated, although mediastinal involvement from any carcinoma can produce a chylothorax. The symptoms of chylothorax are those of the underlying lesion unless the chylothorax is large enough to produce pulmonary symptoms. Since chyle collects within the posterior mediastinum following trauma, the chylothorax does not appear until the mediastinal pleura ruptures, often days after the trauma. The chylous fluid is a milky exudate and, if allowed to stand, a creamy layer forms on top. The lipid content of the fluid is high, as manifested microscopically by sudanophilic fat droplets and a high concentration of neutral fat and fatty acids. Cholesterol content is low, and the fluid contains few cells. Initial therapy is conservative with repeated thoracenteses or tube drainage. Most cases involving trauma require surgical intervention and ligation of the thoracic duct at the site of the rupture. Radiation therapy may be of benefit in some cases when chylothorax is due to malignancy. *Pseudochylothorax* or cholesterol effusion, a milky effusion with high cholesterol and low neutral lipid and fatty acid content, is seen in patients who have longstanding pleural effusions and is often associated with large numbers of degenerating leukocytes and the presence of cholesterol crystals. Treatment is usually not required, but occasionally pleural decortication may be indicated.

Miscellaneous Disorders. *Systemic lupus erythematosus* (SLE) and *rheumatoid arthritis* are frequently associated with pleuritis and pleural effusion. Pleural abnormalities may be the first manifestation of each of these diseases, but most often pleural changes occur after the diagnosis has been established.

SLE may have pleural involvement in over 70 per cent of patients. Sometimes transient episodes of pleuritic pain are the only manifestation, but pleural effusions are seen in up to 50 per cent of cases. They may be the only radiographic abnormality, or there may be associated nonspecific parenchymal infiltrates. The effusions are usually exudates containing varying numbers of leukocytes. Lower than normal concentrations of hemolytic complement and its C3 and C4 components are present, and classic LE cells may be found in the fluid.

Rheumatoid arthritis may result in pleural effusions in approximately 5 per cent of patients. The effusion may be associated with rheumatoid lung disease, but most often it occurs in the absence of other pulmonary changes. The effusions are exudates, often with a predominance of lymphocytes, often have a low pH, and usually contain extremely low concentrations of glucose (less than 15 mg per deciliter and in some cases less than 5 mg per deciliter). Rheumatoid factor may be present, but this is a nonspecific finding. Pleural biopsy may reveal typical rheumatoid nodules, and occasionally palisades of histiocytes, similar to those in rheumatoid nodules, appear in the fluid. In contrast to SLE effusions, rheumatoid pleural effusions may persist for weeks or months and may require repeated thoracenteses.

Subdiaphragmatic abscess resulting from hepatic disease, gastrointestinal perforations, or prior surgery may be associated with pleuritic chest pain, fever, and abdominal findings. Elevation of a hemidiaphragm on the affected side and impaired diaphragmatic motion are characteristic. Exudative pleural effusions, occasionally containing bacteria, and basilar pneumonias are frequent. Treatment includes surgical drainage of the abscess and antibiotics.

Pancreatitis or *pancreatic pseudocysts* may be associated with pleural effusions, most often on the left side, although a significant number are bilateral. Effusions usually are not large. They are exudates, may be blood tinged, and contain levels of amylase that exceed those in serum. Effusions may be due to irritation and inflammation of the diaphragmatic pleura, extension of fluid through diaphragmatic lymphatics, or actual communication of a pseudocyst with the pleural space. The effusion will subside with treatment of the pancreatic problem. Acute pancreatitis may also be a cause of the adult respiratory distress syndrome (ARDS).

Meigs' syndrome is the association of ascites, benign fibroma or other ovarian tumors, and frequently massive and recurrent pleural effusions. The effusion is usually a transudate but may be exudative or serosanguineous. Removal of the tumor relieves the ascites and effusion. The mechanism for the formation of pleural and peritoneal fluid has not been completely explained. The diagnosis should be considered in women with pleural effusion of obscure origin, especially if there is evidence of concurrent ascites and pelvic disease.

Uremia is associated with a polyserositis, which may include the pleural space. The effusions are exudates and often contain varying amounts of blood. At least half the effusions are asymptomatic. Effusions resolve with treatment of the uremia, but repeated thoracenteses may be necessary to control symptoms.

Asbestosis is frequently associated with pleural disease (see Ch. 536). Asbestos is the main cause of pleural plaques, which often appear along diaphragmatic and pericardial pleura. These plaques often calcify 20 to 40 years after exposure and bear no direct relation to amount of asbestos exposure. They cause no functional impairment and do not lead to mesotheliomas. Pleural fibrosis is seen in 10 to 20 per cent of asbestos workers. It is usually bilateral, is not associated with interstitial fibrosis, and may in rare instances lead to functional impairment. Pleural effusion from asbestos is often bilateral, may be recurrent, is an exudate, and is often serosanguineous. There is no direct relation between duration or intensity of exposure and pleural effusions. In contrast to other complications of asbestosis, the latency for pleural effusions is less than 20 years from the initial exposure. Other rare causes of pleural effusions are sarcoidosis, myxedema, hypersensitivity reactions, hepatitis, and amebiasis.

NEOPLASMS OF THE PLEURA. ***Metastatic Tumors.*** Involvement of pleura by malignancies arising elsewhere is common. In middle and older age groups, metastatic disease (through either pleural implants or mediastinal lymphatic obstruction) accounts for 30 to 40 per cent of pleural effusions. Carcinomas of the lung and breast are the neoplasms that most commonly involve the pleura, although virtually any neoplasm may be implicated. Involvement of pleura is considered a sign of inoperability in bronchogenic carcinomas other than superior sulcus tumors. Malignant pleural fluid is usually exudative and may contain blood. Pleural fluid cytology is positive in 20 to 25 per cent of cases, and pleural biopsy provides a diagnosis of malignancy in an additional 25 to 40 per cent of cases. The course of malignant pleural effusions usually involves reaccumulation of fluid despite repeated thoracenteses. Under such circumstances, treatment is aimed at obliterating the pleural space with tube drainage or with one of a number of irritating substances. Intrapleural tetracycline is the present drug of choice, since it produces pleural symphysis in the majority of cases with no systemic and few local side effects. For best results, 1000 mg of the drug is introduced through a chest tube, is left in the pleural space for 24 hours, and then is drained as the pleural surfaces are approximated by suction applied to the tube.

Mesothelioma. Mesothelioma, the main primary pleural tumor, may be benign or malignant. Benign mesotheliomas are rare, have the histologic appearance of a fibroma, and generally present as localized tumor masses. They usually arise from visceral pleura and may reach a rather large size, compressing normal lung and thereby causing symptoms. Parietal pleural lesions may be pedunculated. In either case, benign mesotheliomas appear on roentgenogram as smooth lobulated masses along the pleural surface. Hypertrophic pulmonary osteoarthropathy and clubbing are particularly common in patients with benign mesothelioma. Treatment involves surgical removal. Malignant mesotheliomas are related to asbestos exposure in 80 to 90 per cent of cases, although the dose relationship is a weak one. Smoking is not a factor. These tumors are diffuse and infiltrate the pleura widely, often completely encasing the lung. Symptoms of cough, chest pain, and dyspnea are frequent late in the disease, as are bloody pleural effusions. Although the diagnosis of a malignancy is made readily by the demonstration of malignant cells either in pleural fluid or from a pleural biopsy, distinguishing mesothelioma pathologically from metastatic disease on small tissue samples can be difficult. Prognosis is poor, with median survivals on the order of one year. Surgery is not possible, and radiation and chemotherapy have been largely unsuccessful to date.

Pneumothorax. A pneumothorax is an accumulation of gas within the pleural space. Gas may appear in the pleural space as a result of (1) perforation of the visceral pleura and entry of gas from the lung; (2) penetration of the chest wall, diaphragm, mediastinum, or esophagus; or (3) gas generated by microorganisms in an empyema. Spontaneous rupture of pleura and entry of air from the lung may occur in the absence of known disease (simple pneumothorax) or may occur as a result of parenchymal lung disease (secondary pneumothorax).

Simple spontaneous pneumothorax occurs most commonly in previously healthy men 20 to 40 years of age and is due to rupture of subpleural blebs that appear at the apex of the lung. The cause of these blebs and their predominance in men is not known. The right side is more frequently involved than the left, and recurrence is frequent (30 per cent on the same side, 10 per cent on the opposite side). The clinical presentation involves sudden onset of chest pain with dyspnea appearing in proportion to the size of the pneumothorax. The precipitating event is usually not clear, although some occur during vigorous effort, particularly with rapid large swings in intrathoracic pressure. The pneumothorax may vary in size from minor, being visible only on an expiratory film, to 100 per cent of the hemithorax being filled with air producing collapse of the lung. Small amounts of pleural fluid are present in 25 per cent of simple pneumothoraces. Tension pneumothorax (produced by increasing positive pressures in the hemithorax through a "ball-valve" air leak) is rare but can shift the mediastinum and compromise circulation. Treatment of a simple pneumothorax depends on its size. Small pneumothoraces occupying less than 25 per cent of the hemithorax in asymptomatic individuals can be treated on an outpatient basis without removing the air, since they will reabsorb over a period of seven to ten days. Larger pneumothoraces may be treated by removing air through a small catheter, and pneumothoraces of over 50 per cent or those associated with lung collapse should be treated with a chest tube initially connected to suction and, once the lung is expanded, placed under water seal drainage. The tube should be left in place for two to four days. For recurrent simple pneumothoraces, surgical obliteration of the apical pleural space (scarification, abrasion, or even decortication in certain circumstances) should be undertaken at the time of the second or third episode. Tension pneumothorax requires immediate decompression of the involved side with insertion of a large-bore needle through an intercostal space.

Secondary or *complicated pneumothorax* occurs as a result of trauma or as a result of some other pulmonary disease. Widespread emphysema is the most common pulmonary process producing secondary pneumothorax. Pneumothorax may complicate pulmonary infection by rupture of infected material into the pleural space (pyopneumothorax). Less common pulmonary diseases associated with pneumothorax are bronchial asthma, staphylococcal pneumatoceles, and advanced pulmonary fibrosis. Eosinophilic granuloma is an interstitial disease that is characteristically associated with spontaneous pneumothorax. Pneumothorax may also appear as a complication of mechanical ventilation when high intrathoracic pressures are utilized. In contrast to simple or primary pneumothorax, in which dyspnea and evidence of ventilatory compromise are unusual unless the pneumothorax is large, relatively small pneumothoraces may produce severe respiratory symptoms when superimposed on pre-existing pulmonary disease. Thus, treatment of patients with secondary pneumothorax is more aggressive, with thoracotomy tube drainage being employed more frequently. Persistent pleural leaks (bronchopleural fistulas) and tension pneumothorax are also more frequent with secondary pneumothorax, particularly in those patients who develop a pneumothorax while on mechanical ventilation.

Adams VI, Unni KK, Muhm, JR, et al.: Diffuse malignant mesothelioma of pleura. Diagnosis and survival in 92 cases. Cancer 58:1540, 1986. *A complete clinical, radiologic, and pathologic review of pleural mesotheliomas. Correlation of clinical findings and prognosis.*

Black LF: The pleural space and pleural fluid. Mayo Clin Proc 47:493, 1972. *An excellent discussion of the physiology of normal and abnormal pleural fluid formation. Not much has been added since this article was published.*

Epler GR, McLoud TC, Gaensler EA: Prevalence and incidence of benign asbestos pleural effusion in a working population. JAMA 247:617, 1982. *Puts asbestos pleural effusion in perspective. Reviews diagnostic criteria and epidemiology and emphasizes early onset of pleural effusion as a complication of asbestos exposure.*

Health and Public Policy Committee, American College of Physicians: Diagnostic thoracentesis and pleural biopsy in pleural effusions. Ann Intern Med 103:799, 1985. *A consensus about efficacy and cost effectiveness of various tests used in the evaluation of pleural effusions.*

Light RW, MacGregor MI, Luchsinger PC, et al.: Pleural effusions: The diagnostic separation of transudates and exudates. Ann Intern Med 77:507, 1972. *The "classic" paper that separates transudates and exudates on the basis of pleural fluid to serum ratios of protein and LDH.*

Malden LT, Tattersall MH: Malignant effusions. Q J Med 58:221, 1986. *An extensive review of the pathophysiology, diagnostic considerations, and treatment options for patients with malignant pleural effusions.*

Ryan CJ, Rodgers RF, Unni KK, et al.: The outcome of patients with pleural effusion of indeterminate cause at thoracotomy. Mayo Clin Proc 56:145, 1981. *An interesting study of the natural history of pleural effusions that could not be diagnosed at thoracotomy.*

THE MEDIASTINUM

ANATOMY. The mediastinum is the anatomic space that lies in the mid-thorax. It separates the two pleural cavities and is defined by the diaphragm below and the suprasternal thoracic outlet above. The mediastinum contains several vital structures contiguous to one another in a relatively small space. Thus, abnormalities within the mediastinum, regardless of their cause, can produce a number of serious symptoms. It is convenient for clinical purposes to divide the mediastinum into *anterior, middle,* and *posterior* areas. The anterior mediastinal compartment is bounded posteriorly by the pericardium, ascending aorta, and brachial cephalic vessels and anteriorly by the sternum. This compartment contains the thymus gland, substernal extensions of the thyroid and parathyroid glands, blood vessels, pericardium, and lymph nodes. The middle mediastinal compartment extends from the posterior limit of the anterior compartment to the anterior border of the vertebral bodies. The middle mediastinum contains the heart, great vessels, trachea, main bronchi, esophagus, and phrenic and vagus nerves. The posterior mediastinum extends from the anterior surface of the vertebral bodies to the dorsal chest wall. This compartment contains the vertebral bodies, the descending thoracic aorta, the esophagus, the thoracic duct, the azygous and the hemiazygous veins, the lower portion of the vagus nerve plus the sympathetic chains, and a posterior group of mediastinal nodes.

SIGNS AND SYMPTOMS. *Chest pain, cough, hoarseness,* and *dyspnea* are the most common complaints. Less common symptoms are *stridor, dysphagia,* and *Horner's syndrome.* However, most patients with mediastinal masses are asymptomatic. Occasionally, specific syndromes are associated with primary lesions of the mediastinum. Nearly half of all thymomas are associated with myasthenia gravis (see Ch. 518). Mesotheliomas, fibrosarcomas, and occasional teratomas have been associated with hypoglycemia. Parathyroid tumors may present with hypercalcemia. Neurogenic tumors may result in pressure against the spinal cord, causing a variety of symptoms. Because of the crowding within the normal mediastinum of a large number of structures, more than one organ is likely to be affected by a given disorder. Signs and symptoms of mediastinal disorders are thus nonspecific. The physical findings of mediastinal air or inflammation are specific and discussed below. Physical findings in a patient with a mediastinal mass, however, are unusual unless the mass is large or impinges on a vital structure. Rarely, the mass may be so large that the pleural cavity is obliterated, leading to findings consistent with pleural effusion. Occasionally, a mediastinal tumor may produce superior vena caval obstruction with typical signs of facial edema, dilated neck veins over the thorax, and edema of the upper extremities. A mass can also erode into the trachea, esophagus, or great vessels with life-threatening sequelae.

DIAGNOSIS. Radiographic studies are the most helpful procedures in evaluating patients with mediastinal disorders. A large percentage of such lesions are first detected on routine chest roentgenograms (Fig. 71–1*A*). Computed tomography (CT) has dramatically improved visualization and definition of mediastinal structures and will replace routine tomography in time (Fig. 71–1*B*). The angiographic definition of great vessels and barium esophagograms are often of considerable value in defining mediastinal lesions.

In those patients in whom specific diagnoses cannot be established by radiographic methods, surgical approaches to obtaining tissue for histologic diagnosis are necessary. Anterior and some middle mediastinal lesions can be approached through mediastinoscopy or mediastinotomy. Both procedures provide lymph nodes for histologic and cultural examination without the need for major surgery. Thoracotomy is necessary when tissue from middle and posterior mediastinal lesions is required. Thoracotomy not only provides the opportunity for tissue diagnosis but also allows drainage or definitive resection of specific lesions.

SPECIFIC DISEASES. ***Infections.*** Acute mediastinitis is rare and most often results from endoscopy, surgery, or trauma to the esophagus. Fever, chest pain, widening of the mediastinal shadow by x-ray, and a history of trauma or manipulation of the esophagus suggest the diagnosis. X-ray studies with contrast material may demonstrate esophageal perforation. Complicating pleural effusions are occasionally observed and, if untreated, often develop into an empyema. Repair of the esophageal perforation, surgical drainage of mediastinal abscesses, and antibiotic therapy should be employed. Chronic fibrosing mediastinitis caused by extension of granulomatous disease (especially histoplasmosis) from mediastinal lymph nodes is rare but may cause severe irreversible mediastinal fibrosis with superior vena caval obstruction.

Pneumomediastinum. Air may enter the mediastinum either as a result of a tear in the esophagus or tracheobronchial tree or because of the dissection of air from ruptured alveoli along the peribronchovascular sheath. Rupture of the esophagus usually is associated with instrumentation or trauma. Pneumomediastinum from alveolar rupture may occur spontaneously in individuals with no underlying lung disease or may be a complication of severe diffuse disease or artificial ventilation. In many cases of pneumomediastinum, air will rupture through the mediastinal pleura producing an associated pneumothorax, which may be bilateral. The air may dissect into the subcutaneous tissues of the neck and produce generalized subcutaneous emphysema. In children, the air

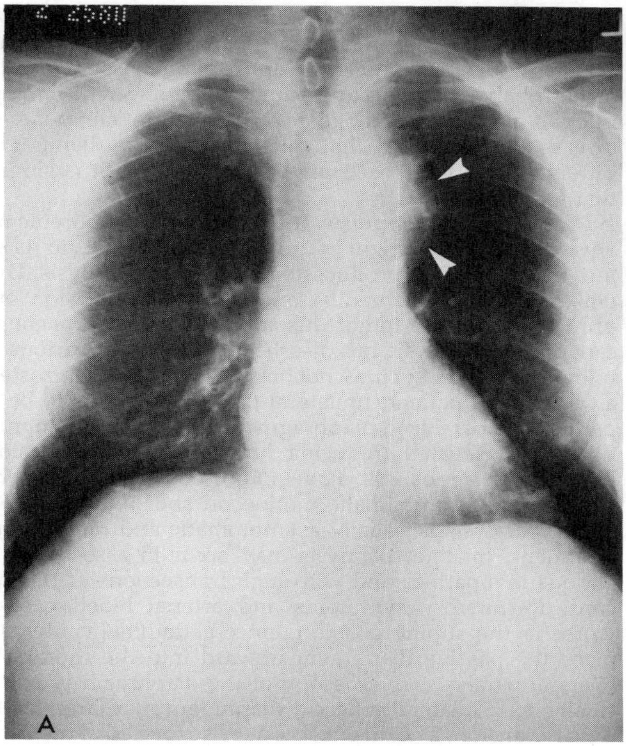

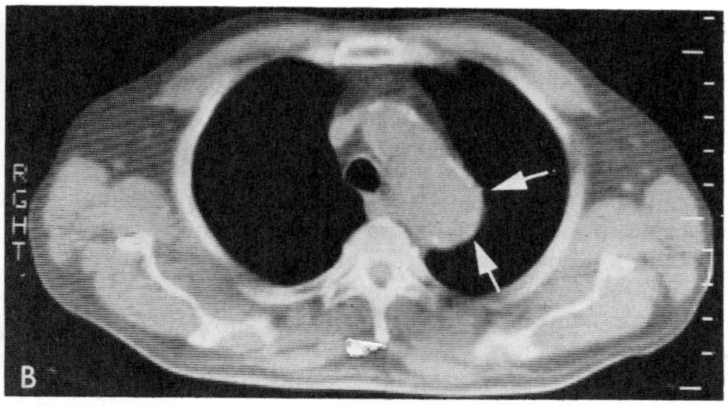

FIGURE 71–1. *A,* Posteroanterior chest roentgenogram of a 61-year-old man with mass noted adjacent to aortic arch (*arrows*). On lateral film the mass projected posteriorly. There was a history of an automobile accident 17 years previously. *B,* CT scan shows large mass projecting from the aorta (*arrows*). Dense calcium can be seen in the wall of this post-traumatic aortic aneurysm, which enhanced with injection of a small bolus of contrast medium (film not shown).

may collect within the mediastinum, compressing the great vessels. Patients with pneumomediastinum may be asymptomatic or at times may develop substernal chest pain indistinguishable from that of myocardial infarction. Physical examination may reveal subcutaneous emphysema in the neck, and auscultation often reveals a mediastinal crunch, a crackling sound synchronous with cardiac systole, best heard over the left sternal border when the patient is upright *(Hamman's sign).* A lateral chest roentgenogram is most effective in demonstrating air in the mediastinum. A simple, spontaneous pneumomediastinum usually subsides without treatment. When pneumomediastinum is severe, complicates airway or esophageal rupture, or involves compression of great vessels, surgical drainage and vigorous treatment of the underlying disease are required.

Tumors. Tumors of the mediastinum are the most common major disorder of this region. In young adults they are often primary in the mediastinum and benign; in older adults they are often malignant and metastatic. Figure 71–2 lists the usual position of common mediastinal tumors. Of primary mediastinal tumors, approximately 20 per cent represent cysts, 20 per cent are neurogenic, 20 per cent are thymomas, 10 per cent are lymphomas, 10 per cent are teratomas, and the remainder are of miscellaneous origin. As noted above, most mediastinal tumors are asymptomatic, but when symptoms do arise they are the result of compression of vital structures within the mediastinum and usually represent malignant lesions. Surgical removal is the treatment of choice of most benign mediastinal tumors, even if asymptomatic, to prevent obstructive symptoms and potential malignant changes. Most malignant tumors are inoperable, although some, such as small cell carcinoma or lymphoma, may respond to radiation therapy or chemotherapy.

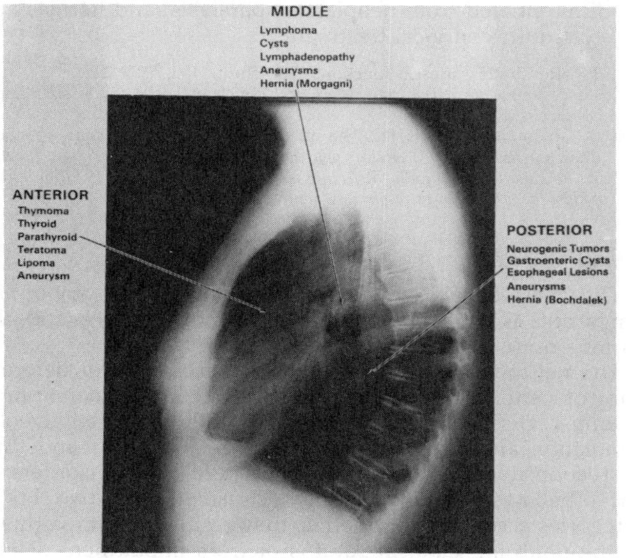

FIGURE 71–2. Locations of mediastinal tumors.

Benjamin SP, McCormack LJ, Effler DB, et al.: Primary tumors of the mediastinum. Chest 62:297, 1972. *A review of nonvascular mediastinal tumors. Many patients were asymptomatic, with masses being discovered on routine roentgenograms.*

Brown LR, Muhn JR: Computed tomography of the thorax: Current perspectives. Chest 83:806, 1983. *An excellent state-of-the-art review of the role that CT scanning plays in diagnosis of mediastinal and other thoracic diseases.*

Pugatch RD, Faling LJ, Robbins AH, et al.: CT diagnosis of benign mediastinal abnormalities. Am J Roentgenol 134:685, 1980. *Makes case for computed axial tomography as the initial procedure and most productive tool for evaluation of mediastinal abnormalities detected on plain chest roentgenogram. Excellent pictures and definition of mediastinal anatomy.*

THE DIAPHRAGM

The diaphragm is an airtight sheet of muscle and tendon lined by parietal pleura on one side and peritoneal membrane on the other. Its muscle fibers arise from the lower ribs and thoracic vertebrae and converge and insert into the margins of the crescentic central tendon. There is a hiatus for each of the principal structures that pass from thorax to abdomen. Motor and sensory fibers reach the diaphragm via the phrenic nerves, with separate innervation to the right and left halves. The diaphragm is the principal muscle of respiration. Diaphragmatic contraction tends to displace abdominal contents downward and to raise the ribs upward and outward, thus creating the negative intrapleural pressure of inspiration.

DIAPHRAGMATIC HERNIAS. Herniation of abdominal or retroperitoneal structures may occur through congenitally weak or incompletely fused areas of the diaphragm, may result from traumatic rupture, or may occur through the esophageal hiatus. The latter accounts for over three fourths of all diaphragmatic hernias and is considered in Ch. 98.

Hernias posteriorly through the foramina of Bochdalek are the most common form of hernia in infancy, occurring more often on the left than the right. The hernial opening may be large because of a virtual absence of the diaphragm owing to failure of its posterolateral portion to close. In this instance, abdominal viscera may extend freely into the left pleural space, producing respiratory distress and requiring immediate surgical repair. When the defect is small, the peritoneum and pleura usually fuse, producing a sac that contains the herniated contents. In adults, the defect is usually small and is discovered on routine chest roentgenogram. The defect is usually posterolateral, and the hernial contents usually contain retroperitoneal fat or the upper pole of the kidney or, rarely, the spleen.

Hernias anteriorly through the foramina of Morgagni are rare and tend to occur in the obese or in patients who have increased intra-abdominal pressure. The hernia commonly presents as an anterior, rounded density in the region of the right cardiophrenic angle. It usually contains omentum, but occasionally stomach, bowel, or liver may appear when hernias are large. Auscultation of borborygmi over the chest, radioisotope scans of the liver, routine gastrointestinal contrast films, and induction of a pneumoperitoneum followed by an upright film of the abdomen may all be useful diagnostic procedures. Therapy of both types of hernias may not be needed, especially when old films demonstrate that the abnormality has been present for a long time. Occasionally surgery is necessary for diagnosis or to relieve strangulation of hernia sac contents.

Traumatic hernias of the diaphragm may result from direct injury to the diaphragm or indirectly from severe abdominal compression. Signs and symptoms may occur immediately owing to extension of abdominal contents into the pleural space with resultant strangulation. More often, a latent period, which may extend for several years, intervenes before either respiratory or abdominal symptoms develop. Diagnosis is accomplished roentgenographically, and treatment is surgical.

DISORDERS OF DIAPHRAGMATIC MOTION. A variety of structural and functional abnormalities interfere with the ability of the diaphragm to develop inspiratory muscle strength. The resulting impairment of diaphragmatic function may be involved in many forms of respiratory failure.

Hiccup. Hiccup, or singultus, is a common disturbance produced by spasm of the diaphragm followed by sudden closure of the glottis during an inspiratory effort. A characteristic sound is produced as the glottis closes, and discomfort may be experienced as thoracic pressure is lowered by continued contraction of the diaphragm. Hiccup is usually of short duration but may persist for days or weeks. Hiccup is most often of unknown cause, presumably resulting from functional gastrointestinal disturbances. Occasionally, hiccups are a sign of serious disease, such as central nervous system disorders (encephalitis, brain stem strokes, tumor), uremia, herpes zoster, and pleural or abdominal processes that invade or irritate the diaphragm. Prolonged hiccups are sometimes thought to be psychogenic in origin. Hiccups usually subside spontaneously or when the initiating disease has been successfully treated. In persistent, debilitating hiccups, local anesthesia or actual crushing of one of the phrenic nerves may be required (crushing theoretically produces paralysis of only several months, but permanent paralysis is frequent).

Diaphragmatic Flutter. This is a rare disorder in which rapid rhythmic contractions of the diaphragm occur at a rate of 1 to 8 per second, lasting for seconds or as long as weeks or months. The contractions produce a cogwheel type of respiration and, when frequent, may hamper gas exchange. They are not accompanied by an inspiratory sound, and one or both halves of the diaphragm may be affected. Etiology is unclear, although psychogenic causes, central nervous system disease, and diseases that might irritate the diaphragm or phrenic nerve have been implicated. Treatment is similar to that for hiccup.

Diaphragmatic Paralysis. Interruption of the phrenic nerve anywhere from its origin in the C3–C5 nerve roots to its entry into the diaphragm produces diaphragmatic paralysis. Unilateral paralysis is frequently associated with invasion of the phrenic nerve by tumor (usually metastatic bronchogenic carcinoma). Paralysis has also been reported in various neurologic disorders such as poliomyelitis and herpes zoster. In an occasional patient, unilateral paralysis appears to be idiopathic. The paralyzed diaphragmatic leaf is not only nonfunctional but elevated, reducing lung volume on the side of paralysis. Diagnosis is made fluoroscopically by observing paradoxical diaphragmatic motion on sniff and cough. Unilateral paralysis is usually asymptomatic and rarely requires treatment. Bilateral paralysis may occur in association with various myopathies and with high transections of the spinal cord. Respiratory symptoms and arterial blood gases are worse in the supine position, since abdominal contents displace the passive diaphragm upward into the thorax. With bilateral paralysis, fluoroscopy of the diaphragm is less conclusive as a bilaterally flaccid diaphragm may drop with rib cage expansion. The diagnosis can be suspected at the bedside by observing inward, instead of outward, motion of the abdomen on inspiration. The diagnosis can be confirmed by recording muscle action potentials or by measuring esophageal and gastric (transdiaphragmatic) pressures on inspiration. Electrical stimulation of the phrenic nerve with measurement of conduction time may be helpful in diagnosing peripheral neuropathy. The hypoventilation of bilateral paralysis often produces respiratory failure. The hypoventilation of bilateral phrenic nerve paralysis can be treated by ventilating the patient on an intermittent or continuous schedule or by implanting and pacing phrenic nerve electrodes.

Eventration. Diaphragm eventration is a localized elevation of the diaphragm resulting from impaired muscle development or local muscle weakness. The diaphragm muscle is either absent or atrophic in the area of eventration. The elevation is usually on the right side of the anteromedial portion of the diaphragm. It most often appears in middle-aged, obese patients. The condition is usually asymptomatic, being recognized on routine chest roentgenograms. It must be differentiated from neoplasms, paralysis, and hernias and rarely requires surgical treatment.

Celli BR: Respiratory muscle function. Clin Chest Med 7:567, 1986. *A comprehensive up-to-date review covering clinical aspects of respiratory muscles clearly and concisely.*

Loh L, Goldman M, Davis JN: The assessment of the diaphragm function. Medicine 56:165, 1977. *A clear and easy-to-read review of diaphragm function and its importance clinically. Reference is made (Q J Med 45:87, 1976) to the role of diaphragm function in respiratory failure.*

THE CHEST WALL

The chest bellows serves to move air in and out of the lungs and is made up of the bony thoracic cage and the various muscles of respiration.

The neuromuscular–chest cage system is a major determinant of ventilatory patterns and of static and dynamic lung volumes. Disease of this system may influence total alveolar ventilation and ventilation-perfusion relationships and thus be responsible for hypoxemia or hypercapnia. Disorders of chest bellows function may be classified into two broad categories according to whether they result from impairment of the neuromuscular apparatus or from impairment of mechanical properties of the chest wall. The former are discussed as individual diseases in Part XXII. Only the latter group will be discussed here.

KYPHOSCOLIOSIS. This deformity of the chest wall is due to a combination of posterior angulation (kyphosis) and lateral angulation and rotation (scoliosis) of the spine. Scoliosis is categorized as to the right or left according to the direction of the convexity of the primary curvature. Idiopathic scoliosis is more frequently to the right in the thorax with a compensatory left curvature in the lumbar region.

The severity of scoliosis may be quantified by measuring the angle between upper and lower portions of spinal curve on a roentgenogram. Greater angles signify more severe deformity and imply greater respiratory impairment. In thoracic kyphoscoliosis the rib cage is distorted so that on the convex side of the spine the ribs are widely separated and rotation of the spine angulates them posteriorly, producing the kyphotic hump. On the concave side, the ribs are crowded and displaced anteriorly. Because of the kyphosis and loss of thoracic height, the lower anterior chest wall tends to bulge forward. Although mild degrees of kyphoscoliosis are common, severe distortion of the chest cage is unusual. Kyphoscoliosis usually begins in childhood but becomes more prominent during the rapid growth years of adolescence. In most cases (80 per cent) there is no discernible etiology; neurologic disorders that influence chest wall muscles and congenital abnormalities account for a small percentage of cases.

Patients are usually asymptomatic in early life. When kyphoscoliosis is severe (angle greater than 90 degrees) or when patients develop pulmonary infections (as a result of locally impaired bronchial clearance mechanisms), dyspnea appears. In these instances, gradual progression, respiratory failure, and cor pulmonale occur with death in the fourth through sixth decades. Patients with mild or moderate kyphoscoliosis (angle less than 50 degrees) who remain free of respiratory infections may have normal life expectancy.

Depending upon the degree of kyphoscoliosis, static lung volumes are reduced with preservation of residual volume; chest wall compliance is reduced, with lung compliance being slightly reduced or normal. Airflow rates are usually reduced only in proportion to the reduction of vital capacity. Studies of regional lung function tend to show variable shifts of ventilation and perfusion owing to the chest wall deformity. Arterial blood gases are also variable. Many patients have mild hypoxemia, secondary to ventilation-perfusion mismatch, but severe hypoxemia and hypercapnia occur only late in the disease and are most commonly associated with superimposed infection.

A variety of methods have been used to restore normal curvature or prevent progressive curvature of the spine. These include surgery, plaster casts, and various types of traction. With most, the cosmetic effect is greater than the physiologic effect, although they may prevent progression of curvature, particularly in those patients with idiopathic kyphoscoliosis. Efforts should be made to prevent airways disease; the patient should discontinue smoking, and respiratory infections should be treated early and vigorously. In patients with severe disease, episodic use of intermittent positive pressure breathing has been found to increase transiently functional residual capacity and total thoracic compliance and may be of value in ambulatory management. Episodes of acute respiratory failure, usually associated with respiratory infections, may require intubation and assisted ventilation. In some patients with chronic respiratory failure, night time ventilatory assistance may be effective in controlling symptoms and respiratory failure. Home oxygen should be used in those patients with severe hypoxemia.

PECTUS EXCAVATUM. This is a congenital deformity of the lower portion of the sternum with symmetric bowing of the anterior ribs. The defect, which is often familial, is thought to be due to a short central tendon of the diaphragm. When the deformity is severe, the heart and mediastinal structures are displaced laterally, but significant functional impairment is rare. Surgical correction is not necessary and is done only for cosmetic purposes.

ANKYLOSING SPONDYLITIS. This disease is characterized by fusion of costotransverse and vertebral joints and may also involve sternomanubrial and clavicular joints (see Ch. 434). The chest cage tends to be fixed in an inspiratory position, with the result that vital capacity is decreased while residual volume and functional residual capacity are increased. Although a small number of patients develop idiopathic upper lobe fibrosis, in most patients gas exchange is normal and respiratory disease is unusual.

FLAIL CHEST. Trauma to the chest that produces multiple anterior rib fractures may lead to instability of a large area of the anterior chest wall. This occurs most commonly in motor vehicle accidents or following cardiopulmonary resuscitation. Paradoxical motion occurs during respiration, with the injured area moving in an opposite direction from the remainder of the chest wall. Hypoxemia is common in flail chest, although alveolar hypoventilation with hypercapnia is rare. Hypoxemia is most often the result either of lung contusion with subsequent ventilation-perfusion mismatch or of breathing at low lung volumes and atelectasis. Artificial ventilation with volume ventilators is not necessary in many cases. Aggressive supportive care with attention to maintaining adequate oxygenation and clearance of airway secretions is the best approach to therapy.

Bergofsky EH: Respiratory failure in disorders of the thoracic cage. Am Rev Respir Dis 119:643, 1979. *A detailed clinical and physiologic review of the chest cage and its disorders. Contains an extensive list of references. Easy reading and "state of the art" for this topic.*

Hoeppner VH, Cockcroft DW, Dosman JH, et al.: Nighttime ventilation improves respiratory failure in secondary kyphoscoliosis. Am Rev Respir Dis 129:240, 1984. *Demonstrates effectiveness of now well-accepted approach to treatment of respiratory failure in patients with chest wall or diaphragmatic paralysis and other mechanical problems.*

Sharkford SR, Smith DE, Zarins CK, et al.: The management of flail chest. Am J Surg 132:759, 1976. *A retrospective review of personal cases and of the literature, establishing that not all patients with flail chest need to be intubated and ventilated.*

72 RESPIRATORY FAILURE

John F. Murray

INTRODUCTION

Adequate respiration consists of the uptake of sufficient amounts of O_2 and the elimination of sufficient amounts of CO_2 to maintain P_{O_2} and P_{CO_2} in arterial blood at their respective normal values. It follows that *respiratory failure* is associated with disturbances in the exchange of O_2 and CO_2 between gas in alveoli and blood in pulmonary capillaries and that these abnormalities must be reflected by changes in the P_{O_2} and P_{CO_2} in arterial blood. Thus respiratory failure is defined as a condition in which arterial P_{O_2} is below the normal range (excluding hypoxemia from intracardiac right-to-left shunting of blood) or arterial P_{CO_2} is above the normal range (excluding respiratory compensation for metabolic alkalosis). This definition, which is physiologically precise as well as clinically applicable, implies that the diagnosis of respiratory failure depends chiefly on laboratory analysis of arterial blood and not on clinical findings.

Respiratory failure is not a disease but a disorder of function that can be caused by a variety of conditions that affect the lungs; in some instances, the lungs are completely normal (e.g., overdose of sedative drugs). Respiratory failure is analogous to heart failure and renal failure, both of which represent the consequences of impaired normal function resulting from numerous disparate diseases.

Respiratory failure is traditionally divided into acute and

chronic varieties, depending on the time it takes for the abnormalities in gas exchange to occur. This arbitrary classification does not take into account the common clinical occurrence of an acute worsening of arterial P_{O_2} and P_{CO_2} in a patient who already has chronic respiratory failure as a result of some underlying disorder. However, the distinction between acute and chronic respiratory failure has important etiologic and therapeutic implications and will be referred to frequently.

PATHOPHYSIOLOGY OF RESPIRATORY FAILURE

In human beings, respiration has been subdivided into four functional processes: *ventilation, diffusion, perfusion,* and *control of breathing*. Each of these contributes uniquely to the maintenance of normal values of P_{O_2} and P_{CO_2} in arterial blood. Therefore, abnormalities in any one of the four processes, if sufficiently severe, will cause respiratory failure; furthermore, in many common respiratory disorders, multiple abnormalities coexist.

Normal Gas Exchange

The physiology of normal gas exchange is described in Ch. 59 and will not be reviewed here. However, understanding what is meant by normal is important, because arterial P_{O_2} varies with age, and both arterial P_{O_2} and P_{CO_2} vary according to the altitude (i.e., the prevailing barometric pressure) at which the person happens to be when the blood specimen is obtained and to the extent of acclimatization. The normal range includes the biologic variabilities among individuals and the analytic variations inherent in the measurements. Because the diagnosis of respiratory failure should be made in the laboratory and not at the bedside, the physician's ability to establish the diagnosis depends on the accuracy of the laboratory tests used to measure P_{O_2} and P_{CO_2}. Normal mean arterial P_{O_2} (Pa_{O_2}) values in subjects 20 years of age or older can be calculated from the regression equation $Pa_{O_2} = 100.1 - 0.323$ (age in years). The normal range of variation is $\pm$ 5 mm Hg from the mean value. Arterial P_{CO_2} does not vary with age and is normally within the range of 40 $\pm$ 5 mm Hg in healthy persons at sea level. Values of P_{O_2} *below* or P_{CO_2} *above* normal limits indicate the presence of respiratory failure.

Abnormal Gas Exchange

The pathophysiology of abnormal gas exchange is also discussed in Ch. 59. Hypoventilation, impaired diffusion, ventilation-perfusion mismatching, right-to-left shunting of blood, and breathing air with a low P_{O_2} all cause arterial hypoxia (a decrease below normal of P_{O_2}); in contrast, for practical purposes, only hypoventilation causes arterial hypercapnia (an increase above normal of P_{CO_2}). In view of the therapeutic importance of recognizing the abnormal mechanism(s) leading to a patient's respiratory failure, each will be reviewed briefly.

HYPOVENTILATION. Alveolar hypoventilation is present when the arterial P_{CO_2} is increased. Furthermore, as arterial P_{CO_2} increases, P_{O_2} decreases *except* when the patient is breathing gas with an enriched concentration of O_2. Because arterial P_{O_2} and P_{CO_2} change in opposite directions by nearly the same amount during hypoventilation, the contribution of hypoventilation to the patient's arterial hypoxia can be readily assessed. (In a 60-year-old person, for example, if P_{O_2} = 50 mm Hg and P_{CO_2} = 70 mm Hg, both have changed from their normal values by the same amount [30 mm Hg] and "pure" hypoventilation is present; in contrast, if P_{O_2} = 30 mm Hg and P_{CO_2} = 70 mm Hg, the change from normal of P_{CO_2} does not account for the entire change in P_{O_2}; therefore, some other cause in addition to hypoxia from hypoventilation must be present.) Arterial hypoxia from alveolar hypoventilation is not associated with an increased alveolar-arterial P_{O_2} difference and is "corrected" by breathing 100 per cent O_2.

IMPAIRED DIFFUSION. Abnormalities of diffusion do not cause arterial hypoxia in persons at rest unless they are extremely severe. Although these occur in occasional patients with respiratory failure, for practical purposes the possible contributions of an abnormality of diffusion to a given patient's arterial hypoxia can be ignored except during exercise or at high altitude. This practice is permissible because diffusion disturbances, even when marked, cause only relatively small increases in the patient's alveolar-arterial P_{O_2} difference, and this abnormality, if it exists, is readily corrected by adding small amounts of O_2 to the inspired air.

VENTILATION-PERFUSION IMBALANCE. When gas exchange units receive more blood flow than ventilation, arterial hypoxia results. Mismatching of ventilation-perfusion is by far the most common cause of arterial hypoxia and can be recognized by giving the patient 100 per cent O_2 to breathe; this causes the alveolar-arterial P_{O_2} difference from pure mismatching that is present while the patient breathes room air to decrease and arterial P_{O_2} to increase to normal values (>550 mm Hg). The importance of breathing 100 per cent O_2 is shown in Figure 72–1; in the presence of a severe ventilation-perfusion disturbance (σ = 2.0 in the figure), even an $F_{I_{O_2}}$ of 0.8 fails to raise P_{O_2} to normal values but 1.0 does. Although a "pure" ventilation-perfusion inequality can lead to CO_2 retention, this is an uncommon cause of hypercapnia because as arterial P_{CO_2} tends to increase, it stimulates peripheral and central chemoreceptors and increases ventilation; this, in turn, reduces P_{CO_2} back to normal values but, owing to the shape of the oxyhemoglobin dissociation curve, does not correct the hypoxia.

RIGHT-TO-LEFT SHUNTS. Shunts of blood from right to left may occur through abnormal anatomic communications in the lung (e.g., pulmonary arteriovenous fistula) but much more frequently by perfusion of lung units that are completely unventilated because they are either collapsed (atelectasis) or filled with fluid (pulmonary edema, pneumonia, intra-alveolar hemorrhage). Regardless of the cause, an alveolar-arterial P_{O_2} difference results that increases when the patient breathes 100 per cent O_2 compared with the value obtained while

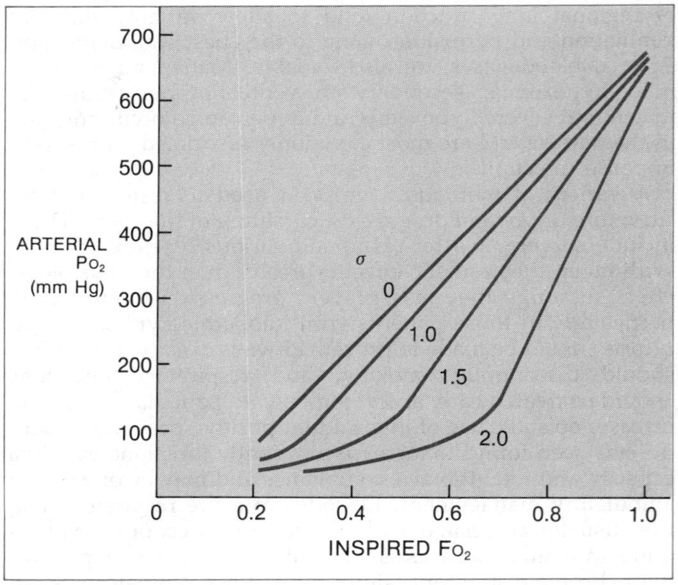

FIGURE 72–1. Graph showing the effects of changing inspired O_2 concentration (F_{O_2}) on arterial P_{O_2} in the presence of varying amounts of ventilation-perfusion inequality. When ventilation and perfusion are evenly matched (σ = 0), the relationship between inspired F_{O_2} and arterial P_{O_2} is linear. As ventilation-perfusion inequalities worsen (σ = 1.0 to 2.0), the effect of breathing a given F_{O_2} is progressively less. (Modified from West JB, Wagner PD: Bioengineering Aspects of the Lung. New York, Marcel Dekker, Inc., 1977. Reprinted with permission of the authors and publisher.)

breathing room air. For reasons similar to those occurring in patients with ventilation-perfusion imbalances, CO_2 retention seldom occurs in patients with right-to-left shunts.

DECREASED INSPIRED P_{O_2}. Expected values of arterial P_{O_2} are corrected for the influence of decreasing barometric pressure; strictly speaking, therefore, the effects of altitude on inspired P_{O_2} and the resulting decreased arterial P_{O_2} are not an abnormal cause of hypoxia, even though the hypoxia may be severe and dangerous. Occasionally, pathologic hypoxia occurs when ambient P_{O_2} is reduced because of combustion of O_2 or because of dilution by some other gas. However, this phenomenon is not of importance when interpreting the results of analysis of arterial blood specimens obtained in the hospital or clinic.

HYPERCAPNIA. In contrast to arterial hypoxia, which may result from five different pathophysiologic derangements, arterial hypercapnia can always be interpreted as signifying alveolar hypoventilation. This is true because arterial P_{CO_2} (Pa_{CO_2}) is governed by the relationship between CO_2 production ($\dot{V}_{CO_2}$) and alveolar ventilation ($\dot{V}_A$): $Pa_{CO_2} = k\dot{V}_{CO_2}/\dot{V}_A$. Normally, however, even when CO_2 production increases markedly, alveolar ventilation increases proportionately and arterial P_{CO_2} is maintained within narrow limits. Thus an increase in arterial P_{CO_2} can always be viewed as respiratory failure in the sense that alveolar ventilation is inadequate to eliminate all the CO_2 being produced at that time. Severe ventilation-perfusion imbalances and right-to-left shunts can produce CO_2 retention, but this is uncommon because, as already emphasized, alveolar ventilation usually increases and corrects the disturbance.

An increase or decrease in P_{CO_2} in the blood has a direct effect on the amount of carbonic acid in the blood and a reciprocal effect on pH. Acute changes in P_{CO_2} have a more profound effect on pH than chronic changes owing to differences in plasma bicarbonate. With acute increases or decreases in P_{CO_2}, there is little change in bicarbonate level and a considerable change in pH; after three to five days of sustained changes in P_{CO_2}, renal compensation has increased plasma bicarbonate in hypercapnia and decreased it in hypocapnia, both tending to restore pH toward normal. Many patients with respiratory failure have mixed respiratory and nonrespiratory acid-base disturbances. Knowledge of the time course of a patient's problem as well as the magnitude of changes in plasma bicarbonate is extremely useful in providing the necessary understanding for appropriate treatment of all components of the disorder.

Right Heart Failure

Acute respiratory failure can cause acute right heart failure (acute cor pulmonale). The normal right ventricle is not a good pressure generator and cannot sustain sudden pressure loads over 40 to 50 mm Hg. Thus acute right heart failure may develop in any condition in which pulmonary vascular resistance increases abruptly; this happens most commonly in patients with multiple pulmonary emboli with obstruction of much of the pulmonary vascular bed (usually >60 per cent). At times, acute cor pulmonale complicates the course of patients with severe bronchial asthma or other forms of marked airways obstruction.

Acute right heart failure may also occur in patients with chronic lung disease during an episode of acute respiratory failure. Most of these patients have right ventricular hypertrophy (chronic cor pulmonale) to begin with, and a subclinical or stable condition is aggravated by the added effects of the superimposed acute lung disease (usually bronchitis or pneumonia). In these patients, right ventricular function is worsened for several reasons: (1) Alveolar hypoxia and acidemia cause pulmonary arterial vasoconstriction; (2) certain lung diseases reduce the cross-sectional area available for perfusion; (3) hyperinflation of the lung increases pulmonary vascular resistance; and (4) arterial hypoxia may depress myocardial contractility. These factors are important to recognize because they are reversible and usually respond well to appropriate treatment of the intercurrent acute disorder.

CAUSES OF RESPIRATORY FAILURE

Because respiratory failure is defined as the presence of arterial hypoxia with or without hypercapnia, it is obvious that a large variety of disorders are capable of producing these abnormalities. For convenience, the multiple causes of respiratory failure can be classified, depending on which component of the respiratory system is involved. Because most of these disorders characteristically cause either acute or chronic respiratory failure, they can be subdivided further into these categories.

Diseases Causing Airways Obstruction

ACUTE. Obstruction may result from acute diseases that involve any portion of the upper and lower airways. The presence of respiratory failure depends on the magnitude and extent of the narrowing. Obstruction of the *extra*thoracic airway (nasopharynx, larynx, extrathoracic portion of the trachea) usually causes stridor, a characteristic alteration of breathing that is associated with harsh, high-pitched respiratory noises that are louder and more pronounced during inspiration than expiration. In contrast, obstruction of the *intra*thoracic airways causes wheezing, an abnormality of breathing in which expiration is louder and longer than inspiration.

Obstruction of the upper airways can result from (1) inflammation-induced swelling of the mucosa secondary to infections, allergic reactions, and, less commonly, thermal or mechanical injuries and (2) impaction of foreign bodies or, occasionally, tumors. Acute obstruction of the upper airways is particularly likely to develop in infants and young children who have smaller and hence more vulnerable upper passages than older children and adults.

Acute obstruction of the lower airways is usually caused by swelling of the mucosa, secretions in the lumen, or bronchospasm. Accordingly, bronchial asthma, infections, bronchiolitis, and the inhalation of chemicals (such as nitrogen dioxide in silo-filler's disease) are important causes of acute respiratory failure.

CHRONIC. Diffuse obstruction may result from disorders originating in large bronchi (bronchiectasis), small bronchi (bronchitis), or the lung parenchyma (emphysema). These abnormalities characteristically progress gradually and lead to chronic respiratory failure. Of considerable importance are the intercurrent episodes of acute disease, usually pneumonia or bronchitis, that complicate the underlying disorder and often worsen the severity of existing respiratory failure.

Diseases Causing Parenchymal Infiltration

ACUTE. The most common cause of acute infiltration of the parenchyma is pneumonia, which usually has an infectious origin but occasionally is caused by inhalation or aspiration of a toxic chemical. Whether acute respiratory failure develops depends on the extent and severity of the disease. Immunologic reactions from drugs, migrating parasites, or leukoagglutinins are uncommon causes of acute respiratory failure but are important because of their special therapeutic requirements.

CHRONIC. There are over 100 different conditions that can cause chronic diffuse parenchymal infiltration. When severe, any of these can cause chronic respiratory failure. As in patients with chronic airways obstruction, patients with chronic infiltrative diseases may have intercurrent episodes of bronchopulmonary infection that cause acute worsening of their underlying respiratory status.

TABLE 72–1. PARTIAL LIST OF CONDITIONS THAT HAVE BEEN ASSOCIATED WITH THE ADULT RESPIRATORY DISTRESS SYNDROME

Shock of any etiology	Inhaled toxins
Infections	O_2 (high concentrations)
Gram-negative sepsis	Smoke
Viral pneumonia	Corrosive chemicals (NO_2, Cl_2, NH_3, phosgene, cadmium)
Bacterial pneumonia	Hematologic disorders
Trauma	Intravascular coagulation
Fat emboli	Massive blood transfusion
Lung contusion	Metabolic disorders
Nonthoracic trauma (including head injury)	Pancreatitis
Liquid aspiration	Uremia
Gastric juice	Paraquat ingestion
Fresh and salt water (drowning)	Miscellaneous
Hydrocarbon fluids	Increased intracranial pressure (including seizures)
Drug overdose	Eclampsia
Heroin	Postcardioversion
Methadone	Radiation pneumonitis
Propoxyphene	Postcardiopulmonary bypass
Barbiturates	
Colchicine	

Diseases Causing Pulmonary Edema

CARDIOGENIC. Pulmonary edema in patients with heart disease may be acute or chronic in onset; both varieties are caused by an increase in the hydrostatic pressure within pulmonary capillaries. Pulmonary edema may follow an acute myocardial infarction or acute left ventricular failure of any cause (hypertensive crises, arrhythmias), or it may be precipitated in patients with valvular or other forms of chronic heart disease by sudden changes in their cardiorespiratory status (from arrhythmias, hypoxemia, or increased systemic blood pressure). Chronic pulmonary edema is found in patients with chronic, usually refractory, heart failure, but even in these patients the amount of edema increases and decreases according to changing hemodynamics and therapy.

INCREASED PERMEABILITY. Acute pulmonary edema can accompany certain conditions that do not involve the heart. The basic pathophysiologic abnormality in most of these disorders appears to be an increased permeability of the pulmonary capillary endothelium. Pulmonary edema resulting from increased permeability is an important and apparently steadily increasing cause of acute respiratory failure, especially in patients who are hospitalized with serious medical or surgical illnesses that initially do not involve the lungs. After a latent period of 6 to 24 hours, these patients develop progressive arterial hypoxia, decreased compliance, and extensive roentgenographic infiltrations; in fatal cases, the lungs are found to be nearly airless, intensely congested, and filled with a proteinaceous edema fluid that also contains large numbers of red blood cells; occasionally, hyaline membranes are found. This constellation of clinical, physiologic, and radiologic findings is known as the *adult respiratory distress syndrome* and has been reported as a complication of many apparently unrelated conditions (Table 72–1). The feature common to all these disorders is the presence of diffuse injury to the alveolar-capillary membrane. Once damage has occurred, probably by many different pathways, and the permeability of the membrane is increased, pulmonary edema follows; thus the clinical, physiologic, and radiologic manifestations are similar, regardless of the cause of the injury. The adult respiratory distress syndrome is described at greater length in Ch. 73.

Pulmonary Vascular Diseases

ACUTE. Pulmonary embolism is usually accompanied by a decreased arterial P_{O_2} and P_{CO_2}, the former from ventilation-perfusion mismatching and the latter reflecting the hyperventilation that nearly always occurs. Pulmonary embolism is also an important cause of worsening respiratory failure in patients with underlying chronic lung disease. Fat emboli and emboli from platelet-fibrin aggregates can cause marked hypoxia by increasing the permeability of the alveolar-capillary membrane and producing severe pulmonary edema.

CHRONIC. Pulmonary vasculitis and recurrent thromboembolism are not common conditions and, when present, usually do not cause respiratory failure until the late stages of the disease. Recurrent thromboembolism occurs in intravenous drug abusers and in patients with chronic peripheral venous thrombi, sickle cell anemia, and schistosomiasis. Pulmonary vasculitis occurs in patients with scleroderma, other collagen diseases, and primary pulmonary hypertension.

Diseases of the Chest Wall and Pleura

ACUTE. The most important cause of sudden respiratory failure from acute disorders involving the thoracic cage is injury to the chest wall. Segmental fractures of several ribs or fractures of ribs on both sides of the sternum can result in a flail chest. Besides the impairment of ventilatory function that results from the unstable chest wall, gas exchange abnormalities are often compounded by contusion of the lung underneath the site of injury. Spontaneous or traumatic pneumothorax is an important cause of acute respiratory failure, which may be severe and which often afflicts otherwise healthy persons.

CHRONIC. Severe idiopathic or acquired kyphoscoliosis can cause chronic respiratory failure, which is often associated with cor pulmonale. Patients with massive pleural effusion(s) or with thickened, constrictive pleural layer(s) may also have chronic respiratory failure.

Disorders of the Neuromuscular System

Disorders of the neuromuscular system are classified according to which part of the effector system is involved, i.e., the brain, neuronal pathways, or muscles of respiration, rather than into acute and chronic varieties. Patients with these disorders often have normal lungs; respiratory failure occurs from inability to ventilate normally.

BRAIN DISORDERS. Probably the most common cause of respiratory failure from impaired function of the central nervous system is the use of sedative drugs or anesthetic agents. Suppression of ventilatory drive from opiates, barbiturates, psychic depressants, alcohol, and a variety of sedative drugs results in hypoxia and hypercapnia that may be life threatening. Ventilatory stimuli can also be depressed by many diseases of the central nervous system, including vascular diseases, tumors, and infections.

SPINAL CORD AND PERIPHERAL NERVE DISORDERS. Injuries to the cervical or high thoracic spinal cord may produce immediate respiratory failure from paralysis of the muscles of respiration. Loss of anterior horn cell function in patients with poliomyelitis was an important cause of acute and chronic respiratory failure but is seldom encountered now because of the widespread use of vaccination. Polyneuritis, whether postinfectious (Guillain-Barré syndrome) or toxic, is an uncommon but important cause of respiratory failure in view of its inherent reversibility.

MUSCULAR DISORDERS. The final effectors in the system that controls breathing are the skeletal muscles of respiration. When these muscles are involved by generalized myopathies, such as muscular dystrophy or myasthenia gravis, respiratory failure results. Respiratory failure in patients with myasthenia gravis occurs during myasthenic or cholinergic crises. In contrast, respiratory failure in patients with muscular dystrophy is nearly always chronic and related to an advanced stage in the progression of the disease.

SLEEP APNEA. Brief periods of apnea occur in normal persons during deep sleep. Much more prolonged episodes associated with severe hypoxia have been documented in patients with massive obesity, chronic mountain sickness, enlarged tonsils, and many other disorders. Apnea results from either failure of ventilatory drive or obstruction of the upper airway. Severe sleep apnea can cause chronic respiratory failure, cor pulmonale, psychosis, and pathologic daytime sleepiness, a condition sometimes called the pickwickian syndrome, with somewhat dubious literary authenticity. Sleep apnea is discussed at greater length in Ch. 457.

CLINICAL MANIFESTATIONS

Given the great variety of disorders that can cause respiratory failure, it is obvious that the clinical manifestations in a given patient depend in large part on which underlying disease he or she has; these are dealt with elsewhere in this book. When respiratory failure ensues and if the blood gas disturbances are sufficiently severe, the signs and symptoms of hypoxia, and possible hypercapnia, become superimposed upon the signs and symptoms of the underlying disease. The clinical manifestations of hypoxia and hypercapnia are nonspecific and usually occur late in the evolution of the clinical problem. This statement underscores the earlier axiom that the diagnosis of respiratory failure is made in the laboratory and not at the bedside.

Hypoxia

The signs and symptoms of acute hypoxia are chiefly caused by abnormalities in central nervous system and cardiovascular function. Characteristic features are impaired judgment and motor instability, a clinical picture closely resembling acute alcoholism. As hypoxia worsens, the brainstem is affected and death results from depression of the medullary respiratory centers. The initial cardiovascular effects of acute hypoxia are tachycardia and increased blood pressure; when hypoxia is very severe, bradycardia, myocardial depression, and shock ensue. Recognizable cyanosis of the lips, mucous membranes, and nail beds usually occurs when the concentration of reduced hemoglobin in the capillaries is >5 grams per deciliter. Accordingly, cyanosis can result from decreases in either arterial PO_2 or blood flow. In patients with lung disease, cyanosis cannot be detected by most physicians until arterial PO_2 is <50 mm Hg; some observers cannot recognize cyanosis unless arterial PO_2 is <40 mm Hg!

In patients with chronic hypoxia, the central nervous system manifestations are drowsiness, inattentiveness, apathy, fatigue, and delayed reaction time. The chronic cardiovascular effects are often minimal, but pulmonary hypertension or even cor pulmonale with signs of right heart failure may be detected on clinical examination. One of the hallmarks of chronic hypoxia is erythrocytosis, which may cause noticeable plethora and changes in the hemoglobin concentration, hematocrit ratio, or red blood cell count. However, the increase in red blood cell mass in many patients with chronic hypoxia is masked by an almost proportionate increase in plasma volume; in these patients, the usual peripheral blood indices of the red blood cell production (hemoglobin, hematocrit) do not reveal the full extent of the erythropoietic response.

Hypercapnia

The physiologic consequences of hypercapnia depend not only on the amount of excess CO_2 in the body but also on the rate at which retention develops. Increases in PCO_2 from acute respiratory failure lead to a constellation of progressive disturbances of central nervous system function: apprehension, confusion, drowsiness, coma, and death. The vascular responses represent a mixture of vasoconstriction, from generalized sympathetic activity, and vasodilation, from local accumulation of CO_2; thus the cardiovascular abnormalities are variable and depend on whether vasoconstrictor or vasodilator influences predominate. There are usually tachycardia and sweating, but blood pressure may be high, low, or normal.

In contrast, if PCO_2 increases slowly, compensation takes place and the clinical consequences may be minimal at values of arterial PCO_2 that would cause death if reached suddenly. There are numerous patients with arterial PCO_2 values over 100 mm Hg who are ambulatory and at times living active lives, although most breathe supplementary O_2 to prevent life-threatening hypoxia. Patients with hypercapnia from chronic respiratory failure frequently complain of headaches and drowsiness; these symptoms are probably attributable to the potent cerebral vasodilating effect of excess CO_2. In addition, patients with chronic hypercapnia may have papilledema, muscular twitching, coarse myoclonic jerky motions, and asterixis. At times, the neurologic findings simulate those of a brain tumor.

TREATMENT OF ACUTE RESPIRATORY FAILURE

The time course of worsening abnormalities varies in patients with acute respiratory failure from almost instantaneous (flail chest, pulmonary embolism) to a gradual crescendo during a period of several hours or even days (respiratory tract infections, bronchial asthma). The demands for treatment and the speed with which it must be provided obviously differ from one patient to another. It is difficult to generalize about such an extremely variable clinical condition, but the principles of treatment of acute respiratory failure are as follows: *first*, establish an airway, administer O_2, and maintain adequate alveolar ventilation; *second*, identify and treat the underlying condition and monitor the patient's progress carefully.

Establish an Airway

The upper airway tends to be occluded in unconscious patients because of relaxation of the oropharyngeal muscles and tongue and the presence of saliva, vomitus, and other secretions. When respiratory arrest occurs away from medical facilities, clear all material from the oropharynx and place the victim on his or her back with the head tilted backward as far as possible and extend the jaw forward. Sometimes these simple maneuvers are all that is required to enable breathing to resume spontaneously. If it does not, start mouth-to-mouth breathing; after three or four quick full breaths without allowing time for deflation to occur, maintain deep breaths once every five seconds until the emergency is over.

An airway can be established by three different methods: an oropharyngeal tube, an endotracheal tube passed via the nose or mouth, and a tracheostomy. Selection of the procedure depends on available facilities and personnel and on the site and severity of the obstruction.

OROPHARYNGEAL AIRWAY. An oropharyngeal airway is valuable in unconscious patients who are breathing spontaneously (e.g., during recovery from general anesthesia, after a cerebrovascular accident). An oropharyngeal airway is also useful in patients who are apneic during emergency resuscitation but who are receiving some form of assisted ventilation (mouth-to-mouth respiration, bag-mask system). Although an oropharyngeal tube is commonly used in these clinical circumstances, its role must be viewed as temporary, either while the patient is waking up or until an endotracheal tube can be inserted.

ENDOTRACHEAL TUBE. The preferred method of establishing an airway in most emergencies is with an endotracheal tube. Once inserted, the tube is used to remove secretions and to provide ventilation. Endotracheal tubes can usually be passed quickly through the nose or, at times, through the mouth into the trachea by an experienced person; the airway is then sealed by inflating a balloon near the tip of the tube. Endotracheal tubes should be used in nearly all patients with acute respiratory failure severe enough to require control of their airways.

TRACHEOSTOMY. Emergency tracheostomy was formerly the only way of quickly establishing an airway in patients with acute respiratory failure. Now, emergency tracheostomy is contraindicated except in one clinical situation: acute obstruction of upper airways (e.g., from foreign bodies, trauma, or inflammation). Otherwise, intubation with an endotracheal tube is the treatment of choice for acute respiratory failure. Tracheostomy, if needed, can be performed electively at a later time in the operating room under ideal conditions. There is virtually no mortality and very little morbidity with an elective tracheostomy, in contrast to the high incidence of complications associated with emergency tracheostomy performed at the bedside.

The decision to convert a satisfactory endotracheal intubation to a tracheostomy is not an easy one and must be individualized in each case. The availability of tubes of inert plastic with low pressure cuffs permits endotracheal tubes to be used for weeks rather than days without prohibitive injury; the main mechanical difference between endotracheal and tracheostomy tubes is the trauma to the vocal cords from the former and problems related to the stoma in the latter. The usual reasons for performing a tracheostomy in a patient with a satisfactory endotracheal tube are (1) failure to control secretions (sometimes it is difficult to suction the lungs adequately, especially the left side, through a long endotracheal tube) and (2) the need for prolonged (i.e., several weeks) intubation for assisted ventilation and/or removal of secretions (these circumstances are uncommon but occur particularly in patients with neuromuscular disease and chest wall injuries).

The presence of a tube and its cuff in the airways can cause necrosis of the mucosa of the trachea; at times the entire airway wall may be eroded with penetration of the esophagus (tracheoesophageal fistula) or a neighboring blood vessel (innominate artery), causing severe hemorrhage. Delayed complications after extubation are caused by damage to the trachea or larynx from the tube or cuff; injury to the vocal cords merely impairs phonation, but serious and life-threatening obstruction to airflow can result from stenosis or malacia of the tracheal wall. These complications should be considered and evaluated in any patient who complains of persisting hoarseness or who develops breathlessness or stridor at any time after endotracheal intubation.

HUMIDIFICATION. Insertion of an endotracheal or tracheostomy tube bypasses the normal source of humidification of the inspired air. When this occurs and unhumidified air or gas mixture is breathed, the result is drying of the mucosa and impairment of mucociliary clearance. Thus as long as the upper airway is bypassed, patients must receive air or a mixture of O_2 that is fully saturated with water vapor at their body temperature. This is easily accomplished if the patient is being ventilated with most commercial ventilators that have heated humidifiers in the circuit. If the patient is breathing spontaneously, humidified gas can be delivered through a T-piece connected to the endotracheal or tracheostomy tube. When proper humidification is carried out, remember that there is *no* insensible water loss through the respiratory tract when evaluating the patient's daily fluid balance.

Administer Oxygen

Acute respiratory failure, by definition, includes decreased arterial P_{O_2}. When respiratory failure is severe, death results from the central nervous system or cardiovascular consequences of hypoxia. During emergencies, supplementary O_2 is given without worrying about the concentration being used; in general, the higher the concentration of O_2, the better. After the patient's emergency condition has stabilized, attention is directed to administering O_2 in the lowest possible concentration required to correct the hypoxia. Any more O_2 than required to raise arterial P_{O_2} to a safe level exposes the patient to the direct toxicity of O_2 on the lung parenchyma and other undesirable effects: suppression of alveolar macrophage function and mucociliary clearance. In patients with chronic obstructive pulmonary disease, especially those with chronic hypercapnia, the administration of O_2 is likely to worsen the CO_2 retention. The further increase in P_{CO_2} can be explained in part by suppression of pre-existing hypoxic ventilatory drive; the remaining increase can be accounted for through the effects of O_2 on tidal volume and the timing of inspiration. In general, the higher the inspired O_2 concentration, the greater the CO_2 retention; this observation underlies the use of "low-flow" O_2 for these patients as described below under Treatment of Chronic Respiratory Failure.

The usual goal of O_2 therapy in acute respiratory failure is to raise arterial P_{O_2} to between 60 and 80 mm Hg. Because these values lie on the flat portion of the oxyhemoglobin dissociation curve, most of the available hemoglobin is saturated with O_2; raising arterial P_{O_2} values even higher adds very little additional O_2 to the blood and may require increases in alveolar P_{O_2} concentrations to toxic levels. At times, especially when the mechanism of arterial hypoxia is right-to-left shunting of blood, arterial P_{O_2} may be considerably less than 60 mm Hg even with the patient breathing 100 per cent O_2. When this occurs, other maneuvers such as addition of end-expiratory pressure are required to raise arterial P_{O_2} and to allow a reduction in inspired O_2 concentration.

There are several ways of giving supplementary O_2 to a patient. Which method is chosen depends on the cause and severity of the arterial hypoxia and convenience to the patient. It is important to emphasize that no method can be relied upon to produce a certain increase in arterial P_{O_2}; the response depends on which physiologic mechanism(s) is responsible for the hypoxia. Thus it is always advisable to monitor the effects of O_2 administration by serial analyses of arterial blood.

NASAL CANNULAS OR PRONGS. The concentration of O_2 in the inspired air can be enriched by nasal cannulas, catheters, or prongs. These devices work well even when patients breathe through their mouths. However, because of the drying effects of unhumidified O_2 on the nasal mucous membranes, if $>$3 to 5 liters per minute is needed to achieve satisfactory arterial oxygenation, other methods of administration are advisable.

VENTURI MASKS. These masks work on the principle of entrainment of a fixed proportion of air that mixes with the O_2 being supplied and results in a constant inspired concentration: 24, 28, 35, or 40 per cent O_2. Although a properly used Venturi mask ensures that the inspired O_2 concentration is constant, the effects on arterial P_{O_2} vary considerably from one patient to another. The mask is somewhat uncomfortable and must be removed for eating and drinking. Because of these disadvantages and high cost, other simpler and cheaper methods usually suffice to deliver relatively low (21 to 41 per cent) concentrations of O_2.

RESERVOIR MASKS. When high concentrations of O_2 (40 to 80 per cent) are needed in patients who are not intubated, reservoir masks are used. To ensure optimal efficiency of operation, the masks must be tight fitting to avoid leaks; because this often causes discomfort, it is difficult to deliver high concentrations of O_2 by reservoir masks for long periods.

OTHER METHODS. Most of the recently developed mechanical ventilators have regulators that can be set to deliver an inspired O_2 concentration that ranges from 21 to 100 per cent. One of the best ways of ensuring that patients actually receive high concentrations of O_2 (60 to 100 per cent) is to use a mechanical ventilator connected to an endotracheal or tracheostomy tube.

Maintain Alveolar Ventilation

Emergency resuscitation after respiratory arrest requires ventilation by mouth-to-mouth respiration or a bag and mask device. As soon as possible thereafter, if the patient does not resume spontaneous breathing, intubation and ventilation by a mechanical ventilator are indicated. Similar considerations apply to patients with acute respiratory failure whose breathing is insufficient to maintain adequate gas exchange. The main indications for mechanical ventilation are ventilatory failure, shown by an elevated or rising P_{CO_2}, or severe refractory hypoxia, shown by a low P_{O_2} that cannot be corrected without high concentrations of O_2 and often end-expiratory pressure. Special indications include the need to produce alkalosis, as in head injuries and certain drug overdoses, to stabilize the thorax, as in traumatic injuries that result in flail chest, or to aspirate secretions, as in bronchopulmonary infections and failure to cough.

MECHANICAL VENTILATION. Two types of mechanical ventilators can be used to provide assisted ventilation: pressure ventilators, in which a certain (adjustable) airway pressure is reached by the machine during each breathing cycle, or volume ventilators, in which a constant (adjustable) tidal volume is delivered to the patient with each breath. Most commercially available ventilators of both types can be set either to cycle automatically or to assist breathing once it is initiated by the patient. Most instruments also provide means of controlling inspiratory and expiratory flow rates. Pressure ventilators were widely used for many years, but almost all hospitals now use volume ventilators, which are more versatile and more reliable.

END-EXPIRATORY PRESSURE. Mechanical ventilators ordinarily raise airway pressure during inspiration and allow it to fall to zero (atmospheric) pressure during expiration; this pattern of assisted ventilation is known as intermittent positive pressure ventilation, or IPPV. At times, it is desirable to add positive pressure to the airway during expiration as well as inspiration to hold the lung at a higher end-expiratory lung volume (functional residual capacity) than it would reach at zero end-expiratory pressure; this pattern of assisted ventilation is known as continuous positive pressure ventilation, or CPPV. Keeping the lung at a high end-expiratory lung volume prevents closure of alveoli and airways during expiration, redistributes pulmonary edema fluid out of alveoli, and often improves arterial Po_2 considerably. Positive end-expiratory pressure (or PEEP) is most useful in patients with the conditions that cause the adult respiratory distress syndrome (Table 72–1).

Although end-expiratory pressure usually results in an improvement in arterial Po_2 and O_2 content, it may also decrease cardiac output by impairing venous return. Accordingly, the actual delivery of O_2 to the tissues of the body may decrease. Thus it is important to monitor both the respiratory and circulatory responses to end-expiratory pressure to determine the optimal amount of pressure and the need for additional therapeutic interventions. Another common and serious hazard of end-expiratory pressure is its tendency to cause spontaneous pneumothorax and pneumomediastinum.

Identify and Treat the Underlying Condition

Acute respiratory failure always has a precipitating cause. Consequently, the cause of the condition should be identified as soon as possible after emergency measures have been started and the patient's condition has stabilized. Usually, the diagnosis can be established easily by a thorough history and physical examination, analysis of the blood and urine, and chest roentgenogram. Helpful auxiliary tests include those that evaluate central nervous system or cardiac function, those that determine the presence of drugs or poisons in the body, and bacteriologic study of secretions and blood.

Treatment obviously depends on the underlying cause, and the reader is referred to the appropriate chapters of this book for information about the therapy of specific pulmonary and other disorders that lead to acute respiratory failure. In all patients with acute respiratory failure, careful attention should be paid to fluid balance. Overhydration is a frequent and serious complication that can usually be avoided by careful attention to fluid replacement and, when needed, monitoring of pulmonary capillary (wedge) pressure.

Many patients cared for in intensive care units are nutritionally depleted at the time of admission or become so soon afterward. Because morbidity and mortality are closely linked to nutritional status, it is important that this be assessed and, when necessary, treated by appropriate enteral or parenteral supplementation.

Monitor the Patient's Progress

The need for monitoring varies from patient to patient according to the response to initial treatment. If the disorder is readily reversible (e.g., bronchial asthma), the patient may respond sufficiently to go home shortly after being seen and treated. Other less rapidly responding conditions causing acute respiratory failure often require hospital care, and seriously ill patients are best treated in special acute care facilities (intensive care units) when available. Intensive care units provide an institutional focus of trained personnel and special equipment for the care of critically ill patients.

All seriously ill patients should have frequent measurements of blood pressure, constant monitoring of heart rate, careful recording of fluid intake and output, and determination of weight daily. Arterial blood gas analysis should be performed as often as needed but usually at least once daily. Special studies include measurement of cardiac output and placement of a Swan-Ganz catheter in the pulmonary artery for determination of pulmonary arterial and wedge pressures and sampling of mixed venous blood; this information is very helpful in guiding fluid replacement and ventilator adjustments, including levels of end-expiratory pressure. In general, wedge pressure values should be maintained in the normal range (5 to 10 mm Hg) and not allowed to increase above 15 mm Hg, especially in patients with the adult respiratory distress syndrome. Less reliance is being placed now, compared with previous years, on values of mixed venous Po_2 as a guide to O_2 delivery, especially in disorders such as sepsis and the adult respiratory distress syndrome. Attention is currently directed at improving O_2 delivery by increasing cardiac output through pharmacologic means or by increasing O_2 content through transfusions of packed red blood cells.

TREATMENT OF CHRONIC RESPIRATORY FAILURE

Patients with chronic lung disease often have sufficient alterations in their arterial Po_2 and Pco_2 values that they are said to be in chronic respiratory failure. Therapeutic regimens for these patients, whose disease is relatively stable, are delivered mainly on an outpatient basis and are designed to meet two objectives: (1) preventing or minimizing the number and severity of the intercurrent complications that would otherwise occur and (2) treating maximally all reversible elements of the underlying disorder. Many of the specific remedies are used for both purposes, and the approaches to preventive and maintenance therapy for patients with the most common chronic lung diseases, asthma, bronchitis, and emphysema, are discussed in Ch. 60 and 61.

Despite emphasis on preventing intercurrent complications, these attacks continue to plague the lives of patients with chronic lung disease. Acute episodes of bronchopulmonary infection, pneumothorax, pulmonary embolism, surgical procedures, and misuse of sedatives all add their effects to those of the underlying lung disease and frequently produce serious disturbances of blood gases. These episodes are potentially life threatening, are usually associated with prolonged morbidity, and frequently require hospitalization. The principles of therapy are to maintain oxygenation while treating all new, presumably reversible, elements of the disease in an effort to restore the patient to his or her former state of health.

Oxygen

Patients with chronic obstructive lung disease and superimposed episodes of acute respiratory failure nearly always have severe hypoxia from a combination of hypoventilation and ventilation-perfusion mismatching. Typical arterial blood values are Po_2 of approximately 30 mm Hg, Pco_2 of 70 mm Hg, and pH of 7.30. Neither the hypercapnia nor the acidemia is life threatening, but the hypoxia is potentially fatal. Thus treatment is directed mainly at alleviating the disturbance in oxygenation; the changes in Pco_2 and pH will return to the ordinary values for that patient as the acute condition improves. In view of the possibility that O_2 therapy may depress ventilation further by withdrawing the hypoxic stimulus to breathe and affecting the pattern of breathing, O_2 is given initially in low concentrations (1 to 3 liters per minute). The goal is to raise Po_2 to satisfactory levels (50 to 60 mm Hg) without depressing ventilation to the extent that unacceptable increases in Pco_2 and decreases in pH (particularly) occur.

The O_2 is usually started at 2 liters per minute, and an arterial blood specimen is analyzed 15 to 30 minutes later to determine the patient's response. Depending on the Po_2 value, the flow of O_2 can be adjusted. If hypoventilation and acidemia result from too much O_2 (e.g., Po_2 80 mm Hg, Pco_2 80 mm Hg, and pH 7.25), the supplementary O_2 should *not* be discontinued but the flow rate should be decreased. This is necessary because the Po_2 decreases much faster than the stimulus to breathe returns, and cardiac arrest or other serious complications of hypoxia may result.

Intubation-Assisted Ventilation

Low-flow O_2 given in the manner described provides satisfactory relief of hypoxia in nearly all instances. Although the goal of low-flow O_2 is an arterial Po_2 of 50 to 60 mm Hg, at times one has to be satisfied with 40 to 50 mm Hg. When oxygenation cannot be achieved without intolerable hypercapnia and acidemia, the decision whether to intubate and ventilate the patient must be made. Experience with intubation and mechanical ventilation in this group of patients has been extremely unrewarding, particularly because of the prolonged need for assisted ventilation once intubation is performed and the poor prognosis for lengthy survival and return to useful life after recovery from the acute episode. Although each case must be considered individually, in general, patients with chronic obstructive pulmonary disease who develop superimposed acute respiratory failure should not be intubated. The major exception to this axiom is the need for ventilator support during the postoperative period. Doxapram (see Respiratory Stimulants, below) often allows administration of "extra" O_2 without depressing ventilatory drive.

Bronchodilators

Most intercurrent episodes of acute respiratory failure in patients with chronic obstructive pulmonary disease are associated with increased airways resistance from the presence of secretions, edema of the mucosa, and bronchospasm. Because it is impossible to discriminate among these, bronchodilator drugs are always included in the treatment regimen to take advantage of the reversibility of whatever element of bronchospasm is present.

When patients seek medical attention for intercurrent attacks, they frequently have already tried—and failed to respond to—oral and aerosolized bronchodilators. In this circumstance, intravenous aminophylline is a useful drug. Aminophylline can be injected slowly in 250-mg or 500-mg boluses, or, if the patient has been hospitalized and prolonged treatment is envisioned, by a loading dose (5.6 mg per kilogram of body weight) and constant sustaining infusion (0.9 mg per kilogram of body weight per hour). These dosages should be reduced in patients who have been receiving aminophylline, who are elderly, or, especially, who have liver disease or heart failure. It is advisable to determine the aminophylline plasma level at the outset in those who have been taking the drug and 24 to 36 hours after the constant infusion regimen has been started to ensure that values are in the therapeutic range (10 to 20 μg per milliliter) and to avoid toxicity.

Selective $beta_2$ sympathomimetic drugs, usually administered by aerosol, are another mainstay of treatment. Because aerosolized drugs fail to penetrate effectively throughout the tracheobronchial system in the presence of airways secretions and severe narrowing, they are given more frequently than is customary, usually at 1- or 2-hour intervals for the first 12 to 24 hours.

The indications for and dosage of corticosteroids in this clinical setting are controversial, although there is an increasing tendency to use these drugs in virtually all patients with asthma or chronic obstructive lung disease whose exacerbation is severe enough to warrant hospitalization. Either methylprednisolone, 60 mg, or hydrocortisone, 100 mg, intravenously every six hours is indicated. Much higher doses of corticosteroids (e.g., methylprednisolone, 15 mg per kilogram of body weight per day in divided doses) have been recommended, but there is no evidence to suggest that these are more efficacious in this clinical setting than the lower doses recommended above.

Antimicrobials

Infections are the most frequent and important cause of acute respiratory failure in patients with chronic underlying lung disease. Intercurrent attacks usually begin as a typical cold, with rhinitis, pharyngitis, and headaches. Shortly afterward, lower respiratory involvement appears with increasing cough, sputum production, purulence, wheezing, and breathlessness. These episodes occur several times a year in most patients with chronic obstructive pulmonary disease. (It should be noted that fever, leukocytosis, and new roentgenographic infiltrations are uncommon in this syndrome.) When airway infection is present, the sputum is not only purulent but usually contains numerous microorganisms detectable by Gram's stain of the secretions. Sputum cultures, however, often fail to reveal pathogenic bacteria, although at times *Streptococcus pneumoniae* and/or *Hemophilus influenzae* may be grown. Regardless of the presence or absence of identifiable pathogens, oral treatment with ampicillin (250 to 500 mg every six hours), a combined preparation of trimethoprim-sulfamethoxazole (160 mg and 800 mg, respectively, every 12 hours), or tetracycline (250 to 500 mg every six hours) frequently results in decreased volume of sputum, thinning of the secretions, change in sputum appearance from purulent to mucoid, and improvement in blood gases.

When pneumonia is present, signified by the presence of new infiltration(s) on the chest roentgenogram, Gram's stain of the sputum is likely to show one bacterial species predominating, and the initial selection of antimicrobials should cover this organism. Therapy can be revised, if necessary, when the results of the sputum cultures are available.

Control of Secretions

Many patients complain of thick tenacious sputum that is troublesome to clear. Although it seems desirable to attempt to alter the character of these secretions to facilitate their removal, there is no clear evidence that it is possible to do so by pharmacologic means. Iodides, enzymes, detergents, and acetylcysteine, administered orally or by aerosol, have been tried extensively, but none has been shown convincingly to be effective. Moreover, each has potential toxic side effects. Similarly, mist tents and ultrasonic nebulizers, once widely used, are seldom employed today. The best way to control secretions is to control infection with antimicrobials and to ensure adequate (but not excessive) hydration by the administration of intravenous fluids.

Patients with troublesome sputum retention may require intermittent nasotracheal suction to control the volume of secretions. Manual or mechanical percussion serves to loosen secretions and enhances their removal in patients who have retained sputum in their airways. Respiratory physical therapy, especially when carried out by a skilled therapist, may result in an increase in arterial Po_2 related to the improvement in the distribution of ventilation from clearance of sputum.

Treatment of Heart Failure

Cor pulmonale is an inevitable complication of severe chronic lung disease. Right ventricular hypertrophy followed by heart failure occurs secondary to the increased work load imposed on the ventricle by the changes in the pulmonary circulation from the effects of lung disease. Resistance to blood flow through the lungs increases when pulmonary blood vessels are destroyed (as in emphysema), obstructed (as in pulmonary thromboembolism), narrowed (from vasoconstriction), or compressed (breathing at high lung volumes), or when the blood is unusually viscous (polycythemia). Patients whose cor pulmonale is well compensated or even inapparent while their chronic lung disease is stable often develop acute right heart failure during intercurrent attacks of acute respiratory failure. Peripheral edema, increased venous pressure, and an enlarged, painful liver are important clues to the presence of acute cardiac decompensation.

Most patients with right heart failure from cor pulmonale, even if severe, have a satisfactory diuresis when put to bed, given O_2, and treated appropriately for their underlying lung disease. Diuretics may make patients feel more comfortable by diminishing peripheral edema and hepatic and gastrointestinal congestion faster than spontaneous diuresis; but if used, the drugs should be administered orally in low doses. Intravenous ethacrynic acid or furosemide can cause excessive renal loss of Cl^- that worsens existing acid-base disturbances and depletes intravascular volume sufficiently to decrease cardiac output and blood pressure. A particularly dangerous situation occurs in patients who already have coexisting nonrespiratory (metabolic) alkalosis often from Cl^--losing diuretics, in addition to their hypercapnia from chronic respiratory failure; when the measures designed to improve ventilation lower arterial P_{CO_2}, the metabolic alkalosis becomes "unmasked" and arterial pH becomes markedly alkaline. When this occurs, the patients can develop cardiac arrhythmias, become comatose, or manifest convulsive seizures or other focal neurologic abnormalities.

If an element of pulmonary edema or pulmonary vascular congestion is present from left heart failure, this may also respond to diuretics. Whether left heart failure can occur secondary to purely right-sided disease is controversial. Of greater importance are coexisting causes of left-sided involvement (e.g., valvular disease, coronary atherosclerosis); furthermore, chronic hypoxia and severe polycythemia may impair left ventricular as well as right ventricular function.

Present evidence indicates that digitalis preparations are not beneficial in patients with cor pulmonale. Also, the use of digitalis is hazardous in patients with chronic respiratory failure owing to the sudden shifts in acid-base balance and electrolyte concentrations that may occur in these patients. Therefore digitalis drugs should be used only in patients with digitalis-responsive arrhythmias or coexisting left heart failure.

Respiratory Stimulants

With few exceptions, respiratory stimulants are obsolete. Nikethamide, picrotoxin, and ethamivan have been replaced by other less hazardous and more efficient methods of maintaining ventilation. Doxapram, a drug that works by stimulating carotid chemoreceptors rather than neurons in the brain, appears to be much safer than centrally acting stimulants. The chief use of doxapram is to minimize or prevent the depression of ventilation, with consequent increase in P_{CO_2} and decrease in pH, that occurs in some hypoxic patients with hypercapnia who are given O_2 to breathe. Almitrine, another drug that stimulates the carotid chemoreceptors but that can be administered orally, is widely used in Europe to improve arterial P_{O_2} in outpatients with chronic respiratory failure. This drug has not been approved by the Food and Drug Administration at the time of publication.

Sedation

All sedative drugs should be avoided in patients with chronic lung disease and intercurrent acute respiratory failure, including diazepam (Valium) and chlordiazepoxide (Librium), which can suppress ventilation. Exceptions to this cardinal rule are made from time to time, but usually only when the patient is being mechanically ventilated and sedation is required to enable breathing synchronous with the machine.

Postoperative Complications

Patients with chronic respiratory failure are high-risk operative candidates. Moreover, the closer the surgical incision to the thorax, the higher the incidence of postoperative complications. Despite this caveat, it is safe to say that virtually *all* patients who have respiratory failure can safely undergo *non*thoracic surgery or *nonresectional* thoracic surgery. Postoperative complications can be anticipated and often prevented by attention to the general principles of care outlined in this chapter. Close observation and monitoring are usually required, and these can best be carried out in an intensive care unit.

Askanazi J (ed.): Nutrition and respiratory disease. Clin Chest Med 7:1, 1986. *Entire issue devoted to contribution of nutritional depletion to respiratory failure and how to prevent and treat it.*

Bone RC (ed.): Respiratory failure. Med Clin North Am 67:549, 1983. *Symposium of 13 articles that cover the most important topics related to respiratory failure.*

Brandstetter RD: The adult respiratory distress syndrome. Heart Lung 15:155, 1986. *Up-to-date review with 94 references.*

Robin ED: The cult of the Swan-Ganz catheter: Overuse and abuse of pulmonary flow catheters. Ann Intern Med 103:445, 1985. *Appropriate cautionary message that applies to all kinds of invasive monitoring devices.*

Zapol WM, Falke KJ (eds.): Acute Respiratory Failure. New York, Marcel Dekker, Inc., 1985. *Collection of comprehensive and authoritative articles with emphasis on respiratory failure following acute lung injury.*

PART VIII
CRITICAL CARE MEDICINE

73 CRITICAL CARE MEDICINE

Philip C. Hopewell

The practice of critical care medicine involves virtually all areas in general internal medicine. Severe illness represents one end of a spectrum of pathophysiologic derangement that shades into less severe illness related to the same organ systems. The same basic diagnostic and therapeutic principles therefore apply. A wide variety of clinical problems are commonly encountered in critical care units, many of which are discussed in other chapters. This section will focus on areas in critical care medicine that are not extensively described elsewhere in this text and on the aspects of medical care that are unique to critical care units.

In the critically ill patient, the interdependence of organ systems must remain in sharp focus. Limited attention to one component of the illness, even if that component is predominant, frequently will yield a therapeutic approach that is detrimental to the patient as a whole. Commonly, management of the critically ill patient presents extremely difficult dilemmas. For example, treatment directed toward reducing the pulmonary capillary wedge pressure in patients with the adult respiratory distress syndrome may adversely affect renal and central nervous system perfusion. Conversely, increasing the pulmonary artery wedge pressure to optimize cardiac output in a patient with ischemic heart disease may result in noncardiogenic pulmonary edema if there has been a pre-existing acute diffuse lung injury. Bronchodilating agents may increase cardiac irritability and therefore cause significant arrhythmias, particularly in the presence of hypoxemia or acid-base disturbances or both. Nephrotoxic antimicrobial agents may be essential in the treatment of sepsis in a patient with pre-existing or acute renal disease. The physician who is primarily responsible for the care of a gravely ill patient often must synthesize an overall diagnostic and treatment strategy that incorporates the views of various consultants with a more narrow focus and reconcile the conflicting effects of their recommendations.

ATTRIBUTES OF A CRITICAL CARE UNIT

A critical care unit is defined by its ability to provide the environment, facilities, and personnel for the care of severely ill patients. The important features required of such a unit are listed in Table 73–1.

TABLE 73–1. UNIQUE FEATURES OF CRITICAL CARE UNITS

1. High nurse-to-patient ratio
2. Ready accessibility of physicians
3. Ability to provide invasive hemodynamic monitoring
4. Availability of respiratory support techniques
5. Ability to provide supervised continuous intravenous infusions of pharmacologic agents

Critical care units may have a general orientation, treating all types of severely ill patients, or be more specialized, accepting only specific categories of patients as defined by the type of illness (for example, burn units), organ system involved (coronary and acute neurologic care units), specialty service designation (medical and surgical units), or patient age (neonatal intensive care units). In addition to the basic attributes listed in Table 73–1, specialized units provide medical personnel specifically skilled in the area of care provided by the unit and have available particular forms of technology with applications generally limited to the category of patients accepted by the unit.

Critical care units usually need administrative policies and procedures that differ from those of standard hospital units. Because of the gravity of illness of their patients, critical care units require clear delineation of administrative and medical lines of authority and responsibility. Likewise, there must be at least general guidelines for admission and discharge of patients, specifically described nursing roles, standing orders, and a program of continuing staff education. The existence of such policies reduces the apparent ambiguity often inherent in the difficult environment of a critical care unit and enables prompt decision making by both physicians and nurses.

Greenbaum DM: Standards for critical care medicine. *In* Shoemaker WC, Thompson WL, Holbrook PR (eds.): Textbook of Critical Care. Philadelphia, W. B. Saunders Company, 1984, pp 1004–1005. *Provides a summary description of facilities, personnel, and services available in critical care units in the United States.*

National Institutes of Health. Consensus development of conference on critical care medicine. Crit Care Med 11:466, 1983. *This report summarizes the discussions of a large consensus development group that addressed issues of critical care unit utilization, organization, training of personnel, and research needs.*

GENERAL PRINCIPLES OF ASSESSMENT OF SEVERE RESPIRATORY DYSFUNCTION

The discussion in this section will focus on the techniques of assessment generally applicable to severely ill patients in whom it usually is neither possible nor desirable to perform elaborate comprehensive assessments of pulmonary function. Patients often cannot cooperate, and measurements made under non–steady-state conditions are generally inaccurate. The basic components of normal respiratory function are discussed in Ch. 59 and the characteristic abnormalities of various types of lung disorders in other chapters of Part VII.

Nonspecific Indicators of Severity

Respiratory rate is perhaps the simplest measurement that can be made. Although influenced by many factors, the respiratory rate provides a general indication of cardiorespiratory function and may be the first clue to impending or early respiratory failure. In addition, periodic counting of respiratory rate serves as a simple monitoring technique.

The degree of pulsus paradoxus correlates with the forced expiratory volume in 1 second (FEV_1) in patients with acute airways obstruction and therefore may indicate the severity of airways narrowing. Similarly, the presence of suprasternal, supraclavicular, and intercostal space retractions also correlates roughly with the degree of airways obstruction.

The mental status of the patient is an important, albeit even more nonspecific, indicator of the status of cardiorespiratory function. Behavioral alterations may reflect changes in the partial pressure of oxygen (Pa_{O_2}) and carbon dioxide (Pa_{CO_2}) in arterial blood.

Measurements of Lung Function

The lung function studies applicable in severely ill patients are rather limited. Depending on the type and severity of illness and the patient's ability to cooperate, one may measure vital capacity (VC), maximal inspiratory pressure (MIP), timed forced expiratory volume, and peak expiratory flow rate (PEFR).

The vital capacity is the maximal volume of air that can be slowly exhaled after maximal inspiration and as such provides an indication of the patient's ventilatory capability (Fig. 59–2). The VC is influenced by the respiratory neuromuscular system, the chest wall, the elastic properties of the lung, and the caliber of the airways. It cannot therefore be used to identify specific abnormalities. Nevertheless, it is particularly helpful in assessing and following patients with neuromuscular illnesses and in evaluating patients being mechanically ventilated to determine if it is feasible to consider weaning from the ventilator. A minimal acceptable VC is 10 to 15 ml per kilogram of body weight.

The maximal inspiratory pressure is somewhat analogous to the VC in the information that it provides and the factors by which it is influenced. However, the ability to generate an acceptable inspiratory pressure, less (more negative) than −20 cm H_2O, does not necessarily imply that the VC will be adequate.

The timed forced expiratory volume, which is usually expressed as the forced expiratory volume in 1 second (FEV_1) over the forced vital capacity (FVC), measures the severity of airways obstruction in patients with asthma or chronic airways obstruction. The measurement may not be possible in patients with severe airways obstruction who have marked tachypnea. However, it does provide the best objective indicator of the degree of airways obstruction and, when measured serially, the response to therapy. Absolute FEV_1 values of less than 0.75 liter or less than 25 per cent of the predicted value are commonly associated with increased Pa_{CO_2} values and hence are indicative of severe obstruction.

Peak expiratory flow rate provides information similar to the FEV_1 in patients with airways obstruction. It has the distinct advantage of not requiring a full inhalation followed by a full forced exhalation, a maneuver that may actually worsen airways obstruction. The PEFR is measured by having the patient slowly inhale and then blow a short forced puff through the flowmeter, a maneuver similar to a cough. Values below 60 liters per minute are indicative of severe obstruction.

Arterial Blood Gas and pH Measurements

The *Pa_{O_2}, Pa_{CO_2}, and arterial pH* provide the most informative indication of integrated cardiorespiratory function. These values are not particularly sensitive to early cardiorespiratory abnormalities and are not specific for the kind of abnormality present, but they provide crucial information in patients with severe dysfunction. The mechanisms of normal gas exchange and its abnormalities are discussed in Ch. 59. This section will focus on the interpretation of arterial blood gas and pH values in the assessment of severely ill patients and how these interpretations can be used to ascertain the pathophysiology and indicate the proper approach to treatment.

HYPOXEMIA. Clinically significant reductions in Pa_{O_2} can result from *hypoventilation*, *mismatching of ventilation to perfusion*, and *shunting*. It is important to determine which of these mechanisms is operative in a given patient.

Hypoventilation as the cause of hypoxemia implies that the lung itself is normal and that the only necessary therapeutic goal is improved ventilation. This type of hypoxemia is characterized by a normal alveolar-to-arterial P_{O_2} difference ($P(A\text{-}a)_{O_2}$). The $P(A\text{-}a)_{O_2}$ can be determined by using the alveolar gas equation (Equation 5) to calculate $P_{A_{O_2}}$ and by measuring Pa_{O_2}. In patients breathing room air, the difference should not be greater than 10 mm Hg, and with an increased fractional concentration of oxygen in inspired gas ($F_{I_{O_2}}$) sufficient to cause a $P_{A_{O_2}}$ of 200 mm Hg or greater, the $P(A\text{-}a)_{O_2}$ should not be greater than 40 mm Hg.

Ventilation-perfusion mismatching and *shunting* can be distinguished by measuring the response to administration of 100 per cent oxygen. The Pa_{O_2} will increase normally to values of nearly 600 mm Hg if the hypoxemia is due purely to mismatching, whereas with a shunt the increase may be markedly reduced, depending on the magnitude of the shunt flow. Figure 73–1 shows the relationship between Pa_{O_2} and $F_{I_{O_2}}$ with different shunt fractions, and Figure 73–2 demonstrates the effect of increasing amounts of mismatching of ventilation to

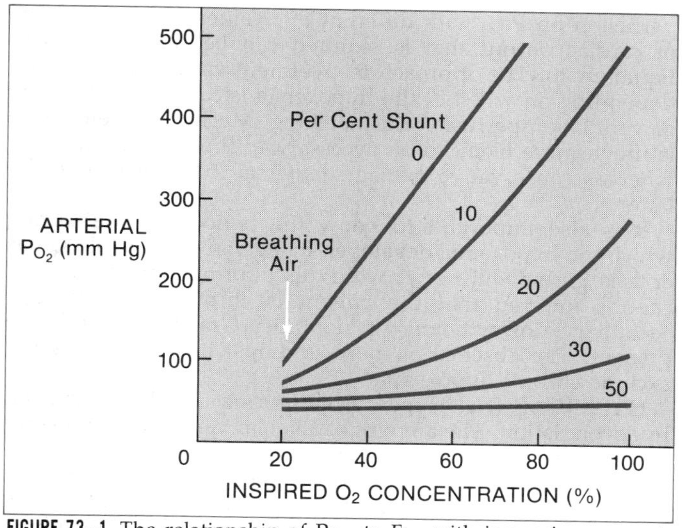

FIGURE 73–1. The relationship of Pa_{O_2} to $F_{I_{O_2}}$ with increasing amounts of shunt. Note that with 30 per cent of the cardiac output being shunted there is only a slight increase in Pa_{O_2} with increasing $F_{I_{O_2}}$ and with 50 per cent shunting, there is no increase in Pa_{O_2}. (From West JR: Pulmonary Pathophysiology: The Essentials. Copyright 1977, Baltimore, The Williams and Wilkins Company.)

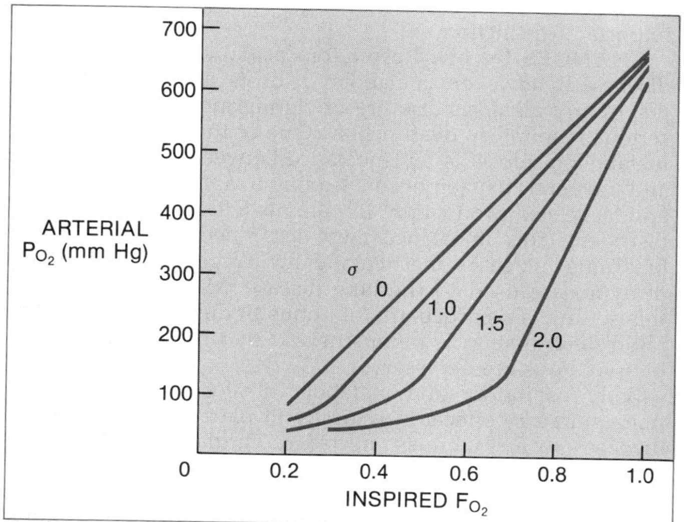

FIGURE 73–2. The relationship of Pa_{O_2} to $F_{I_{O_2}}$ with increasing amounts of ventilation to perfusion mismatching (σ = standard deviation of log normal distribution of ventilation and perfusion). Note that even with marked mismatching the Pa_{O_2} increases to nearly normal values with very high $F_{I_{O_2}}$. (From West JR: Pulmonary Pathophysiology: The Essentials. Copyright 1977, Baltimore, The Williams and Wilkins Company.)

perfusion on Pa_{O_2} with different FI_{O_2} values. The percentage of cardiac output that is shunted can be calculated using Equation 10. The approach to treatment varies considerably, depending on whether the hypoxemia is caused by shunting or ventilation-perfusion mismatching. Mechanical ventilation is much more likely to be necessary in the former situation, whereas conservative management may be sufficient in the latter.

It is also important to know the period of time during which the hypoxemia developed in a given patient. Blood gas criteria per se will not provide this information; however, it can be inferred that the patient is chronically hypoxic if secondary polycythemia or right heart failure or both are present. The absence of these findings, however, does not exclude chronic hypoxemia.

HYPERCAPNIA. Hypercapnia is caused only by alveolar hypoventilation. The amount of alveolar ventilation necessary to eliminate carbon dioxide and maintain a normal Pa_{CO_2} will vary depending on carbon dioxide production in accordance with Equation 1. Alveolar ventilation will in turn be influenced by the amount of wasted ventilation as shown in Equation 4. Thus, increases in Pa_{CO_2} can occur because of increased production of carbon dioxide or increased wasted ventilation or both.

The relationship between Pa_{CO_2} and blood bicarbonate concentration determines the arterial pH, as indicated by the Henderson-Hasselbalch equation (Equation 13). The relationship between Pa_{CO_2} and arterial pH varies, however, depending on the time during which the Pa_{CO_2} has been increased and its rate of increase. Thus, by examining the relationships among Pa_{CO_2}, arterial pH, and $[HCO_3^-]$, the acuteness or chronicity of the carbon dioxide elevation can be inferred. Acute increases in Pa_{CO_2} are accompanied by only small increases in $[HCO_3^-]$ and arterial pH changes in a nearly linear fashion with Pa_{CO_2}. There is approximately a 0.0075 pH unit change in the opposite direction for every 1-mm Hg change in Pa_{CO_2}. Thus, an acute rise in Pa_{CO_2} from 40 mm Hg to 60 mm Hg would be expected to cause a decrease in arterial pH to 7.25. Over a period of one to three days, however, renal bicarbonate retention causes the $[HCO_3^-]$ to increase and buffer the arterial pH change. Thus, for a given change in Pa_{CO_2} the change in arterial pH is much less than when the change occurs acutely. These relationships are shown in Figure 73–3. Obviously the therapeutic implication of an acute as opposed to a chronic change in Pa_{CO_2} makes this an important distinction.

CHANGES IN pH. Respiratory acidosis has already been discussed; however, metabolic acidosis and metabolic and respiratory alkalosis also are of significance in patients with serious respiratory dysfunction. One of the several causes of metabolic acidosis is an imbalance between oxygen delivery and metabolic oxygen needs, leading to anaerobic metabolism and lactic acid production. In patients with severe respiratory disorders, this imbalance may occur because the work of breathing increases the demand for oxygen in the presence of hypoxia caused by the lung disease. Metabolic acidosis in this setting is a particularly ominous finding, suggesting that rapid deterioration is imminent and that prompt therapeutic interventions are necessary.

Both respiratory and metabolic alkalosis have important nonrespiratory effects in critically ill patients. Alkalosis predisposes to arrhythmias, decreases cardiac output, and reduces the seizure threshold. Hypocapnia per se with or without alkalosis reduces cerebral blood flow and may depress the level of consciousness. For these reasons alkalosis should be recognized as an important acid-base disturbance and corrective measures should be taken.

Calculations of Respiratory Variables

A number of equations and calculations are helpful in the assessment of respiratory function. Only brief descriptions of

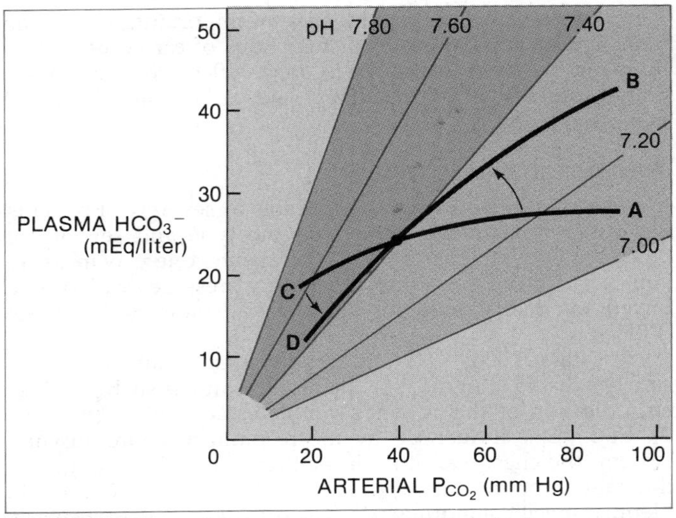

FIGURE 73–3. Effects of acute and chronic variations in Pa_{CO_2} on plasma HCO_3^- and pH. The line connecting points A and C represents the effects of an acute change in Pa_{CO_2} to a value above or below 40 mm Hg. Renal compensation over time results in a shift of the relationship to that represented by the line connecting points B and D as is indicated by the arrows. (From Murray JF: The Normal Lung. 2nd ed. Philadelphia, W. B. Saunders Company, 1986.)

the physiologic principles involved with the equations will be presented in this section.

Representative normal values for selected cardiorespiratory variables are listed in Table 73–2.

EQUATIONS RELATED TO VENTILATION. Arterial P_{CO_2} is related directly to carbon dioxide production ($\dot{V}_{CO_2}$ in milliliters per minute) and inversely to alveolar ventilation ($\dot{V}_A$ in liters per minute) as follows:

$$Pa_{CO_2} = K\frac{\dot{V}_{CO_2}}{\dot{V}_A} \qquad (1)$$

where K is a constant.

The $\dot{V}_A$ is the difference between the tidal volume (V_T in liters) and the wasted or dead space ventilation (V_D) multiplied by the respiratory rate (F in breaths per minute).

$$\dot{V}_A = (V_T - V_D) \times F \qquad (2)$$

Total minute ventilation ($\dot{V}_E$ in liters per minute) is the product of V_T and F.

$$\dot{V}_E = V_T \times F \qquad (3)$$

TABLE 73–2. REPRESENTATIVE NORMAL VALUES FOR SELECTED RESPIRATORY AND HEMODYNAMIC VARIABLES

	Normal
Pa_{O_2}	95 mm Hg
Pa_{CO_2}	40 mm Hg
pH (arterial)	7.40
$P(A\text{-}a)_{O_2}$	<10 mm Hg
O_2 saturation	98%
Ca_{O_2}	19.8 ml/100 ml
$P\bar{v}_{O_2}$	40 mm Hg
$\dot{V}_{O_2}$	240 ml/min
$\dot{V}_{CO_2}$	192 ml/min
R	0.8
Respiratory rate	12
$\dot{V}_E$	6 L/min
V_D	150 ml
V_T	450 ml
V_D/V_T	.33
$\dot{Q}_T$	5 L/min
$\dot{Q}_S/\dot{Q}_T$	<7%
PVR	50–150 dyne sec/cm^5
SVR	800–1200 dyne sec/cm^5
$C\bar{v}_{O_2}$	14.6 ml/100 ml

From these three equations it can be seen that the factors determining the Pa_{CO_2} are VT, VD, F, and $\dot{V}CO_2$.

The volume of wasted ventilation can be calculated from a modification of the Bohr equation:

$$VD = \frac{(Pa_{CO_2} - Pe_{CO_2})}{Pa_{CO_2}} \times VT \quad (4)$$

where Pe_{CO_2} = the partial pressure of carbon dioxide in expired air. The VD so derived is commonly expressed as a ratio of VT. Normal values are from 0.30 to 0.35.

EQUATIONS RELATED TO OXYGENATION. The partial pressure of oxygen in the alveolus (PA_{O_2}) can be calculated from the *alveolar gas equation* as follows:

$$PA_{O_2} = FI_{O_2}\,(PB - 47) - Pa_{CO_2}/R \quad (5)$$

where R = the respiratory exchange ratio ($\dot{V}CO_2/\dot{V}O_2$), PB = barometric pressure, and 47 = the partial pressure of water vapor in mm Hg in fully saturated air at body temperature. The value for R is usually assumed to be 0.8. Having calculated the PA_{O_2}, the $P(A\text{-}a)_{O_2}$ can then be determined, enabling a more precise quantitation of the degree of hypoxemia and mechanisms responsible for it.

Oxygen consumption ($\dot{V}O_2$ in liters per minute) can be estimated fairly accurately from the relationship

$$\dot{V}O_2 = (FI_{O_2} - FE_{O_2}) \times \dot{V}E \quad (6)$$

where FE_{O_2} = the fractional concentration of oxygen in expired air.

Oxygen delivery to the tissues depends not only on Pa_{O_2} but also on arterial oxygen content (Ca_{O_2}) and cardiac output. The Ca_{O_2} (milliliters of oxygen per 100 milliliters of blood) is calculated as follows:

$$Ca_{O_2} = 1.34 \times [Hb] \times \left(\frac{\text{per cent saturation}}{100}\right) + (0.003 \times Pa_{O_2}) \quad (7)$$

where 1.34 is the milliliters of oxygen carried by each gram of hemoglobin, [Hb] = the hemoglobin concentration in grams per 100 milliliters of blood, and per cent saturation = the saturation of hemoglobin with oxygen in arterial blood. The saturation can be measured directly or calculated from the oxyhemoglobin dissociation curve (Fig. 73–4). The constant 0.003 is the amount of dissolved (unbound) oxygen in blood in milliliters per mm Hg Pa_{O_2}.

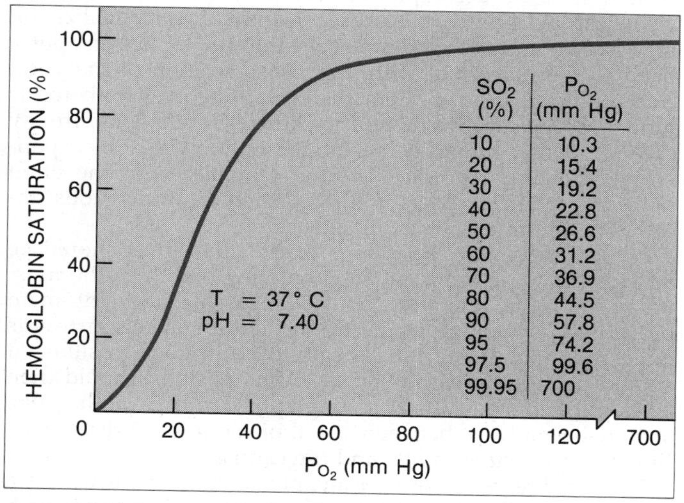

FIGURE 73–4. Relationship of per cent hemoglobin saturation to Pa_{O_2} in man at 37° C and pH 7.40. Note that there is very little increase in hemoglobin saturation for increases in Pa_{O_2} above 60 mm Hg. (From Murray JF: The Normal Lung. 2nd ed. Philadelphia, W. B. Saunders Company, 1986.)

Systemic oxygen transport (SO_2T) in milliliters per minute is calculated as follows:

$$SO_2T = Ca_{O_2} \times \dot{Q}T \quad (8)$$

where $\dot{Q}T$ = cardiac output in liters per minute.

Thus, it can be seen that oxygen delivery to the tissues depends not only on Pa_{O_2} but on [Hb] and $\dot{Q}T$ as well. In evaluating and managing patients with severe respiratory dysfunction, all of these factors need to be taken into account.

The balance between oxygen supply and systemic oxygen demands can be evaluated by calculating the difference between Ca_{O_2} and the content of oxygen in mixed venous blood ($C\bar{v}_{O_2}$). The $C\bar{v}_{O_2}$ is calculated in the same manner as the Ca_{O_2} (Equation 7) but using the oxyhemoglobin saturation value in mixed venous (pulmonary artery) blood.

Using the $\dot{V}O_2$ and the $C(a\text{-}\bar{v})_{O_2}$, the cardiac output can be calculated according to the Fick Principle:

$$\dot{Q}T = \frac{\dot{V}O_2}{C(a\text{-}\bar{v})_{O_2}} \quad (9)$$

The contribution of right-to-left shunting of blood to hypoxemia can be quantitated in patients receiving an FI_{O_2} of 1.0 using the following shunt equation:

$$\frac{\dot{Q}S}{\dot{Q}T} = \frac{Cc'_{O_2} - Ca_{O_2}}{Cc'_{O_2} - C\bar{v}_{O_2}} \quad (10)$$

where $\dot{Q}S$ = the volume of shunted blood, Cc'_{O_2} = an approximation of end capillary blood oxygen content, assuming the Pc'_{O_2} to be the same as PA_{O_2} and calculating the Cc'_{O_2} on the basis of this assumption.

The effect of the per cent shunt on Pa_{O_2} as calculated from this equation is shown in Figure 73–1. This figure illustrates the lack of responsiveness of Pa_{O_2} to increases in FI_{O_2} (PA_{O_2}) once the $\dot{Q}S/\dot{Q}T$ exceeds 30 per cent.

ACID-BASE RELATIONSHIPS. The essential relationships among the factors controlling arterial blood pH are described in the Henderson-Hasselbalch equation:

$$pH = pK + \log \frac{[HCO_3^-]}{[H_2CO_3]} \quad (11)$$

where pK, the dissociation constant, = 6.1 for plasma at 37° C. Because

$$[H_2CO_3] = Pa_{CO_2} \times 0.0301 \quad (12)$$

where 0.0301 is the solubility constant of carbon dioxide in plasma at 37°, Equation 11 can be substituted as follows:

$$pH = 6.1 + \log \frac{[HCO_3^-]}{Pa_{CO_2} \times 0.0301} \quad (13)$$

The relationships among these variables under acute and chronic conditions are shown in Figure 73–3.

LUNG MECHANICS. The stiffness of the lung and chest wall—that is, their resistance to inflation—is termed the *compliance of the respiratory system* (CRS). In patients being mechanically ventilated it is expressed by the following formula:

$$CRS = VT/\text{Pplateau} - PEE \quad (14)$$

where VT is the tidal volume delivered by the ventilator, Pplateau is the inspiratory plateau pressure (see Fig. 73–5), and PEE is the end-expiratory pressure read from the manometer of the ventilator. The effect of airways resistance can be included in the measurement by using the peak inspiratory pressure (Ppeak) rather than Pplateau. This is termed the *effective compliance* (Ceff) or *dynamic compliance*.

$$\text{Ceff} = VT/\text{Ppeak} - PEE \quad (15)$$

Assuming that the compliance of the chest wall is stable, changes in CRS reflect changes in lung mechanical properties,

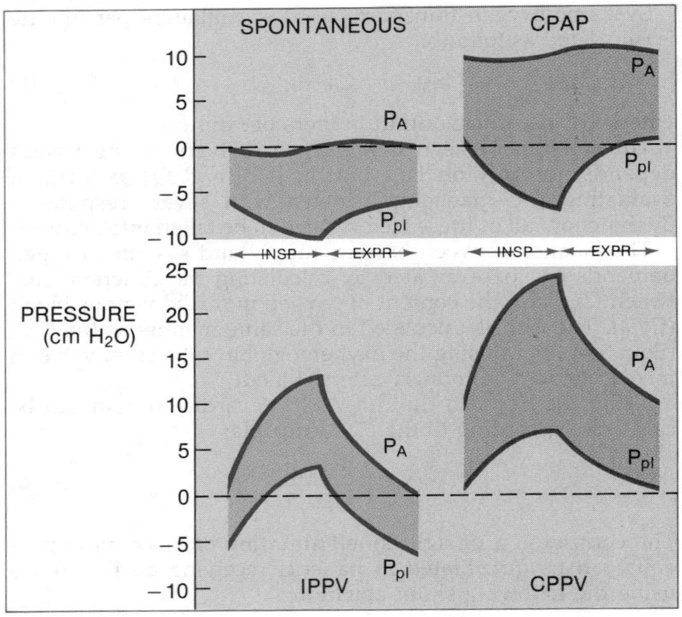

FIGURE 73–5. Schematic representations of airway (P_A) and pleural pressures (P_{pl}) with spontaneous respiration, spontaneous respiration with continuous positive airway pressure (CPAP), intermittent positive pressure ventilation (IPPV), and continuous positive pressure ventilation (CPPV). Note that with CPAP and CPPV, the pressure gradient between the airway and the pleural space is increased compared with spontaneous respiration and IPPV, respectively. (From Hinshaw HC, Murray JF (eds): Diseases of the Chest. Philadelphia, W. B. Saunders Company, 1980.)

whereas changes in Ceff may indicate changes in airways resistance (if inspiratory flow is unchanged) as well as lung compliance.

Murray JF: The Normal Lung. 2nd ed. Philadelphia, W. B. Saunders Company, 1986. *A concise review of normal lung function that provides the basis for an understanding of pulmonary pathophysiology.*

Lemaire F, Harf A, Teisseire BP: Oxygen exchange across the acutely injured lung. In Zapol WM, Falke KJ (eds.): Acute Respiratory Failure. New York, Marcel Dekker, 1985, pp 521–553. *An extensively referenced discussion of the abnormalities in oxygenation that occur in the adult respiratory distress syndrome.*

TECHNIQUES OF RESPIRATORY SUPPORT

External Devices for Administering Oxygen

Supplemental oxygen must frequently be administered by external devices in patients with any cardiorespiratory disorder that results in hypoxemia. The decision to use an external device as opposed to an endotracheal tube depends on the amount of oxygen needed and the potential consequences of failure to provide oxygen should the external device come off. Generally speaking, it is not prudent to rely on external devices for patients with hypoxemia severe enough to require an FI_{O_2} of 0.5 and who could be expected to suffer major consequences should the device not be positioned properly.

A variety of types of delivery systems can be used to provide supplemental oxygen. The choice of a particular method depends on four factors: (1) the amount of oxygen needed, (2) the need for precise control of FI_{O_2}, (3) the need for humidification, and (4) the patient's comfort. *Nasal prongs* are the simplest and most comfortable delivery device. However, the FI_{O_2} provided cannot be quantitated reliably and humidification is poor. *Open face masks or face tents* provide a high flow of well-humidified, premixed air and oxygen with a moderately reliable FI_{O_2} usually set by a Venturi device in a humidifier/mixer. *Tight-fitting face masks* provide higher but generally imprecise concentrations of oxygen. As with nasal prongs, humidification is minimal. The same sort of tight mask fitted with a nonrebreathing valve and a reservoir bag can be used to provide even higher concentrations of oxygen but it is generally uncomfortable and the oxygen is poorly humidified. Positive end-expiratory pressure can also be supplied using a tight mask with an appropriate system of valves. The FI_{O_2} is controlled much more precisely by the Venturi mask, which uses a calibrated Venturi device in the delivery line to provide high flows of gas containing 24, 28, 35, or 40 per cent oxygen. This sort of mask is used for patients with chronic airways obstruction and hypoventilation in whom there is concern that uncontrolled high oxygen concentrations will cause further hypoventilation by reducing ventilatory drive.

Ventilatory Assist Devices

A wide variety of devices can be used to provide ventilatory assistance without resorting to an endotracheal airway and mechanical ventilation. Generally, these devices are of limited usefulness; however, under proper circumstances, some may be quite helpful. Simple ventilators provide intermittent positive pressure ventilation via a mouthpiece but only transiently increase alveolar ventilation and, at least for this purpose, are of little value. External negative-pressure devices such as the cuirass ventilator, which fits over the chest wall and augments ventilation by lowering the pressure around the chest, causing it to expand, may be of value in patients with chronic neuromuscular diseases. Other ventilatory assist devices, including the rocking bed and surgically implanted phrenic nerve pacemakers, are of little general applicability.

Artificial Airways and Airway Management

When it is necessary, mechanical ventilation is best provided, at least initially, through an endotracheal tube passed through the mouth or nose. The oral route has the advantage of being more easily utilized under emergency circumstances, whereas the nasal route is better suited for long-term needs. Tracheostomy should be reserved for patients who will need long-term mechanical ventilation or who cannot tolerate either a nasal or an oral tube. The endotracheal tube should be fitted with a bonded high-volume, low-pressure cuff that will occlude the trachea around the tube, enabling positive pressure mechanical ventilation and preventing aspiration of oropharyngeal contents. Care should be taken to avoid overinflation of the cuff, which predisposes to pressure necrosis of the adjacent tracheal mucosa and to the development of a tracheoesophageal fistula or subsequent tracheal stenosis.

Semielective tube placement in a spontaneously ventilating patient may be accomplished via the nose without direct visualization of the vocal cords; however, direct visualization may be necessary to guide the tube into the larynx. In apneic patients the oral route with direct visualization of the vocal cords must be used. Placement of the tube over a fiberoptic bronchoscope may be helpful in difficult intubations. In any case intubation should be performed only by persons experienced with the procedure who are familiar with the often necessary pharmacologic adjuncts, such as intravenous anesthetics and muscle-relaxing agents.

Immediately after the tube is placed, the lungs should be auscultated to determine if air is entering both hemithoraces. Because of the relatively obtuse angle of the right main bronchus, positioning of the tip of the tube in this airway is quite common. If the tube seems to be in good position, it should be taped securely in place. The position should then be confirmed by a chest radiograph. The tip of the tube should be midway between the thoracic inlet, indicated by the sternoclavicular joints, and the carina.

Complete responsibility for maintenance of the airway in a patient with an endotracheal or tracheostomy tube rests with the persons caring for the patient. The patient can no longer humidify inspired air, cough effectively, or defend the lower airways against airborne microorganisms. Perhaps more important, the patient cannot call for help or unblock the tube should it become obstructed. For all of these reasons, in addition to the gravity of the illness for which the tube was placed, patients with artificial airways should nearly always be managed in a critical care unit.

Nasal or, in occasional circumstances, oral endotracheal tubes can be left in place with no absolute time limit in patients who continue to require mechanical ventilation or airway protection. Tracheostomy may be necessary, however, because of complications, such as infection or soft tissue necrosis in the upper air passages, including the nose. Occasionally, tracheostomy is more effective in facilitating removal of secretions than is an endotracheal tube. In addition, patients may find a tracheostomy more comfortable and may be able to eat and talk with a tracheostomy tube in place.

Endotracheal and tracheostomy tubes bypass the normal humidifying mechanisms in the upper airway; all inspired gas must therefore be fully humidified. Removal of pulmonary secretions using a suction catheter with sterile technique should be performed at regular intervals as determined by the volume of secretions present. All gas delivery circuits in direct communication with the airway should be sterile when connected and changed at least at 48-hour intervals.

Definitive indications for endotracheal intubation that apply to all situations are difficult to determine. Nevertheless, the criteria listed in Table 73–3 seem generally applicable. The decision to perform endotracheal intubation is often based on more subjective criteria and/or observation of the patient's course during a period of time. In each of the listed situations, the potential reversibility of the patient's underlying disorder must be taken into account in determining if intubation is indicated.

Mechanical Ventilation

INDICATIONS. As with endotracheal intubation, the indications for mechanical ventilation are not always easily definable. In general terms, however, mechanical ventilation is clearly necessary in the following situations: (1) progressive hypoxemia that is unresponsive to treatment of its underlying causes and in which external devices cannot provide a sufficiently high $F_{I_{O_2}}$ and (2) progressive hypoventilation with respiratory acidosis that is unresponsive to treatment of the underlying disorder. Less clear indications include: (1) "prophylactic" mechanical ventilation in patients in whom respiratory failure is anticipated, such as after thoracic or upper abdominal surgery and (2) patients who are barely maintaining adequate gas exchange at the expense of expending energy on the considerable work of breathing. Finally, mechanical ventilation is occasionally necessary in patients who require general anesthesia or heavy sedation to allow diagnostic or therapeutic intervention.

TYPES OF MECHANICAL VENTILATORS. The most important variable used to categorize mechanical ventilators is the mechanism determining the point at which the change-over from the inspiratory phase to the expiratory phase takes place (Fig. 73–5). This point may be determined by the volume of gas delivered *(volume-cycled)*, the airway pressure achieved *(pressure-cycled)*, or the elapsed time of inspiration *(time-cycled)*. Both time-cycled and pressure-cycled ventilators have the disadvantage of not necessarily delivering a constant tidal volume. For this reason volume-cycled ventilators are used most commonly. Many ventilators, however, have options that allow the device to be pressure- or time-cycled in addition to a volume-cycling mode.

TABLE 73–3. INDICATIONS FOR ENDOTRACHEAL INTUBATION

1. Need for an $F_{I_{O_2}} > 0.5$ for more than a short time to maintain adequate oxygenation
2. Progressive hypoventilation with respiratory acidosis not responding to conservative management
3. Apnea
4. Loss of airway protective mechanisms
5. Inability to clear secretions
6. Need for heavy sedation or paralysis to control patient for diagnostic or therapeutic interventions

FEATURES OF MECHANICAL VENTILATORS. Mechanical ventilators must have certain essential features in order to provide adequate ventilatory support in different patients with different types of respiratory disorders. Chief among these is the ability to deliver a wide range of tidal volumes (100 to 2000 ml), with an adjustable respiratory frequency (5 to 60) and an accurate adjustable $F_{I_{O_2}}$ (0.21 to 1.0). Additional important features include controls for adjusting the inspiration-expiration ratio (or the inspiratory flow rate) and the inspiratory pressure limit. The device should be capable of operating in an assist (patient-triggered) mode, a controlled (machine-triggered) mode, and an assist-control combination mode. The ventilator must be equipped with devices that monitor exhaled tidal volume, inspiratory pressure, the temperature of the inspiratory gas, and $F_{I_{O_2}}$ and have battery-operated alarms that signal loss of exhaled tidal volume, excessive inspiratory pressure, and reduction in $F_{I_{O_2}}$.

Preferably, ventilators should also have built-in controls for adjusting positive end-expiratory pressure (PEEP), for allowing intermittent mandatory ventilation (IMV), and for providing continuous positive airway pressure (CPAP) in spontaneously breathing patients.

PATTERNS OF VENTILATORY SUPPORT. Two basic patterns of ventilatory support may be employed in the management of patients with respiratory failure: (1) *intermittent positive pressure ventilation* (IPPV) and *intermittent mandatory ventilation* (IMV). The fluctuations in airway pressure that characterize spontaneous and mechanical ventilation are shown in Figure 73–5. The difference between IPPV and IMV is that there is no allowance for spontaneous ventilation with IPPV, whereas with IMV a portion of the patient's ventilation is spontaneous. The use of one or the other of these two patterns is often a matter of the physician's personal preference; however, some guidelines can be provided.

IPPV is clearly indicated in patients who have no spontaneous ventilation, who have severe pain with respiration and/or an unstable chest wall, or in whom the work of breathing represents a significant energy drain.

IMV offers the advantage of maintaining the condition of the respiratory muscles, and for this reason may be useful in patients who do not have chronic processes with pre-existing deconditioned muscles. In addition, patients may find IMV more comfortable than IPPV. Intermittent mandatory ventilation is also useful for patients who have significant reductions of cardiac output with mechanical ventilation, especially with PEEP, in that it may allow greater amounts of PEEP to be used. In patients who are not capable of synchronizing their inspiratory efforts with the ventilator and have a chaotic ventilatory pattern, IMV may allow adequate ventilation without the need for sedation or muscle-relaxing agents. It may also be a useful weaning technique in some situations.

POSITIVE END-EXPIRATORY PRESSURE (PEEP). As illustrated in Figure 73–5, PEEP increases the mean distending pressure across the walls of the airways and alveoli and thereby increases the volume of gas in the lung. This effect is beneficial in disorders characterized by pulmonary edema (usually noncardiogenic in origin) with consequent loss of functioning gas exchange units because of fluid filling or atelectasis. PEEP tends to re-expand collapsed units and to enable gas exchange to take place, thereby reducing intrapulmonary shunting of blood and improving Pa_{O_2}. PEEP can be added to IPPV to produce continuous positive pressure ventilation (CPPV) or to IMV. In addition, it can be used in spontaneously ventilating patients to produce CPAP or expiratory positive airway pressure (EPAP).

Positive end-expiratory pressure is not as clearly beneficial

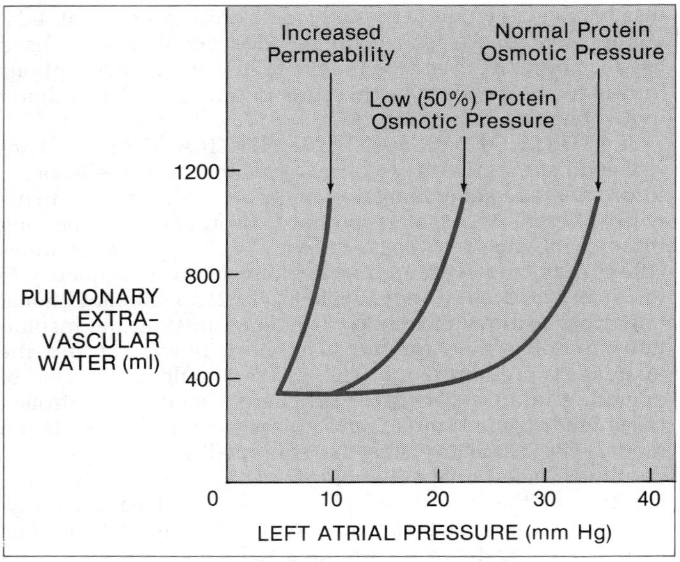

FIGURE 73–6. Schematic representation of the relationship of pulmonary extravascular water volume and left atrial or pulmonary artery wedge pressure. Curve at right represents the relationships when both capillary permeability and plasma protein osmotic pressures are normal; middle curve represents normal permeability but a reduction in plasma protein osmotic pressure of 50 per cent; left curve shows relationship when permeability of the capillaries is increased. (From Hopewell PC, Murray JF: Adult respiratory distress syndrome. In Moser KM, Spragg RG (eds.): Respiratory Emergencies. 2nd ed. St. Louis, The C. V. Mosby Company, 1982.)

and in fact may be harmful in patients with other types of respiratory failure, especially those failures caused by airways obstruction wherein the lung is already overinflated. In such cases further increases in lung volume may be hazardous. This dictum applies not only to CPPV but also to IMV with PEEP and to CPAP. PEEP may also decrease Pa_{O_2} in patients with focal infiltrative processes by increasing blood flow through the abnormal areas.

The conventional levels of PEEP range from 3 cm H_2O to 20 cm H_2O. Higher levels are occasionally used with IMV, but the indications for and the value of high levels of PEEP are not clearly defined.

CONSIDERATIONS IN INITIATING MECHANICAL VENTILATION. Once it is decided to initiate mechanical ventilation, a series of nearly equally important decisions should be made (Table 73–4). Much of the decision making is influenced by the pathophysiology of the underlying disorder for which mechanical ventilation is necessary. This is discussed in subsequent sections of this chapter.

VENTILATOR EMERGENCIES. Patients who are being mechanically ventilated are subject to a variety of potentially disastrous events that can occur suddenly and may be related either to the underlying disorder that made mechanical ventilation necessary or to malfunction of the ventilator or artificial airway. Such occurrences may rapidly be fatal. It is important that persons caring for critically ill patients develop a routine for assessment and management of these situations. The first indication that a problem is developing is usually

TABLE 73–4. DECISIONS IN INITIATING MECHANICAL VENTILATION

Type of ventilator
Pattern of ventilation (IPPV vs. IMV)
Mode (assist, control, or assist/control)
Tidal volume
Frequency
FI_{O_2}
Inspiration:expiration ratio
End-expiratory pressure (PEEP vs. no PEEP)

that the patient is no longer being adequately ventilated, as manifested by patient distress, by activation of the high-pressure or low-VT alarm, or by sudden hemodynamic changes in the patient.

When the high-pressure limit is exceeded, problems that should be suspected include obstruction of the endotracheal or tracheostomy tube, obstruction in the patient's airways, or pneumothorax. Occasionally, migration of the tip of the tube into a mainstem bronchus (usually the right) will cause the high-pressure limit to be exceeded, but this is usually not so dramatic an occurrence. Less commonly, obstruction of the artificial airway may result from overinflation of the cuff with subsequent tube compression or herniation of the cuff over the tip of the tube.

When the high-pressure limit is exceeded and ventilation is ineffective, the first step is to disconnect the patient from the ventilator and begin hand ventilation with an anesthesia bag using an FI_{O_2} of 1.0. At nearly the same time as bagging begins, the artificial airway should be checked for position and for evidence of external obstruction, such as kinking between the ventilator tubing connection and the nose or mouth or in the hypopharynx. If there is no external obstruction, the tube position seems correct, and compression of the bag is still difficult, the next step is to pass a suction catheter through the airway to check its patency and to remove mucous plugs or blood clots that may be causing the obstruction. If the obstruction is not removed, the tube cuff should be deflated to determine if it is causing the problem.

Assuming that the suction catheter can be passed, failure of these maneuvers to relieve the apparent obstruction indicates that the problem is within the patient and may be caused by major airway obstruction that was not removed by suctioning, sudden severe and more peripheral airways obstruction, or pneumothorax. The problem can usually be ascertained by a rapid physical examination of the chest. Tracheal obstruction is manifested by the finding of no or markedly reduced entry of air into the lungs. Mainstem bronchial obstruction is indicated by the absence of entry of air into the lung distal to the obstruction, causing a rocking motion of the chest with the affected side not expanding with inspiration and the unobstructed side being overinflated. Peripheral airways obstruction may be suspected from the patient's history and is usually indicated by wheezing, although with severe bronchoconstriction there may be little air movement and thus little or no wheezing. Pneumothorax in a patient being mechanically ventilated usually becomes a tension pneumothorax, characterized by difficulty with ventilation, reduction in arterial blood pressure, and an increase in central venous pressure. Examination of the chest shows no entry of air on the affected side, but, in contrast to the findings of mainstem bronchial obstruction, the affected side is hyperinflated and hyper-resonant to percussion. If the clinical situation allows, a chest roentgenogram can aid in a definitive diagnosis; however, a chest film showing a large tension pneumothorax may be viewed as being analogous to a 12-lead electrocardiogram in a patient with asystole.

Management of each of these situations is obviously different. Vigorous chest physical therapy and suctioning of the airway usually will remove obstructing mucous plugs or clots. Occasionally emergency fiberoptic bronchoscopy may be necessary. Tension pneumothorax requires prompt intervention to reduce the intrathoracic pressure. In an emergency situation a 14-gauge needle can be placed in the second anterior intercostal space. This will serve to relieve the tension with prompt restoration of the hemodynamic status and ability to ventilate the patient. After the needle is inserted, a chest tube should always be placed. Even if the diagnosis of pneumothorax was mistaken, a chest tube must be placed because of the high probability of lung puncture with the needle.

When the patient is suddenly not receiving adequate ventilation, but the high-pressure limit is not being exceeded, the problems that should be considered are leaks in the ventilator tubing or around the cuff of the artificial airway, ventilator malfunction, or a tracheoesophageal fistula. Again, the first step is to disconnect the ventilator and begin manual ventilation with an FI_{O_2} of 1.0. At the same time, the position of the tube and the inflation of the cuff of the endotracheal or tracheostomy tube should be checked. If the external pilot balloon is deflated, more air should be added. Leaks around the cuff may be caused by breaks in the cuff itself or in the external pilot balloon, or by enlargement of the trachea at the site of the cuff because of pressure on the tracheal wall. Occasionally, an endotracheal tube may be positioned too high in the airway with the cuff at the level of the vocal cords or higher, causing air to leak around the cuff. If the cuff itself is leaking, the tube must be replaced. With some kinds of tubes, the outer pilot balloon may be replaced, if defective, without changing the tube. If the leak is occurring because of tracheal enlargement, the problem may be solved by adding air to the cuff or by changing the level of the cuff within the trachea. If air is added, care should be taken not to exceed a measured intracuff pressure of 20 mm Hg.

Tracheal dilatation is often the precursor of a much more serious problem, formation of a tracheoesophageal fistula. This usually can be prevented by maintaining intracuff pressures of less than 20 mm Hg. When a fistula does develop, however, it is usually catastrophic. Patients with fistulas can sometimes be managed temporarily by placing the tube at a lower level in the trachea with the cuff below the fistula. Definitive management is surgical correction of the fistula.

WEANING FROM MECHANICAL VENTILATION. Patients being mechanically ventilated should be evaluated frequently to determine if their lung function has improved sufficiently to allow weaning from the ventilator and subsequent removal of the endotracheal tube. Factors other than the condition of the lungs play an important role in determining if the patient is ready to be weaned and in the outcome of the weaning process (Table 73–5).

The techniques and the rapidity of weaning vary considerably depending on the nature of the underlying disorders that caused the need for mechanical ventilation. There are some basic criteria that are generally applicable in determining if it is feasible to initiate weaning. First, the patient should be awake and fairly alert. Lung function should be adequate as indicated by the ability of the patient to generate a VC of greater than 10 ml per kilogram of body weight. This ability may also be inferred by the generation of a maximum inspiratory pressure of less (more negative) than -20 cm H_2O. In addition, the patient should not require an FI_{O_2} of greater than 0.5. Additional criteria that may be useful include a resting minute ventilation of less than 10 liters, the ability to double this volume voluntarily, a $P(A\text{-}a)_{O_2}$ less than 350 mm Hg at $FI_{O_2} = 1$, and a V_D/V_T of less than 0.55.

In patients who meet these criteria, weaning can commence. The techniques used include progressive lengthening of periods of spontaneous ventilation with the endotracheal tube attached to a "T-piece," a similar arrangement but with CPAP, and IMV with a progressive reduction in the number of breaths delivered by the ventilator. Patients whose lungs were previously normal and who have required only a short period of mechanical ventilation usually can be weaned and extubated quickly. The weaning process is often much longer in patients with chronic airways obstruction who have required a long period of ventilatory support.

TABLE 73–5. NONPULMONARY FACTORS THAT AFFECT WEANING FROM MECHANICAL VENTILATION

Cardiac function
Nutritional status
Electrolyte balance
Fluid balance
Pain
Mental status

Hudson LD: Diagnosis and management of acute respiratory distress in patients on mechanical ventilators. In Moser KM, Spragg RG: Respiratory Emergencies. St. Louis, C. V. Mosby Company, 1982, pp 202–213. *Describes the differential diagnosis of respiratory distress in patients who are being ventilated mechanically and discusses the steps to be undertaken in evaluation and management.*

Lanken PM: Weaning from mechanical ventilation. In Fishman AP (ed.): Update: Pulmonary Diseases and Disorders. New York, McGraw-Hill Book Company, 1982, pp 366–386. *Presents a comprehensive, well-referenced discussion of weaning. Reviews the basic pathophysiology of respiratory failure, criteria for weaning, and weaning techniques.*

Luce JM, Pierson DJ, Hudson LD: Intermittent mandatory ventilation. Chest 76:678, 1981. *A synthesis of information concerning the physiology and uses of IMV.*

Mushin WW, Rendell-Baker L, Thompson PW, et al.: Automatic Ventilation of the Lungs. 3rd ed. Oxford, Blackwell Scientific Publications, 1980. *The most comprehensive single-source reference on mechanical ventilation and ventilators that exists. Provides detailed technical information on nearly every commercially available positive pressure mechanical ventilator.*

Rizk NW, Murray JF: PEEP in pulmonary edema. Am J Med 72:381, 1982. *A concise updating of thinking concerning the effects of PEEP on lung fluid balance.*

Snider GL, Rinaldo JE: Oxygen therapy in medical patients hospitalized outside the intensive care unit. Am Rev Respir Dis 122(2):29, 1980. *A good description of the indications for and effects of supplemental oxygen with a discussion of the pros and cons of different techniques.*

Welch GW, Rippe JM: Airway Management and Endotracheal Intubation. In Rippe JM, Irwin RS, Alpert JS, et al. (eds.): Intensive Care Medicine. Boston, Little, Brown and Company, 1985, pp 3–16. *A comprehensive description of acute airway management, the indications for and techniques of endotracheal intubation, and complications resulting from intubation.*

PATHOPHYSIOLOGY, ASSESSMENT, AND CRITICAL CARE MANAGEMENT OF SPECIFIC FORMS OF RESPIRATORY FAILURE

The causes of respiratory failure may be categorized by the component of the respiratory system primarily involved and by the time course of the process. Life threatening or fatal respiratory failure may occur as the result of processes involving the respiratory neuromuscular system, the chest wall, the extrathoracic and intrathoracic airways, the lung parenchyma, and the pulmonary vasculature. Each of these produces respiratory failure by a different basic pathophysiologic mechanism and entails different approaches to treatment. In many instances, however, there is a mixture of the mechanisms that are causing respiratory failure. For example, fatigue of the respiratory muscles may be the final event precipitating fullblown respiratory failure in patients with other primary lung disorders. Thus, although the basic approach to management is determined by the major underlying pathophysiologic mechanism, a variety of secondary approaches may be called for as well.

Central Nervous System, Peripheral Nervous System, and Muscular Causes of Respiratory Failure

Processes such as sedative hypnotic drug overdose and brain injuries and infections can reduce or abolish central respiratory drive, resulting in respiratory failure that is characterized predominantly by hypoventilation. The airways and lung parenchyma are unaffected except by atelectasis, which may occur because of a lack of periodic hyperinflations (sighs). Once ventilation is provided, gas exchange is normal unless atelectasis has occurred. The same pathophysiologic pattern can result from high cervical spinal cord injuries, peripheral nervous system disorders such as Guillain-Barré syndrome, or muscular disorders such as myasthenia gravis.

Use of critical care in these instances is dictated by the requirement for careful observation and/or for ventilatory support. Generally ventilatory support is indicated for patients in this category who have hypoventilation that does not respond to initial conservative management.

Measurements of Pa_{CO_2}, Pa_{O_2}, and arterial pH in comatose or sedated patients provide a direct indication of alveolar ventilation and also inferential information on the status of the lung parenchyma. In patients with spinal cord injury or neuromuscular disease, measurements of arterial blood gas tensions and pH are similarly useful, but gas exchange may be well preserved until there is a marked reduction in ventilatory capability. Serial measurements of VC and maximal inspiratory pressure are therefore of value in predicting the likelihood of hypoventilation and the need for ventilatory support. In persons with normal ventilatory control mechanisms, hypoventilation does not occur with a VC of greater than 1 liter. Once the ventilatory capability is reduced to this degree, however, any further decrease is likely to be associated with a sudden increase in Pa_{CO_2}. Similarly, decreases in maximal inspiratory force to less than 20 cm H_2O are indicative of a critical reduction in ventilatory capability and the imminent possibility of hypoventilation. Apart from the direct respiratory consequences of these processes, critical care may be required to provide adequate airway protection and, in the case of drug overdose, to treat other toxic effects such as hemodynamic instability.

The pathophysiologic manifestations in this group of disorders are nearly identical, so that the approach to respiratory support of existing or imminent hypoventilation is the same. An oral or nasal endotracheal tube should be used to provide mechanical ventilation, preferably with a volume-limited ventilator. An initial tidal volume of 10 ml per kilogram of body weight is used in the control mode for apneic patients or in the assist/control mode for patients capable of initiating breaths. The ventilator frequency should be 8 to 10 breaths per minute with an inspiration-expiration ratio of 1:3. The appropriateness of this level of alveolar ventilation must be checked by measuring Pa_{CO_2}, Pa_{O_2}, and arterial pH approximately 10 minutes after initiating mechanical ventilation.

If the gas exchange abnormality is purely hypoventilation, use of supplemental oxygen should not be necessary. However, this is rarely the case. It is good practice to initiate mechanical ventilation using an FI_{O_2} of 1.0; after the initial measurement of Pa_{O_2}, FI_{O_2} should be adjusted downward. PEEP is generally not necessary in this category of illness but may be beneficial in preventing collapse or in re-expanding existing atelectatic areas of the lungs, complications not infrequent in patients with neurologic or muscular disorders.

Weaning from mechanical ventilation and the decision to remove the endotracheal tube should be made in accordance with the guidelines discussed previously. Generally, the weaning and extubation of drug-overdosed patients who do not have complications proceed quite rapidly once they are awake. Patients with chronic neuromuscular disorders present much more of a problem and may require long-term ventilatory support.

Respiratory Failure Caused by Chest Wall Abnormalities

The most frequently encountered cause of this type of respiratory failure is traumatic injury to the chest wall with consequent rib fractures. This is associated with pain that inhibits full lung inflation, with atelectasis, and occasionally with hypoventilation. Multiple ribs fractured in multiple places, in addition to causing pain, can interfere with lung inflation because of the loss of chest wall rigidity and subsequent paradoxic motion of the involved area, so-called *flail chest*. Atelectasis, hypoxemia, and hypoventilation in severe cases characterize the pathophysiologic picture. In addition, the underlying lung is frequently contused, which adds to the abnormalities of gas exchange. Chronic deformities of the chest wall or marked pleural disease also can result in respiratory failure, although in these situations the pathophysiologic alterations are more complex than in injuries to the chest wall and often involve parenchymal and vascular abnormalities as well.

The primary mode of assessment is measurement of arterial blood gas tensions. The basic indications for placement of an endotracheal tube are an inability to maintain adequate oxygenation with external oxygen delivery devices and significant increases in Pa_{CO_2}. The need for ventilatory support may be anticipated in patients who require large doses of narcotic agents to control their pain.

The pattern of mechanical ventilation utilized in patients with chest wall injuries is much the same as that described for patients with neuromuscular disorders. However, because of the greater likelihood of involvement of the lung parenchyma with atelectasis and hemorrhage, a higher V_T (12 to 15 ml per kilogram) and PEEP may be beneficial. The use of PEEP also helps to correct or prevent atelectasis and to stabilize the injured chest wall.

Weaning from mechanical ventilation does not necessarily have to await full stabilization of the chest wall, which can take weeks. Standard criteria can be used as the basis for making decisions concerning weaning and removal of the endotracheal tube.

Respiratory Failure Caused by Airways Obstruction

Impediments in the proximal portion of the airways (e.g., hypopharynx, larynx, and trachea) or generalized narrowing of the peripheral airways can severely obstruct airflow. With proximal obstruction hypoventilation is the major pathophysiologic abnormality. Gas exchange is normal once the obstruction is removed or bypassed. Similarly, hypoventilation is the hallmark of respiratory failure associated with diffuse airways obstruction (i.e., asthma, chronic bronchitis, and emphysema); however, the hypoventilation is invariably associated with hypoxemia due largely to ventilation-perfusion mismatching.

In this latter group of disorders, the primary abnormality is an increased resistance to airflow resulting from intrinsic narrowing of the airways or loss of airway tethering forces, or both. Regardless of the mechanism, the results are hypoxemia caused by mismatching of ventilation and perfusion and hypoventilation resulting from the airways obstruction itself plus fatigue of the respiratory muscles.

Measurements of airflow rates (FEV_1, PEFR) and arterial blood gas tensions are helpful in evaluating the severity of obstruction of airflow, and serial measurements describe the course of the episode and enable quantitation of response to treatment. The interpretation of a given set of arterial blood gas values varies considerably, depending on the time over which the abnormalities develop and their rate of change.

In patients with asthma or chronic airways obstruction, Pa_{CO_2} begins to increase when the FEV_1 is reduced to approximately 750 ml or less, or 25 per cent of its predicted value. With further reductions, Pa_{CO_2} tends to increase rapidly. Increased Pa_{CO_2} values occurring in association with FEV_1's of greater than 750 to 1000 ml may be the result of reduced ventilatory drive or increased production of carbon dioxide in a patient with a limited ability to increase the alveolar ventilation. As previously described, the distinction between acute and chronic hypoventilation can be determined by analyzing the relationships among Pa_{CO_2}, arterial pH, and $[HCO_3^-]$. Acute hypoventilation obviously dictates a more prompt response than chronic partially compensated respiratory acidosis.

The presence of metabolic acidosis is a more ominous finding than pure respiratory acidosis in the setting of airways obstruction. It implies a failure of the oxygen delivery system to provide sufficient amounts of oxygen to meet the demands imposed by the increased work of breathing. Such a situation cannot exist in steady state, and unless these patients rapidly improve, their condition will rapidly deteriorate.

Although hypoxemia invariably is present in patients with severe airways obstruction, the degree of reduction in Pa_{O_2} is generally in itself not sufficient to require respiratory support other than supplemental oxygen via external devices.

One cannot definitively state criteria for placement of an endotracheal tube and use of mechanical ventilation in patients with severe airways obstruction. Arterial blood gas and pH values at a single point in time showing marked acute respiratory acidosis or respiratory plus metabolic acidosis may be sufficient information on which to base the decision to provide mechanical ventilation. More commonly, however, it is necessary to evaluate the patient during a period of time while maximal conservative therapy is being administered and to evaluate the response to therapy. If the blood gas values are worsening or not improving in spite of maximal treatment, mechanical ventilation is the next logical step. In addition to the objective evaluation provided by arterial blood gas and pH measurements, subjective assessments are also of value. Patients who are confused, somnolent, or uncooperative may require ventilatory support because their mental status may indicate an end-organ effect of the blood gas abnormalities and because the patients cannot cooperate with conservative management.

Severe airways obstruction presents a difficult situation in which to apply mechanical ventilation. There is the need to allow adequate exhalation time in the presence of marked expiratory airflow slowing, but also slow inspiratory flows are desirable to optimize the distribution of ventilation and to minimize the airways pressure required to deliver the set V_T. To accomplish these goals, at least early in the course of mechanical ventilation, it is often necessary to sedate the patient to effect a slow respiratory frequency, which results in an appropriate inspiration-expiration ratio. The V_T should be approximately 10 ml per kilogram and the $F_{I_{O_2}}$ adjusted to provide an adequate Pa_{O_2}. As the airways obstruction improves, the need for sedation will decrease. In initiating mechanical ventilation in patients with chronic hypoventilation, it is important not to reduce the Pa_{CO_2} rapidly because it will result in uncompensated metabolic alkalosis. The minute ventilation should be set to reduce the Pa_{CO_2} gradually, allowing the arterial pH to go no higher than 7.50. In general, PEEP should not be used in patients with airways obstruction because it will further distend the already overinflated lungs.

Weaning patients with airways obstruction from mechanical ventilation also may present a difficult problem. Patients with asthma may be weaned and extubated quickly. However, patients with chronic airways obstruction may at best have marginal lung function with persistent retention of carbon dioxide. Generally speaking, the arterial blood gas pattern that is estimated to exist when the patient is "well" should be approximated while mechanical ventilation is still being used. Ideally, weaning can then proceed using previously described indicators. In many instances, however, patients with chronic airways obstruction never meet the objective criteria for weaning and extubation. When this occurs, the decisions in weaning and extubation are based on subjective criteria, such as level of alertness, patient cooperation, and prognosis. These factors obviously cannot be quantitated. Once the patient has demonstrated the ability to ventilate spontaneously for 30 to 60 minutes, the endotracheal tube should be removed.

It is important to try to determine which patients with chronic airways obstruction have a component of reversible respiratory dysfunction and which patients have simply reached the end stage of their disease. Although chronic mechanical ventilation is occasionally used to maintain life in a patient with end-stage chronic airways obstruction, the decision to pursue this course should be carefully considered by the patient, the family, and the physician, preferably before mechanical ventilation is begun.

Disorders of the Lung Parenchyma Causing Respiratory Failure

Disorders of the lung parenchyma can be divided into those that predominantly involve the interstitium and those that involve the alveolar airspaces. Accumulations of fluid in alveoli can be caused by cardiogenic pulmonary edema (left ventricular failure or mitral stenosis) or diffuse injury to the lung causing noncardiogenic pulmonary edema (adult respiratory distress syndrome [ARDS]). A list of the conditions that have been associated with ARDS is provided in Ch. 72.

Both cardiogenic and noncardiogenic pulmonary edema may cause respiratory failure that is characterized by hypoxemia caused by right-to-left intrapulmonary shunting of blood and ventilation-perfusion mismatching. In severe cases retention of carbon dioxide can occur. Although mechanical ventilation may be required in both forms of pulmonary edema, other therapeutic interventions and response to treatment are quite different. This section will focus on pulmonary edema resulting from an increase in the permeability of the alveolar-capillary membrane. Cardiogenic pulmonary edema is discussed in Ch. 43.

ADULT RESPIRATORY DISTRESS SYNDROME (ARDS). A constellation of clinical, radiographic, and pathophysiologic findings that result from diffuse injury to the lung parenchyma defines ARDS. The characteristics of the syndrome are (1) hypoxemia due to intrapulmonary shunting of blood, (2) increased lung stiffness (or decreased compliance), and (3) presence of diffuse infiltration on the chest roentgenogram. The common abnormality that accounts for these features is an increase in the permeability of the endothelium of the pulmonary capillary and the epithelium of the alveolar wall. This allows fluid to leak from the capillary into the alveolus even though the hydrostatic pressure within the capillary is normal; hence, noncardiogenic pulmonary edema results.

The injury to the lung that results in ARDS may be delivered via the airways or via the circulation. In many instances (e.g., aspiration of gastric juice or diffuse pneumonia), the mechanism by which the injury occurs is easily understood. However, in others (e.g., sepsis or pancreatitis), the mechanism is obscure.

Regardless of the type or mechanism of injury, both the pathophysiologic and the pathologic abnormalities are uniform. Grossly, the lung is edematous and hemorrhagic. Microscopic examination reveals intra-alveolar collections of proteinaceous fluid, red blood cells, and often inflammatory cells. Microthrombi or white blood cell aggregates may occasionally be seen in small vessels. After 24 to 48 hours, hyaline membranes line the inner aspects of alveoli and alveolar ducts. These membranes are formed by fibrin that has escaped through the leaking capillaries. Subsequently, as repair of the injury occurs, fibrosis may ensue although this is not an invariable consequence.

The pathophysiologic alterations affect lung volume, mechanical properties of the lung, and gas exchange. Reductions in VC and functional residual capacity (FRC) are characteristic of ARDS and are caused in part by fluid replacing alveolar air. As previously noted, one of the hallmarks of ARDS is the increased stiffness of the lung. This results not only from fluid in the alveoli but probably also from interaction between extravasated protein and surfactant, which increase surface forces at the air-liquid interface. The work of breathing considerably increases because of these effects on lung volume and lung compliance. The major and most frequent gas exchange abnormality is *hypoxemia*. This again is related predominantly to alveolar filling with fluid, causing these units to be the sites of shunting. In other less involved portions of the lung, ventilation-perfusion mismatching occurs and contributes to the hypoxemia.

In severe forms of ARDS, as the process evolves from injury to repair, the gas exchange abnormalities also evolve. Lung fibrosis may result in obliteration of capillaries and coalescence of airspaces to produce an increased V_D/V_T with overall alveolar hypoventilation, as indicated by an increased Pa_{CO_2}.

Definite abnormalities of gas exchange are seen only when the process has advanced to the stage of alveolar flooding.

Thus, such measurements of blood gas tensions are relatively insensitive in assessing the lung injury. Nevertheless, patients who either have or are at risk of developing ARDS should be carefully observed, and Pa_{O_2}, Pa_{CO_2}, and arterial pH should be measured frequently. Early in the course, the critical variable is the Pa_{O_2}. Because patients frequently hyperventilate at this stage, the $P(A\text{-}a)_{O_2}$ should be calculated to provide an accurate index of the course of the process. The occurrence of either respiratory or metabolic acidosis in this setting is an ominous finding. In addition to blood gas tensions, it is often necessary to measure the pulmonary artery wedge pressure both to determine if there is a contribution of cardiogenic pulmonary edema to the process and to serve as a guide for fluid management.

Patients who have fully developed ARDS invariably require mechanical ventilation. The determination of when to intervene with ventilatory support in patients who are at risk of developing ARDS or who have minor abnormalities of pulmonary function that suggest early ARDS may be quite difficult. The occurrence of edema and consequent loss of lung volume tends to be a self-perpetuating cycle, so that it is generally better to provide mechanical ventilation earlier rather than later.

When mechanical ventilation is undertaken, V_T of 12 to 15 ml per kilogram of body weight should be used. Volumes of this magnitude are more effective in preventing or reversing atelectasis. In addition, use of PEEP has a well-documented role in the management of patients with ARDS. The beneficial effect of this pattern of ventilation is mainly attributable to the increase in FRC that it produces. By maintaining a continuously positive distending pressure across the walls of alveoli and airways, PEEP re-establishes their patency allowing gas exchange to resume in these units. Thus, shunting is decreased and Pa_{O_2} is improved.

Use of PEEP is not without hazards: (1) The increase in intrathoracic pressure caused by PEEP may reduce cardiac output. This appears to occur predominantly because of a reduction in venous inflow to the right side of the heart. It is therefore important to assess carefully the effects of PEEP not only on Pa_{O_2} but also on systemic oxygen transport by measuring cardiac output after PEEP is applied and after changes in PEEP. (2) The second potential complication of PEEP is the occurrence of pneumothorax. This seems more likely to occur later in the course of ARDS as architectural rearrangements take place in the lung that weaken its structure.

The application of PEEP may decrease Pa_{O_2} in situations in which there is considerable regional variation in the distribution of lung pathology. This results from shifting blood flow away from the more normal portions of the lung to the more abnormal portions and thereby increasing shunting.

Appropriate use of intravenous fluids is an important component of the management of ARDS. Pulmonary capillary permeability is increased and the regulatory mechanisms that normally tend to protect the lung from fluid overload are impaired. The prevailing capillary hydrostatic pressure therefore assumes an enhanced importance. Thus, administration of fluid, which increases the capillary hydrostatic pressure, tends to increase the amount of water in the lung. The relationship between capillary hydrostatic pressure and lung water content is shown schematically in Figure 73–6.

On the other hand, adequate pulmonary and systemic perfusion may also be important in preventing lung damage, and systemic perfusion is clearly important in maintaining renal, cardiac, and central nervous system functions. Thus, the effects of fluid administration should be carefully monitored with clear endpoints in mind. Rather than using systemic arterial pressure or central venous pressure alone to guide treatment, indexes of end-organ perfusion, such as urine output or mental functioning, should also be monitored. Frequently, at least early in the course of the process, a Swan-Ganz pulmonary artery catheter may be extremely helpful. Sufficient fluid should be administered to maintain perfusion of critical organs with as little effect as possible on the pulmonary artery wedge pressure.

Crystalloid solutions are probably preferable to colloid solutions, at least early in the course of the process when the increase in capillary permeability is most marked. At present there are not sufficient clinical data to support the use of corticosteroids in the treatment of patients who either have or are at risk of developing ARDS.

Pulmonary Vascular Diseases

The major effects of pulmonary vascular obstruction are circulatory rather than respiratory. Nevertheless, both acute pulmonary embolism and chronic pulmonary vasculitis are commonly associated with hypoxemia. In the former it is thought to be caused by microatelectasis producing right-to-left shunting. In the latter, the gas exchange abnormalities probably relate to pulmonary parenchymal abnormalities adjacent to vascular inflammation and result from a mixture of shunting and ventilation-perfusion mismatching.

Both the assessment and the management of the respiratory abnormalities caused by pulmonary vascular disease are directed toward the vascular process itself. Rarely is mechanical ventilation necessary solely because of gas exchange abnormalities caused by pulmonary vascular disease. However, small and occasionally large pulmonary emboli may occur in patients with other respiratory illnesses, thus compounding their cardiorespiratory abnormalities.

Bell RC, Coalson JJ, Smith JD, et al.: Multiple organ system failure and infection in adult respiratory distress syndrome. Ann Intern Med 99:293, 1983. *A prospective study evaluating the role of multiple organ system failure and infection in patients with ARDS. The overall survival rate was 26.2 per cent and was significantly worse in patients who developed central nervous system, gastrointestinal, renal, endocrine, or coagulation disorders and in patients who had infections.*

Cherniack RM: Management of acute respiratory failure in chronic obstructive pulmonary disease. Semin Respir Med 8:158, 1986. *A detailed review of the pathophysiology and management of respiratory failure caused by chronic airways obstruction.*

Hopewell PC, Miller WT: Respiratory failure in status asthmaticus. Clin Chest Med 5:623, 1984. *Presents a review of the pathophysiology, assessment, and management of severe asthma.*

Hopewell PC, Murray JF: Adult respiratory distress syndrome. In Moser KM, Spragg RG (eds.): Respiratory Emergencies. 2nd ed. St. Louis, C. V. Mosby Company, 1982. *A comprehensive review of pathogenesis, pathophysiology, pathology, and management of ARDS.*

Hyers TM: Markers of acute lung injury in humans. Semin Respir Med 8(Suppl):65, 1986. *Describes the current status of our understanding of mediators and markers of acute lung injury.*

Montgomery AB, Stager MA, Carico CJ, et al.: Causes of mortality in patients with the adult respiratory distress syndrome. Am Rev Respir Dis 132:485, 1985. *An analysis of factors causing and contributing to death in patients with ARDS pointing out the importance of sepsis in causing and complicating the syndrome.*

Prewitt RM, Matthay MA, Ghignone M: Hemodynamic management in the adult respiratory distress syndrome. Clin Chest Med 4:251, 1983. *Discusses the important cardiopulmonary interactions in ARDS and optimal management strategies.*

Rinaldo JE, Rogers RM: Adult respiratory distress syndrome: Changing concepts of lung injury and repair. N Engl J Med 306:900, 1982. *An excellent review of ARDS emphasizing the mechanisms by which the lung injury might occur.*

CRITICAL CARE MONITORING

A critical care unit is unique in its ability to provide continuous and often invasive measurements of respiratory and hemodynamic status in severely ill patients. Such monitoring enables early detection of changes in the patient's condition and provides information that both directs therapy and assists in evaluating the response to treatment. The complexity of monitoring systems varies considerably, ranging from simple electrocardiographic monitoring with only a real-time screen display to automated "closed loop" systems wherein the monitored data, through a computer program, serve to regulate intravenous infusions of fluids and drugs. Usually, the kind of system employed relates to the kinds of patients being cared for in the unit.

Respiratory Monitoring

As a minimum, respiratory monitoring should consist of measurement of respiratory rate and periodic measurement of Pa_{O_2}, Pa_{CO_2}, and arterial pH. Respiratory rate can be measured and recorded automatically in nonintubated patients using impedance devices to which alarms can be attached. Both respiratory rate and VT can be monitored in intubated, spontaneously breathing patients using a spirometer and appropriate alarms.

In patients who are being mechanically ventilated, monitoring of respiratory rate, exhaled VT, and airway pressure is essential. Additional monitoring techniques are available but do not yet have a demonstrated role. These include breath by breath measurements of respiratory system compliance and volume-pressure and volume-flow relationships. In addition, multiplexed mass spectrometer-based systems are available for measurement of FI_{O_2} and exhaled carbon dioxide and oxygen. These systems may provide early indications of changes in Pa_{CO_2}, but their usefulness and general applicability remain to be determined.

The transcutaneous PO_2 and PCO_2 that are indirect reflections of Pa_{O_2} and Pa_{CO_2} can be measured continuously using heated skin electrodes. Measurement of transcutaneous PO_2 in infants has proved to be a helpful monitoring technique, but the value of this measurement in adults is uncertain.

Pulse oximeters are noninvasive monitoring devices that measure and record oxyhemoglobin saturation. This technique has proved to be useful in a variety of clinical situations, including weaning from mechanical ventilation and evaluating oxygenation during sleep and during procedures such as bronchoscopy.

Indwelling catheter electrodes for continuous intra-arterial measurement of Pa_{O_2}, Pa_{CO_2}, and arterial pH have been used but still have important technical limitations. More recently, a fiberoptic pulmonary artery catheter for continuous measurement of oxyhemoglobin saturation in mixed venous blood has been developed but does not have a defined role as yet.

Hemodynamic Monitoring

Most critical care units have the basic capacity to monitor and record heart rate and rhythm (usually with a built-in memory and recall capability), venous pressure, pulmonary arterial pressure, and systemic arterial pressure. In addition, many units have the instruments necessary for measurement of cardiac output.

Electrocardiographic monitoring is clearly of value in patients with specific cardiac disorders such as acute myocardial infarction or cardiac arrhythmia. This form of assessment is also essential in patients with any illness severe enough to require critical care. Abnormalities in heart rate or rhythm may signal the worsening of a respiratory condition, electrolyte abnormalities, or a variety of other noncardiac problems. Ideally, the system should have a built-in memory and should be able to display frequency and kinds of arrhythmias occurring in a given period of time. Both high-rate and low-rate alarms are necessary to complete the system.

Continuous *systemic arterial pressure monitoring* is of obvious value, assuming it is performed accurately. Changes in blood pressure can be detected immediately and therefore enable beat by beat assessment of the effects of such maneuvers as changes in ventilatory pattern or infusion of vasoactive drugs. Continuous measurement of the blood pressure decreases the amount of time necessary for staff members to spend with the patient. Finally, an arterial catheter provides ready access to arterial blood for measurement of blood gases.

Each of these advantages has a corollary disadvantage, however. If the equipment is not properly calibrated, an inaccurate reading may be obtained that may result in inappropriate decisions. Beat to beat variations in blood pressure may not warrant specific intervention. In many instances it is better for the nurse to be at the patient's bedside rather than watching a monitor screen. Finally, the presence of an arterial catheter may encourage withdrawal of more blood than is necessary for measurement of blood gases.

The advantages and disadvantages of arterial pressure monitoring must be taken into account in deciding when arterial catheter placement is indicated. In addition to the problems just listed, there are specific complications of arterial catheterization, which are discussed below (see Complications of Hemodynamic Monitoring, Systemic Arterial Pressure).

Given these considerations, the basic indication for monitoring arterial blood pressure is the presence or anticipation of hemodynamic instability as a result of either the disease process or the therapeutic intervention. In patients who require frequent measurement of arterial blood gases, insertion of an arterial catheter may be indicated to provide access to arterial blood.

The usual technique of monitoring systemic arterial pressure is to insert percutaneously a Teflon catheter into an accessible artery. The radial artery of the nondominant hand is usually the vessel of choice. The Allen test should be performed to determine the patency of the palmar arterial arch before insertion of the catheter. The femoral artery is the second choice for placement. The brachial artery, ulnar artery, and dorsalis pedis artery can also be used.

The catheter is connected via a stopcock to a rigid connecting tube that in turn is attached to a transducer. Commonly, a device that continuously flushes the catheter with a small volume of heparinized solution is also connected to the catheter.

Central venous pressure monitoring by a continuous technique is useful in quantitating and following the course of right ventricular failure, right ventricular infarction, tricuspid regurgitation, and cardiac tamponade. In addition, it is useful in evaluating the intravascular volume status of patients who have no pulmonary or cardiac disease.

Under normal circumstances, central venous pressure (CVP) is equivalent to right atrial and right ventricular diastolic pressures and bears a more or less constant relationship to the pulmonary wedge pressure (pulmonary artery wedge pressure [PPAW] = CVP + 6 mm Hg). However, if cardiac or pulmonary disease is present, the CVP does not reflect the left atrial filling pressure (pulmonary artery wedge pressure). In fact, the CVP may provide misleading information leading to erroneous therapeutic decisions.

To monitor CVP a catheter is inserted percutaneously into either the subclavian or the external or internal jugular vein. An antecubital vein may also be used for catheter insertion either percutaneously or via a cutdown. Care should be taken to avoid passing the catheter into the right ventricle where it can cause ventricular arrhythmias. A chest roentgenogram should be obtained immediately after insertion of the catheter to determine its position and to check for pneumothorax or pneumomediastinum (with subclavian and internal jugular sites of catheter insertion).

The instrumentation for measurement of CVP is the same as that described for arterial pressure. The CVP measurements should be interpreted cautiously. In patients who have significant hemodynamic instability, the CVP should not be relied on as an accurate indicator of volume status, especially in the presence of cardiac or pulmonary disease.

In *pulmonary arterial pressure monitoring*, development of the balloon-tipped flotation catheter by Swan and Ganz increased both the ease and safety of catheter placement and, in addition, enabled bedside measurement of the wedge pressure. This catheter, in addition to having a central lumen with a distal opening to measure PPA, has a balloon bonded to the catheter just proximal to the tip and a separate lumen for inflating the balloon. With the catheter properly positioned, inflation of the balloon occludes the vessel in which the tip resides, stopping blood flow and allowing measurement of

TABLE 73–6. INDICATIONS FOR PULMONARY ARTERIAL PRESSURE MONITORING

1. To help distinguish cardiogenic from noncardiogenic pulmonary edema.
2. To provide information in the differential diagnosis of hypotension.
3. To assist in determining the cause of hypoxemia.
4. To characterize the patterns of abnormal cardiac function after myocardial infarction.
5. To monitor the effects of various therapeutic interventions such as vasoactive agents, intravenous fluids, diuretics, digitalis, and CPPV.

the pulmonary artery wedge pressure. In addition to the basic single lumen No. 5 F catheter, there are a variety of modifications. The most versatile version is a No. 7 F size that has, in addition to the distal lumen, a proximal lumen for measurement of CVP and a thermistor near the tip that allows measurement of cardiac output using the thermal dilution technique.

Thus, the Swan-Ganz pulmonary artery catheter provides measurement of PPA, PPAW, CVP, and cardiac output. In addition, blood can be sampled from the pulmonary artery for measurement of oxygen content. The indications for monitoring PPA are listed in Table 73–6.

It is important to recognize the limitations of monitoring PPA. First, because of the effects of oscillations in pleural pressure on the measured intravascular pressure, the values are extremely difficult to determine in persons who are breathing rapidly. Second, the values are altered by PEEP; an accurate absolute value cannot be obtained in a patient in whom PEEP is being used. The measurement has a relative value, however, that can be used comparatively to evaluate a therapeutic maneuver unless the catheter is positioned in a portion of the lung in which alveolar pressure is greater than pulmonary venous pressure alone or PPA and pulmonary venous pressure (an unlikely occurrence). If this occurs, the reading of pulmonary artery wedge pressure will reflect alveolar pressure rather than left atrial pressure. Finally, pulmonary artery wedge pressure will not reflect the left ventricular filling pressure in the presence of mitral stenosis or pulmonary venous obstruction.

To obtain the maximal amount of information from the procedure, a recording of the wave form and pressures should be made as the catheter passes from the superior vena cava to the right atrium, right ventricle, and pulmonary artery. Figure 73–7 shows the normal wave forms encountered during passage of the catheter. Specific abnormal patterns may be seen in patients with tricuspid regurgitation or cardiac tamponade and constriction.

Insertion of the catheter is via the same choice of routes described for insertion of the catheter for measuring CVP. The instrumentation is also the same. The procedure must be performed with continuous electrocardiographic monitoring to allow identification of ventricular arrhythmias induced by the catheter passing through the right ventricle. Because of the possibility of ventricular arrhythmias, lidocaine for immediate intravenous administration must be available. The catheter should be positioned so that a pulmonary artery wedge pressure tracing is seen with 1 ml of air in the balloon (for a No. 7 F catheter with a 1.5-ml capacity balloon). The catheter should then be secured in that position and a chest roentgenogram taken to confirm and record the position and to check for pneumothorax. The PPA tracing should be monitored continuously to detect distal migration and permanent wedging of the catheter, which may cause pulmonary infarction.

Measurements of cardiac output can be obtained easily and routinely using the thermistor-equipped Swan-Ganz catheter. Such measurements complement the pressure measurements described earlier and enable nearly complete characterization of the hemodynamic status of the severely ill patient.

The instrumentation required to perform thermal dilution determinations includes, in addition to the Swan-Ganz catheter, a cardiac output computer that processes the indicator-dilution measurements and calculates cardiac output. Such measurements are not without error, but, using standard techniques, the results are of acceptable accuracy.

Patterns of hemodynamic abnormalities are often of diagnostic value. Using the systemic and pulmonary arterial pressure, CVP, and cardiac output, the resistance across the pulmonary and systemic vascular beds can be calculated as follows:

$$PVR = \frac{\overline{P_{PA}} - \overline{P_{PAW}} \times 80}{\dot{Q}_T}$$

$$SVR = \frac{\overline{P_{SA}} - \overline{P_{RA}} \times 80}{\dot{Q}_T}$$

where PVR = pulmonary vascular resistance, SVR = systemic vascular resistance, $\overline{P_{PAW}}$ = mean pulmonary artery wedge pressure, $\overline{P_{SA}}$ = mean systemic arterial pressure, $\overline{P_{RA}}$ = mean right atrial pressure. Normal values are 50 to 150 dyne-sec per centimeter^5 for PVR and 800 to 1200 dyne-sec per centimeter^5 for SVR.

Using these calculated variables plus the measured vascular pressures and cardiac output, patterns of hemodynamic abnormalities can be determined. Table 73–7 shows the hemodynamic patterns characteristic of the problems most frequently encountered in a critical care unit.

Liebowitz RS, Rippe JM: Arterial line placement and care. In Rippe JM, Irwin RS, Alpert JS, et al. (eds.): Intensive Care Medicine. Boston, Little, Brown and Company, 1985, pp 33–42. *A detailed description of indications, techniques, and complications of systemic arterial catheterization.*

Matthay MA: Invasive hemodynamic monitoring in critically ill patients. Clin Chest Med 4:233, 1983. *An excellent comprehensive review of indications, techniques, interpretation, and pitfalls of hemodynamic monitoring in critical care units.*

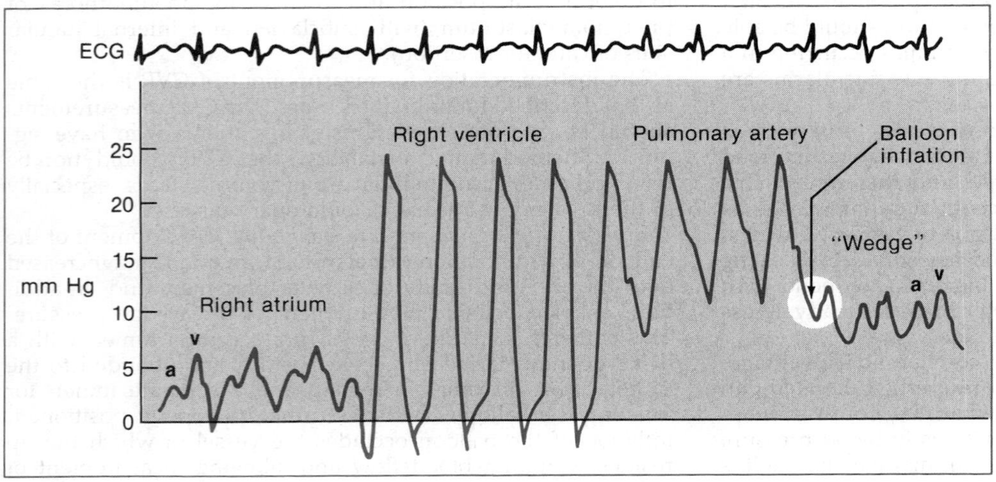

FIGURE 73–7. Tracing of pressures during passage of a Swan-Ganz catheter from the internal jugular vein into the pulmonary artery. Pressures and wave form are normal. (From Matthay MA: Invasive hemodynamic monitoring in critically ill patients. Clin Chest Med 4:233, 1983.)

TABLE 73–7. PATTERNS OF HEMODYNAMIC ABNORMALITIES IN SEVERELY ILL PATIENTS

Situation	$P\overline{SA}$	$P\overline{RA}$	$P\overline{PA}$	$P\overline{PAW}$	$C(a-\bar{v})_{O_2}$	$\dot{Q}_T$	PVR	SVR	$P\bar{v}_{O_2}$
Hypovolemic Shock	↓	↓	↓	↓	↑	↓	↑	↑	↓
Septic Shock	↓	↓	↓	↓	↓	↑	↓	↓	↑
Cardiogenic Shock	↓	↑	↑	↑	↑	↓	↑	↑	↓
Pulmonary Embolism	↓	↑	↑	→↓	↑	↓	↑	↑	↓
Airways Obstruction	→	→↑	↑	→	→	→	↑	→	→
Right Ventricular Infarct	↓	↑	→	↓→↑	↑	↓	→	→↑	→↓
Cardiac Tamponade	↓	↑	↑	↑	↑	↓	→	↑	↓
End Stage Liver Disease	↓	→↓	→↓	→↓	↓	↑	→	↓	↑

$P\overline{SA}$–mean systemic arterial pressure
$P\overline{RA}$–mean right atrial or central venous pressure
$P\overline{PA}$–mean pulmonary arterial pressure
$P\overline{PAW}$–mean pulmonary arterial wedge pressure
$C(a-\bar{v})_{O_2}$–arteriovenous O_2 content difference
$\dot{Q}_T$–cardiac output
PVR–pulmonary vascular resistance
SVR–systemic vascular resistance
$P\bar{v}_{O_2}$–mixed venous P_{O_2}

Sheneff MG, Rippe JM: Central venous catheters. In Rippe JM, Irwin RS, Alpert JS, et al. (eds.): Intensive Care Medicine. Boston, Little, Brown and Company, 1985, pp. 16–33. *An excellent description of the indications, techniques, and complications of central venous catheterization.*

Sprung CL: The Pulmonary Artery Catheter. Baltimore, University Park Press, 1983. *A thorough review of indications, techniques, complications, and clinical applications of pulmonary artery pressure measurements.*

Tooker J, Huseby J, Butler J: The effect of Swan-Ganz catheter height on the wedge pressure–left atrial pressure relationship in edema during positive pressure ventilation. Am Rev Respir Dis 117:721, 1978. *An experimental study that demonstrated that positioning of the catheter tip in the upper lung zones resulted in wedge pressure measurements that were artifactually high.*

COMPLICATIONS OF CRITICAL CARE

The complications of critical care are often difficult to detect and separate from the complications of the illnesses that necessitated the care. Iatrogenic diseases uniquely associated with the technology that constitutes critical care clearly cause significant morbidity and occasionally death, however.

Some complications are straightforward and clearly related to an intervention taking place in a critical care unit, such as ventricular tachycardia occurring during the passage of a Swan-Ganz catheter through the right ventricle. The cause of other untoward events is less easy to discover. For example, cardiac arrhythmias and gastrointestinal hemorrhage are common in patients in critical care units but are not necessarily caused by the sort of care rendered in the unit. Confounding the issue further are errors in management that, because they occur in severely ill patients, may have much graver consequences than the same error would have in a less sick patient on a medical ward.

In addition to patient-related complications, the critical care environment takes its toll on the personnel who work there. The psychologic effects of working under what often are high-pressure conditions can result in nurse or physician "burnout." Moreover, personnel in the unit may be at greater risk for certain organic diseases.

The kinds of complications to which patients are prone relate to the kind of illness they have and to the diagnostic and therapeutic interventions carried out. Respiratory support has its unique complications as does hemodynamic support and monitoring.

Complications of Respiratory Support

Oxygen therapy administered by external devices may be associated with the following adverse effects: (1) discomfort related to the device or to administration of dry gas, (2) fires, and (3) hypoventilation because of uncontrolled administration of oxygen in patients who need a precisely controlled FI_{O_2}. The first of these is not of great consequence and usually is easily managed by changing the device or improving the humidification. Fires related to oxygen delivery equipment may be catastrophic for the patient but fortunately are uncommon and generally preventable by prohibiting smoking where oxygen is being used. The last complication may be related to the wrong choice of an oxygen delivery device or to using too high a concentration of oxygen. It may also be unavoidable because of the pathophysiology underlying the disease. In any case, severe hypoventilation may be prevented by close observation of such patients and measurement of arterial blood gas tensions early in the course of oxygen administration.

Artificial airways may be associated with a number of complications. The placement of an endotracheal tube may cause immediate injury to the structures through which the tube passes—nose, hypopharynx, larynx, or trachea. The tube may be improperly positioned either at the time of placement or as a result of subsequent migration. This can result in the tube being either too low, usually in the right mainstem bronchus, or too high, with the cuff being at the level of the larynx or higher, causing an air leak around the cuff with inadequate ventilation. These problems may be minimized by the use of a tube that is easily visible on a roentgenogram and by taking a chest film immediately after placement or adjustment of the tube. In addition, daily chest roentgenograms should be obtained in patients with endotracheal tubes in place and the position of the tube noted.

Long-term problems from endotracheal tubes include necrosis of the nasal alae or internal nasal structures, sinus infection, retropharyngeal abscess formation, vocal cord damage, and tracheal injury. The tracheal injury may take the form of a tracheoesophageal fistula, which usually develops at the site of the cuff, or subsequent tracheal stenosis, also at the cuff site, that may not become apparent for several months after the tube is removed. Vocal cord or laryngeal injury may be apparent immediately after the tube is removed or may slowly progress over a period of several months.

The proper use of tubes with high compliance and low-pressure cuffs has greatly reduced the risk of injury at the cuff site. To reduce the risk still further, the pressures in the cuff should be checked periodically and kept below 20 mm Hg. The probability of injury at the other sites may be minimized by careful taping and stabilization of the tube, use of an appropriate-sized tube, and careful intubation technique. The tape holding the tube should be changed daily and the nose (if a nasal tube is used) inspected for areas of skin breakdown or necrosis.

Tracheostomy, because it bypasses the upper airway, avoids the problems associated with a tube passing through the aforementioned structures. However, tracheostomy itself has its own unique complications that more than offset its advantages. Early problems include hemorrhage, mediastinal and subcutaneous emphysema, and malpositioning of the tube. Subsequently, soft tissue infection, late hemorrhage, and tracheal stenosis may occur either at the site where the tube cuff impinged on the tracheal wall or, more commonly, at the site of the opening into the trachea. The overall frequency of complications, particularly the occurrence of tracheal stenosis, appears to be greater with tracheostomy than with endotracheal tubes. The frequency of tracheostomy complications can be reduced by careful operative techniques, use of tubes with low-pressure cuffs, effective stabilization of the tube, and meticulous wound care.

Obstruction of either endotracheal or tracheostomy tubes may occur as a result of inspissated secretions or blood clots. This problem may be prevented by adequate humidification of the inspired gas mixture and by frequent suctioning through the tube.

Both endotracheal and tracheostomy tubes are associated with an increased risk of *pulmonary infection*. The presence of the tube considerably compromises the normal mechanisms by which the airways rid themselves of potentially infecting agents. In addition, hospitalized patients, particularly those in critical care units, are much more likely to have colonization of the airways with organisms that are more pathogenic than those usually present. Both aerobic gram-negative organisms and staphylococci tend to replace the normal oropharyngeal flora in critically ill patients. The distinction between airway colonization with these organisms and true pulmonary infection may be quite difficult. Patients with endotracheal or tracheostomy tubes in place should have daily Gram's stains (not cultures) of aspirated sputum. Infection is often heralded by an increasing number of organisms and polymorphonuclear leukocytes present in the sputum with a subsequent increase in abnormalities on the chest roentgenogram and the appearance of or increase in fever. The finding of organisms in the sputum should not in itself be interpreted as indicating infection.

Mechanical ventilation may be associated with complications apart from the artificial airway, for example, *overventilation* and *underventilation, reduction in cardiac output*, and *pneumothorax* and/or *pneumomediastinum*. Use of the guidelines for mechanical ventilation discussed previously in this chapter will minimize the likelihood of either overventilation or underventilation. Nevertheless, Pa_{O_2}, Pa_{CO_2}, and arterial pH must be determined shortly after mechanical ventilation is initiated and after changes in either ventilator settings or the patient's condition.

The mechanisms by which mechanical ventilation and particularly CPPV reduce cardiac output are probably multifactorial, but the major effect seems to be a reduction of right ventricular inflow caused by decreased transmural right ventricular filling pressure. This effect is particularly evident in patients who are hypovolemic and may be offset by volume replacement. High levels of PEEP usually reduce cardiac output in normovolemic as well as hypovolemic patients. When cardiac output is reduced by PEEP, its beneficial effects must be weighed against the potential deleterious effects of further administration of intravenous fluids. In evaluating the usefulness of PEEP in a given patient, the overall effect on systemic oxygen transport should be measured and PEEP adjusted to yield the optimal balance between Pa_{O_2} and cardiac output.

Lung rupture with subsequent pneumothorax or pneumomediastinum probably relates to the increased transmural distending pressure in airways and alveoli. This pressure results in less distention of abnormal alveoli and relative overdistention of the more normal alveoli that can predispose them to rupture. For this reason, as well as to minimize the effects of pressure on cardiac output, the minimal amount of PEEP that is consistent with optimal oxygen transport should be used. Peak airway pressure can be lowered by using inspiratory flows that are as slow as possible while still maintaining an appropriate inspiration-expiration ratio.

Oxygen toxicity is not a complication of mechanical ventilation per se but usually occurs in patients who are being mechanically ventilated with gas mixtures containing high concentrations of oxygen (see Ch. 537). Although it is not clearly determined, the threshold for clinically significant oxygen toxicity seems to be approximately 0.6 atmospheres, the important variable being PI_{O_2} rather than FI_{O_2}. Histologic changes in the lung that are compatible with oxygen toxicity have been noted in persons receiving lower concentrations of oxygen for long periods of time, but the clinical significance of these observations appears to be minimal.

The clinical syndromes produced by hyperoxia include tracheobronchitis, ARDS, and bronchopulmonary dysplasia. *Tracheobronchitis* is usually acute, manifested by substernal chest pain and nonproductive cough occurring after 12 to 24 hours of breathing oxygen at 1 atmosphere. The time course of *ARDS caused by oxygen* is not well defined and probably varies, being influenced by other factors in addition to the FI_{O_2}. *Bronchopulmonary dysplasia* probably does not occur in adults but is common in neonates given high concentrations of oxygen.

The diagnosis of oxygen toxicity is extremely difficult to establish. Patients who require high oxygen concentrations already have sufficient clinical, physiologic, radiographic, and histologic abnormalities to obscure any additional changes caused by oxygen. Thus, at present the diagnosis is usually presumptive.

The prevention of oxygen toxicity rests with the general principle of using as low an inspired oxygen concentration as possible that provides the patient with adequate systemic oxygen transport. From the oxyhemoglobin dissociation curve (Fig. 73–4) it is apparent that at a Pa_{O_2} of 60 mm Hg, hemoglobin is nearly fully saturated. Further increases in Pa_{O_2} add little to oxygen transport. Thus, a Pa_{O_2} of 60 mm Hg, in general, should be regarded as satisfactory. In patients with ARDS the use of PEEP as previously described will often allow reduction of the FI_{O_2}. At present, there are no proved biochemical approaches to the prevention of oxygen toxicity, although several theoretically attractive possibilities exist.

Complications of Hemodynamic Monitoring

There are primarily three types of problems associated with hemodynamic monitoring: local complications associated with vascular access, passage and final positioning of the catheter, and inappropriate decision making based on inaccurate data or misinterpretation of information from the monitoring device. The last complications can best be prevented by proper maintenance of equipment and accurate and frequent calibration checks. As a general rule, monitoring data that are not consistent with the clinical situation or on which crucial therapeutic decisions hinge should not be accepted until the system has been thoroughly checked, zeroed, and calibrated.

SYSTEMIC ARTERIAL PRESSURE. The most frequent complication of systemic arterial blood pressure monitoring is formation of a hematoma at the site of the arterial puncture. This may be prevented or minimized by careful insertion technique, manual application of pressure immediately after insertion, and use of a pressure dressing, with care taken not to compromise distal circulation. Actual laceration of the vessel may require surgical repair.

Peripheral nerve damage may result from direct injury at the time of insertion or from a hematoma. Prevention involves careful insertion technique and measures to reduce the likelihood of formation of a hematoma.

Ischemia distal to the site of catheter insertion may result from arterial obstruction by the catheter itself, because of a clot forming around the catheter or because of embolization from clots on the tip of the catheter. Use of the appropriate-sized catheter will reduce the likelihood of obstruction of flow. Newer materials such as polyamine resins and Teflon are minimally thrombogenic and decrease the risk of a clot forming around the catheter. Also, continuous flush devices that deliver a small constant volume of heparinized solution greatly decrease clotting at the catheter tip or in the lumen.

Local infection at the site of insertion of a percutaneous arterial catheter or in the vessel itself is less common than with venous catheters but nevertheless may be a problem. This risk can be minimized by careful asepsis at the time of catheter insertion, sterile dressings changed daily, and prompt removal of the catheter when it is no longer needed or serving its intended purpose.

CENTRAL VENOUS PRESSURE. The complications of central venous pressure monitoring include problems related to venous access, air embolism, infection, and venous thrombosis. When the subclavian or internal jugular vein is used for venous access, important complications include pneumothorax, hydrothorax, hemothorax, mediastinal hematoma, and subclavian or carotid artery puncture. If the left internal jugular or subclavian vein is used, the thoracic duct may be damaged, resulting in lymph fistula or chylothorax. Brachial nerve injury also may result from attempted subclavian vein catheterization. When an antecubital cutdown is used for central venous catheter placement, the brachial artery or median nerve may be injured. With each of these approaches local or intravascular infection or both and venous thrombosis may occur. If insertion is via a needle, withdrawal of the catheter through the needle may shear the catheter and create embolism of a foreign body.

Prevention of all of these complications is best approached through the use of meticulous insertion technique and maintenance of asepsis. Catheters placed and maintained with strict aseptic technique may be kept in place for long periods of time. However, under standard conditions in severely ill patients, they should not be left in place for more than 48 to 72 hours. A chest roentgenogram should be obtained promptly after catheter placement to look for evidence of pneumothorax or pleural fluid and to check the catheter position. Catheters that have entered the right ventricle should be withdrawn into the superior vena cava.

PULMONARY ARTERY PRESSURE. All of the complications attendant to central venous pressure monitoring may also occur with a pulmonary artery catheter. In addition, problems occur that are unique to this form of hemodynamic monitoring. The most common complication is a disturbance of cardiac rhythm or conduction or both. Premature ventricular contractions occur quite commonly as the catheter passes through the right ventricle. These generally are self-limited, at least with prompt catheter passage, but may occasionally require intravenous administration of 50 to 75 mg of lidocaine. Sustained ventricular tachycardia and ventricular fibrillation may also occur.

The frequency of ventricular arrhythmias can be minimized by inflating the balloon fully during catheter insertion and attempting rapid passage through the right ventricle. Guide wires and central venous catheters should not be advanced into the ventricle. Electrocardiographic monitoring with a visual display and audible signal should always be used during insertion. If ventricular arrhythmias occur, the catheter should promptly be withdrawn from the ventricle. Finally, intravenous lidocaine, a defibrillator, and resuscitation equipment should be immediately available.

During catheter insertion and occasionally after placement, right bundle branch block can develop. This usually does not present a problem unless there was a pre-existing left bundle branch block. In patients with left bundle branch block who need a pulmonary artery catheter passed, it may be advisable first to place a temporary transvenous pacemaker.

Intrapulmonary complications of Swan-Ganz catheters include pulmonary infarction and pulmonary artery rupture. Pulmonary infarction occurs because the tip of the catheter has migrated into and obstructed a peripheral vessel or because of clot propagation at the catheter tip. These can be avoided by continuously monitoring the pulmonary artery pressure to look for a "permanent wedge" pressure tracing. If this is noted, the catheter should be withdrawn to a point where the pulmonary artery wedge pressure appears only after the balloon is inflated with 1 ml of air. Clot propagation is minimized by using the continuous flow device described previously. The likelihood of rupture of the pulmonary artery is also decreased by ensuring that the catheter is positioned properly in a more proximal vessel.

Psychologic Consequences of Critical Care

CONSEQUENCES FOR THE PATIENT. The patient-related psychologic consequences of critical care are difficult to define and quantitate. In many instances what might appear as disordered behavior in a critically ill patient in fact represents an appropriate response to a genuinely threatening situation. In others the behavior is an organic effect of the illness itself; for example, patients with chronic airways obstruction and hypoxemia have been found to have well-defined behavioral alterations. It is only logical to assume, however, that an environment so foreign and so frightening as a critical care unit that operates totally independent of and without concern for any biologic rhythm could in and of itself produce significant psychologic disturbances, especially when superimposed on the effects of critical illness. Pain and discomfort, sensory deprivation—often with beeps, hisses, and buzzes as the major input—erratic and interrupted sleep patterns, immobilization, and total dependence on others are certainly capable of contributing to clouding of consciousness, perceptual distortion, behavioral confusion, and delusional experiences.

Because of the difficulty in identifying and quantitating the psychologic consequences of critical care, specific preventive measures are not so clearly definable as with other complications. However, standard approaches in critical care management of patients should be geared to providing a milieu that is least likely to generate the factors previously cited as contributing to psychiatric syndromes. Patients should be treated as cognizant, intelligent human beings by all staff. Every attempt should be made to incorporate the patient into discussions regarding care. A patient, even one who appears to be comatose, should not be treated as an inanimate object around which an esoteric discussion is held. Monitoring equipment should not be used as a substitute for interpersonal contact. The equipment used and procedures performed should be carefully explained to the patient. Insofar as possible, the day-night sleep cycle should be maintained. Providing the patient with a calendar serves to create or maintain a correct time orientation. A television set in the room may provide more "normal" sensory input serving to over-ride the barrage of alarms and noises from ventilators and other sources. A liberal visiting policy allows needed "outside world" contact and helps to maintain contact with a familiar frame of reference. Sedative drugs and narcotics should be used only for specific indications such as for adequate pain relief. Benzodiazepines (such as diazepam or midazolam) and occasionally haloperidol (Haldol) can be extremely helpful in managing the psychiatric syndromes that do not respond to supportive treatment. Perhaps more important than all of these is the establishment of a pattern of behavior and interaction on the part of the critical care staff that fosters patient trust and confidence.

CONSEQUENCES FOR THE STAFF. Critical care staff members are also subject to the psychologic effects associated with providing care to severely ill patients. A variety of factors have been identified as contributing to the stress on critical care personnel, especially the nursing staff. First, the work is physically demanding and tiring. Second, patients, families, and physicians are emotionally demanding; emotional fatigue becomes superimposed on physical fatigue. The responsibilities are great and the performance expectations high while quite commonly the level of responsibility is not matched by decision-making authority. Such authority is vested in physicians who may have considerably less experience and expertise in critical care than the nurses. Nurses see what they may consider to be errors being made or patients getting worse and they are powerless to intervene in a meaningful way. These sorts of conflicts compound the already heightened emotional tension almost invariably present in critical care units. In addition, there are the genuine sorrow, distress, and sometimes guilt that accompany deaths occurring in the unit.

The important consequences of these factors are that patient care may be compromised and that the turnover of unit personnel is high. Prevention of these sorts of situations is not easy. Many of the problems are inherent in the job. However, provision of clearly defined administrative guidelines describing the lines of authority and responsibility may minimize the conflicts. Likewise, having standard policies that are developed and agreed upon by the nursing and physician staff members provides support for independent nursing action. Nursing administrative policies also have considerable influence on the emotional well-being of the staff. Staffing ratios, hours worked per shift, and work breaks all are important factors that can be manipulated to reduce stress among the critical care staff. Finally, it is important that there be a single physician in charge of the unit through whom "official" communication between the nursing and medical staff takes place and to whom members of each group can present their problems and complaints. This physician, working in concert with the head nurse, can develop mechanisms for dealing with the various stressful situations either as they arise or preferably before they occur.

Fisher AB: Oxygen therapy: Side effects and toxicity. Am Rev Respir Dis. 122:61, 1980. *A concise review of what is known about oxygen toxicity. Discusses approaches to prevention.*

Kieley WF, Procci WR: Psychiatric aspects of critical care. In Zschoche DA (ed.): Comprehensive Review of Critical Care. St. Louis, C. V. Mosby Company, 1981, pp 107–114. *A review of the kinds of psychiatric disorders commonly seen in critically ill patients with a discussion of specific approaches to management.*

Liebowitz RS, Rippe JM: Arterial line placement and care. In Rippe JM, Irwin RS, Alpert JS, et al. (eds.): Intensive Care Medicine. Boston, Little, Brown and Company, 1985, pp 33–42. *A detailed description of indications, techniques, and complications of systemic arterial catheterization.*

Robin ED: The cult of the Swan-Ganz catheter: Overuse and misuse of pulmonary flow catheters. Ann Intern Med 103:445, 1985. *Presents the view that pulmonary artery catheters are vastly overused relative to their proven benefits and complications.*

Seneff MG, Rippe JM: Central venous catheters. In Rippe JM, Irwin RS, Alpert JS, et al. (eds.): Intensive Care Medicine. Boston, Little, Brown and Company, 1985, pp 16–33. *An excellent description of the indications, techniques, and complications of central venous catheterization.*

Spring CL: Complications of pulmonary artery catheterization. In Spring CL (ed.): The Pulmonary Artery Catheter. Baltimore, University Park Press, 1983, pp 73–101. *An extensively referenced discussion of the complications occurring with Swan-Ganz pulmonary artery catheters. Presents the mechanisms by which the complications occur and the means for their prevention.*

Stauffer JL, Olson DE, Petty TL: Complications and consequences of endotracheal intubation and tracheostomy. Am J Med 70:65, 1981. *A prospective study of 150 patients requiring either endotracheal intubation or tracheostomy because of critical illness. Points out that, although the frequency of complications was similar with the two artificial airways, the complications of tracheostomy were much more likely to be severe than those associated with endotracheal tubes.*

SOCIAL AND ETHICAL ISSUES IN CRITICAL CARE

Indications for and Value of Critical Care

Although defining the value of critical care and its indications would not seem to pertain to a discussion of social and ethical issues, this is, in fact, the topic area in which such considerations are most appropriate. The kinds of technology used and techniques involved in critical care are rather easily described in a straightforward scientific manner. The ends achieved by these interventions are not so clearly defined. If the relationship was strictly one between science and health or between medical practice and the patient's well-being, the discussion would be simple. Unfortunately, medical practice and the patient's well-being are not clearly and directly related when the connection is through the medium of a critical care unit. Critical care expensively consumes public resources, and its indications and values are poorly defined. The uses of critical care have therefore become a matter involving serious ethical and public policy considerations.

Critical care units have been utilized more or less in their present form for approximately 25 years, yet their contribution to health has not been quantitated. Studies of patients suspected of having a myocardial infarction have suggested that if there are no early (initial 2 hours in one study and 24 hours in the second) indications of complications, management in a coronary care unit does not offer any advantage over management in a general ward or at home. Unfortunately, no such studies exist for the usual category of patients admitted to a general critical care unit. The available data generally describe features of patients admitted to general critical care units and construct evaluative indexes that can be correlated with prognosis. In theory, patients for whom the index indicates a poor prognosis should not be admitted to a critical care unit because it is highly unlikely that all of the interventions available will produce a favorable result. In practice, most physicians caring for a gravely ill patient want the patient to have every opportunity to survive and will request that critical care be provided almost regardless of ultimate prognosis. This is a dilemma that to date has not been solved.

Some categories of patients such as those with end-stage malignancies or those who are very old should clearly not be treated in critical care units. Mentally competent adults who do not wish to undergo the potential rigors of critical care and so inform their physicians should not be admitted to such a unit. On the other hand, patients with significant cardiac arrhythmias, drug-overdosed patients, patients with reversible neuromuscular diseases, those with severe asthma, and victims of multiple trauma, in general, definitely benefit from critical care.

Death rates in critical care units vary considerably depending on the type of unit and the severity of illness of patients admitted. The apparent overall mortality ranges from approximately 10 per cent to 30 per cent. The mortality is higher if patients have a chronic disease. Patients who require mechanical ventilation do much less well than the group as a whole. In one study the need for mechanical ventilation for 48 hours, independent of the reasons for ventilation, was associated with an in-hospital mortality rate of 64 per cent, a one-year mortality rate of 70 per cent, and a three-year mortality rate of 72 per cent. In another study of patients with acute respiratory failure the mortality rate for those who required mechanical ventilation with an $F_{I_{O_2}}$ of 0.5 or greater for more than 24 hours was 66 per cent; patients who required an $F_{I_{O_2}}$ of 1.0 with a PEEP of 5 cm H_2O or more for 2 hours or an $F_{I_{O_2}}$ of 0.6 and a PEEP of 5 cm H_2O for 12 hours or more had a mortality rate of 92 per cent.

Unfortunately, with the data available, physicians are not able to predict reliably who will benefit from critical care and who will not. For this reason much of the decision making regarding who should be admitted to a critical care unit will in the future probably be conditioned by social (i.e., public policy) and ethical considerations rather than by scientific analyses.

Specific Ethical Issues

The basic precepts of medical ethics are discussed in Ch. 5. In this section specific concerns that arise in critical care are addressed.

THE INFLUENCE OF PATIENT WISHES ON THE CARE GIVEN. The autonomy of a mentally competent patient must be respected. If the patient indicates that a specific intervention such as endotracheal intubation, mechanical ventilation, or cardiopulmonary resuscitation is not to be used, it should not be used. The concern with the patient's competence, however, often clouds the issue and makes the decision less than clear-cut. The physician charged with the care of the patient must thoroughly review the process by which the decision was made with the patient and, when appropriate, with the patient's family. If there is a question in the physician's mind as to the competence of the patient, consultation should be sought.

"DO NOT RESUSCITATE" ORDERS. Orders not to initiate cardiopulmonary resuscitation (CPR) may be written at the request of patients as just discussed or may be initiated by physicians caring for patients when to the best of the physician's knowledge CPR is an intervention that will not be successful in the broad sense of restoring meaningful life. In most instances, such decisions should be discussed with the patient and, when appropriate, with the family. The order should then be written in standard fashion in the order sheet, and a note describing the basis for the order and the discussions that took place with the patient and family should be included in the chart. These orders should be reviewed at least daily because circumstances may change. Such orders clarify the ambiguity that surrounds the decisions concerning critical care for a patient with an irreversible illness and relieve the nurse or uninvolved physicians from the responsibility of deciding not to initiate CPR in such a patient.

So-called "no code" patients may still benefit from critical care. Treating airways obstruction, heart failure, metabolic abnormalities, or arrhythmias may at least temporarily improve the patient's condition, making the existence of "do not resuscitate" orders a moot point.

TERMINATION OF LIFE SUPPORT SYSTEMS. Supportive measures may be discontinued when there is no hope for recovery. Continuation of such measures serves only to prolong the process of dying. Defining the hopeless situation, however, may be difficult. The most straightforward instance is that of brain death. Brain death has been defined by several sets of unambiguous medical criteria (see Ch. 457). The American Bar Association and a number of states have adopted the broader concept that "for all legal purposes a human body with irreversible cessation of brain function, according to usual and customary standards of medical practice, shall be considered dead."

Various prognostic indicators have been developed to allow prediction of the likelihood of recovery after severe brain insults. These provide guidance in instances in which all criteria for brain death are not present.

Black PMcL: Brain death. N Engl J Med 299:338 and 393, 1978. *An extensive review of all aspects of brain death, including legal considerations.*

Chassin MR: Costs and outcome of medical intensive care. Med Care 20:165, 1982. *In addition to discussing costs and outcomes in critical care, this report describes the growth of critical care units in the United States.*

Hill JD, Hampton JR, Mitchell JRA: A randomized trial of home-versus-hospital management for patients with suspected myocardial infarction. Lancet 1:837, 1978. *A report of the only well-designed prospective randomized study of the value of critical care (in this case, coronary care). Demonstrated that if the myocardial infarction was not complicated, hospital care offered no clear advantage over home care.*

Knaus WA, Droper EA, Wayne DP, et al.: Prognosis in acute organ-system failure. Ann Surg 202:685, 1985. *Presents the results of a prospective study relating acute organ-system failure to prognosis in patients admitted to critical care units.*

Lee MA, Cassel CK: The ethical and legal framework for the order not to resuscitate. West J Med 140:117, 1984. *Describes the ethical consideration to be taken into account in determining a patient's resuscitation status and reviews the legal underpinnings of such decisions. Step by step guidelines in implementing the decision process.*

Levy DE, Bates D, Caronna JJ, et al.: Prognosis in nontraumatic coma. Ann Intern Med 94:293, 1981. *Presents the results of a prospective study of 500 patients with nontraumatic coma. Identifies factors that allow early identification of patients in whom recovery is very unlikely.*

Robin ED: A critical look at critical care. Crit Care Med 11:144, 1983. *A provocative discussion of the role of critical care in modern medical care. Presents a plea for objective evaluation of the indications and value of critical care.*

Schmidt CD, Elliott CG, Carmelli D, et al.: Prolonged mechanical ventilation for respiratory failure: A cost benefit analysis. Crit Care Med 11:407, 1983. *Defines the cost and benefits associated with prolonged (48 hours or more) mechanical ventilation primarily in medical patients.*

Waner SH, Adelstein SJ, Cranford RE, et al.: The physician's responsibility toward hopelessly ill patients. N Engl J Med 310:955, 1984. *The report, written by a multidisciplinary group, discusses the role of patients and physicians in determining appropriate levels of care for patients who are hopelessly ill.*

CARDIOPULMONARY RESUSCITATION

Cardiopulmonary resuscitation is the supportive and sometimes definitive treatment applied to persons in whom, for whatever reason, effective cardiac and ventilatory activity has stopped. The situations in which this catastrophic event may occur unexpectedly include primary cardiac arrhythmias, arrhythmias associated with myocardial infarction, drowning, electrocution, acute upper airways obstruction, drug intoxication, and accidental trauma. In addition, cardiorespiratory arrest may result from a variety of underlying disease processes that reduce myocardial oxygen delivery or are associated with marked electrolyte or acid-base disturbances.

There are no data on the annual number of cardiorespiratory arrests occurring in this country. It is estimated, however, that more than 1 million persons have myocardial infarctions each year and that 540,000 persons die annually of coronary artery disease (Ch. 51). The majority of these deaths take place out of the hospital, usually within two hours of the onset of symptoms. These data have suggested that for CPR to be truly effective it should be applied in the community at large rather than being limited to an in-hospital technique. For this reason, a standard program for training lay persons in basic life support was developed and implemented throughout the country. By 1980 over 12 million persons in the United States had received training in basic life support.

In some communities more than 40 per cent of patients with documented ventricular fibrillation occurring out of the hospital have been resuscitated and in some subgroups survival has been as high as 60 to 80 per cent. These rates of success are generally attributed to the intervention of trained bystanders in initiating CPR and maintaining support until paramedical personnel arrive. The rate of survival following in-hospital cardiac arrest is much lower, ranging from 5 to 20 per cent. Different subgroups have markedly different rates, however. In one series patients with evidence of cardiac failure prior to the arrest had only a 2 per cent likelihood of survival and renal failure was associated with 3 per cent survival rate. Only 4 per cent of patients who were homebound before hospitalization in which the cardiac arrest occurred survived. On the other hand 27 per cent of patients who were active before entering the hospital survived.

Pathophysiology of Cardiorespiratory Arrest

SYSTEMIC EFFECTS. Cardiorespiratory arrest results in the cessation of effective delivery of oxygen to body tissues. The immediate effects are the same as those described in the discussion of shock (Ch. 44). Catecholamine release results in peripheral vasoconstriction in an attempt to preserve blood flow to the brain and heart at the expense of cutaneous, muscle, and renal blood flow. Without oxygen, tissue metabolic processes become anaerobic with production of lactic acid, a by-product of anaerobic glycolysis, resulting in systemic metabolic acidosis. The amount of acidosis is determined largely by the balance between oxygen supply and oxygen demand. Thus, hypothermic patients, such as near-drowning victims, because of reduced oxygen needs have less lactate production and less tissue damage. Because there is no circulation or the circulation is much reduced, the lactic acid is not cleared from the tissues. As the hydrogen ion concentration increases, the effectiveness of catecholamines rapidly decreases, resulting in full vasodilation that abolishes the major mechanisms by which the blood volume is preferentially distributed to the brain and the heart. Irreversible damage to these critical organs ensues.

The critical determinants of the outcome of a cardiorespiratory arrest and resuscitation attempts are: (1) the reversibility of the abnormality leading to the cessation of effective cardiac output and (2) the success of the CPR in providing sufficient oxygen to the brain to prevent permanent damage.

CEREBRAL EFFECTS. Oxygen consumption by the brain ranges from 3 to 5 ml per minute per 100 grams of tissue during normal consciousness and cerebral blood flow (CBF) averages 50 to 60 ml per minute per 100 grams of tissue. Aerobic metabolism can be supported by as little as 0.21 ml of oxygen per minute per 100 grams of tissue. Experimentally, CBF carrying a normal amount of oxygen can be reduced to 16 to 18 ml per minute per 100 grams of tissue before electroencephalographic evidence of injury is seen. The determinants of CBF are the mean systemic arterial pressure ($\overline{PSA}$), the cerebrovascular resistance (CVR), and the intracranial pressure (ICP), which determines cerebral venous pressure. Thus,

$$CBF = \frac{\overline{PSA} - ICP}{CVR}$$

Under normal circumstances, CBF increases with increases in Pa_{CO_2} and with hypoxemia (below Pa_{O_2} 50 mm Hg) because of decreases in CVR.

Sudden cessation of blood flow to the brain, as occurs with cardiorespiratory arrest, results in unconsciousness within 10 seconds. Cerebral glycolysis is stimulated seven-fold, but endogenous stores of glucose are inadequate to maintain cellular viability for more than a few minutes. When brain adenosine triphosphate is reduced to 20 per cent of basal levels, which occurs within five minutes of cessation of effective CBF, lactate production ceases and irreversible neuronal damage results. Because oxygen utilization is nonuniform within the brain, some areas such as the frontal and temporal cortexes are more susceptible to ischemia than areas of lower metabolic activity. Restoration of cerebral perfusion after a period of no flow may result in transient increases in ICP, perhaps causing focal hypoperfusion and further ischemic injury.

CARDIAC EFFECTS. Myocardial oxygen consumption ranges from 8 to 10 ml of oxygen per minute per 100 grams of tissue for basal needs in the normally beating, nonischemic heart and 4 to 5 ml of oxygen per minute per 100 grams of tissue during ventricular fibrillation. Assuming normal Ca_{O_2} and an extraction of oxygen of 75 per cent, a myocardial blood flow of approximately 60 ml per minute per 100 grams of tissue would be required to meet oxygen needs in normal sinus rhythm. In ventricular fibrillation this figure would be 25 ml per minute per 100 grams of tissue. Myocardial blood flow (MBF) is determined by the $\overline{PSA}$, the coronary venous sinus pressure approximated by the mean right atrial pressure ($\overline{PRA}$), and the coronary vascular resistance CVR, as follows:

$$MBF = \frac{\overline{PSA} - \overline{PRA}}{CVR}$$

Coronary flow normally occurs during diastole when the aortic valve is closed. Thus, maintenance of coronary perfusion during CPR requires that the aortic valve close normally, that $\overline{PSA}$ remain elevated above $\overline{PRA}$, and that time for coronary filling be allowed. Coronary vascular resistance is likely to be minimal during ventricular fibrillation or asystole; however, in the presence of coronary artery disease, resistance and therefore flow will be nonuniform and probably cause regional ischemia and perhaps infarction. Fortunately, myocardial oxygen needs should also be low.

EFFECTS ON RESPIRATORY MUSCLES. Under normal circumstances the oxygen consumption of the respiratory muscles, primarily the diaphragm, is less than 5 per cent of total body oxygen consumption. However, as the work of breathing increases because of cardiac or pulmonary disorders or metabolic acidosis the oxygen needs of the respiratory muscles increase. In cardiogenic shock the respiratory muscles may become the most metabolically active tissues in the body. Because the oxygen need is increasing at a time when supply is decreasing, the ability of these muscles to maintain their work level may be impaired and hypoventilation may ensue.

Fatigue of the diaphragm may play an important role in augmenting the factors that lead to cardiorespiratory arrest. This suggests also that restoration of respiratory muscle function is an important goal in CPR. Restoration of function depends on improvement in muscle blood flow, which is determined by $\overline{PSA}$, $\overline{PRA}$, and muscle vascular resistance (MVR):

$$MBF = \frac{\overline{PSA} - \overline{PRA}}{MVR}$$

Furthermore, the oxygen needs of the respiratory muscles can be greatly reduced by effective mechanical ventilation.

RENAL EFFECTS. Renal blood flow suffers from the preferential redistribution of cardiac output to the brain and heart when hypotension occurs. Under baseline conditions, renal blood flow is approximately 25 per cent of the normal resting cardiac output and oxygen consumption is 9 to 10 ml of oxygen per minute per 100 grams of tissue. Although autoregulation of renal perfusion tends to maintain blood flow over a wide range of perfusion pressures, in shock the flow is markedly reduced. This may result in cellular injury and acute renal failure even if circulation is properly restored.

Administering Cardiopulmonary Resuscitation

IMMEDIATE INTERVENTIONS. The immediate sequence of events that should be undertaken by the person who first encounters a victim of a cardiorespiratory arrest is listed in Table 73–8. The mechanisms for providing the necessary support will, of course, vary depending on the training of the person or persons on the scene and whether or not the arrest occurs within a hospital.

Artificial Ventilation. An important determinant of success in CPR is the provision of adequate ventilation. The first step is to open the airway and assure its patency. The most common cause of obstruction is the tongue. This may be corrected simply by tilting the head backward and lifting the chin or lower jaw forward. Mouth-to-mouth ventilation can then be applied unless there is a foreign body obstructing the airway. A breath sufficient to make the chest wall rise should be given in 1 to 1.5 seconds.

A resuscitator's exhaled air may provide an FI_{O_2} of approximately 0.17 during mouth-to-mouth ventilation and carbon dioxide will be eliminated because of passive lung deflation. Commonly, however,, gas exchange within the lungs is not normal and significant hypoxemia develops. For this reason supplemental oxygen should be administered as soon as it is available. Both oxygen administration and ventilation can be accomplished via a tight-fitting face mask and ventilation bag, preferably one capable of delivering an FI_{O_2} of 1.0. Endotracheal intubation provides the most reliable closed system of oxygen administration and also protects the airway against the aspiration of gastric contents.

Closed Chest Compression. Closed chest compression should be administered to patients who do not have a palpable pulse. The patient should be supine and on a firm surface. Sufficient pressure should be applied to the lower half of the

TABLE 73–8. IMMEDIATE SEQUENCE OF EVENTS IN CPR

Establish unresponsiveness
Call for help
Position victim
Open airway
Check for foreign body in airway
Institute mouth-to-mouth breathing
Check for pulse
Initiate closed chest compression

sternum to depress it 4 to 5 cm in most adults and 2 cm in children. The pressure should be relaxed after each compression, allowing the sternum to return to its relaxed position. The recommended compression-to-relaxation ratio is 1:1, and the rate of compressions should be a minimum of 80 per minute and 100 per minute if possible. The adequacy of closed chest compression should be determined by attempting to palpate a carotid or femoral pulse produced by the compression.

The mechanism by which closed chest compression causes blood to circulate is not clear. The original "cardiac pump" theory was that by compressing the chest the heart was squeezed between the sternum and the vertebral column, producing a mechanical systole in which right and left ventricular pressures exceed pulmonary artery and aortic pressures, respectively, causing forward blood flow. Release of the pressure caused diastolic filling of the ventricles due to the gradient between the peripheral venous system and the intrathoracic structures.

More recent data suggest that it is the total intrathoracic pressure that causes forward blood flow rather than cardiac compression ("thoracic pump" theory). For example, cough in itself has sustained cardiac output and consciousness in patients with ventricular fibrillation. A variety of experimental studies are consistent with this contention.

INTERMEDIATE INTERVENTIONS. The arrival of persons with more advanced training and equipment marks the second or intermediate phase of CPR. Electrocardiographic monitoring enables proper application of direct current countershock for defibrillation or conversion of ventricular tachycardia. A current of 200 to 360 joules should be used for ventricular fibrillation and 25 to 50 joules for ventricular tachycardias. The current given should be increased if there is no response to the initial shock. In patients with ventricular fibrillation, epinephrine should be administered routinely either intravenously (preferably by a central venous catheter) or via an endotracheal tube before countershock is applied. Epinephrine enhances myocardial contractility, constricts peripheral vasculature, and lowers the defibrillation threshold. This combination of effects operates to improve cerebral and cardiac perfusion and to increase the likelihood of defibrillation occurring. Standard doses are 0.5 to 1.0 mg or 5 to 10 ml of a 1:10,000 dilution. The dose can be repeated at approximately five-minute intervals. Although previous recommendations indicated that calcium chloride was useful in improving myocardial contractility, recent data have not demonstrated its usefulness, and because of theoretic adverse effects, calcium is not recommended for routine administration.

Lidocaine is the initial drug of choice to suppress ventricular ectopy in the setting of cardiorespiratory arrest. The usual dose is approximately 1 mg per kilogram (50 to 75 mg) given intravenously as a bolus injection. Additional boluses of 0.5 mg per kilogram may be given at 10-minute intervals to a total of 3 mg per kilogram. This is then followed by a continuous intravenous infusion of 1 to 4 mg per minute. Other agents that may be useful for ventricular arrhythmias not responsive to lidocaine include bretylium tosylate, procainamide, and verapamil. The doses and uses of these drugs are discussed in Ch. 45.

Atropine sulfate is useful in treating sinus bradycardia or complete heart block because it increases the rate of discharge of the sinus node and improves atrioventricular conduction. The usual dose of atropine sulfate is 0.5 mg administered intravenously and repeated at 5-minute intervals until the desired rate is achieved or a total dose of 2 mg is given.

Isoproterenol may also be used to treat hemodynamically significant bradycardia resulting from heart block that is refractory to atropine. Caution should be exercised in the use of both of these agents in that myocardial oxygen requirements increase with increases in heart rate. Thus, ischemia may be worsened by increasing heart rate above that necessary to provide an adequate cardiac output.

Contrary to previous recommendations, administration of bicarbonate is no longer thought to be beneficial and is not recommended for routine use.

INTERVENTIONS AFTER INITIAL RECOVERY. All patients who have been resuscitated successfully should be transferred as quickly as possible to a critical care unit. As a minimum, electrocardiographic monitoring should be provided. The need for invasive hemodynamic monitoring depends on the causes and consequences of the cardiorespiratory arrest. Often, at least transiently, it is necessary to provide mechanical ventilation. This allows rest and functional recovery of the respiratory muscles and minimizes total oxygen needs. The major determinant of return of brain function is the adequacy of cerebral perfusion during the period of cardiac arrest. Subsequently, after recovery of cardiac function, all factors that influence oxygen delivery to the brain should be evaluated and made normal where possible. Measures to prevent elevation in intracranial pressure (ICP), such as keeping the patient's head elevated, controlling arterial pH and Pa_{CO_2}, and treating seizures and agitation, should be undertaken. The effectiveness of measures designed to minimize brain damage, including the use of barbiturates, calcium channel–blocking agents, and systemic hypothermia, remains to be proven.

REASONS FOR FAILURE. Obviously, not all persons who sustain cardiac arrest can or should be resuscitated. Often the process leading to the arrest is irreversible or the resulting cardiac injury is so severe that it precludes successful resuscitation. In some instances, however, reversible factors may play a major role in the failure of CPR to restore an adequate cardiac output. These factors include severe electrolyte and acid-base disturbances, inadequate oxygenation or ventilation because of faulty technique, hypovolemia, pneumothorax (especially tension pneumothorax), and cardiac tamponade. Abnormalities of electrolyte and acid-base balance as well as inadequate oxygenation and/or ventilation usually manifest themselves as an inability to restore an adequate cardiac rate and rhythm. Hypovolemia, tension pneumothorax, and cardiac tamponade usually cause electromechanical dissociation in which the rate and rhythm of the heart are satisfactory but the cardiac output is inadequate. When electromechanical dissociation is detected, the initial response should be to administer epinephrine. Failure of epinephrine to increase cardiac output should prompt an immediate evaluation for mechanical factors that may be preventing adequate blood flow. If such factors are detected, pericardiocentesis, chest tube placement, or volume replacement may be lifesaving.

American Medical Association: Standards and guidelines for cardiopulmonary resuscitation (CPR) and emergency cardiac care (ECC). JAMA 255:2905, 1986. *This is the basic reference source describing CPR.*

Bedell SE, Delbanco TL, Cook EF, et al.: Survival after cardiopulmonary resuscitation in the hospital. N Engl J Med 309:569, 1983. *Reviews the results of in-hospital CPR and describes factors associated with prognosis.*

Cummins RO, Eisenberg MS: Prehospital cardiopulmonary resuscitation. Is it effective? JAMA 253:2408, 1985. *Presents a summary of the results of bystander-initiated resuscitation and concludes that it leads to improved survival.*

Luce JM, Ross BK, O'Quin RJ, et al.: Regional blood flow during cardiopulmonary resuscitation in dogs using simultaneous and nonsimultaneous compression and ventilation. Circulation 67:258, 1983. *An experimental study of the factors influencing organ blood flow in two forms of CPR.*

PART IX
RENAL DISEASES

74 APPROACH TO THE PATIENT WITH RENAL DISEASE

Thomas E. Andreoli

This chapter provides an overview of the cardinal manifestations of diseases of the kidney or urinary tract, together with a relatively simple classification of these disorders. There are five sections. The first section contains a brief consideration of the cardinal functions of the kidney. A more detailed analysis of renal physiology is presented in Ch. 75. Subsequently the cardinal urinary abnormalities of renal disease are described. The third section enumerates briefly the primary findings in the more common syndromes involving the kidneys and urinary tract, and the fourth section describes the consequences of complete or nearly complete failure of renal function, that is, the uremic syndrome. Finally, the last section considers the relationship between the adaptive response to a reduction in nephron mass and the potential contribution of one of these adaptive responses, renal hyperfiltration, to the pathogenesis of progressive renal disease.

CARDINAL ELEMENTS OF RENAL FUNCTION

URINE FORMATION. The kidneys maintain constancy of the volume and composition of body fluids by forming urine whose composition is ultimately determined by the dietary intake of solute and water and by the rate and kind of metabolic transformation of endogenous and exogenous carbohydrates, proteins, lipids, and nucleic acids. The kidneys also serve as the major route for the excretion of a large number of drugs. The formation of urine serves two purposes: a *regulatory* function, that is, the maintenance of a constant volume and composition for body fluids; and an *excretory* function, that is, elimination of endogenous and exogenous metabolic end-products.

Urine is formed by a sequence of five events:

1. The glomerulus filters approximately 180 liters of extracellular fluid daily across glomerular capillaries and the visceral epithelium of Bowman's capsule, using as a driving force the mean arterial pressure. The glomerular capillary endothelium and basement membrane and the visceral epithelium of Bowman's capsule are freely permeable to water and solutes of relatively low molecular weight (that is, under 6,000 to 8,000 daltons), moderately permeable to large molecular weight species such as myoglobin (molecular weight, approximately 16,000 daltons), and virtually impermeable to macromolecules such as albumin. Filtration is also influenced by molecular charge as well as size. The result is an isotonic, virtually protein-free filtrate whose daily volume is more than ten-fold greater than the volume of extracellular fluid (ECF).

2. The proximal tubule isotonically reabsorbs approximately two thirds of the glomerular filtrate. In the process certain alterations in the composition of tubular fluid are produced by specialized transport mechanisms: the preferential absorption of sodium with bicarbonate rather than chloride; the virtually complete absorption of organic solutes such as glucose and amino acids; and the absorption of organic acids such as uric acid and other nonamino acids in early segments of the proximal nephron, followed by secretion of these acids into tubular fluid in the late proximal nephron. Thus the volume of tubular fluid delivered to the loop of Henle is approximately one third of the volume of glomerular filtrate, has a sodium concentration equal to that of plasma and a bicarbonate concentration about 10 per cent of that in plasma, and contains little or no glucose or amino acids.

3. The loop of Henle dissociates the absorption of sodium and water. The descending limb of Henle passively abstracts water into the hypertonic medullary interstitium, concentrating the tubular fluid. Conversely, the water-impermeable thick ascending limb of Henle actively absorbs approximately 25 per cent of filtered sodium chloride but little water. As a result, about 18 liters of tubular fluid enter the distal convoluted tubule daily. This fluid, which is approximately 10 per cent of the initial glomerular filtrate, is also maximally dilute, having an osmolality of approximately 50 mOsm per kilogram of H_2O.

4. The distal convoluted tubule primarily absorbs sodium under the influence of aldosterone and secretes protons, ammonia, and potassium. Aldosterone regulates sodium absorption in this nephron segment.

5. The collecting duct system regulates the osmolality of urine. When antidiuretic hormone (ADH) is present, water is absorbed across the collecting duct and tubular fluid equilibrates osmotically with the hypertonic medullary interstitium; when ADH is absent, the water permeability of collecting ducts is at a minimum and a dilute urine is excreted.

THE KIDNEY AS AN ENDOCRINE RECEPTOR. Among many hormones that regulate renal function, three are of particular importance: parathyroid hormone (PTH), aldosterone, and antidiuretic hormone (ADH). PTH enhances the absorption of calcium and magnesium and inhibits the absorption of phosphate and bicarbonate in the proximal tubule by increasing intracellular cyclic 3',5'-adenosine monophosphate (cAMP). PTH also stimulates the renal conversion of 25-hydroxycholecalciferol, the major metabolite of vitamin D_3, to 1,25-dihydroxycholecalciferol, which is the major biologically active form of vitamin D_3 (Ch. 245).

Aldosterone and other mineralocorticoids stimulate the rate of sodium absorption in the distal nephron. Aldosterone also increases the rate of net potassium secretion and net proton secretion (and consequently, the rate of bicarbonate regeneration) by the distal nephron.

ADH promotes the formation of a hypertonic urine both by increasing the rate of salt absorption in the thick ascending limb of Henle and by increasing the water permeability of the collecting duct system. Both actions are mediated by ADH-dependent increases in cytosolic cAMP in those renal tubular segments.

THE KIDNEY AS AN ENDOCRINE ORGAN. The kidney plays a major role in prostaglandin production, in the operation of the kallikrein-kinin system, and in the degradation of low molecular weight proteins. The kidney is also the major site for the synthesis of erythropoietin and of renin. Erythropoietin is a glycoprotein produced by renal enzymatic action on a circulating precursor of hepatic origin. The principal action of erythropoietin is to stimulate the rate of red blood cell production by the bone marrow.

Renin is secreted by the granular cells of the juxtaglomerular apparatus in response to reductions in renal perfusion pressure or in effective circulating volume. Renin increases the rate of conversion of angiotensinogen to angiotensin I, which in turn is a precursor of angiotensin II. In turn, angiotensin II is a potent vasoconstrictor agent and a strong stimulus to thirst and to aldosterone production. Thus, the kidney, by way of renin production, plays a central role in the volume repletion reaction.

URINARY MANIFESTATIONS OF RENAL DISEASE (Ch. 76)

HEMATURIA. Hematuria indicates an abnormality in the kidneys or urinary tract, but not the particular form of renal disease. Hematuria of itself is not painful, but the passage of blood clots along the ureter or urethra may produce renal colic or dysuria, respectively. In general, hematuria occurs in the following disorders: (1) systemic disorders such as the hemoglobinopathies, coagulation disorders, sepsis, and, rarely, severe congestive heart failure; hematuria may also occur following severe exercise; (2) inflammatory and necrotizing glomerular diseases; hematuria also occurs in certain types of interstitial nephritis, particularly those that are acute, and in renal infarction; (3) diseases characterized by disruption of the normal structure of the kidneys or urinary tract, as in neoplasms, urolithiasis, trauma, or cystic disease of the kidney; and (4) irritative or inflammatory disorders of the kidneys, ureter, or lower urinary tract, as in pyelonephritis or lower urinary tract infection.

The presence of red blood cell casts indicates that the hematuria is of renal parenchymal origin. Proteinuria in combination with hematuria is a classic indicator of parenchymal renal disease; massive proteinuria (in excess of 3.0 grams per 24 hours) in combination with hematuria is typically, but not exclusively, a characteristic of glomerular disease.

Isolated, painless hematuria in the absence of associated urinary abnormalities such as red cell casts or proteinuria or of systemic disease or obvious entities such as urolithiasis or urinary tract infection generally requires more detailed studies such as renal ultrasonography, CT scanning, arteriography, or renal biopsy. The intent of such studies is the detection either of occult glomerular or interstitial disease or of renal tumors or cysts.

Isolated hematuria may occur in association with entirely normal renal imaging studies, a normal renal biopsy, and negligible proteinuria. This condition, which occurs most frequently in children and is often termed *benign recurrent hematuria of childhood*, is characterized by recurrent bouts of microscopic and gross hematuria. To date, there is no evidence that this disorder, when accompanied by normal glomerular architecture and negative glomerular immunofluorescence, leads to progressive renal disease.

PROTEINURIA. The normal daily rate of urinary protein excretion averages less than 150 mg per 24 hours. In certain instances, notably fever, severe congestive heart failure, and severe exercise, the rate of urinary protein excretion may be increased transiently in the absence of intrinsic renal disease. Furthermore, in young individuals, so-called "postural" proteinuria, defined as transient or consistent proteinuria in the upright but not recumbent position, may occur in the absence of histologically detectable lesions on renal biopsy.

Persistent proteinuria, occurring in both the recumbent and the upright positions and exceeding 750 mg per 24 hours, is a specific indicator of parenchymal renal disease. Proteinuria of less than 2.0 grams per 24 hours occurs commonly either in interstitial or in glomerular disease, but when in excess of 3.0 to 3.5 grams per 24 hours usually indicates glomerular disease and, more specifically, the nephrotic syndrome. However, massive proteinuria may also occur in severe congestive heart failure, in accelerated hypertension, and rarely in acute allergic interstitial nephritis.

URINARY LEUKOCYTES, CASTS, AND BACTERIA. *Pyuria* occurs when more than five to ten white blood cells per high-power field are found in centrifuged samples of the urinary sediment and indicates an inflammatory process within the kidneys or urinary tract. When leukocyte casts are also found, renal parenchymal inflammation is usually present.

Cylindruria, the presence of tubular urinary casts, is traditionally regarded as evidence of renal parenchymal injury. The matrix of most urinary casts is composed mainly of Tamm-Horsfall glycoprotein derived from the renal tubular epithelium. No single type of cast is explicitly diagnostic of any specific disease entity. In general, red cell casts are most often indicative of glomerular injury, white cell casts are suggestive of parenchymal inflammation, and so-called "broad" casts are formed within the region of the collecting duct or dilated nephron segments. The specific significance of granular, epithelial, hyaline, or fatty casts is not always clear.

Significant *bacteriuria* indicates bacterial colonization of urine. The presence of bacteria in freshly collected, clean-voided urine specimens generally correlates closely with bacterial colony counts in excess of 100,000 organisms per milliliter of urine, and a Gram's stain of the urinary sediment of a similarly collected specimen is generally helpful in identifying whether the offending organism is gram-positive or gram-negative.

MISCELLANEOUS URINARY FINDINGS. An evaluation of urinary *cytology*, done conveniently by a Wright's stain of the urinary sediment, is a useful diagnostic test for transitional cell tumors of the renal pelvis or ureter. Similarly, cytologic examination of bladder washings may be helpful in the diagnosis of bladder neoplasia (Ch. 93).

Pneumaturia, the passage of urine mixed with air, can occur in the presence of fistula tracts from either the bowel or the vagina into the bladder. These tracts may follow surgical procedures, pelvic infections, or inflammatory bowel disease. A plain film of the abdomen may also indicate the presence of air in the urinary bladder.

THE MAJOR RENAL SYNDROMES

Renal disorders are often nonspecific in their manifestations, as hematuria, azotemia, hypertension, or metabolic acidosis, for example. The interpretation of a group of findings obtained by history, physical examination, and routine laboratory studies, however, may be used to describe some of the more common syndromes and disorders affecting the kidneys and urinary tract, which are briefly described below.

THE PRERENAL SYNDROMES. The major classes of prerenal disorders are (1) renal hypoperfusion secondary to a reduction in effective circulating volume, and (2) renal ischemia because of occlusive disease in one or both renal arteries. Both sets of disorders are associated with hyperreninemia, but the clinical manifestations of the two diseases differ significantly (Table 74–1).

Renal hypoperfusion secondary to a *reduction in effective circulating volume* may occur in association with true volume contraction; an increase in vascular capacitance, as in sepsis; sequestration of fluid in interstitial compartments, as in ascites and the hepatorenal syndrome; or an inability to transfer fluid from the venous to the arterial limbs of the circulation, as in severe congestive heart failure, constrictive pericarditis, or pericardial tamponade. When the effective circulating volume is sufficiently reduced, the kidneys are hypoperfused, the glomerular filtration rate is reduced, and renin is released.

TABLE 74–1. THE PRERENAL (HYPOPERFUSION) SYNDROMES

Class of Disorder	Major Findings
Reduced Effective Circulating Volume	Oliguria Azotemia Reduced fractional sodium excretion Elevated plasma renin Normotension
Occlusive Renal Artery Disease	Hypertension Elevated plasma renin Azotemia: with severe, bilateral disease or an affected solitary kidney

This results in oliguria, an elevation in serum blood urea nitrogen (BUN) and creatinine concentrations, and a reduced fractional excretion rate for sodium (that is, generally less than 1 per cent). Although plasma renin levels are elevated, the patients are ordinarily normotensive, presumably because the effective circulating volume is decreased.

Renal ischemia produced by *occlusive disease* of the renal arteries results in renin release from the ischemic kidney without a reduction in effective circulating volume and consequently is manifested primarily as hypertension, since pressor activity is elevated while filling of the arterial tree is normal or only slightly reduced. If the renal arterial occlusive disease is limited to one kidney and the contralateral kidney retains normal function, azotemia is absent. However, if the hypertension results in injury to the unaffected kidney, azotemia may ensue. When both renal arteries are involved, azotemia occurs when renal ischemia is sufficiently severe that renal autoregulatory mechanisms are inadequate to maintain an adequate glomerular filtration rate.

THE RENAL PARENCHYMAL SYNDROMES. ***Acute Glomerular Disorders.*** GLOMERULONEPHRITIS AND THE NEPHROTIC SYNDROME (Ch. 81). Two major types of disorders affect the glomerulus: (1) the *acute nephritic syndrome*, characterized mainly by inflammatory and/or necrotizing lesions within glomeruli, and (2) the *nephrotic syndrome*, a predominantly noninflammatory derangement of the glomeruli characterized by an abnormal "leakiness" of the glomeruli to albumin and other macromolecules.

The etiologic, histologic, and clinical characteristics of the glomerulonephritic and nephrotic syndromes overlap to a considerable degree: (1) A given disease process—for example, systemic lupus erythematosus—may produce a mild, focal glomerulonephritis with hematuria, mild proteinuria, but no azotemia; a diffuse proliferative glomerulonephritis with hematuria, proteinuria and severe renal failure; or membranous nephropathy characterized by a relatively pure nephrotic syndrome. (2) Glomerular lesions may evolve; for example, Goodpasture's syndrome can begin as a mild, focal nephritis and progress to a diffuse, necrotic glomerulonephritis. (3) The extent of glomerular injury, as viewed on renal biopsy, correlates generally but inexactly with the severity of the clinical picture. (4) A given pathogenic mechanism—for example, immune complex disease—may in some instances result in acute glomerulonephritis and in other cases in a pure nephrotic syndrome. (5) In certain disorders such as membranoproliferative nephritis, both a nephritic picture and a nephrotic picture may coexist simultaneously.

These diverse glomerular disorders can be somewhat arbitrarily classified by four major patterns that may be defined by the initial presentation of the patient (Table 74–2). Table 74–3, in turn, lists the most common diseases that present as nephritic, nephrotic, and mixed syndromes.

THE MILD ACUTE GLOMERULONEPHRITIS SYNDROMES. In this class of glomerular inflammation, glomerular blood flow is sufficient to maintain the glomerular filtration at a normal or near normal rate. Mild acute glomerulonephritis is characterized by hematuria, red cell casts, modest proteinuria, minimal azotemia, and mild or no edema. Because renal perfusion is not severely compromised, hypertension or salt retention or both are generally absent.

THE DIFFUSE ACUTE GLOMERULONEPHRITIS SYNDROMES. These glomerulonephritic syndromes are usually characterized by diffuse glomerular inflammation and/or necrosis sufficiently severe that hematuria and proteinuria are accompanied by a reduction in filtation rate and, consequently, azotemia of varying degrees. Simultaneously, for reasons that are not well understood, sodium acquisitiveness in acute glomerulonephritis is considerably greater than that expected solely from the reduction in glomerular filtration rate. Plasma albumin is generally normal, so that a significant fraction of retained sodium remains in the vascular compartment and may result in hypertension, plasma volume dilution, circulatory overload, congestive heart failure, and a suppression of plasma renin activity.

NEPHROTIC SYNDROME. In the pure nephrotic syndrome the glomerular filtration barrier is abnormally permeable to macromolecules, so that massive proteinuria occurs even though the filtration rate may be normal. This large urinary loss of protein contributes to the characteristic hypoalbuminemia in such patients. Hypercholesterolemia also occurs and correlates closely with the degree of hypoalbuminemia.

Nephrotic patients are usually salt acquisitive and edematous. In the nephrotic syndromes the reduced plasma oncotic pressure leads to translocation of fluid to the interstitium, a reduced effective circulating volume, and a secondary sodium acquisitiveness and edema. Patients with the pure nephrotic syndrome often are normotensive, rarely develop circulatory overload, and frequently have elevated plasma renin activities. As further evidence for a reduced effective circulating volume, severely nephrotic patients may have postural hypotension even in the presence of anasarca and may have hemoconcentration and renal hypoperfusion with attendant azotemia following excessive diuretic use.

The Interstitial Nephritis Syndromes (Ch. 82). In the interstitial nephritis syndromes, the primary abnormality is damage to the tubulointerstitial system of the kidney with secondary glomerular damage. Thus renal tubular function tends to be deranged disproportionately to reductions in glomerular filtration rate.

Generalized tubulointerstitial disorders often damage the juxtaglomerular apparatus and therefore tend to impair renin production. As a consequence of hyporeninemia, aldosterone production is curtailed. This combination generally results in hyporeninemia, hypoaldosteronism, modest degrees of salt

TABLE 74–2. CLASSIFICATION OF MAJOR GLOMERULAR SYNDROMES

Class of Disorder	Major Derangement	Major Findings
1. Mild Acute Glomerulonephritis	Mild glomerular inflammation	Hematuria, proteinuria Absent or mild azotemia Absent or mild edema
2. Severe Acute Glomerulonephritis	Extensive glomerular inflammation Renal ischemia Primary tubular sodium acquisitiveness	Hematuria, proteinuria Azotemia Plasma volume expansion Hypertension Edema Circulatory overload (if severe)
3. Pure Nephrotic Syndrome	Glomerular protein leak	Massive proteinuria Reduced plasma oncotic pressure Anasarca Normotensive Sensitive to diuretics
4. Mixed Disorders	1 plus 3 or 2 plus 3	Hematuria Massive proteinuria Azotemia (variable) Hypertension (variable) Edema

wasting, hyperkalemia, and hyperchloremic metabolic acidosis. These abnormalities occur even when the glomerular filtration rate is only modestly reduced.

Urinary abnormalities such as hematuria and proteinuria are usually, but not always, relatively modest in patients with tubulointerstitial disease. Three general classes of tubulointerstitial diseases can be defined:

1. *Chronic tubulointerstitial disease* may occur as a consequence of any of a large number of diseases that produce chronic damage to the renal interstitium: chronic hypertension, with progressive ischemia to the renal interstitium; diabetes mellitus, in which microvascular disease within the kidney effects the same end result; occlusive disease of smaller renal vessels, as in sickle cell disease; chronic pyelonephritis; gout; and exogenous toxins, notably illicit alcohol containing lead, and analgesic abuse, particularly the combination of phenacetin and aspirin. Chronic interstitial disease is generally detected in individuals who have modest degrees of sodium wasting, hyperkalemia, metabolic acidosis, and an acid urine. These abnormalities may occur even when only mild degrees of azotemia exist. The plasma renin activity is generally reduced, as are rates of aldosterone secretion. Hematuria and massive proteinuria are not common in chronic interstitial disease.

2. *Acute allergic interstitial disease* occurs when patients are treated with antibiotics, notably penicillin and related drugs, or with nonsteroidal anti-inflammatory agents. In addition to producing electrolyte abnormalities similar to those described above for chronic interstitial nephritis, acute allergic interstitial nephritis may severely reduce glomerular filtration and be associated with marked hematuria and proteinuria and with oliguria.

Oliguria and azotemia associated with acute allergic interstitial nephritis may be difficult to differentiate from that of acute tubular necrosis. In this setting an electrolyte pattern of hyperkalemic, hyperchloremic metabolic acidosis, a reduced plasma renin activity and rates of aldosterone secretion, an elevated fractional excretion rate for sodium, eosinophilia, and the presence of eosinophils in the urine would strongly suggest acute allergic interstitial nephritis.

3. *Acute pyelonephritis*, a form of acute interstitial nephritis due to bacterial invasion of the kidney, usually produces a septic picture with fever, flank pain, leukocytosis, and dysuria (Ch. 86). Factors that predispose to acute pyelonephritis are often present, such as diabetes mellitus, obstructive uropathy, prior instrumentation of the urinary tract, or bacterial endocarditis with septic renal emboli. The most useful clues to the presence of acute pyelonephritis include findings of sepsis, costovertebral angle tenderness, pyuria, leukocyte casts, the presence of bacteria in unspun samples of urine, and positive urine cultures.

Isolated Tubular Defects (Ch. 84). In addition to tubular derangements secondary to diffuse tubulointerstitial disease, there are a number of specific defects of tubular function.

PROXIMAL TUBULAR DEFECTS. *Renal glycosuria* occurs when the glucose threshold of the proximal nephron is reduced. *Renal phosphate wasting* results when the rate of proximal absorption of phosphate is reduced. Similarly, *aminoaciduria* may result from tubular defects that are either generalized or specific. Finally, the rate of bicarbonate absorption by the proximal nephron may be reduced, resulting in profound bicarbonate wasting, a syndrome entitled *proximal renal tubular acidosis* (Ch. 84).

Renal phosphate wasting, renal glycosuria, renal aminoaciduria, and proximal renal tubular acidosis occurring simultaneously constitute Fanconi's syndrome (Ch. 84). These proximal tubular defects may be congenital or may be found in association with heavy metal poisoning of the proximal nephron, notably by copper in Wilson's disease, following exposure to toxic agents such as maleic acid, and in the gammopathies.

POSSIBLE LOOP OF HENLE DEFECT. The pathogenesis of *Bartter's syndrome* has not been elucidated (Ch. 84). Yet it appears that many of the findings of Bartter's syndrome, including profound salt wasting, potassium wasting, and compensatory hypertrophy of the juxtaglomerular apparatus with hyperreninemia, may be the result of a salt-absorptive defect in the thick ascending limb. Most commonly, a clinical syndrome resembling Bartter's syndrome occurs because of surreptitious ingestion of furosemide or furosemide-like diuretics.

DISTAL TUBULAR DEFECTS. *Distal, gradient-limited renal tubular acidosis* represents a specific defect of the distal nephron (Ch. 84). In this disorder the distal nephron is abnormally permeable to protons and cannot therefore maintain an adequately acid urine. In contrast to patients who have tubulointerstitial disease, the classic electrolyte abnormalities in distal, gradient-limited renal tubular acidosis include a tendency to salt wasting, hyperchloremic metabolic acidosis, a urine that is relatively alkaline with respect to arterial pH, and profound hypokalemia. The hypokalemia of distal, gradient-limited renal tubular acidosis is probably a consequence of aldosterone release in response to salt depletion. In contrast to proximal renal tubular acidosis or to the hyperkalemic, hyperchloremic renal tubular acidosis of diffuse tubulointerstitial disease, gradient-limited distal renal tubular acidosis is frequently associated with severe nephrocalcinosis, renal calculi, renal infection, and progressive destruction of renal mass.

Distal, gradient-limited renal tubular acidosis may occur congenitally. The disorder may also occur as a consequence of exposure to exogenous agents, notably amphotericin B and lithium, and in association with the gammopathies.

COLLECTING DUCT DEFECTS. The unique tubular defect of the collecting duct is nephrogenic diabetes insipidus (NDI), in which the collecting duct is refractory to the action of ADH (Ch. 227). Patients with NDI are consistently polyuric, even when large amounts of ADH are administered. The disorder may occur congenitally; in association with certain systemic disorders, such as Sjögren's syndrome and sarcoidosis; and as a result of lithium intoxication or exposure to the antibiotic demethylchlortetracycline.

The Renal Calculus Syndrome. The origin and composition of renal calculi are described in Ch. 90; most renal calculi contain magnesium-ammonium-phosphate, calcium oxalate, uric acid, a combination of calcium oxalate and uric acid, or cystine as their main crystalloids. Of these, all but uric acid stones are radiopaque.

Renal calculi may be asymptomatic and detected only on routine radiographic examination of the kidney, especially isolated calculi that do not move down the urinary tract and staghorn calculi lodged within the renal pelvis. Calculi may obstruct urine flow and consequently lead to pyelonephritis. Therefore, in any patient in whom pyelonephritis is suspected, a careful radiographic and urologic examination for renal calculi is mandatory. *Renal colic* refers to the passage of a renal calculus from the renal pelvis into the ureter characterized by exquisite pain, generally beginning in the flank and radiating into the groin. Patients almost always describe renal colic as the worst pain they have ever experienced. Renal colic is almost invariably accompanied by hematuria, unless the calculus is lodged within a ureter and produces complete unilateral obstruction to urine flow. Under these circumstances, the urine voided by the patient represents red cell–free urine from the unaffected kidney.

Kidney stones are among the more common renal disorders. It is generally prudent, particularly in patients with multiple renal calculi or with a family history of renal calculi, to evaluate the patient for potential underlying causes for stone formation (for example, gout, absorptive hypercalciuria, cystinuria, distal, gradient-limited renal tubular acidosis, or primary hyperparathyroidism). The presence of nephrocalcinosis should alert the physician to the possibility of distal, gradient-limited renal tubular acidosis or to primary hyperparathyroidism.

The patient with renal colic also warrants an evaluation for obstructive uropathy on the affected side and for urinary tract infection. These approaches generally involve culture of the urine, plain films of the abdomen, and, when indicated, ultrasonography of the kidneys, excretory urography, evaluation of parathyroid function, and evaluation for an absorptive hypercalciuric state.

Renal Cystic Disease (Ch. 91). There are three major forms of renal cystic disease: single or multiple cysts, polycystic kidney disease, and microcystic disease of the renal medulla. The clinical characteristics, significance, and clinical presentations of these three kinds of renal cysts vary significantly. There is no evidence that true simple cysts, multiple simple cysts, or polycystic kidney disease progresses to renal neoplasia.

Isolated simple cysts, either single or multiple, form sporadically for unknown reasons within the renal parenchyma, generally within the renal cortex. Single cysts in particular usually cause no symptoms; they are generally detected in one of two circumstances: episodes of renal trauma that provoke cyst rupture and hematuria, or on routine excretory urography. The true single, simple cyst (in contrast to the cystic neoplasm, see below) is innocuous and needs no therapy. *Multiple simple cysts* probably represent an extension of the process described above and are also similarly innocuous unless they encroach on renal parenchyma. Multiple simple cysts should be distinguished from polycystic kidney disease, a disorder with a more ominous prognosis. These two forms of multicystic disease can be distinguished by excretory urography; in individuals with multiple simple cysts, the overall size of the kidney is normal and the calyceal system is not elongated and only minimally distorted.

Adult polycystic kidney disease is a form of nephropathy that is generally inherited by autosomal dominance with incomplete penetrance. If a parent has polycystic kidney disease, approximately one half of the progeny will ultimately develop the disorder, although the time at which polycystic kidney disease becomes manifest is highly variable.

Polycystic kidney disease may present with recurrent bouts of hematuria, renal colic, hypertension, or urinary tract infection because of intrarenal obstruction due to cysts. Many patients with polycystic kidney disease develop renal failure, although the rate and extent of development of renal failure depend on the degree of penetrance of the autosomal dominant trait.

Three factors distinguish between patients with polycystic kidney disease and those with multiple simple cysts: (1) a positive family history consistent with an autosomal dominant trait; (2) enlargement of the kidneys, generally detected as a pole-to-pole diameter in excess of 15 to 17 cm and a cortical thickness in excess of 3 cm; and (3) elongation and deformation of the calyceal structure from the progressive enlargement of the parenchymal cysts.

Microcystic kidney disease of the renal medulla, a disorder of children generally inherited as a recessive trait, is characterized by progressive disruption and destruction of the renal medullary architecture by multiple cysts. The disease is generally detected when young children complain of fatigue and are noted to have mild degrees of proteinuria, anemia, and mild azotemia. The clinical course is characterized by an inordinately high requirement for salt intake in order to maintain blood pressure and an adequate filtration rate and by stunted growth due to chronic illness, to uremia, and to excessive urinary calcium losses. Nephrons are gradually destroyed, usually with progression to end-stage renal disease before the age of 30.

Renal Neoplasia (Ch. 93). Two major classes of renal tumors occur in adults: *renal cell carcinomas* (sometimes called hypernephromas), which originate in the renal cortex, and *transitional cell tumors* of the renal pelvis. Hypernephromas are versatile tumors and are often difficult to diagnose. Many patients present simply with painless hematuria. However, hypernephromas also produce a number of unusual syndromes, including polycythemia, presumably due to excessive erythropoietin production; hypertension, presumably because the neoplasm acts as the equivalent of an arteriovenous fistula and results in renin release by the affected kidney; fever of unknown origin; and hypercalcemia (see Table 93–3).

Transitional cell tumors of the renal pelvis commonly present as hematuria, which may be painless or accompanied by renal colic from the clots that are passed. The systemic manifestations described for hypernephroma are uncommonly found in transitional cell tumors. Examination of urine cytology by a Wright's stain of the urinary sediment may provide a useful diagnostic clue to the presence of these tumors.

Acute Renal Failure (Ch. 78). Acute renal failure refers either to the sudden cessation of urine flow or to sudden oliguria. Acute renal failure caused by acute glomerular disorders is generally evident from the findings described above for the acute glomerulonephritic syndromes. The general approach to the differential diagnosis of individuals with acute renal failure, particularly in hospitalized patients, involves the distinction among three major classes of disorders: (1) the prerenal hypoperfusion syndromes indicated in Table 74–1; (2) intrarenal syndromes, especially acute tubular necrosis and acute allergic interstitial nephritis; and (3) postrenal syndromes, that is, oligoanuria resulting from urinary tract obstruction.

The general approach to these patients involves the following cardinal maneuvers: (1) an assessment of circulatory dynamics; (2) a careful history to assess possible antecedent hypotension or exposure to nephrotoxic agents, coupled with a measurement of the fractional excretion of sodium; and (3) renal ultrasonography to exclude the possibility of obstruction of both kidneys, or obstruction of a solitary kidney, as in an individual with renal agenesis or with renal transplantation. These maneuvers are generally helpful in distinguishing between prerenal, intrarenal, and postrenal causes of oliguria. Invasive hemodynamic monitoring, coupled with a fluid challenge, may still be required to exclude rigorously the possibility of oliguria due to a reduced effective circulating volume. A percutaneous renal biopsy may be needed to distinguish between acute tubular necrosis and acute allergic interstitial nephritis. Renal ultrasonography has reduced strikingly the need for retrograde ureteral catheterization as a means for excluding obstructive uropathy.

TABLE 74–3. MAJOR GLOMERULAR SYNDROMES

Common Presentation	Major Disorders
Acute Nephritic Syndrome	Post-infectious glomerulonephritis
	Vasculitides: SLE
	Polyarteritis nodosa
	Wegener's granulomatosis
	Henoch-Schönlein purpura
	Rapidly progressive glomerulonephritis
	Goodpasture's syndrome
	Hemolytic-uremic syndrome
Nephrotic Syndrome	Minimal change disease (nil lesion)
	Membranous nephropathy
	Focal glomerulosclerosis
	Amyloidosis
	Essential cryoglobulinemia
Nephritic-Nephrotic Syndrome	Membranoproliferative glomerulonephritis
	Type I
	Type II (dense deposit disease)
	Mesangioproliferative glomerulonephritis
	(IgG/IgA nephropathy)
	Diabetic glomerulosclerosis
	(Kimmelstiel-Wilson lesion)

THE POSTRENAL SYNDROMES (Ch. 83). The postrenal syndromes result from obstruction of urine flow at various loci in the urinary tract from the renal papillae to the urethral meatus. Azotemia and oliguria occur in urinary tract obstruction only when the urinary tract is obstructed bilaterally or when obstruction exists in a sole functioning kidney. The degree of azotemia depends upon the extent of the obstruction; partial obstruction may produce only moderate degrees of azotemia, while complete obstruction of the urinary tract obviously produces anuria. Obstruction of urine flow can irreversibly damage the kidneys. If the obstruction is partial or nearly complete, renal function may be preserved for as long as four to five weeks following the onset of obstruction. Obstructive uropathy also carries with it the possible complication of urinary tract infection.

Bilateral ureteral obstruction most frequently occurs at three major sites: (1) the *ureteropelvic junction*, where the obstruction is generally due to scar formation or, less commonly, to renal vessels crossing the ureter; (2) the site where the ureters cross the *pelvic brim*—neoplasms are the primary cause of such obstruction, particularly extensive carcinoma of the cervix; and (3) the *ureterovesical junction*, because of either neoplasm or scar formation. Less commonly, other disorders such as *retroperitoneal fibrosis* or disseminated retroperitoneal lymphoma may cause bilateral ureteral obstruction between the ureterovesical junction and where the ureters cross the pelvic brim. The probability of renal calculi causing bilateral ureteral obstruction is small unless one kidney is already nonfunctional and a stone obstructs the outflow of urine from the other kidney. Prostatic enlargement is a common cause of partial or complete obstruction to urine outflow. In contrast to patients with ureteral obstruction, the urinary bladder distends and often results in overflow urinary incontinence. The patient may therefore present with azotemia secondary to a profound reduction in glomerular filtration and yet have significant volumes of urine flow.

Urinary tract obstruction represents a potentially remediable cause of renal failure; every attempt should be made to exclude obstructive uropathy in individuals who are oliguric or anuric. Renal ultrasonography has simplified this task greatly, since it noninvasively detects whether or not the renal calyces are dilated and the ureters narrowed, as occurs in ureteropelvic junction obstruction; or whether the ureters and renal calyces are both dilated, as occurs in ureterovesical obstruction or urethral obstruction.

RENAL FAILURE: THE UREMIC SYNDROME

The uremic syndrome (Ch. 79) occurs when the functional renal mass is reduced sufficiently that the kidney is no longer able to carry out excretory functions, functions relating to the regulation of the volume and composition of body fluids, functions as an endocrine receptor, and functions as an endocrine organ. The manifestations of *acute* uremia may differ from those of *chronic* uremia, but these differences relate more to the rate of development of renal failure than to fundamental differences in pathophysiology.

Uremia is in part a syndrome of "autointoxication." While the chemical agents responsible for this autointoxication have not been clearly identified, uremic syndromes may be ameliorated by dialysis (which generally removes molecules having molecular weights less than 1,000 to 2,000 daltons), and severe protein restriction may minimize the rate of development of the uremic symptoms. Thus it is plausible to presume that the retention of the end-products of protein metabolism, reflected primarily by the BUN and serum creatinine levels as well as by other factors such as acidosis, are responsible for many of the manifestations of the uremic syndrome.

Uremic symptoms that relate primarily to a reduction in glomerular filtration rate begin to occur when the GFR is reduced below 5 to 10 per cent of normal. The primary findings include central nervous system symptoms ranging from lethargy and confusion to coma and seizures; a bleeding tendency, due at least in part to interference with adequate platelet function; peripheral neuropathy, which is most evident in individuals with long-standing rather than acute uremia; intense pruritus; and asthenia.

In uremia the major electrolyte alterations include hypocalcemia, presumably due to the inability to form 1,25-dihydroxycholecalciferol as renal mass is reduced and to hyperphosphatemia; hyperphosphatemia resulting from a reduction in glomerular filtration rate; and metabolic acidosis, which results from a reduction in the renal excretion of "fixed" acids (that is, incompletely combusted organic acids; and sulfate and phosphate, which represent the end-products of protein and nucleic acid metabolism, respectively).

The occurrence of hyperkalemia among uremic individuals is variable and depends on a number of factors, including the rate of potassium intake, the rate of tissue catabolism, and the rate at which renal failure has evolved. In general, patients in whom the uremic syndrome evolves acutely do not develop adaptive mechanisms (both renal and extrarenal) for potassium elimination and are therefore more prone to develop hyperkalemia. In contrast, individuals who approach end-stage renal disease gradually may often be normokalemic even when the glomerular filtration rate is less than 5 per cent of normal. Two factors may account for this phenomenon: (1) The development of renal disease is accompanied by asthenia and anorexia so that dietary intake of potassium may be minimized; and (2) both renal and extrarenal mechanisms for more efficient potassium excretion are gradually developed.

Uremia, whether acute or chronic, is a catabolic disorder. In individuals with acute renal failure, even extensive hyperalimentation fails to prevent the loss of approximately 0.5 to 1.0 pound daily. In individuals with chronic renal failure, weight loss is more gradual and less easily perceived by patients. But in both acute and chronic renal failure, asthenia and loss of lean body mass are inevitable sequelae.

As the functional renal mass is diminished, erythropoietin production is also reduced. Thus within two to three weeks of the onset of acute renal failure, the combination of diminished erythrocyte production and an accelerated rate of red cell destruction invariably reduces the hematocrit level to the range of 20 to 25 per cent. Similar hematocrits are found in patients with chronic renal failure, particularly prior to dialysis therapy. Polycystic kidney disease represents an exception in that profound reductions of glomerular filtration rate may occur coincident with the maintenance of an hematocrit well in excess of 30 per cent. Presumably, the large renal mass of polycystic kidney disease produces sufficient erythropoietin to maintain an adequate hematocrit.

Two symptoms of uremia are seen commonly in individuals with chronic renal failure but are rare in acute uremia: *peripheral neuropathy* and *renal osteodystrophy*. Peripheral neuropathy almost never develops in individuals with acute renal failure but is common in individuals with long-standing uremia who have not been treated with dialysis. Individuals with acute renal failure do not develop significant bone disease. In contrast, individuals with chronic, severe reductions in glomerular filtration rate and in functional renal mass often have significant bone disease, termed renal osteodystrophy (Ch. 249). At least four factors may contribute to the complex bone disorders in uremia: (1) The synthesis of 1,25-hydroxycholecalciferol in the kidney is reduced with consequent diminished calcium absorption from the gut. (2) The calcium malabsorption leads to secondary hyperparathyroidism, which mobilizes calcium from bone in an attempt to maintain a normal level of serum ionized calcium and in the process produces osteitis fibrosa (Ch. 247). (3) Bone calcium is exchanged for retained protons in buffering the metabolic acidosis of chronic renal failure with partial maintenance of acid-base homeostasis, but at the expense of progressive dissolution of bone. (4) The uremic state impairs protein synthesis in bone and with this the formation of osteoid.

In short, the uremic syndrome results from varying impairment in the ability of the kidney to meet all of its normal metabolic and physiologic obligations: to regulate the volume and composition of body fluids, to excrete the end-products of metabolism, to serve as an endocrine receptor, and to serve as an endocrine organ. Within that framework the particular manifestations of uremia in any given patient will depend largely on the rate at which kidney failure has occurred, the severity of the renal failure (that is, the extent to which residual nephron mass is able to maintain homeostasis), and the homeostatic stresses to which the individual is subjected.

ADAPTATION TO RENAL INJURY AND THE PATHOGENESIS OF PROGRESSIVE RENAL FAILURE

There are two added characteristics of nearly all forms of chronic renal disease that warrant particular consideration. First, nephron loss may be accompanied by *adaptive functional changes* in residual nephrons, which tend to minimize the effects of reducing the functional nephron mass on the chemical composition of blood. This argument, generally termed the *intact nephron hypothesis*, considers that, in chronic renal disease, the function of residual nephrons may be normal or supranormal. Among the cardinal adaptive characteristics described by the intact nephron hypothesis have been an increased glomerular filtration rate per nephron with elevated serum BUN concentrations or increased rates of protein feeding, and an increase in the rate of phosphate excretion per nephron mediated through secondary hyperparathyroidism, such that, in chronic renal failure, serum phosphate levels do not rise until the glomerular filtration rate is reduced to about 30 per cent of normal.

Second, these adaptive responses may ultimately be harmful to the kidney: For example, the maintenance of relatively normal serum calcium and phosphate concentrations in a setting of modest reductions in glomerular filtration rate (that is, to 30 to 40 per cent of normal) by secondary hyperparathyroidism is achieved at the expense of bone dissolution. Likewise, recent observations have provided evidence that increases in protein intake lead to glomerular hyperperfusion and that the elevated glomerular filtration rate produced by this hyperperfusion can result in progressive glomerular sclerosis. Thus, in principle, glomerular hyperperfusion produced by a protein intake that is large in relation to the residual nephron mass could contribute to the progression of chronic renal disease. A corollary to this hypothesis is the possibility that dietary protein restriction early in the course of chronic renal failure might slow the rate of progression of renal disease.

Brenner BM: Nephron adaptation to renal injury or ablation. Physiol 249:F324, 1985. *A detailed analysis of the relation between glomerular hyperfiltration and progressive renal damage.*

Coe FL, Favus MJ: Disorders of stone formation. In Brenner B, Rector F (eds.): The Kidney. 3rd ed. Philadelphia, W. B. Saunders Company, 1986. *A thorough review of the approach to patients with stone disease.*

Huh MP, Kelleher SP: Proteinuria and the nephrotic syndrome. In Schrier RW (ed.): Renal and Electrolyte Disorders. Boston, Little, Brown and Company, 1986. *A thorough review of the pathogenesis and clinical manifestations of proteinuria.*

Swartz RD: Fluid, electrolyte and acid base changes during renal failure. In Kokko JP, Tannen RL (eds.): Fluids and Electrolytes. Philadelphia, W. B. Saunders Company, 1986. *A comprehensive review of the laboratory derangements in renal failure.*

75 STRUCTURE AND FUNCTION OF THE KIDNEYS

Saulo Klahr

This chapter reviews the structure and function of the normal mammalian kidney as a framework for understanding the derangements that occur with kidney disease.

Renal Structure

The kidneys are located retroperitoneally with their upper and lower poles opposite the twelfth thoracic and third lumbar vertebrae, respectively. Because of the presence of the liver, the right kidney is generally inferior to the left. Each adult kidney weighs 130 to 170 grams and measures about 12 by 6 by 3 cm. Through the hilus of the kidney pass a renal artery and vein, lymphatics, a nerve plexus, and the *renal pelvis,* which subdivides into the *three major calices* and subsequently into eight or more *minor calices.* A coronal section of the kidney reveals two distinct regions: the medulla and the cortex. The *renal medulla* is composed generally of 12 to 18 conical masses, the *pyramids.* The base of each pyramid is located on the corticomedullary boundary, and the apex extends toward the renal pelvis, forming the *papilla,* which projects into the minor calix. Each papilla is perforated by the distal end of 15 or more *terminal collecting ducts* (of Bellini). The *renal cortex,* about 1 cm in thickness, covers the base of the pyramids and extends medially between the individual pyramids to form the renal columns (of Bertin).

BLOOD SUPPLY

Generally, each kidney is supplied by a single artery originating from the aorta at the level of the first lumbar vertebra. This artery generally divides into two branches (anterior and posterior) before entering the renal sinus. The anterior branch gives rise to upper, middle, and lower branches *(lobar arteries).* As these arteries enter the renal parenchyma they form the *interlobar arteries* that course toward the cortex along the lateral borders of the medullary pyramids. The interlobar arteries then run across the base of the renal medulla, forming the *arcuate arteries.* The *interlobular arteries,* branching at right angles from the arcuate vessels, course through the cortex to the periphery. They give rise to *afferent arterioles,* each of which ends in a fine capillary bed known as a glomerulus. Thus, the glomerulus is supplied by a single afferent arteriole and drained, in turn, by an *efferent arteriole,* which emerges at the glomerular vascular pole and immediately ramifies into numerous peritubular capillaries that surround the tubular segments of the cortex. The *vasa recta,* which extend medially into the medulla, are the capillaries that originate from efferent arterioles of juxtamedullary glomeruli.

The venous system follows the same pattern as the arterial system, with the capillaries forming venules that unite into interlobular, arcuate, lobular, and ultimately renal veins. Each renal vein drains into the inferior vena cava.

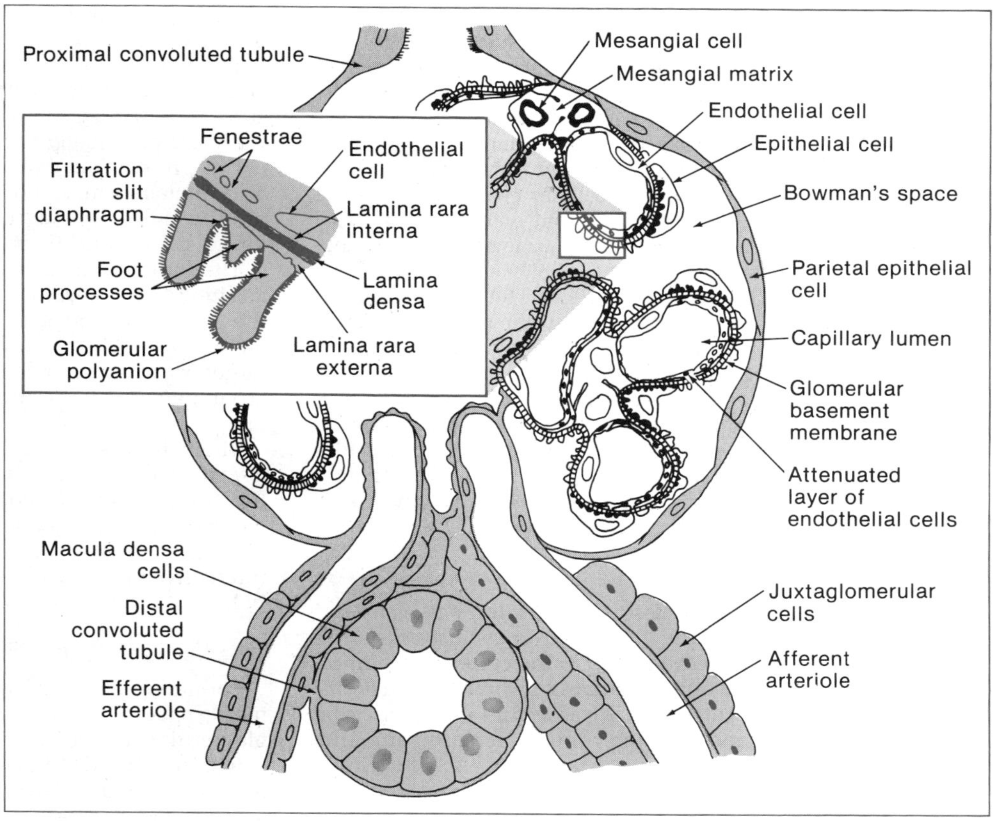

FIGURE 75–1. Schematic representation of the glomerulus, illustrating the three major types of cells (endothelial, epithelial, and mesangial) and the close relationship of the distal convoluted tubule to afferent and efferent arterioles ("juxtaglomerular apparatus"). Notice that there is no basement membrane interposed between the mesangium and the lumen of the capillaries. The inset shows a magnified view of the capillary wall, illustrating the gaps between the endothelial cells (fenestrae), the three layers of the basement membrane, and the foot processes of the epithelial cells. For more details see text.

THE NEPHRON

The nephron is the functional unit of the kidney. There are approximately 1,200,000 nephrons in each human kidney. Each is composed of a malpighian corpuscle (the *glomerulus* and *Bowman's capsule*) and its attached *tubule.* The tubule contains several distinct anatomic and functional segments: proximal tubule, loop of Henle, distal convoluted tubule, and cortical collecting tubule. The junction of cortical collecting tubules form the collecting ducts, which traverse the medulla and terminate at the tip of the papilla. There are two distinct populations of nephrons in the human kidney: those with glomeruli located in the outer cortex *(superficial nephrons)* and those with glomeruli situated near the corticomedullary junction *(juxtamedullary nephrons).* The superficial nephrons, which constitute about 85 per cent of the total nephron population, have short loops of Henle that frequently do not penetrate the medulla. The juxtamedullary nephrons have long loops of Henle that extend into the inner medulla and are in close apposition to the vasa recta.

GLOMERULUS. The glomerulus (Fig. 75–1) is a network of capillaries originating from the afferent arteriole. After dividing into four to eight lobules to form the glomerular tuft, the capillaries rejoin to form the efferent arteriole, which leaves the glomerulus at the vascular pole. The glomerular tuft is surrounded by *Bowman's capsule,* which is an extension of the basement membrane and connective tissue of the proximal tubule. The *urinary* or *Bowman's space* separates the capsule from the glomerular tuft. Bowman's capsule contains a single layer of squamous cells *(parietal epithelial cells),* which undergo an abrupt transition to taller columnar cells typical of the proximal tubule at the urinary pole of the glomerulus. In the glomerular tuft there are three distinct cell types (endothelial, mesangial, and epithelial), a capillary wall (basement membrane), and an interstitial or supporting region (mesangium).

Capillary Wall. The capillary wall contains endothelial cells, a basement membrane, and epithelial cells (see Fig. 75–1). The *endothelial cells* line the capillary lumen. Fenestrae or pores (approximate diameter of 700 Å) covered by thin diaphragms are present in the attenuated endothelium. The *basement membrane,* a structure with an average thickness in the adult of 3200 Å, contains three distinct areas: a central electron-dense *lamina densa* and, on either side, a *lamina rara externa* and *lamina rara interna* (see Fig. 75–1). The major constituents of the basement membrane are collagen and glycoprotein. Thickening of this structure is seen in a number of glomerular diseases. The *visceral epithelial cells,* or *podocytes,* are the largest of the glomerular cells. Extending from the body of the podocyte are primary processes, from which individual *foot processes,* or *pedicels,* project to come into contact with the lamina rara externa of the basement membrane. Between the foot processes is a space (*filtration slit* or *slit pore*) 250 to 400 Å wide, which is covered by a thin membrane, the *filtration slit diaphragm,* which is located approximately 600 Å from the basement membrane. This slit diaphragm is a zipper-like structure composed of rectangular pores (40 to 140 Å in a cross-section). The estimated total area of these pores is approximately 3 per cent of the total surface area of the glomerular capillaries. In renal diseases characterized by proteinuria the pedicels of the podocytes are replaced by a continuous band of cytoplasm adjacent to the lamina rara externa (fusion of foot processes).

The Mesangium. The mesangium, the interstitial portion of the glomerular lobules, is composed of *mesangial cells* (axial or intercapillary) and *mesangial matrix.* The latter is a homogeneous fibrillary material containing mucopolysaccharides and glycoprotein. The mesangial cells, which have phagocytic properties, resemble smooth muscle cells, contain myosin, and usually do not communicate directly with the vascular space. The mesangium is unique in that entry of a substance into the space does not require passage through a capillary basement membrane. In human glomerulonephritis, immune deposits are found in the mesangium, often exclusively.

THE TUBULE. The renal tubule is composed of distinct

anatomic and functional segments: the *proximal convoluted tubule*, the *pars recta* or *straight portion* of the proximal tubule, the *thin descending* and *ascending limbs of Henle's loop*, the *thick ascending limb of Henle's loop*, the *distal convoluted tubule*, the *cortical collecting tubule*, and the *medullary collecting duct*. These segments differ in their location, length, diameter, characteristics of the lining epithelium, including number and size of mitochondria, appearance of intercellular channels, presence of luminal microvilli (brush border), and complexity of basal infoldings. The functional differences among nephron segments are described below.

JUXTAGLOMERULAR APPARATUS. The juxtaglomerular apparatus is a region near the glomerular vascular pole in which the *distal convoluted tubule* and the *afferent* and *efferent arterioles* come into juxtaposition. Here, the cells of the distal tubule become smaller and more numerous *(macula densa)*, and cells derived from the afferent arteriole *(juxtaglomerular cells)* are present between the distal tubule and the vascular pole (Fig. 75–1). These cells may be granular (containing renin) or agranular. Adrenergic nerve endings have been demonstrated in the juxtaglomerular region.

INTERSTITIUM

The interstitial connective tissue of the kidney is scant and consists primarily of *reticular fibers* and *interstitial cells*. It is more prominent in the medulla than in the cortex. In addition to capillaries, the interstitium contains *lymphatics* and *motor* and *sensory nerves*. In interstitial disease this region may be infiltrated by white blood cells and contain increased amounts of connective tissue.

Normal Renal Function

The principal functions of the kidney are summarized in Table 75–1. The kidneys have a central role in the *maintenance of volume and ionic composition of body fluids* (homeostasis). This function is accomplished by regulation of the rate of excretion of water and/or ions. Regulation entails feedback mechanisms that involve participation of the nervous system, the endocrine system, or both. Some of the homeostatic functions of the kidney are concerned with the balance of water, sodium, chloride, potassium, magnesium, phosphate, and hydrogen ions. The large changes in urine volume and composition, which occur in response to alterations in the diet, reflect the adaptability of the kidney to the requirements of homeostasis. There is no fixed normal volume or composition of the urine. Normal homeostatic renal function is defined by the capacity of the organ to vary the volume and composition of the urine over a wide range.

TABLE 75–1. PRINCIPAL FUNCTIONS OF THE KIDNEY

1. Maintenance of volume and ionic composition of body fluids (homeostasis)
2. Excretion of metabolic waste products—e.g., urea, uric acid, creatinine
3. Detoxification and elimination of toxins, drugs, and their metabolites
4. Endocrine regulation of extracellular fluid volume and blood pressure
   a. Renin-angiotensin system
   b. Renal prostaglandins
   c. Renal kallikrein-kinin system
5. Control of red blood cell mass: erythropoietin
6. Endocrine control of mineral metabolism: formation of 1,25-dihydroxycholecalciferol and 24,25-dihydroxycholecalciferol
7. Degradation and catabolism of peptide hormones: insulin, glucagon, parathyroid hormone, calcitonin, growth hormone, etc.
8. Catabolism of low molecular weight proteins: light chains, $beta_2$-microglobulin
9. Metabolic interconversions: gluconeogenesis, lipid metabolism

The kidney is the main route of elimination of fixed (nonvolatile) metabolic waste products *(excretory function)*. These substances usually serve no biologic function, and some of them are potentially toxic. Examples include urea (end-product of protein metabolism), uric acid (end-product of nucleic acid metabolism), and creatinine (end-product of creatine metabolism). The kidney also *eliminates exogenous chemicals (drugs, toxins)* and their metabolites.

The kidney participates in endocrine functions as well. In addition to its capacity to *metabolize and excrete certain hormones*, the kidney is the site of *production* of *renin, erythropoietin, prostaglandins, 1,25-dihydroxycholecalciferol*, and *kinins*. It is the target organ for several hormones (e.g., parathyroid hormone, atrial peptide, antidiuretic hormone, angiotensin, aldosterone).

The kidney is also involved in the *catabolism of small molecular weight proteins* and in *metabolic interconversions* that regulate the composition of body fluids. The ability of the kidney to convert certain organic acids (lactic, alpha-ketoglutaric) to glucose (a neutral substance) is an example of a metabolic interconversion that minimizes potential changes in plasma pH.

GENERAL SCHEME OF FORMATION OF URINE

Formation of urine begins with the ultrafiltration into Bowman's space of a portion of the plasma flowing through the glomerular capillaries.

RENAL BLOOD FLOW. Functionally, the renal circulation is characterized by two capillary beds in series: the glomerular and the peritubular capillaries. The glomerulus has a high intracapillary hydrostatic pressure because it is interposed between two arterioles, i.e., resistive vessels. Therefore, filtration is favored. The second capillary system (peritubular capillaries in the cortex, vasa recta in the medulla) is a high-flow, low-pressure system that acts as a reservoir for tubular reabsorption and secretion.

The kidneys receive 20 to 25 per cent of the cardiac output, or approximately 1.1 liters of blood per minute. In subjects with a physiologic hematocrit of 45 per cent, total renal plasma flow is about 600 ml per minute. Cortical blood flow is about 75 per cent and medullary blood flow 25 per cent of total renal blood flow. Only 1 per cent of the renal blood flow reaches the papilla. As blood flows through the glomerular capillaries, hydrostatic forces translocate about 20 per cent of the plasma volume (120 ml per minute) across the capillary wall into Bowman's space (glomerular filtration). The ratio of glomerular filtration rate (GFR) to renal plasma flow is called the *filtration fraction*.

Renal blood flow is maintained relatively constant (*autoregulation*) even in the face of wide variations (80 to 180 mm Hg) in perfusion pressure (i.e., mean pressure in the renal artery). This is achieved by changes in renal vascular resistance proportional to changes in perfusion pressure. Since the afferent and efferent arterioles determine renal vascular resistance, changes in arteriolar resistance will alter renal blood flow. When blood pressure falls below 80 or rises above 180 mm Hg, autoregulation is no longer operative and renal blood flow changes in proportion to pressure. In autoregulation, it appears that the afferent arteriole can sense transmural pressure and adjust wall tension to keep resistance proportional to pressure. Autoregulation of renal blood flow maintains a constant GFR despite altered perfusion pressure. Although the kidneys are innervated by adrenergic nerve fibers, renal sympathetic tone probably does not play a significant role in regulating renal blood flow under basal conditions. Thus, denervation or alpha- or beta-adrenergic blockers do not alter renal blood flow. However, augmented sympathetic activity (e.g., fright, pain, exercise, norepinephrine, congestive heart failure) increases renal vascular resistance and reduces renal blood flow. Both afferent and efferent arterioles contract, but GFR falls less than renal blood flow, suggesting that catecholamines exert their major effect at the efferent arteriole. Renal blood flow is increased by substances inducing fever (pyrogenic reaction).

GLOMERULAR FILTRATION RATE. The initial step in the formation of urine (ultrafiltration) occurs across the glomerular wall and separates the plasma water and its nonprotein constituents (crystalloids), which enter Bowman's space, from the blood cells and protein (colloids), which remain in the capillary lumen. The rate of glomerular ultrafiltration (GFR) is governed by the differences between transcapillary hydrostatic (ΔP) and colloid osmotic pressures ($\Delta \Pi$). GFR is influenced also by the filtration coefficient (K_f), which is a function of both total capillary surface area and the permeability per unit of surface area. Thus:

$$GFR = K_f (\Delta P - \Delta \Pi) \text{ or } GFR = K_f [(P_{GC} - P_{BS}) - \Pi_{GC}]$$

The difference in hydrostatic pressure (ΔP) between glomerular capillaries (P_{GC}) and Bowman's space (P_{BS}) favors filtration, whereas the colloid osmotic pressure inside the capillaries (Π_{GC}) opposes it. (The colloid osmotic pressure in Bowman's space is normally negligible and can be disregarded.) Hydrostatic pressure (P_{GC}) remains relatively constant along glomerular capillaries; however, the colloid osmotic pressure (Π_{GC}) undergoes a large progressive increase because filtration of "protein-free fluid" results in an increase of protein concentration along the capillary lumen. Hence, the mean effective pressure for ultrafiltration ($\Delta P - \Delta \Pi$) decreases along the glomerular capillary as $\Delta \Pi$ increases. In rats with surface glomeruli, the rise in glomerular capillary Π, as a function of length, is such that effective ultrafiltration pressure becomes zero before the end of the capillary. In other words, *filtration pressure equilibrium* ($P_{GC} = \Pi_{GC} + P_{BS}$) occurs, and filtration ceases before the end of the glomerular capillary. This fact makes GFR highly dependent on the flow rate of plasma entering the glomerulus, because at high flow rates, a slower rise in colloid osmotic pressure (Π_{GC}) occurs. Thus, glomerular filtration takes place across a greater length of the capillary. Hence, increased plasma flow tends to elevate GFR, whereas decreased plasma flow may cause a fall in GFR. As noted previously, renal blood flow and GFR are autoregulated within a wide range of renal arterial pressure. When perfusion pressure falls, the resistance of the afferent arteriole decreases. Thus, glomerular plasma flow and GFR are maintained. Below 80 to 90 mm Hg, renal plasma flow and GFR vary directly with arterial pressure, and the GFR ceases when the pressure falls below 50 mm Hg.

At a physiologic GFR of 120 ml per minute, the filtration rate per nephron (assuming 2,400,000 nephrons in both kidneys) would be 50 nanoliters per minute. However, just as superficial and juxtamedullary nephrons differ anatomically, they also appear to differ functionally. The larger juxtamedullary glomeruli have filtration rates that are about twice as high as the superficial ones. Single-nephron GFR probably is progressively lower in successively more superficial glomeruli. The physiologic implications of this extensive heterogeneity are not clear, although it has been suggested that redistribution of intrarenal blood flow toward deeper nephrons is associated with salt retention, and may contribute to edema in hepatic disease and congestive heart failure.

Alterations by disease states of any of the primary determinants discussed above may modify GFR. Thus, GFR can fall as a result of (1) decreased hydrostatic pressure in glomerular capillaries (marked hypotension); (2) increased hydrostatic pressure in Bowman's space (intratubular or urinary tract obstruction); (3) elevated glomerular plasma oncotic pressure as a consequence of increased concentration of proteins in the systemic circulation (dehydration: vomiting, diarrhea); (4) decreased renal blood flow (glomerular plasma flow), which may lead to filtration equilibrium at a more proximal region along the glomerular capillary, and hence may decrease the total surface area of capillary available for filtration (e.g., congestive heart failure, hepatic disease); or (5) a decrease in the filtration coefficient (K_f) due to a fall in permeability or to a reduction in total surface area available for filtration (intrinsic renal disease: certain nephrotoxins, acute or chronic glomerulonephritis).

Permselectivity of the Glomerular Capillary Wall. The glomerular capillary wall is highly permeable to small solutes and water. Molecules the size of inulin (molecular weight 5200) or smaller are present in the glomerular filtrate at the same concentration as in plasma water. Constituents with increasing *molecular size* exhibit progressively decreasing concentration in the filtrate. For example, albumin (molecular weight 69,000) is filtered to a very limited degree. However, plasma proteins with molecular sizes smaller than albumin are filtered at least to some degree.

In addition to molecular size, *molecular configuration, deformability,* and *net electrical charge* influence the filtration of macromolecules across the glomerular capillary wall. Negatively charged dextrans, of comparable size to albumin (a polyanion), have a clearance similar to that of albumin (less than 1 per cent that of inulin). In contrast, uncharged (neutral) dextran molecules of the same size as albumin are filtered at a much greater rate (20 per cent the rate of inulin), and filtration of cationic (positively charged) dextrans is even greater. Therefore, at constant molecular size, negative charge of the solute restricts and positive charge accelerates its filtration, suggesting that, phenomenologically, glomerular filtration occurs through pores with negative charges. A negatively charged glycoprotein (*"glomerular polyanion"*), predominantly found lining the foot processes of the epithelial cells, has been identified. Loss of these negative charges, in certain glomerular diseases, may lead to increased filtration of albumin.

HOMEOSTATIC AND EXCRETORY FUNCTIONS OF THE KIDNEY

The formation of urine begins with the elaboration of a protein-free plasma ultrafiltrate across the glomerular capillaries *(glomerular filtration).* As this ultrafiltrate flows through the renal tubule, solutes and water are reabsorbed from lumen to blood *(reabsorption).* Other solutes are secreted into the tubular lumen from the blood *(secretion).* In some cases, both processes (reabsorption and secretion) affect a given substance, permitting flexible regulation of its excretion. Quantitatively, about 170 liters of fluid is ultrafiltered daily, of which less than 1 liter to more than 10 liters may be excreted as urine, depending on the water balance of the individual. Large amounts of filtered sodium, chloride, calcium, magnesium, and phosphate are reabsorbed, with the quantity remaining in the final urine varying according to the dietary intake of each one of these solutes. Substances such as glucose, amino acids, and bicarbonate are almost completely reabsorbed and, under physiologic conditions, do not appear in the urine. The contribution of tubular transport to homeostasis is discussed in more detail below.

TUBULAR TRANSPORT. The renal tubule can be divided functionally into three major segments: (1) the proximal tubule, (2) the loop of Henle, and (3) the distal nephron. Although there are physiologic and morphologic subdivisions of these segments, it is possible to ascribe a general function to each. The proximal tubule reabsorbs, rather nonselectively, a large fraction (two thirds) of the glomerular filtrate. The loop of Henle has unique water and solute transport properties and serves to establish a hyperosmolar medullary interstitium that influences the ultimate concentration or dilution of the urine. The distal nephron is the site of fine regulation of water and electrolyte excretion and appears to be the main target of hormones that control these processes. Since the tubule segments are arranged in series, the function of any segment depends not only on its own intrinsic transport characteristics but also on the volume and composition of the fluid delivered to it from the previous segment.

Proximal Tubule. The proximal tubule reabsorbs sodium, several other solutes, and water at a high rate. Active sodium reabsorption and hydrogen ion secretion are the essential processes to which transport of chloride, several organic solutes, and water is coupled by a variety of mechanisms. Fluid transport is isosmotic, so that concentration gradients of solute across the wall are small. Functionally, the proximal tubule can be divided into three segments:

INITIAL PORTION OF THE CONVOLUTED SEGMENT. Sodium reabsorption in this portion occurs through cells and intercellular spaces. Transcellular reabsorption of sodium is active, generating a small transtubular electrical potential (1 to 5 mV, lumen negative) (Fig. 75–2). It requires entry of sodium across luminal (brush border) membranes and extrusion of sodium across basolateral membranes. Entry of sodium across luminal membranes is passive and occurs (1) by diffusion, (2) coupled to the transport of other solutes (e.g., glucose, amino acids, phosphate), and (3) in exchange with H^+ secreted from cell to lumen. Sodium extrusion from cells into the intercellular spaces and across the basolateral membrane is an active (energy-requiring) process that is accomplished by the sodium-potassium pump (Na^+, K^+-ATPase). Transport of sodium into the intercellular channels increases the concentration of solute in these spaces and creates an osmotic pressure gradient favoring the flow of water from lumen to intercellular spaces across the tight junctions that connect, toward the lumen, the lateral boundaries of the epithelial cells. The osmotic flow of water carries salt with it (solvent drag) and leads to bulk reabsorption of sodium.

Preferential reabsorption of bicarbonate resulting from H^+ secretion occurs in this segment, with bicarbonate concentration falling and chloride concentration increasing to an equivalent degree as the fluid flows along this segment of the tubule. The reabsorption of glucose and amino acids is active, is coupled to sodium transport, and is essentially complete in this segment. Some permeant solutes, such as urea, are partially reabsorbed by a passive mechanism because of the increase in their luminal concentration as water is absorbed.

DISTAL TWO THIRDS OF THE CONVOLUTED SEGMENT. The luminal fluid of the last two thirds of the convoluted tubule is characterized by a low concentration of bicarbonate and by the absence of glucose and amino acids. The tubular fluid remains isosmotic with plasma and has the same concentration of sodium as does the filtrate. The concentration of chloride in the lumen, however, exceeds the concentration of chloride in the peritubular capillary. This concentration gradient for chloride favors its diffusion out of the lumen generating a lumen-positive potential (which is on the order of 1 to 3 mV). In experiments in vitro in which luminal and peritubular fluids have identical compositions, active sodium transport occurs. Therefore, sodium reabsorption in this segment occurs by (1) active transport, (2) passive flow (because of the positive luminal potential), and (3) solvent drag.

STRAIGHT SEGMENT (PARS RECTA). This segment is the main site of secretion of organic acids (penicillin, uric acid). Its rate of sodium and fluid transport is slower, and its capacity for glucose and amino acid reabsorption is minimal when compared with that of the convoluted segments. The potential of the lumen is positive, and sodium and chloride are transported by the same mechanisms as in the last two thirds of the proximal convoluted tubule.

Modulation of Reabsorption by the Proximal Tubule. Proximal reabsorption conserves most of the filtered fluid and all of a number of essential solutes. Several factors modulate the transport rate at the proximal tubule and therefore influence the performance of subsequent segments by altering their load.

TRANSTUBULAR PHYSICAL FACTORS. The hydrostatic pressure (P) in the peritubular capillaries is markedly decreased compared with that in the glomerular capillaries. The colloid osmotic pressure (Π) is increased owing to filtration of a "protein-free fluid" at the glomeruli. These "Starling forces" thus favor the uptake of fluid (from the interstitium) by the peritubular capillaries. When Π falls or P rises, the uptake of fluid by peritubular capillaries decreases. This leads to fluid accumulation in the interstitium, increased hydrostatic pres-

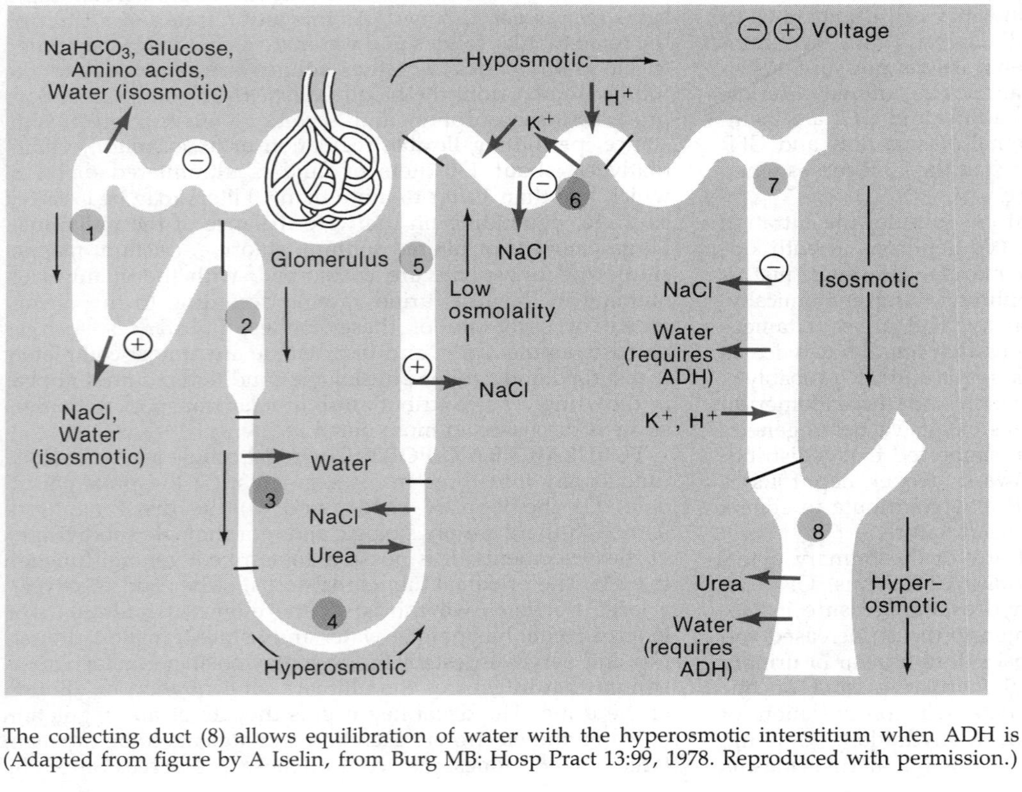

FIGURE 75–2. Schematic representation of the principal processes of transport in the nephron. In the convoluted portion of the proximal tubule (1) salt and water are reabsorbed at high rates, in isotonic proportions. Bulk reabsorption of most of the filtrate (65 to 70 per cent) and virtually complete reabsorption of glucose, amino acids, and bicarbonate take place in this segment. In the pars recta (2) organic acids are secreted and continuous reabsorption of sodium chloride takes place. The loop of Henle comprises three segments; the thin descending (3) and ascending (4) limbs and the thick ascending limb (5). The fluid becomes hyperosmotic, because of water abstraction, as it flows toward the bend of the loop and hyposmotic, because of sodium chloride reabsorption, as it flows toward the distal convoluted tubule (6). Active sodium reabsorption occurs in the distal convoluted tubule and in the cortical collecting tubule (7). This latter segment is water impermeable in the absence of ADH, and the reabsorption of sodium in this segment is increased by aldosterone. The collecting duct (8) allows equilibration of water with the hyperosmotic interstitium when ADH is present. For further details see text. (Adapted from figure by A Iselin, from Burg MB: Hosp Pract 13:99, 1978. Reproduced with permission.)

sure in this space, and a delay in the egress of fluid from the lateral intercellular channels. The limiting junctions of these channels become more permeable, and backflux of fluid (from intercellular spaces to tubular lumen) occurs, thus diminishing net fluid reabsorption. When P falls or Π rises in the peritubular capillaries, as in dehydration, reabsorption of fluid increases.

Glomerular tubular balance refers to a direct relationship between GFR and the prevailing rates of proximal tubular reabsorption and has been ascribed to changes in Π in the peritubular circulation that result from changes in GFR (increases in GFR and hence in filtration fraction lead to a greater protein concentration and increases in Π in the efferent arterioles and peritubular capillaries; a decrease in GFR has the opposite effect). Thus, when GFR increases, a greater amount of fluid is delivered to the proximal tubule; however, the resulting rise in peritubular Π leads to a proportional increase in the reabsorption of fluid in this segment so that the percentage of the filtrate reabsorbed in the proximal tubule remains constant. An alternative mechanism accounting for glomerular tubular balance is a link between fluid reabsorption in the proximal tubule and flow rates of tubular fluid. Increases in GFR, and hence in proximal tubular flow, augment reabsorption; decreases in GFR and in flow decrease reabsorption.

EFFECTS OF HORMONES ON SODIUM REABSORPTION BY THE PROXIMAL TUBULE. Parathyroid hormone reduces sodium and fluid reabsorption in the proximal tubule; catecholamines may stimulate fluid reabsorption in this segment. However, the physiologic significance of these observations has not been established.

Loop of Henle. The loop of Henle, which is interposed between the proximal and distal tubules, is a hairpin-shaped structure extending into the renal medulla (Fig. 75–2). Under physiologic conditions it reabsorbs about 25 per cent of the filtered sodium and chloride and 15 per cent of the filtered water. In consequence, the isotonic fluid entering Henle's loop becomes hypotonic to plasma before entering the distal tubule.

The maintenance of water balance requires the excretion of urine of varied tonicity. The formation of a dilute (hypotonic to plasma) or concentrated (hypertonic to plasma) urine takes place by means of a *countercurrent system* that involves not only the loops of Henle but also the distal tubule, the collecting ducts, and the blood vessels supplying these segments. The excretion of a hypertonic urine involves two basic steps: (1) creation of a hypertonic medullary interstitium and (2) osmotic equilibration of the fluid that enters the medullary collecting duct with the hypertonic interstitium. Antidiuretic hormone (ADH) is required in this latter process. Hypotonic urine is excreted when the fluid that enters the medullary collecting duct does not equilibrate with the hypertonic interstitium owing to low levels or absence of ADH. Only the juxtamedullary nephrons contribute significantly to the production of medullary hypertonicity. However, the fluid from both superficial and deep nephrons drains into the collecting ducts and reaches osmotic equilibrium with the interstitium in the presence of ADH.

In normal human subjects the maximal osmolality of urine that can be achieved is around 1200 mOsm per kilogram. Since the tubular fluid reaches this osmolality by equilibration with the medullary interstitium, it follows that the interstitium must have a similar osmolality. *Countercurrent multiplication* is the process by which the interstitial osmolality is increased from 285 mOsm per kilogram in the cortex (the same osmolality as plasma) to 1200 mOsm per kilogram in the papillary tip. The thin descending and ascending limbs of juxtamedullary nephrons lie in close proximity to each other in the medulla. Flow through them is countercurrent. Fluid obtained from thin ascending limbs has a lower osmolality than fluid obtained from thin descending limbs at comparable levels in the papilla. This is due to functional differences. Whereas the descending limb is highly permeable to water, slightly permeable to urea, and highly impermeable to sodium, the ascending limb is highly permeable to sodium, moderately permeable to urea, and impermeable to water. In normal mammals, the medullary interstitium is hyperosmotic owing to the accumulation of high concentrations of both urea and sodium chloride (see below). This composition and the properties of the two segments of the loop result in quite specific transport processes. The isotonic fluid delivered from the proximal tubule becomes progressively hypertonic as it traverses the thin descending limb owing to net water flow from lumen to interstitium. The highest osmolality of the luminal fluid is achieved at the tip of the loop. This hyperosmolar fluid becomes diluted progressively as it flows up the thin ascending limb, owing to the movement of sodium without water from the lumen to the interstitium. Urea present in the interstitium diffuses inward. However, since the permeability of this segment to sodium chloride is greater than to urea, the net effect is a greater exit of sodium chloride than urea entry, resulting in net addition of solute to the interstitial fluid. In addition, since the thin ascending limb is impermeable to water, the fluid is diluted (hypotonic) with respect to the interstitial fluid at the same level. The thick ascending limb of the loop reabsorbs sodium chloride actively. This segment is essentially impermeable to water, even when ADH is present; therefore, salt transport from lumen to interstitial fluid decreases the osmolality of the luminal fluid and increases the osmolality of the interstitium. This increased osmolality of the outer medullary interstitium promotes the exit of water from the thin descending limb. The function of the thick ascending limb accounts for the countercurrent multiplication that occurs in the renal medulla. Although analysis of the electrochemical gradient (Fig. 75–2) might suggest active chloride transport, there is strong evidence that sodium transport is primary and active and that chloride is moved across the luminal membrane in cotransport with sodium as neutral sodium chloride. The amount of urea present in the fluid of the thick ascending limb is higher than in the fluid entering the thin descending limb. This is due to water abstraction, in excess of urea, out of the latter segment and net urea entry (recycled from the collecting duct) into the thin ascending and descending limbs of Henle's loop.

Urea and sodium chloride contribute most of the 1200 mOsm per kilogram of solute present at the papillary tip during antidiuresis. Antidiuretic hormone plays a critical role in this high interstitial urea concentration. In the cortical collecting duct ADH increases water but not urea permeability. This results, as water is lost from the tubular fluid, in a rise in concentration of urea in the tubular lumen. In the medullary collecting duct, ADH enhances the permeabilities of both water and urea. As water leaves the collecting duct, urea concentration increases further and urea enters the interstitium; it then enters the thin descending (very little) and ascending limbs, increasing the amount of urea in the tubular fluid (see above). The net result is that both urinary and medullary urea concentrations are maintained at high levels in the presence of ADH (antidiuresis).

The fluid emerging from the loop of Henle is virtually always hyposmotic (about 150 mOsm per kilogram) compared with plasma, regardless of the final urine osmolality. With low or absent ADH the luminal fluid in the cortical collecting duct does not equilibrate with the isosmotic cortical interstitium or in the medullary collecting duct with the hypertonic medulla. Hence, the volume of fluid delivered to the tip of the collecting duct is increased and its osmolality decreased compared with plasma. The osmolality of this fluid can be further decreased to as low as 30 mOsm per kilogram by the reabsorption of solute in excess of water in distal tubule and cortical and medullary collecting ducts (see below).

Since the maximal urine osmolality cannot exceed that in

the interstitium, the ability to conserve water by excreting a highly concentrated urine is reduced when the hypertonicity of the medullary interstitium is decreased. This may be due to reduced papillary urea accumulation such as occurs in protein malnutrition, as a consequence of decreased urea production, or due to reduced interstitial sodium chloride accumulation (use of loop diuretics, hypercalcemia). Reduced levels or absence of ADH (diabetes insipidus) or unresponsiveness of the collecting duct to the action of ADH (nephrogenic diabetes insipidus) may prevent equilibration of the fluid in the collecting duct with the hypertonic interstitium, leading to an impairment in water conservation.

Distal Nephron (Distal Convoluted Tubule, Cortical Collecting Tubule, and Medullary Collecting Duct). The distal nephron accomplishes the final and delicate adjustments in the reabsorption of water, sodium, chloride, phosphate, and calcium in response to aldosterone, ADH, and parathyroid hormone.

The *distal convoluted tubule* is defined anatomically as the segment that extends from the macula densa to the site of transition from homogeneous cells to a mixture of dark and light cells (typical of the collecting duct). The distal convoluted tubule is essentially impermeable to water and unresponsive to ADH. Sodium chloride is reabsorbed at a slower rate than in the proximal tubule or in the loop, but against large concentration gradients. The rate of reabsorption is proportional to the load. The transtubular electrical potential, lumen negative, is related to the reabsorption of sodium and varies from –10 in the initial portion to –45 mV in the distal portion. Most of the reabsorption of sodium chloride occurs transcellularly. Potassium is secreted in this segment from peritubular capillary into the lumen (see below). Acidification of the luminal fluid in the distal tubule has been attributed to an active H^+ transport mechanism located at the luminal membrane.

The *cortical collecting tubule* extends from the end of the distal tubule to the corticomedullary junction. Under basal conditions, water permeability is negligible in this segment. It is increased markedly by ADH. Sodium chloride is actively reabsorbed at this level; therefore, in the absence of ADH the luminal fluid osmolality falls further. When ADH is present the luminal fluid equilibrates with the cortical interstitial fluid and becomes isosmotic with plasma; at the same time, luminal urea concentrations rise (see above). The transtubular electrical potential is about 35 mV, lumen negative; it is related to active reabsorption of sodium and is highly dependent on the levels of mineralocorticoids, which increase sodium reabsorption. Potassium and hydrogen are secreted in this segment. Aldosterone increases sodium reabsorption as well as potassium and H^+ secretion in this portion of the nephron (Fig. 75–2).

The *medullary collecting duct* starts at the corticomedullary junction and ends on the surface of the papilla. Water and urea permeabilities are low in the absence of ADH. Continuous sodium chloride reabsorption at this level, in the absence of ADH, results in a further drop in urine osmolality. ADH increases water and urea permeability and allows the equilibration of the luminal osmolality with that of the hypertonic interstitium.

To recapitulate, in the proximal tubule salt and water are transported at high rates, in isotonic proportions. Bulk reabsorption of most of the filtrate (65 to 70 per cent) and virtually complete reabsorption of "metabolically useful" solutes (glucose, amino acids, bicarbonate) take place in this segment. The *loop of Henle* comprises three segments with strikingly different properties of active transport and permeability of water and solute. Because of these properties, the medullary interstitium is made hyperosmolar and acts as the driving force for final water reabsorption. The loop reabsorbs additional sodium chloride (about 25 per cent of that filtered) and water (about 15 per cent of the filtrate) and leaves about 10 per cent of the sodium and 15 per cent of the water to be reabsorbed in the last segments of the tubule.

The distal convoluted tubule and the collecting tubule can establish large sodium gradients between fluid in the lumen and in the peritubular capillary. The collecting ducts, water impermeable in the absence of ADH, become permeable to water in response to the hormone. It is in these segments that the final volume and osmolality of the urine are determined. Salt transport occurs at a slower rate than in the preceding segments but against large concentration gradients. The final regulation of salt excretion takes place in these segments, under the influence of aldosterone. Potassium and H^+ excretion are regulated also in these segments.

ROLE OF THE KIDNEY IN SODIUM CHLORIDE HOMEOSTASIS. Normally the kidney regulates sodium balance (and hence extracellular fluid volume) in a very efficient manner. The daily intake of sodium varies considerably. In the Western world the average diet contains about 170 mEq per 24 hours. About 98 per cent of this amount is excreted in the urine. However, even when the normal daily excretion of sodium is 165 to 170 mEq per day, i.e., sufficient to maintain sodium balance on a relatively high sodium intake, less than 1 per cent of the amount of sodium filtered (140 mEq per liter × 170 liters = 23,800 mEq per day) is excreted in the urine. Thus, maintenance of sodium homeostasis is primarily a function of the renal tubule and reabsorption of filtered sodium; changes in GFR appear to be quantitatively less important. Thus, (1) sizable increases in GFR, not accompanied by extracellular fluid (ECF) volume expansion, do not result in a marked natriuresis because of glomerular tubular balance (see above), and (2) the natriuresis of ECF volume expansion occurs under experimental conditions in which GFR is maintained constant or even decreased experimentally. When a normal subject increases the intake of salt, urine sodium excretion increases progressively, reaching, in three to four days, a steady-state level equal to and offsetting intake. During the interval of adjustment, positive sodium balance occurs, with an accompanying retention of water and consequent gain in body weight. When salt intake is suddenly reduced, the opposite effects are observed. Sodium excretion decreases, reaching a level equal to intake within three to five days with a reduction in total body water and body weight.

Several physiologic mechanisms ordinarily control sodium reabsorption by the kidney to maintain the sodium content of ECF. Changes in sodium mass are not sensed as such, but secondarily as changes in ECF volume. Total ECF volume changes are sensed through their effects on circulatory dynamics ("effective arterial blood volume"). The determinants of effective arterial blood volume are (1) the degree of filling of the arterial tree, which depends in large part on cardiac output, and (2) peripheral vascular resistance, which depends on the compliance of the peripheral vessels and the magnitude of the arterial runoff. Decreases in effective volume (dehydration, hemorrhage, venodilation, venous pooling) lead to renal retention of salt. Increases in effective volume (saline administration, excessive salt intake) lead to a rise in salt excretion by the kidney.

Factors That Influence the Tubular Reabsorption of Sodium. Alterations in effective arterial volume affect handling of sodium by the kidney through the renin-angiotensin-aldosterone system, the sympathetic nervous system, and other less well-defined factors. The last category probably includes changes in intrarenal hydrostatic and oncotic pressures (so-called physical factors), a natriuretic (or salt-losing) hormone, and possibly the distribution of blood flow within the kidneys (Fig. 75–3).

ROLE OF PHYSICAL FACTORS IN THE REABSORPTION OF SODIUM. A fall in effective arterial blood volume (dehydration, hemorrhage) and the consequent decline in blood pressure decrease renal perfusion. In response to reductions in renal perfusion pressure, glomerular plasma flow decreases more

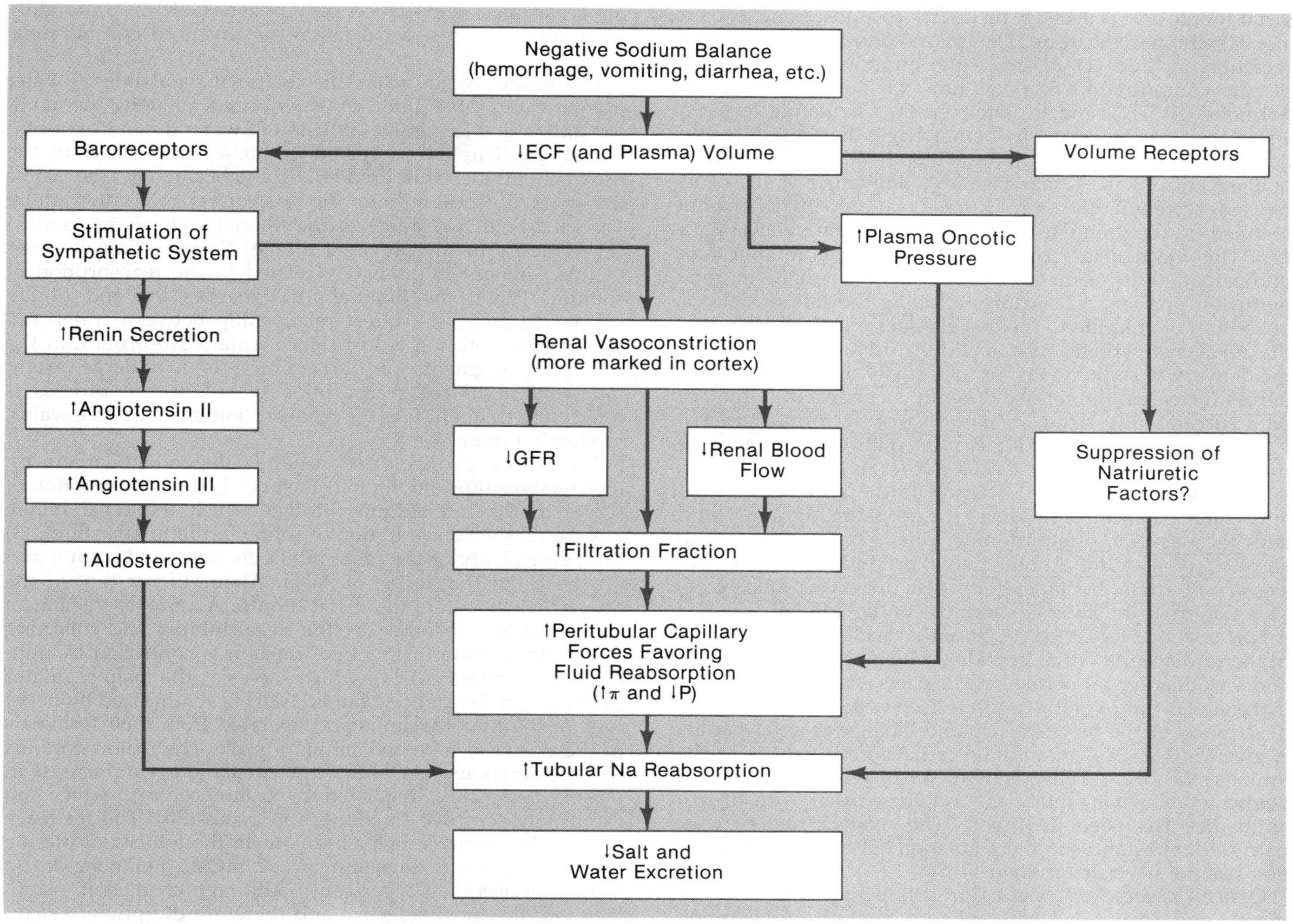

FIGURE 75–3. Mechanisms responsible for increased sodium reabsorption in the renal tubule in response to a negative sodium balance. These mechanisms and the accompanying stimulation of thirst and antidiuretic hormone secretion tend to restore the extracellular fluid (ECF) volume. The arrows indicate a decrease (↓) or an increase (↑). Oncotic pressure and hydrostatic pressure in peritubular capillaries are indicated by Π and P, respectively.

than does glomerular capillary hydrostatic pressure, resulting in a fall in GFR that is proportionally less than the decline in renal plasma flow. This disparity is due to a greater vasoconstriction of efferent compared with afferent arterioles in response to increased levels of catecholamines and angiotensin II in the circulation. The lesser fall in GFR compared with renal plasma flow increases filtration fraction and hence the concentration of protein in the efferent arterioles and peritubular capillaries. In addition, vasoconstriction of the efferent arteriole results in a fall in hydrostatic pressure (P) in the peritubular capillaries. The increase in Π and the decrease in P in the peritubular capillaries augment sodium and water reabsorption along the proximal segments of the nephron. Thus, in response to contraction of effective arterial volume, the glomerular and peritubular microcirculations act in concert to minimize fluid losses by both lowering GFR and augmenting salt and water reabsorption by the tubules (Fig. 75–3).

Expansion of the ECF volume elicits opposite effects. The increase in renal perfusion pressure leads to not only a rise in GFR but also a proportionally greater rise in renal plasma flow; consequently filtration fraction falls. The net effect is a decrease in peritubular protein concentration and hence in Π, with a decrease in reabsorption of fluid by peritubular capillaries. The importance of such physical factors in the normal control of sodium and water reabsorption is not exactly clear. Since alterations in Π and P in the peritubular capillaries influence fluid reabsorption mainly, if not exclusively, in the proximal tubule, it is likely that changes in physical factors are important only when fluid balance deficits or gains are very large (as, for example, with severe hemorrhage or marked expansion of the ECF volume). Whether significant changes in proximal reabsorption occur in response to more modest alterations in fluid balance (as might result, for example, in response to a diet very low or very high in sodium chloride) remains uncertain.

REDISTRIBUTION OF BLOOD FLOW. Another mechanism potentially altering sodium excretion is redistribution of blood flow. It has been suggested that certain nephrons, those with superficially placed glomeruli, have less capacity to reabsorb sodium than others. If so, at any given total GFR, the relative amounts of fluid filtered by the two different nephron populations would be an important determinant of sodium excretion. Redistribution of GFR toward the "high reabsorption nephrons" (juxtamedullary nephrons) would be associated with decreased sodium excretion because of the greater capacity of these nephrons to reabsorb sodium. Despite the attractiveness of this theory, evidence favoring it is scanty.

RENIN-ANGIOTENSIN-ALDOSTERONE. Sodium balance is controlled also by *mineralocorticoid hormones, mainly aldosterone.* Only a small but significant fraction (some 2 per cent) of the filtered sodium is under hormonal control. Yet loss or gain of an amount of sodium equivalent to 2 per cent of the filtered load (about 500 mEq per day) has profound effects on sodium balance. Aldosterone increases sodium reabsorption in the distal tubule and collecting duct. Lack of aldosterone leads to loss of sodium in the urine. The factors controlling aldosterone secretion include (1) plasma concentration of sodium, (2) plasma concentration of potassium, (3) adrenocorticotropic hormone (ACTH), and (4) angiotensin. Circulating levels of angiotensin are increased by hemorrhage, dietary salt restriction, changes in distribution of blood and fluids (venous pooling and edema-forming states), and other states of increased secretion of renin. *Renin* is a proteolytic enzyme secreted by the granular cells of the juxtaglomerular apparatus. The mechanisms controlling its release are not fully understood, but seem to depend on (1) changes in renal perfusion pressure, (2) factors reflecting the rate of delivery of sodium or chloride to the macula densa, and (3) activity of the renal sympathetic nerves. When perfusion pressure or the delivery of sodium falls, or the activity of the sympathetic nerves increases, the release of renin is enhanced. Renin acts on a substrate in plasma, *angiotensinogen,* to form *angiotensin I* (a decapeptide). *Converting enzyme* splits two amino acids from angiotensin I to form *angiotensin II* (an octapeptide). The latter is a potent hormone, central to the regulation of salt and water balance. It produces vasoconstriction and stimulates the secretion of aldosterone, thirst, and the renal reabsorption of sodium. Another split product of angiotensin, *angiotensin III* (a heptapeptide), also increases aldosterone secretion from the zona glomerulosa of the adrenal.

NATRIURETIC HORMONES. A 28–amino acid peptide produced in the cardiac atria (atrial peptide), which has both natriuretic and vasodilating properties, participates in the regulation of extracellular fluid volume and electrolyte balance. A detailed description of the biochemistry and biology of atrial peptide is given in Ch. 224. In addition, a natriuretic substance that inhibits Na^+, K^+-ATPase activity, displaces ouabain that is bound to cellular membranes, and cross-reacts with digoxin antibodies has been described. The relative role of these natriuretic substances in the regulation of renal sodium excretion has not been determined.

OTHER HORMONAL AGENTS. Cortisol, estrogen, growth hormone, and insulin all can enhance sodium reabsorption. Glucagon, progesterone, and parathyroid hormone can decrease it. It is almost certain that when circulating levels of these hormones are elevated (as, for example, estrogen during pregnancy), significant influences occur on sodium reabsorption and thereby excretion. However, there is no evidence that any of them, unlike the factors described previously, are controlled specifically as part of the homeostatic regulation of sodium balance. Of great interest is the possible role played by intrarenally produced substances such as *prostaglandins* and *kinins*. These agents are potent vasodilators and may reduce sodium reabsorption, by altering regional intrarenal vascular resistance or by direct actions on the tubular cells. Their levels change with alterations of sodium balance, but it is not yet clear how extensively they participate in the renal regulation of sodium excretion.

RENAL NERVES. The renal sympathetic nerves play a prominent role in sodium homeostasis by modulating (1) secretion of aldosterone via the renin-angiotensin system, (2) intrarenal physical factors, (3) the reabsorptive activity of the tubular cells themselves, and (4) GFR. Yet, because of the many other known (and potential) factors involved, a transplanted and, therefore, denervated kidney maintains sodium homeostasis quite well.

RENAL REGULATION OF WATER EXCRETION. The capacity to regulate renal excretion of water, independent of solute excretion, maintains the osmolality of body fluids within narrow limits despite wide variations in intake of water. Roughly 170 liters of water is filtered daily. Of this amount, less than 2 liters, or about 1 per cent of the amount filtered, is excreted. Except for setting an upper limit for the amount of water that can be excreted per unit time, GFR is not involved in the regulation of water excretion. This upper limit assumes importance only when GFR is profoundly reduced as in acute renal failure or advanced chronic renal disease.

The tubule is the major site for renal regulation of water excretion. Net absorption of water occurs all along the nephron and is due to passive diffusion of water down its concentration gradient into a region of higher osmolality. In the proximal tubule, this gradient is established by the active transport of sodium into the basolateral and intercellular spaces. About two thirds of the filtered water is reabsorbed isosmotically in the proximal tubule. Reabsorption of water in this segment is intimately related to the reabsorption of sodium. When the luminal fluid reaches the end of the proximal tubule, the direct relationship between water and sodium reabsorption is lost. Since water reabsorption in the remaining segments of the nephron is to a large extent independent of the reabsorption of solute, the process is referred to frequently as the reabsorption of solute-free water, or simply *free water*.

The reabsorption of free water is dependent largely on interrelationships among four factors: (1) the concentration of solute in the interstitium through which the renal tubule passes, (2) the concentration of solute in the tubular fluid, (3) the permeability of the renal tubule to water and solute, and (4) the circulating levels of ADH. About 15 per cent of the filtered water enters the distal tubule. A variable fraction of this water is reabsorbed by the distal tubules and collecting ducts. Absorption of this final fraction is controlled by antidiuretic hormone (ADH), which serves as the main regulator of the osmolality of body fluids. ADH is synthesized by nerve cells in the hypothalamus and liberated from their terminals in the posterior lobe and pituitary stalk. The major stimulus for the secretion of ADH into the circulation is an increase in plasma osmolality, mediated by osmoreceptors, which are exquisitely sensitive to changes in osmolality. The feedback system they provide helps to maintain the tonicity of plasma within a standard deviation of ± 2 mOsm per kilogram (a change of less than 1 per cent). Although changes in osmolality are the most sensitive and therefore the primary regulators of ADH release, alterations in ECF volume can modulate and sometimes override the effects of tonicity. However, secretion of ADH is not increased unless volume loss is greater than 10 per cent. Baroreceptor stimulation appears to mediate the increase in ADH secretion resulting from volume contraction. This effect is potentiated by elevated levels of circulating catecholamines, which act directly on these receptors. Angiotensin II, prostaglandins, and nicotine may also affect ADH release through activation of arterial baroreceptors. When a surfeit of body water develops, ADH release is inhibited and a dilute urine is excreted; when a water deficit is present, free water is reabsorbed and the urine becomes concentrated by mechanisms discussed previously.

The human kidney can dilute urine tenfold with respect to plasma (to about 30 mOsm per kilogram) but can concentrate it to a maximum of only fourfold with respect to plasma (to about 1200 mOsm per kilogram). The daily volume of urine depends on the intake of fluid and can be varied from 600 ml to over 24 liters. When a large load of water is ingested, the following events occur: (1) The osmolar concentration (osmolality) of plasma falls; (2) over the next 15 to 20 minutes ADH levels fall, and as a consequence the flow rate of urine increases, reaching a maximum in 45 to 60 minutes. The maximal increase in urine flow occurs when free water excretion is about 15 per cent of GFR.

ROLE OF THE KIDNEY IN THE PRESERVATION OF POTASSIUM BALANCE. The reader is referred to Ch. 77 for a detailed discussion of potassium balance and potassium distribution in body fluids.

The daily intake of potassium ranges from 50 to 150 mEq. Most of the potassium ingested is absorbed (less than 10 mEq is excreted in the stool); thus, maintenance of balance requires the daily renal excretion of an amount of potassium identical to that absorbed from the gut. Under physiologic conditions, approximately 70 per cent of the potassium filtered is reabsorbed in the proximal tubule. The loop of Henle reabsorbs the remaining 20 to 30 per cent. Distal segments of the nephron can both reabsorb and secrete potassium. The balance between distal reabsorption and secretion determines the net urinary excretion of this cation. On a normal diet (100 mEq per day) the kidneys excrete approximately 90 mEq of potassium per day. The potassium that appears in the urine is secreted in the distal tubule and collecting duct. The secretion of potassium is influenced by the potassium concentration in renal tubular cells and by the magnitude of the electrochemical gradient between cell interior and tubular lumen (see below). The factors that regulate potassium excretion in the urine are summarized in Table 75–2. If potassium intake is increased acutely, renal excretion of potassium can rise more than tenfold. About 50 per cent of the amount administered appears in the urine within 12 hours. The renal response to potassium deprivation is sluggish. Excretion falls to levels of 10 to 15 mEq per 24 hours only after 7 to 14 days of a potassium-free diet. During this interval a deficit of as much as 200 mEq of potassium may be incurred. In adults with increased catabolism (infections, surgery), the renal excretion of potassium may exceed the amount ingested.

Urinary excretion of potassium (Table 75–2) depends on its rate of secretion by the distal tubule. Increased net secretory rates of potassium in this segment could be due to (1) increased active uptake by the peritubular membrane leading to increased cell potassium concentration and increased passive leak across the luminal membrane, (2) increased permeability of the luminal membrane to potassium, (3) decreased active reabsorption of potassium by the luminal membrane, or (4) decreased electrical potential difference across the luminal membrane.

A high concentration of potassium in distal tubular cells is maintained through the action of a Na^+, K^+ exchange pump located in the peritubular membrane. Potassium uptake via this pump is stimulated by high plasma levels of potassium, alkalosis, aldosterone, and increased sodium reabsorption. All factors that raise cell potassium (increased peritubular pump activity, dehydration) favor its diffusion into the lumen. If the cellular potassium concentration falls (potassium deprivation, acidosis, dilution of body fluids), the rate of potassium translocation into the lumen falls and may be less than the potassium uptake across the luminal membrane. Under these conditions, net reabsorption of potassium may replace net potassium secretion.

TABLE 75–2. FACTORS THAT REGULATE POTASSIUM EXCRETION IN THE URINE

Condition		Effect on K^+ Excretion
Dietary K^+	High	Increase
	Low	Decrease
Serum levels of K^+	High	Increase
	Low	Decrease
Levels of mineralo- or glucocorticoid hormones	High	Increase
	Low	Decrease
Tubular fluid or urine flow rate	Fast	Increase
	Slow	Decrease
Sodium excretion in the urine	High	Increase
	Low	Decrease
Most diuretics		Increase
K^+-sparing diuretics (spironolactone, triamterene)		Decrease
Metabolic alkalosis		Increase
Metabolic acidosis		Decrease
Augmented urine excretion of impermeant anions (sulfate, carbenicillin)		Increase

The difference in electrical potential across the entire distal tubular cell is established by the active reabsorption of sodium and is about 50 mV (lumen negative to peritubular fluid). The cell interior is negative (–70 mV) in relation to the peritubular capillary. Thus, the luminal membrane potential difference is about 20 mV (cell negative to lumen). This electrical profile favors a greater leak of potassium across the luminal membrane than across the peritubular membrane. Thus, potassium is pumped into distal tubular cells and then leaks across the luminal membrane into the tubular lumen. Such passive translocation of potassium from the cell into the lumen depends not only on the electrical potential difference across the luminal membrane but also on the chemical concentration gradient. A decrease in luminal membrane potential difference (increased lumen electronegativity) or factors that increase cellular potassium or lower luminal potassium have been shown to augment potassium secretion.

Augmented sodium reabsorption in the distal tubule increases lumen electronegativity, which favors potassium secretion from the cell interior into the tubular fluid. Hence, increased distal sodium reabsorption will favor potassium excretion. For example, diuretic administration increases sodium delivery distally, which, in turn, increases potassium excretion, particularly in patients with secondary aldosteronism. Hyperkalemia increases potassium excretion by two mechanisms: It stimulates aldosterone secretion directly, and it also enhances renal secretion, presumably via increased cell content of potassium. Alkalosis enhances and acidosis depresses potassium secretion, probably by inducing corresponding changes in renal cell potassium. The rates of *distal tubular flow* also influence potassium excretion, presumably because of the rapid dissipation of the concentration of potassium in the tubular lumen at higher flow rates.

ROLE OF THE KIDNEY IN ACID-BASE BALANCE. The reader should consult the section on "Disturbances of Acid-Base Balance" in Ch. 77 for a detailed discussion of acid-base balance. The kidney maintains plasma pH in a physiologic range by regulating the concentration of plasma bicarbonate. This is accomplished by the excretion in the urine of 50 to 100 mEq of H^+ in the form of ammonium (NH_4^+) and titratable acid (the amount of alkali required to titrate the urine to the pH of plasma). Disodium phosphate (Na_2HPO_4) present in the filtrate is converted to NaH_2PO_4, which accounts for most of the titratable acid excreted in the urine. Net excretion of acid (titratable acid + ammonium excretion − bicarbonate excretion) equals the daily production of nonvolatile acids under physiologic conditions. Both the *reclamation* of filtered bicarbonate and the *regeneration* of bicarbonate depend on the secretion of H^+ from the tubular cells into the lumen. The secreted H^+ is generated within the tubular cells by the *carbonic anhydrase*–catalyzed hydration of CO_2 to H_2CO_3, which immediately dissociates into H^+ and HCO_3^-. The H^+ is secreted into the tubular fluid, and the bicarbonate, concomitantly produced intracellularly, enters the peritubular capillary. Thus, H^+ secretion results in addition of bicarbonate to plasma. When the H^+ secreted into the lumen combines with filtered bicarbonate, it forms H_2CO_3, which quickly dissociates to CO_2 and H_2O. As a consequence, a bicarbonate disappears from the lumen, and the net effect is bicarbonate reabsorption (reclamation).

At a physiologic GFR of 170 liters per day and a plasma bicarbonate level of 24 mEq per liter, the reabsorption of over 4000 mEq of bicarbonate requires the secretion of an equivalent amount of H^+, whereas the excretion of net acid requires the secretion of 50 to 100 mEq of H^+ daily (Table 75–3). The process of bicarbonate reclamation operates to reabsorb all the filtered bicarbonate below a critical serum concentration, the *bicarbonate threshold concentration,* which in adult humans is normally about 24 mEq per liter, essentially identical to the concentration of bicarbonate in plasma. When plasma bicarbonate concentration rises above this threshold, renal recla-

TABLE 75–3. ROLE OF THE KIDNEY IN ACID-BASE BALANCE

Function	mEq/24 hr
1. Reabsorption of filtered bicarbonate ("reclamation")	≅ 4000
2. Generation of new bicarbonate (net excretion of acid)	50–100
a. Ammonium excretion	35–65
b. Titratable acid excretion	15–35

mation is incomplete and the excess bicarbonate escapes into the urine, enabling the plasma bicarbonate concentration to return to the threshold level. Under physiologic conditions the virtually complete reabsorption of bicarbonate serves to preserve bicarbonate stores but does not replace the bicarbonate consumed in the buffering of nonvolatile acids. If the secreted H^+ combines with buffers, such as $HPO_4^=$ or NH_3, a new bicarbonate ion (de novo synthesis) is added to the peritubular capillary blood. This results in replacement of the bicarbonate consumed in buffering the daily acid load (Table 75–3).

In the steady state, the net amount of H^+ excreted is equal to the H^+ load, about 50 to 100 mEq per day. At times, net acid excretion is absent or has a negative value. This occurs after ingestion of an alkaline load (bicarbonate or substances that can be metabolized to bicarbonate). Ammonium excretion accounts for two thirds and titratable acid for one third of the urinary excretion of acid. When the daily H^+ load increases (e.g., increased catabolism, infection), the rise in acid excretion by the kidney is usually due to increased ammonium excretion. Ammonia (NH_3), produced within the renal tubular cells from glutamine, diffuses into the peritubular capillary or lumen down its concentration gradient. In the lumen it combines with H^+ to form NH_4^+. As noted, each mole of NH_4^+ excreted will result in the de novo generation of 1 mole of bicarbonate. Thus, when metabolic acidosis develops and the need for regenerating bicarbonate increases, synthesis of ammonia and NH_4^+ excretion usually increase.

Hydrogen secretion occurs in both proximal and distal segments of the nephron. As the concentration of bicarbonate in the lumen decreases, the concentration of H^+ increases, and as a result a limitation is imposed on the net rate of H^+ secretion. The maximal H^+ gradient achievable between cell and collecting duct lumen is about 800:1 (luminal fluid pH of 4.5).

Factors That Regulate the Renal Secretion of Hydrogen Ions. The major factors that influence the renal secretion of H^+ are (1) *effective circulating volume,* (2) *arterial pH and* P_{CO_2}, (3) *plasma concentration of potassium,* and (4) *mineralocorticoids (aldosterone).*

EFFECTIVE CIRCULATING VOLUME. Hydrogen ion secretion is increased by volume depletion (increased sodium reabsorption) and diminished by ECF volume expansion. Hydrogen secretion is stimulated also when significant amounts of nonreabsorbable anions, i.e., sulfate ions, are present in the distal nephron and when sodium reabsorption is enhanced by any mechanism. Thus, the effective circulating volume of the ECF and the amounts of nonreabsorbable anion accompanying sodium through the distal nephron are important determinants of renal H^+ secretion.

ARTERIAL pH AND P_{CO_2}. Net acid excretion is increased with acidosis and decreased with alkalosis. Acidosis, resulting from a decrease in the plasma concentration of bicarbonate (metabolic acidosis) or induced by an elevation in P_{CO_2} (respiratory acidosis), augments H^+ excretion and increases the renal synthesis of bicarbonate. Metabolic alkalosis (increased plasma bicarbonate) or respiratory alkalosis (decreased P_{CO_2}) has the opposite effects. The effects of arterial pH on net acid excretion are most likely mediated by changes in renal tubular cell pH. Elevations in arterial P_{CO_2} increase bicarbonate reabsorption, and a fall in arterial P_{CO_2} reduces bicarbonate reabsorption.

PLASMA POTASSIUM CONCENTRATION. Hypokalemia increases and hyperkalemia decreases bicarbonate reabsorption. These effects are due to changes in intracellular H^+ concentration induced by cation shifts between the ICF and the ECF. In hypokalemia, potassium leaves the cell and is replaced by H^+ and sodium. The increase in intracellular H^+ concentration (intracellular acidosis) leads to the enhanced H^+ secretion and bicarbonate reabsorption associated with potassium depletion. The opposite occurs with hyperkalemia.

ALDOSTERONE. Aldosterone stimulates secretion of both potassium and hydrogen in the distal nephron. Excess of aldosterone may cause metabolic alkalosis, and its deficiency may lead to metabolic acidosis by decreasing H^+ excretion.

ROLE OF THE KIDNEY IN MINERAL HOMEOSTASIS. The kidney regulates the homeostasis of minerals not only by modifying the excretion of phosphate, calcium, and magnesium (see below) but also by influencing the metabolism of vitamin D. Vitamin D_3 (cholecalciferol) is metabolized to 25(OH) cholecalciferol in the liver and subsequently to $1,25(OH)_2D_3$ and $24,25(OH)_2D_3$ in the kidney. The $1,25(OH)_2D_3$ is the calcemic hormone produced in the renal cortex in response to hypophosphatemia or elevated levels of parathyroid hormone (when hypocalcemia occurs), and $24,25(OH)_2D_3$ is produced preferentially when the balance of minerals is normal. The $1,25(OH)_2D_3$ increases absorption of calcium and phosphate from the gut as well as mineral mobilization from bone. The role of $24,25(OH)_2D_3$ is less well defined; it seems to promote bone mineralization and suppress parathyroid hormone release.

REGULATION OF PHOSPHORUS METABOLISM. The kidneys play a major role in maintaining the serum phosphorus concentration within narrow limits, about 3.0 to 4.5 mg per deciliter in adults. On an average diet, 1 gram of phosphorus is ingested daily, of which 700 mg is absorbed and the rest is excreted in the stool. The kidneys filter about 7 grams of phosphorus daily, of which 6.3 grams (90 per cent) is reabsorbed and 700 mg is excreted in the urine. As serum phosphorus and filtered load of phosphorus rise, the capacity to reabsorb phosphorus increases until a transport maximum (Tm) for phosphorus reabsorption is reached when serum phosphorus concentrations are between 6 and 9 mg per deciliter. Under physiologic conditions, about 70 per cent of the filtered phosphorus is reabsorbed in the proximal tubule and 10 to 15 per cent in the distal tubule and collecting ducts; thus, 5 to 20 per cent of the filtered phosphorus is excreted in the urine. In other words, the tubular reabsorption of phosphate (TRP) ranges normally from 80 to 95 per cent.

Numerous factors (the major ones being dietary phosphorus load and the serum levels of parathyroid hormone) affect the reabsorption of phosphorus. Phosphorus reabsorption approaches 100 per cent in patients fed a very low-phosphorus diet. In contrast, patients ingesting 2 to 3 grams of phosphorus daily can excrete 60 to 70 per cent of this amount in the urine. Changes in phosphorus intake affect phosphorus excretion directly and also by altering the levels of ionized calcium that modify the release of parathyroid hormone. Parathyroid hormone decreases phosphorus reabsorption in both proximal and distal segments of the nephron. An excess of parathyroid hormone may increase fractional excretion of phosphorus from a basal value of 10 per cent to 30 per cent or more. In the absence of parathyroid hormone the tubular capacity to reabsorb phosphorus is increased. Additional factors affect phosphorus reabsorption by the kidney. Volume expansion of the ECF, calcitonin, glucocorticoids, metabolic acidosis or alkalosis, and glycosuria increase urinary phosphorus excretion. On the other hand, administration of growth hormone and respiratory acidosis decrease phosphorus excretion. Vitamin D and its metabolites increase phosphorus reabsorption by the kidney.

RENAL REGULATION OF CALCIUM METABOLISM. Serum calcium concentrations in humans are maintained between 9 and 10 mg per deciliter despite wide variations in dietary calcium intake. Total serum calcium consists of ultrafilterable calcium (approximately 60 per cent of the total) and calcium bound to protein, primarily albumin. The ultrafilterable fraction includes both the ionized calcium (50 per cent of the total) and calcium complexed to citrate, bicarbonate, and phosphate, which represents 10 per cent of total serum calcium. Serum calcium levels are maintained relatively constant through modification of calcium absorption from the gastrointestinal tract, changes in renal calcium excretion, and mobilization of calcium from bone.

Approximately 1000 mg of calcium is ingested daily in the diet. About 800 mg appears in the stool (from unabsorbed dietary calcium and intestinal secretion) and 200 mg in the urine. The percentage of dietary calcium absorbed from the intestine increases when calcium intake is low and decreases when it is high. Parathyroid hormone and vitamin D participate in these adaptations. Thus, in patients fed a low-calcium diet, the development of mild and transient hypocalcemia increases the release of parathyroid hormone, which augments the renal conversion of $25(OH)D_3$ to $1,25(OH)_2D_3$. This latter compound increases intestinal calcium absorption and mobilizes calcium from bone, synergistically with parathyroid hormone. Thus, serum calcium returns toward normal. On the other hand, in patients fed a high-calcium diet, the mild hypercalcemia that may occur suppresses the release of parathyroid hormone, leading to decreased activity of the renal 1-hydroxylase enzyme and the preferential production of $24,25(OH)_2D_3$. This metabolite is less efficient than $1,25(OH)_2D_3$ in promoting calcium absorption from the intestine and in mobilizing calcium from the skeleton.

The kidneys filter approximately 10 grams of calcium per day, but usually less than 200 mg appears in the urine. Thus over 98 per cent of the filtered load is reabsorbed. Approximately 55 per cent of the filtered calcium is reabsorbed in the proximal tubule, 20 to 30 per cent in the loop of Henle, 10 to 15 per cent in the distal tubule, and 2 to 8 per cent in the terminal nephron, including the collecting duct. Most maneuvers that decrease sodium and fluid reabsorption in the proximal tubule (infusion of saline, administration of acetazolamide, or mild-to-moderate hypercalcemia) decrease calcium reabsorption in this segment as well. The reabsorption of calcium in the loop of Henle also parallels sodium reabsorption. It is only distal to the loop of Henle that calcium and sodium are influenced separately and independently.

Parathyroid hormone stimulates the renal absorption of calcium and decreases urinary calcium excretion. Acute parathyroidectomy increases calcium excretion despite a fall in total serum calcium and hence in the filtered load of calcium. However, the degree of calciuria declines when the plasma concentration of calcium falls below 7 mg per deciliter. Pharmacologic doses of vitamin D usually increase intestinal absorption of calcium and bone resorption, leading to increases in serum calcium, the filtered load of calcium, and urinary calcium excretion. Metabolic acidosis or phosphate depletion produces hypercalciuria. Both furosemide and ethacrynic acid inhibit sodium and calcium transport in the thick ascending limb of Henle's loop and increase calcium excretion. Chronic administration of thiazides results in natriuresis and hypocalciuria. This effect may be due to contraction of ECF volume and increased calcium reabsorption in the proximal segments. In addition, thiazides may potentiate the effect of parathyroid hormone on calcium reabsorption in the distal segment.

RENAL REGULATION OF MAGNESIUM METABOLISM. Total body magnesium is approximately 2000 mEq (or 25 grams). About 60 per cent of total body magnesium is found in bone. Another 20 per cent is present in muscle. Only a small fraction (about 1 per cent) is present in the ECF. The normal plasma concentration of magnesium in humans is 1.7 to 2.2 mg per deciliter, of which 80 per cent is ultrafilterable and the remainder protein bound. Most of the ultrafilterable magnesium is ionized. Roughly 300 mg or 25 mEq of magnesium is ingested daily in the diet. About two thirds of this amount appears in the stool and one third is eliminated in the urine. The kidney filters about 2 grams of magnesium daily, and approximately 100 mg (5 per cent) appears in the urine; thus, 95 per cent of the filtered magnesium is reabsorbed. Renal excretion of magnesium can be reduced to less than 0.5 per cent of the filtered load during magnesium deprivation. On the other hand, during infusion of magnesium or among patients with advanced chronic renal insufficiency the kidney can excrete 40 to 70 per cent of the filtered magnesium. The proximal tubules reabsorb about 20 to 30 per cent of the filtered magnesium, with 50 to 60 per cent being reabsorbed in the loop of Henle. Expansion of the ECF volume, produced by infusion of saline or chronic administration of mineralocorticoids, reduces the reabsorption of magnesium. A diet deficient in magnesium or the administration of parathyroid hormone enhances the reabsorption of magnesium in the thick ascending limb of Henle's loop. Infusions of calcium, ingestion of alcohol, administration of glucose, diets containing large amounts of magnesium, and diuretics such as furosemide or ethacrynic acid increase the urinary excretion of magnesium.

OTHER NONEXCRETORY FUNCTIONS OF THE KIDNEY

In addition to its role in the secretion of renin and the metabolism of vitamin D already discussed, the kidney has several other nonexcretory functions.

REGULATION OF THE RED BLOOD CELL MASS. *Erythropoietin* promotes the differentiation, proliferation, and maturation of red blood cell precursors in the bone marrow. The site of synthesis of this glycoprotein within the kidney has not been clearly defined, but the juxtaglomerular cells have been implicated. The stimulus to increased erythropoietin production by the kidney appears to be decreased renal oxygen tension or decreased renal perfusion (anemia, hypoxia, renal ischemia) or circulatory alterations induced by vasoconstrictors such as norepinephrine, angiotensin, or vasopressin. Increased erythropoietin levels may be seen in association with renal artery stenosis, renal cysts, renal cell carcinoma, and hydronephrosis and after renal transplantation. Production of erythropoietin decreases with hyperoxia or an excess red blood cell volume.

RENAL METABOLISM OF PLASMA PROTEINS AND PEPTIDE HORMONES. The kidney is an important catabolic site for low molecular weight proteins (less than 50,000) but not for proteins with a molecular weight exceeding 68,000 (e.g., albumin, immunoglobulins).

Low molecular weight proteins are filterable. In the absence of tubular reabsorption they would be excreted quantitatively in the urine. Reabsorption of proteins or their catabolic products by the kidney prevents their loss in the urine, thereby conserving nutritionally important components. The proteins catabolized by the kidney are broken down to amino acids or polypeptides prior to return into the renal venous blood. The kidney, therefore, contributes to the regulation of their concentrations in plasma and precludes extensive loss of protein components in the urine.

In some patients with abnormalities of renal tubular function, low molecular weight proteins may appear in the urine in the absence of albumin owing to decreased tubular reabsorption. Conversely, in patients with reduced GFR the fractional catabolic rate of low molecular weight proteins (lysozyme, ribonuclease, beta$_2$-microglobulins, insulin, proinsulin, gastrin, glucagon, parathyroid hormone, Bence Jones protein, retinol binding protein, and growth hormone) is decreased and their levels in plasma are elevated.

Insulin, parathyroid hormone, and glucagon are catabolized by the kidney by filtration and subsequent tubular reabsorption as well as by peritubular uptake.

The catabolism of albumin, immunoglobulins, and larger

plasma proteins is relatively low, with the kidney accounting for less than 5 per cent of their fractional catabolic rate, unless the nephrotic syndrome is present, in which case albumin catabolism could be significantly increased owing to both urinary losses and increased tubular degradation.

THE KALLIKREIN-KININ SYSTEM. Kallikrein is a peptidase produced in various tissues, including the kidney, which acts on a specific substrate (kininogen) to split off a peptide, kinin. The kinin is destroyed by plasma and tissue peptidases (kininases). Kinins are potent vasodilators. The renal kallikrein-kinin system may constitute a local hormonal mechanism involved in the regulation of renal blood flow and sodium excretion. Renal kallikrein is probably produced by the cortex and excreted into the urine. It acts on a kininogen substrate to produce the potent vasodilator decapeptide (kallidin). Kallikrein excretion is augmented by reduced sodium intake. In contrast, high sodium intake decreases it. Administration of mineralocorticoids increases the excretion of kallikrein, and the increased kallikrein excretion of a low-salt diet is blocked by aldosterone antagonists (spironolactones). However, the role of the renal kallikrein system in sodium homeostasis is not yet established.

RENAL PROSTAGLANDINS. The prostaglandins are 20-carbon unsaturated fatty acids. Both vasodilator prostaglandins (PGE_2, prostacyclin, or PGI_2) and vasoconstrictor substances (thromboxanes) are synthesized in renal cortex (by arteries and glomeruli) and medulla (by interstitial and collecting duct cells) from free arachidonic acid, released from phospholipids. Renal prostaglandins may play a role in control of blood flow and GFR and in sodium and water excretion. They affect renin secretion as well. Prostaglandins may also modulate phosphorus transport and regulate renal ammonia synthesis. Their synthesis is stimulated by bradykinin, angiotensin II, ADH, and catecholamines. The last substances are vasoconstrictors that tend to diminish renal plasma flow. Therefore when constrictor stimuli are operative, renal prostaglandin production may increase, resulting in maintenance of renal blood flow.

Two other pathways of arachidonic acid metabolism have been described recently in the kidney: (1) an NADPH-dependent mono-oxygenase pathway that leads to the formation of 19- and 20-hydroxyeicosatetranoic acid (19-HETE and 20-HETE), 19-ketoarachidonic acid, and 1,20-dicarboxylic acid; and (2) a calcium-dependent lipoxygenase pathway with synthesis of 15-HETE, 12-HETE, and leukotrienes. The physiologic or pathophysiologic importance of these pathways is unknown, but it should be remembered that the HETE's are potent chemotactic compounds and, therefore, may play a role in inflammatory glomerular disease. Leukotrienes are known to contract vascular and nonvascular smooth muscle and enhance vascular permeability. Thus, they may play a role in the control of renal blood flow and GFR.

Brenner BM, Dworkin LK, Ichikawa I: Glomerular ultrafiltration. In Brenner BM, Rector JC (eds.): The Kidney. 3rd ed. Philadelphia, W. B. Saunders Company, 1986, pp 124–144. *A lucid chapter written by investigators who have made important contributions to our understanding of glomerular physiology.*

Dunn MJ: Renal prostaglandins. In Klahr S, Massry SG (eds.): Contemporary Nephrology. Vol III. New York, Plenum Publishing Company, 1985, pp 143–190. *A clear review of the role of arachidonic acid metabolites in health and disease.*

Jackson EK, Branch RA, Margolius HS, et al.: Physiological functions of the renal prostaglandin, renin and kallikrein systems. In Seldin DW, Giebisch G (eds.): The Kidney: Physiology and Pathophysiology. New York, Raven Press, 1985, pp 613–644. *An excellent chapter on intrarenal hormones and their mechanisms of action.*

Klahr S, Hruska KA: Effects of parathyroid hormone on the renal reabsorption of phosphorus and divalent cations. In Peck WB (ed.): Bone and Mineral Research. Vol 2. Amsterdam, Elsevier, 1983, pp 65–124. *A detailed view of phosphorus and calcium reabsorption in the kidney and its control by hormones and other factors.*

Lang F, Messner G, Rehiwald W: Electrophysiology of sodium-coupled transport in proximal renal tubules. Am J Physiol 250 (Renal Fluid Electrol Physiol 19):F953, 1986. *A recent editorial review with up-to-date references on the coupling of sodium transport to that of other solutes.*

Tisher CC, Madsen KM: Anatomy of the kidney. In Brenner BM, Rector JC (eds.): The Kidney. 3rd ed. Philadelphia, W. B. Saunders Company, 1986, pp 3–60. *An authoritative and clearly written review of kidney structure.*

Valtin H: Renal Function: Mechanisms Preserving Fluid and Solute Balance in Health. 2nd ed. Boston, Little, Brown and Company, 1983. *This book presents the essential elements in renal fluid and electrolyte physiology, which every medical student should master.*

76 INVESTIGATIONS OF RENAL FUNCTION

Vincent W. Dennis

Methods are available to assess the functional integrity of the glomerular ultrafiltration barrier; the presence of urogenital inflammation; the overall rate of glomerular filtration; the ability to dilute, concentrate, or acidify urine; and the ability to conserve or to excrete specific solutes. Measurements of certain values in blood and urine detect abnormalities in renal function and may occasionally point to specific etiologies, but a final diagnosis usually requires direct or indirect visualization of the kidneys and urogenital system or morphologic examination of renal tissue.

PROTEINURIA. Increased urinary excretion of protein is one of the most common and most easily detected signs of renal disease. The normal excretion rate of urinary protein is less than 150 mg per 24 hours for adults, but values as high as 300 mg per 24 hours may occur in apparently healthy adolescents. The normal composition of urinary protein includes about 40 per cent albumin, 40 per cent tissue proteins originating from renal and other urogenital tissues, 15 per cent immunoglobulins and their fragments, and 5 per cent other plasma proteins. Abnormalities may occur in both the quantity and the composition of urinary proteins.

Urinary protein is usually detected by a colorimetric test ("dipstick test"), which depends on the ability of proteins, especially albumin, to alter the color reaction of a pH-sensitive dye. Such qualitative tests may detect protein concentrations as low as 15 mg per deciliter and result in a positive test if a normal amount of protein is present in a concentrated volume of urine. Conversely, abnormal rates of protein excretion may remain undetected in large volumes of dilute urine. It is therefore important to have some estimate of the degree of urine concentration when considering the significance of a positive qualitative test for protein. A positive qualitative test for urinary protein usually warrants quantification of the absolute protein excretion rate per 24 hours. Alternatively, the protein-creatinine ratio of a random daytime urine sample correlates well with values from 24-hour collections. The protein-creatinine method is quicker but less precise (Fig. 76–1). Proteinuria usually results from (1) elevated plasma concentration of normal or abnormal proteins, (2) increased glomerular permeability, (3) decreased tubular reabsorption of normally filtered proteins, and (4) alterations in renal hemodynamics (Table 76–1).

Overflow Proteinuria. Changes in plasma protein concentrations may alter the rates of protein excretion by both the normal and the abnormal kidney. This type of proteinuria may occur from the presence in plasma of increased concentrations of proteins not normally present in significant amounts. Examples include light-chain immunoglobulin fragments such as Bence Jones protein associated with plasma cell disorders (see Ch. 163) or myoglobin associated with rhabdomyolysis. The presence of increased concentrations of abnormal proteins in either plasma or urine may be confirmed by electrophoresis. Changes in the concentration of normal plasma proteins may also influence passage across the *abnormal* glomerular capillary wall. For example, increases or de-

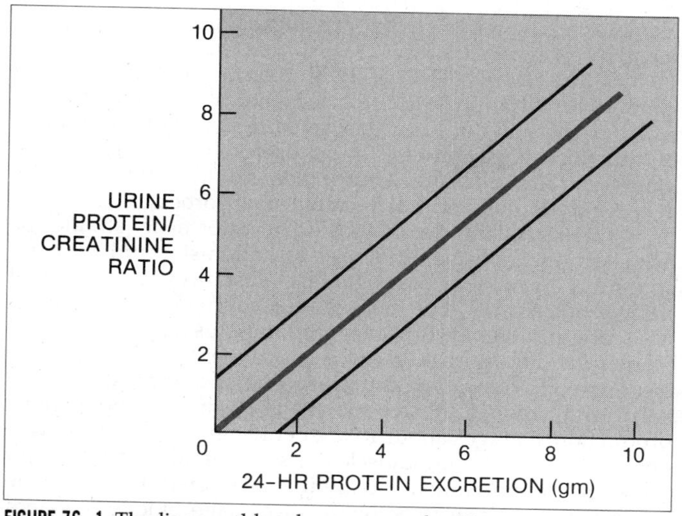

FIGURE 76–1. The lines and bands represent the 95 per cent confidence levels for the relationship between the protein-to-creatinine ratio in a random daytime urine sample to the amount of protein excreted in 24 hours.

creases in the plasma concentration of albumin may increase or decrease its rate of urinary excretion without necessarily indicating improvement or worsening of the renal conditions that led to proteinuria.

Increased Glomerular Permeability. The glomerular capillary wall consists of capillary endothelium, basement membrane, visceral epithelium, and mesangium. Each of these four anatomic components contributes directly or indirectly to the formation and maintenance of the functional ultrafiltration barrier that limits the passage of proteins into the urinary space. The glomerular capillary wall restricts the passage of plasma proteins according to their size (steric hindrance) and surface charge (electrostatic hindrance). At any given molecular size, negative charges on the glomerular capillary basement membrane hinder the passage of negatively charged molecules more than positively charged molecules.

A number of systemic and primary renal diseases may affect one or more glomerular structures and thereby increase the effective permeability of the glomerular capillary wall to proteins. The degree of proteinuria may range from 0.2 to greater than 20 grams per 24 hours. Proteinuria that exceeds about 3 to 5 grams of normal plasma protein per 24 hours provides direct evidence of increased effective permeability of the glomerular capillary wall, since these amounts exceed those that may be filtered by the normal glomerulus and reabsorbed by the renal tubules. Such massive losses of plasma proteins may be responsible for changes in plasma oncotic pressure and thereby set in motion the events that are manifest clinically as the nephrotic syndrome (see Ch. 81).

Because of its low molecular weight and its dominance among plasma proteins, albumin is typically the major urinary protein in this type of proteinuria. However, the relative proportion of albumin in the urine, even if corrected for changes in its proportion in plasma, is lower in some forms of renal diseases than in others. *Selective proteinuria* refers to the ability of the glomerulus to retain higher molecular weight proteins despite increased filtration of low molecular weight proteins. A highly selective proteinuria therefore consists almost exclusively of increased excretion of albumin, whereas a poorly selective proteinuria contains proportionately greater amounts of higher molecular weight proteins and is generally associated with severe disruption of the glomerular capillary wall. This selectivity may be attributed to the glomerulus only if the composition of urinary proteins is not affected significantly by downstream events such as tubular reabsorption. This requirement is presumably met with levels of proteinuria that exceed 3 to 5 grams per 24 hours, but the selectivity pattern of lesser amounts of proteinuria may be significantly influenced by tubular reabsorption. To define glomerular selectivity requires measurements of the relative clearances of specific proteins with increasing molecular weights such as albumin (69,000), transferrin (90,000), gamma globulin (150,000), and alpha$_2$-glycoprotein (820,000). Although attractive in theory and potentially useful as an index of the severity of glomerular damage, the techniques required to characterize the selectivity of proteinuria are generally too laborious and too imprecise to have achieved widespread clinical applicability. Nevertheless, heavy proteinuria characterized by the dominance of albumin and the absence of higher molecular weight globulins is typical of minimal change or nil lesion (see Ch. 81), whereas the detection of a nonselective pattern is highly suggestive of the presence of some other form of otherwise undefined glomerular disease.

Microalbuminuria refers to increases in albumin excretion that are detectable by sensitive immunoassay but not by current standard clinical techniques. The presence of microalbuminuria in diabetics may predict the development of diabetic nephropathy, whereas its absence may forecast a more favorable prognosis.

Tubular Proteinuria. Many polypeptides and low molecular weight proteins normally present in plasma are filtered freely at the glomerulus and are reabsorbed by the tubules. Examples include polypeptide hormones such as insulin, glucagon, and parathyroid hormone and plasma proteins smaller than 20,000 daltons. Once filtered, these proteins are absorbed by specific endocytic processes that bind and engulf the filtered proteins. The presence of tubular disorders, especially injuries that result from various antibiotics or heavy metals (see Ch. 82), may be associated with increased urinary excretion of low molecular weight proteins and relatively slight increases in the excretion of albumin (*tubular proteinuria*). This pattern is in marked contrast to the predominance of albumin in the urine of patients with glomerular disorders. Patients characterized clinically as having tubulointerstitial rather than glomerular diseases have increased urine protein excretion (generally less than 2 grams per 24 hours) and increased renal clearance of beta$_2$-microglobulin, especially relative to albumin. Beta$_2$-microglobulinuria is less likely to occur in those disease processes such as diabetes mellitus that cause proteinuria via effects on glomerular permeability. The clinical significance of tubular proteinuria is unclear at this time because

TABLE 76–1. TYPES OF PROTEINURIA*

Type	Mechanism	Quantity	Molecular Weight	Examples
Overflow	Increased filtration of abnormal plasma proteins across normal glomeruli	Variable (0.2 to >10g)	Low (<40,000)	Bence Jones proteinuria, myoglobinuria
Glomerular	Defective glomerular retention of normal plasma proteins	>3–5 grams	High (>68,000)	Glomerulonephritis, nephrotic syndrome
Tubular	Defective reabsorption of normally filtered plasma proteins	<2 grams	Low (<40,000)	Interstitial nephritis, antibiotic injury, heavy metals
Hemodynamic	Increased filtration and possibly decreased reabsorption	<2 grams	Variable (20,000–68,000)	Transient proteinuria, congestive heart failure, fever, seizures, exercise

*Values >150 mg per 24 hours.

there is still insufficient documentation of correlations between tubular proteinuria and detailed functional, biochemical, and morphologic descriptions of the underlying diseases in which it has been observed.

Proteinuria from Altered Renal Hemodynamics. Changes in protein excretion rate may also occur in response to changes in renal hemodynamics. Exercise, major motor seizures, change to the standing position, fever, and vasoactive agents such as renin, angiotensin, and norepinephrine increase urine protein excretion by mechanisms that seem related to reductions in renal blood flow. Changes in renal blood flow may alter urine protein excretion in normal subjects as well as in those with abnormal rates of protein excretion. Possible mechanisms include local increases in protein concentration within the glomerular capillary, increased effective permeability of the glomerular capillary wall, increased transglomerular hydrostatic pressure, and increased effective filtration area. Hemodynamic increases in urine protein excretion are generally transient or additive to other causes of proteinuria.

LEUKOCYTURIA. The urinary leukocyte excretion rate in apparently healthy individuals ranges between 0 and 300,000 leukocytes per hour; rates greater than 400,000 per hour are generally regarded as abnormal. If appropriate cleansing precautions are used, there is no difference in leukocyte excretion rates between apparently healthy males and females or between urine samples obtained from suprapubic puncture and midstream urine.

In practice, leukocyte excretion rates are estimated indirectly by microscopic examination of urinary sediment resuspended after centrifugation of approximately 10 ml of urine. Abnormal leukocyturia probably exists when more than 5 white blood cells occur per high-power field. However, about 20 per cent of urine specimens from patients excreting more than 400,000 white blood cells per hour may demonstrate fewer than 5 leukocytes per high-power field. The indirect method thus underestimates the prevalence of abnormal leukocyturia, although increased numbers of white blood cells per high-power field appear to correspond well to increased rates of leukocyte excretion. Leukocyturia results frequently from urinary tract infection (see Ch. 86) but may also indicate other causes of inflammation, such as tubulointerstitial diseases (see Ch. 82).

HEMATURIA. The detection of hematuria is aided by the widespread use of the multifunctional "dipstick," which includes a section impregnated with orthotolidine. The test is sufficiently sensitive to detect the equivalent of greater than 10,000 red blood cells per milliliter of urine but is negative in normal individuals despite the wide range of red blood cell excretion rates. A positive orthotolidine test may also occur in the presence of free hemoglobin or myoglobin in urine. Free hemoglobin in the urine generally results from the lysis of red blood cells in the urine, but may also reflect free hemoglobin in the plasma. When indicated, this question can be resolved by direct measurements of plasma hemoglobin and haptoglobin concentrations. Myoglobin in the urine is detected by the differential precipitation of hemoglobin with ammonium sulfate, by spectrophotometry of the ferricyanide derivatives of hemoglobin and myoglobin, by the co-migration on paper electrophoresis of myoglobin with hemoglobin C, or, preferably, by direct immunoassay of myoglobin in plasma or urine. Myoglobinuria is usually accompanied by marked increases in plasma concentrations of creatine phosphokinase (CPK).

As with leukocytes, the presence of red blood cells in urine is quantified in terms of red blood cells per high-power field and is normally 0 to 1 in males but may be slightly higher in females. The persistent presence in males or females of even small numbers of red blood cells in urine is cause for concern and may indicate the presence of a coagulopathy, hemoglobinopathy, renal parenchymal disease, tumor, trauma, or inflammation anywhere along the renal and urinary tract. Hematuria accompanied by proteinuria generally indicates renal parenchymal disease.

GLOMERULAR FILTRATION RATE. Measurements of glomerular filtration rate are used clinically largely as estimates of the mass of functional renal tissue or of the number of functioning nephrons. To be useful in the measure of glomerular filtration rate, a substance should be filtered freely at the glomerulus and not secreted, reabsorbed, catabolized, or synthesized by the kidney. The substance should be harmless, inexpensive, and easy to administer and measure accurately. A number of exogenous substances fulfill some of these requirements, but there is no ideal material of endogenous origin. Overall, however, the most useful indicators of glomerular filtration rate are measurements of the plasma creatinine concentration and creatinine clearance. Creatinine is an end-product of creatine metabolism. Its endogenous production averages about 15 mg per kilogram of body weight per day, correlates with muscle mass, and tends to be constant for a given individual. Creatinine is filtered freely at the glomerulus and is secreted by the proximal tubule to an extent that may increase with elevated plasma concentration. The excretion rate of creatinine thus reflects the combined effects of filtration and secretion, and normally the clearance of creatinine exceeds the glomerular filtration rate. The secretion of creatinine is inhibited by certain drugs such as cimetidine and trimethoprim, which may increase the plasma creatinine concentration without affecting glomerular filtration rate. Ketonemia may cause spurious increases in measurements of plasma creatinine because acetoacetate interferes with certain automated analytic techniques (Table 76–2).

Figure 76–2 shows the theoretic relationship between plasma creatinine concentration and creatinine clearance and the relationship between creatinine clearance and other measures of glomerular filtration rate, such as inulin clearance. The relationship between plasma creatinine and creatinine clearance is described by a rectangular hyperbola. This reflects the mathematical reality that values on the horizontal axis are determined by the reciprocals of values on the vertical axis, since the formula for creatinine clearance includes the serum creatinine concentration in the denominator. To the extent that creatinine clearance and glomerular filtration rate are equivalent, the same ideal relationship should apply between observed glomerular filtration rate and plasma creatinine concentration, but deviations from this ideal occur.

In the normal range, measurements of plasma creatinine concentration include a significant and variable component of noncreatinine chromogen that is not excreted in the urine. This overestimate offsets in part the error introduced by the renal secretion of creatinine, so that in this range creatinine clearances correlate well with other measures of glomerular filtration rate.

In the presence of renal failure, plasma creatinine concentration rises much more so than that of noncreatinine chromogens, and thus measurements of plasma creatinine concentration approach the true creatinine concentration. Moreover, in the presence of moderate degrees of renal failure, the secretory component of creatinine excretion may increase until the glomerular filtration rate falls below about 10 ml per minute. For these reasons, in the presence of moderate renal failure the clearance of creatinine tends to overestimate the glomerular filtration rate. In advanced renal

TABLE 76–2. FACTORS THAT AFFECT PLASMA CREATININE CONCENTRATION WITHOUT CHANGES IN GLOMERULAR FILTRATION RATE

Increase	
Ketonemia	Spurious increase in automated measurements by acetoacetate
Cimetidine, trimethoprim	Inhibition of tubular secretion
Decrease	
Muscle wasting	Reduced creatinine production

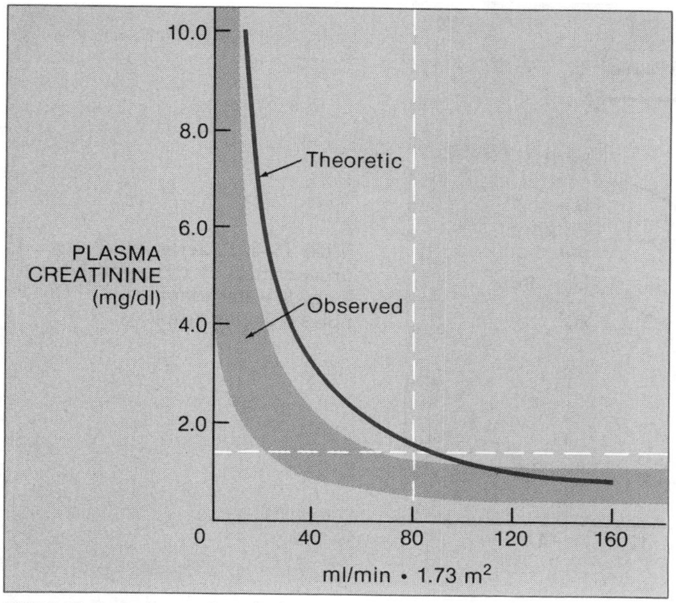

FIGURE 76–2. Relationship between plasma creatinine concentrations and various measures of glomerular filtration rate. The solid line depicts the theoretical relationship between plasma creatinine concentration and creatinine clearance. The color screened area represents the relationship between plasma creatinine and independent measures of glomerular filtration rate. The dashed lines denote the limits of normal values. Note the extent to which normal plasma creatinine values may occur in spite of reduced filtration rates.

failure (glomerular filtration rate less than 10 ml per minute), creatinine clearance again approximates the glomerular filtration rate (Fig. 76–2). Despite these shortcomings, measurements of plasma creatinine concentration and clearance of endogenous creatinine are useful indices of filtration rate largely because of the ease with which repeated observations may be made in individual patients along the course of their disease.

The most accurate measures of glomerular filtration rate in humans are obtained with the use of a number of exogenous substances such as inulin or a variety of radioisotopically labeled compounds such as ^{125}I-iothalamate. Standard clearance techniques for these measurements require injection of the compound to a steady-state plasma concentration and then the timed collection of urine.

The blood urea nitrogen (BUN) concentration is an imperfect quantitative indicator of renal filtration despite its frequent use for this purpose. Urea is synthesized by the liver from ammonia derived from the catabolism of proteins and amino acids. Urea production is therefore variable and is influenced by hepatic as well as dietary conditions. At the kidneys, urea is filtered, reabsorbed, and secreted. Reabsorption dominates, but the rate of reabsorption varies with the degree of hydration. Those conditions, such as dehydration, that tend to increase the renal reabsorption of volume also increase the reabsorption of urea. Accordingly, blood urea nitrogen concentration may increase without any abnormality in renal function. Conversely, in the presence of renal excretory failure and reduced filtration rate, the blood urea nitrogen concentration may be influenced significantly by the degree of dietary protein intake. For these reasons, measurement of plasma creatinine concentration provides a more reliable index of renal filtration rate than the BUN. The BUN is used mainly to quantify the balance between the accumulation and excretion of nitrogenous metabolites (i.e., the degree of uremia), especially in the presence of more than moderate reductions in glomerular filtration rate.

RENAL CONCENTRATING AND DILUTING ABILITY. The total solute concentration of urine is generally assessed clinically by measurement of urinary specific gravity, which relates the weight of a unit volume of urine to an equal volume of water. Because of its simplicity, this technique has persisted despite well-recognized deficiencies. Errors of technique relate primarily to poor calibration of the hygrometer, but even in the absence of faulty technique the specific gravity of urine provides only a rough indication of urine osmolality. For example, urines that contain high concentrations of urea have lower specific gravities than expected for their osmolality, and urines that contain higher density solutes, such as glucose, iodinated contrast material, or protein, have higher specific gravities relative to their osmolalities. Within these limitations, however, there is a useful correlation between the specific gravity and osmolality of urine such that urinary osmolality in milliosmoles per kilogram of water may be estimated as 40 times the increase in specific gravity of urine above the value of water, which is 1.000. Thus, urine with a specific gravity of 1.007 would have an estimated osmolality of 280 mOsm, similar to that of plasma, and urine with a specific gravity of 1.020 would be distinctly concentrated, with an estimated osmolality of 800 mOsm. Nonetheless, measurements of urine specific gravity represent only crude estimates of osmolality, and, when indicated, accurate measures of urine osmolality may be made easily by measurement of freezing-point depression in a cryoscopic osmometer.

Maximal urine concentrating ability is measured by restricting fluid intake until the patient loses a minimum of 3 per cent or a maximum of 5 per cent body weight, or until three consecutive urine specimens show no further increase in osmolality. These results are usually achieved within 16 hours of fluid restriction but may occur much earlier in patients with severe inability to conserve water. Once either one of these end-points is achieved, additional information may be obtained by the subcutaneous administration of 5 units of aqueous vasopressin to determine if any further increase in urine osmolality can be achieved. Normal subjects achieve maximal urine osmolality of 1000 $\pm$ 200 (SD) mOsm without further change after vasopressin. Patients who have complete or incomplete defects in antidiuretic hormone secretion, nephrogenic diabetes insipidus, or psychogenic polydipsia will have abnormal and distinctive patterns of response (Fig. 76–3).

Maximum diluting capacity of the kidney is assessed by the rapid administration of 1200 ml of water by mouth to a fasting subject. The osmolality of three hourly urine specimens is measured and should achieve values lower than 80 mOsm or specific gravity of 1.002. Measurements of the rate or extent of excretion of the administered water are quite variable and are not generally useful. Both maximal diluting and maximal concentrating ability of the kidney may be impaired by diuretics, especially potent loop diuretics such as furosemide and ethacrynic acid, and by diuretic states such as glucosuria.

ACIDIFICATION CAPACITY. The urine is normally more acidic than body fluids because of the endogenous production and renal excretion of nonvolatile acids derived primarily from sulfate and phosphate contained in dietary protein. Even at low pH, however, the amount of acid excreted as free hydrogen ion is negligible, and most hydrogen ion is excreted in the form of ammonium or titratable acids. For these reasons, the pH of a random specimen of urine provides only limited information about renal function and essentially no reliable information about the systemic acid-base status.

Assessment of the renal acidification capacity is accomplished by the *ammonium chloride tolerance test.* The basis of this test is to induce mild metabolic acidosis by the administration of ammonium chloride by mouth and to measure the maximal depression in urinary pH, maximal excretion rate of ammonium and titratable acid, and the percentage of excretion of the administered hydrogen ion equivalent. Because the purpose of the ammonium chloride is to induce metabolic acidosis, its administration is not necessary if acidosis is

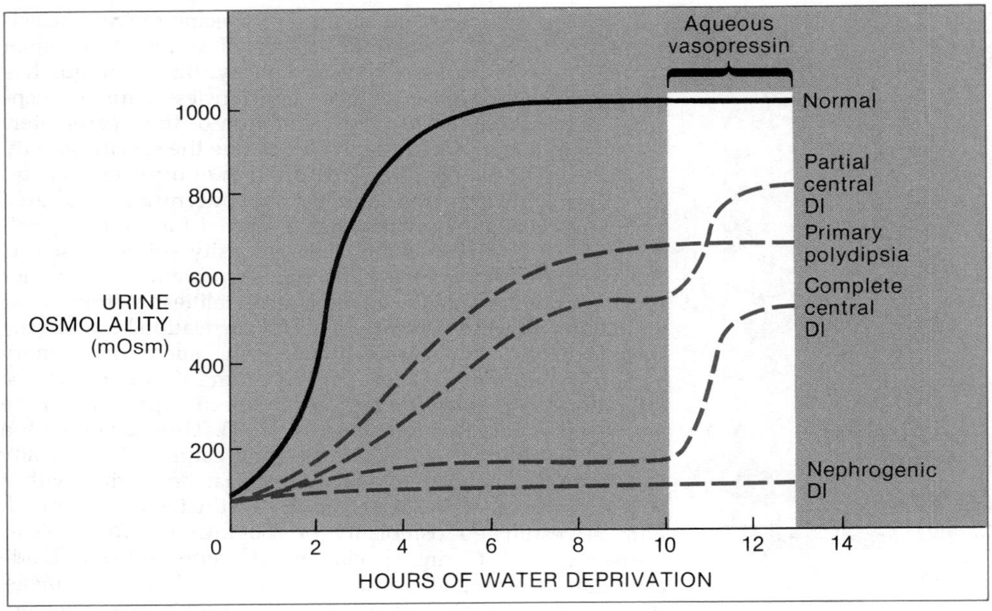

FIGURE 76–3. Patterns of changes in urine osmolality in response to prolonged water deprivation. DI denotes diabetes insipidus.

present spontaneously. Indications for the ammonium chloride test are generally restricted to those conditions, usually suspected abnormalities in distal tubular function, that are associated with only mild reductions in glomerular filtration rate. Ammonium chloride, 0.1 gram per kilogram, is administered by mouth, and urine is collected hourly for six to eight hours. A normal response is to achieve a urinary pH of 5.4 or less and to excrete at least 30 per cent of the administered hydrogen ion equivalent. An abnormal response consists of failure to acidify the urine below pH 5.4 despite a measured reduction in arterial pH. This indicates a defect in maximal acidification capacity. The ammonium chloride tolerance test is not generally performed in patients with renal insufficiency, but, if performed, these patients usually achieve reduction in the urinary pH below 5.4, although there is reduced excretion of ammonium and titratable acid.

URINARY ELECTROLYTES. Measurements of urinary sodium, potassium, and chloride may provide important information but only in a limited set of clinical circumstances. Two types of measurements are made. The absolute daily excretion of sodium, potassium, or chloride (milliequivalents per day) is derived from the electrolyte concentration of a 24-hour collection of urine. Such measurements provide quantification of the daily intake of these electrolytes provided that two requirements are met. First, total body weight must be constant to indicate balance between intake and output. Second, electrolyte excretion must be limited to the urine, and losses via the gastrointestinal tract or skin must be negligible. Under these conditions, the daily excretion of sodium, potassium, or chloride will reflect the dietary intake, but this information has only limited clinical value.

Measurement of the *concentration* of sodium, potassium, or chloride in a random urine sample may provide information of importance in certain circumstances such as the evaluation of hyponatremia, acute oliguria, volume depletion, hypokalemia, and metabolic alkalosis. In the evaluation of hyponatremia, a urinary sodium concentration less than 10 mEq per liter indicates the presence of reduced effective extracellular volume with an appropriate increase in mineralocorticoid and antidiuretic hormone (ADH) activity that leads to the renal retention of sodium and solute-free water. Higher urinary sodium concentrations indicate significant renal losses of sodium such as might occur from diuretics or, less commonly, from mineralocorticoid or glucocorticoid insufficiency or with volume expansion from the inappropriate secretion of ADH. Similarly, in the evaluation of patients with reduced extracellular volume, urinary sodium concentrations greater than 10 to 20 mEq per liter indicate that the kidney is participating in the loss of sodium and volume, perhaps because of renal or adrenal insufficiency, whereas urinary sodium concentrations less than 5 to 10 mEq per liter indicate that losses of sodium and volume are occurring via extrarenal routes.

In the setting of acute oliguria, urine sodium concentration greater than 20 to 40 mEq per liter occurs frequently with acute renal failure or incomplete obstruction, whereas urine sodium concentrations are generally less than 20 mEq per liter in the presence of severe volume depletion (prerenal azotemia), acute glomerulonephritis, congestive heart failure, coexistent liver disease, or acute renal failure from radiocontrast material or acute rejection (Ch. 78). As is often the case, however, these values may be modified by many factors, including the administration of diuretics, and urine sodium concentrations are not generally regarded as sufficiently discriminatory to be useful in the differential diagnosis of acute oliguria.

The urine potassium concentration may be useful in the evaluation of unexplained hypokalemia. In the presence of hypokalemia, urine potassium concentrations greater than 20 mEq per liter indicate significant renal losses such as might occur from diuretics, increased mineralocorticoid activity, or magnesium deficiency. Urine potassium concentrations less than 10 mEq per liter indicate that the hypokalemia may be related to gastrointestinal losses such as may occur from the surreptitious use of laxatives or may indicate changes in plasma potassium concentration without potassium deficits such as may occur with hypokalemic periodic paralysis (see Ch. 516).

Urine chloride concentrations provide important information in the evaluation of metabolic alkalosis. Persistent metabolic alkalosis results most often from the depletion of chloride via the gastrointestinal tract or urine. In the presence of metabolic alkalosis, urine chloride concentrations greater than 10 mEq per liter suggest the presence of diuretic-induced increases in chloride excretion, severe depletion of potassium, Bartter's syndrome, or increased adrenocortical hormone activity. On the other hand, urine chloride concentrations less than 10 mEq per liter point to losses of chloride via extrarenal routes, usually vomiting, and indicate further that the metabolic alkalosis is likely to respond to replacement of volume and chloride.

IMAGING OF THE KIDNEYS AND UROGENITAL TRACT

Imaging techniques of importance in the evaluation of renal abnormalities include roentgenography, ultrasonography, radionuclide studies, and magnetic resonance imaging. These techniques are used (1) to visualize the number, size, and location of the kidneys; (2) to identify the presence and site of obstruction; (3) to detect and to characterize mass lesions; (4) to visualize renal arteries and veins; and (5) to guide percutaneous diagnostic and therapeutic interventions such as biopsy and nephrostomy. The choice of a technique is based on its relative simplicity, its safety, its potential to yield results that for a particular suspected disorder are neither falsely positive (lack of specificity) nor falsely negative (lack of sensitivity), and its potential to provide additional information not already available from previous studies.

ROENTGENOGRAPHIC STUDIES. The most simple radiologic study of the kidneys and urogenital system is the plain roentgenogram of the kidneys, ureter, and bladder (KUB), which will often reveal abnormal calcifications and may reveal renal size if not obscured by overlying bowel. If indicated, tomography may be necessary to determine the renal outlines.

Excretory Urogram. The excretory urogram, also known as the intravenous pyelogram, or IVP, is the standard radiologic method to detect anatomic abnormalities of the kidneys and ureters and to evaluate patients with renal abnormalities. The basic excretory urogram is performed by the intravenous injection of iodinated contrast material, which is filtered at the glomerulus and concentrated within the tubular lumina and collecting system by the renal reabsorption of volume. Visualization of the contrast material within the renal parenchyma yields a *nephrogram*, and visualization within the major collecting system yields a *pyelogram*. Each of these phases is dependent on the amount of radiocontrast material that is delivered to the kidneys and filtered and also on the degree of extraction of volume that concentrates the dye within the parenchyma and collecting system. Modern radiocontrast materials are not secreted. In view of these mechanisms, it is useful to limit hydration prior to an excretory urogram in an effort to increase the intrarenal concentration of the contrast material. In some patients, however, especially those with renal insufficiency, restriction of fluid intake prior to an excretory urogram appears to increase the rate of adverse reaction and is now deemed more harmful than beneficial.

A nephrogram normally appears within one to three minutes after injection of the contrast material. The nephrogram provides an opportunity to determine the number of kidneys, their size and configuration, and the possible presence of inhomogeneous areas or filling defects. In addition, the symmetric and timely appearance of nephrograms bilaterally provides qualitative information on the relative blood flow and filtration rate of each kidney. The pyelogram phase occurs within five minutes after the injection of dye as the nephrogram fades. This phase allows visualization of the caliceal system, ureters, and bladder and provides opportunities to detect abnormalities in shape, size, or drainage that might result from intrinsic defects or from extrinsic compression. Vascular or outflow obstructions may result in marked delays in the onset of both the nephrogram and the pyelogram phases.

Retrograde Pyelography. Retrograde pyelography is the direct injection of radiocontrast material into the ureter and upper urinary tract. The approach to this area is achieved via insertion of a ureteral catheter under direct visualization through cystoscopy. Some form of anesthesia may be required. Although retrograde pyelography was used frequently to assess renal size and to evaluate the possibility of ureteral obstruction in patients who presented with advanced renal failure, these questions are now resolved more readily with ultrasonography. Retrograde pyelography does provide more direct and improved visualization of the ureters and calices, and this visualization is useful in the localization and diagnosis of tumors and obstructions.

Antegrade Pyelography. Direct injection of radiocontrast material into a distended upper urinary tract or cyst may be achieved without the need for general anesthesia by the percutaneous injection of dye. This is performed under fluoroscopy or ultrasonography and requires the presence of a fluid-filled target such as a radiolucent or sonolucent mass. Antegrade pyelography may be useful to distinguish cysts from hydronephrosis.

Interventional Percutaneous Pyeloureteral Techniques. The combination of visualizing techniques such as roentgenographic fluoroscopy or ultrasonography and the availability of percutaneous catheters allows placement of a catheter in the renal pelvis, calices, or perirenal space if these spaces are distended by abnormal collections of fluid. Percutaneous catheter placement allows drainage and irrigation of pyonephrosis, abscesses, and obstructions, and placement of temporary nephrostomy catheters.

Renal Arteriography and Venography. The renal vasculature is visualized with radiocontrast material injected via a catheter introduced usually through the femoral vessels. Renal arteriography is performed most often to evaluate possible renal arterial stenosis as a cause or aggravating factor in systemic hypertension and to evaluate renal mass lesions. In general, cystic mass lesions are devoid of vasculature and may stretch and distort normal renal vessels and calices. Solid tumors are frequently vascular with irregular and erratic vessels that fill early as a blush of contrast material.

Renal venography is limited largely to searches for renal vein thrombosis and venous extension of renal cell carcinoma. Because renal venography requires the injection of dye against usually heavy renal venous outflow, turbulence may on occasion distort the distribution of dye and give the appearance of an intravascular filling defect. For this reason, renal venography is sometimes performed with intra-arterial infusion of epinephrine to reduce renal blood flow.

Digital Subtraction Angiography. Digital subtraction angiography uses high-quality image intensifiers and video camera recordings to visualize major arterial vessels following the rapid intravenous injection of radiocontrast material. Standard x-ray sources are used to produce sequential images at rates of about one per second beginning at the time of injection of radiocontrast material into a central or peripheral artery or vein. Images are intensified electronically, displayed on a video camera, digitized, and stored on magnetic tape in a memory system. Images obtained prior to the arrival of radiocontrast material at a particular vascular region are subtracted electronically from the subsequent images to enhance the contrast between vessels and other tissues. With regard to the detection of renal vascular diseases, digital subtraction venous angiography has an overall accuracy of about 70 to 80 per cent compared with conventional arteriography. Technically successful studies are generally sensitive enough to detect significant renal vascular lesions, but false-positive results may be as frequent as 20 to 30 per cent. Because venous angiography does not require an arteriotomy, it can be performed without hospitalization at considerably less cost than direct arteriography.

Computed Tomography. Computed tomography represents a sophisticated extension of roentgenography and may be performed with or without contrast material. Its usefulness in the evaluation of renal abnormalities consists primarily in its application as a tertiary mode after excretory urograms and ultrasonography to detect and localize mass lesions. Computed tomography may detect cystic masses as small as 0.5 cm in diameter, but the sensitivity is less for noncalcific solid masses (Fig. 76–4). Computed tomography is also useful to detect and evaluate obstruction and dilatation of the major collecting system in patients allergic to iodinated contrast

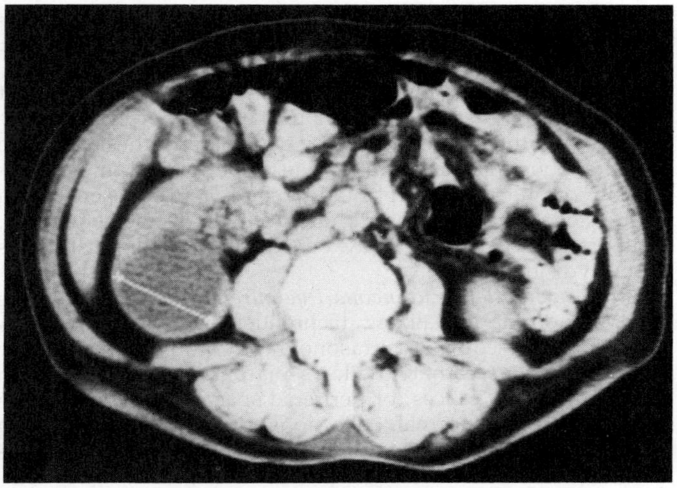

FIGURE 76–4. Computed tomography of the abdomen. The orientation is looking upward from toes to head. The right kidney is visualized at this level, but only a small portion of the left kidney is shown. There is a large, well-demarcated, homogeneous mass (white diagonal) in the right kidney which has the density of water rather than tissue. This is characteristic of a renal cyst.

material or for whom ultrasonography is inconclusive for technical reasons such as interference by bone, calcifications, or gas.

Adverse Effects of Urography. Two types of adverse effects should be considered in relation to the performance of excretory urograms, angiograms, or computed tomography with intravenous contrast material. First, any exposure to radiation is associated with a finite, statistical risk of permanent alteration in DNA. Depending on the question being asked, alternative modes of visualization such as ultrasonography might be considered in certain circumstances, especially those that involve pregnancy or repeated examinations over time.

The second type of adverse effect of excretory urography relates to toxic reactions to the iodinated contrast material. The overall incidence of adverse reactions to intravenous contrast is about 5 per cent for the general population and about 10 per cent for those with any allergies. The most common reactions involve nausea or urticaria; about 10 per cent of reactions will involve life-threatening events such as hypotension, laryngeal edema, or cardiac arrhythmias.

Excretory urography is a remarkably safe procedure, especially when performed in essentially healthy individuals. Not unexpectedly, excretory urography is less safe in individuals who are less healthy. Patients with diabetes mellitus and associated renal abnormalities are at increased risk to develop additional renal injury from excretory urography. Renal function may also deteriorate more frequently following excretory urography in patients with advanced age, marked dehydration, hyperuricemia, proteinuria, and pre-existing azotemia. Perhaps based on one or more of these factors, patients with multiple myeloma are at increased risk to develop adverse reactions to radiocontrast material. Appropriate precautions are indicated: consideration of alternative modes of visualization, attention to optimal hydration, and use of the minimal amount of contrast material consistent with an adequate examination.

ULTRASONOGRAPHY. Ultrasonography represents a major advance in the noninvasive visualization of the kidneys and genitourinary system. The acoustic impedance of a tissue to ultrasonic waves is the product of its density and the velocity of sound in that tissue. Significant differences in acoustic impedance occur among tissues that differ in their content of water, fat, collagen, minerals, and other solids, and interfaces between these tissues will reflect portions of the sound energy back to the transmitting transducer. These reflections are recorded as electrical signals and may be visualized by various display modes. The brightness modulation or B-mode displays echoes as bright dots plotted along the vertical and horizontal axes of an oscilloscope at positions corresponding to their point of origin in the area being scanned and, through so-called gray-scale processing, in degrees of brightness that correspond to their amplitude. So-called "real-time" imaging, or sonofluoroscopy, produces repetitive scans that give the impression of a continuous image.

Sonography can usually allow delineation of the renal outlines and measurement of the longitudinal and transverse dimensions (Fig. 76–5). Difficulties may arise from overlying ribs that may obscure the upper poles or from similarities in the acoustic impedance of perirenal fat and renal cortex such that the renal margins are poorly defined. The structures within the renal parenchyma are sufficiently similar that few intrarenal echoes are produced except by the vascular and caliceal structures of the renal pelvis. Advanced gray-scale examination of the kidney may permit identification of the cortex, medulla, arcuate vessels, and renal pyramids. The ureters are not normally visualized unless distended.

The primary applications of ultrasonography to the evaluation of renal abnormalities include assessment of renal size, especially in the presence of severe renal failure, evaluation of mass lesions detected by excretory urography, examination of the perinephric area, and detection and grading of hydronephrosis. Renal ultrasonography may serve as the primary imaging procedure for patients with unexplained acute renal failure, for diabetics and other individuals at higher risk for adverse reactions to contrast material, in the presence of pregnancy, and to diagnose suspected polycystic kidney disease.

Evaluation of Renal Mass Lesions. Ultrasonography is used widely and effectively in the evaluation of renal mass lesions detected by excretory urography. Fluid-filled cysts as small as 1 to 2 cm in diameter may be detected, but reliable detection

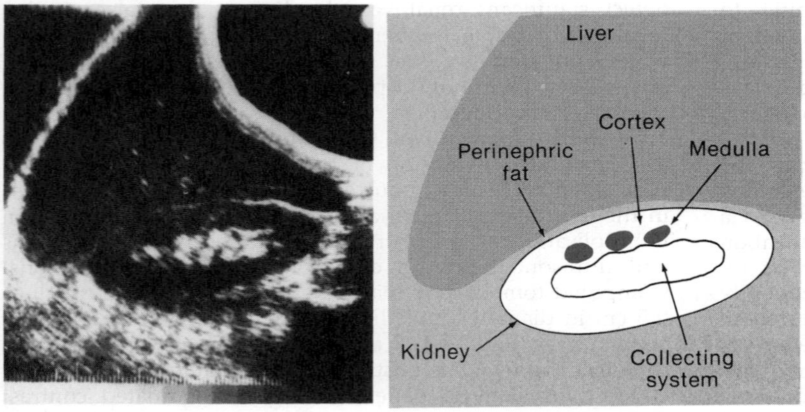

FIGURE 76–5. Ultrasonography and schematic of a normal right kidney. This was obtained anteriorly by transmission through the liver.

and evaluation of consistency generally require lesions greater than 2.5 to 3.0 cm. The primary application of ultrasonography is to describe the ultrasonographic characteristics of mass lesions according to three patterns: cystic, solid, or complex. Cystic lesions are free of internal echoes, have smooth, sharply defined margins, and cause accentuation of echoes from their far wall. Solid lesions have less distinct margins because of attenuation of the signal by solid tissue and also demonstrate internal echoes related to vessels, connective tissue, or hemorrhage. Complex lesions represent features of both patterns. Because of the inherent limitations of the technique, ultrasonographically defined lesions should be described simply as having the *characteristics* of cysts or solids. Physically solid lesions that may appear on ultrasonography as cysts include melanomas, lymphomas, and certain metastases. Localized areas of hydronephrosis may also appear as cysts.

Renal ultrasonography is most nearly diagnostic in adult polycystic kidney disease and severe hydronephrosis. In other instances, ultrasonography should be regarded as informative rather than diagnostic. In the evaluation of renal mass lesions, combinations of ultrasonography, computed tomography (Fig. 76–4), and arteriography may distinguish between benign cysts and potentially malignant solid tumors with remarkable accuracy. Clinical judgment will still be needed to decide whether even a 90 to 95 per cent level of accuracy is sufficient in an individual instance or whether surgery is indicated to obtain a definite diagnosis.

RADIONUCLIDE SCINTILLATION IMAGING. Radionuclide imaging has not achieved a major role in the evaluation of the kidneys and urinary tract. Two advantages of these techniques, however, make them useful in special circumstances. First, radionuclide imaging does not require the injection of radiocontrast material. Second, radionuclide studies are relatively simple and rapid and may be performed repeatedly at intervals of 24 to 48 hours. For these reasons, radionuclide imaging has perhaps its greatest application in the evaluation of patients at high risk for adverse reaction to radiocontrast material and in the evaluation of patients in the period immediately after renal transplantation. Otherwise, these techniques have few advantages over more direct radiologic and ultrasonographic methods.

With regard to the kidneys, radionuclide imaging techniques involve the intravenous injection of an agent labeled with a radionuclide that emits gamma radiation. Use of a scintillation camera allows the performance of dynamic studies that monitor the passage of a radiopharmaceutical agent through the vascular, renal parenchymal, and urinary tract compartments. Static studies examine the local accumulation of radionuclide activity. At present, radiopharmaceuticals of value in studies of the kidney contain either ^{131}I or ^{99m}Tc (technetium).

Static Imaging. Static imaging of the kidney consists of the administration of a radiopharmaceutical agent, usually ^{99m}Tc-glucoheptonate, that accumulates within the renal parenchyma and persists for several hours. Static imaging provides information on the location, size, and contour of functional renal tissue and may reveal areas of inhomogeneity or filling defects.

Dynamic Imaging. Dynamic scintillation imaging consists of the intravenous injection of a radiopharmaceutical agent and the visualization of its course through the vascular, renal parenchymal, and urinary collecting system by external monitoring of regional radioactivity with a scintillation camera. The time course of the appearance and disappearance of radioactivity is recorded in intervals as brief as one second. The radiopharmaceuticals used most frequently include ^{131}I-orthoiodohippurate, which is excreted by secretion with only a small component of filtration, and ^{99m}Tc-diethylenetriamine pentacetic acid (DTPA), which is excreted by filtration only.

The time-activity data observed for the passage of either radionuclide generally delineate three discrete phases. The vascular phase is the first 15 to 60 seconds after injection and consists of a rapid increase in radioactivity in the region viewed by the scintillation camera. The second phase occurs over the next three to five minutes and consists of slower accumulation of regional radioactivity. The third, or excretory, phase refers to the decrease in activity that occurs as the radionuclide is excreted from the region of interest. Unilateral or bilateral disturbances in renal blood flow, renal filtration, renal tubular function, or excretion cause disturbances in the various phases of this renogram. Although some efforts have been made to provide quantification of the various phases, interpretation of renograms still depends for the most part on the recognition of patterns in the scintillation displays. Dynamic imaging is especially useful for comparing excretory function between the right and left kidneys when renal dysfunction is asymmetric, such as may occur with congenital, vascular, or urologic disorders.

MAGNETIC RESONANCE IMAGING. Magnetic resonance imaging (MRI) represents a new and emerging diagnostic technology that uses high magnetic fields and radiofrequencies to construct images. The method avoids the use of ionizing radiation or the administration of contrast material. Imaging depends instead on the water content and the chemical behavior of hydrogen compounds in the tissues themselves. MRI provides images in a tomographic format similar to computed tomography (Fig. 76–6). The technique is very sensitive to blood flow and represents an excellent method for evaluating major vascular structures for patency or tumor involvement.

RENAL BIOPSY

Biopsy of the renal parenchyma by either the percutaneous or the open technique is useful (1) to define the morphologic expression of primary renal diseases, (2) to determine the type and extent of renal involvement by systemic diseases, and (3) to diagnose systemic diseases. The performance of renal biopsy is seldom necessary to *diagnose* systemic diseases. Diseases such as systemic lupus erythematosus, multiple myeloma, and diabetes mellitus, which may have typical but seldom diagnostic morphologic patterns, are diagnosed more

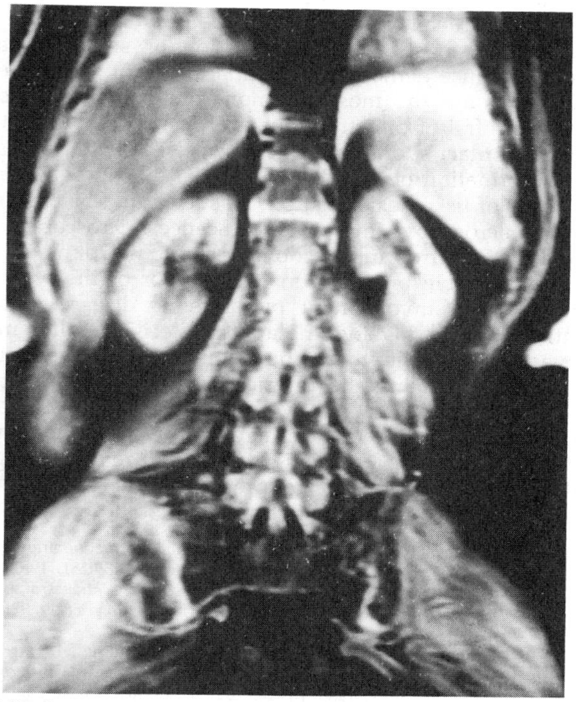

FIGURE 76–6. Magnetic resonance image of two normal kidneys in an elderly woman.

TABLE 76–3. INDICATIONS FOR RENAL BIOPSY

- Presumptive presence of glomerular disease
  - Heavy proteinuria (> 3 to 5 grams per 24 hours)
  - Nephrotic syndrome
  - Acute nephritic syndrome
- Proteinuria with hematuria
- Renal involvement by systemic disease
  - Connective tissue disease
  - Vasculitis
  - Amyloidosis
  - Suspected Goodpasture's disease
- Unexplained acute renal failure
- Persistent acute renal failure (beyond two to four weeks)
- Renal transplantation
  - Acute rejection
  - Chronic rejection
  - Recurrence of original disease

readily by other means. Systemic lupus erythematosus, diabetes mellitus, thrombotic thrombocytopenic purpura, Wegener's granulomatosis, and amyloidosis may on occasion display pathognomonic features on renal biopsy, but of these diseases only amyloidosis is likely to require renal biopsy for diagnosis.

Renal biopsy is performed most frequently via the percutaneous technique. The indications for percutaneous biopsy are listed in Table 76–3; the contraindications are the presence of a single kidney, bleeding disorders, and uncontrolled hypertension. In experienced hands, percutaneous renal biopsy is a safe and effective technique that should provide sufficient tissue in more than 90 per cent of the attempts. Complications occur in 5 to 10 per cent of the attempts, and the most frequent complication is gross hematuria that usually resolves uneventfully in 24 to 48 hours. The formation of a perirenal hematoma may on occasion require surgical evacuation. Microscopic hematuria occurs very frequently and is not generally considered as a complication. Complications that occur less frequently include persistent bleeding, formation of arteriovenous fistula, aggravation of hypertension, and inadvertent biopsy of nonrenal tissue such as muscle, liver, pancreas, spleen, or small bowel. Although fluoroscopy and ultrasonography may on occasion be useful or even necessary to localize the kidney for biopsy, it is not clear that these added maneuvers diminish the occurrence of complications or notably improve the rate of success. Complications of percutaneous renal biopsy occur more often in younger patients and in those with hypertension or small, diseased kidneys. Because hemorrhagic complications of percutaneous renal biopsy are the most common, the patient should be advised to refrain from strenuous exercises, especially lifting, and from contact sports for at least two weeks after biopsy.

The information obtained from a renal biopsy depends on the quality of tissue examination. Tissue should be examined by light microscopy, immunofluorescence microscopy, and, on occasion, electron microscopy. Accurate morphologic definition of possible primary renal disease or of the type and extent of renal involvement by systemic disease is often essential prior to making therapeutic decisions that might involve the use of life-threatening immunosuppressive therapy and to informing the physician and patient about the expected natural history of any renal abnormality. Moreover, for those renal disorders that may be treated ultimately by renal transplantation, knowledge of the nature of the original renal disease is important to predictions of whether that disease is likely to recur in the transplanted kidney.

Buonocore E, Meaney TF, Borkowski GP, et al.: Digital subtraction angiography of the abdominal aorta and renal arteries. Radiology 139:281, 1981. *Along with some early results from a comparison between conventional and digital subtraction angiography, there are some useful insights into relevant technology and procedures.*

Dennis VW, Robinson RR: Clinical proteinuria. In Stollerman GH, Harrington WJ, Lamont JT, et al. (eds.): Advances in Internal Medicine. Chicago, Year Book Medical Publishers, 1986, pp 243–263. *This article provides more detail on the mechanisms and clinical classifications of proteinuria isolated from other renal abnormalities.*

Kokko JP, Tannen RL: Fluids and Electrolytes. Philadelphia, W. B. Saunders Company, 1986. *This monograph is the finest and most thorough exposition of the laboratory evaluation of abnormalities in renal function and electrolyte metabolism. The chapter on clinical interpretation of laboratory values is especially relevant and well-referenced.*

Mogensen CE: Microalbuminuria predicts clinical proteinuria and early mortality in maturity-onset diabetes. N Engl J Med 310:356, 1984. *This article advances the concept of microalbuminuria as a predictor of poor renal prognosis in patients with diabetes mellitus. It also refers to the theories and observations upon which the concept is based.*

Shemesh O, Golbetz H, Kriss JP, et al.: Limitations of creatinine as a filtration marker in glomerulopathic patients. Kidney Int 28:830, 1985. *Data provided in this article represent the modern basis upon which we interpret plasma creatinine values.*

77 DISORDERS OF FLUID VOLUME, ELECTROLYTE, AND ACID-BASE BALANCE

Thomas E. Andreoli

INTRODUCTION

Electrolyte abnormalities often occur as manifestations of underlying illnesses. In turn, fluid and electrolyte abnormalities, of themselves, produce systemic derangements. This chapter considers four major derangements of fluid and electrolyte balance, namely, volume disturbances, osmolality derangements, abnormalities of potassium balance, and acid-base disorders.

In health, the functional capacities of the mechanisms regulating water and electrolyte balance are so large that one can vary the intake of solutes and water over a wide range without developing perceptible metabolic disturbances. But when these mechanisms are impaired, the limits between which solute and water intake can be varied become narrower.

This concept is illustrated schematically in Figure 77–1. The safe range, or the range over which homeostasis is maintained, is bounded at the lower level by the minimal physiologic requirement and at the upper level by the maximal physiologic tolerance. These limits become progressively narrowed in disease. As the degree of functional impairment

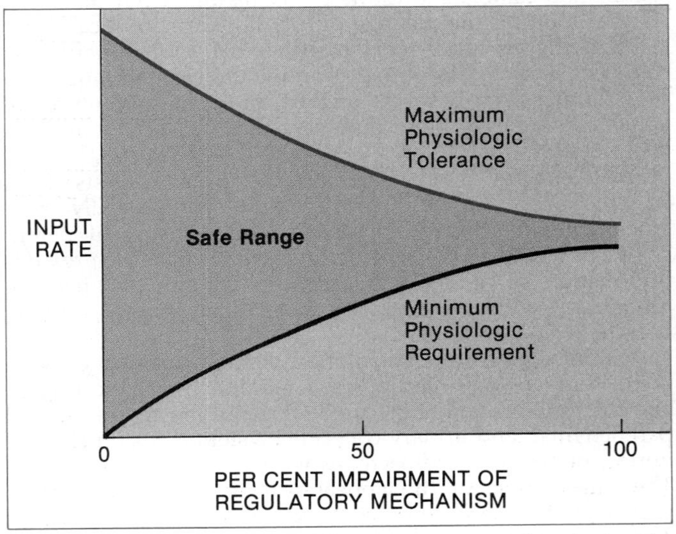

FIGURE 77–1. Upper and lower limits of intake. The safe range, or the range over which homeostasis is maintained, is bounded at the upper level by the maximum physiologic tolerance and at the lower level by the minimum physiologic requirement. Impairment of the regulating mechanism by disease narrows the safe range.

progresses, minimal requirements tend to increase while maximal tolerances tend to decrease. For example, salt intake in normal individuals can vary from approximately 10 mEq per day to several hundred milliequivalents per day without affecting volume homeostasis. In the presence of chronic renal disease, the minimal requirement rises and the maximal tolerance decreases, so that dietary salt intake must be kept within a much narrower range if volume depletion or volume overload is to be avoided.

Volume Disorders

PHYSIOLOGIC CONSIDERATIONS

Protection of extracellular fluid volume is the most fundamental characteristic of fluid and electrolyte homeostasis. It is helpful to use the term *effective circulating volume (ECV)*. The latter cannot be defined in an absolute sense. In operational terms, effective circulating volume may be viewed as adequate filling of the arterial tree, that is, an arterial flow rate sufficient to maintain adequate perfusion of body tissues. The mechanisms regulating volume balance respond primarily to changes in the effective circulating volume.

The Body Fluid Compartments

In healthy adults, body water comprises approximately 60 per cent of body weight and exists in two compartments: The intracellular compartment (ICF) contains two thirds of body water, or 40 per cent of body weight; the extracellular compartment (ECF) contains the remaining one third of total body water; and total blood volume, that is, plasma plus formed elements, constitutes one third of the total ECF volume. This "rule of thirds" for the body fluid compartments is useful in the assessment of most clinically encountered fluid and electrolyte disorders. Thus in a healthy 70-kg man, total body water comprises about 40 liters, of which 25 liters is intracellular. The functional extracellular fluid volume is 15 liters, 5 liters of which is blood; and since the normal hematocrit is 40 to 45 per cent, total plasma volume is approximately 2.75 to 3.0 liters.

More than 95 per cent of total body sodium is extracellular, and sodium and its associated anions, primarily chloride and bicarbonate, constitute the principal solutes of the ECF. Albumin and other macromolecules present in plasma are restricted to the vascular bed and constitute 5 per cent of plasma volume, so that plasma is about 95 per cent water. Since capillaries are freely permeable to water and small solutes, interstitial fluid is a protein-poor, but not entirely protein-free, ultrafiltrate of plasma.

Potassium is the principal cation of intracellular fluid, and nearly 98 per cent of total body potassium is intracellular. The principal anions of intracellular fluid vary among different cells. In muscle cells, they include phosphate, sulfate, and negatively charged macromolecules; and in red blood cells, they are the last-named anions, together with chloride and bicarbonate.

Regulation of Fluid Transfer Among Compartments

The transfer of fluid between vascular and interstitial compartments occurs at the capillary level and is governed by the balance between hydrostatic pressure gradients and plasma oncotic pressure gradients. This relation may be stated by the familiar Starling equation:

$$J_v = K_f\,(\Delta P - \Delta\pi)$$

where J_v is rate of fluid transfer between vascular and interstitial compartments, K_f is the water permeability of the capillary bed, ΔP is the hydrostatic pressure difference between capillary and interstitium, and $\Delta\pi$ is the oncotic pressure difference between capillary and interstitial fluids. Under normal circumstances, interstitial tissue pressure is low and the ΔP term in the Starling equation represents the integrated hydrostatic pressure gradient from arteriolar to venular ends of a capillary. Since interstitial fluid is protein poor, the $\Delta\pi$ term in the Starling equation represents the oncotic pressure of plasma proteins, principally albumin; 5 grams of albumin per deciliter of plasma exerts an oncotic pressure of about 15 mm of mercury.

Protection of Fluid Balance

As noted earlier, protection of the effective circulating volume is the single most fundamental characteristic of body fluid homeostasis. This primacy is underscored by the fact that, in circumstances in which multiple physiologic variables are threatened simultaneously, the homeostatic response invariably protects ECF volume even at the expense of aggravating another electrolyte disorder. For example, a volume-contracted patient who is replenished with water, and not sodium, will retain water and become hyponatremic in an attempt to avoid circulatory collapse. Likewise, the maintenance of metabolic alkalosis in patients who have vomited and are not repleted with salt depends, in part, on an elevated renal absorptive capacity for sodium bicarbonate. The latter maintains fluid balance at the expense of pH homeostasis.

Two cardinal mechanisms protect extracellular fluid volume: alterations in systemic hemodynamic variables and alterations in external sodium and water balance. Both mechanisms maintain filling of the arterial tree and consequently are activated by external fluid losses; by inability to transfer fluid from the interstitium to the venous system, for example, in ascites; or by impaired fluid transfer from venous to arterial systems, for example, in congestive heart failure, pericardial tamponade, or constrictive pericarditis.

The combination of alterations in systemic hemodynamic variables and alterations in external water and solute balance can be termed the integrated volume response (Table 77–1). Significantly, both limbs of the response, that is, systemic hemodynamics and external salt and water balance, are modulated by the same positive effectors and negative inactivators.

There are differences in the two response systems. Tachycardia, peripheral arteriolar vasoconstriction, and peripheral venoconstriction occur within minutes of external fluid losses, whereas renal salt and water conservation lag behind by 12 to 24 hours. The sensitivities of the two limbs also differ. For example, a 2 to 3 per cent decrease in extracellular fluid volume, which amounts to the loss of 40 to 60 mEq of sodium, results in virtual elimination of sodium from the urine but produces negligible changes in systemic hemodynamic factors such as heart rate, blood pressure, or systemic vascular resistance. Since there is 2500 to 3000 mEq of exchangeable sodium in the ECF, the system for conserving renal sodium is remarkably sensitive.

Renal Volume Regulation

Figure 77–2 provides a schematic summary of the renal factors regulating volume homeostasis. In general, the system

TABLE 77–1. THE INTEGRATED VOLUME RESPONSE

	Systemic Hemodynamic Changes	External Salt and Water Balance
Response	Tachycardia ↑ Peripheral resistance ↓ Venous capacitance	Thirst Renal Na^+, water retention
Onset	Minutes	Hours
Major activators	Catecholamines Angiotensin II ADH	Catecholamines Aldosterone ADH
Major inactivators	Prostaglandins Atriopeptin	Prostaglandins Atriopeptin

ADH = Antidiuretic hormone.

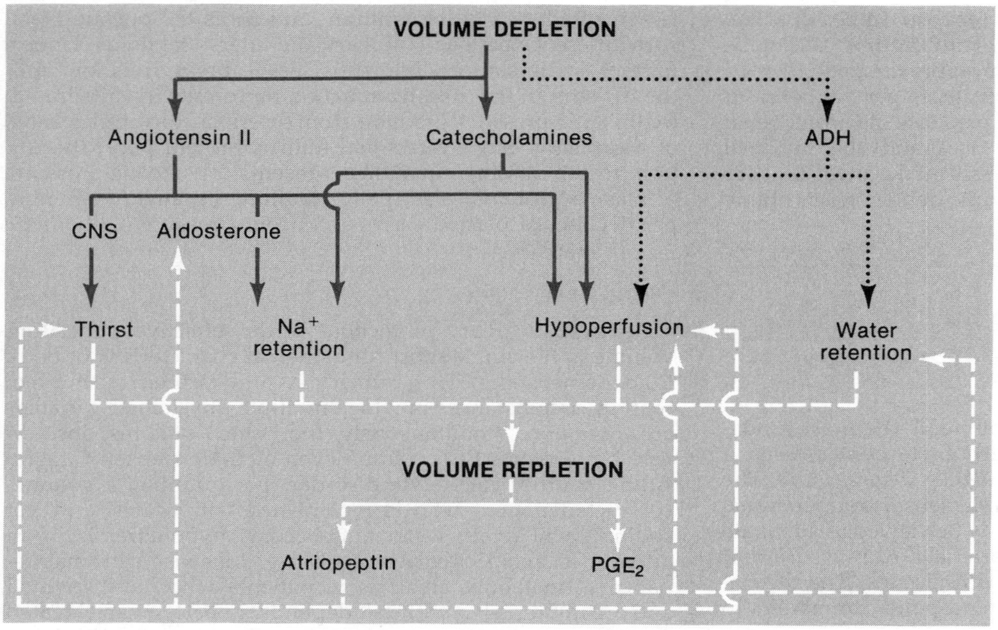

FIGURE 77–2. The volume repletion reaction. The solid arrows indicate positive mechanisms activated when volume depletion is modest; the dotted arrows indicate positive mechanisms activated with severe volume depletion. The dashed lines indicate negative feedback mechanisms.

is characterized by a positive limb, activated by volume contraction, and by negative feedback activated by volume repletion. In Figure 77–2 the solid lines and dotted lines represent volume conservation mechanisms activated by small and severe degrees of volume contraction, respectively; the dashed lines indicate negative feedback mechanisms activated by volume repletion. The separate details of this mechanism are as follows.

SENSING AND EFFECTOR ELEMENTS. Changes in effective ECF volume that exceed acceptable physiologic limits are sensed by baroreceptors located in both the high- and the low-pressure regions of the circulation. The low-pressure baroreceptors are located primarily in the left atrium and in major thoracic veins, whereas the arterial high-pressure baroreceptors are located in the sinus body and aortic arch. Both sets of baroreceptors respond to pressure and stretch stimuli associated with changes in effective circulating volume. Activation of these extrarenal baroreceptors by relatively slight reductions in effective circulating volume results in increased sympathetic nerve activity and in rises in plasma catecholamine activity.

This catecholamine response raises blood pressure by increasing arteriolar resistance and heart rate, while simultaneously decreasing venous capacitance. Increases in arteriolar resistance also reduce capillary hydrostatic pressure and therefore promote fluid transfer from interstitial fluid to the vascular compartment. Within the kidney this increase in arteriolar resistance results in renal hypoperfusion. Moreover, adrenergic nerve terminals are in direct contact with proximal renal tubular epithelial cells, and direct stimulation of renal sympathetic nerves increases proximal tubular sodium absorption.

A second effector mechanism activated by stimulation of extrarenal baroreceptors is release of antidiuretic hormone (ADH). When blood volume is isotonically contracted by more than 8 to 10 per cent, afferent stimuli carried by the ninth and tenth cranial nerves result in nonosmotic ADH release by the neurohypophysis. In turn, ADH enhances renal water conservation and, because the hormone also has potent vasoconstrictor activity, reduces renal perfusion.

In addition to these extrarenal baroreceptors the renal juxtaglomerular apparatus serves as an intrarenal baroreceptor system. Sympathetic nerve stimulation, reductions in afferent arteriolar blood pressure, or reductions in the rates of distal tubular sodium delivery enhance renin release by the juxtaglomerular apparatus. Renal renin release into plasma accelerates the formation of angiotensin II according to the following general scheme:

Renin Substrate
↓ renin
Angiotensin I
↓ pulmonary converting enzyme
Angiotensin II
↓ circulating angiotensinase
Angiotensin III

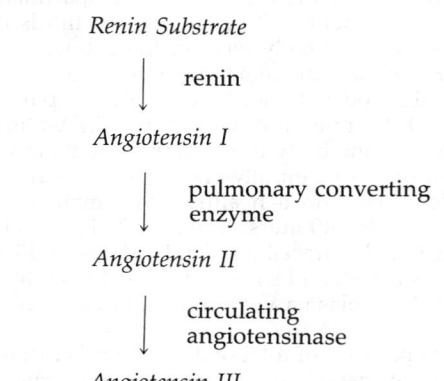

The octapeptide angiotensin II has three major effects on volume conservation: (1) It is a potent pressor agent; on a molar basis, angiotensin II is a more potent vasoconstrictor than norepinephrine. (2) Angiotensin II is the major stimulus to aldosterone secretion and consequently is a key factor modulating renal sodium conservation. (3) The angiotensin II formed in the central nervous system is a potent stimulus to thirst. The heptapeptide angiotensin III is also a potent vasoconstrictor but is not as potent a stimulator of aldosterone secretion as is angiotensin II; angiotensin III also stimulates thirst.

RENAL ELEMENTS. The kidneys respond to slight reductions in effective circulating volume by increasing the rate of proximal tubular sodium absorption without disturbing either glomerular filtration rate or osmoregulatory mechanisms. In normal circumstances, approximately 70 per cent of filtered sodium is absorbed by the proximal nephron. So long as euvolemia persists, the fractional rate of proximal sodium absorption remains constant when the glomerular filtration rate is varied; this constant relation is referred to as *glomerulotubular balance*.

A number of factors modulate glomerulotubular balance in association with changes in effective circulating volume. In empiric terms, this modulation includes a down-setting of glomerulotubular balance in volume-expanded states and an increase in the rate of fractional proximal sodium absorption when filling of the arterial tree is impaired. Among these factors, the hemodynamic regulation of oncotic pressure in peritubular capillaries seems to have a dominant role. At relatively low concentrations, angiotensin II has a vasoconstricting effect on efferent, but not afferent, glomerular arterioles. Therefore this agent, by increasing glomerular filtration fraction, can increase peritubular capillary oncotic pressure and thereby enhance proximal tubular rates of sodium absorption. At high concentrations, angiotensin II, like norepinephrine, produces afferent glomerular arteriolar constriction, which results in reductions in glomerular filtration rate and in renal ischemia.

The kidney responds to modest sodium depletion by increasing the rate of tubular sodium absorption without altering glomerular filtration rate. Glomerulotubular balance is reset upward, so that a greater fraction of glomerular filtrate is absorbed in the proximal nephron; both direct stimulation of renal nerves and the effect of angiotensin II on efferent glomerular arterioles contribute in part to this resetting of glomerulotubular balance. Angiotensin II also provides a second mechanism for renal sodium conservation by increasing the rate of aldosterone secretion, which enhances sodium absorption in the terminal regions of the distal tubule. Finally, increased sodium absorption by more terminal portions of the collecting duct may also be part of the volume repletion reaction. When volume contraction becomes severe, the vasoconstrictive effects of high levels of norepinephrine and angiotensin II tend to reduce both the glomerular filtration rate and the rate of renal sodium excretion.

NEGATIVE FEEDBACK. As indicated in Figure 77–2, atriopeptin and E series prostaglandins (PGE) constitute the principal negative feedback elements of the renal volume regulatory response. The major features of these negative feedback mechanisms are as follows.

Prostaglandins, particularly of the E series, are potent vasodilators. Within the kidney, two cardinal loci of PGE_2 production include renal glomeruli, where angiotensin II activates eicosanoid production and release, and renal medullary interstitial cells, which produce and release PGE_2 in response to increases in medullary osmolality.

As indicated in Figure 77–2, E series prostaglandins suppress renal volume conservation by at least three effects: (1) These agents are natriuretic, although it is not yet established whether the natriuretic effect of prostaglandins is due to changes in renal hemodynamics or to a direct inhibition of tubular sodium absorption. (2) Prostaglandins are potent renal vasodilators and consequently play a major role in protecting the kidneys from ischemia in circumstances such as volume depletion, when levels of the vasoconstrictor agents, angiotensin II and norepinephrine, are increased. (3) PGE_2 is a direct antagonist of the renal tubular effects of ADH and thus impairs renal water conservation.

An important therapeutic principle follows from a consideration of the renal vasodilatory effects of prostaglandins. Specifically, the use of aspirin and other nonsteroidal anti-inflammatory agents should be avoided in circumstances characterized by a high degree of sodium avidity, that is, by a reduction in effective circulating volume. These agents inhibit prostaglandin synthesis and thus reduce the rate of prostaglandin production. Consequently, in sodium-avid states, the use of aspirin or other nonsteroidal anti-inflammatory agents will increase the rate of development of renal ischemia and hence azotemia.

Atriopeptin, or atrial natriuretic peptide, is the second negative feedback element in the renal volume regulatory response. This hormone is released from cardiac atrial storage granules in response to atrial distention; immunoreactive atriopeptin has also been identified within the central nervous system. Atriopeptin is discussed in detail in Ch. 224. In the present context, three actions of atriopeptin have particular pertinence: (1) Centrally released atriopeptin suppresses pituitary ADH release and angiotensin II–mediated thirst. (2) Atriopeptin of cardiac origin inhibits aldosterone secretion and hence renal Na^+ conservation; atriopeptin may also block terminal nephron Na^+ absorption directly. (3) Atriopeptin is a potent vasodilator that increases renal blood flow strikingly. The last-named effect also accounts in part for the natriuretic effects of this peptide.

SUMMARY. When considered in an overall context, two features of the volume repletion reaction illustrated in Figure 77–2 are noteworthy. First, redundant mechanisms protect effective circulating volume. Thus, angiotensin II release, catecholamine release, and ADH release all produce overlapping results.

Second, the magnitude of the volume repletion reaction varies depending on the degree of volume contraction. In modestly volume-contracted states, peripheral vasoconstriction and renal sodium conservation occur, but renal blood flow, glomerular filtration rate, and osmoregulation are unaffected. When volume contraction becomes advanced, nonosmotic ADH release, angiotensin II–mediated thirst, and reductions in the rate of salt delivery to the loop of Henle act in concert to produce hyponatremia. Finally, when catecholamine release and angiotensin II release become sufficiently great that renal blood flow is compromised beyond autoregulatory limits, prerenal azotemia ensues.

VOLUME DEPLETION

DEFINITION. A true hypovolemic state is one in which there is a reduction in total body water, functional ECF volume, and ICF volume; it occurs when the rate of salt and water intake is less than the combined rates of renal plus extrarenal volume losses. In chronic volume-contracted states, input and output may be equal.

ETIOLOGY AND PATHOGENESIS. Three major groups of diseases, occurring individually or in combination, account for most clinically encountered states of true volume contraction. Table 77–2 summarizes these three sets of disorders and the more common specific diseases in each group.

Hormone Deficit. Volume contraction can occur whenever there is loss of ADH or aldosterone. Untreated *diabetes insipidus*, either pituitary or nephrogenic, produces profound volume contraction and hypertonic encephalopathy in patients denied free access to water. Approximately 10 per cent of the glomerular filtrate, or about 18 liters daily, reaches the early distal convoluted tubule. Under normal circumstances, this fluid is hypotonic and, so long as ADH is present, is concentrated by osmotic equilibration with the hypertonic renal medullary interstitium. In diabetes insipidus, a large fraction

TABLE 77–2. MAJOR CAUSES OF VOLUME DEPLETION

Renal Losses	Extrarenal Losses
Hormonal Deficit	**Hemorrhage**
Pituitary diabetes insipidus	**Cutaneous Losses**
Aldosterone insufficiency	Sweating
Addison's disease	Burns
Hyporeninemic hypoaldosteronism	
Interstitial nephritis	
Renal Deficits	**Gastrointestinal Losses**
Specific Tubular Nephropathies:	Vomiting
Renal tubular acidosis	Diarrheal disorders
Proximal	Gastrointestinal fistulas
Distal, gradient-limited	Tube drainage
Bartter's syndrome	
Nephrogenic diabetes insipidus	
Diuretic abuse	
Postobstructive diuresis	
Excessive Filtration of Nonelectrolytes:	
Osmotic diuresis	
Generalized Renal Disease:	
Chronic renal failure	

of hypotonic tubular fluid may escape reabsorption and appear in the urine. Thus the obligatory loss of solute-free water in diabetes insipidus may be as high as 10 to 18 liters daily. Both forms of diabetes insipidus are discussed in Ch. 227.

Addison's disease may impair aldosterone production and hence lead to renal sodium wasting. A second major cause of aldosterone lack occurs in *hyporeninemic hypoaldosteronism*, which may accompany interstitial renal disease. Disorders that damage the renal interstitium, such as hypertension, diabetes mellitus, gout, sickle cell disease, chronic ingestion of lead-containing illicit alcohol, and analgesic abuse, can suppress the ability of the juxtaglomerular apparatus to produce renin. In turn, the low rate of renin secretion results in low rates of aldosterone secretion. Thus hyporeninemic hypoaldosteronism represents a disorder in which impaired aldosterone production results in renal salt wasting, hyperkalemia, and metabolic acidosis. It is not yet known why hyperkalemia, which is a potent stimulus to aldosterone secretion, fails to enhance rates of aldosterone secretion in patients with hyporeninemic hypoaldosteronism.

Renal Deficits. A number of disorders impairing renal tubular sodium or water conservation can lead to volume contraction. For convenience, these derangements may be grouped into three classes.

First, various tubular nephropathies are characterized by specific deficits in salt or water absorption. As mentioned above, nephrogenic diabetes insipidus and interstitial renal disease may produce water or sodium wasting, respectively. Because interstitial renal disease often results in hyperchloremic, hyperkalemic metabolic acidosis, the term "renal tubular acidosis, type IV" is often applied to this disorder. However, the general term "renal tubular acidosis" also includes other sodium-wasting disorders accompanied by hyperchloremic acidosis, such as proximal tubular acidosis, a specific proximal defect in bicarbonate reabsorption, and gradient-limited distal renal tubular acidosis, a specific defect in distal tubular sodium bicarbonate regeneration (Ch. 84).

Alternatively, Bartter's syndrome is a specific tubular nephropathy that results in failure of sodium chloride absorption by distal regions of the nephron; the disorder is accompanied by excessive production of prostaglandins by the renal medullary interstitium and is characterized by sodium chloride wasting, juxtaglomerular hyperplasia, high renin levels, and secondary hyperaldosteronism; the last-named results in hypokalemic metabolic alkalosis.

Inhibition of tubular sodium absorptive processes due to *chronic diuretic abuse* may also lead to salt wasting, volume contraction, and specific metabolic acid-base abnormalities. These abnormalities are discussed below in connection with Table 77–5 (see below). Diuretics such as furosemide and thiazides produce serum electrolyte changes indistinguishable from those of Bartter's syndrome.

Profound but reversible defects in tubular salt and water absorption may occur during *postobstructive diuresis*, that is, shortly after relief of partial or complete urinary tract obstruction. Salt and water losses may also occur in the *diuretic phase* of acute tubular necrosis. However, profound salt and water losses associated with the diuretic phase of acute tubular necrosis are seen uncommonly if extracellular fluid volume is carefully controlled during oliguric acute tubular necrosis.

Third, glomerular filtration of large amounts of nonelectrolytes may produce volume deficits by overwhelming renal tubular reabsorptive capacity for salt and water; in this instance, water losses predominate so that hypernatremia generally occurs. This phenomenon, termed *osmotic diuresis* or *solute diuresis*, occurs in diabetic ketoacidosis, hyperglycemic hyperosmolar coma, or hyperalimentation with large glucose loads in chronically debilitated patients; in patients with burns, in whom there are abnormally high rates of urea production; and during mannitol or glycerol administration to patients with central nervous system disorders requiring reductions of intracranial pressure.

Finally, in *chronic renal failure* of any cause, there is an obligatory loss of sodium. As indicated in Figure 77–1, chronic renal failure of any cause is associated with a significant increase in the minimal physiologic requirement for maintaining sodium balance. The extent of obligatory sodium loss in chronic renal failure is most pronounced in cystic renal diseases, notably medullary cystic disease and polycystic kidney disease (Ch. 91).

Extrarenal Losses. In addition to hemorrhage, two other classes of extrarenal losses account for volume contraction. Simple dehydration may result from increased insensible water loss in *excessive sweating* due to high ambient temperatures or to fever. Because sweat usually contains less than 50 mEq per liter of sodium, the ICF and the ECF share the water loss, and body water osmolality rises while ECF volume loss is modest. *Burns* allow the loss of large amounts of plasma and interstitial fluid through affected areas and therefore can lead rapidly to profound ECF losses.

Finally, gastrointestinal volume losses occur when portions of the 8 to 10 liters of normal gastrointestinal secretions are lost, particularly in secretory diarrheas. Volume depletion is most commonly the consequence of vomiting, gastric drainage, or diarrhea but may occur with any type of bowel fistula. Loss of hydrochloric acid from the stomach may produce metabolic alkalosis, whereas loss of sodium bicarbonate from pancreatic secretions lost through the lower gastrointestinal tract, as in diarrhea, may produce metabolic acidosis.

CLINICAL MANIFESTATIONS. The clinical findings in states of true volume contraction are due both to underfilling of the arterial tree and to the renal and hemodynamic responses to this underfilling. In mild or partially compensated volume contraction, particularly when the latter has occurred gradually, the patient may exhibit nothing more than mild postural giddiness, postural tachycardia, and weakness. In more advanced stages of volume depletion, particularly those occurring acutely, there may be recumbent hypotension, tachycardia, and a reduced urine volume. Finally, when volume contraction is severe, the combination of profound fluid loss and increased sympathetic activity produces circulatory collapse characterized by oliguria, a nondetectable blood pressure (except by Doppler studies), recumbent tachycardia, and cold extremities. In short, mild-to-severe volume contraction may range from minimal symptoms to life-threatening circulatory collapse.

The lack of physical findings does not exclude the presence of mild-to-moderate volume contraction in a given patient. In postoperative patients, 7 to 10 per cent blood volume losses are often accompanied by normal vital signs and by only slight decreases in the central venous pressure or the pulmonary capillary wedge pressure.

Skin turgor and the moistness of mucous membranes are valuable indices to the volume of body water in infants but are unreliable in adults. In young adults, reductions in skin turgor do not occur unless profound volume contraction is present; and normal loss of skin elasticity makes skin turgor difficult to assess in older patients. Likewise, mouth breathing and other factors affect the oral mucosa independently of external volume balances.

The signs and symptoms of volume contraction, regardless of cause, are referable to a reduction in effective circulating volume. Consequently, the clinical findings in volume contraction depend primarily on the interplay among four major factors: the magnitude of the volume loss; the rate of volume loss; the nature of the fluid loss, that is, whether the fluid loss is primarily water, a combined sodium plus water loss, or a blood loss; and finally, the responsiveness of the vasculature to volume reduction. Some simple considerations illustrate these relations.

The clinical manifestations of volume contraction are obviously related intimately to the volume and rate of fluid loss. For example, an acute gastrointestinal hemorrhage of 1 liter of blood can easily result in oliguria, coupled with the signs and symptoms of circulatory collapse, while the hematocrit remains constant. In other words, the hemorrhage is sufficiently acute that fluid flux from the interstitial to the vascular bed makes a negligible contribution to expanding the vascular bed. However, the same amount of gastrointestinal blood loss occurring more slowly—for example, over a one-day period—permits a partial transfer of fluid from the interstitium to the vascular bed and consequently produces a fall in hematocrit; but since the effective circulating volume is at least partially restored by this fluid shift, the volume of urine flow and the hemodynamic response to volume contraction may be minimally affected.

Second, the kind of fluid loss significantly affects the clinical findings in volume contraction. Consider, for example, a 1-liter loss of different kinds of body fluids in a 70-kg man having a total body water of 40 liters and a hematocrit of 45 per cent. The acute loss of 1 liter of predominantly solute-free water, as in diabetes insipidus, produces a 2.5 per cent reduction in blood volume; urine flow and systemic hemodynamics are minimally affected. The acute loss of 1 liter of predominantly extracellular fluid produces a 6.6 per cent reduction in blood volume, since sodium is confined to the ECF; in this circumstance, modest oliguria and recumbent tachycardia ensue. Lastly, the acute loss of 1 liter of blood by hemorrhage reduces blood volume by 20 per cent, thus resulting in profound oliguria and near circulatory collapse.

Finally, peripheral vasoconstriction and tachycardia represent important physiologic responses to volume losses. Consequently, the signs and symptoms of volume contraction, even of modest degree, are amplified appreciably in patients with diminished myocardial reserve or reduced sympathetic nervous system function. The former occurs commonly in cardiomyopathies of any cause or in pericardial tamponade or pericardial constriction. The latter occurs commonly in patients subjected to prolonged bed rest, in diabetic patients with autonomic neuropathy, and as a consequence of therapy with certain antihypertensive drugs.

DIAGNOSIS. The pulse, blood pressure, and changes of these variables with position, together with a clinical estimate of the venous pressure and skin temperature, provide an initial assessment of circulatory dynamics. Because these findings may be inconclusive in moderate degrees of volume contraction, invasive hemodynamic monitoring may be required in critically ill patients who are hemodynamically unstable. In such patients, the central venous pressure may correlate poorly with cardiac output and with pulmonary vascular volume. Measurement of the pulmonary capillary wedge pressure with a Swan-Ganz (flow-directed) catheter may therefore be required.

However, even the pulmonary capillary wedge pressure may remain within normal limits when blood volume has been reduced by 5 to 10 per cent. Consequently, a fluid challenge is useful in the evaluation of critically ill patients in whom a volume deficit is thought to be a contributory factor to a reduced cardiac output. A convenient way of achieving this goal is to administer 500 ml of normal saline over 1 to 3 hours and to measure the change in the pulmonary capillary wedge pressure or the cardiac output, as estimated by thermal dilution.

The cardinal laboratory findings associated with volume contraction follow directly from the volume repletion mechanism summarized in Figure 77–2. The kidney initially responds to a decrease in effective circulating blood volume by reducing urine volume and sodium excretion. Severe degrees of volume contraction also reduce filtration rate and result in prerenal azotemia.

The urinary sodium concentration and the fraction of filtered sodium excreted in the urine, denoted as FE_{Na}, are clinically useful indices of renal sodium avidity. The FE_{Na} is calculated as the urine to plasma sodium concentration ratio divided by the urine to plasma creatinine concentration ratio. In the volume-contracted state, the urinary sodium concentration is generally less than 10 mEq per liter and the FE_{Na} is less than 1 per cent, whereas in acute tubular necrosis, the urinary sodium concentration is greater than 40 mEq per liter and the FE_{Na} is greater than 1 per cent. These indices are useful in the differential diagnosis between acute oliguric tubular necrosis and volume contraction associated with prerenal azotemia, with certain notable exceptions.

The urinary sodium indices are not reliable determinants of volume contraction when there is obligatory renal sodium wasting, as in interstitial nephritis. When volume contraction is due to the renal losses listed in Table 77–2 (except for diabetes insipidus), the urinary sodium concentration and the FE_{Na} may both be elevated even when volume losses are large enough to produce azotemia. The urinary sodium excretion may also be elevated in volume contraction due to upper gastrointestinal losses associated with vomiting or gastric drainage. This occurs during early metabolic alkalosis if the filtered load of bicarbonate exceeds the renal tubular reabsorptive capacity for bicarbonate. During this interval, the urinary chloride concentration is a more reliable index of renal salt avidity. Finally antecedent diuretic therapy may invalidate FE_{Na} measurements.

TREATMENT. The major goal of the treatment of volume contraction is to expand the effective circulating volume by replacing fluid deficits. The type of fluid, the route and rate of fluid administration, and the total amount of fluid to be given will vary with the particular circumstance. For example, a mild, nonpersisting upper gastrointestinal hemorrhage may be treated appropriately by infusion of normal saline, whereas a major, persisting upper gastrointestinal hemorrhage will generally require replacement with whole blood.

The degree to which a given volume of crystalloid solution expands the effective circulating volume depends on solution composition. If glucose metabolism is normal, the infusion of 5 per cent dextrose in water (D_5W) is equivalent to administering solute-free water, which distributes uniformly in total body water. Since less than 10 per cent of total body water is in the intravascular compartment, infusion of 1 liter of 5 per cent dextrose in water expands the intravascular volume by 75 to 100 ml, that is, by about 2 per cent.

Solutions containing sodium as the principal solute preferentially expand the extracellular fluid volume. Infusion of 1 liter of a normal saline solution increases blood volume by about 300 ml, or about 6 per cent; the remaining portion is distributed in the interstitial compartment. Hypotonic sodium-containing salt solutions expand intravascular volume in a manner intermediate between that of 5 per cent dextrose in water and normal saline.

Colloid-containing solutions, such as iso-oncotic albumin solutions and plasma, preferentially expand the intravascular compartment, since large molecules like albumin are mainly restricted to the intravascular space. Finally, blood, which contains formed elements, is the most potent expander of the intravascular space. A unit of packed red blood cells will remain entirely in the vascular bed. A unit of whole blood having a hematocrit of 45 per cent will retain all formed elements in the vascular bed; of the remaining 55 per cent volume of that unit, more than 40 per cent of the plasma will also remain in the vascular bed because of the oncotic effect of plasma proteins.

Three other factors concerning fluid replacement therapy warrant consideration: (1) When large volumes of glucose-containing solutions are given rapidly, an increase in plasma glucose concentration that results in glycosuria produces an obligate renal loss of sodium and water that aggravates volume losses. (2) Iso-oncotic albumin solutions expand intravascular volume rapidly. The half-life of infused albumin in critically ill patients is only four to six hours, however, and the cost of an iso-oncotic albumin solution is approximately 90 times greater than that of an equal volume of normal saline. For these reasons, the use of iso-oncotic albumin solutions should be limited to hemodynamically unstable patients in whom rapid intravascular expansion is critical. (3) Because volume contraction is associated with vasoconstriction, both in the venous and arterial circuits, transient changes in the pulmonary capillary wedge pressure may not reflect accurately the volume status of the patient. During volume expansion, the wedge pressure rises and subsequently falls. The initial pressure elevation is due to fluid infusion into a vasoconstricted, low-capacity vascular bed and should not be misinterpreted to indicate adequacy of volume repletion. The subsequent reduction in wedge pressure coincides with decreases in arterial resistance coupled to increases in venous capacitance.

CIRCULATORY COMPROMISE WITHOUT TRUE VOLUME CONTRACTION

DEFINITION. In the previous section, we considered those disorders characterized by inadequate filling of the arterial tree that occurred because of fluid losses between the patient and the external environment. Clearly, the cardinal signs and symptoms of these disorders are referable to responses accompanying the integrated volume repletion reaction (Fig. 77–2). There are also disorders in which inadequate arterial filling occurs in the absence of external fluid losses. The signs and symptoms of these disorders mimic closely those that characterize true volume contraction.

ETIOLOGY AND PATHOGENESIS. Table 77–3 lists three commonly encountered classes of derangements that may present clinically with tachycardia, acute hypotension, oliguria, azotemia, and a reduced Fe_{Na}. These disorders can be termed "non–volume-contracted circulatory compromise," with the understanding that the term "non–volume-contracted" refers to the absence of body fluid losses between the patient and the external world.

Impaired Cardiac Output. A profound collapse of cardiac output, due to acute myocardial infarction with pump failure (cardiogenic shock) or to acute pericardial tamponade, may clearly result in circulatory collapse. In this instance, failure to fill the arterial tree and to maintain an effective circulatory volume occurs because the heart fails to translocate blood adequately from venous to arterial beds.

Increased Vascular Capacitance. Circulatory collapse and its attendant signs and symptoms will occur when there is a sudden increase in the capacitance of the vascular bed, most notably in the venous part of the circulation. This kind of increase in ratio of vascular capacitance to vascular volume occurs most commonly in sepsis but may also be seen in circumstances in which peripheral vasodilators, particularly those having a postarteriolar locus of action, are administered injudiciously.

TABLE 77–3. CIRCULATORY COMPROMISE WITHOUT EXTERNAL FLUID LOSSES

I. Impaired cardiac output
Acute myocardial infarction
Pericardial tamponade
II. Increased Vascular Capacitance
Septic shock
III. Vascular → Interstitial Fluid Shifts
Acute pancreatitis
Bowel infarction
Rhabdomyolysis
Noncardiogenic pulmonary edema

Vascular-Interstitial Fluid Shifts. Profound hypotension, tachycardia, progressive oliguria, and azotemia are also encountered when there is a rapid translocation of fluid from vascular to interstitial compartments, presumably because of a sudden, profound increase in the permeability characteristics of peripheral capillaries. Some common derangements of this type include infarction of the small or large intestine, extensive tissue trauma, acute pancreatitis, and rhabdomyolysis. An analogous mechanism, namely, a marked increase in the permeability of pulmonary capillaries, is also presumed to account for the formation of noncardiogenic pulmonary edema in the adult respiratory distress syndrome.

DIAGNOSIS AND THERAPY. The diagnosis and therapy of acute myocardial infarction with circulatory collapse and of acute pericardial tamponade are considered in detail in Section IV of this book. It is, however, worth citing certain factors particularly germane to the management of fluid therapy in such patients. In individuals affected either by right ventricular infarction or by pericardial tamponade, maintenance of adequate filling of the systemic arterial tree depends critically on providing a relatively high venous preload to the right side of the heart. Attempts at volume contraction in patients with right ventricular infarcts or pericardial tamponade may exacerbate systemic hypotension. Thus treatment of these disorders generally requires concomitant hemodynamic monitoring with a flow-directed Swan-Ganz catheter to avoid excessive preload to the left side of the heart.

In patients with left ventricular infarction and systemic hypotension, particular attention should be directed to excluding the possibility that antecedent true volume depletion—for example, with prolonged diuretic therapy and salt restriction prior to the myocardial infarction—may be a significant contributor to what otherwise might be mistaken for true cardiogenic shock. The combined findings of acute left ventricular infarction, systemic arterial hypotension, a reduced pulmonary capillary wedge pressure, and an antecedent history of prolonged diuretic therapy, when taken together, indicate that improved systemic hemodynamics may be achieved by cautious attempts at volume expansion carried out in combination with serial measurements of the cardiac output and the pulmonary capillary wedge pressure.

The distinction between hypotension as being due either to true volume contraction or to an increase in the capacitance/volume ratio of the vascular bed, as occurs in sepsis, is often difficult. This distinction is particularly difficult in individuals who have been in intensive care units for prolonged periods of time and in those at high risk for developing sepsis, such as cancer patients treated with potent chemotherapeutic agents. A useful clue to the presence of septic circulatory collapse is the occurrence of warm extremities coupled with hypotension and oliguria, since true hypovolemia, particularly when advanced, is ordinarily accompanied by profound peripheral vasoconstriction and hence cool and often cyanotic extremities.

True hypovolemia and sepsis may also coexist. In such a circumstance, invasive hemodynamic monitoring may be helpful. Both in true hypovolemia and in sepsis, the pulmonary capillary wedge pressure is reduced; but in septic circulatory collapse, the calculated systemic vascular resistance falls, because of peripheral vasodilation, whereas in true hypovolemia, peripheral vasoconstriction ordinarily raises the systemic vascular resistance. The diagnosis of disorders producing rapid transfer of fluids from the vascular bed to the interstitium, such as trauma, acute pancreatitis, or rhabdomyolysis, is generally evident from clinical appraisal.

The treatment of patients with sepsis and an increased vascular capacitance/volume ratio, as well as those individuals with rapid vascular to interstitial fluid shifts, has as a mainstay the administration of sufficient sodium-containing fluids, generally isotonic saline, to permit adequate filling of the arterial tree. This therapy necessarily expands total body water, particularly in the vascular and interstitial compartments. Consequently, during recovery from the underlying disorder, care must be taken to avoid unnecessary expansion of the vascular bed and consequently the risk of volume-mediated cardiac decompensation.

VOLUME EXCESS

DEFINITION. Volume-expanded states are characterized by an increase in total body water, which is accompanied, in most but not all circumstances, by an increase in total body sodium. Total body salt and water may be increased while the effective circulating volume is decreased. In other words, certain volume-expanded states are characterized by dissociation between total body salt and water and the effective circulating volume.

ETIOLOGY AND PATHOGENESIS. Volume expansion occurs whenever the rate of salt or water intake exceeds the rate of renal plus extrarenal losses; in chronic volume expansion, the external salt and water balance may be normal. A convenient way of considering volume-expanded states is to view them in the context of three different classes of physiologic explanations (Table 77–4).

Disturbances in Starling Forces. The most common diseases encountered in which both volume expansion and edema occur are those in which derangements in the Starling forces regulating fluid transfer between capillaries and interstitium tend to promote expansion of the interstitial compartment at the expense of the effective circulating volume. Consequently, renal sodium retention and edema occur. By definition, this group of disorders is characterized by increases in capillary hydrostatic pressure, by decreases in capillary oncotic pressure, or by a combination of these two factors.

Four groups include most edematous states characterized by abnormal Starling forces (Table 77–4). First, the systemic venous pressure may be increased because of primary cardiac disorders, such as right heart failure or constrictive pericarditis. Second, there may occur local elevations in pulmonary or systemic venous pressure, as in left heart failure, vena caval obstruction, or portal vein obstruction. Third, a reduction in plasma oncotic pressure, and consequently a net increase in the tendency for fluid transudation from capillaries to interstitium, accounts plausibly for edema formation in the nephrotic syndrome. Finally, a combination of these factors may be responsible for edema formation. For example, both hypoalbuminemia and portal hypertension are major contributory factors to the development of ascites in hepatic cirrhosis.

Plasma renin activity and aldosterone concentrations in these disorders tend to be elevated, although the results also tend to be variable. In advanced cases of disorders characterized by increases in local or systemic venous pressure, most notably in severe congestive heart failure and in cirrhosis, hyponatremia may occur; this finding represents an ominous prognostic sign. Finally, edema formation due to such derangements of Starling forces may result in the "third space" phenomenon, namely, the sequestration of large volumes of interstitial fluid in regions such as the pleural or peritoneal cavities.

Primary Hormonal Excess. These disorders include those disturbances in which there is unregulated production of mineralocorticoids or ADH. The volume expansion that occurs in states of mineralocorticoid excess, such as primary hyperaldosteronism, is due to sodium retention and is accompanied by a primary, preferential expansion of the ECF and consequently by hypertension. The serum sodium level is generally normal. In the syndrome of inappropriate ADH production (SIADH), primary water retention occurs. Consequently, the volume expansion involves both the ICF and ECF; dilutional hyponatremia is the hallmark of SIADH, whereas hypertension is uncommon. Edema is not characteristic in either of these two disorders. Instead, patients with primary aldosteronism or SIADH reach a volume-expanded steady state in which output equals input.

Primary Renal Sodium Retention. The kidneys may also retain sodium abnormally when the effective circulating volume is normal and there is no effector excess. For example, in acute glomerulonephritis unidentified renal mechanisms are primarily responsible for edema formation. Patients with acute glomerulonephritis retain salt and water and become hypertensive without reductions in glomerular filtration rate or in effective circulating volume. Furthermore, sodium retention and edema develop when plasma renin activity and aldosterone concentration are normal or reduced and when the serum albumin concentration is normal. Thus, the renal tubule may be abnormally avid for sodium in acute glomerulonephritis. Congestive heart failure may occur as a secondary consequence of the volume expansion.

DIAGNOSIS AND TREATMENT. The recognition and management of volume-expanded states depend on proper identification and treatment of the underlying disorder. Clearly, the cornerstones of therapy in volume-expanded states characterized by sodium excess include salt restriction and diuretics. Table 77–5 provides a summary of some of the major diuretics used commonly and certain of their properties. For convenience, these drugs have been classified according to their sites of action in the nephron.

Proximal Diuretics. The cardinal example of a proximal tubular diuretic is acetazolamide, a carbonic anhydrase inhibitor that blocks proximal reabsorption of sodium bicarbonate. Consequently, prolonged use of acetazolamide may lead to hyperchloremic acidosis, in contrast to all other diuretics, which act at loci prior to the late distal nephron. Metolazone, a congener of the thiazide class of diuretics, blocks sodium chloride absorption in two nephron sites by unknown mechanisms. Specifically, in addition to an action on the early distal tubule, metolazone also inhibits proximal tubular sodium chloride absorption. Since the major locus for phosphate absorption is in the proximal nephron, the phosphaturia accompanying metolazone administration exceeds considerably that observed with other thiazide class diuretics.

Loop Diuretics. Loop diuretics, such as ethacrynic acid and furosemide, produce diuresis by inhibiting the coupled entry on Na^+, Cl^-, and K^+ across apical plasma membranes in the thick ascending limb of Henle. The latter is responsible for the reabsorption of approximately 25 per cent of filtered sodium. The natriuretic dose-response characteristics of these diuretic agents are considerably more linear than those of all other currently used diuretics. Consequently, the loop diuretics are, for practical purposes, the most potent diuretics currently available; therefore these drugs are commonly referred to as "high-ceiling" diuretics.

Early Distal Tubule Diuretics. Early distal tubule diuretics, such as thiazide and metolazone, interfere primarily with sodium chloride absorption in the earliest segments of the distal convoluted tubule. The thiazide diuretics appear to exert their effect by blocking sodium entry from tubular fluid across apical plasma membranes into distal tubular cells.

TABLE 77–4. DISORDERS OF VOLUME EXCESS

I. Disturbed Starling Forces	**II. Primary Hormone Excess**
(Reduced effective circulating volume; edema formation)	(Increased effective circulating volume)
Systemic Venous Pressure Increases	Primary aldosteronism
Right heart failure	Cushing's syndrome
Constrictive pericarditis	SIADH
Local Venous Pressure Increases	
Left heart failure	**III. Primary Renal Sodium Retention**
Vena cava obstruction	(Increased effective circulating volume)
Portal vein obstruction	Acute glomerulonephritis
Reduced Oncotic Pressure	
Nephrotic syndrome	
Combined Disorders	
Cirrhosis	

SIADH = Syndrome of inappropriate antidiuretic hormone production.

TABLE 77–5. CHARACTERISTICS OF COMMONLY USED DIURETICS

Diuretic	Primary Effect	Secondary Effect	Complications
I. Proximal Diuretics			
Acetazolamide	↓ Na^+/H^+ exchange	↑ K^+ loss, ↑ HCO_3^- loss	Hypokalemic, hyperchloremic acidosis
Metolazone	↓ Na^+ absorption	↑ K^+ loss, ↑ Cl^- loss	Hypokalemic alkalosis
II. Loop Diuretics			
Furosemide Ethacrynic acid	↓ $Na^+:K^+:2Cl^-$ absorption	↑ K^+ loss, ↑ H^+ secretion	Hypokalemic alkalosis
III. Early Distal Diuretics			
Thiazide Metolazone	↓ Na^+ absorption	↑ K^+ loss, ↑ H^+ secretion	Hypokalemic alkalosis
IV. Late Distal Diuretics			
Aldosterone Antagonists Spironolactone Nonaldosterone Antagonists Triamterene Amiloride	↓ Na^+ absorption	↓ K^+ loss, ↓ H^+ secretion	Hyperkalemic acidosis

With the exception of acetazolamide (which impairs bicarbonate absorption), hypokalemia and metabolic alkalosis may complicate the administration of proximal diuretics, loop diuretics, and early distal tubular diuretics. This occurs because the rate of sodium delivery to terminal distal tubular regions, where a significant fraction of potassium and proton secretion occurs, is a major factor promoting these two processes. Consequently, an increased delivery of salt to the late distal nephron, occasioned by inhibition of sodium reabsorption in the proximal tubule, the ascending limb of Henle, or the early distal tubule, leads to accelerated rates of proton and potassium secretion and consequently to hypokalemia and metabolic alkalosis.

Late Distal Nephron Diuretics. Finally, a group of agents inhibit sodium absorption in terminal regions of the distal tubule and concomitantly suppress indirectly potassium secretion and proton secretion. Spironolactone competes with aldosterone; the primary use of this agent is restricted to conditions of aldosterone excess, either primary or secondary. Alternatively, both triamterene and amiloride operate independently of aldosterone. These agents directly block sodium uptake by late distal tubular cells and concomitantly suppress indirectly both potassium and proton secretion. Accordingly, hyperkalemic, hyperchloremic metabolic acidosis may complicate the injudicious use of spironolactone, triamterene, or amiloride.

One factor common to the treatment of disorders with reduced effective circulating volumes and expanded ECF volumes merits particular consideration. A major factor in edema formation is an increase in the Starling forces promoting fluid translocation from the vascular to interstitial spaces. When potent diuretics are administered to patients with portal hypertension or with hypoalbuminemia, urinary sodium excretion may exceed the rate at which salt and water are transferred from the interstitium to the vascular bed. As a result, vigorous diuretic therapy may result in volume contraction, reduced salt delivery to diluting segments, nonosmotic ADH release, and consequently hyponatremia. In advanced cases of diuretic abuse, hypotension, hemoconcentration, and azotemia also occur.

A like effect occurs in volume-expanded patients, particularly those exhibiting a third space effect and having significant hypoalbuminemia, if relatively large volumes of ascitic fluid are removed by paracentesis. In this circumstance, the transudation of fluid from the vascular space to the interstitial space may result in circulatory collapse.

Campbell WB, Currie MG, Needleman P: Inhibition of aldosterone biosynthesis by atriopeptins in rat adrenal cells. Circ Res 57:113, 1985. *The role of atriopeptin in negative feedback of aldosterone synthesis is discussed.*

Laragh JH: Atrial natriuretic hormone, the renin-aldosterone axis and blood pressure–electrolyte homeostasis. N Engl J Med 313:1330, 1985. *A general discussion of atriopeptin.*

Laski ME: Diuretics—mechanism of action and therapy. Semin Nephrol 6:210, 1986. *A topical summary of diuretic action.*

Lifschitz MD, Stein JH: Hormonal regulation of renal salt excretion. Semin Nephrol 3:196, 1986. *A good review of sodium excretion and its modulation by hormones.*

Needleman P, Greenwald JE: Atriopeptin: A cardiac hormone intimately involved in fluid, electrolyte and blood-pressure homeostasis. N Engl J Med 314:828, 1986. *The role of atriopeptin in negative feedback of volume control is described.*

Reid IA: The renin-angiotensin system and body function. Arch Intern Med 145:1475, 1985. *The role of renin and angiotensin in volume regulation.*

Osmolality Disturbances

PHYSIOLOGIC CONSIDERATIONS

In normal individuals, the serum osmolality is virtually constant from day to day and the serum sodium concentration is an accurate index to body water osmolality. In fact, the normal ranges for serum sodium concentrations or for serum osmolalities in populations of healthy individuals depend on small differences in body water osmolality among individuals, rather than on variations in body water osmolality in a given individual.

It is useful to define "effective ECF osmolality," since the osmoregulatory mechanisms that adjust water balance in normal individuals are determined primarily by changes in cell volume that result from variations in effective ECF osmolality. In dilutional states, the measured and effective ECF osmolalities are approximately equal, since ECF dilution also produces ICF dilution and, at least acutely, cell swelling. Osmoregulatory mechanisms are activated when ECF hypertonicity is due to a solute that is excluded from cells and therefore produces, at least acutely, cell shrinkage; in this case, the measured and effective ECF osmolalities are approximately equal. If the ECF osmolality is increased by solutes such as urea, which penetrate cell membranes readily, acute cell shrinkage does not occur and osmoregulatory mechanisms are not activated. In this case, the measured ECF osmolality is greater than the effective ECF osmolality.

The serum osmolality can be approximated from the following formula:

$$\text{Osmolality} = 2[\text{Na}^+] + \frac{[\text{glucose}]}{18} + \frac{[\text{BUN}]}{2.8}$$

where the glucose and blood urea nitrogen (BUN) concentrations are expressed as milligrams per deciliter and the serum sodium concentration is expressed as milliequivalents per liter. In normal circumstances, glucose contributes 5.5 mOsm per kilogram of H_2O and urea contributes 2 to 6 mOsm per kilogram of H_2O to the serum osmolality. When hyperglycemia occurs, the effective ECF osmolality rises because glucose entry into cells is limited. When azotemia occurs, the effective ECF osmolality does not rise because urea enters cells readily.

Cell Volume Regulation

Starling forces regulate fluid transfer between the ICF and the ECF. Because plasma membranes cannot tolerate even small hydrostatic gradients, the operational Starling forces between ICF and ECF are almost entirely osmotic. Significant changes in cell volume, particularly in the central nervous system, are by themselves potentially lethal. Thus the goals of fluid transport between the ECF and ICF are to maintain constancy of cell volume and to maintain a negligible hydrostatic pressure gradient between cells and the ECF. Since cell membranes are freely permeable to water, these two goals are achieved when the ECF osmolality is normal and intracellular and extracellular osmolalities are identical.

Since cell membranes are partially permeable to sodium and potassium, there is a tendency for sodium to leak into cells and for potassium to leak out of cells. Because impermeant macromolecules account for a large fraction of intracellular anions, passive sodium and potassium movements tend toward a Donnan distribution, in which total intracellular cations would exceed total interstitial cations, in precise analogy to the way in which total plasma water cations exceed total interstitial cations. If these passive cation movements across cell membranes were unopposed, osmotic water movement into cells would tend to produce cell lysis. Consequently, active transport mechanisms are required to balance intracellular and interstitial cation concentrations.

Specifically, both sodium leakage from the ECF into cells and potassium leakage out of cells into the ECF are counterbalanced exactly by active outward sodium transport coupled to active inward potassium transport. These active transport events maintain the intracellular cation (and therefore osmolar) content equal to that of extracellular fluid and also maintain the predominant extracellular and intracellular distributions of sodium and potassium, respectively. Thus because cellular cation pumps balance cellular cation leaks, cells are *operationally* impermeable to sodium and to potassium. Active sodium efflux coupled to active potassium influx is mediated by membrane-bound (Na^+ + K^+)–adenosine triphosphatase (ATPase), and the activity of these cellular cation pumps accounts for more than 50 per cent of the basal caloric consumption.

Cation transport mediated by (Na^+ + K^+)-ATPase is the major factor regulating cell volume when the effective ECF osmolality is normal. When the effective ECF osmolality is increased or decreased, additional processes are required to maintain the constancy of cell volume. These auxiliary mechanisms are of particular importance in minimizing potentially lethal changes in brain volume because of osmotic water shifts into or out of brain cells.

In chronic hypotonic disorders, cell swelling is offset by the loss of potassium chloride from cells. This potassium chloride efflux mechanism appears to be activated by small increases in cell volume produced by ECF dilution. In chronic hypernatremia, brain shrinkage is minimized by the accumulation of additional solutes within brain cells. These latter solutes, often called "idiogenic osmoles," include amino acids and other unidentified solutes. As will be discussed in the section on Treatment, these auxiliary transport processes affect significantly the therapeutic approach to patients with osmoregulatory failure.

Water Balance

The key elements regulating water balance are summarized in Figure 77–3. The solid lines indicate osmoregulatory mechanisms, which, as indicated above, maintain constancy of cell volume. When the effective circulating volume is reduced by more than 10 per cent, volume-mediated stimuli participate in the regulation of water balance. These pathways, indicated by the dotted lines in Figure 77–3, are the same as those shown in Figure 77–3 for extreme volume contraction. Finally,

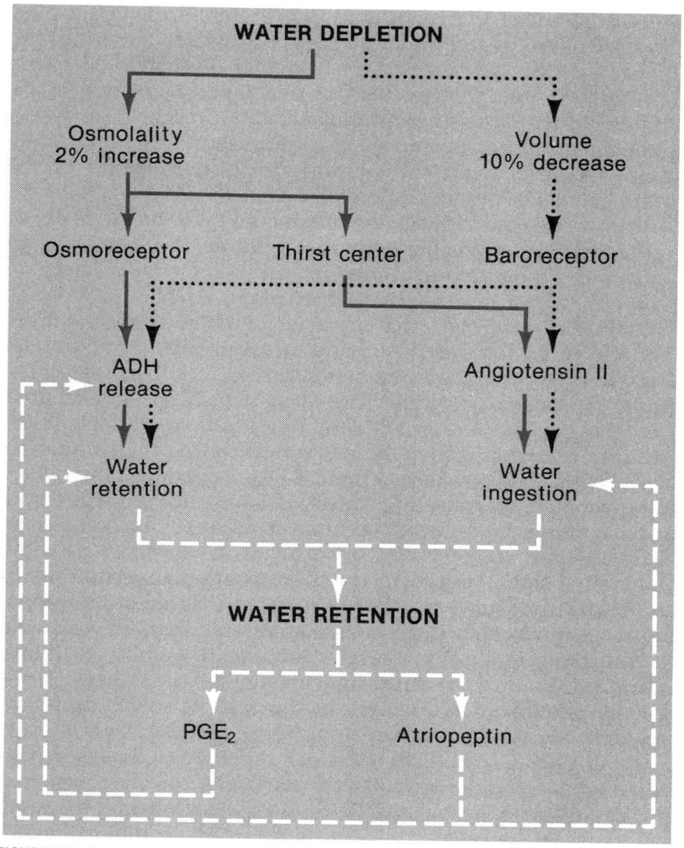

FIGURE 77–3. The water repletion reaction. The solid arrows are positive water conservation processes activated by osmolality increases; the dotted lines indicate volume-activated water conservation. The dashed lines show negative feedback.

the dashed lines in Figure 77–3 indicate the negative feedback limbs activated by water conservation.

SENSORS AND EFFECTORS. Three kinds of *sensor* elements adjust water balance. Two of these, osmoreceptors and the thirst center, respond to small changes in effective ECF osmolality, whereas baroreceptors respond to changes in effective circulating volume. The osmoreceptors are situated in the supraoptic and paraventricular nuclei of the hypothalamus, whereas the thirst center is in the organum vasculosum of the anterior hypothalamus. As little as a 2 per cent increase in effective ECF osmolality produced by solutes such as sodium chloride, but not urea, causes shrinkage of osmoreceptor cells and thirst center cells. The osmoreceptors stimulate the release of the *effector* hormone ADH from storage sites in the posterior pituitary gland. The stimulation of thirst by the thirst centers depends on centrally produced angiotensin II.

When the effective circulating volume is reduced by more than 10 per cent, volume-dependent mechanisms stimulate ADH release. Activation of extrarenal baroreceptors by blood volume depletion produces afferent signals, carried by the ninth and tenth cranial nerves, which result in nonosmotic ADH release. Volume contraction also acts as a potent stimulus to thirst via angiotensin II.

THE ANTIDIURETIC RESPONSE. The cardinal characteristics of the antidiuretic response depend primarily on the integrated activity of two regions of the nephron: the medullary thick ascending limb of Henle, referred to as the diluting segment; and the collecting duct, which may be termed the concentrating segment.

The medullary thick ascending limb absorbs a large amount, possibly as much as 25 per cent, of the filtered load of sodium. Some of this reabsorbed sodium is trapped in the renal medullary interstitium, thus accounting in large part for the hypertonicity of the renal medullary interstitium. However, the medullary thick limb of Henle is also water impermeable. Consequently, salt abstraction from the thick limb of Henle accounts simultaneously for the development of medullary hypertonicity, thus permitting, in the presence of ADH, maximal antidiuresis, and the appearance of maximally dilute urine in early distal convolutions, thus permitting, in the absence of ADH, maximal water diuresis.

In normal individuals, approximately 18 liters daily of tubular fluid reaches the early distal tubule; the osmolality of this fluid is quite dilute, approximately 50 mOsm per kilogram of H_2O. Thus in the total absence of ADH and volume contraction, maximal rates of water diuresis include a urine volume of 18 liters daily having an osmolality of 50 mOsm per kilogram of H_2O. During antidiuresis, ADH increases the water permeability of collecting ducts (Ch. 227). Tubular fluid equilibrates osmotically with the hypertonic medullary interstitium, reducing urine volume, concentrating the urine, and conserving body water. When ADH is absent, the water permeability of collecting ducts is low and absorption of tubular fluid is reduced so that it escapes unchanged as hypotonic urine.

Finally, since collecting ducts are partially permeable to water in the absence of ADH, a reduced volume of hypotonic fluid reaching collecting ducts equilibrates partially with the medullary interstitium, thereby limiting the ability to dilute urine maximally. In some experimental circumstances, sufficiently significant reductions in the rate of solute excretion result in formation of a hypertonic urine when ADH is absent.

NEGATIVE FEEDBACK. Water repletion activates a negative feedback of water conservation by at least two systems, PGE_2 and atriopeptin (Fig. 77–3). PGE_2 is produced by renal interstitial cells in response to increases in medullary osmolality. In turn, PGE_2 impairs water conservation by inhibiting the actions of ADH on nephron segments involved in the antidiuretic response, namely, the medullary thick ascending limb and the collecting duct.

Immunoreactive atriopeptin is elaborated within the central nervous system as well as by secretory granules in cardiac atria. This centrally released atriopeptin is capable of suppressing both ADH release and angiotensin II–stimulated thirst (Ch. 224).

HYPOTONIC DISORDERS

DEFINITION. A hypotonic disorder is one in which the ratio of solutes to water in body fluids is reduced, and the serum osmolality and serum sodium are both reduced in parallel. True hypotonicity must be distinguished from disorders in which the *measured* serum sodium is low while the measured serum osmolality is either normal or increased.

The distinction among these disorders is listed in Table 77–6. The measured serum sodium can be reduced either because there is an increased concentration of small, nonsodium solutes restricted to the ECF or because of a laboratory artifact. In hyperglycemia or excessive mannitol administration these solutes, which are restricted to the ECF, draw water from the cellular compartment. The serum sodium level is therefore reduced even though the serum osmolality may be increased. When a small, nonsodium solute is distributed in total body water, as in ethanol intoxication or in azotemia, the serum osmolality rises but the serum sodium concentration remains normal, resulting in an "osmolar gap."

TABLE 77–6. DISTINCTION BETWEEN APPARENT AND REAL HYPOTONICITY

Condition	Measured Serum [Na]	Measured Serum Osmolality
True hypotonicity	↓	↓
Increased nonsodium ECF solutes		
Hyperglycemia	↓	↑
Mannitol administration	↓	↑
Increased nonsodium ECF and ICF solutes		
Ethanol	normal	↑
Ethylene glycol	normal	↑
Methanol	normal	↑
Isopropyl alcohol	normal	↑
Laboratory artifact		
Hyperlipemia	↓	normal
Hyperproteinemia	↓	normal

TABLE 77–7. HYPONATREMIA REFERABLE TO IMPAIRED RENAL EXCRETION OF WATER

I. Reduced Sodium Delivery to the Diluting Segment	**III. Mixed Disorders**
Starvation	Volume contraction (Addison's disease)
Beer potomania	Edema with deranged Starling forces (congestive heart failure, constrictive pericarditis, and cirrhosis)
? Myxedema	
II. Primary Excess of ADH	
SIADH	
Drug-induced ADH production	
Drug potentiation of ADH action	
Trauma	
Potassium depletion	
? Myxedema	
? Acute intermittent porphyria	

In hyperlipemic or hyperproteinemic states, the volume of water in a given sample of serum sent for laboratory analysis is reduced. The flame photometer measures the total amount of sodium in a correspondingly reduced volume of water per unit volume of serum; therefore the serum sodium level appears low. However, the measured serum osmolality, which is a colligative property of aqueous solutions, is measured as normal, since the actual concentration of sodium per unit volume of water is normal. These instances of spurious hyponatremia are becoming less common as more laboratories adopt the use of ion-selective electrodes to measure the serum sodium concentration.

ETIOLOGY AND PATHOGENESIS. Hyponatremia and simultaneous body water hypotonicity develop whenever water intake exceeds the sum of renal plus extrarenal water losses; in chronic hyponatremia, the net water intake and net water output may be equal. Thus hyponatremia and body fluid hypotonicity occur when there is a primary increase in water ingestion, when the ability of the kidney to dilute urine maximally is limited, or when a combination of these factors is operative.

Dilutional hyponatremia may be the consequence of an absolute increase in water intake that exceeds the ability of a normal kidney to excrete free water, as in *primary polydipsia*, often referred to as psychogenic polydipsia. Patients with this disorder ingest unusually large volumes of water, often in excess of 10 to 15 liters daily, and generally develop mild, clinically asymptomatic hyponatremia. Profound hyponatremia is rare in these patients because the ability of the kidney to excrete large volumes of maximally dilute urine is not impaired.

More commonly, hyponatremia occurs because the ability of the kidney to excrete a maximally dilute urine is reduced. This inability to dilute urine maximally occurs because of (1) reductions in the rate of salt absorption by the diluting segment, that is, the thick ascending limb of Henle; (2) sustained nonosmotic release of ADH; or (3) a combination of these factors. Table 77–7 summarizes these disorders.

Reduced Sodium Delivery to Diluting Segments. These disorders occur when a reduced sodium intake, without significant sodium depletion or ECF volume contraction, decreases the rate of sodium delivery to the diluting segment and consequently impairs the maximal rate of dilute urine formation, the minimal urine osmolality, or both. Beer potomania, although an uncommon disorder, illustrates this mechanism for hyponatremia nicely.

Patients with beer potomania derive a substantial part of their caloric intake from the ingestion of large volumes of beer, which contains little salt or protein. Because sodium and urea are the major urinary solutes, dietary restriction of these solutes, particularly sodium, increases the fractional rate of proximal sodium absorption, diminishes the rate of salt delivery to diluting segments, and in turn limits the daily rate of formation of dilute urine. For example, the minimal urinary osmolality is approximately 50 mOsm per kilogram of H_2O; consequently, the excretion of 15 liters of highly dilute urine requires the excretion of 750 mOsm of solute. If the daily urinary solute excretion falls, the maximal amount of dilute urine formed daily is also reduced. Moreover, partial equilibration of reduced volumes of collecting duct fluid with the renal medullary interstitium impairs even further the daily excretion of dilute urine.

Hyponatremia due to reduced solute intake is not restricted to individuals with beer potomania but may occur during starvation, when intake may be dramatically reduced without parallel reductions in water intake. This form of hyponatremia occurs with increasing frequency in elderly patients in nursing homes who are inadequately supervised.

Patients with beer potomania or starvation are to be distinguished from individuals in whom a reduced effective circulating volume accompanied by an increase in total body water or by a reduction in glomerular filtration rate reduces the rate of salt delivery to diluting segments and collecting ducts (see below). In short, beer potomania and starvation are classic examples in which a reduced rate of delivery to the diluting segment, in the absence of ADH release, blunts significantly urinary diluting power in the absence of profound gains or excesses in total body water.

Primary Effector ADH Excess. THE SYNDROME OF INAPPROPRIATE ADH PRODUCTION (SIADH). In SIADH hyponatremia occurs as a result of sustained endogenous production and release of ADH or ADH-like substances; the effective circulating volume is normal or increased, and there are no other physiologic or pharmacologic stimuli to ADH release. Table 77–8 lists the major causes of SIADH. A similar process may account in part for the hyponatremia seen in myxedema.

Antidiuretic hormone, or a peptide having comparable biologic activity, is produced by tumors. Increased ADH levels, estimated by either bioassay or radioimmunoassay, have also been noted in patients with cranial disorders such as skull fractures, subdural hematomas, subarachnoid hemorrhage, and brain tumors; in acute intermittent porphyria; and possibly in myxedema. Four different patterns of plasma ADH concentrations have been described in patients with SIADH. Figure 77–4 illustrates three of these patterns; the shaded area in Figure 77–4 illustrates the normal relation between plasma ADH levels and serum osmolality. The pattern denoted as "erratic ADH release" in Figure 77–4 accounts for about 37 per cent of patients with SIADH; the hormone is released completely independently of osmotic control. About one third of patients with SIADH have a "reset osmostat"; there is an abnormally low threshold for ADH secretion, but if sufficiently hyponatremic, these patients with SIADH can produce a maximally dilute urine. About 16 per cent of patients with SIADH exhibit the "ADH leak" pattern, namely, sustained ADH production below the osmotic threshold, and normal increases in serum ADH levels with osmotic challenge (Fig. 77–4). Finally, about 14 per cent of patients with SIADH have no detectable abnormality in ADH levels; they fail, for reasons not yet understood, to dilute urine maximally.

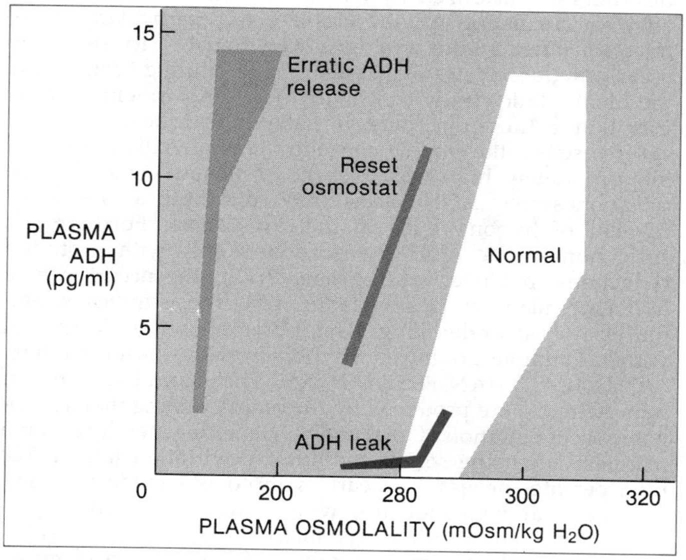

FIGURE 77–4. The patterns of serum ADH abnormalities in SIADH. The shaded areas indicate the normal relation between increases in effective ECF osmolality and ADH levels; the normal osmotic threshold is lower than the normal serum osmolality. The three shaded areas indicate ADH patterns in SIADH. (Adapted from Zerbe R, Strope L, Robertson G: Vasopressin function in the syndrome of inappropriate diuresis. Ann Rev Med 31:315, 1980.)

TABLE 77–8. MAJOR CAUSES OF SIADH

Malignant Neoplasia
Carcinoma: bronchogenic, pancreatic, ureteral, prostatic, bladder
Lymphoma and leukemia
Thymoma and mesothelioma
Central Nervous System (CNS) Disorders
Trauma
Infection
Tumors
Porphyria
Pulmonary Disorders
Tuberculosis
Pneumonia
Ventilators with positive pressure

The typical features of SIADH are listed in Table 77–9. The cardinal results of the sustained water conservation in SIADH are twofold: hyponatremia and volume expansion. In fact, patients with SIADH who are allowed free access to water generally gain about 3 kg in water weight, or, in other words, nearly 10 per cent of body water. In that respect, patients with SIADH differ from those with hyponatremia secondary to salt depletion, Addison's disease, or diuretic excess, since patients with the latter disorders are volume contracted. However, patients with SIADH, although volume expanded, do not develop edema and thus differ in that respect from patients with congestive heart failure or cirrhosis.

When total body water is expanded by about 10 per cent by water conservation in SIADH, a natriuresis occurs even in the face of hyponatremia. Thus the patient with SIADH reaches a steady state in which body water is expanded by water retention and in which natriuresis, even in the face of hyponatremia, prevents edema formation.

The causes for the natriuresis that is characteristic of SIADH are multiple. Volume expansion will result in enhanced release of atriopeptin, which enhances urinary sodium wasting both by enhancing glomerular filtration and probably by suppressing tubular sodium absorption. Second, the volume expansion of SIADH also reduces the rate of proximal tubular sodium absorption, as well as the rate of proximal uric acid absorption.

In short, SIADH is a disorder in which hormone-stimulated water conservation results in hyponatremia, volume expansion, and consequently an increased glomerular filtration rate, tubular sodium wasting, and reduced net tubular absorption of creatinine and uric acid, but no edema formation. These

TABLE 77–9. MAJOR CHARACTERISTICS OF SIADH

Hyponatremia
Volume expansion without edema
Natriuresis
Hypouricemia
Normal or reduced serum creatinine level
Normal thyroid and adrenal function

characteristics are summarized in Table 77–9. Finally, as indicated in connection with Figure 77–4, the urine osmolality in patients with SIADH may be either inappropriately high for the level of serum osmolality or maximally dilute.

OTHER CAUSES OF EXCESSIVE ADH PRODUCTION AND/OR RELEASE. Table 77–7 lists other circumstances in which an increased level of ADH is the primary factor responsible for hyponatremia. A number of commonly used drugs stimulate ADH release: vincristine, cyclophosphamide, carbamazepine, phenothiazines, morphine, barbiturates, chlorpropamide, amitriptyline, thiothixene, and clofibrate. Chlorpropamide also potentiates the effect of ADH on the water permeability of collecting ducts. The posterior pituitary peptide oxytocin (Pitocin) also has an antidiuretic action, although oxytocin is a much less potent antidiuretic agent than vasopressin. Thus the administration of intravenous hypotonic solutions containing oxytocin for the purpose of inducing labor may result in profound hyponatremia. Trauma or surgical stress also stimulates ADH release.

Ordinarily, diuretic-induced hyponatremia is related to volume contraction; this kind of body fluid dilution will be discussed below. Chronic severe potassium depletion induced by diuretics also can result in ADH release, although the mechanisms by which potassium depletion stimulates ADH release are unknown.

Mixed Disorders. Hyponatremia occurs commonly in true volume contraction and in edematous states in which filling of the arterial tree is impaired. The former disorders include patients in whom both ECF and total body water are reduced; the latter group comprises those patients with deranged Starling forces, notably local or systemic increases in venous pressure, which result in inadequate filling of the arterial tree. In both sets of disorders, two factors contribute, individually or in unison, to the pathogenesis of hyponatremia: nonosmotic, volume-mediated ADH release and reductions in the rate of sodium delivery to the diluting segment.

Volume contraction is a potent nonosmotic stimulus to ADH release. Figure 77–5 shows the relations between osmotic and nonosmotic, volume-mediated stimuli and plasma ADH levels in experimental animals; entirely comparable responses occur in humans. Increases in plasma osmolality are related linearly to increases in plasma ADH levels. The relation between blood volume depletion and plasma ADH levels is nonlinear. However, with depletion of more than 7 to 10 per cent blood volume, plasma ADH levels rise sharply and produce an antidiuretic effect even when the plasma osmolality is reduced below normal. In other words, volume-mediated, nonosmotic ADH release occurs primarily when circulatory dynamics are moderately to severely advanced; in that circumstance, volume-mediated stimuli over-ride osmotically mediated ADH release, and hyponatremia ensues.

A second factor that accounts for hyponatremia in volume-contracted states is an inability to dilute urine maximally because the rate of sodium delivery to diluting segments in the thick ascending limb is reduced. This occurs because increased rates of proximal tubular sodium absorption are stimulated by reduced sodium intake or by inadequate filling of the arterial tree in conditions with combined ECF volume expansion and reduced arterial tree filling. The significance of volume contraction as a pathogenic factor in this type of hyponatremia can be gauged by noting that hyponatremia occurs during volume contraction in experimental animals with pituitary diabetes insipidus.

Hyponatremia is a common feature of untreated Addison's disease and occurs because of a combination of circumstances. In mineralocorticoid deficiency, ECF volume contraction, glomerular filtration reduction, enhanced proximal tubular salt absorption, and volume-mediated, nonosmotic ADH release appear to be the major factors responsible for an inability to handle water loads. Glucocorticoid deficiency also impairs the ability to handle water loads. One of the factors responsible

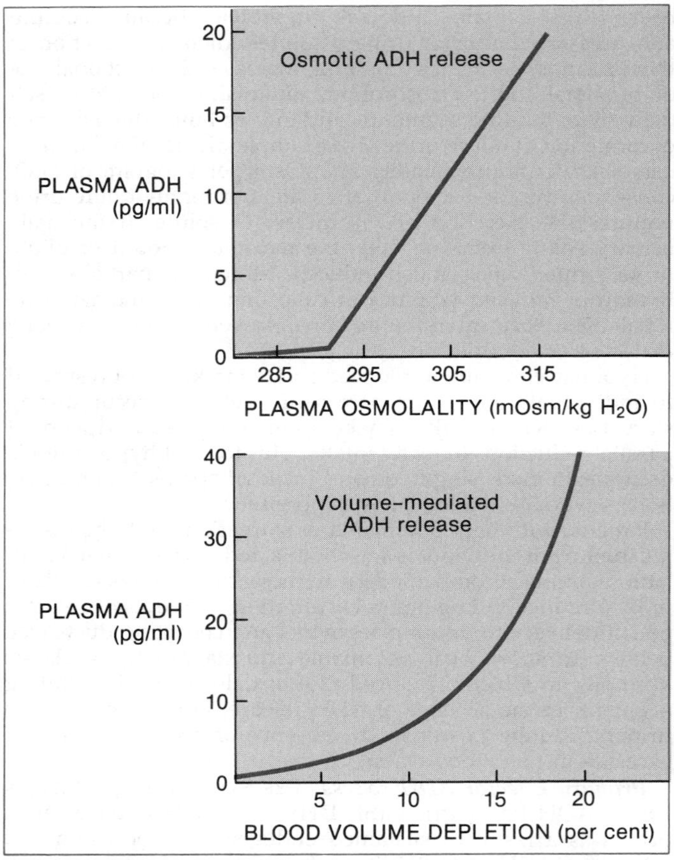

FIGURE 77–5. Relation between plasma ADH concentrations and either effective ECF osmolality (upper plot) or the per cent of blood volume depletion (lower plot). (Adapted from Dunn FL, Brennan TJ, Nelson AE, et al.: The role of blood osmolality and volume in regulating vasopressin secretion in the rat. J Clin Invest 52:3212, 1973.)

for water retention in Addison's disease is nonosmotic ADH release, which results from impaired cardiac function.

Hyponatremia occurs commonly in advanced stages of disorders characterized by edema formation and a reduced effective circulating volume (Table 77–7), particularly in intractable heart failure and advanced hepatic cirrhosis with ascites. Reduced rates of salt delivery to diluting segments of the renal tubule clearly contribute to the impairment in water excretion in these disorders. In patients with heart failure or severe ascites, the plasma concentrations of ADH tend to be inappropriately high with respect to plasma osmolality, so that nonosmotic ADH release may contribute to the development of hyponatremia in these disorders. Furthermore, since nonosmotic ADH release occurs only with profound reductions in blood volume (Fig. 77–5), the occurrence of hyponatremia in congestive failure or cirrhosis indicates profound arterial underfilling. This observation correlates well with the ominous prognosis of hyponatremia in these disorders.

CLINICAL MANIFESTATIONS. The clinical features of hyponatremia are produced by the brain swelling that accompanies acute dilution of total body water and generally become manifest when the serum sodium concentration falls to 120 mEq per liter or less. The early symptoms include lethargy, weakness, and somnolence, which proceed rapidly to seizures, coma, and death as hyponatremia worsens. Untreated acute water intoxication is nearly uniformly fatal and represents a medical emergency. In chronic hyponatremia, central nervous system manifestations are far less common, even when the serum sodium concentration is as low as 100 mEq per liter, because the loss of brain solutes, principally potassium chloride, minimizes brain cell swelling for a given reduction in body water osmolality.

DIAGNOSIS. Hyponatremia should be considered whenever there is a sudden deterioration in central nervous system function, particularly in circumstances such as intractable heart failure, hepatic cirrhosis with ascites, or the administration of large volumes of intravenous fluids. The hyponatremic patient should be evaluated to determine the underlying condition that produced body fluid dilution. This evaluation should include a careful history and physical examination; measurement of the serum creatinine, BUN, and electrolytes; measurement of the urinary sodium concentration, or the FE_{Na}; measurement of serum and urine osmolalities; and, when appropriate, evaluation of thyroid and adrenal function.

The history and physical examination are generally adequate for recognizing disorders such as beer potomania or compulsive water ingestion or for noting the ingestion of drugs that stimulate ADH release or enhance ADH action. The presence of edema is characteristic of individuals in whom hyponatremia occurs because of a reduced effective circulating volume coupled to ECF volume expansion. In myxedema or Addison's disease, the typical clinical or laboratory findings of these disorders are generally present (Ch. 229 and 230).

The most difficult differential diagnosis among hyponatremic disorders involves the distinction between patients who are modestly volume contracted and those who have SIADH. In both circumstances, the serum sodium and the serum osmolality are reduced, whereas the urine osmolality is inappropriately high with respect to the reduced serum osmolality. Nonosmotic water conservation in SIADH and in volume contraction is recognized by the presence of a urine osmolality greater than 120 to 150 mOsm per kilogram of H_2O in association with a reduced serum osmolality. The distinction between the two disorders therefore depends on a clinical and laboratory assessment of effective circulating volume.

Patients who are volume contracted may provide a history of volume losses or of diuretic ingestion and may exhibit the signs of ECF volume contraction discussed previously in the section on Volume Depletion. When the volume losses are due to extrarenal causes, the urinary sodium concentration is less than 10 to 15 mEq per liter and the FE_{Na} is generally less than 1 per cent. The presence of hyperuricemia may also be a useful index to the possibility of ECF volume contraction. Prerenal azotemia may occur if the volume contraction is severe. Patients with SIADH are generally normovolemic or slightly volume expanded and therefore exhibit none of the signs of volume contraction. The serum BUN and creatinine levels are normal, and the serum uric acid level is generally reduced. The urinary sodium concentration usually exceeds 30 mEq per liter, and the FE_{Na} is greater than 1 per cent. Tests of adrenal function yield normal results.

The above studies usually discriminate between SIADH and extrarenal volume contraction. When ECF volume contraction is due to renal salt wasting, urinary sodium losses generally persist unless volume contraction is profound. Moreover, as noted previously (see Volume Depletion), the blood pressure and pulse may be normal in states of modest volume contraction. A useful diagnostic and therapeutic maneuver in this situation is to observe the results of water restriction. When water intake is restricted to 600 to 800 ml daily, patients with SIADH exhibit a highly characteristic response: A 2- to 3-kg weight loss is accompanied by correction of hyponatremia and cessation of salt wasting, usually over a period of two to three days. If weight loss fails to correct both hyponatremia and urinary sodium wasting simultaneously, the diagnosis of SIADH is doubtful. Rather, renal sodium wasting with ECF volume contraction, due to Addison's disease or the other renal salt-losing disorders listed in Table 77–2, is the more probable diagnosis.

TREATMENT. The goal of treatment in hyponatremia is to correct body water osmolality and therefore restore cell volume to normal by raising the ratio of sodium to water in extracellular fluid. The increase in ECF osmolality draws water from cells and therefore reduces their volume. The choice of therapeutic approach, and whether or not net sodium and water balance is adjusted to be positive or negative during therapy, depends on the serum sodium concentration, the rate at which hyponatremia has developed, the clinical status of the patient, and the underlying disorder.

Acute Hyponatremia. Acute hyponatremia associated with a serum sodium concentration below 120 mEq per liter and with central nervous system manifestations requires immediate therapy. In volume-contracted states, the treatment of choice is to raise the serum sodium level to 125 mEq per liter over a six-hour interval by administering hypertonic 3 to 5 per cent saline. Since the desired effect is to correct body water osmolality, the amount of sodium administered must be sufficient to raise total body water osmolality to approximately 250 mOsm per kilogram of H_2O, that is, to approximately twice the desired serum sodium concentration. A convenient formula for calculating this sodium requirement is as follows:

$$[125 - \text{measured serum Na}^+] \times 0.6 \text{ body weight} = \text{required mEq of Na}^+$$

The serum sodium level is in milliequivalents per liter, and the body weight is in kilograms. Since 60 per cent of body weight is water, the formula allows an estimate of the amount of sodium required to raise body water osmolality to 250 mOsm per kilogram of H_2O.

The administration of hypertonic saline solutions is hazardous in volume-expanded, salt-retaining states such as congestive heart failure. Furthermore, in SIADH associated with volume expansion and sodium wasting, hypertonic saline alone is ineffective in correcting hyponatremia because the administered salt is excreted promptly in a relatively concentrated urine.

A preferable alternative is to use normal saline in combination with furosemide administration. The diuretic induces urinary salt loss and therefore reduces the risk of ECF volume expansion. Moreover, the diuresis induced by furosemide is characterized by the excretion of urine having a sodium concentration that is appreciably lower than that in plasma. Consequently, the combination of intravenously administered normal saline with a furosemide-induced diuresis of urine that is dilute with respect to plasma provides an effective way of raising the serum sodium level in SIADH or other volume-expanded states. By adjusting the rates of salt administration to be less than urinary salt losses, reductions in ECF volume can be produced simultaneously.

Rapid elevation of serum sodium concentrations to levels greater than 125 mEq per liter is hazardous. Since loss of brain solute represents one of the compensatory mechanisms for preserving brain cell volume in dilutional states, a serum sodium level of 140 mEq per liter may be relatively hypertonic to brain cells that have become partially depleted of solute as a result of hyponatremia. Consequently, raising the serum sodium rapidly to levels greater than 120 to 125 mEq per liter can result in central nervous system damage.

Chronic Hyponatremia. Mild, asymptomatic chronic hyponatremia is generally managed by correction of the underlying disorder, when the hyponatremia occurs in volume contraction or in salt-retaining states such as congestive heart failure or hepatic cirrhosis with ascites. Chronic hyponatremia in SIADH may be easily corrected by restricting water intake to 800 to 1000 ml daily, provided that patients can adhere to the program of water restriction. An alternative approach involves the use of agents such as lithium or demethylchlortetracycline, which interfere with the renal tubular effects of ADH. However, both agents have other adverse effects. As another alternative, some workers have recommended reducing renal ability for urinary concentration by administering large oral loads of urea, thereby producing a modest osmotic diuresis.

HYPERTONIC DISORDERS

DEFINITION. A hypertonic disorder is one in which the ratio of solutes to water in total body water is increased. All hypernatremic states are hypertonic. In some hypertonic disorders, the increase in effective ECF osmolality is due to nonsodium solutes, for example, uncontrolled hyperglycemia.

ETIOLOGY AND PATHOGENESIS. Hypernatremia develops whenever water intake is less than the sum of renal and extrarenal water losses; in chronic hypertonic states, net water balance may be zero. The most common causes for clinically significant hypernatremia occur as a consequence of three pathogenic mechanisms: impaired thirst; solute or osmotic diuresis; excessive losses of water, either via the kidneys or extrarenally; and combinations of these derangements. These disorders are grouped in Table 77–10 according to the primary pathogenic mechanism. There is also a group of miscellaneous disorders, such as hypokalemia, hypercalcemia, and interstitial renal disease, and chronic renal failure, which either impair partially renal urinary concentrating ability or blunt partially the responsiveness of collecting ducts to ADH. These disorders rarely cause significant hypernatremia and will not be discussed further.

Inadequate Intake of Water. This problem occurs in patients who are comatose or who are otherwise unable to communicate thirst. Because of the exquisite sensitivity of thirst mechanisms to changes in effective body water osmolality, hypernatremia due to inadequate water intake is rare in conscious patients allowed free access to water. Rarely, patients will have a primary thirst deficiency. Patients with Cushing's syndrome or primary hyperaldosteronism commonly have slight elevations in the serum sodium level for unknown reasons.

Finally, "essential hypernatremia" is characterized by a slightly elevated serum sodium level that occurs in the conscious state. The defect in patients with essential hypernatremia appears to be an insensitivity of thirst centers and osmoreceptors to osmotic stimuli. However, both thirst and antidiuresis occur when these patients are volume contracted. Consequently, it has been inferred that volume-mediated stimuli to thirst and ADH release are intact in patients with essential hypernatremia. This disorder may be either congenital or acquired, sometimes in association with histiocytic infiltration of the central nervous system.

Osmotic Diuresis. This is another mechanism for producing renal water losses in excess of sodium losses and therefore hypertonicity. Osmotic diuresis occurs commonly in uncontrolled glycosuria and may occur during mannitol administration for the treatment of increased intracranial pressure. Since these solutes are restricted to the ECF, the serum sodium level is generally reduced in the early stages of osmotic diuresis, and the effective ECF osmolality is increased primarily by the impermeant nonsodium solute. In prolonged osmotic diuresis, net water losses may be sufficiently great that hypernatremia develops. In this circumstance, the increase in effective ECF osmolality is due to the combined effects of hypernatremia and the nonsodium solute. Hypernatremia due to an osmotic urea diuresis can occur if large amounts of protein and amino acids are administered by nasogastric tube, or if tissue catabolism is great, as in burns. In this circumstance, hypernatremia is entirely responsible for the increased effective ECF osmolality.

Hypernatremia may also occur when large amounts of hypertonic sodium solutions are administered, particularly in patients whose renal function is compromised. Two common examples of this condition include the rapid intravenous administration of multiple ampules of sodium bicarbonate during cardiopulmonary resuscitation and the administration of large amounts of sodium bicarbonate to patients with lactic acidosis.

Excessive Water Losses. Impairment of ADH production, release, or action, as in pituitary or nephrogenic diabetes insipidus, respectively, can lead to profound water deficits and to hypernatremia. In such circumstances, the urine volumes are large, the urine osmolality is low, and the net rate of solute excretion is low, in contrast to individuals undergoing osmotic diuresis, in whom rates of urinary solute excretion are elevated.

Striking water losses may also occur with excessive sweating, particularly during rigorous physical activity by untrained individuals exercising in high humidity. This phenomenon plays a major role in the evolution of heat stroke.

Combined Disorders. Finally, hypertonic dehydration may occur as a combination of these events. A common example in modern clinical practice involves the injudicious administration of large amounts of carbohydrate or amino acids by nasogastric tube, coupled with limited amounts of water, to stroke patients unable to communicate thirst.

CLINICAL MANIFESTATIONS AND DIAGNOSIS. Since two thirds of body water is intracellular, primary water losses tend to have modest effects on circulating volume unless fluid losses are profound. Rather, the clinical manifestations are produced by brain shrinkage that results from increases in effective ECF osmolality. Thus the symptoms of hypertonicity produced either by hypernatremia or by impermeant nonsodium solutes such as glucose are referable to the central nervous system and range from somnolence and confusion to coma, respiratory paralysis, and death. The degree of symptomatology varies with the degree of hypertonicity and with the rate at which hypertonicity develops. In acute hypertonicity, symptoms generally appear when the effective ECF osmolality exceeds 320 to 330 mOsm per kilogram of H_2O, and coma and respiratory arrest may occur when the ECF osmolality exceeds 360 to 380 mOsm per kilogram of H_2O. Chronic hypertonicity generally produces fewer central nervous system manifestations, because brain cells accumulate idiogenic osmoles, which minimize the tendency for brain shrinkage.

TREATMENT. The treatment of acute hypernatremia requires the administration of isotonic dilute saline solutions, generally by an intravenous route. The following factors should be borne in mind when treating acute hypernatremia.

In the severely volume-contracted patient with severe hypernatremia, the administration of isotonic saline solutions has two advantages. It provides fluid resuscitation in impending cardiovascular collapse. Moreover, the isotonic salt solution, which is hypotonic with respect to the hypertonic patient, avoids an unnecessary rapid fall in the serum sodium level.

Rapid correction of hypertonicity to a normal serum osmolality is hazardous. Since accumulation of idiogenic osmoles by brain cells is a compensatory mechanism for preserving brain volume in hypertonic disorders, a normal serum osmolality may be relatively hypotonic to brain cells that have accumulated idiogenic solutes. Hence if the serum osmolality is reduced rapidly, central nervous system damage due to brain swelling may occur. A useful guide to circumventing this difficulty is to reduce the serum sodium level by no more

TABLE 77–10. MAJOR CAUSES OF HYPERNATREMIA

- I. **Impaired Thirst**
  - Coma
  - Essential hypernatremia
- II. **Solute Diuresis**
  - Osmotic diuresis: diabetic ketoacidosis, nonketotic hyperosmolar coma, mannitol administration
- III. **Excessive Water Losses**
  - Renal
    - Pituitary diabetes insipidus
    - Nephrogenic diabetes insipidus
  - Extrarenal
    - Sweating
- IV. **Combined Disorders**
  - Coma plus hypertonic nasogastric feeding

than 1 mEq per liter during every two hours of the first two days of treatment.

Finally, if solutions of 5 per cent dextrose in water are administered at a rapid rate, hyperglycemia and osmotic diuresis may occur and hence aggravate the hypertonic state. In this circumstance, the use of a 2.5 per cent dextrose solution in one-quarter normal saline is advisable. This solution has been particularly useful in treating hypernatremia associated with volume contraction in children with pituitary or nephrogenic diabetes insipidus.

Anderson RJ, Chung H-M, Kluge R, et al.: Hyponatremia. A prospective analysis of its epidemiology and the pathogenetic role of vasopressin. Ann Intern Med 102:164, 1985. *A study of the frequency and causes of hyponatremia in hospitalized patients.*

Arieff AI: Hyponatremia, convulsions, respiratory arrest, and permanent brain damage after elective surgery in healthy women. N Engl J Med 314:1529, 1986. *A detailed analysis of the central nervous system complications of acute hyponatremia.*

Ayus JC, Krothapalli RK, Arieff AI: Changing concepts in treatment of severe symptomatic hyponatremia. Am J Med 78:897, 1985. *A review of the controversy surrounding the treatment of hyponatremia and its relation to central pontine myelinolysis.*

Buckalew VM Jr: Hyponatremia: Pathogenesis and management. Hosp Pract 21:49, 1986. *An excellent description of the treatment of hyponatremia.*

Gennari FJ: Serum osmolality—uses and limitations. N Engl J Med 310:102, 1984. *An introduction to the concepts of osmolality and tonicity with guides to the appropriate laboratory evaluation of osmolality disorders.*

Hebert SC, Culpepper RM, Andreoli TE: The posterior pituitary and water metabolism. In Wilson JD, Foster DW (eds.): Williams Textbook of Endocrinology. Philadelphia, W. B. Saunders Company, 1985, pp 614–652. *A complete discussion of the physiology of water metabolism, hypernatremia, and hyponatremia.*

Manning PT, Schwartz D, Katsube NC, et al.: Vasopressin-stimulated release of atriopeptin: Endocrine antagonists in fluid homeostasis. Science 229:395, 1985. *The role of atriopeptin in the negative feedback of water balance.*

Miller M, Dalakos T, Moses AM, et al.: Recognition of partial defects in antidiuretic hormone secretion. Ann Intern Med 73:721, 1970. *A concise guide to testing procedures for states of ADH insufficiency and a rational scheme for interpreting the test results.*

Narins RG, Jones ER, Stom MC, et al.: Diagnostic strategies in disorders of fluid, electrolyte and acid-base homeostasis. Am J Med 72:496, 1982. *A good clinical approach to osmolality disturbances.*

Thompson CS, Andreoli TE: Hyponatremia and hypernatremia. In Callaham ML (ed.): Current Therapy in Emergency Medicine. Philadelphia, B. C. Decker, 1987, pp 739–744. *A practical guide to the diagnosis and treatment of hyponatremia and hypernatremia.*

Zerbe R, Strope L, Robertson G: Vasopressin function in the syndrome of inappropriate diuresis. Ann Rev Med 31:315, 1980. *The patterns of ADH response in SIADH.*

Disturbances in Potassium Balance

PHYSIOLOGIC CONSIDERATIONS

The body contains approximately 3500 mEq of potassium, of which only 60 mEq, or about 2 per cent, is extracellular. In normal circumstances external potassium balance depends mainly on dietary potassium intake and renal potassium excretion; fecal potassium losses are only about 10 mEq per day unless diarrhea is present. Since 98 per cent of potassium is located intracellularly, primarily in skeletal muscle, regulation of the serum potassium concentration depends not only on external potassium balance but also on potassium exchanges between the intracellular and extracellular compartments.

Transfer Between ICF and ECF

The intracellular compartment acts as a large potassium reservoir in series with the small ECF potassium pool. In potassium-depleted states a 1 mEq per liter fall in the serum potassium level requires the loss of about 100 to 200 mEq of potassium; hence the bulk of external potassium loss comes from the cellular compartment. Conversely, if large amounts of potassium are administered acutely, the rise in serum potassium level is less than would be expected if the administered potassium were distributed solely in the ECF. In this situation, cellular uptake of potassium obviously occurs and prevents greater increases in the serum potassium concentration. This ability of cells to accumulate potassium can be enhanced strikingly by chronic administration of high-potassium diets.

A number of *effector* mechanisms regulate the partition of potassium between the ICF and ECF. These include active and passive ionic transcellular transport processes.

ACTIVE TRANSPORT PROCESSES. The cardinal transport process regulating K^+ distribution between ICF and ECF is cell membrane–bound (Na^+ + K^+)-ATPase, which actively transports potassium into cells and therefore counterbalances the passive leak of potassium from cells into interstitial fluid. Insulin is a second effector that promotes potassium transfer from ECF to ICF; this hormone promotes cellular uptake of potassium independently of cellular glucose uptake by increasing (Na^+ + K^+)-ATPase activity. Furthermore, hyperkalemia augments insulin release. Thus hyperkalemia may be the sensor that stimulates release of insulin, which then serves as an effector for potassium entry into cells. Finally, beta-adrenergic agents such as epinephrine and isoproterenol promote cellular uptake of potassium.

PASSIVE TRANSPORT PROCESSES. A number of passive effector mechanisms also regulate the partition of potassium between the ICF and the ECF. Alterations in the pH of ECF reproducibly shift potassium between the ICF and the ECF: Systemic acidosis, whether metabolic or respiratory, promotes potassium efflux from cells, whereas systemic alkalosis, either metabolic or respiratory, promotes cellular potassium uptake. As a general rule, a reduction in plasma pH of 0.1 unit raises the serum potassium level by 0.6 mEq per liter, whereas a plasma pH increase of 0.1 unit produces a similar reduction in serum potassium. The mechanisms for these pH-induced potassium shifts between ICF and ECF are not understood.

Second, cellular shrinkage produced by increases in effective ECF osmolality raises the intracellular potassium concentration and thereby increases the driving force for passive potassium leakage from the ICF to the ECF. This leakage may result in hyperkalemia when large glucose loads are administered to insulin-deficient diabetic patients who also have hyporeninemic hypoaldosteronism; the insulin lack limits cellular re-entry of potassium, and the aldosterone deficiency limits renal potassium excretion. Increases in cell potassium concentrations produced by cellular shrinkage also contribute significantly to the hyperkalemia of diabetic ketoacidosis, because hyperglycemia raises cell potassium levels by cell shrinkage and insulin lack prevents accelerated potassium reentry into cells.

Finally, brain cells and renal tubular cells lose potassium when exposed to chronic ECF hypotonicity. However, muscle cells, which are the largest component of ICF potassium, do not appear to participate in this process. Consequently, hypotonic disorders, by themselves, have little effect on the serum potassium level or on external potassium balance.

Renal Handling of Potassium

The kidneys process potassium strikingly differently from the way in which they process sodium. Sodium excretion involves filtration, partial tubular absorption, and appearance of nonabsorbed sodium as urinary sodium excretion. When dietary sodium intake is varied, there is a prompt adjustment in urinary sodium excretion, either in the upward direction, when sodium intake is increased, or in the downward direction, when sodium intake is curtailed.

In contrast, virtually all dietary potassium, ordinarily about 50 to 200 mEq per day, appears in the urine because of tubular secretion of potassium by terminal nephron segments. These regions of the nephron can increase rates of potassium secretion significantly if dietary potassium intake is augmented; and they carry out net absorption of potassium in kaliopenic states. In other words, these terminal nephron segments

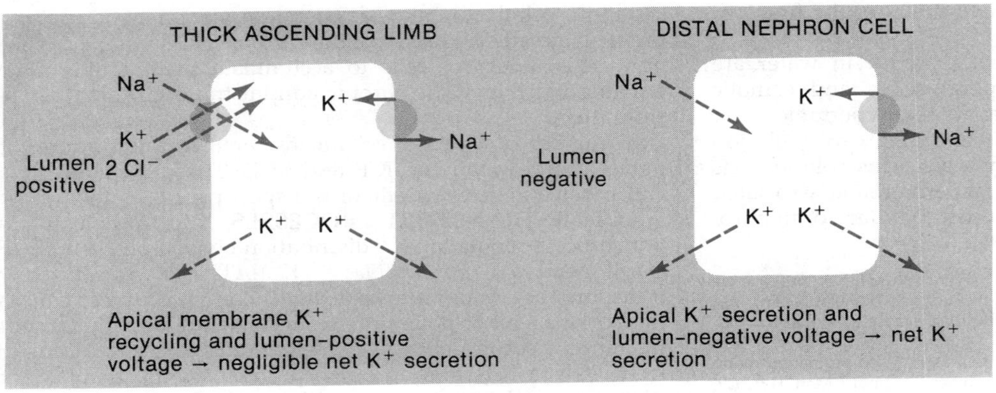

FIGURE 77–6. Handling of potassium in late nephron segments, including the thick ascending limb and the distal nephron. The dashed arrows represent passive transport processes and the solid arrows represent active transport processes. In the thick ascending limb, K^+ recycling into cells by Na^+:K^+:2 Cl^- cotransport and the lumen-positive voltage reduce the rate of net K^+ secretion. Most urinary K^+ comes from net K^+ secretion by terminal nephron segments.

regulate external potassium balance by adjusting *renal output* to balance *intake*.

A convenient way of considering distal nephron handling of potassium, and the ways in which effector mechanisms modulate this process, is shown in Figure 77–6. The dashed lines indicate passive processes, and the solid lines denote active transport processes. Basolateral membranes of all terminal nephron segments, including the thick limb of Henle, the distal tubule, and the collecting duct, share two common characteristics: a passive leakage pathway for K^+ efflux and an active (Na^+ + K^+)-ATPase for cellular K^+ uptake. The apical membranes of these nephron segments also contain passive potassium leakage pathways, which can be blocked by barium. In the thick ascending limb of Henle, apical membranes contain a furosemide-sensitive coupled entry step that involves electroneutral Na^+:K^+:2Cl^- cotransport, driven by the electrochemical sodium gradient between lumen and cells. In distal tubular and collecting ducts, Na^+ entry into cells involves sodium-specific channels that are blocked by amiloride. Thus in the ascending limb, coupled electroneutral sodium entry into cells does not result in luminal electronegativity (in fact, the lumen in the thick ascending limb is electropositive), whereas in the distal tubule and collecting duct, amiloride-sensitive ionic sodium entry produces luminal electronegativity.

The majority of net K^+ secretion occurs in these latter two segments and is driven indirectly by the rate of sodium entry into cells, which increases luminal electronegativity and increases the activity of basolateral (Na^+ + K^+)-ATPase, thus raising cell potassium concentrations. In the loop of Henle, little net potassium secretion occurs, because the lumen is electropositive and because coupled Na^+:K^+:2Cl^- transport from lumen to cells recycles secreted potassium back into cells.

The major elements of the *effector systems* that regulate distal nephron potassium excretion include the rate of distal tubular sodium delivery; dietary potassium intake; plasma pH; aldosterone; impermeant anions; and tubular flow rates. When distal sodium delivery rates are increased, increased sodium entry into cells across apical membranes is accompanied by increased activity of pump (Na^+ + K^+)-ATPase, which tends to raise intracellular potassium concentrations. Second, either an increase in dietary potassium intake or an increase in plasma pH tends, as indicated above, to raise cellular potassium content. Third, urinary excretion of impermeant anions such as sulfate, carbenicillin, or penicillin produces greater luminal electronegativity. Fourth, aldosterone and mineralocorticoids, whose kaliuretic effects may be dissociated from their sodium-sparing effects, increase the permeability of luminal membranes to potassium. These hormones may also augment distal tubular (Na^+ + K^+)-ATPase activity. Among these factors, the rate of aldosterone secretion and the rate of distal salt delivery to terminal nephron segments are the cardinal variables.

Each of the above factors modulates one or another portion of a generalized mechanism, namely, an electrochemical gradient favorable to the passive movement of potassium from tubular cells to urine and consequently for net potassium secretion. Conversely, reductions in sodium delivery, potassium restriction, reductions in plasma pH, and mineralocorticoid lack all reduce the magnitude of passive potassium movement from cells to tubular fluid and therefore tend to decrease net potassium secretion. Finally, increases in tubular flow rates, as in osmotic diuresis, also promote potassium secretion, whereas reductions in tubular flow rates decrease potassium secretion. The mechanism responsible for this effect is unknown.

The net rate of urinary potassium excretion in any given circumstance therefore depends on the interplay of these multiple factors in modulating the common effector mechanism for potassium secretion. For example, mineralocorticoid excess in primary aldosteronism commonly leads to severe potassium wasting. This kaliuresis can be curtailed by dietary sodium restriction and accentuated by dietary sodium loading. Conversely, in hyporeninemic hypoaldosteronism, hyperkalemia may be prevented by insuring a liberal intake of sodium.

The renal adaptation to excess potassium loads occurs over a 24- to 36-hour period. Consequently, hyperkalemia from the ingestion of large oral potassium loads is uncommon in normal individuals. But the renal response to dietary potassium restriction is more sluggish and requires seven to ten days for full development. Even under the latter circumstances, urinary potassium losses are rarely less than 20 mEq daily.

Excitable Tissues and the ICF/ECF Potassium Ratio

The clinical consequences of hypokalemia and hyperkalemia are generally due to changes in the excitable characteristics of heart, skeletal muscle, and smooth muscle. Excitable tissues, such as nerve, heart, and skeletal muscle, share certain common properties. At rest excitable tissues are far more permeable to potassium than to sodium. The cell interior is electronegative with respect to extracellular fluid, and this voltage is largely determined by the logarithm of the ratio of intracellular (K_i) to extracellular (K_o) potassium concentrations. When excitable tissues are suddenly depolarized to their threshold voltage, sodium permeability increases profoundly with an accompanying increase in the sodium to potassium permeability ratio. This sodium entry into the cells of excitable tissues occurs through sodium-specific channels having electronegative sites that are activated by sudden depolarization. During depolarization, rapid sodium entry produces the initial spike of the action potential, and the cell interior becomes electropositive.

This voltage-dependent increase in sodium permeability during depolarization to threshold is the most fundamental characteristic of excitable tissues (except in tissues such as the atrioventricular node, where Ca^{++} influx into cells is responsible for the action potential). If an excitable cell is partially depolarized in the resting state, the rate of rise of action potentials is reduced; the prolonged resting depolarization, by undefined mechanisms, reduces the increase in sodium permeability that accompanies the action potential. This effect of resting depolarization on reducing sodium permeability during action potentials is referred to as inactivation.

Repolarization of excitable cells occurs more slowly than depolarization. During repolarization, potassium permeability rises with respect to sodium permeability, and there is passive potassium efflux from the cell to the ECF. This potassium efflux restores the electronegativity of the cell interior. In nerve and skeletal muscle potassium efflux occurs almost immediately after the initial spike of the action potential. In cardiac muscle potassium efflux follows the absolute refractory period and coincides with the relative refractory period (phase 3) of the cardiac action potential.

Hyperkalemia reduces the K_i/K_o ratio and consequently partially depolarizes electrical tissues at rest. Hyperkalemia also increases the potassium permeability of excitable cells. The results of these changes on cardiac excitation are illustrated in the left hand panel of Figure 77–7. Because partial resting depolarization decreases the rate of sodium entry into cells during excitation, the rate of phase zero depolarization is slower and the peak of phase zero depolarization is markedly reduced. The increased potassium permeability accelerates repolarization and shortens the plateau phase. The net effect of progressive hyperkalemia is therefore to make the heart progressively refractory to excitation.

The effects of hypokalemia on excitable tissues are more complex. Because the K_i/K_o ratio rises in hypokalemia, excitable cells at rest should be hyperpolarized. This occurs initially, but resting depolarization eventually follows, because the high K_i/K_o ratio, by itself, reduces the potassium permeability of excitable cells. The effects of hypokalemia on cardiac muscle fibers are shown in the right hand panel of Figure 77–7. At rest the cell is partially depolarized because the reduced potassium permeability allows the high extracellular to intracellular sodium ratio to make the cell interior less negative. The initial spike of the action potential is less affected than in hyperkalemia because the reduced potassium permeability offsets the reduced sodium permeability during phase zero depolarization. Since potassium efflux determines the rate of repolarization, the reduced potassium permeability prolongs the relative refractory period. The net effect of these changes in cardiac tissue is to increase the likelihood of sinus bradycardia, and, because of a prolonged relative refractory period, the risk of arrhythmia formation. In skeletal muscle the reduction in membrane permeability to potassium produced by hypokalemia leads, in severe hypokalemia, to generalized paralysis.

HYPOKALEMIA AND POTASSIUM DEPLETION

DEFINITION. Chronic hypokalemia generally reflects a reduction in total body potassium. A 1-mEq reduction in serum potassium level generally implies the net loss of 100 to 200 mEq of potassium from the body. In extreme body potassium depletion the serum potassium level may be as low as 1.5 to 2.0 mEq per liter. Acute reductions in serum potassium level without parallel reductions in total body potassium occur when potassium is shifted from extracellular to intracellular compartments.

ETIOLOGY AND PATHOGENESIS. Hypokalemia and simultaneous potassium depletion occur whenever renal plus extrarenal potassium losses exceed potassium intake. In advanced body potassium depletion, intake and output of potassium may be equal. The four major causes for hypokalemia are given in Table 77–11.

Inadequate Intake. Reduced potassium intake may result in potassium depletion and hypokalemia because maximal renal conservation of potassium requires, as indicated above, seven to ten days. During this interval, the net renal potassium loss may be as much as 150 to 200 mEq.

Excessive Renal Losses. Many of the causes for renal potassium wasting can be analyzed in terms of factors that modulate the common effector system for potassium secretion. *Mineralocorticoid excess* accelerates distal tubular potassium secretion (Fig. 77–6). Consequently, hypokalemia occurs regularly in primary hyperaldosteronism, in Cushing's syndrome, and in secondary hyperaldosteronism. *Chronic licorice ingestion* produces a syndrome that mimics primary hyperaldosteronism, because glycyrrhizinic acid, a component of licorice extract, has physiologic properties similar to those of aldosterone.

In *Bartter's syndrome* sodium chloride wasting and secondary aldosteronism may contribute to potassium depletion (Ch. 84). However, potassium depletion in Bartter's syndrome may also occur either when aldosterone secretion rates are normal or following bilateral adrenalectomy. Consequently, it is believed that a tubular defect in potassium handling also contributes to the hypokalemia of Bartter's syndrome.

Most diuretics having a locus of action prior to the late distal tubule (Table 77–5) increase urinary potassium losses. Enhanced sodium delivery to distal nephron segments is the major factor responsible for the kaliuresis produced by these diuretics, and sodium restriction or volume depletion tends to minimize diuretic-induced potassium losses. Carbonic anhydrase inhibitors such as acetazolamide inhibit proximal bicarbonate absorption and thereby accentuate potassium losses. Distal tubular segments are relatively impermeable to

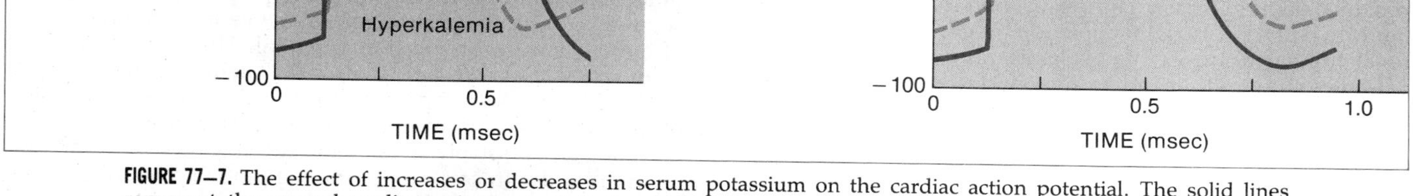

FIGURE 77–7. The effect of increases or decreases in serum potassium on the cardiac action potential. The solid lines represent the normal cardiac action potential; the dashed lines represent the cardiac action potential with either hyperkalemia (*left*) or hypokalemia (*right*).

TABLE 77–11. MAJOR CAUSES OF HYPOKALEMIA

I. Inadequate Intake	III. Gastrointestinal Losses
II. Excess Renal Loss	Vomiting
Mineralocorticoid excess	Diarrhea, particularly secretory diarrheas
Bartter's syndrome	Villous adenoma
Diuresis	IV. ECF → ICF Shifts
Diuretics with a pre–late distal locus	Acute alkalosis
Osmotic diuresis	Hypokalemic periodic paralysis
Chronic metabolic alkalosis	Barium ingestion
Antibiotics	Insulin therapy
Carbenicillin	Vitamin B_{12} therapy
Gentamicin	Thyrotoxicosis (rarely)
Amphotericin B	
Renal tubular acidosis	
Distal-gradient limited	
Proximal	
Liddle's syndrome	
Acute leukemia	
Ureterosigmoidostomy	

bicarbonate; consequently, increased delivery of bicarbonate to distal nephron regions has an impermeant anion effect that increases luminal electronegativity in these nephron regions.

Osmotic diuresis is commonly associated with increased renal potassium losses, because increased tubular flow rates enhance net potassium secretion. In diabetic ketoacidosis renal potassium losses are common. Yet patients with diabetic ketoacidosis and a reduced total body potassium commonly present with hyperkalemia, because metabolic acidosis tends to promote potassium shifts from the ICF to the ECF. Consequently, profound hypokalemia may develop if body potassium is not replenished concomitantly with insulin therapy and ECF volume expansion (Ch. 231).

Potassium depletion is seen frequently in *chronic metabolic alkalosis*. When the alkalosis is associated with volume contraction, secondary hyperaldosteronism results in renal potassium losses. Potassium depletion in chronic metabolic alkalosis is also enhanced if bicarbonaturia is present, because of the impermeant anion effect produced by bicarbonate delivery to terminal nephron segments. In fact, the hypokalemia associated with upper gastrointestinal fluid losses, as in vomiting or nasogastric suction, is primarily the result of the renal potassium losses produced by secondary hyperaldosteronism or bicarbonaturia or both. The potassium losses from the upper gastrointestinal tract are small, since upper gastrointestinal tract fluid contains only about 10 mEq of potassium per liter.

Hypokalemia may develop during therapy with certain *antibiotics*. Carbenicillin or other penicillin-like antibiotics exist as sodium or potassium salts of impermeant anions and promote kaliuresis because they increase net sodium excretion and because of an impermeant anion effect. Amphotericin B increases the permeability of luminal membranes to potassium and therefore promotes potassium secretion. Gentamicin produces potassium losses by unknown mechanisms.

Hypokalemia and potassium depletion are common findings in *distal, gradient-limited renal tubular acidosis* (Ch. 84). Increased distal sodium delivery and the impermeant anion effect produced by bicarbonate wasting account for most of the potassium losses seen in proximal renal tubular acidosis. Consequently, salt restriction, which enhances the rate of proximal sodium bicarbonate absorption in this disorder, also tends to correct potassium depletion. In gradient-limited distal renal tubular acidosis, hypokalemia may be accentuated by volume losses and secondary hyperaldosteronism. Other factors, not yet understood, also contribute to hypokalemia in this disorder. Hyperkalemia, rather than hypokalemia, commonly accompanies the hyperchloremic acidosis of interstitial disease (type IV acidosis).

Liddle's syndrome is a rare tubular disorder characterized by hypokalemia, metabolic alkalosis, hypertension, and normal aldosterone secretion rates. Therapy with triamterene, but not with aldosterone antagonists such as spironolactone, ameliorates the disorder. These findings suggest that terminal nephron sodium avidity and potassium secretion independent of aldosterone are major factors in the pathogenesis of Liddle's syndrome. Thus in operational terms, Liddle's syndrome may be described as distal nephron hyperfunction, in regard to Na^+ absorption and H^+ and K^+ secretion.

Gastrointestinal Losses. These provide the major route for potassium depletion, other than the kidney. As indicated above, potassium depletion associated with vomiting is referable primarily to renal potassium losses. Diarrhea produces significant potassium losses, since diarrheal fluid contains 30 mEq per liter of potassium. The most striking diarrheal potassium losses occur in secretory diarrheas, such as with non–beta islet cell tumors of the pancreas, which produce vasoactive intestinal polypeptide, and in laxative abuse. In both secretory diarrheas and chronic laxative abuse, hypokalemia is probably caused by increased rates of K^+ secretion through apical membrane K^+ channels. Villous adenomas of the colon produce potassium depletion because of excessive colonic K^+ secretion from the adenoma. Hypokalemia is uncommonly seen in inflammatory bowel disease.

ECF-ICF Shifts. Acute hypokalemia with a normal total body potassium may occur because of *potassium shifts* from the ECF to the ICF. In *hypokalemic periodic paralysis*, acute shifts of potassium from the ECF to the ICF produce limb and trunk paralysis. The periodic attacks are often precipitated by high-carbohydrate meals. Patients with the disorder can often abort attacks by exercising affected muscles. The chronic use of acetazolamide can prevent attacks. A condition resembling hypokalemic periodic paralysis occurs with the ingestion of *barium salts* and is endemic in China, where the disorder is referred to as "Pa-Ping." Barium appears to produce hypokalemia by blocking K^+ channels in skeletal muscle and thus blocking efflux of potassium from the ICF to the ECF. *Insulin* therapy and *vitamin B_{12}* therapy also promote potassium shifts from the ECF to the ICF. Hypokalemia can also result rarely from thyrotoxicosis, especially in Asian males, for reasons that are unclear.

CLINICAL MANIFESTATIONS. The clinical effects of potassium deficiency are manifest in one or more organ systems, including skeletal muscle, heart, kidneys, and the gastrointestinal tract. The most serious disturbances are those affecting the neuromuscular system. At serum potassium concentrations in the range of 2 to 2.5 mEq per liter, muscular weakness is likely to occur; with more severe hypokalemia, the patient may develop areflexic paralysis, in which case respiratory insufficiency is an immediate threat to survival. The severity of the neuromuscular disturbance tends to be proportional to the speed with which the potassium level has declined.

Losses of large amounts of potassium from skeletal muscle may be accompanied by rhabdomyolysis and myoglobinuria. Hence, rhabdomyolysis sometimes occurs in military recruits subject to severe exercise, sweating, and ECF volume contraction. The secondary hyperaldosteronism that follows excessive salt loss produces urinary potassium wasting and consequently potassium depletion. Potassium depletion secondary to malnutrition and vomiting is also one of the pathogenic mechanisms in alcoholic rhabdomyolysis.

The electrocardiographic abnormalities of potassium depletion, shown in Figure 77–8, affect primarily repolarization segments of the electrocardiogram, in keeping with the effects of hypokalemia on the action potential. The common electrocardiographic manifestations of hypokalemia include sagging of the ST segment, depression of the T wave, and elevation of the U wave. With marked hypokalemia, the T wave becomes progressively smaller and the U waves show increasing amplitude. In some cases the merging of a flat or positive T wave with a positive U wave may erroneously be interpreted as a prolonged QT interval. Ordinarily, there are no serious clinical consequences from the abnormalities in cardiac exci-

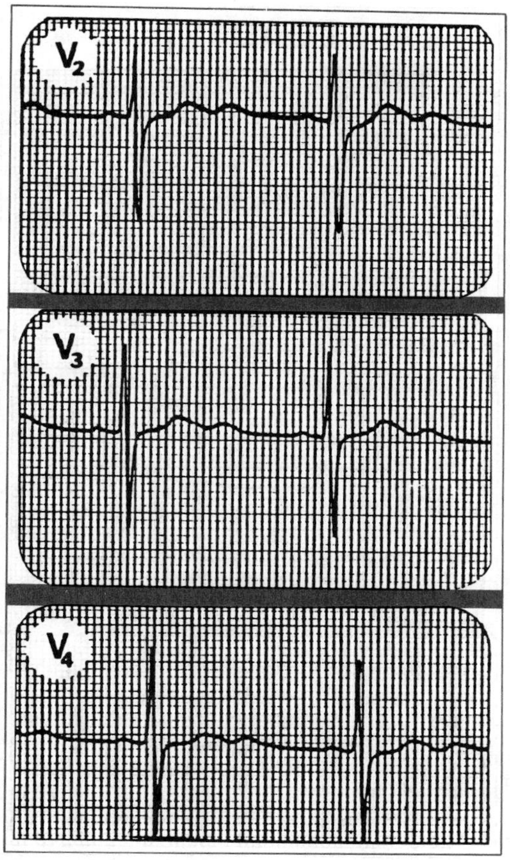

FIGURE 77–8. The electrocardiographic manifestations of hypokalemia. The serum potassium was 2.2 mEq/L. Note that the ST segment is prolonged, primarily because of a V wave following the T wave, and that the T wave is flattened.

tation. In patients treated with digitalis hypokalemia may precipitate serious arrhythmias.

Longstanding potassium depletion may produce renal tubular damage, referred to as hypokalemic nephropathy. Potassium deficiency also affects smooth muscle of the gastrointestinal tract and can result in paralytic ileus.

TREATMENT. The treatment of hypokalemia involves replacement therapy with potassium salts and attempts to correct the underlying disorder. Since diuretic abuse is probably the most common cause for hypokalemia in routine clinical practice, every attempt should be made to identify diuretic ingestion.

Except in extreme circumstances, oral rather than parenteral potassium replacement is prudent. However, when gastrointestinal function is impaired, or when neuromuscular manifestations of hypokalemia are present, parenteral therapy with potassium may be advisable. Since potassium deficits involve both the ICF and the ECF, their correction requires the transfer of administered potassium from the ECF into the ICF. The major problem in parenteral therapy is to avoid intravenous administration of potassium at rates sufficiently great to produce hyperkalemia. A prudent protocol to follow is to add potassium chloride to intravenous solutions at a final concentration of 40 to 60 mEq per liter and to administer no more than 10 to 20 mEq of potassium per hour. Except in unusual circumstances, the total amount of potassium administered daily should not exceed 200 mEq. The serum potassium level should be monitored at appropriate intervals; the frequency of monitoring should be determined by the patient's clinical condition, by the initial serum potassium, by the rate at which the serum potassium changes in a given patient, and by the patient's renal function. Because the electrocardiographic manifestations of hypokalemia are subtle, the electrocardiogram should not be used as a guide to replacement therapy.

Although potassium chloride is the salt of choice for intravenous potassium replacement, oral potassium chloride solutions are not well tolerated because of gastrointestinal irritation. Enteric-coated potassium chloride tablets are to be avoided, because they produce small bowel ulcerations. Oral potassium is administered most conveniently in the form of organic salts such as gluconate or citrate. This form of therapy is, however, not effective in hypokalemic metabolic alkalosis with hypochloremia. In this circumstance, chloride supplementation is required together with potassium replacement and is most easily achieved by administering sodium chloride supplementation.

HYPERKALEMIA AND POTASSIUM EXCESS

DEFINITION. Chronic hyperkalemia can occur with little or no increase in total body potassium. However, acute increases in serum potassium concentrations, produced by potassium shifts from the ICF to the ECF, can occur even when total body potassium is normal or reduced.

ETIOLOGY AND PATHOGENESIS. Hyperkalemia develops whenever the rate of potassium intake or the rate of potassium efflux from cellular to extracellular fluids exceeds the sum of renal plus extrarenal potassium losses. The renal mechanisms for potassium excretion adapt efficiently to increases in the rate of potassium influx to extracellular fluid, particularly from dietary sources. Hence acute or chronic hyperkalemia due to exogenous potassium intake is uncommon, unless renal mechanisms for potassium excretion are compromised. In the latter setting injudicious potassium administration may result in hyperkalemia. This occurs most commonly when intravenous potassium chloride is administered too rapidly; when potassium salts of antibiotics such as penicillin are administered; when transfusions are given with blood that has been stored for long periods of time; or when salt substitutes containing potassium are used. The occurrence of hyperkalemia in these settings usually requires that renal potassium excretion be impaired.

Acute or chronic hyperkalemia occurs most commonly either because of diminished *renal excretion* or because there is a sudden *transcellular shift* of potassium from the ICF to the ECF. The major causes for hyperkalemia listed in Table 77–12 follow this format.

Diminished Renal Excretion. Hyperkalemia may occur in *acute oliguric renal failure* of any cause. In *chronic renal failure* hyperkalemia generally does not occur until the glomerular filtration rate has reached markedly low levels. Hyperkalemia may be precipitated in chronic renal failure, however, either by the development of acidosis or, as indicated above, by the injudicious administration of potassium salts. Hyperkalemia also occurs with little or modest reduction in the glomerular filtration rate, if there is impairment of potassium secretion by terminal nephron regions. This occurs in *Addison's disease,* in *hyporeninemic hypoaldosteronism,* and with the injudicious

TABLE 77–12. MAJOR CAUSES OF HYPERKALEMIA

I. Diminished Renal Excretion	II. Transcellular Shifts
Reduced GFR	Acidosis
Acute oliguric renal failure	Cell destruction
Chronic renal failure	Trauma, burns
Reduced tubular secretion	Rhabdomyolysis
Addison's disease	Hemolysis
Hyporeninemic hypoaldosteronism	Tumor lysis
Potassium-sparing diuretics	Hyperkalemic periodic paralysis
	Diabetic hyperglycemia
	Insulin dependence plus aldosterone lack
	Depolarizing muscle paralysis
	Succinylcholine

GFR = Glomerular filtration rate

administration of *potassium-sparing diuretics* such as triamterene or spironolactone. The tendency toward hyperkalemia in these circumstances can be aggravated by ECF volume contraction, which reduces sodium delivery to terminal nephron segments, or by acidosis, which promotes cellular potassium efflux.

Transcellular Shifts. The second class of disorders causing acute hyperkalemia includes situations in which there is an abrupt shift of potassium from the ICF to the ECF. This occurs in acidosis or in circumstances that result in *cell destruction;* the latter occurs commonly with tissue trauma, burns, rhabdomyolysis, or hemolysis, and with lysis of large masses of tumor cells. As indicated previously, hypokalemia predisposes to rhabdomyolysis. Thus the sudden occurrence of hyperkalemia in potassium-depleted patients is a diagnostic clue to the development of rhabdomyolysis.

Hyperkalemic periodic paralysis is an autosomal dominant disorder in which sudden increases in serum potassium level result in muscle paralysis. The hyperkalemia is often provoked by dietary potassium intake or by exercise. Myotonia occurs commonly in the disorder and appears either between attacks or immediately preceding attacks. The pathogenesis of the disorder is not understood. The acute paralytic attack can be treated by intravenous administration of calcium gluconate or glucose and insulin. Chronic treatment with diuretics such as acetazolamide minimizes the frequency of attacks.

Paradoxical hyperkalemia occurs when *sudden hyperglycemia* develops in insulin-dependent diabetics who also have interstitial renal disease and associated hyporeninemic hypoaldosteronism. The sudden increase in ECF osmolality draws water from cells, raises intracellular potassium concentrations, and therefore promotes passive potassium efflux from cells. The insulin lack minimizes cellular re-entry of potassium, and the aldosterone deficiency blunts renal potassium excretion. Insulin therapy promptly corrects the hyperkalemia. Finally, anesthetic agents or other drugs that cause a *depolarizing muscle paralysis,* such as succinylcholine, promote potassium efflux from muscle cells. The loss of cell electronegativity in this situation increases passive potassium efflux from muscle cells.

Pseudohyperkalemia may occur in thrombocytosis or leukocytosis, because clotting of blood promotes potassium release from these cells and may be identified by noting that the *serum* potassium level is elevated while the *plasma* potassium level is normal. This kind of artifact occurs most commonly in patients with myeloproliferative disorders.

CLINICAL MANIFESTATIONS. The most important clinical manifestations of hyperkalemia relate to alterations in cardiac excitability. For this reason the electrocardiogram is the single most important guide in appraising the threat posed by hyperkalemia and in determining how aggressive a therapeutic approach is necessary.

The electrocardiographic manifestations of hyperkalemia, shown in Figure 77–9, follow directly from the effects of hyperkalemia on cardiac action potentials (Fig. 77–7). The earliest manifestation of hyperkalemia is the development of peaked T waves, which become evident when the serum potassium level exceeds 6.5 mEq per liter. This peaking of the T waves is a manifestation of the accelerated repolarization of the cardiac action potential produced by hyperkalemia. When the potassium concentration exceeds 7 to 8 mEq per liter, diminished cardiac excitability results in prolongation of the PR interval followed by a loss of P waves and widening of the QRS complex. These changes indicate progressive inexcitability of cardiac muscle and are referable to hyperkalemia-induced inactivation of sodium permeability during the initial spike of the action potential. When the serum potassium level exceeds 8 to 10 mEq per liter, the electrocardiogram may develop a sine wave pattern and cardiac standstill can occur.

The correlation between serum potassium concentrations and electrocardiographic abnormalities is approximate at best;

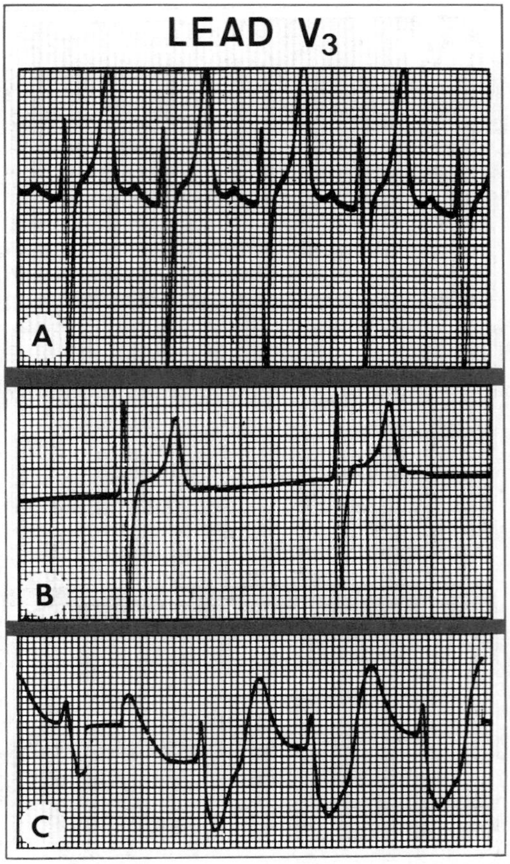

FIGURE 77–9. The effects of progressive hyperkalemia on the electrocardiogram. All of the illustrations are from lead V_3. *A,* Serum K^+ = 6.8 mEq/L; note the peaked T waves together with normal sinus rhythm. *B,* Serum K^+ = 7.7 mEq/L; note the peaked T waves and absent P waves. *C,* Serum K^+ = 8.9 mEq/L; note the classic sine wave with absent P waves, marked prolongation of the QRS complex, and peaked T waves.

in a given patient, progression from peaked T waves to a sine wave pattern may occur rapidly, particularly if the serum potassium concentration rises rapidly. Therefore the development of peaked T waves in conjunction with hyperkalemia should be viewed as a serious disorder; more advanced electrocardiographic manifestations of hyperkalemia should be treated as life-threatening medical emergencies.

TREATMENT. Three kinds of maneuvers are used in the treatment of hyperkalemia: agents such as glucose plus insulin or sodium bicarbonate, which promote the transfer of potassium from the ECF to the ICF; maneuvers that enhance potassium elimination from the body, such as diuretics, exchange resins, or dialysis; and the use of calcium, which does not alter serum potassium concentrations but counteracts the effects of hyperkalemia on cardiac excitability.

Both insulin and sodium bicarbonate promote potassium entry into cells. The administration of 25 grams of glucose, together with 10 units of regular insulin, is an effective way of reducing the serum potassium level rapidly. The glucose may be administered over 30 minutes as a 20 per cent solution, or it may be given as a 50 per cent glucose solution. Insulin promotes potassium entry into cells, and glucose is administered to prevent hypoglycemia. In insulin-dependent diabetic patients in whom sudden hyperglycemia has precipitated the hyperkalemia, insulin administration alone suffices to reduce the serum potassium concentration.

The administration of 40 to 150 mEq of sodium bicarbonate intravenously over a 30- to 60-minute interval also promotes potassium entry into cells, particularly if acidosis is also present. This maneuver should be used with caution in patients with compromised renal function because of the risks of hypernatremia and of ECF volume overload.

None of the maneuvers described above removes potassium from the body. Gastrointestinal potassium losses may be produced by the use of cation exchange resins in the sodium cycle, such as sodium polystyrene sulfonate (Kayexalate). Each gram of the resin contains approximately 1 mEq of sodium and exchanges for about 1 mEq of potassium. This stoichiometry is not precise, since the sodium form of the resin also exchanges for other cations in gastrointestinal secretions, including calcium. In chronic hyperkalemia, 20 grams of Kayexalate may be given three or four times a day in a 70 per cent solution of sorbitol. The sorbitol creates an osmotic diarrhea and enhances resin passage through the gastrointestinal tract. In acute circumstances, Kayexalate may also be administered by enema, generally as 100 grams of resin suspended in 200 ml of 20 per cent sorbitol. The use of chronic Kayexalate therapy in patients with chronic renal failure carries with it the risk of sodium overload.

In settings of extreme hyperkalemic cardiotoxicity, when P waves are absent and the QRS complexes are widened, the administration of calcium gluconate, 10 to 30 ml of a 10 per cent solution over a 10- to 20-minute interval, may be life saving. This approach should be undertaken with constant electrocardiographic monitoring and should be used with extreme caution in patients who have received digitalis. In the latter circumstance, calcium administration may unmask digitalis intoxication, especially if other agents are used simultaneously to reduce the serum potassium level. Calcium salts should not be added to bottles of intravenous fluids containing bicarbonate, because water-insoluble calcium salts will form.

The influence of calcium salts in minimizing the cardiotoxic effects of hyperkalemia may be understood by noting, as described in the section on Physiologic Considerations, that depolarization of excitable tissues by elevating serum K^+ concentrations inactivates sodium channels and that the extracellular sides of these sodium channels are electronegative. Divalent cations such as calcium provide a remarkably effective way of screening these electronegative sites. Thus calcium salts raise the voltage gradient across sodium channels by screening electronegative surface charges of these channels on their extracellular fluid sides and consequently restoring the voltage-dependent excitability of these channels.

Finally, acute hemodialysis or peritoneal dialysis provides another mechanism for potassium removal from the body. This approach is particularly advantageous in acute renal failure; when patients are volume expanded and sodium administration may produce congestive heart failure; or when there is a continued efflux of large amounts of potassium from the ICF to the ECF, as in burns or rhabdomyolysis.

Brown RS: Extrarenal potassium homeostasis. Kidney Int 30:116, 1986. *A summary of cellular uptake processes for potassium.*

Field MJ, Giebisch GH: Hormonal control of renal potassium excretion. Kidney Int 27:379, 1985. *A thorough account of renal potassium handling.*

Ponce SP, Jennings AE, Madias NE, et al.: Drug induced hyperkalemia. Medicine 64:357, 1985. *A summary of drugs that provoke hyperkalemia.*

Tannen RL: Potassium disorders. In Kokko JP, Tannen RL (eds.): Fluids and Electrolytes. Philadelphia, W. B. Saunders Company, 1986. *A complete discussion of hypokalemia and hyperkalemia.*

Tsien RW, Hess P: Excitable tissue—the heart. In Andreoli TE, Hoffman JF, Fanestil DD, et al. (eds.): Physiology of Membrane Disorders. New York, Plenum, 1986, pp 469–490. *A meticulous description of the ionic basis for the cardiac action potential.*

Disturbances in Acid-Base Balance

PHYSIOLOGIC CONSIDERATIONS

The pH of arterial blood and interstitial fluid normally ranges between 7.38 and 7.42 despite wide variations in dietary intake of acids or alkali. The arterial pH range over which cardiac function, metabolic activity, and central nervous system function can be maintained is narrow; the widest range of pH values compatible with life is from 6.8 to 7.8, or an interval of one pH unit.

The major buffer system in extracellular fluid is the bicarbonate–carbonic acid pair. The relation between pH, bicarbonate, and carbonic acid concentrations in ECF may be expressed according to the familiar Henderson-Hasselbalch equation:

$$\mathrm{pH} = \mathrm{pK} + \log \frac{\mathrm{HCO_3^-}}{\mathrm{H_2CO_3}}$$

where pK is the carbonic acid dissociation constant, HCO_3^- is the plasma bicarbonate concentration, and H_2CO_3 is the plasma carbonic acid concentration. The H_2CO_3 concentration is given by $\alpha PaCO_2$, where α is the CO_2 solubility constant, and has a value of 0.03, and $PaCO_2$ is the arterial carbon dioxide tension. Therefore, with a $PaCO_2$ of 40 mm Hg, the Henderson-Hasselbalch equation becomes the following:

$$7.4 = 6.1 + \log \frac{24 \text{ mM/L}}{1.2 \text{ mM/L}}$$

The arterial pH provides a qualitative, but not quantitative, index to total body water acid-base status because, at any given time, about two thirds of an acid or alkali load is buffered by proton shifts into or out of the ICF, respectively. For this reason, some prefer to use the term "acidemia" for acidosis and "alkalemia" for alkalosis to connote that plasma pH measurements provide quantitative information about the pH status of plasma and interstitial fluid and only qualitative information about total body acid-base balance.

A convenient way to consider the total body buffering capacity is as follows. Bicarbonate is predominantly an extracellular anion, and the total ECF bicarbonate content in a 70-kg man having 15 liters of ECF is (24 mEq/liter × 15 liters), or 360 mEq HCO_3^-. However, about two thirds of a given acid or alkali load is buffered within cells. Consequently, the total body buffering capacity, often referred to as the "bicarbonate space," is calculated as:

$$(\text{Arterial } \mathrm{HCO_3^-} \times 0.6 \text{ body weight})$$

that is, using total body water as an index to total buffering capacity. The bicarbonate space is also an index to net acid excess or net base excess. If the arterial HCO_3^- concentration in a 70-kg man is reduced to 15 mEq per liter while the $PaCO_2$ remains constant, the net acid excess (or net base deficit) is $(24-15)$ mEq/liter × 42 liters = 378 mEq. Conversely, if the arterial HCO_3^- concentration rises to 33 mEq per liter while the $PaCO_2$ remains constant, the net base excess (or acid deficit) is 378 mEq.

Proton shifts between the ECF and ICF stabilize the plasma pH against acute fluctuations. But the ultimate maintenance of pH balance requires that input of acid or base into the body be matched by output of acid or base, so that the HCO_3^-/H_2CO_3 ratio and the total bicarbonate content in the ECF remain constant. The cardinal systems involved in these external processes are the kidneys, for bicarbonate balance, and the lungs, for carbon dioxide balance.

Carbon Dioxide Production and Elimination

VOLATILE ACID INPUT. The largest source of endogenous acid production is from combustion of glucose and fatty acids to carbon dioxide and water or, in other words, to a volatile acid. During aerobic glycolysis, that is, cellular respiration, glucose oxidation involves oxygen utilization and carbon dioxide production according to the following reaction:

$$C_6H_{12}O_6 + 6O_2 \rightarrow 6CO_2 + 6H_2O$$

Since red blood cells contain carbonic anhydrase (c.a.), carbon dioxide hydration in erythrocytes yields the following:

$$CO_2 + H_2O \overset{c.a.}{\rightleftarrows} H_2CO_3 \rightleftarrows H^+ + HCO_3^-$$

The protons formed from carbonic acid dissociation are buffered by hemoglobin, whereas bicarbonate leaves red blood cells in exchange for chloride (the familiar chloride shift). In other words, carbon dioxide generation is equivalent to carbonic acid formation, and the bulk of hydrogen ion formed is buffered intracellularly.

A simple way of calculating the daily rate of nonvolatile acid production is to note, from the above reactions, that the production of 1 mole of metabolic water and 1 mole of carbon dioxide represents, through dissociation of carbonic acid, the formation of 1 mole of hydrogen ions.

Since the molecular weight of water is 18, 1 liter of water contains about 55 moles of water. Consequently, the average rate of metabolic water production, about 400 ml daily, yields 22,000 mmol of water and an equal number of carbon dioxide molecules. Thus the rate of volatile acid production amounts to about 22,000 mEq of hydrogen ion daily. The cellular combustion of carbohydrates and fatty acids to carbon dioxide and water is remarkably efficient. Under normal circumstances, organic anions such as lactate and ketoacids, which derive from incomplete combustion of carbohydrates and fatty acids, have plasma concentrations of approximately 5 mEq per liter.

VOLATILE ACID OUTPUT. Pulmonary ventilation excretes the carbon dioxide formed by cellular respiration. During blood transit through the lungs, bicarbonate re-enters red blood cells and combines with protons to form carbonic acid, which dissociates to carbon dioxide and water. The carbon dioxide so formed diffuses freely through red blood cells and alveolar epithelium, so that the rate of carbon dioxide excretion is governed primarily by the rate of minute ventilation.

MODULATION OF RESPIRATION. The prime factors normally regulating alterations in the rate of minute ventilation are subtle changes in cerebrospinal fluid (CSF) pH or arterial pH. Sensor chemoreceptors in central medullary centers or in the carotid body are activated by small reductions in CSF pH or arterial pH, respectively; the pH reduction can result either from carbon dioxide accumulation or from nonvolatile acid accumulation, which reduces the plasma bicarbonate concentration. In most circumstances, central medullary chemoreceptors provide the major impetus to altering ventilatory response, and the carotid body chemoreceptors serve as relatively minor stimuli to ventilation. The medullary respiratory centers therefore serve as the major *effector* mechanism for regulating carbon dioxide output by increasing ventilation rate.

The ventilatory response for carbon dioxide removal involves an increase in both tidal volume and respiratory rate. On an average, for every 1 mEq per liter reduction in plasma bicarbonate produced by metabolic acidosis, increased minute ventilation will produce a 1.2 mm Hg fall in the $PaCO_2$. In most circumstances, the maximum reduction in $PaCO_2$ produced by the hyperventilatory response to severe metabolic acidosis is to a $PaCO_2$ of 12 to 15 mm Hg; hyperventilation to $PaCO_2$ values less than 10 mm Hg in metabolic acidosis almost never occurs. Conversely, an increase in arterial pH reduces the rate of minute ventilation and therefore results in carbon dioxide retention. For increases in plasma bicarbonate concentrations to 35 mEq per liter, the $PaCO_2$ usually remains less than 50 mm Hg. When profound metabolic alkalosis occurs, the $PaCO_2$ may rise further but virtually never exceeds 65 mm Hg.

Renal Bicarbonate Processing

In addition to volatile acid production due to carbon dioxide formation, cellular metabolism also results in the formation of a number of nonvolatile acids. The major source for nonvolatile acid production is the metabolism of sulfur-containing amino acids such as cysteine and methionine, which results in sulfuric acid formation. Consequently, the daily rate of nonvolatile acid production is closely related to dietary protein intake and to the rate of endogenous protein catabolism. Nonvolatile acids also derive from oxidation of phosphoproteins and phospholipids, which results in phosphoric acid formation; nucleoprotein degradation, which yields uric acid; and incomplete combustion of carbohydrates and fatty acids, which produces lactic acid and the ketoacids.

The daily rate of nonvolatile acid production under normal conditions is about 1 mEq per kilogram of body weight. Thus daily nonvolatile acid production would consume the total body fluid buffering capacity in about two weeks, were it not for the fact that the kidneys excrete nonvolatile acids and, in so doing, regenerate bicarbonate. Since the minimal urine pH ordinarily attainable is 5.0 and the amount of nonvolatile acid to be excreted is about 70 mEq daily, renal hydrogen ion excretion, which is equivalent to renal bicarbonate regeneration, occurs mainly as protons trapped in an undissociated form by urinary buffers.

The kidneys also filter large quantities of bicarbonate daily: For a normal plasma bicarbonate concentration of 24 mEq per liter and a glomerular filtration of 180 liters daily, the net amount of bicarbonate filtered daily is approximately 4300 mEq, or about four times the total body buffering capacity. Thus in addition to generating new bicarbonate, the renal tubules must also absorb filtered bicarbonate.

BICARBONATE REABSORPTION. Virtually all filtered bicarbonate is absorbed, together with sodium, by the proximal tubule. Consequently, the rate of proximal bicarbonate reabsorption is modulated by the same *effectors* that regulate proximal sodium absorption. Among these, the effective circulating volume exerts a central effect. Volume expansion, which resets glomerulotubular balance downward, reduces the fractional rate of proximal bicarbonate reabsorption. Conversely, volume contraction raises the bicarbonate threshold by increasing the fractional rate of proximal tubular sodium bicarbonate reabsorption.

Two other *effectors* regulate, in operational terms, the rate of bicarbonate reabsorption. One of these is the arterial $PaCO_2$: High $PaCO_2$ values raise the apparent bicarbonate threshold, whereas low $PaCO_2$ values reduce the rate of bicarbonate reabsorption. This factor accounts for the compensatory increase in plasma bicarbonate concentrations in respiratory acidosis. Second, hypokalemia also increases the rate of bicarbonate reabsorption, presumably by raising the intracellular hydrogen ion concentration. This factor accounts for the fact that, in hypokalemic, hypochloremic metabolic alkalosis associated with volume contraction, alkalosis can persist after volume deficits are restored. In this circumstance, correction of potassium deficits is required for correction of the alkalosis.

BICARBONATE REGENERATION. The excretion of nonvolatile acids and the simultaneous renal regeneration of bicarbonate occur principally in distal nephron segments. Distal renal tubular cells hydrate carbon dioxide to carbonic acid, which dissociates to protons, which are secreted into urine, and bicarbonate anions, which are absorbed into blood. The secreted protons titrate urinary buffers, principally phosphate, while sodium is absorbed. Thus the overall reaction is as follows:

$$\underset{\textit{(filtered)}}{Na_2HPO_4} + H^+ + HCO_3^- \longrightarrow \underset{\textit{(excreted)}}{NaH_2PO_4} + \underset{\textit{(absorbed)}}{NaHCO_3}$$

Titratable acid formation normally accounts for about one third of renal acid excretion. The remaining two thirds of acid excretion is accounted for by ammonia (NH_3) secretion by the following sequence:

$$\underset{\textit{(filtered)}}{NaR} + NH_3 + H^+ + HCO_3^- \longrightarrow \underset{\textit{(reabsorbed)}}{NaHCO_3} + \underset{\textit{(excreted)}}{NH_4R}$$

where NaR is the filtered sodium salt of a nonvolatile acid, NH_3 is ammonia produced by renal tubular cells, and the protons and bicarbonate come from carbon dioxide hydration by tubular cells.

Distal acid excretion and bicarbonate absorption are accompanied by sodium absorption. Consequently, *effector* systems that enhance distal sodium absorption, such as aldosterone or increased rates of sodium delivery to terminal nephron segments, also promote terminal nephron hydrogen ion excretion. Three other *effector* mechanisms also increase the rate of hydrogen ion excretion: (1) Delivery of sodium to terminal nephron segments in association with impermeant anions such as sulfate favors proton movement from tubular cells to lumen. (2) Hypokalemia enhances hydrogen ion excretion, particularly in sodium-acquisitive states, presumably because hypokalemia is accompanied by a fall in intracellular pH. (3) Acidosis stimulates ammoniagenesis by renal tubular cells; consequently, in metabolic acidosis, increases in the rate of renal acid excretion are referable primarily to increased rates of ammonium excretion. In other words, these last-named three effector systems enhance renal acid excretion by creating a favorable situation for proton transfer from tubular cells to urine. Conversely, aldosterone deficiency, alkalosis, or reduced rates of salt delivery to terminal nephron segments reduce renal capacity for acid excretion.

pH Disequilibria Between Plasma and CSF

Central rather than arterial chemoreceptors are the prime sensors for pH-mediated changes in respiration. The ventilatory responses to pH changes mediated by respiratory processes or by metabolic processes therefore differ. The blood-brain barrier is freely permeable to carbon dioxide. Consequently, pH changes produced exclusively by hyperventilation or hypoventilation occur almost simultaneously in arterial plasma and in the CSF, and the respiratory response to primary increases or decreases in $PaCO_2$ occurs almost instantaneously. The blood-brain barrier imposes a lag, however, in the rate at which arterial bicarbonate equilibrates with the CSF. Thus in metabolic acidosis, the arterial pH and bicarbonate concentration fall more rapidly than they do in the CSF; and in metabolic alkalosis, the CSF pH and bicarbonate concentration rise more slowly than they do in arterial plasma. Consequently, in the early stages of acute metabolic acidosis, there may be a one- to three-hour delay in the development of a maximal hyperventilatory response. Conversely, when metabolic acidosis is corrected rapidly, hyperventilation may persist for a few hours because of a delay in the rise of cerebrospinal fluid pH.

An unusual situation relating to this effect occurs in diabetic ketoacidosis and in certain other metabolic acidoses associated with impaired central nervous system function. In these situations, carotid body chemoreceptors, rather than central medullary chemoreceptors, provide the major stimulus to respiration driven by a reduced arterial pH. The rapid correction of ECF acidosis by bicarbonate administration reduces the rate at which carotid body chemoreceptors drive ventilation. When this occurs, $PaCO_2$ levels in plasma and in the CSF rise almost simultaneously; but because of a lag in the rate of bicarbonate entry into the CSF, the CSF bicarbonate/carbonic acid ratio tends to fall. In severe diabetic ketoacidosis, this situation can result in an actual fall in CSF pH simultaneously with a rise in arterial pH produced by intravenous bicarbonate administration.

DEFINITION OF ACID-BASE ABNORMALITIES

The arterial pH is determined by the ratio of the bicarbonate/carbonic acid buffer system, as expressed in the Henderson-Hasselbalch equation. These data also provide an index to total body acid-base balance, because, as indicated in the preceding section, the majority of body buffering occurs within cells. Acid-base disturbances can therefore occur either by altering the serum bicarbonate concentration, referred to as a "metabolic" disorder, or by altering arterial carbon dioxide tension, referred to as a "respiratory" disorder. A convenient way for considering these disturbances is illustrated in Figure 77–10, which illustrates pH isobars (for pH 7.0, 7.4, and 7.8) calculated according to the Henderson-Hasselbalch equation for the bicarbonate concentrations and $PaCO_2$ values listed on the ordinate and abscissa, respectively.

TYPES OF ACID-BASE ABNORMALITIES. The left hand panel in Figure 77–10 shows the directional changes in $PaCO_2$ and bicarbonate concentrations that *initiate* the four basic types of acid-base abnormalities. *Respiratory acidosis* results from hypoventilation and reduces pH by raising the $PaCO_2$. *Respiratory alkalosis* results from hyperventilation and raises pH by reducing the $PaCO_2$. *Metabolic alkalosis* occurs when increases in the plasma bicarbonate concentration raise pH, and *metabolic acidosis* occurs when reductions in plasma bicarbonate decrease pH.

Any of these initial acid-base disturbances activates *compensatory responses,* illustrated in the right hand panel of Figure 77–10, that tend to minimize the pH changes produced by the initial acid-base abnormality. By comparing the directional arrows in the left and right hand panels of Figure 77–10, it becomes evident that the initial disturbance in any of these four acid-base abnormalities tends to displace the arterial pH away from the pH 7.4 isobar and that the compensatory response partially restores arterial pH values toward the pH 7.4 isobar. The arterial pH, $PaCO_2$, and plasma bicarbonate concentrations illustrated in the right hand panel of Figure 77–10 are the values usually observed clinically in the four primary acid-base disturbances.

In respiratory acidosis increased renal bicarbonate reabsorption raises plasma bicarbonate concentrations to offset increases in $PaCO_2$ values. Since the renal response to an increased $PaCO_2$ requires 24 to 28 hours, a given increase in $PaCO_2$ will result in a more severe acidosis acutely rather than chronically. In respiratory alkalosis, renal bicarbonate excretion minimizes the tendency to an increased arterial pH but generally is inadequate to prevent arterial pH increases, particularly in acute hyperventilatory states.

In metabolic acidosis, compensatory hyperventilation can reduce the arterial $PaCO_2$ to 12 to 15 mm Hg, but in severe metabolic acidosis it is never adequate to restore the arterial pH to normal. In metabolic alkalosis, plasma bicarbonate concentrations in excess of 35 mEq per liter result in a compensatory hypoventilation that can raise the $PaCO_2$ to 50 mm Hg. In severe metabolic alkalosis, $PaCO_2$ values as high as 60 to 65 mm Hg may occur, particularly in azotemic patients.

THE ANION GAP. Sodium is the principal cation in extracellular fluids. The sum of plasma chloride plus bicarbonate concentrations is less than the serum sodium concentration; the remaining anions required for electroneutrality, generally not reported with routine serum electrolyte measurements, are referred to as unmeasured anions, or as the anion gap. A convenient formula for calculating the anion gap is the following:

$$\text{Anion gap} = Na^+ - (Cl^- + HCO_3^-)$$

where Na^+, Cl^-, and HCO_3^- are the serum sodium, chloride, and bicarbonate concentrations, respectively. The anion gap includes primarily phosphates and sulfates derived from tissue metabolism; lactate and ketoacids arising from incomplete combustion of carbohydrates and fatty acids; and negatively charged protein molecules, principally albumin. The normal value for unmeasured anions, or the anion gap, is 10 to 12 mEq per liter; albumin and other proteins normally account for about half of the anion gap.

An *increased* anion gap generally indicates the presence of

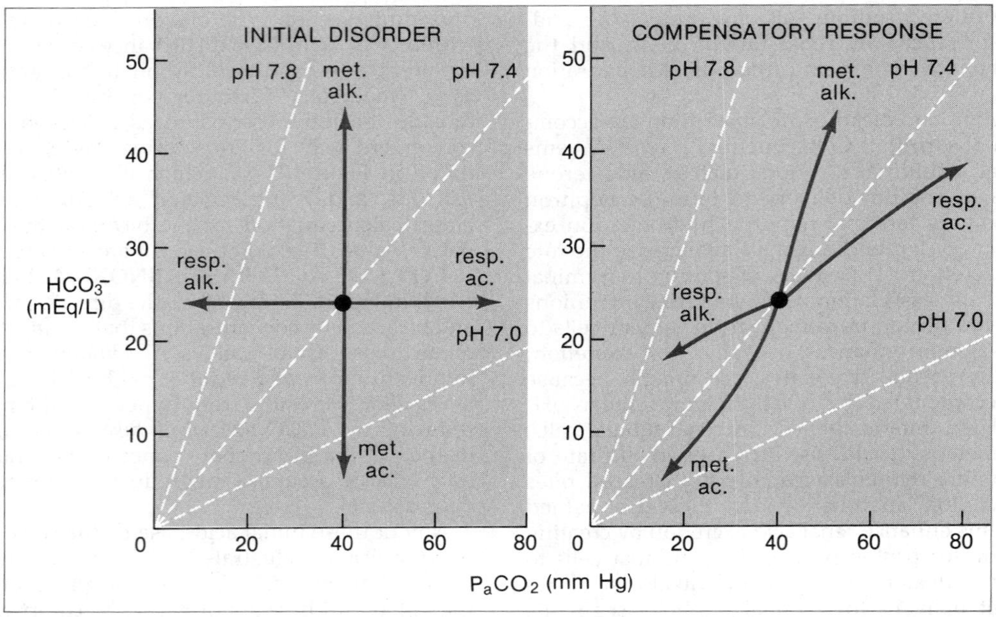

FIGURE 77–10. Schematic frame of reference for considering acid-base disturbances. The dotted lines are the pH isobars for pH values of 7.8, 7.4, and 7.0 computed from the Henderson-Hasselbalch equation for given combinations of arterial bicarbonate values (vertical axes) and arterial carbon dioxide tensions (horizontal axes). The graph on the left shows the initial derangement in HCO_3^- concentrations in metabolic acidosis and metabolic alkalosis and the initial P_aCO_2 derangement in respiratory acidosis and respiratory alkalosis. Note that each of the four changes in either HCO_3^- or P_aCO_2 tends to displace the arterial pH from the pH 7.4 isobar. The graph on the right, labelled compensatory response, indicates the general trend of pH, HCO_3^- and P_aCO_2 changes actually observed in the four primary acid-base disturbances: respiratory acidosis, respiratory alkalosis, metabolic acidosis, and metabolic alkalosis. Respiratory acidosis and alkalosis are accompanied by compensatory renal bicarbonate retention and loss, respectively. Metabolic acidosis and alkalosis are accompanied by compensatory hyperventilation and hypoventilation, respectively. Note that the compensatory response in each of the four acid-base disorders tends to restore arterial pH values toward the pH 7.4 isobar.

metabolic acidosis. The factors responsible for this kind of metabolic acidosis are discussed in the next section.

A *reduced* anion gap provides an index to certain other disorders. The anion gap will be reduced if the sodium concentration falls while the chloride plus bicarbonate concentrations are unchanged or, in other words, when the concentration of another cation in serum is increased while the serum osmolality remains normal. This may occur in multiple myeloma of the immunoglobulin G (IgG) variety, if the myeloma proteins are cationic at pH 7.4. Hyperviscosity syndromes may also result in a reduced anion gap because of a laboratory artifact: When serum is excessively viscous, automatic pumps deliver decreased volumes of serum to a flame photometer, producing artifactual reductions in sodium concentrations. Rarely, lithium intoxication, hypermagnesemia, and hypercalcemia raise nonsodium cation concentrations sufficiently high to reduce the anion gap.

The anion gap will also be decreased if the serum sodium concentration remains normal while the serum chloride plus bicarbonate concentrations are increased. This occurs most commonly in hypoalbuminemia. A low anion gap also occurs in bromide intoxication, since colorimetric techniques for serum chloride determinations give spuriously high values for chloride plus bromide when bromide is present in relatively high concentrations in serum.

METABOLIC ACIDOSIS

ETIOLOGY AND PATHOGENESIS. A convenient way to consider the metabolic acidoses is to divide them into two groups, normal anion gap and increased anion gap metabolic acidoses (Table 77–13). The pathogeneses of these two groups differ appreciably.

NORMAL ANION GAP METABOLIC ACIDOSIS. The metabolic acidoses having a *normal anion gap* result whenever there are abnormally high net bicarbonate losses. This may occur because the kidneys fail to reabsorb or regenerate bicarbonate; because there are extrarenal losses of bicarbonate; or because excessive amounts of substances yielding hydrochloric acid have been administered.

Bicarbonate Losses. Bicarbonate losses occur either when the proximal tubule fails to absorb virtually all filtered bicarbonate, that is, when the apparent bicarbonate threshold is reduced, or when there are losses of bicarbonate from the gastrointestinal tract.

Renal bicarbonate wasting occurs in *proximal renal tubular acidosis*, either alone or as part of Fanconi's syndrome (Ch. 84). The apparent threshold for bicarbonate in this disorder is set below the normal value of 26 mEq of bicarbonate per deciliter of glomerular filtrate and may be as low as 15 to 20

TABLE 77–13. MAJOR CAUSES OF METABOLIC ACIDOSIS

Normal Anion Gap	Increased Anion Gap
I. Bicarbonate Loss Proximal renal tubular acidosis Dilutional acidosis Carbonic anhydrase inhibitors Primary hyperparathyroidism Diarrheal states Small bowel drainage Ureterosigmoidostomy	**I. Reduced Excretion of Inorganic Acids** Renal failure **II. Accumulation of Organic Acids** Lactic acidosis Ketoacidosis: alcoholic diabetic starvation Ingestion: salicylates paraldehyde methanol ethylene glycol
II. Failure of Bicarbonate Regeneration Distal, gradient-limited renal tubular acidosis Hyporeninemic hypoaldosteronism Diuretics: triamterene, spironolactone	
III. Acidifying Salts Ammonium chloride Lysine hydrochloride Arginine hydrochloride Parenteral hyperalimentation	

mEq of bicarbonate per deciliter of glomerular filtrate. Consequently, bicarbonate wasting occurs whenever the plasma bicarbonate level is raised above the apparent renal threshold for bicarbonate.

Attempts to correct the acidosis of proximal renal tubular acidosis by bicarbonate administration are generally unrewarding, because increases in the plasma bicarbonate level produced by administering bicarbonate salts are accompanied by corresponding increases in bicarbonaturia. A promising approach to this disorder involves reducing the effective circulating volume by sodium restriction. This maneuver exploits the fact that ECF contraction resets glomerulotubular balance upward and consequently increases the fractional rate of sodium, and hence bicarbonate, reabsorption by the proximal tubule.

A converse of this situation is sometimes referred to as *dilutional acidosis*. Individuals who are volume expanded reduce the fractional rate of sodium bicarbonate absorption by the proximal tubule and consequently develop mild reductions in plasma bicarbonate concentrations. *Carbonic anhydrase inhibitors* such as acetazolamide inhibit proximal sodium bicarbonate absorption, resulting in metabolic acidosis. *Primary hyperparathyroidism* also reduces the apparent bicarbonate threshold in the proximal tubule; mild degrees of hyperchloremic acidosis are commonly noted in patients with this disorder.

Gastrointestinal bicarbonate wasting can occur in several circumstances. Both pancreatic and small bowel secretions are rich in bicarbonate; pancreatic fluid, for example, has a pH of approximately 8.0. Hence *diarrheal states* and *ileal drainage* can result in significant bicarbonate losses. *Ureterosigmoidostomy* results in metabolic acidosis because the colon can secrete bicarbonate in exchange for chloride. Thus in patients with this surgical procedure, urine reaching the colon is alkalinized by bicarbonate exchange for chloride, thereby producing a net bicarbonate loss.

Failure of Bicarbonate Regeneration. The second major group of disorders producing hyperchloremic acidosis includes those disorders in which the ability of the distal nephron to regenerate bicarbonate is impaired. *Distal, gradient-limited renal tubular acidosis* and chronic interstitial renal disease with *hyporeninemic hypoaldosteronism* are prototypes of this kind of metabolic acidosis (Ch. 84). The nature of these two disorders is, however, different. In gradient-limited distal renal tubular acidosis, proton secretion may be normal, but because the distal tubule is unable to maintain a steep urine to blood proton concentration gradient, secreted protons are recycled back to blood. The administration of large quantities of phosphate salts permits the excretion of large amounts of titratable acid in this disorder, because the pH of the phosphate buffer system is 6.8, that is, relatively high. Potassium wasting and hypokalemia are common in distal gradient-limited renal tubular acidosis, owing at least in part to secondary hyperaldosteronism stimulated by sodium wasting.

In hyporeninemic hypoaldosteronism, which generally occurs in association with interstitial disease, the distal tubular derangements include diminished rates of sodium absorption and diminished rates of proton and potassium secretion. Consequently, sodium wasting and hyperkalemic, hyperchloremic acidosis are the hallmarks of this disorder. Diuretics such as *triamterene, spironolactone, and amiloride*, which interfere with distal tubular sodium absorption, proton secretion, and potassium secretion, also result in hyperkalemic, hyperchloremic metabolic acidosis (Table 77–5).

Acidifying Salts. The third major group of conditions producing hyperchloremic acidosis includes the administration of *acidifying salts* such as ammonium hydrochloride, lysine hydrochloride, or arginine hydrochloride. In each instance, metabolism of the ammonium or of the amino acids leads to hydrochloric acid formation. *Parenteral hyperalimentation* without the administration of adequate amounts of bicarbonate or bicarbonate-yielding solutes (such as lactate or acetate) can also produce hyperchloremic metabolic acidosis. The acidosis occurs because the synthetic amino acids used in hyperalimentation mixtures contain positively charged amino acids such as arginine, lysine, and histidine, which yield proton equivalents when metabolized.

INCREASED ANION GAP METABOLIC ACIDOSIS. Metabolic acidoses characterized by an increased anion gap occur either because the kidneys fail to excrete inorganic acids, such as phosphate or sulfate, or because there is net accumulation of organic acids.

Reduced Acid Excretion. Renal failure, either acute or chronic, results in metabolic acidosis with an increased anion gap due to retention of sulfates and phosphates. In chronic renal failure metabolic acidosis occurs because the net amount of ammonium excreted daily falls as functional renal mass diminishes. The plasma bicarbonate concentration in most patients with chronic renal failure ranges between 16 and 20 mEq per liter. Although this degree of acidosis appears relatively modest, the daily acid load is buffered by bone salts; this buffering may contribute to the osteopenia of chronic renal failure (Ch. 249). In acute tubular necrosis, acidosis occurs because of generalized tubular dysfunction, including impaired net acid excretion. The plasma bicarbonate level generally remains above 16 mEq per liter unless sepsis, profound hypoxia, or extensive tissue necrosis complicates the disorder.

Organic Acid Accumulation. Accumulation of organic acids represents the second major cause for metabolic acidosis with an increased anion gap and is the most common cause for acute metabolic acidosis. Normally, the complete combustion of carbohydrates and fatty acids to carbon dioxide and water is highly efficient and results in the production of approximately 22,000 mEq of hydrogen ion per day. Thus the lungs eliminate, as expired carbon dioxide, more than 300 times as much acid as the 70 mEq of fixed acid excreted daily by the kidneys as titratable acid plus ammonia. Processes that impair cellular respiration, and therefore result in nonvolatile rather than volatile acid production, lead to profound metabolic acidosis. In these circumstances, the interplay of three cardinal factors determines the magnitude of the anion gap acidosis.

One of these is the rate of lipolysis, regulated by insulin, and the rate of glycolysis. Diabetic ketoacidosis is the prototype of such an anion gap acidosis. The second variable is the rate of cellular respiration, which in practical terms is determined by the rate of tissue perfusion with oxygen and the functional state of mitochondria. Lactic acidosis due to hypoperfusion or phenformin thereby is an anion gap acidosis caused by impaired cellular respiration.

The last factor determining the magnitude of the anion gap for such conditions is the extent of renal perfusion, which in turn regulates the proximal renal tubular threshold for organic acid excretion. Thus in diabetic ketoacidosis, volume expansion with normal saline can convert a large anion gap acidosis to a normal anion gap acidosis, not by correcting the underlying metabolic derangement, which requires insulin, but simply by increasing the rate of renal organic acid excretion.

The syndrome of *lactic acidosis* results from impaired cellular respiration. Lactic acid is produced in muscle, red blood cells, and other tissues as a consequence of anaerobic glycolysis. Lactic acid oxidation involves reduction of nicotine adenine dinucleotide (NAD) by lactic acid dehydrogenase *(LDH)* according to the following reaction:

$$\text{Lactate} + \text{NAD} \underset{}{\overset{LDH}{\rightleftharpoons}} \text{pyruvate} + \text{NADH}$$

Cellular respiration involves mitochondrial oxidation of pyruvate and NADH to carbon dioxide and water. When lactic acidosis occurs because of impaired cellular respiration, the lactate to pyruvate ratio (L/P) rises, as does the NADH/NAD ratio. Thus glycolysis in a setting of impaired cellular respiration results in increased production of nonvolatile lactic acid. Lactic acidosis should not be confused with states in which serum lactate levels are elevated with normal L/P and NADH/NAD ratios, as, for example, in vigorous exercise. Lactic acidosis is also characterized by negative serum nitroprusside (Acetest) reactions, since Acetest tablets react with acetoacetic acid and acetone, but not with lactic acid or beta-hydroxybutyric acid. In lactic acidosis the beta-hydroxybutyric acid/acetoacetic acid ratio is elevated in parallel with the increased NADH/NAD ratio.

Lactic acidosis occurs most commonly in disorders characterized by inadequate oxygen delivery to tissues, such as shock, septicemia, and profound hypoxemia. Drug-induced lactic acidosis may occur with phenformin therapy and isoniazid toxicity; in both circumstances, oxygen utilization by tissues is thought to be impaired. Lactic acidosis also occurs in association with leukemia and diabetes mellitus. A negative serum Acetest reaction in patients with diabetes acidosis is a valuable clue to the coexistence of diabetic ketoacidosis and lactic acidosis. There is also a spontaneous, idiopathic form of lactic acidosis in debilitated patients, which is almost uniformly fatal.

A second group of disorders characterized by an anion gap metabolic acidosis includes those disorders in which cellular respiration may not be impaired, but accelerated rates of organic acid production, particularly from lipolysis, result in an increased anion gap. *Alcoholic ketoacidosis* occurs in patients with chronic alcoholism and a recent history of binge drinking, little or no food intake, and recurrent vomiting. Hypoglycemia may be present. The major pathogenic mechanism for alcoholic ketoacidosis is accelerated lipolysis and beta-hydroxybutyric acid production because of reduced insulin secretion. The Acetest reaction is variably positive, and the beta-hydroxybutyrate/acetoacetate ratio is elevated. Lactate utilization is diminished in this disorder. Patients with alcoholic ketoacidosis have beta-hydroxybutyric acid, rather than lactic acid, as the principal nonvolatile acid. *Diabetic ketoacidosis* is the most common cause for metabolic acidosis with an increased anion gap and occurs because of increased rates of ketogenesis due to insulin lack and inadequate carbohydrate combustion. *Starvation* produces metabolic acidosis by essentially the same mechanism: increased hepatic ketogenesis with reduced caloric intake. Thus in a general sense, alcoholic ketoacidosis, diabetic ketoacidosis, and starvation share at least one common feature: accelerated lipolysis and ketogenesis due to insulin lack.

Finally, a number of ingested substances result in severe metabolic acidosis with a large anion gap. *Salicylism* produces a complex set of acid-base abnormalities. Salicylates stimulate ventilation through central mechanisms; the decrease in $PaCO_2$ then results in reductions in plasma bicarbonate concentrations. Since salicylate is a relatively strong acid, the ingestion of large quantities of salicylate can, by itself, contribute to metabolic acidosis and an increased anion gap. Salicylates also interfere with mitochondrial function. As a consequence, a number of as yet unidentified organic acids accumulate in serum and are the major factors responsible for the anion gap acidosis of salicylism.

A number of other agents, including *paraldehyde, methanol,* and *ethylene glycol,* also produce severe metabolic acidosis with organic acid accumulation. In methanol poisoning, formic acid (an end-product of methanol metabolism) accounts in large part for the reduction in serum bicarbonate concentration. In ethylene glycol intoxication, glycolic and lactic acid accumulation accounts for the majority of the reduction in plasma bicarbonate level; however, oxalate deposition in tissues is clearly a major factor in ethylene glycol toxicity. The organic acids responsible for an increased anion gap in paraldehyde intoxication have not been identified.

DIAGNOSIS AND TREATMENT. The diagnosis of metabolic acidosis requires analysis of serum electrolytes and, when indicated, measurement of arterial pH and $PaCO_2$. A cardinal clinical manifestation of metabolic acidosis is hyperventilation, which, when severe, is manifest as Kussmaul's respiration. In patients with chronic metabolic acidosis, however, hyperventilation may be difficult to detect clinically.

Severe metabolic acidosis exerts a negative inotropic effect on the heart, which depends, at least in part, on the fact that acidosis diminishes tissue responsiveness to catecholamines. Thus in lactic acidosis, negative inotropy sets the stage for a potentially lethal chain of events: poor tissue perfusion → lactic acidosis → decreased cardiac function → further reduction in tissue perfusion.

Acidosis also affects the delivery of oxygen to tissues. In acidosis, the Bohr effect shifts the oxyhemoglobin dissociation curve to the right. This compensatory mechanism permits the delivery of oxygen to inadequately perfused tissues. However, the protective characteristics of the Bohr effect may be offset by the effect of pH variation on red blood cell 2,3-diphosphoglycerate (2,3-DPG). Increases in red cell 2,3-DPG also shift the oxyhemoglobin dissociation curve to the right. However, acidosis tends to reduce red blood cell 2,3-DPG; this may offset partially the compensatory Bohr effect and therefore aggravate inadequate tissue oxygenation in acidosis.

Since metabolic acidosis is a manifestation of a variety of different diseases, the treatment of metabolic acidosis varies depending on the underlying process and on the acuteness and severity of the acidosis. Certain general principles serve as useful guidelines for therapy. Those disorders characterized by *failure of bicarbonate regeneration* or *reduced excretion of inorganic acids* represent acidoses in which the kidneys fail to excrete a normal load of nonvolatile acid or, in other words, fail to regenerate approximately 70 mEq of bicarbonate daily. Thus the treatment of these metabolic acidoses requires removal of the offending agent, if patients are receiving triamterene or spironolactone, and the administration of relatively modest amounts of bicarbonate. In chronic renal failure, alkali therapy is generally not required unless the plasma bicarbonate level falls below 16 to 18 mEq per liter. If the acidosis is more severe, bicarbonate supplementation in the form of Shohl's solution (see below) may be instituted. Caution should be exercised to avoid sodium overload or the appearance of tetany, if overalkalinization occurs.

In distal, gradient-limited renal tubular acidosis, the administration of 30 to 60 mEq of bicarbonate daily usually corrects the acidosis. This can be given conveniently in the form of Shohl's solution, which is a mixture of sodium citrate and citric acid; 1 ml of Shohl's solution yields the equivalent of 1 mmol of sodium bicarbonate. Potassium supplementation is also required in the disorder. In children with distal renal tubular acidosis, greater quantities of bicarbonate, in the range of 5 to 14 mEq of alkali per kilogram daily, are usually required to avoid growth retardation.

The therapy of patients with metabolic acidosis due to *external bicarbonate loss* varies with the nature of the disorder. As indicated above, sodium restriction, and an attendant rise in the apparent bicarbonate threshold, may be helpful in treating proximal renal tubular acidosis. In acute metabolic acidosis due to gastrointestinal losses, the net bicarbonate deficit may be roughly calculated, as indicated previously, from the reduction in "bicarbonate space," or total body buffering capacity, as follows:

$$(24 \text{ mEq/L} - \text{measured plasma } HCO_3^-) \times 0.6 \text{ body weight (kg)}$$

Bicarbonate therapy should be instituted when the arterial pH falls below 7.1. It is prudent to administer sufficient sodium bicarbonate intravenously to raise the plasma bicarbonate concentration to 16 mEq per liter over a 12- to 24-hour interval, rather than to repair the entire bicarbonate deficit. Calculation of the bicarbonate deficit in this manner is valid only if there are no further bicarbonate losses. If the latter persist, as in cholera or other types of secretory diarrhea, the daily amount of bicarbonate given to maintain the plasma bicarbonate concentration in the range of 16 mEq per liter may actually exceed the calculated bicarbonate space.

The treatment of acidoses due to *accumulation of organic acids* varies with the disorder. In *lactic acidosis* therapy should be directed toward improving tissue perfusion. Because the disorder results from a failure of conversion of lactic acid and other organic acids to carbon dioxide and water, large amounts of sodium bicarbonate, sometimes in excess of 1000 mEq per 24-hour period, have been used in attempts to avoid lethal acidosis.

The treatment is complicated by the fact that the response to alkali therapy is not predictable. In experimental lactic acidosis, dichloroacetate can raise arterial pH by suppressing endogenous lactic acid production, but bicarbonate therapy worsens the disorder by increasing the rate of splanchnic bed lactate production. Moreover, large amounts of sodium bicarbonate (in the form of ampules containing 44.5 mmol of sodium bicarbonate per 50 ml) can produce cellular shrinkage due to hypertonicity and circulatory overload due to ECF volume expansion.

The treatment of *alcoholic ketoacidosis* generally requires only the administration of saline solutions and glucose. Alkali therapy should not be used unless the metabolic acidosis is in the lethal range. The same considerations apply to starvation ketosis. The insulin release provoked by glucose administration suppresses lipolysis and consequently the overproduction of ketoacids.

In *diabetic ketoacidosis*, insulin therapy promotes glucose utilization and consequently complete oxidation of ketoacids; simultaneously, ketogenesis is reduced. Therefore alkali therapy is ordinarily not required in the disorder. Furthermore, because the hyperventilatory response to acidosis in some diabetic patients is governed by arterial rather than central medullary chemoreceptors, intravenous sodium bicarbonate administration may result in arterial alkalinization, a reduction in the rate of minute ventilation, and a potentially lethal fall in CSF pH. Sodium bicarbonate therapy in diabetic ketoacidosis should therefore be reserved for initial therapy of the disorder when the arterial pH is below 7.0 to 7.1 and cardiac contractility is impaired. Finally, because *salicylates, methanol*, and ethylene glycol are by themselves tissue toxins, appropriate therapy for these disorders includes not only alkalinization but also hemodialysis for removal of the offending agent. Ethanol can be administered to slow the rate of metabolism of methanol to formic acid.

METABOLIC ALKALOSIS

ETIOLOGY AND PATHOGENESIS. The maintenance of the plasma bicarbonate concentration depends on renal bicarbonate reabsorption and renal bicarbonate regeneration (that is, net acid excretion). Consequently, although metabolic alkalosis may be *initiated* by the loss of hydrogen ion from the body—for example, during gastric drainage—the *maintenance* of a sustained metabolic alkalosis requires that the net rate of renal bicarbonate reabsorption or renal bicarbonate generation, or both, be greater than normal. In other words, a steady-state elevation of plasma bicarbonate concentrations to levels greater than 24 mEq per liter requires increased activity of one or more of the effector mechanisms regulating bicarbonate handling by renal tubules. In normal individuals it is therefore difficult to produce metabolic alkalosis by simple alkali loading.

Table 77–14 lists the major clinical causes of metabolic alkalosis. The table includes two disorders in which the apparent threshold for proximal bicarbonate reabsorption is increased, namely, volume contraction and potassium depletion, and disorders that increase net bicarbonate regeneration, including increased rates of distal salt delivery and mineralocorticoid excess, either primary or as a consequence of volume contraction. Table 77–14 also lists Liddle's syndrome, in which the pathogenesis of alkalosis is obscure.

TABLE 77–14. MAJOR MECHANISMS FOR METABOLIC ALKALOSIS

ECF volume contraction
Potassium depletion
Increased distal salt delivery
Mineralocorticoid excess
Liddle's syndrome
Bicarbonate loading (post-hypercapneic alkalosis)
Delayed conversion of administered organic acids

Volume contraction can sustain metabolic alkalosis because of an increase in the apparent rate of bicarbonate reabsorption by the proximal tubule. The most common cause for initiating this kind of alkalosis is hydrochloric acid loss because of vomiting or gastric suction. In the early stages of gastric fluid losses there is a modest sodium bicarbonate diuresis, but urinary sodium chloride excretion is reduced. As volume contraction becomes increasingly severe, sodium conservation occurs and potassium bicarbonate is excreted in an attempt to maintain pH homeostasis. Finally, when potassium depletion becomes severe, urinary sodium plus potassium excretion is sharply reduced and paradoxical aciduria occurs: The urine is acid while the plasma bicarbonate level and pH are both elevated. *Contraction alkalosis* is a frequently misunderstood term; the designation should be reserved for those patients in whom metabolic alkalosis has developed and volume contraction maintains the alkalosis by increasing the apparent proximal tubular threshold for bicarbonate reabsorption. Thus contraction alkalosis is a mirror image of the dilutional acidosis listed in Table 77–13.

Potassium depletion from any cause, when sufficiently severe, can sustain metabolic alkalosis initiated by acid loss, for example, during gastric drainage. Presumably, potassium loss from cells is accompanied by increased hydrogen ion concentrations within cells, including renal tubular cells. Thus potassium depletion, when sufficiently severe, can raise the rate of renal tubular bicarbonate reabsorption and hence maintain a metabolic alkalosis. Consequently, when serum potassium concentrations are reduced to about 2 mEq per liter, metabolic alkalosis due to gastric fluid loss becomes saline resistant but responsive to potassium chloride administration.

Situations in which there occurs *enhanced delivery of sodium chloride* to terminal nephron segments enhance renal acid excretion and therefore lead to metabolic alkalosis by increasing the rate of renal bicarbonate generation. This effect occurs with loop diuretics (Table 77–5), such as furosemide or ethacrynic acid, and with the proximal tubular diuretic metolazone. These diuretics also contribute to the maintenance of metabolic alkalosis by contracting ECF volume and by promoting potassium depletion. Salt wasting is common in *Bartter's syndrome;* metabolic alkalosis due to renal bicarbonate generation is therefore a common feature of the disorder. The administration of large amounts of *impermeant anions* such as carbenicillin also favors distal hydrogen ion secretion. Thus carbenicillin therapy is one of the few circumstances in which an increased anion gap and metabolic alkalosis can be produced simultaneously by the same agent.

Mineralocorticoid excess, either primary or secondary, can also result in metabolic alkalosis because of renal bicarbonate generation. The disorder can occur in volume-expanded patients, for example, in primary hyperaldosteronism, in which the alkalosis is unresponsive to sodium chloride loading; and in patients with a reduced effective circulating volume and secondary hyperaldosteronism. The alkalosis of mineralocorticoid excess occurs primarily because of increased generation of bicarbonate by terminal nephron segments (or, in other words, by increased renal acid excretion) and is clearly accentuated by potassium depletion. *Liddle's syndrome* is a disorder of unknown cause in which metabolic alkalosis, hypokalemia, and hypertension occur because of an increase in sodium avidity by terminal nephron segments, which can be blocked by triamterene therapy.

When viewed in this context, the disorders listed in Table 77–14, with the exception of posthypercapneic alkalosis, result in metabolic alkalosis by two general kinds of mechanisms. First, metabolic alkalosis may be initiated by a loss of acid from nonrenal sources, for example, gastric fluid loss; and the kidney maintains the metabolic alkalosis by raising the rate of proximal tubular bicarbonate reabsorption. This is the primary mechanism responsible for the alkalosis associated with ECF volume contraction or potassium depletion. Second, the generation of metabolic alkalosis may occur intrarenally, because of increased rates of renal bicarbonate generation (or net acid excretion). This appears to be the major factor responsible for the alkalosis accompanying increased rates of salt delivery to the terminal nephron, mineralocorticoid excess, and Liddle's syndrome. Obviously, there may be considerable degrees of overlap. For example, loop diuretics increase rates of salt delivery to terminal nephron segments and therefore enhance bicarbonate generation. However, these agents also produce hypokalemia and ECF volume contraction and as a consequence raise the apparent threshold for bicarbonate reabsorption. Likewise, in primary aldosteronism, increased distal nephron bicarbonate generation as a cause for alkalosis is accentuated by the effects of hypokalemia on bicarbonate reabsorption.

In normal circumstances it is nearly impossible to produce metabolic alkalosis by increasing dietary alkali intake. In certain situations, however, *bicarbonate loading* can produce either a transient or a steady-state alkalosis. One such circumstance is *posthypercapneic alkalosis*. Patients with chronic hypercapnia develop compensatory increases in plasma bicarbonate concentrations: On an average, chronic hypoventilation results in a 0.3 mEq per liter rise in serum bicarbonate level for each 1.2 mm Hg increase in excess of $PaCO_2$ of 40 mm Hg. If ventilatory status is improved acutely, the $PaCO_2$ will fall quickly but the plasma bicarbonate level will remain elevated, particularly if the patient is salt acquisitive because of congestive heart failure or ECF volume contraction. A common way to accentuate posthypercapneic alkalosis is to maintain patients on ventilators having high positive end-expiratory pressures (PEEP), which causes a central-tourniquet effect that reduces cardiac output.

Delayed conversion of *accumulated organic acids* is a second mechanism for producing transient metabolic alkalosis. This may occur after insulin therapy for diabetic ketoacidosis, during the recovery phase of lactic acidosis, and following high-efficiency hemodialysis. In the last-named circumstance, acetate in the dialysis bath is taken up rapidly during dialysis. The accumulated acetate, which represents "potential bicarbonate," is then converted to bicarbonate after dialysis has been completed. Prolonged metabolic alkalosis because of alkali loading is a common feature of the *milk-alkali syndrome*. The alkalosis occurs because of prolonged ingestion of absorbable alkali in patients with impaired renal function due to hypercalcemic nephropathy. Frequent vomiting and attendant ECF volume contraction may also contribute to alkalosis in this disorder.

CLINICAL FEATURES AND DIAGNOSIS. There are no specific signs or symptoms of metabolic alkalosis. Relatively severe metabolic alkalosis can result in cardiac arrhythmias. Severe metabolic alkalosis can also result in severe hypoventilation, especially in patients with reduced renal function. Tetany and increased neuromuscular irritability, which are quite common in acute respiratory alkalosis, are very rare in chronic metabolic alkalosis. Rather, since hypokalemia generally accompanies metabolic alkalosis, muscular weakness and hyporeflexia are often seen in chronic metabolic alkalosis.

The diagnosis is inferred in most cases by routine measurements of serum electrolytes and can be confirmed by arterial blood gas analysis. Hypokalemia is generally present. The finding of an unexplained hypokalemic metabolic alkalosis is suggestive of the presence of Cushing's syndrome due to an extrarenal neoplasm.

The urinary chloride concentration is a useful index for distinguishing metabolic alkalosis due to volume contraction from that due to primary mineralocorticoid excess. In volume-contracted states, the urinary chloride concentration is generally less than 10 mEq per liter. Volume-contracted patients with Bartter's syndrome, or volume-contracted patients taking diuretics, generally have elevated urinary chloride concentrations. The combination of postural hypotension, hypokalemic metabolic alkalosis, and a urinary chloride concentration greater than 20 mEq per liter is therefore suggestive of diuretic abuse or Bartter's syndrome.

TREATMENT. In metabolic alkalosis associated with hypokalemia and volume contraction, appropriate therapy consists of volume expansion with saline solutions and of potassium replacement (see section on Disturbances in Potassium Balance). If the metabolic alkalosis is sufficiently severe that significant hypoventilation is present ($PaCO_2 > 60$ mm Hg), the administration of dilute hydrochloric acid or other acidifying salts, such as lysine hydrochloride or arginine hydrochloride, may be required. The use of these amino acid salts carries with it the risk of hyperkalemia that is in excess of that expected simply from the change in arterial pH, presumably because these agents promote potassium efflux from cells. Neither ammonium chloride, lysine hydrochloride, nor arginine hydrochloride should be used in patients with significant liver disease.

If diuretic abuse can be identified, use of these agents should be discontinued. Indomethacin may correct partially the abnormalities of Bartter's syndrome, although potassium supplementation is almost invariably required. Triamterene is effective in preventing potassium wasting in Liddle's syndrome.

Hypokalemia and metabolic alkalosis due to primary hyperaldosteronism are best treated by potassium chloride supplementation, which tends to correct the metabolic alkalosis partially. Dietary sodium restriction in this disorder also tends to reduce renal potassium wasting. Of course, neither of these maneuvers provides definitive therapy for primary hyperaldosteronism.

MIXED METABOLIC DISORDERS

Mixed metabolic derangements occur commonly. Consequently, the evaluation of metabolic acid-base abnormalities depends on a simultaneous assessment of the anion gap as well as the serum bicarbonate level. Electroneutrality requires that the sum of the principal anions in serum ($Cl^- + HCO_3^-$ + anion gap) equal the serum sodium level. Thus unless the serum sodium level changes, a change in the serum concentration of one or more of these principal anions necessitates a reciprocal change in the remaining anions.

Table 77–15 indicates the pattern of serum anion concentra-

TABLE 77–15. ANION PATTERNS IN METABOLIC ACID-BASE DISORDERS

	Serum Anion Concentrations		
Condition	HCO_3^-	Cl^-	Anion Gap
Simple Disorders			
Hyperchloremic acidosis	↓	↑	nl
Anion gap acidosis	↓	nl	↑
Metabolic alkalosis	↑	↓	nl
Mixed Disorders			
Metabolic alkalosis + anion gap acidosis	nl, ↑ or ↓	↓	↑
Anion gap acidosis + hyperchloremic acidosis	↓	↑	↑
Metabolic alkalosis + hyperchloremic acidosis	nl	nl	nl

nl = normal

tions in single and mixed acid-base disorders. In the single acid-base disturbances, the change in the concentration of one anion is usually balanced by a reciprocal change in one other anion. For example, in hyperchloremic acidosis, the increase in chloride concentration equals the decrease in bicarbonate concentration.

In mixed disorders, the anion patterns are more complex. In a mixed metabolic alkalosis combined with an anion gap acidosis (e.g., diabetic ketoacidosis complicated by vomiting), the identifying pattern is an increased anion gap offset partially or entirely by a reduction in chloride; the serum bicarbonate level is variable. In an anion gap plus hyperchloremic acidosis, the reduction in bicarbonate is offset by increases in both chloride and the anion gap. Finally, in metabolic acidosis combined with hyperchloremic acidosis (e.g., vomiting combined with interstitial nephritis), offsetting changes in serum bicarbonate and chloride concentrations may result in normal anion concentrations.

RESPIRATORY ACIDOSIS

ETIOLOGY AND PATHOGENESIS. Respiratory acidosis occurs whenever there is impairment in the rate of alveolar ventilation. Carbon dioxide elimination involves the following sequence: transfer of carbon dioxide from tissues to the lungs in the form of venous bicarbonate; formation of carbon dioxide within red blood cells by a reversal of the chloride shift, described previously in connection with tissue buffering mechanisms; perfusion of the lungs with systemic venous blood; diffusion of carbon dioxide from pulmonary capillaries to alveoli; and alveolar ventilation. Under normal circumstances, the rate of carbon dioxide hydration within red blood cells and the rate of carbon dioxide diffusion from pulmonary capillaries into alveoli are sufficiently rapid that carbon dioxide accumulation is virtually synonymous with hypoventilation.

Acute respiratory acidosis occurs when there is a sudden depression of the medullary respiratory center, as in narcotic overdose or anesthesia; when there is paralysis of the respiratory muscles, as in profound hypokalemia, neuromuscular disorders (myasthenia gravis), or the administration of agents that impair neuromuscular transmission (aminoglycoside antibiotics); when there is airway obstruction, as in foreign body aspiration or profound bronchospasm; when trauma, such as flail chest, impedes ventilation; and when an acute insult is imposed on a chronic hypercapneic state.

Chronic respiratory acidosis generally occurs in individuals with chronic bronchitis, emphysema, and bullous lung disease; in patients with extreme kyphoscoliosis; and in individuals with extreme obesity (pickwickian syndrome).

The arterial pH and plasma bicarbonate concentrations differ in acute and chronic respiratory acidosis. The compensatory response to carbon dioxide retention is to increase the apparent renal threshold for bicarbonate reabsorption. In general, the plasma bicarbonate concentration rises by approximately 0.3 mEq per liter for every millimeter of Hg increase in the $PaCO_2$ over 40 mm Hg, until the $PaCO_2$ reaches 80 mm Hg. This compensatory increase in plasma bicarbonate concentration requires two to three days for complete expression. Conversely, when chronic hypercapnia is relieved suddenly, there is a two- to three-day lag in renal bicarbonate excretion, resulting in posthypercapneic alkalosis.

These concepts are also useful in evaluating the possibility of mixed acid-base disorders occurring in association with respiratory acidosis. For example, since the rate of compensatory bicarbonate retention is delayed in acute respiratory acidosis, the presence of an elevated plasma bicarbonate concentration in a setting of acute carbon dioxide retention should be an index to the simultaneous occurrence of acute respiratory acidosis and metabolic alkalosis. Likewise, because renal bicarbonate reabsorption is an effective compensatory mechanism for chronic carbon dioxide retention, plasma bicarbonate concentrations below 28 to 30 mEq per liter in patients having chronic $PaCO_2$ values in excess of 50 mm Hg should alert one to the possible coexistence of acute metabolic acidosis and chronic respiratory acidosis.

Since hypercapnia is synonymous with alveolar hypoventilation, patients with carbon dioxide retention are invariably hypoxemic. A compensatory polycythemia occurs commonly in chronic hypercapneic states.

CLINICAL MANIFESTATIONS. The clinical manifestations of respiratory acidosis vary depending on the severity of the disorder and on the rate at which carbon dioxide retention has occurred. Acute increases in $PaCO_2$ values result in somnolence, in confusion, and ultimately in *carbon dioxide narcosis*. Asterixis may also be present. Because carbon dioxide is a cerebral vasodilator, the blood vessels in the optic fundi are often dilated, engorged, and tortuous; in severe hypercapneic states, frank papilledema may occur.

TREATMENT. The only practical treatment for acute respiratory acidosis involves treatment of the underlying disorder and ventilatory support. The possibility of drug abuse should always be considered in otherwise healthy patients who suddenly develop acute respiratory depression; consequently, naloxone (Narcan) therapy should be considered in all comatose patients seen in the emergency room in whom no apparent cause for respiratory depression can be identified.

In patients with chronic hypercapnia who develop sudden increases in $PaCO_2$ values, attention should be directed toward identifying factors such as pneumonia or pulmonary embolism, which may have aggravated the underlying disorder. It should be emphasized again that oxygen therapy in patients with chronic hypercapnia should be instituted with extreme caution, since hypoxemia may be the primary stimulus to respiration in this setting. Consequently, in such patients, sudden increases in the arterial $PaCO_2$ produced by oxygen administration may result in cessation of respiration. The administration of alkalinizing salts has no place in the management of chronic respiratory acidosis.

RESPIRATORY ALKALOSIS

ETIOLOGY AND PATHOGENESIS. Respiratory alkalosis occurs when hyperventilation reduces the arterial $PaCO_2$ and consequently increases arterial pH. Acute respiratory alkalosis is most commonly the result of the hyperventilation syndrome in anxiety. Acute hyperventilation may also occur because of damage to the respiratory centers; in acute salicylism; in fever and septic states; and in association with pneumonia, pulmonary emboli, or congestive heart failure. The disorder may also be produced iatrogenically by injudicious mechanical ventilatory support. Chronic hyperventilation occurs in the acclimation response to exposure to high altitudes (a low ambient oxygen tension), in advanced hepatic insufficiency, and in pregnancy.

During acute hyperventilation, plasma bicarbonate concentrations fall by approximately 3 mEq per liter when the $PaCO_2$ falls to about 25 mm Hg. This fall in plasma bicarbonate level is due largely to proton shifts from the ICF to the ECF and tends to minimize acute changes in arterial pH. In chronic hyperventilation, renal bicarbonate loss provides the compensatory response to the reduction in $PaCO_2$. In experimental studies with dogs, approximately two to four days are required for a maximal renal compensatory response, which involves approximately a 0.4 mEq per liter reduction in plasma bicarbonate concentrations for every millimeter of Hg fall in $PaCO_2$.

Hyperventilation and respiratory alkalosis may also occur, as mentioned previously, following the correction of metabolic acidosis and particularly in diabetic ketoacidosis. In all likelihood, hyperventilation persists in this setting because of the lag in the rate at which plasma bicarbonate concentrations rise with respect to ECF bicarbonate concentrations during correction of metabolic acidosis.

CLINICAL MANIFESTATIONS AND TREATMENT. Chronic hyperventilation may be asymptomatic. The acute hyperventilation syndrome is characterized by light-headedness, paresthesias, circumoral numbness, and tingling of the extremities. Tetany occurs in severe cases. Both the acute metabolic alkalosis and the reduction in ionized calcium contribute to the increased neuromuscular excitability.

The treatment of acute respiratory alkalosis involves correction of the underlying disorder. When severe anxiety provokes the hyperventilation syndrome, air rebreathing with a paper bag generally terminates the acute attack. If this maneuver fails, sedation may also be required.

Gabow PA: Disorders associated with an altered anion gap. Kidney Int 27:472, 1985. *A good summary of anion gap acidoses.*

Gabow PA, Clay K, Sullivan JB, et al.: Organic acids in ethylene glycol intoxication. Ann Intern Med 105:16, 1986. *An analysis of the plasma organic acids in ethylene glycol intoxication, showing significant accumulation of glycolic and lactic acids.*

Graf H: Effects of dichloroacetate in the treatment of hypoxic lactic acidosis in dogs. J Clin Invest 76:919, 1985. *Experimental observations on the beneficial effects of dicholoroacetate therapy in experimental lactic acidosis.*

Halperin ML, Hammeke M, Josse RG, et al.: Metabolic acidosis in the alcoholic: A pathophysiologic approach. Metabolism 32:308, 1983. *An analysis of acidosis in alcoholic patients.*

Hamm L, Jacobson HR: Mixed acid-base disorders. In Kokko JP, Tannen RL (eds.): Fluids and Electrolytes. Philadelphia, W. B. Saunders Company, 1986. *A thorough account of acid-base disturbances.*

Madias NE: Lactic acidosis. Kidney Int 29:752, 1986. *A superb discussion of lactic acidosis.*

Narins RG, Emmett M: Simple and mixed acid-base disorders: A practical approach. Medicine 59:161, 1980. *A good clinical summary of acid-base disturbances.*

Oster JR, Epstein M: Acid-base aspects of ketoacidosis. Am J Nephrol 4:137, 1984. *An account of ketosis and its relation to acidosis.*

Steinmetz PR, Palmisano J: Disorders of proton secretion by the kidney. In Andreoli TE, Hoffman JF, Fanestil DD, et al. (eds.): Physiology of Membrane Disorders. New York, Plenum, 1986. *A complete discussion of renal acidification and renal acidosis.*

78 ACUTE RENAL FAILURE

Jared J. Grantham

DEFINITION

Acute renal failure is a syndrome characterized by a relatively rapid decline in renal function that leads to the accumulation of water, crystalloid solutes, and nitrogenous metabolites in the body. Clinically significant acute renal failure is usually associated with a daily increase in the serum creatinine and urea nitrogen levels (azotemia) greater than 0.5 and 10 mg per deciliter, respectively. *Oliguria,* a rate of urine flow less than 400 ml per day, is commonly observed, but in some cases the urine output may exceed this limit (*nonoliguric* acute renal failure). Complete cessation of urine flow, *anuria,* is relatively uncommon.

ETIOLOGY

Acute renal failure may be seen in a wide variety of clinical settings (Table 78–1). A systematic approach to the causes of acute renal failure facilitates diagnosis in the individual patient. It is important to remember that acute renal failure is a bilateral process, except in patients with only one functioning kidney.

Prerenal

Prerenal causes lead to renal failure by decreasing the effective perfusion of kidney parenchyma. An absolute decrease in blood volume (hypovolemia), the most common prerenal disorder, may be caused by skin, gastrointestinal, and renal losses of water and electrolytes, hemorrhage, and sequestration of fluids in body cavities. In some conditions the kidneys respond as though the blood volume were decreased, when in fact the measured volume is normal or even increased. These oliguric states include congestive heart failure (which may be precipitated by myocardial infarction or dysrhythmia), sepsis, anaphylaxis, and liver failure. Bilateral renal artery occlusion can occur spontaneously owing to emboli from the heart or from an atheromatous aorta. Embolism of atheroma occurs commonly in the course of difficult surgical procedures involving the abdominal aorta.

TABLE 78–1. CAUSES OF ACUTE RENAL FAILURE SYNDROME

Location of Primary Disorder	Clinical Examples
Prerenal	
Absolute decrease in effective blood volume	Hemorrhage, skin losses (burns, sweating), GI losses (diarrhea, vomiting), renal losses (diuretics, glycosuria), fluid pooling (peritonitis, burns)
Relative decrease in blood volume (ineffective arterial volume)	Congestive heart failure, dysrhythmias, sepsis, anaphylaxis, liver failure
Arterial occlusion	Bilateral thromboembolism, thromboembolism of solitary kidney, aortic or renal artery aneurysm
Postrenal	
Ureteral obstruction	Bilateral or solitary kidney (calculi, neoplasm, clot, retroperitoneal fibrosis, iatrogenic)
Venous occlusion	Bilateral or solitary kidney (renal vein thrombosis, neoplasm, iatrogenic)
Intrarenal	
Vascular	Vasculitis, malignant hypertension, vasopressors, eclampsia, microangiopathy, hyperviscosity states, nonsteroidal anti-inflammatory drugs, hypercalcemia, iodinated radiocontrast agents
Glomerulus	Acute glomerulonephritis
Tubular injury	
Ischemia	Profound hypotension, postrenal transplant, vasopressors, microvascular constriction
Intratubular pigments	Hemoglobinuria, myoglobinuria
Intratubular proteins	Myeloma
Intratubular crystals	Uric acid, oxalate, sulfonamides, pyridium
Tubulointerstitial	Interstitial nephritis due to drugs, infection, radiation
Nephrotoxins	Antibiotics (gentamicin, kanamycin, neomycin, amikacin, tobramycin, streptomycin, cephaloridine, amphotericin B); metals (mercury, bismuth, uranium, arsenic, silver, cadmium, iron, antimony); solvents (carbon tetrachloride, glycol, tetrachlorethylene); iodinated contrast agents; streptozotocin, cisplatin

Postrenal

Although quite rare, *bilateral ureteral obstruction* may be due to calculi, shed papillae in analgesic nephropathy, thrombus, neoplasms, and iatrogenic causes. Commonly in bilateral obstruction one kidney is blocked for several days or weeks before obstruction of the contralateral kidney causes acute renal failure. Acute ureteral obstruction of a solitary kidney is seen occasionally. Acute renal failure can be caused by *urethral obstruction* due to prostatic hypertrophy, prostatitis, bladder and prostate tumors, bladder rupture, calculi, and iatrogenic causes. In hospitalized patients with indwelling urinary catheters, the patency and correct placement of the catheter should always be checked in the evaluation of acute renal failure.

Bilateral renal venous occlusion is rare but may be seen in hypercoagulable states, with intra-abdominal neoplasms, or secondary to surgical procedures.

Intrarenal

The renal arterial and arteriolar *blood vessels* may be involved in vasculitis, malignant hypertension, eclampsia, and microangiopathies. Pronounced vasospasm leading to acute renal failure may be seen in scleroderma, during systemic infusions of norepinephrine, secondary to the use of nonsteroidal anti-inflammatory compounds, iodinated radiocontrast agents, or diet pills, or in hypercalcemic states.

Glomerular inflammation (acute glomerulonephritis, Ch. 81) may cause acute renal failure by sharply reducing renal blood flow. *Renal tubules* are susceptible to a number of insults. *Ischemic* injury, sometimes progressing to frank necrosis, may be seen secondary to profound hypotension, especially in elderly persons. Rarely, ischemia may be severe enough to cause irreversible necrosis of renal parenchyma. About one half of kidneys transplanted from cadaver sources undergo oliguric renal failure. The intravenous administration of powerful vasoconstrictors, such as norepinephrine, may cause acute ischemic tubular injury in certain susceptible patients. Renal tubules are susceptible to injury by high levels of urinary pigments (hemoglobinuria, myoglobinuria), especially in the setting of renal hypoperfusion and ischemia. Several serum proteins are potentially nephrotoxic, including kappa and lambda light chains, which may be abundantly excreted in patients with multiple myeloma. Renal tubules may be occluded by uric acid, oxalate, sulfonamide, or pyridium crystals, leading to acute renal failure.

A wide variety of chemicals are potential tubular toxins. Antibiotics of the aminoglycoside class (one of the most common iatrogenic nephrotoxins), streptomycin, cephaloridine, and amphotericin all injure renal tubules when given in excessive doses. These agents are apparently nephrotoxic even at low therapeutic doses in patients who are oliguric or hypotensive or who have underlying renal disorders. The combined effects of aminoglycosides and certain cephalothin drugs appear to be additive in causing acute renal failure. Heavy metal poisoning is seen rarely but may cause acute tubular necrosis and renal failure. Iodinated radiocontrast agents may directly injure renal tubules in patients with underlying disorders such as diabetes mellitus, systemic lupus erythematosus, and chronic renal insufficiency from nearly any cause. Chemotherapeutic agents such as streptozotocin and cisplatin almost routinely cause acute renal injury that may progress to acute renal failure. Phencyclidine, a psychotropic agent, has caused acute renal failure in a few patients.

INCIDENCE

Acute renal failure is a relatively common syndrome. The incidence in the general outpatient population is not known; in one study about 5 per cent of patients on medical and surgical units in a general hospital experienced an episode of acute renal failure. Approximately 60 per cent of cases are related to surgery or trauma; the remainder have medical or obstetric causes. Overall, about one half of cases of acute renal failure in hospitalized patients may be iatrogenic.

PATHOGENESIS

Ischemia and nephrotoxins are the most common causes of acute renal failure listed in Table 78–1. There are at least three important phases in the acute renal failure syndrome due to ischemia or nephrotoxins. In the first, or *initiation* phase, the kidneys are subjected to an insult that produces parenchymal injury (e.g., temporary cessation of renal blood flow; nephrotoxins or pigments; see Table 78–1 and Fig. 78–1). In some patients who are hypovolemic, the initiation phase can be overridden by plasma volume expansion and the acute renal failure syndrome aborted. More commonly, however, the initiation phase causes profound renal vasoconstriction and an initial decrease in renal blood flow. The initiation phase is followed by the *maintenance* phase, during which renal vasoconstriction may persist, thereby decreasing the formation of glomerular filtrate. The hydraulic permeability of the glomeruli is usually decreased, diminishing further the ability of glomeruli to form filtrate. In addition to factors operating within the glomeruli, injury to renal tubules causes the cells to slough from the basement membranes to form casts that can obstruct urine flow. Moreover, the damaged epithelium of the tubules allows the small amount of glomerular filtrate that is formed to leak back into the peritubular capillaries. These four factors, vasoconstriction, decreased glomerular permeability, intratubular obstruction, and tubular back leak of filtrate (Figs. 78–1 and 78–2), operate in concert to depress the effective glomerular filtration rate in the ischemic and nephrotoxic types of acute renal failure listed in Table 78–1.

In some cases the renal blood flow may return to relatively normal levels 24 to 48 hours after the initiation phase. Despite this, the glomerular filtration rate (GFR) remains very low owing to the decreased glomerular hydraulic permeability, tubular obstruction, or tubular back leak of filtrate.

The third stage in the pathogenetic sequence is the *recovery* phase. Provided that the initiating causes remit, healing of renal parenchyma and recovery of function may be expected in most types of acute renal failure.

CLINICAL MANIFESTATIONS

The onset of acute renal failure usually follows the initiating event by an interval varying from a few hours to as long as several days. Patients and physicians usually first notice a reduction in urine volume in the oliguric types of acute renal failure. Facial edema, tight fitting rings, and weight gain reflect the retention of water. Rarely pulmonary edema may be an initial manifestation. Renal pain is uncommon except in association with acute infection, urolithiasis, and tumors. Hematuria is seen in nephritic syndromes and vascular occlusive states but is uncommon in nephrotoxic and transient ischemic states.

The serum creatinine and urea levels rise steadily. In severely oliguric persons of average size the serum creatinine level rises about 1.5 to 2 mg per deciliter per day. When the measured increase in serum creatinine exceeds this range, one should consider hypercatabolic factors; when the measured increase is less, renal clearance of creatinine may be greater than the rate of urine volume flow would suggest. The serum urea nitrogen level usually rises in concert with

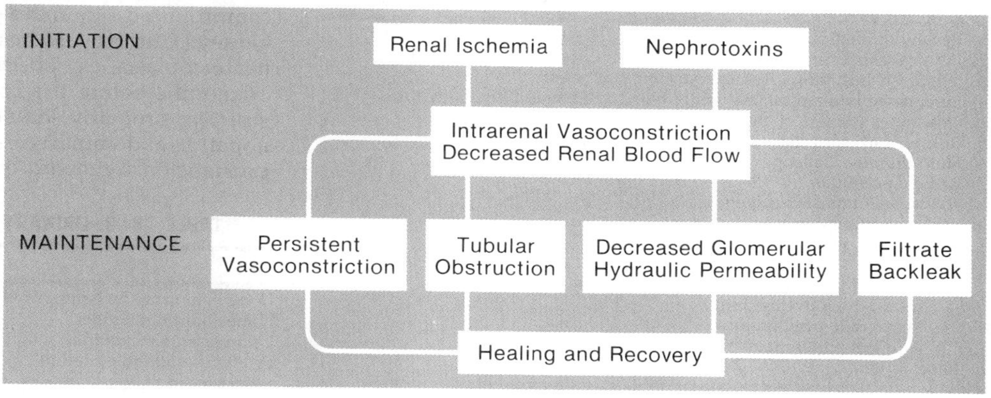

FIGURE 78–1. Pathogenesis of acute renal failure.

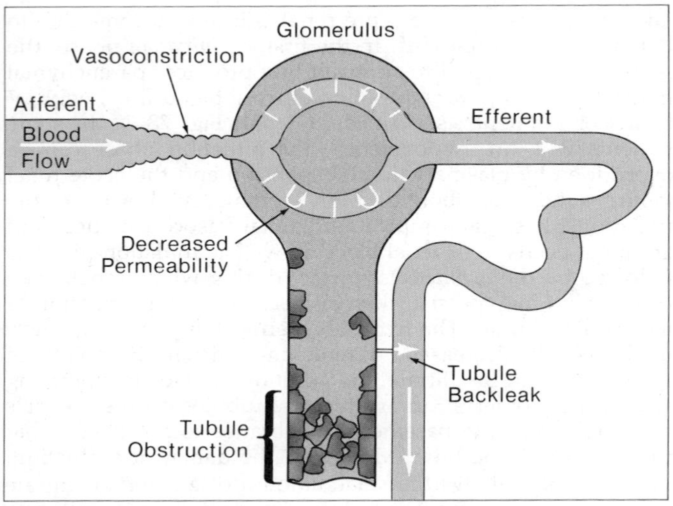

FIGURE 78–2. Possible mechanisms contributing to oliguria in acute renal failure.

the creatinine level. However, urea production is altered by food intake, by tissue catabolism, and by blood within the intestines; consequently, the urea levels do not reflect the performance of the kidneys as well as do creatinine levels.

Hyperkalemia due to inadequate renal excretion of potassium may be life threatening early in the course of acute renal failure. Metabolic acidosis due to inadequate renal excretion of hydrogen ions is seen later on. Hyponatremia may be seen in patients who drink unlimited amounts of water or other fluids. Hypocalcemia, hyperphosphatemia, hyperuricemia, and anemia usually develop after several days unless there are mitigating factors such as rhabdomyolysis and hemolysis. Serum amylase levels may be twice normal in the absence of pancreatitis.

The uremic syndrome develops gradually and, in addition to the features mentioned above, is characterized by the progressive development of anorexia, nausea, vomiting, nervous irritability, hyperreflexia, asterixis, seizures, and coma. Hemorrhagic signs include ecchymoses, gastric and colonic hemorrhage, and pericarditis.

DIAGNOSIS

When renal failure is recognized it is important to determine the probable cause and remediable factors underlying kidney dysfunction. Table 78–2 lists several key components in the diagnostic approach to renal failure.

The initial objective is to determine if the renal failure is acute or chronic. The diagnostic evaluation starts at the patient's bedside. With conversant ambulatory patients the onset of renal dysfunction can usually be determined based on historical changes in urine output (oliguria, polyuria, nocturia), abnormal urine color, and changes in body weight. Chronic renal failure is further indicated by anemia, osteodystrophy, lipiduria, bilaterally small kidneys, neuropathy, and a modestly elevated serum level of uric acid.

In the differential diagnosis of acute renal failure it is important to distinguish among *prerenal*, *postrenal*, and *intrarenal* factors.

TABLE 78–2. DIAGNOSTIC APPROACH TO RENAL FAILURE

1. Review of medical history, clinical setting, medications
2. Physical examination including evaluation of hemodynamic status
3. Urinalysis including careful sediment examination
4. Simultaneous chemical analysis of blood and urine. Osmolality, urea, creatinine, sodium, chloride, potassium, uric acid
5. Bladder catheterization if urethral obstruction suspected
6. Fluid-diuretic challenge
7. Radiologic studies
   - Plain abdominal roentgenogram
   - Ultrasonography
   - Radioisotope scans (pertechnetate ^{99m}Tc, ^{131}I-hippurate)
   - CT scan
   - Pyeloureterography
     - Intravenous pyelography
     - Retrograde pyelography
     - Antegrade (percutaneous) pyelography
8. Renal biopsy

Prerenal Failure

Prerenal failure is suggested by a history of rapid weight loss, flu-like illness, lack of fluid ingestion, bleeding, nasogastric aspiration, diuretic therapy, or orthostatic dizziness. In prerenal failure due to *extracellular fluid volume contraction* the physical examination may reveal orthostatic hypotension and tachycardia, poor venous filling and a "thready" pulse, and peripheral vasoconstriction with cool extremities and dry mucous membranes. When prerenal failure occurs in *euvolemic or hypervolemic* patients, one usually finds signs of congestive heart failure or liver failure, including distended veins, a third heart sound, pulmonary rales and wheezes, ascites, jaundice, and peripheral edema.

Urinary indices (Table 78–3) show concentrated urine (relatively high specific gravity and osmolality), low fractional excretions of sodium and chloride, and a high urine to plasma creatinine ratio. Diuretics can diminish the diagnostic usefulness of urinary indices and should not be used prior to collecting urine for analysis. Urinalysis and urine sediment examination are usually unremarkable except for hyaline casts.

When the physical and chemical findings point to prerenal acute azotemia due to a *decrease in extracellular fluid volume,* a fluid challenge of 500 to 1000 ml of isotonic saline may stimulate urine formation in the average adult. In the author's opinion, mannitol and diuretics are contraindicated in volume-depleted patients with prerenal azotemia. In prerenal azotemia associated with an *expanded extracellular fluid volume,* diuretics may be indicated as part of the general plan to improve cardiac function.

Prerenal azotemia due to occlusion of renal arteries is revealed by radioisotope screening tests and arteriography. Urine output generally is scanty. Urinalysis may show hematuria and proteinuria, and urinary indices show an inability to concentrate urinary solutes (Table 78–3).

Postrenal Failure

Obstruction to the flow of urine may be acute or chronic (see Ch. 83). In most cases of acute obstruction of the *upper tract* the patient notices pain in the flank or lower abdominal regions and fluctuating urine output. *Urethral* obstruction usually causes urinary frequency, dribbling, and lower abdominal fullness. In urinary tract obstruction infected urine is commonly observed.

The onset of renal failure due to obstruction of the urinary drainage system can be difficult to determine. To cause renal failure the urinary drainage from both kidneys must be compromised; alternatively the patient may have only one kidney. Chronic progressive processes, such as retroperitoneal neoplasia, can obstruct the drainage of one ureter weeks or months before the contralateral ureter is obstructed. Obstructive uropathy should be suspected in patients with adenopathy, abdominal scars, palpable bladder, flank tenderness, prostatic enlargement, or pelvic masses with induration.

TABLE 78–3. URINARY INDICES IN ACUTE RENAL FAILURE

Index	Prerenal	Acute Tubular Injury
Urine osmolality mOsm/kg H_2O	> 500	< 350
Urine sodium mEq/liter	< 20	> 40
Urine/plasma creatinine	> 40	< 20
Fractional sodium excretion	< 1	> 1

Urinary findings are nonspecific. The sediment contains leukocytes and erythrocytes in infected patients. The urinary indices are variable. In acute obstruction the indices are identical to those seen in prerenal failure; in obstructions more than two days in duration the indices are similar to those seen in intrarenal tubular injury (Tables 78–2 and 78–3).

When urethral obstruction is suspected bladder catheterization may be diagnostic. With upper tract obstruction ultrasonography in the hands of an experienced radiologist is the most useful diagnostic test. Rarely, acute obstruction of the urinary tract may occur without dilation of the renal pelvis and cannot be detected by sonography. The ^{131}I-hippurate scan is a noninvasive test that is useful for determining the potential for return of renal function in obstructive uropathy. Bilateral upper tract obstruction is usually nonsynchronous. In such cases the hippurate scan shows asymmetric accumulation of the isotope. The kidney showing the most intense uptake of hippurate is the best candidate for return of function after relief of obstruction. Intravenous pyelography is useful to localize the site of obstruction, but adequate renal function is needed to concentrate the contrast material in the urinary tract. Retrograde pyelography should be reserved for those cases in which the noninvasive methods are not available or those in which equivocal results have been obtained. In some cases the CT scan may provide anatomic confirmation of obstruction.

Occlusion of the renal veins is suggested by a history of a hypercoagulable state, pulmonary emboli, hematuria, or proteinuria. Urinary indices are not diagnostic. Radioisotope studies of renal perfusion may be suggestive, but definitive diagnosis depends on renal arteriography or venography.

Intrarenal Failure

Renal failure due to intrinsic dysfunction is suggested by a history of multisystem disease (e.g., SLE, vasculitis), fever, malaise, skin rash, hypertension, gross hematuria, hypotensive episode, or exposure to nephrotoxins.

The urinalysis is an invaluable guide in the diagnosis of intrarenal failure. Acute glomerulonephritis is characterized by hematuria, proteinuria, erythrocyte casts, and granular casts. Lipid bodies and broad waxy casts suggest a chronic process. Pus casts indicate acute or chronic interstitial inflammation. Urinary eosinophils are seen in allergic interstitial nephritis. Crystalluria is observed in urate and oxalate disorders. Physicians should be able to recognize these formed elements in the urine and should personally examine a freshly prepared urine sediment. Acute inflammation of the preglomerular arterioles may or may not be associated with alterations in glomerular capillaries. In the absence of glomerular capillary inflammation the urinalysis reflects ischemic tubular injury due to reduced renal blood flow. Acute tubular injury does not give specific urinary sediment findings, but cellularia, epithelial cell casts, and coarse granular casts should raise the index of suspicion.

Urinary indices (Table 78–3) are very helpful in differentiating between conditions that cause injury to preglomerular arterioles and glomeruli and those that cause acute tubular injury. In the former the indices show a prerenal pattern, whereas in acute tubular injury the fractional excretion of sodium is increased and the urinary osmolality approaches that of plasma. The conditions that may exhibit low or normal fractional sodium excretion at some point in the course of the acute renal failure syndrome are listed in Table 78–4.

Radiologic tests are relatively nonspecific in the evaluation of intrarenal failure. The ^{131}I-hippurate scan shows accumulation of isotope in both kidneys if some renal perfusion is preserved and viable tubules remain. Renal arteriography may show microaneurysm formation in polyarteritis nodosa. Renal biopsy is usually indicated in the evaluation of glomerulonephritis, vasculitis, or interstitial nephritis but is not commonly used when pyelonephritis or acute tubular injury is suspected.

TABLE 78–4. CONDITIONS ASSOCIATED WITH FRACTIONAL SODIUM EXCRETION (FE_{Na}) LESS THAN 1 PER CENT IN ACUTE RENAL FAILURE SYNDROME

Intense Intrarenal Vasoconstriction
1. Iodinated radiocontrast
2. Acute bilateral ureteral obstruction
3. Severe burns
4. Sepsis
5. Pigment excretion (myoglobin, hemoglobin)
6. Nonsteroidal anti-inflammatory drugs
7. Amphotericin B
8. Norepinephrine, dopamine
9. Liver disease
10. Cardiopulmonary bypass
Vascular Inflammation
1. Acute glomerulonephritis
2. Acute vasculitis
3. Renal transplant rejection

TREATMENT

There are at least four major objectives in the treatment of acute renal failure: (a) correct the reversible causes, (b) prevent additional injury, (c) convert oliguric to nonoliguric renal failure, and (d) provide general metabolic support during the maintenance and recovery phases of the syndrome.

Correct Reversible Causes

Prerenal and postrenal factors contributing to renal function should be corrected insofar as is possible. Drugs that interfere with renal perfusion or that are directly nephrotoxic should be stopped. In hypotensive patients the blood pressure should be restored by discontinuing antihypertensive drugs and administering isotonic volume-expanding solutions. In elderly patients with longstanding hypertension, a "normal" blood pressure of 110/70 may in fact be inadequate to generate glomerular filtrate. If there is doubt about the status of the plasma volume, an intravenous challenge of isotonic saline (500 to 1000 ml) is warranted. In the states listed in Table 78–4 associated with a low fractional sodium excretion due to intrarenal vasoconstriction, a volume challenge combined with 40 to 80 mg of intravenous furosemide may reverse the oliguric state, and in some cases prevent the maintenance phase of acute renal failure.

Prevention of Additional Injury

Radiocontrast agents are potentially harmful to patients in the maintenance phase of acute renal failure, and alternative diagnostic methods should be used whenever possible. CT scans are often done with contrast enhancement, and physicians are not always aware of this "hidden" source of iodinated radiocontrast material. Nonsteroidal anti-inflammatory drugs and nephrotoxic antibiotics should be avoided if possible. Drug dosages should be adjusted according to guidelines for renal failure, and plasma drug levels should be monitored when possible.

Convert Oliguria to Nonoliguria

Oliguria in and of itself is not harmful, and a normal urine flow rate does not accelerate the healing process in the acute renal failure syndrome. Nonetheless, experience shows that the management of patients with acute renal failure is simplified and the survival rate may be improved by converting oliguria to nonoliguria with diuretics and fluid administration. A trial of furosemide (2 to 10 mg per kilogram intravenous) is warranted. If urine output exceeding 40 ml per hour is achieved, additional doses of diuretic may be given periodically.

General Support

Conservative management without dialysis may be adequate in many cases. Indwelling urinary catheters should be avoided in uncomplicated cases. Intermittent catheterization using careful sterile technique is usually sufficient in oliguric obtunded patients. In all patients careful attention to fluid status is crucial to successful management. Daily weight measured by a competent assistant or physician is essential in the evaluation of changes in fluid balance. Catabolic patients may be expected to lose about 0.5 kg per day. As a rule of thumb, patients can be allowed to drink a volume of fluid (water, tea, coffee) equal to 500 ml plus the amount of the preceding 24-hour urine output. In febrile patients this fluid limit can be increased. In anorectic patients the fluids are given intravenously.

Sodium, potassium, and chloride are not given to patients in the maintenance phase of acute renal failure, except inadvertently in the food they eat. This may amount to about 1 mEq per kilogram of Na, K, and Cl daily. Protein intake is restricted to 0.7 to 1 gram per kilogram of body weight per day and is principally composed of foods high in essential amino acid content. Carbohydrates and fats are given to insure an adequate caloric intake. In patients who cannot eat, intravenous infusion of essential amino acids and glucose may be necessary, but this regimen contributes a considerable fluid load.

In addition to measurements of daily weight, fluid intake and fluid output, serial determinations of blood pressure (supine and upright), serum electrolytes, creatinine, urea nitrogen, and blood hematocrit are essential for patient management. Hyperkalemia exceeding 6 mEq per liter is a potentially serious complication that can be handled temporarily by ingestion of polystyrene sulfonate exchange resin (25 to 50 grams) in a solution containing sorbitol. Electrocardiographic changes showing widened QRS complexes or AV dissociation demand immediate treatment with intravenous sodium bicarbonate (88 mmol), glucose and insulin (25 units regular insulin per liter of 10 per cent glucose), and calcium gluconate (10 per cent solution, 10 to 30 ml). These measures will generally control the serum potassium level until dialysis can be initiated. (See Ch. 77 for a discussion of hyperkalemia.)

Dialysis may be necessary in certain patients in the maintenance phase of acute renal failure. The indications for dialysis include severe hyperkalemia (serum $K^+ > 6.5$ mEq per liter after treatment), severe metabolic acidosis (serum bicarbonate < 10 mEq per liter after bicarbonate therapy), pulmonary edema due to fluid overload, progressive azotemia (urea nitrogen > 100, creatinine > 10 mg per deciliter), encephalopathy, seizures, bleeding diathesis, pericarditis, and uremic enteropathy.

In uncomplicated cases, peritoneal dialysis may be the most suitable method of treatment. This procedure avoids the wide shifts in blood volume and blood solute composition encountered in hemodialysis, and anticoagulants are not used. Peritoneal dialysis can be used for prolonged treatment if recovery of renal function is slow.

In many cases, one must remove solutes and water from the blood faster than can be achieved by peritoneal dialysis. Also, patients with acute renal failure frequently have preexisting abdominal injuries. In such cases hemodialysis is the preferred dialytic method. One has rapid access to the circulation by percutaneous catheterization of femoral or subclavian veins. Alternatively, external plastic shunts can be placed in adjacent arteries and veins in the lower or upper extremities. In hemorrhagic states, systemic heparinization is not feasible, and regional anticoagulation with citrate or prostacyclin may be necessary.

PROGNOSIS

The prognosis for patient recovery must be viewed from at least two perspectives: (1) patient survival, and (2) recovery of renal function.

Patient Survival

With the advent of modern dialysis techniques few if any patients with the acute renal failure syndrome die of uremia. Death is usually a consequence of the underlying disease that caused the acute renal failure or secondary to trauma and/or sepsis. The mortality rate in traumatized septic patients with acute renal failure is disturbingly high (40 to 80 per cent).

Recovery of Renal Function

The prognosis for recovery of renal function depends on the nature of the underlying disorder that initiated the renal dysfunction. All acute renal failure due to prerenal causes is potentially reversible. In postrenal failure, renal function may be expected to stabilize or improve significantly if the obstruction is relieved.

Acute renal failure due to intrarenal causes has a variable outcome. Glomerulonephritis and vasculitis may respond to immunosuppressive therapy, with complete recovery of renal function. Acute renal failure due to renal tubular injury is usually reversible provided that the cause of ischemia is removed or nephrotoxins are avoided. Recovery of renal function to near normal levels is more likely in nonoliguric than in oliguric patients, and in subjects who have strong images by the ^{131}I-hippurate renal scan. The duration of the period of poor renal function is highly variable. Recovery of renal function takes longer in elderly patients than in young persons. Recovery is also prolonged in patients who develop acute renal failure in addition to a chronic renal disorder that compromises baseline function.

The major improvements in renal function usually appear in the first and second weeks after the beginning of the recovery phase. Some mild defects in renal function may persist for months or years after a bout of acute tubular injury.

PREVENTION

The opportunity for major prevention of acute renal failure is in the hands of physicians and surgeons. As noted, hospital-acquired acute renal failure was seen in nearly 5 per cent of all patients admitted to one general hospital; nearly one half of these cases were iatrogenic.

A few simple measures will diminish the incidence of acute renal failure acquired in the hospital: (1) Patients should be adequately hydrated before receiving iodinated radiocontrast material. (2) Adequate hydration is necessary before certain surgical procedures, specifically repair of abdominal aortic aneurysm and renal transplantation. (3) Adequate hydration is essential before and during chemotherapy using cisplatin and streptozotocin. (4) Pretreatment with allopurinol before chemotherapy of massive tumors will diminish uric acid excretion. (5) Nonsteroidal anti-inflammatory drugs should be avoided in patients with renal diseases. (6) Nephrotoxic antibiotics should be avoided or carefully monitored. (7) Antibiotic combinations that synergistically potentiate acute tubular injury should be avoided (gentamicin and cephalothin, for example).

Bennett WM, Muther RS, Parker RA, et al.: Drug therapy in renal failure: Dosing guidelines for adults. Ann Intern Med 93:62, 286, 1980. *A handy, well-referenced guide to drug dosages in acute renal failure.*

Brezis M, Rosen S, Epstein FH: Acute renal failure. In Brenner BM, Rector FC Jr (eds.): The Kidney. 3rd ed. Philadelphia, W. B. Saunders Company, 1986, pp 735–799. *This is an exhaustive up-to-date compendium with 1003 references.*

Harwood TH, Hiesterman DR, Robinson RG, et al.: Prognosis for recovery of function in acute renal failure. Arch Intern Med 136:916, 1976. *A simple noninvasive radioisotope test (^{131}I-hippurate) is shown to be useful in judging the prognosis for recovery of renal function.*

Hou SH, Bushinsky DA, Wish JB, et al.: Hospital-acquired renal insufficiency: A prospective study. Am J Med 74:243, 1983. *A disturbing study that establishes in one hospital the risk for developing acute renal failure.*

Myers BD, Morna SM: Hemodynamically mediated acute renal failure. N Engl J Med 314:97, 1986. *The clinical patterns of acute renal failure are examined systematically in this excellent paper.*

Porter GA: Nephrotoxic Mechanisms of Drugs and Environmental Toxins. New York, Plenum Press, 1982. *A comprehensive collection of essays by an excellent group of authorities who deal with topics of increasing clinical interest.*

79 CHRONIC RENAL FAILURE

Juha Kokko

INTRODUCTION

Chronic renal failure (CRF) is a functional diagnosis characterized by a progressive and generally irreversible decline in glomerular filtration rate (GFR). It is caused by a large number of diseases. Figure 79–1 summarizes the causes of chronic renal failure in North American patients on chronic maintenance dialysis according to 1978 figures from the National Dialysis Registry. In some geographic locations diabetes and hypertension are more common disease processes leading to dialysis than the National Dialysis Registry indicates for the entire country. In this classification "glomerulonephritis" is not a specific disease but reflects a heterogeneous group of glomerular disorders in which the common expression is renal failure. This chapter considers the pathophysiology and clinical manifestations of CRF, an approach to the patient with CRF, and principles of management.

PATHOPHYSIOLOGY AND CLINICAL MANIFESTATIONS

The clinical constellation of signs and symptoms of end-stage renal failure is known as the "uremic syndrome" (Table 79–1). In the initial phases of advancing renal failure most organ functions remain normal so that the patient often seeks medical attention only when his or her disease has progressed to the uremic stage. Normally, the adult patient is unaware of advancing renal failure until the GFR has decreased to 20 ml per minute. At this phase adherence to strict therapeutic principles is of utmost importance to prevent the complications of CRF. When conservative medical management is no longer adequate, alternative approaches such as dialysis or transplantation (see Ch. 80) must be considered.

The uremic syndrome results from derangements of function of many systems of the body, although the prominence of specific symptoms may vary from patient to patient (Table 79–1). No organ system is spared. The pathophysiology and clinical manifestations of uremia will be discussed by components even though this is arbitrary and not all of them may be present in the same patient. This clinical description will be followed by a short summary of the retained "toxins" that have been considered of importance in the development of the uremic syndrome.

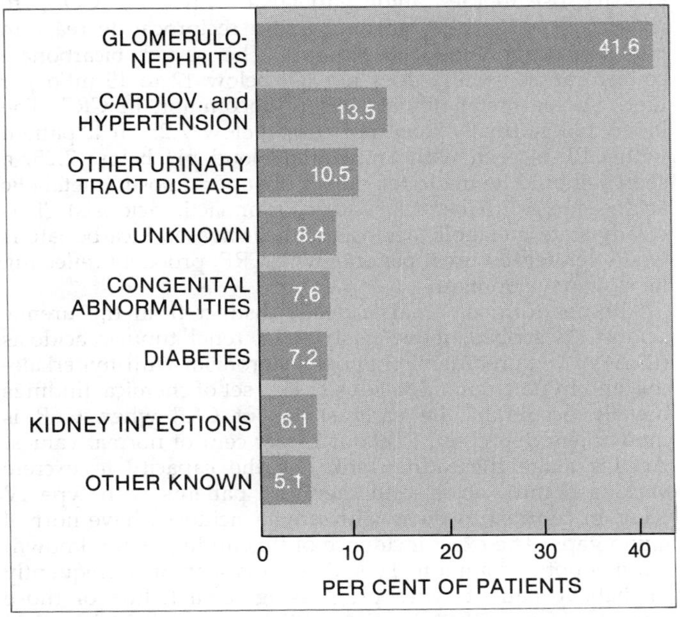

FIGURE 79–1. Histogram of primary renal diseases leading to dialysis. (Data based on National Registry data as represented by Wernman in Dialysis Transplantation 7:1034, 1978.)

TABLE 79–1. THE UREMIC SYNDROME OF CHRONIC RENAL FAILURE*

1. Electrolyte disorders
   a. Potassium: hyperkalemia, total body depletion
   b. Sodium: salt-losing nephropathy, sodium retention
   c. Acidosis: metabolic acidosis with high "anion gap," type IV renal tubular acidosis (hyporeninemic hypoaldosteronism)
   d. Calcium (see Table 249–1): tendency toward hypocalcemia—complicated mix of phosphate retention, second-degree hyperparathyroidism, calcitriol ↓
   e. Magnesium: mild hypermagnesemia
   f. Phosphate: hyperphosphatemia contributes to acidosis and to disorders of calcium metabolism
2. Cardiovascular abnormalities
   a. Accelerated atherosclerosis
   b. Hypertension
   c. Pericarditis
3. Hematologic abnormalities
   a. Anemia: erythropoietin ↓, Fe deficiency
   b. Leukocyte dysfunction
   c. Hemorrhagic diathesis: defective platelet function
4. Increased susceptibility for infections
   a. Impaired cellular immunity
   b. Leukocyte dysfunction
5. Gastrointestinal disorders
   a. Anorexia, nausea, vomiting
   b. GI bleeding
6. Renal osteodystrophy (see Table 249–1)
   a. Osteomalacia
   b. Osteitis fibrosa (secondary hyperparathyroidism)
   c. Osteosclerosis
   d. Osteoporosis
7. Neurologic abnormalities
   a. Central nervous system: insomnia, fatigue, psychologic symptoms
   b. Peripheral neuropathy
8. Myopathy: especially of proximal muscles
9. Impaired carbohydrate tolerance: peripheral resistance to insulin
10. Hyperuricemia: clinical gout is rare
11. Pruritus

*These manifestations occur to differing degrees in individual patients, depending on the severity and duration of renal failure, its cause, and unknown variables in the host.

Components of the Uremic Syndrome

WATER, ELECTROLYTE, AND ACID-BASE METABOLISM IN UREMIA. Renal and extrarenal compensatory mechanisms maintain electrolyte and water metabolism near normal until the late stages of renal failure. However, characteristic changes can occur at that time.

Potassium. The normal human dietary intake of potassium is 1 to 1.5 mEq per kilogram of body weight per day, more than 90 per cent of which is excreted by the kidneys. Essentially all the filtered potassium is normally reabsorbed so that only a small fraction is delivered to the early distal nephron. The potassium excreted in the urine has been largely secreted by nephron segments beyond the macula densa, chiefly by passive diffusion down an electrochemical gradient, and to a lesser extent by active transport processes. In each case intracellular concentration of potassium is important in net potassium secretion. The accumulation of potassium in the distal tubular cells is related to the activity of Na-K-ATPase in the basolateral region of the cell. The greater the activity of this pump, the higher the rise in intracellular potassium and the greater the secretory rate of potassium. The activity of Na-K-ATPase is controlled by diet and mineralocorticoid status (both high-potassium diet and mineralocorticoids lead to high renal Na-K-ATPase). Both normal and uremic subjects adapt to high-potassium diets by increasing potassium excretion per nephron. In addition, the gut increases its ability to secrete potassium in response to a rise in intracellular potassium concentration.

In spite of these adaptive processes, potassium homeostasis in CRF patients is not normal. In advanced CRF the serum potassium concentration tends to be higher than normal even though body stores of potassium are often reduced. Hyperkalemia can be accentuated by trauma, surgery, anesthesia, blood transfusion, increased acidosis, or sudden changes of dietary intake. It can produce the usual spectrum of cardiac abnormalities, but many patients are asymptomatic until cardiac arrest occurs. Occasional patients complain of muscle weakness or paresthesias. The major warning signs are those detected by electrocardiography.

Total body potassium content may be low in CRF: (1) Many patients with CRF have anorexia and reduced dietary intake of potassium. (2) There is greater than normal loss of intracellular potassium to extracellular compartments with subsequent loss from the body. Of special importance is the low intracellular content of potassium in muscle. The low intracellular potassium concentration may reflect a decrease in Na-K-ATPase activity, as well as displacement of intracellular potassium by hydrogen ion. Patients with chronic renal failure tolerate acute increases in serum potassium concentration with less cardiotoxicity than do patients without kidney disease. Vigorous dialysis can restore the intracellular concentration of potassium to normal, suggesting the removal of circulating inhibitor of potassium transport.

Sodium. The kidney has a remarkable capacity to maintain total body sodium content within normal limits until the very end stages of functional deterioration. To accomplish this the remaining nephrons of the CRF patient must excrete a proportionately greater quantity of dietary sodium to maintain total body sodium balance within normal limits. This observation has led to a search for a humoral factor(s) that might be responsible for the increased natriuresis per nephron of the failing kidney.

Sodium excretion can be varied only over a restricted range in renal failure, and this narrows as GFR declines. Nevertheless, most patients remain in sodium balance until their GFR is below 5 ml per minute. Rarely, patients exhibit inappropriate natriuresis; more commonly patients have a tendency toward sodium retention and volume expansion because their dietary intake exceeds the blunted ability of the diseased kidney to excrete the usual sodium load.

SODIUM WASTING. Those patients who have CRF and *salt-losing nephropathy* may lose sodium to the point of extracellular volume contraction and hypotension. These patients will require sufficient dietary salt to prevent their hypotensive symptoms. A wide variety of renal diseases may be associated with salt wasting, but the most common are pyelonephritis, medullary cystic disease, hydronephrosis, interstitial nephritis secondary to analgesic abuse, and milk-alkali syndrome. Presumably in these conditions the collecting ducts are incapable of reabsorbing sufficient quantities of delivered sodium.

SODIUM RETENTION. Some patients are unable to increase sodium excretion to appropriate levels with increases in sodium intake. Most of these patients come to a new steady state with total body weight a few pounds higher than their euvolemic weight. When these patients then receive an extra sodium load they usually excrete it promptly, thus maintaining their new state of volume expansion. They behave as if they have reset their feedback control system for sodium reabsorption. This situation is more common in patients with glomerular than with tubulointerstitial disease. These patients often have the physical findings of expanded extracellular fluid volume: hypertension, peripheral edema, pulmonary congestive state, enlarged heart, and functional flow murmur. The clinical picture is often interpreted as heart failure, and valvular heart disease is suspected erroneously. A small percentage of patients with normal cardiac output become relentless sodium retainers and require hemodialysis for volume control. These patients tend to be diabetic. Surreptitious intake of salt may play a role, but other unknown factors may also be of etiologic significance.

Acid-Base Balance. The kidney normally regulates blood pH within narrow limits by reabsorption (proximal tubule) and regeneration (distal tubule) of bicarbonate or by secretion of hydrogen (distal convoluted tubule and collecting duct segments). When diets high in alkali content are ingested, the kidney excretes less acid; whereas with acid ash diets and endogenous acid production, the kidney reabsorbs and regenerates bicarbonate and secretes hydrogen ion in amounts sufficient to maintain normal pH. A maximally acid urine in the human has a pH of 4.5 to 5.0. However, the total quantity of acid that can be excreted is a function of the amount of buffer that can be excreted. The excreted buffers may be filtered or generated. Quantitatively the most important filtered buffer is phosphate; the most important newly generated buffer is ammonium.

In chronic renal disease with progressively fewer functioning nephrons there is progressively less ammonia produced for the titration of secreted acid. Thus in CRF the urine pH may be maximally acid, but the total amount of hydrogen ion is low. In disease processes that disproportionately affect the medulla, the ability to form maximally acid urine is lost early. Metabolic acidosis, which may be partially compensated by respiratory mechanisms, develops when exogenous intake and endogenous production of acid exceed renal excretory capacity. In metabolic acidosis there is recruitment of extrarenal buffering mechanisms. Either the excess hydrogen ions are buffered by bone salts and other extracellular mechanisms or they enter the cells to be buffered by intracellular mechanisms. These buffering mechanisms allow for maintenance of relatively stable, albeit lower than normal, blood bicarbonate concentrations when the urinary excretion rate cannot keep up with endogenous production of acid. Tissue stores of buffer are partly consumed over long periods of time. Loss of bone salts contributes to the development of osteomalacia and renal osteodystrophy (Ch. 249). With recruitment of the various buffer mechanisms and with a decreased ability of the kidney to excrete various organic acids, there is a progressive rise in the "anion gap" $[Na - (Cl + HCO_3)]$, to around 20 to 24 mEq per liter, and a reciprocal decrease in plasma bicarbonate concentration. The serum bicarbonate concentration usually does not fall below 12 to 15 mEq per liter. Severe metabolic acidosis is uncommon in CRF. The blood pH normally does not drop below 7.25. If a patient with CRF is seen with an arterial blood pH below 7.25, a search should be made for causes of superimposed metabolic acidosis (e.g., diabetic ketoacidosis or lactic acidosis). This steady-state metabolic acidosis with decreased bicarbonate is well tolerated by most patients with CRF, probably reflecting its slow development.

Another form of renal acidosis, distinct from the uremic acidosis described above, is type IV renal tubular acidosis (RTA) or hyporeninemic hypoaldosteronism with hyperkalemia and hyperchloremic acidosis. This set of chemical findings usually occurs in the early stages of CRF when GFR is moderately depressed to about 25 per cent of normal values. At this stage the kidney still has the capacity to excrete various organic acids, and therefore patients with type IV RTA, in contrast to those with uremic acidosis, have normal anion gaps. The exact incidence of this finding is not known, but it is not uncommon. Type IV RTA is seen most frequently in diabetic patients with progressing renal failure or those with predominantly tubulointerstitial disease. It is described further and compared with other types of RTA in Ch. 84.

Chloride. Patients with CRF are unable to regulate chloride excretion. For example, CRF patients excrete greater amounts of sodium when they are given an excess of sodium bicarbonate than following administration of an equivalent amount of sodium chloride. With increased intake of NaCl there is retention of salt and fluid and weight gain. Many CRF patients are in a stable volume-expanded state. The preferential retention of chloride in CRF patients does not usually lead to a reciprocal decrease in bicarbonate concentration, and thus CRF patients tend to be proportionately hyperchloremic with respect to sodium concentration.

Calcium. The total serum calcium concentration in CRF patients is significantly lower than normal, although usually above 7.5 mg per deciliter. Great variability exists, and occasionally the calcium level is very low. CRF patients tolerate the hypocalcemia quite well, and rarely is a patient symptomatic from the decreased calcium concentration. Tetany is surprisingly uncommon. It is occasionally precipitated by the infusion of sodium bicarbonate, but the usual muscle twitching and cramping of CRF are unrelated to hypocalcemia.

CRF patients have decreased intestinal absorption of calcium, and in consequence fecal calcium loss exceeds that of normal subjects. Jejunal and ileal malabsorption of calcium in CRF can be corrected by oral administration of active vitamin D analogues with increases in serum calcium concentrations.

In addition, patients with either acute or chronic renal failure are resistant to the normal calcemic action of parathyroid hormone (PTH). The mechanism of resistance may be secondary to a decreased permissive effect of $1,25(OH)_2D_3$ on bone action of PTH. Renal osteodystrophy is discussed in Ch. 249.

A subgroup of CRF patients develops hypercalcemia after some months on hemodialysis. Most often the hypercalcemia is due to persistent secretion of PTH from glands that have previously undergone hyperplasia. Occasionally these patients become symptomatic with bone pain or exhibit signs of metastatic calcification. Parathyroidectomy may be indicated if other causes of hypercalcemia can be ruled out.

Magnesium. Patients with CRF tend to have modest elevations in serum magnesium concentration when GFR has fallen below 20 per cent of normal. Urinary excretion of magnesium is diminished, but often intestinal magnesium absorption continues normally. Most CRF patients with hypermagnesemia have no associated symptoms or findings. Nevertheless, it is prudent to discontinue magnesium-containing antacids and cathartics in patients with GFR below 20 ml per minute.

Phosphate. The most important determinant of serum phosphate level is the relationship between net reabsorption of phosphate from the gut and excretion of phosphate by the kidney. The serum phosphate concentration is significantly higher than normal in patients with GFR below 20 ml per minute.

The major reason for hyperphosphatemia is decreased excretion of phosphate with advancing renal disease. The retained phosphate is of major pathogenetic importance in the development of the secondary hyperparathyroidism of CRF. It is postulated that in the evolution of CRF there are periodic decreases in phosphate excretion as nephrons progressively drop out. The resultant increases in plasma phosphate concentration lead to reciprocal decreases in serum calcium concentration, increased secretion of PTH, and increased tubular rejection of phosphate. This adaptive mechanism will maintain a normal serum phosphate concentration until GFR has fallen to approximately 20 per cent of normal. However, if usual dietary phosphorus intake continues in patients with far advanced renal disease, these adaptive mechanisms cannot compensate fully and hyperphosphatemia ensues. If dietary phosphorus is decreased in proportion to the decrease in GFR, hyperphosphatemia can be prevented and the expected rise in serum parathyroid hormone blunted. In addition, intestinal absorption of phosphate can be reduced by use of compounds that bind phosphate in the gut in nonabsorbable form.

CARDIOVASCULAR ABNORMALITIES. Cardiovascular complications are common in patients with CRF and can be classified into three main categories: atherosclerosis and hyperlipidemia, hypertension, and pericarditis.

Atherosclerosis. Accelerated atherosclerosis is one of the major factors limiting the longevity of patients with chronic renal failure. Although the plasma lipid pattern may be normal in CRF, the most characteristic abnormality is elevated triglyceride concentrations with normal or slightly elevated plasma cholesterol levels (type IV). A smaller percentage of patients has type IIa or IIb hyperlipoproteinemia. The incidence of elevated triglyceride concentrations is increased in patients maintained on chronic hemodialysis as compared with nondialyzed patients. Cardiovascular death is particularly common after the fifth year of dialysis. There appears to be a positive relationship between the elevation of plasma triglycerides and the increased incidence of occlusive coronary disease. The cause of hypertriglyceridemia in CRF is unknown, but current evidence favors a defect in triglyceride removal rather than an increase in triglyceride production. The most probable cause of the decreased removal rate of very low density lipoproteins is a defect in hepatic lipoprotein lipase activity.

Hypertension. Hypertension is common in chronic renal disease, being present in the majority of patients at the onset of maintenance dialysis. At least two factors contribute to its high incidence in CRF: (1) The tendency toward sodium retention and volume expansion is perhaps the most important. Expansion of the extracellular volume is accompanied by an initial rise of cardiac output, which may persist, followed by a rise in peripheral resistance. Patients with volume-sensitive hypertension may have increasing problems with blood pressure control as they progress into renal failure. (2) Alterations of the renin-angiotensin axis are also important contributors to the pathogenesis of hypertension. Although the absolute plasma values for renin and angiotensin are variable in CRF, plasma renin activity is inappropriately high for the degree of sodium retention in most patients. This view is supported by the efficiency of angiotensin-converting enzyme inhibitors in controlling hypertension and by those few patients whose hypertension can be controlled only by bilateral nephrectomy.

Pericarditis. "Uremic pericarditis" is a term that refers to pericarditis of unknown etiology occurring in association with uremia. Conventionally, pericarditis is not classified as "uremic" if an infectious etiology can be documented. Some authorities have attempted to divide pericarditis in renal failure into two subsets: "uremic" and "dialysis-associated." The former is said to occur in a uremic patient prior to initiation of dialysis, whereas the latter occurs in a uremic patient who is undergoing chronic hemodialysis. However, since the pathologic pericardial characteristics are similar in these two clinical settings and since the etiology has not been identified, the division of pericarditis in renal failure into two distinct subtypes appears arbitrary, and therefore the continued use of the term "uremic pericarditis" seems justified. In the older literature, uremic pericarditis was more commonly seen in nondialyzed patients, whereas currently it is most common in patients who are not dialyzed adequately. It is most likely caused by some unknown biochemical substance. Characteristically, the pericardial fluid is hemorrhagic. The onset of pericarditis is usually signaled by pain, often on the left side of the chest with respiratory accentuation. Pain is often severe and frequently associated with a friction rub. The friction rub can be loud, generalized, and even palpable. Tamponade can occur with signs of falling blood and pulse pressures, raised jugular venous pressure, and poorly perfused extremities. The hemorrhage is thought to originate from sheared pericardial capillaries that have developed in response to uremic inflammation of the pericardium. It is recognized that in previously nondialyzed patients, uremic pericarditis responds to dialysis more rapidly than in patients who develop pericarditis during dialysis. However, the pericarditis in this latter group usually responds to intensification of hemodialysis.

HEMATOLOGIC ABNORMALITIES. Hematologic abnormalities are among the most consistent manifestations of uremia. These abnormalities include anemia, bleeding, and granulocyte and platelet dysfunction.

Anemia. Many patients with CRF have severely reduced hematocrits. Hematocrits in the 20 to 25 per cent range are not uncommon. The manifestations of anemia include pallor, tachycardia, a wide pulse pressure with accentuation by exercise, a systolic ejection murmur best heard over the pulmonary area, and the precipitation of angina pectoris in patients with underlying coronary artery disease.

The primary cause of anemia in CRF is a deficiency of erythropoietin, which is a glycoprotein normally produced in the kidney in response to anoxia. It is responsible for normal red blood cell differentiation from stem cells. The decreased erythropoietin may be the result of destruction of renal parenchyma, the presence of circulating inhibitors, or protein deprivation that in turn decreases erythropoietin production. The result is normochromic, normocytic anemia.

Other factors may contribute to anemia. Many patients on maintenance hemodialysis programs are iron deficient. Iron absorption from the gut may be decreased in CRF patients and restored to normal following hemodialysis. Furthermore, iron deficiency may develop in dialyzed patients because of frequent blood sampling, loss of blood in hemodialysis tubing and coils, and periodic accidental losses from hemodialysis access sites. Red blood cell survival is shortened in uremia, probably due to some extrinsic factor: (1) Red blood cells isolated from uremic patients and infused into nonuremic individuals have a normal life span. (2) Aggressive hemodialysis increases the red blood cell survival to or toward normal. In addition, many patients with CRF have added intrinsic erythrocytic factors contributing to anemia, which include decreased Na-K-ATPase activity, pentose phosphate dysfunction, microangiopathic hemolytic component as a result of hypersplenism, and folate deficiency due to its dialyzability in chronic hemodialysis patients.

Leukocyte Dysfunction. In addition to anemia, there are other hematologic abnormalities in CRF. Although the granulocyte count is usually normal, some patients have a tendency toward granulocytopenia. Moreover, the chemotactic response of granulocytes is subnormal.

Hemorrhagic Diathesis. A hemorrhagic tendency, manifested by epistaxis, menorrhagia, or excessive bleeding or bruising after trauma, is common in late renal failure but seldom life threatening. Whole blood clotting time and prothrombin time are usually normal. Bleeding time may be prolonged, perhaps related to the associated abnormalities of platelet function. Platelets are often decreased in number owing to increased peripheral destruction. In addition, there are functional defects such as decreased adhesiveness and aggregation. These abnormalities are often corrected by hemodialysis and may be secondary to a dialyzable uremic toxin. The hemorrhagic diathesis of uremia is discussed further in Ch. 166 and 167.

INFECTIONS. Most patients with CRF develop serious infections during the course of their disease. Theoretically, this assumed susceptibility to infection could be due to deranged or deficient humoral or cellular immunity, impaired inflammatory reaction, or increased exposure to pathogenic bacteria and viruses. Humoral immunity is, in general, intact. Although exceptions exist, most patients have a normal humoral response to vaccines. Cellular defense mechanisms are often deficient. Skin tests may show impairment of delayed hypersensitivity. Patients with CRF may have low lymphocyte counts, and their lymphocytes do not respond normally to mitogenic stimulation. Abnormal lymphocyte function may be due to some dialyzable factor, since it is nearly normal after vigorous dialysis or after suspension of lymphocytes harvested from uremic patients in nonuremic sera. The neutrophil count is usually normal in chronic renal failure, and it rises appropriately in response to infection. However, a transient decrease may occur following hemodialysis owing to sequestration of leukocytes in pulmonary capillaries. In addition, leukocytes of uremic subjects have a decreased ability to phagocytize bacteria. The chemotactic response of polymorphonuclear leukocytes is also depressed; this function improves with hemodialysis. Additionally, patients on hemodialysis are frequently exposed to bacterial and viral infections. Staphylococcal sepsis is not uncommon. The presumed portal of entry is cutaneous contamination through the arteriovenous hemodialysis access. Gram-negative sepsis also occurs with increased frequency. Often an infected urinary tract can be implicated as the cause. Superinfection with *Candida albicans* is very common, mainly affecting the buccal mucosa. There is a significant increase in frequency of hepatitis in dialysis patients owing to multiple transfusions and increased exposure, secondary to either hepatitis B virus or non-A non-B viruses. The disease is usually asymptomatic, but it can be severe. A significant fraction of CRF patients who contract hepatitis become chronic carriers.

GASTROINTESTINAL DISORDERS. Gastrointestinal symptoms are common in patients with uremia. Their symptoms have varying presentations and may be quite distressing. The most common early symptom is loss of appetite. Many uremic patients then progress to develop nausea and vomiting, sometimes severe enough to cause loss of salt and water leading to volume depletion and negative caloric balance causing weight loss. The specific cause of these symptoms has not been identified.

Gastrointestinal bleeding is also common in uremic patients. Often it is of minor magnitude detected by positive stool guaiacs, but it also can be severe. The gastrointestinal bleeding may be the result of scattered petechiae, ulceration, or other specific lesions. Undoubtedly the platelet defects contribute to the increased frequency of gastrointestinal bleeding characteristic of uremic patients.

OSTEODYSTROPHY. The term "renal osteodystrophy" is an all-inclusive term for the skeletal changes in uremia, which include, in decreasing order of frequency, osteitis fibrosa, osteomalacia, osteoporosis, and osteosclerosis. Osteitis fibrosa is almost universal in terminal renal failure; it may be found in as many as 90 per cent of patients starting regular dialysis, the exceptions being those with rapidly progressive disease and a short experience of uremia. A substantial minority will exhibit abnormal radiographs, but very few will complain of bone tenderness or muscle weakness. Few patients survive more than a year or two on dialysis without evidence of bone disease. The pathogenesis and clinical features of renal osteodystrophy are discussed in greater detail in Ch. 249.

NEUROPATHY. Many patients with CRF have abnormalities in central and peripheral nervous system function. Tiredness, insomnia, and psychologic symptoms, including agitation, irritability, depression, regression, and rebellion, are common. Patients tend to have fewer such symptoms if they are eating a nutritious diet and are well dialyzed. Patients with secondary hyperparathyroidism caused by uremia have abnormal electroencephalograms (EEG) characterized by increased frequency of slow wave activity. Patients with secondary hyperparathyroidism caused by CRF may show improvement in their EEG and psychologic symptoms after parathyroidectomy. The mechanism by which PTH exerts these effects is not known, but in the uremic dog PTH increases brain calcium content and abnormal EEG changes of uremia require elevated levels of PTH. Brain calcium content is higher in patients with CRF than in patients who die without renal failure.

Peripheral neuropathy is also common in CRF. Clinical manifestations include painful paresthesias of extremities, twitchings, "restless leg syndrome," loss of deep tendon reflexes, muscular weakness, and occasional sensory deficits. Lower extremities are involved much more frequently than upper extremities. Diminished deep tendon reflexes and vibratory sense may be found, but the most reliable objective measurement of peripheral neuropathy in CRF is slowing of nerve conduction velocities. Peripheral neuropathy can be drug induced, but its pathophysiology in most patients is unknown. However, symptoms of neuropathy can be improved by prolonging the period of dialysis and by use of membrane dialyzers with larger membrane surface areas. Also, patients on chronic peritoneal dialysis have been said to have fewer symptoms than patients on extracorporeal hemodialysis. These findings suggest that the development of peripheral neuropathy is related to dialyzable uremic toxins of the "middle molecule" range.

MYOPATHY. Muscular weakness develops slowly, but it is common in patients with end-stage renal failure. Proximal muscles are affected more than distal muscles. It is not uncommon to see some wasting of the limb and cervical muscles. There are no distinct histologic features of uremic myopathy. The resting transmembrane potential difference of skeletal muscle cells is abnormally low, and the average mean duration of the action potential is significantly shortened in uremic individuals. In inadequately dialyzed uremic patients intracellular sodium and chloride contents are elevated, whereas potassium content is reduced. These findings are consistent with either increased permeability of the muscle membrane to these ions or a decrease in active efflux of sodium. However, it is doubtful that these are primary muscle membrane abnormalities, since all the abnormalities can be corrected by dialysis. Indeed, resting skeletal muscle membrane responses have been used as an index of adequacy of hemodialysis. Although a number of hormones and factors have been proposed as causal of uremic myopathy, the identity of such a factor(s) remains conjectural.

CARBOHYDRATE METABOLISM. Carbohydrate metabolism is often abnormal in patients with chronic renal failure. Glucose tolerance is reduced as shown by a rapid rise and delayed return to normal of the blood glucose concentration after an oral or intravenous glucose load. Fasting blood glucose values are normal or slightly elevated. This state of impaired glucose tolerance is often termed *uremic pseudodiabetes mellitus.* Severe hyperglycemia does not occur unless the patient receives a large load of glucose, e.g., during peritoneal dialysis with hypertonic glucose solutions. Nevertheless, the requirement for exogenous insulin decreases in insulin-dependent diabetics as renal failure progresses. At least two different mechanisms are responsible for the simultaneous coexistence of abnormal glucose tolerance and a decreased requirement for exogenous insulin: (1) enhanced peripheral resistance to insulin, and (2) a decreased renal clearance of insulin.

Increased peripheral resistance to insulin in uremia is manifested by a diminished forearm uptake of glucose in response to insulin and by elevated concentrations of circulating insulin as compared with normal subjects. A number of possibilities exist to explain the insulin resistance. First, some uremic substances may interfere with the action of insulin, since aggressive hemodialysis decreases exogenous requirements for insulin. Second, potassium deficiency may alter the nature of insulin released from the pancreas. Indeed, proinsulin to insulin ratios rise in nonuremic patients who are potassium deficient. Third, there is decreased binding of insulin to peripheral receptors in CRF. Whatever the reason(s), patients with CRF clearly have some degree of peripheral resistance to insulin.

Insulin is filtered and metabolized by the kidney. With progressing CRF the urinary clearance of insulin approaches GFR, presumably reflecting a decreased uptake of filtered insulin by the proximal convoluted tubule. Nevertheless, blood insulin concentrations rise owing to decreased extraction of insulin by renal tubular epithelial cells. These observations explain the decrease in insulin requirements of diabetics with progressing CRF, but it is also necessary to postulate a degree of peripheral resistance to insulin to explain the carbohydrate intolerance ("uremic pseudodiabetes") of nondiabetic subjects with CRF.

URIC ACID. Approximately two thirds of the total uric acid excretory load is normally removed each day by the kidney. With progression of CRF hyperuricemia is a consistent finding once GFR has decreased to 20 per cent of normal. However, the correlation between the rise of serum uric acid and the severity of chronic renal failure is poor. Only rarely does the serum uric acid concentration rise above 10 mg per deciliter unless dehydration is superimposed. Whether or not the elevated serum uric acid levels hasten the development of end-stage renal disease is not known.

PRURITUS. Generalized pruritus is a frequent symptom of CRF and is occasionally severe and intractable. Usually there are no dermatologic findings. To date no single causative factor has been identified. Implicated factors include some dialyzable product of uremia, high calcium-phosphorus product in extracellular fluid with deposition of calcium salts in the dermal structures, and abnormalities in nerve end-plates. Symptomatic relief has been reported with more frequent dialysis, parathyroidectomy, dietary protein restriction, and exposure to sunburn spectrum of ultraviolet light.

Role of Retained Toxins

The kidney has a remarkable capacity to regulate the excretion of a variety of substances to maintain their blood concentrations at optimal levels. During the evolution of renal insufficiency until GFR is severely compromised this capacity is maintained by adaptive mechanisms whereby the remaining nephrons either metabolize or excrete greater than normal quantities of the substance in question. Adaptive mechanisms do not exist for substances that are freely filtered and neither reabsorbed nor secreted. Urea and creatinine are the classic examples of this group of compounds. Their clearance rates are close approximations of the glomerular filtration rate. However, most substances are not only filtered but also reabsorbed, secreted, or metabolized. In general, the blood concentrations of the latter group of substances do not rise until the later stages of renal disease. Many of the putative uremic toxins belong in this latter group.

The symptoms of uremia are, in part, caused by dialyzable substances that accumulate from failure of their renal excretion. Azotemic patients improve symptomatically after initiation of hemodialysis. No single substance has evolved as the cause of uremic symptoms. Multiple compounds no doubt contribute. The list of the suggested "uremic toxins" is long (e.g., guanidines, amines, phenols, indoles) and beyond the scope of this chapter. Urea and "middle molecules" (presumed polypeptides with molecular weights between 1000 and 1500) have received the most attention and will be discussed here.

UREA. Since blood urea nitrogen rises rapidly with decreasing GFR, and since intravenous injections of urea to animals produced neurologic symptoms, it was only natural to suspect that high urea concentrations produced uremic symptoms. However, this view is no longer held. For example, in studies in which patients were dialyzed for prolonged periods of time against a dialysate with a high concentration of urea, only minimal symptoms of headache, lethargy, emesis, or tremor were noted with postdialysis blood urea concentrations as high as 200 mg per deciliter. This is strong presumptive evidence that the clinical manifestations of chronic renal failure are not secondary to urea itself. In addition some patients have uremic symptoms at serum urea concentrations as low as 60 mg per deciliter. Therefore other factors in end-stage renal disease are of importance in producing uremic symptoms.

"MIDDLE MOLECULAR WEIGHT" TOXINS. The origin of the "middle molecular weight" toxin concept came from the clinical observation that patients who were peritoneally dialyzed had fewer uremic symptoms than patients who were hemodialyzed to the same blood urea concentration with small surface area dialyzers. It was argued that the peritoneum was more permeable to substances in the molecular weight range of 500 to 5000 than were the small pore hemodialyzers. Significant effort has been spent to identify specific compounds in this molecular range that might be toxic. Although a great number of compounds have been identified, there have been few correlative studies to establish "cause and effect" relationships. However, toxic effects of "middle molecules" isolated from uremic serum include inhibitions of hemoglobin synthesis, glucose utilization, lymphoblast transformation, leukocyte phagocytic activity, and nerve conductivity. Although the "middle molecular weight" toxin theory has not been established with certainty, clinical observations are consistent with the view that there are compounds in this molecular weight range that may play a role in the pathogenesis of the uremic syndrome.

APPROACH TO THE PATIENT WITH UREMIA

The principles of approach to the uremic patient are the same as those toward any patient who comes to the attention of the physician. A detailed clinical history is imperative, with special emphasis on urinary tract symptoms such as nocturia, hematuria, dysuria, polydipsia, and polyuria. Also of special importance is a complete history of systemic diseases, of exposure to toxins and infections, and of renal diseases in the family. The medical history will often be of diagnostic significance. The physical examination should emphasize the blood pressure, retina, cardiovascular system, renal examination with auscultation for bruits and palpation of size, rectal examination for size of prostate in males, gynecologic examination for pelvic masses in females, extremity examination for edema and nail bed findings, and neuroskeletal examination for evidence of myopathy, neuropathy, and osteodystrophy. Laboratory tests should include a complete blood count and urinalysis.

Additional studies should be designed to elucidate whether a patient has acute reversible renal failure, acute worsening of CRF resulting from aggravating factors, or a chronic progressive disease. Again, the history is important. It is unlikely that a patient with acute renal disease is asymptomatic with elevations of serum creatinine and blood urea nitrogen above 10 and 100 mg per deciliter, respectively. On the other hand, patients, especially if young, with slowly progressing CRF are often asymptomatic with much higher elevations of serum creatinine and blood urea nitrogen. Thus, if in the absence of other diseases, a patient complains of nausea, vomiting, anorexia, and weakness and the creatinine and blood urea nitrogen are below 10 and 100 mg per deciliter, respectively, the chances are that the patient is suffering from an acute process. Unfortunately exceptions to this rule exist. Also, in chronic renal failure the hematocrit tends to be lower, phosphate concentration higher, uric acid concentration lower, and urine sediment more benign. However, none of these tests is specific enough to differentiate with certainty between acute and chronic renal failure.

X-ray determination of the kidney size can be helpful in determining the chronicity of renal disease. The x-rays can be in the form of plain abdominal films, tomograms, or intravenous urograms (if the blood urea nitrogen is less than 100 mg per deciliter). Of these the plain abdominal film is least expensive, free from complications, and often informative. Renal sonograms can be used to estimate renal size and identify hydronephrosis or cystic masses. If the kidneys are significantly reduced in size, this almost always indicates chronicity and irreversibility. Normal kidney size tends to favor an acute process, although exceptions exist. Chronic renal processes in which kidney size may be normal or larger than normal include polycystic renal disease, amyloidosis, scleroderma, and diabetes mellitus. Thus normal renal size does not rule out a chronic process.

It is also important to differentiate between renal versus extrarenal causes of azotemia. Extrarenal causes of progressive uremia may be either pre- or postrenal. Prerenal causes are those disease processes that decrease the blood flow to the kidneys. This may be due to true extracellular fluid (ECF) volume depletion or to effective volume depletion as seen with cardiac and liver failure. This is discussed in more detail in the management section under "Aggravating Factors." Also, it is imperative to rule out postrenal causes of azotemia, namely, lower or upper urinary tract obstruction. Lower urinary tract obstruction may be diagnosed by having the patient void completely and then measuring the residual urine volume in the bladder via catheterization. The presence of residual urine indicates lower urinary tract obstruction. Occasionally sufficient time has elapsed between voluntary voiding and insertion of the catheter so that "new" urine is formed. When the physician is unsure of the significance of 5 to 10 ml of residual urine, he or she may elect to instill 20 to 40 ml of air into the bladder. If this air is passed (which the patient experiences as a "whistling" sound) during the next voiding, then the bladder can empty completely and lower urinary tract obstruction is ruled out. In males by far the most common cause is an enlarged prostate. Any time a uremic patient is seen with anuria, it is imperative that lower urinary tract obstruction be ruled out, especially if accompanied by symptoms such as hesitancy in initiating the urinary stream, slow urinary stream, and incontinence. Upper urinary tract obstruction can be established by ruling out residual urine in the bladder and demonstrating dilated renal calices, pelvis, and ureter(s) above the obstruction. This can be established by intravenous and retrograde pyelography or by renal sonograms. In addition to the dilated urinary tract systems, delayed visualization and delayed clearance of the dye on intravenous urograms characteristically exist. The most common causes of upper urinary tract obstruction include renal stones, congenital obstruction, and bladder cancer.

Once it has been determined that uremia is secondary to renal parenchymal disease and not due to pre- or postrenal causes, the physician must determine if a treatable form of parenchymal disease is present. The most common forms of treatable renal disease are listed in Table 79–2. The following additional tests may be helpful and are often considered: renal arteriography and renal biopsy. In general, although renal arteriography produces excellent visualization of the kidney,

TABLE 79–2. TREATABLE* TYPES OF PARENCHYMAL RENAL DISEASE

Acute hypertensive nephropathy
Analgesic nephropathy
Hemolytic-uremic syndrome
Hypercalcemic nephropathy
Lupus nephritis
Multiple myeloma
Oxalate nephropathy
Pyelonephritis
Renal vein thrombosis
Wegener's granulomatosis

*The mode of therapy and results in these disease processes are variable. All these processes may present with such severe end-stage renal disease that no form of conservative management is effective.

it is of limited diagnostic value in patients with uremia. It may be helpful in patients suspected of having polyarteritis nodosa, tumors (although uremia is an uncommon association), and renal disease secondary to severe hypertension.

Renal biopsy may give a definitive histologic diagnosis provided it is performed before the disease has progressed to such a degree that the only possible morphologic interpretation is "end-stage kidney disease." Renal biopsy can be performed by a percutaneous route with local anesthesia or as an open biopsy under general anesthesia, but it should be carried out only by those who are trained in its use. The associated morbidity and mortality are low, but the possibility of complications nevertheless exists. For these reasons renal biopsy is probably indicated in only a small number of patients with uremia. While a consensus does not exist among nephrologists, biopsy should not be done unless the physician has strong feelings that the information to be gained will influence management. Contraindications to renal biopsy include uncorrectable bleeding tendencies, severe hypertension, bacteriuria, suspicion of perinephric abscess, hydronephrosis, and extreme obesity. Biopsy is often useful in patients with normal sized kidneys and progressive renal disease if they have (or are suspected to have) nephrotic syndrome, collagen vascular disease (especially systemic lupus erythematosus), tubulointerstitial disease, or rapidly progressive glomerular disease.

MANAGEMENT

The management of CRF patients can be divided conveniently into three separate categories: treatment of aggravating factors, treatment of specific complications of uremia, and consideration of optimal diet and general principles in the long-term follow-up of patients with CRF. We will consider those principles of management that are common to all forms of CRF regardless of etiology.

Aggravating Factors

Patients with CRF are highly susceptible to factors that may cause a deterioration of renal function. These must be sought meticulously and treated immediately so that the underlying renal failure will not be worsened permanently. Table 79–3 lists factors that may rapidly increase the serum creatinine concentration in a patient with previously stable CRF. The relative incidence of these factors causing acute deterioration of renal function is dependent on the demographics of the patient population. Thus, generalized frequency distribution cannot be formulated; however, it is important for the physician to consider each of these general categories as a differential diagnostic possibility when evaluating a patient with progressive renal disease.

TABLE 79–3. AGGRAVATING FACTORS FOR PROGRESSION OF RENAL DISEASE

1. Vascular volume depletion
   a. Absolute: aggressive use of diuretics, gastrointestinal fluid losses, dehydration, etc.
   b. Effective: low cardiac output, renal hypoperfusion with atheroembolic disease, ascites with liver disease, nephrotic syndrome, etc.
2. Drugs: aminoglycosides, prostaglandin synthesis inhibitors in a setting of renal hypoperfusion, diuretics in dosage to cause volume depletion, etc.
3. Obstruction
   a. Tubular: uric acid, Bence Jones protein, etc.
   b. Post-tubular: prostatic hypertrophy, necrotic papillae, ureteral stones, etc.
4. Infections: sepsis with hypotension, urinary tract infections, etc.
5. Toxins: radiographic contrast materials, etc.
6. Hypertensive crises
7. Metabolic: hypercalcemia, hyperphosphatemia, etc.

Volume Depletion. One of the most common causes of rapidly rising serum creatinine concentration in a CRF patient is vascular volume depletion. Vascular volume depletion can be the result of either absolute volume depletion or contraction of the effective arterial blood volume. A common cause of absolute volume depletion is the combination of aggressive use of diuretics coupled with restricted intake of salt and fluids. Another common cause of absolute volume depletion of CRF patients is gastrointestinal loss of fluid from either vomiting or diarrhea. Vascular volume depletion can also be "effective." Effective arterial blood volume (EABV) is a dynamic concept that refers to blood volume that perfuses various volume receptors. Under circumstances of decreased EABV, the renal blood flow decreases. The kidneys of CRF patients are especially sensitive to decreases in renal blood flow. Therefore, aggravating factors that cause decreases in EABV can produce rapid rises in serum creatinine concentrations (Table 79–3). Physical signs of volume depletion should thus be sought. In addition, urinary electrolyte measurements will often suggest volume depletion. Although CRF patients normally have an elevated fractional urinary excretion of sodium and chloride (the degree being dependent on the severity of the decrease in GFR), these patients are able to decrease their fractional excretion of sodium and chloride in response to volume depletion. A decrease in previously determined high fractional excretion of sodium and chloride of 2 per cent (or a decrease in fractional excretion to less than 1 per cent) is highly suggestive of either true or effective volume depletion. Patients with CRF may rapidly and irreversibly decrease their GFR with volume depletion, so it is imperative for treatment, either oral or intravenous fluid replacement, to be started as soon as feasible. Patients with CRF who are not on chronic dialysis should be hospitalized if there is any doubt that adequate volume repletion can be carried out on an outpatient basis.

Drugs. Patients with CRF are often treated with various types of drugs, a number of which are nephrotoxic. Table 79–3 lists the nephrotoxic drugs. Of these, the aminoglycoside antibiotics are a common cause of worsening renal failure. In addition, prostaglandin synthesis inhibitors can decrease the creatinine clearance in CRF patients, especially in a setting of decreased EABV. It is beyond the scope of this chapter to review different drug-related nephrotoxins, but it is prudent to obtain a detailed drug ingestion history whenever a CRF patient with an accelerating rate of renal failure is seen.

Obstruction. Acute (less than a day) or subacute (less than a few weeks) obstruction of the urinary tract can occur from multiple causes in CRF patients. Urinary tract obstruction is conveniently divided into tubular and post-tubular causes. The more common etiologies for tubular obstruction include uric acid crystal deposition (as observed with malignancies) and Bence Jones protein deposition (in association with multiple myeloma). More common causes of post-tubular obstruction include prostatic hypertrophy and/or prostatism; necrotic papillae, especially in patients with diabetes; and ureteral stones. When the clinical symptoms suggest urinary tract obstruction, it is important that prompt diagnostic and therapeutic measures are undertaken. Rapid in-and-out catheterization will rule out bladder obstruction, whereas ultrasonography is useful in ruling out ureteral obstruction. These measures are simple and safe and often will prevent progression of azotemia.

Infection. Urinary tract infections are significantly increased when obstruction is present. The rate of infection rises especially after repeated catheterization. Although infection limited to the urinary tract rarely causes progression of renal failure, nevertheless, specific attention should be directed toward evaluating the degrees of proteinuria, pyuria, and bacteriuria and any changes from baseline abnormalities. Increased proteinuria and exaggerated pyuria suggest urinary tract infection. A culture of clean-voided urine should be done under these circumstances. If infection is documented, specific antibiotics are indicated. Care must be exercised to adjust the drug dosage for the degree of renal failure. A number of antibiotics are nephrotoxic, and the susceptibility to neprotoxicity increases with advancing renal failure. Uremic patients are also more prone to other infections such as pneumonia and sepsis on a de novo basis. These systemic infections, if present, in turn may compromise renal blood flow and result in worsening uremia. The index of suspicion should be high for sepsis in hypotensive CRF patients with urinary tract infection in whom the serum creatinine level is rising.

Toxins. The list of potential nephrotoxins is long. Therefore, it is important to obtain a good history in CRF patients with a rising serum creatinine level. In a hospitalized CRF patient, when the serum creatinine starts to rise rapidly, one must consider exposure to radiocontrast materials. Volume-depleted CRF patients, especially diabetics and patients with multiple myeloma, are susceptible for development of worsening renal disease. Fortunately, the prognosis is quite good if the patients are adequately hydrated.

Hypertensive Crisis. A good percentage of patients with CRF are hypertensive. Indeed, hypertension is one of the significant risk factors that may accelerate the rate of progression of renal disease. Thus strict attention must be paid to adequate control of blood pressure in CRF patients. Occasionally, patients with CRF will develop malignant hypertension with rapidly deteriorating renal function. It is imperative that the blood pressure is controlled rapidly in these patients.

Metabolic. Of the metabolic abnormalities that worsen the progression of renal disease, the rises in calcium-phosphorus products are among the most common. The rise in Ca × P product may not only cause soft tissue calcification but also be a precipitating factor in progression of renal disease. This is especially true in patients with multiple myeloma. An increased Ca × P product may become more frequent with the recent increase in the use of oral $CaCO_3$ to control hyperphosphatemia.

Complications of Uremia

WATER AND ELECTROLYTE ABNORMALITIES. Treatment of altered states of calcium, phosphorus, and bicarbonate balance is discussed in Ch. 249, "Renal Osteodystrophy."

Hyperkalemia. The mean serum potassium is higher than normal, whereas the total body potassium content is lower than normal in CRF. Serum potassium concentrations up to 6 mEq per liter are well tolerated in CRF patients. However, patients with CRF have difficulty in excreting a sudden increase in potassium load. Therefore potassium concentrations above 6 mEq per liter should be treated. One should initially determine whether the hyperkalemia is a result of some aggravating factor such as volume depletion, tissue breakdown, transient worsening of acidosis, action of drugs such as spironolactone or triamterene, fever, or high intake of potassium; or whether hyperkalemia is a consequence of steady metabolic events. If hyperkalemia is of modest degree and due to some aggravating factor, the therapy should be directed toward correcting the source of hyperkalemia. However, if hyperkalemia is severe, paralysis of skeletal muscles and electrocardiographic changes may be present. This represents a medical emergency and requires immediate transfer of potassium intracellularly and rapid excretion of potassium from the body. The treatment of hyperkalemia is described in detail in Ch. 77.

Abnormalities of Sodium Balance. Total body sodium content dictates total extracellular fluid volume. Although fractional excretion of sodium per nephron increases as renal disease progresses, patients with CRF are nevertheless susceptible to both volume contraction and volume expansion. Since even mild volume depletion may affect renal function adversely in CRF patients, it is prudent to maintain these patients in a somewhat expanded state (on the "wet side"). Volume-sensitive hypertension and pulmonary edema will be limiting factors, but it is even more hazardous to keep a patient completely edema free. If a patient should develop orthostatic hypotensive symptoms, salt intake should be liberalized. Ideally, dietary salt intake should be decreased in proportion to the decrease in GFR. Some of the sodium should be given as sodium bicarbonate as described for renal osteodystrophy, below. If the patient is poorly compliant and becomes volume expanded, the use of diuretics such as furosemide or bumetanide is indicated, assuming that underlying kidney function is sufficient to permit a satisfactory clinical response to these drugs. If volume expansion causes severe symptoms and does not respond to conventional techniques, acute peritoneal or hemodialysis is indicated. Hypo- and hypernatremia are treated with the same general principles of water restriction or free water administration as in any other patient. Neurologically symptomatic, life-threatening hyponatremia may require the administration of hypertonic sodium chloride, but this risks potential volume expansion. One should be prepared for the possibility of acute dialysis to remove extra volume.

CARDIOVASCULAR ABNORMALITIES. It is important to control the cardiovascular complications of CRF to realize the potential longevity of chronic hemodialysis. Hypertriglyceridemia and hypertension are the primary risk factors leading to accelerated atherosclerosis and high cardiovascular mortality. It is not clear whether the course of atherosclerotic vascular disease in CRF patients can be altered. Even patients who have undergone successful renal transplantation seem to have an increased incidence of cardiovascular deaths. Nevertheless, it seems advisable to adhere to the same dietary principles in patients with hypertriglyceridemia and CRF as in patients without CRF (see Ch. 50). If clofibrate is used, its dosage level should be decreased proportionately to the degree of renal failure to prevent its adverse side effects.

Hypertension is the result of numerous interrelated factors in CRF patients. It is most commonly volume dependent and volume sensitive. Thus one of the primary objectives is to decrease intravascular volume, an approach that will be sufficient to control hypertension in many patients. If the patient has an adequate urine volume, the judicious use of diuretics together with a decrease in the dietary intake of salt and water is indicated. Of the available diuretics, furosemide and bumetanide are preferred because of their low renal toxicity. Volume can be removed in patients on dialysis by ultrafiltration during the procedure. If volume contraction is not sufficient, then the same general principles apply to the treatment of hypertension as in any other patient (see Ch. 47). Additional drugs such as methyldopa, hydralazine, and beta blockers such as propranolol and metoprolol may be required. Captopril, an oral inhibitor of angiotensin-converting enzyme, has been shown to be particularly useful in some patients. Minoxidil, a direct smooth muscle vasodilator, has also been advocated in a small group of patients with otherwise refractory hypertension. There still exists an extremely small number of patients with malignant hypertension that cannot be controlled by any medical regimen. These patients may respond to bilateral nephrectomy.

The diagnosis of uremic pericarditis requires hospitalization and treatment for fear of impending cardiac tamponade. The best initial therapy is daily dialysis for approximately a week. Indomethacin is not effective in uremic pericarditis. If pericarditis remains refractory to increased frequency of dialysis, intrapericardial injection of nonabsorbable steroids may prove therapeutic. Some patients will require partial pericardiectomy if they develop circulatory impairment that does not respond to medical management.

HEMATOLOGIC ABNORMALITIES. Anemia of CRF

often improves with maintenance hemodialysis. The rise in hematocrit is not due to stimulation of erythropoietin production but rather to the removal of some circulating factor that inhibits the normal response to erythropoietin.

Besides achieving the best possible metabolic status of the patient with either hemodialysis or transplantation, there exist two general considerations for treatment of anemia: long-term medical treatment and transfusion. The general aim of medical treatment is to increase the hematocrit to values as high as possible without secondary side effects. Because patients with CRF, especially those on maintenance hemodialysis, are iron deficient, supplemental iron should be given. Iron can be given daily as a ferrous salt or on a periodic basis as intravenous iron dextran. Oral iron supplementation is inexpensive and is associated with very few side effects. Unfortunately, not all patients rebuild their iron stores to normal even if given 900 mg of ferrous sulfate per day. These patients probably do not absorb iron normally in spite of hemodialysis. They require periodic intravenous iron dextran. There is no consensus on frequency or dosage, and there is the potential of iron overload with hemosiderosis and occasional anaphylactoid reaction. While some patients have a gratifying hematologic response to periodic intramuscular injections of androgens, many patients do not respond at all (especially anephric patients) and many have untoward side effects to androgens. Most CRF patients do not have folate deficiency unless they are receiving maintenance dialysis treatment. Folic acid is dialyzable, and therefore it is standard practice to order small daily doses of folate (1 mg per day orally) in the hope of increasing erythropoiesis.

Clinical trials have been recently carried out with recombinant human erythropoietin for the treatment of uncomplicated anemia in patients with end-stage renal disease. Gratifying and dose-dependent rises in hematocrits occurred in response to intravenous erythropoietin administration when given three times weekly after dialysis. If the results of this study are confirmed, they represent a major breakthrough in treatment of anemia of end-stage renal disease.

The above findings with erythropoietin may change the indications for transfusions. Many CRF patients tolerate extraordinarily low hematocrits surprisingly well. This may be due to increased release of oxygen from hemoglobin during chronic anemia. Nevertheless, before erythropoietin becomes available to all centers, some patients do require periodic transfusions. If patients are unduly tired and unable to do routine tasks, packed red blood cell transfusions can be given in amounts sufficient to abate the symptoms. If such symptoms improve, this provides strong presumptive evidence that the weakness was due to anemia and not to uremia per se. It is rare that transfusions are necessary in CRF patients if the hematocrit is above 20 per cent. However, notable exceptions are provided by patients with angina pectoris. In these patients the physician may be forced to transfuse the patient even at hematocrit values in the low 30's. This situation may become more common as the mean age of dialysis patients increases.

INFECTIONS. Infections are more common in uremic than nonuremic patients. The general approach to the use of antibiotics should be the same in both groups of patients. Ideally, the antibiotic dose should be adjusted by monitoring the serum concentration of the antibiotic. However, this often is not feasible and therefore after an initial normal loading dose, dosage levels must be adjusted for the degree of renal failure if the antibiotic is excreted by the kidney (Table 79–4). Some antibiotics are more nephrotoxic than others, and nephrotoxicity is potentiated by CRF. If drug sensitivities allow a choice in treatment of a given infection, the physician should choose the least nephrotoxic antibiotic that is therapeutic.

RENAL OSTEODYSTROPHY. Hyperparathyroidism, decreased amounts of active vitamin D metabolites, and chronic metabolic acidosis all contribute to the development of renal osteodystrophy as noted above. The goals of treatment are to normalize these abnormalities to the extent possible. Renal osteodystrophy is described in detail in Ch. 249.

NEUROPATHY. No specific treatment exists for either central or peripheral neuropathy. However, both objective and subjective improvement may occur by prolonging the periods of dialysis and by use of larger surface area dialyzers. Also, gratifying improvement of peripheral neuropathy has been noted following successful renal transplantation.

MYOPATHY. No specific therapy exists for myopathy. Patients may improve dramatically with adequate dialysis. Some patients have shown improvement of myopathy following treatment with active vitamin D analogues.

CARBOHYDRATE METABOLISM. Abnormalities of carbohydrate metabolism in the nondiabetic patient are of no or minimal clinical significance. In the diabetic patient, insulin dosages must be adjusted to maintain serum glucose values at normal levels. Often smaller insulin doses will be adequate as CRF progresses.

URIC ACID. Although uric acid levels are consistently elevated in CRF, they are rarely much above 10 mg per deciliter. However, even if the uric acid levels are significantly higher there is little or no evidence to suggest that asymptomatic hyperuricemia should be treated. It is our practice to treat elevated uric acid levels in uremic patients only when there are tophaceous deposits or symptomatic gout. If treatment is elected, allopurinol is the drug of choice, since patients with CRF do not respond to uricosuric agents. The allopurinol dose should be decreased to 100 mg per day in chronic uremic patients due to potential toxic side effects.

PRURITUS. No specific therapy has withstood the test of time in the treatment of pruritus. A few patients get relief following topical application of emulsified oils or the use of oral antihistamine agents. Some patients have benefited from lowering the serum phosphate concentration by phosphate binders. There are reports of beneficial effects of ultraviolet light. Parathyroidectomy has sometimes relieved intractable pruritus.

Diet

An appropriate diet can be critically important in the management of patients in chronic renal failure, for it may provide symptomatic improvement and also may slow the rate of loss of residual renal function. Although nutritional and caloric intake should be individualized for obese and malnourished patients, some general principles are applicable to all patients. In general, the higher the amount of protein in the diet, the higher will be the serum urea concentration. This occurs because amino acids are metabolized to form urea in addition to all other nitrogenous waste products that have been implicated as factors causing the uremic syndrome. Reducing the amount of protein in the diet will lower the blood urea concentration and reduce symptoms. Moreover, the difficulties in controlling serum phosphorus and acidosis will be ameliorated, since a high-protein intake is always associated with a high intake of phosphates as well as other inorganic ions. However, if dietary protein is too low, protein malnutrition will occur with loss of strength, body weight, and muscle mass. This can be avoided if the protein requirements are met by providing 0.6 gram of protein per kilogram of body weight per day, of which at least 60 per cent contains proteins rich in essential amino acids, e.g., eggs, lean meat, and milk. Although a high-calorie intake can improve nitrogen utilization at very low nitrogen intakes, it is not necessary to force large numbers of calories on these patients as long as minimum protein requirements are being met. Providing about 30 kilocalories per day generally suffices, although this may be lowered for obese patients or raised for patients weighing less than their ideal body weight. Accumulated waste products can be reduced even further by lowering the daily protein intake to approximately 20 grams of protein per

TABLE 79–4. ANTIBIOTIC DOSAGE IN CRF

Major Reduction in Dosage	Moderate Reduction in Dosage	Minor or No Reduction in Dosage	Agents That Should Not Be Used
Flucytosine	Ampicillin	Amphotericin B	Bacitracin
Gentamicin	Carbenicillin	Cefotaxime	Chlortetracycline
Kanamycin	Cefazolin	Cefoperazone	Nitrofurantoin
Oxytetracycline*	Cephaloridine	Chloramphenicol	
Streptomycin	Cephalothin	Clindamycin	
Tetracycline*	Cloxacillin	Doxycycline	
Tobramycin	Co-trimoxazole (trimethoprim-sulfamethoxazole)	Erythromycin	
Vancomycin	Methicillin	Isoniazid	
	Moxalactam	Lincomycin	
	Oxacillin	Nafcillin	
	Penicillin G		
	Ticarcillin		

*Although tetracyclines are not significantly nephrotoxic per se, their dosage should be reduced in CRF because of their hepatotoxicity with increased blood levels (especially with chlortetracycline) and because their antianabolic actions cause an increase in blood urea nitrogen disproportionate to the degree of renal failure. If tetracyclines are indicated in renal failure, doxycycline is the drug of choice because it is cleared by hepatic routes.

day, but only if the diet is supplemented with essential amino acids or a mixture of essential amino acids and their alpha-ketoanalogues. Such a regimen will maintain adequate protein nutrition for prolonged periods of time in patients with advanced renal failure. Alpha-ketoanalogues of essential amino acids are aminated in the body to form essential amino acids and hence body protein. Nitrogen, which otherwise would have accumulated as waste products, is therefore used to build body proteins. Low-protein diets in which daily minimum requirements are met and the very-low-protein diet supplemented with mixtures of amino acids and alpha-ketoanalogues may slow the rate of loss of residual renal function and possibly postpone the time when therapy with chronic hemodialysis becomes necessary. Diets should be supplemented with the water-soluble B vitamins plus vitamin C and folic acid; there is no need to supply additional vitamin A or E. Vitamin D should be reserved for treatment of severe renal osteodystrophy. In general, there is no need to place a severe restriction on dietary sodium unless there is hypertension or edema. Most patients with chronic renal failure can readily excrete sodium until renal function is markedly impaired (creatinine clearances less than 10 ml per minute), but they cannot rapidly stop excreting salt when dietary sodium is markedly restricted. For most patients, the diet should contain at least 1.5 to 2 grams of sodium per day. As long as the amount of urine excreted is greater than 1 liter per day, it is unusual to have to restrict potassium in the diet. Using these guidelines, uremic symptoms and the consequences of renal insufficiency can be controlled for most patients. Once

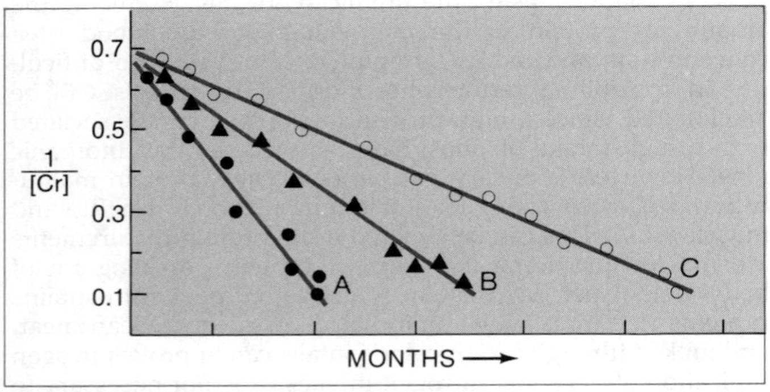

FIGURE 79–2. Plot of reciprocal of serum creatine concentration (vertical axis) against time (horizontal axis) in three hypothetical patients. This is a useful way to determine the rate of predetermined slope reflecting the underlying cause of CRF. For example, patient A reflects rapidly progressing renal failure such as seen with diabetes mellitus, patient B might represent nephrosclerosis secondary to essential hypertension, and patient C might reflect the slower rate of progression of polycystic disease.

chronic hemodialysis becomes necessary, the diet should be altered to meet the added requirements related to dialysis therapy.

General Principles of Follow-up

Patients with CRF should be seen at regular intervals to monitor the progress of their disease. The frequency of these visits will depend upon the presence of other diseases, e.g., hypertension and heart failure, and on how rapidly residual renal function is being lost. All patients should be seen at least every three months, at which time a medical history is taken and a physical examination is performed. In addition, laboratory values including hematocrit, white blood cell count, serum urea nitrogen and creatinine concentrations, and electrolyte values should be obtained. Monitoring the progress of renal insufficiency is generally accomplished by measuring the serum creatinine concentration as an indirect index of GFR. Alternatively, 24-hour urine collections can be obtained to measure creatinine and urea clearances, since the average of these two values gives a close approximation of GFR. For most patients, the loss of residual renal function proceeds at a constant rate; this rate is different for each patient, although generally patients with polycystic renal disease have a slower rate of loss of renal function than those with diabetic nephropathy. To monitor the progress of the disease, the reciprocal of the serum creatinine concentration can be plotted against time for an individual patient, as shown in Figure 79–2. For most patients, this relationship is remarkably linear and can be used to estimate when a patient will become a candidate for maintenance hemodialysis. When the reciprocal of serum creatinine concentration reaches 0.1 or less (a creatinine concentration of 10 mg per deciliter), the patient is close to the time when dialysis becomes necessary. Moreover, a sudden change in the slope of this line can indicate that some other factor, such as obstruction, infection, or uncontrolled hypertension, is accelerating the rate of loss of residual renal function.

Anderson S, Brenner BM: Effects of aging on the renal glomerulus (review). Am J Med 80:435, 1986. *This article reviews nicely the consequences of aging on renal function. It reminds us that the reduction in creatinine clearance with aging is accompanied by a reduction in daily production of creatinine. Thus, the serum creatinine level in the elderly patient does not reflect the same high creatinine clearance as in the younger patient. This becomes of importance in the management of elderly patients receiving nephrotoxic drugs. The article also proposes a provocative hypothesis based on animal studies that limitation of dietary protein intake may delay the age-related loss in renal function.*

Bricker NS: Sodium homeostasis in chronic renal disease. Kidney Int 21:886, 1982. *This article is an examination of factors regulating sodium homeostasis in normal and chronic failure patients.*

Chan MK, Varghese Z, Moorhead JF: Lipid abnormalities in uremia, dialysis and transplantation. Kidney Int 19:625, 1981. *An excellent overview editorial that discusses clearly the complex lipid abnormalities in uremic and dialysis patients.*

DeLuca HF: The vitamin D hormonal system: Implications for bone diseases. Hosp Pract April 1980, pp 57–63. *Dr. DeLuca reviews clearly the factors important in the pathophysiology of renal osteodystrophy, with special emphasis on the central role of vitamin D.*

Eschbach JW, Adamson JW: Anemia of end-stage renal disease. Kidney Int 28:1, 1985. *An excellent editorial review that discusses the mechanisms that contribute to the anemia and treatments that have been proposed for anemia of end-stage renal disease.*

Eschbach JW, Egrie JC, Downing MR, et al.: Correction of the anemia of end-stage renal disease with recombinant human erythropoietin. N Engl J Med 316:73, 1987. *This is an important report of results from phase I and II clinical trials using recombinant human erythropoietin to treat uncomplicated anemia in end-stage renal failure patients undergoing hemodialysis. The authors demonstrate a remarkable dose-dependent rise in hematocrit in response to intravenous erythropoietin given three times weekly after dialysis.*

Giordana C (ed.): Fourth Capri Conference on Uremia. Kidney Int 28(Suppl. 17):S1–S193, 1985. *This supplement represents contributions from 48 leading interdisciplinary specialists on various aspects of uremia. Clinical symptoms, pathogenesis, and treatment of uremia and its complications are discussed in great detail.*

Oldrizzi L, Rugin C, Valvo E, et al.: Progression of renal failure in patients with renal disease of diverse etiology on protein-restricted diet. Kidney Int 27:553, 1985. *This is a long-term study on more than 200 patients with renal disease of diverse etiology in which the authors demonstrate that the administration of protein-restricted diet delays the progression of functional renal deterioration.*

Wineman RJ: End-stage renal disease: 1978. Dialysis Transplantation 7:1034, 1978. *A review of demographic characteristics of end-stage renal disease as derived from the National Dialysis Registry.*

80 TREATMENT OF IRREVERSIBLE RENAL FAILURE

80.1 Dialysis

Robert G. Luke

Each year approximately 1 in 10,000 of the United States population develops end-stage renal disease (ESRD) and requires one of the various forms of renal replacement therapy: chronic hemodialysis in a center or at home; intermittent peritoneal dialysis—usually at home; continuous ambulatory peritoneal dialysis; or transplantation from a live-related or cadaveric donor. Most of the costs of such treatment are covered for almost all of the United States population by the Renal Medicare Program, and by the late 1980's approximately 100,000 patients are expected to participate. The most common causes of end-stage renal disease are chronic glomerulonephritis, nephrosclerosis, chronic pyelonephritis (reflux nephropathy), diabetic glomerulosclerosis, and polycystic kidney disease. The overall incidence of end-stage renal disease is 4.5 times greater in blacks than in Caucasians; hypertensive nephrosclerosis accounts for 33 per cent of the cases in blacks but only 8 per cent in whites.

Choices of renal replacement therapy is dictated by the availability of a live-related donor (best results), the age of the patient (transplantation is less frequently performed over the age of 55 years), and the presence of important systemic extrarenal disease (which may preclude surgery or immunosuppression). Preliminary hemodialysis is usually necessary before transplantation. Home hemodialysis or intermittent peritoneal dialysis requires the support of a partner, an adequate home, self-motivation by the patient, and reasonably stable medical circumstances. Such patients have better rehabilitation and survival rates than those on in-center hemodialysis, but this may relate to patient selection factors. The cost of home dialysis is less than in-center dialysis. In general, patients are best served when all modalities of treatment for end-stage renal disease are readily available and well integrated.

TECHNICAL ASPECTS

As renal excretory function becomes progressively impaired, solutes accumulate in the body and eventually contribute to the uremic syndrome (see Ch. 79) and, ultimately, to death. These solutes, especially those of low molecular weight such as urea, can be removed efficiently from the blood by the process of diffusion across a semipermeable membrane down a chemical concentration gradient (dialysis). Substances higher in concentration in the dialysate than in the plasma, such as bicarbonate, will diffuse into the plasma (Fig. 80–1). The membrane must be nontoxic and compatible with red blood cells, white blood cells, platelets, and plasma proteins. Either a synthetic membrane in the process of extracorporeal hemodialysis or, in peritoneal dialysis, the lining membrane of the peritoneal cavity is used.

Hemodialysis

Membranes of varying hydraulic conductivity and solute permeability can be used in dialyzers of varying surface area and extracorporeal blood volume (100 to 250 ml in adults) to accommodate patients of different sizes, including infants. To remove accumulated sodium chloride and water, ultrafiltration across artificial membranes is induced by a transmembrane hydrostatic pressure, either positive on the blood side or negative on the dialysate side (Fig. 80–1). The removal of over 1 liter of fluid per hour is feasible and predictable based on the ultrafiltration coefficient of the dialyzer. The essential components of a dialysate delivery and monitoring system of an artificial kidney apparatus are shown in Figure 80–2. Blood flow rates of 200 to 300 ml per minute are usual. Heparin is given intermittently or infused continuously (1000 to 10,000 units in total) to prevent clotting of blood in the dialyzer during the usually three- to six-hour procedure; dosage is controlled by the whole blood or activated clotting time.

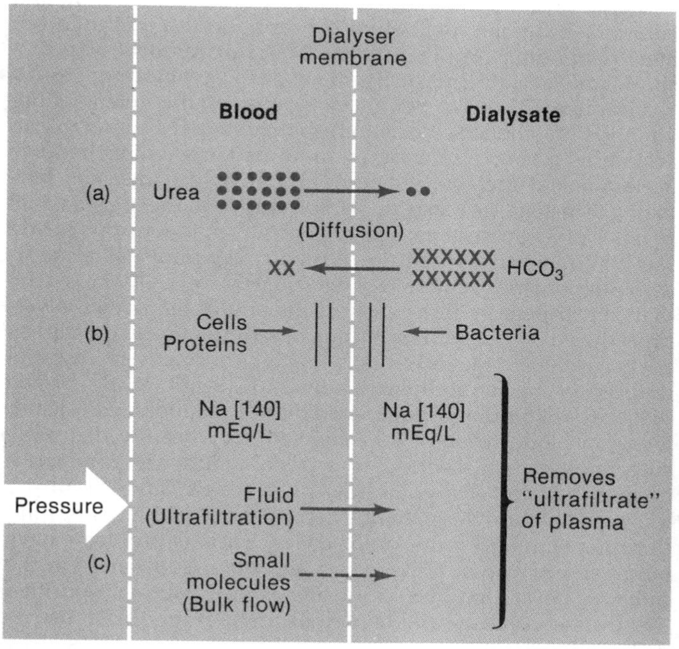

FIGURE 80–1. Mechanisms of removal of solute and fluid during dialysis. (*a*) Diffusion of urea from high concentration in blood into dialysate and of bicarbonate from higher concentration dialysate into lower concentration in the blood of patient with renal failure. (*b*) The dialysis membrane is impermeable to red blood cells and plasma proteins and to bacteria in the dialysate (but not to endotoxins). (*c*) The dialysate sodium is freely diffusible and determines the plasma sodium; fluid is removed by application of a transmembrane pressure (in peritoneal dialysis by increased glucose and hence osmotic pressure in the dialysate). The fluid is accompanied by small molecules such as sodium and chloride by convection (solvent drag).

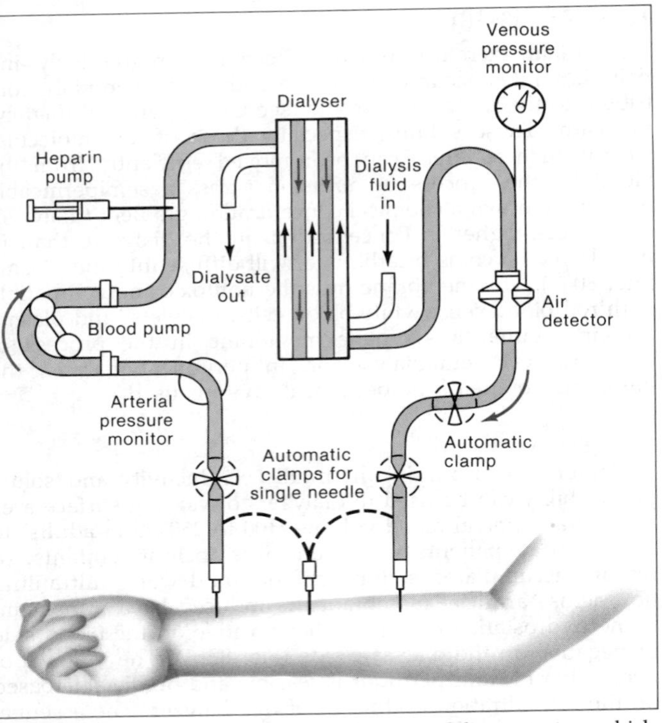

FIGURE 80–2. Essential components of a dialysis delivery system which, together with the dialyzer, makes up an "artificial kidney." In isolated ultrafiltration no dialysis fluid is used (bypass mode). Also shown is the apparatus for using a single needle for inflow and outflow of blood from the patient. (From Keshaviah PR, Shaldon S: In Drukker W, Parsons FM, Maher JF (eds.): Replacement of Renal Function by Dialysis. 2nd ed. Boston, Martinus Nijhoff Publishers, 1983, p. 224.)

Dialysate contains normal serum levels of sodium and chloride, a variable potassium concentration (0 to 4 mEq per liter) depending on the patient's need for removal of potassium, and acetate (normally metabolized to bicarbonate) or bicarbonate (35 mEq per liter) to correct the renal failure patient's metabolic acidosis. Bicarbonate may be preferable to acetate as a source of base in some patients, either because acetate is not metabolized normally (in which case the normally transient increase in "anion gap" in the plasma will persist) or because it may contribute to hypotension during the hemodialysis procedure. A slight respiratory alkalosis is common during dialysis because of loss of CO_2 across the dialyzer. It persists transiently at the end of the hemodialysis procedure because, although the extracellular base deficit has been corrected, the respiratory center continues to respond transiently to intracellular acidosis. Calcium levels in the dialysate—3.5 mEq per liter—are higher than ionized calcium levels in blood to allow a calcium influx from the dialysate, since most patients with chronic renal failure are in negative calcium balance. Dialysate flow rates are usually 500 ml per minute and thus the patient's blood "sees" 120 liters of fluid during a standard four-hour dialysis. Various problems have occurred because of trace metals and other substances in the public water supply, but tap water is now routinely purified by reverse osmosis and/or deionization prior to its use in dialysate.

Peritoneal Dialysis

In peritoneal dialysis clearances of low molecular weight substances are less than for hemodialysis (for example, a urea clearance of 20 to 25 ml per minute versus 150 ml per minute for hemodialysis), but clearance of some larger, perhaps also toxic, substances is greater because of the greater permeability of the peritoneal membrane to these larger molecules and the longer duration of treatment. When required, fluid removal is carried out by means of osmotic movement of water using high concentrations of glucose (1500 to 4500 mg per deciliter) in the dialysate. Exchange volumes during peritoneal dialysis are commonly 1 to 3 liters each hour. Several types of automated machines are available that make dialysate from concentrate, deliver set volumes of fluid into the abdomen, and then allow drainage after a set "dwell" time. The commonest type now in use is the cycler, which is relatively simple, uses commercially prepared dialysate in bottles, and automatically cycles up to a total of 16 liters of dialysate in and out of the abdomen for a period of 8 hours (often overnight). Because peritoneal dialysis is less efficient than hemodialysis, dialysis times are much longer (Table 80–1). Therefore chronic intermittent peritoneal dialysis is practical only for use at home.

Continuous Ambulatory Peritoneal Dialysis (CAPD)

This technique makes use of the fact that small molecular weight solutes reach complete equilibration with peritoneal fluid in four to six hours. Thus the patient exchanges 1.5 to 3.0 liters of sterile dialysate containing hypertonic glucose (1.5, 2.5, or 4.25 per cent) and physiologic electrolytes three to five times a day through a Tenckhoff peritoneal dialysis catheter and is able to maintain adequate removal of solutes and water. Since insulin-dependent diabetics have more complications of vascular access because of their vasculopathy and since regular insulin can be given in the dialysate with excellent control of the blood sugar, CAPD offers advantages to patients with diabetic glomerulosclerosis. In infants and children the higher peritoneal surface area relative to body size also facilitates CAPD. In contrast to poorer dialysis of small molecular weight solutes compared with hemodialysis, dialysis of larger molcules (>500 daltons) is increased (see Table 80–1). Larger "middle molecules" may accumulate in chronic hemodialysis patients and contribute to complications such as pericarditis. Many patients have been managed successfully by CAPD for several years, but technique failure rates remain higher than for chronic hemodialysis, mainly because of problems with the peritoneal catheter or recurrent peritonitis.

CLINICAL USE

During hemodialysis, the major limiting factor for clearance of small molecular weight substances such as urea is the "unstirred layer" barrier to diffusion at the blood-membrane interface. Clearance does not increase significantly beyond blood flow rates of 250 ml and dialysate flow rates of 500 ml per minute. Surface areas of 1.0 to 1.3 square meters are usually adequate to reduce blood urea by about 50 per cent during a three- to four-hour hemodialysis. In contrast, the limitation to clearance of a larger molecular weight substance such as inulin is the permeability of the membrane, and inulin clearance for most commonly used hemodialysis membranes is quite small (Table 80–1). The permeability of the peritoneal membrane (the effective surface area of which is estimated to be between 0.5 and 1 square meter in adults) for larger molecular weight substances is much greater than the artificial membranes, but dialysate flow rates in intermittent peritoneal

TABLE 80–1. TIME-AVERAGED CLEARANCE (ml/min)*

Technique	Weekly Duration	Urea Clearance	B_{12} Clearance	Inulin Clearance
		(60)†	(1350)†	(5200)†
Hemodialysis	3 × 4 = 12 hr	11 (160)‡	2.5 (30)	0.3 (4)
Intermittent PD	4 × 10 = 40 hr	6 (25)	1.5 (7)	1.2 (5)
CAPD	Continuous	7	5	3
Normal kidney	Continuous	60	120	120

*Does not include residual renal function.
†Molecular weight (daltons).
‡Figures in parenthesis are actual clearances during procedure.
PD, peritoneal dialysis; CAPD, chronic ambulatory peritoneal dialysis.

TABLE 80–2. CONTINUOUS AMBULATORY PERITONEAL DIALYSIS (CAPD)

Advantages	Disadvantages
Requires no machine	Peritonitis due to contamination during bag changes*
Maintains constant plasma solutes	Patient time: 4 exchanges at 30 to 40 minutes/7 days per week
Less restricted dietary intake	Loss of protein in dialysate (8 to 12 grams/day)—requires increased protein intake
Less expensive (?)	Hyperlipidemia and obesity (glucose in PD fluid)
No dependence on helpers or nurses	Long-term adequacy of peritoneal membrane as dialyzer (?)
Enhanced mobility	
Better control of blood pressure (?)	
Good control of blood glucose by intraperitoneal insulin in diabetic patients	
Less cardiovascular stress	

*Majority of cases can, however, be treated on an outpatient basis with intraperitoneal antibiotics.

dialysis are much less (35 ml per minute). Thus urea clearance for peritoneal dialysis is much less than for hemodialysis, and inulin clearance is relatively greater (Table 80–1). Peritoneal blood flow has been estimated at 50 to 100 ml per minute and is clearly a factor that may critically limit clearance in states of markedly reduced cardiac output. Unfortunately, the causes of toxicity in the uremic syndrome are poorly understood, so that the ideal dialysis regimen or membrane cannot be defined. Techniques that remove small molecular weight end-products of protein metabolism, such as urea, are quite successful and compatible with prolonged survival and reasonable well-being, however.

Permanent vascular access is usually obtained by creation of an end-to-side arteriovenous fistula in the forearm or insertion of a prosthetic arteriovenous graft when the vessels themselves are inadequate. A permanent indwelling peritoneal catheter is made of radiopaque Silastic 25 cm long and includes an intra-abdominal (located in the pelvis), subcutaneous (with a Dacron felt cuff barrier to bacteria at each end), and external segment. Most ESRD patients continue to be managed, however, by chronic in-center hemodialysis, and only about 20 per cent of all dialysis patients are on some form of home dialysis, including chronic ambulatory peritoneal dialysis. The advantages and disadvantages of the latter technique are outlined in Table 80–2.

Initiation of Dialysis

Before initiating chronic dialysis careful discussion with the patient and family should address the issue of whether such treatment is in the patient's best interest. For example, if there is extensive irremediable extrarenal disease, such as severe cerebrovascular disease or a painful malignancy, it may be wiser to continue conservative treatment only.

Initiation of dialysis should occur when conservative management of chronic renal failure is beginning to be inadequate but before the development of uremic symptoms. In general, dialysis becomes necessary at a creatinine clearance of 4 to 8 ml per minute or a serum creatinine of about 10 mg per deciliter. However the patient's general clinical state is more important than the level of blood urea nitrogen or creatinine. It is especially important to institute therapy before the onset of pericarditis, peripheral neuropathy, or an impaired nutritional state secondary to anorexia or other uremic gastrointestinal symptoms, as subsequent recovery is then quite prolonged and mortality rate increased. Vascular access should be placed, if feasible, a few months before dialysis to allow it to mature adequately. Of the permanent types of access, only the Scribner shunt (a Teflon external connector between the radial artery and a forearm vein) is available for use immediately. If uremia develops abruptly, acute vascular access can be maintained for up to several weeks by an indwelling subclavian vein catheter or intermittently via the femoral vein. Permanent peritoneal access is placed one to two weeks prior to use to prevent fluid leaks, which predispose to peritoneal and subcutaneous infections.

In *diabetic nephropathy* renal failure may accelerate microangiopathic complications—especially retinopathy, gastropathy, and peripheral neuropathy—and many nephrologists therefore prefer to initiate replacement therapy earlier in such patients, perhaps when serum creatinine approximates 5 to 8 mg per deciliter. The progression of diabetic glomerulosclerosis to ESRD at that stage also tends to be quite rapid.

Hypertension is an important complication in most patients who reach end-stage renal disease. Antihypertensive medications can usually be tapered after initiation of dialysis, and blood pressure can be controlled by adjustment of plasma and extracellular fluid volume by ultrafiltration during dialysis and by dietary salt and water restriction. Sympatholytic drugs or drugs that cause postural hypotension are best avoided, since they interfere with the ability to remove fluid adequately by ultrafiltration. A reduction in urinary volume commonly accompanies the onset of dialysis because of lessening of solute osmotic diuresis. The concept of "dry weight" is a clinically important one in a chronic dialysis patient, regardless of modality of therapy. This is the postdialysis weight at which the patient has an acceptable blood pressure and a plasma volume adequate for avoiding symptoms of diminished cardiac output or of pulmonary congestion. Short-term changes in weight are always due to salt and water deficits or excesses, but careful supervision is required to detect changes in body mass in either direction over longer periods. Interdialytic weight gains should not exceed 2 to 3 kg but unfortunately often do so in patients who are not compliant with dietary salt and fluid restrictions.

Most dialysis patients thus have "volume-dependent" hypertension and require antihypertensive medications only if they are noncompliant with salt and water intake. In perhaps 10 per cent of patients, however, blood pressure is "renin dependent," and progressive ultrafiltration is accompanied by persistent rebound hypertension after hemodialysis due to rising circulating levels of angiotensin II. Previously bilateral nephrectomy was sometimes employed to control blood pressure in such patients, but the advent of such potent drugs as captopril and minoxidil has virtually eliminated the need for this procedure. Furthermore, it is especially important to avoid bilateral nephrectomy when some recovery of renal function may occur in time, as after an episode of primary or secondary malignant hypertension or after rapidly progressive glomerulonephritis. Indeed, anephric patients fare less well overall during chronic dialysis because of absence of erythropoietin production and, possibly, of $1,25(OH)_2$ cholecalciferol, and because of loss of residual renal clearance of larger molecular weight substances.

Dialysis disequilibrium describes a syndrome in which confusion, headache, and focal neurologic signs develop owing to more rapid dialysis of solutes from the plasma than from the intracellular compartment, especially from the brain. Thus an osmotic gradient can be set up between brain cells and extracellular fluid and lead to cerebral edema. This complication usually occurs in patients with acute or chronic renal failure and uremic symptomatology and/or a very high blood urea nitrogen (BUN). Short dialysis with a low blood flow usually prevents this problem, which does not occur in maintained chronic dialysis patients and is extremely rare during initiation of any of the forms of peritoneal dialysis because of their lesser efficiency.

Hepatitis B (Hb_sAg) is carried in the plasma of some patients with chronic renal failure, who therefore constitute a serious risk to dialysis staff and other patients, since there is repeated exposure to the patient's blood. Separate dialysis facilities and staff are needed for such patients if home dialysis or transplantation is not feasible. Routine monitoring for Hb_sAg is now performed in patients initially testing negative for the antigen, and active immunization is available and indicated for patients and staff. Non-A, non-B hepatitis also remains an epidemiologic problem.

TABLE 80–3. RELATIVE INDICATIONS FOR PERITONEAL (PD) OR HEMODIALYSIS (HD) FOR MANAGEMENT OF ACUTE RENAL FAILURE

Clinical Circumstance	Comment
1. Recent cerebral surgery, vascular accident or trauma	PD preferred; risk of hemorrhage with heparin and of fluid shifts in brain during HD
2. Hypercatabolic states (e.g., multiple injuries)	HD preferred; PD may not provide adequate clearance of urea, etc.
3. Recent cardiac surgery or myocardial infarction	PD preferred; increased risks of hypotension and arrhythmias with HD
4. Recent abdominal surgery	HD preferred; loss of fluid via incisions during PD; ileus requires surgical placement of PD catheter
5. Acute hemorrhage or severe coagulopathy	PD preferred; but in certain circumstances HD without heparin feasible
6. Complicating severe lung disease	HD preferred; PD may cause atelectasis and impair vital capacity by interfering with movement of diaphragm

Hemodialysis and acute intermittent peritoneal dialysis are also employed in the treatment of acute renal failure, the most frequent cause of which is acute tubular necrosis (see Ch. 78). These patients are often quite ill, and survival is aided by frequent "prophylactic" dialysis to maintain a blood urea nitrogen (BUN) of less than 100 mg per deciliter. The relative merits of hemodialysis and peritoneal dialysis for acute renal failure are outlined in Table 80–3.

Continuous Arteriovenous Hemofiltration

The technique of continuous arteriovenous hemofiltration can be uniquely valuable, especially in patients with acute cardiorenal failure and a low cardiac output. This procedure employs a membrane with a very high ultrafiltration coefficient, which allows fluid and solute removal at low blood perfusion pressures and flow rates. No blood pump or complex monitoring devices are required, and the procedure can be readily performed in an intensive care setting with femoral artery and vein cannulation in very ill, often fluid-overloaded patients in whom hemodialysis or peritoneal dialysis would be very difficult or impossible. Intravenous administration of electrolyte replacement solutions may be necessary with intravenous nutrition if indicated. Heparin is needed.

ROUTINE MANAGEMENT

Patients on chronic hemodialysis usually require a slightly reduced protein intake (0.8 to 1.0 gram per kilogram), but a more stringent control of salt and potassium intake, to maintain satisfactory levels of blood urea nitrogen, potassium, and blood pressure. Hyperkalemia remains a significant cause of death in chronic dialysis patients, usually due to dietary indiscretion. Monitoring of adequacy of dialysis requires assessment both of clinical well-being, including nutritional state, and of BUN and serum electrolytes, including calcium and phosphorus. The BUN reflects urea production rates and is dependent on protein intake and endogenous protein catabolism as well as on adequacy of urea removal by dialysis. Provided nutrition and protein intake are adequate, a BUN less than 90 to 100 mg per deciliter immediately prior to dialysis is usually acceptable. Plasma chemistries are checked monthly, or less often in stable home patients, in the absence of clinical problems. Adequate clearances can usually be achieved by a total of 12 (9 to 15) hours of hemodialysis per week on a thrice-weekly schedule. In most patients supplemental oral base (sodium bicarbonate) is not required; serum HCO_3 should be kept above 20 mEq per liter in the predialysis blood. Dialysis is almost always inadequate to maintain serum phosphorus in an acceptable range (3.5 to 5.0 mg per deciliter) and, as in the conservative management of renal failure, oral aluminum-containing phosphate binders are necessary. Constipation is a frequent result and needs treatment by, for example, the use of an osmotic cathartic such as 70 per cent sorbitol. In some patients, aluminum-containing binders contribute to aluminum-related bone disease; calcium or magnesium carbonate may be used to substitute partially as phosphate binders. Because of loss of water-soluble vitamins, including folic acid, from the blood during dialysis, routine administration of supplements of these substances is necessary. Oral iron is also given because there is a chronic small loss of blood that cannot be returned to the patient at the end of each dialysis. Anabolic steroids such as nandrolone decanoate can improve the red blood cell production in dialysis patients and hence are commonly administered. Recently human erythropoietin, produced by recombinant DNA technology, has been shown to be capable of returning the hematocrit to normal in patients on chronic hemodialysis. This observation has obvious therapeutic implications for the future.

COMPLICATIONS OF CHRONIC DIALYSIS

The major clinical complications experienced by patients on chronic dialysis are renal osteodystrophy, anemia, vascular access infections and thromboses, pericarditis, and ascites (Table 80–4). The major cause of death remains cardiovascular disease, but the high incidence of coronary atherosclerosis probably reflects the risk factors of hypertension and hyperlipidemia (and perhaps of a high calcium-phosphate product) rather than any specific effects of chronic dialysis per se. Dialysis does cause some cardiovascular stress during the procedure owing to ultrafiltration and reduction of plasma volume and to a modest reduction in arterial oxygen levels (by 10 to 20 mm Hg). This latter is due either to hypocarbia secondary to loss of CO_2 across the dialyzer and/or to sequestration of blood leukocytes in alveolar capillaries after the activation of complement by the dialyzer membrane; a transient leukopenia is usual during the first hour of dialysis. Episodes of hypotension and hypoxia secondary to those dialysis effects frequently provoke angina in patients with coronary vascular disease.

Renal osteodystrophy is discussed elsewhere from the standpoint of both pathogenesis and treatment (see Ch. 249). Normal serum levels of calcium, phosphate, bicarbonate, and parathormone should be maintained. Calcium supplements, phosphate binders, and $1,25(OH)_2$ cholecalciferol may be needed. Rarely soft tissue calcification, hypercalcemia, and progressive osteitis fibrosa cystica may necessitate subtotal parathyroidectomy. Osteomalacia usually responds to $1,25(OH)_2$ cholecalciferol, but one resistant type, in which an excess of aluminum is found on bone biopsy, appears to respond only to diminishing bone aluminum by chelating agents such as desoxyferamine.

Anemia is a constant finding. The hematocrit in a well-dialyzed, well-nourished dialysis patient is usually in the range of 25 to 35 per cent. However, in anephric patients it

TABLE 80–4. COMPLICATIONS IN PATIENTS ON CHRONIC DIALYSIS

Accelerated cardiovascular disease	Hepatitis B (Hb_sAg) carrier state
Hypertension	During dialysis
Renal osteodystrophy	Hypotension
Anemia	Cramps
Serositis	Bleeding
Pericarditis	Leukopenia with pulmonary sequestration of WBC's
"Dialysis ascites"	Hypoxia
Pleural effusion	Electrolyte disturbances
Access infections and thrombosis	Dialysis disequilibrium
Dialysis dementia	CAPD
Pseudogout, tenosynovitis	Exacerbation of symptoms of abdominal hernia or back pain
Pruritus	
Poor nutrition	

WBC's, white blood cells.

is usually 12 to 20 per cent. Transfusion is not indicated unless anemia is contributing to symptoms, heart failure, or angina. The major cause of the anemia appears to be lack of erythropoietin together with depression of erythropoiesis by azotemia. As noted above, synthetic human erythropoietin is likely to be available soon for use in man. Iron deficiency anemia is not uncommon and may be indicated by a lowered serum ferritin level. Eosinophilia is quite common in chronic dialysis patients and appears to be of little clinical importance.

Serositis, as manifested by pleural effusion, ascites, or pericarditis, may complicate chronic dialysis. The pathogenesis is not established, although onset often accompanies periods of infection, stress, or protein catabolism. The diagnosis in each case is dependent on elimination of other causes. In general, the abnormal fluid has the characteristics of an exudate and, especially in the case of the pericardial sac, may be hemorrhagic. Patients with pericardial effusion may develop pericardial tamponade, especially during dialysis, when intravascular volume and pressure in the right side of the heart are being reduced. Atrial arrhythmias are also common. If pericardial effusion occurs, dialysis should be carried out daily with very careful control of anticoagulation. If hemodynamic, radiologic, or ultrasonic assessment shows no improvement, surgical treatment by pericardial stripping or medical treatment by pericardiocentesis and insertion of a locally long-acting steroid such as triamcinolone is indicated. "Dialysis ascites" can be an intractable management problem. Poor nutrition and fluid overload often contribute, and insertion of a LeVeen shunt (one-way valve with bacterial filter between peritoneum and vena cava) may be necessary. Tuberculosis is an important differential cause of these complications, and diagnosis is dependent on histologic findings and culture, since anergy is common. Pleural effusion is less common and less troublesome than pericarditis and ascites.

Access infections are commonly due to *Staphylococcus aureus* infection, may be associated with bacteremia or septicemia, or even bacterial endocarditis, and may require excision of the graft. Access problems are the most frequent cause of admission to hospital in the dialysis population. These include thrombosis, aneurysms, and infection of the graft. Arteriovenous fistulas last, on the average, longer than synthetic grafts, but each may function for several, even many, years. Steal syndromes may develop with pain in the hand during dialysis, especially in patients with diabetic vascular disease. Very high blood flows through fistulas may contribute to congestive heart failure, but this is quite unusual.

Dialysis dementia is a progressive fatal disease of the central nervous system associated with speech and motor defects, dementia, and seizures. It is now much less frequent, probably because of improved procedures for preparation of dialysate water and reduction in its aluminum content. Motor paralysis due to peripheral neuropathy is also now rare in well-dialyzed patients.

Pseudogout and *tenosynovitis* occur quite frequently in dialysis patients and respond well to drugs such as indomethacin. *Pruritus* is a troublesome symptom and is sometimes attributable to a high blood calcium-phosphate solubility product or to hyperparathyroidism. In some cases pruritus, despite correction of the above factors, remains resistant to treatment.

The dialysis procedure itself may be complicated by hypotension and muscle cramps; both are related to rates of ultrafiltration and usually respond to injections of small amounts of hypertonic fluids such as 0.3 M NaCl or 20 per cent mannitol. Contributory causes of hypotension are autonomic insufficiency, diminished cardiac function, and hypotensive drugs. In patients who are prone to ventricular ectopy it is important to avoid hypoxia by use of supplemental oxygen and rapid changes in serum potassium by modifying dialysate potassium concentration. This is especially true in patients on cardiac glycosides. Other complications of the dialysis procedure are air embolism, bleeding secondary to heparin, loss of blood due to clotting of the dialyzer, and electrolyte disturbances due to errors in the dialysate. Fortunately these are all now quite unusual. Indeed, death or serious morbidity due to complications of the hemodialysis procedure itself in properly trained or supervised patients is now exceedingly rare.

LIMITATIONS OF DIALYSIS

For chronic dialysis, hemodialysis remains the "gold" standard, and many patients continue to do well after over ten years on this form of treatment. The three-year survival rate for American patients aged 20 to 25 years is 85 to 90 per cent; for those 60 to 65 years, 60 per cent; and for those with diabetic renal disease, 40 per cent. This form of treatment is inherently limited, however, not only because of low clearances (see Table 80–1) but also because the endocrine and regulatory functions of the native kidney are not replaced by the "artificial kidney." Indeed, life saving as it is, the latter term is a misnomer; the patient with an endogenous creatinine clearance of even 15 ml per minute is usually better off than one on maintenance chronic dialysis or CAPD.

Drukker W, Parsons FM, Maher JF: Replacement of Renal Function by Dialysis. Edition 2. Boston, Martinus Nijhoff Publishers, 1983. *This is a complete reference work for all technical and clinical aspects of dialysis.*

Eschbach JW, Egrie JC, Downing MR, et al.: Correction of the anemia of end-stage renal disease with recombinant human erythropoietin: Results of a combined phase I and II chemical trial. N Engl J Med 316:73, 1987. *This is an important new development that may become standard therapy in the future.*

Golper TA: Continuous arteriovenous hemofiltration in acute renal failure. Am J Kidney Dis 6:373, 1985. *This extensive review describes the clinical indications and advantages and disadvantages for continuous arteriovenous hemofiltration (CAVH) and compares it with traditional dialysis therapies for renal failure.*

80.2 Renal Transplantation

William J. C. Amend, Jr.

HISTORICAL PERSPECTIVE. Clinical renal transplantation had its successful beginnings at the Peter Bent Brigham Hospital in 1954 with the successful implantation of a kidney from a healthy identical twin donor into a young patient with chronic renal failure. This predated by some years the technique of chronic, repetitive hemodialysis and offered hope to patients with chronic renal failure. Unfortunately, most patients do not have an identical twin donor. Success in extending this transplantation technique to patients who were genetically dissimilar to their organ donor (the donor being a relative, nonrelative, or cadaver, or even a subhuman primate) had to await the discovery and use of various immunosuppressant techniques.

More recently, advances in organ preservation, knowledge of histocompatibility, tests in vitro involving pretransplant immunologic responses, immunosuppression, and other aspects of patient management have greatly improved the likelihood of transplant functional success. A greater utilization of both dialysis and transplantation has occurred from (1) technical and scientific improvements, (2) physician and patient awareness of treatment availability, and (3) economic support for its clinical applications (through legislative appropriation). At present, approximately 8000 patients per year receive a renal transplant, and approximately 85,000 patients per year receive some form of chronic dialytic support in the United States.

DONOR ASPECTS. Organ transplants can be generally divided into two types: (1) those from a living donor (related or nonrelated) and (2) those from a cadaver donor.

Living Donor. A prospective donor should have no significant medical history and be of an acceptable age (18 to 60 years). High motivation and normal emotional responses are necessary. Preliminary tissue-typing tests are performed, including ABO typing, HLA serotyping (human leukocyte antigen typing), and a direct lymphocyte crossmatch between donor lymphocytes and recipient sera. Biologic relatives are preferred, since there is an increased chance of tissue-typing compatibility. The post-transplant clinical response can be roughly predicted after this histocompatibility testing and with other immune tests performed in vitro (see "Immunologic Aspects," below, and Ch. 425). Finally, the donor undergoes intensive medical testing, culminating in pyelography and renal arteriography. If these medical tests are completely normal, the person can serve as a low-risk donor with the probability of near normalization of renal function following a half-year period of compensatory renal hypertrophy in the remaining kidney. Renal donors have shown little functional deterioration, proteinuria, or hypertension for a subsequent 2 to 20 years.

Cadaver Donor. Cadaver donations come after death from brain trauma, subarachnoid bleeding, or some other sudden, terminal event that occurs in a previously healthy individual. After brain death has been determined, the next of kin is contacted for permission for organ donation. When permission is given, a transplant team or regional organ bank is contacted for organ procurement. Often a cadaver donor serves for multiple organ purposes (i.e., kidney, lung, heart, pancreas, liver). The kidneys are removed and maintained at cold temperatures (4 to 6° C) with either a saline flush solution (cold preservation) or pulsatile perfusion (Belzer technique). While the kidneys are stored, the donor-recipient matching is performed at a histocompatibility laboratory, utilizing lymphocytes from donor lymph nodes obtained during the procurement procedure. These tests must be carried out rapidly (within 6 to 24 hours) in order to utilize the cadaver kidney before irreversible, storage-induced damage occurs. Computer-assisted analysis allows for the selection of recipients from a cadaver-transplant waiting list. This necessary speed of matching is in marked contrast to the methodical pretransplant immune testing (sometimes taking weeks) in live-related donor renal transplants.

RECIPIENT CHARACTERISTICS. The transplant recipient may have end-stage renal failure from a variety of causes. The most common are glomerulonephritis, diabetes mellitus, nephrosclerosis, and polycystic disease. Dialysis patients with severe chronic pulmonary disease, with severe obesity, with known cancer within three years of surgery, or with known active infection are considered unsuitable transplant candidates. Psychologic or compliance problems may be relative contraindications.

Recurrent urinary tract infections, persistently high antiglomerular basement membrane antibody levels, or resistant forms of renin-dependent hypertension often indicate the need for pretransplant bilateral nephrectomy. Also, if ureteral reflux is demonstrated with or without positive urine cultures, preliminary bilateral nephrectomy is performed. Recipients with certain forms of renal disease must be carefully informed regarding the absolute and relative risks of recurrent disease possibilities.

IMMUNOLOGIC ASPECTS. ***Histocompatibility.*** Increasing degrees of genetic similarity between donor and recipient confer upon organ transplants increasing chances for successful transplant function. When the transplant is between identical twins (isografts), there is no genetic disparity and hence no likelihood of rejection. The transplant success in these instances relates to nonrejection factors such as technical problems or the possibility of recurrent disease. More commonly, organ transplants are performed between two genetically dissimilar members of the same species (allografts or homografts).

Histocompatibility is defined as the degree to which the tissues of two individuals are alike. Cell surface antigens (phenotypes appearing on white cells and endothelial cells) are determined by histocompatibility genes, known as the HLA system (Ch. 425). Each genetic locus expresses its phenotypic information independently on human lymphocytes (T and/or B cells). A combination of five genetic loci on the sixth human chromosome is known as the major histocompatibility locus (MHL) and encompasses genotypes for both Class I and Class II antigens.

The antigens of the serologically defined loci (such as A, B, C, and DR) can be determined over six hours, whereas the antigens of the lymphocyte-defined loci (D) are determined by lymphocyte blastogenesis occurring in vitro over three to five days. A haplotype is that genetic information (from adjoining gene loci) that would be carried on any one chromosome. All individuals have leukocyte phenotypes that are made up of two haplotypes for the various HLA antigens.

Prior to a transplant, a patient with kidney failure undergoes tissue typing to assess his or her histocompatibility and to compare this with potential donors. By noting the various A, B, and DR leukocyte phenotypes (and their distribution) in a family, such as in Figure 80–3, it is possible to construct haplotypes involving these three histocompatibility antigens. In the example shown, the patient is a two-haplotype match to one sister, one-haplotype match to two siblings and both parents, and a zero-haplotype match to one sister. The last sibling could be of the same match grade as a randomly obtained, live-unrelated, or cadaver donor. In addition, ABO compatibility is currently felt to be necessary, so that donor selection includes both red-cell and white-cell tissue antigen systems. If there are no compatible relatives who might be a donor, the potential histocompatibility match from a nonrelative (living or cadaver donor) is shown in Figure 80–3.

As noted in Figure 80–4, functional survival of the transplant is excellent when two full haplotypes (HLA-identical) are shared and is less when only one haplotype is shared. Many centers employ pretransplant donor-specific blood transfusions, DST (see below under "Immune Responses"), for one-haplotype as well as zero-haplotype transplants (the latter being completely mismatched, such as a wife-husband match). Thus far, these are as successful as the pairs with the best HLA-match grades. Cadaver kidney transplant results are also depicted in Figure 80–4. HLA A and B locus matching does not improve cadaver-donated graft success rates in most centers in the United States. On the other hand, pretransplant blood transfusions have an important beneficial effect on graft survival. Recently, matching for the DR locus has improved cadaver graft success in some, but not all, regions of the United States. Most importantly, newer immunosuppressive agents, such as cyclosporine, have markedly improved two-year cadaver graft survivals.

Immune Responses. Organ transplants evoke a variety of responses in the recipient. If there has been previous sensitization (from blood transfusions, previous transplants, or pregnancy) a *hyperacute rejection* can immediately occur. This is based on a recipient antibody–donor endothelial cell reaction and resembles a Shwartzman's phenomenon. The result is cortical necrosis with no treatment possible. This is avoided with carefully performed pretransplant donor-recipient lymphocyte crossmatching. This crossmatching must particularly involve a T cell–type crossmatch. Interestingly, despite a positive T cell crossmatch with historic sera (sera from the patient more than one year before transplant), the transplant can be successfully performed as long as more recent sera are negative with the T cell crossmatch.

If a weaker degree of sensitization, perhaps to a minor histocompatibility locus, has occurred, a slightly delayed secondary humoral response can occur. This is termed an *acute-accelerated rejection*, which is pathologically similar to the hyperacute rejection. This likewise is irreversible, but it occurs in a delayed manner two to six days post-transplant.

In the more usual circumstances, the allograft is initially invaded by recipient macrophage and monocyte cells. If antigenic differences to the allograft are noted, these cells will process the antigen with a T lymphocyte and activate this T

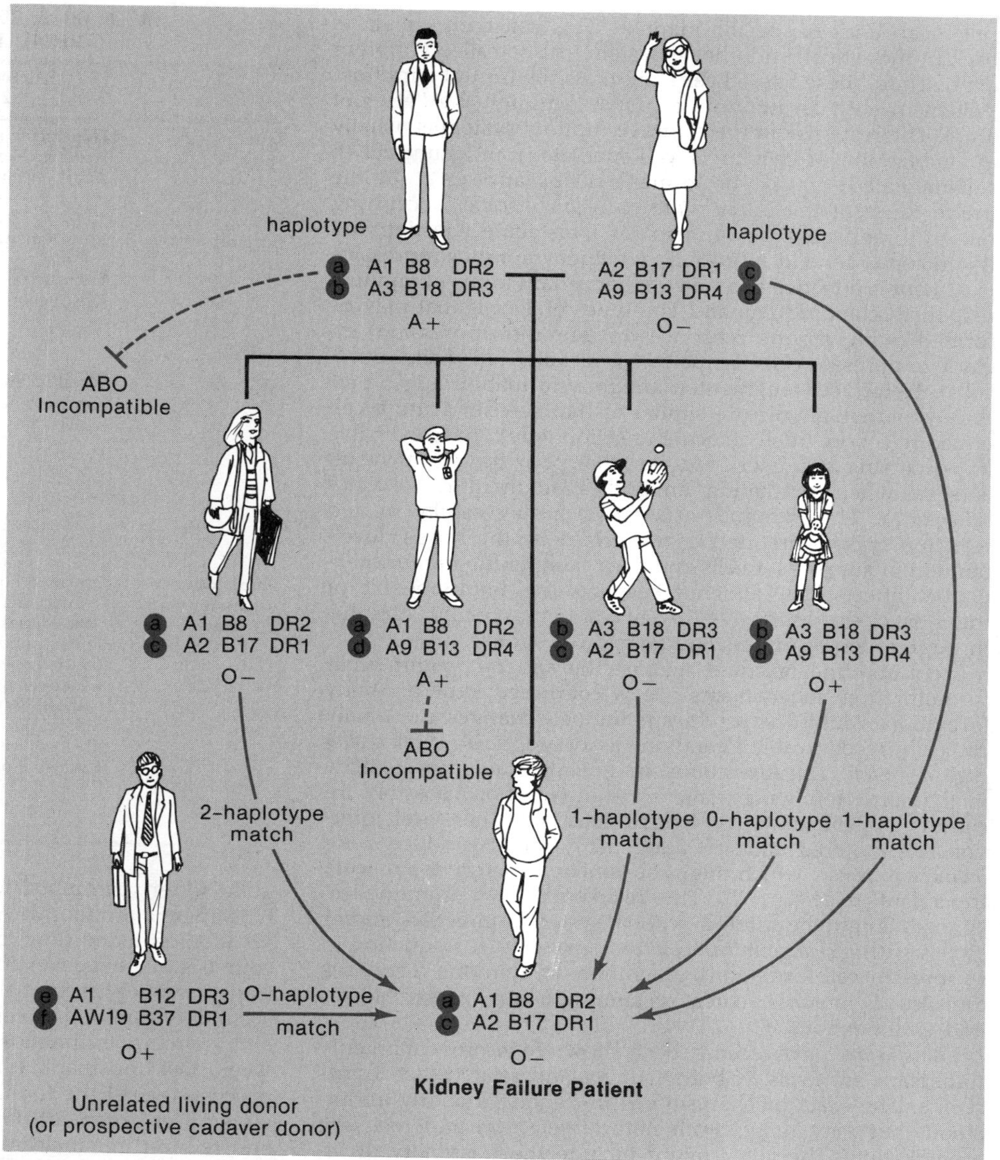

FIGURE 80–3. Family tree of HL-A genotypes and unrelated HL-A genotype.

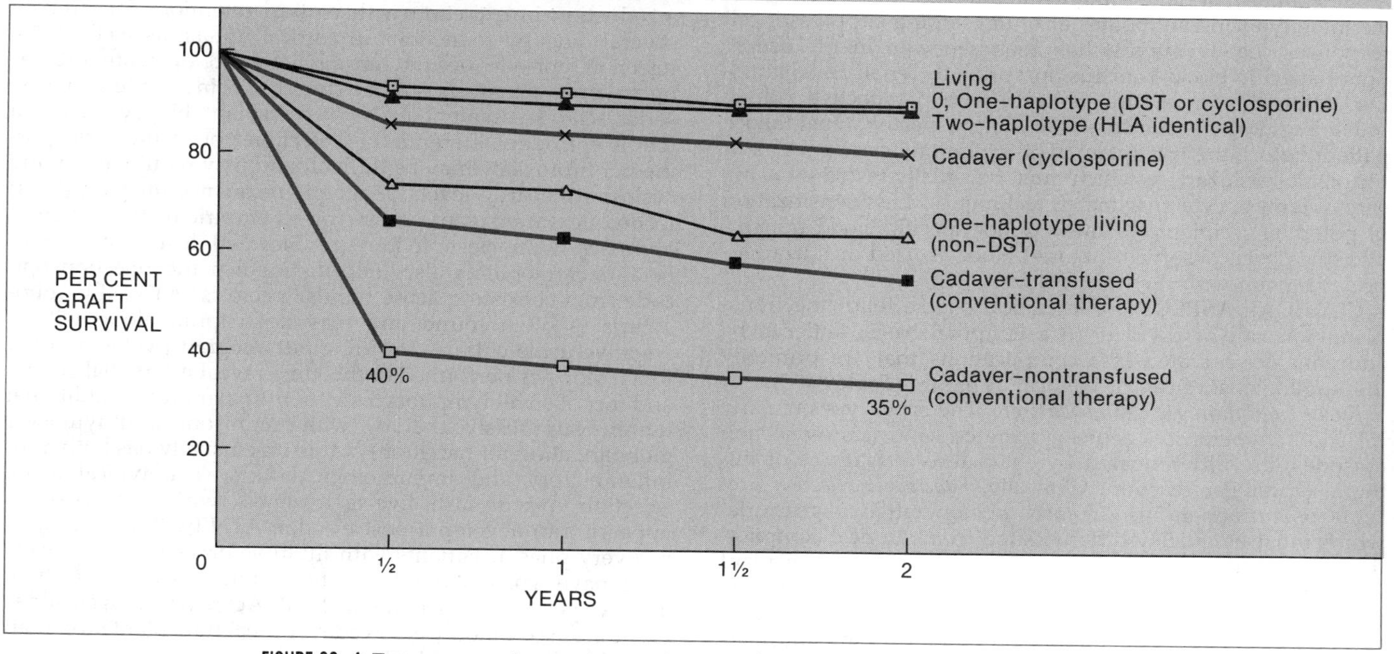

FIGURE 80–4. Two-year renal transplant graft survivals utilizing various transplant strategies.

cell in an antigen-specific manner. This cell then circulates back to the reticuloendothelial system (the so-called "afferent arc"). There these altered cells stimulate the central lymphoid system to elicit an immune response (through the "efferent arc"). The response in the central lymphoid system is usually a combination of cellular (T cell–mediated) and humoral (B cell–mediated) types. The former reaction appears to be the prime cause of the initial *acute transplant rejection*, occurring one to three weeks post-transplant. This acute rejection and its outcome depend in part on whether immunosuppressive treatment is effective and on whether certain forms of immune response cells predominate. The types of T cells that may be formed (with varying responses to immunosuppression) include suppressor cells, helper cells, or killer cells (cytotoxic T cells). Helper cell–augmented antibody formation might produce a pathologic picture similar to that seen in acute accelerated rejection. Such an acute rejection would be irreversible but occurring at a later date. Another poor transplant result is seen when circulating antibodies augment *cell-mediated cytotoxicity*. The immune response in a successfully treated rejection episode is often characterized by the host's development of suppressor cells and their dampening immunoregulatory effects. The allograft becomes less immunogenic or the host less responsive to this antigen-specific stimulus through a poorly understood adaptive response.

Later immune reactions against the allograft might occur through three mechanisms: (1) A continued slow antibody formation would first produce pathologic changes and finally clinically recognizable alterations associated with *chronic allograft rejection*. (2) Alterations in the allograft's antigenicity might occur following some sorts of infection, possibly including cytomegalovirus, Epstein-Barr, or other viral infection. This altered allograft antigenicity might produce a *late immune response*, which might be similar in nature to an acute transplant rejection. (3) The recipient's own immune responses might be altered with a systemic infection and/or illness with a *change in the adaptive response* (e.g., reduction in suppressor cell formation). Alterations in immune responses are already noted in such systemic illnesses as sarcoidosis and viral hepatitis.

Transfusions have recently been shown to improve markedly transplant survivals of both cadaver and related-type transplants. The exact mechanism of this benefit is poorly understood, but may reflect both natural selection and recipient modification. The latter might include the possibility of inducing enhancing antibodies or of developing suppressor cell responses. Lately interest has been renewed in the use of donor-specific blood transfusions prior to renal transplantation. With this procedure, blood from a prospective kidney transplant donor is transfused to the prospective renal failure patient before the transplant. This technique carries a risk of recipient sensitization, which must be serially tested by using careful lymphocyte crossmatch techniques. Less sensitization of potential recipients to these donor-specific blood transfusions has been observed if stored blood is used or if azathioprine is given with the transfusions.

CLINICAL ASPECTS. The clinical course following transplantation can be divided on a temporal basis, and can be additionally separated into complications that are primarily immunologic, surgical, or medical in nature (Table 80–5).

Early Immunologic Complications. The three types of early rejection (hyperacute, acute-accelerated, and acute-rejection episodes) are differentiated by characteristic features of humoral or cellular reaction. Clinically, *hyperacute rejection* presents as intraoperative or early postoperative oligoanuria, which must be quickly differentiated from surgical complications. Renal scan flow studies with pertechnetate or transplant arteriography show nonvisualization. Transplant nephrectomy must be performed. *Acute-accelerated rejection* occurs several days post-transplant and presents as fulminant rejections with fever, oliguria, tenderness, and enlargement of the graft. Often, thrombocytopenia and microangiopathic hemolytic anemia are found. Again, renal scans will reveal little or no allograft blood flow, consistent with cortical necrosis. The course is that of irreversible renal failure, which again requires transplant nephrectomy. This form of rejection represents a secondary humoral or cell-mediated response.

TABLE 80–5. COMPLICATIONS FOLLOWING RENAL TRANSPLANTATION

	Early Complications (< 2 months)	Late Complications (> 2 months)
Immunologic	Hyperacute rejection Acute accelerated rejection Acute rejection	Acute rejection Chronic rejection
Surgical	Procurement/perfusion injury Urinary leak Obstruction	Lymphocele Reflux Obstruction—stone, cicatrization Renal artery stenosis
Medical	Renal failure—acute tubular necrosis, acute rejection	Progressive renal failure or nephrotic syndrome—chronic rejection, recurrent disease Transplant pyelonephritis Hypertension Atherosclerotic events Erythrocytosis
Immunosuppression-related	Impaired host defense—infections Moon facies, obesity Poor wound healing Gastrointestinal bleeding Leukopenia, thrombocytopenia Steroid psychosis Cyclosporine nephrotoxicity Cyclosporine hepatotoxicity	Impaired host defense—infections Moon facies, obesity, hirsutism Aseptic necrosis, osteoporosis Steroid myopathy Hypophosphatemia Cataracts Steroid hyperglycemia Neoplasia Hepatitis, pancreatitis Cyclosporine nephrotoxicity

Acute rejection, the most common type, occurs after the first week post-transplant. It is felt to be a primary, cell-mediated process against the foreign donor cells. It is characterized by allograft enlargement, fever, malaise, oliguria, hypertension, and reduced renal clearances. Renal scans will initially show a reduction in excretion with cortical retention, followed in several days by reductions in cortical uptake as well. If the rejection episode occurs during a period of acute tubular necrosis, its diagnosis may be delayed, being made either by serial scan assessment or by a transplant biopsy during a febrile episode. Differentiating rejection from acute cyclosporine nephrotoxicity may be difficult and may require obtaining cyclosporine drug levels, magnetic resonance imaging (MRI) techniques, transplant biopsy, or an empiric (drug-lowering) approach with close follow-up. Elevated levels of urinary $beta_2$-microglobulins also help distinguish the rejection episode from coexisting acute tubular necrosis (ATN). Lymphocyturia is often found and may be helpful, along with a negative urine culture, in ruling out allograft pyelonephritis. Renal biopsies performed at this time reveal interstitial edema and foci of small lymphocytes in peritubular areas. Additional immunosuppressive therapy (with prednisone, antithymocyte globulin, allograft radiation) at this time usually has both anti-inflammatory and immunologic effects. The typical acute rejection episode lasts five to ten days, with some patients appearing to develop a postrejection ATN (with a prolonged recovery phase). Patients with multiple or severe early rejections have worse allograft functional outcomes (at one, two, and five years) than patients without. Acute rejection episodes occur more commonly after cadaver renal transplantation than after live-donor transplantation.

Early Surgical Complications. After cavader transplantation, there may be initial ATN on the basis of donor-agonal changes, warm ischemia (in excess of 30 minutes), or excessive donor-sympathetic responses at or near the time of the cadaver organ procurement. ATN per se does not affect the eventual transplant outcome. The patient will, however, require post-transplant dialysis. Rarely, storage or perfusion injury can occur. In either case, a technically poor result will occur with suboptimal renal function. In addition, the use of cyclosporine superimposed on this injury may be disadvantageous. These problems are usually not seen with live-donor transplants, since there can be careful preoperative management of the donor's hydration status and a marked reduction in warm ischemic injury. Attentive surgical technique lowers the possibilities of vesicoureteral reflux, of urinary leak from the neocystostomy site, and of lymphocele formation.

Early Medical Complications. Medical problems initially noted post-transplant include continuing renal failure (from ATN or rejection), during which the patient requires dialysis. As noted above, cyclosporine may induce varying degrees of drug-related acute nephrotoxicity. Hypophosphatemia can be seen after normal renal function is regained. Persisting secondary hyperparathyroidism causes exaggerated phosphaturia. This parathyroid hyperplasia usually regresses during the first half-year following successful transplantation. Correction of the patient's anemia or an increase in a diabetic patient's daily insulin requirement gives a favorable transplant prognosis, since the transplanted kidney has already begun normal renal endocrine function.

Immunosuppression commonly used following renal transplantation may include one or a combination of glucocorticosteroids, azathioprine or cyclophosphamide, antithymocyte globulin (either polyclonal or monoclonal antibodies against T cells or T cell subsets), cyclosporine or some other lymphocyte depletion technique such as thoracic duct drainage or, more recently, total lymph node irradiation. All these therapies confer what is termed "nonspecific immunosuppression." Despite different mechanisms of action, generalized impairments of cell- or humoral-mediated immune responses are produced.

Hypercortisolism accounts for many of the undesired side effects and morbidity in renal transplant patients. In the early post-transplant period, poor wound healing, reduced host defenses, psychologic changes, and steroid-induced hyperglycemia are particularly common. Growth may be retarded in children receiving daily glucocorticosteroids. In an attempt to reduce these problems, many transplant patients are shifted to once-daily or alternate-day dose regimens (see Ch. 30). Other immunosuppressive agents also reduce host defenses in a nonspecific fashion. The patient becomes more susceptible to viral, protozoal, fungal, or bacterial infection. Infections, particularly pulmonary, must be aggressively diagnosed and specific treatment rapidly begun. The patient's immunosuppression should be reduced if infection is suspected, even at the potential risk of transplant rejection loss. Bone marrow suppression, liver abnormalities, or hemorrhagic cystitis can also occur from one or more of these antimetabolites. The type and dosage of the drugs must be adjusted with monitoring of these signs and/or with drug blood levels (cyclosporine).

Late Immunologic Complications. Occasionally, an acute rejection process occurs more than two to three months after a transplant. This may occur either spontaneously or more frequently following an abrupt change in immunosuppressant therapy. Usually, rejection processes are more of a chronic, vascular type in the months to years following the transplant. Chronic rejections are clinically asymptomatic and are detected by renal functional abnormalities (progressive azotemia, proteinuria) and often have associated hypertension.

Late Surgical Complications. Late problems are primarily of a urologic type. Vesicoureteral reflux is not seen if the reflux-correcting "tunnel" procedure is employed at the time of transplantation. Lymphoceles may not be detected until years after the transplant and can be associated with partial obstruction, infection, or hypertension. Since allografts are denervated, stone passage is painless and is usually associated only with (temporary) renal impairment, hematuria, or signs of an associated urinary tract infection.

Late Medical Complications. Atherosclerotic disease, already a noteworthy complication of dialysis, is frequently present. Predisposing risk factors include smoking and significant hypertension and lipid abnormalities seen during uremia and dialysis. Opportunistic infectious problems still can occur in long-term situations. Careful evaluation for any post-transplant patient with a febrile illness is necessary. Fungal, protozoal, or viral infections are particularly serious and require rapid diagnosis and supportive therapy. Immunosuppression should be diminished if host resistance is compromised. Aseptic necrosis or osteonecrosis, particularly of weight-bearing joints, is an unfortunate complication seen in 15 per cent of these patients. It principally affects hip, knee, and shoulder joints and is related to pre-existing secondary hyperparathyroidism, in addition to the transplant corticosteroid therapy. Excellent rehabilitation therapy, however, can be provided with arthroplastic surgery. Hypertension frequently occurs after transplantation and may be related to rejection (either acute or chronic), residual kidney or renal pressor mechanisms (from the native kidneys), glucocorticoid or mineralocorticoid effects (cyclosporine per se), urologic abnormalities (lymphoceles or obstruction), or transplant renal artery stenosis. Evaluation of severe hypertension necessitates a urologic and renovascular workup, with the need for selective venous renin measurements from three kidney sites. Infusions of angiotensin-converting enzyme inhibitors might also be important in detecting renin-dependent, angiotensinogenic hypertension.

Certain forms of neoplasms are particularly noted in transplant patients. Cervical dysplasia and carcinoma may be related to herpes type 2 involvement. Excessive cases of immunoblastic lymphoma, leukemia, and cutaneous malignancies have also been noted. However, a generalized increase of malignancies (solid tumors as well as other forms of lymphoproliferative disorders) has not been demonstrated. It is not known whether the immunosuppression lowers tumor surveillance in these patients or whether the allograft alters the patient's own immune response (from a chronic antigen exposure). Rarely, a patient will develop post-transplant erythrocytosis. Such patients should be evaluated to establish the primary nature of this disorder. Often, recurrent phlebotomies are necessary for one to two years. It is felt that the erythropoietin source comes from the native kidneys (nonsuppressed in a nonuremic milieu).

The transplant kidney may develop the nephrotic syndrome with or without clearance deterioration. Usually, particularly if the primary renal disease was nonimmunologic, this is secondary to chronic rejection. By pathologic examination, chronic rejection has elements either of a predominantly arteriolar lesion with an intimal reaction or of a glomerular lesion with generalized basement membrane thickening and mesangial proliferation. Clinically, progressive hypertension and proteinuria are hallmark features of early phases of chronic rejection, with the eventual development of intractable renal failure. On the other hand, patients with certain forms of renal disease (Table 80–6) may be predisposed to recurrence of the original disease in their allografts. This was first noted in a high frequency with identical twin transplants, but must be suspected in all patients with these primary renal diseases. Renal biopsy or immunologic tests must be performed for diagnosis. Treatment of such conditions in the allograft is the same as that of primary disease. Transplant pyelonephritis is characterized by pain and swelling over the transplant and by usual accompanying renal functional dete-

TABLE 80–6. RECURRENT DISEASES OF RENAL ALLOGRAFTS

Primary Disease	Comments
Membranous glomerulonephritis	Same immunologic pattern; appearance is similar to that of chronic rejection
Rapidly progressive glomerulonephritis	Fulminant course in isografts; "crescents" on pathology; graft failure
Anti-GBM* glomerulonephritis	With and without preliminary bilateral nephrectomy; graft failure
Juxtamedullary focal glomerulosclerosis	With and without graft failure
IgA nephropathy	Immunofluorescence with and without graft failure
Membranoproliferative disease	
Type 1	With and without graft failure
Type 2 ("dense deposit")	Graft failure often
Oxalosis	Deposits and graft failure
Cystinosis	Deposits without graft failure
Henoch-Schönlein syndrome	
Hemolytic uremic syndrome	
Diabetes mellitus	Glomerular lesions nodular and diffuse; no graft failure (yet)

*GBM, glomerular basement membrane

rioration. Potential urologic problems should be tested for in this circumstance.

Patients who are positive for hepatitis B surface antigen (before or after the transplant) have a serious probability of developing chronic active hepatitis, cirrhosis, and/or hepatomas. Caution must be taken in recommending transplantation in such patients at the present time.

Transplant patients often regain fertility, and contraceptive advice is indicated. Despite theoretic risks of genetic malformation and a higher incidence of miscarriage and spermatozoal malformation, no severe congenital malformations have been described, and many successful pregnancies have occurred.

Psychologically, much anxiety and depression can occur with transplant- or immunosuppressive-related problems. The glucocorticoids directly affect the emotions of such patients, making the reactive nature of their emotional responses even more labile during such stresses. Despite an otherwise excellent physical status, some patients remain overly concerned that the transplant may "fail." Most patients with well-functioning renal transplants attain a degree of rehabilitation similar to their premorbid status.

Over a period of time, the patient seems to adapt immunologically to the transplant in a poorly understood manner. Even after an initial success of two years or more, there continues to be a relationship between the degree of histocompatibility and the long-range functional prognosis. There is a greater chance of late transplant failure in cadaver renal transplants than in forms of related renal transplants. Also, one-haplotype transplants do less well than fully matched sibling pairs. After an initial two years of transplant success, the T½, or half-life, probabilities for two-haplotype transplants are 34 years, for one-haplotype transplants 10 years, and for cadaver transplants 7.5 years. This analysis is practically important when discussing the long-range prognosis with a transplant recipient. The prognosis of certain patient populations, those with diabetes, for instance, is worsened because of systemic complications in these groups.

When a patient rejects a first renal transplant within the first year, transplant nephrectomy is usually necessary. Rejected foreign tissue left in situ will produce a symptom constellation of fever, allograft tenderness, generalized malaise, cachexia, and weight loss. Transplants that undergo chronic rejection, if well tolerated, may be left in place.

Retransplantation (a second or third time) can be attempted if the first transplant fails. An effort is made to avoid similar histocompatibility antigens in subsequent transplants or at least to assess whether specifically shared lymphocytotoxic antibodies have developed subsequent to the first transplant. A similar clinical course (regarding rejection probabilities) can be anticipated in later transplants, suggesting that the recipients' own immune regulation is an important factor in transplant success. Choosing a different immunosuppressive agent for a second transplant might be important to attain better transplant success.

Prognosis. Three to 5 per cent of patients receiving a cadaver renal transplant are at risk of dying each year. Related-donor transplants have improved the likelihood of patient survival. The risk of death in certain patient groups (transplant recipients with diabetes or other systemic disease) is higher than in those patients who are otherwise healthy. A successful transplant permits the best opportunity for complete rehabilitation of a patient with chronic renal failure.

Calne RY: Organ transplantation: From laboratory to clinic. Br Med J 291:1751, 1985. *An informational recounting of the development of organ transplantation.*

Hunsicker LG: Impact of cyclosporine on cadaveric renal transplantation: A summary. Am J Kidney Dis 5:335, 1985. *A nice review of cyclosporine's beneficial results and toxicity problems. Summarizes many institutions' results.*

Opelz G: Correlation of HLA matching with kidney graft survival in patients with or without cyclosporine treatment. Transplantation 40:240, 1985. *Large collaborative study that emphasizes the role of donor-recipient histocompatibility.*

Strom TB: The improving utility of renal transplantation in the management of end-stage renal disease. Am J Med 73:105, 1982. *A thorough review of the subject, particularly good with the discussion of immunosuppression.*

81 GLOMERULAR DISORDERS

William G. Couser

About 80,000 patients in the United States require hemodialysis or transplantation for chronic renal failure at an annual cost in excess of 2 billion dollars. Two thirds of these have some glomerular disease. First described in the writings of Richard Bright in the early nineteenth century, these diseases have subsequently intrigued many clinician-investigators who have attempted to separate and classify them solely on the basis of clinical manifestations and histopathology. Inconsistent terminology and confusing classification systems proliferated, sufficient to befuddle generations of medical students.

The past two decades have witnessed a marked improvement in this situation: (1) Experimental models of glomerular diseases have been produced by immunizing animals with either renal antigens or various foreign proteins, thus confirming a long-held suspicion that most such diseases have an immunologic basis. (2) The histologic and functional abnormalities in these models were found to be associated with the development of immune deposits in glomeruli, demonstrated by immunofluorescence (IF) and electron microscopy (EM). The widespread application of percutaneous renal biopsy as a routine clinical diagnostic tool has allowed experimental observations to be applied to understanding the pathogenesis of glomerular lesions in humans. In this chapter, glomerular diseases are classified on a clinical basis into three groups: (1) primary renal diseases that usually present with the abrupt onset of hematuria, red cell casts, proteinuria, and decreased glomerular filtration rate (acute nephritic syndrome or glomerulonephritis [GN]); (2) primary renal diseases that usually present with the insidious onset of heavy proteinuria and relatively normal glomerular filtration rate (nephrotic syndrome); and (3) secondary glomerular diseases resulting from renal involvement by a variety of systemic illnesses, which may be either nephritic or nephrotic. This approach has the virtue of simplicity, but it is useful only if its limitations are fully appreciated. Separation between primary and secondary renal diseases is sometimes difficult and arbitrary. For example, IgA nephropathy is recognized as a primary renal disease and Henoch-Schönlein purpura is classified as a secondary one, although they probably represent only differing clinical manifestations of the same process and often overlap. Most of the diseases that present as acute GN may cause the nephrotic syndrome, although they do so uncommonly, and some nephrotic glomerular diseases may occasionally exhibit nephritic features.

IMMUNE MECHANISMS AND THE GLOMERULAR RESPONSE TO INJURY

Two immunologic mechanisms of glomerular disease are generally accepted: (1) Rare patients develop glomerulonephritis due to deposition of antibody to glomerular basement membrane (GBM) antigens, which results in a typical uninterrupted linear staining pattern along all glomerular capillary walls by immunofluorescence microscopy, (see Fig. 81–7). (2) Much more commonly, glomerulonephritis is associated with discontinuous, or granular, deposits of immunoglobulin and complement (see Figs. 81–2*B*, 81–3*B*, and 81–8). These deposits may occur at three sites: (1) within the glomerular mesangium, as in IgA nephropathy, Henoch-Schönlein purpura, and early lupus nephritis; (2) along the subendothelial surface of the capillary wall between endothelial cells and GBM, as seen in more severe forms of lupus nephritis and type I membranoproliferative glomerulonephritis (MPGN); and (3) on the outer, subepithelial surface of the capillary wall, as in membranous nephropathy and the so-called subepithelial "humps" in post-streptococcal glomerulonephritis. Granular, or immune complex, deposits at mesangial and subendothelial sites either can result from the passive glomerular trapping of preformed immune complexes from the circulation or may form in situ owing to initial glomerular localization of free antigens followed by antibody binding to them. Subepithelial immune complex deposits appear to form only on a local basis. Figure 81–1 illustrates schematically how immune deposits at each of these sites are related to normal glomerular structures and some of the morphologic lesions that result.

Several glomerular diseases that are believed to be immunologically mediated do not have immune deposit formation in glomeruli. For example, minimal change nephrotic syndrome (MCNS) exhibits a marked increase in capillary wall permeability without immune deposits or histologic changes; and idiopathic rapidly progressive glomerulonephritis (RPGN) is characterized by severe glomerular inflammatory changes with crescent formation without detectable immune deposits.

The type and severity of histologic and functional glomerular disease induced by immune deposits in glomeruli depend on many factors, including the quantity, composition, and site of the deposits. Most glomerular antibody deposits contain predominantly IgG, which activates complement via the classic complement pathway. When deposits are in mesangial and subendothelial sites they are accessible to circulating inflammatory cells. Chemotactic and immune adherence mechanisms recruit participation of neutrophils and macrophages, and these effector cells cause direct damage to glomeruli by release of proteolytic enzymes and toxic oxygen metabolites. An inflammatory glomerular lesion results, with clinical manifestations that include hematuria, proteinuria, and loss of renal function. IgA deposits activate complement less well and predominantly by the alternate complement pathway. When immune deposits form at a subepithelial site, as in membranous nephropathy, they are not accessible to circulating cells and the resulting lesion is a noninflammatory one, with the nephrotic syndrome apparently induced by a direct effect of the C5b-9, or membrane attack complex, portion of complement on capillary wall permeability. Thus, glomerular immune complex deposits may induce a spectrum of both clinical and histologic manifestations. The clinical consequences range from the acute nephritic syndrome with acute renal failure, as seen in some cases of post-streptococcal glomerulonephritis, to idiopathic nephrotic syndrome with

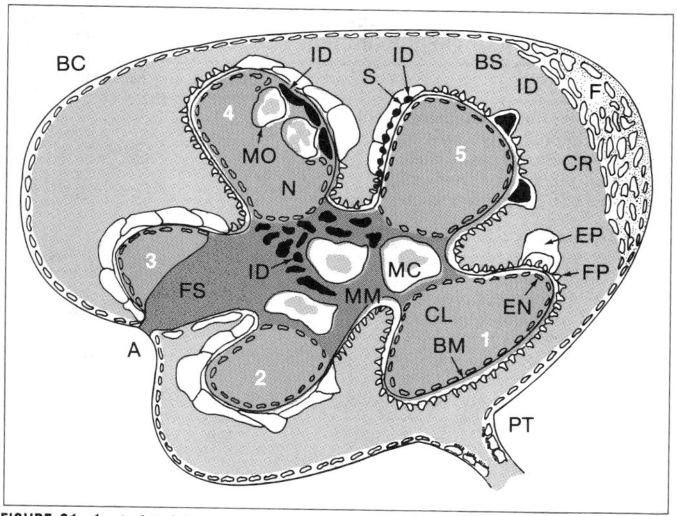

FIGURE 81–1. A highly schematized illustration of a cross-section of a single glomerulus showing normal glomerular architecture and some of the characteristic changes seen in glomerular diseases. One lobule with five capillary loops is illustrated within Bowman's capsule (BC). The capillary loops are supported by the intercapillary mesangium, containing mesangial cells (MC) and mesangial matrix (MM). Note that the normal glomerular capillary wall (loop 1) is composed of three layers: Endothelial cells (EN), basement membrane (BM), and epithelial cells (EP) with epithelial cell foot processes (FP).

Loop 2 illustrates minimal change nephrotic syndrome with only diffuse effacement, or "fusion," of epithelial cell foot processes. Foot process effacement is also seen in other areas where increased capillary permeability with proteinuria would occur. In loop 3 a focal sclerotic lesion (FS) is seen with collapse of the capillary loop and adhesion (A) to Bowman's capsule. Immune complex deposits (ID) are shown in black at three sites: within the mesangial matrix (loop 4); as subendothelial deposits between endothelial cells and basement membrane as seen in class IV SLE and type I MPGN (loop 4); and as the diffuse, finely granular subepithelial deposits of membranous nephropathy (left, loop 5) with intervening "spikes" (S) of basement membrane, or the larger, more widely spaced subepithelial humps (right, loop 5) seen in post-streptococcal glomerulonephritis. Mesangial and subendothelial deposits usually elicit an infiltrate of neutrophils (N) and monocytes (MO) that may displace endothelial cells and directly injure basement membrane, as shown in loop 4. With severe injury, fibrin (F) leakage into Bowman's space (BS) may induce formation of a cellular crescent (CR) composed of proliferating parietal epithelial cells and circulating mononuclear cells as shown from 1 to 3 o'clock. CL = Capillary lumen; PT = proximal tubule.

normal renal function, as in membranous nephropathy. Table 81–1 lists the glomerular diseases, classified by the mechanisms that produce them and with their major clinical presentations noted.

ACUTE GLOMERULONEPHRITIS

Pathophysiology of the Acute Nephritic Syndrome

The terms *acute GN* and *acute nephritic syndrome,* which are synonymous, refer to the abrupt onset of hematuria and proteinuria, usually associated with some impairment in renal function and often with retention of salt and water, leading to hypertension and edema. Virtually all of these abnormalities are present in patients with post-streptococcal GN (PSGN) but are less frequently found in other causes of the acute nephritic syndrome. The most common primary renal diseases that produce the acute nephritic syndrome are summarized in Table 81–2, where their major distinguishing clinical and pathologic features are compared. The syndrome may also result from membranoproliferative glomerulonephritis (MPGN), which is discussed under diseases that cause the nephrotic syndrome, and from glomerular involvement in several of the systemic diseases to be discussed subsequently.

HEMATURIA. Hematuria is the hallmark of the acute

TABLE 81–1. GLOMERULAR DISEASES CLASSIFIED BY IMMUNOLOGIC MECHANISMS AND THEIR PRINCIPAL CLINICAL MANIFESTATIONS

	Nephritis	Nephrotic Syndrome
Anti-GBM Antibody Glomerulonephritis		
With pulmonary involvement (Goodpasture's syndrome)	Yes	Rare
Without pulmonary involvement	Yes	Rare
Complicating membranous nephropathy	Yes	Yes
Immune Complex Glomerulonephritis		
Primary renal diseases		
IgA nephropathy	Yes	Rare
Membranous nephropathy	No	Yes
Type I membranoproliferative glomerulonephritis (MPGN)	Yes	Yes
Idiopathic	Yes	Rare
Associated with systemic diseases		
Postinfectious glomerulonephritis		
Post-streptococcal	Yes	Rare
Following other bacterial, viral, fungal, mycoplasmal, protozoal, spirochetal infections	Yes	Variable
Subacute bacterial endocarditis (SBE)	Yes	Rare
"Shunt nephritis"	Yes	Yes
Visceral abscesses	Yes	No
Collagen vascular diseases		
Systemic lupus erythematosus (SLE)	Yes	Yes
Henoch-Schönlein purpura (HSP)	Yes	Yes
Essential mixed cryoglobulinemia (EMC)	Yes	Yes
Diseases of Undefined but Probably Immune Pathogenesis		
Minimal change–focal sclerosis group	No	Yes
Idiopathic rapidly progressive glomerulonephritis (RPGN)	Yes	Rare
Type II MPGN (dense deposit disease)	Yes	Yes
Vasculitides: Polyarteritis nodosa (PAN)	Yes	Rare
Hypersensitivity vasculitis	Yes	No
Wegener's granulomatosis	Yes	Rare
Hemolytic uremic syndrome (HUS) and thrombotic thrombocytopenic purpura (TTP)	Rare	No

nephritic syndrome. When hematuria is associated with proteinuria (> 500 mg per day) and red blood cell (RBC) casts, it usually reflects an acute glomerular inflammatory process that may have the potential for rapid loss of renal function. RBC's probably reach the urine through breaks or "gaps" in the capillary wall and form casts as they become embedded in concentrated tubular fluid with an increased protein concentration. Hematuria and RBC casts may occasionally be seen in other diseases in which capillary wall disruption occurs, such as malignant hypertension and hereditary nephritis.

PROTEINURIA. In acute GN, proteinuria invariably accompanies hematuria but rarely exceeds 3.5 grams per day and is therefore in the "non-nephrotic" range. Proteinuria in acute GN reflects an increased urinary content of serum proteins due to some combination of three factors: (1) a generalized increase in the permeability characteristics of the glomerular capillary wall itself, (2) altered glomerular hemodynamics, and (3) mechanical disruptions in capillary wall structure. Thus proteinuria in acute GN is "nonselective" and contains serum globulins as well as albumin. The pathophysiology of glomerular protein excretion is discussed in more detail below under "Nephrotic Syndrome."

IMPAIRED RENAL FUNCTION. When glomerular inflammation severe enough to cause hematuria and proteinuria is present, the glomerular filtration rate (GFR) is usually reduced. This may range from a minimal reduction in GFR with normal serum creatinine values to oliguria or anuria requiring dialysis. Multiple factors account for the reduced GFR, including the effects of acute immune injury on glomerular pathophysiology and the development of glomerular intracapillary thromboses, acute tubular necrosis secondary to glomerular ischemia, tubular obstruction by casts, and compression of the glomerular tuft by proliferating epithelial cells forming crescents. The return of renal function to normal depends not only on cessation of the process that initiated the injury but also on the extent of irreversible structural changes that have occurred, such as necrosis, sclerosis, and fibrosis.

HYPERTENSION. Hypertension is a common manifestation of the acute nephritic syndrome in PSGN and may be a presenting sign in older patients. It is largely volume dependent, reflecting impaired renal excretion of sodium and water with reduced levels of plasma renin and aldosterone. Hypertension can generally be controlled by strict adherence to sodium restriction.

EDEMA. Edema in the acute nephritic syndrome, like hypertension, reflects extracellular fluid volume expansion due to renal retention of salt and water. The mechanisms of renal sodium retention in acute GN are poorly understood but include a reduced filtered sodium load as well as enhanced

TABLE 81–2. SUMMARY OF PRIMARY RENAL DISEASES THAT PRESENT AS ACUTE GLOMERULONEPHRITIS

Diseases	Post-streptococcal Glomerulonephritis (PSGN)	IgA Nephropathy	Goodpasture's Syndrome	Idiopathic Rapidly Progressive Glomerulonephritis (RPGN)
Clinical Manifestations				
Age and sex	All ages, mean 7, 2:1 male	15–35, 2:1 male	15–30, 6:1 male	Mean 58, 2:1 male
Acute nephritic syndrome	90%	50%	90%	90%
Asymptomatic hematuria	Occasionally	50%	Rare	Rare
Nephrotic syndrome	10–20%	Rare	Rare	10–20%
Hypertension	70%	30–50%	Rare	25%
Acute renal failure	50% (transient)	Very rare	50%	60%
Other	1–3 week latent period	Follows viral syndromes	Pulmonary hemorrhage; iron deficiency anemia	None
Laboratory Findings	↑ ASO titers (70%) Positive streptozyme (95%) ↓ C3–C9 Normal C1, C4	↑ Serum IgA (50%) IgA in dermal capillaries	Positive anti-GBM antibody	None
Immunogenetics	HLA-B12, D "EN" (9)*	HLA-Bw 35, DR4 (4)*	HLA-DR2 (16)*	None established
Renal Pathology				
Light microscopy	Diffuse proliferation	Focal proliferation	Focal→diffuse proliferation with crescents	Crescentic GN
Immunofluorescence	Granular IgG, C3	Diffuse mesangial IgA	Linear IgG, C3	No immune deposits
Electron microscopy	Subepithelial humps	Mesangial deposits	No deposits	No deposits
Prognosis	95% resolve spontaneously 5% RPGN or slowly progressive	Slow progression in 25–50%	75% stabilize or improve if treated early	75% stabilize or improve if treated early
Treatment	Supportive	None established	Plasma exchange, steroids, cyclophosphamide	Steroid pulse therapy

*Relative risk

sodium reabsorption in either the distal nephron or deep juxtamedullary nephrons. Edema and fluid retention are seen in over 90 per cent of patients with acute PSGN but are less common in other diseases causing the acute nephritic syndrome. Unlike nephrotic edema, edema in the nephritic syndrome is often present in nondependent areas such as eyelids, face, and hands. The key to management is effective sodium restriction, since diuretics may not be effective in the acute stage of GN.

Couser WG: Mechanisms of glomerular injury in immune-complex disease. Kidney Int 28:569, 1985. *A current, in-depth review of the pathogenetic mechanisms that underlie immune glomerular diseases.*

Madaio MP, Harrington JT: Medical intelligence. Current concepts: The diagnosis of acute glomerulonephritis. N Engl J Med 309:1299, 1983. *This short review provides a useful outline of the diagnosis and classification of acute glomerulonephritis, emphasizing the distinctive clinical and laboratory features of each of the diseases that cause the acute nephritic syndrome.*

Whitley K, Keane WF, Vernier RL: Acute glomerulonephritis: A clinical overview. Med Clin North Am 68:259, 1984. *This article reviews the pathogenetic mechanisms, clinical presentations, laboratory features, and renal biopsy findings in each of the major disease entities that cause acute glomerulonephritis.*

Isolated Hematuria

The presence of persistent abnormal hematuria (more than five RBC's per high-power field in more than one fresh-voided urine specimen), without systemic disease, RBC casts, significant proteinuria, or impaired renal function, is a common medical problem that may or may not reflect renal parenchymal disease. It is more common in children and adolescents than in adults. A careful medical and urologic evaluation must be performed with appropriate laboratory, radiologic, and urologic procedures to exclude nonglomerular lesions of the urinary tract such as infection, prostatism, papillary necrosis, polycystic and medullary sponge kidney, renal or urinary tract tumors, arteriovenous malformations, renal stones, blood dyscrasias, and hemoglobinopathies. The "loin pain-hematuria syndrome" is a disorder usually seen in young women taking oral contraceptives who develop recurrent episodes of gross hematuria accompanied by loin pain and mild hypertension in the absence of proteinuria or reduced renal function. The condition appears to be benign and is reversible when oral contraceptives are discontinued.

If no cause of hematuria can be found and no evidence of systemic or renal disease is present, isolated hematuria appears to be a benign entity, and only careful follow-up is indicated. Renal biopsy would be performed in such patients only if evidence of progressive renal disease developed or if the patient required further evaluation for other purposes such as insurance or employment. When such patients do undergo renal biopsy, the results usually reveal a mild, nonprogressive form of glomerular disease, often focal GN with or without mesangial IgA deposits. Only about 20 per cent of such patients will have normal renal biopsies.

Copley JB: Isolated asymptomatic hematuria in the adult. Am J Med Sci 29:101, 1986. *An excellent review of the causes of hematuria and the approach to diagnosis with a useful algorithm for evaluating patients who have only hematuria without proteinuria or renal dysfunction.*

Trachtman H, Weiss RA, Bennett B, et al.: Isolated hematuria in children: Indications for a renal biopsy. Kidney Int 25:94, 1984. *This paper reviews the findings in 76 children and adolescents biopsied for isolated hematuria and identifies a family history of hematuria and episodes of gross hematuria as the best predictors of significant renal pathology.*

Isolated Proteinuria

A more detailed discussion of proteinuria is given in Ch. 76. Like isolated hematuria, non-nephrotic range proteinuria *without* hematuria or decreased renal function may indicate a significant glomerular disease, but usually does not. When increased urinary protein excretion is suggested by qualitative analyses such as the dipstick, it must be confirmed by an accurate measurement of 24-hour protein excretion. Values in excess of 150 mg per day in adults, and 140 mg per square meter per day in children, are regarded as abnormal if an accurate 24-hour urine collection has been obtained. Abnormal protein excretion may be intermittent or persistent (fixed).

INTERMITTENT PROTEINURIA. The most common causes of intermittent proteinuria are *exercise*, assumption of the *upright position* (postural proteinuria), and *fever*. Up to 10 per cent of routine medical admissions may exhibit transient proteinuria. The basis for proteinuria in most of these conditions is probably hemodynamic (see above), although subtle alterations in glomerular architecture have not been excluded. Total protein excretion is usually less than 2.0 grams per day, renal function is normal, and 20-year follow-up studies have shown resolution of the proteinuria in a majority of cases with no evidence of progressive renal disease.

PERSISTENT PROTEINURIA. Persistent or fixed proteinuria can also occur without glomerular disease. *"Overflow" proteinuria* occurs when excess production of filterable, low molecular weight proteins exceeds the tubular reabsorptive capacity, as occurs with the production of lysozyme (molecular weight 14,000) in myelomonocytic leukemia or L-chains in plasma cell dyscrasias such as multiple myeloma. In some cases up to 5.0 grams of L-chains may be excreted daily. Another nonglomerular cause of proteinuria is renal tubular disease in which normal quantities of proteins such as lysozyme or beta$_2$-microglobulin are filtered but not reabsorbed. This can result in urinary excretion of up to 2.0 grams of such proteins daily in a variety of interstitial nephropathies and disorders of tubular function.

Isolated, fixed, non-nephrotic proteinuria of glomerular origin is associated with an increased incidence of hypertension and a somewhat decreased life expectancy in long-term follow-up studies, but progressive renal disease is rare. Renal biopsy in such patients usually reveals some glomerular abnormality. The spectrum of lesions in isolated proteinuria is wide and similar to that discussed above in isolated hematuria. In patients with fixed proteinuria of less than 2.0 grams per day without hematuria, systemic disease, or impaired renal function, renal biopsy is usually not performed unless a change in clinical status occurs or the patient requests a biopsy for other purposes.

Abuelo JG: Proteinuria: Diagnostic principles and procedures. Ann Intern Med 98:186, 1983. *A well-written summary of the different types of proteinuria, their causes and prognosis, with emphasis on the approach to evaluation of patients with mild proteinuria and normal renal function.*

SPECIFIC RENAL DISEASES THAT PRESENT AS ACUTE GLOMERULONEPHRITIS (GN) (see Table 81–2)

The prototype of acute postinfectious GN is post-streptococcal GN (PSGN), but glomerular disease may follow infection with a variety of other bacterial and nonbacterial agents: both gram-positive and gram-negative bacteria, viruses, mycoplasma, fungi, protozoa, helminths, and spirochetes. Many of these associations have been noted only in patients with endocarditis or infected ventriculoatrial shunts. It is important to distinguish between specific postinfectious glomerular diseases such as PSGN and the nonspecific role of many infections, particularly viral illnesses, in producing "exacerbations" of underlying glomerular disease. These exacerbations are usually evidenced by a transient increase in proteinuria and hematuria associated with the infection, usually without an intervening latent period.

Post-Streptococcal Glomerulonephritis (PSGN)

Etiology, Incidence, and Epidemiology. GN occurs only following infection with a group A (beta-hemolytic) streptococcus of nephritogenic M type, usually type 12 in the United States. Streptococcal pharyngitis is the most common antecedent event in the North, and PSGN occurs with a frequency of less than 5 per cent after a latent period of 6 to 20 days (average 10). The disease is often sporadic, occurs in the winter and spring, is more common in males, and is accompanied by serologic evidence of recent streptococcal infection in over 80 per cent of cases. In the South streptococcal pyoderma or impetigo is more common, the attack rate is higher (25 to 50 per cent), the latent period is longer (14 to 21 days, average 20), and the disease affects males and females equally, often occurring in epidemic form in more temperate climates in the summer and fall.

Pathogenesis. Granular immune complex deposits in glomeruli cause the clinical and histologic features of PSGN. The presence of these deposits, hypocomplementemia, and the latent period between infection and the onset of GN suggest that the disease is similar to experimental acute serum sickness, in which acute GN is mediated by formation of glomerular deposits containing antigen and antibody to it eight to ten days following a single injection of antigen. The deposits are thought to reflect glomerular trapping of circulating immune complexes, but they may also form on a local basis. Streptococcal antigens have been identified in glomerular deposits early in PSGN in some patients. The presence of C3 in the deposits and the prominent infiltrate of neutrophils and mononuclear cells in the acute stage suggest a lesion that is mediated by complement, neutrophils, and macrophages.

Pathology. Figure 81–2 illustrates the typical findings in acute PSGN by light microscopy, IF, and EM. The histologic lesion in PSGN is a diffuse (all glomeruli involved) proliferative GN with a marked hypercellularity involving glomerular endothelial and mesangial cells, as well as neutrophils and mononuclear cells with narrowing or occlusion of capillary loops (Fig. 81–2*A*). Proliferation of epithelial cells in Bowman's space results in formation of glomerular "crescents" in severe disease. Extensive crescent formation is seen in about 5 per cent of patients and correlates with a more severe initial disease and reduced likelihood of complete recovery. Coarsely granular deposits of IgG and C3 occur along the glomerular capillary walls and in the mesangium (Fig. 81–2*B*). By EM there are discrete electron-dense subepithelial nodules or "humps" (Fig. 81–2*C*) that persist for about eight weeks. Subepithelial humps are a highly characteristic feature of PSGN, although they may occasionally be seen in other types of bacterial postinfectious GN and type I MPGN.

Clinical Findings. PSGN is the prototype of the acute nephritic syndrome and causes all of the findings discussed above under "Pathophysiology of the Acute Nephritic Syndrome." The disease is most common in children between 3 and 12 years of age, with a mean age of about 7, and is rare in infancy and in adults over 50. The typical presentation of

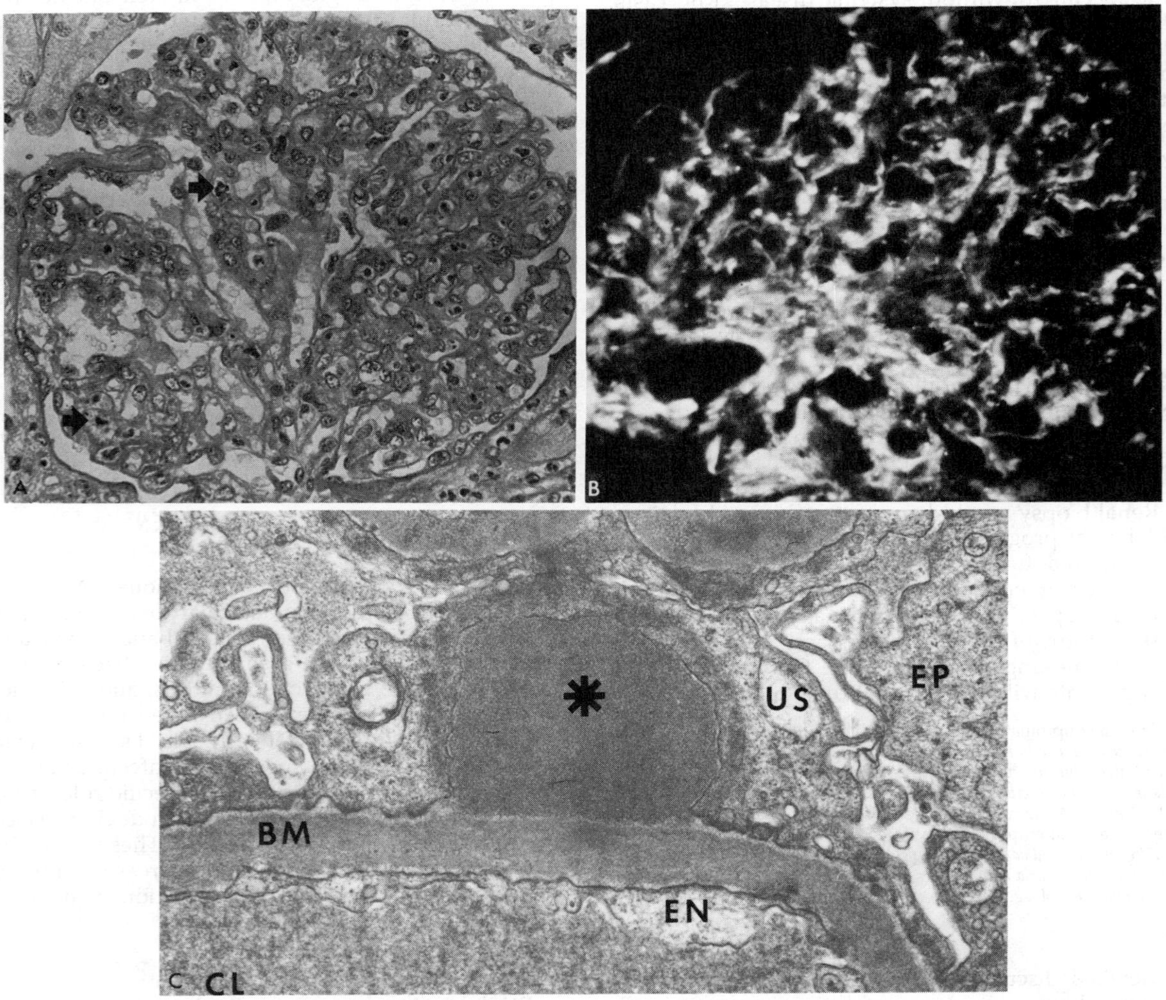

FIGURE 81–2. The renal lesion of post-streptococcal glomerulonephritis (PSGN). *A*, Light microscopic section of a renal biopsy from a patient with acute PSGN showing a marked increase in glomerular cells and infiltration by polymorphonuclear leukocytes (*arrows*) (periodic acid–Schiff stain; × 300). *B*, Immunofluorescent staining for IgG from the same biopsy reveals a coarse granular pattern of deposits on the capillary walls and in the mesangium (× 350). *C*, Electron microscopy in acute PSGN reveals a characteristic electron-dense "hump" on the subepithelial surface (*) with effacement of epithelial foot processes around the deposit. BM = Basement membrane; CL = capillary lumen; EN = endothelial cell; EP = epithelial cell; US = urinary space (× 14,400). (Reproduced with permission from Couser WG, Salant DJ, Stilmant MM. In Flamenbaum W, Hamburger RJ (eds.): Nephrology. Philadelphia, JB Lippincott Company, 1982, pp 265–301.)

PSGN is the abrupt onset of hematuria (90 per cent), which is usually evident as dark or *"smoky" urine,* accompanied by *malaise* and sometimes gastrointestinal symptoms such as abdominal pain, nausea, and vomiting. Central nervous system manifestations may include headaches and occasionally seizures. *Edema* is an early and frequent sign, often in a periorbital distribution most evident on arising and sometimes progressing to peripheral edema and anasarca. *Hypertension* is present in 60 to 70 per cent of patients and reflects renal retention of salt and water with volume overload. Proteinuria is usually present as well. About 20 per cent of hospitalized patients develop nephrotic range proteinuria, usually transiently and during the recovery phase. Renal function is impaired in about 50 per cent of patients.

Prognosis. Three clinical courses can be defined in PSGN: complete recovery, no recovery, or partial recovery with progressive disease. In over 90 per cent of cases complete recovery occurs with spontaneous diuresis in an average of four to seven days. Even patients who require dialysis during the acute phase usually recover spontaneously without specific therapy. Abnormal hematuria and proteinuria may persist for up to two years. Progressive renal disease is a very uncommon consequence of PSGN, however, if renal function returns to normal and proteinuria is less than 500 mg per day.

Fewer than 5 per cent of patients with PSGN have oliguria lasting more than nine days; the prognosis in these patients is worse. Although spontaneous complete recovery has been reported with oliguria or anuria for up to 25 days, this is unusual. Many patients with prolonged oliguria will have a crescentic glomerular lesion. About half of these will still recover spontaneously. In the remainder, the disease behaves like rapidly progressive glomerulonephritis (RPGN) with no recovery at all or with only partial recovery of renal function, which may be followed by persistent proteinuria and progressive renal disease leading to renal failure in months to years. Patients with PSGN who have oliguric renal failure lasting over one week, particularly adults, should undergo a renal biopsy. If extensive crescent formation is found they should be considered for therapy as outlined below under "Treatment."

Laboratory Features. Laboratory findings consist of an abnormal urinalysis, elevated antibodies against streptococcal exoenzymes, and reduced serum complement levels. The urinalysis usually reveals signs of glomerular inflammation with proteinuria, RBC's, white blood cells (WBC's), and casts. RBC casts are present in 60 to 85 per cent of cases when a freshly voided urine is examined. The urine is often concentrated and exhibits biochemical characteristics of prerenal azotemia, including a low urine sodium, indicating severe glomerular disease with good preservation of tubular function.

Beta-hemolytic streptococci are detected by culture in only 25 per cent of untreated patients, but serologic tests generally confirm recent streptococcal infection. The anti–streptolysin O (ASO) titer exceeds 200 Todd units within one to three weeks and may remain elevated for months. An increase in ASO titer may not be seen if penicillin therapy is initiated early or if the antecedent infection was in the skin. Antibodies to other streptococcal enzymes are usually elevated as well. The streptozyme test utilizes five of these antigens in a single assay and is quite sensitive and specific. Over 90 per cent of patients with PSGN have a reduced level of total hemolytic complement or C3 during the first two weeks of illness, with most returning to normal within eight weeks. The pattern of complement component depression suggests alternate pathway activation, with levels of C1q and C4 usually normal.

Diagnosis. The differential diagnosis of acute GN with hypocomplementemia includes other forms of postinfectious GN such as subacute bacterial endocarditis (SBE) or shunt nephritis, systemic lupus erythematosus (SLE), and type I membranoproliferative glomerulonephritis (MPGN). Only MPGN is difficult to exclude by clinical and laboratory criteria. A similar pattern of alternate complement pathway activation is seen in MPGN, a disease that also may occasionally follow streptococcal infection (see p. 597), and MPGN must be considered when nephrotic range proteinuria and hypocomplementemia persist for longer than two months. The diagnosis of PSGN can usually be made by the presence of typical clinical features of the acute nephritic syndrome following a streptococcal infection by an appropriate latent period, and by hypocomplementemia and serologic evidence of recent streptococcal infection. Because patients with PSGN usually recover spontaneously and no specific therapy is indicated, the diagnosis is often made clinically without a renal biopsy. Biopsy is indicated, however, if atypical features are present, such as prolonged oliguria, anuria, persistent hypocomplementemia, the nephrotic syndrome, or clinical or serologic evidence of systemic disease.

Treatment. In most patients with PSGN there is no need for specific therapy, since spontaneous recovery can be anticipated. Antibiotics should be given if cultures are positive for group A streptococci, but penicillin therapy does not alter the incidence or severity of PSGN. Manifestations of sodium retention such as hypertension, edema, and congestive heart failure can usually be managed with careful sodium restriction, but diuretics and antihypertensive agents may be employed if necessary. Dialysis may be required temporarily in some patients, most of whom will still recover normal renal function spontaneously.

There are no data on which to base a recommendation for therapy in patients with prolonged oliguria and a crescentic glomerular lesion on biopsy. Although up to 50 per cent of such patients may recover spontaneously, the prognosis is sufficiently guarded to warrant considering therapy with pulse steroids or plasma exchange as outlined below under RPGN.

Nissenson AR, moderator: Post-streptococcal acute glomerulonephritis: Fact and controversy. Ann Intern Med 91:76, 1979. *An excellent overview of the microbiology, epidemiology, clinical manifestations, laboratory features, pathogenesis, and sequelae of PSGN, with 128 references.*

Rodriguez-Iturbe B: Epidemic poststreptococcal glomerulonephritis. Kidney Int 25:129, 1984. *An excellent review of the pathogenesis, laboratory findings, clinical features, and long-term prognosis in acute post-streptococcal nephritis, with 65 references.*

Glomerulonephritis in Subacute Bacterial Endocarditis (SBE)

Glomerular disease in SBE ranges in severity from the proteinuria and hematuria seen in 70 per cent of patients, usually with normal renal function, to occasional cases of crescentic GN with acute renal failure. It is more common in chronic cases with right-sided cardiac involvement and negative blood cultures, as may occur in patients who abuse drugs. A wide variety of organisms have been implicated, most commonly *Staphylococcus aureus* and *Streptococcus viridans.* A similar syndrome may be seen in patients with infected ventriculoatrial shunts for hydrocephalus (shunt nephritis), often due to *Staphylococcus albus.* Serologic abnormalities are often present, including hypocomplementemia with activation of both the classic and the alternate complement pathways, cryoglobulinemia, and positive rheumatoid factor. Renal biopsy usually demonstrates a focal proliferative GN, often with necrosis and intra-capillary thrombi. Granular deposits of IgG, IgM, and C3 occur in mesangial and subendothelial areas, implicating an immune complex rather than an embolic mechanism in the pathogenesis of the lesion. Renal function usually returns to normal following appropriate antibiotic therapy and eradication of the infection. However, recovery may be slow if the lesion is severe or crescents are present.

Feinstein EI, Eknoyan G, Lister BJ, et al.: Renal complications of bacterial endocarditis. Am J Nephrol 5:457, 1985. *This discussion, with 69 references, of endocarditis and glomerulonephritis in a patient who is an intravenous drug abuser presents a comprehensive review of glomerular disease associated with both endocarditis and drug abuse.*

Neugarten J, Gallo GR, Baldwin DS: Glomerulonephritis in bacterial endocarditis. Am J Kidney Dis 3:371, 1984. *This paper reviews 107 patients with endocarditis and notes that 22 per cent had glomerulonephritis with a spectrum of renal lesions and that* Staphylococcus aureus *was the predominant organism. The relationship among renal lesion, therapy, and prognosis is discussed.*

Glomerulonephritis with Visceral Abscesses

The abrupt onset of acute renal failure associated with proteinuria, hematuria, and red cell casts may occur in patients with a pyogenic visceral abscess. Abscesses are most frequently located in the respiratory tract but have been reported at numerous other sites, including the abdomen and uterus. Endocarditis may be present but usually is not, and blood cultures are commonly negative. In contrast to PSGN, SBE, and shunt nephritis, serologic studies, including complement levels, are usually normal. A variety of bacteria have been implicated. The glomerular lesion is usually a proliferative GN with crescents, and monocytes may be prominent in glomeruli. IF and EM studies usually do not reveal immune deposits, so that the pathogenesis of this lesion is unclear. Recovery of renal function has occurred in about half of the patients reported with acute renal failure who were successfully treated to eradicate the infection, but the overall mortality is quite high.

Beaufils M: Glomerular disease complicating abdominal sepsis. Kidney Int 19:609, 1981. *A detailed review of nonstreptococcal postinfectious glomerulonephritis, including SBE- as well as abscess-related lesions. The frequency with which renal biopsies reveal glomerular disease as a cause of acute renal failure in patients with sepsis is striking, since most such patients would not be as extensively studied in the United States.*

Glomerular Disease in Acquired Immunodeficiency Syndrome (AIDS)

Up to 50 per cent of patients with AIDS have abnormal proteinuria and 10 per cent develop nephrotic syndrome. A variety of glomerular, tubular, and interstitial lesions have been noted, presumably induced by infections, drug exposure, and other factors. However, a majority of patients with nephrotic syndrome have focal glomerular sclerosis (see p. 594). A rapid loss of renal function may occur in this subset of patients.

Rao TKS, Filippone EJ, Nicastri AD, et al.: Associated focal and segmental glomerulosclerosis in the acquired immunodeficiency syndrome. N Engl J Med 310:669, 1984. *This paper documents the significant incidence of proteinuria and nephrotic syndrome in patients with AIDS associated with a lesion of focal segmental glomerulosclerosis usually accompanied by rapid deterioration of renal function.*

IgA Nephropathy (Berger's Disease)

Overview and Incidence. In 1968 Jean Berger reviewed 55 biopsies of children with so-called benign hematuria, idiopathic hematuria, or recurrent hematuria of childhood and noted a high frequency of mesangial IgA deposits and a variety of glomerular lesions, most commonly focal GN. IgA nephropathy is the commonest cause of primary glomerular disease in Europe, Australia, and probably the United States. The disease is now regarded as a monosymptomatic form of *Henoch-Schönlein purpura* (HSP), but clinical manifestations are milder than in HSP and are usually confined to the kidney. HSP is discussed later in this chapter and also in Ch. 166.

Pathogenesis. The pathogenesis of the renal lesion in IgA nephropathy and HSP is not known. It appears to be a consequence of mesangial formation of immune deposits composed predominantly of IgA (see Fig. 81–3*B*). The IgA probably represents the antibody component of an immune complex containing a nonrenal antigen. A similar glomerular lesion may develop in liver disease associated with elevated portal pressure. The glomerular IgA deposits appear to be predominantly polymeric and of mucosal origin, which may reflect the association of disease activity with viral infections of the upper respiratory and gastrointestinal tracts.

Pathology. The typical lesion of IgA nephropathy has a focal distribution, meaning that some glomeruli are involved while others are spared, and is also segmental, with lesions in some glomerular tufts but not others (Fig. 81–3*A*). Mesangial expansion and hypercellularity are common, but the characteristic lesion is a focal and segmental proliferative GN. When crescents are present they are usually small and rarely involve more than 30 per cent of glomeruli. Immune deposits are present diffusely in the mesangium of all glomeruli and contain IgA as the predominant immunoglobulin, accompanied by C3 in 60 per cent and IgG in 30 per cent of cases (Fig. 81–3*B*). C1q and C4 are usually absent, suggesting alternate complement pathway activation. Some patients have deposits along the subendothelial aspect of the capillary wall

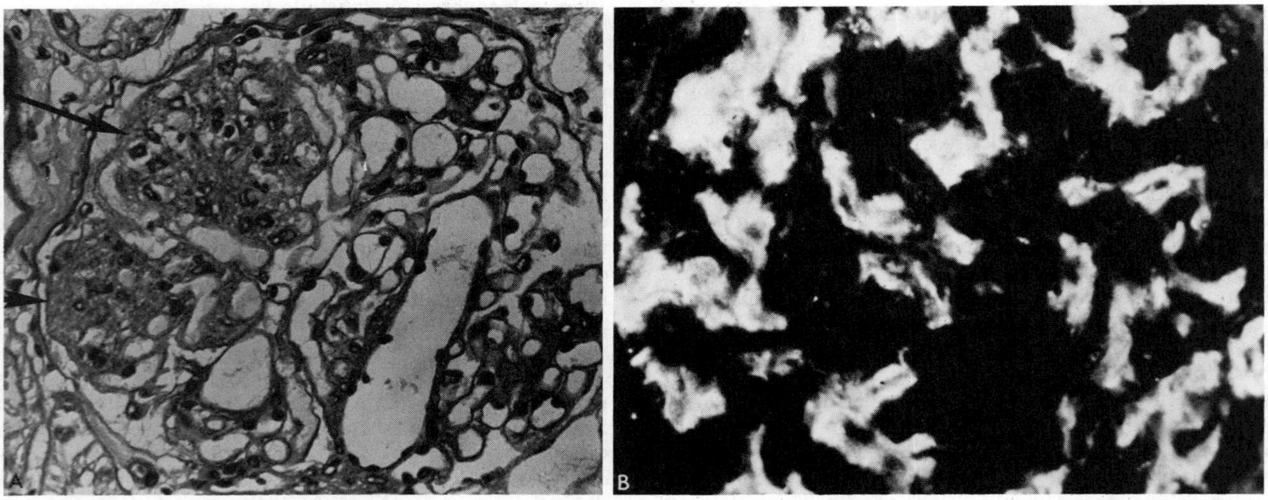

FIGURE 81–3. The renal lesion of IgA nephropathy. *A*, Light microscopic section from a patient with gross hematuria and focal glomerulonephritis due to IgA nephropathy. There is segmental involvement of the glomerulus, which shows mesangial matrix increase and hypercellularity in two lobules (*arrows*). Adjacent lobules are essentially normal (periodic acid–Schiff stain, × 350). *B*, Immunofluorescence microscopy on the same biopsy reveals bright, diffuse staining for IgA in all mesangial areas. No significant capillary wall staining is present. IgG and C3 may be found in a similar pattern but with less intensity (× 450). (Reproduced from Couser WG, Salant DJ, Stilmant MM. In Flamenbaum W, Hamburger RJ (eds.): Nephrology. Philadelphia, JB Lippincott Company, 1982, pp 265–301.)

or in the subepithelial space and generally have more severe disease and more proteinuria.

Clinical and Laboratory Findings and Diagnosis. IgA nephropathy is two to three times more common in males than in females, and most patients present before the age of 35. The classic presentation is with *gross hematuria* that occurs coincident with, or immediately following (24 to 48 hours), a viral upper respiratory infection (50 per cent), flu-like illness (15 per cent), a gastrointestinal syndrome (10 per cent), or other infectious prodrome. Associated findings often include mild fever, malaise, myalgias, dysuria, and loin pain. The remainder of cases are identified during medical evaluation for persistent, asymptomatic hematuria or proteinuria. The absence of a latent period, as well as normal levels of complement and anti-streptococcal antibodies, distinguishes this disease clinically from PSGN. Moreover, other features of the acute nephritic syndrome, including edema and hypertension, are seen in fewer than half of the patients. Only about 25 per cent of patients have impaired renal function during active disease, and the serum creatinine rarely exceeds 3 mg per deciliter. Proteinuria is usually less than 1 gram per day.

Gross hematuria usually lasts only two to six days, but microscopic hematuria often persists between attacks. Fifty per cent of patients will have only a single episode of gross hematuria. The remainder have recurring episodes for many years, usually "triggered" by viral infections.

There are no laboratory findings diagnostic of IgA nephropathy. About half of all patients have elevated serum levels of IgA that do not correlate with disease activity. Circulating immune complexes containing IgA are present intermittently, and deposits of IgA, C3, and fibrin may be present in the dermal capillaries of normal skin. The incidence of this disease is greater in persons with HLA-Bw 35 and HLA-DR4 phenotypes.

Course and Prognosis. Progression to renal failure occurs in 15 to 20 per cent of patients within 6 months, and a 50 per cent death or dialysis rate is projected over 20 years. While there are no clinical or pathologic features that permit accurate prediction of progression, patients who tend to do worse are male, have a prolonged clinical course, develop hypertension or proteinuria exceeding 3 grams per day, or have extensive glomerular sclerosis present on biopsy.

Treatment. No specific form of therapy has been shown to alter the long-term clinical course of this disease. Rigorous control of hypertension is important. Mesangial deposits of IgA occur with a high frequency in renal allografts but rarely compromise graft function.

Boyce NW, Holdsworth SR, Thomson NM, et al.: Clinicopathological associations in mesangial IgA nephropathy. Am J Nephrol 6:246, 1986. *Data are presented on the clinical features and histopathology of 112 patients, emphasizing presenting manifestations and features predictive of long-term course.*

Rodicio JL: Idiopathic IgA nephropathy. Kidney Int 25:717, 1984. *An in-depth review of the differential diagnosis, clinical features, pathology, diagnosis, course, and therapy of IgA nephropathy, with an appended commentary on pathogenesis by Michael P. Madaio, M.D.*

Rapidly Progressive Glomerulonephritis (RPGN)

Overview. The term RPGN is applied to any glomerular disease in which rapid loss of renal function occurs in association with extensive crescent formation in many glomeruli, usually over 50 per cent (Fig. 81–4). Volhard and Fahr first noted the association between crescents and a poor prognosis in 1914, and the term RPGN was first applied by Ellis in 1942.

RPGN may occur in severe cases of a wide variety of glomerular diseases, which are listed in Table 81–3, or it may occur alone as a primary renal disease. The classification system used here is based on pathogenetic mechanisms. Accurate prognosis and selection of appropriate therapy require that the underlying mechanisms be defined. About 20 per cent of cases of RPGN are mediated by anti-GBM antibody deposition and 40 per cent by glomerular immune complex formation (usually in association with some systemic disease process such as PSGN or SLE), and 40 per cent are primary renal lesions with no significant glomerular immune deposits, which are classified here as idiopathic RPGN (Table 81–3).

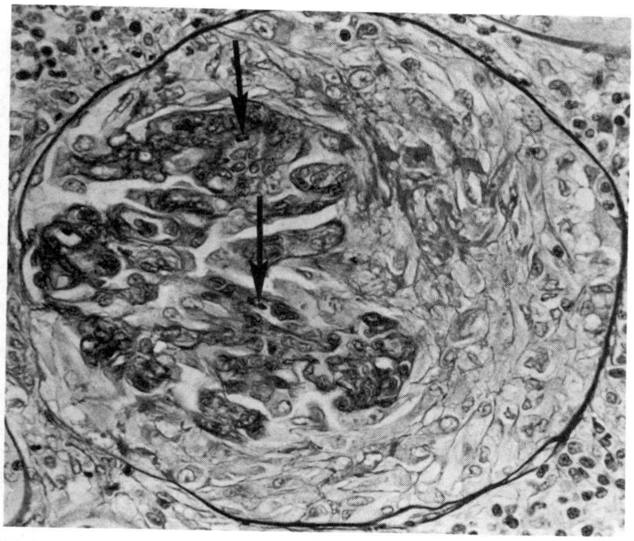

FIGURE 81–4. Light microscopy from a patient with idiopathic RPGN reveals the presence of a large cellular crescent in Bowman's space surrounding and compressing the glomerular capillary. A few polymorphonuclear leukocytes are seen in the glomerulus (*arrows*) (periodic acid–Schiff stain, × 275). (Reproduced from Couser WG, Salant DJ, Stilmant MM. In Flamenbaum W, Hamburger RJ (eds.): Nephrology. Philadelphia, JB Lippincott Company, 1982, pp 265–301.)

RPGN DUE TO ANTI-GBM ANTIBODY. Although much is known of the mediation of immune glomerular injury from studies of experimental anti-GBM nephritis, this mechanism accounts for fewer than 5 per cent of cases of GN seen clinically. Anti-GBM GN is characterized by the abrupt onset of a proliferative GN, usually with crescents, and a characteristic linear deposition of IgG along the GBM by IF (Fig. 81–5). In about two thirds of cases, pulmonary hemorrhage accompanies GN, and the disease is termed Goodpasture's syndrome. The remaining one third of patients have anti-GBM nephritis without pulmonary involvement.

Goodpasture's Syndrome. PATHOGENESIS. The events that initiate anti-GBM antibody production are not known. Anti-

TABLE 81–3. CLASSIFICATION OF RAPIDLY PROGRESSIVE (CRESCENTIC) GLOMERULONEPHRITIS

Type of RPGN	Frequency
Anti-GBM Antibody–Mediated RPGN	20%
Goodpasture's syndrome	
Idiopathic anti-GBM nephritis	
Membranous nephropathy with crescents	
RPGN Associated with Granular Immune Deposits	40%
Postinfectious	
Post-streptococcal glomerulonephritis	
Bacterial endocarditis	
"Shunt" nephritis	
Visceral abscesses, other nonstreptococcal infections	
Noninfectious	
Systemic lupus erythematosus	
Henoch-Schönlein syndrome	
Mixed cryoglobulinemia	
Solid tumors	
Primary Renal Disease	
Membranoproliferative glomerulonephritis	
IgA nephropathy	
Idiopathic "immune complex" nephritis	
RPGN Without Glomerular Immune Deposits	40%
Vasculitis	
Polyarteritis	
Hypersensitivity vasculitis	
Wegener's granulomatosis	
Idiopathic RPGN	

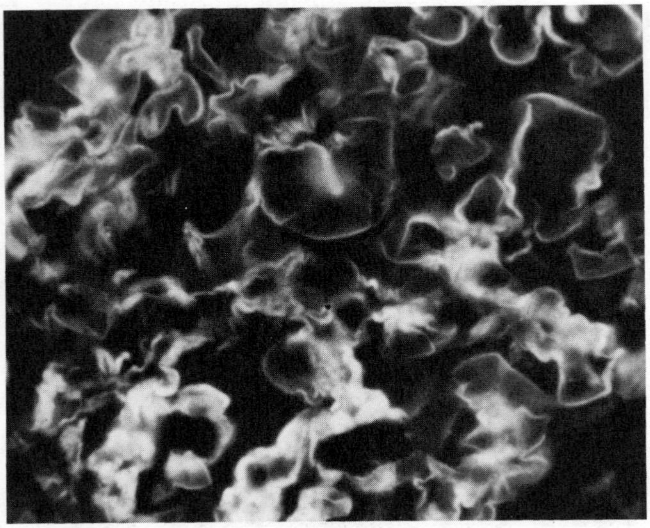

FIGURE 81–5. Immunofluorescence microscopy on a renal biopsy from a patient with Goodpasture's syndrome reveals continuous, uninterrupted, linear deposition of IgG along all capillary walls. This pattern is characteristic of anti-GBM disease (× 450). (Reproduced from Couser WG, Salant DJ, Stilmant MM. In Flamenbaum W, Hamburger RJ (eds.): Nephrology. Philadelphia, JB Lippincott Company, 1982, pp 265–301.)

body reactive with GBM and alveolar basement membrane mediates the glomerular disease in anti-GBM nephritis with and without pulmonary hemorrhage. The development of lung hemorrhage appears to require the presence of prior lung damage to allow antibody deposition. Genetic factors are clearly important in this disease. There is a strong association with HLA-DRw2 (relative risk 15 to 34 times normal). Anti-GBM antibody production is a self-limited event usually lasting several months. Exacerbations of disease associated with increased antibody levels may be triggered by infectious complications. Antibody binding to GBM mediates glomerular injury by mechanisms that involve complement activation and participation of both neutrophils and macrophages. Fibrin deposition in Bowman's space is believed to initiate glomerular crescent formation.

PATHOLOGY. The early histologic lesion in Goodpasture's syndrome is a focal proliferative and necrotizing GN that progresses to diffuse involvement with crescent formation. Extensive interstitial infiltrates may also be present, perhaps due to antibody deposition on tubular basement membranes. There is a characteristic, continuous, linear pattern of IgG deposition along the capillary wall, accompanied by C3 in about 70 per cent of cases (Fig. 81–5). Tubular basement membrane deposits may also occur. EM is not diagnostic.

CLINICAL FEATURES. Goodpasture's syndrome is a disease of young males (6:1 male-to-female ratio) characterized by a triad of *pulmonary hemorrhage, GN,* and *anti-GBM antibody production.* It usually begins with pulmonary hemorrhage manifest as hemoptysis, pulmonary alveolar infiltrates by x-ray, dyspnea, and iron deficiency anemia. The pulmonary symptoms are followed within days to weeks by development of hematuria, proteinuria, and rapid loss of renal function. Over half of patients with Goodpasture's syndrome are azotemic when first seen. Hypertension and fluid retention are uncommon. Preceding flu-like illness or exposure to other pulmonary toxins such as volatile hydrocarbon solvents and cigarettes is common. Until recently, 80 per cent of cases required treatment for end-stage renal disease within one year, although some patients with mild disease recover spontaneously. Up to 30 per cent of patients may die as a consequence of the pulmonary hemorrhage.

LABORATORY FINDINGS AND DIAGNOSIS. The only laboratory finding specific for anti-GBM nephritis is the demonstration of antibody to GBM in the serum or as linear deposits of IgG in glomeruli. The antibody can be detected quickly in serum by indirect IF using normal human kidney substrate in a test that is similar to the fluorescent antinuclear antibody test. The indirect IF assay is positive in 80 to 90 per cent of patients with Goodpasture's syndrome. A more sensitive radioimmunoassay is also commercially available and is positive in over 95 per cent of patients. It is urgent to make a diagnosis and to initiate therapy early in RPGN of all types. An anti-GBM assay, as well as a renal biopsy, should therefore be obtained as soon as possible after the diagnosis of RPGN is suspected. The demonstration of anti-GBM antibody is critical, since a variety of other diseases may result in similar pulmonary and renal manifestations, including SLE, polyarteritis nodosa, Wegener's granulomatosis, and other forms of systemic necrotizing vasculitis.

TREATMENT. As in all forms of RPGN, the success of treatment is critically dependent upon how quickly it is initiated. The overall survival rate in Goodpasture's syndrome has risen from less than 10 per cent 15 years ago to over 50 per cent today owing to earlier diagnosis and detection of milder cases, better general medical care, and probably some improvements in specific therapy for the disease. There is little evidence that oral steroids or immunosuppressive agents alone significantly alter the course of the renal lesion. The pulmonary hemorrhage commonly responds either to high-dose oral prednisone therapy or to intravenous "pulse" methylprednisolone (see treatment of idiopathic RPGN below). However, steroid pulse therapy does not appear to benefit the renal lesion. Most centers now treat anti-GBM disease with vigorous plasma exchange therapy combined with prednisone, 1 mg per kilogram per day, and cyclophosphamide, 2 to 3 mg per kilogram per day. Plasma exchanges of up to 4 liters per day are performed on a daily or alternate-day basis until anti-GBM antibody is no longer detectable in the circulation and disease progression has halted. Therapy may require several weeks. Replacement is with albumin, or, when pulmonary hemorrhage is active, with fresh frozen plasma. Overall survival in anti-GBM nephritis appears to be improved by plasma exchange therapy. However, the response rate in patients who are oliguric on presentation or who have serum creatinines exceeding 6 mg per deciliter is very low, again emphasizing the need for early diagnosis. In patients with end-stage renal disease due to anti-GBM nephritis, renal transplantation appears to be safe if delayed until anti-GBM antibody is no longer detectable in the serum.

Anti-GBM Glomerulonephritis Without Pulmonary Hemorrhage. Some patients have the same anti-GBM antibody–mediated renal disease as seen in Goodpasture's syndrome, but antibody localization does not occur in lungs and pulmonary hemorrhage is therefore absent. The patients are generally older than those with Goodpasture's syndrome (mean age about 50), and males and females are equally affected. In all other respects, the clinical and pathologic findings, course, and treatment are the same as those discussed above for Goodpasture's syndrome. Because such patients present with an idiopathic form of acute RPGN without pulmonary hemorrhage and may respond to plasma exchange therapy, it is important that the possibility of anti-GBM nephritis be considered in all patients who present in this fashion and that circulating anti-GBM antibody studies and renal biopsy be performed early.

Savage COS, Pusey CD, Bowman C, et al.: Antiglomerular basement membrane antibody mediated disease in the British Isles 1980–4. Br Med J 292:301, 1986. *Experience with 71 patients in a single center is reviewed, disclosing two patterns of disease: young women in their twenties with Goodpasture's syndrome and women in their sixties with glomerulonephritis alone. The poor response to plasma exchange in patients with serum creatinine levels exceeding 6 mg per deciliter or in those requiring dialysis is emphasized.*

Walker RG, Scheinkestel C, Becker GJ, et al.: Clinical and morphological aspects of the management of crescentic anti–glomerular basement membrane antibody (anti-GBM) nephritis/Goodpasture's syndrome. Q J Med 543:75,

1985. *This review of 22 patients with anti-GBM nephritis details the clinical features of this disease. Anuria and greater than 80 per cent crescents are identified as poor prognostic signs, and a beneficial effect of plasma exchange is suggested.*

RPGN DUE TO GLOMERULAR IMMUNE COMPLEX FORMATION. Patients with RPGN associated with granular deposits of immunoglobulin and complement in glomeruli account for about 40 per cent of all patients seen with crescentic GN. In most cases the glomerular disease is a manifestation of some well-defined systemic illness such as SLE, Henoch-Schönlein purpura, or other forms of vasculitis, or of another well-defined primary renal disease such as PSGN, MPGN, or, rarely, IGA nephropathy. In all of these disorders the correct diagnosis can usually be made from the associated clinical, laboratory, and pathologic findings. Prognosis depends considerably on the underlying disease. For example, about 50 per cent of patients with RPGN secondary to streptococcal infection will recover spontaneously without specific therapy, while in RPGN due to SLE spontaneous recovery virtually never occurs. Therapy for the glomerular disease per se is the same as that outlined below under treatment for idiopathic RPGN and includes the use of methylprednisolone pulse therapy and/or plasma exchange.

IDIOPATHIC RPGN. ***Pathogenesis.*** RPGN as a primary renal disease is usually not associated with significant glomerular deposits of anti-GBM or immune complexes. The disease mechanism in such patients is undefined but probably immune in nature. Whatever the mechanism leading to capillary wall damage, leakage of fibrin into Bowman's space apparently initiates epithelial cell proliferation and crescent formation. Some of the vague prodromal clinical manifestations, as well as the presence of crescentic GN without immune deposits, are quite similar to findings in several of the vasculitides. This disease may be a form of vasculitis and may share a common pathogenetic mechanism, although inflammatory changes are confined primarily to the glomerular capillaries.

Pathology. There is extensive glomerular crescent formation with circumferential cellular crescents usually involving 50 to 100 per cent of glomeruli (see Fig. 81–4). Earlier cases may show fewer or smaller crescents and later ones reveal more fibrosis of crescents and glomerular obsolescence. There is a rough correlation between the percentage of glomeruli with crescents, the severity of clinical disease, and the prognosis. Changes in the glomerular tuft itself may be minimal. Prominent proliferative changes suggest a postinfectious etiology and a better prognosis. Interstitial changes are frequently prominent, and vasculitis is absent. Fibrinogen and fibrin polymers are present in the crescents. The glomeruli at most show only focal granular deposits of IgM and C3, which are nonspecific. EM may show "gaps" or rupture of the capillary wall but usually does not show immune deposits.

Clinical Manifestations and Diagnosis. Idiopathic RPGN is a disease of older patients (mean age 58). There is a slight male predominance. The disease tends to present in clusters. Many patients have a prodrome that resembles a viral illness with myalgias; arthralgias; loin, back, and abdominal pain; fever; and malaise. Minor hemoptysis is common, and fleeting pulmonary infiltrates may be seen by x-ray. No specific inciting events have been identified. RPGN presents as an acute nephritic syndrome, including *hematuria, proteinuria,* and *rapidly decreasing renal function,* often without hypertension or edema. As in anti-GBM nephritis, the progression of renal disease is usually very rapid, with up to 50 per cent of patients oliguric at the time of presentation and half of these sufficiently uremic to require immediate dialysis. The remaining patients may require dialysis within one to three weeks. At the time of presentation the disease is often relatively acute and potentially reversible.

The laboratory features of idiopathic RPGN are entirely nonspecific. ASO titers, antinuclear and anti-GBM antibodies, circulating immune complexes, and complement levels are normal or negative. The diagnosis is made by renal biopsy in a patient with deteriorating renal function, evidence of glomerular disease in the urine sediment, absence of anti-GBM antibody, and lack of clinical or serologic evidence of other systemic diseases such as SLE.

Treatment and Prognosis. Treatment with oral steroids and/or cytotoxic agents has been of little apparent benefit, and a death or dialysis rate of about 75 per cent in two years is reported. Favorable prognostic factors include a young age at the time of onset, a history of a preceding infectious episode, absence of oliguria and hypertension, serum creatinine below 6 mg per deciliter at presentation, and fewer than 50 per cent crescents in the renal biopsy. Success rates approaching 75 per cent have been reported in patients treated with either methylprednisolone pulse therapy or plasma exchange. Methylprednisolone, 30 mg per kilogram to a maximum of 3 grams, is given intravenously over 20 minutes on a daily or alternate-day basis three times, followed by oral prednisone, 2 mg per kilogram, which is tapered over several months. About 75 per cent of patients, including some who were oliguric and on dialysis, have shown a dramatic response, with a return of renal function to normal or nearly normal levels. Responses have generally been evident within five to ten days and have continued over four to six weeks. However, long-term follow-up data in such patients are limited, and some will progress to renal failure later despite an impressive initial response. Very similar results have been reported in patients treated with intensive plasma exchange (plus prednisone and cyclophosphamide). This treatment is extremely expensive and, compared with pulse therapy, probably has a higher incidence of complications, primarily bleeding and infection. Neither form of therapy has yet been shown in a prospective, controlled study to improve long-term patient or kidney survival over what might be achieved with more conservative measures. Until such data are available, the author's feeling is that both pulse therapy and plasma exchange probably do represent significant advances in the treatment of idiopathic RPGN. Steroid pulse therapy is safer and cheaper and appears to be as effective as plasma exchange. There are no data on the efficacy of cytotoxic drugs in this disease. However, if there is evidence of segmental necrotizing glomerular lesions or systemic manifestations consistent with vasculitis, cyclophosphamide should probably be given concurrently with steroids.

Idiopathic RPGN appears to recur rarely in allografted kidneys.

Couser WG: Idiopathic rapidly progressive glomerulonephritis. Am J Nephrol 2:57, 1982. *This review discusses the classification, clinical features, pathology, pathogenesis, and treatment of idiopathic RPGN in considerable detail, with 159 references.*

Glassock RJ: Natural history and treatment of primary proliferative glomerulonephritis: A review. Kidney Int 28:S136, 1985. *In this review of treatment of several forms of glomerulonephritis, the section on crescentic glomerulonephritis provides a thoughtful and comprehensive review of the literature on treatment of RPGN, with useful guidelines and recommendations.*

Hind CRK, Paraskevakou H, Lockwood CM, et al.: Prognosis after immunosuppression of patients with crescentic nephritis requiring dialysis. Lancet 1:263, 1983. *This paper reviews the experience with plasma exchange and immunosuppression in 48 patients with all forms of RPGN and acute renal failure requiring dialysis. No patients with acute anti-GBM disease responded, while about two thirds of patients with other forms of RPGN, including idiopathic, vasculitic, and Wegener's, showed a sustained improvement in renal function. The urgency of early diagnosis is emphasized.*

NEPHROTIC SYNDROME

The nephrotic syndrome is not a disease; it is a group of signs and symptoms commonly seen in patients with glomerular diseases that are characterized by a marked increase in capillary wall permeability to serum proteins rather than (or sometimes in addition to) glomerular inflammatory changes. The primary abnormality in nephrotic syndrome is the excretion of large amounts (greater than 3.5 grams per day) of protein in the urine. Other manifestations that may occur

TABLE 81–4. SUMMARY OF PRIMARY RENAL DISEASES THAT PRESENT AS IDIOPATHIC NEPHROTIC SYNDROME

	Minimal Change Nephrotic Syndrome (MCNS)	Focal Glomerular Sclerosis (FGS)	Membranous Nephropathy	Membranoproliferative Glomerulonephritis (MPGN)	
				Type I	*Type II*
Frequency*					
Children	75%	10%	<5%	10%	
Adults	15%	15%	50%	10%	
Clinical Manifestations					
Age	2–6, some adults	2–6, some adults	40–50	5–15	
Sex	2:1 male	1.3:1 male	2:1 male	male-female	
Nephrotic syndrome	100%	90%	80%	60%	
Asymptomatic proteinuria	0	10%	20%	40%	
Hematuria	20%	60–80%	60%	80%	
Hypertension	10%	20% early	Infrequent	35%	
Rate of progression	Does not progress	10 years	50% in 10–20 years	10–20 years	5–15 years
Associated conditions	Allergy, Hodgkin's disease	None	Renal vein thrombosis, cancer, SLE	None	Partial lipodystrophy
Laboratory Findings	Manifestations of nephrotic syndrome	Manifestations of nephrotic syndrome	Manifestations of nephrotic syndrome	Low C1, C4, C3–C9	Normal C1, C4, low C3–C9 C3 nephritic factor
Immunogenetics	HLA-B8, B12 (3.5)†	Not established	HLA-DRW3 (12–32)†	Not established	
Renal Pathology					
Light microscopy	Normal	Focal sclerotic lesions	Thickened GBM, spikes	Thickened GBM, proliferation, lobulation	
Immunofluorescence	Negative	IgM, C3 in lesions	Fine granular IgG, C3	Granular IgG, C3	C3 only
Electron microscopy	Foot process fusion	Foot process fusion	Subepithelial deposits	Mesangial and subendothelial deposits	Dense deposits
Response to Steroids	90%	15–20%	May slow progression	Not established	

*Approximate frequency as a cause of idiopathic nephrotic syndrome. About 10 per cent of adult nephrotic syndrome is due to various diseases that usually present with acute glomerulonephritis (Table 81–2).

†Relative risk.

secondary to *proteinuria* include *hypoalbuminemia, edema, hyperlipidemia,* and *lipiduria.* In contrast to the acute nephritic syndrome, the onset of the nephrotic syndrome is usually insidious, gross hematuria and red cell casts are infrequent, and renal function is often normal at the time of presentation.

The list of diseases that may cause the nephrotic syndrome is extensive and includes virtually every disorder that may affect the glomerulus. About one third of adults and 10 per cent of children have the nephrotic syndrome as a manifestation of some systemic disease, usually diabetes, SLE, or amyloidosis. In two thirds of adults, and most children, the nephrotic syndrome is idiopathic and a manifestation of one of three types of primary glomerular disease: minimal change nephrotic syndrome (MCNS) or its variants, membranous nephropathy, or membranoproliferative glomerulonephritis (MPGN). The relative frequencies of these diseases and their identifying characteristics are presented for comparison in Table 81–4. It is important to note that the occurrence of the nephrotic syndrome in patients over 45 may be associated with occult malignancy. The association of Hodgkin's disease with MCNS and of solid tumors of the lung, breast, and GI tract with membranous nephropathy is discussed below. All of the diseases discussed in the section on acute GN can also cause the nephrotic syndrome, although they do not commonly do so.

Pathophysiology of the Nephrotic Syndrome

PROTEINURIA. Glomeruli are normally perfused with plasma containing over 60,000 grams of protein per day, but less than 150 mg of protein is excreted in the final urine. The filtration barrier, which includes the endothelial cells, basement membrane, epithelial cells, and slit diaphragms, restricts the transcapillary passage of proteins on the basis of their size, shape, and electrical charge. The size barrier is primarily at the level of the endothelial cells and GBM. It restricts filtration of molecules between about 18 and 42 Å and effectively prevents filtration of neutral molecules larger than 42 Å. Circulating proteins such as albumin (36 Å) are further restricted from crossing the capillary wall by an electrical charge barrier conferred by the polyanionic sialoprotein coating on endothelial and epithelial cells and heparan sulfate–proteoglycans in the lamina rara externa and interna. Thus, molecules with a net negative charge (anionic) are less freely filtered, or encounter smaller "pores" in the capillary wall, than positively charged (cationic) molecules of the same size. Most serum proteins are anionic at physiologic pH and may be filtered in increased amounts if the charge barrier is reduced, as it is in some glomerular diseases.

Glomerular hemodynamic factors also alter protein filtration. Thus, in situations of reduced renal perfusion, renal blood flow (RBF) may be reduced while GFR is maintained by adaptive changes in other determinants of GFR such as intracapillary hydraulic pressure. Under these circumstances the filtration fraction (GFR/RBF) is increased, resulting in a higher than normal protein concentration at the efferent end of the glomerular capillary. This may produce an increased diffusion of protein across the capillary wall, resulting in proteinuria in the absence of glomerular disease in conditions such as congestive heart failure and other states of reduced renal perfusion (see isolated proteinuria above).

Proteinuria, the hallmark of the nephrotic syndrome, exceeds 3.5 grams per day in adults or 40 mg per square meter per hour in children. Fixed nephrotic range proteinuria with the nephrotic syndrome generally occurs only in the presence of diffuse glomerular disease. The immune mechanisms that may cause an increase in the permselective properties of the glomerular capillary wall may induce a loss of net negative charge on the capillary wall, as appears to occur in MCNS, leading to a marked increase in urinary albumin excretion without significant change in the excretion of other serum proteins *(selective proteinuria).* Other diseases with extensive capillary wall immune deposits, such as membranous nephropathy, or disorders of basement membrane biochemistry or structure, such as those found in diabetes or hereditary nephritis, are associated with apparent structural defects and increased filtration of all serum proteins *(nonselective proteinuria).* Over 40 grams of protein may be excreted in the urine each day in some patients. It is this loss of protein that leads to the other clinical and biochemical manifestations of the nephrotic syndrome.

HYPOALBUMINEMIA. Serum albumin concentration decreases to less than 3.0 grams per deciliter when the rate of urinary protein loss and renal catabolism of filtered albumin (which may exceed 10 grams per day in the nephrotic syndrome) exceeds the rate of hepatic synthesis. Hepatic albumin synthesis is normally 12 to 14 grams per day in adults and may increase in the nephrotic syndrome but can be limited by various factors, including age, poor nutritional status, and liver disease. Thus, some patients may exhibit significant hypoalbuminemia with proteinuria of less than 10 grams per day, while others excreting larger amounts of protein are better able to maintain serum albumin levels.

EDEMA. Edema in the nephrotic syndrome results in part from a reduction in plasma oncotic pressure such that capillary hydraulic pressure exceeds oncotic pressure in peripheral capillaries and fluid leaves the capillaries. Although the reduction in effective circulating volume that occurs may result in increased renal retention of salt and water through normal compensatory mechanisms, over 50 per cent of patients with the nephrotic syndrome have normal or increased plasma volume and normal or low levels of plasma renin during sodium retention, suggesting a primary renal contribution to salt retention in the nephrotic syndrome through mechanisms that remain poorly defined.

HYPERLIPIDEMIA. Hyperlipidemia is common in the nephrotic syndrome and is inversely proportional to the serum albumin concentration. Hypercholesterolemia and elevated phospholipids are the most constant abnormalities observed, but increased levels of low and very low density lipoproteins, triglycerides, and chylomicrons are also seen. The primary mechanism appears to be increased hepatic synthesis of cholesterol, triglycerides, and lipoproteins, but reduced catabolism of these compounds has also been demonstrated.

LIPIDURIA. In a nephrotic urine sediment lipids are seen as free fat, oval fat bodies (degenerated renal tubular epithelial cells containing cholesterol esters), and fatty casts, all of which exhibit a Maltese cross pattern under polarizing light. Lipiduria parallels the level of urine protein excretion rather than the serum lipid levels.

Complications of the Nephrotic Syndrome

The most clinically important metabolic complications of the nephrotic syndrome are severe protein malnutrition, which may require appropriate nutritional supplementation, hypercoagulability with a tendency to form thrombi in both renal and peripheral veins leading to thromboembolic complications, and acute renal failure.

Hypercoagulability is thought to be a consequence of altered clotting factor levels in the nephrotic syndrome, including reduced levels of factors IX, XI, and XII; elevated levels of factors V and VIII, fibrinogen, beta-thromboglobulin, and platelets; a reduction in levels of antithrombin III and antiplasmin; and increased susceptibility of platelets to aggregation. There is a high incidence (10 to 40 per cent) of thrombus formation in renal, pulmonary, and peripheral veins, and occasionally in arteries, with frequent thromboembolic phenomena. The incidence of renal vein thrombosis appears to be particularly high in patients with the nephrotic syndrome due to membranous nephropathy. Routine anticoagulation is not indicated unless emboli occur.

Acute renal failure in the nephrotic syndrome very rarely occurs owing to rapid progression of the underlying renal disease, since most diseases that cause the nephrotic syndrome progress very slowly. However, acute renal failure does occur as a consequence of several potentially treatable disorders superimposed on nephrotic glomerular disease. These include (1) reduced renal perfusion due to low plasma volume, which can result in acute tubular necrosis, particularly following a surgical procedure or biopsy; (2) interstitial renal edema in patients with MCNS and significant peripheral edema, who may develop intrarenal swelling sufficient to produce increased intrarenal pressure, cessation of filtration, and acute renal failure (this may be reversible with diuretic therapy); (3) drug-induced allergic interstitial nephritis, particularly in patients receiving diuretic therapy; (4) bilateral acute renal vein thrombosis; and (5) reduced glomerular perfusion due to nonsteroidal anti-inflammatory drugs, which inhibit synthesis of vasodilatory prostaglandins and reduce glomerular plasma flows in states of volume contraction or diffuse glomerular disease. Nonsteroidal anti-inflammatory agents may also cause acute allergic interstitial nephritis, which may be accompanied by a reversible nephrotic syndrome with a glomerular lesion like that in MCNS.

Other complications that may also be associated with the nephrotic syndrome include reduced levels of IgG (which may dispose to bacterial infection), proximal tubular dysfunction with signs of Fanconi's syndrome, deficiencies of trace metals such as iron, copper, and zinc, and loss of vitamin D with development of osteomalacia and secondary hyperparathyroidism. Measurements of thyroid function such as T_4 radioimmunoassay and T_3 resin uptake may falsely suggest reduced function, but free T_4 and TSH levels are generally normal.

Coggins CH: Management of nephrotic syndrome. In Brenner BM, Stein JH (eds.): Contemporary Issues in Nephrology. Vol 9. New York, Churchill Livingstone, 1982, p 283. *A clear review of the approach to clinical management of each of the systemic manifestations of nephrotic syndrome independent of the glomerular disease that causes them.*

Kaysen GA, Myers BD, Couser WG, et al.: Biology of disease: Mechanisms and consequences of proteinuria. Lab Invest 54:479, 1986. *An in-depth review that correlates the pathophysiology of glomerular protein filtration with observations in patients with nephrotic syndrome and discusses the mechanisms and the consequences of massive urinary protein loss.*

Reineck HJ: Mechanisms of edema formation in the nephrotic syndrome. In Brenner BM, Stein JH (eds.): Contemporary Issues in Nephrology. Vol 9. New York, Churchill Livingstone, 1982, p 31. *A clear and comprehensive analysis of this controversial topic, with suggestions on management.*

Primary Renal Diseases That Present as the Nephrotic Syndrome

Minimal Change Nephrotic Syndrome (MCNS)

As indicated in Table 81–4, MCNS accounts for about 75 per cent of cases of idiopathic nephrotic syndrome in children and up to 20 per cent of adults. Synonyms include minimal change disease, nephropathy or glomerulopathy, lipoid nephrosis, and nil disease.

Pathogenesis. The pathogenesis of MCNS is not known. The disease is characterized by a loss of net negative charge on the capillary wall and can recur promptly in the transplanted kidney, suggesting the presence of a circulating factor that neutralizes or destroys glomerular polyanion, resulting in loss of the charge barrier and a selective type of proteinuria. The association of MCNS with Hodgkin's disease, its responsiveness to steroids and alkylating agents, and the tendency for remission to follow some viral infections, particularly measles, have focused attention on the possibility of an abnormality in T lymphocytes, perhaps involving production of a lymphokine with properties that induce increased glomerular capillary permeability. However, attempts to demonstrate such a substance have not been successful thus far.

Pathology. By definition, the diagnosis of MCNS requires the absence of abnormalities by light microscopy and of immune deposits by IF. Diffuse epithelial cell foot process effacement, or "fusion," is the abnormality usually seen by EM, but some morphologic abnormalities may occur in MCNS, including mild-to-moderate focal or diffuse proliferation of mesangial cells; mesangial deposits of IgM, IgA, or C3 by IF; and the presence of focal glomerular sclerosis (FGS) by light microscopy. In the presence of FGS, response to steroids is poor, and progressive loss of renal function is commonly seen. This has led several authors to consider FGS as a separate disease (see below). However, in some patients the FGS lesion appears to develop late in the course of MCNS and may simply be a histologic marker of a more severe and less responsive form of MCNS mediated by a similar mechanism.

Mesangial proliferation and mesangial IgM deposits may occur together or separately and usually predict a poor (or delayed) response to steroids and an increased possibility of progression. As with FGS, there have been attempts to classify such patients into separate disease categories (mesangial-proliferative GN, IgM nephropathy). When progression occurs in patients with MCNS and mesangial proliferation and/or IgM deposits, glomeruli develop changes typical of FGS.

Clinical Features. The peak incidence of MCNS is in children two to six years of age, in whom it virtually always presents as a full-blown nephrotic syndrome. In childhood, males are affected twice as commonly as females. One third of patients will have a preceding upper respiratory tract infection or other identifiable antecedent event. In the absence of volume contraction, renal function and blood pressure are normal, but up to one third of patients may have a reduced GFR when first seen due to hypovolemia and reduced renal perfusion. Urine protein excretion may exceed 40 grams per day in severe cases, and serum albumin is less than 2.0 grams per deciliter in over 90 per cent of children. The complications of this disease are discussed above under complications of the nephrotic syndrome in general. In addition, there is an association between MCNS and Hodgkin's disease in which the nephrotic syndrome may be the presenting sign of an occult lymphoma. Allergic reactions to nonsteroidal anti-inflammatory agents may produce nephrotic syndrome and MCNS on biopsy, usually associated with interstitial nephritis and reduced renal function.

Laboratory Findings. The laboratory findings in MCNS are those of the nephrotic syndrome of any etiology. Proteinuria is "selective" (greater than 90 per cent albumin) in about 85 per cent of cases. Complement levels are usually normal. A consistent finding is a marked reduction in ASO titers (less than 100 Todd units).

Course and Treatment. Before steroids and modern antibiotics were available the spontaneous remission rate in MCNS was estimated at 25 to 40 per cent. During that era, the mortality rate in children exceeded 50 per cent in five years owing to infections or thromboembolic complications. The mortality rate now is about 7 to 12 per cent in nephrotic children and less than 2 per cent in those who respond to steroids. Some of this improvement reflects the development of effective antibiotics and better general medical care. Steroid therapy has never been shown in a controlled study to improve survival in patients with MCNS. However, the usual dramatic resolution of the nephrotic syndrome following steroid administration, as well as the fact that survival has improved since the presteroid era, has led to the widespread belief that such treatment is beneficial.

Conventional doses of oral prednisone are 60 mg per square meter per day in children and 2 mg per kilogram per day in adults, given daily for four weeks, followed by alternate-day therapy for four more weeks and then a tapering course over four to six months. Within four weeks, 90 per cent of children will have responded, and 90 per cent of adults will respond within about eight weeks. There is little value in continuing steroid therapy beyond eight weeks if abnormal levels of proteinuria persist. The 10 per cent of patients who fail to respond generally have FGS (see below).

Of the steroid responders, roughly 50 per cent will remain free of proteinuria or develop infrequent relapses that respond to steroids, eventually entering permanent remission. The remainder will either become "frequent relapsers" (more than twice a year) or steroid dependent, often with a high incidence of steroid side effects. Some can be managed conservatively with salt restriction, diuretics, and a high-protein diet. In children, the clinical manifestations of the nephrotic syndrome are usually more severe, and steroid toxicity may require the use of an additional drug. Both cyclophosphamide, 2 to 3 mg per kilogram per day (75 mg per square meter per day in children), and chlorambucil, 0.2 to 0.3 mg per kilogram per day, given for 8 to 12 weeks, have been shown to increase the frequency and duration of remission in steroid-sensitive MCNS. However, because of their gonadal toxicity, teratogenic potential, and other side effects, these agents should be used only when both the nephrotic syndrome and steroid side effects are severe. About half of such patients treated with a second drug are reported to be in remission four years later, suggesting that complete remission can be achieved with drug therapy in almost 90 per cent of patients with MCNS.

Hoyer JR: Idiopathic nephrotic syndrome with minimal glomerular changes. In Brenner BM, Stein JH (eds): Contemporary Issues in Nephrology. Vol 9. New York, Churchill Livingstone, 1982, p 145. *This is an excellent and current review of all aspects of MCNS, including the clinical features, pathogenesis, pathology, and treatment.*

Nolasco F, Cameron JS, Heywood EF, et al.: Adult-onset minimal change nephrotic syndrome: A long-term follow-up. Kidney Int 29:1215, 1986. *This paper reviews the clinical course and response to therapy in 89 adults with MCNS and documents a higher incidence of complications and slower response to therapy compared with children with this disease.*

Focal Glomerular Sclerosis (FGS)

Overview. FGS is a histologic lesion found in some patients with otherwise typical MCNS, and it correlates well with steroid resistance and progressive renal failure. Controversy exists regarding whether it should be classified as a separate glomerular disease or should be viewed as one end of a spectrum that ranges from pure steroid-responsive MCNS with no morphologic abnormalities to typical FGS. This spectrum includes patients who have either mesangial proliferation by light microscopy and/or mesangial IgM deposits with or without evidence of FGS. The author favors the views that mesangial proliferation, mesangial IgM deposits, and FGS are part of the MCNS spectrum. However, the clinical features of patients with idiopathic nephrotic syndrome and FGS in early biopsies are sufficiently different from those who do not have these lesions to warrant separate consideration.

Pathogenesis. The etiology and pathogenesis of the lesion of FGS are unknown. Presumably, the basic mechanism underlying the generalized increase in capillary wall permeability may be the same as that in MCNS, and the structural lesion may be the consequence of either the greater severity of this process in such patients or the presence of some additional, as-yet-unidentified factor(s). Experimentally, a marked increase in mesangial trafficking and deposition of circulating macromolecules occurs in association with altered glomerular permeability. Mesangial dysfunction, with loss of contractile properties and regulation of local capillary loop hemodynamics, may precede the development of FGS. This could result in persistent glomerular vasodilatation, hypertension, and hyperfiltration, with consequent structural damage to the capillary wall.

Pathology. The diagnosis of FGS is made by renal biopsy in which sclerotic lesions are seen only in some glomeruli (focal) and within an affected glomerulus are present only in some capillary loops (segmental). The presence of sclerosis involving occasional entire glomeruli (global sclerosis) is a common finding that increases with age in all patients and does not have prognostic significance. The FGS lesion itself is an expansion of the mesangial matrix with wrinkling and collapse of adjacent capillary loops, development of PAS-positive intracapillary hyaline deposits, adhesions to Bowman's capsule, and often foamy cells and focal epithelial cell proliferation (Fig. 81–6). Glomeruli that do not contain the lesion of FGS exhibit changes identical to those of MCNS, indicating that the increase in capillary permeability is a

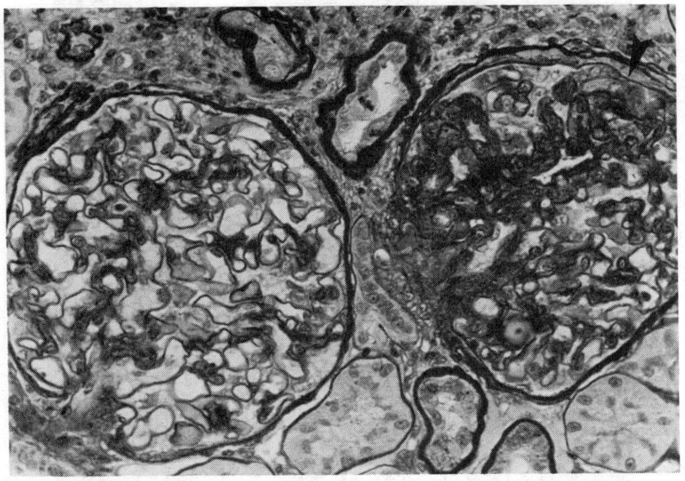

FIGURE 81–6. Renal biopsy from a patient with nephrotic syndrome, FGS, and decreased renal function. By light microscopy the glomerulus on the left appears almost normal with only slight mesangial matrix increase, while the glomerulus on the right is partially sclerotic with an adhesion to Bowman's capsule at one o'clock (*arrowhead*). Two atrophic tubules with thickened basement membranes in the upper part of the field are surrounded by fibrosis and mononuclear cells. (Periodic acid–Schiff stain, × 350.) (Reproduced from Couser WG, Salant DJ, Adler S, et al. In Brenner BM, Lazarus JM (eds.): Acute Renal Failure, Philadelphia, WB Saunders Company, 1983, p 403.)

diffuse one not confined to the areas of sclerotic lesions. Interstitial infiltrates and tubular atrophy usually accompany lesions of FGS. IgM and C3 are frequently deposited nonspecifically in sclerotic lesions and may occasionally be seen more diffusely in the mesangium.

Clinical Features. FGS is present in 5 to 15 per cent of patients with idiopathic nephrotic syndrome and is associated with a higher frequency of hematuria (65 per cent), hypertension (10 per cent), and renal insufficiency (10 per cent) than is seen in MCNS (Table 81–4). Sterile pyuria is also common. Proteinuria is nonselective, presumably reflecting the focal areas of structural damage to the capillary wall associated with lesions of FGS. While most patients have the nephrotic syndrome, a significant minority are detected with asymptomatic proteinuria, a finding that is rarely seen in MCNS. When all of these features accompany the finding of FGS in an early biopsy, only about 20 per cent of such patients will respond to steroid therapy and many of these do not remain steroid responsive. The presence of the nephrotic syndrome, hematuria, hypertension, decreased renal function, and mesangial hypercellularity on biopsy tends to indicate a poor prognosis.

A smaller group of patients appears to have clinically typical MCNS without hematuria or hypertension but shows early lesions of FGS on biopsy. Often such biopsies are obtained later in the course of the disease after several episodes of steroid-responsive nephrotic syndrome, and such patients may remain steroid responsive for many years and progress very slowly or not at all. When all patients with FGS on initial biopsy are studied, only about 40 per cent are in renal failure at the end of ten years.

Laboratory Features. There are no distinctive laboratory abnormalities, except for the increased incidence of hematuria and presence of nonselective proteinuria, that differentiate patients with FGS from those with pure MCNS.

Course and Treatment. Patients with FGS on initial biopsy, especially if hematuria, hypertension, and nephrotic syndrome are present, rarely respond to steroids and progress to renal failure in an average of about ten years. The level of proteinuria is clearly related to prognosis, and 80 per cent of all patients with non-nephrotic proteinuria retain normal renal function for over ten years. About 15 to 20 per cent of all patients with FGS and the nephrotic syndrome will show a response to steroids, sometimes months to years after therapy, a phenomenon that justifies a trial of steroid therapy as outlined above for MCNS in such patients. If steroid responsiveness is present, the prognosis is considerably better, and such patients may behave like those with MCNS. Alkylating agents such as cyclophosphamide and chlorambucil have been shown to increase the frequency and duration of steroid-induced remission in FGS as they have in MCNS. Immunosuppressive drugs may occasionally be effective in steroid-resistant patients.

Patients with FGS who progress to renal failure have a high incidence of recurrent disease in renal transplants. Factors that have been correlated with recurrence include mesangial hypercellularity, a rapidly progressive course (less than three years), and receipt of a well-matched living-related donor transplant. In four antigen matches, the recurrence rate may be as high as 80 per cent, although it is less than 50 per cent for all patients with end-stage renal disease due to FGS. With recurrence, patients develop the nephrotic syndrome within a few hours to one week, accompanied by lesions of FGS in the transplant and usually a shortened graft survival. This phenomenon is important both in emphasizing the necessity for accurate diagnosis of renal disease in patients prior to transplantation and in selecting and counseling potential kidney donors.

Korbet SM, Schwartz MM, Lewis EJ: The prognosis of focal segmental glomerulosclerosis of adulthood. Medicine 66:304, 1986. *This detailed analysis of 46 patients with idiopathic nephrotic syndrome and focal glomerulosclerosis emphasizes clinical features, prognosis, and therapy.*

Southwest Pediatric Nephrology Study Group: Focal segmental glomerulosclerosis in children with idiopathic nephrotic syndrome: A report of the Southwest Pediatric Nephrology Study Group. Kidney Int 27:442, 1985. *This report reviews the clinical features, pathology, response to treatment, and clinicopathologic correlations in 75 children with FGS. The overlap with MCNS and the relatively poor prognosis are emphasized.*

HEROIN NEPHROPATHY. In some centers up to 25 per cent of new cases of FGS and 10 per cent of all cases of end-stage renal disease occur in young adults with a history of parenteral drug abuse, usually including heroin. Other renal lesions such as GN secondary to bacterial endocarditis, hepatitis B–associated membranous nephropathy, large vessel vasculitis, amyloidosis, and interstitial nephritis related to embolized foreign material are also seen in addicts. However, the entity of nephrotic syndrome with FGS, hypertension, and rapidly progressive renal disease appears to be the most common drug-related lesion. A similar lesion may cause nephrotic syndrome in patients with AIDS (see above). Discontinuation of drug use has resulted in stabilization or improvement in renal function in some patients, but no other form of therapy has proved beneficial. The role of the injected drugs or other foreign substances in the pathogenesis of this lesion is not known.

Dubrow A, Mittman N, Ghali V, et al.: The changing spectrum of heroin-associated nephropathy. Am J Kidney Dis 5:36, 1985. *This study of 35 heroin abusers with nephrotic syndrome confirms the presence of FGS as a common underlying lesion but emphasizes the increasing frequency with which amyloid is seen as the cause of nephrotic syndrome.*

Membranous Nephropathy

Overview. Membranous nephropathy is an uncommon disease in childhood but is the commonest cause of idiopathic nephrotic syndrome in adults, in whom it accounts for about 50 per cent of all cases (Table 81–4). As with all other causes of idiopathic nephrotic syndrome, the diagnosis can be made only by renal biopsy.

Pathogenesis. Experimentally, subepithelial immune deposits may result from antibody binding to an epithelial cell membrane antigen or to exogenous antigens that become localized at this site, usually on the basis of charge-charge interactions with glomerular anionic structures. It has not been established which of these mechanisms is the predominant one in humans, but the idiopathic form of membranous nephropathy may be an autoimmune disease. Subepithelial immune deposits appear to induce proteinuria by a mechanism that probably involves the C5b–9, or membrane attack, portion of the complement system.

The role played by inciting agents such as drugs or hepatitis virus in initiating this process is unknown. A strong association exists between idiopathic membranous nephropathy and HLA-DRw3 (relative risk about four), an association also noted in patients who develop membranous nephropathy while taking drugs. Although most cases are idiopathic, some develop in association with a variety of other conditions, including *drugs* (penicillamine, gold, captopril), *infectious agents* (hepatitis B, various parasitic infestations), *SLE*, and *malignancy*, particularly solid tumors of the lung, breast, and gastrointestinal tract. The nephrotic syndrome may be the presenting sign of an otherwise occult neoplasm, and older patients with idiopathic membranous nephropathy should be carefully evaluated for malignancy. An identical lesion occurs in about 15 per cent of patients with SLE and may be the presenting sign of this disease when other systemic and serologic manifestations are absent. Young females who present with what appears to be idiopathic membranous nephropathy must be carefully followed for later development of SLE. Other associations such as those with Sjögren's syndrome, mixed connective tissue disease, diabetes, thyroiditis, syphilis, sarcoidosis, and sickle cell disease are documented but rare.

Pathology. By light microscopy glomeruli may appear entirely normal early, but as the disease progresses, a diffuse thickening of capillary walls occurs without any increase in glomerular cellularity (Fig. 81–7). A silver methenamine stain will usually demonstrate the spike-like extensions of basement membrane between areas of subepithelial deposits, and the subepithelial deposits themselves may be seen with a PAS stain. A diffuse, very finely granular pattern of immune deposits of IgG and C3 is found along the subepithelial surface of all capillary loops (Fig. 81–8). EM demonstrates electron-

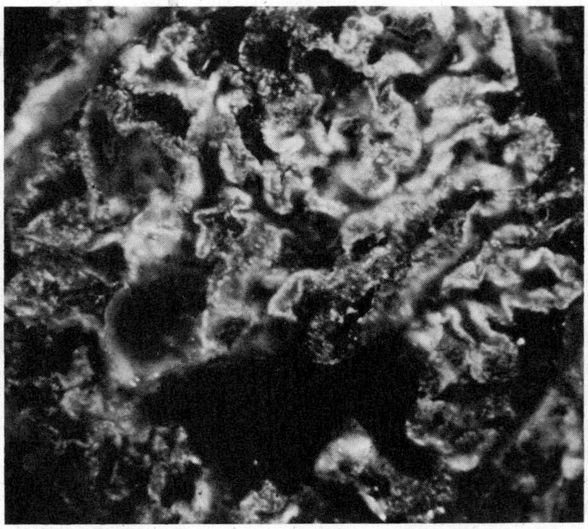

FIGURE 81–8. Immunofluorescence microscopy in membranous nephropathy demonstrates diffuse, finely granular staining of IgG (and C3) on all capillary walls, usually without mesangial deposits (× 400). (Reproduced from Couser WG, Salant DJ, Stilmant MM. In Flamenbaum W, Hamburger RJ (eds.): Nephrology. Philadelphia, JB Lippincott Company; 1982, pp 265–301.)

dense deposits in an exclusively subepithelial distribution with effacement of overlying foot processes (Fig. 81–9).

Clinical Manifestations. The mean age of onset of idiopathic membranous nephropathy in the United States is 40 to 50, and males predominate about 2 to 1. However, the disease has been reported in patients as young as 2 and over 70. Over 80 per cent of patients present with the nephrotic syndrome, but 20 per cent may be seen first with asymptomatic proteinuria. Microscopic hematuria is present in about 60 per cent of cases in adults, but red cell casts are rare. Hypertension is uncommon and renal function is usually normal at the time of presentation. The association of membranous nephropathy with other disease processes has been discussed above under "Pathogenesis."

Two complications of this disease are important: (1) Several patients have been reported to develop a *superimposed anti-*

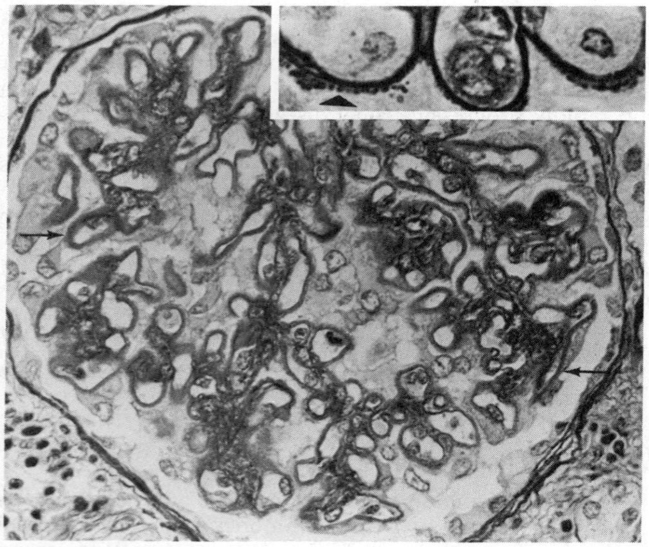

FIGURE 81–7. Light microscopy in early membranous nephropathy shows minimal thickening of the glomerular capillary walls (*arrows*) without any increase in cells or mesangial matrix. In the inset, three capillary loops stained with silver methenamine demonstrate the "spike" of basement membrane between deposits (*arrowheads*) (periodic acid–Schiff stain, × 350; inset: silver methenamine stain, × 900). (Reproduced from Couser WG, Salant DJ, Stilmant MM. In Flamenbaum W, Hamburger RJ (eds.): Nephrology. Philadelphia, JB Lippincott Company, 1982, pp 265–301.)

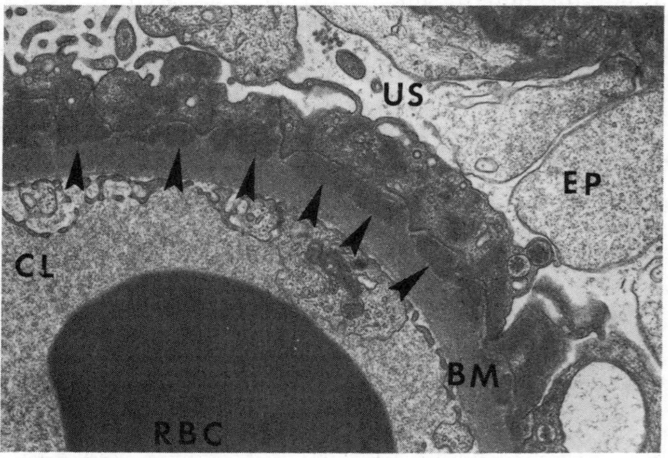

FIGURE 81–9. Electron micrograph of a glomerulus in membranous nephropathy showing many electron-dense subepithelial deposits (*arrowheads*) between the basement membrane and effaced epithelial cell foot processes. A red blood cell is present in the capillary lumen (× 15,000). BM = Basement membrane; CL = capillary lumen; EP = epithelial cell; RBC = red blood cell. (Reproduced with permission from Couser WG, Salant DJ, Adler S, et al. In Brenner BM, Lazarus JM (eds): Acute Renal Failure. Philadelphia, WB Saunders Company, 1983, p. 406).

GBM nephritis with crescent formation and a clinical course similar to that of RPGN. This possibility must be considered in otherwise stable patients who experience a rapid deterioration in renal function accompanied by a nephritic urine sediment. (2) An incidence of *renal vein thrombosis* as high as 50 per cent has been reported in membranous nephropathy. Any patient in whom a thromboembolism is suspected should be studied for renal vein thrombosis and treated with long-term anticoagulation to reduce thromboembolic complications if a venous thrombosis is demonstrated.

Laboratory Studies. There are no laboratory abnormalities specific for idiopathic membranous nephropathy. Because of the frequency of various associated conditions, the laboratory workup should include determinations of antinuclear and anti-DNA antibody, serum complement levels, rheumatoid factor, cryoglobulins, hepatitis B antigen, VDRL, and tests to exclude diabetes. In older patients, a careful clinical and radiologic search for occult malignancy is justified. If the patient has unusual flank pain, hematuria, or a reason to suspect pulmonary emboli, the renal veins should be studied by venography.

Course and Treatment. The disease has a widely variable clinical course with substantial fluctuations in proteinuria and an uncertain prognosis. The spontaneous remission rate is about 25 per cent in adults. Another 25 per cent of patients will have persistent nephrotic range proteinuria for many years but will retain normal renal function. The remaining 50 per cent of adults, and 10 to 15 per cent of children, experience a slowly progressive deterioration of renal function that results in end-stage renal disease in an average of about 15 years, although more rapid progression may be seen. No clinical or pathologic criteria have been identified that will predict the future clinical course in an individual patient.

The variable clinical course in idiopathic membranous nephropathy makes any assessment of benefits from therapy difficult, since large numbers of patients must be followed in a prospective controlled fashion to obtain meaningful data. One such study in adults with idiopathic membranous nephropathy and normal renal function compared treatment with 100 to 150 mg of prednisone every other day for two months with a placebo and demonstrated a slower rate of deterioration in renal function in patients treated with prednisone. Several retrospective studies have reached similar conclusions. Concomitant administration of cytotoxic drugs may further improve these results. Since fewer than 50 per cent of patients will develop progressive disease, the author recommends cytotoxic drugs only in patients with evidence of progressive loss of renal function.

Recurrent membranous nephropathy in a renal transplant is rare but has been reported in several patients who have progressed to end-stage renal disease in a period of four years or less. Recurrence usually has not adversely affected graft survival. Significantly more cases of de novo membranous nephropathy have been reported in renal allografts than cases of recurrence, and the disease is a relatively common cause of the nephrotic syndrome in transplant patients.

Cameron JS: Pathogenesis and treatment of membranous nephropathy (Nephrology Forum). Kidney Int 15:88, 1979. *A very complete and thoughtful discussion of membranous nephropathy by an experienced clinical investigator. It includes a review and discussion of the data on steroid treatment in this disease with Dr. Cecil Coggins.*

Ponticelli C: Prognosis and treatment of membranous nephropathy. Kidney Int 29:927, 1986. *This excellent summary reviews the causes of membranous nephropathy, the factors that influence prognosis, and the data on benefits of therapy. The results of a prospective study by the author suggesting a beneficial effect of treatment with a cytotoxic drug as well as steroids are reviewed and discussed in detail.*

Membranoproliferative Glomerulonephritis (MPGN)

Overview. The term membranoproliferative glomerulonephritis (MPGN) refers to a clinicopathologic entity found primarily in young adults and characterized by idiopathic nephrotic syndrome, hypocomplementemia, and a histologic lesion having the lobular appearance of glomeruli with both thickening of the basement membrane and cellular proliferation. This entity has also been called lobular GN, chronic hypocomplementemic GN, and mesangiocapillary GN. These histologic and clinical features are probably common to at least two separate and perhaps unrelated diseases, which are now referred to as type I MPGN (that with subendothelial immune deposits) and type II MPGN (dense deposit disease). Type I MPGN is about twice as common as type II, and the two diseases cause about 10 per cent of cases of idiopathic nephrotic syndrome in both children and adults (Table 81–4). However, unlike the other glomerular diseases that cause idiopathic nephrotic syndrome, about 20 per cent of patients present with an acute nephritic syndrome, and nephritic features are common in both of these diseases.

Pathogenesis. TYPE I MPGN. Several features of type I MPGN suggest that it is a chronic immune complex GN: (1) the granular deposits of IgG and C3 in a subendothelial and mesangial distribution, (2) the activation of the classic complement pathway, (3) the frequent presence of cryoglobulins and circulating immune complexes, (4) the presence of similar lesions in patients with some forms of postinfectious GN, including shunt nephritis and nephritis associated with chronic hepatitis B antigenemia, and (5) the production of similar lesions in animals immunized chronically with a foreign serum protein. However, the etiology of the disease, the nature of the antigen(s) involved, and the reasons for the chronicity of the process remain unknown.

TYPE II MPGN. This disease does not appear to be an immune deposit disease, and the nature of the dense deposits remains unclear. Despite much study of the unique abnormalities in complement metabolism associated with this disease, and the identification of C3 nephritic factor in the serum, the role of the complement abnormalities, if any, in the pathogenesis of the disease remains undefined. There is no animal model of dense deposit disease, and similar lesions have not been described in other renal diseases.

Pathology. TYPE I MPGN. Light microscopy reveals a diffuse proliferative GN with thickening of the glomerular capillary walls, increase in mesangial cells and matrix, and a lobulated appearance of the glomerulus (Fig. 81–10). The thickened capillary walls are due to subendothelial immune deposits and interposition of mesangial matrix between GBM and endothelium, resulting in a double contour, splitting, or "tram

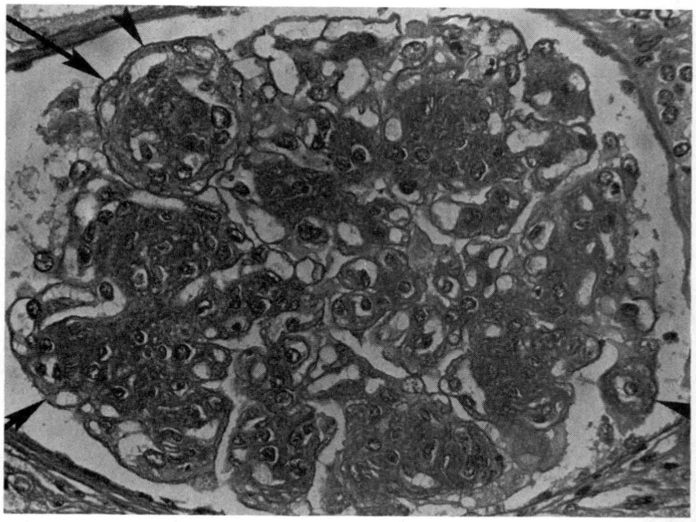

FIGURE 81–10. Light microscopy in membranoproliferative glomerulonephritis shows glomerular hypercellularity, segmental thickening of the basement membrane (*arrowheads*), and lobulation of glomerulus (*arrows*). (Periodic acid–Schiff, × 350.) (Reproduced from Couser WG, Salant DJ, Stilmant MM. In Flamenbaum W, Hamburger RJ (eds.): Nephrology. Philadelphia, JB Lippincott Company, 1982, pp 265–301.)

track" appearance of the capillary walls on silver stain. Crescents are present in less than 10 per cent of cases. Coarsely granular deposits of C3, and often of IgG, IgM, C4, properdin, and fibrin, occur in the mesangium and in peripheral capillary loops in a pattern much like that seen in diffuse proliferative, or class IV, SLE. By EM there are dense subendothelial and mesangial deposits present as well as mesangial matrix interposition with capillary wall thickening and narrowing of the capillary lumen.

TYPE II MPGN. The histologic findings in type II MPGN are very similar to those in type I disease except that crescents are present in up to 30 per cent of patients and correlate with a worse prognosis. The dense deposits may be seen as PAS-positive, ribbon-like deposits within the capillary wall as well as along Bowman's capsule and tubular basement membrane. C3 is present along the margins of these deposits, resulting in a double linear pattern on the capillary walls as well as surrounding deposits of similar material in the mesangium (mesangial rings). Granular immune deposits of IgG are much less common than in type I disease. EM reveals extensive replacement of the lamina densa with homogenous, dark-staining material that may also be seen in the mesangium, Bowman's capsule, and tubular basement membrane.

Clinical Features. There are only minor differences in the clinical manifestations of types I and II MPGN. What follows is a description of patients with the more common type I disease. The differences observed in type II disease are commented on below. MPGN is a disease of children and young adults, rarely seen before age 5 and relatively uncommon after age 30. Males and females are affected approximately equally. The nephrotic syndrome is the presenting sign in about 50 per cent of patients and develops during the course of the disease in over 80 per cent. Up to 20 per cent may present with an acute nephritic syndrome (which is more common in type II), and the remainder are detected with asymptomatic hematuria or proteinuria or both. Preceding upper respiratory tract infections have occurred in about half of patients with type I MPGN and may have been streptococcal. Hematuria is a common feature of the disease. Hypertension is present in one third, and 25 per cent have a reduced GRF on initial presentation.

The clinical course is quite variable. One third of patients develop end-stage renal disease within 6 to 10 years, one third have persistent nephrotic syndrome with relatively stable renal function, and one third have persistent non-nephrotic proteinuria or hematuria. Fewer than 5 per cent experience spontaneous remissions. In the long term at least 50 per cent of patients with type I will reach end-stage renal disease in 15 to 20 years, while type II progresses somewhat more rapidly (6 to 10 years). Poor prognostic signs in individual patients include a reduced GFR at onset, the presence of the nephrotic syndrome, early hypertension, gross hematuria, and the presence of either crescents or sclerosis on a renal biopsy.

Type I MPGN recurs in about 25 per cent of patients who receive renal transplants but rarely interferes with graft function.

The clinical features of type II disease that differ from those of type I include a higher frequency of both the nephrotic syndrome and acute nephritic episodes, a lower frequency of asymptomatic hematuria and proteinuria, more rapid progression to renal failure (probably due to the greater frequency of nephritic episodes), more frequent and persistent hypocomplementemia (see below), and a higher frequency of recurrence in transplants. Type II disease is also associated with partial lipodystrophy in some patients.

Laboratory Abnormalities. Type I MPGN is characterized by fluctuating levels of complement with depression of both classic (C1q, C4) and alternate pathway components at some time in most patients. In type II disease, hypocomplementemia is more frequent and persistent, and only alternate pathway activation is usually seen with a reduction in C3 and other alternate pathway proteins such as properdin and factor B, while classic pathway components are usually normal. Most type II patients have a circulating IgG autoantibody (C3 nephritic factor, or C3 Nef) directed against the C3 convertase of the alternate complement pathway. The definitive diagnosis of either type I or type II MPGN can be made only by renal biopsy with complete IF and EM studies.

Treatment. Improvement or stabilization in renal function in MPGN has been reported with two-year courses of alternate day steroid therapy and with a "cocktail" of drugs including steroids, cytotoxic agents, anticoagulants, and antiplatelet agents. However, side effects of such treatments are significant. Administration of the platelet inhibitor dipyridamole, 225 mg per day, and aspirin, 975 mg per day, significantly reduces the rate of loss of renal function in type I MPGN with minimal side effects. This regimen is the one of most demonstrable benefit and least toxicity at present. Too few patients with type II MPGN have been studied prospectively to be certain that similar results are achieved with that lesion.

Cameron JS, Turner DR, Heaton J, et al.: Idiopathic mesangiocapillary glomerulonephritis. Comparison of types I and II in children and adults and long-term prognosis. Am J Med 74:175, 1983. *An excellent clinical review of 104 well-studied patients that discusses the clinical and laboratory findings in types I and II MPGN, the differences between children and adults, and the long-term prognosis and prognostic features.*

Donadio JV, Anderson CF, Mitchell JC III, et al.: Membranoproliferative glomerulonephritis: A prospective clinical trial of platelet-inhibitor therapy. N Engl J Med 310:1421, 1984. *In a prospective, randomized, double-blind, controlled trial of dipyridamole and aspirin versus plaebo in 40 patients, most with type I MPGN, the author demonstrates better maintenance of renal function in the treated group without significant complications*

West CD: Childhood membranoproliferative glomerulonephritis: An approach to management. Kidney Int 29:1077, 1986. *This review by the investigator who first described this disease in 1965 discusses the clinical characteristics of 51 patients and reviews data on therapy, concluding that long-term steroid therapy is beneficial in altering the natural history.*

GLOMERULAR INVOLVEMENT IN SYSTEMIC DISEASES

The most common systemic diseases resulting in glomerular involvement are the various forms of vasculitis. With the group of diseases referred to as systemic necrotizing vasculitis, a distinction is made between necrotizing vasculitis involving medium-sized and larger vessels (the polyarteritis nodosa group including classic PAN, allergic granulomatosis, and "overlap" syndromes), and necrotizing vasculitis involving small vessels and capillaries (hypersensitivity vasculitis or microscopic PAN plus several well-defined clinical syndromes, including SLE, HSP, and mixed essential cryoglobulinemia). The only other common vasculitic syndrome with significant renal involvement is Wegener's granulomatosis.

Polyarteritis Nodosa (PAN)

Classic PAN, a disease of older adults sometimes associated with drug abuse (particularly amphetamines) and heptitis B antigenemia, is described in detail in Ch. 440. Renal involvement, which occurs in 90 per cent of cases, is usually manifest first as hematuria with an active urine sediment and mild proteinuria. In 70 per cent of cases, the renal lesion is primarily an ischemic one caused by vasculitic involvement of arcuate and interlobular arteries. This is best demonstrated by abdominal angiography and is generally not seen on renal biopsy. Aneurysmal dilatation is present in renal, hepatic, and mesenteric vessels. In 30 per cent of patients, a focal necrotizing GN with crescents may be seen. Both types of glomerular involvement may sometimes occur in the same patient. Immune deposits are generally not found in the glomerulus, and the pathogenesis of the renal disease is uncertain. Renal failure is a major cause of death and either may be a slowly progressive process or develop acutely in association with accelerated hypertenion. In patients with PAN who develop hypertension and acute renal failure, renal cortical necrosis is common, and there is little reversibility. More often, the disease is a slowly progressive one in which vigorous control of hypertension, use of oral steroids, and addition of cytotoxic agents such as cyclophosphamide have achieved five-year survivals of over 80 per cent of patients in uncontrolled studies.

Milder renal lesions may occur in the other two subgroups of this category. In allergic granulomatosis, allergic symptoms, asthma, pulmonary involvement, and eosinophilia are prominent features of the disease. In the overlap syndromes, both allergic manifestations and small vessel involvement may occur in the presence of the classic large vessel involvement seen in PAN.

Balow JE: Renal vasculitis. Kidney Int 27:954, 1985. *A comprehensive review of the classification, pathogenesis, and clinical features of the various forms of systemic necrotizing vasculitis involving the kidney. The utility of angiography in the diagnosis of PAN and the indications for cytotoxic drug therapy are stressed.*

Wegener's Granulomatosis

Wegener's granulomatosis is a granulomatous and necrotizing vasculitis but also involves large vessels, usually of the upper and lower respiratory tract and kidney (see Ch. 441). The disease presents most frequently in the fourth or fifth decade of life and affects more males than females. Presenting signs usually are respiratory and include purulent rhinorrhea, painful sinusitis, otitis, keratoconjunctivitis, oral ulcerations, and multiple bilateral nodular pulmonary infiltrates. Renal involvement eventually develops in over 80 per cent of patients and untreated may result in the death of up to 30 per cent. Early renal involvement is manifest by hematuria, proteinuria, and mild renal impairment with a focal and necrotizing proliferative GN, usually without immune deposits. However, severe diffuse necrotizing and crescentic GN may develop rapidly. Necrotizing granulomatous vasculitis may be seen in biopsies of the respiratory tract but is often not evident in renal biopsies. The presence of granulomas may be the only pathologic finding that distinguishes Wegener's granulomatosis from PAN. Spontaneous improvements in renal disease have not been reported. There are no characteristic laboratory abnormalities in Wegener's granulomatosis. Although the diagnosis can usually be made on clinical grounds, a renal biopsy is generally performed early in the disease to identify potentially severe renal involvement that may be clinically silent and to distinguish Wegener's granulomatosis from other diseases with pulmonary and renal manifestations, such as Goodpasture's syndrome, which would be treated differently. Prognosis and therapy are discussed in Ch. 441.

Fauci AS, Haynes BF, Katz P, et al.: Wegener's granulomatosis: Prospective clinical and therapeutic experience with 85 patients for 21 years. Ann Intern Med 98:76, 1982. *This paper from the NIH describes in detail the clinical manifestations of 85 patients with Wegener's granulomatosis and the treatment protocol now used to induce remissions in over 90 per cent of patients.*

Hypersensitivity Vasculitis (Microscopic PAN, Allergic Vasculitis, Leukocytoclastic Angiitis)

This disease is a form of systemic necrotizing vasculitis of small vessels in which the clinical manifestations do not fall into a well-recognized syndrome such as SLE, HSP, or essential mixed cryoglobulinemia (see Ch. 439). The disease is believed to be a manifestation of immune complex formation in small vessels and frequently follows exposure to some offending antigen such as an infectious agent, drug, or foreign protein by about a seven- to ten-day latent period. However, about half of patients will not have an identifiable antecedent event. The skin is most commonly involved, with palpable purpura. Other frequent manifestations include microangiopathic hemolytic anemia and pulmonary infiltrates with hemoptysis.

Clinical renal involvement is present in about 50 per cent of cases and is usually manifest initially as asymptomatic proteinuria associated with a segmental necrotizing GN or biopsy. Impairment in renal function is present in 20 to 40 per cent of cases, and up to 10 per cent may develop acute oliguric renal failure. On biopsy, these patients generally have extensive necrotizing glomerular lesions with abundant crescent formation and negative IF studies. Treatment considerations are similar to those outlined above for idiopathic RPGN, including high-dose steroid pulse therapy and possibly plasma exchange. There is more evidence to support the use of additional cytotoxic agents, such as cyclophosphamide, in the treatment of RPGN due to vasculitis than is present in idiopathic RPGN.

Serra A, Cameron JS, Turner DR, et al.: Vasculitis affecting the kidney: Presentation, histopathology, and long-term outcome. Q J Med 210:181, 1984. *Fifty-three patients with vasculitis involving the kidney are reviewed. The finding of a segmental necrotizing glomerular lesion accompanied by systemic symptoms such as fever, malaise, or weight loss was considered diagnostic of a small vessel vasculitis. Clinical features in such patients were identical to those who had histologic evidence outside the kidney. The paper is an excellent review of the wide spectrum of clinical manifestations of vasculitis and the frequency of crescentic glomerulonephritis in such patients as well as the relatively poor prognosis.*

Systemic Lupus Erythematosus (SLE)

The current diagnostic criteria and clinical manifestations of SLE are considered in more detail in Ch. 436. This section will discuss only the renal involvement. About 70 per cent of patients will have clinical manifestations of renal disease ranging from microscopic hematuria and proteinuria to an acute nephritic syndrome with acute renal failure and typical nephrotic syndrome. Renal biopsies reveal some abnormalities in most patients.

CLASSIFICATION. The most common classification system used for renal involvement in SLE is the World Health Organization (WHO) classification based on histopathologic criteria (Table 81–5).

Class I (Normal Kidneys). Only very rarely do patients with diagnostic criteria for SLE have entirely normal kidneys by light microscopy, IF, and EM, and they do not have clinical manifestations of glomerular disease.

Class II (Minimal or Mesangial Lupus Nephritis). This is the earliest and mildest form of renal involvement in SLE and is characterized by mesangial deposits of immunoglobulin and C3 with (Class IIB) or without (Class IIA) focal proliferative changes by light microscopy. Clinical manifestations of proteinuria and hematuria are present in most patients, but the nephrotic syndrome and renal insufficiency are very

TABLE 81–5. HISTOLOGIC CLASS, CLINICAL PRESENTATION, AND PROGNOSIS IN SLE NEPHRITIS

Histologic Type	WHO Class	Frequency (%)*	Proteinuria (%)	Nephrotic Syndrome† (%)	Azotemia‡ (%)	Death (%)	Uremic Death (%)
Normal	I	<5					
Mesangial	II	15	68	0	12	18	0
Focal proliferative	III	20	100	15	18	30	11
Diffuse proliferative	IV	50	100	87	75	58	36
Membranous	V	15	100	88	20	38	6

*Per cent of patients biopsied with SLE who show this lesion.
†Proteinuria exceeding 3.0 grams per 24 hours.
‡Serum creatinine exceeding 1.2 mg per deciliter or BUN exceeding 25 mg per deciliter.

uncommon and do not develop unless progression to a more severe lesion occurs, as happens in about 20 per cent of patients. Five-year survival is over 90 per cent, and no specific therapy is indicated for the renal lesion.

Class III (Focal Proliferative Lupus Nephritis). This is a stage in a continuum between mesangial lesions alone and diffuse proliferative lupus nephritis. Focal proliferative changes are present in fewer than 50 per cent of glomeruli, but all glomeruli contain immune deposits of IgG, IgA, C3, and usually IgM and fibrin-related antigens. Deposits are predominantly mesangial, but occasional subendothelial deposits may be seen. All patients have proteinuria, but the nephrotic syndrome and renal insufficiency occur in fewer than 20 per cent and may remit following steroid therapy. Serologic abnormalities including hypocomplementemia are more severe than in Class II disease. Long-term prognosis with this lesion is also good (90 per cent five-year survival). However, there is a relatively high incidence of transformation to Class IV disease, resulting in a reduction in five-year survival to about 70 per cent, with almost half of the deaths occurring from renal failure. The most reliable predictor of progression is probably the presence of subendothelial deposits by EM.

Class IV (Diffuse Proliferative Lupus Nephritis). This is the severest of the glomerular lesions in lupus, with proliferation seen in over 50 per cent of glomeruli, frequently with crescent formation and necrosis. Extensive mesangial and subendothelial deposits contain all immunoglobulins, C3, and fibrin. Mesangial and subendothelial deposits are present by EM, often with subepithelial deposits as well. Proteinuria is seen in all patients, and nephrotic range proteinuria is present in 50 per cent at onset and 90 per cent some time during the course of the disease. Renal function is decreased in 75 per cent at the time of presentation, and serologic evidence of disease activity, including hypocomplementemia, elevated levels of anti-DNA antibody, and circulating immune complexes, is present in most patients. The long-term prognosis for this lesion has improved considerably over the years, with most centers now achieving survival rates of about 75 per cent at five years. The best prognosis is in those patients in whom a remission of the nephrotic syndrome and normalization of serologic parameters are achieved within one year of starting therapy.

Class V (Membranous Lupus Nephritis). About 15 per cent of patients with SLE will develop a glomerular lesion that may be indistinguishable from idiopathic membranous nephropathy with extensive subepithelial deposits of all immunoglobulins and C3. The nephrotic syndrome and a slowly progressive renal disease are common (see Table 81–4). Patients may have undetectable levels of antinuclear antibody at the time of presentation. The incidence of systemic manifestations of SLE and serologic abnormalities in general is also lower in patients with a membranous lesion. The long-term prognosis for patients with this lesion does not differ significantly from those with Class II disease. As in idiopathic membranous nephropathy, there appears to be an increased incidence of renal vein thrombosis. Steroid therapy as discussed under idiopathic membraneous nephropathy is usually recommended.

TREATMENT OF LUPUS NEPHRITIS. In patients with active renal disease and a class III or IV lesion, steroids have a beneficial effect in lupus nephritis. High-dose steroid therapy is given for a period of four to six weeks and subsequently tapered and adjusted according to responses in renal function, serologic parameters, and extrarenal disease. In the presence of crescents and deteriorating renal function, steroid pulse therapy, as discussed above under idiopathic RPGN, may result in more rapid return to maximal renal function. The addition of a cytotoxic agent such as cyclophosphamide to oral steroid therapy may result in better preservation of renal function in a subset of patients with evidence of active Class III or IV disease and mild chronic changes by biopsy. Thus a renal biopsy appears to be useful as a basis for selecting therapy in patients with active lupus nephritis. Administration of cyclophosphamide as a monthly intravenous pulse may provide a therapeutic effect equivalent to a daily oral dose with fewer side effects.

With development of renal failure, disease activity in SLE usually subsides. Renal transplantation has been carried out in a large number of patients without significant problems.

Austin HA, Muenz LR, Joyce KM, et al.: Prognostic factors in lupus nephritis: Contribution of renal histologic data. Am J Med 75:382, 1983. *Newer histologic parameters have been shown to be useful in selecting patients with lupus nephritis who may benefit from administration of a cytotoxic drug in addition to steroids. This paper establishes the value of age, sex, and initial level of renal functions, as well as the chronicity index determined from the renal biopsy, as important prognostic factors in lupus nephritis.*

Austin HA III, Klippel JH, Balow JE, et al.: Therapy of lupus nephritis: Controlled trial of prednisone and cytotoxic drugs. N Engl J Med 314:614, 1986. *This prospective study of 106 patients with active lupus nephritis suggests a beneficial effect of intravenous cyclophosphamide in reducing the risk of end-stage renal disease only in the subset of high-risk patients identified by the presence of chronic histologic changes. The data support the claim that monthly intravenously administered cyclophosphamide is less toxic than a daily dose. This is the best study currently available on the efficacy of cytotoxic drug therapy in lupus nephritis.*

Ballow JE, moderator: Lupus nephritis. Ann Intern Med 106:79, 1987. *This review from a group with extensive experience in the classification and treatment of lupus nephritis summarizes current understanding of the pathogenesis and treatment of renal disease in SLE.*

Henoch-Schönlein Purpura (HSP)

Henoch-Schönlein syndrome, or anaphylactoid purpura, is another systemic necrotizing vasculitis of small vessels in which systemic manifestations include palpable purpura (100 per cent) on the lower extremities and buttocks due to a leukocytoclastic vasculitis of dermal vessels, arthralgias of large joints, usually the knees and ankles (70 per cent), gastrointestinal involvement with colic and bleeding (25 per cent), and renal involvement (see Ch. 167). About 30 per cent of patients have clinical evidence of renal disease in the form of hematuria or acute nephritic syndrome. Except for the systemic manifestations, the disease is very similar in its morphologic and clinical characteristics to IgA nephropathy but is of somewhat greater severity. Typically the disease presents with an acute nephritic syndrome, usually without edema or hypertension, developing within three months of the onset of other systemic manifestations of HSP. Many patients have an infectious episode prior to the onset of renal disease. Up to 25 per cent of adults may develop a severe crescentic lesion with RPGN. The nephrotic syndrome has been reported to develop in over 50 per cent, and progressive renal failure occurs in at least 25 per cent of patients. The renal involvement is much less severe in children. Predictors of progressive disease include presentation with an acute nephritic syndrome, nephrotic syndrome, crescents, and subepithelial deposits or subendothelial "lead-shot" lesions by EM. Most patients have self-limited episodes of renal involvement, usually lasting one week or less. However, recurrences are common.

Laboratory features are not distinctive and do not differ from those described for IgA nephropathy. Renal biopsy may reveal a spectrum of lesions ranging fom focal mesangial proliferation to diffuse crescentic GN, but the most characteristic lesion is a focal necrotizing GN in which necrosis and fibrin deposition are more common than in IgA nephropathy. IF and EM findings do not differ from those in IgA nephropathy with diffuse mesangial deposits of IgA and lesser amounts of IgG and complement. IgA deposits are also present in dermal capillaries of involved or uninvolved skin.

The pathogenesis of HSP is unknown but is presumed to be immunologic and similar to that of IgA nephropathy. Similar immunogenetic associations in the two diseases, as well as the clinical, histologic, and immunopathologic similarities, strongly suggest that a common underlying disease mechanism is involved.

No treatment has been shown to be of benefit in the nephritis of HSP. Short courses of steroids may be useful in controlling systemic manifestations but do not appear to benefit the renal lesion. Patients who develop crescents and a clinical picture of RPGN should be considered for treatment as outlined above under idiopathic RPGN.

Lee HS, Koh HI, Kim MJ, et al.: Henoch-Schönlein nephritis in adults: A clinical and morphological study. Clin Nephrol 26:125, 1986. *This paper provides a detailed analysis of the clinical and morphologic features as well as prognostic variables in 17 adult patients with Henoch-Schönlein nephritis.*

Meadow AR, Glasgow EF, White RHR, et al.: Schönlein-Henoch nephritis. Q J Med 41:241, 1972. *This older article provides an excellent review of the clinical features in a large series of adult patients with HSP.*

Essential Mixed Cryoglobulinemia (EMC)

Low concentrations of mixed cryoglobulins, usually type III with polyclonal IgG and IgM with rheumatoid factor activity, are seen in a variety of immune glomerular disorders, autoimmune diseases, vasculitides, and neoplastic syndromes, in which they rarely produce symptoms (Ch. 439). Type II mixed cryoglobulins, composed of monoclonal IgM rheumatoid factor and polyclonal IgG, are characteristic of a disorder called essential mixed cryoglobulinemia (EMC), in which dependent vascular purpura, Raynaud's phenomenon, arthralgias, weakness, and GN are the principal clinical manifestations. Cryoprecipitates from these patients often contain hepatitis B antigen. The disease is one of middle age and affects females somewhat more often than males.

Renal involvement is present in about 40 per cent of cases and is usually preceded by purpura and arthralgias. The severity of renal disease ranges from microscopic hematuria and proteinuria to an acute nephritic syndrome with acute renal failure. In contrast to most of the other vasculitic syndromes, the nephrotic syndrome is a rather frequent occurrence, and severe hypertension is common. Laboratory abnormalities include a markedly elevated sedimentation rate, cryoglobulins, rheumatoid factor activity, and sometimes an artifactual decrease in levels of early complement components, with C3 and later components often normal. The glomerular lesion is a diffuse proliferative and exudative GN, sometimes accompanied by vasculitis, with large PAS-positive proteinaceous deposits present in many capillaries. The subendothelial capillary deposits are composed predominantly of IgG and IgM, with lesser amounts of C3 and fibrin. In patients with acute nephritic syndrome and renal failure the prognosis is poor. However, in all patients with renal disease, over 50 per cent may recover with or without therapy, and the survival rate at ten years is about 75 per cent. Although steroids and cytotoxic agents alone have not been shown to be of consistent benefit in the renal lesion, plasma exchange therapy may improve the prognosis in patients with severe renal disease.

Tarantino A, DeVecchi A, Montagnino G, et al.: Renal diseases in essential mixed cryoglobulinaemia. Q J Med 197:1, 1981. *A detailed review of the renal manifestations, biopsy findings, and long-term course in 44 patients with EMC and renal disease, emphasizing the spectrum of disease and prognosis.*

Thrombotic Microangiopathy (Hemolytic Uremic Syndrome and Thrombotic Thrombocytopenia Purpura)

Hemolytic uremic syndrome (HUS) and thrombotic thrombocytopenic purpura (TTP) are referred to collectively by some authors as thrombotic microangiopathy. The two disorders can be clinically indistinguishable, probably have a common, although poorly understood, pathogenesis, and respond to similar therapy.

HEMOLYTIC UREMIC SYNDROME (HUS). HUS is a syndrome of microangiopathic hemolyic anemia, thrombocytopenia, and renal impairment, which usually occurs abruptly in children about three to ten days following episodes of gastroenteritis or viral upper respiratory tract infection. Gastroenteritis is often associated with verotoxin producing *Escherichia coli* infections. A similar syndrome occurs less commonly in adults, often associated with complications of pregnancy or during the postpartum period (postpartum acute renal failure) or associated with the use of oral contraceptives. HUS also occurs in adults following treatment with a variety of antineoplastic agents. Acute renal failure develops in up to 60 per cent of children but usually resolves spontaneously within about two weeks with only supportive therapy. Chronic renal failure occurs in only 10 per cent of patients, usually those who suffer loss of renal function in a gradual, progressive manner, who have oliguria lasting longer than two weeks, or who have total anuria. Laboratory features of the disease include microangiopathic hemolytic anemia, thrombocytopenia, increased numbers of reticulocytes, elevated bilirubin levels, reduced haptoglobin levels, and elevated levels of fibrin split products, usually with only minimal laboratory evidence of disseminated intravascular coagulation. In TTP (see below) levels of fibrin split products are less commonly elevated. The glomerular lesion is one of intimal hyperplasia of arterioles and intracapillary fibrin thrombi, sometimes with areas of focal necrosis. The anemia and thrombocytopenia are presumably due to trapping of platelets and destruction of red cells in the areas of capillary thrombosis. The pathogenesis of the syndrome is unknown but probably involves glomerular endothelial cell injury by some as yet unidentified circulating factor, with subsequent fibrin deposition and thrombosis. Decreased endothelial cell production of prostacyclin, a vasodilator and inhibitor of platelet aggregation, has been reported but may be a secondary event.

In typical HUS in children, only supportive therapy, including early dialysis, is required, since the rate of spontaneous recovery is very high. In adults, the prognosis is considerably worse because renal involvement is more severe and development of bilateral cortical necrosis more common. This is particularly true in cases associated with pregnancy and oral contraceptives. No form of therapy has been determined to be effective in HUS, although aspirin, antiplatelet agents, heparin, fresh frozen plasma infusions, and plasma exchange have all been advocated by some authors. In adults with severe disease, treatment with plasma exchange as described below for TTP, in addition to steroids, antiplatelet agents, and aspirin, is probably indicated.

THROMBOTIC THROMBOCYTOPENIC PURPURA (TTP). TTP is clinically and pathologically very similar to HUS (see Ch. 167). The differences that distinguish this end of the spectrum of thrombotic microangiopathy are (1) a more common occurrence in young adults, (2) fever as a frequent manifestation of the disease, (3) neurologic abnormalities that tend to predominate and cause death, and (4) a lesser degree of renal involvement with acute renal failure in only about 10 per cent of cases. Hematuria is the most common manifestation of renal disease. Proteinuria, generally less than 5 grams per day, and a serum creatinine in excess of 2 mg per deciliter occur in about 50 per cent of cases. Histologically the renal lesion is the same as that in HUS. TTP has a considerably worse prognosis than HUS, with about a 75 per cent mortality within three months, and spontaneous recovery is rare.

A wide variety of therapeutic regimens have been employed in TTP, including all of those listed above for HUS as well as intravenous infusion of prostacyclin and vigorous plasma exchange. The most promising results have been obtained with plasma exchange, often in combination with fresh plasma, antiplatelet agents, and steroids, a regimen that has produced rather dramatic clinical remissions in several patients with apparently severe and advanced disease. In refractory cases, splenectomy may confer an additional benefit.

Hakim RM Schulman G, Churchill WH Jr, et al.: Successful management of thrombocytopenia, microangiopathic anemia, and acute renal failure by plasmapheresis. Am J Kidney Dis 5:170, 1985. *This report describes successful treatment of six consecutive adult patients with thrombocytopenic, microangiopathic anemia and renal failure with plasmapheresis as well as fresh plasma and steroids. This approach is the treatment of choice for severe cases of thrombotic microangiopathy.*

Ridolfi R, Bell WR: Thrombotic thrombocytopenic purpura. Report of 25 cases and review of the literature. Medicine 60:413, 1981. *This is a comprehensive review article covering clinical features, renal involvement, pathology, and pathogenesis of TTP, with a detailed approach to therapy and over 200 references.*

CHRONIC GLOMERULONEPHRITIS

Chronic GN is not a separate disease. It represents the progressive stage of any of the primary or secondary glomerular diseases discussed in this chapter prior to development of end-stage renal disease. Thus, PSGN, IgA nephropathy, RPGN, focal glomerular sclerosis, membranoproliferative glomerulonephritis, membranous nephropathy, and SLE, as well as diseases such as hereditary nephritis, may result in chronic GN with progressive loss of renal function, proteinuria, abnormal urine sediments, and diminishing renal size. About 60 per cent of all cases of end-stage renal disease result from some form of chronic GN. In the early stages these lesions can be accurately diagnosed by renal biopsy and sometimes successfully treated. However, in patients with chronic disease, small kidneys, and creatinine clearances below 15 ml per minute, the changes on renal biopsy are rarely diagnostic, and there is little reversible component to the renal damage.

The clinical features of chronic GN are noteworthy only for the frequency with which progressive renal disease is asymptomatic. About 50 per cent of patients will present with advanced renal insufficiency without a clear past history of renal disease. In most patients with chronic renal failure and creatinine clearances below 25 ml per minute, progression to renal failure is inexorable. The rate of progression can be quite accurately predicted from plots of the reciprocal of serum creatinine concentration versus time and is quite consistent for individual patients although not for specific diseases. The clinical manifestations of chronic renal failure are discussed in more detail in Ch. 79.

In end-stage glomerular disease the renal cortex is thin, and glomeruli are acellular, sclerotic, and often replaced by collagenous material. Tubular atrophy, interstitial fibrosis, and cellular infiltrates are widespread. The mechanisms by which acute renal injury leads to progressive loss of renal function have not been well defined. In some acute inflammatory diseases such as RPGN, immune injury may be so severe that glomeruli are irreversibly destroyed by ischemia, necrosis, and thrombosis, resulting in acute renal failure and end-stage renal disease without a chronic or progressive phase. However, in most diseases progression is a much slower process that appears to continue long after the initial disease process has resolved.

The primary mechanisms of progression in glomerular disease may be hemodynamic. Loss of functioning nephron mass from an acute injury results in an adaptive increase in glomerular capillary plasma flow rates and transcapillary hydraulic pressure gradient (*glomerular hyperfiltration*) to maximize the GFR. Increased intraglomerular pressure appears to result in increased capillary permeability to protein and structural glomerular damage when sustained above a certain level over time. The histologic manifestation of this form of glomerular injury is focal glomerular sclerosis—a process that characterizes virtually all progressive renal diseases and results in gradual loss of filtering surface areas. Glomerular hyperfiltration induced experimentally can be substantially modified by restricting dietary protein intake or by treatment with angiotensin-converting enzyme inhibitors, which reduce efferent arteriolar constriction and thereby lower intraglomerular pressure. Thus, changes in dietary protein or specific drug therapy may be beneficial in slowing or halting progression in a variety of chronic renal diseases. The role of these treatments in chronic renal disease has not yet been defined but is the subject of intensive ongoing investigation.

Dunn BR, Anderson S, Brenner M: The hemodynamic basis of progressive renal disease. Semin Nephrol 6:122, 1986. *This paper reviews the experimental basis for postulating that progressive renal disease is hemodynamically mediated and reviews the data suggesting that protein restriction therapy or angiotensin-converting enzyme inhibitors may prevent the loss of renal function in a wide variety of glomerular diseases.*

Glassock RJ, Adler SG, Ward HJ, et al.: Primary glomerular diseases. In Brenner BM, Rector FC Jr (eds.): The Kidney. Philadelphia, W. B. Saunders Company, 1986, p 946. *This chapter presents a detailed discussion of the clinical and pathologic features, course, and therapy of chronic GN and is extensively referenced.*

Oldrizzi L, Rugiu C, Valvo E, et al.: Progression of renal failure in patients with renal disease of diverse etiology on protein-restricted diet. Kidney Int 27:553, 1985. *The study of 78 patients with chronic glomerulonephritis, polycystic kidney disease, and chronic interstitial nephritis documents a significantly reduced rate of loss of renal function in patients treated with protein and phosphorus restriction compared with controls. The results suggest that the beneficial effects of such treatment demonstrated experimentally in animal models probably apply to humans as well.*

82 TUBULOINTERSTITIAL DISEASES AND TOXIC NEPHROPATHIES

T. Dwight McKinney

COMMON FEATURES OF TUBULOINTERSTITIAL DISEASES

Tubulointerstitial disease (tubulointerstitial nephritis or nephropathy, interstitial nephritis) refers to a diverse group of acute and chronic disorders that primarily affect the renal tubules and interstitium. In contrast, in other primary renal diseases, most notably glomerulonephritis, the tubules and interstitium are only secondarily involved. Approximately 30 per cent of all cases of chronic renal insufficiency in the United States result from tubulointerstitial diseases. Usually the cause of tubulointerstitial disease can be identified. Renal function may improve or stabilize with appropriate therapy.

Clinical Manifestations

In tubulointerstitial diseases, functional renal tubular defects, which are present to some degree in advanced renal insufficiency of any cause, are frequently out of proportion to the degree of renal insufficiency as measured by reduction in glomerular filtration rate (GFR). In fact, the finding of such a disproportional loss of tubular compared with glomerular function should lead one to suspect the diagnosis of tubulointerstitial disease (Table 82–1). Urinary concentration in response to water deprivation or exogenous antidiuretic hormone may be reduced, particularly in chronic interstitial nephritis. This may result in decreased maximal urinary osmolarity, polyuria (generally <3 liters per day), and nocturia. Concentration defects, an acquired form of nephrogenic

TABLE 82–1. MANIFESTATIONS OF RENAL TUBULOINTERSTITIAL DISEASES

1. Tubular dysfunction disproportionate to reduction in GFR
2. Tubular abnormalities
   a. Reduced maximal urinary concentrating ability (polyuria, nocturia)
   b. Renal tubular acidosis (hyperchloremic metabolic acidosis)
   c. Partial or complete Fanconi's syndrome
      - Phosphaturia
      - Bicarbonaturia
      - Aminoaciduria
      - Uricosuria
      - Glycosuria
   d. Sodium wasting
   e. Hyperkalemia
3. Renal endocrine deficiencies
   a. Hyporeninemic hypoaldosteronism (hyperkalemia, metabolic acidosis)
   b. Calcitriol deficiency (renal osteodystrophy)
   c. Erythropoietin deficiency (anemia)
4. Urinalysis
   a. May be normal but usually contains cellular elements
   b. Proteinuria is usually modest (<3.5 grams per day) and consists largely of low molecular weight "tubular" proteins such as lysozyme and beta$_2$-microglobulin

diabetes insipidus, may result from interference with the action of antidiuretic hormone on the collecting ducts or anatomic damage or disruption of the medullary structures involved in the urinary concentrating mechanism (Ch. 227). Damage to the proximal tubules may result in excessive urinary excretion of substances normally reabsorbed in this location. Bicarbonaturia (proximal renal tubular acidosis), phosphaturia, aminoaciduria, uricosuria, glycosuria, kaliuresis, and low molecular weight proteinuria may be seen. These losses may cause low plasma levels of some of these substances, particularly phosphate, bicarbonate, and urate. The presence of multiple proximal tubular defects is referred to as Fanconi's syndrome (Ch. 84). In addition to proximal renal tubular acidosis, failure of the distal nephron to acidify the tubular fluid maximally results in classic distal renal tubular acidosis. Hyperkalemic (type 4) distal renal tubular acidosis may also occur. All of these cause a hyperchloremic (normal anion gap) metabolic acidosis (Ch. 77). Hyperkalemia may result from a primary failure of potassium secretion by the distal nephron but more commonly results from decreased renal production of renin and subsequent secondary hypoaldosteronism. Patients with tubulointerstitial disease may also fail to conserve sodium normally. In some, this is due to the hyporeninemic hypoaldosteronism noted above. Renal sodium wasting may result in signs of extracellular fluid volume depletion when sodium intake is restricted and may cause worsening of renal function. With acute and, to a lesser extent, chronic interstitial nephritis, these tubular defects may be accompanied or, indeed, overshadowed by other signs, symptoms, and laboratory abnormalities of renal failure (Ch. 78 and 79).

Diagnosis

A specific diagnosis of tubulointerstitial renal disease can often be made or inferred from historical information, physical examination, or laboratory tests. Renal biopsy is the most definitive method of diagnosis, but this is not always necessary. Pathologic features are discussed below. Radiographic, ultrasonographic, and radionuclide examinations generally show only evidence of acute or chronic renal insufficiency but may provide a specific diagnosis such as urinary tract obstruction or polycystic kidney disease.

Prognosis and Treatment

The prognosis usually depends on the specific cause of tubulointerstitial renal disease as discussed below. General supportive therapy, e.g., treatment of electrolyte disorders, and management of acute and chronic renal failure are discussed in Ch. 78 and 79.

COMMON FEATURES OF TOXIC NEPHROPATHIES

The term toxic nephropathy refers to those renal disorders resulting directly or indirectly from exposure of the kidneys to exogenous chemicals and physical factors, including both drugs and environmental agents, and abnormal concentrations of substances normally present in the body fluids, such as calcium and uric acid. Drug-related renal disease is the most important cause of toxic nephropathy. Toxic nephropathy often results in tubulointerstitial disease, but it is not synonymous with it.

Several factors predispose the kidneys to toxic injury: (1) The kidneys receive approximately 20 per cent of the resting cardiac output and, therefore, are exposed to more blood-borne materials than any other organ except the lungs. (2) The high metabolic rate of the renal tubules required for active transport processes makes them particularly vulnerable to toxic insults. (3) The large glomerular capillary surface area is an available site for trapping immune complexes or for in situ antigen-antibody reactions. (4) Some substances (e.g., aminoglycosides) are selectively concentrated in the renal cortex because of specific transport processes located in the proximal tubules, whereas others (e.g., phenacetin) are concentrated in the medulla owing to the renal countercurrent system. This selective concentration accounts, in part, for the anatomic distribution of damage by some nephrotoxins. (5) Certain substances are converted to less soluble forms with resultant precipitation (e.g., urate to uric acid) consequent to acidification of tubular fluid in the distal nephron. This may lead to tubular obstruction.

Nephrotoxins injure the kidneys in a variety of ways, both direct and indirect (Fig. 82–1). Indirect injury, for example, may result from immunologic reactions or from secondary effects such as drug-induced hypotension or hemolysis. These mechanisms, alone or in concert, may cause an array of renal disorders ranging from isolated functional tubular defects to reversible acute renal failure to progressive end-stage renal disease.

ACUTE INTERSTITIAL NEPHRITIS

Pathology and Pathogenesis

Characteristically, in acute interstitial nephritis (AISN) mononuclear cells infiltrate the interstitium, particularly in the cortex. Eosinophils, especially in cases of drug-related AISN, and occasionally small numbers of polymorphonuclear leukocytes may also be present. Inflammatory cells may invade the tubule walls and, in severe cases, may be associated with areas of tubular necrosis. The infiltrate may be diffuse or patchy; the extent of the infiltrate corresponds in general to the degree of renal functional impairment. In addition to the cellular infiltrate, the renal tubules are separated by interstitial edema, but no fibrosis is present. With prolonged AISN, interstitial fibrosis may develop and the pathologic picture may merge into that of chronic interstitial nephritis. In primary AISN the glomeruli are generally normal, although there may be some mesangial prominence. The predominant mononuclear inflammatory cells in infiltrates are T cells. Both helper/inducer and suppressor/cytotoxic T cells are present, although their relative numbers may vary depending on the specific disease. These observations suggest that both T cell–mediated delayed hypersensitivity reactions and cytotoxic T cell injury may be involved in AISN. In some cases immunoglobulins and complement components are demonstrable in the interstitium and/or tubular basement membrane by immunofluorescence. Rarely, electron microscopy may reveal electron-dense deposits in these areas suggestive of immune complexes. Finally, in occasional cases there may be linear deposition of immunoglobulins and complement in the tubular basement membrane indicative of anti–tubular basement membrane antibodies. There is, therefore, considerable evidence for immune injury mediated by cellular and humoral mechanisms as the cause of AISN. Usually, however, the immunopathogenetic mechanisms involved in a given case of AISN remain unknown.

Etiology

Acute interstitial nephritis may result from a variety of causes (Table 82–2). Drug-related AISN is becoming more frequently recognized as an important cause of acute renal insufficiency, probably because of (1) the more widespread use of renal biopsy, (2) the increasing number of drugs being used, and (3) the characteristic clinical presentation.

DRUG-INDUCED ACUTE INTERSTITIAL NEPHRITIS. The list of drugs that have been implicated as etiologic in AISN continues to expand (Table 82–3). AISN is a rare complication of drug therapy, but because of the frequency with which these agents are used, drugs account for a substantial portion of all cases of acute renal failure.

Penicillins. A number of penicillin congeners may cause AISN, including amoxicillin, ampicillin, carbenicillin, methicillin, mezlocillin, nafcillin, oxacillin, and penicillin G. Meth-

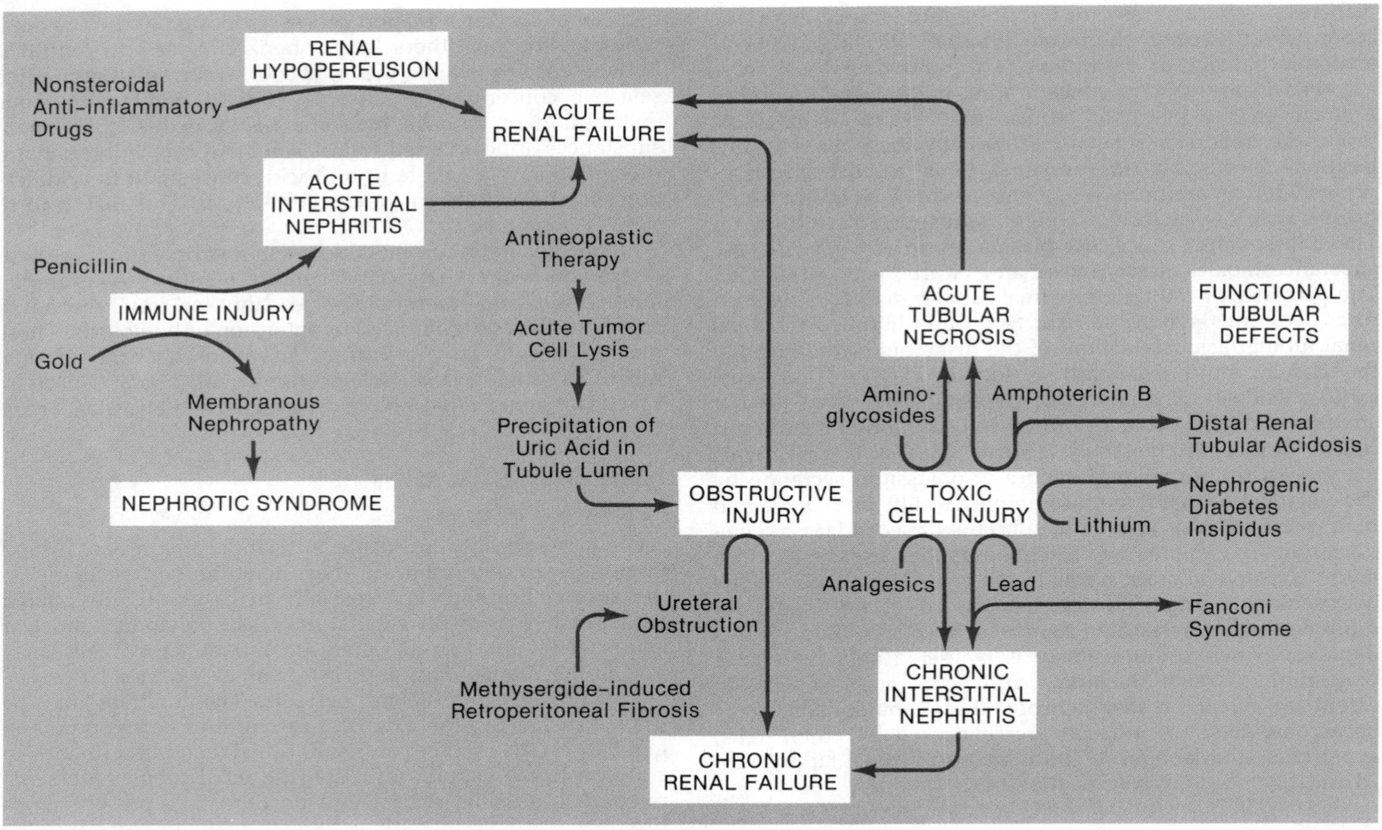

FIGURE 82–1. Types of toxin-induced renal disease.

icillin has been responsible for most reported cases, but the clinical syndrome is similar for the other penicillins. It is reasonable to presume that AISN may occur with any penicillin. Typically, penicillins have been taken for about two weeks prior to the onset of signs and symptoms of AISN, but this time interval has varied from two days to several weeks. The disorder appears to be more frequent in men and children. There is no correlation between the dosage of the drug administered and subsequent development of AISN. In one review of methicillin nephritis, the most frequent manifestations were as follows: hematuria, 97 per cent (this may be gross and associated rarely with red cell casts in the urinary sediment); proteinuria, 94 per cent (usually less than nephrotic range); pyuria, 93 per cent (eosinophiluria is frequently present and strongly suggests the diagnosis of AISN); fever, 87 per cent; eosinophilia, 79 per cent (this may be evanescent); azotemia, 61 per cent in adults and 16 per cent in children (often associated with oliguria); and skin rash, 24 per cent. Serum IgE levels may be elevated. Renal sodium wasting and hyperchloremic metabolic acidosis with hyperkalemia (hyperkalemic distal renal tubular acidosis) may also occur. The pathogenesis of the disorder is uncertain. Binding of penicillin haptens to renal tubule basement membranes may result in formation of anti–tubular basement membrane antibodies, but evidence for this mechanism is not convincing in most patients.

For treatment, the offending drug must be discontinued and another appropriate drug for the underlying infection should be substituted. In the majority of cases this will result in restoration of renal function. Recovery may require several weeks, with some patients needing interval dialysis. A short course of high-dose corticosteroids (60 mg per day of pred-

TABLE 82–2. CAUSES OF ACUTE INTERSTITIAL NEPHRITIS

1. Drug-related (Table 82–3)
2. Systemic infections
   - Brucellosis
   - Cytomegalovirus
   - Diphtheria
   - Infectious mononucleosis
   - Legionnaires' disease
   - Leptospirosis
   - Mycoplasmal pneumonia
   - Polyomavirus
   - Rocky Mountain spotted fever
   - Streptococcal infections
   - Syphilis
   - Toxoplasmosis
3. Primary renal infections
   - Bacterial pyelonephritis (Ch. 86)
   - Renal tuberculosis
   - Fungal nephritis
4. Immune disorders
   - Acute glomerulonephritis associated with anti-tubular basement membrane antibodies and/or secondary interstitial nephritis (Ch. 81)
   - Systemic lupus erythematosus
   - Acute rejection of a renal transplant (Ch. 80.2)
   - Necrotizing vasculitis
5. Other conditions
6. Idiopathic

TABLE 82–3. DRUGS ASSOCIATED WITH ACUTE INTERSTITIAL NEPHRITIS

Antimicrobial Drugs	
Cephalosporins	Para-aminosalicylic acid
Chloramphenicol	Penicillins*
Colistin	Polymyxin B
Erythromycin	Rifampin*
Ethambutol	Sulfonamides*
Isoniazid	Tetracyclines
	Vancomycin
Nonsteroidal Anti-inflammatory Drugs (Table 82–6)	
Miscellaneous	
Allopurinol*	Methyldopa
Antipyrene	Phenindione*
Azathioprine	Phenylpropanolamine
Bismuth	Phenytoin
Captopril	Probenecid
Cimetidine	Sulfinpyrazone
Clofibrate	Sulfonamide diuretics*
Gold	Triamterene

*Most frequent or clinically important.

nisone for one to two weeks) may possibly accelerate the recovery process, but the added risk in patients with underlying infections must be weighed against possible benefits.

Sulfonamides. Both antimicrobial sulfonamides and sulfonamide diuretics (thiazides, furosemide, chlorthalidone, acetazolamide) have been implicated in AISN. Although frequently these are prescribed in combination with other drugs (e.g., sulfamethoxazole plus trimethoprim as antimicrobials and hydrochlorothiazide plus triamterene as diuretics), it is most likely that the sulfonamide moiety of these combinations is responsible for AISN. Typically, evidence for AISN develops several days after therapy is begun, but rechallenge of a patient with a previous past history of sulfonamide-induced AISN may result in signs and symptoms within hours of exposure. The clinical presentation is in many ways similar to that described for the penicillins. Pyuria, hematuria, eosinophilia, and azotemia are frequent. A skin rash is present in a minority of patients. Renal failure may be severe and may require temporary dialysis, but recovery is the rule when the offending drug is discontinued. A brief course of corticosteroids may hasten recovery if no contraindication to their use is present.

Drug-induced AISN should be particularly considered in patients with underlying renal disease, such as nephrotic syndrome, who are treated with sulfonamide diuretics and who experience a more rapid decline in renal function than expected or other manifestations, such as eosinophilia, that suggest an allergic reaction. If diuretic therapy is required in a patient in whom a diagnosis of AISN is made by renal biopsy or presumed to be present based on characteristic clinical findings, a nonsulfonamide diuretic such as ethacrynic acid should be prescribed.

Antituberculous Drugs. A number of patients have developed AISN while receiving chemotherapy for tuberculosis, usually while being treated with more than one agent. Although rifampin, isoniazid, ethambutol, and para-aminosalicylic acid have all been incriminated as causing AISN, the evidence is most compelling for rifampin. AISN appears to occur more often and to be more severe with intermittent therapy with rifampin or after reinstitution of therapy following a drug-free interval than during continuous therapy. Fever, chills, flank pain, and anuria may develop after readministration of a single dose of rifampin. In contrast to other types of acute renal failure, transient hypercalcemia of unknown cause has been reported in several patients developing AISN during therapy for tuberculosis. Discontinuing the offending drugs is generally followed by recovery of renal function, although sometimes rather slowly. Corticosteroids do not appear to be beneficial in hastening recovery of renal function.

Allopurinol. Allopurinol-associated AISN generally develops after several days of treatment (mean interval of three weeks). Most patients have an exfoliative maculopapular skin rash, fever, eosinophilia, and decreased renal function. In addition, most have evidence of acute hepatic injury. Elevations of serum glutamic-oxaloacetic transaminase, sometimes to values in excess of 1000 U per liter, are present in about two thirds of patients. This form of allopurinol toxicity is severe and carries a mortality of approximately 20 per cent. Deaths result from severe systemic reactions, sepsis, gastrointestinal bleeding, or acute hepatic or renal failure. The cause of allopurinol toxicity is uncertain. Clinical and laboratory manifestations suggest a severe systemic hypersensitivity reaction. Most reported patients have been treated with conventional doses of the drug (200 to 400 mg per day), but most have had underlying renal insufficiency prior to development of allopurinol toxicity. Serum concentrations of the major metabolite of allopurinol, oxipurinol, are elevated in renal insufficiency. It may be that hypersensitivity to this or another metabolite may be responsible for the syndrome. In addition, about one half of the reported patients were receiving concomitant diuretic therapy. Whether this represents a causal relationship or merely coincidence is uncertain, as allopurinol is commonly prescribed to treat hyperuricemia that develops with diuretic therapy. Treatment of allopurinol toxicity consists of discontinuing the drug and instituting supportive measures, including dialysis, when indicated. Although corticosteroids have been given to many patients, it is uncertain whether they are efficacious. The incidence of allopurinol toxicity can be reduced by prescribing the drug only for clearly documented indications such as recurrent gouty arthritis or uric acid nephrolithiasis and not for asymptomatic hyperuricemia *per se* (including diuretic-induced hyperuricemia). The dose should be reduced in patients with underlying renal insufficiency.

Other Drugs Associated with AISN. Of the numerous other drugs reported to cause AISN, perhaps the most important are the anticoagulant phenindione and the nonsteroidal anti-inflammatory drugs. For the remainder of the agents listed in Table 82–3, AISN appears to be a very rare complication. Nevertheless, when manifestations characteristic of AISN occur in patients receiving these drugs (or other drugs not listed), the diagnosis of AISN should be entertained. In this setting it may be simplest to discontinue the suspect drug and replace it with an alternative agent. On the other hand, in patients for whom no suitable alternative exists, it may be necessary to confirm or exclude the diagnosis of AISN by renal biopsy.

AISN ASSOCIATED WITH INFECTION. Systemic bacterial, viral, rickettsial, mycoplasmal, and parasitic infections have been associated with AISN. Infections with group A beta-hemolytic streptococci are, perhaps, the most frequent, especially in children. The pathogenesis of AISN related to systemic infection is uncertain. Possibly, renal deposition of antigens related to the infectious agent elicits humoral and cell-mediated immune reactions that result in renal injury as discussed earlier. Many patients with AISN associated with systemic infections have received antibiotic therapy and may have drug-induced AISN (see above). Therapy of AISN due to systemic infections consists of treatment of the underlying infection and supportive therapy. The prognosis for recovery of renal function is usually quite favorable.

Acute bacterial pyelonephritis is a common cause of AISN. The clinical presentation with fever, chills, flank pain, and bacteria is characteristic (Ch. 86). Similarly, renal parenchymal fungal and mycobacterial infections may cause acute renal interstitial inflammation. All of these can result in renal scarring but only rarely cause acute renal failure.

AISN ASSOCIATED WITH IMMUNE DISORDERS. Varying degrees of acute and chronic interstitial nephritis may accompany numerous renal or systemic diseases of presumed immune origin. Several types of glomerulonephritis are associated with interstitial inflammation that may be out of proportion to the degree of glomerular injury (Ch. 81). In some, there may be antibodies to the tubular basement membranes. Although glomerulonephritis is generally the primary renal lesion in systemic lupus erythematosus, interstitial nephritis is the predominant finding in some patients (Ch. 81 and 436). Acute and chronic interstitial inflammation is the hallmark of renal transplant rejection (Ch. 80.2). Renal involvement with necrotizing vasculitis is generally manifest as a focal segmental glomerulonephritis, but in some patients, particularly those with Wegener's granulomatosis, there may be prominent interstitial involvement.

OTHER CONDITIONS ASSOCIATED WITH AISN. Sarcoidosis (Ch. 69), may involve the kidneys in a number of ways, including acute (granulomatous) interstitial nephritis, chronic interstitial nephritis (often associated with hypercalcemia and hypercalciuria), and primary glomerulonephritis. Rarely, AISN may cause acute renal failure in sarcoidosis. There have been isolated case reports of AISN following therapy with recombinant leukocyte interferon.

IDIOPATHIC AISN. In a number of patients with AISN, a specific cause cannot be identified. Some of these have evidence, such as eosinophilia, suggesting a hypersensitivity reaction to an unknown antigen. In addition to acute interstitial inflammation, renal biopsies sometimes demonstrate evidence for anti–tubular basement membrane antibodies. Others have granulomatous interstitial nephritis in the absence of an obvious etiology. The course of idiopathic AISN is variable, with some patients recovering spontaneously or in response to corticosteroid therapy and others progressing to renal insufficiency.

CLINICAL MANIFESTATIONS

In AISN the GFR usually declines abruptly, often producing oliguria. The urinary sediment typically contains numerous leukocytes. In cases of drug-induced AISN, eosinophils are often present as well. Hematuria is ordinarily present, and red blood cell casts, although rare, may be observed. Proteinuria is usually present but modest (<3.5 grams per day), except in AISN due to nonsteroidal anti-inflammatory drugs (see below). The fractional excretion of sodium tends to be high, as it is in most cases of acute tubular necrosis (see Ch. 78). A spectrum of renal tubular defects may be present (Table 82–1). In cases of drug-induced AISN (see above), other manifestations of drug allergy, such as fever, skin rash, and eosinophilia, are frequent. In AISN occurring as part of a systemic process, such as systemic lupus erythematosus, clinical and laboratory manifestations of the primary disease may dominate the clinical presentation. The diagnosis of AISN is established by examination of renal tissue obtained by biopsy (or autopsy). In drug-induced AISN, the diagnosis is often inferred from characteristic clinical and laboratory findings. The outcome of AISN depends on the underlying disease process. In drug-induced disease, renal function generally improves once the offending drug is stopped. Corticosteroid therapy may be beneficial, as discussed above. With prolonged and severe AISN, variable degrees of chronic renal insufficiency may result.

CHRONIC INTERSTITIAL NEPHRITIS

Pathology

Chronic interstitial nephritis (CISN) is characterized pathologically by interstitial fibrosis with atrophy and loss of renal tubules. The glomeruli may be normal but frequently are contracted. There is generally a patchy interstitial infiltrate of chronic inflammatory cells. The renal vasculature may show evidence of associated hypertension. In addition to these general findings, there may be others that suggest a specific disease, such as casts typical of multiple myeloma.

Etiology (Table 82–4)

TABLE 82–4. CAUSES OF CHRONIC INTERSTITIAL NEPHRITIS

1. Persistence or progression of acute interstitial nephritis (Table 82–2)
2. Chronic urinary tract obstruction (Ch. 83)
3. Nephrotoxins
   - Drugs: analgesics, nitrosoureas
   - Endogenous substances: hypercalcemia, hypokalemia, oxalate, uric acid
   - Metals: cisplatin, copper, lead, lithium, mercury
   - Radiation
4. Chronic bacterial pyelonephritis (Ch. 86) or renal tuberculosis (Ch. 302)
5. Immune disorders
   - Chronic glomerulonephritis with interstitial nephritis (Ch. 81)
   - Chronic rejection of a renal transplant (Ch. 80.2)
   - Systemic lupus erythematosus (Ch. 436)
   - Sjögren's syndrome (Ch. 438)
6. Associated with neoplasia or paraproteinemias
   - Leukemia
   - Lymphoma
   - Amyloidosis (Ch. 210)
   - Waldenström's macroglobulinemia (Ch. 163)
   - Cryoglobulinemia (Ch. 81)
   - Multiple myeloma (Ch. 163)
7. Cystic diseases
   - Medullary cystic disease
   - Polycystic kidney disease (Ch. 91)
8. Miscellaneous
   - Diabetes mellitus
   - Sickle cell hemoglobinopathies
   - Vascular diseases
   - Advanced renal failure
   - Idiopathic

CISN may result from persistence or progression of many of the acute forms of interstitial nephritis (Table 82–2) or may evolve without an obvious preceding phase of acute injury. Many of the specific causes of CISN are discussed subsequently; some of the remainder are commented on briefly below.

Urinary tract obstruction (including vesicoureteral reflux), the single most important cause of CISN, is discussed in Ch. 83. Perhaps the second most important group of disorders comprises those caused by nephrotoxins, most of which are discussed later as toxic nephropathies. In addition to exogenous toxins, certain endogenous chemical abnormalities may result in CISN. The major renal complication of *chronic hypokalemia* and potassium depletion is nephrogenic (vasopressin-resistant) diabetes insipidus, which results in mild polyuria, but chronic interstitial nephritis with modest renal insufficiency may also rarely occur. *Hypercalcemia* also produces mild polyuria due to nephrogenic diabetes insipidus. Acute hypercalcemia also acts on the glomeruli and renal vasculature to reduce GRF in a manner largely reversible with correction of hypercalcemia. Chronic hypercalcemia results in nephrocalcinosis and chronic interstitial nephritis with reduced glomerular filtration rate that may be only slowly and incompletely reversible. In addition, nephrocalcinosis may cause distal renal tubular acidosis (Ch. 84). In the absence of urinary tract obstruction, *chronic bacterial pyelonephritis* rarely causes severe renal failure. Renal *tuberculosis* can result in acute and chronic tubulointerstitial disease. Tuberculous ureteral strictures may cause hydronephrosis.

A variety of *immune disorders* may be associated with both acute and chronic interstitial nephritis, including several types of glomerulonephritis (Ch. 81), chronic renal transplant rejection (Ch. 80.2), and systemic lupus erythematosus (Ch. 436). Renal involvement in *Sjögren's syndrome* is usually in the form of CISN. The most common functional abnormalities are distal renal tubular acidosis and urinary concentrating defects (Ch. 438).

Neoplastic and *paraproteinemic* disorders may be associated with CISN. In patients with lymphomas and leukemias, particularly acute lymphoblastic leukemia, neoplastic cells may infiltrate the renal interstitium and cause renal enlargement. Adjacent renal tubules may be compressed and destroyed, but renal function is rarely compromised. Renal disease in patients with *amyloidosis* (Ch. 210), *Waldenström's macroglobulinemia* (Ch. 163), and *mixed cryoglobulinemia* (Ch. 81) usually involves the glomeruli, but, rarely, there may be prominent tubulointerstitial involvement. Renal failure is a common cause of death in patients with *multiple myeloma,* especially in patients with Bence Jones proteinuria (monoclonal immunoglobulin light chain paraproteins). CISN, often associated with cast nephropathy, is the most important cause of renal failure in multiple myeloma. Large, dense eosinophilic casts occur within the tubule lumina, surrounded by a chronic interstitial infiltrate. Renal failure appears to result both from obstruction of the renal tubules by these casts and/or from direct toxic effects of the Bence Jones proteins. In addition to renal insufficiency, multiple myeloma may cause proximal and distal renal tubular acidosis, Fanconi's syndrome, urinary concentrating defects, and the nephrotic syndrome. The last is usually associated with renal amyloidosis. Recovery from renal failure due to CISN with cast nephropathy is rare in contrast to that occurring from other abnormalities in these individuals, particularly hypercalcemia.

Miscellaneous Factors

In *diabetes mellitus* and *sickle cell hemoglobinopathies,* CISN may be accompanied by papillary necrosis. Hyperkalemia and hyperkalemic distal renal tubular acidosis may occur in both. In diabetic patients this is generally due to hyporeninemic hypoaldosteronism. Urinary concentrating defects are particularly common in sickling disorders. Chronic reduction in renal blood flow from a variety of *renal vascular disorders* causes atrophy of both the renal tubules and the glomeruli, along with interstitial fibrosis. *Advanced renal disease* of any etiology results in interstitial fibrosis with mild interstitial inflammation, tubular atrophy, and glomerular sclerosis characteristic of the "end-stage" kidney. Cysts of varying size may also be present. In many causes these changes are so severe that it is not possible to determine whether the underlying cause of renal failure was tubulointerstitial, glomerular, or vascular in origin. In occasional cases of *CISN,* sometimes accompanied by granulomas, no recognized cause can be identified.

Clinical and Laboratory Manifestations

The clinical manifestations may be primarily those of renal tubular functional defects (Table 82–1) or may primarily reflect those of advanced renal failure. Sterile pyuria may be seen, but, in contrast to AISN, eosinophilia and eosinophiluria are not. Historical and laboratory findings may suggest a specific diagnosis, e.g., flank pain and radiographic or ultrasonographic evidence of hydronephrosis suggesting obstructive nephropathy. Clinical presentations unique to certain entities are discussed elsewhere.

TOXIC NEPHROPATHIES (Table 82–5)

Drug-induced acute interstitial nephritis, an important type of nephrotoxic renal injury, is discussed in the preceding section with other causes of acute interstitial nephritis. Other important toxic nephropathies are discussed below.

Analgesic Nephropathy

Chronic interstitial nephritis leading to chronic renal failure may result from excessive consumption of certain analgesic agents. In the United States 2 to 10 per cent of all cases of end-stage renal disease are thought to be due to analgesic nephropathy (AN). In other countries, AN is an even more important cause of chronic renal failure. For example, about 20 per cent of all cases of end-stage renal disease in Australia result from AN. The drugs most commonly associated with AN are phenacetin or acetaminophen (phenacetin is largely converted to acetaminophen soon after ingestion), usually in combination with aspirin. Generally, the offending agents are taken in the form of proprietary drugs, but sometimes they are obtained by prescriptions from physicians. In many countries the availability of phenacetin in proprietary drugs is now greatly restricted.

Pathogenesis and Pathology

Although phenacetin, acetaminophen, and aspirin may be nephrotoxic when consumed in large quantities over extended periods of time, there is some debate about which of these may be the most noxious to the kidney. The combination of acetaminophen or phenacetin with aspirin appears to be more nephrotoxic than either drug alone. Prospective epidemiologic studies show a convincing correlation between the amount of analgesics consumed and the development of renal disease. The generally accepted requirement for the presumptive diagnosis of AN is a cumulative ingestion of 3 kg or more of the above drugs or daily consumption of 1 gram per day for three or more years. In most reported cases of AN, consumption has far exceeded these amounts and has usually consisted of mixtures of phenacetin or acetaminophen and aspirin.

The pathogenesis of AN is still uncertain. Both aspirin and acetaminophen are concentrated within the kidney, and for acetaminophen, and perhaps aspirin, a concentration gradient exists within the kidney from the renal cortex to the medulla. Phenacetin and acetaminophen are metabolized to reactive species that covalently bind to proteins and result in oxidative tissue damage by depleting reducing equivalents such as glutathione. Aspirin may exacerbate this toxicity by inhibition of the hexose monophosphate shunt, which is a major metabolic pathway for maintaining glutathione stores. In addition, aspirin is a potent inhibitor of prostaglandin synthesis. This later action may lead to a reduction in renal medullary blood flow and result in ischemic damage. In addition to aspirin, other nonsteroidal anti-inflammatory drugs that also inhibit prostaglandin synthesis (e.g., phenylbutazone, ibuprofen, and indomethacin) have been associated with papillary necrosis in humans and in experimental animals. The ultimate importance of these other drugs as a cause of chronic interstitial nephritis will require long-term observations, as many of them have been only recently used on a wide scale.

In the initial stages of AN, there is patchy necrosis of interstitial cells, loops of Henle, and capillaries in the inner medulla, with calcium deposition and lipid accumulation in the involved areas. With continued exposure to these drugs, the process progressively involves the outer medulla and often results in total papillary necrosis. In advanced stages, the renal cortex is thin and the renal tubules are atrophic. There is interstitial fibrosis accompanied by a round-cell infiltrate. The glomeruli are initially spared, but later they and the arterioles become sclerotic. If AN is complicated by bacterial infection, focal collections of acute inflammatory cells are evident. The necrotic papillae may remain in situ, often with cavities in them, or they may totally detach from the medulla and slough into the renal pelvis.

Clinical and Laboratory Manifestations

AN is usually associated with a characteristic group of signs, symptoms, and laboratory findings. The diagnosis of AN is often overlooked because patients frequently do not admit to taking analgesics or, if they do, will not provide a true estimate of the amount consumed. When the diagnosis is suspected, therefore, the possibility of AN should be vigorously pursued by discussions with family members or physicians who have cared for the patient previously. AN occurs more frequently in women (usually middle age) with a female to male ratio of 1.3 to 1.6:1. Although patients may consume analgesics for a variety of complaints, especially headaches, more often than not there is no disease that warrants taking large amounts of analgesics. In many patients there is a large psychologic component to their clinical presentation. In some patients there is a family history of heavy analgesic use. Anemia is present in most patients and is frequently more severe than can be attributed to their degree of renal insufficiency. In addition to renal insufficiency, anemia may result from hemolysis or gastrointestinal blood loss due to peptic ulcer disease or gastritis, which also occur commonly. Hypertension is present in about one half of patients, but generally appears after renal disease is obvious. Malignant hypertension occasionally develops.

TABLE 82–5. PROMINENT OR COMMON NEPHROTOXINS

Anticonvulsants: paramethadione, phenytoin, trimethadone
Antihypertensive drugs: captopril, methyldopa
Antimicrobials: aminoglycosides, amphotericin B, cephalosporins, ethambutol, isoniazid, para-aminosalicylic acid, penicillins, rifampin, sulfonamides, tetracyclines
Antineoplastic agents: cisplatin, methotrexate, mitomycin-C, nitrosoureas, radiation
Sulfonamide diuretics: acetazolamide, chlorthalidone, furosemide, thiazides
Endogenous compounds: Bence Jones proteins, calcium, hemoglobin, myoglobin, oxalate, uric acid
Halogenated alkanes, hydrocarbons, and solvents: carbon tetrachloride, ethylene glycol, paraquat, toluene
Iodinated radiographic contrast media
Metals: arsenic, bismuth, cadmium, copper, gold, lead, lithium, mercury
Nonsteroidal anti-inflammatory drugs (Table 82–6)
Miscellaneous compounds: acetaminophen, allopurinol, amphetamines, azathioprine, cimetidine, cyclosporine, heroin, methoxyflurane, methysergide, D-penicillamine, phenacetin, phenindione, silicon

Urinalysis frequently reveals pyuria. Urinary tract infections are present in approximately one half of patients at some point and may be associated with leukocyte casts in the urinary sediment. Sloughing of a necrotic papilla into the urinary tract may be associated with gross hematuria, flank pain (ureteral colic), and passage of tissue in the urine. Proteinuria is generally modest (<2 grams per day), but as the disease progresses, occasional patients develop focal sclerosing glomerulopathy with heavy proteinuria. Generally, progression to end-stage renal failure occurs over a period of several years. An abrupt decline in renal function may accompany ureteral obstruction from sloughed papillae. Renal tubular abnormalities may be reflected by hyperchloremic metabolic acidosis due to decreased renal acidification, mild polyuria with an inability to concentrate the urine above the osmolality of blood due to nephrogenic diabetes insipidus, and an inability to reduce appropriately urinary sodium excretion with sodium deprivation (renal salt wasting).

Early in the course of the disease, the kidneys may be of normal size and contour when evaluated radiographically or by ultrasonography. In the late stages, the kidneys are small with a thin cortex and an irregular surface. A variety of findings on intravenous urography or retrograde pyelography—including caliceal clubbing, papillary cavities, and caliceal filling defects due to the presence of a sloughed papilla (ring sign)—may suggest papillary necrosis. Demonstration of papillary necrosis in the absence of its more common causes (e.g., diabetes mellitus, urinary tract obstruction, often with infection, or sickle cell disease) should suggest AN. Finally, patients with AN are at increased risk for development of transitional cell carcinoma of the urinary tract, particularly of the renal pelvis. The appearance of hematuria should lead to prompt evaluation to exclude a uroepithelial neoplasm. This evaluation should generally include examination of the urine for neoplastic cells, cystoscopy, and retrograde pyelograms.

Prevention and Therapy

Obviously, avoidance of drugs implicated as causes of AN will prevent the disorder. Public education about the dangers of excessive analgesic consumption is important. In Canada removal of phenacetin from proprietary analgesic mixtures has been associated with a decline in the incidence of AN. This has not been the case in Australia, however.

The most important factor in treatment of established AN is cessation of analgesic use. For individuals who habitually abuse analgesics, this requires a great deal of education and encouragement. Often psychologic counseling is needed. For patients with diseases requiring analgesics—e.g., rheumatoid arthritis—alternative forms of therapy are indicated. With cessation of analgesic use renal function will generally stabilize or improve. If renal disease is clearly established and drug use continues, renal function inexorably declines, often to the point of end-stage renal disease, over a period of several years. Urinary tract infections, ureteral obstruction from sloughed papillae, hypertension, and dehydration are conditions that may cause a more rapid decline in renal function, and all should be treated promptly.

Nonsteroidal Anti-inflammatory Drugs

During the last decade, a large number of drugs that inhibit production of the various prostaglandins have been marketed. These agents are referred to collectively as nonsteroidal anti-inflammatory drugs (NSAID'S) (Table 82–6). With more widespread use of these drugs, several renal and electrolyte complications have been recognized.

The functions of renal prostaglandins have yet to be completely elucidated. Nevertheless, vasodilator prostaglandins (PGE_2, PGI_2) appear to be important in maintaining renal blood flow in states of sodium depletion or when "effective" arterial blood volume is low. These states are generally associated with elevated levels of circulating angiotensin II and catecholamines. By causing renal vasodilation, prostaglandins preserve renal blood flow while allowing angiotensin II and catecholamines to maintain systemic blood pressure by increasing systemic vascular resistance. Prostaglandins may also cause a natriuresis, stimulate renin release, and antagonize the effect of antidiuretic hormone. Many of the renal and electrolyte complications of prostaglandin inhibition by NSAID's (Table 82–7) are predictable, based on these recognized functions of the prostaglandins.

TABLE 82–6. NONSTEROIDAL ANTI-INFLAMMATORY DRUGS

Aclofenac	Meclofenamate
Diclofenac	Mefenamate
Fenclofenac	Naproxen
Fenoprofen	Phenylbutazone
Galfenine	Piroxicam
Ibuprofen	Salicylates
Indomethacin	Sulindac
Ketoprofen	Tolmetin

HEMODYNAMICALLY MEDIATED ACUTE RENAL FAILURE. This has been reported in several patients receiving NSAID's, most notably indomethacin. This type of renal failure appears to result from renal hypoperfusion and occurs shortly after drug therapy is instituted. Patients at risk are those with sodium depletion (e.g., from diuretic therapy) or low "effective" arterial blood volumes (e.g., nephrotic syndrome, congestive heart failure, and hepatic cirrhosis with ascites), older individuals, and patients with underlying renal disease. Individuals receiving triamterene may be especially at risk. This type of acute renal failure is usually associated with oliguria and low fractional excretion of sodium (see Ch. 78). The urinary sediment is generally unremarkable. Renal biopsies have shown evidence of acute tubular necrosis. Azotemia generally resolves promptly after discontinuation of the offending drug. Occasional patients, however, require temporary dialysis.

ACUTE INTERSTITIAL NEPHRITIS (AISN). AISN resulting in acute renal failure has been described in several patients in association with NSAID's, particularly fenoprofen. Heavy proteinuria, often in the nephrotic range, is peculiar to this form of drug-induced AISN. In addition to copious proteinuria, there are other features of AISN due to NSAID's that differ from those associated with other drugs. For example, eosinophilia, eosinophiluria, and skin rashes are uncommon. As with other types of drug-induced AISN, however, urinalysis frequently reveals microscopic hematuria and pyuria. In addition to histopathologic changes of AISN (described earlier), electron microscopy of the glomeruli reveals fusion of podocyte foot processes. Unlike hemodynamically mediated acute renal failure, AISN usually appears only after the offending drug has been administered for several days to several months. The disorder usually resolves with discontinuation of the drug, but recovery may not occur until several months later, and interval dialysis may be required. Corticosteroid therapy is believed by many to hasten recovery, and, in the absence of contraindications, it is reasonable to prescribe a short course of high-dose corticosteroids (1 mg per kilogram per day of prednisone) if renal failure is severe and

TABLE 82–7. RENAL AND ELECTROLYTE COMPLICATIONS OF NONSTEROIDAL ANTI-INFLAMMATORY DRUGS

1. Renal failure
    a. Hemodynamic (major risk factors are sodium depletion and low "effective" arterial blood volume)
    b. Acute interstitial nephritis with or without the nephrotic syndrome
    c. Glomerulonephritis associated with diffuse vasculitis
    d. Papillary necrosis with chronic interstitial nephritis
2. Sodium and fluid retention
3. Hyperkalemia, metabolic acidosis (occurs more often in patients with renal insufficiency, sodium depletion, or other factors predisposing to hyperkalemia)

spontaneous recovery does not occur within several days of stopping the drug.

OTHER RENAL COMPLICATIONS OF NSAID's. In addition to the above causes of acute renal insufficiency, *systemic vasculitis* with *glomerulitis* and *papillary necrosis* with chronic interstitial nephritis may occur rarely in association with NSAID's.

RETENTION OF SODIUM (AND FLUID). This is perhaps the most common renal side effect of NSAID's. Although this retention may not present a problem in persons with normal cardiovascular and renal function, it may result in worsening of pre-existing congestive heart failure or hypertension. Finally, inhibition of prostaglandin synthesis may result in *hyperkalemia* and *metabolic acidosis* due to inhibition of renin secretion and secondary hypoaldosteronism. Underlying renal insufficiency, sodium depletion, or concomitant administration of other drugs that predispose to hyperkalemia (e.g., potassium-sparing diuretics) increases the risk for developing the latter electrolyte abnormalities.

Antimicrobial Drugs

Renal damage from penicillin, sulfonamide, and antituberculous antimicrobials usually results from AISN, described earlier. Additional antibiotics may cause renal disease manifested in other ways.

AMINOGLYCOSIDES. The aminoglycosides, excreted primarily by glomerular filtration, accumulate in the renal cortex to levels higher than those in serum. They may cause several renal tubular functional abnormalities, the most clinically relevant of which are potassium and magnesium wasting, which may result in hypokalemia and hypomagnesemia. The most important manifestation of aminoglycoside renal toxicity, however, is acute renal failure. Evidently, this results from both a direct effect of these drugs on glomerular filtration and tubular toxicity causing acute tubular necrosis. Up to 10 per cent of patients receiving aminoglycosides develop some degree of acute renal failure, accounting for 10 to 15 per cent of all cases of this disorder in the United States. Generally, this failure is manifested by a rise in the serum creatinine level after several days of therapy with one of the aminoglycosides. At times, renal failure may become evident only after the drug has been discontinued. Acute renal failure is usually mild and of the nonoliguric variety. However, oliguria and severe renal failure requiring dialysis may be seen.

The most nephrotoxic aminoglycoside is neomycin, which is, therefore, not administered parenterally. It may rarely cause acute renal failure when given orally or by enema to decrease the bowel flora. The least nephrotoxic is streptomycin. Tobramycin and netilmicin are, perhaps, less nephrotoxic than gentamicin and amikacin. Risk factors for development of aminoglycoside toxicity include the dose of drug administered; the length of therapy; simultaneous administration of other potential nephrotoxins, particularly cephalosporins; renal insufficiency; advanced age; extracellular fluid volume depletion; and, possibly, potassium depletion. In older individuals the GFR is normally lower, although this is unaccompanied by an elevated serum creatinine level. Failure to consider this variable when calculating the dose of aminoglycosides is a major (and preventable) factor in production of acute renal failure.

Management of acute renal failure following aminoglycoside administration consists of discontinuing the drug and substituting another appropriate antibiotic, if continued treatment is necessary. Supportive measures are similar to those indicated with acute renal failure of other causes (Ch. 78). The prognosis for recovery of renal function after several days is excellent.

CEPHALOSPORINS. Acute renal failure due to acute tubular necrosis was an important complication of cephaloridine, the first cephalosporin widely used in clinical medicine. Renal failure due to acute tubular necrosis and acute interstitial nephritis may rarely accompany treatment with the newer cephalosporins also. The combination of a cephalosporin and an aminoglycoside carries a risk higher than for either drug alone, requiring close monitoring of renal function when this combination of drugs is used.

TETRACYCLINES. Tetracyclines inhibit protein synthesis and, therefore, shunt amino acids into urea. The enhanced synthesis of urea elevates the blood urea nitrogen (BUN) without a concomitant elevation of serum creatinine or a reduction in GFR. In normal individuals this is of little consequence. In patients with underlying insufficiency, however, the increase in azotemia may be dramatic. With the exception of doxycycline and minocycline, which do not accumulate in renal failure and which require only minor dosage adjustments, tetracyclines should be avoided in individuals with significant renal insufficiency. Demeclocycline causes a dose-related nephrogenic diabetes insipidus. This property has been used to treat some hyponatremic patients, particularly those with the syndrome of inappropriate secretion of antidiuretic hormone. Demeclocycline has been reported to cause acute renal failure, however, when used to treat hyponatremic patients with hepatic cirrhosis. Although the renal failure is reversible, demeclocycline (and other tetracyclines) should be avoided in these patients. Outdated tetracyclines can cause Fanconi's syndrome.

AMPHOTERICIN B. Most patients receiving more than 2 grams of this antifungal agent develop one or more renal abnormalities. Defects in distal nephron function are the first to appear: distal renal tubular acidosis, nephrogenic diabetes insipidus, and renal potassium wasting. These alterations may occur without a reduction in GFR and are generally reversible with discontinuation of the drug. Metabolic acidosis and hypokalemia should be treated with supplemental alkali and potassium salts. Acute renal insufficiency, which may be progressive and incompletely reversible, is a major side effect of amphotericin B. This is dose related and appears to result both from direct renal tubular toxicity and from ischemia due to renal vasoconstriction. Acute renal failure is more likely to occur in patients who are sodium depleted from whatever cause: diuretics, vomiting, and so on. Sodium repletion may protect against amphotericin B nephrotoxicity. Once moderate azotemia is present (BUN $>$ 50 mg per deciliter), consideration should be given to prescribing the drug on alternate days or to temporarily discontinuing therapy until renal function improves. The risk of renal insufficiency has to be weighed, of course, against the severity of the underlying infection and whether alternative antifungal therapy is available.

Radiographic Contrast Agents

Acute renal failure resulting from acute tubular necrosis is an uncommon, but important, complication of iodinated radiographic contrast agents used, for example, in intravenous urography, arteriography, or contrast-enhanced computed tomography. The incidence of acute renal failure associated with these agents has varied in large series from 0 to 13 per cent but is much higher in certain groups of patients. Risk factors include underlying renal insufficiency, diabetes mellitus, older age, dehydration, history of prior acute renal failure following use of contrast agents, multiple contrast procedures in a short period of time, concomitant exposure to other nephrotoxins, and, perhaps, multiple myeloma. In addition, acute renal failure is more likely after administration of larger doses of these agents. Clearly, individuals at highest risk are diabetic patients with renal insufficiency. The incidence of acute renal failure following exposure to these agents in this population of patients may be as high as 75 per cent. In the absence of other risk factors, diabetes *per se* does not appear to pose a major risk. The same is true for multiple myeloma.

The pathogenesis of radiocontrast-induced acute renal failure is uncertain. Several possible mechanisms have been suggested, including ischemia resulting from renal arteriolar vasoconstriction due to the hypertonicity of these agents, tubular obstruction due to precipitation of proteins, and direct tubular toxicity. In addition, as with any drug, anaphylaxis with hypotension is a rare cause of acute renal failure. Patients who develop acute renal failure generally become oliguric within 24 hours of exposure to radiocontrast agents. This usually persists for two to four days, and the peak in serum creatinine elevation typically occurs within seven days. Renal insufficiency is usually moderate and resolves in a few days, but it may be severe and necessitate temporary dialysis. With advanced underlying renal disease, the acute insufficiency may be irreversible. In patients at risk, the serum creatinine concentration should be measured the day after exposure to these agents to determine if nephrotoxicity has occurred. A persistent nephrogram at this time also suggests renal injury.

Prevention of renal failure in patients at high risk includes avoidance of dehydration, minimizing the amount of contrast administered (no more than 0.88 mg of iodine per kilogram of body weight), and using alternative diagnostic methods such as ultrasonography, if possible. Hypertonic mannitol (25 to 50 grams given over one hour) immediately following exposure to radiographic contrast agents may reduce the incidence of acute renal failure in high-risk patients. Treatment of acute renal failure due to contrast agents is similar to that resulting from other etiologies (Ch. 78).

Nephropathies Resulting from Anti-neoplastic Therapy

Several drugs used in the treatment of neoplasia may produce renal toxicity. Some of these may cause isolated abnormalities in renal tubular function, whereas others may produce acute or chronic renal insufficiency. For some of these compounds, renal damage represents the dose-limiting toxicity.

CISPLATIN. Cisplatin and its metabolites are eliminated primarily by urinary excretion. Acute tubular necrosis, which may occur after intravenous administration of the drug, is dose related, being uncommon with single doses less than 50 mg per square meter but occurring in most patients with doses above 100 mg per square meter. The cause of cisplatin toxicity is uncertain, but it appears similar to that produced by other heavy metals (see below). Concomitant administration of cisplatin and other nephrotoxins, such as aminoglycosides, increases the risk of acute renal failure. Generally, azotemia appears a few days after administration of the drug and is usually reversible over a period of two to four weeks. With severe acute renal failure and/or repeated administration of cisplatin, chronic renal insufficiency due to chronic interstitial nephritis may develop. The incidence of acute renal failure due to cisplatin can be reduced by ensuring adequate hydration and establishing a saline diuresis prior to and during administration of the drug and by continuously infusing the drug slowly over several hours or a few days. Hypomagnesemia due to renal magnesium wasting may occur in as many as 50 per cent of patients treated with cisplatin. Hypomagnesemia may be severe, may develop in the absence of renal insufficiency, and may persist for several weeks following cisplatin therapy. Other renal tubular abnormalities, such as potassium wasting, decreased urinary concentrating ability, and low molecular weight proteinuria may also be observed but are generally of little clinical importance.

METHOTREXATE. This folic acid antagonist is eliminated principally by urinary excretion. Nephrotoxicity is rare with low doses (5 to 60 mg per square meter). With high-dose therapy (500 to 7500 mg per square meter), the drug precipitates in the renal tubule lumina and causes acute renal failure from tubular obstruction. Direct tubular toxicity may also play a role. Nephrotoxicity may be reduced by vigorous (intravenous) hydration to maintain a urine flow of greater than 100 ml per hour for several days following high-dose therapy. In addition, the urine pH should be kept above 7 by alkali administration, since methotrexate is more soluble in alkaline solutions. Development of renal insufficiency prolongs the half-life of methotrexate and increases the likelihood of systemic toxicity.

NITROSOUREAS. A number of nitrosoureas used in cancer chemotherapy, including streptozocin, BCNU, CCNU, and methyl CCNU, may produce several types of renal toxicity. Streptozocin may cause proteinuria, sometimes resulting in nephrotic syndrome, due to glomerular injury; acute tubular necrosis leading to acute renal failure; and a variety of renal tubular abnormalities, including proximal renal tubular acidosis, glycosuria, phosphaturia, and aminoaciduria. Proteinuria is generally the first manifestation of renal toxicity. Should this occur, therapy should be withheld and only cautiously restarted if this resolves. Azotemia developing after streptozocin should lead to permanent discontinuation of the drug. The other nitrosoureas given in multiple courses over several weeks have been associated with a very high incidence of chronic renal insufficiency. In one series the majority of patients receiving at least six courses of therapy developed insidious chronic renal insufficiency, sometimes resulting in uremia, without an antecedent episode of acute renal failure and without abnormalities in the urinary sediment. The principal pathologic findings are chronic interstitial nephritis and glomerular sclerosis. Any nitrosoureas should generally be discontinued at the first sign of an otherwise unexplained decrease in renal function.

MITOMYCIN-C. There is a 5 to 40 per cent incidence of nephrotoxicity following mitomycin-C therapy. Toxicity is dose related and generally appears after repeated courses and/or a cumulative dose of 60 mg per square meter. Renal injury is manifested by proteinuria (usually mild) and azotemia. Renal insufficiency may develop gradually or abruptly. In the latter instance, the clinical features are similar to those of the hemolytic uremic syndrome (Ch. 81) and include thrombocytopenia, microangiopathic hemolytic anemia, and acute renal failure. Renal pathologic findings consist of glomerular alterations (mesangial fragmentation, capillary thrombi, and hemorrhage) and thrombosis and fibrinoid necrosis of the arterioles. There is no established therapy except for supportive measures for renal failure developing after administration of mitomycin-C. Renal function should be monitored closely in patients receiving this drug, and therapy should probably be discontinued if otherwise unexplained azotemia occurs.

MISCELLANEOUS ANTINEOPLASTIC AGENTS. Nephrotoxicity has occasionally been reported with other cancer chemotherapeutic agents, including 5-azacytidine, daunorubicin, doxorubicin, mithramycin, dacarbazine, and recombinant leukocyte A interferon. Finally, therapy resulting in massive acute killing of neoplastic cells may cause the tumor lysis syndrome (see below).

RADIATION NEPHRITIS (Also see Ch. 539). Exposure of the kidneys during abdominal irradiation for cancer may subsequently result in damage of varying degree. Manifestations range from mild proteinuria, urinary concentrating defects, and benign hypertension with a reduced GFR to malignant hypertension with end-stage renal failure. Evidence for renal damage occurs several months to years after renal irradiation, and the severity bears a general relationship to the amount of irradiation received. Clinically evident renal injury is uncommon with less than 1000 to 2000 rads but develops in approximately 50 per cent of patients receiving doses higher than this. In the early stage of radiation nephritis, there is tubular necrosis, medial and intimal thickening of the small renal arteries, and damage to the glomerular endothelium. Later, glomerular sclerosis, collagenous thickening of the small renal arteries, and interstitial fibrosis are prominent. It is unclear whether the primary injury is to the renal tubular epithelium or to the vascular endothelium, both tissues being equally sensitive to radiation damage in experimental situations. The incidence of radiation nephritis can be minimized by limiting the total dose of abdominal irradiation in a single course to 2000 rads over two weeks and by shielding the kidneys as much as possible. Malignant hypertension resulting from unilateral radiation nephritis can be cured by nephrectomy.

URIC ACID AND THE TUMOR LYSIS SYNDROME. Patients with certain hematologic malignancies, particularly acute lymphoblastic leukemia and poorly differentiated lymphomas, may rarely develop spontaneous acute renal failure from obstruction of the renal tubules by uric acid. More frequently, this complication occurs following chemotherapy or radiation therapy, which kills cells and releases massive amounts of purine uric acid precursors. The resulting hyperuricemia greatly increases the filtered load of uric acid. Its solubility is exceeded, and precipitation occurs in the renal tubules, often resulting in acute obstructive renal failure. A ratio of urinary uric acid/creatinine concentrations greater than 1:1 suggests the diagnosis of acute uric acid nephropathy. During massive cell lysis, phosphate is also released in large amounts, and hyperphosphaturia with intrarenal precipitation of calcium phosphate may contribute to the renal failure. Hyperkalemia due to release of intracellular potassium may also be observed. Prevention of acute renal failure secondary to massive tumor cell killing includes establishing a urine output of 3 or more liters per 24 hours and treatment with high-dose allopurinol (300 to 400 mg per square meter per day) prior to institution of cytotoxic therapy. The role of urinary alkalinization is uncertain. Although this will increase the solubility of uric acid, a high urine pH will favor precipitation of phosphate salts in the renal tubules. If renal failure occurs despite the foregoing precautions, hemodialysis is indicated for supportive therapy and for removing uric acid. This allows renal function to recover, generally in a few days. Chronic interstitial nephritis (gouty nephropathy), a rare complication of chronic hyperuricemia and gout, is discussed in Ch. 195.

Metal Nephropathies

The diagnosis and treatment of intoxication with trace metals are discussed in detail in Ch. 542. Only certain aspects of this subject related to the kidney are discussed below. Acute intoxication with some metals may cause both acute renal injury with a reduction in GFR and renal tubular dysfunction. With chronic intoxication, the most common form of injury is chronic interstitial nephritis manifested by renal tubular abnormalities with or without reduction in GFR. In certain instances glomerular injury may also occur. Metal intoxication is often treated by chelation therapy. Unfortunately, some of the drugs used for this purpose, e.g., penicillamine, may also be nephrotoxic, as discussed below.

LITHIUM. Lithium carbonate, used in the treatment of affective disorders, causes a variety of renal abnormalities. The most frequent is a form of vasopressin-resistant nephrogenic diabetes insipidus, probably due to decreased production of cyclic adenosine monophosphate (AMP) by collecting ducts in response to the hormone. This is of little consequence in most patients. Polyuria (urine volumes > 3000 ml per day) may result but usually abates when lithium therapy is stopped. The diuretic amiloride may significantly reduce the polyuria associated with lithium. Incomplete distal renal tubular acidosis and mild renal sodium wasting may also result from lithium therapy. Chronic interstitial nephritis is more common in individuals with psychiatric disorders than in the general population. The risk of this nephritis occurring in lithium-treated patients seems to be only minimally higher than in similar but untreated patients. In patients taking lithium, a history of acute lithium intoxication, however, appears to predispose to development of chronic renal insufficiency.

LEAD. Lead poisoning may result from acute exposure, e.g., from ingestion of lead-containing paint, but more often from chronic exposure, e.g., in foundry and battery workers or from consumption of illicit alcoholic beverages or "moonshine"). Acute intoxication, more common in children, is manifested primarily by abdominal colic, hemolytic anemia, and encephalopathy. Acute interstitial nephritis with eosinophilic inclusions in the proximal tubular cells, tubular necrosis with a reduction in GFR, and Fanconi's syndrome may also occur. Whether acute lead intoxication without further exposure results in chronic renal disease in later years is unclear. Chronic lead intoxication causes interstitial nephritis with variable reductions in GFR and renal tubular dysfunction. Some patients develop gout and hypertension as a result of chronic lead intoxication ("saturnine gout"). Some patients with "essential" hypertension and renal failure have excess body burdens of lead. Therefore, chronic lead intoxication should be considered in individuals with the triad of gout, hypertension, and chronic renal insufficiency. A history of exposure to lead should be sought and a $CaNa_2$-EDTA infusion carried out to evaluate lead stores (Ch. 542). Treatment of acute lead intoxication consists of preventing further exposure to the metal, supportive care, and chelation with dimercaptopropanol (BAL) or $CaNa_2$-EDTA. Chronic renal insufficiency resulting from lead may sometimes improve during chelation therapy but may also progress despite this therapy.

MERCURY. Acute intoxication with mercurial salts may cause tubular necrosis and severe renal failure. The strong affinity of mercury for sulfhydryl groups, along with the hypotension that frequently accompanies acute intoxication, probably accounts for the acute renal injury. Acute exposure may occur rarely in industrial settings or with intentional ingestion of mercurial salts. Treatment of acute mercury poisoning with mercurial salts consists of chelation therapy with dimercaptopropanol or penicillamine and supportive care (Ch. 542). Chronic exposure to organomercurials may result in subtle renal damage manifested by increased urinary excretion of low molecular weight proteins and renal tubular enzymes (tubular proteinuria). Chelation therapy is ineffective in removing organomercurials. Chronic exposure to mercurial compounds may also cause the nephrotic syndrome as a result of glomerular damage, most commonly from membranous nephropathy. The pathogenesis of this disorder is uncertain, as mercury is not demonstrable in the glomeruli.

GOLD. Proteinuria may complicate the treatment of rheumatoid arthritis with gold salts, more frequently with parenteral than with oral administration. Proteinuria may develop at any time, but usually after several months of therapy. Rarely, it may be severe enough to result in the nephrotic syndrome associated with membranous nephropathy. It is unlikely that gold *per se* is directly responsible for the glomerular injury, since the metal can be demonstrated in the renal tubules, but not in the glomeruli. Gold may in some way modify an intrinsic protein such that it becomes antigenic and elicits the immune reactions that produce membranous nephropathy. Membranous nephropathy may also occur in patients with rheumatoid arthritis who have not been treated with gold. The appearance of proteinuria in a patient receiving gold should prompt discontinuation of the drug. This will generally result in disappearance of the proteinuria, but this may occur only several months later.

ARSENIC. Arsenic is used in a number of industrial applications and is present in several commercial products such as insecticides. In addition, illicit alcohol may be contaminated with the metal. Gastrointestinal symptoms and peripheral neuropathy are the most prominent manifestations of acute arsenic poisoning, but acute tubular necrosis may also occur. Like mercury, arsenic has a high affinity for sulfhydryl groups of proteins. Cellular damage resulting from this interaction and from hypotension are the most likely causes of acute renal damage. Treatment of arsenic poisoning includes supportive measures and chelation therapy with dimercaptopropanol. Arsine gas may cause acute renal failure secondary to hemoglobinuria from acute hemolysis and from hypotension.

CADMIUM. With chronic low-level exposure—for example, in alkaline battery workers—cadmium accumulates in the renal cortex. This may result in mild proteinuria, of both glomerular and tubular origin, and in early renal insufficiency. The incidence of proteinuria increases with the length of exposure.

MISCELLANEOUS METALS. *Bismuth* has been reported to cause both acute tubular necrosis and the nephrotic syndrome. Acute *copper* poisoning may result in acute tubular necrosis, most likely resulting from hemolysis with hemoglobinuria and from hypotension. Chronic copper accumulation in Wilson's disease (Ch. 205) may be associated with proximal renal tubular acidosis and other components of Fanconi's syndrome and mild renal insufficiency. In rare instances, renal injury has been reported with *antimony, thallium*, and *uranium* intoxication. *Platinum* nephrotoxicity is discussed under cisplatin.

Oxalate

End-stage renal failure from chronic interstitial nephritis and from recurrent nephrolithiasis is the major complication of primary hyperoxaluria and may rarely occur in enteric hyperoxaluria as well (Ch. 182).

Acute intoxication with ethylene glycol is the major cause of acute renal failure due to oxalate. Ethylene glycol is the major component of antifreeze and is usually ingested by desperate alcoholics, by children accidently, or in a suicide attempt. Ethylene glycol is metabolized to several toxic substances, one of which is oxalic acid. Intoxication with ethylene glycol causes acute renal failure, profound metabolic acidosis of the anion gap variety (Ch. 77), and acute central nervous system and pulmonary dysfunction. Renal failure results from massive deposition of oxalate within the renal tubules. This is usually accompanied by large numbers of calcium oxalate crystals in the urinary sediment. Ethylene glycol intoxication is managed by (1) administration of ethyl alcohol to slow the metabolism of ethylene glycol by competing for alcohol dehydrogenase; (2) hemodialysis to remove the parent compound, to allow treatment with sodium bicarbonate therapy, which may be required in amounts that would otherwise result in pulmonary edema and hypernatremia, and to treat acute renal failure; and (3) administration of pyridoxine and thiamine to help shunt ethylene glycol into other metabolic pathways that result in less toxic metabolites. If patients survive acute intoxication, chances for recovery of renal function are good, but many will require temporary dialysis for several days prior to functional renal recovery.

As noted below, acute renal failure accompanying methoxyflurane anesthesia may result, in part, from oxalate.

Captopril

This angiotensin-converting enzyme inhibitor used in the treatment of hypertension and congestive heart failure has been associated with both acute renal failure and the nephrotic syndrome. Acute renal failure has been reported in patients with bilateral renal artery stenosis or stenosis of the renal artery supplying a solitary kidney. Usually captopril-associated acute renal failure is thought to be hemodynamic in origin, resulting from loss of autoregulation of renal blood flow and glomerular filtration rate. Sometimes, however, acute renal failure has been accompanied by skin rash, eosinophilia and eosinophiluria, a constellation of findings strongly suggesting allergic interstitial nephritis. Acute renal failure in both the above settings generally resolves with discontinuation of captopril but may recur upon rechallenge with the drug. Membranous nephropathy with the nephrotic syndrome may also occur in association with captopril therapy. This complication may resolve slowly after discontinuation of the drug. Membranous nephropathy occurring during therapy with captopril and penicillamine (see below) may possibly be related to the active sulfhydryl group that they contain.

D-Penicillamine

Therapy with this drug for metal chelation, rheumatoid arthritis, scleroderma, or cystinuria is complicated by proteinuria in 4 to 7 per cent of patients, often sufficiently severe to result in the nephrotic syndrome. Proteinuria, which may be associated with mild azotemia, usually results from membranous nephropathy (Ch. 81). Rarely, rapidly progressive glomerulonephritis accompanied by pulmonary hemorrhage occurs. Proteinuria generally resolves or decreases when therapy with D-penicillamine is discontinued, but usually only after several months.

Methoxyflurane

This fluorinated anesthetic agent may cause a dose-related postoperative nephrogenic diabetes insipidus and acute renal failure. Similar complications have rarely been reported with enflurane. The initial polyuric acute renal failure may progress to oliguria in severe cases. Renal function may recover after several days, but persistent renal failure, which has required long-term dialysis, may develop. The pathogenesis of methoxyflurane-induced acute renal failure is uncertain. The drug is metabolized to fluoride and oxalate. Although oxalate is nephrotoxic (see above), it is believed that the major toxic product is fluoride, since nephrotoxicity correlates with blood levels of this ion and fluoride produces nephrotoxicity in experimental animals. Volume depletion due to the urinary concentrating defect may also contribute to acute renal failure.

Miscellaneous Nephrotoxins

Exposure to *hydrocarbons*, frequently in the form of paint or glue sniffing, has been associated with a variety of (generally) reversible abnormalities, including azotemia, renal tubular acidosis, Fanconi's syndrome, proteinuria, hematuria, and pyuria. Similar findings may result from exposure to halogenated alkane solvents such as *carbon tetrachloride* and insecticides such as *paraquat*. *Silicon* exposure—for example, in sandblasters—has been implicated in a connective tissue–like disease with multiple serologic abnormalities and progressive renal failure associated with both glomerular and renal tubular pathologic changes that appear to be immune mediated.

Heroin abuse is associated with a variety of glomerular lesions, including amyloidosis, and glomerulonephritis due to bacterial endocarditis or hepatitis B infection. In a number of patients, however, these etiologies cannot be implicated as the cause of the heroin-associated glomerular disease. Most commonly, focal sclerosing glomerulopathy is found, often resulting in the nephrotic syndrome. Heroin-associated nephropathy generally results in progressive renal failure unless abuse of the drug is stopped.

The nephrotic syndrome may occur as a rare complication of *trimethadione* and *methimazole*. *Sulfonamides* and intravenous *amphetamines* may cause systemic vasculitis that results in renal damage from segmental renal infarction or glomerulonephritis (Ch. 81 and 439). Acute renal insufficiency is a major complication of cyclosporine therapy of organ transplantation (Ch. 80.2). *Nifedipine*, like many other drugs, may cause prerenal azotemia because of hypotension but, in addition, may also rarely cause reversible acute renal failure in the absence of a fall in blood pressure and without abnormalities in the urinary sediment.

Retroperitoneal fibrosis as a complication of long-term treatment of migraine headaches with *methysergide* may obstruct the ureters. *Anticoagulant therapy* may cause ureteral obstruction from intraluminal blood clots or from ureteral compression by a retroperitoneal hematoma.

ACUTE AND CHRONIC INTERSTITIAL NEPHRITIS

Adler SG, Cohen AH, Border WA: Hypersensitivity phenomena and the kidney: Role of drugs and environmental agents. Am J Kidney Dis 5:75, 1985. *An excellent review of the various types of immune-mediated renal injury that may result from numerous pharmacologic agents.*

Boucher A, Droz D, Adafer E, et al.: Characterization of mononuclear cell subsets in renal cellular interstitial infiltrates. Kidney 29:1043, 1986. *Using monoclonal antibodies, the authors found that the predominant mononuclear cells in interstitial cellular infiltrates of 33 renal biopsies, including 11 with acute or chronic interstitial nephritis, were T cells. However, the relative proportions of the different T cells subsets varied among the biopsies.*

Cotran RS, Rubin RH, Tolkoff-Rubin NE: Tubulo-interstitial diseases. In Brenner BM, Rector FC Jr (eds.): The Kidney. Edition 3. Philadelphia, W. B. Saunders Company, 1986. *An excellent review of this topic (353 references).*

Lins LE: Reversible renal failure caused by hypercalcemia. Acta Med Scand 203:309, 1978. *In 13 patients with hypercalcemia of differing etiology, there was a direct correlation between serum concentrations of calcium and creatinine before and after treatment of their hypercalcemia.*

McCluskey RT: Immunologically mediated tubulo-interstitial nephritis. In Cotran RS (guest ed.), Brenner BM, Stein JH (eds.): Tubulointerstitial Nephropathy, Vol. 10 of Contemporary Issues in Nephrology. New York, Churchill-Livingstone, 1982, p 121. *A comprehensive review of this subject utilizing both clinical and experimental observations.*

Riemenschneider T, Bohle A: Morphologic aspects of low-potassium and low-sodium nephropathy. Clin Nephrol 19:271, 1983. *This report describes the renal histopathology and clinical findings in 40 patients with chronic hypokalemia of varying etiologies.*

Stone WJ: Renal complications of neoplastic paraproteinemias. In McKinney TD (ed.): Renal Complications of Neoplasia. New York, Praeger, 1986. *A recent review of this subject with emphasis on clinical manifestations and management.*

DRUG-INDUCED ACUTE INTERSTITIAL NEPHRITIS

Ditlove J, Weidmann P, Bernstein M, et al.: Methicillin nephritis. Medicine 56:483, 1977. *In this report the authors describe 4 of their patients with methicillin nephritis and review 68 others previously reported in the literature.*

Galpin JE, Shinaberger JH, Stanley JH, et al.: Acute interstitial nephritis due to methicillin. Am J Med 65:756, 1978. *This report describes 14 cases of methicillin nephritis, 8 of whom were treated with prednisone.*

Hande KR, Noone RM, Stone WJ: Severe allopurinol toxicity. Am J Med 76:47, 1984. *This report describes 7 patients with allopurinol toxicity treated by the authors and reviews another 78 cases from the literature. Dosage guidelines for allopurinol for patients with varying degrees of renal insufficiency are proposed.*

Magil AB, Ballon HS, Cameron EC, et al.: Acute interstitial nephritis associated with thiazide diuretics. Am J Med 69:939, 1980. *This report describes the clinical characteristics and renal biopsy findings in three patients who developed AISN while being treated with a combination of hydrochlorothiazide and triamterene.*

Nessi R, Bonoldi GL, Redaelli B, et al.: Acute renal failure after rifampicin: A case report and survey of the literature. Nephron 16:148, 1976. *One case of acute renal failure that developed after rifampin administration is presented, along with a review of 36 previously reported cases.*

Pusey CD, Saltissi D, Bloodworth L, et al.: Drug associated acute interstitial nephritis: Clinical and pathological features and response to high dose therapy. Q J Med 52:194, 1983. *In this report nine cases of drug-related AISN are described, four of which were associated with sulfonamides. Seven episodes were treated with high-dose methylprednisolone with rapid improvement in renal function.*

TOXIC NEPHROPATHY (GENERAL REFERENCES)

Heptinstall RH: Renal complications of therapeutic and diagnostic agents, analgesic abuse and addiction to narcotics. In Heptinstall RH (ed.): Pathology of the Kidney. Edition 3. Boston, Little, Brown and Company, 1983. *This chapter provides a thorough discussion and representative photographs of the renal histopathology of these toxic compounds.*

Humes HD, Weinberg JM: Toxic nephropathies. In Brenner BM, Rector FC Jr (eds.): The Kidney. Edition 3. Philadelphia, W. B. Saunders Company, 1986. *A recent, extensive, and well-written review with 579 references.*

Roxe DM: Toxic nephropathy from diagnostic and therapeutic agents. Am J Med 69:759, 1980. *A brief summary of this topic with 141 references.*

ANALGESIC NEPHROPATHY

Blohme I, Johansson S: Renal pelvic neoplasms and atypical urothelium in patients with end-stage analgesic nephropathy. Kidney Int 20:671, 1981. *This paper describes 4 cases of renal pelvic carcinoma among 84 patients with end-stage analgesic nephropathy. In addition, urothelial atypia was found in the renal pelvis of 27 of 56 patients whose kidneys were removed immediately prior to or after renal transplantation. No atypia was found in other types of renal disease.*

Buckalew VM Jr, Schey HM: Renal disease from habitual antipyretic analgesic consumption: An assessment of the epidemiologic evidence. Medicine 65:291, 1986. *This paper reviews the worldwide evidence which indicates that habitual analgesic use is an important cause of renal diseases (74 references).*

Eknoyan G, Qunibi WY, Grissom RT, et al.: Renal papillary necrosis: An update. Medicine 61:55, 1982. *A comprehensive review of the various causes of papillary necrosis, including analgesic nephropathy.*

Kincaid-Smith P (ed.): Analgesic nephropathy. Kidney Int 13:1, 1978. *This entire issue is devoted to virtually every aspect of clinical and experimental analgesic nephropathy.*

NONSTEROIDAL ANTI-INFLAMMATORY DRUGS

Carmichael J, Shankel SW: Effects of nonsteroidal anti-inflammatory drugs on prostaglandins and renal function. Am J Med 78:992, 1985. *This paper summarizes in tabular form many cases of the various renal syndromes that have been reported with the NSAID's in current use (146 references).*

Clive DM, Stoff JS: Renal syndromes associated with nonsteroidal anti-inflammatory drugs. N Engl J Med 310:563, 1984. *An excellent review of this topic with 157 references.*

Dunn MJ, Patrono C (eds.): Renal effects of nonsteroidal anti-inflammatory drugs. Am J Med 81(Suppl 2B):1, 1986. *The several papers from the proceedings of this recent symposium deal with most aspects of this topic (1068 references).*

ANTIMICROBIAL DRUGS

Appel GB, Neu HC: The nephrotoxicity of antimicrobial agents. N Engl J Med 296:663, 722, 784, 1977. *This three-part series provides an extensive review of this topic (272 references).*

Heidemann HT, Gerkins JF, Spickard WA, et al.: Amphotericin B nephrotoxicity in humans decreased by salt repletion. Am J Med 75:476, 1983. *This report describes five patients, four of whom were sodium depleted, who developed renal insufficiency with amphotericin B therapy. Sodium repletion was associated with improved renal function, which allowed completion of therapy.*

Humes HD, Weinberg JM, Knauss TC: Clinical and pathophysiologic aspects of aminoglycoside nephrotoxicity. Am J Kidney Dis 2:5, 1982. *This in-depth review discusses both clinical and experimental features of aminoglycoside nephrotoxicity (215 references).*

Perez-Ayuso RM, Arroyo V, Camps J, et al.: Effect of demeclocycline on renal function and urinary prostaglandin E_2 and kallikrein in hyponatremic cirrhotics. Nephron 36:30, 1984. *In this report, five of eight hyponatremic cirrhotic patients given demeclocycline developed acute reversible renal insufficiency with a reduction in GFR from an average of 72 to 31 ml per minute.*

RADIOGRAPHIC CONTRAST–INDUCED NEPHROTOXICITY

Anto HR, Chou SY, Porush JG, et al.: Infusion intravenous pyelography and renal function. Arch Intern Med 141:1652, 1981. *In this report there was a 22 per cent incidence of worsening renal function in 37 patients with underlying renal insufficiency (mean serum creatinine 4.1 ml per deciliter) given 50 grams of mannitol immediately following intravenous urography. This compares with a 70 per cent incidence in a similar group of patients not receiving mannitol previously reported by the same authors.*

Berkseth RO, Kjellstrand CM: Radiologic contrast-induced nephropathy. Med Clin N Am 68:1, 1984. *A comprehensive review of this topic (101 references).*

NEPHROTOXICITY ASSOCIATED WITH ANTINEOPLASTIC THERAPY

Chiuten D, Vogl S, Kaplan B, et al.: Is there cumulative or delayed toxicity from cis-platinum? Cancer 52:211, 1983. *This study of 95 patients receiving repeated courses of cisplatin in doses of 50 to 75 mg per square meter suggests that cumulative nephrotoxicity is low (around 4 per cent) if adequate hydration and diuresis are established prior to and during administration of the drug.*

Giroux L, Bettez P, Giroux L: Mithramycin-C nephrotoxicity: A clinicopathologic study in 17 cases. Am J Kidney Dis 6:28, 1985. *This is a good description of clinical and pathological findings in this disorder.*

Goldberg ID, Garnick MB, Bloomer WD: Urinary tract toxic effects of cancer therapy. J Urol 132:1, 1984. *This brief review provides a concise discussion of the genitourinary complications of radiation therapy, cisplatin, methotrexate, and nitrosoureas.*

Hainsworth JD, Johnson DH, Porter LL: Nephrotoxicity associated with antineoplastic therapy. In McKinney TD (ed.): Renal Complications of Neoplasia. New York, Praeger, 1986. *A recent review of this topic with a particularly extensive discussion of cisplatin nephrotoxicity.*

Hande KR: Hyperuricemia, uric acid nephropathy and the tumor lysis syndrome. In McKinney TD (ed.): Renal Complications of Neoplasia. New York, Praeger, 1986. *A recent comprehensive review of this topic.*

METAL NEPHROPATHIES

Craswell PW, Price J, Boyle PD, et al.: Chronic renal failure with gout: A marker of chronic lead poisoning. Kidney Int 26:319, 1984. *This is one of several recent papers that confirms the association of renal failure, gout, and chronic lead intoxication.*

Cullen MR, Robins JM, Eskenazi B: Adult inorganic lead intoxication: Presentation of 31 new cases and a review of recent advances in the literature. Medicine 62:221, 1983. *This article describes clinical characteristics in 31 patients with lead intoxication resulting from industrial exposure, along with a review of the topic (207 references).*

Falck FY Jr, Keren DF, Fine LJ, et al.: Protein excretion patterns in cadmium exposed individuals. High resolution electrophoresis. Arch Environ Health

39:69, 1984. *In this study, 7 of 39 men chronically exposed to industrial sources of cadmium had mild proteinuria, and 5 had mild elevations of serum creatinine concentrations.*

Gerhardt RE, Crecelius EA, Hudson JB: Moonshine-related arsenic poisoning. Arch Intern Med 140:211, 1980. *This paper reviews 12 cases of arsenic poisoning, 50 per cent of which resulted from "moonshine" ingestion. Five patients with acute or semiacute poisoning had renal damage.*

Johanson GFS, Hunt GE, Duggin GG, et al.: Renal function and lithium treatment: Initial and follow-up tests in manic depressive patients. J Affective Disord 6:249, 1984. *In this study, several renal function tests were serially examined in 61 patients receiving long-term lithium therapy. Twelve per cent of them had a low GFR, which correlated with previous episodes of acute lithium intoxication.*

Katz WA, Blodgett RC Jr, Pietrusko RG: Proteinuria in gold-treated rheumatoid arthritis. Ann Intern Med 101:176, 1984. *In this report 41 of 1283 (3 per cent) patients receiving oral gold treatments for rheumatoid arthritis developed proteinuria. In 9 this was in the nephrotic range. The results suggest that oral gold is less nephrotoxic than parenteral gold therapy.*

Tubbs RR, Gephardt GN, McMahon JT, et al.: Membranous glomerulonephritis associated with industrial mercury exposure. Am J Clin Pathol 77:409, 1982. *This report describes two patients with industrial exposure to mercury who developed biopsy-proven membranous nephropathy with heavy proteinuria. In one case proteinuria resolved after cessation of exposure to mercury, and this correlated with a decline in urinary mercury excretion from high to normal values.*

Wedeen RP: Occupational renal disease. Am J Kidney Dis 3:241, 1984. *This review discusses numerous important aspects of intoxication with several metals and other industrial toxins.*

MISCELLANEOUS NEPHROTOXINS

Bolton WK, Suratt PM, Sturgill BC: Rapidly progressive silicon nephropathy. Am J Med 71:823, 1981. *The clinical and pathologic features of four cases of this syndrome are described.*

Diamond JC, Cheung JY, Fang LST: Nifedipine-induced renal dysfunction. Am J Med 77:905, 1984. *This paper describes four patients with underlying renal insufficiency who had reversible acute declines in renal function during nifedipine therapy in the absence of hypotension.*

Gabow PA, Clay K, Sullivan JB, et al.: Organic acids in ethylene glycol intoxication. Ann Intern Med 105:16, 1986. *This paper describes three patients with ethylene glycol intoxication, acute renal failure, and metabolic acidosis successfully treated by a combination of ethanol infusion and hemodialysis.*

Hricik DE, Browning PJ, Kopelman R: Captopril-induced functional renal insufficiency in patients with bilateral renal artery stenosis in a solitary kidney. N Engl J Med 308:373, 1983. *Eleven patients are described who developed reversible renal insufficiency four days to two months after institution of therapy with captopril.*

Llach F, Descoeudres C, Massry SG: Heroin-associated nephropathy: Clinical and histologic studies in 19 patients. Clin Nephrol 11:7, 1979. *A variety of glomerular lesions were present in these patients, the majority of which resulted in the nephrotic syndrome.*

Ntoso KA, Tomaszewski JE, Jimenez SA, et al.: Penicillamine-induced rapidly progressive glomerulonephritis in patients with progressive systemic sclerosis: Successful treatment of two patients and a review of the literature. Am J Kidney Dis 8:159, 1986.

Streicher HZ, Gabow PA, Moss AH, et al.: Syndromes of toluene sniffing in adults. Ann Intern Med 94:758, 1981. *Clinical features of 25 cases of toluene sniffing are reported. The most prominent renal-electrolyte manifestation was hyperchloremic metabolic acidosis.*

83 OBSTRUCTIVE NEPHROPATHY

Floyd C. Rector, Jr.

Obstruction of the urinary tract may produce profound structural and functional changes in the kidneys and, if uncorrected, may result in complete, irreversible loss of renal function. Early diagnosis and appropriate correction, therefore, are essential for preserving or restoring renal function and preventing the progression to end-stage renal failure. The obstructing lesions may occur at any site in the urinary tract from the renal tubules to the terminal urethra. The clinical presentation is variable, depending on the site of obstruction and whether the obstruction is acute or chronic, complete or partial, unilateral or bilateral, or complicated by urinary tract infection.

INCIDENCE AND ETIOLOGY. In a large series of autopsies the prevalence of hydronephrosis has varied from 3.5 to 3.8 per cent. Clinically significant urinary tract obstruction occurs less frequently than noted at postmortem examination; nevertheless it is a rather common disease in all age groups. Hydronephrosis is a contributing factor to destruction of renal function in 15 to 25 per cent of uremic patients.

TABLE 83–1. CAUSES OF OBSTRUCTIVE UROPATHY

Intraluminal	
Stone	Ureteral tumor
Bladder tumor	Bence Jones proteinuria
Papillary necrosis	Acute urate nephropathy
Clot	
Intramural	
Congenital	
Ureteropelvic dysfunction (10 per cent bilateral)	
Ureterovesical stricture (simple or ureterocele)	
Bladder neck obstruction	
Pinpoint meatus	
Acquired	
Urethral stricture	
Ureteral stricture (tuberculosis, etc.)	
Neurogenic bladder dysfunction	
Extramural	
Prostatic obstruction	
Ureteropelvic juncture—vessels, bands, etc.	
Aortic aneurysm	
Periureteral fibrosis	
Retroperitoneal tumor or nodes	
Extraurinary growth (carcinoma of colon, diverticulitis)	
Pelvic tumor	
Inadvertent ligature	

Obstructive uropathy can result from three general types of obstruction (Table 83–1): (1) mechanical obstruction of the lumen of the urinary tract; (2) functional or anatomic abnormalities of the ureter, bladder, or urethra; or (3) compression from masses or processes extrinsic to the urinary tract. The prevalence of the various causes of obstruction varies with age and sex. The most common causes are congenital abnormalities of the urinary tract (e.g., urethral valves, vesicoureteral reflux, cystocele) in children, pregnancy and pelvic malignancy in women, renal stones in young men, and prostatic hypertrophy in elderly men. Acute ureteral obstruction from calculi results in the hospitalization of 1 out of 1000 Americans each year. Benign prostatic enlargement occurs in 80 per cent of men over 60 years, and 10 per cent of these require surgery for the correction of obstruction. Vesicoureteral reflux is most common in young girls, but also occurs to some extent in approximately 5 per cent of adults. Neurogenic bladder dysfunction is a serious medical problem frequently complicated by incontinence, recurrent urinary tract infection, bladder stones, and hydronephrosis; this disorder can occur secondary to traumatic injuries of the spinal cord or to metabolic and neurologic diseases (diabetes mellitus, multiple sclerosis, myelodysplasia, senile dementia, and vascular disease).

PATHOLOGY AND PATHOPHYSIOLOGY. Obstruction of the lower urinary tract produces profound structural and functional changes in the kidney and, if complete, can irreversibly destroy renal function within four to six weeks. This is the consequence of combined mechanical and hormonal factors (Table 83–2). Superimposition of urinary tract infection or renal immunologic injury (antibody formation secondary to the release of renal antigens into the circulation) will accelerate and intensify this destruction of renal function.

Immediately following obstruction of one ureter, pressures in the pelvis and tubules increase, causing the pelvis and tubules to dilate and the renal papillae to become flattened. Secondary to the increased tubular pressure and dilatation there is a marked decrease in glomerular filtration rate, disruption of the junctional complexes between tubular cells permitting backleak of solutes from tubule lumen to blood, and inhibition of sodium reabsorption and potassium and hydrogen secretion in the distal nephron.

Concomitant with these mechanical changes there is stimulation of prostaglandin production within the kidney. Increased levels of PGI_2 (prostacyclin) stimulate the release of renin (sufficient to cause acute hypertension) and produce

TABLE 83–2. EFFECTS OF OBSTRUCTION ON RENAL FUNCTION

- I. Mechanical
  - A. Increased tubular pressure
    1. Disruption of junctional complexes—increased tubule permeability
    2. Decreased collecting duct Na transport; decreased H^+ and K^+ secretion
    3. Decreased GFR
  - B. Increased renal interstitial pressure
    1. Altered proximal reabsorption
    2. Impaired countercurrent function
- II. Hormonal
  - A. Increased PGI_2 synthesis
    1. Stimulated renin release
    2. Cortical vasodilation
  - B. Increased PGE_2 synthesis
    1. Medullary vasodilation
    2. Inhibition of vasopressin action
    3. Inhibition of aldosterone action
    4. Inhibition of Cl^- transport in thick ascending limb
  - C. Increased thromboxane A_2 synthesis
    1. Cortical vasoconstriction
    2. Decreased number of functioning nephrons
  - D. Retained natriuretic factors in blood
- III. Other
  - A. Decreased glomerular permeability
  - B. Decreased mesangial clearance of immune complexes

vasodilation in the renal cortex. Increased levels of PGE_2 produce vasodilation in the renal medulla, block the action of vasopressin, and further inhibit salt transport in the loop of Henle and distal nephron. As a consequence of these hormonal changes there is an initial rise in renal blood flow, lasting four to six hours. Thereafter, renal blood flow progressively falls to levels of 10 to 15 per cent of normal despite continued increased production of PGI_2 and PGE_2. This fall in blood flow is the result of intense renal vasoconstriction produced by increased levels of the prostaglandin derivative thromboxane A_2, one of the most potent vasoconstrictors known. Associated with these mechanical and hormonal changes the kidney becomes severely ischemic, with many nephrons ceasing to function. The residual nephrons have reduced filtration rates and impaired ability to conserve sodium, secrete potassium, and acidify and concentrate the urine. The tubules progressively atrophy, the medulla is destroyed, and by four to six weeks the cortex consists of only a thin shell of connective tissue with few remaining glomeruli.

If the obstruction is corrected prior to this stage of irreversible renal damage, there may be significant recovery of renal function. Experimental studies in dogs have shown 45 to 50 per cent recovery after two weeks of complete obstruction, 15 to 30 per cent recovery after three to four weeks of obstruction, but no recovery after six weeks of complete obstruction.

In contrast to the changes observed with complete obstruction, with partial obstruction, particularly if bilateral, the renal pelvis may become tremendously dilated, holding 2 to 3 liters of urine, and yet structure and function of the renal cortex may be relatively well preserved. Functionally, filtration rate and blood flow may be only slightly (or moderately) reduced, and the major abnormality may be the inability to concentrate the urine and/or secrete potassium and hydrogen ions.

CLINICAL MANIFESTATIONS OF URINARY TRACT OBSTRUCTION. The clinical manifestations of urinary tract obstruction depend on the site of obstruction and on whether it is acute or chronic. Patients with obstruction below the bladder (prostate, urethra) may have decreased force and caliber of the urinary stream, intermittency, postvoid dribbling, hesitancy, and nocturia. Neurogenic dysfunction of the bladder with incomplete emptying may cause urgency, frequent urination, and urinary incontinence (overflow incontinence). These symptoms, however, do not occur with obstruction at higher levels in the urinary tract. Urinary tract obstruction may also present as asymptomatic hydronephrosis, as renal colic, as either acute or chronic renal failure, or occasionally as a specific renal tubular disorder (Table 83–3).

Pain. The pain associated with urinary tract obstruction is produced by distention of the renal capsule, and the intensity of the pain is related to the rate of distention. With chronic, low-grade obstruction the renal collecting system can be tremendously dilated without producing pain. This form of obstruction will be discovered either accidentally or during the workup for urinary tract infection, renal failure, or renal tubular abnormalities. Occasionally, in patients with chronic asymptomatic hydronephrosis the urinary tract may become acutely and painfully distended during a diuresis induced by large fluid intake (e.g., water, beer). Therefore, intermittent flank pain induced by fluid intake should suggest the presence of urinary tract obstruction. Pain induced by urination should suggest vesicoureteral reflux. Acute obstruction of a ureter with a stone may produce one of the most severe forms of pain encountered in clinical medicine. Usually the pain is located in the lower abdomen or flank, radiating into the groin on the obstructed side.

Renal Failure. Chronic obstruction of one kidney will result in unilateral hydronephrosis if the obstruction is partial, and in a nonfunctioning kidney if the obstruction is complete. Unilateral obstruction will not produce renal failure if the opposite kidney is functional. However, obstruction of a single functioning kidney or bilateral obstruction can give rise to either acute or chronic renal failure.

Acute renal failure secondary to obstruction is usually associated with severe oliguria or anuria, although it may occasionally present as "high output" acute renal failure. Variable output from day to day should suggest the presence of lower urinary tract obstruction. Acute renal failure can arise from sudden occlusion of the lower urinary tract or from widespread intratubular obstruction secondary to precipitation of Bence Jones protein in patients with multiple myeloma or of uric acid in patients with myeloproliferative disorders treated with chemotherapy.

TABLE 83–3. CLINICAL MANIFESTATIONS OF URINARY TRACT OBSTRUCTION

1. Lower tract symptoms: urgency, hesitancy, incontinence, nocturia
2. Chronic hydronephrosis
   - a. Asymptomatic
   - b. Intermittent pain
3. Renal colic
4. Renal failure
   - a. Acute
     - (1) Intratubular
     - (2) Lower tract
   - b. Chronic
     - (1) Hydronephrosis
     - (2) Infection ± lithiasis
     - (3) Interstitial nephritis
     - (4) Reflux nephropathy
     - (5) Papillary necrosis
5. Recurrent urinary tract infection
6. Renal tubule dysfunction
   - a. Concentration defect
     - (1) Nocturia, polyuria
     - (2) Nephrogenic diabetes insipidus
   - b. Distal renal tubular acidosis
   - c. Potassium secretory defect
7. Hypertension
   - a. Acute—renin dependent
   - b. Chronic—volume dependent
8. Polycythemia
9. Postobstructive diuresis

Urinary tract obstruction is an important pathogenetic factor in 15 to 25 per cent of patients with end-stage renal failure and uremia. This progression to chronic renal failure can occur as a consequence of progressive hydronephrosis or by the destructive effects of recurrent urinary tract infections. In fact, it is unusual for chronic, recurrent pyelonephritis to occur in the absence of mechanical problems in the lower urinary tract. Urinary tract obstruction may also produce chronic interstitial nephritis unrelated to infection. Recently, several patients with chronic vesicoureteral reflux have been found to have severe chronic glomerulonephritis. The mechanism is not known.

Infection. Recurrent urinary tract infection may be superimposed on urinary tract obstruction and present with the typical symptoms of fever, flank tenderness, and dysuria. The incidence of urinary tract infection ranges from 8 to 15 per cent in patients with urinary tract obstruction who have not been previously instrumented. Instrumentation (bladder catheters, cystoscopy), neurogenic bladder dysfunction, and bladder stones all increase the incidence of chronic infection. Once infection is established in the obstructed urinary tract, it is extremely difficult to eradicate and may contribute significantly to morbidity and the rate of destruction of renal function.

Tubular Dysfunction. A small percentage of patients may present with renal tubular abnormalities as the principal manifestation of their urinary tract obstruction. The most frequent of these abnormalities is inability to concentrate the urine. Usually, this is characterized by isosthenuria, nocturia, and modest polyuria, but occasionally may express itself as vasopressin-resistant nephrogenic diabetes insipidus with the excretion of large volumes (greater than 4000 ml per day) of dilute urine. The factors contributing to the defect in concentrating ability are destruction of the renal medulla and the antagonistic effects of PGE_2 against the renal action of vasopressin. Occasionally, patients with obstruction may present with renal tubular acidosis of the distal type, characterized by hyperchloremic acidosis with an inability to lower urine pH below 6.0 in response to acid loading. Less commonly, patients with obstruction may present with hyperkalemia secondary to a renal tubular defect in potassium secretion. When hyperkalemia occurs it is invariably associated with hyperchloremic acidosis.

Hypertension. Hypertension occurs in approximately 30 per cent of patients with acute unilateral obstruction. The hypertension tends to be mild and transient (rarely lasting longer than one week) and is caused by increased renin secretion. In general, hypertension is not a feature of chronic unilateral obstruction, although there have been a few cases of high-renin hypertension reported, which were corrected by removal of the obstructed kidney. In contrast, a high percentage of patients with chronic bilateral hydronephrosis have hypertension. These patients do not have elevated renin levels, and the hypertension appears to be the consequence of retained salt and water.

Polycythemia. A rare manifestation of obstructive nephropathy is polycythemia. In the small number of patients in whom this disorder has been observed, the erythrocytosis rapidly resolves following nephrectomy and is thought to be due to abnormal production of erythropoietin by the obstructed kidney.

Postobstructive Diuresis. Following the surgical correction of lower urinary tract obstruction the patient may undergo a marked diuresis ("postobstructive diuresis"). Both clinically and experimentally, postobstructive diuresis is associated with bilateral, but not with unilateral, obstruction. In most instances the diuresis is transient and does not result in significant contraction of extracellular volume. In these cases the diuresis is the consequence of the excretion of salt, urea, other solutes, and water retained during the period of obstruction, and continues until the volume and composition of the extracellular fluid return to normal. In a few instances, however, the diuresis represents a true salt and water wastage, with depletion of extracellular volume and its associated findings (e.g., postural hypotension, tachycardia). A natriuretic factor, normally excreted into the urine, may be retained during periods of bilateral obstruction and causes salt wasting when the obstruction is released. There also appears to be a vasopressin-resistant component to the diuresis, possibly caused by high levels of renal prostaglandins.

DIAGNOSIS AND EVALUATION. Urinary tract obstruction should be suspected in patients who have lower urinary tract symptoms (diminished stream, urgency, hesitancy, incontinence); recurrent urinary tract infections; pain in the flank, groin, or lower abdomen; abdominal masses; or unexplained uremia or oliguric acute renal failure. The patient's history should be evaluated for previous stone disease, drug ingestion, diabetes mellitus, or neurologic disorders. The physical examination should evaluate the abdomen and flanks for pain or masses, the external genitalia, the prostate in men, and the pelvic structures in women. In selected circumstances, postvoiding urine volume measured by bladder catheterization may provide the key to diagnosis. This test, however, must be performed with great care to avoid inducing infection.

In patients presenting with acute oliguric renal failure, other causes of oliguria-anuria must be excluded. These include (1) extracellular volume depletion, (2) renal arterial or venous occlusion, (3) acute glomerular disease or vasculitis, (4) cortical necrosis, (5) acute tubular necrosis, and (6) urinary tract obstruction. Workup of these patients should include history of drug exposure (antibiotics, radiopaque dyes, analgesics, chemotherapy), evidence for multiple myeloma or uric acid nephropathy, and status of extracellular fluid volume. The urine should be carefully examined for red cell casts, renal tubular cell casts (renal failure casts), urate crystals, and red cells. Urine sodium concentration is helpful in that it should be low (less than 10 mEq per liter) in prerenal azotemia, acute glomerular disease, or renal vasculitis, but will be relatively high in acute tubular necrosis and urinary tract obstruction.

The key to the diagnosis of urinary tract obstruction is the demonstration of a dilated urinary collecting system. One of the most useful techniques for identifying dilation of the renal pelvis, particularly in acutely oliguric patients, is ultrasonography. This technique is rapid and noninvasive and avoids the potential hazards of radiocontrast dyes. The intravenous urogram with nephrotomography is also a useful procedure in patients in whom radiocontrast agents are not contraindicated. In the presence of renal failure it is necessary to use a higher dose of dye. In most patients, even those with severe reduction of glomerular filtration rate (GFR), there should be adequate visualization to determine kidney size, whether there are one or two kidneys, and whether the renal pelvis is dilated. If the obstruction is acute, the nephrogram will be delayed but quite dense, whereas if the obstruction is more chronic, the nephrogram will be faint. Delayed films, 24 to 36 hours after dye injection, may be necessary to visualize the renal pelvis and collecting system sufficiently to identify the site of obstruction. More recently, computed tomography has proved useful in identifying urinary tract obstruction and its cause. In performing these tests it must be remembered that the renal pelvis may not be dilated at the time of study if the obstruction is partial and/or intermittent or if the patient is severely volume depleted. In evaluating patients with intermittent flank pain, it is important, therefore, to perform the study at a time when the patient is having pain or after induction of osmotic or water diuresis. In severely ill patients, it is important to correct any deficits of extracellular volume prior to the test.

Once the presence of urinary tract obstruction is established, more complex urologic procedures such as retrograde pyelography, percutaneous antegrade pyelography, cystoscopy, and voiding cystograms may be needed to identify the site of obstruction, the presence of vesicoureteral reflux, and the functional status of the bladder. Renal radionuclide scans are helpful in determining the relative function of the two kidneys and are particularly useful in determining the residual function of a unilaterally obstructed kidney.

TREATMENT. The general aims of therapy are (1) relief from the symptoms of obstruction, (2) prevention or eradication of infection, and (3) preservation of renal function. Obstruction complicated by infection and sepsis is a potentially lethal disease requiring relief of obstruction as soon as possible. Complete obstruction, uncomplicated by infection, is not a medical emergency, but should be evaluated and corrected promptly for optimal preservation of renal function. In this situation uremia, if present, should first be treated by dialysis before proceeding with surgical correction of the obstruction. Elective repair of urinary tract obstruction is indicated in patients with recurrent urinary infections, persistent pain, urinary retention, recurrent bleeding, or progressive renal damage. Simple uncomplicated postvoid residual urine, vesicoureteral reflux, and dilation of the collecting system are not indications for surgery.

The specific method used for relief of obstruction depends on the general status of the patient, whether the situation requires an emergency or elective procedure, the location of the obstruction, whether the obstructing lesion is benign or malignant, whether the obstruction is mechanical or neurogenic, and the functional status of the obstructed kidney.

In the septic patient requiring an emergency procedure, the obstruction can be relieved either by urethral or ureteral catheters or by percutaneous placement of a nephrostomy tube into the dilated renal pelvis. These bypass procedures can also be used electively in the presence of complete obstruction to gain time for diagnostic studies and the evaluation of residual renal function. Occasionally, one may elect to leave these diversion tubes in place permanently. Despite the inevitable urinary infection associated with the presence of these tubes, the patients may survive for years with little or no further loss of renal function. However, whenever possible, the tubes should be removed and a more definitive procedure performed. If the obstructed kidney is nonfunctional and has no chance of recovering function (chronic obstruction or complete acute obstruction for more than three to four months), then nephrectomy may be the most judicious procedure. A discussion of surgical procedures is beyond the scope of this chapter.

Acute obstruction of a ureter with a renal stone is usually transient and will correct spontaneously in 85 to 90 per cent of the cases. If the stone is greater than 5 mm, it may become impacted in the ureter and require surgical removal within a few days. If a stone lodged in the ureter does not produce complete obstruction, one can delay for two to four weeks to see if spontaneous passage will occur. If the stone is not passed, it should then be surgically removed. Manipulation or removal of ureteral stones by a basket catheter is sometimes successful, but this procedure runs the risk of ureteral injury with subsequent stricture.

Functional obstruction secondary to neurogenic bladder is a complicated and difficult management problem. Helpful maneuvers are frequent voiding, double voiding, suprapubic pressure on the bladder during voiding, and the use of cholinergic drugs. Intermittent catheterization may also be used, with the addition of anticholinergic or sympathomimetic drugs to prevent incontinence between catheterizations. More severe cases may require a permanent indwelling catheter or, preferably, surgical reimplantation of the ureters into an ileal conduit.

Klahr S (guest ed.): Obstructive uropathy. In Kurtzman N (ed.): Seminars in Nephrology, Vol II, No 1, March, 1982. *A superb multiauthored review of the physiologic, biochemical, and hormonal changes in the obstructed kidney.*

Klahr S, Buerkert J, Morrison A: Urinary tract obstruction. In Brenner BM, Rector FC (eds.): The Kidney. 3rd ed. Philadelphia, W. B. Saunders Company, 1986, pp 1443–1490. *An extensive review of the pathophysiology of obstructive uropathy written for nephrologists; with 379 references.*

Okegawa T, Jonas PE, DeSchryver K, et al.: Metabolic and cellular alterations underlying the exaggerated renal prostaglandin and thromboxane synthesis in ureter obstruction in rabbits. J Clin Invest 71:81, 1983. *Acute unilateral ureteral obstruction produces an inflammatory reaction in the obstructed kidney with an interstitial infiltrate of monocytes and fibroblasts. These inflammatory cells account for the increased cyclo-oxygenase activity and the exaggerated production of PGE_2 and thromboxane A_2.*

84 SPECIFIC RENAL TUBULAR DISORDERS

Martin G. Cogan

INTRODUCTION

The diverse reabsorptive functions of the kidney are generally segregated such that specific nephron segments are responsible for specific transport functions. As described in Ch. 75, the proximal nephron is responsible for the reabsorption of most of the filtered bicarbonate, glucose, amino acids, uric acid, phosphate, and low molecular weight proteins. The loop of Henle reabsorbs over half the filtered sodium chloride as well as divalent cations. The distal nephron (including the cortical and medullary collecting ducts), under the influence of aldosterone, reabsorbs the final quantity of sodium, secretes hydrogen ions to lower the pH of the urine and titrate buffers, and secretes potassium ions. The terminal collecting ducts can be induced by antidiuretic hormone to permit water reabsorption and thereby cause urinary concentration.

Genetic and acquired conditions exist that can affect one or more of the reabsorptive or secretory transport processes within each of these nephron segments, as illustrated in Table 84–1. Depending on the transport sites affected, these diseases therefore lead to abnormal wastage or retention of specific solutes. For instance, within a given nephron segment, there may be a selective transport defect for a single solute (e.g., bicarbonate in proximal renal tubular acidosis or glucose in renal glycosuria) or for a class of solutes (e.g., dibasic amino acids in cystinuria). Alternatively, those solutes modulated by a specific hormone may be affected by a hormone-deficient or -resistant state (e.g., in hypoaldosteronism or diabetes insipidus). Finally, there are diseases that affect all solutes normally transported by a given nephron segment (e.g., all proximal transported solutes in Fanconi's syndrome). Luminal, cellular, or peritubular components of the overall transport process can be responsible for each of these situations. The following sections, and other chapters (195, 196, 227, 230, 246, and 247) as identified in Table 84–1, describe some of the more common transport defects of the individual nephron segments.

DISORDERS OF PROXIMAL NEPHRON FUNCTION

The proximal nephron is responsible for reabsorbing 80 to 99 per cent of several filtered solutes, including glucose, amino acids, and bicarbonate. Appearance of one or more of these solutes in the urine at normal filtered loads implies a disorder of proximal transport.

Renal Glycosurias

The renal glycosurias are caused by inherited or acquired defects in proximal tubule glucose reabsorption such that glycosuria occurs in the absence of hyperglycemia.

PATHOPHYSIOLOGY. Glucose is reabsorbed across the luminal membrane of the proximal tubule by a stereospecific carrier that requires sodium. The amount of glucose reabsorbed changes in proportion to filtered glucose load until a

TABLE 84–1. CLINICAL SYNDROMES DUE TO NEPHRON TRANSPORT DEFECTS

Proximal Nephron

I. *Selective transport defects*
  A. Renal glycosurias
    1. Primary
    2. Combined:
      a. Glucose/galactose malabsorption
      b. Glucoglycinuria
  B. Renal aminoacidurias
    1. Basic aminoacidurias
      a. General: cystinuria (cystine, lysine, arginine, ornithine)
      b. Specific: hypercystinuria, dibasic aminoaciduria (lysine, arginine, ornithine), lysinuria
    2. Neutral aminoacidurias
      a. General: Hartnup disease
      b. Specific: methioninuria, tryptophanuria, histidinuria
    3. Iminoglycinuria
      a. General (proline, hydroxyproline, glycine)
      b. Specific: glycinuria
    4. Dicarboxylic aminoaciduria
      a. General (glutamic, aspartic acids)
  C. Proximal renal tubular acidosis
    1. Primary: idiopathic or genetic
    2. Transient (infants)
    3. Carbonic anhydrase deficiency, inhibition, alteration
      a. Drugs: acetazolamide, sulfanilamide, mafenide acetate
      b. Idiopathic?
  D. Renal uric acid disorders (see Ch. 195, 196)
  E. Phosphate and calcium disorders (see Ch. 246, 247)
II. *Nonselective transport defects: Fanconi's syndrome*
  A. Primary: idiopathic or genetic
  B. Genetically transmitted systemic diseases
    1. Cystinosis
    2. Lowe's syndrome
    3. Wilson's disease
    4. Tyrosinemia
    5. Hereditary fructose intolerance
    6. Pyruvate carboxylase deficiency
  C. Dysproteinemic states
    1. Multiple myeloma
    2. Monoclonal gammopathy
  D. Secondary hyperparathyroidism with chronic hypocalcemia
    1. Vitamin D deficiency or resistance
    2. Vitamin D dependency
  E. Drugs and toxins
    1. Outdated tetracycline
    2. Methyl-3-chromone
    3. Streptozotocin
    4. Glue
    5. Gentamicin
  F. Heavy metals
    1. Lead
    2. Cadmium
    3. Mercury
  G. Tubulointerstitial diseases
    1. Sjögren's syndrome
    2. Medullary cystic disease
    3. Renal transplantation
  H. Other diseases
    1. Nephrotic syndrome
    2. Amyloidosis
    3. Osteopetrosis
    4. Paroxysmal nocturnal hemoglobinuria

Loop of Henle

I. *Bartter's syndrome*
II. *Drugs*
  A. Furosemide
  B. Bumetanide
  C. Ethacrynic acid

Distal Nephron

I. *Selective transport defects*
  A. Classic distal RTA
    1. Primary: genetic or idiopathic
    2. Genetically transmitted systemic diseases
      a. Ehlers-Danlos syndrome
      b. Hematologic disorders: hereditary elliptocytosis, sickle cell anemia, carbonic anhydrase I deficiency or alteration
      c. Medullary cystic disease
      d. With nerve deafness
      e. Glycogenosis type III
    3. Autoimmune diseases
      a. Hypergammaglobulinemia: hyperglobulinemic purpura, cryoglobulinemia, familial
      b. Sjögren's syndrome
      c. Thyroiditis
      d. Pulmonary fibrosis
      e. Chronic active hepatitis
      f. Primary biliary cirrhosis
      g. Systemic lupus erythematosus
    4. Diseases associated with nephrocalcinosis
      a. Primary hyperparathyroidism
      b. Vitamin D intoxication
      c. Hyperthyroidism
      d. Hypercalciuria: idiopathic or genetic
      e. Hereditary fructose intolerance
      f. Medullary sponge kidney
      g. Fabry's disease
      h. Wilson's disease
    5. Drug or toxic nephropathies
      a. Amphotericin B
      b. Toluene
      c. Glue
      d. Analgesics
      e. Cyclamate
    6. Tubulointerstitial diseases
      a. Chronic pyelonephritis secondary to urolithiasis
      b. Obstructive uropathy
      c. Renal transplantation
      d. Leprosy
      e. Hyperoxaluria
    7. Miscellaneous
  B. RTA of glomerular insufficiency
  C. Hypermineralocorticoid and other potassium secretory disorders (see Ch. 230)
II. *Nonselective transport defects: generalized distal RTA, hyperkalemia, and renal salt wasting*
  A. Primary mineralocorticoid deficiency (see Ch. 230)
  B. Hyporeninemic hypoaldosteronism
    1. Diabetic nephropathy
    2. Tubulointerstitial nephropathies
    3. Nephrosclerosis
    4. Nonsteroidal anti-inflammatory agents
  C. Mineralocorticoid-resistant hyperkalemia
    1. Without salt wasting: genetic
    2. With salt wasting
      a. Childhood forms
      b. Tubulointerstitial nephropathies: methicillin, obstructive nephropathy, transplantation, sickle cell disease
      c. Drugs: spironolactone, amiloride, triamterene

Loop and Medullary Collecting Ducts

I. *Diabetes insipidus* (see Ch. 227)
II. *SIADH* (see Ch. 227)
III. *Other concentrating and diluting disorders*

maximal reabsorptive capacity or "Tm" is reached, as shown in Figure 84–1. Somewhat before saturation is attained, glucose reabsorption is incomplete, representing the "splay" in the response. The initial point of the splay represents that filtered glucose concentration or load, called the "threshold," at which reabsorption no longer equals filtration and glucose appears in the urine. The normal threshold concentration is 200 to 240 mg per deciliter, well above the normal plasma glucose concentration, so little glucose (< 125 mg per day) appears in the urine of a normal individual. The kinetics of glucose reabsorption have been analogized to an enzyme system: The Tm is equivalent to the $\dot{V}max$, whereas the Km is related to the degree of splay. In the two major types of renal glycosurias, either the capacity (type A, $\dot{V}max$ or Tm mutation) or the affinity (type B, Km, or degree of splay mutation) of glucose reabsorption is altered (Fig. 84–1). In either case, the threshold is reduced so glucose is spilled into the urine at a normal plasma glucose concentration. The glycosuria is markedly exaggerated when filtered glucose concentration is elevated by intravenous hypertonic glucose infusion.

SYMPTOMS AND ETIOLOGIES. Renal glycosurias (Table 84–1) are relatively unusual, with an incidence (depending on the stringency of diagnostic criteria) of about 0.2 to 0.6 per

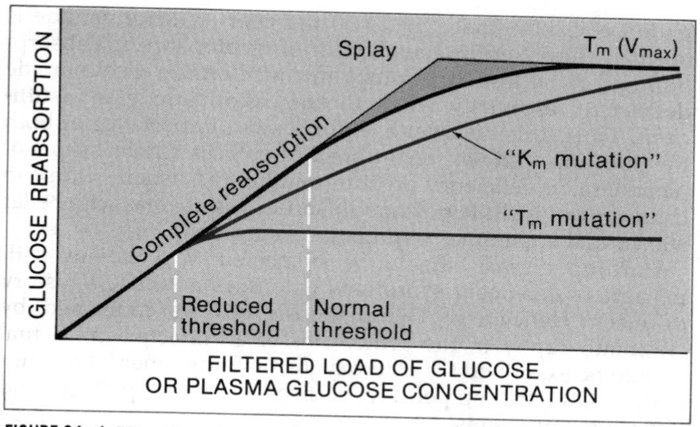

FIGURE 84–1. Kinetics of renal glucose reabsorption and the two variants of renal glycosuria. (Modified from Cogan MG: Disorders of proximal nephron function. Am J Med *72*:278, 1982.)

cent. They are usually inherited in an autosomal recessive manner. Homozygotes have more severe glycosuria than heterozygotes. Usually, but not invariably, V̇max and Km variants of the syndrome are inherited separately. On renal biopsy, there are no consistent pathologic distinguishing features. Unlike the aminoacidurias, there is no coexisting intestinal transport defect for glucose. Renal glycosuria is completely asymptomatic (i.e., affected individuals do not have polydipsia or polyuria).

Intermittent glycosuria is not infrequent during pregnancy (second and third trimesters) and during the terminal phases of chronic renal insufficiency. In both cases, an increase in tubular flow rate, due to an increase in total or just single nephron glomerular filtration rate (GFR), is probably the primary cause of the functional alteration in glucose transport kinetics. In a rare syndrome in children, malabsorption of two sugars, glucose and galactose, in both the jejunum and the kidney causes diarrhea and mellituria.

DIAGNOSIS AND TREATMENT. Diagnosis should be based on finding a urinary glucose excretion of greater than 500 mg per 24 hours (on a diet containing 30 kilocalories per kilogram, of which 50 per cent is carbohydrate) in the absence of hyperglycemia (plasma glucose < 140 mg per deciliter). The glucose oxidase method should be used to confirm that the excreted sugar is glucose in order to exclude other mellituric conditions (pentosuria, fructosuria, sucrosuria, maltosuria, galactosuria, and lactosuria). Appropriate tests to rule out coexistent tubular transport defects (of amino acids, bicarbonate, phosphate, and uric acid) typical of the Fanconi syndrome should be performed, and diabetes mellitus must be excluded, using standard clinical and laboratory evidence. If desired, differentiation of the V̇max or Km variants can be accomplished by glucose loading.

The condition is completely benign with respect to symptoms and to renal functional deterioration. Treatment is unnecessary. Prolonged fasting should be avoided to prevent the unusual complication of hypoglycemia and ketosis.

Cystinuria and Other Renal Aminoacidurias

The renal aminoacidurias are inherited disorders in which one or a group of amino acids are excreted by the kidney (in the absence of hyperaminoacidemia) and are usually also malabsorbed by the intestine (Table 84–1).

GENERAL CONSIDERATIONS. Amino acids are avidly reabsorbed in the proximal nephron so that only about 2 per cent of the filtered amino acid load is excreted in the urine (except for glycine, 5 per cent, and histidine, 8 per cent). In general, most amino acids are transported by a stereospecific carrier across the luminal membrane of the proximal nephron accompanied by sodium and driven by the lumen-to-cell sodium gradient. Under some circumstances, amino acids can also be secreted. Reabsorptive kinetics are similar to those of glucose (Fig. 84–1). Five major luminal membrane carriers for reabsorption exist, each of which transports a specific group of amino acids: basic amino acids (cystine, lysine, arginine, and ornithine); acidic amino acids (glutamic and aspartic acids); neutral amino acids (alanine, serine, threonine, valine, leucine, isoleucine, phenylalanine, tyrosine, tryptophan, and histidine); iminoglycine amino acids (proline, hydroxyproline, and glycine); and beta-amino acids (beta-aminoisobutyric acid, beta-alanine, and taurine). Inherited dysfunction of a carrier results in urinary loss of the entire amino acid group: cystinuria (basic aminoaciduria); dicarboxylic aminoaciduria; Hartnup disease (neutral aminoaciduria); and iminoglycinuria. There is no clinical disorder yet described of beta-amino acid transport. There are also other carriers (> 25 are estimated to exist) that selectively transport only one or several members of a given amino acid group. Disorders of these carriers cause even more selective aminoaciduria: hypercystinuria, histidinuria, and lysinuria.

Many of the amino acid carriers in the proximal nephron are also expressed on the luminal membrane of gastrointestinal epithelial cells. Defective gastrointestinal absorption therefore occurs conjointly with increased renal excretion of the amino acid or acids in question. Amino acid dimers can be normally absorbed by the gut, however, so that nutritional problems arising from amino acid malabsorption are unusual. Furthermore, gut absorption is not so constrained by time as that in the renal tubule, i.e., does not require such rapid efficiency.

For diagnosis of a renal aminoaciduria, a high plasma level of the amino acid must first be excluded. Excessive filtration of an amino acid can overwhelm the tubular transport carrier for it and other members of its amino acid family and result in one or more aminoacidurias. These "overflow" aminoacidurias are discussed in Ch. 187–193. In contrast, the renal aminoacidurias are associated with low or normal levels of plasma amino acid concentrations because the aminoaciduria is due to defective proximal tubular transport.

CYSTINURIA. One of the most common aminoacidurias is *cystinuria* (basic aminoaciduria), an autosomal recessive disease estimated to affect about 1:7000 individuals (between 1:1000 and 1:20,000, depending on the population studied). Urinary spillage of lysine, arginine, and ornithine is asymptomatic. Cystine, however, is the least soluble of naturally occurring amino acids, and it therefore tends to precipitate to form cystine urolithiasis. Cystinuria accounts for about 1 to 2 per cent of all urinary calculi. Stone formation usually becomes manifest during the second and third decades of life, though presentation may occur from infancy to the ninth decade, and males are more severely affected. Cystine stones are yellow-brown and have a granular appearance. Such stones are radiopaque, can create staghorn calculi, and frequently form a nidus for calcium oxalate stone formation. Symptoms include renal colic, which may be associated with obstruction or infection or both. Evidence associating cystinuria with central nervous system disorders has been tenuous. A more general discussion of nephrolithiasis is found in Ch. 90.

The diagnosis of cystinuria should be entertained in any patient with a renal calculus, even if the stone is composed primarily of calcium oxalate (since cystine might have been the formation nidus). The typical hexagonal crystals may be recognized on urinalysis, especially in a concentrated, acidic, early morning specimen. A useful screening test is the cyanide-nitroprusside test, which will detect a cystine excretion rate of about 75 to 125 mg per gram of creatinine. Because of false-positive results, a definitive diagnosis requires thin-layer or ion-exchange chromatography or high-voltage electrophoresis. Excretion rates in an adult of greater than 18 mg of cystine per gram of creatinine confirm the diagnosis. The dibasic amino acids will also be increased in excretion per gram of creatinine: lysine > 130 mg; arginine > 16 mg; and ornithine > 22 mg. Persons with homozygous cystinuria routinely excrete more than 250 mg of cystine per gram of creatinine, usually about 0.5 to 1.0 gram per day. Cystinuria has three allelic variants, classified according to whether coexisting intestinal and renal basic amino acid transport is completely absent (types I and II) or variably reduced (type III) and whether heterozygotes have normal (type I) or supernormal (types II and III) urinary cystine and basic aminoaciduria.

Medical therapy of cystinuria is aimed at decreasing the urinary concentration below the solubility limit of 300 mg of cystine per liter. The most practical approach is to increase fluid intake to about 3 to 4 liters per day. The polyuria must be maintained at all times, including nighttime, when the urine otherwise tends to become concentrated and acidic. Cystine solubility also can be increased by alkalinizing urine pH, but a urine pH of greater than 7.5 is necessary to achieve a salutary effect. Avoidance of excessive intake of methionine, the metabolic precursor of cystine, is a reasonable adjunctive therapy but is ineffective as a sole therapy. When conservative measures fail, D-penicillamine is recommended, usually in a dose of 1 to 2 grams per day. This drug forms a mixed disulfide of penicillamine-cysteine, which is much more soluble than cystine alone. Free cystine excretion then falls to an acceptable level. Unfortunately, penicillamine causes fever and a rash in as many as 50 per cent of patients, and sometimes arthralgias. More severe hypersensitivity reactions also occur, including membranous nephropathy and nephrotic syndrome, pancytopenia or thrombocytosis, epidermolysis, hypogeusia, and a Goodpasture-like syndrome. In some cases the drug can be readministered at a lower dose following an adverse reaction. Pyridoxine should be given as a supplement, since penicillamine can deplete this cofactor. Other investigational agents, such as N-acetyl-D-penicillamine and mercaptopropionylglycine, have been reported to be efficacious. There have been conflicting reports regarding the utility of glutamine administration. Chlordiazepoxide has also been found to reduce cystine excretion.

HARTNUP DISEASE. Hartnup disease, a neutral aminoaciduria, is a rare autosomal recessive disorder (1:16,000 births) in which the clinical presentation is dominated by nicotinamide deficiency. Since up to 50 per cent of nicrotinamide is normally supplied by metabolism of tryptophan, malabsorption and renal loss of tryptophan contribute to nicotinamide deficiency, especially when dietary nicotinamide is insufficient. Thus, this disorder exemplifies the importance of both the intestinal and the renal transport defects. Clinical signs of nicotinamide deficiency are intermittent and usually worse in children and include pellagra in sun-exposed areas, cerebellar ataxia, and sometimes psychiatric disturbance.

Hartnup disease should be suspected in a patient with pellagra or cerebellar symptoms who does not have a history of niacin deficiency. The diagnosis can be confirmed by chromatography of the urine. Sibs of an affected individual should be examined for heterozygosity. Supplemental nicotinamide (40 to 250 mg per day) suffices to prevent pellagra and neurologic problems.

OTHER AMINOACIDURIAS. Less common aminoacidurias lacking clinical manifestations include iminoglycinuria, isolated hypercystinuria (without hyperexcretion of other basic amino acids), isolated glycinuria, and dicarboxylic aminoaciduria. Mental retardation predominates in the rare disorders of hyperdibasic aminoaciduria, isolated lysinuria, histidinuria, and methioninuria.

Proximal Renal Tubular Acidosis (RTA)

Proximal (type II) RTA is a hyperchloremic, hypokalemic metabolic acidosis due to a selective defect in proximal acidification, which is characterized by a normally acidic urine during acidosis but marked bicarbonate wasting when plasma bicarbonate concentration is normalized.

PATHOPHYSIOLOGY. The proximal nephron reabsorbs 85 to 90 per cent of the filtered bicarbonate, predominantly by Na^+/H^+ exchange and the enzymatic degradation of H_2CO_3 to CO_2 and H_2O by carbonic anhydrase (Fig. 84–2). Interference with the normal operation of Na^+/H^+ exchange or of carbonic anhydrase activity will therefore result in excess delivery of bicarbonate to the distal nephron and, because of the limited distal bicarbonate reabsorption capacity, into the urine. Thus, the urinary wastage of 15 per cent or more of the filtered bicarbonate load at a normal blood bicarbonate concentration is pathognomonic of proximal RTA. The excess delivery of the relatively impermeant bicarbonate to the distal

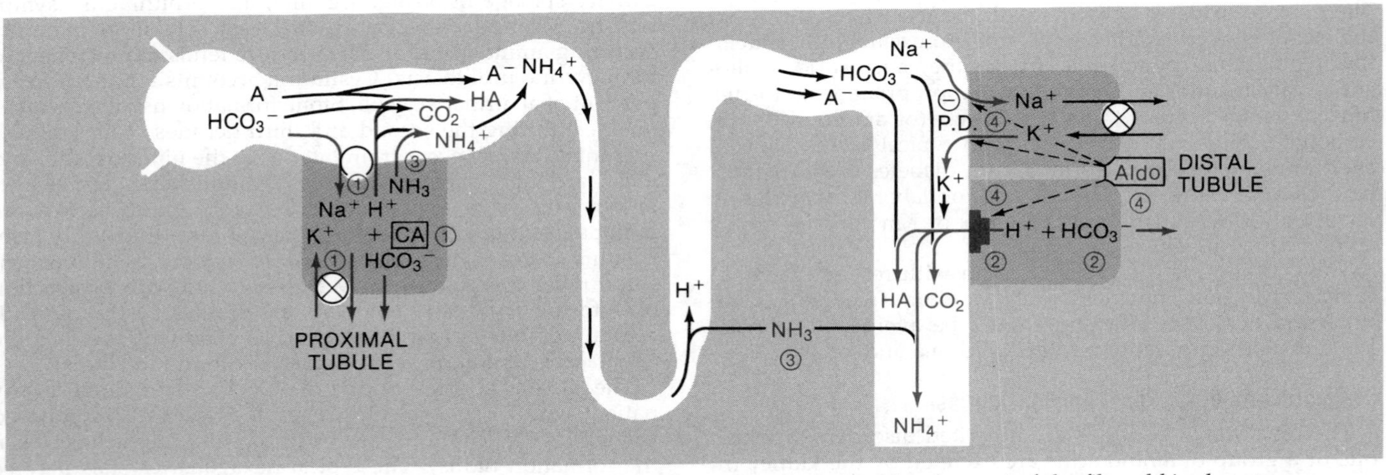

FIGURE 84–2. Sites of impaired renal acidification (RTA). The proximal tubule reabsorbs most of the filtered bicarbonate by hydrogen ion secretion. Proximal acidification is sodium- and carbonic anhydrase–dependent and is energetically driven by the lumen-to-cell sodium gradient. Disorders of proximal acidification, proximal RTA, may result from defects (labelled 1) in the Na^+/H^+ exchanger, carbonic anhydrase activity, or the activity of the basolateral Na^+-K^+ ATPase. The distal nephron is regulated by aldosterone to reabsorb sodium and secrete hydrogen ions. Distal acidification is responsible for titrating both remaining filtered buffer (labelled A^-) to form titratable acids (HA) and proximally produced ammonia (NH_3) to form ammonium (NH_4^+). Disorders of distal acidification include defects of the proton pump or basolateral bicarbonate exit step (labelled 2) in classic distal RTA, of ammonia production or delivery (labelled 3) in the RTA of glomerular insufficiency, or in aldosterone levels or target sites (labelled 4) in generalized distal RTA.

TABLE 84–2. RENAL TUBULAR ACIDOSES

Type	Renal Defect	Plasma [K+]	Proximal Acidification: HCO_3^- Reabsorption (During HCO_3^- Loading)	Distal Acidification: $U_{pH_{min}}$ (During Acidosis)	Distal Acidification: $(U_{NH_4^+} \cdot V) + (U_{TA} \cdot V)$ (During Acidosis)
Proximal (type II)	↓ Proximal acidification	↓	↓	< 5.5	N
Classic distal (type I)	↓ Distal pH gradient	↓	N	> 5.5	↓
Glomerular insufficiency	↓ NH_3 production	N	N	< 5.5	↓
Generalized distal (type IV)	↓ Aldosterone action	↑	N	< 5.5	↓

Abbreviations: $U_{pH_{min}}$ = minimal urinary pH; $(U_{NH_4^+} \cdot V) + (U_{TA} \cdot V)$ = urinary ammonium plus titratable acid excretion; N = normal.

nephron also results in accelerated potassium secretion and hypokalemia. As the plasma bicarbonate concentration and filtered load fall owing to defective proximal bicarbonate reabsorption and subsequent urinary bicarbonate wastage, absolute bicarbonate delivery to the distal nephron progressively decreases. At a certain point, usually when the plasma bicarbonate concentration is 15 to 18 mM, the distal nephron can cope with the delivery out of the proximal tubule. At this stage, bicarbonaturia disappears, urinary pH can be lowered normally, and net acid excretion equivalent to endogenous acid production resumes. Acid-base homeostasis is reestablished at the expense of metabolic acidosis.

SYMPTOMS AND ETIOLOGIES. Manifestations of proximal RTA are attributable to acidemia (growth retardation, anorexia and malnutrition, volume depletion), potassium depletion (muscular weakness, polyuria, nocturia, polydipsia), and disordered calcium/phosphate/parathormone/vitamin D metabolism (osteomalacia and other bone diseases). Proximal RTA is a rare disorder, usually found when carbonic anhydrase is defective or is inhibited or in conjunction with the full Fanconi syndrome (Table 84–1).

DIAGNOSIS AND TREATMENT. Laboratory findings of proximal RTA are those of a hyperchloremic, hypokalemic metabolic acidosis. When the patient is acidemic, the urine is acidic and net acid excretion equals endogenous acid load (Table 84–2). When bicarbonate is infused to normalize the plasma bicarbonate concentration, massive bicarbonaturia results ($\geq$ 15 per cent of the filtered load). Proximal RTA is usually not isolated but rather associated with the full Fanconi syndrome.

Therapy of the underlying disease should be undertaken if possible (e.g., multiple myeloma) or offending drugs or toxins discontinued (e.g., heavy metals). When this is not possible, proximal RTA is treated with large amounts of sodium and potassium bicarbonate. As the plasma bicarbonate concentration rises with treatment, distal bicarbonate delivery increases, causing more potassium wasting and the need for further potassium supplementation. Because of the inability to correct the disorder fully with bicarbonate alone, volume contraction utilizing diuretics is also used to stimulate fractional proximal bicarbonate reabsorption. Therapy with vitamin D is indicated when signs of vitamin D deficiency exist.

Nonselective Proximal Nephron Dysfunction: Fanconi's Syndrome

In the Fanconi syndrome, the entire array of proximal transport functions is impaired, resulting in glycosuria, generalized aminoaciduria, proximal RTA, phosphaturia, and uricaciduria.

PATHOPHYSIOLOGY. The lumen-to-cell sodium gradient provides the driving force in the proximal tubule for the absorption of glucose, amino acids, phosphate, and organic acids and for secretion of hydrogen ions needed to reabsorb bicarbonate. Disruption of this common driving force serves as an attractive hypothesis to explain the global functional impairment of reabsorption of solutes in the proximal tubule observed in the Fanconi syndrome. Collapse of the sodium gradient could arise by several mechanisms: a primary disturbance of the Na^+-K^+ adenosinetriphosphatase (ATPase); increased permeability of the cell to sodium; or reduced metabolic energy due to an abnormality in the redox potential or in intracellular phosphate supply.

In addition to the solutes described above, there is disordered reabsorption, and sometimes depressed serum concentrations, of calcium, magnesium, citrate, and low molecular weight proteins. Enhanced sodium delivery to the distal nephron causes kaliuresis and hypokalemia. Since the proximal nephron is the principal site of conversion of 25-OH vitamin D to 1,25-$(OH)_2$ vitamin D, the circulating level of this latter hormone is also diminished.

SYMPTOMS AND ETIOLOGIES. As a result of the complex disorders of mineral and vitamin D metabolism, the most prominent clinical finding of the Fanconi syndrome is metabolic bone disease, either rickets in children or osteomalacia in adults (see also Ch. 246). Nausea, episodic vomiting, anorexia, and growth retardation in children are frequent. Other clinical findings include symptoms of hypokalemia, such as polyuria and muscle weakness.

Causes of the Fanconi syndrome are listed in Table 84–1. The most common inherited disorder is *cystinosis*, in which cystine accumulates in cells, specifically in lysosomes, of the kidney, liver, gut, lymphoid tissues, conjunctiva, and cornea and in bone marrow–derived cells and fibroblasts. Cystinosis should be distinguished from cystinuria, described above. Cystinosis may present as the Fanconi syndrome, followed by renal failure, in the first two years of life (infantile nephropathic form) or in the adolescent years. It is usually relatively benign if it first appears in adulthood, causing only asymptomatic cystine deposits in the conjunctiva, cornea, and bone marrow. An interesting inducible form of the Fanconi syndrome is *hereditary fructose intolerance* (HFI) caused by a deficiency of aldolase B activity. Ingestion of fructose in affected individuals causes acute symptoms, including nausea, vomiting, abdominal pain, and neurologic dysfunction. Chronic fructose ingestion can cause symptoms associated with the Fanconi syndrome and with liver dysfunction.

In adults, acquired Fanconi's syndrome is most often due to dysproteinemias, heavy metal (especially chronic cadmium or acute lead) exposure, or immunologic diseases (Table 84–1). An older adult presenting with the Fanconi syndrome should be assumed to have multiple myeloma until proven otherwise.

DIAGNOSIS AND TREATMENT. Diagnosis of the Fanconi syndrome is established by finding consequences of the full array of proximal nephron dysfunction: glycosuria, generalized aminoaciduria, proximal RTA, phosphaturia, hypouricemia, hypovitaminosis D, and secondary hypokalemia. Underlying causes of the Fanconi syndrome (Table 84–1) should be sought. Serum and urine electrophoresis should be obtained to rule out multiple myeloma in adults.

Treatment of the Fanconi syndrome itself requires attempts to normalize the electrolyte and vitamin imbalance. Supplements of bicarbonate (up to 15 to 20 mEq per kilogram of body weight daily), potassium, phosphate, magnesium, and vitamin D are necessary. Treatment of the underlying disease, of course, varies widely. Effective results have been reported in the treatment of cystinosis with cysteamine, of Wilson's disease with penicillamine, of hereditary fructose intolerance with fructose restriction, and of heavy metal intoxication with removal from metal exposure or chelation (for lead).

DISORDERS OF FUNCTION OF THE ASCENDING LIMB OF THE LOOP OF HENLE

The thick ascending limb of Henle reabsorbs sodium chloride by means of a luminal Na-K-2Cl system. A lumen-positive potential difference and parallel transport systems effect potassium, calcium, and magnesium reabsorption. Defective reabsorption by the thick ascending limb of Henle occurs during diuretic treatment or in Bartter's syndrome.

Bartter's Syndrome

Bartter's syndrome consists of a constellation of findings including hypokalemia and metabolic alkalosis with hyper-reninemic hyperaldosteronism. Hypertension and edema are absent.

PATHOPHYSIOLOGY. Evidence that dysfunction of the thick ascending limb of Henle is the proximate cause of Bartter's syndrome comes primarily from free-water clearance studies. The pathophysiologic consequences of diminished loop sodium chloride reabsorption is illustrated in Figure 84–3. Mild extracellular volume depletion causes hyper-reninemic hyperaldosteronism and the juxtaglomerular hyperplasia found on renal biopsy. Enhanced sodium chloride delivery to the collecting duct stimulates potassium secretion (exacerbated by concurrent hyperaldosteronism) leading to hypokalemia, as well as hydrogen ion secretion resulting in metabolic alkalosis. Accelerated kinin and prostaglandin (especially PGE_2 and prostacyclin) production occurs and may account for the vascular unresponsiveness to pressors and various other phenomena known to occur in Bartter's syndrome.

SYMPTOMS AND ETIOLOGY. Symptoms of Bartter's syndrome are usually manifested in childhood. Inheritance is autosomal recessive, with a higher penetrance in males. Adult cases have also been reported. Presenting features relate primarily to the hypokalemia, including muscle weakness and a vasopressin-unresponsive urinary concentrating defect, characterized by polyuria, nocturia, and enuresis. Divalent cation wasting and metabolic alkalosis may conspire to cause symptoms characteristic of hypocalcemia, including Trousseau's and Chvostek's signs. The electrolyte abnormalities can also present acutely as intestinal ileus or chronically as growth retardation in children. Affected patients are normotensive and nonedematous, have a normal GFR, and can usually conserve sodium chloride when dietary salt is restricted, though at the expense of signs of moderate extracellular volume compromise.

DIAGNOSIS AND TREATMENT. Other conditions associated with hypokalemia, metabolic alkalosis, and secondary hyper-reninemic hyperaldosteronism must be excluded before making a diagnosis of Bartter's syndrome. Surreptitious vomiting, chronic diarrheal states, or surreptitious diuretic or laxative administration can cause symptoms indistinguishable from those of Bartter's syndrome. These disorders are associated with extracellular volume depletion, and therefore the urinary chloride level is less than 20 mEq per liter, unless diuretics are being actively consumed. Thus, diagnosis of Bartter's syndrome must be preceded by confirmation that urinary chloride concentration is more than 20 mEq per liter and by negative screens for diuretics in the urine and for laxatives in the stool (phenolphthalein test). States of primary hyper-reninism or hypermineralocorticoidism can be readily excluded, since they are usually associated with hypertension.

Therapy of Bartter's syndrome is primarily aimed at ameliorating the hypokalemia by disrupting the renin-angiotensin-aldosterone and kinin-prostaglandin axes. Potassium supplementation, magnesium repletion, propranolol, spironolactone, prostaglandin inhibition, and captopril have all been used, but each has usually been met with incomplete success.

DISORDERS OF DISTAL NEPHRON FUNCTION

The distal nephron, including the distal convoluted tubule and the collecting ducts, is responsible for reabsorbing the final quantity of sodium in the tubule fluid and for secreting potassium and hydrogen ions. Inherited and acquired defects exist for selective or combined disorders of sodium, potassium, and acid-base regulation.

Classic Distal Renal Tubular Acidosis (RTA)

Classic distal (type I) RTA is a hypokalemic, hyperchloremic metabolic acidosis due to a selective defect in distal acidification and is characterized by inability to lower the urine pH normally and therefore by subnormal urinary net acid excretion.

PATHOPHYSIOLOGY. The distal nephron (especially the cortical and medullary collecting ducts) is normally capable of lowering the urine pH fully 2 to 3 pH units below that of blood to titrate filtered buffers (principally phosphate) to form

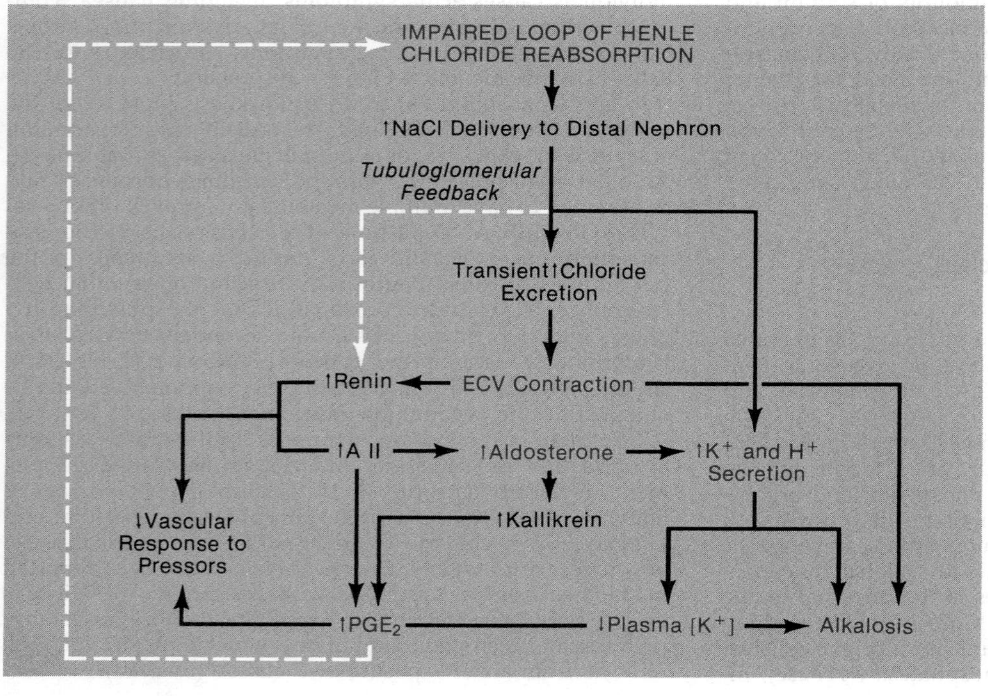

FIGURE 84–3. Pathophysiology of Bartter's syndrome. The primary sodium chloride reabsorptive defect is presumed to reside in the thick ascending limb of the loop of Henle. (From Cogan MG, Rector FC Jr: Acid-base disorders. In Brenner BM, Rector FC Jr [eds.]: The Kidney. 3rd ed. Philadelphia, W. B. Saunders Company, 1986, pp 457–518.)

titratable acids and endogenously produced ammonia to form ammonium (Fig. 84–2). If the distal nephron is incapable of lowering the luminal pH below 5.5 when challenged by metabolic acidosis, a classic distal RTA is present. Because of the inappropriately high urine pH, net acid excretion (titratable acid plus ammonium minus bicarbonate) is subnormal, less than acid production by the body. Accelerated potassium secretion occurs, presumably because there is reduced competition by proton secretion for the electrochemical driving forces in the distal nephron. The acidification defect may result from an insufficient number of proton-secreting pumps in the distal nephron. Alternatively, there may be backleak of acid across the luminal membrane, so that establishment of a pH gradient is prevented even when proton secretion is normal.

SYMPTOMS AND ETIOLOGIES. Distal RTA is found both in infants and children and in adults. Symptoms may be of acidosis or hypokalemia, as described above. Nephrocalcinosis and nephrolithiasis are common, either as a cause or as a result of classic distal RTA. However, bone disease is not as frequent as in proximal RTA. Classic distal RTA may also be genetic (most frequently autosomal dominant) or due to autoimmune diseases, drugs and toxins, and various tubulointerstitial diseases (Table 84–1.)

DIAGNOSIS AND TREATMENT. The findings of hyperchloremic, hypokalemic metabolic acidosis with an inappropriately high urine pH (> 5.5) and diminished net acid excretion confirm the diagnosis (Table 84–2). In individuals with a normal plasma bicarbonate concentration, the failure to lower urine pH to less than 5.5 following an acute acid challenge with NH_4Cl defines the syndrome of incomplete classic distal RTA (see Ch. 77 for details of the NH_4Cl test). Proximal bicarbonate reabsorption as tested by bicarbonate loading is normal. Treatment with alkali is generally very effective. The daily dose of alkali in adults is 1 to 3 mEq per kilogram, to compensate for the normal acid production by the body plus a small amount of urinary bicarbonate wastage. In contrast to proximal RTA, urinary potassium wasting is ameliorated with alkali therapy. Children require more alkali, about 5 to 14 mEq per kilogram per day. Prognosis with respect to stabilization of glomerular filtration rate in adults or growth in children is excellent with provision of adequate alkali therapy.

RTA of Glomerular Insufficiency

This disorder is a normokalemic, hyperchloremic metabolic acidosis associated with moderate renal insufficiency (glomerular filtration rate of 20 to 30 ml per minute), due to deficient ammonia delivery, and is characterized by an appropriately low urine pH but subnormal urinary net acid (ammonium) excretion.

PATHOPHYSIOLOGY. When the GFR falls to about 20 to 30 ml per minute owing to any intrinsic glomerular or tubulointerstitial disease, a normokalemic metabolic acidosis is frequently found. The cause of this acidosis is thought to be either deficient ammonia production or impairment in the urinary trapping of ammonia as ammonium (Fig. 84–2). In either case, proximal bicarbonate reclamation and the ability to lower the urine pH to less than 5.5 are intact, but the failure to generate sufficient acid excretion to equal intake results in systemic acidosis.

SYMPTOMS AND ETIOLOGY. The degree of metabolic acidosis is generally mild, and plasma bicarbonate concentration is usually greater than 15 mEq per liter. The acidemia has been suggested by some investigators to exacerbate the osteodystrophy of progressive renal disease. Although tubulointerstitial diseases are thought to produce this form of RTA more commonly than glomerular diseases, this distinction has been difficult to verify. This hyperchloremic metabolic acidosis should be distinguished from the high anion gap (normochloremic) metabolic acidosis due to retained organic acids that usually occurs when glomerular insufficiency is more severe (GRF < 20 ml per minute). The two acidoses may coexist.

DIAGNOSIS AND TREATMENT. A hyperchloremic, normokalemic metabolic acidosis that occurs when GFR falls to about 20 to 30 ml per minute is typical of the RTA of glomerular insufficiency. Although net acid, specifically ammonium, excretion is subnormal, the urine pH is appropriately acidic (Table 84–2). Mineralocorticoid levels are not diminished. An elevated anion gap (uremic acidosis) is generally seen only when GFR is less than 20 ml per minute. Treatment consists of 1 to 3 mEq per kilogram per day of alkali therapy to compensate for daily acid ingestion and production.

Nonselective Distal Nephron Dysfunction: Generalized Distal RTA, Hyperkalemia, and Renal Salt Wasting

These disorders arise from global dysfunction of the distal nephron due to aldosterone deficiency or antagonism and are characterized by hyperkalemic, hyperchloremic (type IV) metabolic acidosis due to subnormal net acid excretion and frequently by renal salt wasting.

PATHOPHYSIOLOGY. When sodium is reabsorbed in the distal nephron under the influence of aldosterone, luminal sodium concentration can be reduced to very low levels, less than 10 mEq per liter (sometimes ≤1 mEq per liter). Sodium reabsorption creates a lumen-negative potential difference, favoring secretion of potassium and hydrogen ions (Fig. 84–2). Disruption of sodium reabsorption and of potassium and hydrogen secretion may therefore be ascribable to a defect in the integrity of the distal nephron cell, deficient aldosterone production or action, diminished sodium reabsorption, or blunting of the lumen-negative potential by enhanced chloride reabsorption. Any of these processes will lead to diminished total hydrogen ion and potassium excretion and therefore metabolic acidosis with hyperkalemia. The hyperkalemia will also serve to depress renal ammoniagenesis independently, which exacerbates the defect in renal acidification. The ability to reabsorb bicarbonate (a proximal nephron function) and to lower the urinary pH normally (a qualitative distal nephron function at low buffer strength) remains intact (Table 84–2).

SYMPTOMS AND ETIOLOGIES. The symptoms of generalized distal RTA in children or adults usually relate to the acidosis itself or occasionally to the neuromuscular consequences of hyperkalemia. Renal salt wasting can cause extracellular volume depletion and hypotension when sodium chloride intake is reduced. The most common forms of generalized distal RTA are due to reduction in aldosterone level or prevention of its action (Table 84–1). The adrenal synthesis of aldosterone may be directly impaired, as in Addison's disease or in inherited enzymatic defects, such as 18- or 21-hydroxylase deficiencies. More commonly, primary hyporeninemia due to diabetic nephropathy, hypertensive nephrosclerosis, or tubulointerstitial diseases can also reduce aldosterone levels. Finally, end-organ unresponsiveness to mineralocorticoid with high circulating levels of aldosterone can be found in various tubulointerstitial diseases, especially those that have a predilection for the medulla and papilla of the kidney (e.g., analgesic abuse, sickle cell disease, and obstructive nephropathies).

DIAGNOSIS AND TREATMENT: HYPERKALEMIC, GENERALIZED DISTAL RTA. Generalized distal RTA is unique among the hyperchloremic metabolic acidoses in being a hyperkalemic disorder (Table 84–2). Glomerular filtration rate is invariably reduced in the forms associated with hyporeninemia or tubulointerstitial nephropathy but may be at levels (≥ 30 ml per minute) above that typically found in the RTA of glomerular insufficiency.

Treatment of the hyperkalemia and generalized distal RTA is effected with mineralocorticoid (9-α-fludrocortisone 0.1 mg per day) when deficient. When hyporeninemia is the cause, high doses of the synthetic mineralocorticoid are required (up to 0.5 mg per day) because of associated mineralocorticoid resistance. Hypertension can be precipitated with this treatment. Alternatively, providing modest amounts of alkali to compensate for daily acid generation (1 to 3 mEq per kilogram per day) can be used. Treatment of the hyperkalemia by dietary potassium restriction, potassium-wasting diuretics, or cation-exchange resins can also ameliorate or even correct the acid-base disorder.

DIAGNOSIS AND TREATMENT: RENAL SALT WASTING. Renal salt wasting becomes apparent when dietary sodium chloride intake becomes less than the minimal threshold for sodium chloride excretion. In normal persons, abrupt dietary sodium restriction to 10 mEq per day causes urinary sodium excretion to fall to a comparable level (10 mEq per day) within three to five days. Only a transient period occurs in which urinary sodium excretion exceeds intake and slight weight loss occurs ($\leq$ 1 kg). Renal salt wasting is diagnosed when, in response to acute reduction of sodium intake (10 mEq per day), urinary sodium excretion remains inappropriately elevated, typically greater than 50 mEq per day and weight loss is significant ($>$ 3 kg). Progressively severe extracellular volume depletion occurs with development of hypotension and renal insufficiency. This diagnostic maneuver is not without hazard, since symptomatic hypovolemia or hyperkalemia can be precipitated, and should be performed under close supervision.

Therapy for renal salt wasting due to aldosterone deficiency or partial resistance requires physiologic or supraphysiologic mineralocorticoid replacement, as described above. In all other cases, sodium chloride supplementation is indicated to prevent volume depletion in the event sodium intake is curtailed. The dose of sodium chloride prescribed, in the diet plus salt tablets, should exceed that amount of sodium chloride spilled into the urine by the patient when dietary salt was restricted.

GENERAL

Cogan MG: Disorders of proximal nephron function. Am J Med 72:275, 1982. *This paper presents an overview of the physiology, pathophysiologic mechanisms, and clinical disorders of proximal nephron function.*

Sebastian A, Hulter HN, Kurtz I, et al.: Disorders of distal nephron function. Am J Med 72:289, 1982. *This article is a thoughtful, pathophysiologically oriented overview of the various clinical dysfunctions of potassium and hydrogen ion secretion.*

RENAL GLYCOSURIAS

Wen S-F: Glycosurias. In Gonick HC, Buckalew VM Jr. (eds.): Renal Tubular Disorders. New York, Marcel Dekker, Inc., 1985, pp 159–199. *This chapter presents an excellent discussion of the physiology of glucose transport and the pathophysiology and clinical spectrum of the renal glycosurias.*

RENAL AMINOACIDURIAS

Foreman JW, Segal S: Aminoacidurias. In Gonick HC, Buckalew VM Jr. (eds.): Renal Tubular Disorders. New York, Marcel Dekker, Inc., 1985, pp 131–157. *This chapter presents an excellent overview of the physiology of amino acid transport and the clinical spectra of the aminoacidurias.*

Segal S, Thier SO: Cystinuria. In Stanbury JB, Wyngaarden JB, Fredrickson DS, et al. (eds.): The Metabolic Basis of Inherited Disease. 5th ed. New York, McGraw-Hill Book Company, 1983, pp 1774–1791. *This is an authoritative review of the most common of the aminoacidurias.*

FANCONI'S SYNDROME

Brewer ED: The Fanconi syndrome: Clinical disorders. In Gonick HC, Buckalew VM Jr. (eds.): Renal Tubular Disorders. New York, Marcel Dekker, Inc., 1985, pp 475–544. *This is a superb, exhaustive review of the pathophysiology, clinical presentations, and principles of treatment of the multiple causes of the Fanconi syndrome.*

Roth KS, Foreman JW, Segal S: The Fanconi syndrome and mechanisms of tubular transport dysfunction. Kidney Int 20:705, 1981. *An excellent review of the pathogenetic mechanisms of this syndrome.*

BARTTER'S SYNDROME

Gill JR, Bartter FC: Evidence for a prostaglandin-independent defect in chloride reabsorption in the loop of Henle as a proximal cause of Bartter's syndrome. Am J Med 65:766, 1978. *This paper describes in vivo studies pinpointing the tubular site of the reabsorptive defect in Bartter's syndrome.*

Stein JH: The pathogenetic spectrum of Bartter's syndrome. Kidney Int 28:85, 1985. *This article reviews the variety of clinical presentations and current concepts of pathogenesis of this heterogeneous syndrome.*

RENAL TUBULAR ACIDOSIS

Arruda JAL, Kurtzman NA: Mechanisms and classification of deranged distal urinary acidification. Am J Physiol 239:F515, 1980. *This paper provides a critical and insightful examination of the causes of classic and generalized distal RTA.*

Cogan MG, Arieff AI: Sodium wasting, acidosis and hyperkalemia induced by methicillin interstitial nephritis. Evidence for selective distal tubular dysfunction. Am J Med 64:500, 1978. *This article describes the standard evaluation and treatment of a patient with marked renal salt wasting.*

Cogan MG, Rector FC Jr.: Acid-base disorders. In Brenner BM, Rector FC Jr. (eds.): The Kidney. 3rd ed. Philadelphia, W. B. Saunders Company, 1986, pp 457–518. *This chapter is a comprehensive review of acid-base homeostasis including the RTA's.*

Harrington JT, Cohen JJ: Metabolic acidosis. In Cohen JJ, Kassirer JP (eds.): Acid-Base. Boston, Little, Brown & Company, 1982, pp 121–226. *This chapter describes the pathophysiology and clinical manifestations of metabolic acidoses.*

Rector FC Jr., Cogan MG: The renal acidoses. Hosp Pract 15:99, 1980. *This article provides an introduction to the diagnosis and pathophysiology of the hyperchloremic metabolic acidoses.*

Schambelan M, Sebastian A, Biglieri EG: Prevalence, pathogenesis and functional significance of aldosterone deficiency in hyperkalemic patients with chronic renal insufficiency. Kidney Int 17:89, 1980. *This paper provides one of the most comprehensive reviews of the heterogeneous causes of generalized distal (Type IV) RTA.*

85 DIABETES AND THE KIDNEY

Bryan D. Myers

INCIDENCE AND PREVALENCE

Among the 15,000 patients entering chronic dialysis and kidney transplantation programs in the United States each year, the development of end-stage renal failure can be attributed to diabetes mellitus in approximately 25 per cent. Diabetic glomerulopathy, a complex disorder associated with a diffuse expansion of collagenous components of the glomerulus, is the predominant cause of the renal failure. The diabetic patient is also prone to other renal diseases such as pyelonephritis, papillary necrosis, and obstructive nephropathy that occasionally cause or exacerbate renal failure (Ch. 83 and 86). Diabetic patients with glomerulopathy are more susceptible to these associated renal disorders than are those who do not have glomerulopathy. Most victims of end-stage diabetic renal disease have longstanding type I diabetes, defined here as juvenile-onset and insulin-dependent diabetes (see Ch. 231). Patients with type II diabetes, characterized by a more advanced age of onset and not requiring insulin for control of hyperglycemia, are not spared from diabetic glomerulopathy and comprise a substantial minority among diabetic patients in end-stage renal failure programs.

CLINICAL AND LABORATORY FEATURES OF DIABETIC GLOMERULOPATHY

The natural history of diabetic glomerulopathy has been best documented in type I patients. Early abnormalities of glomerular function and structure appear to be invariable in all type I diabetics, but only 30 to 50 per cent will develop a progressive, proteinuric form of diabetic glomerulopathy. The evolution of the glomerulopathy in this subset of type I diabetics may be thought of as a continuum of glomerular injury divisible into three stages (Fig. 85–1). The first stage of occult glomerulopathy cannot be diagnosed by conventional laboratory techniques and lasts for approximately ten years. It is followed by two clinically evident stages of increasingly severe glomerular injury. Both are identified by the presence of proteinuria, while the milder, intermediate second stage

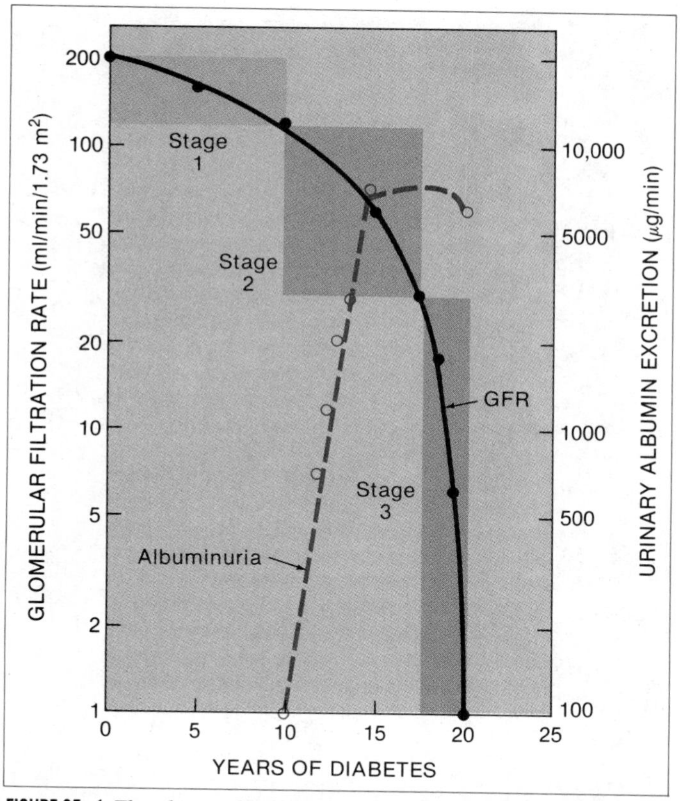

FIGURE 85–1. The glomerular filtration rate (●—●) and albumin excretion rate (○—○) have been plotted against time to chart a hypothetical course typical of diabetic glomerulopathy. The course of the disease has been divided into three stages, which are described in the text.

merges with the advanced third stage with the development of azotemia. The clinical and laboratory features of this prolonged and progressive glomerular disease will be reviewed by each stage separately.

Stage 1—Occult Diabetic Glomerulopathy

During this stage, the type I diabetic patient is devoid of clinical symptoms and signs of glomerulopathy. The most striking laboratory finding is a 20 to 40 per cent *elevation of the glomerular filtration rate* (GFR) above that found in age-matched normal controls. Although ultrastructural alterations can be demonstrated in the glomerular capillary wall and mesangium in the early stages of the disease, they do not appear to account for the observed glomerular hyperfiltration. Striking elevations of GFR in poorly controlled diabetic patients can be lowered within a matter of hours following restoration of normoglycemia. A parallel *increase in renal plasma flow*, measured by the clearance of *p*-aminohippurate, and also reversible by lowering blood glucose levels, points to a hemodynamic basis for the hyperfiltration. Notwithstanding the responsiveness of vasomotor regulation in the kidney to alterations in the metabolic milieu, GFR tends to remain elevated even with good metabolic control of the diabetic state. Not until proteinuria ushers in the intermediate second stage of the glomerulopathy does the GFR fall into the normal range.

The stage 1 glomerular hyperfiltration is accompanied by a subtle increase in the urinary albumin excretion rate that is not measurable by conventional techniques. Healthy adolescents and young adults excrete albumin in their urine at rates of up to 15 μg per minute. Many patients with type I diabetes of short duration excrete albumin at rates in excess of 15 μg per minute but less than the 100 μg per minute, which is roughly the threshold detectable by conventional techniques. This *"microalbuminuria"* is inferred to represent an increase in the transglomerular filtration of albumin rather than a decrease in tubular reabsorption of a normal, filtered albumin load. Microalbuminuria tends to be associated with the most striking degrees of hyperfiltration observed among type I diabetics, suggesting that it may also have a hemodynamic basis. It is exaggerated by exercise, which causes an increase in the intraluminal hydraulic pressure of the glomerular capillaries, and is blunted, although not abolished, by restoration of normoglycemia.

Early in the course of type I diabetes there is a consistent *increase in kidney size*. Hyperfiltration, renal hyperemia and enlargement, and microalbuminuria are all characteristic of this early occult stage, but hypertension, an important complication of diabetic glomerulopathy, is not prevalent. The incidence of hypertension in large diabetic populations without proteinuria is no different from that in nondiabetic populations.

Stage 2—Intermediate Diabetic Glomerulopathy

This stage is heralded by the development of persistent, easily measurable proteinuria. Once proteinuria has become manifest its magnitude tends to reflect the rate of deterioration of glomerular capillary wall function that typifies the second stage of diabetic glomerulopathy. As indicated in Figure 85–1, proteinuria tends to increase exponentially with time and to be related inversely to GFR.

After several years of proteinuria, urinary losses reach nephrotic proportions (> 3.5 grams per 24 hours) and the patient will frequently become edematous. The proteinuria is also paralleled by an increasing prevalence of hypertension. Thus stage 2, intermediate diabetic glomerulopathy, is characterized by *increasing proteinuria, declining GFR*, and the development of *hypertension* and *edema*.

The proteinuria of stage 2 diabetic glomerulopathy has no pathognomonic characteristics, but several features distinguish it from other glomerular diseases: (1) From the onset of the second stage, immunoglobulins and other large plasma proteins are excreted in the urine in large quantities along with albumin, signifying an early loss of barrier size-selectivity in this disorder. (2) Persistent and ultimately massive urinary losses of plasma proteins in stage 2 diabetic glomerulopathy are rarely accompanied by hypoproteinemia. Inasmuch as the conventional definition of the nephrotic syndrome requires hypoproteinemia in addition to massive proteinuria and edema, stage 2 diabetic glomerulopathy does not truly exemplify the nephrotic syndrome. An important role in edema formation is ascribed to reduction of plasma oncotic pressure in patients with the nephrotic syndrome as classically defined; the absence of hypoproteinemia, and hence the maintenance of normal plasma oncotic pressure, in stage 2 diabetic glomerulopathy implicates alternate mechanisms of edema formation. (3) Neither can edema formation, or, for that matter, hypertension, be related to a stimulated renin-angiotensin-aldosterone system. To the contrary, diabetic glomerulopathy is usually associated with an inability to cleave the inactive precursor of renin, with the result that concentrations of active renin in plasma are low and angiotensin production is depressed. Plasma concentration and urinary excretion rate of aldosterone tend also to be depressed, despite the presence of edema. In fact, proteinuric diabetic glomerulopathy probably constitutes the commonest example of hyporeninemic hypoaldosteronism, and such patients not infrequently exhibit the syndrome of generalized distal type IV renal tubular acidosis (see Ch. 84). Thus, both the mechanism by which edema is formed and the basis for the widespread prevalence of hypertension in stage 2 diabetic glomerulopathy remain obscure.

Stage 3—Advanced Diabetic Glomerulopathy

The third, advanced stage represents the terminal 2 or 3 years of what is typically a 20- to 25-year process. Its onset is delineated by the development of *azotemia*. Retention of urea, creatinine, and other nitrogenous compounds will generally become apparent once the GFR has declined to less than one third of normal levels. As with the intermediate stage that precedes it, GFR in the third and terminal stage of diabetic glomerulopathy has been observed to decline at rates approaching 1 ml per minute per month. Thus in the prototypical case illustrated in Figure 85–1, GFR is predicted to decline from a normal value approximating 120 ml per minute at the onset of stage 2 to zero at the end of stage 3 over a period of 10 years. Not only does GFR decline irrevocably, resulting in progressive azotemia but *edema* and *hypertension* tend to worsen in the third and final stage of the disease. Similarly, *proteinuria* continues to be massive and *hypoproteinemia* finally results. Although reduced plasma protein concentration and the lowered GFR serve to lower the filtered protein load, urinary protein excretion rate is maintained at massive levels, reflecting increasing leakiness of the glomerular capillary wall to large plasma proteins.

By the time the third, advanced stage of diabetic glomerulopathy is reached, *widespread microangiopathy* involving the retinae and peripheral nerves is invariable. Although its extent varies among patients, retinopathy is frequently associated with visual impairment sufficient to result in functional blindness. The effects of peripheral and more particularly of autonomic neuropathy may be equally devastating. This is particularly true when autonomic neuropathy results in partial paresis of the bladder. Progressive urinary retention may exacerbate renal insufficiency in stage 3 glomerulopathy by resulting in a superimposed obstructive nephropathy. Obstructive nephropathy in turn may predispose the already vulnerable patient to ascending pyelonephritis and/or ischemic papillary necrosis, thereby compromising renal function even further. (For more detailed discussion of obstructive nephropathy, see Ch. 83.)

Given the prolonged duration of diabetes mellitus, by the time stage 3 glomerulopathy is reached many patients will be 40 years of age or more, an age group in which atherosclerosis, accelerated in part by the presence of longstanding hypertension, will adversely affect several organ systems. Coronary artery disease, cerebrovascular disease and stroke, and peripheral vascular disease are all common in the third stage of diabetic glomerulopathy, and account collectively for the majority of fatalities. The eventual need for substitution therapy in end-stage renal failure programs occurs in a setting, therefore, in which serious extrarenal complications are prevalent and impair the effectiveness of rehabilitation generally achieved by such therapy.

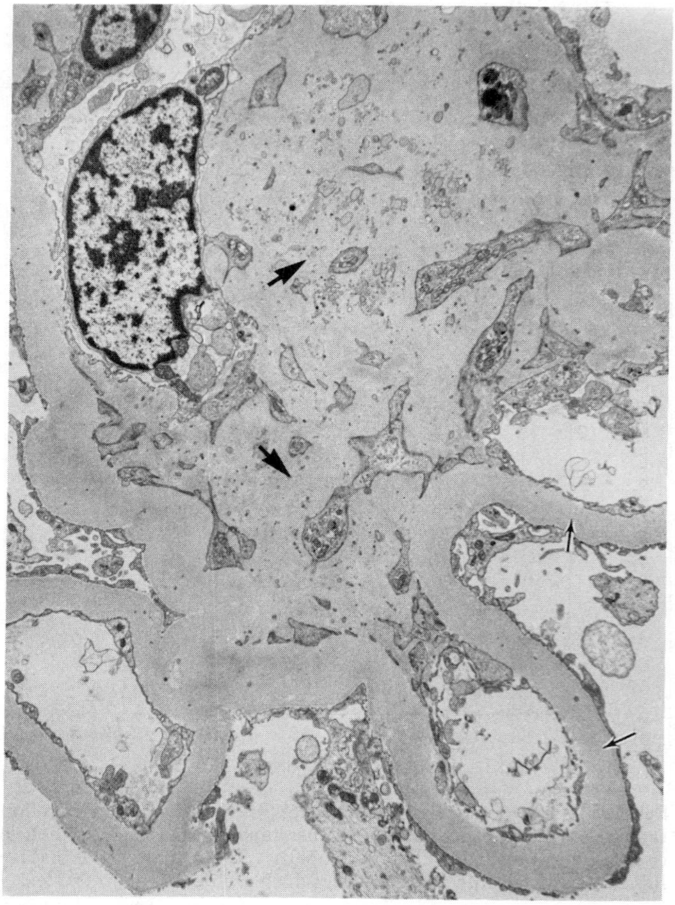

FIGURE 85–2. Electron photomicrograph of a portion of a glomerulus from a patient with proteinuric, diabetic glomerulopathy (magnification × 5000). A striking increase in collagenous components has resulted in (1) widening of the basement membrane of peripheral capillary loops (*small arrows*), and (2) expansion of the matrix of the glomerular mesangium (*large arrows*). The latter alteration is responsible for compressing and ultimately obliterating the glomerular capillary network.

DIAGNOSIS

Proteinuria due to diabetic glomerulopathy is accompanied by typical changes of glomerular histopathology. These include a striking accumulation of matrix components of the mesangium and a widening of the glomerular capillary wall due to a thickened glomerular basement membrane. The former change results in an acellular expansion of the mesangium, which is most commonly diffuse in nature and hence termed diffuse intercapillary glomerulosclerosis. Not infrequently mesangial matrix accumulation occurs in a segmental fashion, resulting in the formation of acellular spherical nodules at the center of single or multiple peripheral glomerular lobules (Fig. 85–2), referred to as nodular glomerulosclerosis. A nodular accumulation of mesangial matrix material, indistinguishable from that observed in diabetic subjects, has been associated with dysproteinemia, notably that associated with a monoclonal proliferation of B lymphocytes or plasma cells. Provided that the latter entity is excluded, however, the finding of diffuse or nodular glomerulosclerosis in a proteinuric diabetic subject is diagnostic of diabetic glomerulopathy.

A diagnosis of diabetic glomerulopathy can be made with a high degree of certainty in a proteinuric diabetic patient, without resort to biopsy, which carries a finite risk for the patient. Background and proliferative retinopathy, for example, are correlated strongly with the presence of diffuse or nodular glomerulosclerosis in a proteinuric diabetic. The diagnostic probability can be further strengthened by using noninvasive imaging techniques, such as ultrasonography or nephrotomography, to demonstrate kidney enlargement. Nephrotoxic acute renal failure caused by contrast agents occurs more commonly in patients with diabetic glomerulopathy than in any other patient category. For this reason nephrotomography (or other radiologic procedures) should be performed without the use of contrast agents whenever possible. The coexistence of retinopathy and nephromegaly in diabetic patients with proteinuria is so constant that the performance of a diagnostic renal biopsy need be considered only when these factors are absent, particularly when the duration of diabetes is less than 10 years. In these circumstances, a renal biopsy has frequently revealed other, and presumably unrelated, primary glomerulopathies such as minimal change nephropathy, membranous glomerulopathy, and proliferative glomerulonephritis (Ch. 81).

PATHOGENESIS AND PATHOPHYSIOLOGY

The diabetic state per se is the presumed forerunner of glomerulopathy. Glomerular basement membrane widening and increased mesangial matrix, the earliest ultrastructural markers of glomerulopathy, are absent at the onset and can be detected only after some years of type I diabetes. An identical sequence has been observed in experimental diabetes induced in a variety of mammalian species with the use of pancreatic beta cell toxins or pancreatectomy.

As in humans, GFR is substantially elevated in the rat with experimental diabetes of short duration. The early hyperfiltration is a consequence of altered vasomotion in the major resistance vessels of the renal cortex. Dilatation of the efferent and especially the afferent glomerular arterioles results in an elevation of glomerular capillary perfusion rate and pressure. By contrast, those determinants of GFR that are intrinsic to the glomerular capillary wall, namely hydraulic conductivity and the surface area available for filtration, are unaltered. Thus hyperfiltration early in the course of diabetes appears to have a purely hemodynamic basis. It remains to be determined which factor or factors associated with the diabetic state are responsible for the deranged renal vasoregulation. Hyperglycemia per se, or elevated levels of vasodilator glucoregulatory hormones such as glucagon and growth hormone, may be implicated. Abnormalities of other hormonal regulators of glomerular perfusion rate and pressure have also been identified. Thus diminished production and activity of angiotensin II, but increased production of vasodilator prostaglandins, by glomerular cells isolated from diabetic rats point to an imbalance in favor of local vasodilatation of renal cortical microvessels. Experimental maneuvers that further increase glomerular overperfusion in the diabetic rat, including surgical reduction of renal mass or feeding a high-protein diet, are followed by heavier proteinuria and more severe glomerulosclerosis than observed in diabetic rats with a normal complement of nephrons and fed conventional rat chow. Conversely, measures that prevent glomerular hyperemia and hypertension—such as partial constriction of the renal artery with a clip, the administration of angiotensin-converting enzyme inhibitor, or dietary protein restriction—largely prevent the development of proteinuria as well as the histopathologic damage observed in diabetic rats not so protected. These findings are taken to indicate that hemodynamic factors serve as a stimulus for an ensuing accumulation of mesangial matrix components and, hence, subsequent glomerulosclerosis.

Whether or not glomerular capillary hypertension and hyperperfusion are unique causes of an accumulation of mesangial matrix components, there seems little doubt that this lesion is responsible for the progressive reduction of GFR that typifies the second and third stages of clinical diabetic glomerulopathy. As shown in Figure 85–2, expansion of the mesangial matrix occurs at the expense of the surrounding glomerular capillary loops, with progressive reduction of the surface area available for filtration. By the time the end of the third stage of diabetic glomerulopathy has been reached, the mesangium will have encroached upon most glomerular capillary loops to the point that they have become almost totally obliterated.

The process by which the glomerular basement membrane becomes widened has been presumed to be responsible for the alteration in the glomerular capillary wall, causing it to become permeable to large plasma proteins. Surprisingly, however, there is no correlation whatsoever between glomerular basement membrane width and proteinuria. While the structural basis of proteinuria remains obscure, the functional nature of the disturbance in glomerular permselectivity has been elucidated by the use of in vivo physiologic techniques in which the clearance of probe filtration markers of graded size has been used to define the size-selective properties of the glomerular filter. One such study has revealed that proteinuria in diabetic glomerulopathy can be accounted for by the development within the glomerular capillary wall of a subpopulation of enlarged, protein-permeable pores. In contradistinction to the diffuse widening of the basement membrane seen by electron microscopy (Fig. 85–2), the enlarged pores can be estimated to be few in number and to behave as isolated defects in the glomerular capillary wall.

PROGNOSIS AND TREATMENT

The profound loss of filtering surface area and the disruption of glomerular membrane pore structure that underlie stage 2 and 3 glomerulopathy in diabetics are unlikely to be reversible. Attempts to maintain blood glucose in such patients in a normal range have failed to prevent or attenuate the progression of renal insufficiency. Meticulous control of hypertension, however, may slow the rate of decline of GFR. Together with antihypertensive therapy, attention to and correction of coexistent cardiac failure, obstructive nephropathy, pyelonephritis, and other events that may lower GFR independently of the glomerulopathy represent the mainstay of therapy of proteinuric glomerulopathy.

On the basis of our current understanding of the pathophysiology and pathogenesis of diabetic glomerulopathy, a strong case can be made for trying to prevent the advent of progressive stage 2 disease by correcting glomerular overperfusion during the first decade of diabetes. The subset of patients most likely to benefit from early, protective therapy is that with microalbuminuria (50 to 200 μg per minute) and an elevated GFR, particularly when associated with ophthalmoscopic evidence of diabetic retinopathy. Measures that are likely to lower glomerular perfusion rate and pressure include restoration of euglycemia by custom-tailored insulin replacement regimens and dietary protein restriction. The rationale for protective therapy is based on purely theoretic considerations, however. Prolonged and carefully controlled trials have yet to be conducted to confirm the efficacy and safety of such measures.

Once end-stage renal failure has supervened, the diabetic patient should be referred for treatment to a dialysis and/or transplantation center (Ch. 79 and 80). Many diabetic patients respond favorably to and enjoy a good quality of life with these modalities of treatment. With special attention to the unique problems of the diabetic patient with renal failure, the survival rates achieved with chronic hemodialysis or with chronic ambulatory peritoneal dialysis, or following renal transplantation, are today approaching those achieved for nondiabetic patients.

Hostetter TH, Rennke HG, Brenner BM: The case for intrarenal hypertension in the initiation and progression of diabetic and other glomerulopathies. Am J Med 72:375, 1982. *A lucid review of the pathophysiology of diabetic glomerulopathy citing virtually every important reference to this subject.*

Hostetter TH, Troy JL, Brenner BM: Glomerular hemodynamics in experimental diabetes mellitus. Kidney Int 19:410, 1981. *An elegant micropuncture study demonstrating the hemodynamic basis for glomerular hyperfiltration in early experimental rat diabetes.*

Luetscher JA, Kraemer FB, Wilson DM: Increased plasma inactive renin in diabetes mellitus. N Engl J Med 312:1412, 1985. *The abnormalities in the renin-angiotensin system in diabetic glomerulopathy are clearly delineated.*

Mauer SM, Steffes MW, Ellis EN, et al.: Structural-functional relationships in diabetic nephropathy. J Clin Invest 74:1143, 1984. *A review of the authors' use of electron microscopy and elegant morphometric techniques to chart the evolution and progression of diabetic glomerulopathy.*

Myers BD, Winetz JA, Chui F, et al.: Mechanisms of proteinuria in diabetic nephropathy: A study of glomerular barrier function. Kidney Int 21:96, 1982. *Modern physiologic techniques and mathematical modeling are used to describe the glomerular capillary wall as an ultrafiltration membrane; the defect in the glomerular filter of proteinuric diabetics is elucidated.*

Omachi R: The pathogenesis and prevention of diabetic nephropathy. West J Med 145:222, 1986. *This summary of a recent medical grand rounds offers a review of the topic with 57 references.*

Viberti GC, Bilous RW, Mackintosh D, et al.: Monitoring glomerular function in diabetic nephropathy. Am J Med 74:256, 1983. *A careful prospective study of the effects of metabolic control on proteinuric glomerulopathy. Its message is pessimistic.*

Zatz R, Meyer TW, Rennke HG, et al.: Predominance of hemodynamic rather than metabolic factors in the pathogenesis of diabetic glomerulopathy. Proc Natl Acad Sci USA 82:5963, 1985. *The protective effect of lowering glomerular pressures and flows on sclerosing diabetic glomerulopathy is well documented.*

86 URINARY TRACT INFECTIONS AND PYELONEPHRITIS

Vincent T. Andriole

DEFINITION

Urinary tract infection refers to both microbial colonization of the urine and tissue invasion of any structure of the urinary tract. Bacteria are most commonly responsible, although yeast, fungi, and viruses may produce urinary infection. Urinary tract infections may be relatively mild, such as the "honeymoon cystitis" syndrome, or catastrophic, such as a perinephric abscess in a diabetic. Urinary tract infections are often categorized by the site of infection, which is convenient for the purpose of discussion. However, it is often not possible to diagnose the various types of infections on clinical grounds alone.

Significant bacteriuria refers to sufficient numbers of bacteria in the urine to denote active infection rather than contamination. A bacteria count over 100,000 organisms per milliliter in a fresh "clean-catch" midstream specimen is a reliable indicator of active urinary tract infection but does not indicate whether the infection is cystitis or pyelonephritis. In addition, women with acute cystitis may have $>10^3$ but $<10^5$ bacteria per milliliter in midstream urine cultures.

Asymptomatic bacteriuria refers to large numbers of bacteria in the urine without producing symptoms. Dysuria and frequency in the absence of significant bacteriuria are common problems among young women. This entity has been called the *acute urethral syndrome* and is often caused by *Chlamydia trachomatis*.

Cystitis and *acute pyelonephritis* are symptomatic infections of the bladder and kidney, respectively. *Perinephric and renal abscesses*, uncommon complications of urinary infections, usually occur in (1) urinary tract obstruction, (2) bacteremia, particularly staphylococcal or candidal bacteremia, and (3) immunocompromised individuals, particularly diabetics.

Complicated infections refer to bacteriuria in association with structural or neurologic defects in the voiding mechanism (vesicoureteral reflux, neurogenic bladder), foreign bodies (stones or indwelling catheter), or intrinsic renal disease (diabetic nephropathy or polycystic renal disease).

Chronic pyelonephritis refers to the pathologic and radiologic findings of chronic cortical scarring, tubulointerstitial damage, and deformity of the underlying calix. Chronic bacterial pyelonephritis can be *active*, which occurs in patients with persistent *complicated* infection, or *inactive*, which consists of focal sterile scars of a past infection. Recurrent infection can result in multiple scars combined with active foci of infection. In the absence of obstruction, reflux, foreign bodies, or an immunocompromised host (notably the diabetic patient), urinary tract infections rarely cause the shrunken, scarred kidneys of end-stage chronic pyelonephritis.

Other disease states can produce renal lesions that mimic "chronic pyelonephritis." Identical characteristics can be observed, in the absence of infection, in patients who suffered from severe vesicoureteral reflux in childhood. This entity, *reflux nephropathy*, refers to the radiographic triad of intrarenal reflux and vesicoureteral reflux, scarring, and loss of parenchymal mass in the absence of other obstructive lesions and can ultimately lead to end-stage renal failure with scarred, shrunken kidneys. "Reflux nephropathy" may result from "autoimmune" renal damage rather than bacterial infection of the kidney. Nevertheless, the combination of recurrent infection and reflux nephropathy can also result in chronic pyelonephritis. *Analgesic nephropathy* may produce papillary necrosis and may also mimic bacterial pyelonephritis on radiography.

PATHOGENESIS

The normal urinary tract is free of bacteria except for some organisms normally present near the external meatus and some staphylococci and diphtheroids normally found in the distal urethra. Urine, as a culture medium, generally supports bacterial multiplication. However, high concentrations of urea and hyperosmolality (which are present in the renal medulla), an acid pH, and urinary organic acid are generally unfavorable to bacterial growth. In addition, the dynamics of the urinary flow (washout) and antibacterial properties of the lining membrane of the urinary tract and of the vaginal and periurethral epithelial cells appear to be important defense mechanisms.

Urinary tract infections result most commonly from ascending transurethral invasion of the bladder by pathogenic gram-negative aerobic bacilli normally present in the large bowel and perineum, particularly of women. Sequentially, bacteria migrate from the anus to the periurethral area and along the urethra into the bladder, where infections occur if the organisms become established. This pathogenic mechanism helps explain the higher rate of urinary tract infection in women, whose urethras are shorter than those of men, and the marked frequency of the urinary infection associated with instrumentation of the urethra and the bladder.

Other pathways from the large bowel to the urinary passages and kidneys include the hematogenous and lymphatic routes. The hematogenous route, a less common mechanism for renal infection, generally, but not always, requires antecedent structural damage to the kidney. Staphylococcal bacteremia can produce multiple microabscesses in the kidney (*renal carbuncle*). Disseminated *Candida albicans* infections in the immunocompromised host can involve the kidney. Finally, septic emboli, particularly in the setting of bacterial endocarditis, represent a classic mode for hematogenously disseminated infection of the kidney.

The renal medulla, because of its unique hypertonicity, is much more susceptible to infection than the cortex. In experimental pyelonephritis, as few as 10 to 100 *Escherichia coli* may produce infection in the medulla, whereas 100,000 are required to infect the cortex. The increased susceptibility of the medulla is thought to be due to impaired leukocyte mobilization and phagocytosis in the hypertonic environment.

Microbial virulence factors are also important in the pathogenesis of symptomatic urinary infections. *E. coli* strains isolated from patients with pyelonephritis are more likely to (1) possess large amounts of K (capsular) antigen, (2) adhere in larger numbers to human urinary epithelial cells, and (3) possess surface pili, than are strains found in asymptomatic bacteriuria. The virulence of *Proteus* species may be related to their urease content and ammonia production.

CLINICAL MANIFESTATIONS

The symptoms of acute urinary tract infections are varied and include frequency, dysuria, burning pain on urination, suprapubic discomfort, passage of cloudy and occasionally blood-tinged urine, fever, costovertebral angle tenderness or flank pain, and rigors. Urinary tract symptoms, particularly dysuria, occur in 20 per cent of women each year, although only half seek medical attention. Approximately equal numbers of these women will have either the acute urethral syndrome (urethritis), bladder bacteriuria (cystitis), or renal infection.

In general, clinical grounds form an uncertain basis for separating patients with the acute urethral syndrome from those with either bladder or renal bacteriuria because frequency, burning, and suprapubic pain are found approximately equally in all three groups of patients. Costovertebral angle tenderness and fever may be present as frequently in patients with the acute urethral syndrome as in those with renal bacteriuria. Rigors occur almost equally (15 per cent) in patients with the acute urethral syndrome and those with cystitis. Similarly, tenderness in the region of one or both kidneys occurs not infrequently in lower urinary tract infections. However, sudden fever to 38.9° to 40.6°C, shaking chills, aching costovertebral or flank pain, and symptoms of sepsis are more characteristic of acute pyelonephritis than of cystitis or urethritis.

Laboratory tests show a polymorphonuclear leukocytosis in both cystitis and pyelonephritis. Pyuria is seen in urethritis, cystitis, and pyelonephritis, but white blood cell casts are more typical of pyelonephritis. Stain of the sediment and urine cultures reveal numerous bacteria, usually gram-negative bacilli. Cultures of blood may also be positive in some cases of pyelonephritis. A simple but convenient way of identifying infection of the urinary tract is by examining the urine (see below): The microscopic presence of bacteria in the urine generally indicates more than 100,000 colonies per milliliter of urine. However, the microscopic absence of bacteria does not exclude the diagnosis of urinary infection.

Impaired renal function or acute hypertension is rarely seen in acute pyelonephritis, but renal concentrating ability may be impaired. Also, subclinical forms of acute pyelonephritis may occur because tests that differentiate "upper" (kidney) from "lower" (bladder) infection may indicate the presence of renal infection in the absence of flank pain or fever. However, the only reliable tests, ureteral catheterization and bladder washout, are considered to be research maneuvers. Search for antibody-coated bacteria in the urine as a marker of renal bacteriuria may be performed, but the sensitivity and specificity of this test are not optimal. Pyelonephritis at times presents with symptoms that do not point to the urinary tract. Some patients may have only backache without demonstrable renal tenderness. Others have upper or lower abdominal pain together with symptoms of disturbed gastrointestinal function. Some complain only of general fatigue.

In the absence of obstructive lesions of the urinary tract or host immunocompromise, as in diabetics, upper or lower urinary tract infections are generally self-limited, lasting 10 to 14 days. When obstruction or host immunocompromise is present, pyelonephritis may be complicated by papillary necrosis, perinephric abscess, or renal carbuncle. These complications should be suspected when persistent flank pain, fever, and leukocytosis are unresponsive to otherwise adequate chemotherapy (see below).

Acute urinary tract infection complicated by pyelonephritis may occur in patients subjected to urethral instrumentation, particularly long-term indwelling catheters. Sepsis from pyelonephritis is a major cause of death in individuals having neurologic disorders requiring long-term indwelling catheters.

DIAGNOSIS

Microscopic Methods

Rapid diagnostic methods are available either (1) by preparation of a Gram's stain of either centrifuged or uncentrifuged urine and examination with an oil immersion lens or (2) by study of either centrifuged or uncentrifuged urine, employing the high-dry objective under reduced light, with or without methylene blue stain. The presence of any bacteria on Gram's stain of centrifuged urine correlates best (97 per cent) with quantitative culture (100,000 bacteria per milliliter of urine). Examination of the unstained sediment for the presence of any bacteria is also very helpful and can be done during routine examination for formed elements. Pyuria, arbitrarily defined as ten or more leukocytes per high-power field in the centrifuged specimen, can also be detected by the leukocyte esterase dipstick test. The presence of pyuria in a midstream urine sample suggests the likelihood of a urinary tract infection. Some erythrocytes may be seen in the urine, and gross hematuria may occur when inflammation in the bladder is intense. Proteinuria is not common in urinary infections, but in fulminant pyelonephritis, as in other severe acute interstitial nephritides, significant degrees of proteinuria may occur transiently.

Significant Bacteriuria

The concept of "significant bacteriuria" was introduced to distinguish between those bacteria that actually multiply in the urine and bacteria that are contaminants. This distinction can be made by knowledge of the site and manner in which the urine is collected from the patient and by enumeration of the number of organisms present in the sample. The criterion of 100,000 or more organisms per milliliter of urine for the diagnosis of significant bacteriuria is an excellent operational definition when the clear-voided method is used, in both males and females, to collect specimens that are processed promptly. However, bacterial counts lower than 100,000 colonies per milliliter may occur in patients with true bacteriuria. Specifically, some women with acute bacterial cystitis, who present with dysuria and frequency (the acute urethral syndrome), may have as few as 100 bacteria per milliliter of urine. Isolation of multiple species from the urine usually indicates contamination, especially in the asymptomatic person.

Urine collected by suprapubic aspiration or bladder catheterization is less likely to be contaminated. In this instance, bacterial counts of fewer than 100,000 organisms per milliliter are likely to be significant.

Bacteriologic Findings

The species of bacteria most likely to be recovered from individuals with bacteriuria depends upon prior history of infection, prior antimicrobial therapy, hospitalization, and instrumentation of the urinary tract. Enterobacteriaceae are the most common organisms identified. *E. coli* accounts for more than 80 per cent of all species recovered in uncomplicated cases, whereas *Proteus*, *Klebsiella*, *Enterobacter*, *Pseudomonas*, enterococci, and staphylococci are more often found in patients who have had previous infection or instrumentation. Occasionally, *Serratia marcescens*, *Acinetobacter*, *Candida albicans*, and *Cryptococcus neoformans* may produce infection of the urinary tract in diabetics and in immunosuppressed or corticosteroid-treated patients. Coliforms are also the most common organisms responsible for the acute urethral syndrome in women who have fewer than 10^5 bacteria per milliliter of urine, although *Staphylococcus saprophyticus* and *Chlamydia trachomatis* are responsible for some cases. Patients with the acute urethral syndrome caused by *Chlamydia trachomatis* have pyuria but sterile bladder urine when cultured with standard bacteriologic media.

Anaerobes are commonly present in the distal urethra and the vagina and are abundant in the gut, but they rarely produce urinary tract infection. Suprapubic aspiration of urine or examination of tissues is needed to prove anaerobic infections. When responsible, anaerobes are usually associated with complicated, longstanding infections.

Radiology

Radiographic evaluation of the urinary tract is undertaken to detect correctable lesions that may contribute to the severity or recurrence of urinary tract infections. Evaluation is indicated in men with any type of urinary tract infection or in instances of documented bacteremia. In women, urography is not indicated unless a complication, such as papillary necrosis, perinephric abscess, renal carbuncle, or tumor, is suspected because the patient is unresponsive to otherwise adequate chemotherapy.

EPIDEMIOLOGY AND NATURAL HISTORY

Bacteriuria in the newborn population has been difficult to study because of problems inherent in urine collection. Cultures of urine obtained by bladder puncture suggest an incidence of 1 to 2 per cent. Infection of the urinary tract in this age group may be part of a generalized, life-threatening gram-negative sepsis and is more common in boys than girls. Symptomatic urinary infections are more prevalent among girls in preschool years and are often associated with obstructive or neurogenic lesions. Urologic investigation is valuable in this age group. *Urologic evaluation is mandatory in males of any age because of the high frequency of structural abnormalities found* (valves, malformation, and obstructive and neurogenic lesions).

The incidence of bacteriuria among school girls is 1 to 2 per cent; it is only 0.03 per cent in boys of the same age. The incidence of bacteriuria in females rises about 1 per cent per decade.

Urinary infection is common after marriage. The pathogenesis of the "honeymoon cystitis" syndrome remains unclear. Physical factors associated with sexual activity in previously sexually nonactive women may play a prominent role. Many patients with "honeymoon cystitis" (up to 50 per cent) will have dysuria due to local irritation rather than infection, and this should be clearly differentiated by culture.

Bacteriuria of pregnancy varies from 2 to 6 per cent, depending upon age, parity, and socioeconomic group. Acute symptomatic pyelonephritis will develop later in pregnancy in approximately 20 per cent of these women. However, there is no evidence that isolated episodes of pyelonephritis in pregnant women lead to chronic urinary tract infections after these women cease childbearing activities. Early detection and treatment of bacteriuria in pregnancy will prevent the emergence of symptomatic infection.

Elderly women may have frequencies of bacteriuria as high as 10 per cent; this rate may increase in hospitalized patients, particularly diabetics. Bacteriuria in the male begins to appear in "prostate years" and is often initiated by instrumentation.

Role of Instrumentation

Bacteriuria persists in 1 to 2 per cent of relatively healthy individuals following a single catheterization; the risk is higher in the debilitated patient and in males with prostatic obstruction. With open indwelling catheter drainage, bacterial colonization exceeds 90 per cent within three to four days. This may lead to life-threatening pyelonephritis and gram-negative sepsis. Fortunately, it is largely preventable by (1) careful criteria for catheterization and (2) use of aseptic closed drainage. The catheter should be removed as soon as it is no longer needed.

Intermittent self-catheterization coupled with abdominal pressure may be of benefit in patients with neurogenic bladders and may result in minimal urinary tract infections.

TREATMENT

The goal of treatment is to eradicate bacteria from the urinary tract in order to relieve symptoms, prevent renal damage, and diminish the likelihood of spread of infections to other sites. Prophylaxis is used to prevent recurrent symptomatic infection. Suppression, although rarely effective, is used to diminish the number of bacteria in the urine or tissue. Indications for therapy depend on the potential of infection to give rise to symptoms or damage to the urinary tract and the likelihood that treatment will be effective (Fig. 86–1).

Asymptomatic Bacteriuria

Asymptomatic bacteriuria should probably not be treated except in those patients who are at high risk of developing symptomatic infections. Thus, treatment of asymptomatic bacteriuria is indicated in pregnant patients to prevent symptomatic illness in the third trimester; in patients who may have major predisposing factors to renal disease, such as diabetic or polycystic kidneys, or who have anatomic or neurologic abnormalities; and in patients who are immunocompromised or who will undergo urologic manipulation. If the treatment fails to eradicate asymptomatic infections in such individuals, further treatment should be reserved for acute symptomatic episodes. In contrast, asymptomatic bacteriuria in females should not be treated in the absence of underlying structural or neurologic lesions, since the likelihood that renal damage will occur is slight. Furthermore, short courses of therapy, when effective, are commonly followed by reinfection. In addition, asymptomatic bacteriuria in patients with indwelling catheter and in the very elderly or nonambulatory patients should not be treated, because the toxicity and expense of therapy may outweigh the risk of disease.

Symptomatic Urinary Tract Infection

Acute uncomplicated episodes of symptomatic bacteriuria localized to the lower urinary tract (bladder or urethra) can be treated effectively with oral single-dose therapy, either amoxicillin, 3 grams, or co-trimoxazole (trimethoprim, 0.32 gram, plus sulfamethoxazole, 1.6 grams), two double-strength tablets. Single-dose therapy will usually fail to eradicate either renal bacteriuria or complicated infections. In addition, single-dose therapy is more effective in suburban compared with inner-city women with cystitis and in women less than 25 years of age compared with women over 40 years of age. Higher cure rates may be achieved in inner-city or older women with trimethoprim, 0.16 gram, plus sulfamethoxazole, 0.8 gram, twice daily for three days. Symptomatic urethritis caused by *Chlamydia trachomatis* should respond to oral doxycycline (100 mg twice daily) or tetracycline (500 mg four times daily) for seven days.

Pyelonephritis requires a 7- to 14-day or longer course of therapy. Complicated infections in which obstruction or a foreign body is not removed may not respond to such a course. Hematogenous pyelonephritis requires specific therapy directed at the invading organism.

The choice of an oral or parenteral agent depends upon the severity of the infection and the patient's ability to take the oral agent. Drugs are selected on the basis of cost, side effects, and antibacterial spectrum. Antimicrobial susceptibility tests should be used to guide therapy of recurrent episodes. Effective oral agents include sulfonamides, tetracyclines, ampicillin, amoxicillin, cinoxacin, cephalosporins, co-trimoxazole, trimethoprim, and nitrofurantoin. The last three drugs are useful in recurrent infections, because emergence of resistant strains occurs infrequently.

The initial attack of urinary tract infection is usually due to *E. coli*, which is sensitive to most antimicrobial agents and therefore may be treated "blindly" with the agents described above with equal success. However, the widespread use of these agents for other infections has decreased their previous reliability. For example, approximately 40 per cent of *E. coli*, including those that are community acquired, are now resistant to ampicillin.

Microscopic examination of urine and urine cultures have been the mainstay for accurate diagnosis of urinary tract infections. Pretreatment urine cultures are probably not essential, however, and are not cost effective in selected young women with acute dysuria and pyuria, in whom the probability of uncomplicated bacterial cystitis is high. These patients respond to short-course empiric therapy. Urine cultures can be reserved for those in whom therapy has failed. In contrast, pretreatment urine cultures should be obtained in symptomatic infants, children, men, and the elderly; patients with suspected pyelonephritis or complicated infection; patients with relapsing infections; those with *symptomatic* catheter- or instrument-associated nosocomial infection; and pregnant women to detect covert bacteriuria of pregnancy.

When therapy is successful, bacteriuria should disappear within 24 hours even if pyuria and symptoms continue. A

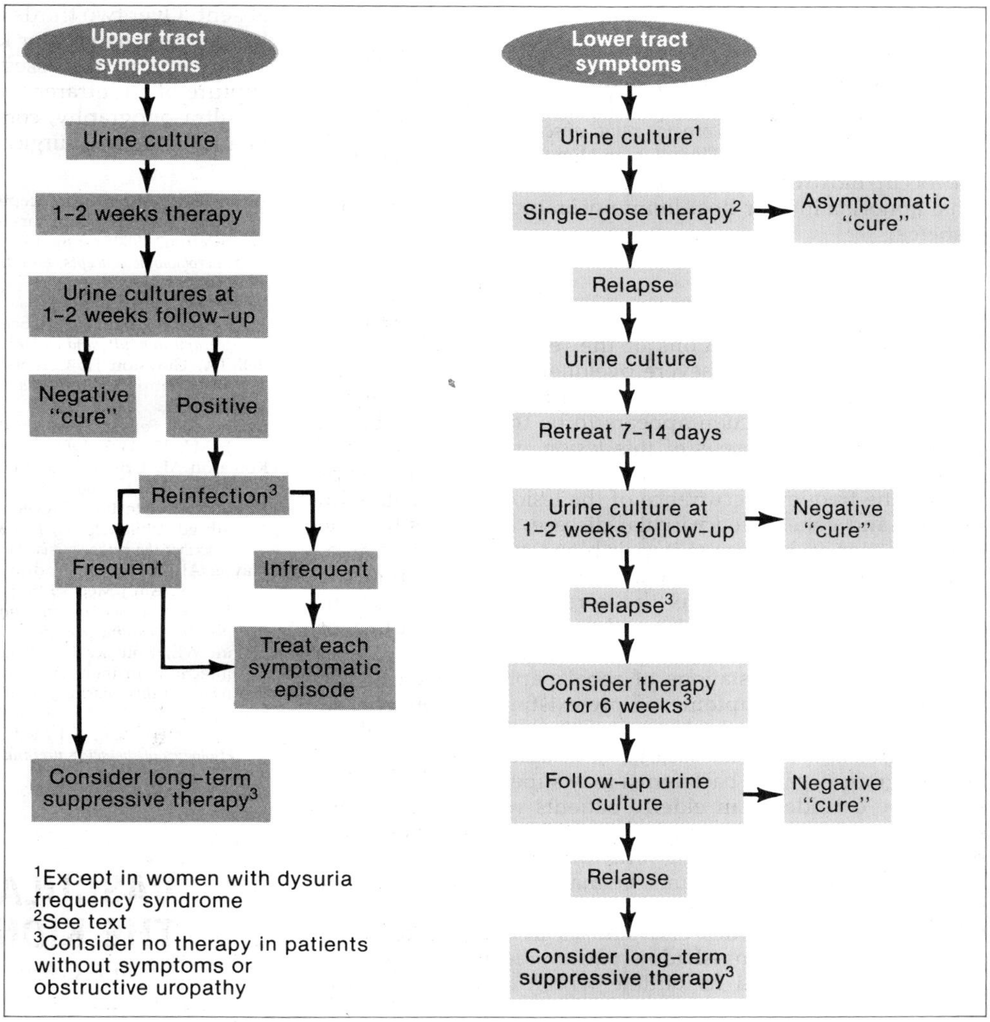

FIGURE 86–1. Management of urinary infections.

repeat urine culture should be obtained after 72 hours of treatment in those patients who have had a pretreatment culture. A positive culture at this time denotes treatment failure. It is important to recognize bacteriologic failure early and to change to another drug. Parenteral agents, such as ampicillin, a cephalosporin, or an aminoglycoside, may be required in some instances or when the patient is too ill to receive an oral agent. A follow-up culture one week after the completion of antimicrobial therapy is recommended to document a cure.

Some authors recommend routine follow-up cultures several times over the ensuing year to detect recurrent bacteriuria, but this practice is prohibitively expensive and difficult to justify on medical grounds in asymptomatic patients.

Recurrent Infections

Recurrence of infection in the few weeks after treatment is usually due to persistence of the same focus, whereas later recurrence, particularly in females, is more often a result of reinfection. Frequent recurrent infections may be managed either by close follow-up and treatment of each episode or by prophylaxis with nitrofurantoin, trimethoprim, or co-trimoxazole as a single bedtime dose.

Urinary antiseptics such as methenamine mandelate or hippurate require an acid urine, preferably at pH 5.5, and are of little value unless their use is accompanied by agents that consistently lower urinary pH, such as high-dose ascorbic acid (1000 mg daily). Methenamine, however, is an effective "suppressant" agent and is best used after infection is eradicated by a more effective drug.

Prophylaxis when given for three to six months is effective for recurrent infections of the reinfection type in women. Cessation of prophylaxis, however, results in a significant incidence of recurrence in individuals having structural abnormalities of the urinary tract or intrinsic renal structural defects. In those circumstances prophylaxis should be reinstituted. Generally, the therapeutic agent should be changed if bacteriuria persists during treatment. This latter circumstance usually means an organism resistant to the agent is now colonizing the urine. Prophylaxis is ineffective in patients with indwelling catheters and will only lead to emergence of resistant bacteria.

The patient should be instructed to drink fluids generously and void frequently. Double voiding in patients with vesicoureteral reflux is recommended. Voiding after sexual intercourse is felt by some to decrease the chance of recurrent infection, but postcoital use of prophylactic agents is probably more effective.

Complicated Infections

Complex urinary infections, i.e., those in the presence of obstructive uropathy, neurogenic bladders, or catheters, are exceedingly difficult to eradicate. They are often best left untreated except for management of acute episodes. Suppressive therapy should be considered ineffective if bacterial populations in the urine are not reduced to less than 1000 per milliliter. The key to management is relief of obstruction or the removal of foreign bodies. Intermittent catheterization has benefited some patients with neurogenic bladders.

COMPLICATIONS

While most urinary infections, including pyelonephritis, are self-limited and easily treated, there are three severe complications of pyelonephritis with which the clinician must be familiar: *renal papillary necrosis*, *renal abscess* (renal carbuncle), and *perinephric abscess*. These complications are uncommon and occur most often in patients with underlying structural renal abnormalities or host immunocompromise (particularly diabetes).

Renal Papillary Necrosis

Renal papillary necrosis, an ischemic necrosis of the renal papilla and adjacent portions of the renal medulla, may be seen in association with severe pyelonephritis, diabetes mellitus, sickle cell anemia, obstructive uropathy, and analgesic abuse. Although infection appears to be the most important factor in the pathogenesis of this lesion, the peculiarities of blood supply of the medulla must also be a factor. This helps explain the frequent occurrence of the lesion in patients with diabetes and generalized vascular disease, as well as the role of obstruction, which must impair blood supply to this area. The zone of necrosis may occur from the extreme tip of the pyramid as far proximal as the corticomedullary junction. Eventually this may slough, with migration of chunks of necrotic tissue down the urinary passages.

The clinical manifestations of renal papillary necrosis are intensification of symptoms of pre-existing pyelonephritis. There may be pain in the lumbar region, colicky pain along the ureteral radiation, hematuria, and high fever. Manifestations of gram-negative bacteremia may supervene. This lesion should be considered in elderly patients with diabetes who show rapid deterioration in clinical status with signs of active pyelonephritis and increasing renal decompensation.

The diagnosis can sometimes be made by finding pieces of renal medullary tissue in the urinary sediment. Pyelography may demonstrate cavities and sinuses in the region of the papillae. The classic ring-shadow pattern results from detachment of a papilla and its outline within the contrast-filled cavity.

Therapy should be directed toward control of infection and measures employed to improve the status of patients who have diabetes mellitus or who are habitual abusers of analgesic agents.

Renal Abscess

Renal abscesses usually occur as a result of extension of a pyelonephritis process. Up to one half of the cases, however, arise from hematogenous spread, by virulent organisms such as *S. aureus*, from a distant focus.

A renal abscess may be identified by intravenous pyelography, ultrasonography, computed tomography, or magnetic resonance imaging. It should be suspected whenever a urinary tract infection fails to respond to an adequate course of appropriate antibiotics. Blood and urine cultures may be negative, so empiric antibiotic regimens may be needed to cover gram-negative rods and staphylococci. Surgical drainage is usually required in addition to parenteral antibiotics, although early diagnosis may eliminate the need for surgery in some patients.

Perinephric Abscess

Perinephric abscesses are notoriously difficult to diagnose. They have an insidious onset, with symptoms usually present for over two weeks at the time of presentation. Fever and unilateral flank pain are common presenting symptoms. The diagnosis should be considered in the evaluation of any patient with a fever of unknown origin. A recent history of urinary tract infection should alert one to the possibility of a perinephric abscess, although this piece of history is often absent. Over two thirds of patients with perinephric abscesses have either diabetes or kidney stone disease.

Perinephric abscesses occur almost exclusively from the rupture of an intrarenal abscess. Diagnosis can be established by ultrasonography, computed tomography, or magnetic resonance imaging. Surgical drainage is mandatory.

Andriole VT: Current concepts of urinary tract infections. In Weinstein L, Fields BN (eds.): Seminars in Infectious Disease, Vol III. New York, Thieme-Stratton, 1980, pp 89–130. *The author's review of practical diagnostic methods, microbiologic concepts, host defenses, clinical syndromes, and treatment of urinary tract infections.*

Bailey RR (ed.): Single Dose Therapy of Urinary Tract Infection. Sydney, Australia, ADIS Health Science Press, 1983. *A multiauthor text on single-dose therapy in adults and children.*

Bell TA, Grayston JT: Centers for Disease Control guidelines for prevention and control of *Chlamydia trachomatis* infections. Ann Intern Med 104:524, 1986.

Jenkins RD, Fenn JP, Matsen JM: Review of urine microscopy for bacteriuria. JAMA 255:3397, 1986.

Komaroff AL: Urinalysis and urine culture in women with dysuria. Ann Intern Med 104:212, 1986.

Kunin CM: Detection, Prevention and Treatment of Urinary Tract Infections. 4th ed. Philadelphia, Lea & Febiger, 1986 (in press). *An excellent text that describes the pathogenesis, management, and prevention of urinary infections.*

Mayrer AR, Miniter P, Andriole VT: Immunopathogenesis of chronic pyelonephritis. Am J Med 75 (Suppl 1B):59, 1983. *Recent studies describing immunologic mechanisms of renal injury and scarring, which produce a histopathologic picture of chronic pyelonephritis.*

Stamm WE, Koutsky LA, Benedetti JK, et al.: *Chlamydia trachomatis* urethral infections in men. Ann Intern Med 100:47, 1984. *An excellent and concise review of this underdiagnosed type of infection.*

Stamm WE, Wagner KF, Amsel R, et al.: Causes of the acute urethral syndrome in women. N Engl J Med 303:409, 1980. *A detailed description of the various etiologies of the acute urethral syndrome in women.*

87 VASCULAR DISORDERS OF THE KIDNEY

Jordan J. Cohen

RENAL ARTERY OCCLUSION

Partial occlusion (stenosis) of the main renal artery, or one or more of its branches, is common and typically results in hypertension. The clinical features of renovascular hypertension are discussed in Ch. 47. This section considers total or nearly total occlusion of the arterial supply to all or a portion of the kidney.

CAUSES (see Table 87–1). Thrombosis in situ rarely occurs in the absence of a severely diseased or damaged vessel. Macroemboli of the renal circulation are far more common as a cause of complete occlusion than are in situ thrombi. (Atheroemboli are considered in the following section.) Approximately 90 per cent of renal artery emboli originate in the heart. Of these, most arise from the left atrium and are a consequence of atrial fibrillation due to arteriosclerotic heart disease. Although 20 per cent of the cardiac output normally goes to the kidney, only 2 to 3 per cent of the systemic emboli derived from the heart lodge in the renal circulation. The number, the size, and the consistency of individual embolic particles vary with the nature of the underlying process and determine the extent of renal involvement. Large emboli can occlude the main renal artery, but, more frequently, embolic material reaches primary or secondary branches of the vessel. Thus, total infarction of the kidney is much less common than is ischemia or segmental infarction. The presence of one or more accessory renal arteries in 20 to 30 per cent of people and of a generally rich capsular circulation also reduces the likelihood of extensive infarction. In most instances, the embolic event involves only one kidney; bilateral emboli and

TABLE 87–1. CAUSES OF RENAL ARTERY OCCLUSION

Thrombosis, in situ
Progressive atherosclerosis
Blunt trauma
Inflammation (e.g., polyarteritis, thromboangiitis obliterans)
Aortic or renal artery aneurysm
Aortic or renal artery dissection
Angiographic catheter
No obvious cause ("spontaneous")
Macroemboli
Atrial fibrillation
Mitral stenosis
Mural thrombus
Atrial myxoma
Infective endocarditis
Prosthetic valve
Paradoxical emboli (patent foramen ovale)
Atheroemboli
Abdominal aorta surgery
Blunt trauma
Angiographic catheters
Anticoagulation (?)
No obvious cause ("spontaneous")

emboli to a solitary kidney do occur and are associated with greater morbidity.

CLINICAL MANIFESTATIONS. Sudden occlusion of a renal artery, whether from embolus or thrombosis, results in a wide spectrum of clinical manifestations in accordance with the caliber of the vessel or vessels involved and with the preexisting status of the renal circulation. Occlusion of a primary or secondary branch of the renal artery in a patient with well-established collateral circulation due to chronic, high-grade stenosis may produce little or no infarction and, hence, few or no signs or symptoms; conversely, occlusion of the main renal artery in an otherwise normal kidney may result in immediate infarction of most of the organ and in a dramatic clinical presentation. Renal infarction typically results in the acute onset of vague, nonspecific flank pain that is described as dull and aching in character. The pain may, however, resemble that due to renal colic, cholecystitis, or pancreatitis. Nausea and vomiting are frequent; gross hematuria is *not* common. The symptoms usually subside within three to four days.

Fever is an infrequent finding at onset but often appears within one to two days. Blood pressure does not usually rise above baseline values. The white blood cell count is usually elevated, and a leftward shift in the differential count is characteristic. Microscopic hematuria is common but may be absent. Striking elevations of serum lactate dehydrogenase (LDH) levels and lesser evaluations of serum glutamic-oxaloacetic transaminase (SGOT) are characteristic. The blood urea nitrogen (BUN) and creatinine levels typically rise transiently in unilateral infarction; more severe and protracted degrees of renal functional impairment, including acute oliguric renal failure, may follow bilateral renal infarction or infarction of a solitary kidney.

DIAGNOSIS. The diagnosis of renal artery occlusion and infarction is often difficult because the clinical findings are frequently meager and nonspecific. As a result less than 1 per cent of autopsy-proven cases may be diagnosed ante mortem. The intravenous pyelogram typically reveals reduced or absent function in the involved kidney or kidneys; retrograde pyelography usually reveals no abnormality. Indeed, a normal retrograde study in a kidney that makes no urine and fails to visualize on intravenous pyelography is virtually diagnostic of arterial occlusion. Radionuclide scanning of the kidney may show segmental perfusion defects or complete absence of perfusion. Definitive diagnosis of renal artery occlusion, however, requires renal angiography. In addition, angiography can often distinguish between embolic and thrombotic occlusion. Angiography should be reserved for those patients in whom the diagnostic information is crucial for making management decisions because the risk of the procedure in this setting is appreciable.

TREATMENT. The choice of therapy of renal artery occlusion varies widely with individual circumstances (Table 87–2). As a rule, unilateral renal artery occlusion should be treated conservatively, especially if a branch vessel or vessels are involved; observation alone or coupled with anticoagulation often results in recanalization and avoids the high risk of surgery. Patients with bilateral occlusion or occlusion in a solitary kidney generally fare better with operative intervention. Although early intervention maximizes recovery of renal function, sufficient time should be taken for stabilizing the patient's underlying medical condition to reduce the operative risk; mortality rates as high as 35 per cent have been reported in patients undergoing acute revascularization procedures. Fibrinolytic therapy followed by anticoagulation can be considered as an alternative to surgery in selected cases. Recovery of renal function is a complex function of the duration and magnitude of the occlusion, the extent of collaterals, the degree of associated cardiovascular disease, and the skill and experience of the operative team. Hemodialysis can be used as a temporizing maneuver if the degree of renal functional impairment warrants. Recovery of renal function has been reported to occur after as long as one month of oliguric renal failure due to renal artery occlusion. Given that irreversible renal damage occurs within 60 minutes of total renal ischemia induced experimentally, such occurrences of recovery after lengthy delay underscore the important role of renal collaterals.

Percutaneous transluminal angioplasty has proved successful as an alternative to surgery for stenotic lesions of the renal artery and shows promise for occlusive lesions as well. Nephrectomy should not be considered unless unequivocal evidence of total infarction is present.

RENAL ARTERY ATHEROEMBOLI

CAUSES. Renal artery atheroembolization is a complication of severe erosive (ulcerative) atheromatosis of the abdominal aorta. Atheroemboli may occur with great frequency in patients with this condition, but, fortunately, in only a small fraction does the process culminate in significant clinical abnormalities. Common events that can trigger the release of cholesterol-laden embolic material from ulcerative plaques are listed in Table 87–1.

CLINICAL MANIFESTATIONS. Atheroemboli characteristically lodge in vessels smaller than the interlobular arteries. As a consequence, macroscopic renal infarction does not usually occur, and the clinical picture is usually bland. The insidious development of renal insufficiency is the mode of presentation in most instances of severe atheroemboli. Hypertension is frequently present and may be severe. Distal embolization in the lower extremities, occasionally associated with livedo reticularis, is frequent. Acute pancreatitis and gastrointestinal bleeding can occur and indicate more widespread embolization. Laboratory findings are nonspecific and give evidence of steady or episodic decline in renal function over a period of days, weeks, or even months. Eosinophilia is common, but its cause is unknown. Urinalysis reveals nothing characteristic and is frequently normal. Kidney size is usually normal or only slightly reduced.

DIAGNOSIS. Diagnosis is made by renal biopsy. Choles-

TABLE 87–2. TREATMENT OPTIONS FOR RENAL ARTERY OCCLUSION

Observation
Anticoagulation
Thrombolytic therapy followed by anticoagulation
Percutaneous transluminal angioplasty
Surgical embolectomy or endarterectomy
Partial or total nephrectomy

TABLE 87–3. CAUSES OF RENAL VEIN THROMBOSIS

Reduced renal blood flow (especially in infants)
Nephrotic syndrome (especially in membranous glomerulopathy)
Renal cell carcinoma
Inferior vena caval thrombosis
External compression (e.g., retroperitoneal fibrosis, tumor)

terol crystals contained in the embolic material are dissolved during routine preparation of the histologic sections, leaving pathognomonic biconvex, cleftlike structures in the occluded vessels.

TREATMENT. No effective therapy is available for this condition. Anticoagulants are *not* helpful and may in fact foster atheroemboli by delaying healing of the atheromatous ulcers in the aorta. Unfortunately, once renal manifestations are evident, the process often progresses unrelentingly to renal failure.

RENAL VEIN THROMBOSIS

CAUSES (see Table 87–3). Renal vein thrombosis in infants is typically an acute catastrophic event triggered by a volume-depleting illness such as profuse diarrhea. The consequences are sudden cessation of renal function, engorgement and enlargement of the kidneys, and ultimate renal infarction and atrophy if venous obstruction is not relieved. Fortunately, acute renal vein thrombosis of such magnitude is rare in older children and adults.

Renal vein thrombosis in adults is typically of insidious onset and is almost always superimposed on an established disease. It occurs most frequently in association with idiopathic nephrotic syndrome, especially that due to membranous glomerulopathy. Predisposing factors may include reduced antithrombin III levels, reduced intravascular blood volume (often aggravated by diuretic therapy), thrombocytosis, and elevated liver-derived clotting factors. Patients with renal cell carcinoma often develop renal vein thrombosis consequent to tumor invasion of the renal vein.

CLINICAL MANIFESTATIONS. In the typical circumstance in which gradual occlusion of the renal vein occurs, the process may progress without any outward sign. Mild abdominal or back pain may be present, but severe pain is uncommon. Pulmonary emboli occur during the course of approximately half of all patients with chronic renal vein thrombosis and are frequently the initial manifestation of the condition. Renal vein thrombosis can also cause unexplained deterioration in renal function in patients with the nephrotic syndrome. Chronic renal vein thrombosis itself results in no characteristic findings on physical examination or laboratory testing. Heavy proteinuria occurs frequently in patients with this condition but reflects the presence of pre-existing nephrotic syndrome; it is not the result of renal vein thrombosis itself.

DIAGNOSIS. The index of suspicion may be heightened greatly by the clinical setting (e.g., recurrent pulmonary emboli in a patient with neophrotic syndrome) or by findings on intravenous pyelography (e.g., large kidneys with splayed calices due to interstitial edema, notching of the upper ureters due to collaterals). Definitive diagnosis, however, requires visualization of the renal vein. Adequate visualization of the main vein can often be obtained with ultrasound, computerized tomography, or magnetic resonance imaging. Selective renal venography may be required for unequivocal visualization of the vessel and its branches.

TREATMENT. Long-term anticoagulation remains the treatment of choice in chronic, subtotal renal vein thrombosis. Fibrinolytic therapy for a few days prior to instituting anticoagulation should be considered in patients with more serious manifestations of renal vein thrombosis (e.g., acute flank pain coupled with a rising serum creatinine level, rapidly recurring pulmonary emboli).

Harrington JT, Kassirer JP: Renal vein thrombosis. Ann Rev Med 33:255, 1982. *An excellent, clinically relevant review.*

Keating MA, Althausen AF: The clinical spectrum of renal vein thrombosis. J Urol 133:938, 1985. *A well-referenced review of historical and modern concepts of the etiology and management of renal vein thrombosis.*

Lessman RK, Johnson SF, Coburn JW, et al.: Renal artery embolism: Clinical features and long-term follow-up of 17 cases. Ann Intern Med 89:477, 1978. *An excellent detailed review and follow-up of one of the larger series of patients with renal artery embolism; emphasizes the nonoperative management.*

Sniderman KW, Sos TA: Percutaneous transluminal recanalization and dilation of totally occluded renal arteries. Radiology 142:607, 1982. *A report of seven patients treated by this technique.*

Stanley JC, Whithouse WMJ: Occlusive and aneurysmal disease of the renal arterial circulation. DM 30:7, 1984. *A readable review emphasizing the diagnosis and therapy of common afflictions of the renal arteries.*

Wagoner RD, Stanson AW, Holley KE, et al.: Renal vein thrombosis in idiopathic membranous glomerulopathy: Incidence and significance. Kidney Int 23:368, 1983. *A well-referenced study of a moderately large series of cases.*

88 RENAL DISEASE IN PREGNANCY

John P. Hayslett

The detection and clinical management of renal disease in the gravid woman is complicated by concern for fetal development and survival, as well as for the health of the patient. In addition, clinical evaluation must account for physiologic changes in volume status and renal function that accompany pregnancy.

RENAL FUNCTION IN PREGNANCY. Pregnancy is characterized by a gradual, cumulative retention of 500 to 900 mEq of sodium and 6 to 8 liters of water, which are distributed between maternal extracellular fluid and the fetus. Despite an expansion in plasma volume of 30 to 45 per cent, mean blood pressure falls approximately 15 per cent owing to a reduction in peripheral vascular resistance. The glomerular filtration rate increases by 30 to 50 per cent by the twelfth week of gestation; the elevation is sustained until term and is position dependent (Fig. 88–1). An evaluation of glomerular filtration rate should take into account expected levels during gestation and should not compare measured values with reported normal values obtained in the nonpregnant individual. Because of the marked position dependence, a convenient way of measuring filtration rate in later pregnancy is with a timed (e.g., four hours) water-loaded creatinine clearance with the woman positioned in the lateral recumbent position.

Owing to the increase in glomerular filtration rate and expanded plasma volume, the levels of creatinine and blood urea nitrogen fall to approximately 0.5 mg per deciliter and 9 mg per deciliter, respectively. Plasma concentrations above 0.8 mg per deciliter of creatinine and 13 mg per deciliter of urea nitrogen should alert the physician to the possibility of renal insufficiency. Plasma osmolality falls from approximately 280 mOsm · kg H_2O^{-1} to 270 owing to a resetting of the osmostat; plasma uric acid falls to 3 to 4 mg per deciliter and plasma bicarbonate to approximately 20 mEq per liter (owing to mild respiratory alkalosis). Glucosuria and aminoaciduria may occur during pregnancy as a result of a transient reduction in the renal threshold of absorption. The ureters dilate during pregnancy and for as long as 12 weeks post partum with no implication of outflow obstruction.

TOXEMIA OF PREGNANCY

DEFINITION. Toxemia, unique to human pregnancy, is characterized by hypertension, edema, and proteinuria. Clinically the syndrome is divided into the stages of preeclampsia and eclampsia, the latter when convulsions have occurred. Onset is usually insidious after the thirty-second week of pregnancy, but it may occur as early as the twenty-fourth

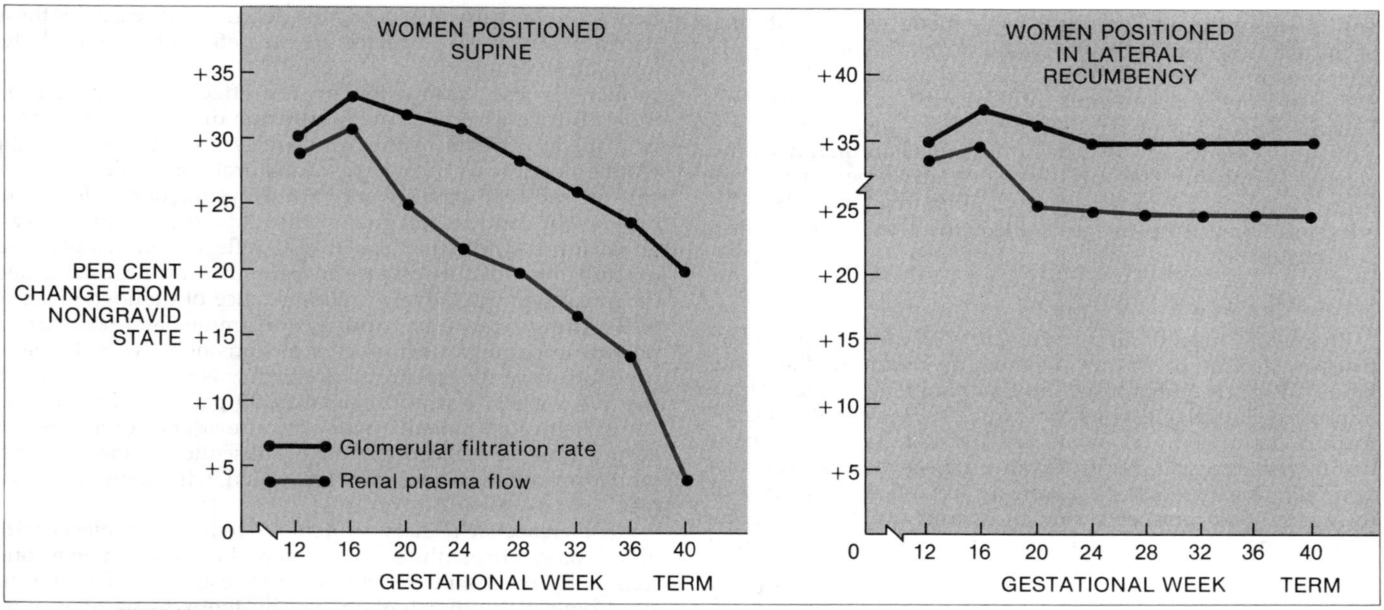

FIGURE 88–1. The early increment of glomerular filtration rate and effective renal plasma flow is position dependent and is sustained if subjects are studied in lateral recumbency. (Adapted from Pippig L: Clinical aspects of renal disease during pregnancy. Med Hyg 27:181, 1969. In Lindheimer MD, Katz AI: Kidney Function and Disease in Pregnancy. Philadelphia, Lea and Febiger, 1977.)

week. In women with a hydatidiform mole, toxemia has been reported to occur in the first trimester. The usual sequence is edema and hypertension, followed by proteinuria, although proteinuria may occasionally precede hypertension. Signs of toxemia spontaneously subside after delivery. Clinical criteria for diagnosis vary depending on changes of blood pressure considered to be abnormal in pregnancy. In general, hypertension in the third trimester is defined by a blood pressure measurement of 140/85 mm Hg or greater if sustained for four to six hours, or an increase of 30 mm Hg or more in systolic blood pressure and 15 mm Hg or more in diastolic pressure above values measured during the early stages of pregnancy. The major differential diagnosis involves a distinction among toxemia, essential hypertension, and primary renal disease, although toxemia can be superimposed on the other two clinical entities.

INCIDENCE. Toxemia of pregnancy occurs worldwide with an incidence that varies between 2 per cent and 25 per cent in different populations. In the United States the quoted incidence is 6 to 7 per cent. Individuals with a poor socioeconomic status are at higher risk for developing the syndrome; the incidence is reduced after introduction of adequate prenatal care with special attention to weight gain and monitoring of blood pressure. The syndrome occurs predominantly in primigravidas and in multiparous women over 35 years of age.

CLINICAL MANIFESTATIONS. Clinical symptoms may include headache, visual disturbances, and apprehension. While diastolic hypertension may be prominent, systolic blood pressure seldom exceeds 160 mm Hg except when associated with underlying hypertension. Funduscopic examination may reveal segmental arteriolar narrowing and a generalized glistening fundus indicative of retinal edema. The ocular changes reflect vasoconstriction. Signs of central nervous system hyperexcitability are regarded as ominous, since they often precede convulsions with a high maternal and fetal death rate. Laboratory findings include a rate of protein excretion usually less than 2 grams per day, but higher levels in the range seen in the nephrotic syndrome may occur. There is a reduction in glomerular filtration rate and renal plasma flow to about 60 per cent of that in pregnancy control subjects. Owing to elevated levels of glomerular filtration rate in normal pregnancy, however, blood urea and serum creatinine levels may not appear to be elevated in toxemic patients, especially if compared with nonpregnant control values. Plasma uric acid levels rise in toxemia to about 5.0 mg per deciliter in mild toxemia and to over 7.0 mg per deciliter in severe states, owing to a fall in its renal clearance. It is suggested that uric acid levels provide a guide for estimating severity of toxemia.

PATHOGENESIS AND PATHOLOGY. The cause of toxemia is not understood. Plasma levels of aldosterone and renin are lower in toxemic women than in normal pregnant individuals but still may be inappropriately high in relation to salt intake and volume status. Many primigravidas who eventually develop toxemia exhibit increased sensitivity to the pressure effects of infused angiotensin many weeks before they become hypertensive. In addition, although a reduction in placental blood flow is found in toxemia, it is not known whether this is a primary change or is secondary to systemic hypertension.

The histopathologic renal changes in toxemia, primarily confined to the glomerulus, are termed *glomerular capillary endotheliosis*. The glomeruli are large and swollen, with encroachment on capillary lumina by swollen and vacuolated endothelial and mesangial cells. Occasionally, small subendothelial deposits and fibrin deposits may be seen, but immunofluorescence studies are negative for deposition of immunoglobulins. The characteristic lesion of endotheliosis seems to be invariably present in toxemia, even in patients with mild clinical preeclampsia, but resolves during an interval of a few weeks or months after delivery.

TREATMENT AND PROGNOSIS. All patients suspected of having preeclampsia should be hospitalized. The majority of patients with mild preeclampsia respond to bed rest and sedation. If they do not, antihypertensive agents are administered, usually in the form of vasodilators and alpha methyldopa. In general there are strong arguments for avoiding diuretic agents in the treatment of hypertension in pregnancy because of risks of reducing placental blood flow. The definitive treatment for toxemia is delivery, which is indicated as soon as fetal maturity is achieved. The occurrence of hyperreflexia or convulsions requires immediate efforts to reduce the level of hypertension and depress central nervous system hyperexcitability. Most obstetric units employ parenteral magnesium sulfate to achieve these aims, along with monitoring of plasma magnesium levels to assure that therapeutic levels of approximately 6 to 8 mEq per liter are maintained.

The remote consequences of toxemia are controversial. Patients with eclampsia in first pregnancies seem not to have a higher incidence of subsequent hypertension than does the general population. The prevalence of late hypertension has been found to be increased in multiparous patients with eclampsia. Preeclampsia does not lead to chronic renal disease post partum.

RENAL PARENCHYMAL DISEASES

Pregnancy may occur in women with pre-existing renal disease; during pregnancy women may acquire the same kinds of disease that exist in the nongravid state. Three important clinical questions concerning these patients warrant further discussion: (1) What are the criteria that help to distinguish preeclampsia from other causes of renal dysfunction? (2) Does pregnancy adversely influence the course of the underlying renal or systemic disease? (3) Does the presence of renal insufficiency or nephrotic syndrome significantly reduce the likelihood for a successful fetal outcome?

DIFFERENTIAL DIAGNOSIS OF RENAL DISEASE IN PREGNANCY. Since the clinical hallmarks of preeclampsia, e.g., hypertension, proteinuria, and edema, are also manifested by most other types of renal parenchymal disease, a diagnostic evaluation cannot be based on these clinical features alone. Preeclampsia does not occur before the twenty-fourth week of gestation, except in hydatidiform mole or multiple gestation pregnancies. The differential diagnosis is therefore simplified if clinical signs of renal disease are known to exist prior to conception or in the early stages of pregnancy. In patients who are not observed until the last trimester of pregnancy, however, identification of the cause of renal dysfunction is often difficult. Multisystem involvement resulting in abnormal liver function tests and coagulation studies suggests preeclampsia. The renal biopsy finding of the pathognomonic changes of preeclampsia provides the only absolute method of confirming the diagnosis of toxemia. When it is necessary to establish the diagnosis, renal biopsy should be performed during the week immediately following delivery. During pregnancy, therefore, management in most cases must rely on a presumed clinical diagnosis. Since the clinical manifestations of preeclampsia usually resolve spontaneously within four to six weeks post partum, persistence of hypertension, proteinuria, or renal insufficiency strongly suggests a primary renal disease.

Information on the relative incidence of the various causes of hypertension and proteinuria during gestation has been reported in a large series of patients in whom the diagnosis was confirmed by renal biopsy performed within six days of delivery. In most of these patients a presumed diagnosis of preeclampsia was made during pregnancy. Among primigravidas the incidence of preeclampsia, primary renal disease, and hypertensive glomerulosclerosis was 83 per cent, 12 per cent, and 5 per cent, respectively. In multiparous patients, in contrast, preeclampsia occurred in only 38 per cent of patients, while renal disease accounted for 26 per cent of cases, and hypertensive renal disease for 24 per cent.

INFLUENCE OF PREGNANCY ON UNDERLYING RENAL DISEASE. Pregnancy does not significantly alter the course of pre-existing primary renal disease due to either glomerular or tubulointerstitial injury in patients with normal or nearly normal renal function. The effect of pregnancy on underlying disease, when renal insufficiency is more severe, (serum creatinine >2.0 mg per deciliter) is less certain because of insufficient data. Although increased proteinuria, often to nephrotic levels, occurs in nearly one half of patients with a glomerulonephropathy, there is no constant relationship between pregnancy and long-term changes in glomerular filtration rate. In general, the course of renal disease in these patients follows the expected course defined by the underlying pattern of injury.

There is less information on the effect of pregnancy on renal disease associated with systemic disorders. Pregnancy in diabetic patients neither accelerates the onset of diabetic glomerulosclerosis nor alters the natural course of renal disease in subjects with signs of renal dysfunction before conception. In contrast, pregnancy may adversely influence systemic lupus erythematosus (SLE), reflected in relapse and exacerbations of this disease in patients with an established diagnosis and a relatively high incidence of de novo onset of SLE during pregnancy and in the immediate postpartum period. In patients with no clinical signs of active SLE before pregnancy the course during pregnancy is relatively mild and the live birth rate is approximately 90 per cent. In contrast, about half of all patients with clinical evidence of active SLE at the time of conception have subsequent exacerbations, which are often severe and associated with increased fetal loss.

An increase in urinary protein excretion in subjects with glomerulonephropathies is common during pregnancy and frequently results in the clinical manifestations of nephrotic syndrome. Sodium retention usually tends to become more severe in the last trimester. In most cases the level of proteinuria spontaneously returns to pregestational levels after delivery. Low birth weight has been reported by some to correlate directly with low serum albumin levels, but this finding has not been seen in all patient series. An increase in the rate of edema formation should be anticipated during the later stages of pregnancy in patients with moderate or severe proteinuria and can be blunted by the introduction of a diet with low sodium content. The use of diuretics in pregnancy is controversial because of the possible induction of reduced placental blood flow. Conservative measures including dietary measures and bed rest are preferred. The judicious use of natriuretic agents may be useful in patients who fail to respond to conservative measures and has not been shown to increase fetal death.

INFLUENCE OF RENAL DISEASE ON FETAL OUTCOME. In the absence of hypertension and severe renal insufficiency, e.g., serum creatinine greater than 2.0 mg per deciliter, the live birth rate is greater than 90 per cent in most patients with primary renal disease. Pregnancies associated with mild to moderate renal insufficiency, however, result in an increased rate of preterm delivery and small-for-gestational-age births. Severe renal insufficiency reduces the incidence of live births to 20 to 50 per cent. Since there is no evidence that pregnancy alters the natural course of primary renal diseases or most types of renal disease due to systemic disease, early termination of pregnancy is not indicated on medical grounds. Clinical management should include control of hypertension and careful monitoring of fetal growth to maximize the likelihood of fetal maturity at birth.

ACUTE RENAL FAILURE IN PREGNANCY

Acute renal failure during pregnancy results from severe injury to tubular epithelial cells due to renal ischemia or to the action of nephrotoxic agents (Ch. 78). The cell injury may be reversible, with an eventual complete restoration of renal function; it may be irreversible and lead to renal cortical necrosis. Renal cortical necrosis is characterized by the development of fibrosis within the cortex in a diffuse or patchy pattern, with relative sparing of the medullary portions of the kidney. Although cortical necrosis is uncommon in nonpregnant individuals, it is a frequent complication of obstetric conditions, especially in subjects beyond the age of 30 years and in association with abruptio placentae. It has been suggested that increased reactivity of the renal vasculature to vasoactive amines in pregnancy and local activation of coagulation may play an important role in the induction of tissue injury leading to cell death.

In addition to the usual causes of acute renal failure, some types of renal insults are unique to pregnancy. Septic abortion and hyperemesis gravidarum may cause renal failure in early pregnancy, while severe preeclampsia, placenta previa, and abruptio placentae are causative factors in the later stages of pregnancy. Clinical management of acute renal failure in pregnancy is comparable to that in nonpregnant patients (Ch. 78). Because of the reported high rate of fetal death, delivery should be performed as soon as the maternal condition has been stabilized and fetal maturity is ascertained. There is inadequate experience with dialysis treatment in gravid patients with acute renal failure to assess its possible usefulness.

Hayslett JP: Pregnancy does not exacerbate primary glomerular disease. Am J Kidney Dis 6:273, 1985. *An analysis of the literature concerning the effect of pregnancy on the underlying renal disease.*

Katz AI, Davison JM, Hayslett JP, et al.: Pregnancy in women with kidney disease. Kidney Int 18:192, 1980. *An analysis of a large series of pregnancies associated with primary renal disease. An excellent source for references.*

Pritchard JA: Management of preeclampsia and eclampsia. Kidney Int 18:259, 1980. *A clear and concise description of the regimen used to treat toxemic women in obstetric units.*

89 HEREDITARY CHRONIC NEPHROPATHIES

Wadi N. Suki

Several genetically transmitted renal disorders of unknown pathogenesis may fall under this heading. This chapter will discuss two of these disorders, Alport's syndrome and the nail-patella syndrome. Some hereditary disorders of renal tubular function are described in Ch. 84. Other genetic disorders that may be associated with renal disease are listed in Table 89–1.

TABLE 89–1. INHERITED RENAL DISEASES*

Disorders of Tubular Function
Proximal tubule
Cerebro-oculorenal syndrome of Lowe
Cystinosis (Fanconi's syndrome)
Cystinuria
Galactosemia
Glycogen storage (von Gierke's) disease
Glycinuria
Hartnup disease
Hepatolenticular degeneration (Wilson's disease)
Hereditary fructose intolerance
Hypophosphatemic vitamin D–resistant rickets
Iminoaciduria
Proximal renal tubular acidosis
Pseudohypoparathyroidism
Renal glucosuria
Distal/collecting tubule
Distal renal tubular acidosis
Nephrogenic diabetes insipidus
Disorders of Renal Structure
Agenesis
Cystic disorders
Hepatocerebrorenal syndrome of Zellweger
Medullary sponge kidney
Medullary cystic disease
Polycystic kidney disease, adult type
Polycystic kidney disease, infantile type
Renal retinal dysplasia
Duplication
Renal malformations with extrarenal anomalies
Biochemical Disorders
Alkaptonuria
Cystinosis
Diabetes mellitus
Glycosphingolipidosis (Fabry's disease)
Hepatolenticular degeneration (Wilson's disease)
Hyperuricemia
Primary hyperoxaluria (oxalosis)
Xanthine oxidase deficiency
Systemic Disorders
Amyloidosis
Asphyxiating thoracic dystrophy (Jeune's disease)
Charcot-Marie-Tooth disease
Laurence-Moon-Biedl syndrome
Osteo-onychodysplasia (nail-patella syndrome)
Hereditary Chronic Nephropathies
Benign recurrent hematuria
Hereditary chronic nephritis
Hereditary chronic nephritis with hyperprolinemia
Hereditary chronic nephritis with thrombocytopathy
Hereditary immune nephritis
Infantile nephrosis

*Includes diseases that affect the kidney secondarily.

ALPORT'S SYNDROME

DEFINITION. Also known as "chronic hereditary nephritis," this syndrome is characterized by the familial occurrence in successive generations of a progressive nephritis, more severe in males, manifested invariably by hematuria and frequently associated with a sensorineural hearing deficit.

GENETICS. The mode of transmission in most kindreds is consistent with autosomal dominant inheritance with discrepant penetrance in the two sexes, males being affected earlier and more severely than females. Male and female offspring of an affected female are at equal risk (1 in 2) for inheriting this disorder, whereas male offspring of an affected male are at a greatly reduced risk (1 in 8) compared with the female (1 in 2). Autosomal recessive and sex-linked dominant inheritances also have been described in certain kindreds, suggesting that this disorder may be genetically heterogeneous.

INCIDENCE AND PREVALENCE. Several hundred kindreds of all races and geographic origins have been described. Alport's syndrome accounts for nearly 5 per cent of patients with end-stage renal disease.

PATHOLOGY AND PATHOGENESIS. Early in the disease the kidneys may be normal or large in size, but they shrink with progression of the disease. Under light microscopy the glomeruli may be normal or show some hypertrophy of epithelial cells and increase in mesangial matrix. Later changes consist of mesangial cell proliferation, thickening and splitting of glomerular and tubular basement membranes, thickening of Bowman's capsule, tubular cell atrophy, interstitial fibrosis, and the presence of foam cells. Electron microscopy characteristically reveals both thinning and irregular thickening of the glomerular and tubular basement membranes, with splitting of the lamina densa into several lamellae separated by lucent zones containing electron-dense round granulations.

The etiology and pathogenesis of Alport's syndrome are unknown. It has been speculated that an inherited deficiency of a collagenous or noncollagenous component of basement membrane may be responsible for thinning and rupture followed by repair and focal thickening.

CLINICAL MANIFESTATIONS. The disease is discovered in 70 per cent of patients by the age of six years, the rest of the cases being discovered at any age thereafter up to and well into adulthood. Persistent or intermittent microscopic hematuria is universally present. Gross hematuria, especially after exercise or respiratory infections, may occur in 60 per cent of affected children but rarely in adults. Proteinuria is present in 70 per cent of patients. It is usually mild but reaches the nephrotic range in 30 to 40 per cent of patients. Sensorineural hearing loss in the high-frequency (4000 to 8000 Hz) range is observed in 40 to 60 per cent of patients, predominantly males. Its detection may require audiometric testing, but it may progress to clinical deafness. Ocular disorders, especially anterior and posterior lenticonus and spherophakia, are seen in 15 per cent of patients. The renal disease may be mild and nonprogressive, especially in women, or may progress with the development of azotemia and hypertension culminating in chronic renal failure and uremia. Progression occurs predominantly in males, with a predilection to those with massive proteinuria, deafness, and lenticonus. Renal failure may occur in childhood or in adulthood, and in affected males usually before age 40 years. Affected females may experience decline of renal function during pregnancy.

In several kindreds patients with classic Alport's syndrome have been reported to have thrombocytopenia with giant platelets manifested clinically by bruising, epistaxis, and gastrointestinal bleeding, and in the laboratory by prolonged bleeding time. A few cases have also been associated with hyperprolinemia (Ch. 191).

DIAGNOSIS. The presence of progressive renal disease in one family member younger than age 50, other than the proband, and the presence of neural hearing loss in the patient or a relative form the basis for the diagnosis of Alport's syndrome in a patient with hematuria with or without proteinuria, azotemia, or hypertension. Differential diagnosis includes benign familial hematuria, a nonprogressive disorder characterized by a uniformly thin glomerular capillary basement membrane; and IgA nephropathy (Berger's disease), a glomerulonephritis with distinctive findings on light, electron, and especially immunofluorescent microscopic examination of the renal glomerulus. The audiometric findings, ocular manifestations, and family history, coupled with the changes in the glomerular and tubular basement membranes, usually should distinguish Alport's syndrome from other renal disorders.

TREATMENT. There is no specific treatment for Alport's syndrome, and no therapy is known to alter its course. Only conventional management of progressive renal disease is available. Peritoneal dialysis or hemodialysis and related or cadaveric donor kidney transplantation have been utilized with degrees of success at least matching those in other renal disorders. In fact, improvement of hearing deficit has been reported after renal transplantation. Recurrence of the renal lesion has not been observed following transplantation, but several patients have developed Goodpasture's syndrome.

NAIL-PATELLA SYNDROME

An autosomal dominant trait also known as osteo-onychodysplasia, this disorder of mesenchymal tissue is characterized by atrophic or absent fingernails, hypoplasia or aplasia of the patella, accessory conical iliac horns, thickening of the scapula, and subluxation of the radial heads at the elbow. In 40 per cent of patients the kidneys may be involved, as manifested by mild proteinuria and rarely hematuria. Occasionally the nephrotic syndrome and progression to renal failure (27 per cent) may be observed. Light microscopy shows glomerular cellular proliferation, mesangial sclerosis, and basement membrane thickening. Electron microscopy reveals areas of rarefaction in the lamina densa of the glomerular basement membrane filled with bundles of curvilinear fibrils having the typical periodicity of collagen. No specific therapy exists for this disorder. Renal transplantation has been carried out without evidence of recurrence of the disease in the transplanted organ.

Bennett WM, Musgrave ME, Campbell RA, et al.: The nephropathy of the nail-patella syndrome. Am J Med 54:304, 1973. *A good description of the renal disorder in the nail-patella syndrome.*

Gubler C, Levy M, Broyer M, et al.: Alport's syndrome. A report of 58 cases and a review of the literature. Am J Med 70:493, 1981. *An excellent review of the clinical and histologic features of Alport's syndrome in children.*

90 RENAL CALCULI

Charles Y.C. Pak

DEFINITION

Renal calculi (kidney stones, nephrolithiasis) are abnormal concretions occurring in the kidneys, consisting of crystalline components and an organic matrix. They are typically located within the calices or pelvis and may become lodged in the ureter or bladder as they are passed. Nephrolithiasis should be differentiated from nephrocalcinosis, which is calcification of renal parenchyma. Stones originating in the bladder (bladder stones) are rare in industrialized countries, although they were common in antiquity and are still frequent in certain countries in Southeast Asia.

Nephrolithiasis affects 1 to 5 per cent of the population, with a recurrence rate in afflicted individuals of 50 to 80 per cent and an annual incidence rate of 0.1 to 0.3 per cent. Calcareous (calcium-containing) renal stones account for 80 to 95 per cent of stones and are principally composed of calcium oxalate and calcium phosphate, usually occurring as mixtures. The remaining stones are composed of uric acid, cystine, magnesium ammonium phosphate (struvite), and, rarely, xanthine (Table 90–1).

ETIOLOGY AND PATHOGENESIS

Renal stones form by an initial crystallization of a nidus (termed nucleation) from a supersaturated urine with subsequent crystal growth and aggregation of the nidus into a macroscopic stone. Kidney stones are not simply masses of crystals. They usually have an organic matrix that gives form, cohesiveness, and sometimes a remarkably regular structure to the stone. At the present time, abnormalities in the amount or composition of stone matrix have not been demonstrated to be important in stone pathogenesis. It is impossible to dissolve the amounts of calcium, oxalate, and phosphate present in normal urine in 1 or 2 liters of distilled water. Obviously, therefore, there are substances present in normal urine that impede crystallization and sustain supersaturation. These normal inhibitors are not fully characterized but seem to include pyrophosphate, citrate, magnesium, and certain organic macromolecules (such as glycosaminoglycans and glycoproteins).

All patients with stones are presumed to have some physiologic derangements that make them susceptible to stone formation, although no cause can be demonstrated by current

TABLE 90–1. COMPOSITION OF RENAL STONES*

Type	Percentage
Calcium oxalate	70
Calcium phosphate	10
Hydroxyapatite	
Brushite	
Tricalcium phosphate	
Carbonate apatite	
Magnesium ammonium phosphate	5–10
Uric acid	< 5
Cystine	1
Xanthine	< 1

*Some stones occur as mixtures. Percentages are calculated for the predominant stone types.

TABLE 90–2. PATHOGENESIS OF NEPHROLITHIASIS

Cause	Percentage of Patients with Stones	Sex Predominance	Stone Composition
Hypercalciuria			
Absorptive hypercalciuria	35–50	Male	Ca oxalate, Ca phosphate
Renal hypercalciuria	5–15	Equivalent	Ca oxalate, Ca phosphate
Fasting hypercalciuria with normal PTH*	5–25	Male	Ca oxalate, Ca phosphate
Primary hyperparathyroidism	4–10	Female	Ca phosphate, Ca oxalate
Hyperoxaluria			
Primary	Rare	Equivalent	Ca oxalate
Enteric	2	Equivalent	Ca oxalate
Hyperuricosuric calcium nephrolithiasis	10 (pure) 30–50 (mixed)	Male	Ca oxalate, Ca phosphate
Hypocitraturic calcium nephrolithiasis			
Renal tubular acidosis	1–10	Equivalent	Ca phosphate, Ca oxalate
Other	10 (pure) 10–50 (mixed)	Male	Ca oxalate, Ca phosphate
Uric acid stone diathesis	3–10	Male	Uric acid, Ca oxalate, Ca phosphate
Cystinuria	1–3	Equivalent	Cystine
Infection lithiasis	< 10	Female	Struvite, carbonate apatite
Low urine volume	< 5 (pure) 10–50 (mixed)	Female	Ca oxalate
No physiologic disturbance	< 5	Female	Ca oxalate

*PTH = parathyroid hormone.

techniques in 3 per cent of patients. These derangements alter urinary concentration of stone-forming constituents and of inhibitors to cause supersaturation and facilitate crystallization (Table 90–2).

Supersaturation of crystalloids can result from (1) too little urine output (a concentrated urine), (2) an absolute increase in the amount of a stone constituent excreted over a period of time, such as calcium, oxalate, or uric acid, or (3) an alteration in urine pH. Low urinary pH (< 5.5) increases urinary saturation of uric acid, whereas high urinary pH raises that of calcium phosphate and magnesium ammonium phosphate.

Reduction in the concentration of inhibitors of crystallization in the urine may be of great importance in stone pathogenesis. Some inhibitors (such as citrate) may be directly measured in urine, providing diagnostic utility. Other inhibitors (such as glycoproteins) that are difficult to analyze can sometimes be assessed indirectly from the overall inhibitor activity against crystallization of stone-forming salts.

Other factors may be important in stone formation. (1) *Stasis*: Most embryonic stones are probably harmlessly washed out in the urine. Stasis allows time for nascent stone to grow. (2) *Heterogeneous nucleation*: Crystallization may begin in a supersaturated solution that is seeded with a crystal of a different (heterogeneous) composition but one that has an analogous surface topography. This process of one crystal growing on the surface of another is known as epitaxy. Many stones are mixed in composition and perhaps represent epitaxial growth. Of greatest practical importance, however, is the fact that calcium oxalate crystals can be nucleated by uric acid or sodium hydrogen urate crystals. This is the presumed cause of the calcium oxalate stone diathesis associated with hyperuricosuria (see below).

HYPERCALCIURIA. As noted, calcium is a constituent of 80 to 95 per cent of kidney stones. Hypercalciuria is the single most frequent abnormality found in patients with stone diathesis. Hypercalciuria is often statistically defined and varies with body size and diet. In general, the normal upper limit for urinary calcium is 300 mg per day on a diet containing 1000 mg of calcium per day (some authorities use a figure of 4 mg per kilogram per day) and 200 mg per day on a diet with a daily composition of 400 mg of calcium and 100 mEq of sodium (urinary calcium tends to parallel urinary sodium so that dietary sodium should ideally be controlled). Hypercalciuria can result from (1) enhanced absorption from dietary sources, (2) primary renal wastage with secondary enhanced absorption, (3) excessive resorption from storage in bone, or (4) a combination of the above (Fig. 90–1). These different forms will be discussed briefly.

Absorptive hypercalciuria, the most common abnormality, is encountered in 35 to 50 per cent of patients with kidney stones. Increased absorption of dietary calcium may rarely occur from excessive ingestion of milk and other dairy products, from vitamin D excess (Ch. 245), or from the altered vitamin D metabolism associated with sarcoidosis (Ch. 69). Absorptive hypercalciuria usually refers, however, to a primary idiopathic increase in intestinal absorption of calcium. The consequent rise in serum calcium concentration tends to suppress parathyroid function (PTH ↓). Hypercalciuria ensues from the increased renal filtered load of calcium and the reduced renal tubular reabsorption of calcium associated with

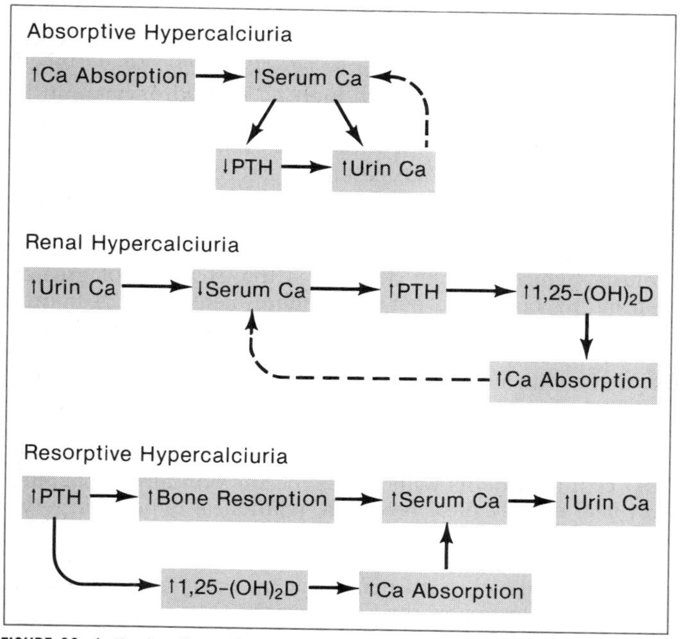

FIGURE 90–1. Pathophysiologic schemes for hypercalciuria. (After Pak CYC: Kidney stones. In Foster DW, Wilson JE [eds.]: Williams Textbook of Endocrinology. Philadelphia, W. B. Saunders Company, 1985, pp 1256–1273.

suppression of the secretion of parathyroid hormone (PTH). Serum calcium is typically maintained within the normal range because of compensatory hypercalciuria. In its usual presentation, the disorder tends to be familial and is believed to occur independently of hypophosphatemia or altered vitamin D metabolism. There is some evidence that it represents a jejunal disease characterized by a selective intestinal hyperabsorption of calcium in this intestinal segment.

Renal hypercalciuria, as a form of "idiopathic hypercalciuria," occurs less commonly than absorptive hypercalciuria and originates from an impaired renal tubular reabsorption (renal leak) of calcium. The ensuing decline in serum calcium causes secondary hyperparathyroidism, which in turn stimulates the renal synthesis of 1,25-dihydroxyvitamin D (Fig. 90–1). Thus, the skeletal mobilization and intestinal absorption of calcium may be secondarily increased, effects that restore serum calcium concentration to normal and further contribute to the hypercalciuria. The possibility that there may be a more generalized disturbance in proximal tubular function is shown by an exaggerated natriuretic response to thiazide and calciuric response to a carbohydrate load.

Resorptive hypercalciuria results from excessive bone resorption, most commonly from the hypersecretion of PTH. Four to 10 per cent of all kidney stones are caused by primary hyperparathyroidism (Table 90–2); conversely, 10 to 40 per cent of patients with primary hyperparathyroidism present with renal stones. The hypercalcemia of hyperparathyroidism causes hypercalciuria by augmenting the renal filtered load of calcium. The intestinal calcium absorption may also be increased secondarily, consequent to parathyroid hormone–dependent stimulation of the synthesis of 1,25-dihydroxyvitamin D; this increased calcium absorption further contributes to the hypercalciuria. Hypercalciuria secondary to net bone resorption is also seen in thyrotoxicosis, multiple myeloma, pseudohyperparathyroidism of malignancy, metastatic disease of bone, and immobilization (acute osteoporosis) and with spontaneous or iatrogenic Cushing's syndrome.

Fasting hypercalciuria with normal levels of serum PTH is neither absorptive hypercalciuria (because of the presence of apparent renal calcium leak) nor renal hypercalciuria (since parathyroid stimulation is lacking). This picture may result from several disturbances. (1) *Enhanced 1,25-dihydroxyvitamin D synthesis*: It may cause parathyroid suppression and an acquired renal calcium leak. (2) *Renal phosphate leak*: It may produce hypophosphatemia and increased synthesis of 1,25-dihydroxyvitamin D. (3) *Combined renal proximal tubular defect*: Renal calcium leak may coexist with high 1,25-dihydroxyvitamin D production occurring primarily or secondarily from renal phosphate leak.

HYPEROXALURIA. Oxalate is the second most common constituent of kidney stones, after calcium (Table 90–1), but the great majority of patients with calcium oxalate stones have no abnormality of oxalate metabolism. Sustained hyperoxaluria, which may be defined as the excretion of greater than 60 mg of oxalate per 1.73 square meters per 24 hours, occurs only (1) in primary hyperoxaluria, a rare genetic disorder described in Ch. 182, (2) in pyridoxine deficiency, (3) rarely with excessive ingestion of ascorbic acid, and (4) from enhanced absorption of dietary oxalate, termed enteric hyperoxaluria.

Enteric hyperoxaluria, which is encountered in approximately 2 per cent of patients with stones, occurs typically in patients with ileal disease (ileal resection, jejunoileal bypass surgery, inflammatory disease of the small bowel). In ileal disease in which there is malabsorption of fat, the intraluminal content of divalent cations, particularly calcium, may be reduced by being bound to unabsorbed fatty acids. Thus, calcium is not normally available to bind and limit oxalate absorption. The resulting enlarged free intestinal oxalate pool increases absorption and renal excretion of oxalate. Oxalate absorption may be stimulated primarily as well, especially in the colon, since patients with ileostomies do not have hyperoxaluria. Low urine volume (from an excessive intestinal loss of fluid) and defective urinary inhibitor activity (from an impaired renal excretion of citrate and magnesium) probably contribute to calcium stone formation in ileal disease.

In hypercalciuria associated with increased calcium absorption (e.g., absorptive hypercalciuria), a mild increase in oxalate excretion to the higher ranges of normal may be found (up to 50 mg per day). The total amount of oxalate absorbed from the gut may be high because more calcium is absorbed and less calcium is available intraluminally to bind oxalate.

HYPERURICOSURIC CALCIUM OXALATE STONE DIATHESIS. Hyperuricosuria may be the only discernible biochemical abnormality associated with calcium oxalate stones (10 per cent), although it often coexists with hypercalciuria (30 to 50 per cent). Most patients with hyperuricosuric calcium oxalate nephrolithiasis do not suffer from clinical gout. The hyperuricosuria is usually dietary in origin, since a history of high purine intake may often be disclosed and normal urinary uric acid excretion values may be restored by purine restriction. Less commonly, hyperuricosuria results from a primary overproduction of uric acid. The urinary pH typically exceeds 5.5, so that dissociated urate rather than uric acid predominates. It is believed that urates facilitate crystallization of calcium oxalate, either directly by inducing heterogeneous nucleation or indirectly by removing macromolecular inhibitors through adsorption.

HYPOCITRATURIA. Citrate reduces urinary saturation of calcium salts by complexing calcium, as well as inhibits the crystallization of these salts. Thus, hypocitraturia would be expected to increase the tendency toward the formation of calcium-containing kidney stones. Hypocitraturia is encountered in any acidotic condition, such as renal tubular acidosis, chronic diarrheal states, thiazide-induced hypokalemia (which causes intracellular acidosis), and ingestion of excessive animal protein (which has a high acid-ash content). Distal (type I) renal tubular acidosis, often in an incomplete form, may first manifest with nephrolithiasis. The cause for stone formation is multifactorial and probably includes hypercalciuria (from induced renal leak of calcium by acidosis), enhanced dissociation of phosphate, an increased saturation of calcium phosphate (from high urinary pH), as well as an impaired inhibitor activity (from defective excretion of citrates). Renal tubular acidosis is described in greater detail in Ch. 84. Hypocitraturia of excessive intestinal alkali loss has been found not only in ileal disease (enteric hyperoxaluria) but also in postgastrectomy states and ulcerative colitis. Hypocitraturia should be suspected in patients with hypercalciuric nephrolithiasis who continue to form stones while on thiazide therapy. Another cause of hypocitraturia is urinary tract infection (probably from bacterial degradation of citrate). The cause for hypocitraturia often remains unknown. Hypocitraturia may occur as a sole abnormality (5 per cent) but is usually associated with other causes of nephrolithiasis (10 to 50 per cent).

URIC ACID STONES. Approximately two thirds to three fourths of the uric acid synthesized in the body is excreted in the urine. The rest is excreted in the intestine and largely destroyed by bacterial degradation. Uric acid excretion varies widely with diet. Urinary values greater than 600 mg per 1.73 square meters per 24 hours after three days of a diet moderately restricted in purine probably represent endogenous overproduction. In the study of patients with kidney stones, it is more important to measure uric acid excretion on the patient's usual diet. In this case, an excretion of more than 750 mg for women and more than 800 mg for men would be considered abnormally high.

Uric acid stones usually form in urines with a pH of less than the dissociation constant for uric acid (5.5), especially when there are absolute increases in uric acid (hyperuricosuria). Thus, the amount of urinary free uric acid is increased. Uric acid stones often occur in primary gout, which may be accompanied by low urinary pH and hyperuricosuria (Ch. 195), or in secondary causes of purine overproduction, such as myeloproliferative states, glycogen storage disease, and malignancy. Chronic diarrheal syndromes (ulcerative colitis, regional enteritis, jejunoileal bypass surgery) may cause uric acid stones by inducing net alkali deficit (thereby reducing urinary pH) and lowering urine volume (thereby augmenting urinary concentration of uric acid). Most patients with uric acid stones do not have clinical gout. Some patients with uric acid stones may also form calcium-containing stones.

CYSTINURIA. A cystine kidney stone forms only in a patient with the genetic disorder cystinuria (Ch. 84). Other forms of aminoaciduria are not associated with the excretion of enough cystine to form stones. Cystinuria is characterized by a disturbance in renal and intestinal handling of lysine, arginine, ornithine, and cystine. Stone formation, occurring in a minority of patients with cystinuria, is the result of an excessive renal excretion of cystine and its low solubility in urine. Cystine solubility is pH dependent; at pH 5, 170 to 300 mg of cystine may be dissolved in each liter of urine, whereas at pH 7.5, 220 to 500 mg of cystine may go into the solution. Many patients with homozygous cystinuria who are prone to cystine stone formation excrete more than 250 mg of cystine per day.

INFECTION. Urinary tract infections with urea-splitting organisms may be associated with renal stones of struvite (magnesium ammonium phosphate) and varying amounts of calcium phosphate. Ammonia formed by enzymatic degradation of urea by bacterial urease undergoes hydration to form ammonium and hydroxyl ions. The resulting alkalinity of urine augments dissociation of phosphate to form more triphosphate ions and reduces the solubility of struvite. Thus, the urinary environment becomes supersaturated with respect to struvite. Although struvite stones may form de novo from infection alone, they may sometimes occur as a complication of other causes of renal calculi, such as hypercalciuria. The presence of a struvite stone is presumptive evidence for concurrent or previous urinary tract infection.

MISCELLANEOUS. A minority of patients (less than 5 per cent) present with low urine volume (< 1 liter per day) without any of the previously mentioned causes. Habitual decreased drinking of fluids may have contributed to stone formation. It has been reported that oxalate exchange in peripheral red blood cells is significantly increased in patients with "idiopathic" calcium oxalate nephrolithiasis and that this disturbance may be corrected by treatment with thiazide or amiloride. The significance of this finding is uncertain, since intestinal absorption and renal excretion of oxalate (given without calcium) are normal, and urinary oxalate is not affected by thiazide in patients with absorptive or renal hypercalciuria.

RENAL STRUCTURAL ABNORMALITIES. Nephrolithiasis may also be found in association with *renal structural abnormalities*, such as ectopic kidney, polycystic kidney, and horseshoe kidney. In this situation, it is generally believed that stones, usually composed of struvite or calcium phosphate, form secondarily to urinary tract infection. Medullary sponge disease is often associated with calcareous renal calculi. There is no convincing evidence that the structural abnormality causes stone formation, since metabolic abnormalities (such as the three forms of hypercalciuria) are usually found in medullary sponge disease, in similar distribution to that of patients without this disease.

IDIOPATHIC STONE DIATHESIS. In less than 5 per cent of patients, no physiologic abnormality can be discerned. The cause for stone formation remains unknown.

CLINICAL MANIFESTATIONS

Patients with renal stones may be asymptomatic; may pass small, sandlike concretions with relatively little pain; or may experience severe symptoms from ureteral obstruction, localized trauma, or infection. Renal colic is the manifestation of ureteral spasm produced by the irritation of a stone and accompanying obstruction. Microscopic hematuria is almost invariably present; gross hematuria, even clots, may sometimes accompany renal colic. Pain may begin in the costovertebral angle or the flank and may migrate toward the groin; sometimes pain moves into, and may be most severe in, the testis or penis in the male. Pain may subside after the stone or clot has passed, but the process may take several hours, even days, if the stone is impacted or if ureteral swelling impedes migration. Women frequently report that the pain of renal colic is more severe than that of labor. Infection arising from stones may lead to fever, flank tenderness, dysuria, and frequency of urination.

DIAGNOSIS

INITIAL SCREEN. The first step in the diagnosis of the cause of a kidney stone is to secure the stone for analysis, if at all possible. The analysis should preferably be carried out by a crystallographic technique, which can sometimes reveal the sequence of stone formation from the central nidus to the periphery.

All patients with renal stones should have a carefully taken history, abdominal roentgenographic examination, urinalysis and culture, and a routine blood screen.

A positive family history of renal calculi suggests absorptive hypercalciuria or, more rarely, cystinuria, primary hyperoxaluria, or type I renal tubular acidosis. Absorptive hypercalciuria should be suspected in middle-aged white men who have a history of recurrent calcium-containing stones and a family history of renal stones. Renal hypercalciuria may be present in patients with a history of recurrent urinary tract infection, especially if the infection preceded the onset of the stone disease. A high-calcium diet may aggravate the stone disease in those with an intestinal hyperabsorption of calcium. Patients with gout may form stones of either uric acid or calcium oxalate. A history of chronic diarrhea, ileal disease, or intestinal surgery should arouse the suspicion of uric acid or calcium oxalate stones (enteric hyperoxaluria or hypocitraturic calcium nephrolithiasis). A high purine intake may cause hyperuricosuria and contribute to stone formation in hyperuricosuric calcium oxalate nephrolithiasis. Acetazolamide may impair renal acidification and cause formation of calcium phosphate stones. Excessive ingestion of vitamin D and of oxalate-rich foods (such as spinach and brewed tea) may increase oxalate excretion.

Calcium-containing stones, struvite stones, and cystine stones are radiopaque. Uric acid stones and the rarely encountered xanthine and 2,8-dihydroxyadenine stones are radiolucent (see Ch. 196). A staghorn calculus suggests a cystine or struvite stone. Positive urine culture for *Proteus, Pseudomonas, Klebsiella,* or *Staphylococcus* in association with an alkaline urine indicates that the stone is probably struvite. On a routine blood screen, primary hyperparathyroidism is suggested by hypercalcemia and hypophosphatemia (Ch. 247); gouty diathesis by hyperuricemia; and defective acidification by the electrolyte picture of hyperchloremic metabolic acidosis.

IN-DEPTH EVALUATION. The objective of in-depth evaluation, applicable particularly to those with recurrent calculi, is to discern the specific metabolic cause for the nephrolithiasis. Ideally, it should include a measure of parathyroid function (serum immunoreactive PTH); 24-hour urinary calcium (on defined diets with respect to calcium and sodium intake); 24-hour urinary calcium, oxalate, uric acid, citrate, total volume, and pH (on random diets); and a measure of renal tubular reabsorption and intestinal absorption of calcium (from urinary calcium levels during fasting and following excessive oral ingestion of calcium). Hypercalciuria should be defined with respect to the particular diet during which urinary calcium is determined as noted above. If the stone is not known to contain calcium, a qualitative test for urine cystine is indicated.

The nature of parathyroid function distinguishes the three forms of *hypercalciuria*. Primary hyperparathyroidism is suggested by parathyroid stimulation in the setting of hypercalcemia, absorptive hypercalciuria by normal or suppressed parathyroid function with normocalcemia and hypercalciuria, and renal hypercalciuria by parathyroid stimulation with normocalcemia and hypercalciuria. The fasting urinary calcium level is invariably increased in renal hypercalciuria and is frequently elevated in primary hyperparathyroidism, whereas it is typically normal in absorptive hypercalciuria. Intestinal calcium absorption is always increased in absorptive hypercalciuria and is often high in renal and resorptive hypercalciurias. Fasting hypercalciuria with normal parathyroid function is suggested by high fasting urinary calcium levels in the setting of normal levels of serum calcium and PTH.

In *enteric hyperoxaluria*, the urinary calcium level is typically low (< 100 mg per day) and the urinary oxalate level is high (often > 100 mg per day). Serum calcium and magnesium levels may be low, parathyroid function may be stimulated, metabolic acidosis may be present, and the urinary citrate level is low (< 320 mg per day). Hypocitraturia is also found in hypocitraturic calcium nephrolithiasis.

Urinary uric acid consistently exceeds 600 mg per day (and often > 750 to 800 mg per day), and pH is greater than 5.5 in *hyperuricosuric calcium oxalate nephrolithiasis*. Urinary pH is usually low (< 5.5) *in uric acid lithiasis* and high (> 7.5) in *struvite lithiasis*. Urine pH is high (> 6.9) in complete type I *renal tubular acidosis* and high normal or high (> 6) in the incomplete form.

TREATMENT

Kidney stones are heterogeneous in pathogenesis and not infrequently are manifestations of a generalized multisystem disorder. By and large, kidney stones cannot be treated medically in the sense of causing their dissolution. The goal of treatment is to stop growth or new formation of stones by correcting the specific underlying physicochemical and physiologic derangements. Stone prophylaxis often entails a prolonged program. It is particularly important, therefore, to ensure patient compliance, few complications, and reasonable costs.

GENERAL TREATMENT. The initial treatment program, applicable to all patients with renal calculi, consists of a high fluid intake to ensure a minimum urine volume of 2 liters per day. At least 3 liters of fluids should be drunk each day, distributed throughout the day. In general, any fluid (with the exception of milk and oxalate-rich tea in certain disorders to be enumerated) may be consumed. In patients with intestinal hyperabsorption of calcium, dairy products and certain calcium-rich foods should be avoided. Oxalate intake should be restricted in patients with calcium oxalate stones. An excessive dietary intake of sodium should be discouraged, since this may enhance calcium excretion. Urinary tract infection should be vigorously treated.

Activity of Stone Diathesis. As noted, as many as 5 per cent of the population may have a kidney stone at some time. Some patients, usually men, have a single calcium oxalate stone in middle life and are not subsequently affected. Clearly, it would not be wise to begin a lifetime program of pharmacologic intervention without some knowledge of the prognosis of the stone diathesis in the individual patient. In the absence of remediable disorders, such as primary hyperparathyroidism, it is often wise following a first stone episode to institute the general measures noted above and then to follow patients carefully with sequential radiographs to document whether new stones are forming or old stones are enlarging before more vigorous measures are instituted.

SPECIFIC MEDICAL TREATMENT. Specific programs may be required when the aforementioned conservative measures are ineffective in controlling stone formation and there is continued activity of stone diathesis.

Treatment of Hypercalciuria. The surgical removal of abnormal parathyroid tissue is clearly the treatment of choice for kidney stones secondary to the hypercalciuria of primary hyperparathyroidism. Following parathyroidectomy, serum 1,25-dihydroxyvitamin D levels, intestinal calcium absorption, and urinary calcium levels decline toward normal. Parathyroidectomy may also ameliorate the extrarenal manifestations of primary hyperparathyroidism, such as bone disease and peptic ulcer disease (Ch. 100). Similarly, the hypercalciuria of vitamin D excess, sarcoidosis, thyrotoxicosis, multiple myeloma, and malignancies may respond to specific therapies directed toward those systemic entities. The main problem is in the management of remaining forms of hypercalciuria. Several agents that have proved to be useful will be individually discussed.

Thiazides (and related compounds such as chlorthalidone) are unique among diuretics in their ability to augment the renal tubular reabsorption of calcium and therefore to reduce urinary calcium. At a dosage of hydrochlorothiazide of 50 mg once or twice a day, or an equivalent amount of related drugs, thiazides represent the treatment of choice for renal hypercalciuria. Thiazides correct the renal leak of calcium and thereby reverse the sequence of parathyroid hyperactivity, increased synthesis of 1,25-dihydroxyvitamin D, and enhanced absorption of intestinal calcium. The urinary saturations of calcium oxalate and calcium phosphate are reduced. Thiazides may be equally effective in the control of absorptive hypercalciuria, at least during the first two years of therapy. However, some patients may show an attenuation of the hypocalciuric response with chronic treatment. Moreover, thiazide therapy may cause hypokalemia and hypocitraturia. To overcome these problems, urinary calcium levels should be monitored, and potassium supplement (preferably as potassium citrate) should be provided.

Sodium cellulose phosphate (Calcibind) should be used only in patients with normophosphatemic absorptive hypercalciuria without bone disease in whom hypercalciuria cannot be controlled by dietary calcium restriction. When given orally, it forms a nonabsorbable complex with calcium that is then excreted in the feces. About 2.5 to 5 grams of this resin with each meal is sufficient to limit the amount of luminal calcium available for absorption and to restore normal urinary calcium levels. This reduces urinary saturation of calcium salts, particularly that of calcium phosphate, without overly stimulating parathyroid function or causing bone disease. Urinary oxalate may increase, because less calcium may be available intraluminally to complex oxalate, so that a moderate dietary restriction of oxalate is recommended. Oral magnesium supplementation should be provided, since this drug also binds magnesium. Sodium cellulose phosphate is contraindicated in primary hyperparathyroidism, in other states of excessive skeletal calcium mobilization, in renal hypercalciuria, and in states of normal intestinal calcium absorption because it tends to stimulate parathyroid function and thereby produces or aggravates bone disease.

Orthophosphates, as neutral or alkaline soluble salts of sodium or potassium or both, are potentially absorbable from the intestinal tract, unlike sodium cellulose phosphate. When given orally (at a dosage of 1.5 to 2.0 grams of phosphorus per day in divided doses), they decrease urinary calcium and increase urinary phosphate levels. They reduce urinary saturation of calcium oxalate, although they may increase that of calcium phosphate. Moreover, urinary inhibitor activity may be increased, probably consequent to the increased renal excretion of inhibitors, such as pyrophosphate and citrate.

Orthophosphates are optimally indicated in the management of renal phosphate leak because of the possibility that they may restore normal levels of serum 1,25-dihydroxyvitamin D and calcium absorption. Orthophosphates are contraindicated in moderate or severe hypercalcemia and in renal failure because of the danger of metastatic calcification and in urinary tract infection because of the danger of struvite or calcium phosphate stone formation.

Treatment of Enteric Hyperoxaluria. Oral administration of large amounts of calcium or magnesium has been recommended for the control of nephrolithiasis of enteric hyperoxaluria. Although urinary oxalate levels may decrease, the concurrent rise in urinary calcium may obviate the beneficial effect of this therapy in some patients. Cholestyramine does not generally cause a sustained reduction in oxalate excretion. A limitation of dietary oxalate intake and potassium citrate therapy (to be discussed) may be helpful in lowering oxalate and increasing citrate levels in urine, respectively. A high fluid intake is essential to overcome intestinal fluid loss.

Treatment of Hyperuricosuric Calcium Nephrolithiasis. This form of hyperuricosuria usually results from a diet high in purine precursors of uric acid. It should therefore be subject to effective dietary therapy. Unfortunately, many patients cannot or do not choose to maintain this dietary restraint. Allopurinol, 300 mg per day orally, will produce normal or subnormal levels of urinary uric acid and thereby may inhibit urate-induced crystallization of calcium oxalate.

Treatment of Hypocitraturic Calcium Nephrolithiasis. In renal tubular acidosis (distal), sodium citrate or potassium citrate (60 to 120 mEq per day in divided doses) may augment citrate excretion (see Ch. 84 for details). In the absence of renal insufficiency, potassium citrate is preferable because it could reduce urinary calcium and correct potassium deficiency. In *chronic diarrheal states,* potassium citrate in a liquid form is recommended to allow for rapid absorption (60 to 120 mEq per day). Hypocitraturia is sometimes very severe and recalcitrant to alkali therapy. In *thiazide-induced hypocitraturia,* potassium citrate (30 to 60 mEq per day in two divided doses in a slow-release tablet form) is generally sufficient to correct both hypokalemia and hypocitraturia. In other causes of hypocitraturia, a sufficient dose of potassium citrate may be provided to restore normal urinary citrate levels. The efficacy of potassium citrate is shown in Figure 90–2.

Treatment of Uric Acid Stones. In uric acid diathesis, administration of potassium citrate may increase urinary pH and create an environment in which uric acid is more soluble. Moderate amounts of alkali (40 to 60 mEq of potassium citrate per day in divided doses), sufficient to raise urinary pH to a range of 6 to 6.5, are recommended. Alkali therapy, especially at high dosages, may be complicated by the formation of calcium stones. The potassium salt rather than sodium salt of bicarbonate or citrate may be preferable in preventing this complication. If hydration and alkali therapy are ineffective, allopurinol should be used to decrease uric acid stone formation. See the discussion in Ch. 195 on gout for more details.

Treatment of Cystinuria (see Ch. 84). If a high fluid intake and alkali therapy are ineffective in reducing cystine concentration below saturation of cystine, D-*penicillamine* (2 grams per day in divided doses) may be required. This compound reduces urinary cystine content by forming a more soluble mixed disulfide with cysteine. Unfortunately, penicillamine treatment may be complicated by serious side effects, including nephrotic syndrome, dermatitis, and pancytopenia. An investigational drug, alpha-mercaptopropionylglycine, may exert similar action on cystine excretion, with apparent reduced toxicity.

Treatment of Struvite (Magnesium Ammonium Phosphate) Stones. If a longstanding effective control of infection with urea-splitting organisms can be achieved, there is some evidence that new struvite stone formation can be averted or some dissolution of existing stones may be achieved. Unfortunately, such a control is difficult to obtain with antibiotic therapy alone. It is difficult to eliminate the infection com-

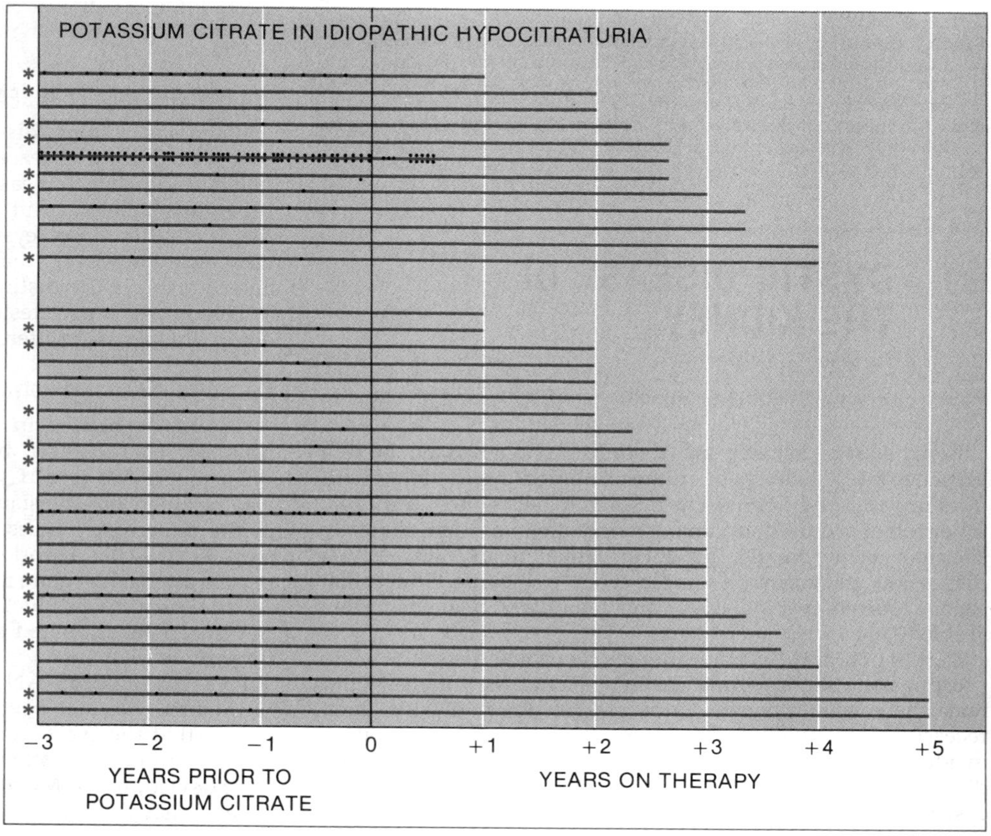

FIGURE 90–2. Effect of potassium citrate therapy on new stone formation. Each line represents one patient. An asterisk before the line indicates the presence of pre-existing stone(s). Each point shows new stone formation.

pletely from an existing struvite stone because the stone often harbors the organisms within its interstices. Even if sterilization of urine is achieved by antibiotic therapy, reinfection often occurs from harbored organisms. Addition of acetohydroxamic acid, a urease inhibitor, at a dosage of 250 mg three times per day, may be more effective in controlling struvite stone formation. If not, surgical removal of stones should be considered.

Surgical Treatment

Removal of stones may become mandatory when nephrolithiasis is complicated by obstruction, infection, gross hematuria, or intractable pain. Dramatic progress has been made in techniques for stone removal. Certain stones may now be removed less invasively via percutaneous nephroscopy and by extracorporeal shock wave lithotripsy. The latter procedure, now widely introduced in the United States, utilizes focused, electrically generated shock waves to fragment stones within a human kidney without incision. Single stones of moderate size ($\leq$ 1 cm in diameter) located in the renal pelvis are particularly amenable to this treatment. The risk of obstruction, pain, and retained fragments is higher for multiple stones and larger stones. Not all stones are amenable to shock wave lithotripsy alone (e.g., staghorn calculi and stones in lower ureter). The criteria for the choice of different methods are undergoing rapid refinement as further experience is gained with new approaches.

Coe FL: Nephrolithiasis: Pathogenesis and Treatment. Chicago, Year Book Medical Publishers, 1979. *A detailed review of current concepts of cause and treatment of calcareous as well as noncalcareous stones.*

Drach GW, Dretler S, Fair W, et al.: Report of the United States cooperative study of extracorporeal shock wave lithotripsy. J Urol 135:1127, 1986. *A review of results of extracorporeal shock wave lithotripsy among 2501 patients undergoing this procedure in the United States.*

Millman S, Strauss AL, Parks JH, et al.: Pathogenesis and clinical course of mixed calcium oxalate and uric acid nephrolithiasis. Kidney Int 22:366, 1982. *A useful review of the intriguing and important interactions of uric acid and oxalate in stone pathogenesis.*

Pak CYC: Kidney stones. In Foster DW, Wilson JD (eds.): Williams Textbook of Endocrinology. Philadelphia, W. B. Saunders Company, 1985. pp 1256–1273. *A comprehensive discussion of the pathogenesis and treatment of renal calculi.*

Pak CYC, Britton F, Peterson R, et al.: Ambulatory evaluation of nephrolithiasis: Classification, clinical presentation and diagnostic criteria. Am J Med 69:19, 1980. *A detailed description of the outpatient protocol that provides diagnostic criteria for different causes of nephrolithiasis.*

Pak CYC, Fuller C, Sakhaee K, et al.: Long term treatment of calcium nephrolithiasis with potassium citrate. J Urol 134:11, 1985. *A detailed study describing mechanism of action and utility of potassium citrate in calcium nephrolithiasis.*

91 CYSTIC DISEASE OF THE KIDNEY

Patricia A. Gabow

Renal cystic diseases are disorders characterized by the presence in the kidneys of epithelium-lined cavities filled with fluid or semisolid debris. The cysts may be single or multiple, inherited or acquired, occurring in infancy or old age, clinically silent or symptomatic, producing renal insufficiency. This discussion will focus on simple cysts, polycystic kidney disease, acquired cystic disease, and medullary cystic disorders (Table 91–1).

Certain clinical settings suggest various disorders. The presence of abdominal masses in a neonate or infant should raise the consideration of autosomal dominant or autosomal recessive polycystic kidney disease. The onset of renal failure in adolescence suggests autosomal recessive polycystic kidney disease or medullary cystic disease. The finding of a solitary cyst in a 50-year-old adult suggests a simple cyst. A history of renal disease in a family raises the possibility of autosomal dominant polycystic kidney disease or medullary cystic disease. Recurrent renal stones can occur in autosomal dominant polycystic kidney disease or with medullary sponge kidneys. The onset of gross hematuria in a patient undergoing chronic hemodialysis raises the possibility of acquired cystic disease.

SIMPLE CYSTS

Simple renal cysts, the most common and clinically least significant of all the cystic disorders, increase in frequency with age (from 0.1 to 4 per cent in children to 50 per cent in the population over 50 years of age). Often the cysts are asymptomatic and are discovered during abdominal imaging studies performed for other reasons. Occasionally patients with simple cysts present with hematuria or flank pain, thereby raising the question of malignancy within the cyst. Evaluation should begin with renal ultrasonography, which in a simple cyst will demonstrate smooth walls, good sound transmission, and no intracystic debris. If the ultrasonographic pattern differs from these characteristics, but the lesion is clearly cystic rather than solid, patients should undergo cyst puncture with ultrasonographic guidance. In this manner, cyst fluid can be obtained for cytology and for measurement of lactic dehydrogenase (LDH) and lipids, and contrast material can be injected to delineate the cyst wall architecture. This approach differentiates simple cysts from malignancy with 96 per cent or greater accuracy (Table 91–2). If the functional and structural characteristics of a cyst suggest malignancy, obviously surgery should be considered. For another discussion of renal masses, see also Ch. 93.

Kleist H, Jonsson O, Lundstam S: Quantitative lipid analysis in the differential diagnosis of cystic renal lesions. Br J Urol 54:441, 1982. *Cyst fluid analysis is discussed.*

Lang E, Johnson B, Chance HL, et al.: Assessment of avascular renal mass lesions: The use of nephrotomography, arteriography, cyst puncture, double contrast study and histochemical and histopathologic examination of the aspirate. South Med J 65:1, 1972.

Mir S, Rapola J, Koskimies O: Renal cysts in pediatric autopsy material. Nephron 33:189, 1983. *Data from autopsy material in 6521 children are presented.*

Zeman RK, Cronan JJ, Rosenfield AT, et al.: Imaging approach to suspected renal mass. Radiol Clin North Am 23:503, 1985. *A comprehensive review of the subject.*

POLYCYSTIC KIDNEY DISEASE

Polycystic kidney disease includes autosomal dominant polycystic kidney disease (ADPKD) and autosomal recessive polycystic kidney disease (ARPKD). These disorders were previously labeled adult polycystic kidney disease and infantile or childhood polycystic kidney disease, respectively. It is now clear, however, that pattern of inheritance rather than age of onset is the distinguishing characteristic. ADPKD not uncommonly is manifested in childhood and even occasionally in infancy or in utero.

Autosomal Dominant Polycystic Kidney Disease (ADPKD)

ADPKD, inherited in an autosomal dominant pattern, is primarily characterized by cyst development and growth of cysts in the kidneys. Cyst formation or outpouchings may also occur in other organs, particularly in the liver, but also in the pancreas, ovaries, gastrointestinal tract, and vascular tree. ADPKD has a worldwide occurrence with 1/200 to 1/1000 people affected. A gene for ADPKD is carried on chromosome 16, but the gene product is not known. Complete penetrance of the gene is estimated to occur by the time the individual is 90 years of age.

PATHOGENESIS AND PATHOLOGY. The pathogenesis of ADPKD has not been established. An early theory suggested that the cysts were "dead ends" of renal tubules that failed to unite with other nephron segments during embryologic development. Microdissection of renal tubules, however, reveals that the cysts are outpouchings occurring at various

TABLE 91–1. CHARACTERISTICS OF RENAL CYSTIC DISORDERS

Feature	Simple Cysts	ADPKD	ARPKD	ACKD	MCD	MSK
Inheritance pattern	None	Autosomal dominant	Autosomal recessive	None	Often present, variable pattern	None
Prevalence	Common, increasing with age	1/400 to 1/1000	Rare	40% in dialysis patients	Rare	Common
Age of Onset	Adult	Usually adults	Neonates, children	Older adults	Adolescents, young adults	Adults
Presenting symptom	Incidental finding: hematuria	Pain, hematuria, infection, family screening	Abdominal mass, renal failure, failure to thrive	Hematuria	Polyuria, polydipsia, enuresis, renal failure, failure to thrive	Incidental, urinary tract infections, hematuria, renal calculi
Hematuria	Occurs	Common	Occurs	Occurs	Rare	Common
Recurrent infections	Rare	Common	Occurs	No	Rare	Common
Renal calculi	No	Common	No	No	No	Common
Hypertension	Rare	Common	Common	Present from underlying disease	Rare	No
Method of diagnosis	Ultrasound	Ultrasound	Ultrasound	CT scan	None reliable	Excretory urogram
Renal size	Normal	Normal to very large	Large initially	Small to normal, occasionally large	Small	Normal

ADPKD = Autosomal dominant polycystic kidney disease; ARPKD = autosomal recessive polycystic kidney disease; ACKD = acquired cystic kidney disease; MCD = medullary cystic disease; MSK = medullary sponge kidney.

points along intact nephrons. Cyst puncture and cyst fluid analysis demonstrate transport characteristics compatible with various nephron segments. For example, some cysts have sodium concentrations similar to that of plasma, whereas others have low sodium concentrations, suggesting that the cysts are of proximal and distal tubular origin, respectively. Exposure to an environmental toxin or bacterial product in a susceptible individual has been postulated with no direct evidence. By electron microscopy polypoid lesions have been noted throughout the cyst walls in both experimental cystic disease and human ADPKD. These polyps have been envisioned as obstructing tubules with retrograde tubular bulging or cyst formation, but this theory fails to explain the extrarenal cysts. In addition, obstructive uropathy does not produce cystic renal changes. The observation of polyp formation suggests that ADPKD is a disorder of altered cell growth. Cell proliferation must occur to provide for the epithelial lining of the renal cysts. The basement membrane has been noted to be abnormally split in ADPKD, suggesting that it is intrinsically abnormal. The concept that ADPKD is a disorder of extracellular matrix formation, i.e., basement membrane and other collagen types, offers the best current pathogenetic explanation for the extrarenal manifestations. The genetic defect may result in both altered cell growth and abnormal matrix formation because of the close inter-relationship of cell growth and cell supporting structure. In fact, cell cultures from cysts of patients with ADPKD demonstrate both altered cell growth and abnormal basement membrane structure.

Kidneys in ADPKD can be normal in size with few cysts, particularly early in the course of the disorder. Ultimately, the kidneys enlarge and may attain the size of a football, weighing as much as 8 kg. The end-stage kidney appears to be virtually replaced by cysts (Fig. 91–1). The cysts can contain clear fluid, purulent-appearing fluid, or blood. The cut surface of the kidney reveals cysts throughout the renal parenchyma (Fig. 91–2).

CLINICAL MANIFESTATIONS. Individuals usually present for screening either because of a family history of the disease or because of symptoms. *Pain* and *hematuria* are the most common clinical manifestations. Flank pain and back pain are more common than abdominal pain. The pain can be constant or intermittent, mild or severe and disabling. Both microscopic and gross hematuria occur. One third of patients will have microscopic hematuria on a random urinalysis. Episodes of hematuria occur in about 30 per cent of patients and are often precipitated by trauma or strenuous exercise. Headaches, gastrointestinal complaints, nocturia, frequency, and polyuria are other presenting symptoms. Some patients also present with renal complications of ADPKD, such as urinary tract infections, renal calculi, or retroperitoneal bleeding.

The extrarenal manifestations of ADPKD are summarized in Table 91–3. The most common extrarenal involvement in ADPKD is that of hepatic cysts, which occur in 40 per cent to 60 per cent of patients. As with renal cysts, hepatic cysts appear to increase in number or size, or both, over time and can eventuate in massive hepatomegaly, but they rarely produce functional impairment. However, hepatic cysts can become infected. Colonic diverticulosis, often resulting in perforation and intra-abdominal abscess formation, has been reported in 83 per cent of patients with ADPKD undergoing chronic hemodialysis treatment, compared with a prevalence of 32 per cent in dialysis patients with other renal disease. Both hiatal and inguinal hernias may be more frequent in

TABLE 91–2. DIFFERENTIATING CHARACTERISTICS OF BENIGN AND MALIGNANT CYSTS

Feature	Benign	Malignant
Color of fluid	Straw color	Turbid or reddish
Cytology of fluid	Normal	Atypical or malignant cells
LDH of fluid	Low	High
Mean total lipid of fluid (mmol/liter)	0.3	13.2
Mean cholesterol of fluid (mmol/liter)	0.18	8.5
Cyst wall	Smooth	Irregular

LDH = Lactate dehydrogenase.

TABLE 91–3. SYSTEMIC INVOLVEMENT IN AUTOSOMAL DOMINANT POLYCYSTIC KIDNEY DISEASE (ADPKD)

I. Genitourinary
   - Polycystic kidney
   - Hypernephroma
   - Renal calculi
   - Ovarian cyst (?)

II. Gastrointestinal
   - Hepatic cysts
   - Pancreatic cysts
   - Diverticuli

III. Cardiovascular
   - Hypertension
   - Cardiac valvular abnormalities
   - Berry aneurysms
   - Thoracic aortic aneurysms

IV. Hematopoietic
   - Erythrocytosis

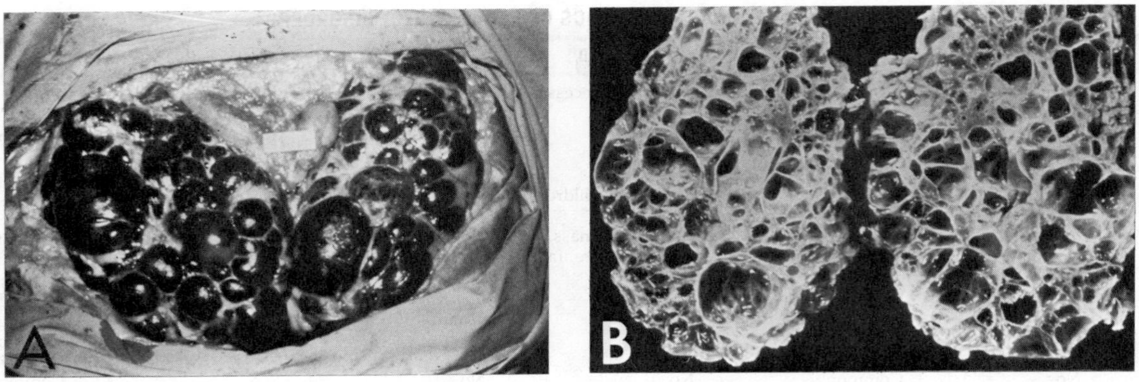

FIGURE 91–1. Autosomal dominant polycystic kidney disease (ADPKD) in situ (*A*) and on cut section (*B*). Note diffuse, bilateral distribution of cysts. (Courtesy of F. E. Cuppage, Kansas City, KS.)

patients with ADPKD. An occasional patient will also demonstrate pancreatic cysts.

Hypertension, the most common cardiovascular manifestation of ADPKD, occurs in 60 per cent of patients before the onset of renal insufficiency. The hypertension does not appear to be related to the renin-angiotensin system. *Berry aneurysms* occur in 10 per cent to 40 per cent of patients with ADPKD; it is not clear what percentage of these actually rupture. No known clinical factors predict which patients with ADPKD are at high risk for rupture. Rarely a subarachnoid hemorrhage is the presenting manifestation of ADPKD. Thoracic aortic aneurysms and cardiac valvular abnormalities (especially aortic and mitral valve involvement, occasionally with myxomatous degeneration) also seem to be increased in prevalence.

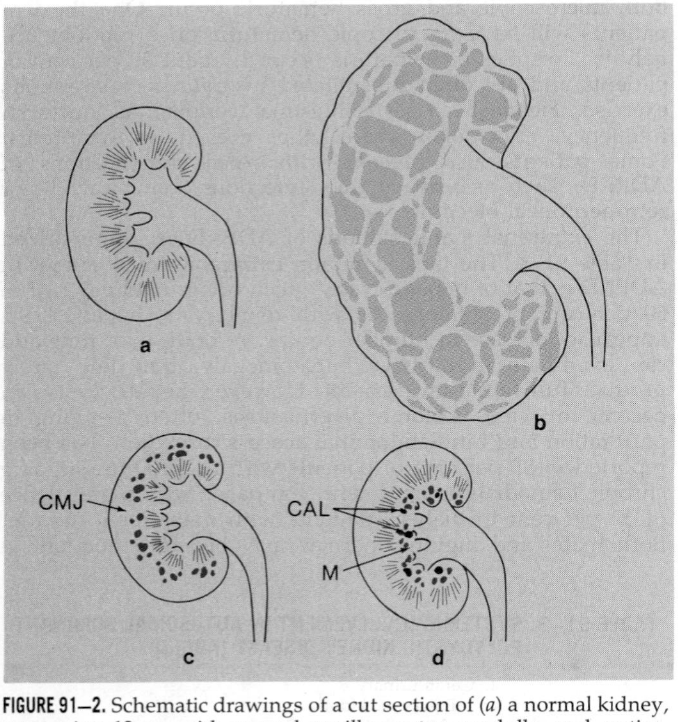

FIGURE 91–2. Schematic drawings of a cut section of (*a*) a normal kidney, measuring 12 cm with normal papilla, cortex, medulla, and corticomedullary junction and (*b*) a kidney from a patient with ADPKD. The kidney is large, measuring 29 cm, and contains cysts throughout the cortex and medulla which vary in size from 1 mm to 5 cm. *c*, A kidney from a patient with medullary cystic disease. The kidney is small, measuring 8 cm, with a scarred surface. The cysts are at the corticomedullary junction (CMJ) and are small, measuring 1 to 5 mm across. *d*, A kidney from a patient with medullary sponge kidney. There are multiple ductal dilatations measuring 1 to 5 mm in diameter, giving the medulla (M) a porous appearance. Some dilatations contain calculi (CAL). (*c* and *d* adapted from Spence HM, Singleton R: What is sponge kidney disease and where does it fit in the spectrum of cystic disorders? J Urol 107:176, 1972.)

Ovarian cysts occur in ADPKD, but the relationship of this common abnormality to the genetic defect is not known. Occasionally patients with ADPKD demonstrate erythrocytosis. This is presumed to reflect increased erythropoietin production by the cystic kidney.

The incidence of bilateral renal malignancy appears to be higher in patients with ADPKD than in the general population. A person with this malignancy may present with asymmetric renal enlargment, increasing frequency or amount of hematuria, and weight loss, but the presence of these symptoms in the absence of malignancy, and the underlying structural abnormalities in the kidney, often make the diagnosis of renal malignancy difficult.

The natural history of renal functional impairment with ADPKD is variable. Renal failure may occur as early as the first decade of life in children with early symptomatic disease, or renal function may be well maintained into the eighth decade. End-stage renal disease rarely occurs before 40 years of age. Approximately 50 per cent of patients have well-preserved renal function at 70 years of age. Renal function is less well maintained in ADPKD patients with hypertension. Other factors that influence long-term prognosis are less well defined.

DIAGNOSIS. The diagnosis of ADPKD depends upon the demonstration of the characteristic bilateral renal cystic involvement, now best established by renal ultrasonography. Not infrequently, screening studies of families will demonstrate only a few unilateral cysts or only one or two cysts in each kidney. This situation requires differentiation of ADPKD from multiple simple cysts (Table 91–4). The patient's age and the presence of extrarenal involvement are most helpful in this instance (Fig. 91–3). Since simple cysts are uncommon in

TABLE 91–4. COMPARISON OF MULTIPLE SIMPLE CYSTS AND EARLY ADPKD

Feature	Multiple Simple Cysts	ADPKD
Family history	No	≈ 60%
Ultrasonographically demonstrable cysts in other family member(s)	No	≈ 90%
Sex distribution	M > F	M = F
Renal size	Normal	Normal to mildly enlarged
Kidneys involved	Usually unilateral, may be bilateral	Usually bilateral, may be unilateral early
Cyst distribution	Cortical	Cortical and medullary
Cyst size	Usually < 2 cm, occasionally larger	< 2 cm early
Blood in cysts	Rare	Common
Hepatic cysts	No	40–60%; likelihood increases with age
Berry aneurysm	No	10–40%
Hypertension	Rare	60%

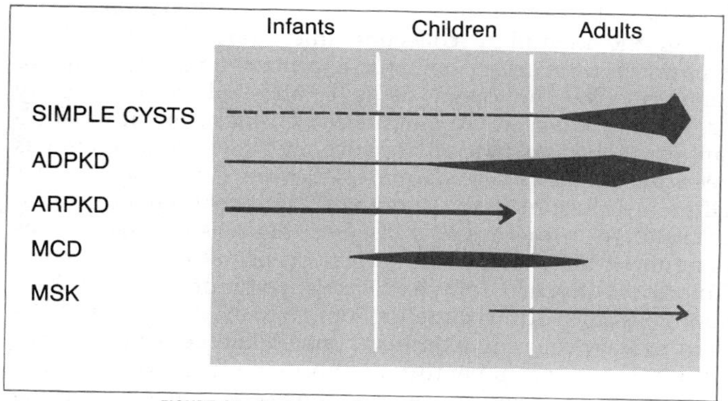

FIGURE 91–3. Ages of renal cystic disease.

children, the finding of any cysts in a child in a family with ADPKD strongly suggests the disorder. In an individual over age 50 with similar ultrasonographic findings, however, the diagnosis is much less certain. The presence of extrarenal involvement, particularly hepatic cysts, lends support to the diagnosis of ADPKD. In the absence of extrarenal involvement, which is often absent early in the course of the disease, the best method of establishing a diagnosis in a patient with only unilateral cysts or very few cysts is follow-up abdominal ultrasonography in two to three years. If renal cystic involvement increases or if extrarenal involvement occurs, the diagnosis of ADPKD can be made. If there is a need for more immediate definitive diagnosis, computerized axial tomography will occasionally reveal more diffuse cystic involvement than is apparent by ultrasonography. The role of magnetic resonance imaging remains to be defined. The finding of a gene linkage with a gene for ADPKD on chromosome 16 opens the possibility in the near future for definitive diagnosis of the gene carrier state prior to the development of gross structural abnormalities.

It is not important to establish the presence of extrarenal involvement in all patients with ADPKD. Currently, routine total abdominal ultrasonography for diagnosis of hepatic, pancreatic, or ovarian cysts is not recommended. Moreover, routine carotid angiography or computerized axial tomography of the head in search of a berry aneurysm is not recommended in asymptomatic patients with ADPKD. Echocardiography need not be performed routinely to assess valvular disease.

TREATMENT. The treatment for patients with ADPKD is generally aimed at preventing complications of the disease and at preserving renal function. First, patients and family members should be educated about the inheritance and manifestations of the disease. Patients with large kidneys should be cautioned about risks of contact sports, since significant renal trauma seems to occur more frequently in structurally abnormal kidneys. Episodes of gross hematuria should be managed conservatively with bed rest, analgesics, and hydration. Urinary tract instrumentation, including Foley catheter placement, should be avoided because of the increased risk of serious urinary tract and renal cyst infections in patients after such instrumentation. Patients suspected of having a urinary tract infection should have urine and blood cultures obtained. Selection of appropriate antibiotic therapy depends on the presumed site of infection. Bladder and renal parenchymal infections can be treated as they are treated in other patients. Failure to respond to appropriate antibiotic treatment suggests cyst infections. In this instance the antibiotic chosen must be one that has been shown to enter cyst fluid. These include chloramphenicol and trimethoprim-sulfamethoxazole.

Hypertension should be aggressively treated. The roles for restriction of phosphorus or protein, or both, or for cyst puncture in the preservation of renal function have not yet been established in ADPKD. Patients should have their blood pressures monitored. A serum creatinine level should be obtained yearly prior to the development of renal insufficiency and at least every six months thereafter. Repeat imaging studies need not be performed unless new clinical symptoms occur. Computerized axial tomography is the method of choice for establishing the diagnosis of complications such as intracystic or retroperitoneal hemorrhage, renal calculi, or renal malignancy. A more general discussion of the treatment of renal failure is found in Ch. 80.

Bach JF, Crosnier J, Funck-Brentano JL, et al.: Liver changes and complications in adult polycystic kidney disease. In Grunfeld (ed.): Advances in Nephrology, Vol. 14. Chicago, Year Book Medical Publishers, 1985, pp 1–20.

Gabow PA, Ikle DW, Holmes JH: Polycystic kidney disease: Prospective analysis of nonazotemic patients and family members. Ann Intern Med 101:238, 1984. *A comprehensive presentation of symptoms, signs, and ultrasonography in a large, young, nonazotemic patient population.*

Grantham JJ, Gardner KD Jr (eds): Polycystic Kidney Disease. Proceedings of the First International Symposium on ADPKD. Kansas City, MO, PKR Foundation, 1985. *Contains many interesting discussions on all aspects of ADPKD.*

Schwab SJ, Bander SJ, Klahr S: Renal infection in autosomal dominant polycystic kidney disease. Am J Med 82:714, 1987.

Welling LW, Grantham JJ: Cystic and developmental diseases of the kidney. In Brenner BM, Rector FC Jr. (eds.): The Kidney. 3rd ed. Philadelphia, W. B. Saunders Company, 1986, pp 1341–1376. *An admirable summary of all cystic disorders in the kidney, with 279 references.*

Wilson PD, Schrier RW, Breckon RD, et al.: A new method for studying human polycystic kidney disease epithelia in culture. Kidney Int 30:371, 1986.

Autosomal Recessive Polycystic Kidney Disease (ARPKD)

Autosomal recessive polycystic kidney disease (ARPKD) is a rare disorder that has been classified into perinatal, neonatal, infantile, or juvenile types based on age of onset. The presenting manifestations include abdominal masses, failure to thrive, and urinary tract infections. The pathogenetic mechanism is not understood. The kidneys are large early in life and may diminish in size with time. The cut surface of the kidney reveals radially oriented fusiform cysts. As in ADPKD, ultrasonography is the diagnostic method of choice. Examination of the parents and, in some instances, liver biopsy of the affected child are necessary to distinguish ARPKD from the childhood presentation of ADPKD. Normal findings on renal ultrasonography in the parents strongly suggest ARPKD. In addition, children with ARPKD, particularly the juvenile form, often have hepatic involvement with hepatic fibrosis, frequently resulting in portal hypertension. Children with ARPKD usually progress to end-stage chronic renal failure before adolescence; in the perinatal form, this occurs within the first few weeks of life. Treatment of the chronic renal failure of ARPKD is similar to that of other childhood renal insufficiency.

Blyth H, Ockenden BG: Polycystic disease of kidneys and liver presenting in childhood. J Med Genet 8:257, 1971. *A discussion of classification of this disorder.*

ACQUIRED CYSTIC KIDNEY DISEASE (ACKD)

Acquired cystic disease refers to the development of cysts in previously noncystic kidneys in patients with end-stage renal disease, almost exclusively in those undergoing dialysis. Forty per cent of patients undergoing chronic dialysis appear to develop this disorder. Most patients have no symptoms attributable to this complication, but some patients develop hematuria, and about 16 per cent of ACKD patients develop renal tumors. Unlike ADPKD or ARPKD, computerized axial tomography is the diagnostic method of choice in ACKD because the kidneys are often small and prone to malignancy. Episodes of hematuria can be treated as in ADPKD. Severe, recurrent hematuria can be treated with renal arterial embolization, as it is not critical to preserve renal parenchyma in dialysis patients. Renal tumors less than 3 cm can be followed with yearly computerized axial tomography; larger tumors require surgery because of their greater propensity for malignancy.

Gehrig JJ Jr, Gottheiner TI, Swenson RS: Acquired cystic disease of end-stage kidney. Am J Med 79:609, 1985. *Excellent review of clinical and pathologic data.*

Levine E, Grantham JJ, Slusher SL, et al.: CT of acquired cystic kidney disease and renal tumors in long-term dialysis patients. Am J Roentgenol 142:125, 1984. *Role of computerized tomography (CT) in assessing ACKD is fully discussed and documented.*

MEDULLARY CYSTIC DISORDERS

Medullary cystic disease and medullary sponge kidney are the most common of the medullary cystic disorders. Medullary cystic disease has also been labeled nephronophthisis, cystic medullary complex, and renal-retinal dysplasia (because of the coincidence of retinitis pigmentosa in some families). Medullary cystic disease is uncommon; only about 300 cases have been reported. A familial pattern appears to be present in a majority of cases. Both autosomal recessive and autosomal dominant patterns of inheritance have been reported. Recessive transmission may occur more often in the childhood presentation of the disease and dominant inheritance more commonly in the adult presentation of the disorder.

PATHOGENESIS AND PATHOLOGY. No pathogenetic theory has been proposed for this disorder. The kidneys are small and generally display some cysts at the corticomedullary junction and in the medulla (Fig. 91–2). An acystic form of the disorder appears to occur. The glomeruli are hyalinized, and the tubules vary in appearance, some being atrophic and others being tortuous. The tubular basement membrane is often irregular with areas that are thickened and others that are thinned and split. The interstitium reveals fibrosis and mononuclear cell infiltrate. This interstitial involvement suggests some as yet undefined relationship with other immune and nonimmune tubulointerstitial disease. It has been postulated that medullary cystic disease may be the end-stage form of other tubulointerstitial disease.

CLINICAL MANIFESTATIONS. A majority of patients present in childhood or early adolescence with polydipsia, polyuria, and enuresis. Often the children demonstrate growth retardation and anemia. The polyuria and enuresis with secondary polydipsia are presumed to reflect a defect in urinary concentrating ability, which apparently occurs early in the disease.

Renal salt wasting has also been suggested to occur in the disorder to a degree in excess of the impaired sodium conservation that accompanies any end-stage renal disease. Certainly the possibility of salt wasting should be considered in a patient with this disorder prior to sodium restriction.

DIAGNOSIS. Diagnosis of the disorder is often difficult. The urinalysis is often unremarkable, and proteinuria is generally minimal. Imaging studies reveal only small end-stage kidneys. Some patients are simply labeled as having "chronic renal failure" or "chronic pyelonephritis." The disorder should be considered in children or young adults who present with renal insufficiency, small kidneys, and a family history of renal disease. No specific treatment exists. Management is the same as that appropriate for any child with renal insufficiency, with attention to growth, bone disease, and, in particular, sodium balance. The possibility of retinal abnormality must also be considered in initial evaluation.

Avasthi PS, Erickson DG, Gardner KD: Hereditary renal-retinal dysplasia and the medullary cystic disease–nephronophthisis complex. Ann Intern Med 84:157, 1976. *The association is described, and the inheritance of medullary cystic disease is described.*

Chamberlin BC, Hagge WW, Stickler GB: Juvenile nephronophthisis and medullary cystic disease. Mayo Clin Proc 52:485, 1977. *Six cases are presented, and literature is reviewed.*

Helczynski L, Landing BH: Tubulointerstitial renal diseases of children: Pathologic features and pathogenetic mechanisms in Fanconi's familial nephronophthisis, antitubular basement membrane antibody disease, and medullary cyst disease. Pediatr Pathol 2:1, 1984.

Steele BT, Lirenman DS, Beattie CU: Nephronophthisis. Am J Med 68:531, 1980. *The clinical data and follow-up information on 21 patients are presented.*

MEDULLARY SPONGE KIDNEY

Medullary sponge kidney is a relatively common disorder affecting between 1/5000 and 1/20,000 individuals. There is no known pathogenetic mechanism. Tubular dilatations occur within the medullary collecting ducts (Fig. 91–2). Patients present with recurrent hematuria, urinary tract infections, or renal calculi. The diagnosis is established with excretory urography, which reveals normal-sized kidneys with medullary ductal ectasia. The appearance on excretory urogram has been described as a "bouquet of flowers" or a paintbrush. Often a plain film of the abdomen will reveal renal calculi or calcification in the cystic areas. For this reason other causes of nephrolithiasis and nephrocalcinosis need to be considered. Coincident hyperparathyroidism is common in medullary sponge kidney, and therefore both serum calcium and 24-hour urinary calcium determinations should be obtained and, if indicated, a serum parathyroid hormone level (see Ch. 247). Conversely, as many as 20 per cent of patients presenting with nephrolithiasis may have medullary sponge kidney. Other clinical manifestations of medullary sponge kidney reflect the structural alterations in the renal papillae that occur in the disease and include a decreased renal concentrating ability, an inability to acidify the urine maximally with an incomplete renal tubular acidosis and an impairment in renal potassium excretion in response to acute potassium loading. However, despite these defects, serum electrolyte concentrations are almost always normal. Treatment includes appropriate management of renal infections and of renal calculous disease (Ch. 86 and 90). Urinary tract obstruction must be considered during acute episodes of renal colic. In the absence of obstruction, renal function remains normal.

Green J, Szylman P, Sznajder II, et al.: Renal tubular handling of potassium in patients with medullary sponge kidney. Arch Intern Med 144:2201, 1984. *Presentation of renal tubular defects in medullary sponge kidney.*

Morris RC, Yamaughi H, Palubinskas AJ, et al.: Medullary sponge kidney. Am J Med 38:883, 1965. *Twenty patients with medullary sponge kidney and some related abnormalities are discussed.*

Parks JH, Coe FL, Strauss AL: Calcium nephrolithiasis and medullary sponge kidney in women. N Engl J Med 306:1088, 1982.

Zawada ET Jr, Sica DA: Differential diagnosis of medullary sponge kidney. South Med J 77:686, 1984. *Differential diagnosis—a case report with excretory urography.*

92 ANOMALIES OF THE URINARY TRACT

Richard D. Williams

Congenital aberrations of the urinary tract occur in over 10 per cent of the population. They vary in severity from lesions incompatible with life to those that are insignificant and detected only incidentally during studies prompted by unrelated causes. Often the anomalies, although not intrinsically detrimental, predispose to infection, lithiasis, and chronic renal failure, which lead to their recognition.

KIDNEY

ANOMALIES OF NUMBER. *Bilateral renal agenesis* is rare (1 in 4800 births), more frequent in males (3 to 1 ratio), and typically accompanied by oligohydramnios, Potter's facies, and pulmonary hypoplasia; this complex results in death within a few days of birth. *Unilateral renal agenesis* is more common (1 in 1100 births), generally involves the left kidney, and is seen more often in males (ratio 1.8 to 1). Renal absence is considered secondary to lack of a ureteral bud. Occasionally, a presumptive diagnosis of unilateral renal absence may be made in males when an ipsilateral vas deferens is absent on palpation. In only 10 per cent of renal agenesis cases is the adrenal absent. Extrarenal tissue or *supernumerary kidneys* are extremely rare (only 60 cases have been described); they are distinct from ureteral and caliceal duplication to be described later.

ANOMALIES OF POSITION (ECTOPIA). These are due to abnormal renal ascent: They include lumbar and pelvic and the less common thoracic or crossed ectopic varieties (Fig. 92–1). As a group they occur in 1 in 900 cases and reach clinical significance only when they are mistaken for tumor during exploratory surgery or because of associated genital anomalies. Anomalies of fusion fall into this same category, since the abnormality leads to lack of ascent; *fused pelvic kidneys* or *horseshoe kidneys* (typically fused at their lower poles) are prevented from normal ascent by the inferior mesenteric artery (Fig. 92–2). These latter two anomalies are associated with recurrent infection and calculi in 10 to 20 per cent of patients and with a high incidence of ureteropelvic junction obstruction. *Nephroptosis* is the descent toward the pelvis of a normally ascended kidney when the upright posture is assumed; it is seen in adults and is perhaps due to poor renal fixation in the retroperitoneum. This condition, which is not an anomaly per se, is usually asymptomatic and rarely, if ever, needs surgical correction. Anomalies of rotation, commonly termed *malrotation,* are due to incomplete ventromedial rotation during ascent and are rarely related to any functional abnormality.

ANOMALIES OF THE RENAL PARENCHYMA. There is a heterogeneous group of cystic and dysplastic lesions of the kidney. The most important group of disorders comprises those that produce cystic abnormalities, described in detail in Ch. 91. *Renal dysplasia* occurs in several forms: (1) *Multicystic kidneys* are malformed, nonfunctioning, generally unilateral, and invariably associated with ipsilateral ureteral atresia. When both kidneys are involved the manifestations and prognosis are similar to those in patients with bilateral renal agenesis. (2) *Segmental dysplasia* or *hypoplasia* is rare; it is not usually associated with significant renal complications, except in the bilateral and generalized form. (3) *Total renal dysplasia* is associated with lower urinary tract obstruction such as *posterior urethral valves* or functional bladder outlet obstruction, as in the *"prune-belly" syndrome.*

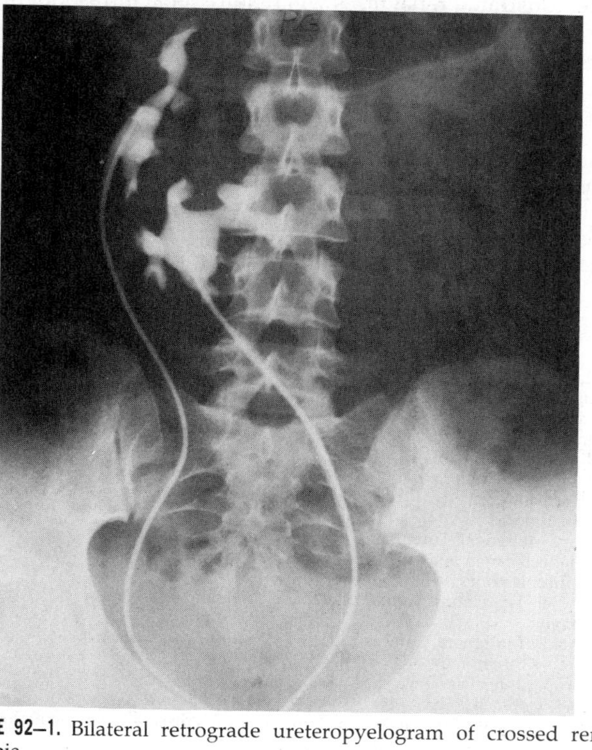

FIGURE 92–1. Bilateral retrograde ureteropyelogram of crossed renal ectopia.

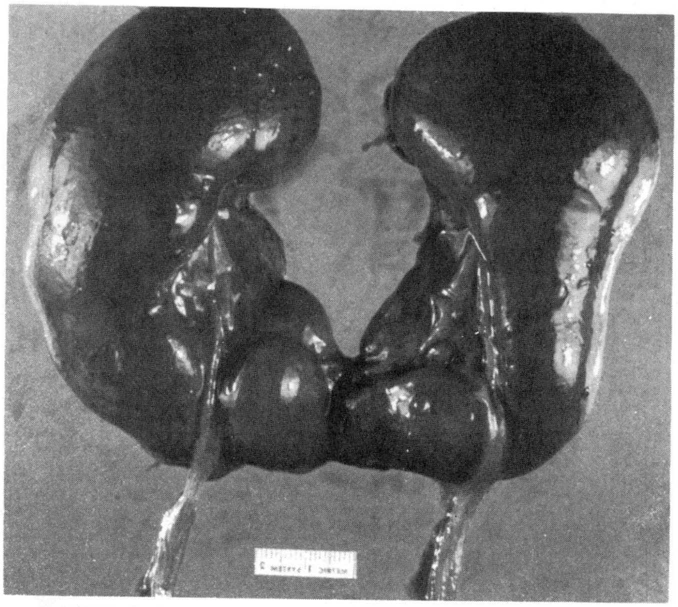

FIGURE 92–2. Gross pathologic specimen of horseshoe kidneys.

RENAL VASCULATURE

Multiple renal arteries occur in 15 to 20 per cent of the population. They are of little significance, except when they are inadvertently injured during an operation or (rarely) when they cause caliceal infundibular obstruction or (more often) *ureteropelvic junction obstruction. Congenital renal artery aneurysms* are infrequent; they are differentiated from acquired lesions by their location at the bifurcation of the main renal artery or at a distal branch point. The lesions require surgical treatment only if resulting hypertension is uncontrolled or if they are calcified and/or have a diameter of more than 2.5 cm. *Congenital arteriovenous fistulas* are rare but may result in hematuria, hypertension, and/or cardiac failure (if large), necessitating surgical intervention.

COLLECTING STRUCTURES AND URETER

Caliceal anomalies include *diverticuli, hydrocalycosis, megacalycosis,* and *infundibular stenosis.* They are clinically important only when urinary stasis results in recurrent infection and/or stone formation. *Ureteropelvic junction obstruction* is one of the more frequent causes of hydronephrosis in childhood (Fig. 92–3). Bilaterality is not unusual and the condition is often asymptomatic; however, flank pain (particularly following diuresis), urinary infection, and gross hematuria (following minor trauma) are frequent findings on presentation. Relief of symptoms as a rule follows surgical repair (pyeloplasty), although normalization of the radiologic abnormality is infrequent.

Ureteral duplication is the most common ureteral anomaly; it may be incomplete, with the duplicated ureters combining to form only one entrance per side into the bladder, or complete, with two or more ureters coursing toward the bladder on one or both sides. Most often all completely duplicated ureters enter the bladder. The ureter from the upper pole is always placed inferior in the bladder to that of the lower pole and often drains in an ectopic site, such as the bladder neck, prostate, or seminal vesicle in the male or midurethra in the female. The ureter from the lower pole often obtains poor implantation within the bladder, which may result in vesicoureteral reflux and possibly recurrent infection and hydroureteronephrosis. Ureteral ectopia can also occur in the absence of duplication but results in similar sequelae.

Ureteral reflux may be unrelated to duplication but due to an abnormal implantation of the ureter into the bladder with a resulting poorly developed trigone and deficient lower

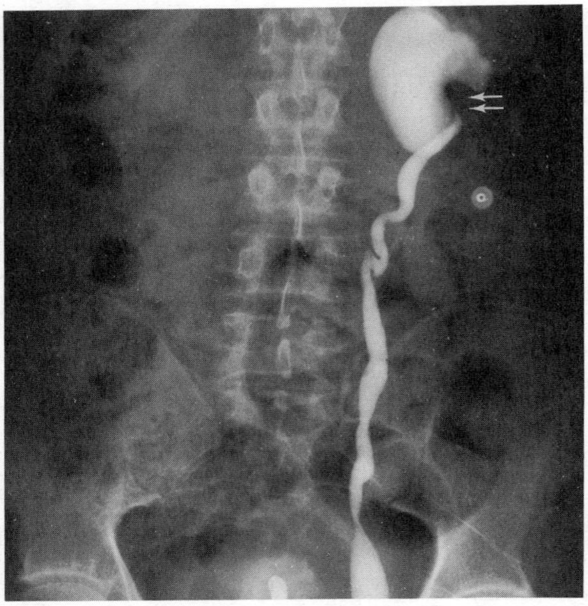

FIGURE 92–3. Retrograde ureteropyelogram showing ureteropelvic junction obstruction due to an aberrant lower pole renal artery (*arrows*).

ureteral muscle. This condition can cause recurrent urinary infection in children; however, surgical reimplantation is necessary only in severe cases. Other ureteral anomalies include *ureterocele,* a congenital distal ureteral meatal stenosis; *megaloureter,* an abnormality of the ureteral musculature allowing massive ureteral dilatation, often without caliceal distortion; *ureteral valves; ureteral diverticuli;* and *retrocaval ureter,* an anomaly of the formation of the vena cava causing the ureter to course behind the cava.

BLADDER

Anomalies of the bladder are very infrequent and include (1) *complete absence* (agenesis), which results in a persistent cloaca; (2) *duplication,* which may be complete with separate ureteral openings drained by separate urethras, or incomplete with a septum or hour-glass deformity; (3) *urachal* anomalies, which may appear as a patent connection to the umbilicus, a *diverticulum* at the dome of the bladder, or a *urachal cyst* along the course of the partially obliterated urachus; and (4) *exstrophy,* which is the most common severe anomaly of the bladder. Exstrophy represents a midline defect in closure of the bladder wall, lower abdominal muscles, pubic bones, and anterior urethra *(epispadias).* The *"prune-belly" syndrome* is a complex anomaly in which absence of the abdominal muscles is associated with bilateral cryptorchidism, ureteral dilatation and reflux, and an irregular capacious bladder with a dilated proximal urethra.

URETHRA

Hypospadias is the most common urethral anomaly in males (1 in 300 live births). The lesion results from failure of ventral fusion of the urogenital folds. It may present as a ventrally displaced meatus on the distal penile shaft or, in more severe forms, with the meatus opening more proximal on the shaft or in the perineum. These latter forms are often associated with a ventral penile chordee. Isolated *epispadias* (failure of dorsal closure of the urethra) occurs in males or females and is usually associated with incontinence. Congenital *urethral strictures* are infrequent. Although *meatal stenosis* is common, it is thought to be acquired, inasmuch as it generally is seen only in circumcised boys. Congenital *urethral diverticuli* are not rare, yet they generally are small and of no consequence. Finally, *megalourethra,* a markedly dilated anterior urethra, often associated with poor development of the erectile corpora, is rarely seen.

Arey LB: Developmental Anatomy. 7th ed. Philadelphia, W.B. Saunders Company, 1974. *The most complete text describing the derivation of congenital anomalies.*

Perlmutter AD, Retik AA, Bauer SB: Anomalies of the upper urinary tract. In Harrison et al.: Campbell's Urology. 5th ed. Philadelphia, W.B. Saunders Company, 1986, p 1665. *A complete and well-referenced treatise of the subject.*

93 TUMORS OF THE KIDNEY, URETER, AND BLADDER

Richard D. Williams

Benign and malignant renal tumors are either primary in the kidney and its surrounding connective tissue or collecting structures, or secondary (involving the kidney from adjacent organs or distant sites of origin). By definition, any mass within the kidney is a "renal tumor," but only solid masses are considered in this chapter. Cystic lesions of the kidney are discussed in Ch. 91. A classification of renal tumors is presented in Table 93–1.

APPROACH TO THE PATIENT WITH A RENAL MASS

In the past, most renal masses were detected on excretory urograms (IVP) during an evaluation prompted by signs or symptoms of disease (Table 93–2). Surgical exploration was often necessary for definitive diagnosis and treatment. Today, there are multiple new modalities for the accurate diagnostic study of renal masses, and because of their sensitivity an increasing number of incidental renal masses are being identified in asymptomatic patients. A systematic algorithmic approach should result in less than 10 per cent of renal masses being indeterminate prior to surgery (Fig. 93–1). Its use will often obviate the requirement for surgical definition.

The IVP with nephrotomography is still the study of first choice and can accurately define 75 per cent of renal masses. A demonstrated renal mass will require renal ultrasonography (US) to determine more accurately whether the mass is cystic or solid. If the mass fulfills all US criteria for a simple cyst (65 per cent of renal masses) there is little need for further workup, inasmuch as US is over 95 per cent accurate (Ch. 91). In the symptomatic patient, however, further workup, including needle aspiration cytology or computed tomographic (CT) scan or both, may be appropriate. When a mass is suspected on IVP but not confirmed on US (15 per cent of cases), either an isotopic scan of the renal cortex (DMSA) or renal CT is required, particularly in symptomatic patients.

TABLE 93–1. CLASSIFICATION OF RENAL TUMORS

Benign Tumors
Adenoma
Oncocytoma
Mesoblastic nephroma
Hamartoma-angiomyolipoma
Leiomyoma
Hemangioma
Primary Malignant Tumors
Renal cell carcinoma (adenocarcinoma)
Nephroblastoma (Wilms' tumor)
Urothelial carcinoma (renal collecting system and pelvis)
Sarcoma
Secondary Malignant Tumors (Direct Extension or Metastatic)
Adrenal carcinoma
Retroperitoneal sarcoma, pancreas, colon
Lung, stomach, breast
Reticuloendothelial—lymphoma and Hodgkin's disease, and hematologic—leukemia and multiple myeloma

TABLE 93–2. PRESENTING SYMPTOMS, LABORATORY FEATURES, OR PHYSICAL FINDINGS IN PATIENTS WITH RENAL CELL CARCINOMA

Finding	Occurrence (%)
Hematuria	50–60
Elevated erythrocyte sedimentation rate (ESR)	50–60
Abdominal mass	24–45
Anemia	21–41
Flank pain	35–40
Hypertension	22–38
Weight loss	28–36
Pyrexia	7–17
Hepatic dysfunction	10–15
Classic triad (gross hematuria, flank pain, and palpable abdominal mass)	7–10
Hypercalcemia	3–6
Erythrocytosis	3–4
Acute varicocele	2–3

Data from Skinner DG, et al.: Diagnosis and management of renal cell cancer. Cancer 28:1165, 1971; Chisholm GD: Nephrogenic ridge tumors and their syndromes. Ann NY Acad Sci 230:402, 1974; Fallon B: Renal parenchymal tumors. *In* Culp DA, Loening SA (eds.): Genitourinary Oncology. Philadelphia, Lea & Febiger, p 202, 1985.

If the mass on US is solid or complex (20 per cent of cases), a renal CT scan (both with and without intravenous injection of iodine contrast) has replaced renal arteriography as the next diagnostic step. CT is as accurate as, and obviates the potential morbidity of, angiography in defining renal masses. Contrast enhancement of the usually highly vascular renal cancer on a CT study leaves little doubt as to the nature of a solid mass. In addition, CT can give sufficient local staging information to allow definitive surgical management. When contrast enhancement is coupled with areas of a negative CT number (relative tissue density in Hounsfield units) typical of fat, a diagnosis of angiomyolipoma is appropriate and no further workup or immediate treatment will be required. In indeterminate cases, arteriography or needle aspiration cytology or both may be needed to define the diagnosis further; however, in these unusual cases, final definition will likely require surgery.

In general, the nature of primary renal parenchymal masses in adults will be readily defined via this algorithm. Another advance that might further shape the algorithm suggested above is magnetic resonance imaging (MRI). MRI is nearly equal to CT in diagnosing renal masses but is better in local tumor staging (defining perirenal fat, para-aortic nodal and adjacent organ extension, and intravascular tumor thrombi). With the advent of paramagnetic agents capable of contrast-like enhancement, MRI may permit differentiation between tumor types.

Cronan JJ, Zeman RK: Renal mass imaging: The internist's role. Am J Med 81:1026, 1986. *A succinct discussion of the imaging modalities available for renal mass evaluation, including cost and efficacy considerations.*

Cronan JJ, Zeman RK, Rosenfeld AT: Comparison of computerized tomography, ultrasound and angiography in staging renal cell cancer. J Urol 127:712, 1982. *A definitive study showing CT to be the most accurate modality for staging renal cell carcinoma (RCC).*

Hricak H, Demas BE, Williams RD, et al.: MRI in the diagnosis and staging of renal and perirenal neoplasms. Radiology 154:709, 1985. *The initial report correlating pathologic data and MRI findings in renal cancer.*

Richie JP, Garnick MD, Seltzer D, et al.: CT scan for diagnosis and staging of renal cell cancer. J Urol 129:1114, 1983. *A substantial series of patients studied by CT with surgical correlation results.*

BENIGN RENAL TUMORS

Renal adenoma is the most common benign solid parenchymal lesion. Those under 3 cm in size have been designated as "benign," yet they tend to occur in circumstances similar to lesions larger than 3 cm (which are considered cancerous), i.e., in patients above 40 years of age, with a male to female ratio of 2 or 3 to 1. Small "renal adenomas" (< 3 cm) are virtually indistinguishable histologically from renal adenocarcinomas and a few have in fact metastasized. Since the biology

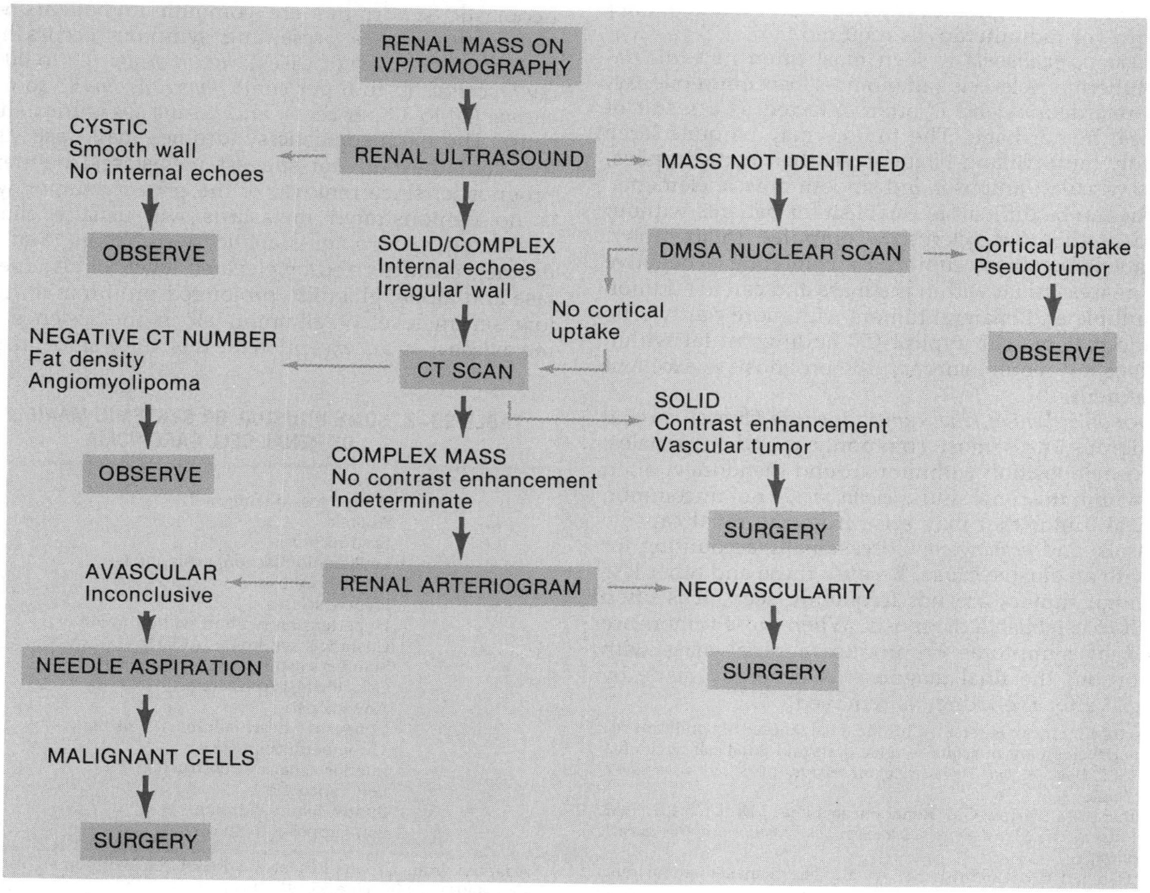

FIGURE 93–1. Algorithm for the work-up of a renal mass.

of these small tumors cannot be predicted preoperatively, most urologic oncologists consider them to be malignant and recommend radical nephrectomy. Trials of a subtotal nephrectomy in highly selected lesions are appropriate, however, since there are surprisingly good survival rates following partial nephrectomy for renal cancer in solitary kidneys and after subtotal nephrectomy in bilateral disease, and since the frequency of diagnosis of small, asymptomatic renal tumors is increasing because of the liberal use of CT scanning.

Renal oncocytoma, a subtype of adenoma accounting for 5 to 7 per cent of renal tumors, has a characteristic pale brown gross appearance and contains cells with an acidophilic cytoplasm. These tumors, although sometimes several centimeters in size, are generally asymptomatic. The typical spoke-wheel pattern on angiography is not sufficiently specific to exclude a malignant lesion preoperatively, and therefore treatment continues to be radical nephrectomy.

Acquired renal cystic disease is a new entity described in up to 45 per cent of patients with end-stage renal disease after three years of chronic hemodialysis. Approximately 10 per cent of these patients develop renal tumors that vary histologically from benign adenomas and oncocytomas to renal cell carcinomas. The tumors tend to be multiple and bilateral. The metastatic rate of these tumors is only about 6 per cent. The etiology is thought to be due to a poorly excreted, nondialyzable metabolite, since the entity has been described in patients with renal failure but who are not yet on dialysis. These tumors tend to present with gross hematuria. It is recommended that all patients be screened by annual renal ultrasonography after three years of chronic dialysis.

Mesoblastic nephroma, a benign congenital renal tumor of early childhood, must be distinguished from the highly malignant nephroblastoma, or Wilms' tumor. Unlike the latter, however, the mesoblastic nephroma is commonly diagnosed at birth or within the first few months of life. The prognosis is excellent; complete surgical resection is curative, and neither chemotherapy nor radiotherapy is required.

Hamartoma-angiomyolipoma is seen most often in adult patients with tuberous sclerosis (adenoma sebaceum, epilepsy, and mental retardation) and is often detected as a result of retroperitoneal hemorrhage. The tumors may be quite large and commonly multiple and bilateral. As their name implies, they contain vascular, adipose, and smooth muscle elements. The diagnosis can be difficult to establish for patients without the stigmata of tuberous sclerosis. Computed tomography, however, can define these tumors by exhibiting a negative CT number in areas of fat within the mass and can in addition delineate multiple and bilateral tumors with more clarity. The asymptomatic patient with typical CT findings of fat within the tumor does not require surgery; the prognosis is excellent without treatment.

A variety of *other benign renal tumors* include *fibroma*, a renal medullary fibrous mass most commonly found in females; *lipoma*, adipose deposition within or around the kidney, often perihilar or within the renal sinus; *leiomyoma*, a not uncommon retroperitoneal tumor that may arise from the renal capsule or renal vessels; and *hemangioma*, occasionally accounting for hematuria with an elusive cause. Because these and other less common benign tumors are not frequently seen, it is often quite difficult to establish a diagnosis. When these tumors are accompanied by symptoms or produce a renal mass with caliceal distortion, the final diagnosis is generally made by the pathologist after the kidney is removed.

Bretan PN, Busch MP, Hricak H, et al.: Chronic renal failure: A significant risk factor in the development of acquired renal cysts and renal cell carcinoma. Cancer 57:1871, 1986. *A complete review of the reported cases with discussion of the probable causes.*

Lieber MM, Tomera KM, Farrow GM: Renal oncocytoma. J Urol 125:481, 1982. *An excellent discussion of the diagnosis, pathology, and treatment of this recently recognized entity.*

Oesterling JE, Fishman EK, Goldman SM, et al.: The management of renal angiomyolipoma. J Urol 135:1121, 1986. *An excellent discussion of presenting findings and conditions for conservative management.*

PRIMARY MALIGNANT TUMORS

RENAL CELL CARCINOMA. Renal cell carcinoma is the most common renal malignancy in adults, accounting for 6 per cent of all malignancies and approximately 7500 deaths per year in the United States. The tumor is also called renal adenocarcinoma, Grawitz' tumor, hypernephroma, and nephrocarcinoma, although renal cell carcinoma (RCC) has become a universally accepted designation. RCC appears to arise from cells of the proximal convoluted tubule. Risk factors include pipe and cigar smoking and maleness (ratio of 2 or 3 to 1). Persons with HLA antigen types BW44 and DR8 may be more prone to develop renal cancer, and evidence suggests that oncogenes localized to the short arm of chromosome 3 may have etiologic implications. RCC is occasionally familial and is more common in patients with von Hippel-Lindau disease, horseshoe kidneys, adult polycystic kidney disease, and acquired renal cystic disease from renal failure. Histologically, RCC is of three varieties: the classic "clear cell" type characterized by uniformly large, cholesterol-laden cells with small nuclei and rare mitoses; a granular cell type exhibiting a darker staining cytoplasm containing numerous mitochondria, and more numerous mitoses; and an uncommon spindle cell (sarcomatoid) variety that has fusiform cells and variability in cell size.

Clinical Manifestations. The classic presenting triad of *hematuria*, *flank pain*, and a *palpable abdominal mass* is seen in less than 10 per cent of patients and among those only with far advanced local tumors (Table 93–2). Gross or microscopic hematuria alone, however, is present in approximately 60 per cent of patients with RCC. The detection of renal tumors in asymptomatic patients has increased, but 30 per cent of patients continue to have local extension or metastatic disease at the time of diagnosis. Because of its protean manifestations and propensity for curious metastatic sites, RCC has been dubbed the "internist's tumor" (Table 93–3). Indeed, paraneoplastic syndromes are common in patients with RCC: *pyrexia* (fever as a presenting symptom occurs in approximately 15 per cent of cases), *hypertension* (20 to 40 per cent), *erythrocytosis* (3 to 6 per cent), *hypercalcemia* (3 to 6 per cent), *anemia* (20 to 40 per cent), and *hepatic dysfunction* (10 to 15 per cent). The paraneoplastic syndromes may raise suspicion of RCC but they do not suggest metastases; neither are they prognostic, since removal of the primary tumor when there is no demonstrated metastasis will usually eliminate the associated syndrome. Hepatic dysfunction (Stauffer's syndrome), characterized by elevated levels of alkaline phosphatase and alpha$_2$-globulin, prolonged prothrombin time, and a low serum level of albumin, all in the absence of hepatic metastases, is an exception to this rule, since in such cases

TABLE 93–3. SOME UNUSUAL OR SYSTEMIC MANIFESTATIONS OF RENAL CELL CARCINOMA

Fever
Weight loss, inanition
Anemia
Erythrocytosis
Leukemoid reaction, eosinophilia
Thrombocytosis
Hypercalcemia
Hypertension (with or without renin ↑)
Cushing's syndrome (ACTH)
Stauffer's syndrome (hepatopathy)
Galactorrhea (prolactin)
Amyloidosis
Congestive heart failure (A-V fistula)
Thrombophlebitis
Inferior vena cava obstruction
Left varicocele
Budd-Chiari syndrome
von Hippel–Lindau disease

Adapted from Cronin RE, et al.: Renal cell carcinoma: Unusual systemic manifestations. Medicine 55:191, 1976.

ACTH = adrenocorticotropic hormone; A-V = arteriovenous.

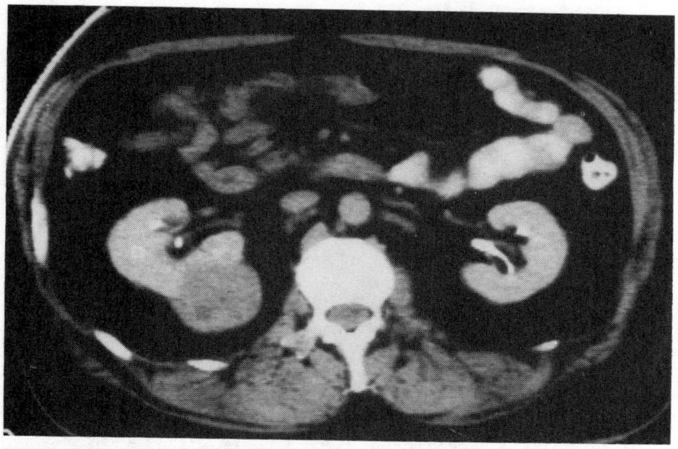

FIGURE 93–2. Contrast-enhanced abdominal CT scan showing renal cell cancer in the right kidney.

there is an unexplained high recurrence rate after definitive treatment of localized disease.

Diagnosis. There is no specific diagnostic laboratory test for RCC. The physician must often suspect RCC in patients with unexplained constitutional symptoms. The diagnostic evaluation relies on the algorithm previously described for investigation of renal mass (Fig. 93–1). A mass suspected on IVP with nephrotomograms should be confirmed by ultrasonography. If it is solid on US, an abdominal CT scan will, in approximately 95 per cent of cases, be sufficient to establish the diagnosis (Fig. 93–2). MRI can also establish the diagnosis and be useful for staging (Fig. 93–3). A renal vein or caval thrombus is common and may change the surgical approach to treatment, so the presence of a thrombus should be determined by ultrasonography, CT scanning, or MRI. In equivocal cases a venacavogram may be necessary for definition and/or determination of the cephalad extent of the thrombus before operation. The CT scan may be capable of determining local extension and/or local lymph node involvement, although it has not been found to be specific enough in most cases to obviate exploratory surgery for confirmation.

Staging and Treatment. It is important to determine the presence of metastases before determining therapy. No benefit has been ascribed to removal of the primary tumor in patients with known metastases unless the patient is symptomatic, the metastasis is solitary and amenable to resection, or a promising medical therapeutic protocol is planned (see below). Spontaneous regression of metastases following surgical removal of the primary tumor is calculated at 0.5 per cent, whereas the surgical mortality is nearly 2 per cent. The primary metastatic sites beyond the ipsilateral adrenal and local lymph nodes are lung and long bones. A chest roentgenogram and CT and a radionuclide bone scan are routine staging modalities. Lymphangiography has not been helpful in staging RCC patients.

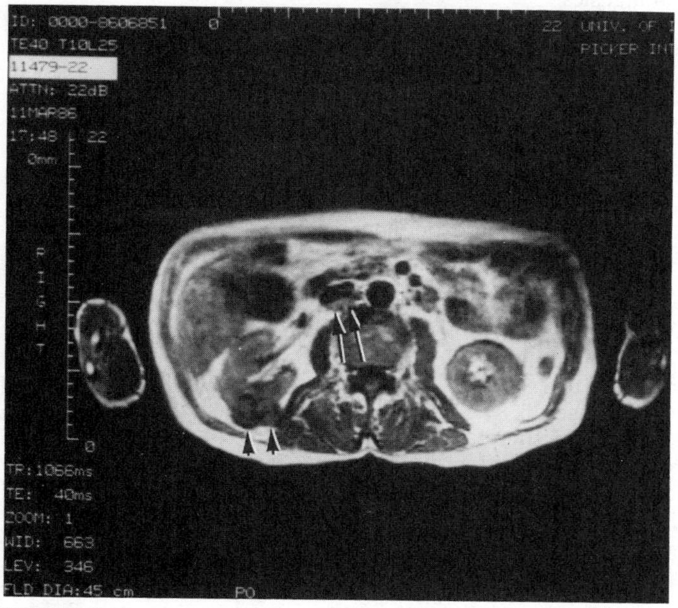

FIGURE 93–3. Transaxial MRI showing a renal cancer in the right kidney (*short arrows*) and a tumorous retroperitoneal lymph node (*long arrows*).

TABLE 93–4. STAGING SYSTEM FOR RENAL CARCINOMA

Stage I	Tumor confined to the renal parenchyma
Stage II	Tumor involving the perinephric fat or adrenal but confined within Gerota's fascia
Stage III A.	Tumor thrombus in renal vein or vena cava
B.	Tumor involving regional nodes
C.	Tumor involving lymph nodes and renal vein or vena cava
Stage IV	Tumor extending into adjacent organs (liver, colon, pancreas, duodenum) or distant metastases

Therapy of RCC depends entirely on the staging system summarized in Table 93–4. In patients with Stages I, II, and III A, treatment consists of a radical nephrectomy, which includes removal of the kidney and ipsilateral adrenal intact within its surrounding fascia, as well as removal of a possible intracaval thrombus. The local hilar lymph nodes will be included, but a formal para-aortic node dissection is not warranted. The prognosis for patients so treated approximates a 50 to 70 per cent five-year survival. Patients with lymph node involvement (Stage III A, C) have a 15 to 35 per cent five-year survival, and those with distant metastases (Stage IV) generally have less than a 5 per cent five-year survival.

Treatment of metastatic disease has included radiotherapy, chemotherapy, and immunotherapy, with none of these modalities emerging as clearly beneficial in effecting long-term survival. Hormonal therapy with medroxyprogesterone has less than a 5 per cent response rate. A variety of other hormonal agents, including testosterone, tamoxifen, nafoxidine, and estramustine, have similarly shown few responses. Approximately 20 per cent of patients with metastatic RCC were reported to respond to vinblastine. Immunotherapy with bacille Calmette-Guérin (BCG), *Corynebacterium parvum*, and xenogeneic immune ribonucleic acid (RNA) has been tried with limited success. Recent trials of recombinant alpha-interferon are reported to show up to a 30 per cent response rate with an occasional complete remission. An additional form of immunotherapy entails production of augmented autologous lymphocytes (LAK cells) by incubation with interleukin-2 in vitro. LAK cells are then reinfused into the patient. Early results show greater than 80 per cent response rate in patients with pulmonary metastases, but the toxicity of the treatment is great, and the durability of remissions is unknown. Although radiation therapy is not important in primary treatment, it can provide short-term control of symptomatic bone metastases.

Cronin RE, Kaehny WD, Miller PD, et al.: Renal cell carcinoma: Unusual systemic manifestations. Medicine 55:291, 1976. *This article presents eight cases with unusual aspects of RCC and contains a comprehensive review of the literature.*

DeKernion JB: Treatment of advanced renal cell cancer—traditional methods and innovative approaches. J Urol 130:2, 1983. *A superb and inclusive review of the treatment of disseminated RCC.*

Garnick MB, Richie JP: Renal neoplasia. In Brenner BM Rector FC, Jr (eds.): The Kidney. 3rd ed. Philadelphia, W. B. Saunders Company, 1986, pp 1533–1550. *An excellent general review of renal cell carcinoma, sarcomas of renal origin, and Wilms' tumor, with 141 references.*

Holland JM: Cancer of the kidney—natural history and staging. Cancer 32:1030, 1973. *The classic article on RCC containing a complete description of the staging system.*

Niedhart JA: Interferon therapy for the treatment of renal cancer. Cancer 57 (suppl):1696, 1986. *Complete review of the interferon treatment studies for RCC.*

Richie JP, Garnick MD: Primary renal and ureteral cancer. In Rieselbach RE, Garnick MB (eds.): Cancer and the Kidney. Philadelphia, Lea & Febiger,

1982, pp 662–706. *An excellent general review in a book devoted to the interrelationships of neoplastic diseases and renal disease; 185 references.*

Rosenberg SA: The adoptive immunotherapy of cancer using the transfer of activated lymphocytic cells and interleukin-2. Semin Oncol 13:200, 1986. *The initial report of the LAK cell therapy of human malignancies.*

NEPHROBLASTOMA. Nephroblastoma (Wilms' tumor) is the most common malignant neoplasm of the urinary tract in childhood. It is diagnosed in one third of cases when the child is under the age of two and in two thirds of cases when the child is under the age of four.

Clinical Manifestations and Diagnosis. The tumor is palpable in as many as 80 per cent of cases, often noted by a parent. Pain is initially present in 50 per cent of cases, hematuria (usually microscopic) in 10 to 20 per cent, and hypertension in approximately 60 per cent. The diagnosis is established first by IVP, which commonly shows caliceal distortion. Calcification within the mass occurs in 10 to 15 per cent of cases. Abdominal ultrasonography or CT scans are useful to determine tumor extension and the possibility of bilaterality (this occurs in approximately 10 per cent of patients). Arteriography is rarely utilized.

If there still is doubt about the differential diagnosis (after the studies just described are done), measurement of urine vanillylmandelic acid should help rule out neuroblastoma. The metastatic workup should be directed to the lungs, liver, and opposite kidney. A chest roentgenogram and CT and an abdominal CT are sufficient. Nephroblastoma, as is the case with RCC, often produces a tumor thrombus in the inferior vena cava, which may have to be delineated by venacavography. Abdominal ultrasonography is also a reasonable alternative to establish this possibility.

Treatment. The development of successful treatment of nephroblastoma (Wilms' tumor) is rightfully heralded as one of the most significant advances in cancer therapy of the past few years. The prognosis has improved from a 25 per cent survival in the 1960s to a current rate of over 85 per cent disease-free survival, if there is no distant dissemination or unfavorable histology.

The initial treatment of nephroblastoma is complete surgical removal of the primary tumor and kidney, even when there are metastases. A transabdominal approach will allow the safest access and the necessary visibility of the liver, para-aortic nodes, and contralateral kidney for complete staging. Occasionally radiotherapy or chemotherapy may be required preoperatively to decrease the bulk of massive tumors. Combined therapy is indicated postoperatively in all patients but is dependent upon accurate staging, completeness of surgical extirpation, and tumor histology. A tumor confined to the kidney in children under two years of age requires only postoperative administration of actinomycin D and vincristine, whereas for all others the best results are obtained with radiation therapy to the tumor bed plus administration of actinomycin D and vincristine. Doxorubicin is also an active agent in the treatment of this disease. Additional areas of current investigation are (1) radiation therapy and the addition of doxorubicin to vincristine and actinomycin D for patients with extensive local disease and favorable histology, and (2) radiation therapy with triple drug versus quadruple drug (addition of cyclophosphamide) for cases with unfavorable histology (anaplasia or sarcomatous elements). Wilms' tumor may occasionally be seen in adults; similarly, RCC occurs but rarely in children.

D'Angio GJ, Evans A, Breslow N, et al.: The treatment of Wilms' tumor: Results of the second National Wilms' Tumor Study. Cancer 47:2302, 1981. *A follow-up of the first NWTS report establishing improved results with complete staging and chemotherapy only in younger patients.*

UROTHELIAL TUMORS. Malignant tumors of the urothelial lining of the urinary tract include those involving the collecting structures of the kidney (renal pelvis and calices), ureter, and bladder. These tumors are transitional cell cancers (TCC) in over 90 per cent of cases, with an occasional squamous cell carcinoma (often in association with chronic inflammation due to stone formation in the upper tracts and with *Schistosoma haematobium* infestation in the bladder) and rarely adenocarcinoma (commonly associated with embryologic hindgut remnants such as a persistent urachus in the dome of the bladder). TCC tends to be multifocal, occurring bilaterally in the upper tracts in a few cases but with an increasing frequency of simultaneous occurrence or recurrences in the ureter and particularly in the bladder. In each location there is a strong association of TCC with cigarette smoking, exposure to certain industrial chemicals (particularly aromatic amines), and chronic abuse of phenacetin-containing analgesics.

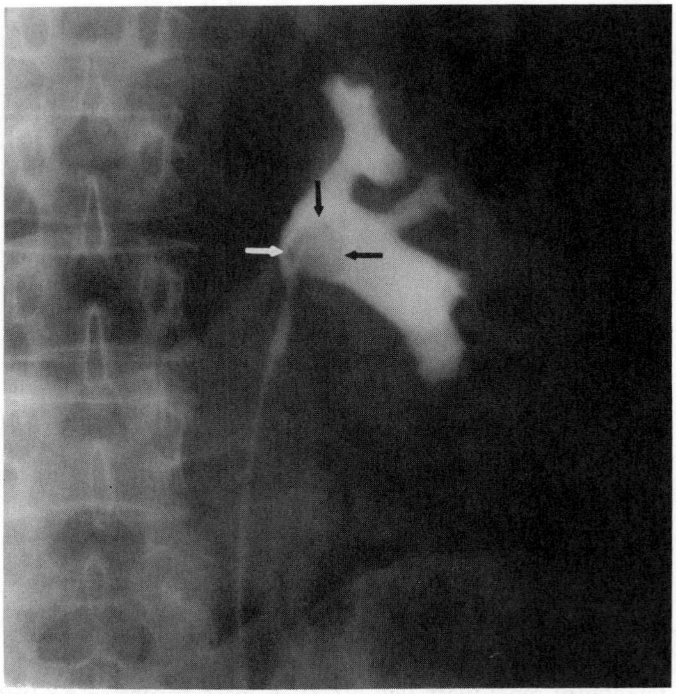

FIGURE 93–4. Retrograde pyelogram showing a transitional cell cancer in the pelvis of the right kidney (*arrows*). (Reproduced with permission from Williams RD: Renal, perirenal, and ureteral neoplasms. In Gillenwater JY, Grayhack JT, Howards SS, et al.: Adult and Pediatric Urology. Chicago, Year Book Medical Publishers, 1987.)

TCC of the Renal Pelvis and Calices. Clinical Manifestations and Diagnosis. The presenting finding is gross or microscopic hematuria in more than 60 per cent of cases. In contrast to RCC, constitutional symptoms and paraneoplastic syndromes are few. Generally the diagnosis is made by the finding of a filling defect in a calix, infundibulum, or renal pelvis on IVP (Fig. 93–4). Ultrasonography can be utilized to eliminate the possibility of a nonopaque calculus. Examination of the urine by an experienced cytologist can be diagnostic of TCC, although the site will be undetermined. Cystoscopy with retrograde pyelography, including ureteral wash or brush cytology, may be required to establish the diagnosis. Ureteroscopy may be useful in equivocal cases. CT scanning may be useful in determining local extent of tumor but is usually unnecessary. Arteriography is generally not diagnostically useful. The tumors tend to metastasize to lung and bone, and therefore a chest roentgenogram and CT and a bone scan are often indicated. Since these tumors tend to be multifocal, careful preoperative scrutiny of the opposite side of the urinary tract (on IVP) and of the bladder and urethra by direct cystourethroscopy is recommended.

Treatment and Prognosis. Treatment of renal urothelial cancer is radical nephroureterectomy, with removal of the entire ureter. Because 40 to 50 per cent of patients will have or develop similar tumors within the bladder, direct cystourethroscopy is a necessary postoperative routine, usually done quarterly the first year, twice the second year, and then annually.

Most of these tumors are low grade and noninvasive, and the five-year tumor-free survival rate after complete removal of the ipsilateral upper tract is more than 90 per cent. Patients with high-grade and/or invasive lesions, however, have a poor prognosis (<15 per cent five-year survival). Chemotherapeutic combinations, which have begun to show activity in TCC of the bladder, are also efficacious in metastatic TCC of the upper tracts (see below).

TCC of the Ureter. Clinical Manifestations and Diagnosis. These tumors are most often detected secondary to gross or microscopic hematuria, but occasionally present with renal colic due to obstructing blood clots. Diagnosis is commonly made by the finding of a ureteral filling defect on IVP. If the ureter is totally obstructed with a resultant lack of contrast excretion, cystoscopy with retrograde ureterography or ureteroscopy is required to demonstrate the lesion. As in renal pelvis TCC, ureteral urine or brush cytology can be diagnostic. Abdominal CT scans can aid in local staging, as can chest roentgenograms, and CT and bone scanning assist in detecting distant metastases.

Treatment and Prognosis. Prognosis is determined by the histologic grade of the lesion and the depth of invasion. Selected low-grade lesions may be successfully treated by segmental resection, particularly in patients with renal insufficiency or a solitary kidney, but the definitive approach remains nephroureterectomy, as in renal pelvis TCC. Prognosis of low-grade noninvasive lesions is greater than 70 to 80 per cent five-year survival, but for the higher grade, usually invasive lesions the prognosis is dismal. Treatment of metastatic disease is rarely successful; however, as with TCC of the renal pelvis, the newer combinations of chemotherapy are promising (see below).

TCC of the Bladder. Bladder cancer affects over 20,000 people and accounts for nearly 10,000 deaths annually in the United States. Men are affected at least twice as often as women.

Clinical Manifestations and Diagnosis. Hematuria occurs at presentation in 68 per cent of patients and classically is total (throughout the stream) whether microscopic (as tested by a three-glass test) or gross. The degree of hematuria does not parallel the size of the lesion. Bladder irritability (frequency and dysuria) in the absence of infection is also a common (25 per cent) presenting complaint, particularly in males.

Intravenous pyelography is not sufficiently sensitive to detect small bladder tumors, but it is helpful in detecting upper tract TCC in the 10 per cent of patients with simultaneous lesions and in predicting bladder wall invasion in patients with concomitant unilateral ureteral obstruction. Urine cytology may establish the diagnosis of TCC but not the site. Definitive diagnosis requires cystoscopy and transurethral bladder biopsy under anesthesia, at which time a bimanual examination can predict whether the tumor has extended beyond the bladder wall. Metastases are local into adjacent pelvic structures and lymph nodes and distant to lungs and bones, and therefore staging of deeply invasive tumors is by chest roentgenograms, CT of the chest and abdomen, and bone scanning.

Treatment and Prognosis. Nearly 80 per cent of bladder TCC's are low grade and noninvasive (stage 0) or invade only into the lamina propria (stage A). Patients with such lesions have an 85 per cent five-year survival rate when treated by complete transurethral resection of the tumor(s). The lesions tend toward multiple recurrences in more than 50 per cent of patients and therefore cystoscopic surveillance is a mandatory postoperative routine. Intravesical chemotherapy with thiotepa, doxorubicin, mitomycin-C, or more recently BCG has been used successfully for prophylaxis in patients with multiple or recurrent superficial low-grade tumors, resulting in an approximate 50 per cent reduction in recurrences. Importantly, only about 20 per cent of patients presenting with superficial bladder TCC will subsequently develop high-grade and/or invasive disease.

Unfortunately, 80 per cent of patients with invasive bladder TCC are found so at initial presentation. In patients with deeply invasive disease, stage B_1 refers to superficial muscle invasion, stage B_2 to deep muscle invasion, and stage C to full-thickness bladder wall invasion. In the absence of metastases current best efforts at cure of invasive disease require pelvic lymphadenectomy and radical cystectomy (complete removal of the bladder and prostate in males and the bladder, urethra, and uterus in females). This approach affords a 50 to 60 per cent five-year survival rate in patients with stage B_1, B_2 or C disease. Patients with pelvic lymph node (stage D_1) or distant metastases (stage D_2) have less than a 15 per cent five-year survival rate.

Metastatic disease is difficult to treat, but combination chemotherapy with vinblastine, methotrexate, and cisplatin with or without doxorubicin is showing a durable 30 per cent complete remission rate. This significant advance, if consistent, may alter the surgical approach to bladder TCC in the future.

SARCOMAS. Renal sarcomas are rare; they include rhabdomyosarcoma, liposarcoma, fibrosarcoma, osteogenic sarcoma, and, most commonly, leiomyosarcoma (60 per cent). In general, sarcomas are quite malignant and usually detected at a late stage, and thus have a poor prognosis. The diagnosis approach is similar to that for RCC. Treatment is surgical with wide local excision; however, local recurrence and subsequent distant metastases are the rule.

Droller MJ: Transitional cell cancer: Upper tracts and bladder. In Walsh PC, Gittes RF, Perlmutter AD, (eds).: Campbell's Urology. Philadelphia, W. B. Saunders Company, 1986, pp 1343–1440. *A detailed and complete discussion of uroepithelial cancer diagnosis and treatment.*

McCarreen JP, Mullis D, Vaughn ED: Tumors of the renal pelvis and ureter: Current concepts and management. Semin Urol 1:75, 1983. *A definitive review of upper tract urothelial cancer.*

Myers F, Palmer J, Harrigan J: Chemotherapy of disseminated TCC. In Williams RD (ed.): Advances in Urologic Oncology. New York, Macmillan, 1987. *A discussion of cisplatin/methotrexate/vinblastine chemotherapy showing a 40 to 50 per cent overall complete remission/partial remission rate.*

SECONDARY MALIGNANT TUMORS

Tumors of the lung, stomach, and breast most commonly metastasize to the kidney, but the metastases are usually clinically silent except for microscopic hematuria. More than 50 per cent of patients with primary lung cancer have renal metastases at autopsy. Routine use of staging abdominal CT in a variety of primary malignancies is expected to increase the premorbid diagnosis of secondary renal tumors. Adjacent tumors of the adrenal, colon, and pancreas, and sarcomas may spread contiguously into the kidney. Reticuloendothelial tumors, such as lymphoma and Hodgkin's disease, and hematologic malignancies, such as leukemia and multiple myeloma, may infiltrate the kidney, but this type of renal involvement is almost never primary or symptomatic. Other forms of renal involvement in multiple myeloma are described in Ch. 163.

PART X
GASTROINTESTINAL DISEASES

94 INTRODUCTION

Marvin H. Sleisenger

Digestive diseases in the United States account for a large part of the economic burden of illness, of total days of illness among adults, of all admissions to general hospitals, and of all major surgical operations. The prompt recognition of digestive disease and its treatment are thus plainly important. In order best to discharge this responsibility, knowledge of the pathophysiologic basis for signs and symptoms of gastrointestinal disease is most helpful. This introduction to the chapters on gastrointestinal diseases will be concerned with this broad subject.

APPROACH TO THE PATIENT WITH GASTROINTESTINAL DISEASE. In the approach to a patient with gastrointestinal disease the physician must obtain an accurate history of illness, correctly interpret the principal symptoms of digestive disease, conduct a thorough physical examination in which findings often characteristic of specific gastrointestinal diseases and syndromes are assiduously sought, and make intelligent use of laboratory tests and other diagnostic aids. An accurate history of digestive disease requires attention to details that mark the duration of the disability, establishing relationships between the waxing and waning of symptoms and external factors such as stress, eating, or fasting. Understanding the pathophysiologic basis of symptoms and signs helps greatly to establish the location, nature, and urgency of the problem.

The majority of patients with digestive disease have had their illness for years. The common diseases are chronic: *acid-peptic disease* affecting the esophagus, stomach, or duodenum; *alcoholic disease* of the *liver* and *pancreas; calculous biliary tract disease; inflammatory bowel disease; postprandial dyspepsia; irritable bowel;* and *cancer* of the stomach, intestines, pancreas, or liver. To be sure, some gastrointestinal diseases may be acute and even catastrophic; the *acute abdomen* is a general phrase of importance in both medical and surgical practice.

THE VALUE OF A THOROUGH HISTORY. The duration of symptoms in patients with digestive diseases ranges from moments to decades. In an emergency room a physician may be called to see a previously healthy person suffering the symptoms and displaying the signs of an acute intra-abdominal disorder requiring a rapid decision about whether surgery is indicated. The next patient seeking care may be an elderly person with a problem of four or more decades' duration. This patient is also ill but does not appear to be. Differences exist in the incidences of digestive problems in patients' families, in their reactions to stress, in their dietary habits, in the degree of involvement of other organ systems, and in the degree to which their illnesses affect general health and activity.

The natural history of many gastrointestinal diseases is marked by characteristic patterns of symptoms. Complaints often have a particular intensity, a periodicity (time of day, month, or season), and a relationship to fatigue, stress, eating, or drinking alcohol. For example, patients with irritable bowel tend to have low-grade, nagging, cramplike lower abdominal distress for decades. The distress may be aggravated by certain foods and may wax and wane with the appearance and disappearance of stress. Although the discomfort may be intense at times, its intensity contrasts with the acute, sudden, and excruciating pain of the patient with an acutely obstructed small intestine, ureter, or common bile duct; a perforated duodenal ulcer; a dissecting aneurysm; or an acutely ischemic small intestine. Pain of gastrointestinal disease may be intermediate between acute and chronic, and between severe and mild, e.g., the epigastric distress of duodenal ulcer. It rarely incapacitates and is usually relieved quickly with appropriate therapy. However, a change in these characteristics, i.e., increased duration and less relief with antacids, may signal a possible penetration and deserves special attention. Complications are common in the natural history of many other gastrointestinal diseases. The patient with longstanding irritable bowel may also have diverticulosis and suddenly rupture a diverticulum. Knowledge of the natural history of digestive diseases is essential to understanding changes in patterns of symptoms, particularly pain.

The *locus* and *timing* of the distress are important in determining which organ of the digestive tract is affected. Upper abdominal discomfort related to meals usually means that the stomach, duodenum, gallbladder, or pancreas is the site of the problem. Periumbilical pain one-half hour or so postprandially may indicate that the small intestine is involved. When the discomfort is in the lower abdomen and is associated with an abnormal bowel habit or rectal bleeding or is relieved by bowel movement or flatus, the colon is likely to be at fault. The *nature* of the pain is also important. Aching pain is characteristic of ulcer disease, boring pain of pancreatic disease, and cramping pain of both small and large intestines.

The presence of associated symptoms is important in evaluating gastrointestinal disease. Fever, arthritis, conjunctivitis, uveitis, and erythema nodosum may all be associated with the diarrhea of chronic inflammatory bowel disease. Continuing weight loss and evidence of malnutrition with vitamin deficiencies usually reflect a serious organic disease; however, such malnutrition may result from anorexia, early satiety, or forced vomiting often associated with laxative abuse in order to lose weight (*bulimia*), all related to neuropsychiatric problems (Ch. 13). Type and location of pain, presence of diarrhea, a relationship of symptoms to diet and alcohol, and history of prior surgery all help the clinician better to define the disease underlying the malnutrition and possible malabsorption. The historical facts associated with *weight loss* due to digestive disease are crucial for correct diagnosis. Is anorexia due to depression or physical illness? If the appetite is normal, is decreased intake due to *dysphagia, nausea, early satiety,* or *fear* of postprandial symptoms? Some individuals lose weight, despite good appetite and adequate food intake, because of *malabsorption* or *occult intra-abdominal malignancy.* The chronic alcoholic may get enough calories from ethanol to supply energy needs and may not lose weight; however, his or her diet lacks important ingredients such as essential amino acids and fatty acids, vitamins, minerals, and electrolytes.

EMOTION AND STRESS. *Emotion* and *stress* play a large role in many gastrointestinal disorders. Patients who are massively obese or who have *anorexia nervosa* or *bulimia* are emotionally disturbed, and their eating habits are expressions of the disturbance extended over prolonged periods of time. These aberrant eating habits may represent bizarre conscious or unconscious attempts to lose weight or somehow to resolve personal or family conflicts. No clear association among personality, stress, and the pathogenesis of duodenal ulcer has been established. Nevertheless, it is clear that recurrence of symptoms can often be correlated with emotional tension.

It has long been held that emotion plays a role in the pathogenesis of ulcerative colitis, but patients with this disease have not been shown to have an abnormal prevalence of psychiatric illness or an abnormal number of "critical life incidents." There is a higher incidence of both psychoneurotic behavior and critical life incidents in patients with irritable bowel than in those with ulcerative colitis.

A personality disorder often underlies the habitual abuse of alcohol, found in many patients with diseases of the digestive system. No amount of effort in treating the esophagus (reflux esophagitis), stomach (erosive gastritis), pancreas (acute and chronic pancreatitis), or liver (acute alcoholic hepatitis, cirrhosis) will favorably affect the clinical course of these patients without attention to the basic problem.

THE PHYSICAL EXAMINATION: COMMON SIGNS OF GASTROINTESTINAL DISEASE. Certain signs of serious illness must be sought on physical examination of patients with complaints of digestive disease. The abdominal findings in patients with acute abdominal problems that require immediate surgery are discussed in Ch. 115.

Evidences of Malnutrition. Malnutrition is common in serious gastrointestinal diseases. It is characterized principally by signs of weight loss, mainly disappearance of fat depots and decreased muscle mass. Malnutrition is often associated with signs of *vitamin* and *mineral deficiencies.* Erythroderma, glossitis, cheilosis, muscle tenderness, angular stomatitis, bronzing of exposed skin, nasolabial seborrhea, dementia, and peripheral neuropathy all reflect deficiency of B soluble vitamins. Glossitis, peripheral neuropathy, and lemon-tinted pallor may reflect vitamin B_{12} deficiency. Rough skin may be due to hyperkeratosis follicularis (vitamin A deficit?) or perifolliculitis of vitamin C deficiency. Petechiae, ecchymoses, or other evidences of easy bruising may reflect vitamin K deficiency. Pallor and glossitis may be due to folate deficiency while pallor, lingual atrophy, koilonychia, and splenomegaly point to iron deficiency. Petechiae and ecchymoses may reflect vitamin K deficiency; failure to grow, kyphosis, and skeletal deformities are evidences of vitamin D lack. Xerophthalmia results from insufficient vitamin A. Deficiencies of trace metals may be suspected on physical examination. Copper and zinc deficiencies are associated with loss of taste acuity, and zinc deficiency with severe dermatitis, hyperpigmentation, as well as alopecia and evidence of dementia. Central nervous system damage, due principally to deficiency of vitamin B_1 and ranging from recent ophthalmoplegia and confusion to dementia and cerebellar ataxia, may be noted, particularly in alcoholics.

Patients with *protein deficiency* not only lose subcutaneous fat and muscle mass but also may have edema; decreased turgor and dyspigmentation of skin; dryness, brittleness, and lightening of hair; hepatomegaly; and mental dullness. Inadequate protein intake slows growth of children and impairs bone integrity in adults. Protein malnutrition caused by gastrointestinal disease is usually not selective, being coupled with subnormal caloric intake, and this is called *protein-calorie malnutrition.* Lack of essential fatty acids leads to skin eczema.

Other Important Signs. Physical signs pointing to disease in a particular organ system are also important. Thus, jaundice, hepatomegaly, splenomegaly, ascites, and spider angiomas all indicate chronic and severe liver disease. Palpable abdominal masses may be found in patients with *pancreatic pseudocyst, malignancies* of the gastrointestinal tract, *Crohn's disease,* intraperitoneal *abscesses, lymphoma, dissecting aortic aneurysms,* malignant extrahepatic biliary tract obstruction (*enlarged gallbladder*), or *lacerated* or *infarcted spleens.* Abdominal distention with evidence of gas-filled loops of bowel is often noted in patients with malabsorption resulting from diffuse proximal small bowel disease or from conditions associated with bacterial overgrowth.

Fever may be present during periods of inflammatory activity in patients with acute and chronic inflammatory disease of the gut, pancreatitis, cholecystitis, cholangitis, lymphoma, abscesses (intra-abdominal, hepatic, retroperitoneal, and perirectal), and acute progressive infarction of the bowel. The duration of fever varies and reflects the nature of the underlying disease. For example, fever is present for hours in acute suppurative cholangitis or acute small bowel infarction, and for days or even weeks in alcoholic hepatitis, Crohn's disease, pancreatitis with extensive necrosis or sepsis, abscesses (including liver), or lymphoma.

PATHOPHYSIOLOGIC BASIS FOR COMMON SYMPTOMS OF GASTROINTESTINAL DISEASE. An understanding of the pathophysiologic basis of the important symptoms of digestive disease will help in their correct interpretation and thus in arriving at an effective plan for diagnosis and treatment.

Anorexia. Disturbances of appetite, such as *anorexia* and *early satiety,* are common in digestive disease. *Hunger* is the desire for food accompanied by unpleasant epigastric sensations. *Appetite* is the desire for food after hunger ceases. *Satiety* is the loss of the desire to eat after ingesting food. The control of both hunger and satiety is complex, involving neurotransmitters, including neuropeptides, which regulate hypothalamic centers that control hunger and satiety. Cholecystokinin (CCK) peptides, released after feeding, elicit satiety, whereas opioids (endorphins, enkephalins), norepinephrine ($alpha_2$) pancreatic polypeptides, growth hormone–releasing factor, as well as other gut-brain peptides, stimulate eating.

Gastric distention and delayed gastric emptying inhibit feeding, probably via the actions of CCK, glucagon, and somatostatin. In turn, hormonal action depends upon intact vagal afferent innervation of the stomach. The factors that initiate hunger and affect appetite and satiety and are related to release of neuropeptides in gut and brain are not clearly defined but may include arteriovenous (A-V) glucose gradients, sugar intake, physical activity, and behavior.

The causes of anorexia are both physical and psychologic. *Anorexia nervosa* is a psychologic disorder in which appetite virtually does not exist and hunger is greatly reduced. Anorexia, of course, is associated with many organic diseases, intestinal and extraintestinal. In many patients anorexia is clearly associated with continuing intra-abdominal pain or fever; in others, with chronic or recurrent nausea. In those with cancer of the stomach or pancreas but without pain, its basis is not known.

Hyperphagia. The complex factors underlying excessive feeding include (1) inability to regulate energy intake according to nutritive value for the food, (2) cultural influences, (3) possible failure of normal response to feeding, i.e., failure of release of peptides that delay gastric emptying or defective receptor mechanism for them, and (4) a hypothalamic lesion, although this has not as yet been demonstrated in humans. Another group, usually young females, will alternate cramming of food and induced vomiting (*bulimia*) with periods of anorexia.

Abdominal Pain. The most frequent symptom that brings a patient with digestive disease to the physician is pain, most commonly abdominal, but not infrequently located in the chest or back. Pain warns the patient of possible imminent tissue damage and is usually caused by anoxia, inflammation, or stretching of smooth muscle or organ capsules. Pain from the viscera and peritoneum is mediated by the sympathetic nervous system. The afferent endings are located in the smooth muscle of hollow organs, in the peritoneum, and in organ capsules. These afferents are identified with dermatomes, which correspond with segments of the spinal cord. They travel with afferents from the periphery. This association is the basis of *referred pain* to extra-abdominal structures.

Pain originating from hollow viscera is called *visceral;* it is midline, dull, and often associated with nausea. The location depends upon the organ involved. Pain from the esophagus is usually felt over the site but occasionally in the suprasternal notch. Pain from the stomach and duodenum is epigastric or to the right of the midline in the epigastrium. Jejunal and ileal pain is often periumbilical, although distal ileal pain may be perceived in the right lower quadrant. Colonic pain is lower abdominal in location, often poorly localized. Pain from the gallbladder and common bile duct is in the right upper quadrant or epigastrium; when severe, it is often felt in the midline of the upper back. Pancreatic pain is midline or to the left of the epigastrium and often radiates through to the midline of the upper back.

Pain may be felt at a site distant from the organ involved, either by referral or by involvement of neighboring structures. Thus, an abscess in the lower abdomen over the psoas may refer its pain to the hip or groin; spasm of the esophagus may lead to pain felt down the inner aspect of the left upper arm, as in the pain of myocardial ischemia. The pain in the trapezius ridge areas of the shoulders may be associated with irritation of the diaphragmatic pleura by an inflammatory process such as a subdiaphragmatic abscess. The physician must be familiar with the common areas of pain reference and with the influence on pain patterns of involvement by contiguity.

Intra-abdominal pain is often due to *inflammation* or *ischemia.* Edema and spasm narrow the involved segment; smooth muscle proximal to the narrowed gut stretches, causing pain. In addition, ischemia and inflammation lower the pain threshold by releasing local bradykinin, serotonin, histamine, prostaglandins, and lactic acid. Pain is due in part also to the stretching of smooth muscle in blood vessels. Sensory nerve fibers may be directly involved by a tumor (e.g., paraspinal sensory nerve roots may be entrapped by cancer of the pancreas, other retroperitoneal malignancies).

Initially *visceral* pain is felt in the midline and is dull in character regardless of the organ involved. As inflammation or ischemia progresses, the pain will shift gradually to the site of the organ affected. Thus, in a matter of hours the pain of acute appendicitis shifts from the midline to the right lower quadrant, and that of cholecystitis from the midline to the right upper quadrant.

The patient's behavior during the pain is important in correct interpretation. Pain caused by stretching of smooth muscle of the gut, ureter, or common bile duct is colicky. The patient tends to be restless, and the pain is not aggravated by movement. The patient with peritoneal irritation, on the other hand, prefers to lie quietly, since jarring or movement exacerbates the pain.

FACTORS AFFECTING INTENSITY AND PERCEPTION OF PAIN. The patient's description of pain is influenced by neural, psychologic, and cultural factors. Perception is reduced by environmental stress, as in battle, probably owing to release of enkephalins. Likewise, depression blunts perception. The neural influences reside within the spinal cord, particularly the dorsal horns, which integrate central and peripheral impulses with those of pain, altering them before they reach the brain. Perception is also affected by cultural influences, ranging from demonstrativeness to stoicism. Finally, age affects pain perception. Patients in the eighth decade and beyond often have a significant rise of pain threshold. Degree of discomfort is often disproportionately low even with sepsis, perforation, and infarction in this group.

Vomiting. Vomiting is the rapid evacuation of gastric contents in retrograde fashion from stomach through mouth. It must be distinguished from *rumination,* the asymptomatic regurgitation of food, rechewing, and reswallowing. It is immediately due to a forceful contraction of the abdominal muscle with the cardia and mouth open. It is most often the final stage of a three-part act. The first is *nausea,* a most unpleasant feeling, difficult to define but universally recognizable. Gastric motor activity is diminished, and duodenal pressure increases with reflux of duodenal contents into the stomach. Nausea is followed by *retching,* which comprises spasmodic respiratory movements opposed by expiratory contractions of the abdominal muscles and raises the cardia of the stomach, an important preparatory maneuver to evacuation, which is the third stage. Paraphenomena of vomiting include hypersalivation, some reverse peristalsis of the small intestine, evidences of abnormal vagal stimulation (principally bradycardia), and the urge to defecate. Vomiting is controlled by bilateral vomiting centers in the dorsal portions of the lateral reticular formation of the medulla, activated by so-called chemoreceptor trigger zones (CTZs) located near the postrema.

Drugs and ionizing radiation cause nausea and vomiting by stimulating the chemoreceptor trigger zones; this pathway also mediates the nausea and vomiting of motion sickness, uremia, diabetic ketoacidosis, and use of general anesthetics. Vagal afferents may also stimulate the vomiting centers, bypassing the chemoreceptor trigger zones. Examples include distention of the smooth muscle of the gut, particularly when sudden; substances noxious to the mucosa of the stomach such as copper sulfate or mustard; and irritation and inflammation of the peritoneum. Thus, a large number of diseases and disorders that affect the intestine, bile ducts, ureters, and peritoneum are associated with nausea and vomiting. The symptom complex is often nonspecific and not helpful in differential diagnosis of intra-abdominal disorders. Additional pathways to the vomiting center are stimulated by noxious smells and tastes, but the location of the involved supramedullary receptors is not known. Apparently, many different pathways in the brain stem as well as different neurotransmitters are involved in the multiple stimuli that cause nausea and vomiting.

TYPES OF VOMITING. Important features of vomiting that may characterize a particular category of underlying disease are its amount, duration, content, and relationship to meals.

When a patient vomits during or immediately after a meal, it is most likely to be psychogenic, although such vomiting, particularly after a heavy meal, may be due to edema and spasm of the pylorus associated with a pyloric canal ulcer. (However, in these latter cases, the patient often has pain that is relieved by emesis, in contrast to failure of pain relief by vomiting in patients with cancer of the pancreas or biliary tract disease, for example.) Vomiting an hour or more after a meal is more compatible with gastric outlet obstruction, acute pancreatitis, or motility disorder of the stomach (diabetic neuropathy, postvagotomy). Vomiting of material eaten many hours previously also fits in the category of organic obstruction. Often patients with chronic outlet obstruction will have large, dilated stomachs and on examination will be noted to have a succussion splash. This sign is important in distinguishing psychogenic from organic obstruction in chronic vomiting. Alcoholics, pregnant women, and uremic persons have nausea and vomiting early in the morning on arising. Some patients with increased intracranial pressure may have vomiting unassociated with meals or nausea; classically, it has been described as projectile or forceful, although this is by no means always the case.

Large amounts of vomitus, food and secretions, usually

TABLE 94–1. COMMON DISEASES AND DISORDERS ASSOCIATED WITH NAUSEA AND VOMITING

Psychogenic
Drug-induced
Intra-abdominal problem:
Colic, sepsis, perforated viscus
Inflammation: ischemia
Toxins and poisons (ingested, inhaled, injected)
Metabolic disorders and diseases
Gastric outlet obstruction
Duodenal and high small bowel obstruction
Intracranial diseases
Viral gastroenteritis
Cyclic vomiting, childhood
Pregnancy
Due to pain, intra-abdominal or extra-abdominal

indicate nearly complete or complete obstruction. This may also result, however, from severe gastric atony and dilatation, or, in rare instances, from hypersecretion of gastric juice in the Zollinger-Ellison syndrome without outlet obstruction.

QUALITY OF VOMITUS. *Content* of the vomitus is important in the determination of the underlying disorder. Undigested food indicates a gastric outlet obstruction. If there is blood in the vomitus, an inflammatory or malignant disease of the stomach should be suspected. Vomitus without bile indicates that the problem is prepyloric, whereas consistent appearance of bile suggests that the problem is postpyloric. The presence of bile may signify only that the increase in pressure in the duodenum was sufficiently great that, with a relaxed pylorus, duodenal contents entered the stomach preceding evacuation. Large-volume vomitus of high acidity (pH 1.5 or less) suggests gastrinoma, although outlet obstruction with an active duodenal ulcer may have a similar output and pH.

Odor may also be helpful. A fecal smell to vomitus suggests lower intestinal obstruction, a fistula between the stomach and colon or between the upper small intestine and colon, or bacterial overgrowth of the stomach or small intestine (long-standing obstruction).

Nausea and vomiting that follow the recent onset of a persisting abdominal pain provide a clue to a likely important event within the abdomen, an event that often requires hospitalization and, in some cases, surgery.

CLASSIFICATION OF DISEASES AND DISORDERS ASSOCIATED WITH VOMITING. The major categories of disorders associated with vomiting are summarized in Table 94–1.

Psychogenic vomiting, a chronic and complex disturbance, takes place immediately after eating or during the meal. It is often self-induced and, although chronic, is compatible with good health over many years. It is frequently associated with anorexia nervosa or follows the binge eating of bulimia.

The clinical entities associated with nausea and vomiting that command immediate attention are *intra-abdominal, intracranial,* and *metabolic diseases.* In the abdomen they include gastric outlet obstruction; intestinal obstruction; gastrointestinal inflammation; perforation of a viscus; peritonitis; pancreatitis; abscess; acute distention of smooth muscle in bile ducts, the ureter, and the small intestine; and acute ischemia. In general, nausea and vomiting often follow severe pain, extra-abdominal as well as intra-abdominal. In addition, ileus of the intestine and stomach, and acute gastric dilatation with atony, no matter what the cause, are often associated with nausea and vomiting. In these instances, organic outlet obstruction or intestinal obstruction cannot be demonstrated.

Intracranial disease causing increased intracranial pressure (tumor, hematoma), many *toxic* and *metabolic encephalopathies* (including infection), migraine headache, and *gastric neuropathies* are examples of neurologic diseases associated with vomiting.

In medical practice nausea and vomiting are most commonly *drug induced.* The list of offending drugs is lengthy; most drugs are capable of causing nausea and vomiting in susceptible individuals. Whether the afferent stimuli originate from the action of drugs on the gastrointestinal tract or from the direct effect of drugs on the chemoreceptor zone is not clear in most instances. Anticholinergic agents, however, may cause vomiting by inhibiting motor activity in patients with partial outlet obstruction. The most common causes of gastric outlet obstruction are chronic ulcer disease of the pylorus or duodenum and antral carcinoma.

COMPLICATIONS OF VOMITING (Fig. 94–1). The major consequences of prolonged vomiting include *dehydration, hypokalemia,* and *alkalosis.* Dehydration is due to fluid loss. Hypokalemia results from exchange of sodium for potassium in the renal tubule in an effort to conserve sodium lost in vomitus, from diminished potassium intake, and from loss of potassium in the vomitus. Alkalosis follows loss of hydrogen ions in the vomitus and is exacerbated by a contraction of extracellular fluid, with noncommensurate loss of bicarbonate and shift of hydrogen into cells resulting from potassium deficiency. So-

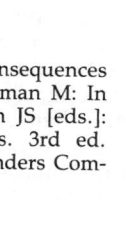

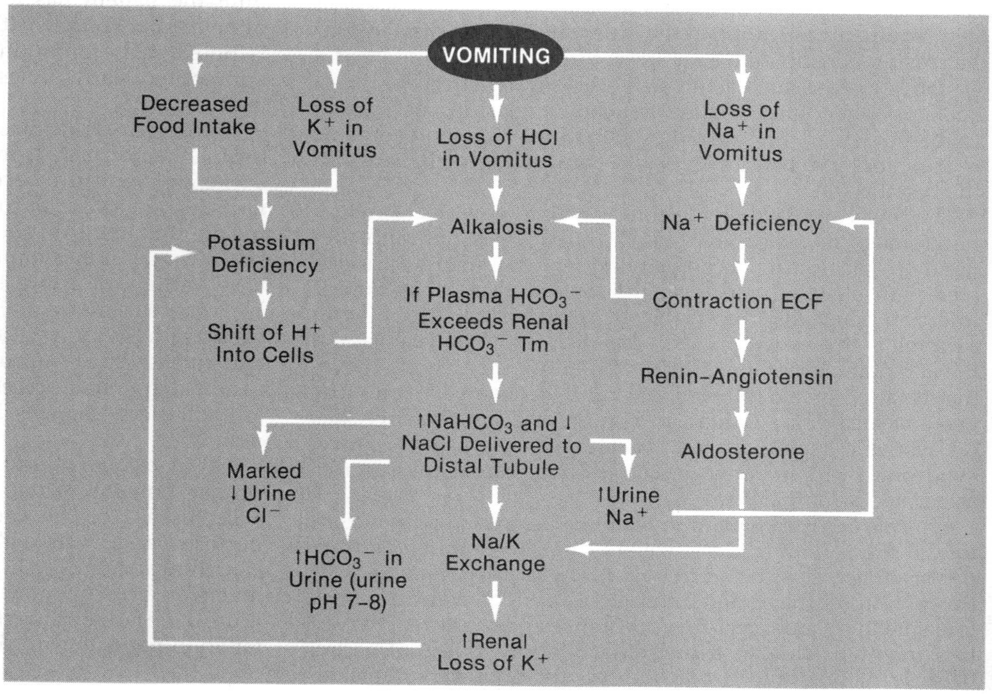

FIGURE 94–1. Metabolic consequences of vomiting. (From Feldman M: In Sleisenger MH, Fordtran JS [eds.]: Gastrointestinal Diseases. 3rd ed. Philadelphia, W. B. Saunders Company, 1983.)

dium depletion results from loss of sodium in the vomitus and, in some instances, renal loss of sodium. Urine is concentrated; a variable amount of bicarbonate is lost, depending upon whether or not the renal transport maximum (Tm) for bicarbonate is exceeded. The urinary excretion of sodium, potassium, and chloride is low if the Tm for bicarbonate is not exceeded. On the other hand, if the Tm for bicarbonate is exceeded, sodium, potassium, and bicarbonate will be high in the urine, and urine chloride will be low.

Signs and symptoms that result from the metabolic consequences of vomiting include muscle weakness, polydipsia, impaired urinary concentration, and abdominal distention (caused by hypokalemia); muscle cramps, weakness, somnolence, and even stupor (caused by hyponatremia and marked dehydration); and hypotension and low urinary output (caused by dehydration and intravascular volume contraction).

Change in Bowel Habit: Constipation and Diarrhea. Normal bowel habit ranges from one bowel movement per one to three days to three to four stools per day. Generally patients readily discern significant changes in their own pattern. Some persons may have only one stool per week or longer for many years. Severe constipation may be lifelong, as in congenital aganglionosis of the colon (Hirschsprung's disease). The definition of diarrhea is also difficult. It is not based entirely on numbers of bowel movements, although patients with diarrhea most frequently have more than three bowel movements per day. The definition most often used is based on volume—a daily stool bulk that exceeds 150 ml. A patient may have three or more small bowel movements a day but not be considered to have diarrhea. The physician who is consulted for long-standing constipation or diarrhea is obliged to investigate the complaint. Hitherto undiagnosed chronic treatable disease may be found.

Change in bowel habit must always be taken seriously even if it has occurred gradually over many months or even years. The recent onset of constipation or diarrhea may represent a reaction to stress, a change in diet, an enteric infection, malignancy of the colon, or a result of a metabolic disease. The majority of patients with nonorganic causes of constipation (bowel movement frequency of less than two per week) will increase the number of movements to three or more if placed on a high-fiber diet. A few patients will complain of lifelong inability to have bowel movements without vigorous catharsis or enemas. Such patients may also have megacolon and require investigation of the innervation of the distal colon. Increasing constipation may be a chronic manifestation of a systemic disease such as myxedema or of the effects of drugs such as phenothiazines or anticholinergics. A decreasing caliber of stool, on the other hand, may connote organic obstruction and may be due to a constricting malignancy of the distal colon.

The onset of diarrhea of more than a few weeks' duration necessitates investigation (see Ch. 103). Its significance depends in part on its accompanying features. Thus, if associated with bleeding and fever in a recent traveler, an enteric infection (shigellosis or amebiasis) is suggested. At the other extreme is the individual with diarrhea for many years and a bowel habit characterized by several loose, nonbloody movements after breakfast each day and occasionally after the evening meal. This individual appears healthy, is active, has no systemic symptoms, and most likely has irritable bowel syndrome (IBS). In between these extremes are many diseases associated with diarrhea.

Chronic diarrhea may or may not be associated with weight loss. If the patient is losing weight, the question of *malabsorption syndrome* must be addressed (see Ch. 104). Patients with this syndrome have abnormal stools—bulky, light in color, foul smelling, and greasy in appearance and character. Weight loss might be due to associated anorexia or fear of eating because of discomfort following meals, both symptoms resulting possibly from an inflammatory or malignant disease of the intestine, liver, or pancreas. Does the diarrhea persist despite the patient's abstaining from eating? If so, a secretory tumor of the pancreas, thyroid, or enterochromaffin tissue may be responsible. On the other hand, if the diarrhea is ameliorated by restricting food and fluid and if the stool water prior to such restriction has contained lower than normal concentrations of sodium and potassium, a disorder causing so-called osmotic diarrhea must be suspected. It results from the intraluminal generation of osmotically active material from unabsorbed disaccharides, hexoses, fatty acids, and amino acids. The bacterial metabolites of these substances are osmotically active, drawing fluid into the lumen of the intestine. The amount and rate of transit are such that the colon cannot reabsorb most of the water and electrolyte presented to it. A more extensive discussion of the pathophysiology of diarrhea and its differential diagnosis is presented in Ch. 103.

Gastrointestinal Bleeding. Gastrointestinal bleeding may be gross or occult. Gross bleeding may be caused by a variety of disorders, including erosions of the stomach; tears and varices of the lower esophagus; peptic ulcer of the lower esophagus, stomach, duodenum, or jejunum; angiodysplasia or other vascular anomalies (telangiectasia, blue rubber nevi, and so on); tumors of the stomach and small intestine (particularly leiomyomas); sudden, severe ischemia of the small or large intestine; diverticula of the colon; or rupture of arterial aneurysms or of bypass aortic grafts into the gut lumen. The bleeding may be dramatic clinically, particularly if bright red blood has been vomited or passed in large quantities from the rectum. Many patients, particularly those with bleeding from the upper tract (stomach, duodenum, and proximal jejunum), note only black tarry stools (melena). Regardless of the character of the bleeding, the patient's condition is determined by the amount and rapidity of loss. Most often such persons require hospitalization, emergent study, and appropriate treatment, including emergency surgery (see Ch. 114).

CARDIOVASCULAR RESPONSES TO ACUTE GASTROINTESTINAL HEMORRHAGE. Tachycardia is the earliest response to loss of blood volume in otherwise healthy persons, and it is accentuated by change in position from lying to standing. With continuing hemorrhage diastolic hypotension appears. At first it is evident only when the patient assumes an upright or standing posture; later it is present without change in position. A fall in diastolic blood pressure is not ordinarily noted until the patient has lost in excess of 20 to 25 per cent of intravascular volume within a few hours. Systolic hypotension is noted with continuing hemorrhage and also will not be appreciated early unless the patient assumes an upright posture.

The decreased cardiac output of significant acute gastrointestinal hemorrhage is manifested in the skin as coolness and a clammy moisture, occasionally with peripheral cyanosis. Decreasing cardiac output and cerebral ischemia cause confusion, agitation, or obtundation. With the upright posture, patients may note symptoms of blurred vision, roaring in the ears, vertigo, or a dizzy sensation; in severe cases or in later life, patients may suffer syncope. The aging brain is very sensitive to hypoperfusion and, hence, anoxia. In the elderly and those with compromised cerebral circulation, hypoperfusion may initiate cerebral thromboses. Even in those who are still alert, changes in the electroencephalogram may be noted.

Fall in cardiac output is often accompanied by changes in cardiac function. Thus, patients with significant arteriosclerotic disease of the coronary arteries may develop angina pectoris, and even without pain ischemic changes on the electrocardiogram such as ST segment depression or T wave inversion are common. On occasion the patient suffers an acute myocardial infarction. Oliguria is a common manifestation in patients with severe blood loss from the gastrointestinal tract. At onset of bleeding, urinary osmolality and specific gravity are increased and sodium concentrations are usually less than 20 mEq per liter. With severe shock and marked renal hypoperfusion, acute cortical or tubular necrosis may supervene. The gastrointestinal tract itself is not immune from the manifestations of a severe decrease in cardiac output brought about by hypovolemia. The liver is not severely injured unless hypotension is severe and prolonged. However, the tubular gastrointestinal tract (particularly the small bowel beyond the ligament of Treitz), cecum, transverse colon, and descending colon, may suffer the effects of ischemia (see Ch. 106). Nonocclusive ischemia of these areas of the tubular gastrointestinal tract can be associated with a rapid deterioration of the patient.

With occult bleeding, patients may or may not have other symptoms indicative of disturbance in a particular part of the gastrointestinal tract. Many elderly persons complain of the effects of a progressive anemia. Unexplained iron deficiency with stools containing occult blood in such patients often reflects carcinoma of the cecum and right colon. Between these extremes are patients who intermittently pass small amounts of blood by rectum. These are patients who must be suspected of having malignancy, ischemia, or inflammatory disease of the distal colon. Chronic occult bleeding in elderly persons, particularly those with aortic valve disease, may be due to angiodysplastic lesions of the gut, particularly of the cecum and right colon.

Intestinal Gas. Patients are frequently bothered by symptoms caused by intestinal gas. These are *eructation*, the distress of *bloating* with borborygmi, and *excessive flatus*.

The major intraluminal gases are nitrogen (N_2), carbon dioxide (CO_2), and methane (CH_4); all these gases but N_2 are produced in the bowel lumen. About 600 ml of gas is passed per rectum per day, of which over 400 ml is produced enterically. The amount of hydrogen and CO_2 depends to a significant degree upon the diet. Unabsorbed carbohydrate and protein, particularly greens and vegetables, are broken down by colonic bacteria to yield hydrogen and carbon dioxide. CH_4 is produced by only about one third of the adult population.

Although complaints referable to intestinal gas have classically been attributed to excessive air swallowing, it is clear that this habit is not responsible for a major contribution either to the amount of intestinal gas or to the symptoms. Normally, swallowed air is quickly expelled. It may cause distress in only a very limited number of persons who do not normally expel it.

ERUCTATION (BELCHING). Air that is expelled by belching is usually that recently swallowed into the esophagus. Repeated belching may on occasion be associated with serious organic disease, particularly with gastric outlet obstruction or gastric dilatation. The vast majority of patients who belch frequently in order to relieve distress are overanxious (constantly swallowing air, thus the word "aerophagia").

ABDOMINAL DISTRESS OF DISTENTION (BLOATING). Bloating and "gas pains" have classically and erroneously been thought to be due to excessive gas. In fact, abnormal intestinal motor activity usually accounts for these symptoms. Usually, the intestinal contents move along in an orderly fashion, stimulated particularly by eating. Disorders of motility both in the small bowel and in the colon may move gas faster than normal. However, there may be areas of resistance to rapid passage owing to organic disease or, more commonly, to motor dysfunction associated with spasm, noted particularly in the irritable bowel syndrome. Bowel proximal to a narrowed area dilates, whether narrowing is a stricture or spasm, stretching the smooth muscle and eliciting pain of a cramping nature. Organic causes of disturbed motility may also underlie these symptoms, e.g., progressive intestinal obstruction caused by a stricture or tumor. Recent onset of these complaints always warrants thorough investigation.

The *irritable bowel syndrome* is associated with a motor disturbance and often with abdominal bloating. The discomfort of these patients may indeed be due to gas, albeit in normal amounts. It may be alleviated by dietary exclusion of gas-forming foods, including lactose, thus relieving complaints of many years to decades.

EXCESSIVE FLATUS (GAS PER RECTUM). Excessive flatus results from ingesting foods notorious as substrates for gas formation, from an overgrowth of gas-producing bacteria in the gastrointestinal tract, or from malabsorption of carbohydrates (e.g., lactase deficiency). Patients have excessive gas resulting from bacterial action on unabsorbed carbohydrate in the colon (or in the small gut if there is bacterial overgrowth), with release of hydrogen as the most important gas but also of CO_2. Only about one third of normal individuals produce intestinal methane, but a larger number (80 per cent) of patients with cancer of the colon do so. Methane production presumably reflects a special bacterial colonization of the colon. Some patients have normal amounts of flatus per day but complain of increased frequency of flatus following a meal. This complaint is most likely due to a hyperactive gastrocolic reflex, which characterizes many patients with irritable bowel syndrome.

Patients who pass more than a normal amount of gas may complain of bloating and pain. Analysis of flatus demonstrates unusually high percentages of hydrogen and carbon dioxide. Whether it is due to a particular disease of the small intestine, pancreatic insufficiency, bacterial overgrowth of the small intestine, or lactase deficiency requires definition. Excessive colonic production of gas also may be caused by the ingestion of abnormal amounts of fruit and vegetables which contain nonabsorbable carbohydrates, and may respond to dietary restriction of lactose, legumes, and wheat.

Jaundice. Jaundice is due to elevated levels of either conjugated or unconjugated bilirubin in plasma and extracellular fluid. It is a common and important sign of disease of the liver or biliary tract, or of hemolysis. Hyperbilirubinemia may result from excessive production of bilirubin (hemolysis), reduced excretion of bilirubin into the bile (liver disease), or obstruction of the flow of bile into the intestine (biliary tract disease). Rarely jaundice is caused by hereditary diseases producing defects in the hepatic uptake of bilirubin or its glucuronidation. Impaired capacity to secrete conjugated bilirubin into the bile may also be due to inherited metabolic defects. The pathophysiology of bilirubin metabolism is discussed in greater detail in Ch. 118.

Jaundice is not usually detectable in natural light below plasma bilirubin levels of 2 to 2.5 mg per deciliter. Jaundice caused by conjugated bilirubin is associated with dark urine, since conjugated bilirubin is water soluble and therefore excreted in the urine. On the other hand, nonconjugated bilirubin is lipid soluble and protein bound so that it is not excreted in the urine.

The most common cause of jaundice is injury to the hepatocyte by virus, toxin, or drug. The clinical significance of jaundice in a patient therefore depends to a large extent on its duration, intensity, and relationship to possible infection or drug use, and on the presence or absence of factors that may cause obstruction (cholelithiasis). Gradual obstruction of the extrahepatic ductal system with progressive jaundice in an elderly person not taking hepatotoxic drugs and with no evidence of viral infection most frequently indicates *choledocholithiasis*, malignancy of the bile ducts (*cholangiocarcinomas*), or a *periampullary malignancy*. In jaundice due to choledocholithiasis, serum bilirubin rarely exceeds 12.0 mg per deciliter but is commonly much higher with periampullary or bile duct malignancies. *Pruritus* is common in many patients with jaundice; it may be due to severe intrahepatic cholestasis, extrahepatic obstruction, recurrent jaundice of pregnancy, or primary biliary cirrhosis.

Low-grade fever (100° to 101°F) usually accompanies viral or alcoholic hepatitis and, occasionally occurs in so-called *sclerosing cholangitis*, but is dramatically high (102° to 104°F) in cholangitis due to choledocholithiasis. Careful search on physical examination for evidences of liver disease is crucial in evaluating patients with jaundice. The presence of masses, particularly of a palpable gallbladder, indicating long-standing progressive common bile duct obstruction by cancer (*Courvoisier's sign*), is a most important finding. In many instances, the routine laboratory examinations, including liver function tests, are of great help but must be interpreted with caution. The differential diagnosis of jaundice may require use of the specialized diagnostic techniques discussed in Ch. 95 and 96.

Most patients with gastrointestinal disease complain of one (or more) of the symptoms and demonstrate some of the signs that have been discussed. The significance attached to these signs and symptoms determines which road to diagnosis and treatment will be taken. This approach to patients ensures intelligent reference to detailed descriptions of the clinical possibilities and leads to wise choices of tests and procedures. In the chapters that follow, symptoms and signs will be more fully described in terms of specific diseases of the various organs constituting the digestive system, and a wide range of diagnostic tests and procedures will be included. In this way the science of medicine and gastroenterology is brought to bear on good patient care.

Baile CA, McLaughlin CL, Della-Fera MA: Role of cholecystokinin and opíoid peptides in control of food intake. Physiol Rev 66:172, 1986. *A comprehensive review of the complex regulation of food intake with emphasis upon the role of neuropeptides that act upon hypothalamic centers.*

Sleisenger MH, Fordtran JS: Gastrointestinal Disease. 4th ed. Philadelphia, W. B. Saunders Company, 1988. Chapters 1, 9, 10, 14, 15, 17, 20, 22, 25, and 28.

95 DIAGNOSTIC IMAGING PROCEDURES IN GASTROENTEROLOGY

Susan D. Wall

With the development of increasingly complex diagnostic imaging procedures in gastroenterology, the importance of direct communication with the consulting radiologist has increased. Clinical information regarding each diagnostic question is essential to tailoring the studies; none are "routine." In addition to conventional plain films of the abdomen and barium examination of the gastrointestinal tract, radiographic procedures of interest to the gastroenterologist include computed tomography, ultrasonography, endoscopic retrograde cholangiopancreatography, percutaneous transhepatic cholangiography, enteroclysis, radionuclide scanning, and magnetic resonance imaging.

COMPUTED TOMOGRAPHY

The faster scan time (two to three seconds) and higher spatial resolution available with current computed tomography (CT) have improved greatly the images of the alimentary tract as well as of the pancreas (Fig. 95–1), liver, and gallbladder. Computed tomography continues to be an important modality for the investigation of possible hepatic tumor, pancreatic carcinoma, and retroperitoneal adenopathy. Less well known is its contribution to the evaluation of the acute abdomen. When the diagnosis is unclear, CT is helpful in diagnosing possible pancreatitis (Fig. 95–2), perforated viscus, and subdiaphragmatic abscess and in assessing the extent of Crohn's disease or bowel ischemia. It can detect extraluminal abscess associated with appendicitis and diverticulitis (Fig. 95–3) and can sometimes help in the decision regarding surgical versus nonsurgical management. Computed tomography also can detect free intra- (Fig. 95–4) or retroperitoneal air and small amounts of contrast material that have extravasated from the gastrointestinal tract (Fig. 95–3); it provides excellent visualization of the mesentery. It is the modality of choice for evaluation of suspected complications of pancreatitis, such as abscess, pseudocyst, and colonic or mesenteric inflammation.

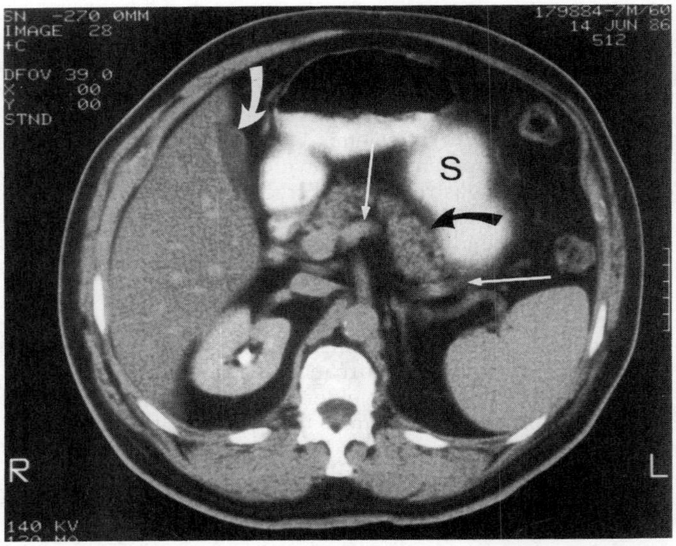

FIGURE 95–1. Normal computed tomogram. One cm thick transverse image (supine, patient's right to reader's left) is at the level of the pancreas (*black arrow*), which is behind the contrast filled stomach (S). The splenic artery is posterior to the splenic vein (*straight white arrows*), which abuts the posterior margin of the tail and neck of the pancreas. The density of the right kidney is enhanced because of intravenous contrast material. *Curved white arow* points to gallbladder.

Percutaneous fine needle aspiration (PFNA) with CT guidance can diagnose pancreatic carcinoma, primary and metastatic tumor of the liver, and sometimes tumor involvement of enlarged lymph nodes. False-negative results occur, but this procedure often obviates the need for diagnostic laparotomy. Furthermore, PFNA can diagnose suspected abscess (Fig. 95–3), which can be variable and nonspecific in its radiographic appearance. Percutaneous drainage of intra-abdominal or pelvic abscess with CT guidance is a nonsurgical treatment option for selected patients; it can palliate others until surgery is performed.

Computed tomography sometimes replaces barium contrast examination as the initial study of the gastrointestinal tract. Barium examination, which provides mucosal detail and delineation of the intraluminal contour, cannot demonstrate thickening of the wall and causes severe artifact on CT images, precluding the possibility of a diagnostic study. Moreover, even unsuspected disease in the gastrointestinal tract, both primary and secondary, often is detected initially with CT. Assessment of thickening of the esophageal, gastric, and bowel wall is possible with current CT, and surrounding organs may also be evaluated, especially regarding inflammatory processes such as diverticulitis, appendicitis, Crohn's disease, pancreatitis, and possible perforated ulcer. Computed tomography has limited value in the regional staging of gastrointestinal malignancies because of its limited accuracy in determining tumor invasion into adjacent tissues. Indications for preoperative evaluation of patients with rectosigmoid colon carcinoma, for example, include suspected extensive disease or complications such as perforation. Computed tomography is more helpful in determining recurrence postoperatively. A baseline study is performed two to four months after resection, with follow-up comparison studies every six months for two years. New or enlarging masses in the pelvis

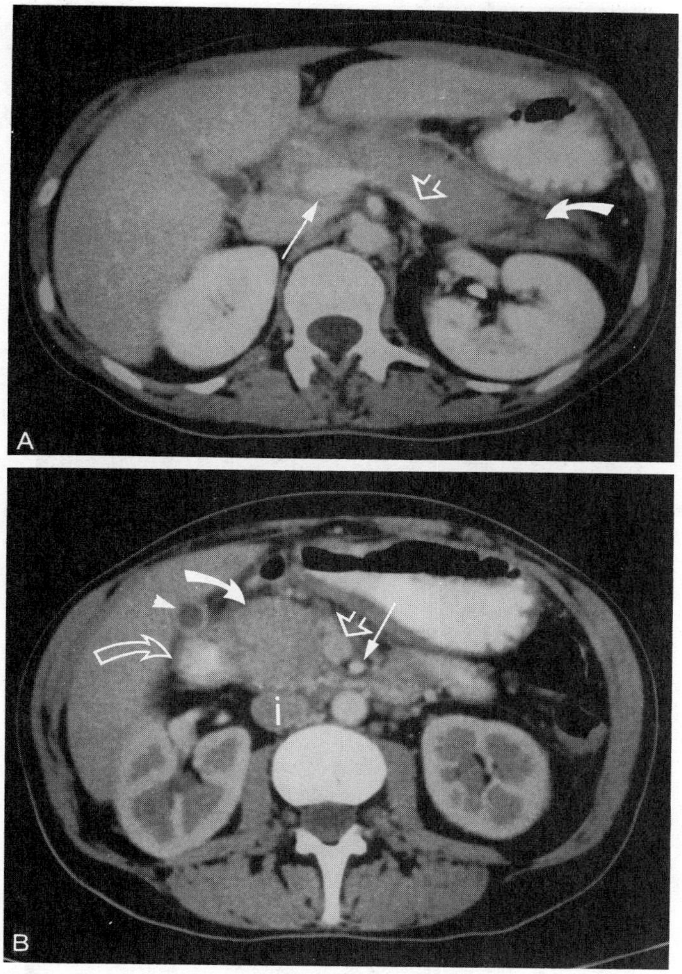

FIGURE 95–2. Computed tomography of pancreatitis. *A*, The body and tail of the pancreas are enlarged. Ill-defined area of low density (*curved arrow*) in the pancreatic parenchyma represents early finding of developing pseudocyst. The enhanced splenic vein (*open arrowhead*) and splenoportal confluence (*straight arrow*) delineate the posterior margin of the pancreas. *B*, The head of the pancreas (*closed curved arrow*), which is swollen, is surrounded by the contrast-filled duodenum (*open curved arrow*) laterally and the inferior vena cava (i) posteriorly. The gallbladder (*closed arrowhead*), superior mesenteric vein (*open arrow*), and superior mesenteric artery (*straight arrow*) are seen. Early intravenous bolus enhancement of the kidneys provides cortical-medullary differentiation.

suggest recurrent tumor; CT-guided biopsy can be performed for tissue diagnosis.

Bret PM, Fond A, Casola G, et al.: Abdominal lesions: A prospective study of clinical efficacy of percutaneous fine-needle biopsy. Radiology 159:345, 1986. *An excellent prospective study and discussion of the influence of percutaneous fine needle biopsy on diagnostic workup, therapeutic choice, and cost benefit.*

Quint LE, Glazer GM, Orringer MB, et al.: Esophageal carcinoma: CT findings. Radiology 155:171, 1985. *A review of the literature and report of their findings; the latter indicates low accurary of staging CT.*

Thompson WM, Halvorsen RA, Foster WL Jr, et al.: Preoperative and postoperative CT staging rectosigmoid carcinoma. Am J Roentgenol 146:703, 1986. *An excellent review of the literature and of their experience.*

ULTRASONOGRAPHY

Abdominal ultrasonography (US) is noninvasive, requires no ionizing radiation, and can be performed with a portable unit. In experienced hands it has excellent results; operator dependence is decreasing as equipment improves. Ultrasonography is superior to other modalities in differentiating cystic from solid lesions and is highly sensitive in detecting ascites. Because of the superb ability to demonstrate gallstones (Fig. 95–5), US has replaced oral cholecystography for the diagnosis

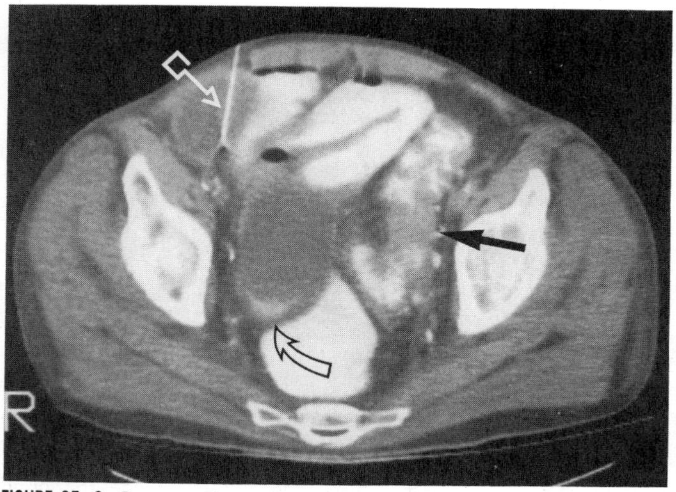

FIGURE 95–3. Computed tomography of diverticular abscess. Percutaneous fine-needle aspiration (*boxed white arrow*) of pelvic fluid collection diagnosed abscess in this patient with thickening of the wall of the sigmoid colon (*straight black arrow*) and diverticulitis. Note second fluid collection with small amount of contrast material (*curved black arrow*) extravasated from the diseased colon. Abscesses were drained percutaneously until the patient was well enough for surgery.

of cholelithiasis. It is an effective and efficient first examination for suspected liver tumors. Ultrasonography is the primary screening examination for hepatobiliary disease and often is the only study needed. Dilatation of the intra-and extrahepatic biliary system can be detected (Fig. 95–6), but the distal common bile duct often is not seen adequately with US. Similarly, the tail or body of the pancreas or both are well visualized less often than the head, principally because of interference by the overlying gas-filled bowel. Ultrasonography, which plays a complementary role with CT in many diseases, often is the preferred modality when follow-up examination is needed, as in pancreatic pseudocyst, abdominal aortic aneurysm, and drained fluid collections. Percutaneous fine needle aspiration and drainage procedures can be performed with ultrasonographic guidance, sometimes with greater ease and less cost compared with CT.

Recent advances in ultrasound involve the application of a transducer to an exposed organ at surgery or through an

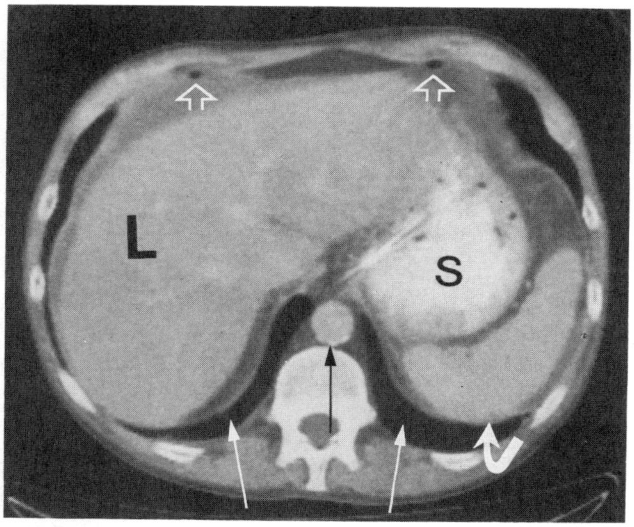

FIGURE 95–4. Computed tomography of pneumoperitoneum. Two small collections of free intraperitoneal air (*open arrows*) are seen in the nondependent areas of the upper abdomen in this patient with colon perforation. Note the air-filled lungs (*straight white arrows*), spleen (*curved arrow*), stomach (S), and liver (L). The aorta (*black arrow*) is anterior to the spine.

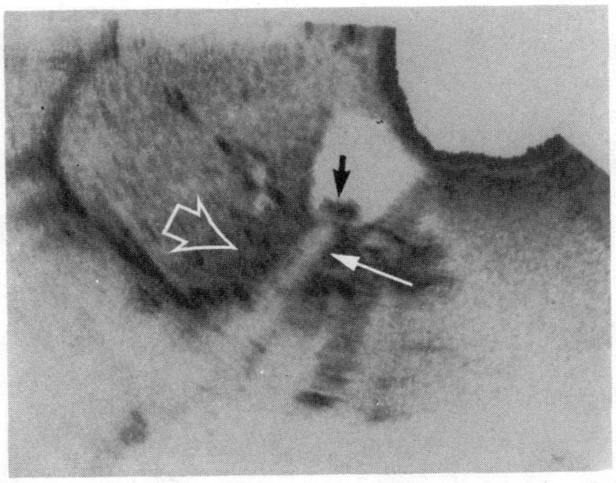

FIGURE 95–5. Ultrasound of cholelithiasis. Sagittal image (patient's head to reader's left) demonstrates a single gallstone (*black arrow*). The sound waves easily pass through the fluid (bile) in the gallbladder—hence the "posterior acoustical enhancement" (*open arrow*) characteristic of a cystic structure. The echogenic stone impedes the sound waves—hence the "posterior shadowing" (*straight white arrow*) characteristic of a gallstone. This "static" ultrasound image produces black echoes on white background.

endoscope. Ultrasonography has facilitated the intraoperative search for pancreatic islet cell tumor and occasionally finds unsuspected multiple tumors. Endosonography requires an end-viewing fiberoptic gastroscope, which is modified to incorporate a transducer. Although still in the developmental stage, this new imaging procedure has been shown to demonstrate the thickness of the esophagus, stomach, and duodenum and to identifv both diffuse and focal intramural lesions. It may also be valuable for diagnosis of early pancreatic lesions.

Cummings S, Papadakis M, Melnick J, et al.: The predictive value of physical examination of ascites. West J Med 142:633, 1985. *Excellent comparison of ultrasonography and physical examination in detecting ascites with a useful list of references.*

Gordon SJ, Rifkin MD, Goldberg BB: Endosonographic evaluation of mural abnormalities of the upper gastrointestinal tract. Gastrointest Endosc 32:193, 1986. *A good presentation of some of the early work with this procedure.*

Jeffrey RB Jr, Laing FC, Wing VW: Extrapancreatic spread of acute pancreatitis: New observations with real-time US. Radiology 159:707, 1986. *A succinct comparison of US and CT in acute pancreatitis with state of the art equipment by experts in the field.*

ENDOSCOPIC RETROGRADE CHOLANGIOPANCREATOGRAPHY

Endoscopic retrograde cholangiopancreatography (ERCP) is performed with the fluoroscopic guidance of the radiologist.

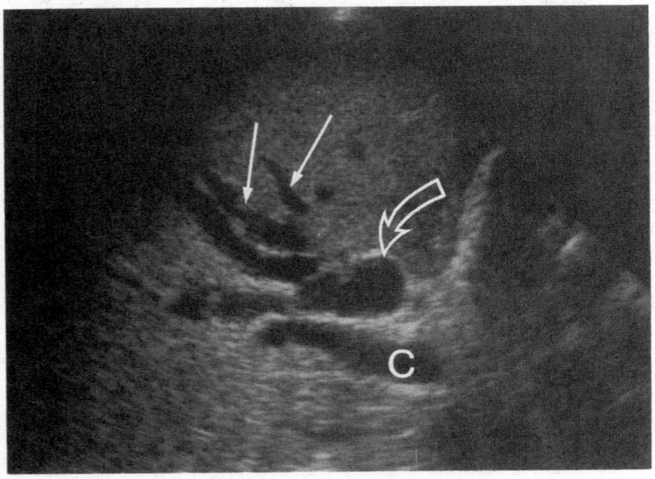

FIGURE 95–6. Ultrasound of dilated bile ducts. Dilatation of the intrahepatic (*straight arrows*) and extrahepatic (*curved arrow*) bile ducts is well demonstrated on the sagittal ultrasound image of a patient with distal biliary obstruction. (C indicates the inferior vena cava.) This real-time ultrasound image produces white echoes on black background.

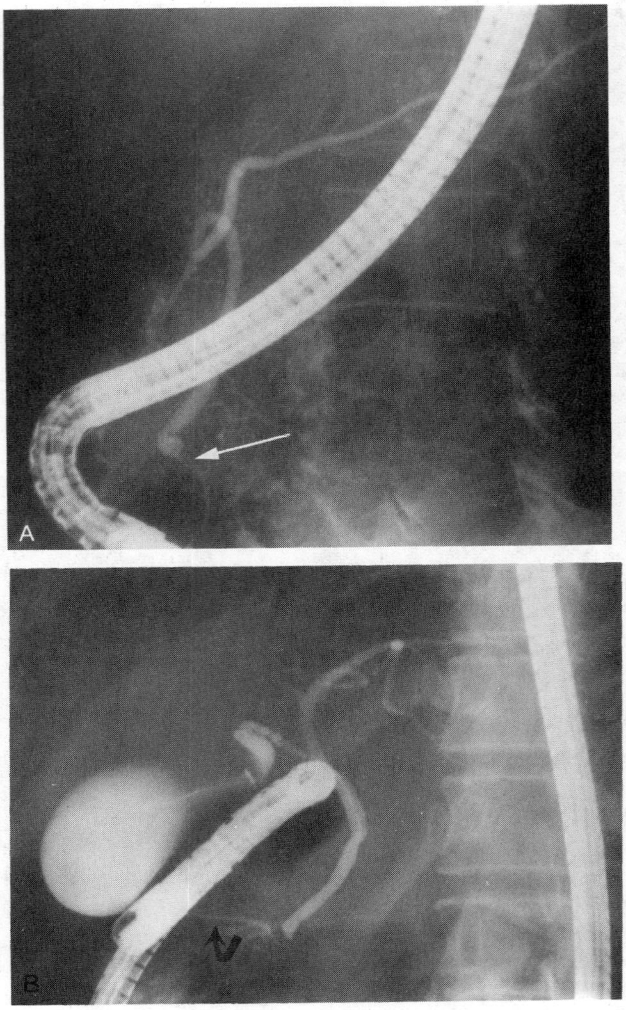

FIGURE 95–7. Normal endoscopic retrograde cholangiopancreatogram. *A*, Normal pancreatogram. The cannula (*arrow*) at the tip of the fiberoptic endoscope has been inserted into the papilla of Vater under direct visualization and the pancreatic duct opacified. *B*, Normal cholangiogram. The gallbladder, cystic duct, common hepatic duct, and common bile duct are visible. *Arrow* indicates cannula in the papilla of Vater.

The papilla of Vater is visualized through a fiberoptic endoscope, and the common bile duct or the pancreatic duct or both are cannulated. Water-soluble iodinated contrast material is injected, and images are taken of the opacified biliary tree or pancreatic duct (Fig. 95–7). ERCP is performed specifically to evaluate the pancreatic duct or follows US or CT demonstrating distal biliary obstruction. When a constricting or obstructing lesion is seen in the distal common bile duct, biopsy or papillotomy can be performed. A further discussion of ERCP is contained in Ch. 76.

TRANSHEPATIC CHOLANGIOGRAPHY

Percutaneous transhepatic cholangiography is used to visualize the intra- and extrahepatic biliary tree following CT, US, or ERCP that has demonstrated proximal obstruction of the common hepatic or common bile duct. It is performed by injecting water-soluble iodinated contrast material through a flexible 23-gauge needle introduced percutaneously into the intrahepatic biliary tree under fluoroscopic guidance. After the biliary tree is opacified, multiple radiographs are taken in order to characterize the suspected site of blockage or narrowing (Fig. 95–8). This study provides the surgeon with the best demonstration of possible anastomotic sites of the biliary tree in the porta hepatis. Serious complications such as bile peri-

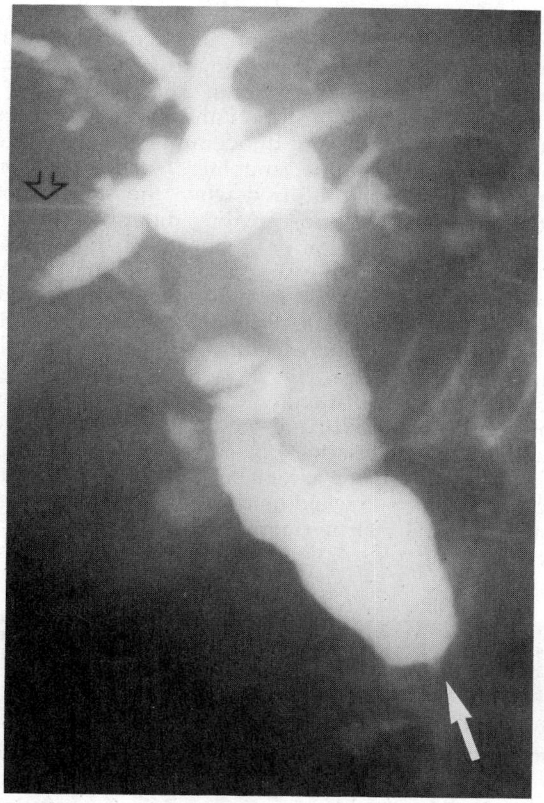

FIGURE 95–8. Percutaneous transhepatic cholangiogram. Dilatation of the biliary tree is demonstrated after percutaneous puncture and opacification of a dilated intrahepatic duct with a long 23-gauge needle (*open black arrow*). The distal common bile duct is abruptly narrowed and obstructed (*white arrow*) owing to cholangiocarcinoma.

tonitis or intraperitoneal hemorrhage occur in less than 2 per cent of cases. Biliary obstruction can be treated in patients who are poor surgical risks by several interventional procedures, including percutaneous stricture dilatation, percutaneous drainage, or insertion of a biliary endoprosthesis. The last procedure can be performed percutaneously or via an ERCP in conjunction with a percutaneous transhepatic technique.

Lammer J, Neumayer K: Biliary drainage endoprostheses: Experience with 201 placements. Radiology 159:625, 1986. *An excellent discussion of procedure, complications, and patient tolerance.*

ENTEROCLYSIS

Procedures used to study the small bowel include the "dedicated" small bowel follow-through, single- and double-contrast enteroclysis, and the peroral pneumocolon. Examination of the small bowel should not accompany most studies of the esophagus, stomach, and/or duodenum because the high-density barium used for the latter interferes with visualization of detail of the small bowel, especially the jejunum. Consequently, lesions that are present may be seen poorly or may be missed, and often it is nearly impossible to exclude abnormality. Hence, the traditional "upper gastrointestinal series with small bowel follow-through" is no longer the optimal examination for small intestinal disease. An exception to this is the patient in whom the terminal ileum is the only suspected site of involvement. In this case, the peroral pneumocolon may be the most precise approach. It is performed with introduction of insufflated air per rectum when orally administered thin barium has reached the cecum. With reflux of air across the ileocecal valve, double-contrast images of the terminal ileum are obtained.

Enteroclysis, also known as small bowel enema, refers to the direct introduction of contrast material after intubation of the first loop of jejunum or, less optimally, the distal duodenum. It allows for a controlled rate of delivery of contrast material independent of gastric emptying and thus optimizes luminal distention. The double-contrast method uses air or methylcellulose to provide fine detail to the folds of the small bowel. Enteroclysis has been advocated as the most accurate method for the detection of focal lesions in the small bowel. However, it is comparable to a dedicated (tubeless) small bowel study for the detection of lesions due to Crohn's disease and tumor and is only slightly more sensitive for adhesions. A dedicated small bowel study does not immediately follow examination of the esophagus, stomach, or duodenum; it is performed with frequent, intermittent spot films by the radiologist. Enteroclysis, which is more lengthy and requires more expertise by the radiologist, is tolerated less well by the patient and, most importantly, involves a much greater radiation exposure.

Ott DJ, Chen YM, Gelfand DW, et al.: Detailed per-oral small bowel examination vs. enteroclysis. Part I: Expenditures and radiation exposure, and Part II: Radiographic accuracy. Radiology 155:29, 1985. *An excellent comparison study of these two modalities; the enteroclysis technique was single contrast.*

Wolf KJ, Goldberg HI, Wall SD, et al.: Peroral pneumocolon: The usefulness in evaluating the normal and abnormal ileocecal region. *A study of 170 patients; demonstrates its value in detecting ulcerations, edematous mucosa, and cobblestone patterns.*

RADIONUCLIDE IMAGING

Acute cholecystitis is usually due to obstruction of the cystic duct by a calculus. Scanning with technetium-labeled iminodiacetic acid (^{99m}TcHIDA), which is excreted by the hepatobiliary system, is valuable when such a diagnosis is in question. Visualization of the liver, bile ducts, gallbladder, and bowel occurs within 60 minutes of injection in normal, fasting patients (Fig. 95–9). Visualization of the gallbladder excludes the diagnosis of obstruction of the cystic duct. Nonvisualization of the gallbladder with normal visualization of the common bile duct and bowel indicates cystic duct obstruction (Fig. 95–10). Nonvisualization of both the gallbladder and the bowel can occur in conditions involving cholestasis without cystic duct obstruction, such as hepatocellular disease, total parenteral nutrition, and obstruction of the distal common bile duct. Ultrasonography is more sensitive regarding the detection of gallstone but is less accurate in the diagnosis of acute cholecystitis.

Gastric mucosa secretes ^{99m}Tc pertechnetate. It can be used to detect ectopic gastric mucosa, especially in Meckel's diverticulum and sometimes in Barrett's esophagus. Ectopic gastric mucosa is present in most symptomatic Meckel's diverticula and in nearly all that bleed, but only half of the bleeding Meckel's diverticula in adults are detected by this study. False-positive results are common. This method of detecting Meckel's diverticulum is far more useful in children.

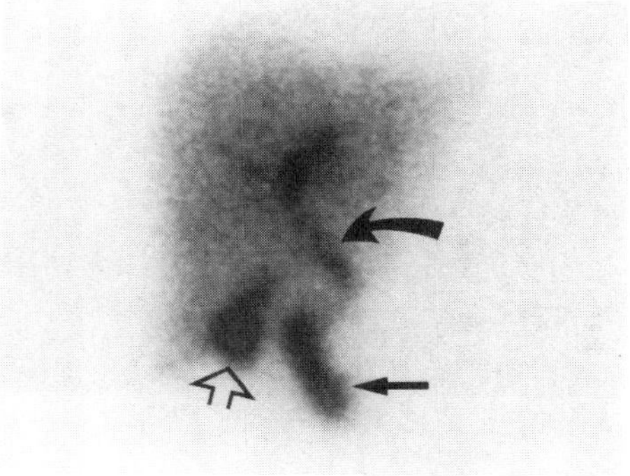

FIGURE 95–9. Normal Tc HIDA scan. Technetium-99m labeled iminodiacetic acid (HIDA) has been excreted by the liver in this normal, fasting patient. Within 60 minutes of intravenous injection, there is visualization of the common bile duct (*curved arrow*), gallbladder (*open arrow*), and duodenum (*straight arrow*).

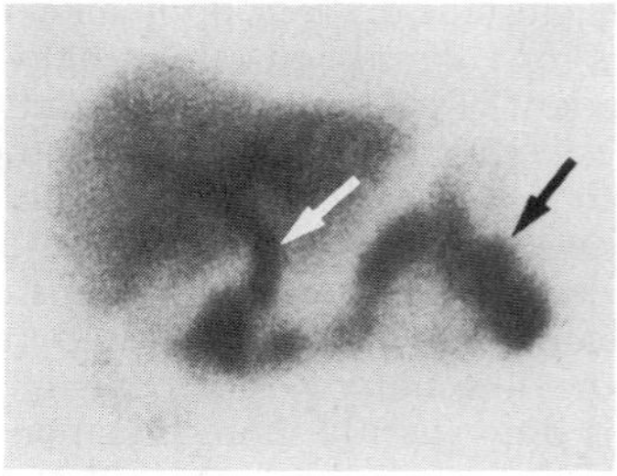

FIGURE 95–10. Tc HIDA of acute cholecystitis. Visualization of the common bile duct (*white arrow*) and small bowel (*black arrow*) without visualization of the gallbladder indicated obstruction of the cystic duct in this fasting patient with acute cholecystitis.

There are two nuclear medicine procedures available for the detection of acute and chronic gastrointestinal bleeding sites, both of which rely upon the extravasation of the radionuclide into the intestinal lumen. Injected ^{99m}Tc sulfur colloid remains in the circulation only briefly, and therefore its use requires active bleeding (approximately 2 ml per minute) at the time of the study. This disadvantage, which is shared with angiography, does not apply to ^{99m}Tc-labeled autologous erythrocytes because they remain in circulation. With the latter procedure, intermittent bleeding of 10 to 20 ml per hour may be detected on delayed views. The reliability of both procedures is greater for the colon and small bowel than for the esophagus, stomach, and duodenum because of overlapping structures in the upper abdomen. *Angiography* for gastrointestinal hemorrhage is used when the site of bleeding cannot be identified by endoscopy or radionuclide imaging or when transcatheter infusion or embolization therapy is indicated. Visceral angiography of most abdominal pathologic conditions has been replaced by other diagnostic procedures, but it is indicated still in the evaluation of vascular occlusive disease, in polysystemic vasculitis, and preoperatively for hepatic tumors.

Disorders of gastric motility are not well evaluated by barium radiographic techniques because these techniques are not quantitative, are relatively insensitive, and are not physiologic. Procedures using radiolabeled food with continuous gastric monitoring may yield quantitative data such as gastric half-emptying time. Furthermore, with radionuclide imaging, gastric emptying of solids versus liquids can be assessed simultaneously.

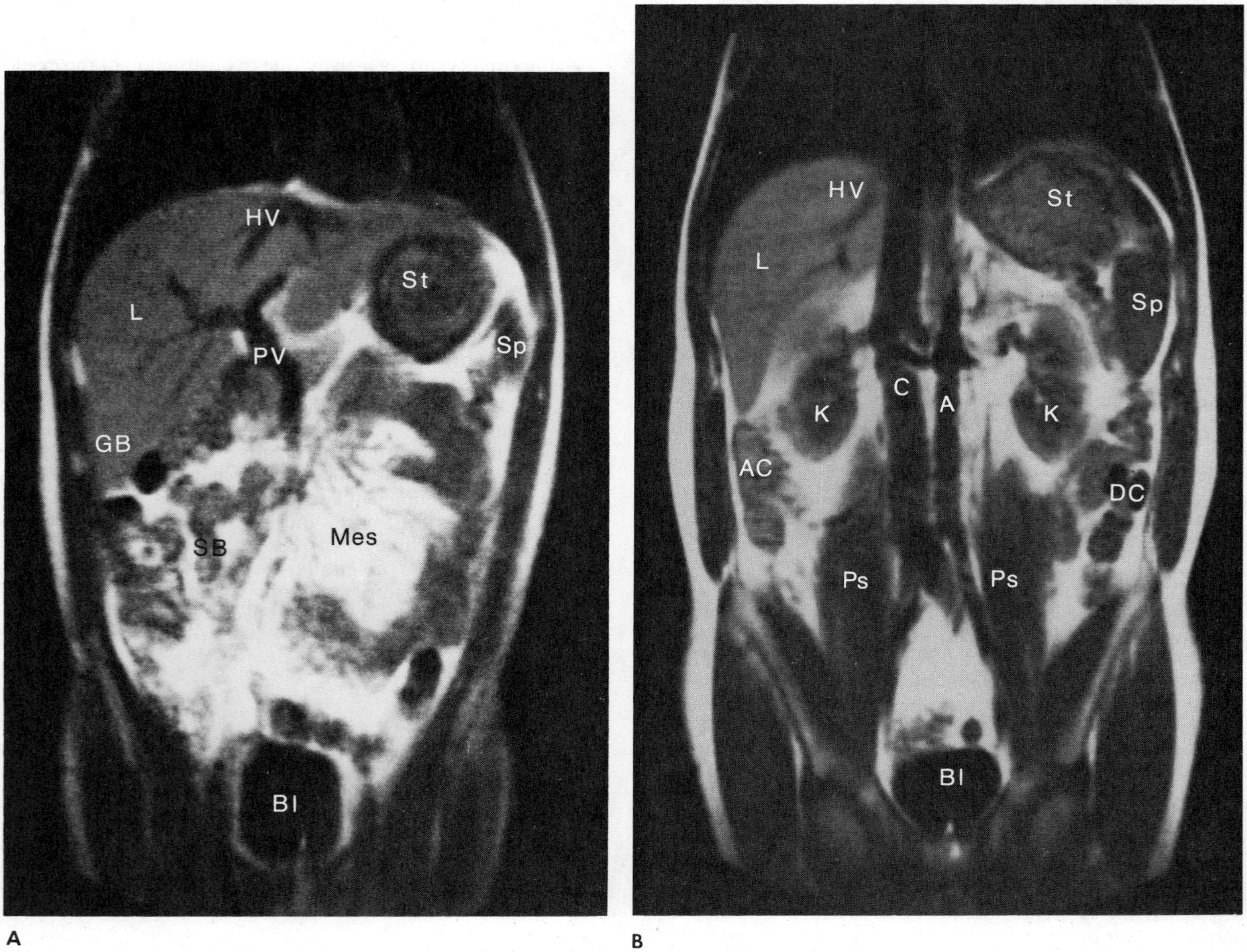

FIGURE 95–11. Normal abdominal magnetic resonance. *A*, T1 weighted coronal image of the anterior abdomen demonstrates the liver (L), spleen (Sp), stomach (St), gallbladder (GB), hepatic veins (HV), portal vein (PV), small bowel (SB), mesentery (Mes), and urinary bladder (B1). *B*, T1 weighted coronal image of the posterior abdomen demonstrates the inferior vena cava (C), aorta (A), kidneys (K), ascending colon (AC), descending colon (DC), and psoas muscles (Ps) in addition to the structures noted in the anterior abdomen in *A*. (Courtesy of General Electric Company, Milwaukee, WI.)

Intravenous injection of indium 111–labeled leukocytes is sometimes indicated in the febrile patient, especially if symptomatic less than two weeks with an acute inflammatory process of uncertain origin. This technique has a sensitivity of 85 to 90 per cent and a specificity of 90 to 95 per cent. Importantly, for the detection of abscess, it can be performed with a portable unit for the patient too ill to go to the radiology department for other imaging procedures.

Liver scanning with ^{99m}Tc-sulfur colloid is used for the assessment of size, shape, and position; identification of space-occupying lesions such as tumor, abscess, or hematoma; and evaluation of hepatocellular disease. Sensitivity for the detection of primary and metastatic tumor is comparable to that of CT (which is slightly more accurate) and that of US (which is slightly less sensitive). The newer technique of liver scanning with SPECT (single photon emission computed tomography) imaging produces three-dimensional cross-sectional tomographic images and eliminates the overlapping influences of the surrounding radioactivity. Thus, the sensitivity for small (2 cm) space-occupying lesions is increased.

Arnstein NB, Shapiro B, Eckhauser FI, et al.: Morbid obesity treated by gastroplasty: Radionuclide gastric emptying studies. Radiology 156:501, 1985. *A study of 50 postgastroplasty patients by experts in radionuclide imaging.*

Kudo M, Hirasa M, Takakuwa H, et al.: Small hepatocellular carcinomas in chronic liver disease: Detection with SPECT. Radiology 159:697, 1986. *Comparison with US, CT, angiography, and alpha-fetoprotein.*

Schwartz MJ, Lewis JH: Meckel's diverticulum: Pitfalls in scintigraphic detection in the adult. Am J Gastroenterol 79:611, 1984. *A review of 37 Meckel scan studies in addition to their own experience; emphasis on adults.*

MAGNETIC RESONANCE IMAGING

A very brief and simplified summary of the physics of magnetic resonance (MR) imaging is presented here as a background. Hydrogen nuclei (protons) have a dipole moment and therefore behave as would a magnetic compass. In MR scanning, the protons align with the strong magnetic field but are easily perturbed by a brief radiofrequency (RF) pulse of very low energy and then are altered in their alignment. As the protons return to their orientation with the magnetic field, they release energy of a radiofrequency that is strongly influenced by the biochemical environment. T1 and T2 relaxation times are a description of the released energy, which is detected, mathematically analyzed, and displayed as a two-dimensional proton-density map according to the "signal intensity" of each tissue. Because the water molecule contains two hydrogen nuclei, changes in distribution of water in tissue, as well as its overall concentration, strongly influence the "intensity" of the MR signal. Hence, MR can provide superior contrast differentiation of tissues with varying amounts of water compared with conventional radiographic modalities, which depend only upon the attenuation of the roentgenographic beam. In addition, fat emits a strong signal because of the abundance of lipid protons. Other advantages of MR include its noninvasiveness, lack of ionizing radiation, and ability to image directly in transaxial, sagittal, coronal (Fig. 95–11), and nonorthogonal planes. Its disadvantages include cost, limited availability, slow scanning time, and problems associated with the powerful magnetic field. The last-named precludes imaging patients with a cardiac pacemaker or metallic clips on intracranial blood vessels. Moreover, critically ill patients cannot easily be monitored because of limited access to the patient during the study and because the strong magnetic field prohibits the presence of resuscitative equipment made of metal.

Physiologic motion limits the diagnostic capability of MR in

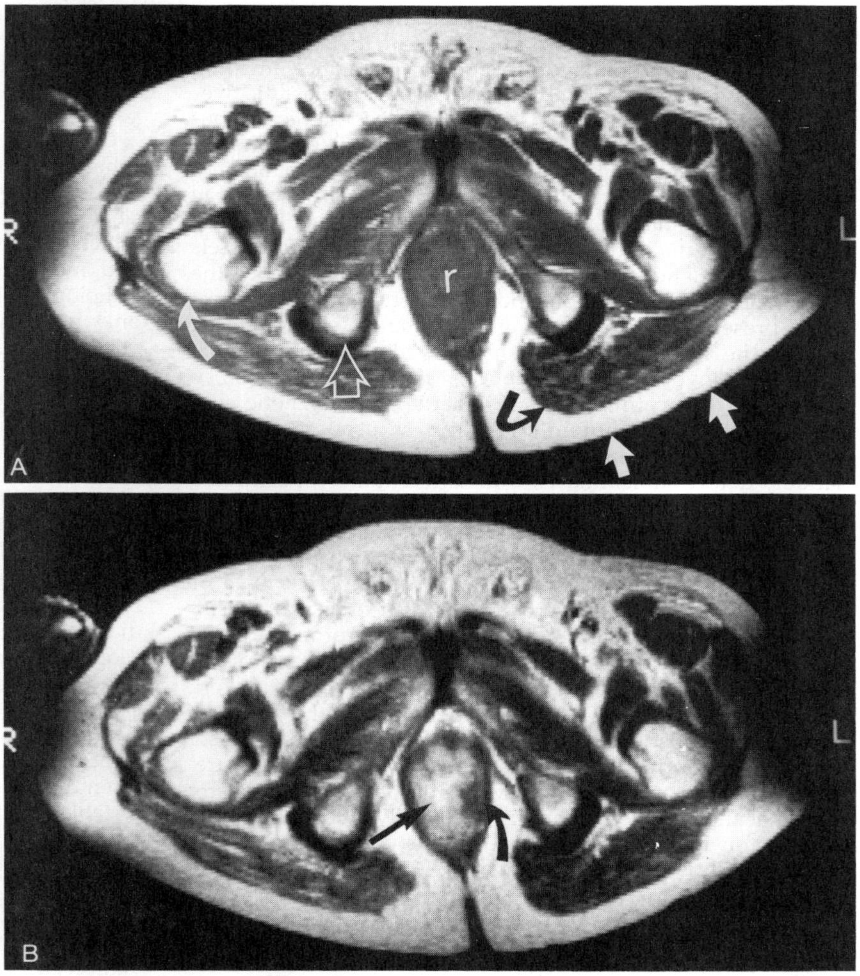

FIGURE 95–12. Magnetic resonance of rectal tumor. *A*, Transverse T1 weighted image (TR = 0.5 sec, TE = 30 msec) demonstrates thickening of the rectum (r) due to cloacogenic carcinoma, which is isointense with the surrounding uninvolved muscle. Normal structures demonstrated include the gluteus muscle (*curved black arrow*), which is emitting a low-intensity signal, subcutaneous fat (*white arrows*), which is emitting a high-intensity signal, the right ischium (*open arrow*) and the right femoral head (*curved white arrow*). *B*, T2 weighted image of the same area demonstrates a relative increase in the signal intensity of the tumor (*straight arrow*) because of prolongation of its T2 relaxation time. It now can be differentiated from the adjacent, noninvolved muscle (*curved arrow*), which has retained a normal low-intensity signal. (Courtesy of Diasonics, San Francisco, CA.)

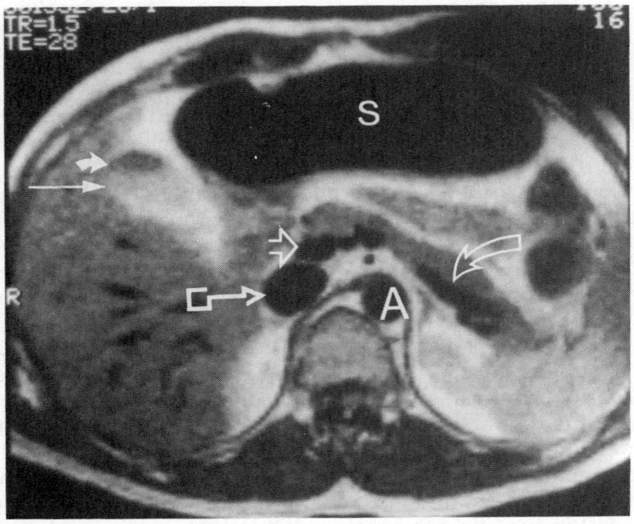

FIGURE 95–13. Magnetic resonance of normal gallbladder. Transverse MR image (TR = 1.5 sec, TE = 628 msec) demonstrates layering of nonconcentrated bile (*closed curved arrow*) (low signal intensity) upon concentrated bile (*straight arrow*) (high signal intensity) within the gallbladder. Note the absence of signal from the air-distended stomach (S) and the patent blood vessels including the splenic vein (*open curved arrow*), portal vein (*open arrow*), aorta (A), and inferior vena cava (*boxed arrow*). (Courtesy of Diasonics, San Francisco, CA.)

the abdomen. With current imaging times of minutes (as opposed to a few seconds for CT), respiration and peristalsis cause blurring and artifact, especially of pancreatic and bowel images. New techniques are being developed to decrease the scan time to seconds. Thereafter, MR imaging may become valuable for the mesenteric alimentary tract. Currently, it images well only the fixed portions, as in the rectum (Fig. 95–12) and distal esophagus. Magnetic resonance imaging may have a greater sensitivity to primary and metastatic liver tumors compared with CT, US, and nuclear medicine; but whether it has greater specificity has not been established. Magnetic resonance can sometimes differentiate hepatic neoplasia from fatty infiltration, either diffuse or focal, with the use of chemical shift imaging, a specifically modified imaging technique. Magnetic resonance can also image blood vessels noninvasively and as such may be useful to evaluate the patency of surgical shunts for portal hypertension. The effect of the presence of a paramagnetic substance, such as ferric iron, on the T1 and T2 relaxation times alters the MR signal intensity of involved tissue. Hence, MR can detect hemosiderosis and hemochromatosis. Similarly, paramagnetic substances such as gadolinium-DTPA can be used as contrast-enhancing agents. Magnetic resonance can image the gallbladder, detect cholelithiasis, and differentiate concentrated from nonconcentrated bile (Fig. 95–13). With further development, it may become the procedure of choice for assessing not only morphology but also function of the gallbladder and for diagnosing acute cholecystitis.

Magnetic resonance spectroscopy (MRS) of tissue specifically localized by imaging techniques is a new procedure that is still in the research stage of development. It has not yet achieved clinical applicability in the abdomen, but early work indicates some promise of diagnostic value in the study of high-energy phosphate metabolism (^{31}P) and in imaging sodium (^{23}Na), fluorine (^{19}F), and carbon (^{13}C). Such a procedure, which would facilitate the in vivo study of the biochemistry of normal and diseased organs, is technically more demanding than proton imaging. Because of great potential clinical impact, research is progressing rapidly.

Bernardino ME, Steinberg HV, Pearson TC, et al.: Shunts for portal hypertension: MR and angiography for determination of patency. Radiology 158:57, 1986. *Demonstrates MRI to be an accurate, noninvasive method of determining shunt patency and presence of collateral vessels.*

Evens RG, Jost RG, Evens RG Jr: Economic and utilization analysis of magnetic resonance imaging units in the United States in 1985. Am J Roentgenol 145:393, 1985. *A study of the utilization, costs, and revenue for users of MRI in 1985.*

Lee JKT, Heiken JP, Dixon WT: Hepatic metastases studied with MR and CT. Radiology 156:423, 1985. *Good discussion of a comparative study with up-to-date references; results suggest MRI indicated for clarification of equivocal or negative CT findings.*

Pykett IL: NMR imaging in medicine. Sci Am 246:78, 1982. *An excellent, understandable review of the physical principles of MRI.*

von Schulthess GK, Higgins CB: Blood flow imaging with MR: Spin-phase phenomena. Radiology 157:687, 1985. *A concise examination and analysis of the current concepts regarding MRI flow imaging.*

ACKNOWLEDGMENT: I wish to express my appreciation to Michael P. Federle, M.D., for helpful review of this manuscript. S.D.W.

96 GASTROINTESTINAL ENDOSCOPY

Jack A. Vennes

Remarkable progress in optical engineering and in fiberoptics during the past two decades has revolutionized the management of many gastrointestinal disorders. Fiberoptic techniques were initially used primarily for diagnosis, but increasingly they have been used for therapy. Excellent optical resolution and tip control permit direct visualization of mucosal abnormalities, with photographic record as desired. End-viewing instruments are adapted to visualize all mucosal surfaces of the esophagus, stomach, and duodenum or, alternatively, the entire colon. An internal channel permits routine aspiration, air insufflation, mucosal biopsy, or cytologic examination. Various therapeutic devices can also be precisely directed. Side-viewing instruments are used for visualizing the ampulla of Vater and for cannulation of the biliary and pancreatic ductal systems for contrast visualization.

Coincident with the development of fiberoptic techniques, other new diagnostic and often therapeutic modalities have also been developed using radiographic, ultrasound, or nuclear scanning. The problem is often to decide, therefore, which of these diagnostic and therapeutic alternatives is best and most cost effective for patients. Proper sequencing of radiologic, ultrasonic, nuclear, and endoscopic techniques is only gradually becoming clear and is often determined by factors of cost, morbidity and locally available skill and experience.

The diagnostic accuracy and therapeutic success of most procedures are dependent on operator skill and experience. Inexperience not infrequently results in increased complications—including the complication of an erroneous diagnosis. Endoscopic training programs are generally available, integrated with the disciplines of gastroenterology or colorectal or general surgery.

Endoscopy is contraindicated if there is severe cardiac or respiratory failure or a probable perforated viscus or if the diagnostic results are unlikely to affect management. Endoscopic procedures should be carefully discussed with patients in advance for reassurance. Procedures done by trained personnel are generally well tolerated after light parenteral sedation and analgesia. Topical pharyngeal anesthesia usually improves acceptance of upper tract endoscopy and indeed is often the only medication required for safe, minimally uncomfortable examinations with modern small-caliber endoscopes.

ESOPHAGOGASTRODUODENOSCOPY

Endoscopic examination of the entire esophagus, stomach, and duodenum (EGD) is accomplished with routine examination to the deep descending duodenum. All mucosal sur-

TABLE 96–1. INDICATIONS FOR ESOPHAGOGASTRODUODENOSCOPY (EGD)

A. Upper abdominal distress that persists despite an appropriate trial of therapy
B. Upper abdominal distress associated with signs suggesting serious organic disease (e.g., anorexia and weight loss)
C. Dysphagia or odynophagia
D. Esophageal reflux symptoms that are persistent or progressive despite appropriate therapy
E. Persistent vomiting of unknown cause
F. Other system disease in which the presence of upper gastrointestinal pathologic conditions might modify other planned management; examples include patients with a history of gastrointestinal bleeding who are scheduled for renal transplantation, long-term anticoagulation, and chronic nonsteroidal therapy for arthritis
G. Radiographic findings of:
   1. A neoplastic lesion, for confirmation and specific histologic diagnosis
   2. Gastric or esophageal ulcer
   3. Evidence of upper tract stricture or obstruction
   4. Mass
H. Gastrointestinal bleeding:
   1. As the first procedure in most actively bleeding patients
   2. When surgical therapy is contemplated
   3. When rebleeding occurs after acute, self-limited blood loss
   4. When portal hypertension or aortoenteric fistula is suspected
   5. For endoscopic therapy of upper gastrointestinal bleeding
   6. For presumed chronic blood loss and iron deficiency anemia when colonoscopy findings are negative

From Appropriate Use of Gastrointestinal Endoscopy. American Society for Gastrointestinal Endoscopy, 1986.

faces are visualized, and photographic records are often made of visually recognized abnormalities. Histologic and cytologic diagnosis can be made as indicated.

COMPLICATIONS. Complications from EGD are rare with modern small-caliber, flexible instruments but do occur. A morbidity of 0.13 per cent and a mortality of 0.0004 per cent have been reported. During or following endoscopic examination, perforation has occurred in the upper esophagus near the cricopharyngeus, through Zenker's diverticula, and through areas of tumor. Use of sedative or analgesic drugs may transiently suppress respiration, especially in elderly patients or those with severe obstructive pulmonary disease. Aspiration during endoscopy is very unlikely unless there is vomiting due to massive bleeding or gastric outlet obstruction. Cardiovascular complications, sepsis, prolonged bleeding, or thrombophlebitis from intravenous medications occur rarely.

INDICATIONS. Indications for diagnostic EGD are listed in Table 96–1. Esophagogastroduodenoscopy is most often indicated in the evaluation or discovery of possible acid-peptic disease, malignancy, or gastrointestinal bleeding. Endoscopy used "just in case" disease is found leads to overutilization, but blind management of a presumed disease without diagnostic confirmation often turns out to be underutilization. Both extremes are frequently cost *in*effective. Therapeutic use of endoscopic techniques will be briefly discussed with each procedure in this chapter.

Patients frequently seek medical help for upper abdominal discomfort and associated dyspeptic symptoms of relatively recent onset. If other findings indicative of serious disease are absent, a trial of therapy may be indicated as a first diagnostic test. Much less than 1 per cent of such patients have a malignancy as the cause of their dyspepsia. Most will respond to a trial of therapy directed toward their presumed acid-peptic problem. Esophagogastroduodenoscopy is therefore indicated for the perhaps 30 per cent of patients with dyspeptic symptoms that continue despite therapy for 14 days.

Irritable bowel syndrome does not usually require endoscopy, but there are occasional exceptions. Other problems that usually do not require endoscopy include intermittent dyspepsia, heartburn responding to medical therapy, and asymptomatic or uncomplicated hiatus hernia. Uncomplicated duodenal bulb ulcer seen on radiograph that responds to therapy does not usually require endoscopy unless symptoms recur quickly.

Acid-Peptic Disease

Acid-peptic disease, i.e., reflux esophagitis, gastric ulcer, duodenal ulcer, and duodenitis, can be strongly suspected on the basis of the history, but one cannot confidently predict the specific site or pathologic condition. Symptoms of reflux esophagitis are quite specific, but other gastroduodenal lesions frequently coexist (Ch. 98). The presence of esophageal reflux symptoms correlates well with the presence of endoscopic findings and less well with histologic findings. Local symptoms in the mid or lower esophagus are usually predictive of disease location, whereas high substernal symptoms may be due to disease anywhere in the esophagus. Gastric or duodenal ulcers are usually symptomatic, but in patients with previous gastric or duodenal ulcer, asymptomatic recurrences are discovered in 5 per cent or more of patients who have had endoscopy in long-term studies.

Esophagogastroduodenoscopy is more sensitive and specific than radiographic studies of the upper gastrointestinal tract, although neither is infallible. Radiographic studies are least sensitive in evaluating lesions without apparent depth, such as flat stomal postgastrectomy ulcers, giant duodenal ulcers involving an entire wall of the duodenal bulb, or erosive esophagitis.

Cancer

Malignant lesions of the upper gastrointestinal tract are generally evident as exophytic masses protruding into the lumen (Ch. 101). Flat, infiltrative lesions do occur occasionally, however. In the esophagus, such lesions may resemble a benign stricture, and in the stomach (linitis plastica), the primary features are stiffness and poor distensibility. Malignancy may occasionally present as ulceration, accurate evaluation of all esophageal and gastric ulcers is therefore mandatory and challenging. At least 75 per cent of malignant ulcers are correctly identified, by endoscopic visual criteria, as asymmetric folds or nodules that randomly form the crater rim and extend irregularly into surrounding mucosa. Malignant tissue is often seen as multihued. Benign ulcers are typically smoother with more crater depth and with more symmetry and less randomness, and a zone of erythema is present at the junction of the crater and rim.

Histologic and cytologic data should be added to the evaluation of all suspicious lesions and most gastric ulcers. This results in a sensitivity (positive when disease is present) and specificity (negative when disease is absent) of 95 per cent. Brush or lavage cytology is a particularly important adjunct in evaluating the smooth, infiltrative esophageal stricture or the linitis plastica gastric lesion or the occasional superficial, spreading, flat gastric cancer. Primary gastric lymphoma may present as an ulcer, ulcerated mass, or large, asymmetric folds. Specific histologic features are frequently present only in submucosal tissue.

Mucosal polyps are rare in the stomach and rarer still in the duodenum and esophagus. Submucosal or intramucosal polypoid defects overlain with normal mucosa are usually pancreatic rests or leiomyomas and can be left in place. Adenomatous polyps have premalignant potential, which increases with size. All polypoid lesions should be endoscopically visualized, with biopsy or removal with snare cautery. Multiple small, hyperplastic polyps are not premalignant and need not all be removed, and no surveillance is indicated. Adenomas should be excised endoscopically when feasible. Very large lesions may require surgical removal. Surveillance is indicated after removal of gastric adenomatous polyps.

Other upper gastrointestinal malignancies originating in the pancreas or biliary tree do not usually extend into gastric or duodenal mucosa, and they require other diagnostic studies (see below). Ampullary carcinoma is usually visible *if* the papilla of Vater is adequately seen via a conventional end-viewing endoscope or a side-viewing instrument (see below).

Upper Gastrointestinal Bleeding (see Ch. 114)

Esophagogastroduodenoscopy is the most informative procedure when further information is indicated for management of the acutely bleeding patient, particularly if it is done within 12 hours of admission. Information obtained includes (1) location and identity of the bleeding source; (2) whether bleeding is continuing; (3) whether bleeding is arterial; (4) which of multiple lesions is bleeding; and (5) whether a visible vessel is present in an ulcer base. These endoscopic observations are available in 85 per cent of patients with acute bleeding and influence prognosis and management decisions. There is no evidence that endoscopy initiates further bleeding. A precise diagnosis of the source of gastrointestinal bleeding would seem to be the logical basis for an improved outcome; however, controlled clinical studies have not shown this to be true. Endoscopic methods for controlling active bleeding are proving effective in current controlled trials. When indications for these techniques become clearer, more early endoscopy of acute bleeding will likely be indicated.

The source of chronic gastrointestinal blood loss or iron deficiency anemia in men is usually discovered in the colon. Esophagogastroduodenoscopy may be indicated by history suggesting upper tract sources or after negative findings on colonoscopy.

Therapeutic Applications of Esophagogastroduodenoscopy

Therapeutic endoscopic procedures commonly carried out in the upper gastrointestinal tract include removal of foreign bodies, dilation of benign or malignant esophageal strictures, sclerotherapy of bleeding esophageal varices, and electrocoagulation of focal bleeding lesions. Foreign bodies in the esophagus or stomach can usually be removed by techniques that employ snares, forceps, and protective overtubes to prevent soft tissue injury or aspiration. Impaction of food may occur because of an underlying esophageal abnormality, and careful esophagoscopy after removal of food may reveal a benign or malignant stricture or may suggest a motility disorder.

Esophageal strictures found to be benign on careful evaluation can be successfully dilated. If the course of the esophagus is tortuous, if the stricture is tight and does not admit the endoscope, or if epiphrenic diverticula are present, dilation is safely done over a guide wire passed under fluoroscopic control. Tapered bougies, metal olives, or inflatable balloons of progressively increasing diameter may be passed over the wire. Following this, endoscopy and biopsy are done to assess whether there is a malignant lesion. Less complex strictures that only partially occlude the lumen may, after endoscopy, be safely dilated with tapered bougies without wire guidance and without further endoscopy. A maintenance dilation schedule with individualized intervals and techniques is important.

Management of malignant esophageal strictures is directed to the goal of allowing the patient to swallow food, liquids, and oral secretions. The options available include surgery, radiation therapy, or such endoscopic procedures as repeated esophageal dilation, dilation and endoscopic placement of a stent across the malignant narrowing (or across a tracheoesophageal fistula), or use of laser energy to restore the lumen by tumor destruction. All of these latter procedures have quite good reported results; all require skill for success and safety; and all can be done without prolonged hospitalization. Local skills are often valid determinants. Quality survival time is usually brief, but 85 to 90 per cent of patients can be helped.

Several endoscopic measures have proved effective in controlling upper gastrointestinal bleeding. Endoscopic variceal sclerosis by intravariceal and perivariceal injection of various sclerosants controls the acute variceal hemorrhage of portal hypertension in 90 per cent of patients. Prophylactic sclerosis may also prevent future hemorrhage. The effect of either acute or prophylactic sclerotherapy on long-term survival is currently undergoing prospective controlled testing.

Focal nonvariceal bleeding can often be controlled using electrocoagulation with monopolar or bipolar current delivery or combined electrocoagulation and thermal heater probe techniques or laser photocoagulation. Argon or neodymium yttrium aluminum garnet (YAG) laser energy is carried through the endoscope via a flexible wave guide and converted to thermal energy when precisely directed to an absorptive (bleeding) area. Bleeding is controlled in up to 90 per cent of lesions, including those with brisk arterial bleeding, but rebleeding rates are significant with all methods. Laser equipment is expensive and not portable. Perforation, though of low risk, is a definite hazard with all techniques. Eighty-five per cent or more of upper gastrointestinal bleeding stops spontaneously; how then shall we select those patients who need endoscopic control of bleeding? A visible vessel in the ulcer base, a fresh adherent clot, or continuing active bleeding are all observable risk factors for further bleeding (and risk of death) and are indications for endoscopic therapy, most frequently with electrocoagulation or heater probe techniques. Surgical management will continue to be required for some whose bleeding is excessive.

Percutaneous endoscopic gastrostomy (PEG) is a useful method for providing selected patients with long-term enteral feeding. Candidates are those with a functioning gut and chronically inadequate oral intake. Some may have recurrent aspiration secondary to upper esophageal dysfunction. Specific indications include neurologic disorders that affect the swallowing mechanism or that result in diminished food intake secondary to a decreased sensorium or cancer of the pharynx or upper esophagus that does not totally obstruct (so that an endoscope can be passed). Percutaneous endoscopic gastrostomy is not indicated in postgastrectomy patients or in those with midline abdominal scar, severe, uncorrectable coagulopathy, or respirator dependency. The decision to initiate chronic enteral feeding can be a difficult one, involving the wishes of patient and family and the gravity of the underlying disease. Once the decision is made, however, PEG is a simple and safe method.

COLONOSCOPY AND FLEXIBLE SIGMOIDOSCOPY

The entire colon is now routinely accessible to high-resolution viewing with biopsy, brush cytology, polypectomy, and photography of observed lesions. Much has been learned of the polyp-cancer progression, and significant control of colon cancer is within cost-effective reach of the trained endoscopist.

COMPLICATIONS. Diagnostic colonoscopy has a complication rate of 0.5 per cent, which rises to 1 per cent when polypectomy is added, with hemorrhage and perforation being the principal complications.

INDICATIONS. The indications for colonoscopy are listed in Table 96–2. As with EGD, colonoscopic examination is primarily used to evaluate possible cancer, inflammation, and bleeding. The procedure is contraindicated in the presence of fulminant colitis; acute, severe diverticulitis; or probable perforated viscus. Colonoscopy is generally not indicated for stable irritable bowel syndrome, acute diarrhea, upper gastrointestinal bleeding, or rectal bleeding with an anorectal source on anoscopy or sigmoidoscopy. Other nonindications include routine follow-up of inflammatory bowel disease (except as noted in Table 96–2) and routine preoperative examination of patients undergoing elective abdominal surgery for noncolonic disease.

Flexible sigmoidoscopy (FFS) is usually carried out with 60-cm instrumentation, although a 35-cm endoscope is available. Training requirements are less rigorous than those for colonoscopy. Indications for flexible sigmoidoscopy are listed in Table 96–3. At least 60 per cent of colon cancers and potential

TABLE 96–2. INDICATIONS FOR COLONOSCOPY

A. Evaluation of an abnormality on barium enema that is likely to be clinically significant, such as a filling defect or stricture
B. For discovery and excision of colonic polyps:
   1. When polyps are seen on barium enema radiograph
   2. When neoplastic polyps are detected by proctosigmoidoscopy
C. Evaluation of unexplained gastrointestinal bleeding:
   1. Clinically significant hematochezia
   2. Melena with a negative upper gastrointestinal workup
   3. Presence of unexplained fecal occult blood
D. Unexplained iron deficiency anemia
E. Surveillance for colonic neoplasia
   1. Examination to "clear" entire colon of synchronous cancer or neoplastic polyps in a patient with a treatable cancer or neoplastic polyp
   2. Follow-up examination at two- to three-year intervals after resection of a colorectal cancer or neoplastic polyp and an adequate initial "clearing" colonoscopy
   3. Patients with a strongly positive family history of colonic cancer
   4. In patients with chronic ulcerative colitis: colonoscopy every one to two years with multiple biopsies for detection of cancer and dysplasia in patients with:
      a. Pancolitis of greater than seven years duration
      b. Left-sided colitis of over 15 years duration (no surveillance needed for disease limited to rectosigmoid)
F. Chronic inflammatory bowel disease of the colon if more precise diagnosis or determination of the extent of activity of disease will influence immediate management
G. Therapeutic colonoscopy, as control of bleeding or colonic decompression

From Appropriate Use of Gastrointestinal Endoscopy. American Society for Gastrointestinal Endoscopy, 1986.

colon cancers (neoplastic polyps) are located in the rectosigmoid and lower descending colon and thus are in reach of the "screening" FFS. Flexible sigmoidoscopy has the same contraindications as colonoscopy and is generally not indicated when colonoscopy is indicated (see Table 96–3). Flexible sigmoidoscopy is specifically not indicated for polypectomy because colonoscopy is needed, and full colonic preparation is necessary to prevent possible explosions during electrocautery. Preparation for FFS is simple, using two enemas, whereas preparation for colonoscopy requires a two-day liquid diet preparation or total gut lavage with large volumes of an isotonic solution. The place for FFS is assured as a more comfortable, more productive replacement for rigid proctosigmoidoscopy at nearly equivalent cost.

Polyps and Cancer of the Colon (see Ch. 107)

Colonoscopy to evaluate the possibility of colon cancer or its precursor polyps is usually indicated after an abnormality is detected by barium enema or proctosigmoidoscopy or if there is unexplained lower gastrointestinal bleeding. If occult blood is detected in the interior of a passed stool, colonoscopy will identify an age-related 20 to 30 per cent incidence of adenomatous polyps and 8 to 15 per cent incidence of cancers. During active bleeding, colonoscopy may encounter technical difficulties in accurately locating the bleeding source. Repeat colonoscopy may be necessary after cessation of bleeding for accurate colonic assessment.

After endoscopic removal of neoplastic polyps or after resection of colon cancer, continued surveillance is indicated, since the patient is now identified as being at risk for later colon cancer. A "clearing" examination may be optionally done within 12 months to be certain no polyps or cancers were missed at the first examination. Thereafter, follow-up examination every three years will detect new lesions before they become infiltrating carcinomas, since the process from polyp inception to infiltrating cancer appears to take up to seven years. The only way to rule out cancer within a polyp is to remove it completely for histologic examination. Other conditions associated with increased risk for cancer also require surveillance (Table 96–2).

TABLE 96–3. INDICATIONS FOR FLEXIBLE FIBEROPTIC SIGMOIDOSCOPY (FFS)

A. Screening of asymptomatic patients at risk for colonic neoplasia
B. Evaluation of suspected distal colonic disease when there is no indication for colonoscopy
C. Evaluation of the entire colon in conjunction with barium enema radiographs

From Appropriate Use of Gastrointestinal Endoscopy. American Society for Gastrointestinal Endoscopy, 1986.

Most colonic polyps are hyperplastic and are not premalignant. In neoplastic polyps, cancer risk increases with increasing dysplasia and villoglandular transformation and also with size. Pedunculated polyps with an uninvolved stalk and with cancer confined to the mucosa can be cured by snare cautery removal. Most colonoscopists remove all polyps greater than 5 mm in diameter. Polyps less than 5 mm may be neoplastic; coagulation or a coagulation biopsy technique during colonoscopy is used to remove them.

Inflammatory Bowel Disease (see Ch. 105)

Most patients with inflammatory bowel disease do not require colonoscopy for diagnosis. At times, however, colonoscopy may provide unique and important information. Differentiation between granulomatous colitis (Crohn's disease) and ulcerative colitis is usually possible with colonoscopy and multiple biopsies. The anatomic extent of disease can be determined. The presence or absence of inflammatory bowel disease can be determined more accurately when clinically suspected despite absence of radiographic or sigmoidoscopic findings.

Diagnostic colonoscopy in ulcerative colitis is at times necessary to evaluate a stricture or a mass seen on barium enema. Occasionally, strictures are malignant with submucosal tumor spread. Pseudopolyps are not premalignant and need not be histologically examined. Polyps may be neoplastic or malignant, however, and those that are larger than 1 cm in diameter and are friable and irregular in color or configuration should be biopsied. In surveillance examinations of patients with ulcerative colitis, multiple biopsies are obtained throughout the involved colon. When moderate-to-severe dysplasia is consistently found, colectomy is usually recommended.

Polypectomy is the main therapeutic use of colonoscopy. Endoscopic control of bleeding is not usually feasible. Electrocautery of angiodysplastic lesions in the cecum and ascending colon has been successful, but new lesions may appear within months. Dilation of anastomotic strictures by balloons passed over a guide wire or through the endoscope is occasionally useful.

ENDOSCOPIC RETROGRADE CHOLANGIOPANCREATOGRAPHY (ERCP)

The side-viewing endoscope and the technique for identifying and cannulating the ampulla of Vater allow for radiographic study of both the common bile duct and the pancreatic duct in 80 to 90 per cent of attempts (Figs. 96–1 and 96–2). Failure may result from anatomic distortions due to prior surgery, tumor infiltration, or the duodenal edema of acute pancreatitis.

COMPLICATIONS. In 1 per cent of patients, acute pancreatitis follows ERCP, usually beginning within two hours of the procedure as a clinically mild complication. Biliary sepsis occurs less commonly but is more serious and even life threatening. Introduction of even a few bacteria into a semiclosed space—bile duct, gallbladder, pancreatic pseudocyst—may occasionally have serious septic consequences. Organisms may be introduced from the unsterile gastrointestinal tract or from instruments. Stringent cleaning and disinfection techniques are mandatory, including periodic cultures of equipment. Sepsis is prevented by prompt surgical, endoscopic, or transhepatic decompression within 24 hours of ERCP, plus judicious use of appropriate parenteral antibiotics.

INDICATIONS. Indications for ERCP are listed in Table 96–4. Endoscopic retrograde cholangiopancreatography is generally not helpful in evaluating abdominal pain of obscure origin in the absence of objective findings suggesting pan-

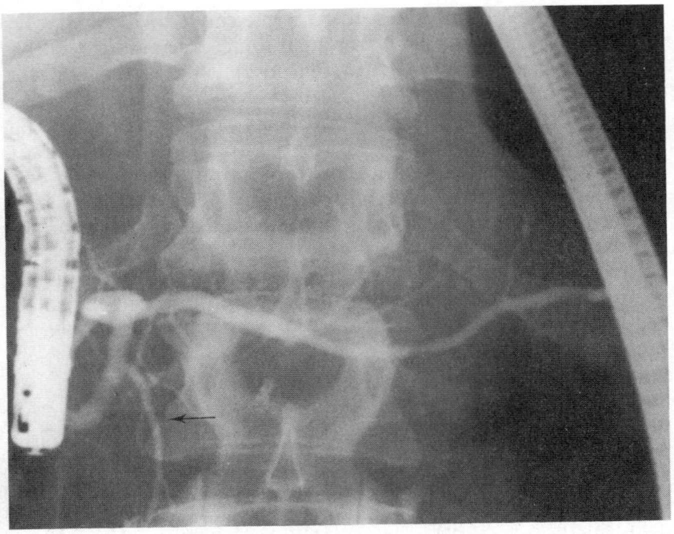

FIGURE 96–1. Normal pancreatogram, endoscopic retrograde cholangiopancreatography. The main pancreatic duct tapers normally from the tail near the hilum of the spleen to the papillary orifice (obscured by the tip of the endoscope). Lateral branches, partially filled with contrast, are of fine caliber and straight, draining the main gland and the uncinate process (*arrow*).

creatic or biliary disease. Known or suspected gallbladder disease is not an indication for ERCP in the absence of evidence for bile duct involvement. Study of patients with acute pancreatitis is usually deferred until a second episode has established its recurrent nature, unless there is evidence to suggest gallstone disease. Pancreatic malignancy clearly demonstrated on CT or ultrasound need not be further evaluated with ERCP except for stent placement.

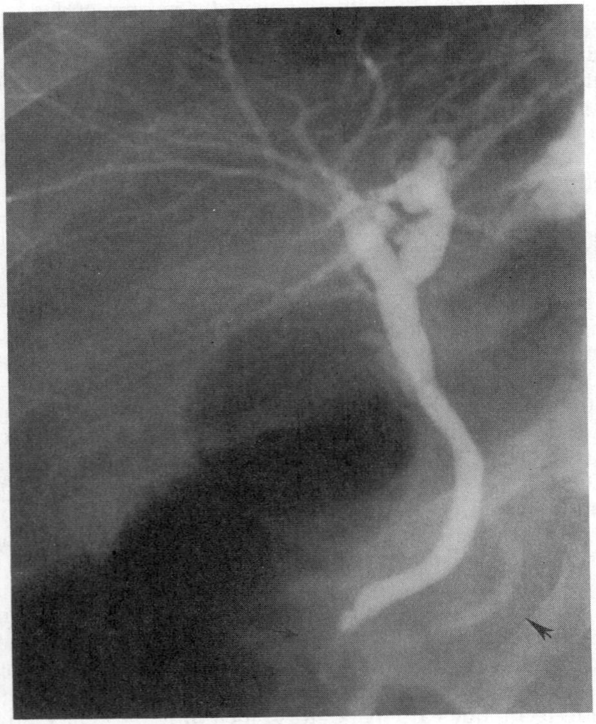

FIGURE 96–2. Normal cholangiogram. The normal-caliber, smoothly tapering intrahepatic ducts are well outlined with contrast, draining into right and left hepatic ducts. The cystic duct stump, remnant of previous cholecystectomy, divides the common hepatic duct above from the common bile duct below as they course medially around the black air-filled duodenum. The intramural duct is faintly visible (*small arrow*), terminating at the papilla. The main pancreatic duct is faintly visible medially (*large arrow*).

TABLE 96–4. INDICATIONS FOR ENDOSCOPIC RETROGRADE CHOLANGIOPANCREATOGRAPHY (ERCP)

A. Evaluation of the jaundiced patient suspected of having treatable biliary obstruction
B. Evaluation of the patient without jaundice (with or without prior cholecystectomy) whose clinical presentation suggests bile duct disease
C. Therapeutic pancreatic or biliary endoscopy, e.g., endoscopic sphincterotomy, balloon dilatation of strictures, stent placement across strictures; these procedures frequently require follow-up endoscopy
D. Evaluation of signs or symptoms suggesting pancreatic malignancy when results of ultrasound (US) and/or computed tomography (CT) are equivocal or normal
E. Evaluation of recurrent or persistent pancreatitis of unknown etiology
F. Preoperative evaluation of the patient with chronic pancreatitis
G. Evaluation of possible pancreatic pseudocyst undetected by CT or US and for known pseudocyst prior to planned surgical therapy

From Appropriate Use of Gastrointestinal Endoscopy. American Society for Gastrointestinal Endoscopy, 1986.

Other tests besides ERCP provide diagnostic evidence of pancreatic and biliary disease: percutaneous transhepatic cholangiography (PTC), computed tomography (CT), and ultrasound (US). Transabdominal fine-needle aspiration cytology with CT, US, or ERCP guidance is also helpful, as malignant cells are found by this means in 85 per cent of patients with pancreatic cancer.

In evaluating suspected biliary obstruction, a cholangiogram is usually obtained prior to therapy (Fig. 96–3). When the patient has fever, pain, and icterus, choledocholithiasis is suspected with high clinical accuracy. One may then proceed directly to cholangiography by PTC or preferably by ERCP if endoscopic sphincterotomy is planned. Ultrasound is usually obtained to assess ductal dilatation, but this is of limited value, as calculi often reside in undilated ducts.

When the presence of extrahepatic obstruction and its etiology are less certain, US as the initial study provides useful information at reasonable cost. For example, a normal gallbladder without calculi makes choledocholithiasis unlikely. Masses in the pancreas, bile duct, or porta hepatis, diffuse pancreatic enlargement, or grossly dilated bile ducts direct an appropriate specific disease evaluation.

Ultrasound and CT have improved greatly in their ability to detect pancreatic malignancy (Ch. 109). Equivocal results at times require confirmation by ERCP. Cut-off or stenosis of pancreatic duct and often of bile duct (double duct sign) is a

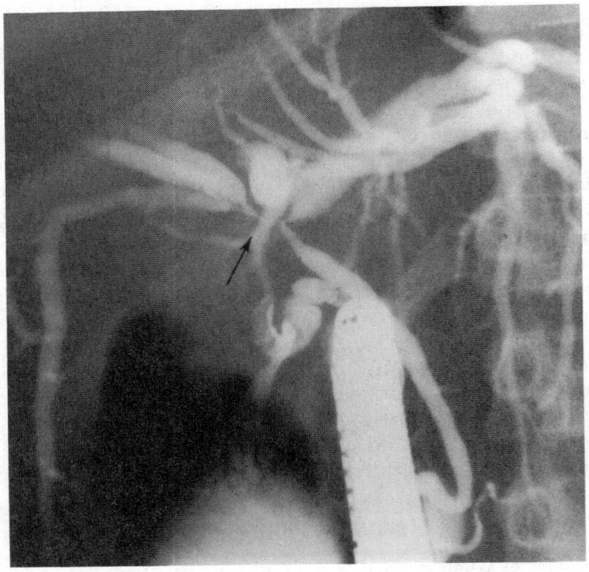

FIGURE 96–3. Retrograde cholangiogram: bile duct cancer. Multiple strictures at the bifurcation of the common hepatic duct (*arrow*) are due to a primary bile duct cancer (Klatskin tumor). Intrahepatic ducts are dilated and partially obstructed. The extrahepatic ductal system distal to the tumor is of normal caliber, here seen coursing medial to the endoscope.

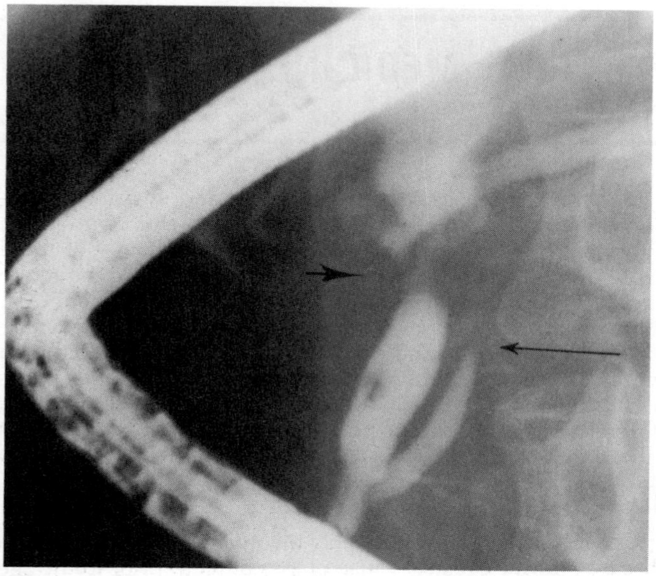

FIGURE 96–4. Pancreatogram and cholangiogram: pancreatic cancer. Both ducts are outlined by retrograde instillation of contrast at the bottom of the picture. Both the common bile duct (*large arrow*) and the pancreatic duct (*small arrow*) are strictured in the classic "double duct sign" of pancreatic cancer.

reliable ERCP finding suggestive of carcinoma (Fig. 96–4). Patients with chronic pain and suspected chronic pancreatitis who are surgical candidates should have preoperative pancreatography and cholangiography to assess patency of the main pancreatic duct and to assess possible stricture of the intrapancreatic bile duct. Differentiating chronic pancreatitis from pancreatic cancer may be difficult, as the pancreatic duct is often dilated and tortuous with dilated, stubby lateral branches (Fig. 96–5). Downstream stricturing in the pancreatic head is the hallmark of malignancy, however.

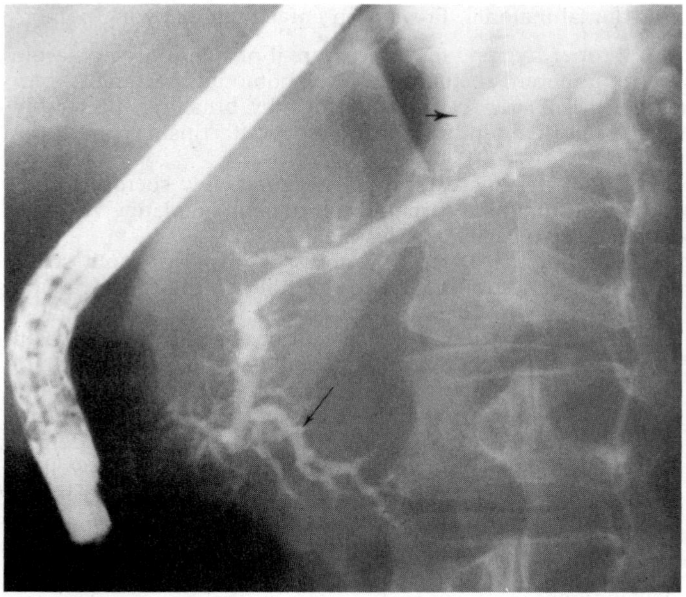

FIGURE 96–5. Pancreatogram: chronic pancreatitis. The main pancreatic duct is moderately dilated and unobstructed. The lateral branches are dilated, tortuous, and stubby. The duct from the uncinate process is prominent (*small arrow*). A small pseudocyst (*large arrow*) is barely visible overlying the spine in this oblique view. Filling defects in the main pancreatic duct may be calculi or air bubble artifact. With progression of the disease the main pancreatic duct may become more tortuous and dilated.

Therapeutic Applications of Endoscopic Retrograde Cholangiopancreatography

By endoscopic retrograde sphincterotomy (ERS), soft tissues and sphincter fibers of the papilla and intraduodenal portion of the common bile duct are divided with electrocautery to relieve ductal obstruction due to common duct stones or papillary stenosis. Endoscopic retrograde sphincterotomy has assumed a major role in the management of choledocholithiasis and offers a relatively safe and simple alternative to surgical management.

Biliary obstruction is relieved by ERS in 85 to 90 per cent of attempts. Complications of hemorrhage, pancreatitis, perforation, and cholangitis occur in 3 to 8 per cent of cases with a mortality rate of 0.4 per cent. Late complications of restenosis or re-formed stones occur in 1 to 8 per cent of patients.

Endoscopic retrograde sphincterotomy is now widely considered the therapy of choice for patients with symptomatic stones in the common bile duct. The procedure is often carried out immediately following ERCP as soon as the presence of stones in the duct is confirmed. It is clearly safer and cheaper than surgery in these generally elderly patients and more successful than percutaneous transhepatic extraction. Cholangitis and gallstone pancreatitis usually respond dramatically to decompression. About 40 per cent of patients with symptomatic choledocholithiasis have never had cholecystitis, and therefore their gallbladders are intact. Almost all contain calculi. After removing duct calculi with ERS, should the gallbladder be electively removed to preclude further cholecystitis or migration of stones into the now open biliary tree? Or may the gallbladder be left in place and removed only as future symptoms dictate? Experience with patients at high surgical risk suggests the safety and success of waiting, as the probability of cholecystitis does not exceed 5 to 10 per cent per year in these generally elderly patients.

Papillary stenosis is a poorly defined disorder or group of disorders in which recurrent biliary colic or occasionally pancreatitis are thought to result from fibrosis or sphincter dysfunction. Diagnostic criteria include a dilated bile duct, slow ductal drainage, cholestasis following painful episodes, and elevated basal sphincter of Oddi pressure during manometry. The problem arises most commonly in women who have had a cholecystectomy either for cholelithiasis or for biliary colic–like pain without stones. Endoscopic retrograde sphincterotomy is often curative for carefully selected patients with papillary stenosis.

Placement of plastic stents across biliary strictures is the second major therapeutic extension of ERCP. Most strictures are caused by inoperable pancreatic or bile duct carcinoma, and other treatment options are surgical or transhepatic decompression. A catheter containing a guide wire is introduced through the stricture, and a stent is passed over the catheter. The proximal end is left in the duodenum, bile drainage is restored, and barbed flaps prevent dislodgment of the stent. The procedure is successful in 90 per cent of attempts. Present-day stents remain patent for five months or more and can be rather easily replaced.

LAPAROSCOPY

Laparoscopy permits direct inspection of much of the anterior abdominal space. A pneumoperitoneum is created and a (usually) rigid or flexible laparoscope is introduced through a puncture in the abdominal wall, with the patient under local anesthesia and mild sedation. The procedure is well tolerated; complications of bleeding or bowel perforation occur in only 0.1 to 0.2 per cent. When it is clinically important to assess focal or diffuse liver disease, laparoscopy, by combining assessment of gross appearance and guided biopsy, is 90 per cent accurate, substantially better than percutaneous blind liver biopsy. This is true whether the disease is diffuse (cirrhosis) or focal (metastatic nodules). More than two thirds of the liver and variable parts of the gallbladder, spleen, peritoneum, and diaphragm can usually be visualized. The colon and small bowel are variably open to inspection.

The major indications for laparoscopy are (1) inspection and guided biopsy of the liver in suspected diffuse or focal disease, when the information will affect therapy and (2) evaluation of exudative ascites (malignancy versus inflammation). Determination of the presence or absence of abdominal metastases may be important in assessing operability. The procedure is contraindicated in the presence of acute peritonitis, intestinal obstruction, severe coagulopathy, infection of the abdominal wall, or severe ascites in patients with portal hypertension.

FUTURE OF ENDOSCOPY

Endoscopic instrumentation is approaching optimal size and optical resolution, in both conventional and emerging electronic video endoscopy equipment. The number of skilled endoscopists has increased so that precise diagnostic studies are generally available to most patients.

Fiberoptics are contributing enormously to management of gastrointestinal disease and will continue to do so. A clearer understanding of the colonic polyp-cancer progression will likely be available in the next few years. Colonoscopic polypectomy will play a key role in altering the course of this major malignancy. It is likely that nearly all cases of common duct stones will be treated endoscopically, until such time as extracorporeal lithotripsy for bile stones becomes generally available and successful. Measures for successful control of gastrointestinal bleeding are greatly improving. Their influence on mortality should soon become clear.

Optimal management of patients with benign or malignant biliary obstruction is not clearly dependent on a single technique. Endoscopists, radiologists, and surgeons working together will likely evolve an integrated approach with indications for each of several options.

Cello JP, Grendell JH, Crass RA, et al.: Endoscopic sclerotherapy versus portacaval shunt in patients with severe cirrhosis and variceal hemorrhage. N Engl J Med 311:1589, 1984. *The effect of sclerotherapy on short- and long-term outcome is not clear at present.*

Decker W, Tytgat GN: Diagnostic accuracy of fiberendoscopy in detection of upper intestinal malignancy: A follow-up analysis. Gastroenterology 73:710, 1977. *Review of fiberendoscopic studies in 1005 patients revealed an overall correct endoscopic interpretation in 92.7 per cent of 135 patients with gastric malignancy. Diagnosis was correct in 98.8 per cent, owing largely to the number of biopsies (GTR >10) in gastric ulcer patients.*

Dolley CP, Larson AW, Nigel HS, et al.: Double contrast barium meal and upper gastrointestinal endoscopy. Ann Intern Med 101:538, 1984. *In the best controlled study to date comparing endoscopy and barium meal radiographs, endoscopy was more sensitive (92 per cent versus 54 per cent) and specific (100 per cent versus 92 per cent).*

Ferrucci JT, Mueller PR: Interventional radiology of the biliary tract. Gastroenterology 82:974, 1982. *Relief of biliary obstruction is best handled with a team approach involving interventional radiologist, endoscopist, surgeon, and ultrasonographer. Radiologic techniques are discussed.*

Gilbert DA, Silverstein FE, Tedesco FJ, et al.: The national ASGE survey on upper gastrointestinal bleeding. Gastrointest Endosc 27:94, 1981. *A comprehensive, valuable review of collated experience with 2225 patients.*

Kahn K, Greenfield S: Endoscopy in the evaluation of dyspepsia. Ann Intern Med 102:266, 1985. *A clear and important statement of the Clinical Efficacy Assessment Project of the American College of Physicians concerning the diagnostic use of a trial of therapy.*

Proceedings of the NIH Consensus Workshop on Upper Gastrointestinal Bleeding. Dig Dis Sci (suppl):1, 1981. *Papers on the value of endoscopy in upper gastrointestinal bleeding that were used as background for the consensus workshop outlining the role of endoscopy in this condition.*

Scharschmidt BF, Goldberg H, Schmid R: Approach to the patient with cholestatic jaundice. N Engl J Med 308:1515, 1983. *A reasoned approach to this problem, which currently has several contending "solutions."*

Utilization Committee: Appropriate Use of Gastrointestinal Endoscopy. Manchester, MA, American Society for Gastrointestinal Endoscopy, 1986. *The source of the tables used in this chapter and a clear consensus statement on the current status of gastrointestinal endoscopy.*

Vennes JA: Management of calculi in the common duct. Semin Liver Dis 3:162, 1983. *Discussion of present-day evaluation of choledocholithiasis and management with endoscopic sphincterotomy.*

97 ORAL MEDICINE

Sol Silverman, Jr.

Many oral diseases representing local and systemic conditions must be recognized by the physician for appropriate treatment or referral. Signs and symptoms of many of these diseases, as well as effective management, can be quite variable. Fortunately, most oral diseases are benign and noncontagious. Many of the conditions are progressive, making correct diagnosis and early treatment important factors in minimizing morbidity. Precancerous lesions and malignancies occur frequently enough to be of constant concern in the differential diagnosis. Some of the most common and clinically important oral diseases will be reviewed briefly in this chapter.

DENTAL CARIES

Caries (tooth decay) is possibly the most widespread human disease and the greatest cause of loss of teeth prior to the age of 35.

ETIOLOGY. Bacteria, substrate, and a susceptible tooth are required for the carious lesion. Although a variety of microorganisms can be responsible for dental decay, the most important appear to be certain streptococcal strains. Substrate for bacterial growth is a critical factor, primarily carbohydrates in the form of sucrose have been shown to be most harmful in promoting dental plaque, bacterial growth, and the carious lesion. Most natural teeth are susceptible to decay unless preventive measures are instituted.

SIGNS AND SYMPTOMS. Early decay can be detected by careful clinical examination and x-ray evaluation. When the lesion becomes moderately advanced, missing tooth structure, surface softness, discoloration, and sensitivity become apparent.

MANAGEMENT. Treatment requires removal of the carious material by instrumentation and replacement by a suitable dental material. Prevention entails the following points.

1. Proper hygiene to reduce dental plaque (polysaccharide matrix adherent to tooth surface promoting bacterial proliferation). This can be accomplished by brushing, preferably with a fluoride dentifrice, vigorous mouth rinsing, and flossing.
2. Diet (reducing carbohydrates, preferably sucrose-source foods) to minimize a major component of plaque and the most effective bacterial substrate.
3. Fluoride, to produce a more acid-resistant tooth structure, to enhance tooth remineralization, and to interfere with bacterial growth. A fluoride supplement of approximately 1 mg daily during tooth development has been shown to be an effective means of reducing dental decay. The amount of fluoride depends upon that occurring in the communal water supply and the amount of water consumed daily. Daily fluoride mouth rinses and topical applications by the dentist also are very effective supplements for children, as well as for adults who continue to have caries problems. This is particularly true in adults with reduced saliva (e.g., as occurs with Sjögren's syndrome, irradiation effects, drug-induced xerostomia). Fluoride ingestion does not increase the risk for development of cancer.

Newbrun E: Sugar and dental caries: A review of human studies. Science 217:418, 1982. *Studies reviewed indicate that frequent or high intake of sugary foods predisposes to dental decay.*

DENTAL ABSCESS

If the carious process (bacterial infection with tooth decalcification) progresses to the dental pulp, pulpitis (inflammation of the dental pulp) ensues. Spontaneous sensitivity and reactions to temperature changes are often the first signs. The pulpitis may be reversible if the carious process is removed; however, if it continues, abscess formation takes place. The abscessed tooth is manifested by pain that may be spontaneous, in response to temperature changes or to pressure. Dental abscesses can sometimes be caused by deep fillings or trauma, which initiates the pulpal inflammatory process.

DIAGNOSIS. The abscessed tooth is classically diagnosed by its tenderness to slight percussion, reactivity to heat, and a periapical radiolucency visualized in dental x-rays. Progression of the abscess can lead to severe pain, swelling, lymphadenopathy, and fever. The discomfort may be continuous or intermittent, and cannot always be localized to the offending tooth.

Occasionally abscess formation is not accompanied by symptoms and is detected by routine x-ray examination. In these cases the dental abscess or granuloma often converts into a cyst or may develop a fistular tract, establishing chronic low-grade drainage ("gumboil" or parulis).

Ludwig's angina can be a rare complication if appropriate drainage, removal of the infectious source, or effective antibiotics are not instituted.

MANAGEMENT. Emergency care involves drainage, antibiotics (preferably penicillin, with erythromycin being used in penicillin-sensitive individuals), and analgesic drugs. Definitive treatment is by endodontic therapy (root canal filling) or extraction.

PERIODONTAL DISEASE

This condition is the most common cause for the loss of teeth beyond the age of 35. Periodontal disease is manifested by the loss of dental bone support (alveolar process of mandible and maxilla), which creates dental pockets (gingival and bony crevices around the teeth). This further promotes accumulation of bacteria and debris, calculus formation, worsening of the inflammatory process, further acceleration of bone loss, and loosening of the teeth. This process may be accompanied by gingivitis, purulent exudates, swelling, and pain.

ETIOLOGY. Although the most common cause of periodontal disease is poor hygiene (formation of plaque and calculus), in some individuals causative factors remain unknown. Bacterial toxins and inflammation are the common denominators, and immunologic mechanisms have been implicated. Inheritance does not play an important role. In addition to staining tooth structure, tobacco usage has been shown to increase the risk for gingivitis, periodontal disease, and earlier loss of teeth. Diabetes also encourages periodontal disease by suppressing local cell systems that control bacterial proliferation and inflammation. Associations between periodontal disease and other metabolic diseases, gastroenteropathies, and nutritional deficiencies have not been established. The loss of bone through the aging process is a common denominator, and periodontal disease in younger persons is extremely rare, even with poor hygiene.

DIAGNOSIS. Early periodontal disease may go unrecognized, since it is often asymptomatic and without clinically obvious signs. As periodontal disease continues, however, it usually can be detected by gingival erythema and swelling, tooth mobility, and a gingival exudate associated with discomfort or pain. Periodontal disease is confirmed by examination for dental pockets and more accurately assessed by loss of bone seen in x-rays. Certain conditions, such as histiocytosis, hypophosphatasia, and the Papillon-Lefèvre syndrome, can simulate precocious periodontal disease when the jaw bones are affected and teeth are lost prematurely.

PREVENTION AND TREATMENT. Optimal home care (brushing, rinsing, and flossing) and periodic dental office prophylaxes (curettage and polishing) are extremely important factors in removing the causative dental plaque (similar but not identical to plaque causing dental caries). For advanced periodontal disease, surgical alterations of gingiva and alveolar bone, as well as splinting teeth together, may be helpful in slowing or preventing further deterioration. In acute flares, hydrogen peroxide mouth rinses (3 per cent H_2O_2 with equal parts warm water) and antibiotics (preferably penicillin) are usually effective. Although a nutritious diet is important, this will not prevent periodontal disease. Effective human vaccines are not yet available.

Joseph CE, Farnoush A: Current concepts of periodontitis. J Calif Dent Assoc 12:43, 1984. *Assessment of causative factors, pathogenesis, and control of periodontal disease.*

ACUTE GINGIVITIS

This condition, often referred to as acute necrotizing ulcerative gingivitis (ANUG) and Vincent's infection, does not follow any epidemiologic patterns, and there is no evidence that it is contagious. With proper microbiologic testing methods, it does seem to be often associated with fusiform and spirochete organisms. Poor oral hygiene and suboptimal nutrition are frequently found. ANUG can mimic gingival changes occasionally seen in individuals with blood dyscrasias or viral infections.

DIAGNOSIS. The condition is usually characterized by its acute nature associated with pain, fetid oral odor, and gingival ulcerations (Fig. 97–1). There may be associated tendency toward bleeding. Most often there is no associated fever or lymphadenopathy, but malaise may be present.

The diagnosis is established by ruling out other, more serious systemic disease and by response to treatment. This condition differs from chronic gingivitis, which may be asymptomatic and due to poor home care, irritating fillings, or pocket formation (incipient periodontal disease).

TREATMENT. The most conservative approach is by improving oral hygiene, hydrogen peroxide mouth rinses (3 per cent H_2O_2 mixed with equal parts warm water), and dental prophylaxis. Adequate nutrition is important, and antibiotics are useful in cases of fever, lymphadenopathy, or severe oral signs and symptoms. Penicillin is the drug of choice (1000 to 1500 mg daily), with erythromycin in similar dosages an alternative. If good home care is continued, recurrence is unlikely.

When ANUG does not respond to treatment, other diseases must be considered, requiring more extensive laboratory tests. Diseases such as erythema multiforme, lichen planus, pemphigoid, and pemphigus may mimic a chronic or subacute gingivitis. In these instances a biopsy will assist the diagnosis and corticosteroids will control signs and symptoms.

APHTHOUS ULCERS

Aphthous ulcers (canker sore, ulcerative stomatitis) occur in up to 40 per cent of the population. There appears to be a

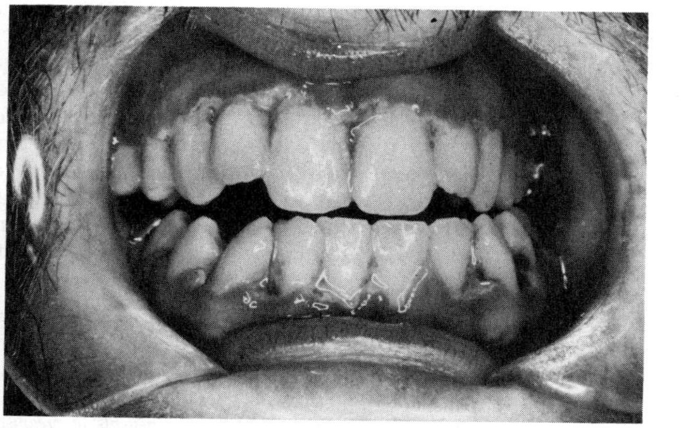

FIGURE 97–1. Acute necrotizing ulcerative gingivitis. Note typical necrosis of marginal gingiva. These signs, associated with pain and fetid odor, were present for one week.

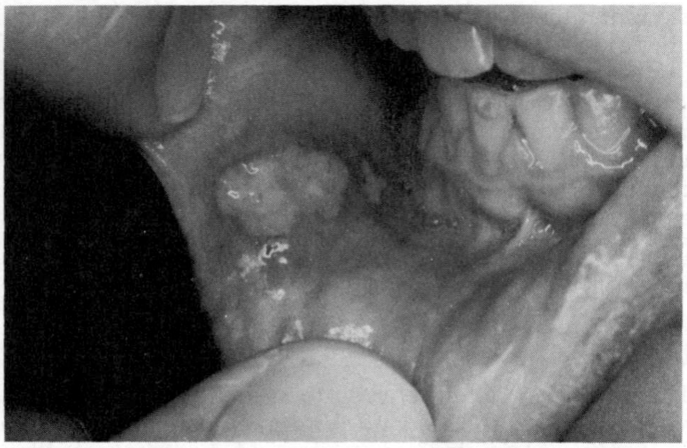

FIGURE 97–2. Aphthous ulcers. These idiopathic ulcerations usually do not exceed 5 to 6 mm in size and heal in 10 to 14 days. This large (major) aphthous ulcer had been present for one month and did not heal for two months.

genetic tendency, since offspring of parents with aphthous ulcers have a greater risk for developing them. Aphthae usually appear by age 20 and without sex preference. There is a tendency to have fewer and less severe attacks as time progresses. Viral, bacterial, or other causative agents have never been proved; immunologic factors are being implicated. Certain foods, fever, and stress may bring on attacks in predisposed persons.

DIAGNOSIS. The diagnosis of aphthae is made by clinical appearance and history. Most commonly they appear as shallow, pseudomembrane-covered ulcerations with a surrounding erythematous halo. They are often tender and heal spontaneously in one to two weeks. Aphthae may occur as multiple small ulcers, or sometimes they appear as single large ulcerations (major aphthae), which usually incur more pain and a longer healing period (Fig. 97–2). This implies a difference in the host and not the disease. Some patients will never be free of ulcers; as one ulcer heals, others occur.

Blood examination or smears are not helpful. Biopsies show nonspecific inflammation and ulceration; the initial inflammatory cell is the lymphocyte. The larger lesions can mimic more serious diseases, since the inflammatory process involves underlying musculature, causing more induration and pain.

Aphthous ulcers may be associated with inflammatory bowel disease and Behcet's syndrome. In the differential diagnosis care must be taken not to confuse aphthae with the oral manifestations of erythema multiforme, erosive lichen planus, primary herpetic stomatitis, pemphigoid, pemphigus, drug reactions, and mucosal manifestations of blood dyscrasias.

TREATMENT. Frequently, special treatment is unnecessary. Empirical approaches, using bland mouth rinses, topical preparations, vitamins, and mild sedatives and analgesics, may be helpful in some persons. The most effective management is by administering short courses of corticosteroids systemically. Frequently less than 40 mg prednisone daily for two to three days will give adequate control of signs and symptoms (this also confirms the inflammatory nature of aphthae). The dosage and duration of corticoid treatment may vary with individual patients and their characteristic patterns of disease. Vaccines and antibiotics have not proved beneficial.

Olson JA, Greenspan JS, Silverman S Jr: Recurrent aphthous ulcerations. J Calif Dent Assoc 10:53, 1982. *Comprehensive review of clinical features, pathogenesis, and management.*

Silverman S Jr, Lozada-Nur F, Migliorati C: Clinical efficacy of prednisone in the treatment of patients with oral inflammatory ulcerative diseases: A study of fifty-five patients. Oral Surg 59:360, 1985. *Benefits of prednisone treatment were shown by comparing time-dosage schedules, reduction of signs and symptoms, and drug side effects.*

ORAL HERPETIC INFECTIONS

Herpes simplex virus (HSV) infects the mouth in a variety of ways. Diagnostic techniques are usually impractical, and treatment is supportive. Evidence for a contagious nature is lacking. A history of these lesions has not been associated with an increased risk for cancer.

COLD SORE (HERPES LABIALIS). The most common bothersome lesion is the cold sore. In the prone individual the latent virus is activated by an external irritant (cold, fever, trauma) and yields the characteristic vesicle or vesicles that subsequently scab and usually take one to three weeks to heal. The lesion is not associated with any rise in HSV antibody titer, and no effective preventive or therapeutic agents (vaccines, vitamins, ointments, and antivirals) are available. Therefore, an empirical approach with which any patient gets the best result is still indicated (see Ch. 533). In more severe attacks, acyclovir, 1200 to 2000 mg daily, may be helpful.

RECURRENT INTRAORAL HSV. Intraoral recurrent herpetic lesions should not be confused with recurrent aphthous ulcers. Recurrent herpetic infections are rare and only occur on the gingiva or hard palate. They are usually characterized by shallow, small, irregular erosive lesions on an erythematous mucosa. Pain is usually no more than moderate, and the lesions are usually self-limiting in seven to ten days.

PRIMARY HERPETIC GINGIVOSTOMATITIS. Primary herpetic gingivostomatitis is the most acute form of oral herpetic infection. Usually 90 per cent of the population is infected before puberty, but most persons do not develop noticeable lesions or complaints. Signs and symptoms can include ulcerations on an erythematous and edematous mucosa (Fig. 97–3). This is often accompanied by lymphadenopathy, fever, and malaise, which can be confused with more serious illnesses. The condition is self-limiting; signs and symptoms usually become progressively severe for one week and disappear by the end of the second week. Treatment is supportive with antipyretic-analgesic agents, rest, and nutritional supplements.

During the course of disease, HSV antibody titer rises at least four-fold and confers lifelong immunity. Blood tests usually show only a slight lymphocytosis. Cytologic smears show pseudogiant cells (squamous) typical of the herpetic infection.

Approximately 10 per cent of adults, as shown by seroepidemiologic study, either did not become infected in childhood or have not developed adequate antibodies. Therefore, this infection is not limited to children. Adult infections of primary herpetic gingivostomatitis are usually more severe than the childhood form. Both forms can be mistaken for more severe diseases such as erythema multiforme, infectious mononucleosis, blood dyscrasias, and pemphigus. Persons who are

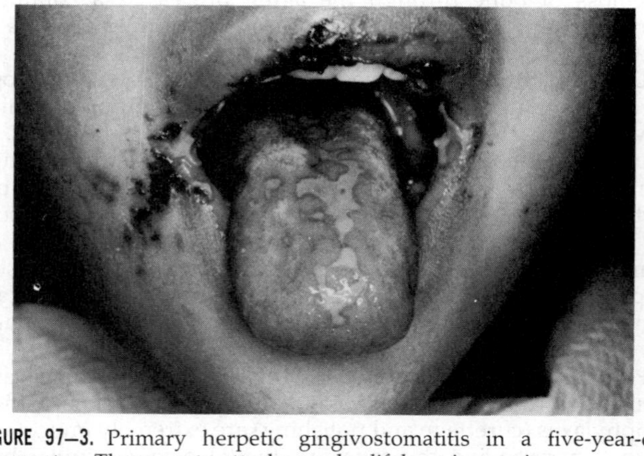

FIGURE 97–3. Primary herpetic gingivostomatitis in a five-year-old youngster. These acute attacks render lifelong immunity.

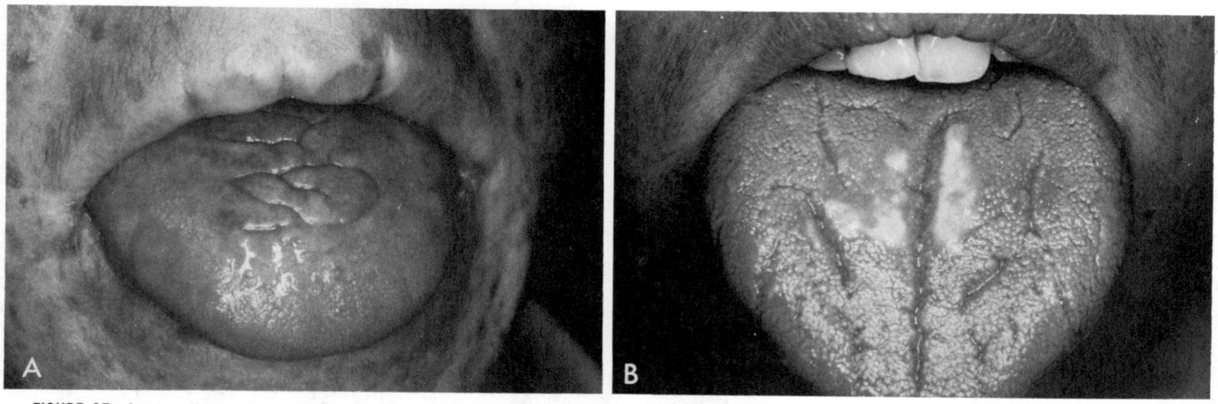

FIGURE 97–4. Candidiasis of tongue. *A*, Note depapillation and angular cheilitis. This patient had an idiopathic iron deficiency anemia. *B*, Note painful white surface colonies. This attack followed a course of antibiotics.

immunosuppressed, e.g., cancer and kidney transplant patients, have an increased risk for developing a primary herpetic stomatitis. Acyclovir (1200 mg daily per os or intravenously) has proved effective in controlling these conditions.

Hirsch MS, Schooley RT: Treatment of herpesvirus infections. N Engl J Med 309:963, 1983. *Reviews HSV infections and management.*

CANDIDIASIS (Moniliasis, Thrush)

Candida albicans (see Ch. 375) is a normal oral flora resident in about 30 to 40 per cent of the population. For unclear reasons, the fungi can become overpopulated and produce clinical signs and symptoms. Most frequently oral candidal infections are associated with antibiotic use (suppressing oral bacterial flora and making more carbohydrate substrate available), diabetes mellitus, xerostomia, immunosuppression, and the wearing of dentures (poor hygiene).

DIAGNOSIS. Oral candidiasis is often recognized by complaints of generalized mouth discomfort. It may be acute or chronic. While examination frequently reveals the typical surface creamy white fungal colonies, often the manifestation is that of irregular or widespread erythema (Fig. 97–4). Occasionally there will be erosive changes. Angular cheilitis is a common finding.

Since the clinical appearance is often only suggestive, smears or cultures (to observe pseudomycelia and spores) may be required to confirm the diagnosis. If biopsies are obtained, special staining with the periodic acid–Schiff (PAS) method may show the fungus, which grows in the most superficial epithelial stratum.

TREATMENT. The first step in treatment is to rule out underlying factors, such as hyperglycemia, xerostomia, and anemia. Hydrogen peroxide–saline mouth rinses (3 per cent H_2O_2 diluted with equal parts warm saline) are helpful. Specific treatment includes orally dissolving nystatin vaginal troches (100,000 units three or four times daily). Nystatin suspension is not as effective, since the contact time with the oral mucosa is much less. Clotrimazole tablets (10 mg dissolved orally five times daily) appear to be equally or more effective than the nystatin. Ketoconazole (200 mg per os daily with food) offers an effective alternative to oral dissolution, which some individuals find objectionable. The angular cheilitis is most effectively treated with Mycolog II cream (nystatin-triamcinolone). Oral candidiasis does not appear to be contagious or related to infections at other sites. Unless the underlying cause is identified and corrected, oral infections can recur.

Mackowiak PA: The normal microbial flora. N Engl J Med 307:83, 1982. *Reviews microbial florae and their interrelationships in health and disease.*

Renner RP, Lee M, Andors L, et al.: The role of *C. albicans* in denture stomatitis. Oral Surg 47:323, 1979. *Reviews biology of oral* Candida, *techniques for measurement and differential diagnosis of clinical appearance. Increased fungal infections were shown in denture wearers.*

ORAL FINDINGS IN ACQUIRED IMMUNODEFICIENCY SYNDROME (AIDS)

Oral signs and/or symptoms of the acquired immunodeficiency syndrome (AIDS) or the AIDS-related complex (ARC) may be the first evidence or complaint indicating the possibility of AIDS virus (HIV) infection. The most common oral infection is chronic candidiasis. This is suspected when there is no other explanation (e.g., dentures, diabetes, leukemia, medicines) other than the possibility of HIV infection and immunosuppression in high-risk individuals (see Ch. 346). A unique white lesion, termed hairy leukoplakia, which occurs almost exclusively on the lateral borders of the tongue in homosexual and bisexual males, is a sign of HIV infection and indicates a high risk for developing AIDS (Fig. 97–5). The Epstein-Barr virus has been isolated from the lesion. Oral Kaposi's sarcoma (KS), often asymptomatic, has been found in over half of the patients with skin KS and sometimes as the sole lesion of KS. It can occur on any oral mucosal surface (predominantly on the palate) as a flat or raised lesion (Fig. 97–6). Other oral findings that should arouse suspicion of HIV infection include progressive periodontal disease (loss of gingival tissue and alveolar bone) for which there is no other obvious explanation; unusually frequent or extensive oral aphthae and herpes simplex lip lesions (cold sores); unilateral mucosal or facial skin vesicles of varicella zoster; cytomegalovirus-induced xerostomia; increased number of allergies usually manifested by mucosal or skin rashes; and condyloma acuminatum (venereal warts), which may occur on any mucosal surface and appear as papillomas.

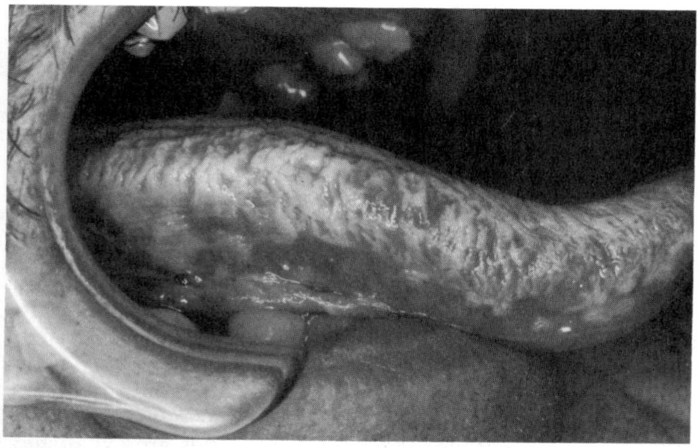

FIGURE 97–5. Hairy leukoplakia in a 31-year-old homosexual male. This unique tongue lesion almost always indicates AIDS virus infection and a high risk for developing AIDS. This patient was diagnosed as having pneumocystic pneumonia four months later.

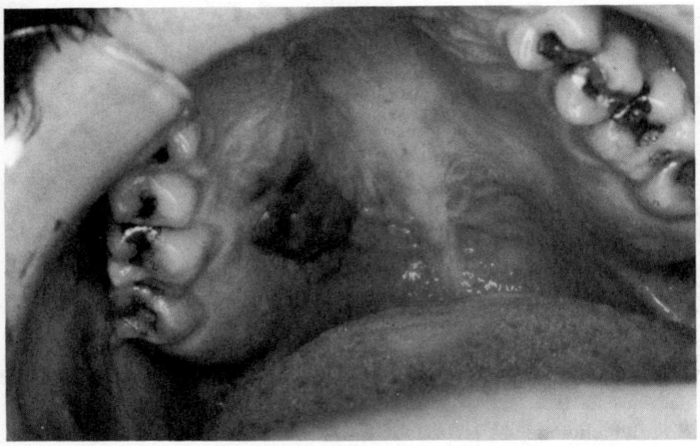

FIGURE 97–6. This exophytic vascular-appearing growth on the palate is a biopsy-proved Kaposi's sarcoma in a 29-year-old homosexual male.

Silverman S Jr, Migliorati CA, Lozada-Nur F, et al.: Oral findings in people with or at high risk for AIDS: A study of 375 homosexual males. J Am Dent Assoc 112:187, 1986. *A study of 375 homosexual-bisexual males, describing and illustrating oral signs and symptoms of ARC and AIDS and discussing risks and control measures.*

GLOSSITIS

Inflammatory conditions of the tongue are moderately common and quite variable. Asymptomatic glossitis may be due to the aging process (atrophy of the filiform papillae) or due to such idiopathic conditions as geographic tongue (glossitis migrans) and median rhomboid glossitis (central papillary atrophy). Occasionally glossitis may reflect a blood dyscrasia or a variety of debilitating diseases involving malnutrition. By careful clinical examination, history, and ruling out other diseases, the asymptomatic atrophic tongue can usually be classified.

Complex clinical problems may be associated with patients having symptomatic glossitis (glossopyrosis, glossodynia). Frequently examination of the tongue will not reveal any specific lesions or depapillation. The symptoms are often a manifestation of anxiety or depression. Occasionally the glossitis may be due to a drug reaction. Xerostomia or dehydration may be causative factors, and candidiasis must be ruled out. Rarely, anemia or hyperglycemia may induce these changes. Glossitis is not caused by poor oral hygiene, dentures, or other tooth-related problems. Tobacco use may contribute to the discomfort, as may certain foods. In many cases the etiology remains unknown, and by default they are classified as psychogenic.

MANAGEMENT. Approach to the patient with a symptomatic tongue usually involves a careful history and consideration of discontinuing or altering drugs. Tobacco must be discontinued, at least temporarily. Blood dyscrasias and hyperglycemia should be ruled out with the appropriate tests. Inspection for any obvious dental or oral pathologic condition is in order, and these should be corrected even though it is unlikely that they may play a role. Occasionally a malignancy of the tongue may create these symptoms, therefore, a careful examination must be performed. Reassuring a patient that there is no sign of malignancy is sometimes an important part of management. Candidiasis should be eliminated by appropriate cultures or smears or by instituting a short trial of antifungal agents.

A systematic pharmacologic approach, including placebos, vitamins, tranquilizers, and antidepressant agents, may be utilized after the other diagnostic approaches are exhausted. Occasionally sialogogues (pilocarpine or bethanechol) or anti-inflammatory agents (corticoids) are helpful. If all these approaches fail and a diagnosis cannot be established, then any acceptable supportive therapy may be attempted, e.g., hypnosis, biofeedback, or even periodic recall visits for reassurance.

Dreizen S: The telltale tongue. Postgrad Med 75:150, 1984. *Reviews diseases of the tongue with reference to cause, appearance, and management.*

LEUKOPLAKIA–ERYTHROPLAKIA

These terms designate white and red patches that may occur on any oral mucosal surface (Fig. 97–7). There may be associated discomfort, and an etiologic factor is not always apparent.

MANAGEMENT AND DIAGNOSIS. The first practical approach is to remove all irritants, such as tobacco use, ill-fitting dentures, poor hygiene, spicy or hot foods, and any other potentially injurious habits, in order to see if the lesions are reversible. If not, representative biopsies should be obtained. Most often leukoplakia will be a manifestation of benign hyperkeratosis and erythroplakia a reflection of epithelial atrophy and inflammation. If a lesion cannot be classified as any specific disease entity, then at the very least it should be followed closely because of the risk for malignant transformation (thus the term precancerous lesion). If the biopsy indicates dysplasia, then a more aggressive attempt should be made to remove these lesions surgically. A red component also increases the risk for malignant transformation. Carbon dioxide laser resection or evaporation has been an effective surgical modality. Removal does not guarantee permanent control or cancer prevention.

DIFFERENTIAL DIAGNOSIS. Occasionally a white- and/or red-appearing oral lesion may already be squamous carcinoma. Alternatively, it may represent a classifiable benign lesion such as lichen planus, erythema multiforme, or pemphigoid. In these latter conditions, topical or systemic corticosteroids will help confirm the diagnosis by at least partial control of the lesion. For leukoplakia and erythroplakia, corticosteroids, keratinolytic agents, vitamin A, and other approaches have not been uniformly effective.

Silverman S Jr, Gorsky M, Lozada F: Oral leukoplakia and malignant transformation. A follow-up study of 257 patients. Cancer 53:563, 1984. *Describes profiles and establishes risk factors in patients with precancerous oral lesions.*

ORAL CANCER

Cancer of the mouth accounts for about 4 per cent of all cancers. The tongue is the most common site, although it may occur in any mouth site. More than 90 per cent are squamous carcinomas, commencing in the oral epithelial lining. The average age of onset approximates 60 years, and there is a 2 to 1 male to female prevalence. Oral cancer occurs in all ethnic groups.

ETIOLOGY. The increased risk and cause-effect relationship among tobacco use, alcohol consumption, and mouth

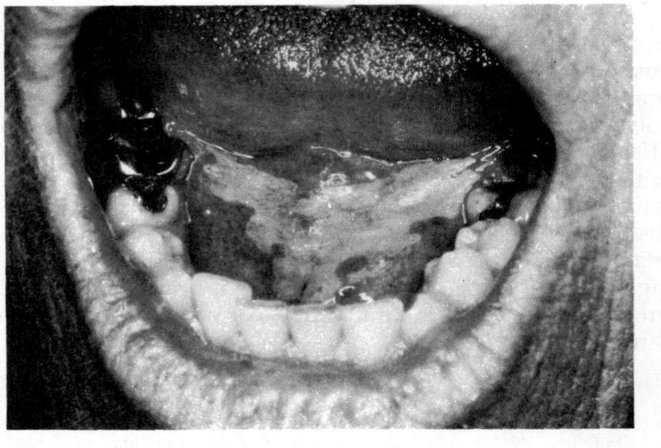

FIGURE 97–7. Leukoplakia of floor of mouth. This lesion, which was asymptomatic, had been present for four years. The cause was related to cigarette smoking.

cancer have been well documented. Abstinence is significant in preventive measures. Since patients with one oral cancer have an extremely high risk for developing second head and neck malignancies (about 20 per cent), discontinuation of tobacco and alcohol is critical. Although various forms of oral irritation, food carcinogens, and herpesvirus have been implicated, studies have not confirmed an associated risk factor.

DIAGNOSIS. There are no reliable signs or symptoms associated with mouth cancer. This causes delay by the patient in seeking professional advice, and conversely the varied features often delay diagnostic procedures. The most common finding is that of a painful ulceration associated with induration. Early malignant changes often can appear as essentially asymptomatic white and/or red surface patches. Patients often describe these changes as lumps or irritations.

Biopsy is the only acceptable method of diagnosis. Exfoliative cytology and vital staining with toluidine blue (1 per cent aqueous toluidine blue, decolorized with 1 per cent acetic acid) are useful adjuncts to clinical opinion when biopsy is delayed or extent of disease is being determined.

TREATMENT. The survival rate for oral cancer is relatively poor, in most studies averaging less than 50 per cent. This is usually due to late detection, promoting lesions that are locally extensive with diffuse margins, large tumor volume, and spread to the neck (cervical lymphadenopathy). While spread to neck nodes is rather common, approximating 50 per cent, involvement of other organ systems occurs in less than 15 per cent of advanced cases.

Curative therapy utilizes radiation and surgery. Often these modalities are used in combination, which seems to increase cure rates slightly, although also increasing morbidity. In advanced cases chemotherapy is also used (most effective drugs include methotrexate, bleomycin, and cisplatin); the sequences, dosages, and combinations vary.

REHABILITATION. Rehabilitation is essential, since treatment often compromises appearance, function, and attitude. For surgical defects maxillofacial prosthetic appliances are very effective. Paraprofessionals are useful in improving speech and swallowing defects. Radiation, which is frequently used, alters saliva and taste, interfering with oral comfort and nutrition. Dietary consultation can often assist food acceptance. Xerostomia usually can be improved by the administration of pilocarpine, 5 mg four times a day, or bethanechol, 50 mg three times a day, if more conservative methods (sugarless gum or candy drops) are unsuccessful. Supplements of elemental zinc (up to 100 mg daily) have improved taste perception in some patients. Jaw bone and mucosal necrosis is also increased with radiation, and special care must be taken regarding dental procedures, extractions, and other forms of dental trauma. The risk is proportional to the radiation dosage, becoming most critical above 6500 rads. Antibiotics and time will often control the necrosis; however, surgery is sometimes required.

Silverman S Jr, Greenspan D: Early detection and diagnosis of oral cancer. J Calif Dent Assoc 13:29, 1985. *Comprehensive review of epidemiology, survival, and early detection and diagnosis; tables and photos.*

98 DISEASES OF THE ESOPHAGUS

Charles E. Pope II

CLINICAL SYMPTOMATOLOGY

The esophagus would seem to be a relatively simple portion of the gastrointestinal tract. Its duty, the transport of solids, liquids, and gas, usually is performed unobtrusively. The structure of the esophagus is not complex. Yet malfunction can lead to such trivial complaints as heartburn or overwhelming clinical problems such as aspiration, obstruction, and hemorrhage. A good clinical history will often be the most valuable diagnostic test. The laboratory diagnosis of esophageal malfunction often exceeds our therapeutic capabilities.

Esophageal disorders can be expressed by a group of symptoms that are unique to this organ. The esophagus also shares other symptoms with the rest of the gastrointestinal tract. The clinician should concentrate on the unique symptoms, as further investigations will usually uncover an esophageal cause.

DYSPHAGIA. Consciousness of bolus arrest during swallowing, even if transient, indicates esophageal dysfunction. The patient will usually use the term "sticks," "hesitates," "pauses," or "hangs up" and will often indicate the site of arrest with a finger.

Bolus arrest closely associated with the act of swallowing is dysphagia. The sensation of a substernal lump present one-half hour after eating is not dysphagia. Most patients consider mild dysphagia a normal phenomenon. "I just swallowed something that was too big." Thus, often they will not spontaneously mention the presence of dysphagia unless questioned closely.

A specialized type of dysphagia occurs when the bolus cannot be propelled from the mouth or hypopharynx into the esophagus, so-called "transfer dysphagia." This type of dysphagia is most commonly related to neurologic disease or to pharyngeal muscle weakness.

The sensation of dysphagia is localized to the suprasternal notch or substernally. The exact location of the sensation is of little use in pinpointing the site of bolus arrest. Dysphagia for a liquid bolus usually indicates an esophageal motor disorder. Dysphagia for solids can be seen either with an organic obstruction (stricture or cancer) or secondary to esophageal motor disorders.

The patient's response to dysphagia can also provide useful information about the cause of dysphagia. If the bolus must be regurgitated, and if an attempt to force the bolus down with water is met by a sudden return of the fluid, then an organic obstruction should be suspected. If the patient is able to force the bolus down by posturing, by performing a Valsalva's maneuver, by repeated swallowing, or by ingesting fluid, then a motor disorder is more likely. Inexorable progression of dysphagia over months usually signals the presence of organic narrowing, either a lumen-obliterating carcinoma or a stricture caused by active peptic esophagitis.

Dysphagia is never an expression of a pure psychiatric disorder; it is not a manifestation of hysteria. Some patients with well-established esophageal disease such as achalasia will report that their dysphagia is often worse at a time of severe emotional tension. Such observations have led many patients (and unfortunately some physicians) to believe that dysphagia is a matter for the psychiatrist rather than the gastroenterologist. Such an opinion can lead to subsequent embarrassment or tragedy, especially if an esophageal carcinoma is overlooked.

ODYNOPHAGIA. Pain upon swallowing, odynophagia, is another cardinal symptom of esophageal disease. Bolus arrest producing dysphagia can sometimes progress to a sensation of pain as esophageal obstruction continues. However, odynophagia usually occurs during the transit of the bolus and disappears once the swallowed material has left the esophagus. It may be mild in intensity so that the patient is merely aware of the location of the swallowed bolus. This is most commonly seen in patients with reflux disease. It can be of such intensity that the patient will refuse to swallow any solids or liquids and will expectorate saliva. Odynophagia can be seen after involvement of the mucosa by *reflux*, by *radiation*, or by *viral* or *fungal infections*. Odynophagia can be an uncommon manifestation of carcinoma or of a localized ulcer caused by a lodged tablet. Odynophagia thus localizes a process to the esophagus but gives no clue to pathogenesis.

HEARTBURN (PYROSIS). Heartburn or pyrosis is the most common manifestation of esophageal disease, so much so that it is difficult to recruit "normal" subjects, if strict histories are taken to eliminate any who have ever had heartburn. The term "burning" rather than "pain" is usually used, although heartburn can increase in intensity until it is perceived as pain. Patients commonly illustrate heartburn with a movement of the open hand up and down the sternum. This is in contrast to the stationary tightly clenched fist of angina pectoris. Heartburn is usually relieved, even if only temporarily, by taking antacids. A constant burning, unrelieved by antacids, may well be of esophageal origin, but it does not represent heartburn. Heartburn is often worse after recumbency or lifting; and may follow overeating or alcoholic indiscretion.

REGURGITATION. Regurgitation of fluid contents into the mouth often accompanies heartburn. Sometimes such regurgitation is associated with eructation; often it accompanies bending over, lifting, or lying down at night. The bitter regurgitated fluid is often described as yellow-brown or green. Regurgitation at night may lead to stridor or to wheezing, a hoarse voice, and other respiratory symptoms from unrecognized reflux. Less commonly, regurgitated fluid is not from the stomach or duodenum, but from fluid retained in an *achalasic esophagus* or in a large *pharyngeal diverticulum*. An uncommon but fascinating process that can be confused with regurgitation is *rumination*. In this condition, recently eaten food is propelled back into the mouth from the stomach by a strong contraction of the abdominal wall musculature. The food commonly is rechewed, reswallowed, and again returned to the mouth (Ch. 215).

ESOPHAGEAL COLIC. In addition to the discomfort from severe reflux, which can advance from heartburn into pain, abnormal motor activity of the esophageal muscle can cause severe pain clinically indistinguishable from angina pectoris in terms of intensity, radiation, relationship to exercise, and even response to nitroglycerin. Chest pain of esophageal origin can radiate directly through to the back and is often found in patients who also notice dysphagia. Esophageal colic can last from five to ten seconds to hours.

HEMATEMESIS. Although vomiting blood is less specific for esophageal disease than are many of the symptoms listed above, hematemesis can signal the presence of esophageal varices, of mucosal ulceration resulting from esophageal reflux, of a rent of the mucosa of the lower esophagus, or, uncommonly, of an ulcerating carcinoma or leiomyoma of the esophagus. Although bleeding from the esophagus may be life threatening, more often it is a slow ooze, usually caused by esophageal reflux disease, which presents clinically as an iron deficiency anemia.

Berk JE (ed.): Bockus' Gastroenterology. 4th ed. Philadelphia, W. B. Saunders Company, 1985, pp 666–850. *Reference textbook chapters on esophagus. Good source for recent references.*

Pope CE II: Chapters on the esophagus. In Sleisenger MH, Fordtran JS (eds.): Gastrointestinal Disease. 4th ed. Philadelphia, W. B. Saunders Company, (in press). *Reference textbook on esophageal disease.*

GASTROESOPHAGEAL REFLUX DISEASE

DEFINITION. Gastroesophageal reflux disease (GERD) refers to the varied clinical manifestations of reflux of stomach and duodenal contents into the esophagus. It is preferable to the term "reflux esophagitis" because the latter expression tends to mean different things to the clinician, the endoscopist, and the pathologist. Although it may be associated with a sliding hiatus hernia, "symptomatic hiatus hernia" is a term that tends to put the emphasis on the wrong anatomic entity and pathophysiology. Gastroesophageal reflux disease can be characterized by any combination of symptoms and radiologic, endoscopic, or pathologic changes. In its milder manifestations, it is a common disease; its most florid state is uncommon but may be life threatening.

PATHOGENESIS. Several factors must work in concert to produce clinical effects of esophageal reflux. All persons will demonstrate short bursts of reflux if monitored with an intraesophageal pH probe over 24 hours. This reflux is seen postprandially and usually in the upright position. Those in whom reflux has produced symptoms or pathologic changes will demonstrate more prolonged episodes of reflux, which tend to occur at night. The factor or factors that cause this difference are not known. However, important differences between persons with and without reflux might help explain these findings.

The *lower esophageal sphincter* (LES) is a specialized bundle of circular muscle at the lower end of the esophagus with different physical and pharmacologic characteristics when compared with the circular muscle above and below it. There is a tendency for mean LES pressure to be significantly lower in subjects with GERD compared with normal persons, but LES pressures are not very useful in predicting whether reflux is present in an individual patient unless the pressure is very low. The most common event associated with reflux appears to be an *inappropriate relaxation of the lower esophageal sphincter*, i.e., LES relaxation unassociated with either swallowing or the distention of the esophageal body by refluxed fluid. Thus, two abnormalities of LES may be associated with reflux: a sphincter with very low tone, as measured by lower esophageal sphincter pressure, or inappropriate relaxation of a normally competent sphincter.

Several factors are important in removing refluxed material. The upright position facilitates esophageal emptying by gravity. Peristaltic waves initiated by swallowing or by esophageal distention help remove the refluxed material. Acid placed within the esophagus is cleared less well by patients with GERD than by normal subjects, even though the manometric tracings seen in both groups seem identical. Clearing occurs in two phases. The bulk of the fluid is returned to the stomach by a peristaltic contraction; the remainder of the acid film clinging to the esophageal wall is neutralized by swallowed saliva.

The composition and perhaps the quantity of the refluxed material also play a role in the production of GERD. Gastric acid and pepsin seem clearly important in the pathogenesis of GERD. Bile salts and possibly pancreatic enzymes may be responsible in those patients in whom acid is absent. The combination of bile salts plus acid is more injurious to the esophagus than either agent alone. Other less well-studied factors such as altered or abnormal esophageal mucus, swallowed saliva of high bicarbonate content, and diminished resistance of the esophageal mucosa to digestion may be important in determining the amount of mucosal damage in GERD.

Esophageal squamous epithelium reacts to reflux by an increase in the basal cell or germinative layer. The dermal pegs are increased in height and may become more vascular. If the process becomes more severe, the epithelial layer is destroyed, with the appearance of microulcers and classic signs of inflammation in the lamina propria, such as infiltration with polymorphonuclear leukocytes and edema. Even deeper lesions cause first submucosal, then muscular inflammation and fibrosis, resulting in an esophageal stricture. Why reflux is so common, yet inflammation and stricture formation so relatively uncommon, is not known.

Other conditions can be associated with the pathogenesis of reflux. Reflux during pregnancy, once thought to be due to the increased abdominal pressure from the fetus, may be due mainly to diminished LES strength caused by extra estrogen and progesterone. Weight gain also tends to aggravate reflux through an unknown mechanism. As expected, resection of the lower esophageal area for cancer or myotomy for achalasia can lead to severe postoperative reflux (see below).

ROLE OF HIATUS HERNIA. The presence of a hiatus

hernia is now considered to be much less of a factor in GERD than previously thought. Some radiologists find hiatus hernias in a large percentage of patients, no matter what the reason for the examination. Others rarely demonstrate a hiatus hernia. It is not appropriate to spend a great deal of time trying to define whether a hiatus hernia is present or absent in dealing with most patients with GERD. The important entity to investigate is reflux, not hiatus hernia.

SYMPTOMS OF GASTROESOPHAGEAL REFLUX DISEASE. *Heartburn* is the most common manifestation of GERD. It can vary from an occasional mild burning after overeating to an ever-present, severe discomfort that severely limits a patient's lifestyle. It may be accompanied by *regurgitation* of gastric contents either into the mouth or into the respiratory tree. This latter group of patients may complain of nocturnal wheezing, hoarseness, a need to clear the throat repeatedly, and a sensation of deep pressure at the base of the neck. This group of symptoms may be the primary clinical presentation and more prominent than the classic symptoms of GERD.

Dysphagia is often present in those with significant GERD. Although dysphagia may be severe and even mark the onset of stricture formation, it usually is mild and must be carefully sought. Dysphagia of GERD is for solids, and the dysphagia is usually overcome by swallowing repeatedly or by washing down the bolus with some water. Dysphagia without anatomic strictures has been noted in about three fourths of patients scheduled for antireflux surgery. Many patients with GERD will not complain of bolus arrest, but rather of being aware of the location of each solid morsel as it travels down the esophagus.

Blood loss may result from esophageal erosion and shallow ulcers. Rarely producing life-threatening hemorrhage, the erosions are much more likely to weep quietly over a prolonged period of time, producing iron deficiency anemia. Some of these patients have very few other clinical manifestations of GERD, and the condition is discovered by endoscopy during an evaluation of occult gastrointestinal bleeding. Patients who vigorously and repeatedly abuse alcohol seem prone to develop severe erosive esophagitis with bleeding; this lesion heals with abstinence from alcohol without other major antireflux therapy.

DIAGNOSIS. The history and clinical manifestations of GERD are the most important diagnostic aids in the establishment of the diagnosis; objective testing is used to quantify the extent and severity of the process. In the evaluation of an individual, questions to be answered dictate the appropriate test.

Does reflux exist and, if so, to what degree? This question might arise either if another condition such as pulmonary disease is present and a causal relationship is being sought, or if some idea of the frequency and extent of reflux is important. Reflux during a barium swallow in adults is uncommon unless vigorous provocative maneuvers are employed. When spontaneous reflux of barium is seen, it usually denotes free reflux. Children reflux barium more easily than do adults. The pH probe can be used either for short-term studies of 15 to 30 minutes or for more prolonged periods (24 hours). If repeated bursts of reflux are demonstrated during a 15-minute period, then severe reflux is present. At the same time, the ability of the esophagus to clear itself of refluxed acid can be evaluated. Usually a manometric catheter is attached to the pH probe in order to locate it in the esophagus; this catheter can also estimate the LES pressure. Only very low values of LES pressure such as 1 to 2 mm Hg (normal, about 20 mm Hg) are of prognostic value.

Twenty-four–hour pH monitoring can be performed with a portable unit, which allows the patient to follow an almost normal lifestyle. During the prolonged monitoring period, the relationship between symptoms (heartburn, pain, wheezing) and episodes of reflux can be ascertained, and calculations can be made of the number of episodes of reflux and the amount of time the esophagus is acidified.

Reflux can be measured noninvasively by scanning of the esophageal area with a gamma camera after placing a solution of ^{99m}Tc sulfur colloid in the stomach. An abdominal binder is used to stress the gastroesophageal junction if free reflux is not seen. This technique seems to be of most value in infants and children, who tolerate esophageal tubes very poorly.

Could reflux be responsible for the patient's symptoms? This question might be asked if pain is the predominant symptom rather than more classic heartburn. This question can be answered with the same catheter assembly used to measure LES pressure and acid reflux. After a five-minute period of dripping normal saline through one of the pressure catheters whose opening has been localized to the upper esophagus, this infusion is changed to 0.1 N hydrochloric acid without the patient's knowledge. Reproduction of the symptoms within 30 minutes of acid infusion (usually four to five minutes into the infusion) and rapid disappearance of the symptom with a switch back to saline infusion suggests an esophageal cause of the discomfort.

As another approach, the patient is asked to signal the time of discomfort during prolonged pH monitoring of the esophagus. If the patient signals discomfort at the same time that reflux is demonstrated by the pH probe, then a causal relationship is made more likely. Prolonged pH monitoring is not used widely clinically because of the expense of hospitalization. The development of portable pH monitors has made this approach more feasible.

What has reflux done to the esophageal mucosa? A barium swallow will detect gross changes such as stricture formation or a deep esophageal ulcer but will miss the much more common shallow ulcerations and erosions. These will be detected by direct inspection with the endoscope. Only discrete lesions such as erosions and ulcerations should be taken as proof of esophageal damage; such endoscopic findings as erythema, edema, or friability are subject to wide interobserver variation. If the mucosa appears absolutely normal, as it is in approximately one third of patients with moderate-to-severe symptoms of GERD, a suction biopsy can demonstrate the changes of reflux.

A logic tree of how these tests might be used is shown in Table 98–1. A patient whose symptoms are severe enough to seek medical attention might be screened with a barium swallow. Uncommonly, reflux will be demonstrated, a stricture found, or a deep ulcer seen. This might lead to immediate endoscopy for more complete evaluation. If a patient presents with hematemesis and reflux symptoms, endoscopy might appropriately be used as the first step. After first evaluation, it is appropriate to begin therapy (see Treatment, below). Only if there is a poor response to therapy should an acid perfusion test be used to confirm the diagnosis. At the same time, the presence of reflux can be checked, an estimate of LES pressure and acid clearance obtained, and the presence or absence of peristaltic waves determined.

More intensive therapy should be instituted at this point. If it fails and the patient is still symptomatic, endoscopy can be employed to see if gross disease is still present in the face of maximal therapy. If the appearance of the mucosa is normal grossly in the presence of overwhelming symptoms, suction biopsies can be obtained to search for objective evidence of reflux damage. This scheme will restrict extensive testing to those who have failed medical therapy and who are presumably candidates for surgical treatment. This algorithm can be modified if the patient has blood loss or severe dysphagia. Endoscopy should follow a screening barium radiographic examination of such patients.

COMPLICATIONS OF GASTROESOPHAGEAL REFLUX DISEASE. ***Esophageal Stricture.*** Of the many who complain of symptoms of GERD, only a few will develop esophageal

TABLE 98–1. DIAGNOSIS OF REFLUX

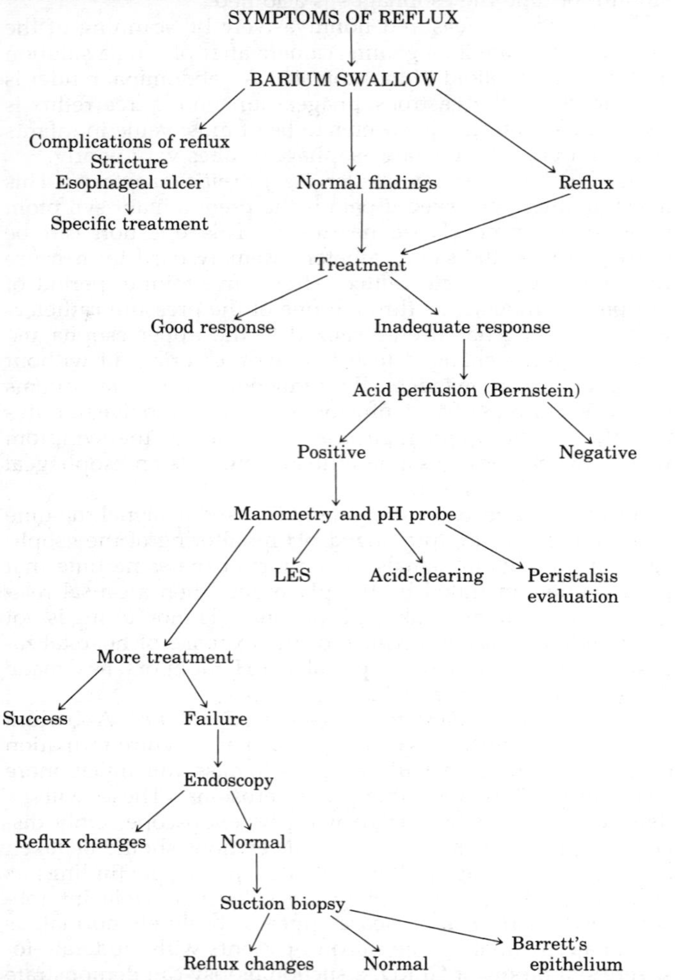

strictures. Usually beginning at the lower end of the esophagus, strictures may migrate over years to the midesophagus or higher. Columnar epithelium will be found below the stricture. Presumably those who develop strictures have had deep circumferential ulceration of the esophageal mucosa due to reflux damage. Instead of healing with only minimal submucosal and muscular fibrosis, these patients develop esophageal obstruction with a narrowed esophageal lumen. If reflux can be controlled, these strictures will disappear.

Dysphagia is the clinical hallmark of esophageal stricture formation. Unlike the relatively mild dysphagia seen in uncomplicated GERD, the dysphagia in patients with strictures tends to be constant and slowly progressive, causing the patient to alter the type of food taken. If a bolus becomes arrested in the stricture, it is usually necessary for the bolus to be regurgitated back into the mouth before further intake of food or fluids is possible.

Strictures are most easily evaluated by barium swallow. Sometimes the extent of the strictured area is overestimated unless the esophagus below the stricture can be fully distended by barium. For mild strictures, the ingestion of a bread or marshmallow bolus can draw attention to slight luminal narrowing when the bolus impacts there. Once demonstrated, endoscopy with biopsy and/or brush cytology is in order to make certain that the stricture is benign.

Esophageal Ulcer. In addition to the more common shallow ulcerations, deep esophageal ulcers may complicate severe GERD. These ulcers, which retain barium and usually project outside the wall of the esophagus, characteristically produce severe and unrelenting pain, often with radiation of the pain through to the back. Brisk hemorrhage is another manifestation, from erosion either through to an esophageal artery or, more catastrophically, into the nearby aorta. The presence of an ulcer can be suspected on a barium swallow and confirmed endoscopically. The ulcer is usually found to reside in columnar (Barrett's) epithelium.

TABLE 98–2. CLINICAL FEATURES OF PULMONARY ASPIRATION

1. Onset of "asthma" in patients over 30 years without a family history of asthma or industrial exposure
2. Nocturnal or early morning cough
3. Nocturnal wheezing
4. Hoarseness, especially on arising
5. The need to clear the throat repeatedly
6. A feeling of constant pressure deep in the neck

Columnar Epithelium. In some patients who have suffered severe esophageal ulceration as a result of GERD, the healing epithelium is replaced not with squamous epithelium but with a specialized columnar epithelium. The junctional zone between squamous and columnar epithelium can progress orad over years. Columnar epithelium is found at and below midesophageal strictures and around deep esophageal ulcers, although it can be found on routine biopsy of patients with severe GERD. Its major clinical importance is not only as a marker of severe reflux but also as a precursor for adenocarcinoma of the esophagus (see under Esophageal Tumors).

Pulmonary Aspiration. If refluxed material breaches the upper esophageal sphincter, it may easily spill into the larynx and tracheobronchial tree. Some patients react to such a spill with intense respiratory stridor. Others seem to tolerate the presence of refluxed contents in the larynx and tracheobronchial tree with milder laryngeal or respiratory symptoms. It is even possible that the gastric contents do not have to reach the larynx, instillation of acid in the esophagus of susceptible individuals while they are in the upright posture can be shown to cause closing of small bronchial airways, presumably by a vagal reflex.

None of the clinical features of pulmonary aspiration (Table 98–2) is pathognomonic. Taken together they point toward reflux and aspiration as a possible etiology. Diagnostic proof of the relationship is difficult with current techniques. Radioisotopes placed in the stomach have been demonstrated the next morning to be in the lungs by gamma camera scanning, but this cannot be demonstrated in the majority of patients. Only correction of reflux with subsequent disappearance of pulmonary symptoms can prove the relationship.

TREATMENT OF GASTROESOPHAGEAL REFLUX DISEASE AND ITS COMPLICATIONS. ***Medical Management.*** Most mildly symptomatic patients with reflux and some moderately afflicted individuals can be helped by manipulations designed to alter the frequency or type of esophageal reflux. Many patients respond to the simple measures outlined in Table 98–3. Elevation of the head of the bed by 6 to 8 inches is the simplest and most effective form of therapy. Twenty-four–hour pH monitoring has shown that this simple measure decreases the frequency and length of reflux epi-

TABLE 98–3. TREATMENT OF GASTROESOPHAGEAL REFLUX DISEASE

Simple Measures

1. Elevation of head of the bed
2. Avoidance of food and fluid intake before bedtime
3. Reduction of fat in diet
4. Liquid antacid (aluminum hydroxide, magnesium hydroxide) one and three hours after meals and at bedtime
5. Avoidance of cigarettes and alcohol
6. Weight loss

Measures for Resistant Cases

1. Alginic acid–antacid (Gaviscon), 15 ml four times a day
2. Bethanechol (Urecholine),* 10 or 25 mg four times a day
3. Metoclopramide (Reglan),* 10 mg three times a day
4. Cimetidine,* 300 mg four times a day
5. Ranitidine,* 150 mg twice a day

*This use is not listed in the manufacturer's directive.

sodes. The use of pillows to elevate the thorax does not work well, as patients tend to roll off the pillows during the night. A foam rubber wedge can be used if the bed frame cannot be moved. Avoiding food and fluid for at least three hours before retiring decreases the amount of material available for reflux at night. Avoidance of food that the patient finds distressing, such as fatty foods, chocolate, and onions, makes sense but has never been subjected to clinical trial.

Neutralization of acid is approached by taking 30 ml of aluminum hydroxide–magnesium hydroxide antacid one and three hours after meals and at bedtime. In recalcitrant cases, hourly antacids may be tried, with substitution of pure aluminum hydroxide gel to control diarrhea produced by the magnesium ion. Most patients will not tolerate such a regimen for long.

An attempt should be made to have the patient stop smoking, drinking alcohol, and overeating. Most patients, however, apparently prefer to suffer with reflux symptoms rather than to give up these mainstays of life.

If these simple measures are not effective, more vigorous treatment is indicated. Alginic acid–antacid, 15 ml after each meal and at bedtime, is more effective than placebo and as effective as antacids. It is worth trying, but often will not control symptoms of severe reflux. Bethanechol* is a parasympathomimetic agent that can be used in doses of 10 or 25 mg four times a day. Metoclopramide,* 10 mg three times a day, can be helpful, but central nervous system side effects can limit its usefulness. Cimetidine,* 300 mg four times a day, or ranitidine,* 150 mg twice a day, although not approved for therapy of heartburn, improves symptoms significantly when compared with placebo.

Surgical Management. In a patient in whom adequate trial of medical management as outlined above has not brought good results in a six-month period, and in whom there is good objective evidence of reflux, surgical correction of reflux should be considered. Current surgical therapy, regardless of exact techniques, attempts to restore sphincter competence by surrounding the lower end of the esophagus with a cuff of gastric fundal muscle. This is done either completely, as in the Nissen fundoplication, or partially (Hill repair, Belsey repair).

It is difficult to choose one operation or method over another, as most published surgical reports do not carefully define the exact indications for the operation, the length and type of preoperative medical management, or the use of objective tests pre- and postoperatively. Follow-up tends to be short and incomplete; the postoperative assessments are usually made by those responsible for choosing or operating upon the patients. Therefore, no firm statement can be made about the true efficacy of surgery in the correction of reflux.

A surgeon experienced in the techniques of antireflux surgery is necessary for good postoperative results. Technique is all important. Although some individual surgeons have enviable postoperative results, antireflux surgery has a relatively poor reputation in many medical communities. Currently, a conservative approach toward antireflux surgery seems indicated.

Treatment of Complications. Esophageal strictures, if only mildly symptomatic, can be handled by careful attention to dietary intake, improvement of dentition, and institution of medical therapy. Techniques of dilation have proliferated in recent years, but they still require an experienced operator. Short, simple strictures can be dilated with weighted rubber or Teflon dilators (Hurst, Maloney). Tortuous or angulated strictures are more easily approached over a previously placed guide wire. This, in turn, can be passed through an endoscope or under radiographic control. Graded steel olives (Eder-Peustow), a dilator with graded increases of size (Celestin), or a balloon with a fixed maximal diameter (Cooke) can be passed over the previously placed wire. Alternatively, a balloon of fixed maximal diameter can be passed through the large channel of an endoscope during diagnostic endoscopy, and dilation can be done under direct vision. Once the lumen is restored to a diameter of 13 to 15 mm, most patients swallow without difficulty. If the stricture is stable and requires dilation only every four to six months, nothing else is necessary.

*This use is not listed in the manufacturer's directive.

Some patients will not tolerate dilation or require vigorous dilation every three to four weeks. This is an indication for definitive antireflux operation, following which the stricture may regress. Unfortunately, many strictures persist after attempts at antireflux surgery. Esophageal replacement by colon, jejunum, or stomach is a surgical maneuver of last resort; such procedures have relatively high morbidity and mortality. Those afflicted by strictures often have significant lung and cardiovascular disease that makes them unsuitable operative candidates.

If a patient has a peptic stricture that does not respond to dilation and if surgery is deemed too risky because of the patient's age or condition, irradiation of the stomach may be tried. Fifteen hundred rads to the stomach is usually well tolerated and produces anacidity for weeks to months after therapy is completed. Acid production usually returns at a later date, but often at a lower level. This procedure sometimes facilitates dilation of the stricture.

Esophageal ulcers also represent a major therapeutic problem. Although cimetidine therapy may heal an ulcer, antireflux surgery, if tolerated, is a more reliable mode of treatment. If not, gastric radiation can be employed as in esophageal stricture.

Columnar epithelium may be premalignant. There is no way short of esophageal resection to make certain that the epithelium can be removed. Adequate antireflux therapy will cause regression of columnar epithelium in a rare patient, but further study is necessary before antireflux surgery can be recommended as a treatment for columnar epithelium. The effect of long-term cimetidine therapy on recurrence of either esophagitis or the columnar epithelium is not known.

Treatment of the pulmonary complications of reflux depends on the age of the patient. Infants who present with recurrent bronchitis can be treated by postural methods and by thickening the formula. In adults, attention to posture at night is most important (see above). Since diagnostic methods that establish a direct causal relationship between reflux and lung disease are lacking, caution is advised in offering surgery to those who present with primary pulmonary problems and in whom reflux is demonstrated.

Castell DO, Wu WC, Ott DS: Gastroesophageal Reflux Disease. Mt. Kisco, NY, Futura Publishing Company, 1985, pp 1–324. *Monograph with good literature review.*

Spechler SJ, Goyal RK: Barrett's esophagus. N Engl J Med 315:362, 1986. *Up-to-date review of columnar epithelium.*

MOTOR DISORDERS OF THE ESOPHAGUS

DEFINITION AND PATHOGENESIS. The muscular tube of the esophagus is guarded at both ends by specialized bundles of muscle, the upper and lower esophageal sphincters (UES, LES). Material from the oropharynx is injected at a high velocity (in the case of liquids), and precise coordination is required to link the muscles of the oropharynx, UES, body of the esophagus, and LES into a functional unit. Failure of any or all of these components will result in an esophageal motor disorder.

Failure of the oropharyngeal and UES units can be caused either by primary muscle disease such as *myotonia dystrophica* or *dermatomyositis* or by neurologic lesions involving the innervation of these muscle groups. *Brain stem infarcts, multiple sclerosis*, and *amyotrophic lateral sclerosis* serve as examples for the latter process.

The pathogenesis of motor abnormality of the esophageal

body is less well understood. The striated muscle that constitutes the upper one quarter to one third of the body can be affected by primary muscle disease, such as *myotonia dystrophica*, or by metabolic disease affecting muscle function, such as *hypothyroidism*. The smooth muscle seems more resistant to muscular disease, but the intrinsic nervous network can be involved in *Chagas disease* and *achalasia*. In the latter disease, there is infiltration of Auerbach's plexus with lymphocytes or actual disappearance of the neuron cell bodies in the plexus.

The motor disorders of the body of the esophagus have historically been classified as *achalasia* or *diffuse spasm*. In achalasia, dysphagia and esophageal retention predominate; the radiograph shows a dilated esophagus with a distal beak, and manometry reveals a high pressure in the LES with no or incomplete relaxation as well as only simultaneous low-amplitude contractions in response to a swallow. Diffuse spasm has been characterized as a clinical syndrome of esophageal colic or dysphagia or both; segmental contractions seen by radiograph; and a manometric picture of some peristaltic waves interspersed with periods of slight simultaneous elevation of the baseline pressure in several leads surmounted by simultaneous contractions. Another common manometric abnormality is high-amplitude, long-duration waves that are peristaltic and can be associated with either esophageal colic or dysphagia or both (nutcracker esophagus). There are many variations of these "classic" diseases, and progression from diffuse spasm to achalasia has been documented in the same individual. Many nonspecific motor disorders of the esophagus do not fit these syndromes. The pathophysiology of these nonspecific disorders has not been described. It seems best at the present state of knowledge to be descriptive of the features of a motor disorder without being too precise about an actual name of the disorder.

SYMPTOMS. The type of symptom produced is a function of the level and extent of the problem. *Weakness of the oropharyngeal musculature* may cause *transfer dysphagia*—the inability to propel a solid or liquid bolus from the pharynx to the esophagus. Patients are aware usually that they cannot begin the act of deglutition. Solids are usually more trouble than liquids. Palatal weakness may lead to *nasal regurgitation* of fluids or to *laryngeal aspiration* because of muscular failure to seal off the larynx. Such weakness may be signaled by a nasal quality of the voice.

Incoordination of UES relaxation has been suggested as a cause of transfer dysphagia and for the production of Zenker's diverticulum, but current high-fidelity methods fail to show such incoordination. Transfer dysphagia accompanied by a prominent cricopharyngeal impression on a barium swallow ("cricopharyngeal achalasia") similarly shows no defect in relaxing or in timing when studied by modern manometric methods.

Motor disorders in the body of the esophagus produce either *dysphagia* or *pain*, or both. The dysphagia may be intermittent or continuous. It may be manifest both for solids and for liquids. It is rare for the arrested material to be regurgitated; often posturing (throwing the shoulders back and extending the neck) or a Valsalva maneuver will help the material pass into the stomach.

Pain or esophageal colic is the other major clinical presentation of motor disorders. The pain is usually substernal, described as a feeling of pressure or aching, radiating to the back as well as to the neck, jaw, and arms. It can range in intensity from a transient discomfort to an overwhelming, agonizing pain similar to that of a major myocardial infarction or dissecting aortic aneurysm. The pain may last for only five to ten seconds or may be present for hours. The differentiation between angina pectoris and esophageal colic may be impossible on clinical grounds; both may be related to exercise, have the same intensity and distribution, and respond to sublingual nitroglycerin.

Failure of the lower esophageal sphincter may present with two separate symptom complexes. If the sphincter fails to relax on deglutition (as occurs in achalasia), there will be dysphagia and retention of contents in the body of the esophagus. This failure, coupled with loss of peristalsis (achalasia), leads to marked esophageal retention, regurgitation, and overflow of esophageal contents into the tracheobronchial tree. If there is primary muscle failure of the sphincter, as occurs in *scleroderma*, massive reflux and the consequences of GERD will follow.

DIAGNOSIS. A careful history is essential in choosing the correct diagnostic tools for evaluating esophageal motor disorders. If the difficulty is thought to be in the oropharynx and upper esophageal sphincter, a cineradiograph would offer the most information. The cine film allows for frame-by-frame analysis of this rapidly moving portion of the gastrointestinal tract. Incoordination of tongue and palate, unilateral pharyngeal weakness, and aspiration of small amounts of barium into the trachea on swallowing can be shown. Air double-contrast examinations of the pharynx can elucidate an unsuspected hypopharyngeal carcinoma. A diverticulum or prominence of the cricopharyngeal muscle can also be seen. Manometric examination of the hypopharynx and upper esophageal sphincter has not been helpful.

Radiology offers the best chance of diagnosis when the motor disorders have relatively static changes. In achalasia the body of the esophagus commonly dilates with retention of food, secretions, and barium (Fig. 98–1). Special attention can be paid to the terminal end of the esophagus. In achalasia, there is a smooth, tapering beak. Any irregularity of this beak should lead to a vigorous search for an infiltrating neoplasm of the cardia, which can exactly mimic achalasia clinically and radiologically.

If the esophageal muscle is atonic, as is seen in far-advanced scleroderma, barium and even air will be retained for long periods of time in the supine position. Assumption of the upright position will rapidly clear the barium from the esoph-

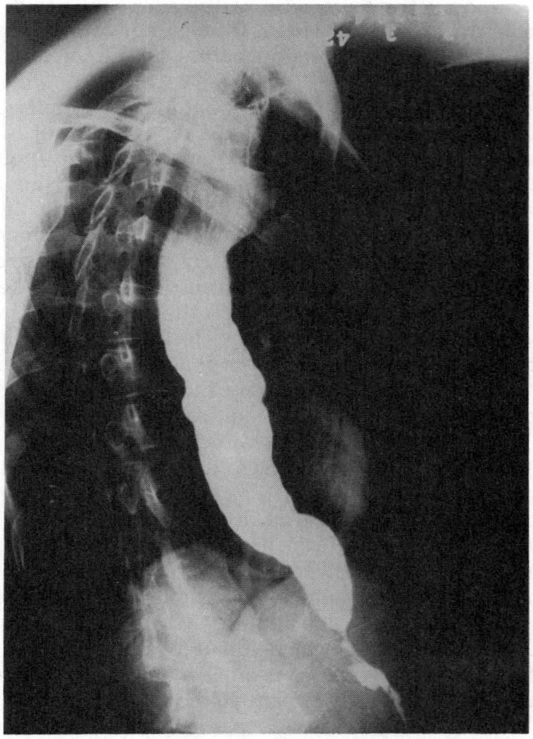

FIGURE 98–1. Radiologic appearance of achalasia. The esophageal body is dilated and terminates in a narrowed segment. (Courtesy of Dr. FE Templeton. From Pope CE II: In Sleisenger MH, Fordtran JS [eds.]: Gastrointestinal Disease. 3rd ed. Philadelphia, W. B. Saunders Company, 1983.)

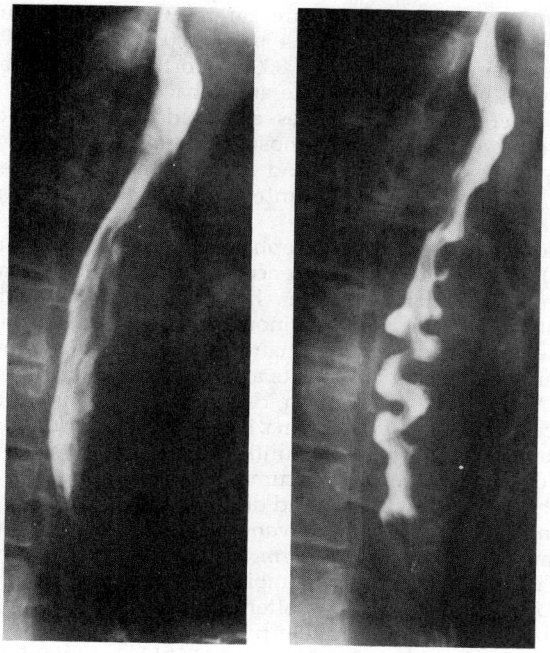

FIGURE 98–2. Radiologic appearance of diffuse spasm. Two spot films were taken within 10 seconds of each other. A fairly normal appearance on the left changes rapidly to an appearance of numerous contractions. (Courtesy of Dr. CA Rohrmann. From Pope CE II: In Sleisenger MH, Fordtran JS [eds.]: Gastrointestinal Disease. 3rd ed. Philadelphia, W. B. Saunders Company, 1983.)

agus and leave a double-contrast view of a dilated esophagus.

The radiologist has more difficulty when the motor abnormality is more intermittent (Fig. 98–2). Such a radiologic appearance is not always evidence for a clinically important motor disorder; elderly patients will often show similar radiologic findings and yet be totally asymptomatic.

Manometric examination allows more prolonged evaluation of esophageal motor function and is the only method that allows lower esophageal sphincter function to be directly determined. Normally, a swallow causes a peristaltic wave to be detected sequentially by pressure detectors spaced along the esophagus. Aperistalsis (no response to a swallow), simultaneous single or multiple contractions, prolonged contractions of high amplitude and low velocity, and spontaneous activity not related to swallowing can be recorded. Some of the "classic" patterns associated with diseases are shown in Figure 98–3. Many subjects present with dysphagia and/or chest pain in different patterns. It is best to describe the radiologic and manometric findings in the individual patient and then try to relate them to the classic syndrome most closely resembled. Also, one syndrome (diffuse spasm) may progress over time to another (achalasia).

Manometric examination can be of special benefit in the evaluation of chest pain if the patient happens to have an attack of chest pain during the examination. If the chest pain is accompanied by motor activity that allows the manometrist to predict onset, intensity, and disappearance of the chest pain by watching the manometric tracing, the diagnosis of an esophageal origin of chest pain is firmly established. Similarly, if pH is being simultaneously monitored and the episodes of chest pain correlate closely with drops in intraesophageal pH, an esophageal origin of pain is likely. Conversely, if typical chest pain occurs but there is no change in motor activity or pH over control values, an esophageal cause of pain is unlikely. Unfortunately, such definitive statements can be made only in about 20 per cent of the patients examined.

Pharmacologic stimulation of the esophagus has been employed for diagnostic purposes using such agents as mecholyl, pentagastrin, bethanechol, and ergonovine, but no universally successful stimulus has yet been found. The possibility of serious coronary ischemia or cardiac arrhythmia with ergonovine limits the usefulness of this agent.

Endoscopy has little usefulness in the evaluation of most motor disorders except for inspection of the cardia with a retroflexed view from the stomach to rule out an infiltrating carcinoma. Possibly transport of radionuclides as measured by a gamma camera will aid in the detection and evaluation of motor disorders.

FIGURE 98–3. Idealized manometric patterns. *A,* The normal swallow consists of a progressive wave with a wave of short duration and rapid rise time in the striated upper esophagus. The lower esophageal sphincter shows a fall in pressure coincident with swallowing. *B,* In achalasia the striated muscle sometimes but not always produces a typical wave. The smooth muscle portion of the esophagus has a simultaneous low-amplitude contraction that follows the striated muscle contraction. The elevated pressure in the LES shows either incomplete or no relaxation. *C,* Diffuse spasm shows an elevation of the baseline after swallowing, on top of which are superimposed repetitive simultaneous contractions. LES pressure may be high and relaxation may terminate prematurely. *D,* High-amplitude, long-duration waves (nutcracker esophagus). The wave is peristaltic but of high amplitude. Duration is increased and velocity of propagation may be decreased. *E,* Scleroderma. Striated muscle contraction is normal, but the amplitude of contraction in the smooth muscle is reduced or may be absent. Sphincter pressure is low.

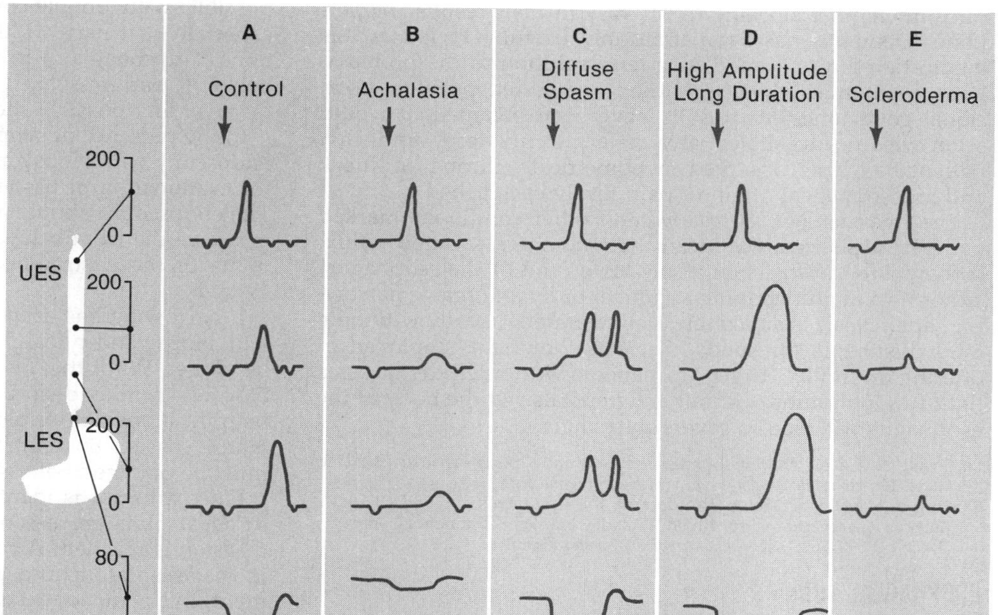

TREATMENT. Of the various motor disorders of the esophagus, only *achalasia* seems amenable to relief. Since the problem in achalasia is one of obstruction of the lower end of the esophagus by a sphincter that will not relax, all forms of therapy are directed at relief of this obstruction. Short-term improvement in clinical symptoms and in scintigraphic esophageal emptying may occur with isosorbide dinitrate, a long-acting nitrate, or with nifedipine, a calcium channel blocker. The place of long-term pharmacologic management of achalasia has not been established. Dilation with a large Hurst bougie may give temporary relief; a few patients have been maintained for long periods of time with weekly self-dilations. Much more effective is brisk dilation with a pneumatic bag under radiographic control. This should be performed by an expert, since the rate of perforation even in good hands is about 5 to 15 per cent. Bag dilation is preferable initially for all patients.

Surgery is reserved for those in whom bag dilation fails or those who do not wish to be exposed to the risk of perforation. Direct section of the lower esophageal sphincter muscle (myotomy) is carried out, sparing some gastric muscle fibers to prevent postoperative reflux (Heller procedure). Amazingly, after both bag dilation and myotomy, manometry reveals return of normal peristalsis in 20 per cent of those with achalasia. This observation is difficult to explain in view of the degeneration of Auerbach's plexus in the intramural nervous network, thought to explain the pathogenesis of this disease.

Treatment of most other motor disorders is much more difficult. Patients with diffuse spasm can be given nitroglycerin or anticholinergics, but the results are disappointing. Balloon dilation has also been suggested to be of benefit in diffuse spasm, but it is difficult to understand how stretching of the lower esophageal sphincter segment would benefit a process that involves the entire esophageal body. Division of all the circular muscle with a long myotomy has been tried, but the long-term results of this procedure are not always favorable.

Treatment of other nonspecific motor disorders associated with chest pain can be equally frustrating. Prescribing sublingual nitroglycerin is justifiable. If it is ineffective, long-acting nitrate therapy will probably not work. Anticholinergic drugs will benefit only a few. Preliminary reports on the use of calcium channel blocking drugs vary in their results. Meperidine (Demerol) has been uniformly useful. Obviously this medication is not a good long-term solution to the problem. Long myotomies have been tried in selected patients; occasional good long-term results have been obtained. It would seem wise not to subject any patient to myotomy until that patient had been observed manometrically during an attack and an esophageal origin of pain firmly established.

The treatment of *scleroderma* and other conditions marked by aperistalsis revolves mostly around the associated reflux. If there is no obstruction at the lower end of the esophagus, either by a malfunctioning sphincter or by an organic narrowing, aperistalsis is amazingly well tolerated, usually with only mild dysphagia for solids. Caution should be employed in offering antireflux surgery to patients with scleroderma, as a tight fundoplication without any peristalsis in the body of the esophagus will lead to severe dysphagia.

Blackwell JN, Castell DO: Oesophageal chest pain: A point of view. Gut 25:1, 1984. *Review of the esophagus as a source of anginal pain.*

Ouyang A, Cohen S: Motor disorders of the esophagus. In Berk JE (ed.): Bockus' Gastroenterology. 4th ed. Philadelphia, W. B. Saunders Company, 1985, pp 690–704. *Good current review of motor disorders.*

ESOPHAGEAL TUMORS

ETIOLOGY AND PATHOGENESIS. Carcinoma of the esophageal epithelium, both squamous cell and adenocarcinoma, is by far the most common and important tumor of the esophagus. Benign neoplasms (leiomyoma, papilloma, and fibrovascular polyps) are rarer by far. Squamous cell cancer has an incidence of 4 per 100,000 in males (United States), rising to 130 per 100,000 in North China. It is associated with both alcohol intake and tobacco smoking in countries where these substances are used. Esophageal cancer occurs more commonly in those who have developed squamous cancers of the head and neck, in those with lye strictures, and in patients with untreated or inadequately treated achalasia.

Adenocarcinoma of the esophagus arises in columnar (Barrett's) epithelium. The sequence of dysplasia, adenoma formation, and adenocarcinoma has been demonstrated. The actual incidence of adenocarcinoma in a patient with columnar epithelium is probably less than the original estimate of 10 to 15 per cent but still represents a significant problem.

SYMPTOMS. In Western countries, the most common clinical symptom of carcinoma is *progressive dysphagia* over a six- to eight-month period until only liquids can be taken. The obstruction reflects circumferential involvement of the esophageal wall by tumor and does not occur until the cancer is biologically rather far advanced. The dysphagia may be accompanied by a *steady, boring pain,* which signals mediastinal involvement and inoperability. In the Orient but not in the United States, pain is often a relatively early sign of a localized and thus resectable tumor. Unexplained persistent chest pain should always be investigated by a careful double-contrast radiographic view of the esophagus or by endoscopy.

More advanced lesions manifest themselves with *halitosis, weight loss,* and *coughing after drinking fluid.* The last-named symptom is caused either by near-complete esophageal lumen obstruction with overspill into the larynx or by the development of a tracheoesophageal fistula. Hoarseness from involvement of the recurrent laryngeal nerve by tumor and hematemesis are unusual symptoms. Nail bed clubbing can be seen with both benign and malignant tumors.

Since dysphagia is the most common presenting symptom of neoplasm of the esophagus, the physician is responsible for making absolutely certain that cancer is not the cause of dysphagia. Early diagnosis affords the only chance for cure. Early diagnosis allows the patient, family, and physician to plan better all aspects of the patient's future.

DIAGNOSIS. The clinical suspicion of a cancer of the esophagus should lead immediately to an esophagogram, possibly with double-contrast techniques. Any irregularity, especially if it narrows the lumen, mandates further evaluation. If dysphagia is present, the radiologist should give a bolus of barium-soaked bread or a large marshmallow to discover any possible sites of arrest.

In the presence of symptoms but a normal barium swallow, endoscopy with biopsy and brushing of any suspicious lesion for examination of tissue and of exfoliated cells is indicated. The endoscopist should always obtain a good retroflexed view of the cardia from below to make certain that an adenocarcinoma of the gastroesophageal junction has not been overlooked.

If narrowing has been seen by barium swallow, endoscopy with biopsy and cytologic brushings of the involved area must be done. With the fiberoptic endoscope, numerous blind biopsies from as deep in the lesion as possible will be most helpful. Biopsy of visible tissue will often reveal only inflammatory tissue. Sometimes as many as eight or nine biopsies must be obtained before tumor is recovered.

Once a tumor is identified, certain procedures in addition to chest films are essential for staging before a therapeutic decision is reached. A careful physical examination for nodal metastases, bronchoscopy for evidence of tracheal involvement, liver function tests plus ultrasound for evidence of liver metastases, and computed tomographic (CT) scanning for mediastinal nodal involvement, esophageal wall thickness, and liver metastases are necessary before the final therapeutic plan is decided upon. A chest roentgenogram is mandatory.

TREATMENT. The ideal form of treating cancer of the esophagus, either for cure or for palliation, has not yet been developed. No series exists in which patients were carefully staged with the best noninvasive methods available and then randomized to different treatment modalities.

Surgical resection of squamous cell carcinoma and adenocarcinoma of the lower one third of the esophagus is preferred in most centers if the patient does not have widespread metastases. Surgery offers the benefit of rapidly restoring esophagogastric continuity. Perhaps only one quarter of all patients presenting to a medical-surgical center will have a resectable tumor; of these patients 20 per cent will not survive the operative period, and five-year survival will be only 5 to 10 per cent, even with extensive resections. Long-term survival cannot be predicted in the individual case by the operative findings. There is growing enthusiasm for palliative resection with restoration of gastrointestinal continuity with stomach or colon. Surgical results in China and Japan, with hospital deaths of 5 per cent and five-year survivals of 20 to 30 per cent, are better than those quoted for the United States. Whether this represents better technical skill, a different type of patient, or earlier diagnosis is not certain.

Radiotherapy is employed in lesions of the upper one third of the esophagus and often in middle third tumors as well. This form of therapy has little hospital mortality, although it carries some short-term and long-term morbidity. With ideal home situations, radiotherapy can be carried out on an outpatient basis. Approximately 40 per cent of tumors cannot be destroyed with conventional 6000-rad therapy. Combination of pre- and postoperative radiation with resective therapy has been employed, but there is no good evidence that such combined therapy is better. Adenocarcinomas occasionally respond to radiotherapy but are not as radiosensitive as squamous cell carcinomas.

When obvious extraesophageal spread is present, palliation with bougienage to restore and maintain an adequate esophageal lumen may be done. If performed with a guide wire under fluoroscopic guidance, such therapy is not hazardous in skilled hands. If dilation does not offer lasting relief, then a Silastic tube can be placed perorally for relief of esophageal obstruction. Such tubes are also of great benefit in the treatment of a malignant tracheoesophageal fistula. Another promising approach is the destruction of intraluminal tumor and restoration of an adequate lumen by laser therapy or an intraluminal heat-coagulating probe.

Choice of therapy will depend on the location and size of the lesion, presence or absence of spread, cell type, and the skills of the medical community. Until an adequate randomized trial after adequate staging is carried out, choice of treatment modality will continue to be a matter of preference.

Earlam R, Cunha-Melo JR: Oesophageal squamous cell carcinoma. Br J Surg 67:381, 457, 1980. *Two articles present exhaustive literature reviews of surgical and radiotherapy of esophageal carcinoma.*

Livstone EM: General considerations of tumors of the esophagus. In Berk JE (ed.): Bockus' Gastroenterology. 4th ed. Philadelphia, W. B. Saunders Company, 1985, pp 818–840. *Review of diagnostic and therapeutic considerations in esophageal carcinoma.*

OTHER CONDITIONS

RINGS AND WEBS. During early development, the lumen of the esophagus becomes completely obliterated and then is recanalized to form the adult hollow viscus. A failure of this process leads to atresia or a residual web. Such webs usually occur in the upper esophagus, often with eccentric openings; occasionally they are multiple. A much more common web or ring is located in the terminal esophagus, has a symmetric opening, and is usually at the junction between squamous and the normal transitional or columnar epithelium of the stomach (Fig. 98–4). This latter ring (Schatzki's ring) can be demonstrated in many individuals if cine studies of the lower esophageal zone are used. It produces symptoms infrequently but in a characteristic manner. An acquired web located in the postcricoid area is sometimes associated with iron deficiency anemia.

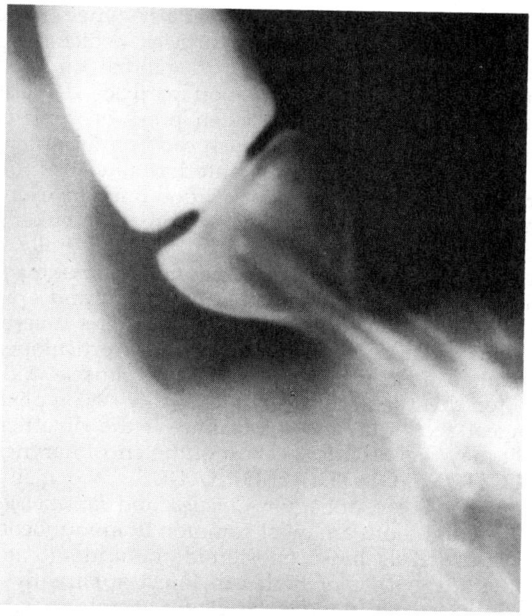

FIGURE 98–4. Lower esophageal ring (Schatzki's ring). This ring consists of a symmetric thin web located in the terminal esophagus. (From Pope CE II: In Sleisinger MH, Fordtran JS [eds.]: Gastrointestinal Disease. 3rd ed. Philadelphia, W. B. Saunders Company, 1983.)

All these types of webs or rings cause dysphagia for solids, and the impacted bolus usually has to be regurgitated. The lower esophageal ring (Schatzki's ring) has a characteristic clinical presentation that allows the diagnosis to be made by history. Every three to four months, after a bolus of meat or bread, the patient will complain of dysphagia and total inability to swallow solids or liquids. The bolus will be regurgitated, and then the patient can continue to eat normally. If the patient comes to the emergency room with an impacted bolus of meat, nothing will be seen after the impacted bolus is removed with the operating endoscope, and the disorder will be labeled as "hysterical dysphagia." The lower esophageal ring is not well seen with the rigid endoscope, as the lower portion of the esophagus cannot be distended enough to force the ring into prominence.

Treatment of all webs involves mechanical disruption either with a dilator or with the endoscope. Treatment of iron deficiency anemia is said to cause the postcricoid webs to disappear. Only very rarely will a surgical approach to a web or ring be necessary.

DIVERTICULA OF THE ESOPHAGUS. Zenker's diverticulum of the pharynx is not anatomically an esophageal diverticulum, as its neck is above the upper esophageal sphincter muscle, but custom has dictated its inclusion in description of esophageal diverticula. An epiphrenic diverticulum usually occurs on the right side of the esophagus just above the lower esophageal sphincter. Other diverticula are at the level of the carina and are known as traction diverticula, although traction by scar tissue is rarely demonstrated. Scleroderma is occasionally associated with numerous wide-mouthed diverticula scattered along the length of the esophagus. Large-amplitude motor waves have been associated with midbody diverticula and either achalasia or motor incoordination with epiphrenic diverticula.

Symptoms vary widely; many diverticula are found by accident during barium examination of the esophagus. If a patient with dysphagia is found to have a diverticulum, it is difficult to tell whether the diverticulum or the associated motor disorder is the cause. Zenker's diverticulum often has a classic symptom complex, particularly when it becomes large. It retains saliva and food particles, which may either be aspirated or cause repeated postprandial throat clearing with production of liquid and food particles. Patients with this type of diverticulum can often press on the neck and empty the diverticulum. The pouch can become so large that it can compress the esophagus anteriorly and obstruct it. In the presence of diverticula great caution must be exercised in passing tubes into the esophagus or stomach. Zenker's diverticulum is a special problem, since tubes naturally enter it rather than the esophageal opening, and the risk of perforation into the mediastinum is great. Traction and epiphrenic diverticula do not require treatment. Zenker's diverticulum, if large, may require diverticulectomy or diverticulopexy with coincident section of the cricopharyngeus muscle. Most techniques for diverticulectomy automatically accomplish cricopharyngeal section at the same time. If the diverticulum is small, it may regress after section of the cricopharyngeus.

INFECTIONS OF THE ESOPHAGUS. Two major infections involve the esophagus: *Candida* and *herpesvirus* infections. Although both are most common in immunocompromised hosts such as those on steroids or undergoing cancer chemotherapy, either or both can infect apparently healthy hosts. Both can be found incidentally at autopsy or during endoscopy for other indications. Most commonly, infection of the mucosa leads to odynophagia of rather marked degree. Dysphagia for both solids and liquids usually accompanies the odynophagia and can be of such intensity that weight loss is rapid.

Although the radiograph occasionally reveals a shaggy mucosa in the case of monilial involvement, and occasionally even a stricture, endoscopy is the best method of detecting and confirming infectious involvement. *Candida* can present as isolated white plaques, which can be confused with glycogenic acanthosis, or progress to form confluent ulcerations with an overlying membrane. Herpesvirus tends to produce isolated ulcers, but extensive involvement can produce confluent ulcerations. Biopsy of the ulcerated area usually shows either invasive hyphae of *Candida* or characteristic nuclear changes of the squamous cells when herpesvirus is present. Cytologic washings occasionally demonstrate the same change.

Treatment depends on correct identification of the etiologic agent. For *Candida* infection, an assessment of the degree of severity is needed. For mild disease, topical therapy with 250,000 units of nystatin (Mycostatin) every two hours will suffice. For more serious infections, low-dose intravenous amphotericin therapy has been successful, the dose being individualized on the basis of weight and renal status. Treatment with miconazole and ketoconazole appears promising. For severe esophageal infections, ketoconazole should be given in doses of 200 mg to 400 mg per day for eight to ten days. Herpesvirus infection is treated symptomatically with viscous lidocaine.

ESOPHAGEAL INJURIES. ***Caustic Ingestion.*** Caustic burns of the esophagus occur in children by accident; adults usually suffer such burns because of suicide attempts. Lye crystals, and especially liquid lye preparations for drain cleaning, are the most common cause. The speed of lye injury is so great that attempts to neutralize the caustic are futile. Detergents and Clorox also find their way into the esophageal lumens of both children and adults. The history is all important, but the degree of esophageal injury still must be assessed endoscopically as an emergency. Significant esophageal damage has been seen even without oral burns; conversely, oral burns do not necessarily mean that the material has reached the esophagus. If there is no esophageal reaction after apparent caustic ingestion, further care directed toward the esophagus will not be necessary.

The accepted therapy of a definite lye or caustic burn remains unsupported by clinical trials. For burns with solid lye or other solid agents, steroids have been recommended, at an initial dose of 80 mg per day, tapering to 20 mg per day until esophageal healing. Most clinicians also use broad-spectrum antibiotics such as ampicillin, 500 mg four times a day. If liquid lye has been the damaging agent, serious consideration of emergency esophagogastrectomy is in order, as lesser measures have met with unacceptably high mortality.

Damage by Medication. A new form of iatrogenic illness of the esophagus has recently become evident. Ingested pills tend to lodge in the esophagus and damage the mucosa in a localized area. Tetracycline, doxycycline, ascorbic acid, and quinidine have all been indicted, and the list will undoubtedly grow. Normal individuals can retain small capsules in the esophagus, even when swallowing in the upright position. The clinical syndrome consists of steady burning or chest pain, accompanied by local odynophagia, all occurring four to six hours after ingestion of one of the offending capsules or tablets. Endoscopy (not clinically necessary) usually shows a localized mucosal ulcer, which heals without a scar within a week. Symptomatic therapy is adequate, but prophylaxis seems to be a more practical idea. Pills of the offending class should be taken in the upright position with several swallows of water.

Esophageal Trauma. The esophagus is well protected by the thoracic cage, but can be involved either by blunt trauma (automobile accidents) or by penetrating missiles (gunshots, knives). Often the surgeon's attention is directed toward more life-threatening damage to heart, lungs, or major blood vessels, and it is understandable that a rent in the esophagus may thus be overlooked. This unfortunate oversight, however, will be followed by mediastinitis, which may worsen an already grave situation. Iatrogenic perforation with endoscope, dilator, or, very rarely, nasogastric tube leads to a similar complication.

Vomiting itself can cause esophageal injury, either mucosal (*Mallory-Weiss*) or through-and-through rupture (*Boerhaave's syndrome*). The mucosal lesion first described by Mallory and Weiss has been recognized much more frequently since the advent of rapid emergency endoscopy with fiberoptic endoscopes. Classically, the patient has repeated attacks of retching, productive at first of gastric contents, and later of bright red blood. One quarter of patients shown to have a Mallory-Weiss tear have no prior history of vomiting. The tear is usually in the gastric mucosa just below the gastroesophageal junction, although it can extend through the junction and up into the esophageal mucosa. Diagnosis of this condition is almost always made at endoscopy; the rent is usually seen as the endoscope is being withdrawn from the stomach into the esophagus. The majority of such lesions heal with conservative therapy. Angiographic or surgical therapy is necessary in less than 5 per cent.

Vomiting can also cause a complete tear in the esophageal wall. Unlike the Mallory-Weiss lesion, the tear in Boerhaave's syndrome is located above the gastroesophageal junction on the left side. It usually follows vomiting, but other marked increases in intra-abdominal pressure such as lifting a heavy weight or straining at stool have been associated with a tear. The clinical diagnosis can be extremely difficult; often patients with esophageal rupture are thought to have a myocardial infarct, pneumothorax, a perforated viscus, or pancreatitis. Air in the mediastinum or the rapid appearance of a hydrothorax on the left usually leads to the correct diagnosis.

The diagnosis of esophageal perforation can usually be established by a cautious radiographic examination with water-soluble material. Barium may be used only if a rent is not demonstrated by the water-soluble agent. Immediate surgical repair is the accepted method of treatment of esophageal perforation. In those too ill for surgery, treatment consists of nasogastric suction, antibiotics, and subsequent mediastinal drainage if necessary.

Pope CE II, McDonald GB: Rings and webs; Diverticula; Involvement of the esophagus by infections, systemic illnesses, and physical agents. In Sleisenger MH, Fordtran JS (eds.): Gastrointestinal Disease. 4th ed. Philadelphia, W. B. Saunders Company (in press). *Textbook review of these various conditions.*

99 GASTRITIS

Charles T. Richardson

DEFINITION. Inflammation of the stomach mucosa may be diffuse and involve all parts of the stomach or localized to the fundus and body or antrum (see Fig. 100–1). Even within a specific area (e.g., the antrum), inflammation may be diffuse or localized. Gastritis is classified as acute or chronic primarily on the basis of histologic and/or endoscopic findings and long-term clinical follow-up. Acute gastritis is believed to be a self-limited disease, whereas chronic gastritis by definition persists for long periods of time.

ACUTE GASTRITIS

ETIOLOGY. Nonsteroidal anti-inflammatory drugs (such as aspirin), ethanol, bile salts, and pancreatic enzymes damage the gastric mucosa and are believed to cause both acute and chronic gastritis (see Chronic Gastritis, below). How these chemical agents cause gastritis is not known. They are thought to disrupt the so-called "gastric mucosal barrier" (the ability of gastric mucosa to restrict movement of hydrogen ions from lumen to mucosa), thereby allowing back-diffusion of acid and pepsin, and in this manner to contribute to the development of gastritis. Inhibition of prostaglandin synthesis by nonsteroidal anti-inflammatory drugs also may be a factor in the pathogenesis of acute gastritis in patients who are treated with these drugs.

Acute gastritis also occurs in the setting of severe medical or surgical illnesses such as respiratory failure, sepsis, renal failure, hypotension, or trauma. This form of acute gastritis is called "stress"-induced gastritis and may produce "stress" bleeding. Mucosal ischemia is believed to be an important factor in the pathogenesis of "stress"-related gastritis. Gastric acid is also likely to be involved, since in experimental models mucosal damage does not occur in the absence of acid. Bile and pancreatic juices also may be contributing factors.

Infectious agents cause some forms of acute gastritis. An example is a rare but fulminant and often fatal form of acute bacterial gastritis called acute phlegmonous gastritis. Streptococci are most commonly the cause, although staphylococci, *Escherichia coli,* and *Proteus* have been cultured from stomachs of patients with acute phlegmonous gastritis.

Gastric *Campylobacter*-like organisms (GCLO) are found in some patients with either acute or chronic gastritis. Although evidence suggests that these organisms cause gastritis, a cause-and-effect relationship has not been firmly established, since these same bacteria have been found also in gastric mucosa of normal humans.

An epidemic form of acute gastritis has been reported to be associated with decreased gastric acid secretion (hypochlorhydria). Since gastritis occurred in a number of different persons who were in contact with each other over a relatively brief period of time, an infectious etiology was suspected. In fact, some investigators have postulated that this acute gastritis with hypochlorhydria was due to GCLO.

Additional causes of acute gastritis include roentgen irradiation, ingestion of corrosive substances, and ingestion of staphylococcal exotoxin.

CLINICAL MANIFESTATIONS. Patients with acute gastritis secondary to aspirin, other nonsteroidal anti-inflammatory drugs, or "stress" may have hematemesis and/or melena and pain, nausea, and vomiting. This form of acute gastritis is called acute hemorrhagic or erosive gastritis. At times, bleeding can be so severe that patients develop hypotension or shock. In contrast, other patients with acute gastritis secondary to nonsteroidal anti-inflammatory drugs may have minimal gastrointestinal bleeding detected only by testing stools for occult blood.

Finding acute gastritis on biopsy does not necessarily mean that a patient has clinically important disease, since as many as 30 per cent of otherwise healthy, asymptomatic persons can have acute gastritis on biopsy. Also, some forms of acute gastritis with known cause, such as acute irradiation gastritis, are not associated with symptoms. However, patients with other causes of gastritis may have symptoms. For example, some patients with epidemic gastritis with hypochlorhydria have epigastric pain, nausea, and vomiting.

The physical examination in patients with acute gastritis is usually normal unless bleeding or other illnesses such as liver disease or arthritis are present. If bleeding occurs, the patient may have a reduced hematocrit, increased blood urea nitrogen, and a positive nasogastric aspirate or stool guaiac test for blood. Unless there are concomitant diseases, other laboratory studies are usually normal (see Ch. 114).

DIAGNOSIS. Most clinically significant forms of acute gastritis are associated with mucosal abnormalities that can be visualized at endoscopy (Table 99–1). For example, in acute gastritis secondary to aspirin or "stress," the gastric mucosa often appears congested, and petechial hemorrhages, erosions, and superficial ulcerations cover the mucosal surface. These changes may be diffuse, although the fundus and body are most severely affected.

In the strictest sense, the diagnosis of acute gastritis is made by the pathologist from the histologic findings of the biopsy specimen. Inflammatory cells (usually neutrophils and mononuclear cells) infiltrate the lamina propria, whereas the glandular areas are distorted by edema and hemorrhage. Exudate often fills the gastric pits and/or glands (pit and/or gland abscesses). In severe forms of gastritis (e.g., aspirin- or "stress"-induced), focal sloughing of surface epithelial cells can occur, producing superficial erosions and ulcerations.

NATURAL HISTORY. The major feature differentiating acute from chronic gastritis is the tendency for mucosal changes in acute gastritis to revert to normal. The time over which this occurs depends on the type of acute gastritis and on the method used to detect the endpoint. For example, in acute hemorrhagic gastritis the endoscopic appearance of the gastric mucosa may revert to normal within 24 to 48 hours after bleeding has stopped. Histologic reversion to normal may require a longer period of time.

Some patients with epidemic gastritis with hypochlorhydria have had moderate-to-severe gastritis on biopsy from 2 to 5 months after initial diagnosis and moderate gastritis even up to 12 months. Acute gastritis is a reversible lesion, but histologic abnormalities may persist for months in some forms. Whether acute gastritis progresses to chronic gastritis in some patients is not known.

TREATMENT. Most patients with acute gastritis do not require treatment. For example, acute gastritis found on biopsy in asymptomatic, healthy persons need not be treated. Treatment with antacids may be warranted in symptomatic patients who have a histologic diagnosis of acute gastritis and in whom other causes of symptoms have been excluded. Since there have been no controlled clinical trials evaluating antacids in the treatment of acute gastritis, the effectiveness and dosage are not known. Bismuth-containing compounds

TABLE 99–1. TYPES OF GASTRITIS, METHOD OF DIAGNOSIS, AND ENDOSCOPIC, BARIUM X-RAY, AND/OR HISTOLOGIC FINDINGS

Types of Gastritis	Method of Diagnosis*	Endoscopic, Barium X-ray, and/or Histologic Findings
Acute		
Drug-induced (salicylates or other nonsteroidal anti-inflammatory drugs or alcohol)	Endoscopy	Congested mucosa with petechial hemorrhages and erosions.
	Histology	Neutrophils and mononuclear cells infiltrate the lamina propria; edema and hemorrhage distort the glands; inflammatory cells fill the pits and glands, forming small abscesses.
Stress-induced (secondary to severe medical or surgical diseases or trauma)	Endoscopy	Erythema, petechial hemorrhages, and erosions cover most of the mucosa.
	Histology	Inflammatory cells (primarily neutrophils) infiltrate the lamina propria; edema and hemorrhage distort the glands; pit and gland abscesses and focal sloughing of surface cells can be seen.
Chronic		
Superficial	Histology	Inflammatory cells (neutrophils, lymphocytes, plasma cells, and a few eosinophils) are limited to the gastric pits and upper lamina propria.
Atrophic	Histology	Inflammatory cells are located superficially but also invade deeper into the lamina propria; thinning of the mucosa with loss of glandular elements and intestinal metaplasia may occur.
Gastric atrophy	Histology	More severe form of atrophic gastritis; a marked reduction in mucosal thickness with loss of parietal and chief cells occurs; only a few inflammatory cells are present.
Special Types		
Giant hypertrophic	Endoscopy or barium x-ray	Large folds are usually confined to the fundus and body but may involve the antrum.
	Histology	Hyperplasia of mucus, parietal, and chief cells; large cystic spaces containing mucus are often seen.
Eosinophilic	Endoscopy or barium x-ray	Rigid, nondistensible antrum and/or thickened mucosal folds are usually seen.
	Histology	Eosinophils infiltrate the lamina propria, submucosa, and muscular layers.
Granulomatous	Endoscopy or barium x-ray	Involved portions of the stomach are narrowed and rigid.
	Histology	Granulomas are found in the mucosa and submucosa and occasionally can be found in the muscular layer and serosa.

*Some clinicians and investigators believe that gastritis is always a histologic diagnosis and that the findings on endoscopy and barium radiography only suggest what the pathologist might find on the histologic stain.

are believed to eradicate GCLO from gastric mucosa. Therefore, some investigators have advocated using Pepto-Bismol to treat patients suspected of having GCLO-induced gastritis.

Patients with acute hemorrhagic gastritis present special therapeutic problems. Many of these patients experience severe upper gastrointestinal bleeding that requires treatment, including fluid and blood replacement and nasogastric lavage. Since acid and pepsin probably play a role in the pathogenesis, it seems reasonable to reduce gastric acidity and concomitantly peptic activity with antacids and/or cimetidine or ranitidine. Recent results suggest that sucralfate also may be useful in preventing "stress"-induced ulceration and bleeding. Surgical therapy is to be avoided if at all possible because of its inordinately high morbidity and mortality.

Initially, an antacid (usually 30 ml of a liquid aluminum-magnesium preparation) is prescribed every hour during the day and night; higher doses or more frequent administration may be needed in some patients. A combination of antacid plus cimetidine or ranitidine has been recommended by some physicians. Measurement of intragastric pH every hour and administration of medications in doses to keep intragastric pH above 3.5 have been suggested. Such a regimen prevents "stress"-induced ulcerations and bleeding in a large percentage of critically ill patients and is recommended in treating such patients; however, there is no evidence that maintaining pH above 3.5 controls bleeding or assists in healing acute hemorrhagic gastritis once it occurs.

CHRONIC GASTRITIS

CLASSIFICATION. Chronic gastritis is usually classified on the basis of mucosal histology and/or the anatomic portion of the stomach involved. Although endoscopic and radiologic criteria for classifying chronic gastritis have been reported, gastric mucosal biopsy is the most reliable means of diagnosis. Biopsies should be obtained from several different areas, since chronic gastritis may be a localized disease.

HISTOLOGY. Chronic gastritis is divided into superficial gastritis, atrophic gastritis, and gastric atrophy (Table 99–1). When inflammatory cells are limited to the gastric pits and upper lamina propria, gastritis is classified as superficial. In atrophic gastritis inflammatory cells invade deeper into the lamina propria and glandular epithelium. Lymphoid follicles may also be seen. As the disease progresses, thinning of the mucosa occurs with loss of glandular elements. In some patients intestinal metaplasia develops with loss of parietal and chief cells and development of goblet cells, absorptive cells, and intestinal villi. Finally, in patients with gastric atrophy, parietal and chief cells are absent, mucosal thickness is reduced markedly, and only a small number of inflammatory cells are present.

LOCATION. Chronic atrophic gastritis has been divided into Type A and Type B, based primarily on the anatomic portion of the stomach involved and the presence or absence of parietal cell antibodies. In Type A gastritis the fundus and body of the stomach are involved, whereas the antrum is relatively normal. Parietal cell antibodies are found in a large percentage of patients, and pernicious anemia may develop. On the other hand, in Type B gastritis the antrum is involved primarily, although inflammation is found frequently in the fundus and body. Parietal cell antibodies do not occur. Immunologic, functional, and clinical differences between these two types of gastritis will be discussed below.

ETIOLOGY. The causes of chronic gastritis are unknown. Radiation injury, nutritional deficiencies, endocrine disorders, and infectious diseases have been postulated but not proved to cause chronic gastritis. Gastric *Campylobacter*-like organisms (GCLO) have been found in association with histologic evidence of chronic gastritis, but a cause-and-effect relationship has not been established (see Acute Gastritis, above). Repeated insults to the gastric mucosa by mechanical, thermal, or chemical agents have also been thought to cause chronic musocal changes. Long-term alcohol or aspirin ingestion may lead to chronic gastritis, although this has not been clearly established.

Reflux of duodenal juice into the stomach is believed to irritate gastric mucosa and perhaps lead to chronic gastritis. Lysolecithin, which is formed when phospholipase A from pancreatic juice reacts with lecithin from bile, appears to be the most damaging constituent of refluxed duodenal juice. Lysolecithin, bile, and pancreatic juice are postulated to initiate the process leading to gastritis by removing the mucus layer from the epithelial surface. This leads to damage of the "mucosal barrier," allowing diffusion of gastric acid and pepsin into the mucosa. This, in turn, leads to further mucosal damage.

Immunologic injury may play a role in the pathogenesis of chronic gastritis in some patients. Patients with atrophic gastritis of the fundus and body (Type A gastritis) usually have antibodies against parietal cells, and some, but not all, of these patients develop pernicious anemia. Approximately 90 per cent of patients with pernicious anemia have parietal cell antibodies. Many also have antibodies to intrinsic factor, which may be of two types: (1) a blocking antibody, which reacts with the vitamin B_{12}–intrinsic factor binding site and blocks the binding of vitamin B_{12} and intrinsic factor; or (2) a binding antibody, which can react either with intrinsic factor alone or with intrinsic factor–vitamin B_{12} complex.

Antibody to gastrin-producing cells occurs in a few but not all patients with gastritis primarily involving the antrum (Type B gastritis). This finding adds further support for the role of immunologic abnormalities in the development of chronic gastritis. These patients do not have parietal cell or intrinsic factor antibodies and do not develop pernicious anemia.

Whether parietal cell and other cellular antibodies lead to mucosal destruction or whether they are markers of mucosal damage caused by other mechanisms is not known. Repeated injection of cellular antibodies can lead to gastric atrophy and decreased acid secretion in laboratory animals, suggesting that development of antibodies may be the initiating event. Serum of some patients with pernicious anemia has been found to contain an autoantibody that is cytotoxic to canine gastric mucosal cells. On the other hand, patients with adult-onset hypogammaglobulinemia can develop gastric atrophy and pernicious anemia even though they do not have antibodies to parietal cells or intrinsic factor.

Genetic influences also have been implicated in the development of chronic gastritis. Family members of patients with pernicious anemia have a higher incidence of atrophic gastritis, achlorhydria, vitamin B_{12} malabsorption, and parietal cell and intrinsic factor antibodies than does the general population. The role of genetics in patients with chronic gastritis who do not have pernicious anemia has not been adequately explored.

Theoretically, gastric atrophy could also develop from the absence of a mucosal trophic factor such as gastrin, urogastrone, or epidermal growth factor, or from end-organ resistance to one of these factors. So far, there are no studies evaluating these possibilities.

CLINICAL MANIFESTATIONS. As with acute gastritis, many patients with chronic gastritis and no other underlying disease are asymptomatic and have a normal physical examination. For example, it is rare for patients with pernicious anemia to have symptoms related to gastritis or gastric atrophy. Symptoms such as nausea, vomiting, and epigastric pain can occur in patients with chronic gastritis; however, studies have shown a poor correlation between presence or absence of symptoms and histologic evidence of gastritis. Thus a biopsy diagnosis of chronic gastritis should not be used as the sole explanation for upper gastrointestinal symptoms, and other causes such as peptic ulcer disease, gastric cancer, or cholelithiasis should be excluded.

Other clinical findings in patients with chronic gastritis relate to abnormalities in laboratory studies. Gastric acid secretion usually is lower than normal and is especially low or absent in patients with atrophic gastritis or gastric atrophy. Decreased secretion of pepsin also occurs. Patients with gastritis involving the fundus and body but sparing the antrum (Type A gastritis) usually are hypo- or achlorhydric and have elevated serum gastrin concentrations presumably secondary to an alkaline antral pH (sometimes as high as in patients with Zollinger-Ellison syndrome). When gastritis involves the antrum primarily (Type B gastritis), acid secretion is usually diminished but serum gastrin concentration is in the normal range.

In patients with pernicious anemia, the vitamin B_{12} absorption test (Schilling test) is abnormal when performed in the absence of exogenous intrinsic factor, and in untreated patients signs and symptoms of vitamin B_{12} deficiency may develop. Some patients with pernicious anemia have clinical and laboratory evidence of other diseases such as Hashimoto's thyroiditis, hypothyroidism, hyperthyroidism, insulin-dependent diabetes mellitus, or vitiligo.

NATURAL HISTORY. Chronic gastritis is a longstanding disease that increases in frequency with advancing age. The process in an individual patient is thought to progress over time from superficial gastritis to chronic atrophic gastritis to gastric atrophy, but this has not been established. It is also not known whether all patients who later in life are found to have gastric atrophy initially had superficial gastritis. In one study, patients with chronic superficial gastritis were followed for 10 to 20 years. Superficial gastritis persisted, relatively unchanged, in half of the patients, whereas progression to atrophic gastritis occurred in most of the remainder. Reversion to normal was also noted in a few patients.

Associations have been reported between chronic gastritis and gastric polyps, benign gastric ulcer, and gastric cancer. Although benign gastric ulcers usually occur in an area of chronic superficial or atrophic gastritis, it is not known whether gastritis precedes and perhaps leads to gastric ulcer formation or whether gastritis develops in response to ulceration. Gastric cancer may occur more frequently in patients with both Types A and B gastritis; however, numerically the incidence is higher in Type B.

TREATMENT. Most patients with chronic gastritis do not require treatment for the following reasons: (1) the pathogenesis of chronic gastritis is poorly understood; thus, it is difficult to design rational therapy; (2) most patients with chronic gastritis are asymptomatic; and (3) there is no evidence that therapy prevents sequelae such as gastric atrophy, pernicious anemia, or cancer.

Although pernicious anemia cannot be prevented, it seems reasonable to follow patients with known gastric atrophy for development of either signs or symptoms of pernicious anemia or low serum B_{12} levels. Glucocorticoid therapy can partially reverse the gastric mucosal changes in patients with pernicious anemia, but chronic therapy with steroids is impractical and dangerous.

Patients with pernicious anemia should be evaluated for other diseases such as thyroid disease or diabetes mellitus, and their relatives should be screened for pernicious anemia. Whether or not patients with pernicious anemia and/or gastric atrophy should be screened periodically for gastric cancer is controversial.

SPECIAL TYPES OF GASTRITIS

GIANT HYPERTROPHIC GASTRITIS. Several relatively uncommon clinical syndromes are characterized by gastric mucosal hypertrophy. These syndromes are usually included under the heading of giant hypertrophic gastritis, although inflammatory cells are not always present. The most commonly recognized syndrome is *Menetrier's disease*, which is characterized by gastric mucosal hypertrophy, hyposecretion of gastric acid, increased loss of protein from the stomach, edema, weight loss, and occasionally pain, nausea, and vomiting. Another syndrome, *hypertrophic hypersecretory gastropathy*, is similar but is associated with hypersecretion of acid. These syndromes are more commonly found in men than in women and usually occur between the ages of 30 and 50, although a childhood variety has been described. Gastric atrophy and parietal cell antibodies have been reported as late developments in a few patients.

Diagnosis is based on clinical findings, appearances of large mucosal folds on upper gastrointestinal x-ray series or endoscopy, and histologic appearance of mucosal biopsies (Table 99–1). Large mucosal folds are usually limited to the fundus and body of the stomach, although the antrum may be involved. Mucosal biopsy reveals hyperplasia of all three glandular elements—parietal, chief, and mucus-secreting cells. Because of the enlarged folds, other diseases such as Zollinger-Ellison syndrome, infiltrating carcinoma, lymphoma, or amyloid must be excluded.

In some patients medical therapy with anticholinergic drugs has led to reduced gastric secretion, decreased protein loss, and clinical improvement. Cimetidine also has been reported to decrease protein loss, although the mechanism is unknown. One or both of these therapies should be tried prior to surgical intervention. Some patients have been treated successfully with vagotomy and pyloroplasty. In a few patients, persistent, severe protein loss or recurrent gastrointestinal hemorrhage may necessitate total gastrectomy.

EOSINOPHILIC GASTRITIS (GASTROENTERITIS). Eosinophilic infiltration of the gastrointestinal tract can involve the stomach and/or small intestine. Peripheral eosinophilia also commonly occurs. The pathogenesis is poorly understood, although allergic or immunologic factors are thought to be involved. Both IgE-mediated and IgE-independent mechanisms have been implicated.

Gastric involvement is usually limited to the antrum. On biopsy eosinophils infiltrate the mucosa and the muscular layer (Table 99–1). This leads to antral rigidity and thickening of mucosal folds. Delayed gastric emptying and/or gastric outlet obstruction may occur. On x-ray it is often difficult to differentiate eosinophilic gastritis from granulomatous disease or neoplasm. Clinically, patients usually present with pain, nausea, and vomiting. Occasionally, eosinophils may invade the serosa, leading to ascites.

Eosinophilic gastritis is often a self-limited disease, but in some patients symptoms persist or recur. Corticosteroid therapy has been useful in alleviating obstructive signs and symptoms as well as ascites.

GRANULOMATOUS GASTRITIS. Granulomas can be found in the stomach as part of generalized diseases such as tuberculosis, histoplasmosis, sarcoidosis, syphilis, or Crohn's disease, or may be limited to the stomach and unassociated with other diseases. Two examples of the latter are eosinophilic granuloma (a separate disease from eosinophilic gastritis) and isolated (idiopathic) granulomatous gastritis.

On upper gastrointestinal x-ray the involved portions of the stomach appear rigid and narrowed and the x-ray appearance is often similar to that of malignancy (Table 99–1). The antrum is most often involved, although granulomas can be found also in the mucosa of the body and fundus. Mucosal biopsies reveal granulomas in the mucosa and submucosa, and in surgical specimens granulomas have been found in the muscular layer and serosa. Ulcerations may also occur. Because of the malignant appearance on x-ray, cancer must be ruled out in all patients by multiple biopsies and/or cytology.

Because of problems with differentiating granulomatous gastritis from malignancy, the condition in most patients is diagnosed at the time of surgery. If the diagnosis of granulomatous gastritis is made preoperatively, a search should be made for a primary disease and therapy should be tailored to the specific disease (e.g., tuberculosis). If an etiology cannot be found and malignancy has been excluded, the patient should be observed for several weeks, since spontaneous resolution of isolated granulomatous gastritis has been reported. If resolution does not occur, surgical therapy is indicated.

GASTRITIS FOLLOWING GASTRIC SURGERY. Gastritis is a common histologic and endoscopic finding after either a subtotal gastrectomy or antrectomy has been performed for peptic ulcer disease. This form of gastritis is often referred to as bile reflux or alkaline gastritis, reflecting the theory that it is caused by the reflux of bile or pancreatic juice or both into the gastric remnant. Features believed to be compatible with the diagnosis include (1) epigastric pain, heartburn, nausea, and vomiting (often vomiting of bile-containing material) and/or weight loss; (2) presence of bile in the gastric remnant; (3) endoscopic evidence of gastritis; and (4) histologic evidence of gastritis. None of these features, however, are specific for the diagnosis. For example, such symptoms frequently occur following ulcer surgery with or without histologic or endoscopic evidence of gastritis. Furthermore, histologic or endoscopic changes can occur in postoperative patients who are asymptomatic. The presence of bile in the gastric remnant also does not mean necessarily that patients have bile-induced gastritis, because it is very easy for bile and other duodenal contents to reflux into the gastric remnant. Thus, caution should be exercised in making the diagnosis of bile reflux gastritis.

Cholestyramine or aluminum hydroxide antacids, as bile acid–binding agents, have been given to patients with postgastrectomy gastritis but usually do not alleviate symptoms or reverse the histologic appearance of gastritis. As noted, bile acids alone may not be responsible for symptoms associated with "bile reflux gastritis"; other substances such as pancreatic secretions may be needed. Corrective surgery has consisted of procedures designed to divert duodenal contents away from the gastric remnant. The most commonly used operation is called a Roux-en-Y diversion. Some, but not all, studies have shown this procedure to be successful in relieving symptoms in some patients. Thus, surgery should be reserved for patients with incapacitating symptoms.

Meyer JH: Reflections on reflux gastritis (editorial.) Gastroenterology 77:1143, 1979.

Miller TA: Stress erosive gastritis. In Moody FG, Carey LC, Jones RS, et al. (eds.): Surgical Treatment of Digestive Disease. Chicago, Year Book Medical Publishers, 1986, pp 203–215. *A review of the pathophysiology, methods of prophylaxis, and the medical and surgical treatment of stress erosive gastritis.*

Peura DA, Johnson LF: Cimetidine for prevention and treatment of gastroduodenal mucosal lesions in patients in an intensive care unit. Ann Intern Med 103:173, 1985. *Results of this study demonstrate that cimetidine is better than placebo at treating mucosal abnormalities already present in the stomach or duodenum and is better than placebo in preventing mucosal disease from occurring in patients who are critically ill and who are in an intensive care unit.*

Priebe HJ, Skillman JJ, Bushnell LS, et al.: Antacid versus cimetidine in preventing acute gastrointestinal bleeding: A randomized trial in 75 critically ill patients. N Engl J Med 302:426, 1980. *Antacid was better than cimetidine for protecting seriously ill patients from developing acute upper gastrointestinal tract bleeding.*

Sauerbruch T, Schreiber MA, Schussler P, et al.: Endoscopy in the diagnosis of gastritis: Diagnostic value of endoscopic criteria in relation to histological diagnosis. Endoscopy 16:101, 1984. *Histologic examination of biopsy specimens obtained from the stomach is a better method for diagnosing gastritis than endoscopic appearance.*

Weinstein WM: Gastritis. In Sleisenger MH, Fordtran JS (eds.): Gastrointestinal Disease. 4th ed. Philadelphia, W. B. Saunders Company, 1987.

100 PEPTIC ULCER

100.1 Pathogenesis

Charles T. Richardson

DEFINITION

Ulcers are defects in the gastrointestinal mucosa that penetrate the muscularis mucosa. This distinguishes them from superficial erosions that do not extend through the muscularis mucosa. Peptic ulcers usually occur in the stomach, pylorus, or duodenal bulb but also can develop in the esophagus and the postbulbar duodenum. In patients with markedly increased acid secretion (as in Zollinger-Ellison syndrome) ulcers sometimes develop in the distal duodenum and jejunum.

Peptic ulcers occasionally occur in the ileum in or near Meckel's diverticula.

Originally, all ulcers in the upper gastrointestinal tract were believed to be caused by the aggressive action of hydrochloric acid and pepsin on the mucosa. Thus they became known as "peptic ulcers." Although acid and pepsin are secreted by most patients with benign ulcers, they are not the only causes of ulcers. Ulcers probably result from several different pathogenetic mechanisms. In general, ulcers occur when luminal aggressive factors overcome opposing mucosal defenses. Mechanisms believed important in the pathogenesis of ulcer disease are discussed in greater detail below.

NORMAL PHYSIOLOGY

STRUCTURE. The stomach is divided into four anatomic regions: the cardia, fundus, body, and antrum (Fig. 100–1). *Parietal cells,* which secrete acid, and *chief cells,* which secrete pepsinogen, are located primarily in the fundus and body, although a few are found in the antrum. *Gastrin (G) cells* are located in the antrum.

Gastric mucosa is made up of a series of pits and glands (Fig. 100–2). The pits contain surface epithelial cells, whereas the glands contain mucous, parietal, endocrine, and chief cells. Normal gastric juice is a mixture of parietal secretion (acid and intrinsic factor) and nonparietal secretions (mucus, bicarbonate, sodium, potassium, and pepsinogen).

CONTROL OF GASTRIC SECRETION. Three endogenous chemicals (acetylcholine, gastrin, and histamine) stimulate acid secretion (Fig. 100–3): (1) *Acetylcholine,* believed to be a neural transmitter, is released by vagal efferent neurons. Vagal stimulation of acid secretion occurs when humans see, smell, taste, chew, or think about appetizing food. Local neurons within the wall of the stomach also release acetylcholine and are activated when the stomach is distended. (2) *Gastrin* is a hormone responsible for acid secretion. Protein in food is the most potent stimulant of gastrin release, but vagal stimulation, calcium, other cations such as magnesium and aluminum, and alkalinization of the antrum also release gastrin. Gastrin release is inhibited by acid within the lumen of the antrum. (3) *Histamine* stimulates acid secretion via a paracrine mechanism. Mastlike cells that contain histamine are located in the lamina propria of the stomach in close proximity to parietal cells. When histamine is liberated from mast cells, it diffuses through intercellular spaces to reach parietal cells. Gastrin or acetylcholine or both may release histamine from mast cells. Acetylcholine, gastrin, and histamine are believed to act on receptors on parietal cell membranes to cause acid secretion (see Ch. 100.3, on medical therapy of peptic ulcer disease).

Mechanisms within parietal cells that lead to acid secretion are not well defined. It is believed that cyclic adenosine monophosphate (AMP) is important in the mediation of histamine-stimulated acid secretion, while calcium entry into parietal cells is believed to play a role in acetylcholine-stimulated secretion. A hydrogen/potassium adenosine triphosphatase (ATPase) enzyme is located on the luminal surface of parietal cells (Ch. 100.3). This enzyme serves as a proton pump, which is the final step in secretion of hydrogen ions.

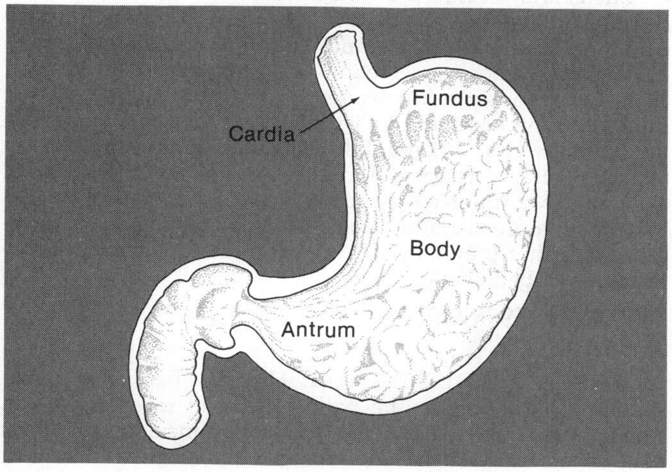

FIGURE 100–1. Anatomic divisions of the stomach.

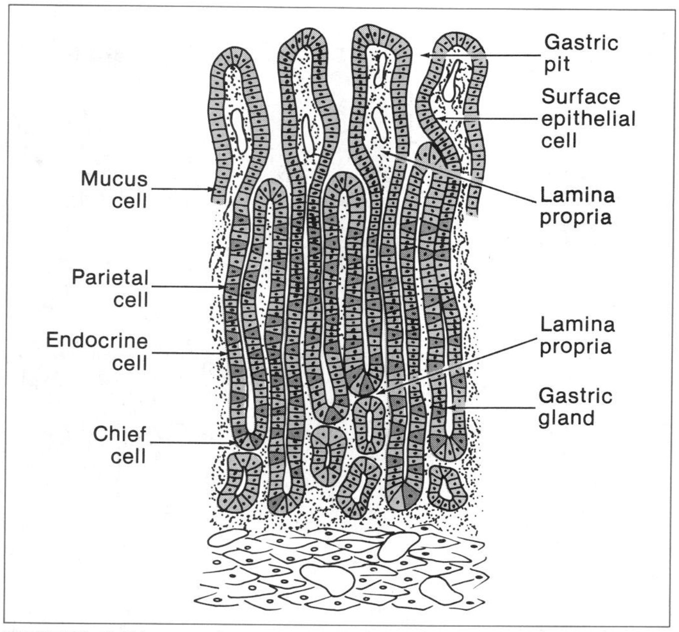

FIGURE 100–2. Diagram demonstrating the cell types lining the pits and glands of the gastric mucosa.

PRODUCTS OF GASTRIC SECRETION. In the pathogenesis of peptic ulcer the two most important products of gastric secretion are hydrochloric acid and pepsin.

Secretion of Acid. Basal acid output (BAO) is the amount of acid secreted under fasting or unstimulated conditions. Peak acid output (PAO) or maximum acid output (MAO) is acid secreted in response to an injection of either pentagastrin or histamine, the maximal amount of acid that a normal subject or patient with ulcer disease can secrete. MAO reflects the number of parietal cells in an individual, and the ratio of BAO to MAO represents the fraction of parietal cell mass functional under basal conditions. Thus, if a patient has an increased amount of gastrin, acetylcholine, or histamine near

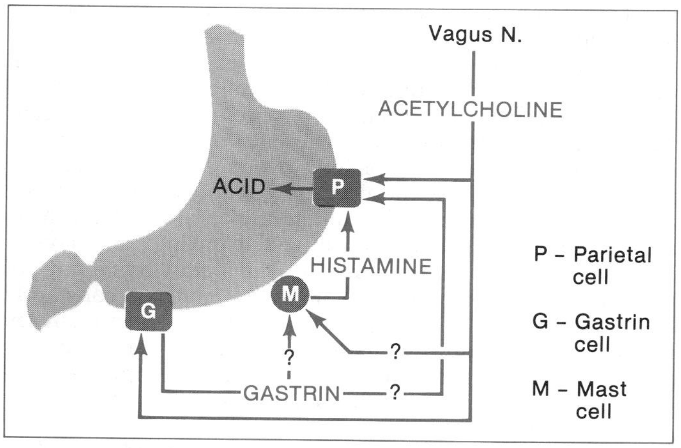

FIGURE 100–3. Model illustrating the chemical stimulants of acid secretion. Acetylcholine originates in the vagus nerves; gastrin is released from gastrin cells in the antrum; and histamine is liberated from mast cells in the lamina propria of the gastric mucosa.

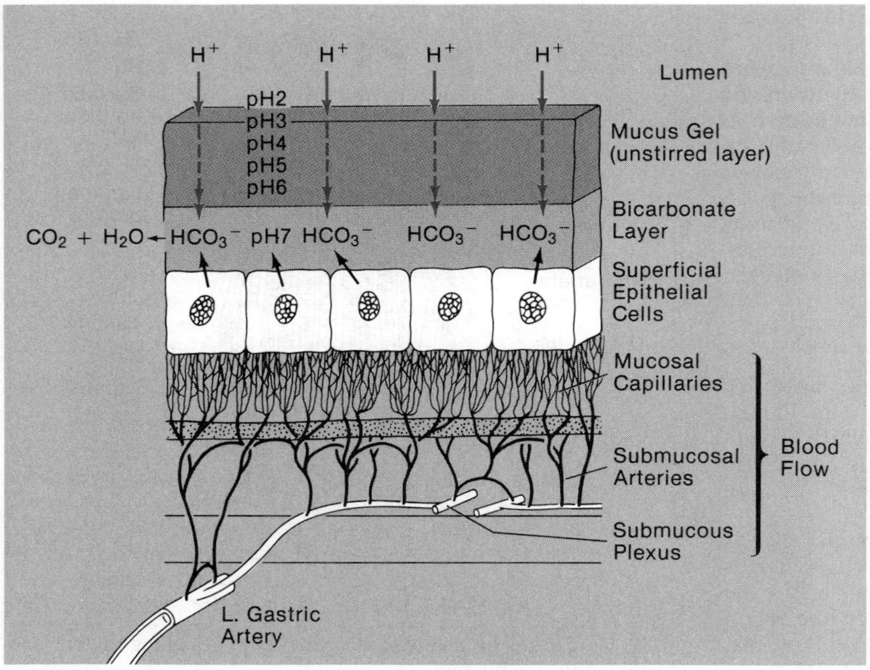

FIGURE 100–4. Model illustrating mechanisms maintaining mucosal integrity. Superficial epithelial cells secrete mucus and bicarbonate, which aid in maintaining a pH gradient between lumen and mucosa and protect the underlying epithelial cells from damage by acid and pepsin. Epithelial cell renewal and mucosal blood flow also are believed to be important mechanisms in maintaining mucosal integrity.

parietal cells or if there is increased sensitivity of parietal cells to normal amounts of these stimulants, BAO will be increased, as will the BAO/MAO ratio. Such a patient is said to have a basal acid hypersecretory state (see below).

Upper and lower limits of normal acid secretion are shown in Table 100–1. Men secrete more acid than women. This can be explained, in part, by differences in body size, but men secrete more acid than women even when corrections are made for weight and lean body mass.

Secretion of Pepsin. Pepsin is secreted into the lumen as an inactive precursor, pepsinogen. Pepsinogen secretion usually accompanies acid secretion. Although mechanisms controlling pepsinogen secretion are less well understood, cholinergic stimulation is believed to be a major mediator. Once pepsinogen is secreted into the gastric lumen, it is converted by acid to pepsin, the active enzyme. The optimal pH for conversion of pepsinogen to pepsin ranges between 1.8 and 3.5.

MAINTENANCE OF NORMAL MUCOSAL INTEGRITY. Several mechanisms are believed important in protecting gastric and duodenal mucosa from damage by acid, pepsin, bile, pancreatic enzymes, and other possible aggressive factors. These defensive mechanisms include mucus, bicarbonate, mucosal blood flow, and cell renewal. Endogenous prostaglandins currently are the most likely candidates as mediators to control these defensive mechanisms.

Mucus. This secretory product is a gel that forms a thin, protective coat over superficial mucosal cells (Fig. 100–4). Mucus has several functions: (1) to protect underlying cells from mechanical forces of digestion; (2) to lubricate the mucosa, assisting movement of food over mucosal surfaces; (3) to retain water within the mucous gel and thereby provide an aqueous environment for underlying cells; and (4) to form an unstirred layer impeding, but not blocking, diffusion of hydrogen ions from the lumen to the apical membrane of epithelial cells. Under normal conditions, mucus is constantly being produced but also is being removed continuously by mechanical forces during mixing and grinding of food and by pepsin, which degrades mucus into soluble glycoprotein subunits. However, secretion and degradation of mucus remain in equilibrium.

Bicarbonate. A bicarbonate-rich fluid is secreted by surface epithelial cells in the stomach and duodenum and also by Brunner's glands in the duodenum. Although some bicarbonate reaches the lumen, much of the secreted bicarbonate remains below or within the mucous layer (Fig. 100–4). Thus, the mucosal surface is in contact with fluid that contains a high pH relative to the lumen of the stomach. Under normal conditions, hydrogen ions are neutralized by bicarbonate (producing carbon dioxide and water) as they diffuse through the mucous gel layer. A pH gradient is thus established between the lumen and surface epithelial cells.

Mucosal Blood Flow. The rich blood supply of the stomach and duodenum is important in maintaining normal mucosal integrity. Gastric and duodenal mucosae are supplied by arborizing mucosal capillaries that traverse the glandular area of the stomach and duodenum. Beneath the muscularis mucosa, an extensive system of submucosal arteries and a submucous plexus of arteries and veins regulate the blood supply to surface epithelial cells (Fig. 100–4).

Cell Renewal. Normal cell renewal is also an important factor in maintaining mucosal integrity. Cells are constantly dying and are being replaced by new cells. In order for this system to function normally, there must be a balance between cell loss and cell renewal. Disruption of this steady state may lead to mucosal damage.

Endogenous Prostaglandins. Prostaglandins of the E, F, and I types are found in the gastric and duodenal mucosa. When administered exogenously, prostaglandins stimulate secretion of mucus and bicarbonate and increase mucosal blood flow. Prostaglandins also may have a trophic effect on the mucosa. Duodenal mucosal prostaglandins appear to stimulate basal duodenal bicarbonate secretion and its response to luminal acid. Exogenously administered prostaglandins protect the mucosa of animals against a variety of noxious agents, including boiling water, ethanol, bile acids, and aspirin, a property termed "cytoprotection." On the basis of such studies of exogenously administered prostaglandins, it is presumed that endogenous prostaglandins also possess cytoprotective properties and that they may help regulate the defensive mechanisms described above.

ABNORMALITIES IN PATIENTS WITH DUODENAL OR GASTRIC ULCERS

GENETIC PREDISPOSITION. Heredity has been postulated to play a role in the pathogenesis of ulcer disease in some patients. Several families with a high incidence of ulcers have been described. The mechanism or mechanisms whereby genetic factors contribute to ulceration in these families is unclear. Originally, it was believed that familial aggregations of ulcer disease represented polygenic inheritance because the genetics of peptic ulcer could not be explained by a single autosomal, sex-linked, dominant, or recessive defect. Polygenic or multifactorial disorders are believed to be caused by the interaction of several genes with environmental factors. Thus, the hereditary component in ulcer disease was believed to reflect the combined contribution of many different genes in an individual patient. More recently, polygenic inheritance has seemed less likely than genetic heterogeneity. In this form of inheritance a number of genetically determined abnormalities share a common clinical manifestation—in this case, the ulcer crater. A number of rare genetic syndromes are associated with peptic ulcer disease. Multiple endocrine neoplasia I syndrome is the most common example (Ch. 241). Additionally, several pathophysiologic abnormalities believed to be associated with increased acid and pepsin secretion or increased gastric emptying have been discovered and several of these have been found in "ulcer families." For example, in several families an increased level of serum pepsinogen I was inherited as an autosomal dominant trait. Since serum pepsinogen I concentrations reflect chief cell mass and correlate with maximum acid output, members of these families may have developed ulcers because of either increased pepsin or acid secretion or increased secretion of both. Other abnormalities, such as those leading to diminished mucosal defense, may be inherited also. The true importance, if any, of hereditary factors in the pathogenesis of peptic ulcer disease in most patients has not been established.

ABNORMALITIES IN SECRETION OF ACID AND PEPSIN. Approximately 30 to 40 per cent of patients with duodenal ulcer disease have acid secretion rates above the upper limits of normal shown in Table 100–1. The remainder have values within the normal range. Since pepsinogen secretion usually accompanies acid secretion, approximately the same percentage of ulcer patients will have increased or normal pepsinogen secretion.

Most patients with gastric ulcers have either normal or lower than normal acid secretion rates. Only a minority of patients with gastric ulcer disease (for example, a few patients with Zollinger-Ellison syndrome) have secretion rates above the normal range. The fact that most gastric ulcer patients have normal or lower than normal acid secretory rates does not exclude acid and pepsin as the cause of gastric ulcer disease in an individual patient but suggests that other factors may be involved (see below). This same concept applies to patients with duodenal ulcers who have normal rates of acid secretion. In fact, the exact role acid or pepsin or both play in the pathogenesis of either gastric or duodenal ulcers is not known. It is assumed that acid is involved in the pathogenesis of ulcer disease in patients with higher than normal rates of acid secretion (see below).

There are three known mechanisms for increased basal acid secretion: (1) increased stimulation by *gastrin* (Zollinger-Ellison syndrome, retained antrum syndrome, and antral gastrin [G] cell hyperplasia or hyperfunction); (2) increased stimulation by *acetylcholine* (vagal hyperfunction); and (3) increased *histamine* stimulation (systemic mastocytosis or basophilic leukemia). Other causes of basal hypersecretion may exist, but so far they have not been described. Ulcers presumably occur in patients with these disorders because of increased levels of acid and pepsin. All of the currently recognized syndromes causing increased basal acid secretion are rare. Of the group Zollinger-Ellison syndrome is the most common and will be discussed separately (see Ch. 100.6).

TABLE 100–1. UPPER (ULN) AND LOWER (LLN) LIMITS OF NORMAL ACID SECRETION IN HEALTHY MEN AND WOMEN

	Acid Output (mmol/hr)*			
	Basal	*Peak*	*Maximum*	Basal/Maximum
Men (N = 172)				
ULN	10.5	60.6	47.7	0.31
LLN	0	11.6	9.3	0
Women (N = 76)				
ULN	5.6	40.1	31.2	0.29
LLN	0	8.0	5.6	0

*Acid output (volume of gastric juice times concentration of acid) is measured in 15-minute intervals and is expressed in mmol/hr. Basal acid output is the sum of acid secreted during four 15-minute periods. Peak acid output is the sum of the highest two 15-minute periods after pentagastrin or histamine stimulation multiplied by two. Maximum acid output is the sum of four 15-minute intervals after pentagastrin or histamine stimulation.

REFLUX OF BILE AND PANCREATIC JUICE. Bile acids, lysolecithin, and pancreatic enzymes are believed to be aggressive factors that lead to ulceration in some patients, especially some of those with gastric ulcers. It has been postulated that duodenal contents reflux into the stomach causing gastritis that, in turn, predisposes to gastric ulceration. Some patients with gastric ulcers may have an incompetent pyloric sphincter that allows reflux of bile or pancreatic enzymes or both into the stomach.

Two mechanisms have been proposed whereby bile and pancreatic juice may damage gastric mucosa: first, alteration of mucus overlying surface epithelial cells, reducing its protective effect; and second, damage to the so-called gastric mucosal barrier (the ability of the stomach to maintain electrical and hydrogen ion concentration gradients between lumen and blood). When these protective mechanisms are disrupted, the mucosa becomes more permeable to the damaging effects of acid and pepsin. Although bile and pancreatic juice have been postulated as the cause of ulcers in some patients, a cause-and-effect relationship has not been clearly established.

ABNORMALITIES OF MUCOSAL DEFENSE. Little is known at the present time about how disruptions in mucosal integrity may lead to ulceration, although there are several theoretic ways in which this might occur. For example, some patients may secrete *reduced amounts of mucus* or *structurally abnormal mucus*. Both could lead to a weaker mucous gel layer.

Diminished blood flow may lead to cell injury and ulceration in some patients. Gastric mucosal ischemia is believed to be a factor in the pathogenesis of acute mucosal injury, as occurs in patients with severe medical or surgical illnesses (stress ulceration). Whether similar reductions in blood flow contribute to the development of chronic gastric or duodenal ulcers is not known. There are fewer collateral blood vessels on the lesser curvature of the stomach compared with the greater curvature. Whether this anatomic difference in blood supply leads to reduced blood flow to the lesser curvature with subsequent ulceration in some patients is not known, but most gastric ulcers do occur on the lesser curvature.

Decreased bicarbonate secretion is a theoretic possibility as a cause for diminished mucosal defense. Gastric bicarbonate secretion has been measured in patients with duodenal ulcer disease and found not to be significantly different from that in normal subjects. However, results of a recent study suggest that bicarbonate secretion from the duodenum may be decreased in duodenal ulcer patients. Reduced pancreatic bicarbonate secretion into the lumen of the duodenum could lead to increased acidity in the duodenal bulb with subsequent duodenal ulceration. There is no evidence, however, that patients with pancreatic insufficiency have a higher incidence of duodenal ulcers. The role of possible *abnormalities in cell renewal* in the pathogenesis of peptic ulcer is entirely speculative at the present time.

Prostaglandin content in gastric or duodenal mucosa might be diminished, leading to abnormalities of mucosal defense (see above). The preliminary studies have led to conflicting reports, however, so that it is impossible at this time to evaluate adequately the possible role of endogenous prostaglandins in the pathogenesis of gastric or duodenal ulcers.

EMOTIONAL STRESS. The mechanism or mechanisms by

which emotional stress might contribute to ulcer disease in some patients are unclear. Certain emotions such as hostility, resentment, guilt, and frustration are associated with increased gastric acidity. Furthermore, basal acid secretion has been reported to increase during stressful interviews and prior to surgery in ulcer patients or before difficult school examinations in healthy subjects. Patients have been described who developed acid hypersecretion and gastric ulcer disease during periods of severe emotional stress. With alleviation of stress, acid secretion diminished and symptoms and ulcerations disappeared. Thus, it appears that certain emotions can cause increased acid secretion that in turn may lead to ulceration in certain patients. Emotional stress may alter factors that maintain mucosal integrity and thereby result in ulcers because of decreased mucosal defense. Although emotional stress is likely to be a factor in the pathogenesis of ulcer disease in some patients, its exact role is uncertain.

DELAYED GASTRIC EMPTYING. For a number of years delayed gastric emptying was believed to be a major factor in the pathogenesis of gastric ulcer disease. It was postulated that delayed gastric emptying caused retention of food in the stomach; in turn, this retention led to increased gastrin release, higher rates of acid secretion, and gastric ulceration. Prolonged gastric emptying, perhaps due to antral hypomotility, was also believed to cause stasis and delayed clearing of duodenal contents (bile and pancreatic enzymes) that had refluxed into the stomach. This in turn could damage gastric mucosa, cause gastritis, and lead to ulceration. Neither of these proposed pathogenetic mechanisms was ever established. Currently delayed emptying is believed to be related to ulceration in only a minority of patients.

EXOGENOUS FACTORS. The most important exogenous factors that have been associated with peptic ulcer disease are cigarette smoking and the use of nonsteroidal anti-inflammatory drugs. The possible association with adrenocorticosteroid therapy, infectious agents, alcohol or caffeine is more tenuous.

Cigarette Smoking. Whether cigarette smoking is related to the pathogenesis of ulcer disease is unclear, although epidemiologic data suggest an association between the two: (1) Smoking is more common among patients with ulcers than among control subjects. (2) There is a positive correlation between the quantity of cigarettes smoked and the prevalence of ulcer disease. (3) Death due to peptic ulcer disease is more likely among patients who smoke than among those who do not. (4) Duodenal ulcers are less likely to heal in cigarette smokers than in nonsmokers. (5) Duodenal ulcers recur more frequently in smokers than in nonsmokers. Whether this applies also to patients with gastric ulcers is not known.

Two mechanisms have been postulated whereby smoking may lead to ulceration: reduction of pyloric sphincter pressure and decreased pancreatic bicarbonate secretion. Smoking has been shown to reduce pyloric sphincter pressure in some patients with gastric ulcers. This, in turn, may lead to increased duodenogastric reflux of bile and pancreatic enzymes into the stomach with subsequent damage to the gastric mucosa. Nicotine reduces pancreatic bicarbonate secretion and may thereby lead to duodenal ulcers by impairing neutralization of acid by bicarbonate in the duodenal bulb. There is no proof, however, that either of these mechanisms actually causes ulceration.

Nonsteroidal Anti-inflammatory Drugs. These medications inhibit prostaglandin synthesis and cause decreased mucus and bicarbonate secretion, diminished mucosal blood flow, and perhaps reduced cell renewal. Aspirin and other nonsteroidal anti-inflammatory drugs cause superficial mucosal erosions in the stomach, presumably by reducing the factors believed important in maintaining mucosal integrity. It is unclear, however, whether these drugs also cause chronic gastric or duodenal ulcers. Chronic gastric ulcers seem to occur more frequently in patients taking large doses of aspirin than in control populations, but a definite relationship between the intake of aspirin and other nonsteroidal anti-inflammatory drugs and the development of chronic ulcers has never been established. These drugs may play a role in the pathogenesis of chronic gastric ulcers in some patients. Their role in the development of duodenal ulcers seems less likely.

Adrenocorticosteroid Therapy. An association between treatment with glucocorticoids (especially prednisone) and peptic ulcer disease has been both supported and denied in conflicting studies. Any relationship between steroid therapy and ulcer disease remains controversial, therefore.

Infectious Agents. Cytomegalovirus (CMV) has been isolated from gastric ulcers in a few patients receiving immunosuppressive drugs and in patients with post-transfusion CMV mononucleosis. *Candida albicans* also has been found in gastric ulcers in several patients. Whether these organisms caused the ulcers or whether the organisms were there secondarily is not known. Herpesviruses have never been isolated from gastric or duodenal ulcers, but one study indicated that antibodies to Herpesvirus type I occurred more frequently and in higher titers in patients with duodenal ulcers than in control subjects.

Gastric *Campylobacter*-like organisms (GCLO) have been associated with acute and chronic gastritis (see Ch. 99). Some postulate that these organisms may be related to the pathogenesis of gastric or duodenal ulcers, but such a relationship remains to be established.

Alcohol or Caffeine-Containing Beverages. Even though both of these substances stimulate acid secretion, there is no evidence that either causes gastric or duodenal ulcers.

Grossman MI (ed.): Peptic Ulcer. A Guide for the Practicing Physician. Chicago, Year Book Medical Publishers, 1981. *This book is an objective review of information relative to the pathogenesis of peptic ulcer disease, including the role of environmental and hereditary factors.*

Miller TA: Protective effects of prostaglandins against gastric mucosal damage: Current knowledge and proposed mechanisms. Am J Physiol 245:G601, 1983. *An excellent review of mechanisms that maintain normal mucosal integrity, the regulation of these mechanisms, and some of the ways in which alterations in these mechanisms may lead to mucosal diseases.*

Richardson CT: Gastric ulcer. In Sleisenger MH, Fordtran JS (eds.): Gastrointestinal Disease. 4th ed. Philadelphia, W. B. Saunders Company, 1987. *The factors involved in the pathogenesis of gastric ulcer are discussed.*

Soll AH: Duodenal ulcer diseases. In Sleisenger MH, Fordtran JS (eds.): Gastrointestinal Disease. 4th ed. Philadelphia, W. B. Saunders Company, 1987. *The pathophysiologic abnormalities found in various groups of duodenal ulcer patients are discussed.*

100.2 Epidemiology, Clinical Manifestations, and Diagnosis

Lawrence R. Schiller

EPIDEMIOLOGY

Peptic ulcer disease is a common disorder; 5 to 10 per cent of all individuals develop peptic ulcer in their lifetime. Although ulcer disease is a common cause of morbidity, it is a relatively rare cause of death. The annual prevalence of symptomatic peptic ulcer disease in the United States is approximately 18 per 1000 adults, but the current mortality rate is only 2.5 per 100,000. Approximately 350,000 new cases of ulcer present each year in the United States.

Ulcer incidence varies by site, sex, and age. Symptomatic duodenal ulcer is more common than symptomatic gastric ulcer in both men (5.5 to 1) and women (2.8 to 1). Men are twice as likely as women to develop a duodenal ulcer but equally likely to develop a gastric ulcer; sex differences may be narrowing, however. Duodenal ulcer usually first produces symptoms between the ages of 25 and 55 years (peak occurrence at age 40) and gastric ulcer most commonly between 40 and 70 years of age (peak occurrence at age 50).

Hospitalization and mortality rates for peptic ulcer disease seem to be declining in the United States, suggesting that the prevalence of peptic ulcer may be declining. It is unclear whether this reflects an actual change in the prevalence of peptic ulcers, a change in the criteria for hospitalization, or a change in the way mortality data are recorded. Studies from other countries suggest that morbidity and mortality from ulcer disease vary widely with geography and may not be declining with time. Before 1900 duodenal ulcer was a rarity and gastric ulcer was a disorder diagnosed mainly in young women. The reasons for reported changes in prevalence and sex incidence with time and for geographic differences are not known.

SYMPTOMS

DYSPEPSIA. Peptic ulcer usually presents as a painful upper abdominal disorder with the constellation of symptoms known as *dyspepsia*. Dyspepsia is poorly defined by both patients and physicians and often includes such symptoms as nausea, vomiting, anorexia, and fullness and bloating in addition to pain or discomfort. Most patients thought to have ulcers because of "typical dyspepsia" are not found to have peptic ulcer by radiography or endoscopy but instead have other diseases or are classified as having "non-ulcer" (functional) dyspepsia.

A list of clinical features and their frequency in gastric ulcer, duodenal ulcer, and "non-ulcer" dyspepsia is provided in Table 100–2. It is impossible to differentiate these conditions from each other or from other diseases producing upper abdominal symptoms, such as cholelithiasis, by any one clinical feature. In practice physicians make the correct diagnosis on the basis of history in patients with dyspepsia less than 50 per cent of the time. In contrast, the use of structured questionnaires and computer-generated multivariate analysis of clinical findings has been remarkably successful in predicting diagnoses in patients with upper abdominal symptoms (80 to 90 per cent correct). This suggests that information leading to a correct diagnosis is contained within the history, but that physicians may be obtaining or analyzing the data incorrectly.

PAIN. The clinical diagnosis of ulcer disease has usually been based on the location of pain, its character, and the factors aggravating or alleviating it. For example, ulcer pain is classically described as being located in the epigastrium and as burning or gnawing in character. Pain in this location also occurs in a majority of patients with "non-ulcer" dyspepsia, however, and pain of this character actually occurs in a minority of patients with either gastric or duodenal ulcer (Table 100–2). Some patients describe ulcer pain as a cramping sensation not unlike hunger pangs, but descriptions of the character of pain are often hard to obtain in an unbiased way and are difficult to assess. Typical ulcer pain is said to be relieved by ingestion of food or antacids, but this is also quite variable. A better predictor of the presence of peptic ulcer (especially duodenal ulcer) is an episodic pattern of pain. Individual episodes of pain usually are short lived, lasting for minutes rather than hours. Episodes of pain usually occur in clusters lasting from days to weeks, interspersed with long symptom-free periods. Some patients with ulcer report annual recurrences of pain during particular seasons such as spring or fall.

The cause of ulcer pain remains unknown. Ulcer pain is usually attributed to increased acidity at the ulcer site and the relief of pain to a decrease in luminal acidity. This theory is consistent with the typical onset of pain several hours after a meal, when gastric emptying has reduced the buffering capacity of gastric contents and intraluminal acidity rises. Attempts to induce pain by perfusing the ulcer site with acid have not uniformly produced pain, however. In several studies ingestion of placebo with no buffering capacity was as effective as ingestion of active antacid in relieving ulcer pain. In addition, ingestion of food sometimes worsens pain. Alternative mechanisms for the production of ulcer pain have been proposed, such as abnormal gastric or duodenal motor function, but are similarly unproved.

COMPLICATIONS. Peptic ulcers frequently fail to produce dyspepsia or pain and therefore may present de novo as a complication, such as bleeding, obstruction, or perforation. These are discussed in Ch. 100.5.

TABLE 100–2. CLINICAL FEATURES OF GASTRIC ULCER, DUODENAL ULCER, AND "NON-ULCER" DYSPEPSIA*

Clinical Feature	Gastric Ulcer (%)	Duodenal Ulcer (%)	"Non-ulcer" Dyspepsia (%)
Features of pain:			
Primary pain location			
Epigastric	67	61–86	52–73
Right hypochondrium	6	7–17	4
Left hypochondrium	6	3–5	5
Radiation to back	34	20–31	24–28
Frequently severe	68	53	37
Gnawing pain	13	16	6
Clusters (episodic)	16	56	35
Occurs at night	32–43	50–88	24–32
Within 30 min of food	20	5	32
Increased by food	24	10–40	45
Food relief	2–48	20–63	4–32
Not related to food or variable	22–53	21–49	22–65
Relief by alkali	36–87	39–86	26–75
Anorexia	46–57	25–36	26–36
Weight loss	24–61	19–45	18–32
Nausea	54–70	49–59	43–60
Vomiting	38–73	25–57	26–34
Heartburn	19	27–59	28
Fatty food intolerance	—	14–72	53
Bloating	55	49	52
Belching	48	59	60

*From Soll AH, Isenberg JI: Duodenal ulcer disease. In Sleisenger MH, Fordtran JS (eds.): Gastrointestinal Disease. 3rd ed. Philadelphia, W.B. Saunders Company, 1983, pp 625–672.

PHYSICAL EXAMINATION

The physical examination is usually not helpful in uncomplicated peptic ulcer disease. Epigastric tenderness is an insensitive and nonspecific finding and correlates poorly with the presence of an active ulcer crater. When ulcer disease is complicated by obstruction, perforation, penetration, or bleeding, important physical findings may be present (see Ch. 100.5).

Rarely, peptic ulcer is associated with multisystem syndromes that may produce physical findings. For instance, systemic mastocytosis, stiff skin syndrome, pachydermoperiostosis, and multiple lentigenes–ulcer syndrome may have cutaneous findings. Ulcer-tremor-nystagmus syndrome and amyloidosis may produce both peptic ulcer and neurologic findings.

DIAGNOSTIC VISUALIZATION

The initial diagnosis of ulcer depends on visualizing the ulcer crater by radiography or endoscopy. Radiography is well tolerated (even in patients in fragile condition), readily available, and comparatively inexpensive, making it an excellent screening test. However, radiography may miss as many as 20 per cent of peptic ulcers. Endoscopy is more accurate and allows directed biopsy and cytologic study of suspicious lesions but cannot always be done safely in uncooperative patients or those whose condition is unstable. In the United States, where endoscopy currently costs from three to five times as much as radiography, upper gastrointestinal radiographs, preferably with both single-contrast and double-contrast techniques, are often the initial diagnostic test. In symptomatic patients with no radiographic abnormalities or with equivocal evidence of ulcer, endoscopy can establish or exclude the diagnosis of active ulcer disease. In situations in

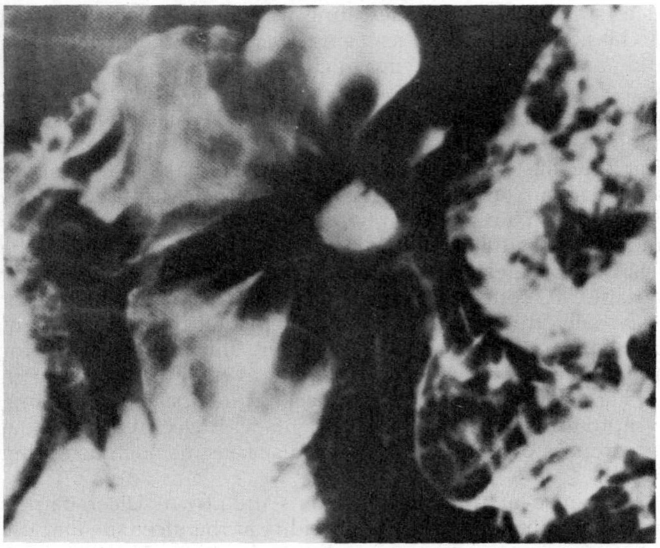

FIGURE 100–5. Duodenal ulcers are recognized when barium is retained within an ulcer niche. In this example barium has collected in an ulcer at the base of the duodenal bulb along the posterior wall. Folds radiate to the margin of this ulcer. (From Goldberg HI: In Sleisenger MH, Fordtran JS [eds.]: Gastrointestinal Disease. 2nd ed. Philadelphia, W. B. Saunders Company, 1978.)

which there is little difference in cost between endoscopy and radiography, endoscopy is preferable in the investigation of patients with dyspepsia because of its greater sensitivity in diagnosis.

DUODENAL ULCER. If a duodenal ulcer is demonstrated radiographically (Fig. 100–5), no further diagnostic evaluation is necessary and treatment can be started. Since duodenal ulcers are rarely malignant, endoscopic biopsy is not necessary. Follow-up examinations to assess healing of a duodenal ulcer need not be done routinely. However, if symptoms fail to subside with therapy, endoscopy should be done to prove the diagnosis of ulcer before considering surgery (see Ch. 100.4)

GASTRIC ULCER. If a gastric ulcer is found on the radiograph (Fig. 100–6), malignancy should be rigorously excluded, particularly if there is any suspicion by the radiologist that the ulcer may be malignant. Malignancy should be suspected if (1) the ulcer is located completely within the gastric wall or in an intraluminal mass, (2) there is nodularity of the ulcer base or of adjacent gastric mucosa, (3) there are no folds radiating to the ulcer margin, or (4) the ulcer is large. Malignancy can best be excluded by direct endoscopic visualization of the gastric ulcer to obtain brush cytologic specimens and to obtain a minimum of six to eight punch biopsy specimens for careful pathologic examination. This approach will lead to an accurate diagnosis in more than 95 per cent of cases. Some investigators recommend that patients with radiographically benign-appearing gastric ulcers not have endoscopy initially but that malignancy be excluded by repeating a radiographic study or by endoscopy after a period of therapy to prove that the ulcer has healed completely. Whether initially endoscoped and found benign or not, all gastric ulcers should be followed to healing. This can be done best by endoscopy after treatment for 8 to 12 weeks to allow healing to occur. Surgery may be needed to exclude malignancy in nonhealing gastric ulcer even if multiple endoscopic biopsies yield negative results (Ch. 100.4).

LABORATORY STUDIES

SERUM GASTRIN LEVELS. Radioimmunoassay of gastrin is useful in screening patients with known ulcer disease for Zollinger-Ellison syndrome and other rare hypersecretory states. The reasons for identifying these patients are (1) they may have a more severe course marked by excessive complications such as bleeding, obstruction, or perforation; (2) therapy is different, particularly surgical therapy (see Ch. 100.4); (3) associated but undiagnosed diseases of other organs, such as multiple endocrine neoplasia type I, may cause morbidity; and (4) gastrinomas associated with Zollinger-Ellison syndrome may be malignant and cause death from metastasis. Early recognition of Zollinger-Ellison syndrome makes possible effective control of symptoms and sometimes allows resection of tumor and cure of the disease (Ch. 100.6).

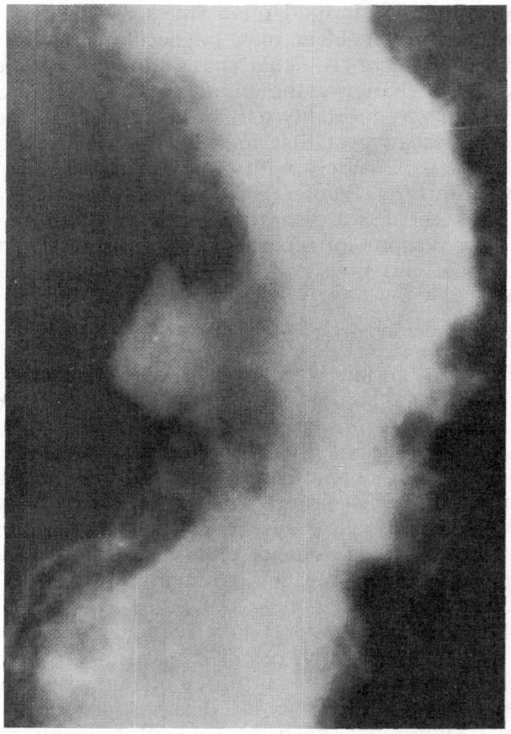

FIGURE 100–6. This ulcer of the lesser curve of the stomach demonstrates several features typical of benign gastric ulcers: The ulcer crater projects beyond the contour of the gastric wall, the margin of the ulcer crater is sharply defined and smooth, the ulcer is surrounded by a broad lucent band—an ulcer collar—resulting from edema at the ulcer orifice, and mucosal folds radiate from the ulcer collar. (From Goldberg HI: In Sleisenger MH, Fordtran JS [eds.]: Gastrointestinal Disease. 2nd ed. Philadelphia, W. B. Saunders Company, 1978.)

Measurement of serum gastrin concentrations in all patients with peptic ulcer disease is not cost effective because the incidence of Zollinger-Ellison syndrome is low (less than 1 per cent of patients with peptic ulcer disease). Table 100–3 lists the selective clinical situations in which obtaining a fasting serum gastrin level may be useful, although even with this selectivity the likelihood of identifying a patient as having Zollinger-Ellison syndrome is low.

If fasting serum gastrin concentrations are elevated (> 200 pg per milliliter) in patients not taking medications that alter intragastric pH, gastric acid secretion should be measured in

TABLE 100–3. CLINICAL SITUATIONS IN WHICH MEASUREMENT OF SERUM GASTRIN LEVELS IS INDICATED

Family history of peptic ulcer
Ulcer associated with hypercalcemia or other manifestations of multiple endocrine neoplasia type I
Multifocal peptic ulcer
Peptic ulceration of postbulbar duodenum or jejunum
Peptic ulceration associated with diarrhea*
Chronic unexplained diarrhea*
Enlarged gastric folds on upper GI x-ray
Before surgery for "intractable" ulcer
Recurrent ulcer after ulcer surgery

*Not due to antacid ingestion.
GI = Gastrointestinal.

order to prove that gastrin levels are not elevated in response to hypochlorhydria or achlorhydria, such as that due to pernicious anemia, atrophic gastritis, gastric cancer, or vagotomy. A finding of high serum gastrin levels and increased basal acid output limits the differential diagnosis to only a few entities (Table 100–4). If both fasting gastrin levels and basal acid secretion are very high (> 1000 pg per milliliter and > 15 mmol per hour, respectively), a diagnosis of Zollinger-Ellison syndrome is likely.

When fasting gastrin levels or basal acid outputs or both are less markedly elevated and the diagnosis of Zollinger-Ellison syndrome is unclear, the response of serum gastrin concentration to an intravenous injection of secretin may be helpful. In individuals with Zollinger-Ellison syndrome, intravenous injection of pure Secretin-Kabi, 2 U per kilogram of body weight, results in a prompt and pathognomonic rise of gastrin of > 200 pg per milliliter within two to ten minutes. Patients with other hypergastrinemic conditions (Table 100–4) and normal individuals do not show this elevation. Gastrin secretion rises with calcium infusion also, but this rise is less reliable diagnostically than that following injection of secretin.

Differentiation of other rare hypergastrinemic syndromes (Table 100–4) can be made on the basis of (1) history of ulcer surgery (retained antrum syndrome, discussed in Ch. 100.4) or small bowel resection, (2) demonstration of gastric outlet obstruction by radiography or endoscopy, (3) laboratory evidence of renal failure, or (4) response of serum gastrin levels to a meal. Patients with antral G cell hyperplasia or hyperfunction more than double their already elevated fasting gastrin levels after ingestion of a protein meal. Patients with Zollinger-Ellison syndrome do not usually have this exuberant response to a meal.

ACID SECRETORY TESTING. Gastric acid secretion is measured by placing a vented nasogastric tube in the gastric antrum under fluoroscopic guidance and aspirating gastric juice with a suction pump. By measuring the volume and acid concentration (determined either by titration to pH 7.0 or indirectly from pH measurements), the quantity of acid secreted by the stomach can be calculated. Basal acid output (BAO) is defined as the amount of acid produced during four consecutive 15-minute periods. Vmax for acid secretion is estimated by injecting a maximally effective dose of gastric secretagogue. Pentagastrin (6 μg per kilogram), the biologically active carboxyl-terminal fragment of gastrin, is preferred for this purpose. Histamine or betazole (Histalog) can also be used. Stimulated secretion is expressed as peak acid output (PAO, the sum of the two highest consecutive 15-minute periods after injection multiplied by 2) or as maximal acid output (MAO, the sum of four consecutive 15-minute periods after injection). Values for acid secretion in healthy subjects and ulcer patients are shown in Table 100–1. In the absence of hypergastrinemia, measurement of gastric acid secretion is usually unnecessary in patients with peptic ulcer. Basal and peak acid output are increased in duodenal ulcer patients as a group (see Ch. 100.1), but knowledge of the level of acid secretion has no therapeutic implications for the individual patient at present. Measurement of acid secretion rates is sometimes useful preoperatively so that postoperative values can be compared and the effect of the operation on acid secretion can be assessed (see Ch. 100.4). When ulcer disease occurs in the presence of achlorhydria, malignancy should be suspected.

TABLE 100–4. CAUSES OF INCREASED FASTING SERUM GASTRIN CONCENTRATIONS AND INCREASED BASAL ACID OUTPUT

Zollinger-Ellison syndrome
Retained antrum syndrome
Massive small bowel resection (?)
Chronic gastric outlet obstruction (?)
Renal failure
Antral G cell hyperplasia or hyperfunction

TABLE 100–5. COMMON DISEASES THAT MAY PRODUCE EPIGASTRIC PAIN SIMULATING PEPTIC ULCER

Myocardial infarction
Pleurisy
Pericarditis
Esophagitis
Cholecystitis
Pancreatitis
Irritable bowel syndrome

DIFFERENTIAL DIAGNOSIS

Peptic ulcer can usually be distinguished from painful intestinal disorders that customarily produce discomfort in the periumbilical or lower quadrants of the abdomen (e.g., appendicitis or diverticulitis). Disorders affecting the viscera of the upper abdomen or chest are more difficult to differentiate from peptic ulcer disease (Table 100.5). Differentiation of these disorders can often be made by considering the acuteness of pain, lack of response to eating or antacids, changes of pain with changes in position, radiation of pain, and the presence of physical findings such as rebound tenderness, all of which are atypical in uncomplicated peptic ulcer disease. Because ulcer disease is common and ulcer symptoms are often variable, however, peptic ulcer must be considered as a possible cause of abdominal symptoms even in patients with atypical symptoms.

FUNCTIONAL DYSPEPSIA. *Functional dyspepsia* ("non-ulcer" dyspepsia) is diagnosed when a symptomatic individual is not found to have an ulcer or other structural disease, such as cholelithiasis. Women in their twenties are especially likely to have this condition. The causes of this syndrome are unknown. It is likely that several different problems can lead to dyspepsia. It has been estimated that 20 to 30 per cent of patients with this diagnosis eventually develop peptic ulcer; therefore, some of these patients may really have evanescent ulcers that evade diagnosis. Some of these patients have a disruption of normal gastric motor function. Gastrokinetic agents such as metoclopramide or domperidone have been found to reverse both symptoms and motor dysfunction in some of these patients. Longer clinical trials are needed before such therapy can be generally recommended for patients with functional dyspepsia.

GASTRIC CANCER. Many patients with gastric cancer present with dyspepsia (Ch. 101). This diagnosis should be considered in particular when dyspepsia is associated with weight loss or evidence of occult gastrointestinal blood loss in an elderly individual or when radiographic or endoscopic appearances of gastric ulcer are suspicious for malignancy. However, a diagnosis of cancer should also be considered in any individual with a benign-appearing gastric ulcer, since roughly 2 to 5 per cent of such ulcers contain foci of gastric carcinoma.

MISCELLANEOUS DISORDERS. A variety of other diseases can produce dyspepsia that may mimic that of peptic ulcer. These conditions include *infiltrative diseases* of the stomach such as hypertrophic gastritis, tuberculosis, syphilis, Crohn's disease, and other granulomatous gastritides (see Ch. 99); *duodenal obstruction* by polyps, webs, or an annular pancreas; and *intestinal parasitosis* by *Giardia* or *Strongyloides*. More common diseases causing dyspeptic symptoms include *biliary tract disease* and *pancreatitis*. These can often be differentiated from ulcer disease by history, but tests such as sonography, cholecystography, and serum amylase determinations are usually necessary to confirm their diagnosis.

Bonnevie O: Changing demographics of peptic ulcer disease. Dig Dis Sci 30(Suppl. Nov. 1985):8S, 1985. *Well-referenced review of changing trends in ulcer disease from a European perspective.*

Cotton PB, Shorvon PJ: Analysis of endoscopy and radiography in the diagnosis, follow-up and treatment of peptic ulcer disease. Clin Gastroenterol 13:383, 1984. *Thoughtful and detailed analysis of the role of radiography and endoscopy in ulcer patients.*

de Dombal FT: Analysis of foregut symptoms. In Baron JH, Moody FG (eds.): Butterworth's International Medical Reviews, Gastroenterology 1, Foregut. London, Butterworth & Co, Ltd, 1981, pp 49–66. *Excellent review of new approaches to foregut symptoms, including multivariate analysis.*

Kurata JH, Haile BM: Epidemiology of peptic ulcer disease. Clin Gastroenterol 13:289, 1984. *Precise analysis of current statistics with discussion of epidemiologic problems.*

Lagarde SP, Spiro HM: Non-ulcer dyspepsia. Clin Gastroenterol 13:437, 1984. *Wide-ranging review of this diffuse syndrome.*

Thompson WM, Kelvin FM, Gedgaudas RD, et al.: Radiologic investigation of peptic ulcer disease. Radiol Clin North Am 20:701, 1982. *Review of state of the art for radiology of peptic ulcer with many excellent examples.*

100.3 Medical Therapy

Walter L. Peterson

In the healthy human stomach and duodenum there is an effective balance between the potential of gastric acid and pepsin to damage mucosal cells and the ability of these cells to protect themselves from injury. Disruption of this balance leads to peptic ulcers. In some patients the imbalance occurs primarily because of acid (and pepsin) hypersecretion, in others primarily because of some abnormality in mucosal defense, and in still others because of both mechanisms. However, once an ulcer has formed, healing may be promoted by manipulating either factor, regardless of which was primarily responsible for the ulcer. For example, although aspirin is believed to produce a gastric ulcer by disrupting mucosal defense in some way, the ulcer may be treated by a drug that reduces gastric acidity, such as cimetidine.

Therapeutic agents for peptic ulcer disease can be classified as those that act primarily by reducing levels of acid and pepsin in the gastric lumen and those that act primarily by enhancing mucosal defense. Since pepsin's activity is pH dependent, reduction of acidity reduces peptic activity simultaneously.

DRUGS THAT REDUCE GASTRIC ACIDITY

Gastric acidity may be reduced either by inhibiting secretion of acid from parietal cells or by neutralizing acid that has been secreted.

INHIBITION OF ACID SECRETION. Secretion may be reduced either by blocking the interaction of histamine or acetylcholine with their receptors on parietal cells (histamine *H_2-receptor antagonists* or *antimuscarinic drugs*) or by interfering with the intracellular machinery of the parietal cell (*prostaglandins* or *substituted benzimidazoles*) (Fig. 100–7).

H_2-RECEPTOR ANTAGONISTS. The effects of histamine are mediated through H_1 and H_2 receptors. H_1 receptors are located in the smooth muscle of the bronchus and small bowel, and H_2 receptors are located on parietal cells and the uterus. H_1 receptors are blocked by classic antihistamines such as diphenhydramine (Benadryl), while H_2 receptors are blocked by specific H_2-receptor antagonists. All such drugs effectively lower both fasting and food-stimulated gastric acid secretion.

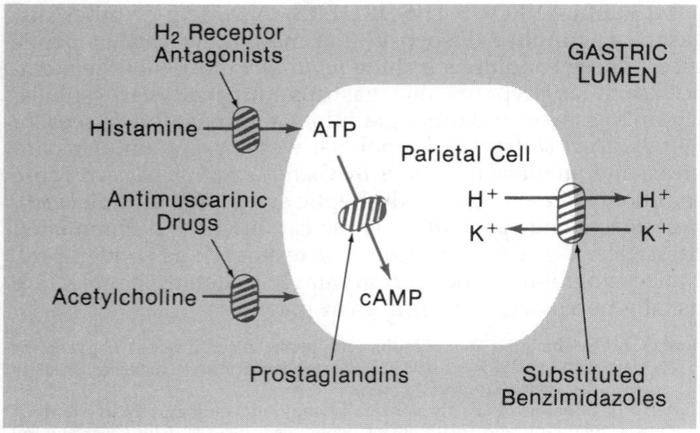

FIGURE 100–7. Sites of action of four drugs employed to inhibit acid secretion.

The first commercially available H_2-receptor antagonist was *cimetidine* (Tagamet), whose structure, like histamine, contains an imidazole ring. Side effects with cimetidine, which are uncommon and almost always reversible, include mental confusion (especially in elderly patients with hepatic or renal insufficiency), gynecomastia, impotence, and interaction with other commonly prescribed drugs. Cimetidine competitively antagonizes the metabolism (via the cytochrome P-450 system) of warfarin, theophylline, propranolol, phenytoin, chlordiazepoxide, and diazepam. Although blood levels of these drugs rise when given concomitantly with cimetidine, the clinical importance of such rises is unsettled. *Ranitidine* (Zantac), which possesses a furan ring, is the second H_2-receptor antagonist to gain widespread human use. Its putative advantages over cimetidine include a five- to tenfold increase in potency, and to date fewer reported side effects. It does not cross the blood-brain barrier well and therefore may not cause mental confusion. Although it has less of an effect on the cytochrome P-450 system, it may also interfere with the metabolism of drugs. *Famotidine* (Pepcid), containing a thiazole ring, is yet another H_2-receptor antagonist that is now available.

ANTIMUSCARINIC DRUGS. The classic antimuscarinic drugs reduce fasting and food-stimulated acid secretion by about 50 per cent and 30 per cent, respectively. However, these drugs also block other muscarinic receptors and produce unwanted side effects such as drowsiness, blurred vision, and urinary hesitancy. The centrally active tricyclic antidepressant drugs trimipramine and doxepin also possess antimuscarinic properties. Pirenzipine is a tricyclic antimuscarinic compound that does not cross the blood-brain barrier and therefore has no antidepressant activity or central nervous system side effects. Pirenzipine (not available in the United States) is believed to block certain types of muscarinic receptors (e.g., those controlling acid secretion) at doses that do not block other muscarinic receptors (e.g., those controlling heart rate and smooth muscle contraction). Thus, acid secretion can be controlled by doses of drug too small to produce side effects such as tachycardia and bladder atony.

PROSTAGLANDINS. Several methylated analogues of prostaglandins E_1 and E_2 have been shown to reduce gastric acid secretion, probably by interfering with generation of cyclic adenosine monophosphate (cAMP) in the parietal cell. Diarrhea occurs in about 10 per cent of patients treated with these agents, although it is usually mild and self-limited. Concern has also been voiced that prostaglandins may induce abortions. At the time of writing, none of the prostaglandin analogues has been approved for use in the United States.

SUBSTITUTED BENZIMIDAZOLES. Drugs of this class, the prototype of which is omeprazole,* are extremely potent inhibitors of gastric acid secretion. These drugs inhibit H^+/K^+ adenosine triphosphatase (ATPase), an enzyme found at the acid secretory surface of parietal cells that mediates final transport of hydrogen ions (via exchange with potassium ions) into the gastric lumen (Fig. 100–7). There is a prolonged duration of action, even when blood levels of drug are undetectable. Studies are underway to determine clinical efficacy and safety profiles in humans. In animals given high doses of omeprazole, gastric carcinoid tumors have developed. These tumors are likely a result of the profound hypergastrinemia that results from the prolonged achlorhydria induced by omeprazole.

NEUTRALIZATION OF GASTRIC ACID. Antacids react with hydrochloric acid to form a salt and water, thereby

*Investigational drug.

reducing gastric acidity. Sodium bicarbonate, a classic antacid, is not recommended for long-term use because of its short duration of action and its propensity to produce alkalosis and sodium retention. Neither is calcium carbonate suggested for therapy of peptic ulcer because it may cause acid rebound (sustained hypersecretion of gastric acid after antacid has emptied from the stomach) and may cause the milk-alkali syndrome. Antacids most widely recommended are those containing varying proportions of magnesium and aluminum hydroxide. Serious side effects with these two compounds are uncommon. However, antacids containing proportionately larger amounts of magnesium hydroxide often produce diarrhea, whereas those with large amounts of aluminum hydroxide may produce constipation. All antacids can result in "taste fatigue" for individual patients. Most antacids used today are relatively low in sodium content.

Beyond individual preferences for antacid flavors, patients with ulcer may choose any of the commercially available magnesium and aluminum hydroxide antacids as long as neutralizing capacity is considered. Most clinical studies with antacids specify doses in terms of in vitro neutralizing capacity (for example, 140 mmol seven times per day), and antacids vary in potency. Table 100–6 lists several commonly prescribed antacids with the volume required to neutralize 70 to 140 mmol of hydrochloric acid in vitro.

DRUGS THAT ENHANCE MUCOSAL DEFENSE

Mucosal protection is more of a conceptual term than one with a firm definition because it is not known exactly what constitutes "mucosal defense." Mucus, bicarbonate secretion, and blood flow may all play roles, and some of the drugs that "enhance mucosal defense" may indeed affect these variables. However, a more general description of these drugs is that they exert a beneficial effect on an ulcer *without affecting luminal gastric acidity*. Since they do not belong in the first group, they fall by default into the second group.

SUCRALFATE. Sucralfate (Carafate) is the aluminum hydroxide salt of a sulfated disaccharide, sucrose octasulfate. The exact mechanisms of action are not understood. It has been suggested that sucralfate (1) forms a viscous shield over an ulcer crater, preventing acid from reaching regenerating ulcer tissue, (2) adsorbs bile acids or pepsin or both in the lumen, or (3) stimulates the generation of local prostaglandins. The drug should not be taken at the same time as food, antacids, or other medications. Binding with food or antacids may limit the effectiveness of the drug, and binding by sucralfate of the other medications may limit their absorption.

PROSTAGLANDINS. Prostaglandins play a poorly defined role in mucosal integrity, but their absence may permit development of ulcers of the stomach and duodenum. However, when given exogenously in doses that do not affect acid secretion, prostaglandin analogues do not promote ulcer healing. It may well be that the properties of prostaglandins that maintain "mucosal integrity" have little to do with ulcer healing.

TABLE 100–6. VOLUMES (IN ML) OF SEVERAL COMMONLY PRESCRIBED LIQUID ANTACIDS REQUIRED TO NEUTRALIZE 70 OR 140 MMOL OF HYDROCHLORIC ACID

	70 mmol	140 mmol
Maalox Therapeutic Concentrate Mylanta II	15	30
Gelusil II	20	40
Maalox Mylanta Gelusil Riopan Alternagel*	30	60
Amphojel*	50	100

*Aluminum hydroxide antacids.

BISMUTH. Tripotassium dicitrato-bismuthate (DeNol), a complex bismuth salt, chelates with protein (e.g., necrotic ulcer tissue) at acidic pH levels. Its mechanism of action is unknown, although recent evidence suggests it is bactericidal for *Campylobacter pyloridis*, an organism that may play a role in some patients with peptic ulcer disease. Side effects are minor. The drug in liquid form has an unpleasant odor and, like all bismuth compounds, it will darken stools. DeNol is unavailable in the United States at the time of writing.

LICORICE EXTRACTS. Carbenoxolone is a synthetic derivative of glycyrrhetic acid, a substance found in licorice. It appears to promote ulcer healing by several mechanisms. The drug produces thick mucus, inhibits peptic activity (independent of pH), and may actually increase the longevity of mucosal cells. Because carbenoxolone possesses licorice's aldosterone-like side effects (salt retention, hypertension, hypokalemia), it is not the preferred drug for peptic ulcer therapy; it is unavailable in the United States.

TREATMENT OF PATIENTS WITH PEPTIC ULCER

At this writing, five drugs are available in the United States as first-line therapy for patients with peptic ulcers: cimetidine, ranitidine, famotidine, antacids, and sucralfate. One or more of the prostaglandin analogues may soon be available. Because of their side effects, currently available antimuscarinic drugs should be used as adjunctive therapy only. While selecting one of the first-line drugs, a physician should also be aware of several factors that at one time or another have been considered important in ulcer therapy.

COMPLEMENTARY FACTORS IN PEPTIC ULCER THERAPY. Factors to consider in this category include diet, smoking, alcohol or analgesic use, sedatives, and the need for hospitalization.

Diet. Diet therapy was once the standard in the treatment of peptic ulcer disease. Now, it is clear that no specific diet is of proven benefit in ulcer therapy. Patients should avoid whatever foods cause them discomfort but otherwise eat whatever they like. Because food, especially milk, stimulates acid secretion, between meal or bedtime snacks should be taken in moderation.

Smoking. There are many important reasons (other than the presence of a peptic ulcer) to encourage patients to stop smoking. However, data are very persuasive that patients who do not smoke heal ulcers more often and more rapidly than those who smoke. The mechanism of this adverse effect on peptic ulcers is not known, although components of cigarettes may reduce endogenous generation of prostaglandins.

Alcohol. There is no evidence that alcohol ingestion retards ulcer healing. Nevertheless, because alcohol damages gastric mucosa, patients with ulcers who choose to drink should be advised to drink in moderation.

Analgesics. Drugs that inhibit prostaglandin synthesis (aspirin, nonsteroidal anti-inflammatory drugs) can produce gastric ulcers and therefore patients with this disorder should stop the drugs if possible. Although the evidence that these drugs cause duodenal ulcer is unconvincing, patients with refractory or bleeding duodenal ulcer should be advised not to take them.

Sedatives. Although emotional stress may play a role in the pathogenesis of peptic ulcers in some patients, routine use of sedative drugs is of no proven benefit in ulcer therapy.

Hospitalization. Hospitalization should be reserved for patients with complications of ulcer disease (bleeding, perforation, penetration, obstruction) (see Ch. 100.5) or patients with ulcer pain refractory to routine medical management. In other situations, hospitalization is not warranted and has not been shown to lead to more rapid healing.

TREATMENT OF PATIENTS WITH UNCOMPLICATED DUODENAL ULCER. In selecting a drug with which to treat a patient with duodenal ulcer (or gastric ulcer, see below), four factors must be considered: effectiveness, safety, convenience, and cost (Table 100–7).

Effectiveness. All available drugs are equally effective in hastening healing of duodenal ulcer when compared with placebo, with approximately 70 per cent of patients experiencing ulcer healing by four weeks and 90 per cent by six weeks. Each also promptly relieves ulcer pain, although often not significantly better than placebo.

Safety. Although side effects do occur with these drugs, they are uncommon and usually not serious. As examples, one can anticipate diarrhea occurring with large doses of magnesium hydroxide antacid or one may need to monitor serum levels of some drugs (e.g., theophylline or phenytoin) when taken in conjunction with cimetidine. Sucralfate is theoretically the safest, since it is not absorbed.

Convenience. Antacids have been proved effective in United States studies only when large doses of a liquid antacid are taken seven times daily, an inconvenience for many patients. Sucralfate must be taken four times daily on an empty stomach. The H_2-receptor antagonists with their once-a-day dosing are clearly the most convenient.

Cost. Cost varies according to the regimen and the locale where the drug is purchased. As shown in Table 100–7, antacid in large doses is the most expensive regimen in Dallas, followed by ranitidine, famotidine, sucralfate, and cimetidine.

Recommendation. Patients should initially be treated with adequate doses of a single drug. Cimetidine, ranitidine, and famotidine are the first-line drugs of choice, primarily because of convenience. Sucralfate and antacids are just as effective as H_2-receptor antagonists but are somewhat less convenient. Prostaglandins may offer yet another option. Treatment should continue for four to six weeks, and if the patient is symptom free, the medication is stopped. Documentation of ulcer healing by radiography or endoscopy is unnecessary in the patient with routine duodenal ulcer.

APPROACH TO PATIENTS WITH DUODENAL ULCER IN WHOM FIRST-LINE THERAPY FAILS. Failure of first-line therapy for duodenal ulcer is defined as the development of a complication (bleeding, perforation, penetration) while the patient is on therapy or persistence of ulcer symptoms after several weeks of therapy. For patients who do not require surgery, there are several alternatives for continued medical therapy. These options include changing to a different drug, increasing drug dosage, combining two drugs, or any combination of these. There are no adequate data to support any of these particular approaches.

If symptoms persist after one or more changes in medical therapy, surgery should be considered (see Ch. 100.4). However, before it is performed, the patient should undergo endoscopy to verify the existence of an unhealed ulcer, compliance with the medication regimen should be established, and the Zollinger-Ellison syndrome should be excluded. A period of medical therapy in a hospital may benefit some patients with peptic ulcer disease of this severity.

TREATMENT OF PATIENTS WITH GASTRIC ULCER. Cimetidine, ranitidine, and famotidine will each lead to complete healing in 85 per cent of benign gastric ulcers by eight weeks (Table 100–7). Liquid antacids in doses of 70 mmol (15 to 50 ml) seven times daily produce results comparable to those with cimetidine, although once again the inconvenience of such a regimen may be a disadvantage. Results of sucralfate therapy are currently being evaluated.

Because 2 to 3 per cent of benign-appearing gastric ulcers harbor a malignancy (not a problem with duodenal ulcer), special efforts are taken to make sure that the ulcer is benign and that it heals completely. Assuming that endoscopic biopsies were taken at the time of initial diagnosis and showed no evidence of malignancy, proof of healing can be obtained by either radiography or endoscopy. Unless the ulcer was very large initially, it will usually heal in eight weeks. If the ulcer is unhealed at this time, repeat endoscopic biopsies should be taken to confirm the benignity of the ulcer and if no evidence of tumor is found, medical therapy should be continued for another four to eight weeks. Since very few ulcers that have not healed after eight weeks of therapy will ultimately heal if the same dose of medication is continued, either the dose of drug should be increased or antacids should be added. A specific duration for continued therapy should be specified (e.g., another four or eight weeks), after which the patient should be operated upon if the ulcer has not healed.

TABLE 100–7. COMPARISON OF DRUGS TO TREAT DUODENAL (DU) AND GASTRIC (GU) ULCERS

Drugs	Dose	Regimen	Effective for Healing of DU	Effective for Healing of GU	Approximate Cost to Patient for 30-Day Course‡
1. *H_2-Receptor Antagonists*					
Cimetidine	300 mg	q.i.d.	Yes	Yes	$49
	400 mg	b.i.d.	Yes	Yes*	$48
	800 mg	h.s.	Yes	Yes*	$51
Ranitidine	150 mg	b.i.d.	Yes	Yes	$54
	300 mg	h.s.	Yes	Yes*	$59
Famotidine	40 mg	h.s.	Yes	Yes*†	$57
2. *Antacids*§					
Liquid	35 mmol	1 and 3 h p.c.	Yes†	NT	$15
	70 mmol	1 and 3 h p.c. and h.s.	NT	Yes	$36
	140 mmol	1 and 3 h p.c. and h.s.	Yes	NT	$72
Tablet	30 mmol	1 h p.c. and h.s.	Yes†	Yes†	$6
3. *Sucralfate*	1 gram	q.i.d.	Yes	Probably*	$49
	2 gram	b.i.d.	Yes*†	NT	$49
4. *Prostaglandins*					
Arbaprostil**	100 μg	q.i.d.	Yes*	NT	Not yet available
Enprostil**	35μg	b.i.d.	Yes*	Yes*	Not yet available
Misoprostol**	50 μg	q.i.d.	No	No	Not yet available
	100 μg	q.i.d.	Yes*	Probably*	Not yet available
	200μg	q.i.d.	Yes*	Yes*†	Not yet available
	400 μg	b.i.d.	Yes*	NT	Not yet available

*Not approved by United States Food and Drug Administration at time of writing.
†Not studied in United States.
‡Mean of four drugstores in Dallas, Texas (in July 1986; famotidine, February, 1987).
§Maalox Therapeutic Concentrate (Rorer, Inc.): 35 mmol per 7.5 ml liquid; 30 mmol per one tablet.
**Investigational drug.
No antacid has been approved by the United States Food and Drug Administration for treatment of peptic ulcer.
NT = Not tested; h.s. = hora somni; p.c. = post cibum.

LONG-TERM MAINTENANCE THERAPY. Once an ulcer has healed with full-course therapy, long-term treatment with any of the H_2-receptor antagonists, antacids, or sucralfate will significantly reduce the high incidence of recurrent ulcer (as high as 70 to 80 per cent in one year). However, not every patient requires such therapy. Patients who have bled from an ulcer should receive maintenance therapy in the hope that rebleeding will not occur and that surgery will not be necessary. Maintenance therapy is also given to those patients with frequent or especially severe recurrences for whom surgery might otherwise be considered. Unless a patient is a poor operative candidate, surgery is recommended if the ulcer recurs during maintenance therapy.

TREATMENT OF PATIENTS WITH ZOLLINGER-ELLISON SYNDROME. Patients with Zollinger-Ellison syndrome (ZES) pose a special problem. Because of constant gastrin-induced hypersecretion of acid, they are always at risk of ulceration and ulcer complications. The treatment is discussed in Ch. 100.6.

Berstad A, Weberg R: Antacids in the treatment of gastroduodenal ulcer. Scand J Gastroenterol 21:385, 1986. *Up-to-date review of studies using various doses of antacids to treat peptic ulcer.*

Feldman M: Inhibition of gastric acid secretion by selective and nonselective anticholinergics. Gastroenterology 86:361, 1984. *Scholarly discussion of pharmacology of anticholinergic drugs.*

Hawkey CJ, Rampton DS: Prostaglandins and the gastrointestinal mucosa: Are they important in its function, disease, or treatment? Gastroenterology 89:1162, 1985. *Extensive review of all aspects of prostaglandins as they relate to gastroduodenal disease.*

Lauritsen K, Rune SJ, Bytzer P, et al.: Effect of omeprazole and cimetidine on duodenal ulcer. N Engl J Med 312:958, 1985. *Illustrates the results achievable in treatment of duodenal ulcer when acid secretion is profoundly suppressed.*

Pounder RE: Duodenal ulcers that will not heal. Gut 25:697, 1984. *Complete, practical approach to the ulcer that does not heal with first-line therapy.*

Richardson CT: Gastric ulcer. In Sleisenger MH, Fordtran JS (eds.): Gastrointestinal Disease. 4th ed. Philadelphia, W. B. Saunders Company (in press). *Includes a detailed discussion of clinical results with therapeutic agents for gastric ulcer.*

Soll AH: Duodenal ulcer. In Sleisenger MH, Fordtran JS (eds.): Gastrointestinal Disease. 4th ed. Philadelphia, W. B. Saunders Company (in press). *Presents for duodenal ulcer what the preceding reference does for gastric ulcer.*

Strum WB: Prevention of duodenal ulcer recurrence. Ann Intern Med 105:757, 1986.

100.4 Surgical Therapy

Richard C. Thirlby

INDICATIONS

Peptic ulcers can be managed medically in most patients. However, surgery may be required to treat patients with complications of ulcers (hemorrhage, perforation, or obstruction) or patients with intractable ulcer disease. The decision to operate for intractability is difficult and is made primarily on subjective criteria. The physician and the patient must decide when pain and multiple ulcer recurrences become intolerable or intractable. Patients should be considered candidates for surgery when medical therapy has failed. Failure of medical therapy occurs when an ulcer does not heal on medication, when ulcers recur during maintenance medical treatment, or after multiple ulcer recurrences. Pain, interruption of livelihood or lifestyle, and history of major complications all influence the decision to refer patients for surgery. Pain per se is not an indication. Endoscopy should be performed before surgery to document the presence of an active ulcer in a patient with intractable pain, because the pain may arise from another cause.

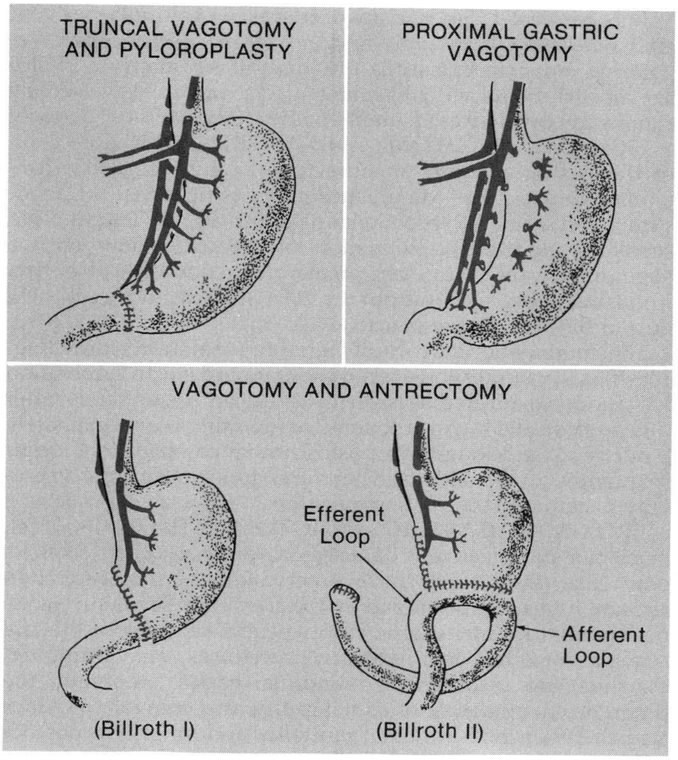

FIGURE 100–8. Model illustrating surgical procedures for peptic ulcer disease.

SURGICAL PROCEDURES

SUBTOTAL GASTRECTOMY. Subtotal gastrectomy (65 to 75 per cent gastrectomy) was the standard operation for duodenal ulcer disease for many years. This procedure was effective in preventing ulcer recurrence in 90 to 95 per cent of cases, but the incidence of long-term postoperative complications was excessive (Table 100–8). This procedure is no longer recommended for treating patients with duodenal ulcers but is occasionally necessary in treating patients with gastric ulcers (see below).

TRUNCAL VAGOTOMY AND PYLOROPLASTY. Vagotomy eliminates cephalic (vagal) stimulation of acid secretion and reduces basal acid output by 80 to 90 per cent and maximal (peak) acid output by 50 to 60 per cent. Truncal vagotomy also denervates the antral pump mechanism, leading to delayed gastric emptying. This can be overcome by adding a drainage (gastric emptying) procedure to vagotomy either as a pyloroplasty (Fig. 100–8) or a gastrojejunostomy.

Operative mortality with vagotomy and pyloroplasty is less than 1 per cent (Table 100–8). Even when this procedure is performed as an emergency, operative mortality is relatively

TABLE 100–8. SURGICAL PROCEDURES FOR TREATMENT OF PEPTIC ULCER DISEASE

	Operative Mortality		Late Postoperative Complications					Incidence of Recurrent Ulcers
			Dumping		*Diarrhea*			
	Elective	*Emergency*	*Mild**	*Severe*	*Mild**	*Severe*	*Weight Loss*	
Subtotal gastrectomy	1%	10%	60%	5%	15%	0%	50%	5–10%
Truncal vagotomy and pyloroplasty	<1%	<7%	20%	2%	20%	2%	5–39%	7–10%
Truncal vagotomy and antrectomy	1%	9–15%	30%	2–5%	20–30%	2%	10–42%	1%
Proximal gastric vagotomy	0.1%	1%	0.5%	0%	1–2%	0%	0–5%	10%

*Nearly all patients have some change in bowel habits. Numbers are averages of many series and reflect clinically important symptoms.

low in contrast to an operative mortality of 9 to 15 per cent after emergency vagotomy and antrectomy (see below). Vagotomy and pyloroplasty is the surgical treatment of choice for most patients with bleeding ulcers and is also used by some surgeons to treat patients with intractable ulcer disease.

TRUNCAL VAGOTOMY AND ANTRECTOMY. Resection of the gastric antrum, or antrectomy, removes gastrin-containing mucosa and diminishes the gastric phase of food-stimulated acid secretion. Antrectomy alone reduces acid secretion, and the combination of an antrectomy with a vagotomy leads to an even greater reduction of acid output (reducing basal acid output by 90 per cent and peak acid output by 70 to 80 per cent).

The combination of truncal vagotomy and antrectomy (Fig. 100–8) is frequently considered the standard elective operation for duodenal ulcer disease because ulcers recur rarely after this procedure. However, operative mortality is approximately 1 per cent, and long-term postoperative complications occur frequently (Table 100–8). Therefore, proximal gastric vagotomy is gaining favor in some centers.

PROXIMAL GASTRIC VAGOTOMY. The parietal cell mass can be selectively denervated (proximal gastric vagotomy) (Fig. 100–8) while antral innervation and motor function remain intact. This operation reduces acid secretion while maintaining normal gastric emptying. Since many of the late sequelae of other acid-reducing procedures (e.g., dumping, diarrhea) are secondary to abnormal gastric emptying, the theoretic advantage of proximal gastric vagotomy is to reduce acid secretion with minimal mortality and long-term postoperative morbidity (Table 100–8).

Proximal gastric vagotomy is probably not indicated in patients with gastric outlet obstruction, active pyloric channel ulcers, prepyloric ulcers, or actively bleeding ulcers. Complicated peptic ulcer disease (history of bleeding or perforation) or high acid outputs do not contraindicate this procedure. Proximal gastric vagotomy is becoming the operation of choice in many hospitals for patients undergoing elective operations for duodenal ulcers.

SPECIAL CONSIDERATIONS IN PATIENTS WITH GASTRIC ULCERS

The indications for operation and the surgical management of gastric ulcers are the same as for duodenal ulcers except that gastric cancer is a concern in patients with nonhealing gastric ulcers. If endoscopy with multiple biopsies and brush cytology specimens indicates that a gastric ulcer is benign, cancer is excluded with 95 to 98 per cent certainty (see Ch. 101). However, if an ulcer has not healed after 12 weeks of medical management (15 weeks in patients with initial ulcers > 2.5 cm in diameter), surgery is usually indicated to exclude the possibility of cancer.

While proximal gastric vagotomy is currently the procedure of choice for most patients with duodenal ulcers, antrectomy alone with resection of the ulcer is indicated in most patients with gastric ulcers (Fig. 100–8). Sometimes a subtotal gastrectomy is necessary to remove all of the gastric ulcer–prone epithelium. Vagotomy may not be necessary, because many patients with gastric ulcers have normal or low acid secretion rates. Some patients, on the other hand, also have duodenal ulcers or prepyloric gastric ulcers and require vagotomy in addition to an antrectomy.

LATE POSTOPERATIVE COMPLICATIONS

POSTPRANDIAL DUMPING. This can occur whenever the pyloric mechanism is disrupted by pyloroplasty, gastroduodenostomy (Billroth I) (Fig. 100–8), or gastrojejunostomy (Billroth II). The dumping syndrome rarely develops after proximal gastric vagotomy (Table 100–8). The syndrome is transient in most patients and can usually be managed by dietary manipulations (see below).

TABLE 100–9. DIETARY TREATMENT OF DUMPING SYNDROMES AND POSTVAGOTOMY DIARRHEA

1. Follow low-carbohydrate, high-protein, high-fat diet.
2. Avoid refined carbohydrates and concentrated carbohydrates such as sugar, jelly, cake, pie, pudding, candy; substitute complex carbohydrates such as starch.
3. Eat six small meals a day.
4. Drink fluids between meals rather than immediately before or during meals.
5. Eat slowly.

Postprandial dumping syndrome is divided into early and late symptoms. *Early* symptoms occur immediately after a meal and are both intestinal (nausea, vomiting, epigastric pain, diarrhea, and dyspepsia) and vasomotor (flushing, dizziness, tachycardia, and diaphoresis). The initiating event is believed to be rapid gastric emptying, and symptoms may be caused by several pathophysiologic events: (1) duodenal or jejunal distention produced by the food bolus, (2) contraction of circulating blood volume due to displacement of fluid into the hyperosmolar solution in the gut (especially after consumption of refined carbohydrates), and (3) release of vasoactive hormones (serotonin, bradykinin, vasoactive intestinal peptide).

Late postprandial dumping symptoms occur one to three hours after a meal and are believed to result from hypoglycemia. The mechanism is presumed to be a rapid rise in blood glucose after ingestion of a large carbohydrate meal. This leads to an exaggerated insulin response followed by reactive hypoglycemia.

Treatment of the dumping syndrome is largely dietary (Table 100–9). Medications such as serotonin antagonists or antimuscarinic drugs are ineffective in most patients. Reconstructive surgery aimed at slowing the transit of food through the small intestine using reversed intestinal segments or Roux-en-Y jejunal interposition may be indicated in the 2 to 5 per cent of patients who are severely disabled (Fig. 100–9).

POSTVAGOTOMY DIARRHEA. Diarrhea is common following gastric surgery, especially when vagotomy is included. In 20 to 30 per cent of patients, diarrhea is clinically important and in 2 per cent it is incapacitating (see Table 100–8). The pathogenesis is unclear, and diagnosis of postvagotomy diarrhea should not be made without excluding *inflammatory bowel disease, lactose deficiency, celiac sprue,* or other causes of diarrhea, because gastric surgery may unmask previously silent diseases.

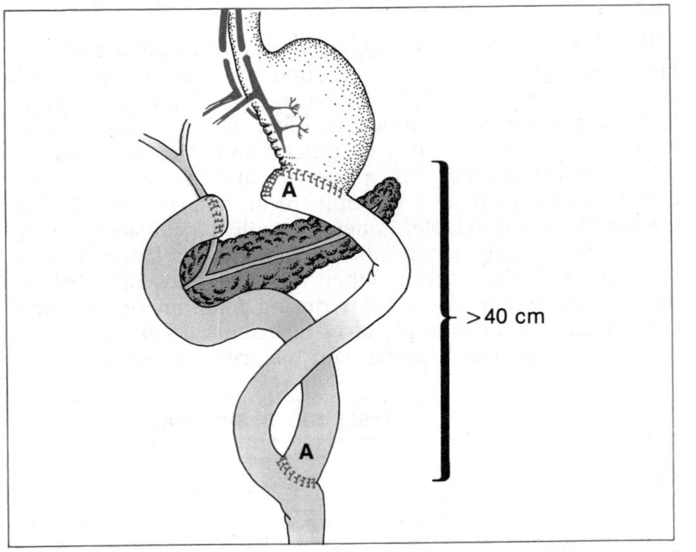

FIGURE 100–9. Model illustrating truncal vagotomy, antrectomy, and Roux-en-Y gastrojejunostomy (see text). Jejunum is divided at A-A' with distal end (A) anastomosed to stomach. Pancreaticobiliary secretions are thus diverted from the stomach by at least 40 cm of interposed intestine (pancreaticobiliary secretions shown in red).

Treatment of postvagotomy diarrhea is largely dietary (Table 100–9). Medications (antidiarrheal agents, opiates, cholestyramine, and aluminum hydroxide–containing antacids) may be helpful in some patients. Approximately 2 per cent of patients will require reoperation (using reversed intestinal segments) to control disabling diarrhea.

WEIGHT LOSS. Weight loss occurs frequently after antrectomy (see Table 100–8). In general, it develops in proportion to the extent of gastric resection and occurs most commonly after a Billroth II gastrojejunostomy (see Fig. 100–8). Weight loss after gastric surgery most commonly results from inadequate caloric intake. Early satiety resulting from a small gastric remnant may cause patients to limit meal size. Fear of eating because of postprandial symptoms or diarrhea may also prevent patients from consuming adequate calories. Other causes of weight loss include bacterial overgrowth that can occur in the afferent limb (blind loop) of a Billroth II anastomosis (see Fig. 100–8), relative pancreatic insufficiency, and in rare cases celiac sprue. Bacterial overgrowth leads to hydrolysis of conjugated bile salts and also damage to small intestinal absorptive cells. In turn, this causes malabsorption of fat, fat-soluble vitamins, and other nutrients. Bacteria also utilize vitamin B_{12}; this may lead to B_{12} deficiency.

Antibiotics or surgical conversion of a Billroth II to a Billroth I anastomosis will reduce bacterial overgrowth and may restore vitamin B_{12}, fat, and fat-soluble vitamin absorption toward normal. Converting a Billroth II to a Billroth I anastomosis also may increase absorption by better mixing of food with pancreatic secretions, which further reduces malabsorption. Weight loss and malabsorption may be helped also by dietary manipulations (Table 100–9), antidiarrheal drugs, pancreatic enzymes, or a gluten-free diet in patients with celiac sprue.

ANEMIA. Anemia after surgery for ulcer disease can be caused by deficiency of iron, vitamin B_{12}, or folate. Iron deficiency is frequent after gastric resection. Malabsorption of iron and bleeding from recurrent ulcers or peristomal gastritis contribute to iron deficiency. Vitamin B_{12} deficiency may occur either because of atrophic gastritis (loss of parietal cells that secrete intrinsic factor) or because of bacterial overgrowth in the afferent loop of a Billroth II anastomosis (see Fig. 100–8). Folate deficiency is uncommon and presumably is caused by malabsorption of folate from food and by decreased ingestion of dietary folate.

Evaluation of anemic patients after surgery for peptic ulcer requires measurements of serum iron, B_{12}, and folate and assessment of stool for occult blood. Parenteral administration of vitamin B_{12} (1000 μg per month intramuscularly) and oral or intravenous iron (Imferon) may be required if deficiencies are documented. If bacterial overgrowth is suspected in patients with a Billroth II anastomosis, antibiotics (e.g., tetracycline, 250 mg four times daily) may be helpful.

ALKALINE REFLUX GASTRITIS AND ESOPHAGITIS. Reflux of duodenal contents, particularly bile, into the gastric remnant is believed to cause gastritis and esophagitis (see Ch. 99). Symptoms include continuous, burning abdominal pain, nausea, and vomiting of bile-containing material. Establishing reflux and inflammation as the cause of symptoms is difficult, since many asymptomatic postgastrectomy patients have similar endoscopic or histologic findings. No test definitively confirms that the symptoms are caused by reflux.

Results of medical treatment with drugs that bind bile salts (cholestyramine or aluminum hydroxide–containing antacids) are poor. Roux-en-Y jejunal interposition prevents reflux of duodenal contents into the gastric remnant and esophagus and may relieve symptoms in some patients (Fig. 100–9). However, it is difficult to select patients who may benefit from this operation, because the diagnosis is often in doubt.

AFFERENT LOOP SYNDROME. This can occur in patients who have a Billroth II–type gastroenterostomy (Fig. 100–8). Symptoms occur when pancreatic and biliary secretions collect in a partially obstructed afferent loop, causing distention and pain. Eventually, the fluid bypasses the partial obstruction, rushes into the stomach, and provokes vomiting. Thus, the symptom complex is characterized by postprandial cramping epigastric pain followed by projectile vomiting. Pain is relieved after vomiting. The vomitus is voluminous, contains bile, and does not contain food because food has left the stomach and passed through the efferent loop. Management of severe symptoms requires operative revision of the gastrojejunal anastomosis.

POSTOPERATIVE RECURRENT PEPTIC ULCER

Postoperative ulcers can develop in the stomach, the duodenum, or the jejunum in patients with a Billroth II gastrojejunostomy (marginal ulcer) (Fig. 100–8). The incidence varies for the different operations (Table 100–8). The clinical presentation is characterized by pain in only one half of patients, and complications, especially bleeding, are frequent. Diagnosis of postoperative recurrent ulcer is best made by endoscopy because upper gastrointestinal barium studies are poor at identifying postoperative ulcers, particularly after a Billroth II gastrojejunostomy.

Incomplete vagotomy is responsible for postoperative recurrent ulcers in the majority of patients. Other uncommon causes include *Zollinger-Ellison syndrome, retained antrum syndrome, ulcerogenic drugs* (aspirin or other nonsteroidal anti-inflammatory drugs), *silk surgical sutures* at the anastomosis, or *antral G cell hyperplasia*. Serum gastrin concentrations should be measured in all patients with recurrent ulcers to rule out Zollinger-Ellison syndrome (see Ch. 100.6) or retained antrum syndrome.

Sham feeding is the best test for diagnosis of incomplete vagotomy (see Ch. 100.1). An appetizing meal is presented to a patient, and the meal is chewed but not swallowed. Acid output is measured during the test by aspirating gastric secretions through a nasogastric tube. Acid output induced by sham feeding greater than 10 per cent of pentagastrin-stimulated peak acid output implies intact vagal innervation of the stomach. The insulin test, or Hollander test, of vagal function is no longer recommended because it is dangerous; hypoglycemic seizures, strokes, myocardial infarction, and deaths have been reported. It is also less reliable and less specific than the sham feeding test.

Until recently, the treatment of postoperative recurrent ulcers caused by incomplete vagotomy was surgical. The advent of histamine H_2-receptor antagonists has made medical management the first choice. Postoperative recurrent ulcers will heal with standard doses of histamine H_2-receptor antagonists in 60 to 90 per cent of patients, and reoperation may not be necessary. Lifetime maintenance therapy (cimetidine, 400 to 800 mg, or ranitidine, 150 mg, at bedtime) is required in most patients to prevent further recurrence and complications. The indications for reoperation in patients with recurrent ulcer secondary to incomplete vagotomy are (1) failure to heal with cimetidine or ranitidine, (2) recurrence on maintenance therapy with H_2-receptor antagonists, (3) a complication (bleeding, obstruction, or perforation) associated with recurrent ulcer, or (4) noncompliance with long-term medical therapy. The choice of reoperation should be individualized. If sham feeding confirms incomplete vagotomy, transthoracic revagotomy usually should be performed if the patient has had an emptying procedure such as pyloroplasty or a type of gastroenterostomy such as Billroth I or II at the initial operation. Antrectomy may be indicated in some patients who have had only a vagotomy as their initial procedure.

Herrington JL, Davidson J, Shumway SJ: Proximal gastric vagotomy: Follow-up of 109 patients for 6–13 years. Ann Surg 204:108, 1986. *Long-term follow-up on 109 patients after proximal gastric vagotomy. The incidence of side effects was very low, and the recurrent ulcer rate was 9.2 per cent.*

Herrington JL, Scott HW, Sawyers JL: Experience with vagotomy-antrectomy and Roux-en-Y gastrojejunostomy in surgical treatment of duodenal, gastric and stomal ulcers. Ann Surg 199:590, 1984. *Report of a large experience with Roux-en-Y gastrojejunostomy in the treatment of patients with postoperative recurrent ulcer, postgastrectomy syndromes, and complicated duodenal ulcer.*

Jordan PH Jr: Operations for peptic ulcer disease and their early postoperative complications. In Sleisenger MH, Fordtran JS (eds.): Gastrointestinal Disease. 4th ed. Philadelphia, W. B. Saunders Company (in press). *A general review of the surgical treatment of peptic ulcer disease, including indications for surgery and a description of the operations.*

Knight CD, VanHeerden JA, Kelly KA: Proximal gastric vagotomy: Update. Ann Surg 197:22, 1983. *Seven-year experience with proximal gastric vagotomy in 298 patients evaluated and treated in the Mayo Clinic.*

100.5 Complications

Mark Feldman

Approximately one of three patients with peptic ulcer disease experiences *bleeding*, *perforation*, or *obstruction* at some point in the course of his or her disease. A complication may be the first manifestation, or it may occur later. Patients with a peptic ulcer in the pyloric channel or postbulbar duodenum, with combined duodenal and gastric ulcer, and with Zollinger-Ellison syndrome are especially likely to experience complications.

BLEEDING

Bleeding is the most common complication of peptic ulcer disease, occurring in 15 to 20 per cent of patients with duodenal ulcer and 10 to 15 per cent of patients with gastric ulcer. Risk of bleeding is unrelated to duration of ulcer disease; one of four patients will have no history of ulcer disease when he or she presents with bleeding. The mortality rate for a single bleeding episode (5 to 10 per cent) has not changed in the past several decades.

Hemorrhage results from erosion of the ulcer into a blood vessel. The most common sign of acute bleeding is melena, with or without hematemesis. Although these symptoms usually indicate major blood loss (> 1000 ml), melena may occur with loss of as little as 50 to 75 ml of blood. In some patients with major hemorrhage, gastrointestinal transit of blood may be so rapid that the stool is bright red or maroon. Moreover, a nasogastric aspirate may not contain blood if active bleeding from a duodenal ulcer does not reflux into the stomach. Thus, the combination of hematochezia and a bloodless nasogastric aspirate can occur in patients with bleeding peptic ulcer. The hemoglobin and hematocrit on admission may not reflect the severity of bleeding if sufficient time has not elapsed to allow for compensatory hemodilution. Therefore, the severity of acute bleeding is better assessed by the blood pressure and pulse rate. A systolic blood pressure of less than 100 mm Hg and a pulse rate of more than 100 beats per minute, both taken with the patient supine, suggest major blood loss, as do a fall in blood pressure of greater than 10 mm Hg and an increase in pulse of more than 20 beats per minute after the patient assumes an upright position.

Peptic ulcer is the commonest source of acute upper gastrointestinal bleeding (accounting for 40 to 50 per cent of cases). The differential diagnosis, however, includes esophagogastric varices, erosive and hemorrhagic gastritis, and Mallory-Weiss laceration. Less common causes include benign and malignant gastric neoplasm, esophagitis, duodenitis, vascular anomaly (e.g., angiodysplasia and arteriovenous malformation), and aortoenteric fistula, usually in patients with a prosthetic aortic graft. Peptic ulcers may also cause chronic or intermittent bleeding, resulting in iron deficiency anemia. In such instances, it is mandatory to exclude other causes of chronic blood loss, such as colonic cancer, before attributing the bleeding to a peptic ulcer.

Certain factors may, if present, adversely affect clinical outcome in patients with bleeding peptic ulcers: (1) severe, continuing hemorrhage (arbitrarily defined as the need for three or more units of blood in the first 24 hours or six or more units in the first 48 hours after pre-existing losses have been replaced); (2) early rebleeding, usually occurring within 3 to 5 days of initial stabilization; (3) age greater than 60 years; (4) associated diseases, especially involving the cardiovascular system, lungs, and liver (particularly active alcoholic liver disease); (5) history of ingestion of nonsteroidal anti-inflammatory drugs; and (6) endoscopic visualization of a blood vessel or clot in the base of the ulcer.

Various therapeutic measures have been employed in patients with bleeding ulcers, including nasogastric suction, antacid therapy, and inhibition of gastric acid–pepsin secretion with intravenous or oral histamine H_2-receptor antagonist drugs. None of these measures, alone or in combination, has been proved to stop active bleeding, to prevent rebleeding, to decrease need for surgery, or to reduce mortality. As an exception H_2-receptor antagonists may be modestly effective in patients with bleeding gastric ulcers.

Ulcers that are actively bleeding or that have endoscopic stigmata of recent bleeding are sometimes treated endoscopically using electrodes (monopolar, bipolar, heater probes) or laser (argon, neodymium: yttrium aluminum garnet). Unfortunately, the efficacy of these modalities has not yet been adequately documented by controlled clinical trials. Endoscopic therapy of actively bleeding ulcers may someday replace surgical therapy in many patients.

Continuous bleeding from an ulcer or major bleeding that recurs in the hospital commonly is an indication for surgery. Urgent surgery is required in approximately 15 per cent of patients with bleeding peptic ulcers, carrying with it a mortality rate two- to threefold higher than that of elective surgery. Emergency surgical therapy for bleeding duodenal ulcer consists of suture ligation of the bleeding vessel, along with either (1) truncal vagotomy and pyloroplasty or (2) truncal vagotomy and antrectomy. The procedure of emergency vagotomy and pyloroplasty has a higher in-hospital rebleeding rate than truncal vagotomy and antrectomy but a lower operative mortality rate. For bleeding gastric ulcer, the distal stomach, including the ulcer, is usually resected. If the ulcer is quite proximal in the stomach, the ulcer is usually biopsied and oversewn, followed by distal gastrectomy. Emergency surgery stops bleeding in 90 to 95 per cent of cases. In poor surgical candidates, angiography with arterial embolization using Gelfoam or autologous clot may stop bleeding.

Following discharge from the hospital, a patient has a 30 to 50 per cent chance of bleeding again from an ulcer, a twofold or greater risk than for the overall population of patients with peptic ulcers. This enhanced risk remains approximately the same after a second or third bleeding episode. The severity of the initial bleeding event is not correlated with the severity of subsequent bleeding. Chronic medical therapy or surgery does not clearly reduce the subsequent risk of rebleeding.

PERFORATION

An ulcer may penetrate the wall of the duodenum or stomach, resulting in (1) *free perforation*—rupture into the peritoneal cavity with spillage of duodenal or gastric contents; (2) *penetration*—erosion into and confinement by a solid organ, such as pancreas, liver, or spleen; or (3) *fistula formation*—extension into a hollow viscus, such as the common bile duct, pancreatic duct, gallbladder, or intestine.

Free perforation occurs in 6 to 11 per cent of patients with duodenal ulcer and in 2 to 5 per cent of patients with gastric ulcer, usually during the course of known peptic ulcer disease. Free perforation occurs more commonly in men, in elderly patients, and in patients who ingest nonsteroidal anti-inflammatory agents. Duodenal ulcers that bleed are more often posterior; duodenal ulcers that perforate are usually anterior. A duodenal ulcer may occasionally perforate posteriorly into the lesser sac and cause back pain rather than signs of generalized peritonitis. Most perforated gastric ulcers arise from the lesser curvature. In approximately 10 per cent of cases, peptic ulcer perforation is complicated by significant bleeding.

Free perforation characteristically causes sudden, severe, constant abdominal pain that reaches maximal intensity rapidly. The pain is initially present in the upper abdomen but quickly becomes generalized. Movement exacerbates the pain so that the patient prefers to lie on his or her back without moving. Marked abdominal tenderness to palpation and diffuse, boardlike rigidity of the abdominal wall musculature are present. Hypotension and tachycardia usually occur owing to intraperitoneal fluid losses. Hemoconcentration and leukocytosis are usually present, whereas fever often is absent. The serum amylase level is mildly elevated in one of six patients. Upright abdominal or chest radiographs show free air (pneumoperitoneum) in approximately 75 per cent of cases. If pneumoperitoneum is not evident and there is clinical suspicion of perforation, it may be helpful to insufflate 400 to 500 ml of air into the stomach through a nasogastric tube and then to obtain upright radiographs of the chest and abdomen (pneumogastrography) or to administer a contrast agent such as meglumine diatrizoate (Gastrografin) through the tube or by mouth. A definite diagnosis of perforated peptic ulcer often is not established until surgery is performed. The differential diagnosis of perforated ulcer is discussed in Ch. 100.2.

The presentation of free perforation may be atypical: (1) A perforation may close rapidly with only minimal contamination of the peritoneal cavity and with rapid, spontaneous clinical improvement. (2) Abdominal pain and physical findings may be less impressive in elderly patients and in patients with neurologic or psychiatric problems or both. Such patients may present with unexplained shock. (3) Fluid may leak into the peritoneal cavity slowly and collect in the right paracolic gutter, resulting in a clinical presentation simulating that of acute appendicitis.

Treatment of free perforation is usually surgical. In most cases, surgery is carried out to establish the diagnosis and to patch the perforation with a piece of omentum (Graham's closure). Whether definitive ulcer surgery should be carried out also at the time of patching a perforation is controversial. Many physicians will perform parietal cell vagotomy, truncal vagotomy and pyloroplasty, or truncal vagotomy and antrectomy for perforated duodenal ulcer (or distal gastrectomy for perforated gastric ulcer) if there has been a long history of ulcer disease or previous ulcer complications. If perforation occurred more than 8 to 12 hours earlier, definitive surgery is usually not performed because of extensive peritoneal soiling. If a perforated gastric ulcer is not resected, the ulcer should be biopsied because 10 per cent of perforated gastric ulcers are malignant. Medical therapy of free perforation, usually reserved for high-risk patients, consists of nasogastric suction, intravenous fluids, and systemic broad-spectrum antibiotics. Some patients whose perforation appears to have become sealed off and who are improving rapidly can also be treated medically.

Mortality from free perforation is approximately 5 to 15 per cent for duodenal ulcer and somewhat higher for gastric ulcer, especially if the gastric ulcer is near the cardia. The most important factors associated with a poor outcome in perforated duodenal ulcer are longstanding (> 48 hours) perforation prior to surgery; preoperative shock; serious concurrent illnesses, and, possibly, old age.

Penetration into solid organs such as the pancreas occurs with unknown frequency, since penetration can be diagnosed with certainty only at surgery or autopsy. These patients almost always have a long history of ulcer disease and usually present with intractable ulcer pain. Serum amylase and lipase levels may be elevated with posterior penetrating ulcers.

A *fistula*, an uncommon form of perforation, from a duodenal ulcer usually extends into the common bile duct; one from a gastric ulcer usually extends into the colon or duodenum. Patients with duodenocholedochal fistula may be asymptomatic but have air in the biliary tree, or they may present with cholangitis and abnormal liver function tests. The fistula is usually demonstrated by an upper gastrointestinal series, in which case barium refluxes from the duodenal bulb into the biliary tree. The fistula may close during medical treatment, although surgery may be required in some cases. Gastrocolic or gastrojejunocolic fistula caused by perforated gastric ulcer is often associated with ingestion of nonsteroidal anti-inflammatory drugs. These patients may present with diarrhea and malabsorption. The usual treatment is surgical. A gastric ulcer in the antrum may also perforate into the duodenal bulb, resulting in two or even three channels from the stomach to the duodenum.

OBSTRUCTION

Gastric outlet obstruction occurs in approximately 5 per cent of patients with duodenal or gastric ulcer and is especially common if the ulcer is located in the pyloric channel. Obstruction is caused by edema, smooth muscle spasm, fibrosis, or a combination of these processes. Obstruction usually occurs after ulcer disease of many years duration but may occasionally occur as the initial manifestation. Mortality rates from obstruction in peptic ulcer disease are 7 to 26 per cent, depending on the age of the patient and the presence or absence of associated diseases.

Obstruction delays gastric emptying and commonly causes nausea, vomiting, epigastric fullness or bloating, anorexia, early satiety, and a fear of eating (sitophobia). Significant weight loss may result. Epigastric pain is frequent and may be relieved temporarily by vomiting. Symptoms have usually been present for weeks or months. Vomiting, which may be delayed an hour or more after eating, is often copious and may contain undigested food but usually no bile. Physical examination may reveal volume depletion (hypotension, tachycardia, and dry skin and mucous membranes), visible peristalsis in the epigastrium, or a succussion splash over the stomach.

Any of the following objective measurements support the diagnosis of gastric retention: (1) aspiration of more than 300 ml of gastric fluid four or more hours after a meal (a large-bore tube may be necessary for measuring this), (2) aspiration of more than 200 ml of gastric fluid the morning after an overnight fast, or (3) removal of more than 400 ml of gastric fluid 30 minutes after instilling 750 ml of isotonic saline into the empty stomach (*saline load test*). Gastric retention may be appreciated on a plain abdominal radiograph (large, dilated stomach containing solid debris) and documented by an upper gastrointestinal series or radionuclide scintigraphy. Gastric retention is not always caused by gastric outlet obstruction. It may result from gastric atony, as in diabetic gastroparesis, from vagotomy, or as a side effect of medications. Gastric outlet obstruction, which is caused by peptic ulcer disease in 80 to 90 per cent of cases, can usually best be established by endoscopy. The other common cause is carcinoma of the antrum. Less common causes include gastric lymphoma, pancreatic carcinoma, pancreatitis, hypertrophic pyloric stenosis, eosinophilic gastritis, Crohn's disease, antral caustic stricture, antral polyp, and annular pancreas.

Laboratory studies usually reflect intravascular volume depletion (hemoconcentration, prerenal azotemia) and a hypokalemic, hypochloremic metabolic alkalosis due to vomiting. If extensive weight loss has occurred, hypoalbuminemia, cutaneous anergy, and a low serum transferrin concentration may be present. The urine is usually concentrated and contains less than 10 mEq of chloride per liter, but the urinary sodium concentration and pH are variable, depending on the renal tubular threshold for bicarbonate reabsorption.

Therapy of gastric outlet obstruction has three goals: gastric decompression and resolution of obstruction; replacement of fluids and electrolytes; and nutritional support. Gastric decompression is accomplished by continuous nasogastric suction for at least 72 hours. With prolonged obstruction, gradual gastric dilation occurs, and this interferes with the contractile function of gastric smooth muscle. Electrolyte disturbances such as hypokalemia can also contribute to gastric motor dysfunction. Saline load tests, performed serially, may have prognostic value. For example, a return of more than 300 ml after 24 hours of nasogastric suction suggests that obstruction will not resolve and that surgery may be required. After 72 hours, a return of less than 200 ml is a favorable sign and usually indicates that the tube can be removed and the patient can be fed liquids. Intravenous fluids and electrolytes are given to replace pre-existing and current losses. Isotonic saline containing 10 to 20 mEq of potassium chloride per liter is satisfactory in most cases. Losses of gastric acid from continuous gastric aspiration can be curtailed by administering H_2-receptor antagonists (cimetidine or ranitidine) intravenously. If suction is carried out for only a few days, 5 per cent dextrose solution administered intravenously, along with soluble vitamins, may suffice. If prolonged suction proves necessary, parenteral intravenous hyperalimentation should be instituted. This is especially valuable if the patient has lost significant lean body mass.

Approximately 50 per cent of patients with obstruction respond acutely to medical management. This response is related to the relative degrees of edema, spasm, and fibrosis, because edema and spasm may resolve. Obstruction relieved by medical therapy not infrequently occurs again within the next several years, requiring surgery at that time. Medical therapy may be effective for many years, however, so that it may be prudent to attempt it initially rather that to proceed directly to surgery in all patients. If obstruction does not resolve in three to seven days, surgery is usually necessary. There is controversy over which operation is best: truncal vagotomy and antrectomy, truncal vagotomy and drainage (pyloroplasty or gastrojejunostomy), or subtotal gastrectomy. Some surgeons are reluctant to perform truncal vagotomy for fear of postoperative gastric atony, although this complication is uncommon. Gastrojejunostomy (without gastric resection or truncal vagotomy) is associated with a high rate (30 to 40 per cent) of recurrences of ulcer. Nonsurgical dilation of the obstructed pylorus using balloons passed through an endoscope is a newly introduced therapy, the long-term efficacy of which remains to be established.

Collier D St J, Pain JA: Non-steroidal antiinflammatory drugs and peptic ulcer perforation. Gut 26:359, 1985. *Demonstrates an association between ingestion of these drugs and perforation in patients older than 65.*

Collins R, Langman M: Treatment with histamine H_2 antagonists in acute upper gastrointestinal hemorrhage. Implications of randomized trials. N Engl J Med 313:660, 1985. *Reviews data from 27 randomized trials, emphasizing end points of rebleeding, need for operation, and death.*

Fleischer D: Endoscopic therapy of upper gastrointestinal bleeding in humans. Gastroenterology 90:217, 1986. *Comprehensive and critical review of current modalities for endoscopic therapy of upper gastrointestinal bleeding, including bleeding ulcers.*

Graham D: Complications of peptic ulcer disease and indications for surgery. In Sleisenger MH, Fordtran JS (eds.): Gastrointestinal Disease. 4th ed. Philadelphia, W. B. Saunders Company (in press). *Comprehensive review with extensive references.*

Hogan RB, Hamilton JK, Polter DE: Preliminary experience with hydrostatic balloon dilation of gastric outlet obstruction. Gastrointest Endosc 32:71, 1986. *Uncontrolled study suggests that endoscopic dilation can delay or prevent surgery in most patients with gastric outlet obstruction, although long-term follow-up was short (4 to 14 months).*

Koo J, Lam SK, Boey J, et al.: Gastric acid secretion and its predictive value after vagotomy for perforated duodenal ulcer. Scand J Gastroenterol 18:929, 1983. *Controlled study of 101 patients with perforated duodenal ulcer found an ulcer recurrence rate of 3 per cent after proximal gastric vagotomy, 6 per cent after truncal vagotomy and pyloroplasty, and 43 per cent after simple closure without vagotomy.*

Lieberman DA, Keller FS, Katon, RM, et al.: Arterial embolization for massive upper gastrointestinal tract bleeding in poor surgical candidates. Gastroenterology 86:876, 1984. *Reviews embolization techniques in treating high-risk patients with bleeding ulcers.*

Peoples JB: Peptic ulcer disease and the nonsteroidal anti-inflammatory drugs. Am Surg 51:358, 1985. *Retrospective study suggests that patients with bleeding ulcers require surgery and die more often if they have been receiving these drugs prior to admission.*

100.6 Zollinger-Ellison Syndrome

Charles T. Richardson

DEFINITION

The Zollinger-Ellison syndrome is defined by both chemical and clinical criteria: (1) an increased serum gastrin concentration, (2) an increased basal acid output, (3) an increased ratio of basal to peak (pentagastrin-stimulated) acid output, and (4) the presence of peptic ulcer disease or diarrhea or both. Not all patients with an elevated serum gastrin concentration and hypersecretion of acid have tumors that can be identified at surgery. Presumably, such patients have tumors that are too small to be found at exploratory laparotomy, or they have hyperplasia of the islets of Langerhans, a condition known as microadenomatosis.

CLINICAL MANIFESTATIONS

Zollinger-Ellison syndrome can develop at any age; it occurs most frequently, however, between ages 35 and 65 years and more commonly in men than in women.

Abdominal pain resulting from an ulcer is the most common clinical finding. Ulcers usually occur in the duodenal bulb but also may develop in the postbulbar duodenum, jejunum, stomach, or esophagus. Complications of ulcer disease, such as bleeding or perforation, occur in 40 to 50 per cent of patients at some time during their course and may be the presenting manifestation. *Diarrhea* is a frequent complaint and may precede ulceration in some patients or occur without ulcers in others (5 to 10 per cent). *Fat malabsorption* (steatorrhea) is occasionally noted.

About 20 to 30 per cent of patients with Zollinger-Ellison syndrome have multiple endocrine neoplasia (MEN I) syndrome and thus have a hereditary form of peptic ulcer disease (Ch. 241). These patients may have parathyroid or pituitary tumors and clinical findings such as hypercalcemia, renal stones, or increased prolactin levels. It is unlikely that peptic ulcer disease occurs with increased frequency in association with parathyroid adenomas except in patients who also have MEN I syndrome.

In some patients, Cushing's syndrome can develop as a result of either pituitary disease or ectopic adrenocorticotropic hormone (ACTH) production by gastrinomas. Patients with ectopic ACTH production frequently have metastatic gastrinoma, for example, in the liver.

PATHOPHYSIOLOGY

Peptic ulcers in patients with Zollinger-Ellison syndrome presumably result from increased secretion of acid and pepsin driven by excessive amounts of circulating gastrin. Gastrin also has a trophic effect on parietal (acid-secreting) cells that leads to an increased parietal cell mass. Since parietal cell mass correlates with maximum acid output, some patients with Zollinger-Ellison syndrome also have increased maximum (peak) acid outputs.

Diarrhea results almost exclusively from the large volumes of fluid secreted by the stomach and is relieved in most patients by aspirating gastric juice via a nasogastric tube or more conveniently by treating patients with histamine$_2$ (H_2)-receptor antagonists (see below). Independent of stimulating acid secretion, gastrin may also play a role in the development of diarrhea by reducing intestinal absorption of water and electrolytes.

Steatorrhea may occur for several reasons. First, acid damages small bowel epithelial cells. This, in turn, causes a mucosal defect that limits transport of fat and perhaps other nutrients across the mucosa. Second, pancreatic lipase is inactivated by acid. This leads to decreased breakdown of triglycerides and contributes to fat malabsorption. Third, acid may decrease the amount of conjugated bile acids in the duodenum and upper jejunum. This results in inadequate formation of micelles, this, in turn, may lead to fat malabsorption.

DIAGNOSIS

Zollinger-Ellison syndrome should be suspected in patients who have (1) ulcers in unusual locations, such as the postbulbar duodenum or jejunum, (2) ulcers that persist despite medical treatment, (3) ulcers and diarrhea, (4) abnormally large gastric folds or thickened duodenal and/or jejunal folds, (5) ulcers and manifestations of other endocrine tumors such as renal stones, (6) a family history of ulcer disease, and (7) recurrent ulcers after ulcer surgery.

These criteria call for measurement of the serum gastrin concentration (Table 100–3). If the level is abnormally high, a gastric analysis should be performed. Zollinger-Ellison syndrome is a likely diagnosis if the serum gastrin level is elevated, basal acid output is increased (>10.6 mmol per hour in men and 5.6 mmol per hour in women), and the ratio of basal to peak acid output (pentagastrin stimulated) is greater than 0.40:1.0. The diagnosis can be confirmed by performing a secretin stimulation test (see Ch. 100.2). This test is especially helpful in patients with serum gastrin concentrations or basal acid outputs that are only slightly increased. A positive secretin test, along with an increased serum gastrin concentration and basal acid output, establishes the diagnosis of Zollinger-Ellison syndrome in over 95 per cent of patients.

Tumors are found at surgery in 40 to 70 per cent of patients with Zollinger-Ellison syndrome and are usually located in the pancreas. Tumors have also been found in the duodenum, stomach, greater omentum, transverse mesocolon, and other areas of the peritoneal cavity. Computerized axial tomography (CT) is useful in detecting gastrinomas and therefore should be performed in patients suspected of having the Zollinger-Ellison syndrome. A positive CT scan is almost always correct, whereas a negative CT scan is less reliable. Angiography is a helpful adjunct to CT if a laparotomy is planned but is not indicated in every patient with the Zollinger-Ellison syndrome. Since some gastrinomas have been found in the stomach or duodenum, upper endoscopy also should be performed to look for tumors. Techniques such as intraoperative sonography or transhepatic venous sampling to measure gastrin from tributaries draining the pancreas or duodenum have been helpful in some centers in localizing tumors, but these tests are not available in most hospitals.

THERAPY

For many years total gastrectomy was the treatment of choice for patients with Zollinger-Ellison syndrome and in some hospitals remains the treatment of choice. All of the acid-secreting mucosa as well as the antrum is removed, with subsequent cure of peptic ulcers and diarrhea. However, many of the late postoperative complications that occur in patients with ordinary peptic ulcer disease develop after total gastrectomy (see Ch. 100.4). Furthermore, in some centers mortality is higher with total gastrectomy than with other surgical procedures for ulcer disease.

With the advent of H_2-receptor antagonists, it has become possible to treat patients medically. Antagonism of the H_2-receptor with either cimetidine, ranitidine, or famotidine effectively reduces acid secretion in most patients and decreases symptoms related to the disease. However, larger than normally prescribed doses, as well as more frequent administration, are often required. For example, 600 mg of cimetidine every four hours or 300 mg of ranitidine every eight hours may be necessary to reduce acid secretion adequately.* A few patients have required even larger and more frequent doses of cimetidine or ranitidine. For example, a few patients have required as much as 5 to 10 grams of cimetidine daily. The dose of cimetidine or ranitidine may be reduced by treating patients concomitantly with an antimuscarinic drug such as glycopyrrolate or isopropamide (see Fig. 100–7), since antimuscarinic drugs have been shown to enhance the inhibitory effect on acid secretion of H_2-receptor antagonists. A new drug, omeprazole, is currently being tested for treating patients with Zollinger-Ellison syndrome. This compound is a potent inhibitor of acid secretion, and in many patients, acid secretion can be inhibited by taking the drug once daily (see Ch. 100.3).

Medical treatment with H_2-receptor antagonists is not ideal for two reasons: First, complications of ulcer disease have occurred in some patients, and second, medical therapy does not provide an opportunity to search for resectable tumors, more than half of which are believed to be malignant. Because of this, a reasonable approach to treating patients with Zollinger-Ellison syndrome is laparotomy to search for resectable tumors present in about 20 to 30 per cent of patients, followed by medical therapy with H_2-receptor antagonists.

Vagotomy may be combined with H_2-receptor antagonists in some patients to reduce acid secretion and to add to the inhibitory effect of cimetidine or ranitidine. Treatment with H_2-receptor antagonists is still necessary, although the dose of medication can sometimes be reduced. Regardless of the therapy used (tumor search followed by medical therapy alone or medical therapy combined with vagotomy), close follow-up to ensure compliance with the regimen is mandatory.

*May exceed maximum recommended daily dose.

Jensen RT, Doppman JL, Gardner JD: Gastrinoma. In Brooks, F, Dimagno E, Gardner JD, et al.: The Exocrine Pancreas: Biology, Pathology and Disease. New York, Raven Press, 1986, pp 727–745. *An excellent review of the clinical manifestations, diagnosis, and treatment of patients with Zollinger-Ellison syndrome.*

Jensen RT, Gardner JD, Raufman J-P, et al.: Zollinger-Ellison syndrome: Current concepts and management. Ann Intern Med 98:59, 1983. *A review of the literature relative to diagnosis and treatment of Zollinger-Ellison syndrome, including the experience with patients treated at the National Institutes of Health.*

McGuigan JE: The Zollinger-Ellison Syndrome. In Sleisenger MH, Fordtran JS (eds.): Gastrointestinal Disease. 4th ed. Philadelphia, W. B. Saunders Company (in press). *A review of the pathophysiology, diagnosis, and treatment of Zollinger-Ellison syndrome.*

101 NEOPLASMS OF THE STOMACH†

Sidney J. Winawer

The majority of gastric neoplasms are malignant, in contrast to the colon, where the reverse is true. Although gastric carcinoma is steadily decreasing in the United States, it still represents a major public health problem throughout the world. In some countries it is the most frequent cancer and the leading cause of death from cancer. In the United States gastric carcinoma is responsible for 90 to 95 per cent of malignant disease of the stomach. Approximately 5 per cent of all primary gastric malignancy is Hodgkin's disease (HD) and non-Hodgkin's lymphoma, particularly the latter, since HD rarely involves the stomach as a primary site. The sarcomas, including leiomyosarcoma, liposarcoma, neurogenic sarcoma and fibrosarcoma, are all relatively rare malignant tumors that may involve the stomach. Leiomyosarcoma of the stomach represents about 1 per cent of gastric cancers.

†This revised chapter was originally written by Paul Sherlock, to whom this is dedicated.

CARCINOMA OF THE STOMACH

EPIDEMIOLOGY. The incidence of gastric cancer varies markedly in different areas of the world. It is extremely common in Japan, Latin America west of the Andes, some parts of the Caribbean, and Eastern Europe; moderately common in Finland, Austria, and Czechoslovakia; and uncommon in the United States, Australia, New Zealand, and other Anglo-Saxon countries. Colorectal cancer tends to be rare where gastric cancer is common and vice versa. The low incidence in the United States is a recent development, since gastric cancer was the most common known cancer in the United States 40 to 50 years ago. Other countries that previously had a high incidence have also begun to show a decrease. The reasons for this are unknown. Environmental factors are considered important in the etiology of gastric cancer, as evidenced by populations migrating to areas of either low or high risk and taking on the risk of the area of migration. Japanese moving to Hawaii have a decreased incidence of gastric cancer in subsequent generations, and there is a further reduction with migration to the mainland. The incidence of colonic cancer increases with this migration.

ETIOLOGY. *Dietary influences* are thought to be important, but without direct proof. Consumption of barbecued meals, smoked or pickled fish and sauces, and alcohol and deficiencies of magnesium and vitamin A have all been postulated but unproved as causes of gastric cancer (Table 101–1).

Nitrosamines are powerful carcinogens for animals. They can be formed easily from common, secondary, tertiary, and quaternary amines by combining these with nitrite (the nitrosation reaction). This reaction can take place under varying conditions of pH and temperature, so that nitrosamines may be formed in the soil, under conditions of food storage, during food preparation such as frying bacon, or in the body. Bacteria may play a role by catalyzing the amine nitrite union or by reducing nitrate to nitrite. Thus the achlorhydric stomach is considered a favorable site for nitrosamine synthesis. The necessary amines can be found in many foods and medications, whereas nitrate and nitrites are found naturally in food and water and are present in food preservatives. Ascorbic acid (vitamin C) blocks the nitrosation reaction in the test tube. The increased intake of vitamin C and refrigeration have been postulated to be responsible for the decrease in gastric cancer in this country over the last few decades, but the nitrite hypothesis itself remains to be validated.

Blood group A is associated with a higher incidence of gastric cancer even in areas of the world where gastric cancer is rare. This fact and the aggregation of gastric cancer in certain families have raised the possibility of a genetic component.

Pernicious anemia had been considered a premalignant condition. However, the prior high incidence of gastric cancer seen in this disease is no longer seen. This may be a reflection of the progressively decreasing incidence of gastric cancer being observed worldwide. Although atrophic gastritis is usually seen in association with gastric cancer, this disorder is extremely common, and the vast majority of such patients never develop cancer.

Adenomatous polyps of the stomach, especially those larger than 2 cm, may occasionally give rise to carcinoma. Most stomach polyps are hyperplastic and do not become malignant.

TABLE 101–1. DIETARY FINDINGS FROM CASE CONTROL STUDIES OF GASTRIC CANCER*

Positive Association	Negative Association
Salted fish	Vegetables
Pickled vegetables	Fruit
Salty foods	Milk
Smoked fish	Meat
Starchy foods	Squash
Cabbage, potatoes	Eggplant
Cooked cereals	Lettuce
Bacon	Celery
	Animal fat

*United States (including Hawaii), Japan, Norway, England, and Israel.

Subtotal resection for benign disease results in chronic atrophic gastritis from either bile reflux or removal of the gastrin trophic factor. This has been shown to produce gastric cancer in animals. It has also been shown to result in gastric cancer after a ten-year interval in persons living in countries at increased risk for gastric cancer, especially in men, who are at higher risk than women.

Immunologic deficiencies, particularly the common variable type, may cause a predisposition to gastric cancer.

Gastric ulcer does not transform into cancer. Cancer foci may be present in association with an ulcer, however. All gastric ulcers must be suspected of having small areas of malignancy even when the ulcer appears benign by radiograph or endoscopy. Biopsy and cytologic examination will reveal the true nature of the lesion.

INCIDENCE AND PREVALENCE. It is estimated that there were 23,000 new cases of gastric cancer and 14,000 deaths from gastric cancer in the United States in 1986. Although this is a substantial number, a dramatic decline in the incidence of stomach cancer has occurred here and in many other countries. The magnitude of the decline varies. In the United States the age-adjusted mortality rate for males dropped from 28 per 100,000 in 1930 to 9.7 per 100,000 in 1967. The rate of decline has been the steepest among United States whites and in the older age group of all race-sex categories. Carcinoma of the stomach occurs most frequently between the ages of 50 and 70 years and is rare in patients younger than 30 years. The incidence and mortality rise steeply with age. Rates are higher in males than females by 2 to 1. The incidence of gastric cancer is higher for United States blacks than whites, but the marked difference noted earlier in the century is diminishing. Risk of gastric cancer is greatest among those of low socioeconomic status.

PATHOLOGY. Carcinoma of the stomach is adenocarcinoma that usually is manifested pathologically in one of four ways (Fig. 101–1): (1) Most often it appears as a bulky mass with deep central ulceration projecting into the lumen and invading the wall. (2) The tumor may infiltrate and narrow a portion of the lumen, most often in the antrum. Less commonly, the infiltration extends throughout the entire stomach,

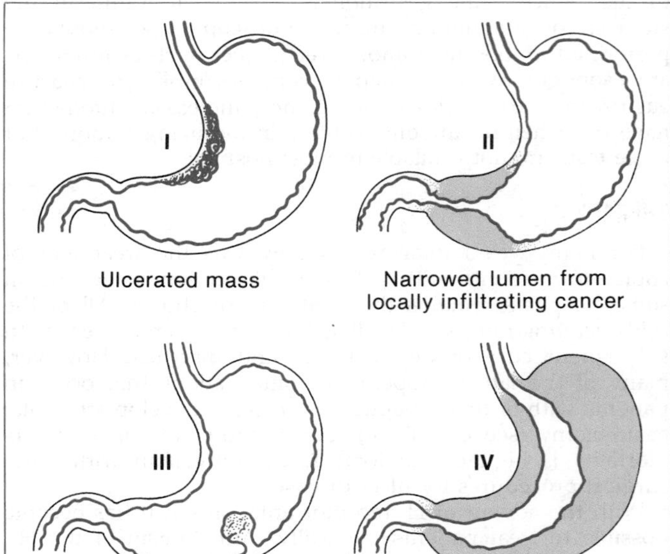

FIGURE 101–1. Diagrammatic representation of various presentations of gastric carcinoma.

resulting in *linitis plastica*—a fixed, nondistensible stomach with absence of normal folds and a narrowed lumen. (3) Polypoid or exophytic carcinoma with or without a stalk may occur and be difficult to distinguish from a benign polyp on radiograph. (4) More rarely, carcinoma of the stomach may occur as a superficially spreading tumor involving only the mucosal surface and producing a granular appearance. This is unlike linitis plastica, which extends through the entire thickness of the wall.

Gastric carcinomas may be well-differentiated adenocarcinomas or may be so anaplastic as to resemble diffuse histiocytic lymphoma or sarcoma. A true carcinoma in situ is rarely found and is confined entirely to the glands. This is more commonly seen at the surface of large adenomatous polyps of the stomach.

In about 75 per cent of patients with carcinoma of the stomach the tumors are found in the distal third. The lymphatic flow from such tumors is in the direction of the subpyloric nodes and porta hepatis and along both curvatures. The tumor very rarely spreads to the pancreaticolineal nodes, in contrast to proximal and midstomach lesions. Celiac and pancreatic nodal involvement occurs from lesions in all areas. In addition to invasion of lymph nodes, gastric carcinoma invades local structures: the lower end of the esophagus by submucosal spread, the pancreas, the transverse colon, the peritoneum, and, rarely, the duodenum. Hematogenous spread results in pulmonary, pleural, liver, brain, and bone metastases.

CLINICAL MANIFESTATIONS (Table 101–2). Early carcinoma of the stomach is frequently asymptomatic. *Anorexia* and *weight loss* are nonspecific symptoms and not well correlated with the size of the tumor. *Early satiety*, particularly with linitis plastica; *bloating; dysphagia; epigastric distress;* or more severe epigastric boring pain may be later symptoms. *Vomiting* is commonly a later symptom that may be caused by pyloric obstruction but may occur with other levels of obstruction. Vomiting also occurs without obstruction and may be secondary to the motility disturbance that a fixed mass in the wall produces. The pain is similar to that of peptic ulcer in about one fourth of patients, particularly when the tumor has ulcerated. In most patients, however, the pain usually occurs after eating and is not relieved by foods or antacids. Boring pain radiating to the back may indicate penetration of the tumor into the pancreas.

Dysphagia may occur with more proximal lesions, particularly when they have invaded the area around the cardioesophageal junction or spread submucosally to the esophagus, which is common in fundal lesions. Weakness and fatigue from *anemia* caused by chronic occult blood loss are common, although massive bleeding and hematemesis are unusual. Angina pectoris, congestive heart failure, and cerebral ischemia may occur because of the anemia. Perforation occurs in a small percentage of patients and can simulate peptic ulcer. When the tumor metastasizes, symptoms will depend upon organ involvement and may include jaundice, diarrhea, bone pain, cough, fever, hiccups, central nervous system disturbances, and abdominal bloating from ascites.

Physical examination during the early stages of gastric carcinoma may be completely unremarkable. Later there may be signs of weight loss and anemia. When the tumor has disseminated, hepatomegaly from metastases, jaundice, or ascites from peritoneal implants may be present. Splenomegaly may occur if the portal or splenic vein is invaded. A palpable *epigastric mass* is present in less than one half of patients and usually, but not always, indicates extensive involvement. Left supraclavicular adenopathy (Virchow's node), a nodular perirectal wall (Blumer's shelf), or umbilical nodules give evidence of metastatic spread.

TABLE 101–2. ADENOCARCINOMA OF THE STOMACH

Associated With	Clinical Manifestations
Environment—geographical differences	Anorexia, early satiety, weight loss
Diet—? nitrosamines	Dysphagia, vomiting, weakness
Blood group A—genetic	Epigastric distress to severe, boring pain
Atrophic gastritis	Anemia, occult blood in stools
Adenomatous polyps (>2 cm)	Epigastric mass, signs of metastases
Subtotal resection for benign ulcer disease in high-risk countries	Rare—Virchow's node, Blumer's shelf, Trousseau's syndrome, acanthosis nigricans

Several extragastric signs may precede the detection of an underlying malignancy. These include recurrent thrombophlebitis (Trousseau's syndrome); acanthosis nigricans, a verrucous, hyperpigmented, elevated skin lesion involving primarily the flexor spaces of the body; neuromyopathy characterized by localized sensory and/or motor disturbances; and profound central nervous system involvement with abrupt onset of confusion, memory defects, hostility, or ataxia. More detailed descriptions of the paraneoplastic syndromes are contained in specific chapters in Part XIII.

Laboratory studies usually disclose iron deficiency or megaloblastic anemia if the tumor is associated with untreated pernicious anemia. *Occult blood in the stool*, even with a single determination, is present in about one half of the patients. Most patients have gastric acid present but in reduced amounts. A few have achlorhydria after maximal stimulation with pentagastrin. A few have hypersecretion, especially with antral tumors. Therefore the presence of acid does not ensure that carcinoma is not present. Abnormalities in liver function, particularly a markedly elevated alkaline phosphatase and 5'nucleotidase level, suggest liver metastases. Microangiopathic hemolytic anemia has been reported in several patients with gastric cancer. Rarely, protein-losing enteropathy occurs with ulcerated carcinomas of the stomach.

DIAGNOSIS. ***Roentgenologic Diagnosis.*** Most gastric cancers will be suspected on roentgenologic examination. The standard upper gastrointestinal series has been refined to include barium contrast studies capable of detecting very small lesions. With the gastric mucosa covered by a thin layer of barium and distended with air or gas, multiple projections are taken, which outline almost the entire stomach surface. Refinement of technique can be accomplished by using high-density barium, CO_2, simethicone for gas dispersion, and glucagon to induce gastroparesis. With such methods films showing fine detail may be produced and small mucosal lesions visualized.

The radiologist is usually able to define the characteristics of a benign versus malignant lesion and is on occasion even able to suggest a histologic diagnosis. For example, lymphoma of the stomach may be suspected by the extensive involvement, multiple shallow ulcerations, and giant rugal hypertrophy caused by infiltrative disease, and by the fact that the duodenum may be involved in the neoplastic process. A gastric ulcer often gives difficulty, but radiologic accuracy is in the range of 80 per cent. Characteristic radiographic signs that suggest a malignant lesion are the presence of an ulcer in a mass, irregular folds stopping short of the ulcer crater, and an irregular ulcer base. It is essential to determine the nature of the ulcer by endoscopy with biopsy and cytology when any doubt exists. Generally the location of an ulcer is not too important in determining malignancy. Ulcers on the greater and lesser curvatures have about equal frequency of malignancy. Rigidity, loss of distensibility, unchanging contour, and irregular peristalsis are characteristic of a malignant lesion; when extensive infiltration from linitis plastica is present, a "leather bottle" appearance may result.

Endoscopy with Biopsy and Cytology. Fiberoptic endoscopy has increased the diagnostic yield over radiology alone. When combined with biopsy and brush cytology, the diagnostic accuracy is in the range of 95 to 99 per cent in various series. About one half of early gastric cancers present as small ulcerations; some have slight elevation or depression of the adjacent mucosa. The next most common type is a small polyp. Appearance at endoscopy may be misleading. Directed tissue sampling techniques, such as biopsy or brush cytology, should be used on any suspicious area, whether it is raised, depressed, or ulcerated. With more advanced carcinoma a specific tissue diagnosis can also be achieved with high accuracy by directed biopsy and cytology. The use of endoscopy to diagnose malignancies of the stomach is described in greater detail in Ch. 96.

Other Techniques. Maximal gastrin-stimulated gastric acid determination defines achlorhydria. This is less important now with fiberoptic endoscopy, biopsy, and cytology.

Elevation of carcinoembryonic antigen (CEA) is a late finding in gastric carcinoma but can define metastatic disease before it is clinically evident. The immunologic detection of fetal sulfoglycoprotein antigen (FSA) in the gastric juice of patients with cancer has been noted. The sulfoglycoprotein of carcinomatous gastric juice often has blood group A glycoprotein, which has been associated with gastric cancer.

TREATMENT. At present *surgery* provides the only satisfactory curative treatment for gastric cancer. The high frequency of regional node metastases plays a major role in the choice of the surgical procedure and the results of various therapeutic efforts. When the tumor is localized in the distal portion of the stomach, the omentum as well as nodes in the region of the porta hepatis and the pancreatic head are dissected, and a generous subtotal gastrectomy is performed. For tumors in the pars media and the proximal stomach, total gastrectomy may be indicated to obtain an adequate margin and for dissection of the predictable lymphatic spread in all directions. Distal pancreatectomy and splenectomy are usually necessary. There is little doubt that operative mortality is greater after total gastrectomy than after subtotal resection, and the procedure should be avoided whenever possible.

With extensive bleeding or obstruction, a palliative limited subtotal gastric resection can be done even in the presence of residual cancer. Palliative total gastrectomy should almost never be done. Resection of recurrent cancer in the gastric remnant may be of palliative value even when a cure is not obtained.

Chemotherapy is often suggested for unresectable gastric adenocarcinoma in an effort to decrease symptoms and prolong survival. The most widely used drug has been 5-fluorouracil (5FU), with an overall partial response rate of 15 to 20 per cent. Other agents such as mitomycin-C, doxorubicin (Adriamycin), and the various nitrosoureas have also been used as single agents with varying response. Combined use of several agents has not proved to be more effective than single agents so far.

Adjuvant chemotherapy following apparently curative surgery is an attractive concept for gastric carcinoma because of its high recurrence rate. Micrometastases are undoubtedly frequently present after surgery, and it has been postulated that chemotherapy might be most effective against such minimal disease. However, multiple trials with single agents have not been successful. Several trials using adjuvant chemotherapy with combinations of agents are in progress and may provide an answer to this very important question, although to date no effective adjuvant program has been demonstrated.

Radiation therapy is generally unsatisfactory, since gastric carcinomas are usually radioresistant. Occasionally palliation may be obtained for persistent bleeding, obstruction, or pain. An occasional patient with inoperable gastric carcinoma has had prolonged survival with radiation therapy. A controlled study combining 5FU with radiation therapy for inoperable metastatic disease resulted in a synergistic effect in both response rate and survival. Further studies are needed utilizing this combination modality.

Patients with gastrointestinal cancer frequently have complications associated with their disease or its treatment that require vigorous supportive treatment. Many aspects of the patients' general condition require consideration and treatment, including the management of infection; anemia; gastrointestinal bleeding; fluid and electrolyte loss secondary to vomiting, diarrhea, or fistula formation; disabling ascites; pain; and poor nutrition. Endoscopic LASER treatment is also being evaluated as a palliative approach to keeping the lumen open in unoperated upon or recurrent cancer in order to maintain nutrition. Total parenteral nutrition is being utilized more frequently to supply the daily caloric requirement of patients with gastric cancer. Preoperative and postoperative use of this modality enables patients to withstand the rigors of surgery and to tolerate more effectively the postoperative period, including the use of chemotherapy.

PROGNOSIS. The five-year survival rate depends upon whether or not adjacent lymph nodes contain cancer. The presence of perigastric lymph node metastases indicates a less than 15 per cent chance for survival. Early diagnosis plays a role in prognosis because a long period of time between the onset of cancer and its diagnosis favors lymphatic spread. In the Japanese studies, resection of gastric cancer limited to the mucosa and submucosa had a more than 80 per cent cure rate; when disease was limited to the mucosa, cure rate was 90 to 95 per cent. Linitis plastica and infiltrating lesions have a very poor prognosis compared with polypoid or exophytic disease.

PREVENTION. Until we learn more of the etiologic factors in gastric carcinoma we cannot practice primary prevention. We can only practice a limited degree of secondary prevention, i.e., detect the disease at an earlier stage in minimally symptomatic people in order to prevent its devastating consequences. The mass survey approach utilized in Japan is not practical in the United States because of the relatively low incidence of gastric cancer.

LYMPHOMA OF THE STOMACH (Ch. 158 and 160)

Primary lymphoma represents about 5 per cent of all primary malignant tumors of the stomach, and non-Hodgkin's lymphoma accounts for most of these. It is extremely rare for Hodgkin's disease (HD) to involve the stomach as a primary lesion. Patients with lymphoma are generally about a decade younger than those with carcinoma of the stomach, and males are affected most frequently. Pain is the most frequent symptom, and mild anemia is common, owing to gastrointestinal bleeding (which on occasion can be massive). A palpable mass is the most common presenting physical finding. Studies of maximal stimulation of gastric acid secretion have not been done in a large group of patients, but achlorhydria seems to be unusual. Secondary lymphoma involving the stomach is common in the course of disseminated lymphoma but is difficult to diagnose.

Lymphoma of the stomach frequently presents radiographically as a bulky mass and less frequently as a diffusely infiltrating tumor—the most common form of secondary lymphoma—giving the appearance of large folds on upper gastrointestinal series, frequently associated with multiple nodular defects and ulcerations. Lymphoma of the stomach often resembles superficially spreading carcinoma, linitis plastica, or solitary adenocarcinoma. Gastroscopy with directed biopsy and brush cytology gives a higher yield than was previously appreciated. Exophytic lesions provide a diagnosis in about 88 per cent of cases; the infiltrative type does not yield as high an accuracy.

Pseudolymphoma is a gastric lesion that may be confusing. This diffuse or discrete lesion is an atypical inflammatory response in the region of benign gastric ulcers. It is frequently difficult for the pathologist to differentiate pseudolymphoma from a true lymphoma.

In patients with lymphoma of the stomach there is a significant incidence of nontumorous lesions such as stress ulcer, hemorrhagic gastritis, and monilial gastritis. Therefore in such patients with upper gastrointestinal bleeding or other symptoms referable to the stomach, it is important that a careful diagnostic approach be undertaken to determine the possible nontumor cause of the sign or symptom.

Treatment of primary lymphoma of the stomach is usually surgical resection followed by 3600 to 4000 rads of radiotherapy, particularly if lymph nodes are involved. Some have advocated radiotherapy alone because of the marked sensitivity of lymphoma to radiation. If lymphoma involves the stomach secondarily, radiotherapy or chemotherapy or both are indicated. The five-year survival following surgery for primary lymphoma of the stomach is in the range of 50 per cent for non-Hodgkin's lymphoma and less for HD, suggesting that HD is already disseminated when initially found in the stomach. The best prognosis for primary tumors occurs with small lesions confined to the stomach, differentiated into tumor follicles without lymph node involvement and with only superficial infiltration of the wall.

OTHER MALIGNANT TUMORS OF THE STOMACH

Leiomyosarcoma of the stomach represents about 1 per cent of gastric cancers and may present with a large intramural mass with central ulceration. Systemic symptoms are minimal, but massive bleeding or a palpable mass of which the patient is aware may be the presenting complaints. The tumor may be slow growing; five-year survival following resection is in the range of 50 per cent. Metastases to the liver and nodes are common, but these patients have a better prognosis than those with other metastatic tumors. Liposarcoma, fibrosarcoma, myxosarcoma, and neurogenic sarcoma are extremely rare and present with symptoms similar to those of leiomyosarcoma. Neurogenic sarcoma can be associated with von Recklinghausen's disease.

Metastatic disease to the stomach from other sites is not common but may simulate primary gastric cancer. Malignant melanoma and breast and lung carcinomas are the most frequent offenders. In breast cancer the metastatic lesions may be ulcerative, of linitis plastica type, or polypoid.

LEIOMYOMAS AND BENIGN TUMORS

Leiomyomas are commonly found at postmortem examination but are rarely of clinical significance. They occur equally in men and women, and are usually found in the midportion and antrum of the stomach. They may grow toward the mucosa, encroach on the lumen, and cause mucosal effacement and secondary ulceration. They may grow in the direction of the serosa, producing a mass that is predominantly extrinsic. Simultaneous inward and outward growth results in a dumbbell shape. These features are also characteristic of leiomyosarcomas, and differentiation on radiography or gastroscopy is difficult. Bleeding is common and epigastric pain may simulate peptic ulcer disease. On roentgen examination the findings are usually an intramural filling defect with or without secondary ulceration. Gastroscopic examination reveals effaced but normal mucosa overlying the mass. Central ulceration may be seen.

Asymptomatic leiomyomas need not be removed while symptomatic lesions are excised locally.

Neurofibroma occasionally associated with von Recklinghausen's disease, neuroma, lymphangioma, ganglioneuroma, lipoma, carcinoid, and hamartoma associated with Peutz-Jeghers syndrome all may involve the stomach. About 10 per cent of hamartomas of the stomach and duodenum in Peutz-Jeghers syndrome become malignant.

ADENOMAS

Adenomas of the stomach are relatively rare lesions. Most polyps of the stomach are hyperplastic, not neoplastic, and do not become malignant. Adenomatous polyps are the usual neoplastic type of polyp. These are more frequent in men than in women and are generally seen in patients over 50. Bleeding, dyspepsia, and nausea are the most common symptoms, but most patients are asymptomatic. The diagnosis may be strongly suspected when a rounded smooth defect in the stomach on upper gastrointestinal series or a mass covered by mucosa with or without a stalk is detected by radiograph or endoscopy.

The size of polyps strongly influences management. It is rare for a polyp under 2 cm to show malignant change. In view of their potential for malignancy (present and future), polyps larger than 2 cm or polyps of any size causing significant symptoms should be removed. Pedunculated polyps can now be safely removed by cautery-snare technique via the fiberoptic endoscope. For sessile polyps more than 2 cm in diameter, a segmental gastric resection may be necessary to rule out carcinoma. If carcinoma is diagnosed histologically at the time of surgery, subtotal gastric resection should be done. Multiple gastric polyps are usually hyperplastic and of no significance.

TUMORS OF THE DUODENUM

Adenocarcinoma of the duodenum is rare but is more common than lymphoma, which, in turn, arises more commonly in the jejunum and ileum. The second and third portions of the duodenum are the usual sites of adenocarcinoma except when associated with Crohn's disease, in which it is in the ileum. Cancer in the duodenal bulb is exceedingly rare. Adenocarcinoma of the duodenum more frequently affects men and develops at a younger age than carcinoma of the stomach or colon. The tumor tends to grow into the lumen or to invade the wall of the duodenum. Cramping abdominal pain, anorexia, weight loss, vomiting, and melena are common. Jaundice or fever may result from obstruction of the ampulla of Vater or the common bile duct when the carcinoma involves the second portion of the duodenum. The tumor may simulate benign postbulbar ulceration. The diagnosis is usually made by radiologic examination and confirmed by endoscopy. Pancreaticoduodenectomy is necessary. Five-year survival ranges between 4 and 15 per cent.

Lymphoma, leiomyosarcoma, carcinoid, metastatic cancer, and benign tumors may involve the duodenum, and these are discussed in more detail in Ch. 107. In general, these lesions are manifested as an intramural and submucosal mass with the exception of lymphoma and metastatic cancer, which frequently are exophytic and ulcerate. Any tumor, benign or malignant, may occur in a diverticulum at the descending portion of the duodenum. Aberrant pancreatic tissue may produce a submucosal filling defect in the duodenum, which may resemble a neoplastic lesion. Also, hyperplasia or adenoma of Brunner's glands may produce multiple polypoid defects in the duodenal bulb and is frequently associated with hypersecretion, duodenal ulcer and, rarely, Zollinger-Ellison syndrome. A prominent ampulla of Vater may resemble a neoplastic lesion radiographically. Endoscopy may be necessary to clarify the situation.

Brooks JJ, Enterline HT: Primary gastric lymphomas. A clinicopathologic study of 58 cases with long-term follow-up and literature review. Cancer 51:701, 1983. *A large series of primary gastric lymphomas with long-term follow-up (average 12.8 years). Five- and ten-year survival rates were 57 and 46 per cent, respectively. Statistically significant prognostic variables were smaller tumor size, superficial mural invasion (submucosal only), and pathologic stage I disease.*

Correa P: Clinical implications of recent developments in gastric cancer pathology and epidemiology. Semin Oncol 12:2, 1985. *A comprehensive review of etiologic factors in gastric cancer. Worldwide epidemiology, risk factors, mucosal abnormalities, and genetics are discussed.*

Douglass HO, Nava HR: Gastric adenocarcinoma—management of the primary disease. Semin Oncol 12:32, 1985. *Excellent review of the overall management of patients with gastric cancer, including surgery and postoperative supportive care. Pathology and preoperative staging are also discussed.*

Kurtz RC, Lightdale CJ, Winawer SJ, et al.: Endoscopy and gastrointestinal neoplasm: Diagnosis and management. Curr Probl Cancer 5:4, 1980. *This monograph describes the techniques and applications of endoscopy in patients with cancer of the gastrointestinal tract, including the stomach. Great technical progress has been made in recent years.*

Le Chevalier T, Smith FP, Harter WK, et al.: Chemotherapy and combined modality therapy for locally advanced and metastatic gastric carcinoma. Semin Oncol 12:46, 1985. *An overview of recent results. Response rates are still disappointing, and combination protocols have not as yet been dramatically better.*

Ming SC: Gastric carcinoma. A pathological classification. Cancer 39:2475, 1977. *The classification described provides a simple basis for evaluation of various aspects of gastric cancer.*

O'Brien MJ, Burakoff R, Robbins EA, et al.: Early gastric cancer, clinicopathologic study. Am J Med 78:195, 1985. *Early gastric cancer as seen in United States patients is discussed. The disease is not seen often in the United States because of late diagnosis but is the same disease as early gastric cancer seen in Japan.*

Phillips JC, Lindsay JW, Kendall JA: Gastric leiomyosarcoma: Roentgenologic and clinical findings. Am J Dig Dis 15:239, 1970. *The typical clinical and roentgenologic findings are reviewed in 11 patients. The tumors were predominantly exogastric lesions. Ulcerations were present in five cases. Hemorrhage, fever, abdominal pain, and a palpable abdominal mass are helpful clinical points.*

Schafer LW, Larson DE, Melton LJ, et al.: Risk of development of gastric carcinoma in patients with pernicious anemia: A population-based study in Rochester, Minnesota. Mayo Clin Proc 60:444, 1985. *This study demonstrates the present lack of significant risk of gastric cancer in patients with pernicious anemia. The prior association was probably related to the higher incidence of gastric cancer worldwide. The risk for gastric cancer is no longer being expressed in this population.*

Shiu MH, Papacristou DN, Kurloff C, et al.: Selection of operative procedure for adenocarcinoma of the midstomach. Ann Surg 192:730, 1980. *This paper demonstrates the varying survival following different types of surgery for gastric cancer. Early-stage cancers seemed to benefit from an elective, more radical procedure.*

Sonenberg A: Endoscopic screening for gastric stump cancer—would it be beneficial? Gastroenterology 87:489, 1984. *This paper provides a current perspective as well as a review of recent literature. Gastric stump cancer is a real entity but is expressed primarily in individuals living in countries at high risk for gastric cancer.*

Winawer SJ, Posner G, Lightdale CJ, et al.: Endoscopic diagnosis of advanced gastric cancer. Factors influencing yield. Gastroenterology 69:1183, 1975. *Diagnostic yield was higher for exophytic lesions than for infiltrative tumor, and directed brush cytology alone was more productive than directed biopsy alone. Combination of infiltrative character and location in antrum or cardia often resulted in nondiagnostic biopsy and cytology specimens.*

102 DISORDERS OF GASTROINTESTINAL MOTILITY

Sidney Phillips

Normal Motility of Stomach, Small Intestine, and Colon

MOTILITY AND OVERALL FUNCTIONS OF THE BOWEL. Motility embraces all movements of the gastrointestinal tract and its contents. As such, the subject encompasses contractions of smooth muscle, the intraluminal pressures thereby developed, and the transit of contents that results from gradients of pressure. Movements of chyme along the bowel are modified by the actions of specialized segments of intestine and the spincters, and the whole is integrated by neural and humoral levels of control. Motility is best understood teleologically, i.e., as a process that facilitates the nutritive functions of the gut.

After solid food is chewed and moistened by saliva, it moves rapidly, in small boluses, into the stomach. Acting as a simple conduit, the esophagus is well served by strong bands of smooth muscle, integrated toward propulsive peristaltic motility, that push solid food to the stomach, even against the forces of gravity. Moreover, the lower and upper esophageal sphincters prevent acid-peptic reflux from corroding the esophageal mucosa and entering the bronchial tree. (Ch. 98 covers esophageal function and disease in detail.)

The stomach has three major functions: (1) accommodating meals of variable volumes, (2) grinding of solid food into small particles, and (3) the finely tuned process of gastric emptying. This last function is an important control of the load of chyme presented to the small bowel for digestion and absorption. Thus, the gastric fundus exhibits "receptive relaxation," a decrease in basal tone that is mediated by vagal reflexes and that reduces pressure in the body and fundus during a meal. Receptive relaxation provides accommodation for that meal, and food remains in the stomach for acid-peptic digestion to proceed. Later in the postcibal period basal tone returns; this increase in intraluminal pressure facilitates emptying of the liquid phase of mixed meals. Meanwhile, the antrum has developed strong, rhythmic peristaltic contractions that propel food to the prepyloric antrum. Solids are ground against the terminal antrum, triturated, and retropelled to the proximal antrum for another cycle of grinding. The pylorus allows only small solids (<1 mm) to pass through with the meal; larger solids are retained and emptied between meals. By a combination of these forces and the integrated action of duodenal musculature, pressure gradients are developed whereby gastric emptying is controlled very precisely. Sensitive receptors in the duodenal mucosa respond to intraluminal fat and hydrogen ions or hypertonicity of the contents, setting in motion a feedback mechanism that brakes emptying. In this way, contents entering the duodenum are prepared for their subsequent contact with pancreaticobiliary secretions. These controls are disturbed most dramatically when the pylorus is destroyed surgically; dumping syndromes or gastric stasis may be unfortunate, and all too common, sequelae.

Transit through the small bowel is steady but slow, a series of gentle to-and-fro movements of chyme, well suited to the mixing of food with digestive enzymes. Further, exposure of digestive products to the absorptive cells is maximized. Moreover, a normal pattern of motility is important in maintaining relative sterility of the small bowel. Disordered motility leads to bacterial overgrowth ("blind loop syndrome") and a malabsorption syndrome (see Ch. 104).

The colon can be thought of as two functional entities. The proximal half dehydrates its contents, removing salt and water very effectively. In addition, it stores feces, which undergo bacterial biotransformation by the fecal flora. Some components of dietary fiber can be digested only in this way. The motor activity of this segment subserves these functions of storing and mixing via its back-and-forth movements and mixing waves (haustra). The distal colon and rectum store formed stools until evacuation is convenient. The necessary propulsion and excretion are achieved by coordination of peristaltic contractions and voluntary elevations of intra-abdominal pressure. The anal sphincters relax in concert with these propulsive forces.

GASTROINTESTINAL SPHINCTERS. In physiologic terms, a sphincter is an area of high intraluminal pressure within the bowel. Sphincters separate areas of lower pressure and thus are able to modify the flow of intestinal contents. Sphincters respond to distention or changes of pressure within the adjacent bowel by either tightening or relaxing. Sphincters may be recognized anatomically by the presence of specialized bands of muscle (upper esophageal sphincter) or may be associated with no clearly defined or unique tissue (lower esophageal sphincter) (see Ch. 98). The pylorus has a concentrated bundle of circular muscle characteristic of a sphincter, but it contracts and relaxes in concert with adjacent bowel. Functionally, the pylorus is not clearly distinct from the antrum or duodenum and can be considered as having only certain characteristics of a "sphincter." The ileocecal junction has the appearance of a valve but can function like a sphincter. One of its important roles is to prevent reflux of fecal flora into the small intestine. The anal sphincters are well developed anatomically and function as true sphincters.

ELECTRICAL AND MECHANICAL CORRELATES OF MOTILITY. Contractions of smooth muscle cells are determined by the state of polarization-depolarization of the cell membranes, contraction occurring only when action potentials ("spikes") are superimposed on an appropriate background level of depolarization. Throughout the stomach and intestines a baseline fluctuation of basal electrical activity is present in the muscularis, as measured by extracellular electrodes embedded in the muscle layers. This omnipresent "basic electrical rhythm" (BER, slow wave or pacesetter potential) originates at specific sites ("pacemakers") located in the proximal stomach, proximal duodenum, and midcolon. The potentials so generated, at 3 per minute in stomach, 12 per minute in duodenum, and 3 to 12 per minute in the colon, spread distally along muscle bundles, thus establishing a maximal frequency at which the smooth muscle can contract. In other words, antral pacesetters of 3 per minute establish this as the maximal rate of antral contractions. The corresponding rate in the proximal duodenum is 12 per minute, but this rate slows progressively, in a caudad direction along the bowel, so that the terminal ileal rate is 8 to 9 per minute. When spike discharges are present on any slow wave complex, adjacent smooth muscle contracts (Fig. 102–1). At each level, not all pacesetter potentials have action potentials; in other words, the smooth muscle may contract at its maximal rate, not contract at all, or exhibit any intermediate level of activity. The state of fasting or feeding is a major determinant of the degree of muscular activity that actually occurs. The colonic pacemaker is probably located in the transverse colon, and pacesetter potentials spread distally and proximally. Such a system may well provide the basis for to-and-fro movement in the colon, allowing storage, desiccation, and fermentation in the cecum.

FASTING AND POSTCIBAL MOTILITY. The fasting bowel is not quiescent; it exhibits cycles of contractility that are interrupted by food. With a periodicity of approximately two hours, an intense burst of motor activity begins in the stomach, in which every pacesetter potential has an action potential associated with it. This wave of activity passes caudally through duodenum, jejunum, and ileum. The velocity of this "front" is such that on reaching the ileum another "front" (or migrating motor complex) originates in the stomach. At any single locus, a cycle of activity lasts approximately 2 hours during fasting, each intense burst of motility lasting 5 to 15 minutes. The remainder of the 2-hour cycle is taken up with quiescence (lasting about 1 hour—"phase I"), intermittent contractile activity (about 45 minutes—"phase II"), and then the migrating complex ("phase III"). The migrating complex has been described by Code as the "interdigestive housekeeper." The function proposed is one of sweeping secretions, desquamated cells, and food residue distally in preparation for another meal. Food interrupts the cycle, replacing it with the "fed pattern" of intermittent contractions (similar to phase II) that last for 4 to 10 hours. Whereas transit is rapid in phase III of fasting, it is slower after a meal.

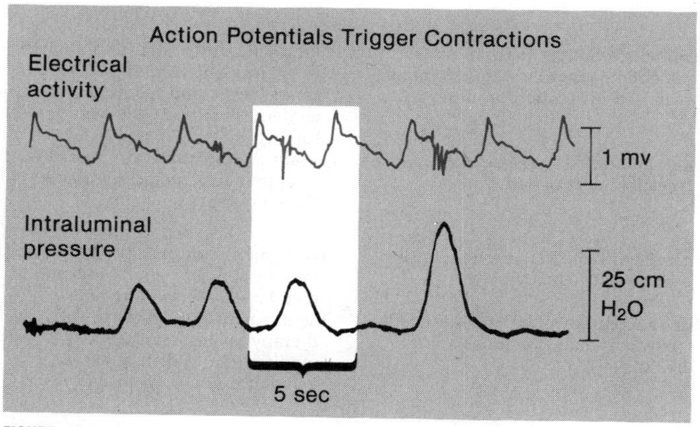

FIGURE 102–1. Simultaneous electrical and mechanical activity in the canine jejunum. The electrical signal was recorded from an extracellular electrode in the tunica muscularis; it shows a regular cycle of depolarization-repolarization at 12 to 14 cycles per minute. Superimposed on some of these cycles (basic electrical rhythm, slow wave, or pace-setter potential) are more rapid oscillations (fast waves, spikes). When spiking occurs, the smooth muscle contracts, causing intraluminal pressure to rise (lower tracing).

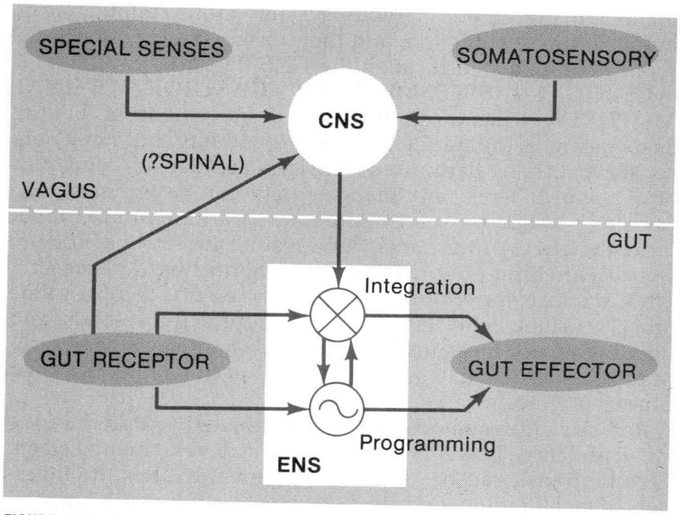

FIGURE 102–2. Scheme for the control of intestinal motility. Possible stimuli for gut receptors include wall tension, serosal inflammation, and luminal chemoreceptors. The signals are integrated and programmed by the enteric nervous system within the bowel and then act on effector tissues (smooth muscle, absorptive, or secretory cells). The vagus nerves are 80 to 90 per cent afferent and other, less well-defined, pathways go via abdominal ganglia and the spinal cord to the CNS. Input from the special senses is best demonstrated by the cephalic phase of gut function. The somatosensory input is illustrated by altered intestinal motility in response to cold or pain stress. (From Wingate DL: Viewpoints on Digestive Diseases, Vol 17, No 5, November, 1985. Reproduced with permission of the publishers, American Gastroenterological Association.)

CONTROL OF GASTROINTESTINAL MOTILITY. The cholinergic system has important control of the proximal gut. Vagal denervation impairs receptive relaxation of the stomach and, by reducing gastric accommodation to large volumes, speeds the emptying of liquids. Vagal denervation also diminishes the important duodenal "brake" on gastric emptying. Antral contractions are also weakened by vagotomy, and hence the grinding and emptying of solids are reduced. The sympathetic nervous system becomes more important in the distal bowel, particularly in the coordination of rectal contractions and relaxation of the anal sphincters. A third system ("noncholinergic-nonadrenergic") also exists, although the exact neurotransmitters responsible for it are as yet unclear. Among the candidates are adenosine triphosphate (ATP) ("purinergic"), dopamine-like compounds, and neuropeptides. A number of peptides can alter gastrointestinal motility, but whether they have physiologic roles is unclear. Cholecystokinin-pancreozymin contracts the gallbladder and intestinal smooth muscle. Other stimulating hormones include gastrin and motilin, and inhibitory hormones include secretin, glucagon, vasoactive intestinal polypeptide, and gastric inhibitory polypeptide.

Neurohumoral control of gut motility is coordinated ultimately by interactions between the enteric nervous system (nerve cells and axons of the intramural plexuses), the intra-abdominal ganglia, and the central nervous system. An important new concept is the autonomy of the enteric nervous system ("mini-brain" in the gut), which is, in turn, modulated by the central nervous system (CNS) (Fig. 102–2). Recognition of these different levels of control gives a basis for a general separation of intestinal dysmotility into those conditions originating in the enteric nervous system, those resulting from more central dysfunction, and those originating in the special senses but mediated through the CNS (Fig. 102–2).

CLINICAL ASSESSMENT OF GASTROINTESTINAL MOTILITY. Measuring the rate of movement of barium suspensions is the traditional index of motility, but not a very satisfactory one. Barium suspensions are dense, behave as liquids, and hence are inappropriate for determining the transit of water or solids. Moreover, barium, unlike food, lacks the effect of nutrients. As a result, the study of barium transit is helpful only when gross abnormalities are present. Similar criticism pertains to the gastric emptying of a saline "meal" (saline load test). Gastric emptying of solids and liquids is best measured by external gamma camera techniques, using suitably labeled markers of the liquid and solid phases of "meals."

Radionuclide methods can also be applied to transit of the small and large bowel but are still in the developmental stage. Colonic transit can be assessed conveniently after the ingestion of small radiopaque markers; stools can be radiographed to determine mouth-to-anus transit times, or abdominal radiographs may be used to quantify transit through different segments of the colon. The arrival time of a bolus of fermentable carbohydrate in the cecum can be identified by the excretion of hydrogen in the breath. Hydrogen is generated in the body only by bacterial fermentation of carbohydrate. In this way, mouth-to-cecum transit times can be measured noninvasively. The measurement of intraluminal pressures by transducers or water-filled catheters is used extensively in the diagnosis of esophageal and anorectal disease. Application of these techniques to the stomach, small intestine, and colon is restricted largely to research studies.

Christensen J: Motility of the colon. In Johnson LR (ed.): Physiology of the Gastrointestinal Tract. 2nd ed. New York, Raven Press, 1987. *Complete review with reference to basic mechanisms; includes some material on pathophysiology of disease.*

Meyer JH: Motility of the stomach and gastroduodenal junction. In Johnson LR (ed.): Physiology of the Gastrointestinal Tract. 2nd ed. New York, Raven Press, 1987. *Comprehensive review of the physiology of the region; contains all major references to basic mechanisms.*

Sarna SK: Cyclic motor activity; migrating motor complex: 1985. Gastroenterology 89:894, 1985. *Extensive review of intestinal motility, with emphasis particularly on the basic mechanisms and control of fasting patterns. Contains all important references.*

Wingate DL: Backwards and forwards with the migrating complex. Dig Dis Sci 26:641, 1981. *Complete historical and scientific review of small intestinal motility with emphasis on the normal physiology. Referenced extensively.*

Disorders of Gastroduodenal Motility

PYLORIC STENOSIS: GASTRIC OUTLET OBSTRUCTION

ETIOLOGY AND PATHOGENESIS. A transient syndrome occurs when acute peptic ulcers involve the pyloric canal. A chronic, cicatricial condition often complicates recurrent ulceration in the pyloroduodenal region, and vomiting may be severe. Carcinoma is also a cause of gastric outlet obstruction.

TABLE 102–1. COMMON DISORDERS OF GASTROINTESTINAL MOTILITY

Disorder	Suggested Mechanisms	Clinical Features	Treatment and Comments*
Stomach			
Congenital			
Hypertrophic pyloric stenosis	Hypertrophied, nonpropulsive muscle, neuronal agenesis	First-born males; vomiting without bile	Ramstedt's operation is curative
Postoperative			
Gastroparesis	Poor mechanical drainage; vagotomy	Early: excessive gastric aspirations; late: easy satiety, bezoars	Radiology and endoscopy to rule out mechanical obstruction; soft diet; cholinergic drugs; metoclopramide, 10 mg q.i.d.†
Dumping syndrome	Rapid gastric emptying; hypovolemia; hypoglycemia; inappropriate release of gastrointestinal peptides	Early: weakness, dizziness, palpitations, diarrhea; late: features of hypoglycemia	Dry diet; reduced sugar intake; rest after meals; surgery may be required
Others			
Gastroparesis (idiopathic or diabetic)	Diminished motor fronts; ? pylorospasm	Fullness; nausea; vomiting; bezoars	Juvenile diabetics; soft diet; drug treatment with metoclopramide or cholinergic drugs
Small Bowel			
Adynamic ileus	Postoperative; electrolyte disturbances; peritonitis	Vomiting; abdominal distention	Intestinal decompression; maintenance of fluid and electrolyte balance; correction of cause
Mechanical obstruction	Bands; hernias; tumors, etc.	Proximal: vomiting, pain, minimal distention; distal: lower abdominal pain with distention prominent	Plain radiographic films of abdomen; fever, feculent vomiting, leukocytosis, and rebound tenderness indicate the need for surgery
Pseudo-obstruction	(See Table 102–2 for causes)	Older patients with features of intestinal obstruction	Therapy of idiopathic form usually disappointing; metoclopramide, cholinergics[2]
Large Bowel			
Constipation	(See Table 102–3 for causes)	Decreased frequency or quantity of stool; stools usually hard	Investigations toward specific cause; therapy toward patient education, diet; laxatives used judiciously
Irritable bowel syndrome	Disorder of small bowel and large bowel motility	Pain; altered bowel habit; associated "psychosomatic" manifestations likely	Organic disease to be ruled out; therapy is reassurance, modification of diet, and avoidance of chronic use of drugs
Megacolon			
Congenital	Absence of intramural nerve plexuses ("aganglionosis")	Obstipation, meconium ileus from birth; rectum empty; narrow segment on barium radiograph	Diagnosis by manometry and rectal biopsy; corrected by surgery
Acquired	Secondary to constipation	History of constipation; older age groups; rectum full	Disimpaction of feces; treatment of constipation

*It is essential in all suspected disorders of gastrointestinal motility to rule out mechanical obstruction or organic disease as a cause for symptoms.

†Two new "prokinetic" drugs (Domperidone, Cisapride) are unavailable in the United States at the time of writing. Both show promise as alternative therapies of gastroparesis and pseudo-obstruction.

In infants, hypertrophy of pyloric muscle may occur, leading to severe degrees of obstruction. Hypertrophic pyloric stenosis occurs rarely in adults, although in later life it is difficult to distinguish a specific "hypertrophic syndrome" from the multiple, variable manifestations of chronic peptic ulcer disease.

Congenital Hypertrophic Pyloric Stenosis

INCIDENCE. This lesion occurs in two to four infants per 1000 live births, is more common in firstborn children, and is four to five times more frequent in males. A familial incidence is reported, as is an increased incidence in twins. Some degree of muscle spasm is present, since partial relaxation may occur during anesthesia or with the use of anticholinergic drugs. The morphology of the affected muscle may be similar to that of Hirschsprung's disease (see later); neurons are sparse or absent, but nerve fibers are present.

CLINICAL MANIFESTATIONS. The infant usually seems normal at birth, but regurgitation is noted at one to three weeks post partum and rapidly progresses to projectile vomiting, dehydration, and weight loss but without anorexia. The vomitus contains no bile. Gastric peristalsis may be visible, and the hypertrophied pylorus may be palpable in the epigastrium.

DIAGNOSIS. The radiologic appearances are characteristic: an elongated, narrow pylorus surrounded by the hypertrophied muscle, which may be seen as a soft tissue shadow. In adults, the pyloric region may protrude proximally into the antrum, resembling a uterine cervix at endoscopy.

TREATMENT. After correction of acid-base and electrolyte imbalance, a trial of anticholinergics and small feedings is justified in milder examples, but surgical correction will usually be necessary. Pyloromyotomy in the fashion of Ramstedt is performed; a simple longitudinal incision of the circular muscle suffices, with an excellent prognosis. In adults, resection of the pylorus and distal antrum with vagotomy is usually advisable.

POSTOPERATIVE DISORDERS

Surgical therapies for peptic ulcer disease often result in profound alterations of the finely tuned process of gastric emptying (see also Ch. 100). The most radical surgical procedures for peptic ulceration resect the antrum and pylorus, thus removing the physical effect of the distal stomach in the grinding of solid food, as well as removing the pyloric sieve. The lesser procedure of total gastric vagotomy is usually combined with pyloroplasty or gastroenterostomy ("drainage"), since reduced antral grinding in the vagotomized stomach leads to retention of solids. If the "drainage" maneuver is less than adequate, stagnation of solids may occur, although, at the same time, gastric emptying of liquids may be excessively rapid. This "dumping" of liquids is readily explicable by impairment of vagally innervated receptive relaxation of the proximal stomach, a process that permits storage of volume without undue elevation of intragastric pressure. Thus, after gastric surgery many disorders of gastric emptying are encountered, including rapid emptying of liquids (dumping syndrome), reduced emptying of solids (gastroparesis), or a combination of both. Certain mechanical complications of gastroenterostomy are also recognized, including obstruction of afferent jejunal loops and intussusception of jejunal limbs into the gastric remnant. The least traumatic surgical procedure, proximal gastric vagotomy, reduces gastric hypersecretion by denervation of the parietal cells alone. Innervation of the antrum and pylorus being preserved, gastric emptying is minimally affected.

Diagnostic steps for the patient with postoperative problems include a careful history, which must determine the exact temporal relationship of symptoms to meals, degree of nausea, nature of vomitus, and ability to handle liquid or solid diet. Barium meal examination is often unhelpful, testing as it does only the emptying of a dense liquid without nutrient content. However, failure to empty some barium by 30 minutes or retention of most barium at six hours signals a severe abnormality. Endoscopy may reveal fasting retention of foods or solid masses (bezoars) in the stomach and is useful to exclude mechanical obstruction. This common and confusing syndrome can be better evaluated by the use of gamma-labeled mixed meals monitored by external gamma cameras, thus allowing selective evaluation of emptying patterns for labeled liquids and solids.

Dumping Syndrome

DEFINITION, CLINICAL FEATURES, AND INCIDENCE. This symptom complex of sweating, weakness with orthostatic features, tachycardia, and sometimes diarrhea following meals occurs transiently in one third or more of patients after gastric surgery. Although most common and severe after gastric resection and gastroenterostomy (Billroth II), it may complicate any operation for peptic ulceration. Symptoms appear as soon after surgery as patients begin a regular diet. Although usually subsiding by 3 to 12 months after surgery, symptoms may persist and be debilitating. Liquid meals, especially those containing large amounts of carbohydrate, are most likely to evoke symptoms. Patients learn that recumbency minimizes symptoms and often discover that avoidance of sugars and desserts helps.

ETIOLOGY AND PATHOGENESIS. No other syndrome in gastroenterology has received more scrutiny and yet yielded so little uniform information as to its cause and rational treatment. Hypovolemia caused by pooling of interstitial fluid in the gut (as a result of uncontrolled entry of hyperosmolar fluids into the small bowel), hypoglycemia, and hormonal imbalance have received most attention. Among the humoral agents incriminated are serotonin and neurotensin. The symptoms can be mimicked in some patients by depletion of extracellular volumes (and corrected by volume expansion), by hypoglycemia, and by distention of a balloon in the small intestine.

DIAGNOSIS. The diagnosis is established by the characteristic history and the exclusion of other diseases likely to produce similar symptoms. Radiology and endoscopy of the upper gastrointestinal tract are required to rule out organic or mechanical problems.

TREATMENT. Reassurance that the symptoms will subside with time will often be sufficient treatment. Patients should be advised to eat small meals, separating fluids from the more solid components of major meals. Lying down after large meals may help, as will avoidance of sweetened drinks and desserts. The prognosis is good with regard to major incapacitation, although minor symptoms may continue indefinitely if certain combinations of diet and activity are pursued.

Gastroparesis and Bezoars

DEFINITION AND PATHOPHYSIOLOGY. Many patients demonstrate mild degrees of gastric retention of solids after gastric surgery, although few (<10 per cent) have major problems. Motility studies reveal diminished phase III activity ("motor fronts") in the stomach but normal cyclic activity in the small bowel.

CLINICAL MANIFESTATIONS. Postprandial fullness, nausea, and vomiting are the major features. Occasionally, solid material may completely obstruct the stoma or the esophagus. The most important consequence, however, is superficial ulceration of the stomach, which often bleeds.

DIAGNOSIS. Bezoars are detected by barium meal examination or endoscopy. The latter procedure has additional therapeutic potential, since boluses can be broken up mechanically and washed into the small intestine or removed by gastric lavage. Barium studies reveal intraluminal filling defects, often of massive dimensions.

TREATMENT. Physical disruption of bezoars by endoscopy, repeated gastric lavage, or both will be helpful. Chemical disruption by papain or cellulase has been successful also. Patients should then be advised to chew their food well and avoid large amounts of raw fruit and vegetables. Metoclopramide can accelerate the delayed emptying of solids after gastric surgery, although most studies report only short-term benefits. Metoclopramide (10 mg) or bethanechol (5 mg) has been shown experimentally to stimulate gastric contractions and to speed emptying of solids.

PROGNOSIS. In general, dietary measures and gradual recovery of gastric contractile function can be expected to alleviate symptoms. In some patients, however, a permanent change in eating patterns is required.

Intussusception

Jejunal intussusception into the stomach may occur after Billroth II gastric resection or, less often, after gastroenterostomy. Although it is sometimes asymptomatic, pain and gastric outlet obstruction may result. The radiologic picture of a "coiled spring" filling defect and the endoscopic appearances are characteristic. When intussusception is severe, surgical correction is required.

GASTROPARESIS DIABETICORUM

DEFINITION AND INCIDENCE. Severely impaired gastric emptying without evidence of mechanical obstruction is a well-recognized complication of diabetes mellitus. It is unknown whether lesser degrees of gastric stasis are responsible for milder symptoms and the variable control of blood sugar so common in diabetics with longstanding disease.

PATHOGENESIS AND CLINICAL FEATURES. The cause is unknown, but autonomic denervation of the proximal gut seems likely. Patients may be of any age and either sex and are usually "juvenile-onset" diabetics whose disease is of more than ten years' duration. Retinopathy, nephropathy, and other complications are common. The pathophysiologic features are an absence of phase III activity "fronts" in the distal stomach and increased tone across the pylorus, with the motor pattern of the small bowel being normal. Nausea, vomiting, poor and variable control of blood sugar levels, and weight loss are the major presenting symptoms. Esophageal reflux, esophagitis, and even repeated episodes of Mallory-Weiss syndrome from vigorous vomiting may be seen.

DIAGNOSIS. The clinical picture is characteristic, but mechanical obstruction must be excluded by radiology and upper gastrointestinal endoscopy. Fluoroscopy may suggest reduced antral contractions or display retained food and secretions.

TREATMENT AND PROGNOSIS. Dietary management with soft foods well cooked and chewed should be instituted, since pharmacologic maneuvers provide little long-term benefit. Metoclopramide is certainly the best agent available at this time. Unfortunately, drug resistance is common, and long-term benefit is less common. Cholinergic agents (bethanechol 5 to 10 mg) are worthy of trial but are not often effective. Surgical treatment (e.g., gastroenterostomy) may be attempted, but only temporary benefit should be anticipated.

IDIOPATHIC GASTROPARESIS

DEFINITION AND INCIDENCE. Otherwise healthy persons may develop symptoms suggestive of gastroparesis, sometimes acutely in association with a flulike illness. Vomiting in nonbacterial gastroenteritis (e.g., those caused by parvoviruses or Norwalk and Hawaii agents) is accompanied by slow gastric emptying. Some patients diagnosed as having psychogenic vomiting actually have impaired motility and gastric emptying.

PATHOGENESIS AND CLINICAL FEATURES. Abnormalities of the gastric pacemaker potential have been reported in some persons with delayed emptying. Electrogastrography can be performed, using intraluminal or external electrodes, "tachygastria" and other arrhythmias have been noted. The abnormal electrical potentials in turn lead to a failure to develop "spikes" and adequate contractions of smooth muscle. Gastric retention, more often for solids than liquids, causes bloating, nausea, and vomiting.

DIAGNOSIS. Mechanical obstruction and peptic ulceration must be excluded carefully, but it is still uncertain how often those pathophysiologic disturbances are present in patients with "nonulcer dyspepsia."

PROGNOSIS AND TREATMENT. Most examples are transient, perhaps in association with a viral illness. Occasionally, when the problem is chronic, surgery has been required. Some evidence suggests that prostanoids are implicated in "tachygastria" and trial of a nonsteroidal anti-inflammatory drug should be considered.

MISCELLANEOUS CONDITIONS

Gastric diverticula are uncommon, single, and asymptomatic. True diverticula are always located in the upper quarter of the stomach, usually on the posterior wall. Their only significance is in their diagnostic confusion with peptic ulcers or ulcerating neoplasms. Endoscopy may be required for this differentiation. Pseudodiverticula are scarred areas of dilatation, usually in the prepyloric antrum, in association with peptic ulcer disease.

Gastric volvulus is torsion of the stomach along its long axis, the esophagogastric junction and pylorus remaining fixed. Large hiatal hernias or diaphragmatic defects may be predisposing factors. An acute volvulus is often an abdominal emergency, particularly if the gastric blood supply is compromised. The chronic form is more common, bloating, regurgitation, dysphagia, and pain may occur and the diagnosis is made radiologically. Surgical treatment is required for acute volvulus and for severe symptomatic chronic volvulus.

Acute dilatation of the stomach is best considered as a localized form of paralytic ileus (see below); it is seen after abdominal operations or immobilization in body casts, during diabetic ketoacidosis, or as an acute side effect of anticholinergics. Distention of the stomach may become massive if nasogastric suction is not instituted, and mucosal bleeding may lead to "coffee-ground" emesis.

Aerophagia is a normal accompaniment of swallowing but may be exaggerated in anxious persons, leading to epigastric bloating. Bloating often induces patients to attempt repeated belches, each of which perpetuates the swallowing of gas. Organic disease must be excluded, and the chewing of gum and ingestion of carbonated beverages should be avoided.

Malagelada J-R, Camilleri M, Stanghellini V: Manometric Diagnosis of Gastrointestinal Motility Disorders. New York, Thieme-Stratton, 1986. *A monograph on the diagnosis of motility disorders but dealing also with normal physiology and the pathophysiology of the common and uncommon disorders of motility. The bibliography is extensive and will guide the reader into any area.*

Meyer JH: Chronic morbidity after ulcer surgery. In Sleisenger MH, Fordtran JS (eds.): Gastrointestinal Disease. 4th ed. Philadelphia, W. B. Saunders Company, 1988. *Comprehensive review of all the major problems encountered after gastric surgery. Includes pathophysiology, clinical features, and treatment.*

Disorders of Small Bowel Motility

INTRODUCTION

Normally, progression of food through the small intestine is slow and steady. Although the "head" of a barium meal may reach the terminal ileum in one to two hours, mean transit time (for 50 per cent of a meal) is slower and the "tail" is even more delayed. The only documented examples of intestinal hurry are in patients with "short bowel syndrome," seen after extensive resection of the small bowel, and the malabsorption that accompanies jejunoileal bypass. In these conditions, the major defect is inadequate contact between chyme and the digestive-absorptive surface (see Ch. 104).

The chronic stasis of delayed transit through the small intestine, from any cause, is often accompanied by an overgrowth of intestinal flora, since normal motility helps maintain the relative sterility of the small bowel. The *"blind loop syndrome"* can be produced experimentally by ganglionic blocking drugs (nonobstructive or adynamic ileus) and by partial mechanical obstruction. The blind loop syndrome occurs clinically (1) in conditions causing stasis (chronic obstruction, giant jejunal diverticula, and surgical blind pouches), (2) when a fistula is present between the colon and the upper bowel, and (3) with disturbances of the interdigestive motor complex (see Ch. 104).

ILEUS: ADYNAMIC AND MECHANICAL

DEFINITION AND ETIOLOGY. Ileus signifies impairment of caudad transit of intestinal contents. It can be subdivided into two broad categories: (1) adynamic or paralytic and (2) mechanical. The difference between these categories is important clinically: Mechanical causes are usually treated surgically, whereas adynamic ileus requires medical management. Adynamic ileus occurs in association with abdominal surgery or external trauma, when the peritoneum is exposed to irritants (bacterial toxins, bile, blood, pancreatic enzymes, or intestinal contents), in severe electrolyte imbalance, and after intra-abdominal vascular accidents. The etiopathogenesis is unknown, although disordered sympathetic tone is presumed. Ileus can also be induced by ganglionic blocking drugs.

Mechanical obstruction may occur at any level of the small bowel or colon; it can be separated pathogenetically into lesions lying outside the bowel (e.g., adhesive bands, obstructed hernias), those within the wall (e.g., intramural tumors, hematomas, strictures), and those within the lumen (e.g., epithelial tumors, foreign bodies, intussusception).

PATHOPHYSIOLOGIC CONSEQUENCES. The proximal bowel distends, and its function becomes compromised. In experimental obstruction of the canine small intestine, absorption from distended bowel segments diminishes after 6 to 12 hours and is replaced by secretion of sodium and water. Increased intraluminal pressure, elevation of portal venous and lymphatic pressures, ischemia, and the toxic effects of rapid bacterial multiplication in the involved segment are among the mechanisms proposed to account for these changes.

Once obstruction is established, edema, petechial hemorrhages, and finally necrosis and gangrene develop in the bowel wall. These changes are most pronounced when occlusion or strangulation of the vasculature occurs, as in closed-loop obstruction, which produces exceedingly high intraluminal pressure. Excessive permeability of the damaged intestinal mucosa allows proteins to leak from blood into the intestinal lumen; conversely, bacteria and their toxins enter the damaged and permeable mucosa. Peritonitis, therefore, frequently complicates untreated obstruction. Additional injury to ischemic mucosa may be caused by compounds in the intestinal lumen, including pancreatic enzymes, bile acids, and bacterial enterotoxins. The sequence whereby untreated obstruction leads to irreversible shock and death is uncertain. Extracellular fluid volume depletion, free perforation of the bowel, bacterial toxins, gram-negative septicemia, and splanchnic vasoconstriction all have been implicated. The general role of bacteria is well established experimentally, since mortality from obstruction is reduced in newborn or germ-free animals, or when broad-spectrum antibiotics have been given previously.

Hypovolemia, hyponatremia, and hypochloremia are the major abnormalities observed. During the course of ileus, several liters of extracellular fluid may become sequestered in the intestine. Experimental obstruction of the distal small bowel results in leakage of as much as 50 per cent of the plasma volume into this "third space." Additional fluid may accumulate in the peritoneal cavity. Plasma concentrations of electrolytes are initially normal, since the fluid lost is isotonic, but the patient usually drinks sodium-poor fluid, so that hyponatremia develops. Severe vomiting depletes chloride, and alkalosis may be prominent in obstruction of the upper intestine. Impairment of renal function secondary to hypovolemia and starvation, with consequent ketosis, may combine to produce mild acidosis.

CLINICAL MANIFESTATIONS. The symptoms and signs depend on the level of obstruction, its duration, and whether the cause is obstructive or adynamic. Paralytic ileus may cause little pain and be manifested only by abdominal distention and vomiting. Increased volumes of aspirate obtained from nasogastric suction and oliguria may be early manifestations of paralytic ileus in the patient already under close observation, e.g., postoperatively. The symptoms of mechanical obstruction are vomiting, cramping abdominal pain, distention, and obstipation. When obstruction is episodic, relief may be heralded by watery, voluminous stools. When proximal, obstruction produces earlier vomiting, epigastric or midabdominal pain, and minimal distention. Distal obstructive lesions are associated with less vomiting, lower abdominal pain, and more prominent abdominal distention with obstipation. Physical signs are those of the metabolic disorder, particularly extracellular dehydration and hypovolemia, abdominal distention with variable tenderness, and a mass that might indicate the underlying lesion. Bowel sounds are high pitched, frequent, and rushing in mechanical obstruction. Adynamic ileus has lesser physical signs; distention is prominent, but tenderness is less pronounced unless the ileus is associated with peritonitis. Bowel sounds are infrequent to absent early in ileus in contrast to mechanical obstruction. Bowel sounds may disappear later in the course of mechanical obstruction.

DIAGNOSIS. Plain abdominal radiographic films are vital for diagnosis, to determine the level of obstruction, and to distinguish mechanical from adynamic ileus. Air-fluid levels in obstructed bowel will be seen in upright or lateral decubitus films. Mechanical obstruction often also demonstrates a sharp demarcation between dilated bowel above and collapsed bowel below the point of obstruction. Such a transition is not seen in ileus, in which dilatation is uniform throughout small and large intestines.

Colonic gas shadows are recognized by the presence of haustra, which are asymmetric and do not extend across the entire diameter of the bowel. Valvulae conniventes of the small bowel are regular, symmetric shadows across the entire diameter. Contrast material will pool above an obstruction and should not be given by mouth. Proctosigmoidoscopy and a barium enema, without preparation, can be performed cautiously when the obstruction is thought to be in the colon. Other diagnostic measures to determine a cause of ileus should then be considered. Overall metabolic evaluation will include measurements of serum electrolytes and the status of acid-base balance, blood urea, hematocrit, and serum protein levels, as well as careful monitoring of urine volume.

TREATMENT. The primary goals of therapy for ileus or obstruction are (1) intestinal decompression, (2) restoration or maintenance of fluid and electrolyte balance, and (3) treatment of the cause. Most instances of adynamic ileus are transient, and a medical approach can achieve all three goals. However, when the obstruction is mechanical, initial decompression is achieved by intubation, but definitive decompression and removal of the obstruction usually require surgery.

Nasogastric aspiration is usually sufficient for decompression, because this removes air before it reaches the intestine. Fluid replacement is aimed at replacing the lost water, sodium, chloride, and potassium. Alkalosis or acidosis should be corrected. Central venous pressure should be monitored to assure adequate replacement as well as to avoid fluid overload, particularly in patients with compromised cardiovascular reserve. Repeated observations are made of serum electrolytes as well as blood pressure, urinary output, and hematocrit. When fever, leukocytosis, or signs of peritonitis suggest perforation or strangulation, appropriate antimicrobials are administered to suppress growth of intestinal bacteria. Strangulation with impending gangrene demands surgery within six hours.

Jones RS: Intestinal obstruction, pseudo-obstruction, and ileus. In Sleisenger MH, Fordtran JS (eds.): Gastrointestinal Disease. 4th ed. Philadelphia, W. B. Saunders Company, 1988. *A more detailed description of the causative lesions, clinical features, and practical management of obstruction of the small and large intestines.*

INTESTINAL PSEUDO-OBSTRUCTION

DEFINITION. Pseudo-obstruction implies a syndrome with clinical features akin to mechanical obstruction but for which there is no obstructive lesion. When the episode is single and transient, pseudo-obstruction is more appropriately included among examples of adynamic ileus. Thus, the term should be applied to chronic or recurrent episodes of obstruction. The underlying causes are either unknown or untreatable diseases, and pseudo-obstruction has a poor prognosis.

ETIOLOGY. So-called "primary idiopathic pseudo-obstruction" has no known cause. It affects families, and the defect appears to be transmitted as an autosomal dominant trait. Relatives of patients with the syndrome may have only radiologic and manometric evidence of abnormal intestinal motility or the full-blown disease. Primary pseudo-obstruction can be subdivided into (1) hollow visceral myopathy and (2) autonomic neuropathies. Pseudo-obstruction also occurs as a manifestation of other diseases (Table 102–2), termed secondary intestinal pseudo-obstruction.

PATHOGENESIS. The pathophysiology of both primary and secondary forms is unknown, but the mechanisms are probably diverse. Category 1 of Table 101–2 includes diseases in which the smooth muscle itself is directly replaced by infiltrates, fibrous tissue, or other noncontractile elements. Category 2 lists diseases in which intramural nervous tissue is involved, either destroyed (Chagas' disease) or histologically intact but functionally disturbed ("ganglioneuromatosis"). Category 2 also includes diseases with extensive denervation, as when there is other evidence of autonomic dysfunction with involvement of the urinary bladder (diabetes mellitus and other neuropathies). Disturbances of hormonal regulation of intestinal function may also occur as a paraneoplastic syndrome. Certain drugs as listed in Table 102–2 may occasionally be associated with pseudo-obstruction.

TABLE 102–2. CAUSES OF SECONDARY INTESTINAL PSEUDO-OBSTRUCTION*

1. Diseases involving intestinal smooth muscle ("intestinal myopathies")
Collagen vascular diseases
Scleroderma
Dermatomyositis
Polymyositis
Systemic lupus erythematosus
Amyloidosis
Primary muscular diseases
Myotonic dystrophy
Progressive muscular dystrophy
2. Neurologic diseases ("intestinal neuropathies")
Chagas' disease
Hirschsprung's disease
Familial autonomic dysfunction
Parkinson's disease
3. Endocrine diseases
Hypothyroidism
Diabetes mellitus
Hypoparathyroidism
Pheochromocytoma
4. Drug effects
Phenothiazines, tricyclic antidepressants, antiparkinsonian drugs, ganglion blockers, clonidine
5. Miscellaneous associations
Ceroid deposits in bowel
Nontropical sprue
Jejunal diverticulosis

*Modified, with permission of the authors, from Faulk DL, Anuras S, Christensen J: Gastroenterology 74:922, 1978.

CLINICAL MANIFESTATIONS. Patients with pseudo-obstruction may be of any age but, as anticipated from the nature of the underlying causes, are more often middle aged or older. The clinical presentation may vary from one of persistent symptoms of moderate severity to more acute episodes of pain, distention, and vomiting, closely mimicking the more common circumstance of mechanical obstruction. The symptoms and signs are those of retarded transit and stagnation of intestinal contents, a variable spectrum of dysphagia, regurgitation, vomiting, distention, obstipation, diarrhea, and malabsorption. Abdominal pain is quite variable also and, when prominent, makes differentiation from mechanical obstruction quite difficult. Manifestation of neuromuscular incoordination of other systems, notably the urinary bladder, may be present, as may the features of any underlying disease. Severe and chronic pseudo-obstruction may produce malnutrition and inanition.

DIAGNOSIS. The diagnosis of pseudo-obstruction requires the painstaking exclusion of mechanical obstruction. Free flow of contrast must be demonstrated after a barium meal with small bowel follow-through and with a barium enema. Failure to recognize a correctable mechanical obstruction may have grave consequences. The differentiation of pseudo-obstruction from slowly progressive distal obstruction (as, for example, with carcinoid tumors, radiation enteritis, and other fibrosing lesions) can also be quite difficult. Adjunctive evidence of a generalized disorder of muscle function can be obtained from motility studies of the esophagus, from cystometric studies, and from clinical evidence of underlying disease. When malabsorption is present, other causes of steatorrhea must be excluded. In some instances, exploratory laparotomy cannot be avoided, and full-thickness biopsy of involved intestine can be helpful.

TREATMENT. Pharmacologic treatment of pseudo-obstruction, although rational, has generally been unrewarding. Cholinergic agents and metoclopramide have the most appeal but are usually ineffective; hormones such as cholecystokinin-pancreozymin and a related peptide, cerulein, have also been tried with poor results. Corticosteroids have not augmented motility or reduced steatorrhea. Elevated serum levels of prostaglandins have been reported, as has partial relief with indomethacin. However, in an uncommon disease with an unpredictable natural history, any therapeutic information is largely anecdotal. Acute episodes require nasogastric suction and parenteral fluids, sometimes leading to parenteral alimentation. When a "blind loop syndrome" is present, antibiotics can be helpful. Surgical resection of more severely affected segments can help very occasionally but should not be entertained lightly; each laparotomy merely increases the likelihood of adhesive obstruction, further confusing an already complex problem. The prognosis is poor, and some patients have required total (home) parenteral nutrition.

Anuras S, Mitros FA, Sofer RT, et al.: Chronic intestinal pseudo-obstruction in young children. Gastroenterology 91:62, 1986. *Report of eight children with symptoms beginning between the ages of a few weeks to five years. All had marked dilatation of the entire intestine and megacystis. The disease was variable among individual examples, but, in most, the smooth muscle appeared normal.*

Schuffler MD, Baird HW, Fleming CR, et al.: Intestinal pseudo-obstruction as the presenting manifestation of small-cell carcinoma of the lung. Ann Intern Med 98:1983. *A carefully studied and well-documented example of a paraneoplastic neuropathy of the gastrointestinal tract. Though a rare syndrome, it exemplifies one of the multiple mechanisms of motor control that can be disturbed by disease.*

Snape WJ Jr: Pseudo-obstruction and other obstructive disorders. Clin Gastroenterol 11:3, 1982. *Succinct review of pathophysiology and clinical features of the syndrome. Contains all major original references.*

DIVERTICULA OF THE SMALL INTESTINE

Duodenal diverticula are common and only rarely of any significance. Although a few examples of ulceration and bleeding have been documented, duodenal diverticula are of little diagnostic significance in upper gastrointestinal hemorrhage. Jejunal diverticula are important when stasis and bacterial overgrowth occur, resulting in the "blind loop syndrome" (see Ch. 104).

Meckel's diverticulum is the most common congenital abnormality of the gut, occurring in 2 per cent of the population. Meckel's diverticula are situated 30 to 90 cm proximal to the ileocecal sphincter on the antimesenteric wall of the ileum. Although usually 5 to 7 cm in length, they can be much longer. Gastric mucosa is present within the lumen in about one third of these diverticula. They are usually asymptomatic, but occasionally bleed, perforate, become inflamed, or obstruct the ileum. The presence of gastric mucosa and the capacity of this tissue to take up selectively radioisotopes of technetium form the basis of a diagnostic test using external gamma-camera scintillography. The diverticulum "lights up" and can be occasionally identified in this way.

Disorders of Colonic Motility

INTRODUCTION

The colon's multiple functions—desiccation of feces, bacterial metabolism of unabsorbed materials, storage of stools, and voluntary defecation—are served by a complex pattern of motility. The walls of the cecum and ascending and transverse colons show radiologic indentations ("haustra") that correspond to low-pressure mixing waves, as recorded by intraluminal pressure transducers. These waves are thought to provide a "back-and-forth" mixing that facilitates reabsorption of salt and water. This motor pattern probably also increases the digestive potential for bacterial enzymes on dietary fiber. Transit through the descending colon is more rapid, although feces are stored in the sigmoid region. Entry of stools into the rectum triggers a coordinated sequence of rectal events, voluntary elevations of intra-abdominal pressure, and relaxation of the anal sphincters whereby controlled and voluntary defecation is possible.

Dietary fiber, components that are resistant to digestion by mammalian enzymes, may modify colonic motor function. Modern analytic techniques have now identified the important components of fruits, vegetables, and the outer shells of cereals that constitute fiber. The major components of fiber are celluloses (large, unbranched polymers of glucose), hemicelluloses (highly branched polymers of five-carbon sugars), pectins (gel-forming carbohydrates), and lignins (noncarbohydrate polymers of phenylpropanes). The differing chemical compositions within each of these classes and wide variations among the natural sources of fiber in foods contribute to the variable clinical effects of different fibers. In most instances, fiber decreases transit time through the colon and increases fecal bulk while undergoing some degree of digestion by the fecal flora. Gases (hydrogen, carbon dioxide, and, in one third of adults, methane) and organic anions (butyrate, propionate, acetate) are generated. Undigested components of fiber have physical effects on feces by entrapping ions and water within their complex matrices. Fiber deficiency has been incriminated in several colonic diseases, including simple constipation, diverticulosis, hemorrhoids, and carcinoma of the colon.

Vahovny GV, Kritchevsky D: Dietary Fiber in Health and Disease. New York, Plenum Press, 1982. *A simple but comprehensive monograph that contains much that will be useful for clinicians wishing to know more about modern views on fiber. Excellent chapters on "what is fiber," physical properties of fiber in the bowel, and effects of fiber on colonic function.*

SIMPLE CONSTIPATION: LAXATIVES AND THEIR ABUSE

DEFINITION. Most normal adults experience brief episodes of constipation when their living habits change abruptly. Normal frequency of stools is approximately three or more per week; moreover, defecation should be painless, not require undue straining, and be satisfyingly complete. Patients may complain of constipation if any of these criteria is not fulfilled. In order to determine whether a patient has constipation, stool frequency and fecal weight should be measured over a period of two weeks during which the intake of fiber in the diet is adequate and no constipating drugs are being taken. On such a schedule a stool should be passed with ease at least every other day.

ETIOLOGY. Constipation is a symptom and not a disease. The major causes are listed in Table 102–3. In many instances a combination of factors will be present, e.g., diets that contain little fiber, complicated by drugs that constipate, being ingested by an individual who is debilitated, with poor muscular tone, and who has a poor habit for defecation. Clearly, the list of underlying causes in Table 102–3 dictates that constipation that continues despite the program outlined above must be evaluated carefully.

PATHOGENESIS. The major abnormality is slow transit of feces through the colon, an abnormality that can be documented best by observing the time required for small radiopaque pellets to be excreted. There is no evidence that fluid absorption by the colon is excessive, except to the degree that augmented absorption can be explained by slower transit. In some persons, stools are held up at the rectal outlet, since the muscles of the pelvic floor and anal sphincter fail to relax during defecatory efforts. In most instances of secondary constipation, a pathogenic mechanism cannot be specified.

CLINICAL MANIFESTATIONS AND DIAGNOSIS. Many symptoms are falsely attributed to constipation; these include halitosis, distention, belching, rectal gas, abdominal discomfort, headache, and even temper tantrums. However, severe fecal impaction can cause intestinal obstruction with spurious ("overflow") diarrhea, stercoral ulceration with bleeding, and even acute abdominal crises. Features of underlying disease may be present by history or on physical examination. Other

TABLE 102–3. MAJOR CAUSES OF CONSTIPATION

1. **"Functional causes"**
   - Fiber-deficient diets
   - Inadequate evacuatory habits
   - Variants of "irritable bowel syndrome"
   - Psychoses and mental deficiency
   - Debilitation and extreme old age
2. **Colonic diseases**
   - Chronic obstructive lesions (e.g., tumors, strictures)
   - Ulcerative proctitis
   - Collagen vascular diseases with muscular abnormalities
3. **Rectal diseases**
   - Stricture (e.g., ulcerative colitis, postsurgical)
   - Painful conditions (fissure, abscess)
   - Prolapsed rectal mucosa
   - Rectocele
4. **Neurologic diseases**
   - Hirschsprung's disease
   - Ganglioneuromatosis
   - Chagas' disease
   - Intestinal pseudo-obstruction
   - Spinal cord injuries and disease
   - Parkinson's disease
   - Cerebral tumors and cerebrovascular disease
5. **Metabolic diseases**
   - Porphyria
   - Hypothyroidism
   - Hypercalcemia
   - Pheochromocytoma
   - Uremia
6. **Drugs**
   - Analgesics, antacids (calcium and aluminum compounds), anticholinergics, anticonvulsants, antidepressants, bismuth salts, ganglion blockers, heavy metal poisonings, drugs for parkinsonism and psychotherapy

physical findings may include tenderness of the colon to abdominal palpation and sigmoidoscopic visualization of melanosis coli, a superficial, brown pigmentation of the rectal mucosa that is seen in persons who use anthraquinone laxatives habitually. Abuse of laxatives can have other serious sequelae (see below).

TREATMENT. When treatable diseases are excluded, it is important to educate the patient about the colon's functions. Establishment of a daily ritual, aided by an increase in dietary fiber through use of fruit and vegetables or the addition of psyllium hydrophilic colloids (Metamucil), should be the major approach. Patients need to be told that such agents are not cathartics and that a prompt evacuation will not follow their use. The patient should gradually increase a regular (three times daily) dosage of psyllium hydrophilic colloids until an effect is achieved and then continue that dosage. One teaspoonful (7 grams) of powder three times a day may suffice, as an example. Chronic use of more potent laxatives should be avoided. In fecal impaction, enemas may soften and dislodge hard feces; suppositories and "wetting agents" may also help. When all else fails, manual removal, under appropriate sedation, may be necessary.

Laxatives are classified conventionally into several classes: (1) Osmotic agents are poorly absorbed molecules that retain water in the bowel lumen through osmotic pressure. Sulfates, phosphates, and magnesium salts are in this category. (2) Stool softeners, such as dioctyl sodium sulfosuccinate, are thought to be "wetting agents," although they also stimulate fluid secretion in a way similar to the next class. (3) "Stimulant laxatives," which vary in potency from the relatively mild to the powerful purgatives, include phenolphthalein, senna, the biguanides, and castor oil. All these drugs stimulate intestinal secretion of fluid and also augment propulsive motor activity. (4) Bulking agents are derivatives of plant fiber. For regular use, only this last class can be considered totally harmless. The major stimulants can destroy intramural nerve plexuses in the large bowel, causing "cathartic colon." This serious sequel of lifelong laxative abuse features a radiologic appearance similar to that of ulcerative colitis, a "pipestem" colon lacking haustra and with abnormal propulsive activity. Laxative abuse can also cause major electrolyte imbalance, mild steatorrhea, and a protein-losing enteropathy.

Binder HJ: Pharmacology of laxatives. Ann Rev Pharmacol Toxicol 17:355, 1977. *Succinct review of classification of laxatives, including sections on influence of laxative on fluid absorption and secretion, intestinal motility, and side effects of laxative abuse.*

Devroede GJ: Constipation: Mechanisms and management. In Sleisenger MH, Fordtran JS (eds.): Gastrointestinal Disease. 4th ed. Philadelphia, W. B. Saunders Company, 1988. *This is the most complete scientific evaluation of constipation. By focusing on the important underlying diseases, the author develops a strong approach that will not always be needed for simpler examples. But valuable understanding of this common and variable symptom will arise from careful review, and the clinician wishing to understand this common symptom will gain much from such review.*

IRRITABLE BOWEL SYNDROME

DEFINITION AND INCIDENCE. The key features of the irritable bowel syndrome are abdominal discomfort, alterations of bowel habit, and no demonstrable organic cause. It is the most common gastrointestinal disorder in Western societies, constituting up to 50 per cent of all referrals for subspecialty opinion. It is more common in women than men and occurs in the middle years of life. Numerous terms are applied to the syndrome, but several are inappropriate and even harmful. The entity is not an inflammation, and thus "mucous" or "spastic" *colitis* is incorrect. Functional diarrhea is sometimes considered as a separate entity, although irritable bowel syndrome may be characterized by episodes of diarrhea, often alternating with constipation.

ETIOLOGY AND PATHOGENESIS. Although causative mechanisms are unknown, it is likely that the syndrome includes a number of entities for which specific causes will eventually be uncovered. For example, the definition of lactase deficiency has allowed some patients who earlier would have been designated as having irritable bowel to receive a specific diagnosis and therapy. Psychologic and social stresses are often present in patients with irritable bowel syndrome and may be related in a temporal sense to exacerbations of symptoms. They are thought to be at least aggravating factors but may be causative.

Investigations of the pathophysiology have centered on motility studies of the colon. The colonic neuromusculature is abnormally sensitive to stress in the irritable bowel syndrome. Thus, although basal contractions are not very different from normal, meals, emotional stresses, mechanical distention, and pharmacologic stimuli elicit greater numbers of more powerful contractions. In the sigmoid colon, higher intraluminal pressures have been incriminated as a mechanism for pain and the development of diverticula and muscular hypertrophy. Studies of colonic myoelectrical activity reveal an increased incidence of waves at a rate of three per minute and fewer at six per minute, when compared with control subjects. More sensitive methods have uncovered abnormalities of muscle function in the esophagus and small intestine. Thus, it seems likely that the pathophysiology may involve an "irritability" of the entire gut in some persons.

CLINICAL FEATURES. Particular traits of personality have been attributed to patients with irritable bowel syndrome. They are often rigid, methodical persons who are conscientious, with obsessive-compulsive tendencies. Depression and hysteria are the most common psychiatric illnesses.

Abdominal pain is the most common complaint. This pain may be of any type or severity but characteristically is not severe enough to interfere with sleep. Pain is often related to meals, sometimes suggesting peptic ulcer disease, and possibly triggered in the colon by the "gastrocolic reflex." Pain may be relieved by passing flatus, which is often thought by the patient to be excessive in amount. Variants of irritable bowel syndrome include the "splenic flexure syndrome," in which colonic gas appears to be localized to that region. In fact, volumes of intestinal gas are not increased in the irritable bowel syndrome, rather, the patient is overly sensitive to normal volumes of gas or to intestinal distention by balloons. Some disturbance of bowel habit is always present as diarrhea, constipation, or a variable pattern. Stools are described as marbles, pellets, and "rabbity" mucus and undigested food are described but are of no significance. Bleeding is not a feature unless hemorrhoids are also present, and weight loss does not occur unless depression is a major feature. Associated features—emotional lability, lethargy, headaches, and benign cardiovascular symptoms—are likely psychosomatic manifestations. The program of investigation, which includes stool analysis, clinical laboratory surveys, proctosigmoidoscopy, and barium enema, is designated to eliminate underlying organic disease.

TREATMENT AND PROGNOSIS. Sympathetic explanation of the nature of the disorder and a careful exclusion of other diseases of the colon with subsequent reassurance are keys to successful management of these patients. A positive approach can be taken, irritable bowel syndrome is *not* a "wastebasket" but a disorder of intestinal function with an as yet unknown pathogenesis. Drug therapy should be avoided if at all possible. Psychoneuroses may require treatment, and severe pain may require a non-narcotic analgesic. Anticholinergic spasmolytics may also be helpful, and episodes of diarrhea may require treatment with antimotility agents. Constipation should be explained and treated with hydrophilic colloids and diet (see above). Patients should eliminate foods from the diet *only* when a specific food predictably increases symptoms and when exclusion of that food has been shown to help. The rigid use of a "low-residue" diet has no place and may well aggravate many features of the syndrome. The disorder is chronic, and it is unlikely to be modified greatly by any single measure. The aim should be to reduce symptoms to a tolerable level that interferes minimally with the patient's normal activities.

Connell AM: Motility and its disturbances. Clin Gastroenterol 11:3, 1982. *Excellent monograph with chapters covering irritable bowel syndrome, emotions and the gastrointestinal tract, and diverticular disease.*

Thompson WG: The Irritable Bowel. Gut 25:305, 1984. *An extensive review with 112 references. It summarizes well current views on the prevalence, pathophysiology, diagnosis, and treatment of this very common disorder.*

DIVERTICULOSIS COLI

DEFINITION AND INCIDENCE. Colonic diverticula are outpouchings of mucosa through the muscular layers and therefore contain no smooth muscle in their walls. They occur in close proximity to the teniae coli, where the muscular coats of the colon are perforated by an arteriole. The prevalence of colonic diverticula increases with age above 30 to 40 years, and they are present in over 50 per cent of octagenarians in the United States. Since most patients remain asymptomatic, simple diverticulosis is more an anatomic abnormality than it is a disease. However, the term "diverticular disease" is often applied to a spectrum that extends from uncomplicated diverticula, which are thought by some to be variants of the irritable bowel syndrome, to the serious complications of diverticula: bleeding, perforation, and diverticulitis (see Ch. 115).

PATHOGENESIS. Diverticula with muscle hypertrophy seem to be related to spasm of colonic muscle with raised luminal pressures and muscular hypertrophy in the sigmoid colon. "Simple" diverticula have no associated hypertrophy of muscle or evidence for high intraluminal pressures. The former or "spastic" type has been related both to irritable bowel syndrome and to a deficiency of fiber in the Western diet. Fiber is thought to protect by increasing fecal bulk, which, in turn, increases the diameter of the colon. By Laplace's law, the smaller the radius of a cylinder, the greater the pressure generated at a given tension. It is proposed that heightened pressure herniates mucosa and submucosa through the wall of the colon at points of intrinsic weakness. The fiber theory rests to a large extent on the increased incidence of spastic diverticulosis in Western society when compared with societies in which more fiber is ingested. This theory is supported by the increased incidence of diverticulosis in the past century, associated with increasing refinement of the Western diet. The pathogenesis of "simple" diverticula is unknown.

CLINICAL FEATURES. Most patients with diverticula are asymptomatic. When diverticula are present in patients with irritable bowel syndrome, it is virtually impossible to determine their role in the cramping left lower quadrant pain, constipation, or alternating constipation and diarrhea of which these individuals complain. Episodes of more severe distress, lasting for hours or a few days, are classified clinically as *acute diverticulitis*. Although tenderness and a sausage-shaped mass may be noted in the left lower quadrant, fever and leukocytosis characteristic of diverticulitis are absent in bouts of "diverticular disease." On occasions, however, there will be clinical overlap between the symptoms of "diverticular disease" and those of diverticulitis. Bleeding of two types can be seen with diverticula, those with or without diverticulitis. Minimal or occult bleeding may complicate either form of the disease. Significant gross bleeding is seen most often in asymptomatic patients and is less common in those with diverticulitis.

DIAGNOSIS. The diagnosis of diverticula in the colon is by barium enema examination. The diverticula are seen as outpouchings, particularly in the sigmoid colon. Muscular spasm and hypertrophy may be present, giving a "sawtooth," asymmetric pattern to the barium column. In appropriate cases evidence of diverticulitis should be sought—i.e., extraintestinal flow of barium, indicating chronic perforation of the bowel. The differential diagnosis from carcinoma can be difficult, or impossible in some instances. Proctosigmoidoscopy may be painful but may reveal diverticula, luminal spasm, and fixed angulation of the sigmoid from prior disease.

TREATMENT. The only plausible program for treating diverticula of the colon is designed to increase stool bulk; the aim is to prevent constipation and the development of high pressures within the lumen of the colon. Bran, hydrophilic colloids, and dietary supplements of vegetables and fruits should be used. However, the clinical success of these programs is still uncertain. Spasmolytic anticholinergics and nonopiate analgesics may be needed. Narcotics increase intraluminal pressure and should be avoided. During follow-up visits an assessment must be made as to whether the episodes of pain represent diverticulitis, since this diagnosis raises the question of surgical treatment if recurrences are frequent. (For a discussion of treatment of diverticulitis see Ch. 98.)

Almy TP, Howell DA: Diverticular disease of the colon. N Engl J Med 302:324, 1980. *This medical progress article gives an excellent summary of current knowledge concerning the pathogenesis, clinical picture, and treatment of colonic diverticula. It also supplies 119 pertinent references.*

MEGACOLON: CONGENITAL (HIRSCHSPRUNG'S DISEASE) AND ACQUIRED

DEFINITION. Hirschsprung's disease is colonic dilatation resulting from a functional obstruction of the rectum, where there is a congenital absence of intramural neural plexuses ("aganglionosis") and a "narrow segment." Acquired megacolon may be secondary to any of the causes of constipation discussed under that heading and may be assumed if colonic dilatation was not present at an earlier examination.

INCIDENCE. Congenital aganglionosis occurs in one of each 5000 live births, is five to ten times more common in boys, and is more common in sibs of probands and in children with Down's syndrome or other congenital abnormalities. Acquired megacolon occurs in the young, the very old, and the infirm.

PATHOGENESIS. Aganglionosis is due to arrest of the caudad migration of cells from the neural crest, cells that are destined to develop as intramural plexuses; thus, the aganglionic segment always extends from the internal anal sphincter a variable distance proximally. In most instances, the aganglionic segment is within the rectum and sigmoid colon; involvement of very short segments, only in the region of the anal sphincters, has also been described. The aganglionic segment is permanently contracted, causing dilatation proximal to it. Pressure studies of the anorectal segment demonstrate an absence of normal relaxation of the internal sphincter in response to rectal distention. This abnormality is absent in acquired megacolon, which has no specific pathogenesis but is merely the extreme end-result of severe constipation of many possible causes.

CLINICAL MANIFESTATIONS AND DIFFERENTIAL DIAGNOSIS. Children with congenital megacolon have obstipation, intestinal obstruction, and meconium ileus in the first days of life. Later in life the presentation is less dramatic. It does not then mimic acute intestinal obstruction, but is characterized by severe constipation and recurrent fecal impactions. Although most children have difficulty before the second month of life, very short segment aganglionosis may not cause severe symptoms until after infancy.

Congenital megacolon must be differentiated from other causes of neonatal intestinal obstruction, particularly intestinal atresia and imperforate anus. The differential diagnosis from acquired megacolon is also important. Fecal incontinence is common in acquired megacolon but does not occur in Hirschsprung's disease. Other underlying causes of severe constipation (Table 102–3) should also be sought. Digital examination of the rectum shows the rectum to be empty in congenital megacolon; barium enema usually confirms the absence of stool from the rectal ampulla and will demonstrate the narrowed distal segment in three fourths of patients. In acquired megacolon, dilatation of the bowel extends as far distal as the anal sphincter. Definitive diagnosis of Hirschsprung's disease is made by the absence of ganglion cells from Meissner's and Auerbach's plexuses, as seen in a full-thickness biopsy of the rectum. Hirschsprung's disease can be excluded when ganglion cells are seen within Meissner's submucosal plexus in more superficial biopsies; however, failure to see ganglion cells may be due to faulty technique, and their absence from punch or suction biopsies is not diagnostic of congenital megacolon.

TREATMENT. When a diagnosis of congenital megacolon is established, the treatment of choice is definitive surgery, although preliminary decompression by a colostomy may be necessary to relieve acute obstruction. In other instances, decompression can be achieved by a regular program of enemas. A number of surgical approaches are well established, and the procedure of choice should be left to the surgeon.

Treatment of acquired megacolon is medical. It involves disimpaction of feces by laxatives and enemas, a retraining of bowel habits, and behavioral modifications.

Phillips SF: Megacolon: Congenital and acquired. In Sleisenger MH, Fordtran JS (eds.): Gastrointestinal Disease. 4th ed. Philadelphia, W. B. Saunders Company, 1988. *A description of congenital and acquired megacolon in children, including clinical features, diagnosis, and treatment.*

MOTOR DYSFUNCTION IN SPINAL CORD TRANSECTION

DEFINITION. Whether due to trauma or intrinsic neurologic disease, cord transection causes a predictable disturbance of gastrointestinal motility, the recognition and management of which is key to adequate acute and long-term management of these patients.

PATHOGENESIS. The exact level of denervation and the rapidity of onset, instantaneous in many traumatic transections but slower with some intrinsic diseases, will modify the clinical picture. However, three clinical stages can be generally recognized.

CLINICAL FEATURES AND TREATMENT. In the acute stage of spinal shock, motility, transit, and evacuation are markedly depressed. Although most emphasis has been placed upon the symptoms of obstipation and abdominal distention, acute gastric dilatation and paralysis of the small intestine can also be serious complications. This phase, which lasts usually only a few days, may require nasogastric suction, rectal decompression, and the use of stimulants (e.g., neostigmine [Prostigmin*], 0.3 to 0.5 mg). During a second stage, automatic reflex activity of the bowel is established. By this time, the functions of the upper gut are usually nearly normal, but emptying of the colon may require suppositories or digital removal to reinforce reflex defecation. In the chronic stage of "reconditioning," bulking agents, stool softeners, and a program featuring planned attempts at defecating will be required. Postprandial timing and a sitting posture will be helpful at this point. The anal sphincteric reflexes are retained in most paraplegics.

Guttmann L: Spinal Cord Injuries: Comprehensive Management and Research. 2nd ed. Oxford, Blackwell Scientific, 1976. *The most comprehensive discussion of pathophysiology, clinical features and practical therapy of this problem; written by the pioneer of systematic care for spinal injuries.*

*This use is not listed in the manufacturer's directive.

Drugs That Modify Intestinal Motility

Whether or not diarrhea should be equated with rapid movement of contents through the bowel and constipation with slow transit, drugs that are used to treat these conditions are often assumed to alter motility and, hence, to modify absorption. Few reliable data are available, however, to support the concept that rapid transit impairs absorption, or the reverse. Indeed, dual effects seem more likely; thus, antidiarrheals of proven efficacy, such as the opiates, slow transit and may also have primary effects on epithelial function to enhance absorption. Some newer drugs that modify intestinal motility and transit have been introduced recently, but some are still under investigation and are not freely available in the United States at the time of writing.

AGENTS THAT REDUCE MOTILITY AND/OR TRANSIT

1. **Muscarinic blockers of the belladonna-atropine class** ("anticholinergics") have been used traditionally to reduce gastric secretion and intestinal motility. They reduce antral propulsion, delay gastric emptying, and block contractions in the small and large intestines. Some synthetic compounds (e.g., dicyclomine) are suggested to have more specific effects on "spastic" smooth muscle. Most of these drugs have generalized side effects (e.g., ophthalmologic, or on the urinary tract) that limit their usefulness.
2. **Opiates** are effective antidiarrheals, but they actually increase contractile activity in the small intestine. They stimulate propulsive activity initially and briefly, but transit is slowed later. Decreased propulsion despite increased numbers of contractions presumably reflects the stimulation of nonpropulsive, segmenting patterns of motility. Newer antidiarrheals, such as loperamide and diphenoxylate, are thought to act mainly peripherally when given by mouth, without much central opiate effect. Central effects are seen when they are administered parenterally or in large doses.
3. **Alpha-2 adrenergic agonists,** such as clonidine and lidamidine, have antidiarrheal potential. They modify the balance between absorption and secretion of fluids but also reduce motility and slow transit. Their pharmacologic actions include considerable potential for cardiovascular side effects (postural hypotension), especially if the agent (e.g., clonidine) crosses the blood-brain barrier.
4. **Neuropeptides.** Glucagon relaxes and inhibits intestinal smooth muscle and is used often in diagnostic procedures such as intestinal endoscopy and radiology. A brief action and the need for parenteral administration limit its therapeutic utility. Somatostatin inhibits the release of other gastrointestinal peptides, reduces intestinal secretion, and slows transit. It has been used successfully to control the symptoms of the carcinoid syndrome (Ch. 243).
5. **Calcium channel blockers** act at the level of the smooth muscle cell and are being tested for the treatment of "spastic" conditions such as diffuse esophageal spasm and the pain of irritable bowel syndrome.

AGENTS THAT ENHANCE MOTILITY AND/OR TRANSIT

1. **Traditional agents** include those that increase acetylcholine-like activity at the level of the smooth muscle cell, either by anticholinesterase (neostigmine) or choline-like (bethanechol) activity. Durations of action are brief; generalized effects on multiple systems must be anticipated; and they have limited clinical utility, although bethanechol has been used to correct slow gastric emptying.
2. For the treatment of slow transit, including constipatiuon, a novel class of drugs ("prokinetics") has emerged. They appear to act peripherally, possibly through enhancing the release of acetylcholine, although the precise mechanisms are still unclear. **Metaclopramide** normalizes slowed gastric emptying and has proved useful in the treatment of diabetic gastroparesis. Drug resistance has limited its long-term utility, and it has little action on the distal small bowel or colon. **Domperidine**, which has antidopaminergic properties, has effects that are also confined largely to the stomach and duodenum. **Cisapride** has been tested extensively in Europe

and appears more likely to provide broader stimulation of the small and large bowels.

3. The traditional "stimulant laxatives" promote propulsive motility, especially in the colon. The mechanisms of action are unclear, and long-term use may lead to permanent changes in the enteric nervous system and colonic atony.

Burks TF: Actions of drugs on gastrointestinal motility. In Johnson LR (ed.): Physiology of the Gastrointestinal Tract. New York, Raven Press, 1981. *Classic pharmacologic treatment of the subject, extensively referenced for background and basic sciences.*

First International Cisapride Investigators' Meeting. Digestion 34:137, 1986. *A group of 50 preliminary reports on the use of this novel stimulant of intestinal motility, which appears to act from esophagus to colon.*

103 DIARRHEA

Guenter J. Krejs

Diarrhea is defined as the presence of stool liquidity (instead of formed or soft stool) and an increase in daily stool weight, the upper normal limit of which is 200 grams in industrialized societies. Diarrhea is usually associated with increased stool frequency (more than three bowel movements per day) and is often accompanied by urgency, perianal discomfort, and incontinence. Some patients may have increased frequency and liquidity of stools, however, when their daily stool weights are less than 200 grams. Since diarrhea results from a disturbance in the normal flow and transport of gut fluids, the normal physiology of absorption in the digestive tract will first be considered.

NORMAL PHYSIOLOGY

DELIVERY, FLOW, AND ABSORPTION RATES. During fasting, the intestine contains very little fluid, but when three normal meals per day are eaten, about 9 liters of fluid are delivered to the proximal duodenum. Approximately 2 liters of this fluid are from ingested food and liquids, the rest being digestive secretions.

The volume of chyme that passes through different segments of the small bowel depends on the type of food that has been eaten. For example, meals containing high concentrations of sugar are hypertonic, and when such meals are ingested, the volume of material passing through the jejunum is even greater than the volume that enters the proximal duodenum. On the other hand, after isotonic or hypotonic meals (such as a meal of steak, potatoes, and tea), the volume of fluid traversing the jejunum is much less than that which was delivered to the duodenum. (These considerations are especially important in patients who have had gastric surgery or intestinal resection.) In either case, the osmolality of chyme is adjusted toward that of plasma as fluid travels through the duodenum and upper jejunum, and by the time chyme reaches the ileum, most of the dietary sugars, amino acids, and fats have been absorbed. Fluid arriving at the ileum is mainly an isotonic salt solution and therefore similar in its ionic composition to plasma. The ileum absorbs much, but not all, of this salt solution. About 1 liter per day of this isotonic unabsorbed ileal fluid enters the colon. Although ileal fluid resembles plasma with regard to its sodium and potassium concentrations, the concentrations of chloride and bicarbonate are quite different, being approximately 70 and 60 mEq per liter, respectively.

The colon can absorb 2 to 4 liters of isotonic salt solution per day (even more in patients with secondary hyperaldosteronism associated with salt depletion). The presence of nonabsorbable and osmotically active solutes from the diet and from bacterial action, a relatively slow rate of absorption from the rectosigmoid, and timely bowel movements prevent complete fluid absorption and desiccation of the fecal mass. About 100 ml of fluid is excreted in the feces; its sodium and chloride concentrations are about 50 mEq per liter, while the potassium concentration is about 90 mEq per liter. This fluid also contains a high concentration of volatile fatty acids (from bacterial action on nondigestible carbohydrates), which dissipate most of the unabsorbed or secreted bicarbonate ions and which often cause stool fluid to be hypertonic to plasma. Since the gastrointestinal tract does not have a diluting mechanism, the osmolality of fecal fluid is never less than the osmolality of plasma.

To summarize, daily volumes of fluid traversing the duodenum are 9 liters, traversing the ileocecal valve area are 1 liter, and traversing the anal sphincter are 0.1 liter. Stated in another way, the small bowel absorbs 8 liters of fluid per day and empties 1 liter into the colon, and the colon absorbs 0.9 liter. Theoretically 2 to 4 liters of fluid would have to be delivered to the colon per day before diarrhea would ensue, provided that delivery rates were steady, the fluid contained no abnormal solutes, and colon function was normal. Unfortunately, the latter qualifications do not apply in many gastrointestinal diseases.

TRANSPORT PHYSIOLOGY. The mechanisms responsible for fluid absorption differ in different regions of the gut and in different species. According to the model for the ileum shown in Figure 103–1, the brush border membrane contains a carrier that facilitates the simultaneous entry of Na^+ and glucose into the cells; Na^+ cannot enter without glucose. A separate pair of exchange carriers works together to facilitate the simultaneous and electrically neutral entry of Na^+ and Cl^-. Na^+ enters in exchange for H^+, and Cl^- enters in exchange for HCO_3^-. If these two exchange carriers operate at the same rate, Na^+ and Cl^- are absorbed in equal amounts, and H^+ and HCO_3^- are secreted in equal amounts and react in the lumen to form CO_2 and water. However, the anion carrier usually operates more rapidly than the cation carrier, and there is a net secretion of HCO_3^-. (This accounts for the high concentration of HCO_3^- and the low concentration of Cl^- in fluid that the ileum delivers to the colon.) Once inside the cell (via either the Na^+/H^+ exchange or the Na^+-glucose carrier), Na^+ is pumped out of the cell across the basolateral membrane by a pump that is probably an Na^+-K^+ adenosine triphosphatase (ATPase). Chloride and glucose exit the basolateral membrane by facilitated or passive diffusion.

Sodium pumping at the basolateral membrane causes a potential difference (PD) across the mucosa (serosal side positive). However, the tight junctions between small bowel mucosal cells (the "shunt pathway") are "leaky," and passive diffusion of anions (in the absorptive direction from lumen to plasma) or cations (in the secretory direction) readily dissipates the PD. Therefore, the residual PD across small bowel mucosa is only 2 to 4 mV.

Colonic cells and colonic transport are somewhat different. The brush border membrane apparently has a carrier for Na^+ that is not influenced by glucose or other actively absorbed nonelectrolytes (glucose is not absorbed in the colon). There is no convincing evidence for Na^+-H^+ exchange, but the brush border membrane appears to have an anion exchange carrier that facilitates chloride absorption and bicarbonate secretion. The tight junctions are "tight," so the electrical gradient generated by the basolateral membrane pump is sustained. The PD is, therefore, about 30 mV (serosal side positive).

Potassium movement in all regions of the gut is passive, in response to electrochemical gradients. Thus, passive potassium absorption in the colon is retarded (owing to the high lumen negative PD), and the potassium concentration in fecal fluid is much higher than in plasma (up to 100 mEq per liter). Water movement throughout the gut is passive, secondary to osmotic pressure gradients generated by active solute transport.

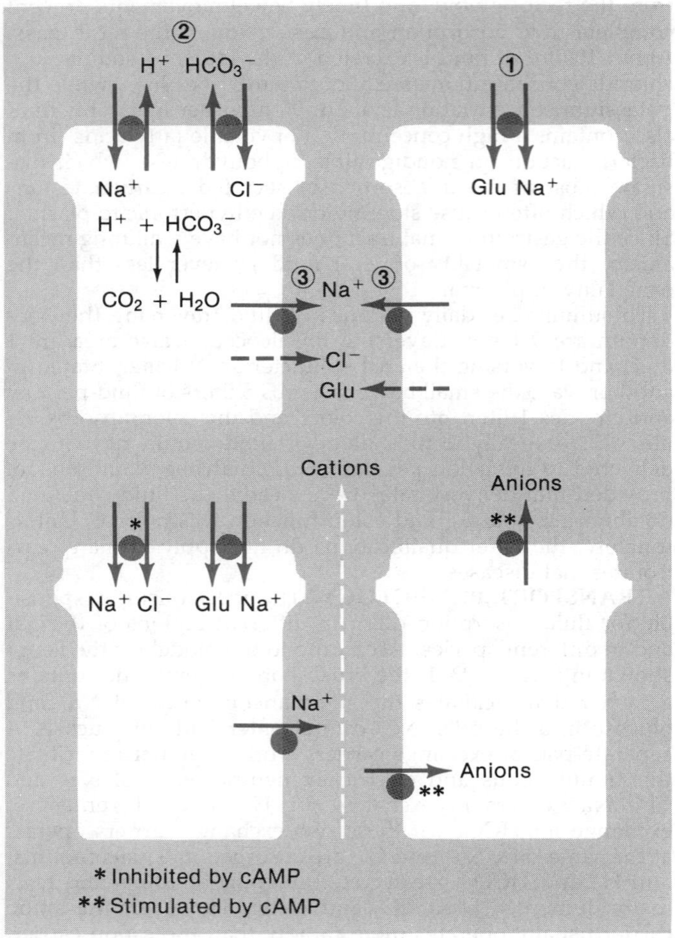

FIGURE 103–1. *Top*, Active transport mechanisms in the human ileum. *1*, Brush border glucose-sodium carrier. *2*, Double exchange carriers for neutral NaCl entry. *3*, Basolateral membrane sodium pump. *Bottom*, Model of cyclic AMP–mediated change in intestinal transport. Active anion secretion is stimulated (**), and there is inhibition of neutral NaCl entry across the brush border membrane (*). The glucose-sodium entry carrier and the basolateral membrane sodium pump are intact. Cations are secreted passively via the tight junction pathway.

NORMAL SMALL BOWEL SECRETION. Small intestinal cells normally secrete as well as absorb electrolytes and water, with the secretory rate normally being of less magnitude than the absorptive rate, so that the net effect of small bowel transport processes is absorption of fluid. (Although it is possible that the same cell might both absorb and secrete, the putative small bowel secretion probably originates in crypt cells, whereas absorption takes place from villous cells.) This is an extremely important concept, because it means that a hormone or toxin might reduce net absorption rate in either of two ways: (1) by stimulating secretion, and (2) by inhibiting absorption. In either case, the observed effect is reduced absorption. Similarly, a hormone or a toxin might cause small bowel secretion by stimulating active secretion, so that it overwhelms the normal absorptive process; or a hormone or a toxin could cause secretion by inhibiting absorption, so that the normal small bowel secretion is unmasked. In fact, many toxins and hormones appear capable of both stimulating secretion and inhibiting normal absorption (see below). In patients with diarrhea caused by toxins or hormones, it is difficult to ascertain which of these factors is predominant.

In the colon, absorption takes place from the surface epithelial cells. There is no evidence for or against a normal colonic secretion.

PATHOPHYSIOLOGY OF DIARRHEA

Diarrhea may result from one or more of the following four mechanisms. There is, in addition, a miscellaneous group for which a single mechanism cannot currently be identified:

1. Poorly absorbable, osmotically active solutes in the intestinal lumen.
2. Active ion secretion.
3. Deranged intestinal motility.
4. Altered mucosal morphology or loss of absorptive surface.
5. Miscellaneous (several mechanisms or pathophysiology not clearly understood).

Osmotic Diarrhea

Osmotic diarrhea is caused by the accumulation of nonabsorbed solutes in the gut lumen. There are three main subtypes: (1) ingestion of poorly absorbable solutes, such as saline purgatives; (2) maldigestion of ingested food, such as in lactase deficiency; and (3) failure of a mucosal transport mechanism, such as in glucose-galactose malabsorption (Table 103–1). Being osmotically active, these solutes cause water and salts to be retained within the intestinal lumen, resulting in diarrhea.

Osmotic diarrhea stops when the patient fasts (or stops ingesting the poorly absorbable solute). Furthermore, the fecal fluid has a large solute gap, i.e., normal electrolytes do not account for much of the fecal fluid osmolality (fecal solute gap = [osmolality] − 2[(Na^+) + (K^+)]; the factor of 2 is to account for anions in stool water). An exception is congenital chloridorrhea, in which unabsorbed chloride prevents water absorption. In chloridorrhea the chloride concentration in fecal fluids exceeds the sum of the concentration of sodium and potassium. Such fecal fluid analysis is performed on supernatant stool water following centrifugation of a stool sample in a test tube (30 minutes at 2000 g). In most instances, electrolytes and osmolality will provide meaningful information only if the stools are liquid enough that at the end of centrifugation the supernatant stool water constitutes at least one third of the total sample. In osmotic diarrhea resulting from carbohydrate malabsorption, the concentration in stool of short-chain fatty acids is high, and thus the pH is low (pH 4.0 to 6.0). In some instances it is necessary to measure magnesium (normal less than 12 mM), sulfate (normal less than 5 mM), and phosphate (normal less than 12 mM) in stool water to identify the cause of osmotic diarrhea, especially in surreptitious laxative abuse.

Normal fecal fluid, which can be isolated from stool by dialysis methods, often has a modest solute gap (mainly because of unabsorbed carbohydrates and their bacterial products). Therefore, the presence of a solute gap is suggestive of osmotic diarrhea only if stool volume losses are substantially higher than normal. For example, a modest osmotic gap with

TABLE 103–1. CAUSES OF OSMOTIC DIARRHEA

1. *Ingestion of poorly absorbable solutes*
Magnesium sulfate, sodium sulfate, citrate-containing laxatives
Some antacids—$Mg(OH)_2$
Mannitol, sorbitol (chewing gum, diet candy)
2. *Maldigestion*
Disaccharidase deficiencies (lactose, sucrose-isomaltose, trehalose intolerance)
Gastrocolic fistula, jejunoileal bypass, short bowel syndrome
Postgastrectomy, postvagotomy state
Chronic intestinal ischemia
Lactulose therapy
3. *Mucosal transport defects*
Glucose-galactose malabsorption
Chloridorrhea
Congenital sodium diarrhea
General malabsorption in diffuse disease of small bowel mucosa

a stool weight of only 200 grams per 24 hours would not by itself be suggestive of osmotic diarrhea.

Secretory Diarrhea

The net effect of a secretory stimulus on intestinal mucosa can be either inhibition of absorption or a net luminal gain (secretion) of water and electrolytes. This sequence of net movement changes may follow a dose-response curve, with a low secretagogue dose (e.g., circulating vasoactive intestinal polypeptide concentration) inhibiting intestinal water and ion absorption and a high dose causing net secretion. On a cellular level, both processes can occur at the same time, with inhibition of villus absorption and enhancement of crypt secretion in the small bowel.

Secretory diarrhea is recognized clinically by certain features: Stools are large in volume and watery (more than 1 liter per day), and diarrhea persists with fasting. The stool osmolality can be totally accounted for by normal ionic constituents: $([Na^+] + [K^+]) \times 2$ equals stool osmolality, which is close to the osmolality of plasma. Table 103–2 gives the major causes of secretory diarrhea. A few examples are discussed in detail.

ENTEROTOXIN-INDUCED SECRETION. The classic disease in this category is Asiatic cholera (Ch. 287). Intestinal secretion is caused by cholera toxin; the morphologic appearance of intestinal mucosa, however, remains normal. An increase in intracellular cyclic adenosine monophosphate (cAMP) in cholera mediates active ion secretion by the enterocytes (Fig. 103–1*B*). Patients may lose 10 to 20 liters of watery stool per day. Mortality was high prior to the introduction of oral rehydration solutions. This therapy is successful because glucose-stimulated sodium absorption remains normal despite ongoing secretion.

Enterotoxigenic *Escherichia coli* strains can produce one or more of at least three types of toxins (one heat-labile and two heat-stable toxins). Intestinal secretion caused by these toxins is responsible for many episodes of acute diarrhea, including traveler's diarrhea (Ch. 289). Enterotoxin is produced by a large number of other bacteria, some of which are also capable of tissue invasion (*Campylobacter jejuni, Yersinia enterocolitica, Salmonella, Shigella, Clostridium difficile, Staphylococcus aureus, Klebsiella pneumoniae, Aeromonas, Plesiomonas*).

PANCREATIC CHOLERA SYNDROME (Ch. 233). High circulating levels of VIP (vasoactive intestinal polypeptide) cause intestinal water and electrolyte secretion that results in large-volume diarrhea. In adults, VIP production usually comes from tumors originating in pancreatic islet cells, whereas in children these tumors are often ganglioneuromas or ganglioneuroblastomas. The disease can be mimicked by prolonged intravenous VIP infusion in healthy subjects. This syndrome is also known as Verner-Morrison syndrome, VIP-oma syndrome, or watery diarrhea-hypokalemia-hypochlorhydria (WDHH) syndrome. Diarrhea disappears when plasma VIP levels return to normal following tumor resection. Fifty per cent of patients have metastatic disease at diagnosis, however, so that resection is not possible.

In one study of patients with pancreatic cholera, mean daily stool weights averaged 4224 grams during a regular diet and 1817 grams during fasting. Hypokalemia and metabolic acidosis due to large fecal potassium and bicarbonate losses are prominent features, whereas hypochlorhydria is variable. Cosecretion of calcitonin, pancreatic polypeptide, PHM (peptide histidine methionine), or helodermin by these tumors has been found in a number of patients.

IDIOPATHIC SECRETORY DIARRHEA. Patients with this syndrome present with the large-volume secretory diarrhea and other clinical features of pancreatic cholera, but no evidence of tumor or of an abnormally elevated concentration of a circulating secretagogue can be found. These patients undergo extensive negative investigations that often include exploratory laparotomy. Autopsy examination may also be unrevealing, and the etiology remains unknown. Both the severity of this syndrome and the prognosis vary widely. Spontaneous resolution of the diarrhea may occur after several months. A few patients respond to opiates.

CARCINOID SYNDROME (Ch. 243). Diarrhea is a common manifestation of the carcinoid syndrome, occurring in about 70 to 80 per cent of patients. In most patients, intestinal secretion can be demonstrated. Serotonin and substance P elicit intestinal water and ion secretion in experimental animals, and these agents are often elevated in the plasma of patients with the carcinoid syndrome. In other patients, the diarrhea appears episodic and possibly associated with the hypermotility that can be demonstrated when serotonin is given intravenously to normal volunteers. In addition, other contributing causes for diarrhea may be (1) bile salt catharsis if ileal resection was required for tumor removal, (2) lymphatic obstruction due to tumor mass, or (3) subacute intestinal obstruction as a consequence of bowel wall fibrosis induced by the tumor.

MEDULLARY CARCINOMA OF THE THYROID (Ch. 229). Diarrhea occurs in 30 per cent of patients with medullary carcinoma of the thyroid and may precede the presence of a palpable thyroid mass. Circulating calcitonin is the major mediator of intestinal secretion in this syndrome. Since this tumor may be part of multiple endocrine neoplasia syndromes (Ch. 241), first-degree relatives need to be investigated by measuring basal and postprovocation (intravenous pentagastrin) plasma calcitonin concentrations. Other than in medullary carcinoma of the thyroid, calcitonin is also found in high concentrations in the plasma and tumor tissue of a number of patients with endocrine pancreatic tumors (VIPoma, somatostatinoma), but usually it is not the predominant peptide.

ZOLLINGER-ELLISON SYNDROME (Ch. 100). The secretory diarrhea that occurs in gastrinoma (Zollinger-Ellison syndrome) has a unique pathophysiology. Due to the gastric hypersecretion caused by high concentrations of circulating gastrin, an excessive load of acidic fluid enters the small bowel and overwhelms the intestinal absorptive capacity. In such patients, daily delivery of up to 24 liters of acidic fluid to the jejunum can occur in the fasting state. Although the percentage of decrease in luminal flow rates in the intestine is similar to that in healthy subjects, the remaining fecal volume is often still in excess of 1 liter per day. Other factors that may play a role in causing diarrhea in gastrinoma are the functional

TABLE 103–2. INTESTINAL SECRETION: DIARRHEAL SYNDROMES AND CORRESPONDING SECRETORY STIMULI

Diarrheal Syndromes	Secretory Stimulus
Traveler's diarrhea, Asiatic cholera	Enterotoxins (*Escherichia coli, Vibrio cholerae*)
Laxative abuse	Laxatives (phenolphthalein, senna, bisacodyl)
Pancreatic cholera syndrome	Vasoactive intestinal polypeptide
Medullary carcinoma of the thyroid	Calcitonin
Carcinoid syndrome	Serotonin, substance P
Zollinger-Ellison syndrome	Gastrin
Secreting villous adenoma of the rectum	Prostaglandins
Small intestinal obstruction	Intestinal distention
Diarrhea in patients with portal hypertension plus severe hypoalbuminemia	Increased hydrostatic vascular pressure and tissue pressure
Congenital chloridorrhea (intestinal secretion in some instances); lethal familial protracted diarrhea	Congenital mucosal ion transport defects
Giardiasis, strongyloidosis, amebiasis	Unknown mechanism activated by protozoa
Idiopathic chronic secretory diarrhea (pseudopancreatic cholera syndrome)	Unknown
Collagen vascular diseases (scleroderma, systemic lupus erythematosus, mixed connective tissue disease)	Unknown
Intestinal lymphoma	Unknown

or morphologic impairment of the mucosal brush border by the abnormal acid milieu, the direct effect of excessive gastrin on the small bowel mucosa (reducing absorption), and inactivation of pancreatic lipase by the acidic fluid, causing a mild degree of steatorrhea. Low intraluminal pH may also cause some of the primary bile acids to become insoluble, leading to a reduction of micelle formation and a mild degree of steatorrhea.

BILE ACID DIARRHEA. Watery diarrhea in cholerrheic enteropathy results from the secretory effect of malabsorbed bile acids on colonic mucosa. Interruption of the normal enterohepatic circulation of bile acids can be caused by three types of bile acid malabsorption. Type I is due to ileal disease or resection. Type II, which is less common, consists of a selective ileal transport defect for bile acids. Type III is bile acid malabsorption in the postcholecystectomy and postvagotomy state. Cholestyramine is the treatment of choice for Type I and Type II bile acid diarrhea. Patients with Type III are rarely found to have secretory concentrations of fecal bile acids and rarely respond to cholestyramine.

Deranged Intestinal Motility

On a priori grounds, three major derangements might cause diarrhea: (1) Abnormally reduced peristalsis may allow bacterial overgrowth in the small bowel. (2) "Intestinal hurry" may reduce contact time between the small bowel mucosa and its contents and thus result in delivery of abnormally large and qualitatively abnormal fluid loads to the colon. This occurs in spite of the fact that absorption in the small bowel is normal per unit of time. (3) Premature emptying of the colon caused by an abnormality of its contents, or by intrinsic colonic "irritability" or inflammation, results in a reduced contact between luminal contents and colonic mucosa and therefore increased volume and liquidity of the stools.

Some diarrheal diseases due, at least in part, to deranged motility are irritable bowel syndrome, malignant carcinoid syndrome, postvagotomy diarrhea, diarrhea resulting from diabetic neuropathy, diarrhea resulting from thyrotoxicosis, and the diarrhea associated with postgastrectomy dumping syndrome. Abnormal motility may also contribute to acute diarrhea caused by infections. Stool analysis in diarrhea due to a motility disturbance may be consistent with that in osmotic diarrhea if nutrient absorption is impaired in the small bowel or may resemble that in secretory diarrhea, if, following nutrient absorption, the ileocecal transit volume remains largely unabsorbed. Alternatively, a mixed pattern can exist, with electrolytes accounting for an osmolality equal to that of plasma and an additional component making stool water hyperosmolar, owing mainly to bacterial metabolism of malabsorbed carbohydrates in the collection unit following passage of the stool. Irritable bowel syndrome and fecal incontinence will be discussed in more detail.

IRRITABLE BOWEL SYNDROME. In the United States, up to 50 per cent of all patients seen by primary care physicians for digestive tract problems have irritable bowel syndrome. Diarrhea is usually referred to as functional diarrhea, since no obvious cause can be found on extensive routine clinical testing. On special investigations, altered myoelectric activity in the large bowel and a significant acceleration in small bowel transit have been demonstrated in patients with irritable bowel syndrome and diarrhea. At the present time, however, it is unclear what clinical relevance these findings may have in the diagnostic and therapeutic management of such patients.

Although functional diarrhea as part of the irritable bowel syndrome is generally considered a diagnosis by exclusion, this does not mean that extensive testing is necessary when one is initially confronted with such a patient. Rather, a positive diagnosis can often be made at the first interview. This is based mainly on a typical history: abdominal pain of long duration (often for several years), discomfort and pain in different areas of the abdomen, bloating associated with various so-called food intolerances, and alternating diarrhea and constipation. Functional diarrhea may show a temporal relation to meal intake, and nocturnal diarrhea is typically absent. Furthermore, signs of systemic disease, such as weight loss, are usually absent. Classically, patients are female and in their 20's and 30's, and a history of emotional conflict, stress, or anxiety is common.

In functional diarrhea, stool weight rarely exceeds 500 grams per day (normal less than 200 grams). In a patient who complains of an increased frequency of defecation, a normal or nearly normal 24-hour stool weight may be the first clue to fecal incontinence, a diagnosis often confused with functional diarrhea.

INCONTINENCE. Most patients whose major disability is due to fecal incontinence present to their physician with "diarrhea." Either they are embarrassed to mention the incontinence, or they interpret it as a manifestation of severe diarrhea. If patients do mention incontinence, the physician also usually attributes it to voluminous diarrhea. In most instances, however, these patients are suffering primarily from a defect in the continence mechanisms rather than from severe diarrhea. As a matter of fact, quantitative stool collections usually reveal rather small fecal volumes, even though stools are soft to liquid in consistency. In any case, the major problem in most such patients is in the anal continence mechanisms. The most frequent causes for sphincter dysfunction are previous anal surgery for fissures, fistulas, or hemorrhoids; episiotomy or tear during childbirth; anal Crohn's disease; and diabetic neuropathy.

Anal sphincter training may improve sphincter function and reduce the frequency of incontinent episodes. It is also important to establish the cause of diarrhea if possible, since effective therapy of the diarrhea will usually prevent further incontinence. Symptomatic therapy with opiate drugs is helpful in some patients. There is recent interest in surgical treatment for incontinence, but no good prospective studies have been done. No therapy for incontinence in patients with diarrhea, whether involving drugs, biofeedback, or surgery, has included objective data that convincingly establish its benefit.

Morphologic Alterations

Efficient intestinal absorption requires that the intestinal mucosa be intact with a well-functioning blood supply and intact neural connections. A large number of diseases can cause diarrhea by disrupting the normal anatomy of the intestine (Table 103–3).

VIRAL GASTROENTERITIS. It is estimated that every year 5 million children less than two years of age will die in

TABLE 103–3. DIARRHEA DUE TO DISRUPTION OF STRUCTURAL INTEGRITY OF THE INTESTINE

Viral gastroenteritis
Bacterial infection with tissue invasion
Sprue (tropical, nontropical, collagenous)
Whipple's disease
Radiation enteritis
Drugs (e.g., chemotherapeutic agents)
Amyloidosis
Collagen vascular diseases (systemic lupus erythematosus, scleroderma, mixed connective tissue disease)
Inflammatory bowel disease (Crohn's disease, ulcerative colitis, microscopic and collagenous colitis)
Eosinophilic gastroenteritis
Intestinal lymphoma
Ileocecal tuberculosis
Intestinal ischemia, mesenteric vasculitis
Diverticulitis
Pelvic inflammatory disease
Acquired immunodeficiency syndrome (AIDS)

developing countries as a consequence of acute diarrhea. Rotavirus is responsible for at least 50 per cent of these infections. The pathogenesis of viral diarrhea is thought to be as follows. The virus enters the absorptive epithelial cells on the tip of the villus, and these cells are sloughed off. Crypt cells then move quickly to replace the lost enterocytes. These cells, however, are immature and cannot absorb effectively. Their sucrase and lactase activities are low, whereas adenylate cyclase activity and cAMP content are normal (in contrast to cholera, in which sucrase and lactase activities are normal and adenylate cyclase activity and cAMP content are increased). There is no enhanced water and electrolyte secretion in viral gastroenteritis; however, sodium-stimulated glucose absorption is markedly diminished. Malabsorption of water, electrolytes, and nutrients results until the infection subsides and mature enterocytes again coat the surface of the villus.

SPRUE (Ch. 104). The changes associated with sprue involve villous atrophy and a marked diminution in the effective absorptive surface of the bowel. When studied with intestinal perfusion techniques, such patients demonstrate jejunal secretion. This can be expected from the observation that the mucosa in total villous atrophy consists only of crypts, and crypts normally secrete fluid and electrolytes. Diarrhea is a result of fat and carbohydrate malabsorption. Typically, there is no diarrhea when these patients fast, suggesting that the colon reabsorbs the small bowel secretions. In rare cases patients with sprue have severe secretory diarrhea; a stool output as high as 5 liters a day has been observed.

RADIATION ENTERITIS. Acute radiation enteritis usually occurs within the initial weeks of radiation exposure and is characterized by abdominal cramping, diarrhea, nausea, and vomiting. With the passage of time, symptoms abate, and a quiescent period ensues. The average onset of further symptoms is one year, but symptoms may occur at any time. Malabsorption of varying degree for bile acids, fat, carbohydrate, and vitamin B_{12} is observed. Interference with absorption occurs owing to infiltration of the mucosa by inflammatory cells and luminal narrowing of the submucosal arterioles with fibrin plugs. Disturbances in motility due to the effects of radiation on the muscularis propria can also contribute to the diarrhea. Late-appearing structural changes with intermittent obstruction, mucosal ulceration, and fistula formation may also lead to diarrhea. Medical therapy with antidiarrheal agents, broad-spectrum antibiotics for bacterial overgrowth, and prednisone rarely provides total control of symptoms. Ultimately, 15 per cent of patients will require surgical intervention, such as segmental resection or fistula closure.

LOSS OF ABSORPTIVE SURFACE. The diarrhea that results from intestinal resection may be on the basis of the region removed (e.g., ileum, with its special transport sites for active bile acid absorption) or of the length of bowel resected. At least 50 per cent of the small bowel is required in order to avoid diarrhea and malnutrition associated with the short bowel syndrome.

AIDS (ACQUIRED IMMUNODEFICIENCY SYNDROME) (Ch. 346). Small intestinal morphologic alterations and consequent malabsorption and diarrhea are common among patients with the acquired immunodeficiency syndrome. Infectious agents (*Giardia, Salmonella, Cryptosporidium,* and *Stronglyoides*) and Kaposi's sarcoma can cause gastrointestinal disturbancs in AIDS. There remains a group of patients, however, who do not have identifiable infectious or parasitic agents or Kaposi's sarcoma but who still manifest diarrhea, malabsorption, and weight loss. Such patients have abnormal D-xylose and fat absorption. Duodenal biopsies reveal blunting of the villi and an inflammatory infiltrate in the lamina propria. This condition is referred to as AIDS enteropathy. Other patients with AIDS may demonstrate a histiocytic infiltrate (pseudo-Whipple's disease) containing numerous acid-fast organisms. *Mycobacterium avium intracellulare* has been isolated in these patients.

TABLE 103–4. MISCELLANEOUS CAUSES OF DIARRHEA

Drugs
Diuretics, cardiac glycosides, propranolol, quinidine, colchicine, antibiotics, methotrexate, 6-mercaptopurine, 5-fluorouracil, guanethidine, ethanol
Endocrine disorders
Addison's disease, hypoparathyroidism
Neurologic diseases
Tabes dorsalis, multiple sclerosis, myelitis, encephalitis, heat stroke, Charcot-Marie-Tooth disease, myotonia dystrophica, orthostatic hypotension
Toxicologic disorders
Lead poisoning
Immunoglobulin deficiency
Allergy
Systemic mastocytosis

MICROSCOPIC COLITIS. Some patients with chronic diarrhea demonstrate inflammation of colonic mucosa despite a normal appearance of the colon on barium enema and colonoscopy. The histologic changes consist of excess neutrophils and round cells in the lamina propria, cryptitis, and reactive changes of surface epithelial cells. When colonic absorption is measured in these patients by perfusion techniques, water and electrolyte absorption is either abolished or abnormally low. Thus, the normal ileocecal transit volume (1 liter per day) remains largely unabsorbed, and stool weights are typically in the range of 400 to 800 grams per day.

Miscellaneous Causes of Diarrhea

Table 103–4 gives a list of diseases in which several of the discussed mechanisms may cause diarrhea or in which the pathophysiology is not clearly understood.

DIAGNOSIS

Although the cause of diarrhea is obvious in many clinical situations, in many others it is not. Here we are concerned with a diagnostic approach to the patient with diarrhea in whom the cause is unknown.

History and Physical Examination

When the stools are consistently large in volume, the underlying cause of diarrhea is likely to be located in the small bowel or in the proximal colon. By contrast, in small-volume diarrhea, in which the patient has frequent urges to defecate but passes only small amounts of feces or mucus, the disorder is usually in the left portion of the colon and rectum. Passage of blood mixed in with the diarrheal stool usually indicates inflammation of the mucosa, less often a neoplasm. Passage of nonbloody mucus suggests irritable bowel syndrome, as does a history of small-volume diarrhea alternating with constipation. Frothy stools and excessive flatus suggest fermentation of unabsorbed carbohydrates. Excessively foul stools suggest putrefaction of unabsorbed amino acids. Visible oil or fat indicates severe steatorrhea. Fecal soiling (incontinence) suggests an anal sphincter defect. Diarrhea in a patient with features of anorexia nervosa suggests laxative abuse.

There are, of course, many other pertinent facts obtainable from the history, including previous surgery, drug intake (Table 103–4), symptoms of systemic illness, travel, and related illnesses in family members. In chronic and recurrent diarrhea, an association of exacerbation of diarrhea with emotional stress should be sought, an association that may suggest irritable bowel syndrome. The patient's sexual history should be discussed, as male homosexuals have a high incidence of shigellosis, giardiasis, other intestinal infections, and the usually recognized venereal diseases. Diarrhea may be the presenting manifestation of AIDS.

The physical examination may provide clues to the cause of diarrhea. Some physical findings, as well as other clinical associations that may assist in the diagnosis of diarrhea, are listed in Table 103–5.

TABLE 103–5. CLUES TO DIAGNOSIS OF DIARRHEA FROM OTHER SYMPTOMS, SIGNS, AND LABORATORY TESTS

Symptom or Sign Associated with Diarrhea	Diagnoses To Be Considered
Arthritis	Ulcerative colitis, Crohn's disease, Whipple's disease
Liver disease	Ulcerative colitis, Crohn's disease, bowel malignancy with metastasis to liver
Fever	Ulcerative colitis, Crohn's disease, amebiasis, lymphoma, tuberculosis
Marked weight loss	Malabsorption, inflammatory bowel disease, cancer, thyrotoxicosis
Eosinophilia	Eosinophilic gastroenteritis, parasitic disease
Lymphadenopathy	Lymphoma, Whipple's disease, AIDS
Neuropathy	Diabetic diarrhea, amyloidosis
Postural hypotension	Diabetic diarrhea, Addison's disease, idiopathic orthostatic hypotension
Flushing, large liver	Malignant carcinoid syndrome
Proteinuria	Amyloidosis
Perianal disease or right lower quadrant abdominal mass	Crohn's disease
Purpura	Celiac disease
Peptic ulcer	Zollinger-Ellison syndrome, antacid therapy, gastrocolic fistula
Following cholecystectomy	Bile acid malabsorption
Frequent infections	Immunoglobulin deficiency, AIDS
Immunodeficiency	Giardiasis, nodular lymphoid hyperplasia, celiac sprue
Hyperpigmentation	Whipple's disease, celiac disease, Addison's disease
Good response to corticosteroids	Ulcerative colitis, Crohn's disease, Whipple's disease, Addison's disease, pancreatic cholera, eosinophilic enteritis
Good response to antibiotics	Bacterial overgrowth in small intestine, tropical sprue, Whipple's disease, celiac disease

Diagnostic Tests

ROUTINE EXAMINATION OF STOOL. Unless the diagnosis is readily apparent from the history and physical examination, certain relatively simple studies on the stool should routinely be performed. Regardless of the clinical classification, the information obtained will usually narrow the diagnostic possibilities.

Stain for Pus. The presence or absence of intestinal inflammation can often be ascertained by examination of a stained stool specimen. Wright's or methylene blue stains are satisfactory. The presence of large numbers of white blood cells is diagnostic of inflammation. The presence of rare, scattered white cells is within normal limits.

In patients with acute or traveler's diarrhea, pus in the stool suggests invasion of the mucosa by *Shigella, E. coli, Entamoeba histolytica, Salmonella, Campylobacter,* gonococci, or other invasive organisms. In general, shigellosis and invasive *E. coli* infections cause more pus than *Salmonella* and *E. histolytica* infections. Antibiotic-related colitis may or may not be associated with pus. Diarrhea caused by noninvasive organisms that produce enterotoxins (toxigenic *E. coli,* for example), viruses, and *Giardia* is not associated with pus in the stool.

In patients with chronic and recurrent diarrhea or diarrhea of unknown etiology, pus suggests colitis of some type—idiopathic ulcerative colitis, Crohn's colitis, antibiotic-associated colitis, amebic colitis, ischemic colitis, or tuberculous colitis. Pus is especially abundant in idiopathic ulcerative colitis and tends to be less so in amebic colitis. It is usually absent in microscopic colitis. Absence of pus on a single examination does not, of course, absolutely rule out any of these entities. Radiation-induced disease of the large or small bowel and Crohn's disease limited to the small intestine may or may not be associated with pus in the stool. Pus is not present in the stools of patients with irritable bowel syndrome, most causes of malabsorption syndrome, laxative abuse, viral gastroenteritis, and giardiasis.

Occult Blood. Occult (or gross) blood in association with diarrhea usually indicates inflammation and therefore usually has the same significance as pus in the stools (see above). When blood is present in diarrheal stools that do not contain pus, one should consider neoplasms of the colon, heavy metal poisoning, and acute ischemic damage to the gut.

Sudan Stain for Fat. If excess fat is evident on Sudan stain, steatorrhea is probably present, and the various causes of malabsorption syndromes should be considered (see Ch. 104). Most such patients will have chronic and recurrent diarrhea; steatorrhea in a patient with acute or traveler's diarrhea suggests giardiasis.

Alkalinization. A pink color following alkalinization of a stool or urine sample indicates phenolphthalein ingestion as the cause of diarrhea. The test is so easily and quickly done, and the significance of a positive result is so great, that it should be carried out routinely in female patients with chronic diarrhea. Surreptitious laxative ingestion is rarely seen in males.

OTHER TESTS. Evidence of systemic illness will have obvious implications in the etiology of diarrhea (Table 103–5). For instance, a history of flushing and diarrhea will lead to determination of urinary 5-hydroxyindole acetic acid (Ch. 243). The order in which tests are carried out, assuming that further tests are necessary, will vary according to the physician's intuition regarding a particular patient. Certain of the diagnostic tests deserve brief discussion here.

Search for Infectious and Parasitic Organisms. It is important to complete the examination for parasites and to have adequate bacterial cultures in progress prior to examination of the patient with radiologic contrast media because barium interferes with successful demonstration of pathogens. Failure to find *Giardia* in stool samples is not strong evidence against giardiasis; sometimes it is necessary to examine duodenal fluid in order to demonstrate this organism. *Cryptosporidium* can be revealed by acid-fast stain of feces subjected to a flotation technique for concentration. Special culture methods are required if the presence of infection by *Gonococcus, Campylobacter,* or *Yersinia* is to be established. A microimmunofluorescent test with monoclonal antibodies can be used on a rectal mucosal smear to assess for chlamydial proctitis. Serologic tests for amebae and lymphogranuloma venereum may assist in the diagnosis in some patients. Finally, tests for clostridial toxin in fecal fluid will help in the diagnosis of pseudomembranous colitis.

Proctosigmoidoscopy. Proctosigmoidoscopy is helpful in establishing the presence or absence of mucosal inflammation. In antibiotic-associated diarrhea, it may reveal pseudomembranes. Proctosigmoidoscopy is often essential in patients with chronic and recurrent diarrhea and in patients with diarrhea of unknown etiology. The findings are especially apt to be abnormal in those whose stools contain pus or blood or both; they are usually normal in patients with diarrhea caused by the various malabsorption syndromes.

Proctosigmoidoscopy to investigate diarrhea should be done without enemas, laxatives, or suppositories. Such preparation may wash away exudate, distort the mucosa, induce trauma, and possibly obscure evidence of disease or create the false impression of disease. In almost all instances, fecal matter can easily be aspirated or pushed aside, and since most abnormalities are diffuse, fecal matter does not interfere greatly with a satisfactory examination. The presence of solid stool in the rectum of a patient who supposedly has diarrhea is also revealing, suggesting that an acute diarrhea is subsiding, that the patient may have irritable bowel syndrome, that the diarrhea is an illusion, or that the diarrhea is secondary to fecal impaction.

Since proctitis may not be evident grossly, even to the experienced eye, mucosal smears should always be obtained and stained for pus. The mucosa should be carefully examined for melanosis coli, although melanosis may be present microscopically even if it is not present grossly.

Rectal Biopsy. Biopsy can often be helpful in the evaluation of patients with diarrhea. The main disorders that might be detected by biopsy, but not by smears and stool examination, are amyloidosis, Whipple's disease, microscopic colitis, granulomatous inflammation, melanosis coli, intestinal spirochetosis (other than that caused by *Treponema pallidum*), and schistosomiasis. Biopsy is indicated in patients with diarrhea of unknown origin, especially in a search for melanosis coli and unsuspected colitis that may not have been evident grossly. It is the opinion of this author that irritable bowel syndrome should not be diagnosed until after a rectal mucosal smear has shown that pus is not present and a rectal biopsy is found to reveal no abnormality. The biopsy should be taken from the posterior wall of the rectum on a valve. Although the risk is uncertain, some clinicians believe that a rectal biopsy with large forceps predisposes to a colonic perforation if a barium enema is done within ten days of the biopsy.

Quantitative Fecal Fat. Collected stools (usually for 72 hours) should be quantitatively analyzed for fat content (1) when malabsorption is suggested by the history and physical examination, (2) when the qualitative test for fecal fat is positive, or (3) routinely in patients with diarrhea of unknown origin. If steatorrhea is present, the differential diagnosis of malabsorption syndrome can be pursued (see Ch. 104). Of course, the results of this test must be interpreted with knowledge of the approximate intake of dietary fat. Stool weight in grams (which is equivalent to stool volume in milliliters) should also be noted and recorded (see below).

Twenty-four–hour Stool Volume. For reasons indicated under History and Physical Examination above, knowledge of stool volume helps localize the region of the intestine that is most likely responsible for diarrhea, and in several instances specific information on stool volume is of great diagnostic help. For example, stool volumes greater than 500 ml per day are rarely seen in patients with irritable bowel syndrome, and stool volumes of less than 1000 ml per day provide evidence against pancreatic cholera syndrome. In addition, very large measured stool volumes will alert the physician to the need for vigorous fluid replacement therapy.

Collection of 24-hour stool specimens is easy to do in the initial phases of a diarrhea workup, prior to barium radiographs, enemas, or other preparations. With a little effort, it can be accurately done on an outpatient basis. If a record of stool frequency is kept, the average volume of each stool can be calculated, and the results may give useful insight.

In special instances, e.g., in diarrhea of unknown origin, it is useful to measure stool electrolytes and osmolality and to determine whether or not the diarrhea persists during a 48-hour fast (while the patient is given glucose and salt solutions intravenously). These results will help establish whether the diarrhea is secretory or osmotic in type (see Pathophysiology, above). If the osmolality of stool water is less than 250 mOsm per kilogram, water has been added to the stool to simulate diarrhea. A sodium concentration in fecal water that is higher than that of plasma indicates contamination by urine.

Vasoactive Intestinal Polypeptide (VIP) and Other Circulating Agents. The pancreatic cholera syndrome should be considered if diarrhea of unknown origin has lasted longer than four weeks, is secretory in type, and is severe (more than 1 liter per day and/or associated with hypokalemia and salt and water depletion), and if surreptitious laxative abuse and organic disease of the gastrointestinal tract have been excluded. The incidence of this syndrome is 1 in 10 million population per year. Only in this rare subgroup of patients is serum assay for VIP, PHM, and calcitonin likely to be helpful. Other gastrointestinal hormones such as pancreatic polypeptide (PP) may be elevated in plasma and serve as markers of endocrine pancreatic malignancy. In the United States, Dr. O'Dorisio's laboratory (Columbus, Ohio) and, in England, Dr. Bloom's laboratory (London) offer a gastrointestinal hormone profile that can be obtained from a single plasma sample. Blood needs to be drawn in iced tubes containing ethylenediamine tetra-acetic acid (EDTA) with aprotinin added to inhibit serum peptidases (aprotinin [Trasylol], 0.5 ml [5000 Kallikrein Inactivator Units] per 10 ml of blood). After immediate centrifugation in a refrigerated centrifuge, plasma is stored at −25°C or lower until sent in a frozen state on dry ice to the appropriate laboratory.

Therapeutic Trials. In some instances therapeutic trials are indicated as diagnostic tests. (Obviously, in most instances, the results must be considered suggestive rather than conclusive.) These trials may include pancreatic enzymes, antibiotics (also as part of the Schilling test), metronidazole or quinacrine (for giardiasis), cholestyramine (for bile acid malabsorption), indomethacin (for prostaglandin synthetase inhibition), and various diets (lactose free, carbohydrate free, low fat, and avoidance of any specific food to evaluate the unlikely possibility of food allergy).

THERAPY

The most satisfactory therapy is to cure the underlying disease. When this is not possible, certain drugs may ameliorate the disease and thus reduce the severity of diarrhea (prednisone for inflammatory bowel disease is an example). In a few instances, the disease cannot be ameliorated, but there is fairly specific therapy for the diarrhea, such as cholestyramine for bile acid malabsorption.

At present, unfortunately, in many patients the disease process responsible for diarrhea cannot be satisfactorily suppressed, and specific therapy is lacking. Supportive and symptomatic therapy is required in such instances.

Fluid Replacement

The most important aspect of therapy in acute and traveler's diarrhea, and in some patients with chronic diarrhea, is prevention or correction of salt and water depletion. This can be done by oral ingestion of liquids and salty foods, oral glucose-saline solutions, or intravenous fluid therapy, as dictated by the clinical situation. Two points deserve emphasis. First, soft drinks, tea, and citrus juices contain little, if any, sodium chloride (even Gatorade contains only 23 mEq per liter of sodium chloride). Second, oral glucose-saline solutions or liquids plus salty foods will actually worsen the diarrhea (in terms of stool volume) as they help correct fluid depletion. The oral rehydration solution recommended by the World Health Organization contains the following in millimoles (grams) per liter; glucose, 111 (20); NaCl, 60 (4); KCl, 20 (2); $NaHCO_3$, 30 (2); and osmolality is 331 mOsm per kilogram. In some patients, particularly those with short bowel syndrome, a high sodium concentration is needed in the oral rehydration solution to achieve a positive sodium and fluid balance. To prevent hypertonicity of such a solution, glucose is best given as a polymer. Glucose polymer consists of linear chains of mostly five to nine glucose units and is obtained from hydrolysis of starch. Glucose polymer is available as Polycose (Ross Laboratories, Columbus, Ohio) or Moducal (Mead Johnson, Evansville, Indiana) and in England as Caloreen (Roussel Ltd., Wembly Park, England). Glucose polymer is readily hydrolyzed in the gut lumen, providing glucose to the sodium-glucose carrier in the brush border. The solution contains the following in millimoles (grams) per liter: glucose polymer, 20 (20); NaCl, 120 (7), KCl, 10 (1); and osmolality is 280 mOsm per kilogram. Various flavoring substances can be added to this solution (e.g., Kool Aid).

Avoidance or Treatment of Perianal Discomfort

Helpful therapy consists of the following: (1) avoidance of soap, toilet paper, washcloths, and towels; (2) gentle washing with warm water on absorbent cotton after each bowel movement, followed by gentle, thorough drying with absorbent cotton; (3) if seepage is present, absorbent cotton retained next to the anal orifice and held in place by snug underwear; (4) sitz baths for 10 minutes two or three times a day; and (5) hydrocortisone creams (1 per cent). In addition to these measures, patients may obtain relief by additional gentle cleaning with soft pads containing witch hazel (Tucks). Locally applied anesthetic ointments may be transiently helpful, but ointments restrict perspiration and anesthetics may irritate the perianal skin, so these agents should be used only for short periods of time. It is important to recognize specific treatable conditions, such as perianal moniliasis.

Opiates

Codeine, diphenoxylate with atropine (Lomotil), and loperamide reduce urgency, bowel movement frequency, and stool volume in a wide variety of acute or chronic diarrheal illnesses. This is not to say that they have a beneficial effect in every patient; but they do in most, so that when groups of patients are studied, both stool frequency and stool volume are reduced to a statistically significant extent. Of the three drugs, loperamide and codeine are usually somewhat superior to diphenoxylate; loperamide may have less tendency than codeine to cause addiction. Codeine, however, is much less expensive. In chronic diarrhea, the drugs may be given once a day in a maximally tolerated dose or several times daily in smaller doses.

Opiate drugs are generally thought to reduce diarrhea through reducing the propulsive activity of the gut and thereby reducing stool frequency. This mechanism might also enhance contact time between intestinal mucosa and luminal contents. Assuming that at least part of the gut mucosa is in an absorbing and not a secretory state, this would allow greater absorption of fluid and thereby reduce stool volume. In vitro opiates have also been reported to stimulate sodium chloride absorption and to have antisecretory action against several secretagogues. These effects cannot be demonstrated in clinical situations using therapeutic doses of opiate drugs.

Opiates should not be used in patients with severe ulcerative colitis with impending toxic megacolon, and there is evidence suggesting that they may prolong the diarrhea in shigellosis and perhaps in diarrheal diseases caused by other invasive bacteria and in antibiotic-associated diarrhea. These reservations notwithstanding, opiates are often of benefit in the symptomatic relief of diarrhea in patients with less severe ulcerative colitis and with many acute infectious diarrheal illnesses. Obviously, they should be prescribed only when diarrhea is causing significant disability.

There are rare case reports suggesting that opiate drugs can be a cause of paradoxical diarrhea.

Bismuth Subsalicylate

Bismuth subsalicylate may prevent infection with enterotoxin-producing *E. coli* organisms. In addition, this agent will bring mild symptomatic relief in patients with acute infectious diarrhea, whether bacterial or viral in origin. The mechanism of the effect is unknown. The dose is 30 to 60 ml every 30 minutes for eight doses. Patients should be warned that this medication may turn their stools black. If the patient is on other medications, possible drug interaction should be considered.

Antibiotics in Acute and Traveler's Disease (Ch. 289)

For at least two reasons, antibiotics should not usually be used. First, in most patients they will not shorten the duration of illness. Second, their use risks the development of antibiotic-associated diarrhea or colitis, superimposed on whatever was causing the diarrhea initially. This greatly confuses the problem if the diarrhea becomes chronic.

In mild disease (small-volume diarrhea, no chills or fever, no blood or pus in the stool), antibiotics should not be prescribed unless a specific indication emerges from the bacteriology and parasitology laboratory. In patients who are severely ill, especially if they have blood or pus in the stool, antibiotic therapy aimed at shigellosis is reasonable, pending the result of stool culture.

Antisecretory Drugs

A specific and potent inhibitor of intestinal secretion is not available. On the basis of in vitro observations and individual case reports, a number of agents can be tried on an empiric basis. Phenothiazines inhibit secretion caused by cholera toxin and *E. coli* enterotoxins; aspirin, indomethacin, and other nonsteroidal anti-inflammatory agents reduce secretion mediated by prostaglandins (inhibition of prostaglandin synthesis); glucocorticoids decrease mucosal inflammation and enhance NaCl absorption (increase in Na-K-ATPase activity); nicotinic acid, clonidine, lidamidine,* and lithium carbonate may increase intestinal NaCl absorption (inhibition of adenylate cyclase), and cromoglycate may inhibit release of mediators of allergic reaction in the intestine. When diarrhea is due to circulating agents (VIPoma, carcinoid), a somatostatin analogue given subcutaneously may abolish diarrhea by decreasing secretagogue release from tumor tissue.

Bo-Linn GW, Vendrell DD, Lee E, et al.: An evaluation of the significance of microscopic colitis in patients with chronic diarrhea. J Clin Invest 75:1559, 1986. *First description of microscopic colitis as a separate disease entity. Patients reveal abolished water and electrolyte absorption during colonic perfusion studies.*

Field M, Fordtran JS, Schultz SG (eds.): Secretory Diarrhea. Bethesda, Md., American Physiological Society, 1980. *Sixteen chapters by different experts on various aspects of the pathophysiology of secretory diarrhea. The emphasis is on basic research, although there is a highly original chapter on the pharmacology of antidiarrheal drugs.*

Krejs GJ (ed.): Diarrhoea. Clin Gastroenterol 15, No 3, 1986. *Thirteen chapters on the pathophysiology and clinical investigation of diarrhea. Contains re-evaluation of criteria for defining secretory diarrhea and extensive description of* diarrhée motrice *(diarrhea due to motility derangement).*

Krejs GJ: VIPoma syndrome. Am J Med (in print). *An extensive description of pancreatic cholera syndrome, the most prominent example of secretory diarrhea caused by a circulating agent.*

Krejs GJ, Fordtran JS: Diarrhea. In Sleisenger MH, Fordtran JS (eds.): Gastrointestinal Disease. 3rd ed. Philadelphia, W. B. Saunders Company, 1983, pp 257–279. *A detailed description of the physiology of the human intestinal tract with regard to water and electrolyte movement and the pathophysiology of chronic diarrhea.*

Lambert HP (ed.): Infections of the GI tract. Clin Gastroenterol 8, No 3, 1979. *Twelve excellent chapters by different experts dealing with the pathophysiology of diarrhea, viral infections, pathogenic mechanisms in bacterial diarrhea,* E. coli, Shigella, *food poisoning, typhoid and paratyphoid fever,* Campylobacter *enteritis, traveler's diarrhea, antibiotic-associated colitis, antibiotic resistance, and antimicrobial agents. The book contains much practical and clinically useful information.*

Read NW, Krejs GJ, Read MG, et al.: Chronic diarrhea of unknown origin. Gastroenterology 78:264, 1980. *A detailed account of the clinical problems encountered in patients with intractable and difficult-to-diagnose chronic diarrhea.*

Santangelo WC, Krejs GJ: Gastrointestinal manifestations of the acquired immunodeficiency syndrome. Am J Med Sci 292:328, 1986. *Complete review of enteric infections, parasitic infestations, enteropathy, gastrointestinal bleeding, and neoplasms in patients with AIDS.*

*Investigational agent.

104 MALABSORPTION

Phillip P. Toskes

The malabsorption syndrome refers to a clinical condition in which a number of nutrients and minerals are not normally absorbed; almost always, however, lipids fail to be normally absorbed. At times the absorption of a single nutrient may be selectively impaired. A sound knowledge of normal absorptive processes allows the physician to pursue a logical approach to the diagnosis and treatment of the patient with malabsorption.

NORMAL ABSORPTION OF NUTRIENTS

Absorption is the integration of those processes whereby the products of digestion pass from the lumen of the intestine through the small intestinal enterocyte to appear in the general circulation via the lymphatics or the portal vein. Although the digestive process is initiated by acid and pepsin within the stomach, the exocrine pancreas has the major role in digesting fat, carbohydrate, and protein by its secretion of lipase, amylase, and proteases. Fat is eventually broken down to monoglycerides and fatty acids; carbohydrate, to disaccharides and monosaccharides; and proteins, to peptides and amino acids. These forms of nutrients are absorbed through the intestinal enterocyte. The villi and microvilli of the small intestine provide an enormous area for absorption. The motility of the intestine and the contraction of the microvilli allow molecules to pass through an "unstirred layer" adjacent to the microvilli.

Nutrients pass through the enterocyte by several processes: active transport, passive diffusion, facilitated diffusion, and endocytosis. Active transport and passive diffusion are the main mechanisms whereby nutrients pass through membranes. *Active transport* moves nutrients against a chemical or electrical gradient, requires energy, is carrier mediated, and is subject to competitive inhibition. *Passive diffusion* does not require energy and allows nutrients to pass through a membrane according to chemical concentration and electrical gradients. Passive diffusion, best typified by water absorption, is not carrier mediated and does not demonstrate competitive inhibition. *Facilitated diffusion* is similar to passive diffusion but may be carrier mediated and may be subject to competitive inhibition. *Endocytosis* is a process whereby nutrients are engulfed by parts of the cell membrane. Although endocytosis may be most important in the neonatal period, this absorptive mechanism may also occur to some extent in the adult and may be involved in the absorption of antigens.

Absorption of nutrients may be regionalized (Table 104–1). Although many nutrients can be absorbed throughout the small intestine, each nutrient has a major site of absorption. When areas of the intestine are damaged or resected, the remaining intestine usually adapts effectively to absorb the nutrients that would normally have been absorbed by those areas. Two noteworthy exceptions to this adaptation process are cobalamin (vitamin B_{12}) and bile salts. If the distal ileum has been resected, the subject can *never* actively absorb these two nutrients again. This has important clinical implications, especially for cobalamin. Patients who have had their distal ileum resected must receive monthly parenteral cobalamin or they will develop macrocytic anemia and neuropathy secondary to cobalamin deficiency (Ch. 136).

TABLE 104–1. REGIONALIZATION OF NUTRIENT ABSORPTION

Nutrient	Major Site of Absorption
Fat	Proximal small intestine
Protein	Mid small intestine
Carbohydrate	Proximal and mid small intestine
Iron	Proximal small intestine
Calcium	Proximal small intestine
Folic acid	Proximal and mid small intestine
Cobalamin (vitamin B_{12})	Distal small intestine (ileum)
Other water-soluble vitamins	Proximal and mid small intestine
Bile salts	Distal small intestine (ileum)
Water and electrolytes	Small intestine and colon (especially cecum)

Fat Absorption

Dietary fat is ingested largely as long-chain triglycerides, the absorption of which is a complex process involving the pancreas, liver, small intestine, and lymphatics (Fig. 104–1). Nevertheless, the process is very efficient; the coefficient of fat absorption is greater than 93 per cent, i.e., less than 7 per cent of ingested fat escapes absorption and appears in the stool per day. A breakdown in any one of these steps (Fig. 104–1) leads to malabsorption of fat (steatorrhea). A thorough knowledge of this physiologic process allows a logical approach to be pursued in the evaluation of the patient with steatorrhea.

Some triglyceride digestion begins in the stomach by lingual and gastric lipases. Triglyceride is emulsified in the stomach, and fat is slowly emptied into the duodenum, where its entry and that of acid release cholecystokinin-pancreozymin and secretin. As a result, the pancreas secretes enzymes and bicarbonate, and the gallbladder contracts to release bile salts. Bicarbonate maintains the pH of the intestinal lumen above 4, allowing pancreatic lipase to be effective in hydrolysis of triglycerides to yield free fatty acids and monoglycerides. Another pancreatic protein, colipase, facilitates the interaction between lipase and triglyceride for effective lipolysis. Fatty acids and monoglyceride interact with conjugated bile salts to form molecular aggregates or micelles (Fig. 104–1). A critical concentration of bile salts for micelle formation (5 to 15 μmol per milliliter) is maintained by a very efficient enterohepatic circulation of bile salts. Although the total bile salt pool is only 2 to 4 grams, 95 per cent of bile salts is actively absorbed in the ileum and returned to the liver by the portal venous system. Each day 20 to 30 grams of bile salts recirculate in this enterohepatic circulation. Only about 200 to 600 mg of bile salts is excreted in the feces per day and must be replaced by hepatic biosynthesis from cholesterol.

Micellar fat passes through the "unstirred" water layer covering the surface of the enterocyte. Because of their solu-

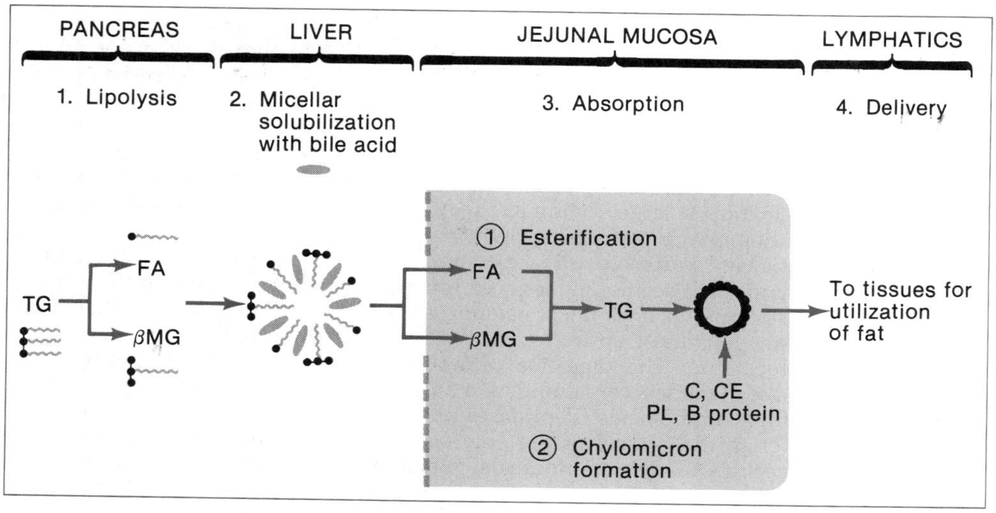

FIGURE 104–1. Schematic of intestinal absorption, showing the participation of the pancreas, liver, and intestinal mucosal cell in fat absorption. (From Wilson FA, Dietschy JM: Gastroenterology 61:911, 1971. Copyright 1971, The Williams & Wilkins Company, Baltimore.)

bility in the lipid-rich surface membrane, the fatty acids and monoglycerides are released and diffuse into the enterocyte. Fatty acid–binding protein (low molecular weight cytosolic protein) avidly binds long-chain fatty acids in the enterocyte and transports them to the smooth endoplasmic reticulum, where they are re-esterified with monoglyceride to form triglyceride. Absorbed cholesterol is also largely esterified with fatty acids for optimal transport. The intestine must also synthesize phospholipids and specific proteins (apoproteins) in order to incorporate these nonpolar lipids into lipoproteins, the major transport vehicles for fat transport in lymph and plasma (Ch. 183). These polar components are added to the surface of the lipid droplet, producing lipoproteins called chylomicrons. Chylomicrons are concentrated in the Golgi apparatus and then discharged through the lateral basal portion of the cell to the interstitium and mesenteric lymph to be delivered via the thoracic duct to the vena cava.

Medium-chain triglycerides (C-6 to C-12 fatty acids) are absorbed quite differently and more effectively than are long-chain triglycerides (C-16 to C-18 fatty acids) described above. Medium-chain triglycerides (MCT) (1) are more completely hydrolyzed by pancreatic lipase, (2) do not require bile salts for absorption, (3) can be directly taken up into the enterocyte and hydrolyzed by a mucosal lipase to fatty acids, (4) do not need to be re-esterified, (5) are not incorporated into lipoproteins, and (6) can pass directly into the portal venous system, transported as fatty acids bound to albumin. These characteristics of MCT allow its therapeutic use to improve fat absorption in a number of diseases in which dietary triglyceride absorption is impaired.

Fat-soluble vitamins (A, D, E, K) are absorbed after micellar solubilization and are transported into lymph with chylomicrons. In the case of vitamin A, the free vitamin is esterified within the enterocyte with palmitic acid, transported via chylomicrons in the lymph and stored as retinol palmitate in the liver. Vitamin metabolism is described more fully in Ch. 217.

Carbohydrate Absorption

Carbohydrate is ingested in the form of starch, sucrose, and lactose. Salivary and pancreatic amylases hydrolyze starch to oligosaccharides and disaccharides. All carbohydrate must be digested to a final monosaccharide product before it can be absorbed. Disaccharides are split by membrane-bound disaccharidases located on the microvilli of the enterocyte. Lactose is digested by lactase to glucose and galactose; sucrose, by sucrase to glucose and fructose, and maltose by maltase to two molecules of glucose. These monosaccharides are then transported through the enterocyte to the portal blood. Glucose and galactose are absorbed by active transport requiring sodium. Fructose is transported by facilitated diffusion. Glucose is transported into the enterocyte, probably bound along with sodium to a protein carrier. These monosaccharides are transported out of the cell by active sodium extrusion across the basolateral aspect of the enterocyte via a sodium pump.

Protein and Amino Acid Absorption

The digestion of dietary protein is initiated in the stomach by acid and pepsin but is largely completed by pancreatic proteases, both endopeptidases (trypsin, chymotrypsin, elastase) and exopeptidases (carboxypeptidase). Pancreatic proteases secreted in inactive forms (zymogens) must be activated. Enterokinase from the small intestinal mucosa activates trypsin from trypsinogen, and trypsin then activates all of the other protease precursors. The digestive products of pancreatic proteases are peptides containing two to six amino acids as well as single amino acids. Peptidases on the microvillus membrane or in the cytosol of the enterocyte further hydrolyze oligopeptides to free amino acids, which are directly absorbed in the portal vein.

The L forms of amino acids are actively transported in the enterocyte by specific energy-requiring, sodium-dependent processes. There are several specific transport systems for amino acids: (1) the dibasic amino acid system, which is often abnormal in cystinuria, (2) the neutral amino acid system, which is abnormal in Hartnup disease; (3) the iminoglycine system, and (4) the dicarboxylic acid system. Intact di- and tripeptides are also actively transported across the enterocyte membrane without hydrolysis by peptidases on the microvillus membrane. These peptides are hydrolyzed in the cytosol of the enterocyte to amino acids, which are then released into the circulation.

Water and Electrolyte Absorption

Over 7 liters of water (both ingested and reabsorbed from intestinal secretion) is absorbed by the small intestine per day through the process of passive diffusion. Absorption of water often follows that of glucose and electrolytes in order to maintain isotonicity of intraluminal contents.

Sodium is actively transported linked to an exchange with H^+ in the jejunum and ileum and with Cl^- and HCO_3^- in the ileum. Na^+ transport is enhanced by glucose absorption in the jejunum (via the glucose-Na^+ carrier on the microvillus membrane) and by solvent (water) drag. Some Na^+ also moves down a gradient across the mucosa, i.e., by passive diffusion. Changes in the concentration of sodium in the lumen depend on relative rates of exchange of both sodium and water between blood and lumen. Potassium passively diffuses from the lumen of the proximal small intestine and into the lumen of the distal small intestine.

Calcium Absorption

Calcium is actively absorbed in the duodenum largely regulated by the active form of vitamin D_3—1,25-dihydroxycholecalciferol (calcitriol). Vitamin D_3 from the diet is metabolized first by the liver (25-hydroxylation) and then by the kidney (1-hydroxylation) to form 1,25-dihydroxycholecalciferol (1,25[OH]$_2$D$_3$) (Ch. 245). This process is influenced by parathyroid hormone levels, which are regulated by plasma levels of ionized calcium. Calcitriol stimulates the synthesis of calcium-binding protein, alkaline phosphatase, and a calcium-activated ATPase—all involved in active calcium transport. Absorption of vitamin D, a fat-soluble vitamin, is often impaired in the malabsorptive syndromes such that calcium absorption is diminished. Fatty acids within the lumen of the intestine may also directly impair absorption by binding calcium. In turn, the unavailability of ionized calcium in the lumen leads to excessive absorption of oxalate and a resulting propensity to form calcium oxalate kidney stones.

Iron Absorption (Ch. 135)

The average intake of iron from dietary sources is 15 to 25 mg per day, of which 0.5 to 2.0 mg is normally absorbed. Iron is absorbed as inorganic iron (cereals, vegetables) or as heme iron (meat). For optimal absorption, inorganic iron must be released from dietary components to soluble iron complexes in the intestinal lumen. Gastric acid enhances the absorption of inorganic iron (both Fe^{+++} and Fe^{++}) by facilitating its chelation with sugars, amino acids, bile, and ascorbic acid. Such iron complexes remain in solution at the alkaline pH of the duodenum—the major site of iron absorption. Inorganic iron is absorbed from the intestinal lumen by the mucosa and then transported to the blood by mechanisms that are still not clear. A mucosal regulatory system keeps much of the iron trapped within the enterocyte, to be excreted into the feces depending on the need for iron, as determined by body stores of iron or by the rate of erythropoiesis. Organic iron (heme iron) is absorbed more efficiently than is inorganic iron. Heme is split from globin and absorbed as an intact metalloporphyrin at an alkaline pH. Iron is released from heme by heme oxygenase intracellularly. In plasma, iron is transported bound to transferrin, a specific globulin, to various tissues for use or storage.

Iron absorption is increased in iron deficiency, pregnancy, idiopathic hemochromatosis, and any conditions in which there is active erythropoiesis. Absorption is decreased in chronic infection and after the ingestion of large amounts of iron. Diffuse disease of the duodenum such as nontropical sprue may impair iron absorption and lead to iron deficiency.

Folic Acid Absorption

Dietary folic acid is conjugated with glutamyl peptides, prior to its absorption, these polyglutamates must be deconjugated to monoglutamates by folic deconjugase, an enzyme found on the microvillus membrane. Folate monoglutamates are absorbed by active transport at low concentrations of folate and by passive diffusion at high concentrations of folate. Folic acid undergoes an enterohepatic circulation. Since its body stores are limited, the major cause of folate deficiency is poor dietary intake of fresh fruits and vegetables. Folic acid deficiency may also occur if there is extensive damage to the proximal small intestine (e.g., nontropical sprue) or secondary to the use of a number of medications (sulfasalazine, phenytoin, trimethoprim) that inhibit its absorption. Other causes of folate deficiency are listed in Table 136–1.

Cobalamin (Vitamin B_{12}) Absorption (Ch. 136)

The current concept of cobalamin absorption and transport is depicted in Figure 104–2. Cobalamin, found in animal protein, is released from protein in the stomach by the synergistic action of both acid and pepsin. Cobalamin initially binds to a cobalamin-binding protein (R binder or cobalophilin), also secreted by the stomach. The cobalophilin-cobalamin complex is degraded by pancreatic proteases within the duodenal lumen, with release of cobalamin to bind with gastric intrinsic factor (a glycoprotein secreted by the parietal cells). After intrinsic factor binds cobalamin, the intrinsic factor–cobalamin complex passes down the small intestine until it reaches the distal 60 cm of the ileum, where it binds to a specific receptor of the brush border. In the absence of the terminal ileum, intrinsic factor–mediated cobalamin absorption ceases, although large doses of cobalamin (milligram in contrast to microgram amounts) may lead to adequate absorption by passive diffusion throughout the gastrointestinal tract.

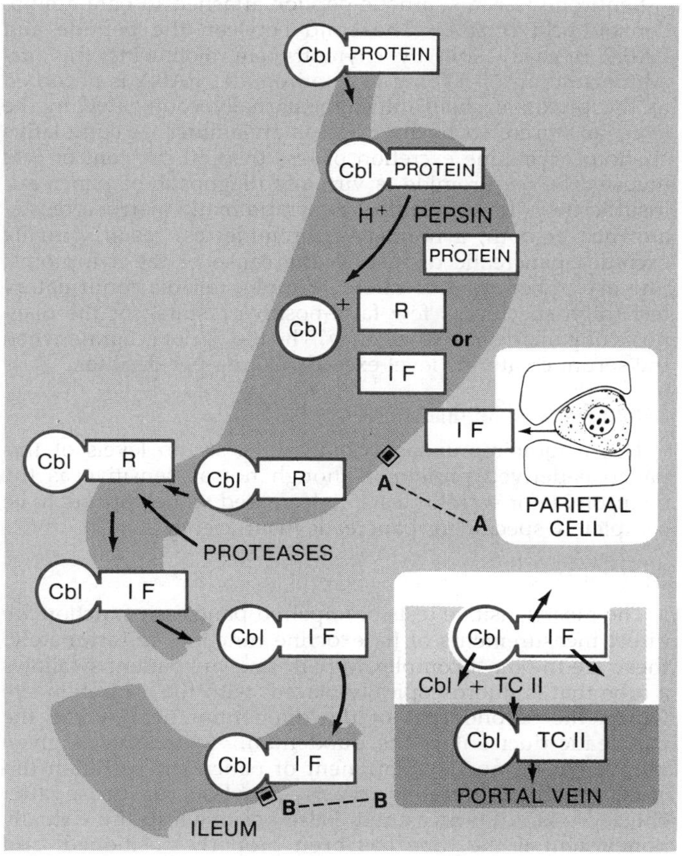

FIGURE 104–2. Cobalamin absorption and transport. Cbl = Cobalamin, R = R-protein or cobalophilin, IF = intrinsic factor, TC II = transcobalamin II. (From Toskes PP: J Clin Gastroenterol 2:287, 1980.)

Intrinsic factor does not enter the ileal cell and is not absorbed. Transcobalamin II (TCII), the most important transport protein for cobalamin, picks up cobalamin in the ileal mucosa and promotes its uptake by tissues throughout the body. The TCII-cobalamin complex enters tissues via endocytosis, with cobalamin being released by lysosomal proteolysis.

At equilibrium, the majority of circulating cobalamin is attached to cobalophilin, which is also found in saliva, gastric secretions, intestinal secretions, semen, and tears. It also moves continuously in an enterohepatic circulation. The function of the ubiquitous cobalophilins is unclear, but they may prevent or retard the absorption and dissemination of a variety of cobalamin analogues, either produced by bacteria or even found within multivitamin supplements.

CLASSIFICATION AND CLINICAL MANIFESTATIONS OF MALABSORPTION

Causes of Malabsorption

Table 104–2 divides the causes of the malabsorption syndrome into nine categories, based upon its pathophysiology (Fig. 104–1). Some conditions have multiple reasons for malabsorption but are arbitrarily classified under one major category. The differential features and management of important types of this syndrome are detailed later in the chapter.

Clinical Manifestations

Patients with the malabsorption syndrome usually present with diarrhea, weight loss, and malnutrition. These patients often complain that their stools are bulky, greasy, and excessively malodorous and that they float and are difficult to flush down the toilet. Steatorrheal stools float not because of their fat content but because of their high gas content. Patients with severe malabsorption, as exemplified by that secondary to pancreatic insufficiency, may complain of oil seeping out of the rectum. The symptoms and signs of malabsorption are varied and involve a number of organ systems. Patients may demonstrate one or more of these manifestations depending on the severity of their malabsorption. The different symptoms and signs that such patients may show and the causes of these symptoms and signs are detailed in Table 104–3. These aspects of the history and physical examination are crucial in evaluating a patient with malabsorption.

DIAGNOSIS OF MALABSORPTION

Although there may be selective malabsorption of nutrients, most patients with clinically relevant malabsorption have steatorrhea. Consequently, documentation of steatorrhea is important and is the cornerstone of the diagnostic evaluation of patients with malabsorption. The only truly reliable means to document the presence of steatorrhea is the quantitative chemical analysis of fat in a 72-hour stool collection while the patient is ingesting a high-fat diet (at least 100 grams per day). On such a diet normal subjects excrete less than 7 grams of fat per day (coefficient of absorption of >93 per cent). Unfortunately, the quantitative fecal fat determination is cumbersome to perform and difficult to obtain in most hospitals.

TABLE 104–2. CLASSIFICATION OF THE MALABSORPTION SYNDROME

1. Impaired digestion
   a. Primary pancreatic exocrine insufficiency
   b. Gastric surgery (Billroth I and II, vagotomy, and pyloroplasty)*
   c. Gastrinoma*
2. Reduced bile salt concentration
   a. Liver disease
   b. Small intestine bacterial overgrowth (scleroderma, diabetes mellitus, primary motility disturbances, postgastrectomy, achlorhydria)*
   c. Ileal disease or resection*
3. Abnormalities of intestinal mucosa
   a. Disaccharidase deficiency
   b. Impaired monosaccharide transport
   c. Folate or cobalamin deficiency
   d. Nontropical sprue
   e. Nongranulomatous ileojejunitis
   f. Amyloidosis
   g. Crohn's disease*
   h. Eosinophilic enteritis
   i. Radiation enteritis*
   j. Abetalipoproteinemia
   k. Cystinuria
   l. Hartnup disease
4. Inadequate absorptive surface
   a. Short bowel syndrome
   b. Jejunoileal bypass*
5. Infection
   a. Tropical sprue
   b. Whipple's disease*
   c. Acute infectious enteritis
   d. Parasitic infections
6. Lymphatic obstruction
   a. Lymphoma*
   b. Tuberculosis
   c. Lymphangiectasia
7. Cardiovascular disorders
   a. Congestive heart failure
   b. Constrictive pericarditis
   c. Mesenteric vascular insufficiency
8. Drug-induced
   a. Cholestyramine
   b. Neomycin
   c. Colchicine
   d. Phenindione
   e. Irritant laxatives
9. Unexplained
   a. Carcinoid syndrome
   b. Diabetes mellitus*
   c. Adrenal insufficiency
   d. Hyper- and hypothyroidism
   e. Mastocytosis
   f. Hypogammaglobulinemia

*= Multiple reasons for malabsorption.

Furthermore, the documentation of steatorrhea only indicates that the patient has the malabsorption syndrome—it does not indicate the pathophysiology or confer a specific diagnosis.

Table 104–4 details some alternative tests (other than the quantitative fecal fat determination) that can be employed to detect the presence and the cause of malabsorption in a given patient. The tests are categorized into screening tests and those that are more specific in localizing the site of the malabsorption. It is usually necessary to utilize a number of malabsorptive tests to establish the cause of the malabsorption.

Qualitative Stool Fat

The microscopic examination of stool for the presence of fat is a helpful test if performed properly and if the patient is ingesting a high-fat diet. Two specimens of stool are placed on two slides. To the first slide, two drops of water and two drops of 95 per cent ethyl alcohol are added, followed by two drops of a fat stain (e.g., Sudan III). The specimen is microscopically examined for orange neutral fat (triglyceride) globules. The globules should be larger than a red cell and should be numerous per high-power field. To the second slide, several drops of 36 per cent acetic acid are added, then several drops of Sudan III. The slide is heated until it begins to boil. Microscopically, the presence of large orange globules or spicules represents free fatty acids. Part 1 is positive in patients with pancreatic insufficiency, detecting undigested triglyceride; part 2, in patients with small bowel disease, detecting free fatty acids. Figure 104–3 demonstrates a positive part 1 test in a patient with pancreatic insufficiency. There is a 25 per cent false-negative rate when steatorrhea is mild, i.e., <10 grams per 24 hours. The false-positive rate is about 15 per cent. This test is simple to perform and inexpensive.

Urinary D-Xylose Test

The urinary xylose excretion test distinguishes between malabsorption due to small intestinal disease and that due to pancreatic exocrine insufficiency. A five-hour urinary excretion of 5 grams or greater is normal following the oral administration of 25 grams of D-xylose to a well-hydrated subject. Decreased xylose absorption and excretion are found in patients with damage to the proximal small intestine and in bacterial overgrowth in the small intestine (the bacteria catabolize the xylose). Patients with pancreatic steatorrhea usually have normal xylose absorption. As with any urinary excretion test, decreased renal function or incomplete collection of the urine may invalidate the test. Impaired renal function is most important when evaluating an elderly patient who may not have obvious renal disease, but whose creatinine clearance may be low. Decreased urinary xylose values may also be seen in patients with ascites. Although a blood level of 30 mg per deciliter or greater one hour after ingestion of xylose may indicate normal absorption, there appears to be a great deal of overlap between control subjects and those with malabsorption.

Bentiromide Urinary Excretion Test

Bentiromide is a synthetic peptide attached to para-aminobenzoic acid (PABA) The bond between the peptide and PABA is easily split by chymotrypsin. Following the oral administration of 500 mg of bentiromide, PABA is absorbed in the proximal small intestine, partially conjugated in the liver, and excreted in the urine as arylamines. A cumulative six-hour arylamine excretion of less than 50 per cent of that ingested as bentiromide is virtually diagnostic of pancreatic insufficiency. In a patient with symptomatic diarrhea or steatorrhea or both, a normal bentiromide test result virtually excludes pancreatic disease as the cause of the symptoms. The use of bentiromide offers a simple, reliable confirmatory test (high specificity, few false-positive results) for the diagnosis of pancreatic insufficiency. The test is not accurate when the serum creatinine level exceeds 2.0 mg per deciliter.

Serum Trypsin-like Immunoreactivity (TLI)

TLI, a radioimmunoassay, measures serum levels of this pancreas-derived protein. Although not as sensitive as the bentiromide or secretin tests, a decreased value appears to be completely specific for pancreatic insufficiency.

Secretin Test

The most sensitive tests of impaired pancreatic function are direct measurements of its exocrine function; unfortunately, these are the most complex to perform. The patient swallows a tube that is fluoroscopically placed, with the aspiration site within the second part of the duodenum near where the pancreatic duct enters the duodenum. A hormone is given intravenously, and a component of pancreatic secretion (bicarbonate after secretin; trypsin, amylase, or lipase after cholecystokinin) is measured. False-positive tests are virtually nonexistent if the tube has been properly positioned, and false-negative tests are not relevant because the secretin test will invariably be abnormal if the steatorrhea is secondary to pancreatic insufficiency.

TABLE 104–3. SYMPTOMS AND SIGNS OF MALABSORPTION

History	Pathophysiology	Physical Examination	Pathophysiology
Diarrhea	Increased secretion and impaired absorption of water and electrolytes, unabsorbed dihydroxy bile acids, unabsorbed fatty acids	Pallor	Anemia secondary to iron, folate, or cobalamin deficiency
Greasy, bulky, malodorous stools that are difficult to flush	Increased fat in stool	Glossitis, stomatitis, cheilosis	Iron, folate, cobalamin, and other vitamin deficiencies
Oil seeping from rectum	Unabsorbed triglyceride (pancreatic insufficiency)	Ecchymosis, purpura	Vitamin K malabsorption
Weight loss despite good appetite	Loss of calories from malabsorption	Acrodermatitis	Zinc and fatty acid deficiency
Excessive flatus	Fermentation of unabsorbed carbohydrates by colonic bacteria	Dehydration, hypotension	Water and electrolyte malabsorption
Diffuse abdominal pain	Inflammation or infiltration of tissue (pancreatic insufficiency, Crohn's disease, lymphoma)	Edema	Protein malabsorption (decreased serum albumin)
Postprandial (30 minutes after eating) midabdominal pain	Intestinal ischemia	Peripheral neuropathy	Cobalamin deficiency
Abnormal bruisability	Vitamin K malabsorption		
Weakness and fatigue	Protein, electrolyte, fat, iron, folate, cobalamin malabsorption		
Milk intolerance	Lactase deficiency		
Bone pain	Calcium and protein malabsorption		
Tetany, paresthesias	Calcium and magnesium malabsorption, cobalamin deficiency (paresthesias only)		
Night blindness	Vitamin A malabsorption		
Nocturia	Delayed absorption of water, hypokalemia		
Amenorrhea	Protein malabsorption		

TABLE 104–4. TESTS FOR MALABSORPTION

Test	Normal Values	Comments Relevant to Patients with Malabsorption
Screening Tests		
1. Serum carotene	>0.06 mg/dl	Decreased; very good test if poor oral intake has been excluded
2. Serum calcium	9.0 to 10.5 mg/dl	Decreased, not very sensitive
3. Serum cholesterol	150 to 250 mg/dl	Decreased, not very sensitive
4. Serum albumin	4.0 to 5.2 mg/dl	Decreased, not very sensitive
5. Serum magnesium	1.7 to 2.0 mEq/liter	Decreased, not very sensitive
6. Prothrombin time	Control value	Increased, not very sensitive
7. Qualitative stool fat	No fat globules per hpf*	Numerous fat globules per hpf; part 1 for neutral fats, part 2 for split fats (see text)
Specific Tests		
1. Serum iron	80–150 μg/dl	Malabsorbed in proximal small bowel disease
2. Serum folate	5–21 ng/ml	Decreased in proximal small bowel disease, may be increased in bacterial overgrowth
3. Serum cobalamin (vitamin B_{12})	200–900 pg/ml	Malabsorbed in distal small bowel disease, pernicious anemia, bacterial overgrowth, chronic pancreatitis
4. Urinary D-xylose	>5 grams/5 hr	Decreased in small bowel disease and bacterial overgrowth, normal in pancreatic disease
5. Bentiromide test	Arylamine excretion >57% in 6 hr	A value of <50 per cent is diagnostic of pancreatic insufficiency
6. Serum trypsin–like immunoreactivity (TLI)	29–80 ng/ml	A value of <20 ng/ml is specific for pancreatic insufficiency
7. Secretin test	HCO_3^- conc >80 mEq/liter Vol >1.8 ml/kg/hr	Most sensitive test of pancreatic function
8. ^{57}Cyanocobalamin urinary excretion test	>8% 24 hr	Decreased in pernicious anemia, chronic pancreatitis, bacterial overgrowth, ileal disease
9. Urine 5-HIAA	1.7–8.0 mg/24 hr	Markedly elevated in carcinoid syndrome, minimally elevated in any kind of malabsorption
10. Breath tests		
a. ^{14}C-xylose	<0.0013% of administered dose as breath $^{14}CO_2$ at 30 min	Elevated in bacterial overgrowth
b. cholyl-1-^{14}C-glycine	<1% of administered dose as breath $^{14}CO_2$ at any interval over 4 hr	Elevated in bacterial overgrowth or bile acid malabsorption
c. Lactulose H_2	<10 ppm rise in breath H_2 over baseline at any interval for 120 min	Elevated in bacterial overgrowth; increase in fasting breath H_2 suggests bacterial overgrowth; up to 27% of subjects may not have flora that produces H_2
d. Lactose-H_2	<20 ppm rise in breath H_2 over baseline at any interval for 180 min	Elevated in lactase deficiency
11. Small intestinal culture	≤10^5 organisms per ml jejunal secretions	>10^5 organisms per ml jejunal secretions indicates bacterial overgrowth
12. Small intestinal biopsy	See Figure 104–4	See Table 104–7

*hpf = High-power field, 5-HIAA = 5-hydroxyindoleacetic acid.

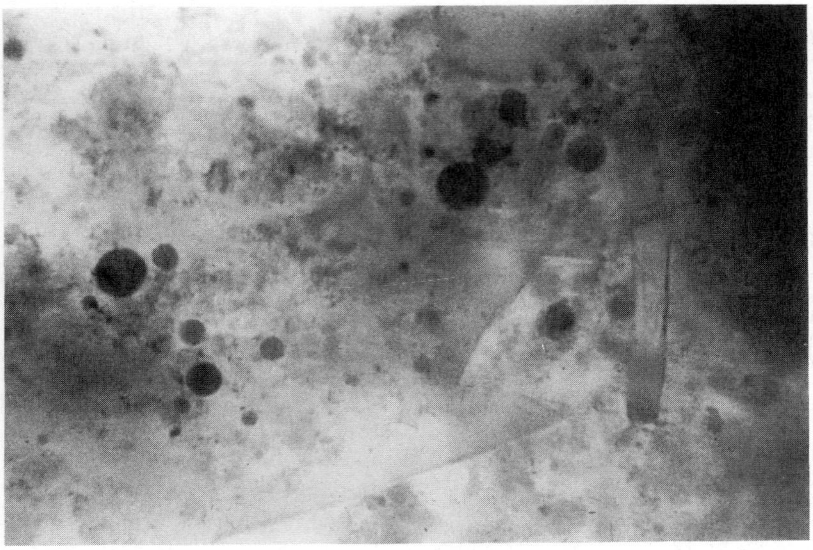

FIGURE 104–3. Positive fecal fat stain. Note the many globules of undigested triglycerides.

Tests for Cobalamin (Vitamin B_{12}) Absorption (Ch. 136)

In the Schilling test, 1.0 μg of ^{57}Co-cyanocobalamin is administered orally, followed by 1000 μg of nonlabeled cobalamin given intramuscularly to help "wash out" that fraction of the isotope that has been absorbed. If the subsequent 24-hour urinary excretion of the radioactivity is less than 8 per cent of that administered, cobalamin malabsorption is present. There are four common clinical causes of cobalamin malabsorption, which can be sorted out by a differential Schilling test (Table 104–5). If an abnormal test result improves with the concomitant administration of hog intrinsic factor or pancreatic extract (six to eight conventional tablets or three enteric-coated microsphere capsules), the cobalamin malabsorption is secondary to pernicious anemia or exocrine pancreatic insufficiency, respectively. If cobalamin malabsorption still persists, the tests should be repeated after four days of antimicrobial therapy (metronidazole, 250 mg three times daily). If the malabsorption of labeled cobalamin is corrected by this therapy, bacterial overgrowth was the etiology. Metronidazole is the antimicrobial agent of choice because anaerobes such as *Bacteroides* are usually responsible for the cobalamin malabsorption. If the malabsorption still persists, damage to the ileal receptor (Crohn's disease, ileal resection, lymphoma, Imerslund's syndrome) is probably present and the patient must always receive a monthly injection of cobalamin (100 μg). In the face of renal impairment, 4 ml of plasma may be obtained eight hours after the administration of labeled cobalamin. A value greater than 0.6 per cent of the orally administered dose is considered normal.

There are two caveats concerning the Schilling test: (1) Severe cobalamin deficiency itself may damage the ileum such that the ileal receptors may not bind the intrinsic factor–cobalamin complex. This may confuse interpretation of the Schilling test. Thus, it is advisable to wait until one week of cobalamin therapy (100 μg per day intramuscularly) has been completed before performing the differential Schilling test. (2) Two other clinical conditions are associated with cobalamin deficiency—cobalamin deficiency secondary to lack of intake (as in complete vegetarians) and the failure to absorb food-bound cobalamin because of decreased acid secretion—that are not associated with an abnormal Schilling test (Table 104–5). The patient's history is the key to the former, and a test of protein-bound cobalamin absorption will detect the latter.

Breath Tests

Two breath tests are reliable enough to receive routine clinical use—the lactose-H_2 breath test for detecting lactase

TABLE 104–5. THE DIFFERENTIAL SCHILLING (^{57}CO-CYANOCOBALAMIN) TEST

	Stage 1: Free Cobalamin	Stage 2: Free Cobalamin and Intrinsic Factor	Stage 3: Free Cobalamin and Pancreatic Extract	Stage 4: Free Cobalamin and Antibiotics	Comment
Pernicious anemia	Abnormal	Normal	Abnormal	Abnormal	In face of severe cobalamin deficiency, test should be performed only after a week of cobalamin therapy
Chronic pancreatitis	Abnormal	Abnormal	Normal	Abnormal	Although cobalamin malabsorption is common, cobalamin deficiency is rare
Bacterial overgrowth	Abnormal	Abnormal	Abnormal	Normal	Anaerobicidal antibiotic is needed
Ileal disease	Abnormal	Abnormal	Abnormal	Abnormal	Once receptor is permanently damaged, cobalamin malabsorption is permanent
Complete vegetarian* (vegan)	Normal	Normal	Normal	Normal	Cobalamin deficiency secondary to poor intake, absorption normal
Hypo- or achlorhydria*	Normal	Normal	Normal	Normal	Absorption of cyanocobalamin (free B_{12}) does not depend on acid; food B_{12} (protein-bound) does; must employ protein-bound cobalamin absorption test

*Cobalamin deficiency with normal Schilling test.

TABLE 104–6. BREATH TESTS FOR BACTERIAL OVERGROWTH

Procedure	Simplicity	Sensitivity	Specificity	Safety
^{14}C-xylose	Excellent	Excellent	Excellent	Good
Cholyl-1-^{14}C-glycine	Excellent	Fair	Poor	Good
Lactulose-H_2	Excellent	Fair–good	Fair	Excellent

Modified from King CE, Toskes PP: The use of breath tests in the study of malabsorption. Clin Gastroenterol 12:591, 1983.

deficiency and the ^{14}C-xylose breath test for the diagnosis of small intestine bacterial overgrowth.

The *lactose-H_2 breath test* has replaced the lactose intolerance test because of superior sensitivity and specificity. Lactose (1 gram per kilogram) is administered orally, and an increase in breath H_2 of more than 20 ppm over basal breath H_2 indicates lactose malabsorption. This test depends upon the release of H_2 from unabsorbed lactose by bacterial metabolism.

The *^{14}C-xylose breath test* is a sensitive and specific test for bacterial overgrowth. Following the oral administration of xylose (1 gram, 5 to 10 μCi), breath $^{14}CO_2$ concentration is monitored at 30 and 60 minutes, with an increase of $^{14}CO_2$ at 30 minutes being the most reliable assessment. Neither false-negative nor false-positive results appear to be a clinically significant problem. Xylose is catabolized by gram-negative aerobes, which are always part of the overgrowth flora, whereas other breath tests often utilize substrates that are catabolized by gram-negative anaerobes, which may or may not be present in the overgrowth of bacteria. The small dose of xylose (1 gram) is either catabolized by the overgrowth flora or absorbed in the proximal bowel, leaving very little xylose to "dump" into the colon, causing a possible false-positive result. An abnormal xylose breath test indicates, similar to a culture, the presence of increased numbers of bacteria within the lumen of the proximal small intestine. Whether or not the abnormal test indicates that therapy is necessary is a decision the clinician must make. Table 104–6 lists two other breath tests used to diagnose bacterial overgrowth, both of which suffer from inadequate sensitivity and specificity.

A ^{14}C-triolein breath test has received some use as a test of fat absorption, but it does not appear to separate control subjects from those with malabsorption very reliably, especially if the steatorrhea is not severe.

Culture of the Small Intestine

The proximal small intestine of normal subjects has less than 10^5 organisms per milliliter of jejunal fluid—usually less than 10^3, largely streptococci and staphylococci, and only an occasional coliform or *Bacteroides*. The ileocecal area is a transition zone with both a qualitative and a quantitative change toward the pattern that is found in the colon. In the colon, there is a marked increase in both aerobes ($>10^7$ organisms per milligram of stool) and anaerobes ($>10^{10}$ organisms per milligram of stool). The qualitative change is also remarkable, with a preponderance of anaerobes (*Bacteroides, Clostridium,* enterococci) and coliforms (*Escherichia coli, Klebsiella*). In small intestine bacterial overgrowth, the small intestine becomes populated with a colon-like flora. Cultures should be considered suspicious if more than 10^3 organisms per milliliter are present (especially when anaerobes are identified) and clearly abnormal when more than 10^5 organisms per milliliter are present.

Biopsy of the Small Intestine

Biopsy of the small intestine is an important test in the evaluation of malabsorption presumed to be secondary to disease of the small intestine itself. Most instruments (Rubin's tube, Crosby's capsule, Carey's capsule) utilize a blind suction biopsy technique, but biopsies can be obtained endoscopically as well. Figure 104–4 illustrates the findings of a normal biopsy. Note the long, frondlike villi. The lining columnar epithelium is regular with basal orientation of the nuclei. There is not much cellular infiltration of lamina propria. The villus/crypt ratio favors the villus, with villus height normally being three to four times the height of the crypts.

For contrast, note Figure 104–5, which represents a biopsy from a patient with nontropical sprue (adult celiac disease). There is total villus atrophy, elongated crypts, and a dense infiltration of chronic inflammatory cells in the lamina propria, and at higher magnification the surface epithelial cells are cuboidal, not columnar. Total villus atrophy, as shown in Figure 104–5, is almost always nontropical sprue (adult celiac disease), but it is not a specific lesion, since it may occasionally be observed in other diseases such as lymphoma, Whipple's disease, tropical sprue, ileojejunitis, or bacterial overgrowth. Table 104–7 lists disorders associated with abnormalities in the biopsy of the small intestine and points out that there are very few disorders in which multiple biopsies are consistently abnormal and diagnostic, i.e., a diagnostic diffuse lesion.

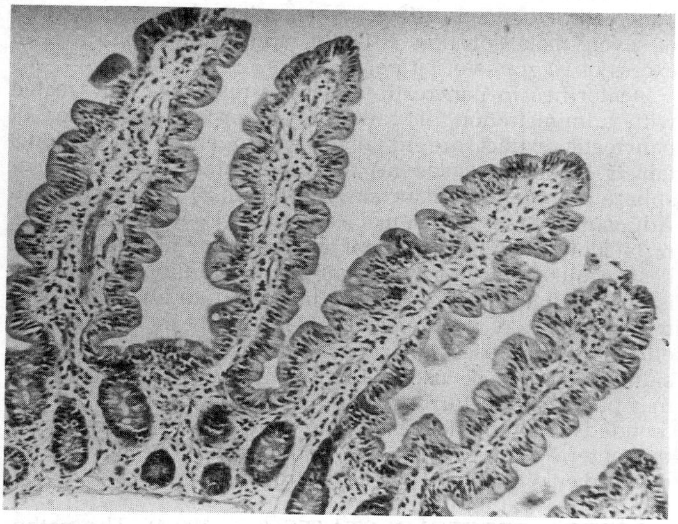

FIGURE 104–4. Appearance of normal small intestine on biopsy.

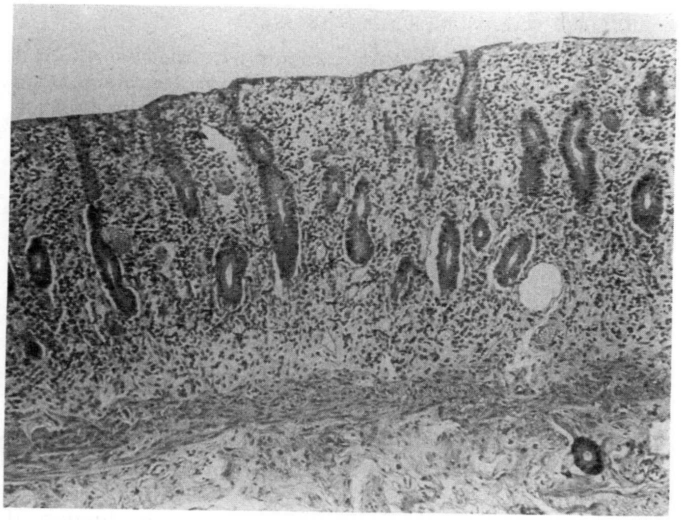

FIGURE 104–5. Small intestinal biopsy from a patient with nontropical sprue showing total villus atrophy.

TABLE 104–7. VALUE OF SMALL INTESTINAL BIOPSY

I. Conditions in which the biopsy is consistently abnormal and diagnostic:
- Abetalipoproteinemia
- Immunodeficiency syndrome
- Whipple's disease

II. Conditions in which the biopsy is diagnostic but the lesion is often patchy:
- Amyloidosis
- Capillariasis
- Coccidiosis
- Crohn's disease
- Cryptosporidiosis
- Eosinophilic enteritis
- Giardiasis
- Lymphangiectasia
- Lymphoma
- Mastocytosis
- Strongyloidiasis

III. Conditions in which the biopsy is often abnormal but not diagnostic:
- Bacterial overgrowth
- Cobalamin (vitamin B_{12}) deficiency
- Celiac sprue (nontropical)
- Drug enteritis
- Folate deficiency
- Infectious gastroenteritis
- Protein-calorie malnutrition
- Radiation enteritis
- Tropical sprue
- Unclassified sprue
- Zollinger-Ellison syndrome

IV. Conditions in which the biopsy is invariably normal:
- Functional bowel disease
- Liver disease
- Pancreatic disease
- Primary disaccharidase deficiency
- Ulcerative colitis

TABLE 104–8. ALGORITHM FOR EVALUATION OF MALABSORPTION

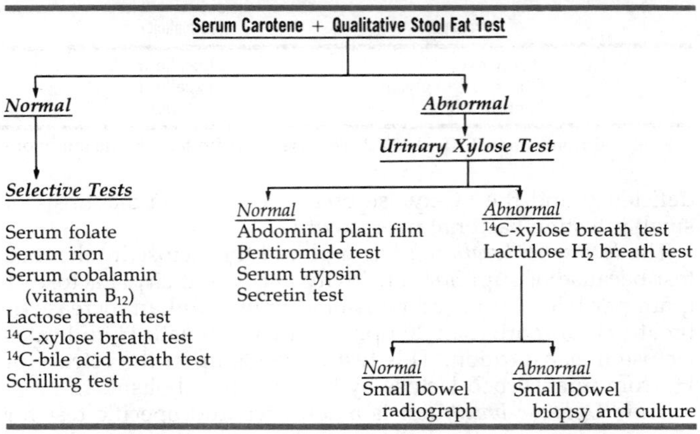

Gastrointestinal Radiology

With the possible exception of pancreatic calcification on plain film of the abdomen, radiographs of the intestinal tract do not play a primary role in the diagnostic evaluation of malabsorption. Function tests as described previously are more sensitive and more specific and afford the patient little, if any, radiation exposure. The radiation exposure received from a small bowel series may be considerable. The traditional signs of malabsorption on small bowel radiographs—segmentation or clumping of the barium (moulage sign)—were noted when thick barium was used in contrast to the thin barium commonly employed now. Small bowel radiographs are most frequently used now to determine why bacterial overgrowth has occurred (e.g., the presence of diverticula or dilation of the small intestine in scleroderma) or to confirm a clinical diagnosis of Crohn's disease.

Algorithm for Evaluation of Malabsorption

An algorithm for evaluating patients with malabsorption is presented in Table 104–8. The algorithm complements a thorough history and physical examination. A serum carotene determination and a microscopic fat stain of the stool are the best screening tests and together will detect the presence of steatorrhea about 85 per cent of the time, especially if the patient is excreting more than 15 grams of fat per day. Once steatorrhea has been confirmed, the clinician should ask whether the steatorrhea is secondary to pancreatic disease or to small bowel disease. The urinary xylose test helps differentiate between these two categories. If xylose absorption is normal, tests of pancreatic function should be pursued. If diffuse calcification of the pancreas is present on a plain film of the abdomen, there is likely to be approximately 80 per cent damage to the exocrine pancreas. The bentiromide test has about the same sensitivity as plain film calcification and will be abnormal 80 to 90 per cent of the time if the steatorrhea has a pancreatic cause. A serum trypsin level will complement the bentiromide test, adding specificity to the evaluation. If these simple tubeless tests of pancreatic function are not diagnostic, a direct tube test like the secretin test should be performed.

If the xylose test is abnormal, small bowel tests should be performed. A breath test (^{14}C-xylose, lactulose H_2) will detect bacterial overgrowth. If normal, a small bowel radiograph, culture, and biopsy should be done, with the radiograph suggesting the site to be biopsied. If steatorrhea is not present, tests designed to detect selective malabsorption of single nutrients can be pursued (lactose H_2 breath test, the Schilling test, and so on).

The algorithm is logical and cost effective, emphasizing inexpensive, noninvasive, outpatient evaluation. A specific diagnosis can often be made for less than $300 with minimal or no discomfort to the patient. If more complicated tests are needed, such as the secretin test or small bowel biopsy, the expense and discomfort to the patient will increase. The algorithm also emphasizes initial testing for the more common causes of malabsorption (pancreatic insufficiency, bacterial overgrowth) and delayed testing for less common disorders (nontropical sprue, Whipple's disease, and so on).

DIFFERENTIAL FEATURES AND TREATMENT OF INDIVIDUAL FORMS OF THE MALABSORPTION SYNDROME

Numerous disorders can be associated with malabsorption (Table 104–2). Although there may be specific therapy for individual disorders (gluten-free diet for nontropical sprue, pancreatic enzymes for pancreatic insufficiency), there are many nonspecific therapies for malabsorption (Table 104–9).

Impaired Digestion

PANCREATIC EXOCRINE INSUFFICIENCY (Ch. 108). Pancreatic exocrine insufficiency is a relatively common cause of severe malabsorption. It is not rare to note steatorrhea in excess of 50 grams of fat per day.

Steatorrhea in pancreatic disease is relatively well treated with administration of pancreatic extract. Large doses of pancreatic extract are required: six to eight conventional tablets (Viokase, Cotazym) or three enteric-coated, microsphere preparations (Pancrease, Cotazym-S) with each meal. Adjuvant therapy (sodium bicarbonate, H_2-receptor antagonists) along with conventional tablet therapy may lead to the best results by raising duodenal pH. The adjuvant of choice is sodium bicarbonate (650-mg tablet before and after each meal) because of its effectiveness, low cost, and lack of side effects at this dose. Antacids containing calcium or magnesium are not to be used as adjuvant therapy because they may increase steatorrhea. Adjuvant therapy is not recommended with enteric-coated preparations, for it may cause the enteric coat to open up within the stomach and the released enzymes may then be destroyed by gastric acid before they can enter the duodenum.

POSTGASTRECTOMY STATES (Ch. 100.4). The pathogenesis of the malabsorption noted in patients with gastric surgery (Billroth I, Billroth II, vagotomy and antrectomy, vagotomy and pyloroplasty) is multifactorial: (1) loss of reservoir function with rapid emptying and dispersion of food through the small intestine, thereby diluting the normal output of pancreatic enzymes; (2) postcibal asynchrony, i.e., in a patient who has undergone a Billroth II procedure, food may get to the jejunum before bile salts and pancreatic enzymes do; and (3) occurrence of stasis, leading to bacterial overgrowth of the small intestine. Postgastrectomy steatorrhea is usually mild (<10 grams of fat per day) but occasionally may be marked. Severe steatorrhea in this setting is usually the result of bacterial overgrowth or rarely is secondary to pancreatic insufficiency. Because the duodenum (the major site for calcium and iron absorption) is bypassed when a Billroth II procedure is performed, clinically significant problems related to calcium and iron malabsorption may result.

TABLE 104–9. AGENTS USED IN THE TREATMENT OF MALABSORPTION

1. **Calcium**
   Oral: Requires 1200 mg elemental calcium daily as
   a. Calcium gluconate (91 mg Ca^{++}/gm), 5–10 gm 3 times per day *or*
   b. Calcium carbonate (500 mg Ca^{++}/tablet)1–2 gm per day in divided doses *or*
   c. Calcium carbonate, 2 tablets supplied as Caltrate or 2½ tablets as Os-Cal 500
   Intravenous: Calcium gluconate injection (10% solution, 9.1 mg Ca^{++}/ml), 10–30 ml administered slowly)
2. **Magnesium**
   Oral: Magnesium gluconate, 500-mg tablets (20 mg Mg^{++}/tablet), 1–4 gm daily in divided doses
   Intramuscular: (20% sol.) 10 ml 2–3 times daily
   Intravenous: Magnesium sulfate, 0.5 per cent sol., up to 1000 ml at a rate not faster than 1.0 mEq/min
3. **Iron**
   Oral: Ferrous sulfate, 325 mg (65 mg elemental iron) 3 times daily
   Intramuscular: Imferon must be calculated according to severity of anemia; detailed instructions accompany preparation
4. **Cyanocobalamin** (vitamin B_{12})
   Intramuscular: 100 μg daily for 2 weeks, then 100 μg monthly
5. **Folic acid**
   Oral: 5 mg daily for 1 month; maintenance 1 mg daily
6. **Vitamin B complex**
   Any multivitamin preparation that contains US RDA amounts; use 2 tablets daily; intramuscular preparations are available for severe deficiencies
7. **Fat-soluble vitamins**
   a. Vitamin A
   Vitamin A capsules (25,000 units per capsule), 100,000–200,000 units daily in severe deficiencies; maintenance, 25,000–50,000 units daily. *Caution:* Vitamin A toxicity can occur with recommended doses if hypertriglyceridemia is present
   b. Vitamin D
   Vitamin D (as vitamin D_2 or D_3), 30,000 units daily; dosage varies considerably depending on response as determined by level of serum calcium and urinary calcium
   c. Vitamin K
   Oral: Menadione, 4–12 mg daily; vitamin K tablets (Mephyton), 5–10 mg daily
   Intravenous: Acute bleeding episodes: vitamin K (Mephyton), 50-mg ampule administered slowly over 10-min period; repeat in 8–12 hr if prothrombin time has not returned to normal
8. **Cholestyramine**
   4-gm pk, 1–2 pk before breakfast and lunch
9. **Medium-chain triglyceride** (MCT oil)
   Administer 60% of fat intake as MCT oil, 40% as dietary long-chain triglyceride
10. **Human albumin, salt poor** (0.25 gm/ml)
    Intravenous administration of 50–100 gm daily for 3–7 days to elevate a severely depressed serum albumin level
11. **Immune serum globulin** (0.165 gm/ml)
    Intramuscular injection of 0.05 ml/kg each 3–4 wk in patients with hypogammaglobulinemia and recurrent infection
12. **Adrenocorticosteroids**
    Prednisone, 40–60 mg daily for 2 wk, then decrease by 5 mg each week to maintenance of 5–15 mg daily
13. **Antidiarrheal agents**
    Oral: Diphenoxylate hydrochloride (Lomotil), 5.0 mg (2 tablets) initially and after each loose bowel movement, not to exceed 8 tablets daily; loperamide hydrochloride (Imodium), 2-mg capsules, 2 capsules initially and then 2 capsules after each loose bowel movement, not to exceed 8 capsules daily
14. **Drugs for parasites**
    Oral: Metronidazole (Flagyl), 250-mg tablet 3 times daily for 1 wk, or quinacrine hydrochloride (Atabrine), 100-mg tablet 3 times daily for 1 wk for *Giardia lamblia.* Thiabendazole (25 mg/kg/day): strongyloidiasis, 2–3 days; *Capillaria phillipinensis,* 30 days; *A. duodenale, N. americanus,* 25 mg/kg/day twice daily for 2 days.

GASTRINOMA (Ch. 100.6). Multiple mechanisms contribute to the malabsorption observed in patients with a gastrinoma (Zollinger-Ellison syndrome). The extreme hypersecretion of acid irreversibly inactivates lipase, causing a secondary pancreatic insufficiency. In addition, this acid environment precipitates bile salts and may cause abnormal small bowel histologic findings. All of these abnormalities have been shown to revert to normal after effective therapy with large doses of H_2-receptor antagonists (cimetidine or ranitidine).

Reduced Concentration of Bile Salts

LIVER DISEASE. Steatorrhea (usually mild) may occur in acute or chronic liver disease, presumably owing to impaired synthesis and excretion of conjugated bile salts. Patients with liver disease who manifest clinically significant steatorrhea should have their pancreatic function evaluated, since these patients will often have pancreatic exocrine insufficiency responsive to pancreatic extract therapy. Metabolic bone disease (bone pain, spontaneous pathologic fractures) resulting from malabsorption of calcium and vitamin D may occur, particularly in those with biliary cirrhosis (Ch. 246).

BACTERIAL OVERGROWTH. Overgrowth of bacteria within the small intestine accompanied by nutrient malabsorption is called the stasis, stagnant loop, or blind loop syndrome. The normal subject usually has sparse bacterial growth in the proximal small intestine (see section on Diagnosis—Culture of the Small Intestine). In the stasis syndrome, the proximal small intestinal flora resembles that of the colon and the overgrowth flora competes with the human host for ingested nutrients. The resultant malabsorption is due to a disturbed intraluminal environment (catabolism of carbohydrate by gram-negative aerobes, deconjugation of bile salts by anaerobes, binding of cobalamin by anaerobes) and patchy damage to the small intestinal enterocyte, perhaps secondary to toxins secreted by the overgrowth flora.

In healthy persons, bacteria within the small intestine are controlled by the cleansing motion of the small intestine, gastric acid secretion, and luminal immunoglobulins. Any alteration of these protective factors may lead to bacterial overgrowth (Table 104–10). In the past, bacterial overgrowth was thought to be related largely to blind loops and other structural abnormalities. Now the emphasis is on motor disturbances, often with no structural abnormality, and on states of decreased acid secretion. Indeed, bacterial overgrowth is one of the major, if not the major, cause of clinically significant malabsorption in the elderly, who often have both decreased acid secretion and a motility disturbance of the small intestine.

The diagnosis has become much more practical with the development of noninvasive breath tests (see section on Diagnosis—Breath Tests, Tables 104–4 and 104–6). This has greatly increased the awareness of this syndrome. Intestinal cultures have been expensive, awkward to perform, and usually not utilized extensively in clinical practice.

In the past, treatment was often empiric, not based on a firm diagnosis but dictated by a clinical impression. Broad-spectrum antibiotics (tetracycline) were prescribed for 7 to 10 days and the clinical response monitored. Up to 60 per cent of the anaerobes (*Bacteroides*) now may be resistant to tetra-

TABLE 104–10. CLINICAL CONDITIONS ASSOCIATED WITH BACTERIAL OVERGROWTH

- **I. Gastric proliferation of bacteria**
  - Hypo- or achlorhydria, especially when combined with motor or anatomic distrubances
- **II. Small intestinal stagnation**
  - Anatomic
    - Afferent loop of Billroth II partial gastrectomy
    - Duodenal or jejunal diverticulosis
    - Surgical blind loop (end-to-side anastomosis)
    - Surgical recirculating loop (side-to-side anastomosis)
    - Obstruction (stricture, adhesion, inflammation, cancer)
  - Motor
    - Scleroderma
    - Idiopathic intestinal pseudo-obstruction
    - Derangements of interdigestive motor complex
    - Diabetic autonomic neuropathy
- **III. Abnormal communication between proximal and distal gastrointestinal tract**
  - Gastrocolic or jejunocolic fistula
  - Resection of ileocecal valve
- **IV. Miscellaneous**
  - Hypogammaglobulinemia
  - Chronic pancreatitis

Modified from King CE, Toskes PP: Small intestine bacterial overgrowth. Gastroenterology 76:1035, 1979.

cycline. It behooves the physician to establish the diagnosis firmly, for the antibiotics needed may have serious side effects.

The mainstays of therapy are antimicrobial therapy and nutritional support. If there is a surgically correctable cause of the overgrowth, surgery should be performed if possible. Most patients with overgrowth do not have a surgically correctable cause (e.g., they have scleroderma, diverticulosis, or diabetes) and must receive lifelong antimicrobial and nutritional therapy.

A ten-day course of a cephalosporin (Keflex), 250 mg four times a day, and metronidazole (Flagyl), 250 mg three times a day, is very effective in suppressing the flora and correcting malabsorption. Tetracycline is an alternative, but the resistance problem must be appreciated. If these fail, chloramphenicol (50 mg per kilogram per day in four divided doses) is also very effective. Anaerobicidal agents by themselves (metronidazole, clindamycin) do not seem to be as effective as the combination of an aerobicidal and an anaerobicidal agent.

Three therapeutic patterns occur. Usually a ten-day course of an effective antimicrobial program will correct the malabsorption for months; some patients may need cyclic therapy (one week out of every six); rarely a patient may need continuous therapy for several months. Antibiotic sensitivity assays of the overgrowth flora are not recommended because of the multitude of organisms present.

Nutritional therapy (especially with medium-chain triglyceride oil) is very important but often ignored. Medium-chain triglyceride administration is ideal therapy for this condition, since this form of fat does not need bile salts for absorption. Other agents such as cobalamin, vitamin D, and calcium are given in doses detailed in Table 104–9.

ILEAL DISEASE OR RESECTION. Disease of the distal ileum leads to an interruption of the enterohepatic circulation of conjugated bile acids, resulting in a diminished bile acid pool and steatorrhea. The degree of steatorrhea is proportional to the amount of diseased or resected intestine. When less than 100 cm of intestine is damaged or resected, proximal to the ileocecal valve, the steatorrhea is mild and choleretic diarrhea tends to be the most frequent problem. The malabsorbed bile acids dump into the colon and impair water and electrolyte absorption. When more than 100 cm of small intestine is resected, the steatorrhea is large owing to a number of factors, including a diminished bile acid pool, loss of the absorptive function of the ileum, and bacterial overgrowth (loss of the ileocecal valve). Choleretic diarrhea can usually be managed with cholestyramine (Table 104–9).

Abnormalities of the Intestinal Mucosa

DISACCHARIDASE DEFICIENCY AND MONOSACCHARIDE MALABSORPTION. The most common disaccharide deficiency is lactose deficiency, which may be primary or secondary. Primary lactase deficiency is common throughout the world, with 60 to 90 per cent of American Indians, black Americans, and Asians being deficient with varying degrees of lactose intolerance. Only 5 to 15 per cent of Caucasians are lactase deficient. Any disease that damages the enterocyte may lead to secondary lactase deficiency.

Lactase-deficient subjects are intolerant to milk, experiencing bloating, abdominal cramps, and diarrhea. The lactose within milk cannot be hydrolyzed to glucose and galactose. It remains in the intestinal lumen, where it is fermented by bacteria, producing organic acids, which increase the osmotic load, inducing shifts of water into the intestinal tract. The end result is distention of the intestine and diarrhea.

Primary lactase deficiency may not manifest itself until adulthood, yet the reason for this delayed appearance is not clear. Subtotal gastrectomy or pyloroplasty and vagotomy may unmask the condition by increasing the load of ingested lactose on the jejunal mucosa. Although the diagnosis is often made by taking a history, the lactose-H_2 breath test is the best way to document lactose intolerance (see Diagnosis section and Table 104–4). Treatment of primary lactase deficiency is through avoidance of milk products or through the ingestion of one to two capsules of Lactrase when dairy products are ingested. Lactrase, derived from *Aspergillus oryzae,* is commercially available.

Sucrase deficiency is quite rare. In afflicted patients, diarrhea occurs after ingesting sucrose. Elimination of sucrose, dextrins, and starches from the diet is effective.

Monosaccharide (glucose-galactose) malabsorption is a rare disorder present from birth. All sugars metabolized to glucose or galactose cannot be tolerated. Therapy consists of utilizing fructose as a source of sugar.

NONTROPICAL SPRUE (ADULT CELIAC DISEASE, CELIAC SPRUE, GLUTEN-SENSITIVE ENTEROPATHY). Nontropical sprue is a disease of unknown etiology characterized by malabsorption resulting from gluten-induced damage to the differentiated villus epithelial cells of the small intestine. Gluten is a high molecular weight protein found in wheat, rye, oats, and barley. The mechanism for this toxic effect is not known, but the most accepted theory at present is that metabolites of gluten initiate an immunologic reaction in the enterocyte. The enterocyte is often strikingly damaged, and biopsy of the small intestine demonstrates characteristic changes (see Fig. 104–5 and discussion of small bowel biopsy in Diagnosis section). Malabsorption is secondary to the impaired transport of nutrients through the damaged enterocyte. In addition, a net secretory state for water and electrolytes has been noted in the jejunum, and pancreatic exocrine function may be secondarily diminished owing to a decreased release of secretin and cholecystokinin from the damaged small bowel mucosa.

Genetic factors appear important in this disease. Nontropical sprue is closely linked to two histocompatibility antigens, HLA-B8 and HLA-DW3. These antigens are present in 60 to 90 per cent of patients with this disease and in only 20 to 30 per cent of the general population. An additional antigen has been found on the surface of B lymphocytes in 70 to 80 per cent of patients with nontropical sprue and in 15 per cent of normal controls. The same antigen is present in 100 per cent of the patients' parents. Perhaps these antigens evoke antibodies to gluten, which result in the binding of gluten to the enterocyte with subsequent mucosal damage.

Patients with nontropical sprue usually have severe malabsorption—steatorrhea, diarrhea, weight loss, and many of the other symptoms and signs detailed in Table 104–3. Symptoms typically begin in infancy, disappear in late childhood, and reappear in the third to sixth decade of life. The proximal small intestine is usually the most severely damaged, and the symptoms, signs, and laboratory evaluation reflect this (Tables 104–3 and 104–4). At times, the clinical presentation may be quite subtle, e.g., anemia secondary to iron deficiency or bone pain from osteomalacia without obvious diarrhea or steatorrhea. Small bowel biopsy is essential in this disease, for a diagnosis of nontropical sprue commits the patient to a very restricted diet indefinitely.

The cornerstone of therapy is the withdrawal of all gluten from the diet, i.e., all grains must be eliminated except rice and corn. Most patients will respond to dietary restriction with a remarkable decrease in symptoms and signs within a few days to a week. In some patients, however, it may take months before a significant improvement is noted. Function tests such as urinary xylose excretion return to normal within a few weeks of gluten withdrawal. Post-treatment biopsies demonstrate marked improvement in most patients and completely normal histologic findings in many. The patient with the characteristic syndrome and biopsy findings who does not respond to gluten withdrawal is usually not adhering to the diet. Some patients may have the characteristic clinical picture and flat biopsy and in reality are not responding because they have another disease such as Whipple's disease, nongranulomatous ileojejunitis, giardiasis, lymphoma, or collagenous sprue. Collagenous sprue, a variant of nontropical sprue, demonstrates not only the characteristic changes in the small intestinal biopsy but also masses of eosinophilic hyaline material in the lamina propria. Such patients have a poor prognosis. Corticosteroid therapy (Table 104–9) or parenteral hyperalimentation may be needed in some patients.

Small bowel lymphoma and carcinoma in general seem to be increased in patients with nontropical sprue. The appearance of abdominal pain in a patient with sprue should suggest lymphoma. Whether or not these complications are fewer in those who adhere strictly to a gluten-free diet is controversial.

Two other associated abnormalities in patients with sprue are (1) ulcers of the jejunum and ileum with abdominal pain, bleeding, and perforation, which are unresponsive to therapy, and (2) dermatitis herpetiformis. Some patients with this skin lesion may have latent sprue. The dermatitis is pruritic, vesicular, and papular and responds to sulfone treatment. Sulfone does not improve the intestinal lesion, but some of these lesions may respond to gluten withdrawal.

NONGRANULOMATOUS ILEOJEJUNITIS. This disease has features of both Crohn's disease and nontropical sprue, even a flat small intestinal biopsy. There is an abrupt onset with fever, abdominal pain, at times splenomegaly, and elevated white count—all suggesting lymphoma. Malabsorption may be profound, resulting in a therapeutic trial of steroids and a gluten-free diet—often to no avail.

CROHN'S DISEASE (Ch. 105.2). Malabsorption in Crohn's disease results from several problems: (1) decreased absorptive surface from active disease or surgical resection, (2) bile salt depletion from ileal disease, and (3) bacterial overgrowth secondary to dilatation of the bowel and resection of the ileocecal valve.

EOSINOPHILIC ENTERITIS. Peripheral blood eosinophilia and infiltration of the gastrointestinal tract by eosinophils characterize this disease. Three patterns of involvement are seen: (1) involvement of the muscle layers of the stomach and small intestine causing obstruction, (2) involvement of the mucosa of the small intestine causing malabsorption, and (3) involvement of the subserosa causing ascites. Most patients have no evidence of allergy or food sensitivity. Corticosteroids and occasionally surgery are employed successfully.

RADIATION ENTERITIS (Ch. 115 and 539). Radiation injury to the intestine may lead to malabsorption from (1) extensive mucosal damage, (2) lymphangiectasia from lymphatic obstruction, and (3) bacterial overgrowth. Malabsorption may occur shortly after exposure to radiation or years later. Most patients with clinically significant malabsorption appear to respond to therapy for bacterial overgrowth.

ABETALIPOPROTEINEMIA (Ch. 183). This rare disease represents a defect in chylomicron formation. The intestinal cells are lacking apoprotein B, and therefore fat absorption cannot occur normally. Biopsy of the small intestine shows the epithelial cells to be engorged with fat even after an overnight fast. The clinical manifestations are steatorrhea, neurologic disease (ataxia, retinitis pigmentosa), very low serum cholesterol and triglyceride levels, and "spiny red cells" (acanthocytes). Therapy consists of substitution of dietary fat with medium-chain triglyceride and administration of fat-soluble vitamins, especially vitamin E.

Inadequate Absorptive Surface

SHORT BOWEL SYNDROME. Extensive resection of the small intestine is usually performed for Crohn's disease, intestinal infarction, or trauma. Acute hyperalimentation in these patients has been life-saving, and the ability of the remaining gut to adapt for increased nutrient absorption by hypertrophy of residual small intestinal villi is remarkable. Patients do rather well despite extensive resection if approximately 90 to 100 cm of duodenum and jejunum and the terminal ileum (intact ileocecal valve) remain.

Treatment consists of parenteral hyperalimentation for weeks to months until evidence exists that the remaining gut is functional. Gradual introduction of oral feedings, high in protein content, vitamins, and minerals, as well as medium-chain triglyceride (MCT), forms the basis for maintenance therapy. Antidiarrheal agents and cholestyramine may help (Table 104–9). Occasionally, pancreatic extract therapy and H_2-receptor antagonists are necessary to treat the transient acid hypersecretion and secondary pancreatic insufficiency that may occur. Steroids may increase water absorption. Finally, some patients must receive hyperalimentation at home indefinitely.

JEJUNOILEAL BYPASS. Some patients with morbid obesity have had a surgical procedure performed (14 inches of proximal jejunum is anastomosed to 4 inches of terminal ileum) that induces malabsorption. In addition to many of the problems detailed above in the short bowel syndrome, other serious complications occur, such as oxalate kidney stones, intestinal pseudo-obstruction, cirrhosis, and arthritis. Because of these complications, the operation has been abandoned.

Infection

TROPICAL SPRUE. The pathogenesis of this malabsorptive disorder occurring in tropical regions (Far East, India, Caribbean) is poorly understood. An overgrowth of coliforms within the jejunum has been demonstrated in these patients. Such organisms have been shown to elaborate an enterotoxin that induces fluid secretion. Tropical sprue is not a true bacterial overgrowth, since anaerobes (particularly *Bacteroides*) are conspicuously absent. Malabsorption of many nutrients occurs, especially folic acid, cobalamin, and fat. The intestinal biopsy does not demonstrate total villus atrophy, but rather nonspecific changes in the villi (shortening, thickening) and cellular infiltration of the lamina propria. Successful therapy has been achieved with cobalamin, folic acid, or antibiotics. A two-month course of a broad-spectrum antibiotic (e.g., tetracycline, 250 mg orally four times daily) and folic acid, 5.0 mg daily, is most effective. In those patients with cobalamin deficiency, 1000 μg of cobalamin should be given intramuscularly for two consecutive days. Improvement of malabsorption following therapy with folic acid or cobalamin alone casts doubt upon infection as the sole etiology.

WHIPPLE'S DISEASE. Patients (usually male) who present with Whipple's disease manifest steatorrhea, weight loss, abdominal pain, nondeforming arthritis, fever, peripheral lymphadenopathy, and neurologic abnormalities (nystagmus, ophthalmoplegia, cranial nerve defects). Protein-losing enteropathy may be present because of lymphatic obstruction.

Small bowel biopsy is diagnostic, demonstrating heavy infiltration of the mucosa and lymph nodes by macrophages that stain positive with periodic acid–Schiff reagent (PAS). Biopsy of the small intestine also shows blunting of villi and dilated lymphatics. The macrophages are filled with rod-shaped bacilli, which disappear after antibiotic therapy and reappear prior to an exacerbation of the disease. Although these rodlike structures resemble bacilli, no bacteria have been consistently cultured from patients with this disease—hence the bacterial etiology of Whipple's disease has not been proved.

Untreated, this is a fatal disease. These patients should be treated for at least a year and probably indefinitely. The antibiotic of choice appears to be trimethoprim-sulfamethoxazole, 500 mg given orally four times daily.

Lymphatic Obstruction

LYMPHOMA (INTESTINAL). Malabsorption occurs in patients with intestinal lymphoma from (1) mucosal invasion, (2) lymphatic obstruction, and (3) bacterial overgrowth secondary to dilatation of the bowel with stasis. Antibiotic therapy will often completely correct the clinical manifestations of malabsorption (diarrhea, steatorrhea), suggesting that bacterial overgrowth is an important cause of malabsorption in these patients. Abdominal pain, fever, and steatorrhea are principal complaints; lymphadenopathy and hepatosplenomegaly are uncommon. The small bowel biopsy may mimic nontropical sprue but not respond to a gluten-free diet. The diagnosis is usually made by the finding of malignant lymphoid cells in the mucosa or submucosa via small bowel biopsy or by full-thickness biopsy at surgery. As many as 10 per cent of patients with nontropical sprue may develop lymphoma.

LYMPHANGIECTASIA. Primary or congenital lymphangiectasia is characterized by diarrhea, mild steatorrhea, edema, enteric loss of protein (protein-losing enteropathy), and abnormal dilated lymphatic channels on small intestinal biopsy (Fig. 104–6). The main clinical feature of this disorder, which affects primarily children and young adults, is asymmetric edema secondary to the hypoplastic peripheral lymphatics and chylous effusions. Lymphocytopenia and depressed serum protein levels are a result of the protein-losing enteropathy. The hypoplastic lymphatics lead to an obstruction in lymph flow, increased pressure within lymphatics, dilated lymphatic channels in the intestine, and finally rupture of the lymphatic channels, discharging lymph into the bowel lumen. Therapy is directed to decreasing lymph flow via a low-fat diet and substitution of dietary fat with medium-chain triglycerides (MCT), which are transported by the portal venous system rather than the lymphatic system.

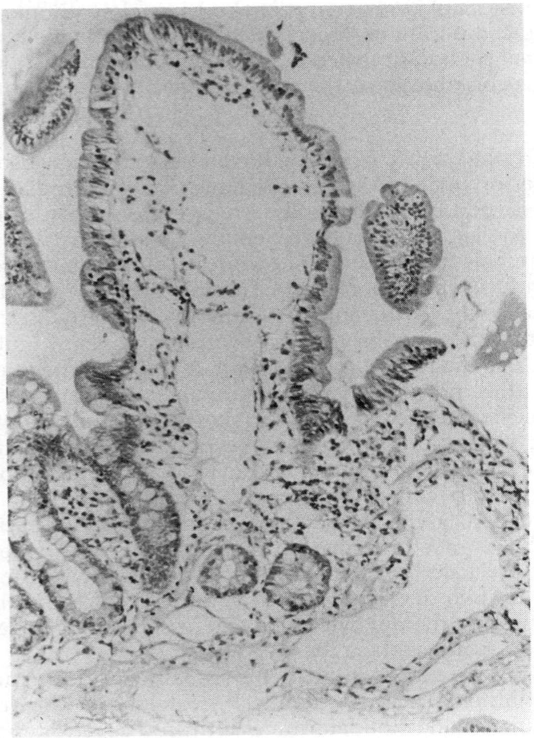

FIGURE 104–6. Small intestinal biopsy from a patient with intestinal lymphangiectasia. Note the dilated lymph channels (clear spaces).

Although protein-losing enteropathy is a hallmark of intestinal lymphangiectasia, many other disorders can also cause enteric protein loss. The mechanisms are multifactorial: (1) exudation of protein through inflamed or engorged mucosa (gastric cancer, hypertrophy of gastric mucosa, ulcerative colitis), (2) loss of protein because of abnormal enterocytes (nontropical sprue, scleroderma), and (3) passage of proteins into the intestine secondary to increased pressure within lymphatics (lymphangiectasia, constrictive pericarditis, lymphoma).

Enteric protein loss can be detected by intravenously administering various labeled macromolecules and measuring the radioactivity in the feces. These tests are cumbersome to perform and not readily available. Recently, $alpha_1$-antitrypsin has been used as a marker for this disorder. $Alpha_1$-antitrypsin (similar size as albumin) can be measured in the feces by immunodiffusion.

Cardiovascular Disorders

Any disorder causing poor perfusion of the intestine may lead to steatorrhea. Atherosclerosis and vasculitis may both affect the mesenteric blood supply.

Drug-Induced Malabsorption

This entity is not very common and usually produces clinically insignificant malabsorption. Steatorrhea secondary to therapy with cholestyramine and neomycin is thought to be a result of precipitation of bile salts. The mechanism or mechanisms of most drug-induced malabsorption is not well understood.

Unexplained Malabsorption

Other than that in diabetes and perhaps in the carcinoid syndrome, the malabsorption occasionally observed in endocrine disorders (adrenal insufficiency, thyroid disease) is not at all understood. In diabetes, malabsorption may result from neuropathic changes (diarrhea) or bacterial overgrowth (steatorrhea). In systemic mast cell disease, there may be massive infiltration of the small intestine with mast cells, blunting of intestinal villi, and marked acid hypersecretion (Ch. 427). Malabsorption, however, does not appear to correlate well with any of these abnormalities. Hypogammaglobulinemia is at times associated with severe malabsorption. Although the pathogenesis is not well defined, such patients may have giardiasis, bacterial overgrowth, and histologic abnormalities of the small intestine (patchy villus atrophy, nodular lymphoid hyperplasia). Plasma cells are absent within the intestine.

Malabsorption in the Elderly

Elderly patients may develop malabsorption from any of the disorders listed in Table 104–2, but bacterial overgrowth appears to be the most common cause of clinically significant steatorrhea in this population. The elderly often have decreased gastric acid secretion and abnormalities in intestinal motility that predispose them to malabsorption from bacterial overgrowth. The hypo- or achlorhydria may lead to cobalamin (vitamin B_{12}) deficiency from malabsorption of food-bound cobalamin (Table 104–5). Such patients may be treated effectively just with tablets of cyanocobalamin (unbound B_{12}), since they have intrinsic factor in adequate amounts. Recognition of this problem may avoid parenteral administration of cobalamin.

Malabsorption in the Acquired Immunodeficiency Syndrome (AIDS) (Ch. 346)

Patients with AIDS often have diarrhea, malabsorption, and weight loss. Although these patients often have enteric infections and intestinal involvement with Kaposi's sarcoma, there are significant numbers of patients with AIDS who have malabsorption without these two abnormalities. In some patients with AIDS, biopsy of the small intestine demonstrates large numbers of histiocytes within the lamina propria. Although such findings on biopsy may be confused with Whipple's disease, in patients with AIDS these histiocytes contain acid-fast bacilli, representing *Mycobacterium avium-intracellulare.* Still other patients with AIDS have malabsorption with the only abnormality found being that of a nonspecific mild-to-moderate chronic inflammatory response in the small bowel biopsy. The malabsorption in this last group of patients may be due to bacterial overgrowth or other unidentified enteric infections.

Cole SG, Kagnoff MF: Celiac disease. Ann Rev Nutr 5:241, 1985.

Florent C, L'Hirondel C, Desmazures C, et al: Intestinal clearance of α_1-antitrypsin: A sensitive method for the detection of protein-losing enteropathy. Gastroenterology 81:777, 1981. *New method of documenting protein-losing enteropathy.*

Gaskin KJ, Durie PR, Hill RE: Colipase and maximally activated pancreatic lipase in normal subjects and patients with steatorrhea. J Clin Invest 69:427, 1982. *Points out the importance of colipase.*

Gillin JS, Shike M, Alcock N, et al: Malabsorption and mucosal abnormalities of the small intestine in the acquired immunodeficiency syndrome. Ann Intern Med 102:619, 1985. *Good discussion of causes of malabsorption in patients with AIDS.*

Keinath RD, Merrell DE, Vlietstra R, et al: Antibiotic treatment and relapse in Whipple's disease. Long-term follow-up of 88 patients. Gastroenterology 88:1867, 1985. *Current discussion of therapy in this disease.*

King CE, Toskes PP: Comparison of the 1-gram ^{14}C-xylose, 10-gram lactulose-H_2, and 80-gram glucose-H_2 breath tests in patients with small intestine bacterial overgrowth. Gastroenterology 91:1447, 1986.

King CE, Toskes PP: Small intestine bacterial overgrowth. Gastroenterology 76:1035, 1979. *Comprehensive review of the subject.*

King CE, Toskes PP: The use of breath tests in the study of malabsorption. Clin Gastroenterol 12:591, 1983. *Thorough overall review of clinical usefulness of these tests.*

Montgomery RD, Haboubi NY, Mike NH, et al.: Causes of malabsorption in the elderly. Age Ageing 15:235, 1986.

Simon CL, Gorbach SL: The human intestinal microflora. Dig Dis Sci (Suppl) 31:147, 1986.

Sleisenger MH, Fordtran JS (eds.): Gastrointestinal Disease. 4th ed. Philadelphia, W. B. Saunders Company, 1988, Ch. 18, 19, 57, 61, 66–68. *Normal absorption and malabsorption in well-referenced text of gastroenterology.*

Toskes PP: The bentiromide test for pancreatic exocrine insufficiency. Pharmacotherapy 4:74, 1984. *Review of worldwide experience with this noninvasive test of pancreatic function.*

Weser E, Fletcher JT, Urban E: Short bowel syndrome. Gastroenterology 77:572, 1979. *Excellent review of this important problem.*

Westergaard H: The sprue syndromes. Am J Med Sci 290:249, 1985.

105 INFLAMMATORY BOWEL DISEASE

105.1 Introduction

Irwin H. Rosenberg

The term *inflammatory bowel disease* is broadly used to refer to idiopathic chronic inflammatory diseases of the intestine, principally *ulcerative colitis* and *Crohn's disease.* Ulcerative colitis, as the name implies, is an inflammatory, ulcerating process of the colon; Crohn's disease is a transmural granulomatous enteritis that may involve any part of the intestine, but primarily the distal small intestine and colon. These two conditions of unknown etiology share a number of clinical, epidemiologic, immunologic, and genetic features, including extraintestinal complications and response to treatment. Therefore, they are often considered together despite distinguishing clinical and pathologic features. These diseases may represent different pathologic responses to a common cause, or they may turn out to be unrelated in etiology and pathogenesis. These two major forms of inflammatory bowel disease will be discussed separately for convenience, but it will prove useful to compare and contrast them throughout.

105.2 Crohn's Disease

Irwin H. Rosenberg

DEFINITION. *Crohn's disease* is a subacute and chronic inflammatory process of unknown cause that may involve any part of the intestinal tract, especially the distal ileum, colon, and anorectal region. Although earlier reports are suggestive, Crohn's disease was first clearly described as an inflammatory condition of the terminal ileum by Burrill Crohn and his colleagues in 1932 and called *regional ileitis.* Shortly thereafter reports of similar transmural granulomatous inflammation of portions of the small and large bowel made the term "regional enteritis" more appropriate. A similar granulomatous inflammation of the colon, distinguishable from ulcerative colitis, was subsequently described and termed "Crohn's disease of the large intestine." The pattern in over 50 per cent of patients with Crohn's disease is *ileocolitis,* which involves the distal small bowel with variable, segmental involvement of the colon. *Ileitis* is a common designation for Crohn's disease confined to the ileum. *Crohn's colitis* refers to predominant involvement of the colon.

EPIDEMIOLOGY. Like ulcerative colitis, Crohn's disease is more common in northern Europe and the United States, less frequent in central Europe and the Middle East, and infrequent in Asia and Africa. Crohn's disease has a prevalence roughly half that of ulcerative colitis. The incidence and prevalence of Crohn's disease rose gradually through the 1960's and 1970's. The incidence has stabilized in most European and North American countries. In the United States this disease affects 50,000 to 100,000 patients at any time, with 5000 to 10,000 new cases diagnosed each year. The incidence of Crohn's disease is approximately equal in males and females. The age of onset profile of Crohn's disease is shown in Figure 105–1. Crohn's disease is uncommon before age ten; the peak incidence occurs in the next two decades and declines thereafter. A later peak of incidence has been reported at 55 to 60 years, but whether this represents a true secondary peak or the effect of hospitalization for other disorders (e.g., ischemic bowel) remains uncertain.

American blacks and American Indians are at less than one fifth the risk of the white population for inflammatory bowel disease. There is growing evidence that the incidence of inflammatory bowel disease in blacks is rising. In Japan the incidence of inflammatory bowel disease has been relatively low, but now is rising steadily. The prevalence of Crohn's disease is six times higher for Jewish men and three times higher for Jewish women. The incidence of inflammatory bowel disease among Jews in Israel is lower than that of Jews in the United States or in northern Europe. Israeli Jews of European (Ashkenazic) ancestry are at considerably greater risk than are Jews of Mediterranean or Middle Eastern (Sephardic) ancestry. Inflammatory bowel disease occurs with equal frequency in urban and rural populations. Some of these demographic features are summarized in Table 105–1.

FAMILIAL-GENETIC PATTERN. There are definite famil-

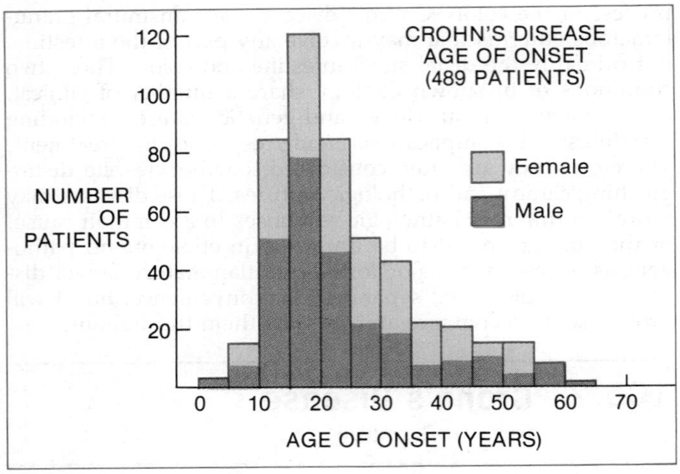

FIGURE 105–1. Age of onset of 489 patients with Crohn's disease. (From Rogers BHG, Clark LM, Kirsner JB: J Chron Dis 24:743, 1971.)

ial clusters of patients with both ulcerative colitis and Crohn's disease. In one large series, 17.5 per cent of patients had a positive family history for a similar disorder. As many as five members in a single family with inflammatory bowel disease have been reported. Three fourths of family clusters involve either ulcerative colitis or Crohn's disease, but in one fourth of such families both ulcerative colitis and Crohn's disease are found in the same pedigree. Disease concordance has occurred in some, but not all, monozygotic twins.

ETIOLOGY AND PATHOGENESIS. Both Crohn's disease and ulcerative colitis are diseases of unknown etiology. The patterns of prevalence described above suggest both host and environmental factors. Individual susceptibility factors are suggested by the specific ethnic patterns of occurrence and the phenomenon of family clustering. Familial occurrence might also represent exposure of the patient and family members to common environmental factors. Parallel trends in disease incidence with increasing technologic development in Asia as well as Europe and the United States also suggest environmental factors. Some of the many and disparate theories of the etiology of Crohn's disease will be reviewed briefly.

Psychogenic Factors. Significant emotional events have often seemed to be temporally related to the onset or exacerbation of inflammatory bowel disease, leading to the hypothesis that psychogenic factors are important in its etiology or pathogenesis. The nervous system may profoundly influence the motor, secretory, vascular, and metabolic functions of the digestive system, but it is difficult to postulate that these variables would lead to the type of segmental involvement or transmural inflammation often seen in Crohn's disease. Psychogenic factors are probably important in their contribution to symptomatic exacerbations.

Infectious Origin. From the time of the first descriptions of this condition, etiologic interest has emphasized possible bacterial or other microbiologic causes. The similarity of the inflammatory response to that with mycobacterial infection, the fever and toxemia in some patients, and the response of some to antimicrobial therapy have been recurrent clinical observations. Sporadically, microbial isolates have been made from tissues of patients with Crohn's disease, most recently cell wall–deficient mycobacteria and ribonucleic acid (RNA) viruses. However, evidence for an etiologic role for any of these agents has been lacking. Earlier reports of transmission of an infectious agent or agents in animal models or of viral isolations have not been confirmed by multicenter trials using standardized methods and interlaboratory exchanges of tissue homogenates. *Yersinia enterocolitica* infection can produce an acute ileitis, and *Campylobacter* and *Clostridium difficile* have been reported in association with exacerbations of Crohn's disease, but these agents are not implicated in the etiology. Nevertheless, the search for microbiologic agents represents one current approach to understanding the etiology of the inflammatory bowel diseases.

TABLE 105–1. DEMOGRAPHIC FEATURES OF CROHN'S DISEASE

Worldwide distribution
More common in whites than nonwhites
Increased frequency among European stock
More common among Jews (especially Ashkenazic) than non-Jews (3 to 6 times)
Most frequent age of onset: 15 to 30 years
Aggregation in families

Modified from Donaldson RM Jr: In Sleisenger MH, Fordtran JS (eds.): Gastrointestinal Disease. 3rd ed. Philadelphia, W. B. Saunders Company, 1983.

Immunologic Factors. Whether or not microorganisms are directly implicated in the etiology of these diseases, they may be involved in their pathogenesis in concert with altered immune mechanisms. Some of the extraintestinal manifestations of inflammatory bowel disease suggest the presence of antigen-antibody complexes in these sites. Serum concentrations of the major immunoglobulin classes follow no predictable pattern among patients with ulcerative colitis or Crohn's disease and fail to show a consistent relationship to the state of activity or severity of the diseases. Circulating lymphocytes from patients with inflammatory bowel disease may be cytotoxic to cultures of human fetal or adult colonic epithelial cells. Responses of circulating lymphocytes to nonspecific mitogens are generally intact, especially in patients with ulcerative colitis. Some abnormalities of proportions or numbers of circulating B and T lymphocytes, particularly T-suppressor cells, have been reported. None of these immunologic changes has been clearly shown to be implicated in the etiology or pathogenesis of inflammatory bowel disease. Lymphocytes and macrophages isolated from the intestinal tissue itself tend to show "inappropriate" immune responses, perhaps genetically determined, which are thought to result in a persistent, and thus pathologic, local mucosal response to unidentified antigens. Whether these abnormalities in the behavior of macrophages and regulatory T lymphocytes are central or peripheral to the etiopathogenesis of Crohn's disease remains the challenging question.

MEDIATORS OF INFLAMMATION. Endogenous mediators, such as prostaglandins and leukotrienes, participate in the inflammatory/metabolic responses in Crohn's disease. Increased amounts of these highly active agents have been measured in the involved tissues of patients, thereby providing a rationale for the use of drugs that might blunt the action of known mediators of inflammation or of fat-modified diets to limit availability of their fatty acid precursors.

PATHOLOGY. Crohn's disease may involve any segment of the alimentary canal or any combination of segments. There are, however, pathologic changes that characterize the inflammatory process in any segment of involved bowel. The involved portion of the bowel, usually the distal ileum and adjacent right colon, is thickened and hyperemic with some serosal fibrin deposition and adhesions between adjacent loops of bowel (Fig. 105–2). The adjacent mesentery is commonly thickened with migration or "creeping" of mesenteric fat onto the serosal surface of the bowel. Mesenteric lymphatics are engorged, and mesenteric lymph nodes are commonly enlarged and matted.

Diseased segments of bowel wall are thickened. The mucosa may be nearly normal or only mildly hyperemic, or there may be elongated linear ulcerations, usually in the long axis of the bowel. In more advanced cases the mucosal architecture is destroyed by multiple ulcerations, with only small islands of mucosa remaining. Numerous aphthoid ulcers may be present in the mucosa. Deep ulcers or clefts may extend into the thickened and edematous submucosa and sometimes through to the serosal surface.

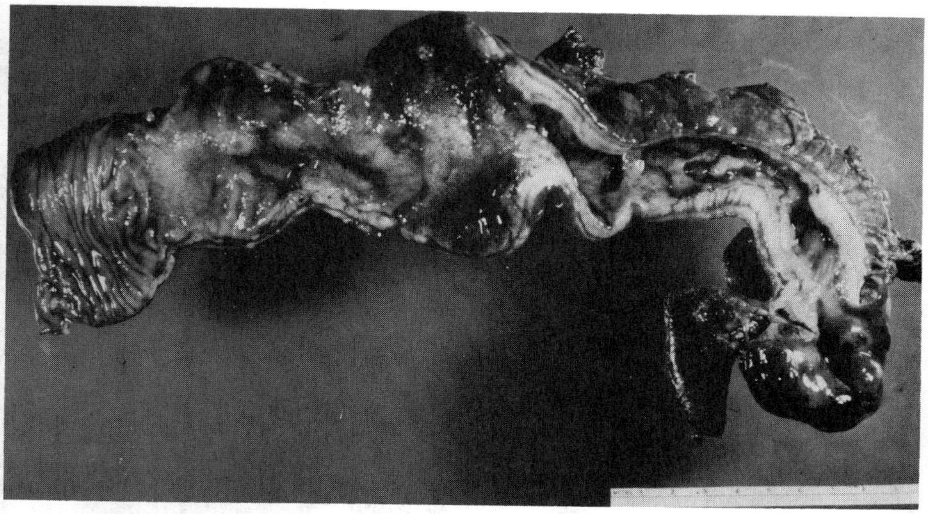

FIGURE 105–2. Resected specimen of ileum showing thickening of the wall, loss of normal mucosa, scarring, and stricture in Crohn's disease. "Creeping fat" is visible on the serosal surface.

Fistulas form readily in this setting of a transmural inflammation when deep ulcerations and fissures combine with obstruction and stenosis to form a penetrating, pressure-relieving pathway to adjacent and adherent loops of bowel or other viscera, and sometimes to the abdominal wall. Ileoileal, ileosigmoid, and ileocecal communications are most common, but communication with other parts of the gastrointestinal tract, including the stomach, duodenum, and gallbladder, has been reported. Fistulas may also occur from the intestine to the urinary bladder, the renal collecting system, and the female genital tract, most often the vagina.

The inflammatory process involves all layers of the bowel and consists of infiltration of lymphocytes, histiocytes, and plasma cells with characteristic aggregation to form noncaseating granulomas. Focal granulomas are found in about half of the cases; in the remainder, well-defined lymphoid aggregates are found.

These pathologic changes and their progression correlate with many of the important clinical manifestations of Crohn's disease. Abdominal pain and cramps reflect the narrowed lumen and partial obstruction that result from thickening of the bowel wall. Diarrhea may represent disordered mucosal absorptive-secretory function or abnormal motility of either small or large bowel. The transmural inflammation increases adherence of loops of bowel, producing signs of peritoneal irritation and the formation of abdominal masses.

CLINICAL PRESENTATION. When Crohn's disease affects primarily the distal small intestine (*Crohn's ileitis* or *regional enteritis*), the most characteristic clinical pattern emerges. A young person, usually in the second or third decade, will present with a period of episodic abdominal pain, largely postprandial and often periumbilical, occasionally with low-grade fever and mild diarrhea. Such episodes often remit spontaneously but recur with increasing frequency and severity, with pain eventually localizing to the right lower quadrant.

The *abdominal pain* often has the characteristics of partial intestinal obstruction, made worse by eating and improved by rest, local heat, and fasting. The effect of early ileitis on bowel habits may be variable. *Diarrhea* is rarely more severe than four or five stools daily, and rectal bleeding is uncommon. *Weight loss* is frequent. In children growth retardation and delayed sexual maturation may be the presenting clinical features in Crohn's disease. The patient may be aware of *tenderness in the right lower quadrant* and even of a palpable mass in that region. The similarity of this presentation to that of acute appendicitis commonly results in an abdominal exploration, and diagnosis is then made surgically. When the involvement of the small intestine is more diffuse in the syndrome of jejunoileitis, the presentation may include more diffuse abdominal pain and more prominent weight loss, growth retardation, and sometimes peripheral edema.

In Crohn's colitis or ileocolitis the presentation is characterized by lower abdominal, crampy pain worsened by eating, by diarrhea, and by fever. Crohn's colitis tends to be more subtle in onset than ulcerative colitis and thus may not be diagnosed until anemia or other systemic complications predominate.

One third of all patients with Crohn's disease and one half with Crohn's colitis develop perirectal or perianal fistulas with pain, mass, purulent drainage, and often fever. Perianal complications may represent communication of a fistulous tract from the small bowel along the presacral gutter to the perirectal area but more commonly are a complication of deep, penetrating ulceration in Crohn's colitis of the lower colon. When drainage is impaired, local abscess formation occurs.

Extraintestinal manifestations such as arthritis, ankylosing spondylitis, and erythema nodosum may precede or strongly influence the presenting syndrome. These extraintestinal manifestations of Crohn's disease will be discussed subsequently.

DIAGNOSIS. The diagnosis of Crohn's disease may be delayed for months or even years in patients whose symptoms are subtle and insidious and in those in whom extraintestinal manifestations focus attention away from the bowel. Crohn's disease should be suspected in patients of any age, but particularly in those in the younger age groups, when there is a history of recurrent episodes of abdominal pain worsened by eating, and a change in bowel habits with intermittent or persisting diarrhea. The presence of pain, tenderness, and a mass in the right lower quadrant should strongly heighten the suspicion of this diagnosis. A history of weight loss is common. In addition, unexplained arthritis, perianal disease, recurrent fevers, or, in children, cessation of normal growth should raise the question of Crohn's disease even if gastrointestinal symptoms are minimal.

Physical Examination. A moderately ill patient may be pale, underweight, and febrile (temperature seldom greater than 38°C). An abdominal examination often demonstrates tenderness or a mass in the right lower abdominal quadrant. The bowel sounds may be hyperactive. Examination of the extremities may reveal signs of large joint arthritis or, rarely, clubbing. Uveitis, iritis, and skin manifestations (see below) may occasionally be present. Peripheral edema may reflect protein depletion. Examination of the rectum and perianal area may identify perianal fistulas, fissures, or an abscess. A purulent vaginal discharge in a woman with Crohn's disease is strongly suggestive of enterovaginal fistula.

Radiographic Examination. The diagnosis of Crohn's dis-

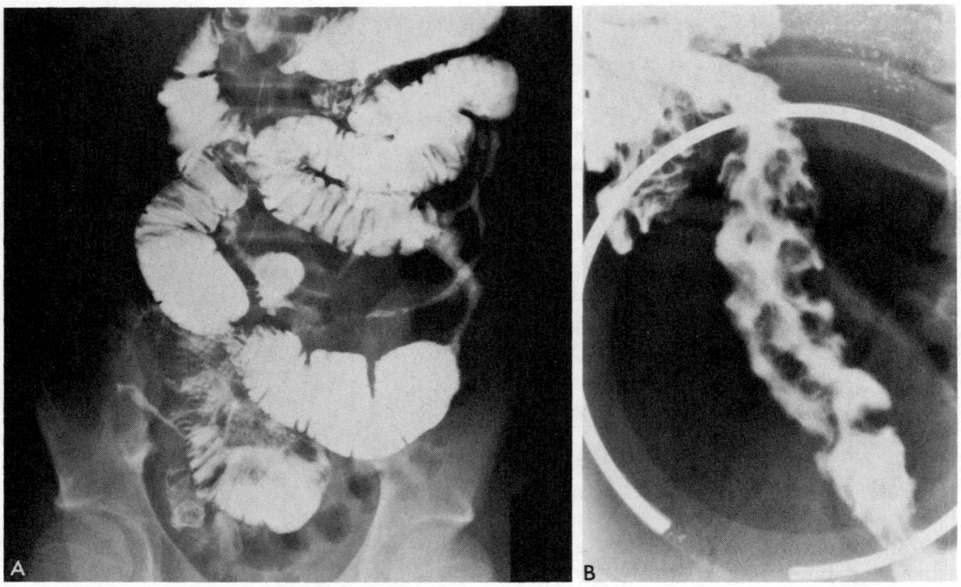

FIGURE 105–3. *A*, Small bowel radiograph in Crohn's disease demonstrating extensive jejunoileitis with areas of narrowing and mucosal damage alternating with "skip areas" of more normal bowel. *B*, Cobblestone appearance of the terminal ileum in Crohn's disease.

ease depends in considerable measure on the presence of characteristic radiographic findings in the bowel. The abdominal plain film may demonstrate dilated loops of small bowel in the presence of partial obstruction. The diagnosis depends, however, upon upper and lower intestinal barium contrast studies (Figs. 105–3 and 105–4). Characteristic changes on the small bowel roentgenogram include segmental narrowing, obliteration of the normal mucosal pattern with or without evidence of ulceration, enteroenteric fistula formation, or the classic "string sign" of the contrast medium shown on segmental films of the terminal ileum, particularly when changes are localized to the most distal small bowel and the adjacent right colon (Fig. 105–3).

Most radiologists prefer air contrast radiography of the colon to delineate the presence or extent of disease in the large bowel (Fig. 105–4). In 85 per cent of patients with Crohn's disease of the large bowel, there will also be involvement of the distal small bowel, which is best demonstrated by antegrade barium studies as described above. It is important to distinguish between "backwash ileitis" associated with ulcerative colitis and true mucosal involvement of ileal Crohn's disease. In Crohn's colitis there is a characteristic asymmetric and segmental pattern with areas of disease separated by areas of apparently normal colonic tissue.

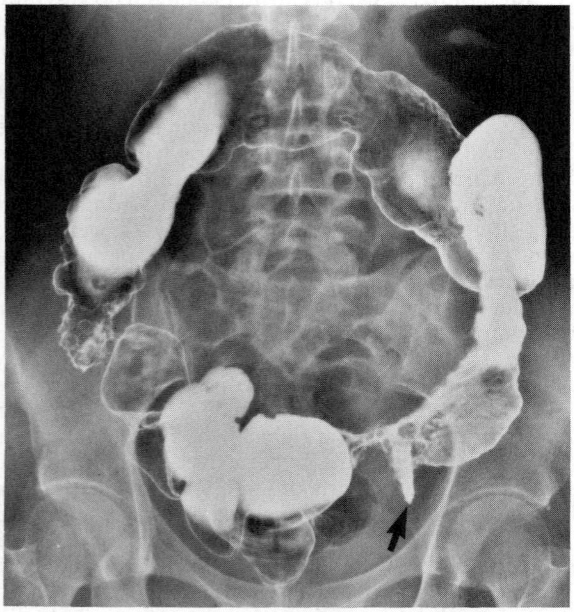

FIGURE 105–4. Typical Crohn's colitis demonstrated by air-contrast exam. Note asymmetric involvement, loss of normal haustral markings, and early fistula in the sigmoid region (*arrow*).

The most subtle changes in the small bowel are thickening and edema of the valvulae conniventes. Earliest changes in the large bowel are the appearance of small aphthous ulcers on air-contrast examinations. Loss of haustral markings may be a subtle early finding. Mucosal ulcers are likely to be longitudinal. When severe ulcerative disease is present, the alternation of ulcers with regenerating mucosa produces the "cobblestone" appearance (Fig. 105–3*B*). As the disease progresses, there is increasing scar formation with total loss of mucosal pattern and narrowing of the segments of involved bowel. The presence of fistulous tracts from one loop of bowel to another can often be demonstrated. The presence of distinctly narrowed segments of bowel need not be taken as clear evidence of cicatricial and irreversible obstruction. These findings are often manifestations of severe edema and thickening of the bowel and may improve substantially following treatment. The newer technique of enteroclysis—instillation of barium directly into the small bowel by tube—may add precision to small intestinal studies.

Laboratory Diagnosis. No laboratory test is diagnostic for Crohn's disease. Anemia may result from blood loss or iron or folate deficiency. Sedimentation rate and other acute phase reactants, including serum orosomucoid, may be elevated. Examination of the stool may reveal the presence of occult blood and increased fat. Fecal leukocytes call attention to inflammatory processes as a basis for the diarrhea. A low serum albumin reflects malnutrition and increased enteric protein loss. Low serum calcium or magnesium may be seen in patients with severe diarrhea and steatorrhea. An abnormal Schilling test of vitamin B_{12} absorption reflects extensive disease or resection of the ileum. Other tests of intestinal absorption, including the quantitative fecal fat, xylose absorption test, and lactose absorption test, are helpful in assessing the extent and severity of disease. Analyses of the circulating levels of iron, folate, vitamin B_{12}, 25-hydroxy vitamin D, and plasma zinc may demonstrate evidence of micronutrient depletion.

Proctosigmoidoscopy. In contrast to ulcerative colitis, the rectum is uninvolved in more than half of the patients with Crohn's disease. Proctosigmoidoscopy may simply show mild erythema associated nonspecifically with diarrhea. Rarely, a biopsy of the normal-appearing rectum will reveal inflammatory changes and even granuloma, but such biopsies are not a necessary part of the diagnostic evaluation.

Colonoscopy. Colonoscopy may be valuable in determining the extent and severity of colonic involvement and in evaluating strictures or polypoid masses. Colonoscopic biopsies are helpful for verification of the diagnosis in difficult cases.

LOCAL COMPLICATIONS. Chronic, transmural inflammation of the bowel with progressive scarring leads to a number of local complications. Hemorrhage is uncommon, but *chronic blood loss* leading to iron deficiency often occurs. Local scarring and narrowing of the bowel lead to *intestinal obstruction* of varying severity. Free *intestinal perforation* occurs rarely; more often there is fistulous communication between loops of bowel or into matted mesentery, which presents as a tender, inflammatory mass with fever. Fistulas can occur to any abdominal viscus, as previously noted.

Perianal fistulas and related fissures and abscesses affect nearly half of all patients with Crohn's disease. Indurated, nonhealing rectal fissures, draining perianal fistulas, or local abscesses may cause local pain, fever, and progressive perineal distortion. Abscesses must be drained, with special attention to the integrity of the anal sphincter muscles and the threat of fecal incontinence. A judicious and persistent combination of bowel rest and dietary, drug, and surgical therapy is required (see Treatment).

MALABSORPTION AND NUTRIENT-LOSING ENTEROPATHY. Predictably, malabsorption is found largely in those patients with extensive inflammatory involvement or following partial resection of the small intestine. The ileum is the major site of absorption of both vitamin B_{12} and bile salts. Ileitis may therefore result in malabsorption of this vitamin as well as steatorrhea on the basis of the interrupted enterohepatic circulation of bile salts. Malabsorption of fat-soluble vitamins, including vitamin D, and of water-soluble vitamins, such as folate, has been reported in Crohn's disease. There is a tendency, especially in those who have had resection of the ileocecal valve, to develop bacterial overgrowth, which further contributes to malabsorption. Enteric protein loss through the damaged epithelium may be an important contributor to protein and associated trace metal depletion. The reader is referred to Ch. 103 for a more extensive discussion of malabsorption.

SYSTEMIC AND EXTRAINTESTINAL COMPLICATIONS (see Table 105–2). ***Nutritional Complications.*** Nutritional complications are common in inflammatory bowel disease. The majority of patients admitted to the hospital will exhibit some degree of nutritional depletion. Assessment of the nutritional status should be part of the initial evaluation of the patient in order to recognize and treat nutritional complications early. Deficiencies of protein, calories, minerals, vitamins, and trace metals are well documented in both Crohn's disease and ulcerative colitis. These deficiencies may result from inadequate dietary intake, malabsorption, or intestinal loss of protein, as noted above. In addition, increased nutritional requirement relating to the chronic inflammatory response and faster cell turnover in the diseased gut is probable but less well documented.

Growth Retardation. Retarded skeletal growth, often with a delay in sexual maturation, is frequently observed in children whose onset of Crohn's disease occurs before puberty. In some patients a slowing or arrest of linear growth occurs years before the diagnosis of Crohn's disease is made and may be the condition that brings the patient to medical attention. The pathogenesis of growth retardation is complex. No hormonal deficiencies have been demonstrated in these patients. Corticosteroids administered daily in high doses for colitis or Crohn's disease may suppress growth in some patients. Lower doses or alternate-day steroid therapy may allow restoration of normal growth by suppressing the activity of the disease. Abnormalities of intestinal absorption have not been prominent in those patients carefully studied. Caloric insufficiency is of central etiologic importance and usually results from a dietary intake that is limited by the young patient in response to abdominal pain and diarrhea. Protein, vitamin, and mineral deficiencies are less regular.

TABLE 105–2. EXTRAINTESTINAL MANIFESTATIONS OF THE INFLAMMATORY BOWEL DISEASES

Nutritional and metabolic abnormalities
Weight loss, growth retardation in children
Hypoalbuminemia—nutritional, protein-losing enteropathy
Vitamin deficiencies
Deficiencies of calcium, magnesium, or zinc
Hematologic abnormalities
Anemia—bleeding, Fe deficiency, folate deficiency
Leukocytosis, thrombocytosis
Skin and mucous membrane
Pyoderma gangrenosum
Erythema nodosum
Stomatitis with multiple aphthous ulcers
Musculoskeletal
Ankylosing spondylitis, sacroiliitis (HLA-B27 associated)
Peripheral arthritis of large joints
Osteoporosis, osteomalacia
Hepatic and biliary manifestations
Fatty liver
Pericholangitis
Sclerosing cholangitis
Cirrhosis
Gallstones
Carcinoma of the bile ducts
Renal complications
Kidney stones—uric acid, calcium oxalate
Obstructive uropathy
Fistulas to urinary tract
Amyloidosis (rare)
Eye complications
Conjunctivitis, episcleritis, uveitis
Iritis

Hepatobiliary Complications. Hepatobiliary complications of Crohn's disease (and of ulcerative colitis) include a spectrum from clinically inapparent histologic abnormalities through progressive and sometimes life-threatening liver disease. The possibility that chronic or intermittent portal bacteremia or the return from the gut to the liver of toxic metabolic products, such as lithocholic acid, may be responsible for hepatic injury has been suggested but not proved. Neither viral hepatitis after blood transfusion nor drug toxicity can account for a significant proportion of liver disease in these patients. *Fatty infiltration* of the liver is found in virtually all biopsy or autopsy specimens of patients with inflammatory bowel disease. Abnormalities other than fatty infiltration are found in the majority of liver specimens obtained by needle biopsies in patients with inflammatory bowel disease: *pericholangitis* (50 to 70 per cent), *chronic active hepatitis, cirrhosis,* extrahepatic obstruction associated with *primary sclerosing cholangitis,* and, most rarely, *carcinoma of the bile ducts.* Fewer than 25 per cent of such patients will have increased alkaline phosphatase activity; jaundice is even less common. However, when serious or progressive liver disease is present histologically, liver function tests are usually abnormal.

Pericholangitis refers to a lymphocytic inflammatory response in the entire portal triad, not only periductal as the name implies. Most patients with pericholangitis demonstrated by biopsy are asymptomatic, and the majority have normal liver function tests. Some may have recurring episodes of cholestasis, jaundice, and pruritus with increased serum alkaline phosphatase. In a few patients the full picture of ascending cholangitis, shaking chills, fever, and jaundice will occur. Recurrent right upper quadrant pain may cause diagnostic confusion with gallstone disease, which is also more common in patients with Crohn's disease. Occasionally, pericholangitis will progress to cirrhosis. Those patients with pericholangitis found incidentally on liver biopsy at the time of surgery without a history of cholangitis or hepatic function abnormalities are likely to have a benign course without progressive hepatic deterioration.

Sclerosing cholangitis is an uncommon inflammatory and sclerosing lesion of extra- and intrahepatic bile ducts causing biliary obstruction and recurrent cholangitis. Its relationship to pericholangitis is uncertain. In some patients inflammation extends from the portal triads to the intra- and extrahepatic ducts. The extent of anatomic abnormality is best determined by endoscopic retrograde cholangiography. Corticosteroids are often used to suppress inflammation, and antibiotics are used to treat episodes of cholangitis. Promising results have recently been reported with low-dose methotrexate therapy. In some patients adequate bile drainage may have to be established surgically. Carcinoma of the bile ducts, although extremely rare in Crohn's disease, is sometimes seen in the setting of sclerosing cholangitis.

Gallstones develop with increased frequency in patients with Crohn's disease whether or not bile duct abnormalities exist. This tendency is often attributed to bile salt malabsorption in the diseased ileum, leading to a diminished bile salt pool and a relative increase in the ratio of cholesterol to bile salts in bile.

Renal Complications. Renal complications in Crohn's disease include *obstructive uropathy, nephrolithiasis, fistulas* to the renal collecting system, and rarely, *amyloidosis.* Fistulas from the bowel to the renal excretory system may present as the passage of gas or fecal material in the urine. The diagnostic changes may be more subtle and simply involve recurrent episodes of pyuria or infection. Right-sided hydronephrosis resulting from cicatricial and inflammatory obstruction of the right ureter may be asymptomatic, and some advocate the regular use of ultrasonography in the full evaluation of the patient with Crohn's disease. Corrective surgery by unsheathing of the right ureter may prevent progressive destruction of the right kidney.

The most common renal complication is *nephrolithiasis.* There is an increased incidence of uric acid stones in both Crohn's disease and ulcerative colitis, probably related to increased cell turnover and the excretion of a concentrated urine of increased acidity. The most frequent type of kidney stone in patients with Crohn's disease, however, is composed of calcium oxalate as its main crystalloid. Patients with extensive disease of the distal small intestine, particularly those who have had resections of the distal small bowel, have excessive absorption of dietary oxalate and low urinary excretion of citrate and are therefore at increased risk for the formation of calcium oxalate stones (see Ch. 90 for more details).

Miscellaneous Complications. Both *peripheral arthritis* and *spondylitis* occur in Crohn's disease as in ulcerative colitis, affecting approximately 10 to 20 per cent of patients. Osteoporosis, especially in patients who receive high doses of corticosteroids, is common even though usually asymptomatic. Osteomalacia usually reflects subclinical vitamin D deficiency. *Erythema nodosum* is seen in approximately 9 per cent of patients with Crohn's disease, but *pyoderma gangrenosum* and *erythema multiforme* are rare. Ocular complications include *episcleritis, uveitis,* and *iritis* in 3 to 4 per cent of patients.

DIFFERENTIAL DIAGNOSIS. The classic presentation of Crohn's disease with a characteristic history, a palpable right lower abdominal mass, and typical radiographs offers little diagnostic challenge. The presentation, however, may be highly variable. With an acute onset, Crohn's disease may be mistaken for appendicitis, particularly in a young person with right lower quadrant rebound tenderness and leukocytosis. Diarrhea, however, is uncommon in appendicitis. If progression of symptoms and signs is rapid and the opportunity to diagnose Crohn's disease by the typical radiographic findings is not feasible, exploration may be necessary. An *appendiceal abscess* is particularly difficult to distinguish from a mass associated with Crohn's disease by radiography.

Infection by *Yersinia enterocolitica* causes an acute or subacute mesenteric adenitis and may produce diarrhea, abdominal pain, and fever. Infection by *Campylobacter fetus* may resemble acute or subacute colitis. Successful diagnosis requires attention to the specific requirements for culturing these organisms. Distinction of Crohn's disease from *ileocecal tuberculosis* or from fungal infections involving the bowel is usually possible on epidemiologic grounds. Intestinal tuberculosis is rare in the United States and western Europe and is usually seen in native-born Americans only in the presence of extensive pulmonary tuberculosis. Persons raised in areas where milk-borne tuberculosis is common often have ileocecal tuberculosis without pulmonary disease.

Benign lymphoid hyperplasia of Peyer's patches in the ileum is seen on barium radiographs in children and young adults in a setting of infection or fever. This benign condition is distinguishable from Crohn's disease on radiographic grounds, since no mucosal abnormality or luminal narrowing occurs.

Patients with a more chronic course present a more extensive differential diagnosis. *Nongranulomatous ulcerative jejunoileitis,* another inflammatory condition of the small bowel of unknown etiology, has more prominent malabsorption, nutrient-losing enteropathy, and nonspecific shallow small bowel ulcers on intestinal biopsy. This distinction in rare cases, however, requires exploration and surgical biopsies.

Lymphoma or *lymphosarcoma* of the small bowel may produce a picture similar to that of Crohn's disease. Once initiated, the symptoms of this malignant process are usually more persistent and more rapidly progressive than those of Crohn's disease. Palpable abdominal masses tend to be firmer. A diffuse nodularity of the bowel without segmental narrowing characteristic of Crohn's disease on small bowel series suggests abdominal lymphoma. Occasionally *carcinoid* of the ileum or other malignancies will be extensive and invasive enough to be mistaken for Crohn's disease by radiography.

Radiation enteritis involving the distal ileum and colon after pelvic irradiation for carcinoma is distinguished from Crohn's disease mainly by history.

Eosinophilic gastroenteritis may present with diarrhea, malabsorption, and protein-losing enteropathy, but the pattern of the intestinal involvement demonstrated by radiographic or endoscopic techniques, peripheral blood eosinophilia, and positive findings on intestinal biopsy are distinguishing features.

When Crohn's disease involves the duodenum or stomach, it may be mistaken for duodenal ulcer disease, or even the Zollinger-Ellison syndrome when there are multiple ulcerating lesions. The pain pattern tends to be different in these conditions. Crohn's disease causes more persistent or postprandial abdominal pain and symptoms of obstruction. Endoscopy and biopsy in addition to radiographic findings may be helpful in distinguishing these conditions from Crohn's disease.

For distinction between Crohn's ileitis and backwash ileitis associated with ulcerative colitis and for the differentiation of Crohn's colitis and ulcerative colitis, the reader is referred to Table 105–3.

TREATMENT. There is no known cure for Crohn's disease. Treatment is empiric and is directed at alleviating the symptoms and manifestations of the disease. Symptomatic remissions may occur during therapy, or even in its absence, but the disease is lifelong, and surveillance by the physician must be a continuing process. In addition to medical and sometimes surgical management, general support is very important, including attention to the psychologic stresses imposed by the disease on the patient and the family. In addition, the physician must anticipate, identify, and, when possible, prevent the common nutritional and metabolic complications described above.

Medical Management. Medical management of Crohn's disease requires a comprehensive assessment of the clinical status of the patient. It is particularly important to determine the extent and severity of the disease, largely by radiologic and

TABLE 105–3. A COMPARISON OF THE CLINICAL AND PATHOLOGIC FEATURES OF CROHN'S COLITIS AND ULCERATIVE COLITIS

Feature	Crohn's Colitis	Ulcerative Colitis
Intestinal		
Malaise, fever	Common	Uncommon
Rectal bleeding	Sometimes	Common
Abdominal tenderness	Very common	May be present
Abdominal mass	Very common (especially with ileocolitis)	Not present
Abdominal pain	Very common	Unusual
Fistulas	Very common	Very uncommon
Endoscopic		
Rectal disease	Occasionally	Very common
Diffuse, continuous, symmetric involvement	Uncommon	Very common
Aphthous or linear ulcers	Common	Very unusual
Cobblestoning	Common	Very unusual
Friability	Unusual	Very common
Radiologic		
Continuous disease	Uncommon	Very common
Ileal involvement	Very common	"Backwash ileitis"
Asymmetry	Very common	Uncommon
Strictures	Common	Uncommon
Fistulas	Very common	Uncommon
Pathologic		
Discontinuity	Common	Uncommon
Rectal involvement	Uncommon	Common
Intense vascularity	Uncommon	Common
Ileal involvement	Common	Nonexistent
Aphthous ulcers	Common	Very uncommon
Transmural involvement	Common	Very uncommon
Lymphoid aggregates	Common	Uncommon
Crypt abscesses	Uncommon	Very common
Granulomas	Common	Uncommon
Linear clefts	Common	Uncommon

proctoscopic methods, and to assess the presence or absence of the complications. Only on the basis of this complete information, and a knowledge of the patient as an individual, can a full program of nutritional, drug, and supportive therapy be rationally planned. The physician-patient relationship is challenging and critical.

Nutritional Treatment. Nutritional assessment is based on a careful diet history to determine the extent of calorie insufficiency, to document weight loss, and to analyze nutritional status on the basis of body measurements and laboratory tests. In prepubertal patients assessment of growth pattern is a critical part of the evaluation.

For ambulatory patients dietary goals should be set that are adequate for the nutritional needs of the patient, but that minimize stress on the inflamed and often narrowed segments of bowel. Evidence of lactose intolerance should be sought by history and, when possible, confirmed by *blood* or *breath test analysis* (see Ch. 104). Removal of lactose-rich foods, such as milk and ice cream, in the lactase-deficient patient may have a prompt symptomatic benefit. In many patients with cramping and diarrhea, decreasing the intake of fiber-containing foods may be beneficial, and in those with steatorrhea a decrease of fat intake to 70 to 80 grams per day may substantially improve diarrhea. Attention to restoration of an adequate diet must always accompany these deletions.

The hospitalized patient presents a different management problem. More than half of such patients suffer from deficiencies of calories, protein, certain vitamins, and minerals. Most such patients take an inadequate diet limited by the worsening of intestinal symptoms after eating. One approach in such patients is to put the inflamed and narrowed bowel "at rest" by removing the stimulus of food intake on intestinal secretion and motility. Many patients derive symptomatic benefit from partial rather than total bowel rest with the delivery of nutrients enterally in the form of low residue–defined formula diets. Rarely can adequate nutritional maintenance be achieved by the oral intake of these formula diets alone owing to limitations of palatability. The use of small-caliber nasogastric tubes for continuous or intermittent drip provides a well-tolerated alternative means of delivery that is often associated with a marked decrease in bacterial flora, stool frequency, and symptoms. In more severely ill patients, and in those who cannot tolerate enteral feeding or who lack adequate intestine for absorption, total parenteral nutritional support is used increasingly.

For the severely malnourished patient, total parenteral nutrition can be used to achieve nutritional repletion during the diagnostic investigation, to prepare the nutritionally depleted patient for surgery, and, when required, to maintain the patient through the postoperative period. For the patient with a short bowel disability following major intestinal resections, total parenteral nutrition can be used in the immediate postoperative period or even for prolonged nutritional support at home until the adaptive responses permit oral nutritional maintenance. In patients with fistulas total parenteral nutrition and bowel rest may lead to closure of the fistulas with sustained remission in 20 to 50 per cent of patients. The combination of nutritional support therapy and corticosteroids appears more effective than either modality alone.

Specific attention to vitamin and mineral depletion will help in the management of anemia and bone disease and should aid the healing process and the overall sense of well-being. Calcium and magnesium losses may be particularly high in the presence of poor intake, severe diarrhea, and steatorrhea. Vitamin D deficiency may lead to metabolic bone disease in Crohn's disease patients, particularly after intestinal resection. This deficiency can usually be corrected with adequate amounts of oral vitamin D, approximately 4000 IU daily. Vitamins can usually be replaced by a therapeutic multivitamin preparation containing three to five times the normal daily requirement. Zinc deficiency should be considered, especially in patients with prolonged and severe diarrhea who may require replacement therapy. In patients on parenteral nutrition, addition of trace metals to parenteral fluids is mandatory.

Therapy in Growth-Retarded Patients. The young patient whose growth is retarded presents a special challenge. In some patients the institution of a medical regimen, including sulfasalazine or corticosteroids, preferably on an alternate-day regimen, will suppress symptoms and disease activity sufficiently to improve dietary intake and restore growth. Restoring normal nutrition is crucial to success of medical therapy. Nutrition may be restored by total parenteral nutrition, including episodic administration at home, or by administering a defined, minimal-residue formula diet by enteral tube. Surgery, timed to permit a maximal growth spurt during puberty, is recommended by some for intractable disease in ulcerative colitis or Crohn's ileocolitis unresponsive to medical management. In such instances the possibility of a period of relative freedom from symptoms and potential growth restitution must be balanced against the strong likelihood of recurrence of Crohn's disease and the need for repeated resections later.

Sulfasalazine. Containing a sulfonamide, sulfapyridine, and salicylate in azo linkage, sulfasalazine is the most commonly used drug in inflammatory bowel disease. Sulfasalazine in the usual dose of 3 grams a day orally has been established by means of a national cooperative study as effective treatment for the management of exacerbations of Crohn's disease, particularly of Crohn's disease of the colon. Sulfasalazine in combination with prednisone was not better than prednisone alone in treatment of an acute exacerbation of Crohn's disease. The effectiveness of sulfasalazine in Crohn's disease limited to the small intestine remains in question. No drug regimen has been proved to reduce recurrences of Crohn's disease after clinical remission, whether spontaneous, induced by drugs, or after resective surgery. Still, in many centers sulfasalazine therapy, once instituted, is maintained. Side effects of sulfasalazine treatment are discussed in Ch. 105.3.

Newer Drugs Containing 5-Aminosalicylate (5-ASA). Increasingly, 5-ASA is recognized as the active moiety of sulfasalazine. Topical 5-ASA is equivalent to sulfasalazine in resolving rectal inflammation. Oral preparations of 5-ASA designed to deliver the drug to the lower bowel by slow-release tablets or by azo linkage to other compounds have yielded encouraging initial results and are used increasingly, especially in sulfasalazine-sensitive patients. Major trials are in progress in America and Europe.

Antimicrobial Therapy. Despite the fact that no specific microbiologic agent has been implicated in the etiology or pathogenesis of Crohn's disease (see above), antibiotics are often used empirically in this inflammatory disorder. Parenteral antibiotics are commonly used in the acutely ill patient with fever and signs of peritoneal irritation and sometimes as an adjunct in programs for bowel rest or with corticosteroid therapy. The use of antibiotics, including tetracycline and trimethoprim-sulfamethoxazole, in ambulatory patients with Crohn's disease has yielded some promising results, but these observations require confirmation in controlled trials.

Metronidazole has a broad spectrum of activity against anaerobic bacteria that predominate in the gastrointestinal tract and are present in markedly increased numbers in inflammatory bowel diseases. Metronidazole has been used as an adjunct in the management of perianal fistula in Crohn's disease with reported success. A recent controlled trial has demonstrated the efficacy of metronidazole, 10 mg per kilogram per day in divided doses, in the management of acute exacerbations of Crohn's disease.

Corticosteroid Therapy. Corticosteroids are used to suppress inflammation in the bowel and the coincident systemic manifestations of inflammation. The decision to use corticosteroids in Crohn's disease is one that should be made with care. Prednisone in doses of 0.25 to 0.75 mg per kilogram for four months is usually effective in the treatment of an exacerbation of Crohn's disease, but prolonged corticosteroid use does not seem to prevent exacerbations of the disease. Therefore, the usual practice is to treat the acute exacerbation with 40 to 60 mg of prednisone per day for two to four weeks followed by tapering doses as symptoms permit. Some patients, unable to be tapered off prednisone, may continue to take low doses for protracted periods. In prepubertal patients it is particularly important to give corticosteroids on an alternate-day regimen, if at all possible, to reduce growth retardation. Such an alternate-day regimen should be used when possible even in adult patients. Novel corticosteroid preparations for topical use with better therapeutic to toxicity ratios are largely of interest in the treatment of ulcerative colitis.

Immunosuppressive Therapy. Azathioprine* and 6-mercaptopurine* have been used with encouraging results in the management of patients with Crohn's disease. In Crohn's disease, as well as in ulcerative colitis, the use of daily doses of 1.0 to 1.5 mg per kilogram has permitted the lowering of corticosteroid doses without symptomatic exacerbation in controlled trials. As a single agent, however, azathioprine demonstrated no superiority over a placebo in a four-month trial. When 6-mercaptopurine is used for longer periods, it may be effective in the management of some patients with Crohn's disease if sufficient time is allowed for the immunosuppressive effects to be accomplished. Toxic side effects may limit the use of these agents, especially in women of childbearing age (see Ch. 176).

Antidiarrheal Drugs. Patients may be symptomatically improved by drugs given to diminish intestinal motility and diarrhea. Loperamide, diphenoxylate, tincture of opium, or paregoric can be used to reduce diarrhea in Crohn's disease. Anticholinergic drugs are helpful in some patients in diminishing stool frequency. All these antimotility drugs should be used carefully, with special attention to narcotic dependence in the case of codeine, paregoric, and opium. Symptoms of obstruction may be exacerbated with all of these drugs.

Surgery for Ileitis or Ileocolitis. Surgical resection of bowel involved in Crohn's disease is occasionally required but is undertaken with reluctance because of the high rate of recurrence of the disease. In one study recurrence after resection of the involved distal small bowel or ileum and adjacent colon was 50 per cent in 5 years, 75 per cent in 10, and 91 per cent in 15. Still there is a prominent place for surgery in the management of many patients with Crohn's disease. Surgery is clearly indicated for high-grade intestinal *obstruction* unresponsive to medical therapy, for *perforation*, and for *fistulas* to other abdominal organs such as the bladder. Patients lacking these clear indications may undergo resective surgery for *intractable disease* with the knowledge that recurrence is likely but still seeking temporary symptomatic relief. Surgery in the adolescent with growth retardation has been discussed earlier. The most common operation is resection of the involved portions of the terminal ileum with an ileocolonic anastomosis. Such an anastomosis should retain as much of the right colon as possible, since the right colon may be critical in determining the extent of debility from postiliectomy diarrhea.

Surgery for Crohn's Colitis. Indications for surgery in Crohn's colitis are similar to those for ulcerative colitis (see Ch. 105.3). Uncontrolled bleeding, perforation, and toxic dilatation are rarer than in ulcerative colitis but may occasionally demand acute surgical intervention. Most commonly surgery is performed for clinical intractability of the disease despite full medical management. Intractability usually means inability to work or function socially despite therapy, inadequate growth and development in children, unresolved perianal complications, or unremitting systemic complications such as iritis or liver disease. The surgical approach may be that of total proctocolectomy and resection of involved terminal ileum with ileostomy, or a subtotal colectomy with ileosigmoid, ileorectal, or ileoanal anastomosis. For any resection with internal anastomosis, recurrence rate is in excess of 75 per cent in ten years. In many patients a period of several years of relative freedom from symptoms without ileostomy makes ileorectal or ileosigmoid anastomosis the surgical approach of choice. For patients with extensive involvement of colon, including the rectum, total proctocolectomy with ileostomy is usually performed. The need for surgical revision of the ileostomy, usually caused by complications resulting from recurrent inflammatory disease, may be as high as 40 per cent in five years. The actual rate of recurrence of Crohn's disease after ileostomy is uncertain but is probably less than 15 per cent in five years. Thus Crohn's colitis, in contrast to ulcerative colitis, is not cured by total proctocolectomy.

PROGNOSIS. Crohn's disease exacts a very substantial cost in altered patient lifestyle and in regular, often intensive medical care. A pattern of remissions and exacerbations is usual. Although disease-free intervals may extend for years and, rarely, for decades, the most characteristic and discouraging feature of Crohn's disease is its almost relentless tendency to recur despite intensive medical treatment or after surgery. The benefits of some years free of symptoms after surgical resection are substantial in many patients. About 50 per cent of patients require surgical treatment eventually. Surgery is rarely if ever curative, however, so every effort should be made to manage all aspects of the patient's illness. Overall mortality attributed to Crohn's disease or its complications ranges from 5 to 18 per cent in various reports. It is lower in patients with disease limited to the small intestine.

The outlook for patients with Crohn's disease has improved steadily with advances in general and supportive treatment. Further progress may be expected as our understanding of the etiology of Crohn's disease increases.

*This use is not listed in the manufacturer's directive.

Donaldson RM Jr: Crohn's disease. In Sleisenger MH, Fordtran JS (eds.): Gastrointestinal Disease. 4th ed. Philadelphia, W.B. Saunders Company,

1988. *Excellent, balanced review of all phases of Crohn's disease, supplemented by illustrative radiographs and 129 references.*

Gitnick G: Evidence for infectious agents in IBD. In Gitnick G (ed.): Current Gastroenterology, Vol 7. Chicago, Year Book Medical Publishers, 1987.

Greenstein AJ, Janowitz HD, Sachar DB: The extraintestinal complications of Crohn's disease and ulcerative colitis: A study of 700 patients. Medicine 55:401, 1976.

Hanauer S: New Drug Therapies for inflammatory bowel disease. In Gitnick G: Current Gastroenterology. Vol 7. Chicago, Year Book Medical Publishers, 1987.

Kirsner JB, Shorter RG: Recent developments in "nonspecific" inflammatory bowel disease. N Engl J Med 306:775, 837, 1982. *An authoritative review with emphasis on concepts of etiopathogenesis.*

Mendeloff AL: The epidemiology of inflammatory bowel disease. Clin Gastroenterol 9:259, 1980. *A comprehensive review and critique comparing the behavior of Crohn's disease and ulcerative colitis in a volume devoted to inflammatory bowel disease.*

The National Cooperative Crohn's Disease Study. Gastroenterology 77:825, 1980. *Twelve articles summarizing the results of a cooperative study, clinical characteristics, drug therapy, diagnostic studies, complications, and adverse reactions.*

105.3 Ulcerative Colitis

Bernard Levin

DEFINITIONS. Ulcerative colitis is a chronic disease of unknown etiology characterized by inflammation of the mucosa and submucosa of the large intestine. The inflammation usually involves the rectum down to the anal margin and extends proximally in the colon for a variable distance.Terms in common usage refer to the anatomic extent of the disease: *pancolitis* for involvement of the entire colon; *ulcerative proctitis* or *proctosigmoiditis* for diseases limited to the rectum or rectosigmoid; and *left-sided colitis* for disease of the descending colon.

Ulcerative colitis has an estimated incidence of 2 to 7 cases per 100,000 and a prevalence of 40 to 100 cases per 100,000 population in the United States. For ulcerative proctitis both the incidence and prevalence are roughly comparable to those for colitis. Although both Crohn's disease and ulcerative colitis are being increasingly recognized, there is no evidence that the incidence of ulcerative colitis is actually increasing. In the United States between 200,000 and 400,000 persons suffer from inflammatory bowel diseases, with about 30,000 new cases diagnosed each year. Ulcerative colitis affects women more frequently than men and exhibits a bimodal age distribution, with a first peak of incidence between the ages of 15 and 20 years and a secondary small peak at ages 55 to 60 (Fig. 105–5). The incidence of ulcerative colitis in blacks may be as low as one third that in whites, and its incidence among Jews is about three to five times greater than among non-Jews.

FAMILIAL AND GENETIC FEATURES. There is an increased familial incidence of inflammatory bowel disease, both for ulcerative colitis and for Crohn's disease, but without a clear-cut pattern of inheritance. In one study about 4 per cent of a control population had a family history of inflammatory bowel disease, whereas 11 per cent of those with chronic inflammatory bowel disease had a family history of these disorders. The onset of disease in patients from affected families occurred at a lower age than in those without family histories.

Patients with inflammatory bowel disease and ankylosing spondylitis have a likelihood of 50 to 90 per cent of possessing the histocompatibility antigen HLA-B27, whereas the antigen is found in 6 to 9 per cent of the control population. The antigen is present in even higher prevalence in patients with spondylitis without inflammatory bowel disease (see Ch. 434). An increased incidence of ankylosing spondylitis has been reported in relatives of patients with ulcerative colitis or Crohn's disease. These findings continue to arouse interest in genetic factors in the pathogenesis of chronic inflammatory bowel disease.

ETIOLOGY AND PATHOGENESIS. The etiology of chronic ulcerative colitis is unknown. Furthermore, no satisfactory animal model of the human disorder has been discovered.

Psychogenic Factors. Considerable debate has occurred about the role of psychosomatic factors in the initiation and further development of ulcerative colitis. Once the illness has become manifest, it is often impossible to distinguish its influences on behavior from the patient's premorbid personality. Any illness characterized by severe diarrhea, rectal bleeding, and a variety of constitutional symptoms, especially when occurring in a young, previously healthy person, constitutes a stressful situation and can destroy a patient's self-confidence. Regressive behavior may result. Hospitalized children with colitis are often compulsively neat, demanding, and immature for their age. Adults may exhibit exaggeration of dependency needs during periods of active disease. Conflicting data exist about the occurrence of significant life-stress crises at the time of onset of the disease.

Infectious Agents. Ulcerative colitis is characterized by an inflammatory reaction in the bowel resembling that caused by known microbiologic pathogens such as *Shigella*. However, no organism has been reproducibly demonstrated to be responsible for the condition. Nevertheless, microbial infection remains a possible cause because of the recent recognition of bacterial causes of enteritis and colitis (*Yersinia enterocolitica* and *Campylobacter fetus jejuni*). The possible role of viral agents in the etiology of inflammatory bowel disease is discussed in more detail in relation to Crohn's disease (see Ch. 105.2).

Immunologic Factors. An immunologically mediated pathogenetic mechanism is suggested by the frequent presence of personal and family histories of atopic diseases in patients with ulcerative colitis and the concomitant presence of conditions such as erythema nodosum, arthritis, uveitis, and vasculitis. Circulating anticolon antibodies have been described in ulcerative colitis, but these remain of unknown significance. The beneficial effects of corticosteroid therapy for ulcerative colitis are consistent with its immunosuppressive as well as its anti-inflammatory effects.

Some of the extraintestinal manifestations of ulcerative colitis such as skin rashes, arthritis, and vasculitis suggest immune complex deposition. Activation of the alternative complement pathway in ulcerative colitis is suggested by the observations of normal or elevated levels of C3PA and markedly reduced levels of properdin convertase in sera from patients with extraintestinal complications of the disease.

Antilymphocyte antibodies have been found in up to 40 per cent of patients with ulcerative colitis and in up to 50 per

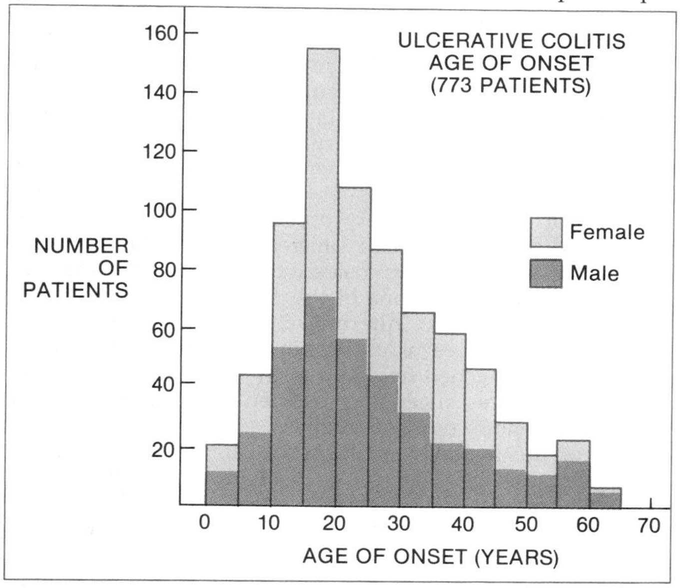

FIGURE 105–5. Age of onset in 773 patients with ulcerative colitis. (From Rogers BHG, Clark LM, Kirsner JB: J Chron Dis 24:743, 1971.)

cent of family members and unrelated household contacts of patients with inflammatory bowel disease. In contrast, these antibodies were found in only 4 per cent of control family members. Lymphocytotoxic antibodies have been found in sera from patients with inflammatory bowel disease and from their unaffected spouses more frequently than sera from age-matched controls and their spouses. Such data suggest exposure to a common environmental agent, but genetic factors must also be implicated, since there is an increased prevalence of lymphocytotoxic antibody in sera from consanguineous relatives without household contact as well.

The T lymphocytes of patients with inflammatory bowel disease do not proliferate normally when stimulated with autologous non–T cells, and suppressor T cell generation is also impaired in these patients. Such failure of suppression may create a "permissive environment," allowing abnormal responses to antigens.

Observations of immunologic events at the intestinal mucosal level have suggested decreased spontaneous antibody secretion in intestinal mononuclear cells compared with peripheral blood mononuclear cells, which showed increased synthesis and secretion of IgG, IgM, and IgA. This suggests the possibility that a primary mucosal immunodeficiency in the bowel of patients with inflammatory bowel disease weakens the mucosal barrier, thereby facilitating both a local inflammation and a heightened systemic immune response.

PATHOLOGY. Pathologic changes in the colon in ulcerative colitis readily predict the clinical features of the disease. In 75 per cent of patients disease involves only the left side of the colon. In the remainder, the entire colon is involved (pancolitis). Extensive vascular engorgement and mucosal ulceration result in bleeding. The damaged mucosa is less able to absorb sodium and water, and watery diarrhea results. Iron deficiency anemia results from blood loss, and hypoalbuminemia may reflect transmucosal loss of protein. The histologic changes in ulcerative colitis are nonspecific, but the chronicity and distribution pattern are characteristic.

Ulcerative colitis involves primarily the mucosa of the colon. Unlike the segmental lesions of Crohn's disease, the mucosa is inflamed continuously, occasionally terminating at some point in the colon where the abnormality gradually changes to a normal appearance over a distance of a few centimeters. The involved mucosa is red and granular and bleeds diffusely. The macroscopic lesions may progress from small, petechial ulcerations to deeper, linear ulcers separated by islands of inflamed but intact mucosa. In severe cases, large areas of the colon may be denuded.

The inflammatory process begins with increased numbers of inflammatory cells in the lamina propria: plasma cells, lymphocytes, monocytes, eosinophils, and polymorphonuclear leukocytes. Capillary dilatation causes hyperemia and vascular engorgement. Polymorphonuclear cells accumulate near the tips of the crypts of Lieberkühn. The crypt epithelium shows degenerative changes or even frank necrosis, with extension of the inflammatory process into the surrounding tissue causing characteristic microabscesses (Fig. 105–6). These crypt abscesses may coalesce by lateral enlargement to produce shallow ulcerations of the mucosa extending down to the lamina propria. Alternatively, the mucosa may be undermined on three sides, leaving an area of ulceration adjacent to an attached fragment of the mucosa. Such resulting mucosal excrescences may be seen as pseudopolyps on radiologic or endoscopic examination.

Some of the features of ulcerative colitis result from the attempts of the inflamed colon to regenerate or repair the destroyed crypts. Regenerating crypts become distorted, branching, and diminished in number and contain goblet cells. Highly vascular granulation tissue may develop in denuded areas. Collagen may be deposited in the lamina propria, and the muscularis mucosae may hypertrophy.

The alternating processes of superficial ulceration and granulation followed by re-epithelialization can lead to the development of polypoid excrescences. These are inflammatory polyps (pseudopolyps) that are not neoplastic. Longstanding disease gives rise to hyperplasia of the muscularis mucosae, and this change, accompanied by postinflammatory fibrosis, causes shortening of the colon. The haustrations are lost, and the large bowel has the appearance of a smooth tube. Strictures may be caused by the localized fibromuscular hyperplasia; a distinction must be made between these and malignant strictures.

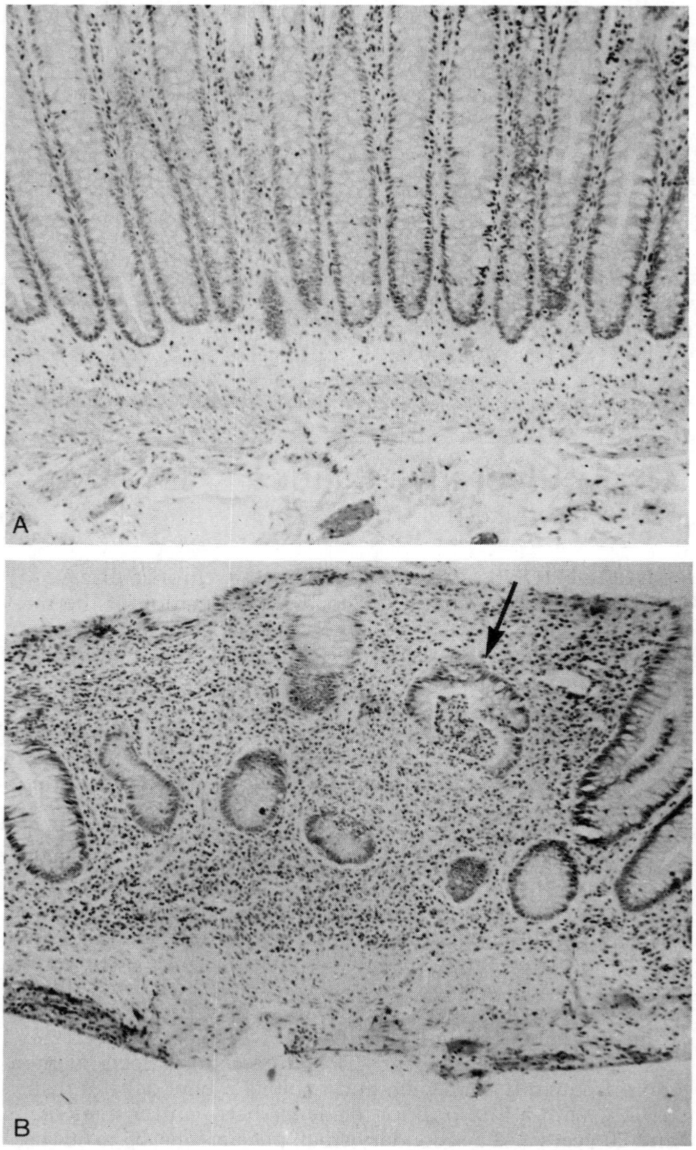

FIGURE 105–6. Rectal biopsies from (*A*) a normal patient and (*B*) a patient with ulcerative colitis. In *B*, note mucosal atrophy, branching of a gland, cellular infiltration, and crypt abscess (*arrow*). × 100. (From Cello JP: In Sleisenger MH, Fordtran JS [eds.]: Gastrointestinal Disease. 3rd ed. Philadelphia, W. B. Saunders Company, 1983.)

In the most severe cases, the inflammation can involve the submucosa and even the serosa and lead to perforation. In toxic dilatation of the colon, a particularly severe and acute form of this disease, the diameter of the lumen of the colon is greatly increased and the bowel wall is thinned, with a serious risk of spontaneous perforation.

CLINICAL MANIFESTATIONS AND COURSE. The five most common symptoms of ulcerative colitis are *rectal bleeding, diarrhea, abdominal pain, weight loss,* and *fever*. The patient is usually in the second, third, or fourth decade of life at the onset of symptoms. Ulcerative colitis may begin in a subtle manner or with catastrophic suddenness. Patients may relate the acute onset of symptoms to a recent emotional upset, to an upper respiratory infection, or occasionally to oral antibiotic therapy.

When signs and symptoms of colonic inflammation (including malaise, lower abdominal discomfort, and an increased number of bowel movements with rectal bleeding) are not marked, the designation *mild ulcerative colitis* is often used. This form of the disease, which accounts for roughly half of all patients with ulcerative colitis, is less likely to be recognized and may not be diagnosed for months or even years. The mortality is negligible, and the long-term prognosis for these patients does not differ from that of a control population. The development of colonic cancer in mild ulcerative colitis is about one seventh of that occurring in the more severe forms of the disease.

Moderate ulcerative colitis describes a more abrupt onset of the disorder, typically associated with four to five loose and bloody bowel movements per day. In this form of the disease, which accounts for about 30 per cent of ulcerative colitis, abdominal cramps may be severe and may awaken the patient at night. Low-grade fever, fatigue, and malaise may be prominent symptoms, as may some of the extracolonic manifestations (see below). The patient may have anorexia and weight loss. Some patients with moderate colitis may become progressively worse, with increasingly severe diarrhea, bleeding, and fever. The immediate mortality in patients with moderate colitis is low because of the efficacy of corticosteroid therapy, but the long-term prognosis for avoiding colectomy is guarded. Exacerbations of the disease often occur and may require intensive medical management over extended periods. The risk of developing cancer of the colon is increased and probably affects this group most significantly.

Severe or fulminant ulcerative colitis presents usually in a dramatic fashion with *profuse diarrhea, rectal bleeding,* and *fever,* which may be as high as 39°C. This form of the disease occurs in about 15 per cent of patients with ulcerative colitis. Abdominal cramps, rectal urgency, and profound weakness are common presenting symptoms. Intermittent nausea, anorexia, and weight loss are also present. Occasionally patients with initially less severe disease may worsen and present a picture of fulminant colitis. Physical examination reveals an acutely ill, pale, weak, and febrile patient. Tachycardia, hypotension, and even shock may be present. Examination of the abdomen reveals generalized tenderness; localized tenderness, especially with "rebound," signals the onset of peritoneal irritation. This suggests that the inflammatory process has extended beyond the mucosa. Absence of bowel sounds should suggest the diagnosis of toxic dilatation, and this serious complication must be carefully excluded.

TOXIC DILATATION OF THE COLON (TOXIC MEGACOLON). In severe ulcerative colitis, the patient may become gravely ill with signs and symptoms of a general toxic state associated with abdominal pain, distention, rebound tenderness, and dilatation of the diameter of the colon on plain abdominal roentgenograms to 6 cm or greater (Fig. 105–7). In a patient with severe active colitis, toxic megacolon may be precipitated by a barium enema examination (and its antecedent preparation), potassium depletion, or anticholinergic or narcotic medication. The complication may also develop spontaneously. Medications that may decrease colonic motility should be avoided in these patients. Severe inflammation disrupts the neural and muscular elements that maintain normal tone. This allows the intraluminal pressure to expand the colon well beyond its normal width. Bacteria overgrow and are thought to produce toxins that intensify the complication and contribute to the hazard of peritonitis. Diffusion of these toxic products into the systemic circulation contributes to the toxic state.

Clinical signs include fever, tachycardia, dehydration, and abdominal tenderness and distention. The loss of bowel sounds is a significant finding. The colon is found to be dilated with severe mucosal disease demonstrated by a plain film of the abdomen (Fig. 105–7). Marked leukocytosis, hypokalemia, anemia, and hypoalbuminemia are frequently present. The mortality rate in toxic dilatation of the colon may be as high as 20 to 30 per cent. Intensive medical therapy with early colectomy can decrease mortality (see Treatment).

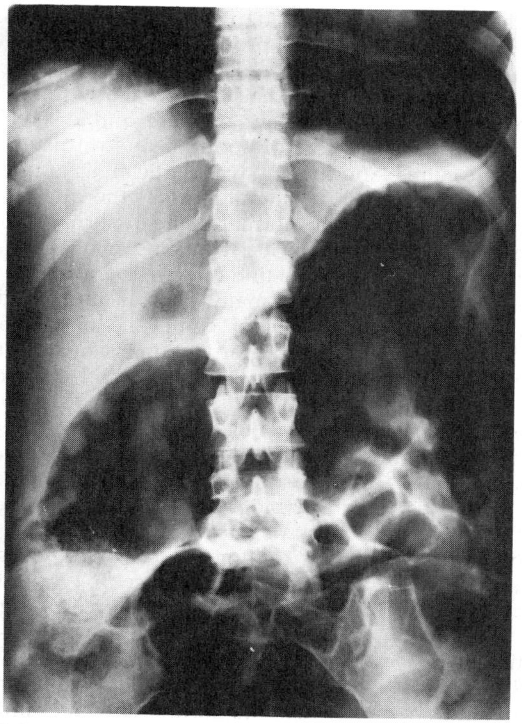

FIGURE 105–7. Plain film of the abdomen from a patient with ulcerative colitis and toxic megacolon. Note that the air in the colon silhouettes an irregular colonic mucosa. (From Cello JP: In Sleisenger MH, Fordtran JS [eds.]: Gastrointestinal Disease. 3rd ed. Philadelphia, W. B. Saunders Company, 1983.)

DIAGNOSIS. The diagnosis of ulcerative colitis is usually made on the basis of its clinical features, the demonstration of inflammation of the rectal and sigmoidal mucosa on proctosigmoidoscopy, and the exclusion of specific infections by appropriate stool culture and examination for parasites. The diagnosis may be supported by radiologic examination, fiberoptic colonoscopy, and rectal biopsy.

Proctosigmoidoscopy. This is the most reliable diagnostic study in ulcerative colitis because the observer may inspect the mucosa directly. This examination is indicated in every patient with rectal bleeding. At the same time, fresh stool samples may be obtained for culture and microscopy to determine the presence of fecal leukocytes or trophozoites. The mucopurulent exudate should be aspirated, mixed with a drop of warm saline, and examined microscopically for motile, hematophagous trophozoites of *Entamoeba histolytica.* It is important to exclude the diagnosis of amebiasis before beginning corticosteroid therapy.

The gross appearance of the rectal mucosa is nonspecific in acute colitis. Specific causes such as shigellosis and *Campylobacter* infections should be excluded by cultures obtained at the time of proctosigmoidoscopy. Particularly, but not exclusively, in patients with prior antibiotic therapy acute colitis may be caused by the enterotoxin of *Clostridium difficile.* Such patients may have endoscopic features of pseudomembranous colitis (see Ch. 279). It is preferable to avoid enemas prior to proctosigmoidoscopy in a patient suspected of having ulcerative colitis because they may confuse by irritating normal rectal mucosa and by aggravating mild abnormalities. Despite its name, in the early phases ulcerative colitis does not produce visible ulcers, but rather the red, diffusely bleeding, granular mucosa looks as though it has been gently sandpapered. Edema and erythema produce a markedly reddened, swollen mucosa with a diminished vascular pattern, the changes of hyperemia, petechiae, and fragility.

In moderate colitis, purulent exudate and discrete small ulcers appear. Gross pus and spontaneous diffuse bleeding mark severe colitis, and there may be large areas of ulceration. After appropriate therapy in mild cases, the appearance of the rectum may return to normal or near normal; however, repeated attacks with attempts at healing may cause loss of the normal vascular pattern, fine or coarse granularity of the mucosa, blunting of the normally sharply angulated rectal valves, and inflammatory polyps composed of tags of damaged mucosa and heaped-up granulation tissue. After many cycles of inflammation and healing, the bowel may scar and become stenosed.

Rectal Biopsy (Fig. 105–6). A biopsy usually is not necessary to make the diagnosis of ulcerative colitis if the clinical and sigmoidoscopic features are typical. However, there may be certain instances in which biopsy is helpful: (1) to exclude other forms of colitis such as Crohn's disease of the colon, pseudomembranous colitis, or amebic colitis; (2) to search for mucosal dysplasia in cancer surveillance in patients with longstanding colitis; or (3) to confirm equivocal sigmoidoscopic findings in a patient with a history suggestive of ulcerative colitis.

Radiography. The patient who is ill with moderate or severe colitis should not be subjected to barium enema examination. In such patients radiologic examination is unnecessary for diagnosing ulcerative colitis and may be dangerous. Preparation of the patient by use of cathartics and enemas will worsen the condition significantly.

In the acutely ill patient the plain abdominal film should be employed in the initial evaluation. The extent of disease can be predicted by observing the patterns of fecal residue in the colon as well as the mucosal outline and haustral patterns. Failure to recognize early a grave complication such as toxic megacolon increases the risk of morbidity and mortality. The diagnosis of toxic dilatation is made on both clinical and radiographic grounds. Patients suspected of having toxic megacolon (fever, abdominal tenderness and distention, decreased or absent bowel sounds) may be seen on plain film to have dilatation of the midtransverse colon to a diameter of 6 cm or more (Fig. 105–7).

Barium enema examination may provide the following important information: (1) When sigmoidoscopy confirms the diagnosis of colitis, and after specific infectious causes have been excluded, it helps to determine the extent and severity of the mucosal lesions. If the sigmoidoscopy is negative in a patient with rectal bleeding and diarrhea, barium examination will be helpful in making the diagnosis of another cause such as neoplasm, Crohn's disease of the colon, or ischemic colitis. (2) In patients with equivocal findings at sigmoidoscopy or on a rectal biopsy, it may demonstrate features of ulcerative colitis more proximally. (3) The barium enema may detect complications such as colonic cancer in patients with longstanding colitis.

The postevacuation film of a single-contrast barium enema also provides information about mucosal detail. Unless the double-contrast (barium and air) technique is used, however, fine mucosal abnormalities may be overlooked and the extent of the involvement underestimated.

In the acute stage of ulcerative colitis, fine granularity reflects mucosal edema and hyperemia. As the disease progresses, superficial erosions develop and adherent barium produces a stippled appearance. Tiny ulcerations may be seen as these enlarge, and "collar-button"–like projections appear that involve the colon circumferentially. As the disease progresses, the normal colonic mucosal surface is lost; however, it may regenerate with healing. Inflammatory polyps may appear as rare or numerous intraluminal filling defects (Fig. 105–8). The inflammatory process also may affect the muscular layers of the colon, producing a smooth, foreshortened colon without haustra. After recovery from a first attack, haustral markings may reappear. After longstanding mucosal and submucosal thickening in some patients with ulcerative proctitis or colitis, the presacral space may enlarge. This is seen best on a lateral view of the barium-filled rectum.

A small bowel follow-through radiographic study should be performed after acute symptoms are controlled to help exclude the diagnosis of Crohn's disease. In ulcerative colitis involving the entire colon, the ileocecal valve may be dilated and incompetent. The terminal ileum may be dilated, but discrete ulceration is seen only when Crohn's disease is present.

Colonoscopy. Colonoscopy has little place in the diagnosis of acute ulcerative colitis and may be hazardous because of the risks of perforation and hemorrhage. Since the entire colon may be examined by colonoscopy, it is extremely useful in the patient who does not have acute and severe symptoms when the diagnosis and extent of inflammatory bowel disease are uncertain. Colonoscopy is most commonly used in obtaining multiple biopsies in patients with longstanding colitis in a search for neoplastic changes.

DIFFERENTIAL DIAGNOSIS. Numerous other causes of diarrhea must be considered in the differential diagnosis of ulcerative colitis, but the clinical presentation, sigmoidoscopic findings, and radiologic features are used to make a definite diagnosis. The differential diagnosis of rectal bleeding includes hemorrhoids, colonic adenomas and carcinomas, angiodysplastic lesions, bleeding disorders, and diverticular disease. The differential diagnosis of gastrointestinal bleeding is discussed in greater detail in Ch. 114.

Viral infections, bacillary dysentery, and toxigenic strains of *Escherichia coli* may cause acute colitis and occasionally simulate ulcerative colitis. Diarrhea is a prominent symptom of these diseases, but rectal bleeding is uncommon except in *shigellosis*, which rarely lasts more than a few days. *Campylobacter* infections may closely mimic nonspecific ulcerative colitis. Their diagnosis is particularly important, since these infections respond well to appropriate antibiotic therapy. *Salmonella* infections may present as an acute or subacute diarrheal disorder. *Yersinia enterocolitica* produces an acute

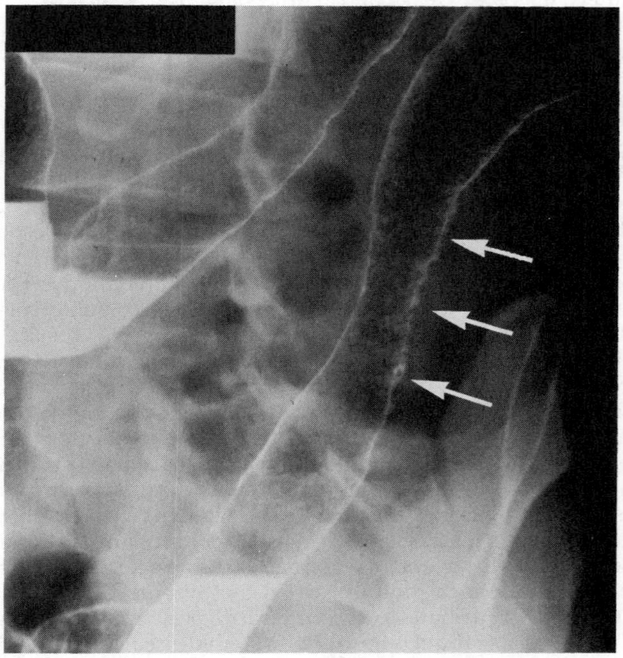

FIGURE 105–8. Double-contrast enema in patient with active ulcerative colitis with discrete collar button ulcers (*arrows*) in an anhaustral and diffusely granular colon.

bacterial ileitis and mesenteric adenitis, which more closely resemble an acute attack of Crohn's disease.

Ischemic colitis is more common in elderly individuals and often causes a segmental form of colitis. Typically, roentgenographic features of "thumbprinting" caused by intramural hemorrhage are observed. Infarction of the colon, affecting primarily the right side of the colon, may be seen in young women taking oral contraceptives. This clinical picture of acute lower abdominal pain, fever, and rectal bleeding may resemble acute ulcerative colitis, but the course will help distinguish this entity.

Amebiasis may occasionally be difficult to distinguish from ulcerative colitis in its early phases. A history of foreign travel may be elicited but is not essential. Mild, diffuse hyperemia on sigmoidoscopic examination is not uncommon. Later, distinctive features include discrete large ulcers with overhanging edges. Fresh preparations of mucopus must be examined for the presence of trophozoites (see Ch. 390).

Gonococcal proctitis may present with rectal burning and diarrhea, a mucopurulent discharge, or bleeding. On sigmoidoscopic examination, generalized redness and edema of the rectal mucosa may be indistinguishable from ulcerative proctitis. The rectal discharge should be cultured for gonococci.

Pseudomembranous colitis is usually associated with a preexisting history of antibiotic use. This condition is generally related to the growth of *Clostridium difficile*, which produces a toxin that can be identified in stools. In patients with pseudomembranous colitis, proctoscopic examination reveals raised, initially small, yellowish plaques on intensely red and later ulcerated mucosa. The plaques may be covered by mucus, which must be swabbed off before the plaque can be seen. The mucosa bleeds when the membrane is stripped.

The following diseases also may cause rectal inflammation: *histoplasmosis, leukemic* and *lymphomatous infiltration, solitary ulcer syndrome, malakoplakia,* and *lymphogranuloma venereum.* The last-named disorder presents with the passage of blood, mucus, and pus from the rectum, but patients also may have perianal fistulas and inguinal adenopathy. Patients with *radiation proctitis* will have a history of radiation therapy for cancer of the cervix, prostate, or testis, but the proctoscopic appearance is indistinguishable from that of nonspecific ulcerative colitis. It is important to recognize that the workup of homosexual patients with proctitis or colitis should include a search for common and uncommon viral, bacterial, and parasitic pathogens.

The most difficult differential diagnosis is that between ulcerative colitis and Crohn's disease of the colon. *Crohn's colitis* presents with diarrhea but usually not with rectal bleeding. Crohn's colitis also is frequently associated with perianal lesions. Characteristic features of these two diseases are compared in Table 105–3. Clinical data, endoscopic examinations, and barium enemas can differentiate Crohn's disease of the colon from ulcerative colitis in 80 to 85 per cent of patients with inflammatory bowel disease. In approximately 15 to 20 per cent of patients differentiation is not possible, and the type of colitis remains undetermined. The differentiation is useful in that it affects the approach to treatment and the assessment of prognosis.

LOCAL COMPLICATIONS. Local complications include hemorrhoids, anal fissures, perianal or ischiorectal suppuration, rectovaginal fistulas, and rectal prolapse. These complications appear most frequently when diarrhea is severe. Anal fissures improve with control of the colitis. Perirectal abscesses and rectal fistulas heal with incision and drainage of abscesses and unroofing of fistulous tracts.

More significant complications include massive hemorrhage, colonic strictures, inflammatory polyps, adenomatous polyps, adenocarcinoma, and toxic dilatation. *Massive hemorrhage* occurs in about 5 per cent of patients. Prompt replacement of circulating blood volume, correction of hypoprothrombinemia, and early colectomy if bleeding is uncontrollable are the principles of management of this condition.

Colonic strictures are seen in some patients on barium examination or during colonoscopy. Occasionally these apparent strictures may be due to spasm and will disappear after the intravenous administration of glucagon. It is essential to ensure that strictures are benign by colonoscopic biopsy and brushing cytology. Nevertheless it is not always possible to exclude a deeply infiltrating carcinoma by these means, and colectomy should be considered if any doubt exists about the diagnosis. *Inflammatory polyps* do not require removal except in cases in which it is impossible to distinguish them grossly from true adenomas. *Adenomatous polyps*, when identified, should be removed at the time of colonoscopy. Their association with carcinoma of the colon is of particular significance in the patient with longstanding colitis, and the patient's colon warrants careful evaluation for the presence of other adenomas or carcinoma (see Ch. 107).

Carcinoma of the large bowel occurring as a complication of ulcerative colitis is correlated with the extent of disease and its duration. The overall prevalence of cancer in all patients with ulcerative colitis is between 3 and 5 per cent. For those with pancolitis and a duration of disease greater than ten years, the risk is 10 to 20 times greater than that of the general population (see Fig. 107–4). In children ulcerative colitis usually involves the entire colon; more adults have disease limited to the distal colon. The risk of developing cancer is similar in both children and adults with universal disease, viz. 13 per cent after 15 years, 23 per cent after 20 years, and 42 per cent after 25 years of the disease. Some authorities have suggested that the risk of complicating cancer is much lower and that most published studies are from referral centers with a markedly biased patient composition.

The patients who develop colonic cancer are often in a quiescent stage of their illness, and diagnosis often is delayed because the symptoms of bleeding or diarrhea may be attributed initially to a recurrence of the colitis. The tumors in colitis may be flat and small and not detectable even by expert colonoscopic and radiologic techniques. The prognosis of carcinoma of the colon in ulcerative colitis tends to be worse than that developing in the absence of colitis, because the diagnosis is often made late and the lesions are often multifocal and display a high grade of malignancy.

Some physicians advocate elective proctocolectomy after 10 to 12 years of the active ulcerative colitis to avoid progression to colonic cancer. The patient, however, may be very reluctant to undergo this procedure, particularly if the colitis or the side effects of medication are minimal. In biopsies obtained at proctoscopy or colonoscopy, the presence of epithelial dysplasia (neoplastic change) in the mucosa may provide an early indication of increased vulnerability to colonic cancer. Multiple biopsies are required and interpretation by an experienced pathologist is essential. These issues are discussed in detail in Ch. 107.

EXTRAINTESTINAL COMPLICATIONS (see Table 105–2). Two characteristic skin lesions occur in ulcerative colitis: *pyoderma gangrenosum* and *erythema nodosum. Erythema nodosum* is characterized by the appearance of dull, red, raised, painful nodules usually on the skin of the legs. This lesion, which is more common in women than in men, is roughly correlated with the activity of the mucosal disease and is likely to develop when arthritis also accompanies the attack of colitis. It is seen in both ulcerative colitis and Crohn's disease. *Pyoderma gangrenosum* is seen in 5 per cent of patients with ulcerative colitis and is characteristic of that disease. The lesion starts with the appearance of a furuncle on the skin and later appears as a painful, indurated area surrounded by violaceous, undermined skin. Topical and systemic corticosteroids have been used to suppress the colonic inflammation with a parallel improvement of the lesions of pyoderma gangrenosum. Favorable responses to dapsone (Avlosulfon) therapy also have been reported.

There are two separate types of *joint involvement* in ulcerative colitis and Crohn's disease: (1) sacroiliitis with or without ankylosing spondylitis and (2) a specific form of peripheral arthritis. The prevalence of *ankylosing spondylitis* in chronic ulcerative colitis and Crohn's disease varies from 1.6 to 12.6 per cent, at least 30 times more common than in the general population. The symptoms of ankylosing spondylitis are pain and stiffness in the spine with loss of normal lumbar lordosis. *Sacroiliitis* may be symptomatic or associated only with mild pain in the region of the sacroiliac joints. On routine radiologic examination, changes compatible with sacroiliitis were identified in approximately 20 per cent of patients with ulcerative colitis and Crohn's disease. When spondylitis occurs unassociated with ulcerative colitis, the histocompatibility antigen HLA-B27 is found in roughly 90 per cent of patients. Seventy-five per cent of patients with ankylosing spondylitis who have simultaneous inflammatory bowel disease have this antigen. The *peripheral arthritis* associated with both Crohn's disease and ulcerative colitis occurs in about 10 to 12 per cent of patients with both conditions. The arthritis is a transient, acute, painful swelling that usually affects one or more large joints and is accompanied by a sterile serous joint effusion. The knees are commonly affected, but any joint may be involved. Arthritis rarely precedes the onset of the inflammatory bowel disease but may begin at any time during its course. It is more common in patients with extensive bowel involvement and at times of a flare-up of intestinal symptoms. Peripheral arthritis is more common in patients with perianal disease.

There appears to be a *hypercoagulable state* in ulcerative colitis, with reported increases in the platelet count and in the plasma levels of factor V, factor VIII, and fibrinogen. This may account for the enhanced susceptibility to thromboembolic phenomena exhibited by these patients.

Conjunctivitis, iritis, and/or episcleritis occur as complications in 3 to 10 per cent of patients with ulcerative colitis or Crohn's colitis (and a smaller percentage of those with regional enteritis). Iritis is the most important because of its threat to vision. There is a high incidence of iritis in patients with both spondylitis and colitis. Iritis presents as a red, painful eye with discomfort increased in the dark owing to pupillary dilatation. *Stomatitis* with multiple aphthous ulcers may occasionally be severe.

The incidence of *kidney stones*, particularly urate stones, in patients with ulcerative colitis is approximately twice that in the normal population. Following colectomy and ileostomy, the incidence of urate stones may be as high as 20 times normal. Prevention is best achieved by ensuring adequate hydration and reducing urine acidity but may on occasion require the use of allopurinol (see Ch. 90).

Hepatobiliary complications of both ulcerative colitis and Crohn's disease range from asymptomatic *pericholangitis* to *sclerosing cholangitis, chronic active hepatitis* and *cirrhosis*, and *bile duct carcinoma*. The *nutritional abnormalities* commonly seen in patients with ulcerative colitis are usually not as severe as those seen with Crohn's disease, but growth retardation is not unusual (see Ch. 105.2).

TREATMENT. Management of the patient with ulcerative colitis requires a comprehensive review of the patient's medical, nutritional, and psychologic needs. Ulcerative colitis tends to follow an acute relapsing course with quiescent intervals in some patients, during which the rectal mucosa may appear normal. No method other than colectomy is known to cure ulcerative colitis. During remission treatment is designed to prevent relapse. In patients with chronic active inflammation, therapy is intended to suppress inflammation.

General Therapy. Dietary and nutritional decisions are important in the management of ulcerative colitis and of Crohn's disease (see Nutritional Treatment in Ch. 105.2). The fiber content of the diet should be reduced during periods of diarrhea. In lactose-intolerant patients restriction of lactose intake (avoidance of dairy products) may ameliorate the diarrhea. Alternatively, bacterial lactase is commercially available and may be used to reduce the lactose content of milk to well tolerated levels. Nutritionally balanced, minimal-residue liquid nutritional formulas are available and are acceptable as supplements to most patients. In the severely ill, catabolic patient, parenteral alimentation may be employed to put the bowel at rest, largely to prepare patients for colectomy or for the postoperative recovery period.

The causes of anemia may be multiple and may include the anemia of chronic illness (see Ch. 135), blood loss with resulting iron deficiency, or folate deficiency. Oral iron may be poorly tolerated, necessitating the use of parenteral iron. Folate deficiency is associated with sulfasalazine therapy as well as with inadequate dietary intake owing to reduction in folate-containing foods such as fresh fruits and leafy vegetables.

In the patient with mild or moderate colitis, agents to reduce diarrhea may be useful. These include diphenoxylate with atropine (2.5 to 5 mg), codeine (15 to 30 mg), deodorized tincture of opium (6 to 10 drops), paregoric (4 to 8 ml), or loperamide (2 to 4 mg) before meals and at bedtime. Tincture of belladonna (10 drops) four times a day and other anticholinergics may be used to decrease abdominal cramps. Extreme care must be exercised in the use of these medications in the moderately ill patient because of the risk of precipitating toxic dilatation.

Nonspecific measures include attention to psychologic stresses in the patient's life, often involving interactions with close relatives. Patients should be encouraged to have adequate amounts of rest and sleep. As with any other chronic illness, patient education is important in enabling the patient and family to understand the nature of the disease and its effects on the individual. Formal psychiatric counseling is reserved for a minority of patients, although most benefit from a sympathetic, supportive relationship with their physicians, which may involve modest amounts of psychotherapy.

Therapy for Severe Acute Colitis. Early diagnosis and recognition of this condition are important in reducing mortality. An early decision between intensive medical treatment and immediate surgery may be necessary, particularly if there is evidence of perforation or of peritonitis, or if there is uncontrollable hemorrhage. Toxic dilatation is perhaps the most threatening type of acute severe ulcerative colitis. Failure of toxic dilatation to respond to medical management within 24 to 36 hours is ominous, since the mortality of such patients is very high unless colectomy is performed. Adequate replacement of circulating plasma volume with crystalloid, plasma, and blood is essential. Broad-spectrum antibiotics (cefoxitin or imipenem-cilastin) and intravenous corticosteroids are used. Hydrocortisone, 300 mg intravenously daily, is effective but may cause sodium and water retention. Alternatives include intravenous prednisolone, 60 mg daily, or methylprednisolone, 48 mg daily, in four divided doses.

Successful treatment depends on prompt recognition, early surgical consultation, and intensive resuscitative, antibacterial, and anti-inflammatory therapy. Important measures include intravenous fluids, plasma, blood, nasogastric suction, antibiotics, and intravenous corticosteroids. It is essential that the patient be re-evaluated every four to six hours by the physician and surgeon, and that plain abdominal films be obtained twice daily. Failure to respond to maximal therapy within 24 to 36 hours makes prompt surgical intervention essential. Usually the surgeon will choose to perform an abdominal colectomy with ileostomy, leaving the rectum in place for a subsequent operation when the patient has recovered from this severe episode. Early surgical intervention has resulted in decreased mortality in the acute phase. Overall mortality (in both medically and surgically treated patients) is high, between 12 and 30 per cent. About one fifth of patients with toxic dilatation require surgery after failure to respond to medical treatment. Patients who do not undergo surgical therapy during the attack of toxic dilatation often require elective surgery within 6 to 12 months because of subsequent failure of medical therapy.

If the patient with severe ulcerative colitis does not respond to full treatment within five to ten days, many clinicians advise colectomy (even in the absence of toxic megacolon) as soon as the patient's general condition has been stabilized. Postoperative mortality can be reduced by earlier operation, by correction of malnutrition, and by appropriate antibiotic therapy.

If the patient's general condition responds to maximal therapy and there is improvement in the sigmoidoscopic appearance of the rectal mucosa, oral feeding can commence along with the use of oral corticosteroids. If liquids are tolerated well, solid foods are added gradually as tolerated. Sulfasalazine, 2 to 4 grams orally daily, is usually then added. The oral corticosteroid dose should initially be about 40 mg of prednisone a day. If the clinical response continues to be satisfactory, this dose can be reduced by 5 mg daily every week to a dose of 20 mg of prednisone daily. This dose should be administered for a period of six to eight weeks before it is slowly tapered. Slow reductions in dosage sometimes help individual patients to withdraw eventually from this medication. Repeated brief courses of steroids for treatment of recurrences do not cause as many disabling side effects as does continuous use. Alternate-day dosage is associated with fewer side effects, but this regimen may have diminished symptomatic benefit in some patients. An alternate-day regimen may be of particular value in prepubertal children to avoid the growth suppression of large daily doses of corticosteroids.

Moderate-to-Mild Acute Colitis. For mild or moderate attacks of colitis, hospitalization is usually not required. In addition to the general measures already described, sulfasalazine is used with or without corticosteroids, depending on the severity of diarrhea and systemic symptoms. For mildly symptomatic colitis with predominantly left-sided disease, oral sulfasalazine and topical corticosteroid therapy are often satisfactory.

Corticosteroid can be applied locally to the rectal and colonic mucosa as hydrocortisone (100 mg) administered in 100 ml of saline either by enema or by slow rectal infusion. This volume of fluid always reaches the sigmoid colon, but the proximal spread is variable. Approximately one third is absorbed systemically. Suppositories and foam can be used for disease confined to the rectum. Newer nonabsorbed topical corticosteroid preparations diminish systemic side effects.

Sulfasalazine is largely unabsorbed and is metabolized by colonic bacteria to sulfapyridine and 5-aminosalicylic acid. The 5-aminosalicylic acid may exert a therapeutic effect by interfering with prostaglandin synthesis, a mediator of inflammation. Synthesis of prostaglandin E_2 by cultured rectal mucosa from patients with colitis and prostaglandin synthetase activity of the rectal mucosa are increased in active colitis. Adverse reactions to sulfasalazine, including headaches, arthralgias, nausea, skin rashes, and mild hemolysis, occur in up to 15 to 20 per cent of patients. More severe blood dyscrasias, high fever, leukopenia, and agranulocytosis are rare. A reversible loss of fertility may occur in some patients. Many of these side effects occur in patients taking 4 grams or more of sulfasalazine per day; reduction to a dose of 2 to 3 grams is often effective. Sulfapyridine is acetylated in the liver after absorption before being excreted in the urine. Many of the patients with adverse effects are genetic slow acetylators. Sulfasalazine is effective in treating moderate colitis, and continued treatment lessens the frequency of recurrent attacks. Newer compounds, such as sustained-release 5-aminosalicylic acid, have been devised to transport this compound into the colon without sulfapyridine.

Active Chronic Colitis. For patients with chronic symptoms resulting from persistent inflammation, topical corticosteroids in addition to sulfasalazine and antidiarrheal preparations are used. Azathioprine* may be of benefit in the rare patient who is dependent on corticosteroids and for whom surgical management is inappropriate. In general, there is a reluctance to use azathioprine in children or in adults who have not completed their families in view of the mutagenic potential of the drug. The aim in quiescent colitis is to prolong remission. Sulfasalazine (2 to 3 grams per day orally) has been demonstrated to be effective. The newer 5-aminosalicylic acid formulations may also be useful in such patients.

Surgical Therapy. Proctocolectomy with construction of an ileostomy cures ulcerative colitis and leads to a remission or improvement in many of the peripheral manifestations. Absolute indications for subtotal or total colectomy are (1) *perforation*, with or without abscess formation; (2) *colonic carcinoma*, for which total proctocolectomy and lymph node dissection are required; and (3) *massive hemorrhage*. Relative indications are as follows: (1) Severe acute colitis with or without toxic dilatation of the colon (toxic megacolon), with failure to respond to maximal therapy. The current trend is toward earlier surgical intervention in this group of patients after restoration of plasma volume, administration of antibiotics, corticosteroids, and total parenteral nutrition for as long as possible preoperatively. In the absence of toxic dilatation many clinicians are willing to wait for seven to ten days before advising surgery. It is indefensible to extend medical therapy in a patient who continues to bleed and who has high fever, tachycardia, severe diarrhea, depleted intravascular and extravascular volumes, hypoalbuminemia, and electrolyte depletion. (2) Failure of medical management. The patient with chronic symptoms or frequent relapses over a period of five years or longer, particularly in the face of corticosteroid-induced complications, has the promise of improved quality of life after proctocolectomy and ileostomy. Although this decision is particularly difficult in children, it should not be delayed, since the risk of growth retardation in children is great (see Growth Retardation, Ch. 105.2). (3) Suspicion of cancer. In a patient with extensive colitis of long duration the presence of dysplastic changes or a mass lesion with overlying dysplasia may be used as a basis for recommending proctocolectomy. Other considerations may include chronic symptoms or the presence of a highly suspicious persisting stricture even after endoscopic biopsy and cytology have failed to reveal malignancy.

The internist, surgeon, and stoma therapist all play an important role in the pre- and postoperative education and management of the patient with proctocolectomy and ileostomy. The mortality of elective proctocolectomy is approximately 1 to 3 per cent. Over two thirds of patients have no postoperative complications such as hemorrhage, intra-abdominal sepsis, or intestinal obstruction. Between 10 and 15 per cent of patients with a standard ileostomy (Brooke) following proctocolectomy will require some form of surgical revision of the stoma. The reoperation rate for the continent ileostomy (Kock) is as high as 20 to 30 per cent in some series, and postoperative complications and dysfunction not requiring operation are common. The continent ileostomy is contraindicated in Crohn's disease, in fulminating ulcerative colitis, in cases of diagnostic uncertainty, in emotionally unstable patients, and when experienced surgeons are unavailable. Other, rare complications include impotence (less than 2 per cent, in contrast to a universal incidence after an abdominoperineal resection for carcinoma of the rectum) and damage to the ureters. Healing of the perineal wound may be delayed for up to six months. Patients who are about to undergo or have undergone proctocolectomy with ileostomy will benefit from referral to groups such as the Ileostomy

*This use is not listed in the manufacturer's directive.

Association or Ileoptomists. Ingenious procedures have been developed with the goal of preserving rectal muscle and anal sphincter function. These include ileoanal anastomosis after construction of an ileal reservoir in the pelvis. Particularly in the young, intelligent patient, such procedures may be useful alternatives to the conventional ileostomy.

ULCERATIVE COLITIS AND PREGNANCY. About one third of patients with inactive ulcerative colitis have exacerbation and about two thirds with active disease have worsening of their condition either during pregnancy or in the early postpartum period. For those with continuing active colitis the worsening is likely to occur in the first trimester. When the first attack of ulcerative colitis occurs during pregnancy or the postpartum period, symptoms are often severe. About 10 per cent of pregnancies in women with ulcerative colitis will terminate in spontaneous abortions.

The general diagnostic and therapeutic measures previously described apply to pregnant patients. Radiographic studies should be minimized and proctoscopy performed only when necessary, especially during the first trimester. The usual indications for corticosteroid therapy apply. Sulfasalazine therapy during pregnancy has not been reported to have adverse effects on the fetus. Azathioprine is not used during pregnancy, although no adverse effects upon the fetus have been reported. Therapeutic abortion has little place in the management of pregnant patients with ulcerative colitis except for the rare instances of women in the first trimester who are desperately ill and are likely to lose the child. Women with quiescent ulcerative colitis should not be discouraged from pregnancy. In the presence of active colitis, pregnancy should be postponed until control of the colitis has been achieved for at least one year.

ULCERATIVE PROCTITIS. Ulcerative proctitis probably represents ulcerative colitis limited to the rectum. Typically the patient presents with mild or moderate rectal bleeding, rectal tenesmus, and an increased number of bowel movements. Symptomatic episodes recur periodically several times a year.

The macroscopic and microscopic features are similar to those described previously for ulcerative colitis, although only the distal 3 to 10 cm of the rectum may be involved. On sigmoidoscopy there is usually a sharp line of demarcation between the distal inflammatory process and normal proximal rectal or lower sigmoid mucosa.

Therapy includes the general measures described for ulcerative colitis, with the use of sulfasalazine, 2 to 3 grams per day by mouth, and topical corticosteroids. Commonly used preparations include enemas containing 100 mg of hydrocortisone or 40 mg of methylprednisone, administered once daily. Steroid suppositories (25 mg of hydrocortisone) or steroid foam (90 mg of hydrocortisone per dose) may be inserted into the rectum once or twice daily. Newer forms of therapy include topical 5-aminosalicylic acid and nonabsorbable corticosteroids. Response to treatment is usually very satisfactory, although occasional patients may remain symptomatic despite intensive therapy.

PROGNOSIS OF ULCERATIVE COLITIS. The outlook for recovery from a first attack of ulcerative colitis is very good. Mortality, which is about 5 per cent, occurs almost exclusively in those who have a severe form of the disease involving the entire colon. The mortality is higher in patients over 60 years, approximately 17 per cent, compared with 2 per cent in patients between ages 20 and 59. Toxic megacolon has a mortality rate of about 20 per cent. Death generally results from the complications of massive hemorrhage, systemic infections, pulmonary embolism, or associated cardiac disorders. Better medical therapy and earlier colectomy for patients who do not respond to medical therapy have improved the overall acute prognosis.

After the first attack about 10 per cent of patients will have a remission lasting up to 15 years or more. An additional 10 per cent will experience continuously active colitis. The remainder (80 per cent) experience remissions and exacerbations of their disease over the ensuing years irrespective of the severity of the initial attack. About one fifth of patients with ulcerative colitis require proctocolectomy at some stage in their illness. After the first postoperative year, the long-term prognosis for patients with colectomy for ulcerative colitis is similar to that of the general population. With continuous improvements in medical and surgical management, the outlook for both survival and quality of life continues to improve.

Allan RN, Keighley MRB, Alexander-Williams J, et al. (eds.): Inflammatory Bowel Disease. Edinburgh, Churchill-Livingstone, 1983. *A multiauthored, well-referenced book covering all aspects, with representation from North America and Britain.*

Cello JP: Ulcerative colitis. In Sleisenger MH, Fordtran JS (eds.): Gastrointestinal Disease. 4th ed. Philadelphia, W. B. Saunders Company, 1988. *An excellent general review with an extensive bibliography.*

Dozois RR (ed.): Alternatives to continent ileostomy. Chicago, Year Book Medical Publishers, 1985. *A detailed consideration of newer surgical alternatives in the management of ulcerative colitis.*

Faintuch JS, Levin B, Kirsner JB: Inflammatory bowel disease and malignancy. CRC Crit Rev Oncol Hematol 2:323, 1985. *An extensive review of the association of neoplasia with ulcerative colitis and Crohn's disease.*

Hanauer SB, Kirsner JB (eds.): Inflammatory Bowel Disease: A Guide for Patients and Their Families. New York, Raven Press, 1985. *A useful text for the education of patients and family members with helpful, common-sense advice.*

Kirsner JB, Shorter RG (eds.): Inflammatory Bowel Disease. Philadelphia, Lea & Febiger, 1987. *An in-depth monograph with chapters by leading authorities on incidence trends, pathology, etiology, and medical and surgical therapy.*

Riddell RH, Goldman H, Ransohoff DF, et al.: Dysplasia in inflammatory bowel disease: Standardized classification with provisional clinical applications. Hum Pathol 14:931, 1983. *A definitive description of colonic dysplasia, including an illustrative atlas.*

106 VASCULAR DISEASES OF THE INTESTINE

James H. Grendell

ANATOMY, PHYSIOLOGY, AND PATHOPHYSIOLOGY OF THE MESENTERIC CIRCULATION

The intra-abdominal portions of the digestive tract receive their blood supply almost entirely from three relatively large arteries arising from the aorta. The anatomy of these vessels, including their anastomotic interrelationships and potential for collateral formation, determines the consequences of acute or chronic vascular occlusion.

The celiac axis, the most cephalad of the three major arteries, usually originates at a level between the twelfth thoracic and the first lumbar vertebrae, passing next to the median arcuate ligament of the diaphragm (Fig. 106–1). Its branches supply the liver and biliary structures (hepatic artery), spleen (splenic artery), and the stomach (left gastric and gastroepiploic, short gastrics, and branches of the gastroduodenal, including the right gastroepiploic). The gastroduodenal artery gives rise to the superior pancreaticoduodenal arteries, which not only provide part of the blood supply to the pancreas and duodenum but also form anastomoses with the inferior pancreaticoduodenal arteries, which are derived from the superior mesenteric artery. These interconnections, the pancreaticoduodenal arcades, are an important potential route for collateral blood flow between the celiac and the superior mesenteric arteries.

The superior mesenteric artery originates behind the pancreas at the level of the first lumbar vertebra, just caudal to the celiac axis (Fig. 106–2). In addition to the inferior pancreaticoduodenal arteries, the superior mesenteric artery gives rise to branches supplying the small and large intestines from the distal duodenum to the distal transverse colon. These intestinal branches form a series of three or four arcades before entering the wall of the intestine as arteriae rectae. Although

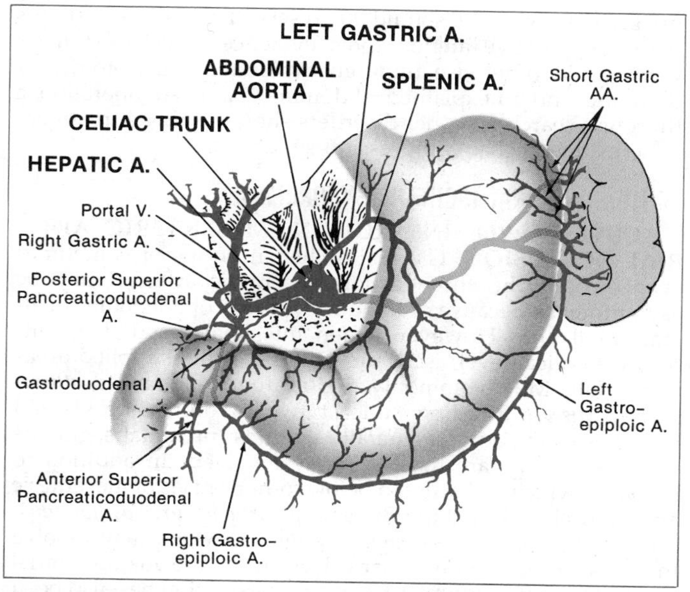

FIGURE 106–1. Arterial supply to the stomach and duodenum, showing major branches of the celiac axis and the superior portion of the pancreaticoduodenal arcades. (From Grendell JH, Ockner RK: In Sleisenger MH, Fordtran JS [eds.]: Gastrointestinal Disease. 3rd ed. Philadelphia, W. B. Saunders Company, 1983.)

there is considerable potential for collateral flow within the primary and secondary arcades, the arteriae rectae appear to represent end-arteries, and few, if any, important anastomotic connections are present within the bowel wall itself. Accordingly, selective occlusion of these more distal vessels, as may occur in vasculitis, may lead to segmental infarction.

The inferior mesenteric artery, the smallest of the three major arteries, supplies the distal transverse colon, the descending and sigmoid colon, and the proximal portions of the rectum.

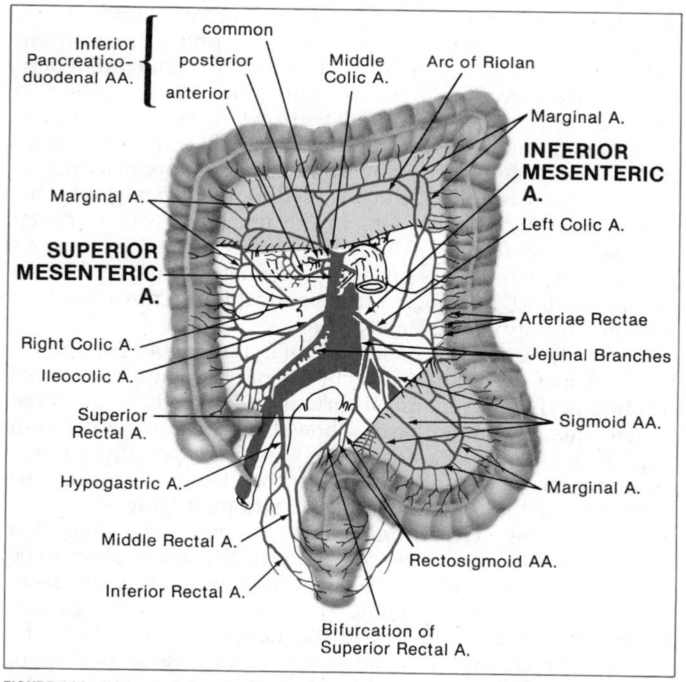

FIGURE 106–2. Arterial supply to the small and large intestines, showing the inferior portion of the pancreaticoduodenal arcades and the anastomoses between superior and inferior mesenteric arteries (arc of Riolan or "meandering mesenteric," and the marginal artery). (From Grendell JH, Ockner RK. In Sleisenger MH, Fordtran JS [eds.]: Gastrointestinal Disease. 3rd ed. Philadelphia, W. B. Saunders Company, 1983.)

Its branches form a series of arcades ending in arteriae rectae similar to what is found in the superior mesenteric artery's distribution. Branches of the inferior mesenteric artery connect with those of the superior mesenteric artery via the arc of Riolan ("meandering mesenteric artery") and the marginal artery (Fig. 106–2), and with the inferior and middle rectal branches of the hypogastric (internal iliac) arteries.

In general, veins parallel arteries in the smaller branches and for portions of the main mesenteric trunks. However, rather than entering the vena cava directly, the superior mesenteric and splenic veins join to form the portal vein, which enters the liver after receiving additional blood from the gastric circulation via the coronary vein. The inferior mesenteric vein usually drains into the splenic vein.

The blood supply to the intra-abdominal portion of the gastrointestinal tract is richly endowed with anastomotic interconnections that help protect against the consequences of occlusive vascular disease. If the occlusive process is chronically progressive, these interconnections usually permit sufficient collateral flow to maintain intestinal viability. In fact it is possible for *all* of the intra-abdominal digestive tract to be adequately supplied by only one of its three primary arterial sources. Conversely, the collateral supply may be only marginally adequate or nonexistent in certain areas, such as the arteriae rectae and intramural arteries. Also potentially vulnerable are the "watershed" areas in the distal transverse colon and splenic flexure and at the junction of the superior and middle portions of the rectum, where branches of the inferior mesenteric artery anastomose with branches of the superior mesenteric and hypogastric arteries, respectively. This may, in part, explain why segmental infarction of the colon occurs most commonly in the region of the splenic flexure and rectosigmoid.

The mesenteric circulation is regulated by three different means: (1) *Intrinsic regulation* or local modulation of blood flow occurs in response to changes in arteriolar transmural pressure or to alterations in tissue oxygenation in order to maintain adequate blood flow and oxygen delivery. Examples of this include the vasodilatation observed after brief periods of arterial occlusion (reactive hyperemia) and during digestion of a meal (functional hyperemia). Functional hyperemia may also, in part, be due to the effects of regulatory gastrointestinal peptides. (2) *Extrinsic neurologic regulation* of intestinal blood flow is mediated by sympathetic postganglionic fibers originating from the splanchnic nerves, which cause constriction of arteries and arterioles and a reduction in intestinal blood flow. Continued stimulation of these nerves, however, leads to a partial or in some cases complete recovery of flow (autoregulatory escape). (3) *Circulating endogenous and exogenous agents* may affect mesenteric blood flow. Increased arteriolar resistance is caused by α-adrenergic agonists, vasopressin, angiotensin II, prostaglandin F_2, and digitalis glycosides. Vasodilatation and increased blood flow result from the actions of β-adrenergic agonists, prostaglandin E_2, and the gut hormones cholecystokinin, gastrin, and glucagon.

The microcirculation of the intra-abdominal digestive organs is controlled by (1) the arteriole that, as the major site of resistance, is the most important local determinant of overall mesenteric blood flow, and (2) the precapillary sphincter, which determines capillary perfusion.

Several factors are important in determining the extent, severity, or possible reversibility of ischemic processes or events. The first of these is the abruptness of a vascular occlusion; more gradually occlusive processes may permit development of collaterals. A second factor is size and configuration of a vessel; emboli most commonly enter the large, obliquely situated superior mesenteric artery. A third factor is the level of involvement of a localized occlusive process. Vasculitis involving arteriae rectae or intramural arteries does not allow for development of collateral blood flow and may result in ischemia of a limited segment of intestine.

Intestinal ischemia may occur in hypoxic or low cardiac output states in the absence of an anatomic obstruction to blood flow (nonocclusive intestinal infarction). It is postulated that this may result from (1) the formation of toxic superoxide anions, (2) loss of the protective function of small intestinal brush border glycoproteins against the deleterious effects of luminal pancreatic proteases and bacterial toxins, or (3) shunting of oxygen from the villus tip caused by a countercurrent exhange resulting from the arrangement of blood vessels in the villus.

CHRONIC INTESTINAL ISCHEMIC SYNDROMES

ABDOMINAL ANGINA. This uncommon syndrome is due to severe atherosclerosis involving at least two of the three major arterial supplies to the intestine. There is usually a history of intermittent dull or cramping midabdominal pain characteristically beginning 15 to 30 minutes after eating and lasting for 1 to 2 hours. This is the period of increased intestinal blood flow and oxygen consumption required for digestion and absorption. Patients may also have lost a substantial amount of weight owing mainly to a decrease in food consumption resulting from fear of the pain associated with eating. Mild-to-moderate malabsorption may also be present. Physical examination usually uncovers evidence of atherosclerotic disease involving other vessels. The presence or absence of an abdominal bruit is not of diagnostic value. A presumptive diagnosis may be made on the basis of a strongly suggestive history and the angiographic demonstration of significant (> 50 per cent) narrowing of at least two of the three major arteries. Often there is evidence of collateral flow. Many patients who are asymptomatic, however, may show similar angiographic findings. Surgical treatment has included bypass, endarterectomy, and reimplantation procedures with significant relief of symptoms in most patients. Percutaneous transluminal angioplasty has also been employed successfully and offers the possibility that nonoperative approaches may also prove useful in some patients. As many as 50 per cent of patients with acute mesenteric arterial occlusion (see below) give a history suggestive of previous abdominal angina. Successful treatment of chronic intestinal ischemia may prevent such a catastrophic outcome.

CELIAC COMPRESSION SYNDROME. Recurrent abdominal pain in some individuals has been found to be associated with narrowing of the celiac axis alone. These patients, generally younger women in otherwise good health, complain of epigastric pain of variable frequency and duration. The pain may or may not be related to meals and is infrequently accompanied by nausea and vomiting. An epigastric bruit that does not radiate to the lower abdomen is the only physical finding that has been frequently described. Lateral views of the celiac axis during angiography demonstrate narrowing near its origin. At surgery this has usually been ascribed to compression by the median arcuate ligament of the diaphragm. In some cases, however, the stenosis has been reported to be due to neurofibrous tissue of the celiac ganglion or to intimal narrowing of the vessel itself. Surgical therapy has involved either division of the obstructing structure or bypass grafting, usually with relief of symptoms. The symptoms have recurred with time in some patients. The validity of this syndrome is a matter of considerable controversy for several reasons: (1) similar degrees of celiac axis narrowing have been found incidentally at angiography or autopsy in a substantial number of patients without symptoms of this syndrome, and (2) stenosis of the celiac axis alone would not be expected to result in symptomatic intestinal ischemia because of mesenteric collateral vessels. Some investigators believe that the pain is not truly ischemic but may arise in the celiac ganglion, which is removed or disrupted by most surgical treatments for this syndrome. Resolution of this controversy will require more precise clinical and pathophysiologic definition of the syndrome, including detailed follow-up studies. Surgery should be reserved for those patients with preoperative angiographic evidence of celiac stenosis who would otherwise undergo exploratory laparotomy for disabling and unexplained abdominal pain. At operation a thorough search for other disorders should precede treatment for presumed celiac compression syndrome.

ACUTE INTESTINAL ISCHEMIC SYNDROMES

ACUTE BOWEL INFARCTION: MESENTERIC ARTERIAL OCCLUSION. Gradual occlusion of one or sometimes even two of the three major mesenteric arteries may be asymptomatic because of the development of adequate collateral circulation. However, when intestinal blood flow falls below a critical level, ischemic necrosis of the supplied areas will result. Most commonly this is due to advanced *atherosclerotic disease* affecting at least two of the major visceral branches of the aorta. Generally the most proximal segments of these arteries are most severely involved. In addition to *embolism,* which is discussed below, other causes of mesenteric arterial occlusion include dissecting *aortic aneurysm, fibromuscular hyperplasia,* and *systemic vasculitides,* which may involve the mesenteric arteries at any level from the major arterial trunks to the intramural arteries. An association has also been reported with the use of *oral contraceptives.*

Diagnosis. The early diagnosis of acute intestinal infarction is often difficult. The history usually is not very helpful, but evidence of "abdominal angina" (see above) or other conditions predisposing to thrombosis may aid in the evaluation. Patients frequently have *severe abdominal pain* that initially may be colicky in nature and periumbilical in location. Bowel sounds not only may be present but may even be hyperactive. At this stage the patient's complaint of pain often appears out of proportion to physical findings or laboratory studies. As ischemia progresses, pain becomes constant and poorly localized. Systemic manifestations become prominent and severe, including *tachycardia, hypotension, fever, leukocytosis, acidosis,* and the presence of *blood* in nasogastric aspirate, vomitus, or stool. It has been suggested, on the basis of small numbers of patients and experimental animal studies, that elevations in serum and peritoneal fluid phosphate concentration may be sensitive indicators of intestinal infarction. Because an elevation in serum phosphate concentration in this setting is often associated with extensive bowel injury, acute renal insufficiency, and acidosis, it implies a poor prognosis. Abdominal radiographs usually show evidence of an *ileus* with distended, thick-walled loops of bowel and air-fluid levels (Fig. 106–3). Gas in the intestinal wall or portal vein is a late finding. Ultimately, when ischemic necrosis becomes transmural, signs of *peritonitis,* including bloody peritoneal fluid, appear. At this point, the prognosis (with or without surgery) is extremely poor.

The early diagnosis of bowel infarction depends upon a high index of suspicion and exclusion of other intra-abdominal conditions that can manifest virtually identically (e.g., acute pancreatitis, perforated viscus, bowel obstruction). A decision regarding extensive radiographic studies, especially angiography, in patients with suspected bowel infarction must be individualized. For the patient in whom hypotension, acidosis, or signs of peritonitis are present, suggesting that perforation may have already occurred, the information to be obtained from further studies may not justify the necessary delay in surgical management. However, earlier in the course, angiography may help define the nature and extent of the occlusive process or, in the absence of major vessel occlusion, suggest the diagnosis of nonocclusive infarction. Interpretation, however, is often difficult and clinical judgment is based only in part on angiographic findings. Computed tomography shows promise of becoming a rapid, noninvasive means of confirming the diagnosis of acute bowel infarction by identifying characteristic changes in the appearance of the bowel wall and mesentery.

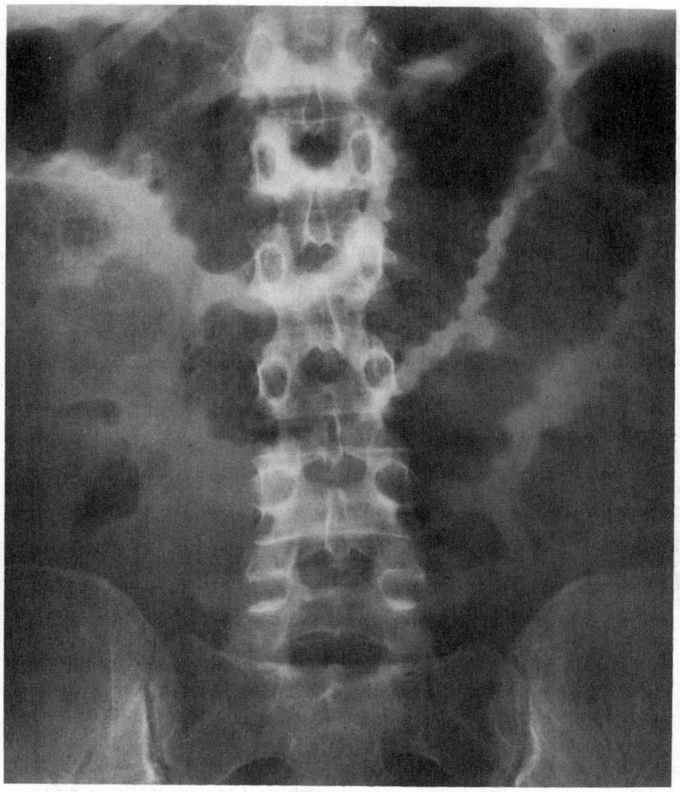

FIGURE 106–3. A supine abdominal x-ray in a patient with acute infarction of the small intestine showing dilated loops of small bowel with irregular thickening of the bowel wall.

Treatment. Initial supportive therapy, aimed at stabilization of the patient's condition prior to surgery, includes nasogastric suction, replacement of fluid and electrolyte deficits, administration of broad-spectrum antibiotics after blood cultures have been obtained, and cardiopulmonary support, if needed. As soon as the patient's condition is adequately stabilized and the diagnosis strongly suspected, prompt surgical exploration should be performed. At surgery, resection of necrotic bowel is the primary objective. An attempt may be made to revascularize the remaining viable intestine by bypass graft or endarterectomy if the patient's condition is sufficiently stable to perform the additional surgery.

At the time of operation it is important but sometimes difficult to define the limits of viable bowel in order to resect completely irreversibly diseased intestine while at the same time avoiding unnecessary development of the short bowel syndrome. It is often necessary to perform a "second-look" operation 12 to 36 hours after the initial exploration to identify and resect any additional bowel that in the interim proves to be nonviable. Infarction of large segments of intestine carries essentially a 100 per cent mortality rate without surgery. Even with surgery the mortality rate is > 50 per cent in most series because of delay in diagnosis or because of other complicating factors such as advanced age or atherosclerotic disease involving other vital organs.

Mesenteric vasculitis (e.g., as may occur in lupus erythematosus, polyarteritis nodosa, dermatomyositis, rheumatoid vasculitis, and Henoch-Schönlein purpura) may cause segmental intestinal infarction not conforming to the distribution of the major arteries. Vascular occlusion may not be demonstrable angiographically if only intramural arteries and arterioles are involved. Although some patients may require emergency surgery for intestinal necrosis and perforation, these complications are less common than with occlusions of the major arteries or their principal branches. In some cases the acute episode may resolve spontaneously, which may leave the patient with a segmental stricture demonstrable by barium contrast studies.

MESENTERIC ARTERY EMBOLISM. Emboli to the mesenteric circulation most commonly involve the superior mesenteric artery because of its size and the oblique angle of its origin from the aorta. These emboli usually arise from mural thrombi in the heart in patients with atherosclerotic or valvular heart disease but may also arise from vegetations of bacterial endocarditis, atrial myxomas, valvular prostheses, or atherosclerotic plaques in the thoracic or upper abdominal aorta, either spontaneously or during angiography. Patients may have a history of previous embolic episodes or exhibit evidence of simultaneous peripheral embolization (e.g., to the brain or extremities). Typically patients described the *abrupt onset of severe midabdominal cramping pain,* accompanied by vomiting or diarrhea. Although patients may feel and appear severely ill, early in the course objective physical findings are sparse. If the diagnosis is not made promptly and appropriate treatment undertaken, a mesenteric embolus will lead to bowel infarction. Angiography may demonstrate mesenteric artery occlusion in the absence of collateral circulation, indicating the acute nature of the process. Computed tomography may also strongly suggest the diagnosis early in the course of the disease in a patient with acute onset of abdominal pain of unknown source. Following supportive measures as needed to stabilize the patient's condition, immediate exploration with embolectomy and resection of any infarcted bowel is indicated. A "second-look" procedure will sometimes be necessary. The characteristic setting in which mesenteric embolism occurs, as well as its abrupt onset, offers a greater opportunity for early diagnosis and treatment. For this reason, and because the patients generally are younger, the prognosis is more favorable than for most nonembolic causes of bowel infarction. Some patients who are successfully treated by embolectomy without need for bowel resection may develop a transient malabsorption syndrome persisting for several months.

NONOCCLUSIVE INTESTINAL INFARCTION. In some patients clinical findings suggestive of mesenteric arterial occlusive disease or embolism occur without a demonstrable obstruction to arterial flow. This syndrome, now recognized with increasing frequency, usually occurs in the setting of severe congestive heart failure, shock, hypoxia, or a recent myocardial infarction. In addition, it has been reported following cocaine ingestion, possibly related to α-adrenergic stimulation due to the drug. The clinical course often evolves more slowly than is seen with occlusive processes. Occasionally a precipitating event is not identifiable. The use of α-adrenergic vasoconstrictors (and possibly digitalis glycosides) may also contribute to the development of this process. Because of its high degree of metabolic activity, the mucosa has the greatest requirement for intestinal blood flow of the various layers of the bowel wall. Thus it will show the earliest evidence of ischemic injury. At times, it may be the only portion to undergo hemorrhagic infarction. However, infarction may ultimately become transmural and occur in a patchy and irregular distribution, not conforming to the area supplied by a major vessel. Early angiography is useful to exclude a major vessel occlusion, which would usually require vascular surgery. In at least 50 per cent of such patients angiography reveals irregular narrowing of the major arterial branches and arcades (due to spasm) and impaired filling of the intramural vessels. Therapy consists of supportive measures and surgical exploration to resect infarcted bowel if the patient's situation suggests the need for this. Selective infusion of vasodilators into the mesenteric circulation has been suggested, but its therapeutic efficacy remains to be established. This syndrome generally carries a very poor prognosis, primarily because it is usually associated with shock or severe cardiopulmonary disease.

ISCHEMIC COLITIS. Ischemic injury to the colon may be

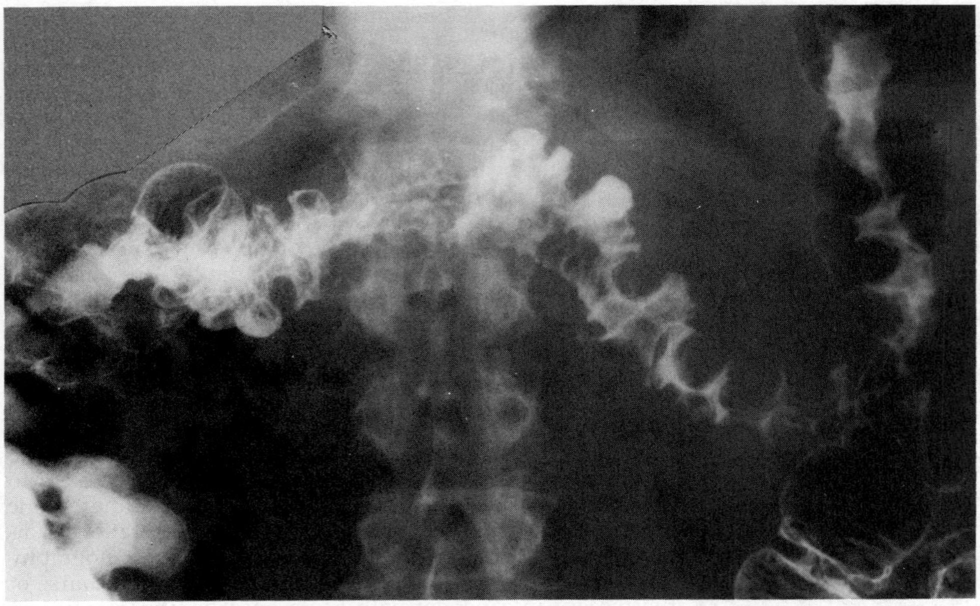

FIGURE 106–4. A barium enema in a patient with ischemic colitis showing narrowing and "thumbprinting" (nodular indentations of the bowel wall) in the distal transverse colon. This is one of the "watershed" areas of the colon between two adjacent arterial supplies (superior and inferior mesenteric arteries) where ischemia is more likely to develop.

caused by advanced atherosclerosis or interruption of the colonic blood supply during surgery (e.g., abdominal aortic aneurysmectomy, aortoiliac reconstruction, abdominoperineal resection) or may occur in association with "hypercoagulable" states, amyloidosis, vasculitis, ruptured aortic aneurysm, colorectal cancer, or the use of oral contraceptive agents. In addition, nonocclusive colonic ischemia may occur in states of low cardiac output or hypoxia. Nonocclusive colonic ischemia may be mediated primarily by the renin-angiotensin system, to which the colonic vasculature appears to be remarkably sensitive. The syndrome of ischemic colitis may be quite variable in its extent, severity, and prognosis. However, extensive infarction and perforation appear to be infrequent. Localized or segmental ischemia is more common, particularly affecting those areas of the colon that lie on the "watershed" between two adjacent arterial supplies, i.e., the splenic flexure (superior and inferior mesenteric arteries) and the rectosigmoid (inferior mesenteric and internal iliac arteries). Characteristically, patients over the age of 50 are most often affected with *abrupt onset of lower abdominal cramping pain, rectal bleeding*, and, to variable degrees, *vomiting* and *fever*. Some patients give a history of similar symptoms occurring intermittently for weeks to months before presentation. Left-sided abdominal tenderness and peritoneal signs may be present, as well as evidence of generalized atherosclerotic disease. Sigmoidoscopy may be normal; may show evidence of mild, nonspecific proctitis; or may reveal a spectrum of findings, including multiple discrete ulcers, blue-black hemorrhagic submucosal blebs, or an adherent pseudomembrane. Angiography generally has not proved useful in the diagnosis of patients in this setting. The differentiation of ischemic colitis from infections of the colon, diverticulitis, and idiopathic inflammatory bowel disease (ulcerative colitis, Crohn's disease of the colon) may be very difficult. Initial management consists of general supportive measures, including antibiotics. In those patients in whom perforation or infarction of the colon appears likely, early surgical exploration is indicated; however, many patients will improve without surgery. Subsequent barium enema will often show a characteristic picture of intramural hemorrhage and edema, including "thumbprinting," tubular narrowing, and "sawtooth" irregularity (Fig. 106–4). Some patients will proceed to complete resolution of the clinical process and radiographic abnormalities. Others will develop a residual stricture that eventually may require surgical resection.

MESENTERIC VENOUS THROMBOSIS. This condition, which accounts for about 5 to 15 per cent of patients with intestinal ischemia, almost always involves the superior mesenteric vein. It is associated with a variety of conditions: stasis in the mesenteric venous bed (portal hypertension, congestive heart failure), abdominal neoplasms, intra-abdominal inflammation (peritonitis, abscess, inflammatory bowel disease), abdominal surgery and trauma, a variety of presumed hypercoagulable states (antithrombin III deficiency, polycythemia vera), and use of oral contraceptives. Occasionally a predisposing condition is absent. Patients may have abrupt onset of a clinical picture indicative of acute bowel infarction; however, many others have a more gradual course with development of progressive abdominal discomfort over a period of weeks. Physical findings are nonspecific. The presence of a small amount of bloody peritoneal fluid is typical and may be an important clue to the diagnosis in patients with a subacute clinical course. Selective superior mesenteric angiography shows intense spasm of the arteries to the involved segment of bowel and absence of venous drainage.

Following initial supportive care to stabilize the patient's condition, an operation should be performed to resect infarcted or severely ischemic bowel. Reconstructive venous surgery is not generally possible. Because there is about a 25 per cent rate of recurrent thrombosis within the first several weeks postoperatively, anticoagulation is recommended except in patients who have underlying disease processes that would make this too hazardous. A "second-look" operation to search for recurrent thrombosis may also be required if there is unexplained clinical deterioration following initial surgery. In general, the prognosis is more favorable than for patients with mesenteric arterial disease, with reported mortality as low as 20 per cent.

MISCELLANEOUS DISORDERS

INTRAMURAL INTESTINAL HEMORRHAGE. This may follow abdominal trauma or may occur in the setting of ischemic bowel injury, vasculitis, or bleeding diatheses. Some patients have a picture suggesting a perforated viscus (severe abdominal pain, tenderness, leukocytosis), but most have cramping abdominal pain and vomiting suggestive of partial or complete bowel obstruction. Hematemesis or melena and fever may be present. Occasionally a palpable abdominal mass caused by the presence of a hematoma may be noted. Barium studies of the small intestine typically show a "stacked coins" or "thumbprint" appearance. Usually intramural intestinal hemorrhage can be managed conservatively with nasogastric suction, intravenous hydration and electrolytes, and correction of an underlying coagulopathy, when possible. In those patients with high-grade or unremitting intestinal obstruction, or in whom signs of peritonitis develop (suggesting perforation), surgery is necessary.

PARAPROSTHETIC-ENTERIC AND AORTOENTERIC FISTULAS. Following aortic aneurysmectomy and other procedures in which vascular prostheses are placed in the abdomen or retroperitoneum, fistulas may form between the graft and adjacent bowel. This may occur as early as several weeks postoperatively but in most cases is delayed by at least two years. This complication usually results from local infection or damage to the intestine or its blood supply at surgery, with subsequent erosion of the bowel wall by the graft. Patients may present with massive upper or lower gastrointestinal bleeding or both that may be rapidly fatal without emergency surgery. In a number of patients, however, bleeding may be initially intermittent, resembling that from a number of more common lesions. In these patients, early consideration of this diagnosis with urgent evaluation by upper endoscopy, radiolabeled red blood cell studies, computed tomography, and/or angiography may be required to establish the diagnosis and need for surgical intervention.

Unoperated upon abdominal aortic aneurysms and aneurysmal dilatations of other major abdominal arteries may erode into the gastrointestinal tract, causing upper or lower gastrointestinal bleeding or both of various degrees of severity.

SUPERIOR MESENTERIC ARTERY SYNDROME. This uncommon syndrome of postprandial epigastric pain, distention, and vomiting has been attributed to compression of the third portion of the duodenum between the superior mesenteric artery anteriorly and the fixed retroperitoneal structures posteriorly. This has been described as occurring most commonly in individuals who have lost a substantial amount of weight or are of "asthenic habitus," and in children with rapid growth in the absence of corresponding weight gain or who have been fixed in a position of hyperextension by a cast following spinal injury or surgery. Barium contrast studies show distention of the proximal duodenum, and lateral aortograms or abdominal sonograms have shown a narrowing of the angle between the aorta and the superior mesenteric artery. The differential diagnosis includes generalized disorders of gastrointestinal motility, such as scleroderma, and anorexia nervosa. Recommended treatment has included the use of small feedings and elemental diets with the patient lying prone or on the left side in the knee-chest position after eating. In refractory cases duodenal mobilization or duodenal-jejunal bypass has reportedly been effective in relieving symptoms. Since apparent compression of the duodenum by the superior mesenteric artery does not prove clinically significant obstruction, the diagnosis of this syndrome must be made only after other possible causes of duodenal stasis have been excluded. This entity is frequently overdiagnosed unless strict diagnostic criteria are employed.

VASCULAR MALFORMATIONS INCLUDING ANGIODYSPLASIA. Hemangiomas of the small intestine are very uncommon vascular tumors found throughout the bowel, particularly the jejunum. They represent one of the causes of gastrointestinal bleeding that may be very difficult to locate. These lesions are most reliably diagnosed by abdominal angiography.

Vascular malformations can occur in the gastrointestinal tract in association with diseases involving the skin, such as the *hereditary hemorrhagic telangiectasia (Osler-Weber-Rendu) syndrome, blue rubber bleb nevus syndrome*, and the *CREST syndrome* (calcinosis, Raynaud's phenomenon, esophageal hypomotility, sclerodactyly, and telangiectasia). In addition, vascular malformations may occur as a primary process *(angiodysplasia, vascular ectasia)* chiefly involving the colon but also occurring in the stomach or small intestine. This latter process is being increasingly recognized as a frequent cause of lower intestinal bleeding, especially in patients over the age of 60. An association of angiodysplasia with aortic stenosis has also been reported but not fully established. Angiodysplastic lesions of the stomach and small intestine may be the most common source of upper gastrointestinal bleeding in patients with chronic renal failure.

Angiodysplastic lesions consist of ectatic, tortuous submucosal veins and groups of ectatic mucosal vessels lying just under the gastric, intestinal, or colonic epithelium or at times on the luminal surface unprotected by any intestinal epithelium. The etiology of these lesions remains uncertain. One theory suggests that they develop as a result of chronic low-grade obstruction of the submucosal veins as they penetrate the muscularis propria; another theory proposes that these lesions develop because of chronic mucosal ischemia.

Larger vascular malformations, including some primary angiodysplastic lesions, may be visualized by selective mesenteric arteriography. Many of these lesions are small and are best demonstrated by endoscopy. Such lesions are present in a large number of older individuals without apparent gastrointestinal blood loss. For those patients who have chronic or recurrent gastrointestinal blood loss without other apparent cause, surgery has been recommended if vascular malformations could be identified and localized (e.g., right colectomy for lesions in the cecum). This approach is often unsatisfactory, and bleeding may recur either because some lesions in other parts of the gastrointestinal tract may not have been appreciated at the initial evaluation or because new lesions may subsequently develop. For these reasons, nonoperative endoscopic approaches have been developed to obliterate vascular malformations by such techniques as laser photocoagulation, electrocoagulation, or thermal coagulation (heater probe).

Baur CM, Millay DJ, Taylor CM, et al.: Treatment of chronic visceral ischemia. Am J Surg 148:138, 1984. *Illustrates the efficacy of surgical treatment for abdominal angina in properly selected patients.*

Cello JP, Grendell JH: Endoscopic laser treatment for gastrointestinal vascular ectasias. Ann Intern Med 104:352, 1986. *Demonstrates the effective use of nonoperative therapy for this disorder.*

Cooke M, Sande MA: Diagnosis and outcome of bowel infarction on an acute medical service. Am J Med 75:984, 1983. *Highlights the difficulty of differentiating bowel infarction from other intra-abdominal catastrophes.*

Croft RJ, Menon GP, Marston A: Does "intestinal angina" exist? A critical study of obstructed visceral arteries. Br J Surg 68:316, 1981. *A provocative report demonstrating the difficulty in relating gastrointestinal symptoms to angiographic findings.*

Federle MP, Chun G, Jeffrey RB, et al.: Computed tomographic findings in bowel infarction. Am J Roentgenol 142:91, 1984. *This report demonstrates the potential value of computed tomography in the diagnosis of vascular diseases of the intestine.*

Grendell JH, Ockner RK: Vascular diseases of the bowel. In Sleisenger MH, Fordtran JS (eds.): Gastrointestinal Disease. 4th ed. Philadelphia, W.B. Saunders Company, 1988. *A comprehensive survey including pathophysiology, diagnosis, and management.*

Hines JR, Gore RM, Ballantyne GH: Superior mesenteric artery syndrome: Diagnostic criteria and therapeutic approaches. Am J Surg 148:630, 1984. *Emphasizes the importance of strict diagnostic criteria to avoid overdiagnosis of this entity.*

Kiernan PD, Pairolero PC, Hubert JP Jr, et al.: Aortic graft–enteric fistula. Mayo Clin Proc 55:731, 1980. *A detailed review of clinical features, management, and prognosis.*

Rogers DM, Thompson JE, Garret WV, et al.: Mesenteric vascular problems: A 26-year experience. Ann Surg 195:554, 1982. *This article describes an extensive surgical experience with a variety of vascular diseases of the intestine.*

Zuckerman GR, Cornette GL, Clouse RE, et al.: Upper gastrointestinal bleeding in patients with chronic renal failure. Ann Intern Med 102:588, 1985. *Demonstrates the importance of angiodysplastic lesions as a source of upper gastrointestinal bleeding in patients with chronic renal failure.*

107 NEOPLASMS OF THE LARGE AND SMALL INTESTINE

Sidney J. Winawer

NEOPLASMS OF THE LARGE INTESTINE

Adenocarcinoma of the large intestine is a worldwide health problem of major importance, especially in western countries. The incidence of this cancer in the United States is more than 145,000 per year; more than half of those affected will die of their disease within five years of the time of diagnosis. With the exception of skin cancer, cancer of the colon, along with lung cancer and breast cancer, is one of the three leading malignancies in this country in terms of annual new cases. New concepts and new technologies for diagnosis and treatment of this cancer have evolved over the past few years, providing opportunities for earlier detection and improved survival.

The colon is the site of a variety of other malignant tumors. Its second most common primary malignant tumor is the epidermoid or squamous cell carcinoma of the anal canal and rectum. Other primary malignant tumors that can involve the colon include lymphomas, leiomyosarcomas, and malignant carcinoid tumors as well as direct invasion by tumors from adjacent sites such as stomach, uterus, ovary, and prostate. Rarely tumors from such sites as breast and lung metastasize to the colon.

The most frequent tumors that involve the large intestine are adenomas, which are present in as many as 30 to 40 per cent of asymptomatic patients over the age of 40. A variety of other benign tumors, including lipomas, leiomyomas, and benign carcinoid tumors, occur in the colon. Of these all are rare except for lipomas of the ileocecal valve. Adenomas of the large intestine will be discussed first because of their frequency and their association with cancer of the colon.

Polyps of the Colon

A polyp in a generic sense is any lesion that arises from the surface of the gastrointestinal tract and protrudes into the lumen (Fig. 107–1). Polyps are usually defined pathologically as overgrowths of epithelial tissue that may be either hyperplastic or neoplastic, benign or malignant, and of various histopathologic subtypes. They are noted clinically in the large bowel as negative shadows in the lumen demonstrated by barium enema or by direct visualization during proctosigmoidoscopy or colonoscopy. They may be single or multiple, pedunculated (on a stalk) or sessile (flat and without a stalk), and sporadic in occurrence or part of a dominantly transmitted familial polyposis syndrome. Their importance lies in their frequency, their occasional production of symptoms (bleeding), and most of all their potential for malignant transformation. They are to be distinguished from pseudopolyps, which have an inflammatory mass in association with normal epithelium.

PATHOLOGY. In addition to carcinoma of the large intestine, which may present as a polypoid mass, four distinct types of benign polyps arise from colonic epithelium: (1) hyperplastic (metaplastic), (2) tubular adenomas, (3) villous adenomas, and (4) mixed type. *Hyperplastic polyps*, which account for about 25 per cent of all polyps and for most of the polyps of the rectum, tend to be small and asymptomatic, and are not considered to be neoplastic, based on the histologic criteria of normal cellular differentiation and a sharp line of demarcation between the polyp and the normal mucosa. *Neoplastic polyps* or adenomas have the same distribution in the colon as do cancers of the colon and account for most of the polyps above the area of the rectum. They are usually less than 1 cm in diameter (75 per cent), may be sessile or pedunculated, and represent localized neoplastic tumors of colonic epithelium. Histologically they have abnormal cellular differentiation and exhibit predominantly tubular structure. *Villous adenomas* typically are spongy, exophytic, and larger than adenomatous polyps (60 per cent > 2 cm). They exhibit a predominantly glandular pattern representing overgrowth of poorly differentiated cells from the base of the crypts of Lieberkühn. They have a high association with malignant transformation. *Mixed type adenomas* contain both tubular and villous components, and the villous component tends to increase with the size of the polyp.

RELATIONSHIP OF COLONIC ADENOMAS TO CANCER. The evidence that links benign adenomas (the neoplastic polyps classified as adenomas, mixed or villous) to adenocarcinoma of the colon is compelling: (1) the epidemiology of adenocarcinomas and adenomas of the colon is similar wherever studied in the world; (2) adenocarcinomas of the colon occur in the same anatomic distribution as adenomas of the colon; (3) the risk for colorectal cancer is high in patients with a prior history of adenomas, but is lower if adenomas are removed; (4) as adenomas grow in size, the frequency of finding cancer in the adenoma increases; (5) residual adenomatous tissue can sometimes be found in colorectal cancers on pathologic examination; and (6) the association of cancer and adenomas is particularly strong in the inherited colorectal cancer syndromes, with adenocarcinomas having been documented to have arisen from the underlying adenomas. In brief, there is now very little doubt that colorectal cancer arises from an antecedent premalignant tumor of the colon, the benign adenoma.

The premalignant nature of adenomas is related to size and

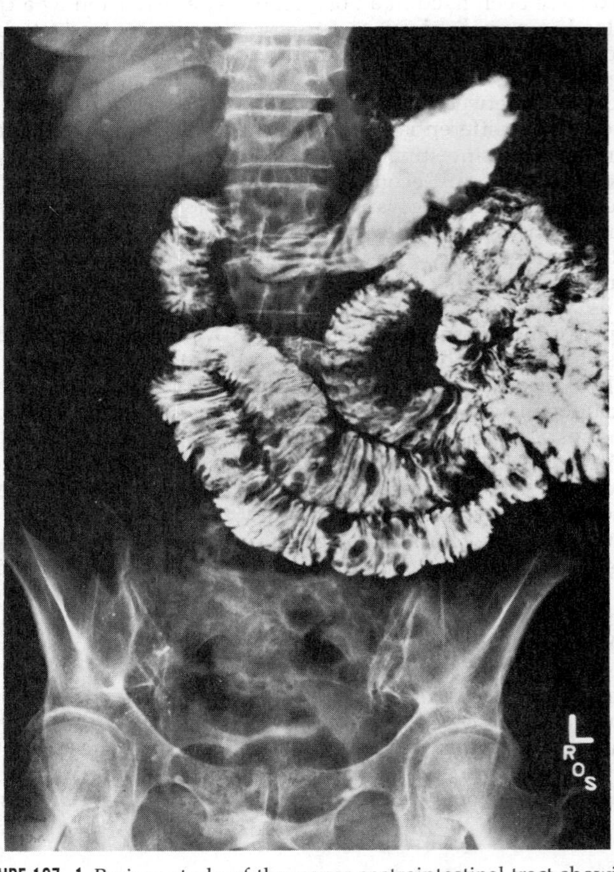

FIGURE 107–1. Barium study of the upper gastrointestinal tract showing multiple polyps of the small bowel in a patient with Peutz-Jeghers syndrome.

histology. The frequency of cancer in adenomas is 1 per cent in adenomas less than 1 cm in size; 10 per cent in adenomas between 1 and 2 cm in size; and 30 per cent in adenomas greater than 2 cm in size. The relationship of cancer to adenomas is much greater in adenomas with villous components than in adenomas without villous components. Cancer in adenomas is usually well differentiated and occurs most commonly in the tip of the adenoma without invasion of the muscularis mucosae. These are called in situ or focal cancers and are not immediately dangerous. Less commonly, cancers in adenomas invade the muscularis mucosae, and therefore have the potential to grow down the stalk, invade lymphatics, involve adjacent lymph nodes, and metastasize.

The occurrence of adenomas signifies an important transformation of the colonic mucosa to a premalignant state. Thus, it is understandable that additional adenomas often concurrently exist (synchronous adenomas) and others will appear subsequently (metachronous adenomas). The synchronous rate for adenomas is 50 per cent, and the metachronous rate is 30 to 40 per cent. Synchronous and metachronous rates for colorectal cancers are 1.5 to 5 per cent and 5 to 10 per cent, respectively. Multiple adenomas appear to be associated with a higher frequency of metachronous adenomas and metachronous cancers.

CLINICAL MANIFESTATIONS. Most polyps are asymptomatic. When symptoms do occur, they most frequently result from *bleeding* (hematochezia or iron deficiency anemia, depending on the location of the polyp and the rate of blood loss). When polyps are very large they may rarely cause *abdominal pain* from partial intestinal obstruction or from induced intussusception. Villous adenomas may rarely result in *watery diarrhea* with severe potassium depletion or in excessive secretion of mucus with loss of sufficient protein to produce hypoalbuminemia (an unusual form of "protein-losing enteropathy").

TREATMENT AND FOLLOW-UP. Because of the association of polyps with cancer of the colon, it is recommended that they be removed when identified.

Colonoscopic Polypectomy. Pedunculated polyps of any size can be removed by cautery snare through the colonoscope (see Fig. 96–3). Sessile polyps smaller than 2 cm can generally also be removed by cautery snare through the colonoscope. Controversy exists as to whether sessile polyps larger than 2 cm should be removed by colonoscopy or by surgery. Although large sessile polyps can be excised segmentally via the colonoscope, this approach is challenged because many of them already are cancerous, the risk of complications during removal is significantly increased, and the completeness of removal is uncertain. Since there is also risk involved in surgery, each case must be individualized. Suspicion that a polyp may be a polypoid adenocarcinoma warrants a biopsy and brushing for cytology. If the diagnosis of carcinoma is confirmed, surgery is indicated. Benign-appearing polyps are totally excised, not biopsied, and the entire polyp is submitted for pathologic examination. Polyps up to 7 or 8 mm in size can be removed by a combination of biopsy and fulguration. This is a particularly rapid and effective means for treating these small lesions.

After endoscopic polypectomy the patient must be followed periodically. Usually a repeat colonoscopy is performed one year later to search for missed synchronous lesions, and then approximately every three years thereafter to search for metachronous lesions. If the patient has multiple adenomas, colonoscopy is often done annually for several years.

Focal cancer in an adenoma demands special consideration. If the cancer is in the tip of the polyp and has not penetrated the muscularis mucosae, no further surgery need be done. If the cancer has penetrated the muscularis mucosae and lymphatic invasion has been demonstrated, if the cancer is poorly differentiated, or if it has extended down to the line of cautery, then follow-up laparotomy and segmental resection are indicated. In such circumstances there will be approximately a 5 per cent frequency of regional lymph node metastases.

Inherited Polyposis Syndromes of the Large and Small Intestines

There are a number of heritable syndromes characterized by polyposis of the intestine with or without additional extraintestinal manifestations. Some of these syndromes have a greatly increased frequency of cancer, and some have a slightly increased frequency of cancer.

Familial polyposis of the colon, an autosomal dominant trait, is characterized by multiple adenomas of the large intestine and rarely of the ileum as well (Fig. 107–2). In this disorder, which occurs approximately once each 8000 births, hundreds and sometimes thousands of polyps develop throughout the entire colon, beginning in childhood. Virtually all patients with familial polyposis develop carcinoma of the colon by age 40, so subtotal colectomy should be carried out early in adult life in affected persons. An intensive survey of other family members must be conducted because of the inheritance pattern; some cases occur without a family history and probably represent spontaneous mutations.

Gardner's syndrome is a dominantly transmitted disorder characterized by the triad of adenomas of the colon, bone tumors (osteomas), and soft tissue tumors (lipomas, sebaceous cysts, fibromas, fibrosarcomas) (Fig. 107–3*A*). Other associated features include retroperitoneal fibrosis, pigmented ocular fundus lesions, supernumerary teeth, and a tendency toward the development of carcinomas of the thyroid, adrenal, and duodenum in the region of the ampulla of Vater. There may be osteosclerosis of the skull in addition to the osteomas of the mandible and maxillary regions. The colonic polyps resemble those of familial polyposis and have the same potential for malignancy. The treatment is therefore subtotal colectomy and a careful survey for other affected members of the family.

Turcot's syndrome represents the rare association of adenomas of the colon with a variety of tumors of the central nervous system. The polyps have a high frequency of malignant transformation. The central nervous system lesions have included medulloblastoma, ependymoma, and glioblastoma. The mode of transmission is thought to be autosomal recessive, although this is unclear.

Peutz-Jeghers syndrome is a rare familial disorder, with autosomal dominant transmission, characterized by multiple intestinal polyposis and mucocutaneous pigmentation (Fig. 107–3*B*). The polyps, which occur in the small intestine, large intestine, and stomach, are mostly hamartomas rather than true adenomas and as such have a low potential for malignant transformation. It is estimated that 2 to 3 per cent of patients with this syndrome develop adenocarcinoma of the intestinal tract, with the small intestine being more frequently involved than the colon. Pigmentation is particularly marked in the buccal mucosa, in the hard and soft palate, on the lips, on the soles of the feet, on the dorsum of the hands, and around the mouth and nostrils. More rarely exostoses, ovarian tumors, and polyps of the bladder and nose have been described. Surgical removal of gastric and small bowel polyps is reserved only for complications such as bleeding or intestinal obstruction. True adenomas can occur in the colon in this disorder. These can usually be removed endoscopically.

Generalized juvenile polyposis refers to a familial syndrome with autosomal dominant transmission characterized by hamartomatous polyps in the colon and rectum and to a lesser extent in the small intestine and stomach. Symptoms usually begin in the first decade of life with bleeding, diarrhea, and abdominal pain. There are no extraintestinal manifestations. There seems to be an increased incidence of carcinoma of the intestine in the families with generalized juvenile polyposis, probably from true adenomas that occur with higher frequency in these families.

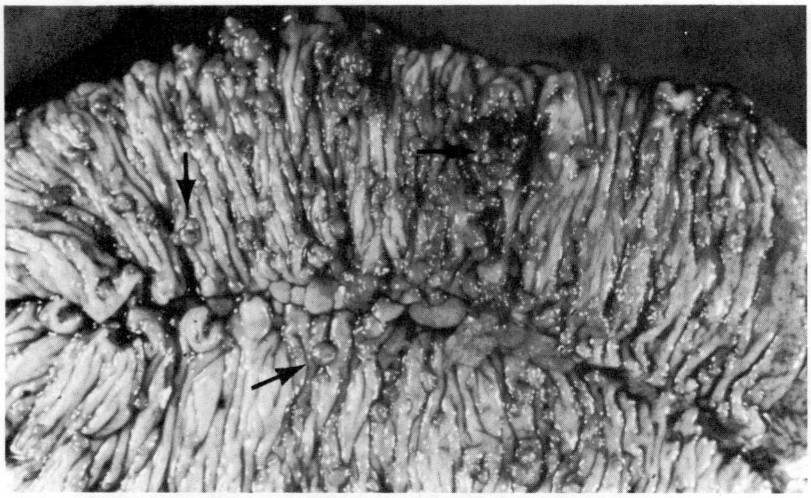

A

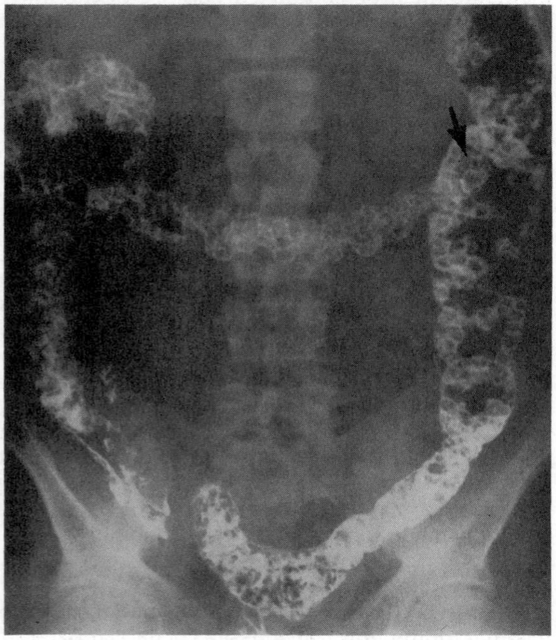

B

FIGURE 107–2. *A*, Patients with familial polyposis have multiple adenomatous polyps carpeting the colon, as demonstrated in this gross specimen. Note that the colon is diffusely studded with sessile and occasional pedunculated adenomatous polyps (*arrows*). Many of the larger polyps contain villous elements, and occasionally villous adenomas are found. Although no carcinoma was seen in this patient, nearly all patients will eventually develop colorectal carcinoma if surgery is not performed. *B*, This barium enema examination of a patient with familial polyposis represents diffuse studding of the large bowel with adenomatous polyps. Note the marked variation in size of these polyps. Although this patient did not have osteomas or soft tissue tumors, the barium enema is similar to that seen in Gardner's syndrome. (From Boland CR, Kim YS: In Sleisenger MH, Fordtran JS [eds.]: Gastrointestinal Disease. 3rd ed. Philadelphia, W. B. Saunders Company, 1983.)

Cronkhite-Canada syndrome refers to the rare association of generalized intestinal polyposis, dystrophy of the fingernails, alopecia, and cutaneous hyperpigmentation. The polyps are hamartomas; no familial association has been clearly established.

Adenocarcinoma of the Colon

EPIDEMIOLOGY. Colorectal cancer is more prevalent in the developed countries, suggesting a relationship to economic development. Its incidence is high in North America, New Zealand, and Europe and low in South America, Africa, and Asia. The United States has one of the highest rates of colorectal cancer in the world. Migrants to a particular geographic area assume the colonic cancer risk of that area. This is well illustrated by the higher incidence of the disease among blacks in America compared with those in Africa, in Puerto Ricans who have migrated to the mainland compared with those in Puerto Rico, and in first- and second-generation Japanese immigrants to Hawaii and the mainland United States compared with Japanese in Japan. In the United States the incidence of colorectal cancer is higher in the north than in the south, in urban areas compared with rural areas, and in whites compared with blacks. There is a slightly increased risk among certain occupations such as factory wood-workers.

ETIOLOGY. Migrant studies strongly suggest that *environmental factors*, particularly *diet*, are important in the etiology of colorectal cancer. There is a low incidence of appendicitis, adenomas, diverticulosis, ulcerative colitis, and colorectal cancer in the South African Bantu and other African populations in which diets contain more fiber and less animal fat than is the case with diets in more developed areas. High-fiber diets produce rapid intestinal transit so that any potential carcinogen is in contact with the mucosa for a shorter period of time. The various components of fiber may bind carcinogens or cocarcinogens or increase intraluminal bulk, and thereby dilute carcinogens. A direct association between *increased fat and animal protein* intake (particularly beef) in the western diet and the rising incidence of colonic cancer has been suggested. In Japan, the intake of fat (mostly unsaturated) provides only 12 per cent of the total caloric intake; in the United States fat intake represents 40 to 44 per cent of the total caloric intake. It has been postulated that the western diet with its high beef and fat content favors the establishment of bacterial flora capable of producing enzymes such as beta-glucuronidase and azoreductase, resulting in increased metabolism of acid and neutral sterols to carcinogens and cocarcinogens. Studies are in progress concerning putative mutagens in feces, including nitrosamide, which has been demonstrated in the feces of persons on high-beef diets. Reduction in mutagenicity

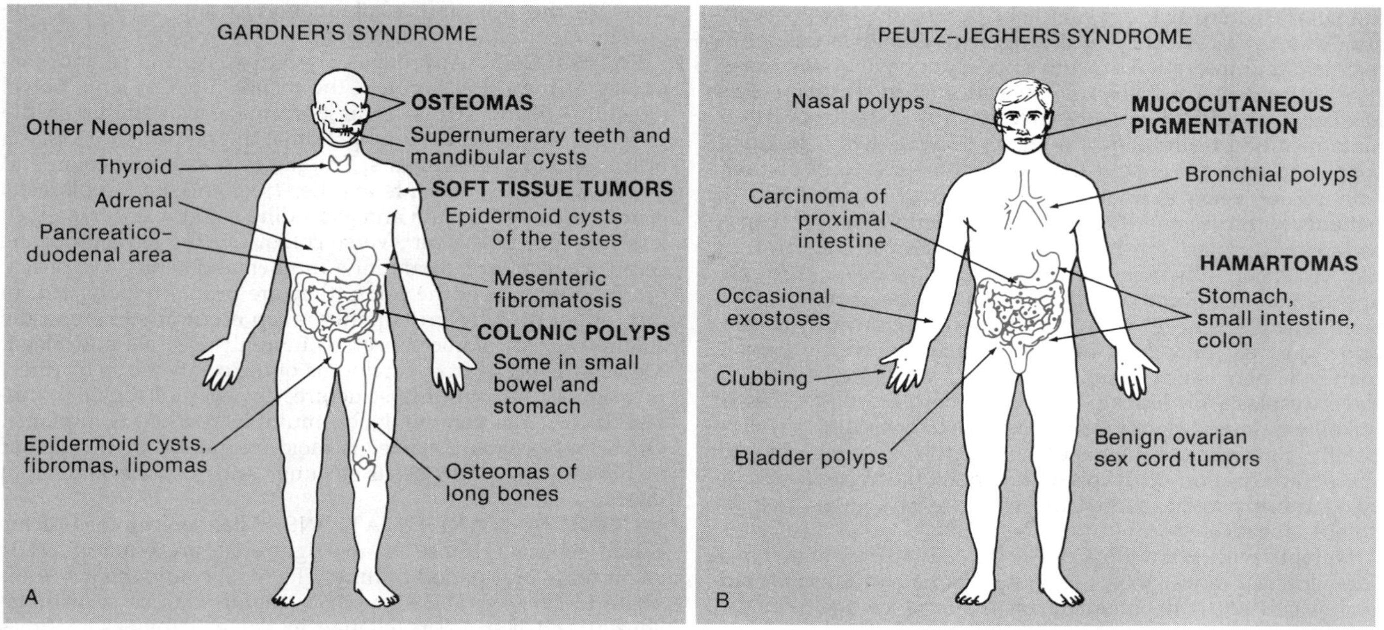

FIGURE 107–3. *A*, Schematic representation of Gardner's syndrome. The triad of colonic polyposis, bone tumors, and soft tissue tumors (heavy print) are the primary features; other features are indicated in lighter print. *B*, Schematic presentation of the Peutz-Jeghers syndrome. Mucocutaneous pigmentation and benign gastrointestinal polyposis (heavy print) are the primary features of this syndrome. Lighter print shows the secondary features. (From Boland CR, Kim YS: In Sleisenger MH, Fordtran JS [eds.]: Gastrointestinal Disease. 3rd ed. Philadelphia, W. B. Saunders Company, 1983.)

and in levels of nitrosamide in the stool has been noted in patients on high doses of ascorbic acid and alpha-tocopherol. Dietary calcium has recently been shown possibly to offer protection against colorectal cancer. The mechanism of this protection either may be a direct effect on the mucosal cells or may be the result of the combination of calcium with fatty acids and bile acids, thereby eliminating their toxic effect on the mucosa. Obviously much remains to be learned about the proposed relationship of diet to colorectal cancer, concerning both the validity of the association and the chemical link between diet and the induction of neoplastic transformation.

SUSCEPTIBILITY. In addition to general risk factors that influence susceptibility on a broad basis (Table 107–1), there are a number of specific factors that affect risk in the individual (see accompanying table). One of these factors is age. The risk for colorectal cancers begins to increase slightly at age 40 and more sharply at age 50, doubling with each decade and reaching a maximum at age 75. Additional risk factors include a prior history of colorectal cancer or adenoma, a prior history of female genital cancer, underlying ulcerative colitis of long standing, and a family history of one of the inherited colon cancer syndromes (see below).

Prior Colonic Cancer or Adenoma. Patients who have had one colorectal cancer are at increased risk for a subsequent colorectal cancer (metachronous lesion) occurring at a future time from the initial or index lesion. A prior adenoma of the colon also increases risk for subsequent colorectal cancer. The association of adenomas and cancer of the colon has been previously discussed in detail.

TABLE 107–1. COLORECTAL CANCER RISK FACTORS*

Standard Risk:	Age over 40, men and women
High Risk:	Inflammatory bowel disease
	History of female genital or breast cancer
	History of colonic cancer or adenoma
	Peutz-Jeghers syndrome
	Familial polyposis syndromes
	Family cancer syndromes
	Hereditary site-specific colonic cancer
	History of juvenile polyps
	Immunodeficiency disease

*From Stearns MW Jr (ed.): Neoplasms of the Colon, Rectum, and Anus. New York, John Wiley & Sons, 1980, pp 9–22. Reprinted with the kind permission of the publisher.

Ulcerative Colitis. One third of deaths related to chronic ulcerative colitis (CUC) are due to colorectal cancer, which occurs in an overall incidence 7 to 11 times greater in patients with CUC than in the general population. The risk of cancer in ulcerative colitis can be related to two recognized variables: (1) the duration of active colitis, and (2) the anatomic extent of colonic involvement by the pathologic process.

The relationship between duration of ulcerative colitis and the cumulative risk of colorectal cancer for both adults and children is shown in Figure 107–4. In adults the risk begins to rise after seven years, and 20 per cent of patients with cancer and CUC develop their malignancies between seven and ten years from the onset of colitis. Extent of colonic involvement by CUC also affects risk for cancer. Pancolitis carries a greater risk than colitis confined to the left side of

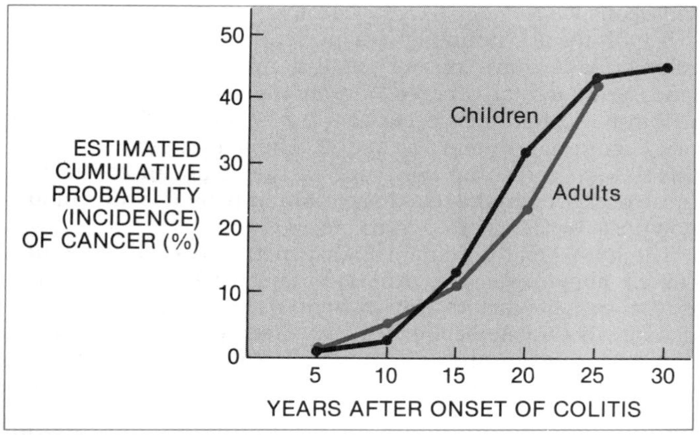

FIGURE 107–4. Estimated cumulative incidence with time of cancer complicating ulcerative colitis in adults and children with panproctocolitis. (From Stauffer JQ: In Sleisenger MH, Fordtran JS [eds.]: Gastrointestinal Disease. 2nd ed. Philadelphia, W. B. Saunders Company, 1978.)

the colon, where risk appears later, approximately 15 years after onset. Colitis confined to the rectosigmoid carries minimal risk, and ulcerative proctitis appears to have no increased risk for cancer. The high risk for cancer in ulcerative colitis has been considered by some investigators to be an overestimate resulting from referral of many patients with ulcerative colitis and cancer to centers that have reported the association.

In recent years a small subgroup (10 to 15 per cent) of patients with longstanding CUC has been identified by biopsy as having dysplasia of the colonic mucosa as an indicator for risk of cancer. When severe (high-grade) dysplasia is found, approximately 50 per cent of patients will be found to have simultaneous cancer; with moderate (low-grade) dysplasia, approximately one third of patients have cancer. Approximately 80 per cent of patients with CUC and colorectal cancer have dysplasia on biopsy. Although there are difficulties in histologic interpretations and dysplastic changes may be patchy, nevertheless the general concept is an important one; the demonstration of dysplasia has potential value in identifying those patients with CUC who are at greatest risk for colorectal cancer.

Patients with granulomatous colitis are also at higher risk for colorectal cancer than the general population, but considerably less so than patients with CUC. Once again, risk is related to the duration of disease.

Heredity and Colonic Cancer. Inherited predisposition to colonic cancer can be divided into two major categories: the polyposis type (familial polyposis, Gardner's syndrome, juvenile polyposis, Peutz-Jeghers syndrome, and Turcot's syndrome) and the nonpolyposis types (site-specific colonic cancer, the familial cancer syndromes, and Muir's [Torre's] syndrome). The familial polyposis syndromes have been discussed previously.

When it is stated that certain patients with a heritable predisposition to colonic cancer belong to a "nonpolyposis group," it is meant only that the colon is not carpeted by a myriad of small polyps. There is increasing evidence, however, that even in this group colorectal cancer develops from adenomas as in the familial polyposis syndromes. These adenomas are either single or multiple but if multiple are only in small numbers. Three major patterns are seen in this group: (1) Cancer confined to the colon and rectum (site-specific). In site-specific colonic cancer the transmission from generation to generation is only for colorectal cancer. (2) Multifocal cancer involving other sites in the gastrointestinal tract or the female sex organs (ovary, uterus, and breast) as well as the colon and rectum. This is sometimes called the "family cancer syndrome." (3) Muir's (Torre's) syndrome, a rare disorder resulting in multiple adenocarcinomas and epidermoid carcinomas in many organs in association with a large number of sebaceous cysts.

All of these "nonpolyposis syndromes" associated with colonic cancer have an autosomal dominant mode of inheritance with a high degree of penetrance. Multiple cancers within the colon often occur at a young age (under 40), with risk beginning as young as age 20. The majority of cancers in this group are on the right side of the colon, in contrast to those occurring in the usual patient or in patients with familial polyposis or Gardner's syndrome.

The autosomal dominant high-penetrance syndromes discussed above are rare. An important question is to what extent genetic factors are present in the vast majority of people who develop colonic cancer. There is a threefold excess of colonic cancers among first-degree relatives of patients with colonic cancer. Studies have suggested that most colonic cancer is genetically transmitted as an autosomal dominant low-penetrance disease. Environmental factors, especially diet, then modulate the expression of the disease in genetically susceptible individuals. This susceptibility or predisposition is first manifest as abnormalities in mucosal phenotypic expression of cell proliferation and cell differentiation, later by the appearance of adenoma, and finally by the development of adenocarcinoma.

PATHOLOGY. Approximately 50 per cent of adenocarcinomas of the colon occur in the distal 25 cm of large bowel (Figs. 107–5 and 107–6). This percentage was higher in the past, but there has been a "proximal migration" of neoplasia in the colon in recent years. The distal descending colon and upper sigmoid represents another frequent site of colorectal cancer, as do the cecum and ascending colon. Cancer is much less frequent in the transverse colon. On the left side of the colon, cancers are commonly annular and tend to obstruct; on the right side of the colon, they are primarily polypoid. In fact, either of these gross patterns can occur anywhere in the colon, and all colonic cancers commonly ulcerate and bleed. Metastatic spread from carcinoma of the colon occurs by direct invasion of surrounding structures, by way of regional lymphatics, or less commonly by multiple peritoneal implants. Of distant organs the liver is most frequently involved, but metastases may also occur to lung, and to bone and brain rarely.

CLINICAL MANIFESTATIONS. Adenocarcinomas of the colon, especially those on the right side, are often clinically silent for a long period of time. The most common symptoms relate to *bleeding* (anemia with its manifestations or hematochezia) and *obstruction* (change in bowel habits, sometimes pain). When the lesion is in the right colon, the bleeding is often occult, since the blood tends to be well mixed with stool and therefore escapes notice. Tumors of the cecum and ascending colon rarely obstruct, at least early in their course, so that a change in bowel habits or pain is less useful as an early symptom. Polypoid lesions of the left side of the colon may be associated with frequent and sometimes loose stools. With obstructing left-sided lesions, changes in bowel habits are usually those of gradual but progressive constipation, tenesmus, or a reduction in stool caliber, and hematochezia is much more frequent. Because of the frequency of tumor ulceration and bleeding, testing chemically for occult blood is an excellent survey technique and leads to an earlier diagnosis with a greater chance for cure. The general symptoms of malignancy—weakness, malaise, anorexia, weight loss—are frequent but nonspecific. Adenocarcinoma of the colon may present with a localized perforation, which becomes sealed off, or with signs of peritonitis (fever, generalized discomfort, rebound tenderness) when the perforation enters freely into the abdominal cavity. An abdominal mass or the signs and

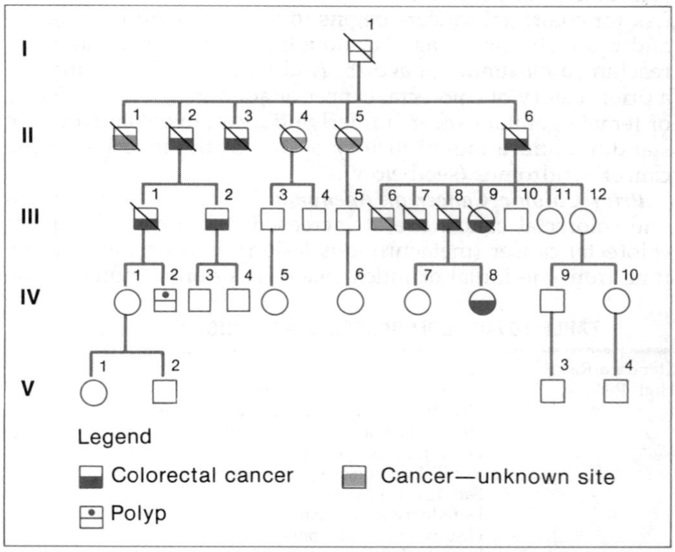

FIGURE 107–5. Pedigree of family with high prevalence of colorectal cancer. (From Kussin SZ, et al.: Am J Gastroenterol 72:448, 1979. Reprinted with permission of the publishers of the American Journal of Gastroenterology.)

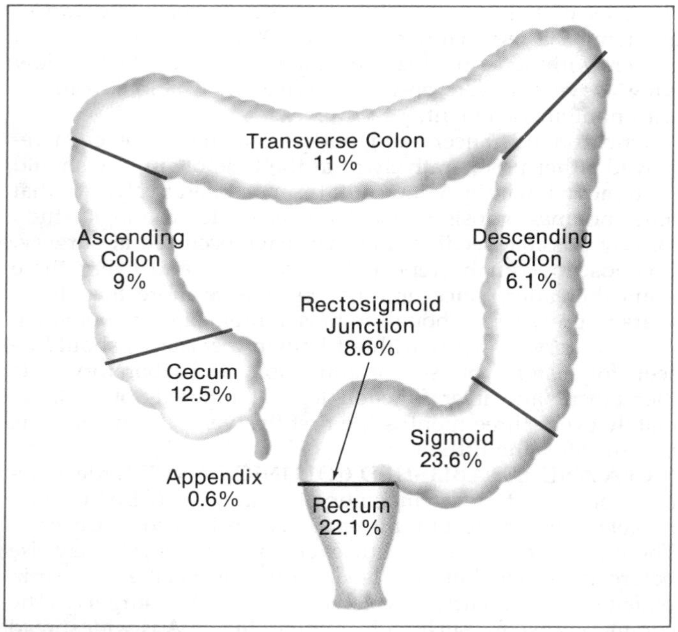

FIGURE 107–6. Distribution of large bowel cancer by anatomic segment according to the third national cancer survery (segment unspecified). (From Shottenfeld D, Fraumeni J Jr [eds.]: Cancer Epidemiology and Prevention. Philadelphia, W. B. Saunders Company, 1982, pp 703–727.)

symptoms of metastasis to the liver may be the earliest complaints.

Cancers at the mucocutaneous junction or in the anal canal or rectum may present with rectal bleeding, change in bowel habits, mass, or perineal pain. These can also present with symptoms referable to invasion of adjacent organs, including hematuria, urinary frequency, and vaginal fistulas.

DIAGNOSIS. ***Differential Diagnosis.*** The diagnosis of colorectal cancer must be considered when patients present with a change in bowel habits, a recent decrease in caliber of the stool, rectal bleeding, unexplained abdominal pain, or iron deficiency anemia. Overall the most common causes for bright red rectal bleeding are non-neoplastic, but the frequency of neoplastic lesions as the cause for bleeding increases progressively over age 40 and is especially high in those with a family history of colonic cancer. Bright red rectal bleeding can also be caused by angiodysplasia of the colon, diverticulosis, and a variety of other benign and malignant tumors of the colon (see Ch. 114).

A change of bowel habits can be produced by many other neoplastic lesions as well as by several benign disorders. Change in the character of the stool to a pellet type with more difficulty in passage is as common in progressive diverticular disease and muscle hypertrophy of the colon as in colonic malignancy (see Ch. 102). Diarrhea and incontinence can be a manifestation of many colonic and small intestinal diseases in addition to colorectal cancer. A recent change in bowel habits in one who has always had regular bowel habits, particularly if the person is at risk for colorectal cancer, clearly raises the possibility of a colonic neoplasm. The character of rectal bleeding cannot distinguish benign from neoplastic disorders. Blood appearing only on the toilet paper is indeed most commonly from hemorrhoids or a fissure, but it can also be from rectal cancer. Although a profuse bleeding episode is more likely to be the result of angiodysplasia, diverticulosis, ulcerative colitis, or ischemic colitis, it may be due to a large ulcerating neoplasm of the right colon.

Metastatic Colonic Cancer. Metastases of colonic cancer may be present before resection or may occur after it, producing different patterns of symptoms. Metastases to liver with progressive hepatomegaly may produce pain from distention of the liver capsule. Spread within the pelvis can result in pressure on the urinary bladder, obstruction of the rectosigmoid, sciatic nerve pain, and sometimes small bowel obstruction. Metastases to lung and bone are usually silent until very advanced. Intra-abdominal metastases may produce multiple areas of small and large bowel obstruction. Implants on the peritoneum sometimes cause ascites. Metastatic lesions can also occur in the skin, within the subcutaneous tissues, in suture lines, and within the bowel lumen. Intraluminal recurrences of colorectal cancer are unusual and follow surgery performed under adverse circumstances such as obstruction, or a low anterior resection for rectal cancer that leaves only a very narrow distal margin free of tumor. When tumor recurs within the colon, it more commonly is an intra-abdominal growth from the serosa into the lumen.

Diagnostic Approach. The history, physical examination, and common laboratory tests are essential for early diagnosis of colonic cancer. The history should combine the patient's symptoms with important clues such as the prior removal of an adenoma or even of a colorectal cancer, a history suggesting ulcerative colitis, or a family history suggesting one of the inherited colonic cancer syndromes. Physical examination may reveal evidence for Peutz-Jeghers syndrome, soft tissue tumors suggesting Gardner's syndrome, or the possibility of Muir's syndrome, and will provide clues as to any possible spread of the tumor to the liver, peripheral nodes, or skin. The digital rectal examination is important to determine the presence of a low-lying tumor or of perianal or pelvic disease. Laboratory testing might reveal iron deficiency anemia, occult blood in the stool, or an abnormality of liver function. Evaluation of the patient would also include a chest roentgenogram to search for pulmonary metastases.

When patients have symptoms or signs of colorectal cancer, the digital rectal examination should be followed by either proctoscopy and barium enema or colonoscopy. Proctoscopy may be performed with a rigid instrument, but this has had poor patient acceptance and physician application. Flexible sigmoidoscopes are more comfortable for the patient and have produced a much higher diagnostic yield because of the more complete insertion (see Ch. 96). A double-contrast barium enema is more revealing of mucosal lesions than the single-column study. In a well-prepared patient the majority of colorectal cancers can be detected by the combination of these two techniques. A barium enema should not be ordered without a prior proctoscopy, since there may be a distal lesion that could be obstructive and result in a perforation during the examination if the radiologist is not alerted to its presence. In addition, the patient may not have a neoplastic lesion but may have another disease, such as ulcerative colitis, which can readily be diagnosed by proctoscopy. If this disease is very active, a barium enema may in fact be undesirable.

Colonoscopy will be successful in uncovering lesions not detected by the barium enema, especially polyps but also cancers. Colonoscopy is also desirable in patients who have had an abnormality detected by barium enema. If the lesion detected radiologically appears to be cancer, it should be located endoscopically and confirmed by biopsy. In addition, a search for synchronous lesions and polyps should be carried out. If the lesion seen on radiographs is clearly an obstructing cancer of the left side, then colonoscopy is not necessary and may actually be hazardous. When the barium enema has uncovered only a polyp, colonoscopy can be utilized to remove the polyp, to search for other polyps, and to rule out an associated malignancy.

During colonoscopy, tissue sampling would include not only biopsies but also brushings for cytology, which increases the sensitivity of tissue diagnosis. In longstanding ulcerative colitis, biopsies are useful to look for dysplasia as an indication of premalignancy. These are obtained from the cecum to the rectum.

TREATMENT. ***Surgery.*** The goal of treatment for primary malignant neoplasms of the colon is to remove them as completely as possible. The best hope for cure is surgical removal of the segment of colon harboring the neoplasm, including omentum with lymph nodes. Cancers of the right and left colons are treated by hemicolectomies; cancer of the sigmoid and upper rectum above 5 cm from the anal verge is resected anteriorly with removal of a wide margin of normal colon above and below the tumor. In low anterior resections, the surgeon wishes to leave 2 to 3 cm of tumor-free margin distal to the tumor. Lesions within 4 cm of the anal verge are usually treated by a combined abdominal-perineal resection (APR). It is desirable to do a lower anterior resection rather than an APR if at all possible, since APR is not associated with increased survival and leaves the patient with a permanent colostomy. The availability of staplers allows the surgeon to do a low anterior resection of tumors closer to the anal verge than previously possible.

Epidermoid cancers in the anal canal may be treated by local excision if superficial. If deeper, an APR is required. A period of preoperative radiation and chemotherapy in these cases will usually shrink the tumor and improve the likelihood of successful resection.

Patients may require surgery for palliation as well as for cure. Obstruction usually requires a colostomy, followed at a later time by closure of the colostomy. In most patients with obstruction, however, a primary resection and colostomy can usually be accomplished in one stage. Carcinoma that has perforated also is usually treated by primary resection and colostomy with later closure of the colostomy. Patients with obvious metastatic disease may require surgery for their tumor if it bleeds or obstructs significantly. Palliative treatment with radiation and/or chemotherapy of the metastases may then proceed.

Radiation Therapy. Radiation may be used preoperatively and in patients who have evidence of recurrent disease, especially in the pelvis, or localized recurrences intra-abdominally. Adjuvant use of radiation and chemotherapy in rectal cancer has been associated with a longer tumor-free interval after surgery.

Chemotherapy. Chemotherapy of colorectal cancer is used primarily for metastatic disease. Unfortunately, chemotherapeutic agents are usually unsuccessful in the treatment of adenocarcinoma of the colon. 5-Fluorouracil (5-FU) has been disappointing because of its poor efficacy. Most combination agent trials have not been very encouraging for adenocarcinoma of the colon. For epidermoid cancers of the anal canal, the combination of mitomycin C and 5-FU in sequence with radiation has been effective in producing tumor regression preoperatively. Chemotherapy is most effective for liver metastases and is not as effective as radiation for pelvic recurrence or an isolated single mass. Current trials suggest that there may be some benefit for adjuvant chemotherapy in patients with rectal cancer judged histologically to be at high risk of recurrence, but as yet no benefit has been demonstrated for patients with colonic cancer. There has also been interest in direct infusion of the liver with floxuridine (FUDR) and other agents through a surgically placed catheter connected to a pump implanted subcutaneously. The efficacy of this method compared with systemic chemotherapy has not been demonstrated conclusively.

Most other primary malignancies of the colon are treated by resection. Metastatic disease to the colon may require surgery for obstruction or bleeding. Disseminated cancers involving the colon, such as lymphoma, melanoma, or breast cancer, usually require systemic treatment for the primary tumor.

PROGNOSIS AND FOLLOW-UP. The overall ten-year survival for patients after surgery for colorectal cancer is approximately 42 per cent. The survival correlates directly with the stage of the disease: cancer confined to the mucosa, 80 to 90 per cent ten-year survival; cancer extending through all areas of the bowel wall, 60 to 80 per cent; and cancer involving the regional lymph nodes, 30 to 40 per cent. Rectal cancers with node involvement, especially when they are low lying, have a lower ten-year survival than colonic cancers with node involvement.

Synchronous cancers and polyps that have not been removed either preoperatively or at the time of surgery should be removed within a few months postoperatively. At that time the anastomosis is usually brushed for cytologic study for any possible seeding that may have occurred at surgery. Colonoscopy can be repeated a year later and every three years thereafter, since new polyps require more than three years to grow large enough to have a premalignant potential. After surgery, patients without known metastases should be seen for history, physical examination, and laboratory tests (hematocrit and liver function test) at intervals of approximately every three months the first five years, then every six months after the fifth year.

CEA AND ESTABLISHED COLONIC CANCER. Measurement of circulating carcinoembryonic antigens (CEA) is not a reliable screening test for the early diagnosis of colonic cancer. There is some indication, however, that CEA levels may rise before any other clinical or laboratory abnormalities appear in patients with recurrent colonic cancer after surgery. The common cause for such an increase in the CEA is widespread metastatic disease, particularly involving the liver. In a few patients, however, rising CEA may reflect a small, localized, potentially resectable intra-abdominal metastasis. Although still investigational, it has been suggested that the CEA measurement be performed every three months. If a significant rise in the CEA is detected, the patient should undergo an intensive investigation, including liver function tests, computed tomographic scan, colonoscopy, and chest radiographs; if all are negative, a "second-look" exploration could be considered to search for a localized, potentially resectable intra-abdominal metastasis. In patients who have a rising CEA with negative workup there is an 80 per cent chance of finding recurrent tumors, 30 per cent of which are resectable. However, this approach has, as yet, not been of demonstrated effectiveness and must be viewed as controversial and investigational. Re-exploration and resection of recurrences have not been shown to prolong survival.

PREVENTION OF COLORECTAL CANCER. Prevention may be defined as (1) primary, the identification and eradication of agents in the environment that produce colorectal cancer, and attempted control of genetic factors; and (2) secondary, the identification and eradication of premalignant lesions, and the detection and resection of cancer while it is still curable. No effective primary preventive measures are yet available. Despite the previously cited evidence that diet may be related in some way to the evolution of colorectal cancer, there is no current proof that proscription of any diet in favor of a low-fat and high-fiber regimen would be effective.

Secondary prevention as defined above has been more rewarding with the introduction of better methods of screening for early cancer or premalignant adenomas. Effective screening requires the application of relatively simple and inexpensive tests to a large number of people in order to identify those who are likely to have disease. There are several critical questions to consider in any screening program: (1) What are the expected benefits in terms of survival of those patients whose disease is discovered by screening tests and treated, and in terms of the possible mortality reduction from colorectal cancer in the entire screened population? (2) Can high-risk subgroups be identified? (3) Are effective screening tests available? (4) Are community health resources adequate for the diagnostic workup and treatment of persons with positive screening tests? (5) What are the costs, patient compliance, and risks of screening?

It is justifiable to consider screening for colorectal cancer in the United States, since it is a high-risk country by worldwide epidemiologic standards. It is assumed that earlier diagnosis would lead to longer survival. In general, screening programs that have been in progress for colorectal cancer have demonstrated earlier staging and better survival of patients with cancer detected through screening but have not had sufficient time to prove that the screened group has a lower mortality from colorectal cancer. Screening for rectosigmoid cancer with periodic sigmoidoscopy may lead to earlier detection and improved long-term survival and even to a less than expected incidence of cancer at this anatomic site, probably because of identification and eradication of polyps. Screening for colorectal cancer can be classified in two ways: general screening of patients at average risk, and screening of patients in high-risk subgroups.

Average-Risk Patients. In average-risk groups (all of those not in one of the defined high-risk groups), suggested screening includes testing stool specimens for occult blood annually with impregnated guaiac slides and by sigmoidoscopy every three to five years. Guaiac solutions, Hematest, and benzidine have been discarded because of too many false-negative and false-positive results. Testing with six slides over a period of three days, with the patient making smears from two different parts of the same stool each day while on a high-fiber, meat-free diet, has resulted in detection of early colorectal cancer. Current trials using this approach have been promising but need further time for long-term results. This test is useful only in totally asymptomatic patients and should not be used as a substitute for clinical judgment in patients who have symptoms of neoplastic disease or who have already reported a history of rectal bleeding. The effective utilization of this test requires follow-up studies of patients who have positive tests, positive being defined as one or more positive slides. Diagnostic workup must include colonoscopy to search for lesions that are missed by the barium enema and an upper gastrointestinal series if no colonic neoplasm is detected. Approximately 30 per cent of patients with positive tests will have neoplastic lesions, mostly adenomas but also colorectal cancers. The stool blood test in its present form will detect 70 to 80 per cent of colorectal cancers present. More specific sensitive fecal occult blood tests using immunologic methods and quantitative assays for human hemoglobin are being evaluated. The fecal occult blood test is not very sensitive for rectosigmoid tumors and therefore is complemented by sigmoidoscopy. Rigid sigmoidoscopes have been used; however, flexible scopes of 30 to 60 cm in length have been tested and appear to increase the yield of polyps and cancers and provide a more comfortable examination.

High-Risk Groups. GENETIC. Familial polyposis requires early surgery. Patients with a family history of polyposis or Gardner's syndrome should have sigmoidoscopy at least annually beginning at puberty. Female patients with a history of genital or breast cancer should have periodic fecal occult blood testing and sigmoidoscopy, beginning as soon as they are identified. Patients with site-specific colonic cancer or the family cancer syndrome must be examined with barium enema and/or colonoscopy beginning at age 20, since one cannot comfortably rely only on fecal occult blood testing in these very high-risk patients. A reasonable screening approach would be a fecal occult blood test annually and colonoscopy every three to five years. The search would be primarily for adenomas, for which the colonoscope is much more sensitive than radiography. The number of patients with nonpolyposis inherited colonic cancer syndromes is not known. It has been estimated that these patients account for 1000 to 5000 cases of colorectal cancer annually.

PRIOR ADENOMA OR COLONIC CANCER. Patients with a prior history of adenoma or colonic cancer should be examined periodically by colonoscopy. Once the colon has been cleared of all synchronous lesions, screening every three years is sufficient, since excisable metachronous lesions usually do not develop sooner and often require years to evolve.

ULCERATIVE COLITIS. No well-established data exist on the optimal detection of cancer early in ulcerative colitis or granulomatous colitis, or at what intervals screening should be conducted. One suggestion is that multiple biopsies be obtained by colonoscopy once a year or once every other year after the patient has had universal colitis for 7 years or left-sided colitis for 15 years. If moderate or severe dysplasia is seen on these biopsies and confirmed in several specimens at several examinations, total colectomy should be considered. Patients with granulomatous colitis should be evaluated endoscopically if they have a change in their symptoms or develop a stricture (which may harbor a tumor).

NEOPLASMS OF THE SMALL INTESTINE

EPIDEMIOLOGY. Cancer is rare in the small intestine; only about 2000 cases occur in the United States each year. Small bowel cancer, like cancer of the large intestine, is more common in developed Western countries than in underdeveloped countries. With rare exceptions, the incidence for males is higher than that for females.

ETIOLOGY AND RISK FACTORS. Some cancers originating in the small intestine are related to pre-existing premalignant states, such as Crohn's disease of the small intestine or gluten-sensitive enteropathy. Small intestinal cancer may rarely develop from polyps of the Peutz-Jeghers syndrome or from polyps in patients with familial polyposis or Gardner's syndrome. The incidence of small bowel malignancy, especially lymphoma, is also increased in patients with various hereditary syndromes involving decreased humoral or cellular immunity. Lymphoma is by far the most common malignancy complicating celiac disease. A particular type of small intestinal lymphoma, called Mediterranean lymphoma, is endemic in the Middle East, affecting Sephardic Jews, Arabs, Armenians, and Iranians; environmental factors in the area have not been adequately studied.

Several hypotheses have been suggested to explain this striking rarity of small intestinal malignancies, especially adenocarcinomas, compared with adenocarcinomas of the colon. The bacterial population of the colon, quantitatively much greater than that of the small intestine, may convert bile acids or other products to carcinogens. Ingested carcinogens may be diluted in the small intestine by the large volume of liquid present there. Also, the transit time through the small bowel is much faster than through the colon, limiting the exposure of the small intestinal epithelium to carcinogens. The rapid cell proliferation of the small intestinal mucosa may also be important in preventing malignancy.

PATHOLOGY. Four types of neoplasms, adenocarcinomas, carcinoids, lymphomas, and leiomyosarcomas, account for over 95 per cent of malignant small bowel tumors. The most common tumor of the small intestine is asymptomatic benign carcinoid, most often found at postmortem examination. The most common tumor detected clinically in the small intestine is metastatic malignancy (lymphoma, melanoma, and carcinoma of the breast, kidney, ovary, and testicle). Adenocarcinomas are most common in the proximal small intestine, and carcinoids and lymphomas are most common in the distal small intestine.

CLINICAL MANIFESTATIONS. Small carcinoid tumors are asymptomatic, but larger carcinoid tumors can obstruct or bleed. The vast majority of symptomatic carcinoid tumors produce features of the carcinoid syndrome; the primary tumor of the small intestine is asymptomatic (see Ch. 243). Leiomyosarcomas often cause bleeding, and lymphomas present with a spectrum of clinical manifestations, including intestinal obstruction, bleeding, fever and malabsorption. Adenocarcinomas have characteristic clinical presentations, depending on their location: in the postbulbar area they may simulate peptic ulcer disease; in the periampullary area they can obstruct the common bile duct, causing jaundice; and beyond the periampullary area they can obstruct the bowel.

Adenocarcinomas of the distal small bowel usually develop as a complication of Crohn's disease and are most often found at surgery in patients operated on for longstanding Crohn's disease and obstruction. The clinical manifestation of benign polyps of the small intestine is usually bleeding. Most, however, are silent.

DIFFERENTIAL DIAGNOSIS. Tumors of the small intestine that present with bleeding or obstruction of the small bowel must be differentiated from many other causes of these symptoms. Bleeding can be secondary to Meckel's diverticulum, vascular anomaly, or duodenal ulcer, among other diagnoses. Obstruction can be due to adhesions, internal hernias, volvulus, or strictures. Obstructive jaundice can be due to tumors in the area of the ampulla as well as to carcinoma of the pancreas, bile duct cancer, impacted common duct stone, acute pancreatitis, and many other causes. Investigation of a patient with suspected small bowel tumor depends on the location and the clinical presentation. Patients presenting with atypical duodenal ulcer disease usually require upper gastrointestinal radiographs. Patients presenting with obstructive jaundice usually require sonography and either percutaneous transhepatic cholangiography or endoscopic retrograde cholangiopancreatography (ERCP). Those with small intestine obstruction require a period of decompression followed by radiologic study of the small bowel. Where tumors are accessible to direct visualization, such as the terminal ileum by colonoscopy and ileoscopy, or the upper duodenal area by upper gastrointestinal endoscopy, the procedures should be performed to confirm the presence of tumor and to obtain a tissue diagnosis.

THERAPY. Treatment is primarily surgical for adenocarcinomas, leiomyosarcomas, and malignant carcinoids. Primary lymphoma of the small intestine is usually treated surgically, although in poor-risk patients radiation therapy may provide the same benefit. Radiation therapy may be used postoperatively if there is evidence of spread beyond the bowel wall. If the lymphoma of the small intestine is part of a disseminated process, then chemotherapy is usually the treatment of choice (see Ch. 158).

PROGNOSIS AND PREVENTION. The prognosis of small intestinal adenocarcinomas is generally poor, with survival extremely low for the majority of patients. The prognosis for leiomyosarcoma and primary lymphomas of the small bowel is good if the lesion can be entirely removed by surgical resection, but this is rarely possible. Patients with malignant carcinoid tumors may survive for long periods, even after extensive metastases (see Ch. 243).

So little is known of the etiology of carcinoid tumors and leiomyosarcomas of the small bowel that no speculation regarding their prevention can be made. Primary small intestinal lymphomas could possibly be decreased in the Middle East by public health measures that decrease the high incidence of chronic bowel inflammation and parasitic infestation in this area. Diagnosis and treatment of celiac disease may reduce the frequency of superimposed malignancies. Surgical resection, rather than bypass, for Crohn's disease may decrease the incidence of adenocarcinoma in this high-risk group. In Peutz-Jeghers and multiple polyposis syndromes, adenomas in the duodenum could be monitored and potentially removed endoscopically.

GENERAL REVIEW

Bresalier R, Kim YS: Malignant neoplasms of the small and large intestine. In Sleisenger MH, Fordthan JS (eds.): Gastrointestinal Disease. 4th ed. Philadelphia, W. B. Saunders Company, 1988.

Winawer SJ, Enker WE, Lightdale CJ: Malignant tumors of the colon and rectum. In Berk JE (ed.): Bockus Gastroenterology. 4th ed. Philadelphia, W. B. Saunders Company, 1985, pp 2531–2574.

EPIDEMIOLOGY

Schottenfeld D, Winawer SJ: Large intestine. In Schottenfeld D, Fraumeni J Jr (eds.): Cancer Epidemiology and Prevention. Philadelphia, W. B. Saunders Company, 1982, pp 703–727. *A critical overview of the present concepts in the worldwide epidemiology of large bowel cancer.*

ETIOLOGY

Weisburger JH, Reddy BS, Spingarn NE, et al.: Current views on the mechanism involved in the etiology of colorectal cancer. Burkitt DP: Fibre in the aetiology of colorectal cancer. Goldin B: The role of diet and the intestinal flora in the etiology of large bowel cancer. In Winawer SJ, Schottenfeld D, Sherlock P (eds.): Colorectal Cancer: Prevention, Epidemiology, and Screening. Progress in Cancer Research. Vol. 13. New York, Raven Press, 1980, pp 19–41. *This series of papers reviews the evidence for the three major factors (fat, fiber, and bacterial flora) currently felt to be important in the etiology of colorectal cancer.*

RISK

Burt RW, Bishop DT, Cannon LA, et al.: Dominant inheritance of adenomatous colonic polyps and colorectal cancer. N Engl J Med 312:1540, 1985.

Devroede G: Risk of cancer in inflammatory bowel disease. In Winawer SJ, Schottenfeld D, Sherlock P (eds.): Colorectal Cancer: Prevention, Epidemiology, and Screening. Progress in Cancer Research. Vol. 13. New York, Raven Press, 1980, pp 325–334. *This paper carefully examines the relative risk among the subgroups of patients with inflammatory bowel disease.*

Kussin SZ, Lipkin M, Winawer SJ: Inherited colon cancer: Clinical implications. Am J Gastroenterol (State of the Art) 72:448, 1979. *A review of the literature of inherited colonic cancer with a focus on the possible link of genetic factors to sporadic cancer.*

DIAGNOSIS

Hunt RH, Waye JD (eds.): Colonoscopy. Techniques, Clinical Practice and Colour Atlas. England, Chapman and Hall, 1981. *A comprehensive treatise by various authors on technique and practical application.*

TREATMENT

DeCosse JJ (ed.): Clinical Surgical International. Large Bowel Cancer. Vol 1. New York, Churchill-Livingstone, 1981. *The subject of treatment is extensively covered in this book.*

CARCINOEMBRYONIC ANTIGEN (CEA)

Zamcheck N: Current status of CEA. In Winawer SJ, Schottenfeld D, Sherlock P (eds.): Colorectal Cancer: Prevention, Epidemiology, and Screening. Progress in Cancer Research. Vol. 13. New York, Raven Press, 1980, pp 219–234. *The current status of CEA in the follow-up of patients after surgery is discussed in detail in this paper by one of the senior investigators in the field.*

PREVENTION

Gilbertsen VA, Nelms JM: The prevention of invasive cancer of the rectum. Cancer 41:1137, 1978. *Unique long-term study demonstrating the impact of proctosigmoidoscopy on the natural history of rectosigmoid cancer.*

Lipkin M, Newmark H: Effect of added dietary calcium on colonic epithelial–cell proliferation in subjects at high risk for familial colonic cancer. N Engl J Med 313:1381, 1985.

Rozen P, Winawer SJ: Secondary prevention of colorectal cancer: An international perspective. Basel, Karger, 1986. *A compendium of papers from worldwide programs, including screening.*

Sherlock P, Lipkin M, Winawer SJ: The prevention of colon cancer. A combined clinical and basic science seminar. Am J Med 68:917, 1980. *Screening is examined from the viewpoint of the spectrum of risk, with heavy emphasis on markers being investigated in high-risk groups.*

Simon JB: Occult blood screening for colorectal carcinoma: A clinical review. Gastroenterology 88:820–837, 1985. *An update of screening issues and screening program results.*

Winawer SJ, Fleisher M, Baldwin M, et al.: Current status of fecal occult blood testing in screening for colorectal cancer. Cancer 32:100, 1982. *A comprehensive review of the background and status of fecal occult blood testing.*

SMALL INTESTINE

Lightdale CJ, Koepsell TD, Sherlock P: Small intestine. In Schottenfeld D, Fraumeni JF Jr (eds.): Cancer Epidemiology and Prevention. Philadelphia, W. B. Saunders Company, 1982, pp 692–702. *An excellent review of various epidemiologic and etiologic aspects of small intestinal tumors.*

108 PANCREATITIS

Michael D. Levitt

The pathogenesis of pancreatitis remains obscure and treatment is therefore supportive rather than specific. Only in the area of diagnostic procedures have there been major recent advances. The physician can now diagnose acute and chronic pancreatitis accurately, but the ability to influence the course of the disease has progressed little during the past ten years.

NORMAL ANATOMY AND PHYSIOLOGY OF EXOCRINE PANCREAS. The exocrine pancreas consists of acinar cells that synthesize digestive enzymes. These enzymes reside in zymogen granules within the cells and are deposited into the central ductule of the acinus. The ductules coalesce to form larger ducts, finally draining into the main pancreatic duct (Wirsung), which empties into the duodenum at the ampulla of Vater. Pancreatic secretion is stimulated by two hormones produced in the duodenum: (1) *secretin*, which is released in response to acid in the duodenum, stimulates a pancreatic juice high in volume and [HCO_3^-]; (2) *cholecystokinin-pancreozymin* (CCK-PZ), which is released in response to fatty acids and amino acids in the duodenum and results in a secretion rich in enzymes.

The enzymes secreted by the pancreas are grouped into those that digest starch (amylase), fat (lipases), and protein (trypsin and other proteolytic enzymes). The proteolytic enzymes are secreted in an inactive form, thus preventing autodigestion of the pancreas. Trypsinogen is activated to trypsin in the duodenal lumen, and trypsin then activates the other proteolytic enzymes. Protease inhibitors in the pancreas and pancreatic juice provide additional protection against autodigestion.

CLASSIFICATION OF PANCREATITIS. Pancreatitis is classified as acute or chronic by clinical pathologic criteria. Clinically, an attack of pancreatitis is defined as *acute* if the patient becomes asymptomatic following recovery, whereas in *chronic* pancreatitis the patient has persistent pain or insufficient exocrine or endocrine pancreatic secretion. The term *relapsing* denotes recurrent attacks that may occur in either acute or chronic pancreatitis. The pathologic findings in acute pancreatitis range from mild interstitial edema (which may not warrant the designation of pancreatitis), to acute inflammatory infiltrate, to necrosis and hemorrhage with virtually complete destruction of the gland. Since laparotomy is contraindicated in acute pancreatitis, pancreatic pathology is seldom documented by examination of tissue. Chronic pancreatitis is characterized by the disappearance of acinar tissue and the presence of fibrosis, calcification, and cyst formation. Pancreatitis will occur in roughly 0.5 per cent of the population and accounts for about 1 death annually per 100,000 population.

ACUTE PANCREATITIS

PATHOGENESIS. The final common pathway of acute pancreatitis is thought to be autodigestion by activated enzymes. The exact mechanism that provokes this process of autodigestion remains speculative. There is an association between pancreatitis and the clinical conditions listed in Table 108–1. Familiarity with these conditions is useful clinically, since the diagnosis of pancreatitis is often suggested by the coexistence of one of these states, and the prevention of recurrent pancreatitis usually hinges on the elimination of the predisposing condition. No cause of acute pancreatitis is uncovered in about 15 per cent of cases. In the United States, the majority of patients with acute pancreatitis have *alcoholism* or *gallstones* as an etiologic factor.

TABLE 108–1. ETIOLOGIC FACTORS IN PANCREATITIS

Alcoholism
Biliary tract disease
Trauma—postoperative, abdominal injuries, post-ERCP
Infections—mumps, coxsackievirus and echovirus, mycoplasma, parasitosis
Metabolic—hyperlipidemia, hyperparathyroidism, pregnancy, uremia, postrenal transplant
Drugs
Multiple reports
Immunosuppressive—corticosteroids, azathioprine, L-asparaginase
Diuretics—thiazides, furosemide, ethacrynic acid
Miscellaneous—phenformin, oral contraceptives, tetracycline
Rare or questionable reports
Acetaminophen, isoniazid, rifampin, propoxyphene
Vascular—shock, lupus erythematosus, periarteritis, atheromatous embolism
Mechanical—pancreas divisum, ampullary stenosis, ampulla of Vater tumor, duodenal diverticula, duodenal Crohn's disease, duodenal surgery
Penetrating duodenal ulcer
Familial

Alcoholic pancreatitis develops in susceptible persons after heavy ethanol ingestion for many years. Chronic alcoholism may produce proteinaceous plugs in the small pancreatic ducts, causing atrophy of the acini drained by the obstructed duct. These chronic, irreversible pathologic changes antedate the first attack of acute pancreatitis, and 10 per cent of alcoholics develop pancreatic insufficiency without a recognized acute attack. The factors triggering the superimposition of an acute attack on this chronic process are not understood.

Gallstone pancreatitis is virtually always associated with fecal excretion of gallstones, whereas a much lower frequency of fecal stones is found in patients with gallstones who do not have pancreatitis. Thus, passage of a gallstone through the ampulla of Vater creates conditions favorable to the development of pancreatitis. This condition is not simply obstruction, since ligation of the ampulla does not cause pancreatitis. Rather, some factor such as reflux of biliary or duodenal contents or stimulation of pancreatic secretion appears necessary to produce pancreatitis. This "large duct" form of pancreatitis differs from the "small duct" type observed in alcoholics, in that the former seldom leads to chronic pancreatitis or pancreatic calcifications and is cured by cholecystectomy.

Postoperative pancreatitis, the third most commonly identified cause of acute pancreatitis, may follow any type of abdominal surgery. Biliary tract procedures and retroperitoneal node dissections have the highest incidence of this complication.

Hypertriglyceridemia, often with lactescent serum, occurs in about 15 per cent of patients with acute pancreatitis. Many of these patients are alcoholics who have an underlying abnormality of lipid metabolism, which is particularly pronounced during the acute attack. The apparent decrease in frequency of attacks of pancreatitis following dietary therapy for hypertriglyceridemia suggests that hyperlipidemia is a cause of pancreatitis.

Vascular insufficiency of the pancreas is a more common cause of pancreatitis than is generally recognized. Pancreatitis (usually asymptomatic) was observed in postmortem examination of 10 per cent of patients who died with hemorrhagic shock. Pancreatitis is a well-recognized complication of ischemia resulting from vasculitis or cholesterol emboli.

Pancreas divisum is a common (5 per cent) anatomic variant in which the portion of the pancreas (tail, body, and part of head) derived from the embryologic dorsal pancreas is drained through the duct of Santorini and the minor papilla rather than via the duct of Wirsung and the ampulla of Vater. Pancreas divisum occurs in 20 to 25 per cent of patients with otherwise unexplained pancreatitis. Presumably, this variant drainage is sometimes inadequate, although sphincterotomy of the minor ampulla has yielded only equivocal benefit in the prevention of pancreatitis.

Drugs have been linked to the development of pancreatitis (Table 108–1). This linkage is generally rather weak with the exception of antimetabolites such as L-asparaginase, which is associated with a 10 per cent frequency of pancreatitis. Frequently it is difficult to exclude the possibility that pancreatitis is a complication of the disease for which the drug was prescribed. For example, the high frequency of pancreatitis reported in patients taking diuretics may reflect the increased incidence of pancreatitis in patients with various forms of vascular disease.

Pancreatitis may be inherited as an autosomal dominant trait, which often begins in childhood. This type of pancreatitis has an increased incidence of late-developing pancreatic carcinoma.

CLINICAL PRESENTATION. The hallmark of acute pancreatitis is *abdominal pain*. This diagnosis should be considered in every patient presenting with abdominal discomfort. The time from onset to peak intensity of the pain ranges from seconds to hours. The pain, which tends to be steady rather than colicky, varies in intensity from minor to agonizing. At the onset of the attack, the pain is often localized to the epigastrium and left upper quadrant but as the attack progresses, it becomes diffuse and radiates to the back. The back pain results from retroperitoneal irritation and is partially relieved by flexing the trunk. Acute pancreatitis may be relatively painless, and massive hemorrhagic necrosis of the gland, frequently in postoperative patients, may be an unexpected postmortem finding. *Vomiting* occurs in 70 to 90 per cent of the cases, but often brings about only minimal relief of the abdominal discomfort. The past medical history is important, since pancreatitis is usually associated with one of the underlying conditions listed in Table 108–1, and there frequently is *a previous history* of similar attacks of pain.

Nonspecific physical findings include fever, tachycardia, and hypotension. *Abdominal tenderness* is virtually always present; however, abdominal guarding and rigidity may be surprisingly slight, given the apparent distress of the patient. Although rarely palpable on initial examination, an abdominal mass subsequently develops in 10 to 20 per cent of patients. Occasionally, in hemorrhagic pancreatitis, retroperitoneal blood dissects into the flanks or around the umbilicus, producing Grey Turner's or Cullen's sign, respectively.

History and physical examination are seldom diagnostic of acute pancreatitis, and the differential diagnosis includes all causes of abdominal pain. Features favoring the existence of pancreatitis include a left upper quadrant component of the pain (as opposed to the right-sided nature of gallbladder pain), steady pain (as opposed to the colic of bowel disease), vomiting that does not relieve pain (the discomfort of gastritis and bowel obstruction are transiently relieved by vomiting), and abdominal rigidity less than that expected for pain (perforated peptic ulcer has marked rigidity). The absence of a condition associated with pancreatitis (Table 108–1) reduces the possibility of pancreatitis, whereas a previous history of documented pancreatitis is the single most reliable indicator that the present attack is also due to pancreatitis.

LABORATORY TEST. ***Amylase.*** In few disease states does the diagnosis rely so heavily on a single laboratory determination as is the case with acute pancreatitis and the measurement of serum amylase. The patient with abdominal pain and an elevated serum or urine amylase level is usually considered to have pancreatitis, whereas a patient with identical symptoms and physical findings but normal amylase levels seldom is diagnosed as having pancreatitis. The sensitivity and specificity of the amylase measurements cannot be evaluated, since the actual presence or absence of pancreatitis is seldom verified by some independent, more reliable technique.

Amylase is produced in large quantity by the pancreas, salivary glands, and certain malignant tumors, and in lesser quantity by the fallopian tubes and lungs. Normally, most of the amylase secreted by the pancreas and salivary glands enters and is confined to the gut. A small fraction enters the plasma, accounting for the normal serum amylase activity, of which about two thirds is salivary isoamylase and one third pancreatic isoamylase.

In pancreatitis, increased quantities of pancreatic amylase escape into the lymph and blood flow of the pancreas. An increase in pressure in the pancreatic duct owing to obstruction or injection of contrast material during endoscopic retrograde cholangiopancreatography (ERCP) causes amylase to regurgitate into the plasma usually with little or no accompanying inflammation.

Amylase is cleared from the plasma with a half-life of about two hours, about 20 per cent being excreted in the urine. Two thirds of the amylase filtered by the glomerulus is normally reabsorbed or catabolized by the renal tubule.

A variety of conditions other than pancreatitis may cause an elevated serum amylase level. Inflammation or trauma to the salivary glands causes excessive release of salivary amylase into the serum. Chronic, unexplained elevations of serum amylase activity are almost always due to increases in salivary-type isoamylase, although there is usually no clinical evidence of salivary gland disease. In mesenteric infarction and perforated peptic ulcer, amylase from the intestinal lumen may leak into the circulation. These conditions must always be differentiated from pancreatitis in patients with abdominal pain and hyperamylasemia. Ruptured ectopic pregnancy, ovarian cysts, and various forms of pulmonary disease have also been reported to be associated with elevations of serum amylase. A chronic, very high serum amylase level may result from the production of amylase by metastatic tumors originating in the lung, reproductive tract, or pancreas. Serum amylase levels may also be elevated because of slow clearance from the blood. Uncomplicated renal failure is commonly associated with serum amylase values up to two times normal; higher levels suggest associated pancreatitis. Macroamylasemia is an asymptomatic state in which amylase is bound to serum proteins, thus forming a complex that is slowly cleared from the serum. Confusion results when the macroamylasemic patient has associated abdominal pain.

The rate of excretion of amylase in the urine is increased out of proportion to the serum amylase level in pancreatitis and may be elevated when the serum amylase is normal. This disproportionate elevation apparently results from the inhibition of tubular reabsorption of amylase in acute pancreatitis; thus, a greater portion of the filtered amylase appears in the urine. Although a more sensitive indicator of pancreatitis than is the serum level, the urinary amylase may be falsely normal when renal failure complicates pancreatitis. Spuriously elevated values occur in virtually all the nonpancreatitic conditions that cause hyperamylasemia (except macroamylasemia and renal disease) and in a variety of conditions with proximal renal tubular malfunction, including thermal burns, diabetic acidosis, and postoperative states.

Serum amylase originates from a variety of organs in addition to the pancreas, but serum lipase, trypsin, or pancreatic isoamylase is derived almost entirely from the pancreas. These enzymes, although technically more difficult to measure than amylase, may therefore provide in the future a more specific and sensitive indicator of pancreatitis.

The appropriate interpretation of amylase measurements may be summarized as follows. The patient with an acute attack of abdominal pain and an elevated serum amylase activity in all likelihood has acute pancreatitis, provided that perforated ulcer and bowel infarction are excluded. An elevated urinary amylase with a normal serum amylase is suggestive, but less diagnostic, of pancreatitis. The height of the amylase elevation does not correlate with the severity of the pancreatitis. For example, extremely high values, which return to normal over one to two days, are often associated with the passage of common duct stone and minimal, if any, inflammation of the pancreas. Elevation of amylase activity beyond 7 days is usually associated with relatively severe pancreatitis, and a protracted clinical course and elevation for more than 14 days suggest the possibility of a pseudocyst or pancreatic ascites. Chronic elevations of serum amylase activity associated with mild or no abdominal symptoms are seldom due to pancreatic disease but rather to renal failure, macroamylasemia, salivary hyperamylasemia, or tumor hyperamylasemia. Serum isoamylase assay can readily distinguish pancreatic from salivary hyperamylasemia. Serum lipase levels can also be used to distinguish pancreatic from salivary hyperamylasemia, since lipase is not produced by the salivary gland.

Other Laboratory Tests. The leukocyte count is usually elevated. Early in the course of acute pancreatitis, the hematocrit often rises to supranormal levels owing to *hemoconcentration* resulting from the massive loss of serum into the peritoneal and retroperitoneal spaces. *Hyperglycemia* often occurs, possibly resulting from increased glucagon and/or decreased insulin release. The serum in pancreatitis is frequently lactescent, and for unknown reasons the serum amylase level is frequently normal in this situation. *Hypocalcemia* is indicative of severe pancreatitis and is postulated to result from sequestration of calcium in soaps in areas of fat necrosis. In addition, there is a probable failure of the usual mechanisms that regulate calcium homeostasis. The presence of any of these nonspecific findings—elevated hematocrit, hyperglycemia, hypocalcemia, or hyperlipemia—in a patient with abdominal pain should always arouse suspicion of acute pancreatitis. Methemalbuminemia results from the extravascular destruction of hemoglobin and is the only laboratory finding that directly indicates that the pancreatitis is hemorrhagic. Evidence of cholestasis (elevated serum bilirubin and alkaline phosphatase) occurs in as many as 25 per cent of patients with acute pancreatitis, owing to compression of the common bile duct as it passes through the edematous pancreas. The cholestasis usually clears spontaneously in seven to ten days.

Roentgenograms. Roentgenograms of the abdomen should be obtained to rule out the presence of free air, signifying a perforation. In pancreatitis nonspecific ileus is usually observed. Somewhat more specific for pancreatitis, but not diagnostic, are localized gas collections in loops of bowel overlying the pancreas.

Imaging Techniques. Until recently, the pancreas could be only indirectly visualized radiographically via its impression of other viscera. The development of techniques to visualize the pancreas directly by means of ultrasound, computed tomography (CT), and ERCP has marked a great advance.

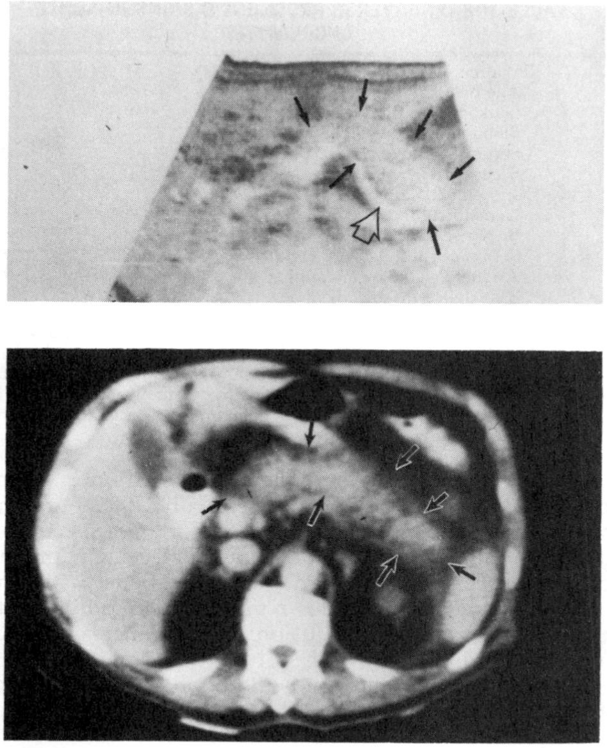

FIGURE 108–2. Diffusely enlarged pancreas of acute pancreatitis demonstrated by ultrasound (*above*) and computed tomography (*below*). The large arrow on the sonogram points to the splenic vein. (Courtesy of Dr. Henry I. Goldberg, Department of Radiology, University of California at San Francisco.)

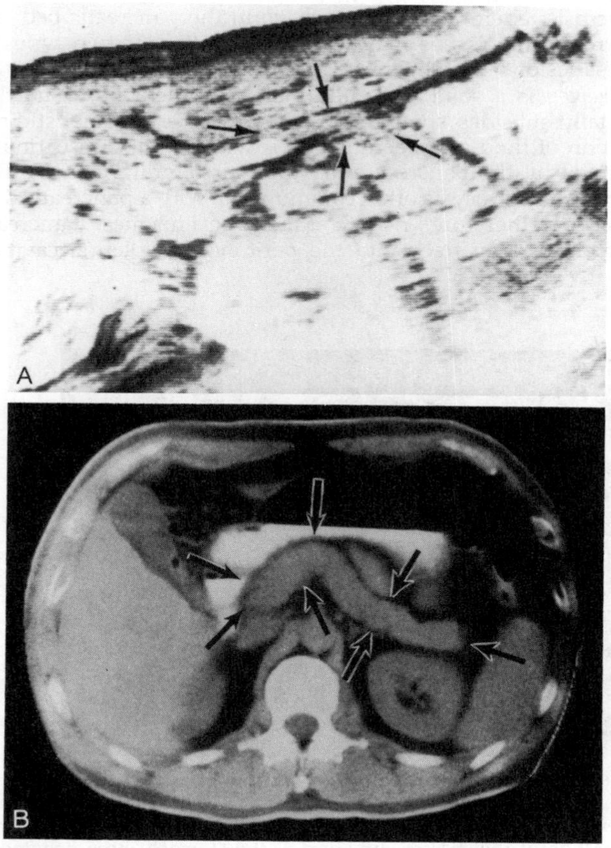

FIGURE 108–1. Normal pancreas demonstrated by ultrasound (*A*) and computed tomography (*B*). (Courtesy of Dr. Eugene P. DiMagno, Mayo Medical School, Rochester, Minnesota.)

Computed tomographic scanning demonstrates a diffusely enlarged pancreas in over 90 per cent of patients during an acute attack of pancreatitis, whereas ultrasound is less sensitive owing to problems with overlying gas (Figs. 108–1 and 108–2). Computed tomography is not required for the diagnosis of pancreatitis in most patients and should be reserved for very ill patients in whom the diagnosis is in doubt. This procedure is particularly valuable in the deteriorating patient who might have a gut perforation or infarction, since the pancreas appears normal in such patients, in contrast to the distinctly abnormal scan in severe acute pancreatitis. Endoscopic retrograde cholangiopancreatography exacerbates acute pancreatitis and is contraindicated during an acute attack.

TREATMENT. About 50 per cent of patients with acute pancreatitis have relatively mild and self-limited disease and probably would recover without benefit of medical therapy; 40 per cent are quite ill but survive their attack; and 10 per cent succumb despite the best of therapy. Virtually all deaths occur during the first or second attack of acute pancreatitis, recurrent attacks having a very low mortality rate. It is frequently difficult to judge the severity of the attack during the initial stages; therefore most patients with acute pancreatitis should be hospitalized, with a possible exception being the patient having recurrent attacks of chronic pancreatitis.

A number of objective measurements (Table 108–2) have been found to correlate with a poor prognosis.

Surgical intervention during the acute, symptomatic stage of pancreatitis is associated with a greater morbidity and mortality than is medical therapy, so the initial treatment of acute pancreatitis should be medical rather than surgical. Medical therapy is largely symptomatic and supportive, and there is little evidence that the acute inflammation of the pancreas is altered by this therapy. Meperidine should be used for pain relief because of the theoretic problem of spasm of the sphincter of Oddi with morphine. In severe pancreatitis, as much as 6 to 10 liters of plasma and blood may be

TABLE 108–2. ADVERSE PROGNOSTIC SIGNS IN ACUTE PANCREATITIS*

On admission:
Age over 55
Leukocyte count over 16,000/mm^3
Blood glucose over 200 mg/dl
Serum LDH over 350 IU/liter
Serum GOT over 250 sigma Frankel U/dl
During initial 48 hours:
Hematocrit decrease over 10%
BUN rise over 5 mg/dl
Serum calcium below 8 mg/dl
Arterial P_{O_2} below 60 mm Hg
Base deficit over 4 mEq/liter
Estimated fluid sequestration over 6 liters

*If fewer than three of these signs are present, mortality is negligible (<1 per cent) and few are seriously ill. If more than four signs are present, mortality may be 25 per cent and an additional 50 per cent of patients are seriously ill.

LDH = lactate dehydrogenase; GOT = glutamic-oxaloacetic transaminase, BUN = blood urea nitrogen.

sequestered in the retroperitoneal and peritoneal spaces. Prompt replacement of these losses with colloid or whole blood is probably the single most important aspect of the initial medical therapy. Such volume replacement probably accounts for recent sharp declines in the frequency with which acute renal failure complicates pancreatitis. In addition, this therapy helps maintain perfusion of the pancreas, a factor that seems to diminish the severity of experimental pancreatitis. Cautious insulin therapy is indicated for marked hyperglycemia, and intravenous calcium may be required for hypocalcemia.

For years, the major objective of therapy for acute pancreatitis was to "put the pancreas at rest" by reducing the humoral stimuli to pancreatic secretion. To this end, the patient received no oral alimentation, and gastric suction was carried out to prevent gastric HCl from entering the duodenum, thus minimizing secretin release. This therapy was based on limited evidence of benefit in experimental pancreatitis and on the clinical observation that the abdominal pain of pancreatitis appeared to subside more rapidly following the initiation of nasogastric suction. Two controlled studies in mild to moderately severe pancreatitis failed to demonstrate any significant benefit from nasogastric suction, and in such patients this form of therapy is optional. The value of suction in severe hemorrhagic pancreatitis has not been confirmed; however, the associated ileus that invariably complicates severe pancreatitis provides a strong indication for nasogastric suction.

TABLE 108–3. COMPLICATIONS OF ACUTE PANCREATITIS

Pancreatic—phlegmon, pseudocyst, abscess, ascites, hemorrhage
Contiguous organs—portal venous thrombosis, bowel necrosis, intraperitoneal bleeding, obstruction of common duct
Systemic
Cardiovascular—hypotension, nonspecific ST-T changes, pericardial effusion
Pulmonary—pleural effusion, shock lung, atelectasis
Renal—acute renal failure
Gastrointestinal—gastritis
Hematologic—disseminated intravascular coagulation
Metabolic—hypocalcemia, hyperglycemia, hypertriglyceridemia
Fat necrosis—subcutaneous, bone
Central nervous system—psychosis

The use of peritoneal dialysis to remove toxins in the peritoneal cavity should be considered when the patient's condition deteriorates despite standard medical therapy. A randomized trial of peritoneal dialysis showed striking short-term benefit in severe pancreatitis; however, late deaths due to sepsis resulted in similar overall mortalities for the dialyzed and control groups.

A number of therapies have been shown to be ineffective in controlled studies: proteolytic enzyme inhibitors such as aprotinin (Trasylol), glucagon to reduce pancreatic secretion, anticholinergics to reduce gastric and pancreatic secretion, and prophylactic antibiotics to prevent infection in the pancreatic bed.

COMPLICATIONS. The most important complications associated with acute pancreatitis are listed in Table 108–3. In the absence of these complications, recovery usually occurs in one to two weeks. A frequent cause of death during the first few weeks of the illness is the development of the *adult respiratory distress syndrome* (ARDS) secondary to increased alveolar capillary permeability. Prompt recognition and treatment with O_2 and positive end-expiratory pressure (PEEP) breathing appear to be lifesaving in some of these patients. Necrosis, edema, and hemorrhage in the pancreatic bed and surrounding tissues may lead to formation of two types of mass lesions, which can be differentiated by sonography. A *phlegmon* is a solid, inflamed mass of pancreatic tissue that usually subsides spontaneously. A *pseudocyst* is a cystic collection of fluid and necrotic debris whose walls are variously formed by the pancreas and other surrounding organs (Fig. 108–3). Pseudocysts often communicate with a pancreatic duct and are, therefore, rich in pancreatic enzymes. Pancreatic secretions may track into the peritoneal or pleural cavities,

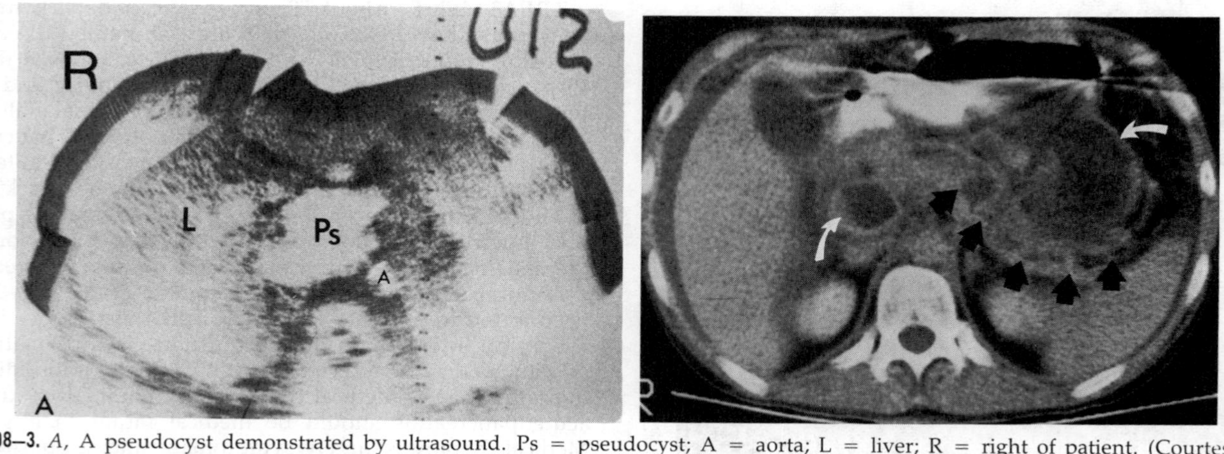

FIGURE 108–3. *A*, A pseudocyst demonstrated by ultrasound. Ps = pseudocyst; A = aorta; L = liver; R = right of patient. (Courtesy of Dr. Dennis A. Sarti, Dept. of Radiological Sciences, University of California at Los Angeles, and Radiology 125:789, 1977.) *B*, A CT scan through the region of the tail, body, and head of the pancreas demonstrates the presence of two pancreatic pseudocysts (*curved white arrows*). The larger of the two extends from the tail of the pancreas anteriorly to compress a portion of the greater curvature of the stomach, here denoted by contrast material in the dependent portion and an air/fluid level. The smaller of the two is well circumscribed and located in the head of the pancreas. Both pseudocysts are of low CT density and well-described margins. In addition, the pancreatic duct (*black arrows*) is dilated and irregular in contour, a finding typical of a chronic pancreatitis. (Courtesy of Dr. Henry Goldberg, University of California at San Francisco.)

resulting in pancreatic ascites or a pleural effusion. The pancreatic origin of these fluids is established by the finding of a fluid amylase concentration many-fold higher than that of serum. A serious complication of either phlegmons or pseudocysts is the development of an *abscess*, which is usually heralded by increasing pain, hectic fever, and leukocytosis. Immediate surgical drainage of the lesion is indicated, since nonoperative therapy carries a mortality of nearly 100 per cent.

Large pseudocysts are usually palpable, but smaller cysts are detected only by sonography or CT scanning. Many pseudocysts (particularly the smaller ones) are relatively asymptomatic and resolve spontaneously; some pseudocysts (usually the larger ones) cause marked discomfort and have the potentially lethal complications of hemorrhage or perforation. It is usually safe to follow smaller, asymptomatic pseudocysts or larger, uncomplicated cysts that are diminishing in size. The cyst that is expanding or causing appreciable discomfort should be drained, either surgically via anastomosis of the cyst to the gut or percutaneously via a needle. The indications for the traditional surgical as opposed to the newer percutaneous procedures remain to be determined. Complications of abscess, hemorrhage, or rupture require immediate surgical intervention.

It is very important to prevent the recurrence of acute pancreatitis by the treatment of conditions listed in Table 108–1. Abstinence from ethanol frequently does not prevent the progression of alcoholic pancreatitis but may reduce the frequency and severity of attacks. Studies to rule out the presence of gallstones are mandatory, since cholecystectomy in such patients nearly always prevents subsequent attacks. Cholecystectomy usually should be carried out after the subsidence of symptoms but during the initial hospitalization. Treatment of hypertriglyceridemia with a low-calorie, low-fat diet, as well as abstinence from alcohol, seems to prevent some subsequent attacks of hyperlipemic pancreatitis. Hypercalcemia as the cause of pancreatitis may be obscured during the acute attack and should be excluded by a serum calcium determination following recovery. Endoscopic retrograde cholangiopancreatography should be performed in patients who have had more than one attack of otherwise unexplained pancreatitis. Lesions, potentially correctable by surgery, that may be detected by ERCP include small gallstones missed by sonography, an isolated stricture in the main pancreatic duct, an undetected pseudocyst, pancreas divisum, or ampullary stenosis.

CHRONIC PANCREATITIS

ETIOLOGY. Chronic pancreatitis may be associated with most of the conditions listed in Table 108–1, with the exception of gallstone disease, which produces only recurrent acute attacks. Alcoholism is by far the most common cause of chronic pancreatitis in the United States; in some parts of the world, protein-calorie malnutrition is the major cause.

PATHOPHYSIOLOGY. In chronic alcoholism (with or without superimposed acute pancreatitis), proteinaceous plugs in the pancreatic ducts apparently lead to atrophy of the acinar tissue, fibrous tissue replacement, and dilatation of the ductular system. Calcification of these ductular plugs accounts for the diffuse, stippled calcification of the pancreas observed in about 30 per cent of patients. Pseudocysts are also a frequent finding. The normal secretion of pancreatic enzymes far exceeds that required for digestion, and malabsorption occurs only when enzyme secretion falls to less than 10 per cent of normal. Clinically significant malabsorption of fat-soluble vitamins is relatively rare in pancreatic insufficiency (as compared with small bowel mucosal disease), since normal lipolysis is relatively unimportant for the absorption of the fat-soluble vitamins. The pathophysiology of pancreatic malabsorption is discussed in detail in Ch. 104. Impaired glucose tolerance is common, but diabetic ketosis and coma are rare. The vascular, neurologic, and renal complications of diabetes mellitus are seldom seen in the hyperglycemia of chronic pancreatitis. Cobalamin malabsorption occurs in about 50 per cent of patients with chronic alcoholic pancreatitis, because of failure to digest cobalamin-binding proteins, but pernicious anemia is relatively uncommon.

CLINICAL MANIFESTATIONS. *Pain* is the predominant symptom in about 90 per cent of patients. It may take the form of recurrent acute attacks often superimposed on a background of low-grade abdominal pain or relatively constant pain usually aggravated by food ingestion. The discomfort is most often epigastric and in the left upper quadrant with radiation to the back and is characteristically relieved by forward flexion of the trunk. Physical examination of the abdomen usually reveals less abdominal tenderness than expected in view of the often disabling pain of which the patient complains.

As the disease progresses, insufficient pancreatic secretion results in *malabsorption* manifested by the passage of bulky, foul-smelling stools. The failure to digest triglycerides may result in the passage of fat droplets that float as a visible scum on the toilet water, a finding that indicates that the steatorrhea is due to pancreatic insufficiency rather than small bowel mucosal disease. The combination of malabsorption and poor oral intake often leads to appreciable weight loss. Malabsorption is described more extensively in Ch. 104.

Less common clinical manifestations of chronic pancreatitis include cholestasis caused by compression of the common duct as it passes through the head of the pancreas; subcutaneous fat necrosis presenting as erythematous, tender nodules, usually on the lower extremities; and intramedullary fat necrosis, causing bone pain. The complications of chronic pancreatitis are listed in Table 108–4.

DIAGNOSIS. The diagnosis of chronic pancreatitis usually requires no additional laboratory confirmation in the alcoholic patient with a past history of acute pancreatitis who subsequently develops chronic abdominal pain and steatorrhea. When the patient presents with chronic abdominal pain and steatorrhea without previous history of acute pancreatitis, the usual diagnostic problem is to distinguish chronic pancreatitis from carcinoma of the pancreas. Diffuse, stippled pancreatic calcification is observed radiographically in about 30 per cent of patients with chronic pancreatitis and is virtually diagnostic. Sonography or CT scanning should be the next step to rule out the presence of a solid, localized pancreatic mass suggesting carcinoma and to demonstrate calcifications not seen with a survey abdominal film. Pancreatic exocrine insufficiency is most readily documented by the bentiromide test. Bentiromide is a peptide linked to para-aminobenzoic acid (PABA) via a bond that is split by chymotrypsin. Free PABA is absorbed from the gut and excreted in urine. If diarrhea or steatorrhea is due to pancreatic insufficiency, PABA is not liberated from ingested bentiromide, and hence urinary excretion of PABA is subnormal. If the existence of chronic pancreatitis remains in doubt, it may be useful to measure pancreatic secretory function by collecting duodenal aspirate during secretin stimulation. Pancreatic secretion in chronic pancreatitis usually has decreased [HCO_3^-] and low output of enzymes; however, similar results may be observed in

TABLE 108–4. COMPLICATIONS OF CHRONIC PANCREATITIS

Pseudocyst formation
Pancreatic abscess
Obstruction of the common bile duct
Diabetes mellitus
Drug addiction
Exocrine insufficiency
Peptic ulcer
Fat necrosis—bone pain, subcutaneous tender nodules

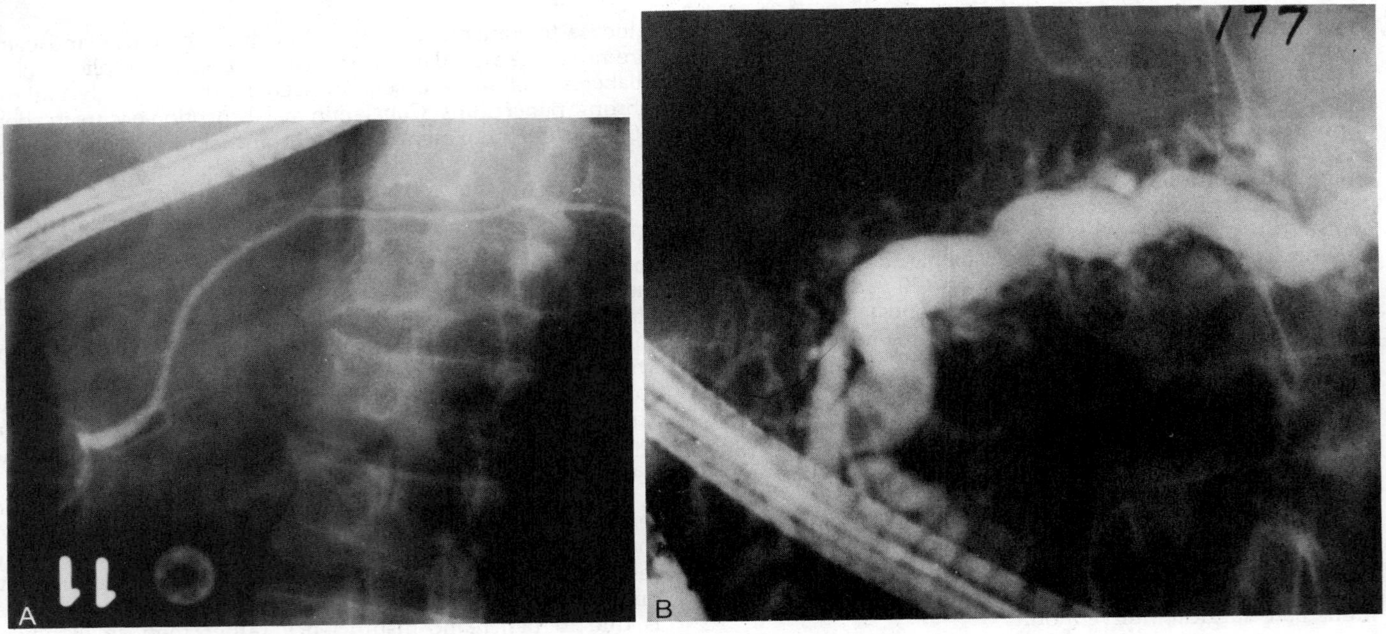

FIGURE 108–4. Normal pancreatic ductogram as demonstrated by ERCP (*A*), contrasted with dilatation of ductal system in chronic pancreatitis (*B*). (Courtesy of Dr. Stephen E. Silvis, Chief, Specialized Diagnostic and Treatment Unit, Medical Service, Veterans Administration Medical Center, Minneapolis, MN.)

carcinoma of the pancreas. Endoscopic retrograde cholangiopancreatography is almost always diagnostic in chronic pancreatitis. The main pancreatic duct is found to be irregularly strictured and dilated ("chain of lakes"), and the major branches have a "beaded" appearance owing to dilatation (Fig. 108–4). In pancreatic carcinoma a localized stricture of the main duct is observed, with dilatation distal to the stricture.

TREATMENT. Chronic symptomatic pancreatitis denotes irreversible pathologic damage to the pancreas. Although the course of the disease may not be modified, the conditions that predispose to pancreatitis (particularly alcoholism) should be eliminated if possible.

Pain. Pain is the predominant problem of most patients with chronic pancreatitis. In fact, there are few benign diseases associated with such persistent, disabling pain for which current medical or surgical therapy is so unsatisfactory. The cause of the pain is unclear, although its frequent relation to food ingestion suggests that pancreatic secretion plays a role. Large doses of pancreatic supplements appear to reduce the pain of some patients, presumably via a negative feedback on pancreatic secretion. Efforts should be to treat with nonaddicting analgesics, such as salicylates or acetaminophen. Unfortunately, most patients with chronic pancreatitis sooner or later become addicted to narcotics and the withdrawal of the narcotics is difficult to achieve. Dietary regimens or other forms of medical manipulation are rarely useful in the management of the pain. Fortunately, as the pancreatitis "burns out" the pain often gradually disappears, leaving exocrine and endocrine deficiency as the major clinical problems.

Because of the inadequacy of medical therapy, a variety of surgical procedures have been employed for the treatment of the pain of chronic pancreatitis. If the patient has a localized stricture of the main pancreatic duct or a pseudocyst, resection of the pancreas distal to the stricture or drainage of the cyst may produce remarkable improvement. However, most patients do not have such surgically treatable lesions. Although widely employed in the past, sphincterotomy and various procedures designed to interrupt the pain fibers from the pancreas appear to be of limited value. The Puestow procedure is designed to allow free drainage of the entire pancreatic duct into the small bowel. The main pancreatic duct is "filleted" along its entire linear extent, and a loop of jejunum is then anastomosed longitudinally over the opened duct. There is disagreement as to the benefit derived from the Puestow procedure. At best, not more than two thirds of patients obtain some pain relief, and most studies have not taken into account the decreasing pain that is part of the natural history of chronic pancreatitis.

Exocrine Deficiency. A second problem associated with chronic pancreatitis is malabsorption and diarrhea caused by deficient secretion of pancreatic enzymes. This problem can be controlled, although absorption is frequently not normalized, by the administration of 4 to 8 capsules of a pancreatic enzyme preparation with each meal. A low pH in the stomach irreversibly denatures the pancreatic enzyme. Therefore if malabsorption does not respond to pancreatic supplements, the additional administration of antacids or cimetidine to raise the pH of the stomach will enhance delivery of active enzyme into the duodenum and improve absorption. The treatment of pancreatic exocrine deficiency is described in greater detail as part of the general approach to patients with malabsorption (see Ch. 104).

PROGNOSIS. Few patients die of chronic pancreatitis per se. The incidence of carcinoma of the pancreas is, at most, only slightly increased above normal, except in the familial form of pancreatitis. Thus, the prognosis is largely a function of the associated alcoholism or of other diseases that may be associated with chronic pancreatitis.

Arvanitakis C, Cooke AR: Diagnostic tests of exocrine pancreatic function and disease. Gastroenterology 74:932, 1978. *Extensive review and bibliography of exocrine pancreatic function tests.*

Ettien JT, Webster PD III: The management of acute pancreatitis. Adv Intern Med 25:169, 1980. *Excellent review and bibliography of treatment of acute pancreatitis.*

Field BE, Hepner GW, Shabot MM, et al.: Nasogastric suction in alcoholic pancreatitis. Dig Dis Sci 24:339, 1979. *Controlled study showing no benefit from nasogastric suction in acute pancreatitis.*

Husband JC, Meire HG, Kreel L: Comparison of ultrasound and computer-assisted tomography in pancreatic diagnosis. Br J Radiol 50:855, 1977. *Compares the images of the ultrasound and computed tomography in acute and chronic pancreatitis.*

Isaksson G, Ihse I: Pain reduction by an oral pancreatic enzyme preparation in chronic pancreatitis. Dig Dis Sci 28:97, 1983. *Provides data on controlled trial of pancreatic supplements for control of pain of chronic pancreatitis.*

Ranson JH: The surgical treatment of acute pancreatitis. NY Acad Med Bull 58:601, 1982. *Review of surgical intervention in acute pancreatitis.*

Ranson JHC, Rifkind KM, Turner JW: Prognostic signs and nonoperative peritoneal lavage in acute pancreatitis. Surg Gynecol Obstet 143:209, 1976.

Evaluates the prognostic significance of various clinical and laboratory findings in acute pancreatitis.
Sarles H: Chronic calcifying pancreatitis—chronic alcoholic pancreatitis. Gastroenterology 66:604, 1974. *Review of pathogenesis of chronic, alcoholic pancreatitis.*
Soergal KH: Acute pancreatitis. Grendell JH, Cello JP: Chronic pancreatitis. In Sleisenger MR, Fordtran JS (eds.): Gastrointestinal Disease. 4th ed. Philadelphia, W. B. Saunders Company, 1988. *Excellent review of acute and chronic pancreatitis.*
Winship D, et al.: Pancreatitis: Pancreatic pseudocysts and their complications. Gastroenterology 73:593, 1977. *Review of etiology, diagnosis, course and treatment of pseudocysts.*

109 CARCINOMA OF THE PANCREAS

John P. Cello

DEFINITION. Carcinoma of the pancreas is an insidiously developing, relentlessly progressive, and nearly universally fatal malignancy arising in the epigastric retroperitoneum. Over 90 per cent of carcinomas of the pancreas are adenocarcinomas, derived from the simple cuboidal epithelium of the pancreatic duct. Five per cent of adenocarcinomas of the pancreas are of islet cell origin, often manifested early by the secretion of hormones. These islet cell malignancies are discussed in Ch. 233. Even rarer forms of pancreatic malignancy include acinar cell, epidermoid, adenocanthomas, sarcomas, and cystadenocarcinomas.

INCIDENCE AND EPIDEMIOLOGY. Carcinoma of the pancreas is responsible for over 24,000 new cases of cancer and 20,000 cancer-related deaths annually in the United States. This accounts for 5 per cent of all cancer-related deaths among both men and women. It is the second most common tumor of the digestive system (after colonic cancer) and the fourth most common cause of cancer deaths (after lung, breast, and colonic cancer). Men are more frequently afflicted than women (2:1 in most clinical studies). Although carcinoma of the pancreas may be seen in patients at any age, the mean age of onset is the seventh and eighth decades of life.

For unknown reasons, the age-adjusted mortality rate from carcinoma of the pancreas has been increasing in Western society over the past half century, whereas carcinoma of the stomach has decreased sharply in incidence. Pancreatic cancer is higher than expected among New Zealand Maoris, native Hawaiians, blacks, diabetics, and urban dwellers in higher latitudes.

Cigarette smoking is the strongest environmental factor associated with an increased risk for pancreatic cancer. The odds ratios for male and female smokers developing pancreatic cancer are 3:1 and 2:1, respectively, when compared with nonsmokers. Other environmental factors reported to increase the risk of pancreatic cancer include meat consumption; high fat intake; exposure to oil refining, gasoline, and paper manufacturing; and possibly asbestos in drinking water. A negative correlation has been suggested between pancreatic cancer and increased consumption of raw fruits and vegetables. There is little to suggest an association with either alcohol abuse or coffee consumption.

PATHOPHYSIOLOGY AND CLINICAL MANIFESTATIONS (see Table 109–1). Ductal adenocarcinoma of the pancreas is characterized pathologically by a dense fibrotic or desmoplastic reaction producing a compact, hard mass of tissue. The pancreas lacks a mesentery. It lies adjacent to the bile duct and other vital porta hepatis structures and is surrounded by duodenum, stomach, and colon; the most common clinical manifestations of pancreatic cancer are those related to the encroachment of these adjacent structures. There are few characteristic signs or symptoms that immediately point to a diagnosis of pancreatic cancer. At the time of diagnosis more than half of the patients complain of constant, dull *epigastric abdominal pain* occasionally going to the back. This usually implies invasion of adjacent retroperitoneal organs or splanchnic nerves. *Insidious weight loss* with anorexia and occasionally with a curious aversion for meats, accompanied by a metallic taste in the mouth, diarrhea, weakness, and vomiting, may also be seen. *Vomiting* may indicate gastric or duodenal invasion or extensive peritoneal metastases. *Hematemesis* and *melena* are occasionally noted by patients with duodenal or gastric involvement as the tumor erodes into these richly vascularized adjacent structures. *Jaundice* is noted in over 50 per cent of patients, the vast majority of whom have large tumor masses arising from the head of the pancreas encasing the distal common bile duct. On rare occasions, however, a small focal mass in the head of the pancreas will obstruct the distal common bile duct and produce early jaundice. About one quarter of the patients with pancreatic malignancy have a large, hard, palpable abdominal mass noted at the time of presentation. Occasionally, the jaundice and weight loss may be accompanied by a palpable, distended gallbladder *(Courvoisier's sign),* which is suggestive of the obstructing periampullary lesion. Patients with carcinoma of the pancreas may also have *thrombophlebitis, psychiatric disturbances,* or *diabetes mellitus.*

TABLE 109–1. SYMPTOMS AND ROUTINE LABORATORY TESTS IN CARCINOMA OF THE PANCREAS

Symptoms*	Percentage	Laboratory Test†	Percentage Abnormal
Abdominal pain	74	Alkaline phosphatase	82
Jaundice	65	5′-Nucleotidase	71
Weight loss	60	LDH	69
Diarrhea	27	SGOT	64
Weakness	21	Albumin	60
Constipation	8	Bilirubin	55
Hematemesis/melena	7	Amylase	17
Vomiting	6		
Abdominal mass	1		

*Modified from Anderson A, Bergdahl L: Am Surg 42:173, 1976.
†Modified from Fitzgerald PJ, Fortner JG, Watson RC, et al.: Cancer 41:868, 1978.
LDH = lactate dehydrogenase; SGOT = serum glutamic-oxaloacetic transaminase.

DIAGNOSIS. The insidious development of pancreatic malignancy without characteristic signs or symptoms and its low five-year survival rate have given rise to the search for newer, more sensitive and specific diagnostic tests. More patients with pancreatic cancer will have *anemia* resulting from nutritional deficiency, indolent blood loss into the bowel, or the anemia of "chronic disease." An *elevated erythrocyte sedimentation rate* is common, as is the presence of blood in the stools on chemical testing. On occasion, the obstructive jaundice together with blood loss into the duodenum may produce a characteristic *silver-colored stool.*

Serologic biochemical tests cannot definitively make or exclude the diagnosis of pancreatic malignancy (see Tables 109–1 and 109–2). On occasion, patients with pancreatic malignancy will have *elevated serum amylase* due to associated pancreatitis. *Elevation of serum alkaline phosphatase* (often greater than five to ten times the upper limits of normal values) occurs commonly in patients with pancreatic malignancy and is due either to distal common bile duct obstruction or to multiple hepatic metastases. In patients with bile duct obstruction, relentlessly progressive *hyperbilirubinemia* is noted, with the direct-reacting fraction predominant.

An array of serologic markers for the detection of pancreatic cancer has been reported with sensitivities ranging from 10 to 88 per cent. None of these markers can or should be used to make or exclude a diagnosis of pancreatic cancer. The most promising at present are carcinoembryonic antigen (CEA), galactosyltransferase isoenzyme II (GT-II), and antibody CA-19–9. An elevated serum level of CEA has been noted in over

TABLE 109–2. EVALUATION OF SENSITIVITY AND SPECIFICITY OF TESTS FOR PANCREATIC CANCER

	Ultrasound Positive in*	CT Positive in	ERCP Positive in	CEA Positive in	GT-II Positive in
Pancreatic cancer	64%	79%	93%	34%	67%
Other malignancies	13%	7%	0	26%	55%
Benign diseases	1%	4%	0	2%	2%

*"Positive in" refers to an imaging result suggestive of pancreatic cancer or an abnormally high serum level of CEA or GT-II. (Modified from Podolsky D, McPhee MS, Alpert E, et al.: N Engl J Med 304:1313, 1981.)

CT = computed tomography, ERCP = endoscopic retrograde cholangiopancreatography; CEA = carcinoembryonic antigen; GT-II = galactosyltransferase isoenzyme II.

70 per cent of patients with pancreatic malignancy. Elevation of CEA is not, however, specific for either pancreatic cancer or gastrointestinal tract malignancies in general (see Ch. 172). Elevated CEA levels are noted in patients with cirrhosis, chronic pancreatitis, renal failure, and some nongastrointestinal malignancies. Sixty-seven per cent of patients with pancreatic cancer had elevated GT-II levels in one study; however, 55 per cent of patients with other cancers and 2 per cent of patients with chronic pancreatitis also had elevated serum levels of this enzyme.

Nearly 90 per cent of patients with pancreatic cancer are reportedly positive for a serum mucin antigen detected by monoclonal antibody 19–9 (CA-19–9). A specificity of 95 per cent has been suggested, i.e., 95 per cent of patients *without* pancreatic cancer have negative results on the CA-19–9 antibody test. Other serologic and skin test markers for pancreatic cancer are promising, yet incompletely evaluated: pancreatic cancer–associated antigen (67 per cent sensitivity), oncofetal pancreatic antigen (88 per cent sensitivity), and skin test reactivity to Thomsen-Friedenreich antigen (88 per cent sensitivity).

The *upper gastrointestinal tract series* may demonstrate widening of the "C-loop" of the duodenum and mass indentation along the medial aspect of the descending duodenum in patients with cancer of the pancreatic head. Anterior displacement of the stomach and/or displacement of the ligament of Treitz from the greater curvature of the stomach may be noted radiographically in patients with carcinoma of the pancreatic body or tail. The upper gastrointestinal series is, however, a poor screening test in making an early diagnosis of pancreatic malignancy, especially in patients with carcinoma of the body and tail of the pancreas. Barium radiography will also interfere with computed tomographic (CT) scanning and thus should not be done initially in patients who are suspected of having pancreatic disease, either benign or malignant.

The abdominal imaging techniques of ultrasound and computed tomography (CT) (see Ch. 95) have markedly enhanced our ability to visualize the pancreas. Pancreatic malignancy is characteristically seen on *ultrasound* and *CT scanning* as either an asymmetrically or a uniformly enlarged and nonhomogeneous pancreas. In addition to the mass enlargement of the pancreas, marked dilation of the extrahepatic and intrahepatic bile ducts will be readily apparent in patients with bile duct obstruction (see Fig. 95–6). Metastases to the liver and peripancreatic lymph nodes may also be detected by either ultrasound or CT scanning. The sensitivity and specificity of both ultrasound and CT scanning in pancreatic cancer exceed 90 per cent. The larger mass lesions will almost certainly be demonstrated by both ultrasound and CT. However, the lower limits of resolution in both techniques are in the range of 1 to 2 cm; thus small, potentially resectable pancreatic cancers, especially those not altering the contour of the gland, may be overlooked. Nonetheless, these two tests are the most helpful in identifying patients with pancreatic disease and, when combined with cytologic studies, can establish the diagnosis of pancreatic cancer in the majority of instances (see below).

Many invasive diagnostic procedures are available for investigating tumors of the pancreas (see Ch. 95). *Angiography* will usually demonstrate displacement of the pancreatic arcades or tumor encasement of celiac, splenic, gastroduodenal, or superior mesenteric arteries. Moreover, the venous phase of the angiogram may demonstrate occlusion of the splenic vein and portal vein. With *secretin or cholecystokinin (CCK) stimulation of the pancreas*, the volume of pancreatic juice that can be collected via a duodenal sump (Dreiling) tube is characteristically decreased, but the bicarbonate and trypsin concentrations remain normal. *Transhepatic cholangiography* (THC) in patients with pancreatic malignancy obstructing the common bile duct will usually demonstrate a long, irregular, tapered segment of the common bile duct as it passes through the pancreatic malignancy. The radiographic findings are similar to those shown for cholangiocarcinoma in Figure 95–8. Difficulty may be encountered, however, in differentiating malignant stricturing of the distal common bile duct caused by pancreatic malignancy from that produced by scarring in a patient with chronic pancreatitis.

Endoscopic retrograde cholangiopancreatography (ERCP) provides the only means of directly opacifying the pancreatic duct (see Ch. 96). Since most pancreatic cancer is ductal adenocarcinoma, even small mass lesions will occlude branches of the main pancreatic duct. The characteristic finding of an abrupt cutoff of the pancreatic duct or the stricturing of both pancreatic and common bile duct (so-called "double duct sign") is virtually diagnostic of pancreatic carcinoma (Fig. 109–1).

Intraoperative transduodenal biopsy was previously the only means of obtaining tissue for histologic demonstration of malignancy. *Cytologic study of fluid* collected during ERCP may demonstrate malignant cells in the majority of patients. *Guided*

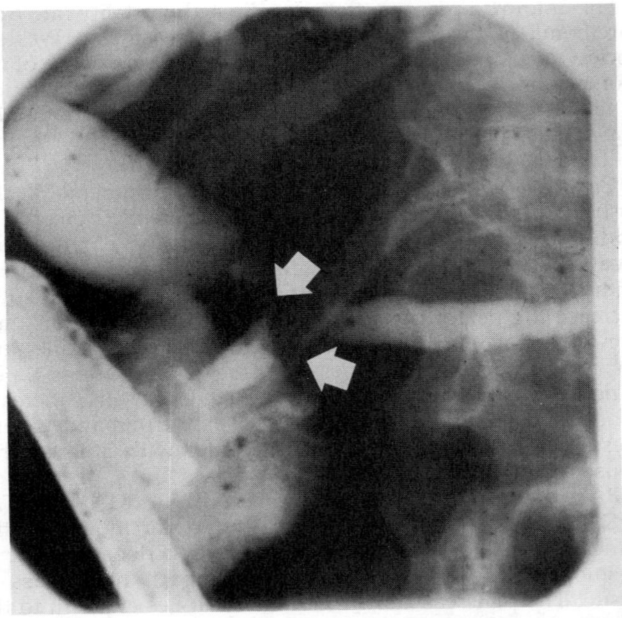

FIGURE 109–1. Endoscopic retrograde cholangiopancreatography (ERCP) in carcinoma of the head of the pancreas. A classic "double duct sign" is seen with stricturing of both the distal common bile duct and pancreatic duct (*arrows*). A markedly enlarged proximal common bile duct is filled with contrast material. A 2-cm pancreatic adenocarcinoma was successfully removed by Whipple's resection. However, death occurred within six months of recurrent disease.

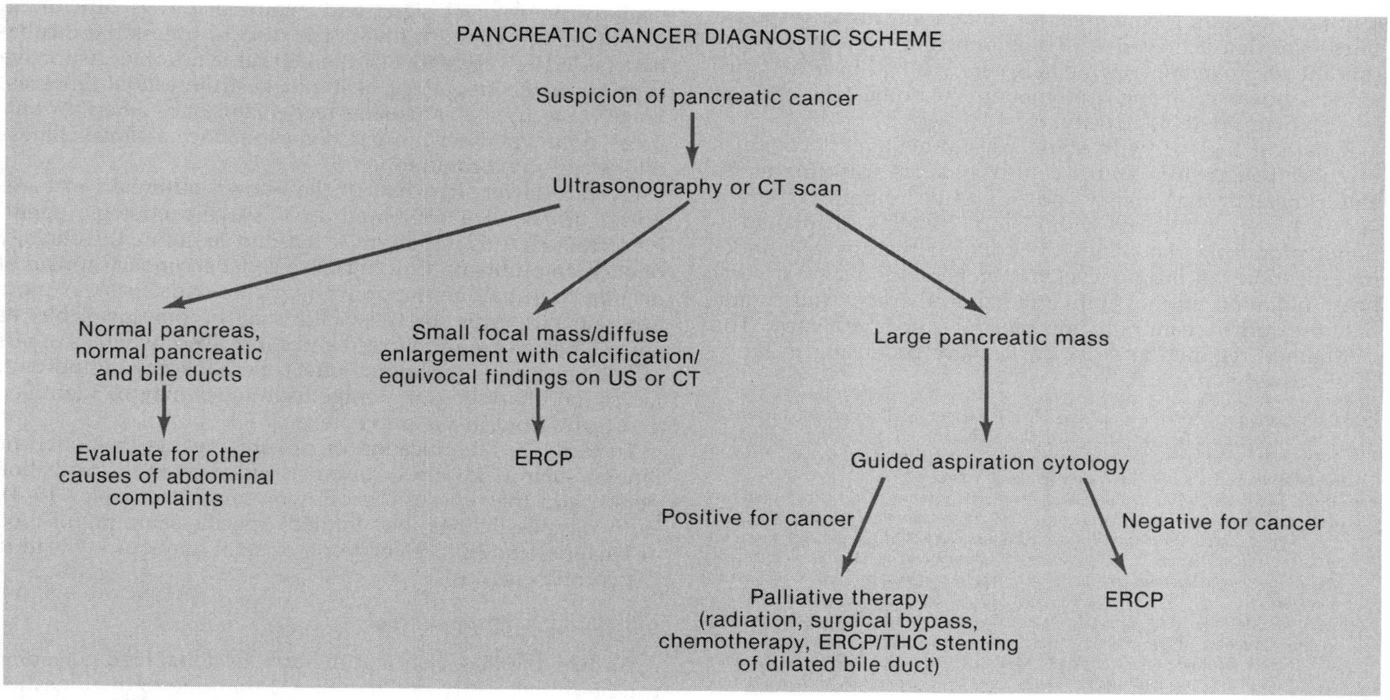

FIGURE 109–2. Suggested approach to the patient with the suspicion of pancreatic cancer. The initial evaluation should include adequate noninvasive imaging by either ultrasonography or computed tomography.

fine-needle aspiration cytology of the pancreas is now possible using either ultrasound or CT guidance. In most series, 80 to 90 per cent sensitivity and 100 per cent specificity in the presence of pancreatic cancer have been demonstrated.

LOGICAL USE OF DIAGNOSTIC METHODS. A schematic approach to the diagnosis of pancreatic cancer is summarized in Figure 109–2. In the patient who is suspected of having pancreatic malignancy, ultrasound should be performed first. If the ultrasound scan is inadequate in visualizing the pancreas, a CT study should then be done. In those patients with an accessible pancreatic mass (the situation in most patients with pancreatic cancer), a guided aspiration biopsy or cytologic examination of the mass lesion should be performed, using either ultrasound or CT guidance. In those patients with histologic or cytologic confirmation of malignancy, appropriate therapy may be initiated. For those patients with large pancreatic mass lesions but negative cytologic studies, an ERCP should be performed to demonstrate ductal changes of either pancreatic cancer or chronic pancreatitis. In patients with small focal enlargement or pancreatic calcification, ERCP should be performed to differentiate focal pancreatic disease such as malignancy from either chronic pancreatitis or a normal gland. A normal ultrasound scan and/or CT with a normal ERCP (all of which can and should be done on an outpatient basis) virtually excludes pancreatic cancer.

DIFFERENTIAL DIAGNOSIS. There are no characteristic signs or symptoms of carcinoma of the pancreas, especially for a cancer arising in the body or tail of the gland. In patients *without* jaundice, the vague abdominal pains, anorexia, weight loss, and malaise are all nonspecific and may be difficult to distinguish from those in patients with gastric ulcer, gastric cancer, other intra-abdominal malignancies, chronic pancreatitis, and even severe depression. In a reliable elderly patient, however, these complaints should lead to a suspicion of pancreatic or other malignancy. Epigastric abdominal masses from pancreatic cancer should be distinguished from an enlarged left hepatic lobe, gastric or colonic masses, large omental metastases, and pancreatic pseudocyst or chronic pancreatitis.

Most patients with carcinoma of the pancreatic head have obstructive jaundice. Other periampullary malignancies such as ampullary, duodenal, and cholangiocarcinomas and porta hepatis node metastases should be differentiated from pancreatic cancer, since they may have better prognoses than pancreatic cancer following radical surgery. Benign conditions causing obstructive jaundice, such as common bile duct gallstones, chronic pancreatitis, or bile duct strictures, must always be clearly differentiated from malignant obstruction of the bile duct. Intrahepatic cholestasis from drugs, toxins, hepatitis, abscess, cirrhosis, and even alcoholic hepatitis must be distinguished from extrahepatic cholestasis, usually by employing biochemical tests and noninvasive imaging techniques.

THERAPY. Despite the technical advances mentioned above, pancreatic cancer usually manifests clinically at a nonresectable stage of disease. Pancreatic cancer is usually treated by combinations of surgery, chemotherapy, and radiation therapy. Whipple's resection (pancreaticoduodenectomy) or subtotal or total pancreatectomy should be reserved for patients with small focal mass lesions without any evidence of involvement of adjacent vascular structures or distal metastases. The operative mortality of Whipple's procedure is 20 per cent, with a mean five-year survival of only 5 per cent. Mean survival in an unselected series of patients undergoing Whipple's resection is not significantly better than with the palliative biliary bypass alone. Total pancreatectomy, combining the en bloc resection of pancreas and spleen, may improve mean survival when compared with palliative bypass and Whipple's resection. In symptomatic patients with large, bulky tumor masses obstructing the common bile duct, palliative surgical bypass with a choledochojejunostomy or cholecystojejunostomy should be considered. Percutaneous transhepatic or endoscopic retrograde stenting of the common bile duct may likewise palliatively decompress the dilated biliary tree. These last two techniques, in experienced hands, should be employed, rather than laparotomy palliative duct decompression, in poor-risk surgical patients with large, bulky tumors.

Single-agent chemotherapy offers limited palliation but no improved survival in patients with nonresectable pancreatic cancer. Combination chemotherapy, employing agents such as 5-fluorouracil (5-FU), mitomycin C, streptozocin, and doxorubicin in varying combinations, offers improved response rates over that achieved with single-drug treatment. No significant improvement in median survival has been demonstrated, however, using combination chemotherapy, often at levels of considerable toxicity.

Radiation therapy with standard supravoltage techniques provides palliation in 70 per cent of patients with nonresectable pancreatic malignancy and can result in improved mean survival when compared with historic controls. Several additional promising modalities of radiation therapy are under investigation, including cyclotron-generated heavy particle beam radiation, intraoperative radiation therapy, and combination external beam radiation plus 5-FU chemotherapy. The last-named regimen appears particularly promising in terms of improved survival.

Cello JP: Carcinoma of the pancreas. In Sleisenger MH, Fordtran JS (eds.): Gastrointestinal Disease. 4th ed. Philadelphia, W. B. Saunders Company, 1988. *This recent review covers the general topic of carcinoma of the pancreas and contains an extensive and up-to-date list of 54 references.*

Fitzgerald PJ, Fortner JG, Watson RC, et al.: The value of diagnostic aids in detecting pancreas cancer. Cancer 41:868, 1978. *Thorough analysis is made of the diagnostic accuracy of invasive and noninvasive tests in 184 patients suspected of having pancreatic cancer. CT scanning, celiac angiography, alkaline phosphatase, and ^{75}Se-selenomethionine, in that order, had the highest percentage of correct diagnoses.*

Podolsky D, McPhee MS, Alpert E, et al.: Galactosyltransferase isoenzyme II in the detection of pancreatic cancer: Comparison with radiologic, endoscopic and serologic tests. N Engl J Med 304:1313, 1981. *GT-II was the most sensitive (67 per cent) and specific (98 per cent) for discriminating between benign and malignant pancreatic disease. As a single test, only ERCP was more sensitive than GT-II. When GT-II was combined with ultrasound or with CT, sensitivities of 92 and 88 per cent, respectively, were noted.*

Van Dyke JA, Stanley RJ, Berland LL: Pancreatic imaging. Ann Intern Med 102:212, 1985. *Review of the available imaging techniques of the pancreas. Computed tomography is the best for initial evaluation of the patient with suspected pancreatic disease. No single test will always provide all necessary diagnostic information.*

110 FOOD POISONING

David F. Altman

Food poisoning, which may be defined as clinical syndromes arising from the ingestion of food that either is contaminated or is itself toxic, may cause illness in three distinct ways: (1) by contamination of food with microorganisms or their products (most common); (2) by its contamination with poisonous chemicals; or (3) by ingestion of poisonous plants or animals.

As the gastrointestinal tract is the mode of entry for these various contaminants, most illnesses associated with food poisoning involve some form of gastroenteritis, with either upper or lower gastrointestinal manifestations predominating. Other syndromes are often identifiable by extraintestinal (particularly neurologic) signs and symptoms. It is difficult to identify single cases of foodborne disease unless the incubation period is very short or the clinical syndrome distinctive because of the frequency of minor gastrointestinal illnesses. Foodborne disease is usually recognized only when an outbreak occurs and several persons experience a similar illness after ingesting a common food.

Overall, fewer than half of the known outbreaks of foodborne disease are attributed to a specific etiologic agent. Nevertheless, it is important to attempt to define the etiology of such an outbreak. Prophylaxis against secondary spread of an infection may be important (e.g., in shigellosis). A more accurate prognosis for the victim may become available, as some illnesses are self-limited and short-lived, whereas others may have a chronic residual effect. Perhaps most important, faulty food handling or storage techniques may be identified and further outbreaks prevented.

To facilitate identification of possible agents in foodborne illness, such syndromes can be classified by their incubation period and the type of clinical symptoms (see Table 110–1). With the possibilities thus limited, specific sampling of food or bacteriologic cultures of blood or stool may quickly lead to the correct diagnosis.

BACTERIAL FOOD POISONING

As an aid to diagnosis and therapy, bacterial food poisoning can be conveniently classified as (1) that due to the ingestion of living microorganisms, (2) that due to the ingestion of a toxin produced by microorganisms in food prior to its ingestion, or (3) that due to enterotoxins produced in the gut by pathogens only after their ingestion.

The most important "infectious" types of food poisoning, requiring ingestion of living organisms, are *Salmonella* gastroenteritis and *Shigella* dysentery, which are dealt with in Ch. 284 and 285, respectively. Other organisms responsible in this way include *Campylobacter jejuni, Escherichia coli, Vibrio cholerae, Vibrio parahaemolyticus, Bacillus cereus,* and *Clostridium perfringens.* In addition, epidemics of listeriosis transmitted by food and a foodborne outbreak of streptococcal pharyngitis have both been reported.

The "toxin" type of food poisoning most often identified is due to *Staphylococcus aureus.* The syndrome of botulism caused by ingestion of the toxin produced by *Clostridium botulinum* is discussed in Ch. 280.

Staphylococcal Food Poisoning

ETIOLOGY. This form of food poisoning is caused by an enterotoxin produced by multiplying staphylococci before the contaminated food is ingested. Nearly all strains known to elaborate enterotoxins are coagulase-positive *Staphylococcus aureus;* however, some coagulase-negative strains have also been incriminated. The two major sources of contamination are human carriers (usually nasal or skin) and cows with mastitis, the former accounting for nearly 90 per cent of

TABLE 110–1. CLINICAL INDICATORS OF THE ETIOLOGY OF FOODBORNE ILLNESS

	Mean Incubation Period			
Predominant Symptomatology	*< 2 Hours*	*2–7 Hours*	*8–14 Hours*	*> 14 hours*
Upper intestinal	Heavy metals	*S. aureus* *B. cereus*		
Lower intestinal			*C. perfringens* *B. cereus*	*V. cholera* Enterotoxic or invasive *E. coli* *Shigella* spp. *V. parahaemolyticus* *Salmonella*
Both upper and lower gastrointestinal				*V. parahaemolyticus*
Extragastrointestinal, i.e., some gastrointestinal plus others, usually paresthesias or other abnormal sensory complaint	Scombrotoxin Shellfish toxin Mushroom toxin (early)	Ciguatoxin	Mushroom toxin (delayed)	*C. botulinum*

outbreaks. Staphylococcal food poisoning requires not only contamination of food with the microorganisms but also a period of some hours during which they may multiply, as may occur during slow cooling after cooking or if food is held at ambient temperature. Subsequent reheating may destroy the organism but not the remarkably heat-resistant toxin, and it is the latter that causes the clinical illness.

PATHOGENESIS, CLINICAL MANIFESTATIONS, AND TREATMENT. Little is known about the mode of action of the enterotoxins. In experimental animals they cause destruction of gastrointestinal mucosal cells and evoke an inflammatory response. Effects on other organ systems, including the emetic centers in the brain, also have been postulated. Symptoms usually begin two to four hours after ingestion of the toxin, heralded by salivation and followed rapidly by nausea, vomiting, abdominal cramping, and diarrhea. The illness usually is short, rarely lasting 24 hours, and often is subsiding by the time medical attention is sought. It may occasionally be life-threatening, especially in the elderly or in persons with other serious illness. Therapy is supportive and symptomatic, the primary goal being to restore extracellular fluid volume with parenteral fluids as necessary. Antibiotic therapy may worsen the course of the illness.

PREVENTION. Proper food handling is essential for the prevention of staphylococcal food poisoning. Sanitary measures and personal hygiene can prevent contamination of the food to some degree. More importantly, food handlers must recognize that enterotoxin is not produced at ordinary domestic refrigerator temperatures. Foods should not be left to cool slowly, especially in large containers, and should be taken from the refrigerator (and reheated, if required) immediately before serving.

Clostridial Food Poisoning

ETIOLOGY. *Clostridium perfringens* type A has been the third most common bacterial cause of food poisoning in the United States for the last several years. Clostridial poisoning typically occurs in fairly large outbreaks. The organism is ubiquitous, being found in most samples of raw meat, human and animal feces, flies, soil, and dirt from kitchens. Both heat-sensitive and heat-resistant strains have been known to cause outbreaks. The conditions necessary for an outbreak generally include the cooking of meat, poultry, or beans at a temperature (usually less than 100° C) high enough to kill vegetative forms but insufficient to destroy heat-resistant spores. Oxygen is driven out of the food, thereby lowering the oxidation-reduction potential of the medium. During slow cooling the spores germinate, encouraged by the relatively anaerobic environment and the rich supply of amino acids and other growth factors. If the food is not reheated to a temperature high enough to inactivate the recently multiplied organism, ingestion may result in illness.

PATHOGENESIS AND CLINICAL MANIFESTATIONS. Ingestion of living organisms is necessary for the production of clostridial food poisoning, but the pathogenesis of the clinical manifestations remains to be defined. Several toxins have been suggested, but none is clearly responsible for human disease. The incubation period is usually 8 to 12 hours after ingestion, but may be as long as 24 hours. The usual symptoms are abdominal cramps and diarrhea; vomiting is rare, as are headache, chills, and fever. The illness is self-limited, rarely lasting more than 24 hours. Treatment rarely is necessary and should always be confined to efforts at symptomatic relief. The few deaths recorded have been in elderly or debilitated patients.

PREVENTION. Food is best served immediately after cooking. If it is to be kept, it should be cooled rapidly. Cooked meat should always be kept either cold, below 5° C, or hot, over 60° C. This is especially true of food prepared in large batches.

Vibrio parahaemolyticus Food Poisoning

V. parahaemolyticus is a gram-negative facultative anaerobe found in marine water and fauna throughout the world. It lives in sediment of coastal and estuarian waters during cold winter months. As the temperature rises in spring and summer, the organism leaves the sediment and colonizes animal life, especially shellfish and crustaceans. Not all strains are pathogenic.

The pathogenesis of the illness is not clearly defined, and different serotypes may produce disease by different mechanisms. The presence of fecal leukocytes and occasionally bloody diarrhea implies bacterial invasion and damage of the gut mucosa.

Virtually all outbreaks of *V. parahaemolyticus* food poisoning have occurred during warm months of the year and have been associated with the ingestion of raw or improperly refrigerated seafood. Although originally described in Japan, cases have occurred in other parts of Asia and on the Atlantic, Gulf, and Pacific coasts of the United States. The incubation period is usually between 12 and 24 hours, but has been as long as 96 hours. Explosive watery diarrhea is present in more than 90 per cent of cases, with nausea, vomiting, and abdominal cramps as common accompaniments. Fever, headache, and chills occur less often. The diagnosis is suspected when a typical illness occurs after eating seafood, and is confirmed by recovery of the organism from stool. Treatment is rarely necessary, as the illness infrequently lasts more than two days. However, in protracted cases, antibiotic treatment with tetracycline or ampicillin may shorten the illness.

Prevention depends on the recognition both of the potential for contamination of seafood with *V. parahaemolyticus* during warm months and of the predisposition of organisms to multiply under conditions of inadequate refrigeration. Cooked seafood may also become cross-contaminated when stored under proper conditions with a raw source.

Bacillus cereus Food Poisoning

Bacillus cereus, an aerobic, motile, spore-forming, gram-positive rod, has been increasingly recognized as a cause of foodborne disease. There appear to be two separate clinical forms of the disease. An emetic form, clinically identical to staphylococcal food poisoning, is associated with contaminated fried rice. A diarrheal form has a longer incubation period and predominantly lower gastrointestinal symptoms, reminiscent of *Clostridium perfringens* food poisoning. Cell-free filtrates derived from *B. cereus* strains responsible for this latter form of illness stimulate the adenylate cyclase–cyclic adenosine monophosphate (cAMP) system in intestinal epithelial cells, and their activity is destroyed by heat, thus resembling cholera enterotoxin. The illnesses are usually mild and self-limited, and antibiotics are not indicated. No fatalities have been reported. As the organism commonly occurs in soil and in many dried or processed foods, careful food handling is most important in prevention of the disease. *B. cereus* may be found in uncooked rice, for example, and heat-resistant spores may survive boiling. If the rice is left unrefrigerated, the spores may then germinate and produce toxin. Flash frying or rewarming before serving is often not sufficient to destroy the preformed, heat-stable toxin. The disease thus can be prevented by prompt refrigeration of boiled rice.

Blake PA: Diseases of humans (other than cholera) caused by vibrios. Ann Rev Microbiol 34:341, 1980. *A comprehensive review of clinical and microbiologic aspects of Vibrio-caused disease.*

Centers for Disease Control: Foodborne disease outbreaks, annual summary, 1982. In CDC Surveillance Summaries, 35:7ss, 1986. *An annual compendium of reports of foodborne diseases in the United States, with analysis of vehicles of transmission and contributing factors to contamination for each type of infection identified.*

Holmberg SD, Blake PA: Staphylococcal food poisoning in the United States: New facts and old misconceptions. JAMA 251:487, 1984. *Information on the epidemiology and clinical characteristics of this entity.*

Horowitz MA: Specific diagnosis of foodborne disease. Gastroenterology 73:375, 1977. *A clinician's guide to the clinical and epidemiologic differential diagnosis of foodborne diseases.*
Schlech WF III, Lavigne PM, Bortolussi RA, et al.: Epidemic listeriosis—evidence for transmission by food. N Engl J Med 308:203, 1983. *This is a thorough account of a heretofore suspected but unproved type of food-related illness.*
Terranova W, Blake PA: *Bacillus cereus* food poisoning. N Engl J Med 298:143, 1978. *A brief but comprehensive review of the various forms of this illness.*

CHEMICAL FOOD POISONING

Food poisoning caused by chemicals may be related either to the accidental contamination of food prior to its preparation or during storage or to a food additive or preservative. Thus various forms of metallic poisoning, discussed in Ch. 542, can occur when food, particularly acid liquids, comes in contact with certain metals, especially cadmium, copper, tin, or zinc.

The so-called Chinese restaurant syndrome, in which individuals develop sensations of burning skin, facial pressure, chest pressure, and headaches 10 to 20 minutes after eating certain Chinese foods (especially won ton soup), has been attributed to the use of monosodium L-glutamate (MSG). The symptoms appear to be a pharmacologic effect of MSG, obeying a dose-effect relationship, but with a widely variable threshold for an oral dose.

Sodium nitrite, widely used as a preservative in smoked meats, has been blamed for the "hot dog headache" seen in some persons. In addition, because of its metabolism to nitrosamines it is suspected to be a potential carcinogen, although evidence for this is inconclusive.

Food additives such as aspartame and pesticides have been incriminated as a cause of foodborne disease. Although the former have not been conclusively identified as the source of illness, outbreaks of the latter have been documented. A recent episode of contamination of watermelons by aldicarb caused gastrointestinal and neurologic symptoms in over 1000 individuals.

Schaumburg HH, Byck R, Gerstil R, et al.: Monosodium L-glutamate: Its pharmacology and role in the Chinese restaurant syndrome. Science 163:826, 1969. *A careful analysis of MSG pharmacology and its dose-effect relationships.*

POISONOUS ANIMALS AND PLANTS

Fish and Shellfish Poisoning

Vertebrate fish may contain various toxins capable of causing human illness. Most commonly this is due to toxin contained in musculature (ichthyosarcotoxins), of which nine types have been described. The most common fish poisonings worldwide—ciguatera, scombroid, and puffer fish poisoning—are attributable to ichthyosarcotoxins.

Two forms of shellfish poisoning, paralytic and neurotoxic, have been described. These are caused by toxins derived from dinoflagellates contaminating the shellfish.

CIGUATERA FISH POISONING. Ciguatera fish poisoning is caused by ciguatoxin, a lipid-soluble, heat-stable substance for which chemical structure has not been determined. More than 400 fish species have been implicated, generally bottom-dwelling shore fish found in temperate and tropical zones.

The onset of the illness usually occurs one to six hours after, but may be as soon as a few minutes or as long as 30 hours after, ingestion of toxic fish. Gastrointestinal symptoms, including abdominal cramps, nausea, vomiting, and diarrhea, predominate at the outset, along with numbness, pruritus, and paresthesias of the lips, tongue, and throat. Paresthesias may later involve the extremities, and in severe cases there may be abnormal temperature sensations, cranial nerve palsies, hypotension, bradycardia, and even respiratory paralysis. Acute symptoms usually subside within a few days and require only symptomatic, supportive therapy. The return of pruritus with alcohol ingestion is thought to be almost pathognomonic of this syndrome. Weakness and sensory disturbances may persist for months or years.

SCOMBROID FISH POISONING. Scrombroid fish poisoning is the only form of ichthyosarcotoxism in which toxins are formed by the action of bacteria, in this case particularly *Proteus morgani*, on fish flesh. The chemical nature of the scombrotoxin is unknown, but it is thought to consist of histamine and related substances. Most fish that have caused outbreaks are members of the suborder *Scombroidea*, most commonly mahi-mahi, tuna, mackerel, and bonito. Symptoms begin within a few minutes of ingestion and resemble those of a histamine reaction: flushing, headache, dizziness, abdominal cramps, nausea, vomiting and diarrhea, and occasionally urticaria and generalized pruritus. The illness has a median duration of four hours in the reported outbreaks. Antihistamines have provided symptomatic relief, which has been reported to be rapid and complete with intravenous cimetidine. Production of the toxin is inhibited by proper refrigeration, perhaps reflecting the temperature optimum of 20 to 30° C for the enzymatic conversion of histidine to histamine. Improper refrigeration of fresh-caught fish has been observed in most outbreaks of this illness.

PUFFER FISH POISONING (TETRODOTOXIN POISONING). Many puffer fish found in the Pacific, Atlantic, and Indian Oceans are inherently toxic. The tetrodotoxin found in their viscera is a neurotoxin, and its effects are nearly identical to the saxitoxin that produces paralytic shellfish poisoning (see below).

PARALYTIC SHELLFISH POISONING. Paralytic shellfish poisoning is caused by the ingestion of bivalve mollusks contaminated with the neurotoxin of the dinoflagellates *Gonyaulax catanella* or *Go. tamarensis.* Although a "red tide," related to "blooming" of the dinoflagellates, has been associated with paralytic shellfish poisoning, not all red tides are toxic, and some outbreaks have occurred in the absence of a red tide. The toxin of *Go. catanella,* saxitoxin, appears to act by blocking the propagation of nerve and muscle action potentials.

The illness begins within 30 minutes of ingestion of a toxic mollusk and is characterized by paresthesias of the mouth, lips, face, and extremities and by nausea, vomiting, and diarrhea. In more severe cases, muscle weakness or paralysis and respiratory embarrassment may occur. Deaths, though rare, have occurred within the first 12 hours. Treatment consists of a cathartic or enema in severe cases to remove unabsorbed toxin. Gastric lavage may be used if vomiting has not occurred. Mechanical ventilatory assistance may be required.

NEUROTOXIC SHELLFISH POISONING. *Gymnodinium breve* is a toxic dinoflagellate that causes a red tide off both the Gulf and Atlantic coasts of Florida. Within three hours of the consumption of shellfish contaminated with this toxin, patients experience paresthesias, abnormal temperature sensations, ataxia, nausea, vomiting, and diarrhea. The disease is self-limited and milder than paralytic shellfish poisoning. No deaths have been reported.

MUSHROOM POISONING

Of the more than 2000 identified species of mushrooms, fewer than 50 are poisonous. However, even expert mycologists may have difficulty identifying poisonous species. Moreover, with the increased interest in "organic" foods and in the hallucinogenic substances found in certain species, poisoning from the ingestion of wild mushrooms has been increasing in frequency.

The principal toxin is amanitine, which contains cyclic octapeptides. Phalloidin, another putative toxin, appears to have some hepatocellular toxicity, but mushrooms with phalloidin but without amanitine have been consumed without ill effect. Amanitine selectively inhibits nuclear ribonucleic acid (RNA) polymerase II. Mushrooms containing these toxins belong to the genera *Amanita* and *Galerina*. *Amanita verna* (the "destroying angel"), *A. virosa*, and *A. phalloides* (the "death cap") are the species most often associated with mushroom poisoning in the United States, and *A. phalloides* accounts for more than 90 per cent of such deaths in Europe.

Symptoms of *A. phalloides*–type mushroom poisoning characteristically occur in three stages. The first is characterized by the abrupt onset of abdominal pain, nausea, vomiting, and diarrhea 6 to 24 hours after ingestion. This may be accompanied by severe fluid and electrolyte disturbances and fever. The second stage, occurring during the next 24 to 48 hours, involves worsening of hepatic and renal function despite resolution of the initial symptoms. Finally, during the third and fourth days after ingestion, hepatic and renal function deteriorates, accompanied occasionally by cardiomyopathy and coagulopathy, convulsions, coma, and death. The mortality rate is between 40 and 90 per cent.

The diagnosis of mushroom poisoning may be difficult. The delayed onset of symptoms may cause patients not to associate the illness with the ingestion of wild mushrooms. The mushroom toxins can be detected in gastric aspirate, vomitus, or stool by thin-layer chromatography in some laboratories. Treatment remains supportive, including renal dialysis when indicated. Thioctic acid has been used experimentally since 1968 as an antidote for *A. phalloides*–type mushroom poisoning, but this treatment now appears to be ineffective. There has been a report of a successful orthotopic liver transplantation in a child, but timing of surgery and availability of a suitable donor will continue to make this rarely possible.

Plant Alkaloids, Mycotoxins, and Other Poisonings

These various forms of food poisoning remind us of historic knowledge of the pharmacologic effect of plant alkaloids and other toxicants found naturally in foods. Although formerly used with therapeutic intent, plant alkaloids are now more often ingested accidentally and often in large doses. Reports now appear of digitalis intoxication from home-brewed teas made with foxglove or oleander, diarrhea from senna tea, which contains the stimulant cathartic anthraquinone, and liver failure from *Senecio longilobus*, which contains highly hepatotoxic pyrrolizidine alkaloids. Other highly toxic plants include *Atropa belladonna* (deadly nightshade) and *Datura stramonium* (thorn apple, jimson weed), whose berries and seeds can cause an atropine effect, *Conium maculatum* (hemlock), which contains several alkaloids with severe central nervous system depressant effects, and *Phytolacca americana* (pokeweed), whose leaves and berries have strong emetic properties.

Lathyrism, a slowly progressive spastic paraplegia, is associated with the ingestion of sweet peas of the species *Lathyrus sativus*. Large amounts of this may be ingested during famines in Africa and Asia. The toxic principle appears to be beta-aminoproprionitrile. Interestingly, this substance, when given to poultry and other experimental animals, causes degeneration of the aortic media, with resulting dissecting aortic aneurysms or aortic rupture. This effect is not seen in humans.

Mycotoxins may contaminate some moldy foods. Ergotism, characterized by intense vasospasm, is the most familiar syndrome caused by this ingestion. Other mycotoxins, including aflatoxin, have been identified. This product of *Aspergillus flavus* contaminates grains stored in warm, damp areas, and has been associated with the development of hepatocellular carcinoma. Small amounts of aflatoxin have been found in commercial peanut butter in the United States.

Hughes JM, Merson MH: Fish and shellfish poisoning. N Engl J Med 295:1117, 1976. *A thorough review of the pathophysiology and clinical manifestations of this group of illnesses.*

Olson KR, Pond SM, Seward J, et al.: *Amanita phalloides*–type mushroom poisoning. West J Med 137:282, 1982. *This is a comprehensive review of the clinical manifestations of mushroom poisoning, the various species involved, and a brief guide to their identification. Therapeutic options are presented.*

Poisoning associated with herbal teas. MMWR 26:257, 1977. *Case reports and discussions of several types of herbal poisonings.*

Wogan GN: Mycotoxins. Ann Rev Pharmacol 15:437, 1975. *A review of the current understanding of the pharmacology and health impact of mycotoxins.*

111 DISEASES OF THE RECTUM AND ANUS

David F. Altman

DISEASES OF THE RECTUM

INTRODUCTION. The rectum primarily serves a storage function by allowing convenient disposition of fecal waste. Most diseases of the rectum involve some inflammatory change that alters neuromuscular control over defecation and results in symptoms of constipation or diarrhea, tenesmus, and urgency.

The sigmoidoscope and forceps biopsy instruments are most useful to examine the rectum. In contrast, the barium enema gives poor resolution in the rectum and therefore is unreliable as a primary diagnostic tool. Sigmoidoscopy using flexible fiberoptic instruments permits more of the rectum and sigmoid to be examined with decreased patient discomfort.

PROCTITIS. Inflammatory disease of the rectum may be caused by radiation injury, trauma from a foreign body, ischemia or infection, or other processes. Chronic inflammatory disease of unknown etiology, perhaps related to more generalized inflammatory bowel diseases, is a frequent occurrence.

INFECTIOUS PROCTITIS. Inflammatory disease in the rectum may be caused by several infectious agents. The syndromes of bacillary dysentery and amebiasis are discussed in Ch. 285 and 390, respectively. Venereally transmitted diseases, especially gonorrhea, syphilis, lymphogranuloma venereum (LGV), and non–LGV chlamydial serotypes, may involve the rectum primarily (see Ch. 306, 307, and 310). These diseases have their greatest impact in the male homosexual population; e.g., asymptomatic rectal carriage of gonorrhea may be detected in up to two thirds of tested subjects, and frequent sexual contact permits rapid spread of the infection.

Diagnosis of anorectal gonorrhea is best made by obtaining culture material with a sterile cotton swab inserted approximately 2.5 cm into the anal canal, swept around a peripheral arc for ten seconds, and then inoculated immediately on selective growth medium. Rarely, disseminated gonococcal infection with bacteremia has been reported after anorectal gonorrhea. Treatment is the same as for other localized gonococcal infections (see Ch. 306).

Herpes simplex virus is known to cause an acute proctitis in homosexual men. Anorectal pain and discharge are the most common presenting complaints, and these are often accompanied by constipation, tenesmus, and hematochezia. Neurologic involvement, with urinary bladder dysfunction, paresthesias, erectile difficulties, and gluteal or thigh pain, is also seen. Proctoscopy will often show an acute distal proctitis with ulcerations. Rectal biopsy shows acute inflammation, and intranuclear inclusions, if seen, confirm the diagnosis. Treatment is supportive and symptoms resolve spontaneously, although there may be periodic recurrences.

NONSPECIFIC ULCERATIVE PROCTITIS. Nonspecific ulcerative proctitis most commonly produces symptoms of rectal bleeding, tenesmus, and often a mucosanguineous anal discharge. The bleeding seldom is severe, and patients with diarrhea often describe no increase in stool volume but rather frequent passage of small amounts of mucus or blood. Systemic symptoms, such as fever and weight loss, rarely occur. Indeed, the patient usually feels remarkably well in spite of the primary complaints noted above. Extraintestinal manifestations of inflammatory bowel disease, especially arthritis, uveitis, and dermatitis, also are rare. The diagnosis is made when (1) sigmoidoscopy reveals inflammation of the rectal mucosa with a clearly demarcated upper border above which the mucosa is normal, (2) the remainder of the colon and small intestine is found to be normal by barium radiograph and/or colonoscopy, and (3) a rectal biopsy demonstrates changes indistinguishable from those of chronic ulcerative colitis.

Differential diagnosis includes Crohn's ileocolitis, radiation proctitis, and infectious disease of the rectum, especially bacillary dysentery, amebiasis, lymphogranuloma venereum, and gonorrheal proctitis. A detailed history and physical examination, appropriate cultures of stool and rectal mucus, biopsy, and serologic studies for chlamydiae should suffice to distinguish among these possibilities.

Treatment is primarily that used for more generalized inflammatory bowel disease, with the exception that systemic corticosteroids are rarely or never used. Topical corticosteroids, administered once or twice daily either as suppositories or as enemas, often provide a satisfactory response. Sulfasalazine or other poorly absorbed sulfa preparations may also be used either orally or rectally. With treatment the disease usually runs a course with periodic exacerbations. Rectal strictures may occur, but carcinoma of the rectum seems to be only a small risk. However, biannual sigmoidoscopy is warranted to follow the course of the illness. Fewer than 15 per cent of patients with ulcerative proctitis develop diffuse ulcerative colitis.

FECAL IMPACTION AND STERCORAL ULCER. Incomplete evacuation of feces over an extended period of time may result in the formation of an obstructing mass of firm stool in the distal colon or rectum. *Fecal impaction* occurs most often in children with undiagnosed congenital megacolon or psychiatric disorders, in patients with painful anal diseases, and in elderly, debilitated, or sedentary persons. Patients may complain only of a sensation of fullness in the lower abdomen, anorexia, and malaise. Liquid stool above the fecal mass may distend the proximal colon and then pass around the obstruction. This may be misinterpreted as diarrhea, and inappropriate treatment may be instituted. The diagnosis is most easily made on digital rectal examination, but when the impaction is located more proximally in the sigmoid colon, only an abdominal mass may be felt.

A large fecal impaction usually requires both administration of enemas and mechanical disimpaction digitally. Treatment consisting of saline enemas and oral mineral oil is usually successful once the fecal mass has been broken up. More extraordinary enema solutions have included milk and molasses in equal volumes and water-soluble radiographic contrast material. Warm oil or soapsuds enemas rarely are necessary; in fact, they may be injurious to the rectal mucosa.

Fecal impactions may be associated with the development of intestinal obstruction, volvulus, megacolon, or rectal prolapse. Colonic perforation can occur spontaneously, usually during the attempted passage of the fecal mass. More often, perforation is iatrogenic and is signaled by the onset of fever, abdominal pain and distention, or shock shortly after disimpaction. Surgical treatment is required, and without early diagnosis mortality is high.

Stercoral ulcers in the rectum and colon probably result from pressure necrosis produced by the fecal mass. The ulcer is irregular and has a dark gray or purple outline. Biopsies reveal little inflammation. The ulcer heals rapidly after the mass is removed, but complications of bleeding or perforation have been reported.

Prevention of recurrent impaction is essential. In patients with illness predisposing to the development of impaction, prophylaxis may consist of the use of stool-wetting or bulk-forming agents. Mild laxatives may also be used when necessary.

SOLITARY RECTAL ULCER. Discrete, usually single ulcerations of unknown cause may develop in the rectum as well as in other areas of the colon. Solitary ulcer of the rectum is commonly a chronic condition in which the patient complains of painless passage of blood and/or mucus with stool and, less frequently, of dull rectal pain. In contrast, ulcers in the proximal colon usually cause acute abdominal pain. Although this condition has been called solitary ulcer, sigmoidoscopy reveals multiple lesions in 30 per cent of patients. Usually located 7 to 10 cm from the anal verge, the ulcers are shallow and occasionally have heaped-up or nodular borders. The ulcers may be round, linear, or irregular in outline and average 2 cm in diameter. They are chronic, lasting many years, and no treatment has been uniformly successful. Fortunately, complications are rare. The cause of solitary rectal ulcers has not been established. Trauma does not appear to be a major factor. Possibly the ulcer is related to the unusual entity *colitis cystica profunda,* with the ulcer resulting from rupture or cystic degeneration of heteroptic colonic mucosa. Solitary rectal ulcer must be distinguished from other diagnostic possibilities requiring more specific therapy, particularly carcinoma, Crohn's disease, and lymphogranuloma venereum. Biopsy of the rim of the ulcer is most helpful in diagnosis.

PROCTALGIA FUGAX. Proctalgia fugax is episodic severe rectal pain, probably related to spasm of the coccygeus and levator ani muscles. Anorectal infection, fracture of the coccyx, or chronic prostatitis may cause symptoms that mimic those of proctalgia fugax. Chronic trauma from poor sitting posture is said to be causative, but psychologic factors often are prominent. The pain is severe, lasting up to 45 minutes, and even may awaken the patient from sleep. The physical examination is generally normal except for muscle tenderness detected on digital rectal examination. Warm baths, muscle massage, and improvement of posture often constitute successful therapy. In most patients, the symptoms resolve spontaneously over a period of months to years.

Trauma to the coccyx can result in severe pain, termed *coccygodynia.* This may also be related to muscle spasm secondary to the trauma. The diagnosis is made by eliciting pain during movement of the coccyx, and treatment consists of administration of warm sitz baths, massage of the spastic muscles, tranquilizers such as diazepam, and local anesthetic injections.

Chronic ischemia of the rectum may also cause severe anorectal pain accompanied by fecal incontinence and rectal bleeding. This is most often seen in patients over age 50 and may follow anal surgery. Arteriography may show inferior mesenteric artery occlusion or a vascular steal.

Devroede G, Vobecky S, Masse S, et al.: Ischemic fecal incontinence and rectal angina. Gastroenterology 83:970, 1982. *A brief but comprehensive description of this entity, including histology, radiography, and rectal manometry.*

Goldberg M, Hoffman GC, Wombolt DG: Massive hemorrhage from rectal ulcers in chronic renal failure. Ann Intern Med 100:397, 1984. *Reports of the occurrence of solitary rectal ulcers in patients with chronic renal failure.*

Goodell SE, Quinn TC, Mkrtichian PA-C, et al.: Herpes simplex virus proctitis in homosexual men: Clinical, sigmoidoscopic and histopathological features. N Engl J Med 308:868, 1983. *This series of articles provides an overview of the etiology, diagnosis, and management of anorectal infections seen in homosexual men.*

McMillan A, Lee FD: Sigmoidoscopic and microscopic appearance of the rectal mucosa in homosexual men. Gut 22:1035, 1981. *In a study of 100 men who practiced anal intercourse, the authors demonstrated the presence of proctitis on both gross and histologic inspection, without microorganisms identified.*

Quinn TC, Goodell SE, Mkrtichian PA-C, et al.: *Chlamydia trachomatis* proctitis. N Engl J Med 305:195, 1981.

Rompalo AM, Stamm WE: Anorectal and enteric infections in homosexual men. West J Med 142:647, 1985. *A comprehensive review of the particular infectious problems of this population.*

Thompson WG: Proctalgia fugax in patients with the irritable bowel, peptic ulcer, or inflammatory bowel disease. Am J Gastroenterol 79:450, 1984. *A current review of the clinical presentation that also dispels the association with irritable bowel syndrome.*

DISEASES OF THE ANUS

By virtue of its strategic location and function, diseases of the anus occasion many complaints. Examination of the anal canal is best performed by external inspection, with the glutei spread and the patient bearing down, and with an anoscope. Most patients with common anal disorders can be well cared for without surgery or referral to a proctologist.

HEMORRHOIDS. Hemorrhoids are dilated vessels of the hemorrhoidal plexuses in the anal canal and lower rectum. By age 50, fully 50 per cent of people have hemorrhoids. *Internal hemorrhoids* arise from the superior (internal) hemorrhoidal venous plexus and are covered by rectal mucosa. *External hemorrhoids* are dilatations of the inferior (external) hemorrhoidal plexus and are covered with pain-sensitive anoderm and perianal skin. The pathogenesis of hemorrhoids remains controversial. They are not varicose veins of the rectum. The upright human posture may combine with downward pressure from defecation to cause enlargement of hemorrhoidal vessels. This effect may be enhanced when prolonged straining stretches the pelvic muscles and diminishes muscle tone, thereby causing a failure of retraction of the anal cushion after defecation. Manometric studies of the anal sphincters in patients with internal hemorrhoids often show elevated resting pressures and abnormal low-frequency pressure waves undulating at less than two cycles per minute. These changes are found in 40 per cent of patients with hemorrhoids but in only 5 per cent of people without hemorrhoids. It has been postulated that these pressure changes contribute to the development of the hemorrhoids.

Hemorrhoids are usually asymptomatic but may cause bleeding, prolapse, or a mucous anal discharge. Pain is not caused by hemorrhoids except when they thrombose. Chronic bleeding from internal hemorrhoids may be severe enough to cause iron deficiency. Prolapse of an internal hemorrhoid usually is mild, but eventually the hemorrhoid may become irreducible, leading to thrombosis. The differential diagnosis is not difficult; however, rectal bleeding should not be attributed to hemorrhoids until completion of the anorectal examination, including sigmoidoscopy.

Conservative therapy, consisting of warm sitz baths and stool softeners, usually suffices for hemorrhoids that cause only scant bleeding or minimal discomfort. Internal hemorrhoids that bleed persistently or prolapse are most successfully treated with sclerosis by the submucosal injection of a sclerosing agent (e.g., 5 per cent phenol in oil) into the tissue at the upper pole of the hemorrhoid (not into the hemorrhoid itself). Elastic band ligation has been widely used with success, but several cases of fatal sepsis after this procedure have raised concern. Photocoagulation of hemorrhoids is a new and very promising technique. These measures are not appropriate for the pain-sensitive external hemorrhoids. When these thrombose, the clot can be excised under local anesthesia. If pain is subsiding when the patient comes for treatment, simple therapy with analgesics, sitz baths, and stool softeners will usually suffice. Ointments and suppositories widely advertised for therapy of hemorrhoids have at best limited value.

ANORECTAL ABSCESS AND FISTULA. *Anorectal abscesses* are infections of the tissue spaces in and adjacent to the anorectum. Clinical features, dependent on the size and location of an abscess, usually include a throbbing, constant pain either in the perianal area or higher in the rectum. A large abscess may produce fever. The abscess is palpated externally near the anus or internally by digital rectal examination. These abscesses are classified according to their location in the anatomic spaces. The perianal abscess, just beneath the anal skin, is the most common. Other sites include the ischiorectal fossa, the intermuscular plane between the internal and external sphincters, the pelvirectal space above the levator ani and below the pelvic peritoneum, and the retrorectal space. Infection usually arises in an anal crypt. Patients with Crohn's disease, hematologic disorders, and other immune-deficient states are particularly susceptible to the development of anorectal abscesses. Prompt surgical drainage of the abscess is the treatment of choice.

Anorectal fistulas, hollow fibrous tracts lined by granulation tissue and connecting the anal canal or rectum with the perianal skin, may result from the rupture or surgical drainage of an anorectal abscess. Such fistulas may also develop from tuberculosis, Crohn's disease, carcinoma, radiation therapy, lymphogranuloma venereum, and anal fissures. Patients complain of the constant and irritating drainage of pus, blood, mucus, and occasionally stool. Treatment requires both control of the underlying disease and surgical fistulotomy.

ANAL FISSURE. An anal fissure is a longitudinal elliptical or rounded defect that occurs in the anoderm (usually in the posterior midline) and that extends into the anal canal as far as the pectinate line. The cause is most often anal trauma, usually the passage of a large, firm stool. The patient complains of severe tearing or burning anal pain and occasionally of the passage of a few drops of blood. In a patient with a chronic anal fissure, a swelling at the lower end of the fissure, the "sentinel pile," may be perceived as an anal mass. Chronic spasm and inflammation can lead to anal stenosis. Observation of fissures out of the midline or of multiple fissures should raise the question of inflammatory bowel disease, carcinoma, tuberculosis, syphilis, or other venereal disease. Most fissures heal spontaneously, and local anesthetics, sitz baths, and stool softeners give good results in most cases. Chronic fissures may require surgical excision or sphincterotomy.

PRURITUS ANI. Itching of the perianal skin is a symptom, not a diagnosis. The causes are many and varied. Principal categories of etiologies include anorectal diseases (e.g., fistulas, fissures, neoplasms); dermatologic diseases (psoriasis, eczema, lichen planus, seborrheic dermatitis); contact dermatitis (including reaction to agents commonly used to treat the pruritus); infections and parasites (especially pinworms, scabies, and pediculosis); inappropriate hygiene (either insufficient or excessive); and systemic diseases, especially diabetes mellitus and chronic liver disease. Also, many patients are thought to have pruritus on the basis of irritant stools. Normal feces are weakly acid, and diarrheal stools tend to be alkaline, which may be irritating to perianal skin. Specific therapy of one of the aforementioned conditions is the preferred approach; however, most patients require a general regimen, including avoidance of topical agents, laxatives, and tight underclothing, and careful hygiene after defecation with use of nonmedicated talcum powder if necessary. Occasionally, patients benefit from the sparing application of 1 per cent hydrocortisone to the skin, especially at night, when the symptoms seem to be worst. Anecdotal reports suggest benefit from the use of *Lactobacillus acidophilus* preparations or malt soup extract (Maltsupex) to produce a more acid colonic flora.

ANAL MALIGNANCY. Epidermoid carcinomas of the anus of various histologic types (e.g., squamous cell, basal cell, cloacogenic) constitute about 2 per cent of cancers of the large bowel. Homosexual men who practice anal-receptive intercourse may be at increased risk for this neoplasm. The lesions tend to spread widely both directly into the perianal structures and via lymphatic and hematogenous metastases. Bleeding, pain, and a mass are the usual presenting symptoms. Pruritus, mucoid drainage, and change in bowel habits may also occur. Surgical excision is necessary except in the anoderm well below the pectinate line, where small lesions may respond to irradiation. Overall five-year survival rates of 60 per cent have been reported for surgically treated patients.

Other malignancies more rarely seen in the anus include malignant melanoma, mucinous adenocarcinoma, and extramammary Paget's disease. Each of these may produce trivial symptoms and may have widely metastasized by the time of discovery. Wide surgical excisional biopsy must be performed for a suspected lesion. Abdominoperineal resection is still the treatment of choice, but its impact on survival in melanoma is unclear.

Kaposi's sarcoma of the perianal skin, anus, and rectum may occur, particularly as a manifestation of the acquired immune deficiency syndrome (AIDS). In fact this may be the earliest manifestation of the syndrome. Symptoms are rare, as is clinically significant bleeding. Local therapy of isolated lesions with radiation has been successful in selected cases, but this does not address the problem of the underlying immune defect.

FECAL INCONTINENCE. Anal sphincter dysfunction can be a most devastating result of perianal disease, anal surgery, or certain neurologic diseases. Various surgical reconstructive techniques have been employed with some success. Operant conditioning, using biofeedback techniques, has been highly successful in some individuals, and the long-term result has been good.

Bush RA, Owen WF Jr: Trauma and other noninfectious problems in homosexual men. Med Clin North Am 70:549, 1986. *A comprehensive review of these problems, their diagnosis, and treatment.*

Lieberman DA: Common anorectal disorders. Ann Intern Med 101:837, 1984. *An excellent review of pathogenesis, diagnosis, and treatment.*

112 DISEASES OF THE PERITONEUM

Michael D. Bender

ANATOMY AND PHYSIOLOGY. The peritoneum is a continuous mesothelial membrane that lines the abdominal cavity and its contained viscera. The peritoneal cavity is subdivided by peritoneal reflections and mesenteric attachments into several compartments or recesses, which are clinically important because they determine the location and spread of pathologic processes such as abscesses and metastases. The omentum, a double layer of fused peritoneum, plays an important role in peritoneal defense mechanisms by closing perforations, containing infection, and providing blood supply. The microvascular anatomy of the peritoneum consists of long, straight vessels arranged in two layers at right angles to each other, which helps account for the efficiency of the peritoneal membrane as an exchange interface.

The visceral peritoneum does not contain pain receptors; afferent stimuli are transmitted via the visceral autonomics. In contrast, the parietal peritoneum is supplied by spinal nerves that also innervate the abdominal wall. As a result, irritation of the parietal peritoneum produces well-localized somatic pain, whereas irritation of the visceral peritoneum produces a less well-defined discomfort that is poorly localized. The diaphragmatic portion of the peritoneum is supplied by the phrenic nerve centrally and by intercostal nerves peripherally. As a result, pain caused by diaphragmatic irritation may be referred either to the shoulder or to the thoracic and abdominal wall.

The peritoneal surface, a semipermeable membrane, allows for the passive diffusion of water and solutes between the abdominal cavity and the subperitoneal vascular (blood and lymphatic) channels. In general, water and solutes of molecular weight less than 2000 are absorbed from the peritoneal cavity via the blood vascular system; larger molecules and particulate substances enter the lymphatics. Movement of particles from the peritoneal cavity into the subdiaphragmatic lymphatics is facilitated by discontinuities that exist between the peritoneal mesothelial cells and the lymphatic endothelial cells. Basement membranes are scanty or absent so that particles of substantial size may move freely from the abdominal cavity into the subdiaphragmatic lymphatics, a process that may be facilitated by respiratory motion of the diaphragm itself. Water and electrolytes equilibrate rapidly (within two hours) between the blood vascular compartment and the free peritoneal cavity. *Net* fluid movement from the abdominal cavity into the plasma occurs at a maximal rate of approximately 30 to 35 ml per hour both in normal persons and in patients with portal hypertension and ascites. This rate cannot be exceeded despite vigorous diuresis; rather such diuresis only serves to remove fluid from other body compartments, and may cause hypovolemia. The importance of transperitoneal fluid exchange is also illustrated in peritonitis, in which fluid movement into the peritoneal cavity caused by increased vascular permeability can be rapid and massive and may lead to hypotension and shock.

The peritoneum heals readily after damage. Peritoneal injuries normally heal without the formation of adhesions, but in the presence of infection, ischemia, or foreign bodies, adhesions may result. In these situations, fibrinogen released into the peritoneal cavity is converted to fibrin, and then to fibrous adhesions.

DIAGNOSIS. The cardinal symptoms of peritoneal disease are *abdominal pain* and *ascites*. More variable in their occurrence are fever, distention, nausea and vomiting, and altered bowel habits. Direct tenderness, rebound tenderness, and involuntary spasm of the abdominal musculature are the major signs of peritoneal irritation. These signs and symptoms may be minimal or absent in the elderly or debilitated patient and will vary, depending on the location, cause, and acuteness of the underlying process. Because of this, peritoneal disease should be considered in any patient whose abdominal pain is difficult to diagnose.

Radiographically, ascites may be manifested by abdominal haziness, separation of bowel loops, or widening of the flank stripe on plain abdominal films. Otherwise, peritoneal disease reflects itself indirectly on barium contrast studies. Angulation, separation, or rigidity of bowel loops may indicate visceral peritoneal involvement. *Ultrasonography* and *computed tomography* may be useful in demonstrating relatively small amounts of peritoneal fluid, and especially in distinguishing free fluid from cystic masses. Computed tomography also has occasionally been successful in the demonstration of peritoneal implants and in the examination of the retroperitoneum.

If ascites is present, *abdominal paracentesis* is essential to establish its cause (see below). *Peritoneal biopsy*, particularly with the Cope needle, is a relatively simple and safe bedside technique that may yield a positive diagnosis of neoplastic or infectious causes in 50 to 60 per cent of cases. *Peritoneoscopy*, performed under the proper circumstances by a physician experienced in this technique, can be accomplished with little morbidity or mortality. A successful examination may obviate the need for exploratory surgery and may permit biopsy under direct vision of involved portions of the peritoneum or liver. If a diagnosis cannot be made in a patient with obvious peritoneal disease by means of the aforementioned procedures, *exploratory laparotomy* may be necessary.

ASCITES

CLINICAL FEATURES. The accumulation of fluid within the peritoneal cavity is a common clinical finding with a wide range of causes. Its pathophysiology varies with the cause; possible factors are outlined in Table 112–1. The pathophysiology of ascites associated with portal hypertension is considered in Chapter 127.

Small amounts of ascites may be asymptomatic, but as it

TABLE 112–1. FACTORS IN ASCITES FORMATION

Cirrhotic Ascites
- Increased portal venous hydrostatic pressure
- Decreased portal venous colloid osmotic pressure
- Increased hepatic lymph formation
- Decreased renal sodium excretion
- Decreased renal free water excretion

Noncirrhotic Ascites
- Increased subperitoneal capillary permeability
- Decreased peritoneal lymphatic drainage
- Leakage from disrupted abdominal viscera

increases the patient becomes aware of abdominal distention and a sense of fullness and discomfort. Larger amounts of ascites, especially if the abdomen is tensely distended, may cause respiratory distress, anorexia, nausea, early satiety, pyrosis, or frank pain. Body weight may vary, depending on the state of nutrition and the underlying disease process. On physical examination the flanks bulge, and a fluid wave may be demonstrable. Shifting dullness is somewhat more sensitive but may be nonspecific. Although it is difficult to detect less than 1.5 to 2 liters of fluid, placing the patient on his or her hands and knees and percussing flatness over the dependent abdomen (puddle sign) may demonstrate smaller amounts. Indirect evidence such as penile or scrotal edema, umbilical herniation, or pleural effusion may suggest the presence of ascites.

The diagnosis of ascites may be facilitated by plain abdominal films, ultrasonography, or computed tomography.

EVALUATION OF ASCITES FLUID. Once the diagnosis of ascites is made by examination, imaging techniques, or paracentesis, laboratory analysis of the fluid removed is essential to determine its cause. Evaluation of ascites fluid consists of routine studies to characterize the fluid and other studies that may be chosen depending on the clinical situation, as noted in Table 112–2.

Fluids with protein concentrations *exceeding 3 grams per 100 ml* are designated exudates, and below these values, transudates. Other characteristics that may help separate transudates from exudates include ascites-lactate dehydrogenase (LDH), and ascites-serum protein and LDH ratios. The *serum-ascites albumin gradient,* which reflects the oncotic pressure gradient between the vascular bed and the ascitic fluid, is elevated in association with increased portal pressure, whereas a low gradient occurs in conditions in which portal hypertension is not a factor in the genesis of ascites. Tests that help distinguish transudates from exudates, and their common causes, are listed in Table 112–3. Although this classification is useful, exceptions in both directions occur not infrequently. For this reason, ascitic fluid chemistries must be interpreted only in the context of all other clinical and laboratory findings.

TABLE 112–2. LABORATORY ANALYSIS OF ASCITIC FLUID

Test	Abnormal Values	Clinical Situations
Red cell count	> 10,000/mm³	Routine
White cell count and differential	> 500/mm³	Routine
Total protein*	> 3 gm/dl	Routine
LDH*	> 200 IU/liter	Routine
Albumin†	< 1.1	Routine
Bacterial culture	+	Routine
Acid-fast, fungal culture	+	History or findings of Tbc; cirrhosis; immunosuppressed patient
Cytology	+	Neoplasm
Amylase‡	Ascites > serum	Pancreatitis, alcoholism, cirrhosis
Glucose‡	Ascites < serum	Tuberculosis, neoplasm, secondary bacterial peritonitis
Triglycerides‡	Ascites > serum	Chylous (milky) ascites
Starch granules (polarizing microscopy)	+	Postoperative abdominal pain
pH§	< 7.35	Spontaneous bacterial peritonitis
Lactate§	> 25 mg/dl	Spontaneous bacterial peritonitis
CEA	> 10 ng/ml	Adenocarcinoma
Hyaluronic acid¶	> 0.25 mg/ml	Mesothelioma

*Simultaneous blood value for ratio.
†Serum albumin − ascites albumin = gradient. See text.
‡Simultaneous blood value for comparison.
§Also abnormal in neoplastic, tuberculous, and pancreatic ascites.
¶Liquid chromatographic method.
LDH = lactate dehydrogenase; CEA = carcinoembryonic antigen, Tbc = tuberculosis.

A large number of red cells suggests the diagnosis of neoplasm, especially hepatocellular or ovarian carcinoma. Other causes of bloody ascites include tuberculosis, trauma, perforated viscus, and spontaneous bleeding associated with cirrhosis. An ascitic fluid leukocyte count of more than 500 per cubic millimeter is strongly suggestive of a peritoneal inflammatory process, such as infection or tumor infiltration. A predominance of polymorphonuclear leukocytes suggests acute bacterial infection, whereas lymphocytes and monocytes characterize chronic inflammatory disease, especially tuberculosis, but there are exceptions. Cytologic examination is essential if malignancy is suspected and may be expected to yield accurate results in more than half of cases. Samples of fluid should be cultured for bacteria, acid-fast bacilli, or fungi in the appropriate clinical setting, such as fever, undiagnosed pain, or deterioration in a patient with cirrhosis. Other chemical determinations that may be helpful in diagnosis are listed in Table 112–2.

TREATMENT: GENERAL CONSIDERATIONS. Although small or moderate amounts of ascites are often only esthetically displeasing, ascites frequently has a detrimental effect on the overall sense of well-being of the patient. Massive ascites may require urgent removal for severe abdominal discomfort, respiratory distress, cardiac dysfunction, or ulceration or impending rupture of an umbilical hernia. Paracentesis is the method of choice for rapid removal of fluid, as it rapidly reduces intra-abdominal pressure and improves cardiac performance. The risk to the patient of a single, large paracentesis of 2 to 5 liters is minimal and is not associated with a change in plasma volume in cirrhotic patients with edema. One should not hesitate to remove ascites in sufficient volume to treat the complications of tense ascites noted above, but repeated paracentesis to control ascites is rarely warranted.

In patients with intractable, disabling, massive ascites that does not respond to repeated paracentesis or diuretic therapy, peritoneovenous shunting has been successful. Because of numerous complications, careful consideration must be given before recommending peritoneovenous shunting (see Ch. 127). Details of nutritional and diuretic management of ascites are discussed in Chapter 127.

DIFFERENTIAL DIAGNOSIS OF ASCITES. More than 90

TABLE 112–3. DIAGNOSIS OF TRANSUDATIVE VERSUS EXUDATIVE ASCITES

	Transudate	Exudate
Protein	< 3 gm/dl	> 3 gm/dl
LDH	< 200 IU/liter	> 200 IU/liter
Protein ascites/serum ratio	< 0.5	> 0.5
LDH ascites/serum ratio	< 0.6	> 0.6
Albumin gradient*	> 1.1	< 1.1
Common causes	Congestive heart failure Constrictive pericarditis Inferior vena cava obstruction Budd-Chiari syndrome Cirrhosis Nephrotic syndrome Hypoalbuminemia	Neoplasm Tuberculosis Pancreatitis Myxedema Vasculitis

*Serum albumin − ascites albumin.
LDH = lactate dehydrogenase.

TABLE 112–4. CAUSES OF ASCITES NOT ASSOCIATED WITH PERITONEAL DISEASE*

- I. **Portal hypertension**
  - A. Cirrhosis
  - B. Hepatic congestion
    - 1. Congestive heart failure
    - 2. Constrictive pericarditis
    - 3. Inferior vena cava obstruction
    - 4. Hepatic vein obstruction (Budd-Chiari syndrome)
  - C. Portal vein occlusion
- II. **Hypoalbuminemia**
  - A. Nephrotic syndrome
  - B. Protein-losing enteropathy
  - C. Malnutrition
- III. **Miscellaneous**
  - A. Myxedema
  - B. Ovarian disease
    - 1. Meigs' syndrome
    - 2. Struma ovarii
    - 3. Ovarian overstimulation syndrome
  - C. Pancreatic ascites
  - D. Bile ascites
  - E. Chylous ascites
  - F. Urine ascites and nephrogenic ascites

*From Bender MD, Ockner RK: In Sleisenger MH, Fordtran JS (eds.): Gastrointestinal Disease. 3rd ed. Philadelphia, W. B. Saunders Company, 1983.

per cent of patients with ascites have *cirrhosis, neoplasm, congestive heart failure,* or *tuberculosis*. Causes of ascites may be divided into diseases not involving the peritoneum (Table 112–4) and diseases of the peritoneum (Table 112–5). Of those cases not associated with peritoneal disease, cirrhosis is by far the most common (Ch. 126). Portal hypertension caused by diseases of the heart and great veins accounts for a substantial number of patients with ascites of obscure origin. Included in this group are patients with congestive heart failure, constrictive pericarditis, and inferior vena cava and hepatic vein obstruction (Budd-Chiari syndrome). Clinically, patients with these conditions may not be readily distinguishable from those with hepatic cirrhosis; a high index of suspicion is necessary, and special procedures may be required in order to establish or exclude the diagnosis.

TABLE 112–5. DISEASES OF THE PERITONEUM

- I. **Infections**
  - A. Bacterial peritonitis
  - B. Tuberculous peritonitis
  - C. Fungal diseases
    - 1. Candidiasis
    - 2. Histoplasmosis
    - 3. Coccidioidomycosis
    - 4. Cryptococcosis
  - D. Parasitic diseases
    - 1. Schistosomiasis
    - 2. Enterobiasis
    - 3. Ascariasis
    - 4. Strongyloidiasis
    - 5. Amebiasis
- II. **Neoplasms**
  - A. Secondary malignancy
  - B. Mesothelial hyperplasia and benign mesothelioma
  - C. Primary malignant mesothelioma
  - D. Pseudomyxoma peritonei
- III. **Granulomatous peritonitis**
  - A. Exogenous
  - B. Endogenous
  - C. Iatrogenic
- IV. **Sclerosing peritonitis**
- V. **Miscellaneous**
  - A. Vasculitis
  - B. Familial paroxysmal peritonitis (familial Mediterranean fever)
  - C. Eosinophilic gastroenteritis
  - D. Whipple's disease
  - E. Gynecologic disease
    - 1. Endometriosis
    - 2. Deciduosis
    - 3. Gliomatosis
    - 4. Leiomyomatosis
    - 5. Dermoid cyst
    - 6. Melanosis
  - F. Splenosis
  - G. Peritoneal lymphangiectasia
  - H. Peritoneal cysts
  - I. Peritoneal encapsulation

*Modified from Bender MD, Ockner RK: In Sleisenger MH, Fordtran JS (eds.): Gastrointestinal Disease. 3rd ed. Philadelphia, W. B. Saunders Company, 1983.

Hypoalbuminemia of any cause, including nephrotic syndrome and protein-losing enteropathy, may be associated with a classically transudative ascites.

Various endocrine conditions may be associated with ascites. These include *myxedema,* in which the fluid is typically protein rich, and diseases of the ovary, among them *Meigs' syndrome,* in which transudative ascites is associated with ovarian fibroma or cystadenoma, struma ovarii, ovarian edema, and "ovarian overstimulation syndrome."

Pancreatic ascites usually occurs in the presence of chronic pancreatitis or pseudocyst. The most common etiologic factors are alcohol and trauma. The ascites fluid amylase concentration is elevated, often to extremely high levels. Diagnosis of ductal disruption and pseudocyst leakage is usually possible with endoscopic retrograde pancreatography. Drainage of the pseudocyst and repair of duct injury often have been effective in managing this complication, particularly in traumatic cases. In the chronic alcoholic with pancreatic ascites, a trial of conservative management is indicated before surgery is undertaken. Leakage of bile may be associated with the development of *bile ascites,* a condition for which surgical repair of the biliary tract is usually necessary. This situation is not necessarily associated with the fulminant clinical picture of fever, leukocytosis, and peritonitis, i.e., *bile peritonitis,* which appears to result from superimposed infection.

Chylous ascites is due to the presence of lipoproteins and chylomicrons in the peritoneal cavity and is the result of lymphatic obstruction or leakage. These lipid-rich particles impart a turbidity to the fluid that facilitates its diagnosis. However, not all turbid abdominal fluids are "chylous." Establishment of the diagnosis requires direct evidence that the turbidity is indeed the result of neutral lipid, a determination best made by analysis of the fluid for triglyceride concentration. Other turbid abdominal fluids may be due to cellular debris and are designated *pseudochylous ascites,* a condition occasionally associated with abdominal neoplasm or infection. The differential diagnosis of true chylous ascites depends upon its chronicity and the age of the patient. *Chronic chylous ascites* in adults is caused in over 80 per cent of cases by abdominal neoplasm, usually lymphoma, with associated obstruction and disruption of the abdominal lymphatics resulting from extensive lymph node involvement. Inflammatory causes include tuberculosis, pancreatitis, cirrhosis, and adhesions. *Acute chylous ascites* ("chylous peritonitis") is associated with abrupt onset of abdominal pain. In some cases, this syndrome is due to trauma, intestinal obstruction, or rupture of a chylous cyst, but identifying a specific cause may not be possible even at laparotomy. In children, congenital malformations of the lymphatics, including intestinal lymphangiectasia, account for a higher proportion of the cases of chylous ascites. Treatment of chylous ascites depends on the underlying cause. General measures include (1) the use of low-fat diets with medium-chain triglyceride supplementation (these are transported by the portal vein rather than the lymphatics); (2) total parenteral nutrition, to achieve bowel rest and allow healing of damaged lymphatics; and occasionally (3) peritoneovenous shunting, if other measures are unsuccessful.

Urine ascites may result from trauma to the urinary tract, high-grade obstruction caused by posterior urethral valves in the neonate, or renal transplantation. Ascites also may occur in a few patients maintained on chronic hemodialysis. The cause appears to reflect a number of factors including prior peritoneal dialysis or infection, fluid overload, hypertension, poor nutrition, or hypoalbuminemia. Management may be difficult, but if aggressive dialysis does not help, renal transplantation seems to offer the best chance of relieving chronic ascites.

INFECTIONS OF THE PERITONEUM

ACUTE BACTERIAL PERITONITIS. Bacterial peritonitis most commonly results from perforation of an abdominal viscus caused by trauma, obstruction, infarction, neoplasm, foreign bodies, or primary inflammatory disease (Ch. 54). Peritonitis may also be associated with chronic indwelling catheters used for chronic ambulatory peritoneal dialysis, peritoneovenous shunting, and intraperitoneal chemotherapy. The peritoneum has several defense mechanisms in response to bacterial contamination: (1) Bacteria may be cleared from the peritoneum via the diaphragmatic lymphatics. (2) Opsonins, polymorphonuclear leukocytes, and macrophages enter the peritoneal cavity, where phagocytosis of bacteria can occur. (3) The peritoneum and omentum can contain localized infections and enclose small visceral perforations, in part by exudation of fibrin-containing fluid.

Regardless of etiology, abdominal pain, nausea, vomiting, tachycardia, and fever are usually present. The severity of these symptoms is related to the extent of contamination; in generalized peritonitis, shock is often present and may be profound, whereas signs and symptoms may be minimal if infection is localized. In severe cases, there may be exquisite, diffuse direct and rebound tenderness and rigidity of the abdomen; bowel sounds are usually diminished or absent, and distention may be present. Despite its dramatic presentation, recognition of acute peritonitis may be difficult in those patients in whom the clinical manifestations are masked or suppressed, such as the elderly patient or those receiving corticosteroids. In these patients, a high index of suspicion is necessary, since minor or isolated signs such as tachycardia or unexplained hypotension may herald peritonitis.

Laboratory findings are nonspecific and may include leukocytosis, hemoconcentration (from fluid loss into the peritoneum), and subdiaphragmatic air or distended intestinal loops on plain abdominal films. In debilitated or obtunded, elderly patients, *peritoneal lavage* may help establish or rule out the presence of peritonitis. One liter of fluid is instilled through a peritoneal dialysis catheter; a positive lavage fluid contains more than 500 white blood cells per cubic milliliter of fluid or more than 50,000 red blood cells per milliliter or, on Gram's stain, reveals bacteria.

The principal systemic complications of peritonitis are septicemia, shock, ileus, and widespread organ failure, including respiratory, renal, hepatic, and cardiac failure. Local complications include wound infection, abscess, anastomotic breakdown, and fistula formation.

The initial management of peritonitis includes restoration of fluid and electrolyte balance, institution of nasogastric suction to reduce distention and improve pulmonary function, oxygen, analgesics to control pain, and early antibiotic therapy. In advanced peritonitis, polymicrobial aerobic and anaerobic organisms are usually found, requiring broad-spectrum coverage. A frequently used regimen combines an aminoglycoside for aerobes with clindamycin or metronidazole for anaerobes. Cephalosporins are popular for their low toxicity and broad-spectrum coverage, especially the third-generation compounds such as cefoxitin and ceftazidime, which provide broad aerobic and anaerobic coverage (see Ch. 28). Total parenteral nutrition may be necessary in severe peritonitis with major catabolic losses.

In patients who are seen early after a recognized perforation of a viscus and who are good operative candidates, early surgery is usually indicated. In a few patients who are very poor operative risks, it may be desirable to attempt to control the process nonoperatively and to encourage its localization by antibiotic drugs and other conservative measures. Localized abscesses so formed may be drained later when circumstances are more favorable.

Despite the use of antibiotics, modern anesthesia, and intensive support systems, the mortality of generalized peritonitis remains at 50 per cent. Factors adversely affecting prognosis include older age, malnutrition, shock, and organ failure.

ABDOMINAL ABSCESSES. Intra-abdominal abscesses form from a collection of necrotic tissue, bacteria, and white blood cells contained in one of the spaces of the peritoneal cavity and walled off from the rest of the peritoneal cavity by inflammatory adhesions. The contamination is almost invariably derived from endogenous gut flora that escapes as a result of inflammatory perforation, ischemia, traumatic injury, or a surgical procedure. Abscesses within the abdomen localize in three distinct areas: the subphrenic spaces, the intermesenteric area (including the paracolic gutters and interloop areas), and the pelvis. The subphrenic and pelvic localizations reflect the dependent position of these spaces in the recumbent patient and the effect of diaphragmatic movement in drawing fluid up into the subphrenic spaces.

The diagnosis of intra-abdominal abscesses is often a difficult challenge, particularly in immunologically depressed patients with malignancy or malnutrition or patients receiving perioperative antibiotics; all of these may mask clinical signs of sepsis. Fever is the most reliable finding. Other signs and symptoms include malaise, pain, nausea, vomiting, anorexia, tachycardia, abdominal tenderness, and abdominal distention. A subphrenic localization is suggested by thoracic symptoms and signs, including dyspnea, chest pain, decreased breath sounds, dullness, and radiologic evidence of impaired diaphragmatic motion, pleural effusion, or atelectasis. Pelvic localization is suggested by urinary or rectal symptoms and careful vaginal or rectal examination. Leukocytosis with a left shift in the differential count, the usual finding, may be absent. Elevated bilirubin or hepatic enzymes may be a clue to the presence of intra-abdominal sepsis. In summary, a high degree of suspicion is important, and the possibility of an abdominal abscess should be suggested by otherwise unexplained fever, sepsis, leukocytosis, ileus, poor postoperative recovery, or organ dysfunction.

Diagnosis is facilitated by imaging procedures. Plain films may reveal nonmovable gas bubbles, often with air-fluid levels, and barium contrast studies may suggest a mass by displacement of normal structures. Ultrasonography, computed tomography, and gallium citrate 76 or indium 111 leukocyte labeling are newer modalities to diagnose and visualize abscesses. Of these, computed tomography is the most sensitive and specific. Occasionally the diagnosis is made only at the time of abdominal exploration.

Antimicrobial therapy usually suppresses the process and helps to contain it but may also obscure its recognition. Prior computed tomography–guided percutaneous aspiration, with Gram's stain and culture of the obtained fluid, may quickly confirm the presence or absence of an abscess and expedite selection of the proper antibiotic.

Appropriate drainage is indispensable for treatment of an intra-abdominal abscess. Computed tomography–guided percutaneous drainage has increasingly been utilized but may be less successful in abscesses associated with multiple cavities, viscous debris, or a source of continued contamination, such as a perforated viscus or fistula. If percutaneous drainage is inappropriate, surgical drainage should be undertaken.

PRIMARY (SPONTANEOUS) BACTERIAL PERITONITIS. Bacterial peritonitis may occur in the absence of an acute intra-abdominal precipitating factor. In this circumstance, the offending organism may not be enteric, and the syndrome is more likely to occur in patients who have pre-existing ascites, impaired immunologic defenses, or a cause for bacteremia such as localized infection elsewhere in the body or indwelling catheters. A widely recognized example of this circumstance is the child with nephrotic syndrome and ascites who develops primary peritonitis. The pathogenesis is probably hematogenous seeding of the peritoneum, particularly suggested by the frequent identification of extra-abdominal pathogens such as *Streptococcus pneumoniae*. The mortality rate associated with this entity has diminished considerably during recent decades because of the availability of antimicrobial drugs.

More common is spontaneous bacterial peritonitis in patients with advanced, decompensated cirrhosis and ascites. This syndrome is discussed in Chapter 127.

OTHER INFECTIONS. *Tuberculous peritonitis* is discussed in detail in Ch. 302. This disorder may present in a variety of ways, ranging from an acute abdomen to an insidiously developing, otherwise unexplained ascites resembling cirrhosis. Accordingly, its presence should be suspected in all patients with ascites, particularly in patients from endemic areas, in cirrhotic patients, and in immunosuppressed patients. Fewer than half of the patients have active disease elsewhere in the body, and tuberculosis skin testing and appropriate cultures of ascites fluid for tubercle bacilli should be regarded as routine in the evaluation of ascites. The diagnosis is strongly suggested by a high percentage of lymphocytes in the abdominal fluid and may be confirmed by means of a positive culture, peritoneal biopsy, laparoscopy, or, if necessary, exploratory laparotomy. The very satisfactory response of this condition to appropriate chemotherapy adds to the importance of early diagnosis.

Fungal and parasitic diseases may be associated with peritoneal involvement and occasionally with ascites. The most common fungal peritonitis is due to *candidiasis*, which may occur after contamination of the peritoneal cavity caused by perforated ulcer, trauma, surgery, or peritoneal dialysis. Other disorders, including histoplasmosis, coccidioidomycosis, cryptococcosis, ascariasis, amebiasis, and schistosomiasis, are quite uncommon, but deserve consideration in otherwise unexplained cases of peritoneal disease with or without ascites.

TUMORS OF THE PERITONEUM

SECONDARY CARCINOMATOSIS. Secondary malignancy is the most common form of neoplastic involvement of the peritoneum. More than 75 per cent of such tumors are classified as adenocarcinoma, mainly from ovary, pancreas, and colon, but peritoneal involvement by sarcoma, lymphoma, leukemia, carcinoid, and multiple myeloma has been described. Ascites formation in these patients appears to result from the combination of increased capillary permeability and obstruction of channels that drain the peritoneal cavity by way of the subdiaphragmatic lymphatics. The clinical picture is usually that associated with advancing malignancy, including weakness and weight loss, and variable complaints referable to the abdomen such as pain, distention, nausea, or vomiting. Radiographic findings may include angulation, fixation, or displacement of intestinal loops, or submucosal edema reflecting lymphatic obstruction. Ultrasonography or computed tomography may help confirm the presence of ascites and associated mass lesions. On abdominal paracentesis, the fluid obtained usually has a high LDH and protein content (more than 3.0 grams per deciliter); cellular composition is variable, and occasionally the fluid is grossly bloody (see Tables 112–2 and 112–3). The diagnosis is made by cytology in approximately 50 per cent of patients, and, if that is negative, by computed tomography–guided percutaneous biopsy or peritoneoscopy. Occasionally surgical exploration may be necessary.

Malignant ascites formation is a grave prognostic sign, with few patients surviving beyond six months after onset. Treatment of this condition involves the intraperitoneal administration of antitumor agents, including alkylators, antimetabolites, or radioactive isotopes. The standard intracavitary treatments use a small drug volume, but recent trials have used a large volume (2 liters) administered through a semipermanent indwelling catheter to allow for uniform drug distribution, high local drug levels, and repetitive treatments. Intra-abdominal quinicrine or other sclerosing agents have occasionally been successful in producing a fibrous serositis, thereby obliterating the free peritoneal space and reducing further fluid exudation, but the usefulness of this approach is limited by the frequent occurrence of fever, nausea, vomiting, and abdominal pain.

Salt restriction and diuretics may be tried but are often unsuccessful. Paracentesis is useful, and removal of large volumes may be well tolerated; although it may reduce body protein stores, it is often indispensable for patient comfort. In selected patients, peritoneovenous shunting affords palliation in 75 per cent of cases.

PRIMARY MESOTHELIOMA. The mesothelium may undergo hyperplasia or metaplasia, and rare benign cystic and papillary mesotheliomas have been described, but most mesothelial neoplasms are malignant. Primary mesotheliomas are tumors arising from the epithelial and mesenchymal elements of the mesothelium. Approximately 25 per cent involve the peritoneum, often in association with the more frequent pleural localization. Exposure to asbestos is the most established etiologic factor (see Ch. 536), although it is unclear if asbestos fibers produce peritoneal disease by passage from the intestinal lumen, penetration of the diaphragm, or via retrograde lymphatic transport.

Mesothelioma is most common in males over the age of 50 and is associated with the gradual onset of abdominal pain and distention, anorexia, nausea, vomiting, weight loss, and ascites. Blood counts and chemistries are rarely helpful, and barium contrast films reveal nonspecific findings. Ultrasonography and computed tomography demonstrate ascites in sheetlike masses that may suggest the diagnosis. Paracentesis yields an exudate that may be hemorrhagic, and high fluid hyaluronic acid concentrations suggest the diagnosis. Peritoneoscopy reveals extensive studding of peritoneal surfaces with nodules and plaques. However, laparotomy is often necessary to provide adequate biopsies and rule out a primary neoplasm. Even with biopsy or cytologic specimens, the variable histologic characteristics of epithelial and mesenchymal elements may make it difficult to differentiate from other malignancies.

The prognosis of peritoneal mesothelioma is exceedingly poor, with a median survival of about one year after diagnosis. Death usually results from cachexia or obstruction rather than metastatic disease. Tumor response and increased survival have been reported after chemotherapy (especially doxorubicin) and/or radiotherapy. Intensive combination therapy with surgical debulking, whole abdominal radiotherapy, and intraperitoneal doxorubicin and cisplatin may provide substantial palliation in selected, early cases.

PSEUDOMYXOMA PERITONEI. Pseudomyxoma peritonei is a rare condition in which the peritoneal cavity becomes distended with a mucinous, semisolid, translucent material. The two major causes of this "mucinous ascites" are mucinous cystadenomas and cystadenocarcinomas of the ovary and appendix, although other tumors of the genitourinary and gastrointestinal tract have been associated with the process. Extensive pseudomyxoma is invariably associated with cystadenocarcinomas, although they may be low grade.

The condition usually presents as an increase in abdominal girth with little in the way of other clinical signs of disease. At surgery, the abdominal cavity is found to contain gelatinous material existing in a variety of states, including cystic masses, lying freely without apparent attachment or anchored to the peritoneal surface. If the tumor is indeed malignant, it appears to be low grade and rarely metastasizes. As a result, the course of the disease is prolonged and is characterized by recurrent episodes of intestinal obstruction and fistula formation. Surgical removal of the ovary, appendix, and as much mucin as possible and intraperitoneal instillation of an alkylating agent are usually indicated.

GRANULOMATOUS PERITONITIS. The peritoneum responds to a wide variety of stimuli with a granulomatous inflammatory reaction. *Exogenous* causes include mycobacteria, parasites, fungi, or organic material; *endogenous* causes are rare and include keratin in squamous tumors, meconium, sarcoidosis, and Crohn's disease. The most common etiology is *iatrogenic*, due to contamination at the time of surgery from starch, talc, cotton, or wood fibers used in surgical gloves, gowns, or drapes. *Starch granulomatous peritonitis* presents two to nine weeks postoperatively with pain, tenderness, fever, distention, nausea, and vomiting, and may suggest adhesions or abscesses. If it is considered, the diagnosis can be made by demonstrating starch granules in peritoneal fluid. Short-term indomethacin or corticosteroids often speeds recovery.

SCLEROSING PERITONITIS. This unusual form of peritonitis manifests with symptoms of intestinal obstruction caused by the encasement of the entire small bowel in a fibrotic membrane or "cocoon." It has been reported following peritoneovenous shunting, chronic ambulatory peritoneal dialysis, practolol (but not other beta blockers) administration, intraperitoneal chemotherapy and as an idiopathic form in young females. The etiology is unclear but may involve toxins or subacute infections that stimulate fibroblast proliferation.

MISCELLANEOUS DISEASES OF THE PERITONEUM. The peritoneal membrane may be affected by a wide variety of systemic diseases, including systemic lupus erythematosus (see Ch. 436) and other collagen vascular diseases, Whipple's disease (see Ch. 104), familial Mediterranean fever (see Ch. 209), and eosinophilic gastroenteritis. Rarely, unusual tissues deposit on the peritoneum, which may cause low grade peritoneal symptoms or be mistaken for metastatic carcinoma. Examples include endometrial, decidual, glial, and splenic tissue. Several other unusual conditions affecting the peritoneum have been described (Table 111–5).

Antman KH, Pomfret EA, Aisner J, et al.: Peritoneal mesothelioma: Natural history and response to chemotherapy. J Clin Oncol 1:386, 1983. *A concise report of 23 patients from two oncology centers with a large experience in mesothelioma.*

Bastani B, Sharietzadeh MR, Dehdashti F: Tuberculous peritonitis—report of 30 cases and review of the literature. Q J Med 56:549, 1985. *Presents clinical data from Iran, as well as a thorough review of clinical statistics from studies over the last 20 years.*

Bender MD, Ockner RK: Ascites. In Sleisenger MH, Fordtran JS (eds.): Gastrointestinal Disease. 4th ed. Philadelphia, W. B. Saunders Company, 1988.

Bender MD, Ockner RK: Diseases of the peritoneum, mesentery and diaphragm. In Sleisenger MH, Fordtran JS (eds.): Gastrointestinal Disease. 4th ed. Philadelphia, W. B. Saunders Company, 1988. *A broad review, extensively referenced.*

Hau T, Haaga JR, Aeder MI: Pathophysiology, diagnosis, and treatment of abdominal abscesses. Curr Probl Surg 21:1, 1984. *A comprehensive monograph covering all aspects of abdominal abscesses, including current perspectives on percutaneous drainage.*

Press OW, Press NO, Kaufman SD: Evaluation and management of chylous ascites. Ann Intern Med 96:358, 1982. *An analysis of 28 cases from one institution, seen over 20 years.*

Weaver DW, Walt AJ, Sugawa C, et al.: A continuing appraisal of pancreatic ascites. Surg Gynecol Obstet 154:845, 1982. *Reviews a series of 42 alcoholic patients with chronic pancreatitis. Preoperative endoscopic retrograde cholangiopancreatography (ERCP) is emphasized to plan the surgical approach.*

113 DISEASES OF THE MESENTERY AND OMENTUM

Michael D. Bender

GENERAL CLINICAL FEATURES. Patients with mesenteric disease usually have nonspecific symptoms such as abdominal pain, distention, or intestinal obstruction. The most frequent physical finding is a mass, which may be mobile. There are no specific laboratory findings, but mesenteric disease may be suspected if calcifications, displacement of bowel loops, or pressure deformities are observed radiographically. Ultrasonography and computed tomography are useful in identifying mesenteric and omental masses. However, definitive diagnosis usually depends on direct inspection and biopsy, either surgically or by peritoneoscopy.

MESENTERIC INFLAMMATORY DISEASE. This syndrome includes a spectrum of conditions ranging from acute inflammation to a chronic fibrosing process associated with intestinal obstruction, ascites, and steatorrhea. Included are such conditions as "mesenteric panniculitis" and "retractile mesenteritis." The cause of this syndrome is not known, but it is believed to represent the sequel to some inciting event such as trauma, infection, or ischemia in the mesentery. Fat necrosis occurs, evoking an inflammatory reaction with subsequent scarring and granuloma formation.

The condition is most commonly seen in males and in late adulthood. The acute syndrome ("mesenteric panniculitis"), which constitutes the presentation of 60 per cent of cases, is characterized by recurring abdominal pain, weight loss, nausea, vomiting, and fever. In most patients, a tender abdominal mass is palpable; leukocytosis may or may not be present. The remaining 40 per cent of cases are identified by the discovery of a mass on examination or at surgery. Radiographic examination is nonspecific, showing the effects of an abdominal mass and variable scarring that includes displacement and separation of intestinal loops with angulation, stenosis, and extrinsic compression. In some patients the condition evolves into a more chronic process ("retractile mesenteritis"), characterized by continuing pain, fever, weight loss, and various signs of intestinal obstruction, ascites, and steatorrhea. At surgery, the small bowel mesentery is found to be the principal site of involvement; it is thickened and fibrotic, particularly at the root. Resection of the mass is often not possible, and generally should not be attempted. Microscopically in mesenteric panniculitis there is infiltration of adipose tissue by foamy macrophages and lymphocytes, with fat necrosis, fibrosis, and calcification. In retractile mesenteritis, the thickening and fibrosis are more pronounced, and there is less evidence of acute necrosis and inflammation. Infrequently, the mesocolon or parietal peritoneum may be involved, or the process may occur in association with retroperitoneal fibrosis.

Most patients seem to have prolonged survival and become asymptomatic after a period of months to years. A minority exhibits the more chronic symptoms noted earlier. The role of corticosteroids is uncertain; although they may be effective in the management of those patients in whom acute symptoms predominate, there is no evidence that they affect the long-term prognosis or progression of the disease. In 15 per cent of patients, malignant lymphomas develop; the basis for this apparent association is not known.

MESENTERIC AND OMENTAL CYSTS AND TUMORS. Mesenteric cysts usually develop as the result of anomalies in the mesenteric lymphatic system but may also be of mesothelial origin. They may spontaneously wax and wane in size; usually they do not cause symptoms in patients less than 10 years of age. Symptoms are related to the size and position of the cyst, which on physical examination is nontender, round, and mobile. Spontaneous rupture, hemorrhage, or infection may occur, but these complications are unusual. Treatment consists of surgical enucleation or excision.

Mesenteric tumors are rare and usually arise from the cellular elements normally present in the mesentery. They include fibromas, myxomas, lipomas, and other less common neoplasms of mesenchymal or neural origin. Most are well-differentiated, low-grade fibrosarcomas that produce symptoms such as pain, weight loss, abdominal mass, and compression of adjacent organs. They may be treated successfully by surgical excision. Others are more highly malignant and may metastasize distantly. *Mesenteric lymphoid tumors* also occur, and certain of these have been associated with unexplained abnormalities in iron metabolism with hypochromic microcytic anemia. *Metastatic tumors* of the mesentery are more common than primary tumors and are usually due to enlarged lymphomatous or carcinomatous lymph nodes.

Tumors of the omentum, unlike those of the mesentery, are chiefly muscular in origin (leiomyomas, leiomyosarcomas). About 40 per cent of these are malignant and cause symptoms by virtue of local invasion and development of an abdominal mass; distant metastasis is unusual.

MISCELLANEOUS DISEASES. *Torsion of the omentum* is an acute surgical condition that mimics acute appendicitis or cholecystitis. It usually occurs in patients over age 30 and causes right-sided abdominal pain with nausea, vomiting, fever, leukocytosis, and occasionally a mass. Omentectomy is indicated. *Idiopathic primary omental infarction* presents a similar clinical picture and is invariably diagnosed only at laparotomy. *Mesenteric fibromatosis* (desmoid tumor) is a benign, noninflammatory fibrous proliferation of the mesentery, which occurs mainly in patients with familial polyposis of the colon or Gardner's syndrome.

Bender MD, Ockner RK: Diseases of the peritoneum, mesentery and diaphragm. In Sleisenger MH, Fordtran JS (eds.): Gastrointestinal Disease. 4th ed. Philadelphia, W. B. Saunders Company, 1988. *A broad review, extensively referenced.*

Vanek VW, Phillips AK: Retroperitoneal, mesenteric and omental cysts. Arch Surg 119:838, 1984. *Surveys the literature and gives a complete overview of cystic lesions.*

114 GASTROINTESTINAL HEMORRHAGE

Walter L. Peterson

Gastrointestinal (GI) hemorrhage is a common clinical problem. Despite increased availability of intensive care units and improved methods of diagnosis, mortality from upper gastrointestinal hemorrhage is still approximately 10 per cent, which represents almost no decline over the past 30 years. The most likely reason for this observation is that the efficacy of available therapy is little better today than 30 years ago. This is especially true for the group of patients who account for the largest share of overall mortality, i.e., those with bleeding esophageal or gastric varices. This chapter describes general considerations in the management of the patient with gastrointestinal hemorrhage. The important goals in this regard are (1) hemodynamic stabilization of the patient, (2) cessation of bleeding by the least invasive technique possible, and (3) prevention of recurrent hemorrhage. The overall approach to the patient with GI hemorrhage is shown in Figure 114–1.

RECOGNITION OF GASTROINTESTINAL HEMORRHAGE

PRESENTING SIGNS AND SYMPTOMS. Patients with GI hemorrhage have either obvious efflux of blood from the GI tract or no external manifestation (i.e., occult bleeding). Efflux of blood is manifested as (1) *hematemesis,* in which bright red or "coffee-ground" material is vomited; (2) *melena,* which is black, tarry, sticky, odoriferous stool;* and (3) *hematochezia,* the passage of bright red or maroon stool. Occult bleeding may occur with (1) signs and symptoms of *hypovolemia;* (2) *anemia,* either symptomatic or detected only by routine laboratory screening; or (3) chemical evidence of *occult blood* in the stool.

OBJECTIVE CONFIRMATION. Objective evidence that blood has entered the GI tract may be obtained by examining the gastric aspirate or stool for blood. If blood is not grossly evident, a chemical test for occult blood—for example, Hemoccult—can be performed on a stool specimen. False-positive results occur 1 to 2 per cent of the time. Vitamin C may produce false-negative tests. The hematocrit should always be measured to substantiate blood loss from any source or site, although the hematocrit may be normal immediately after an acute bleeding episode (see below).

*Melena must not be confused with dark stools produced by iron or bismuth compounds.

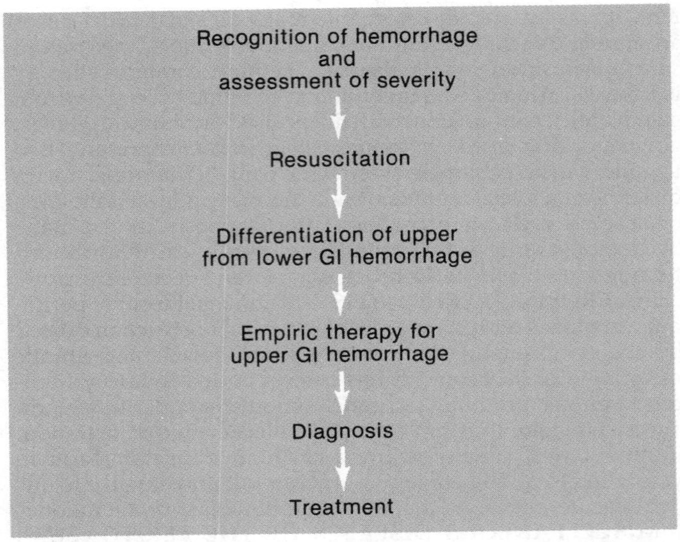

FIGURE 114–1. Approach to the patient with gastrointestinal hemorrhage.

RAPIDITY AND MAGNITUDE OF HEMORRHAGE. After confirming that a patient is bleeding (or recently has bled), the physician must determine whether it is continuing, determine its rapidity and magnitude, and begin resuscitation. These are important steps that must precede any concern for the site of gastrointestinal hemorrhage, whether upper or lower.

The rapidity of hemorrhage is gauged initially by the manner in which bleeding is manifested. Hematochezia or repeated episodes of copious hematemesis suggest brisk hemorrhage, as does inability to clear the nasogastric aspirate of bright red blood with gastric lavage. The ultimate measure of rapidity of hemorrhage remains the amount and rapidity of blood transfusions required to restore and maintain the vascular volume.

The magnitude of hemorrhage can be estimated by the clinical presentation. Melena can be produced experimentally by as little as 100 to 200 ml of blood, although in clinical practice the presence of melena almost always indicates at least 500 ml of blood loss. Upper gastrointestinal (UGI) bleeding manifested by hematochezia suggests losses of 1000 ml or more. By contrast, as little as 25 ml blood loss will produce a guaiac-positive stool.

Acute blood losses greater than 1000 ml are more accurately estimated by evidence of hypovolemia manifested by tachycardia, hypotension, or a fall in blood pressure upon change of position (orthostatic hypotension). These signs must be evaluated with knowledge of the physiologic compensatory responses following an acute GI hemorrhage (see below). To interpret these signs too literally may lead to underestimation of the severity of the hemorrhage, a cardinal danger in the management of such patients.

PATHOPHYSIOLOGY OF ACUTE BLEEDING. The hematocrit and blood pressure measured initially in a bleeding patient reflect four basic factors: (1) pre-existing blood volume, (2) the volume of blood lost, (3) the rate at which it is lost, and (4) the extent of endogenous volume replacement. Following loss of 20 per cent of the circulating blood volume (1000 ml), there is an immediate fall in blood pressure, a rise in heart rate, and peripheral vasoconstriction. The hematocrit initially remains unchanged. Only as fluid enters the vascular space from extravascular compartments does the hematocrit fall and blood pressure rise. The heart rate may soon return to normal or actually fall below normal and may therefore be an unreliable sign of the severity of a hemorrhage. As noted, the level of the hematocrit depends on the rapidity and completeness of dilution of the remaining blood as well as the severity of the hemorrhage. An isolated hematocrit reading, unless low, is of little help.

The blood pressure is the most important sign of the state of blood volume and most accurately mirrors the severity of the situation. However, it is also affected by the patient's age, pre-existing blood pressure, and ability to mobilize fluid. For example, a dehydrated patient who bleeds acutely may be unable to restore volume. The resulting blood pressure will be low and the hematocrit may remain normal or high. A low hematocrit, low blood pressure, or rapid heart rate usually indicates a severe hemorrhage. A normal hematocrit, normal blood pressure, or normal heart rate must be interpreted with caution.

INITIAL THERAPY

RESUSCITATION. Initial therapy (resuscitation) is independent of the source of bleeding. Rather, it is dependent on the rapidity and magnitude of hemorrhage. Generally, patients should be placed in an intensive care unit unless it is clear that the bleeding is mild or chronic and the patient does not require resuscitation. It is also prudent to obtain surgical consultation to follow the patient through resuscitation, diagnosis, and therapy, so that rapid surgical assistance is available if needed. Resuscitation is directed toward supporting the vascular volume and providing adequate tissue oxygenation. Large intravenous catheters should be inserted, at times into a large central vein, and fluids begun. The physician must remember that the dilutional effect of exogenous fluids will lower the hematocrit. Nasal oxygen (2.0 to 3.0 liters per minute) may be necessary, particularly for elderly persons or those with cardiac or pulmonary disease. Urine output and systemic blood pressure should be closely monitored and, if necessary, central venous or pulmonary wedge pressures as well. Blood is sent for typing and crossmatching as well as for other laboratory data (especially determinations of clotting factors). An electrocardiogram and chest radiograph should be obtained and, to record the patient's progress, a flow sheet for fluids, vital signs, and other values is initiated.

The blood products administered depend upon the rapidity of hemorrhage and the resources of individual blood banks. Patients with active bleeding should receive whole blood if possible; but if packed red blood cells must be used to treat active bleeding, fresh frozen plasma should be given with every 4 to 6 units.

In patients whose plasma volume has been restored from extravascular compartments, packed red blood cells are sufficient. Packed cells are indicated especially in elderly patients with chronic bleeding who are in shock and in whom whole blood may produce vascular volume overload. Fresh frozen plasma should be given to patients whose bleeding has ceased only if there are demonstrated needs. For example, patients with cirrhosis may have special needs for clotting factors present in fresh frozen plasma.

When and how much blood is transfused varies from patient to patient and is dependent upon several factors. These include the volume of blood lost, the presence or absence of continuing hemorrhage, the chronicity of blood loss, and the patient's clinical response to blood loss. For example, a young patient may tolerate without transfusion a hematocrit of 25 per cent or less quite well, especially if bleeding has been chronic; on the other hand, an older patient, at the same hematocrit, may have postural hypotension, confusion, or angina pectoris and require transfusion. Patients with continuing hemorrhage usually require blood regardless of the absolute hematocrit level. A hematocrit of 30 per cent has proved to be a satisfactory level to achieve with transfusions. Nevertheless, the requirements for numbers of units of blood must often be determined individually, based on the patient's clinical status.

DISTINGUISHING BETWEEN UPPER AND LOWER GASTROINTESTINAL HEMORRHAGE

As restorative therapy is begun, thought should be given to whether the source of bleeding is from the upper or lower gastrointestinal tract. Hematemesis connotes a source of bleeding above the ligament of Treitz. Melena results from the breakdown of blood during its transit through the intestinal tract. The longer blood remains in the GI tract, the more likely melena will occur. Therefore, melena occurs most often from upper GI bleeding lesions and only occasionally from bleeding sites as distal as the right colon. Hematochezia represents either a very rapid, massive (1000 ml) UGI hemorrhage or, more likely, a lower intestinal source. Hypovolemia, anemia, or occult stool blood may be manifestations of either upper or lower GI hemorrhage. To confirm or detect a UGI source, a nasogastric tube is placed. A bloody aspirate is diagnostic of UGI hemorrhage; a clear aspirate effectively rules out active bleeding from the esophagus and stomach. When the gastric aspirate is negative for blood, the source of bleeding is usually lower GI, but an actively bleeding postpyloric lesion (such as duodenal ulcer) may still be present. Obviously the nasogastric aspirate may be negative if bleeding has ceased.

Other findings in UGI bleeding include hyperactive bowel sounds, leukocytosis, low-grade fever, and elevation of the blood urea nitrogen (BUN). Elevation of the BUN in acute UGI bleeding probably represents a combination of (1) absorption of a high protein load (approximately 15 grams of globin plus plasma proteins per 100 ml of blood) with resulting increased synthesis of urea and (2) hypovolemia with reduced renal perfusion.

EMPIRIC THERAPY FOR UPPER GASTROINTESTINAL HEMORRHAGE

If the patient is suspected of having UGI hemorrhage, a nasogastric tube is placed to document that its source is esophageal, gastric, or (in many cases) immediately postpyloric and to gauge the rapidity of bleeding. If the aspirate is a flow of fresh blood, this tube is withdrawn and is replaced with a large-bore orogastric tube for gastric lavage. Large volumes (500 to 1000 ml) of iced saline or tap water are lavaged through the orogastric tube, although room temperature fluids may function as well. The fluid is removed from the stomach by gravity drainage, avoiding excess suction, which can damage the gastric mucosa. Gastric lavage serves several purposes: the rate of bleeding is gauged, blood clots are evacuated, and hemostasis may be promoted. Although cause and effect have not been proved, gastric lavage is associated with cessation of such bleeding in 85 to 90 per cent of patients. No therapeutic intervention, including cimetidine, has been shown to improve upon the results obtained with lavage alone. The amount of lavage fluid required varies from patient to patient. Gastric contents will clear in some with 1 to 2 liters of fluid, whereas in others 10 or more liters may be required.

If bleeding does not subside during lavage, levarterenol (Levophed, 8 mg in 100 ml of normal saline) may be instilled into the stomach through the nasogastric tube. Such local vasoconstrictor therapy may be effective as a stopgap measure, although no controlled evidence is available to prove its effectiveness.

If hemorrhage ceases during lavage, empiric therapy should be begun for the most common cause of UGI hemorrhage in the nonalcoholic—i.e., peptic ulcer. One such approach is to maintain gastric pH as close to neutrality as possible during the initial 24 to 72 hours when recurrent hemorrhage is most likely. This may be accomplished by blocking acid secretion with an H_2-receptor blocking agent and monitoring gastric pH hourly. Hourly doses of supplemental antacids (beginning with 30-ml aliquots of an aluminum-magnesium preparation) are then instilled through the nasogastric tube to maintain the pH near 7. When a particular dose of antacid is found that will reliably maintain the pH near 7, the nasogastric tube can be withdrawn and antacids given orally. After three days, therapy is continued with standard doses of ulcer medication (see Ch. 100).

DIAGNOSTIC APPROACH TO DETERMINE THE SPECIFIC CAUSE OF HEMORRHAGE

To this point in a patient's course, attention has been directed toward establishing that GI hemorrhage has occurred, determining its rapidity and magnitude, localizing the source as upper or lower GI, and initiating resuscitation. During this time, it is important to obtain a careful history and perform a thorough physical examination. Although the information obtained often provides only valuable clues, it may at times be diagnostic. The subsequent approach to treatment depends on whether or not bleeding continues or ceases with initial therapy.

UPPER GASTROINTESTINAL HEMORRHAGE. Helpful historic information includes prior episodes of bleeding, associated illnesses (e.g., cirrhosis), medications taken (especially analgesics and anticoagulants), or prior abdominal surgery (for peptic ulcer or for placement of aortic vascular prostheses). Has the patient experienced epistaxis or hemoptysis? Does the patient tell of dyspepsia, heartburn, or retching prior to hematemesis, which may indicate peptic ulcer, reflux esophagitis, or a Mallory-Weiss mucosal tear, respectively? On physical examination, the physician should look for cutaneous manifestations of underlying diseases such as Osler-Weber-Rendu syndrome, Ehlers-Danlos syndrome, pseudoxanthoma elasticum, and the blue rubber bleb nevus syndrome. Is there adenopathy to suggest malignancy? Or jaundice, palmar erythema, spider angiomas, or hepatosplenomegaly to suggest cirrhosis?

If Hemorrhage Continues Despite Initial Therapy. If bleeding continues even after vigorous gastric lavage, further therapy may be invasive and will differ depending upon the actual source of bleeding. Therefore, rapid, accurate diagnosis is required and is best achieved with panendoscopy. In the occasional situation in which bleeding is so brisk as to preclude visualization by endoscopy, and if time will allow, arteriography will often delineate an actively bleeding arterial site. If none is found, venous bleeding from varices is inferred. Arteriography offers the additional advantage of permitting infusion of vasoconstrictor drugs or embolization of a substance such as Gelfoam into the offending vessel as a means of treatment. Barium studies of the UGI tract are not appropriate in this setting, because only potential bleeding sites can be seen and because the contrast material may hinder further diagnostic procedures such as endoscopy or arteriography.

Rapid bleeding from fistulization of an aortofemoral bypass graft into the duodenum is a special situation. The nasogastric aspirate is often clear, but melena or marked hematochezia suggests a UGI site. In a patient with an aortofemoral graft, endoscopy of the esophagus, stomach, and proximal duodenum should be done immediately to exclude a bleeding site other than a graft-enteric fistula. The fistula itself, if present, is rarely seen at endoscopy. Arteriography may not reveal the bleeding from the graft and should not be done. Immediate surgery is indicated in patients with grafts if no other site of hemorrhage is visualized.

If Hemorrhage Ceases with Initial Therapy. In most patients (85 per cent or more), hemorrhage ceases with initial therapy or is not active at the time of admission and urgent diagnosis is not required. Most patients should undergo either a barium UGI series or panendoscopy for diagnostic evaluation. The UGI series is a safe, inexpensive procedure that will detect most UGI malignancies and many peptic ulcers. This is especially true if a double-contrast radiographic examination is performed. Panendoscopy is more specific and sensitive, and hence a more accurate diagnostic tool (especially for superficial bleeding lesions). Clinical settings in which endoscopy is the preferable diagnostic test are shown in Table 114–1.

Angiography is rarely indicated in patients who cease bleeding, for it will detect only abnormal vascular patterns that are rare and may or may not be the actual source of bleeding. Nevertheless, in selected cases of UGI bleeding in which UGI radiographs and endoscopy are unrevealing, arteriography may be helpful (see The Diagnostic Dilemma, below).

LOWER GASTROINTESTINAL HEMORRHAGE. Remote and recent historical points that are important in assessing lower gastrointestinal hemorrhage include a prior history of rectal bleeding (hemorrhoids, diverticulosis, or polyps), a recent change in stool caliber (colonic cancer), acute abdominal pain with bleeding (ischemic colitis), or recurrent or bloody diarrhea (inflammatory bowel disease). A history of familial colonic polyposis or of an aortofemoral bypass graft would also be very important. On physical examination, one should palpate for abdominal masses, look for external hemorrhoids, and note any masses present on digital rectal examination. Inflammatory bowel disease or familial polyposis may have extracolonic manifestations involving skin, bones, or joints (see Ch. 105 and 107).

If Hemorrhage Continues Despite Initial Therapy. Anoscopy and proctosigmoidoscopy can detect lesions involving the lower 20 to 25 cm of the colon, such as hemorrhoids, polyps, inflammatory bowel diseases, ischemic colitis, or rectosigmoid cancer. On many occasions, however, all that can be seen is blood coming from somewhere above the level reached by the instruments. While an angiography team is being assembled, it is reasonable to perform a quick upper endoscopy to exclude a postpyloric bleeding site in the UGI tract. If endoscopy is negative, and if bleeding persists, angiography will sometimes localize the site of lower intestinal bleeding, although perhaps not the specific lesion (see above for the approach to possible bleeding from aortofemoral grafts). This is especially helpful in patients bleeding from diverticula or vascular anomalies. Intra-arterial infusions of vasopressin may even stop the bleeding before surgical intervention is required. Barium enema examination should not be performed, as it will preclude subsequent angiography. Colonoscopy is difficult in the face of continuing hemorrhage, but may be performed if bleeding slows to an ooze.

Detection of intestinal extravasation of a radioisotope such as technetium 99m (^{99}Tc)–labeled sulfur colloid is a noninvasive means to localize active bleeding. ^{99}Tc sulfur colloid is rapidly cleared from the blood by the liver and spleen, which means that bleeding may be detected only a short time. Attachment of ^{99}Tc to the patient's own red blood cells avoids this problem. While important therapeutic decisions should probably not be based solely on the results of radionuclide scanning until more experience has been gained, this technique may provide clues to the location of bleeding and may at the least be a helpful screening test prior to arteriography.

TABLE 114–1. CLINICAL SETTINGS FOR ENDOSCOPY IN PATIENTS WITH UGI BLEEDING*

1. Radiologic technique is inadequate
2. Patient has had gastric resection
3. Endoscopic or surgical therapy is planned
4. More than one lesion may be present (especially in patients with varices)
5. Vascular graft is in place

*These are settings in which endoscopy is preferable to a barium UGI series.

If Hemorrhage Ceases with Initial Therapy. Patients whose bleeding ceases spontaneously during resuscitation should in most instances undergo colonoscopy at the earliest convenient time. This is the quickest, most convenient, and most accurate means of making a diagnosis. If colonoscopy is not performed, the patient should undergo proctoscopy and then be observed for 48 hours before further diagnostic evaluation. A barium enema is not performed before this time for fear of being unable to utilize arteriography (because of residual barium) should hemorrhage recur. After 48 hours a barium enema may be obtained. In some patients, the results of the barium enema, when coupled with the clinical findings, may complete the evaluation. In others, colonoscopy may be performed (after cleansing the colon) to confirm or biopsy lesions detected by barium enema, to exclude other sources of bleeding in the large number of patients who may have diverticulosis as an incidental finding, and to detect mucosal lesions or small polyps missed by barium enema. Patients who experience recurrent hemorrhage during the first 48-hour period may require angiography or, if bleeding again ceases or slows, colonoscopy, if not yet performed. If evaluation of the patient with presumed lower GI bleeding is unrewarding, UGI sources should be excluded with an UGI series and possible endoscopy; lesions below the ligament of Treitz but above the terminal ileum may be sought with a small bowel series (see The Diagnostic Dilemma, below).

SPECIFIC CAUSES OF HEMORRHAGE AND THEIR TREATMENT

The causes of GI bleeding are shown in Table 114–2. The ligament of Treitz is generally considered the dividing point for upper and lower GI lesions. However, because jejunal and ileal lesions are so rarely the cause of GI bleeding, lower GI bleeding almost always comes from the colon.

UPPER GASTROINTESTINAL HEMORRHAGE. The three most common causes of serious upper gastrointestinal bleeding are peptic ulcer, acute mucosal lesions, and esophageal varices.

Peptic ulcer (gastric, duodenal, or postsurgical anastomotic ulcers) will in most cases require urgent surgery if bleeding does not cease. In some patients, surgery may be precluded, or at least delayed, by application of one of the available endoscopic modalities to coagulate the bleeding lesion thermally. Unfortunately, use of such techniques is not based on clear results from controlled clinical trials. Only laser therapy has been well studied, and results are conflicting. If bleeding ceases, therapy after the first three days (see above) is the same as for nonbleeding ulcers, i.e., antacids, sucralfate, or histamine H_2-receptor antagonists (see Ch. 100). Use of endoscopically delivered thermal therapy to prevent rebleeding in selected patients remains unsettled. *Acute mucosal lesions* (esophagitis, gastritis, or Mallory-Weiss tears) that continue bleeding often respond to intra-arterial infusions of vasoconstrictor drugs such as vasopressin, thereby precluding the need for surgery. Such treatment, of course, necessitates catheterization of visceral arteries, usually the celiac. In some centers embolic therapy with blood clot or Gelfoam is also used. If bleeding ceases, acute mucosal lesions are treated with measures to reduce gastric acidity, although Mallory-Weiss lesions usually require no specific therapy. If aspirin is believed to be the cause of acute gastric mucosal bleeding, other analgesics should be substituted. This should be done cautiously, since most other analgesics (with the exception of enteric-coated aspirin) also may cause mucosal bleeding. "Stress" gastritis can be prevented in patients predisposed to this lesion by the prophylactic administration of frequent, large doses of a potent antacid.

TABLE 114–2. CAUSES OF GI BLEEDING

Upper GI	Upper or Lower GI	Lower GI
Duodenal ulcer	Neoplasms	Hemorrhoids
Gastric ulcer	Carcinoma	Anal fissure
Anastomotic ulcer	Leiomyoma	Diverticulosis
Esophagitis	Sarcoma	Meckel's diverticulum
Gastritis	Hemangioma	Ischemic bowel disease
Mallory-Weiss tear	Lymphoma	Inflammatory bowel disease
Esophageal varices	Melanoma	Solitary colonic ulcer
Hematobilia	Polyps	Intussusception
Menetrier's disease	Arterial-enteric fistulas	
	Vascular anomalies	
	Osler-Weber-Rendu	
	Blue rubber bleb nevus	
	CREST syndrome	
	Arteriovenous malformations	
	Angiodysplasia (vascular ectasia)	
	Hematologic diseases	
	Elastic tissue disorders	
	Pseudoxanthoma elasticum	
	Ehlers-Danlos	
	Vasculitis syndromes	
	Amyloidosis	

Continuing hemorrhage from *esophageal or gastric varices* is a condition for which no therapy has been convincingly shown to be satisfactory. A low-dose, constant intravenous infusion of vasopressin* (0.1 to 0.4 unit per minute) is often recommended. This therapy may be no better than placebo at stopping variceal bleeding. Use of vasopressin may also result in unwanted side effects of arterial vasoconstriction, including mesenteric ischemia and angina pectoris. Concomitant use of nitroglycerin may reduce the incidence of side effects. Balloon tamponade will often stop the bleeding but at a substantial risk of esophageal perforation or pulmonary aspiration. Because emergent or even urgent surgery for variceal hemorrhage carries with it an extremely high mortality in patients with cirrhosis of the liver, new techniques such as transhepatic obliteration of varices or endoscopic sclerotherapy have been developed. Because the transhepatic angiographic technique requires puncture of a diseased, easily bleeding liver, and because there are more endoscopists available than angiographers, endoscopic sclerotherapy has more or less been given pre-eminence. Although controlled data are scarce, it appears that urgent endoscopic sclerotherapy will stanch variceal bleeding most of the time. If hemorrhage has ceased, and depending upon the individual circumstances, consideration may be given to means of preventing future episodes of hemorrhage. Propranolol, a beta-blocking agent that lowers portal pressure, has been suggested as one form of long-term therapy to prevent recurrent variceal bleeding. However, reductions in portal pressure are often trivial, and controlled trials do not uniformly show efficacy. More reliable is portal vein decompressive surgery, which prevents recurrent bleeding in a large proportion of patients. Hepatic encephalopathy often occurs after portal vein decompression, however, so many experts recommend obliteration of the varices via repeated endoscopic injections of varices with a sclerosing solution. This technique reduces the incidence of recurrent esophageal (but not gastric) variceal bleeding without interrupting portal blood flow to the liver.

Malignant lesions producing UGI hemorrhage are usually treated surgically, while rare *vascular lesions* such as Osler-Weber-Rendu syndrome or angiodysplasia may respond either to experimental thermal obliteration with endoscopic electro- or laser coagulation or, if localized, to segmental surgical resection.

LOWER GASTROINTESTINAL HEMORRHAGE. *Hemorrhoids* are treated medically with sitz baths and lubricating suppositories, by banding, or surgically, depending on the severity and frequency of bleeding episodes (see Ch. 111). *Ischemic colitis, inflammatory bowel disease,* and *cancer* only rarely produce bleeding severe enough to necessitate immediate surgery and are managed as they would be if hemorrhage had not been the presenting symptom. Hemorrhage from *diverticulosis* that continues after initial therapy may respond to intra-arterial vasopressin therapy. If not, diagnostic arteriography may localize the bleeding site to permit segmental colonic resection rather than subtotal colectomy. *Vascular*

*This use is not listed in the manufacturer's directive.

anomalies located by arteriography may also respond to intra-arterial vasopressin. Indication for elective surgical resection of diverticula or vascular anomalies that cease bleeding either spontaneously or with vasopressin depends upon the severity and frequency of bleeding episodes.

THE DIAGNOSTIC DILEMMA

The diagnostic approach just described for patients with gastrointestinal hemorrhage will fail to disclose a diagnosis in many patients. Fortunately such failure is not detrimental to most, particularly during a period of observation. Nevertheless, failure to locate and define the source of bleeding jeopardizes patients with multiple episodes of hemorrhage that require repeated hospitalizations and blood transfusions, particularly high-risk elderly patients with a potentially curable lesion.

There are at least three reasons for failure to diagnose the bleeding lesion. First, it may be in a location that is relatively inaccessible to standard radiographic procedures and endoscopy. The best example is a lesion of the small bowel, i.e., a middle GI lesion. Second, there may be single or multiple lesions that are potential bleeding sites, and documentation of the one responsible may be virtually impossible. Third, the lesion responsible for the hemorrhage may be overlooked because of its subtle manifestation or because diagnosticians are unfamiliar with the lesion.

Lesions of the small bowel include tumors, vascular anomalies, and Meckel's diverticula. An infusion small bowel series, in which a tube is positioned in the third portion of the duodenum to allow a controlled, steady infusion of barium, permits the radiologist to follow the column of barium more closely than with the standard small bowel series. Tumors of the small bowel may be detected with this technique. If this procedure is unrewarding, visceral angiography may detect abnormal vascular patterns of tumors or vascular anomalies, although contrast material will not enter the lumen unless bleeding is active (at least 0.5 ml of blood loss per minute). Meckel's diverticula are sources of bleeding primarily in young patients and may at times be localized by using a technetium isotopic scan. This test is often difficult to interpret.

Confirmation that a lesion is actually the site of hemorrhage requires either endoscopy or arteriography performed while the patient is bleeding. In the UGI tract this may be of particular importance in patients with esophageal varices, whereas in the lower GI tract it is important in the patient with suspected bleeding from diverticulosis or angiodysplasia. For example, a patient may present with a lower GI hemorrhage that ceases spontaneously. Barium enema and/or colonoscopy disclose only diverticula. If the patient at a later time has another hemorrhage, arteriography may demonstrate that a diverticulum is bleeding in a particular area of the colon, or it may disclose a lesion such as angiodysplasia that was overlooked on colonoscopy. The role of radionuclide scanning in patients whose conditions present a diagnostic dilemma remains to be settled.

Vascular anomalies are subtle lesions with which many physicians may be unfamiliar. These range from the hereditary telangiectasias of Osler-Weber-Rendu to angiodysplasia, which may account for an important proportion of GI hemorrhage in elderly patients. This lesion is believed to be an acquired one that develops as part of the aging process. In theory, many years of low-grade obstructions of submucosal veins ultimately lead to small arteriovenous communications in the mucosa and submucosa. This lesion was originally recognized by arteriography as a cause of bleeding in the cecum and may be responsible for a substantial proportion of bleeding episodes previously ascribed to right-sided diverticula. Because many of these malformations are submucosal, they cannot alway be seen by colonoscopy or at surgery.

Angiodysplasias arising in the mucosa have been described endoscopically as bright red, flat, and fernlike. These vascular lesions have been found both in the cecum and in the UGI tract. As more endoscopists become familiar with this lesion, it will likely become a more frequently listed cause of both upper and lower gastrointestinal hemorrhage in the elderly.

Angiodysplasia localized to the cecum and ascending colon may be treated with right hemicolectomy. In fact, some investigators suggest resection after the first episode of hemorrhage. An alternative form of therapy is thermal coagulation, using electrocoagulation or laser. This technique would appear especially useful when there are multiple, widely scattered lesions or when they are present in the UGI tract and surgical resection would result in undesirable postoperative complications.

Fleischer D: Endoscopic therapy of upper gastrointestinal bleeding in humans. Gastroenterology 90:217, 1986. *An up-to-date review with extensive bibliography.*

Flesicher D: Etiology and prevalence of severe persistent upper gastrointestinal bleeding. Gastroenterology 84:538, 1983. *A nice evaluation of severe upper gastrointestinal bleeding.*

Graham DY, Smith JL: The course of patients after variceal hemorrhage. Gastroenterology 8:800, 1981. *Demonstrates the dismal prognosis for variceal bleeders.*

Larson DE, Farnell MB: Upper gastrointestinal hemorrhage. Mayo Clin Proc 58:371, 1983. *An in-depth review of all aspects of upper gastrointestinal bleeding with excellent reference list.*

Lieberman DA, Keller FS, Katon RM, et al.: Arterial embolization for massive upper gastrointestinal tract bleeding in poor surgical candidates. Gastroenterology 86:876, 1984. *One of the largest series of severe bleeders treated with arterial embolization.*

Peterson WL: Gastrointestinal bleeding. In Sleisenger MH, Fordtran JS (eds.): Gastrointestinal Disease. 4th ed. Philadelphia, W. B. Saunders Company, 1988. *A much expanded, fully referenced review of gastrointestinal bleeding.*

Rector WB: Drug therapy for portal hypertension. Ann Intern Med 105:96, 1986. *Scholarly review of pharmacologic agents used to treat variceal bleeding.*

Rutgeerts P, Van Gompel F, Geboes K, et al.: Long term results of treatment of vascular malformations of the gastrointestinal tract by Neodymium Yag laser photocoagulation. Gut 26:586, 1985. *One of the largest published experiences with laser treatment of vascular anomalies.*

Zinner MJ, Zuidema GD, Smith PL, et al.: The prevention of upper gastrointestinal tract bleeding in patients in an intensive care unit. Surg Gynecol Obstet 153:214, 1981. *The best study of prophylactic prevention of "stress" bleeding.*

115 MISCELLANEOUS INFLAMMATORY DISEASES OF THE INTESTINE

Marvin H. Sleisenger

Acute Appendicitis (Including the Acute Abdomen)

DEFINITION. Appendicitis is acute inflammation of the vermiform appendix. It is rare before the age of two and reaches a peak incidence in the second and third decades. The vast majority of patients are between the ages of 5 and 30. Although incidence of the disease declines after the age of 40, the annual incidence is about 1.5 per thousand for males and 1.9 per thousand for females between the ages of 17 and 64. The disease is important because it is common and curable; it therefore constitutes the most important entity in the differential diagnosis of the acute abdomen.

PATHOLOGY. Usually, the appendix is swollen, hyperemic, warm, and covered with exudate. However, in the early stages it may appear only slightly discolored and, in the late stages, gangrenous with perforation. Microscopically, the picture ranges from some acute inflammatory cells in the lumen and mucosa to acute inflammatory changes transmurally with superficial mucosal ulcerations; in advanced stages, one or more perforations may be noted, particularly in patients over the age of 60.

ETIOLOGY AND PATHOGENESIS. Although the vast majority of cases have no obvious cause for obstruction, identifiable etiologies include *calculi, Enterobius vermicularis, Kaposi's sarcoma, Burkitt's lymphoma, adenocarcinoma, schistosomiasis,* and *carcinoid tumors.* The initiating event in acute appendicitis appears to be obstruction, followed by increased intraluminal pressure, reduced venous drainage, thrombosis, hemorrhage, edema, and bacterial invasion of the wall. The appendiceal artery (an end-artery) becomes occluded and perforation results.

Calculi are thought to be the most common cause of the initial obstruction. A small percentage of inflamed appendices contain a radiologically demonstrable calculus, compared with 2.7 per cent of normal ones. Gangrene and perforation are more common in appendices with calculi. The calculi are composed of inspissated fecal material, calcium phosphate–rich mucus, and inorganic salts. Although fecaliths are more common in populations eating a low-fiber diet, the incidence of appendicitis is decreasing in the West, and 70 per cent of patients with acute appendicitis do not have calculi. Whether the increasing use of high-fiber diets underlies this reduction of incidence is not yet proved.

CLINICAL PICTURE AND DIAGNOSIS. The duration of appendicitis is usually 12 to 48 hours from onset to hospitalization. Over 95 per cent of patients complain of *pain* at onset, classically referred to the epigastric or periumbilical areas and later localizing in the right lower quadrant. This sequence, however, is not found in all patients and is notably absent in *retrocecal appendicitis.* Further, in a significant number of patients, particularly women in the late second or third trimester of pregnancy, the pain will not localize clearly to the right lower quadrant, being either diffuse or in the lower abdomen. In *pelvic appendicitis* the pain may be in the left lower quadrant. When retrocecal, the pain may be referred to the thigh or right testicle. Dysuria is present frequently in both types of appendicitis.

Pain referred to the midepigastrium is due to stretching of the organ during early inflammation. Initially it is vague and mild, but it gradually increases over about four hours and may be colicky. It tends to subside, and when the process has reached the serosa and the peritoneum, it localizes over the site of disease. In some patients distress appears to be alleviated at the time of perforation; after perforation, localization of pain will depend on whether or not the process is quickly walled off locally. Thus if the spreading infection is not contained, generalized abdominal discomfort of variable severity will result. *Anorexia* and *nausea* (with or without vomiting) are the second and third most frequent symptoms. In almost all instances, pain precedes the appearance of these other complaints, and its principal feature is *persistence.* About 10 per cent of patients will have constipation; diarrhea is uncommon. Temperature usually ranges between 38 and 38.6°C; higher levels usually indicate perforation.

PHYSICAL EXAMINATION. The findings on physical examination depend not only upon the stage of the inflammation but also upon the age of the patient. Tenderness to palpation is the most common (99 per cent), important, and reliable sign; indeed, without it, diagnosis is unlikely. It is usually confined to McBurney's point (one finger) in the right lower quadrant, corresponding to the usual location of the organ. However, although rectal tenderness is present in about one third of patients, it may be so severe as to indicate pelvic peritonitis and thus probable *pelvic appendicitis.* On initial examination in a minority of patients, a mass may be felt in the right lower quadrant or in the pelvis or transrectally. Localized rebound pain is found in 75 per cent. Generalized rebound tenderness indicates diffuse peritonitis. Bowel sounds may be present or absent; absence associated with distention and generalized rebound tenderness is consistent with perforation and diffuse peritonitis. The patient with acute appendicitis often does not seem ill. The physician must not be deceived; the diagnosis rests upon persisting pain and localized tenderness.

On occasion, tenderness may be elicited in the case of retrocecal appendicitis by stretching the psoas by hip extension. Very rarely, because of the odd location of the appendix, tenderness may be in the right upper quadrant or even the left lower quadrant.

LABORATORY FINDINGS. Laboratory studies consistently show a leukocytosis with an increase in polymorphonuclear cells—over 10,000 per cubic millimeter and greater than 75 per cent, respectively. Urinalysis is usually normal; however, about 15 per cent of patients have either a slight amount of protein or mild pyuria or hematuria. Presence of a calcified fecalith in the right lower quadrant on flat film of the abdomen is helpful, but it is present in only a small percentage of patients. Other findings on flat film include possible obliteration of the right psoas shadow, right lower quadrant sentinel loop ileus, and a right lower quadrant soft tissue mass with or without gas bubbles. With perforation and generalized peritonitis, fluid in the peritoneal cavity and obliteration of the peritoneal lines may be noted.

DIFFERENTIAL DIAGNOSIS OF APPENDICITIS AND OF THE ACUTE ABDOMEN. Appendicitis is first on the list of conditions causing acute abdominal pain that require surgery or immediate consultation with a surgeon. Computerized tomography (CT) is now increasingly used in diagnosis, demonstrating swelling, perforation, and fecaliths in a high proportion of cases, and appears to be more helpful than a plain film early in the disease. About 15 per cent of patients operated upon for acute appendicitis will have a normal appendix; in view of the gravity of unoperated upon disease, this figure is entirely acceptable. Here a few principles regarding the acute surgical abdomen in the setting of the differential diagnosis of acute appendicitis will be reviewed.

Pain Characteristics. Conditions associated with pain of sudden onset include *perforated viscus,* more commonly a *peptic ulcer* or a *colonic diverticulum,* or, rarely, a *carcinoma of the colon* or *acute ischemia* (although acute ischemia does not always cause acute or severe pain in the elderly); the onset of pain in *acute small bowel obstruction, choledocholithiasis, ureteral obstruction, rupture of an abdominal aortic aneurysm,* and *dissection of the abdominal aorta* may also be abrupt. The more gradual onset of pain usually indicates an inflammatory lesion—*cholecystitis, acute pancreatitis, diverticulitis,* and *appendicitis.* However, the pain of diffuse *inflammatory bowel disease* is not localized as it is in appendicitis, except as a consequence of perforation or fistulization in Crohn's disease. The pain of pelvic inflammatory disease is usually associated with menstruation and has been present for 24 or more hours, whereas appendicitis pain is more often intermenstrual and rarely is suffered so long except with perforation.

The type and radiation of the pain also help in differential diagnosis. For example, evidence of irritation of the diaphragm may be found on the right in *acute cholecystitis* and on the left in *acute pancreatitis*; sudden, severe pain referred to the tips of the shoulders, associated with diffuse intra-abdominal pain and, later, distention, is more typical of perforated viscus, particularly *peptic ulcer. Ureteral obstruction* causes pain that is frequently referred to the genitalia or groin. Steady, continuous pain is more characteristic of inflammation, as in appendicitis; on the other hand, intermittent or crampy pain is more characteristic of *obstruction of a hollow viscus* such as the gallbladder or small bowel.

Pain precedes nausea and vomiting in *appendicitis;* on the other hand, vomiting may be an early symptom of *acute cholecystitis* or *acute pancreatitis.* Bile-stained vomitus associated with acute cramping upper abdominal pain suggests *small bowel obstruction*; blood in the vomitus points toward a mucosal lesion proximal to the third portion of the duodenum. Relief of pain by vomiting suggests *gastric outlet obstruction*. Vomiting, of course, may accompany any intra-abdominal conditions, particularly if the patient is in great pain and has ileus or generalized peritonitis.

Physical Findings. Physical examination of the patient with an acute abdomen is of great importance, and the range of findings expected in acute appendicitis has been discussed. Unlike many causes of acute and severe abdominal pain, *mesenteric ischemia* is not associated with notable abdominal tenderness for six or more hours after onset. Localized tenderness and temperature elevation associated with continuing pain over a period of hours reflect either *localized peritonitis*, with or without perforation, or *vascular necrosis* of an ischemic organ. In such instances, the temperature is approximately 38.5 to 39.5°C. Higher temperatures are more often associated with urinary tract infections or bacterial pneumonias. Marked epigastric tenderness in a patient with a steadily increasing boring type of epigastric pain for several hours, particularly if accompanied by falling blood pressure, suggests *acute pancreatitis*. A rapidly rising pulse rate strengthens this possibility but is present with *perforation of a viscus*, a *gangrenous bowel*, or *rupture of an aneurysm*, as well.

Diffuse peritonitis is reflected by resistance of movement and change in position because of accentuation of pain; on the other hand, colic caused by *obstruction* of bile ducts, ureter, or small bowel early in its course is associated with restless movement. Later, in biliary tract and small bowel obstruction, infection and compromise of the blood supply may ensue and will cause the appearance of signs of localized tissue necrosis and peritonitis. The abdomen should be carefully examined for scars of previous surgery that may now underlie an *intestinal obstruction* caused by adhesions; hernias must be sought. A succussion splash indicates marked *gastric outlet obstruction*. A large, pulsatile midabdominal mass points to *dissection of the abdominal aorta*. *Rupture of an aortic aneurysm* is usually very sudden; pain is brief, since shock quickly supervenes. Abdominal examination reveals distention.

In examining the patient with an acute abdomen, the physician should palpate in that quadrant that is farthest removed from the site of distress. The important findings that indicate a surgical condition include persistent, localized tenderness with unequivocal rebound, indicating localized peritonitis, and guarding. Guarding must be interpreted circumspectly, because it may be voluntary or involuntary. If it is the latter, underlying peritoneal irritation is likely. Generalized involuntary guarding is a classic finding for a perforated intra-abdominal viscus. The presence of an abdominal mass not previously noted, particularly when associated with other findings of inflammation, gangrene, or perforation, is very strong evidence for a surgical condition. Likewise, free air in the abdominal cavity, as evidenced by distention, absence of bowel sounds, and absence of liver dullness in the setting of acute abdominal pain, reflects a perforated viscus. Bowel sounds may be more active and high pitched in early obstruction or continuously active in diffuse acute inflammation (nonsurgical) of the small bowel. With increasing distention of small bowel loops, the sounds become less frequent and more high pitched. Bruits are an important finding, because they may reflect the presence of *arterial aneurysms*, the dissections of which may be the cause for the abdominal pain.

Rectal examination is crucial in differential diagnosis. Unequivocal tenderness indicates pelvic inflammation, and a mass usually reflects the presence of an abscess. As noted above, this examination often reveals positive findings in *acute appendicitis*. A glove specimen of stool must always be examined for occult blood. In females with acute abdominal pain, pelvic examination is essential to complement a careful gynecologic history.

Laboratory Aids in Diagnosis. The laboratory examination, consisting of urinalysis, complete blood count, serum electrolytes, blood urea nitrogen (BUN) and creatinine, serum amylase, radiographic examination of the abdomen and chest, and sonography of the abdomen, is essential in the differential diagnosis of the acute abdomen.

A *polymorphonuclear leukocytosis* strongly substantiates an acute intra-abdominal process with inflammation or necrosis; a low hematocrit reflects a disorder that is also capable of producing bleeding—*mucosal ulcerations, intestinal carcinoma, ischemia*, or *dissecting aneurysms*. An elevated hematocrit and BUN suggest dehydration, usually caused by vomiting and deficient fluid intake.

Urinalysis is vital in differential diagnosis, because the presence of pyuria, particularly white cell casts and bacteria on the smear of urinary sediment, is strong evidence for urinary tract infection and interdicts surgical exploration. Microscopic hematuria (numerous red cells) suggests stone or tumor of the genitourinary tract; red cell casts, on the other hand, suggest glomerulitis. A few scattered white and red cells may be seen in the sediment of about 20 per cent of patients with acute appendicitis. Examination of a *stool specimen* for blood and white blood cells is indicated in patients with right lower quadrant pain, fever, and *diarrhea*. *Salmonella* enterocolitis (and other bacterial infections) may be confused with acute appendicitis.

Important blood chemistries are *serum amylase*, elevation of which usually reflects acute pancreatitis; however, it may not be elevated in chronic relapsing pancreatitis, and it is elevated in other conditions such as *perforated peptic ulcer, strangulated obstruction* of the small bowel with perforation, *acute cholecystitis, cholangitis, acute renal failure*, and *ruptured tubal pregnancy*.

Visual Aids in Diagnosis. Roentgenologic examinations of importance include chest and flat films of the abdomen and CT scans, including contrast films with water-soluble, iodine (1 to 2 per cent)-containing substances. Radionuclide studies and ultrasonography are often useful as well. The flat and upright films of the abdomen may show free air in the peritoneal cavity, reflecting a perforation of a hollow viscus (80 per cent of cases are due to perforated ulcer, followed by perforated diverticulum and appendicitis). They also support the diagnosis of acute small bowel obstruction, indicate the likelihood of calculus disease of either gallbladder or urogenital tract, outline a large obstructed stomach, and reveal a variety of soft tissue masses that may reflect cysts or abscesses. Collections of extraintestinal gas often point to abscesses; occasionally, the biliary tree may be outlined by air, thus revealing a fistula to bowel. Diffuse calcification of the region of the pancreas indicates chronic pancreatitis. As noted, calculi in the right lower quadrant may rarely help in the diagnosis of acute appendicitis. Flat film of the abdomen also may yield findings characteristic of acute pancreatitis, including "sentinel" loops and a "cut-off" of the colon. A cross-table lateral view will outline an abdominal aortic aneurysm. A routine chest radiograph is essential in order to reveal free intraperitoneal air under the diaphragm, to demonstrate pneumonia, or to show an elevated diaphragm on the left with or without pleural effusion and partial atelectasis, as noted in acute pancreatitis, or on the right, reflecting subphrenic abscess.

Sonography is particularly helpful in demonstrating gallstones, obstruction of the extrahepatic biliary tract (dilated intrahepatic ducts), collections of fluid including abscesses, defects in the liver, and obstruction of the urinary tract. Ultrasonography may also indicate *colonic diverticulitis, Crohn's disease, intramural hemorrhage*, or *intussusception* by revealing a thickened bowel wall. It may also help in diagnosing *"closed loop" obstruction*.

Computerized tomographic scans are increasingly used in difficult cases, especially when flat films and sonograms are not helpful. Computerized tomography may detect choledocholithiasis, the swollen pancreas of acute pancreatitis; inflammatory pseudocyst of the pancreas; intra-abdominal abscess; enlarged lymph nodes; subcapsular hematomas of liver, spleen, or kidney; dissection of the aorta; colonic diverticulitis; and with contrast, perforated or thickened bowel of Crohn's disease or cancer.

Radionuclides given intravenously may help by visualizing the gallbladder (technetium 99m, labeled iminodiacetic acid or derivative compounds) or by localizing an intra-abdominal abscess (gallium citrate 67). Visualization of the gallbladder by technetium 99m scan renders the diagnosis of acute cholecystitis highly unlikely. Radiolabeled agents may also detect localized inflammation and abscess. Gallium 67 collects in granulocytes and mononuclear cells; indium 111–labeled white cells of the patient are given intravenously. These agents are most useful when CT scanning and ultrasonography yield negative findings in the search for an inflamed organ or mass.

Nonsurgical conditions that cause acute abdominal pain are important in the differential diagnosis of acute appendicitis. Chief among these are *pyelonephritis, pneumonia, pulmonary infarction, acute myocardial infarction,* and *pericarditis,* all of which may cause acute upper abdominal pain. Acute distention of the liver and its capsule resulting from *acute right heart failure* may simulate *acute cholecystitis; acute hepatitis,* viral or toxic (including alcohol), may closely simulate acute biliary tract disease. In these instances, however, an enlarged, tender liver will be felt. Further, serum glutamic-oxaloacetic transaminase (SGOT) determinations will be markedly elevated. (However, acute obstruction of the common duct with cholangitis may transiently raise SGOT to levels of 1000 units or more for 24 to 48 hours.)

Systemic diseases, such as *sickle cell disease, acute intermittent porphyria, tabes dorsalis, heavy metal poisoning,* and *diabetic neuropathy,* all may present pictures simulating an acute surgical abdomen.

Acute pancreatitis usually is characterized by pain of many hours' to days' duration, associated with a history suggestive of biliary tract disease or indicative of acute and chronic alcoholism, and in its early stages abdominal tenderness is usually localized to the epigastrium. Markedly elevated plasma amylase (within 48 hours of onset) will help establish the diagnosis. Elevation of serum bilirubin above 3.0 mg per deciliter and of alkaline phosphatase indicates obstruction of the common bile duct, and occasionally ultrasonography or CT scan, in addition to indicating obstruction, may help in establishing choledocholithiasis as the cause of the pancreatitis.

SPECIAL CONSIDERATIONS IN DIFFERENTIAL DIAGNOSIS OF ACUTE APPENDICITIS. Great care must be extended to establish the diagnosis of this condition in the very young and very old. Children with diffuse abdominal pain that is preceded by anorexia, nausea, and vomiting and is often associated with diarrhea are more likely to have *acute infectious gastroenteritis,* in some cases due to *Yersinia enterocolitica, Campylobacter,* or *Salmonella.* Acute enteric infection with *Salmonella* must always be suspected, particularly in young adults with right lower quadrant pain, fever, and diarrhea. *Acute mesenteric adenitis,* presumably caused by viral illnesses and often associated with diffuse abdominal pain, is frequently confused with acute appendicitis in children. The difficulty is in those patients in whom there is some right lower quadrant tenderness and slight elevation of the white count. In such instances a diagnosis must be established at operation, because it is far safer to undertake a negative exploration than to neglect removal of an acutely inflamed appendix. Clinical differentiation of acute appendicitis from *Meckel's diverticulitis* is impossible. The acute onset of *Crohn's disease* involving terminal ileum may be very difficult to distinguish from acute appendicitis, although such patients usually have cramping abdominal pain and diarrhea.

In young women diagnosis is confused by problems in the reproductive system, such as *ruptured graafian follicles, twisted ovarian cysts, ectopic pregnancy, dysmenorrhea, ruptured endometrioma,* and *acute pelvic inflammatory disease. Ruptured ectopic pregnancy* is usually of dramatic suddenness and is often associated with shock and massive blood loss; these findings in a pregnant woman make the diagnosis virtually certain. The *ruptured graafian follicle* is noted in midcycle; fever and leukocytosis are uncommon. Tenderness on moving of the cervix on vaginal examination points toward a *twisted ovarian cyst,* the pain of which is out of proportion to the general well-being of the patient. The pain of *gonococcal salpingitis* is more diffuse, and tenderness is not so well localized as in appendicitis. Localized pain and tenderness in a pregnant woman whose pregnancy remains normal and who is not bleeding indicate probable appendicitis.

The differential diagnosis of appendicitis in the elderly may also be difficult. The classic picture is seldom noted, the history may be inadequate or misleading because of infirmity or the effects of medication, and the appendix perforates early. Findings on physical examination are usually not as dramatic, and, despite complications, fever may be only slightly elevated. Accuracy in diagnosis of patients over 60 years of age is below 70 per cent, and the incidence of perforation without a localized or generalized peritonitis at surgery is nearly 70 per cent—more than twice as high as all other age groups combined.

In elderly patients the principal problems in differential diagnosis are *cholecystitis, diverticulitis, mesenteric thrombosis, intestinal obstruction, incarcerated hernia,* and *perforated ulcer.*

Right-sided acute diverticulitis may simulate acute appendicitis in every respect. In a few instances, *left-sided diverticulitis* may localize tenderness to the right lower quadrant, because the sigmoid is often more redundant in the elderly. The patient also may have an episode of diarrhea associated with cramping or steady lower abdominal pain, slight temperature elevation, and, later, evidence of moderate-to-complete large bowel obstruction. When differential diagnosis is difficult, a cautiously administered barium enema or a CT scan with contrast may help greatly in excluding acute diverticulitis as the cause of the problem.

In all instances, elderly patients must not be subjected to the risk of exploration falsely. Accordingly, all efforts should be extended to make certain that *acute myocardial* or *pulmonary infarction, pneumonia,* or other systemic disease or toxin, in addition to intra-abdominal conditions that do not require immediate surgery, are not responsible for acute abdominal pain simulating appendicitis.

TREATMENT. Unless strongly contraindicated, the only therapy for acute appendicitis is surgical removal of the appendix. Since mortality correlates with perforation and, except in elderly patients, perforation correlates with duration of symptoms, early diagnosis and appendectomy are essential for the lowest acceptable morbidity and mortality for the disease. To avoid the catastrophe of unoperated-upon acute appendicitis, normal appendices may have to be removed in 20 to 25 per cent of patients.

In patients in whom complications (*perforation, peritonitis,* and *abscess*) have already occurred or are suspected, dehydration must be corrected; continuous nasogastric suction should be started; and gentamicin, 1.0 to 1.5 mg per kilogram, clindamycin, 1.6 to 2.5 grams, and metronidazole, 2.0 grams, given parenterally per day in divided doses, should be administered prior to surgery.

Patients with obvious acute appendicitis for whom no surgeon is available may be treated with head-up position of the bed; intravenous fluids; gentamicin, 1.0 to 1.5 mg per kilogram, clindamycin, 1.6 to 2.4 grams, and ampicillin, 2.0 grams, intravenously in divided doses daily; and nasogastric suction. The chance for recovery in otherwise healthy individuals with this program is surprisingly good. However, these patients must be scheduled for appendectomy six weeks later, or appendicitis is likely to recur.

MORBIDITY AND MORTALITY OF SURGERY. Overall, about 15 per cent of patients with acute appendicitis develop complications postoperatively; this figure is about 35 per cent in those with perforation and localized peritonitis at the time of surgery and is 70 per cent in those with perforation and generalized peritonitis. The complications include *wound infection, intra-abdominal abscess,* mechanical *small bowel obstruction, fecal fistula,* and, much more rarely, *intraperitoneal hemorrhage. Pylephlebitis* is extremely rare (1 in 1000).

The overall mortality of acute appendicitis ranges from 0.18 to 1.6 per cent and is due principally to the inter-related factors of age and perforation. Indeed, mortality over the age of 60 ranges from 6.4 to 14 per cent. The cause of death in this group may be attributed equally to septic and nonseptic complications.

Alvarado A: A practical score for the early diagnosis of acute appendicitis. Ann Emerg Med 15:557, 1986. *Predictive factors for diagnosis in order of importance are localized tenderness in the right lower quadrant, leukocytosis, migration of pain, shift to the left in the neutrophils, temperature elevation, nausea, vomiting, anorexia, and direct rebound pain.*

Brender JD, Marcuse EK, Koepsell TD, et al.: Childhood appendicitis: Factors associated with perforation. Pediatrics 76:301, 1985. *Delay in treatment—the interval between first recognized symptoms of abdominal pain and surgery—was most predictive of perforation. A treatment delay of more than 36 hours was associated with a 65 per cent or greater incidence of perforation.*

Lau WY, Fan ST, Yiu TF, et al.: Acute appendicitis in the elderly. Surg Gynecol Obstet 161:157, 1985. *A prospective study of 104 patients more than 60 years old with appendicitis. Showed clinical features similar to those of the younger patient; however, the elderly patient may have little or no pain, and the incidence of appendiceal perforation is increased.*

Schrock TR: Acute appendicitis. *In* Sleisenger MH, Fordtran JS (eds.): Gastrointestinal Disease. 4th ed. Philadelphia, W. B. Saunders Company, 1988. *A concise yet comprehensive article on every aspect of the subject. A handy reference.*

Way LW: Abdominal pain and the acute abdomen. *In* Sleisenger MH, Fordtran JS (eds.): Gastrointestinal Disease. 4th ed. Philadelphia, W. B. Saunders Company, 1988. *An excellent chapter containing all important information on diagnosis of the acute abdomen, identifying the cause and the accepted approaches to management.*

Diverticulitis of the Colon

DEFINITION. *Diverticulitis* of the colon is a focal inflammation in the wall of the apex of a diverticulum, most commonly of the sigmoid, caused by inspissated feces. It is more common in those with multiple diverticula that have appeared at an early age. Peridiverticulitis results from necrosis with micro- or macroperforation. An abscess then forms, its size depending on the size of the rupture; small ones may subside with scarring, while larger abscesses involve pericolonic tissue and may even dissect along, or within, the bowel wall. Occasionally they rupture into contiguous organs (bladder, ureter, vagina, and small bowel).

CLINICAL PICTURE. The predominant clinical symptoms of diverticulitis are *pain* and *fever*. The pain is usually prominent and is frequently constant. Most commonly, it is localized in the left lower quadrant, because the sigmoid and descending colon are the sites of the largest number of diverticula. The patient may have a few loose stools or become constipated, and only rarely is rectal bleeding noted. Bleeding from diverticula is not associated with inflammation and perforation. It is usually bright red and may be copious. Bleeding colonic diverticula must be differentiated from ischemic colitis, acute amebic and *Shigella* dysenteries, *ulcerative colitis,* and *tumors of the colon* (see Ch. 114). When the perforation and sepsis are of sufficient magnitude, the patient may also have chills with fever as high as 39 to 39.5°C. Usually, however, the fever is low grade, between 38 and 39°C.

Although the pain may be somewhat intermittent and even colicky at onset, it usually becomes steady and is of the same quality as noted in acute appendicitis. Indeed, acute diverticulitis has often been referred to as "left-sided appendicitis." The patient may seek medical help after only a few hours or, when the situation is not so severe, after a few days of lingering but nagging lower quadrant pain and low-grade fever. Rarely, a *diverticulum of the right colon* will perforate, causing right lower quadrant pain with fever, closely simulating appendicitis. Diagnosis is usually made at laparotomy.

Physical examination is extremely important in establishing the diagnosis. Since the process usually quickly involves the serosal surface and peritoneal cover, marked, localized tenderness will be found, both direct and rebound. Frequently, a tender mass may be discerned. When present for more than a few days, this mass may be astonishingly firm, even hard, and the distinction grossly from carcinoma is almost impossible. The abdomen is often slightly distended. Rectal examination also will be painful, because inflamed bowel is often within reach of the finger; also, a mass may be palpable if a sizable abscess has formed.

In some instances the patient will have complications of diverticulitis; *dysuria, pyuria, pneumaturia,* or *passing gas or feces through the vagina.* These symptoms are due to perforation of bladder or vagina by the diverticulitis (colovesical and colovaginal fistulas). The vast majority of these patients, usually elderly, do not relate these symptoms to a prior attack of severe pain. The presenting symptom may be septic fever, caused by pericolic, pelvic, or subdiaphragmatic abscess. The inflammatory process may penetrate other pelvic organs, but such fistulization is often clinically undramatic. Rarely, the diverticulum perforates freely. In this instance the signs of free perforation are evident—that is, distention of the abdomen, generalized rebound tenderness, and absent bowel sounds. It is unusual also for diverticulitis to cause persistent colonic obstruction (see below).

DIAGNOSIS. Diverticulitis should be suspected particularly in patients with known diverticula who develop fever, leukocytosis, and signs of pericolic and peritoneal inflammation in the left lower quadrant. The diagnosis is even more likely if a mass is palpable. Fever between 38.5 and 39°C is also compatible with the diagnosis; when the process is more extensive and with formation of a *pericolic abscess* and its complications, the temperature is usually over 39°C, and the white count is proportionately higher. Urinalysis will reflect varying degrees of involvement of the urinary tract by this septic process; that is, with mild ureteral irritation a few red and white cells may be seen in the urinary sediment, but with direct involvement of the ureter or invasion of the ureter or the bladder, the urine may be frankly septic and contain large numbers of red cells.

Some patients suffer much left flank pain owing to *hydronephrosis* resulting from obstruction of the ureter by a *pericolic abscess.* An intravenous pyelogram shows no function or an obstructed kidney on the left, and a sonogram or CT scan demonstrates unilateral hydronephrosis.

The use of radiographs is of crucial importance in the diagnosis, especially a flat film of the abdomen. Evidence of pericolic perforation and abscess formation may be suspected from collections of air and fluid in the left lower quadrant. Free air may be seen under the diaphragm in instances of free perforation. Sonography may reveal a localized thickening of the wall of the involved colon. Computerized tomographic scans are particularly helpful by showing inflamed pericolic fat in nearly all cases, the involved diverticula in 85 per cent, and thickening of the bowel wall in 75 per cent. Sonography, CT scan, or scintigraphy (gallium citrate 67) may localize an abscess. A fistula to the bladder or ureteral obstruction may be seen with ultrasonography or by CT scan.

Sigmoidoscopy should be carefully performed with minimal preparation. Air insufflation should not be used, and the importance of the examination is to exclude other conditions (see below). Usually with diverticulitis the instrument cannot be passed beyond the rectosigmoid junction, which is occluded by fixation, angulation, and spasm.

Clinicians debate the advisability of using a barium enema

in the diagnosis of diverticulitis, particularly in its acute phase. The concern is that the increased intraluminal pressure may cause perforation. The history, physical examination, laboratory information, flat film of the abdomen—and, in many cases, ultrasonography or CT scan—are sufficient to make the clinical diagnosis in most instances. Barium enema should await some subsidence of the acute phase of the illness. The exceptions to this dictum are those instances in which the *acute ischemic colitis* of the left colon and perforation of a left colonic carcinoma cannot otherwise be excluded. Colonoscopy or flexible sigmoidoscopy also is not indicated unless the diagnosis is not clear and the patient has gross rectal bleeding, since the techniques often do not reveal the perforated diverticulum.

The roentgenographic features characteristic of diverticulitis are the presence of barium outside a diverticulum, the delineation of a pericolic mass (Fig. 115–1), or the demonstration of a fistula originating in the colon. In some instances the distinction between diverticulitis and carcinoma or Crohn's disease may be difficult (see below). The presence of irregularity, thickening, or even a sawtooth appearance of the bowel is not sufficient to make the diagnosis of diverticulitis, because these are typical for diverticula without perforation.

After diagnosis of diverticulitis has been established, ultrasonography should be done to ascertain whether or not obstructive involvement of the urinary tract is present, particularly on the left side. In some instances, as noted above, urinary symptoms may be the predominant feature, and ultrasonography or radiographic examination of the urinary tract may have to be performed early.

DIFFERENTIAL DIAGNOSIS. For many years symptoms of *diverticulosis* have been attributed incorrectly to *diverticulitis. Diverticulosis* may periodically be associated with marked local tenderness, a palpable sigmoid loop, and some degree of large bowel obstruction, and thus the picture suggests diverticulitis. However, such patients do not have fever, the localized tenderness gradually recedes, the white count is not elevated, and there is no evidence of involvement of contiguous organs. Barium enema will reveal an irregular luminal contour with a narrowed sigmoid, possibly even a so-called "sawtooth" appearance of the mucosa. Barium must be noted outside the diverticulum, a fistula seen, or evidences of a pericolic or intramural mass detected before the diagnosis of diverticulitis is definitely made.

Carcinoma of the colon must be distinguished from diverticulitis because of similarity of age during which both diverticulitis and cancer of the colon appear. The differential diagnosis is especially difficult, because in about 25 per cent of patients with diverticulitis the lumen is narrowed, suggesting carcinoma. Differentiation from cancer is more difficult if diverticulitis has appeared insidiously. Chronic obstruction, more persistent rectal bleeding, and weight loss are more characteristic of *cancer*. However, the tumor may be obscured on barium enema in 50 per cent of patients with diverticula. Localized tenderness with rebound, leukocytosis, and fever support the diagnosis of diverticulitis. In some cases, however, it may be impossible to distinguish the two conditions, especially when the barium enema has features common to both—i.e., a mass, luminal irregularities, and partial obstruction. In such patients CT scan with contrast and colonoscopy may be very helpful in excluding cancer. Rapid disappearance of the obstruction strongly suggests diverticulitis. In some patients correct diagnosis can be made only at surgery, and, in a few, only from surgical biopsy or by the disappearance of the occlusion following colostomy.

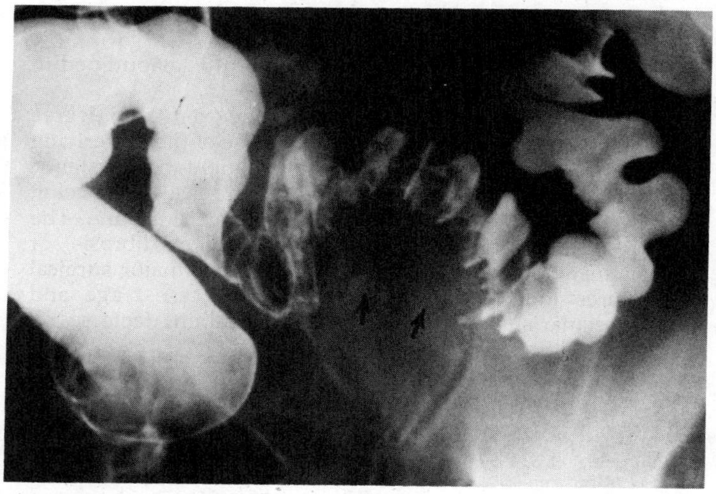

FIGURE 115–1. A paracolic mass that deforms and displaces the sigmoid lumen is delineated in a patient with diverticulitis and a palpable left lower quadrant mass. (From Almy TP, Naitove A: In Sleisenger MH, Fordtran JS [eds.]: Gastrointestinal Disease. 3rd ed. Philadelphia, W. B. Saunders Company, 1983.)

Crohn's disease of the colon may be difficult to exclude in the face of marked luminal narrowing or multiloculated channels parallel to the bowel wall on radiograph. Clinically, although both may produce pain, partial obstruction and lower abdominal mass, some rectal bleeding, fever, and leukocytosis, the past history differs. The patient with Crohn's colitis usually will have had previous episodes of lower abdominal pain, fever, and diarrhea. Sigmoidoscopy may reveal the rectum to be involved with granulomatous disease. Also, evidence elsewhere in the bowel of granulomatous disease, such as cobblestoning, long intramucosal sinus tracts, and skip areas, will help in the differential diagnosis (see Ch. 105).

Ischemic colitis of the left colon in elderly patients may produce signs and symptoms of bowel necrosis and localized peritonitis that are difficult to distinguish from diverticulitis. In these instances, gross rectal bleeding is prominent, and a barium enema is of crucial importance, because so-called "thumbprinting" will be found in ischemic colitis, especially in the area of the splenic flexure and descending colon (see Ch. 106).

TREATMENT OF DIVERTICULITIS. Patients with low-grade fever and no evidence of mass, fistula, or obstruction may be treated with clear liquids by mouth and ampicillin (2.0 grams) or a cephalosporin (4.0 to 6.0 grams) per day in divided dosage intravenously. If the patient has fever of 39° C or more or has a tender mass or other evidence of greater extent of infection, gentamicin, 1.0 to 1.5 mg per kilogram, clindamycin, 1.6 to 2.4 grams, and metronidazole, 2.0 grams, are given parenterally in divided doses daily. In such patients nasogastric suction and intravenous fluids are given to maintain intravascular volume, urinary output, and electrolyte balance. About 50 per cent of complicated cases will require surgery. Surgical consultation must be obtained early in all cases in which a mass is palpable or when there is suspicion of peritonitis or involvement of a contiguous organ.

Most patients respond well to this type of therapy with abatement of the fever, tenderness, and evidence of partial obstruction. Long-term therapy becomes identical with that for diverticulosis (see Ch. 102).

COMPLICATIONS AND INDICATIONS FOR SURGERY. Surgical intervention is necessary for the complications of diverticulitis, such as an *enlarging mass* despite therapy, *generalized peritonitis, persisting intestinal obstruction,* or the development of a *fistula*, most commonly to the urinary bladder and rarely to other contiguous structures, such as the left hip, infecting joint or bone. In unusual cases, acute diverticulitis may bleed massively, requiring laparotomy. If possible, a one-stage procedure is carried out; if not, a temporary colostomy is established after resection of a fistula or drainage of a septic area. More definitive resection and reanastomoses are carried out later. Elective surgery is indicated for recurrent attacks of diverticulitis and for the inability to exclude a carcinoma as-the cause for persisting deformity after recovery from the acute phase.

Almy TP, Howell DA: Diverticular disease of the colon. N Engl J Med 302:324, 1980. *A marvelously lucid update of every aspect of the subject.*

Almy TP, Naitove A: Diverticula of the colon. In Sleisenger MH, Fordtran JS (eds.): Gastrointestinal Disease. 4th ed. Philadelphia, W. B. Saunders Company, 1988. *A complete description of etiology, pathogenesis, and clinical pictures and complications of colonic diverticula, including diverticulitis.*

Hulnick DH, Megibow AJ, Balthazar EJ, et al.: Computerized tomography in evaluation of diverticulitis. Radiology 152:491, 1984. *CT scanning was very helpful in the diagnosis of 43 cases with demonstration of inflamed pericolic fat in 98 per cent of cases, of the involved diverticula in 84 per cent, and of a thickened wall in 70 per cent.*

Radiation Enterocolitis

Damage to the small intestine and colon may result from radiation therapy for abdominal and pelvic malignancy.

INCIDENCE. Incidence of severe radiation injury varies between 2.5 and 25 per cent of patients treated with radiotherapy for pelvic and intra-abdominal malignancy. Minor degrees of damage are common, as evidenced by impaired ileal absorption of conjugated bile acids in many women who are irradiated for pelvic cancer. It is noted most commonly after the total dosage exceeds 5000 rads. Transient histologic inflammatory change may, however, be found in the rectal mucosa of nearly 75 per cent of individuals receiving such therapeutic irradiation. The small intestine is more frequently affected than the rectum.

PATHOGENESIS AND PATHOLOGY. Damage results from interference with replication of radiosensitive epithelial cells, particularly of the crypt, leading to varying degrees of damage to the mucosal surface. Often it is reversible if dosage is not too great or treatment is not prolonged. Such damage may follow dosage of less than 5000 rads. Damage to the mesothelial cells of the small submucosal arterioles results in varying degrees of occlusion and mucosal transmural necrosis. Accordingly, hyperemia and ulceration of the mucosa are frequent. With extreme damage, diffuse edema is followed by extensive fibrosis with multiple strictures and irreversible damage. Such serious damage is more common in diabetics, in those with previous abdominal surgery, and in patients with serious vascular disease.

The pathologic changes range from diminution of crypt cell mitosis and shortening of villi of the small intestine to varying degrees of hyperemia, edema, and inflammatory cell infiltration of the mucosa. Mucosal thickness decreases. Progress of damage is marked by crypt abscesses, sloughing of epithelial cells, and, later, mucosal ulcerations, diffuse or localized, are found. Two to 12 months after radiotherapy, the damage to the blood vessels becomes prominent. In these instances, repair of acute damage does not ensue. The mucosa and submucosa become progressively ischemic and fibrotic. *Abscesses* and *fistulas* may form with sinus tracts between loops of intestine and between intestine and neighboring organs. A more general discussion of radiation injury is found in Ch. 539.

CLINICAL PICTURE. Symptoms may appear early, that is, during the first or second week of therapy, or late, that is, six months or more after completion of therapy. Early, diarrhea and mild rectal bleeding may appear, resembling ulcerative colitis. Sigmoidoscopy reveals an edematous mucosa that may be friable; in more extreme instances, the acute changes also reveal a patchy or diffusely necrotic mucosa.

Later, symptoms of radiation include gross rectal bleeding, decrease in stool caliber, and progressive difficulty in defecation with marked constipation, all indicating severe rectal involvement. Small intestinal symptoms result from either fibrosis and obstruction or fistulization and abscess formation. These serious complications are clinically apparent, on the average, 20 to 24 months after the insult. Those with fistulas are more likely to have synchronous lesions; areas most severely affected are the mid and distal small intestine and the rectosigmoid. If the damage is especially diffuse, malabsorption may be noted, as described in Ch. 104.

DIAGNOSIS. Diagnosis of *radiation enteritis* is suspected with any of the aforementioned symptoms in patients who have received significant radiation. Sigmoidoscopy shows a picture that ranges from variable degrees of edema to a markedly inflamed and necrotic mucosa. Multiple telangiectases are common, as is rectal stricture. Since most cases are fairly clear cut, biopsy is usually not indicated.

Barium studies of the intestine are not specific and range from changes of diffuse edema and spasm to diffuse fibrosis with strictures, fistulas, and ulceration in more severe cases. Thus the picture may resemble localized malignancy in the colon or diffuse granulomatous disease in the small intestine. Long strictured areas may also be noted, however, in the colon.

Differential diagnostic usefulness of small vessel angiography of the intestine in radiation enteritis remains to be confirmed.

TREATMENT. Improving methods for monitoring radiotherapy and delivering rads in small increments will probably reduce the incidence of this complication; however, the increasing incidence of malignancy and of the efficacy of radiotherapy will probably increase the total number of such patients.

Symptoms caused by early reaction consist of mild diarrhea and perhaps some minimal bleeding that can be managed by reduction of dose by 10 per cent, with the judicious use of tranquilizers, anticholinergic drugs, local analgesics, agents that increase stool bulk, and warm sitz baths for those with rectal involvement. An elemental diet free of gluten, milk protein, and lactose may benefit patients with early radiation reaction. If watery diarrhea is a problem, treatment with cholestyramine (4 to 6 grams per day) to bind bile salts may help greatly. If rectal bleeding is prominent, treatment with steroid retention enemas should be initiated as in ulcerative colitis (see Ch. 105). If the bleeding is more significant, transfusions may be required and even, possibly, surgery. Rectal strictures may be dilated, provided that it is early in their course and they are not extensive. Lubricants and stool softeners are often helpful; however, the progress to symptomatic occlusion of the lumen may necessitate proximal colostomy. Fistulas should be resected and abscesses drained. Resection of bowel and anastomoses are hazardous in view of the impaired blood supply, and anastomoses should always be made to uninvolved intestine.

In patients with malabsorption, treatment is as outlined in Ch. 104.

PROGNOSIS. Prognosis depends on the extent and degree of damage, the age of the patient, the course of the underlying malignancy, and whether or not the patient has systemic vascular disease. Unfortunately extensive disease of the colon usually means significant disease in the small intestine. The prognosis is guarded in those with ulceration, fibrosis, or fistulas in whom repeated resections or other major surgical procedures must be carried out. In such cases, age and cardiovascular status are also crucial determining factors.

Earnest DH, Trier JS: Radiation enterocolitis. In Sleisenger MH, Fordtran JS (eds.): Gastrointestinal Disease. 4th ed. Philadelphia, W. B. Saunders Company, 1988. *A comprehensive discussion of the radiation damage to small and large gut.*

Galland RB, Spencer J: Radiation-induced gastrointestinal fistulae. Ann R Coll Surg Engl 68:5, 1986. *Of 70 patients with radiation enteritis, 10 (14 per cent) had 14 radiation-induced fistulas. The median latent period between radiotherapy and presentation of the fistula was 20 months. The fistulas were often multiple and/or associated with other radiation-induced lesions, patients presenting with fistulas being significantly more likely to have synchronous lesions compared with those who presented with strictures.*

Galland RB, Spencer J: Surgical management of radiation enteritis. Surgery 99:133, 1986. *This study of 70 patients with 63 strictures, 14 fistulas, 12 perforations, and 8 bleeds shows that use of nonirradiated bowel for at least one end of an anastomosis significantly improves the results of resection of irradiated bowel.*

Small Intestinal Ulceration: Isolated and Diffuse

ISOLATED NONSPECIFIC ULCERS

This inflammatory disease of unknown etiology is rare. About 75 per cent are ileal and 25 per cent jejunal. Often they are multiple. These ulcers may be caused by ingestion of enteric-coated potassium chloride. Such ulceration may also be associated with *vascular disease* (systemic lupus erythematosus, polyarteritis nodosa, rheumatoid arthritis), *hematologic disorders, granulomatous diseases, trauma, infections, Behçet's syndrome,* and *neoplasia.*

The clinical picture consists of periumbilical colicky pain and perhaps nausea and vomiting. Frequently, however, the patient presents with small bowel obstruction, bleeding, or perforation. Duration of illness is usually weeks to months but may be years. Accordingly, examination may show signs of obstructions, or peritonitis may be present.

Laboratory investigation is normal unless the patient has been bleeding or has had protracted vomiting; plain films of the abdomen are of great value if small bowel is obstructed or has perforated. Barium contrast studies in the uncomplicated cases are most often unrevealing, although in rare instances ulceration and narrowing may be noted. Upper endoscopy may reveal the ulcer or ulcers if located in the high jejunum.

Treatment for the disease is conservative if no complications have occurred. If the involved segment is bleeding, perforated, or stenotic, it should be resected.

Boydstun JS, Gaffey TA, Bartholomew LG: Clinico-pathological study of non specific ulcer of small intestine. Dig Dis Sci 26:911, 1981. *Comprehensive review of the Mayo Clinic's experience with 29 patients.*

Thomas WE, Williamson RC: Nonspecific small bowel ulceration. Postgrad Med J 61:587, 1985. *Good report of clinical and radiologic features of this entity.*

DIFFUSE ULCERATION OF JEJUNUM AND ILEUM

Diffuse ulceration of the small bowel may be found in *gluten-sensitive enteropathy (celiac sprue), lymphoma, idiopathic chronic ulcerative enteritis* (also known as *chronic ulcerative nongranulomatous jejunoileitis*). It may also be found after oral administration of flucytosine. Patients with *gluten-sensitive enteropathy* may develop diffuse ulceration of jejunum and ileum, usually signaling a rapid decline in their clinical course despite elimination of gluten from the diet, with increased diarrhea, malabsorption, and, in some patients, perforation or hemorrhage. In instances of mild degrees of ulceration, steroids may induce remission; however, the majority are refractory to medical therapy and require appropriate resection of involved gut. Mortality in this group is high. The condition in patients with lymphoma and diffuse ulceration also is often refractory to resection and radiotherapy.

Chronic ulcerative enteritis and *eosinophilic gastroenteritis* affect the small intestine, usually in patients under 50. They are characterized by diarrhea, weight loss, variable degrees of malabsorption, and protein-losing enteropathy. *Chronic ulcerative enteritis* is a much graver illness, often with fever, ascites and edema, a rapidly progressive course unresponsive to steroids, and a high mortality. The etiology is unknown. Biopsy, peroral or at laparotomy, reveals nonspecific diffuse inflammation and mucosal ulcers. Prednisolone, 60 to 100 mg intravenously daily over two to three weeks, may be associated with remission in about one half of these patients. Infection, intraperitoneal or systemic, is the common cause of death.

Eosinophilic gastroenteritis may be localized to stomach, small intestine, or colon—so-called *eosinophilic granuloma.* It consists of infiltration by sheets of eosinophils into the submucosal and muscle layers. It is associated with systemic illnesses or peripheral eosinophilia and appears in the fourth to sixth decades. Steroids are often effective, but surgery may be indicated. *Universal eosinophilic gastroenteritis,* on the other hand, is a disease of younger persons, is often associated with allergies, always has a peripheral eosinophilia (greater than 20 per cent), affects stomach and small intestine diffusely, and is associated with diarrhea, crampy pain, weight loss, hypoalbuminemia, and often occult bleeding. Rarely, it responds to elimination of certain foods, particularly fish or meat. Most patients, however, require treatment with steroids, usually short-term (ten days to two weeks), but some may require long-term administration of 10 mg of prednisolone daily.

Bayless TR: Small intestinal ulceration: Isolated and diffuse. In Sleisenger MH, Fordtran JS (eds.): Gastrointestinal Disease. 4th ed. Philadelphia, W. B. Saunders Company, 1988. *Excellent clarification and description of isolated and diffuse ulceration of the small gut.*

Heyman, IN: Allergic disorders of the intestine and eosinophilic gastroenteritis. In Sleisenger MH, Fordtran JS (eds.): Gastrointestinal Disease. 4th ed. Philadelphia, W. B. Saunders Company, 1988. *A concise review of eosinophilic disease of the gut.*

PART XI

DISEASES OF THE LIVER, GALLBLADDER, AND BILE DUCTS

116 CLINICAL APPROACH TO LIVER DISEASE

Robert K. Ockner

The liver plays a central and varied role in many essential physiologic processes. It is the sole source of albumin and many other plasma proteins, and of blood glucose in the postabsorptive state; it is the major site of lipid synthesis and source of plasma lipoproteins; and it is the principal organ in which a wide variety of endogenous and exogenous substances such as ammonia, steroid hormones, drugs, and toxins undergo biotransformation. To the extent that biotransformation "detoxifies" or inactivates a substance, the liver may be viewed as serving a regulatory or protective function for the whole organism; to the extent that such biotransformation results in the formation of toxic products, as in the case of certain drugs, the liver may bear the brunt of their adverse effects.

The clinical manifestations of liver diseases are also varied. Moreover, the clues by which the clinician may be first alerted to the existence of liver disease, even when advanced, may be subtle, consisting of seemingly trivial information gleaned during a careful history (e.g., increased fatigue, or the reversal of sleep pattern or personality change of early hepatic encephalopathy), physical examination (e.g., prominence of breast tissue and small testes in a man with cirrhosis, or excoriation reflecting pruritus), or routine laboratory screening tests (e.g., mild decreases in one or more of the formed elements of the blood because of portal hypertension–associated hypersplenism). Careful assessment is equally important in the patient with obvious liver disease, to address more complex questions. For example, does what seems to be acute hepatitis in fact represent relapse of previously subclinical chronic hepatitis, or delta-agent (hepatitis D) infection in a hepatitis B carrier? (See Ch. 121.) Or does the deteriorating course of a patient with known cirrhosis represent the natural progression of the disease, or a superimposed common bile duct stone, adverse drug reaction, or hepatocellular carcinoma?

HISTORY. Some very *nonspecific symptoms* may be important evidence of liver disease, including fatigue, malaise, fever, change in sleep pattern or behavior, diminished libido, anorexia, weight loss, nausea, and vomiting. *Pruritus* is an important symptom of *cholestasis* (impaired bile secretion), and may be present in the absence of jaundice. *Jaundice* is often first noted by family members or friends, and, especially in dark-skinned individuals, may appear first as a yellow discoloration of the conjunctivae (*"scleral icterus"*). Since jaundice in most forms of liver and biliary disease reflects cholestasis (see below), such patients will often observe that stool color lightens while urine gets darker as the excretion of "bile pigments" is diverted from bile to urine. Right upper quadrant *abdominal discomfort* or *pain* may reflect a rapidly enlarging liver with distension of Glisson's capsule because of acute hepatic inflammation or congestion, an acutely inflamed gallbladder, common bile duct obstruction by an impacted gallstone, or abscess or tumor in the liver or adjacent areas.

The history may provide important clues to the presence of *complications of liver disease,* especially those reflecting *portal hypertension* and *portal-systemic shunting*. Early hepatic *encephalopathy* may cause subtle changes in affect or sleep pattern. More overt symptoms include episodic somnolence, confusion, combativeness, ataxia, incoordination, or obtundation. A history of *abdominal swelling* suggests ascites, and may be most easily recalled by the patient as a change in the fit of clothing, possibly associated with *edema*. Ascites may also occur in many other conditions, including hepatic vein or inferior vena cava occlusion, congestive cardiac failure and constrictive pericarditis, and a wide variety of neoplastic and inflammatory processes (see Ch. 112). A history of *gastrointestinal bleeding* in a patient with liver disease may suggest esophageal varices, but can also reflect other lesions such as *gastritis, Mallory-Weiss syndrome,* and *peptic ulcer*.

The history is of major importance in the identification of potentially significant *etiologic* or *predisposing factors*. Viral hepatitis is suggested by a history of contact with jaundiced persons, exposure to persons known to have hepatitis or to a common source of hepatitis, ingestion of uncooked or partially cooked shellfish, prior blood transfusion, work with subhuman primates, employment in certain health professions (especially in dialysis or transplantation units), accidental inoculation, sexual promiscuity (especially in the homosexual community), sharing of needles, travel to geographic areas with inadequate public health programs, and consumption of water or uncooked vegetables in such areas. Foreign travel may also suggest parasitic disease such as amebic liver abscess. Q fever hepatitis may occur in individuals in proximity to livestock. Exposure to drugs, ethanol, and other potential dietary, occupational, or environmental toxins must be reviewed in detail. The information obtained may require supplementation or corroboration by family members or other close associates, especially in regard to ethanol consumption. It is often possible to document previous liver function through recourse to *medical records,* and this is particularly useful in evaluating the chronicity of liver disease. A *family history* of jaundice, liver disease, or neonatal jaundice may suggest an inherited disorder such as Wilson's disease, $alpha_1$-antitrypsin deficiency, or hemochromatosis.

PHYSICAL EXAMINATION. Scleral *icterus* may be detected at a serum bilirubin concentration as low as 2.0 to 2.5 mg per deciliter. Although *spider telangiectasias,* most prominent around the shoulders and upper trunk, and *palmar erythema* are nonspecific and may be present to a limited extent in normal subjects (especially women in pregnancy), they are potentially important signs of liver disease, and usually imply chronicity. Excoriations reflect pruritus and suggest significant cholestasis, not necessarily accompanied by jaundice. *Xanthomas* and *xanthelasmas* are not specific for hepatobiliary disease, but may be a sign of prolonged cholestatic hypercholesterolemia. Changes in hair pattern, gynecomastia, and small or soft testes may reflect the *hormonal changes* that accompany cirrhosis in men. Prominence of cutaneous veins in the epigastrium or around the umbilicus may indicate a *portal-systemic collateral circulation* and, therefore, portal hypertension.

Examination of the heart and lungs may provide evidence of congestive cardiac failure, constrictive pericarditis, or diseases of the lungs or pleura that may be associated with liver dysfunction, cause pain referred to the abdomen, or reflect processes involving the subdiaphragmatic regions such as tumor or abscess.

Examination of the *liver* should include documentation of its *size*, and is best recorded both as the distance to which the lower edge extends below the costal margin, and its overall vertical span as determined by percussion. These dimensions should be related to a reproducible landmark such as the midclavicular line. The *form* and *consistency* of the liver should be noted: e.g., smooth, with a sharp edge; nodular and rock-hard; firm with a rounded and irregular edge. A rapidly decreasing liver size during the course of severe acute hepatitis may be a sign of massive hepatic necrosis. An abdominal mass, tenderness, or muscular spasm may suggest secondary involvement of the liver or biliary passages by a neoplastic or inflammatory process. *Ascites*, most readily detected as dullness or bulging in the flanks, fluid wave, or shifting dullness, may be caused by advanced liver disease, or superimposed infectious or neoplastic processes.

A diffusely tender and enlarged liver suggests hepatitis or congestion, whereas tenderness in a relatively limited area at or below the lower margin in the region of the interlobar fissure may reflect acute cholecystitis. A visible or palpable gallbladder is abnormal and may be an important sign of primary gallbladder pathology, or of cystic or common bile duct obstruction, the latter usually neoplastic in jaundiced patients (Courvoisier's sign). Splenomegaly may be the first evidence of portal hypertension of any cause, or may reflect primary splenic pathology such as neoplasm or infection.

Neurologic evaluation is of particular importance with respect to signs of hepatic encephalopathy. These are discussed in detail in Ch. 128, but, as noted, these may be very subtle, consisting initially of a personality change, a mild confusional state, or lethargy. A *flapping tremor* (asterixis), characteristic of metabolic encephalopathy of any cause, is usually present in more obvious cases. In advanced hepatic encephalopathy almost any form of neurologic abnormality may be present, including seizures, lateralizing signs, and abnormal posturing. Despite this, it is essential in patients with liver disease to consider other causes of central nervous system pathology such as the effects of ethanol, sedatives or other toxins, hypoglycemia, trauma, hemorrhage, infection, and primary or secondary neoplasms.

Schiff L, Schiff E (eds.): Diseases of the Liver. Philadelphia, J. B. Lippincott Company, 1982.

Sherlock S: Diseases of the Liver and Biliary System. Oxford, Blackwell Scientific Publications, Ltd., 1985.

Wright R, Millward Sadler GH, Alberti KGMM, et al. (eds.): Liver and Biliary Disease. 2nd ed. London, W. B. Saunders Company, 1985.

Zakim D, Boyer T (eds.): Hepatology: A Textbook of Liver Disease. Philadelphia, W. B. Saunders Company, 1982.

Four current and comprehensive textbooks that serve to introduce the topic and provide literature references dealing with the broad field of hepatobiliary structure, function, and disease.

117 HEPATIC METABOLISM IN LIVER DISEASE

Robert K. Ockner

Intermediary metabolism may be profoundly disturbed in liver disease, and in some instances the resulting changes may overshadow the underlying disease process.

CARBOHYDRATE METABOLISM. Except during the absorption of dietary carbohydrate, maintenance of blood glucose levels depends entirely on the liver. Two distinct mechanisms are involved: *glycogenolysis* and *gluconeogenesis*. In glycogenolysis, glucose is released from hepatic glycogen by the enzyme phosphorylase, converted to its active form by the interaction of glucagon or epinephrine with specific liver cell surface receptors and subsequent activation of glycogen phosphorylase kinase via the calcium messenger system. Insulin, conversely, stimulates the incorporation of glucose into hepatic glycogen. Normal hepatic glycogen stores are sufficient to sustain blood glucose concentrations in the absence of exogenous carbohydrate for only about 24 hours; beyond that, maintenance of blood glucose in the fasting state depends entirely on hepatic gluconeogenesis. Gluconeogenesis, i.e., the de novo synthesis of glucose, largely from lactate, pyruvate, and amino acid precursors, is stimulated by glucagon and epinephrine and inhibited by insulin.

Thus, the normally functioning liver is responsive to a continually changing nutritional and hormonal milieu. During the fed state (relative glucose and insulin excess), glucose production (gluconeogenesis and glycogenolysis) is minimal; instead, dietary glucose either is stored as glycogen or is converted to fatty acids *(lipogenesis)*, largely to be secreted from the liver in the form of triglyceride-rich lipoproteins and destined for storage in adipose tissue. In the fasting state, the process is reversed, and relative glucagon excess with respect to insulin favors energy consumption rather than energy storage. Thus, liver glycogen is mobilized, and gluconeogenesis is increased; glucose is no longer diverted to lipogenesis, but is exported into plasma. The decrease in fatty acid synthesis is associated with increased fatty acid oxidation, which becomes the principal energy source for the liver.

In liver disease, disturbances in glucose homeostasis usually produce *hypoglycemia* or *glucose intolerance*. Mild hypoglycemia (blood glucose concentrations between 45 and 60 mg per deciliter) occurs in about 50 per cent of patients with uncomplicated acute viral hepatitis. As a rule, these patients are not hyperinsulinemic; rather, hypoglycemia may reflect several hepatic abnormalities, including diminished glycogen stores, diminished glycogenolytic response to glucagon, diminished gluconeogenesis, and impaired repletion of hepatic glycogen during the fed state. In most cases, the hypoglycemia is not clinically significant, but in very severe acute liver injury of any cause, such as virus- or drug-induced massive hepatic necrosis or Reye's syndrome, hypoglycemia may be an important component of the syndrome of acute liver failure. Hepatic hypoglycemia may also occur in the absence of overt liver damage. For example, *alcoholic hypoglycemia* classically occurs in persons whose only important source of calories over a period of days is ethanol; hypoglycemia in this setting reflects both a depletion of hepatic glycogen stores and inhibition of gluconeogenesis by ethanol. Hypoglycemia should be considered in the differential diagnosis of altered mental status in any patient with significant acute liver disease or exposure to ethanol or other toxins.

Glucose intolerance, on the other hand, is more typically associated with chronic liver disease and cirrhosis. Plasma insulin concentrations tend to be high, suggesting a state of *insulin resistance*. Both insulin receptor number and binding affinity have been found to be diminished in peripheral blood monocytes, suggesting a more generalized receptor defect. In addition, insulin resistance may in part reflect increased plasma glucagon concentrations and in part a diminished insulin effect on the liver because the hormone is diverted to the peripheral circulation via portal-systemic shunts. Regardless of the mechanism, the glucose intolerance associated with chronic liver disease, per se, is rarely of clinical significance. Occasionally, patients with chronic liver disease may also have other disorders such as *hemochromatosis* and *chronic pancreatitis*, in which *diabetes mellitus* may contribute to glucose intolerance.

LIPID METABOLISM. The liver plays a central role in the metabolism of fatty acids and other lipids and lipoproteins. Of the total daily turnover of plasma nonesterified fatty acids (free fatty acids) derived from adipose tissue, about one third enter the liver, where they are esterified to triglycerides or other esters, or undergo oxidation, largely in the mitochondria. The balance between esterification and oxidation is closely regulated, as is the rate of de novo fatty acid synthesis. In the fasting state, fatty acid synthesis is inhibited, whereas fatty acid oxidation is increased at the expense of the esterification pathways. In the fed state, de novo fatty acid synthesis and esterification are favored, whereas oxidation is diminished. Exclusive of dietary sources and de novo synthesis, a total of approximately 60 to 70 grams of plasma nonesterified fatty acid (>200 mmol) is taken up by the liver each day in the average adult, and in the fasting state fatty acids are the major energy source for the liver. Interference with hepatic fatty acid metabolism may either cause or be caused by clinically significant abnormalities of hepatic structure and function.

Fatty liver usually reflects excess accumulation of triglyceride, which may be deposited as large vacuoles displacing the nucleus, or as small droplets, in which the nucleus remains central. It may be viewed as an imbalance between the rate of triglyceride biosynthesis on the one hand, and the rate of triglyceride disposition (primarily secretion into plasma in the form of very low density lipoproteins) on the other. This imbalance may result from many factors that can affect either or both sides of the equation. Conditions associated with large vacuolar fatty liver include obesity, protein-calorie malnutrition (e.g., kwashiorkor, jejunoileal bypass), diabetes mellitus, corticosteroid therapy, and ethanol ingestion (see Ch. 126). Small-droplet fat accumulation (see below) is characteristic of obstetric fatty liver (acute fatty liver of pregnancy), Reye's syndrome, Jamaican vomiting sickness, and tetracycline and valproic acid hepatotoxicity and, occasionally, is ethanol related. Accumulation of triglyceride in the liver cell is usually associated with hepatomegaly and reflects abnormal liver function, but does not *by itself* appear to cause severe, progressive, or lasting liver damage.

Conversely, interference with fatty acid oxidation at any of several stages may have profound consequences. For example, *alcoholic ketosis* is attributed to an ethanol- or acetaldehyde-mediated impairment of the tricarboxylic acid cycle, resulting in incomplete oxidation of the products derived from beta-oxidation of fatty acids. A far more profound derangement of hepatic function is caused by hypoglycin, a low molecular weight compound present in the unripened fruit of the ackee tree and the cause of *Jamaican vomiting sickness*. In this disorder, hypoglycin metabolites are converted to coenzyme A thioesters and to carnitine derivatives. Since these cannot be metabolized further, they effectively sequester the cellular carnitine pool. Fatty acid oxidation is inhibited, and there is a corresponding decrease in ATP production and gluconeogenesis. Continuing fatty acid esterification under these conditions leads to a form of fatty liver characterized by *small-droplet fat* deposition, associated in severe cases with liver failure and hypoglycemia. Despite the histopathologic and clinical similarities among this entity and *Reye's syndrome*, *obstetric fatty liver*, and *tetracycline* and *valproic acid hepatotoxicity*, in none of these latter conditions has the pathogenesis been fully elucidated.

Another clinically important aspect of hepatic lipid metabolism concerns the synthesis of *cholesterol* and *bile acids* and the excretion of biliary lipids. The liver is the major source of endogenously synthesized cholesterol (approximately 0.5 gram per day). Together with cholesterol of dietary origin, this newly synthesized cholesterol enters a "metabolically active" hepatic cholesterol pool, from which is derived the cholesterol destined for secretion into bile or into plasma (in lipoproteins), for synthesis of liver cell membranes, and for conversion to bile acids. Bile acid synthesis accounts for the disposition of approximately half of the total daily turnover of cholesterol and, as such, is an important determinant of body cholesterol stores. Relative rates of secretion of bile acids, cholesterol, and phosphatidyl choline (lecithin) into bile are important factors in the pathogenesis of cholesterol gallstones, but the mechanism(s) by which the secretion of these substances is effected and controlled is incompletely understood.

AMINO ACID AND PROTEIN METABOLISM. Except for the immunoglobulins, most plasma proteins, including albumin, clotting factors, transferrin, alpha$_1$-antitrypsin, and the nonalimentary lipoproteins, are synthesized in the liver. The synthesis of each is controlled by specific regulatory mechanisms. In all cases, however, synthesis and secretion are dependent on the integrity of many aspects of cell function, including the transcriptional mechanisms in the nucleus, the translational mechanisms in the rough endoplasmic reticulum, and the secretory mechanisms in the Golgi apparatus. Despite these common features, individual proteins are affected differently in liver disease. This nonuniformity may result from several factors such as the availability of an essential *nutritional* component (e.g., the vitamin K–dependent clotting factors), *hormonal* influences (e.g., very low density lipoproteins), *genetic* determinants (e.g., ceruloplasmin or alpha$_1$-antitrypsin), the effects of drugs or toxins (e.g., the warfarin-like anticoagulants or ethanol), or the response of selected proteins such as fibrinogen (and other "acute phase reactants," including C-reactive proteins, ceruloplasmin, haptoglobin, and transferrin) to inflammatory processes. In addition, the *kinetics* of synthesis and turnover of a particular protein are major determinants of response of its plasma concentration to acute liver injury. In general, plasma concentrations of proteins of which the turnover is rapid (e.g., clotting factors, plasma half-time of hours to days) are more likely to be depressed by severe acute liver injury than are those of proteins that turn over more slowly (e.g., albumin, plasma half-time of 2½ to 3 weeks). Finally, *catabolism* of certain plasma proteins may be accelerated (e.g., clotting factors in *disseminated intravascular coagulation*, or albumin in *protein-losing enteropathy*). For these reasons, although liver disease generally tends to depress the plasma concentration of proteins of hepatic origin, plasma concentration of such proteins may not accurately reflect the severity of the liver disease in a given patient. Interpretation of the prothrombin time, partial thromboplastin time, and serum albumin concentrations in the evaluation of liver disease is discussed in Ch. 119.

Amino acids, in addition to their obvious importance in protein synthesis, also participate in other reactions in the liver. Of special significance is the role of certain amino acids as precursors for gluconeogenesis, as discussed above. Amino acids may undergo *transamination,* in which the alpha-amino group is transferred to an alpha-keto acid, as in the alanine transaminase (ALT)–mediated deamination of alanine to pyruvate; the resulting transfer of the amino group to alpha-ketoglutarate converts this acceptor to glutamate. Alternatively, amino acids may undergo *oxidative deamination*; in this case, an alpha-keto acid is formed as the amino group is converted to ammonium ion and, ultimately, to urea (see below).

BIOTRANSFORMATION AND DETOXIFICATION. The liver is the major site of chemical modification of a wide variety of exogenous drugs and toxins, as well as endogenous substances such as hormones. The reactions potentially involved are numerous and, in many instances, involve the cytochrome P-450–dependent microsomal mixed function oxidase system. The basic principles of drug disposition are discussed in Ch. 24, but several aspects warrant special emphasis in the context of liver function and disease. First, while biotransformation of an endogenous or exogenous substance may *inactivate* it or render it more suitable for urinary or biliary excretion, there are many examples of compounds upon which activity or toxicity is conferred by this process. A number of clinically significant hepatotoxins are *activated* in this way, and there is good evidence that some "idiosyncratic" hepatic drug reactions may reflect individual differences in drug metabolism rather than an immunologic response (see Ch. 122). Second, diseases of the liver may seriously impair the biotransformation of exogenous substances, thereby resulting in an *increased sensitivity* to certain drugs (e.g., sedatives and opiates), or may enhance the biologic effect of endogenous hormones (e.g., contributing to the feminizing effects of chronic liver disease) or toxins (e.g., diminished hepatic conversion of ammonia to urea in hepatic encephalopathy). Finally, one substance may significantly influence the hepatic biotransformation of another. Examples of this particular form of *drug-drug interaction* include the well-recognized induction of the microsomal drug-metabolizing system by prior administration of phenobarbital and its inhibition by various toxins.

A particularly important hepatic detoxification pathway converts *ammonium ion* to urea via the Krebs-Henseleit *urea cycle*, in which ornithine, citrulline, argininosuccinate, and arginine are intermediates and which involves both mitochondrial and cytosolic components (see Fig. 192–1). Glutamate, formed from NH_4^+ and alpha-ketoglutarate, is the principal NH_2 donor. Ammonium ion is produced in abundance in the intestinal tract, especially the colon, by the bacterial degradation of luminal proteins and amino acids and of endogenous urea, 25 per cent of the daily production of which diffuses into the intestinal lumen. The NH_4^+ so formed diffuses into the portal circulation and is transported to the liver, where it is converted to urea by the mechanism described above. As discussed in Ch. 128, *hepatic encephalopathy* in part reflects the failure of this important detoxification process (or of analogous pathways for other *enterogenous toxins*) because of extensive acute liver cell necrosis or direct entry of portal blood into the peripheral circulation via spontaneous or surgically created portal-systemic shunts.

Arias IM, Popper H, Schachter D, et al.: The Liver: Biology and Pathology. New York, Raven Press, 1982. *An in-depth and well-documented presentation of many more basic aspects of normal and abnormal hepatic structure and function.*

Popper H, Schaffner F (eds.): Progress in Liver Diseases. Vol. 8. Orlando, Grune & Stratton, 1986. *Authoritative reviews of several basic and clinical aspects of liver function in health and disease.*

Zakim D, Boyer T (eds.): Hepatology: A Textbook of Liver Disease. Philadelphia, W. B. Saunders Company, 1982.

118 BILIRUBIN METABOLISM AND HYPERBILIRUBINEMIA

Bruce F. Scharschmidt

BILIRUBIN METABOLISM (See Fig. 118–1)

BILIRUBIN CHEMISTRY. Bilirubin consists of four pyrrole rings linked by three carbon bridges. Unconjugated bilirubin is virtually water-insoluble at physiologic pH because its –COOH and –NH groups are involved in strong intramolecular hydrogen bonds and are therefore unable to interact with water. These intramolecular hydrogen bonds are disrupted by conjugation of the –COOH groups with glucuronic acid as occurs in the liver cell, thus greatly enhancing the aqueous solubility of the molecule and altering its biologic properties. In contrast to the more polar water-soluble conjugates, relatively nonpolar unconjugated bilirubin diffuses across most biologic membranes such as the blood-brain barrier, placenta, and intestinal and gallbladder epithelium. It is excreted in bile in only trace amounts. Thus, hepatic conjugation confers upon bilirubin the properties that permit its elimination from the body and thereby prevents damage to the central nervous system. Exposure of bilirubin to light appears reversibly to convert unconjugated bilirubin to one of several isomers that are also unable to form intramolecular hydrogen bonds, and hence have increased water solubility. These photoisomers are excreted by the liver without conjugation; this may be the primary mechanism by which phototherapy lowers serum bilirubin concentration in neonatal hyperbilirubinemia.

BILIRUBIN FORMATION. Bilirubin is formed by selective cleavage of the heme ring at the alpha-methene bridge. Daily bilirubin production in adults averages about 4 mg per kilogram, of which about 70 per cent results from degradation of the heme moiety of hemoglobin in senescent erythrocytes. Most of the remainder results from the breakdown of nonhemoglobin hemoproteins in the liver, principally the cytochromes P-450. A minor fraction of bilirubin production results from premature destruction of newly formed erythrocytes in the bone marrow or circulation. In certain clinical disorders (e.g., megaloblastic anemia) destruction of young or developing erythroid cells is increased and may account for a substantial proportion of total bilirubin production. The most common cause of increased bilirubin production is increased breakdown of hemoglobin heme resulting from hemolysis.

Senescent erythrocytes are normally sequestered and degraded in the mononuclear phagocytic cells of the spleen, liver, or bone marrow. In contrast, the heme moiety of methemalbumin, methemoglobin, free hemoglobin, and haptoglobin-bound hemoglobin is taken up and catabolized by hepatic parenchymal cells. Microsomal heme oxygenase, the heme-cleaving enzyme, is most abundant in the liver, spleen, and bone marrow and exhibits substrate-mediated induction by heme or hemoglobin. The conversion of heme to biliverdin,

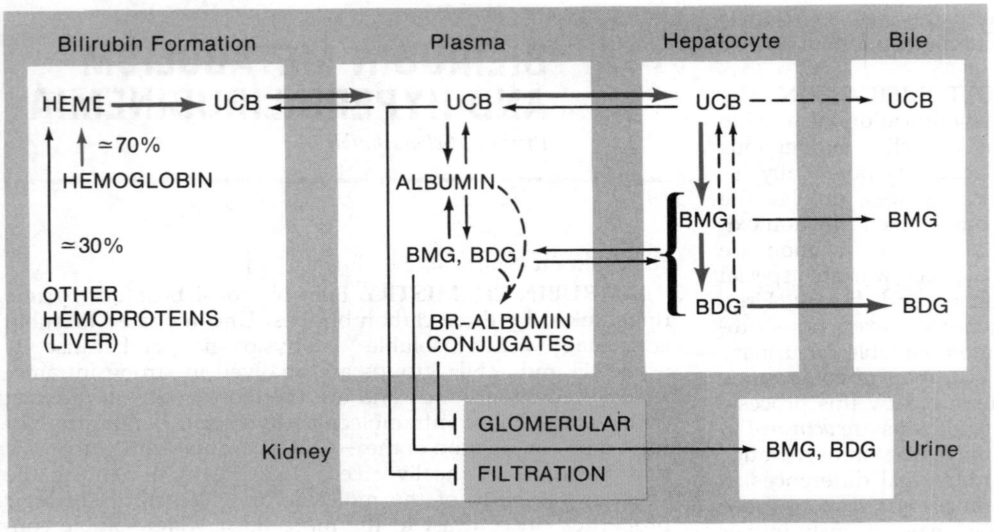

FIGURE 118–1. Overview of bilirubin metabolism. Unconjugated bilirubin (UCB) formed from the breakdown of hemoglobin heme and other hemoproteins is transported in plasma reversibly bound to albumin and is converted in the liver to bilirubin monoglucuronide (BMG) and diglucuronide (BDG), the latter being the predominant form secreted in bile. BMG and BDG together normally account for less then 5 per cent of serum bilirubin. In the presence of hepatobiliary disease, BMG and BDG accumulate in plasma and appear in urine. Bilirubin glucuronides in plasma also react nonenzymatically with albumin and possibly other serum proteins to form protein conjugates, which do not appear in urine and have a plasma half-life similar to that of albumin.

which is rate limiting for bilirubin formation, is followed by reduction of biliverdin to bilirubin by cytosolic biliverdin reductase. The reason mammals convert nontoxic, water-soluble biliverdin to water-insoluble bilirubin is unclear. Bilirubin, unlike biliverdin, is able to cross the placenta, however.

BILIRUBIN BINDING TO PLASMA PROTEINS. Unconjugated bilirubin is bound reversibly to albumin at a primary high affinity site (10^8 M^{-1}). At plasma concentrations exceeding its molar equivalence with albumin (about 35 mg per deciliter), bilirubin also binds to at least two low-affinity sites. A variety of compounds, including certain sulfonamides, penicillin derivatives, furosemide, and radiographic contrast media, may displace bilirubin from its albumin-binding sites and increase the risk of kernicterus in neonates. Presumably because of its tight albumin binding and low water solubility, unconjugated bilirubin is not excreted in urine. Conjugated bilirubin is somewhat less tightly bound to albumin than is bilirubin. It is filtered to a greater extent at the glomerulus, is incompletely reabsorbed by the renal tubules, and therefore does appear in the urine in small amounts in patients with conjugated hyperbilirubinemia.

In addition to the reversible binding to albumin just described, another bilirubin fraction binds very tightly, perhaps covalently, to albumin. This pigment fraction (called delta-bilirubin, biliprotein) has a serum half-life of about 17 days, similar to that of albumin. It has been detected only in patients with conjugated hyperbilirubinemia, in whom it may constitute a substantial proportion of direct-reacting fraction as measured by conventional assays (see below). The identification of this protein-bound fraction helps explain the occasionally slow resolution of hyperbilirubinemia in patients convalescing from hepatitis or in whom biliary obstruction has been relieved, as well as the disappearance of bilirubinuria in these patients prior to the resolution of jaundice.

HEPATIC BILIRUBIN TRANSPORT. Uptake of bilirubin and other substances tightly bound to protein is facilitated by large fenestration in the cells of the sinusoidal lining that permits plasma proteins to enter the space of Disse and directly contact the hepatocyte plasma membrane. Uptake of bilirubin and other organic anions such as sulfobromophthalein across the sinusoidal membrane of the hepatocyte displays several features characteristic of carrier-mediated transport, including saturability and competition. Uptake of albumin-bound bilirubin by the putative membrane carriers may indeed be facilitated by transient binding of the albumin-bilirubin complex to the cell surface. Once inside the liver cell, bilirubin and other organic anions appear to bind to cytoplasmic proteins such as ligandin. Ligandin, which constitutes 2 per cent of cytoplasmic protein in human liver, may alter net uptake by reducing bilirubin efflux back into plasma. In addition to transport through the cytoplasm, bilirubin may be directly transferred from the plasma membrane to the membranes of the endoplasmic reticulum, where conjugation occurs.

In the process of conjugation, the carboxyl groups of one or both propionic acid side chains of bilirubin are esterified, usually with glucuronic acid. Glucose and xylose conjugates are formed in trace amounts only. Formation of bilirubin monoglucuronide and diglucuronide is catalyzed by microsomal UDP-glucuronyltransferase. Transport of conjugated bilirubin from the hepatocyte into bile, like the uptake step, seems to show saturability and competition and therefore is presumably carrier mediated. Excretion and/or conjugation, but not uptake, appears to be rate limiting for overall bilirubin transport from blood to bile. Bilirubin diglucuronide predominates in human bile (70 to 80 per cent), with the isomeric monoglucuronides present in small amounts.

ENTEROHEPATIC CIRCULATION. Absorption of conjugated bilirubin from the gallbladder and small intestine is negligible. In the terminal ileum and colon, bilirubin is converted by bacterial enzymes into colorless urobilinogens and related products, including urobilins. Most urobilinogen that is absorbed from the intestine is re-excreted in bile and ultimately in feces; a small fraction appears in urine. Urobilinogen is absent from the bile and urine of patients with complete biliary obstruction; however, fecal and urinary urobilinogen levels correlate poorly with bilirubin production rate and are of little clinical utility. In addition to urobilins, the normal brown color of stool may reflect the presence of nonbilirubin pigments, perhaps of plant origin, which are also excreted in bile and undergo enterohepatic circulation.

CONCENTRATION IN PLASMA. About 95 per cent of circulating bilirubin in healthy adults is unconjugated. In contrast, circulating bilirubin in patients with hepatocellular or biliary tract disease consists predominantly of monoconjugates and diconjugates. The conventional diazoassay, which is employed in most clinical laboratories, tends to overestimate total plasma bilirubin concentration in patients with hepatobiliary disease, perhaps because of the detection of protein-bound pigment, i.e., delta-bilirubin. Moreover, determination of conjugated bilirubin based on measurement of the direct-reacting fraction is frequently in error. Nonetheless, for practical clinical application, conventional laboratory techniques are generally adequate. Plasma bilirubin concentration, which ranges normally between 0.3 and 1.0 mg per deciliter, varies directly with bilirubin production and inversely with hepatic bilirubin clearance. Thus it is possible to interpret all forms of hyperbilirubinemia in terms of increased production and/or decreased clearance.

INHERITED DISORDERS OF BILIRUBIN METABOLISM

The hereditary disorders of hepatic bilirubin metabolism constitute a heterogeneous group of disorders characterized by impaired ability of the liver to transport or conjugate bilirubin (Table 118–1). The common and benign entity of *Gilbert's syndrome* and the exceedingly rare and almost uniformly lethal Type I *Crigler-Najjar syndrome* represent opposite ends of this spectrum. Routine tests of liver function are generally normal in all these disorders, but a variety of abnormalities in the hepatic handling of bilirubin and other cholephilic anions such as sulfobromophthalein have been described. Many of these disorders, including Gilbert's syndrome, the *Dubin-Johnson syndrome*, and *Rotor's syndrome*, may be mistaken for acquired hepatobiliary disease. They are all of interest because of the insight they provide into hepatic bilirubin transport and conjugation.

GILBERT'S SYNDROME. Because of its frequency (up to 7 per cent of the population), Gilbert's syndrome is the disorder most likely to be encountered by the clinician. Mild unconjugated hyperbilirubinemia is recognized most commonly during the second and third decades of life because of the presence of scleral icterus, often first noted with fasting or as an incidental laboratory finding. Although a variety of nonspecific symptoms have been described, it is unlikely that any significant symptoms are attributable to Gilbert's syndrome itself. Gilbert's syndrome results from a decrease in the hepatic clearance of unconjugated bilirubin, probably due to impaired conjugation. Up to one half of patients with Gilbert's syndrome have a very slight decrease in red cell survival detectable by ^{51}Cr labeling. The principal clinical importance of this disorder is that it may be confused with more serious acquired hepatobiliary disease. From a practical standpoint, the diagnosis of Gilbert's syndrome is made by demonstrating low-grade unconjugated hyperbilirubinemia in a patient with a normal physical examination and otherwise repeatedly normal laboratory tests of liver function. Normal concentrations of bile acids in serum are also helpful in excluding liver disease. Liver biopsy demonstrating normal histology is almost never necessary. An exaggerated hyperbilirubinemic response to fasting, lipid withdrawal, or nicotinic acid administration has been found to be helpful by some investigators, but these tests are neither sensitive nor specific enough to warrant routine use. In patients with overt hemolysis, direct measurement of hepatic bilirubin clearance may be necessary to establish the diagnosis. Gilbert's syndrome and the other inherited disorders of hepatic bilirubin metabolism are outlined in Table 118–1.

BENIGN RECURRENT CHOLESTASIS. In contrast to the inherited disorders in which hepatic bilirubin metabolism or excretion is selectively impaired, this entity is characterized by recurrent attacks of cholestasis manifested by pruritus, conjugated hyperbilirubinemia, and elevated serum levels of alkaline phosphatase and bile salts. Individual attacks may persist from weeks to months, do not result from biliary obstruction, and typically remit spontaneously. Attacks frequently begin in childhood, recur at highly variable intervals, and do not generally lead to cirrhosis or decreased longevity. The etiology of this disorder is unknown, but an inherited basis is postulated because of its early age of onset and familial nature.

There are also inherited forms of hemolytic anemia (e.g., hereditary spherocytosis), which may produce modest unconjugated hyperbilirubinemia due to increased bilirubin production. These disorders are discussed in detail in Ch. 138.

ACQUIRED HYPERBILIRUBINEMIA

HEMOLYSIS. Hemolysis increases bilirubin production and generally produces low-grade unconjugated, indirect-

TABLE 118–1. THE HEREDITARY DISORDERS OF HEPATIC BILIRUBIN METABOLISM

	Gilbert's Syndrome	Type I Crigler-Najjar Syndrome	Type II Crigler-Najjar Syndrome	Dubin-Johnson Syndrome	Rotor's Syndrome
Incidence	Up to 7% of population	Very rare	Uncommon	Uncommon	Rare
Inheritance	? Autosomal dominant	Autosomal recessive	? Autosomal dominant	Autosomal recessive	Autosomal recessive
Defect(s) in bilirubin metabolism	Decreased hepatic UDP-glucuronyl-transferase activity, (?) slow hepatic bilirubin uptake, associated mild hemolysis in up to 50% of patients	Absence of hepatic UDP-glucuronyltransferase activity	Markedly decreased or undetectable UDP-glucuronyltransferase activity	Impaired biliary excretion of conjugated bilirubin	Impaired biliary excretion of conjugated bilirubin
Plasma bilirubin concentration (mg/dl)	≤3 in absence of fasting or hemolysis, predominantly unconjugated	17–50, usually >20, all unconjugated	6–45, usually <20, all unconjugated	1–25, usually <7, about 60% conjugated	1–20, usually <7, about 60% conjugated
Clinical sequelae	None	Death in infancy from kernicterus in almost all cases	Usually none, rarely kernicterus	Probably none	Probably none
Plasma sulfobromophthalein disappearance rate	Mildly abnormal in some patients (45-min retention <15%)	Usually normal	Usually normal	Slow initial disappearance with frequent secondary rise (45-minute retention <20%)	Markedly slowed, no secondary rise (45-minute retention 30–50%)
Oral cholecystography	Normal	Normal	Normal	Faint or nonvisualization	Usually normal
Hepatic histology (light microscopy)	Normal, occasionally increased lipofusion	Normal	Normal	Coarse pigment in centrolobular cells	Normal
Reduction of plasma bilirubin concentration by phenobarbital	Yes	No	Yes	Minimal	Unknown
Diagnosis	Clinical and laboratory findings, response to fasting occasionally helpful, liver biopsy not usually necessary	Clinical and laboratory findings, lack of response to phenobarbital	Clinical and laboratory findings, response to phenobarbital	Clinical and laboratory findings, sulfobromophthalein disappearance, urinary coproporphyrin excretion	Clinical and laboratory findings, sulfobromophthalein disappearance
Treatment	None necessary	None uniformly effective	Phenobarbital if bilirubin concentration markedly elevated	None available, avoid estrogens (may worsen jaundice)	None available

reacting hyperbilirubinemia. Because of the enormous reserve of the hepatic bilirubin transport mechanism, hepatic bilirubin clearance remains constant, and plasma bilirubin concentration increases linearly with bilirubin production rate in most individuals. Since the bone marrow cannot increase erythrocyte production more than about eight-fold, ongoing *steady-state hemolysis* by itself cannot account for a sustained increase in plasma unconjugated bilirubin concentration above 4 to 5 mg per deciliter. Concentrations consistently exceeding this indicate hepatic dysfunction irrespective of the presence of hemolysis. In contrast, *acute hemolysis*, even in patients with normal hepatic function, may produce elevations in total plasma bilirubin concentration that greatly exceed 5 mg per deciliter.

INEFFECTIVE ERYTHROPOIESIS. Bilirubin production is increased and hence the plasma concentration of unconjugated, indirect-reading bilirubin may be elevated in a variety of disorders associated with ineffective erythropoiesis. Markedly increased ineffective erythropoiesis is the basis of the rare disorder known as *shunt hyperbilirubinemia* or *idiopathic dyserythropoietic jaundice*.

FASTING HYPERBILIRUBINEMIA. Fasting causes an increase in the plasma concentration of unconjugated, indirect-reacting bilirubin owing primarily to a decrease in hepatic bilirubin clearance. This effect may be particularly marked in patients with Gilbert's syndrome and the Type II Crigler-Najjar syndrome. Both dietary composition and total caloric intake are important, since a normocaloric but lipid-free diet produces a response similar to that observed with complete fasting, and the effect of complete fasting is reversed by feeding small amounts of lipid. The mechanism of the decrease in hepatic bilirubin clearance with fasting is unclear. A slight increase in bilirubin production contributes to fasting hyperbilirubinemia.

POSTOPERATIVE HYPERBILIRUBINEMIA. Postoperative hyperbilirubinemia (>2 mg per deciliter), also called postoperative intrahepatic cholestasis or postoperative jaundice, usually occurs in patients who have undergone major surgery. The incidence of postoperative hyperbilirubinemia is about 15 per cent following open heart surgery compared with about 1 per cent after elective abdominal surgery and may be increased in patients with pre-existing liver disease. Hyperbilirubinemia, usually predominantly conjugated, occurs from one to ten days after surgery, can become quite marked, and is typically accompanied by a two- to four-fold elevation of the alkaline phosphatase and 5′-nucleotidase with minimally abnormal transaminase levels and prothrombin time. The etiology of the hyperbilirubinemia is probably multifactorial, with both increased bilirubin production (from breakdown of transfused erythrocytes and resorption of hematomas) and impaired hepatic excretory function (from hypotension, hypoxemia, or bacteremia) being potentially important contributing factors. Postoperative hyperbilirubinemia is usually benign and resolves as the overall condition of the patient improves. It is important to distinguish it from postoperative jaundice caused by biliary obstruction or hepatocellular necrosis resulting from shock, anesthetic injury, or post-transfusion hepatitis. The latter is typically accompanied by markedly abnormal transaminase levels and prothrombin time.

DIFFUSE HEPATOCELLULAR INJURY. Hyperbilirubinemia associated with disorders such as viral hepatitis reflects one aspect of a global insult to hepatocellular function. The hyperbilirubinemia is of importance primarily as an index of the severity of hepatocellular injury. In unusual cases in which hyperbilirubinemia seems disproportionate to the hepatic injury, as reflected by serum transaminase levels and prothrombin time, a search for causes of increased bilirubin production (e.g., hemolysis) or decreased hepatic bilirubin clearance (e.g., infection) is worthwhile.

MISCELLANEOUS. Mild unconjugated hyperbilirubinemia is occasionally found in a variety of unrelated conditions. *Cyclic premenstrual unconjugated hyperbilirubinemia* appears related to serum progesterone levels. Administration of *chenodeoxycholic acid* and certain drugs such as *propranolol, rifampin,* and *probenecid* has been associated with apparently mild, reversible unconjugated hyperbilirubinemia in some instances due to reaction of the drug or a metabolite with the diazo reagent.

Fevery J, Blanckaert N: What can we learn from analysis of serum bilirubin? J Hepatol 2:113, 1986. *A brief synopsis of the interpretation of serum bilirubin measurements in relation to current concepts of bilirubin metabolism, the recent development of newer assays, and the recognition of the protein-bound bilirubin fraction.*

Ostrow JD (ed.): Bile Pigments and Jaundice: Molecular, Metabolic, and Medical Aspects. New York, Marcel Dekker, 1986. *A series of 24 exhaustively referenced monographs covering all aspects of bilirubin metabolism, which, collectively, represent the most comprehensive and authoritative treatment of this subject currently available.*

Weiss JS, Gautam A, Lauff JJ, et al.: The clinical importance of a protein-bound fraction of serum bilirubin in patients with hyperbilirubinemia. N Engl J Med 309:147, 1983. *A concise description of the protein-bound fraction—in whom it occurs and what it means.*

119 LABORATORY TESTS IN LIVER DISEASE

Robert K. Ockner

Unlike tests employed in the clinical evaluation of other organ systems (e.g., arterial blood gases, creatinine clearance, plasma hormone assays), "liver function" tests for the most part are highly empirical, and often do not indicate either the integrity of liver function or the severity of a disease process. Despite this, and provided that their limitations are recognized, they may be useful in screening for hepatobiliary diseases, diagnostic evaluation, and following the course of the disease. In this chapter, the generally available laboratory tests for the diagnosis of hepatobiliary disease are discussed with regard to physiology, pathophysiology, and clinical usefulness.

BILIRUBIN. The metabolism of bilirubin and its measurement are discussed in detail in Ch. 118.

TRANSAMINASES. *Transaminases (aminotransferases)* catalyze the transfer of amino groups from aspartate or alanine to alpha-ketoglutarate. The enzymes are named either by the products of the reaction (glutamic and oxalacetic, or glutamic and pyruvic transaminases, SGOT or SGPT, respectively) or, as is currently preferred, by the amino-group donor (aspartate or alanine transaminases, AST or ALT, respectively). Specific isozymes of AST are present in liver cell mitochondria and cytoplasm, whereas ALT is confined to the cytoplasm. Increased serum transaminase activity in liver disease is assumed to reflect leaking from injured cells. Transaminases are not present in appreciable concentrations in urine. Although they are present in bile, activity there does not reflect that in serum, and clearance of these enzymes from plasma does not depend on secretion into bile or urine. Since the mechanisms and determinants of transaminase entry into or clearance from plasma are not fully defined, interpretation of serum activity is necessarily empirical. Generally the height of the transaminase activity reflects the severity of hepatic necrosis, but there are important exceptions. In even the most severe forms of acute *alcoholic hepatitis*, for example, levels seldom exceed 200 to 300 IU per liter. In contrast, serum transaminase activities of 1000 IU or more are often present in mild uncomplicated acute *viral hepatitis* or sudden high-grade *biliary obstruction*, as may occur during passage of a gallstone. Conversely, initially elevated serum transaminase activities may fall as the clinical course of massive hepatic necrosis deteriorates, suggesting that the liver is so severely damaged that little enzyme activity remains.

Despite these caveats, the serum transaminase activities may be helpful in certain circumstances: First, they are useful as *screening tests* for liver disease. Although AST levels may be increased in diseases of other organs (e.g., myocardium and skeletal muscle), values more than ten times the upper limit of the normal range usually reflect hepatic or biliary pathology. Moreover, the ALT is relatively specific for hepatobiliary disease. In the context of other clinical and laboratory findings, identification of the source of increased serum transaminase activity is not usually difficult. Second, it is distinctly uncommon for the AST to exceed 15 times the upper limit of normal in bile duct obstruction, except when it occurs suddenly, or is associated with cholangitis. Third, in contrast to most other forms of parenchymal liver disease, in which the ALT activity usually equals or exceeds the AST, in *alcoholic hepatitis* this relationship is reversed, and this may be useful diagnostically. Finally, transaminase values are often useful in monitoring the course of acute or chronic parenchymal liver disease, although, as noted, they are potentially misleading in certain circumstances.

ALKALINE PHOSPHATASE. This group of enzymes is present in many tissues, including liver, bile ducts, intestine, bone, kidney, placenta, and leukocytes; hepatic alkaline phosphatase itself appears heterogeneous. The phosphatases catalyze the release of inorganic phosphate from a phosphate ester substrate, at alkaline pH. Their biologic function is unknown, except for an apparent relationship to bone deposition. Normally, serum alkaline phosphatase activity reflects mainly the liver and bone isozyzmes. In some persons, especially those of blood types O or A who are secretors of the ABO red cell antigens and are positive for the Lewis antigen, intestinal alkaline phosphatase may account for 20 to 60 per cent of total serum activity. In the later stages of pregnancy, the placental contribution may be substantial. A number of less common sources of alkaline phosphatase have been identified. These include a variant associated with hepatoma, and the so-called *Regan isozyme*. The latter is apparently identical to the placental enzyme, but originates in a variety of tumors, especially lung; it also may be detected rarely in the serum of normal subjects.

Serum alkaline phosphatase activity may be increased in many conditions not associated with hepatobiliary disease, including bone disorders, pregnancy, normal growth, and occasionally the presence of malignancy not involving either bone or liver (e.g., the Regan isozyme), and for this reason the organ or tissue of origin must be identified. In some cases, this is obvious because of other clinical and laboratory findings. When the source is less apparent, several methods have been used to differentiate hepatobiliary from other isozymes, such as heat stability or electrophoretic separation of isozymes. Most practical and available is the measurement of the serum *5′-nucleotidase, leucine aminopeptidase*, or *gamma-glutamyl transpeptidase* activities, which tend to parallel that of alkaline phosphatase in hepatobiliary disease, but do not usually increase in bone disease. However, the first two of these may increase during pregnancy (see below).

Serum hepatobiliary alkaline phosphatase activity is usually increased in bile duct obstruction, parenchymal disease, or infiltrative or mass lesions of the liver. This increased serum activity reflects increased enzyme synthesis rather than decreased biliary excretion or leakage from damaged cells. Although the highest levels usually occur with bile duct obstruction, very high values may also be associated with intrahepatic cholestasis or infiltrative or mass lesions. On the other hand, it is most unusual for the serum alkaline phosphatase activity to remain relatively normal in the presence of significant bile duct obstruction, especially in association with jaundice. Conversely, increased alkaline phosphatase may be the only clinically apparent abnormality in bile duct stricture or in lesions that produce obstruction of a single hepatic lobe or segment. As many as one third of patients with isolated elevations of serum hepatobiliary alkaline phosphatase activity may have no demonstrable underlying liver or biliary disease.

LEUCINE AMINOPEPTIDASE, 5′-NUCLEOTIDASE, AND GAMMA-GLUTAMYL TRANSPEPTIDASE. Leucine aminopeptidase (LAP) is a ubiquitous cellular peptidase, whereas 5′-nucleotidase (5′-NT) is a plasma membrane enzyme that cleaves the inorganic phosphate from adenosine 5′-phosphate or inosine 5′-phosphate. The serum activity of both enzymes usually increases in cholestasis, and their major clinical value is that they may be of help in identifying the source of elevated serum alkaline phosphatase activity.

Since these enzymes may be increased in late pregnancy, they are most useful in the nonpregnant patient. Although elevated serum activity of either of these enzymes suggests a hepatobiliary origin of increased alkaline phosphatase, the converse is not true, and liver alkaline phosphatase occasionally may be increased while the others remain normal.

Gamma-glutamyl transpeptidase (GGTP) is present in many tissues. It increases in serum not only in hepatobiliary disease but also after myocardial infarction, in neuromuscular diseases, in pancreatic disease in the absence of biliary obstruction, and during the ingestion of ethanol and other inducers of hepatic microsomal enzymes. The GGTP has been proposed as a sensitive screening test for hepatobiliary disease, and for the monitoring of abstinence from ethanol. This test may be used to identify the source of an alkaline phosphatase increase, but it offers no clear advantage over the other available tests.

ALBUMIN AND GLOBULIN. *Albumin* is synthesized exclusively in the liver at a rate of 100 to 200 mg per kilogram of body weight per day. The synthetic rate is influenced by systemic or liver disease and by nutritional state, thyroid hormone, glucocorticoids, plasma colloid osmotic pressure, and toxins such as ethanol and carbon tetrachloride. The mechanism of albumin degradation in health is not known; the rate is increased in exfoliative dermatitis, severe burns, nephrotic syndrome, and protein-losing enteropathy. Thus, albumin concentration, which reflects the balance between synthesis and degradation or loss, may be importantly influenced by factors other than the functional state of the liver, and therefore this test is not specific. On the other hand, if other factors can be excluded, hypoalbuminemia may be an important sign of liver disease, and serum albumin concentration may be a useful, albeit slowly responsive, indicator of changing hepatic function. Although hypoalbuminemia reflects diminished synthesis in some patients with cirrhosis and ascites, in others synthesis is normal and hypoalbuminemia is caused by a redistribution among the extracellular fluid compartments, including the peritoneal cavity.

Serum globulins are of limited diagnostic utility in hepatobiliary diseases. As a group, they are heterogeneous with respect to site and regulation of production, physical properties, and physiologic function. Their concentration, as measured by serum protein electrophoresis or salt fractionation, may be influenced by a wide variety of hepatic and extrahepatic factors and disease states. The mechanism for their increased serum concentration in liver disease is not fully understood, but probably is multifactorial, and may include stimulus to increased antibody production resulting from increased entry of bacterial antigens into the systemic circulation, or release of antigenic material from injured liver cells. An important exception to this generalization is the finding of a diminished concentration of the alpha$_1$-globulin fraction as demonstrated by serum protein electrophoresis. Since approximately 85 per cent of this fraction is accounted for by alpha$_1$-antitrypsin, a decrease in its concentration may be an important sign of an

$alpha_1$-antitrypsin deficiency, an inherited disorder associated with neonatal hepatitis, cirrhosis, and pulmonary emphysema (see Ch. 125). Elevated IgM concentrations are common in primary biliary cirrhosis, but other clinical, laboratory, and imaging procedures are of greater diagnostic value. Diffuse increases in globulin concentrations are commonly seen in cirrhosis and may be especially pronounced in HbsAg-negative chronic active hepatitis (see Ch. 123).

PROTHROMBIN TIME. This test, usually performed by the one-stage (Quick) method, measures the rate at which prothrombin in citrated plasma is converted to thrombin in the presence of added calcium, tissue thromboplastin, and activated clotting factors. It depends on the plasma concentration not only of prothrombin but also of other clotting factors synthesized in the liver, including V, VII, X, and fibrinogen. Prothrombin time (or, expressed as a percentage of a standardized control sample, prothrombin content) may be abnormal if plasma concentrations of prothrombin itself or of the other important factors are reduced below a critical level. This may reflect an increased rate of degradation, as in disseminated intravascular coagulation, a decreased rate of synthesis, or both.

Synthesis of fibrinogen, prothrombin and of factors V, VII, IX, X, XI, XII, and XIII occurs in the liver. Synthesis of prothrombin and factors VII, IX, and X depends on an adequate supply of *vitamin K,* which activates preformed polypeptides in the liver by stimulating the synthesis of the calcium-binding residue, gamma-carboxyglutamic acid. Thus, an abnormal prothrombin time that reflects decreased production of these factors may be caused rarely by *inherited abnormalities* and much more commonly by *vitamin K deficiency, liver disease,* or both. Vitamin K is abundant in many foods, and a portion of the vitamin that is produced by intestinal bacteria may also be available to the host. Thus, deficiency of the vitamin is most often caused by one of the *malabsorption syndromes,* including biliary obstruction and other causes of cholestasis. Rarely, it may reflect antimicrobial suppression of intestinal bacteria. Any acute or chronic liver disease may cause an abnormal prothrombin time if the synthesis of essential clotting factors is impaired. In acute liver disease, hypoprothrombinemia often indicates an unfavorable prognosis.

An abnormal prothrombin time may be of diagnostic value in the evaluation of the jaundiced patient. In general, when it is prolonged on the basis of vitamin K deficiency alone, e.g., because of cholestasis-induced malabsorption, it will return to near normal levels within hours after parenteral administration of vitamin K. In contrast, when clotting factor synthesis is diminished because of parenchymal liver disease, response to vitamin K may be slight or absent. Unfortunately, for several reasons this simple and attractive diagnostic approach does not always reliably differentiate obstructive from parenchymal liver disease. First, hypoprothrombinemia may reflect more then one factor, e.g., biliary obstruction associated with parenchymal liver disease or disseminated intravascular coagulation. Second, vitamin K malabsorption and a prolonged but correctable prothrombin time may result from cholestasis of any cause, including parenchymal disease such as primary biliary cirrhosis, cholestatic hepatitis, and drug-induced cholestasis. Finally, a partial response to vitamin K administration may be misleading. Because of these shortcomings, the response to an abnormal prothrombin time to parenteral vitamin K administration must be interpreted in the context of other available information.

The *partial thromboplastin time* is used to assess the "intrinsic" clotting mechanism, and reflects the activity of all clotting factors except for platelet factor 3, factor XIII, and factor VII. For this reason, the test is complementary to the prothrombin time and may indicate deficiencies of other clotting factors or the presence of a circulating anticoagulant.

SERUM LIPIDS AND LIPOPROTEINS. Parenchymal liver disease and bile duct obstruction may be associated with significant abnormalities in serum lipids and lipoproteins. In acute parenchymal liver disease, there may be loss of the $alpha_1$-lipoprotein band normally present on serum lipoprotein electrophoresis, reflecting abnormal composition and physical properties of the high-density lipoproteins. There may also be a transient hypertriglyceridemia, reflecting the presence in serum of abnormal low-density lipoproteins rich in triglycerides. These changes appear attributable in part to deficient activity of plasma lecithin: cholesterol acyltransferase (LCAT), an enzyme of hepatic origin that esterifies plasma cholesterol. The changes are transient, and with resolution of the acute liver injury, plasma lipids and lipoproteins return to their previous state.

In cholestasis the serum concentrations of unesterified cholesterol and phospholipids are increased, and the development of xanthomas and xanthelasma is related to the severity and duration of this abnormality. Of the increased plasma unesterified cholesterol, a major fraction is accounted for by the presence of an abnormal low-density lipoprotein, designated *LPX.* LPX consists mainly of unesterified cholesterol and phosphatidyl choline (lecithin), in a 1:1 molar ratio, with a small amount of protein, largely a mixture of albumin and the C apolipoproteins. In negative-staining electron microscopy, LPX assumes the shape of a disc that may form rouleaux. The similarity of the lipid composition of LPX to that of bile (primarily free cholesterol and lecithin), together with other evidence, suggests that it represents the entry into plasma either of biliary lipid or of lipid from the hepatocyte normally destined for secretion into bile. LPX is not currently of value in the differential diagnosis of jaundice. Its concentrations are correlated with the far simpler determination of plasma-free cholesterol concentration, but not with other tests of liver function.

MITOCHONDRIAL ANTIBODY. In approximately 90 per cent of patients with primary biliary cirrhosis, serum contains antibodies directed against a lipoprotein component of the inner mitochondrial membrane. The antibodies are neither organ nor species specific, and are demonstrated by immunofluorescent techniques employing rat kidney, liver, and stomach and human thyroid, stomach, and kidney. They include the three main immunoglobulin classes and are complement fixing. In patients with primary biliary cirrhosis, the titer is not related to the increased level of serum IgM or the stage or severity of the disease.

Mitochondrial antibodies are also present in up to 25 per cent of patients with chronic active hepatitis and postnecrotic cirrhosis and in 7 to 8 per cent of asymptomatic relatives of patients with primary biliary cirrhosis. They are rarely present in extrahepatic biliary obstruction. A small percentage of patients with nonhepatic diseases may also exhibit positive tests; these include the collagen-vascular disorders, thyroiditis, myasthenia gravis, Addison's disease, autoimmune hemolytic anemia, and chronic biologic false-positive reactions for syphilis. Several types of mitochondrial antibodies have thus far been identified; M_2 is the type usually found in primary biliary cirrhosis. Mitochondrial antibodies are demonstrable in only 0.4 to 0.7 per cent of the general population.

In the differential diagnosis of jaundice the mitochondrial test is useful in two respects. First, a negative result renders the diagnosis of primary biliary cirrhosis unlikely but does not exclude it. Second, because of its rarity in extrahepatic biliary obstruction, a positive result tends to suggest parenchymal liver disease, but it does not exclude bile duct obstruction. Since the incidence of gallstones in patients with primary biliary cirrhosis is approximately 40 per cent, and is also increased in other forms of cirrhosis, the mitochondrial antibody test cannot be regarded as a reliable basis for distinguishing "medical" from "surgical" jaundice.

ANTINUCLEAR AND SMOOTH MUSCLE ANTIBODIES. Either or both of these tests may be positive in a variable percentage of patients with chronic active hepatitis, usually among those cases not associated with hepatitis B infection. They have also been demonstrated in a minority of patients with primary biliary cirrhosis. As is true of the mitochondrial antibody, these factors are neither organ nor species specific. They probably do not play a role in pathogenesis. The presence of these antibodies in serum may suggest but does not differentiate among chronic hepatitis, postnecrotic cirrhosis, or primary biliary cirrhosis, and clearly does not exclude a bile duct lesion.

TESTS FOR HEPATITIS VIRUS INFECTION. These tests and their clinical significance are discussed in Ch. 121.

URINE AND STOOL EXAMINATIONS. The presence of bilirubin in urine indicates that a significant fraction of plasma bilirubin is conjugated, and is strong evidence of hepatobiliary disease. Jaundice in the absence of bilirubinuria indicates an exclusively unconjugated hyperbilirubinemia, i.e., reflecting hemolysis, ineffective erythropoiesis, or an inherited disorder of bilirubin conjugation. For several reasons, urine and fecal *urobilinogen* determinations usually do not provide useful information in the evaluation of hepatobiliary disease (see Ch. 125). Testing of stool for occult blood is essential, and may provide the first evidence of an alimentary tract lesion related or unrelated to hepatobiliary disease, a bleeding diathesis, or an explanation for the appearance of hepatic encephalopathy. In selected cases, depending on the clinical circumstances, stool culture or examination for ova and parasites may provide information of importance in the diagnosis of liver disease.

HEMATOLOGIC TESTS IN LIVER DISEASE. Diseases of the liver may be associated with a wide variety of hematologic abnormalities, including qualitative and quantitative changes in the formed elements, and in clotting function. The abnormalities depend not only on the etiology of the liver disorder but also on whether it is acute or chronic, or associated with complications such as liver failure or portal hypertension.

In acute liver disease not associated with liver failure, major changes in the formed elements are uncommon and consist primarily of mild anemia, reflecting either low-grade hemolysis or marrow depression. Macrocytosis may be present. Slight leukopenia is not uncommon and often is associated with atypical lymphocytes.

Rarely, a severe aplastic anemia may complicate acute viral hepatitis, especially non-A, non-B. The pathogenesis is unknown, the prognosis is very poor, and treatment is largely ineffective. In other forms of acute liver disease, hematologic abnormalities, e.g., marrow suppression, may be caused by toxins such as ethanol or drugs. Zieve's syndrome also occurs in the alcoholic. It consists of hemolytic anemia and hypertriglyceridemia; the basis for this association is not understood. Coagulopathy may complicate massive hepatic necrosis, reflecting depressed hepatic synthesis of clotting factors or disseminated intravascular coagulation.

In chronic liver disease, a number of abnormalities of the erythrocytes may be present. Target cells, often associated with cholestasis, result from an expansion of the cell membrane, with relative preservation of the cholesterol-phospholipid ratio. Spur cells (acanthocytes) are most often found in advanced cirrhosis, usually alcoholic, and reflect a more profound relative and absolute increase in membrane-free cholesterol.

Red cells, white cells, and platelets may be decreased in patients with portal hypertension, primarily because of hypersplenism. A number of other abnormalities may be present, but to a large extent these are caused by associated nutritional, pathologic, or pharmacologic influences. Examples include iron deficiency, megaloblastic, and sideroblastic anemias.

LIVER BIOPSY. Performed by a blind technique or under direct vision during laparoscopy, this procedure is of value in the diagnosis of diffuse or localized parenchymal diseases (e.g., cirrhosis, chronic hepatitis, hemochromatosis) and hepatomegaly. Because bile duct obstruction is often associated with nonspecific parenchymal changes, biopsy is not ordinarily a preferred initial diagnostic procedure in the evaluation of the patient with cholestatic jaundice. Rather, imaging and cholangiographic methods are more rewarding in this setting. Liver biopsy requires the cooperation of the patient, except in infants, and normal clotting function. Relative or absolute contraindications include the presence of biliary sepsis, right pleural disease, ascites, coagulopathy, and high-grade bile duct obstruction.

IMAGING TECHNIQUES AND CHOLANGIOGRAPHY. These techniques are discussed in detail in Ch. 95. In the following chapter, their utility is considered briefly in the context of the diagnosis of jaundice.

Arias IM, Popper H, Schachter D, et al.: The Liver: Biology and Pathobiology. New York, Raven Press, 1982. *An in-depth and well-documented presentation of many more basic aspects of normal and abnormal hepatic structure and function.*

Popper H, Schaffner F (eds.): Progress in Liver Diseases. Vol. 8. Orlando, Grune & Stratton, 1986.

Wright R, Millward-Sadler GH, Alberti KGMM, et al. (eds.): Liver and Biliary Disease. 2nd ed. London, W. B. Saunders Company, 1985.

Zakim D, Boyer T (eds.): Hepatology: A Textbook of Liver Disease. Philadelphia, W. B. Saunders Company, 1982. *A comprehensive textbook. Provides references dealing with hepatobiliary structure, function, and disease.*

120 APPROACHES TO THE DIAGNOSIS OF JAUNDICE

Robert K. Ockner

Jaundice may be caused by a wide range of disorders (Ch. 118). Excluding hemolysis, ineffective erythropoiesis, and congenital errors of bilirubin metabolism (any of which may be present *in addition to other causes*), jaundice can be broadly classified as *intrahepatic* or *extrahepatic*. Included among the intrahepatic causes are (1) hepatocellular diseases such as viral or drug-induced acute or chronic liver disease, (2) various metabolic and infiltrative disorders such as anoxia, Wilson's disease, and metastatic tumor, and (3) disorders of the intrahepatic biliary system such as primary biliary cirrhosis, intrahepatic sclerosing cholangitis, and congenital disorders associated with cystic dilatation of the smaller bile ducts. Extrahepatic causes of jaundice, i.e., large bile duct obstruction, include choledocholithiasis, bile duct strictures, chronic pancreatitis with bile duct compression, and tumors affecting the bile duct itself or critically situated contiguous structures such as lymph nodes in the porta hepatis, the ampulla of Vater, or the head of the pancreas.

In view of the magnitude and diversity of the differential diagnosis, the clinical approach must be equally broad. A careful history and physical examination are of paramount importance, emphasizing a search for clues that might suggest a cause such as exposure to a jaundiced person or a potentially toxic drug (viral or drug-induced hepatitis), an antecedent history of pruritus and xanthelasma (chronic cholestasis such as primary biliary cirrhosis), recurrent abdominal pain and nausea (gallstone disease), chronic ulcerative colitis (sclerosing cholangitis), or epigastric pain, weight loss, and distended gallbladder (cancer of the head of the pancreas). Routinely available laboratory studies are also helpful (see Ch. 119). In general, serum aminotransferase activities do not exceed 10 to 15 times the upper limit of normal in patients with bile duct obstruction, unless there is superimposed bacterial cholangitis or the obstruction occurs suddenly, and is high grade. In the latter instance, usually associated with impaction of a gallstone in the common bile duct, the aminotransferase level, which may exceed 1000 IU, usually also falls quite rapidly (over a few days) toward normal. Alkaline phosphatase activities usually exceed two to three times normal, but very high values may be seen in both intrahepatic and extrahepatic processes. Elevation of serum cholesterol tends to suggest chronic cholestasis but is of little help in differential diagnosis. Amylase activity may be elevated because of pancreatitis induced by passage of a gallstone that also causes bile duct obstruction, or may reflect pancreatitis of some other cause that secondarily causes compression of the intrapancreatic portion of the distal common bile duct. Hepatitis serologies may help in diagnosis, but obstructive biliary disease may be superimposed on chronic parenchymal liver disease such as chronic hepatitis B or cirrhosis.

Despite the seemingly limitless number of diagnostic possibilities and of permutations and combinations of clinical and laboratory findings, the clinical evaluation (that based on history, physical examination, and routine laboratory tests) is quite accurate and serves to identify correctly the cause of jaundice in 80 to 85 per cent of cases. It is for confirmation of these clinical diagnoses (when needed) and for the elucidation of the clinically more obscure processes that other diagnostic procedures are available. The availability and accuracy of these procedures have increased dramatically in recent years, and the decision regarding their proper use has become a critically important part of the judgmental process involved in the management of these problems.

The diagnostic approach to the jaundiced patient does not lend itself readily to generalizations or inflexible algorithms. Rather, a host of highly individual factors must be taken into account. These include the evolving clinical course and current status of the patient; the differential diagnosis; the availability, reliability, and safety of diagnostic procedures in a given institution; and the experience and judgment of a consulting surgeon. Despite these reservations, some general guidelines are valid in many instances and may serve, with appropriate modification, as the basis for an approach to diagnosis.

First, as noted above, the diagnosis in most patients will be obvious or strongly suggested by routine clinical and laboratory findings. For example, if the patient appears to have viral or drug-induced acute hepatitis, if this presumptive diagnosis is supported by appropriate laboratory studies, and if the patient is doing well, more elaborate or invasive studies are usually unnecessary as continuing observation and follow-up studies will suffice.

Second, if more information is needed in a patient with unexplained cholestatic jaundice, *liver biopsy* is often not helpful, since in many cases of parenchymal cholestasis the histopathology is nonspecific. Moreover, parenchymal liver disease not only does not exclude biliary tract disease but may in fact predispose to it (e.g., the increased incidence of gallstones in cirrhosis). Thus, although biopsy can be performed with reasonable safety in the presence of bile duct obstruction, in most cases it will not be the initial diagnostic procedure of choice.

Of the available radiographic and imaging procedures, *ultrasound scanning* and *computed tomography* are attractive because they are noninvasive and provide accurate information concerning caliber of the bile ducts. Because of its lesser cost, the absence of radiation exposure, and its ability to detect stones in the gallbladder accurately, ultrasonography may be preferred. However, these two tests suffer from a finite, albeit small error rate (both false positives and false negatives) in the diagnosis of bile duct obstruction. This is not unexpected in view of the fact that these techniques provide information as to the *caliber* of the bile duct; the presence or absence of biliary obstruction can only be *inferred.* Clearly, the syndrome of biliary tract obstruction is so varied that the relationship between completeness and duration of the obstructive process on the one hand and the caliber of the ducts on the other must also vary. For these reasons, the noninvasive tests, although useful in initial assessment, may not be definitive.

Direct cholangiography is currently the most reliable approach to the nonoperative diagnosis of cholestatic jaundice. It may be accomplished either percutaneously, with the Chiba ("skinny") needle, or endoscopically. In most centers, the probability of duct visualization with the percutaneous transhepatic technique approaches 100 per cent in the presence of bile duct obstruction. The success rate with parenchymal jaundice is variable but generally lower. The procedure is rapid and simple, is readily performed in most institutions, and involves minimal cost and technical experience. For these reasons, percutaneous transhepatic cholangiography represents the best combination of accuracy, speed, low risk, and low cost, and therefore is suggested as the single most valuable of the currently available invasive techniques (see also Ch. 95).

Endoscopic retrograde cholangiography, although more demanding of patient and physician, more expensive, and more time consuming, nonetheless has a definite place. It can be safely performed in the patient with abnormal clotting function, whereas the percutaneous study cannot. It may demonstrate duct pathology when the percutaneous approach has failed, and may be especially suitable in those patients in whom the intrahepatic bile ducts are not dilated, or in whom there may be associated pancreatic disease. Finally, it may permit a direct therapeutic approach in certain cases, e.g., endoscopic sphincteroplasty and stone extraction for patients with retained impacted common bile duct stones or gallstone-associated pancreatitis. Each of these procedures carries with it certain risks, which are discussed in Ch. 96.

Niederau C, Sonnenberg A, Muelle J: Comparison of the extrahepatic bile duct size measured by ultrasound and by different radiographic methods. Gastroenterology 87:615, 1984. *An interesting comparison among commonly used techniques with evidence for some important differences.*

Scharschmidt BF, Goldberg HI, Schmid R: Approach to the patient with cholestatic jaundice. N Engl J Med 308:1515, 1983. *A concise summary, useful approach, and comprehensive bibliography.*

Vennes JA, Bond JH: Approach to the jaundiced patient. Gastroenterology 84:1615, 1983. *A balanced editorial addressing the clinical problem in general and two accompanying articles in particular.*

121 ACUTE VIRAL HEPATITIS

Robert K. Ockner

DEFINITION. Acute viral hepatitis is caused by any of several agents and presents as a spectrum of syndromes ranging from entirely subclinical and inapparent to rapidly progressive and fatal. In most cases, it is self-limited and uncomplicated, but, depending on the viral agent involved, there is a variable incidence of clinically significant extrahepatic manifestations or of progression to chronic liver disease. These diseases represent an infection by a viral agent with relative or absolute predilection for the hepatocyte. After a variable incubation period, viral replication in the liver cell approaches a maximum, followed by the appearance of viral components in body fluids and/or excreta, liver cell necrosis with an associated inflammatory response, changes in laboratory tests of liver function, and symptoms and signs of liver damage. The immunologic response of the host appears to play an important but not fully defined role in pathogenesis.

ETIOLOGY. Viral hepatitis is caused by three major agents and several minor ones. The vast majority of cases are accounted for by hepatitis viruses A and B, and the so-called non-A, non-B agents, of which there appear to be at least two. Selected characteristics of each are summarized in Table 121–1, and each is considered in greater detail below. The

TABLE 121–1. CHARACTERISTICS OF COMMON CAUSATIVE AGENTS OF ACUTE VIRAL HEPATITIS

	Hepatitis A	Hepatitis B	Hepatitis D	Hepatitis Non-A, Non-B (Two or More Agents)
Causative agent	27 nm RNA virus	42 nm DNA virus; core and surface components	36nm hybrid particle with HBsAg coat	Apparent similarities to hepatitis B virus
Transmission	Fecal-oral; H_2O-, food borne	Parenteral inoculation, or equivalent; direct contact	Similar to HBV	Same as for B; epidemic form attributed to HAV-like agent
Incubation period	2–6 weeks	4 weeks–6 months	Similar to HBV	2–20 weeks
Period of infectivity	2–3 weeks in late incubation and early clinical phases	During HBsAg positivity (occasionally only with anti-HBc positivity)	During HDV RNA or anti-HDV positivity	Unknown
Massive hepatic necrosis	Rare	Uncommon	Yes	Uncommon
Carrier state	No	Yes	Yes	Yes (? for epidemic form)
Chronic hepatitis	No	Yes	Yes	Yes (not for epidemic form)
Prophylaxis (see text)	Hygiene; immune serum globulin	Hygiene; hepatitis B immune globulin; vaccine	Hygiene; HBV vaccine	Hygiene; ? immune serum globulin; avoid commercial blood

delta (δ) agent (hepatitis D) may cause an acute or chronic hepatitis syndrome limited to those individuals with simultaneous or pre-existing hepatitis B virus infection (see below). Other viral agents that cause an acute hepatitis syndrome include the Epstein-Barr virus (infectious mononucleosis), cytomegalovirus, herpes simplex, yellow fever, and rubella; the clinical disorders caused by these agents are considered in greater detail elsewhere in the text.

PATHOLOGY. The lesion of ordinary acute hepatitis A, B, and non-A, non-B consists of focal necrosis of individual hepatocytes associated with a mononuclear inflammatory response, and expanded portal areas that are infiltrated predominantly by lymphocytes and in which bile ducts may be especially prominent (bile duct "proliferation"). There is often a variable, but usually minor, degree of necrosis of hepatocytes bordering the portal areas (so-called periportal hepatitis or piecemeal necrosis). Necrosis of an individual liver cell, whether periportal or within the lobule, is usually reflected in its replacement by a cluster of mononuclear cells, or it may be represented by balloon degeneration or by a shrunken cell with homogeneously eosinophilic cytoplasm and a condensed pyknotic nucleus ("acidophil body"). The regular pattern of the cords of hepatocytes is disrupted, mitotic figures and cholestasis are common, and Kupffer cells are prominent. Although these features are characteristic of typical acute viral hepatitis, they are not specific, individually or collectively. Thus, the same overall pattern of injury is seen in certain forms of drug-induced liver disease, and its individual components are seen in many processes of diverse etiology and duration. Mononuclear cell portal infiltrates, periportal hepatitis, and bridging or confluent necrosis may be especially prominent in chronic forms of hepatitis.

More severe variants of the acute necrotic process include "bridging" necrosis, "confluent" or "submassive" necrosis, and massive necrosis. In these, the necrotic process simultaneously involves contiguous groups of cells rather than single cells in isolation. As a result, there may be variable collapse or condensation of stroma. Bridging necrosis, so named because the continuous zones of necrosis may extend between (i.e., "bridge") adjacent portal and/or central areas, may be a necessary, if not sufficient, antecedent to evolution to a subacute form of hepatitis with progressive deterioration of liver function leading over several months to death in liver failure, or to chronic hepatitis or to cirrhosis. Such a predisposition is not conclusively established, however. Thus, bridging necrosis is compatible with complete clinical and histologic recovery and therefore does not per se constitute evidence of chronic or progressive liver disease.

Submassive and massive hepatic necrosis are reflected in a more severe clinical course and a less favorable prognosis. Massive necrosis, in which broad areas of hepatocytes are destroyed, with condensation of stromal elements and portal structures (bile ducts and vessels), is usually manifested clinically as fulminant hepatic failure (see Ch. 128). This syndrome is characterized by severely deranged liver function, hepatic encephalopathy, and a high case fatality rate. In survivors, however, despite the severity of the acute process, a chronic course is unusual, and liver histology typically returns nearly to normal.

In the recovery phase there is regeneration of hepatocytes and a largely complete restoration of normal lobular architecture. It is distinctly uncommon for the healing that follows a circumscribed acute hepatitis to be accompanied by fibrous scar formation or by nodular regeneration. In the latter, hepatocytes cluster in an abnormal configuration lacking a central vein and other components of the normal lobular architecture. These two manifestations of an *abnormal* healing process (fibrosis and nodular regeneration) are the essential components of cirrhosis, a form of chronic liver disease that almost always reflects ongoing injury and repair rather than a single acute event.

CLINICAL AND LABORATORY MANIFESTATIONS. The earliest symptoms of acute viral hepatitis typically are nonspecific, predominantly constitutional and gastrointestinal. They may include malaise, fatigue, anorexia, nausea, vomiting, and arthralgias, and may suggest a "flu" or upper respiratory syndrome to both patient and physician. Classically, the patient may describe a loss of taste for coffee or cigarettes. Fever, if present, is usually mild. Abdominal discomfort may reflect an enlarged tender liver. Arthritis occurs in 10 to 15 per cent of cases; in hepatitis B it appears to represent immune complex deposition, but it also occurs with similar frequency in hepatitis A, in which immune complexes have not been demonstrated. Urticaria may occur occasionally.

After a period of several days to a week or more, the prodromal phase may lead to an icteric phase. The earliest clinical manifestation of a rising serum concentration of direct-reacting bilirubin is bilirubinuria, followed by a lightening of stool color, scleral icterus, and, in light-skinned individuals, frank jaundice. Constitutional symptoms often abate during the icteric phase, especially in children, in whom the disease is characteristically less severe. In adults, the gastrointestinal components of the prodrome may persist or even increase for a time. If cholestasis worsens, pruritus may cause increasing discomfort.

Physical findings are variable and depend on the stage of the illness. The only objective finding during the prodrome, apart from mild fever, may be an enlarged and tender liver, associated in perhaps 20 per cent with splenomegaly. Jaundice may or may not appear; indeed, it is likely that the vast majority of cases remain anicteric. Excoriations reflect the intensity of pruritus. Spider nevi occasionally develop during an acute hepatitis, but since their appearance is unusual, it should suggest the possibility of a more chronic process.

Laboratory studies are highly variable, but almost by definition the clinical onset is accompanied by rising activities of serum transaminases; usually the ALT (SGPT) exceeds the AST (SGOT). An elevated serum bilirubin is predominantly direct reacting; very high concentrations, e.g., greater than 15 to 20 mg per deciliter, indicate a severe lesion or may reflect associated hemolysis. The alkaline phosphatase is usually moderately increased, whereas serum albumin concentration may decrease slightly. A diffuse hyperglobulinemia is common. Prothrombin time is prolonged in more severe cases, and a persisting or increasing prolongation is an unfavorable prognostic sign. Mild and clinically insignificant hypoglycemia occurs in perhaps 50 per cent of cases; more profound hypoglycemia may complicate fulminant hepatic failure. Hematologic tests are also quite variable. Usually the total leukocyte count is normal or slightly decreased and atypical lymphocytes may be present. In more severe cases, total leukocytes may be increased, with relative or absolute neutrophilia. Hemoglobin and hematocrit are usually relatively normal, but occasionally there may be a coincidental hemolytic process, and rarely the course is complicated by aplastic anemia. Urinalysis is usually nonspecific except for the presence of bilirubin.

An important aspect of the laboratory approach to acute viral hepatitis is the etiologic serodiagnosis. Although establishing a specific etiologic diagnosis will not usually influence management, it may have a bearing on prognosis, and is particularly useful epidemiologically and for the immunization of contacts. These tests are considered below, in the discussions of hepatitis A, hepatitis B, hepatitis D, and prevention.

After an icteric phase lasting usually from several days to several weeks, the patient enters a convalescent phase in which there is gradual improvement in symptoms and laboratory tests. The healing process may require several weeks, during which time residual weakness and malaise are common. Normalization of laboratory tests is usually complete within four months. Persistence of abnormalities beyond six months suggests that the process may have become chronic; in this circumstance, liver biopsy may be indicated if there is no evidence of continuing improvement.

COMPLICATIONS AND EXTRAHEPATIC MANIFESTATIONS. The two most important complications of acute viral hepatitis are massive hepatic necrosis (fulminant hepatitis) and progression to chronic hepatitis. Fortunately, these are uncommon, especially in hepatitis A, in which chronicity does not occur and massive necrosis is less common than in hepatitis B and non-A, non-B.

Massive hepatic necrosis with fulminant hepatic failure occurs in fewer than 1 per cent of cases of acute viral hepatitis and is usually signaled by deepening jaundice, increasing prothrombin time, and hepatic encephalopathy, which, in its earliest stages, may appear only as a subtle personality change. Serum transaminase levels may remain high, but in many cases will fall, often in association with a decrease in liver size. These changes are assumed to reflect extensive loss of parenchymal mass and, in the presence of other evidence of a deteriorating course, are unfavorable prognostic signs. The diagnosis and management of acute hepatic failure and encephalopathy are considered in greater detail in Ch. 128.

Evolution to chronic hepatitis is a more common complication of acute hepatitis B, D, and non-A, non-B. It is suggested by persistence of abnormal serum transaminases, with or without other laboratory abnormalities and clinical symptoms, beyond an arbitrarily selected endpoint. Authorities differ as to where that endpoint belongs; guidelines range from four to twelve months, but most would accept six months as reasonable. Clearly, however, judgments must be individualized as to when an acute process becomes chronic (or, more pragmatically, when investigations such as liver biopsy should be performed). For example, as long as the patient continues to show evidence of clinical and laboratory improvement, there is little to be gained from a more vigorous diagnostic or therapeutic approach. Conversely, evidence suggestive of chronic liver disease (e.g., signs of portal hypertension or progressive deterioration of laboratory tests) appearing before six months may justify earlier diagnostic intervention. Since many of the histopathologic features associated with chronic hepatitis also may be components of an acute process, however, liver biopsies obtained too early in the course may be difficult to interpret and potentially misleading. Chronic hepatitis is also considered in the discussions of hepatitis B, D, and non-A, non-B, below, and in greater detail in Ch. 123.

The *cholestatic hepatitis syndrome* occurs occasionally as a complication of acute viral hepatitis. Patients may exhibit a relatively prolonged course dominated by cholestatic features, including pruritus, dark urine, light stools, direct-reacting hyperbilirubinemia, and elevation of alkaline phosphatase. Some of these cases are associated with hepatitis A virus infection. Almost without exception, however, the prognosis is favorable. The major problem in management posed by this variant is its occasionally difficult differentiation from biliary obstruction and the possible need to exclude disorders such as gallstones, stricture, and tumors by means of appropriate imaging and cholangiographic techniques. Brief corticosteroid therapy may be useful symptomatically and is well tolerated, but has no long-range impact.

Aplastic anemia may very rarely complicate the icteric or convalescent phase of acute viral hepatitis, especially non-A, non-B. Its pathogenesis is unknown, and its prognosis poor. Among the relatively few survivors, there is no clear evidence of a beneficial effect of glucocorticoids or anabolic steroid treatment. Other formed elements may also be depressed, and pancytopenia, agranulocytosis, and thrombocytopenia have been reported.

Extrahepatic manifestations of acute viral hepatitis also include *arthralgias* and *arthritis*, and *urticaria*. These are usually most prominent during the prodromal phase and, in hepatitis B, appear to reflect deposition of immune complexes. They also may occur in non-A, non-B hepatitis. Other manifestations of hepatitis B infection, such as *glomerulonephritis* and *vasculitis*, are also associated with immune complex deposition and are discussed in Ch. 81 and 63, respectively. A tentative association of *essential mixed cryoglobulinemia* with hepatitis B infection also has been reported. *Pancreatitis* is found in 12 to 40 per cent of cases of fatal acute viral hepatitis, and serum amylase activity may be elevated in up to 30 per cent of nonfatal cases; the true overall incidence and mechanism of pancreatitis in viral hepatitis are not known. Myocarditis, pneumonitis, and other extrahepatic manifestations are rare, and in their presence other systemic disorders should be considered.

SPECIFIC ETIOLOGIC CATEGORIES OF VIRAL HEPATITIS

HEPATITIS A. This form of hepatitis also has been referred to as infectious hepatitis, short-incubation hepatitis, or MS-I hepatitis. The causative agent (hepatitis A virus) is a 27-nm diameter RNA virus that is readily and almost exclusively transmitted via the fecal-oral route. In this important respect it differs significantly from hepatitis B, D, and most cases of non-A, non-B. Accordingly, when the etiology of water-borne, point-source, food-handler–related, and institutional hepatitis outbreaks has been defined, hepatitis A almost invariably has been implicated. An epidemic form of non-A, non-B hepatitis may also be spread by contaminated water supplies. In addition, hepatitis A occurs sporadically and is spread by direct person-to-person contact; there appears to be an increased incidence among promiscuous homosexuals. Spread of hepatitis A in day care centers may involve not only children but also the staff and the families of affected children. Although parenteral transmission is theoretically possible, it must occur rarely. The incidence of the disease appears to correlate in a general way with personal hygiene and the efficacy of public health measures, as suggested by the apparent influence of socioeconomic status on the incidence of

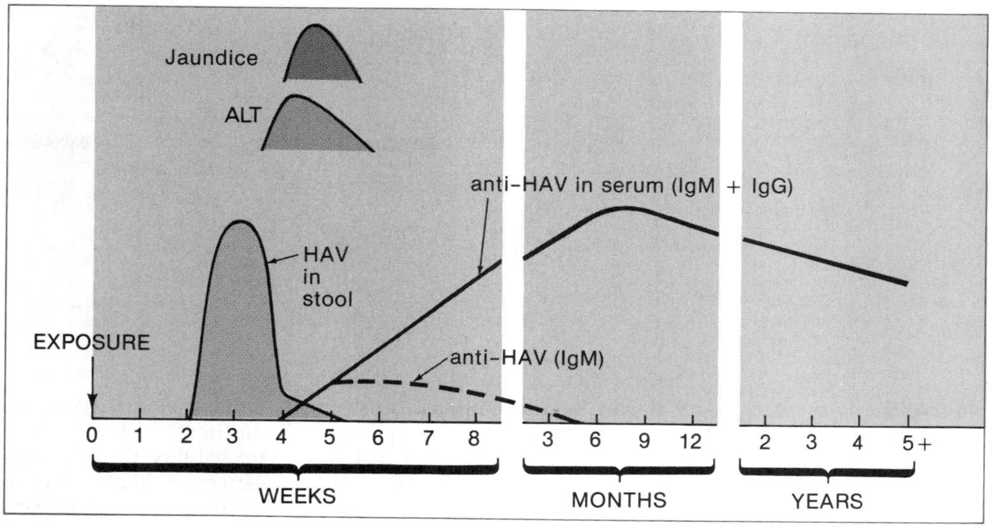

FIGURE 121–1. Sequence of clinical and laboratory findings in a patient with hepatitis A. Fecal shedding of virus is brief in duration, and ends with the appearance of anti-HAV in serum. IgM anti-HAV may persist in serum for a year or more after the acute illness. (From Krugman S, Gocke DJ: Viral Hepatitis. Philadelphia, W. B. Saunders Company, 1978.)

hepatitis A antibodies (anti-HAV), which averaged 45 per cent in one study of an urban population in the United States and approximated 90 per cent in residents of Costa Rica. There is no evidence for the existence of a chronic form of hepatitis A or a carrier state. The "reservoir" for the virus appears to consist of the large number of clinically inapparent acute cases, as well as those persons in the late incubation period of overt hepatitis A in whom shedding of virus occurred prior to the clinical onset.

Hepatitis A infection typically has an incubation period of two to six weeks. Fecal shedding of virus occurs during the final week of the incubation period and the prodromal phase, and declines as serum transaminases reach maximal levels (Fig. 121–1 and Table 121–1). Although there is a transient viremia during this interval, parenteral transmission of the disease is very rare. Viral shedding in stool declines as antibody (anti-HAV) appears in serum. Initially, antibody is predominantly of the IgM class, but an IgG antibody soon appears, and after several weeks to a few months the IgM antibody disappears. The IgG antibody perisists in serum for many years; its exclusive presence indicates prior experience with, and immunity to, the hepatitis A virus. The presence of the IgM antibody, on the other hand, almost always indicates current or very recent infection (Table 121–2), although occasionally this antibody may persist for up to one year or more. Shedding of virus is limited to a two- to three-week period. An IgA antibody to HAV appears in the feces of patients at about the time fecal shedding of virus ceases and persists for several weeks.

The acute illness itself is quite diverse in its clinical manifestations and course. The majority of cases probably are clinically inapparent, especially in children, or are perceived as a nonspecific "flu" syndrome. Jaundice, when it occurs, is usually mild. Symptoms usually subside, and serum transaminases return to normal within three to four months. Hepatitis A virus infection has been implicated in some cases of acute cholestatic hepatitis. Rarely, hepatitis A causes massive hepatic necrosis and fulminant hepatic failure, but this complication is much less common than in hepatitis B and non-A, non-B.

The ease with which hepatitis A is transmitted among contacts and via water and food, as well as the demonstrated efficacy of immune serum globulin in prevention or amelioration of the disease, underscores the value of individual and public health measures to control the spread of infection. The application of these to the management of the individual patient and his or her contacts is discussed below.

HEPATITIS B. In marked contrast to hepatitis A, hepatitis B virus infection may cause a wide variety of acute or chronic hepatic and extrahepatic diseases, as well as a chronic carrier state. Its presentation as an acute hepatitis is typical of those cases that previously were designated serum hepatitis, homologous serum jaundice, long-incubation hepatitis, or MS-II hepatitis, although it is now apparent that many of these cases may also represent non-A, non-B hepatitis (see below). The hepatitis B virus (HBV) differs in almost every respect from hepatitis A (Tables 121–1 and 121–2; Fig. 121–2). The complete infective virion, or *Dane (HBV) particle,* is a DNA virus of 42 nm diameter, consisting of antigenically distinct surface and core components. The *surface coat* is largely lipid and protein, and may exist in serum or other body fluids either as a component of the Dane particle or as separate 20-nm diameter spheres or cylinders. Its major antigenic determinant (hepatitis B surface antigen, HBsAg) includes several

TABLE 121–2. SEROLOGIC TESTS IN VIRAL HEPATITIS

Agent	Terminology	Definition	Significance
Hepatitis A (HAV)	Anti-HAV	Antibody to HAV	
	IgM type		Current or recent infection or convalescence
	IgG type		Current or previous infection; indicates immunity
Hepatitis B (HBV)	HBsAg	HBV surface antigen	Positive in most cases of acute or chronic infection
	HBeAg	e antigen; HBV core component	Transiently positive in acute hepatitis, and in some chronic cases; reflects Dane particle concentration and infectivity
	Anti-Hbc (IgM or IgG)	Antibody to HBV core antigen	Positive in all acute and chronic cases and in carriers; thus, marker of HBV infection; not protective; IgM anti-HBc reflects active virus replication
	Anti-HBe	Antibody to e antigen	Transiently positive during convalescence and in some chronic cases and carriers; not protective; reflects low infectivity and possible integration of HBV DNA into host genome
	Anti-HBs	Antibody to surface antigen	Becomes positive late in convalescence in most acute cases; protective
Hepatitis D (HDV)	Anti-HDV (IgM or IgG)	Antibody to HDV antigen	Similar to anti-HBc in indicating infection; not protective

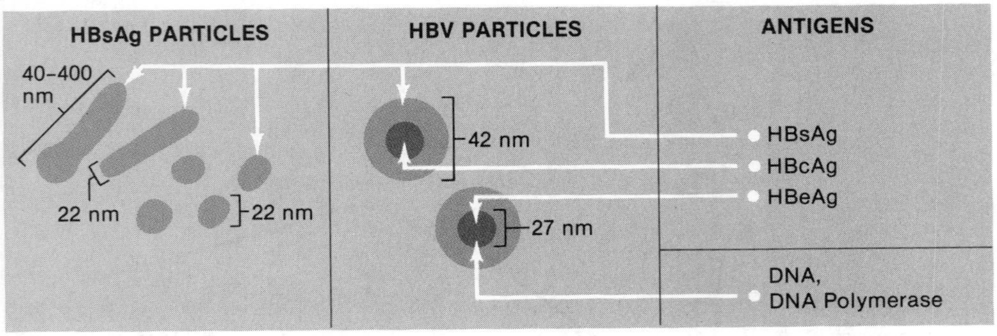

FIGURE 121–2. Forms of HBV in plasma, showing location of the various components and antigenic determinants. (From Koff RS: In Sanford JP, Luby JP [eds.]: The Science and Clinical Practice of Medicine. Infectious Diseases. Vol. 8. New York, Grune & Stratton, 1981, by permission.)

subtypes (d, y; w, r), and it can be detected by sensitive radioimmunoassay techniques in the serum of at least 75 per cent of infected persons during the acute disease (Fig. 121–2). The hepatitis B virus *core* consists of circular DNA, DNA polymerase, and other determinants, which include the hepatitis B core antigen (HBcAg) and two or three related e antigens (HBeAg). The biologic significance of HBcAg and HBeAg is not fully understood, but they are structurally related, and each elicits a humoral antibody response (anti-HBc and anti-HBe, respectively) during the course of the hepatitis B infection, which may be of diagnostic or prognostic significance. HBV-DNA can be detected in serum by molecular hybridization, is the most sensitive test for the presence of infective virus, and may be more widely employed in the near future.

In contrast to hepatitis A, *transmission* of hepatitis B by the fecal-oral route is relatively unimportant; infection may follow oral ingestion, but large doses appear necessary. Instead, the virus is present in virtually all body fluids and excreta, and transmission of this disease occurs primarily via parenteral routes. Therefore, it usually requires either overt inoculation (e.g., transfusion, or injection via a contaminated needle) or intimate personal contact (e.g., between sexual partners, patients and health professionals, and mother and newborn infant). The disease occurs with an increased frequency among sexual partners of acutely infected individuals, as well as among chronically exposed persons, including health professionals and patients exposed to blood and blood products (e.g., workers and patients in clinical laboratories, dialysis and oncology units), the sexually promiscuous (especially male homosexuals), drug users who share needles, and handlers of primates (which are susceptible to infection). In urban centers, hepatitis B may account for up to 50 per cent of sporadic cases of acute hepatitis, even in the absence of documented parenteral inoculation. This attests to the importance of person-to-person contact in the spread of this disease.

Unlike hepatitis A, hepatitis B infection may be chronic, either in association with demonstrable liver disease or in otherwise seemingly healthy carriers. Less than 1 per cent of the general population of the United States and Western Europe is HBsAg-positive. This low incidence contrasts with incidence of anti-HBs of about 10 per cent in the same population, providing additional evidence that in most patients with acute hepatitis B the infection is self-limited and followed by immunity, and only infrequently leads to chronic liver disease or a carrier state. The incidence of HBsAg positivity is much higher in less-developed areas (up to 15 per cent) and among certain subpopulations with increased exposure and/or impaired immunity, such as patients with Down's syndrome, leprosy, or lymphoproliferative disorders; addicts; and patients undergoing dialysis. In addition to acute cases, therefore, these chronically infected individuals constitute the "reservoir" that serves to perpetuate the virus. Historically, it is likely that transmission of the disease has occurred not so often via overt parenteral inoculation but rather via sexual contact or from mother to newborn. In the latter instance (*vertical transmission*), i.e., in infants born to mothers with acute or chronic infection, there is a high probability that the neonate will acquire the disease. This is especially likely when the mother develops acute hepatitis B in late pregnancy or early post partum or has chronic hepatitis. Transmission appears to correlate with the presence of HBeAg in maternal serum, reflecting the concentration of Dane particles. Characteristically, these infants remain chronically infected for many years, either as "carriers" or with a persisting low-grade and chronic hepatitis. They are probably at increased risk of developing hepatocellular carcinoma (see Ch. 129). Vertical transmission may be an important mechanism by which the reservoir of the virus is sustained from generation to generation.

The *incubation period* of acute hepatitis B, as defined by the appearance of clinical symptoms, varies between four weeks and six months, with an average of about 50 days. If the incubation period is defined instead in terms of the interval between exposure and the first *serologic* evidence of viremia, it may be as brief as two weeks, especially after exposure to large parenteral doses. Two weeks to two months prior to the clinical onset, HBsAg becomes detectable in serum (see Fig. 121–3 and Table 121–2). At about the time of the clinical onset and the rise in serum transaminase activities anti-HBc becomes detectable. Initially, an IgM anti-HBc is present in high titer and persists for several months to one year; thereafter IgG anti-HBc predominates. In chronic HBV infections, IgM anti-HBc is likely to be detectable during periods in which the virus is actively replicating. IgG anti-HBc persists for up to several years after acute hepatitis and is present in all chronic carriers. It appears to play no role in host defenses; rather, it serves as a reliable marker of hepatitis B infection currently or within the preceding few years. The Dane particle markers (HBeAg and DNA polymerase) usually become detectable in serum prior to the increase in transaminase. The duration of HBsAg positivity is highly variable. It may persist for a few days to two to three months; persistence beyond this time may indicate a chronic course. Characteristically, HBsAg becomes undetectable prior to the appearance of anti-HBs. This antibody can be demonstrated in 80 to 90 per cent of patients, usually late in convalescence, and indicates relative or absolute immunity. Its appearance generally suggests a successful response to the infection, but there are exceptions to this in certain patients with chronic hepatitis (see Ch. 123).

Several important qualifications should be noted in interpreting the results of hepatitis B serologic tests. First, in a significant number of patients with acute hepatitis B the serum is negative for HBsAg, presumably because the antigen is very low in titer or evanescent. For this reason, a single negative HBsAg test does not exclude the diagnosis. Anti-HBc is more sensitive in this regard and may be the only serologic indication of hepatitis B infection. A negative test for anti-HBc effectively excludes the diagnosis. On the other hand, a positive test for anti-HBc in an HBsAg-negative serum could merely reflect a prior episode of hepatitis B. These HBsAg-negative, anti-HBc–positive patients may be classifi-

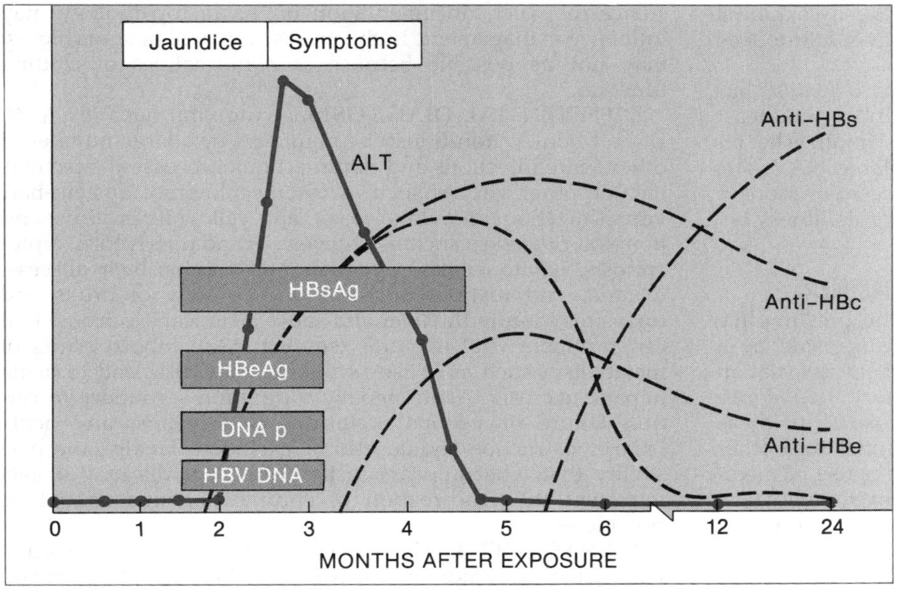

FIGURE 121–3. Sequence of clinical and laboratory findings in a patient with acute hepatitis B, followed by recovery. HBsAg-emia is the initial manifestation. "Dane particle markers" (HBeAg, DNA polymerase, and HBV DNA) precede the ALT rise and are transient. Anti-HBc (IgM, then IgG) appears during the acute illness; after the disappearance of anti-HBsAg and before the appearance of anti-HBs, anti-HBc may be the only marker of hepatitis B infection. (Adapted from Hoofnagle J, Schafer DF: Serologic markers of hepatitis B virus infection. Semin Liver Dis 6:4, 1986.)

able on the basis of the anti-HBs: if this test is positive early in the course of an acute hepatitis, it is evidence against the diagnosis of acute hepatitis B. Detection of IgM anti-HBc suggests recent acute or chronic HBV infection during a phase of active virus replication, as noted above. In those IgM-anti-HBc–negative subjects in whom HBV infection appears to have antedated the acute illness, the possibility of superimposed infection by hepatitis D (delta-agent), a non-A, non-B virus, or other causes of an acute hepatitis syndrome must be considered.

The *clinical course* of acute hepatitis B is more variable and usually more prolonged than that of hepatitis A. It is also more often associated with extrahepatic manifestations, including urticaria and other rashes, arthritis, and, much less commonly, glomerulonephritis and vasculitis. The immune complexes that appear to cause these extrahepatic manifestations consist of HBsAg, anti-HBs, and complement components. Glomerulonephritis and vasculitis are also associated with chronic hepatitis B infection and are not necessarily accompanied by apparent liver disease. Indeed, up to one third of all cases of polyarteritis nodosa may be caused or associated with hepatitis B virus infection.

Approximately 90 per cent of patients with acute hepatitis B recover completely and become HBsAg negative. Fewer than 1 per cent develop massive hepatic necrosis, but this complication is more common than in hepatitis A. Of the 10 per cent of patients who remain HBsAg positive beyond three or four months, in a significant number the antigen will clear over a period of six months to a year or more without evidence of chronic hepatitis developing. Many of those with prolonged HBsAg positivity, however, appear destined either to become chronic carriers or to develop chronic persistent or chronic active hepatitis (see Ch. 123).

HEPATITIS D (DELTA-AGENT). Infection with this unusual agent may be regarded as a complication of hepatitis B. The delta-agent is an incomplete RNA virus that requires antecedent or simultaneous HBV infection to infect the host cell. The agent exists in plasma in a coat of HBsAg and is present in the nuclei of infected hepatocytes. HDV infection is reflected by the presence of anti-HDV antibody (IgM acutely; IgG chronically) or HDV RNA in serum. Almost invariably the serum is positive for HBsAg and anti-HBc and, in most, anti-HBe. It is most commonly found among intravenous drug addicts and recipients of multiple transfusions. In subjects who are acutely and simultaneously infected with HBV and HDV there is no apparent increase in the probability that chronic hepatitis will ensue. In individuals chronically infected with HBV, however, superimposed acute HDV infection usually also becomes chronic and is associated with the histopathologic findings of chronic active hepatitis. Acute HDV infection may cause fulminant hepatic failure.

HEPATITIS NON-A, NON-B. A large number of cases of acute viral hepatitis are caused by at least two other agents. Progress is being made in the identification of these agents, but it still is not possible to document the infection on a routine basis. Consequently, the designation non-A, non-B remains appropriate, since these forms of hepatitis are essentially diagnoses of exclusion.

Non-A, non-B hepatitis is the major cause of *post-transfusion hepatitis*. It occurs in approximately five to ten cases per 1000 transfusions and can be transmitted in whole blood, packed cells, platelets, plasma, and especially clotting factor concentrates. The incidence of post-transfusion hepatitis B has been greatly reduced by screening of donors for HBsAg. Non-A, non-B also is a common cause of hepatitis in needle users and accounts for 20 per cent or more of sporadic cases, i.e., those not associated with obvious contact or parenteral inoculation. A significant number of those cases of hepatitis previously referred to as serum hepatitis or homologous serum jaundice actually represented non-A, non-B hepatitis infections. Conversely, it is also now clear that some cases of "non-A, non-B" hepatitis actually represent HDV infection. Moreover, certain monoclonal antibodies may detect HBsAg in cases otherwise negative for this determinant and therefore are classified as non-A, non-B.

Hepatitis B and non-A, non-B also have many similar clinical manifestations. Thus, the incubation period of non-A, non-B hepatitis is longer than that of hepatitis A, ranging from two to twenty weeks, with an average of eight weeks. The acute illness is also quite variable. The incidence of massive hepatic necrosis appears comparable to that of hepatitis B, and together these two categories account for the great majority of cases.

Finally, post-transfusion and sporadic non-A, non-B hepatitis is associated with both an apparent carrier state (inferred from the fact that it may be transmitted by blood from apparently healthy donors) and chronic hepatitis. The incidence of chronic hepatitis after non-A, non-B transfusion hepatitis approaches 50 per cent. In some of these patients the disease is mild and may spontaneously subside or remit after a year of more, but in others the process may exhibit a progressive course and lead to cirrhosis and liver failure (see Ch. 123).

In recent years, an *epidemic form of non-A, non-B hepatitis* has been described, associated with outbreaks in India, Southeast Asia, Burma, North Africa, and the Soviet Union. The responsible agent appears morphologically similar to HAV. The illness is associated with a mortality of 10 per cent or more in pregnant women. There is no evidence that this illness becomes chronic.

GENERAL APPROACHES TO DIAGNOSIS AND MANAGEMENT

DIAGNOSIS. In its classic presentation, the presumptive diagnosis of acute viral hepatitis is readily suggested by a compatible history and physical examination, in association with laboratory evidence of hepatocellular injury, i.e., significantly increased serum transaminases. Because all of these features are nonspecific, however, it is essential that other possible etiologic factors be considered, such as use of medications or illicit drugs, alcohol, exposure to environmental or industrial toxins, and the possible acquisition of unusual infections as suggested by travel or residence in rural or less well developed areas. Exposure to viral hepatitis itself is suggested by contact with jaundiced persons or persons known to have developed hepatitis, sexual promiscuity (especially among male homosexuals), transfusion of blood or blood products, or the sharing of needles by drug users. Among health professionals, workers in dialysis and oncology units, surgeons, dentists, and clinical laboratory technicians are at increased risk, as is anyone in direct contact with blood blood products, or other body fluids. Despite the importance of a careful inquiry into these possible risk factors, many patients with acute viral hepatitis will report no significant exposures.

A careful and complete physical examination will help establish the diagnosis (tender hepatomegaly is the most common finding) and help exclude other processes that occasionally mimic acute viral hepatitis, such as acute hepatic congestion, disseminated sepsis or liver abscess, or biliary tract disease with or without cholangitis.

Serodiagnosis of viral hepatitis is now possible, with certain limitations (see above). A positive test for the IgM class of anti-HAV or a rising titer of total anti-HAV is strong evidence for acute hepatitis A. Conversely, if the test for anti-HAV is negative well into the convalescent phase, the diagnosis is excluded. A single positive test for anti-HAV is of little diagnostic value, since this could reflect a previous infection.

Although an acute hepatitis syndrome associated with HBsAg positivity has been taken as presumptive evidence for acute hepatitis B, none of the tests generally available at this time permits early and unequivocal diagnosis or exclusion of this entity. An important exception is that the presence of anti-HBs early in the course of acute hepatitis tends to exclude acute HBV infection. Since the classic pattern in which both HBsAg and anti-HBc are positive acutely may not be present in all cases (although anti-HBc itself is virtually always positive), a single negative test for HBsAg does not definitively exclude acute hepatitis B. Medical records, if available, may be of help by providing information about prior liver function tests, hepatitis serologies, or blood donation. Since donated blood has been screened routinely for HBsAg since 1972, such information may be quite helpful in the evaluation of hepatitis B serologies. As tests for the non-A, non-B agents become available, accurate serodiagnosis of hepatitis syndromes will be greatly facilitated.

If a *liver biopsy* is performed, it may demonstrate the pathologic features of acute viral hepatitis. However, these are nonspecific, and in the vast majority of cases biopsy is not indicated. Its use should be reserved for patients in whom the diagnosis is uncertain or in whom there is concern regarding chronicity or a deteriorating course, or any circumstance in which documentation of the histopathology may influence management. In the most severely ill patients biopsy may not be possible because of abnormalities of clotting function.

DIFFERENTIAL DIAGNOSIS. Acute viral hepatitis A, B, D, and non-A, non-B may be mimicked by a large number of other acute infections and noninfectious processes. Infections include other viruses such as cytomegalovirus, Epstein-Barr virus (infectious mononucleosis), and yellow fever virus; and nonviral processes such as Q fever, secondary syphilis, leptospirosis, salmonellosis, pyogenic and amebic liver abscess, malaria, and toxoplasmosis. A wide variety of drugs and toxins may injure the liver and cause a clinical syndrome that can resemble viral hepatitis (see Ch. 122). Inborn errors of metabolism such as Wilson's disease may also lead to acute hepatic necrosis. Acute hepatic congestion secondary to cardiac failure or venous occlusion, cholecystitis, and acute biliary obstruction should also be excluded. Finally, the possibility that what appears to be acute hepatitis may in fact represent the exacerbation of chronic hepatitis should be considered.

MANAGEMENT. There is no specific treatment for acute viral hepatitis. Major emphasis is placed on symptomatic and supportive care and on the prevention of transmission. Prevention is considered in detail below.

Most patients with acute viral hepatitis do not require hospitalization and are appropriately managed at home. Rest is advisable, but strict confinement to bed is not necessary beyond what is dictated by the patient's own sense of fatigue and malaise. No specific dietary measures are indicated, but most patients find a low-fat, high-carbohydrate diet more palatable. During the most severe phases of the illness, anorexia and nausea may be so extreme that oral intake of any kind is minimal. In such instances, attention to fluid balance is important, and it may be necessary to advise the intake of small amounts of clear fluids at frequent intervals. Although there is an appropriate reluctance to administer medication to the patient with liver disease, judicious use of small doses of antinausea agents such as hydroxyzine, trimethobenzamide, and even prochlorperazine is occasionally necessary and usually well tolerated. As the patient's symptoms decrease and appetite improves, intake can be liberalized, usually according to taste. Alcoholic beverages should be avoided throughout the course of the acute illness. Ambulation and activity may be increased as symptoms and laboratory tests improve; the most useful advice is that such activity should be limited so as to avoid causing fatigue. The decision to return to employment or school must take into consideration the patient's symptoms, the strenuousness of the work, and the potential for transmission of the disease; this, in turn, is a function of the viral etiology and the closeness of contact with others. In general, transmission is quite unlikely after two to three weeks in hepatitis A, whereas spread of hepatitis B or non-A, non-B ordinarily requires direct person-to-person contact.

Hospitalization is indicated for those patients in whom severe nausea and vomiting prevent maintenance of adequate fluid balance, in whom there is evidence of progressive deterioration, especially with encephalopathy or prolongation of prothrombin time, or in whom invasive diagnostic studies are indicated.

There is no convincing evidence to justify the use of corticosteroids in acute hepatitis, regardless of its severity. The management of fulminant hepatitis poses special problems in patient monitoring and support and is discussed in detail in Ch. 128.

PREVENTION. The entire area of hepatitis prophylaxis has been dramatically changed by the availability of an effective vaccine for hepatitis B. In this vaccine, the immunizing antigen is HBsAg, prepared from donor sera or, more recently, by recombinant DNA technology employing yeast; an appropriate immune response is reflected by the appearance of anti-HBs. Hepatitis A virus has been propagated in tissue culture, and a vaccine may also be available in the near future for this disease. Finally, continuing progress in the identification, isolation, and characterization of non-A, non-B viral hepatitis agents suggests the possibility of active immunization, although not for some time. Pending the advent of generally available and effective vaccines for all of the viral causes of acute hepatitis, prevention must depend mainly on personal hygiene and public health measures directed at minimizing the exposure of potentially susceptible individuals, and on the appropriate use of passive immunization.

The use of public health and hygienic measures rests on the premise that body fluids and excreta of infected individuals are potentially infective. Clearly there are certain exceptions, depending on the specific virus involved, the clinical stage of the infection, the amount of potentially infective material involved, and the nature of the exposure. For example, because of the ease with which hepatitis A is spread via the fecal-oral route, contact of such patients with others should be minimized, and their excreta and essentially all materials handled by them during their brief period of infectivity should be carefully disposed of. In contrast, hepatitis B and D are not commonly spread via the fecal-oral route. Although excreta are to be regarded as infective in these patients, the more important concern is transmission via puncture by contaminated needles (or equivalent exposure to infective material) or intimate personal (sexual) contact, especially during the period of HBsAg positivity. Non-A, non-B hepatitis in the United States more closely resembles hepatitis B in its transmissibility, but common-source outbreaks analogous to those caused by hepatitis A virus have recently been documented in India, Southeast Asia, Burma, North Africa, and the Soviet Union (see above). Because of these differences among the agents and differences in the approach to passive immunization, serologic diagnosis of the acute viral hepatitis case is useful, even though most patients with these disorders may be expected to do well regardless of etiology. In practice, however, rapid serodiagnosis is not always possible, and for this reason certain generalizations regarding the early management of the patient and his or her contacts are appropriate and are discussed below, along with measures for specific agents.

Hepatitis A. Since the infection is spread primarily via the fecal-oral route, including transmission by handling food, in drinking water, and potentially by fomites, strict attention to hygiene on the part of the patient and his or her attendants, whether in home or hospital, is of utmost importance during the period of viral shedding (Fig. 121–1). Direct body contact should be limited to that necessary for care; attendants should wear gloves, and careful handwashing is appropriate. Food, utensils, clothing, linen, needles, and excreta should be handled separately and carefully, also by gloved attendants. The virus is readily inactivated by boiling or by exposure to formalin, chlorine, or ultraviolet irradiation. In the hospital setting, strict isolation is not usually required for cooperative and informed patients with hepatitis A. In the home, similar measures should be implemented to the extent possible.

Close contacts of patients with hepatitis A should receive passive immunization with immune serum globulin as soon as possible, preferably within the first few days. The official recommended dose is 0.02 ml per kilogram up to a maximum of 2 ml, although up to 5 ml has been advocated. This would apply to immediate family members, sexual contacts, or others with whom the patient has been in close contact during the presumed period of infectivity. Casual contacts in the workplace or school probably do not require passive immunization unless there is reason to suspect mutual handling of food, beverages, or contaminated items. On the other hand, it is important to inquire about other possible cases among work or classroom associates. If there is reason to suspect a possible point-source outbreak, then all similarly exposed persons should receive immune serum globulin and appropriate epidemiologic information obtained.

The mode of transmission of hepatitis A also renders its prevention a matter of concern for those who intend to travel in areas where public health and sanitation measures may be suboptimal. In such circumstances, drinking water, fresh fruits and vegetables, and shellfish may be contaminated and should be avoided if possible. For these persons, administration of a standard dose (0.02 ml per kilogram) of immune serum globulin may be expected to afford protection for up to three months; for longer periods, a dose of 0.05 ml per kilogram is recommended and should be repeated at four- to six-month intervals.

Hepatitis B. Although this agent is less readily transmitted via the fecal-oral route, due consideration should be given to the general hygienic measures outlined for hepatitis A, in both home and hospital. Transmission ordinarily requires direct contact with the patient or the equivalent of a parenteral inoculation of infective material. Thus, in the home, children are far less likely than the spouse to acquire hepatitis B from an acutely infected adult. In the hospital, strict isolation may not be necessary if excreta, needles and other medical supplies, and personal utensils are identified, carefully handled, and discarded.

Passive immunization with immune serum globulin enriched in anti-HBs (hepatitis B immune globulin, or HBIG) is protective against hepatitis B infection in certain circumstances and when used in accordance with established guidelines. Because this material is expensive, it should not be used indiscriminately. At present, its use is officially recommended in the following specific situations:

1. Inoculation of material known to be contaminated with the hepatitis B virus, e.g., inadvertent puncture of a health professional by a needle from an HBsAG-positive patient, or accidental transfusion of HBsAg-positive blood or blood products.
2. Splash of HBsAg-positive material into the eye or on an open skin wound or eruption, as may occur in a laboratory accident or during a surgical or diagnostic procedure.
3. Ingestion of HBsAg-positive material, as may occur during a laboratory pipetting accident.
4. Sexual partners of patients with *acute* hepatitis B (partners of patients with chronic hepatitis B presumably have been previously exposed) within 14 days of contact.
5. Infants born to HBsAg-positive mothers, especially those who have had acute hepatitis B during the final trimester of pregnancy or first two months post partum, or who are positive for both HbsAg and HBeAg at the time of delivery.

The rational use of HBIG depends on two essential components. First, it must be documented that the material to which the person has been exposed contains HBsAg, and this requires identification of the source and appropriate serologic confirmation. For example, accidental puncture of the skin by one of several used needles in a disposal container effectively precludes meeting this requirement and, therefore, the use of HBIG. Second, the exposed person must actually be at risk. If, at the time of exposure, he or she is already positive for HBsAg (i.e., infected) or anti-HBs, (i.e., immune if the s/n value by radioimmunoassay exceeds 10), nothing will be gained from the administration of anti-HBs (HBIG). Ideally, therefore, the serologic status of both "donor" and "recipient" should be documented before the decision to administer HBIG is made. In practice, however, this is not usually possible within the few days' interval after exposure in which HBIG appears to be most effective. As a practical alternative to this dilemma, one possible approach is to immediately obtain serum from both the donor and the person at risk. Pending results of the HBsAg assays, the latter may be given 5 ml of ordinary immune serum globulin. HBIG may be administered later, if indicated by the test results. This approach represents a compromise between the need to institute early passive immunization on the one hand and to avoid indiscriminate use of HBIG on the other, and at a cost that is small relative to that of the HBIG itself. Other approaches are possible. In the family situation, the value of administering HBIG to the spouse remains controversial, but it is generally accepted that its use is not required for children, since they are at low risk.

Hepatitis B Vaccine. As noted, a safe and effective vaccine has been developed for the prevention of hepatitis B. It became generally available in the summer of 1982, after extensive field trials in the homosexual population, in which there is a high incidence of hepatitis B and a high and predictable rate of acquisition of the infection owing to frequent and promiscuous sexual contacts in certain segments of this population. The vaccine consists of highly purified and triple-inactivated HbsAg obtained from the serum of chronic carriers. More recently a recombinant vaccine utilizing HBsAg synthesized in yeast has become available. The vaccine is administered in three 20 μg-doses: initially and one month and six months later, and usually elicits production of anti-HBs in the recipient. Intramuscular injection is important, and is more likely effective with deltoid than with gluteal administration. (Smaller doses are used for children, and larger doses for dialysis and immunocompromised patients.) The vaccine is safe, but caution is recommended by the manufacturer for use in pregnant women. Although most subjects who have completed the three-dose immunization are protected against hepatitis B infection, there are important exceptions, especially among immunosuppressed subjects. The duration of this protection probably is of the order of five years, and is indicated by an anti-HBs titer of s/n >10 by radioimmunoassay.

The vaccine is recommended for use in high-risk groups and individuals. These include, but are not limited to, health professionals (especially those with high exposure risk such as surgeons, dentists, and dialysis workers), susceptible dialysis patients, and those subject to multiple transfusions (e.g., hemophiliacs), certain residents and staff of custodial care institutions, parenteral illicit drug users, heterosexual and household contacts of HBsAg carriers, Alaskan Eskimos, and sexually active and promiscuous male homosexuals. Available evidence suggests that it is also effective, when the first vaccine dose is combined with HBIG, in the passive-active immunization of health professionals after accidental needle stick, and in infants born to HBsAg-positive mothers. The cost-effectiveness of screening of potential vaccine recipients (e.g., anti-HBs determination) varies with the circumstance. In general, in those groups in which prevalence of hepatitis B is relatively low, screening is not cost effective, whereas it is useful in groups with a high prevalence (e.g., the homosexual community). For most health professionals, screening is marginally cost effective and depends on the prevalence of hepatitis B infection in the particular subgroup. In any case, it is established that administration of the vaccine to individuals already infected or immune is without harmful sequelae.

Hepatitis D. There is no established method for active or passive immunization. Since HDV infection requires simultaneous or antecedent HBV infection, prevention of HBV, e.g., by the vaccine, protects against HDV. Since previously infected HBV subjects are at risk for HDV infection, care should be taken to minimize exposure to HDV-containing materials, e.g., HBV-positive serum or secretions.

Hepatitis Non-A, Non-B. There is at present no generally available means of documenting exposure to, or infection by, this group of agents, but it appears to be transmitted in a manner that more closely resembles that of hepatitis B than hepatitis A. Thus close personal contact and parenteral inoculation appear necessary, suggesting that prophylactic measures suitable for hepatitis B are appropriate.

A problem largely confined to non-A, non-B hepatitis at present is that of post-transfusion hepatitis. The single most effective means of reducing the incidence of this disorder is the exclusion of blood obtained from commercial (paid donor) sources. There is a correlation between both elevated aminotransferase activity and anti-HBc positivity in donor unit plasma and the probability of post-transfusion hepatitis in a recipient, and exclusion of such units is desirable. The possible role of pre-exposure (i.e., pretransfusion) immune serum globulin in the prevention of the disorder remains unclear, and at present immune serum globulin is not officially recommended for its prevention.

Alter HJ (ed.): Hepatitis. Semin Liver Dis 6:1, 1986. *A minisymposium in which clinically relevant aspects of acute and chronic hepatitis are discussed by a group of recognized experts.*

Centers for Disease Control: Postexposure prophylaxis of hepatitis B. Ann Intern Med 101:351, 1984. *A summary of official recommendations.*

Dienstag JL: Non-A, non-B hepatitis. Gastroenterology 85:439, 743, 1983. *A thorough consideration of putative agents and summary of clinical, epidermiologic, and prophylactic aspects.*

Favero MS, Maynard JE, Leger RT, et al.: Guidelines for the care of patients hospitalized with viral hepatitis. Ann Intern Med 91:872, 1979. *Specific recommendations based on established concepts of epidemiology. A useful guide.*

Gregory P: Steroid therapy in severe viral hepatitis. N Engl J Med 294:681, 1976. *Convincing evidence that corticosteroids are not helpful, and potentially harmful in severe acute viral hepatitis.*

Health and Public Policy Committee, ACP: Hepatitis B vaccine. Ann Intern Med 100:149, 1984.

Jacobson IM, Dienstag JL: The delta hepatitis agent: Viral hepatitis, type D. Gastroenterology 86:1614, 1984. *Excellent and well-referenced editorial that summarizes concepts and progress toward the understanding of basic and clinical aspects of this newer facet of hepatitis B infection.*

Popper H, Schaffner F (eds.): Progress in Liver Diseases. Orlando, Grune & Stratton, 1986. *Several current and authoritative summaries of various aspects of acute hepatitis.*

Vyas GN, Dienstag JL, Hoofnagle JH (eds.): Viral Hepatitis and Liver Disease. Orlando, Grune & Stratton, 1984. *Proceedings of a March 1984 International Symposium. Progress and concepts in virtually all aspects of the field are presented, discussed, and referenced.*

122 TOXIC AND DRUG-INDUCED LIVER DISEASE

Robert K. Ockner

DEFINITION AND GENERAL PRINCIPLES OF DIAGNOSIS AND MANAGEMENT

Pharmacologic and chemical agents may produce a wide variety of acute or chronic liver diseases. At the one extreme they may take the form of asymptomatic and seemingly inconsequential abnormalities in liver function, whereas at the other they may include fatal acute massive hepatic necrosis or progressive chronic hepatitis, cirrhosis, and liver failure. This spectrum of histopathologic changes, clinical and laboratory features, and prognosis therefore is as broad as that of all other forms of liver disease. Several characteristics of these disorders create special problems for the clinician. First, the mere *association* of a given drug with disturbed liver function does not necessarily imply causality, either in an individual case or in general, and this problem accounts for much of the uncertainty in the field. Second, in a specific instance it may be unclear whether liver dysfunction is caused by a drug, by the underlying disorder for which the implicated drug is being used, by some other concurrent treatment, or by an independent process. Furthermore, in most forms of drug-induced liver injury, there exist important yet poorly understood differences in individual susceptibility. Although some of these differences may be immunologically mediated, this has not been established, and other factors such as differences in drug metabolism are probably of greater significance. Finally, not only may the histopathologic changes seen in drug-induced liver injury be very similar to those of other common entities such as viral hepatitis or biliary obstruction, but some drugs may produce more than one kind of lesion.

Since most forms of drug-induced liver injury are not associated with a specific histopathology, diagnosis must depend chiefly on the history of exposure, consistent clinical, laboratory, and (when appropriate) biopsy findings, and improvement subsequent to removal of the presumed toxin. For those agents that produce small-droplet lipid deposition, such as tetracycline or valproic acid, or those that produce prominent centrilobular necrosis, such as acetaminophen (especially when associated with significant blood levels of the drug), the diagnosis can be made with reasonable certainty on the basis of laboratory and biopsy findings. In most instances, however, unequivocal diagnosis cannot be made without demonstration of recurrent liver damage in response to rechallenge with the implicated drug. With rare exceptions, however, this maneuver is not justified; moreover, for those agents that cause a viral hepatitis–like reaction (e.g., halothane or isoniazid), there is the distinct possibility of a severe or even fatal outcome. Although assumption of such risks may be necessary on rare occasions, in most instances some degree of diagnostic uncertainty is acceptable as long as alternative drugs are available.

The appropriate management of drug-induced liver disease consists of discontinuation of the implicated drug(s) and supportive care for acute hepatitis or liver failure as needed. Only in acetaminophen hepatoxicity is there convincing evidence that specific pharmacologic intervention is beneficial (see below). There is no clear evidence that corticosteroids are of value in the treatment of drug-induced liver disease, although they may suppress systemic manifestations, especially when there is an associated serum sickness–like syndrome. Complications of hepatic adenomas, whether or not estrogen-associated, may require a surgical approach.

HISTOPATHOLOGIC CLASSIFICATION OF DRUG-INDUCED LIVER DISEASE

The classification shown in Table 122–1, although useful conceptually, should not obscure the fact that a given agent may cause more than one form of liver injury. For example, isoniazid may produce a nonspecific focal hepatitis, an acute viral hepatitis–like lesion, or chronic active hepatitis, whereas oral contraceptives may cause hepatocellular cholestasis or liver cell adenoma and have been implicated in hepatic vein thrombosis.

ZONAL NECROSIS. Zonal necrosis is most commonly produced by hepatotoxins that cause a predictable and dose-related injury that also can be produced in laboratory animals. Examples include the centrilobular necrosis associated with *carbon tetrachloride* and *acetaminophen* toxicity. For these and some other agents, toxicity depends on their conversion in the liver cell to a toxic derivative. Despite the predictability and dose dependency that characterize this class of agents, there are significant differences in individual susceptibility, in part reflecting differences in rates of conversion to toxic products. The acute lesion either is fatal or is followed by essentially complete recovery. A similar lesion may result from chronic exposure, but it is not certain that this leads to progressive liver disease and cirrhosis.

TABLE 122–1. CLASSIFICATION OF DRUG-INDUCED LIVER DISEASE

Category	Examples
Predictable hepatotoxins with zonal necrosis	Acetaminophen, carbon tetrachloride
Nonspecific hepatitis	Aspirin, oxacillin
Viral hepatitis-like reactions	Halothane, isoniazid, phenytoin
Cholestasis	
Noninflammatory	Estrogens, 17α-substituted steroids
Inflammatory	Chlorpromazine, antithyroid agents
Fatty liver	
Large droplet	Ethanol, corticosteroids
Small droplet	Tetracycline, valproic acid
Granulomas	Phenylbutazone, allopurinol
Chronic hepatitis	Methyldopa, nitrofurantoin
Tumors	Estrogens, vinyl chloride
Vascular lesions	6-Thioguanine, anabolic steroids

NONSPECIFIC HEPATITIS. Nonspecific hepatitis consists of isolated foci of liver cell necrosis and inflammation, without the characteristic features of viral hepatitis. It also appears to exhibit a variable dose dependency. Neither the mechanism of the injury nor the basis for individual differences in susceptibility is known. Examples include *aspirin* and *oxacillin*.

VIRAL HEPATITIS–LIKE REACTIONS. These may mimic the broad spectrum of clinical, histopathologic, and prognostic variants of viral hepatitis, from an acute uncomplicated process, to bridging or submassive necrosis, to fatal massive necrosis. Examples include *halothane, isoniazid, ketoconazole, methyldopa, sulfonamides,* and *phenytoin*. There are marked differences in individual susceptibility to this form of injury, accounting for its sporadic occurrence and for the common belief that it represents a form of drug allergy. Although there appears to be a specific antibody to hepatocyte surface membranes in the serum of patients with severe halothane hepatitis, it is not certain whether this is important in pathogenesis or represents a secondary immune response to membrane antigens exposed during the halothane-induced injury. Furthermore, in the hepatitis associated with isoniazid and phenytoin, there is strong evidence that cell injury is mediated by a toxic drug metabolite. Thus, differences in individual susceptibility need not imply an immunologic mechanism, but may reflect the influence of genetic, dietary, environmental, or pharmacologic factors on drug metabolism.

CHOLESTASIS. Cholestasis is a very common manifestation of drug-induced liver injury and takes two distinct forms. In the first, caused principally by *natural and synthetic estrogens* and by *17 alpha-substituted androgenic and anabolic steroids*, there is usually little or no evidence of hepatocellular necrosis or a substantial inflammatory response. The injury is most simply viewed as the impaired secretion of bile by the liver cell, probably reflecting a direct steroid effect on the physical properties of cellular membranes or the activities of enzymes involved in this process. Although large doses may minimally impair bile secretion in most subjects, certain persons seem especially sensitive. These differences in individual susceptibility clearly are not allergic, and appear at least in part genetically determined. The lesion is completely and rapidly reversible.

In the second form of cholestatic injury, there is significant hepatocellular necrosis and portal and lobular inflammation; acidophil bodies and eosinophils are variably present. Systemic features, including fever, rash, and arthralgias, are not uncommon. This form of injury is produced by a broad group of agents, including the *phenothiazines, oral hypoglycemic* and *antithyroid* agents, and the *macrolide antibiotics* (e.g., erythromycin estolate). Its prognosis is generally favorable and complete recovery may be expected, except in very few individuals in whom chlorpromazine leads to a prolonged but ultimately resolving cholestatic course; rarely, the reaction may prove fatal. Marked differences in individual susceptibility associated with systemic features have suggested drug allergy as the basis for this form of injury. Chlorpromazine, however, is converted to a number of variably toxic metabolic products; this may account not only for the frequently abnormal liver function observed in patients receiving large doses for prolonged periods but also for the smaller number who develop the overt inflammatory and necrosing cholestatic lesion.

FATTY LIVER. Fatty liver usually represents the accumulation of triglyceride within the hepatocyte, and also may occur in two forms. In the most common, associated with *ethanol, corticosteroids, protein-calorie malnutrition, obesity, uncon-*

trolled diabetes mellitus, and after *jejunoileal bypass,* the fat accumulates in large droplets that displace the liver cell nucleus and confer upon it an adipocyte-like appearance. Despite this distortion, liver function may be well preserved.

A much less common pattern is seen in association with *tetracycline* or *valproic acid* hepatotoxicity, and occasionally with alcoholic liver disease, and superficially resembles that seen in *Reye's syndrome, obstetric fatty liver,* and *Jamaican vomiting sickness.* It consists of fat deposited in smaller droplets throughout the liver cell, the nucleus remaining central. This pattern is usually associated with significant, occasionally fatal, disturbances in liver function.

GRANULOMAS. Granulomas are found in the liver in certain forms of drug-induced liver injury, and may be associated with extrahepatic granulomas and prominent systemic features. Included among the agents responsible are *phenylbutazone, quinidine, allopurinol, phenytoin, halothane,* and *hydralazine.*

CHRONIC HEPATITIS. Chronic hepatitis has been associated with an increasing number of drugs, including *amiodarone, dantrolene, isoniazid, methyldopa, nitrofurantoin, oxyphenisatin, perhexilene maleate, phenytoin, propylthiouracil, sulfonamides, acetaminophen,* and *aspirin.* Although these agents more often cause acute liver injury, prolonged use may occasionally result in a chronic progressive process leading in some instances to cirrhosis. In many cases, the lesion is largely or completely reversible, but in severe cases this may require many months after the drug is discontinued. Rarely, progressive liver failure and death may ensue despite cessation of the drug. *Ethanol* abuse occasionally is associated with a lesion similar to that of chronic active hepatitis.

TUMORS. Tumors caused by drugs and other chemical agents may be of several types, including *hepatic adenoma (and possibly hepatocellular carcinoma)* associated with *oral contraceptive* use, and *angiosarcoma* caused by prolonged exposure to *vinyl chloride* monomer or Thorotrast. The mechanisms by which these tumors are produced are not known, but their clinical and laboratory features generally resemble those of similar tumors occurring "spontaneously." A possible exception is the apparently greater size, vascularity, and tendency to sudden hemorrhage of hepatic adenomas associated with oral contraceptive use (see Ch. 129).

VASCULAR LESIONS. Vascular lesions of several kinds occasionally are caused by drugs. Oral contraceptives have been implicated as a cause of hepatic vein thrombosis. Hepatic *veno-occlusive disease,* a process that affects the smaller tributaries of the hepatic vein, has been associated with the use of *antitumor agents,* including *6-thioguanine* and *cytarabine* as well as with ingestion of *pyrrolidizine alkaloids,* e.g., from plants of *Senecio* and *Crotalaria* species ("bush tea poisoning"). *Oral contraceptives* and *anabolic steroids* have been identified as causes of *peliosis hepatis,* a condition in which the liver lobule contains extrasinusoidal blood-filled spaces; this lesion is also seen in certain chronic wasting neoplastic and inflammatory diseases.

SELECTED EXAMPLES OF DRUG-INDUCED LIVER DISEASE

ACETAMINOPHEN. Hepatotoxicity caused by acetaminophen is a classic example of a predictable, dose-dependent form of zonal necrosis. This readily available agent has been used with increasing frequency in suicide attempts. It causes death in acute liver failure, often associated with renal failure, and usually with doses in excess of 10 to 15 grams. Within several hours patients develop nausea, vomiting, and hypotension. This initial phase may then subside and the patient may exhibit few symptoms, but over the next 24 to 48 hours there appears clinical and laboratory evidence of progressive deterioration of liver function.

The injury apparently is caused by toxic products of acetaminophen biotransformation; above threshold levels these toxic products overwhelm the capacity of detoxification mechanisms (e.g., conjugation with glutathione or other acceptors) and appear to react directly with critical cell constituents or lead to the formation of highly reactive free radicles. The rate of formation of these toxic products reflects not only drug dose but also the activity of the cytochrome P-450–dependent microsomal drug metabolizing system. When the activity of this pathway has been stimulated by inducers such as phenobarbital or ethanol, increased amounts of toxic product are formed. The activity of this pathway and the availability of endogenous acceptors such as glutathione are probably important determinants of individual differences in susceptibility to acetaminophen toxicity. In addition, glutathione is important in many and diverse aspects of cell function; thus, depletion of this critically important substance may have major adverse effects apart from its unavailability to combine with toxic drug metabolites.

Although acute toxicity usually requires a dose in excess of 10 to 15 grams, the clinical history is quite unreliable as the basis for assessing prognosis in a given case. Far more useful is the acetaminophen plasma level: When it exceeds 200 mg per liter at four hours, 100 mg per liter at eight hours, or 50 mg per liter at 12 hours after ingestion, severe liver damage may occur. Subsidence of the early gastrointestinal symptoms is not necessarily a favorable prognostic sign, and measurement of the plasma concentration is important both for prognosis and for treatment. Treatment of the higher-risk patients with *N*-acetylcysteine within the first ten hours after ingestion may significantly improve chances for survival. *N*-acetylcysteine has been thought to act by providing additional cysteine for glutathione synthesis, but other possible mechanisms are not excluded. The recommended dose of *N*-acetylcysteine (Mucomyst) is 140 mg per kilogram orally initially, followed by maintenance doses of 70 mg per kilogram every four hours for a total of 72 hours. (In Britain, an intravenous preparation is available and is administered as follows: 150 mg per kilogram initially over 15 minutes, 50 mg per kilogram over the next four hours and 100 mg per kilogram over the next 16 hours.) In all cases, supportive care is also indicated, and early gastric aspiration may permit recovery of a substantial portion of the ingested dose. In survivors, recovery is virtually complete; there is no evidence of chronic progressive liver disease, but in some cases serum bile acid concentrations may be increased, and there may be residual hepatic fibrosis.

In addition to the acute effects of a massive overdose, acetaminophen may also cause liver injury when taken for a long time at doses within the therapeutic range (3 to 8 grams per day). On liver biopsy, either centrilobular necrosis or a picture suggestive of chronic hepatitis may be found. This injury is fully reversible after the drug is discontinued.

ASPIRIN. Usually in doses in excess of 3.0 grams per day, aspirin may cause abnormalities in serum transaminases and other liver function tests, associated with a biopsy picture of either a nonspecific or chronic hepatitis. Not unexpectedly, these effects are seen most often in patients with diseases such as juvenile and adult rheumatoid arthritis and systemic lupus erythematosus, in which long-term high-dose salicylate therapy may be employed. The mechanism of the injury is not known, but its clear-cut dose dependency suggests a toxic effect of either aspirin or a product of its biotransformation.

The diagnosis of aspirin hepatotoxicity should be suspected in any subject with abnormal liver function on a regimen of high-dose salicylate therapy. Serum salicylate concentrations will usually be found to exceed 20 mg per deciliter. The injury is rapidly and completely reversible when salicylates are discontinued. A potential source of confusion may arise when liver functions are abnormal in a patient with features of "autoimmune" disease and a liver biopsy suggestive of chronic active hepatitis. If the patient is taking salicylates and the serum salicylate concentration is compatible, this constellation of findings should suggest salicylate hepatotoxicity and should be managed accordingly, before giving consideration to corticosteroid treatment for chronic active hepatitis.

There has been recent concern regarding aspirin treatment of viral syndromes in children and its possible etiologic or contributory role in the development of Reye's syndrome. While a causal relationship has not been established, currently available epidemiologic evidence is sufficiently convincing to justify avoidance of aspirin in these circumstances.

CHLORPROMAZINE. This agent characteristically produces a cholestatic reaction, associated with variable local and systemic symptoms, including fever, anorexia, nausea, abdominal discomfort, and, occasionally, rash. On biopsy, a hepatocellular and canalicular cholestasis is found, together with a significant but variable lobular and portal inflammatory infiltrate and liver cell necrosis. The sporadic occurrence of this reaction, and its systemic features and frequently associated eosinophilia, have suggested "drug allergy." However, chlorpromazine may cause a form of toxic liver injury. Thus, among those using this drug in high doses or for prolonged periods, there is a high incidence of abnormal liver function tests. Furthermore, in acute animal experiments, chlorpromazine at doses approximating those used clinically causes an acute dose-related impairment of bile secretion. Finally, certain chlorpromazine metabolites have been shown to affect adversely several factors necessary for the formation of bile. Individual differences in susceptibility to chlorpromazine cholestasis may reflect corresponding differences in the rate of formation of the more toxic metabolites.

The prognosis of chlorpromazine cholestasis is generally favorable. Rarely, patients may exhibit a prolonged course resembling primary biliary cirrhosis despite discontinuation of the agent, but in these cases eventual recovery, even after three to four years, also is the rule. Fatal hepatic necrosis is rare. Therapeutic intervention is not indicated, other than discontinuation of the drug and symptomatic support (e.g., cholestyramine or colestipol for puritus); if cholestasis is prolonged, replacement of fat-soluble vitamins may be necessary.

ERYTHROMYCIN ESTOLATE. The lauryl sulfate salt of propionyl erythromycin may cause a cholestatic reaction with components of inflammation and necrosis of liver cells. A similar reaction occasionally has been associated with erythromycin ethylsuccinate and erythromycin propionate. Erythromycin estolate hepatotoxicity often presents as an acute syndrome of a right upper-quadrant pain, fever, and variable cholestasis, and there are several well-documented cases in which such patients were subjected to major surgery for presumed cholecystitis or cholangitis. The prognosis for the hepatic lesion is uniformly excellent, but the reaction may be expected to recur if the drug is readministered. The mechanism of the injury is unknown.

HALOTHANE. This anesthetic agent is now generally accepted as a rare cause of a viral hepatitis-like reaction and, even more rarely, of fatal massive hepatic necrosis. The mechanism of the injury is unknown. An immunologic basis has been invoked because most clinically apparent cases occur in persons with a history of prior exposure to halothane or a related agent, and because antibodies to hepatocyte surface membranes can be demonstrated in patients' serum (see above). On the other hand, halothane is predictably hepatotoxic in animals when circumstances favor its metabolism via reductive pathways, and its incidence appears to be higher among individuals with genetically determined impairment of enzymatic mechanisms for detoxifying harmful drug metabolites. Halothane hepatitis usually becomes evident approximately seven to ten days after anesthesia, but with repeated exposures the interval between administration of halothane and the clinical onset decreases. The course is indistinguishable from that of viral hepatitis, and the hepatitis may terminate fatally within days, or the patient may progress to rapid and complete recovery or exhibit a more prolonged course with eventual recovery. Despite earlier evidence to the contrary, single-exposure halothane hepatitis does not appear to lead to chronic hepatitis.

ISONIAZID (INH). The overall incidence of clinical hepatitis among persons taking *isoniazid* (INH) for single drug chemoprophylaxis against tuberculosis approximates 1 per cent, with a case fatality rate of about 10 per cent. Clinically and histologically, the disease resembles the wide spectrum of viral hepatitis, and may appear as a relatively mild acute process, a subacute or chronic hepatitis, or fatal massive necrosis. There is an important age effect on incidence, which may exceed 2 per cent among persons over the age of 50. Most cases become manifested within two to three months after the start of the drug, but the onset may be delayed for up to 12 months. Despite earlier reports to the contrary, there seems to be no apparent relationship between acetylator status (rapid as opposed to slow acetylators) and risk of hepatotoxicity.

In addition to the 1 per cent overall incidence of overt hepatitis, there is approximately a 10 to 20 per cent incidence of subclinical liver injury, manifested by mild to moderate increases in serum transaminase activity reflecting a focal nonspecific hepatitis. The laboratory abnormalities associated with this lesion appear nonprogressive and will subside in most patients despite continued administration of the drug.

The mechanism of neither of these two forms of expression of isoniazid hepatotoxicity is fully understood. However, there is evidence that a toxic metabolite may be involved. There is no evidence to suggest "drug allergy"; indeed, patients with isoniazid hepatitis usually lack clinical manifestations, such as skin rash and arthralgias, which might suggest drug allergy.

The clinical presentation of isoniazid hepatitis may be nonspecific, consisting initially of a "flu" syndrome or low-grade fever. For this reason, any patient receiving isoniazid should be followed at regular intervals and advised to report intercurrent symptoms. If these are found to be associated with clinical or laboratory evidence of disturbed liver function, the drug should be discontinued, pending further evaluation. A more difficult question concerns the appropriate management of the patient with an asymptomatic transaminase elevation early in the course of isoniazid treatment. Since there is at least a 90 per cent probability (especially in younger patients) that this finding reflects a transient and self-limited event rather than significant hepatitis, it is not generally recommended that liver function tests be routinely monitored in patients taking isoniazid. However, a several-fold elevation in transaminase levels in a patient over 35 years of age, even in the absence of symptoms, must be regarded as potentially serious and may be sufficient to justify discontinuation of the drug. As a general rule, the risk-benefit ratio for isoniazid chemoprophylaxis rises rapidly after age 35. In this group it is often best to err on the side of caution in deciding whether to employ chemoprophylaxis and by stopping the drug when in doubt regarding possible hepatotoxicity.

The management of suspected isoniazid hepatitis, apart from discontinuing the drug, is supportive. Fulminant hepatic failure should be treated as described in Ch. 128. There is no evidence that corticosteroids are of value in either acute or chronic forms of the disease.

RIFAMPIN. This antituberculous agent may cause liver injury. It reversibly impairs the hepatic uptake of bilirubin and sulfobromophthalein from plasma; it is also an inducer of the microsomal cytochrome P-450–dependent drug-metabolizing system. This latter effect has been cited as the mechanism by which rifampin may cause an unusually precipitous and severe form of isoniazid hepatitis when the two agents are administered together, but this possible drug interaction is not conclusively established. Rifampin itself has been implicated as a cause of acute hepatitis, but in most reported cases isoniazid was also being used; thus, the true incidence of rifampin hepatitis is unknown.

METHYLDOPA. This drug appears to be the only important antihypertensive agent with a significant incidence of hepatotoxicity. It is similar to isoniazid in that minor and apparently inconsequential abnormalities in liver function occur in perhaps 5 per cent of subjects, whereas overt acute or chronic hepatitis is much less common. There is a high incidence of serologic indicators of altered immunity in users of this drug, but hepatic injury does not correlate with Coombs' test positivity and may be mediated by a toxic drug metabolite. Most reported cases have resembled acute viral hepatitis, but this agent is also important among the growing list of drugs implicated as causes of chronic active hepatitis.

ORAL CONTRACEPTIVES. These hormonal agents have been associated with several adverse effects on the hepatobiliary system: (1) hepatocellular cholestasis, (2) hepatic vein thrombosis, (3) liver cell neoplasia, and (4) increased predisposition to cholesterol gallstone formation.

The *cholestatic effects* of oral contraceptives are largely attributable to the estrogenic component. Among oral contraceptive users, the majority exhibit subtle disturbances in bile secretory function (e.g., as demonstrated by measurement of the transport maximum for sulfobromophthalein), whereas only a few develop clinical cholestasis, with associated pruritus and jaundice. Histologically, there is usually little or no inflammation or hepatocellular necrosis. The syndrome is completely reversible, usually within two to three months, when the pill is discontinued. An entirely analogous situation may occur during the later stages of pregnancy, in which subclinical or mild cholestasis is common (e.g., mild pruritus), whereas clinically overt cholestasis ("recurrent intrahepatic cholestasis of pregnancy") is unusual and resolves rapidly after parturition. Cholestasis of pregnancy can be reproduced by subsequent administration of estrogens; it may be caused by a direct physical effect of the natural or synthetic estrogen on membrane components important in the bile secretory process. The obvious marked individual differences in susceptibility to this effect, although clearly not related to "drug allergy," are not well understood. The possible importance of genetic factors is suggested by the higher incidence of this problem among women with the Dubin-Johnson syndrome, the substantial differences in its incidence among descendants of certain Indian tribes in Chile, apparently unrelated to current location, diet, or other environmental factors, and the recent documentation of the familial occurrence of recurrent cholestasis of pregnancy.

Treatment of oral contraceptive-induced cholestasis consists of discontinuation of the drug, and symptomatic support (e.g., bile acid sequestrants for pruritus) as needed. Resolution should be rapid and complete; persistence of abnormalities beyond two or three months, or worsening at any time after the pill is discontinued, suggests the possibility that the agent may have simply unmasked some pre-existing clinically inapparent condition, and additional diagnostic evaluation may be indicated.

Farrell G, Prendergast D, Murray M: Halothane hepatitis. Detection of a constitutional susceptibility factor. N Engl J Med 313:1310, 1985. *Evidence for a genetically determined predisposition to halothane hepatitis based on impaired drug metabolism.*

Goldman IS, Winkler ML, Raper SE, et al.: Increased hepatic density and phospholipidosis due to amiodarone. AJR 144:541, 1985. *CT abnormalities in patients with histologically documented amiodarone hepatotoxicity.*

Kaplowitz N, Aw TY, Simon FR, et al.: Drug induced hepatotoxicity. Ann Intern Med 104:826, 1986. *A useful current review of mechanisms and clinical aspects of drug hepatotoxicity.*

Lewis JH, Zimmerman HJ, Benson GD, et al.: Hepatic injury associated with ketoconazole therapy. Analysis of 33 cases. Gastroenterology 86:503, 1984. *A summary and analysis of reported cases to date with histologic documentation and useful guidelines.*

McMaster KR, Hennigas GR: Drug-induced granulomatous hepatitis. Lab Invest 44:61, 1981. *A summary of implicated agents, with histopathologic documentation.*

Ockner RK: Drug-induced liver disease. In Zakim D, Boyer T (eds.): Hepatology. Philadelphia, W. B. Saunders Company, 1982, pp 691–722. *A classification and summary of pharmacologic agents that may cause liver injury, including consideration of mechanisms and clinical aspects.*

Seeff LB, Cuccherini BA, Zimmerman HJ, et al: Acetaminophen hepatotoxicity in alcoholics. A therapeutic misadventure. Ann Intern Med 104:399, 1986. *This paper and an accompanying editorial by M. Black and J. Raucy provide and review evidence regarding the mechanism by which alcohol use increases susceptibility to acetaminophen hepatotoxicity.*

Zimmerman HJ (ed.): Drug-induced liver disease. Semin Liver Dis 1:89, 1981. *A useful, multiauthored summary of advances and perspectives.*

Zimmerman HJ: Hepatotoxicity. The Adverse Effects of Drugs and Other Chemicals on the Liver. New York, Appleton-Century-Crofts, 1980. *A comprehensive and authoritative source. Well organized, readable, and thoroughly referenced.*

Zimmerman HJ: Hepatotoxic effects of oncotherapeutic agents. In Popper H, Schaffner F (eds.): Progress in Liver Diseases. Orlando, Grune & Stratton, 1986, vol 8, pp 621–642. *A useful and current summary, thoroughly referenced.*

123 CHRONIC HEPATITIS

Robert K. Ockner

GENERAL CONSIDERATIONS

DEFINITION. Chronic hepatitis is a sustained inflammatory process in the liver lasting more than six months to one year. It encompasses a wide spectrum of syndromes of diverse etiology, pathogenesis, histopathology, and clinical manifestations. In most, there is a variable element of hepatocellular necrosis. In its more severe forms, this inflammatory and necrotic process may lead to collapse of stromal elements, distortion of the lobular architecture, and a reparative process consisting of fibrosis and nodular regeneration (i.e., cirrhosis). The cell necrosis is associated with an inflammatory response that may be predominantly portal, periportal, or lobular in its distribution.

ETIOLOGY. Chronic hepatitis (Table 123–1) can be caused by *hepatitis B* (with or without superimposed hepatitis D) and *non-A, non-B* virus infection, *drugs* and *toxins* (see below and Ch. 122), and *inborn errors of metabolism* such as *Wilson's disease* and *alpha$_1$-antitrypsin deficiency*. In addition, there are one or more poorly understood types of *unknown etiology* in which clinical and laboratory features suggest but do not prove an immunologically mediated process.

CLINICAL AND LABORATORY MANIFESTATIONS AND DIAGNOSIS. Patients with chronic hepatitis may be entirely asymptomatic and exhibit only minimal abnormalities in routine laboratory tests, or may be incapacitated by progressive liver failure and the complications of portal hypertension. At any given time, the clinical and laboratory features may not correlate well with histopathology or long-term prognosis. For this reason, and because concepts of the natural history and response to treatment are changing for some of these disorders, decisions regarding diagnosis, management, and prognosis are often difficult and uncertain.

TABLE 123–1. CAUSES OF CHRONIC HEPATITIS

Chronic viral infections	
Hepatitis B	
Hepatitis B with superimposed hepatitis D	
Hepatitis non-A, non-B	
Drugs and toxins, including	
Acetaminophen	Nitrofurantoin
Amiodarone	Oxyphenisatin
Aspirin	Perhexilene maleate
Dantrolene	Phenytoin
Ethanol	Propylthiouracil
Isoniazid	Sulfonamides
Methyldopa	
Wilson's disease	
Alpha$_1$-Antitrypsin deficiency	
Idiopathic (? "autoimmune")	

These aspects of the various chronic hepatitis syndromes are considered in greater detail in the balance of this chapter.

PATHOLOGY. In most forms of chronic hepatitis there is a prominent portal inflammatory reaction, consisting mainly of mononuclear cells, especially small lymphocytes and plasma cells. There is also variable necrosis and inflammation involving hepatocytes immediately adjacent to the portal area. In this *periportal hepatitis* (or *"piecemeal necrosis"*) the inflammatory process invades the peripheral portions of the hepatic lobule, so that individual liver cells or nests of cells are isolated within the inflammatory zone. Periportal hepatitis is not specific for chronic hepatitis, and often is present in uncomplicated acute hepatitis and several other processes. For this reason it does not necessarily reflect a chronic or progressive process, and its significance can be judged only in the context of associated pathologic and clinical findings.

The lobular architecture may be substantially disrupted, as indicated by extension of the portal inflammatory and necrotic process into the lobule to a depth sufficient to span adjacent portal and/or central areas, i.e., *"bridging necrosis."* Although bridging necrosis can occur as part of an otherwise uncomplicated and self-limited acute hepatitis, it reflects a more severe injury that has a greater propensity to lead to progressive deterioration over a period of weeks to months (*"subacute hepatic necrosis"*) or to chronic active hepatitis and cirrhosis. Thus, its presence, or the presence of submassive necrosis or significant fibrosis in a patient with liver disease lasting more than six months, suggests a chronic and progressive process. Paradoxically, among survivors of the most extreme forms of acute liver injury, i.e., massive hepatic necrosis, chronic progressive liver disease is uncommon. Although the classification of chronic hepatitis that follows is based on histopathology, overlap is common, and differentiation of one from the other may be difficult.

CHRONIC PERSISTENT HEPATITIS

DEFINITION AND PATHOLOGY. Chronic persistent hepatitis is a nonprogressive inflammatory process largely confined to the portal areas. There is little or no periportal or lobular hepatitis; significant fibrosis and cirrhosis are absent. Of the small number of patients with acute hepatitis B whose illness becomes chronic, most will be found to have this lesion, and it is the most common form of chronic hepatitis. By definition, the diagnosis of persistent hepatitis is not appropriate if there is significant stromal collapse, fibrosis, or nodular regeneration.

CLINICAL AND LABORATORY MANIFESTATIONS. Chronic persistent hepatitis may be entirely asymptomatic or associated with nonspecific symptoms, including fatigue, anorexia, abdominal discomfort, or right upper-quadrant pain. Extrahepatic manifestations such as arthritis, glomerulonephritis, and vasculitis are rare. Jaundice, if present, is usually very mild. Physical findings are usually limited to palmar erythema, a few spider telangiectasias, and mildly tender hepatomegaly; the spleen occasionally is slightly enlarged. By definition, complications of advanced liver disease and portal hypertension, such as evidence of a collateral circulation, ascites, and encephalopathy, are absent.

Laboratory abnormalities are also mild, and include moderate increases in serum transaminases, bilirubin, and globulins. Albumin concentration and prothrombin time are usually normal. The serum is positive for HBsAg in perhaps 20 to 30 per cent of patients; other serologic tests such as mitochondrial, smooth muscle, and antinuclear antibodies are usually negative.

DIAGNOSIS, PROGNOSIS, AND MANAGEMENT. In any patient with persisting abnormalities of liver function, ethanol or other potential hepatotoxins should be discontinued, at least temporarily, to determine their possible etiologic significance. Because its clinical and laboratory features are totally nonspecific, the diagnosis of persistent hepatitis cannot be made without liver biopsy, but even biopsy does not always make it possible to distinguish this syndrome with certainty from chronic active hepatitis. In particular, HBsAg-positive individuals are subject to worsening of their hepatitis during a "reactivation" in which active virus replication is spontaneous or induced by immunosuppressive agents.

The outlook for persistent hepatitis usually is favorable, in that progression to cirrhosis or liver failure does not occur. However, the syndrome may last for ten years or more, and may cause continuing or intermittent discomfort or disability. Because of the difficulties inherent in the biopsy diagnosis of this group of disorders, continuing observation is important. Evidence of significant clinical deterioration may indicate the presence of a more serious process such as chronic active hepatitis, cirrhosis, or hepatocellular carcinoma and would be reason to consider repeating the liver biopsy. No specific treatment is indicated or available for chronic persistent hepatitis. Symptomatic and nutritional support is appropriate, and exposure to potential hepatotoxins should be avoided. For patients in whom alcohol has been excluded etiologically, small amounts of alcoholic beverages are permissible if they do not cause worsening of symptoms or laboratory tests. A form of chronic persistent hepatitis may be found in those patients in whom corticosteroid treatment of idiopathic or "autoimmune" chronic active hepatitis has induced a remission. The prognosis of this variant is less favorable, since about 50 per cent of such patients may have relapse after steroid therapy is discontinued.

CHRONIC LOBULAR HEPATITIS

This is a less well defined variant of chronic hepatitis in which the predominant lesion is a scattered single-cell necrosis in the lobule, with a relatively minor portal inflammatory component. It is, in effect, a variant of chronic persistent hepatitis, appearing not to progress to cirrhosis or liver failure except in those subjects in whom the disease becomes more active. Aside from those few patients in whom hepatitis B infection is present (with or without hepatitis D), a specific etiology is not identifiable.

CHRONIC ACTIVE HEPATITIS

DEFINITION. This is the most serious form of chronic hepatitis because of its potential for progression to cirrhosis and liver failure. It has been designated by a number of other essentially synonymous terms, such as *lupoid hepatitis, autoimmune hepatitis, plasma cell hepatitis, chronic aggressive hepatitis,* and *chronic active liver disease.*

ETIOLOGY. Approximately 20 per cent of cases are associated with, and presumably caused by, *chronic hepatitis B infection,* with or without superimposed hepatitis D infection (see Ch. 121). Chronic active hepatitis may also follow non-A, non-B hepatitis. Drugs that can cause the syndrome include *amiodarone, dantrolene, isoniazid, methyldopa, nitrofurantoin, oxyphenisatin, perhexilene maleate, phenytoin, propylthiouracil,* and *sulfonamides.* Long-term use of *acetaminophen, aspirin,* and *ethanol* occasionally may cause similar changes, as may *Wilson's disease* and *alpha$_1$-antitrypsin deficiency.* In a large number of cases the etiology is unknown, although many of this group exhibit clinical features and serologic abnormalities suggestive of autoimmunity. Despite such suggestive evidence, however, a truly "autoimmune" basis for chronic hepatitis has not been conclusively established, and in many instances phenomena that might be considered to reflect such a mechanism are also found in that form of the disease associated with hepatitis B virus infection. With time, specific etiologies may be identified for additional subsets of chronic active hepatitis.

PATHOLOGY. The syndrome is characterized by expansion of portal areas, which are infiltrated by lymphocytes and plasma cells, by periportal hepatitis, and by a variable degree of bridging necrosis, collapse, and fibrosis. In one third or more of patients, macronodular cirrhosis is present at the time of diagnosis. Except for the characteristic features of $alpha_1$-antitrypsin deficiency, which can be demonstrated by histochemistry, the various causes of chronic active hepatitis cannot be differentiated from one another on the basis of pathology.

CLINICAL MANIFESTATIONS. The course of chronic active hepatitis may be highly variable. The onset is usually insidious, but in perhaps one third of cases may resemble an acute hepatitis. It may affect all age groups and both sexes. However, HBsAg-negative cases occur mainly in young adult females, often associated with a more severe course and autoimmune features, whereas HBsAg-positive cases are more common in males and are often minimally symptomatic. Patients may be asymptomatic or may exhibit a wide range of local or constitutional symptoms typical of liver disease, such as fatigue, malaise, fever, anorexia, jaundice, or ascites.

Extrahepatic manifestations are often quite prominent and at times may dominate the clinical picture, especially in young females. These include amenorrhea, various skin rashes, glomerulonephritis, polyserositis, thyroiditis, vasculitis, Sjogren's syndrome, pneumonitis, depression of the formed elements of the blood, and an apparently increased incidence of ulcerative colitis.

Physical findings may also be quite variable. Patients may exhibit only a few spider telangiectasias, possibly with mild enlargement of liver and/or spleen, and may or may not be jaundiced. In advanced cases with cirrhosis, patients may have ascites, evidence of collateral circulation, or encephalopathy. In young women, acne and hirsutism may reflect the hormonal effects of chronic liver disease. Evidence of other extrahepatic manifestations may also be prominent, as noted above.

LABORATORY FINDINGS. Transaminases are usually increased over a range from minimally abnormal to in excess of 1000 IU. Globulins usually are diffusely increased, and the albumin value often is low. The alkaline phosphatase is usually only slightly to moderately increased; major increases should suggest the possibility of biliary tract disease or infiltrative or mass lesions. Prothrombin time generally reflects the severity of the disease, but may also be influenced by vitamin K deficiency. Because of their variability, the laboratory tests often poorly reflect the pathologic process; for this reason they do not always provide a reliable basis for the assessment of natural history or response to treatment.

Chronic active hepatitis is often characterized by the presence of a number of unusual but nonspecific immunoglobulins in serum, especially in patients who are negative for HBsAg. These include smooth muscle antibodies (positive in about two thirds), antinuclear antibodies (about one half), and antimitochondrial antibodies (about one third). Antibodies to a liver plasma membrane protein also have been demonstrated; their significance is unknown.

DIAGNOSIS. Diagnosis of chronic active hepatitis requires liver biopsy. In addition to the pathology, it is essential to establish a specific etiology, if possible, e.g., chronic hepatitis B infection, drugs, ethanol, Wilson's disease, or $alpha_1$-antitrypsin deficiency. Exposure to drugs and toxins usually can be identified by means of a careful history, including, when appropriate, questioning of family members or friends.

A positive test for HBsAg suggests that hepatitis B virus infection is causative, but even in these persons drugs, toxins, or superimposed hepatitis D also should be considered. Conversely, some cases of chronic active hepatitis may be caused by hepatitis B virus despite HBsAg-negative serum (in these patients serum usually has been positive for anti-HBc, but it may not be possible to definitively establish or exclude the diagnosis except by demonstrating the presence of HBV DNA in serum or liver by molecular hybridization). In some patients with chronic hepatitis B, a relapse—either spontaneous or following immunosuppressive therapy—may be followed by an apparent remission associated with seroconversion from HBe-positive to anti-HBe-positive and loss of other Dane particle markers from serum. This seroconversion is considered to represent a change from an actively replicative to a nonreplicative or integrated state of the HBV DNA. However, patients in this latter phase of the disease are still subject to reactivation of their disease, either spontaneous or resulting from immune suppression. Wilson's disease should be excluded in any patient with chronic hepatitis who is under the age of 40. Appropriate tests for this purpose include slit-lamp examination for Kayser-Fleischer rings, and measurement of serum ceruloplasmin and urinary copper excretion. If all tests are negative, additional studies are not necessary; when the suspicion persists, measurement of liver copper concentration or incorporation of radioactive copper into serum ceruloplasmin may be necessary (see Ch. 205). $Alpha_1$-antitrypsin deficiency can be excluded by protease-inhibitor phenotyping of serum and, in liver biopsy specimens, by the presence of PAS-positive material in hepatocytes after diastase treatment of the tissue section.

The *different diagnosis* includes *chronic persistent hepatitis, postnecrotic cirrhosis,* and some cases of *primary biliary cirrhosis* in which clinical and pathologic features may resemble those of chronic active hepatitis.

TREATMENT. Treatment of chronic active hepatitis not attributable to drugs, Wilson's disease, or $alpha_1$-antitrypsin deficiency has been studied in several large clinical trials. The great majority of patients included for study were symptomatic and had clinically obvious liver disease, and most were negative for HBsAg; however, criteria for inclusion, treatment programs, controls, and duration of follow-up differed substantially among the studies.

Generally, *corticosteroids,* with or without low-dose azathioprine, improve laboratory test results, reduce symptoms, suppress the inflammatory response seen on biopsy, and decrease short-term and long-term morbidity and mortality Thus, in the Mayo Clinic study, a favorable clinical, biochemical, and histologic response was seen initially in 56 per cent of patients, whereas spontaneous improvement occurred in only 20 per cent of placebo-treated controls; early mortality and progression to cirrhosis were also decreased. Similarly favorable results were observed in studies conducted at other institutions.

Despite this seemingly beneficial overall response, several factors that importantly influence the natural history and response to treatment must be considered in making the decision to institute a chronic treatment program with potentially significant adverse effects. First, corticosteroid therapy is not indicated for chronic hepatitis B (with or without hepatitis D), as these patients do not benefit and their status may even deteriorate as a result. Second, chronic hepatitis does not usually progress to cirrhosis or liver failure in the absence of bridging necrosis on liver biopsy; the absence of such changes would weigh significantly against the use of corticosteroids. Third, there is no evidence that corticosteroids are of benefit in asymptomatic chronic active hepatitis. Fourth, since the reported series contain an unknown number of patients with chronic non-A, non-B hepatitis, and since the natural history of this disorder is highly variable, it is difficult to assess the impact of corticosteroids in this group, although the presence or absence of "autoimmune" features seemed to be of little consequence in the Mayo Clinic series. Finally, since many patients with chronic active hepatitis would fail to meet the criteria for inclusion in some of the published series, any decision regarding their treatment is necessarily an extrapolation from a limited study population.

In view of this substantial uncertainty concerning the value of corticosteroids in certain subsets of chronic active hepatitis, it is very difficult to make broadly applicable recommendations as to their use. In general, however, an initially favorable response would most likely be expected in a young, HBsAg-negative female with progressive disease characterized by prominent symptoms and autoimmune features and no recent transfusion or other exposure to non-A, non-B hepatitis. Since there appear to be exceptions, such decisions must be individualized.

In the Mayo Clinic study, an initial daily dose of 60 mg of prednisone or of 30 mg of prednisone combined with 50 mg of azathioprine, tapering gradually over several weeks to months to a daily maintenance dose of 20 mg of prednisone or 10 mg of prednisone plus 50 mg of azathioprine, was found to be most effective. The azathioprine was of no value when given alone, but permitted use of the lower prednisone dose, thereby reducing the incidence of significant steroid-related complications, which otherwise approximated 60 per cent. Alternate-day treatment was less effective. If a favorable response is not observed within two to three months, treatment should be discontinued.

Patients being treated for chronic active hepatitis should be examined and have their liver function checked periodically. The possible side effects of drug treatment should be monitored and liver biopsies should be repeated at intervals of six months to one year, depending on the circumstances. Return of liver enzymes to a level less than twice the upper limit of normal, together with a liver biopsy showing subsidence of the inflammatory and necrotic process to a picture similar to that of persistent hepatitis, is considered a successful response and warrants an attempt gradually to discontinue treatment. In about 50 per cent of patients, this attempt will succeed and additional corticosteroid treatment will not be needed. In the remainder, evidence of relapse may suggest the need for reinstitution of therapy.

Unfortunately the disease may eventually progress to cirrhosis despite an apparently favorable clinical response, especially in those patients in whom repeated recurrences of activity require treatment over a period of three years or longer. Over these longer intervals the advisability of continued corticosteroid therapy must be judged not only on the basis of symptoms and laboratory and biopsy findings but also in recognition of the possibility of diminishing returns in the face of increasing risks. The possible effectiveness of other experimental approaches to the treatment of chronic active hepatitis, including the use of interferon and adenine arabinoside in chronic hepatitis B, remains to be determined.

SPECIAL CLINICAL PROBLEMS

Two circumstances are encountered in clinical practice with sufficient frequency that they deserve particular comment with reference to diagnostic approach and management.

UNEXPECTED INCREASE OF SERUM TRANSAMINASES. The advent and common use of multiphasic laboratory screening techniques have led to the identification of individuals in whom transaminase activities are abnormal but who lack clinical evidence of liver disease. If the abnormal finding is confirmed, and if it does not reflect muscle or other extrahepatic disease, it may have either of two possible implications: (1) It may reflect a subclinical acute process (e.g., acute viral hepatitis), or (2) it may reflect a chronic process (e.g., chronic toxic or viral hepatitis). If the patient is asymptomatic or nearly so, a period of observation is appropriate, and follow-up studies and hepatitis serologies should be obtained. Alcohol and potentially hepatotoxic drugs and toxins should be avoided. Improvement would presumably reflect resolution of a self-limited process or the response to removal of a toxin, e.g., ethanol. Worsening of the results may herald the clinical onset of a more overt syndrome, the proper evaluation of which would depend on the circumstances. Persistence of the abnormality beyond six to twelve months may reflect a chronic hepatitis and may justify liver biopsy.

HEPATITIS B SURFACE ANTIGEN POSITIVITY. Approximately 0.1 to 0.2 per cent of the population of the United States is positive for HBsAg. At any given time, most of these persons exhibit no overt evidence of liver disease and are designated carriers. The meaning of the term *carrier* varies, however, and has been used to include all chronically positive individuals, or only those who have no apparent liver disease.

The practical question of significance concerns the management of the patient with a positive test. If the result is confirmed, it could indicate (1) a subclinical acute hepatitis B, (2) chronic hepatitis (persistent or active) or cirrhosis, or (3) a "healthy" carrier state. Although differentiation of these conditions may require liver biopsy, HBsAg-positive persons who have no clinical or laboratory evidence of liver disease usually have normal or nonspecific biopsy findings. For the few among this group of *asymptomatic persons with normal liver function tests* who may have chronic active hepatitis on biopsy, there is no evidence that corticosteroid treatment is indicated. Therefore, these individuals can be followed at intervals without first obtaining a liver biopsy. Those HBsAg-positive persons who do have clinical and/or laboratory signs of liver disease should be managed in accordance with the severity and duration of the process; persistence of the abnormalities beyond six months may suggest a chronic hepatitis and the need for liver biopsy.

Alter HJ (ed.): Hepatitis. Semin Liv Dis 6:1, 1986. *A minisymposium in which clinically relevant aspects of acute and chronic hepatitis are discussed by a group of recognized experts.*

Bonino F, Smedile A: Delta agent (type D) hepatitis. Semin Liv Dis 6:28, 1986. *A summary of this unusual agent prepared by workers in the unit where it was first identified.*

Czaja AJ: Natural history, clinical features and treatment of autoimmune hepatitis. Semin Liv Dis 4:1, 1984. *A summation of the Mayo Clinic experience.*

Czaja AJ, Davis GL, Ludwig J, et al.: Autoimmune features as determinants of prognosis in steroid-treated chronic active hepatitis of uncertain etiology. Gastroenterology 85:713, 1983. *Follow-up data in chronic non-B disease, indicating little difference between patients with and without "autoimmune" features.*

Czaja AJ, Ludwig J, Baggenstoss AH, et al.: Corticosteroid-treated chronic active hepatitis in remission. Uncertain prognosis of chronic persistent hepatitis. N Engl J Med 304:1, 1981.

Davis GL, Czaja AJ, Ludwig J: Development and prognosis of histologic cirrhosis in corticosteroid-treated hepatitis B surface antigen-negative chronic active hepatitis. Gastroenterology. 87:1222, 1984. *A useful observation, based on the Mayo Clinic experience, that histologic cirrhosis in these patients may not have major effects on prognosis.*

Davis GL, Hoofnagle JH, Waggoner JG: Spontaneous reactivation of chronic hepatitis B virus infection. Gastroenterology 86:230, 1984. *A series of cases in which clinically significant reactivation was not preceded by immunosuppressive therapy.*

Gregory P: Interferon in chronic hepatitis B. Gastroenterology 90:237, 1986. Sherlock S, Thomas HC: Treatment of chronic hepatitis due to hepatitis B virus. Lancet 2:1343, 1985. *Two concise overviews of the current status of antiviral therapy.*

Hoofnagle JH, Dusheiko GM, Seeff LB, et al.: Seroconversion from hepatitis B e antigen to antibody in chronic type B hepatitis. Ann Intern Med 94:744, 1981. *Information on natural history and possible implications of spontaneous changes in the e-anti-e system with time.*

Liaw Y-F, Chu C-M, Chen T-J, et al.: Chronic lobular hepatitis: A clinicopathological and prognostic study. Hepatology 2:258, 1982. *A generally benign disorder warranting no specific treatment.*

Scott J, Gollan JL, Samourian S, et al.: Wilson's disease presenting as chronic active hepatitis. Gastroenterology 74:645, 1978. *A thorough clinical and pathologic description of 17 patients presenting with features of chronic active hepatitis. Emphasis is placed on the often difficult problem of different diagnosis.*

Scullard GH, Smith CI, Merigan TC, et al.: Effects of immunosuppressive therapy on viral markers in chronic active hepatitis B. Gastroenterology 81:987, 1981. *Evidence that viral replication may be potentiated.*

Sherman M, Shafritz DA: Hepatitis B virus and hepatocellular carcinoma: Molecular biology and mechanistic considerations. Sem Liv Dis 4:98, 1984. *A useful summary of the continually evolving concepts in this important area.*

Vyas GN, Deinstag JL, Hoofnagle JH (eds.): Viral Hepatitis and Liver Disease. Orlando, Grune & Stratton, 1984. *Proceedings of a March, 1984, international symposium. Concepts in virtually all aspects of the field are presented, discussed, and referenced.*

124 PARASITIC, BACTERIAL, FUNGAL, AND GRANULOMATOUS LIVER DISEASE

Bruce F. Scharschmidt

PARASITIC DISEASE OF THE LIVER AND BILIARY TRACT

The parasitic disorders of humans are discussed in detail in Part XIX. Those parasitic disorders that commonly involve the liver and biliary tract are outlined in Table 124–1. With respect to diagnosis, the most important first step is a carefully obtained history of travel or residence in an endemic area and potential exposure to the parasite. For example, prior travel or residence in Central Africa or the Middle East in a patient with hepatomegaly and portal hypertension suggests the diagnosis of *schistosomiasis.* In East Asia, prior ingestion of raw or undercooked freshwater fish in a patient with biliary disease should raise the possibility of *clonorchiasis* or opisthorchiasis. A history of cattle or sheep raising in a patient being investigated for hepatic mass should suggest *echinococcosis* and interdict the use of needle biopsy until the possibility of a cystic lesion has been excluded. Ingestion of uncooked freshwater plants (e.g., watercress) from cattle- or sheep-raising areas may be an important clue to the presence of *fascioliasis,* and a history of contact with pet cats and dogs, particularly puppies, is typically obtained from patients with *toxocariasis.*

Tender hepatomegaly and eosinophilia are commonly present during the invasive phase of many helminthic disorders, including *ascariasis, toxocariasis, strongyloidiasis, schistosomiasis,* and *fascioliasis,* yet the diagnosis may not be suspected until weeks, months, or even years later when complications resulting from the presence of eggs or the adult parasite appear. At this time, eosinophilia may no longer be present. Except in echinococcosis, serologic and skin tests are of limited value in the helminthic disorders, and the diagnosis generally requires demonstration of larvae or ova in feces or tissue.

Protozoan disorders also frequently involve the liver, and *malaria* is among the most common causes of hepatomegaly worldwide. However, hepatic involvement in malaria and in most protozoan infections represents a relatively minor component of the overall clinical disorder. The outstanding exception is *amebiasis,* of which hepatic amebic abscess is the most life-threatening manifestation (see Liver Abscess, below). In comparison to the helminthic disorders, protozoan infections are less frequently accompanied by eosinophilia and can more often be diagnosed by serologic tests.

Treatment of the helminthic disorders is discussed in Ch. 392 to 413. In addition to eradication of the parasite, biliary tract surgery may be necessary in patients with ascariasis, clonorchiasis, opisthorchiasis, or fascioliasis who develop complications such as biliary obstruction, infection, or stone formation. Patients with schistosomiasis and recurrent life-threatening hemorrhage caused by esophageal varices may be candidates for portacaval anastomosis. However, all adult worms should be eradicated prior to such surgery to prevent systemic dissemination of ova. The treatment of amebic liver abscess is discussed later in this chapter. Treatment of other protozoan disorders involving the liver is discussed in Ch. 381 to 391.

MYCOTIC LIVER DISEASE

Hepatic involvement is frequently absent or constitutes a minor component of mycotic disease in man, but virtually all fungal infections, when disseminated, can involve the liver. These include histoplasmosis, cryptococcosis, mucormycosis, aspergillosis, coccidioidomycosis, North and South American blastomycosis, candidiasis, sporotrichosis, and actinomycosis. Hepatic pathologic changes may include granulomas, hepatocellular necrosis, and abscesses. The manifestations, diagnosis, and treatment of mycotic disease are discussed in detail in Ch. 368 to 379.

HEPATIC MANIFESTATIONS OF SYSTEMIC BACTERIAL INFECTION

Many systemic infections can be accompanied by minor abnormalities of standard liver function tests and, less commonly, jaundice. Since these changes typically occur in the absence of demonstrable invasion of the hepatic parenchyma by the infecting organism(s), they are generally attributed to the hepatic effects of various toxins. For example, bacterial endotoxin has been implicated in the cholestasis occasionally associated with gram-negative bacterial infections. Staphylococcal exotoxin(s) appears responsible for the cholestasis that sometimes accompanies the toxic shock syndrome. Fever and hypoxemia also adversely affect liver cell function. Infection by gram-positive cocci (particularly pneumococcus), gram-negative cocci (e.g., gonococcus), and gram-negative bacilli (particularly *Escherichia coli* infections in infants) may all be accompanied by jaundice. The jaundice and/or abnormal liver function tests in these patients resolve with successful treatment of the infection, and the importance of these abnormalities lies primarily in the fact that they may be mistaken for other disorders such as viral hepatitis or biliary tract obstruction.

In addition, certain organisms can affect the liver directly. Hepatic invasion by streptococci or salmonellae is a rare cause of liver dysfunction and a hepatitis-like illness. Gonococcal perihepatitis *(Fitz-Hugh-Curtis syndrome)* typically occurs in women with concomitant or recent pelvic inflammatory disease and causes an acute inflammatory reaction in the hepatic capsule accompanied by right upper quadrant pain and fever. "Violin-string" adhesions between the anterior abdominal wall and liver surface may result. *Treponema pallidum* may also invade the liver, and secondary syphilis is accompanied by a hepatitis-like illness in up to 10 per cent of cases. Hepatitis associated with secondary syphilis differs from most other forms of acute hepatic injury in that it is typically associated with markedly increased alkaline phosphatase activity in serum.

LIVER ABSCESS

Pyogenic Liver Abscess

DEFINITION. A pyogenic liver abscess is a macroscopic collection of pus within the hepatic parenchyma that results from bacterial infection.

ETIOLOGY. Enteric flora (particularly *Escherichia coli* and *Klebsiella*) and pyogenic gram-positive cocci (particularly *Staphylococcus aureus*) are common causes of pyogenic liver abscess. With appropriate culture techniques, anaerobic bacteria have been isolated from one half or more of pyogenic abscesses, and multiple bacterial species are present in up to two thirds of cases. While mycotic and mycobacterial infections are unusual causes of macroscopic hepatic abscesses in healthy individuals, systemic candidiasis with multiple hepatic abscesses has been recognized with increasing frequency in patients with leukemia and neutropenia. Failure to isolate any organism from a presumed pyogenic abscess occurs relatively frequently and may reflect inappropriate sample handling or culture technique or misdiagnosis of an amebic abscess.

INCIDENCE. Liver abscess is an uncommon disorder, accounting for less than 1 per cent of most necropsy series. This relative infrequency is somewhat surprising when one

TABLE 124–1. COMMON PARASITIC DISEASES OF THE LIVER AND BILIARY TRACT

Disorder (Organism)	Principal Endemic Areas	Nature of Hepatic Involvement: *Pathophysiology*	*Manifestations*	*Diagnosis*
Helminthic disorders				
Ascariasis (*Ascaris lumbricoides*)	Worldwide; most common in underdeveloped areas of Asia, Africa, and tropics	Initially larvae carried to liver by portal blood; later, adult worms may enter the biliary tree from the intestine and deposit eggs	Occasional hepatomegaly and fever during larval migration; later, granuloma formation, biliary obstruction, biliary colic, cholangitis, and stone formation	Identification of ova in feces
Toxocariasis (*Toxocara canis, T. cati*)	North and South America, Europe, India	Larval migration in hepatic parenchyma (visceral larva migrans)	Hepatomegaly, granuloma formation	Identification of larvae in tissue, serologic testing
Strongyloidiasis (*Strongyloides stercoralis*)	Tropics	Larval invasion of liver with hyperinfective syndrome (rare)	Granuloma formation	Identification of larvae in stool or duodenal juice, filarial complement fixation test
Echinococcosis (*Echinococcus granulosus, E. multilocularis*)	Worldwide	Growth of larval form (hydatid cyst) in liver	Signs and symptoms of a hepatic mass, cyst rupture, secondary infection, rarely portal hypertension with *E. multilocularis*	Serologic tests, including hemagglutination and complement fixation
Schistosomiasis (*Schistosoma mansoni, S. japonicum*)	East Asia, Central Africa, Middle East, and South America	Adult worms live in portal venous system, eggs carried to liver by portal blood	Granuloma formation, hepatomegaly, portal hypertension and its complications	Identification of eggs in feces or tissue (e.g., rectal mucosa, liver)
Clonorchiasis (*Clonorchis sinensis*)	East Asia	Worms grow and deposit eggs in bile ducts	Granuloma formation, biliary obstruction and infection, stone formation, cholangiocarcinoma	Identification of ova in stool
Opisthorchiasis (*Opisthorchis felineus, O. viverrini*)	Europe, Asia, and Thailand	Worms grow and deposit eggs in bile ducts	Similar to clonorchiasis	Identification of ova in stool
Fascioliasis (*Fasciola hepatica*)	Worldwide	Larvae migrate through hepatic parenchyma to the bile ducts	Hepatomegaly and fever during invasive phase; later, biliary obstruction and infection	Identification of ova in stool
Protozoan disorders				
Amebiasis (*Entamoeba histolytica*)	Worldwide	Invasion of hepatic parenchyma	Signs and symptoms of hepatic abscess, extension and rupture into adjacent structures	Serologic tests, including gel diffusion precipitin and indirect hemagglutination, for tissue invasion; sigmoidoscopy and stool examination for intestinal infection
Malaria (*Plasmodium falciparum, P. vivax, P. ovale, P. malariae*)	Africa, Asia, Central and South America	Pre-erythrocytic (all types) and exoerythrocytic stages (except *P. falciparum*) present in liver	Centrolobular necrosis with acute *P. falciparum* infection, hepatosplenomegaly with chronic malaria	Identification of plasmodia in blood smear
Visceral leishmaniasis (*Leishmania donovani*)	Mediterranean basin, Asia, Africa, South America	Infection of mononuclear phagocytic cells of liver and other organs	Hepatosplenomegaly, fever	Identification of parasite in tissue, serologic testing
Toxoplasmosis (*Toxoplasma gondii*)	Worldwide	Parasite multiplication in liver	Hepatosplenomegaly	Serologic tests, including indirect fluorescent antibody test and Sabin-Feldman dye test; isolation of organism from tissue or body fluid
Trypanosomiasis (*Trypanosoma brucei, T. gambiense, T. rhodesiense*) (*T. cruzi*)	Tropical Africa; South and Central America	Hepatic involvement during acute systemic phase	Hepatosplenomegaly, hepatocellular necrosis and jaundice occasionally with *T. rhodesiense* infections	Identification of parasite in blood, tissue, or cerebrospinal fluid; serologic testing

considers the large blood flow to the liver and its strategic position between the portal and systemic circulations.

PATHOGENESIS. The most common predisposing cause for pyogenic hepatic abscess is currently biliary tract disease, including acute cholecystitis as well as disorders leading to obstruction of the ductal system. Infection in areas drained by the portal venous system (e.g., appendicitis, diverticulitis, Crohn's disease) may also result in pylephlebitis and pyogenic hepatic abscess, but this occurs less frequently now than in the preantibiotic era. Other causes include direct extension from adjacent structures other than the biliary tree (subphrenic or perinephric abscess), penetrating or blunt abdominal trauma, septicemia, and infection arising in necrotic primary or secondary tumor deposits. In many cases, no predisposing cause is apparent. Pyogenic liver abscesses may be single or multiple. Multiple small abscesses occur particularly frequently in association with pylephlebitis, biliary tract obstruction with cholangitis, and septicemia.

CLINICAL MANIFESTATIONS. The symptoms of hepatic abscess are usually those of a systemic febrile illness lasting from several days to weeks, although multiple small abscesses related to cholangitis or septicemia tend to appear dramatically and suddenly. No characteristics of the fever pattern reliably distinguish hepatic abscesses from abscesses elsewhere in the body. In addition to fever and symptoms of chronic illness, such as weight loss and anorexia, patients may complain of abdominal pain or distension. Jaundice is present in up to 20 per cent of cases and often indicates concomitant biliary tract disease with cholangitis. Extension or rupture into the pleural, pericardial, or peritoneal space occurs less commonly with pyogenic than with amebic abscesses.

The most common physical findings are hepatomegaly and

right upper quadrant tenderness. However, unlike the liver in acute hepatitis, a point of maximal tenderness may be demonstrable by palpation or percussion. Even without extension into the pleural space, basilar rales may be present, or the right hemidiaphragm may be elevated or fixed.

DIAGNOSIS. Routine laboratory studies are not particularly helpful. As with any abscess of comparable duration and severity, leukocytosis and anemia are frequently present. Alkaline phosphatase is elevated in most cases, and other liver function tests may be normal to mildly abnormal. Marked hyperbilirubinemia is uncommon.

Radiologic studies are frequently useful. Roentgenograms of the chest reveal abnormalities such as elevation of the right hemidiaphragm, basilar atelectasis, or pleural effusion in about half of cases. While radionuclide scanning detects most larger abscesses, ultrasonography is probably more sensitive in identifying smaller lesions and may help distinguish abscesses from simple cysts or tumors. Computed tomography is also capable of detecting even small lesions; however, the appearance of abscesses on computed tomography and ultrasonography is quite variable, and the distinction between abscess and tumor cannot always be made reliably by any imaging method.

Blood cultures have been positive in up to 60 per cent or more of reported cases and should be obtained routinely when a hepatic abscess is suspected. On the basis of clinical findings and chest roentgenograms, pyogenic liver abscesses are most commonly mistaken for pneumonia, hepatitis, cholecystitis, or cholangitis.

TREATMENT. When a hepatic abscess is strongly suspected on the basis of clinical, laboratory, and radiologic findings, blood cultures should be drawn and antibiotic therapy begun. Antibiotics should be chosen to include coverage for gram-negative enteric bacteria and anaerobic organisms as well as possibly for enterococci or *S. aureus*. If amebic abscess is a possibility, empiric therapy for this disorder (e.g., metronidazole) should be included.

Although surgical drainage of large solitary abscesses has long been the accepted approach to therapy and is still strongly recommended by many authorities, there are now several reported series of patients treated successfully without surgery. If such a nonoperative approach is chosen, accessible lesion(s) should be aspirated both to confirm the diagnosis and to obtain material for Gram's stain and culture. Aspiration is best performed under sonographic or computed tomographic guidance and should be performed after the beginning of antibiotic therapy and institution of appropriate supportive measures (Fig. 124–1). It is appropriate to drain as much of the abscess content as possible at the time of the diagnostic aspiration, and consideration should be given to leaving in a drainage catheter. Antibiotic therapy should be modified as necessary on the basis of the results of cultures of blood or abscess content. Antibiotics are generally administered parenterally for the first 10 to 14 days and continued for a total of four to six weeks. Even in patients successfully treated by this approach, abnormalities on radionuclide scanning or sonography may persist for months.

Surgical consultation is appropriate for all patients in whom hepatic abscess is strongly suspected, even if the nonoperative approach just outlined is elected, because emergency surgery may be necessary in patients who fail to respond to this treatment or in patients who suffer complications from percutaneous aspiration or drainage. For patients with multiple small abscesses not amenable to surgical drainage, antibiotic administration with attempted aspiration of the largest, most accessible lesions is the only therapy possible, and antibiotics must frequently be administered for several months in such cases. Conversely, surgical intervention is necessary for patients in whom the abscess(es) is due to a predisposing surgical disorder such as intra-abdominal sepsis or biliary tract obstruction. Percutaneous drainage of the biliary system may also be at least temporarily used in the latter group (see Ch. 130).

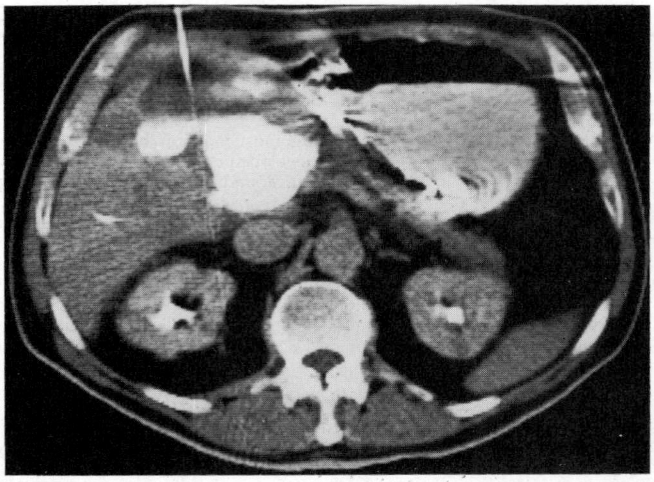

FIGURE 124–1. Computed tomogram showing CT-directed needle aspiration of a liver abscess. The needle is seen as the thin dense linear object entering the liver from the anterior abdominal wall. Contrast material has been introduced into the abscess cavity through the needle in order to outline the extent of the abscess.

PROGNOSIS. The prognosis for patients with pyogenic hepatic abscesses has improved considerably since antibiotics have become available, but this remains a serious illness with reported mortality ranging from 10 to 60 per cent. The prognosis is adversely affected by the presence of multiple abscesses that cannot be surgically drained, advanced age, underlying malignant disease, or extension or rupture into the pleural, pulmonary, or pericardial cavities.

Amebic Liver Abscess

INCIDENCE. In developed countries, such as the United States, liver abscess is most commonly of bacterial origin. In contrast, amebic liver abscess predominates in areas of the world in which sanitation is poor and is a relatively common disorder in some countries. The factor(s) that predisposes to liver abscess in a patient with intestinal amebiasis is unknown. A more general discussion of amebiasis is found in Ch. 390.

CLINICAL MANIFESTATIONS. The clinical and laboratory features of amebic liver abscess are very similar to those of pyogenic liver abscess. Clues to the presence of an amebic as opposed to a pyogenic abscess include age less than 50 years, recent travel to an endemic area, and the absence of any evident intra-abdominal or biliary disease. Approximately 10 per cent of patients have symptoms of more than two weeks' duration, and occasionally symptoms have been present for months. While fever and leukocytosis are typical features of an amebic abscess, very high fever and a leukocyte count in excess of 20,000 per cubic millimeter may represent clues to secondary bacterial infection. Less than one half of patients have a history of recent diarrhea suggestive of intestinal amebiasis, and *Entamoeba histolytica* is identified in the stool of only one third of patients with an abscess. Extension of the abscess into the pleural space commonly causes cough, dyspnea, pleurisy, or even symptoms of a bronchohepatic fistula. Overall, extension or rupture into the pleural, pericardial, or peritoneal cavity occurs in up to 10 per cent of patients. Rupture into the pericardial or peritoneal cavity is particularly frequent with abscesses in the left lobe.

DIAGNOSIS. Routine laboratory studies, chest roentgenogram, radionuclide scan, ultrasound examination, and computed tomography reveal abnormalities very similar to those of pyogenic abscess. Although amebic abscesses are most commonly solitary and located in the right lobe, they may be multiple and can occur in other locations.

Serologic testing is extremely valuable in the diagnosis of amebic liver abscess. Indirect hemagglutination, the standard test performed by the Parasitology Division of the Centers for Disease Control in Atlanta, is positive in more than 90 per cent of patients with amebic liver abscess, and antibody titers remain elevated for many years. The gel diffusion precipitin test, which is available in most state laboratories and many local hospitals, is similarly positive in more than 90 per cent of cases, but reverts to negative in most patients within one year after successful treatment. This fact can be an advantage in distinguishing active disease from past infection.

TREATMENT. For patients with an amebic abscess, medical therapy alone is usually sufficient. Metronidazole (750 mg three times daily for ten days) is the drug of choice, and some authorities recommend that an intestinal amebicide such as diiodohydroxyquin (650 mg three times daily for 20 days) be given in addition. Chloroquine (500 mg daily for 10 weeks) is reportedly equally effective, but the long duration of treatment and lack of efficacy against intestinal amebae render it less desirable. A variety of alternative regimens also exist, including a single-day drug treatment regimen (see Ch. 390). Most patients report rapid symptomatic improvement after both forms of therapy and are afebrile by the end of the first week. However, since metronidazole is also effective against anaerobic bacteria present in pyogenic liver abscesses, a favorable therapeutic response to this agent cannot, by itself, be considered proof of an amebic versus a pyogenic abscess. Rare treatment failures have been reported, and it is particularly important in such cases to make sure that any concomitant intestinal infection has been eradicated. The role of needle aspiration in the treatment of amebic abscess is controversial. Some advocate it routinely and report excellent results; however, there are no controlled studies to support the therapeutic value of aspiration, and most patients recover with medical therapy alone. Aspiration should be undertaken only by skilled personnel, after appropriate medical therapy has been begun, and is probably most appropriate for patients with impending rupture as evidenced by increasing pleural or pericardial reaction or progressive hepatic enlargement, particularly with abscesses in the left lobe for patients in whom the diagnosis is uncertain and for patients who fail to respond to appropriate therapy within three to four days. Surgery is rarely necessary.

PROGNOSIS. The prognosis in uncomplicated amebic abscess is excellent with appropriate medical therapy, the mortality being as low as 1 per cent in some series. With extension or rupture into the pleural, pericardial, or peritoneal space, the mortality increases sharply. The presence of jaundice is associated with a higher incidence of complications and a higher mortality. Even after successful treatment, resolution of the radionuclide scan defect caused by an amebic abscess may require many months.

GRANULOMATOUS DISEASE OF THE LIVER

ETIOLOGY. The liver is one of the most frequent sites in the body for granuloma formation. By virtue of its large number of mononuclear phagocytic cells and strategic location, the liver clears the circulation of many substances, including microorganisms, antigens, and immune complexes. In addition, the liver is the major site of metabolism of many drugs and toxins. These factors help account for the 2 to 10 per cent incidence of granulomas found in liver biopsies.

Hepatic granulomas have been reported in association with a wide variety of infectious and other systemic illnesses, hepatobiliary disorders, and drugs or exogenous agents (Table 124–2). Since granulomas are not a rare finding in liver biopsy material, it is possible that some of the reported associations are spurious. The relative frequency with which various underlying disorders have been associated with hepatic granulomas varies with the patient population under study. Sarcoidosis, tuberculosis, and, more recently, drug reactions have accounted for the largest proportion of patients in the United States and Western Europe.

TABLE 124–2. HEPATIC GRANULOMAS (REPORTED ASSOCIATIONS)

Infections
- Bacterial, mycobacterial, spirochetal
  - Tuberculosis
  - Atypical mycobacteria
  - Tularemia
  - Brucellosis
  - Leprosy
  - Typhoid fever
  - Granuloma inguinale
  - Syphilis
  - Whipple's disease
  - Listeriosis
  - Melioidosis
  - BCG immunotherapy
  - Cat-scratch disease
- Viral
  - Infectious mononucleosis
  - Cytomegalovirus
  - Chickenpox
  - Influenza B
  - Lymphogranuloma venereum
- Rickettsial
  - Q fever
- Fungal
  - Coccidioidomycosis
  - Histoplasmosis
  - Cryptococcosis
  - Actinomycosis
  - Blastomycosis
  - Aspergillosis
  - Nocardiosis
  - Torulopsosis
  - Candidiasis
- Parasitic
  - Amebiasis
  - Giardiasis
  - Schistosomiasis
  - Clonorchiasis
  - Fascioliasis
  - Toxocariasis
  - Ascariasis
  - Toxoplasmosis
  - Strongyloidiasis
  - Ancyclostomiasis
  - Tongue worm (Pentastomida)

Hepatobiliary disorders
- Primary biliary cirrhosis
- Chronic active hepatitis
- Granulomatous hepatitis
- Jejunoileal bypass

Systemic disorders
- Sarcoidosis
- Wegener's granulomatosis
- Vineyard sprayer's lung
- Inflammatory bowel disease
- Chronic granulomatous disease
- Allergic granulomatosis
- Granulomatous arteritis-polymyalgia rheumatica
- Melanoma
- Hodgkin's disease
- Lymphoma

Exogenous agents
- Phenylbutazone
- Alpha-methyldopa
- Sulfonamides
- Carbamazepine
- Hydralazine
- Procainamide
- Quinidine
- Allopurinol
- Phenytoin
- Halothane
- Penicillin
- Nitrofurantoin
- Chlorpromazine
- Chlorpropamide
- Clofibrate
- Oral contraceptives
- Beryllium
- Copper sulfate
- Parenteral foreign material (starch, talc, silicon, etc.)

PATHOLOGY. Granulomas in the liver, as elsewhere, consist of a compact collection of mature mononuclear phagocytes. In well-developed granulomas, these phagocytic cells take the form of epithelioid cells. Giant cells and necrosis are frequent additional features, but their presence is not necessary for the pathologic diagnosis of granuloma. Although the morphologic features of the granuloma itself are seldom characteristic enough to permit a determination of etiology, this is occasionally possible (e.g., acid-fast bacilli in tuberculosis, ova in schistosomiasis, larvae in toxocariasis, fibrinoid ring plus central clear space in Q fever, birefringent granules in starch granuloma or in foreign substance injection as with parenteral drug abuse). The location of the granuloma or the presence of coexisting parenchymal liver disease may also be helpful, as in granulomatous arteritis and primary biliary cirrhosis.

CLINICAL MANIFESTATIONS. The predominant clinical manifestations are generally those of the underlying disorder. In many of the entities listed in Table 124–2, hepatic dysfunction either is not detectable or constitutes a minor component of the illness. Hepatomegaly is present in more than one half of all patients, whereas splenomegaly is less frequent. In the absence of a primary hepatobiliary disorder, peripheral stigmata (vascular spiders, palmar erythema) and complications (portal hypertension, ascites, encephalopathy) of chronic liver disease are uncommon. Serum alkaline phosphatase and transaminase levels are mildly to moderately elevated in up to two thirds of patients, and hyperbilirubinemia occurs in approximately one quarter of the cases. However, these generalizations do not apply to many individual cases. For example, portal hypertension is a frequent complication of schistosomiasis, and rare patients with sarcoidosis have striking cholestasis and jaundice.

DIAGNOSIS. Because hepatic granulomas are associated with a variety of disorders, many of which are infrequently encountered in clinical practice, the differential diagnosis of granulomatous disease of the liver is one of the most challenging problems in medicine. The histopathologic features and location of the granuloma(s) seldom indicate the etiology, and cultures of the biopsy specimen are usually negative. For example, acid-fast bacilli are demonstrable by appropriate stains in 10 to 25 per cent of biopsies from patients with extrapulmonary tuberculosis, and culture is also infrequently positive. In most cases, the finding of hepatic granulomas serves mainly to direct attention to the broad class of diseases known to cause a granulomatous response in the liver, and the specific diagnosis depends on cultures and/or biopsies from other sites, serologic tests, or skin tests. The generally low frequency with which liver biopsy yields a specific diagnosis, however, appears not to apply to patients with the acquired immune deficiency syndrome. Preliminary reports suggest that atypical mycobacteria and other organisms are detected by stain and culture in a high proportion of such patients with fever and abnormal biochemical studies.

The workup of the patient with hepatic granulomas should begin with a careful interview, probing previous illnesses, travel, occupational and environmental exposures, and drug use or abuse. Physical examination should include careful inspection of the skin and palpation of lymph nodes. A chest roentgenogram is valuable in detecting sarcoidosis and tuberculosis as well as certain fungal diseases. Serial thin sections of the biopsy material with special stains should be obtained to increase the likelihood of detecting acid-fast bacilli, fungi, ova, or foreign material. Bacterial, mycobacterial, and fungal cultures of the biopsy material as well as blood and possibly bone marrow should be obtained when the biopsy is performed as part of an investigation of fever. The appropriateness of additional tests, cultures, and biopsies depends upon the individual clinical circumstances. Despite a thorough search, a satisfactory cause for the granuloma(s) is not discovered in 20 per cent or more of cases. Such patients in whom no satisfactory explanation for the hepatic granulomas can be found and who have fever of unknown origin have been designated as having idiopathic *granulomatous hepatitis*. The existence of granulomatous hepatitis as an entity distinct from sarcoidosis has been disputed.

TREATMENT AND PROGNOSIS. The treatment is that of the underlying disorder. When the underlying disorder can be successfully treated or an offending drug or exposure terminated, clinical and biochemical evidence of liver dysfunction typically disappears. The granulomas themselves, however, may persist for a variable time, depending on the rapidity with which the inciting agent is removed. Patients with idiopathic granulomatous hepatitis have generally responded favorably to administration of corticosteroids. However, this approach should not be undertaken until a thorough search has failed to reveal a cause for the granulomas and generally after a trial of antituberculous therapy has failed.

Berger LA, Osborne DR: Treatment of pyogenic liver abscesses by percutaneous needle aspiration. Lancet 1:132, 1982. Herbert DA, Rothman J, Simmons F, et al.: Pyogenic liver abscesses: Successful nonsurgical therapy. Lancet 1:134, 1982. McCorkell, Niles NL. Pyogenic liver abscesses: Another look at medical management. Lancet 1:803, 1985. *These three articles summarize the results of nonoperative management.*

Conter RL, Pitt HA, Tompkins RK, et al.: Differentiation of pyogenic from amebic hepatic abscesses. Surg Gynecol Obstet 162:114, 1986. *A comprehensive review of 82 patients with emphasis on differential diagnosis and management.*

Drugs for parasitic infections. Med Letter 24:5, 1982. *A concise summary of this topic.*

Elliot DL, Tolle SW, Goldberg L, et al.: Pet-associated illness. N Engl J Med 313:985, 1985. *A succinct summary of a variety of parasitic, bacterial, rickettsial, and other infectious disorders (including many affecting the liver) with emphasis on clinical features and diagnosis.*

Harrington PL, Gutierrez JJ, Ramirez-Rhondra CH, et al.: Granulomatous hepatitis. Rev Infect Dis 4:638, 1982. *An exhaustively referenced and thorough review of the disorders associated with hepatic granulomas.*

Katzenstein D, Rickerson V, Braude A: New concepts of amebic liver abscess derived from hepatic imaging, serodiagnosis, and hepatic enzymes in 67 consecutive cases in San Diego. Medicine 61:237, 1982. *A pertinent review that distinguishes acute from chronic cases.*

Orenstein MS, Tavitian A, Yonk B, et al.: Granulomatous involvement of the liver in patients with AIDS. Gut 26:1220, 1985. *Report of a small series of patients with AIDS in whom liver biopsy was found to be a high yield procedure for establishing the presence of mycobacterial infection.*

125 INHERITED, INFILTRATIVE, AND METABOLIC DISORDERS INVOLVING THE LIVER

Bruce F. Scharschmidt

The liver is involved in a variety of inherited, infiltrative, and metabolic disorders. Most of the disorders included in this chapter, e.g., Wilson's disease, hemochromatosis, the glycogen and lipid storage diseases, and amyloidosis, are discussed here only with respect to their hepatic involvement. A more comprehensive treatment of these entities can be found elsewhere in this textbook.

ALPHA$_1$-ANTITRYPSIN DEFICIENCY

Alpha$_1$-antitrypsin (A_1AT) deficiency is an inherited disorder associated with a decreased concentration of A_1AT in serum (see Ch. 61). This glycoprotein, which is found in other body fluids as well as in serum, inhibits a variety of proteolytic enzymes, including pancreatic trypsin, chymotrypsin, and elastase, as well as certain proteases produced by leukocytes and macrophages. It is normally present in a concentration of about 200 mg per deciliter in serum, where it accounts for 90 per cent of total antitrypsin activity and a major portion of the alpha-1-globulin fraction. A_1AT production is controlled by codominant alleles, and more than 25 different alleles have been identified by starch gel electrophoresis of serum. The most common allele at the P_i (protein inhibitor) locus is termed M (allele frequency 0.94 to 0.95 in the United States). The most important variant is Z, since P_iZZ accounts for virtually all patients with severe A_1AT deficiency. The liver plays a critical role in the pathophysiology of the disorder, as evidenced by the observation that A_1AT levels return to normal after liver transplantation and the P_i phenotype converts to that of the donor.

Severe A_1AT deficiency is associated with early-onset emphysema in some individuals, liver disease in others, and occasionally both liver and lung disease. The pathogenesis of the disorder is unclear; the deficiency state, by itself, is not sufficient to produce disease. About 10 per cent of individuals with P_iZZ phenotype develop overt liver disease in childhood and have signs and symptoms of cholestasis in the first few days to weeks of life. In a minority of infants, cholestasis persists or worsens and is associated with liver failure and death in a few years. Cholestasis typically remits by six months in the remaining patients, about half of whom nevertheless develop cirrhosis. The long-term prognosis for these children is uncertain. An as yet undefined proportion of infants with P_iZZ phenotype who do not develop neonatal cholestasis have also been shown to have elevated transaminase levels in serum and fibrosis or cirrhosis on liver biopsy. Severe deficiency, P_iZZ phenotype, is associated with a several-fold increase in the risk of developing both cirrhosis and hepatocellular carcinoma, particularly in males. Heterozygous A_1AT deficiency (phenotypes MZ and SZ) may also be associated with an increased incidence of liver disease and cancer, although the link is less clear than for severe deficiency.

The diagnosis of A_1AT deficiency can be suspected from serum protein electrophoresis and confirmed by measurement of A_1AT in serum either as trypsin inhibitory activity or by immunoassay. However, definitive diagnosis requires determination of protease inhibitor phenotype by starch gel electrophoresis or isoelectric focusing. This is particularly true of individuals with heterozygous A_1AT deficiency who may have serum levels of A_1AT in the low normal range. Patients with the Z allele, with or without liver disease, also exhibit characteristic rounded eosinophilic cytoplasmic inclusions in periportal hepatocytes. These inclusion bodies are immunologically related to A_1AT but differ in certain amino acids as well as in their content of sialic acid and other sugars. Importantly, such eosinophilic inclusions have been recently described as an apparently acquired defect in patients with alcoholic liver disease and are thus not diagnostic of inherited A_1AT deficiency. There is currently no specific therapy for this disorder; however, a number of patients have successfully undergone transplantation with favorable results (Ch. 128).

WILSON'S DISEASE

Wilson's disease is an autosomal recessive disorder with a prevalence worldwide of about 1 in 30,000 (see Ch. 205). Its clinical and pathologic manifestations result from excessive accumulation of copper in many tissues, including the brain, liver, cornea, and kidneys. Although the primary genetic defect remains undetermined, impaired biliary copper excretion rather than enhanced absorption is the cause of the copper accumulation. Unfortunately the diagnosis of this treatable disorder is often missed or delayed because of its rarity and diverse presentations. Hepatic disease is a common initial clinical manifestation in childhood and adolescence and may take the form of a self-limited illness resembling viral hepatitis, fulminant hepatic failure, or chronic active hepatitis; thus, biochemical screening for Wilson's disease is imperative in all patients under the age of 35 years who have liver disease of uncertain etiology. A majority of patients with fulminant hepatic failure die despite initiation of D-penicillamine therapy. Hemolysis represents an important clue to the presence of Wilson's disease and predisposes to the development of cholelithiasis. Neurologic manifestations typically appear between the ages of 12 and 30 years and are almost invariably accompanied by the presence of Kayser-Fleischer rings.

The diagnosis and treatment of Wilson's disease are discussed in detail in Ch. 205; however, certain points merit special emphasis here. First, while the combination of an abnormally low ceruloplasmin level in serum and Kayser-Fleischer rings establishes the diagnosis, about 15 per cent of patients having Wilson's disease presenting with hepatic manifestations have serum ceruloplasmin concentrations in the low normal range, and about one half of patients who seek medical help with chronic active hepatitis or fulminant hepatic failure have not yet developed Kayser-Fleischer rings. If the diagnosis of Wilson's disease is uncertain, a biopsy should be performed for quantitative copper determination. If coagulation abnormalities preclude a biopsy, measurement of incorporation of orally administered radiolabeled copper into ceruloplasmin or measurement of serum copper or urinary copper excretion may be useful.

HEMOCHROMATOSIS

Hemochromatosis is among the more common genetic disorders, with a calculated homozygous frequency of about 1 in 300 to 1 in 400 in certain high prevalence areas. The molecular basis of the underlying defect responsible for enhanced intestinal iron absorption remains undetermined. Males homozygous for the hemochromatosis allele, which is in close linkage with HLA-A3 on chromosome 6, show progressive accumulation of hepatic iron, and clinical evidence of disease usually develops in the fourth, fifth, or sixth decades of life. Most homozygous females do not develop clinical evidence of disease, presumably because of iron loss through menses and pregnancy. Heterozygotes may also show abnormal accumulation of hepatic iron, but the absolute amounts present are much less than in homozygotes, and clinical evidence of iron overload rarely develops.

Hepatic iron overload is most commonly manifested as moderate to marked hepatomegaly with initially well preserved liver function. Esophageal varices, ascites, and impaired hepatic synthetic function are present in more advanced cases. Other important clinical features include abnormal skin pigmentation, glucose intolerance, cardiac involvement, hypogonadism, and arthropathy. Hepatocellular carcinoma develops in up to one third of patients. These classic manifestations are present in only a minority of homozygotes. Indeed, there is considerable variability in the expression of the disorder, and it is possible that some homozygotes never develop overt disease. With appropriate phlebotomy therapy hepatic function frequently improves, and there are case reports that suggest regression of apparent cirrhosis.

Screening for hemochromatosis is probably best accomplished by measurement of transferrin saturation and serum ferritin. A saturation exceeding 50 per cent is present in nearly all homozygotes over 20 years of age, and a value less than 50 per cent largely precludes the diagnosis. However, the positive predictive value of a transferrin saturation exceeding 50 per cent is relatively low. In contrast, a transferrin saturation exceeding 80 per cent is a more reliable indicator of hemochromatosis, and a large study in Utah suggests that a transferrin saturation greater than 62 per cent most reliably separates homozygotes from heterozygotes and normal persons. Serum levels of ferritin are a generally accurate reflection of tissue iron stores and exceed 1000 ng per ml in most patients. However, occasional families with hemochromatosis and normal serum ferritin levels have been described and, conversely, serum ferritin is typically increased out of proportion to tissue iron stores in patients with hepatocellular necrosis. If either of these tests suggests iron overload, liver biopsy with quantitative iron determination and histochemical stains for iron should be performed. A variety of noninvasive methods for measurement of hepatic iron have been proposed for use in patients who cannot undergo a liver biopsy. Dual-energy computed tomography appears particularly promising, and nuclear magnetic resonance and magnetic susceptibility measurement are also undergoing evaluation. Hemochromatosis is discussed in detail in Ch. 206.

STORAGE DISEASES

The glycogen storage diseases may present as disorders of the liver as well as of the heart and musculoskeletal system. Hepatomegaly is a prominent feature of most of these disorders, whereas splenomegaly is found primarily in Type IV and less commonly in Type III. Patients with Type I and III glycogen storage disease frequently survive childhood and may be encountered by the physician treating adults. Patients with type I glycogen storage disease apparently have an increased incidence of hepatic adenoma as well as hepatocellular carcinoma. Portacaval anastomosis may improve growth and reverse certain metabolic abnormalities in selected Type I patients, although the mechanism for these beneficial effects is uncertain. The glycogen storage diseases are discussed in detail in Ch. 179. In addition to glycogen, the liver abnormally stores fatty acids, cholesterol, or complex lipids in the lipid storage disorders as well as various mucopolysaccharides and mucolipids. Although hepatomegaly is common to most of these disorders, the clinical consequences are attributable to involvement of the nervous and musculoskeletal systems.

PROTOPORPHYRIA

Protoporphyria is a disorder characterized by increased protoporphyrin content in erythrocytes, plasma, feces, and liver. It is inherited as an autosomal dominant trait and results from a deficiency of heme synthase (ferrochelatase), the enzyme that catalyzes the formation of heme from protoporphyrin and iron. It is most conveniently diagnosed by demonstrating an elevated level of erythrocyte protoporphyrin. Protoporphyria is usually a mild disorder manifested by mild photosensitivity and, rarely, hemolysis. Hepatobiliary complications include pigment gallstones and infrequent hepatic failure. About 18 cases of hepatic failure associated with protoporphyria have been reported. The hepatic failure, typically heralded by cholestasis, is associated with and presumably results from massive hepatic accumulation of birefringent crystals of protoporphyrin. Interruption of the enterohepatic circulation of protoporphyrin with cholestyramine or activated charcoal has been reported to deplete hepatic protoporphyrin deposits and restore liver function to normal in some patients with mild disease, but the value of such treatment in patients with severe cholestasis and established hepatic failure is unknown. Oral iron therapy has also been reported to decrease protoporphyrin production in a single patient. At present there is no way of identifying the small proportion of patients with protoporphyria who will develop significant hepatic disease.

CYSTIC FIBROSIS

In infants with cystic fibrosis, amorphous eosinophilic material in bile ducts and ductules, presumably representing inspissated secretions, may produce cholestasis (see Ch. 66). Later manifestations include cholangitis, fibrosis, and obstructive biliary cirrhosis. Up to 20 per cent of patients who survive to adolescence have cirrhosis with portal hypertension, and bleeding from esophageal varices represents a significant cause of morbidity in this older age group. Patients who have bled from varices and have good pulmonary function are candidates for shunt surgery. Since liver disease with portal hypertension has even been reported as a first manifestation of cystic fibrosis, the diagnosis should be considered in a young patient with otherwise unexplained liver disease.

AMYLOIDOSIS

Amyloid deposition in the liver is common in amyloidosis of all types (see Ch. 168). Hepatomegaly is present in approximately one half of patients with systemic amyloidosis; splenomegaly is present in about 10 per cent of patients; and mild elevation of the serum alkaline phosphatase is the most common biochemical abnormality. Cutaneous stigmata of chronic liver disease (e.g., spider angiomas, palmar erythema) and portal hypertension are unusual. Intrahepatic cholestasis with marked elevation of the serum bilirubin and alkaline phosphatase concentrations occurs in about 5 per cent of patients. The diagnosis of amyloidosis can usually be established without resorting to liver biopsy.

SARCOIDOSIS

Hepatic involvement in sarcoidosis represents a continuum from the presence of asymptomatic granulomas to cases in which hepatic involvement represents a prominent part of the overall clinical picture (see Ch. 69). Approximately two thirds to three quarters of patients with sarcoidosis have hepatic granulomas, making the liver one of the most commonly involved organs in this disease, and liver biopsy is often of value in establishing the diagnosis of sarcoidosis.

About 20 per cent of patients with sarcoidosis have hepatomegaly, and up to 40 per cent have abnormal liver function tests, most commonly a mild elevation of the level of alkaline phosphatase. Overt hepatic involvement is present in fewer than 20 per cent of patients. This may take several forms, including (1) hepatomegaly, generally with splenomegaly, and multiple abnormal liver function tests; (2) chronic cholestasis, which may closely mimic primary biliary cirrhosis; and (3) portal hypertension and its manifestations. The characteristic histologic feature of hepatic sarcoidosis is the presence of granulomas, frequently located in portal tracts. Chronic portal tract inflammation, hepatocyte poikilocytosis and anisocytosis, fibrosis, and even cirrhosis may be accompanying findings. Little information is available regarding the response of these hepatic lesions to corticosteroids, but a therapeutic trial is justified if significant symptoms are present and tuberculosis and other disorders producing hepatic granuloma have been excluded.

ENTERIC BYPASS

Hepatic disease related to enteric bypass surgery has typically been reported in patients who have had extensive bypass procedures for treatment of marked obesity. Jejunocolic bypass, an early operation, has now largely been abandoned because of a high incidence of complications, including cirrhosis and hepatic failure. Hepatic abnormalities are also common following jejunoileal bypass and may take several forms. Fatty change is present in up to two thirds of markedly obese patients prior to bypass surgery, and hepatic lipid content increases during the period of weight loss. Cirrhosis ensues in up to 5 per cent of patients, and death from liver failure accounts for a substantial proportion of the early postoperative mortality of 2 to 4 per cent. Histologic features may mimic those of alcoholic liver disease, including the presence of alcoholic hyalin. Longer-term follow-up studies suggest that hepatic abnormalities may not appear until several years after surgery in some patients.

The pathogenesis of these hepatic changes is unclear. Weight loss itself does not account for the progressive postoperative fat accumulation, since this does not occur in nonoperated obese patients who lose weight through dietary measures. However, hepatic disease resembling alcoholic hepatitis and even cirrhosis have been described in abstinent patients with obesity who have not undergone bypass surgery. Protein depletion, leading to a kwashiorkor-like state, may contribute to the fatty change. Increased production in the gut of potentially toxic substances may also play a role. For example, increased delivery of chenodeoxycholate to the colon results in increased production of the potentially hepatotoxic bile salt, lithocholate. The bypassed segment may also serve as a site for bacterial overgrowth and production of potentially toxic bacterial products.

Laboratory studies of hepatic function are frequently abnormal in the first few postoperative months following bypass surgery even in the absence of serious liver disease. Conversely, the absence of abnormal hepatic function tests or clinical evidence of liver disease during the first postoperative year does not preclude the possible later development of significant liver disease. Deterioration of synthetic or excretory function as evidenced by an abnormal prothrombin time that does not respond to vitamin K administration, hypoalbuminemia, or hyperbilirubinemia is an ominous sign. Biopsy is the only reliable way of assessing the severity of hepatic disease, and some advocate follow-up biopsies in all patients. Serious and persistent hepatic disease is an indication for reestablishing normal bowel continuity, which may be required in up to 25 per cent of patients. Currently, alternative procedures such as gastroplasty, which are associated with fewer hepatic and metabolic complications, are preferred in the morbidly obese patients.

INFLAMMATORY BOWEL DISEASE

Liver function tests may be transiently abnormal in up to one half of patients with chronic ulcerative colitis and less commonly in Crohn's disease, but significant and persistent biochemical abnormalities are present in fewer than 10 per cent of patients. A variety of histologic abnormalities have been described in these patients. *Pericholangitis* is defined as portal tract inflammation with or without periductular fibrosis in association with inflammatory bowel disease. Direct cholangiography has revealed sclerosing cholangitis in a substantial proportion of patients with pericholangitis. Moreover, the hepatic histologic changes in patients with radiologically documented sclerosing cholangitis are indistinguishable from those of pericholangitis in association with radiologically normal bile ducts (see Ch. 105). Thus, the term *small duct sclerosing cholangitis* has been suggested as preferable to pericholangitis to describe the heterogeneous collection of bile duct abnormalities seen in patients with inflammatory bowel disease and radiologically normal bile ducts. While portal bacteremia or other enteric toxins have been postulated to play a role in the pathogenesis of small- and large-duct sclerosing cholangitis associated with inflammatory bowel disease, such a cause-and-effect relationship between the bowel disease and these lesions does not account for the variable temporal relationship between the two and the often very mild bowel disease. A variable response of bile ducts and colon to some common factor better accounts for these clinical findings. Other hepatic abnormalities in patients with inflammatory bowel disease have included fatty change, chronic active hepatitis, cirrhosis, amyloidosis and granulomas.

No specific therapy is available for these hepatic abnormalities. Treatment should be directed at the underlying bowel disease, although this does not reliably produce improvement in the hepatic disorder. Progression of serious liver disease in ulcerative colitis is not consistently altered by colectomy, so this approach cannot be generally recommended.

TOTAL PARENTERAL NUTRITION

Total parenteral nutrition has been associated with a spectrum of hepatic abnormalities, including mild elevations in alkaline phosphatase and transaminase levels, cholestasis with jaundice, and, rarely, progressive hepatic disease resulting in death. Liver biopsy in these patients has frequently revealed fatty change, cholestasis, and mild periportal inflammation, with fibrosis or cirrhosis found in a minority. Some of these abnormalities have been due to the underlying disease or complicating infection, but total parenteral nutrition, by itself, can produce elevated serum bile salt levels and occasionally hyperbilirubinemia in both infants and adults. The degree of abnormality appears related to the duration and amount of parenteral alimentation. In infants, cholestasis associated with parenteral nutrition also increases in frequency with decreasing gestational age and birth weight, and adults with the short-bowel syndrome appear particularly at risk for severe liver disease. Hepatic function generally returns gradually to normal after total parenteral nutrition is discontinued. Modifying the infusate by lowering the caloric-nitrogen ratio or decreasing the total caloric intake has reportedly produced improvement in some patients, but this has not been systematically studied, and no one component of the parenteral formula has been clearly implicated as causative. Total parenteral nutrition also appears to predispose patients to the development of gallstones and cholecystitis, and these possibilities should be kept in mind when one is evaluating a patient receiving parenteral nutrition for hepatobiliary disease.

PREGNANCY

Liver size and liver histology remain normal during uncomplicated pregnancy. Serum levels of alkaline phosphatase and leucine aminopeptidase typically rise in the second and third trimesters and are of placental origin; aminotransferase and bilirubin levels are normal.

EFFECT OF PREGNANCY ON COEXISTING LIVER DISEASE. In the United States and Western Europe, pregnancy does not appear to alter the course of acute viral hepatitis. In underdeveloped countries, however, viral hepatitis in pregnancy, particularly during the third trimester, appears to run a more severe course and is associated with an unusually high incidence of fulminant hepatic failure with high fetal and maternal mortality. Pregnancy has not been shown to alter the course of chronic persistent or chronic active hepatitis, although maternal and fetal morbidity and mortality may be increased because of variceal bleeding and postpartum hemorrhage. Vertical transmission of hepatitis B virus infection occurs commonly when the mother contracts acute hepatitis B during the third trimester or is a chronic carrier (particularly if she also is HBeAg positive), and it is important that the infant receive appropriate passive and active prophylaxis at delivery (see Ch. 121).

LIVER DISEASES ASSOCIATED WITH PREGNANCY. *Hyperemesis gravidarum* of sufficient severity to require hospitalization may be accompanied by minor abnormalities in standard liver function tests. *Acute fatty liver of pregnancy* can be defined as a syndrome of acute hepatic dysfunction that develops in late pregnancy, is associated with microvesicular fat accumulation in hepatocytes, and resolves with delivery. It typically becomes apparent after the 30th week of gestation and is manifested initially by constitutional symptoms, often with abdominal pain, followed in many instances by overt evidence of hepatic failure, including encephalopathy and jaundice. In the past, intravenous tetracycline therapy was incriminated in some cases, but this is rarely true at present. The only known treatment is termination of the pregnancy. Early reports suggested that the disorder was associated with a very high mortality rate, but more recent reports suggest that there is a spectrum of disease severity and that milder cases without frank hepatic failure occur and have a favorable prognosis. It also appears that acute fatty liver may, at least in some instances, fall within the spectrum of hepatic dysfunction associated with *pre-eclampsia* or *eclampsia,* as these two disorders occasionally share certain features, including onset in late pregnancy, increased incidence in young primiparas, the presence of coagulopathy, hypertension, and proteinuria, and resolution upon delivery. Focal necrosis and, rarely, hepatic rupture may occur in women with *eclampsia. Cholestasis of pregnancy* generally occurs in the last four months of gestation (range 7 to 39 weeks). It is characterized by pruritus, sometimes followed by jaundice. It typically resolves within two weeks of delivery and frequently recurs in subsequent pregnancies or with administration of oral contraceptives. Serum alkaline phosphatase and bile salts are increased, and hyperbilirubinemia may be present. Serum transaminase is also frequently mildly increased. Although generally considered a benign condition, cholestasis of pregnancy has been associated with an increased incidence of premature labor and postpartum hemorrhage.

CIRCULATORY DISTURBANCE

Hepatic function and histology are commonly altered in patients with cardiovascular disease. Disorders associated with an elevation of systemic venous pressure typically produce hepatic venous congestion manifested by hepatomegaly, minor abnormalities of liver function tests, and centrolobular congestion without necrosis. Longstanding hepatic congestion may lead to cardiac cirrhosis with fibrous bands joining centrilobular areas (see Ch. 126). When hypotension is superimposed, even transiently, on hepatic congestion, severe centrilobular to midzonal necrosis, transaminase levels exceeding 1000 units, marked hyperbilirubinemia, and hypoprothrombinemia may result. Differentiating this disorder from viral hepatitis may be difficult, since the clinical features are similar and hepatic dysfunction often is not recognized until several days after the resolution of the circulatory failure. Unlike viral hepatitis, however, serum transaminase levels frequently fall very rapidly and may approach normal within days. If the circulatory insult is brief, patients usually recover from their hepatic injury uneventfully. Fatal fulminant hepatic failure has been reported, however. A similar form of acute hepatic injury is occasionally seen in persons without preexisting cardiovascular disease who suffer severe or prolonged hypotension or in patients with severe isolated left-sided heart failure.

Alagille D: α-1-Antitrypsin deficiency. Hepatology, 4:11S, Jan-Feb Suppl. 1984. *A concise review of the clinical course of 45 children with neonatal cholestasis and A_1AT deficiency.*

Bassett ML, Halliday JW, Powell LW: Genetic hemachromatosis. Semin Liver Dis 4:217, 1984. *A concise, practically oriented, and well-referenced review.*

Eriksson S, Carlson J, Velez R: Risk of cirrhosis and primary liver cancer in alpha-1-antitrypsin deficiency. N Engl J Med 314:736, 1986. *Report of an autopsy study conducted in Sweden that provides the clearest evidence to date that this disorder predisposes to cirrhosis and liver cancer.*

Hocking MP, Duerson MC, O'Leary P, et al.: Jejunoileal bypass for morbid obesity. Late follow-up in 100 cases. N Engl J Med 308:995, 1983. *A summary of complications in patients with intact bypasses followed for more than five years.*

Kaplan MM: Acute fatty liver of pregnancy. N Engl J Med 313:367, 1985. *A short review focusing on practical clinical issues.*

McCullough AJ, Fleming CR, Thistle JL, et al.: Diagnosis of Wilson's disease presenting as fulminant hepatic failure. Gastroenterology 84:161, 1983. *This article summarizes the clinical features of this presentation of Wilson's disease and the value of various tests other than liver biopsy in making the diagnosis.*

O'Leary J: Hepatic complications of jejunoileal bypass. Semin Liver Dis 3:203, 1983. *A comprehensive review with pertinent references.*

Stanko R, Nathan G, Mendelow H, et al.: Development of hepatic cholestasis and fibrosis in patients with massive loss of intestine supported by prolonged parenteral nutrition. Gastroenterology 92:197, 1987. *Report of a small series of patients that suggests that the short-bowel syndrome predisposes to severe liver injury in patients undergoing parenteral alimentation.*

Wee A, Judwig J: Pericholangitis in chronic ulcerative colitis: Primary sclerosing cholangitis of the small bile ducts? Ann Intern Med 102:581, 1985. *A review of the spectrum of hepatobiliary disease seen in 107 patients with ulcerative colitis with emphasis on the relationship between histologic abnormalities noted on liver biopsy and sclerosing cholangitis.*

Zakin D, Boyer TD: Hepatology. Philadelphia, W. B. Saunders Company, 1982. *Consult chapters 12, 33, 42, 43, 44, and 48 for authoritative, and well-referenced reviews of the disorders discussed briefly in this chapter.*

126 CIRRHOSIS OF THE LIVER

Thomas D. Boyer

GENERAL CONSIDERATIONS. Cirrhosis is an irreversible alteration of the liver architecture, consisting of hepatic fibrosis and areas of nodular regeneration. When the nodules are small (less than 3 mm), uniform, and encompass one lobule, the term micronodular or unilobular cirrhosis is applied. In macronodular or multilobular cirrhosis the nodules exceed 3 mm, vary in size, and encompass more than one lobule. Frequently, features of both micronodular and macronodular cirrhosis are present in the same liver. Etiologic diagnosis may be impossible from the gross and microscopic appearance of the cirrhotic liver and must therefore be based on history, physical examination, biochemical and serologic tests, and histochemical stains. The causes of cirrhosis are listed in Table 126–1.

Patients with cirrhosis may have one of two general types of manifestations: (1) signs or symptoms related to hepatocellular necrosis, which are similar to those of acute hepatitis and include jaundice, nausea and vomiting, and tender hepatomegaly; or (2) signs or symptoms of the complications of cirrhosis, which are largely due to the rise in intrahepatic vascular resistance that leads to portal hypertension and its complications (ascites, formation of portal-systemic collaterals, encephalopathy, splenomegaly, and bleeding esophageal and gastric varices). Other, less specific manifestations of cirrhosis include gynecomastia, spider angiomas, parotid hypertrophy, and testicular atrophy. Patients frequently present a mixed picture with features of both hepatocellular necrosis and portal hypertension.

TABLE 126–1. CAUSES OF CIRRHOSIS

Drugs and toxins	***Metabolic***
Alcohol	Wilson's disease
Methyldopa	Hemochromatosis
Methotrexate	Erythropoietic protoporphyria
Isoniazid	Pediatric—alpha$_1$-antitrypsin deficiency, galactosemia, hereditary fructose intolerance, glycogen storage disease Type IV, tyrosinosis
Perhexiline maleate	
Amiodarone	
Oxyphenisatin	
Infections	
Hepatitis B and non-A non-B	***Cardiovascular***
Syphilis (tertiary)	Chronic right heart failure
Schistosoma japonicum	Budd-Chiari syndrome
Biliary Obstruction	Veno-occlusive disease
Carcinoma (pancreatic or bile duct)	***Miscellaneous***
Chronic pancreatitis	Chronic active hepatitis
Common duct stones	Primary biliary cirrhosis
Strictures	Sarcoidosis
Cystic fibrosis	Jejunoileal bypass
Biliary atresia	Neonatal hepatitis
Sclerosing cholangitis	***Cryptogenic***

Agents that cause cirrhosis may have systemic effects as well. Extrahepatic features may dominate the clinical picture with little or no evidence of liver disease. For example, patients with alcoholic liver disease frequently have complaints referable to the central nervous system, peripheral nerves, heart, muscles, and gastrointestinal tract. Patients with disease such as primary biliary cirrhosis may have prominent eye and skin disorders. Patients with hemochromatosis may present with diabetes mellitus or arthritis, and patients with Wilson's disease, with central nervous system dysfunction, before liver disease becomes apparent. Thus, cirrhosis is frequently a subclinical illness, and a high index of suspicion may be necessary to establish a correct diagnosis.

ALCOHOLIC LIVER DISEASE

DEFINITION AND INCIDENCE. Alcoholic liver disease, a frequent and serious sequela of the chronic abuse of ethanol, occurs singly or intermingled in three forms: *fatty liver, alcoholic hepatitis*, and *cirrhosis*. Alcohol is the most common cause of liver disease in the Western world. Alcoholic cirrhosis is discovered in 1.6 to 9.9 per cent of all necropsies in the United States. The peak incidence is in patients 40 to 55 years of age; however, patients in their twenties may be seen with advanced alcoholic liver disease. The male to female ratio is 2:1.

ETIOLOGY AND PATHOGENESIS. *The relationship between alcohol abuse and cirrhosis* is well established. The incidence of cirrhosis and the per capita consumption of alcohol are directly related; countries with the greatest alcohol consumption also have the highest incidence of cirrhosis. Neither the pattern of drinking (spree versus daily) nor the type of alcoholic beverage consumed appears to be important in the genesis of liver disease. The single most important factor is the average daily consumption of ethanol. Levels of daily ethanol consumption exceeding 40 to 80 grams (36 to 72 oz of beer, 4.5 to 9 oz liquor, 15 to 30 oz of wine) for 10 to 15 years are associated with an increase in the incidence of cirrhosis. Women may be more susceptible to the toxic effects of ethanol than men, and a lower daily consumption of ethanol by women may lead to cirrhosis. As the daily level of alcohol consumed rises, the time required for the development of cirrhosis is reduced.

Ethanol is a hepatotoxin. Administration of alcohol to humans or animals leads to the development of fatty liver (hepatic steatosis). The mitochondria and endoplasmic reticulum of hepatocytes are altered morphologically and functionally. Ethanol also causes lactic acidemia, hyperuricemia, and hypoglycemia. Many of the effects of ethanol reflect its metabolism, which is catalyzed primarily by the cytosolic enzyme alcohol dehydrogenase as shown:

$$\underset{\text{Ethanol}}{CH_3CH_2OH} \xrightarrow[\text{NAD}^+ \longrightarrow \text{NADH} + \text{H}^+]{\text{Alcohol dehydrogenase}} \underset{\text{Acetaldehyde}}{CH_3CHO}$$

(Other metabolic pathways via a microsomal ethanol oxidizing system or a catalase system appear to be of minor importance, except perhaps at high ethanol concentrations.) The acetaldehyde formed from ethanol is then oxidized to acetate by acetaldehyde dehydrogenase with NAD^+ as a cofactor. The lack of the active high affinity form of acetaldehyde dehydrogenase (50 per cent of Japanese) leads to high blood levels of acetaldehyde following ethanol ingestion. The high levels of acetaldehyde in these individuals are associated with flushing, vasodilatation, tachycardia, and aversion to ethanol. The limiting step in the rate of metabolism of ethanol is the availability of the cofactor NAD^+, which is converted to NADH during the aforementioned two reactions. This increased reducing potential in the cell favors the conversion of pyuvate to lactate. When blood levels of ethanol are high (more than 200 mg per deciliter), the resulting lactic acidemia decreases the clearance of urate by the kidneys and hyperuricemia develops. At lower levels of ethanol ingestion (blood level $\leq$ 150 mg per deciliter) increased production of urate is the cause of hyperuricemia. Inhibition of gluconeogenesis and fasting hypoglycemia may also follow ethanol abuse (Ch. 117). Fatty acid oxidation is impaired, and the esterification of fatty acids to triglycerides is increased. The latter effects, acting in concert with less well defined events, lead to the development of a fatty liver. The metabolism of ethanol may lead to increased levels of acetaldehyde in the blood and probably within the hepatocyte. Acetaldehyde is a reactive molecule and may interact with proteins and membrane lipids, causing alterations in their structure and function, which may lead to cell injury and death.

The metabolic effects of ethanol are relatively well understood, but the mechanism by which it causes chronic liver disease is not. There is evidence for impaired protein synthesis and secretion, mitochondrial injury, lipid peroxidation, cellular hypoxia, and cell-mediated and antibody-mediated cytotoxicity, but the relative importance of each of these in producing sustained cell injury is unknown.

Ethanol fed to animals receiving an otherwise balanced diet has not been shown to cause alcoholic hepatitis. In addition, only 10 to 20 per cent of alcoholics and about 50 per cent of ethanol-fed baboons develop cirrhosis despite similar levels of ethanol ingestion. Thus, *genetic, nutritional*, or *environmental* factors may act in concert with ethanol to cause liver disease.

Malnutrition is a common finding in alcoholics who have both poor diet and reduced intestinal absorption of dietary nutrients. Administration of ethanol to patients with active alcoholic liver disease does not appear to impair recovery if the patients also receive a balanced, high-calorie diet. Lesions identical to those of alcoholic hepatitis may develop following jejunoileal bypass for obesity, a condition in which protein malnutrition is common. Thus, malnutrition appears to potentiate the adverse effects of alcohol. Other factors, such as simultaneous exposure to other hepatotoxins, may also be important in the genesis of liver injury. Alcoholism and alcoholic liver disease are more common in certain populations, in twins, and within families, but there is no evidence of a genetically determined abnormality in the metabolism of ethanol that renders them more susceptible to liver injury.

DIAGNOSIS. The diagnosis of alcoholic liver disease should be considered in any patient who consumes more than 40 grams of ethanol daily. Tender hepatomegaly, fever, and jaundice are suggestive of alcoholic hepatitis, whereas ascites and venous collaterals suggest cirrhosis. Many patients, however, will lack any distinctive clinical features such that a firm diagnosis cannot be established without liver biopsy. In addition, up to 20 per cent of patients with clinical features of alcoholic liver disease are found on liver biopsy to have another type of hepatic disorder.

PATHOLOGY, CLINICAL PRESENTATION, AND THERAPY. Alcohol causes three major pathologic lesions and clinical illnesses: *fatty liver, alcoholic hepatitis, and cirrhosis*. Each of these may occur as an isolated event, or they may be present in any combination in a single patient. Therefore, although the three lesions will be described as single entities, many patients have all three and will have a mixed clinical picture. The histologic pattern is not specific for alcohol alone, but may also be found in the livers of patients who have undergone jejunoileal bypass for obesity, or as an unusual accompaniment of obesity or diabetes mellitus. Patients treated with the vasodilator perhexiline maleate or the antiarrhythmic drug amiodarone also may develop a lesion identical to alcoholic liver disease.

Fatty Liver. *Fatty liver* is the most common biopsy finding in alcoholics. The fat, either centrilobular or diffuse in location, is present in large droplets, which occupy most of the volume of the hepatocyte. Occasionally the fat is present in small droplets, resembling the lesion of Reye's syndrome or fatty liver of pregnancy. Patients with fatty liver are usually asymptomatic, but on occasion they may have abdominal pain, icterus, or vague gastrointestinal complaints. The liver is enlarged and may be tender, but is of normal consistency. Ascites, venous collaterals, and the stigmata of chronic liver disease, if present, are not attributable to the fatty liver per se, but reflect more serious lesions. The laboratory tests are only mildly abnormal in fatty liver. Jaundice, when present, is usually mild (bilirubin below 5 mg per deciliter), although intense cholestasis occasionally develops in patients with fatty liver. The AST, if elevated, is only modestly so (less than five times normal). The serum albumin and globulin are abnormal in about 25 per cent of patients. Patients with alcoholic fatty liver alone have an excellent prognosis. Withdrawal of the alcohol leads to a rapid resolution of the clinical illness and histologic lesion (fat disappears within three to six weeks). On rare occasions, these patients die suddenly from multiple fat emboli to the lungs.

Alcoholic Hepatitis. *Alcoholic hepatitis* (acute sclerosing hyaline necrosis) is a serious sequela of alcoholism because it may lead to hepatic failure or to cirrhosis. The pathologic lesion is most severe in central areas, and consists of hepatocellular necrosis and the triad of (1) *alcoholic hyalin*, (2) *infiltration by polymorphonuclear leukocytes*, and (3) *increased intralobular connective tissue* with or without occlusion of the hepatic venules and sclerosis of terminal hepatic (central) veins. Alcoholic hyalin (Mallory body) is an eosinophilic intracellular aggregate of proteinaceous material that is characteristically perinuclear in location. The origin of alcoholic hyaline is uncertain although it may be formed by intermediate filaments. It is present in only 30 per cent of liver biopsies in which the diagnosis of alcoholic hepatitis can be made on clinical and other histologic criteria. Alcoholic hyalin is not specific for alcoholic liver disease, since it has also been found in the livers of patients with Wilson's disease, primary biliary cirrhosis, hepatocellular carcinoma, and diabetes mellitus, as well as following jejunoileal bypass. Central vein sclerosis may be severe enough to cause a severe outflow block and portal hypertension in the absence of cirrhosis.

The clinical features of alcoholic hepatitis range from absence of symptoms to hepatic failure. Patients commonly complain of anorexia, nausea, vomiting, abdominal pain, and weight loss. Tender hepatomegaly is present in at least 80 per cent of patients. Ascites, jaundice, fever (temperature 37.2 to 39.4°C), splenomegaly, and encephalopathy are common but not invariable. Although fever is common, bacterial infection should be excluded since such patients are at an increased risk for developing pneumonia, urinary tract infections, sepsis, and bacterial peritonitis. The AST is frequently elevated; however, the degree of elevation is modest (less than 10 times normal) although on occasion it can exceed 15 times normal. The ALT may be normal and is almost always less than the AST. The AST/ALT ratio frequently exceeds two. This is in contrast to viral hepatitis, in which the AST frequently exceeds 15 to 25 times normal and the ALT is equal to or greater than the AST. Hyperbilirubinemia is common (60 to 90 per cent) in alcoholic hepatitis, and it may be marked (20 to 30 mg per deciliter). The alkaline phosphatase is usually elevated to less than three times normal, but an occasional patient has a cholestatic picture in which the alkaline phosphatase is unusually high. Prolongation of the prothrombin time, hypoalbuminemia, and hyperglobulinemia may be present. The white blood cell count frequently is elevated (>10,000) and may exceed 30,000 to 40,000 per cubic millimeter. Patients with alcoholic hepatitis may develop the hepatorenal syndrome, and a rising BUN and creatinine are poor prognostic signs.

Treatment for alcoholic hepatitis is nonspecific. Patients should receive a well-balanced diet, high in calories (2500 to 3000 kcal). Protein should be included in the diets unless encephalopathy is present. Anorexia is frequent, and tube or intravenous alimentation may be necessary. Improvement in the patient's nutritional state may be associated with more rapid resolution of the liver test abnormalities; however, the effect of nutritional support on survival is unclear. Prednisone has not been shown to decrease the morbidity or mortality in patients with mild to moderate disease. Use of steroids to treat patients with severe alcoholic hepatitis is controversial and cannot be recommended on the basis of available evidence. Propylthiouracil, penicillamine, anabolic steroids, and colchicine have also been used in the treatment of alcoholic hepatitis, but without documented success.

The *prognosis* for patients with alcoholic hepatitis is much worse than for those with fatty liver. Some patients who stop drinking may have complete resolution of the lesion. In most patients, however, alcoholic hepatitis persists (with clinical improvement), progresses to cirrhosis, or leads to hepatic failure and death. The hospital mortality for patients with severe disease (who cannot have biopsy or who have encephalopathy) exceeds 40 per cent, whereas for those with milder disease the expected death rate is 10 per cent or less.

Alcoholic Cirrhosis. *Alcoholic cirrhosis* usually consists of micronodules of regular size, but it can be macronodular or of a mixed type. Micronodular cirrhosis is not specific for alcoholic liver disease. Histologically, dense bands of connective tissue join portal and central areas. Scarring is most severe in the central regions, and collagen may deposit in the space of Disse. In addition, alcoholic hepatitis frequently coexists, as well as varying amounts of cholestasis, iron, and fat.

Clinically, cirrhosis is an asymptomatic disease in 10 to 20 per cent of patients. It is also commonly present in association with alcoholic hepatitis, and signs of acute liver injury may dominate the clinical picture. Patients may also have ascites, gastrointestinal bleeding, or encephalopathy. These major sequelae of cirrhosis are discussed in detail in the next chapter (Ch. 127). The liver may be large or small and usually has a firm consistency. Spider angiomas, palmar erythema, parotid enlargement, testicular atrophy and gynnecomastia (men), menstrual irregularities (women), and muscle wasting are frequently found; however, these findings are not specific for alcoholic cirrhosis. Upper abdominal pain associated with bloody ascitic fluid, right upper quadrant bruit, or a friction rub over the liver suggests hepatocellular carcinoma.

The *laboratory abnormalities* present in patients with cirrhosis may be similar to those of alcoholic hepatitis. The AST is normal to mildly elevated, and bilirubin is only slightly increased unless the picture is complicated by alcoholic hepatitis, hemolysis, sepsis, hepatic failure, or carcinoma. Anemia is a common finding. The cause of the anemia is multifactorial, including blood loss, folate and pyridoxine deficiency, hemolysis, and the toxic effect of ethanol on the bone marrow. Hypersplenism or bone marrow suppression by ethanol may lead to thrombocytopenia or leukopenia. The serum sodium and potassium may be low in patients with ascites. Hypomagnesemia and hypophosphatemia are common, as is a mild respiratory alkalosis. The BUN and creatinine are increased in patients who have been treated with excessive diuretics or who are developing hepatorenal failure.

The *treatment* of alcoholic cirrhosis is also nonspecific. Deficiencies of vitamins (folate, thiamine, pyridoxine, vitamin K) and minerals (magnesium, phosphate) should be corrected. The sodium content of the diet need not be reduced unless there is sodium retention by the kidneys. Protein restriction is necessary only when there is clinical evidence of hepatic encephalopathy.

The *prognosis* for patients with alcoholic cirrhosis is dependent upon two features: presence of complications and continued abuse of alcohol. Patients without ascites, jaundice, or gastrointestinal bleeding have a better prognosis than those with these complications. Continued alcohol abuse reduces the expected five-year survival to only 40 per cent, whereas it is 60 per cent or greater in those who abstain.

Bosron WF, Li T-K: Genetic polymorphism of human liver alcohol and aldehyde dehydrogenases, and their relationship to alcohol metabolism and alcoholism. Hepatology 6:502, 1986. *A review of the genetics of these two enzymes and how studies of their polymorphism may help us to understand the inherited nature of alcoholism.*

D'Amico G, Morabito A, Pagliaro L, et al.: Survival and prognostic indicators in compensated and decompensated cirrhosis. Dig Dis Sci 31:468, 1986. *Analysis of variables associated with a poor prognosis in alcoholic and nonalcoholic cirrhosis.*

Galambos J: Cirrhosis. Philadelphia, W. B. Saunders Company, 1979. *An excellent monograph that reviews cirrhosis and its complications.*

Lieber C: Alcohol and the liver: 1984 update. Hepatology 4:1243, 1984. *A review of all of the factors that have been thought to play a role in the pathogenesis of alcoholic liver disease.*

PRIMARY BILIARY CIRRHOSIS

DEFINITION AND ETIOLOGY. Primary biliary cirrhosis, a cholestatic disorder, develops because of progressive destruction of small and intermediate-sized intrahepatic bile ducts. The extrahepatic biliary tree and larger intrahepatic bile ducts are patent. The cause of primary biliary cirrhosis is unknown. The injury to the bile ducts is thought to be on an immunologic basis, as there is a high frequency of serum autoantibodies, elevated levels of immunoglobulins (especially IgM), circulating immune complexes, and a reduced cell-mediated immune response in patients with this disease. In addition, the injured bile ducts are surrounded by lymphocytes and, on occasion, by granulomas. These findings, however, are nonspecific and do not establish the etiologic agent or agents responsible for the disease. Genetic factors may also be important, as the disease has been described in a mother and daughter, in siblings, and in twins. In addition, the incidence of positive tests for antimitochondrial antibodies in relatives of patients with primary biliary cirrhosis is increased. The high female preponderance suggests that estrogens or progesterone may be important in the pathogenesis of this disease.

PATHOLOGY. Primary biliary cirrhosis is characterized by progressive, nonsuppurative, destructive cholangitis, which occurs in four histopathologic stages: *ductal, ductular, scarring*, and *cirrhotic*. The lesions in the first two stages are distributed unevenly and may therefore be absent in needle biopsies of the liver. The characteristic lesion (ductal or Stage 1) consists of damaged interlobular and septal bile ducts surrounded by a dense infiltrate of lymphocytes and plasma cells. Well-formed granulomas are frequently seen near the injured bile ducts. In Stage 2 (ductular) of the disease, bile ductules proliferate and bile ducts are reduced in number. Portal fibrosis may be present or absent, and granulomata are found less often than in Stage 1. Later, as the inflammation subsides, scarring increases, most marked in portal areas with fibrous septa extending into the lobule (Stage 3). When cirrhotic (Stage 4), the liver may lose all of the characteristic lesions. Bile ducts are few in both Stages 3 and 4, and this paucity of bile ducts may be the only clue to the diagnosis of primary biliary cirrhosis. In one quarter of the cases, alcoholic hyalin is identifiable in the biopsy. Histologic features of chronic active hepatitis may also be present, leading to difficulties in diagnosis.

CLINICAL MANIFESTATIONS (Table 126–2). Ninety per cent of patients with primary biliary cirrhosis are female. The disease has been found in patients as young as 23 and as old as 72; however, the majority of patients are of ages 40 to 60. The onset is usually marked by *pruritus*, or by discovery of asymptomatic hepatomegaly. Sometimes the first abnormality is an elevated alkaline phosphatase noted on an automated screening panel. The itching may start during pregnancy or with the use of birth control pills. Following delivery or withdrawal of the medication, the itching usually continues; this is in contrast to *cholestasis of pregnancy*, in which pruritus resolves following parturition. Itching leads to excoriative dermatitis and thickening and darkening of the skin. Hepatomegaly and less frequently splenomegaly may be found at the time of diagnosis. *Jaundice* rarely precedes the onset of pruritus and may follow it by several years. *Portal hypertension* and *hepatic failure* are usually late events, and ascites or bleeding esophageal varices are uncommon presenting features. *Hypercholesterolemia*, secondary to the decreased biliary excretion of cholesterol, may be severe enough to produce xanthomas. *Osteomalacia* or more commonly *osteoporosis* may develop in these patients. The cause of the bone disease is incompletely understood; however, malabsorption of vitamin D and calcium are important pathogenic factors. Copper accumulates in the livers of patients with primary biliary cirrhosis because it cannot be efficiently secreted into the bile. The levels of hepatic copper may reach levels equal to those found in Wilson's disease, and rarely *Kayser-Fleischer rings* have been described.

ASSOCIATED DISEASES. Primarily biliary cirrhosis is associated with a variety of disorders. *Sjögren's syndrome* with dryness of the eyes and mouth is present in at least 70 per cent of patients when specific tests (Schirmer test, buccal biopsy, and others) are used (Ch. 438). These same patients may have hyposecretion by the pancreas. *Scleroderma* and the *CREST syndrome* (calcinosis, Reynaud's phenomenon, esophageal hypomotility, sclerodactyly, telangiectasia) are both increased in frequency in patients with primary biliary cirrhosis. The prevalence of *arthritis*, both seropositive and seronegative, is increased in these patients. *Thyroid autoantibodies* are found in about 25 per cent of patients, and in the antibody-positive patients thyroid dysfunction (primarily hypothyroidism) is common. *Renal tubular acidosis* also is present in patients with primary biliary cirrhosis. The pathogenesis of the renal tubular acidosis is unknown, but it may be secondary to deposition of copper in renal tubules.

LABORATORY FINDINGS. The *alkaline phosphatase* is elevated in almost all patients with primary biliary cirrhosis, although it may be normal in asymptomatic patients. The elevation is usually two to six times normal, but can be more than ten times normal. The serum bilirubin is usually normal or mildly elevated until the later stages of the disease are reached. Serum bile acids and cholesterol are increased frequently. Serum *immunoglobulin M* levels are increased in 75 per cent of patients with primary biliary cirrhosis. The finding, however, is not specific. Hypoprothrombinemia and hyocalcemia may be present and reflect deficiencies of vitamins K and D. The serum transaminases are normal to mildly elevated. Eighty-four to ninety-eight per cent of patients with primary biliary cirrhosis have *circulating antimitochondrial antibodies*. This antibody is directed toward an antigen in the inner mitochondrial membrane. The antibody is neither species nor organ specific. Antimitochondrial antibodies may be present in patients with HBsAg-negative chronic active hepatitis, cryptogenic cirrhosis, and collagen vascular diseases; however, test results are normal in patients with extrahepatic obstruction unless they also have primary biliary cirrhosis or chronic active hepatitis. A small percentage of patients (5 to 30 per cent) with primary biliary cirrhosis have antinuclear antibodies in their serum.

TABLE 126–2. CLINICAL FEATURES OF PRIMARY BILIARY CIRRHOSIS

Signs and Symptoms	Laboratory
Female preponderance (> 90%)	Antimitochondrial antibodies (> 90%)
Pruritus	Elevated alkaline phosphatase, cholesterol, IgM, serum bile acids, and bilirubin
Jaundice	***Associated Diseases***
Skin hyperpigmentation	Sjögren's syndrome
Hepatosplenomegaly	Scleroderma/CREST syndrome
Xanthelasma/xanthoma	Arthritis
Bleeding diathesis (vitamin K deficiency)	Autoimmune thyroiditis
Bone pain (osteoporosis/ osteomalacia)	Renal tubular acidosis
Ascites/variceal hemorrhage (late)	

DIAGNOSIS. The diagnosis of primary biliary cirrhosis is established by finding a positive antimitochondrial antibody test and the characteristic pathology (Stage 1 or 2) on liver biopsy. It may be necessary to exclude extrahepatic obstruction in some patients in whom the diagnosis of primary biliary cirrhosis cannot be made with certainty, as *extrahepatic biliary obstruction* can clinically mimic primary biliary cirrhosis. Also, patients with primary biliary cirrhosis have an increased incidence of gallstones, which may cause biliary obstruction. Biliary tract disease may be excluded by either transhepatic or endoscopic retrograde cholangiography.

THERAPY AND PROGNOSIS. No specific therapy for primary biliary cirrhosis is available. Corticosteroids are not known to be effective in this disease and will aggravate the bone disease. D-Penicillamine, azathioprine, and colchicine have been used in the treatment of primary biliary cirrhosis. D-Penicillamine cannot be recommended because its use is associated with numerous complications without improvement in survival. Recently, treatment with colchicine has been shown to improve liver tests but not hepatic histology as compared to placebo-treated controls. Further experience is required in the use of colchicine before it can be recommended.

The treatment of primary biliary cirrhosis is directed toward its complications and includes correction of specific deficiency states and reduction in the pruritus. Dietary fat may be reduced to 40 grams daily to decrease steatorrhea and improve calcium absorption. Medium-chain triglycerides are absorbed directly into the portal vein without the presence of intraluminal bile salts, and these may be given as a dietary supplement. If the prothrombin time is prolonged, vitamin K (10 mg) is given intramuscularly every four weeks. The osteomalacia may be preventable through such measures as exposure to sunlight (10 to 20 minutes daily) and dietary supplementation with vitamin D and calcium. The serum 25(OH)D level should be measured, and, if low, it should be increased to the normal range with oral vitamin D. If the serum 25(OH)D levels fail to increase with vitamin D therapy, then oral 25(OH)D, 100 to 200 μg daily, may be given. Hepatic osteomalacia, but not osteoporosis, responds to treatment with metabolites of vitamin D. During the administration of vitamin D or its metabolites, the serum and urine calcium must be monitored closely to prevent development of hypercalcemia. See Ch. 246 and 250 for further discussion of osteomalacia and osteoporosis, respectively. Patients with thyroid antibodies should be tested for hypothyroidism.

The cause of the pruritus is unknown, but it may be secondary to increased tissue levels of bile salts. Cholestyramine and colestipol are anion exchange resins that bind bile salts in the intestines, preventing their reabsorption in the terminal ileum. Eight to twelve grams of cholestyramine is given daily in divided doses with breakfast and dinner. Fat-soluble vitamins should not be given at the same time as the resin. The hypercholesterolemia may also respond to cholestyramine therapy. Clofibrate should not be used in these patients, as there may be a paradoxical increase in the serum cholesterol.

Patients with primary biliary cirrhosis who are asymptomatic have a good prognosis, with a ten-year survival similar to age-matched controls. Patients who present with symptoms have, in contrast, an average life expectancy of 5.5 to 11 years. The development of jaundice, ascites, or cirrhosis is associated with a poor prognosis.

Kaplan M: Primary biliary cirrhosis. N Engl J Med 316:521, 1987. *A succinct Medical Progress article with an excellent bibliography of 124 references. A good place to start.*

Kaplan M, Alling DW, Zimmerman HJ, et al.: A prospective trial of colchicine for primary biliary cirrhosis. N Engl J Med 315:1448, 1986. *Sixty patients were treated for up to two years with either colchicine or a placebo. Treatment with colchicine led to an improvement in liver tests but did not affect symptoms or progression of the liver lesions.*

Roll J: A new treatment for primary biliary cirrhosis? Gastroenterology 89:1195, 1985. *An excellent discussion of the treatment and prognosis of patients with primary biliary cirrhosis.*

Roll J, Boyer J, Barry D, et al: The prognostic importance of clinical and histologic features in asymptomatic and symptomatic primary biliary cirrhosis. N Engl J Med 308:1, 1983. *Defines the clinical and pathologic features that predict survival.*

Warnes T: Treatment of primary biliary cirrhosis. Semin Liver Dis 5:228, 1985. *A review of the treatment of the disease and its complications.*

SECONDARY BILIARY CIRRHOSIS

DEFINITION, ETIOLOGY, AND PATHOLOGY. Secondary biliary cirrhosis is an uncommon sequela of longstanding obstruction of the biliary tree. Obstruction is usually present for more than one year (mean of about six years) before cirrhosis develops; however, intervals as short as four months from the onset of obstruction (jaundice) to the diagnosis of cirrhosis have been reported. Cirrhosis or fibrosis may also develop in the absence of jaundice in patients with prolonged partial biliary tract obstruction as may be seen in chronic pancreatitis. In adults, obstruction is due to gallstones, strictures, carcinoma, chronic pancreatitis, or sclerosing cholangitis. In children, biliary atresia and cystic fibrosis are common causes of secondary biliary cirrhosis.

The liver is usually enlarged and dark green. The surface is granular or occasionally nodular. The lobular pattern is usually preserved until the cirrhosis is advanced. The portal tracts are widened owing to fibrosis and proliferation of bile ducts. The hepatic parenchyma may contain bile plugs, infarcts, or lakes. There is focal hepatocellular necrosis. As the cirrhosis progresses, the fibrous septa extend into the hepatic parenchyma, forming pseudolobules. In advanced cirrhosis, there is nodular regeneration.

CLINICAL MANIFESTATIONS. *Jaundice* is common but not invariable, and the level of jaundice may fluctuate. Patients with strictures or stones may have suffered recurrent bouts of cholangitis or biliary colic. *Pruritus* is also a common complaint and may precede the onset of icterus. If the pruritus is severe, itching may lead to thickening and darkening of the skin. Xanthelasma and xanthomas may appear. *Steatorrhea* with diarrhea may be a major complaint, and *bone disease* may develop owing to malabsorption of vitamin D and calcium. Splenomegaly is common. Ascites and gastrointestinal bleeding develop later in the course of the disease and are uncommon presenting complaints.

LABORATORY TESTS. The serum bilirubin is usually moderately increased (3 to 15 mg per deciliter). The alkaline phosphatase is also almost always increased; however, in 25 to 30 per cent, the elevation is less than twice normal. The AST is usually elevated, but the elevations are moderate. The prothrombin time may be prolonged and may improve with vitamin K administration. Hypoalbuminemia and hyperglobulinemia may also be present. Serum cholesterol and bile acids are frequently increased. *Lipoprotein X*, an abnormal lipoprotein, is found commonly in patients with extrahepatic obstruction (see Ch. 119). Lipoprotein X is also present in other forms of liver disease, and its absence does not exclude extrahepatic obstruction. Elevations of the white blood cell count in patients with extrahepatic obstruction suggest the presence of cholangitis or a hepatic abscess.

THERAPY AND PROGNOSIS. Relief of the biliary obstruction is the only specific form of treatment. In patients in whom the obstruction cannot be relieved, the correction of vitamin deficiencies and the use of cholestyramine to relieve itching, as outlined for the treatment of primary biliary cirrhosis, is warranted. In addition, there may be recurrent episodes of cholangitis requiring antibiotic treatment.

The prognosis for patients with carcinoma is poor, with most dying because of the malignancy and not because of the liver disease. The mortality for patients with benign obstructions (stone or stricture) depends on whether or not the obstruction can be relieved. When the obstruction cannot be relieved, mortality is high; however, survival may be prolonged (years) before the patient dies from hepatic failure or bleeding esophageal varices. Surgical relief of the biliary obstruction improves survival, although ascites and esophageal varices may develop later. The development of these complications, usually many years after apparently successful surgery, may be due to subclinical recurrence of partial biliary obstruction.

Littenberg G, Afroudakis A, Kaplowitz N: Common bile duct stenosis from chronic pancreatitis: Clinical and pathologic spectrum. Medicine 58:385, 1979. *Reviews the effects of the liver biliary obstruction secondary to chronic pancreatitis.*

CRYPTOGENIC CIRRHOSIS

DEFINITION AND ETIOLOGY. Cryptogenic (macronodular or postnecrotic) cirrhosis is any cirrhosis for which the etiology is unknown. The liver contains little or no necrosis or inflammation and has no diagnostic pathologic lesions (for example, alcoholic hepatitis). It lacks any specific lesions demonstrable by histochemical stains, e.g., $alpha_1$-antitrypsin or iron; and specific serologic tests, e.g., HBsAg, anti-HBc, AMA, and ceruloplasmin, are normal. It is assumed that most cases represent the end-stage of a previously active, chronic, or recurrent hepatitis, but alcoholic and other chronic liver diseases give rise to a very similar form of coarsely nodular cirrhosis. Cases previously called cryptogenic cirrhosis have been reported to be due to type B hepatitis despite the absence of detectable levels of HBsAg in the plasma. In these cases, HBV antigens or free or integrated HBV DNA was demonstrable in the liver cells. It is unclear, however, what role HBV infection played in the development of cirrhosis in this group of patients. Cryptogenic cirrhosis should become a less frequent diagnosis as our understanding of the causes of liver disease increases and we develop tests for agents such as non-A non-B hepatitis.

PATHOLOGY. The size of the liver is variable and its surface distorted by large regenerative nodules (macronodular), which may be several centimeters in diameter. The liver between the nodules appears to be collapsed and fibrotic. The microscopic appearance of the liver is one of regenerative nodules separated by connective tissue. The portal areas may be infiltrated by mononuclear cells, but the liver cells are well preserved, and active hepatocellular necrosis or hepatic steatosis is minimal or absent.

CLINICAL MANIFESTATIONS. Cryptogenic cirrhosis may remain clinically silent for many years and frequently is discovered unexpectedly, often during the evaluation of an unrelated condition. When the disease becomes "clinically manifest," its signs and symptoms are usually nonspecific (malaise, lethargy) or related to portal hypertension and include ascites, splenomegaly, hypersplenism, or bleeding esophageal varices. The liver frequently is of normal size or small. Splenomegaly is common; spider angiomas, ascites, and abdominal wall venous collaterals may also be present. Serum transaminases and bilirubin are usually normal to slightly increased. Hyperglobulinemia is common and may be the only laboratory abnormality.

DIAGNOSIS. Cryptogenic cirrhosis is a diagnosis of exclusion and is based on histologic and clinical evidence of cirrhosis in the absence of a definable etiology (see Table 126–1). Wilson's disease and hemochromatosis, although uncommon, are specifically treatable and should therefore be carefully excluded (see Ch. 205 and 206). A small number of patients with cryptogenic cirrhosis may have chronic hepatitis B infection despite the absence in the serum of detectable levels of HB_sAg. Measurement of anti-HB_c may be helpful in identifying these patients. Testing for antimitochondrial antibodies, ANA, and an LE preparation will help exclude primary biliary cirrhosis and chronic active hepatitis. Alpha$_1$-antitrypsin deficiency may be excluded by appropriate histochemical stains and serologic tests (see Ch. 125). Findings of hepatic congestion on biopsy may be indicative of occult cardiac disease or hepatic vein occlusion. A previous history of alcoholism may be the only evidence for alcohol as the cause of the cirrhosis.

TREATMENT AND PROGNOSIS. Specific therapy for this type of cirrhosis is lacking. Complications such as ascites, encephalopathy, and gastrointestinal bleeding should be managed as discussed in Ch. 114, 127, and 128. Patients who have asymptomatic cirrhosis may do quite well with a good five-year prognosis; however, the onset of ascites or bleeding esophageal varices is a poor prognostic sign.

CARDIAC CIRRHOSIS

ETIOLOGY. Cardiac cirrhosis is an uncommon complication of severe, prolonged, recurrent right heart failure of any cause, although it is usually due to rheumatic heart disease (mitral or aortic stenosis with tricuspid regurgitation), cardiomyopathy, or constrictive pericarditis.

PATHOLOGY. The gross appearance of the liver in acute hepatic failure is one of alternating red and pale areas (nutmeg liver). The red areas are congested central areas of the hepatic lobule, whereas the pale areas are the preserved hepatocytes. With recurrent bouts of heart failure, the centrilobular hepatocytes atrophy and fibrosis develops. The fibrosis is most marked in the central areas, and with time fibrous septa extend out into the rest of the lobule. Regenerative nodules develop later, and they arise from the periphery of the hepatic lobule.

CLINICAL MANIFESTATIONS, DIAGNOSIS, AND THERAPY. The clinical picture is usually dominated by the cardiac disease. Differentiation of patients with acute hepatic congestion from those with cardiac cirrhosis is difficult, as the clinical features are similar (see Ch. 125). The liver may be small or enlarged and firm. When tricuspid regurgitation is present, the absence of hepatic pulsation suggests cirrhosis. Ascites and splenomegaly are common. The bilirubin is usually only mildly increased, and either the unconjugated or conjugated pigment may predominate. The AST is often moderately elevated, but may be normal if the heart failure is controlled. The prothrombin time may be prolonged, and in the presence of significant liver disease Coumadin and related anticoagulants should be used with caution. The diagnosis of cardiac cirrhosis is established by performing a liver biopsy. However, in most situations, this is not warranted.

Reduction in the incidence of rheumatic fever and tuberculosis as well as advances in cardiovascular surgery in the Western world have made cardiac cirrhosis an uncommon disease. Its prognosis depends largely upon the course of the cardiac disease. If the latter can be successfully treated, hepatic function improves and liver disease stabilizes.

Dunn GD, Hayes P, Breen K, et al.: The liver in congestive heart failure: A review. Am J Med Sci 265:174, 1973. *Reviews both acute and chronic heart failure and their effects on the liver.*

127 MAJOR SEQUELAE OF CIRRHOSIS

Thomas D. Boyer

PORTAL HYPERTENSION

ANATOMY AND PHYSIOLOGY OF PORTAL VENOUS SYSTEM. The portal venous system begins in the capillaries of the intestines and terminates in the hepatic sinusoids. The portal vein is formed by the confluence of the superior and inferior mesenteric veins and splenic vein.

The liver receives about 1500 ml of blood each minute, two thirds of which is provided by the portal vein. The hepatic artery provides 40 to 60 per cent of the oxygen supply to the liver. The liver offers little resistance to the flow of blood, and the pressure within the sinusoids is low (less than 5 mm Hg above the pressure in the inferior vena cava). Since the veins in the portal system lack valves, increased resistance to flow at any point between the splanchnic venules and the heart will increase pressure in all vessels on the intestinal side of the obstruction.

DEFINITION AND PATHOGENESIS. Portal hypertension represents an increase in the hydrostatic pressure within the portal vein or its tributaries. This is manifested clinically by the development of *portal-systemic collaterals, splenomegaly*, and/or *ascites*. Since portal hypertension may be present in the absence of clinical findings, it may be detectable only by measurement of pressures in the portal system. Pressures within the hepatic sinusoids may be measured by catheterizing the hepatic veins (wedged hepatic vein pressure) or the portal vein pressure may be measured directly by transhepatic or umbilical vein catheterization or at surgery. Portal hypertension is present when the wedged hepatic vein pressure is more than 5 mm Hg higher than the inferior vena cava pressure. Although generally considered to be a progressive disorder, portal hypertension may in fact decrease as the liver disease improves, i.e., alcoholic hepatitis. Portal hypertension also can be an acute and transient phenomenon, as may occur with acute right heart failure. Since the pressure in any vascular system is directly proportional not only to resistance but also to flow, portal hypertension may result from either increased blood flow in the portal vein or increased resistance to flow within the portal venous system.

Increased portal venous blood flow is an unusual cause of portal hypertension for two reasons: (1) Increases in portal vein flow cause a reflex decrease in hepatic artery blood flow, thereby tending to maintain relatively normal sinusoidal pressure. (2) The outflow resistance from the liver is so low that increases in portal vein flow must be very large to cause a significant increase in portal venous pressure.

Increased resistance to venous flow is the most common mechanism for the development of portal hypertension. Liver disease accounts for the majority of cases; however, occlusion of the portal or hepatic veins and cardiac disease also cause increased resistance to flow and increases in portal pressure. The diseases causing portal hypertension are listed in Table 127–1 and are discussed below.

CLINICAL MANIFESTATIONS. The clinical presentation

TABLE 127–1. CAUSES OF PORTAL HYPERTENSION

Increased hepatic blood flow
Splenomegaly not due to liver disease
Arteriovenous fistula
Diseases of cardiovascular system
Portal vein occlusion
Splenic vein occlusion
Hepatic vein occlusion
Veno-occlusive disease
Web lesion or thrombosis of inferior vena cava
Congestive heart failure–constrictive pericarditis
Liver diseases
Cirrhosis—all causes
Congenital hepatic fibrosis
Schistosomiasis
Idiopathic portal hypertension
Sarcoidosis
Alcoholic hepatitis
Partial nodular transformation

of portal hypertension depends to a certain extent upon its cause. Essentially all forms may present with either *bleeding esophageal varices* or *splenomegaly* with or without *hypersplenism*. In portal vein thrombosis, as the liver is normal, ascites and jaundice are unusual. *Ascites* and other signs of hepatic disease (jaundice, spiders, encephalopathy) are common clinical features of cirrhosis. Occlusion of the hepatic veins almost always leads to development of ascites and varying degrees of hepatic dysfunction. Thus, the clinical findings may be important clues to the cause of the portal hypertension.

The development of portal-systemic collaterals is the major complication of portal hypertension. Several vessels may form collaterals. The veins that lie in the mucosa of the gastric fundus and esophagus are of greatest clinical interest because, when dilated, they form gastric and esophageal varices (Fig. 127–1). The remnant of the umbilical vein may also dilate. If

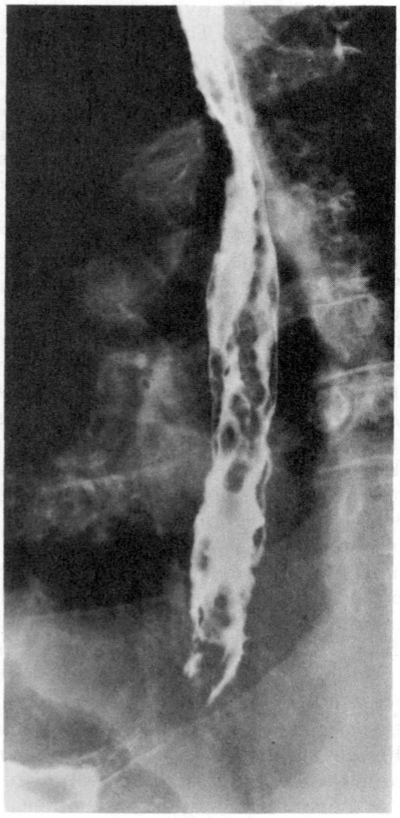

FIGURE 127–1. Barium esophagogram, demonstrating large varices involving the lower two thirds of the esophagus. (Courtesy of T. Munyer. From Zakim D, Boyer TD [eds.]: Hepatology: A Textbook of Liver Diseases. Philadelphia, W. B. Saunders Company, 1983.)

flow through this vessel becomes great enough, a loud venous hum may be audible over the path of the umbilical vein (Cruveilhier-Baumgarten syndrome). The umbilical vein enters the left portal vein, and therefore, if a venous hum is present, the cause of the portal hypertension must be intrahepatic or in the hepatic veins or inferior vena cava. Large collaterals also may form between the splenic and renal (chiefly left) veins. Dilated abdominal wall veins are common in patients with portal hypertension and are especially prominent when the patient stands. The hemorrhoidal veins may also act as collaterals. Varices may also form in unusual locations within the intestines (e.g., ileostomies, upper small bowel, and ascending, descending, and sigmoid colons), and these may bleed.

DISEASES CAUSING PORTAL HYPERTENSION (see Table 127–1). *Arteriovenous fistulas* may form between an artery and the portal vein or one of its tributaries as a consequence of abdominal trauma, liver biopsy, carcinoma (either intrahepatic or extrahepatic), or rupture of an arterial aneurysm (e.g., splenic). An upper abdominal bruit or a palpable thrill at surgery suggests this diagnosis in any patient with portal hypertension. The fistula can be localized by celiac angiography and is usually surgically correctable.

Splenomegaly resulting from hematologic diseases such as polycythemia rubra vera and myelofibrosis or an infiltrative process such as Gaucher's disease may, in rare instances, lead to portal hypertension. The enlarged spleen receives high blood flows from the splenic artery, leading to high flows within the splenic vein which are thought to cause the rise in portal pressure. These diseases also frequently involve the liver and the infiltrative process may increase intrahepatic resistance. However, the principal event in the genesis of the portal hypertension appears to be the high portal vein blood flow, since splenectomy usually cures the portal hypertension.

Splenic vein thrombosis may be caused by pancreatitis, abdominal trauma, or a locally invasive tumor. Pressure is increased only in areas drained by the splenic vein, whereas pressure in the portal vein is normal. The diagnosis should be suspected in a patient with gastric or esophageal varices but a normal liver biopsy, and is established by celiac angiography. Splenectomy is curative.

Portal vein thrombosis may develop following abdominal trauma or intra-abdominal sepsis, or in association with cirrhosis or hepatocellular carcinoma. In the majority of cases, however, the cause is unknown. This is primarily a disease of children, although adults may also develop portal vein thrombosis. The diagnosis is again suggested by the presence of portal hypertension in a patient with a normal liver biopsy. The diagnosis is established by angiography. Thrombi also may be identified using ultrasound or by CT scan. The surgical management of these patients may be difficult because of the absence of a patent vein to use for making a portal-systemic shunt.

Thrombosis of the hepatic veins (Budd-Chiari syndrome) may follow abdominal trauma or the use of birth control pills, or may occur in patients with diseases such as polycythemia rubra vera and paroxysmal nocturnal hemoglobinuria, which have an associated hypercoagulable state. Patients with hepatic vein thrombosis may develop an acute, subacute, or chronic illness in which abdominal pain and ascites are the major features. The liver is usually enlarged and tender. Elevations of the serum transaminases and bilirubin are usually mild, although they can be increased significantly in patients who have an acute illness. The initial clinical diagnosis is usually cirrhosis, and the correct diagnosis is not suspected until centrilobular congestion is seen on liver biopsy. Catheterization of the inferior vena cava and hepatic veins is a useful test in the evaluation of this condition. The presence of thrombi in the inferior vena cava can be established. The diagnosis of hepatic vein thrombosis is made by finding the characteristic pathology on liver biopsy, excluding cardiac disease that causes a similar histologic lesion, and inability to catheterize the hepatic veins. The outlook for patients with hepatic vein thrombosis is poor, with mortality of 50 to 90 per cent. The use of side-to-side portacaval shunts in these patients has been thought to prolong survival. Further experience is required before the proper role of this procedure can be evaluated. The use of anticoagulants has not been shown to affect survival.

Veno-occlusive disease (nonthrombotic occlusion of hepatic venules) also causes a Budd-Chiari–like syndrome. Veno-occlusive disease develops in patients who have ingested plants containing pyrrolidizine alkaloids, who have been treated for malignant disease with certain chemotherapeutic agents, or following bone marrow transplantation. It also is a common pathologic finding in patients with alcoholic hepatitis and cirrhosis. The disease is thought to be due to a toxic injury to the endothelium of the affected vessels. The occluded venules may be present in a liver biopsy, and an abnormal vascular pattern is found when contrast material is injected into the hepatic veins.

Thrombi, tumor, or a membrane in the inferior vena cava may obstruct the hepatic veins and give a clinical picture similar to that of hepatic vein thrombosis, with the additional features of peripheral edema and stasis dermatitis. Membranous obstruction near the terminus of the inferior vena cava has been described in all areas of the world but is most frequently observed in South Africa and the Orient. These patients also have a high incidence of hepatocellular carcinoma. The reasons for this latter association are unclear. Catheterization of the inferior vena cava will identify the obstructing lesion. Removal of the membrane surgically is sometimes possible and leads to resolution of the portal hypertension. Thrombectomy is usually not helpful.

Cirrhosis causes portal hypertension by increasing the intrahepatic vascular resistance. The increased resistance is thought to occur because of compression of vessels by regenerative nodules, distortion and reduction of the sinusoidal bed, and narrowing of portal vessels by the fibrous tissue. In alcoholic liver disease, serious portal hypertension may develop without cirrhosis. In some patients with acute alcoholic hepatitis, there is progressive obliteration of the central veins with resultant centrilobular fibrosis. These patients develop a severe outflow block, which leads to the formation of ascites or esophageal varices.

Portal hypertension due to noncirrhotic portal fibrosis may occur in four conditions. In *schistosomiasis,* the adult worm resides in the intestinal venules. The eggs are shed into these vessels and are swept into the portal vein and into the liver, where they lodge in and obstruct the portal venules. The host's immune response to the eggs leads to periportal fibrosis and the development of portal hypertension. (Schistosomiasis is discussed more fully in Ch. 400.) *Idiopathic portal hypertension* (Banti's syndrome) is a disease in which there is portal hypertension, no cirrhosis, and a patent portal vein. The liver biopsy may be normal, or there may be fibrosis in the periportal areas and in the space of Disse. The disease process is progressive, with the liver eventually becoming small and fibrotic. A similar clinical picture may be seen in patients exposed to arsenic, vinyl chloride, and copper salts. *Congenital hepatic fibrosis* also causes portal hypertension without cirrhosis. In the portal areas, there is marked hyperplasia of the bile ducts and stellate fibrosis. This condition may be present in association with cystic liver disease and Caroli's disease (intrahepatic ductal ectasia), with an associated polycystic renal lesion in many patients. The development of portal hypertension is the major consequence of this form of liver disease, as hepatic function is well maintained. Hepatic *sarcoidosis* may rarely lead to hepatic fibrosis and portal hypertension.

DIAGNOSTIC APPROACH TO PORTAL HYPERTENSION. Portal hypertension should be suspected in any patient with ascites or splenomegaly, and its presence is established when portal-systemic collaterals are found. One may find collaterals on physical examination (dilated abdominal wall or umbilical veins), or they may be identified in the esophagus or stomach by a gastrointestinal series or by endoscopy. It is important that the etiology of portal hypertension be identified, since some causes (splenic vein thrombosis) may be curable. A liver biopsy will provide useful information as to the presence of liver disease; central venous congestion suggests hepatic vein thrombosis or cardiac disease. If the biopsy is not diagnostic, then catheterization of the hepatic veins may be performed. Elevated pressure will establish the presence of liver disease. Also, inferior vena cava or hepatic vein thrombosis may be found during catheterization of the hepatic veins. If the wedge pressure is normal, then the cause of the portal hypertension is (1) occlusion of the portal vein or its tributaries, (2) liver disease that involves the periportal areas and portal venules (schistosomiasis or idiopathic portal hypertension) and therefore does not increase the wedge pressure, or (3) increased flow in the portal vein. Celiac angiography will usually differentiate among this group of patients. Ultrasonography or computed tomography may also be used to identify thrombi in the portal vein.

BLEEDING ESOPHAGEAL AND GASTRIC VARICES

PATHOGENESIS. Hemorrhage from esophageal varices is a major complication of portal hypertension. The mortality in adult patients with cirrhosis varies from 30 to 60 per cent for each bleeding episode. The varices form because of increased pressure in the portal vein. Bleeding from varices may occur when the portal pressure exceeds 11 to 12 mm Hg above inferior vena cava pressure. However, not all patients with pressures above these levels have bleeding varices. The tension on the vessel wall is greater in large as compared to small varices for a given level of pressure. Therefore, large varices are more likely to rupture and bleed than are smaller ones; reflux esophagitis and ascites do not appear to be important in the genesis of bleeding.

CLINICAL MANIFESTATIONS. The most common presentation is hematemesis. The bleeding may be massive with the rapid development of shock, or the bleeding may stop spontaneously only to recur later. On occasion, the patient may only complain of hematochezia or melena without an antecedent history of hematemesis. Features suggesting underlying liver disease such as hepatomegaly, ascites, or jaundice may be present or absent, depending on the etiology of the portal hypertension and the activity of the underlying hepatic disease.

DIAGNOSIS AND TREATMENT. The care of the patient with gastrointestinal bleeding is discussed in detail in Ch. 114. The restoration of the patient's blood volume takes precedence over all other therapy and diagnostic tests. The blood volume should be corrected rapidly but not excessively, since overexpansion may lead to the development of ascites or renewed bleeding. Proof that esophageal or gastric varices are the source of hemorrhage depends on endoscopy, since, even in those with known varices, 30 to 50 per cent will be bleeding from other lesions (especially gastritis).

The bleeding from varices in many patients stops without any specific therapy. The *medical management* of patients who continue to bleed includes *vasopressin, endoscopic sclerosis of varices,* and *balloon tamponade.* Long-term therapy with *propranolol* for the prevention of variceal hemorrhage is controversial and cannot be recommended.

Vasopressin, a potent vasoconstrictor, is believed to act by constricting the splanchnic arterioles, which results in a fall in portal flow and thus a drop in portal pressure. This drug should be given only to patients who can be carefully monitored, preferably in an intensive care unit. Vasopressin is infused into a peripheral vein at a rate of 0.2 to 0.4 unit per minute. This therapy will provide temporary control in about

60 per cent of patients. Unfortunately, about half of those initially controlled will have rebleeding, and the use of vasopressin has little effect on morbidity or mortality. The intravenous use of somatostatin or combined use of vasopressin and nitroglycerin may be as effective as vasopressin alone in controlling variceal hemorrhage, with fewer side effects. Further experience is required before these newer forms of therapy can be recommended. The gastric and esophageal varices lie in the mucosa of the gastric fundus and esophagus and are therefore susceptible to *balloon tamponade*. Tamponade is best accomplished by inserting a tube that has a gastric and an esophageal balloon (Sengstaken-Blakemore tube). Once placed in the stomach, the gastric balloon is inflated and pulled into the cardia of the stomach, tamponading the varices. If bleeding does not stop, then the esophageal balloon is inflated. This therapy is effective in controlling hemorrhage in 70 to 90 per cent of patients. There is a significant risk of aspiration during balloon tamponade, and 50 to 60 per cent of the patients will hemorrhage again. During endoscopy, the *direct injection of esophageal varices* with sclerosing agents has been described as a method for the control of acute bleeding and for the long-term management of these patients. Repeated injections over several weeks are required to obliterate the varices, and rebleeding during this period is common. Once they are obliterated the rate of rebleeding from the varices is reduced, and survival may be improved. Endoscopic sclerotherapy is associated with serious side effects and requires further clinical experience before its role in the management of bleeding varices is established.

In *surgical therapy* for portal hypertension the high pressure portal system is anastomosed to the low pressure systemic venous system to create a *portal-systemic shunt*. There are two basic types of shunts. One is *nonselective*, in that the entire portal-venous system is decompressed. The end-to-side and side-to-side portacaval and mesocaval shunts are nonselective. *Selective* shunts decompress only the varices. The pressure remains high in the portal vein, and portal flow into the liver is preserved. Thus the varices are decompressed with minimal disruption of the normal hepatic circulation. The distal splenorenal shunt is of this type. The selective shunt may cause less encephalopathy than the nonselective types of shunts without improving survival.

Portal-systemic shunts have been used in four clinical situations: (1) *Hypersplenism* is not an indication for a portal-systemic shunt, because the reduction in formed elements in the blood is usually not of clinical significance. (2) The *prophylactic shunt* is made in patients with cirrhosis and varices but who have never bled. Prophylactic shunts shorten survival compared to unoperated controls, with death from hepatic encephalopathy and liver failure. Thus prophylactic shunts should not be performed. (3) *Emergency shunts* may be used to control hemorrhage in actively bleeding patients. However, the operative mortality may exceed 50 per cent, so that emergency shunts should be used rarely and in a select group of patients. The indications for this operation are still controversial. (4) *Therapeutic portal-systemic shunts* are used in patients who have bled at least once from varices. Operations in these patients have been shown to effectively stop further bleeding from varices. Unfortunately, the patient's survival is not improved significantly because of an increased incidence of hepatic encephalopathy and liver failure when compared to unoperated controls. Possibly these results could be improved upon by better selection of patients for the operations. As might be expected, the majority of patients with poor hepatocellular function, i.e., those who are jaundiced with hypoalbuminemia, ascites, encephalopathy, and poor nutrition, tolerate a portal-systemic shunt less well than do patients without these complications of liver disease. Patients with more severe liver disease may well be better managed by sclerosis of their varices than by shunt operations. The choice of therapy (sclerosis or shunt) for bleeding varices in patients with well-compensated cirrhosis is controversial. The morbidity and mortality from bleeding esophageal varices will remain high until current therapies are refined and new ones developed.

Benhamou J-P, Lebrec D: Portal hypertension. Clin Gastroenterol 14:1, 1985. *A multiple-authored review of portal hypertension and the treatment of bleeding varices.*

Boyer TD: Portal hypertension and its complications. In Zakim D, Boyer TD (eds.): Hepatology: A Textbook of Liver Disease. Philadelphia, W. B. Saunders Company, 1982, pp 464–499. *A current review of portal hypertension and its causes.*

Conn HO: Vasopressin and nitroglycerin in the treatment of bleeding varices: The bottom line. Hepatology 6:523, 1986. *An editorial that reviews the use of vasoconstrictors in the management of variceal hemorrhage.*

Groszmann R, Atterbury C: The pharmacological therapy of portal hypertension. Adv Intern Med 31:341, 1985. *An up-to-date review of the use of vasoconstrictors, vasodilators, or β-blockade for the treatment of bleeding varices.*

Mitchell MC, Boitnott JK, Kaufman S, et al.: Budd-Chiari syndrome: Etiology, diagnosis and management. Medicine 61:199, 1982. *An excellent review of hepatic vein thrombosis.*

Smith JL, Graham D: Variceal hemorrhage: A critical evaluation of survival analysis. Gastroenterology 82:968, 1983. *A careful evaluation of survival following an episode of hemorrhage from varices.*

The Copenhagen Esophageal Varices Sclerotherapy Project: Sclerotherapy after first variceal hemorrhage in cirrhosis: A randomized multicenter trial. N Engl J Med 311:1594, 1984. *A large trial that demonstrates a decrease in rebleeding and an improvement in survival in patients who survived long enough to have their varices obliterated.*

ASCITES

DEFINITION. Ascites is the presence of excess fluid in the peritoneal cavity. It is most frequently due to cirrhosis, but there are numerous other causes (see Ch. 112), and it cannot be assumed that the appearance of ascites is indicative of cirrhosis. For this reason, patients with a recent onset of ascites must be thoroughly evaluated to establish its cause.

PATHOGENESIS (Table 127–2). Ascites forms in patients with portal hypertension because of changes in the formation and reabsorption of hepatic and splanchnic lymph and because of alterations in the metabolism of salt and water by the kidneys.

Splanchnic Lymph Formation. Increases in portal venous pressure cause a rise in the pressure within the splanchnic capillaries, resulting in loss of fluid into the interstitial space. The capillaries of the intestine restrict the loss of protein to the interstitial space, and an oncotic gradient develops between the capillary and the extravascular space. This oncotic gradient returns the majority of the fluid to the capillary, and any fluid loss is usually removed by the intestinal lymphatics. For this reason, diseases that elevate the pressure only in the splanchnic bed, e.g., portal vein thrombosis, causes ascites uncommonly.

Hepatic Lymph Formation. In the noncirrhotic liver the endothelial lining of the hepatic sinusoids is discontinuous and does not effectively restrict plasma protein loss with even slight increases in sinusoidal pressure. Thus, in contrast to the intestines, the oncotic gradient between the sinusoids and extravascular space is small, and much of the fluid entering the interstitial space is not returned to the vascular space. These large amounts of fluid lost into the interstitial space must be returned to the vascular space via hepatic lymphatics. When the rate of formation of lymph exceeds the rate of removal, then fluid "weeps" out of the lymphatics and into

TABLE 127–2. FACTORS IN THE PATHOGENESIS OF CIRRHOTIC ASCITES

1. Increased hydrostatic pressure in hepatic sinusoids and splanchnic capillaries.
2. Overproduction of hepatic and splanchnic lymph secondary to (1), leading to a transudation of lymph into peritoneal space.
3. Limited or reduced reabsorption of water and protein by peritoneal lymphatics.
4. Sodium retention by the kidney secondary to hyperaldosteronism, increased sympathetic activity, alterations in metabolism of prostaglandins and kinins, and altered renal hemodynamics.
5. Impaired renal water excretion, in part caused by increased levels of ADH.

the peritoneal cavity. Diseases that cause marked elevations of the sinusoidal pressure, e.g., congestive heart failure and hepatic vein thrombosis, therefore commonly cause ascites with a high protein content. With cirrhosis the situation is more complex in that there is "capillarization" of the sinusoids such that an oncotic gradient forms between plasma and lymph. Large amounts of lymph are formed by the cirrhotic liver with overflow into the peritoneal space; however, the protein content of this fluid is low.

Peritoneal Reabsorption. The peritoneum plays an active role in the reabsorption of the ascitic fluid. Water and protein are reabsorbed by the lymphatics in the peritoneal membrane. The intra-abdominal pressure and character of the peritoneum are important factors in determining the rate of removal. The amount of fluid removed by the peritoneal lymphatics is variable but usually does not exceed 800 to 1000 ml every 24 hours.

Renal Function. An important factor in the genesis of ascites is the *retention of sodium* by the kidney. During the formation of ascites there is a positive sodium balance despite a total body sodium that is greater than normal. The pathogenesis of the sodium retention by the kidney is understood poorly; however, there is increased reabsorption of sodium by both proximal and distal tubules. The increased reabsorption of sodium may be mediated, in part, by increased plasma levels of aldosterone, increased sympathetic activity, and alterations in the renal production of prostaglandins and kinins. Reduced renal blood flow resulting from vasoconstriction also leads to enhanced sodium reabsorption.

CLINICAL MANIFESTATIONS AND DIAGNOSIS. Patients with ascites complain of increasing abdominal girth. The presence of ascites on physical examination is suggested by the findings of shifting dullness, a ballotable liver, or a fluid wave. Small amounts of ascites may be identified by abdominal ultrasound. Once the presence of ascites is suspected, diagnostic paracentesis should be performed. The character of the ascitic fluid in cirrhosis is variable; however, 80 to 90 per cent of patients have an ascitic fluid protein concentration of less than 2.5 grams per deciliter. The ascitic fluid lactic dehydrogenase and albumin concentrations are also low. The ascitic fluid white blood cell count is less than 500 per cubic millimeter in 90 per cent of patients with cirrhosis, and mononuclear cells predominate (>75 per cent).

MANAGEMENT. Resolution of the acute hepatic injury, following withdrawal of ethanol or a specific course of therapy, may reduce portal hypertension, and ascites may resolve spontaneously. In many patients, however, ascites is chronic and specific therapy is warranted. Accumulation of ascitic fluid occurs only in patients who are in positive sodium balance; therefore, *restricting sodium intake* will diminish or stop the accumulation of ascitic fluid. Diets containing 250 to 500 mg of sodium (10 to 20 mEq) are adequate to achieve sodium balance in most patients. The kidney is also unable to excrete a water load normally in some patients with ascites, in part because of high blood levels of antidiuretic hormone. *Fluid restriction* (1000 to 1500 ml daily) is sometimes necessary, therefore, to prevent hyponatremia. Many patients do not lose their ascites or edema with sodium restriction, and the use of *diuretics* becomes necessary. Spironolactone and triamterene act on the distal tubule and cause natriuresis with sparing of potassium. Spironolactone, 150 to 400 mg daily, causes diuresis in patients with mild to moderate sodium retention. Furosemide, thiazides, and ethacrynic acid are more potent diuretics and cause both natriuresis and potassium wasting. Furosemide, 40 to 80 mg daily, in combination with spironolactone or triamterene, causes diuresis in most patients with ascites. All diuretics cause a loss of fluid from the plasma. This fluid is then replaced by the reabsorption of ascitic or edema fluid. The rate of fluid lost should therefore not exceed the rate at which the ascites and edema fluids may be reabsorbed. The maximal rate of reabsorption of ascitic fluid varies widely; however, fluid losses of 1 kg daily in patients with edema and ascites and 0.3 to 0.5 kg daily in those with only ascites are well tolerated. The BUN and electrolytes must be monitored for the development of azotemia and hypokalemia. The use of diets very low in sodium (250 to 500 mg) is possible in the hospital; however, this is rarely possible in an outpatient setting. Therefore, preceding discharge from the hospital, the patient's sodium intake should be increased (1 to 2 grams daily) and diuretics adjusted so that he or she is still in negative sodium balance.

A few patients with cirrhosis will not respond to diuretic therapy. Treatment in the hospital with increasing doses of diuretics leads to azotemia or hepatic encephalopathy. Other patients are controlled in the hospital but, upon discharge, rapidly reaccumulate their ascitic fluid. If these patients are incapacitated by the ascites, they may be candidates for other therapies. The *peritoneovenous (LeVeen) shunt* consists of a tube placed subcutaneously between the peritoneal cavity and the superior vena cava. There is a pressure-activated one-way valve that allows peritoneal fluid to enter the vascular space but prevents the backflow of blood into the tube. This shunt may be effective in controlling ascites; however, its use is associated with episodes of disseminated intravascular coagulation, sepsis, and frequent shunt thrombosis, thus limiting its application only to patients who have severe and incapacitating ascites. Even in this latter group of patients, its use is controversial. The shunt should not be used in patients whose condition can be managed by other therapies. Repeated *abdominal paracentesis* of 1 to 2 liters of ascitic fluid is a poor form of long-term therapy for resistant ascites. Patients presenting with massive ascites and difficulty in breathing, however, may be improved dramatically by the removal of 1 to 2 liters of fluid. Attempts to increase the venous oncotic pressure by infusions of albumin or plasma are not likely to cause sustained diuresis and are an expensive form of therapy.

SPONTANEOUS BACTERIAL PERITONITIS. Patients with cirrhosis and ascites may develop spontaneous bacterial peritonitis. There is no obvious cause for the peritonitis, i.e., perforation of the bowel, and it appears to occur because of bacterial seeding of the ascitic fluid via the lymph or blood or by bacteria traversing the bowel wall. The frequency of this complication in patients with ascites may be increasing, and its early recognition is essential (mortality exceeds 60 to 90 per cent even if treated). Patients with very low ascitic fluid protein levels (less than 1 gram per deciliter) appear to be at greater risk for developing peritonitis. The clues to the diagnosis are the presence of fever, abdominal pain or tenderness, or decreased bowel sounds in a patient with ascites. The diagnosis should also be suspected in patients with the sudden onset of hepatic encephalopathy or hypotension. Patients may be asymptomatic and the diagnosis suggested only by finding an elevated ascitic fluid white blood cell count, or by a positive ascitic fluid culture. The diagnosis is established by abdominal paracentesis, which should be performed in patients with onset of new ascites or in those with a change in their clinical course. The ascitic fluid white blood cell count is usually above 500 per cubic millimeter (93 per cent of cases), and more than 50 per cent of the cells are polymorphonuclear leukocytes. The ascitic fluid pH also is lower than the blood pH. Bacteria may be identified on Gram's stain. The ascitic fluid and blood should be cultured and treatment instituted before the results of culture are known, as delays in therapy may increase mortality. The organisms most frequently cultured are Enterobacteriaceae (mainly *E. coli*) and Group D streptococci, *Streptococcus pneumoniae*, and *Streptococcus viridans*. Other bacteria are cultured less frequently, and anaerobic bacteria are uncommon isolates. Initial antibiotic therapy should therefore include both an aminoglycoside and ampicillin or a newer cephalosporin antibiotic. The response to therapy is monitored by the fever pattern and by changes in the ascitic fluid white blood cell count. If therapy is effective, the ascitic fluid white blood cell count falls and the predominant cell again becomes mononuclear. Antibiotic therapy is continued for 10 to 14 days.

HEPATORENAL SYNDROME

DEFINITION AND PATHOGENESIS. The hepatorenal syndrome (functional renal failure) is a decrease in renal function that develops in a patient with serious liver disease in whom all other causes of renal dysfunction are excluded. The kidneys lack serious pathologic lesions. If the liver disease improves, normal renal function returns. The pathogenesis of the hepatorenal syndrome is unknown. There is intense intrarenal vasoconstriction and redistribution of blood flow. In addition, the plasma levels of renin and aldosterone are increased. These changes may be due to reduced "effective" plasma volume in some patients.

CLINICAL MANIFESTATIONS. Patients developing the hepatorenal syndrome frequently have severe hepatic disease and therefore are jaundiced and have other signs and symptoms of liver disease. Almost all of the patients with this syndrome have ascites. The illness is marked by oliguria. The urine is usually free of protein, and the urine sediment is normal. The urine sodium level is low (<10 mEq per liter), the urine-plasma creatinine ratio is high (>30:1), and the urine-plasma osmolality ratio is greater than 1.0. These urine findings are different from those of acute tubular necrosis, in which the urine sodium content is high (>30 mEq per liter), the urine-plasma creatinine ratio is low (<20:1), and the urine is isosmotic to plasma. The progression of the renal failure is variable, with some patients having a complete loss of renal function over several days, whereas in others the serum creatinine slowly increases over several weeks as the liver function gradually worsens.

DIFFERENTIAL DIAGNOSIS. Patients with liver disease may develop renal failure for a variety of reasons. These patients commonly receive diuretics and may develop prerenal azotemia. Renal function will improve with withdrawal of the medication. Acute tubular necrosis may occur following an episode of hypotension (bleeding or sepsis) or during fulminant hepatitis and can be distinguished from hepatorenal failure by the urine findings. Drugs (antibiotics, especially aminoglycosides, and nonsteroidal anti-inflammatory medications) may cause worsening of renal function in patients with cirrhosis. Acute pyelonephritis, with or without papillary necrosis, may also cause renal failure in patients with liver disease.

THERAPY AND PROGNOSIS. Specific causes of renal failure should be looked for and excluded. Any medications that are potential nephrotoxins should be withdrawn. A brief trial of plasma expansion with monitoring of urine output and serum creatinine may be attempted, to exclude hypovolemia as a cause of the renal failure. The volume of fluid infused should be limited (1000 ml), as overexpansion of the plasma volume may precipitate variceal hemorrhage. Infusions of vasodilators may transiently improve renal function; however, this does not improve survival. Uremia may be treated by dialysis; again, overall survival is not improved. The use of peritoneovenous shunts in these patients is being investigated, but their efficacy is as yet unproven. The prognosis for patients with the hepatorenal syndrome is poor, with over 90 per cent dying during hospitalization, usually from liver failure or complications of portal hypertension. Definitive therapies must await a better understanding of the pathogenesis of this syndrome.

Boyer T, Goldman I: Treatment of cirrhotic ascites. Adv Intern Med 31:359, 1985. *Discusses the overall management of cirrhotic ascites, including the role of the peritoneovenous shunt.*

Epstein M: Peritoneovenous shunt in the management of ascites and the hepatorenal syndrome. Gastroenterology 82:790, 1982. *An authoritative review of the good and bad effects of the peritoneovenous shunt.*

Epstein M (ed.): The Kidney in Liver Disease. 2nd ed. New York, Elsevier Biomedical, 1982. *A complete review of the renal functional alterations in liver disease. Multiple authors contributed to this work.*

Hoefs JC, Canawati HN, Sapico FL, et al.: Spontaneous bacterial peritonitis. Hepatology 2:399, 1982. *Describes the clinical features and hospital course of patients with spontaneous peritonitis.*

Reynolds T: Rapid presumptive diagnosis of spontaneous bacterial peritonitis. Gastroenterology 90:1294, 1986. *An expert's discussion of the value of the newer tests that have been proposed to be of value in the diagnosis of spontaneous bacterial peritonitis.*

128 ACUTE AND CHRONIC HEPATIC FAILURE AND HEPATIC TRANSPLANTATION

Bruce F. Scharschmidt

THE SYNDROME OF HEPATIC ENCEPHALOPATHY

DEFINITION AND SIGNIFICANCE. Hepatic encephalopathy (also called hepatic coma or portal-systemic encephalopathy) represents a constellation of neurologic signs and symptoms accompanying advanced, decompensated liver disease of all types and/or extensive portal-systemic shunting. Recognition of these signs and symptoms often represents an important clue to the presence of deteriorating liver function or superimposed complications. In addition, repeated neurologic evaluation of the encephalopathic patient provides valuable information regarding the patient's course and prognosis.

PATHOGENESIS. The pathogenesis of hepatic encephalopathy remains unclear. The encephalopathy is at least partially attributable to toxic materials that are derived from the metabolism of nitrogenous substrate in the gut and that bypass the liver through anatomic or functional shunts. This is the origin of the term *portal-systemic encephalopathy*, often used interchangeably with hepatic encephalopathy. *Ammonia* and *mercaptans* result from the degradation of urea or protein and sulfur-containing compounds, respectively, and both can produce coma when administered in large doses to animals. The presence of mercaptans in the breath of some encephalopathic patients probably accounts for the characteristic sweetish musty odor termed *fetor hepaticus*. Ammonia-induced changes in central nervous system metabolism include depletion of glutamic and aspartic acids and ATP. While often present in increased amounts in the blood or cerebrospinal fluid or both, the absolute concentration of ammonia, ammonia metabolites including glutamine, and mercaptans correlates only roughly with the presence or severity of encephalopathy. *Gamma-aminobutyric acid*, the principal inhibitory neurotransmitter in the mammalian brain, is also produced in the gut and is present in increased amounts in the blood of patients and animals with hepatic failure. A role for gamma-aminobutyric acid in hepatic encephalopathy is supported by the observation that visual evoked potentials in animals with hepatic failure mimic those of benzodiazepine-induced or barbiturate-induced coma, but differ from those of comatose states caused by administration of ether, ammonia, or mercaptans. A separate hypothesis holds that accelerated entry of *aromatic amino acids* into the central nervous system results in decreased synthesis of normal neurotransmitters such as norepinephrine and enhanced synthesis of *false neurotransmitters* such as octopamine. Other compounds such as short-chain *fatty acids* are also present in blood in increased amounts and have been proposed as potentially toxic. Finally, there is impaired integrity of the *blood-brain barrier* in animals with acute hepatic failure. It is possible that hepatic encephalopathy may represent the synergistic effects of a number of toxins acting on an unusually susceptible nervous system.

TABLE 128–1. STAGES OF HEPATIC ENCEPHALOPATHY

Stage 0	Subclinical encephalopathy associated with impaired psychomotor function
Stage I	Varied manifestations, often diagnosed in retrospect, including apathy, lack of awareness, anxiety, restlessness, slowed thinking, reversal of sleep rhythm
Stage II	Lethargy, drowsiness, disorientation, incontinence
Stage III	Deep somnolence (but patient can at least transiently be aroused), incoherent speech
Stage IV	Coma; patient may (Stage IVA) or may not (Stage IVB) respond to painful stimuli

NEUROLOGIC MANIFESTATIONS. The personality and mental changes of hepatic encephalopathy are frequently divided into stages (Table 128–1). Although this staging of encephalopathy is generally useful, marked individual variations occur, and many patients do not show an orderly progression of symptoms. Moreover, the clinical grading scale is relatively insensitive. Standardized testing has revealed psychomotor abnormalities in a high proportion of patients with cirrhosis in whom conventional neurologic examination is normal. Such *subclinical encephalopathy* is potentially important inasmuch as it may be associated with impaired functional capacity, including job performance and ability to drive an automobile. Patients with hepatic encephalopathy also display a characteristic spectrum of abnormal neurologic signs. Early signs may include asterixis, myoclonus, hyperactive muscle stretch reflexes, facial grimacing, and blinking, as well as primitive reflexes such as suck, snout, and grasp. As encephalopathy progresses, extensor toe responses, clonus, and decerebrate or decorticate posturing may be observed. Generalized flaccidity with absence of reflexes occurs preterminally.

In addition to the acute, reversible signs and symptoms already mentioned, rare patients with longstanding liver disease and portal-systemic shunting develop *irreversible neurologic dysfunction* characterized by tremor, rigidity, slurred speech, oral-facial dyskinesia, choreoathetosis, and ataxic gait. Spastic paraparesis is another rare manifestation of advanced chronic liver disease and portal-systemic shunting.

As with other types of metabolic encephalopathy, asymmetric neurologic findings are unusual, and brainstem reflexes such as the pupillary light response, oculovestibular response, and oculocephalic response are typically preserved until very late. Thus, asymmetric neurologic signs or abnormal brain stem reflexes may suggest a structural lesion of the central nervous system such as a subdural hematoma. Seizures are also uncommon in the absence of alcohol withdrawal and should alert the clinician to the possibility of a structural lesion or hypoglycemia. The disappearance of pupillary reactivity, of the oculocephalic or oculovestibular response, or of deep tendon reflexes is associated with a very poor prognosis in all types of metabolic encephalopathy, including hepatic encephalopathy (but excluding drug overdose). Electroencephalographic changes are sensitive indicators of hepatic encephalopathy but are not specific for this disorder. They include symmetric slowing observed initially over the frontal areas with later spreading laterally and posteriorly.

DIAGNOSIS. The diagnosis of hepatic encephalopathy is based upon the presence of compatible neurologic signs and symptoms in a patient with advanced liver disease and exclusion of other possible causes of the neurologic abnormalities. Routine laboratory studies, including electrolytes, calcium, blood urea nitrogen, creatinine, glucose, and standard liver function tests, are of help primarily in excluding other causes of metabolic encephalopathy and evaluating the presence and severity of hepatic disease. Toxicologic screening is also appropriate when ingestion of sedatives or toxins capable of altering neurologic function is suspected. Blood ammonia and cerebrospinal fluid levels of glutamine correlate only roughly with mental status and are therefore of limited value in most circumstances. Structural lesions such as a subdural hematoma are often a consideration and may require special radiologic studies. Other causes of encephalopathy such as the Wernicke-Korsakoff syndrome, sepsis, or meningitis must also be excluded, depending on the clinical circumstances.

TREATMENT. ***Identification of Precipitating Factors.*** The management of patients with hepatic encephalopathy is largely supportive. A thorough search should be made to detect and correct factors that may precipitate or aggravate encephalopathy (Table 128–2). All nonessential drugs should be stopped—particularly sedatives and potentially hepatotoxic agents. For the occasional patient who demonstrates manic disorientation as an early manifestation of encephalopathy, soft restraints are preferable to sedative hypnotic agents.

Decreasing Production and Absorption of Enteric Toxins. Therapy should also be directed at decreasing the production of putative toxins that result from enteric bacterial metabolism of nitrogenous substrates. The level of blood urea nitrogen should be lowered if possible since urea diffuses into the gut and is a substrate for ammonia production. Gut cleansing should be accomplished by enema, and oral administration of cathartics such as magnesium citrate is appropriate unless lactulose (see below) is administered. It is also generally appropriate to restrict dietary protein to about 40 grams per day in mildly encephalopathic patients and eliminate it in patients with more advanced or progressive encephalopathy. Several additional points regarding protein merit consideration. First, *vegetable protein* appears somewhat less likely to induce encephalopathy than animal protein and may be useful in the long-term management of patients with chronic or recurrent encephalopathy. Second, since protein-calorie malnutrition may play a role in the pathogenesis of alcoholic hepatitis, judicious administration of 40 to 80 grams of protein, with careful observation, may be appropriate for such patients even in the presence of encephalopathy. Finally, while oral or parenteral administration of *branched-chain amino acids* has been reported to be beneficial in the treatment of hepatic encephalopathy, controlled trials have not provided clear evidence of efficacy, and their use is not generally recommended.

In addition to these measures aimed at decreasing nitrogenous substrate, production of enteric toxins should be further inhibited by oral administration of a poorly absorbable antibiotic, such as neomycin in a dose of 1 to 2 grams every six hours, or by administration of lactulose. Lactulose is neither metabolized nor absorbed in the upper small bowel and is metabolized by ileal and colonic bacteria to organic acids. It is as effective as neomycin in lowering blood ammonia and reversing encephalopathy in patients with chronic liver disease. The mechanisms of action of lactulose may include increased bacterial assimilation of ammonia, decreased ammonia production, and possibly trapping of ammonia as NH_4^+ or ammonia precursors in the bowel lumen made more acidic by its metabolism. Lactulose therapy is commonly initiated by administering 50 ml of the syrup orally every two hours until diarrhea ensues. Thereafter, the dose is decreased to that amount necessary to produce two to four soft stools per day. Lactulose can also be given by retention enema. Concom-

TABLE 128–2. HEPATIC ENCEPHALOPATHY—COMMON PRECIPITATING FACTORS

Deterioration in hepatic function
Drugs (sedative or potentially hepatotoxic agents)
Gastrointestinal hemorrhage
Increased dietary protein
Azotemia
Hypokalemia
Infection
Constipation
Anesthesia and surgery
Hypoxia
Diuretics (hypokalemia, alkalosis, and hypovolemia)

itant administration of neomycin and lactulose may be useful in selected patients.

FULMINANT HEPATIC FAILURE

ETIOLOGY. Fulminant hepatic failure is defined as hepatic failure with Stage III or IV encephalopathy developing in less than eight weeks in a patient without pre-existing liver disease. It develops most commonly as a complication of viral hepatitis (usually B; B with superimposed delta; non-A, non-B; less commonly A), but may also result from exposure to a potentially hepatotoxic drug (e.g., acetaminophen) or anesthetic (halothane), exposure to a frank hepatotoxin (e.g., carbon tetrachloride), or from certain less common hepatic disorders (e.g., acute hepatic vein occlusion, acute fatty liver of pregnancy) and infections (herpes simplex virus). Reye's syndrome may present a similar clinical picture; however, it differs from most forms of fulminant hepatic failure in its presumed pathogenesis, its rarity beyond the second decade of life, and by the accumulation of microvesicular fat in hepatocytes. Wilson's disease may also present as acute hepatic failure and is particularly important to recognize because it is potentially treatable (see Ch. 205). Finally, a small group of patients exist in whom the duration of illness prior to the onset of encephalopathy may range from eight weeks to several months, but in whom, as in patients with fulminant hepatic failure, there is no evidence of previous liver disease. Serologic evidence of viral infection or toxic exposure is often lacking, and such *late-onset acute hepatic failure* (also called subacute hepatic necrosis or subacute hepatitis) is frequently attributed to non-A, non-B hepatitis. Apart from the somewhat slower tempo of their illness, these patients exhibit a clinical course and prognosis similar to patients who meet standard criteria for fulminant hepatic failure.

DIAGNOSIS. The diagnosis of fulminant hepatic failure requires the presence of Stage III or IV encephalopathy in a patient with severe, acute liver disease. Synthetic function of the liver as reflected by the prothrombin time is nearly always markedly abnormal. Serum bilirubin concentration is less helpful, since some patients may become very ill rapidly and progress to coma before the serum bilirubin is markedly elevated. Serum transaminase levels are usually elevated early in the illness but do not reliably distinguish between fulminant hepatic failure and acute hepatitis without encephalopathy.

TREATMENT. A thorough search should be made to detect and correct factors that may precipitate or aggravate encephalopathy (Table 128–2); however, encephalopathy in fulminant hepatic failure primarily reflects the severe nature of the underlying liver injury, and correcting potential precipitating factors is less likely to produce objective benefit than it is in patients with encephalopathy complicating chronic liver disease. Special attention must be directed to those complications that frequently occur in patients with fulminant hepatic failure. *Hypoglycemia* is common and results from impaired glycogenolysis and gluconeogenesis. Frequent monitoring of blood glucose is necessary, and administration of a 10 per cent dextrose solution is advisable. *Hyponatremia,* which is typically due to a combination of impaired renal clearance of free water and administration of excessive free water in the form of dextrose solutions, may require water restriction. *Hypokalemia,* which increases renal ammonia production, should be corrected. *Azotemia* frequently occurs and may result from hypovolemia, hepatorenal syndrome, or acute tubular necrosis. Hypovolemia should be corrected when present. Survival in patients with fulminant hepatic failure and either the hepatorenal syndrome or acute tubular necrosis does not appear to be improved by dialysis. In the patient with severe hypoprothrombinemia and serious *bleeding,* administration of fresh frozen plasma is appropriate in addition to measures directed more specifically at the source of hemorrhage. The risk of gastrointestinal bleeding in patients with fulminant hepatic failure has been shown to be reduced by prophylactic administration of the H_2-receptor antagonist cimetidine. However, on the basis of studies in other critically ill patient groups, prophylactic administration of antacids is probably more effective and generally advisable. There is no evidence that heparin improves survival in patients with *disseminated intravascular coagulation* with hepatic failure. The risk of pulmonary, genitourinary, and other *infections* should be minimized by proper positioning of the patient to prevent aspiration and by judicious use of genitourinary and intravenous catheters. *Bacteremia* is a frequent complication of fulminant hepatic failure, with streptococci, *Staphylococcus aureus,* and *Escherichia coli* being the most commonly isolated organisms. *Hypoxemia* is commonly present even in the absence of obvious pulmonary pathology; it may result from both functional right-to-left shunting and ventilation perfusion imbalance and should be corrected by administration of oxygen. *Endotracheal intubation* should be performed for normal indications in fulminant hepatic failure and should be considered with onset of coma to prevent aspiration. *Pulmonary edema* may occur in the absence of left-sided heart failure and may require mechanical ventilation with positive end-expiratory pressure. *Hypotension* is common even in the absence of sepsis or bleeding and results from reduced systemic vascular resistance. However, pressors are often ineffective or only transiently effective. *Respiratory alkalosis* is a common early finding and requires no treatment. *Metabolic acidosis,* which occurs rarely and may be due to lactic acid accumulation, should be treated with bicarbonate. *Cerebral edema* is present in over half of patients dying of fulminant hepatic failure and may result in intracranial herniation. Moreover, in conjunction with systemic hypotension, it reduces cerebral perfusion and may cause brain death. Corticosteroids do not appear to be of benefit, but a single controlled study suggests that direct monitoring of intracranial pressure and treatment of intracranial hypertension with mannitol significantly improve survival. Treatment of clinically evident intracranial hypertension, manifested by unequal or abnormally reactive pupils, myoclonus, and/or decerebrate posturing, is certainly appropriate. Unfortunately, clinical signs may be an insensitive way of detecting intracranial hypertension. The decision regarding invasive intracranial pressure monitoring must thus be carefully individualized.

Experimental Measures. Because the mortality of fulminant hepatic failure is high even with optimal supportive care, a variety of other forms of therapy have been tried. Some of these—*corticosteroid administration, exchange transfusion,* and administration of *L-dopa* or *hepatitis B hyperimmune globulin* (for hepatitis B)—have been shown to be ineffective by controlled prospective clinical trials. Similar controlled observations for the remaining measures, which include *charcoal hemoperfusion, amino acid infusion, plasmapheresis, hemodialysis, total body washout, cross circulation* with a human volunteer or baboon, or *extracorporeal perfusion* through a human cadaver liver, pig liver, or baboon liver, are not available. However, the reported uncontrolled observations strongly suggest that these experimental forms of therapy offer *no advantage* over conventional supportive care.

PROGNOSIS. The short-term prognosis for patients with fulminant hepatic failure that progresses to coma is poor, the average reported survival being about 20 per cent. In contrast, the outlook for those patients who do survive an episode of fulminant hepatic failure with coma is quite good. Virtually all patients have returned to their previous state of health within two to three months, and follow-up liver biopsies have usually demonstrated no or minimal abnormalities. Patients with persistent biochemical or histologic abnormalities have frequently been found to have had pre-existing liver disease or to have continuing exposure to toxic or infectious agents, as for example through parenteral drug abuse.

CHRONIC LIVER DISEASE WITH ENCEPHALOPATHY

ETIOLOGY. Hepatic encephalopathy may also occur in patients with chronic liver disease, usually cirrhosis with portal-systemic shunting. Some patients with cirrhosis may be chronically encephalopathic. In most, however, encephalopathy tends to occur acutely and intermittently. In this latter group, the occurrence of encephalopathy reflects a worsening of hepatic function and/or the presence of one or more precipitating factors (Table 128–2).

DIAGNOSIS. As with fulminant hepatic failure, diagnosis requires the presence of signs and symptoms compatible with hepatic encephalopathy in a patient with underlying chronic liver disease. Routine tests of liver function are typically abnormal but are of little value in differential diagnosis. Unlike fulminant hepatic failure, encephalopathy in patients with chronic liver disease may be accompanied by only minimally abnormal liver function tests. A markedly elevated or rising prothrombin time in an encephalopathic patient with known chronic liver disease suggests superimposed acute hepatocellular necrosis. It is extremely important in patients with chronic alcoholic liver disease to exclude other causes of metabolic encephalopathy (e.g., hypoglycemia, alcohol intoxication, Wernicke-Korsakoff syndrome), meningitis, or structural lesions such as subdural hematoma.

TREATMENT. Unlike fulminant hepatic failure, encephalopathy in the patient with chronic liver disease is frequently not due to acute hepatocellular necrosis, but rather results from one or more potentially reversible precipitating factors. The essential first step in the management of these patients is to identify and, when possible, correct such factors as are outlined in Table 128–2. Additional general measures as outlined earlier for the treatment of hepatic encephalopathy should be undertaken. A small number of patients with chronic hepatic encephalopathy fail to respond to standard measures, and preliminary clinical studies suggest that administration of ornithine salts of branched-chain keto acids or bromocriptine may be helpful in this selected patient group.

The complications and additional supportive care required for these patients are similar to those described for fulminant hepatic failure. Overall, however, the severity and frequency of complications (e.g., hypoglycemia) are less than with fulminant hepatic failure. The various forms of experimental therapy that have been tried in fulminant hepatic failure also have no established role in the management of patients with chronic liver disease with encephalopathy.

PROGNOSIS. Because encephalopathy in patients with chronic liver disease is frequently precipitated by potentially reversible factors, the short-term prognosis is better than in fulminant hepatic failure. Most patients survive the acute episode, particularly if the encephalopathy is not attributable to a sudden deterioration of hepatic function. However, because the underlying chronic liver disease is commonly irreversible and slowly progressive, the long-term prognosis is guarded.

TABLE 128–3. LIVER TRANSPLANTATION*

Hepatobiliary Disease	Per Cent of Total Patients	Per Cent One-Year Survival After 1983
Nonalcoholic cirrhosis	41	60
Hepatobiliary tumors	20	†
Biliary atresia	17	87
Metabolic disorders	7	66
Sclerosing cholangitis	6	78
Alcoholic cirrhosis	4	†
Hepatic vein occlusion	3	71
Fulminant hepatic failure and miscellaneous	2	†

*Based upon an analysis of 279 patients undergoing liver transplantation at several centers during 1983 and 1984.

†Too few patients for meaningful subgroup analysis

HEPATIC TRANSPLANTATION

Between 1963, when the first human liver transplantation was performed, and 1980, only about 300 such procedures were performed worldwide. Since 1980, more than 1000 liver transplantations have been performed, the number of liver transplant centers has increased from 3 to more than 30, and the results of transplantation have improved dramatically.

INDICATIONS AND RESULTS. Liver transplantation merits consideration in any patient with liver disease that is progressive, irreversible, not otherwise treatable, and sufficiently advanced that quality of life and lifespan are likely to be significantly improved. Table 128–3 summarizes the types of liver disease for which transplantation has most commonly been performed and the actuarial one-year survival in cohorts after 1983. Adults with nonalcoholic cirrhosis have repre-

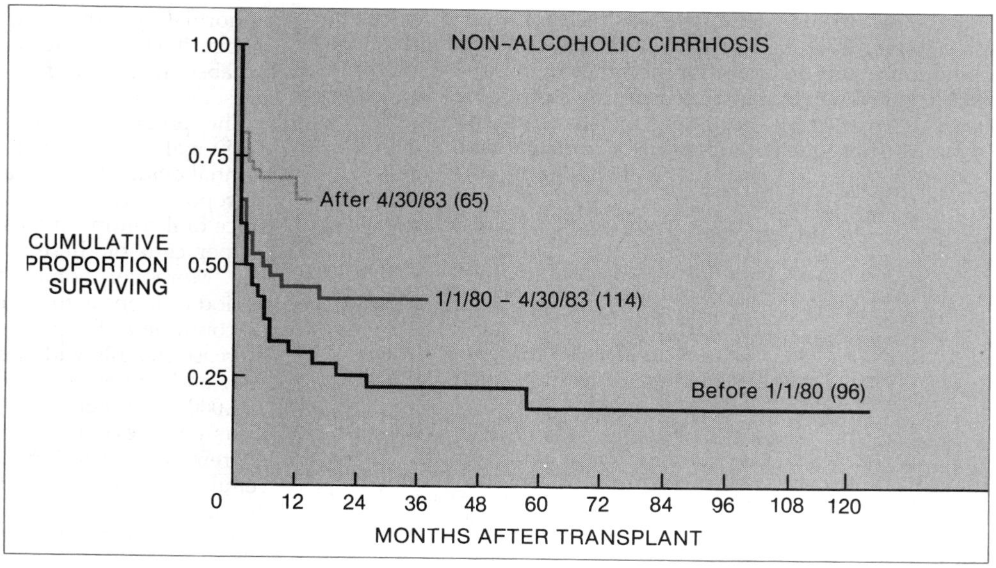

FIGURE 128–1. Actuarial survival of three consecutive cohorts of patients with non-alcoholic cirrhosis undergoing liver transplantation at several centers through August, 1984. The number of patients in each cohort is in parentheses.

sented the largest group of transplant recipients, and as with most other types of nonmalignant hepatobiliary disease, the results of transplantation have improved significantly. The recent improvement in survival likely reflects several factors, including the use of cyclosporin, newer surgical techniques, better supportive care, and the selection of patients with less advanced disease. These advances have greatly decreased postoperative mortality (Fig. 128–1). Most individuals ($\geq$ 80 per cent) who survive the first three postoperative months live at least three years, and the quality of life for such individuals has been good, with about 80 per cent able to resume their former activities. Other diseases for which transplantation has yielded encouraging results have included biliary atresia, metabolic disorders (predominantly alpha$_1$-antitrypsin deficiency and Wilson's disease), sclerosing cholangitis, and hepatic vein occlusion. In contrast to nonmalignant disease, the results of transplantation for malignant hepatobiliary disease have been poor overall and have improved relatively little, with half or more of patients who survive the postoperative period dying of recurrent disease. The appropriateness of transplantation for most such patients thus remains controversial, as it does for patients with alcoholic liver disease. Relatively few patients with fulminant hepatic failure have undergone transplantation. However, preliminary reports of transplantation in this setting have been encouraging, particularly for patients whose disease is less fulminant and spans several weeks to months rather than days (see above.).

Contraindications to liver transplantation include the presence of extrahepatic malignant disease, serious and irreversible extrahepatic disease, active alcoholism, and portal vein thrombosis. Patients with hepatitis-B-virus–related liver disease and evidence of ongoing viral replication (see Ch. 123) have generally experienced recurrent disease in the donor liver and have therefore also been considered poor candidates.

Between 10 and 30 per cent of patients require a second or even third transplant because of failure of the first graft. Such graft failure is most commonly attributable to postoperative complications such as vascular thrombosis, primary graft nonfunction, or rejection; recurrence of the original disease accounts for few cases of graft failure.

TIMING OF TRANSPLANTATION. Tests for precisely measuring hepatic reserve are not available, and the prognosis for an individual patient is often hard to predict. Thus the timing of transplantation for an otherwise appropriate candidate is often difficult to judge. Survival of ambulatory patients undergoing transplantation is greater than that of those who are critically ill at the time of operation. The costs of transplantation are considerably less as well. Thus, it is reasonable to consider liver transplantation and obtain appropriate consultation when deterioration becomes evident. This is particularly true when one is contemplating a procedure (e.g. biliary tract reconstruction, portacaval anastomosis) that might compromise subsequent candidacy for transplantation.

Busuttil RW, Goldstein LI, Danovitch GM, et al.: Liver transplantation today. Ann Intern Med 104:377, 1986. *A well-referenced review that focuses on the UCLA experience and deals with patient selection, operative technique, postoperative care, and results.*

Canalese J, Gimson AE, Davis C, et al.: Controlled trial of dexamethasone and mannitol for the cerebral oedema of fulminant hepatic failure. Gut 23:625, 1982. *A controlled study reporting improved survival with aggressive monitoring of intracranial pressure and treatment with mannitol.*

Conn HO, Leevy CM, Vlahcevic ZR, et al.: Comparison of lactulose and neomycin in the treatment of chronic portal-systemic encephalopathy. A double-blind controlled trial. Gastroenterology 72:573, 1977. *A skillfully designed prospective study in patients with cirrhosis and chronic portal-systemic encephalopathy. Provides useful information regarding clinical assessment of encephalopathy as well as administration of lactulose and neomycin.*

Flute PT: Clotting abnormalities in liver disease. In Popper H, Schaffner F (eds.): Progress in Liver Diseases. New York, Grune & Stratton, 1979, pp 301–322. *A concise review of the role of the liver in blood clotting with emphasis on practical applications.*

Gimson AES, O'Grady J, Ede RJ, et al.: Late onset hepatic failure: Clinical, serological and histological features. Hepatology 6:288, 1986. *A complete characterization of patients without known prior liver disease in whom the total duration of illness exceeds eight weeks. Has a useful reference list.*

Jones EA, Schafer DF: Fulminant hepatic failure. In Zakim D, Boyer TD (eds.): Hepatology: A textbook of Liver Disease. Philadelphia, WB Saunders Company, 1982, pp 415–445. *An exhaustively referenced review of the pathogenesis and treatment of hepatic encephalopathy in the setting of rapidly deteriorating hepatic function. An excellent entry point into the literature.*

Plum F, Hindfelt B: The neurological complications of liver disease. In Vinken PJ, Bruyn GW (eds.): Handbook of Clinical Neurology. Amsterdam, North Holland Publishing Company, 1976, pp 349–377. *The clinical description of neurologic abnormalities is a particularly valuable part of this comprehensive review.*

Scharschmidt BF: Human Liver Transplantation: An analysis of 819 patients from eight centers. In Thomas HC, Jones EA (eds.): Recent Advances in Hepatology. New York, Churchill-Livingston, 1986, pp 175–189. *A comprehensive summary of the results of liver transplantation at several centers in the United States and Western Europe, with a brief consideration of costs and issues regarding patient selection.*

Summary of National Institutes of Health Consensus Development Conference on Liver Transplantation. Hepatology 4:1s–107s, 1984. *This conference, which had a major positive impact upon the field of liver transplantation, reviewed the indications for liver transplantation and results of the procedure in various patient groups.*

Uribe M, Marquez MA, Ramos GG, et al.: Treatment of portal-systemic encephalopathy with vegetable and animal protein diets: A control cross-over study. Dig Dis Sci 27:1109, 1982. *A controlled study of different protein sources with important practical details regarding diet.*

129 HEPATIC TUMORS

Bruce F. Scharschmidt

BENIGN HEPATIC TUMORS

Hepatocellular Adenoma

Hepatocellular adenomas occur almost exclusively in women. These tumors are most frequently detected during the childbearing years, particularly the third and fourth decades of life, but are occasionally found in postmenopausal women as well. Adenomas most commonly occur in the right lobe of the liver, are solitary in about one third of the cases, and are often quite large, with up to one half being 10 cm or more in diameter. Hepatocellular adenomas are usually well circumscribed, may be surrounded by a pseudocapsule, and often show areas of bile stasis, hemorrhage, and necrosis. Microscopically, these tumors consist of a monotonous array of normal to slightly atypical hepatocytes without portal tracts or bile ducts. Kupffer cells are markedly reduced in number or absent, and a few arteries and thin-walled veins are present.

The preponderance of this tumor in women suggests a hormonal role in its pathogenesis, and there is strong circumstantial evidence implicating oral contraceptives. The number of reported cases of this tumor has increased dramatically since oral contraceptives were introduced in 1960, and nearly 90 per cent of these are associated with oral contraceptive use. Moreover, some adenomas have clearly regressed in a period of months to years after use of oral contraceptives was discontinued. The risk of developing this tumor appears to increase steadily with increasing duration of oral contraceptive use, and the annual incidence is estimated to be 3 to 4 per 100,000 in women who have taken oral contraceptives continuously for several years. Although not generally regarded as a premalignant lesion, there are instances in which hepatocellular carcinoma appears to have arisen in an hepatocellular adenoma.

Symptomatic patients with hepatocellular adenomas present with signs and symptoms of an abdominal mass, tumor infarction, intratumor hemorrhage (pain, fever, leukocytosis), or, in about one third of cases, tumor rupture (pain, hemoperitoneum, circulatory collapse). The mortality in this last group is approximately 20 per cent. Because the true incidence of these tumors is unknown, the actual proportion that ruptures cannot be determined.

Because Kupffer cells are infrequent or absent, hepatocellular adenomas usually appear as a defect ("cold spot") on technetium 99m–sulfur colloid scans. The angiographic appearance is typically hypervascular, often with areas of hypovascularity. The management of hepatocellular adenomas is a matter of some debate. In patients taking oral contraceptives that can be discontinued, a several-month period of observation with repeated radionuclide scans is justifiable, particularly if the location, size, or number of tumors would make resection hazardous. Surgery is appropriate for most persistent resectable lesions.

Focal Nodular Hyperplasia

Focal nodular hyperplasia, which shows a female to male predominance of 2:1 to 7:1, has also been referred to as pseudotumor, focal cirrhosis, and hepatic hamartoma. Despite distinctive pathologic features, focal nodular hyperplasia and hepatocellular adenoma have often been confused in the medical literature. Unlike hepatocellular adenoma, a firm link between focal nodular hyperplasia and oral contraceptives has not been established. Focal nodular hyperplasia generally is a solitary tumor in the right lobe. It has a characteristic grossly lobulated appearance on cut section, which is produced by a central fibrous core with septa radiating in a stellate pattern. Hemorrhage and necrosis are rare. Microscopically, these fibrous septa contain bile ductules and inflammatory cells and are surrounded by normal or slightly atypical hepatocytes as well as Kupffer cells.

Unlike hepatocellular adenomas, focal nodular hyperplasia does not usually produce symptoms and is generally found incidentally at surgery or necropsy. In up to 20 per cent of the cases, it presents as an upper abdominal mass. Portal hypertension has been reported in association with multiple lesions, and rupture is rare. Because these tumors contain Kupffer cells, they frequently take up technetium 99m–sulfur colloid normally and may appear as voids, hot spots, or some combination of these on scan. Occasionally they exhibit uniform uptake of isotope equivalent to that of normal liver and are not visualized by technetium 99m–sulfur colloid scan. They are characteristically hypervascular on angiography with a visible capillary blush. Since focal nodular hyperplasia has no known malignant potential, asymptomatic lesions can be followed nonoperatively. If the lesion is encountered unexpectedly at surgery, simple wedge biopsy is appropriate if complete excision would be difficult.

Hemangioma

Cavernous hemangioma is probably the most common benign hepatic tumor, with a 0.4 to 7.3 per cent incidence in necropsy series and a predominance in females. The great majority of hemangiomas are asymptomatic and are found incidentally at surgery or necroscopy. These lesions can, however, present with signs and symptoms of an abdominal mass, infarction, rupture, or thrombocytopenia and hypofibrinogenemia.

Hemangiomas typically appear as a cold spot on conventional scans with technetium 99m–sulfur colloid; enhanced activity with blood pool scanning is frequently found and is highly specific. Their presence can occasionally be suspected on plain roentgenogram of the abdomen by the presence of calcified spicules radiating from the center of the lesion. The angiographic appearance of dense and persistent tumor staining is virtually diagnostic. Computed tomographic studies with rapid sequential imaging following the bolus injection of intravenous contrast material may also provide diagnostically useful information as may magnetic resonance imaging. Because of the accuracy of these imaging techniques in distinguishing hemangioma from a vascular carcinoma or angiosarcoma, resection is not usually necessary to establish a diagnosis, being necessary only for large symptomatic lesions. There are also case reports of regression following radiotherapy or hepatic artery ligation.

Other Benign Tumors

A variety of less common benign liver tumors may also occur in adults. They usually produce no symptoms unless very large. Included in this group are *bile duct adenomas, bile duct cystadenomas, fibromas, lipomas, leiomyomas, mesotheliomas, teratomas,* and *myxomas. Nodular regenerative hyperplasia* is a condition characterized by multiple nodules of varying size arising in a noncirrhotic liver. The nodules are composed of liver plates that are two cells thick. An association with rheumatoid arthritis, Felty's syndrome, CREST syndrome, oral contraceptives, and a variety of drugs is reported. The most common manifestation of nodular regenerative hyperplasia is portal hypertension.

MALIGNANT HEPATIC TUMORS

Hepatocellular Carcinoma

EPIDEMIOLOGY. In the United States and Western Europe, hepatocellular carcinoma (hepatoma) is increasing in incidence but remains relatively uncommon, accounting for less than 1 per cent of all causes of death at autopsy and 2.5 per cent or less of all malignant growths. In certain other areas of the world, including parts of sub-Saharan Africa, Southeast Asia, Japan, Oceania, and Greece, hepatocellular carcinoma is among the most frequent malignant tumor and is an important cause of overall mortality. Hepatocellular carcinoma is predominantly a disease of males and usually arises in a cirrhotic liver. The risk appears to be greatest in cirrhosis associated with hemochromatosis and hepatitis B virus infection, low in primary biliary cirrhosis and Wilson's disease, and intermediate in alcoholic and cryptogenic cirrhosis. Chronic hepatitis B virus infection may predispose to hepatocellular carcinoma: (1) The aforementioned areas of the world in which hepatocellular carcinoma is most prevalent are the same areas in which hepatitis B virus infection is most common. (2) Serologic evidence of hepatitis B virus infection is much more common in patients with hepatocellular carcinoma than in controls, an observation that has been made in all parts of the world, including the United States. (3) The incidence of hepatocellular carcinoma is about one hundredfold higher in individuals with hepatitis B virus infection than in noninfected controls. (4) Analysis of tumor tissue in patients with serologic evidence of hepatitis B virus infection has indicated the presence of hepatitis B virus integrated into the host genome. (5) Woodchucks and ducks infected with viruses that are related to the human hepatitis B virus also develop hepatocellular carcinoma.

Epidemiologic evidence has also suggested a link between hepatocellular carcinoma and ingestion of aflatoxins, mycotoxins produced by *Aspergillus flavus,* a mold that can grow in warm moist areas and contaminate peanuts and stored grains. Case reports have also suggested a link between hepatocellular carcinoma and alpha$_1$-antitrypsin deficiency and administration of androgenic steroids, Thorotrast, and possibly estrogenic steroids in the form of oral contraceptives (Table 129–1).

CLINICAL FEATURES. The most common presenting features of hepatocellular carcinoma are *abdominal pain,* the presence of an *abdominal mass,* and *weight loss.* Hepatocellular

TABLE 129–1. HEPATOCELLULAR CARCINOMA

Incidence From 1–7 per 100,000 to > 100 per 100,000 in high-risk areas	**Common Clinical Presentations** Abdominal pain Abdominal mass Weight loss Deterioration of liver function
Sex 4:1 to 8:1 male predominance, except fibrolamellar carcinoma	**Unusual Manifestations** Bloody ascites Tumor emboli to lung Obstructive jaundice Obstruction of hepatic or portal veins Bloody ascites Metabolic (erythrocytosis, hypercalcemia, hypercholesterolemia, carcinoid syndrome, sexual changes, hypoglycemia, acquired porphyria)
Associations Cirrhosis Hepatitis B virus infection (usually with cirrhosis) Hemochromatosis (with cirrhosis) Aflatoxin ingestion Thorotrast α_1-Antitrypsin deficiency (?)	
Suggestive Clinical or Laboratory Findings Hepatic bruit or friction rub α-Fetoprotein ↑ (> 400 ng/ml)	

carcinoma may also present with rupture and hemoperitoneum, obstructive jaundice, unexplained deterioration in a patient with cirrhosis, or a variety of paraneoplastic syndromes, including erythrocytosis, persistent fever, hypercalcemia, and hypoglycemia. Hepatomegaly is present in about two thirds of patients. Other suggestive physical findings include the presence of a bruit, hepatic friction rub, or bloody ascites. Hepatocellular carcinoma may invade and obstruct the portal and hepatic veins and metastasizes most often to regional lymph nodes and the lungs. Alpha-fetoprotein levels in serum greater than 1000 ng per milliliter or progressively rising levels are highly suggestive of hepatocellular carcinoma. Unfortunately, only a minority of patients with hepatocellular carcinoma in most parts of the world, including the United States, have elevations of this magnitude, and low level elevations up to about 200 ng per milliliter are relatively nonspecific. For this reason, alpha-fetoprotein has proved disappointing in the screening of high-risk populations. Hepatocellular carcinomas typically fail to take up technetium 99m–sulfur colloid, but accumulate gallium 67 normally on radionuclide scan, and they generally appear as an irregular hypervascular mass with tumor "staining" and arterial displacement and/or encasement on angiography.

TREATMENT AND PROGNOSIS. The results of current treatment for hepatocellular carcinoma are discouraging. In the United States, median survival from the time of diagnosis is about six months. Because of the advanced stage of the disease at the time of diagnosis and the frequent coexistence of severe liver disease, only a small fraction of patients are candidates for hepatic resection. The presence of coexisting cirrhosis in a patient with well-preserved hepatic function does not altogether preclude surgery; however, such patients are unlikely to tolerate more than limited resection of a localized tumor. Prospective screening of high-risk patients in Japan has resulted in detection of earlier, smaller tumors and resulted in a higher proportion of tumors being resectable. While patients undergoing resection of such early tumors have shown remarkably high survival rates up to 3 years, the median period of asymptomatic growth of such tumors is about 3 years, and the utility of aggressive population screening and early surgery is as yet unclear. Adriamycin alone or in combination with other agents has produced objective tumor response in up to 50 per cent of patients, but has minimally affected survival. Radiation therapy has also yielded disappointing results. Hormonal therapy has been tried, but experience with this approach is too limited to judge its value. As discussed in Ch. 128, the results of liver transplantation for unresectable hepatocellular carcinoma have been disappointing, with a three-year survival of about 15 per cent.

A variant of typical hepatocellular carcinoma termed *fibrolamellar carcinoma* differs from the typical form of the disease in that it usually occurs in young adults without underlying cirrhosis, lacks the usual male predominance, is associated with a longer survival when untreated, and has been cured surgically in between 10 and 30 per cent of cases.

Other Primary Hepatic Malignancies

Cholangiocarcinoma occurs much less frequently than hepatocellular carcinoma and shows an association with clonorchiasis and opisthorchiasis in the Far East and with sclerosing cholangitis. It may present with obstructive jaundice when it involves major ducts in the area of the hepatic hilum. Truly mixed hepatocellular cholangiocarcinomas are rare. Angiosarcoma, an unusual tumor associated with vinyl chloride exposure as well as arsenic and Thorotrast administration, frequently causes thrombocytopenia and has a propensity to rupture, causing hemoperitoneum and circulatory collapse. Other unusual primary hepatic malignant tumors of adults include cystadenocarcinoma, squamous carcinoma, and hepatoblastoma.

As with hepatocellular carcinoma, treatment of these malignant hepatic tumors has been unsatisfactory. Resection is seldom possible. Of patients with cholangiocarcinoma who have undergone liver transplantation, the three-year survival has been about 7 per cent.

Tumors Metastatic to Liver

The liver and lung are the most frequent sites of metastatic cancer, and metastases constitute the largest group of hepatic tumors in adults. Necropsy studies have demonstrated hepatic metastases in more than half of patients with primary malignant tumors having portal venous drainage (e.g., stomach, colon, and pancreas). Other solid tumors that frequently metastasize to the liver include melanoma and tumors of the lung, oropharynx, and bladder. Next to the spleen, the liver is also the most common extranodal site of involvement by Hodgkin's disease, the non-Hodgkin's lymphomas, and malignant histiocytosis (histiocytic medullary reticulosis).

DIAGNOSTIC APPROACH TO THE PATIENT WITH A SUSPECTED HEPATIC NEOPLASM

Most hepatic neoplasms present as a right upper quadrant or epigastric mass. Additional clinical features that may provide clues regarding the specific type of tumor have been noted above and include pre-existing cirrhosis (hepatocellular carcinoma), portal or hepatic vein thrombosis (hepatocellular carcinoma), oral contraceptive use (hepatocellular adenoma), abdominal pain with hemoperitoneum and hypotension (hepatocellular adenoma; less commonly angiosarcoma, hepatocellular carcinoma, hemangioma), and unusual systemic manifestations (hepatocellular carcinoma). Cholangiocarcinoma and hepatocellular carcinoma can cause biliary obstruction, but this may potentially result from strategically located tumors of all types.

Physical examination most commonly reveals hepatomegaly or a discrete mass. The presence of a bruit or friction rub may suggest hepatocellular carcinoma but is not specific. Elevations of alkaline phosphatase and transaminase levels are the most common biochemical abnormalities. In general, however, liver function tests are not particularly helpful in diagnosis and may be entirely normal in some patients. Uncommon biochemical abnormalities in patients with hepatocellular carcinoma include the presence of a variant alkaline phosphatase, erythrocytosis, or hypercholesterolemia. A markedly elevated and/or progressively rising alpha-fetoprotein level is strongly suggestive of hepatocellular carcinoma.

Examination of tissue is ultimately required for the unequivocal diagnosis of hepatic tumors. In a patient with a known extrahepatic malignant tumor and clinical or biochemical evidence of hepatic metastases, radionuclide scanning or ultrasonography is a reasonable first step. The finding of single or multiple defects is consistent with metastatic disease, and a percutaneous biopsy can be expected to recover tumor in 50 to 75 per cent of such cases. Two biopsies performed through the same skin site and cytologic examination of the tissue core and aspirated fluid appear to enhance the yield without increasing the risk of bleeding. In patients with lymphoreticular malignant disease, percutaneous biopsy is less sensitive in demonstrating hepatic involvement than wedge biopsy obtained at laparotomy, and histologic evidence of hepatic involvement may be found even in the absence of clinical, biochemical, or radionuclide scan abnormalities.

The workup in suspected primary hepatic tumor must be individualized on the basis of the relative risks and benefits of establishing a diagnosis. Ultrasound examination or computed tomography, particularly following intravenous injection of iodinated contrast material, appears to be more sensitive than radionuclide scanning in the detection of small tumors and may be useful also in excluding a cyst. Angiography may occasionally permit a definite diagnosis, as with a hemangioma, and is helpful in assessing resectability. Because of the rapidly evolving capabilities of current imaging procedures, radiologic consultation is helpful in selecting the most appropriate method.

In a patient who is a candidate for operation and who has an apparently resectable lesion of uncertain or suspicious nature based on imaging studies, preoperative biopsy is usually not indicated. Two additional factors must be taken into account when assessing the appropriateness of a preoperative biopsy. First, needle biopsy of primary lesions such as hemangioma, angiosarcoma, and possibly hepatocellular adenoma is potentially dangerous owing to their propensity to hemorrhage, and biopsy of a possible echinococcal cyst is contraindicated. Second, definitive diagnosis of hepatocellular adenoma and focal nodular hyperplasia, which consist predominantly of normal or minimally abnormal hepatocytes, may be difficult from examination of a needle biopsy alone. In the patient who is not a candidate for surgery or in whom information regarding tumor type will importantly influence decisions regarding further evaluation and therapy, a diagnosis can often be established by needle biopsy. Compared with percutaneous biopsy, a laparoscopic approach facilitates directed biopsy of visible tumor deposits and may permit control of bleeding. Inspection of the liver at laparoscopy for evidence of cirrhosis or tumor deposits not evident from radiologic studies may also aid in determining the resectability of a lesion. A directed percutaneous aspiration biopsy has also yielded excellent results in certain centers. Non-neoplastic lesions that may mimic hepatic tumors include regenerative nodules, anomalous hepatic lobulation, cysts, and abscesses.

Kerlin P, Davis GL, McGill DB, et al.: Hepatic adenoma and focal nodular hyperplasia: Clinical, pathologic, and radiologic features. Gastroenterology 84:994, 1983. *A concise review comparing and contrasting these two common benign hepatic neoplasms.*

Kew MC: Hepatic tumors. Semin Liver Dis 4:89, 1984. *A concise and well-referenced review.*

Locker GY, Doroshow JH, Zwelling LA, et al.: The clinical features of hepatic angiosarcoma: A report of four cases and a review of the English literature. Medicine 58:48, 1979. *A review of information about this unusual tumor.*

Malt RA: Surgery for hepatic neoplasms. N Engl J Med 313:1591, 1985. *A brief and very practical summary of this topic.*

Nagasue N, Yukaya H, Ogawa Y, et al.: Hepatic resection in the treatment of hepatocellular carcinoma: Report of 60 cases. Br J Surg 72:292, 1985. *A particularly valuable summary of the results of surgery for early lesions in a generally cirrhotic patient population.*

Sheu J-C, Sung J-L, Chen D-S: Growth rate of asymptomatic hepatocellular carcinoma and its clinical implications. Gastroenterology 89:259, 1985. *A nearly unique report of sequential imaging of non-resected early tumors that has implications regarding screening programs for patients at high risk for hepatocellular carcinoma.*

Shinagawa T, Ohto M, Kimura K, et al.: Diagnosis and clinical features of small hepatocellular carcinoma with emphasis on the utility of real-time ultrasonography: A study in 51 patients. Gastroenterology 86:495, 1984. *A review of the clinical features, biochemical abnormalities, and utility of conventional imaging techniques in the diagnosis of hepatocellular carcinomas less than 5 cm in diameter.*

130 DISEASES OF THE GALLBLADDER AND BILE DUCTS

Peter F. Malet and Roger D. Soloway

Biliary tract disorders result from a variety of congenital, inflammatory, metabolic, infectious, and neoplastic conditions. These conditions often present in subtle ways and can pose challenging diagnostic problems. Ongoing improvements in diagnostic and therapeutic techniques have allowed the clinician to diagnose biliary tract disease more quickly and to treat patients more effectively.

NORMAL PHYSIOLOGY OF BILE FORMATION

Bile is an isotonic aqueous mixture consisting primarily of electrolytes, proteins, bile salts, cholesterol, phospholipids, and bilirubin. Secretion across the canalicular membrane of the hepatocyte accounts for about two thirds of total bile flow. Bile salt–dependent secretion comprises about one half of canalicular bile formation, while the other half is termed bile salt independent and consists mainly of electrolytes. The remaining one third of bile flow is an alkaline fraction generated by the epithelial cells lining the bile ducts; ductular secretion is stimulated by secretin, cholecystokinin, and gastrin. An as yet unquantitated contribution to canalicular bile flow consisting mainly of water and electrolytes occurs by way of the interhepatocytic space (paracellular pathway). The total volume of bile produced ranges from 500 to 800 ml per day.

Under basal (fasting) conditions, tonic contraction of the sphincter of Oddi diverts about half of the flow of hepatic bile into the gallbladder; the other half flows into the duodenum assisted by phasic peristaltic action of the sphincter. The gallbladder actively reabsorbs Na^+, Cl^-, and HCO_3^+ and passively resorbs H_2O. It is capable of concentrating bile tenfold within about four hours. The gallbladder mucosa secretes H^+ and mucin.

Cholecystokinin, released from the intestinal mucosa after meals by fat, amino acids, and H^+, simultaneously stimulates the gallbladder to contract and the sphincter of Oddi to relax, emptying bile into the duodenum.

Bile salts are synthesized by hepatocytes (Fig. 130–1) from cholesterol by a multistep process, the rate-limiting step of which is catalyzed by 7 alpha-hydroxylase, which is under inhibitory feedback control. Cholate and chenodeoxycholate, the two *primary* bile salts (that is, they are synthesized in the liver), are conjugated with either glycine or taurine before secretion to improve solubility. Bile salts are secreted by active transport across the biliary canalicular membrane. After entering the proximal small intestine, bile salts aid in fat absorption by forming *micelles* (Ch. 104) and then are largely reabsorbed in the mid and distal small intestine. Bile salts that reach the colon are partially deconjugated, which makes them more lipid soluble and facilitates their reabsorption. Cholate and chenodeoxycholate are also partially converted by bacterial 7 alpha-dehydroxylation to the *secondary* bile salts, deoxycholate and lithocholate, respectively. Deoxycholate is absorbed from the colon, reconjugated in the liver, and excreted in bile. Lithocholate is poorly reabsorbed; it is sulfated as well as reconjugated during hepatic transfer. Sulfation increases aqueous solubility and further reduces intestinal reabsorption. The average bile salt composition of bile is 35 per cent chenodeoxycholate, 35 per cent cholate, 25 per cent deoxycholate, 2 per cent ursodeoxycholate, and 2 per cent lithocholate. Each is conjugated with either glycine or taurine in a

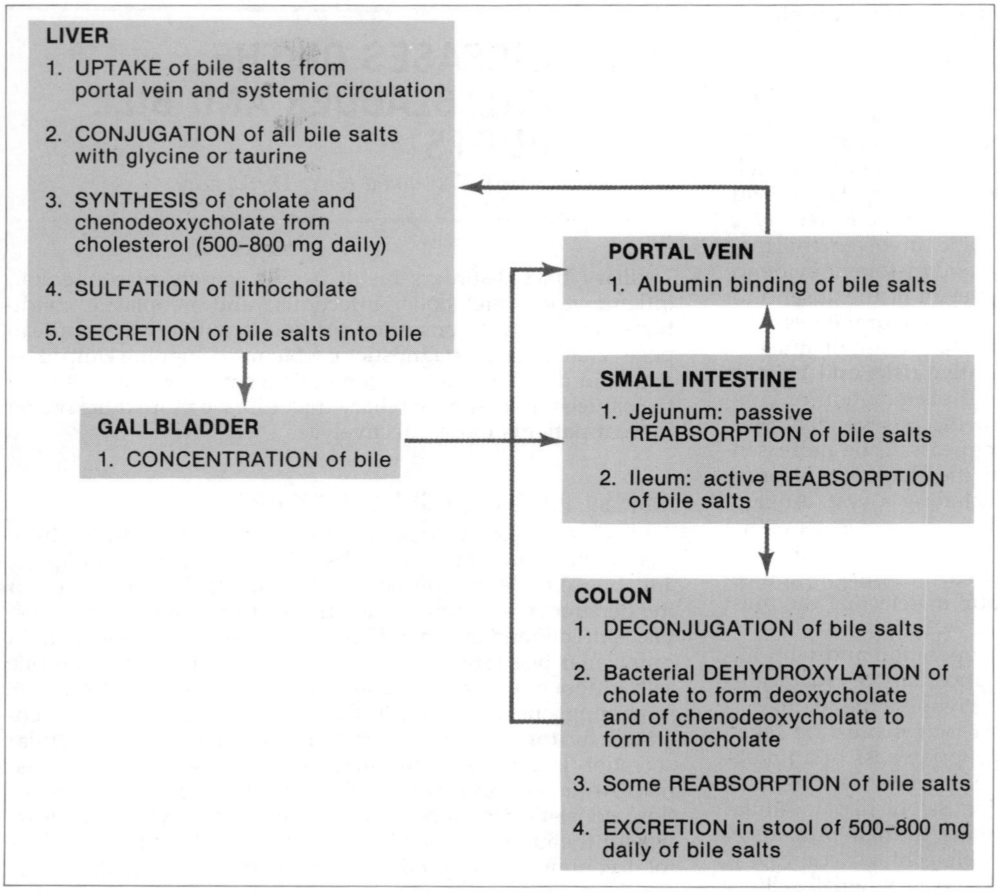

FIGURE 130–1. The major steps in the enterohepatic circulation of bile salts. This cycle provides for conservation of bile salts by an effective reabsorption mechanism in the intestine.

ratio of 2 to 3:1. Bile salts are secreted in the form of micelles containing phospholipids (mainly lecithin), and cholesterol. These lipids account for 90 per cent of biliary solids.

Intestinal reabsorption of bile salts, which is about 95 per cent for a single passage, occurs by passive diffusion throughout the intestine and by active transport within the terminal ileum. The reabsorbed bile salts are largely bound to albumin in portal blood and are then almost completely removed by the hepatocytes in a single passage through the liver sinusoids. The bile salt pool, normally 1.8 to 3.0 grams, passes through the liver and intestine two or three times during each meal, producing six to nine cycles daily (i.e., each day about 20 to 25 grams of bile salts enter the duodenum); this cycling is termed the *enterohepatic circulation*. During an average day involving three meals, bile salts are in continuous motion with peaks of secretion during and following meals. At night, when the majority of the secreted hepatic bile eventually enters the gallbladder, and there is no stimulus for gallbladder contraction, the intestinal concentration of bile salts is much lower. Conservation of bile salts in this enterohepatic circulation is so efficient that only 15 to 25 per cent (500 to 600 mg) of the bile salt pool must be replaced by hepatic synthesis of new bile salts daily. If the efficiency of enterohepatic conservation is impaired by conditions such as biliary fistula, ileal Crohn's disease or ileal resection, hepatic synthesis of bile salts increases. The maximal synthetic rate (5 grams per day) will be insufficient to restore intraluminal concentrations to normal if external losses exceed this amount.

Bile salts are *amphophiles*, possessing water-soluble and fat-soluble sides. In an aqueous medium they are distributed randomly until a critical concentration (about 2 mM) is reached, at which point spontaneous aggregation forms multimolecular structures called micelles. In micelles the bile salt molecules line up with their hydrophilic portions facing the solvent (water) and their hydrophobic portions facing each other (Fig. 130–2). The hydrocarbon center of the micelle can incorporate biliary lecithin and cholesterol, and the entire aggregate remains water soluble. The addition of lecithin expands micellar size and enhances the ability of bile salt micelles to incorporate other lipids. In addition, a variable amount of cholesterol is carried in lecithin-cholesterol vesicles. The ultimate cholesterol-carrying capacity of bile depends on the relative amounts of bile salts and lecithin as well as the total lipid concentration.

Besides electrolytes, other solutes in bile are bilirubin that has been conjugated in the liver with glucuronic acid (Ch. 118), proteins, and cations such as calcium, iron, copper, and zinc, and low concentrations of the end-products of drug and hormone metabolism.

PATHOPHYSIOLOGY OF GALLSTONE DISEASE

In Western cultures about 75 per cent of gallstones are composed principally of cholesterol (*cholesterol gallstones*) and 25 per cent of calcium bilirubinate and other calcium salts (*pigment gallstones*). Overall, about 15 per cent of gallstones are radiopaque, about two thirds of which are pigment and one third are cholesterol stones. The symptoms caused by gallstones are the same regardless of the chemical composition and to a large extent are independent of size. Stones can cause pain and jaundice by passage through the cystic and common bile ducts or can cause pain by intermittently becoming impacted in the neck of the gallbladder.

CHOLESTEROL GALLSTONES. Cholesterol stones are usually yellow green to tan and are round or faceted. They may be single or multiple; most range in size from 1 mm to 3 to 4 cm. Cholesterol accounts for 50 to 100 per cent of stone weight, the remainder consisting of mucin glycoproteins and less than 10 per cent calcium bilirubinate and/or other calcium salts. These stones occur three times as frequently in women as men, the difference beginning at puberty and declining after menopause. The incidence is higher with multiparity and with the use of birth control pills, which suggests an

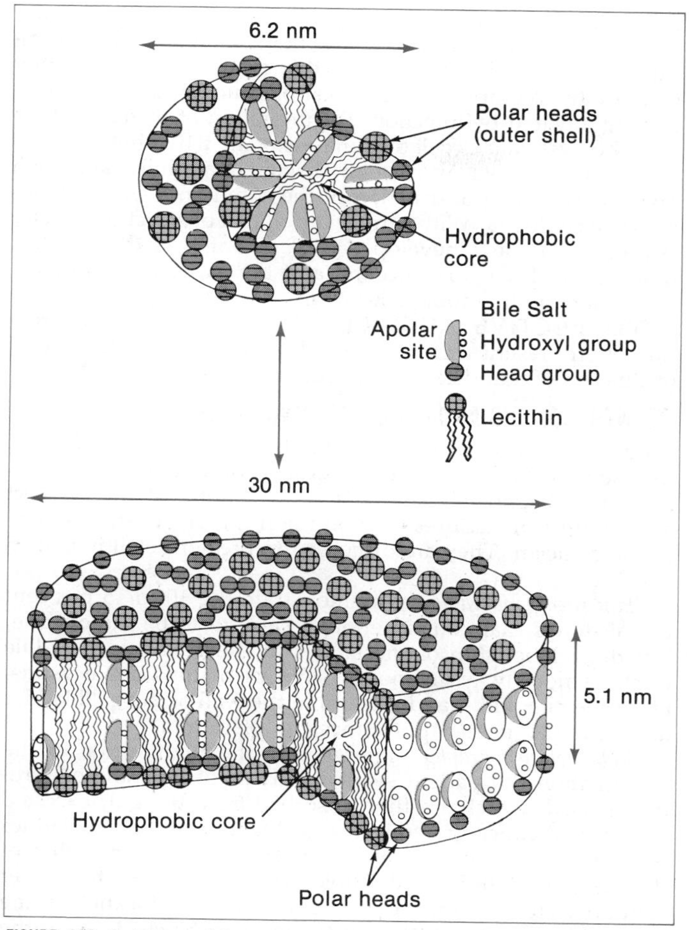

FIGURE 130–2. Dimorphic structure of a biliary mixed lipid micelle, which has been shown to exhibit a sphere → disc transition, depending upon whether the solution is bile salt–rich (sphere) or lecithin-rich (*disc*). The lecithin-rich micelle is larger and capable of dissolving and transporting a much larger amount of cholesterol. The transition depends upon the bile salt–lecithin molar ratio present in the micelle but may also be influenced by other constituents present in native bile. Bile salt molecules in both micellar forms are thought to form pairs (dimers) to avoid contact of the hydroxyl groups (*small clear circles*) with the nonpolar environment of the micellar core. (Adapted with permission from Muller K: Biochemistry 20:404, 1981. Copyright 1981 American Chemical Society.)

influence of female sex hormones. The incidence in blacks, whites, and American Indians increases in that order. About 75 per cent of American Indian women over the age of 25 years and 90 per cent of those over age 60 are affected. In the United States 20 per cent of 75-year-old men and 35 per cent of 75-year-old women have stones at autopsy. Environmental and dietary influences are important. For example, the incidence of gallstones in blacks in Africa is much lower than in blacks in the United States.

Cholesterol, which is insoluble in water, is normally carried in bile within bile salt-lecithin micelles. A completely clear micellar solution of bile is one in which cholesterol is completely solubilized. A prerequisite for cholesterol gallstone formation is an excess of cholesterol in relation to micellar carrying capacity, a condition that may result from decreased bile salt or increased cholesterol concentration in bile. When the cholesterol-solubilization capacity of micelles is exceeded, cholesterol forms either a *metastable* solution, which is clear initially but forms crystals and becomes cloudy after standing, or a *supersaturated* solution, which is visually turbid, containing either liquid or solid crystals of cholesterol.

Bile of patients with gallstones has relatively more cholesterol than that of normal persons, although the overlap is great. In patients with gallstones, bile is supersaturated with cholesterol as it emerges from the liver, implicating the hepatocytes rather than the gallbladder as the cause of the abnormality. In some patients with gallstones the total bile salt pool is decreased in size, and the hepatocytes have decreased amounts of the enzyme 7 alpha-hydroxylase. These observations suggest that diminished bile salt secretion is a factor in the genesis of lithogenic bile in some patients. Another factor, particularly associated with obesity, is increased cholesterol secretion into hepatic bile.

The relationship between cholesterol and bile salt output is hyperbolic, so that when bile salt secretion declines, the cholesterol-bile salt ratio climbs and the bile becomes more lithogenic. During fasting, bile salts are sequestered in the gallbladder, hepatic secretion of bile salts declines, the rate of cholesterol secretion persists, and the bile becomes more lithogenic. Supersaturation of bile with cholesterol is therefore common after overnight or prolonged fasting. Normal human bile probably contains *solubilizing* or *antinucleating factors,* for example, apolipoprotein A-1, that prevent cholesterol crystallization.

Cholesterol saturation of bile appears to be a necessary but not a sufficient condition for cholesterol gallstone formation. Supersaturated bile from patients without gallstones does not form cholesterol crystals, even on prolonged incubation, while bile of identical lipid composition from patients with stones usually contains or forms such crystals. The gallbladder is considered to be important in gallstone formation, possibly by supplying a nidus (*nucleating factor*) for crystallization, such as mucin glycoproteins or other smaller proteins secreted by the epithelium, or by providing an area of stasis to facilitate precipitation. For example, stone formation occurs predominantly in the gallbladder, and cholesterol gallstones rarely recur after cholecystectomy.

PIGMENT GALLSTONES. Pigment stones are subdivided into two categories, black and brown stones, on the basis of differing compositional and clinical characteristics.

Black pigment stones are much more common in the West and are usually under 1 cm, irregular in shape, and featureless on cross-section. They form in the gallbladder and are composed of calcium bilirubinate, bilirubin polymers, calcium phosphate and carbonate, and mucin glycoproteins. There is no relationship between black stones and obesity, parity, saturation of bile with cholesterol, or bile salt pool size. Rather, old age and less than ideal weight are associated with black stone formation in the general population. The great majority of patients with black stones have no underlying disease, but patients with cirrhosis and hemolytic diseases are predisposed to develop these stones. There is no sexual predisposition; American Indians are rarely, and Scandinavians infrequently, affected. The concentration of unconjugated bilirubin is increased in the bile of some patients with these stones.

Brown pigment stones (calcium bilirubinate) have layers of calcium bilirubinate alternating with cholesterol and calcium salts of fatty acids. Bilirubin is thought to precipitate with calcium because beta-glucuronidase of bacterial, biliary epithelial, or hepatic origin deconjugates bilirubin diglucuronide to less soluble bilirubin monoglucuronide or unconjugated bilirubin. The fatty acids of biliary lecithin may be similarly precipitated as calcium salts because of hydrolysis by phospholipases. These stones are much more common in the Orient; the incidence decreases with the westernization of the culture and diet. They can form in the gallbladder and/or in intrahepatic or extrahepatic biliary ducts (Table 130–1). In Western nations they form primarily in the common bile duct years after cholecystectomy for cholesterol or black pigment stones. Unlike in the West, in the Orient stones frequently recur after removal and are associated with massive dilatation of the biliary tract and accompanying cholangiohepatitis (re-

TABLE 130–1. CONDITIONS ASSOCIATED WITH A PROPENSITY FOR GALLSTONE FORMATION

1. **Cholesterol**
   Obesity
   Ileal disease or resection
   Multiparity
   Drugs: clofibrate, estrogens
   Race: American Indian
   Cystic fibrosis
2. **Black pigment**
   Old age
   Cirrhosis
   Hemolysis
   Intravenous hyperalimentation
3. **Brown pigment**
   Oriental cholangiohepatitis
   Sclerosing cholangitis
   Caroli's disease
   Choledochal cysts
   Duodenal diverticula (perivaterian)

current pyogenic cholangitis), often resulting in secondary biliary cirrhosis and hepatic failure.

DISSOLUTION OF GALLSTONES. Attempts have been made to dissolve cholesterol gallstones by reversing some of the above pathogenetic mechanisms. Chenodeoxycholate (CDC), 12 to 15 mg per kilogram per day orally, will dissolve a substantial proportion of radiolucent cholesterol gallbladder stones within two years. CDC causes the bile to become unsaturated by mechanisms that are still unclear. Problems with CDC therapy include diarrhea and hepatoxicity. Ursodeoxycholate has a similar therapeutic effect, but is less hepatotoxic and diarrheogenic. These compounds are ineffective for dissolution of pigment stones, of radiopaque stones, of stones in gallbladders nonopacified by oral cholecystography, and of stones in obese patients. Candidates for dissolution treatment are mildly to moderately symptomatic patients who are bad risks for surgery because of other illnesses. Stones will usually dissolve in one or two years in 30 to 40 per cent of patients who receive CDC in a dose of 12 to 15 mg per kilogram daily. Ursodeoxycholate therapy achieves the same success rate in about half the time. Relative contraindications to therapy include chronic liver diseases, chronic diarrhea, and peptic ulcer disease. Women who may become pregnant should not be treated because of the potential (though not proven) for harmful effects of CDC on the fetus. When treatment is discontinued after initial dissolution, gallstones re-form in up to 50 per cent of patients within five years.

Current research into new methods of gallstone dissolution includes direct instillation of methyl-tert-butyl ether into the gallbladder lumen by percutaneous transhepatic catheter placement. This technique usually dissolves cholesterol gallstones within one to two days. Another technique undergoing study is extracorporeal shock-wave lithotripsy in which gallstones are fragmented into fine particles, using a technique that is similar to that already successfully used for renal stone fragmentation.

PATHOPHYSIOLOGY OF BILIARY OBSTRUCTION

Obstruction caused by a stone is the primary cause of all manifestations of gallstone disease. Obstruction of the cystic duct by gallbladder stones distends the gallbladder, producing biliary pain. If the obstruction persists, acute cholecystitis may ensue. The intermediary steps from obstruction to acute inflammation are discussed later. Whether complications such as empyema or perforation develop depends on whether secondary infection occurs. Cholecystectomy cures cholecystitis, but cholecystostomy, which only relieves the obstruction, will eliminate all the clinical manifestations of the disease.

Obstruction of the common duct may produce pain, jaundice, pruritus, infection, and biliary cirrhosis. Surgical procedures that decompress the duct upstream from the stone eliminate these manifestations. The situation in the ductal system differs from that in the gallbladder, however, because when ductal pressure exceeds about 25 cm/H_2O, bile is refluxed into blood. Pressures in this range and even higher commonly accompany mechanical obstruction and are probably aggravated by infection. Regurgitation of ductal bacteria into the systemic circulation may explain why cholangitis is often accompanied by systemic bacteremia, chills, and high fever. Fortunately obstruction of the common duct by stones is rarely complete. With unrelieved ductal obstruction, biliary cirrhosis gradually develops. Three months is the shortest time in which cirrhosis occurs, and the earliest cases follow neoplastic (high-grade) obstruction.

OBSTRUCTIVE JAUNDICE. Patients with biliary obstruction often present with jaundice. The approach to the clinical evaluation of jaundice is described in detail in Ch. 120.

ROENTGENOLOGIC AND OTHER IMAGING TESTS

Biliary disease usually results from obstructive lesions; radiologic techniques, if successful in outlining the system, are often diagnostic. The choice and timing of these direct and indirect procedures depend upon the diagnostic strategy of the clinician. They are discussed in greater detail in Ch. 95 and 116.

Plain roentgenograms can demonstrate the 10 to 15 per cent of gallstones that contain enough calcium to be radiopaque, but the relationship of the stones to the gallbladder or bile ducts is not always obvious. Emphysematous cholecystitis, air in the bile ducts, and calcium in the wall of the gallbladder also have diagnostic appearances on plain films.

Oral cholecystography requires that the night prior to the examination the patient swallow tablets of iopanoic or tyropanoic acid, which are then absorbed from the gut, excreted in bile, and concentrated in the gallbladder. If the gallbladder is opacified, stones in the lumen are shown as radiolucent defects (Fig. 130–3). Oral cholecystography is 90 to 95 per cent accurate in detecting gallstones. Nonopacification of the gallbladder occurs if the cystic duct is blocked or if the diseased gallbladder mucosa cannot concentrate the contrast material. The gallbladder may not be opacified for several reasons not related to gallbladder disease: if the patient has been vomiting, if the patient has been fasting for several days immediately before taking the tablets, or if absorption by the gut or excretion by the liver is faulty. If extrabiliary causes of a nonopacified gallbladder are excluded, nonopacification is 95 per cent reliable in indicating gallbladder disease.

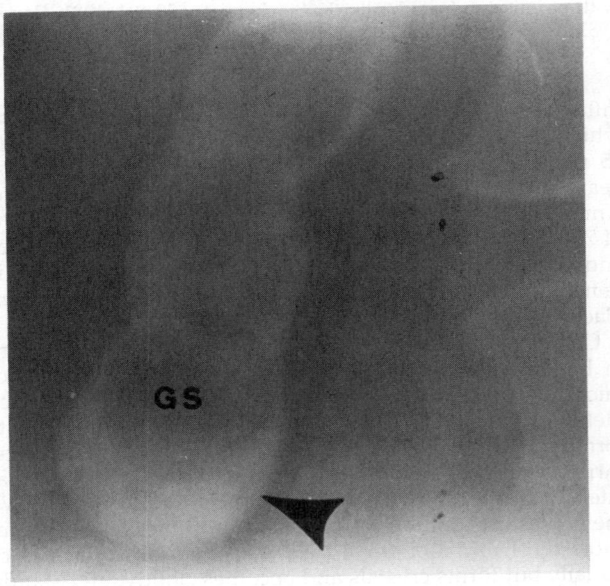

FIGURE 130–3. Oral cholecystogram showing a gallbladder (*arrowhead*) opacified by an orally administered contrast agent. The gallbladder is filled with four large round gallstones (GS).

Ultrasonography of the biliary tree may demonstrate gallstones or dilatation of the intrahepatic or extrahepatic ductal system (Fig. 130–4). It also has the advantage of being able to examine, if indicated, the liver and pancreas at the same time. Real-time ultrasonography is very reliable in detecting gallbladder stones (false positives are uncommon); it should be used as the first test for screening for gallstones. Unfortunately, less than one third of common duct stones are identified. Ductal dilatation is detected in about 90 per cent of cases of proven obstruction. Ductal dilatation usually indicates distal obstruction by neoplasm, stricture, or stone. The correlation between dilatation and obstruction is inexact because (1) the ducts may be dilated from previous disease or surgery although currently unobstructed, (2) cirrhosis or scarring from previous cholangitis may stiffen the ducts enough to prevent dilatation, and (3) lesions characterized by intermittent obstruction (e.g., common duct stones, stricture) may produce dilation followed by spontaneous decompression; ducts may appear undilated if the patient is examined after the duct has spontaneously decompressed.

Percutaneous transhepatic cholangiography (PTC) involves direct percutaneous puncture of an intrahepatic duct by a needle inserted through the eighth or ninth right intercostal space into the center of the liver. An abnormal clotting mechanism, significant ascites, and severe cholangitis are contraindications. PTC has proved particularly valuable in diagnosing gallstones within the intrahepatic biliary tract, biliary strictures, and neoplastic obstruction of the bile ducts (Fig. 130–5). A technically successful study can be obtained in nearly all patients with dilated ducts and in 70 per cent of patients with normal-sized ducts.

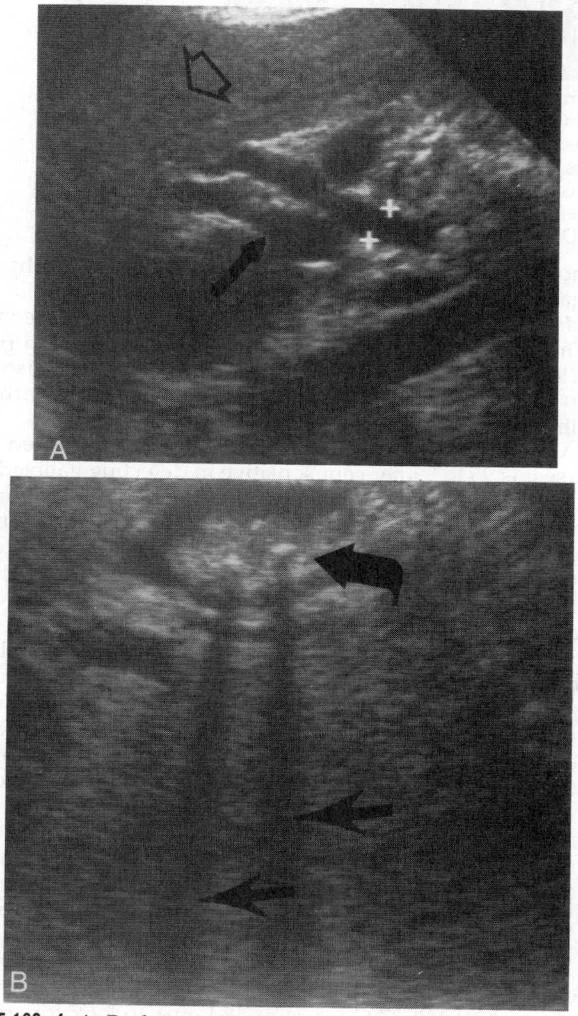

FIGURE 130–4. *A,* Real-time ultrasonography of the extrahepatic biliary tract showing a dilated common bile duct (the width of the duct measured between the two white crosses is 9 mm); the portal vein is seen as the anechoic area (*solid arrow*) directly beneath the common bile duct. The liver parenchyma is indicated by the arrowhead. *B,* Ultrasonography of a gallbladder containing gallstones and sludge (*curved arrow*) that appear as echogenic foci within the gallbladder lumen. The gallstones exhibit acoustic shadowing (*lower two arrows*), that is, paucity of echoes distal to the stones due to blockage of the echo waves by the solid stones. (Courtesy of Dr. Peter Arger.)

Endoscopic retrograde cholangiopancreatography (ERCP) involves cannulation of the common bile duct and pancreatic duct through the ampulla of Vater via the endoscope (see Fig. 95–7). With experience, a successful study of one or both ducts is possible in 80 to 90 per cent of attempts. ERCP is particularly useful in patients with normal-sized bile ducts or in whom pancreatic disease as a cause of bile duct obstruction is strongly suspected.

Both PTC and ERCP are usually contraindicated in active cholangitis unless a therapeutic maneuver is planned because as ductal pressure increases during injection of the contrast material, severe uncontrollable sepsis may be produced. Patients undergoing either of these procedures should usually receive premedication with antimicrobial agents regardless of whether there is a history of cholangitis.

Radionuclide imaging of the biliary tree may be accomplished by intravenous injection of a ^{99m}Tc-labeled derivative of iminodiacetic acid (e.g., HIDA, PIPIDA, or DISIDA). Normally, a high-quality image of the biliary tree appears within 30 minutes after administration of the radionuclide agent (see Fig. 95–9). This test is becoming the procedure of choice in verifying the diagnosis of acute cholecystitis. Filling of the ducts but not of the gallbladder supports the diagnosis of cholecystitis due to obstruction of the cystic duct by a stone. A false-negative study is rare; however, false-positive (nonfilling) studies are seen in patients with severe illnesses such as pancreatitis and cholestatic liver disease and in those receiving intravenous hyperalimentation. Ultrasonography is more useful in detecting common bile duct obstruction than is radionuclide imaging.

Computed tomography is usually performed after evidence of biliary ductal disease has been ascertained by ultrasonography or cholangiography. It is useful in defining pancreatic causes of biliary tract obstruction, in detecting paraductal lymph node enlargement, and in examining the liver for abscesses, intrahepatic ductal dilatation, and neoplasms.

CLINICAL CATEGORIES OF GALLBLADDER AND BILIARY TRACT DISEASES

Asymptomatic Gallstones

Approximately 60 to 80 per cent of patients in the United States with gallstones are asymptomatic, based on surveys using ultrasonography. In the past, patients with asymptomatic gallstones were advised to have a cholecystectomy. The trend now is to observe such patients and not to recommend surgery. Such asymptomatic patients may therefore be followed expectantly with prophylactic cholecystectomy reserved for the following two exceptions: (1) *diabetics,* because their mortality from acute cholecystitis is 10 to 15 per cent, mainly as a result of the coexisting diabetic complications, such as cardiovascular disease, and (2) patients with *calcified gallbladders,* often associated with carcinoma of the gallbladder. Asymptomatic patients with gallstones have approximately an 18 per cent chance of developing biliary pain in 20 years, and only 3 per cent will require cholecystectomy. Mortality from gallstone disease is low when a conservative plan is used of treating only those who present with typical biliary pain. Even with symptomatic patients, the decision to perform surgery is not always clear-cut. Patients with infrequent mild pain may prefer not to undergo cholecystectomy, or the physician may be hesitant to recommend surgery because of serious coexisting illnesses. Such patients may be

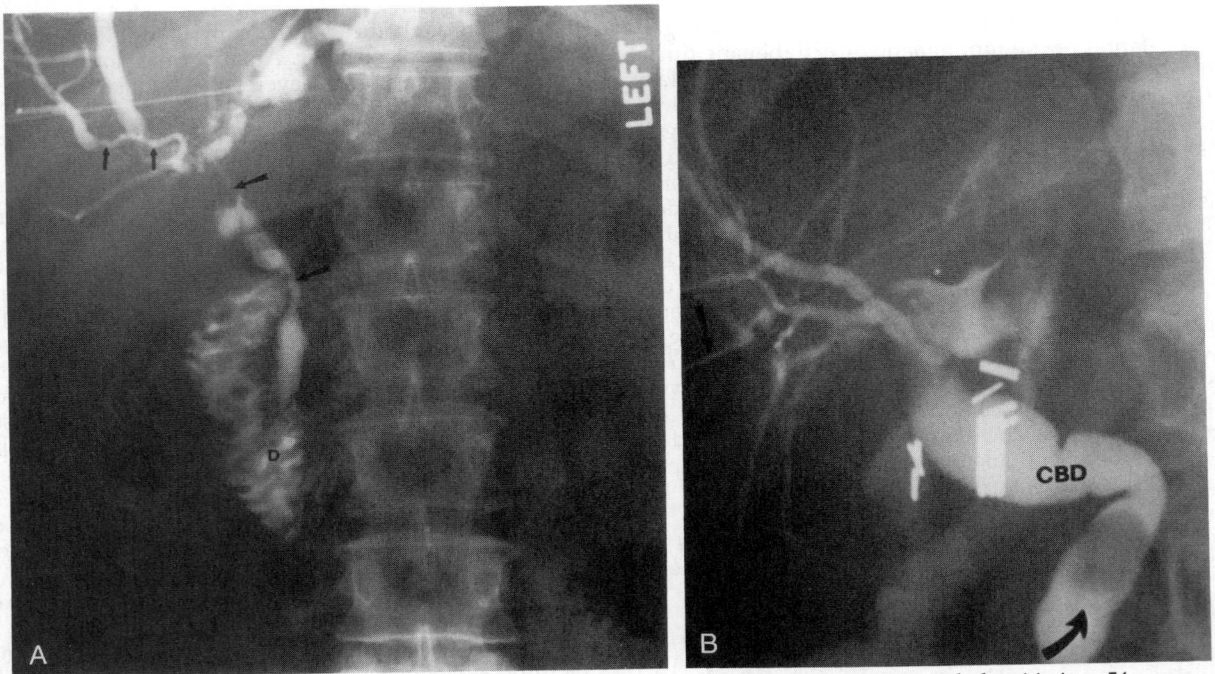

FIGURE 130–5. *A*, Percutaneous transhepatic cholangiogram demonstrating primary sclerosing cholangitis in a 54-year-old woman with a long history of Crohn's disease and biochemical evidence of cholestasis. There are strictures (*arrows*) scattered throughout her intra- and extrahepatic biliary tract; dye is seen to flow into the duodenum (D). *B*, Percutaneous transhepatic cholangiogram (skinny needle used for dye injection is indicated by arrow on left) showing a 1.5 × 2.0 cm gallstone (*curved arrow*) in the distal common bile duct (CBD) causing dilatation of the extrahepatic biliary tract. The metallic clips are from a prior cholecystectomy. The patient presented with a three-day history of RUQ pain and jaundice with a total bilirubin of 5.6 mg per deciliter. (Courtesy of Dr. Gordon McLean.)

suitable candidates for medical dissolution with chenodeoxycholate.

Symptomatic Gallstones

PATHOLOGY. The pathologic findings in the gallbladder wall and the clinical manifestations of gallstone disease often correlate poorly. In some patients the gallbladder is severely affected as the result of previous attacks of acute cholecystitis, with shrinking, scarring, and thickening of the wall, adhesions to adjacent viscera, and patchy replacement of the mucosa by granulation tissue or collagen. Nonopacification following oral cholecystography is frequent in such patients. At the other extreme the gallbladder may be grossly normal with only slight thinning of the mucosa, mild patchy scarring and inflammation, and a normally visualized oral cholecystogram. The term *chronic cholecystitis* is a descriptive pathologic term for such changes although it has been used to describe the clinical manifestations of chronically symptomatic gallstones.

CLINICAL MANIFESTATIONS. Symptomatic gallstones commonly produce a steady pain most often located in the epigastrium or right upper quadrant, thought to be caused by gallbladder distension arising from transient obstruction of the cystic duct by a gallstone. The onset of pain takes only a few minutes; it quickly reaches a plateau in intensity that may range from moderate to excruciating. After 30 minutes to several hours the pain subsides gradually. The pain usually does not wax and wane like intestinal colic; hence the preferred term is *biliary pain,* not biliary colic. Nausea and vomiting may accompany the attack, and only a vague residual ache or soreness may remain after the acute pain has dissipated. Tenderness, muscular guarding, a palpable mass, fever, and leukocytosis are absent, distinguishing this condition from acute cholecystitis. Many patients have simultaneous pain referred to the back near the scapula or to the right shoulder area. Attacks may occur daily or as seldom as once every few years. Dyspepsia, intolerance to fatty food, flatulence, heartburn, and belching may occur, but are not helpful diagnostically because they often occur in persons with normal gallbladders.

Hydrops (mucocele) of the gallbladder refers to its distension with mucus (white bile) and gallstones; it may develop from cystic duct obstruction. Hydrops produces constant discomfort in the right upper quadrant and a palpable mass without the clinical findings of acute cholecystitis.

DIAGNOSIS. Real-time *ultrasonography* is the preferred test because it is 95 to 99 per cent sensitive in detecting gallbladder stones. It also has the advantage of allowing examination of the common bile duct, pancreas, and liver at the same time without radiation exposure. An oral cholecystogram after a double dose of contrast material (that is, taken on the two nights prior to the examination) will identify 90 to 95 per cent of gallstones. If nonopacification occurs and liver function and intestinal absorption are normal and other extrabiliary causes are excluded, gallbladder disease can be inferred with a high degree of certainty. In about 5 to 10 per cent of patients with gallstones, opacification of the gallbladder will be adequate during oral cholecystography, but calculi will not be demonstrated, either because the stones are too small to be seen or because they are of the same radiographic density as the contrast medium.

In patients with typical biliary pain in the absence of demonstrable gallstones by cholecystography or ultrasonography, examination of bile for crystals may prove helpful. A sample of bile is obtained from an orally placed duodenal tube and is examined microscopically for the presence of cholesterol crystals. If no crystals are seen initially the bile can be incubated at 37°C for 24 or 48 hours to look for crystal formation. The significance of calcium bilirubinate crystals is uncertain. In the presence of what seems to be biliary pain, a positive duodenal drainage test is highly suggestive that tiny stones are present or, in a few cases, that cholesterolosis is present.

The *differential diagnosis* includes other common causes of chronic abdominal symptoms such as peptic ulcer, reflux esophagitis, esophageal spasm, and pancreatitis, which may have manifestations similar to those of gallstones. Radicular pain from spinal lesions or rib pain from bone lesions may mimic biliary pain. Angina pectoris may cause pain thought to be abdominal, just as biliary pain may be felt in the precordial region. Postprandial pain or discomfort may result from the irritable bowel syndrome or intestinal tumors.

COMPLICATIONS. *Choledocholithiasis* is the most common complication, affecting about 15 per cent of patients with cholecystolithiasis. The incidence of common duct stones increases with advancing age. Patients with symptomatic gallstones often eventually develop an attack of *acute cholecystitis.* About two thirds of patients with acute cholecystitis have previously had symptomatic gallstones. Mirizzi's syndrome results from extrinsic compression of the common hepatic or common bile duct by a large stone passing through the cystic duct. Obstructive jaundice may develop. Calcification of the gallbladder (*porcelain gallbladder*) is an uncommon condition, but of special significance because of its frequent association with carcinoma of the gallbladder. The diagnosis is made from the radiographic demonstration of an eggshell-like rim of calcium in the gallbladder wall. Adenocarcinoma of the gallbladder is found mainly in elderly patients with cholelithiasis, most of whom have had biliary symptoms for many years.

TREATMENT. Dietary changes, anticholinergics, and antispasmodics have no effect on the course of the disease, but they sometimes provide temporary symptomatic relief. Analgesics should be used for relief of pain. *Cholecystectomy* is the treatment of choice. At operation the common bile duct is inspected, a cholangiogram is obtained, and the common duct is explored if there is evidence of choledocholithiasis.

Cholecystectomy relieves symptoms from gallstones; the postcholecystectomy syndrome is discussed later in this chapter. Loss of the gallbladder does not impair gastrointestinal function. The mortality in elective cholecystectomy is less than 0.5 per cent. In patients over 70 years of age, however, mortality rises to 2 to 3 per cent; most of the postoperative deaths are a result of pre-existing cardiopulmonary diseases.

Acute Cholecystitis

PATHOGENESIS. Acute cholecystitis is the result of cystic duct obstruction and chemical irritation rather than of bacterial infection. Filling the gallbladder of a dog with concentrated bile and obstructing the cystic duct produce acute inflammation. If the gallbladder is empty or distended with physiologic saline solution instead of bile, cystic duct obstruction is tolerated without inflammation. Obstruction is associated with the release of phospholipase from the gallbladder epithelium that can hydrolyze lecithin, releasing lysolecithin, an epithelial toxin. Simultaneously the epithelial barrier coating of mucin glycoproteins may be acutely disrupted, making the epithelium susceptible to injury by the detergent action of the concentrated bile salts.

Bacterial infection is secondary to biliary obstruction rather than being primary. Bacteria are not present in the gallbladders of asymptomatic or chronically symptomatic patients with cholesterol or black pigment gallstones. Early in acute cholecystitis, the gallbladder bile is sterile, but within a week after onset, bacteria may be present in bile in over 50 per cent of cases. Although infection is secondary, it may be ultimately responsible for the most serious sequelae of acute cholecystitis–empyema, gangrene, and perforation.

Acalculous cholecystitis, accounting for less than 5 per cent of cases, is more common in men and in patients with unrelated sepsis. Most cases have been associated with prolonged fasting after major trauma, e.g., war or automobile accident injuries, surgical operations, or severe burns. Rare cases are caused by *Salmonella typhosa*, polyarteritis nodosa, or ischemia of other causes. At operation the bile is viscous and full of sludge. Gangrene and perforation are more frequent, and the outcome is generally worse than in acute calculous cholecystitis.

PATHOLOGY. Early inflammation with subserosal edema, mucosal ulcerations, and submucosal hemorrhages progresses slowly to cellular infiltration of the wall after three to four days, which reaches its greatest intensity at the end of the first week. During the second week, patchy mural gangrene, small intramural abscesses, and collagen deposition appear. Resolution of the acute changes takes another week or more.

The term *empyema* describes the rare entity of a pus-filled gallbladder characterized clinically by a septic form of acute cholecystitis. Gangrene and perforation are most common in the fundus where the blood supply is meager or in the neck where stones become impacted. With perforation, gallbladder contents may spill into the free abdominal cavity (bile peritonitis) or, more often, are confined by adhesions (pericholecystic abscess). Sometimes an adherent viscus is penetrated, forming a cholecystenteric fistula through which the gallstones and pus may be discharged. Fistulization is most frequent with the duodenum, but jejunal and colonic fistulas have been described.

CLINICAL MANIFESTATIONS. An attack of acute cholecystitis begins with *abdominal pain* that increases gradually in severity. The pain is usually located in the right subcostal region from the start, but it sometimes begins in the epigastrium or left upper quadrant and then shifts to the region of the gallbladder as inflammation progresses. Two thirds or more of patients have had previous episodes of typical biliary pain. Early in the attack the patient may expect the symptoms to subside spontaneously as had happened before with similar pain, and medical aid is often not sought until 48 hours or more. Referred pain may be experienced in the back at the scapular level. Patients in their 70's and 80's may have few or no localizing symptoms.

Anorexia, nausea, and vomiting are often present, but vomiting is rarely severe enough to be confused with bowel obstruction and is generally less than in acute pancreatitis. In the absence of complications, chills are rare, and the temperature is about 38°C. Chills and high temperature suggest suppurative cholecystitis or associated cholangitis.

The right subcostal region is tender to palpation, and involuntary muscle spasm generally limits the examination. If the patient takes a deep breath while the subhepatic area is being palpated, heightened tenderness arrests inspiration (*Murphy's sign*).

In somewhat less than a quarter of the patients, a distended, tender gallbladder can be distinctly felt, an important finding that confirms the suspected diagnosis. The gallbladder cannot be felt in the rest of the patients because of obesity, rigidity of the abdominal wall, deep subhepatic location, or because it is small and shrunken from previous inflammation. Other related conditions characterized by a tender mass in the same area are pericholecystic abscess, acute cholecystitis complicating carcinoma of the gallbladder, torsion of the gallbladder, or gallbladder distension in obstructive cholangitis.

About 20 per cent of patients with acute cholecystitis have *mild jaundice* caused by edema of the nearby common duct or more likely by common duct stones. Rarely a tumor of the bile ducts is the underlying cause.

With treatment, improvement is usually noticeable within the first 12 to 24 hours, and the signs and symptoms gradually subside over three to seven days. Persistent severe pain, a rise in temperature or leukocyte count ($>$ 10,000 per cubic millimeter), and appearance of shaking chills or of more severe local or generalized abdominal tenderness all indicate progression of the disease and suggest the need for surgery.

Empyema (suppurative cholecystitis) can produce systemic toxicity and mild increases in bilirubin, alkaline phosphatase, and the transaminases and may herald perforation. If this severe infection is controlled with antimicrobial drugs, a large tender gallbladder may remain palpable for several weeks, and return of well-being is similarly prolonged.

DIAGNOSIS. The diagnosis is strongly suggested by the clinical manifestations just described. Roentgenograms of the abdomen may show calcified gallstones or an enlarged gallbladder. Ultrasonography is probably the simplest and most reliable method of detecting gallbladder stones in these patients. Oral cholecystography is diagnostically unreliable because of unpredictable absorption and excretion of the contrast agent.

Radionuclide scanning following intravenous administration of ^{99m}Tc DISIDA or related compounds is the procedure of choice to verify a clinical impression of acute cholecystitis. If the gallbladder fills, the diagnosis of acute cholecystitis is quite unlikely. If the bile duct fills but the gallbladder does not, the diagnosis is strongly supported.

In the differential diagnosis, acute pancreatitis, acute appendicitis, and penetrated or perforated peptic ulcer are the conditions that most often cause major problems. Furthermore, acute cholecystitis and acute pancreatitis may coexist.

In women, *gonococcal perihepatitis* (Fitz-Hugh-Curtis syndrome), caused by intra-abdominal spread of the infection from the reproductive tract to the right upper quadrant, may be mistaken for acute cholecystitis, but adnexal tenderness is usually present on pelvic examination. A cervical smear usually reveals gonococci, and the patients are younger, often have higher temperature, and are in less distress than would be expected with cholecystitis. Shoulder pain and a friction rub over the liver, common in the Fitz-Hugh–Curtis syndrome, are not found in uncomplicated acute cholecystitis.

Acute hepatitis, either viral or alcoholic, sometimes produces marked right upper quadrant pain and tenderness. A history of recent binge drinking, high transaminase levels, and liver biopsy aid differentiation. Pneumonitis, pyelonephritis, and acute cardiac disease (particularly right-sided failure) all on occasion may cause acute pain suggestive of cholecystitis.

The use of ^{99m}Tc DISIDA will distinguish between the unusual location of pain in these disorders and acute cholecystitis.

TREATMENT. Most patients with acute cholecystitis will improve with either expectant treatment or cholecystectomy performed during the acute attack. In general, the decision regarding the kind of treatment should include the following considerations (Fig. 130–6): (1) whether the diagnosis is secure, (2) whether biliary complications have occurred or appear imminent, and (3) the overall condition of the patient (operative risk).

Upon the patient's admission to the hospital, nasogastric suction should be started if the patient has significant vomiting, and fluids should be given intravenously to correct dehydration. In many elderly patients the acute biliary condition may aggravate pre-existing cardiac, pulmonary, or renal disease and produce a more ominous prognosis if surgery is delayed or if adequate treatment is not given.

Antimicrobials are of principal value to prevent bacteremia and to treat suppurative complications. If the patient is seen shortly after symptoms begin, and if local signs and symptoms are mild, antimicrobial therapy need not be given. Otherwise, an antimicrobial regimen with coverage for gram-negative aerobes as well as enterococci is preferred. One that is often used is ampicillin plus gentamicin given parenterally. In seriously ill patients, such as those with empyema or perforation, it is wise to also add an antimicrobial with anaerobic coverage, such as clindamycin.

Cholecystectomy is generally considered the optimal therapy for acute cholecystitis, but only after the diagnosis is confirmed and the patient adequately prepared for operation. Many physicians still prefer to reserve surgery during the acute attack for those patients who develop complications and for those who become worse or fail to improve. Although this is still common practice, about 25 per cent of patients managed in this way require urgent operation for worsening disease. For patients who respond to nonoperative management, interval cholecystectomy is generally recommended. The timing of cholecystectomy in such patients has been debated, but the trend is to perform surgery later during the same hospitalization.

About 30 per cent of patients are good surgical risks; in these patients the diagnosis is obvious within 12 to 24 hours, and cholecystectomy can be scheduled promptly. Another 30 per cent are good surgical candidates, but the diagnosis is not quite firm. In this situation, a ^{99m}Tc DISIDA scan should be obtained to verify the clinical impression. Another 30 per cent of patients will have serious coexistent cardiac, respiratory, or other disease for which treatment takes precedence. The cholecystitis should be treated expectantly while the other problems are being corrected. Progression of local abdominal findings requires continued re-evaluation, balancing the risks of operation with the risks of continued delay.

About 10 per cent of patients require emergency surgery

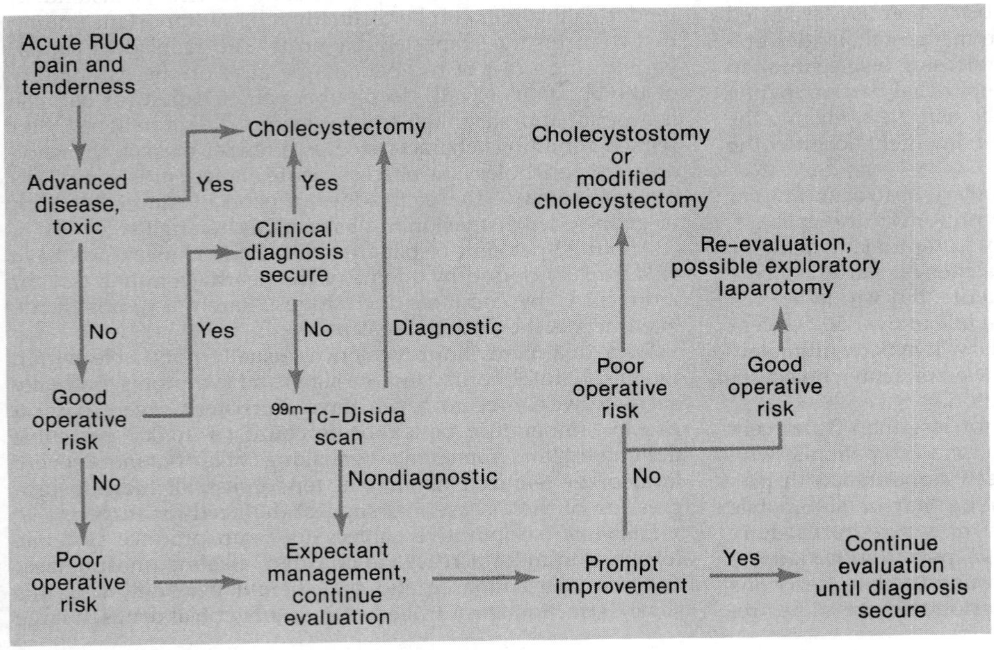

FIGURE 130–6. Schema for managing patients with right upper quadrant pain and tenderness who are thought possibly to have acute cholecystitis. This approach is based on a policy of early operation for appropriate patients and distinguishes between patients who are good versus poor operative risks.

for complications present on admission or that appear later during observation and medical management. When emergency operation becomes necessary, cholecystostomy may sometimes be preferable to cholecystectomy in the seriously ill patient. In this procedure the fundus is incised, stones and pus are removed from the lumen, and the organ is decompressed by catheter drainage, allowing the acute infection to resolve. Patients who recover should undergo cholecystectomy six to eight weeks later. Those who continue to be poor surgical risks may be followed expectantly if postoperative cholecystography shows that the gallbladder and common duct contain no residual stones. If stones are present, interventional radiologic techniques can be used to remove gallbladder stones through the cholecystomy tract after four to six weeks of tract maturation, and endoscopic sphincterotomy can be utilized to remove ductal stones. In seriously debilitated patients the cholecystostomy tube can be left in place indefinitely.

After the cholecystostomy tube is removed from a patient whose biliary system contains no calculi, within the first year about 50 per cent of patients develop new stones. Eventually 90 per cent of patients will again develop stones.

COMPLICATIONS. ***Emphysematous Cholecystitis.*** In emphysematous cholecystitis, a rare variant of acute cholecystitis, gas of bacterial origin can be seen in the gallbladder lumen and adjacent tissues. Clinically, emphysematous cholecystitis causes the same signs and symptoms as acute cholecystitis. Men are affected twice as frequently as women, about 30 per cent of patients have diabetes mellitus, and the gallbladder is acalculous in about half the cases. Gas does not develop until 24 to 48 hours after the attack begins, at which time a radiolucent halo outlines the lumen, and an air-fluid level may be seen on upright films. Subserosal and then pericholecystic emphysema appear with time. Differential diagnosis of the radiographic findings includes cholecystenteric fistula and appendiceal, perinephric, or subhepatic abscess. In about half the cases the gas-forming organisms are clostridia, and the rest are *Escherichia coli*, streptococci, and other bacteria of intestinal origin. Treatment is the same as for acute cholecystitis, but the somewhat more aggressive nature of emphysematous cholecystitis and the association with diabetes mellitus usually require prompt surgery.

Perforation. Perforation is usually manifested by greater sepsis and more marked abdominal signs. Perforation may take any of three forms: (1) free perforation into the abdominal cavity, (2) localized (contained) perforation with pericholecystic abscess, and (3) perforation into another viscus with fistula formation.

Free perforation, which has a 25 per cent mortality, is the least common type. It usually occurs early in the attack, often within the first three days, suggesting that when gangrene develops this quickly it cannot be walled off by adjacent viscera or the omentum. Clinically, free perforation classically causes toxicity with high temperatures (greater than 39°C), leukocytosis (over 15,000 per cubic millimeter), and diffuse abdominal tenderness and rigidity. In more than half the cases the correct diagnosis is unsuspected until laparotomy or autopsy, because a clear-cut history of preliminary right upper quadrant pain is often lacking. Treatment consists of intravenous antimicrobial therapy and emergency laparotomy with cholecystectomy.

Localized perforation most often appears in the second week of the attack at the peak of the inflammatory reaction. The diagnosis should be suspected with increasing local signs, especially when a mass suddenly appears. In most cases cholecystectomy can be performed, but in a severely ill patient cholecystostomy and drainage of the abscess may be wiser.

Fistula Formation. A fistula usually involves the nearby second portion of the duodenum or, less commonly, the colon, jejunum, stomach, or common bile duct. Rare fistulas have entered the renal pelvis or bronchus or extended through the abdominal wall (empyema necessitatis). After intestinal fistulization the contents of the gallbladder are discharged into the gut, often aborting the acute attack. Clinically, the fistula itself may not be suspected because it produces no unique findings; many are discovered incidentally later. In the absence of biliary obstruction a cholecystenteric fistula is not necessarily of pathophysiologic significance. Cholecystocolonic fistulas may cause malabsorption from diversion of bile or from bacterial overgrowth in the upper gut.

Gallstone Ileus. If a particularly large gallstone enters through the fistula, it may obstruct the intestine, a condition called gallstone ileus. The stone, passing through a cholecystenteric fistula, most often enters the gut in the duodenum, less commonly in the jejunum, ileum, colon, or stomach. It is often assumed that the initial event responsible for fistula formation is an attack of acute cholecystitis, but only 30 per cent of patients with gallstone ileus give a history of recent right upper quadrant pain. After entering the gut, the gallstone moves downsteam until it encounters an area of intestinal lumen too narrow to accommodate. Gallstones, usually more than 2.5 cm in diameter, most frequently obstruct the terminal ileum; they will block the colon only if its lumen has been narrowed by intrinsic disease.

On physical examination the findings are those of small-bowel obstruction. Infrequently the large stone can be felt as a mass on abdominal, vaginal, or rectal examination, but it is rarely correctly identified. Roentgenograms usually show air in the biliary tree if the films are carefully examined, and in some cases a radiopaque gallstone can be identified at the leading edge of the obstruction. Treatment consists of removing the obstructing gallstone through a small enterotomy. It is generally wise to leave the biliary disease undisturbed initially, because elderly patients tolerate long procedures poorly, and nothing much is gained by repairing the fistula primarily. Postoperatively, many patients remain asymptomatic, and the fistula may even close spontaneously; for them, expectant management is best. Some patients may require cholecystectomy later because of symptoms related to gallstones.

The mortality is 15 to 20 per cent because of delay in diagnosis and because of cardiopulmonary complications.

PROGNOSIS. The mortality in acute cholecystitis of 5 to 10 per cent is almost totally confined to patients over 60 years of age with serious associated disease. Suppurative complications are more common in the elderly, who can tolerate them least. In most instances, localized perforation can be managed satisfactorily at operation. Free perforation is considerably more ominous (25 per cent mortality), but is rare.

Choledocholithiasis and Cholangitis

In Western countries choledocholithiasis is usually the result of passage of gallstones formed in the gallbladder into the common duct. About 10 to 15 per cent of patients with asymptomatic cholecystolithiasis are thought to develop choledocholithiasis on this basis. Once in the common duct the stones may pass into the duodenum without causing symptoms. The frequency of this event is not known, but is probably greatly underestimated. Less commonly, stones form in a dilated duct behind a longstanding obstruction caused by a stricture or ampullary stenosis. About 5 per cent of patients with choledocholithiasis have no gallbladder stones; in such cases it is assumed that all the gallbladder stones escaped into the duct or, more rarely, that the stones formed primarily in the common duct. Stone type helps to determine site of origin: Cholesterol or black pigment stones more likely form in the gallbladder, while almost all brown pigment stones in patients in Western countries form in the bile ducts.

CLINICAL MANIFESTATIONS. The natural history of choledocholithiasis is incompletely known (Fig. 130–7). About 30 to 40 per cent of patients are asymptomatic at the time of

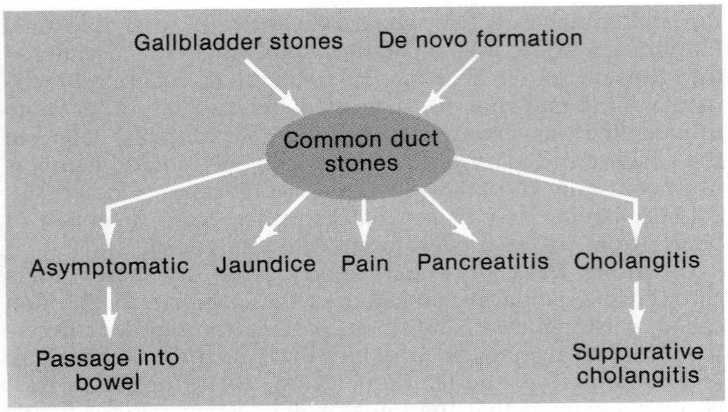

FIGURE 130–7. Natural history of choledocholithiasis. In most cases, common duct gallstones originate in the gallbladder. In some cases, particularly after the gallbladder has been surgically removed, stones may form in the common duct. The majority of stones in the common duct remain asymptomatic and may either remain in the duct without causing symptoms, pass into the bowel through the ampulla of Vater and be excreted in stool, or eventually result in symptoms, the most common of which are indicated. The exact frequency of each of these occurrences is not known.

diagnosis, implying a relatively benign course in many cases. How often asymptomatic stones remain undetected is, of course, unknown. Obstruction by stones of the biliary or pancreatic ducts may produce any of the following syndromes: biliary pain, jaundice or increased alkaline phosphatase alone (without pain), cholangitis, pancreatitis, or a combination of these. Secondary hepatic effects of persistent obstruction include biliary cirrhosis or hepatic abscesses.

Intermittent cholangitis, consisting of biliary pain, jaundice, and fever and chills (*Charcot's triad*), is the most common presenting symptom complex. In the absence of previous biliary surgery it is almost diagnostic of choledocholithiasis in Western countries. Intermittency of symptoms is quite characteristic, a manifestation of intermittent partial obstruction. Whenever pain, chills with fever, and jaundice fluctuate together over a span of a few days or a week, cholangitis from biliary obstruction is almost certainly the cause. In a typical attack, chills may precede the other symptoms, and bilirubinuria may follow. Epigastric or right upper quadrant pain, indistinguishable from biliary pain caused by gallbladder stones, is steady and very severe. Pain may be referred to the right infrascapular area, the upper back, the right shoulder, or even the precordium, suggesting coronary artery or esophageal disease.

The severity of fever and chills varies widely from the usual mild transient illness to overwhelming sepsis with shock (see Suppurative Cholangitis, below). In the average case, the temperature rises to 38.5 to 40°C, preceded by chills and positive blood cultures. Localized tenderness in the subcostal region may be associated with extreme guarding and rigidity, but more often the local findings are minimal or intermittent and are usually less severe than in acute cholecystitis.

In most cases of common duct obstruction caused by stones the gallbladder does not become distended, because it is scarred and inelastic, and the obstruction is recent, partial, or transient, the obverse of Courvoisier's law, i.e., a distended nontender gallbladder in a jaundiced patient signifies neoplastic obstruction of the bile duct.

DIAGNOSIS. In cholangitis the leukocyte count averages 15,000 per cubic millimeter, but may go much higher in severe cases. Bilirubin values are usually in the range of 2 to 4 mg per deciliter and are uncommonly higher than 10 mg per deciliter. Elevated serum alkaline phosphatase and 5′-nucleotidase levels are usually greater than three times the upper limit of normal. The AST generally remains below 200 units; however, transiently it may exceed 1000 units. In these instances the prompt drop of the AST level within 48 hours allows differentiation from viral hepatitis and suggests the diagnosis of obstruction.

The demonstration of gallbladder stones does not necessarily imply that stones in the bile ducts are responsible for the cholangitis. The same conditions considered for the patient with chronically symptomatic gallstones must be excluded for the patient with biliary pain caused by ductal calculi. In patients who have had cholecystectomy, differentiation between choledocholithiasis and biliary stricture as the cause of cholangitis usually depends on radiologic demonstration of the ducts. When the presenting syndrome is painless cholestatic jaundice, other causes, especially periampullary and biliary neoplasms, must be considered. With neoplastic obstruction, the bilirubin averages about 15 to 20 mg per deciliter and rarely fluctuates. Although jaundice from stones may be as intense, the level of bilirubin is characteristically less than 10 mg per deciliter, and it may rise and fall episodically. The diagnosis of intrahepatic cholestasis from causes such as drugs, viral hepatitis, or pregnancy should follow the schema outlined in Ch. 120. In such cases, opacification of normal bile ducts by PTC or ERCP may ultimately be required. Gallstone disease is common in cirrhosis, so choledocholithiasis and alcoholic liver disease may coexist.

Common duct stones may cause acute pancreatitis indistinguishable clinically from that resulting from alcohol or other causes and unaccompanied by specific signs of biliary disease (Ch. 108). Pancreatitis caused by biliary calculi, despite numerous attacks, rarely progresses to pancreatic calcification, chronic pain, and pancreatic insufficiency, as so often occurs in the alcoholic variety. Gallstone disease should be ruled out in every patient with acute pancreatitis, because further damage during such an episode and future attacks can be avoided if the gallstones are removed.

TREATMENT. The potential seriousness of cholangitis warrants hospitalization for diagnosis and treatment. After blood cultures are obtained, antimicrobial drugs effective against enteric organisms are given by the parenteral route. A regimen consisting of an aminoglycoside plus ampicillin for mild attacks with the addition of clindamycin in severe infection is usually successful. Failure to obtain a rapid response may mean that the organisms were not susceptible to the initial drugs, justifying the addition of another drug or a shift from the initial regimen on the basis of the result of cultures and drug susceptibility tests. The margin between mild and severe illness is small; antimicrobial therapy should be expected to control the acute attack within 48 to 72 hours, and if there is no improvement or worsening after this period, emergency surgery or endoscopic sphincterotomy must be considered seriously.

More than 90 per cent of patients respond satisfactorily to treatment, allowing an orderly attempt at diagnosis. Ultrasonography should be performed first to detect ductal dilatation. Direct opacification of the ducts can be attempted by PTC or ERCP. Both kinds of direct cholangiography are potentially hazardous in active cholangitis and should be postponed if possible until infection is well controlled; then one proceeds only under the protection of antimicrobial therapy. However, decompression of the bile duct using a percutaneous transhepatic catheter or by endoscopic sphincterotomy may provide the control needed when there is evidence of duct obstruction.

Deciding between endoscopic and surgical approaches to the management of choledocholithiasis should be on a case by case basis. If the gallbladder is present, cholecystectomy is performed and the common duct is opened and emptied of stones. A T tube is usually left in the duct to decompress biliary pressure in the postoperative period and to provide a route for subsequent cholangiography. With accurate diagnosis and treatment, choledocholithiasis is cured by cholecystectomy and choledocholithotomy. Recurrent ductal stone formation occurs infrequently except when the duct has become markedly dilated.

Selected patients with choledocholithiasis may be satisfactorily treated by endoscopic sphincterotomy. By means of the side-viewing duodenoscope, a wire (papillotome) is passed into the bile duct and the sphincter divided by electrocautery. Common duct stones 1.5 cm or smaller will usually pass into the duodenum. This technique may be unsuccessful with large stones or when the common duct is greatly dilated. Bleeding and pancreatitis are the principal complications, but are infrequent. Mortality in the procedure is less than 1 per cent in experienced hands. When endoscopic sphincterotomy is successfully used for cholangitis in patients with gallbladder stones, there is debate about whether to perform cholecystectomy at a later date. In our opinion this decision should be based on whether the patient subsequently develops symptoms referable to the gallbladder stones.

RETAINED COMMON DUCT STONES. The methods for detecting duct stones at operation are about 95 per cent reliable, which means, unfortunately, that a few are overlooked only to be discovered on postoperative T-tube cholangiograms. There are two approaches to remove residual stones without another laparotomy. Neither method should be tried until four to six weeks postoperatively to allow for maturation of the T-tube tract. One technique depends on the ability of mono-octanoin (glyceryl-1-mono-octanoate) to dissolve cholesterol gallstones. Mono-octanoin is infused into the duct at 5 ml per hour; care must be exercised to avoid producing pressures in the duct greater than 30 cm H_2O during infusion. The retained stones disappear in about one half of patients within a four- to eight-day treatment period. There is no solvent known to be effective against black pigment stones. Mono-octanoin has been partially successful for brown pigment stones.

Instrumental extraction is somewhat simpler and faster and is the treatment of choice. Under image-intensification fluoroscopy the T tube is pulled out, a Dormia ureteral basket is passed into the duct, and the stone is grasped and withdrawn. The best plan usually is to try instrumental extraction first and dissolution if it fails. If neither mechanical extraction nor chemical dissolution is successful, endoscopic sphincterotomy may allow the stone to pass into the duodenum. If that technique is unsuccessful, reoperation is necessary.

SUPPURATIVE CHOLANGITIS. The most severe form of cholangitis, suppurative cholangitis, involves the same causative factors as the "nonsuppurative" form, but differs in that obstruction is complete, ductal contents become purulent, and clinically the manifestations of sepsis overshadow those of cholestasis. Hypotension and mental changes such as lethargy or confusion appear in addition to right upper quadrant pain, chills, fever, and jaundice. Some elderly patients may be hypothermic and have minimal clinical signs. Because infection in the face of the high-grade obstruction progresses so rapidly the serum bilirubin does not reach very high levels before the patient becomes moribund from sepsis. Costly delays in diagnosis are frequent, a consequence of failure to recognize the significance of mild icterus and abdominal pain in a patient with sepsis. All but a few cases involve complications of choledocholithiasis, the others occurring with biliary stricture or neoplastic obstruction, usually from bile duct carcinoma with or without sclerosing cholangitis.

Laboratory tests reveal evidence of cholestasis with bilirubin values between 2 and 5 mg per deciliter and elevated serum levels of alkaline phosphatase, 5′-nucleotidase, and transaminases. The leukocyte count varies from subnormal to 40,000 per cubic millimeter. Hypoglycemia may sometimes be present.

Tenderness to palpation is present in the right upper quadrant, but rigidity is uncommon. In some cases secondary cholecystitis develops, and an enlarged tender gallbladder may be found on abdominal examination. Ultrasonography may show dilated bile ducts. Diagnosis rests on recognizing the evidence of biliary obstruction and its relationship to the sepsis and on verifying the initial impression by ultrasonography. After initial resuscitation—consisting of intravenous infusions, antimicrobial drugs (gentamicin or tobramycin plus ampicillin and clindamycin parenterally), and measures to restore cardiac, pulmonary, or renal function—decompression of the duct by emergency laparotomy, percutaneous transhepatic catheter placement, or endoscopic sphincterotomy offers the only hope of saving the patient. Biliary stents have been placed endoscopically to reduce obstruction and systemic sepsis.

At surgery when choledochotomy is performed, pus often squirts from the duct as a result of the high pressure. If the patient's condition permits, thorough exploration can be carried out to correct the obstruction by removing stones, repairing a stricture, or bypassing a tumor. Insertion of a T tube proximal to the obstruction is sufficient in patients who are unable to tolerate a longer operation, but sometime later it will be necessary to perform a second more definitive procedure before the T tube can be removed. The mortality is about 50 per cent, resulting from septic shock, renal or respiratory failure, acute hepatic insufficiency, or a combination of these complications.

Other Causes of Bile Duct Obstruction

Duodenal and pancreatic tumors are common causes of obstruction in the middle-aged or elderly. These important diseases are discussed in Ch. 107 and 109. Common bile duct obstruction may also be caused by a variety of uncommon disorders such as sclerosing cholangitis in patients with ulcerative colitis or by Oriental cholangiohepatitis in immigrants from Southeast Asia. Rare causes are compression by neoplastic paraductal lymph nodes or by duodenal Crohn's disease.

SCLEROSING CHOLANGITIS. Sclerosing cholangitis, a condition of unknown cause, consists of benign nonbacterial chronic inflammatory narrowing of the bile ducts. The entire ductal system is involved in most cases; less commonly the process may be confined to the extrahepatic or intrahepatic portion. The ratio of males to females is 3:2, and the peak incidence occurs in the third and fourth decades. More than half of the cases are associated with *ulcerative colitis* (Ch. 105) and, to a lesser extent, *regional enteritis*. The severity of sclerosing cholangitis does not parallel the activity of the colitis, and colectomy does not improve the cholangitis. Other much less commonly associated diseases are retroperitoneal fibrosis and Riedel's thyroiditis.

The initial complaint may be jaundice or pruritus, although more cases are being discovered at an asymptomatic stage. There may be mild upper abdominal pain and sometimes fever, but a clinical picture resembling bacterial cholangitis is uncommon in the absence of previous surgical exploration or instrumentation of the ducts. Hepatomegaly may be present in some cases; when secondary cirrhosis develops, ascites or splenomegaly may be found.

Jaundice may be constant or fluctuating, and bilirubin values are usually in the range of 2 to 10 mg per deciliter. The alkaline phosphatase is always increased, usually greater than three times the upper limit of normal, and remains increased despite variations in clinical manifestations. Transaminases are usually mildly increased. Antimitochondrial antibodies are normal.

Percutaneous transhepatic cholangiography or preferably endoscopic retrograde cholangiopancreatography is required to establish the diagnosis. The radiographs show diffuse or focal irregular ductal narrowing with intervening areas of normal caliber or dilatation; this "beaded" appearance is characteristic. Some patients develop gallstones behind the strictured areas as a result of stasis; these are usually brown pigment gallstones. Localized strictures may be difficult to distinguish from ductal carcinoma.

Treatment with corticosteroids or immunosuppressants has not been proved to be generally effective, but a few patients do respond. A trial of treatment is advocated by some experts. Cholestyramine is useful for pruritus. Antimicrobials are necessary if bacterial cholangitis develops.

In symptomatic patients the aim of therapy is to relieve biliary obstruction. If a segmental stricture is present, balloon dilatation can be attempted either percutaneously or, if the lesion is in the common bile duct, endoscopically. This involves the insertion into the bile duct of a balloon-tipped catheter; inflation of the balloon stretches the narrowed area and allows greater bile flow. Balloon dilatation may have to be repeated intermittently to provide sustained relief of obstruction; there is the risk of inducing bacterial cholangitis, particularly with the endoscopic approach. Percutaneous catheter drainage is another option, but often does not provide adequate drainage of all obstructed areas in diffuse disease. Surgical therapy is warranted in some cases to provide stenting in diffuse disease or to bypass severe distal common bile duct disease. Significant palliation follows surgery in most cases, but is not usually permanent. Most patients have episodic remissions and exacerbations, during which secondary biliary cirrhosis develops. Liver transplantation is now an option for those with advanced disease. Death may follow uncontrollable biliary sepsis with hepatic abscesses, liver failure, or bleeding from esophageal varices.

STRUCTURAL ABNORMALITIES. *Choledochal cysts* occasionally produce their initial clinical manifestations in young adults, presenting with jaundice, pain, or cholangitis. Diagnosis requires direct ductal visualization with PTC or ERCP; computed tomography or ultrasonography can provide information about surrounding structures. The most definitive surgical procedure is excision of the cyst, followed by Roux-en-Y choledochojejunostomy.

Caroli's disease, consisting of saccular intrahepatic bile duct dilations, most often becomes symptomatic in patients between the ages of 20 and 50 years, because of intrahepatic stone formation and cholangitis. Two forms are recognized: (1) disease of the ducts only and (2) ductal disease associated with hepatic fibrosis and medullary sponge kidney (more common). The latter patients often have complications of portal hypertension before cholangitis or obstructive jaundice appears. Antimicrobial therapy may control attacks of cholangitis, and surgical procedures to facilitate ductal emptying or to extract stones may help in some cases, but the intrahepatic anomaly cannot be definitively corrected unless lobectomy is possible for single lobe involvement.

PANCREATITIS. Pancreatitis can produce transient jaundice by obstruction of the distal common duct where it is surrounded by pancreatic tissue. Prolonged obstruction can result from pressure by an adjacent pseudocyst or entrapment of the distal common bile duct in severe pancreatic scarring from *chronic pancreatitis.* Diagnosis may be delayed in alcoholic patients in whom elevated alkaline phosphatase or bilirubin values are usually attributed to hepatocellular disease. Persistent elevation of the alkaline phosphatase value in an alcoholic should raise suspicion of the possibility of biliary obstruction, particularly if pancreatic calcification is present on plain abdominal radiographs. Jaundice resulting from chronic pancreatitis requires choledochoduodenostomy or Roux-en-Y anastomosis of jejunum to the common bile duct.

HEMOBILIA. Hemobilia classically presents with biliary pain, obstructive jaundice, and occult or gross intestinal bleeding. Most cases are caused by hepatic injury from external or operative trauma, with secondary bleeding into the ductal system. Other causes include biliary or hepatic neoplasms, ductal rupture of a hepatic artery aneurysm, hepatic abscess, and gallstones, or it may follow percutaneous needle biopsy of the liver or cholangiography. Hemobilia following trauma is best treated by hepatic artery ligation, which is well tolerated except when there is advanced parenchymal disease; otherwise, direct management of the causative lesion is necessary.

PARASITIC DISEASE. An *echinococcal hepatic cyst* can rupture into the ducts and can give rise to biliary colic, jaundice, and cholangitis (Ch. 397). *Ascariasis* may produce biliary colic, jaundice, and cholangitis by worm invasion into the bile ducts from the duodenum (Ch. 406).

ORIENTAL CHOLANGIOHEPATITIS. Oriental cholangiohepatitis or *recurrent pyogenic cholangitis* is a common form of recurrent cholangitis in the Orient associated with brown pigment gallstone formation throughout the biliary tract. The cause is unclear, but the parasite *Clonorchis sinensis* is found in very few cases so does not seem to be a major causative factor. Most patients present with acute cholangitis; those with recurrent cholangitis may develop liver abscesses, biliary–enteric fistulas, or sepsis. In advanced cases, one (usually the left) or both lobar ducts may become honeycombed with scars or abscesses, producing atrophy of the hepatic parenchyma.

Direct cholangiography is necessary for a definitive diagnosis. Sphincteroplasty or choledochojejunostomy is usually performed to remove stones and sludge and provide adequate biliary drainage. Cholecystectomy or partial hepatic resection is required when the gallbladder or localized hepatic segments are involved.

BILIARY STRICTURE. Biliary stricture almost always results from *surgical injury* to the duct and usually follows cholecystectomy rather than procedures on the duct itself such as common duct exploration. Biliary stricture may also result from external trauma or scarring produced by choledocholithiasis.

The symptoms resemble those of cholangitis with choledocholithiasis. Differential diagnosis includes all the various causes of obstructive jaundice and cholangitis. Laboratory evidence consists of leukocytosis and elevated serum levels of bilirubin, alkaline phosphatase, and transaminases. The jaundice and cholangitis are generally mild and transient, and infection generally responds promptly to antimicrobial therapy. Diagnosis can be made with visualization of the biliary tract by either PTC or ERCP. With persistent obstruction over several years, secondary biliary cirrhosis or multiple intrahepatic abscesses may develop.

In almost all cases an attempt should be made to repair the stricture surgically by creating a new unobstructed conduit between normal duct on the hepatic side of the lesion and the proximal intestine rather than attempting direct end-to-end anastomosis of the duct after excision of the lesion. The overall success rate of these operations is about 75 per cent with an operative mortality of 10 per cent.

Balloon catheter dilatation of a short stricture at the time of either PTC or ERCP may be useful in some patients, particularly those who are poor operative risks.

Carcinoma of the Gallbladder

In the United States there are approximately 2500 deaths annually from carcinoma of the gallbladder, a number equal to the mortality from benign disease of the biliary tract. Gallbladder cancer accounts for 1 per cent of all cancer deaths and 3 per cent of gastrointestinal malignant disease. Women are affected more frequently than men by a ratio of 3 to 1, and the average age is 70 years. Because 70 to 80 per cent of cases occur in patients with gallstones, cholelithiasis is thought to be etiologically important, but the mechanism involved is unclear. Gallbladder cancer develops in fewer than 1 per cent of patients with cholelithiasis. The disease is five to ten times more frequent in American Indian populations.

Almost all gallbladder carcinomas are *adenocarcinomas;* the earliest spread is usually by metastasis to the hilar lymph nodes and adjacent hepatic parenchyma followed by direct extension to the liver and hilar structures. Distant metastases appear relatively late.

Patients have one of the following clinical pictures: (1) unremitting deep jaundice from common duct and hepatic involvement; (2) acute cholecystitis, usually with a palpable mass; (3) chronic intermittent right upper quadrant pain; and 4) advanced disseminated carcinoma. The diagnosis is not often considered preoperatively, but in some instances clinical clues are present. In about two thirds of patients a mass can be felt, and in one third there is local tenderness. In all but a few cases the gallbladder is not opacified during oral cholecystography, and even when it is, the tumor can rarely be demonstrated. The diagnosis can be suspected on ultrasound study if an intraluminal gallbladder mass is identified that does not change with position. The differential diagnosis is that of a cholesterol polyp or of a stone adherent to the gallbladder wall. Pathologic studies indicate that all apparent tumor would be removed in 25 per cent of cases by cholecystectomy, resection of a rim of adjacent liver, and dissection of the common duct lymph node chain. Even in this favorable group the five-year survival rate is 5 per cent. Most patients live for only a few months after the diagnosis.

Benign Tumors and Pseudotumors of the Gallbladder

Adenomyomatous hyperplasia, also called *adenomyomatosis*, is the most common of the benign tumors and pseudotumors of the gallbladder; there is hyperplasia of the mucosa with formation of intramural diverticula. The cause is unknown. Typically, neoplastic or inflammatory changes are absent. Adenomyomatosis is usually diagnosed by oral cholecystography as a diffuse, segmental, or focal sessile filling defect with a central umbilication and small peripheral opaque areas representing diverticula. Most often adenomyomatosis is asymptomatic. A few cases are associated with typical biliary pain that can be cured by cholecystectomy.

Cholesterolosis (strawberry gallbladder) is a condition of unknown cause characterized by an accumulation of cholesterol and other lipids in macrophages in the gallbladder mucosa. Unlike cholesterol gallstones, it does not appear to be necessarily related to biliary supersaturation with cholesterol. *Cholesterol polyps* are a focal form of cholesterolosis consisting of a core of macrophages filled with cholesterol covered with epithelium located at a villous tip. Generally, multiple polyps are present. The polyp is attached to the mucosa by a fragile stalk that can easily be broken. Cholesterol polyps appear on oral cholecystography or ultrasonography as a fixed filling defect on the gallbladder wall that does not change with position; in contrast to gallstones, no acoustic shadowing is seen on ultrasonography. Unless cholesterol polyps are present, cholesterolosis is difficult to detect by oral cholecystography. Most patients with cholesterolosis are asymptomatic. Some patients have concomitant gallstones and, if symptoms are present, they are attributed to the gallstones. Those few patients with cholesterolosis without gallstones who have typical biliary pain are often relieved by cholecystectomy.

Papillary and nonpapillary adenomas are benign neoplasms of the gallbladder. They are much less common than cholesterol polyps. Most adenomas are pedunculated; about two thirds are multiple. They appear as filling defects on oral cholecystography. Carcinoma in situ is found in about 5 per cent of adenomas, but the relationship between gallbladder adenomas and carcinoma is not clear.

Tumors of the Bile Duct

The main cause of early morbidity from tumors of the bile duct is biliary obstruction with gradual hepatocellular damage or secondary hepatobiliary infection. Tumors of the bile ducts are rarely benign. Papilloma, the most frequent, is often multifocal and therefore difficult to cure. Adenomas and granular cell tumors are localized, but are often difficult to treat surgically without radical excision. This section will be directed primarily to discussion of malignant tumors, but many of the same principles of pathophysiology and diagnosis will apply to the rare benign tumors.

Except for a rare squamous cell tumor, malignant bile duct tumors are adenocarcinomas with either a scirrhous or a papillary pattern. Grossly, three types of pathologic presentations occur: *focal stricture, diffuse thickening,* and *nodular mass*. The first two varieties can easily be mistaken for a benign process such as post-traumatic stricture or sclerosing cholangitis. In many cases, spread is confined to local lymph node metastases or hepatic invasion for months or years before there is more widespread abdominal or systemic involvement. The common hepatic duct or common bile duct is the site of origin in about two thirds of the cases. The eponym *Klatskin tumor* is often used to refer to adenocarcinoma at the bifurcation of the common hepatic duct. In contrast with carcinoma of the gallbladder, cholelithiasis is found in only one third of patients, and men slightly outnumber women. The average age at diagnosis is 70 years. A number of cases have been reported in younger patients with ulcerative colitis. Since some of these patients have previously undergone colectomy, it is thought that elimination of the diseased colon is not protective. Sclerosing cholangitis is a recognized complication in these same patients and may have identical clinical features, especially when it primarily affects the extrahepatic bile ducts. Caroli's disease and choledochal cysts are also associated with the development of carcinoma in a small percentage of cases. In the Orient, infestation with *Clonorchis sinensis* probably contributes to the higher incidence of bile duct carcinoma.

CLINICAL MANIFESTATIONS. The typical patient presents with unremitting severe jaundice, mild deep-seated upper abdominal pain, and weight loss. Pruritus is reported by many, usually but not always after the onset of jaundice. Pain, present in more than half the patients, is not colicky and tends to be steady; fever and chills are absent. Hepatomegaly without splenomegaly is found on abdominal examination. Tumors of the common duct sparing the cystic duct often produce in addition to jaundice a distended nontender palpable gallbladder (*Courvoisier's law*).

The serum bilirubin value exceeds 10 mg per deciliter in most cases, with a mean between 15 and 20 mg per deciliter. Complete obstruction of the ductal system results in a bilirubin value of 30 mg per deciliter or higher. The alkaline phosphatase is almost always increased, often more than ten-fold, and AST may be slightly elevated, although rarely higher than 200 units per liter. Obstruction of the right or left hepatic system alone causes a 10- to 30-fold increase in alkaline phosphatase with normal levels of bilirubin. Serum proteins are most often normal. The prothrombin time may be prolonged, but responds to parenteral vitamin K. Serum cholesterol is usually increased and averages about 400 mg per deciliter.

DIAGNOSIS. Ultrasonography or computed tomography shows dilatation of the intrahepatic bile ducts. Transhepatic or retrograde cholangiography demonstrates marked ductal dilatation and the site of the block.

The differential diagnosis includes primary biliary cirrhosis and drug-induced cholestatic jaundice. In neither of these conditions does the bilirubin generally reach levels over 12 to 15 mg per deciliter. Xanthelasma, found often with primary biliary cirrhosis, is only rarely seen with neoplastic obstruction. Antimitochondrial antibodies can be demonstrated in the serum of most patients with primary biliary cirrhosis. Sclerosing cholangitis, usually associated with chronic inflammatory bowel disease, is characterized by intermittent attacks of pain, jaundice, and fever. It also shows a characteristic pattern on transhepatic cholangiography or ERCP although it may be difficult to distinguish focal disease from carcinoma.

Choledocholithiasis and postoperative biliary stricture are less likely to present with deepening jaundice and weight loss. The jaundice fluctuates, is milder, and is usually associated with fever. PTC or ERCP will help to differentiate these diseases.

TREATMENT. Unfortunately, complete excision of the tumor is often impossible, because nonexpendable anatomic structures are involved early. Nevertheless, a few cures can be expected when radical surgery is judiciously employed, and palliation is often lengthy and of excellent quality.

Distal lesions require radical pancreaticoduodenectomy (Whipple's procedure) for complete removal. Because this operation has a 15 per cent mortality, it should be performed only if no gross tumor would be left behind. Tumors of the midportion of the common bile duct are sometimes amenable to complete resection. Localized tumors of the bifurcation of the hepatic duct can sometimes be treated by excision, even though microscopic deposits of tumor usually remain in the bed of the dissection. Reconstruction involves use of a Roux-en-Y hepaticojejunostomy. Radiotherapy with either external beam or intraluminal rods may provide some benefit.

For tumors with local or distant spread the goal is palliation. The treatment of choice is percutaneous or endoscopic stenting of the biliary tract with catheters having multiple portholes above and below the point of bile duct obstruction. Either type of tube can be changed periodically to prevent plugging. Distal tumors can be bypassed by cholecystojejunostomy or other types of biliary-enteric anastomoses.

PROGNOSIS. Cure is achieved in 5 to 10 per cent, and many patients survive in good condition for several years or more following palliative excision. If biliary drainage can be maintained with a tube, patients with unresectable lesions occasionally do well for a year of two. Death eventually results from hepatic replacement with tumor or intrahepatic sepsis from recurrent ductal obstruction.

Postcholecystectomy Syndrome

After cholecystectomy, 10 per cent of patients continue to have significant abdominal symptoms. In most patients the explanation for continued postoperative symptoms is that the gallstone disease was not the cause of their preoperative complaints. Patients with typical biliary pain are more often relieved by cholecystectomy than are those with the vague symptoms of fatty food intolerance, dyspepsia, or flatulence. Postcholecystectomy complaints can often be attributed to overlooked disease such as choledocholithiasis, pancreatitis, peptic ulcer, esophageal or small-bowel disease, or irritable bowel syndrome. These possibilities must be investigated by appropriate studies.

Stenosis of the sphincter of Oddi (ampullary stenosis), biliary dyskinesia, neuroma of the cystic duct stump, and other cystic duct remnant lesions are conditions that have returned to clinical favor as causes of the postcholecystectomy syndrome along with objective tests for detection such as ERCP with manometry.

Renewed interest in ampullary stenosis and biliary dyskinesia has followed the development of methods to perform endoscopic sphincterotomy. Early results suggest that a minority of patients with episodic typical biliary pain in the absence of stones have hypertension, dysmotility, and/or stenosis of the sphincter of Oddi. The appearance of a narrowed sphincter alone is insufficient to document either stenosis or dyskinesia. A provocative test has been used that involves injection of morphine (10 mg) and neostigmine methylsulfate (1 mg) intramuscularly. Pain and a rise in serum amylase levels are indications of ampullary stenosis. The results of this test, however, do not correlate with sphincter of Oddi pressures, and the test is sometimes positive in normal subjects. Clinicians should remain skeptical about a diagnosis of ampullary stenosis when the principal finding is abdominal pain. The diagnosis is more secure in patients with recurrent pancreatitis, increase of transaminases, cholangitis, and/or a dilated bile duct whose sphincter appears tight radiographically and will accept only a small probe. Treatment consists of division of the sphincter at operation or transendoscopically. Patients with recurrent pancreatitis should have an operative pancreatic septectomy in addition—division of that portion of the pancreas separating the distal common bile duct and pancreatic duct, thereby dividing that portion of the sphincter that extended onto the pancreatic duct.

Convincing evidence has been submitted to document the importance of each of the aforementioned conditions in specific cases. Dyskinesia of the sphincter without stenosis is very difficult to establish as a cause of the syndrome. Perhaps further data from manometric studies will elucidate a relationship between motor abnormalities and postoperative pain. In the management of such patients with chronic abdominal pain thought to be due to dyskinesia in the absence of objective findings, treatment can be tried with nitrates, anticholinergics, or calcium channel blockers. If this is unsuccessful, consideration can be given to endoscopic sphincterotomy, although its efficacy remains uncertain. Exploratory laparotomy has a low rate of success for diagnosis, and surgical correction of minor variations in the gut anatomy usually fails to cure.

Broughan TA, Sivak MV, Hermann RE: The management of retained and recurrent bile duct stones. Surgery 98:746, 1985. *Endoscopic sphincterotomy is preferable to surgery in a majority of cases.*

Brandy-Rauf PW, Pincus M, Adelson S: Cancer of the gallbladder. A review of 43 cases. Human Pathol 13:48, 1982. *A review of the clinicopathologic findings, epidemiology, and natural history of this virtually incurable disease.*

Chitwood WR Jr, Meyers WC, Heaston DK, et al.: Diagnosis and treatment of primary extrahepatic bile duct tumors. Am J Surg 143:99, 1982. *Covers the subject in detail.*

Cohen S, Soloway RD (eds.): Gallstones. New York, Churchill Livingstone, 1985. *A 341-page multiauthored book with 20 chapters covering virtually all aspects of gallstone disease. The first reference to use to get an authoritative perspective on a specific topic relating to stones.*

Delchier J-C, Benfredj P, Preaux A-M, et al.: The usefulness of microscopic bile examination in patients with suspected microlithiasis: A prospective evaluation. Hepatology 6:118, 1986. *Seeing cholesterol crystals in bile is highly correlated with the presence of small gallbladder stones that may be undetectable by radiologic techniques.*

Gracie WA, Ransohoff DF: The natural history of silent gallstones: The innocent gallstone is not a myth. N Engl J Med 307:798, 1982. *The best article to date describing a group of truly asymptomatic gallstones.*

Grundy SM: Mechanism of cholesterol gallstone formation. Sem Liv Dis 3:97, 1983. *A comprehensive review of the biochemistry leading to cholesterol stone formation, with 105 references.*

Jarvinen HJ, Hastbacka J: Early cholecystectomy for acute cholecystitis. A prospective randomized study. Ann Surg 191:501, 1980. *This controlled trial demonstrates the advantages of early surgery over expectant management for acute cholecystitis.*

Maton RN, Iser JH, Reuben A, et al.: Outcome of chenodeoxycholic acid (CDCA) treatment in 125 patients with radiolucent gallstones. Medicine 61:86, 1982. *Factors influencing efficacy, withdrawal, symptoms and side effects, and postdissolution recurrence.*

Sauerbruch T, Delius M, Baumgartner G, et al.: Fragmentation of gallstones by extracorporeal shock waves. N Engl J Med 314:818, 1986. *Whether or not this becomes the wave of the future awaits more studies.*

Scharschmidt BF, Goldberg HI, Schmid R: Current concepts in diagnosis: Approach to the patient with cholestatic jaundice. N Engl J Med 308:1515, 1983. *Excellent review of the most efficient approach to distinguishing intrahepatic from extrahepatic cholestasis.*

Silvis SE: What is the postcholecystectomy syndrome? Gastro Endoscopy 31:401, 1985. *A succinct editorial outlining what is and what is not known about this condition.*

Somjen GJ, Gilat T: Contribution of vesicular and micellar carriers to cholesterol transport in human bile. J Lipid Res 26:699, 1985. *Both the classically described micelles and the more recently described non–bile salt containing cholesterol vesicles are important in solubilizing cholesterol in bile.*

Trotman BW, Soloway RD: Pigment gallstone disease: Summary of the National Institutes of Health International Workshop. Hepatology 2:879, 1982. *Good starting point for understanding pigment stone disease, with 60 references.*

Wiesner RH, LaRusso NF: Clinicopathologic features of the syndrome of primary sclerosing cholangitis. Gastroenterology 79:200, 1980. *A review of 50 patients with sclerosing cholangitis.*

PART XII
HEMATOLOGIC DISEASES

131 INTRODUCTION
David G. Nathan

This introduction is primarily intended to provide a general background to diagnostic hematology and marrow function. The remaining chapters in Part XII emphasize fundamental physiologic principles and provide descriptions of relatively common hematologic disorders with the hope that the entire Part will influence the reader to consider such diseases broadly and systematically.

The nonmalignant disorders of erythrocytes, phagocytes, and platelets, including their precursors and progenitors, are initially discussed. Then follows a description of the acute and chronic proliferative disorders that involve the cells of the marrow and lymphoid systems, a series of chapters that ends with a discussion of bone marrow transplantation. The final chapters of Part XII are devoted to a review of the disorders of the fluid phase of blood coagulation and the vascular purpuras.

DIAGNOSTIC HEMATOLOGY. The circulating blood cells are the products of the terminal differentiation of recognizable precursors. In fetal life hematopoiesis occurs throughout the reticuloendothelial system. In the normal adult, the process of terminal differentiation of the recognizable precursors of erythrocytes, granulocytes, and platelets occurs exclusively in the marrow cavities of the axial skeleton with some extension into the proximal femoral and humeri, but the space is highly expandable when the demand for blood cell production is accelerated (Fig. 131–1).

Observations of differentiated blood cells by enumeration and relatively simple morphologic studies of properly prepared blood films provide the essential cornerstone of diagnostic hematology. Automated blood counts and cell sizing now provide both reproducibility and enhanced diagnostic capacity. For example, early red cell production failure may be heralded by unexpected macrocytosis. Peripheral blood cell morphology offers insight into the rate of effective hematopoiesis; the state of marrow nutrition with respect to vitamin B_{12}, folic acid, and iron; the presence of acquired and congenital disorders of the membrane; the energy metabolism or the hemoglobin of erythrocytes that leads to their accelerated destruction; the differential diagnosis of infections; the presence of allergic reactions; the acquired or congenital abnormalities of intracellular organelles; and the invasion of the marrow by malignant cells or infectious agents. The contributions of morphologic techniques to hematologic diagnosis depend entirely upon the adequacy of specimen preparation and the skill of the observer. Egregious errors are made when diagnostic pronouncements are based on inadequate material. The slavish enumeration of individual cells is rarely of aid without careful overall inspection and positive searches for diagnostic clues that are relevant to the case at hand. Morphology can be particularly misleading if the observer does not understand that many kinds of disorders induce similar changes in shape, particularly in the red cells.

Although circulating lymphocytes appear to be terminally differentiated cells, they are instead capable of rapid proliferative responses to appropriate stimuli during which they

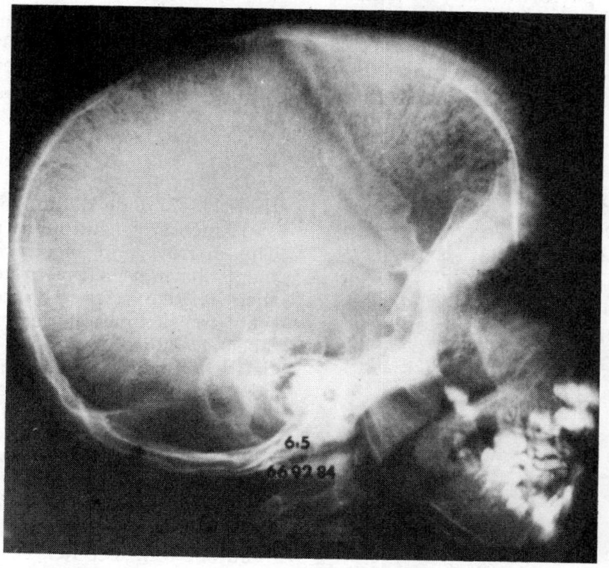

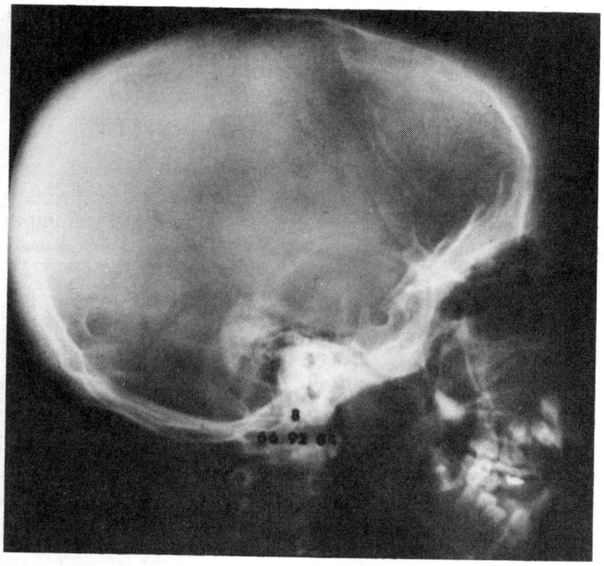

FIGURE 131–1. Roentgenograms of the skull of a patient with homozygous beta thalassemia at the age of 6½ years (*left*), before splenectomy and transfusion therapy, and at the age of eight years (*right*), after splenectomy and transfusion therapy to control anemia. Note the marked "hair-on-end" appearance in the left-hand radiograph, signifying expansion of the marrow space. (From Nathan DG: N Engl J Med 286:586, 1972.)

resume the appearance of relatively undifferentiated precursors. At this stage they are often called atypical, even though this blastic transformation is entirely appropriate. The functional subsets of lymphoid cells are not readily demonstrable by inspection, although "killer" lymphocyte function may be associated with larger cells that contain granules. Obtaining that important information requires studies of lymphocyte function and studies with specially prepared antibodies reactive with lymphocytes.

Well-prepared marrow films and biopsy specimens also contribute important information such as total marrow cellularity, the presence of invading malignant cells or infectious granulomas, the adequacy of the numbers of megakaryocytes, the ratio of myeloid to erythroid precursors, the state of marrow cell nutrition, the presence of abnormal storage cells, and even the deposition of abnormal crystals. In brief, the blood lends itself to biopsy and to structural, chemical, and functional studies far more readily than does any other human organ. Its cellular elements are diverse, bearing in common only a joint ancestral cell, origin in the marrow, and the property of being transported through vessels suspended in plasma.

PRECURSORS OF CIRCULATING BLOOD CELLS. ***Erythrocytes.*** Much of the progress of differentiation of erythroid precursors can be appreciated morphologically, particularly the onset of hemoglobin synthesis and the maturation and extrusion of the nucleus. During this process each proerythroblast may give rise to approximately eight erythrocytes. The transit time from proerythroblast to emergence of reticulocytes is approximately five days. The transit time may decrease during anemic stress to as little as two days by means of skipped divisions. The red cells that emerge under conditions of stress are macrocytic and may contain as much as 25 per cent fetal hemoglobin (F cells). They may also bear additional fetal characteristics, particularly the presence of i antigen on their surfaces. More quantitative analyses of the transit of erythroid precursors during the process of maturation may be appreciated from the use of radioactive iron that, when injected intravenously, accumulates preferentially in the newly synthesized ferritin of proerythroblasts and ultimately emerges in peripheral blood incorporated into reticulocyte hemoglobin. The use of surface scanning following infusion of ^{59}Fe-labeled transferrin reveals the site as well as the rate of intramedullary erythropoiesis. This is largely an investigative and not a clinical tool except for cases in which the anatomic site of erythropoiesis needs to be determined, such as in myeloid metaplasia. A qualitative assessment of erythroid precursor activity throughout the body may be gained from injection of indium chloride and marrow scintigraphy. Indium-111 binds to transferrin and is incorporated into immature marrow erythroid precursors. Body scanning then reveals the distribution of marrow.

Granulocytes. The process of intramedullary granulocyte maturation involves changes in nuclear configuration and the accumulation of specific intracytoplasmic granules. A model that describes the production and kinetics of neutrophils is shown in Figure 131–2 (see also Ch. 148). It is highly compartmentalized. The relatively small peripheral blood pool is divided into two compartments in equilibrium, the circulating and the marginating pools. These pools provide entrance into the tissues. The level of peripheral cells is buffered by an immense marrow reserve of identifiable precursors, some of which are in the mitotic compartment and some in the maturing and storage compartment. The kinetics of proliferation of these recognizable precursors have been studied using labeled precursors of DNA. These so-called labeling indices, from which estimates of cell cycle times can be derived, have served as important approaches to the study of pharmacology and toxicity of chemotherapeutic agents.

Platelets. The differentiation of committed megakaryocytes, the precursors of platelets, involves a nuclear endoreduplication phenomenon which produces 16N and 32N megakaryoblasts. The endoreduplication ceases at the stage of the mature megakaryocyte. Platelet shedding from megakaryocytes is accomplished by the formation of multiple demarcation membranes within the cytoplasm of the cell, usually visible only by electron microscopy. Although the platelet appears at first to be a simple tissue fragment, its functions are diverse and hemostatically versatile. It must selectively adhere to abnormal surfaces and then sequentially secrete, aggregate, fuse, and retract to ensure a firm platelet-fibrin plug. In the process it assists in the coagulation cascade, synthesizes prostaglandins, and releases ADP and a variety of other substances of known and unknown function.

Lymphocytes. The geography of lymphocyte precursor maturation and differentiation is considerably more complex than that of the other hematopoietic cells. Primitive lymphoid precursors of B cell origin arise in the marrow, spleen, and lymph nodes where they continue their maturation and differentiation. Primitive T cell precursors arise in the marrow, travel to the thymus where they undergo further differentiation, and are finally exported to the spleen, lymph nodes, and marrow where they establish their final residence and perform many of their functions. Both T and B cells enter the peripheral blood circulation, which delivers them to tissue sites at which their functions may be required or their unbridled activity may cause disease (see Ch. 417). T cells previously "educated" in the thymus give rise to progeny that survive

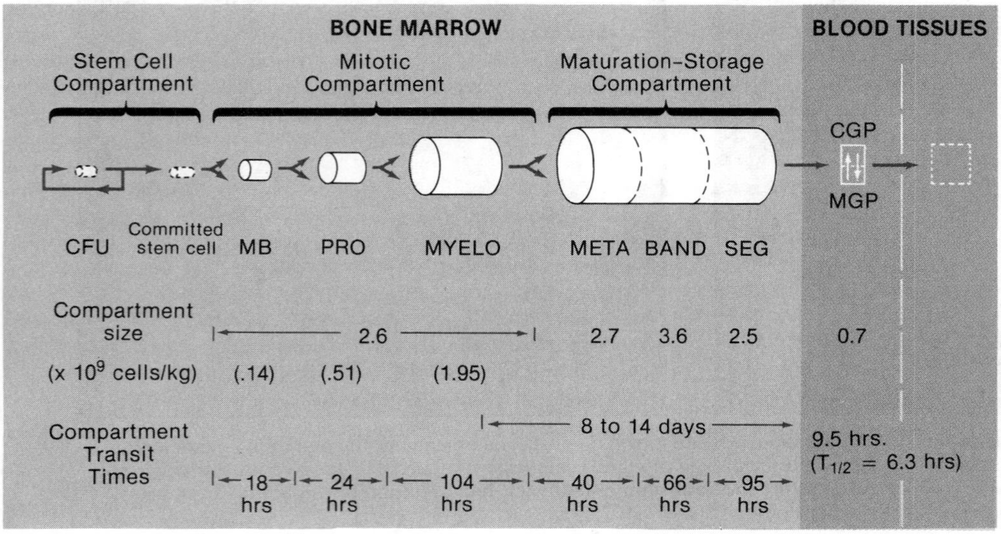

FIGURE 131–2. Model of the production and kinetics of neutrophils in man. The marrow and blood compartments have been drawn to show their relative sizes. The compartment transit times as derived from labeling studies with DF^{32}P and tritiated thymidine are shown on the next to last line and the last line. The less obvious symbols in the figure include CGP, the circulating granulocyte pool; MGP, the marginating granulocyte pool; CFU, the tripotential stem cell; MB, myeloblast; and PRO, promyelocyte. (From Wintrobe MM, Lee RG, et al.: Clinical Hematology. 7th ed. Philadelphia, Lea & Febiger, 1974, p 244.)

for the life of the individual. Circulating lymphocytes represent only a tiny fraction of the total lymphocyte pool. Analysis of these circulating cells may not reflect the nature of the total pool.

HEMATOPOIETIC PROGENITORS. The recognizable marrow precursors of the differentiated peripheral blood cells tend to occupy the attention of hematologists, but they are rarely primary causes of the hematopoietic cytopenias. It is true that various toxins or nutritional deficiencies can so seriously damage the orderly progression of precursor differentiation that effective production of fully differentiated blood cells is embarrassed. In general, however, deficient or excessive production of blood cells is due to abnormalities of *undifferentiated progenitor cells.* They must themselves undergo vital processes of maturation and amplification to give rise to the recognizable precursors of circulating differentiated blood cells.

Progenitor Maturation. Pluripotent stem cells are few in number, but the initial stages of their development lead to committed progenitors of the lymphoid and myeloid systems (Fig. 131–3). These committed progenitors are destined to produce the differentiated, recognizable precursors of the specific types of blood cells. Pluripotent stem cells are capable of slow but indefinite self-renewal, whereas the committed progenitor cells are not capable of indefinite self-renewal. They "die by differentiation," and their numbers depend on influx from the pluripotent stem cell pool. The committed erythrocyte, phagocyte, and platelet progenitors and the precursors to which they give rise emerge as the result of the maturation of a tripotential progenitor usually called CFU-S for the spleen colony-forming unit described by Till and McCulloch in mice. They observed hematopoietic colonies in the spleens of lethally irradiated mice rescued with bone marrow cells of histoidentical donors. The spleen colonies contained megakaryocyte, granulocyte, and erythroid precursors. A small fraction of CFU-S is found to be replicating or in the act of DNA synthesis at any one time. As more committed progenitors are formed, the fraction of these cells undergoing DNA synthesis increases. These increasingly committed progenitors include CFU-M, the progenitors of megakaryoblasts; CFU-GM, progenitors of phagocytic precursors; and BFU-E, the erythroid burst-forming units that ultimately give rise to erythroid precursors. This last-named process of maturation ultimately leads to erythroid colony-forming units, CFU-E, the immediate progenitors of proerythroblasts. The process of maturation of erythroid progenitor cells is accompanied by the increasing size and increased sensitivity to erythropoietin, a hormone produced largely in the kidney in response to anemia or hypoxia, and in the liver, particularly in fetuses. Its deficiency contributes to the anemia

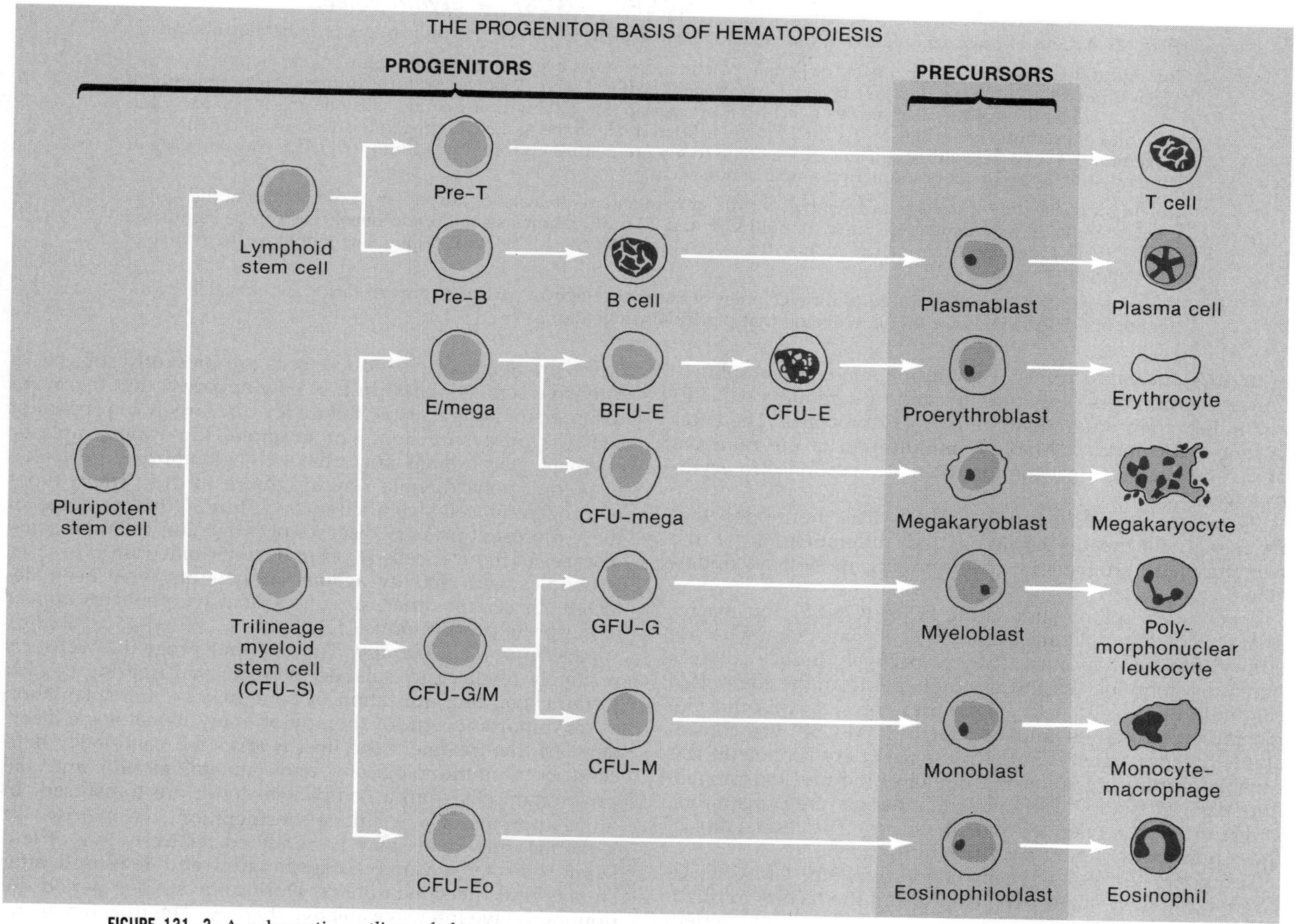

FIGURE 131–3. A schematic outline of the progenitor basis of hematopoiesis. Note the progressive restriction in the potential for terminal differentiation of the progenitors as they mature from left to right in the drawing. They finally form the recognizable marrow precursors from which the circulating blood cells, shown on the far right, are derived. Not shown in this outline is the process of self-renewal of fractions of the progenitor cell populations, particularly the immature progenitors. Also not shown is the progressive amplification of progenitors and precursors as they mature and differentiate. The bipotential erythroid-megakaryocyte progenitor shown in this drawing and referred to in the text has been demonstrated in the mouse, but not definitely in man.

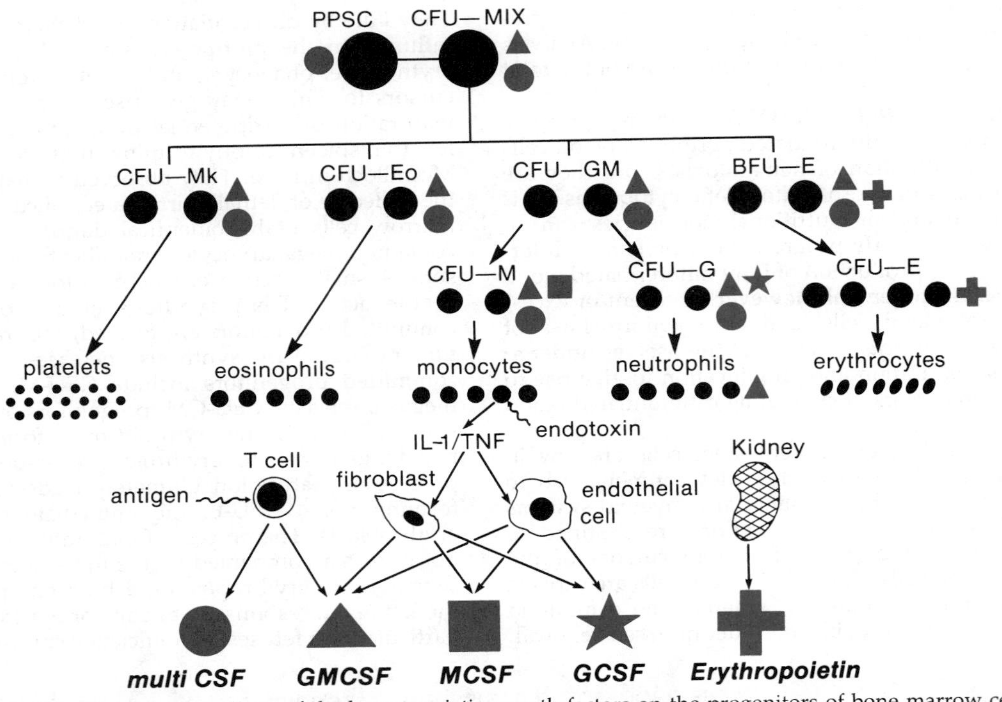

FIGURE 131–4. Cells of origin and effects of the hematopoietic growth factors on the progenitors of bone marrow cells.

The figure demonstrates the hierarchy of hematopoietic progenitors beginning with the pluripoietic stem cell (PPSC) which differentiates to form the first myeloid cell progenitor (CFU mix). This cell, in turn, differentiates randomly to form the progenitors of megakaryocytes (CFU-Mk), of eosinophils (CFU-Eo), of granulocytes and macrophages (CFU-GM), and of erythroid cells (BFU-E). CFU-GM further differentiate to the monocyte progenitor (CFU-M) and neutrophil progenitor (CFU-G), and BFU-E further differentiate to a more mature erythroid progenitor (CFU-E). At each stage of differentiation of progenitors, numerical amplification occurs.

The origin of the growth factors and symbols for the growth factors themselves are shown at the bottom of the figure. T cells stimulated with antigen give rise to multi CSF and GMCSF. Fibroblasts and endothelial cells can be stimulated by IL-1 or TNF derived from mature monocytes to produce GMCSF, MCSF, and GCSF. The kidney is the source of erythropoietin.

Those progenitors that are induced to form colonies of marrow cells by a particular growth factor are indicated by the symbol of the growth factor that is active on that particular progenitor.

of uremia. Increased levels of erythropoietin cause amplification of the numbers of mature erythroid progenitors (CFU-E) and induce their differentiation to proerythroblasts. The latter produce reticulocytes. Marked amplification of the numbers of mature erythroid progenitors occurs in response to erythropoietin.

Progenitor Regulation (Fig. 131–4). The hormones that regulate both the amplification and differentiation of the hematopoietic progenitors are beginning to become understood.

Granulocyte colony-stimulating factor (G-CSF) and macrophage colony-stimulating factor (M-CSF) have somewhat restricted functions in man. They respectively induce colonies of mature granulocytes and macrophages from the committed colony-forming cells with which they interact. Granulocyte-macrophage colony-stimulating factor (GM-CSF) has considerably broader activity. In the presence of erythropoietin it is capable of inducing colonies from all of the myeloid progenitors derived from CFU-S onto the most mature progenitors, and it induces accelerated hematopoiesis. The availability of these hormones offers new vistas in therapy.

The genes for four of them—erythropoietin, GM-CSF, G-CSF, and M-CSF—have been cloned and the factors purified. All are glycoproteins. The last three are produced by interleukin 1–stimulated fibroblasts and endothelial cells (the framework cells of marrow) and by activated T cells.

Progenitors and Marrow Failure. The hematopoietic progenitors can be detected in the null cell fraction of peripheral blood and in the mononuclear Ia^+ cell fraction of marrow. Interactions of progenitor cells and the various factors produced by neighboring inducer cells are presently subjects of intensive scrutiny because it is now apparent that the major disorders of bone marrow failure are due largely to progenitor cell loss or dysfunction. For example, the various aplastic anemias, paroxysmal nocturnal hemoglobinuria, the leukemias, and polycythemia vera are the results of various types of progenitor cell dysfunction or failure. Whether some of these represent primary diseases of progenitor cells and some diseases of inducer cells is yet to be determined. In rare cases antibodies with activity against progenitors have been detected. In certain other cases abnormal lymphocytes appear to suppress progenitor cell function.

Progenitor Cell Therapy. The fact that progenitor cells are relatively resistant to isolation, storage, and freezing has led to the expanding utilization of bone marrow transplantation as an important form of therapy of many hematologic disorders. In this treatment the host is rendered completely deficient both immunologically and hematologically, and the progenitor cells from a compatible donor are transfused. In other approaches now under consideration, the marrows of leukemic individuals may be rendered relatively free of leukemic cells by a variety of techniques and reinfused after storage into the same donors. During the storage period the donors receive intensive ablative therapy. The frozen marrow cells are then infused to reconstitute hematopoietic function.

MARROW ANATOMY. Although most cases of bone marrow failure and malignancy are due to disorders of progenitors, the total microenvironment in which progenitors, inducer cells, and precursors interact to form mature differentiated peripheral blood cells is complex and subject to severe dys-

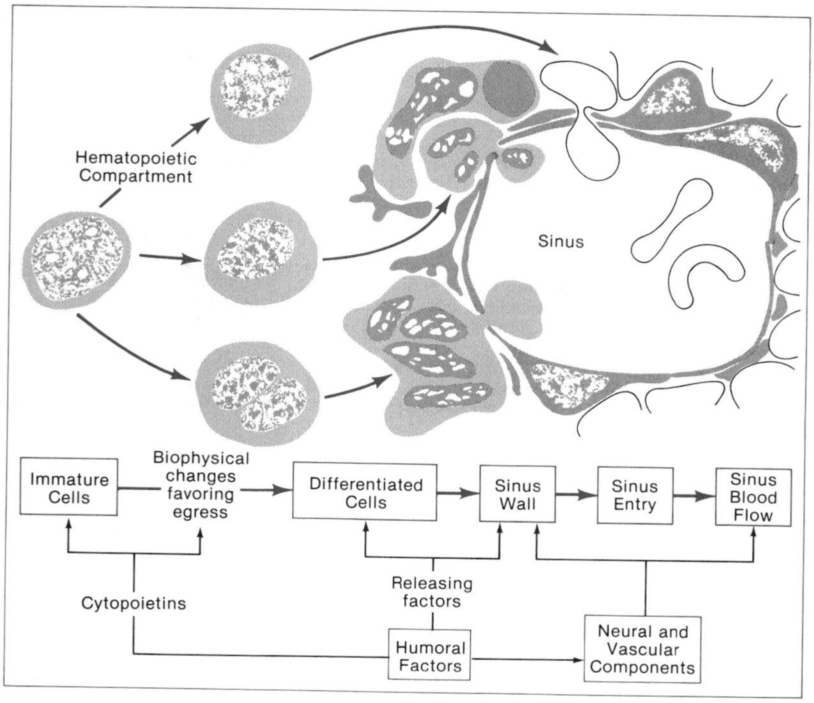

FIGURE 131–5. A schematic diagram of the factors that may be involved in controlling the release of marrow cells. The central relationship between the hematopoietic compartment and the marrow sinus is depicted. The drawing highlights the similarity of the egress process for the three major hematopoietic cells: reticulocytes in the top pathway, granulocytes and monocytes in the center pathway, and platelets in the lower pathway. Immature cells undergo biophysical changes under the influence of cytopoietins that favor egress. In the case of reticulocytes, enucleation precedes egress. This is shown by the solid black inclusion in the perisinal macrophage representing nucleophagocytosis antecedent to digestion of the erythroblast nucleus. The cytoplasmic protrusion of the megakaryocyte presumably detaches itself from the cell and will further fragment into platelets in the circulation. (From Lichtman MA, Chamberlain JK, Santillo PA: In Silber R, LoBue J, Gordon AS [eds.]: The Year in Hematology, 1978. New York, Plenum Medical Book Company, 1978, p 274.)

function. This is an obvious problem in myelofibrosis, or in infectious granulomatosis of the marrow. But certain other forms of bone marrow failure, such as aplastic anemia itself, may also be due to more subtle forms of microenvironmental failure. The marrow cavity is a vast network of vascular channels or sinusoids that separate groups of hematopoietic cells, including fat cells. The hematopoietic cells are found in the intrasinusoidal spaces. Clumps of megakaryocytes are found adjacent to marrow sinuses. They shed platelets, the fragments of their cytoplasm, directly into the lumen. This reduces the requirement for movement of bulky megakaryocytes, a mobility characteristic of the granuloid and erythroid differentiated precursors as they approach the point at which they egress from the marrow. The vascular and hematopoietic compartments are lined by reticular cells that form the adventitial surfaces of the vascular sinuses and extend cytoplasmic processes to create a lattice for the mesh of endothelial cells and fibronectin on which blood cells are found. The lattice is illustrated by reticulin stains of marrow sections and scanning electron photomicrographs. A schema of the egress of cells from marrow is shown in Figure 131–5.

KINETICS OF HEMATOPOIESIS. The marrow microenvironment supporting the progenitors and precursors must provide for the normal steady-state rates of renewal of the cellular elements of blood. Under homeostatic conditions, the production rates precisely equal destruction rates. The average life span of a human red cell is approximately 120 days. This means that approximately 5×10^4 red cells must be produced per day per microliter of blood in an adult. The average life span of platelets is seven to ten days for a daily production rate of 2×10^4 platelets per microliter of blood. The white blood cell compartment exhibits more complex kinetics. Granulocytes are rapidly turned over with an approximate intravascular life span of 6 to 12 hours in humans. To maintain a level of circulating granulocytes of 5×10^3 per microliter requires a daily production that is roughly comparable to that of red cell and platelet production, approximately 2×10^4 cells per microliter of blood. At the opposite extreme in terms of life span is the lymphocyte, which can exhibit lifetimes measured in months, or even years. This long life span of lymphocytes suggests that the daily renewal of certain lymphocyte progenitors occurs at a rate substantially lower than that of the progenitors of the other formed elements of blood.

The various symptoms of complete marrow failure are closely related to the life span and the turnover of the peripheral cells of the blood. Thus, patients with complete marrow failure initially lose granulocytes and therefore usually present with enhanced susceptibility to infection. Petechial bleeding caused by platelet deficiency rapidly follows, and finally pallor and symptoms of anemia occur. Loss of circulating lymphocytes and cellular immune function is an unusual event in such circumstances.

The turnover of red cells and platelets can be measured for diagnostic purposes, using $Na_2{}^{51}CrO_4$ as a labeling agent. Both the red cell and the platelet life spans can be estimated and the site of the red cell destruction determined. This can be a useful maneuver in decisions regarding splenectomy.

CONCLUSIONS. Modern cell biology and molecular genetics have revolutionized hematology, changing it from a largely descriptive field to a remarkable amalgamation of diagnostic and therapeutic ventures. The realization that differentiated marrow precursors arise from a population of lymphoid-appearing cells that have a fascinating developmental biology of their own has led to reclassification of the marrow failure syndrome and to new approaches to therapy, particularly with bone marrow transplantation. In addition, inquiries into the kinetics of progenitors and differentiated precursors have encouraged more rational approaches to the chemotherapy of malignant diseases. As approaches to the actual isolation of progenitors are developed, enumeration of these cells will soon be as commonplace as the evaluation of precursors and mature cells. This kind of enumeration will require specific antibodies and diagnostic instruments that are taking their places as standard aspects of the hematology of this era.

Burakoff SJ, Lipton JM, Nathan DG: Recapitulation of the immune response and hematopoietic system in bone marrow transplantation. In Nathan DG (ed.): Bone Marrow Transplantation. Clin Haematol 12:695, 1983. *A brief up-to-date review of regulation of hematopoiesis in two volumes devoted to basic and clinical aspects of marrow transplantations.*

Donahue, RE, Wang EA, Stone DK, et al.: Stimulation of hematopoiesis in primates by continuous infusion of recombinant human GM-CSF. Nature 321:872, 1986. *Purified recombinant human GM-CSF elicits dramatic leukocytosis and substantial reticulocytosis when infused into healthy monkeys and had a similar effect in one immunodeficient pancytopenic animal.*

Lipton JM, Nathan DG: The anatomy and physiology of hematopoiesis. In Nathan DG, Oski F (eds.): Hematology of Infancy and Childhood. 3rd ed. Philadelphia, W. B. Saunders Company, 1987. *A general review of the anatomy and physiology of normal hematopoiesis, emphasizing new developments in molecular and cellular biology as they relate to blood cell formation.*

Metcalf D: The molecular biology and functions of the granulocyte-macrophage colony-stimulating factors. Blood 67:257, 1986. *An up-to-date comprehensive review of the molecular biology and multiple in vitro effects of murine and human growth factors, their relationships, receptors, and possible role in leukemia.*

Nathan DG, Housman DE, Clarke BJ: The pathophysiology of hematopoiesis. In Nathan DG, Oski F (eds.): Hematology in Infancy and Childhood. 2nd ed. Philadelphia, W. B. Saunders Company, 1980. *A general review of hematopoiesis emphasizing physiology and clinical correlations.*

Sieff CA: Hematopoietic growth factors. J Clin Invest 79:1549, 1987. *A brief review of the currently known growth factors.*

Sieff CA, Emerson SG, Donahue RE, et al.: Human recombinant granulocyte-macrophage colony-stimulating factor: A multilineage hematopoietin. Science 230:1171, 1986. *In addition to its effect on granulocyte-macrophage progenitors, GM-CSF also induces colonies derived from erythroid and multipotent progenitors.*

Weiss RE, Reddi AH: Appearance of fibronectin during the differentation of cartilage, bone and bone marrow. J Cell Biol 88:630, 1981. *Contains an excellent array of photomicrographs of developing marrow cells within a fibronectin framework.*

132 INTRODUCTION TO THE ANEMIAS

Alan S. Keitt

Humans live in tenuous equilibrium with their life blood. Elaborate mechanisms have evolved to extract the nutrients for blood formation from available food stores and to conserve them by efficient recycling. The transition from hunter-gatherer to agricultural societies resulted in the replacement of most readily absorbable heme iron in the human diet by poorly absorbable iron in grains, thus rendering this balance precarious for a large part of the world's population. Other evolutionary strategies have concentrated genes for various red cell abnormalities that enhance survival in malarial areas but at the cost of producing anemia within a large minority of the population of these regions. Parasitic infestations and frequent pregnancies produce stress on iron balance in the same underdeveloped and populous areas. As a result of these combined nutritional, genetic, and parasitic factors, the global hematocrit is by no means optimal; anemia is perhaps the most frequent and significant worldwide health problem. Anemia does not have the same impact on the population of western societies, but it remains a cardinal indicator of disease and requires careful consideration and treatment.

Although defined by numbers, anemia is in reality a *process* that evolves within a clinical context. For the experienced hematologist, this clinical context is analogous to habitat for the ornithologist. A brief glance through the binoculars is often sufficient to identify the microspherocytes of autoimmune hemolytic anemia in a patient known to have systemic lupus erythematosus just as one instantly recognizes a wood duck in the woods because that is where it belongs. In the same vein, an unfamiliar stray may be noticed by the alert observer when it occurs outside of its usual clinical context. The importance of habitat in hematologic diagnosis cannot be overemphasized and is often neglected in the current proliferation of sequential algorithms for the diagnosis of anemia. Such constructions, which are based primarily on laboratory data, may fail to take into account changes occurring over time and often provide only a single point of entry to the process of anemia.

The great majority of anemias are diagnosed and treated by nonhematologists. Except for the primary blood dyscrasias, the diagnostic classification of the anemias is relatively simple and logical. The pathophysiologic classification, presented in Table 132–1, is most useful because it stresses the underlying mechanisms of the anemias and therefore helps one to predict some of the key diagnostic tests that are discussed below.

TABLE 132–1. PATHOPHYSIOLOGIC CLASSIFICATION OF ANEMIAS

I. **Hypoproliferative anemias**
   A. Marrow aplasias (Ch. 133)
   B. Myelophthisic anemia (Ch. 133)
   C. Anemia with blood dyscrasias
   D. Anemia of chronic disease (Ch. 134)
   E. Anemia with organ failure (Ch. 134)
      1. Renal failure
      2. Hepatic failure
      3. Hypothyroidism
      4. Hypopituitarism
II. **Maturation defects**
   A. Cytoplasmic
      1. Hypochromic anemias (Ch. 135)
   B. Nuclear
      1. Megaloblastic anemias (Ch. 136)
   C. Combined
      1. Myelodysplastic syndromes
III. **Hyperproliferative anemias**
   A. Hemorrhagic (Ch. 134)
      1. Acute blood loss
   B. Hemolytic (Ch. 137)
      1. Immune hemolysis (Ch. 139)
      2. Primary membrane defects (Ch. 138)
      3. Hemoglobinopathies (Ch. 143)
      4. Enzymopathies (Ch. 138)
      5. Toxic hemolysis—physical-chemical (Ch. 139)
      6. Traumatic or microangiopathic hemolysis (Ch. 139)
      7. Hypersplenism (Ch. 164)
      8. Parasitic infections (Ch. 139)
IV. **Dilutional anemias**
   A. Pregnancy
   B. Splenomegaly

DEFINITIONS OF ANEMIA

STATISTICAL CONSIDERATIONS. Anemia is defined as a reduction in either the volume of red blood cells (termed the hematocrit or packed cell volume [PCV]) or the concentration of hemoglobin in a sample of peripheral venous blood when compared with similar values obtained from a reference population. Normal values for red blood cell measurements are given in Table 132–2. By convention the normal range is defined to include 95 per cent of a reference population that is assumed to have a normal (gaussian) distribution. In this definition 2.5 per cent of "normal individuals" will fall below this arbitrary statistical limit and be classified as anemic. Some of these individuals in the general population will be truly anemic while others are *statistical outliers*. Unfortunately this statistical definition of anemia may fail to detect truly anemic patients whose hematocrits have decreased significantly without leaving the defined normal range. Here the only valid reference figure is a previous hematocrit in that individual.

RED CELL MASS. Anemia can be more rigorously defined as a reduction in red cell mass (a misnomer for the total volume of circulating erythroid cells in the body). Red cell mass can be accurately measured by isotope dilution using

TABLE 132–2. SELECTED HEMATOLOGIC VALUES IN NORMAL INDIVIDUALS OF VARIOUS AGES*

Age	Hemoglobin (gm/dl) mean (−2SD)	Hematocrit (%) mean (−2SD)	MCV (μ^3) mean (−2SD)
1–3 days	18.5 (14.5)	56 (45)	108 (95)
0.5–2 yrs	12 (10.5)	36 (33)	78 (70)
12–18 yrs			
Male	14.5 (13)	43 (37)	88 (78)
Female	14.0 (12)	41 (36)	90 (78)
18–49 yrs			
Male	15.5 (13.5)	47 (41)	90 (80)
Female	14 (12.0)	41 (36)	90 (80)

*Values selected from Dallman PR: In Rudolph A (ed.): Pediatrics, 16th ed. New York, Appleton-Century-Crofts, Inc., 1977, p 1111. The values were derived by Coulter Counter. Values in parentheses represent two standard deviations below the mean, or the lower limit of normal assuming a normal distribution.

^{51}Cr-labeled red cells, a procedure usually employed to establish increased red cell mass, i.e., erythrocytosis, rather than anemia. This measurement is occasionally useful for assessing anemia in patients with marked splenomegaly in whom the peripheral hematocrit underestimates the true red cell mass (see below).

EFFECTS OF AGE, SEX, AND ALTITUDE. Developmental changes in hematocrit are most evident during the first year of life (see Table 131–2). Adult levels of hematocrit are reached by late childhood in females. The higher hematocrit of males as compared with females begins at puberty as a result of stimulation of hematopoiesis by androgenic hormones.

Whether the hematocrit normally declines with aging is controversial. With age the cellularity of the bone marrow is progressively replaced by fat and in men over 60 the incidence of anemia increases progressively as well. Some studies show similar trends in women. Iron deficiency and chronic diseases are common in this age group but seem not to account entirely for the increased incidence of anemia. Mild anemia in the elderly, therefore, must still be considered as an indicator of potential ill health, but investigation of these patients frequently fails to indicate a precise etiology.

The hematocrit is increased in individuals living at high altitudes as an appropriate response to diminished oxygen content of the atmosphere and blood. This effect can be noticed above 4000 feet where significant desaturation of hemoglobin begins. The definition of anemia therefore requires adjustment to the altitude at which the individual lives.

COMPENSATION FOR ANEMIA

INCREASED PLASMA VOLUME. Initial symptoms of patients with anemia are related to efforts by the body to compensate for the diminished oxygen supply. Later symptoms of progressive anemia reflect failure of these compensatory mechanisms. The symptoms and signs differ markedly depending on the acuteness of onset of the anemia. The abrupt loss of 30 per cent of the circulating blood volume in a patient with gastrointestinal hemorrhage will result in marked postural hypotension, a fall in cardiac output, shunting of blood from skin to central organs, thirst, and air hunger (Ch. 114). In contrast, the gradual loss of 30 per cent of the circulating red cell mass in a patient with iron deficiency may occur without any symptoms at all. The major difference lies in the blood volume, which is maintained by a proportionate increase in plasma volume as a compensatory response in most chronic anemias but is compromised in acute hemorrhage. Because the central blood volume is maintained until very late in the course of a progressive chronic anemia, such *patients are susceptible to volume overload by transfusions.* The injudicious administration of whole blood and even packed red cells may precipitate acute congestive heart failure in a previously well compensated individual.

INCREASED CARDIAC OUTPUT. In chronic anemias cardiac output increases to circulate fewer red cells through the tissues more frequently. This process is abetted by the diminished viscosity of blood at low hematocrits but is ultimately limited by the capacity of the heart to respond to the increased work. An early sign of failing compensation in gradual-onset anemias is postural hypotension, which may be associated with palpitations, dizziness, throbbing headaches, and dyspnea on exertion.

REDUCED AFFINITY OF HEMOGLOBIN FOR OXYGEN. In anemia the oxyhemoglobin dissociation curve usually shifts in a manner to increase the quantity of oxygen released in tissues without appreciably altering the quantity of oxygen bound in the lungs (see Fig. 140–3). Red cell 2,3-diphosphoglycerate (2,3-DPG) regularly increases in anemic patients to mediate this effect. Maximum elevation of RBC 2,3-DPG increases oxygen delivery only about 30 per cent, but this is a highly efficient form of compensation requiring no significant expenditure of energy.

ASSESSMENT OF SYMPTOMS IN ANEMIA. Anemia is usually insidious in its onset and has no specific symptoms to alert the physician to its presence. Unusual fatigue is the earliest and most common complaint, but other more subtle changes such as loss of libido or alterations in mood or sleep patterns may be elicited prior to the awareness of the more typical cardiovascular symptoms mentioned above. The level of anemia at which symptoms occur is highly variable among individuals as would be expected from the widely differing degrees of physical activity, physical conditioning, circulatory adequacy, and sensitivity or stoicism of the population. In otherwise healthy individuals symptoms are usually present when the hemoglobin falls below 7 or 8 grams per deciliter.

Exceptions to this general rule are not infrequent. An occasional patient with a gradual-onset anemia may deny all symptoms despite a hemoglobin of 5 grams per deciliter. Conversely, and more commonly, patients with mild anemia of 9 or 10 grams of hemoglobin per deciliter may complain bitterly of fatigue and lassitude. A careful search for underlying systemic disease or depression is warranted in these patients. Finally, because oxygen transport is much more compromised by impaired circulation than by diminished oxygen-carrying capacity per se, patients with vascular or cardiac disease may become symptomatic with milder degrees of anemia. For example, angina, claudication, transient ischemic attacks, and cardiac failure can occur or be exacerbated with relatively mild anemia. In essence, each organ within each patient sets its own functional definition of anemia.

EVALUATION OF THE ANEMIC PATIENT

The remainder of this chapter outlines in considerable detail a systematic approach to the anemic patient. This involves the construction and interpretation of an initial data base derived from careful assessment of the clinical context, key physical findings, and certain basic laboratory tests. The confirmatory diagnostic procedures for specific types of anemia are detailed in the other chapters of this section and will be mentioned only briefly here. Good practice dictates that this initial data base be collected and analyzed prior to the random ordering of procedures or consultations, since it will provide definitive diagnoses in a surprisingly large number of patients and point toward efficient diagnostic approaches in most of the others.

How to Assess the Clinical Context

The answers to six basic questions provide the essential information with which to include or exclude the great majority of anemias.

1. *Is the patient truly anemic?*

The answer to this seemingly trivial but in fact crucial question requires an awareness of all of the aforementioned factors that can affect the normal hematocrit as well as appreciation of the insidious nature of mistakes in sampling and measurement of blood. An isolated low hematocrit in an otherwise completely normal clinical context bears repeating before an intensive investigation is undertaken.

Does the decreased hematocrit reflect a true decrease in red cell mass? Congestive heart failure and iatrogenic fluid overload commonly cause *dilutional anemia* that disappears once diuresis is obtained. In patients with *giant splenomegaly,* red cells may be concentrated in the enlarged spleen and diluted in an increased plasma volume that is in general proportional to their degree of splenomegaly. Both maldistribution and dilution contribute to the frequently observed reduction in peripheral venous hematocrit in such individuals who may have a normal red cell mass. This phenomenon should be distinguished from hypersplenism in which the red cells (or other elements) are destroyed by the spleen. In contrast, dehydrated or severely burned patients may have significant anemia that is masked by diminished plasma volume.

2. Is the anemia inherited or acquired?

Heritable forms of anemia are almost always intrinsic to the red cell or marrow while acquired anemias more often result from extrinsic factors. This distinction, often of fundamental aid in diagnosis, is by no means always simple because of the episodic nature and variable severity of many genetic disorders, particularly those involving red cells. An inherited susceptibility to hemolysis, for example, may require exposure to an oxidant drug or severe infection for anemia to occur (e.g., G6PD deficiency in blacks). Patients may be unaware of mild to moderate lifelong anemias until they have a routine blood test or develop symptoms during pregnancy or after a severe febrile infection.

A positive *family history* suggests an inherited red cell disorder. Because of the concentration of genes for certain hemoglobinopathies and enzyme defects in various African, Mediterranean, and Oriental populations, detailed information concerning *racial background* is pertinent. Clustering of involvement on one side of the family may give clues to autosomal dominant or sex-linked modes of transmission, while a history of consanguinity may accompany autosomal recessively transmitted diseases. The absence of family history by no means excludes a genetic mechanism of transmission, even in dominantly inherited disorders such as hereditary spherocytosis, which may arise by *spontaneous mutation* in a significant number of cases. The absence of congenital anemia can be implied in regular blood donors who will have been screened by the blood bank prior to each donation.

3. Is there evidence for blood loss?

Iron deficiency anemia is the most common anemia in the general population; in the developed western societies it almost always results from blood loss. Because of the frequency of iron deficiency a careful search for blood loss is mandatory in the initial evaluation of an anemic patient. Women of reproductive age are at particular risk because of the combined iron losses of menstruation (estimated at 20 to 30 mg per month) and pregnancy (estimated at 500 mg). Estimation of menstrual loss is difficult and requires specific questioning concerning the frequency of periods, the duration of heavy flow, the frequency of changing pads or tampons, and the appearance of clots.

Gastrointestinal bleeding caused by ulcers, cancers, anomalous vessels, and parasites is a frequent source of blood loss. The gastrointestinal route is virtually the only significant occult source of bleeding. Thus iron deficiency is a frequent presenting manifestation of otherwise unsuspected gastrointestinal pathology, which must be carefully sought once bleeding has been documented.

A number of causes of blood loss that are frequently forgotten are listed below:

Diagnostic phlebotomy. Hospitalized patients, especially children and patients receiving intensive care, may undergo extensive phlebotomy. Individuals with low iron stores (most menstruating females) are at risk for developing iron deficiency as a result, while patients with other marrow impairments will be slow to make up the loss.

Regular blood donation.

Soft tissue bleeding after trauma or surgery. Fractured hips in the elderly are notorious for copious tissue bleeding. Iron is not readily salvaged from such hematomas.

Urinary loss of hemosiderin in chronic intravascular hemolysis.

Pulmonary bleeding in idiopathic pulmonary hemosiderosis.

Bleeding in patients with *hemostatic defects* including hemophilias and hereditary hemorrhagic telangiectasia.

A useful ancillary question that may uncover the presence of iron deficiency relates to the frequent ingestion of starch, clay, or ice. Craving for non-nutritive material, or *pica*, is common in patients with iron deficiency. In black cultures, clay has been a favorite substance since antiquity, and starch seems to be a modern equivalent. Another favorite material is ice, crushed or in cubes, which is also used by whites. Not all individuals who use these materials are iron deficient: there is a cultural as well as a physiologic component. Curiously, the craving for such substances often disappears within 24 hours of treatment with medicinal iron. Iron deficiency is more extensively discussed in Ch. 136 and 206.

4. Is there evidence for hemolysis?

Hemolytic anemias are considerably less common than are the anemias of iron deficiency or chronic disease and may be more difficult to recognize. Inherited disorders of the red cell show a very wide spectrum of severity for reasons that are not entirely clear. The more severe cases, which are encountered in hospitals and hematology clinics, are easily recognized. In milder cases, however, the patient may be unaware of the disease.

The answers to several questions are important for the initial data base. First, the patient should be asked if he has ever had *jaundice*, or yellowing of skin or eyeballs, and if he has ever had hepatitis. The key to suspecting inherited hemolytic anemias is the presence of constant or episodic jaundice. While the hepatic conjugating mechanism can handle a considerable increase in bilirubin production consequent to the breakdown of hemoglobin, the exacerbation of hemolysis occurring during severe febrile infections often causes visible jaundice. This combination frequently leads to the misdiagnosis of recurrent hepatitis. However, not all patients with intrinsic red cell defects give this history—some are able to handle the bilirubin load without visible jaundice.

Second, the patient should be asked if he has ever noticed *darkening of the urine* resembling tea or cola. Bile is characteristically absent from the urine in patients with hemolysis because the predominant form of bilirubin in the plasma is unconjugated and is tightly bound to albumin (Ch. 118). However, during periods of increased hemolysis, alternate products of bilirubin degradation called *dipyrroles* sometimes appear in the urine, causing considerable darkening in its color. For most patients, dark urine means concentrated urine so that specific questioning concerning the color is essential in order to exclude simple dehydration. Other causes of dark urine include hemoglobinuria in patients with moderate to severe intravascular hemolysis and biliuria in patients with liver or biliary tract disease. A careful search for symptoms of *gallbladder disease* in the patient or the family is warranted because of the frequency with which patients with chronic hemolytic disorders develop pigment stones.

As *exceptions*, megaloblastic anemias and severe dyserythropoietic states, which show marked *ineffective erythropoiesis* (also termed intramedullary hemolysis) can also cause jaundice. Similarly, resorption of large *tissue hematomas* may suggest hemolysis because of the resulting anemia and jaundice.

5. Has the patient been exposed to medication or toxins that can result in anemia?

The frequency with which individuals ingest or inhale medications and recreational drugs and the ubiquitous nature of chemical toxins require that a careful search be made for such exposures in an anemic patient. Drug-induced anemias (lumping together both medications and chemical toxins) may be associated with marrow aplasia, maturational defects, and hemolysis by both direct or immune-mediated mechanisms. While it is frequently difficult to establish cause and effect between a given chemical and anemia, certain drugs are notoriously involved, and a history of their use should always be sought. *Alcohol* is probably the most common toxin associated with anemia. The various categories and some specific agents are listed in Table 132–3.

6. Is there a systemic illness or any nonhematologic organ dysfunction?

Assessment of the habitat within which an anemia arises

TABLE 132–3. DRUGS THAT MAY CAUSE ANEMIA

I. **Agents associated with marrow aplasia* (see Table 133–3)**
- Antineoplastic drugs—antimetabolites, alkylating agents
- Antimicrobials—chloramphenicol, quinacrine
- Anticonvulsants—phenytoin, tridione
- Insecticides
- Solvents—benzene
- Anti-inflammatory drugs—phenylbutazone, gold

II. **Agents associated with hemolytic anemia**
- Oxidant drugs*
  - Antibiotics—sulfasalazine, sulfones, nitrofurantoins, nalidixic acid
  - Antimalarials—primaquine
  - Analgesics—acetanilid, pyridium
  - Miscellaneous compounds—methylene blue, naphthalene, phenylhydrazine, fava beans
- Immune mediated
  - Penicillin, stibophen, alpha methyldopa, quinine, etc.

III. **Agents causing maturation defects**
- Alcohol
- Folate antagonists—trimethoprim, triamterene, methotrexate
- Heme synthesis antagonists—INH, lead

IV. **Agents causing gastrointestinal blood loss**
- Aspirin, nonsteroidal anti-inflammatory agents

*Hemolytic primarily in G6PD-deficient individuals.

requires a careful search for systemic illness or organ dysfunction.

The Anemia of Chronic Disease (ACD). Most patients with *active inflammatory disease* or *advanced malignant disease* show a characteristic mild to moderate anemia. The severity of the anemia is in general related to the intensity of the inflammation or the extent of malignant spread, although occasionally relatively localized tumors may present with prominent systemic symptoms and anemia. Weight loss, fever, and night sweats may indicate underlying systemic inflammation. Chronic infections such as subacute bacterial endocarditis and active inflammatory processes such as *rheumatoid arthritis* and inflammatory bowel disease are almost always associated with ACD. The diagnosis of ACD and its differentiation from iron deficiency are discussed in Ch. 134.

Nonhematologic Organ Dysfunction. Patients with diminished renal, hepatic, or endocrine function are often anemic. The pathogenesis of these anemias is multifactorial, and there are relatively few constant distinguishing features. In each case, a significant degree of organ failure must be present to result in anemia. Therefore they are relatively easily excluded by simple measurement of renal, hepatic, thyroid, or pituitary function.

Anemia Associated with Immune Dyscrasias. Red blood cell production and destruction are intimately modulated by the immune system (Ch. 130). It is thus not surprising that immune dysfunction, due either to dysregulation or neoplasms or both, is commonly complicated by anemias. Autoimmune hemolytic anemia is classically associated with systemic lupus erythematosus or with B cell neoplasms, particularly chronic lymphocytic leukemia or diffuse large cell (histiocytic) lymphomas. The hallmark of this combination is a *positive Coombs test* (Ch. 137). Another B cell neoplasm, *multiple myeloma,* commonly presents with anemia due to marrow invasion or suppression or both. Thus the triad of skeletal symptoms (usually low back pain), renal dysfunction, and anemia should always prompt a search for myeloma (see Ch. 163).

The Physical Examination

As in the evaluation of any systemic disorder, a complete physical examination is essential in the patient who presents with anemia. However, particular attention should be paid to the presence of certain key findings that are of help in classifying the anemia (Table 132–4).

TABLE 132–4. PHYSICAL FINDINGS IN VARIOUS ANEMIAS

Physical Finding	Associated Anemia
Skin	
Jaundice	Hemolysis, liver disease
Petechiae	Blood dyscrasia, autoimmune hemolysis with ITP
Telangiectasia	Iron deficiency
Spider angiomas	Liver disease
Facies	
Frontal bossing, maxillary prominence, hypertelorism	Severe congenital hemolysis
Eyes	
Scleral icterus	Hemolysis, liver disease
Retinal hemorrhages	Severe anemia of any cause
Retinal detachment	SC hemoglobinopathy
Mucous Membranes	
Glossitis	Vitamin B_{12}, folate, or iron deficiency
Angular cheilosis	Iron deficiency
Lymph Nodes	
Generalized adenopathy	Malignant lymphoma, blood dyscrasias
Cardiac	
Valvular murmurs	Traumatic hemolysis with iron deficiency, bacterial endocarditis with ACD
Abdominal	
Splenomegaly	Hypersplenism, chronic leukemias, hemolysis, etc.
Hepatomegaly	Liver disease
Pelvic and Rectal	
Hemorrhoids, masses	Blood loss, iron deficiency
Extremities	
Symmetric joint deformity	Rheumatoid arthritis, ACD, and iron deficiency
Congenital anomalies	Constitutional marrow aplasias
Leg ulcers	Chronic hemolysis, esp. sickle cell disease
Myopathy	Rare red cell enzymopathies (deficiency of phosphofructokinase)
Neurologic	
Diminished vibration, position sense, dementia	Vitamin B_{12} deficiency
Neuropathy	Lead poisoning
Mental retardation, spastic paresis	Rare red cell enzymopathies (deficiency of triosephosphate isomerase)

The Initial Laboratory Data Base

An essential minimum laboratory data base, most of which is obtained on every hospitalized patient, includes a complete blood count (or hemogram), an examination of the peripheral blood smear (usually performed as part of the leukocyte differential), examination of the stool for occult blood, and a reticulocyte count. These readily available procedures provide powerful and sometimes definitive diagnostic information.

THE HEMOGRAM. Modern automated cell counters provide a great deal of information to the physician for remarkably little effort by the laboratory. These instruments are designed to detect the passage of individual blood cells through either an electrically charged aperture or a laser beam. The resulting change in impedance or in light scatter as the cell passes is counted and quantitated. The size of the impedance change is proportional to the size of the cell causing it. Thus both the number and size distribution of cells are measured, which allows for derivation of the total volume of red cells (the hematocrit), as well as separation between cells of different sizes (red cells and platelets).

Red Cell Indices. The mean corpuscular volume (MCV) is the most useful of the red blood cell indices. Most hematologists consider the range of MCV's between 80 and 100 cubic microns as normal, although the actual range defined by statistical criteria is somewhat narrower.

The MCV provides a convenient basis for separating anemias into groups that are microcytic (less than 80 cubic microns), normocytic (80 to 100 cubic microns), and macrocytic (greater than 100 cubic microns). This classification is useful but limited by the fact that the great majority of anemic patients fall within the normocytic group and must be distinguished by other means.

MICROCYTOSIS. Microcytosis (see Table 132–5) almost always reflects *defective cytoplasmic maturation* due to impaired heme synthesis, as in iron deficiency, or defective globin synthesis, as in the thalassemias. Carriers of beta-thalassemia trait have MCV's that are almost always less than 80 and usually less than 70 cubic microns (Ch. 142). The alpha-thalassemia traits are often somewhat milder, with MCV's in the 70's. Moderate to severe iron deficiency is also associated with a decreased MCV. In patients with iron deficiency, the microcytosis is in rough proportion to the degree of anemia, whereas in carriers of thalassemias the microcytosis may be much greater with only mild or no anemia. Severe inflammatory disease can induce iron-deficient erythropoiesis in ACD. While the anemia is usually normocytic, occasionally in such patients the anemia is quite microcytic despite normal or increased iron stores. Other causes of reduced MCV include defects in heme synthesis such as occur in lead poisoning or inherited sideroblastic anemia (Table 132–5).

MACROCYTOSIS. Macrocytosis (see Table 132–5) usually reflects *aberrant nuclear maturation* or is a consequence of stressed erythropoiesis. Values for MCV of 130 cubic microns or more occur in severe megaloblastic anemias due to deficiency of vitamin B_{12} or folate (Ch. 136). Many moderate to severe hemolytic disorders are also macrocytic because of the presence of large prematurely released reticulocytes, which have been called shift cells (see next section).

Combinations of factors that cause macrocytosis and microcytosis, when they occur in the same patient, not infrequently create *exceptions* to these rules. For example, the rather common occurrence of alpha-thalassemia in blacks can mask the macrocytosis seen in pernicious anemia. Similarly, *combined nutritional deficiency* of iron and vitamin B_{12} or folic acid, such as often occurs during *pregnancy* or in *alcoholics*, can result in severe anemia with a normal MCV. Here the key to the diagnosis may rest in the accompanying leukocyte abnormalities of hypersegmentation.

Primary marrow diseases, especially aplastic anemias and refractory anemias associated with myelodysplastic syndromes, commonly have a moderately elevated MCV. Many moderate or severe hemolytic disorders are also macrocytic because of the presence of large prematurely released reticulocytes.

The mean corpuscular hemoglobin (MCH) and mean corpuscular hemoglobin concentration (MCHC), which are derived indices, provide ancillary information concerning cell size and hemoglobin content but are rarely as helpful as the MCV. The Coulter apparatus is relatively insensitive to elevation of the MCHC that is known to occur in spherocytic disorders.

TABLE 132–5. MICROCYTIC AND MACROCYTIC ANEMIAS

Microcytosis (MCV < 80μ^3)	Macrocytosis (MCV > 100μ^3)
Iron deficiency	Megaloblastic anemias
Thalassemias	Chemotherapy* (esp. hydroxyurea)
Anemia of chronic disease (usually normocytic)	Reticulocytosis*
	Aplastic anemias*
Sideroblastic anemias* Hereditary Lead poisoning	Hypothyroidism*
	Sideroblastic anemias* Acquired
Severe red cell fragmentation Burns* Hereditary pyropoikilocytosis	Myelodysplasias* Chromosome (5q−) deletion

*In many cases MCV may be borderline or within the normal range.

The Leukocyte and Platelet Count. Anemia should always be assessed in relation to total marrow function. Anemia with a diminished leukocyte and platelet count—*pancytopenia*—suggests primary marrow disease, megaloblastic anemia, or hypersplenism. A bone marrow study is frequently needed to establish the diagnosis of pancytopenia (see Table 133–3).

THE RETICULOCYTE COUNT. A reticulocyte is a young cell newly released from the bone marrow. Normal circulating reticulocytes in a nonanemic individual are morphologically indistinguishable from more mature red cells and must be counted after staining with new methylene blue. The percentage of cells showing bluish clumps or strands of RNA in 500 or 1000 total cells is referred to as the reticulocyte count. The normal reticulocyte circulates for approximately 24 hours before maturing and may spend a brief portion of that time in the spleen. Because normal red cells survive for an average of 120 days, the normal reticulocyte count is approximately 1 per cent (range 0.5 to 1.8 per cent). Anemia of any cause, by decreasing the denominator of the fraction by which the reticulocyte percentage is derived, will increase the count. For this reason the count is customarily corrected to a "normal" hematocrit of 45 per cent:

$$\text{Corrected retic count} = \text{retic count} \times \text{patient Hct}/45$$

Additional corrections of the reticulocyte count have been proposed that take into consideration the increased time of maturation of the "shift" reticulocytes released prematurely from the marrow in severe anemia. These may circulate for considerably longer than 24 hours, but are also subject to a variable period of sequestration in the spleen. The uncertainty associated with estimating true reticulocyte maturation time in the circulation makes the interpretation of an elevated count a semiquantitative exercise.

While *reticulocytosis is a hallmark of hemolytic anemia,* it gives no information about longevity of red cells; rather it reflects entirely the ability of the marrow to respond. Reticulocytosis is most readily interpreted by several measurements over a significant time span. This allows one to assess whether the hematocrit is rising and the reticulocytosis is sustained. Persistent reticulocytosis of 5 per cent or greater (corrected) with a stable hematocrit over several weeks is highly suggestive of a continuing hemolytic process.

Young patients with congenital hemolytic anemias are at risk from transient suppression of marrow function by viral infection (see Ch. 133). They may have an *aplastic crisis* with a precipitous fall in hematocrit and a low reticulocyte count or absence of reticulocytes. Prompt diagnosis and treatment (by transfusions) of this life-threatening complication of chronic hemolysis depends on recognizing this *exception* to the general correlation between hemolysis and reticulocytosis.

Reticulocytosis with a rising hematocrit suggests either a transient hemolytic episode, such as might occur in G6PD deficiency with an exposure to an oxidant drug, or recovery from blood loss. Recovery of marrow function after reversible suppression, such as correction of vitamin B_{12} or folic acid deficiency, will also cause marked transient reticulocytosis with a rising hematocrit.

A markedly decreased corrected reticulocyte count of less than 0.5 per cent implies a primary suppression of the marrow rather than just inadequate response to anemic stress. The causes of marrow failure are discussed in Ch. 133. Severe reticulocytopenia (0.1 per cent or less) implies aplasia of the marrow, either aplastic anemia or its variant pure red cell aplasia. Reticulocyte counts are sometimes expressed as an absolute number, rather than as a percentage. A normal value represents 1 per cent of 5 million red cells or approximately 50,000 reticulocytes per cubic millimeter. Levels below 20,000 reticulocytes per cubic millimeter represent severe reduction in marrow output.

In the great majority of anemias that represent varying combinations of marrow inadequacy and peripheral loss or destruction of red cells, reticulocytes fall in an indeterminate range within the extreme values given above.

EXAMINATION OF THE PERIPHERAL BLOOD SMEAR. The diagnostic information to be gained from an educated appraisal of the blood morphology exceeds that of any other simple laboratory test. In addition to abnormalities in red cells, abnormal leukocytes or platelets can also contribute valuable diagnostic information. It would be misleading to claim that most anemias can be diagnosed from the peripheral smear alone. However, the large number of anemic processes that can be *excluded* by the smear as well as the frequency of definitive abnormalities make it highly useful.

When looking at a peripheral blood smear from a patient with anemia: (1) It is crucial to be aware of the treacherous effects of *artifact* on red blood cell morphology. Routine differential counts and platelet estimations are frequently performed on blood smears that are totally inadequate for evaluation of red cells. (2) One must seek not only the particular abnormal red cell that may give a clue to diagnosis, but also must *evaluate the background morphology* in which it arises. The frequency of poikilocytosis in anemia is such that one can find almost any cell one wishes by looking long enough. Thus several schistocytes found in association with numerous other abnormal shapes are insufficient evidence that traumatic hemolysis is a major cause of the anemia. Marked poikilocytosis usually represents either the effects of dyspoiesis due to nutritional or dysplastic disorders of the marrow or fragmenting accidents to red cells that occur in the circulation. The distinction between these alternatives is often difficult and may depend on ancillary data including marrow examination. In contrast, a particular abnormality such as spherocytosis when it occurs as a significant minority finding in an otherwise relatively normal cell population assumes more significance. (3) It should be noted that *splenectomy* greatly enhances the range of morphologic diversity in almost any anemia.

A list of relatively specific aberrations in red cell morphology and their associated anemias is given in Table 132–6.

TABLE 132–6. USEFUL FINDINGS FROM PERIPHERAL BLOOD MORPHOLOGY

Abnormalities in Red Cell Morphology	Associated Conditions
A. Hypoproliferative group	
Normal smear	Aplasias, ACD
Rouleaux	Myeloma
Burr cells	Renal failure
Blasts	Blood dyscrasias
Teardrops, nucleated RBC	Myelophthisic anemias
Extreme poikilocytosis	Myelodysplasias
B. Maturation defect group	
Hypochromia, microcytes	Iron deficiency
Targets (occasional)	Thalassemias
Elliptocytes (occasional)	
Oval macrocytes	
Hypersegmented neutrophils (>5% PMN's with 5 or more lobes)	Vitamin B_1- or folate deficiency
Prominent basophilic stippling	Lead poisoning, sideroblastic anemias
C. Hyperproliferative group	
Polychromasia ± nucleated RBC	Hemolysis, response to anemic or hypoxic stress
Sickle forms	Sickle cell disease or variants
Microspherocytes (smooth)	Hereditary spherocytosis, autoimmune hemolytic anemia
Microspherocytes (rough = echinocytes)	Glycolytic enzyme defects esp. postsplenectomy
"Bite" cells—Heinz bodies (special stain)	Oxidant hemolysis, G6PD deficiency
Schistocytes	Traumatic or microangiopathic hemolysis
Target cells (predominant)	HbC and E syndromes
Extreme microspherocytosis with budding	Burns, hereditary pyropoikilocytosis
D. Changes not usually associated with anemia	
Howell-Jolly bodies	Hyposplenism
Target cells	Obstructive jaundice
Elliptocytosis (predominant)	Hereditary elliptocytosis (may be hemolytic)

TABLE 132–7. INDICATIONS FOR BONE MARROW EXAMINATION IN ANEMIA

Presence of circulating nucleated red cells
Pancytopenias
Absence of reticulocytes
Presence of circulating blasts
Monoclonal gammopathies
Definitive estimation of marrow iron stores
Suspicion of sideroblastic anemia
Moderate to severe anemia of unknown cause
Combined nutritional deficiencies

TESTING OF STOOLS FOR OCCULT BLOOD. Gastrointestinal bleeding is a frequent cause of iron deficiency anemia and, furthermore, it may indicate the presence of *carcinoma of the colon* or another malignant tumor. Examination of the stools for occult blood is therefore an essential part of the initial data base on every anemic patient. The most widely used procedure for occult fecal blood is the Hemoccult test, which depends on the presence of peroxidase activity of the heme in the sample. The test is sensitive enough to detect approximately 5 ml of blood in a 24-hour sample of stool, but difficulties arise if bleeding is *intermittent* or if the blood does not permeate the stool evenly (sampling error). Bleeding from the upper gastrointestinal tract and oral doses of vitamin C diminish the sensitivity of the test. Hydrating the stool smear with a drop of water before developing approximately doubles the sensitivity. Red meat and certain raw vegetables with high levels of endogenous peroxides, such as broccoli, may cause false positive tests.

A single negative glove or stool specimen is insufficient to exclude gastrointestinal bleeding as a cause of iron deficiency. At least three samples, and preferably six, should be tested on separate days, and one should never be satisfied with a negative result when there is no other explanation for iron deficiency.

Examination of the Bone Marrow in Evaluation of Anemias

The most common anemias—those associated with blood loss, chronic disease, hemolysis, or nutritional deficiency—do not normally require an examination of the marrow for definitive diagnosis. The available tests for assessing the sufficiency of iron, vitamin B_{12}, and folic acid in serum, when coupled with assessment of response to a therapeutic trial, are generally quite sufficient for simple deficiencies. Difficulties arise, however, in the complex case in which combined deficiencies or chronic disease is present. Since nutritional anemias, particularly in patients with alcoholism, are often multiple, marrow examination may be the only means to establish the adequacy of iron stores in this setting. Similar problems arise in iron deficiency when combined with chronic inflammatory disease such as active rheumatoid arthritis.

Virtually all of the other indications for marrow examination involve the suspicion of a *primary blood dyscrasia* or the invasion of the marrow space by an *extrinsic tumor or infection.* Exami-

TABLE 132–8. SOME USEFUL ANCILLARY TESTS WHEN THE INITIAL DATA BASE IS UNREVEALING

Coombs' test
Sedimentation rate
Creatinine
Liver function tests
Thyroid profile
Serum protein electrophoresis
Serum iron and transferrin

TABLE 132–9. LABORATORY APPROACH TO DIAGNOSIS OF CAUSE OF ANEMIA

Hematocrit	RBC Mass	Retics (corrected)	MCV	Smear	Other	Marrow	Diagnostic Group
↓ (Verify)	↓	↑ (Clinical assessment; Exclude hemodilution)	NL or ↑	Table 132–6 Group C	± Jaundice	Rarely indicated	Hyperproliferative Hemolytic
↓	↓	↑	NL or ↑	Table 132–6 Group C	Acute bleed	Not indicated	Hyperproliferative Hemorrhagic
↓	↓	NL or ↓	↑	Table 132–6 Group B	± Pancytopenia	Megaloblastic	Nuclear maturation defect—B_1-folate deficiency
↓	↓	NL or ↓	NL	Table 132–6 Group A	See Table 132–8	See Table 132–7	Hypoproliferative
↓	↓	NL or ↓	↓	Table 132–6 Group B	Iron studies NL or ↑	↑ Iron stores ± sideroblasts	Cytoplasmic maturation defect—thalassemias, etc.
↓	↓	NL or ↓	↓	Table 132–6 Group B	Chronic blood loss	↓ Iron stores	Cytoplasmic maturation defect—iron deficiency
↓	↓	↓ ↓	↑	Normal	± Pancytopenia	Empty or loss of erythroid precursors	Hypoproliferative — aplasias

nation of aspirated smears in general gives superior cytologic information while the core biopsy provides crucial information concerning the overall cellularity, as well as the presence of fibrosis, tumor, or granulomas. Both procedures are complementary and are best performed together when the diagnosis is in doubt.

Firm indications for marrow examination in anemia are listed in Table 132–7.

USE OF LABORATORY DATA IN EVALUATION OF ANEMIAS. Careful assessment of the initial data base will almost always reveal diagnostic clues to follow. A list of useful ancillary procedures when no hints can be extracted from the data base are given in Table 132–8. In Table 132–9 a rational approach to the laboratory evaluation of anemias is summarized, with reference back to the previous tables in this chapter. The definitive diagnostic approaches to the various disorders are described in the accompanying chapters.

TREATMENT OF ANEMIAS

Therapies for the various causes of anemia are detailed in subsequent chapters. Some general therapeutic principles and common therapeutic errors are pertinent to this introduction. Therapy for anemia may be *specific*, as in the replacement of deficient iron, vitamin B_{12}, or folate; *diagnostic*, as in the therapeutic trial; or *symptomatic*, as in the administration of blood transfusions. It is a mark of good practice to carefully distinguish these differing therapeutic situations.

Specific therapy requires a definitive diagnosis, the absence of which converts it into a therapeutic trial. Therapeutic trials of iron or vitamin B_{12} are consistent with good practice, provided that the response is documented quantitatively and the cause of any deficiency found is thoroughly investigated. Duration of treatment must be correlated with response and based on a thorough understanding of continuing requirements and body stores to avoid harm to patients. For example, patients may continue using iron supplements for years after a course of therapy and become at risk for iron overload. Conversely, the cessation of cobalamin therapy after a full response is obtained in pernicious anemia, a lifelong disease, will inevitably lead to a potentially damaging recurrence. Probably the most frequent error in the treatment of anemia is the excessive use of specific remedies, e.g., iron or cobalamin, for questionable symptomatic indications.

Symptomatic treatment of anemia with blood transfusions must be undertaken within the same constraints as for any other medical disorder—that is, for *real symptoms* that outweigh the *real hazards* of therapy. Deviations from good practice most often involve (1) overestimation of the benefits of transfusion in a compensated patient, particularly when symptoms relate more to an underlying disease than to the anemia per se, and (2) underestimating the life-threatening risks of transfusion, both circulatory and infectious. Thus the sporadic use of small-volume transfusions for symptomatic indications is rarely consistent with good practice.

Blood volume. In Mollison PL: Blood Transfusion in Clinical Medicine. Oxford, Blackwell Scientific Publications. 7th ed. 1983, pp 65–92. *A gold mine of information concerning the many factors influencing blood volume in health and disease. Much of this material is not generally referenced in hematology texts.*

The approach to the patient with anemia. In Wintrobe MM: Clinical Hematology. Philadelphia, Lea and Febiger. 8th ed. 1981, pp 529–558. *A more leisurely approach to the subject with the usual comprehensive perspective and extensive historical references that have characterized this work throughout its many editions.*

133 ANEMIA DUE TO BONE MARROW FAILURE

Alan S. Keitt

The hematopoietic system consists of primitive migratory pluripotential stem cells, their progeny, and certain habitats to which these cells are attracted to undergo differentiation. The organization of these habitats is determined by specialized supporting cells that provide a framework in which the hematopoietic and lymphoid cells may operate. These organs are components of the reticuloendothelial system, named for the fibroblastic and endothelial cells that make up their supporting matrix. They share certain homologies in their vascular architecture, namely a system of cords and sinuses, which are lined by the supporting cells. In subprimates and during fetal life, all of the reticuloendothelial organs may harbor active hematopoietic tissue. In mature primates, however, the liver, spleen, and lymph nodes assume other specialized functions, and only the bone marrow continues to support effective hematopoiesis.

Marrow failure may arise by two basically distinct mechanisms: the aplastic and myelophthisic anemias. The *aplastic anemias* represent failure of the stem cell to undergo differentiation, either because of intrinsic damage, or interruption of its interactions with the particular cast of supporting cells that comprise its microenvironment. The *myelophthisic anemias* result from loss of essential habitat for hematopoiesis due to destruction of the macroenvironment of the bone marrow by neoplastic or inflammatory tissue. This latter group will be considered briefly in a separate section at the end of this chapter.

THE APLASTIC ANEMIAS

Definition

APLASTIC ANEMIA. This refers to a diverse group of potentially severe marrow disorders characterized by peripheral pancytopenia and a marrow that is largely devoid of hematopoietic cells but that retains the basic marrow architecture or stroma with replacement of hematopoietic cells by large amounts of fat. Aplastic anemia has been classified as *severe* when at least two of the following three criteria are present: (1) anemia with a corrected reticulocyte count <1 per cent, (2) neutrophils <500 per cubic millimeter, (3) platelets <20,000 per cubic millimeter. In addition, marrow hypocellularity must be present (estimated as <25 per cent of marrow space).

UNICELLULAR APLASIAS. Isolated deficiencies of each of the main hematopoietic cell lines, i.e., pure red cell aplasia (PRCA), occur somewhat less commonly than typical aplastic anemia. In some instances the unicellular aplasias may progress to frank aplastic anemia with pancytopenia, but a significant number of other cases will remain "pure." The unicellular aplasias exhibit relatively normal cellularity of the bone marrow with selective dropout of one set of precursors. These disorders presumably arise from failure of a "committed" rather than a pluripotential stem cell. There is no clear means at the present time of separating these disorders from those in which recognizable precursors of a given cell line occur in the marrow in the absence of mature forms. It is likely that these disorders are part of a spectrum of autoimmune cytopenias in which the target cells have differing degrees of maturation.

CONSTITUTIONAL APLASIAS. Inherited forms of the disease, both pancellular and unicellular, have been designated as constitutional aplasias. These frequently arise in combination with various congenital anomalies and probably involve fundamental intrinsic abnormalities of stem cells.

Etiology

The multiple causes and diverse associations of the various bone marrow failure syndromes are classified in Table 133–1. Approximately 50 per cent of cases arise de novo and are thus considered idiopathic. The remaining cases are associated with exposure to an extremely diverse array of chemicals or ionizing radiation or occur in the context of a neoplastic, autoimmune, or infectious disease. Such associations do not necessarily imply a causal relationship with the aplasia. There is little apparent clinical difference between the idiopathic and secondary forms of the disease.

DRUG-RELATED APLASIAS (Table 133–2). ***Dose-Dependent Aplasias.*** Chemotherapeutic agents used in the treatment of various neoplasms are virtually uniform in their cytotoxicity for hematopoietic stem cells. The resulting aplasia is usually reversible, and its severity depends on the amount of drug

TABLE 133–1. CLASSIFICATION OF THE ETIOLOGY OF APLASTIC ANEMIA AND RELATED DISORDERS

I. Aplastic Anemias	
A. *Acquired*	
Idiopathic	Radiation
Autoimmune	Infections—hepatitis
Drugs (Table 133–2)	Pregnancy
Toxic chemicals	Paroxysmal nocturnal hemoglobinuria
B. *Constitutional*	
Familial or congenital	
Fanconi's anemia	
Dyskeratosis congenita	
II. Unicellular Aplasias	
A. *Pure red cell aplasia*	
1. Acquired	
Thymoma	Autoimmune
Idiopathic	Drugs and toxins
2. Constitutional	
Diamond-Blackfan anemia	
B. *Agranulocytosis/granulocytopenia*	
1. Acquired	
Idiopathic	Felty's syndrome
Drugs and toxins	Thymoma
2. Constitutional	
Congenital	
Familial-benign, severe, cyclic	
C. *Thrombocytopenia*	
1. Acquired	
Idiopathic	
Autoimmune-systemic lupus erythematosus	
Drugs and toxins	
2. Constitutional	
Amegakaryocytic thrombocytopenia (associated with congenital anomalies)	
Autosomal recessive thrombocytopenia	

exposure. Agents that are cycle specific such as cytosine arabinoside and methotrexate act preferentially on the more mature stem cells, which are known to have a higher mitotic rate than the more primitive pluripotential stem cells. As a result, patients manifest pancytopenia prior to the depletion of the pluripotent stem cells on which ultimate marrow regeneration depends. Other agents such as busulfan and the nitrosoureas attack both cycling and noncycling stem cells and therefore can lead to prolonged or irreversible aplasia unless used with great caution. Certain other drugs that are not used for cancer chemotherapy show reversible, dose-related marrow suppression as an adverse side effect. These include phenytoin, phenothiazines, thiouracil, methicillin, and chloramphenicol.

Idiosyncratic Aplasias. Another large group of seemingly unrelated drugs, which may or may not show dose-related marrow suppression, is associated with the rare occurrence of disastrous aplasia in a small number of sensitive individuals. The prototype of this group is *chloramphenicol*, for many years the leading cause of idiosyncratic drug-related aplastic anemia. Chloramphenicol has restricted usage in developed countries, but it is still widely available and heavily used in Third World countries, where accurate assessment of fatalities is unavailable.

In contrast to the dose-dependent aplasias, idiosyncratic reactions may occur weeks or months after exposure to small amounts of chloramphenicol. The frequency of this reaction is estimated between 1:24,000 and 1:40,000 of the exposed population. Even the use of topical ophthalmic solutions has been associated with aplasia. A latent period does not always occur; the rapid development of severe aplasia during therapy is not uncommon.

Chloramphenicol also manifests reversible dose-related marrow suppression primarily affecting erythroid precursors probably as a result of its inhibition of mitochondrial protein and heme synthesis. This effect of chloramphenicol is associated with prominent vacuolization and sideroblastic changes in developing erythroblasts.

There is evidence from studies of identical twin concordance that some patients who develop severe idiosyncratic aplasia from chloramphenicol have an underlying genetic susceptibility. The nature and frequency of this putative sensitivity is unknown. The management and prognosis of chloramphenicol-related aplasia does not differ from that of other idiosyncratic drug reactions or of the idiopathic form of the disease and will be discussed subsequently. Drugs that have been associated with the development of marrow aplasias are listed in Table 133–2.

ENVIRONMENTAL TOXINS (Table 133–2). Solvents and insecticides comprise the major group of toxins that have been linked to aplastic anemia. Of these, benzene is the most important and has received the most experimental attention. *Benzene* appears to have heterogeneous effects on marrow function and may induce various combinations of aplasia, myelofibrosis, or frank leukemia. The abnormalities in marrow function may arise during or years after exposure to benzene. Most recognized cases have resulted from rather heavy and prolonged industrial exposures. Aplastic anemia after glue sniffing probably relates to the presence of benzene derivatives in glues.

INFECTIONS. ***Hepatitis.*** Severe aplastic anemia may follow an episode of apparent viral hepatitis. The association seems to be with non-A, non-B hepatitis and is twice as common in males as in females, usually occurring in patients under 20 years of age. The hepatitis is not unusually severe, whereas the subsequent aplasia is often quite severe and has a high mortality.

Parvovirus. Selective transient loss of erythroid precursors in the marrow with reticulocytopenia is a well-recognized occurrence in patients with congenital hemolytic anemias and has been termed *aplastic crisis.* Although the suppression of erythropoiesis is self limited, the rapid fall of hematocrit that is a result of the short lifespan of the remaining red cells may induce severe life-threatening anemia. Human parvovirus infection has been linked to aplastic crisis in hereditary spherocytosis and sickle cell anemia, and the virus has been shown to selectively inhibit erythroid progenitors in cell cultures. The association with parvovirus appears quite specific. The apparent tropism of the virus for the erythroid stem cell has rekindled speculations concerning a viral etiology for aplastic anemia.

TABLE 133–2. CHEMICAL AND PHYSICAL AGENTS ASSOCIATED WITH THE DEVELOPMENT OF PANCYTOPENIA AND A HYPOPLASTIC MARROW*†

ANTINEOPLASTIC AGENTS: alkylating agents, antimetabolites, antimitotic agents, antibiotics, radiation
ANTIMICROBIAL AGENTS: *chloramphenicol, organic arsenicals, quinacrine,* streptomycin, penicillin, methicillin, oxytetracycline, chlortetracycline, sulfonamides, sulfisoxazole (Gantrisin), sulfamethoxypyridazine (Kynex), amphotericin B
ANTICONVULSANTS: mephenytoin (Mesantoin), *trimethadione (Tridione),* phenacemide (Phenurone), phenytoin, ethosuximide (Zarontin), carbamazepine (Tegretol)
ANTITHYROID DRUGS: carbethoxythiomethylglyoxaline (Carbimazole), methylmercaptoimidazole (Tapazole), potassium perchlorate, propylthiouracil
ANTIDIABETIC AGENTS: tolbutamide, chlorpropamide, carbutamide
ANTIHISTAMINES: tripelennamine (Pyribenzamine)
ANTIRHEUMATIC AGENTS: *phenylbutazone, gold compounds,* acetylsalicylic acid, indomethacin, penicillamine, colchicine
SEDATIVES AND TRANQUILIZERS: meprobamate, chlorpromazine, promazine, chlordiazepoxide (Librium), mepazine
MISCELLANEOUS: acetazolamide (Diamox)
TOXIC CHEMICALS: solvents (*benzene,* glue, toluene, carbon tetrachloride), insecticides (chlorophenothane [DDT], parathion, chlordane, pentachlorophenol), bismuth, mercury, arsenic, colloidal silver

*Adapted from Wintrobe MM: Clinical Hematology. 8th ed. Philadelphia, Lea & Febiger, 1981. Drugs associated with 20 or more reported cases are in italics.

†Additional drugs that are associated only with agranulocytosis are not listed here (see Ch. 150).

PRELEUKEMIA. Most forms of marrow aplasia, both acquired and congenital, have been associated with the occasional development of acute leukemia. One characteristic sequence of events occurs in children who present with typical aplastic anemia but respond rapidly to corticosteroid therapy. These patients ultimately relapse with typical acute lymphocytic leukemia of childhood. Rarely, acute myeloid leukemias may arise after years of mild or moderate marrow aplasia, particularly in patients with exposure to benzene or radiation.

Pathogenesis

The pathogenesis of aplastic anemia remains elusive. The diversity of the clinical contexts in which it arises (Table 133–1) and the heterogeneity of responses to different therapies suggest that several or perhaps many different mechanisms are involved. Two dominant hypotheses have emerged: (1) a *primary stem cell failure,* i.e., an intrinsic defect of the hematopoietic stem cell that renders it unable to differentiate (such a lesion could arise by exposure of a susceptible individual to an environmental chemical, by viral infection of the stem cell, or by other unknown mechanisms); (2) an *immunologically mediated attack* either on the stem cell itself or on other components of the complex network of cells and factors that are necessary for normal hematopoiesis (reviewed in Ch. 131). It predicts that in some cases, continued suppression of the marrow would prevent simple replacement of stem cells by marrow transplantation.

EVIDENCE FOR DEFECTIVE STEM CELLS. Approximately one half of patients with aplastic anemia who have received marrow transplants from an *identical twin* have had engraftment with rapid, complete, and sustained recovery of marrow function. The simplest interpretation of these dramatic therapeutic results is that the donor marrow has replaced absent or defective stem cells in the patient, since external factors, such as antibodies, would presumably attack the new cells as well. The data give no information about the nature of the original stem cell lesion, however.

EVIDENCE FOR IMMUNE-MEDIATED MARROW FAILURE. In the remainder of the attempted transplants between identical twins, the donated marrow is rejected by the aplastic recipient. In most of these patients, however, grafting can be subsequently carried out after a course of cyclophosphamide therapy, and they then show sustained and complete recovery of marrow function. What cyclophosphamide does in these patients is unclear: (1) It might eliminate a population of immune cells and interrupt an immune reaction against the donor stem cells, or (2) it might eliminate residual defective stem cells from preferred architectural "niches" that are essential for normal stem cell differentiation, allowing access of the donor stem cells to these particular microenvironmental sites.

Antilymphocyte Globulins. Antilymphocyte globulins (ALG) or antithymocyte globulins (ATG), complex heteroantisera raised in animals against thymic lymphocytes, can significantly ameliorate the course of aplastic anemia in many patients. The clinical responses, which are obtained in 30 to 65 per cent of patients, are incomplete; they may occur after several months of therapy, and cytopenias may persist. However, transfusion requirements are often abated, and the granulocyte and platelet counts may rise above the critical levels necessary to prevent infection or bleeding. These antisera are generally assumed to act by immunosuppression, but they also bind to many hematopoietic cells and may have other targets that are not presently defined. Unfortunately, different antisera vary considerably in efficacy, and there is no current method to assay the active components by means other than in vivo therapeutic trials in humans.

In Vitro Studies. Colony growth in normal marrow in vitro cultures is suppressed by various mononuclear cell fractions, usually containing T cells, derived from some patients with aplastic anemia. The interpretation of these results is complicated, however, by the presence of alloimmunization consequent to transfusion therapy of these patients. When alloimmunization is absent (no previous transfusion or in identical twin coculture experiments), inhibition is observed more rarely (10 to 15 per cent) than was initially supposed. As other evidence for the role of cellular immune suppression, erythroid and granulocytic colonies can be grown from marrows of some patients with aplastic anemia only after removal of T cells.

Unicellular Aplasias. Autoimmunity is clearly important in causing some of the unicellular aplasias, particularly in pure red cell aplasia (PRCA). This disease often arises in patients with other manifestations of immune dysfunction. Thymoma, hypogammaglobulinemia, monoclonal gammopathy, antinuclear antibodies, and Coombs-positive hemolysis have all been reported in association with PRCA. Serum inhibitors of erythropoiesis have been described using marrow culture techniques. Immunoglobulin fractions derived from affected patients have shown specific staining of erythroblast nuclei by immunofluorescence as well as complement-dependent cytolysis of erythroblasts. These patients also frequently respond to combinations of prednisone or Cytoxan; reduction in the post-treatment level of serum inhibitor has been demonstrated in some instances. *Transient erythroblastopenia of childhood,* a self-limited form of PRCA, is also associated with antibody-mediated marrow suppression.

SUMMARY. Marrow aplasia syndromes are associated with agents that are known to be both cytotoxic and leukemogenic (e.g., alkylating agents, benzene, and ionizing radiation) as well as with constitutional disorders that may also terminate in acute leukemia (e.g., Fanconi's anemia). This implies that intrinsic genetic damage to stem cells may occur that prevents normal differentiation. The degree to which the proliferative potential of these damaged stem cells is preserved may then determine whether aplasia or leukemia ensues. This apparent dichotomy is reminiscent of the effects of retroviral infections of immune cells that can induce either malignant transformation or selective aplasia of the same cell type. Marrow failure in other cases seems to be associated with inhibition of normal stem cell differentiation as a result of cellular or humoral autoimmunity. It is premature to invoke immune marrow suppression in most patients with aplastic anemia simply because they respond to ALG.

Incidence

Fortunately aplastic anemia is rare. The incidence of idiopathic aplastic anemia was 11 new cases per million population per year in Sweden from 1973 to 1977. This is about one-fourth the incidence of acute leukemia in the general population. There is a fivefold increase in the incidence of this disease after the age of 65 years. Aplastic anemia seems to be more common in the Orient, although this has not been firmly established.

Clinical Description

ONSET. The clinical features of the disease relate almost entirely to the effects of inadequate numbers of functional peripheral blood cells. The onset is usually insidious but may be dramatic, depending on the severity and rapidity with which the aplasia progresses. Bleeding manifestations may be the first indication of severe disease. These include gingival bleeding, epistaxis, and petechial hemorrhages, all of which are characteristic of severe thrombocytopenia. Fatigue and pallor are usually noted at presentation. Infections frequently begin with bacterial invasion of vulnerable areas of the gastrointestinal tract, namely, the oropharynx or the rectum. Opportunistic infections are unusual at presentation, but may occur in patients with very low lymphocyte counts and after immunosuppressive therapy. Systemic symptoms are not prominent unless there is extensive infection, and weight loss is unusual.

PHYSICAL EXAMINATION. Pallor is frequent; its absence in a patient with the acute onset of petechial hemorrhages is much more likely to be associated with immune thrombocytopenic purpura. Retinal hemorrhages are not uncommon and correlate with the severity of anemia rather than thrombocytopenia. The spleen is not enlarged; splenomegaly strongly suggests an underlying blood dyscrasia or hypersplenism rather than marrow aplasia. The constitutional forms of marrow aplasia (Fanconi's anemia, dyskeratosis congenita, Diamond-Blackfan anemia, and others) are frequently associated with congenital anomalies that should be carefully noted. The onset of marrow disease in some of the constitutional disorders may occur in the second or third decade so they must be considered in the differential diagnosis of aplasia in the young adult or adolescent.

Diagnosis

The diagnosis of aplastic anemia is usually straightforward. It is based on the combination of peripheral cytopenias with the characteristic empty marrow replaced with fat.

PERIPHERAL BLOOD FINDINGS. The basic structural framework of the marrow remains relatively intact, so the peripheral red cells do not show marked abnormalities except for a tendency toward macrocytosis. Nucleated red cells occur rarely in simple aplasia; their presence raises the possibility of a myeloproliferative or myelophthisic process instead. The total lymphocyte count may be normal, but is often very low in severe cases and after therapy with steroids or other immunosuppressive agents.

BONE MARROW FINDINGS (Fig. 133–1). The empty marrow replaced by fat is the key diagnostic feature. Residual foci of mainly erythropoietic tissue are often found, however, that can alter the impression of aspirated material. A large-needle biopsy (>1 cm) is an essential adjunct in evaluating the degree of aplasia. If a single biopsy and aspirate are equivocal, repeating is warranted.

Assessment of marrow cellularity is at best semiquantitative, and the degree of hypocellularity has not been shown to correlate well with prognosis. This probably results from unavoidable heterogeneity of sampling this large organ. Benign lymphoid nodules may be found; this finding must not be confused with involvement by malignant lymphoma. The unicellular aplasias arise in the setting of normal marrow cellularity with absence of a single cell line. In some cases of PRCA, as in agranulocytosis, immature precursors may be found in the absence of any mature forms.

ANCILLARY STUDIES. Because of the frequent association of paroxysmal nocturnal hemoglobinuria (PNH), the *Ham test* or *sucrose hemolysis test* is frequently performed in patients with marrow aplasia, especially if there is any degree of reticulocytosis (Ch. 137). Occasional patients have had hypogammaglobulinemia; therefore, measurement of serum immunoglobulins is warranted. A search for *thymoma* should be performed by computed tomography in patients with pure red cell aplasia. When there is a question of a constitutional aplasia, skeletal and renal radiographs are indicated to assess the presence of congenital anomalies.

DIFFERENTIAL DIAGNOSIS. A list of causes of peripheral pancytopenia is presented in Table 133–3. The most important distinction to be made in assessing aplastic anemia is to exclude the presence of leukemia, which may occasionally be characterized by marked marrow hypocellularity and pancytopenia. Splenomegaly, circulating immature cells, and increased marrow reticulin all suggest a primary blood dyscrasia or myelofibrosis rather than simple aplasia.

Management

INITIAL ASSESSMENT. A general approach to the initial assessment and subsequent management of patients with

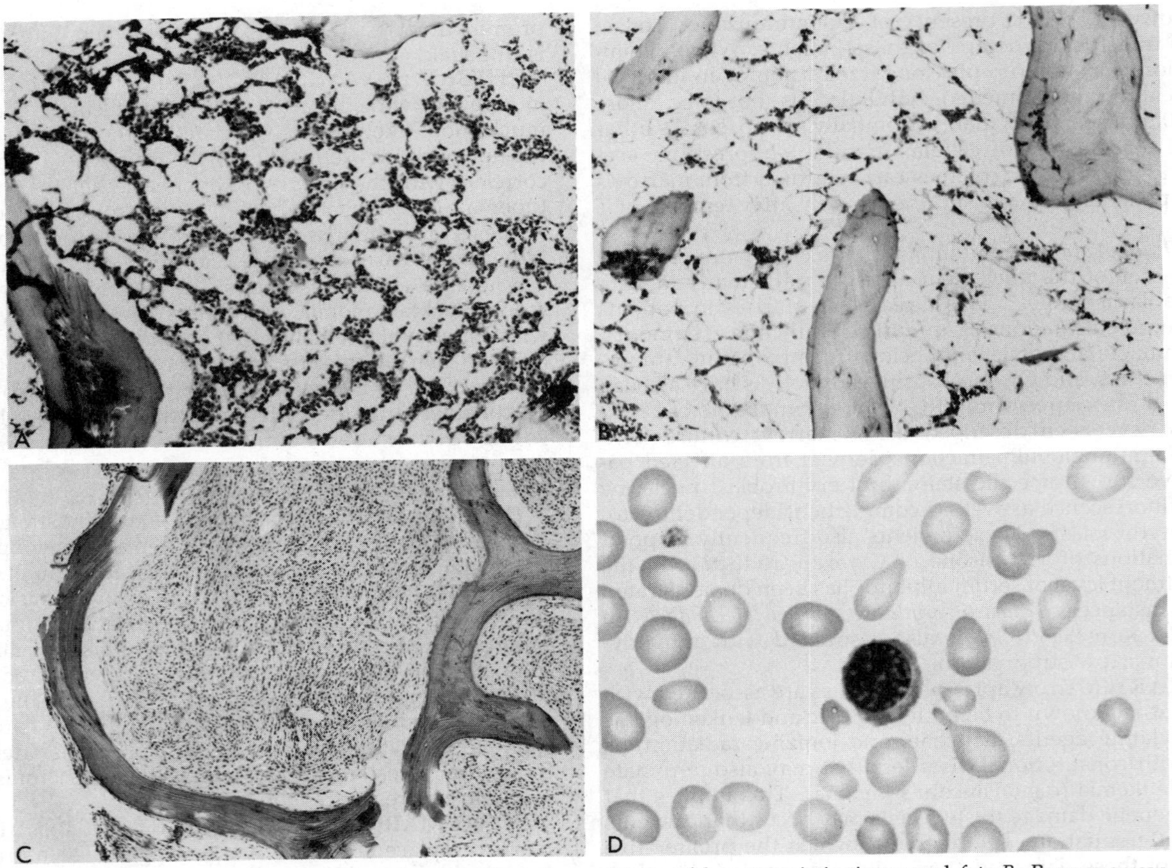

FIGURE 133–1. *A*, Normal bone marrow biopsy. Note even mixture of hematopoietic tissue and fat. *B*, Bone marrow biopsy from a patient with aplastic anemia. Note the increase in fat at the expense of normal hematopoietic tissue. *C*, Bone marrow biopsy from a woman with metastatic breast carcinoma. Note the dense fibrosis. *D*, Peripheral smear from a patient with idiopathic myelofibrosis. Note frequent teardrop forms and the nucleated red cell.

aplastic anemia is presented in Figure 133–2. The most important first task, once the diagnosis is firm, is to assess severity. When severe disease is present, or judged to be imminent when blood counts are falling, *rapid action is essential.* After the initial assessment it is usually best to refer the patient to a center that is experienced in handling the formidable problems associated with the evaluation and care of this disease. The disease is sufficiently rare that new patients are extremely valuable for the important clinical trials that will guide future therapy. Of course, any potentially toxic drugs should be discontinued, and the patient should be removed from any environmental source of marrow toxins during the assessment period.

THERAPY DIRECTED AT REVERSAL OF APLASIA. ***Bone Marrow Transplantation.*** Indications for bone marrow transplantation are being redefined as experience grows with the use of ALG. Transplant candidates must have an HLA-compatible donor, usually a sibling, which markedly limits the use of the procedure. The results of transplantation are excellent in patients under the age of 20 years who have not previously received a transfusion; it is the preferred therapy for this group. The incidence of graft-versus-host disease with its attendant morbidity and mortality becomes unacceptable in patients over age 40. The details of the procedure and the results in aplastic anemia are reviewed in Ch. 165.

Antilymphocyte Globulin. ALG, administered as a single series of injections over a one- to two-week period, improves survival in patients with severe aplastic anemia. The characteristics of the response have been described above (see Pathogenesis). Serum sickness is noted in all patients. Responses have been noted in idiopathic aplasia as well as in aplasia associated with drugs or hepatitis. Older patients respond at least as well as do younger ones.

These encouraging results seem to offer improved survival for the majority of patients with the disease who lack a compatible donor. Use of ALG is still experimental therapy, and the optimal preparation of the reagent, the appropriate use of adjunctive therapies, and the long-term effects on survival remain to be established.

Androgens. As the only available therapy in the era before marrow transplantation and ALG, androgens have been widely used. They have also been incorporated into a number of the ALG trials as adjunctive therapy. It is not clearly established that androgens induce remissions in severe aplastic anemia more frequently than they occur spontaneously. With less severe aplasia, however, androgens may improve the hematocrit and lessen transfusion requirements. In occasional patients who are androgen dependent relapse has occurred repeatedly when androgens are discontinued. Granulocyte and platelet responses are much less common than is a rise in hematocrit. Both the injectable forms of testosterone enanthate* (5 to 8 mg per kilogram once weekly) and synthetic oral agents, e.g., oxymetholone (2 to 4 mg per kilogram daily) have shown responses. Toxicity is significant; both groups of drugs cause masculinization with hirsutism, acne, fluid retention, and clitoral enlargement. The oral agents are associated with additional hepatic toxicity, including cholestatic jaundice and hepatocellular carcinoma.

TABLE 133–3. CAUSES OF PANCYTOPENIA

A. Aplastic anemias (Table 133–1)	D. Megaloblastic anemias
B. Myelophthisic anemias (Table 133–4)	E. Myelodysplastic syndromes
C. Hypersplenism	F. Overwhelming sepsis

*This use is not listed in the manufacturer's directive.

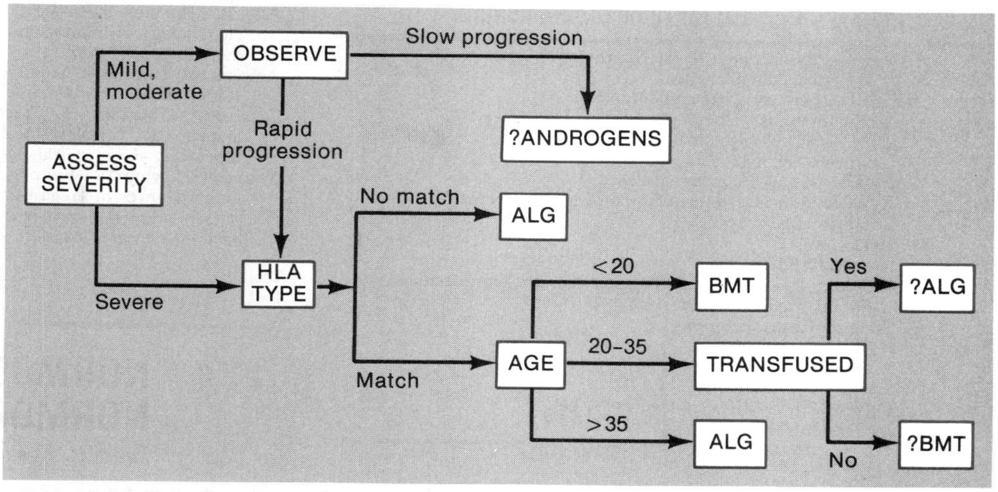

FIGURE 133–2. Schematic approach to the management of aplastic anemia. ALG = Antilymphocyte globulins ± androgens or high-dose steroids. BMT = Allogenic bone marrow transplantation. ? = Optimal therapy in doubt.

High-Dose Corticosteroids. Very high doses of methylprednisolone (100 mg per kilogram per day over a one- to two-week period) have been used in combination with ALG without a notable effect on the observed response rate. Methylprednisolone alone has given responses equivalent to those of ALG alone, including some complete remissions. Because of the marked immunosuppression of such doses and the risk of opportunistic infections in these already granulocytopenic patients, this treatment should be used with caution. It may prove to be a valuable form of therapy when access to transplantation and ALG is unavailable.

Pure Red Cell Aplasias. Immunosuppression has a more clearly defined role in the treatment of unicellular aplasias, especially in pure red cell aplasia. Combinations of cyclophosphamide and other cytotoxic agents and prednisone have induced excellent remissions in PRCA, but the disease eventually recurs in most individuals. About one third of patients with PRCA and thymoma have had remissions after thymectomy.

SUPPORTIVE CARE. Supportive care has assumed an increasingly important role in survival of aplastic anemia patients both before and after various therapeutic interventions.

Transfusions. *Transplant candidates should have transfusion only when absolutely necessary because of the risk of sensitization and subsequent graft rejection.* The number of donors should be restricted, and *family members must be avoided* until the question of transplantation is decided. Complete phenotyping of major and minor red cell antigens should be performed prior to transfusion. This will aid in the detection of red cell alloantibodies should they develop after repeated transfusions. The use of frozen red cells diminishes the development of leukocyte alloantibodies, but washed, leukocyte-poor packed cells are a more widely available and usually satisfactory substitute. Additional aspects of long-term transfusion therapy, including the use of iron chelators to reduce iron overload, are discussed in Ch. 141.

Platelet transfusions are of undoubted value to the bleeding patient, but their continued use is limited by the development of alloantibodies that render the patient refractory to random donor platelets. Such patients may benefit from platelets obtained by pheresis of an HLA-compatible donor. The onset of such refractoriness is highly variable, and nearly half of patients seem to tolerate random donor platelet support for long periods.

Aplastic patients frequently tolerate very low platelet counts with only cutaneous bleeding in the form of petechiae and traumatic ecchymoses. While conventional teaching has held that a count below 20,000 is the threshold value for a high risk of bleeding, it may in fact be much lower. Platelets should be reserved for actual bleeding episodes or when cerebral hemorrhage is suspected. Patients with demonstrable increments after transfusions may reasonably be given prophylaxis as the count falls below 5000 or 10,000 per cubic millimeter. Platelets should be irradiated to avoid graft-versus-host disease if immunosuppressive therapy is given.

General Measures. Suppression of menstruation by appropriate hormonal manipulation is indicated for females with excessive blood loss. *Aspirin and all antiplatelet medications should be avoided.* Low doses of prednisone (10 to 15 mg) appear to decrease capillary bleeding in severely thrombocytopenic patients. Scrupulous attention to aseptic technique in administering intravenous infusions, avoidance of intramuscular injections, careful attention to handwashing by personnel, and isolation from obviously infected visitors are important. Rigid adherence to "reverse isolation" impedes proper nursing care without a corresponding benefit in reducing infections, which are largely acquired from endogenous or ubiquitous flora. Management of these infections in the compromised host is discussed in Ch. 258.

Prognosis

Patients with aplastic anemia appear to fall into two major subgroups: (1) a severely affected group as previously defined with a high mortality (perhaps as high as 96 per cent with no treatment) by six months, and (2) a mildly to moderately affected group with a considerably better outlook. Before the era of bone marrow transplantation and intensive supportive care the overall mortality in all patients was from 55 to 75 per cent. Survival in marrow transplant patients with severe aplasia who had a matched sibling donor ranges from 40 to 80 per cent and is adversely affected by increasing age and prior tranfusions. Graft-versus-host disease is the major factor in morbidity and mortality in these patients (Ch. 165). Long-term survival in ALG-treated patients is not established, but one- and two-year survival is approximately equivalent to that in the marrow transplant patients.

MYELOPHTHISIC ANEMIAS

Myelophthisis is an archaic term for any pathologic process that obliterates the normal marrow architecture. The microcirculatory anatomy of the marrow normally retains developing hematopoietic cells within extravascular spaces, called *cords*, until they are sufficiently mature to gain access to the general circulation by crossing the cordal-sinusoidal boundary. If this delicate network is disrupted, abortive attempts at hematopoiesis occur, which result in the release of immature blood cells into the peripheral blood. The presence of circulating nucleated red blood cells, myelocytes, or blasts and giant platelets is termed *leukoerythroblastosis*. This is a frequent although not invariable accompaniment of myelophthisis (Fig.

TABLE 133–4. CAUSES OF MYELOPHTHISIS

A. Neoplastic Infiltration of the Marrow	
1. Hematologic malignancies	
	Leukemias—acute and chronic
	Lymphomas–Hodgkin's and non-Hodgkin's
	Plasma cell myeloma
	Hairy cell leukemia
2. Nonhematologic malignancies	
	Carcinomas–esp. breast, prostate, lung, stomach
	Neuroblastoma
B. Myelofibrosis	
1. Primary (idiopathic)	
2. Secondary–chronic myeloid leukemia, cancers, vasculitis (lupus, rheumatoid arthritis)	
C. Granulomatous infections	
1. Tuberculosis	
2. Fungi	
D. Metabolic Abnormalities	
1. Lipid storage diseases–Gaucher's, etc.	
2. Osteopetrosis	

133–1). Transient leukoerythroblastosis may occur without myelophthisis under conditions of extreme erythropoietin-mediated marrow stress such as acute hemorrhage, abrupt hypoxemia, or severe chronic hemolysis.

The pathologic processes that cause myelophthisis can be usefully divided into four general categories (Table 133–4). *Metastatic carcinoma* has replaced tuberculosis as the most commonly associated condition. Many of these neoplastic marrow processes incite an intense fibrotic reaction that may obscure the malignant cells. The hematopoietic disorders that are most likely to cause myelofibrosis, idiopathic myelofibrosis, and chronic myelogenous leukemia are associated with marked megakaryocytic hyperplasia. Acute leukemias and well-differentiated lymphoid neoplasms, although they may totally replace the normal marrow, only rarely elicit a leukoerythroblastic response, for reasons that are not entirely clear.

The diagnosis of myelophthisis is frequently suggested by the presence of *nucleated red blood cells* or other immature forms on the peripheral smear. The total leukocyte and platelet count may be decreased if marrow replacement is extensive; however, there may be marked leukocytosis in idiopathic myelofibrosis or when a leukemoid reaction occurs. *Teardrop-shaped red cells* are commonly present along with other poikilocytes (Fig. 133–1). Occasionally the diagnosis is suggested by abnormal bone films showing focal lytic or blastic lesions, or a more widespread increase in bone density as in idiopathic myelofibrosis.

Definitive diagnosis of myelophthisis depends on adequate examination of the bone marrow (Fig. 133–1). *Because the aspirate is characteristically "dry," a needle or surgical biopsy is essential.* The marrow involvement is often patchy, and residual areas of normal or hyperplastic marrow may be found. Demonstration of increased reticulin fibers in the marrow biopsy with silver stains is a useful adjunct in myelofibrotic conditions. A careful search for malignant cells embedded within the fibrotic tissue should always be performed.

The therapy of myelophthisic anemias is entirely dependent on the recognition and appropriate treatment of the underlying pathologic process. Successful treatment of breast or prostatic carcinomas, either by cytotoxic or hormonal agents, can lead to complete resolution of the myelophthisis and recovery of normal marrow function. A dramatic example of the reversibility of the myelophthisic process has been demonstrated in the childhood disease osteopetrosis. This condition has been linked to an inherited defect in the mononuclear phagocytic system that is manifested by decreased osteoclast function. The resulting overgrowth of bony trabeculae that obliterates the marrow space can be completely reversed by bone marrow transplantation with restoration of normal hematopoiesis.

Alter BP: The bone marrow failure syndromes. In Nathan DG, Oski FA (eds.): Hematology of Infancy and Childhood. 3rd ed. Philadelphia, W.B. Saunders Company, 1987.

Ammus SS, Yunis AA: Acquired pure red cell aplasia. Am J Hematol 24:311, 1987. *Concise, well-referenced review.*

Gewirtz AM, Hoffman R: Current considerations of the etiology of aplastic anemia. CRC Crit Rev Oncol Hematol 4:1, 1985. *A current review emphasizing the various sources of data concerning the immune etiology of aplastic anemia.*

Young NS, Levine AS, Humphries RK (ed.): Aplastic Anemia; Stem Cell Biology and Advances in Treatment. New York, Alan R. Liss, Inc., 1984. *State-of-the-art reviews of current theories of pathogenesis and treatment by all of the most active investigators of aplastic anemia. The single most useful volume to date.*

134 NORMOCHROMIC NORMOCYTIC ANEMIAS

James P. Kushner

The normocytic normochromic anemias are those in which the average cell size (mean corpuscular volume; MCV) and the average cell hemoglobin concentration (mean corpuscular hemoglobin concentration; MCHC) are normal. These anemias occur in association with a large number of diseases, and the mechanisms responsible for the anemia are quite diverse. Frequently the anemia is only a minor manifestation of a systemic disease of much more serious consequence. The anemia, however, may be the first detected evidence of disease, and the finding of anemia may lead to studies resulting in correct diagnosis of an underlying disorder.

In spite of their highly variable causes, it is possible to approach normocytic normochromic anemias with a classification scheme that can direct the diagnostic investigation (Table 134–1). Central to this classification is the determination of whether the bone marrow is responding appropriately to a given degree of anemia. Normally functioning bone marrow can accelerate the rate of erythropoiesis up to eightfold. Accelerated erythropoiesis by normal bone marrow is reflected by an increase in the reticulocyte count. Reticulocytosis can be detected on routinely stained smears by the finding of a population of large polychromatophilic red cells. When reticulocytosis is pronounced the MCV may be moderately elevated because of the contribution of the large young erythrocytes to the measurement of the average cell size. Reticulocytosis is a manifestation of an appropriate marrow response to hemolytic anemia (see Ch. 137) and to acute posthemorrhagic anemia. These two conditions can generally be differentiated on clinical grounds.

When evidence of accelerated erythropoiesis in response to anemia is *not* found, it is likely that the underlying disorder

TABLE 134–1. CLASSIFICATION OF THE NORMOCYTIC NORMOCHROMIC ANEMIAS

I. Anemia with appropriate marrow response
- A. Acute posthemorrhagic anemia
- B. Hemolytic anemia (may be macrocytic when there is pronounced reticulocytosis) (Ch. 137–139)

II. Anemia with impaired marrow response
- A. Marrow hypoplasia
  - 1. Aplastic anemia (Ch. 133)
  - 2. Pure red cell aplasia (Ch. 133)
- B. Marrow infiltration
  - 1. Infiltration by malignant cells
  - 2. Myelofibrosis (Ch. 154)
  - 3. Inherited storage diseases
- C. Decreased erythropoietin production
  - 1. Kidney disease
  - 2. Liver disease
  - 3. Endocrine deficiencies
  - 4. Malnutrition
  - 5. Anemia of chronic disease (Ch. 135)

is directly or indirectly affecting the bone marrow. Intrinsic marrow disease should be strongly suspected when leukopenia and thrombocytopenia are also found, or when morphologic abnormalities are found on the blood smear. These morphologic abnormalities include nucleated red cells, teardrop-shaped poikilocytes, immature granulocytes, and large platelets or megakaryocyte fragments (dwarf megakaryocytes). Marrow aspiration and biopsy are nearly always indicated in the face of these findings.

When anemia is found in association with an impaired marrow response and no signs of intrinsic marrow disease are detected, it is likely that an underlying disease is producing an indirect effect on red cell production. Renal disease, liver disease, and a variety of endocrine disorders indirectly affect erythropoiesis in association with a reduction of erythropoietin production. The pathogenesis of the anemia of chronic disease may also involve this mechanism, in addition to the defect in the mobilization of reticuloendothelial iron stores (Ch. 135).

ACUTE POSTHEMORRHAGIC ANEMIA

DEFINITION. The anemia caused by loss of a large volume of blood may occur as a result of trauma or because of an underlying disease that affects blood vessels or the coagulation mechanism. Bleeding may be obvious when profuse hemorrhage occurs from a body orifice or from an external wound. If bleeding occurs within a body cavity, tissue space, or the gastrointestinal tract, the nature of the problem may not be immediately appreciated (Ch. 114). The manifestation of hemorrhage depends on the rate and magnitude of the bleeding and the time elapsed between the acute hemorrhage and the first clinical observations.

CLINICAL MANIFESTATIONS AND DIAGNOSIS. The characteristic sequence of events following a single acute hemorrhage can be divided into two phases. The first, lasting up to three days, reflects the volume of blood loss and is dominated by the manifestations of hypovolemia. Anemia may not be detected by measurement of the hematocrit or hemoglobin. The second phase occurs after the body has restored the blood volume to normal or near normal and is characterized by the findings of anemia and reticulocytosis.

As outlined in Table 134–2, a normal individual can rapidly lose up to 20 per cent of the blood volume without any signs or symptoms. Limited signs of cardiovascular distress appear with losses up to 30 per cent of the blood volume, but shock gradually appears only when the blood loss exceeds 30 to 40 per cent of the blood volume. As the plasma volume and red cell mass are reduced in proportional amounts, the hematocrit and hemoglobin fail to reflect the magnitude of blood lost.

TABLE 134–2. CLINICAL MANIFESTATIONS OF ACUTE BLOOD LOSS IN OTHERWISE HEALTHY INDIVIDUALS

Percentage of Blood Volume Lost	Amount Lost (ml)	Clinical Manifestations
10–20	500–1000	Usually none; vasovagal syncope may occur in 5%; tachycardia in response to exercise; mild postural hypotension may be noted
20–30	1000–1500	Few changes supine; light-headedness and hypotension commonly occur when upright; marked tachycardia in response to exertion
30–40	1500–2000	Blood pressure, cardiac output, central venous pressure, urine volume reduced even when supine; thirst, shortness of breath, clammy skin, sweating, clouding of consciousness and rapid, thready pulse may be noted
40–50	2000–2500	Severe shock, often resulting in death

Clinical signs and symptoms must be used initially to estimate the degree of blood volume depletion and in planning emergency treatment. When blood loss is more gradual, the plasma volume may be restored by endogenous mechanisms, and very large volumes of blood can be lost without clinical manifestations of shock.

Anemia is first detected following expansion of the plasma volume. In recumbent patients most of the plasma volume expansion has occurred by 24 hours; this expansion mainly is caused by movement of water and electrolytes into the intravascular space. In ambulatory patients plasma volume expansion occurs more slowly, mainly through the mobilization of albumin from extravascular sites. The hematocrit may not reach the minimum value until three or four days after the hemorrhagic episode. Erythropoietin secretion is stimulated shortly after the appearance of the anemia, and hyperplasia of marrow erythroid elements then begins.

Reticulocytosis is usually detected three to five days after the hemorrhagic episode, and maximal reticulocyte counts are reached at six to eleven days. The degree of reticulocytosis is related to the magnitude of hemorrhage but rarely exceeds 14 per cent. During the period of maximal reticulocytosis, polychromatophilia and macrocytosis can be detected on the peripheral blood smear, and the MCV may become transiently increased. If the initial evaluation is done during this state, the findings may be mistaken for those of hemolytic anemia. Differentiation from hemolytic anemia may be difficult if bleeding has occurred into a body cavity or tissue space, because resorption of blood from these areas often results in an increased production of unconjugated bilirubin and even mild jaundice. In contrast to the reticulocyte response both the platelet count and the leukocyte count may rise dramatically within hours of hemorrhage. Platelet counts as great as 1000×10^9 per liter may be detected within one to two hours, and leukocyte counts of 20 to 35×10^9 per liter may be reached by two to five hours. Elevated platelet and leukocyte counts generally return to normal within three to five days.

TREATMENT. During the hypovolemic phase therapy should be directed at stopping the hemorrhage, combating shock, and restoring the blood volume. Restoration of the blood volume may be achieved by intravenous infusion of crystalloid (electrolyte) solutions; colloid solutions of plasma protein, albumin, or dextran; or fresh whole blood. Complete reliance on fresh whole blood in the emergency situation is unwise for several reasons. First, large amounts of type O Rh-negative whole blood are required. If typing and cross-matching are done prior to transfusion, there may be a dangerous delay in therapy. Second, allergic transfusion reactions may restrict volume expansion or even produce plasma volume contraction. For the emergency situation crystalloid solutions are preferred.

A nonprotein crystalloid solution with a sodium concentration approximating that of plasma is the most widely used fluid therapy for hemorrhagic shock. Ringer's lactate, Ringer's acetate, or normal saline supplemented with 90 mmol of sodium bicarbonate (2 ampules) per liter may be used. Crystalloid solutions containing large amounts of glucose should be avoided, as they may induce osmotic diuresis, further depleting the vascular volume. An initial infusion of two to three times the volume of the estimated blood loss is administered. When larger volumes of crystalloid solutions are administered, peripheral edema often develops, as these solutions are rapidly distributed throughout the intravascular and extravascular compartments.

The use of protein-containing solutions (albumin or fresh frozen plasma) has been supported by some who claim that increasing the oncotic pressure within the vascular space is beneficial. There is little evidence to support this contention, as protein is extravasated into interstitial spaces throughout the body in patients in shock. Dextran solutions have been widely used in the treatment of hemorrhagic shock, but there is no convincing evidence to suggest they are superior to crystalloid solutions in acute emergencies. Acute renal failure has occurred in a few patients receiving dextran solutions. Dextran may cause difficulty in cross-matching and may interfere with platelet adhesiveness and the normal coagulation cascade.

The administration of 3 liters of a crystalloid solution over 15 to 20 minutes will generally resuscitate any patient in hemorrhagic shock if the hemorrhage has been arrested. Continued signs and symptoms of hypovolemia indicate continued bleeding and usually indicate the need for surgical intervention to control the hemorrhage.

Once the emergency has been dealt with, the bleeding lesion identified, and the bleeding stopped, attention can be directed to the anemia. The anemia itself rarely requires specific therapy and provision of a high-protein diet and oral iron supplementation will suffice in most cases. Blood transfusions may be reserved for those situations in which rapid correction of the anemia is required, as in preparation of the patient for surgery.

Billhardt RA, Rosenbush SW: Cardiogenic and hypovolemic shock. Med Clin North Am 70:853, 1986. *An up-to-date review of the crystalloid versus colloid controversy in the acute management of hypovolemic shock.*

Mollison PL: Blood Transfusion in Clinical Medicine. 7th ed. Oxford, Blackwell Scientific Publications, 1983. *The "bible" for detailed analysis of the measurement of blood volume and its restoration by transfusions.*

OTHER NORMOCYTIC NORMOCHROMIC ANEMIAS

ANEMIA OF CHRONIC RENAL INSUFFICIENCY. In contrast to the anemia found in association with most chronic diseases, the anemia associated with renal failure may be quite severe. Many factors may contribute to the anemia. Folate may be lost into the dialysate in patients receiving long-term dialysis therapy. Iron deficiency may develop because of blood loss from the genitourinary or gastrointestinal tracts or into the hemodialysis coil. Microangiopathic hemolytic anemia may occur in patients with renal failure because of malignant hypertension, or in the hemolytic-uremic syndrome. In the absence of any of these mechanisms the degree of anemia correlates roughly with the increase in the blood urea nitrogen and creatinine. Although red cell survival may be moderately shortened, the mechanism underlying the anemia is mainly reduced red cell production. Failure of the erythropoietin-secreting function of the kidney appears to be responsible for the impaired marrow response to the anemia.

Blood transfusions are infrequently required. The hematocrit rarely drops below 15 per cent, and most patients tolerate this degree of anemia remarkably well. Long-term dialysis therapy may result in a modest reduction in the degree of anemia, provided that folate or iron deficiency does not develop as a complicating factor. Androgens may be useful for patients who do not tolerate anemia well and require repeated transfusions. Weekly intramuscular injections of nandrolone decanoate (100 mg) or the oral administration of fluoxymesterone* (10 to 30 mg per day) have proved effective in reducing transfusion requirements. The administration of human erythropoietin derived from recombinant DNA has proved extremely effective in treating the anemia of chronic renal disease in early studies of patients maintained by hemodialysis. Following a successful renal homograft, normal and even supranormal hematocrit values may be achieved.

ANEMIA IN CIRRHOSIS AND OTHER LIVER DISEASE. Anemia is a frequent manifestation of liver disease; the pathogenetic mechanisms responsible may be more varied than those underlying the anemia of chronic disease. The anemia is generally normocytic and normochromic but occasionally it may be mildly macrocytic. It is unusual for the MCV to exceed 115 fl in the absence of advanced folate deficiency with frank megaloblastic changes in the marrow. Etiologic factors implicated in the pathogenesis of the anemia associated with liver disease include chronic alcoholism and its effect on erythropoiesis; iron deficiency due to blood loss from gastritis, peptic ulcer, varices, and deficient coagulation factors; sequestration of erythrocytes and other formed elements of the blood by the enlarged spleen resulting from portal hypertension; exaggeration of the degree of anemia because of the increased plasma volume associated with cirrhosis; and alterations in the lipid composition of erythrocyte membranes.

*This use is not listed in the manufacturer's directive.

ANEMIAS ASSOCIATED WITH ENDOCRINE DISORDERS. Anemia frequently accompanies disorders of the pituitary gland, the thyroid gland, the adrenal glands, and the gonads. In general the anemia is mild and by itself produces few symptoms. Reduced tissue oxygen requirements as a result of the endocrine disturbance may result in diminished renal production of erythropoietin. Loss of the stimulating effect of androgens on erythrocyte production may be a factor in some cases. Endocrine disorders tend to begin insidiously; the early symptoms are generally no more specific than fatigue and lassitude. When initial laboratory testing reveals anemia, the diagnostic studies may be directed to the hematopoietic system. Unless endocrine disease is included in the differential diagnosis of a normocytic normochromic anemia, the primary diagnosis may be overlooked.

Anagnostou A, Kurtzman NA: Hematological consequences of renal failure. In Brenner BM, Rector FC (eds.): The Kidney. 3rd ed. Philadelphia, W. B. Saunders Company, 1986. *A comprehensive treatise on the subject, with over 500 references.*

Eichner ER: The hematologic disorders of alcoholism. Am J Med 54:621, 1973. *A review of the hematologic effects of the pathogenetic agent responsible for most cases of advanced liver disease.*

Eschbach JW, Egrie JC, Downing MR, et al.: Correction of the anemia of end-stage renal disease with recombinant human erythropoietin: Results of a combined phase I and II clinical trial. N Engl J Med 316:73, 1987. *A clinical study demonstrating the efficacy of erythropoietin in the treatment of the anemia of end-stage renal disease.*

Williams WJ, Beutler E, Erslev AJ, et al. (eds.): Hematology. 3rd ed. New York, McGraw-Hill Book Company, 1983. *Extensive references to the anemias associated with renal and endocrine disorders.*

135 HYPOCHROMIC ANEMIAS

James P. Kushner

Anemias associated with a subnormal average cell hemoglobin concentration (mean corpuscular hemoglobin concentration; MCHC) are classified as hypochromic. When the average cell size (mean corpuscular volume; MCV) is also reduced the anemia is classified as hypochromic, microcytic. Hypochromia and microcytosis can be detected either by examination of the stained blood smear or by calculation of the erythrocyte indices (Table 135–1). The widespread use of electronic cell counting equipment makes available the erythrocyte indices at the same time that anemia is usually detected by the finding of subnormal values for the hemoglobin concentration and the volume of packed red cells (generally referred to as the hematocrit).

The developing erythrocyte requires iron, protoporphyrin, and globin for the biosynthesis of hemoglobin. Hypochromic

TABLE 135–1. RED CELL INDICES* IN HYPOCHROMIC AND MICROCYTIC ANEMIAS

	MCV (fl)	MCHC (gm/dl)	MCH (pg)
Normal	83–96	32–36	28–34
Hypochromic	83–100	28–31	23–31
Microcytic	70–82	32–36	22–27
Hypochromic-microcytic	50–79	24–31	11–29

*Variations in the methods for measuring the red blood cell count, the volume of packed red cells, and the hemoglobin concentration could change the values slightly.

TABLE 135–2. CLASSIFICATION OF ANEMIAS CHARACTERIZED BY DEFICIENT HEMOGLOBIN SYNTHESIS AND THE PRESENCE OF HYPOCHROMIC ERYTHROCYTES

I. **Disorders of iron metabolism**
  A. Iron deficiency anemia
  B. Anemia of chronic disease
  C. Hereditary atransferrinemia
  D. Congenital hypochromic-microcytic anemia with iron overload (Shahidi-Nathan-Diamond syndrome)

II. **Disorders of porphyrin and heme synthesis: sideroblastic anemias**
  A. Acquired sideroblastic anemias
    1. Idiopathic refractory sideroblastic anemia
    2. Complicating other diseases
    3. Associated with drugs or toxins—ethanol, INH, lead
  B. Hereditary sideroblastic anemias
    1. X chromosome–linked
    2. Autosomal recessive

III. **Disorders of globin synthesis**
  A. The thalassemias (Ch. 142)
  B. Hemoglobinopathies characterized by unstable hemoglobins (Ch. 144)

anemias, characterized by deficient hemoglobin synthesis, can be divided into three groups, depending on which of the three components required for hemoglobin biosynthesis is deficient (Table 135–2).

IRON DEFICIENCY ANEMIA

DEFINITIONS. Iron deficiency anemia occurs when body iron stores become inadequate for the needs of normal erythropoiesis. Body iron stores must be exhausted before red cell production is restricted; therefore, anemia occurs at a late stage of iron deficiency. In its fully developed form iron-deficient erythropoiesis is characterized by hypochromia and microcytosis of the circulating erythrocytes, low plasma iron and ferritin concentrations, and a transferrin saturation of about 15 per cent or less. Iron deficiency anemia is a sign of disease and is not in itself a complete diagnosis.

PREVALENCE. Iron deficiency is the most common cause of anemia throughout the world, although it is difficult to define precisely its prevalence. Published studies vary in the reported incidence of iron deficiency because of differences in the criteria used to identify iron deficiency as well as in the nature of the population sampled in terms of age, sex, economic status, and local environmental factors. In parts of Africa and India, where marginal dietary intake and excessive iron loss due to intestinal parasites are present together, over half the population may suffer from iron deficiency anemia.

In most developed countries about 3 per cent of men, 20 per cent of women, and over 50 per cent of pregnant women are deficient in iron as judged by plasma iron levels. As judged by serum ferritin levels, iron stores are greatly reduced in about 25 per cent of children, 30 per cent of adolescents, 30 per cent of menstruating women, 60 per cent of pregnant women, and 3 per cent of men.

IRON METABOLISM. The total iron content of a healthy human subject remains within relatively narrow limits. Loss of iron from the body is precisely matched by absorption of iron from food. Iron loss is not due to "excretion" in the usual sense but rather to loss of intact cells containing iron.

TABLE 135–3. DISTRIBUTION OF IRON IN THE BODY

Compound	Iron Content (mg) Men (70 kg)	Iron Content (mg) Women (50 kg)	Per Cent of Total Body Iron Men	Per Cent of Total Body Iron Women
Hemoglobin	2670	1500	69.6	73.1
Myoglobin	350	220	9.1	10.7
Heme enzymes	8	7	0.2	0.3
Transferrin	6	5	0.2	0.2
Ferritin-hemosiderin	800	320	20.9	15.7
Total	3834	2052	100.0	100.0

Epithelial cells from the gastrointestinal and urinary tracts, and from the skin, account for the normal daily iron loss in men of about 1 mg. In women, menstrual flow, childbearing, and lactation are additional routes of iron loss.

The body iron content in normal adult men is about 50 to 55 mg per kilogram of body weight and in women is about 35 to 40 mg per kilogram. This difference reflects the high incidence of iron deficiency in women and does not indicate any fundamental differences in iron metabolism between the sexes. Most of the body iron is found in hemoglobin, with smaller amounts in myoglobin and iron storage compounds (Table 135–3). Only a minute portion is found in plasma, where it is bound to transferrin.

The metabolism of iron is dominated by its role in hemoglobin synthesis. Iron incorporated into hemoglobin is utilized over and over again through an internal cycle, the *iron cycle* (Fig. 135–1). The plasma iron compartment, in which iron is bound to the transport protein transferrin, is central to this cycle. Iron moves from the plasma to erythroid precursor cells in the marrow. These cells synthesize hemoglobin and, with maturation, are released into the circulation. At the end of their 120-day lifespan the red cells are ingested by macrophages, principally in the splenic sinusoids, and the iron is extracted from the hemoglobin by the enzyme heme oxygenase. A small portion of this iron is stored in macrophages as ferritin or hemosiderin, but most is returned to the plasma where it becomes bound to transferrin, completing the cycle. In the normal adult male about 30 mg of iron completes the iron cycle daily. One to 2 mg of iron leaves the plasma daily and enters the liver and other tissues where it is utilized for the synthesis of other hemoproteins such as cytochromes and myoglobin.

ABSORPTION. The average intake of iron in the meat-containing diet in the United States is about 10 to 30 mg per day, but much greater variations occur in different parts of the world. Only 5 to 10 per cent of dietary iron (about 1 mg) is absorbed daily in order to balance precisely the amount lost. The amount of iron absorbed can increase up to fivefold if body iron stores are depleted or if erythropoiesis is accelerated. The amount absorbed decreases in states of iron overload or if there is erythroid hypoplasia. Total body iron balance is thus regulated at the absorptive step; the precise mechanism by which this control is accomplished has not been defined. Iron is absorbed chiefly in portions of the

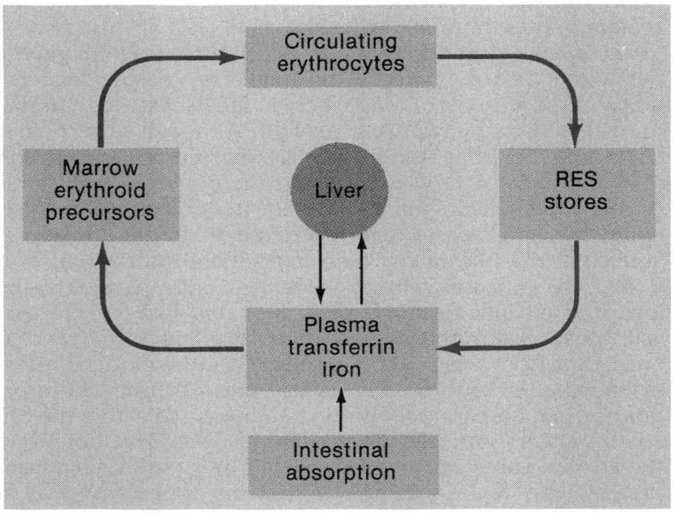

FIGURE 135–1. The internal iron cycle. In the plasma, iron bound to transferrin is transported to the marrow where it is transferred to developing red blood cells and incorporated into hemoglobin. The mature red blood cells are released into the circulation and after 120 days are ingested by macrophages in the reticuloendothelial system (RES). Here the iron is extracted from hemoglobin and returned to plasma, completing the cycle.

intestine proximal to the midjejunum, and very little is absorbed in more caudal intestinal segments.

Iron is absorbed by two distinct pathways in humans, one for iron in heme and the other for iron in ferrous and ferric iron salts. Heme iron is derived from the hemoglobin, myoglobin, and other heme proteins in foods of animal origin. Exposure to the acid and proteases of gastric juice liberates the heme from its apoprotein. Heme is rapidly taken up by gastrointestinal epithelial cells, and the iron is made available by enzymatic degradation of the porphyrin macrocycle. The absorption of heme iron is influenced very little by other dietary components.

The "bioavailability" of nonheme dietary iron, however, varies greatly. Availability is dependent on the oxidation state and solubility of the iron and the presence of chelating substances in the diet. Factors modifying the form in which iron is presented to the intestinal mucosal cell play an important role in the amount of iron that can be absorbed. At the acidic pH normally found in the stomach, both ferrous and ferric iron are soluble. Patients who have undergone gastrectomy, or who are achlorhydric for other reasons, demonstrate impaired absorption of iron. Cimetidine, a potent inhibitor of gastric acid secretion, may also impair the absorption of dietary iron. In the duodenum, as the pH rises, ferric iron is readily converted to insoluble ferric hydroxides. Agents such as ascorbic acid may promote iron absorption by reducing some ferric iron to ferrous iron, which remains soluble at neutral pH. Dietary constituents such as citrate may enhance the solubility of inorganic iron and hence enhance absorption. Phytates, neutral detergent fibers, and other substances present in cereals, grain, and corn impair iron absorption by binding iron as relatively insoluble complexes.

The clinical significance of the various luminal factors that influence iron absorption may be minimal in United States society, where the diet provides relatively large amounts of heme iron. In developing countries, however, diets are generally characterized by low meat content and high content of grains and vegetables. Such diets, with low heme iron content and high content of substances that impair nonheme iron absorption, may not meet the iron demands of many individuals. The manipulation of dietary iron content by large scale iron supplementation programs has been instituted in both developed and underdeveloped countries. The incidence of iron deficiency in the population is decreased by such programs, but the risks to individuals predisposed to iron loading remain to be determined (Ch. 206).

The uptake of iron from the intestinal lumen is both energy dependent and regulated. The uptake of ^{59}Fe by duodenal mucosal cells in iron-deficient individuals exceeds that in normal subjects by two- or three-fold. Although correction of the anemia in iron-deficient subjects by red cell transfusion does not decrease iron uptake, repletion of body iron stores restores the kinetics of iron uptake to normal. Once iron enters the mucosal cell it must be transported to the serosal surface of the intestine, where iron enters the plasma. Iron within the mucosal cell can have two fates. One is to be incorporated into ferritin within the cytosol of the mucosal cell. Most ferritin iron does not ultimately reach the plasma, but is lost from the body when the intestinal mucosal cell is sloughed after its three- to four-day lifespan. Iron not incorporated into mucosal cell ferritin is transported across the cell and ultimately appears in plasma as ferric iron bound to transferrin. The process of intracellular transport has not been precisely defined. Although transferrin appears to play a central role in iron absorption, other mechanisms must also be available, because the rare patients with congenital atransferrinemia show no evidence of deficient absorption.

TRANSPORT. Transferrin, the iron transport protein in plasma, is a glycoprotein with an approximate molecular weight of 80,000. The liver is the major source of transferrin synthesis and the protein is equally distributed in the intravascular and extravascular spaces. Transferrin is capable of binding two iron atoms in the ferric state. In normal subjects the plasma concentration of transferrin is about 2.5 to 3.0 grams per liter. Plasma transferrin is usually quantified in terms of the amount of iron it will bind, a measure called the *total iron-binding capacity* (TIBC). In normal subjects only about one third of the available transferrin binding sites are occupied (TIBC = 33 per cent). Although there is a diurnal variation in plasma iron concentration, with the highest values in the morning and the lowest in the evening, no diurnal variation occurs in the TIBC. Although a number of genetically determined electrophoretic variants of transferrin have been demonstrated, all subtypes appear to function normally as iron transport proteins.

Transferrin has no known function other than as a transport protein and is reused for many cycles of iron transport. With the exception of very small amounts of iron in ferritin, all the iron in plasma is carried by transferrin. The affinity of transferrin for iron is sufficiently high that, theoretically, less than one free iron atom might be present in a liter of blood.

Significant physiochemical differences exist between the two iron-binding sites of transferrin when iron uptake and release are studied in vitro. In spite of these differences the two iron-binding sites function equivalently in the delivery of iron to cells in vivo. The two iron-binding sites are located on separate "halves" of the molecule but about 40 per cent of the amino acid sequence in the two halves is identical. This homology lends credence to the theory that transferrin arose from a duplication of a gene for an antecedent iron transport protein with a single iron-binding site. The evolutionary advantage of the doubled structure may be the reduction of losses in the glomerular filtrate.

CELLULAR UPTAKE. The initial event in the transfer of iron to cells is binding of diferric transferrin to specific, high-affinity receptors on the cell surface. When receptors are lost because of cell maturation (as occurs in developing erythrocytes in vivo) or artificial manipulations in vitro, the ability of the cell to take up iron from transferrin is lost. As cellular iron uptake is directly proportional to the number of transferrin cell surface receptors, it follows that cells with a high iron demand should have large numbers of receptors. The biosynthesis of hemoglobin by erythroid cells has a high iron requirement, and the human reticulocyte may have as many as 300,000 receptors per cell. Developing erythroid cells in the bone marrow may have even more.

In the process of iron uptake by cells the transferrin receptor–diferric transferrin complex is internalized into an acidic, nonlysosomal vesicle (Fig. 135–2). At the acidic pH of the vesicle, iron is readily dissociated from diferric transferrin, but the resulting apotransferrin remains bound to the receptor. The transferrin receptor–apotransferrin complex is transported back to the cell surface where, at neutral pH, the apotransferrin is liberated and becomes available for another cycle of iron binding and release.

Once iron enters the cell, two events occur. One is the delivery of iron to the mitochondria, where it is enzymatically incorporated into protoporphyrin to form heme. The other is the incorporation of iron into ferritin. Ferritin iron is a storage form of iron and is probably not utilized by the cell for heme synthesis. Ferritin iron may, however, be recycled for use by other cells.

STORAGE. Iron-free apoferritin is a spherical protein made up of 24 subunits that surround a central cavity. The central cavity of each apoferritin molecule can potentially store more than 4000 molecules of iron. When iron is present in the central cavity, the protein is termed ferritin. The importance of ferritin as an iron storage compound is emphasized by the wide distribution of structurally similar ferritins in both plant and animal tissues.

A number of isoferritins with differing isoelectric points have been demonstrated. Two different ferritin subunits exist,

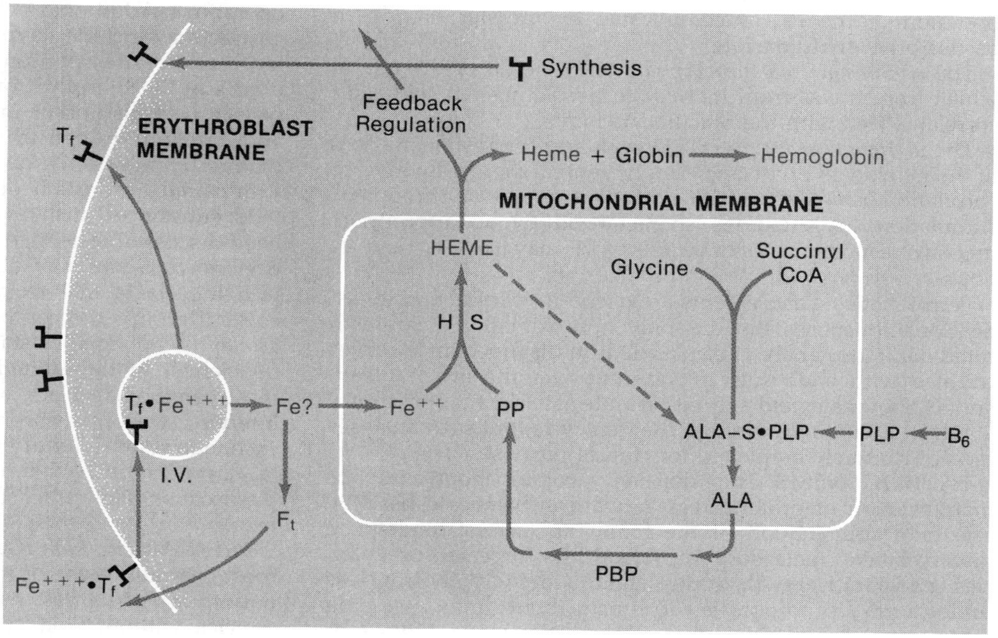

FIGURE 135–2. Diagrammatic representation of heme biosynthesis within the erythroblast. The relationships between the iron pathway, the porphyrin biosynthetic pathway, the vitamin B_6 pathway, and the synthesis of transferrin receptors are illustrated. The biosynthesis of porphyrins is dependent upon the availability of pyridoxal phosphate as a cofactor at the rate limiting Δ-aminolevulinic acid synthase step. The biosynthesis of heme requires both protoporphyrin and iron. Iron uptake is dependent upon the interaction of diferric transferrin with high affinity cell surface receptors. Receptor synthesis is regulated by heme; when heme synthesis is impaired, more receptors are synthesized and the cell takes up more iron. T_f represents transferrin receptors for diferric T_f, I.V. the acidic, nonlysosomal intermediate vesicle, Fe^{+++} ferric iron, PP protoporphyrin, PBP porphyrin biosynthetic pathway, ALA Δ-aminolevulinic acid, ALA-s Δ-aminolevulinic acid synthase, PLP pyridoxal-5′ -phosphate, and B_6 vitamin B_6.

termed H (the major subunit of heart ferritin) and L (the major subunit of liver ferritin). These may be present in differing quantities within a given ferritin molecule, leading to heterogeneity. The H and L subunits are derived from different genetic loci.

Ferritin meets the requirement of cells for an efficient form of iron storage. It has a large capacity to store iron, maintains a reserve storage capacity (few ferritin molecules are iron replete), and can quickly both take up and release iron. Ferritin aggregates are visible by light microscopy in developing erythroid cells when bone marrow smears are stained with Prussian blue. These "siderotic granules" are found in the cytosol of normal developing erythroblasts and are absent in erythroblasts obtained from subjects with iron deficiency anemia.

Small amounts of iron-poor ferritin (mostly apoferritin) circulate in plasma and can be accurately measured by a widely available radioimmunoassay. Under most conditions the concentration of ferritin in the plasma correlates directly with body iron stores. Normal values range from 12 to 325 ng per milliliter with a mean of about 125 for men and 55 for women. The concentration of ferritin in iron-deficient individuals is less than 10 ng per milliliter, whereas in individuals with iron overload the concentration is proportional to the increase in tissue storage iron.

Hemosiderin is an insoluble iron aggregate with a ratio of iron to protein that is high. It is derived from ferritin; however, the reactions leading from ferritin to hemosiderin have not been resolved. Iron in hemosiderin disappears from tissues after repeated venesections, but the mechanism by which iron is mobilized is unknown.

THE MACROPHAGE. While net iron uptake occurs through the intestinal mucosa, most transferrin-bound iron (over 95 per cent) reflects iron recycled from damaged or aged red blood cells by macrophages in the spleen and other organs. Within the macrophage the membrane of ingested erythrocytes is disrupted and the iron in hemoglobin is oxidized to the trivalent state, forming methemoglobin. The heme and globin are dissociated and the iron liberated from hemin (ferric-protoporphyrin) by the microsomal enzyme heme oxygenase, yielding iron and biliverdin. In order to meet a variable demand for iron, macrophages maintain a storage pool in ferritin and hemosiderin. Under normal conditions the amount of iron entering the macrophage approximates that leaving and there is little interchange between iron newly liberated from hemin and iron in the storage pool. Iron from recently destroyed erythrocytes passes quickly through the macrophage and appears in the plasma bound to transferrin.

When the red cell mass is expanding and erythrocytes are being produced more rapidly than they are being destroyed (e.g., following an acute hemorrhage), iron is mobilized from macrophages. The amount of iron leaving the macrophage under these conditions exceeds that entering. When red cell destruction exceeds production (e.g., in aplastic anemia), the amount of iron entering the macrophage exceeds that leaving and iron is deposited in stores. The control mechanism coupling the rate at which iron leaves the macrophage to the rate of erythrocyte production is unknown. Mobilization of iron from the storage pool is interfered with by infection, inflammation, and malignancy; such interference may be responsible for the anemia associated with chronic disease.

FERROKINETICS. Ferrokinetic studies, based on tracking ^{59}Fe as it moves from the plasma transferrin to the bone marrow and into circulating erythrocytes, make it possible to assess rates of both effective erythropoiesis and ineffective erythropoiesis. The term *ineffective erythropoiesis* refers to the production of defective erythrocytes that are destroyed before they leave the marrow (or very shortly thereafter). A small proportion of erythropoiesis is ineffective even in normal subjects, but in conditions such as megaloblastic anemia, thalassemia, and sideroblastic anemias, ineffective erythropoiesis becomes greatly exaggerated. The plasma ^{59}Fe disappearance, expressed as the half-life (t½), is normally between 60 and 120 minutes. More rapid disappearance (a shorter t½) is found in iron deficiency and conditions with accelerated erythropoiesis (such as polycythemia and hemolytic anemias). A long t½ indicates erythroid hypoplasia. The *plasma iron transport rate* (PIT) is a measure of the rate at which iron leaves the plasma. The PIT is a good index of total erythropoiesis, whether effective or ineffective. The PIT correlates well with the total nucleated red cell mass and the rate of red cell production. However, when erythropoiesis is reduced, or when the degree of transferrin saturation is high, the interpretation of the PIT is complicated by transfer of iron to tissues other than marrow.

The *erythrocyte iron turnover rate* (EIT) measures the rate at which iron moves from marrow to circulating red cells, and correlates well with the reticulocyte index.

The *marrow transit time* (MTT) evaluates the responsiveness of the marrow to erythropoietin. In general there is an inverse correlation between the MTT and the degree of erythropoietic stimulation. In situations characterized by an appropriate marrow response to anemia the MTT may be less than 24 hours.

Ferrokinetic measurements are useful for clinical and investigational purposes but are only approximations. Sophisticated computer analysis of plasma iron disappearance curves coupled with body surface counting over the liver, spleen, and sacrum may yield a more accurate assessment of the rates at which iron moves through the iron cycle, but such analyses are not routinely employed for clinical purposes.

PATHOGENESIS. Iron deficiency comes about as a late manifestation of prolonged negative iron balance caused by one or a combination of the following factors: inadequate dietary intake, malabsorption, blood loss, repeated pregnancies, and rapid growth during childhood. As daily iron loss under normal conditions is very small (about 1 mg), assigning the cause of iron deficiency in adults to inadequate intake or malabsorption implies chronicity measured in years. Iron losses that occur from the gastrointestinal tract or through excessive menstrual bleeding are far more important factors. Factors leading to negative iron balance can be divided into two broad categories: decreased iron uptake and increased iron loss (Table 135–4).

Decreased Iron Uptake. The daily dietary iron requirement for healthy adult men is about 5 to 10 mg. For premenopausal women the daily dietary requirement is higher, roughly 7 to 20 mg daily. In the United States the average diet contains about 6 mg per 1000 calories. The average man therefore consumes more iron than needed but many women subsist on a marginal iron uptake. Because of the adequacy of their diets and their larger iron stores, males in the United States rarely develop iron deficiency solely on the basis of an inadequate dietary intake of iron. Even in women some factor in addition to poor diet is usually necessary before overt anemia develops.

Gastric acid facilitates the absorption of ferric iron in the diet (although it has little effect on heme iron or ferrous iron), and iron deficiency is a frequent complication following gastric operations. Additional factors that impair iron absorption after gastrectomy include rapid intestinal transit and bypass of the most active sites of iron absorption in the duodenum (as occurs in the Billroth II or Polya procedures). Malabsorption of iron may also occur in patients with adult celiac disease, and rarely iron deficiency anemia may be the dominant manifestation of celiac disease.

TABLE 135–4. FACTORS PRODUCING NEGATIVE IRON BALANCE AND IRON DEFICIENCY

I. Decreased iron uptake
- A. Inadequate diet
- B. Impaired absorption
  1. Achlorhydria
  2. Gastric surgery
  3. Celiac disease
  4. Pica

II. Increased iron loss
- A. Gastrointestinal bleeding (Ch. 114)
  1. Neoplasm
  2. Duodenal and gastric ulcers
  3. Hiatal hernia
  4. Gastritis from salicylates, other drugs, or toxins
  5. Diverticulosis
  6. Ulcerative colitis and regional enteritis
  7. Hookworm
  8. Meckel's diverticulum
  9. Hemorrhoids
  10. Arteriovenous malformations
- B. Menometrorrhagia
- C. Repeated blood donations
- D. Repeated pregnancies
- E. Hemoglobinuria due to chronic intravascular hemolysis
- F. Hereditary hemorrhagic telangiectasia
- G. Idiopathic pulmonary hemosiderosis
- H. Disorders of hemostasis

Impaired absorption of iron because of interactions with food substances such as phytates and vegetable fibers has been discussed. The ingestion of unusual substances, a practice known as *pica,* may also impair iron absorption. Although pica may be a manifestation of iron deficiency, in certain cultural groups the compulsive ingestion of substances such as clay (geophagia) or starch (amylophagia) may lead to iron deficiency. In the United States the practice appears to be most common in black women in the southern states. Clay interferes with iron absorption by acting in the gut as an ion exchange resin. Laundry starch is a carbohydrate with a very low iron content. When it is consumed in large quantities to the exclusion of other foods, a dietary deficiency of iron results.

Increased Iron Loss. Gastrointestinal bleeding is by far the most common cause of iron deficiency in men and is second only to menstrual loss as a cause in women. Repeated pregnancies without iron supplementation are a less common cause of iron deficiency in women.

Although any hemorrhagic lesion of the gastrointestinal tract may cause iron deficiency (Table 135–4), those most likely to do so are associated with chronic occult bleeding and the steady loss of small amounts of blood. To estimate the effect of blood loss on iron balance it is convenient to consider that 1.0 ml of blood contains about 0.4 mg iron. A steady blood loss of as little as 4 to 5 ml per day (1.6 to 2.0 mg iron) can result in negative iron balance and depletion of iron stores over several years. Failure to detect occult blood in the stool, even after repetitive testing, does not exclude gastrointestinal blood loss as the cause of iron deficiency. *Iron deficiency in men and in postmenopausal women must be considered to result from blood loss unless some other cause can be proven.* This is a critical dictum because iron deficiency anemia may be the first sign of a cancer of the gastrointestinal tract, and the anemia may lead to the diagnosis when the tumor is in an operable stage. Carcinoma of the cecum, for example, is often clinically silent until the symptoms of anemia appear.

Blood loss from erosive gastritis due to aspirin ingestion is becoming an increasingly frequent cause of iron deficiency. Chronic ingestion of as few as two aspirin tablets daily may lead to blood loss of up to 4.5 ml per day.

CLINICAL MANIFESTATIONS. Iron deficiency anemia is not a disease; it is a sign of disease. In some patients, iron deficiency anemia is discovered incidentally when the presenting signs and symptoms are those of the disease that led to the deficiency. In some patients signs and symptoms of both the underlying disease and the iron deficiency are found together. In others only the symptoms of iron deficiency are present and the disease leading to the deficiency is occult.

The onset of iron deficiency anemia is insidious and the progression of symptoms is gradual. Patients are often able to accommodate quite well to the anemia and may continue to perform strenuous work with few symptoms. Fatigue, irritability, palpitations, dizziness, breathlessness, and headache are all common complaints of symptomatic individuals with anemia of any type and do not in themselves suggest iron deficiency as the cause of the anemia. However, some clinical findings do specifically suggest the presence of iron deficiency.

Chlorosis, a peculiar greenish pallor of iron-deficient adolescent girls, was frequently described in the decades between 1890 and 1910, although now is rarely noted. Oral lesions associated with iron deficiency include angular stomatitis (ulcerations or fissures at the corners of the mouth), atrophy of the lingual papillae, and varying degrees of glossitis. *Ozena* (chronic atrophy of the nasal mucosa associated with a foul-smelling discharge) occurs in some patients with iron deficiency anemia, particularly in southeastern Europe. Thinning and flattening of nails and finally the development of spoon-shaped nails (koilonychia) have been described in patients with advanced iron deficiency.

The association of dysphagia, angular stomatitis, and lingual abnormalities with iron deficiency anemia (Plummer-Vinson or Paterson-Kelly syndrome) is rarely noted in the United States but is quite common in Great Britain and Scandinavia. The dysphagia is due to the development of a mucosal web at the juncture of the hypopharynx and esophagus. Multiple webs may develop, usually extending from the anterior wall of the esophagus into the lumen. Occasionally they may encircle the lumen, forming a cufflike structure. In other patients a stricture with or without a web may be found, drastically constricting the opening into the esophagus at the level of the cricoid cartilage. Relief of the dysphagia requires rupturing of the webs or dilatation of the stenosis, because repletion of the iron stores alone is not effective. Other gastrointestinal complaints such as anorexia, pyrosis, flatulence, nausea, belching, and constipation are common in association with advanced iron deficiency anemia.

Pica, as already mentioned, can be a cause of iron deficiency but it also may be a striking manifestation of iron deficiency. The ingestion of ice (pagophagia) is particularly common. Many patients compulsively eat one or other food items; oddly, the object of the unnatural dietary craving usually contains very little iron.

The spleen is slightly enlarged in about 10 per cent of patients with iron deficiency anemia. There are no specific pathologic changes in the organ and the splenomegaly recedes with correction of the iron deficiency. Neuralgic pains, numbness, and tingling without objective neurologic abnormalities are reported by 15 to 30 per cent of patients and rarely iron deficiency anemia may lead to increased intracranial pressure, papilledema, and the clinical picture of pseudotumor cerebri.

LABORATORY FINDINGS. The degree of anemia is variable and depends upon the duration of iron-limited erythropoiesis. Because of the hypochromia the hemoglobin concentration is usually reduced to a greater degree than the hematocrit. The mean corpuscular volume (MCV), mean corpuscular hemoglobin (MCH), and mean corpuscular hemoglobin concentration (MCHC) are all usually reduced. The degree of change in the red cell indices is related to both the duration and the severity of the anemia. Average values for patients with hemoglobin concentrations of 8 to 9 grams per deciliter are MCV of 74 fl, MCHC 28 grams per deciliter, and MCH of 20 pg.

A well-stained blood smear reveals an increase in the area of central pallor in the individual red corpuscles (hypochromia), microcytes, and marked variations in cell size (anisocytosis) and shape (poikilocytosis) (Fig. 135–3 and Color plate 2*D*). The plasma iron concentration is generally less than 50 μg per deciliter, and the total plasma iron-binding capacity (the transferrin concentration) is greater than 350 μg per deciliter. As a result the transferrin saturation is less than 15 per cent. The plasma ferritin concentration is generally less than 10 ng per milliliter. The last enzymatic reaction leading to the biosynthesis of heme (the ferrochelatase or heme synthase reaction) requires both iron and protoporphyrin as substrates. In iron deficiency excess protoporphyrin accumulates in the developing erythrocyte and is retained by the circulating erythrocytes. As a result the free erythrocyte protoporphyrin (FEP) is increased, generally about five times normal (normal range, 30 to 80 μg per deciliter of red cells).

Both the percentage and the absolute number of reticulocytes are usually normal. The osmotic fragility of the erythrocytes may be normal, but more often there is increased resistance to hemolysis in hypotonic salt solutions. Although the leukocyte count is usually normal, in very chronic iron deficiency a slight decrease in the absolute number of granulocytes may be seen. The platelet count is usually elevated to levels of about two to three times normal and returns to normal after therapy. Rarely, in severe, longstanding iron deficiency anemia, mild thrombocytopenia may be noted.

Examination of the bone marrow is generally not required to establish a diagnosis of iron deficiency anemia. An exception is the clinical situation when suspected iron deficiency coexists with a chronic disease. Although anemias associated with chronic disease may mimic iron deficiency (see below), they can be distinguished by examination of the marrow. In iron deficiency the marrow is usually normocellular and there is mild erythroid hyperplasia. Macrophage iron is absent or severely reduced. Fewer than 10 per cent of the marrow normoblasts contain siderotic granules visible with Prussian blue staining. In the anemia of chronic disease macrophage iron stores are normal or increased; however, as in iron deficiency, very few normoblasts contain siderotic granules.

The sequence of laboratory changes in slowly developing iron deficiency is fairly predictable. Initially, as iron stores are depleted, the serum ferritin concentration falls. At the earliest stage of iron deficiency the transferrin concentration rises, the plasma iron concentration falls, and the FEP increases. When

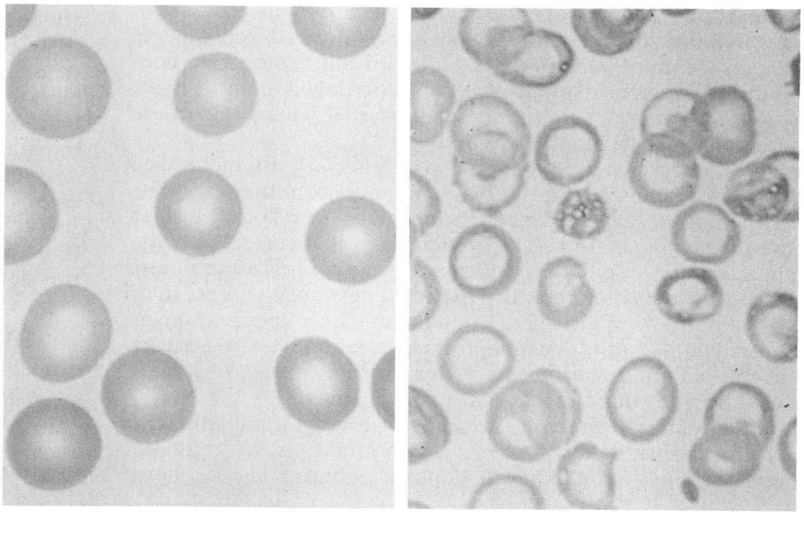

FIGURE 135–3. Blood smear from a patient with advanced iron deficiency anemia (*right*) and from a normal subject (*left*). The red cells from the iron-deficient subject are poorly hemoglobinized (hypochromic), smaller than normal (microcytic), and vary in size and shape (anisocytosis and poikilocytosis). (Wright's stain, × 1000.)

anemia first appears the morphology of the circulating erythrocytes and the erythrocyte indices are generally normal. As the anemia progresses the morphology becomes clearly hypochromic and microcytic and the indices reflect this.

TREATMENT. *Every effort must be made to recognize and if possible correct the underlying cause.* This should be possible in most patients. A simpler goal is correcting the anemia and replenishing body iron stores.

Iron is highly effective in treating iron deficiency but has no other legitimate therapeutic use. Iron exerts no beneficial effect on any of the anemias not caused by iron deficiency. A large number of preparations containing iron have been promoted for the oral treatment of iron deficiency, but none has any advantage over simple ferrous salts (ferrous sulfate, ferrous gluconate, and ferrous fumarate). Ferrous sulfate is the standard preparation for oral use. A daily dose of about 200 mg of elemental iron produces an optimal response. This dose is achieved with three ferrous sulfate tablets (each tablet contains 60 mg of elemental iron) given in divided doses with or just after a meal. Iron is best absorbed when the stomach is empty, but gastric irritation is extremely common when iron is taken this way. In spite of some reduction in absorption when iron is taken with meals, the gain in patient compliance is worth this slight disadvantage. Enteric-coated preparations, designed to reduce gastric irritation by retarding dissolution of the iron, cannot be recommended because with them the most actively absorbing regions of the intestine are bypassed and absorption is markedly reduced. Although large doses of ascorbic or succinic acid will increase iron absorption as much as 20 to 30 per cent, they add greatly to the expense of therapy.

Some patients given oral iron therapy complain of gastrointestinal symptoms (nausea, epigastric pain, cramps, diarrhea); however, it is rare that these symptoms are severe enough to require discontinuation of therapy. Gastric symptoms appear to be dose related and patients intolerant of full therapeutic doses may be able to take a dose of 120 mg per day. Gastric symptoms may be minimized by gradually increasing the dose during the first week of therapy. Regardless of the form of oral therapy used, it is important to continue treatment for 6 to 12 months after the anemia has been corrected. The prolonged therapy allows for repletion of iron stores.

When adequate doses of iron are given, there is often a rapid subjective improvement with a reduction of fatigue, lassitude, and other nonspecific symptoms. This response may occur within two or three days, before any evidence of a hematologic response can be detected. An increase in the number of reticulocytes is the first sign of hematologic response, and a maximal value of 5 to 10 per cent is usually achieved after about ten days of therapy. The height of the reticulocyte peak and the rate of hemoglobin regeneration are proportional to the severity of the anemia. With only slight to moderate degrees of anemia a pronounced reticulocyte response cannot be expected. Although the hemoglobin concentration increases more rapidly at low levels than at high, it takes about two months to reach normal values regardless of the starting level.

It is not rare to encounter patients said to have iron deficiency anemia unresponsive to oral iron therapy. The following possible explanations for failure to respond to iron should be considered: (1) The diagnosis is incorrect and the anemia is not due to iron deficiency; (2) a complicating illness is present that dampens the expected response to iron therapy; (3) the patient failed to take the iron preparation as prescribed; (4) an ineffective iron preparation was prescribed; (5) the patient is continuing to lose iron in excess of intake; and rarely (6) there is malabsorption of iron.

Parenteral iron therapy should be reserved for patients who (1) are unable to tolerate iron compounds given orally, (2) repeatedly fail to heed instructions or are incapable of following them, (3) are losing blood at a rate too rapid to be compensated by oral iron intake, (4) have a disorder such as ulcerative colitis or regional enteritis in which symptoms may be aggravated by oral iron therapy, or (5) are unable to absorb iron from the gastrointestinal tract.

Iron-dextran complex (Imferon) containing 50 mg of iron per milliliter is the preparation of choice for parenteral administration. The total dose required to correct the anemia and to replenish stores can be calculated by the following formula:

$$\text{Iron to be injected (mg)} = [15\text{-patient's Hb (gm/dl)}] \times \text{body weight (kg)} \times 3$$

Iron-dextran can be given intramuscularly or intravenously. Intravenous administration does not appear to have a higher incidence of adverse effects than the intramuscular route. Anaphylactic reactions are rare (0.1–0.6 per cent), but fever, arthralgia, myalgia, and regional adenopathy occur in about 5 per cent of patients. Intramuscular injections should be made into the upper outer quadrant of the buttock, and the skin displaced laterally prior to injection to prevent staining of the skin by reflux of the dark-brown iron solution along the injection path. A test dose of 0.5 ml should be given initially to test for hypersensitivity. Generally 2.5 ml is injected into each buttock (total 5 ml or 250 mg of iron) daily. Intravenous administration permits larger doses to be given in a single injection; thus the discomfort and inconvenience of repeated intramuscular injections can be avoided. After testing for hypersensitivity, 10 ml (500 mg of iron) of undiluted iron-dextran may be administered over about a five-minute period. In Great Britain and Europe it is usual to administer the entire dose calculated by the formula in a single intravenous infusion. A 1:20 dilution of iron-dextran in saline is prepared and administered at an initial flow rate of 20 drops per minute. After five minutes, if no side effects are observed, the rate is increased to 40 to 60 drops per minute. Dextrose solutions should not be used as a diluent because the incidence of superficial phlebitis may be as high as 25 per cent with this vehicle.

PROGNOSIS. The prognosis in iron deficiency relates only to the underlying disorder causing the anemia. Patients rarely if ever die of iron deficiency anemia itself, but may die of the underlying cause. Recurrence of iron deficiency anemia after treatment is common, emphasizing the importance of identifying and effectively treating the cause of the iron deficiency.

HYPOCHROMIC ANEMIAS NOT CAUSED BY IRON DEFICIENCY

Once iron deficiency has been excluded as the cause of a hypochromic anemia, a limited number of diagnostic possibilities remain. A presumptive diagnosis is generally possible after analysis of the history and physical examination and the basic hematologic parameters. If the diagnosis remains obscure, a useful approach is to segregate the diagnostic possibilities on the basis of an accurate determination of the serum iron. When the serum iron is reduced to levels at which the transferrin saturation is less than about 15 per cent, only iron deficiency and the anemia of chronic disease need be considered.

Hypochromic anemias due to defects in globin biosynthesis (the thalassemias and hemoglobinopathies characterized by unstable hemoglobins) are discussed in Ch. 142 and 144.

THE ANEMIA OF CHRONIC DISEASE

The anemia of chronic disease is not always hypochromic; however, because of its association with hypoferremia, it is best discussed under the heading of hypochromic anemias. Although the anemia of chronic disease is usually normocytic and normochromic, hypochromia and even microcytosis may be the dominant morphologic abormalities. When microcytosis is present it is usually not as marked as in iron deficiency. The MCV rarely falls below 72 fl.

DEFINITION. A mild-to-moderate anemia frequently accompanies chronic infections, inflammatory diseases such as rheumatoid arthritis, and cancers. Since these are so common, the anemia of chronic disease is frequently encountered and may be second only to iron deficiency anemia in overall incidence. The anemia of chronic disease is defined by the presence of a chronic disease, anemia, and hypoferremia despite abundant quantities of iron in macrophage stores.

ETIOLOGY AND PATHOGENESIS. Three factors seem to interact in the pathogenesis of the anemia: (1) impaired flow of iron from macrophages to plasma, (2) decreased erythrocyte lifespan, and (3) inadequate marrow response to the mild hemolysis.

Characteristically, the serum iron is decreased, total iron binding capacity is reduced (a point often useful in differentiating the anemia from iron deficiency anemia), and transferrin saturation is subnormal. Injection of ^{59}Fe-labeled red cells (or labeled hemoglobin) reveals rapid clearance by reticuloendothelial cells but defective reutilization of the iron for new hemoglobin synthesis. In bone marrow aspirates stained for iron there is an increase in hemosiderin and ferritin in the macrophages; however, the number of red cell precursors containing siderotic granules is reduced. A decrease in the amount of iron available for heme biosynthesis results in the production of hypochromic erythrocytes and, as in iron deficiency, an increase in free erythrocyte protoporphyrin (FEP) to levels of three to five times normal. In contrast to iron deficiency anemia the FEP increases slowly and does not become clearly abnormal until significant anemia has developed. A humoral factor has been implicated in the pathogenesis of the abnormal iron metabolism. This factor, termed *leukocyte endogenous mediator* (LEM), is released from neutrophils and macrophages during phagocytosis or after stimulation by bacterial toxins. LEM is a low molecular weight protein that, when injected into experimental animals, produces the abnormalities of iron metabolism that characterize the anemia of chronic disease.

The erythrocyte lifespan is about 80 days rather than the normal 120 days. When red cells from a patient with the anemia of chronic disease are transfused into normal subjects they survive normally. Conversely, normal red cells have a shortened survival when transfused into patients with anemia. This suggests that an extracorpuscular factor is involved in the pathogenesis of the hemolysis. However, no such factor has yet been identified. Normally the bone marrow should be able to compensate for such a modest reduction in erythrocyte survival. Failure of the marrow to do so implies that impaired production capacity is important in the pathogenesis of the anemia. The marrow response to anemia is under the control of erythropoietin. In patients with the anemia of chronic disorders erythropoietin levels are usually lower than expected for the degree of anemia. The marrow, however, is capable of responding appropriately to erythropoietin when the hormone is injected or when erythropoietin production is stimulated by hypoxia or cobalt administration. The precise mechanism causing failure of erythropoietin release in response to the slowly developing anemia is unknown.

The three basic abnormalities are interrelated in the pathogenesis of the anemia. For example, the response to erythropoietin suggests that the hormone directly or indirectly affects the block in iron metabolism. It appears that balance is eventually reached among the three factors, and thus the anemia is only mild to moderate and does not generally progress to the point at which transfusion therapy is required.

CLINICAL MANIFESTATIONS. Because this type of anemia occurs in association with so many diseases, the clinical manifestations vary widely. Although the signs and symptoms of the underlying disorder usually overshadow those of the anemia, in occasional patients the anemia is the first sign of the underlying disease.

DIAGNOSIS. The anemia develops during the first few months of the underlying illness and rarely progresses thereafter. The hematocrit generally remains constant in a range between 25 and 40 per cent. The red cell morphology is usually normal as is the reticulocyte count. The characteristic iron determinations are a transferrin saturation less than 15 per cent with a normal serum ferritin. In the marrow there is a decrease in the number of erythroid precursors containing cytoplasmic iron granules (sideroblasts), but reticuloendothelial cells contain normal or increased iron stores. Despite the hemolysis, the usual manifestations of increased blood destruction are absent. The serum bilirubin and the excretion of urobilinogen are generally normal.

TREATMENT. Correction of the anemia depends upon successful treatment of the underlying disease. Blood transfusions are not usually necessary because the anemia is generally mild to moderate and is not progressive. Therapy with cobalt, androgenic steroids, and corticosteroids offers more potential for harm than good. The block to iron flow cannot be bypassed and the administration of oral or parenteral iron is of no benefit. When bleeding causes superimposed iron deficiency, the administration of iron will restore hemoglobin levels to those of the underlying chronic disorder but not back to normal.

SIDEROBLASTIC ANEMIA

DEFINITION. When hypochromic anemia is associated with hyperferremia and increased transferrin saturation, a diagnosis of sideroblastic anemia is suggested. The sideroblastic anemias are a heterogeneous group of disorders associated with various defects in the porphyrin biosynthetic pathway. Porphyrin biosynthetic defects lead to diminished synthesis of heme, which in turn may be associated with an increase in cellular iron uptake (Fig. 135–2). The sideroblastic anemias are characterized by the association of anemia with the presence of an abnormal erythroid precursor in the marrow. The abnormal precursor, the ringed sideroblast, is a normoblast containing excessive deposits of iron within mitochondria. These iron-laden mitochondria, because of their perinuclear distribution, account for the Prussian blue–positive granules forming a full or partial ring around the nucleus of the ringed sideroblast (Color plate 2*H*). Normal sideroblasts contain one to four Prussian blue–positive ferritin aggregates in the cytoplasm and no visible iron in mitochondria.

PATHOGENESIS AND CLASSIFICATION. Mitochondrial iron excess appears to be a consequence of defective heme synthesis. A population of hypochromic erythrocytes, common to all the sideroblastic anemias, is morphologic evidence of the synthetic defect. Other common characteristics include abnormalities in porphyrin biosynthesis; an increase in total body iron stores; an increase in the serum iron concentration, often to the point of complete saturation of transferrin; and kinetic evidence of ineffective erythropoiesis. It is customary to divide the sideroblastic anemias into two groups, depending on whether the disorder appears to be acquired or inherited (Table 135–2).

Acquired Sideroblastic Anemias

IDIOPATHIC REFRACTORY SIDEROBLASTIC ANEMIA. This acquired disease of older adults has an unknown pathogenesis. The anemia develops insidiously and is often discovered during a routine examination. The anemia is usually slightly macrocytic. Examination of the peripheral blood smear reveals two populations of erythrocytes. One is entirely normal and the other is macrocytic and quite hypochromic with prominent basophilic stippling. Leukocyte and platelet counts are usually normal but leukopenia is occasionally noted and either moderate thrombocytopenia or thrombocytosis has been reported. FEP is increased, but the precise enzymatic defect(s) in porphyrin biosynthesis has not been defined. About 30 to 40 per cent of patients have a palpable spleen. Therapy with pyridoxine or folic acid is not successful and only rare patients respond to androgens. The median survival for patients with idiopathic refractory sideroblastic anemia is about ten years; most patients require no therapy. Transfusion therapy should be kept to a minimum because the chronic administration of erythrocytes has led to transfusional hemochromatosis. Therapy with daily subcutaneous infusions of deferoxamine may be of value to selected patients who require repeated transfusion. The condition in about 10 per cent of patients eventually shows evidence of transformation to acute leukemia. No reliable indicators predict the likelihood of leukemic transformation. The closest association between the development of leukemia and the presence of ringed sideroblasts is noted when sideroblastic anemia occurs following chemotherapy for a variety of malignant disorders. Alkylating drugs such as cyclophosphamide, nitrogen mustard, and melphalan are the most common offenders.

SIDEROBLASTIC ANEMIA COMPLICATING OTHER DISEASES. Acquired sideroblastic anemia associated with other diseases and with drugs or toxins is quite common; however, the anemia is usually only mild. Inflammatory diseases such as rheumatoid arthritis, neoplasms, and a variety of primary hematologic disorders have all been associated with a secondary sideroblastic anemia. The treatment, course, and prognosis are all related to the nature of the associated disease.

SIDEROBLASTIC ANEMIA ASSOCIATED WITH DRUGS OR TOXINS. Sideroblastic anemia is a common complication in hospitalized alcoholics. Withdrawal of alcohol results in a reticulocytosis and disappearance of the ringed sideroblasts within five to ten days. *Alcohol* may cause sideroblastic anemia by interfering with pyridoxine metabolism and thus indirectly affecting the activity of Δ-aminolevulinic acid synthetase, the rate-limiting enzyme in the porphyrin biosynthetic pathway. This mechanism likely also underlies the sideroblastic anemia occasionally seen in association with the administration of the antituberculous agent *isonicotinic acid hydrazide* (INH). The sideroblastic anemia that occurs in *lead poisoning* is caused by the inhibition by lead of the enzyme that converts Δ-aminolevulinic acid to porphobilinogen (Δ-aminolevulinic dehydratase) and the enzyme heme synthetase (ferrochelatase). As a result of these two enzymatic defects it is possible to screen for lead poisoning by detecting either increased urinary excretion of Δ-aminolevulinic acid or a markedly increased FEP.

Hereditary Sideroblastic Anemias

Hereditary sideroblastic anemia is almost always a disease of males and is most likely inherited as an X-linked recessive trait. Although the anemia is usually detected in the late teenage years, in rare cases the anemia is found first in either infancy or adult life. The anemia is severe (average blood hemoglobin 6.5 grams per deciliter) and the red cell indices indicate marked microcytosis and hypochromia. The inherited defect in some way involves the interaction between Δ-aminolevulinic acid synthetase and its cofactor pyridoxal phosphate. Individuals with hereditary sideroblastic anemia are not pyridoxine deficient; however, large amounts of vitamin B_6 produce partial correction of the anemia.

Beutler E, Fairbanks VF: The effects of iron deficiency. In Jacobs A, Worwood M (eds.): Iron in Biochemistry and Medicine II. New York, Academic Press, 1980, pp 394–428. *An extensive review of both the hematologic and nonhematologic manifestations of iron deficiency.*

Jacobs A (ed.): Disorders of iron metabolism. Clin Hematol 11:1, 1982. *A collection of review articles covering basic physiology, clinical diagnosis, and patient management of iron deficiency, sideroblastic anemias, and iron overload.*

Miescher PA, Jaffe ER, Finch CA (eds.): Semin Hematol vol. 19, no. 1, 1984. *An issue of a respected review journal devoted to the clinical aspects of iron deficiency and excess.*

Ward JH, Kushner JP, Kaplan J: Iron: Metabolism and clinical disorders. In Fairbanks VF (ed.): Current Hematology and Oncology. New York, John Wiley & Sons, 1984, vol 3, pp 1–50. *A review of basic iron metabolism with an extensive list of references.*

Williams WJ, Beutler E, Erslev AJ, et al. (eds.): Hematology. 3rd ed. New York, McGraw-Hill Book Company, 1983. *A comprehensive textbook of hematology with an excellent presentation of basic iron metabolism and its application to clinical medicine.*

Wintrobe MM, Lee GR, Boggs DR, et al. (eds.): Clinical Hematology. 8th ed. Philadelphia, Lea & Febiger, 1981. *The oldest standard textbook of hematology with an exhaustive description of the clinical manifestations of iron deficiency anemia.*

136 MEGALOBLASTIC ANEMIAS

William S. Beck

DEFINITION. Megaloblastic anemia (often a pancytopenia) is due to impaired DNA synthesis and is manifested by a readily recognized pattern of morphologic changes in bone marrow and blood cells that include giantism of these cells—and indeed of all proliferating cells in most cases—and various evidences of retarded cell division. The anemia is ordinarily macrocytic—i.e., the mean corpuscular volume (MCV) exceeds 100 cu μm—although not all macrocytic anemias are megaloblastic.

ETIOLOGY. Megaloblastic anemia is easily diagnosed in most cases. The differential diagnosis of the underlying disorder, however, may be more difficult because defective DNA synthesis can have many causes. It is convenient to divide the megaloblastic anemias into three major etiologic categories: (1) those that are associated with cobalamin (vitamin B_{12}) deficiency and respond to cobalamin therapy, (2) those that are associated with folate deficiency and respond to folic acid (pteroylmonoglutamate) therapy, and (3) those unresponsive to cobalamin or folic acid therapy. Deficiencies of cobalamin and folate may themselves have a great many specific causes. Pernicious anemia, for example, is but one cause of cobalamin deficiency. Accurate differential diagnosis is important because it guides the choice of therapy and usually discloses a significant underlying disorder.

The major etiologic categories and their underlying causes are summarized in Table 136–1. Cobalamin deficiency and folate deficiency are by far the most common categories. Together with iron deficiency anemia they constitute the bulk of the so-called nutritional anemias, which are among the most common of human ills. Both vitamin deficiencies lead to tissue coenzyme deficiencies that are usually corrected easily by repletion of the lacking vitamin. Hematopoiesis then reverts from megaloblastic to normoblastic. Other mechanisms obviously account for the megaloblastic anemias that are unresponsive to therapy with cobalamin and folic acid.

The approach to a patient suspected of megaloblastic anemia should proceed through several orderly steps. First, it is determined from the reticulocyte count and other tests whether a macrocytic anemia is due to bone marrow failure or erythrocyte loss or destruction. If marrow failure, the presence of megaloblastosis is established by demonstrating in blood and bone marrow the characteristic morphologic features to be described below. The broad etiologic category is then elucidated with serum vitamin assays and other procedures to be discussed. One then seeks a specific causal mechanism, administers specific treatment, and observes the response to treatment.

PATHOGENESIS AND PATHOLOGY OF MEGALOBLASTIC ANEMIA. The following discussion deals with the general features of megaloblastic anemia per se, irrespective of cause. The features of cobalamin and folate deficiency, irrespective of cause, and the major disorders responsible for these deficiencies will then be discussed.

TABLE 136–1. ETIOLOGIC CLASSIFICATION OF THE MEGALOBLASTIC ANEMIAS

Category	Etiologic Mechanisms
I. Cobalamin deficiency	
A. Decreased ingestion	Poor diet, lack of animal products, strict vegetarianism
B. Impaired absorption	1. Intrinsic factor deficiency
	Pernicious anemia
	Gastrectomy (total and partial)
	Destruction of gastric mucosa by caustics
	Anti-IF antibody in gastric juice
	Abnormal intrinsic factor molecule
	2. Intrinsic intestinal disease
	Familial selective malabsorption (Imerslund's syndrome)
	Ileal resection, ileitis
	Sprue, celiac disease
	Infiltrative intestinal disease (e.g., lymphoma, scleroderma)
	Drug-induced malabsorption
	3. Competitive parasites
	Fish tapeworm infestations (*Diphyllobothrium latum*)
	Bacteria in diverticula of bowel, blind loops
	4. Chronic pancreatic disease
C. Increased requirement	Pregnancy
	Neoplastic disease
	Hyperthyroidism
D. Impaired utilization	Enzyme deficiencies
	Abnormal serum cobalamin binding protein
	Lack of transcobalamin II
	Nitrous oxide administration
II. Folate deficiency	
A. Decreased ingestion	Poor diet, lack of vegetables
	Alcoholism
	Infancy
B. Impaired absorption	Intestinal short circuits
	Steatorrhea
	Sprue, celiac disease
	Intrinsic intestinal disease
	Anticonvulsants, oral contraceptives, other drugs
C. Increased requirement	Pregnancy, infancy
	Hyperthyroidism
	Hyperactive hematopoiesis
	Neoplastic disease, exfoliative skin disease
D. Impaired utilization	Folic acid antagonists: methotrexate, triamterene, trimethoprim
	Enzyme deficiencies
E. Increased loss	Hemodialysis
III. Unresponsive to cobalamin or folate therapy	
A. Metabolic inhibitors	Purine synthesis: 6-mercaptopurine, 6-thioguanine, azathioprine
	Pyrimidine synthesis: 6-azauridine
	Thymidylate synthesis: methotrexate, 5-fluorouracil
	Deoxyribonucleotide synthesis: hydroxyurea, cytosine arabinoside, severe iron deficiency
B. Inborn errors	Lesch-Nyhan syndrome
	Hereditary orotic aciduria
	Deficiency of formimino-transferase, methyltransferase, etc.
C. Unexplained disorders	Pyridoxine-responsive megaloblastic anemia
	Thiamine-responsive megaloblastic anemia
	Erythremic myelosis (Di Guglielmo's syndrome)

Mechanism of Megaloblastosis. Megaloblasts contain an increased amount of RNA and a normal or slightly increased amount of DNA per cell, the former presumably accounting for the cytoplasmic basophilia (blue color) in Wright's-stained smears. Thymidine is readily incorporated into their DNA. Hence, DNA synthesis can occur. There is, however, impairment of a critical step in the pathway of DNA synthesis—the synthesis of thymidylate (dTMP). In addition, there is a sharp increase in intracellular dUMP and dUTP levels and thus of the dUTP/dTTP ratio. As a result there is significant misincorporation of uracil into DNA. Much of this uracil is removed by an "editorial" enzyme system, but lack of available dTTP blocks final DNA repair. Hence, DNA is fragmented and DNA replication and cell division are blocked, while synthesis of RNA and protein proceed normally. Prolongation of this state results in permanent loss of the capacity for cell division and eventual cell death. In megaloblastic bone marrow the degree of impairment of DNA synthesis varies from cell to cell and from cell series to cell series. Usually, it is more severe among erythrocyte precursors than granulocyte precursors.

Morphology of Megaloblastic Cells (Color plate 2*F*). The features characteristic of the megaloblastic state are seen most vividly in the Wright's-stained smear of aspirated bone marrow. Among *erythrocyte precursors* megaloblastic changes occur at all stages of development. They are larger than corresponding cells of the normoblastic series and often have a higher than normal ratio of cytoplasmic area to nuclear area. Promegaloblasts, the most immature of the series and the most easily recognized, display brilliantly colored, deeply basophilic (blue), granule-free cytoplasm and lavender-tinted chromatin with a distinctive open and fine-grained texture that contrasts with strand-like pronormoblast chromatin. As the cell matures, the chromatin retains its odd texture and is slow to form coarse deeply basophilic clumps. Development of a dense pyknotic nucleus like that of an orthochromatic normoblast either fails to occur or is delayed. With the appearance of hemoglobin, the apparent maturity of the cytoplasm contrasts sharply with the apparent immaturity of the nucleus—a feature termed nuclear-cytoplasmic asynchronism. All of these changes are less well developed in mild or incipient megaloblastic anemias or in megaloblastic anemias associated with iron deficiency.

Granulocyte precursors may also display nuclear-cytoplasmic asynchronism and enlargement, most strikingly at the metamyelocyte stage. A "giant metamyelocyte" has ragged chromatin and a relatively large nucleus, sometimes of bizarre shape, that takes stain poorly and may be pinched off in several places, in anticipation perhaps of later hypersegmentation (Color plate 2*E*).

The *bone marrow* is extremely cellular, especially when anemia is severe. Megaloblastic changes may be seen in all cell lines, although major changes may be limited to the erythroid cells (Color plate 2*F*). Many mitotic figures (i.e., cells in metaphase) are found among them. The myeloid/erythroid ratio typically falls from 3 to about 1. Megaloblastic granulopoiesis is more evident in infection, in which increased granulocyte production has been stimulated. Unless iron deficiency is present, iron in reticulum cells is increased.

In the *blood*, erythrocytes usually display striking variations in size and shape and are normochromic (unless iron deficiency coexists) and macrocytic, with MCV's ranging from 100 to more than 140 cu μm. Macro-ovalocytes, large oval-shaped erythrocytes up to 14 μm in diameter, are usually present (Color plate 2*E*). The reticulocyte count is often lower than normal, both in absolute and relative (percentage) terms. Erythrocyte changes become more severe as the anemia worsens. When the hematocrit is low (<20 per cent), nucleated red cells may appear in the blood.

Many neutrophils have more than four segments; occasionally some have up to 16 segments. Hypersegmented neutrophils, or macropolycytes, may be quite large. This is a significant finding, because it is not masked by coexisting iron deficiency and in folate deficiency tends to occur before bone marrow cells are overtly megaloblastic. Hypersegmentation is probably due to abnormalities of nuclear division and chromatin.

Megaloblastosis actually occurs in all proliferating body cells, which share the underlying defect in DNA synthesis.

Thus epithelial cells of buccal mucosa, stomach, and vagina all display typical morphologic and biochemical abnormalities. These changes in many patients with cobalamin and folate deficiency account for such phenomena as glossitis (and mouth soreness), secondary gastric atrophy (and dyspepsia), and secondary malabsorption.

Pathophysiologic Features of the Megaloblastic State. Whatever its cause, megaloblastic anemia is associated with two pathophysiologic abnormalities: ineffective erythropoiesis and moderate hemolysis.

Ineffective erythropoiesis is indicated by (1) the marked increase in marrow erythroid precursors and the high ratio of erythroid precursors to released erythrocytes; (2) increase in plasma iron turnover to three to five times the normal level, despite the fact that iron uptake by individual erythroid precursors is normal; (3) decreased rate of reappearance of labeled plasma iron in blood erythrocytes; and (4) various signs of intramedullary destruction of megaloblasts. These include increased production of "early-labeled peak" bilirubin and endogenous carbon monoxide, phagocytosis of megaloblastic erythroid precursors by marrow reticulum cells, and high serum levels of lactic dehydrogenase (isozymes 1 and 2, which come from erythroid percursors) and muramidase (from leukocyte precursors). Other findings are slight to moderate increases in serum bilirubin, iron, and iron saturation, and decreases in haptoglobin (owing to ongoing hemolysis) and, in some patients, serum uric acid (owing to decreased DNA synthesis). Even when serum uric acid is not depressed, it usually rises sharply soon after the start of specific therapy.

Intramedullary hemolysis results from this ineffective erythropoiesis. A substantial degree of extramedullary hemolysis also occurs. Erythrocyte lifespan is moderately decreased (to one-half to one-third normal) when patient erythrocytes are infused into normal subjects, classic evidence of an intracorpuscular defect. Decreased survival of normal erythrocytes infused into untreated patients suggests the presence of an extracorpuscular defect as well.

Inadequate production of myeloid cells accounts for the neutropenia of megaloblastic anemia. Elevated serum muramidase levels reflect the increased rate of intramedullary myeloid cell destruction. Thus, the mechanism of leukopenia is ineffective granulopoiesis. Ineffective thrombopoiesis also occurs; its pathophysiology parallels that of ineffective erythropoiesis and granulopoiesis. A decreased rate of platelet production (despite the presence of megakaryocytes) accounts for the mild to moderate thrombocytopenia observed in many patients with megaloblastic anemia.

Unless iron deficiency is present, ineffective erythropoiesis is associated with features suggesting iron overload: increased plasma iron and iron saturation, increased plasma iron turnover, decreased incorporation of plasma iron into circulating hemoglobin, accumulation of iron in marrow reticulum cells, and increased iron stores in the liver (hepatic siderosis) and other tissues.

MEGALOBLASTIC ANEMIA OF COBALAMIN DEFICIENCY

Classic studies of pernicious anemia led directly or indirectly to much of our early knowledge of cobalamin. Until the demonstration by Minot and Murphy in 1926 of the successful treatment of pernicious anemia by feeding liver, the disease was often fatal. Potent liver extracts soon replaced oral liver, but difficulties plagued investigators attempting to purify the anti-pernicious anemia principle of liver. Cobalamin was finally discovered in 1948 when proportionality was found between the nutrient activity of liver extracts in cultures of *Lactobacillus lactis* Dorner and their therapeutic activity in pernicious anemia. The resulting microbiologic assay rapidly facilitated purification and identification of the vitamin.

Metabolic and Nutritional Aspects of Cobalamin. Cobalamin is synthesized only by certain microorganisms. Wherever it is found in nature, it can be traced to microorganisms growing in soil, sewage, intestine, or rumen. Animals thus depend ultimately upon microbial synthesis for their cobalamin supply. Foods in the human diet that contain cobalamin are essentially those of animal origin: meat, liver, fish, eggs, and milk. The average daily diet in Western countries contains 5 to 30 μg of cobalamin, of which only 1 to 5 μg (the minimal daily requirement) is absorbed. Total body content is 2 to 5 mg in an adult man; approximately 1 mg is in the liver. Hence, a deficiency state will not develop for several years after cessation of cobalamin absorption.

The cobalamin molecule (Fig. 136–1) includes a porphyrin-like moiety (termed *corrin*) and a central cobalt atom. The four cobalamins of importance in animal cell metabolism are *cyanocobalamin* (CN-Cbl) and its analogue *hydroxocobalamin* (OH-Cbl), and two coenzyme forms—*adenosylcobalamin* (AdoCbl) and *methylcobalamin* (MeCbl). In adenosylcobalamin, a 5′-deoxyadenosyl moiety is the ligand of cobalt. This compound, the main storage form of cobalamin in liver, is the coenzyme of *methylmalonyl CoA mutase*, an enzyme catalyzing the final step in the pathway of propionic acid metabolism, in which methylmalonyl CoA is converted to succinyl CoA. This is the major AdoCbl-dependent reaction in animal tissues. Methylcobalamin, which occurs in small amounts in liver but is the major cobalamin in serum, is the coenzyme for the conversion of homocysteine to methionine (Fig. 136–2). This methyltransferase enzyme serves primarily as a means for converting N^5-methyltetrahydrofolate (N^5-methyl FH_4) to tetrahydrofolate (FH_4).

Impairment of DNA synthesis in cobalamin deficiency has been attributed to slowing of the cobalamin-dependent pathway of methionine synthesis. This sequesters folate as N^5-methyl FH_4, a form that is unavailable to the critical thymidylate synthetase reaction. This theory, the so-called methylfolate trap theory, is supported by the occurrence in cobalamin deficiency of elevated serum folate (N^5-methyl FH_4) levels. Folate coenzymes in tissues are in the form of polyglutamates. The enzyme converting folate (folylmonoglutamate) to folylpolyglutamate is most active with FH_4 as substrate and is relatively inactive with N^5-methyl FH_4. When the latter form accumulates in cobalamin deficiency, it is unavailable for conversion to folylpolyglutamate, and thymidylate synthetase is further deprived of its essential cofactor. This situation accounts for depressed levels of folylpolyglutamates in cobalamin-deficient tissues.

Cobalamin in food is liberated by peptic enzymes and acid in gastric juice. The vitamin is then bound by one or more proteins in gastric juice. Electrophoresis reveals two binders or classes of binders in gastric juice, one with slow and one with rapid mobility, that have been designated *S-proteins* and *R-proteins*, respectively (Table 136–2). One of the binding proteins in gastric juice is intrinsic factor (IF), a glycoprotein of molecular weight 44,000 that binds a molecule of cobalamin with high affinity. Secretion of IF parallels HCl secretion by the parietal cells in man. R-cobalamin complexes may be

TABLE 136–2. MAJOR COBALAMIN-BINDING PROTEINS

Source	Protein(s)	Function	Class*
Gastric juice	Intrinsic factor (IF)	Promotes absorption of cobalamin in ileum	S
Gastric juice	"Haptocorrin(s)"	May be involved in formation of IF-cobalamin; binds cobalamin analogues	R
Plasma	Transcobalamin I (TC I)	May participate in plasma transport of cobalamin	R
Plasma	Transcobalamin II (TC II)	Promotes entry of cobalamin into cells	S
Plasma (and granulocytes)	Transcobalamin III (TC III)	Unknown	R

* R = rapid; S = slow. Based on electrophoretic mobility.

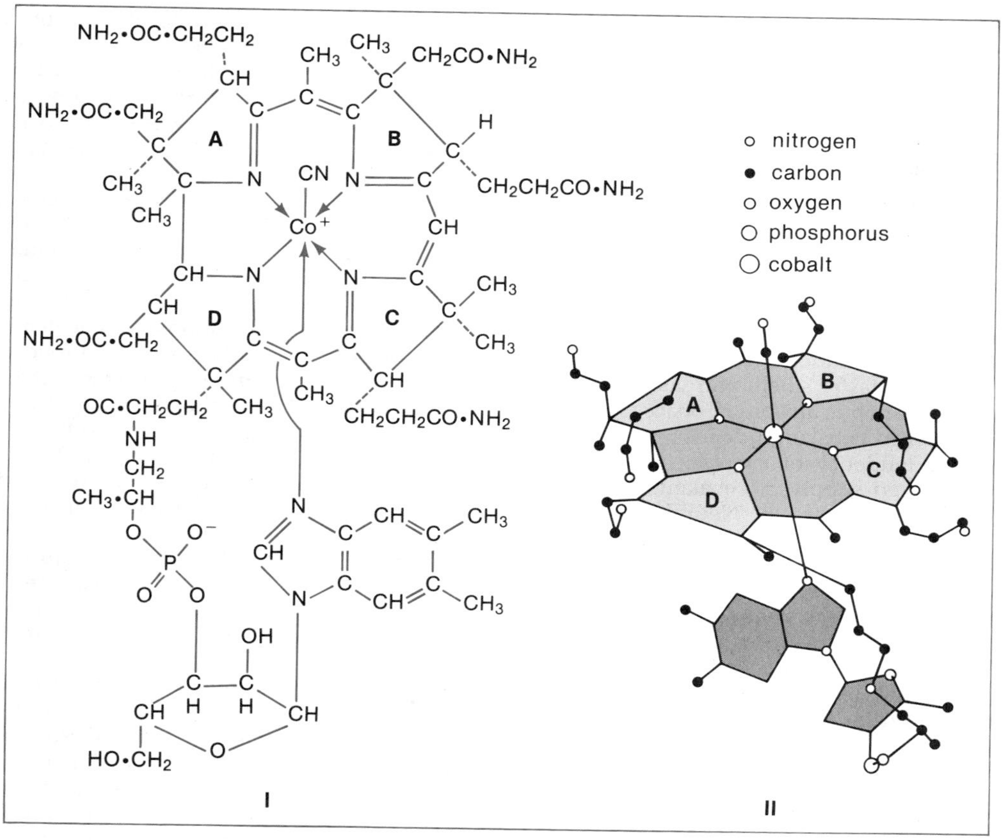

FIGURE 136–1. Chemical structure of cyanocobalamin. *Formula I,* Molecular structure. *Formula II,* Semidiagrammatic representation of three-dimensional structure showing relations of planar and nucleotide moieties. Hydrogen atoms and a number of oxygen atoms are omitted. (Adapted from Beck WS: N Engl J Med *266*:708, 1962.)

converted to IF-cobalamin with the participation of pancreatic proteases. The stable IF cobalamin complex encounters specific mucosal receptors in the microvilli of the ileum that bind to a specific site on the IF molecule. Attachment requires neutral pH, Ca^{++}, or other divalent cations, but no energy. Cobalamin is transferred into the ileal cell and ultimately transferred to portal vein blood. Thus, IF is essential for the intestinal absorption of ingested cobalamin.

Two types of anti-IF antibodies occur. "Blocking" antibodies prevent binding of cobalamin by IF and show little species specificity. "Binding" antibodies combine with IF-cobalamin and with free IF without impairing its ability to bind cobalamin. Both types of antibodies occur in sera of some patients with pernicious anemia.

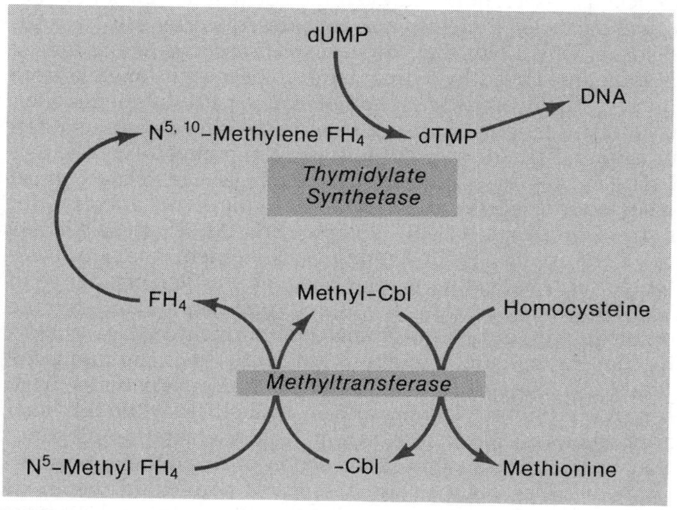

FIGURE 136–2. Diagram of relationship between N^5-methyl FH_4: homocysteine methyltransferase and thymidylate synthetase. In cobalamin deficiency, folate is sequestered as N^5-methyl FH_4. This ultimately deprives thymidylate synthetase of its folate coenzyme ($N^{5, 10}$-methylene FH_4) and thereby impairs DNA synthesis.

Binding proteins, which occur in serum, leukocytes, saliva, gastric juice, milk, and virtually all body cells, promote uptake of cobalamin by mitochondria and other organelles within cells.

Normal plasma contains 175 to 725 pg per milliliter of cobalamin (normal range varying with method and laboratory). All of it is protein-bound. The three major cobalamin-binding proteins of plasma are designated *transcobalamin I* (TC I), *transcobalamin II* (TC II), and *transcobalamin III* (TC III). They have only two known functions: TC II transports cobalamins through cell membranes, and all three prevent loss of cobalamins in urine, sweat, and other body secretions.

Serum cobalamin levels are most conveniently and accurately measured with a radioisotope dilution assay with IF as a binding agent. The results parallel those obtained using the microbiologic assays of the past. There are other cobalamin analogues in serum that will interfere with the assay if the less specific R proteins, rather than IF, are used as binders. The presence of these analogues raises many interesting questions. What is the source and fate of these analogues? Do they have pathophysiologic significance? Is it one of the roles of R-proteins, especially those of gastric juice, to bind these compounds (which may be of dietary origin) to minimize their absorption in the intestine?

Cobalamin Deficiency. The clinical picture of human deficiency includes the nonspecific manifestations of megaloblastic anemia and its sequelae—e.g., megaloblastosis, slowly progressing anemia, glossitis, increased serum lactic dehydrogenase—that occur as well in folic acid deficiency (and are described above), *plus* certain specific features that make possible the diagnosis of cobalamin deficiency, irrespective of the underlying cause. These include neurologic abnormalities, decreased serum cobalamin level, methylmalonic aciduria, and a characteristic response to cobalamin therapy and lack of response to therapy with physiologic doses of folic acid.

Neurologic symptoms occur late in some but not all patients. Curiously, they can occur in the absence of megaloblastic anemia. The neurologic syndrome, typical of cobalamin deficiency and not seen in folate deficiency, classically consists of symmetric paresthesias (tingling and numbness) in feet and fingers, with associated disturbances of vibratory sense and proprioception, progressing to spastic ataxia with *subacute combined system disease* of the spinal cord, i.e., degenerative changes of the dorsal and lateral columns. In fact, the picture is more often chronic than subacute and more varied and complex. The ankle jerks are usually absent, and there is often a severe loss of postural sense. There are extensor plantar reflexes. Clinical signs include cerebral abnormalities, irritability, somnolence, "megaloblastic madness," and perversion of taste, smell, and vision with central scotomas and occasional optic atrophy. Tobacco amblyopia, a curious visual disorder in cobalamin-deficient smokers, has been attributed to the tendency of cyanide in tobacco smoke to convert a diminished supply of cobalamin coenzymes to metabolically inert cyanocobalamin. Neurologic involvement is associated with a defect in myelin synthesis. Its mechanism is still unknown. Several theories have been proposed, among them chronic cyanide intoxication, and the synthesis and incorporation into myelin of abnormal fatty acids produced as a result of competition between acetyl CoA and accumulated methylmalonyl CoA in the biosynthetic pathway of fatty acids. In its early stages the neurologic syndrome can be reversed by cobalamin therapy. In time, however, such chronic manifestations as spinal cord disease become irreversible.

A decreased serum cobalamin level is decisive diagnostic evidence. Clinical signs generally appear when the serum level is below 80 to 100 pg per milliliter. Serum folate is increased when serum cobalamin is depressed unless there is coexisting folate deficiency. Methylmalonic aciduria is also a sensitive index of cobalamin deficiency except in rare cases in which it is due to an inborn error of metabolism. It does not occur in folate deficiency. Normal subjects excrete only traces of methylmalonate, i.e., 0 to 3.5 mg per 24 hours. Levels are variably elevated in cobalamin deficiency, sometimes to more than 300 mg per 24 hours. In practice, assay of urinary methylmalonate is rarely necessary.

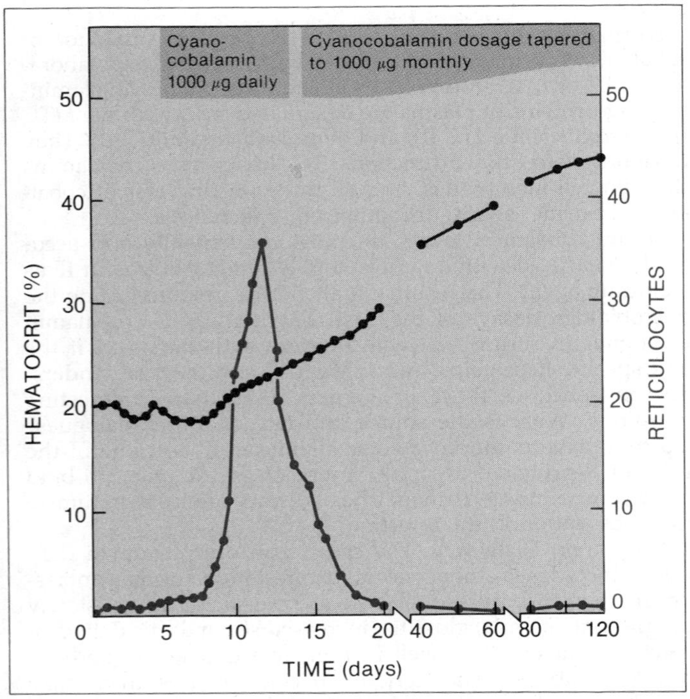

FIGURE 136–3. Time course of reticulocyte count and hematocrit level during treatment of pernicious anemia with cyanocobalamin. (Adapted from Beck WS, Goulian M: In DiPalma J [ed.]: Drill's Pharmacology in Medical Practice. 4th ed. New York, McGraw-Hill Book Company, 1971.)

Cobalamin therapy produces within hours an improved sense of well-being. An abrupt reticulocyte crisis begins several days after the start of therapy (Fig. 136–3). Reversal of clinical abnormalities then ensues. A partial response follows large (i.e., pharmacologic) doses of folic acid (5 mg per day), although the hematocrit is not fully restored to normal, and patients previously without neurologic symptoms may suffer an acute onset of such symptoms. However, small (i.e., physiologic) doses of folic acid (200 to 400 μg per day) produce no response in cobalamin deficiency, whereas they produce good responses in folic acid deficiency.

Specific Deficiency Syndromes. Deficiency of cobalamin, as of all vitamins, may result from inadequate intake, abnormally increased requirements, or impaired utilization in the tissues (see Table 136–1). Deficiency of cobalamin results from poor diet only rarely. Reported instances have occurred mainly in vegetarians who also avoid dairy products and eggs. Most often deficiency is the result of diminished intestinal absorption from various causes. The most common cause is pernicious anemia, discussed below, in which a gastric mucosal defect decreases IF synthesis. Other and less common causes include total (occasionally subtotal) gastrectomy; pancreatic disease, in which lack of proteases in the duodenum appears to interfere with formation of IF-cobalamin; overgrowth of intestinal bacteria in the blind loop syndrome, strictures, anastomoses, diverticula, and other conditions producing intestinal stasis; infestation with the cobalamin-utilizing fish tapeworm *Diphyllobothrium latum* (once a common condition in Scandinavian countries); and organic disease of the ileum that interferes with cobalamin absorption despite the presence of adequate IF. Cobalamin deficiency resulting from increased requirements occurs mainly in pregnancy, presumably arising from the superimposition of fetal demands upon a background of poor nutrition. Impaired utilization of cobalamin occurs in various genetic defects, involving deletions or defects of methylmalonyl CoA mutase, TC II, and enzymes in the pathway of cobalamin adenosylation.

PERNICIOUS ANEMIA

Once a fatal disease and now the physician's favorite for its rich history, scientific importance, and cheerful prognosis, pernicious anemia is an atrophic gastropathy that leads to deficient IF secretion and eventual cobalamin deficiency. Because pernicious anemia was first described by Thomas Addison of Guy's Hospital, the term *addisonian pernicious anemia* is sometimes used to distinguish true pernicious anemia from the regrettably named non-addisonian pernicious anemia (i.e., cobalamin deficiency arising from such other causes as ileitis or acquired gastric atrophy following inflammatory gastritis).

The incidence of pernicious anemia is age related, most cases occurring after the age of 40. Typically, it affects older north Europeans of fair complexion. An exception is its apparent predilection for young black women. A genetic basis for pernicious anemia is suggested by its high incidence in Scandinavians, a relatively inbred population, and by the occurrence of the disease or related abnormalities (e.g., achlorhydria) in patients' families. An underlying autoimmune process is suggested by the fact that many patients have serum binding or blocking anti-IF antibodies. Although such antibodies can block IF function if they enter the intestine, they are not responsible for cessation of IF synthesis. Anti-IF antibodies also occur in the absence of pernicious anemia in the serum of patients with diabetes mellitus, thyroid disease, and other diseases. Serum from pernicious anemia may also contain antibodies against gastric parietal cell cytoplasm and thyroid acinar cell cytoplasm. Pernicious anemia occurs frequently in patients with thyrotoxicosis, Hashimoto's thyroiditis, and several other diseases (hypogammaglobulinemia, vitiligo, rheumatoid arthritis, and gastric carcinoma). Most hematologists have the impression that the incidence of pernicious anemia is decreasing.

Clinically, there is a slow onset of megaloblastic anemia and laboratory signs of cobalamin deficiency. If untreated, the patient may eventually develop neurologic symptoms. Diagnostic features are achlorhydria after histamine stimulation and decreased levels of IF in gastric juice as revealed by direct assay in vitro (which is performed routinely in Europe but infrequently in the United States) or by decreased cobalamin absorption in an in vivo test of cobalamin absorption. In the absorption test known as the *Schilling test*, a fasting patient ingests 0.5 microcurie (0.5 to 2.0 μg) [^{57}Co]cyanocobalamin at time zero. A dose (1 mg) of unlabeled cyanocobalamin is injected at two hours, and radioactivity is measured in a 24-hour urine collection. If excretion of radioactivity is low, the test is repeated (in no less than five days) by the same procedure, except that 60 mg of hog IF is given orally with the radioactive cobalamin. If poor excretion and therefore presumably poor absorption was due to IF deficiency, the result with the addition of exogenous IF should be normal. If excretion is still low, ileal disease may be suspected. Renal disease with impaired glomerular filtration may delay excretion of radioactivity in the Schilling test. Since the Schilling test includes an injection of cobalamin it is a therapeutic commitment if therapy has not already been initiated.

Juvenile pernicious anemia includes four entities: (1) true pernicious anemia, which occurs infrequently between ages 2 and 14; (2) congenital IF lack, with no other abnormality of gastric secretion and no anti-IF antibody; (3) production of biologically inert IF (one case reported); and (4) familial selective malabsorption of cobalamin (Imerslund's syndrome) with normal absorption of other nutrients and normal gastric secretion of IF and HCl. The Schilling test reveals decreased cobalamin uncorrected for IF. Presumably, there is a defect of specific mucosal receptors for IF-cobalamin.

Therapy. Therapy consists in the parenteral administration of cobalamin (hydroxocobalamin or cyanocobalamin) in amounts that are ultimately sufficient to provide the 2 to 5 μg needed for the daily requirement and to replete liver stores and other reservoirs, which normally contain 2 to 5 mg of cobalamin. Because of its low cost and lack of toxicity, doses in excess of need are generally given. Parenterally administered cobalamin is bound to plasma proteins and cellular binding sites. If much more than 100 μg is given parenterally in a single dose, delay in encountering vacant binding sites promptly leads to renal excretion of unbound vitamin. Since hydroxocobalamin is bound more tightly by binding proteins than cyanocobalamin, it is less rapidly excreted by the kidney and more effective in achieving high serum cobalamin levels. Hypokalemia sometimes develops early in the course of treatment, especially in severely deficient patients, as a result of a sudden increase in the need for potassium in young red cells abruptly returning to normal hematopoiesis. The following treatment schedule is used in my clinic: (1) 500 to 1000 μg intramuscularly daily for two weeks; (2) the same dose twice weekly for an additional four weeks or until the hematocrit is normal; and (3) the same dose once monthly for the lifetime of the patient. A dosage schedule of 500 to 1000 μg every two weeks for six months is recommended for patients with neurologic manifestations. Neurologic symptoms persisting beyond 12 to 18 months are usually irreversible.

Oral cobalamin–IF preparations are not recommended, since the condition often becomes refractory to therapy. Oral therapy with cobalamin alone (500 to 1000 μg daily) should be reserved for the occasional patient who for some reason cannot receive parenteral therapy. This mode of therapy depends on intestinal absorption by passive diffusion, a process that is often unpredictable. Patients receiving oral medication who feel well may decide to stop their medication. The patient with pernicious anemia should understand that he or she must be treated for life.

Since the response to cobalamin occurs within 48 to 72 hours, it is seldom necessary to subject the patient to the risks, discomfort, and expense of blood transfusion.

There is no need for iron therapy in pernicious anemia unless there is evidence of associated iron deficiency or reason to suspect that tissue iron reserves are deficient—as, for example, in women of early middle age who may have had heavy menstrual losses or several pregnancies. In such cases, hemoglobin and erythrocyte regeneration is delayed until iron is given. There is no need to administer folic acid or ascorbic acid in addition to the cobalamin, provided that the patient has an adequate diet. As long as cobalamin is given, folic acid therapy causes no harm. It is commonly elected to administer both cobalamin and folic acid to distressed patients with severe megaloblastic anemia without awaiting the diagnostic workup. In this situation, as in all cases of megaloblastic anemia, it is mandatory to obtain serum samples for vitamin assays before therapy starts.

With the exception of hereditary methylmalonic aciduria, cobalamin deficiency of whatever cause is the only valid indication for cobalamin therapy. It has been recommended, nevertheless, for many disorders in which there is no evidence of deficiency, especially for various types of neuropathy, liver disease, dermatologic disorders, and allergies, and as a "tonic" or appetite stimulant. The usefulness of cobalamin in these circumstances has not been proved, and its use for such purposes is not recommended.

MEGALOBLASTIC ANEMIA OF FOLATE DEFICIENCY

Converging lines of nutritional research led to the discovery of folic acid in the mid 1940's. In 1948 crystalline folic acid was obtained from liver and its structure confirmed by organic synthesis. Although experimental folic acid deficiency was known to produce megaloblastic anemia, it was not immediately recognized that folic acid is not the anti-pernicious anemia principle of liver, which was identified a year later. Confusion arose when folic acid therapy produced notable reticulocyte responses in pernicious anemia. Hemoglobin regeneration was incomplete, however, and relapses and neurologic complications occurred during treatment. Liver extracts active in pernicious anemia were then found by direct assay to contain little or no folic acid. Thus, it was recognized that cobalamin deficiency is the basis of the megaloblastic anemia of pernicious anemia and that folate deficiency is a distinctive cause of megaloblastic anemia.

Metabolic and Nutritional Aspects of Folic Acid. Folic acid is the trivial name for *pteroylmonoglutamic acid* (Fig. 136–4), parent compound of the large family of compounds known collectively as folate or folates. The molecule contains three moieties: a pteridine derivative, a *p*-aminobenzoic acid residue, and an L-glutamic acid residue. The first two combined constitute pteroic acid; hence folates are pteroylglutamates.

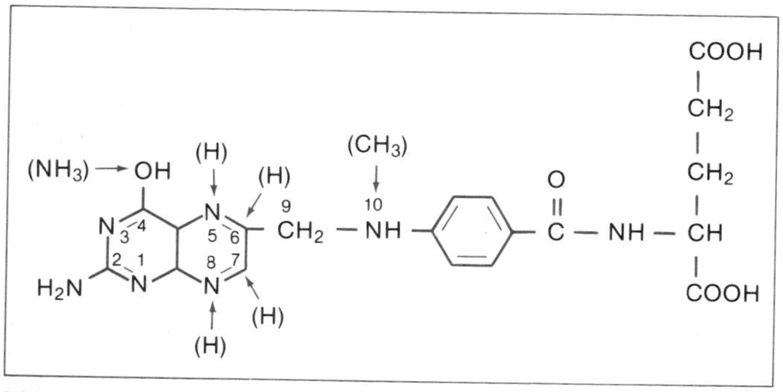

FIGURE 136–4. Chemical structure of folic acid (pteroylmonoglutamic acid). Substituents in parentheses are attached at the sites shown in the several folate derivatives described in the text. (From Beck WS [ed.]: Hematology. 4th ed. Cambridge, Mass., MIT Press, 1985.)

Folic acid occurs in nature largely in the form of folylpolyglutamates, in which multiple glutamic acid residues are attached by peptide linkages to the gamma-carboxyl group of the preceding glutamic acid residue. The synthetic folic acid used therapeutically is folylmonoglutamate. However, folylmonoglutamates are converted in cells to polyglutamates, which are apparently the true coenzymes of folate-dependent enzymes.

Folic acid occurs at three levels of oxidation: folic acid (F); 7,8-dihydrofolic acid (FH_2); and 5,6,7,8-tetrahydrofolic acid (FH_4). Reduction of F to FH_4 is a necessary prerequisite to the participation of folic acid in enzyme reactions. In this reduction, F is reduced to FH_2, which is then reduced to FH_4. In animal cells both reactions are catalyzed by a single NADPH-linked enzyme, *dihydrofolate reductase*, which is notably sensitive to inhibition by folate analogues containing a 4-amino group (Fig. 136–4) such as aminopterin and amethopterin, later renamed methotrexate (MTX).

The folate family consists largely of FH_4 derivatives bearing one of several "one-carbon" substituents on N^5 or N^{10} (or both). Specific enzymes interconvert many of these compounds. Folate derivatives differ in their ability to support various microorganisms. The major form of folate in human serum is N^5-methyl FH_4 (a monoglutamate), which is assayed with *Lactobacillus casei*. Satisfactory isotope dilution assay procedures are now available for the assay of serum folate.

In metabolism, FH_4 is a catalytic self-regenerating acceptor-donor of one-carbon units in anabolic and catabolic reactions involving one-carbon transfers. A number of metabolic systems in animal tissues are known to require folate coenzymes. Impairment of thymidylate synthesis is the key event in folate deficiency that produces major clinical manifestations (see Fig. 135–2). Methylation of deoxyuridylate to thymidylate, catalyzed by the enzyme thymidylate synthetase, is an essential step in the biosynthesis of DNA. Impairment of thymidylate synthesis in folate deficiency slows DNA synthesis with resulting megaloblastic transformation. Folate also participates in the breakdown of histidine and its catabolic product, formiminoglutamic acid (abbreviated FIGlu). Interference with this system in folate deficiency has no morbid effects, but it provides the basis for a diagnostic test for folate deficiency. When insufficient FH_4 is present to accept the formimino group, FIGlu accumulates in the urine, where it is easily detected.

Green vegetables are rich sources of folate, the richest being asparagus, broccoli, spinach, and lettuce, each of which contains more than 1 mg of folate per 100 grams dry weight. Folates are also found in liver, kidney, yeast, and mushrooms. An average daily American diet, prepared without special precautions, contains approximately 200 μg of folate by *Streptococcus faecalis* assay and an additional 400 to 500 μg of folate that is active only with *Lactobacillus casei*. Excessive cooking, particularly with large amounts of water, can remove or destroy a high percentage of the folate in foods. The minimal daily adult requirement for folic acid, or its derivatives, is 50 to 200 μg. Body reserves of folic acid are relatively much smaller than those of cobalamin. When a subject receiving a normal ration is switched to a daily intake of 5 μg per day, megaloblastic anemia develops in about four months. Folic acid requirements are increased during growth, in pregnancy, and in various diseases.

Folate Deficiency. The clinical picture of human folate deficiency includes nonspecific manifestations of megaloblastic anemia that are similar to those observed in cobalamin deficiency—megaloblastosis, glossitis, increased serum lactic dehydrogenase—*plus* certain specific features that make possible the diagnosis of folate deficiency, irrespective of the underlying cause. These include decreased serum folate levels (normal, 6 to 15 ng per milliliter), decreased red cell folate levels (normal, 150 to 600 ng per milliliter of cells), and full clinical response to therapy with physiologic doses of folic acid. Features suggestive but not diagnostic of folate deficiency in a patient with megaloblastic anemia are lack of neurologic changes of the type seen in cobalamin deficiency, normal serum cobalamin and urine methylmalonic acid levels, and a history of circumstances almost certain to lead to folic acid deficiency, e.g., poor diet, malabsorption, or alcoholism.

Specific Deficiency Syndromes. As shown in Table 136–1, the major categories of folate deficiency are those due to decreased intake, increased requirements, and impaired utilization. Decreased intake is by far the most common. Because body folate reserves are small, deficiency develops rapidly in persons with an inadequate diet. As noted, excessive cooking may also promote deficiency, especially among peoples who live on finely divided foods such as rice. Megaloblastic anemia occuring in chronic liver disease is usually due to folate deficiency resulting from poor diet and impaired hepatic storage of folate. The macrocytic anemia accompanying liver disease is often normoblastic and unresponsive to folic acid therapy. Nutritional folate deficiency is often associated with multiple vitamin deficiencies. In such patients, a history of gross dietary inadequacy is usually easy to obtain. Folate is normally absorbed in the upper third of the small intestine and commonly malabsorbed in nontropical sprue (celiac disease) as described in Ch. 103. Tropical sprue is a malabsorptive disorder of unknown etiology that occurs frequently and endemically in the tropics—notably the West Indies, the Indian subcontinent, and Southeast Asia. It can be acquired by residents of temperate climates who go to the tropics, sometimes persisting long after return from the tropics. It may be due in part to deficiency of dietary folate, the malabsorption resulting from secondary gastrointestinal changes. Treatment with folic acid alone usually reverses all abnormalities, including defective folate absorption. Other causes of malabsorption are noted in Table 136–1. Low serum folate levels in patients receiving phenytoin (Dilantin) have been attributed to reversible drug-induced malabsorption of folylpolyglutamate. Oral contraceptives block deconjugation of folylpolyglutamate in certain women.

Pregnancy increases requirements for folate. Although true anemias of pregnancy are commonly due to iron deficiency or multiple nutritional deficiencies, two thirds of anemic pregnant women are folate deficient. Its frequency is attributable both to meager folate reserves and to the fact that pregnancy increases daily requirements for folate five- to tenfold, especially in the last trimester. The presence of multiple fetuses, poor diet (a frequent result of anorexia or nausea), infection, and lactation may further increase requirements. The capacity of the fetus to take up folic acid (and other nutrients) at the expense of the mother, even when the available supply is markedly reduced, is quite remarkable. Folic acid supplementation is desirable during pregnancy not only because requirements are increased but also because there is a suspected association between severe folate deficiency and such complications of pregnancy as abruptio placentae, embryopathology, spontaneous abortion, and bleeding. The folate requirement also rises sharply in hemolytic anemias associated with acute or chronic overactivity of the bone marrow and in most neoplastic diseases, especially metastatic cancer and the leukemias. The deficiency presumably reflects competitive utilization of the vitamin by tumor cells, a phenomenon that resembles the pre-emption of maternal nutrients by a fetus.

Impaired utilization of folate is caused by administration of 4-aminopteroylglutamates, aminopterin and methotrexate, powerful inhibitors of dihydrofolate reductase that can deplete folate coenzymes in tissues within hours. Citrovorum factor (leucovorin, folinic acid, N^5-formyl FH_4) effectively counteracts the actions of MTX by bypassing the inhibited reductase and is useful in the treatment of toxicity.

Therapy. Folic acid is usually administered orally in 1 mg tablets. Oral therapy is satisfactory for most needs. Even in the presence of intestinal malabsorption, the relatively large doses used ordinarily permit sufficient absorption to achieve repletion. The usual dose is 1 to 2 mg daily, although doses in excess of 1 mg are seldom necessary. Folic acid in these doses also partially corrects the hematopoietic and gastrointestinal manifestations of cobalamin deficiency. Neurologic abnormalities, however, may progress with disastrous results. This is the principal danger in the uncritical use of folic acid. Therapy for four to five weeks is usually adequate to replenish stores and correct anemia. Therapy is continued until diet or underlying problems are corrected. In some patients (e.g., those with malabsorption, chronic hemolysis, chronic exfoliative skin disease, or renal failure requiring hemodialysis), it must continue indefinitely.

A parenteral preparation containing 5 mg per milliliter of the sodium salt may be used in severely ill patients, in certain cases of malabsorption, or in patients incapable of taking oral medication. Citrovorum factor is available as a parenteral therapeutic preparation. Its main clinical indication is severe intoxication by folic acid antagonists that block folate reduction. In the absence of such inhibition, little is accomplished by treating folate deficiency with this compound instead of folic acid.

MEGALOBLASTIC ANEMIA UNRESPONSIVE TO COBALAMIN OR FOLIC ACID

Megaloblastic anemia is occasionally unaccompanied by cobalamin or folic acid deficiency and fails to respond to therapy with either vitamin. In some cases, folate or cobalamin deficiency coexists with megaloblastic anemia but is not responsible for it. Most of these occurrences arise in three situations (see Table 136–1): therapy with an antimetabolite drug that inteferes with DNA synthesis (common), inborn error of metabolism (rare), and refractory megaloblastic anemia of undetermined etiology, which is probably due to somatic mutation leading to loss of an enzyme in the pathway of DNA synthesis. Except for various dysplastic features, megaloblasts in the bone marrow of these patients generally resemble those in vitamin-deficiency megaloblastic anemia. The defect in all is probably an impaired capacity to duplicate DNA at a normal rate. Drug-induced megaloblastosis is potentially reversible. However, those cases caused by genetic error or acquired refractory megaloblastosis are irreversible and unfortunately difficult to treat with any but supportive measures.

Beck WS: Metabolic aspects of vitamins B_{12} and folic acid. Erythrocyte disorders—anemias related to disturbance of DNA synthesis (megaloblastic anemias). In Williams WJ, Beutler E, Erslev AJ, et al. (eds.): Hematology, 3rd ed. New York, McGraw-Hill Book Company, 1983, pp 311–331, 434–465. *Sections of a standard hematology text that covers the megaloblastic anemias in detail. Extensive bibliographies.*

Castle WB: The conquest of pernicious anemia. In Wintrobe MM (ed.): Blood, Pure and Eloquent. A Story of Discovery, of People, and of Ideas. New York, McGraw-Hill Book Company, 1980, pp 283–318. *An engrossing historical essay by the one who in 1929 discovered intrinsic factor.*

Chanarin I, Deacon R, Lumb M, et al.: Cobalamin-folate interrelations: A critical review. Blood 66:479, 1985.

Shane B, Stokstad ELR: Vitamin B_{12}–folate interrelationships. Ann Rev Nutr 5:115, 1985. *These two reviews, published almost simultaneously reflect somewhat different views of a puzzling old problem: Why do cobalamin-deficient patients respond as they do to folate therapy? The answer is still not certain. Excellent bibliographies.*

Lindenbaum J: Status of laboratory testing in the diagnosis of megaloblastic anemia. Blood 61:624, 1983. *A brief guide to available methods. I agree with everything in it except the remarks on the deoxyuridine suppression test.*

Rosenberg LE: Disorders of propionate and methylmalonate metabolism. In Stanbury JB, Wyngaarden JB, Frederickson DS, et al. (eds.): The Metabolic Basis of Inherited Disease. 5th ed. New York, McGraw-Hill Book Company, 1983, p 474. *A thorough review of a group of inborn errors that may cause laboratory findings that could confuse an observer who is not alert to the possibilities. 191 references.*

137 HEMOLYTIC DISORDERS: INTRODUCTION

Manuel E. Kaplan

PATHOPHYSIOLOGY OF HEMOLYSIS. Human red blood cells normally survive for approximately 120 days after they are released from the bone marrow as reticulocytes, being destroyed only after they have become senescent. With advancing cell age the activities of various red cell enzymes decline, and the cells become denser and less deformable. Phagocytic cells of the spleen and liver are believed to recognize and destroy effete red cells, although splenectomy does not extend the red cell lifespan beyond 120 days.

A hemolytic disorder is defined as premature destruction of red cells, which may occur either because inherently defective red cells are produced or because noxious factors are present in the intravascular environment. Intrinsic abnormalities that predispose to hemolysis may occur in the red cell membrane or in its contained hemoglobin or enzymes. These are, for the most part, genetically determined. In contrast, the environmental abnormalities that prejudice red cell survival are almost all acquired. A classification of the causes of hemolytic anemia is given in Table 137–1.

To measure red cell survival, anticoagulated venous blood is incubated with radioactive chromium (^{51}Cr) to label intracellular hemoglobin and is then reinfused. Normally 50 per cent of the injected ^{51}Cr activity disappears from the blood ($t\frac{1}{2}$) in 29 ± 3 days rather than at 60 days, because ^{51}Cr is an imperfect label and slowly elutes from the red cells. Nevertheless, the results of such studies are clinically informative because rates of hemolysis are reliably quantified and the sites of red cell destruction can be identified by external scanning utilizing a collimated gamma scintillation counter.

CONSEQUENCES OF HEMOLYSIS. Accelerated destruction of red cells may occur intravascularly or, more commonly, after the cells have been culled from the circulation (sequestered).

Intravascular Hemolysis. Following intravascular hemolysis, hemoglobin is released into the plasma and is bound by haptoglobin, an alpha-globulin synthesized by the liver. The haptoglobin concentration of blood, normally about 100 mg per 100 ml, reflects the rate of haptoglobin synthesis and catabolism. Haptoglobin synthesis is usually diminished in

TABLE 137–1. CLASSIFICATION OF THE CAUSES OF HEMOLYTIC ANEMIA

- **I. Congenital hemolytic disorders (see Ch. 138)**
  - A. Membrane defects
  - B. Enzyme defects
    - 1. Embden-Meyerhof pathway defects
    - 2. Hexose monophosphate shunt defects
  - C. Hemoglobin defects
    - 1. Structural (hemoglobinopathies) (see Ch. 143)
    - 2. Synthetic (thalassemias) (see Ch. 142)
  - D. Other
- **II. Acquired hemolytic disorders (see Ch. 139)**
  - A. Sequestrational hemolysis (hypersplenism)
  - B. Immune hemolytic disorders
    - 1. Alloimmune
    - 2. Autoimmune
    - 3. Drug-induced
  - C. Paroxysmal nocturnal hemoglobinuria
  - D. Due to toxins and metabolic abnormalities
  - E. Due to red cell parasites
  - F. Due to red cell trauma

patients with parenchymal liver disease and may be increased in various inflammatory disorders, in which it acts as an acute phase protein. Free (uncomplexed) haptoglobin has a half-life of approximately four days. In contrast, hemoglobin-haptoglobin complexes are removed from the plasma within minutes, primarily by hepatic reticuloendothelial cells that catabolize both components of the complex. Haptoglobin catabolism usually exceeds haptoglobin synthesis in patients with significant intravascular hemolysis, and plasma haptoglobin levels fall, frequently to undetectable levels. If the quantity of hemoglobin entering the plasma exceeds the binding capacity of haptoglobin, hemoglobin appears in the glomerular filtrate, primarily as a 32,000 dalton alpha-beta dimer. The dimers are readily absorbed by cells of the proximal tubules that convert heme iron into ferritin and hemosiderin. After the tubular cells are sloughed, hemosiderin can be detected in the urinary sediment with a Prussian blue stain. Hemoglobinuria, which occurs only when the filtered load of alpha-beta dimer exceeds the absorptive capacity of the tubular cells, connotes rapid intravascular hemolysis. Persistent urinary loss of hemosiderin or hemoglobin or both may result in iron deficiency.

Hemoglobin in the plasma is unstable. Its heme prosthetic groups tend to dissociate and bind either to hemopexin, a beta-globulin, or to albumin, forming methemalbumin. Neither of these heme-protein complexes appears in the urine unless significant proteinuria is present. Because heme-hemopexin complexes are cleared rapidly from the blood, serum levels of hemopexin, like haptoglobin, are typically reduced or absent in the presence of significant intravascular hemolysis.

Erythrocytes contain high concentrations of the enzyme lactic dehydrogenase (LDH). Consequently, very high LDH levels are found in patients with intravascular hemolysis.

Extravascular Destruction. In most hemolytic disorders red cell destruction occurs extravascularly rather than intravascularly. Red cells are sequestered primarily within the spleen or liver or both and are phagocytized in situ. Although only a small fraction of the hemoglobin they contain escapes into the plasma, plasma haptoglobin levels characteristically fall, particularly when hemolysis is longstanding. However, plasma hemoglobin levels do not rise significantly, and no hemoglobinuria or hemosiderinuria occurs. Serum LDH levels are usually elevated, but not to the degree seen in intravascular hemolysis.

Hemoglobin derived from hemolyzed red cells is normally catabolized by reticuloendothelial cells to unconjugated, indirect-reacting bilirubin. As each heme tetrapyrrole ring is opened, one molecule of carbon monoxide is elaborated. The rate of formation of endogenously produced carbon monoxide has been used to quantify red cell destruction in vivo. However, this may not accurately reflect the rapidity of hemolysis since ineffective erythropoiesis (destruction of immature red cells in the bone marrow) also contributes to carbon monoxide formation. Unconjugated bilirubin produced by phagocytic cells is bound by albumin. The concentration of unconjugated bilirubin in the serum of a patient reflects the quantity of heme catabolized and the rate at which the liver is able to convert it into the direct-reacting, water-soluble product (Ch. 130). Serum levels of conjugated bilirubin are typically normal in patients with uncomplicated hemolytic disorders. Bilirubinuria does not occur unless the patient has concomitant hepatocellular or biliary disease.

Bone Marrow Response. The loss of circulating red cells results in an erythropoietic stimulus to the bone marrow proportional to the decline in the oxygen-carrying capacity of the blood. The normal bone marrow responds by increasing commensurately its erythropoietic activity. When examined morphologically, bone marrows of patients with hemolysis characteristically exhibit erythroid hyperplasia. Consequently, unless an underlying neoplastic disorder such as leukemia or lymphoma is suspected, diagnostic bone marrow studies are usually not indicated. The intensity of the marrow's erythropoietic response to hemolysis, which may reach a maximum of approximately eight times normal, is reflected by reticulocytosis in the peripheral blood. The reticulocyte percentage alone does not adequately reflect the degree of marrow compensation. This may be more reliably gauged by calculating the reticulocyte index (patient hematocrit times percentage reticulocytes/normal hematocrit). In some patients sustained reticulocytosis may compensate fully for the increased red cell destruction, and there is no anemia. More commonly, bone marrow compensation is incomplete so that anemia, of greater or lesser severity, supervenes. If bone marrow function is compromised by such factors as infection or folate deficiency the reticulocyte count will fall and the anemia will rapidly worsen because of the ongoing hemolytic process.

DIFFERENTIAL DIAGNOSIS OF HEMOLYTIC DISORDERS. ***The Diagnosis of Hemolysis.*** The presence of hemolysis as the cause of anemia is generally not difficult to establish. The clinical diagnosis is usually based on the presence of sustained reticulocytosis in a patient exhibiting no evidence of blood loss or of increasing hemoglobin concentration. Some or all of the following findings may occur:

1. *Evidence of enhanced marrow response:* polychromatophilia, reticulocytosis, marrow erythroid hyperplasia.
2. *Evidence for excessive release of red cell components:* (a) plasma—unconjugated bilirubin ↑, LDH ↑, haptoglobin ↓, hemopexin ↓, methemalbumin +, free hemoglobin ↑; (b) urine—hemosiderin +, hemoglobin +.
3. *Evidence of decreased red cell survival:* Decreased ^{51}Cr red cell t½.

The problem remains to determine the cause of the hemolytic process (see Table 137–1). Hemolysis is caused either by an abnormality of the red cell or an abnormality in its environment, the circulatory system in which the red cell resides. Red cell abnormalities associated with hemolysis may be congenital (genetically determined) or acquired. Congenital red cell defects resulting in hemolysis may involve the cell membrane, erythrocyte enzymes, or the contained hemoglobin. Acquired red cell defects that predispose to hemolysis may occur (1) under conditions of grossly abnormal (dysplastic) red cell maturation (such as marked deficiencies of iron, B_{12}, or folate) with bone marrow production and elaboration into the circulation of severely misshapen erythrocytes, and (2) in paroxysmal nocturnal hemoglobinuria (Ch. 139). More commonly, acquired hemolytic disorders are due to the presence in the circulation of such noxious factors as red cell antibodies, immune complexes containing activated complement components, chemical or metabolic "toxins," or parasites.

Clinical Findings. A patient with hemolysis may present with diverse complaints and physical findings that reflect the rapidity, underlying etiology, and pathophysiologic mechanism of red cell destruction. Patients with congenital hemolytic disorders are frequently anemic and intermittently jaundiced early in life. Usually a suggestive family history of anemia, jaundice, cholelithiasis, splenomegaly, and/or therapeutic splenectomy can be elicited. A significant proportion of patients with acquired hemolysis have an identifiable underlying disease such as systemic lupus erythematosus (SLE) or chronic lymphocytic leukemia (CLL). Patients with rapidly falling hemoglobin values resulting from hemolysis of any cause commonly complain of fatigue, palpitations, breathlessness, postural dizziness, and worsening of pre-existing angina. Physical examination typically discloses pallor, mild jaundice, and frequently splenomegaly. Other signs and symptoms referable to specific underlying disease may also be present: joint discomfort in SLE, painful acrocyanosis in cold agglutinin disease, lymphadenopathy in CLL.

Laboratory Findings. Patients with significant hemolysis

TABLE 137–2. MORPHOLOGIC ABNORMALITIES OF RED CELLS IN VARIOUS HEMOLYTIC DISORDERS

	Hemolytic Disorder	
Abnormality	*Congenital*	*Acquired*
Permanently sickled cells	Sickle cell anemia	—
Fragmented cells (schistocytes)	Unstable hemoglobins (Heinz body anemias)	Microangiopathic processes Prosthetic heart valves
Spur cells (acanthocytes)	Abetalipoproteinemia	Severe liver disease
Spherocytes	Hereditary spherocytosis	Immune, warm antibody type
Target cells	Thalassemia Hemoglobinopathies (Hb C)	Liver disease
Agglutinated cells	—	Immune, cold agglutinin disease

typically exhibit reticulocytosis with polychromasia on peripheral smear, unconjugated hyperbilirubinemia, serum haptoglobin levels ranging from decreased to absent, erythroid hyperplasia of the bone marrow, and elevated serum LDH levels. In fact, as noted earlier, these findings form the basis of diagnosing an anemia as being hemolytic. Hemoglobinemia, hemoglobinuria, and hemosiderinuria occur only when rapid intravascular hemolysis is present. Significant intravascular red cell destruction occurs in relatively few situations, e.g., G6PD deficiency, certain infections (*Clostridium welchii*, falciparum malaria), paroxysmal nocturnal hemoglobinuria, paroxysmal cold hemoglobinuria, incompatible transfusions, and as a result of traumatic disruption of red cell membranes by excessive heat or mechanical stress.

The morphologic appearance of red cells is frequently abnormal in patients with hemolysis. Occasionally the abnormalities are so typical that they indicate the correct diagnosis (Table 137–2).

Further Studies. The overall clinical picture for which a patient with hemolysis seeks medical help is usually sufficiently informative to suggest a rational diagnostic approach. Frequently useful laboratory studies to elucidate the cause of a presumed congenital hemolytic process include osmotic fragility test, G6PD and pyruvate kinase screening tests, and hemoglobin electrophoresis. For a presumed acquired hemolytic disorder a direct antiglobulin (Coombs') test is invariably indicated and, less frequently, Ham's test for paroxysmal nocturnal hemoglobinuria.

TREATMENT OF HEMOLYTIC ANEMIA. Only general supportive measures will be discussed here since effective therapy usually requires definition of the cause and pathophysiologic mechanisms underlying the specific disease processes, as described in the subsequent two chapters.

Severely anemic patients should be placed at temporary bed rest to reduce cardiac output. Nasal oxygen may afford symptomatic relief. Transfusions with packed red cells should be utilized to correct hemodynamic abnormalities rather than to treat low hemoglobin or hematocrit values. To avoid iatrogenically induced hypervolemia, transfusions should be administered slowly. The physician must consider the potential dangers of transfusions, particularly in patients with autoimmune hemolytic disorders (see Ch. 139).

To maintain accelerated erythropoiesis patients with chronic hemolysis requires extra quantities of folic acid. Therefore, daily oral supplementation with folic acid, 1 to 2 mg per day, is recommended. The serum cobalamin concentration should be measured if concomitant cobalamin deficiency is suspected. When it is low, parenteral vitamin B_{12} should also be administered.

SPECIFIC HEMOLYTIC DISORDERS. The purpose of this brief introduction is merely to provide a background of the common pathophysiology of the hemolytic anemias as well as a general classification (Table 137–1). The anemias are discussed more extensively in Ch. 135 and 136. Specific hemolytic diseases resulting from intracorpuscular abnormalities (usually caused by genetic abnormalities of the red cell membrane, of red cell enzymes, or of hemoglobin) are presented in the following chapter. Chapter 139 summarizes the acquired hemolytic disorders.

138 HEREDITARY DEFECTS IN THE MEMBRANE OR METABOLISM OF THE RED CELL

Samuel E. Lux

MEMBRANE DISORDERS

Normal Red Cell Membrane

Structure

Membrane Lipids. The red cell membrane, or *ghost*, is a mixture of phospholipids, unesterified cholesterol, and glycolipids, arranged in a bilayer, and traversed randomly by transmembrane protein channels and receptors. The phospholipids are asymmetrically arranged. Choline phospholipids (phosphatidyl choline and sphingomyelin) are found primarily in the outer half of the bilayer; amino phospholipids (phosphatidyl serine and phosphatidyl ethanolamine) and phosphatidyl inositols are confined to the inner half. The mechanism that maintains this arrangement is poorly understood, but there is evidence that the membrane skeleton (see below) is involved. It is probably important to sequester amino phospholipids, since their exposure triggers coagulation and causes red cells to adhere to phagocytes. The lipids are mobile in the plane of the membrane. This gives the membrane properties of a viscous two-dimensional fluid.

Membrane Proteins. The red cell membrane contains 10 to 15 major proteins and innumerable minor ones (Fig. 138–1). The proteins fall into two classes. (1) *Integral membrane proteins* traverse the bilayer, interact with the hydrophobic lipid core, and are tightly bound. They include functionally important transport proteins (e.g., protein 3) and glycoprotein surface antigens (e.g., glycophorin). (2) *Peripheral membrane proteins* are confined to the cytoplasmic membrane surface and include structural proteins, such as spectrin and actin, and some red cell enzymes (e.g., glyceraldehyde-3-phosphate dehydrogenase). These proteins bind to each other and to anchoring sites on integral proteins.

The major peripheral membrane proteins form a two-dimensional protein network that laminates the cytoplasmic membrane surface (Fig. 138–1). The principal components of this *membrane skeleton* are spectrin, actin, protein 4.1, and ankyrin. *Spectrin*, the major skeletal protein, contains two long, flexible chains that are aligned in parallel and twisted about each other. These dimers interact at their "head" end to form tetramers or higher-order oligomers (spectrin self-association) (Fig. 138–1). At the opposite ("tail") end, spectrin binds to *short filaments of actin*. This interaction is greatly strengthened by *protein 4.1*, which attaches to spectrin near the actin-binding site. Because multiple spectrins can bind to each actin filament, the spectrin-actin-4.1 complex is a molecular junction that allows spectrin filaments to branch and form a two-dimensional membrane skeleton. The skeleton is anchored to the overlying lipid bilayer by *ankyrin*, which binds to spectrin near the self-association site and links it to the cytoplasmic portion of protein 3 (Fig. 138–1). Interactions between protein 4.1 and some of the glycophorins and between various skeletal proteins and membrane lipids probably also occur, but are less well characterized.

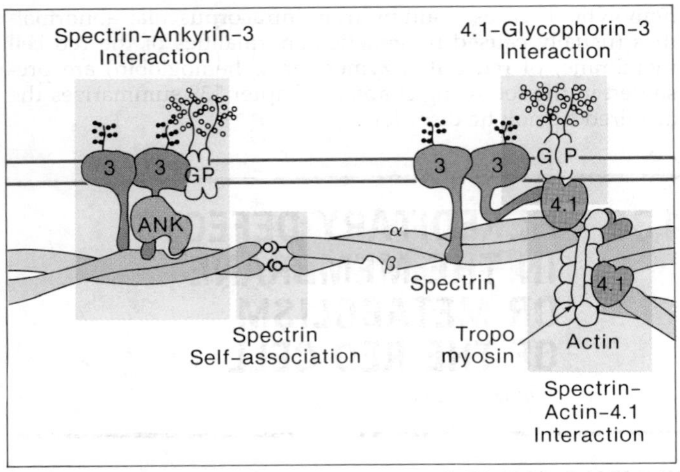

FIGURE 138–1. Schematic illustration of the organization of the major proteins of the red cell membrane and membrane skeleton.

Major Functions

Membrane Strength and Durability. In humans the red cell must be flexible enough to negotiate splenic and capillary channels less than half its diameter and still be strong and durable enough to survive the turbulent journey through the heart approximately 500,000 times during its 120-day lifespan. These properties are *determined by the membrane skeleton*. The membrane spontaneously vesiculates when spectrin and actin are selectively extracted or when spectrin is denatured (at 49°C). Mice with hereditary deficiencies of spectrin have extremely fragile red cells that rapidly fragment in the circulation, leading to marked spherocytosis and severe hemolysis.

Maintenance of Cell Volume. The red cell controls its volume and water content by regulating its intracellular concentration of Na^+ and K^+. This is possible because the membrane is relatively impermeable to cations. Normally, small passive cation leaks are balanced by the active transport of Na^+ outward and K^+ inward. These ion movements are powered by a pump that is fueled by the membrane enzyme *Na^+, K^+-ATPase*. Normally this system maintains intracellular Na^+ and K^+ at about 10 mEq per liter and 100 mEq per liter, respectively. The pump is regulated by the intracellular Na^+ concentration and has considerable ability to compensate for an increased leak of Na^+ into the cell. If this capacity is surpassed and the inward leak of Na^+ exceeds the K^+ leak out, red cells gain cations and water and swell. Unfortunately the pump does not compensate nearly as well to a decrease in intracellular K^+. Any increase in the outward leak of K^+ relative to Na^+ (normally $K^+[out]:Na^+[in] = 2:3$) leads to loss of total monovalent cations and water and results in cellular dehydration.

Calcium Homeostasis. Excessive intracellular Ca^{++} is very deleterious, and the red cell actively extrudes it with an efficient, calmodulin-regulated calcium pump that is driven by a *Ca^{++}-ATPase*. Intracellular Ca^{++} is normally almost undetectable (about 0.1 μM). If ATP levels fall below about 20 per cent of normal or if Ca^{++} leakage exceeds the capacity of the pump, Ca^{++} accumulates and changes the red cell from a biconcave disc to an echinocyte—a spiculated sphere with numerous short, regular projections. Elevated intracellular Ca^{++} also causes a selective loss of K^+ and water. The result is a crenated, dehydrated, almost indeformable cell that is highly susceptible to splenic sequestration and destruction.

Anion Exchange. Physiologically the red cell is a critical component of CO_2 transport. Red cells normally convert tissue CO_2 to HCO_3^- and carry the HCO_3^- to the lungs where they exchange it for Cl^-. The process is massive and requires a large number of transport channels (~1 million per red cell). These are formed by *protein 3* (Fig. 138–1).

Interactions Between Red Cells and the Spleen

Red cells that enter the spleen must squeeze their 7-μ wide bodies through narrow elliptical fenestrations that separate the splenic cords and sinuses to return to the circulation (Ch. 164). Normal red cells make this journey about 120 times per day and complete it in about 30 seconds, but abnormal cells may be detained for minutes to hours in the hypoxic, acidic, hypoglycemic environment of the splenic cords. This taxing metabolic stress is often fatal for old or defective erythrocytes.

Red cells are detained in the spleen if they are rigid or if they are coated with proteins such as IgG1, IgG3, or C3b that bind to receptors on splenic macrophages. Probably other, less well defined, changes in the red cell surface also attract phagocytes and lead to red cell death. Increased rigidity may result from (1) increased cytoplasmic viscosity (e.g., sickled cells and other dehydrated red cells); (2) intracellular rubbish (e.g., Heinz bodies); (3) membrane rigidity (e.g., secondary to oxidative cross-linking of the membrane skeleton); or (4) a decrease in the red cell surface-volume ratio.

Surface-Volume Ratio: Osmotic Fragility Test

Spherocytes are caused by a decrease in the surface-volume ratio of the red cell. Target cells form when this ratio is increased. Because the area of the red cell membrane is fixed (i.e., the membrane is not stretchable), the cell becomes progressively more rigid as its spheroidicity increases. Surface-volume ratio is assessed clinically by the *unincubated osmotic fragility test*. This test measures the ability of red cells to swell in a graded series of hypotonic solutions. Spherocytes are osmotically fragile; that is, they can tolerate less osmotic swelling than normal cells before they hemolyze. Target cells are osmotically resistant.

Hereditary Spherocytosis (HS)

Hereditary spherocytosis is an inherited hemolytic anemia characterized by osmotically fragile, partially spherical, spectrin-deficient red cells that are selectively trapped by the spleen. The disease occurs in all races, but is particularly common in northern Europeans, where the prevalence is about 1 in 5000. There are at least two patterns of inheritance: 75 per cent of the families show a classic autosomal dominant pattern. Most of the remainder have a nondominant (probably autosomal recessive) form.

Pathogenesis. Hereditary spherocytes transfused into normal subjects show impairment of survival, demonstrating clearly that they are intrinsically defective. The primary physiologic defect appears to be membrane instability. Red cell membranes from some HS patients fragment more easily than normal when stressed. This weakness suggests a defect of the membrane skeleton.

All HS red cells are spectrin deficient. Either quantitative or qualitative defects may occur in this major skeletal protein. The degree of spectrin deficiency correlates closely with the degree of spherocytosis, as measured by osmotic fragility, and with the severity of hemolysis and response to splenectomy. In general, patients with dominant HS have only mild deficiency (spectrin content 75 to 90 per cent of normal) and mild to moderate hemolysis. Patients with recessive HS often have a more severe deficit; sometimes so severe (30 to 50 per cent of normal) that it produces life-threatening, transfusion-dependent hemolysis.

In a subset of patients with dominant HS (perhaps 5 to 10 per cent) a qualitative defect in the beta chain of spectrin is also present. About 40 per cent of the spectrin molecules *lack the ability to bind protein 4.1*. (This is close to the expected proportion in the dominant form of HS, since only one of the two beta-spectrin genes will be abnormal.) The defective spectrin binds poorly to actin, weakening the skeleton. Red cells from these patients are also spectrin deficient, presumably because the mutant spectrin is catabolized more rapidly than normal. It is not yet known whether the decreased

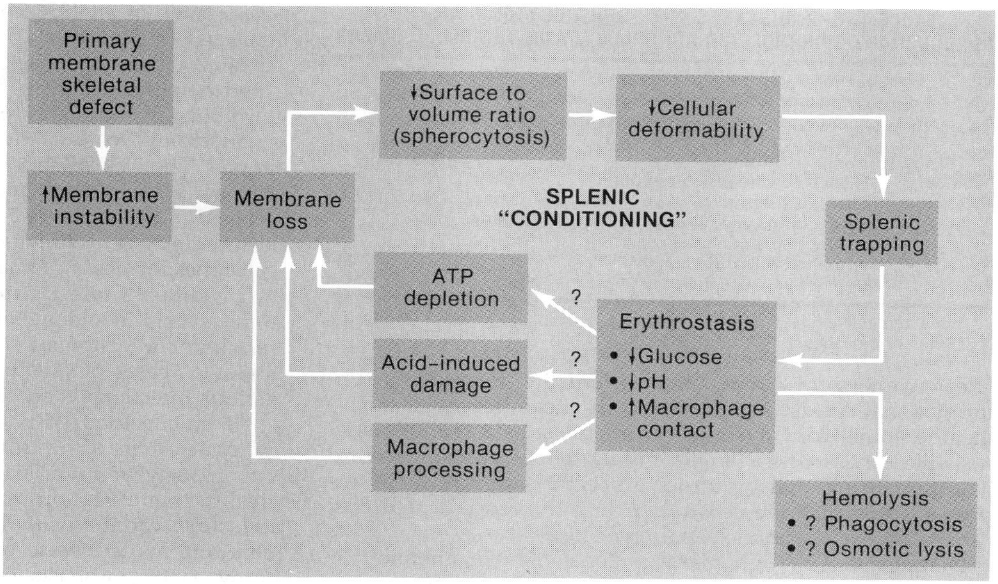

FIGURE 138–2. Currently favored model of the pathophysiology of hereditary spherocytosis.

spectrin observed in other HS patients is due to analogous, unidentified structural defects or whether it results from decreased synthesis of an otherwise normal protein.

It is speculated that HS red cells gradually lose the portions of lipid bilayer that overlie spectrin-deficient regions, and become progressively more spherocytic as they age in the circulation (Fig. 138–2). Eventually they are detained in the splenic cords where, for unknown reasons, their membrane loss is accentuated by the toxic cordal environment. This *"splenic conditioning"* can be mimicked in vitro by incubating red cells in the absence of glucose for 24 hours. Under these conditions hereditary spherocytes lose membrane fragments more rapidly than do normal red cells. This is the basis of the *incubated osmotic fragility test*. In vivo, conditioned spherocytes are prevalent in the splenic pulp, and some escape into the peripheral circulation as the characteristic HS hyperchromic microspherocytes. These impaired cells form the hyperspherical tail on osmotic fragility curves. Undoubtedly many HS red cells never escape the conditioning process. Those that do are especially susceptible to recapture and destruction by the spleen.

Clinical Features (Table 138–1). The hallmarks of HS are *anemia*, *jaundice*, and *splenomegaly*. The disease may present at any age. In neonates excessive jaundice is frequent (~50 per cent) and sometimes requires an exchange transfusion. After the neonatal period most patients develop partially compensated hemolysis with mild to moderate anemia (Hb = 9 to 11.5 grams per deciliter), intermittent mild jaundice (especially during viral infections), and splenomegaly. *Clinical severity can vary widely*, sometimes even within the same family. A small proportion of patients have life-threatening hemolysis and are transfusion dependent. A much larger proportion, roughly 25 per cent, have unusually mild disease. In these patients marrow erythropoiesis is sufficient to balance the modest rate of spherocyte destruction, and there is no anemia, little or no jaundice, and minimal splenomegaly. However, severe hemolysis and anemia may develop with illnesses that cause the spleen to hypertrophy, such as infectious mononucleosis. Hemolysis may also be exacerbated by long-term intensive physical activity, possibly because of increased splenic blood flow. Finally, in old age, when bone marrow function becomes sluggish, previously well compensated splenectomized patients may become dangerously anemic.

TABLE 138–1. HEREDITARY SPHEROCYTOSIS

Clinical Manifestations	Laboratory Features
Anemia	Reticulocytosis
Splenomegaly	Spherocytosis
Intermittent jaundice	Elevated MCHC
From hemolysis	Increased osmotic fragility
From biliary obstruction	(especially incubated osmotic fragility test)
Aplastic crises	
Often dominant inheritance	Normal Coombs' test
Rare manifestations	Decreased red cell spectrin
Leg ulcers	
Spinal cord dysfunction	
Myocardiopathy	
Good response to splenectomy	

Complications. ***Crises.*** The clinical course is interrupted in most patients by periodic crises, characterized by worsening anemia. *Hemolytic crises* are the most frequent, but usually are mild and clinically insignificant. They are presumably secondary to the reticuloendothelial hyperplasia that accompanies many infections. *Aplastic crises* are less prevalent, but are often severe enough to threaten heart failure and require transfusion. They are frequently caused by a human parvovirus that invades hematopoietic stem cells and inhibits their growth. The infection typically presents in young children as a febrile illness or as fifth disease, a viral exantham; however, some older children and adults are also susceptible to the virus and aplastic crises. *Megaloblastic crises* occur when dietary intake of folic acid is inadequate for the increased needs of the erythroid HS bone marrow. This need is particularly acute during pregnancy. To prevent megaloblastic crises, all HS patients should receive daily supplements of folic acid (1 mg per day).

Gallstones. Untreated older children and adults with HS often develop bilirubinate gallstones secondary to increased bilirubin production. Only 5 per cent of children less than 10 years old are affected, but the prevalence rises to 40 to 50 per cent in the second to fifth decades and 55 to 75 per cent thereafter. The frequency after age 30 parallels the frequency in the general population, which suggests that gallstones in HS patients form primarily in the second and third decades. Ultrasonography is the most reliable method for detecting bilirubin stones. Only 50 per cent are radiopaque. Concern about cholecystitis and biliary obstruction is the major impetus for splenectomy in most patients. It is unfortunate, therefore, that there are no accurate data on the prevalence of these complications in patients with bilirubin stones to help assess the indications (risk-benefit ratio) for operation.

Other Complications. Occasional adult patients with HS develop gout, indolent ankle ulcers, or a chronic erythematous dermatitis on the legs. All of these complications disappear

TABLE 138–2. DISEASES WITH SPHEROCYTOSIS AS THE PREDOMINANT MORPHOLOGIC ABNORMALITY ON THE BLOOD SMEAR

Common
Hereditary spherocytosis
Immunohemolytic anemias (warm antibody type)
ABO incompatibility in neonates
Uncommon to rare
Hemolytic transfusion reactions
Clostridial sepsis
Severe burns and other red cell thermal injuries
Spider, bee, and snake venoms
Acute red cell oxidant injury*
Severe hypophosphatemia

*Acute red cell oxidant injury is common, but spherocytosis is rarely the predominant morphology.

after splenectomy. Rarer but potentially interesting syndromes that coexist with HS have also been described. These include spinal cord dysfunction, manifest as a multiple-sclerosis-like illness, and a familial myocardiopathy. In this regard it is tantalizing that erythrocyte spectrin appears to be expressed only in three cells other than the red cell: neurons, cardiac myocytes, and skeletal myocytes.

Diagnosis. Although many patients are not anemic, the *reticulocyte count is always increased* prior to splenectomy (except during an aplastic crisis). It is a much more dependable sign of hemolysis than is hyperbilirubinemia, since indirect bilirubin levels are elevated in only 50 to 60 per cent of patients. *Spherocytosis*, the hallmark of the disease, is the other most reliable finding (Color plate 2*K*). However, spherocytes are a frequent artifact in normal blood smears, so the physician must take care to examine only areas of the smear in which the red cells are well separated and some cells with central pallor are evident. Spherocytosis is also observed in a variety of other conditions (Table 138–2); however, with the exception of certain *immunohemolytic anemias* (which can be excluded with a Coombs test), most of these do not present any diagnostic difficulty.

In 20 to 25 per cent of patients, classic microspherocytes are sparse, and it may be difficult to recognize spherocytosis from the blood smear alone. In these patients the *unincubated* osmotic fragility (OF) test will sometimes be normal or only slightly increased, since it simply quantifies what is visible on the smear. The *incubated* OF, however, is almost always abnormal and is the most reliable available diagnostic test. HS red cells are somewhat dehydrated and therefore have an *increased mean corpuscular hemoglobin concentration (MCHC)*. An MCHC level of 36 or greater is present in 50 per cent of HS patients and is useful confirmatory evidence of the disease. Since spectrin deficiency appears to be the primary defect, a direct assay of red cell spectrin content should be the most accurate test; however, at present this measurement is available in only a few research laboratories.

Once HS is diagnosed *a careful search for the disease should always be made in all close relatives*. It is tragic to see HS become symptomatic in elderly patients with a poor operative risk, whose condition could have been discovered earlier.

Treatment. *Splenectomy* dependably blunts both red cell conditioning and hemolysis in HS and is the recommended therapy. Following surgery, spherocytosis persists because the basic red cell defect is unchanged, but conditioned microspherocytes disappear and changes typical of the postsplenectomy state (Howell-Jolly bodies, target cells, siderocytes, and acanthocytes) become evident on the blood smear. During the operation the surgeon must be careful to search for accessory spleens, which occur in 20 to 30 per cent of patients. Recurrence of hemolysis due to regrowth of an accessory spleen is occasionally observed after years or even decades.

Splenectomy increases susceptibility to sepsis from pneumococci and certain other encapsulated bacteria. The major issues today are who should undergo splenectomy and how should they be treated postoperatively. It is impossible to answer either question absolutely. In general, *we recommend splenectomy for all HS patients with either anemia or significant hemolysis* (reticulocyte counts repeatedly greater than 5 per cent). We defer splenectomy in patients with mild compensated hemolysis, but if these patients subsequently develop bilirubin gallstones and require cholecystectomy, we advocate splenectomy to prevent the recurrence of common duct stones. The risk of sepsis after splenectomy is very high in infancy and early childhood; splenectomy should therefore be delayed until the age of 5 or 6 years. There is no evidence that further delay is useful, and it may be harmful, since the risk of gallstones increases dramatically after the age of 10 years.

It is difficult to estimate accurately the risk of postsplenectomy sepsis in older children and adults. The incidence of fulminant infection in splenectomized adults appears to be about 0.2 cases per 100 person-years, and the incidence of all serious infections is about 7 cases per 100 person-years.

All splenectomized patients should receive *polyvalent pneumococcal vaccine* (Pnu-Immune 23 or equivalent, 0.5 ml subcutaneously or intramuscularly), preferably given preoperatively. Immunization with meningococcal and *Hemophilus influenzae* vaccines should also be considered, especially in children. We advocate prophylactic antibiotics after splenectomy, with emphasis on protection against pneumococcal sepsis (i.e., Pen-Vee K or equivalent, 6 to 8 mg per kilogram twice daily), at least for the first two years after surgery when the incidence of infection is greatest. This is a controversial issue that depends on patient compliance, bacterial resistance in the local community, and a host of other factors.

All unsplenectomized patients with HS (and other hemolytic anemias) should receive *folic acid* (1 mg per day) to sustain erythropoiesis and prevent megaloblastic crises.

Hereditary Elliptocytosis (HE)

Hereditary elliptocytosis, usually inherited as an autosomal dominant trait, is relatively common (~1:2500), particularly in its nonhemolytic form. Clinically the disease is more heterogeneous than is HS (Table 138–3). All types of HE are due to defects in the membrane skeleton. A number of specific molecular defects have been defined, some of which are discussed in the following sections.

Common HE

This most prevalent form of HE (~90 per cent of cases) is usually caused either by defects in the head end of spectrin that interfere with spectrin self-association or by the partial

TABLE 138–3. HEREDITARY ELLIPTOCYTOSIS

Clinical Manifestations	Laboratory Features
Common HE	
Asymptomatic Dominant inheritance: one parent with HE Variants: Some neonates with moderately severe hemolytic anemia and HPP-like smear. Converts to typical common HE by 1 to 2 years Some patients with mild chronic hemolysis	Blood smear: elliptocytes, few or no poikilocytes No anemia, little or no hemolysis (reticulocytes = 1 to 3%) Normal osmotic fragility Often defect in spectrin self-association or partial deficiency of protein 4.1
Hereditary Pyropoikilocytosis	
Anemia Splenomegaly Intermittent jaundice Aplastic crises Recessive inheritance: both parents normal or one or both parents with HE Good response to splenectomy	Blood smear: bizarre poikilocytes, fragments, spherocytes, ± elliptocytes Reticulocytosis Increased osmotic fragility Decreased red cell heat stability Marked defect in spectin self-association
Spherocytic HE	
Anemia Splenomegaly Intermittent jaundice Dominant inheritance pattern Good response to splenectomy	Blood smear: rounded elliptocytes, ± spherocytes Reticulocytosis Increased osmotic fragility

absence of protein 4.1. Practically it is little more than a morphologic curiosity. Most patients have no anemia or splenomegaly and only mild hemolysis (reticulocyte counts of 1 to 3 per cent). The blood smear shows prominent elliptocytosis (usually >40 per cent; normal <15 per cent). Osmotic fragility is normal. A few cases (10 to 20 per cent) have moderate hemolysis and are classified as sporadic hemolytic variants. The reason for this variation is unknown.

In general, patients with common HE require no therapy; but they may develop significant hemolysis if the spleen hypertrophies in response to various stimuli (e.g., infectious mononucleosis, cirrhosis). In addition, the physician must be alert for *transient neonatal hemolysis*. Neonates in some HE families (particularly black families with a defect in spectrin self-association) have moderately severe hemolytic anemia with marked red cell budding, fragmentation, and poikilocytosis. The relative paucity of elliptocytes may create diagnostic confusion; however, the diagnosis is easily made from family studies, since one of the parents will have common HE. Hemolysis gradually declines in these infants during the first year or so of life, and the disorder evolves into typical common HE. This curious phenomenon is unexplained. Presumably it reflects a difference in the fetal red cell or the circulatory system of the newborn that augments the primary defect in spectrin self-association.

Hereditary Pyropoikilocytosis (HPP)

This rare autosomal recessive disorder is characterized by moderately severe hemolytic anemia, marked red cell fragmentation, and *bizarre poikilocytosis*. It is most common in blacks. When heated for short periods, HPP red cells fragment (and their isolated spectrin denatures) at 45 to 46°C instead of the normal 49°C. This *exceptional heat sensitivity* constitutes the primary test for the disease. Hemolysis decreases after splenectomy, the treatment of choice, but the bizarre red cell morphology and heat sensitivity are unchanged. HPP is related to common HE in that all HPP patients have a *defect in spectrin self-association* that is qualitatively identical to the defect in common HE, but more severe. In addition, patients with HPP often have first-degree relatives with HE. A current hypothesis is that HPP patients are either homozygous for common HE, homozygous for a related "silent" mutation, or doubly heterozygous for common HE and the putative silent gene defect.

Spherocytic HE

This variant (~10 per cent of cases) is clinically and pathophysiologically similar to hereditary spherocytosis. It is inherited in an autosomal dominant pattern. The primary molecular defect is unknown. Patients typically have moderate hemolysis, mild anemia, and splenomegaly. Elliptocytes are less prominent and are more rounded than in typical common HE. Spherocytes are often evident and occasionally may predominate; however, at least one family member will usually have clear-cut elliptocytosis. Patients with this form of HE, like those with HS, have osmotically fragile red cells and respond dramatically to splenectomy.

Hereditary Defects in Membrane Permeability

Hereditary Xerocytosis

In this rare, autosomal dominant disorder of red cell membrane permeability the ratio of K^+ loss to Na^+ gain exceeds the normal ratio of 2:3; as a result, total cation content and cell water decrease. This occurs as a secondary event in a variety of conditions (e.g., sickle cell disease and glycolytic enzyme deficiencies). Morphologically, dehydrated red cells are typically either targeted or contracted and spiculated. Because dehydration increases intracellular viscosity, these cells are relatively rigid and risk splenic sequestration and hemolysis.

Hereditary Hydrocytosis (Hereditary Stomatocytosis)

In this rare autosomal dominant disease, an inherited defect in Na^+ permeability causes massive Na^+ influx, which overwhelms the Na-K pump and leads to an increase in intracellular cations and water. In some families this results in severe hemolysis. In others, for unknown reasons, hemolysis is much milder. Patients with the severe variant respond well to splenectomy. The partially swollen red cells appear on blood smears as stomatocytes (i.e., red cells with a mouthlike band of pallor across the center of the stained cell). Stomatocytes are much more frequently seen as an acquired defect, without hydrocytosis, cation changes, or hemolysis, in patients with acute alcoholism or with various types of liver disease.

ENZYME DEFICIENCIES

Normal Red Cell Metabolism

Reticulocytes have no nuclei and lose their mitochondria and microsomes as they mature; consequently, mature red cells consume little oxygen and do not synthesize protein. Glucose, the main metabolic substrate of the cells, is metabolized via two major pathways: the *Embden-Meyerhof pathway* and the *hexosemonophosphate shunt* (Fig. 138–3).

The Embden-Meyerhof (EM) Pathway

Approximately 90 to 95 per cent of metabolized glucose is converted to lactate via the EM pathway. This is the *major pathway of ATP synthesis in mature red cells*. Only two moles of ATP are generated from glycolysis per mole of glucose consumed, very inefficient compared to cells that possess mitochondria and an active Krebs cycle (that generates 38 moles of ATP per mole of glucose). Nevertheless the meager amount of ATP produced permits renewal of 150 to 200 per cent of the total red cell ATP every hour. Red cell ATP is used to transport monovalent cations and calcium, to phosphorylate various proteins, to synthesize glutathione, to salvage nucleotides, and to produce the glucose phosphates needed to fuel glycolysis.

The EM pathway is also the major source of red cell NADH. This cofactor is essential for the maintenance of heme iron in the reduced state, an enzymatic process that is mediated by *NADH methemoglobin reductase*. Oxidation of heme iron to Fe^{+++} produces methemoglobin, which does not transport oxygen (Ch. 146).

Red cells have a uniquely high concentration of *2,3-diphosphoglycerate (2,3-DPG)*; only traces of this metabolic intermediate are present in other cells. This intermediate, formed by the Rapaport-Luebering shunt (Fig. 138–3), decreases the oxygen affinity of hemoglobin and increases oxygen delivery to peripheral tissues (Ch. 140).

Hexose Monophosphate (HMP) Shunt

Approximately 5 to 10 per cent of utilized glucose is normally directed through the HMP shunt. This pathway is the *major source of NADPH* in human red cells: Two moles of NADPH are produced for each mole of glucose metabolized. Under conditions in which the oxidation of NADPH is accelerated, diversion of glucose through the shunt can increase up to 10- or 20-fold.

The most important reactions associated with NADPH oxidation are those related to glutathione. Red cells contain relatively high concentrations (2 mM) of *reduced glutathione (GSH)*, a tripeptide (gamma-glutamylcysteinylglycine) that is synthesized by mature red cells (Fig. 138–3). GSH protects red cells from injury by oxidants such as superoxide anion (O_2^-), hydrogen peroxide (H_2O_2), and hydroxyl radical ($OH^{\bullet}$), which are produced continuously in normal red cells as by-products of the oxidation of heme by its dangerous oxygen cargo. Large amounts of oxidants are generated by activated phagocytes (e.g., during infections) and by red cells in the

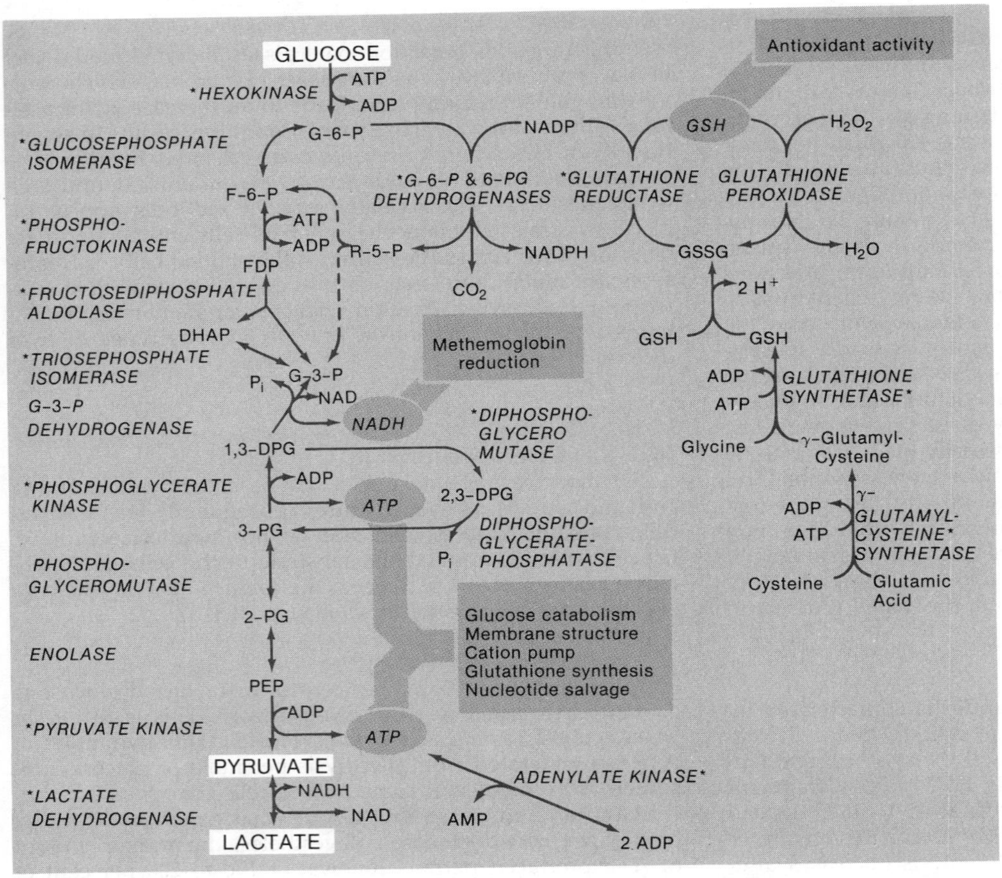

FIGURE 138–3. Glycolytic pathways and glutathione metabolism in the human erythrocyte. Asterisks indicate enzymes for which severe deficiency has been established. (From Valentine WN: Hemolytic anemia and inborn errors of metabolism. Blood 54:549, 1979. Reprinted by permission.)

presence of certain drugs. Injury to cell lipids and proteins occurs if these agents accumulate. Normally this is prevented by GSH. Detoxification of H_2O_2 can occur spontaneously, but it is enhanced by *glutathione peroxidase*. Catalase also degrades H_2O_2, but under physiologic conditions it is less important. In these reactions GSH is converted to *oxidized glutathione (GSSG)* and to mixed disulfides with protein thiols (Fig. 138–3). GSH levels are restored by *glutathione reductase*. In the process, NADPH is oxidized to NADP, which stimulates the HMP shunt, regenerating NADPH. This tight coupling of the HMP shunt with glutathione metabolism normally protects red cells from oxidant injury.

Defects in the HMP Shunt or Glutathione Metabolism

Almost all HMP shunt defects are due to *glucose-6-phosphate dehydrogenase* deficiency, the most common enzyme abnormality associated with hemolytic anemia. It affects millions of people throughout the world. In contrast, pyruvate kinase deficiency, the most common glycolytic defect, affects only hundreds to thousands of patients.

Glucose-6-Phosphate Dehydrogenase (G6PD) Deficiency

Pathophysiology. Defects in the HMP shunt or glutathione metabolic pathways impair the ability of red cells to defend themselves against oxidative assault. Oxidants produced by infections or oxidant drugs are normally detoxified by GSH, but GSH levels are not maintained in G6PD deficiency because of the diminished ability to generate NADPH. As a consequence the oxidants are free to damage vital cell constituents. Oxidation of hemoglobin produces the functionless *methemoglobin* and intracellular precipitates of denatured hemoglobin that are known as *Heinz bodies*. Heinz bodies are not visible in ordinary Wright's stained blood smears, but are revealed with supravital stains such as *methyl violet*. They attach to the membrane and damage it in poorly defined ways. In vitro, this causes increased membrane leakiness to cations, decreased osmotic fragility, and decreased deformability. In vivo, Heinz bodies are "pitted" from circulating red cells by the spleen and thus are more plentiful in splenectomized patients. "*Bite cells*," that is red cells with a localized invagination, possibly at the site of Heinz body removal, appear in the circulation during acute hemolytic episodes. Red cells with a submembranous hemoglobin-free area, "*blister cells*," may also be seen. In addition to damage from Heinz bodies, G6PD-deficient red cells suffer oxidative cross-linking of spectrin and peroxidation of membrane lipids. Spectrin cross-linking decreases membrane flexibility and promotes splenic trapping. Lipid damage may be responsible for the intravascular hemolysis seen during acute hemolytic episodes.

More than 150 G6PD variants are now known, but only a few of these are common. The normal enzyme is termed $G6PD^B$ or Gd^B. It is present in about 70 per cent of American blacks and in more than 99 per cent of whites. Gd^{A+} is a normal variant found in about 20 per cent of American blacks. It has a greater electrophoretic mobility than Gd^B because of substitution of an asparagine for an aspartic acid in the amino acid sequence. Gd^{A-}, the most common variant associated with hemolysis, is found in about 10 per cent of American blacks and in many African black populations. It has the same electrophoretic mobility as Gd^{A+}, but its catalytic activity is decreased. Gd^{Med}, the second most common abnormal variant, is found in peoples of the Mediterranean area (Italians, Greeks, Sardinians, Sephardic Jews, Arabs, etc.), in India, and in southeastern Asia. Its electrophoretic mobility is normal, but its catalytic activity is markedly reduced. Gd^{Canton}, a relatively common variant in Oriental populations, produces a clinical syndrome similar to Gd^{A-}.

As normal red cells age in vivo, the activity of intracellular Gd^B decays slowly with a half-life of about 60 days (Fig. 138–4). Despite this loss of active enzyme, older normal red cells retain enough activity to produce NADPH and maintain GSH in the face of almost all oxidant stresses. The defect in Gd^{A-} results in a *labile enzyme* that disappears with a half-life of about 13 days. *Young red cells thus have normal enzyme activity, while older red cells are grossly deficient.* As a consequence of this heterogeneity, hemolysis is self-limited in individuals with Gd^{A-}.

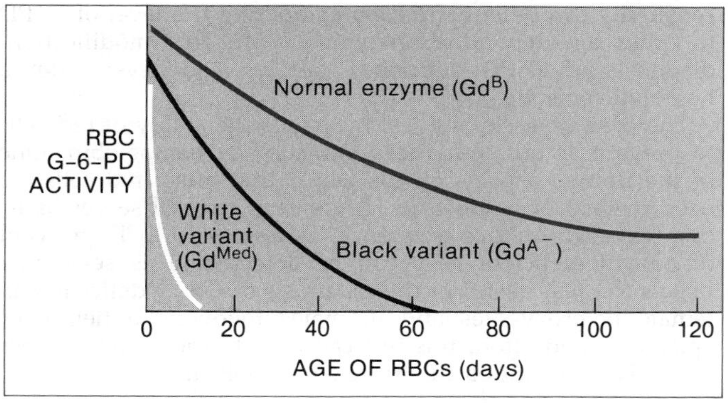

FIGURE 138–4. Intracellular decay of red cell G-6-PD as a function of cell age. The top curve shows the decay rate for Gd^B, the normal enzyme. The middle and lower curves show the greater than normal decay rates for the unstable Gd^{A-} and Gd^{Med} variants. Note that only the oldest Gd^{A-} red cells are markedly G-6-PD deficient and susceptible to hemolysis, whereas nearly all Gd^{Med} erythrocytes are vulnerable. Note also that after the most deficient Gd^{A-} red cells have been destroyed, the average G-6-PD level in the remaining cells will be near normal. This explains why G-6-PD assays after a hemolytic episode often fail to disclose the defect in Gd^{A-} males. (From Lux SE: Hemolytic anemias. Metabolic disorders. In Beck WS (ed.): Hematology. 4th ed. Cambridge, MA, The MIT Press, 1985, p 223. Reprinted with permission.)

This is shown graphically in Figure 138–5, which depicts the course of primaquine-induced hemolysis in an individual with Gd^{A-}. Acute hemolysis with hemoglobinuria and decreased ^{51}Cr red cell survival develops when the drug is first administered, but this is followed by a recovery phase in which anemia and reticulocytosis abate and red cell survival improves despite continued administration of the drug. The reason is that once the oxidant-sensitive older red cells are destroyed, the remaining young cells are oxidant resistant. Since only about 50 per cent of the cells are oxidant sensitive to begin with in Gd^{A-}, the bone marrow can compensate by simply doubling its output. This apparent drug resistance persists as long as the offending drug is continuously administered. Note, however, that if the drug is stopped for two to three months, older red cells will survive and accumulate, and the patient will again become drug sensitive.

Gd^{Med} is considerably more unstable than Gd^{A-} (Fig. 138–4). Very little activity is present in mature red cells. Despite this, chronic hemolysis does not occur, which must indicate that endogenous oxidant stresses are normally very low. When threatened by infections or oxidant drugs, however, these patients are at much greater risk because virtually their entire red cell population can be destroyed.

Clinical Features (Table 138–4). The most dramatic clinical presentation is acute intravascular hemolysis. These patients typically develop hemoglobinemia (pink to brown plasma), hemoglobinuria (red-brown to black urine), and jaundice acutely with an infection or within one to three days of exposure to an oxidant drug. In severe cases abdominal or back pain may be prominent. Symptoms of acute anemia (dizziness, headache, palpitations, dyspnea) may also develop. Heinz bodies and increased levels of methemoglobin appear in the red cells, and some bite cells and blister cells may be seen on the blood smear. In many cases, however, the red cell morphology is relatively normal. More often hemolysis is less dramatic, and a modest decline of hemoglobin (3 to 4 grams per deciliter) occurs, without hemoglobinuria or prominent symptoms. These episodes are easily overlooked unless the physician is alert.

The discovery of G6PD deficiency followed the observation that black soldiers developed explosive hemolysis after receiving primaquine for malaria. Subsequently, numerous other oxidant drugs were implicated as causative agents, some of which are listed in Table 138–5. The most common cause of hemolysis, however, is *infection*. Virtually every type of infection has been associated. One speculation is that oxidants generated by warring phagocytes trigger hemolysis by impinging on neighboring G6PD-deficient red cells. Hemolysis can also be precipitated by diabetic ketoacidosis and is exacerbated by uremia, because of an acquired inefficiency in the operation of the HMP shunt.

Severe hemolytic episodes occasionally follow exposure to *fava beans* (Italian broad beans) or their pollen, probably caused by divicine and isouramil, oxidant pyrimidine derivatives that are present in high concentrations in the beans. This rare phenomenon occurs mainly in individuals with Gd^{Med}; it is not seen in Gd^{A-}. This, and the fact that not all patients with Gd^{Med} are susceptible, indicates that other unknown factors must be involved.

In some patients with rare variants of G6PD, *chronic hemolysis* occurs in the absence of obvious oxidants. These cases are characterized by enzymes that are unable to maintain basal NADPH production. Variants generally have either a high K_m for NADP or a low K_i for NADPH.

Genetics. The gene for G6PD is located on the X chromosome, so its inheritance is sex linked. Males have one type of G6PD; females can have two types. For example, 70 per cent

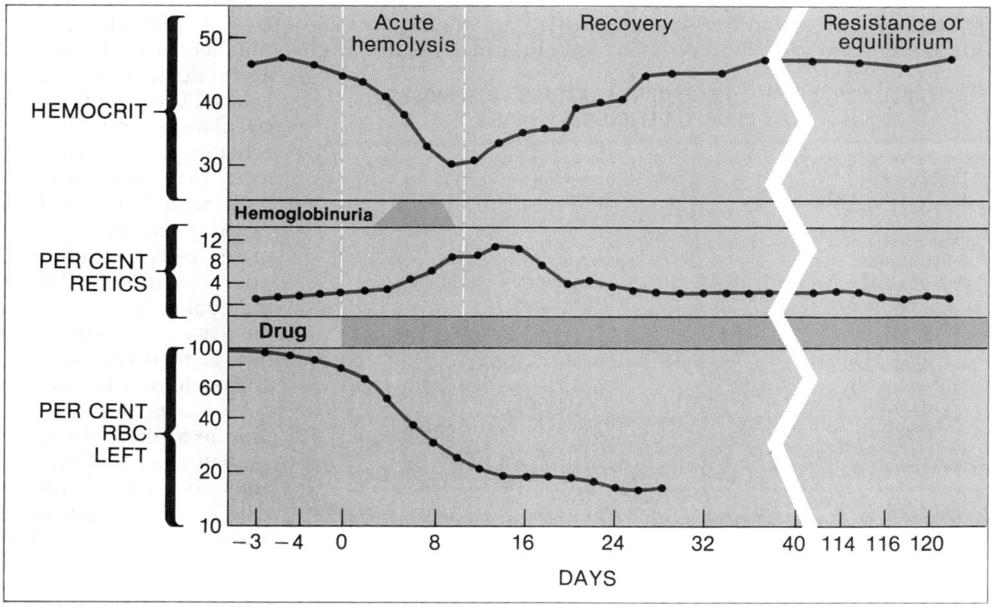

FIGURE 138–5. Course of drug-induced hemolysis in an individual with Gd^{A-}. Note that hemolysis abates and apparent resistance to the drug develops after the initial hemolytic episode due to repopulation with young red cells. (Adapted from Alving AS: Bull World Health Organ 22:621, 1960. Reprinted with permission.)

TABLE 138–4. CLINICAL COMPARISON OF THE TWO COMMON FORMS OF G6PD DEFICIENCY

	Gd^{A-}	Gd^{Med}
Frequency	Common in black populations	Common in Mediterranean populations
Chronic hemolysis	None	None
Degree of acute hemolysis	Moderate	Severe
G6PD defect	Old red cells	All red cells
Hemolysis with:		
Drugs	Unusual	Common
Infection	Common	Common
Need for transfusions	Rare	Sometimes

of black males have Gd^{B}, 20 per cent have Gd^{A+}, and 10 per cent have Gd^{A-}. Black females, however, can be heterozygous for any two of these enzymes. According to the *Lyon hypothesis*, only one X chromosome is active in any somatic cell; thus any given red cell in heterozygous females is either normal or deficient. Mean enzyme activity in females who are heterozygous for G6PD deficiency may be normal, moderately reduced (usual), or grossly deficient, depending on the degree of lyonization. Deficient cells in heterozygous females are just as susceptible to oxidant injury as enzyme-deficient cells in males; however, the overall magnitude of hemolysis is less because of the smaller population of vulnerable cells.

Despite the disadvantages of a gene for G6PD deficiency, it remains common in many geographic areas. Its prevalence has been attributed to a selective advantage it is believed to provide against malaria caused by *Plasmodium falciparum*. This proposal is supported by a large body of data, including epidemiologic studies and observations in heterozygous females demonstrating the resistance of cells containing the abnormal enzyme to malarial infection.

Diagnosis. Several tests for the diagnosis of G6PD deficiency are currently available. Their sensitivity varies and their usefulness is determined by the clinical situation (sex of patient, type of G6PD deficiency, and proximity to the hemolytic episode).

Commonly used screening tests are based on NADPH-mediated dye decolorization or on the reduction of methemoglobin in the presence of methylene blue. These tests are of limited sensitivity, since 30 to 40 per cent of the cells must be abnormal for the deficient state to be detected. This criterion may not be met in patients with Gd^{A-} or Gd^{Canton} after a severe hemolytic episode, since most of their enzyme-deficient, older red cells will have been destroyed.

Definitive assay of the enzyme depends on direct spectrophotometric measurement of NADPH production. This test is more sensitive than the screening tests, but still requires 20 to 30 per cent deficient cells for an abnormal result. The sensitivity can be enhanced by comparing the level of G6PD to other age-dependent enzymes. With this modification, diagnosis of G6PD deficiency can be made even after a hemolytic episode.

The cyanide-ascorbate test measures the ability of red cells to prevent ascorbate-induced oxidation of hemoglobin. One of the unique aspects of this test is that intact red cells are used instead of hemolysate. Thus each red cell serves as its own cuvette. As a consequence, as few as 10 to 15 per cent of enzyme-deficient cells can be detected. This sensitivity makes the test useful in the diagnosis of G6PD deficiency in female heterozygotes and in males following a hemolytic episode. In addition, this test can detect other abnormalities of the HMP shunt or glutathione metabolism.

TABLE 138–5. DRUGS COMMONLY LEADING TO HEMOLYSIS IN G6PD DEFICIENCY*

Antimalarials	*Analgesics*
Primaquine	Acetanilid
Quinacrine (Atabrine)	Acetylsalicylic acid†
	Acetophenetidin (Phenacetin)†
Sulfonamides	*Sulfones*
Sulfanilamide	Diaminodiphenylsulfone (Dapsone)
Salicylazosulfapyridine (Azulfidine)	
Sulfisoxazole (Gantrisin)†	*Miscellaneous*
Other Antibacterials	Dimercaprol (BAL)
Nitrofurantoin (Furadantin)	Naphthalene (moth balls)
Nitrofurazone (Furacin)	Methylene blue†
Chloramphenicol†	Vitamin K (water-soluble analogues)†
Para-aminosalicylic acid	
Nalidixic acid	Ascorbic acid†

*A more comprehensive list of drugs implicated in oxidant hemolysis appears in Beutler E: Pharmacol Rev 21:73, 1969.

†Hemolysis is infrequent and generally requires a high concentration of the drug. Probably a risk in Gd^{Med} but not in Gd^{A-} or Gd^{Canton}.

Other Defects

Abnormalities of GSH metabolism, the first line of defense against oxidants, can also be associated with hemolysis. Defects in either *glutathione synthetase* or *gamma-glutamylcysteine synthetase*, the two enzymes responsible for the synthesis of GSH, occur in rare patients. Erythrocytes lacking either of these enzymes have very low levels of GSH. Clinically the disorders are similar to G6PD deficiency; they are characterized by mild to moderate hemolytic anemia that is sensitive to drugs. Chronic neurologic disease also occurs in some patients with glutathione synthetase deficiency, but it is not certain that the enzyme disorder and neurologic defect are causally related.

Inherited deficiencies of *GSSG reductase* are thought to exist, but they are rare, and no case of hemolysis due to this disorder has been proved. Many individuals (including all newborn infants) are relatively deficient in *GSH peroxidase*, but they do not have excessive hemolysis. This probably reflects the fact that nonenzymatic reduction of peroxide by GSH occurs at a significant rate.

Defects in Glycolysis

General Features. Abnormalities in nearly every glycolytic enzyme have been described, but pyruvate kinase (PK) deficiency accounts for about 90 per cent of the cases associated with hemolysis.

Almost all of the glycolytic defects are inherited in an autosomal recessive pattern. Hemolysis is observed in homozygotes. Heterozygotes are normal, although their red cells contain less than normal amounts of enzyme. Phosphoglycerate kinase (PGK) deficiency is an exception, since this enzyme is located on the X chromosome.

Hemolysis due to glycolytic defects is thought to be due to lack of ATP. However, red cell ATP concentrations are often not decreased because (1) the mean cell age is very young and reticulocytes have high ATP levels; (2) defective cells with low ATP content are probably removed promptly from the circulation; and (3) ATP may be compartmentalized within reticulocytes, in which case a decline in ATP at one critical locus may be sufficient to cause cell injury.

Clinical Features. Hemolysis is chronic and is not affected by drugs. *Splenomegaly* is usually present because of stagnation of red cells in this organ. The acidic, hypoxic, and nutrient-poor environment of the spleen is an added insult to the metabolically abnormal cells. Thus the hemolytic rate often decreases after splenectomy. In most cases red cell morphology is relatively unremarkable prior to splenectomy. After splenectomy the blood smear typically contains a small number of *dense spiculated red cells*, but this is not invariable or unique to these disorders.

Diagnosis. Definitive diagnosis requires spectrophotometric enzyme assays performed under a variety of conditions (i.e., with varying substrate and cofactor concentrations) to detect enzymes with abnormal kinetics. Measurements of glycolytic intermediates may reveal subtle enzyme abnormalities, since the concentration of an intermediate usually increases proximal to a defect and decreases distal to it.

Pyruvate Kinase (PK) Deficiency

PK catalyzes one of the major reactions responsible for ATP production in glycolysis; it is not surprising, therefore, that deficiency of this enzyme causes hemolytic anemia. Hemolysis can be mild and completely compensated or severe enough to require frequent transfusions. The distal glycolytic block in PK deficiency causes a two- to three-fold increase in red cell 2,3-DPG, which enhances tissue oxygenation and may minimize some of the physiologic consequences of the anemia. In most cases hemolysis improves following splenectomy, although the effect is not as dramatic as in diseases like hereditary spherocytosis. The improvement is related to the fact that PK-deficient reticulocytes depend on mitochondrial oxidative phosphorylation as an ATP source. In vitro incubation of PK-deficient reticulocytes under hypoxic conditions or with inhibitors of oxidative phosphorylation causes ATP levels to fall. The cells subsequently gain Ca^{++}, lose K^{+} and water, and become rigid. PK-deficient reticulocytes sequestered in the hypoxic splenic cords presumably undergo similar degeneration. Even when anemia improves following splenectomy, reticulocytes may rise to levels of 50 to 70 per cent. This *paradoxical reticulocytosis* is due to increased reticulocyte survival once the adverse metabolic environment of the spleen is removed.

Defects in Red Cell Nucleotide Metabolism

Deficiency of *pyrimidine-5′-nucleotidase* is the third or fourth most common enzyme deficiency leading to hemolysis. This enzyme degrades pyrimidine nucleotides to cytidine and uridine, which can diffuse out of the cell. Lacking this activity, red cells accumulate partially degraded messenger and ribosomal RNA, and up to 5 per cent of the cells develop *prominent basophilic stippling*. Apparently the basophilic stippling in lead poisoning is produced by a similar mechanism, since pyrimidine-5′-nucleotidase is markedly inhibited by lead. Patients with an inherited (autosomal recessive) deficiency of this enzyme have chronic, moderately severe hemolytic anemia. The mechanism of hemolysis is unknown. Splenomegaly is common, but splenectomy produces little discernible benefit.

Finally, a rare disorder characterized by *overproduction of adenosine deaminase* illustrates the importance of ATP in red cell integrity. In affected patients, excessive deamination of adenosine apparently reduces the amount of this purine sufficiently to impair ATP synthesis. A chronic hemolytic anemia results. The disorder seems to be caused by hyperefficient translation of an adenosine deaminase mRNA that is present in normal amounts and produces a qualitatively normal enzyme. This extraordinary result suggests that a defect will be found in the 5′ untranslated region of the mRNA that enhances binding of the message to ribosomes or initiation factors.

Agre P, Asimos A, Casella JF, et al.: Inheritance pattern and clinical response to splenectomy as a reflection of erythrocyte spectrin deficiency in hereditary spherocytosis. N Engl J Med 315:1579, 1986. *By comparing red cell spectrin content with clinical manifestations in 33 HS patients, the authors find that the dominant form of the disease is milder than the nondominant form and that spectrin content correlates closely with spheroidicity, hemolytic rate, and response to splenectomy.*

Becker PS, Lux SE: Hereditary spherocytosis and related disorders. Clin Haematol 14:15, 1985. *Review of the etiology and clinical features of HS.*

Blood cell cytoskeleton: I. Red cell membrane skeleton. Semin Hematol vol 20, no 3, 1983. *Monograph of excellent reviews on normal membrane structure and function and disorders of the membrane skeleton.*

Lux SE: Disorders of the red cell membrane. In Nathan DG, Oski FA (eds.): Hematology of Infancy and Childhood. 3rd ed. Philadelphia, W. B. Saunders Company, 1987. *Comprehensive (1100 references) review of all inherited and many acquired diseases of red cell membranes. Also covers normal membrane structure and function.*

Luzzatto L, Testa U: Human erythrocyte glucose-6-phosphate dehydrogenase: Structure and function in normal and mutant subjects. Curr Topics Hematol 1:1, 1978. *Excellent review of G6PD and G6PD deficiency.*

Palek J: Hereditary elliptocytosis and related disorders. Clin Haematol 14:45, 1985. *A comprehensive review of the etiology and clinical features of HE and HPP.*

Red blood cell membrane. Clin Haematol vol 14, no 1, 1985. *Monograph of excellent reviews covering diseases of the red cell membrane, including HS, HE, permeability defects, PNH, sickle cell anemia, thalassemia, and the red cell storage lesion. Not much information on the normal red cell membrane.*

Schwartz PE, Sterioff S, Mucha P, et al.: Postsplenectomy sepsis and mortality in adults. JAMA 248:2279, 1982. *The only good epidemiologic study of postsplenectomy sepsis. Indicates that the risk of serious infection is much lower than previously thought.*

Valentine WN: Hemolytic anemia and inborn errors of metabolism. Blood 54:549, 1979. *Excellent review of the biochemical and clinical abnormalities in the glycolytic enzyme deficiencies.*

139 ACQUIRED HEMOLYTIC DISORDERS

Manuel E. Kaplan

Hemolysis resulting from congenital, intrinsic defects of the red cell has been discussed in Ch. 138. Hemolysis can also result from a variety of acquired abnormalities of the erythrocyte and of the circulatory system in which it functions (see Table 137–1). In these disorders red cells are usually formed normally but are destroyed prematurely as a result of immunologic, physical, or chemical injury. The general manifestations of the acquired hemolytic anemias do not differ from those resulting from inherited intracorpuscular defects.

SEQUESTRATIONAL HEMOLYSIS (HYPERSPLENISM)

By virtue of its unique vascular architecture, the normal spleen carefully sieves circulating red cells (Ch. 164). Arterial blood enters the spleen via arterioles in the white pulp. In the red pulp these arterioles communicate with either endothelial-lined sinuses or with closed, nonendothelialized cords that contain numerous fixed macrophages. To re-enter the venous circulation, red cells in the splenic cords must squeeze through narrow (3μ) fenestrations between epithelial cells that line the splenic sinuses. Poorly deformable red cells are unable to meet this challenge and are destroyed by splenic cord macrophages. The splenic filtration barrier does not significantly jeopardize the survival of normal nonsenescent red cells. However, when the spleen becomes enlarged, it may randomly entrap and destroy normal red cells. This pathologic process is called *hypersplenism*. The differential diagnosis of splenomegaly is discussed in Ch. 164. In patients with hypersplenism the rapidity of hemolysis is poorly correlated with overall spleen size. Indeed, patients with marked splenomegaly may show little or no reduction in red cell survival.

Hypersplenism is best treated by effectively managing the underlying disease process. Splenectomy is rarely indicated; the procedure should be limited to transfusion-dependent patients who are reasonable operative risks and whose condition is refractory to medical therapy. Splenectomized individuals, particularly the young (under age ten), are statistically more likely to develop fulminant bacterial or protozoal infections and are less able to mount an effective primary (IgM) immune response to certain antigens. Consequently the indications for splenectomy and its inherent risks should be carefully weighed before it is recommended.

IMMUNE HEMOLYTIC ANEMIAS

MECHANISMS OF IMMUNE HEMOLYSIS. In patients with immune hemolysis red cell destruction results from the binding of antibodies or complement components or both to the erythrocyte membrane. This may occur as a result of autoimmunization, of alloimmunization, or of exposure to certain drugs.

TYPES OF ANTIBODIES. Antibodies destroy red cells in vivo by mechanisms that are largely determined by their structure, concentration, and immunologic properties (complement fixing activity, the optimal temperature at which they are active) as well as the density and topographic distribution of the membrane antigens with which they combine. IgM red cell antibodies are generally agglutinating, complement fixing, and active at colder temperatures. In contrast, most IgG red cell antibodies are fully active at 37°C, have little or no agglutinating activity, and vary in their ability to fix complement. IgA red cell antibodies usually occur in conjunction with IgG and/or IgM red cell antibodies, have little complement-fixing activity, and destroy red cells poorly.

ROLE OF COMPLEMENT. Most IgM and some IgG red cell antibodies after combining with membrane antigens, activate the classic complement pathway. C1 binds to the Fc region of immunoglobulin heavy chains, develops esterase activity (C1s), and splits C4 into two fragments, C4a and C4b (Ch. 418). Nascent C4b may covalently attach to the red cell membrane and bind C2, which is then cleaved into C2a and C2b by C1s. The C4b, 2a complex acts as the classic pathway C3 convertase, binding and dissociating C3 into C3a and C3b. Nascent C3b may also covalently bind directly to the red cell membrane where it completes assembly of the classic pathway C5 convertase (C4b,2a,3b). After binding to C3b, C5 is cleaved by C2a, thereby activating the terminal "membrane attack complex" (C5-9) of the complement cascade. Insertion of activated terminal complement components into the red cell membrane results in osmotic destabilization of the membrane with egress of hemoglobin from the cell. If complement activation continued unimpeded, life-threatening intravascular hemolysis would invariably ensue. However, the process is restrained by inhibitors and inactivators of complement normally present in the plasma (factor I, factor H, C4-binding protein) and within the red cell membrane itself [CR1 (the receptor for C3b present in plasma immune complexes) and DAF (decay-accelerating factor)]. Red cells bearing covalently bound fragments of activated complement, i.e., C4b, C3b, and C3bi (C3b cleaved by factor I), are removed from the circulation and may be prematurely destroyed, primarily by hepatic macrophages bearing complement receptors (CR1 and CR3). A more detailed description of complement is contained in Ch. 418.

HEMOLYSIS WITHOUT COMPLEMENT ACTIVATION. Red cells sensitized with IgG antibodies that fail to fix complement are sequestered and destroyed primarily within the splenic cords. Here they come into prolonged and intimate contact with macrophages bearing membrane receptors for the Fc component of the IgG molecule. The sensitized cells may be damaged by a cytotoxic process (ADCC), or be totally engulfed, or undergo partial phagocytosis. Partially phagocytized red cells may reseal their membranes and, having lost proportionately more membrane than cytoplasm, assume a microspherocytic configuration. In the cells that survive and re-enter the circulation, their abnormal shape testifies to their previous encounter with splenic macrophages. These spherocytic cells are particularly vulnerable, since their deformability has been impaired and they retain significant membrane antibody.

DETECTION OF ANTIBODIES. The presence of red cell antibodies may be suspected from the appearance of freshly collected venous blood. IgM antibodies induce prompt red cell agglutination at room temperature. IgG antibodies are usually nonagglutinating but may so markedly reduce the negative charge (zeta potential) normally present on red cell surface that the cells are strongly aggregated by fibrinogen and other plasma macromolecules.

The *direct antiglobulin (Coombs') test* is most frequently used to detect immunoproteins present on the red cell membrane. This test measures the ability of a polyspecific antiserum that contains antibodies specific for human immunoglobulins and complement components to agglutinate a washed, dilute suspension of the patient's red cells. More precise identification of the membrane-bound immunoproteins may help to delineate the etiology and pathophysiologic mechanisms underlying a patient's hemolytic disorder. Consequently, when a positive direct antiglobulin test is obtained using a polyspecific reagent, the patient's red cells should be tested with various monospecific antisera that detect individual immunoglobulin classes or complement components. Almost all patients with immune hemolytic disorder exhibit a positive direct antiglobulin reaction. In the small percentage of patients (<5 per cent) in whom this test is negative, more sensitive immunologic techniques may disclose increased concentrations of red cell-associated immunoproteins.

The *indirect antiglobulin test* detects serum antibodies capable of attaching to normal red cells. The serum is first incubated with a panel of serologically defined normal red cells. After the cells are washed, membrane-associated immunoprotein is sought by the antiglobulin reaction. Although in clinical situations the direct and the indirect Coombs' tests are frequently ordered together, only the former provides unequivocal evidence of an immune hemolytic process.

HEMOLYSIS DUE TO ALLOANTIBODIES. Alloantibodies capable of destroying transfused, but not autologous, red cells are products of immunologic responses to (1) bacteria that normally colonize the large intestine (giving rise to so-called natural antibodies that cross-react with allogeneic erythrocyte antigens), (2) transfused, imperfectly matched red cells, or (3) antigens of fetal red cells that entered the maternal circulation during pregnancy or at delivery.

Alloimmune red cell antibodies present in a patient's serum may be detected by agglutination of normal cells or by the indirect antiglobulin reaction. Since these antibodies have specificity for nonself antigens, they are harmless unless the patient is transfused with allogeneic red cells bearing the immunizing antigen. Consequently, it is crucial that these antibodies be detected in patients requiring transfusions and in pregnant women. In the latter, IgG red cell alloantibodies that gain access to the fetal circulation may induce erythroblastosis fetalis.

AUTOIMMUNE HEMOLYTIC ANEMIAS. Autoimmune hemolytic disorders are characterized by antibodies with specificity for autologous red cell antigens. The pathophysiologic mechanisms that result in autoantibody production are not fully understood. B lymphocyte clones capable of producing autoantibodies to red cells probably exist in everyone. They do not normally synthesize detectable quantities of autoantibody because their activities are suppressed by immunoregulatory T lymphocytes. If this suppressor mechanism is deranged, red cell autoantibodies may be produced in quantities sufficient to trigger red cell destruction. Certain diseases—infections, neoplasms, or collagen-vascular disorders—appear to stimulate the development of autoimmune hemolysis. The hemolytic disorders that result are therefore categorized as secondary. In primary or idiopathic autoimmune hemolytic disorders no underlying or predisposing diseases can be detected.

AUTOIMMUNE HEMOLYTIC DISEASE DUE TO IgG WARM-REACTING ANTIBODIES

CLINICAL MANIFESTATIONS. ***Disease Associations.*** In approximately 40 per cent of patients IgG-mediated autoimmune hemolytic anemia occurs secondary to an underlying disease, usually neoplastic or collagen-vascular in origin. Chronic lymphocytic leukemia and, less frequently, other lymphoproliferative disorders are the most commonly associated malignant disorders. There is a well-documented relationship between ovarian teratoma and warm autoimmune hemolytic anemia. Systemic lupus erythematosus is the most frequently associated collagen-vascular disorder; less common are systemic sclerosis and rheumatoid arthritis. Occasional patients with ulcerative colitis present with warm autoimmune hemolysis.

Symptoms and Signs. Since the rate of red cell destruction, degree of anemia, and presence of underlying disease differ from patient to patient, a highly variable clinical picture can result. If hemolysis occurs suddenly, the patient usually presents with symptoms and signs related to severe anemia, i.e., pallor, fatigue, exertional dyspnea, dizziness, and palpitations. When hemolysis is more gradual, the anemia is usually less severe, and the patient may be relatively asymptomatic. On physical examination mild jaundice and splenomegaly are commonly present.

Laboratory Findings. The degree of anemia is variable, and there are usually normal numbers of white cells and platelets. In occasional patients significant thrombocytopenia, neutropenia, or both occurs in conjunction with immune hemolysis *(Evans' syndrome).* The mean corpuscular volume (MCV) may be increased, sometimes strikingly so (> 115 fl). When spherocytosis is prominent, the mean corpuscular hemoglobin concentration (MCHC) is usually elevated. The peripheral blood film typically discloses rouleaux formation, significant anisocytosis and poikilocytosis with numerous microspherocytes, and increased numbers of large polychromatophilic reticulocytes. Nucleated red cells may be present, particularly when hemolysis is rapid. The reticulocyte count is almost always elevated. Other typical laboratory findings include hyperbilirubinemia of the unconjugated type, serum haptoglobin that is diminished to absent, normal or slightly elevated plasma hemoglobin levels, and no urine hemosiderin. The direct antiglobulin test discloses only IgG or IgG and complement (C3dg). The indirect antiglobulin test may be positive or negative, a positive result implying that the red cell autoantibody has been produced in excess. Antibody eluted from the patient's red cells may exhibit specificity for well-defined red cell antigens, particularly in the Rh system. More commonly the eluted antibody is found to be a "panagglutinin," reacting with all normal red cells tested.

DIFFERENTIAL DIAGNOSIS. Since underlying diseases are present in almost half the patients with warm autoimmune hemolytic anemia, appropriate diagnostic studies to define them should be undertaken. The possibility of a lymphoproliferative disorder, a collagen-vascular disease, or drug-induced immune hemolysis must be considered. If the hemolytic disorder appears to be acquired but the direct antiglobulin test is negative, a previously undiagnosed congenital hemolytic process, paroxysmal nocturnal hemoglobinuria, and various nonimmunologic causes of hemolysis (hypersplenism, microangiopathy, etc.) must be considered. If there is no evidence for these, the patient may have an immune hemolytic process that can be demonstrated only by immunologic studies more sensitive than the antiglobulin test. Alternatively, this may be inferred from a patient's objective clinical response to an empiric therapeutic trial of steroids.

TREATMENT. If an underlying disease process is identified and treated, marked improvement of the accompanying hemolysis frequently results. Mild hemolysis may require no therapy.

Glucocorticoids. Patients with more rapid hemolysis should be treated with oral steroids equivalent to 1 to 2 mg of prednisone per kilogram per day, in single daily or divided (thrice daily) doses. If the patient is very symptomatic because of severe anemia, initial treatment with intravenous hydrocortisone, 400 to 800 mg per day, may be preferred followed by daily oral prednisone in divided doses. Improvement will usually occur within five to ten days, evidenced by increasing hemoglobin and hematocrit levels and decreasing reticulocytosis. At this time steroid therapy can be given as a single daily dose. Over the succeeding three to four weeks, the daily steroid dosage can usually be tapered, at five- to seven-day intervals, to a daily dose of approximately 20 mg of prednisone. During this time blood counts and reticulocyte counts should be checked periodically. Thereafter, the dose of steroids should be decreased more slowly, every two to three weeks, by 5 mg per day as long as the reticulocyte count does not rise significantly and the hemoglobin level remains stable. In occasional patients it may be possible to discontinue steroids entirely without exacerbating the hemolysis. More commonly, significant hemolysis persists and patients require daily maintenance steroid therapy, 5 to 15 mg of prednisone, or 10 to 30 mg on alternate days, which results in fewer undesirable side effects (Ch. 30).

The mechanism of the corticosteroid effect in warm autoimmune hemolytic disorders is not fully understood. Steroids appear to diminish the number, and possibly the binding strength, of monocyte and macrophage Fc receptors, thereby decreasing the ability of these cells to bind and destroy IgG-sensitized red cells. Prolonged therapy with steroids may suppress antibody synthesis; however, this effect certainly does not explain the prompt, frequently dramatic clinical improvement seen in most patients.

If the response to corticosteroid therapy is unsatisfactory, i.e., if (1) hemolysis and anemia are not significantly improved within two weeks after initiating high-dose steroid therapy or (2) unacceptably large daily doses of steroids (> 15 to 20 mg of prednisone) are required to maintain hematologic improvement, other therapeutic approaches must be considered.

Splenectomy. ^{51}Cr red cell survival and sequestration studies should be performed, if possible, before splenectomy is undertaken. Typically they will disclose significantly reduced RBC survival ($t\frac{1}{2}$ = 5 to 15 days), and the spleen will be the major, if not exclusive, site of red cell destruction. In such a patient splenectomy is advisable and should result in marked hematologic improvement. Occasionally significant hemolysis persists after splenectomy. This usually results from intense red cell sensitization with IgG autoantibody and characteristically responds to small maintenance doses of steroids. If ^{51}Cr sequestration studies reveal the liver to be a major site of red cell destruction, the direct antiglobulin test usually discloses complement (C3dg) as well as IgG. Splenectomy results in less effective control of hemolysis in such patients, favorable responses being achieved in only 30 per cent. Consequently a trial of immunosuppressive therapy may be preferred prior to splenectomy.

Immunosuppressive Drugs. At present either oral azathioprine* (Imuran), 50 to 200 mg per day, or cyclophosphamide* (Cytoxan), 50 to 150 mg per day, is the immunosuppressive agent most frequently employed in patients with warm immune hemolytic anemia. Responses are variable and usually not very dramatic. However, their use in patients whose conditions are refractory to steroids may permit reduction in the excessive steroid dosages required for maintenance.

Transfusion. Before hemolysis is adequately controlled by steroid therapy, severely anemic patients may require red cell transfusions. Transfusion carries an increased risk when the patient has a positive indirect antiglobulin test because donor-patient compatibility cannot be ensured by cross-matching techniques. The serum of such a patient frequently contains a panagglutinating autoantibody reactive with red cells from all prospective donors. More importantly, the serum autoantibody may mask the presence of a red cell alloantibody that may be capable of provoking intravascular hemolysis of transfused red cells. To distinguish these possibilities, patient red cells from which autoantibody has been eluted are used to absorb the autoantibody from the patient's serum. The absorbed serum is then tested for alloantibody activity with potential donor cells. In addition, blood banks usually attempt to identify possible blood group specificity of antibody eluted from a patient's red cells and of the serum antibody. Following these studies, donor red cells "most compatible" with the patient are selected for transfusion. Usually patients with

*This use is not listed in the manufacturer's directive.

warm autoimmune hemolysis can be safely transfused when these precautions are taken. Donor cells should be administered slowly, with the patient being closely observed for symptoms and signs suggestive of a possible hemolytic transfusion reaction, the diagnosis and treatment of which are described in Ch. 147.

COURSE AND PROGNOSIS. In patients with secondary autoimmune hemolytic disorders the clinical course and ultimate prognosis are generally determined by the underlying disease process. Autoimmune hemolysis due to warm IgG antibodies is usually well controlled by corticosteroid therapy or splenectomy or both. Uncontrollable hemolysis resulting in death rarely occurs. All evidence of the disease may disappear in some patients. More commonly a positive direct antiglobulin test persists, and the patient experiences recurrent episodes of hemolysis that may require steroid therapy. Splenectomized patients are generally more stable hematologically than are patients managed by medical therapy alone. Major causes of death include thromboembolic complications and sequellae of chronically impaired host defense mechanisms caused by corticosteroids, splenectomy, or immunosuppressive drugs.

AUTOIMMUNE HEMOLYTIC DISEASE DUE TO COLD-REACTING ANTIBODIES

Cold-reacting red cell antibodies combine most avidly with erythrocyte membrane antigens at grossly subphysiologic temperatures (0 to 4° C). They exhibit characteristic "thermal amplitudes," i.e., maximum temperatures beyond which they are unable to combine effectively with their antigens. Pathologically significant cold antibodies produce clinical hemolysis because they retain significant immunologic reactivity at temperatures that are achievable in vivo (30 to 32° C). Thus, if the thermal amplitude of a red cell antibody does not extend to 30° C, the antibody will have no relevance pathophysiologically. IgM cold-reacting antibodies occur most commonly. Because they strongly agglutinate red cells in the cold, they are designated as *cold agglutinins*. Rare IgA cold agglutinins have been described; however, these antibodies do not produce hemolysis in vivo because they lack complement-fixing activity. Cold-reacting IgG red cell autoantibodies are occasionally encountered. They are intensely complement fixing and produce the disease picture of paroxysmal cold hemoglobinuria.

COLD AGGLUTININ DISEASE. ***Pathophysiology.*** IgM cold agglutinins are normally present in low titer in human serum. They have no known function and may represent byproducts of polyclonal immunologic responses to viruses and other microorganisms. Cold agglutinins in serum are detected and quantified by the cold agglutinin titer, i.e., the maximal serum dilution, at 4° C, that retains red cell agglutinating activity. Normal cold agglutinins are harmless because they are present in low titers (≤ 1:32) and exhibit low thermal amplitudes. Usually, but not always, the higher the patient's cold agglutinin titer, the higher the thermal amplitude of the cold antibody, and the greater the probability that the patient will experience hemolysis.

The synthesis of polyclonal cold agglutinins may increase in response to certain infections, especially mycoplasma, viral (EB, cytomegalovirus), and protozoal (trypanosomiasis, malaria) infections. Titers usually peak within two to three weeks of onset, but rarely do antibody concentrations rise sufficiently to provoke clinically apparent hemolysis.

Cold agglutinin disease occasionally appears in patients with lymphoproliferative disorders, particularly histiocytic lymphoma. Indeed, hemolytic anemia may be the initial manifestation of the lymphoma. In these patients the cold agglutinins are predictably monoclonal, containing either kappa or lambda light chains. Occasionally the antibody may be present in such high concentrations that it is detectable as a spike on serum protein electrophoresis.

TABLE 139–1. RELATIONSHIP BETWEEN COLD AGGLUTININ STRUCTURE AND SPECIFICITY IN VARIOUS DISEASES

Structure	Specificity: *Anti-I*	*Anti-i*	*Anti-PR*
Polyclonal/oligoclonal (κ + λ)	*Mycoplasma pneumoniae*	Infectious mononucleosis	
Monoclonal			
κ	Idiopathic cold agglutinin disease	Lymphoma	Idiopathic cold agglutinin disease
λ		Lymphoma	

Idiopathic cold agglutinin disease occurs most frequently in elderly patients in whom, by definition, no underlying infectious or neoplastic process can be identified. The cold agglutinin is almost always monoclonal kappa IgM.

Cold agglutinins react with polysaccharide components of red cell membrane glycolipids and glycoproteins immunochemically related to human ABO blood group antigens. Some of these polysaccharide antigens are better expressed on adult erythrocytes (designated I) and others on fetal red cells (i). Cold agglutinins that react significantly more strongly with adult red cells are said to exhibit anti-I specificity, whereas those that combine better with fetal (cord) erythrocytes show anti-i specificity. I and i are not alleles, and both antigens are usually expressed on adult, as well as on fetal, red cells. However, the red cells of rare, otherwise normal, individuals express only one or the other. Very infrequently patients with cold agglutinin disease have antibodies that exhibit exclusive anti-I or anti-i reactivity. Some cold antibodies that react equally well with adult and cord cells fail to agglutinate red cells pretreated with proteolytic enzymes and are said to show anti-PR specificity. Identification of the major reactivity of a cold agglutinin (anti-I, -i, or -PR) and its clonal diversity may be clinically informative, since cold agglutinins produced in various diseases show different characteristic patterns of reactivity (Table 139–1).

Mechanisms of Hemolysis. High thermal amplitude cold agglutinins bind to red cells in the cooler portions of the circulation and initiate agglutination and complement activation via the classic pathway. Complement-mediated intravascular hemolysis may ensue. However, this occurs minimally, or not at all, in most patients because propagation of the complement cascade is effectively aborted before membrane damage occurs. Activation of the earlier components of the classic pathway (C1, 4, 2, and 3), as previously described, results in the binding of nascent C3b to the red cell membrane (EC3b). EC3b is so rapidly cleaved by the plasma C3 inactivator (factor I) that it is unable to effectively support activation of the membrane attack components of complement (C5–9). Factor I activity is significantly enhanced by cofactors in the plasma (factor H) and in the red cell membrane itself (CRI). EC3b is progressively cleaved into EC3bi and ECdg, which are not able to support further complement activation. Indeed, C3dg appears to inhibit binding of additional cold agglutinin to the red cell membrane. Although significant intravascular hemolysis is prevented, red cells bearing C3b or C3bi are prematurely removed from the circulation and may be prematurely destroyed, primarily by hepatic macrophages.

Clinical Manifestations. In patients with postinfectious cold agglutinin disease, hemolysis is usually self-limited and mild. In contrast, idiopathic and lymphoma-associated cold agglutinin syndromes are accompanied by persistent hemolysis that is usually worse in winter. After exposure to cold, the patient may experience a picture of painful acrocyanosis, similar to Raynaud's phenomenon, induced by intense red cell autoagglutination. Unlike Raynaud's, there is usually no antecedent blanching or reactive hyperemia, and local gangrene does not occur. Severe chilling may accelerate hemolysis to such a degree that hemoglobinuria results.

Diagnosis. On physical examination the patient may be mildly jaundiced. As the patient's blood is drawn, the red cells may clump so rapidly that the blood appears to clot even in the presence of an anticoagulant. Warming of the anticoagulated blood to 37° C rapidly restores its normal appearance. Electronically measured blood counts are frequently inaccurate because of the intense autoagglutination at room temperature. The red count and MCV measurement are particularly affected, leading to distortion of the calculated hematocrit. This situation should be recognized by alert laboratory personnel. Not uncommonly the reticulocyte count is only mildly increased; this suggests suboptimal bone marrow compensation. The cold agglutinin titer is invariably elevated, and the direct antiglobulin test discoses C3dg. Typically, serum haptoglobin levels are decreased, and lactic dehydrogenase (LDH) concentrations increased.

Treatment. When an underlying disease process is identified, it should be treated appropriately. Patients should be told to avoid exposure to the cold and to dress warmly. Treatment with daily chlorambucil,* 2 to 4 mg orally, decreases the hemolysis in some patients with idiopathic cold agglutinin syndrome, probably by reducing the synthesis of cold agglutinin. Glucocorticoids and splenectomy are generally of no benefit. If rapid hemolysis persists despite treatment, it may be advisable for the patient to move to a warmer climate. Although transfusions are not absolutely contraindicated, they should be avoided unless the patient is critically ill, i.e., exhibiting symptoms and signs of vascular decompensation (tachyarrhythmias, angina, congestive failure) or cerebral hypoxia (confusion, visual disturbances, etc.) that respond poorly to bed rest and oxygen therapy. In addition to the transfusion-associated risks previously described in patients with warm autoimmune hemolysis, the following dangers must be considered: (1) Transfused compatible red cells will be hemolyzed as rapidly, or even more rapidly, than the patient's own red cells; the latter, having membrane-associated C3dg, may be more resistant to additional IgM cold agglutinin binding. By increasing the numbers of circulating red cells at risk of complement-mediated destruction, transfusion may exacerbate intravascular hemolysis with hemoglobinemia and hemoglobinuria. This may further jeopardize the patient's renal function and predispose to thromboembolic complications, red cell stroma being thrombogenic. (2) Although theoretically hazardous, the actual danger of transfusing refrigerated donor blood to a patient with cold agglutinin disease has been debated. Some experts strongly advise that a properly functioning, in-line blood warmer be utilized. However, uncontrolled warming of donor erythrocytes may be more hazardous to the patient than the slow administration of refrigerated blood. (3) The usual risks of transfusion therapy (Ch. 147) must be considered. By expanding the patient's blood volume, transfusion may exacerbate congestive heart failure. Transmission of non-A, non-B hepatitis, cytomegalovirus, or HIV infection may occur. When transfusions are administered the patient must be kept warm, a limited volume of red cells (designed to alleviate life-threatening symptoms, not simply to improve the hemoglobin concentration) should be infused slowly, and the patient's response must be monitored carefully.

PAROXYSMAL COLD HEMOGLOBINURIA (DONATH-LANDSTEINER HEMOLYTIC ANEMIA). Paroxysmal cold hemoglobinuria (PCH) is an exceedingly rare autoimmune hemolytic disorder caused by IgG cold-reacting antibodies directed against the ubiquitous P blood group antigen. It was first described in patients with tertiary syphilis who, following exposure to cold, developed paroxysms of chills, fever, headache, and diffuse pain in the abdomen, back, and legs accompanied by hemoglobinuria. PCH now much more commonly occurs as a complication of various viral infections. In this context, hemolysis is rarely paroxysmal, and a history of cold exposure is seldom obtained. Consequently it has been proposed that the syndrome be renamed Donath-Landsteiner hemolytic anemia in honor of the investigators who first described the offending antibody. The diagnosis of PCH (Donath-Landsteiner hemolysis) is made by demonstrating the presence in the patient's serum of a cold hemolysin, an IgG, nonagglutinating antibody, that activates complement so efficiently that intravascular hemolysis results. Normal red cells are mixed with the patient's serum and a source of complement and chilled (0 to 4° C). Thereafter the cell suspension is incubated at 37° C. The appearance of hemolysis is presumptive evidence of the Donath-Landsteiner antibody. The patient's direct Coombs' test is usually weakly positive for IgG and complement. When PCH accompanies a viral infection, hemolysis is usually transient, requiring only supportive therapy and protection of the patient from cold. If hemolysis recurs or becomes chronic, it may respond to treatment with glucocorticoids or to immunosuppressive drugs such as cyclophosphamide.*

IMMUNE HEMOLYSIS DUE TO DRUGS. A number of drugs, or their in vivo metabolic derivatives, may cause immune hemolytic anemia. Three distinct mechanisms have been described:

1. *Drug binding to red cells.* When administered intravenously, certain immunogenic drugs, exemplified by penicillin, bind tightly to erythrocyte membranes. If drug-specific antibodies are produced, they attach to red cells at membrane sites occupied by the drug. In the case of penicillin-induced immune hemolysis, the offending antibody is characteristically IgG and is noncomplement fixing. In vivo, it binds to penicillin-modified red cells and induces their destruction by a mechanism essentially identical to that seen in warm autoimmune hemolytic anemia, i.e., IgG-sensitized red cells are sequestered primarily within the spleen and destroyed by Fc receptor-bearing macrophages. The direct antiglobulin test discloses only IgG. The antipenicillin specificity of the red cell antibody can be demonstrated by indirect antiglobulin testing. IgG eluted from the patient's red cells, as well as antibody that may be present in the patient's serum, fails to combine with normal erythrocytes unless the cells have been pretreated with penicillin. Since hemolysis promptly ceases soon after penicillin is discontinued, corticosteroid therapy is usually unnecessary.

2. *Innocent bystander hemolysis.* Other drugs that induce immune hemolytic anemia in humans (sulfonamides, phenothiazines, quinine, quinidine, etc.) are bound primarily by plasma proteins rather than red cells. Although they are weakly immunogenic, in some patients they stimulate the synthesis of drug-specific, complement-fixing antibodies. As a result, the patient's erythrocytes are bathed in plasma containing drug-antibody immune complexes that activate complement. The nascent C3b generated by these complexes may covalently bind to the red cell membrane. Membrane-bound C3b facilitates activation of the alternative complement pathway by binding factor B, which is then cleaved into Bb by factor D, a proteolytic enzyme normally present in plasma. C3b,Bb complexes represent the alternative pathway C3 convertase, cleaving plasma C3 and thereby generating additional nascent C3b that may covalently bind to the red cell membrane. The C3b,Bb,C3b complexes, acting as the alternative pathway C5 convertase, cleave C5, thereby triggering activation of the terminal (C5-9) membrane attack complex of complement. This process, if unsuccessfully opposed by the complement inactivators and inhibitors previously described, will result in life-threatening intravascular hemolysis. Even if activation of the membrane attack complex is effectively prevented, red cells bearing C4b, C3b, and C3bi are at risk of sequestration and destruction by hepatic macrophages. The direct antiglobulin test reveals only membrane-associated

*This use is not listed in the manufacturer's directive.

complement cleavage products, primarily C3dg (the small C3 fragment that remains covalently bound to the red cell membrane after degradation of C3bi by factor I). Efforts to elute immunoprotein from the patient's red cells are usually unsuccessful. The indirect antiglobulin test is characteristically negative; however, if the offending drug, or an appropriate metabolic derivative, is added to normal erythrocytes suspended in the patient's serum with a source of complement, hemolysis may occur, and Coombs' testing of the nonhemolyzed cells may disclose membrane-associated complement fragments. After the drug is discontinued, hemolysis generally subsides promptly, and patients usually require no additional therapy.

3. *Drug-induced autoimmune hemolytic anemia.* A pure IgG direct antiglobulin test appears in approximately 15 per cent of patients undergoing long-term treatment with methyldopa (Aldomet). However, only 10 per cent of these Coombs-positive patients develop clinically apparent hemolysis. Antibodies eluted from the patients' red cells combine readily with normal erythrocytes in the absence of methyldopa, thereby displaying true autoimmune reactivity. Patients treated with levodopa or mefenamic acid (Ponstel), a nonsteroidal anti-inflammatory drug, may develop similar erythrocyte autoantibodies. By unknown mechanisms these agents probably interfere with immunoregulatory processes that suppress the synthesis of red cell autoantibodies. Moreover, it is not clear why hemolysis occurs in only a small percentage of Coombs'-positive methyldopa-treated patients. The mechanism of cell destruction appears identical to that seen in warm autoimmune hemolytic anemia, i.e., splenic sequestration and red cell destruction by Fc receptor-positive macrophages. Hemolysis usually subsides within one to three weeks after methyldopa is discontinued but a positive direct antiglobulin test may persist for many months. Although the hemolysis responds to steroid therapy, it is rarely required. If methyldopa is readministered to a patient who has fully recovered from methyldopa-induced hemolyis, no anamnestic autoimmune response usually occurs. Hemolysis may recur, but only after a prolonged treatment period.

PAROXYSMAL NOCTURNAL HEMOGLOBINURIA

Paroxysmal nocturnal hemoglobinuria (PNH) is an acquired hemolytic disorder resulting from the proliferation of an abnormal clone of stem cells whose progeny are uniquely susceptible to complement-mediated membrane damage. Its etiology is not known. Since patients with PNH are unusually prone to develop aplastic anemia or acute leukemia, it may represent a "preneoplastic" transformation of hematopoietic stem cells. The disease is quite rare; however, it is probably underdiagnosed because its manifestations are frequently protean. It occurs with greatest frequency in early adulthood, but has been described in young children and in the very elderly.

PATHOPHYSIOLOGY. PNH red cells, granulocytes, and platelets are inordinately sensitive to the lytic effects of complement. The patient's peripheral blood frequently contains two or three subpopulations of red cells differing in their sensitivity to complement (I = normally sensitive cells, II = cells of intermediate sensitivity, and III = very sensitive cells). When PNH red cells are exposed to complement activated in vitro by either the classic or the alternative pathway, PNH II and III cells bind much greater quantities of C3b than do normal red cells. The rate of red cell destruction in vivo correlates well with the proportions of circulating red cells that are PNH II and III.

Spontaneous limited in vivo activation of the alternative complement pathway appears to occur normally. This may result in covalent binding of C3b to the red cell membrane. As previously described, membrane-bound C3b exerts positive feedback on the alternative complement pathway through factors B and D to generate additional nascent C3b available for coupling to the membrane; the assembled C3b,Bb,C3b complexes, representing the alternative pathway C5 convertase, cleave C5, thereby activating the C5-9 membrane attack complex. If unsuccessfully restrained by the complement inactivator/inhibitor substances normally present in plasma and red cell membrane, such complement activation would result in intravascular hemolysis. Normal red cell membranes contain a glycoprotein, designated decay-accelerating factor (DAF), that inhibits assembly of the C3 convertase (C3b,Bb). PNH I and II red cells are deficient in DAF, which may account, in large part, for their marked susceptibility to complement-mediated hemolysis. Similarly, platelets and granulocytes from PNH patients are DAF deficient and also exhibit abnormal sensitivity in vitro to complement activation.

Although the in vivo survival of PNH platelets has been reported to be normal, their enhanced susceptibility to complement activation may underlie the thrombotic diathesis commonly seen in these patients. Functional abnormalities of the PNH granulocyte have also been described.

CLINICAL MANIFESTATIONS. The diagnosis of PNH must be considered in all patients with chronic hemolysis, particularly when associated with hemoglobinuria, pancytopenia, or unusual veno-occlusive events. During episodes of rapid hemolysis, patients commonly experience diffuse abdominal and back pain that has been attributed to ischemia resulting from microcirculatory thrombi. Not infrequently major thromboses occur involving the hepatic, splenic, portal, or cerebral veins. On physical examination pallor and scleral icterus are common. The degree of anemia is highly variable ranging from mild to severe. The reticulocyte count may be inappropriately low, given the severity of the anemia. The MCV may be normal, slightly increased, or diminished, depending upon the degree of reticulocytosis and the presence of accompanying iron deficiency due to prolonged urinary loss. Mild thrombocytopenia and granulocytopenia occur commonly. The peripheral blood smear reveals no autoagglutination, spherocytosis, or red cell fragmentation. The direct antiglobulin test is usually negative. Bone marrow cellularity varies from markedly hypoplastic to profoundly hyperplastic, and iron stores are usually reduced or absent. Erythroid elements predominate, and cell maturation is typically normoblastic.

Because red cell destruction occurs intravascularly, the serum LDH is elevated, serum haptoglobin levels are reduced or absent, and hemosiderinuria is present. Frank hemoglobinuria usually occurs only intermittently and is most apparent after periods of sleep, when the urine is concentrated.

DIAGNOSIS. The diagnosis of PNH requires that the patient's red cells show excessive susceptibility to complement-mediated hemolysis in vitro. This is most frequently demonstrated by mixing the red cells with freshly collected normal human serum that has been mildly acidified *(Ham's test)*. Hemolysis, which results from activation of the alternative pathway, is highly specific but unfortunately Ham's test is too insensitive to detect all patients with PNH. The simpler sucrose hemolysis test, which results in complement activation via the classic pathway, is much more sensitive than Ham's test, but is less specific, with positive results occurring in some patients with myeloproliferative disorders. Low levels of neutrophil alkaline phosphatase and red blood cell acetylcholinesterase occur commonly in PNH patients, but are nonspecific. Occasionally these measurements are used to confirm the diagnosis.

Other causes of intravascular hemolysis and hemoglobinuria that should be considered in the differential diagnosis include (1) hemolytic transfusion reactions, (2) paroxysmal cold hemoglobinuria, (3) red cell hemolysins such as those present in snake venoms and *Clostridium welchii* exotoxin,

(4) traumatic intravascular hemolysis as occurs in thrombotic thrombocytopenic purpura or march hemoglobinuria, and (5) G6PD deficiency (Ch. 138).

TREATMENT. Erythropoiesis may be enhanced with folic acid, iron, and androgen therapy. In some patients iron administration may provoke increased hemolysis and hemoglobinuria. This may be prevented by prior transfusion and probably results from the destruction of increased numbers of newly produced, complement-sensitive reticulocytes. Androgen administration may significantly improve the anemia. A six- to eight-week trial of oral fluoxymesterone or oxymesterone (5 to 50 mg per day), or of intramuscular nandralone decanoate (25 to 200 mg once weekly), is usually sufficient to identify androgen-responsive patients.

Steroid therapy (equivalent to 0.25 to 1 mg of prednisone per kilogram per day) significantly slows acute hemolytic episodes in some patients, and prolonged administration of low-dose steroids may reduce ongoing hemolysis. Daily steroids should not be administered except in life-threatening situations because of their unacceptable side effects and the increased danger of overwhelming bacterial or fungal sepsis. Alternate-day prednisone therapy, in dosages ranging from 15 to 40 mg, has been reported to improve more than 50 per cent of patients so treated.

Most patients with PNH eventually require blood transfusions. Initially donor red cells survive normally and suppress the production of the patient's abnormal red cells resulting in marked clinical improvement. Following repetitive transfusions, however, patients are prone to develop hemosiderosis and to produce alloantibodies to red cell, neutrophil, platelet, and even to plasma protein antigens. Once alloimmunization has occurred, further transfusion therapy is difficult, since it may be followed by rapid destruction of recipient (as well as of donor) red cells. Even compatible transfusions may trigger increased hemolysis of patient red cells and hemoglobinuria, probably because the donor packs contain small quantities of activated complement. If evidence of increased hemolysis follows transfusion of packed donor red cells, only washed red cells or frozen and reconstituted red cells should be administered.

PNH patients may require anticoagulation because they are susceptible to major thromboembolic events. Since heparin therapy has been reported to exacerbate hemolysis in some patients, it must be used with caution. Vitamin K antagonists can usually be employed without difficulty, but it is not clear whether continuous prophylactic anticoagulation with Coumadin derivatives is clinically beneficial.

Bone marrow transplantation has successfully eradicated the PNH clone in selected patients.

PROGNOSIS. The course of PNH is exceedingly variable. Most patients survive fewer than ten years from the time of diagnosis. In a small percentage of patients all disease manifestations spontaneously subside, possibly reflecting disappearance of the aberrant clone. More commonly, patients experience waxing and waning hemolysis, which may be exacerbated by immunologic stress such as infection, transfusion, and immunization. Thrombotic events, primarily venous, account for much of the morbidity and mortality. With time, marrow function progressively deteriorates, and a clinical picture more closely resembling aplastic anemia may gradually ensue. In approximately 5 per cent of patients the disease evolves into acute myeloblastic leukemia.

HEMOLYSIS CAUSED BY CHEMICALS

A number of chemicals may directly interact with and injure red cells, resulting in hemolysis. These toxins range in complexity from inorganic cations (arsenic and copper) and simple organic compounds such as chloramine to complex biologic substances produced by microorganisms, plants, and lower animals. Arsenic and copper injure red cells probably by binding to membrane sulfhydryl groups. Copper-induced hemolysis has been observed in hemodialyzed patients, and may be responsible for the transient hemolytic episodes observed in patients with Wilson's disease.

Purification of urban water supplies with alum and chlorine results in the generation of chloramine, a potent oxidant. If chloramine is not efficiently removed from tap water that is used for hemodialysis, it may swiftly induce methemoglobin and Heinz body formation, resulting in rapid hemolysis.

Amphotericin B is a lipophilic fungal product that binds avidly in vitro to red cell membrane lipids. In occasional patients it may provoke hemolysis, presumably by altering red cell membrane stability.

Clostridium welchii, spiders, and snakes produce potent lipolytic toxins capable of damaging red cell membrane integrity, thereby provoking intravascular hemolysis. Marked spherocytosis of circulating red cells is commonly seen. Hemolysis of uncertain etiology may accompany severe infection with other bacteria *(Streptococcus pneumoniae, Escherichia coli, Staphylococcus aureus).* Castor beans and certain species of mushrooms contain hemolysis-inducing toxins.

HEMOLYSIS CAUSED BY METABOLIC ABNORMALITIES

SPUR CELL HEMOLYTIC ANEMIA. Patients with a significant hepatocellular disease are frequently anemic. Blood loss, folate deficiency, alcohol-induced marrow dysfunction, and hypersplenism may contribute to the etiology of the anemia. However, in a small percentage of patients with end-stage cirrhosis, a clinical picture of rapid hemolysis develops with the appearance of numerous acanthocytes (spiculated, occasionally spur-shaped red cells).

Pathophysiology. Red cell membrane cholesterol and phospholipids exist in dynamic equilibrium with plasma lipids. In many patients with severe parenchymal liver disease, abnormal plasma lipoproteins appear to unload cholesterol and phospholipids onto the erythrocyte membrane. As a result the membranes spread and the cells thin out to become target cells. The molar ratio of cholesterol to phospholipids in target cells is normal, and these cells usually survive normally. In patients with spur cell hemolytic anemia, excess cholesterol accumulates in the red cell membrane unaccompanied by parallel increases in phospholipids. This may be caused by an abnormal circulating low-density lipoprotein containing an increased ratio of free cholesterol:phospholipids. Red cell deformability is markedly reduced, and the cells are prematurely destroyed within the congested, hypertrophied spleen.

Clinical Manifestations. Patients with spur cell hemolytic anemia characteristically exhibit marked splenomegaly and signs of advanced cirrhosis including jaundice, ascites, varices, and neurologic manifestations of hepatic encephalopathy. The anemia is usually severe, perhaps in part because of concomitant gastrointestinal blood loss. The peripheral smear contains numerous acanthocytes and polychromatophilic reticulocytes. The direct antiglobulin test is negative. Red cells are sequestered by the spleen and have shortened survival.

Diagnosis. The presence of a significantly elevated reticulocyte count and numerous spur cells on peripheral smear in a patient with end-stage cirrhosis is diagnostic of this syndrome. When normal compatible red cells are incubated with the patient's plasma in vitro, they become acanthocytic.

Prognosis and Treatment. Spur cell hemolytic anemia carries an exceedingly poor prognosis, almost all patients dying within months because of the associated liver disease. The beneficial effects of transfusion are limited since normal cells survive no better than autologous cells in these patients. Splenectomy may slow the rate of hemolysis in selected patients but is exceedingly hazardous because of the severity of the liver disease.

HYPOPHOSPHATEMIA. Hemolysis may occur in patients

with profoundly depressed serum phosphorus levels (< 1 mg per 100 ml) (Ch. 207). Hypophosphatemia of this degree occurs primarily in severely malnourished patients, particularly when they consume excessive quantities of phosphate-binding antacids. Erythrocyte ATP levels fall, the cells become poorly deformable, and hemolysis occurs primarily within the spleen.

HEMOLYSIS CAUSED BY RED CELL PARASITES

MALARIA. *Malarial infections,* particularly with *Plasmodium falciparum,* are probably the most common cause of hemolytic anemia worldwide (Ch. 381). Merozoites parasitize red cells and utilize for their own purposes hemoglobin, enzymes, and substrates, thereby metabolically depriving infected erythrocytes. As a result, the osmotic fragility and cation permeability of parasitized red cells are altered. Infected red cells may display new membrane antigens; this may help to explain the positive direct antiglobulin tests reported in some patients with falciparum malaria. Red cell destruction appears to occur primarily in the spleen and splenomegaly is almost universally present in patients with chronic malarial infection. Rarely, rapid intravascular hemolysis with hemoglobinuria (blackwater fever) occurs soon after antimalarial therapy is initiated. It is not clear whether the infection or the drug plays the more important role in this phenomenon.

BABESIOSIS. *Babesia* are protozoans that parasitize red cells of many animal species (Ch. 389). Several cases of babesia-induced hemolytic anemia have been reported in humans, the disease being particularly fulminant in previously splenectomized individuals. Such patients may present with thrombocytopenia, disseminated intravascular coagulation, and renal insufficiency. Although wood ticks are the usual vector, the disease may be transmitted by transfusion of infected red cells. The disease has been reported most frequently in the northeastern United States (Martha's Vineyard and Nantucket). Intraerythrocytic parasites can usually be seen in Giemsa-stained peripheral blood films.

BARTONELLOSIS. *Bartonella bacilliformis,* a bacterial species endemic to South America, grows on the surface of red cells rather than within them (Ch. 301). The disease is transmitted by the bite of the sand fly. Hemolysis is acute in onset and rapid, the red cells being sequestered by both liver and spleen. The peripheral blood smear typically discloses rod-shaped organisms on the erythrocyte surface and large numbers of normoblasts and reticulocytes. The infection responds well to treatment with penicillin, tetracyclines, streptomycin, or chloramphenicol.

HEMOLYSIS RESULTING FROM TRAUMA TO RED CELLS

When subjected to excessive mechanical stress, circulating red cells may hemolyze. The forces responsible may be generated extracorporeally or intravascularly. For example, fragmentational hemolysis may result from excessive intravascular shear stress originating in critically narrowed heart valves, pathologic shunts (arterial or arteriovenous), cardiac valve prostheses, poorly endothelialized vascular surfaces, or microvascular thrombi. In these situations hemolysis is characteristically accompanied by morphologic evidence of red cell fragmentation. Similarly red cell membranes may be injured by heat with resulting hemolysis. Temperatures higher than 49° C destabilize the normal human red cell membrane. Red cells, when heated in vitro, are observed to undergo membrane budding and fragmentation. Patients who have suffered extensive burns may show evidence of profound red cell membrane damage with prominent spherocytosis on peripheral smear. In some cases hemoglobinemia and hemoglobinuria occur. The major syndromes of traumatic hemolysis will be summarized briefly.

MARCH HEMOGLOBINURIA. As red cells circulate through narrow vessels overlying the bones of the hands and feet, they may be traumatized by repetitive, relatively uncushioned forces generated by prolonged marching, running, karate blows, and a variety of other activities. Intravascular hemolysis accompanied by hemoglobinemia and hemoglobinuria may result. Interestingly, no red cell morphologic abnormalities are apparent in the peripheral blood film during, or immediately following, the physical activity that precipitated the hemolytic episode.

FRAGMENTATIONAL HEMOLYSIS DUE TO CARDIAC PATHOLOGY OR ABNORMALITIES OF LARGE VESSELS. Cardiac abnormalities involving primarily the left side of the heart, where pressures are high, may predispose to hemolysis. These include aortic stenosis (acquired and congenital), severe aortic regurgitation, and ruptured sinus of Valsalva. Significant red cell fragmentation may also occur as a result of traumatic arteriovenous fistulas, or therapeutic aortofemoral bypass procedures. In patients with these abnormalities hemolysis is usually mild.

More rapid hemolysis occurs, not uncommonly, in patients who have received prosthetic heart valves. Hemolysis is more likely to occur with aortic rather than mitral prostheses, artificial valves rather than those of biologic (porcine) origin, metallic valves rather than Silastic, cloth-covered valves, and with defective or poorly functioning valves that exhibit ball variance or paravalvular leaks.

Clinical Manifestations. Rapid intravascular hemolysis accompanied by hemoglobinemia and hemoglobinuria occurs in occasional patients. More commonly, patients present with increasing anemia, reticulocytosis, and numerous fragmented red cells (schistocytes) on peripheral blood film. Findings typical of significant intravascular hemolysis are usually present, i.e., haptoglobin levels that are low to absent, increased serum LDH concentrations, and hemosiderinuria. Prolonged urinary iron loss may result in iron deficiency. Although the direct Coombs' test is usually negative, a positive result has been found in a few patients with prosthetic heart valves for reasons that are not understood.

Treatment. Patients should be advised to limit their physical activities in an effort to reduce cardiac output and thereby to slow the rate of hemolysis. Oral iron, 300 mg of ferrous sulfate three times a day, should be given to correct iron deficiency, or rarely parenteral iron (iron-dextran) or transfusions may be required. If the rate of hemolysis necessitates recurrent transfusion, it may be preferable to replace the prosthesis.

FRAGMENTATIONAL HEMOLYSIS DUE TO ABNORMALITIES WITHIN THE MICROCIRCULATION (MICROANGIOPATHIC HEMOLYTIC DISORDERS). ***Pathophysiology.*** Red cells may be fragmented when they are forced to flow through small vessels that have been partially occluded by microthrombi. Excessive shear forces are generated as the cells encounter and become tethered to fibrin strands, which may bisect and fragment the erythrocytes. The microthrombi may be formed as a result of (1) an underlying coagulopathy, i.e., disseminated intravascular coagulation (DIC), (2) injury to the vascular endothelium, or (3) unknown mechanisms. Pathophysiologic processes that trigger DIC commonly induce endothelial injury as well; however, the reverse is frequently not true. Diseases associated with diffuse microvascular pathology may involve none of the characteristic findings of DIC. Consequently, in many patients with microangiopathic hemolytic disorders, the predominant etiologic factor (i.e., coagulation or vascular injury) can be discerned.

DIC results when procoagulant is introduced into the systemic circulation (Ch. 167). Coagulation factors are consumed, thrombus formation occurs, and fibrinolytic mechanisms are secondarily activated. Patients with significant DIC characteristically have thrombocytopenia, abnormally prolonged plasma coagulation studies (prothrombin time, activated partial thromboplastin time) reflecting decreased concentrations of certain clotting factors (particularly V, VIII, and fibrinogen), and increased plasma concentrations of fibrin degradation products, which may prolong the thrombin time. DIC may be triggered by infections, particularly with gram-negative organisms, amniotic fluid embolism, and disseminated neoplasms that synthesize and elaborate potent procoagulants (Trousseau's syndrome). Although patients with severe DIC may be critically ill, hemolysis is usually mild.

Diffuse or localized vascular lesions may induce red cell fragmentation, e.g., cavernous hemangiomas (Kasabach-Merritt syndrome), renal allografts undergoing rejection, malignant hypertension, eclampsia, vasculitic processes (rickettsial infections, periarteritis nodosa, Wegener's granulomatosis), and disseminated neoplasms. The severity of hemolysis ranges from mild to severe. Coagulation abnormalities mimicking those of DIC are usually absent.

Thrombotic thrombocytopenic purpura (TTP) (Ch. 166), the hemolytic uremic syndrome (Ch. 81), and mitomycin C-induced hemolytic uremic syndrome of adult cancer patients are highly fatal disorders of unknown etiology that closely resemble one another clinically. Patients with these disorders develop rapid fragmentational hemolysis, thrombocytopenia, and renal failure. Early there is little or no laboratory evidence of DIC despite the presence of diffuse microvascular thrombi.

Diagnosis. The diagnosis of a microangiopathic hemolytic disorder is based on the demonstration of schistocytes, grossly misshapen, sharply angulated erythrocytes that occasionally appear helmet shaped (Color plate 2*J*), usually in association with reticulocytosis, serum haptoglobin levels that are diminished to absent, increased serum LDH concentrations, and hemosiderinuria. Hemoglobinemia and hemoglobinuria occur less frequently.

Hemolysis may be accompanied by significant thrombocytopenia, with or without laboratory evidence of DIC (i.e., the prolonged prothrombin, partial thromboplastin, and thrombin times are typically incompletely corrected when an equal volume of normal plasma is mixed with that of the patient). When severe DIC is present, the plasma concentrations of fibrin degradation products are characteristically elevated, and coagulation Factors V, VIII, and I (fibrinogen) are usually decreased.

Treatment. Treatment of the patient with microangiopathic hemolysis must be highly individualized and may be very complex. Efforts should be made to reverse the underlying triggering mechanism (i.e., withdrawal of potentially offending drugs, treatment with antibiotics, etc.) and the patient supported with red cell transfusions, platelet packs, and cryoprecipitate as required. Occasional patients may benefit from anticoagulation with heparin to disrupt the vicious cycle of clotting and fibrinolysis. Vigorous plasma exchange (plasmapheresis combined with infusion of normal plasma) may induce dramatic clinical remissions in TTP. Although antiplatelet drugs and high-dose adrenocorticoid therapy are frequently employed, their efficacy is less certain.

IMMUNE HEMOLYTIC ANEMIA

Nydegger UE, Kazatchkine MD: The role of complement in immune clearance of blood cells. Springer Semin Immunopathol 6:373, 1983. *An interesting and perceptive review of complement activation and complement receptors and their roles in immunologically mediated destruction of peripheral blood cells.*

Petz LD, Branch DR: Drug-induced immune hemolytic anemia. In Chaplin H (ed.): Methods in Hematology. Vol. 18. New York, Churchill Livingstone, Inc., 1985, pp 47–94. *An exhaustive but readily assimilable review of the pathophysiologic mechanisms underlying drug-mediated immune hemolysis and of laboratory techniques useful in the diagnosis of this problem.*

Rosse WF: Autoimmune hemolytic anemia. Hosp Pract 20:105, 1985. *A brief but superb summary of the pathophysiology of autoimmune hemolysis.*

Sokol RJ, Hewitt S: Autoimmune hemolysis: A critical review. CRC Crit Rev Oncol Hematol 4:125, 1985. *A comprehensive and well-integrated review of the pathophysiology, clinical manifestations, and treatment of autoimmune hemolytic disorders.*

PAROXYSMAL NOCTURNAL HEMOGLOBINURIA

Rosse WF: Treatment of paroxysmal nocturnal hemoglobinuria. Blood 60:20, 1982. *A brief review of the treatment of PNH by a physician who has had vast clinical experience with this disease.*

Rosse WF, Parker CJ: Paroxysmal nocturnal haemoglobinuria. Clin Haematol 14:105, 1985. *A probing analysis of the membrane abnormality(ies) in PNH and of the pathophysiologic implications of complement activation on the red cell membrane.*

OTHER

Bowdler AJ: Splenomegaly and hypersplenism. Clin Haematol 12:467, 1983. *A thoughtful, comprehensive review of a topic that has generated controversy for many years.*

Cooper RA: Hemolytic syndromes and red cell membrane abnormalities in liver disease. Semin Hematol 17:103, 1980. *An excellent review of the pathophysiologic mechanisms of red cell membrane changes in liver disease.*

140 HEMOGLOBIN STRUCTURE AND FUNCTION

Alan N. Schechter

The interior of the normal erythrocyte contains a 5 mM solution of hemoglobin, corresponding to about 280 million hemoglobin molecules per cell. Each molecule is a tetramer composed of two pairs of polypeptide chains to which four heme moieties are bound. The ability of the hemoglobin molecule to bind oxygen reversibly allows the erythrocyte to transport oxygen from the lungs to the tissues. The complex structure of the hemoglobin molecule allows it to bind, transport, and release oxygen with extraordinary efficiency. As a result of advances in molecular biology during the last several decades, the relationship between the structure and function of hemoglobin is very well understood. It is now possible to explain the pathophysiology of diseases related to hemoglobin at the molecular, and even atomic, level.

STRUCTURE. The normal hemoglobins of the adult are hemoglobins A (about 97 per cent of the total), A_2 (about 2 per cent), and F (about 1 per cent). The protein, or globin, of each of these is composed of two α polypeptide chains and in addition two β (in hemoglobin A), two δ (in hemoglobin A_2), or two γ (in hemoglobin F) polypeptide chains. An additional α-like globin, the ζ chain, and an additional β-like globin, the ϵ chain, have been discovered. These chains, with the α and γ chains, form hemoglobins that are detected in the early embryo: hemoglobin Gower 1 ($\zeta_2\epsilon_2$), hemoglobin Portland ($\zeta_2\gamma_2$), and hemoglobin Gower 2 ($\alpha_2\epsilon_2$).

The sequence of appearance, and sometimes disappearance, of the six polypeptide chains known to be synthesized by human beings is illustrated in Figure 140–1. The factors that control the sequential appearance of these polypeptides are poorly understood. The "switching" process from one hemoglobin to another is mainly related to the age of the fetus or infant and has not been clearly shown to be determined by the site of erythropoiesis, humoral factors, or the appearance of different clones of cells.

The chromosomal arrangements of the genes for these six polypeptide chains are shown in Figure 140–2, the α-like genes on chromosome 16 and the β-like genes on chromosome 11. The genes for the α chains appear in two functional copies that code for identical polypeptides. Of the two ζ genes, only the one on the 5′ (left) of the gene cluster appears to be functional. Chromosome 11 seems to have but one functional copy of the β, δ, and ϵ genes but two copies of the γ gene.

The sequence of nucleotides in the regions of DNA corresponding to these genes and in many of the regions separating them has been determined. The nucleotide sequences of the genes that specify amino acids in each of the polypeptides are interrupted by stretches of DNA, or intervening sequences, that do not code for amino acids in the hemoglobin

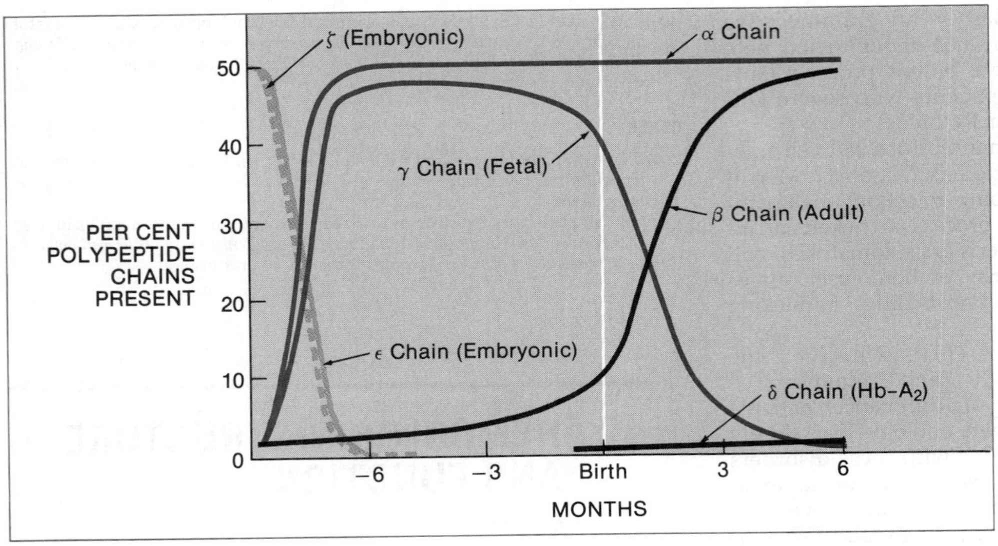

FIGURE 140–1. A diagram of the relative abundance of various human globin chains during development. (From Bunn HF, Forget BG: Hemoglobin: Molecular, Genetic, and Clinical Aspects. Philadelphia, W. B. Saunders Company, 1986.)

molecule (Ch. 141). The elucidation of the anatomy of the human hemoglobin genetic region at this level of detail is providing information about regulatory genetic functions as well as structural genetic elements, as described in Ch. 142.

While globin messenger RNA synthesis reaches a maximum in the early erythroblast series, globin polypeptide synthesis reaches a peak at about the level of the polychromatophilic erythroblast and continues into the reticulocyte stage. There appears to be little enzymatic processing of the globin polypeptides, except for removal of the amino-terminal methionine residue. Each cell contains three or more types of polypeptide chains, and they combine roughly in proportion to their concentrations. As long as synthesis of α (and α-like) chains and β (and β-like) chains is balanced, as it is in the normal person, the hemoglobin in the red cell is formed of two pairs of chains and is largely stable for the lifespan of the erythrocyte. If chain synthesis or degradation is unbalanced as in certain diseases, discussed in Ch. 142, then surplus chains will accumulate. Excess α chains remain monomeric, whereas the excess β chains form tetramers (β_4, hemoglobin H), as do the excess γ chains (γ_4, hemoglobin Barts). All of these surplus chains are unstable compared to normal hemoglobin and precipitate within the erythrocyte, shortening its lifespan and thus causing hemolytic anemias.

The heme prosthetic groups are in four largely hydrophobic pockets, one being formed in each globin polypeptide chain by the amino acid side chains of polypeptide helices on either side of the heme and of other helices at the interior. The iron atoms are at the center of the porphyrin molecules, bound in a square array to the four nitrogen atoms of each pyrrole ring. In addition, the iron is tightly bound to the nitrogen atom of the imidazole side chain of the histidine residue on a nearby helix (the "proximal" histidine). Oxygen or other small molecules such as carbon monoxide bind on the opposite or "distal" side of the heme in a very compact pocket formed by a number of amino acid side chains.

The nonaqueous environment around the iron atom allows it to remain in the ferrous state even in the presence of oxygen molecules, and imparts to the iron-oxygen bond a coordination character that makes its strength intermediate between a noncovalent and a covalent bond. This property is important in allowing the reversibility of oxygen binding. Despite this, some oxidation to the ferric form occurs naturally. A methemoglobin-reduction system exists in the erythrocyte, utilizing reduced nicotinamide adenine dinucleotide and the enzyme methemoglobin reductase, to keep the iron atoms in the ferrous form. This system, and other related enzymatic pathways, will be discussed in more detail in Ch. 146.

FUNCTION. In the range from normal arterial P_{O_2} values (100 mm Hg) to normal tissue P_{O_2} values (thought to be around 40 mm Hg), hemoglobin oxygen saturation decreases from about 100 per cent to about 75 per cent (see Fig. 140–3). Much more oxygen can be released if a further fall in tissue P_{O_2} values occurs. The great physiologic benefit of hemoglobin results from both the sigmoidal shape of the oxygen-binding curve and the fact that the hemoglobin tetramer has relatively

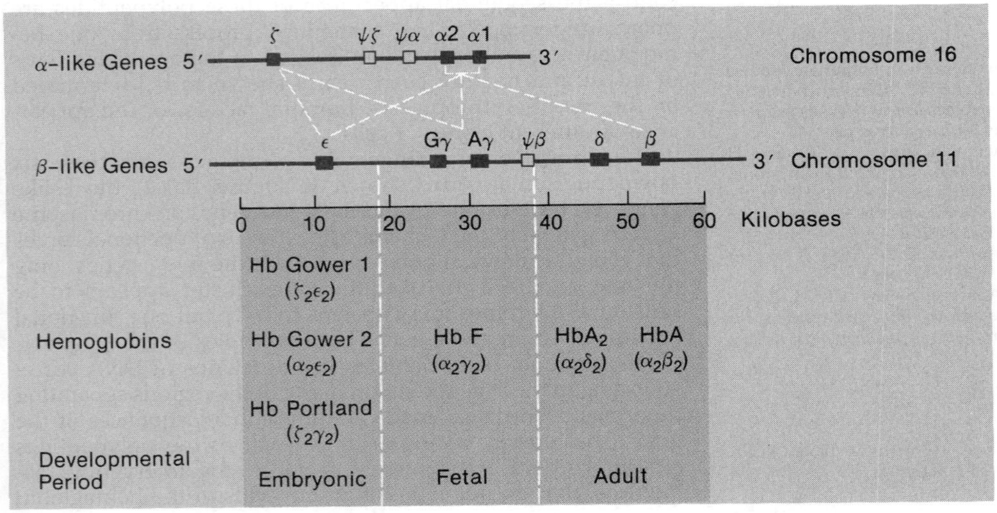

FIGURE 140–2. A diagram of the arrangement of the clusters of human α-like and β-like globin genes on chromosomes 16 and 11 and the embryonic, fetal, and adult hemoglobins that result from the combinations of the various globin chains encoded by these genes. The ψ genes are similar to globin genes but do not code for protein. Distances along the chromosome are expressed in terms of 1000 nucleotide pairs (a kilobase).

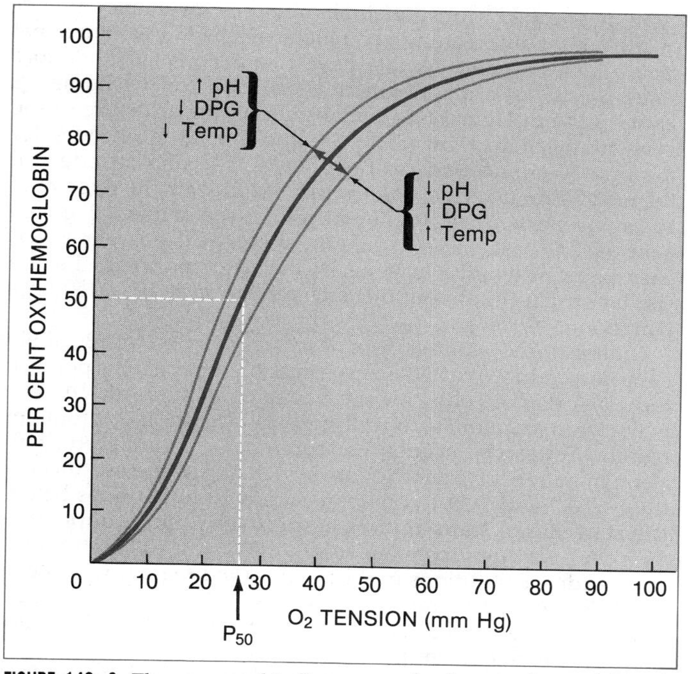

FIGURE 140–3. The oxygen binding curve for human hemoglobin A under physiologic conditions (*dark curve*). The affinity will be shifted by changes in pH, DPG concentration, and temperature as indicated. P_{50} represents the oxygen tension at half saturation. (From Bunn HF, Forget BG: Hemoglobin: Molecular, Genetic, and Clinical Aspects. Philadelphia, W. B. Saunders Co., 1986.)

reduced oxygen affinity (or "shift to the right") as compared to its own subunits or to myoglobin. This allows efficient discharge of oxygen in peripheral tissues.

The normal, relatively low oxygen affinity of hemoglobin is due to the interactions of the subunits with each other and to the binding of protons (the Bohr effect) and the molecule 2,3-diphosphoglyceric acid (DPG) to the hemoglobin tetramer. For reasons that are not completely understood, tetramers of hemoglobin composed of pairs of unlike chains have reduced oxygen affinity as compared to the subunits alone. In the pH region from 7.4 to 7.0, the binding of protons—which increases as pH is lowered—further decreases the oxygen affinity of hemoglobin, i.e., it shifts the oxygen equilibrium curve further to the right (Fig. 140–3). This results in more oxygen being released at a given Po_2, which is very useful since the pH is reduced in the tissues as compared to the capillaries of the lung. Thus the Bohr effect promotes oxygen delivery.

DPG, which is normally roughly equimolar with hemoglobin in the erythrocyte, binds reversibly to the region of the hemoglobin tetramer formed by the amino-terminal ends of each of the β chains. One molecule of DPG binds to each hemoglobin tetramer. The binding affinity of DPG for deoxygenated hemoglobin is much greater than for oxygenated hemoglobin. DPG thus stabilizes the deoxygenated form of hemoglobin, increases its concentration relative to the oxygenated form, and so decreases the overall oxygen affinity, i.e., it causes a shift to the right of the oxygen equilibrium curve (Fig. 140–3). DPG binding to deoxygenated hemoglobin is proportional to its concentration in the erythrocyte, and thus oxygen affinity is inversely related to DPG levels. Variation in intracellular DPG, by mechanisms only poorly understood, appears to be a major physiologic mechanism for adjusting oxygen transport in the human being.

The binding of carbon dioxide to hemoglobin as carbamino complexes also lowers oxygen affinity. This process, however, is a relatively minor one in the red cell, and it is estimated that only 10 per cent of metabolically produced carbon dioxide is transported in this manner.

The sigmoidal nature of the oxygen equilibrium curve itself contributes greatly to the efficiency of hemoglobin by causing a release of much oxygen over a narrow range of tissue Po_2 values. (Roughly 250 million molecules of oxygen per red cell are released to the tissues in each cycle.) The shape of the binding curve is due to interactions or cooperativity within and between the dimers of the hemoglobin tetramer. The basis for these interactions at the level of individual atomic groups is still the subject of much debate, but the overall picture seems clear. Deoxygenated hemoglobin exists in a well-defined arrangement of each polypeptide chain with respect to the heme group (tertiary structure) and with respect to each other (quaternary structure), called the T or tense form. Oxygenated hemoglobin has a significantly changed tertiary and quaternary structure, called the R or relaxed form. As oxygenation of each hemoglobin tetramer proceeds, the change in structure occurs in a relatively all-or-none manner, rather than being a gradual structural transition. This property leads to the cooperative or sigmoidal oxygen equilibrium curve.

The trigger for this structural transition is the binding of oxygen to the iron atoms and the resulting changes in the sizes and positions of these iron atoms and the orientations of the heme groups themselves within the polypeptide chains. The most direct result of these changes in the iron atoms and the heme groups is to lead to movements of the proximal histidine residues and the helices to which they are attached. These movements, in turn, cause further changes in the arrangement of the globin polypeptides and interactions among amino acid side chains, within and between subunits. The final result is that the stable quaternary structure of the oxygenated hemoglobin is significantly different from that of the deoxygenated form. The deoxygenated and the oxygenated forms of human hemoglobin have been studied in detail by x-ray crystallography. As described in Ch. 145, this information has been extremely useful in understanding the molecular basis for altered function in certain hemoglobins. In addition, the molecular basis of the polymerization of deoxygenated sickle hemoglobin is explicable with this information, as described in Ch. 143.

Bunn HF, Forget BG: Hemoglobin: Molecular, Genetic, and Clinical Aspects. Philadelphia, W. B. Saunders Company, 1986. *The best single reference to all aspects of the study of hemoglobin.*

Dickerson RE, Geis I: Hemoglobin: Structure, Function, Evolution, and Pathology. Menlo Park, CA, Benjamin/Cummings Publishing Company Inc., 1983. *A sophisticated and magnificently illustrated introduction to hemoglobin structure and function.*

Fermi G, Perutz MF: Haemoglobin and Myoglobin: Atlas of Molecular Structures in Biology. New York, Oxford University Press, 1981, vol 2. *An introduction to information and conclusions from the structure.*

Honig GR, Adams JG: Human Hemoglobin Genetics. New York, Springer-Verlag, 1986. *The first comprehensive treatise on this rapidly moving field of great clinical relevance.*

Perutz MF: Molecular anatomy, physiology and pathology of hemoglobin. *In* Stamatoyannopoulous G, Nienhuis AW, Leder P, et al (eds.): Molecular Basis of Blood Diseases. Philadelphia, W. B. Saunders Company, 1987. *A rigorous but comprehensive analysis of normal and abnormal hemoglobin function in terms of the molecular structure.*

141 HEMOGLOBIN SYNTHESIS

Arthur W. Nienhuis

The red cell is one of the uniquely specialized cells in the body. Lacking a nucleus and therefore devoid of any proliferative potential or even the ability to renew its own protein constituents, the red cell is totally adapted to carrying oxygen and carbon dioxide for its brief lifespan of approximately 120 days. The red cell's unique membrane constituents give it flexibility, allowing passage through even the narrowest capillaries and egress from the red pulp into the sinusoids of the spleen. The oxygen and carbon dioxide transport properties of the red cell depend on its content of hemoglobin. Hemoglobin amounts to more than 95 per cent of the cytoplasmic protein of the red cell; each cell contains 30 pg (approximately 280 million molecules) of this protein. In this chapter we will consider briefly the mechanism of hemoglobin synthesis, beginning with an outline of the flow of genetic information from gene to protein. Also germane are the mechanisms by which red cells come to contain hemoglobin to the virtual exclusion of most other proteins.

FLOW OF INFORMATION FROM GENE TO PROTEIN. ***Chromatin Structure.*** The nuclei of human cells contain chromatin, a complex of histone core particles called nucleosomes around which the DNA double helix is coiled. Nonhistone chromosomal proteins are thought to play a role in establishing higher order structures of chromatin so that the relatively vast amount of DNA may be packed into a cell's small nucleus. Furthermore, nonhistone proteins are thought to include regulatory factors which establish the structure of a restricted number of genes in a specialized cell to allow their exclusive expression. For example, the globin genes in erythroid cells have been shown to be in an active conformation, whereas in brain cells the globin genes are included among those genes whose conformation in chromatin render them inaccessible for transcription. The nature of these regulatory factors and the manner in which they interact with specific genes to promote their expression have only recently become accessible to experimental study.

Gene Structure. The DNA sequences that encode for a specific protein are not co-linear with the messenger RNA (mRNA) for that protein. Rather the coding portions of the gene, now called exons, are interrupted by a variable number of introns or intervening sequences of DNA. All functional globin genes studied to date have two introns and therefore three exons, as is diagrammatically shown for the human β globin gene in Figure 141–1. Considering the structure of the gene from left to right (5′ to 3′), the first exon encodes for the first 30 amino acids of β globin, the second encodes for the next 74 amino acids, and the last encodes for the remaining 42 amino acids. The smaller intron in the human β globin gene is 130 base pairs in length, whereas the larger is 850 base pairs in length. In general, the α globin genes have a similar structure, although the larger intron is only 150 base pairs long.

Globin mRNA Metabolism. Transcription of the β globin gene to produce its RNA copy probably begins at a point in the DNA that encodes for the 5′ end of mature mRNA. The major transcriptional control signals are in the promoter region. Conserved sequences required for accurate and efficient initiation of transcription by RNA polymerase include the "ATA" and "CAT" boxes at 31 and 76 nucleotides before the start site of transcription, respectively, and a duplicated "CACA" box just upstream from "CAT" (Fig. 141–1). Single nucleotide substitutions in these conserved regions have been identified in thalassemia globin genes (Ch. 142); these mutations cause decreased globin gene expression leading to deficient hemoglobin synthesis.

The entire gene, including its two introns, is copied into a co-linear RNA molecule. Transcription continues beyond those sequences represented in globin mRNA. The nucleotide sequence, "AATAAA," serves as a signal for cleavage of the

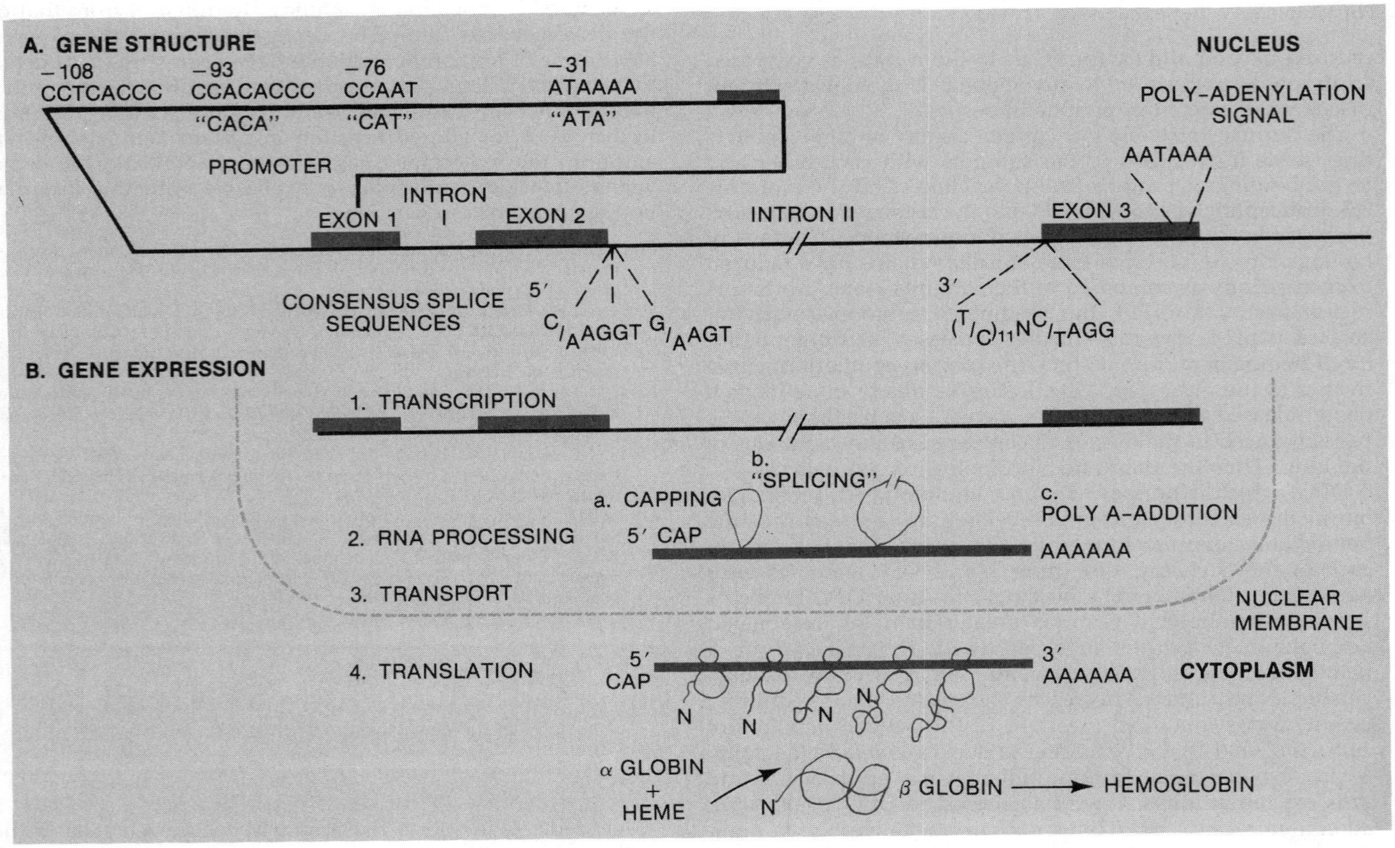

FIGURE 141–1. Structure and expression of the normal human β globin gene. The three exons encode for β globin; these coding sequences are interrupted by two introns or intervening sequences. Certain segments of the promoter region ("boxes") are conserved in many globin genes. The actual sequence of these "boxes" in the β globin gene promoter is shown. The splice sequences shown represent the consensus of those found at many exon-intron boundaries. Those actually found in the β globin gene resemble the consensus sequence but are not identical. C = cytosine, T = thymine, A = adenine, and G = guanine. The processes involved in gene expression include transcription of the gene, processing of the primary RNA transcript, transport of the mRNA from nucleus to cytoplasm, and translation of the mRNA into β globin.

transcription product and addition of a series of adenines to form the poly-A track. The primary transcription product, the β globin mRNA precursor, is a 1600–1700 nucleotide molecule. During transcription, it is also modified at the 5′ end by addition of a guanosine diphosphate residue and several methyl groups in a series of reactions referred to as capping (Fig. 141–1).

The DNA sequences found at the exon-intron boundaries, when transcribed into RNA, serve as signals for precise and efficient splicing of the RNA transcript. Comparison of more than 100 exon-intron boundaries has lead to the identification of the consensus splice sequences shown in Figure 141–1. The dinucleotides "GT" and "AG" at the 5′ and 3′ ends of introns, respectively, are obligatory for functional splicing. The other nucleotides are not invariant and therefore are referred to as *consensus* nucleotides. As discussed in Ch. 142, single nucleotide substitutions in either obligatory or consensus nucleotides at the exon-intron boundaries of thalassemia globin genes cause abnormal RNA splicing, and therefore globin mRNA deficiency. Normally, processing is efficient and rapid; 95 per cent of precursor molecules are thought to become mature mRNA within only a few minutes of their synthesis. Approximately 100 molecules of precursor are present in each erythroblast compared with 20,000 to 50,000 molecules of mRNA.

Globin mRNA Structure. The mature mRNA is 600 to 650 nucleotides in length. Beginning from the cap site, the first 40 to 50 nucleotides represent an untranslated part of the mRNA. The initiation codon (AUG) signals the point at which the beginning of protein synthesis occurs. The next 423 (α) or 438 (β) nucleotides specify the protein sequence of the globin. Next is the terminator or stop codon, UAA in α and β globin mRNA, followed by 80 to 100 nucleotides that make up the 3′ untranslated part of the mRNA and then the poly-A track.

The genetic code is the combination of all possible codons that may specify the 20 amino acids that occur in protein. Four nucleotides can be put together in 64 different triplets or codons. The genetic code is degenerate in the sense that all codons are used; each amino acid is specified by more than one codon. Each codon requires a separate transfer RNA (tRNA) to allow it to be translated during protein synthesis.

Protein Synthesis. To translate mRNA into protein, the small and large ribosomal subunits are required along with several protein initiation, elongation, and termination factors and a complement of tRNA molecules. The initiator tRNA carries the amino acid methionine. Protein synthesis begins when this tRNA binds to an initiation factor and then subsequently is bound to the ribosome as specified by its anticodon, TAC, which interacts with the initiator codon. The codon next in line in both human and α and β globin mRNA is GUG, which specifies valine. A tRNA for valine is bound to the ribosome as its anticodon, CAC, recognizes the valine codon in mRNA. A peptide bond is then formed between methionine and valine. The mRNA is then translocated on the ribosome, and the next codon is ready to be read. This series of reactions continues until the terminator codon is encountered, at which point the ribosomal subunits and a completed globin molecule are released from the mRNA by the action of a termination factor. Each mRNA molecule may serve simultaneously as a template for the synthesis of several globin molecules. The protein synthesis mechanism appears to be quite general; no specific factors are required to translate a particular mRNA.

The globins undergo a number of postsynthetic modifications. Removal of the methionine residue, donated by the initiator tRNA, occurs on the polyribosome before synthesis of the globin polypeptide is complete. After assembly into hemoglobin, nonenzymatic glycosylation reactions give rise to a variety of minor electrophoretic variants. The extent of these reactions is proportional to the lifespan of the erythrocyte and to mean blood glucose levels. The major glycosylated form is designated hemoglobin A_{1C}. It has a glucose molecule linked by means of Schiff base to the amino-terminus of the β chain. Since glycosylation varies directly with blood sugar level, measurements of such modified hemoglobins can be used to evaluate control of diabetes mellitus. Perhaps even more important, these modifications of hemoglobin may be the prototype of many other nonenzymatic glycosylation reactions, which could be the pathophysiologic mechanism for damage to various intracellular and extracellular proteins leading to the complications of diabetes mellitus.

IRON ACCUMULATION AND HEMOGLOBIN SYNTHESIS. To obtain the considerable amount of iron required for hemoglobin synthesis, the red cell utilizes membrane receptors specific for the iron transport protein transferrin. The transferrin receptor complex is transiently internalized into the red cell within an endocytic vesicle. The pH within the vesicle is lowered by active ion transport, thereby releasing iron from transferrin. The receptor-apotransferrin complex is then returned to the cell surface, where apotransferrin is released. Synthesis of protoporphyrin is by a series of reactions catalyzed by enzymes found in relatively high concentrations in erythroblasts (see Ch. 203). Excess iron is stored as ferritin and may later become available for heme synthesis or be transferred from erythroid to phagocytic cells in bone marrow.

Nascent or partially completed globin chains may bind heme while still on the polyribosome as soon as that portion of the globin that binds heme is synthesized and folded into an appropriate conformation. The assembly of the individual globins into the hemoglobin tetramer occurs spontaneously by virtue of both their complementary surfaces and their high concentrations within the developing erythroblasts.

Heme has important roles in the process of hemoglobin synthesis in addition to being an essential component of the hemoglobin molecule. Heme deficiency leads to inactivation of a critically required initiation factor, leading to a marked reduction in the rate of protein synthesis. Furthermore, heme may stimulate the synthesis and accumulation of globin mRNA directly and thus may have a regulatory role in modulating globin gene expression.

PRODUCTION OF HEMOGLOBIN DURING ERYTHROBLAST DEVELOPMENT. The erythroblasts in the bone marrow exhibit a series of amplification divisions during which globin mRNA accumulation and hemoglobin synthesis occur (Fig. 141–2). Thus from a very limited number of progenitor stem cells with high proliferative potential are produced a large number of highly specialized but terminally differentiated red cells.

Only 0.1 to 0.5 per cent of the total RNA synthesized in the earliest erythroblasts is globin mRNA, yet the globin mRNA species ultimately represents 95 per cent of the total mRNA present in reticulocytes. This remarkable accumulation of globin mRNA to the exclusion of other mRNA molecules appears to be the result primarily of two factors. First, globin mRNA is remarkably stable during erythroid differentiation. Indeed, there seems to be no degradation of globin mRNA following its synthesis until the reticulocyte stage of maturation. In contrast other mRNA species decay with a half-life of approximately 20 hours and are destabilized to decay even faster toward the end of erythroblast maturation. Also, during the later phases of erythroid maturation, synthesis of other mRNAs declines precipitously, whereas that of globin mRNA appears to continue until just prior to nuclear exclusion. Thus the remarkable stability and the continued synthesis of globin mRNA during all phases of erythroid maturation appear to account for its accumulation to the exclusion of other mRNA species.

MECHANISM OF PRODUCTION OF SPECIFIC HEMOGLOBINS. Fetal red cells contain predominantly Hb F, whereas adult red cells contain Hb A (see Ch. 140). Selective

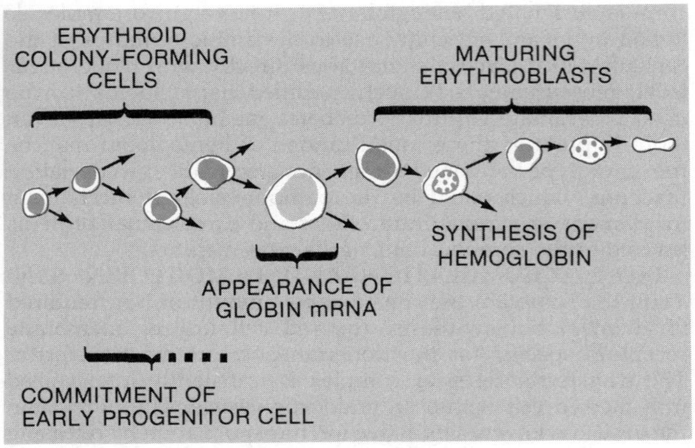

FIGURE 141–2. Regulation of hemoglobin synthesis during erythropoiesis. Two general classes of cells are the precursors of circulating red cells. Erythroblasts at various stages of maturation may be recognized within the bone marrow; these cells and circulating reticulocytes are engaged in hemoglobin synthesis. Erythroid stem cells, the progenitors of erythroblasts, are present within the bone marrow in very small numbers but may be detected by virtue of their ability to form colonies of erythroblasts in semi-solid media in vitro. As discussed in the text, current evidence suggests that commitment to expression of either the γ or β globin genes occurs in erythroid stem cells prior to the initial appearance of globin messenger RNA.

expression of the γ and β genes appears to be modulated at the level of transcription. The precursor to β globin mRNA is present in a lower concentration in fetal erythroblasts than is the precursor to γ mRNA, whereas in adult erythroblasts the β globin mRNA precursor is present in considerably higher concentration than that for γ mRNA. Thus, the pattern of hemoglobin synthesis accurately reflects the relative accumulation of the two mRNA species. Several clues suggest a molecular mechanism(s) that might regulate the transcription of individual globin genes. Nuclease sensitivity studies have shown that the promoter regions of expressed genes are "open" in chromatin, allowing for protein-DNA interactions. The DNA sequences of the promoter region of the individual globin genes are distinctly different, allowing for specific interaction with nonhistone nuclear proteins involved in gene regulation. The frequency of methylation of cytosine residues, a postsynthetic modification of DNA, varies inversely with gene expression and could further alter the interaction of promoter regions with regulatory proteins. Much effort is currently directed at identification of these putative regulatory molecules.

Factors that influence the relative level of expression of individual globin genes appear to be exerted on very primitive erythroid stem cells. Experimental analysis of colonies of erythroblasts formed in vitro indicate that those which develop from the stem cells in fetal liver make Hb F, whereas colonies developing from stem cells in adult bone marrow make predominantly, but not exclusively, Hb A. Thus the primitive stem cells appear to become committed at some very early stage in their differentiation with respect to the pattern of hemoglobin synthesis in their progeny erythroblasts.

Karlsson S, Nienhuis AW: Developmental regulation of human globin genes. Ann Rev Biochem 54:1071, 1985. *A comprehensive review of current knowledge about globin gene structure, expression, and regulation, with particular emphasis on the mechanisms of hemoglobin switching during development.*

Nienhuis A, Wolfe L: The thalassemias: Disorders of hemoglobin synthesis. In Nathan D, Oski F (eds.): Hematology of Infancy and Childhood. 3rd ed. Philadelphia, W. B. Saunders Company (in press). *A detailed account of thalassemic disorders, with a more extensive discussion of gene expression and hemoglobin synthesis than that included here.*

Stamatoyannopoulos G, Papayannopoulou T, Brice M, et al.: Cell biology of hemoglobin switching: I. The switch from fetal to adult hemoglobin formation during ontogeny; Papayannopoulou T, Nakamoto B, Kurachi S, et al.: Cell biology of hemoglobin switching: II. Studies on the regulation of fetal hemoglobin synthesis in human adults. In Stamatoyannopoulos G, Nienhuis AW (eds.): Hemoglobins in Development and Differentiation. New York, Alan R. Liss, Inc., 1981. *These detailed reviews by major contributors to the problem of hemoglobin switching and erythroid stem cell differentiation should be consulted by those with a serious interest in this topic.*

142 THE THALASSEMIAS

Arthur W. Nienhuis

The thalassemias are hereditary anemias that occur because of mutations that affect the synthesis of hemoglobin. In β thalassemia there is deficient synthesis of β globin, whereas in α thalassemia there is deficient synthesis of α globin. Reduced synthesis of one of the two globin polypeptides leads to deficient hemoglobin accumulation, resulting in hypochromic and microcytic red cells. These red cell abnormalities are the most constant and characteristic features of this group of disorders. Table 142–1 contains a clinical classification of the thalassemias presented in the order in which they will be discussed in this chapter.

The incidence and prevalence of these conditions is highly variable. Most common is thalassemia trait, a mild, clinically insignificant anemia that apparently protects individuals from malaria (see below), and therefore through natural selection it has become extremely common in certain parts of the world. Thalassemia trait generally represents the heterozygous form of either α or β thalassemia. Hence where thalassemia trait is common, homozygous, more severely affected patients will be found frequently. In the United States, the incidence of β thalassemia is highest among ethnic groups originating from the Mediterranean area, parts of Africa, and Asia, whereas the incidence of α thalassemia is highest among those from Asia. Generally the incidence of thalassemia trait in these ethnic groups is 3 to 5 per cent. Approximately 1000 patients with more severe forms of thalassemia are known in the United States.

SEVERE β THALASSEMIA (Cooley's Anemia)

Severe β thalassemia occurs in patients who are homozygous for mutations that lead to a decrease in β globin synthesis. Because both β globin genes are affected, there is marked deficiency in β globin synthesis, but α globin synthesis continues at an approximately normal rate. Accumulation of a large excess of α chains for which there are no β chains with which to combine has several serious deleterious effects. α Globin is highly insoluble and forms large intracellular inclusions. These interfere with the cell cycle in the bone marrow, retard the passage of red cells from the bone marrow, and reduce the survival of red cells in the circulation by virtue of membrane damage and splenic trapping. Marked ineffective erythropoiesis is the hallmark of this disorder because α

TABLE 142–1. CLINICAL CLASSIFICATION OF THE THALASSEMIAS

I. Severe β thalassemia (Cooley's anemia)	Severe anemia, growth retardation, hepatosplenomegaly, bone marrow expansion, and bone deformities
A. Thalassemia major	Transfusion-dependent
B. Thalassemia intermedia	No regular transfusion requirement
II. Thalassemia trait (α or β)	Mild anemia with microcytosis and hypochromia
III. Hb H disease (α-thal)	Moderately severe hemolytic anemia, icterus, and splenomegaly
IV. Hydrops fetalis (α-thal)	Death in utero caused by severe anemia
V. Silent carrier (α or β)	Hematologically normal

inclusions interfere with erythroblast maturation, leading to intramedullary death of many red cell precursors. Severe anemia stimulates erythropoietin production, leading to erythroid stem cell and erythroblast proliferation. The vastly expanded erythroid cell mass results in osteoporosis with a potential for pathologic fractures. Extramedullary hematopoiesis is also often seen, and compression of vital structures, particularly the spinal cord, may occur as a consequence. Because of marrow expansion and bony deformities of the skull and facial bones, patients with severe β thalassemia often have an abnormal appearance with prominent epicanthal folds referred to as a chipmunk facies.

Patients with severe β thalassemia may be divided into two groups on the basis of their requirement for blood transfusion. Those with thalassemia major have an absolute requirement for blood without which severe anemia leads to death in infancy or early childhood. In contrast, patients with thalassemia intermedia are able to maintain their hemoglobin at 6 to 7 grams per deciliter without transfusion. This level is compatible with fairly normal growth and development, and many of these patients survive into adulthood.

Thalassemia Major

CLINICAL FEATURES. At birth patients with thalassemia major are nearly normal hematologically, since γ globin synthesis is normal and Hb F production is therefore adequate. However, as the switch from Hb F to Hb A is completed during the first year of life, the deficiency in β globin production becomes evident. By six to nine months of age, severe anemia reflected by pallor, poor growth, or inadequate food intake leads the anxious parents to bring the infant to the physician, at which time examination reveals the presence of marked hepatosplenomegaly. The hemoglobin may be 3 to 6 grams per deciliter, and the red cells exhibit the characteristic severe microcytosis, hypochromia, and fragmentation (Color plate 2G). Demonstration of thalassemia trait (see below) in both parents is usually sufficient to establish the diagnosis. Study of the infant's blood shows absence of or low Hb A, a large amount of Hb F, and an increase in the amount of Hb A_2 to 4 to 10 per cent of the total (normal <2.5 per cent). Biosynthetic studies, a tool of the research laboratory, may be employed to show the deficiency of β globin production.

CLINICAL COURSE. Prior to the use of regular blood transfusions, these children were grossly deformed because of expansion of the marrow spaces of the skull (see Fig. 130–1). Severe osteoporosis led to pathologic fractures, and anemia caused weakness and inanition. Death by two to three years of age was common. Blood transfusions were initially given infrequently for palliation, but gradually physicians interested in this condition came to recognize that regular transfusion to nearly normal hemoglobin levels could be used to suppress all disease manifestations. Growth and bone development are normal in children who have undergone hypertransfusion, and in fact they are virtually indistinguishable from other children if the hypertransfusion regimen is started at a very early age. If transfusions are given less frequently, the patient may exhibit some stigmata of the untreated disorder—bony deformities, growth retardation, and hepatosplenomegaly.

THE PROBLEM OF IRON OVERLOAD. Because humans have a very limited ability to excrete iron, regular blood transfusions inevitably lead to a vast accumulation. Each unit of packed red cells contains approximately 200 mg of iron, so that by the age of 12 the average thalassemic, having received 125 to 150 units of packed cells, will have accumulated 25 to 30 grams of excess iron. This amount compares to the normal 3 to 4 grams found in adults, 75 per cent of which is present in red cells as hemoglobin. Even in the patient with thalassemia intermedia who has not had transfusions, excess iron absorption leads inevitably to the manifestations of hemochromatosis, although at a later age than in the patient with transfusion-dependent thalassemia. Excess iron deposition occurs in virtually all organs. Most cells have a considerable ability to cope with this extra iron by making ferritin and its partial degradation product hemosiderin. Nonetheless, cell damage occurs by virtue of iron-catalyzed peroxidation of membrane lipids and release of the enzymes from lysosomes rendered labile by their content of hemosiderin granules. Thus tissue hemosiderosis (excess iron) leads ultimately to the clinical condition of secondary hemochromatosis. The liver, endocrine glands, and particularly the heart are the primary target organs (see Ch. 206).

Liver dysfunction is mild in the thalassemic patient with secondary hemochromatosis. Typically the liver is enlarged several centimeters below the right costal margin, and the transaminases are two to four times above the normal limits. Despite a 20- to 30-fold increase in iron concentration over normal, liver biosynthetic function as reflected by the concentration of serum albumin and various clotting factors is preserved. Fibrosis, invariably present on liver biopsy, may progress to frank cirrhosis anatomically, but clinical evidence of cirrhosis is rare.

As noted above, the course of adequately tranfused thalassemic patients is essentially normal until the age of 10 to 12. Then growth failure is a frequent and distressing complication for both the child and parents. The mechanism for this growth failure is not known; growth hormone levels are generally normal, but the serum somatomedin concentration may be low. Failure of growth is accompanied by lack of pubescence. Primary hypogonadism is exceedingly common. The mechanism is usually a failure of the pituitary to produce adequate amounts of FSH and LH. Diabetes mellitus, hypothyroidism, and, rarely, hypoparathyroidism with tetany are additional complications that may occur particularly in patients who are in their late teenage years or early 20's.

Cardiac disease in the patients with severe β thalassemia may take three forms: pericarditis, congestive heart failure, and cardiac arrhythmias. Recurrent attacks of acute pericarditis are manifested by chest pain, often pleuritic and affected by a change of position, accompanied by fever and occasionally a pericardial friction rub. These attacks are usually self-limited, lasting four to seven days. Treatment consists of bed rest, aspirin, and other anti-inflammatory agents such as indomethacin in appropriate doses. Rarely constrictive pericarditis may require a pericardectomy.

Congestive heart failure is to be expected ultimately in patients with secondary hemochromatosis unless death occurs early by virtue of cardiac arrhythmias. Careful echocardiographic studies have suggested that iron deposition begins by the age of five to six years. By ten or twelve years, when the patient has received more than 100 units of blood, left ventricular dysfunction may be demonstrated by radionuclide cineangiography during the physiologic stress of exercise. Clinical congestive heart failure is usually a late complication; most patients die within twelve months of the onset of definite evidence of heart failure. Treatment with digoxin in doses adequate to achieve therapeutic blood levels may be quite helpful. Appropriate use of diuretics and vasodilator therapy may be extremely useful in providing palliation and extending the lifespan of these patients.

Atrial and ventricular ectopy is present in 24-hour electrocardiographic recordings in virtually all patients who have received more than 150 units of packed red cells. High grade ventricular ectopy with couplets, short runs of ventricular tachycardia, and multiple ventricular foci are of ominous prognostic significance. Ectopy may be extremely distressful to the patient, particularly at night when it is often most severe. Tachyrhythmias such as ventricular tachycardia and/or ventricular fibrillation occur despite therapy and are frequent causes of death in patients with severe thalassemia undergoing regular transfusions. The pharmacologic treatment of cardiac arrhythmias is described in Ch. 45.

The prognosis of patients with thalassemia major is determined by the cardiac disease. The average age of death is 17 years, although a few patients may survive to their mid-20's. Because of this grim prognosis, a considerable effort has been focused on attempts to reduce the iron burden in these patients.

THE ROLE OF SPLENECTOMY. Splenic enlargement is frequent and often causes functional hypersplenism as manifested by an increasing transfusion requirement. Careful documentation of the patient's needs will often alert the physician to the development of hypersplenism as the need for blood rises. An average patient on a hypertransfusion regimen designed to maintain the hemoglobin at a level greater than 10 grams per deciliter will require 250 ml of packed cells per kilogram per year. If substantially more blood is required, the spleen should be removed. Leukopenia and thrombocytopenia, if present, are indicators of the presence of hypersplenism and should lead to prompt splenectomy.

The complication of splenectomy in this patient population is a risk of sudden overwhelming sepsis by encapsulated organisms. For this reason delay of splenectomy until after the age of four is highly desirable. Splenectomized patients should receive Pneumovax and may be placed on a regimen of daily penicillin prophylaxis. More important, each patient should be given a small supply of a broad-spectrum antibiotic such as ampicillin to be taken orally in appropriate doses if a high temperature develops and immediate medical attention cannot be obtained.

CHELATION THERAPY. The only drug available for use in removal of iron is deferoxamine (Desferal). This drug has an extremely high affinity for trivalent iron, and despite extensive clinical use it appears to be relatively free of serious toxicity. Its disadvantages are that it must be given parenterally and that it has a very short serum half-life. Thus most drug, given as a single intramuscular injection, is rapidly excreted without binding any iron. To maximize the efficacy of the drug, a technique has been devised to administer it subcutaneously by using a small mechanical infusion pump. A needle is inserted into the subcutaneous tissue of the abdomen, and the drug is infused very slowly over a period of eight to twelve hours. With 1.5 to 2.0 grams of Desferal, two to three times more iron may be removed than by a single daily intramuscular injection. Often daily excretion of 30 to 40 mg of iron may be achieved in older patients and may lead to overall negative iron balance despite continued transfusion therapy, provided that the drug is used at least five times per week. This regimen will retard the rate of iron accumulation in the liver and reduce liver fibrosis.

Clinical evidence indicates that cardiac disease may be delayed. Indeed, reversal of established congestive heart failure with documented left ventricular dysfunction has been observed in patients treated intensively with intravenous deferoxamine. This may be accomplished by placement of a Hickman catheter. Well-motivated patients may be taught to administer the drug daily by the intravenous route in doses of 3 to 4 grams per day given over 18 to 20 hours. Gastrointestinal disturbances and reversible renal dysfunction have been observed. Reduction of dose eliminates these complications. The greatest probability of successfully preventing iron damage is in patients in whom treatment is begun early, preferably by the age of five years. Vitamin C in small doses (150 to 250 mg per day) given orally may increase the amount of iron excretion in response to deferoxamine infusions, although some evidence suggests that this agent may enhance tissue iron toxicity, particularly to the heart, and therefore it should be used with caution in older patients.

Thalassemia Intermedia

Those patients with severe β thalassemia who maintain their hemoglobin levels above 6.0 to 7.0 grams per deciliter have a generally better prognosis. Individual patients with thalassemia intermedia generally have large amounts of Hb F, significant amounts of Hb A_2, and variable amounts of Hb A in their red cells. Iron accumulation may occur because of increased gastrointestinal absorption and ultimately may lead to secondary hemochromatosis with endocrine and cardiac dysfunction, but most patients with thalassemia intermedia survive into adulthood and many have children. Splenectomy may become necessary if evidence of hypersplenism is present. Osteoporosis may be severe, as these patients' erythroid mass is not suppressed. A disabling form of arthritis has been described. Large masses of erythroid tissue in extramedullary sites may cause organ dysfunction. Particularly distressing is spinal cord compression with paraplegia, although usually local radiation will reverse this condition. Any or all of these complications may ultimately lead to the use of a regular transfusion regimen in patients with thalassemia intermedia despite their marginally adequate hemoglobin levels. Such treatment has the added benefit of preventing the disfiguring facial abnormalities.

Genetically this condition is heterogeneous. Often the red cells of both parents exhibit stigmata of thalassemia trait, although frequently one parent may be a silent carrier of the thalassemia gene (see below). In such persons the impairment of β globin synthesis is so mild that the red cells are normal, but when the abnormal β gene is paired with another affected by a more severe β thalassemia mutation, thalassemia intermedia results. Elucidation of any thalassemia mutations at the molecular level has revealed marked quantitative variability ranging from 50 to 100 per cent reduction of β globin mRNA production (see below). Many patients are doubly heterozygous for two different mutations. The clinical heterogeneity of the β thalassemias reflects the many combinations of mutations that may be present in individual patients. Other genetic modifiers of the β thalassemia phenotype include α thalassemia mutations and genetic variants characterized by increased Hb F production. Coinheritance of an α thalassemia gene decreases α globin production leading to partial correction of the highly deleterious imbalance in α and β biosynthesis. Increased γ globin synthesis resulting in increased Hb F production compensates directly for deficient β globin production.

THALASSEMIA TRAIT

CLINICAL CHARACTERISTICS. Common to both α and β thalassemia is a condition referred to as thalassemia minor or trait. This condition generally occurs in individuals who are heterozygous for a mutation affecting α or β globin synthesis (see below). Characteristically the red blood cells are small and contain less hemoglobin than normal; the mean corpuscular volume averages 65 cubic microns (range 56 to 74), whereas the mean corpuscular hemoglobin averages 21 pg (range 20 to 23). Normal values for these parameters are 88 ± 5 and 30 ± 2, respectively. The total red cell count is often increased to 10 to 20 per cent above the normal range, so that anemia, if present, is mild. Rarely the packed cell volume may be as low as 30 per cent; values of 32 to 38 per cent are more typical. Splenomegaly is said to occur but is distinctly unusual, and other causes should be sought if this physical finding is present. No clinical symptoms may be attributed to the presence of thalassemia trait.

DIFFERENTIAL DIAGNOSIS. A characteristic feature of β thalassemia trait is an elevation of the level of Hb A_2. This minor hemoglobin accounts for only 2 or 3 per cent of the total in normal red cells, but in thalassemia trait it may be elevated in the range of 4 to 8 per cent in more than 90 per cent of persons with this condition. Similarly, the level of Hb F is often elevated to 1.5 to 2.5 per cent, although in rare types of thalassemia trait it may be as high as 10 to 15 per cent. In normal red cells, Hb F accounts for less than 1 per cent of the total. The minor hemoglobins, Hb A_2 and Hb F, are either normal or slightly decreased in patients with α thalassemia.

The differential diagnosis of thalassemia trait includes a consideration of iron deficiency. This diagnosis can be excluded only by measurement of the serum iron, total iron binding capacity, and serum ferritin. If these values are normal in patients whose red cells are severely microcytic, but in whom anemia, if present, is mild, the diagnosis of thalassemia trait can be considered established. The distinction between α and β thalassemia depends on the measurement of the minor hemoglobins. If these are normal, the diagnosis of α thalassemia is most likely, although rare subjects with β thalassemia also have normal levels of Hb A_2 and Hb F.

GENE FREQUENCY. Thalassemia trait is thought to protect persons from malaria, particularly during the early years of life when immunity is not yet established and fatal cerebral malaria caused by *Plasmodium falciparum* may occur. This selective advantage accounts for the high frequency of thalassemia genes in regions where malaria has been endemic for the past two millennia. These include the Mediterranean basin particularly, but also large parts of Asia and Africa. The gene frequency may be as high as 20 per cent in certain populations.

HEMOGLOBIN H DISEASE

PATHOPHYSIOLOGY. An anemia of moderate severity characterized by hypochromia, microcytosis, striking red cell fragmentation, and the presence of a fast migrating hemoglobin on electrophoresis occurs in patients who have a moderately severe deficiency in α globin production. The genetics of this condition will be considered later in this chapter. The fast migrating "hemoglobin" has the globin subunit composition β_4. It may account for up to 30 per cent of the total hemoglobin in these patients. Because the β_4 tetramer exhibits no cooperativeness and has an extremely high oxygen affinity, it is functionally useless in oxygen transport. Thus patients with a significant amount of Hb H functionally have a more severe anemia than measurement of the hemoglobin concentration might suggest.

Hb H is an unstable tetramer. Thus as the red cell ages and loses its ability to withstand oxidative stress, Hb H may precipitate, forming inclusions that cause hemolysis. Oxidant drugs such as the sulfonamides may exacerbate hemolysis. Because the β_4 tetramer is soluble during the early phases of the red cell's lifespan, erythropoiesis in the bone marrow is effective and the anemia is generally not as severe as that seen in patients with β thalassemia who have an equivalent impairment in β globin production.

CLINICAL FEATURES. The average patient with Hb H disease maintains gainful employment, marries, and reproduces. Usually the anemia is moderate with a hemoglobin concentration of 7 to 10 grams per deciliter, although occasional patients may have more severe anemia. Moderate splenomegaly is often present. Splenectomy may be considered, but the occurrence of severe postoperative thrombocytosis with a propensity for recurrent pulmonary emboli makes this procedure inadvisable except in patients with unequivocal clinical evidence of hypersplenism as manifested by leukopenia, thrombocytopenia, and a worsening anemia or a transfusion requirement in a previously stable patient. Other therapeutic measures include prescription of folic acid, avoidance of oxidant drugs and iron salts, prompt treatment of infection, and judicious use of transfusions. Acquired Hb H disease has been described as a complication in patients with various forms of myeloproliferative and myelodysplastic disorders. In such patients, treatment and prognosis are related to the primary disorder.

HYDROPS FETALIS

The birth of stillborn infants from parents who both have α thalassemia trait reflects the severest form of α thalassemia. These infants are grossly edematous or hydropic because of congestive heart failure that occurs as a result of severe anemia. Their failure to produce any α globin results in the production of only Hb Barts (γ_4) and Hb H (β_4) during the later parts of gestation. Both these hemoglobins are nonfunctional in oxygen transport, so that once the embryonic hemoglobins disappear from the circulation early in fetal development, life is no longer possible. A high incidence of toxemia of pregnancy has been noted in mothers of hydropic infants. Prenatal diagnosis of this condition is possible (see below) and should be followed by prompt termination of the pregnancy.

SILENT CARRIER

The silent carrier state was first recognized among the α thalassemia syndromes. One parent of a patient with Hb H disease usually has all the features of α thalassemia trait, whereas the other has normal-appearing red cells with no anemia. Similarly, progeny of persons with Hb H disease fall into two groups: those having α thalassemia trait, and those with apparently normal hemoglobin production. In the silent carrier, the defect in α globin synthesis is so mild that no impairment in hemoglobin synthesis is evident, although when the mutation is paired genetically with a more severe impairment of globin synthesis, e.g., α thalassemia trait, Hb H disease occurs. A similar silent carrier state has also been described among the β thalassemia syndromes. Thalassemia intermedia occurs in those who inherit one thalassemia gene from a silent carrier and a second from a person with thalassemia trait.

THE GENETICS OF THE α THALASSEMIA SYNDROMES

As described in Ch. 140, the α globin genes in humans are duplicated. Thus two genes are found on each chromosome 16, making a total of four in each diploid cell. Four clinical states are seen in α thalassemia: silent carrier, thalassemia trait, Hb H disease, and hydrops fetalis. These conditions occur in persons who have one, two, three, or four α globin genes affected by mutations that reduce α globin synthesis.

The most frequent mutation that leads to α thalassemia is gene deletion. In the silent carrier one of the two genes on one chromosome 16 is missing, whereas the other two genes on the other chromosome 16 are normal. α Thalassemia trait can occur by two mechanisms. Persons who have two chromosomes with only one α gene will exhibit α thalassemia trait. This form is most common in the black population. Hb H disease is distinctly uncommon in this population, since offspring of two persons each of whom is homozygous for the one α gene chromosome can only have α thalassemia trait and not Hb H disease. In the Oriental population, α thalassemia trait occurs most commonly in those who lack both α genes on one chromosome and have the normal two on the other. Mating of such a person with a silent carrier who has one chromosome having only one α gene can lead to children with Hb H disease. Hydrops fetalis occurs among offspring of parents both of whom are heterozygous for chromosomes lacking both normal α globin genes.

In addition to the deletion mutations, many nondeletional types of α thalassemia have been described. Molecular characterization of several has revealed a diversity of defects involving RNA splicing, polyadenylation, mRNA translation, or α globin stability. These mutations are similar to those in β thalassemia globin genes; their effects on RNA metabolism will be discussed in more detail in the next section.

THE MOLECULAR GENETICS OF THALASSEMIA

The β thalassemia mutations may be separated into two classes: β^+ thalassemia, in which there is synthesis of a small amount of normal β globin, and β^0 thalassemia, which in the homozygote is manifested by no β globin production at all.

Similarly, nondeletional types of α thalassemia may abolish (α^0) or decrease (α^+) alpha globin production. Many mutations having specific effects on gene expression have been characterized by molecular cloning, DNA sequencing, and functional characterization. Each of the several steps in RNA metabolism—transcription, processing, transport, and mRNA translation—has been found to be affected by one or more individual mutations. The variable quantitative effect of the individual mutations on globin production has been clarified by these molecular studies.

PROMOTER MUTATIONS. Five globin genes, each of which has a single nucleotide substitution in the promoter region, have been isolated from different individuals with β thalassemia. Three of the mutant genes have substitutions in the "ATA" box (see Fig. 141–1). These mutations reduce promoter function to 20 to 25 per cent of normal, but some β globin mRNA is produced from these genes; hence they cause β^+ thalassemia. The other two promoter mutants characterized to date have substitutions at 86 or 87 nucleotides from the start site for transcription in the first of the conserved "CACA" boxes.

SPLICING MUTATIONS. These are among the most common of mutations that cause thalassemia. Figure 142–1 contains a few illustrative examples classified by the manner in which they affect splicing of the globin mRNA precursor. Mutations that occur within the splice junction sequence decrease or abolish normal splicing at that site and often are accompanied by splicing at other sites that are not normally used. A substitution in the invariant GT, as shown in the example (Fig. 142–1*A*), abolishes splicing, making this a β^0 gene, whereas substitutions in consensus nucleotides at the splice junction have a quantitative effect on splicing and hence are β^+ mutations.

An interesting class of mutations consists of those that create an alternate site for splicing. These may occur within introns or, as shown in the examples in Figure 142–1*B*, within coding sequence (exons). These substitutions occur within regions of the precursor RNA molecule that resemble the consensus splice junction sequence (see Fig. 141–1), but lack some critical element necessary for splicing. Nucleotide substitutions that add that element to the potential splice junction sequence lead to its activation, causing abnormal splicing and hence a thalassemic effect. Substitution of A for T in codon 24 of the β globin gene does not alter the amino acid sequence (GGT and GGA both encode for glycine), but creates an alternative splicing site. The other two mutations illustrated in Figure 142–1*B* (Hb E and Hb Knossos) alter both protein structure and the splicing pattern. Such structural mutants that are also characterized by decreased synthesis are referred to as *thalassemic hemoglobinopathies*.

A class of mutations that has interesting implications for control of splicing is made up of those that create an alternate site and also activate cryptic splice sites remote from the mutation. There is a potential or cryptic splice site in the β globin gene transcript that matches the consensus splice junction sequence nearly perfectly, and yet this site is used rarely if ever during normal splicing. Use of an alternative site, created by a thalassemia mutation, apparently alters the secondary structure of the precursor RNA molecule, leading to splicing at the otherwise cryptic site (Fig. 141–1*C*).

A POLYADENYLATION MUTATION. The sequence "AATAAA" is one of the signals that leads to cleavage of the globin gene transcript and addition of the poly-A track (see Fig. 142–1). An α thalassemia gene isolated from an individual with Hb H disease has G substituted for A, altering the polyadenylation signal to "AATAGA." Most of the RNA transcript is not processed correctly and is prematurely degraded, although a small amount of normal α globin mRNA is produced by this mutant gene. Thus it is an α^+ thalassemia gene.

MUTATIONS THAT AFFECT mRNA TRANSLATION.

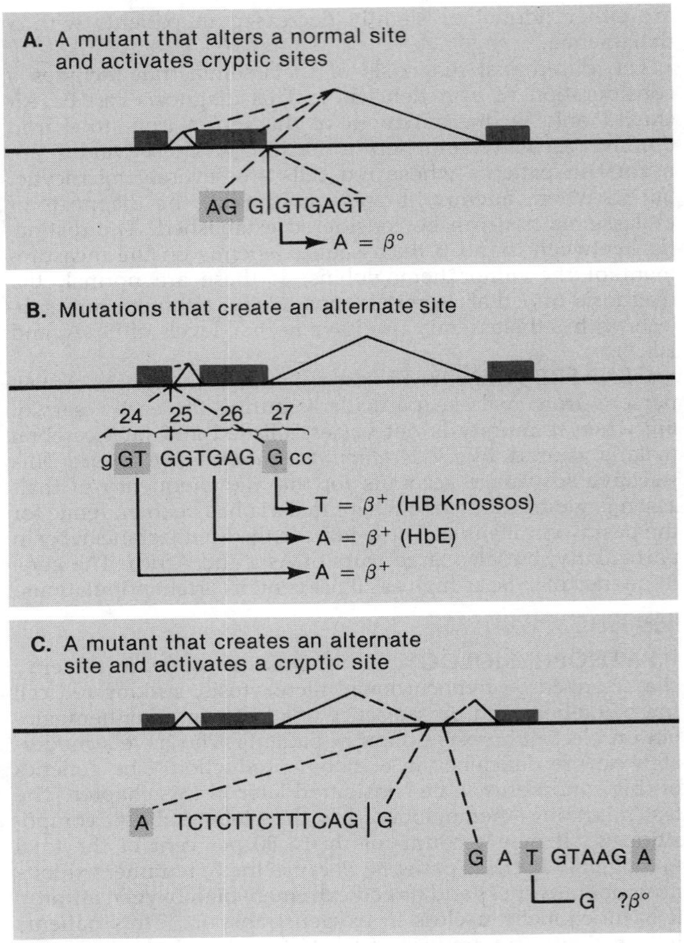

FIGURE 142–1. Thalassemia mutations that alter the splicing of the β globin gene transcript. *A*, The nucleotides, guanine (G) and thymine (T), are obligatory for normal splicing. Replacement of the G with adenine (A) abolishes normal splicing and leads to abnormal splicing at otherwise cryptic sites. *B*, Several different mutations at this position in the transcript create an alternate site that leads to abnormal splicing. This segment of the normal transcript includes the obligatory dinucleotide, GT, and matches the consensus sequence in all but the nucleotides in the boxes. Single nucleotide substitutions activate this otherwise inactive site. *C*, A substitution toward the end of intron II creates an alternate splice site. A normally cryptic site further upstream in the intron is also involved in a splicing reaction with exon 2–intron II splice junction, resulting in formation of a processed globin RNA that retains a portion of the sequence transcribed from intron II. Therefore, it cannot be translated into β globin.

Among the more common mutations in thalassemia genes are those that lead to premature termination of mRNA translation. Single nucleotide substitutions or small deletions that alter the mRNA reading frame introduce codons that signal the termination of protein synthesis on the abnormal mRNA. For example, substitution of thymine for cytosine in codon 39 introduces the stop codon UAG at that position. This abnormal β globin mRNA can be read only through codon 38, yielding a small, nonfunctional remnant of β globin. Premature termination mutations cause β^0 (or α^0) thalassemia.

Common mutations that cause α thalassemia are chain termination mutations. As described in Ch. 141, the completed globin molecule is released from the polyribosome when the protein synthetic apparatus encounters the normal terminator codon UAA. A single nucleotide change in this terminator codon will convert it to a codon that is functional for the insertion of any one of several amino acids, depending on the exact nucleotide that is substituted. In this case protein synthesis continues into the part of the mRNA that is usually untranslated, leading to the synthesis of a protein that may be as many as 30 amino acids longer than normal. Such an elongated α globin is found in Hb Constant Spring. This protein accounts for only 1 to 2 per cent of the total α globin in the cells of patients with Hb Constant Spring and their red cells exhibit the stigmata of thalassemia trait.

MUTATIONS THAT AFFECT GLOBIN STABILITY. Certain mutations may alter globin sequence and lead to instability and thus have a thalassemic effect despite a normal rate of synthesis of the mutant globin. Among the more dramatic of this class of mutations is one that leads to substitution of leucine for proline at position 125 of the α globin found in Hb Quong Sze. This mutation was discovered upon sequencing of the abnormal α gene and evidence of $\alpha^{\text{Quong Sze}}$ instability was subsequently obtained in vitro. Because of its marked instability, $\alpha^{\text{Quong Sze}}$ could not be detected in the red cells of the affected individual. Hb Quong Sze, like Hb E, is another of the thalassemic hemoglobinopathies characterized by both deficient net globin production and a structural abnormality.

DELETION MUTATIONS. Deletions causing α thalassemia have been described earlier. Small deletions that leave one of the two α globin genes intact on a chromosome are classified as α^+ mutations, while large deletions that remove both α genes are considered α^0 mutations. In contrast to α thalassemia, in which gene deletion is the most common mutation, gene deletion is rarely the mechanism for β thalassemia. A few patients of Indian ancestry have been found to have a deletion that has removed the 3′ half of the β globin gene and a small amount of flanking DNA. A special kind of deletion has resulted in the δβ fusion gene present in a few Italian patients who produce Hb Lepore. An unequal crossover during meiosis has led to the fusion gene that encodes for a globin that has the N-terminal sequence of δ globin and the C-terminal sequence of β globin. This globin is produced in very small amounts; hence this gene leads to thalassemia trait or thalassemia major in heterozygotes or homozygotes, respectively.

Several large deletions that have removed two or more genes from the β cluster have been characterized. The β thalassemia mutations have resulted in loss of the δ and β genes; the $^{A}\gamma\delta\beta$ thalassemia deletions include the $^{A}\gamma$ gene in addition. Two interesting forms of γδβ thalassemia have resulted in loss of all but the β gene, and yet this β gene does not function. These observations suggest that the DNA sequences remote from a gene can nonetheless influence its expression. Two deletions have resulted in loss of the entire β-like gene cluster.

MUTATIONS THAT INCREASE Hb F PRODUCTION

About 1 per cent of the hemoglobin in adult blood is Hb F. This fetal hemoglobin is found in 2 to 10 per cent of red cells; these cells—called F cells—contain roughly 4 to 8 pg of Hb F and 24 to 28 pg of adult hemoglobin. As discussed in Chapter 141, these F cells originate during the differentiation of erythroid progenitor cells. F cell number and therefore Hb F levels are genetically determined in man.

Increased Hb F in individuals who are homozygous for β thalassemia mainly reflects amplification of the F cell population. In the bone marrow, those erythroblasts producing small amounts of γ globin have less of an excess in α globin synthesis and therefore are more likely to survive and leave the bone marrow. By this mechanism, the 1 per cent of γ synthesis in the bone marrow cell population may be amplified 10- to 40-fold in the peripheral blood. Of more interest from the aspect of gene control are those mutations that alter Hb F production by genetic mechanisms.

There are two general classes of deletion mutations that increase Hb F production in adults. The δβ thalassemia mutations are characterized by production of 5 to 12 per cent of Hb F in heterozygotes, while *hereditary persistence of fetal hemoglobin* (HPFH) deletion mutations are characterized by production of 25 to 30 per cent. Most of the red cells in heterozygous individuals with HPFH contain Hb F, whereas heterozygotes with δβ thalassemia mutations have Hb F in only 25 to 30 per cent of their red cells. These mutations have been carefully characterized structurally in an attempt to define the basis at the DNA level for these differing phenotypes. Twenty-eight mutations have been studied, but no common patterns have emerged, with one exception. Deletions that remove the left side of the cluster (ε and γ genes) also inactivate the remaining intact β gene, whereas deletions that remove the right-hand portion of the cluster (δ and β genes) increase expression of the remaining γ globin genes. Removal of sequences within the cluster that normally modulate gene expression or movement of "activating" sequences into the cluster by virtue of deletion are other possible mechanisms that may lead to increased Hb F production as a consequence of these deletions.

Another category of mutations that cause HPFH leave the β-like gene cluster intact and therefore are referred to as *nondeletion mutations*. Nondeletion HPFH mutations are characterized by a heterogeneous distribution of Hb F in red cells (heterocellular) in contrast to the pancellular distribution of Hb F in heterozygotes with the deletion types of HPFH. There may be many different heterocellular HPFH mutations; genetic studies indicate that at least some are not linked to the β-like gene cluster. Five different point mutations within the γ globin gene promoter region have been discovered in individuals with nondeletion HPFH.

PRENATAL DIAGNOSIS

Because of the serious consequences of severe β thalassemia (Cooley's anemia), prenatal diagnosis of this condition with subsequent therapeutic abortion is thought by many to be highly desirable. Two general strategies have made this a feasible undertaking. The first approach is based on the fact that small amounts of β globin synthesis may be detected in the early mid-trimester fetus (see Ch. 140). In fetuses who have inherited two genes for β thalassemia, no β globin or very small amounts are produced at a time when normal fetuses are producing approximately 10 per cent β globin. By using sophisticated obstetric techniques, blood may be obtained from the umbilical vein and used for biosynthetic measurements of the globin synthetic pattern. Absence of or low β globin synthesis occurs in homozygous fetuses, whereas intermediate levels are found in heterozygotes. This strategy has been widely applied in parts of Greece and Italy and has led to a significant reduction in the incidence of the severe form of β thalassemia in certain populations.

A second strategy for prenatal diagnosis relies on the study of DNA prepared from amniotic fluid cells of potentially affected persons. The globin genes in such DNA samples may be characterized by the techniques referred to as restriction endonuclease mapping. The DNA is digested with an enzyme that cuts at a specific nucleotide sequence. Among the million or so fragments generated from human DNA are those few that include the globin genes. The DNA is resolved electrophoretically, transferred to a nitrocellulose paper, and annealed to a radioactive probe specific for globin gene sequences. Depending on the enzyme used, a characteristic set of fragments containing globin gene sequences is generated. In persons who have inherited a mutation reflected by deletion of all or part of a globin gene, a change in a position of a particular fragment will serve to indicate the presence of such a mutation. Many cases of α thalassemia and rare cases of β thalassemia may be diagnosed in this way.

More widely applicable to the prenatal diagnosis of thalassemias are so-called restriction enzyme polymorphisms. A single nucleotide change, in an area within or remote from the globin gene, may result in loss of a restriction endonuclease site and therefore a change in the migration position of a particular fragment containing globin gene sequences. Such a polymorphism, in Hpa I site, was first described by

Kan (1978) in individuals who had inherited the gene for sickle hemoglobin. Other polymorphisms have been discovered and have been found useful for diagnosis of β thalassemia. The unique association or linkage of the Hpa I polymorphism with the β^s gene is unusual; most polymorphisms occur in association with both normal and abnormal β globin genes. Hence a different method of analysis is required rather than simple characterization of a single restriction endonuclease site.

Several restriction endonuclease sites—each of which is polymorphic, either present (+) of absent (−)—may be used to define the haplotype of the β globin gene region on a specific chromosome. Eighty to 90 per cent of the time a single mutation is associated or linked to a single set of restriction endonuclease polymorphisms, a single haplotype. Once the haplotype associated with a particular mutation in an ethnic group is known, haplotype analysis may be used to define the frequency of that mutation in that group. The normal β globin gene is found linked to all haplotypes. Hence, simple haplotype analysis cannot be used for prenatal diagnosis directly. Extensive family studies or study of DNA from an affected or completely normal child is necessary before haplotype analysis can be applied for prenatal diagnosis in that family.

An alternative approach utilizing DNA analysis for prenatal diagnosis is now feasible because several frequent mutations have been defined by DNA sequencing. Synthetic oligonucleotide probes, one specific for the normal gene and one specific for a particular abnormal gene, can be used to discriminate between the normal and abnormal genes in amniotic fluid DNA. This method is simple and direct but requires that several probes be available for each of the mutations that occur frequently in the population for whom prenatal diagnosis is offered. Technical innovations to increase sensitivity and specificity and the ready synthesis of specific probes will undoubtedly make this the method of choice for prenatal diagnosis in the future.

The application of prenatal diagnosis requires appropriate screening and identification of persons at risk. Thalassemia trait can usually readily be identified by virtue of the morphologic changes in the red cells. Confirmation of the diagnosis depends on measurement of hemoglobin A_2 and Hb F.

EXPERIMENTAL THERAPY

Knowledge of globin gene structure and regulation has suggested a means to activate the structurally normal but inactive γ globin genes in individuals with severe β thalassemia. Increased γ globin synthesis is desirable because it partially compensates for the deficiency of β globin production and decreases the relative excess of α globin. DNA is modified after synthesis by methylation of cytosine residues. Expressed genes are relatively undermethylated compared to unexpressed DNA sequences. For example, the γ globin genes are undermethylated in fetal erythroid cells, but after the switch to adult hemoglobin synthesis the γ globin genes are fully methylated in adult erythroid cells. 5-Azacytidine* inhibits DNA methylation and has been shown to activate genes in tissue culture cells and in experimental animals. Administration of 5-azacytidine to patients with severe β thalassemia under defined experimental protocols has resulted in increased γ globin synthesis and improvement in red cell production and survival. The effect is transient, lasting only two to three weeks. Reluctance to administer a potentially carcinogenic and toxic drug for longer periods has limited the use of 5-azacytidine to experimental studies of a few severely affected patients. Nonetheless these encouraging results have prompted a search for other effective and less toxic drugs that may make pharmacologic stimulation of the γ globin genes a useful approach for treatment of severe β thalassemia.

*Available from the National Cancer Institute.

Cure of severe β thalassemia can be achieved by bone marrow transplantation from an HLA-identical, unaffected sibling. Several patients have already been cured by this method. This procedure carries a 10 to 40 per cent risk of death or significant graft-versus-host disease (GVHD). Transplantation in infancy, preferably before transfusions are given, increases the probability of successful engraftment and reduces the risk of this disease. However, adequate transfusion therapy and effective chelation may provide 20 or more years of good-quality life for newborns. Thus, the availability of bone marrow transplantation raises a significant ethical dilemma for parents and physicians. In the future, refinements in the treatment of GVHD and transplantation techniques may permit wider application of bone marrow transplantation as treatment for patients with severe β thalassemia.

Insertion of intact globin genes into the bone marrow cells of patients with severe forms of thalassemia has become a feasible research objective. Gene transfer mediated by retroviral vectors is highly efficient and has resulted in the insertion and expression of genes in experimental animals. Many problems remain to be overcome before this strategy becomes clinically feasible, however.

Alter BP: Antenatal diagnosis of thalassemia: A review. Ann NY Acad Sci 445:393, 1985. *A comprehensive description of the methods and results of prenatal diagnosis and its impact on the incidence of severe β thalassemia.*

Ley TJ, Griffith P, Nienhuis AW: Transfusion hemosiderosis and chelation therapy. Clin Haematol 11:437, 1982. *This detailed review describes the pathogenesis of transfusional hemochromatosis and summarizes evidence related to the beneficial effects achieved with chelation therapy.*

Nienhuis AW, Ley TJ, Humphries RK, et al.: Pharmacological manipulation of fetal hemoglobin synthesis in patients with severe beta-thalassemia. Ann NY Acad Sci 445:198, 1985. Ley TJ, Nienhuis AW: Induction of hemoglobin F synthesis in patients with beta thalassemia. Ann Rev Med 36:485, 1985. *Reviews of the results achieved by using drugs in an effort to stimulate fetal hemoglobin synthesis for therapeutic benefit in patients with thalassemia.*

Nienhuis AW, Wolfe L: The thalassemias: Disorders of hemoglobin synthesis. In Nathan DG, Oski F (eds.): Hematology of Infancy and Childhood. Philadelphia, W. B. Saunders Company (in press). *This chapter contains a more detailed exposition of the thalassemia syndromes with a comprehensive account of molecular basis of these disorders and current status of prenatal diagnosis.*

Orkin SH, Kazazian HH Jr, Antonarakis SE, et al.: Linkage of β thalassemia mutations and β globin gene polymorphisms with DNA polymorphisms in human β globin gene cluster. Nature 296:627, 1983. Trisman R, Orkin SH, Maniatis T: Specific transcription and RNA splicing defects in five cloned β thalassemia genes. Nature 302:591, 1983. *These are two classic papers that describe strategies used to identify mutations, to determine their frequencies in populations in which thalassemia genes are common, and to characterize these mutations as to their functional consequences.*

Thomas ED, Sanders JE, Buckner CD, et al.: Marrow transplantation for thalassemia. Ann NY Acad Sci 445:417, 1985. Lucarelli G, Polchi P, Izzi T, et al.: Marrow transplantation for thalassemia after treatment with busulfan and cyclophosphamide. Ann NY Acad Sci 445:428, 1985. *Two papers that represent accounts by leaders in this field of efforts to use bone marrow transplantation to achieve a permanent cure in patients with severe β thalassemia.*

Weatherall DJ, Clegg JB: The Thalassemia Syndromes. 3rd ed. Oxford, Blackwell Scientific Publications, Ltd, 1981. *This superb monograph describes the clinical aspects, genetics, and interactions of the various thalassemia syndromes. It should be consulted by anyone with a serious interest in thalassemia.*

143 SICKLE CELL ANEMIA AND ASSOCIATED HEMOGLOBINOPATHIES

Bernard G. Forget

DEFINITION. The sickle cell syndromes are due to the inheritance of a gene for a structurally abnormal β-globin chain subunit of adult hemoglobin, the β^S-chain of Hb S ($\alpha_2\beta^S{}_2$). The structural abnormality of the β^S-globin chain consists of a single amino acid substitution or replacement: valine instead of the normal glutamic acid at position number 6 of the β-polypeptide chain. Hb S can be found in the heterozygous state (Hb AS or sickle cell trait), in the homozygous state (Hb SS, sickle cell anemia, or sickle cell disease), in association with other structural hemoglobin variants (i.e., Hb SC and SD disease), in association with β-thalassemia (Hb S/β-thalassemia or sickle/β-thalassemia syndromes), or in association with the thalassemia-like disorder termed hereditary persistence of fetal hemoglobin (Hb SF or Hb S/HPFH). The structural abnormality of Hb C, a nonsickling hemoglobin, also consists of a single amino acid substitution at residue number 6 of the β-globin chain: in the β^C-chain lysine replaces glutamic acid. Clinical syndromes associated with the inheritance of Hb C include Hb SC disease and homozygous Hb C disease.

PREVALENCE AND GENETICS. The sickle cell syndromes are particularly prevalent in black persons of African or Afro-American ancestry. However, the gene is also found at a lower frequency in persons of Mediterranean ancestry (southern Italians, Sicilians, and Greeks), in Saudi Arabia, and in India. The highest gene frequencies occur in equatorial Africa, in the so-called malaria belt. The heterozygous state for Hb S (sickle cell trait) probably confers a biologic advantage against infection with falciparum malaria, and for this reason the gene frequency for Hb S has achieved high levels through natural selection in geographic areas of endemic malaria. In the United States the prevalence of the sickle cell trait in blacks is 8 to 10 per cent and the number of homozygous persons approaches 50,000, or 1 in 400 births. In certain areas of western Africa (Ghana and Nigeria), the prevalence of Hb AS can reach 25 to 30 per cent. The prevalence of Hb AC in black Americans is approximately 3 per cent. Gene-mapping studies, using restriction endonuclease analysis of cellular DNA to identify polymorphisms of nucleotide sequence in the DNA around the β^s globin gene, have disclosed an unexpected heterogeneity of polymorphisms linked to the sickle β-globin genes in different individuals, suggesting multiple independent origins of the sickle gene.

PATHOPHYSIOLOGY. Disease in the sickle syndromes results from aggregation or polymerization of Hb S molecules inside erythrocytes, which causes (1) chronic compensated hemolytic anemia, (2) chronic and progressive tissue and organ damage, and (3) acute painful vaso-occlusive crises. These clinical phenomena are directly related to the physicochemical behavior of the intracellular Hb S molecules and result from alterations of red cell rheology and, possibly, changes in the red cell membrane.

The polymerization process occurs only when the Hb S molecule is in the deoxy conformation (see Ch. 140). When Hb S is in the oxy conformation it has essentially normal physicochemical properties. In the deoxy conformation, Hb S molecules can aggregate with one another into long polymers and are aligned to form a gel of liquid crystals that are also called tactoids. The polymerization process goes through a number of stages, as illustrated diagrammatically in Figure 143–1. In the process of nucleation, Hb S molecules form small aggregates, which then grow by addition of successive Hb S molecules. The larger aggregates then align themselves to form linearly arranged fibers that constitute a paracrystalline gel. These fibers can be detected as helical electron-dense tube-like structures by electron microscopy (Fig. 143–1). The end result of the polymerization process is the transformation of the intracellular contents of the red cell from a fluid liquid to a viscous gel. The amount of Hb S polymer within red cells increases progressively as the percentage of oxygen saturation of the hemoglobin decreases. The viscous polymer decreases the flexibility of the erythrocyte and thus impairs its transit through the microcirculation. When the amount of polymer

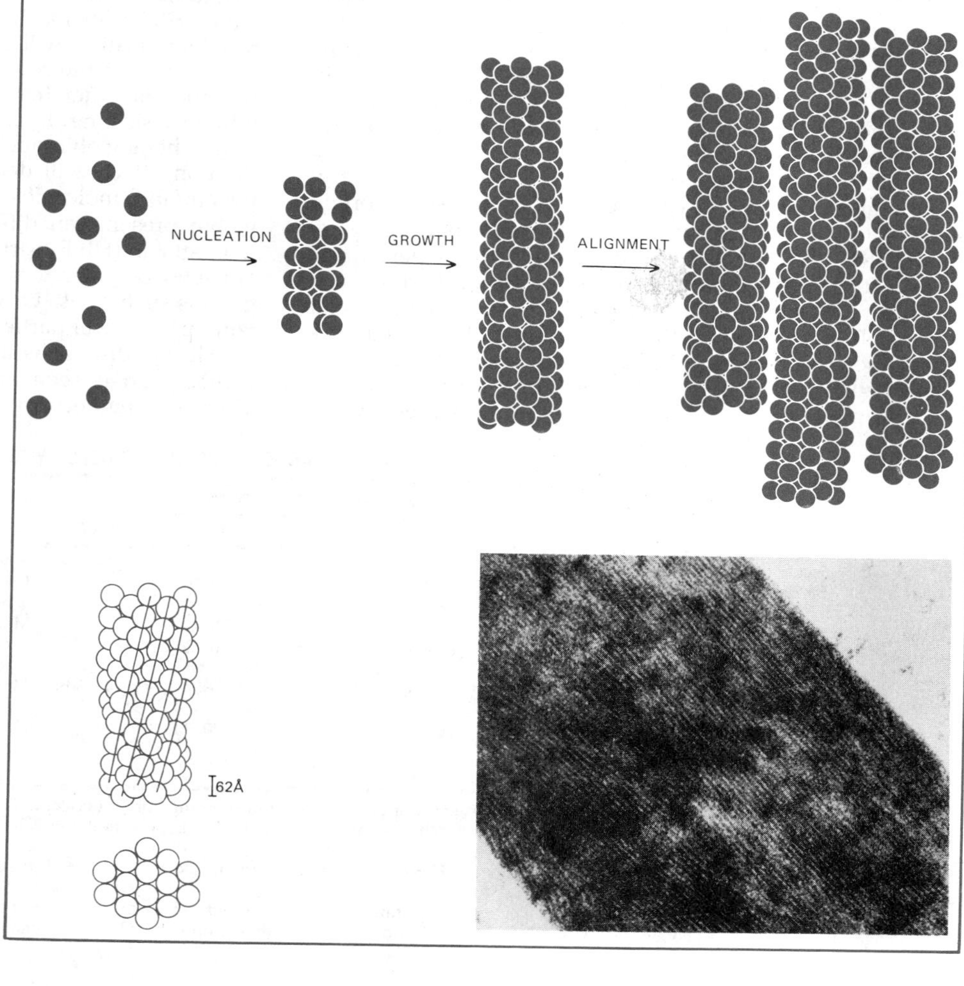

FIGURE 143–1. *Top*, Schematic representation of mechanism of deoxyhemoglobin S polymerization. Each circle represents a deoxyhemoglobin S tetramer: $\alpha_2\beta_2^s$. *Lower left*, Molecular model, based on electron microscopy, of the helical arrangement of deoxyhemoglobin S tetramers in a fiber of polymerized Hb S molecules; side view (above) and cross section or end-on view (below). *Lower right*, Electron micrograph (longitudinal section) of deoxyhemoglobin S gel in a sickled erythrocyte.

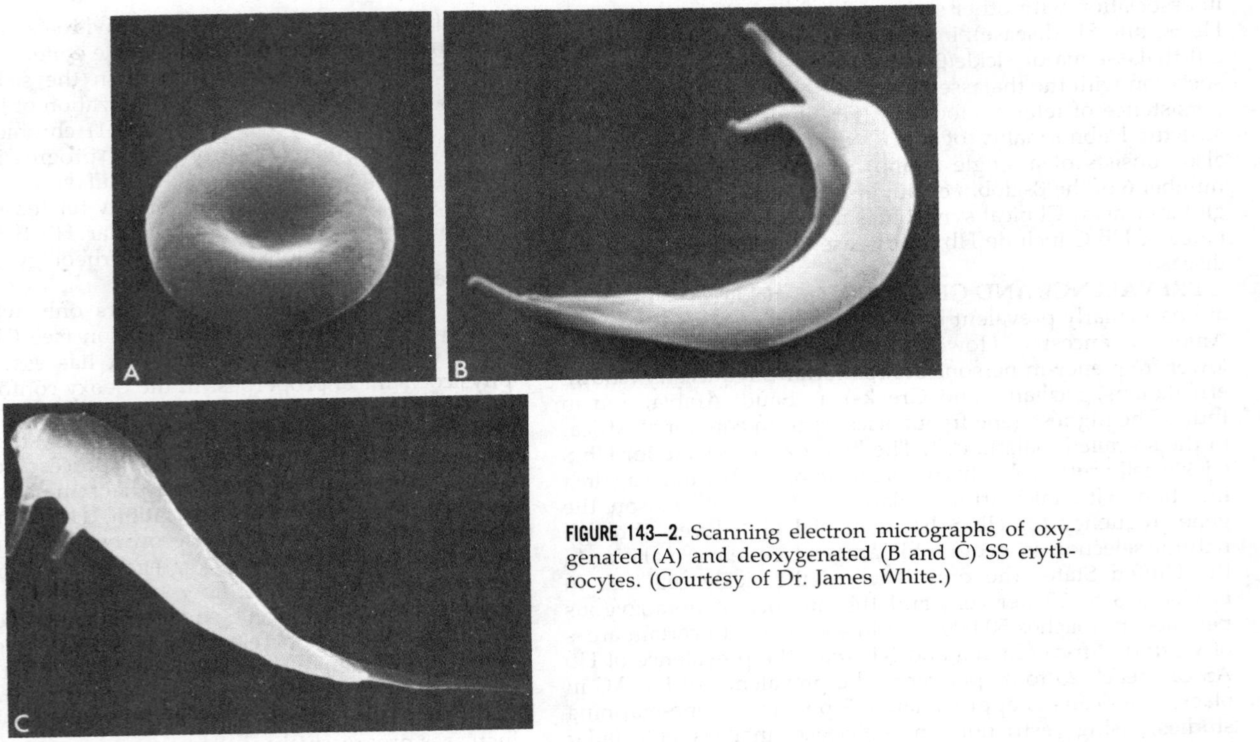

FIGURE 143–2. Scanning electron micrographs of oxygenated (A) and deoxygenated (B and C) SS erythrocytes. (Courtesy of Dr. James White.)

is sufficiently high, the red cells may assume the typical sickle or holly leaf shape associated with sickled erythrocytes (Fig. 143–2). The shape change of the erythrocyte is a passive phenomenon in which the red cell membrane conforms to the shape that is assumed by the intracellular gel of polymerized hemoglobin. The polymerization phenomenon is reversible: With reoxygenation of the Hb S molecules the aggregated molecules disassociate, the gel becomes liquid, and the erythrocyte, if it has sickled, can return to its normal shape, as long as the red cell membrane has not become altered to form an irreversibly sickled cell (see below).

A number of factors can influence the rate and degree of Hb S aggregation in red cells. One of the most important determinants is the concentration of Hb S and of total hemoglobin within the red cell. In general the higher the percentage of Hb S, the more severe the sickle syndrome. Factors such as cellular dehydration that increase the mean corpuscular hemoglobin concentration (MCHC) will greatly facilitate polymerization by increasing the opportunity and frequency of contact between Hb S molecules. The importance of hemoglobin concentration on polymerization is underscored by the clinical observation that the coinheritance of α-thalassemia together with sickle cell anemia is generally (but not universally) associated with less severe hemolysis. The milder clinical course of Hb S/β-thalassemia is also thought to be due in part to the associated hypochromia. The length of time during which Hb S remains deoxygenated is also very important; Hb S polymerization will be enhanced with any increase in the transit time of the red cell through the microcirculation. The presence of other hemoglobins within the red cell can also influence sickling. In general, at a constant MCHC, any other non-S hemoglobin molecules in the red cell, by a simple dilution effect, will decrease the opportunity of contact between Hb S molecules. In addition, the type of non-S hemoglobin present can differentially affect polymerization: Fetal hemoglobin (Hb F) participates much less readily than normal Hb A in polymer formation, whereas certain mutant hemoglobins such as Hb O Arab and Hb D, although nonpolymerizing per se, will participate in gelation more readily than Hb A. Hb SC disease is associated with a more severe clinical course than is seen in sickle cell trait for two reasons: (1) There is a higher proportion of Hb S in SC than in AS cells

TABLE 143–1. DIFFERENTIAL DIAGNOSIS OF SICKLE CELL SYNDROMES

Genotype	Clinical Condition	Hemoglobin Electrophoresis Findings					Other Associated Findings
		Hb A	*Hb S*	*Hb A_2*	*Hb F*	*Hb C*	
AS	Sickle cell trait	55–60%	40–45%*	2–3%	~1%	—	Asymptomatic; no anemia
SS†	Sickle cell anemia	0	85–95%	2–3%	5–15%	—	Usually clinically severe; Hb F distributed heterogeneously among red blood cells
S/β⁰-thal	Sickle cell/β-thalassemia	0	70–80%	3–5%	10–20%	—	Moderate severity; splenomegaly in over half of the cases; Hb F distributed heterogeneously among red blood cells; hypochromia and microcytosis
S/β⁺-thal	Sickle cell/β-thalassemia	10–20%	60–75%	3–5%	10–20%	—	
SC‡	Hb SC disease	0	45–50%	2–3%	~1%	45–50%	Moderate severity; splenomegaly; many target cells on blood smear
SF (S/HPFH)	Sickle/hereditary persistence of fetal hemoglobin	0	70–80%	1.5–2%	20–30%	—	Uniform distribution of Hb F among all red cells; asymptomatic; no anemia

*Persons with associated α-thalassemia trait have lower levels of Hb S, usually in the range of 26 per cent. The finding of a (nonsickling) hemoglobin with the mobility of Hb S but in much lower amounts (5 to 15 per cent) is suggestive of the Hb Lepore trait (see Ch. 142). Hypochromia and microcytosis are usually associated with these conditions.

†Hb SD disease gives similar electrophoretic findings at pH 8.6, but can be distinguished from Hb SS disease by hemoglobin electrophoresis in citrate agar at pH 6.1.

‡Hb S–O Arab and Hb SE diseases give similar electrophoretic findings at pH 8.6, but can be distinguished from Hb SC disease by hemoglobin electrophoresis in citrate agar at pH 6.1. Hb A_2 comigrates with Hb C at pH 8.6 and can be quantitated only by column chromatography.

(Table 143–1); and (2) cells containing Hb C have a higher than normal MCHC, thus facilitating Hb S polymerization. Finally, acidosis can enhance polymerization by decreasing oxygen affinity (see Ch. 140) and thereby increasing the amount of deoxy Hb S in the red cell.

The polymerization phenomenon results in two major red cell disturbances. The first relates to the flow properties of red cells containing substantial amounts of polymerized Hb S. Such cells are much less deformable than normal red cells, and their flow through the microcirculation is greatly retarded. A second major disturbance is damage to the red cell membrane as a result of repeated episodes of aggregation and melting of Hb S polymers. Sickle red cells are "leaky." They tend to lose K^+ and water and eventually become dehydrated, the resulting increase in MCHC probably enhancing further polymerization. The red cell membrane becomes altered in other ways such that it may assume a rigid, abnormal conformation, thus forming an irreversibly sickled cell (or ISC), even when the hemoglobin is not in the aggregated state. As a result of the intracellular polymerization of Hb S, of the increase in MCHC, and of the membrane changes, the red cells become rigid and are sequestered and prematurely destroyed within the reticuloendothelial system. This series of events constitutes the basis for the shortened red cell survival and hemolytic anemia that invariably accompany sickle cell anemia. Occlusion of the microvasculature by viscous erythrocytes leads to ischemia and eventual infarction of the tissue downstream from the obstruction, results in organ damage, and may be the cause of the characteristic painful "crises."

CLINICAL MANIFESTATIONS. ***Sickle Cell Trait.*** Persons who are heterozygous for Hb S are essentially asymptomatic. They should not have any anemia attributable to the hemoglobinopathy. Any anemia in such persons should be investigated for other secondary causes. Symptoms resulting from vaso-occlusion occur only in extreme circumstances of severe hypoxia such as flying in unpressurized aircraft. However, a universal finding in sickle cell trait is microinfarction of the renal medulla presumably owing to the ambient hyperosmolarity that is thought to lead to dehydration of the red cells, an increased MCHC, and sickling; as a result, in affected persons the urine is unconcentrated and isosthenuria is manifested. Painless hematuria can also occasionally be attributed to microinfarction of the renal medulla, although the other usual causes should be ruled out before painless hematuria in persons with sickle cell trait is attributed to the sickling phenomenon.

Sickle Cell Disease. THE ANEMIA. Patients homozygous for Hb S invariably have a chronic compensated hemolytic anemia of variable severity. In general the hematocrit ranges between 20 and 30 per cent and the hemoglobin between 6.5 and 10 grams per deciliter. The hemolysis is compensated by increased erythropoiesis manifested as an elevated reticulocyte count in the range of 10 to 25 per cent. Mild jaundice and indirect hyperbilirubinemia are also present as a reflection of the hemolysis. The degree of the anemia is usually stable in a given patient, although occasional hypoplastic or aplastic crises can occur owing to suppression of erythropoiesis at the time of infectious episodes and result in a rapid decrease in the reticulocyte count and a precipitous drop in the hemoglobin and hematocrit levels. Infection with a particular parvovirus has been implicated in the pathogenesis of aplastic crises. Another cause of rapid worsening of the anemia is the acute splenic sequestration crisis (a sudden pooling of large volumes of blood in the spleen) that can occur in younger patients with sickle cell anemia before autoinfarction of the spleen or in older patients with Hb SC disease and Hb S/β-thalassemia in whom the spleen is not infarcted and may in fact be enlarged. There is some controversy whether or not a hyperhemolytic state can be associated with sickle cell anemia. From what is known of the basis for the hemolysis in this condition, there is no pathophysiologic mechanism for variable or accelerated hemolysis resulting from sickling alone. In general, the anemia and hemolysis in sickle cell disease do not increase or worsen during vaso-occlusive painful crises. If hemolysis suddenly worsens, one should look to other secondary causes that may be responsible, such as an associated glucose-6-phosphate dehydrogenase deficiency and exposure to an oxidant stress from drugs or an acute infection. Finally, in patients with marginal nutritional status and increased requirements, such as during pregnancy, folic acid deficiency can develop and aggravate the anemia—the so-called megaloblastic crisis of sickle cell disease.

VASO-OCCLUSIVE CRISES. The major disabilities suffered by patients with sickle cell anemia are related to painful vaso-occlusive crises and to secondary end-organ damage as a direct consequence of the sickling phenomenon and occlusion of the microvasculature of one or another organ, most commonly the bones of the trunk and extremities. The episodes are characterized by sudden onset of excruciating pain in the back, chest, or extremities. There is frequently no identifiable precipitating event, although infections may be associated with the onset of the episode. Other predisposing factors include dehydration, acidosis, or increased hypoxia as during a pulmonary infection. A low grade fever may be associated with the painful attacks, although not necessarily. In general, the onset of fever will occur one or two days after the onset of pain and will parallel the degree of tissue necrosis resulting from the ischemic infarction. The painful attacks last for variable periods, ranging from a few hours to a few days depending on the extent of the vaso-occlusive phenomenon and the rapidity with which treatment is initiated and is successful in reversing the occlusive episode. In general there are no external signs such as heat, swelling, or tenderness of the soft tissues over the affected bones. However, if the bone infarction occurs in proximity to a joint, an effusion can develop. Bone infarction may be difficult to differentiate from osteomyelitis, and definitive diagnosis of the latter must ultimately rely on positive bacterial cultures from aspirated material.

When the vaso-occlusive process occurs in the vasculature (including large vessels) of organs other than bones, the clinical manifestations are primarily related to damage of the affected organ. Common acute vaso-occlusive clinical syndromes include cerebrovascular accidents (i.e., hemiplegia and seizures) caused by involvement of the cerebral vasculature; the acute chest syndrome associated with occlusion of the pulmonary vessels, which can be difficult to differentiate from acute pulmonary infarction caused by emboli or from acute pulmonary infections; hepatic crisis, with marked hyperbilirubinemia and other abnormal liver function tests, which can be difficult to differentiate from acute hepatitis or choledocholithiasis; priapism resulting from vaso-occlusion within the corpus cavernosum; and acute renal papillary infarction with hematuria and/or obstruction of the urinary collecting system.

More chronic complications include refractory skin ulcers of the leg, usually in the vicinity of the medial malleolus, an area that has poor collateral circulation; and variable degrees of renal insufficiency resulting from the combination of repeated infarctions and infectious episodes. All patients manifest the inability to concentrate the urine and have isosthenuria. Microinfarction in the peripheral retina is initially asymptomatic, but may lead to the formation of new blood vessels that are fragile and can hemorrhage, causing retinal detachment and blindness. For this reason periodic eye examinations are important to recognize and treat the early asymptomatic lesion before it progresses to the point of causing visual disturbances. Finally, repeated bone infarcts in the vicinity of joints can lead to secondary degenerative arthritis, and gradual infarction of the head of the femur results in aseptic necrosis of the hip.

OTHER CLINICAL MANIFESTATIONS. Clinical manifestations of

sickle cell anemia not directly related to the sickling phenomenon include increased susceptibility to infections, cholelithiasis, and abnormal growth and development. The increased susceptibility to infections is probably related at least in part to absence of splenic function and in some cases to an abnormality of the properdin opsonization pathway. In early childhood, septicemia and meningitis caused by encapsulated organisms such as *Streptococcus pneumoniae* and *Hemophilus influenzae* are common. In later life common infectious episodes include recurrent pneumonias, urinary tract infections, and osteomyelitis. The predisposition to osteomyelitis is probably related to the repeated bone infarcts that can form a nidus for infection. Although osteomyelitis caused by *Salmonella* occurs almost exclusively in patients with sickle cell anemia or one of the other sickle cell syndromes, *Staphylococcus aureus* is still the most common causative organism of osteomyelitis in these syndromes.

Cholelithiasis is very common, and can be manifested at a young age; it is caused by the chronic hemolysis that results in increased bilirubin production. Episodes of cholecystitis and choledocholithiasis can easily be confused with abdominal and hepatic sickle cell crises. The causes of delayed growth and development are poorly understood. Delayed puberty can result in late closure of the epiphyses and an asthenic habitus.

SICKLE/β-THALASSEMIA AND HB SC DISEASE. The anemia and the hemolysis are less severe in the other sickle syndromes, such as Hb SC disease and sickle/β-thalassemia, in which there is somewhat less propensity for sickling than in homozygous Hb SS disease. The degree of anemia is strongly related to the extent of intracellular Hb S polymerization. In these conditions the anemia frequently ranges between hemoglobin levels of 10 and 12 grams per deciliter, and the reticulocyte counts are usually less than 10 per cent, frequently in the range of 5 per cent.

In general the vaso-occlusive manifestations resulting from sickling are also less frequent and less severe in Hb SC disease and in sickle/β-thalassemia than in sickle cell anemia, although all of the complications previously described for sickle cell anemia can also occur in these conditions. However, in contrast to sickle cell anemia, splenomegaly in adults is usually present in these syndromes, and splenic infarcts and acute splenic sequestration crises can occur. The ocular complications of sickling also tend to occur more frequently in Hb SC disease than in sickle cell anemia and can in fact be the presenting symptoms. There is also increased frequency of aseptic necrosis of the femoral head in Hb SC disease. Sickle/β^0-thalassemia, in which Hb A is totally absent, is generally more severe than sickle/β^+-thalassemia and can be as clinically severe as sickle cell anemia.

DIAGNOSIS. The diagnosis of the various sickle syndromes relies on two types of tests: (1) screening tests to detect the presence of Hb S on the basis of its physicochemical properties, and (2) more definitive tests for the precise diagnosis of the particular genetic syndrome involved.

Two types of screening tests for the detection of Hb S are in current use. Both tests simply detect the presence of some Hb S in erythroid cells but do not differentiate sickle cell trait from the other sickle syndromes. The standard "sickle cell preparation" consists of mixing blood with a solution of sodium metabisulfate, which totally deoxygenates the blood and thus induces sickling that can be observed under the microscope. A second screening test is a solubility test which consists of mixing blood with a solution of high ionic strength and observing the mixtures for turbidity; normal hemoglobin will give a clear solution, whereas any Hb S in the solution will precipitate to give a turbid solution through which one cannot see the lines of an indicator card. Both tests, if properly done, are highly specific and accurate. The solubility test has the advantages that a microscope is not needed and that the test solution is relatively stable.

Once Hb S is detected by screening tests, hemoglobin electrophoresis should be carried out for precise diagnosis of the sickle syndrome. Table 143–1 summarizes the results obtained by hemoglobin electrophoresis in the various sickle cell syndromes as well as other associated clinical and laboratory findings that are useful in the differential diagnosis. In general, routine hemoglobin electrophoresis at pH 8.6 will suffice to establish the diagnosis. However, a few exceptions to this rule require additional tests to confirm or establish the suspected diagnosis. Because other hemoglobin variants can have the same electrophoretic mobility as Hb S at pH 8.6, electrophoresis in citrate agar at pH 6.1 should be performed to confirm the diagnosis (see Table 143–1). The distinction between Hb SS disease and Hb S/β^0-thalassemia can be very difficult to establish, since electrophoretic findings are similar in both cases. The Hb A_2 level should be elevated in Hb S/β-thalassemia, but precise quantitation of Hb A_2 in the presence of Hb S is sometimes unreliable. Findings that should establish the diagnosis of Hb S/β^0-thalassemia rather than Hb SS disease include (1) the presence of hypochromia and microcytosis indicated by low MCV and MCH; (2) family study showing that one parent or an offspring has β-thalassemia trait rather than sickle cell trait; (3) experimental studies of globin chain synthesis using labeled amino acid precursors (see Ch. 142), demonstrating decreased synthesis of β^S chains relative to α chains (β^S/α = 0.5 to 0.6); and (4) gene-mapping studies to distinguish between β^A and β^S globin genes in the patient's DNA (see Fig. 143–3). The rare but interesting syndrome of Hb S/HPFH will also give hemoglobin electrophoretic findings similar to those of Hb SS disease, but with an unusually high level of Hb F in the range of 30 per cent. Such patients, however, are not anemic and should be asymptomatic. The diagnosis can be confirmed by family study showing the absence of sickle cell trait and presence of heterozygosity for HPFH in a parent or offspring. Study of the distribution of Hb F within individual red cells, using the acid elution test of Betke and Kleihauer, will show uniform distribution of Hb F in Hb S/HPFH but heterogeneous distribution of Hb F in Hb SS disease. Inheritance of Hb D (another relatively common β-chain hemoglobinopathy in blacks) along with Hb S can also mimic homozygosity for Hb S, since Hb D comigrates with Hb S on electrophoresis at pH 8.6. Hb SD disease is not as clinically severe as sickle cell disease, and the diagnosis can be established by performing hemoglobin electrophoresis at neutral or acid pH, which separates the two hemoglobins. Similarly, Hb SC disease can be confused with the inheritance of Hb S along with a second hemoglobin variant that has a similar electrophoretic mobility to Hb C at pH 8.6, such as Hb O Arab or Hb E. These syndromes can be distinguished from Hb SC disease by electrophoresis in citrate agar at pH 6 to 7.

The peripheral blood smear in individuals with Hb SS disease shows variable numbers of irreversibly sickled cells (ISC's), usually ranging between 5 and 10 per cent. In general the number of ISC's is relatively stable for a given patient, and there is a rough correlation between the numbers of ISC's and the severity of the hemolytic anemia. There is no correlation between the number of ISC's and the frequency or presence of vaso-occlusive crises. The peripheral blood smear, in addition to ISC's, will usually show variable numbers of target cells and occasional Howell-Jolly bodies owing to absence of spleen function. Other hematologic findings related to functional asplenia include the presence of target cells and somewhat elevated leukocyte counts and platelet counts. Examination of the peripheral blood smear can also be helpful in differential diagnosis of the sickle syndromes. In general, significant numbers of ISC's will be found essentially only in homozygous SS disease and not in the other sickle syndromes. Large numbers of target cells are characteristic of the inheritance of Hb C in either the heterozygous or the homozygous state (Color plate 2*I*).

TREATMENT. Despite extensive knowledge of the molecular basis and physical chemistry of the polymerization and sickling phenomena, there is still no specific molecular therapy available for the treatment or prevention of sickling. A number of compounds have been tested, and new compounds continue to be sought, that might interfere with sickling in vivo and be useful clinically. Unfortunately no such compound is currently available. Another potential molecular approach to the prevention of sickling would be to reactivate or increase fetal hemoglobin synthesis in the majority of the erythroid cells of affected patients to render them similar to the red cells of patients with Hb S/HPFH, a clinically mild syndrome. Successful enhancement of Hb F levels in patients with sickle cell anemia and homozygous β-thalassemia (see Ch. 142) has been accomplished by the administration of the chemotherapeutic agents 5-azacytidine* and hydroxyurea to a small number of patients. The rationale for 5-azacytidine therapy resided in the findings that the drug causes demethylation of DNA and that active genes are usually hypomethylated, whereas the inactive fetal γ-globin genes of adults are hypermethylated. However, other mechanisms related to cell toxicity, cell selection, and changes in gene expression resulting from disruption of the cell cycle probably also contribute to the increased levels of Hb F following administration of chemotherapeutic agents. These therapies should be considered highly investigational at this time and restricted in their general applicability until the long-term toxicity of these drugs, including carcinogenicity, is established.

The cornerstones of therapy in sickle cell anemia have therefore not changed in recent years and continue to consist of the administration of the following supportive measures: large volumes of intravenous fluids (preferably hypotonic and alkaline); analgesics to control the pain; when indicated, antibiotics to treat any associated bacterial infection; and oxygen to treat hypoxemia. When administering fluids to patients with sickle cell anemia, one should remember that these patients have a fixed renal water loss owing to inability to concentrate urine and that they are frequently dehydrated on presentation because of associated infection and fever. The amounts of intravenous fluids administered should therefore be increased to two to three times what would be considered a normal maintenance volume. Patients with sickle cell disease are frequently hypoxic because of chronic pulmonary disease. Even though they do not appear to be cyanotic, monitoring of arterial P_{O_2} is important, especially if there is an associated chest syndrome, and oxygen should be administered if there is significant hypoxemia. In the absence of arterial hypoxemia, oxygen therapy is probably not beneficial in the treatment of vaso-occlusive crises and may result in suppression of erythropoiesis. The role of alkali is controversial, and certainly if the patient is mildly acidotic, this acidosis should be corrected since it can potentiate the propensity of deoxy Hb S molecules to aggregate.

The role of blood transfusions and partial exchange transfusions is controversial in the treatment of acute vaso-occlusive crises of sickle cell disease. In general there is very little rationale for performing partial exchange transfusions simply for a painful vaso-occlusive crisis in a nonvital organ. Nevertheless such treatment may be occasionally indicated to interrupt an unusually prolonged painful crisis or when a patient is virtually continually disabled by frequent recurrent crises. In cases of life-threatening vaso-occlusive episodes or when there is a threat of severe organ damage as in acute cerebrovascular accidents and priapism, partial exchange transfusions should be promptly carried out because no other effective form of therapy is available. It is also generally agreed that patients who have suffered one cerebrovascular accident are likely to have recurrent life-threatening or debilitating episodes, and a course of long-term maintenance blood transfusions to prevent recurrent sickling is indicated in such cases. Such a program should probably be associated with phlebotomies prior to transfusion and/or the institution of an iron chelation program to prevent or delay the complications of iron overload (see Ch. 142). Use of transfusions during pregnancy is controversial. It is common practice in many centers to give transfusions to pregnant women with sickle cell syndromes during the latter half of pregnancy to prevent fetal wastage and postpartum complications. However, a controlled study has not documented that this practice is clearly beneficial. Finally, it is also general practice for patients with clinically significant sickle cell syndromes to receive a partial exchange transfusion to lower the Hb S value to less than 50 per cent prior to general anesthesia for surgical procedures because of the risk of a fatal or incapacitating sickling episode in the event of an anesthetic accident or transient hypoxia. With the exception of the hypoplastic crises and acute sequestration crises, blood transfusions are not usually required to maintain hemoglobin levels above 6.5 to 7 grams per deciliter, and transfusions are not required on a long-term basis simply to treat the anemia.

Because of the high risk of septicemia and other serious infections caused by *Streptococcus pneumoniae*, young children with sickle cell anemia should receive prophylactic oral penicillin. This approach has been shown to be highly effective in reducing morbidity and mortality in pediatric populations. Pneumococcal vaccines may provide additional protection against such infections.

PROGNOSIS. The prognosis of patients with sickle cell syndromes is variable. A significant number of infants with sickle cell anemia and Hb SC disease may die in the first two to three years because of overwhelming sepsis and/or acute splenic sequestration crises. Cord blood–screening programs and identification of affected individuals with subsequent close medical follow-up, including prophylactic penicillin, should prevent or decrease the incidence of these early fatalities. For the group of patients who survive the early years, improved general medical care has substantially prolonged survival in the last two decades. There are reports of patients surviving to the fifth and sixth decades, although the mean survival is probably to the fourth decade, with death resulting from cardiopulmonary complications and/or renal insufficiency. Other causes of death include sepsis and cerebrovascular accidents. In general, patients with Hb S/β-thalassemia and Hb SC disease have longer survival than patients with sickle cell disease, although there are unexplained cases of relatively mild disease with homozygous inheritance of Hb S.

PREVENTION. Sickle cell disease and other clinically significant sickle syndromes can be prevented in two general ways. First, genetic counseling of identified heterozygotes can alert couples at risk about the possibility of having affected offspring. However, no matter how good the program of genetic counseling and education, it rarely significantly affects the reproductive behavior of identified carriers and generally has little impact on the overall incidence of the disease.

An alternative approach is the availability of prenatal diagnostic services for pregnancies at risk for sickle cell anemia and other sickle hemoglobinopathies. Prenatal diagnosis for sickle cell anemia has gone through many stages in recent years, including fetal blood sampling by fetoscopy for assays of hemoglobin synthesis and analysis by gene-mapping techniques of DNA from amniotic fluid cells, obtained after amniocentesis, for restriction fragment length polymorphisms shown to be linked to the sickle gene by prior study of DNA from family members. A restriction endonuclease enzyme (*Mst* II) can distinguish between a sickle and a nonsickle β-globin gene because the recognition site for this enzyme is specifically abolished by the nucleotide base substitution that is associated with the sickle mutation (Fig. 143–3). Thus the most reliable and acceptable method for prenatal diagnosis of sickle cell anemia is analysis of fetal DNA by the enzyme *Mst*

*Investigational agent available from the National Cancer Institute.

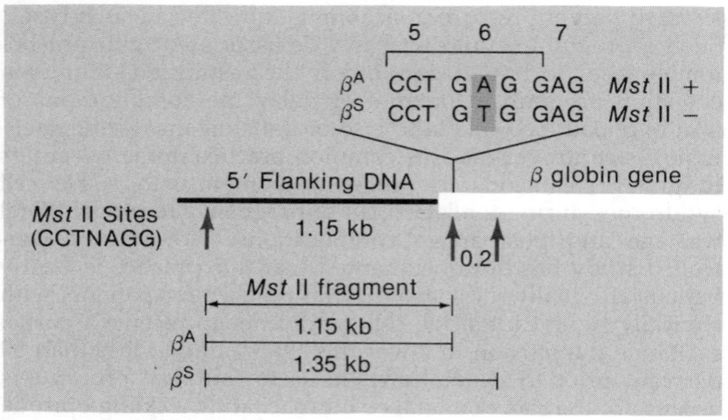

FIGURE 143–3. Direct identification of the sickle cell mutation in cellular DNA by restriction endonuclease digestion using the enzyme *Mst* II. The diagram shows the flanking region and 5′ portion of the beta globin structural gene. Arrows indicate the *Mst* II sites, including the one corresponding to amino acid portions 5, 6, and 7. The 1.15 kilobase (kb) fragment is seen in normal DNA, and the 1.35 kb fragment is seen in sickle DNA.

II. Although amniotic fluid cells obtained after 14 weeks of gestation are currently the source of DNA, it is likely that biopsy of trophoblastic villi in the first trimester will eventually be proved safe and replace amniocentesis.

HOMOZYGOUS Hb C DISEASE. Individuals homozygous for Hb C usually have a mild to moderate hemolytic anemia characterized by splenomegaly and large numbers of target cells on peripheral blood smear. Occasionally intraerythrocytic crystals of Hb C can be visualized in fixed blood smears. The clinical manifestations and general laboratory findngs are those of any mild chronic hemolytic anemia. Diagnosis is established by hemoglobin electrophoresis.

Bunn HF, Forget BG: Sickle cell disease—clinical and epidemiological aspects; and molecular basis of sickle cell disease. In Hemoglobin: Molecular, Genetic and Clinical Aspects. Philadelphia, W. B. Saunders Company, 1986, pp 502–554. Platt O, Nathan DG: Sickle cell disease. In Nathan DG, Oski FA (eds.): Hematology of Infancy and Childhood. 3rd ed. Philadelphia, W. B. Saunders Company, 1987 (in press). *Comprehensive chapters in hematology textbooks covering the pathophysiology as well as the clinical manifestations and therapy of sickle cell disease.*

Dean J, Schechter AN: Sickle–cell anemia: Molecular and cellular bases of therapeutic approaches. N Engl J Med 299:752, 804, 863, 1978. Schechter AN, Noguchi CT, Rodgers GP: Sickle cell disease. In Stamatoyannopoulos G, Nienhuis AW, Leder P, Majerus PW (eds.): Molecular Basis of Blood Diseases. Philadelphia, W. B. Saunders Company, 1987. *Detailed reviews of the physical chemistry and pathophysiology of sickling.*

Fleming AF (ed.): Sickle Cell Disease: A Handbook for the General Clinician. New York, Churchill Livingstone, 1982. Serjeant GR: Sickle Cell Disease. New York, Oxford University Press, 1985. *Comprehensive and detailed clinical descriptions of the manifestations of sickle cell anemia.*

144 UNSTABLE HEMOGLOBINS

Ronald F. Rieder

DEFINITION. The abnormal human hemoglobins manifest their presence by a variety of clinical syndromes of differing severity. One class of mutants, the unstable hemoglobins, is characterized by an increased tendency of the hemoglobin molecule to undergo denaturation. This increased rate of denaturation results in congenital Heinz body hemolytic disease of varying severity.

PATHOGENESIS. The complex three-dimensional arrangement of the four polypeptide subunits of the hemoglobin molecule is maintained primarily by hydrogen bonding and hydrophobic interactions between different amino acids (see Ch. 140). Amino acid substitutions that weaken these forces holding the molecule together result in decreased thermal stability and an increased tendency for hemoglobin to precipitate, especially when exposed to oxidant compounds. Approximately 100 hemoglobin variants have now been described with such amino acid substitutions. The largest group of unstable hemoglobins consists of those with structural alterations that affect the strength of binding of the heme group to the protein by eliminating a specific heme-globin bond or by altering the configuration of the hydrophobic heme pocket. In some of these hemoglobins the binding of the heme group is so weakened that spontaneous loss of heme groups occurs. Hemoglobin Gun Hill has a deletion of a stretch of five amino acids, including the proximal histidine (β92), which normally forms a covalent bond with the heme iron atom; as a result the β chains of hemoglobin Gun Hill lack heme groups. In other unstable hemoglobins there is interference with the helical structure that provides rigidity to the polypeptide chains. Finally, the structural stability and the physiologic function of hemoglobin depend upon the tetrameric arrangement. In several abnormal hemoglobins an amino acid substitution results in the loss of a hydrogen bond that normally serves to stabilize and reinforce an interchain linkage. In unstable hemoglobin Philly the replacement of tyrosine by phenylalanine results in the loss of a single interchain hydrogen bond, permitting greater ease of separation of the α and β chains and denaturation of the hemoglobin. Hemolysis caused by an unstable hemoglobin is a direct result of the intracellular precipitation of hemoglobin to form multiple insoluble aggregates (Heinz bodies), which attach to the red cell membrane (Fig. 144–1). Clearance from the circulation of erythrocytes containing such inclusion bodies by the reticuloendothelial system or removal of inclusions from the cells by pinching off ("pitting") with reduction in red cell membrane and resultant increased fragility is responsible for decreased red cell life span.

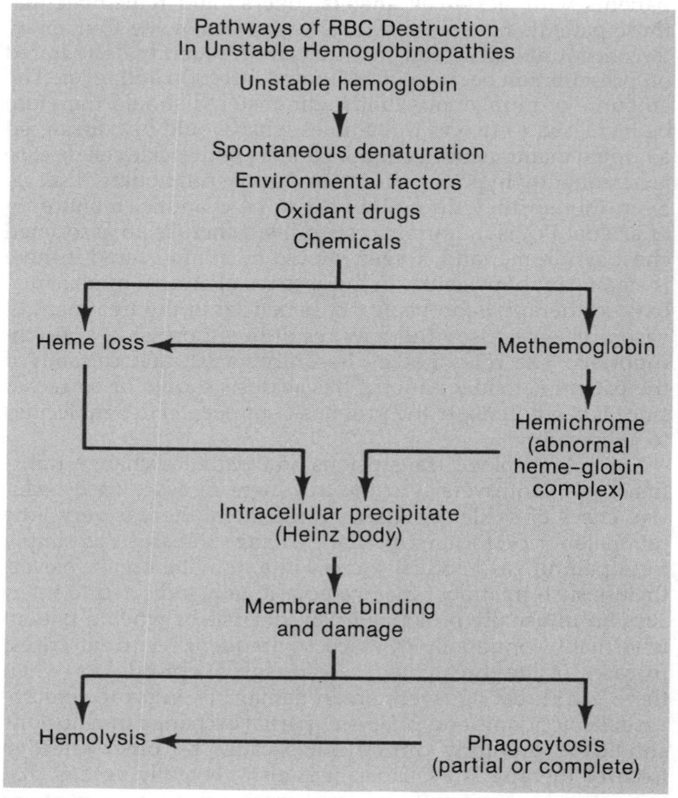

FIGURE 144–1. The presumed mechanisms by which denaturation of hemoglobin leads to erythrocyte destruction are outlined. The rate of travel through the various pathways probably differs for different hemoglobin variants and for a variety of stresses to which the protein is subjected.

CLINICAL MANIFESTATIONS. These disorders are inherited as autosomal dominant traits. Only heterozygotes have been found. The severity of the clinical presentation of patients with unstable hemoglobins is quite varied; some subjects have chronic hemolytic anemia, whereas others with less labile hemoglobins exhibit only mild compensated hemolysis with normal hemoglobin levels. However, exposure of even such mildly affected subjects to a variety of oxidant drugs and chemicals, many of which in large doses can cause methemoglobinemia in normal persons (see Table 146–2), can result in an acute severe hemolysis with the development of pronounced anemia, striking reticulocytosis, and sudden jaundice. Bouts of acute hemolysis may also occur spontaneously during bacterial and viral infections. Some affected subjects exhibit dark urine (pigmenturia) during periods of hemolysis owing to the presence of poorly characterized heme breakdown compounds called dipyrroles.

DIAGNOSIS. Diagnosis of an unstable hemoglobin depends upon the demonstration of a mutant hemoglobin with an increased tendency to precipitate. Intraerythrocytic inclusion bodies (Heinz bodies) can frequently be demonstrated during periods of hemolysis by staining the peripheral blood with a vital dye such as new methylene blue or brilliant cresyl blue. If absent from the circulating red cells, Heinz bodies may appear after incubation of the blood in vitro for two hours at 37° C in the presence of the dye. Instability of the hemoglobin can be demonstrated in hemolysates by formation of a large precipitate with a decrease in the concentration of soluble hemoglobin after heating to 50° C, or to 37° C in the presence of 17 per cent isopropanol. Since similar hemolytic episodes can occur after drug administration in subjects with glucose-6-phosphate dehydrogenase deficiency, this condition should be considered in the differential diagnosis. Hemoglobin electrophoresis may show an abnormal hemoglobin band frequently amounting to less than 25 per cent of the total hemoglobin. Occasionally because of marked preferential destruction of the abnormal molecular species, the unstable hemoglobin may be present in the peripheral blood as only a small percentage of the circulating hemoglobin. Some of the reported unstable hemoglobins are the result of the exchange of one uncharged amino acid for another. Since no alteration in total charge occurs, such mutant hemoglobins may migrate in the same electrophoretic position as hemoglobin A and are therefore difficult to detect by electrophoresis.

TREATMENT. Treatment of subjects with unstable hemoglobins mainly consists of the avoidance of drugs capable of inducing hemolysis (see Table 146–2). Subjects with chronic compensated hemolysis may benefit from prophylactic folic acid administration. Transfusions are required only during periods of profound acute hemolytic anemia. Splenectomy has been helpful when hypersplenism has developed. Special attention should be paid to the possible development of serious hemolytic anemia during episodes of infection.

Bunn HF, Forget BG: Hemoglobin: Molecular, Genetic and Clinical Aspects. Philadelphia, W.B. Saunders Company, 1986. *This authoritative, well-illustrated monograph covers all aspects of human hemoglobins and its disorders. Chapter 13 is devoted to unstable hemoglobin variants.*

Hirano M, Ohba Y, Imai K, et al.: Hb Toyoake: β142(H2O) Ala→Pro. A new unstable hemoglobin with high oxygen affinity. Blood 57:697, 1981. *Chronic hemolytic jaundice, splenomegaly, but no anemia in a subject with an unstable hemoglobin that also has high oxygen affinity.*

Juričić D, Ruždić I, Beer Z, et al.: Hemoglobin Leiden (β6 or 7 (A3 or A4) Glu→0) in a Yugoslavian woman arisen by a new mutation. Hemoglobin 7:271, 1983. *An example of the way a modern hematology laboratory can investigate a mutant hemoglobin.*

Winslow RM, Anderson WF: The hemoglobinopathies. *In* Stanbury JB, Wyngaarden JB, Fredrickson DS, et al. (eds.): The Metabolic Basis of Inherited Disease. 5th ed. New York, McGraw-Hill Book Company, 1983, pp 1666-1710. *This is a comprehensive treatment of the genetics, structure, function, and clinical properties of the various types of abnormal hemoglobins.*

145 ABNORMAL HEMOGLOBINS WITH ALTERED OXYGEN AFFINITY

Ronald F. Rieder

DEFINITION. The ability of hemoglobin to function as a useful means of transporting oxygen depends upon its becoming fully loaded with oxygen in the lungs and unloading a proportion of this oxygen in the tissues at partial pressures of oxygen that are compatible with cell function and viability. A change in the structure of the hemoglobin molecule can affect this respiratory function. An increase in oxygen affinity can impair the ability of the pigment to donate its oxygen to the cells, whereas a decrease in affinity can prevent it from picking up enough oxygen as it passes through the pulmonary circulation. This affinity for oxygen is frequently expressed as the partial pressure of oxygen at which hemoglobin is half-saturated (P_{50}). Many mutant hemoglobins have some degree of alteration of oxygen-binding properties, but only a few have clinically significant defects. Some of these hemoglobins have increased oxygen affinity (decreased P_{50}), whereas others have a decreased capacity for binding oxygen (increased P_{50}).

PATHOGENESIS. During the process of oxygenation and deoxygenation, hemoglobin undergoes reversible structural changes that involve alterations in the three-dimensional configuration of the individual polypeptide chains, as well as shifts in the way the four chains are arranged in the $\alpha_2\beta_2$ tetramer. When fully deoxygenated, hemoglobin is said to be in the T or tense state and has a relatively low affinity for oxygen. Conversely, when hemoglobin is fully oxygenated, it is in the R or relaxed state and has a high affinity for oxygen. This intramolecular reorganization with its resultant change in oxygen affinity is reflected in the physiologically important sigmoidal shape of the hemoglobin-oxygen dissociation curve (see Ch. 140).

The complex stereochemical changes in molecular structure are accomplished by considerable relative movement of the α and β globin chains along the $\alpha_1\beta_2$ interface and of the C-terminal regions of the β chains. Hydrogen bonds, hydrophobic interactions, and salt bridges between amino acids are broken and new ones are formed during these R-T transitions.

Genetic mutations that affect amino acids situated at the $\alpha_1\beta_2$ interface or that otherwise alter molecular structure to interfere with the R-T equilibrium may affect the respiratory function of hemoglobin. Thus an amino acid substitution that destabilizes the T or low O_2 affinity state would tend to favor the R state and increase the oxygen affinity of a mutant hemoglobin. In abnormal hemoglobin Kempsey, asparagine replaces aspartic acid at position β99. Asparagine, unlike aspartic acid, cannot form the hydrogen bond with tyrosine at α42 that normally stabilizes the deoxyhemoglobin conformation. As a result hemoglobin Kempsey has a high oxygen affinity. In contrast in hemoglobin Kansas, threonine replaces asparagine at position β102. Threonine cannot form the hydrogen bond with aspartic acid at α94 that normally stabilizes the R or high affinity state. Therefore hemoglobin Kansas is shifted toward the T state and has a low oxygen affinity.

2,3-Diphosphoglycerate (2,3-DPG) acts as a physiologic modulator of hemoglobin oxygen affinity and binds to specific amino acid sites on the protein. 2,3-DPG increases the P_{50} (lowers the oxygen affinity), and mutations that inhibit bind-

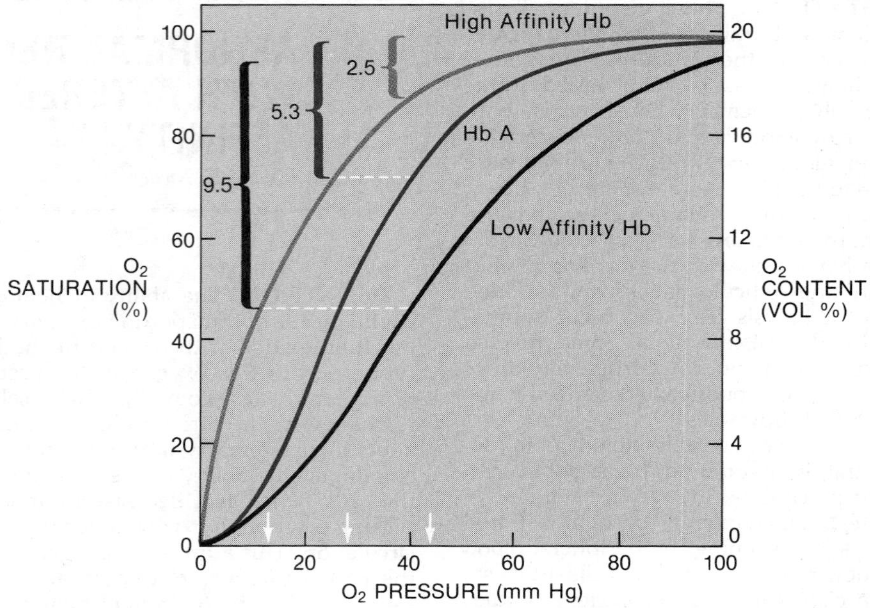

FIGURE 145–1. Hemoglobin-oxygen dissociation curves are illustrated for normal hemoglobin (Hb A) and for model abnormal hemoglobins with high and low oxygen affinities. On the abscissa is indicated the partial pressure of oxygen in millimeters of mercury. On the left ordinate the saturation of hemoglobin with oxygen is indicated as a percentage; on the right ordinate the oxygen content of the hemoglobin is expressed as volumes per cent. The three inverted arrows show the P_{50} for the three hemoglobins (the partial pressure of oxygen at which the hemoglobin is 50 per cent saturated). This value is lowest for the high-affinity hemoglobin. As the partial pressure of oxygen drops from 100 (arterial) to 40 (tissues), hemoglobin desaturates, giving up a portion of its bound oxygen; the numbers on the brackets indicate the amount of oxygen unloaded by the three hemoglobin types expressed in volumes per cent. Note that the high-affinity hemoglobin delivers less than half the oxygen that Hb A gives to the tissues, resulting in tissue anoxia, increased erythropoietin secretion, and erythrocytosis. Conversely, the low-affinity hemoglobin is even more efficient than Hb A in supplying the tissues with oxygen resulting in diminished erythropoietin production and anemia.

ing of this small molecular weight effector result in hemoglobin with increased oxygen affinity.

CLINICAL MANIFESTATIONS. Most of the abnormal hemoglobins with detectable alterations in oxygen-binding characteristics are only minimally affected and of no physiologic significance. However, mutant hemoglobins with greatly increased oxygen affinity tend to unload much less oxygen to the tissues, and this results in relative tissue hypoxia. As a result erythropoietin secretion is increased and erythropoiesis is stimulated with a rise in hematocrit value (Fig. 145–1). Thus subjects with high affinity hemoglobins may have *erythrocytosis.* The disorder is frequently familial and is inherited as an autosomal dominant. No increase in white blood cell or platelet counts occurs. Plasma concentrations of erythropoietin are normal when the subject is polycythemic, but if the hematocrit level is lowered to normal by phlebotomy, an increase in erythropoietin production can be detected.

In subjects with mutant hemoglobins having moderately lowered oxygen affinity, the increased tendency of the hemoglobin to unload oxygen results in enhanced delivery to the tissues. Such persons therefore require less hemoglobin to provide the same volume of oxygen and as a consequence frequently have decreased hematocrit values. In this situation the usually *mild anemia* is not a pathologic condition but is a physiologic response to the increased availability of oxygen at the tissue level.

In some subjects with a hemoglobin with greatly decreased oxygen affinity, *cyanosis* is present owing to the marked inability of the mutant hemoglobin to bind oxygen. Hematocrit values in such cases are normal.

Even in the presence of markedly abnormal hemoglobin function, subjects with hemoglobins with altered oxygen affinity usually are asymptomatic.

DIAGNOSIS. The presence of a hemoglobin with high oxygen affinity should be considered in any patient who has isolated erythrocytosis unaccompanied by increased leukocyte and platelet proliferation (see Ch. 153). After eliminating causes such as the presence of hypoxemia with secondary erythrocytosis as well as other causes of increased erythropoietin secretion, evidence for an abnormal hemoglobin should be sought. Hemoglobin electrophoresis may reveal an abnormal hemoglobin band, but several of the high affinity hemoglobins have electrophoretic mobilities identical to hemoglobin A. An oxygen-hemoglobin dissociation curve should be determined on whole blood and especially on isolated hemoglobin. The latter can eliminate any contribution of diminished or increased 2,3-DPG levels. By adding back 2,3-DPG to the purified hemoglobin, evidence for diminished 2,3-DPG binding can be detected. A low affinity hemoglobin should be considered in instances of unexplained cyanosis with normal arterial oxygen tension.

TREATMENT. Aside from either erythrocytosis or mild anemia, subjects having these functionally defective hemoglobins are usually asymptomatic and no treatment is indicated. Cyanosis accompanying the rare hemoglobins having very low affinity for oxygen is only a cosmetic problem.

Bunn HF, Forget BG: Hemoglobin: Molecular, Genetic and Clinical Aspects. Philadelphia. W. B. Saunders Company, 1986. *This authoritative, well-illustrated monograph covers all aspects of human hemoglobin and its disorders. Ch. 14 provides an in-depth discussion of hemoglobinopathies with abnormal oxygen binding.*

Charache S, Catalno P, Burns S, et al.: Pregnancy in carriers of high-affinity hemoglobins. Blood 65:713, 1985. *Female carriers of three different high affinity hemoglobins demonstrated no increase in either fetal wastage or intrauterine growth retardation.*

Moo-Penn WF, McPhedran P, Bobrow S, et al.: Hemoglobin Connecticut β21(B3)(Asp→Gly): A Hemoglobin variant with low oxygen affinity. Am J Hematol 11:137, 1981. *This hemoglobin with low oxygen affinity was found in three generations of a family and was associated with mild anemia in several individuals.*

Moo-Penn WF, Schneider RG, Shih T-B, et al.: Hemoglobin Ohio (β142A1a→Asp): A new abnormal hemoglobin with high oxygen affinity and erythrocytosis. Blood 56:246, 1980. *This high affinity hemoglobin was found in three members of a family, all of whom exhibited erythrocytosis.*

146 METHEMOGLOBINEMIA AND SULFHEMOGLOBINEMIA

Ronald F. Rieder

METHEMOGLOBINEMIA

DEFINITION. The reversible oxygenation and deoxygenation of hemoglobin at physiologic partial pressures of oxygen require that the heme iron of deoxyhemoglobin remain in the ferrous (Fe^{+2}) form. In methemoglobin the iron atom is oxidized to the ferric (Fe^{+3}) form, rendering the molecule incapable of binding oxygen. When hemoglobin is oxygenated during the process of respiration, an electron is partially transferred from the ferrous iron atom to the bound oxygen molecule. Thus in oxyhemoglobin iron possesses some of the characteristics of the ferric (Fe^{+3}) state, whereas the oxygen takes on the characteristics of the superoxide (O_2^-) anion. Under normal circumstances upon deoxygenation of the hemoglobin molecule the electron is returned to the iron atom and the O_2 molecule is released. Interference with the return of the electron to the iron atom results in the formation of methemoglobin. Normally approximately 3 per cent of the hemoglobin is spontaneously oxidized to methemoglobin each day, but the concentration is maintained below 1 per cent by its reconversion to hemoglobin by metabolic processes. A shift in this equilibrium can result in increased amounts of methemoglobin in the peripheral blood and the development of cyanosis. Enzymatic reducing systems in the red cells are responsible for the maintenance of the heme iron of hemoglobin in the ferrous state. An enzyme variously termed NADH-methemoglobin reductase, NADH-dehydrogenase, NADH-diaphorase, or erythrocyte cytochrome b_5 reductase is responsible for over 90 per cent of the hemoglobin reducing capacity of the erythrocyte under physiologic conditions, catalyzing the transfer of an electron from NADH to oxidized cytochrome b_5:

$$\text{NADH} + \text{Fe}^{+3} - \text{cytochrome } b_5 \xrightarrow{\text{reductase}} \text{NAD}^+ + \text{Fe}^{+2} - \text{cytochrome } b_5$$

Flavine adenine dinucleotide may participate as a prosthetic group on the reductase. Reduced cytochrome b_5 then directly interacts with methemoglobin to result in its reduction to ferrous hemoglobin:

$$\text{Fe}^{+2} - \text{cytochrome } b_5 + \text{Fe}^{+3} - \text{hemoglobin} \rightarrow \text{Fe}^{+3} - \text{cytochrome } b_5 + \text{Fe}^{+2} - \text{hemoglobin}$$

The reconversion of NAD to NADH depends upon the Embden-Meyerhof glycolytic pathway, primarily at the reaction in which glyceraldehyde-3-phosphate is converted to 1,3-diphosphoglycerate by the enzyme glyceraldehyde phosphate dehydrogenase. An NADPH-dependent methemoglobin reductase is present within the erythrocyte, but normally there is no linked physiologic electron carrier available which is capable of directly donating an electron to reduce methemoglobin. However, when provided with an artificial electron carrier such as methylene blue, this enzyme is of great importance in the therapy of acute toxic methemoglobinemia (see below). Ascorbic acid and reduced glutathione are capable of directly reducing methemoglobin, but these reactions occur quite slowly.

CLASSIFICATION (Table 146–1). Methemoglobinemia may be hereditary or acquired. Hereditary methemoglobinemia may result from an abnormality in the metabolic processes that normally reconvert methemoglobin to hemoglobin (see above) or from an inherited abnormality of the hemoglobin molecule conducive to methemoglobin formation. Acquired methemoglobinemia results from exposure to certain chemical agents that increase the formation of methemoglobin.

TABLE 146–1. TYPES OF METHEMOGLOBINEMIA

A. Congenital
  1. Defective enzymatic reduction of Fe^{+3}-hemoglobin to Fe^{+2}-hemoglobin
     a. NADH–methemoglobin reductase (cytochrome b_5 reductase) deficiency
     b. Cytochrome b_5 deficiency
  2. Abnormal hemoglobins resistant to enzymatic reduction (M hemoglobins)

B. Acquired
  1. Excessive (toxic) oxidation of Fe^{+2}-hemoglobin
     a. Environmental chemicals
     b. Drugs

Hereditary Methemoglobinemia Caused by Defective Reduction of Methemoglobin

More than 100 subjects with hereditary methemoglobinemia resulting from NADH-methemoglobin reductase deficiency have been described, and several abnormal variant enzymes differing in catalytic activity, structural stability, and electrophoretic mobility are known. The disorder is inherited as an autosomal recessive trait. It occurs with unusually high frequency in Alaskan Eskimos and Indians, Navajo Indians and Puerto Ricans. In certain families with this disorder there has been an associated mental deficiency with neurologic defects. In this form of the disorder the enzyme deficiency is not restricted to the erythrocytes but is widely distributed, including the brain. Patients with methemoglobinemia have persistent slate-gray cyanosis. In contrast to deoxyhemoglobin, which produces cyanosis only when present at levels above 5 grams per deciliter, methemoglobin at a concentration of only 1.5 to 2 grams per deciliter produces significant cyanosis. Homozygotes usually have methemoglobin levels of 15 to 25 per cent, but no deleterious effect is apparent at this concentration. At concentrations of methemoglobin up to 40 per cent, some symptoms of fatigability and malaise have been described. The patients have been characterized as being more blue than sick. No clubbing or cardiopulmonary disease is present, and mild compensatory erythrocytosis has been noted only occasionally. Heterozygotes for the enzyme deficiency have normal concentrations of methemoglobin, but manifest increased susceptibility to the methemoglobin-producing properties of various oxidant drugs and chemicals (Table 146–2). Recently, congenital methemoglobinemia due to deficiency of cytochrome b_5 has been described.

DIAGNOSIS. Persistent cyanosis without hypoxia should suggest the possibility of methemoglobinemia. The peripheral blood is reddish brown and does not become bright red when exposed to oxygen. Methemoglobin has a characteristic absorption peak at 630 nm, which disappears upon addition of cyanide. Several assays are available to quantitate the level of NADH-methemoglobin reductase in erythrocytes, and stain-

TABLE 146–2. DRUGS AND CHEMICALS HAVING TOXIC EFFECT ON HEMOGLOBIN MOLECULE

	Hemoglobin Derivative Observed	
Agent	*Methemoglobin*	*Sulfhemoglobin*
Acetanilid, phenacetin	+	+
Nitrites (amyl, sodium, potassium, nitroglycerin)	+	+
Trinitrotoluene, nitrobenzene	+	+
Aniline, hydroxylamine, dimethylamine	+	+
Sulfanilamide	+	+
Para-aminosalicylic acid	+	
Dapsone	+	
Primaquine, chloroquine	+	
Prilocaine, benzocaine, lidocaine	+	
Menadione, naphthoquinone	+	
Naphthalene	+	
Resorcinol	+	
Phenylhydrazine	+	+

ing procedures can reveal an abnormal enzyme with altered electrophoretic mobility.

TREATMENT. Treatment of congenital methemoglobinemia caused by reductase deficiency is generally not required, but cosmetic improvement of the cyanosis can be achieved by treatment with methylene blue, 100 to 300 mg per day orally, or ascorbic acid, 500 mg per day orally. Riboflavin, 20 mg per day orally, is also effective. Methylene blue has the disadvantage of producing blue urine. Large doses of ascorbate may lead to oxalate stone production.

Hereditary Methemoglobinemia Due to Abnormal (M) Hemoglobins

Several variant hemoglobins have substitutions in the amino acids that line the heme crevice of the globin chain and contact the porphyrin group or the iron atom. These mutations affect the configuration of the polypeptide chain surrounding the heme group, alter the hydrophobic environment, and often weaken the binding of the porphyrin to the protein. Some of these variant hemoglobins are unstable and lose heme (see Ch. 144), and others are permanently fixed in the methemoglobin state (M hemoglobins). In four of the five described M hemoglobins a histidine is replaced by a tyrosine whose hydroxyl group forms a stable complex with iron in the ferric state. The hemoglobin is thus fixed in the oxidized form. The methemoglobin reductase system of the erythrocyte is ineffective in reducing these abnormal methemoglobins.

CLINICAL MANIFESTATIONS. Subjects inheriting an M hemoglobin are cyanotic but are usually otherwise unaffected by the trait. Mild chronic hemolysis has been observed in association with hemoglobin M Hyde Park, which has a tendency to lose heme and is slightly unstable. The disorder is inherited in a dominant pattern, and families have been reported in which the condition has been noted in several generations.

DIAGNOSIS. The blood has a brown appearance and does not become bright red upon agitation in air. Neither does the addition of cyanide produce the change to the red color that occurs upon such treatment of normal methemoglobin. In subjects with β-chain mutations approximately 50 per cent of the hemoglobin is affected, whereas 20 to 25 per cent of the circulating hemoglobin is methemoglobin in persons with an α Hb M. The presence of an abnormal methemoglobin can be detected by spectrophotometric analysis. The normal absorption peaks of methemoglobin at 630 and 502 nm are shifted to slightly lower wavelengths in the M hemoglobins. In addition, the M hemoglobins have an altered electrophoretic migration; separation from Hb A is most easily demonstrated if first the hemolysate is completely converted to methemoglobin with ferricyanide. No treatment is required for this condition, and methylene blue and ascorbic acid administration are ineffective for significant conversion to reduced hemoglobin.

Acquired or Toxic Methemoglobinemia

A variety of chemical agents and drugs are able to accelerate the oxidation of hemoglobin and produce a significant methemoglobinemia in otherwise normal individuals (Table 146–1). Many of these agents occasionally induce sulfhemoglobinemia and can cause hemolysis in subjects with unstable hemoglobins or glucose-6-phosphate dehydrogenase deficiency. Often these compounds are unable directly to induce the oxidation of hemoglobin in vitro, and thus their toxicity in vivo is probably a result of conversion to intermediate forms that are direct oxidants. Nitrates have been implicated in methemoglobinemia in infants as a result of the use of contaminated well water in the preparation of feeding formulas. They must be converted to nitrite to produce methemoglobinemia. Such conversion may occur as a result of the action of bacteria in the gastrointestinal tract. The ability of drugs to produce large amounts of methemoglobin depends upon overwhelming the normal pathway in the red cell responsible for maintenance of hemoglobin iron in the ferrous state. In normal subjects large doses of drugs are generally necessary. When the activity of the methemoglobin-reducing system is depressed, susceptibility to these agents is increased. Thus heterozygotes for NADH-methemoglobin reductase variants and newborn infants who normally have low levels of the enzyme until about four months of age are very susceptible to the development of methemoglobinemia. Normal doses of primaquine and dapsone have caused methemoglobinemia in enzyme-deficient adults. Menadione, naphthalene, and aniline dyes used by laundries to mark diapers have been implicated in the induction of methemoglobinemia in very young infants. On the other hand, such agents as prilocaine and sulfanilamide have commonly been reported to cause methemoglobinemia in normal persons.

CLINICAL MANIFESTATIONS. Methemoglobinemia induced by drugs is usually an asymptomatic condition, and any associated ill effects are generally due to other actions of these chemicals. However, severe acute methemoglobinemia with levels of methemoglobin greater than 60 to 70 per cent have been associated with collapse, coma, and death. Affected patients develop severe cyanosis, and upon examination the blood is chocolate brown.

DIAGNOSIS. Diagnosis depends upon demonstration of the presence of methemoglobin (see above) and identification of the causative agent. Erythrocyte reductase levels should be measured to rule out enzyme deficiency.

TREATMENT. With mildly affected patients treatment, aside from discontinuing the offending agent, is not required, and the methemoglobin will be reduced spontaneously to ferrous hemoglobin over a period of two to three days. For severely affected patients therapy with methylene blue is effective. One to 2 mg per kilogram of a 1 per cent solution of methylene blue in saline is administered intravenously over 10 minutes. If there is no adequate response within an hour, a second dose may be administered. This treatment generally results in the prompt conversion of methemoglobin to hemoglobin. Such therapy is not effective in subjects with glucose-6-phosphate dehydrogenase deficiency resulting in inactivity of the hexose monophosphate shunt pathway for the production of NADPH, which is required for the reconversion of oxidized methylene blue to reduced or leuko-methylene blue. Exchange transfusion may be required in severely symptomatic patients. Oral ascorbic acid should not be used in the treatment of acute toxic methemoglobinemia, since its speed of action is slow.

Bunn HF, Forget BG: Hemoglobin: Molecular, Genetic and Clinical Aspects. Philadelphia. W. B. Saunders Company, 1986. *This authoritative, well-illustrated monograph covers all aspects of human hemoglobin and its disorders. Ch. 15 covers the M hemoglobins and Ch. 16 discusses the other forms of methemoglobinemia.*

Jaffé ER: Methaemoglobinemia. Clin Haematol 10:99, 1981. *Review emphasizing enzyme deficiency.*

Mansouri A. Methemoglobinemia. Am J Med Sci 289:200, 1985. *Detailed review covering all forms of methemoglobinemia.*

Schwartz JM, Reiss AL, Jaffe ER: Hereditary methemoglobinemia with deficiency of NADH cytochrome b_5 reductase. In Stanbury JB, Wyngaarden JB, Fredrickson DS, et al. (eds).: The Metabolic Basis of Inherited Disease. 5th ed. New York, McGraw-Hill Book Company, 1983, p 1654. *Authoritative, detailed review of all aspects of the inherited enzyme deficiency.*

SULFHEMOGLOBINEMIA

DEFINITION. Sulfhemoglobin is an incompletely characterized greenish-brown hemoglobin derivative found in the blood of some subjects after exposure to large amounts of various drugs or organic chemicals. The pigment causes cyanosis, makes the blood reddish brown, and has a characteristic optical absorption spectrum with a peak at 620 nm that is not abolished by the addition of cyanide. The precise structure of the abnormal pigment is not known except that a sulfur atom is incorporated into the porphyrin ring.

PATHOGENESIS. Abnormal pigments with similar optical absorption characteristics have been noted in the blood of patients after ingestion of toxic doses of acetanilid, phenacetin, and other drugs, as well as after exposure to large amounts of aromatic amino and nitro compounds. The mechanism for the production of sulfhemoglobin in vivo is not understood. Many of the same compounds that have been noted to cause methemoglobinemia in some patients have been implicated in the appearance of sulfhemoglobin in others (see Table 146–1). Neither the reason for the appearance of one hemoglobin derivative rather than the other nor the relationship in vivo to sulfur is clear. Chronic constipation with the production of excess hydrogen sulfide in the gut has been postulated but never proved to be a contributing factor.

CLINICAL MANIFESTATIONS. Cyanosis is the characteristic feature of subjects with sulfhemoglobinemia. As little as 0.5 gram per deciliter produces a slate-gray discoloration of the skin and mucous membranes. This amount of sulfhemoglobin is much less than the 1.5 and 5 grams per deciliter required for methemoglobin and reduced hemoglobin to cause cyanosis. Patients generally experience no ill effects from the condition, and asymptomatic persons with as much as 10 grams per deciliter have been described.

DIAGNOSIS. Positive identification of sulfhemoglobin as the cause of cyanosis in a patient can be made by observing the characteristic optical absorption spectrum of a hemolysate before and after the addition of a small amount of potassium cyanide. Isoelectric focusing has also been used.

TREATMENT. Treatment consists primarily of identifying the causative agent and eliminating further contact. Reconversion of sulfhemoglobin to hemoglobin is not possible. In symptomatic cases exchange transfusion would be indicated. After cessation of contact with the offending agent, production of sulfhemoglobin ceases, and the compound is eliminated from the blood over a period of weeks during the normal course of erythrocyte aging and clearance from the circulation.

Park CM, Nagel RL: Sulfhemoglobinemia. Clinical and molecular aspects. N Engl J Med 310:1579, 1984. *This is a report of a thoroughly studied case, accompanied by an excellent discussion of diagnosis, chemistry, and pathophysiology.*

147 BLOOD TRANSFUSION

Herbert A. Perkins

A standard unit of blood donated for transfusion consists of 450 ml of blood mixed with 63 ml of a solution that contains citrate to prevent clotting, and glucose, phosphate, and adenine for optimal preservation of red cell viability. Without adenine, storage of red cells is limited to 21 days; with adenine, 35 days is acceptable. Nonviable cells are quickly removed from the circulation of the recipient; the remainder are restored to biochemical normality and live out the rest of their usual life span (up to 120 days).

INDICATIONS FOR BLOOD TRANSFUSION

Blood transfusions have the potential for many harmful side effects. Therefore, blood should never be transfused when the risks to the patient outweigh the expected benefit, or when more specific and safer therapy (e.g., iron, B_{12}) is available. When blood transfusions are indicated, only that fraction of the blood that the patient requires should be administered. Most blood donations are separated into components after collection: red blood cells, platelet concentrates, and/or cryoprecipitates and plasma. The plasma may be subsequently fractionated to provide albumin, gamma globulin, and coagulation factor concentrates.

This discussion will be restricted to the use of red blood cell concentrates and whole blood. The indications for transfusion of platelet concentrates are discussed in Ch. 166, for leukocytes in Ch. 150, and for cryoprecipitates and coagulation factor concentrates in Ch. 167.

The patient who is anemic but has a normal blood volume should receive only red blood cells; therefore whole blood transfusions are rarely justifiable on a medical service. Acute hemorrhage is more common on the surgical services, but even here whole blood is inappropriate in most situations. Patients with acute hemorrhage often have a relatively greater deficit of red cells than of plasma. Transfusing red cells until the blood volume is normalized will result in a higher hematocrit and, in turn, greater oxygen-carrying capacity than would an equal volume of whole blood. Moreover, the usual bleeding patient who loses less than 20 to 25 per cent of the blood volume (1000 to 1500 ml in an adult) can be transfused with red cells supplemented by electrolytes instead of whole blood with no impairment of recovery. It is common practice in many hospitals to provide red cells, not whole blood, for the first three units crossmatched for routine surgery. Whole blood is of greatest value when there has been massive acute blood loss creating need for large-scale red cell and volume replacement.

RED BLOOD CELLS. A variety of red blood cell components can be prepared. These are listed in Table 147–1, together with their usual packed cell volume (PCV) and the proportion of red blood cells (RBC), white blood cells (WBC), and plasma of the original whole blood that remains in the final product.

Red blood cells, often called packed red blood cells, should be the primary component for the treatment of chronic anemia or hemorrhage. This component contains all the red cells of the original unit with enough plasma so that it will flow reasonably rapidly through an intravenous needle.

Red blood cells in additive solution may be stored for 42 days. Preservative solution containing adenine is added after most of the plasma has been removed.

Leukocyte-poor red blood cells are given to patients who have had prior febrile reactions to transfusions caused by recipient alloantibodies reacting with donor leukocytes. Leukocyte-poor red blood cells may be prepared by (1) centrifuging blood with removal of the buffy coat, (2) washing red blood cells with removal of the buffy coat, or (3) transfusing through a special filter red cells that have been refrigerated and then centrifuged to pack the leukocytes into clumps (the spin, cool, filter technique). Removal of 85 to 90 per cent of the donor leukocytes is sufficient to prevent febrile reactions in at least 90 per cent of alloimmunized patients. As much as 20 per cent of red cells may be lost to achieve this level of leukocyte depletion, and the final hematocrit varies with the exact procedure.

Washed red blood cells are rarely indicated. They are required only when a recipient has had prior severe reactions to donor plasma proteins. Although they have often been recommended for patients with paroxysmal nocturnal hemoglobinuria, recent evidence indicates that they are rarely necessary. Washed red blood cells should not be considered to be leukocyte poor unless the washing process was modified to remove the buffy coat.

TABLE 147–1. RED BLOOD CELL COMPONENTS

Component	PCV (%)	RBC (%)	WBC (%)	Plasma (%)
RBC	75	100	100	20
RBC in additive solution	60	100	100	5
Leukocyte-poor RBC				
Centrifuged	95	80	15	5
Washed	75	90	10	0
Spin-cool-filter	75	85	15	20
Washed RBC	75	95	50	0
Frozen RBC	75	90	5	0

Frozen red blood cells are also washed and leukocyte poor by the time they have been readied for transfusion. Red cell loss is inevitable, and the procedures involved are time consuming and expensive. Red blood cells, when prepared with glycerol, can be stored in the frozen state for as long as three years; therefore the most important reason to freeze red cells is for preservation of a type so rare that it would otherwise be unavailable for the patient who must receive it. Frozen red cells are also useful for the patient with antibodies to donor leukocytes so strong that he or she has an uncomfortable febrile reaction to leukocyte-poor red cells.

PROVIDING COMPATIBLE BLOOD FOR TRANSFUSION

BLOOD GROUPS. The external surfaces of all blood cells and plasma proteins contain very large numbers of antigenic determinants whose structures are programmed by genes. Many of these genetic loci have multiple possible alleles, with the result that all blood transfusions expose the recipient to a large number of foreign immunogens. Fortunately, most of these antigenic determinants are poor immunogens or result in antibodies that have no notable clinical effect. In routine transfusions, it is usually sufficient to avoid incompatibility for only three antigens (A, B, and D), all on the red blood cells.

The red blood cell antigenic determinants are divided into blood groups, each blood group consisting of the alleles of a single genetic locus. The most important red blood cell group is the ABO group, with two antigens: A and B. The primary importance of the ABO blood group in transfusion therapy is based on two facts: (1) Anti-A and anti-B are regularly present ("naturally occurring") in the plasma of persons who lack the corresponding antigen on their red cells (Table 147–2), presumably because of previous immunization to crossreacting antigens in bacteria and foods. (2) Anti-A and anti-B are almost always present in high concentration, activate the full complement cascade, and are capable of intravascular destruction of an almost unlimited number of incompatible red blood cells.

The second important red cell blood group is Rh. This is important because one of the antigenic determinants in this group (D) is an unusually potent immunogen, and 15 per cent of Caucasoids lack the D antigen. The term *Rh-positive* indicates the presence of D; *Rh-negative* indicates its absence. There are a large number of additional Rh gene products, but only a few of these commonly stimulate production of alloantibodies: C, E, c, and e. C and c resemble alleles, as do E and e, in that one—but not both—is the product of each normal Rh gene. There is no allele for D, but the symbol "d" is used to indicate its absence.

Altogether, more than 300 different antigenic determinants have been identified on human red blood cells. Some of these have been assigned to blood groups; others have not. In addition to the Rh antigens mentioned, additional important red cell immunogens are found in the Kell, Duffy, and Kidd systems. Antibodies to the Rh, Kell, Duffy, and Kidd antigens are not "naturally occurring" and are found after prior transfusions or pregnancies. Typing donors for these antigens (other than D) is necessary only when the recipient has formed the corresponding antibody. Antibodies to certain other red cell antigens (e.g., M, Lewis, P, I) are relatively common and often naturally occurring, but since these antibodies are generally inactive at body temperature, they are rarely of clinical significance.

COMPATIBILITY TESTING. A hospital transfusion service must type the red blood cells of the patient for A, B, and D and confirm the typing of the donor. Further tests are performed to ensure that the patient has not formed "unexpected" antibodies, i.e., antibodies other than the expected anti-A or B. The search for unexpected antibodies is carried out in two ways: (1) Antibody screening involves testing the serum of the patient with a small number of red cells selected to contain among them all of the antigens which commonly cause trouble. (2) Compatibility testing, or crossmatching, tests the patient's serum with red blood cells from the units intended for transfusion. If unexpected antibodies are detected which appear likely by their specificity and characteristics to impair the survival of transfused red cells containing the corresponding antigen, red cells to be transfused must lack the antigen. In general, a positive crossmatch contraindicates transfusion; exceptions should be approved by someone thoroughly knowledgeable about the possible effects of the antibodies detected.

TABLE 147–2. THE ABO GROUP

Red cell type	O	A	B	AB
Possible genotypes	OO	AA or AO	BB or BO	AB
Antibodies in serum	Anti-A and B	Anti-B	Anti-A	None
Frequency in Caucasoids	45%	40%	10%	5%

EMERGENCY TRANSFUSION. Under normal circumstances, transfused red cells are of the same ABO type as those of the recipient; but in urgent situations when ABO-identical red cells are not available, ABO-compatible red cells may be transfused. For example, type O red cells can be given to a recipient of any ABO type, and the type AB recipient can receive red cells of any ABO type. Whole blood should be avoided in these circumstances, since the anti-A and/or anti-B of the donor plasma may destroy recipient red cells.

If Rh negative red cells are not available for an Rh-negative recipient, Rh-positive cells may be transfused in an emergency, but only if the recipient has no anti-D in his or her serum. Special effort should be made to avoid transfusion of Rh-positive cells into Rh-negative recipients who are females and not yet past the childbearing age. The recipient has approximately a 70 per cent chance of being immunized to D, and a subsequent pregnancy with an Rh-positive fetus is very likely to result in severe hemolytic disease of the newborn. If Rh-positive red cells must be transfused into an Rh-negative female of reproductive age, Rh immunoglobulin treatment may prevent immunization.

With sudden massive hemorrhage, it may be necessary to transfuse blood without all of the usual preliminary tests. Type O Rh-negative blood is often reserved for such situations on the grounds that it is likely to be compatible with all recipients. Such blood is in limited supply, however, and it takes only a few minutes to determine the ABO and Rh types of the recipient. Meanwhile, electrolytes or colloid (e.g., albumin) can be used to maintain the patient's circulation. The usual in vitro compatibility tests can be waived if the emergency is sufficiently great, but there must be written documentation of the urgency.

HAZARDS OF BLOOD TRANSFUSIONS

The many potential complications of blood transfusion are listed in Table 147–3.

HEMOLYTIC REACTIONS. Hemolytic reactions correctly attract the most attention, since they can result in serious morbidity or death. Almost all immediate hemolytic transfusion reactions are caused by ABO mismatches, and the cause of the error is almost always clerical. The most common error is incorrect labeling of the patient sample taken for compatibility testing. The patient must be identified without error at the time of sampling, and the correct label must be applied to the crossmatch tube before leaving the patient's side. The other major source of the trouble is transfusion of a unit other than the one intended for that patient. The donor blood label, crossmatch slip, and patient identification must be crosschecked carefully before the transfusion is started.

The most dangerous antibodies are those which activate the complete complement cascade, resulting in intravascular hemolysis. Other antibodies (e.g., Rh, Kell) merely become attached to the red cell, in some instances with subsequent attachment of complement components C3 and C4. The

TABLE 147–3. HAZARDS OF BLOOD TRANSFUSION

1. Hemolytic reactions
2. Chill-fever reactions
3. Contaminated blood
4. Noncardiac pulmonary edema
5. Post-transfusion thrombocytopenic purpura
6. Transmission of disease
   a. Hepatitis
   b. Malaria
   c. Syphilis
   d. Cytomegalovirus
   e. Acquired immunodeficiency syndrome (AIDS)
7. Allergic reactions
   a. Urticaria
   b. Anaphylaxis
8. Circulatory overload
9. Air embolism
10. Hemosiderosis (see Ch. 142)
11. Massive transfusion problems
12. Graft-versus-host disease

coated red cells may then be destroyed in the reticuloendothelial system by macrophages, which have receptors for the Fc portion of IgG molecules and the C3 and C4.

Intravascular hemolysis (such as that caused by anti-A or anti-B) results in release of free hemoglobin into the plasma, binding of hemoglobin to haptoglobin with subsequent removal of the complex, hemoglobinuria once haptoglobin has been saturated, and later rise of serum bilirubin and possibly methemalbumin. Extravascular hemolysis (typical of Rh antibodies) occurs primarily in the spleen, takes place more slowly, and may be limited by saturation of the reticuloendothelial system. Hyperbilirubinemia is the major laboratory abnormality.

The clinical symptoms associated with hemolytic transfusion reactions are highly variable and range in severity from death to shortened survival of the transfused cells unaccompanied by symptoms. The most frequent complaints are chills, fever, and aching in various parts of the body. Oliguria or anuria caused by acute renal failure may follow these symptoms or in some cases may be the first recognized sign that a hemolytic transfusion reaction has occurred. If the patient is under anesthesia, incompatible red cells may continue to be infused until the magnitude of the intravascular antigen-antibody reaction activates disseminated intravascular coagulation. Under anesthesia, then, generalized bleeding and an unexpected drop in blood pressure may be the first evidence of a hemolytic reaction.

Delayed hemolytic reactions may be recognized when the recipient receives a large volume of red cells containing an antigen to which he was previously immunized. The antibody may have become undetectable by the time of the current crossmatch and too weak to cause a reaction at the time of transfusion. Anamnestic increase in antibody concentration to high levels occurs with obvious effects five to ten days after transfusion. The recipient's hemoglobin falls rapidly, and he or she becomes jaundiced. At this point, the alloantibody is usually easily detectable.

When a hemolytic transfusion reaction is suspected, the transfusion must be stopped and the blood container and attached tubing returned to the laboratory accompanied by a new blood and urine sample from the patient. The laboratory will test for evidence that hemolysis has occurred, recheck the identity of all samples, and retest samples obtained before and after the reaction for evidence of incompatibility. If an antibody is identified, blood lacking the corresponding antigen may then be transfused.

The patient's fluid intake and output must be monitored, and he or she should be well hydrated, avoiding circulatory overload. If oliguria occurs, diuretics may be prescribed. The primary danger comes from rising serum potassium; therefore serial monitoring of electrolytes and electrocardiograms is mandatory. Dangerous levels of potassium may be combated by methods described in Ch. 77. Acute renal failure in these cases is self-limited, and full recovery can be expected, barring complications, if electrolytes remain under control at all points.

NONHEMOLYTIC FEBRILE TRANSFUSION REACTIONS. Febrile reactions to blood transfusions are far more likely to have been caused by recipient alloantibodies to donor leukocytes than to donor red cells. Alloantibodies to leukocytes develop at some time in at least 20 per cent of women as a result of pregnancy and in 70 to 90 per cent of multitransfused persons. Donor white cells reacting with recipient antibodies will cause a febrile response in proportion to the number of incompatible cells and the rate at which they are transfused.

Mild reactions cause fever alone. If the fever rises rapidly, shaking chills may occur. Severe reactions may be associated with vomiting and collapse. These reactions can be very uncomfortable but are unlikely to cause prolonged morbidity or mortality per se. The febrile response is completed within 12 hours.

If red cell incompatibility has been eliminated as the cause of the reaction, confirmation that white cells were responsible can be obtained by demonstrating antibodies to leukocytes in the serum of the recipient or by showing that the reactions can be prevented by transfusing leukocyte-poor red cells. If leukocyte-poor red cells fail to reduce symptoms adequately, frozen red cells should be tried.

CONTAMINATED BLOOD. Some bacteria are almost inevitably introduced into a small proportion of blood units collected for transfusion, but most fail to multiply at 4°C storage or are killed through the bactericidal effect of blood leukocytes and antibodies. The dangerous organisms are those which grow preferentially at 4°C. These are gram-negative rods which produce endotoxin. If blood heavily contaminated with endotoxin is transfused, shock, generalized bleeding, and death are almost inevitable. Confirmation of the diagnosis is accomplished by a Gram stain of the donor blood.

These contaminated blood reactions are extremely rare, and published reports suggest that many of them could have been prevented by inspection of the blood before transfusion. Contamination of a unit of blood should be suspected if the blood is of abnormal color, if there is evidence of excessive hemolysis, or if clots are readily demonstrable.

NONCARDIAC PULMONARY EDEMA. Rarely blood transfusion has been associated with sudden onset of dyspnea with radiologic evidence of pulmonary opacities. In many of these cases donor antibodies reacting with recipient leukocytes have been detected.

POST-TRANSFUSION THROMBOCYTOPENIC PURPURA. Thrombocytopenic purpura may occur suddenly seven to ten days after transfusion in association with recipient antibodies to donor platelets. In most cases the antibody has been anti-$P1^{A1}$, and the recipient has been a $P1^{A1}$-negative female with a history of pregnancies. The patient's own platelets are destroyed by mechanisms that are unclear, and the thrombocytopenia may last for a number of weeks. The most effective treatment has been plasma exchange, presumably through removal of the alloantibody to platelets.

TRANSMISSION OF DISEASE. *Hepatitis* remains the most serious unsolved problem in blood transfusion therapy. It is probable that clinically evident hepatitis follows at least 1 per cent of all transfusions and that ten times as many subclinical cases may occur. Hepatitis B has been greatly reduced by eliminating blood donors who are positive for HBsAg, but it still accounts for at least 10 per cent of post-transfusion cases. Unsuspected hepatitis A is unlikely in a healthy blood donor, because infection with this virus does not result in a chronic carrier state. Non-A non-B hepatitis accounts for almost all of the remaining 90 per cent of cases. Cytomegalovirus explains a minute percentage, and EB virus almost none.

Until the non-A non-B virus(es) is identified and tests to

detect it are available, post-transfusion hepatitis is best prevented by elimination of paid blood donors and other high-risk groups. Elimination of donor units either with anti-HBcAg or an increased level of alanine transferase may reduce the frequency of non-A, non-B post-transfusion hepatitis.

Malaria remains a rare but definite problem despite deferral of blood donors for three years if they have had malaria or have taken prophylaxis. A six-month deferral appears adequate if the donor had exposure to a malaria area but did not take prophylaxis. (Prophylaxis may only prolong the incubation period.)

Syphilis is rarely transmitted at present because of early detection and treatment of infected cases. Regulations still require a serologic test for syphilis on all blood donations, although it serves little purpose and unnecessarily excludes donors with biologic false-positive tests and with previous adequately treated syphilis.

Cytomegalovirus transmission by blood transfusion may have serious consequences in immunosuppressed patients such as premature newborn infants and marrow transplant recipients.

Acquired immunodeficiency syndrome (AIDS) may be transmitted by transfusion of whole blood, red blood cells, platelets, or plasma. The relatively rare occurrence of this complication is overshadowed by the public's concern about the high mortality of this disease. Recipients of clotting factor concentrates were at unusually high risk, but such concentrates are now heat treated to kill the AIDS virus. The risk of AIDS from blood transfusion has been reduced to very low levels by elimination of donors from groups at risk for AIDS and by testing all donations for antibody to the AIDS virus.

ALLERGIC REACTIONS. Urticaria may occur in as many as 3 to 5 per cent of transfusions but is rarely of serious concern and can usually be controlled or prevented by antihistamines. The very rare anaphylactoid reactions are characterized by flushing, tachycardia, wheezing, dyspnea, fall in blood pressure, and unconsciousness. One death has been reported. Most if not all such reactions are caused by recipient antibody to donor IgA globulin. Almost all of the involved recipients have no detectable IgA in their sera and have formed antibodies reacting with all IgA preparations (class specific). Rare persons with normal IgA have produced alloantibodies to an IgA allotype. IgA is absent from the serum of 1 in 900 blood donors; 25 to 50 per cent of these donors have antibodies to IgA. Anaphylactoid reactions are so rare in comparison as to suggest that most of the detected antibodies are not of clinical significance.

Patients with previous anaphylactoid reactions associated with anti-IgA should receive only blood products which lack IgA. Red blood cells can be washed free of plasma proteins. Plasma products should be from donors who lack IgA.

If an anaphylactoid reaction occurs, transfusion should be stopped and intravenous antihistamine given. In most cases, epinephrine and corticosteroids will also be required.

CIRCULATORY OVERLOAD. This is a common side effect of transfusion, especially serious if the patient is in danger of heart failure. The risk is minimized by the use of concentrated components. If the need for red cells is great but the patient is in heart failure, it may be advisable to remove blood from the recipient, discarding the plasma and returning the red cells supplemented with red cells from other donors.

AIR EMBOLISM. This is rarely a problem but if a large amount of air enters the bag as the transfusion set spike is inserted, subsequent external pressure on the bag can embolize air.

MASSIVE TRANSFUSION PROBLEMS. Transfused blood has been altered during collection and storage, and additional problems occur when the volume and rate of blood transfusion introduce abnormalities faster than they can be corrected by the recipient.

Bleeding tendency: Blood stored more than 24 hours is essentially devoid of viable platelets, and dilutional thrombocytopenia becomes possible after transfusion of a volume of blood more than one and a half to two times the blood volume of the recipient. Disseminated intravascular coagulation (DIC) is a frequent complication of conditions requiring massive transfusion. Restoration and maintenance of normal blood volume are essential prerequisites to control of DIC. It will usually be necessary to replace platelets (concentrates), fibrinogen (cryoprecipitates), and possibly other plasma coagulation factors (fresh-frozen plasma).

Citrate intoxication: Although depression of ionized calcium is inevitable when large amounts of citrated blood are rapidly transfused, the recipient has a number of compensating mechanisms. Correction of the hypocalcemia with intermittent intravenous calcium solutions is almost never necessary and may be dangerous.

Hypothermia is a serious risk when large volumes of cold blood are rapidly transfused. Ventricular fibrillation may result. This should be prevented by warming the blood either immediately prior to or during transfusion.

Microaggregates in stored blood can be removed during transfusion using special filters. However, there is no evidence that these filters are required for the usual small volume transfusions, and there is no agreement that microaggregates are harmful during massive transfusion.

Hyperkalemia and *acidosis* are primarily of concern in the transfusion of newborn infants. In fact, the massively transfused adult usually has a low plasma potassium level despite the increased levels of potassium in the plasma of the transfused blood.

GRAFT-VERSUS-HOST DISEASE (GVHD). This is a rare but increasingly recognized complication of blood transfusion. Engraftment of stem cells in the donor blood can result if the immunologic responses of the recipient are sufficiently impaired. Immunocompetent donor lymphoid cells are responsible for GVHD. Recipients with congenital deficiencies of T lymphocytes and those prepared for a marrow transplant are at greatest risk. Others at risk include some patients whose immune apparatus has been suppressed to more than the usual degree by antineoplastic therapy. The risk of engraftment increases with the number of mononuclear cells in the transfused blood component. Granulocyte concentrates appear to carry the highest risk.

The clinical signs of GVHD are nonspecific: dermatitis, gastrointestinal disturbances, and liver dysfunction. The best supportive evidence for GVHD is obtained by demonstrating that the recipient's blood carries genetic markers other than his or her own. HLA typing is most useful for this purpose.

Engraftment can be prevented by irradiating blood prior to transfusion. Doses of 1500 to 5000 rads are used and have no demonstrable effect on red cell viability or on platelet and granulocyte function. Except for patients with severe combined immunodeficiency disease and those prepared for marrow transplantation, the indications for irradiation of blood prior to transfusion are not well established.

SUMMARY. Blood transfusion is a very effective form of therapy but with potential serious side effects. Decisions to transfuse must always consider the risk-benefit ratio. The components prescribed must be appropriate for the indications and selected, when necessary, to avoid repetition of previous transfusion reactions.

The majority of complications of blood transfusion can be avoided by using the patient's own blood whenever possible. Autologous donations may be predeposited prior to elective surgery. Intraoperative salvage of extravasated blood can recover red cells for transfusion.

Mollison PL: Blood Transfusion in Clinical Medicine. 7th ed. Oxford, Blackwell Scientific Publications, 1983. *This is the "bible" of transfusion medicine, emphasizing the laboratory aspects. The answers to most of your questions can be found here; if you need more detailed information, Mollison has probably provided the references.*

Petz LD, Swisher SN: Clinical Practice of Blood Transfusion. New York, Churchill Livingstone, 1981. *This text addresses transfusion problems from the point of view of the clinician, providing not only the necessary background but also addressing specific clinical situations.*

148 FUNCTION OF NEUTROPHILS AND MONONUCLEAR PHAGOCYTES

Bernard M. Babior

Neutrophils and mononuclear phagocytes are essential components of the host defense system. Both are made in the bone marrow, and both accomplish most of their purposes through the act of eating (Gr. *phagein* to eat). Mononuclear phagocytes are versatile cells whose functions include the destruction of invading pathogens, the elimination of debris from the bloodstream and from sites of tissue damage, the remodeling of normal tissues, and the assignment of targets to lymphocytes. Neutrophils, on the other hand, are single-mindedly dedicated to the destruction of invading pathogens.

THE NEUTROPHIL

ORIGIN. Like other cells in the circulation, neutrophils originate from pluripotential stem cells that reside in the bone marrow. Depending on environmental influences, a pluripotential stem cell is capable of giving rise to the committed progenitors of any of the blood cells. Under the influence of a small group of peptides known as *colony-stimulating factors,* this stem cell will proliferate and differentiate to produce a population of neutrophils.

The route from a committed progenitor to a neutrophil involves a series of precursors, some of which can be recognized under the microscope. The earliest identifiable neutrophil precursor is a myeloblast, a relatively large cell with a rim of pale blue cytoplasm surrounding a large nucleus containing dispersed chromatin and multiple nucleoli. As the cell progresses through later stages of differentiation, the chromatin condenses and the nucleoli are lost, while at the same time the cytoplasm acquires its characteristic granules. The various neutrophil precursors are listed in Figure 148–1.

Through the myelocyte stage, neutrophil precursors divide as well as differentiate (Fig. 148–1). These proliferative forms are said to constitute the *mitotic compartment* of the neutrophil precursor pool. Later precursors, which do not divide, constitute the *nonmitotic compartment*. This is also called the *storage compartment,* because cells in this compartment can be released into the bloodstream in response to infections or other stresses. As a rule, the only elements released from the storage compartment are neutrophils and bands. If the stress is sufficiently severe, however, a few metamyelocytes may be liberated as well.

A newly committed stem cell requires approximately eight to ten days to become a mature neutrophil and enter the circulation. In the bloodstream, neutrophils are distributed about evenly between two rapidly exchanging pools: the *circulating pool,* composed of neutrophils suspended freely in the circulating blood, and the *marginated pool,* consisting of cells that have settled onto the endothelium of the capillaries and postcapillary venules. Once having entered the circulation, neutrophils leave for the tissues randomly and rapidly; their half time in the bloodstream is only six hours. In the tissues, however, the cells may sojourn for days.

STRUCTURE. The neutrophil is a terminally differentiated, nondividing cell that is well equipped to perform its function of killing microorganisms. The cell is packed with granules whose contents are used for the destruction and degradation of target microorganisms. The granules are of two types: *azurophil,* which contain proteases and other hydrolytic enzymes, a group of microbicidal peptides known as defensins, and a Cl^--oxidizing enzyme known as myeloperoxidase; and *specific,* which contain among other things a collagenase and an enzyme that releases C5a from the complement component C5. The nucleus is a vestigial structure that can no longer replicate its DNA. The plasma membrane contains an element of the neutrophil's killing apparatus as well as sensors that locate and identify the microorganisms against which the neutrophil acts. The cytoskeleton of the neutrophil is a complex system of tubes and fibers that is responsible for the orderly movement of this highly motile cell.

FUNCTION. Neutrophils undergo radical and abrupt changes in behavior in response to external stimuli. These changes include aggregation, degranulation (i.e., the discharge of granule contents through the plasma membrane), and the initiation of oxidant production. They are provoked by many stimuli, the most important of which are target microorganisms and chemotactic factors at high concentration (see below). These behavioral changes convert the neutrophil from a placid resident of the bloodstream to a powerful weapon. A cell that has undergone these changes is known as an *activated neutrophil.* The destruction of a microorganism by a neutrophil can be divided into three stages: finding the microorganism, ingesting it, and finally killing it and disposing of its remains.

Chemotaxis. The neutrophil finds its target through a chemical sense that enables the cell to detect certain substances known as *chemotactic factors.* These chemotactic factors are continuously released at sites where microorganisms have invaded tissues, diffusing away to set up a concentration gradient. Neutrophils in the circulation are able to sense this gradient and travel toward its source. They begin their journey by marginating on the capillary and postcapillary endothelium. They then migrate outward through the vessel walls, penetrating the subendothelial basement membrane by local digestion, presumably with collagenase. Once outside the

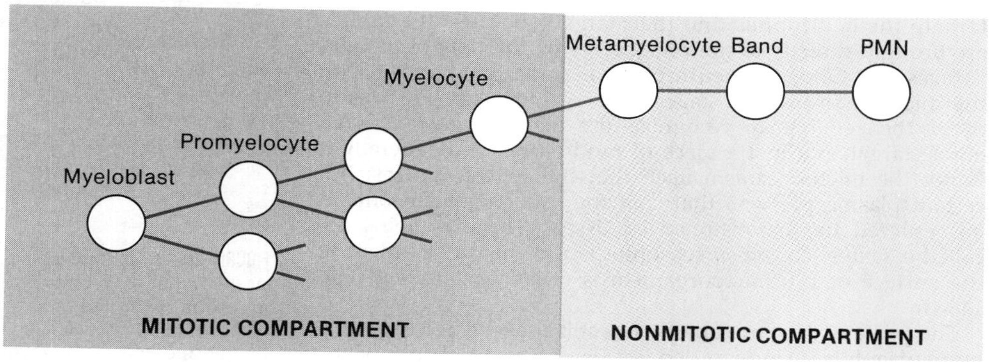

FIGURE 148–1. Neutrophil precursor pool.

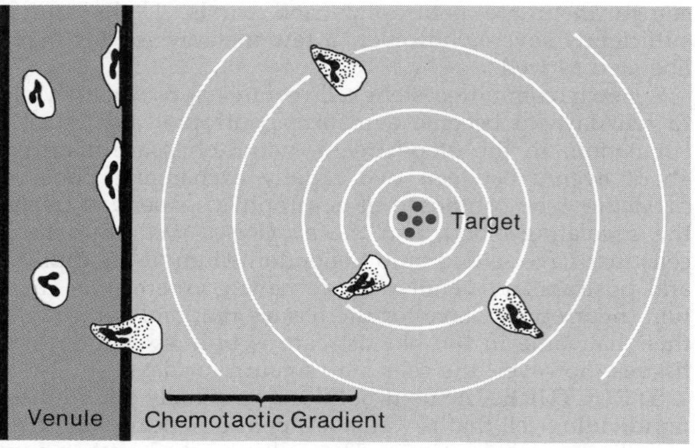

FIGURE 148–2. Chemotaxis. Neutrophils in the venule undergo margination in response to chemotactic factor, then leave the vessel by migrating between the endothelial cells (diapedesis) and travel up the chemotactic gradient toward the target.

capillaries, they continue their directed migration, eventually reaching the site of origin of chemotactic factors—that is, the region of tissue that has been invaded by microorganisms. This process of migrating up a chemical gradient toward the source of the chemical is known as *chemotaxis* (Fig. 148–2).

Neutrophils are able to respond to a very large number of chemotactic factors, but three appear to be of primary importance: (1) *N-formylated oligopeptides,* (2) the complement fragment *C5a,* and (3) a product of arachidonate oxidation known as *leukotriene* B_4 (LTB_4). These chemotactic factors are produced both by the invading microorganisms (N-formylated oligopeptides and C5a) and by the neutrophils themselves (C5a and LTB_4). N-formylated oligopeptides are intermediates in bacterial protein synthesis and are released from bacteria that have been damaged or killed. C5a is produced by the complement system when it interacts with microorganisms and also by activated neutrophils through the release of the C5-splitting enzyme of the specific granules. LTB_4 is also produced by activated neutrophils, which manufacture it by liberating and oxidizing arachidonic acid from endogenous phospholipids. The production of C5a and LTB_4 by activated neutrophils lends a self-reinforcing character to the process of chemotaxis, since neutrophils that have arrived at a site of inflammation are activated to generate chemotactic factors that attract more neutrophils to the inflamed region.

Bacteria in the circulation are thought to be handled primarily by the mononuclear phagocytes (see below). Neutrophils, however, may play a role in clearing the circulation of microorganisms that enter the bloodstream suddenly and in large numbers. During such episodes of bacteremia, the complement system is activated, releasing C5a into the circulation. Neutrophils react to this pulse of C5a by marginating in the pulmonary capillaries where they may act temporarily (15 to 30 minutes) as a filtration system, removing microorganisms from the blood as they pass through the pulmonary circulation. In this special situation, chemotaxis is not needed to help the neutrophils find their targets, because the targets are brought directly to the phagocytes by the flow of blood.

Ingestion. Once the neutrophil has come into contact with the microorganism, the stage is set for ingestion. For this to occur the cell has to recognize the microorganisms as an edible target, not just a piece of random debris. Generally it is not the microorganism itself that the cell recognizes, but certain plasma proteins that coat the microorganism once it has entered the bloodstream or tissue. These proteins are called *opsonins* (Gr. *opson* seasoning), and their attachment to the surface of the microorganism is called *opsonization* (Fig. 148–3).

The proteins that are able to opsonize targets for ingestion by neutrophils include antibodies belonging to certain of the IgG subclasses (opsonizing antibodies) and the complement component C3b. Opsonizing antibodies bind to the microbial surface by means of a simple antigen-antibody reaction. C3b binds to the microbial surface by a more complex process that involves the activation of the complement system through either the classic pathway (initiated by the antigen-antibody complex) or the alternative pathway (initiated by certain complex carbohydrates found on microbial surfaces) (see Ch. 418). One of the steps in complement activation by either of these pathways is the cleavage of component C3 into two pieces: C3a, a small fragment that induces capillaries and venules to dilate and become leaky, and C3b, the large opsonizing fragment. Immediately upon release, this opsonizing fragment locks onto the target through a covalent bond. The opsonized target then attaches to the neutrophil surface by means of these opsonins, which are recognized and bound by receptors in the neutrophil membrane: the Fc receptors, which recognize complexes between antigen and opsonizing antibody, and the C3 receptors, which recognize particle-associated C3b.

The attachment of the target to the neutrophil surface is the signal for ingestion (Fig. 148–4). The membrane in the region of the attached particle invaginates into the cell, carrying the particle in with it. When the particle is fully internalized, the invagination closes at its neck to form a vesicle, which detaches from the inner surface of the cell membrane and is released into the cytoplasm of the neutrophil. The end result of the phagocytic event is that a particle initially attached to the surface of the neutrophil is translocated to the cell's interior enclosed in a vesicle lined with what was originally a portion of the neutrophil plasma membrane. This vesicle, known as the *phagocytic vesicle,* is the site of killing of the ingested organism.

Killing. Killing involves two separate actions on the part of the neutrophils: *degranulation* and the *activation of the respiratory burst.* Degranulation refers to a process whereby the granule membrane fuses with another cellular membrane, releasing the granule contents into the compartment on the opposite side of the other membrane (Fig. 148–5). In the case of azurophil granules, degranulation occurs almost exclusively into the phagocytic vesicles, so that the actions of the azurophil granule contents are directed almost entirely against the ingested microorganism. Specific granules degranulate into both the phagocytic vesicles and the external environment, so their contents exert effects exterior to the neutrophils as well as on the ingested microorganisms. Some of the constituents of each of these granules are listed in Table 148–1, together with their actions.

The *respiratory burst* refers to a sequence of metabolic events the purpose of which is the production of potent microbicidal oxidants through the partial reduction of oxygen. The burst

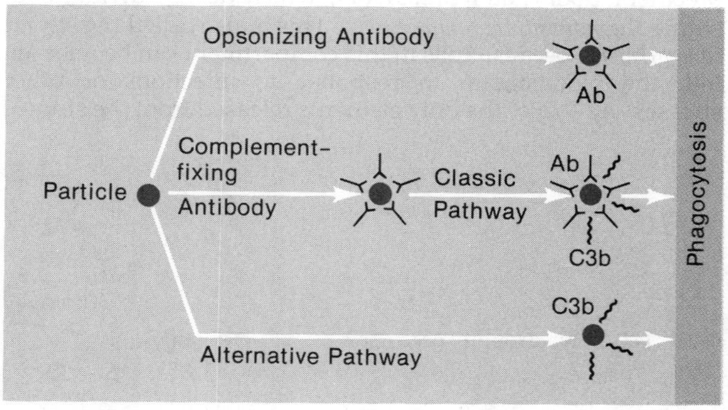

FIGURE 148–3. Opsonization. The coating of a particle by a plasma protein that is recognized by neutrophil receptors as a signal for ingestion is termed *opsonization.* Two classes of proteins are capable of opsonizing particles for ingestion by neutrophils: opsonizing antibodies and complement component C3b.

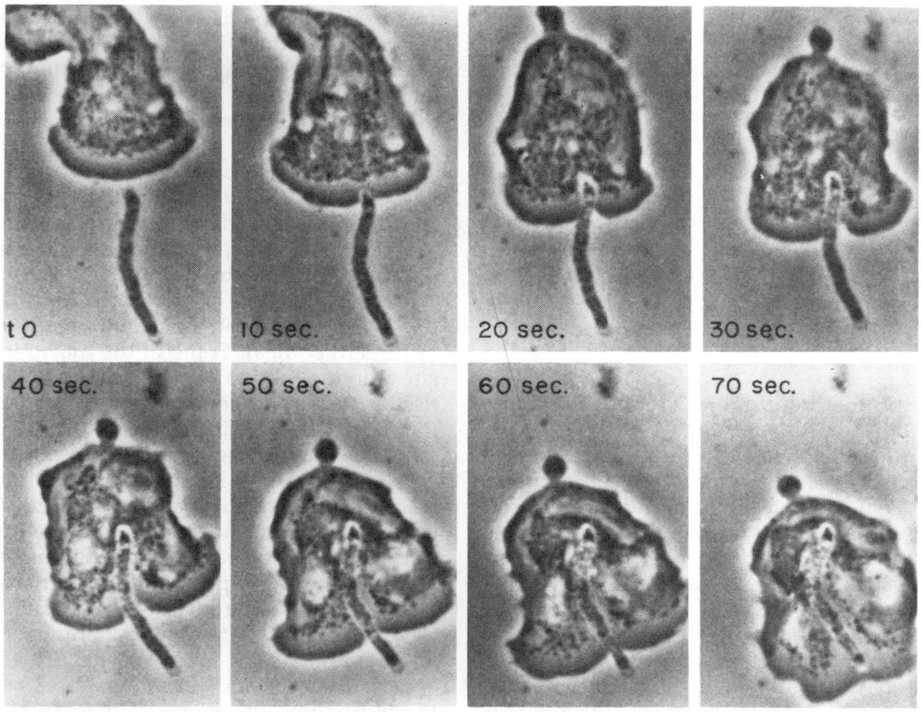

FIGURE 148–4. Ingestion of a target microorganism by a neutrophil. (Reproduced from Hirsch JG: Cinemicrophotographic observations of granule lysis in polymorphonuclear leucocytes during phagocytosis. J Exp Med 116:827, 1962, by copyright permission of the Rockefeller University Press.)

is activated by the same stimuli that provoke degranulation of the specific granules—primarily contact with ingestible particles and exposure to chemotactic factors at high concentrations. These stimuli activate a plasma membrane-bound oxidase dormant in resting cells that catalyzes the one-electron reduction of oxygen to superoxide (O_2^-) at the expense of NADPH (Fig. 148–6). Most of the O_2^- reacts with itself to yield H_2O_2, while at the same time NADPH is regenerated by way of the hexosemonophosphate shunt. These events have nothing to do with respiration as it is usually understood, but they acquired the name *respiratory burst* because of the large increase in neutrophil oxygen uptake that is associated with their onset.

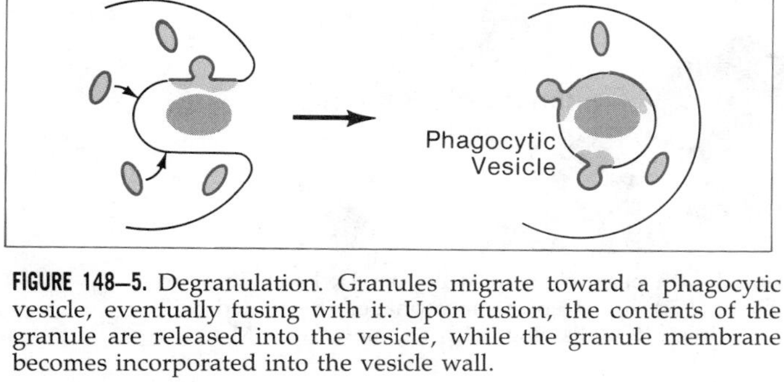

FIGURE 148–5. Degranulation. Granules migrate toward a phagocytic vesicle, eventually fusing with it. Upon fusion, the contents of the granule are released into the vesicle, while the granule membrane becomes incorporated into the vesicle wall.

The microbicidal oxidants are derived from the H_2O_2: (1) A portion of the H_2O_2 is used to oxidize Cl^- to the highly microbicidal hypochlorite ion (OCl^-), a reaction catalyzed by myeloperoxidase, an enzyme delivered into the phagocytic vesicle from the azurophil granules. (2) Another portion of the H_2O_2 is converted to the exceedingly reactive hydroxyl radical (OH•) in a metal-catalyzed reaction with O_2^-. These and related oxidants attack and kill ingested microorganisms by oxidizing their cellular constituents.

MONONUCLEAR PHAGOCYTES

Mononuclear phagocytes and neutrophils are closely related. Both are descended from the same ancestor, and both share many functions, including the unusual ability to ingest particles as large as half or more their own diameter. There

TABLE 148–1. CONTENTS OF NEUTROPHIL GRANULES

Component	Function
I. Azurophil granules	
Acid hydrolases (glycosidases, phospholipases, acid proteases)	Degradation of ingested material
Neutral proteases (cathepsin G, elastase)	Destruction of inflamed tissue?
Lysozyme	Digestion of bacterial cell wall
Defensins	Oxygen-independent bacterial killing
Myeloperoxidase	Oxygen-dependent bacterial killing
II. Specific granules	
Lysozyme	Digestion of bacterial cell wall
Cobalamin-binding protein	Binding of bacterial cobalamin analogues
Apolactoferrin	Binding of free iron, control of granulopoiesis
Collagenase	Digestion of connective tissue
C5-splitting enzyme	Release of C5a
III. Indeterminate	
Bactericidal/permeability-increasing protein	Killing of gram-negative bacteria

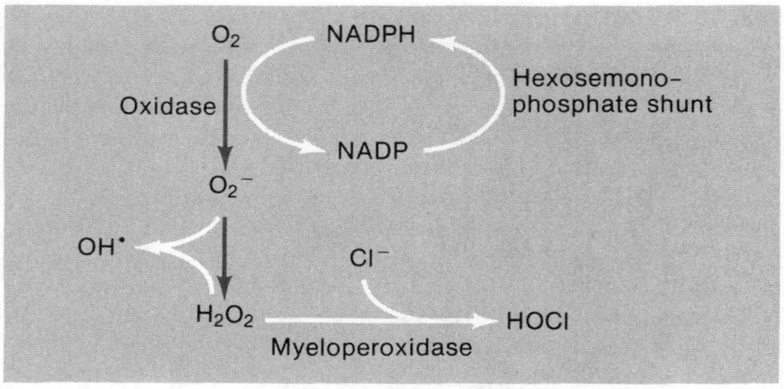

FIGURE 148–6. The respiratory burst.

is, however, only one type of neutrophil, whereas there are many varieties of mononuclear phagocytes.

ORIGIN. All mononuclear phagocytes are derived from a single circulating precursor: the monocyte. This cell and the neutrophil both arise from a single pluripotential stem cell. In the course of differentiation, this stem cell first makes a general commitment to the phagocyte lineage. Later its descendants commit themselves further, some to the neutrophil and others to the monocyte line.

In the monocyte line, the first recognizable precursor is the *monoblast*. In normal marrow, this cell is indistinguishable from a myeloblast; it can be identified, however, in marrow from patients with monocytic leukemia. The next stage is the *promonocyte*, a somewhat larger cell with cytoplasmic granules and an indented nucleus containing finely divided chromatin. Finally, the fully developed *monocyte* appears. It requires about five days to go from a monoblast to a mature circulating monocyte.

STRUCTURE AND FURTHER DIFFERENTIATION. Larger than the neutrophil, and with a large horseshoe-shaped nucleus containing dispersed chromatin, the mature monocyte has cytoplasm that is filled with granules whose contents include hydrolytic enzymes and other proteins necessary for the cell's activities. Unlike the neutrophil, the monocyte seems to have retained a limited capacity to divide and in addition is able to undergo considerable further differentiation.

Monocytes are able to diversify into the many types of cells that constitute the mononuclear phagocyte system. Monocytes circulate in the bloodstream for a time ($t\frac{1}{2}\sim12$ hours) and then enter the tissue, where they differentiate into mature macrophages that live for weeks to months. The properties of these macrophages are characteristic for the tissues in which they reside. Those in the liver, for example, are the Kupffer cells, spidery phagocytes that bridge the sinusoids separating adjacent plates of hepatocytes (Fig. 148–7*A*). Those in the lungs are the large ellipsoidal alveolar macrophages (Fig. 148–7*B*). These and other tissue macrophages are listed in Table 148–2. Little is known about the factors responsible for the various patterns of mononuclear phagocyte differentiation seen in different tissues.

Macrophages are important components of the inflammatory reactions elicited by noxious agents (e.g., microorganisms or foreign bodies). Some of the macrophages that appear at a site of inflammation have been recruited from the surrounding tissues, while others are derived from monocytes that have migrated there from the bloodstream. Once at the inflamed site, the macrophages are exposed to certain stimuli (e.g., *gamma-interferon*, a T lymphocyte product formerly known as macrophage-activating factor, and *lipopolysaccharide*, from the cell walls of gram-negative organisms) which induce them to undergo a sequence of functional and morphologic changes whose purpose appears to be to enable them to deal more effectively with the inciting agent. Initially the cells increase in size, accumulate many new granules, and begin to secrete large quantities of certain specific proteases, including collagenase, elastase, and plasminogen activator, a component of the fibrinolytic system (see Ch. 157). Their capacity for phagocytosis is increased, as is their ability to degrade ingested material. The cells become stickier and more motile and develop the ability to manufacture lethal oxidizing agents. Most important, their microbicidal power is greatly increased, with the result that they become capable of killing pathogens that they were unable to deal with in their former state. Cells that have attained this heightened degree of microbicidal potency are known as *activated macrophages*.

If the inciting agent has not been eliminated within the first few days, the activated phagocytes begin to aggregate into a granuloma. Continued stimulation leads to additional growth of the aggregated cells and further augmentation in secretory capacity; the phagocytes have now turned into epithelioid cells, the characteristic constituents of mature granulomas. Eventually giant cells appear, arising through the fusion of epithelioid cells with each other and with newly arrived macrophages. With the elimination of the inciting agent, the

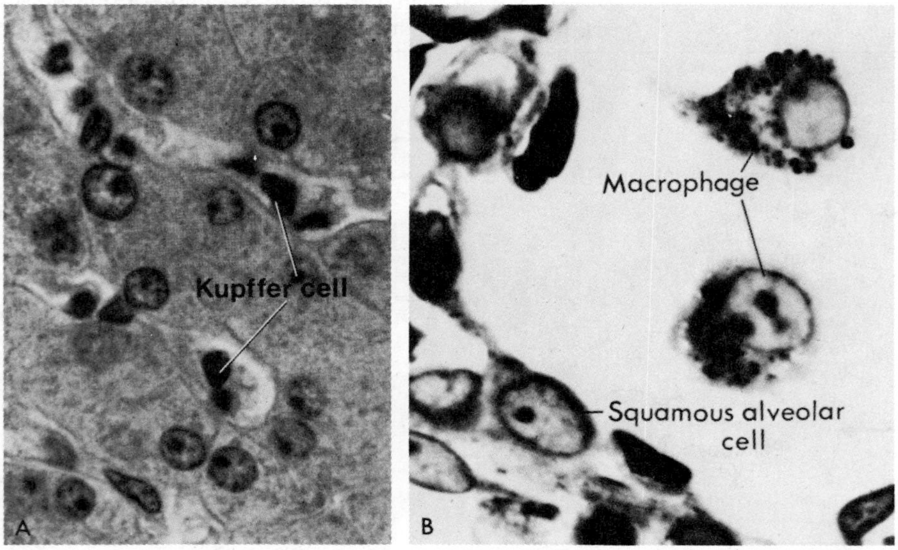

FIGURE 148–7. Some tissue macrophages. *A*, Kupffer cell. (Reprinted with permission from Popper H: Liver Structure and Function. New York, McGraw-Hill Book Company, 1957, p 97.) *B*, Alveolar macrophage. (Reprinted with permission from Sorokin SP: The respiratory system. In Weiss L, Greep RO: Histology. 4th ed. New York, McGraw-Hill Book Company, 1977, p 765.)

TABLE 148–2. TISSUE MACROPHAGES

- Fixed
  - Kupffer cells
  - Microglial cells (central nervous system)
  - Macrophages of spleen, lymph nodes, and bone marrow sinusoids
  - Mesangial cells (kidney)
  - Osteoclasts
- Wandering
  - Macrophages of serosal cavities (pleural, peritoneal, pericardial)
  - Alveolar macrophages

inflammatory process resolves and the macrophages disappear. What becomes of them is not known.

FUNCTIONS. Mononuclear phagocytes carry out three basic functions: secretion, ingestion, and interaction with lymphocytes.

Secretion. Mononuclear phagocytes secrete into the extracellular environment a large number of substances, some protein and others nonprotein in nature (Table 148–3). Lysozyme is secreted by mononuclear phagocytes regardless of their state of activation, whereas proteases active at neutral pH ("neutral proteases") are secreted only by activated cells. Other substances such as O_2^- (superoxide) and leukotrienes are secreted under even more specialized circumstances.

Ingestion. Mononuclear phagocytes received their name from their ability to ingest. These cells use the ability for two separate purposes: to eliminate waste and debris (scavenging) and to kill invading pathogens.

SCAVENGING. Mononuclear phagocytes play a highly important role as general scavengers. They dispose of effete or worn-out cells, remove foreign material from the bloodstream, and clean up debris at sites of infection or tissue damage.

Cell disposal by mononuclear phagocytes is best exemplified by their role in the elimination of outdated red cells. These red cells develop a "senescence antigen" that is recognized by an opsonizing antibody in the circulation. The opsonized cells are then eliminated by splenic macrophages, which internalize and degrade them by a process of phagocytosis, degranulation, and digestion similar to that described for neutrophils. The hemoglobin is converted to bilirubin, iron, and amino acids by lysosomal proteases and other enzymes as described in Ch. 118, while the lipids and complex carbohydrates of the red cell membrane are degraded by lysosomal lipases and glycosidases. Other effete cells are presumably dealt with in a similar manner.

Foreign material is removed from the bloodstream primarily by mononuclear phagocytes in the liver and spleen. In these two organs, the blood is forced to flow through a dense network of mononuclear phagocytes, which ingest foreign matter encountered in the stream. Bacteria and bacterial breakdown products (e.g., lipopolysaccharide) that enter the bloodstream from the large intestine are removed principally by the Kupffer cells of the liver, because these are the first mononuclear phagocytes encountered by the gastrointestinal venous drainage.

Dead cells and tissue fragments are presumably ingested and degraded at sites of infection or tissue damage by macrophages recruited to the damaged area. Ingestion may be aided by circulating fibronectin, a plasma protein that is able to opsonize denatured collagen for phagocytosis by macrophages. The activated macrophages secrete into the environment neutral proteases that are able to break down damaged connective tissue (collagenase, elastase) and fibrin mesh (plasminogen activator), clearing the way for the reconstruction of the injured tissues.

Mononuclear phagocytes also eliminate from the circulation denatured proteins, protein fragments, and certain native proteins (e.g., activated clotting factors). Some proteins are eliminated through *pinocytosis*, a process in which the material to be eliminated is taken into the cell along with a minuscule quantity of plasma via a tiny invagination of the cell membrane that buds off and enters the cytoplasm as a pinocytotic vesicle. (Mononuclear phagocytes are constantly engaged in pinocytosis; they take in and process several times their own volume of plasma every day.) Other proteins are eliminated by *receptor-mediated endocytosis*, a process similar to pinocytosis except that the ingested protein is bound to a surface receptor before internalization. The lipids of atherosclerotic lesions are derived in part from lipoproteins that had been taken into macrophages by receptor-mediated endocytosis.

KILLING. Like neutrophils, mononuclear phagocytes are able to kill invading microorganisms. Killing by both types of phagocytes involves the same general sequence of events—an initial encounter between the phagocyte and the target microorganism, ingestion, and finally the destruction of the target—but the events differ in detail between the two cell types. Neutrophils, for example, generally find their targets by migrating up a chemotactic gradient, while many mononuclear phagocytes (the fixed tissue varieties such as Kupffer cells and splenic macrophages) have their targets brought to them by the bloodstream. Those mononuclear phagocytes that find their targets by chemotaxis (e.g., monocytes) respond to a wider variety of attractants than neutrophils do. Monocytes, for instance, are attracted by lymphocyte-generated chemotactic factors that have no effect on neutrophils. With respect to ingestion, mononuclear phagocytes can take up particles opsonized by IgE as well as IgG; neutrophils will take up only the latter. Mononuclear phagocytes are also equipped with a mannose receptor that enables them to take up certain bacteria and other particles without the need for opsonization. As to microbial killing, mononuclear phagocytes lose their myeloperoxidase as they develop from monocytes into macrophages, so that oxygen-dependent killing by mature macrophages is accomplished by oxidants that can be generated in the absence of myeloperoxidase (e.g., hydroxyl radical).

Mononuclear phagocytes play a particularly important role in defending against nonviral pathogens that live and grow intracellularly (Table 148–4). For the destruction of these pathogens, macrophage activation is critical. The pathogens are readily killed by activated macrophages, but they are able to infect and multiply within unactivated macrophages, eventually killing them and spreading to infect fresh macrophages. Little is known about how the pathogens evade the microbicidal system of the unactivated macrophages.

TABLE 148–3. SUBSTANCES SECRETED BY MACROPHAGES

Substance	State of Macrophage	Additional Stimulus Needed
Lysozyme	Resident, activated	None
Neutral proteases	Activated	None
Collagenase		
Elastase		
Plasminogen activator		
Interleukin 1	Resident, activated	Lymphokine, endotoxin, others
Superoxide	Activated	Contact with particles or appropriate soluble stimulus
Leukotrienes	Resident, activated	
Complement components		

TABLE 148–4. INTRACELLULAR PATHOGENS AGAINST WHICH MACROPHAGES PLAY A SPECIAL ROLE

- Bacteria
  - *Brucella*
  - *Listeria*
  - *Legionella*
  - *Salmonella*
- Mycobacteria and systemic fungi
  - *Coccidioides immitis*
  - *Histoplasma capsulatum*
  - *Mycobacterium tuberculosis*
  - Others
- *Chlamydia*
- *Rickettsia*
- Protozoan parasites
  - *Leishmania*
  - *Trypanosoma*
  - *Toxoplasma*

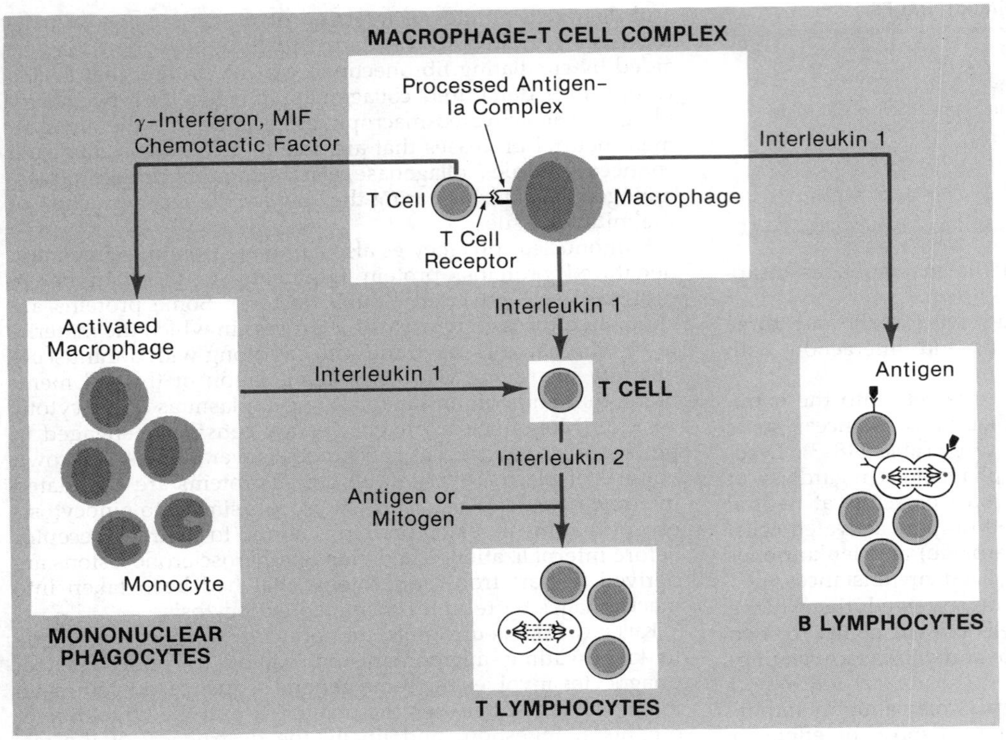

FIGURE 148–8. Macrophage-lymphocyte interactions. The macrophage, acting in its capacity as an "accessory cell," presents antigen to a T cell equipped with specific receptors that recognize the Ia-antigen complex on the macrophage surface. The T cell to which the antigen has been presented undergoes activation and begins to secrete lymphokines. These lymphokines include γ-interferon, macrophage-immobilizing factor (MIF), and monocyte chemotactic factor; they cause macrophages to accumulate and undergo activation at the site of the initial macrophage–T cell interaction. Macrophages so activated secrete interleukin 1, a potent mediator capable among other things of inducing the proliferation of both B and T lymphocytes. B cells are directly stimulated by interleukin 1 to proliferate and to differentiate into antibody-secreting plasma cells. T cells, however, proliferate under the influence of a mediator known as interleukin 2 (T cell growth factor), itself a T cell product; interleukin 1 promotes the proliferation of T lymphocytes indirectly by inducing them to secrete interleukin 2.

Mononuclear phagocytes, particularly activated macrophages, are also able to kill malignant cells in vitro. The extent to which they perform this antitumor function in vivo is unknown.

Interactions Between Mononuclear Phagocytes and Lymphocytes. The activation of mononuclear phagocytes by gamma-interferon is one of a series of mutually potentiating interactions between mononuclear phagocytes and lymphocytes that take place at sites of inflammation (Fig. 148–8). Both T cells and B cells participate in these interactions.

The interaction with T lymphocytes begins with a particular type of physical encounter between a T cell and a mononuclear phagocyte. When an antigen-bearing particle is ingested by a mononuclear phagocyte, the antigen is for the most part completely destroyed. A small portion of the antigen, however, is processed to fragments that appear on the surface of the cell in association with the class II histocompatibility antigen known as Ia (the Ia antigen is one of the products of the major histocompatibility complex [see Ch. 417] that controls immune responses to such challenges as foreign proteins, virally infected cells, and tissue allografts). If a T lymphocyte bearing an appropriate receptor should encounter this antigen-primed mononuclear phagocyte, it will recognize the antigen-Ia complex and bind to the phagocyte, and both cells will begin to secrete immunologic mediators. In this interaction, the mononuclear phagocyte is referred to as an *accessory cell* and is said to have "presented" the antigen to the lymphocyte.

The immunologic mediators secreted by the T lymphocytes are called *lymphokines*. They include gamma-interferon, macrophage inhibitory factor, and monocyte chemotactic factor. Their net effect is to cause the accumulation and activation of mononuclear phagocytes in the region where the initial interaction took place between the antigen-bearing phagocyte and its complementary T lymphocyte. Mediators secreted by mononuclear phagocytes are known as *monokines*. One of these is called *interleukin 1;* among its other effects (for a list, see Table 148–5), it stimulates the proliferation of T lympho-

TABLE 148–5. SOME ACTIONS OF INTERLEUKIN 1

Site of Action	Effect
T lymphocytes	Secretion of interleukin 2 (T cell growth factor)
B lymphocytes	Proliferation, secretion of immunoglobulins
Hepatocytes	Production of acute-phase reactants
Hypothalamus	Fever
Muscle	Catabolism of protein

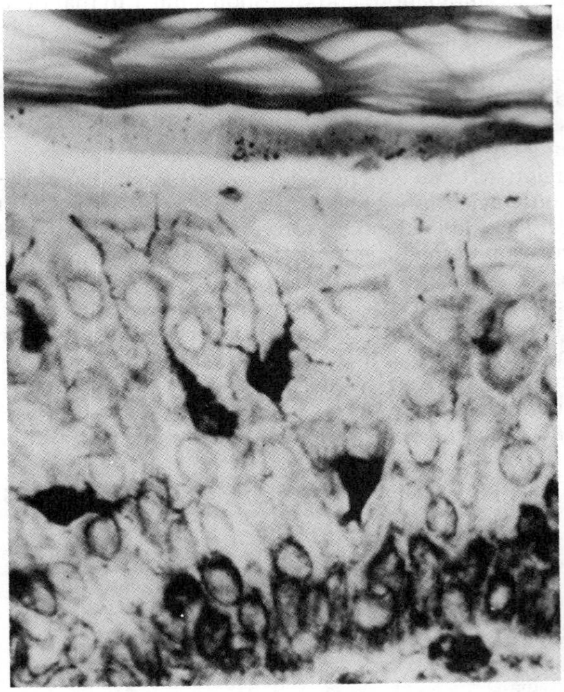

FIGURE 148–9. Langerhans cells in the skin. The darkly stained cells in the acanthocyte layer are the Langerhans cells. Their characteristic branching dendrites are easily seen. (Reproduced with permission from Breathnach AS, Wolff K: Structure and development of the skin. In Fitzgerald TB, Eisen AZ, Wolff K, et al.: Dermatology in General Medicine. 2nd ed. New York, McGraw-Hill Book Company, 1979, p 56.)

cytes indirectly by causing them to secrete *interleukin 2* (also known as T cell growth factor), a substance that promotes their own growth. Another monokine, called *cachectin* or *tumor necrosis factor,* may be responsible for the weight loss seen in patients with chronic wasting illnesses such as tuberculosis and certain forms of cancer.

Macrophages also act upon B lymphocytes. They are not needed for the presentation of antigen to B cells, because B lymphocytes carry surface immunoglobulins that directly recognize the antigens against which the cells are programmed. Rather, the macrophages exert their effects after the antigen-recognition step. They operate through interleukin 1, which they secrete and which causes the antigen-primed B cells to proliferate and differentiate into antibody-secreting plasma cells.

Dendritic Cells. Antigens also appear to be presented by *dendritic cells.* These cells are widely distributed, being found in the follicles of the lymph nodes and spleen, in the thymus, and in the skin, where they are known as *Langerhans' cells* (Fig. 148–9). Like the antigen-presenting class of mononuclear phagocytes, they carry the Ia antigen on their surfaces. They are, however, incapable of phagocytosis. Their role in antigen presentation is not clear, in particular whether they present new antigens or participate only in anamnestic responses and immunologic memory.

Adams DO, Hamilton TA: The cell biology of macrophage activation. Annu Rev Immunol 2:283, 1984. *A complete and clearly written review of this sometimes confusing topic.*

Gallin JI, Fauci AS (eds.): Advances in Host Defense Mechanisms. New York, Raven Press, 1982, vol 1: Phagocytic Cells. *A compilation of authoritative articles on many aspects of phagocyte function. Neutrophils, eosinophils, and mononuclear phagocytes are discussed.*

Ganz T, Selsted ME, Szklarnek D, et al.: Defensins. Natural peptide antibiotics of human neutrophils. J Clin Invest 76:1427, 1985. *The structure and properties of these recently discovered antimicrobial agents.*

Metcalf D: The molecular biology and functions of the granulocyte-macrophage colony-stimulating factors. Blood 67:257, 1986. *An up-to-date survey of this rapidly moving field.*

Steinman RM: Dendritic cells. Transplantation 31:151, 1981. *A short review of dendritic cell structure and function.*

Unanue ER: Cooperation between mononuclear phagocytes and lymphocytes in immunity. N Engl J Med 303:977, 1980. *A concise discussion of the interactions between macrophages and lymphocytes.*

Unanue ER: Antigen presenting function of the macrophage. Annu Rev Immunol 2:395, 1984. *Recent developments in this area, including current views of antigen processing.*

Williams GT, Williams WJ: Granulomatous inflammation: A review. J Clin Pathol 36:723, 1983. *An excellent review of the development and function of granuloma.*

149 DISORDERS OF NEUTROPHIL FUNCTION

Bernard M. Babior

Disorders of neutrophil function are relatively common. For the most part, they are minor manifestations of systemic diseases, rarely diagnosed and of little clinical significance. There are a few disorders, however, in which neutrophil function is defective enough to lead to serious clinical problems. Most of these are inherited disorders in which particular elements of neutrophil function are almost totally deficient.

The principal clinical manifestation of a serious disorder of neutrophil function is the repeated occurrence of major bacterial infections in the affected patient. Such recurrent bacterial infections are most commonly associated with severe neutropenia (<500 neutrophils per cubic millimeter) or an abnormality affecting the immunoglobulins or complement components. In an occasional patient, however, repeated bacterial infections cannot be accounted for by abnormalities in the neutrophil count, the immunoglobulins, or the complement system. In such a patient, a qualitative abnormality in neutrophil function is likely to be at the root of the problem.

TABLE 149–1. SCREENING FOR ABNORMALITIES OF NEUTROPHIL FUNCTION

Examination of blood film
Rebuck skin window test
NBT test
Special stains: myeloperoxidase, alkaline phosphatase

EVALUATING NEUTROPHIL FUNCTION

A complete evaluation of neutrophil function, including motility, granule content and function, respiratory burst activity, and bacterial killing, requires the services of a specialized laboratory. Screening for functional abnormalities, however, can be carried out relatively simply (Table 149–1). Morphologic abnormalities such as the large malformed granules of Chédiak-Higashi disease can be detected by *examination of a blood film* under the microscope. Chemotaxis and locomotion can be estimated by means of a *Rebuck skin window,* a test in which migration of phagocytes onto a glass coverslip applied to a superficial abrasion is measured over time. The respiratory burst is evaluated by the *NBT test,* in which cells attached to a glass slide are activated in the presence of nitroblue tetrazolium (NBT), a dye that precipitates as a mass of deep blue granules onto any cell that is engaged in the production of O_2^- (superoxide). Neutrophil enzymes can be detected by *special stains for myeloperoxidase and alkaline phosphatase.* One or more of these tests will be abnormal in most symptomatic disorders of neutrophil function.

ACQUIRED DISORDERS

In acquired disorders of neutrophils, functional abnormalities are generally incomplete. Accordingly, signs and symptoms due to neutrophil dysfunction are uncommon in these conditions.

ADHESION (Table 149–2). In the normal course of events, neutrophils undergo frequent alterations in their adhesiveness. These alterations are often expressed as changes in the size of the marginated pool (see Ch. 148). *Corticosteroids* and *epinephrine* reduce neutrophil adhesiveness, releasing the cells from the marginated pool into the circulating pool. Conversely, C5a or agents that cause the release of C5a (e.g., an episode of gram-negative bacteremia) increase neutrophil adhesiveness, causing cells to aggregate into clumps. These tend to be trapped in small vessels, particularly in the lungs.

Besides costicosteroids and epinephrine, certain drugs, notably *aspirin* and *alcohol,* cause decreased adhesiveness of neutrophils. With these agents the decrease in adhesiveness is apparent on testing in vitro, but is not associated with demargination. Evidently neutrophil adhesiveness covers a broader range of functions than merely the ability to attach to an endothelial cell.

In patients undergoing *hemodialysis,* neutrophil counts fall sharply, rising a few minutes later to values that exceed the predialysis counts. Pulmonary symptoms may accompany these changes in neutrophil counts. The fall in the neutrophil count and the accompanying pulmonary symptoms occur because C5a is released when the complement system is

TABLE 149–2. ACQUIRED ALTERATIONS OF NEUTROPHIL ADHESIVENESS

1. Decreased adhesiveness
   - A. With demargination
     - Corticosteroids
     - Epinephrine
   - B. Without demargination
     - Aspirin
     - Alcohol
2. Increased adhesiveness
   - A. Bacteremia
   - B. Hemodialysis

TABLE 149–3. CONDITIONS ASSOCIATED WITH DEPRESSED NEUTROPHIL CHEMOTAXIS

Diabetes mellitus	Anergy
Uremia	Hodgkin's disease
Cirrhosis of liver	Leprosy
Severe burns	Sarcoidosis
Bacterial infections	Hypophosphatemia
	Neonates

activated by the passage of blood over the dialysis membrane, causing neutrophils to marginate and be trapped in the lungs. The subsequent neutrophilia reflects the release of cells from the marrow storage pool, possibly another effect of complement activation.

CHEMOTAXIS. Depressed neutrophil chemotaxis is seen in a large number of conditions (Table 149–3). In some of these conditions, chemotactic depression is caused by a circulating inhibitor, while in others the neutrophils themselves are defective. These chemotactic abnormalities contribute in only a minor way to the decreased resistance to bacterial infections characteristic of many of these disorders.

MYELOGENOUS LEUKEMIA AND MYELODYSPLASIA. Variable functional abnormalities are seen in neutrophils from patients with these conditions. Cells in chronic myelogenous leukemia are very sluggish, showing markedly reduced motility and chemotaxis. Granules are often abnormal in number and type (specific granules, for example, may be absent), the respiratory burst is frequently attenuated, and bacterial killing may be depressed. These cells, however, make up in numbers what they lack in function, so infections are unusual in patients with chronic myelogenous leukemia.

In patients with *acute myelogenous leukemia,* neutrophils may arise from residual normal stem cells or by differentiation of the leukemic clone; in the latter case, the neutrophils may show abnormalities similar to those seen in chronic myelogenous leukemia. *Myelodysplasia* is a disease in which hematopoiesis is taken over by a nonmalignant but defective stem cell that gives rise to inadequate numbers of functionally abnormal blood cells. Bilobed nuclei (pseudo Pelger-Huët anomaly) and abnormal granulation are typical of myelodysplastic neutrophils. In both acute myelogenous leukemia and myelodysplasia, bacterial infections are frequent, but their frequency is due more to neutropenia than to functional abnormalities of the phagocytes.

CONGENITAL DISORDERS

CHRONIC GRANULOMATOUS DISEASE. Chronic granulomatous disease (CGD) is the name given to a family of inherited disorders in which phagocytes are unable to express a respiratory burst (Ch. 148). Most cases of the disease are transmitted in an X-linked fashion, but a substantial minority have an autosomal recessive pattern of inheritance. The disorder is caused by a gross impairment in the function of the O_2^--forming NADPH oxidase, whose activity is profoundly reduced in cells from patients with CGD. In some patients the biochemical lesion responsible for the impairment in oxidase activity is in the enzyme itself, while in other patients the lesion affects the system that activates the enzyme. It has not yet been possible to correlate the biochemical lesion with the mode of inheritance of the disorder.

Clinical Picture. The clinical picture of CGD is one of recurrent severe bacterial infections that are slow to heal and difficult to treat. The infections include sinusitis, pneumonia, and abscesses that usually involve the deep subcutaneous tissues, lymph nodes, or liver. Infections generally begin in infancy or early childhood, although the disease is occasionally detected in adolescence or later. In its unmodified form, the course of CGD is characterized by frequent hospitalizations for repeated and protracted infections caused by bacteria that the defective phagocytes are unable to kill (mostly *Staphylococcus aureus* and enterobacteria), with death from infection occurring in the first or second decade. With chronic antibiotic prophylaxis, however, the course of the disease has changed. Hospitalization is much less frequent, and survival seems to be prolonged, but patients develop serious complications due to imperfectly suppressed infections—strictures of the bladder and gastrointestinal tract, for example, and chronic lung disease with fibrosis and bronchiectasis. Death often results from infections by fungi, particularly *Aspergillus.*

Diagnosis. The diagnosis is made by neutrophil function studies. Most of these are normal, but those that measure the respiratory burst are severely deranged: The NBT test is negative (i.e., few if any cells are stained by formazan precipitates) (Fig. 149–1), and O_2^- production and other manifestations of the respiratory burst are greatly reduced or absent. Many microorganisms are handled in a normal fashion by CGD neutrophils (including pneumococci and streptococci, accounting for the rarity of pneumococcal and streptococcal infections in CGD patients), but those, such as *S. aureus,* whose destruction is particularly dependent on oxidant production by phagocytes are poorly killed by these defective cells. In CGD carriers the size of the respiratory burst is decreased by about half, so suspected carriers can often be identified by quantitation of the burst. Female carriers of X-linked CGD are particularly easy to detect. Because these carriers are mosaics, only a fraction of their neutrophils are able to make O_2^-; the NBT test stains only that fraction, leaving the rest of the cells unstained.

A picture similar to CGD has been seen in a few patients with exceptionally severe *glucose-6-phosphate dehydrogenase* (G6PD) *deficiency.* G6PD is essential for the production of NADPH, the reducing agent used by the O_2^--forming oxidase. In neutrophils that are severely deficient in G6PD, the levels of NADPH may be so low that the O_2^--forming oxidase is starved for substrate, so the cells cannot express an adequate respiratory burst.

Treatment. Management of CGD consists of long-term prophylaxis (trimethoprim-sulfamethoxazole at a trimethoprim dose of 5 to 10 mg per kilogram per day is satisfactory) and vigorous treatment of acute infections with antibiotics in adequate doses, plus surgery if indicated. Leukocyte transfusions may be helpful. Complications should be treated as conservatively as possible, although surgery may be required. Bone marrow transplantation has been performed in a few instances, but with its widely known hazards and the improvement in the outlook of CGD resulting from the use of long-term prophylaxis, marrow transplantation must be regarded as a last resort. Families of CGD patients should be investigated to ascertain the mode of transmission of the disease, and genetic counseling should be offered to them. In pregnant carriers, CGD may be diagnosed prenatally through NBT tests of fetal blood. The recent cloning of the gene responsible for X-linked CGD should soon provide safer methods for the prenatal diagnosis of this condition based on molecular biologic techniques.

CHÉDIAK-HIGASHI DISEASE. Chédiak-Higashi disease is an autosomally inherited defect in the production of lysosomes, the membrane-enclosed granular organelles that are found in almost every type of cell. Normally these organelles are oval bodies of relatively uniform size, but in Chédiak-Higashi disease they are very irregular both in size and shape, ranging from tiny spheres to huge malformed bodies many times larger than normal. The molecular lesion responsible for Chédiak-Higashi disease is unknown, although there is some evidence that the condition may result from an abnormality in microtubule function.

Clinical Picture. The clinical features of Chédiak-Higashi disease result from the malfunction of three types of lysosome-containing cells: the melanocytes, the platelets, and the phagocytes. Melanocyte dysfunction leads to *partial albinism,* a uniform but incomplete loss of pigment from the irises, skin, and hair that can be detected even at birth. The platelet defect

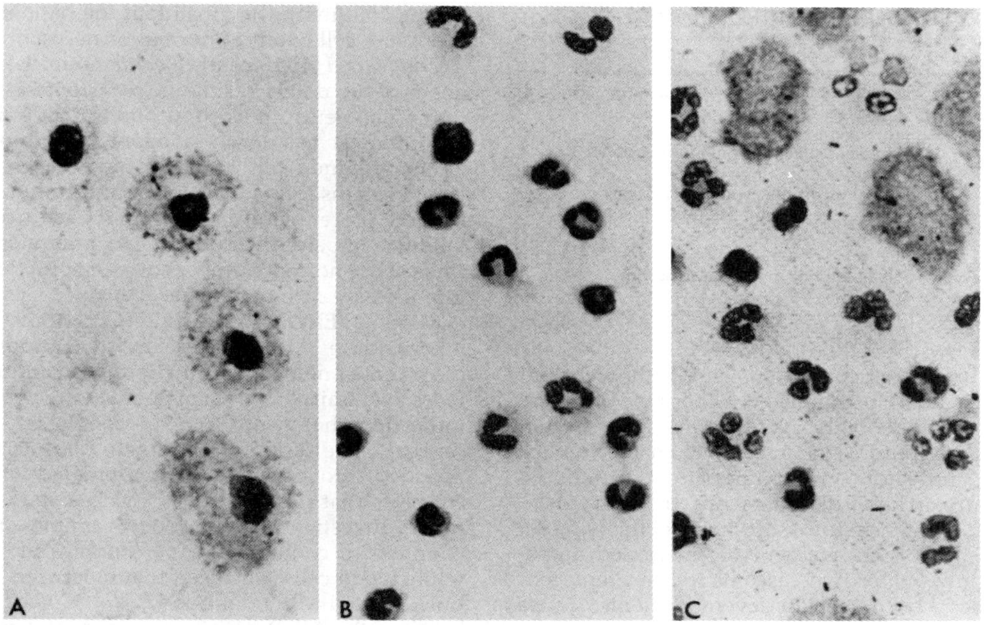

FIGURE 149–1. The NBT test in CGD. Left, normal; center, CGD; right, carrier of x-linked CGD, showing an NBT-positive and an NBT-negative population of neutrophils. (Reprinted with permission from Babior BM, Crawley CA: Chronic granulomatous disease and other disorders of oxidative killing by phagocytes. In Stanbury JB, Wyngaarden JB, Fredrickson DS, et al. [eds.]: The Metabolic Basis of Inherited Disease. 5th ed. New York, McGraw-Hill Book Company, 1983, p 1956.)

causes a mild *bleeding disorder* associated with a prolonged bleeding time. The most serious clinical problems, however, are caused by the abnormalities in the phagocytes. These lead to *marked lowering of resistance to bacterial infections,* so that Chédiak-Higashi patients suffer from frequent deep tissue abscesses as well as recurrent attacks of severe bacterial sinusitis and pneumonia. These infections are difficult to treat and often lead to death in the first or second decade.

Chédiak-Higashi patients who survive into their teens or later are confronted with a further clinical problem, probably the most serious of all. In most of these patients the disease ultimately evolves into a fatal form known as the accelerated phase. This is a peculiar lymphoma-like illness in which the lymph nodes, liver, spleen, and bone marrow become infiltrated with small lymphocytes recently identified as T cells. The lymphocytes look perfectly benign, but they behave in a malignant fashion, causing the infiltrated organs to enlarge and producing through marrow infiltration and splenomegaly a rapid, relentless, and ultimately fatal progression of the mild granulocytopenia seen in the stable phase of the disease. Death from pancytopenia generally occurs within a few months after the onset of the accelerated phase.

In Chédiak-Higashi disease, the white blood cell count is typically low (2000 to 3000 per cubic millimeter), a result of ineffective granulopoiesis (destruction of granulocytes before they leave the marrow). The low white cell count is an important factor in the low resistance to infection that characterizes this condition. Neutrophil chemotaxis and degranulation are depressed, but phagocytosis and the respiratory burst are normal. Bacterial killing is defective, probably because the abnormality in degranulation impedes the delivery of microbicidal substances into the phagocytic vesicles.

Diagnosis. The diagnosis is made by demonstrating under the microscope the presence of giant granules (lysosomes) in neutrophils and eosinophils, a feature that is virtually pathognomonic of Chédiak-Higashi disease (Fig. 149–2) (Color plate 3*B*). The diagnosis of the accelerated phase depends on finding the characteristic lymphocytic infiltrate in a biopsy of the involved tissue.

Treatment. The management of the early stage of Chédiak-Higashi disease amounts to the management of the infectious complications. Prophylactic antibiotics (trimethoprim-sulfamethoxazole at the dose given previously) should be used, and infections should be treated vigorously with appropriate antibiotic therapy. Ascorbic acid (20 mg per kilogram per day) has corrected the microbicidal defect in some but not all patients with Chédiak-Higashi disease. Treatment of the accelerated phase is unsatisfactory; splenectomy has been tried, as has chemotherapy with a variety of agents, but neither has proved to be of any benefit. Marrow transplantation has also been used in Chédiak-Higashi disease, though the indications for transplantation (e.g., the question of transplantation in early childhood as opposed to transplantation for the accelerated phase) are not yet clearly established.

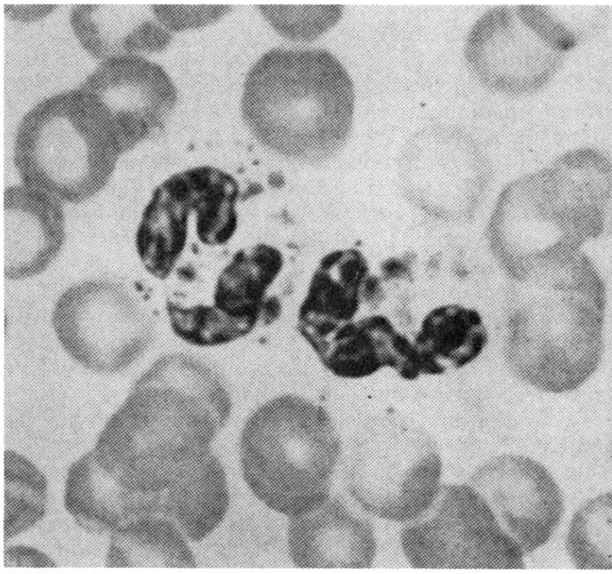

FIGURE 149–2. Neutrophils in Chédiak-Higashi disease, showing the giant granules that are the hallmark of the disease. (Reprinted with permission from Windhorst DB, Zelickson AS, Good RA: Chédiak-Higashi syndrome hereditary gigantism of cytoplasmic organelles. Science 151:81–83, 1966.)

TABLE 149–4. DISORDERS OF NEUTROPHIL MOTILITY

Disorder	Distinguishing Features
Job's syndrome	Cold abscesses, eosinophilia, greatly increased IgE
Juvenile periodontitis	Early severe gingival inflammation, systemic infections only in occasional patients
Leukocyte glycoprotein deficiency	Omphalitis or other infections in newborn, delayed separation of umbilical stump, leukemoid reactions
Congenital absence of specific granules	Abnormal segmentation of nucleus, alkaline phosphatase decreased or absent

DISORDERS OF NEUTROPHIL MOTILITY (Table 149–4). There are a number of conditions in which recurrent abscesses or other bacterial infections occur because of severe impairment in neutrophil mobility. Neutrophils from affected patients migrate poorly onto a glass coverslip in the Rebuck skin window test and show grossly impaired chemotaxis when tested in vitro. These disorders are thought to be inherited, although evidence for their heritability is often weak. For most of them (e.g., congenitally increased microtubule assembly), only one or two cases have been reported. A few, however, have been seen in several patients. These will be discussed here.

Job's Syndrome. This is a condition in which reduced neutrophil motility is associated with bacterial respiratory tract infections and cold staphylococcal abscesses (i.e., abscesses lacking much of the swelling and redness associated with inflammation), eosinophilia, and greatly increased levels of IgE. Patients characteristically have very high blood levels of an antistaphylococcal IgE antibody. Neutrophils from these patients show greatly reduced chemotaxis if assayed immediately after isolation, but chemotaxis returns to normal if the cells are stored for a few hours in the absence of serum prior to assay. This finding suggests that the abnormality lies in the serum, not the cells. The nature of the abnormality is unknown, although a monocyte-derived chemotactic inhibitor has been suggested as the cause of the condition.

Juvenile Periodontitis. In this familial disease neutrophils show a chemotactic defect that is thought to be caused by a serum abnormality. Serious gingival inflammation develops in late childhood or adolescence, similar to but more severe than that seen in normal middle-aged adults with poor dental hygiene. Affected individuals will often have lost many of their teeth by the time they are 30 years old. Among the organisms infecting the gums of such patients is *Capnocytophaga*, an anaerobic bacillus that secretes a potent inhibitor of neutrophil chemotaxis. The antichemotactic agent enters the bloodstream, where in a few patients with juvenile periodontitis it reaches concentrations that impair systemic host defenses and result in repeated bacterial infections. Elimination of the *Capnocytophaga* by means of long-term administration of antibiotics and vigorous local therapy will correct the impairment in host defenses and normalize the patient's resistance against bacterial infections.

Leukocyte Glycoprotein Deficiency. In this inherited disease a chemotactic defect is caused by absence or abnormality of a group of membrane glycoproteins required for normal interaction between neutrophils and surfaces. The first indication of this condition may be delayed separation of the umbilical stump. Patients are subject to recurrent infections, particularly with *Pseudomonas*. The first infection may occur in the newborn as an omphalitis. Infections are generally accompanied by a neutrophilic leukemoid reaction in which the white count may exceed 100,000. The diagnosis can be made with commercially available antibodies (e.g., Mol [Coulter Immunology], OKM1 [Ortho]), which bind to normal but not glycoprotein-deficient white cells. Vigorous and prolonged therapy is necessary for successful treatment of infections in leukocyte glycoprotein deficiency. Prophylactic antibodies are indicated in this condition; they maintain the patient's health and keep the white cell count at normal or near-normal levels.

Congenital Absence of Specific Granules. In this disorder a chemotactic defect results in recurrent severe bacterial infections. The neutrophils show abnormalities in nuclear segmentation, most frequently a bilobed nucleus (the Pelger-Huët anomaly), and stain poorly or not at all for alkaline phosphatase. Proteins located in the specific granules (e.g., cobalamin-binding protein) are absent from the neutrophils, and bacterial killing is impaired. Under the electron microscope the neutrophils show normal numbers of azurophil granules, but specific granules are rare or absent.

MYELOPEROXIDASE DEFICIENCY. Deficiency of myeloperoxidase (MPO) is the most common of the inherited disorders of neutrophil function. Transmitted as an autosomal recessive trait, it is estimated to affect one person in 500, indicating that nearly one person in ten is a heterozygous carrier. Once thought to be quite rare, its true incidence was revealed through the use of automated white cell differential counters that rely on the peroxidase stain to identify neutrophils. Investigations of blood samples reported by these counters to contain high percentages of "large unidentified white blood cells" revealed that most were from patients with unsuspected MPO deficiency.

Clinically, MPO deficiency is almost completely silent. The only problem that can be attributed to it is an increase in the severity of *Candida* infections seen in a few MPO-deficient patients with coincident diabetes mellitus. The original misconception about the incidence of MPO deficiency can probably be explained by the very low incidence of clinical disease in patients with this condition.

MPO-deficient neutrophils show characteristic functional abnormalities. Chemotaxis, phagocytosis, and degranulation are normal, but the respiratory burst is prolonged because of an increase in the survival of the O_2^--forming oxidase, which is typically destroyed by a myeloperoxidase-dependent process during the course of the respiratory burst. Bacterial killing by MPO-deficient cells is delayed, but eventually reaches completion, indicating that the myeloperoxidase-independent oxidants generated by the deficient cells kill more slowly but just as effectively as the myeloperoxidase-dependent oxidants of normal cells. The completeness of bacterial killing by MPO-deficient cells contrasts with the extensive failure of bacterial killing in CGD, and it explains why bacterial infections are such a serious problem in the latter but not the former condition.

The diagnosis is made from a peroxidase stain of the blood film. The stain normally shows activity in three types of cells: neutrophils, monocytes, and eosinophils. In MPO deficiency the activity is missing from neutrophils and monocytes. Eosinophils, however, stain normally, since their peroxidase is different from the myeloperoxidase found in neutrophils and monocytes and is not affected in myeloperoxidase deficiency. Peroxidase levels can be quantitated spectrophotometrically if desired, but this is usually unnecessary.

No treatment is required for MPO deficiency.

Anderson DC, Schmalstieg FC, Shearer W, et al.: The severe and moderate phenotypes of heritable Mac-1, LFA-1, P150,95 deficiency: Their quantitative definition and relation to leukocyte dysfunction and clinical features. J Infect Dis 152:668, 1985. *A thorough discussion of the clinical and laboratory features of leukocyte glycoprotein deficiency.*

Babior BM, Crowley CA: Chronic granulomatous disease and other disorders of oxidative killing by phagocytes. In Stanbury JB, et al. (eds.): The Metabolic Basis of Inherited Disease. 5th ed. New York, McGraw-Hill Book Company, 1983, pp 1956–1985. *A relatively recent review on disorders of oxygen-dependent killing by neutrophils, including CGD, MPO deficiency, and others.*

Boogaerts MA, Nelissen V, Roelant C, et al.: Blood neutrophil function in primary myelodysplastic syndromes. Br J Haematol 55:217, 1983. *A thorough study of neutrophil dysfunction in myelodysplasia.*

Curnutte JT, Babior BM: Chronic granulomatous disease. Adv Hum Genet 16:229, 1987. *A review of chronic granulomatous disease emphasizing the molecular basis for the disorder. Includes a description of the cloning of the gene for X-linked CGD.*

Donabedian H, Gallin JI: The hyperimmunoglobulin E recurrent infection (Job's) syndrome. A review of the NIH experience and the literature. Medicine 62:195, 1983. *A detailed clinical study of Job's syndrome.*

Gallin JI, Fauci AS (eds.): Advances in Host Defense Mechanisms. New York, Raven Press, 1982, vol 1: Phagocytic Cells. *A multiauthor volume containing several chapters on various abnormalities of neutrophil function.*

Gallin, JI, Wright DG, Malech HL, et al.: Disorders of phagocyte chemotaxis. Ann Intern Med 92:520, 1980. *A brief survey of conditions associated with defective neutrophil chemotaxis and motility.*

Klebanoff SJ, Clark RA: The Neutrophil: Function and Clinical Disorders. Amsterdam, Elsevier/North Holland Biochemical Press, 1978. *This comprehensive treatise includes detailed discussions on many abnormalities of neutrophil function. Separate chapters are devoted to CGD, MPO deficiency, and Chédiak-Higashi disease. Exhaustively referenced.*

Rebuck JW, Crowley JH: A method for studying leukocyte function in vivo. Ann NY Acad Sci 59:759, 1955. *How to perform and interpret the Rebuck skin window test.*

Wolff SM, Dale DC, Clark RA, et al.: The Chédiak-Higashi syndrome: Studies of host defenses. Ann Intern Med 76:293, 1972. *A discussion of Chédiak-Higashi disease emphasizing the abnormalities in neutrophil function seen in this condition.*

150 LEUKOPENIA

Grover C. Bagby, Jr.

The peripheral blood white cell count ranges from 5.0 to 10.0 × 10^9 per liter in normal individuals. Circulating leukocytes consist of heterogeneous cell types (neutrophils, monocytes, basophils, eosinophils, and lymphocytes), each of which serves a unique purpose and each of which represents a different fractional component of the total peripheral leukocyte population. A rational discussion of leukopenia must therefore focus on specific leukocyte types. Nor can a normal white blood cell count assure that substantial and serious deficiencies of leukocyte components do not exist. Patients may be severely neutropenic or lymphocytopenic despite total white blood counts that fall within the normal range. If there is a reason to order a white blood count, that reason is generally sufficient to justify performance of a differential count as well.

NEUTROPENIA

DEFINITION. Neutropenia exists when the peripheral neutrophil count is less than 2.0 × 10^9 per liter. Because the normal range in blacks and Yemenite Jews is somewhat lower, neutropenia in these populations is defined as counts less than 1.5 × 10^9 per liter. The role of the neutrophil in phagocytic defense of the host is generally met if the neutrophil count is above 1.0 × 10^9 per liter. If the neutrophil count drops below this number, particularly when the count falls below 0.5 × 10^9 per liter, the incidence of serious, recurrent, and difficult-to-treat infections rises markedly.

ETIOLOGY AND PATHOGENESIS. The multiple causes of neutropenia in pathophysiologic terms are best described in the context of the normal processes of neutrophil production and traffic. Such a description also simplifies the diagnostic and therapeutic approaches to patients with neutropenia. Neutrophils arise from a pool of marrow precursor cells through serial divisions and synchronous maturation steps (Fig. 150–1). The rate of neutrophil production is astonishingly high; more than 10^{11} cells per day. The bone marrow component of the neutrophil's life consists of a mitotic pool and a storage pool, the latter containing cells that no longer divide. Released after a few days in the bone marrow, neutrophils circulate freely for only a matter of hours before crawling into the extravascular space. For unknown reasons, half of the neutrophils in the peripheral blood are "marginated" along the endothelium and therefore are not measured in the white blood cell count. Accordingly, the true peripheral blood content of neutrophils, consisting of the circulating and the marginated pools, is ordinarily twice that measured by the neutrophil count (Fig. 150–1).

A simple etiologic classification of neutropenia can be derived from the three-compartment model, representing abnormalities in (1) the marrow compartment, (2) the peripheral blood compartment, (3) the extravascular compartment, or (4) combinations of the above (Fig. 150–2).

Abnormalities in the Marrow Compartment. Abnormalities in the marrow account for the majority of neutropenias in clinical practice. Failure of the marrow compartment can occur as a result of direct injury, in which case the marrow usually contains fewer than normal hematopoietic cells, or from maturation defects of hematopoietic cells, principally characterized by normal or increased numbers of morphologically abnormal hematopoietic cells. In either case, neutropenia most frequently occurs along with abnormalities in the number of platelets and red cells. Marrow injury can occur as a consequence of a variety of diseases (Fig. 150–2).

Drug-induced injury is most common (Table 150–1). Antineoplastic and immunosuppressive agents are generally *designed* to inflict injury on a proliferative population of cells; myelo-

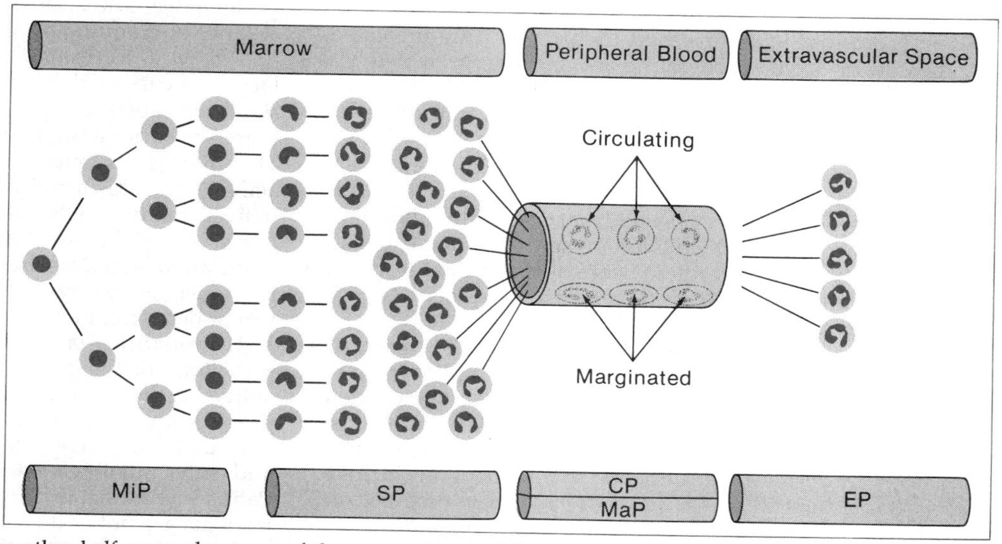

FIGURE 150–1. Production and distribution of neutrophils involves three compartments. Stem cells, committed progenitor cells, and morphologically recognizable precursor cells proliferate and mature (differentiate) under the influence of a variety of humoral regulatory factors, including GM-CSF and G-CSF. These phenomena occur in the "mitotic pool" (MiP). Once the cells reach the intermediate maturation stage known as the metamyelocyte, they stop proliferating but continue differentiating to bands and segmented neutrophils. These cells, although capable of leaving the marrow if needed, generally spend about five days in the marrow, in the "storage pool" (SP). The neutrophils then enter the blood. Half of those cells in the blood circulate and can be measured in a blood sample by counting—the "circulating pool" (CP)—but the other half move about out of the main column of flowing blood, probably in close association with vascular endothelial cells. These latter cells are components of the "marginated pool" (MaP). After their brief sojourn in the peripheral blood, the neutrophils invade the extravascular compartments of most organs, where they are either utilized as defenders or garbage disposal systems or die within one or two days.

Marrow

ABNORMALITIES IN THE BONE MARROW COMPARTMENT

1. Bone Marrow Injury
   A. Drugs
      Cytotoxic and noncytotoxic agents
   B. Radiation
   C. Chemicals
      Benzene, DDT, dinitrophenol, arsenic, bismuth, nitrous oxide
   D. Certain congenital and hereditary neutropenias
   E. Immunologically mediated (largely seen in patients with rheumatic disorders)
      Cytotoxic T cell-mediated (T)
      Antibody-mediated (Ab)
      Mechanisms that require both T and Ab
   F. Infection
      Viral (hepatitis, parvovirus, AIDS)
      Bacterial (*M. tuberculosis, M. kansasii)*
   G. Bone marrow replacement (infiltrative diseases)
      Malignancies (lung, breast, prostate, stomach, lymphomas, and lymphoid leukemias)
      Fibrosis
      Agnogenic myeloid metaplasia
      Long-standing polycythemia vera
      Chronic myelogenous leukemia
      Radiation injury
      Injury from chronic cytotoxic drug therapy
      Acute megakaryocytic leukemia

2. Maturation Defects
   A. Acquired
      Folic acid deficiency
      Vitamin B_{12} deficiency
   B. Neoplastic and other clonal disorders
      Congenital neutropenias
      Acute nonlymphocytic leukemia
      Myelodysplastic syndromes
      Paroxysmal nocturnal hemoglobinuria

Peripheral Blood

ABNORMALITIES IN THE PERIPHERAL BLOOD COMPARTMENT

1. Shift of neutrophils from the circulating to the marginated pool (known as pseudoneutropenia)
   A. Hereditary or constitutional benign pseudoneutropenia
   B. Acquired
      Acute: Severe bacterial infection, frequently associated with endotoxemia
      Chronic: Protein-calorie malnutrition, malaria
2. Intravascular sequestration
   A. In lung (complement-mediated leukoagglutination)
   B. In spleen (hypersplenism)

Extravascular

ABNORMALITIES IN THE EXTRAVASCULAR COMPARTMENT

1. Increased utilization
   A. Severe bacterial, fungal, viral, or rickettsial infection
   B. Anaphylaxis
2. Destruction
   A. Antibody-mediated (rheumatic disorders, drugs)
   B. Hypersplenism

FIGURE 150–2. The causes of neutropenia, arranged according to the compartment in which the abnormality usually resides. The approach to the neutropenic patient should begin by determining which of the three major compartments is likely at fault.

suppressive toxicity is the rule but is generally predictable and dose related. Drugs that are well tolerated in the majority of patients, however, can induce either marrow injury or peripheral neutrophil destruction in certain patients. These drug-induced reactions can result from direct drug-mediated cytotoxicity or from an immune mechanism in which (1) neutrophils are destroyed in extravascular sites (e.g., the penicillins) or (2) the marrow compartment is injured (e.g., procainamide, chloramphenicol, dapsone).

Radiation may result in acute self-limited and chronic marrow injury. Chronic radiation-induced injury can also result in the later development of myelodysplasia and nonlymphocytic leukemia, both of which often present with neutropenia. *Benzene* toxicity can also result in acute or chronic neutropenia and, like radiation-induced marrow failure, is associated with a high risk of acute nonlymphocytic leukemia.

Immune-mediated abnormalities may injure the marrow, either by autoantibody-mediated or by T lymphocyte–mediated mechanisms. Most patients with immune-mediated leukopenia have concurrent rheumatic or autoimmune diseases. *Infection* of the marrow per se is unusual, and most often does not result in neutropenia; some exceptions include mycobacterial infection (especially *Mycobacterium* tuberculosis and M. kansasii) and certain viral infections.

Marrow invasion by abnormal cells can result in neutropenia. Carcinoma of the prostate, breast, stomach, and lung, as well as malignant hematopoietic disorders, can occupy enough of the medullary space to cause global marrow failure. Similarly, fibroblasts can proliferate in certain disease states to the extent that they dominate the marrow (Fig. 150–2).

Maturation arrest can result in bone marrow failure in the absence of granulopoietic hypocellularity. In *folate* and *vitamin B_{12} deficiency,* for example, the marrow is loaded with granulocyte precursors that, because of the effects of the deficiency states on nuclear replication, fail to mature normally and therefore suffer a high rate of intramedullary death (Ch. 136). The marrow is hypercellular, and hematopoiesis goes on actively, but this activity belies the inability of the marrow to deliver mature cells effectively—hence the term *ineffective hematopoiesis.* Certain congenital neutropenias also represent maturation abnormalities, as do the acute nonlymphocytic leukemias, myelodysplastic syndromes, and paroxysmal nocturnal hemoglobinuria.

Abnormalities in the Peripheral Blood Compartment. Perturbations of the peripheral blood compartment result from shifts in the circulating pool (Figs. 150–1 and 150–2). In *pseudoneutropenia,* neutrophil production and utilization are normal, but the size of the marginated pool is unusually large and substantially greater in size than the circulating pool. Patients with stable hereditary or constitutional pseudoneutropenia are not at increased risk of infection unless a neutrophil function abnormality coexists. Acquired pseudoneutropenia often occurs as an acute or subacute response to systemic infections. It is generally associated with acute

TABLE 150–1. DRUGS THAT CAUSE NEUTROPENIA

Antiarrhythmics	Procainamide, propranolol, quinidine
Antibiotics	Chloramphenicol, penicillins, sulfonamides, trimethoprim-sulfa, PAS, rifampin vancomycin, isoniazid, nitrofurantoin
Antimalarials	Dapsone, quinine, pyrimethamine
Anticonvulsants	Phenytoin, mephenytoin, trimethadione, ethosuximide, carbamazepine
Hypoglycemic Agents	Tolbutamide, chlorpropamide
Antihistamines	Cimetidine, brompheniramine, tripelennamine
Antihypertensives	Methyldopa, captopril
Antiinflammatory Agents	Aminopyrine, phenylbutazone, gold salts, ibuprofen, indomethacin
Antithyroid Agents	Propylthiouracil, methimazole, thiouracil
Diuretics	Acetazolamide, hydrochlorothiazide, chlorthalidone
Phenothiazines	Chlorpromazine, promazine, prochlorperazine
Immunosuppressive Agents	Antimetabolites
Cytotoxic Agents	Alkylating agents, antimetabolites, anthracyclines, vinca alkaloids, *cis*-platinum, hydroxyurea, actinomycin D
Other Agents	Recombinant alpha interferon, allopurinol, ethanol, levamisole, penicillamine

changes in other compartments (Fig. 150–3) and resolves when the infection is appropriately treated or spontaneously abates.

Abnormalities in the Extravascular Compartment. Phagocytes and their precursors respond to infections in a highly coordinated and regulated fashion. The cellular responses are largely controlled by two granulopoietic factors, GM-CSF and G-CSF, and include (1) a rather prompt increase in the rate of production of neutrophils in the mitotic compartment, a response mediated by a complex network of cellular and humoral regulatory interactions, (2) the early release of neutrophils from the marrow storage pool to the peripheral blood pool, (3) an increase in the rate of neutrophil egress from the peripheral blood pool to the invaded tissue or tissues, and (4) increased phagocytic and bactericidal activity of the neutrophils. Rarely, increased demand for neutrophils in the extravascular compartment can lead to transient neutropenia, especially in patients with severe infections (Fig. 150–3). In such cases the acute demand for neutrophils completely utilizes the marrow storage pool before it can be restored by increased proliferative activity. The neutrophil count generally rises within a few days. The bone marrow is highly effective in responding to infectious events so that the demand for neutrophils almost never exceeds the capacity of the mitotic pool to supply them. In contrast, neutrophil consumption in patients with autoimmune neutropenia and hypersplenism can outstrip marrow production. Whether this reflects absence in such patients of the complete humoral stimulatory mechanisms that evolve in the infected host, or whether the rate of destruction in these patients actually exceeds the rate of utilization in patients with infections, is not known.

In summary, the causes of neutropenia are heterogeneous and best categorized in pathophysiologic terms (Fig. 150–3).

CLINICAL MANIFESTATIONS. Neutropenia can occur in a wide variety of systemic diseases (Fig. 150–2), the manifestations of which may dominate the clinical picture. Many neutropenic patients remain asymptomatic, most often those whose neutrophil count exceeds 1.0×10^9 per liter or those whose neutropenia is acute and self-limited in duration. When symptoms do occur, they generally result from recurrent, often severe, bacterial infections. This is not surprising in view of the pivotal importance of the neutrophil in the defense of the host against microorganisms (Ch. 148).

This risk of bacterial infection increases significantly as the peripheral neutrophil count falls below 1.0×10^9 per liter but is greatly increased at levels below 0.5×10^9 per liter. The degree to which monocytosis compensates for neutropenia may modify the risk. I have observed a patient with such severe congenital neutropenia that no neutrophil has ever been seen in her blood over a 12-year period. Her leukocyte count is, however, normal because of marked monocytosis; the frequency of infections in this patient has been low.

Lungs, genitourinary system, oropharynx, and skin are the most frequent sites of infection in neutropenic patients. The infecting organisms are the usual pathogens for the given anatomic site. In patients who have recurrent infections and require prolonged and recurrent antibacterial therapy, un-

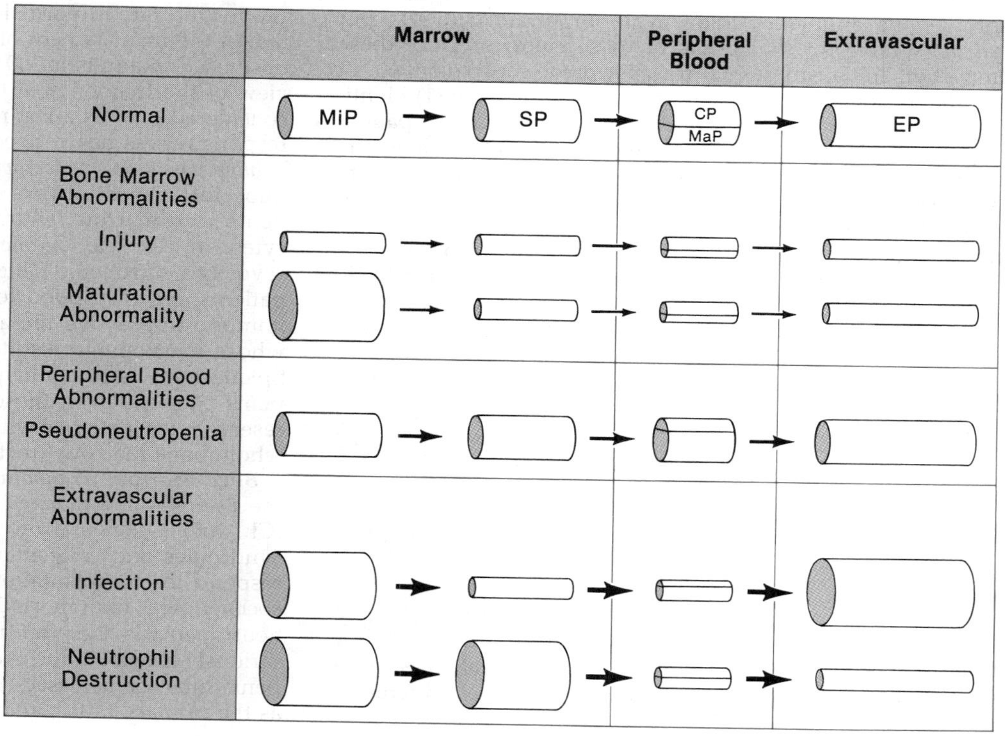

FIGURE 150–3. Pathophysiologic mechanisms of neutropenia. The size of a given compartment is represented by the size of the corresponding cylinder. The number of cells leaving a compartment for the next compartment can vary substantially, but flow between compartments is unidirectional. Notice that, in every case, the circulating neutrophil pool is small, but the size of the other pools is variable. In marrow injury there is a global decline in the size of all pools. A maturation abnormality, however, is characterized by an increase in the number of precursor cells that do not mature. Pseudoneutropenia is characterized by a movement of circulating neutrophils to the marginated pool. In severe infections the acute demand for neutrophils in the infected extravascular site results in a transient loss of storage pool neutrophils before the hypercellular (but as yet immature) mitotic compartments can renew the storage pool. Finally, excessive destruction of neutrophils can result in neutropenia.

usual organisms can colonize and subsequently cause infection. The antibiotic history of patients is important to obtain. *The usual signs and symptoms of infection are often diminished or absent in patients with neutropenia because the cell that mediates much of the inflammatory response to infection is absent.* Thus, neutropenic patients with severe bilateral bacterial pneumonia can present with minimal infiltrates demonstrable by the chest radiograph and nonpurulent sputum; patients with pyelonephritis may not exhibit pyuria; patients with bacterial pharyngitis may not have purulence in the oropharynx; and patients with severe bacterial infection of the skin may present only with erythroderma rather than furunculosis. In the neutropenic patient, infections that in an otherwise normal individual might have been well localized become quickly disseminated. Therefore, not only is the infected neutropenic patient a diagnostic problem, but, in addition, any given infection is more apt to be widespread at the time of diagnosis.

DIAGNOSIS. The diagnostic evaluation of neutropenia is influenced by its severity and the clinical setting in which it occurs. The evaluation in patients with neutrophil counts of less than 0.5 to 1.0 × 10^9 per liter should obviously proceed briskly. The patient with fever, sepsis, or both, in whom neutropenia is discovered for the first time presents a particularly difficult problem. In such patients it is impossible to determine immediately whether the neutropenia antedated sepsis, a situation with both prognostic and therapeutic implications, or whether the neutropenia is merely a short-lived response to the infection itself (Fig. 150–3). Examination of the peripheral blood smear and differential white blood count can be helpful in such cases. If the blood film has been prepared promptly after obtaining the sample, vacuolization of neutrophil cytoplasm correlates well with the presence of bacterial infection. An increase in the fraction of circulating band forms to levels above 20 per cent suggests that marrow granulopoietic activity is responding appropriately (Fig. 150–4). It is then presumed either that the marrow is recovering from injury or that the neutropenia is derived from a transient shift to the marginated pool or to the extravascular compartment.

The diagnostic evaluation of neutropenia must first address the question of the severity of the disorder and then whether the patient has fever, sepsis, or both. The patient with sepsis and severe neutropenia should be treated promptly with intravenous antibiotics following appropriate cultures, but *without waiting* for the results of those cultures. Once these important initial questions are answered, the remainder of the diagnostic evaluation can proceed (Fig. 150–5): (1) identifying any potential drugs and toxins to which the patient might have been exposed, (2) determining, if possible, the chronicity of the neutropenia, (3) ascertaining whether there have been recurrent infections, (4) identifying any underlying systemic disease that might be causative, and (5) examining the blood counts and blood morphology and bone marrow (the latter is usually indicated) to determine the most likely pathophysiologic explanation. The latter is important even if a specific, likely causative, underlying disease is promptly identified. Felty's syndrome, for example, is a well-recognized cause of neutropenia, but there are at least two separate pathophysiologic mechanisms in groups of these patients, one mediated by antineutrophil antibodies, the other by T lymphocyte–mediated bone marrow failure. Each mechanism has different therapeutic implications.

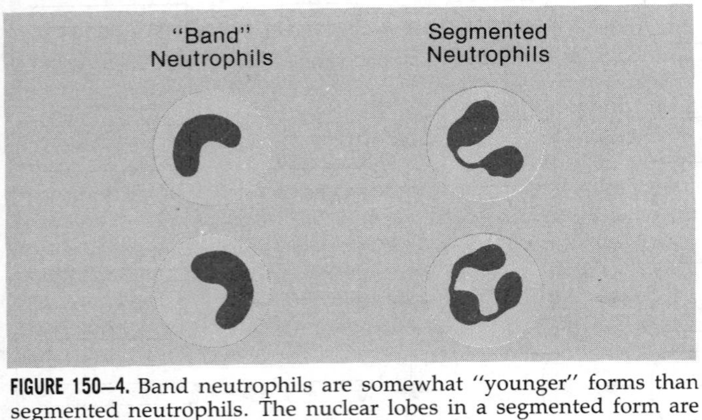

FIGURE 150–4. Band neutrophils are somewhat "younger" forms than segmented neutrophils. The nuclear lobes in a segmented form are separated by fine filaments absent in the band.

One approach to the neutropenic patient is shown in algorithmic form in Figure 150–5. Once the severity of the neutropenia is determined, careful examination of the peripheral blood counts and blood smear is in order. Patients with selective neutropenia are approached differently from those with additional deficiencies of platelets and red cells, although drugs or toxins may be involved in either category. Patients with selective neutropenia but with no drug or toxin exposure, no history of recurrent sepsis, and no underlying chronic inflammatory or autoimmune disease may have stable and benign neutropenia. This category includes some cases of familial and congenital neutropenia and pseudoneutropenia. Any patient with selective neutropenia with a history of sepsis or toxin exposure should have a bone marrow examination to assess (1) the degree of cellularity of each compartment (storage and mitotic pools), (2) the differentiation stages found in each pool, and (3) whether any morphologic abnormality exists in the hematopoietic cells.

In patients with pancytopenia or bicytopenia, bone marrow examination, which must include not only aspiration but biopsy as well, is almost always indicated. The only regular exception to this rule would include patients with unambiguous evidence of vitamin B_{12} or folate deficiency (Ch. 136).

TREATMENT. Rational treatment of the neutropenic patient follows diagnosis and generally involves treatment of the underlying disease or discontinuation of suspected toxins or drugs. The nature of the specific therapy naturally depends on the pathophysiology of the neutropenia in a given patient.

Treatments Specifically Designed to Increase the Neutrophil Count. Trials of the few agents available for the purpose of increasing the neutrophil count must be considered only in patients with severe neutropenia and a history of infections and should be attempted only after the potential risks involved are explained to the patient.

Lithium carbonate, an agent that increases the neutrophil production rate in normal individuals, rarely has been effective in the management of chronic bone marrow failure. The dose used in adults is 300 mg by mouth three times daily. In view of the frequency of toxicity, trials of therapy should be considered only as a last resort. No test to predict individual responsiveness has yet been developed.

Immunosuppressive therapy, including glucocorticoids or azathioprine, almost always elicits a favorable response in patients with marrow failure mediated by cytotoxic T lymphocytes. In vitro clonogenic cultures of bone marrow cells in severely neutropenic patients can aid in the identification of patients apt to respond to such therapy. Some responses to immunosuppressive therapy have also occurred in patients whose neutropenia resulted from antineutrophil antibodies. Splenectomy is rarely helpful in the management of neutropenic patients, even those with Felty's syndrome. It is now reserved for patients with unambiguous hypersplenism in whom bone marrow function is normal.

Bone Marrow Transplantation. In severe aplastic anemia the role of bone marrow transplantation is well established (Ch. 165). Other marrow failure states (e.g., myelodysplastic syndromes and congenital neutropenias) may also prove to respond to transplantation. Allogeneic transplantation is associated with high mortality; its use in patients with **selective** neutropenia is therefore uncertain. Before transplantation is seriously considered, the duration and severity of the neutropenia must be assessed; marrow failure must be established as the primary cause; and immunologically mediated marrow

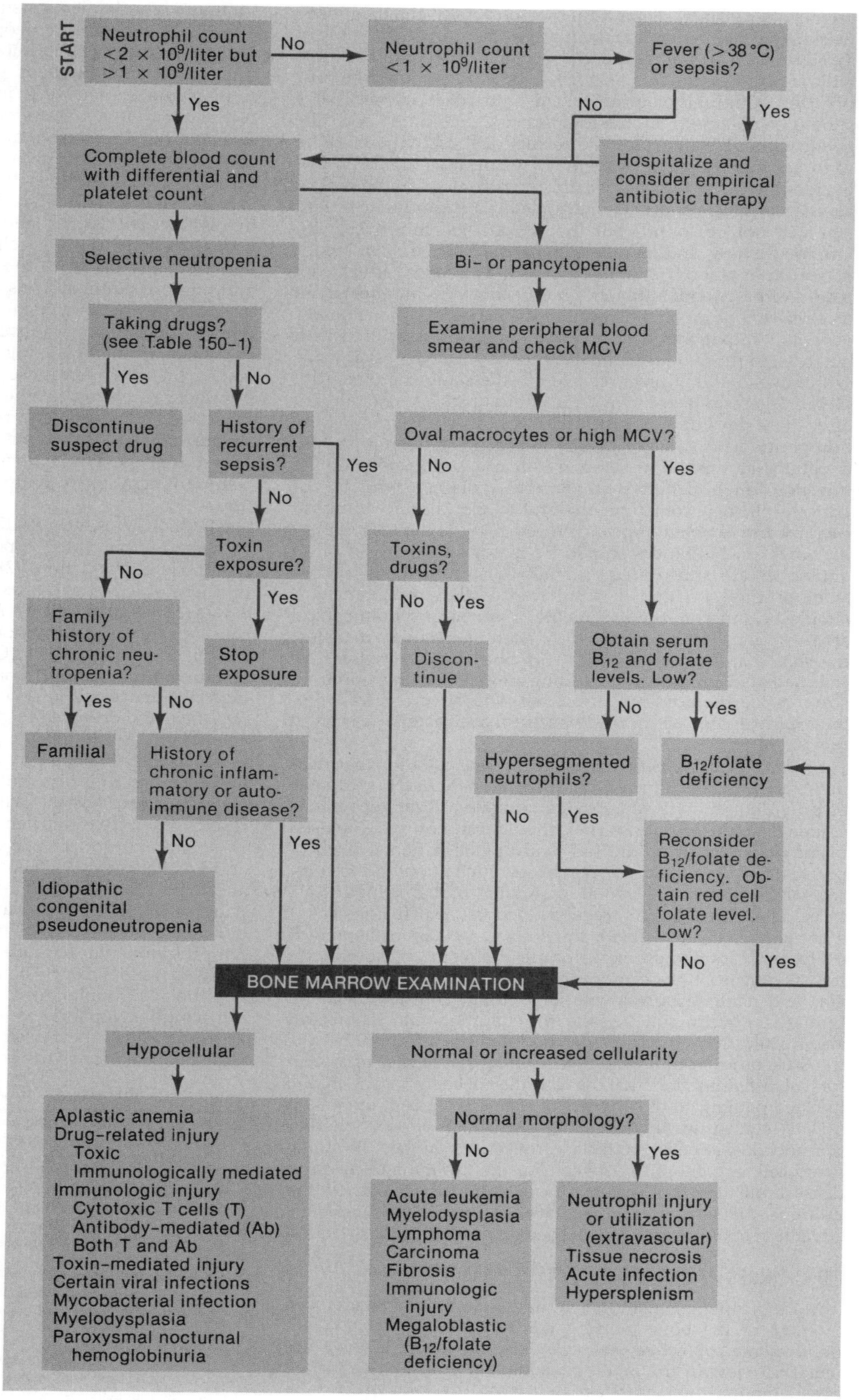

FIGURE 150–5. An algorithm for the evaluation of patients with neutropenia.

failure should be ruled out. If the patient has an identical twin, transplantation might be attempted with fewer constraints, but allogeneic transplantation should always be reserved for individuals with severe and symptomatic neutropenia caused by marrow failure.

Treatment of the Infected Neutropenic Patient. Each patient with neutropenia should understand the function of neutrophils, the consequences of neutrophil deficiency, and the importance of communicating with his or her physician the moment signs and symptoms of infection occur. If a neutropenic patient is afebrile and there is no sepsis, the diagnostic workup should generally take place in the outpatient clinic to avoid unnecessary exposure to nosocomial infections. Patients with severe neutropenia and fever, however, should be hospitalized. Cultures of urine, blood, and other relevant sites should be obtained, but broad-spectrum antibiotics should be given without waiting for the results of these cultures. One of three responses will be seen: (1) A causative organism will be identified, in which case the spectrum of antimicrobial agents can be appropriately narrowed. (2) A candidate organism will not be found, but the patient still improves with empiric therapy. In this type of setting a full course of broad-spectrum antibiotics should be given. Moreover, after a full course of parenteral antibiotics has been given, another seven to fourteen days of oral antibiotics should be considered, especially in patients with invasive infections associated with necrosis, in those whose initial response was slow, or in those with infections that have recurred in the same anatomic site. (3) No organism is found and the clinical picture is not altered after three days of empirical treatment. This unsettling situation occurs with some regularity in practice. The approach to a patient at this point depends on the seriousness of the infection. In a patient with localized disease who is not critically ill, it is sometimes helpful to discontinue empirical therapy and to obtain repeat cultures. If the patient is critically ill, however, antibiotics should be discontinued *only* if other antibiotics are substituted. Among those antibiotics to consider in this situation is amphotericin B. Amphotericin B should be added to the therapeutic regimen in certain clinical settings, i.e., for patients with acute leukemia, diabetes, dysphagia and/or esophagitis, endophthalmitis, or defective cell-mediated immunity (including those receiving immunosuppressive therapy) and for those who have received prolonged treatment with broad-spectrum antibacterial agents in the recent past.

Neutrophil transfusions, when used specifically for the treatment of seriously infected neutropenic patients, are capable of providing enough phagocytes to make a difference in the course of some infections. They should not, however, be used prophylactically in uninfected neutropenic patients. Neutrophils survive briefly in the peripheral circulation and tissues, so that they must be given at least daily, probably for at least three days. The decision to use neutrophil transfusions is not a trivial one. White cells for transfusion are expensive and, if preformed antibodies exist in the recipient, a number of transfusion reactions can occur, including fever, chills, myalgia, and acute dyspnea with or without transient bilateral pulmonary infiltration. These same clinical manifestations can also result from invasion of the sites of infection by the transfused neutrophils and their subsequent release of mediators of inflammation that have hitherto been absent in the infected patient. In the absence of clear-cut signs of hypersensitivity (e.g., urticaria), therefore, one cannot be sure whether the infection is being better controlled or whether the transfused cells are being destroyed. For this reason a decision to discontinue neutrophil transfusions cannot be made on the grounds that such reactions have occurred. Each patient's adverse response must be approached individually.

DEFICIENCIES OF OTHER CIRCULATING PHAGOCYTES

Monocytopenia, eosinopenia, and basophilopenia are seen in most of the bone marrow failure states associated with neutropenia. Selective *monocytopenia,* however, is very unusual. In view of the heterogeneous and critical roles played by the monocyte-macrophage in normal physiology (Ch. 148), complete failure of monocyte production for a period of more than nine to ten months (the estimated lifespan of tissue macrophages) may be incompatible with life.

Eosinopenia and *basophilopenia* are more common than monocytopenia in clinical practice and most often represent redistributional mechanisms resulting from stress, including acute infections, widespread neoplasms, and severe injury (e.g., burns). A variety of humoral factors, including glucocorticoids, prostaglandins, and epinephrine, are released in such settings and are known to induce eosinopenia. In view of the consistency of this stress response, if a patient with sepsis does **not** have eosinopenia, one should consider that adrenal cortical insufficiency or a primary myeloproliferative syndrome may coexist.

LYMPHOCYTOPENIA. The life cycle of the neutrophil involves a well-defined and limited set of compartments and a unidirectional flow of cells from the marrow to the blood and from the blood to the tissues. Lymphocyte production and traffic are difficult to assess: (1) Both T and B lymphocytes replicate in heterogeneous anatomic sites, including the lymph nodes, spleen, tonsils, and bone marrow; (2) lymphocytes are capable of leaving and then later re-entering a given compartment. Given these variables, it is surprising that the lymphocyte counts in the peripheral blood are so tightly regulated; normal counts range from 2 to 4 $\times$ 10^9 per liter. Approximately 20 per cent of these are B lymphocytes, and 70 per cent are T lymphocytes. Lymphocytopenia is defined as a peripheral blood lymphocyte count below 1.5 $\times$ 10^9 per liter.

ETIOLOGY AND PATHOGENESIS. Lymphocytopenia can result from three types of abnormalities: (1) those of lymphocyte production, (2) those of lymphocyte traffic, and (3) those of lymphocyte loss and destruction (Table 150–2).

Reduced Production of Lymphocytes. The most common cause of reduced lymphocyte production in the world is *protein-calorie malnutrition* (Ch. 214). The immunologic paresis resulting from malnutrition contributes substantially to the high incidence of infection in malnourished populations. *Radiation* and *immunosuppressive agents,* including alkylating agents and antithymocyte globulin, can induce lymphocytopenia by injuring the progenitor pool and inhibiting replication of more well differentiated cells. A variety of *congenital lymphocytopenic immune deficiency states* exist, some of which result in selective deficiencies of B lymphocytes, some of T cells, and in other cases, combined deficiencies of both T cells and B cells (Ch. 419). The mechanisms by which production and maturation of B and T lymphocytes are impaired in these patients are heterogeneous; many are ill defined. Immune deficiency states can clearly exist even in the absence of lymphocytopenia, because of abnormal lymphocyte function or selective deficiency of one component of the circulating lymphocyte population. Certain *viruses* are capable of inducing lymphocytopenia; some of these agents infect lymphoid cells and cause their destruction. Such viruses include measles, polio, varicella zoster, and HIV (the acquired immuno-

TABLE 150–2. CAUSES OF LYMPHOCYTOPENIA

Abnormalities of lymphocyte production
Protein-calorie malnutrition
Radiation
Immunosuppressive therapeutic agents
Congenital immunodeficiency states
Wiskott-Aldrich syndrome
Nezelof's syndrome
Adenosine deaminase deficiency
Viral infections
Hodgkin's lymphoma (?)
Widespread granulomatous infection (mycobacterial, fungal)
Alterations in lymphocyte traffic
Acute bacterial infection, trauma, stress, glucocorticoids
Viral infection
Widespread granulomatous infection
Hodgkins lymphoma (?)
Lymphocyte destruction or loss
Viral infection
Antibody-mediated lymphocyte destruction
Protein-losing enteropathy
Chronic right ventricular failure
Thoracic duct drainage or rupture

deficiency syndrome [AIDS] virus) (Ch. 346). HIV does not frequently cause lymphocytopenia but does infect the helper ($T4^+$) subset of T lymphocytes and destroys them, a process that results in a marked decline in the absolute numbers of helper ($T4^+$) T cells in the peripheral circulation. Patients with untreated Hodgkin's disease occasionally have lymphocytopenia, especially during the late stages of the disease and with the least favorable histologic subtypes (Ch. 160).

Alterations in Lymphocyte Traffic. Alterations are common and most frequently represent transient responses to a variety of stressful events, including bacterial infections and trauma. These responses are likely mediated by high levels of endogenous glucocorticoids that induce rapid declines in circulating levels of B and T lymphocytes. The lymphocytopenic response to this type of steroid results from a self-limited shift of lymphocytes away from the peripheral blood compartment. Lymphocyte values generally return to normal within 24 to 48 hours. For this reason the transient declines induced by endogenous steroid production are not associated with functional immunologic deficiency. Certain viruses can also bind to lymphocyte populations and cause their departure from the blood compartment into other sites.

More persistent lymphocytopenia has been described in patients with widespread granulomatous disease, a phenomenon that is likely multifactorial, deriving from both inhibition of production and alterations of traffic. Patients with these disorders are often difficult to treat. Establishing a cause-and-effect relationship between the infection and lymphocytopenia is difficult when one considers that the reverse might just as easily be true; consider, for example, the frequency of mycobacterial infection in patients with AIDS.

Increased Destruction of Lymphocytes. Lymphocytopenia can occur as a result of *viral infection,* as outlined above. In some patients lymphocytopenia results from *antilymphocyte antibodies*. As was the case in patients with immunologically mediated neutropenia, the majority of such individuals have underlying autoimmune or rheumatic diseases. Losses of viable lymphocytes can also occur because of *structural defects* in sites of high-density lymphocyte traffic, e.g., via thoracic duct fistulas. In such patients, both T cells and B cells decline in the peripheral blood. Loss of lymphocytes from intestinal lymphatics can occur in protein-losing enteropathies, severe congestive heart failure, or primary diseases of the gut or intestinal lymphatics (Table 150–2).

CLINICAL MANIFESTATIONS AND DIAGNOSIS. There are no specific clinical manifestations of lymphocytopenia per se. The signs and symptoms present in patients with lymphocytopenia are those characteristic of the disease with which the cytopenia is associated. Whether the patient exhibits signs of immunologic deficiency depends on the pathophysiology of the disorder, the duration of the disease, which subsets of lymphocytes are affected most significantly, and the degree to which cellular or humoral immunity is functionally perturbed. Accordingly, unless the clinical setting is clearly one in which transient lymphocytopenia is likely, the approach to diagnosis should involve comprehensive assessment of the integrity of the immune apparatus. Specifically, the subsets of lymphocytes remaining in the circulating blood should be identified and should at least include B cells, helper–inducer T cells, and cytotoxic–suppressor T cells. In addition, quantitative immunoglobulin levels should be measured in the serum, and a series of skin tests performed to detect deficiencies of cell-mediated immunity.

TREATMENT. Because lymphocytopenia ordinarily represents a response to an underlying disease, primary attention must be paid to establishing the nature of that disease and instituting therapy for it. Patients whose lymphocytopenia is accompanied by hypogammaglobulinemia may require immune globulin replacement therapy (Ch. 419). The treatment of severe deficiencies of cell-mediated immunity remains experimental. Responses have been described with transplantation of allogeneic marrow, fetal liver, or thymic epithelial cells.

Abdou NI, Chaiyakiati N, Balentine L, et al.: Suppressor cell mediated neutropenia in Felty's syndrome. J Clin Invest 61:738, 1978. Bagby GC, Gabourel JD: Neutropenia in three patients with rheumatic disorders. Suppression of granulopoiesis by cortisol sensitive thymus dependent lymphocytes. J Clin Invest 64:72, 1979. Bagby GC, Lawrence HJ, Neerhout RC: T - lymphocyte mediated granulopoietic failure: In-vitro identification of prednisone responsive patients. N Engl J Med 309:1073, 1983. *Neutropenic patients with rheumatic and autoimmune diseases had been, until the appearance of these reports, almost as a reflex, classified in pathophysiologic terms as having excessive destruction and/or hypersplenism. The above studies demonstrate that in many patients, immunologically mediated failure of the granulopoietic marrow is the explanation. The third paper documents that among such patients, resolution of neutropenia often occurs upon treatment with immunosuppressive agents.*

Jacob HS, Craddock PR, Hammerschmidt D, et al.: Complement-induced granulocyte aggregation. An unsuspected mechanism of disease. N Engl J Med 302:789, 1980. *This work documents very well the rapidity with which complement-induced aggregation can account not only for neutropenia but for significant respiratory dysfunction as well.*

Lelezari P, Jiang A-F, Yegen L, et al.: Chronic autoimmune neutropenia due to anti-NA2 antibody. N Engl J Med 293:744, 1975. *Despite the difficulties in documenting shortened survival of a cell whose survival is intrinsically short, this paper presents good evidence that chronic neutropenia can be mediated by antibodies directed at antigens expressed by neutrophils.*

Metcalf D.: The molecular biology and functions of the granulocyte macrophage colony-stimulating factors. Blood 67:257, 1986. Donahue RE, Wang EA, Stone DK, et al.: Stimulation of hematopoiesis in primates by continuous infusion of recombinant human GM-CSF. Nature 321:872, 1986. *Since the introduction of the colony-growth assays in 1966, much has been learned about the regulation of phagocyte production by humoral factors. Metcalf's investigative group has shown impressively sustained activity on this subject. This comprehensive and up-to-date paper is one worth reading for a number of reasons, not the least of which is the real possibility that recombinant CSF's will be useful therapeutic agents in certain patients with neutropenia. Indeed, the paper by Donahue et al. documenting the in vivo effects of one of the recombinant factors, GM-CSF, in primates is the first in what will soon be a long list of publications relevant to the therapeutic value of recombinant factors.*

Williams WJ, Beutler E, Erslev AJ, Lichtman MA: Hematology. 3rd ed. New York, McGraw Hill Book Company, 1983. Spivak JL: Fundamentals of Clinical Hematology. 2nd ed. Philadelphia, Harper & Row Publishers, 1984. Wintrobe MM, Lee RE, Boggs DR, et al.: Clinical Hematology. 8th ed. Philadelphia, Lea & Febiger, 1981. *Each of these textbooks of hematology includes a number of chapters on phagocyte and lymphocyte production, traffic, distribution, and function. The reviews of leukopenia are comprehensive, and reference lists are encyclopedic.*

Young GAR, Vincent PC: Drug-induced agranulocytosis. Clin Haematol 9:483, 1980. *This is a concise and comprehensive review of the pathophysiology and clinical features of drug-induced neutropenia.*

151 LEUKOCYTOSIS AND LEUKEMOID REACTIONS

Grover C. Bagby, Jr.

Circulating leukocytes consist of neutrophils, monocytes, eosinophils, basophils, and lymphocytes. Any one or all of these cell types can rise to abnormal levels in peripheral blood in response to various stimuli. Each type of leukocyte is produced in response to specific growth factors. The term *leukocytosis*, an increase in the total leukocyte count to a level above 11.0×10^9 per liter, is less meaningful clinically than are terms that identify the type of leukocyte that is predominantly increased. The terms *neutrophilia* (neutrophilic leukocytosis), *monocytosis*, *lymphocytosis*, *eosinophilia*, and *basophilia* suggest specific diagnostic considerations.

Leukocytosis is a common finding in acutely ill patients. When the leukocyte count exceeds 25 to 30×10^9 per liter, it is termed a *leukemoid reaction*. Leukemoid reactions generally reflect the response of healthy bone marrow to signals that evolve in the patient under the influence of trauma, inflammation, and similar stresses. Leukemoid reactions are *not* synonymous with *leukoerythroblastosis*, which indicates the presence of abnormally immature white cells and nucleated red cells in the peripheral blood irrespective of the total

TABLE 151–1. CAUSES OF LEUKOERYTHROBLASTOSIS

- **Normal Marrow**
  - Severe acute hemolytic anemia
  - Acute infection in hyposplenic patients
- **Abnormal Marrow**
  - Multiple fractures
  - Marrow infiltration
    - Tuberculosis
    - Fungal disease
    - Fibrosis
    - Malignant cells (carcinoma, sarcoma, lymphoma, myeloma, acute leukemia)
  - Chronic myeloproliferative disorders
    - Agnogenic myeloid metaplasia
    - Chronic myelogenous leukemia
  - Other disorders
    - Osteopetrosis
    - Gaucher's disease
    - Amyloidosis
    - Paget's disease of bone
    - Severe tissue hypoxia

leukocyte count. Leukoerythroblastosis is less common than leukemoid reactions but often, especially in the adult patient, reflects serious marrow dysfunction (Table 151–1). Consequently the finding of leukoerythroblastosis represents a clear indication to perform bone marrow aspiration and biopsy, unless the clinical setting is acute severe hemolytic anemia, sepsis in a patient with hyposplenism, or massive trauma (with multiple fractures).

NEUTROPHILIA

PATHOPHYSIOLOGY. There are three major anatomic sites of neutrophil traffic: the bone marrow, the peripheral blood, and the extravascular space (Fig. 151–1). Traffic moves unidirectionally from marrow to blood to extravascular space. The number of neutrophils within each site can be independently regulated. The number of neutrophil precursors in the marrow mitotic pool (MiP) is largely influenced by the granulopoietic growth factors: granulocyte-macrophage colony-stimulating factor (GM-CSF), granulocyte colony-stimulating factor (G-CSF), and macrophage colony-stimulating factor (M-CSF, also known as CSF-1). These factors, the products of three separate genes, one on the long arm of chromosome 5, function not only to stimulate the growth and differentiation of granulocyte and/or macrophage progenitor cells but also to assist in activating neutrophils. The marrow storage pool is sufficient to provide the periphery with neutrophils for about five days in the steady state, even if it were unsupported by the MiP. Neutrophils are released from the storage pool into the circulating pool in response to a variety of physiologic stresses, including endogenous glucocorticoids (Fig. 151–1*B*). Peripheral neutrophils are normally equally divided between the circulating pool and the marginated pool. Neutrophilia can therefore result from a shift of neutrophils from the marginated to the circulating pool—"demargination" (Fig. 151–1*C*). This response is rapid and can be induced by injections of epinephrine. In patients with acute inflammatory illnesses, both storage pool release and demargination usually occur together (Fig. 151–1*D*).

A complex regulatory network of mononuclear phagocytes, stromal cells, lymphocytes, and granulocyte progenitors and their progeny responds to acute inflammatory events by augmenting production of the critically important CSF's (Fig. 151–2). The CSF's act on the granulopoietic progenitors to increase mitosis, which expands the storage pool and consequently increases the size of the blood and extravascular pools (Fig. 151–1*E*). This new state persists until the inflammatory process is resolved.

CAUSES. Neutrophilia (neutrophil counts greater than 7.5 $\times 10^9$ per liter), a common finding in clinical practice, usually reflects the inflammatory response to acute or subacute illnesses (Fig. 151–2, Table 151–2). Indeed, while the presence of neutrophilia should initiate a search for the cause of this response, it should also be viewed as a sign that the patient is likely responding appropriately to the stimulus.

When neutrophilia occurs in the absence of evidence of acute inflammation or illness, three conditions should be

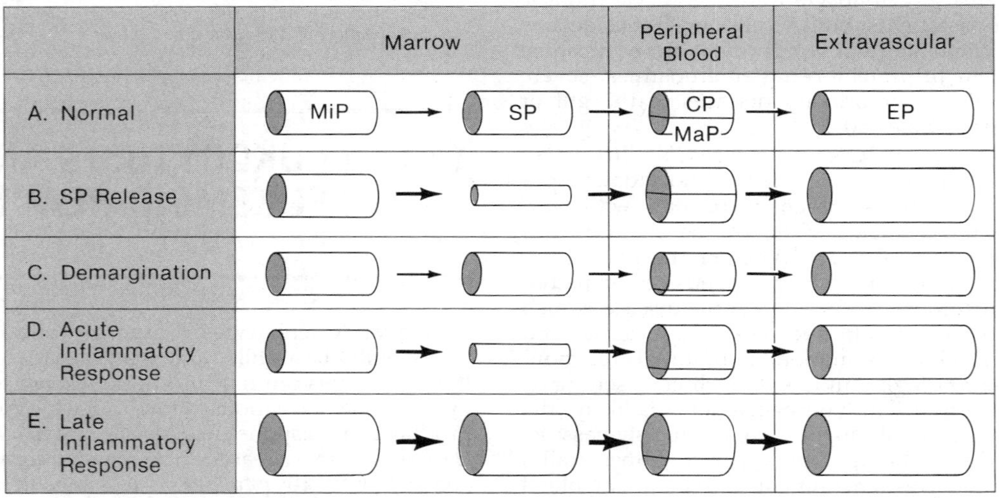

FIGURE 151–1. Pathophysiologic mechanisms of neutrophilia. In this figure the size of a given compartment is represented by the size of a given cylinder. The number of cells leaving a compartment for the next compartment is reflected by the size of the arrows between compartments. *A*, MiP = The mitotic pool of granulocyte precursor cells; SP = the granulocyte storage pool; CP = the circulating granulocyte pool; MaP = the marginated pool; EP = the extravascular pool. Notice that, in every case, the circulating neutrophil pool is large, but the size of the other pools is variable. *B*, A variety of stresses on the organism can result, perhaps through the action of glucocorticoid hormones, in the release of storage pool granulocytes. This occurs commonly as an acute response to acute infections. *C*, The circulating granulocyte pool can also increase in size by virtue of a shift of neutrophils from the marginated to the circulating pool. The demargination response can be regularly elicited by the administration of epinephrine and can also result from a variety of stresses, including acute infection. *D*, With most bacterial infections and other inflammatory processes, the acute demand for neutrophils in the infected extravascular sites results in the simultaneous release of storage pool neutrophils and demargination. *E*, Once the hematopoietic growth factor released in response to the inflammatory stimulus (see Fig. 151–2) has induced a few days of proliferation in the mitotic pool, the content of granulocytes in all pools increases and delivery to the tissues becomes maximal.

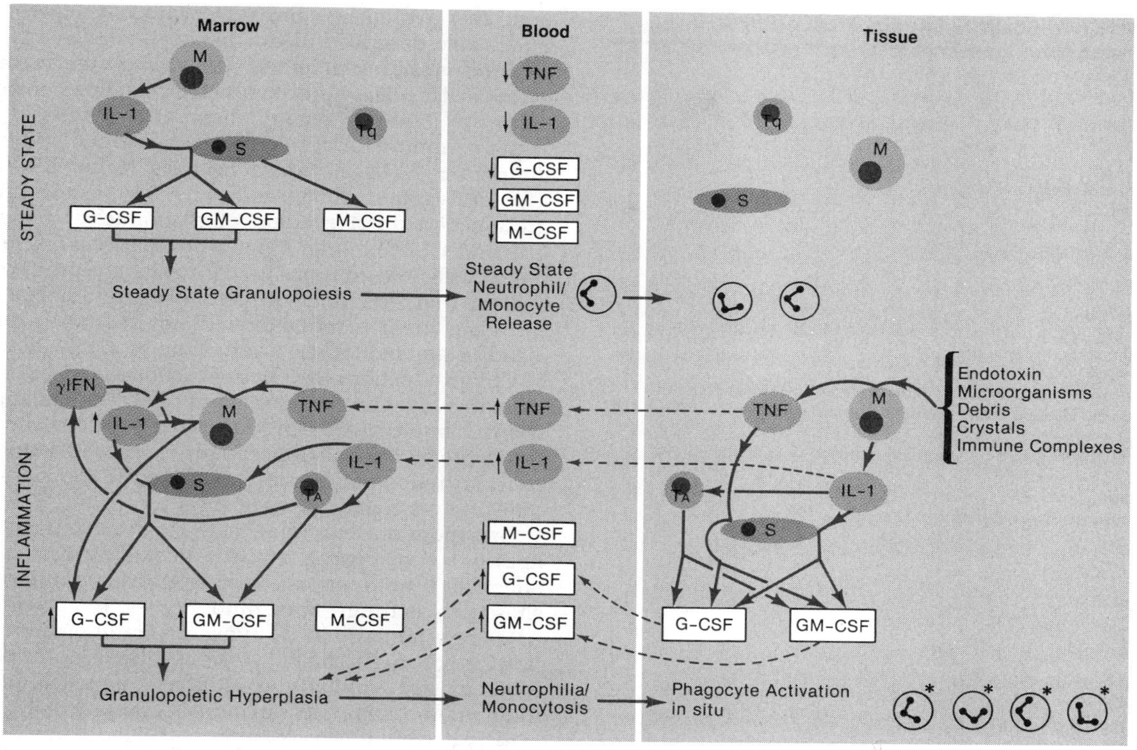

FIGURE 151–2. An intercellular regulatory network controls the production and function of phagocytes in inflammation. The figure represents the likely mechanisms by which neutrophil production and function are enhanced by inflammation. The cells (with nuclei) labeled M, S, and T represent monocytes/macrophages, stromal cells (fibroblasts and endothelial cells), and T lymphocytes, respectively. Tq are quiescent T cells (not activated), and Ta are activated T cells. Two monokines, interleukin-1 (IL-1) and tumor necrosis factor alpha (TNF), are represented by circles labeled IL-1 or TNF. The three lineage-specific granulopoietic growth factors—granulocyte colony stimulating factor (G-CSF), granulocyte/macrophage CSF (GM-CSF), and macrophage CSF (M-CSF)—are represented by rectangles. Relative concentrations of monokines and CSF's are reflected by the size of the circles or rectangles, respectively. In the steady state, stromal cells of the marrow produce all three CSF's. The production of G-CSF and GM-CSF by stromal cells even in the steady state may be under the influence of IL-1 produced by marrow macrophages and monocytes. Blood levels of monokines and growth factors are low. Production of these factors in uninflamed tissues is probably undetectable. In states of inflammation, however, the activation of macrophages by microorganisms, endotoxin, immune complexes, crystals, etc., results in the production of both TNF and IL-1. Both induce the expression of G-CSF and GM-CSF genes by stromal cells and activated T lymphocytes. IL-1 also induces G-CSF expression in macrophages. Production of CSF's in the tissue results in activation of phagocytes in that locale and in increased blood levels of both monokines (the inducers of growth factor expression), and the growth factors themselves. Macrophages, stromal cells and activated T lymphocytes in the marrow also respond to these monokines by producing G- and GM-CSF which stimulate increased growth and differentiation of granulocyte precursors with consequent granulocytic hyperplasia and neutrophilic leukocytosis.

considered: (1) Certain agents such as glucocorticoids, lithium chloride, or epinephrine commonly produce neutrophilia. (2) Malignant tumors may express certain of the CSF genes inappropriately and thereby increase CSF blood levels. When such cancers are effectively treated the neutrophilia resolves. (3) The chronic myeloproliferative disorders—chronic myelogenous leukemia, agnogenic myeloid metaplasia, essential thrombocytosis, and polycythemia rubra vera—may result in substantial neutrophilia. Patients with these diseases can present with few symptoms. When there is an acute inflammatory illness it is most prudent to await its resolution before seeking to rule out one of the myeloproliferative disorders.

DIAGNOSIS. The diagnostic approach to patients with neutrophilia is presented as an algorithm in Figure 151–3. Notice that the diagnostic path leads quickly to the performance of bone marrow aspiration and biopsy for patients with leukoerythroblastosis. In patients without leukoerythroblastosis, neutrophilic leukocytosis generally results from acute toxic, inflammatory, or traumatic stresses, and it is usually best simply to observe the course of neutrophilia to determine its degree of linkage with the underlying disease. If the underlying disease resolves and the neutrophilia does not, other less common explanations must be pursued.

Neutrophil Morphology. Neutrophil morphology can lead to early diagnosis (Fig. 151–3). Toxic granulation of neutrophils, the presence of Döhle bodies, and the presence of vacuoles in the neutrophil cytoplasm suggest that overt or subclinical inflammation, exposure to a toxin, trauma, or neoplasia exists. Because glucocorticoids induce prompt eosinopenia and basophilopenia, these cells are almost universally absent in the blood of the acutely injured or infected patient. Thus their presence should indicate that: (1) the acutely ill patient may have concomitant adrenal cortical insufficiency, (2) the neutrophilia derives from the inappropriate production of GM-CSF (generally by malignant cells), or (3) the neutrophilia is one manifestation of a hematopoietic neoplasm (a chronic myeloproliferative disorder, myelodysplastic syndrome, or certain of the acute nonlymphocytic leukemias).

Leukocyte Alkaline Phosphatase. Leukocyte alkaline phosphatase (LAP) activity is restricted to the neutrophil. Simple histochemical techniques are used to measure LAP levels in neutrophils of the peripheral blood. When neutrophilia represents a reaction to an acute illness, the LAP levels usually increase substantially. In chronic myelogenous leukemia (CML), however, the LAP score is markedly decreased. A

TABLE 151–2. COMMON CAUSES OF NEUTROPHILIA

Infections
- Bacteria
- Viruses
- Fungi
- Parasites
- *Rickettsiae*

Rheumatic and Autoimmune Disorders
- Rheumatoid arthritis
- Vasculitis
- Autoimmune hemolytic anemia
- Colitis
- Gout

Neoplastic Disorders
- Pancreatic, gastric, bronchogenic and renal cell carcinoma; melanoma
- Any cancer metastatic to bone marrow
- Hodgkin's disease
- Chronic myeloproliferative disorders (chronic granulocytic leukemia, agnogenic myeloid metaplasia, essential thrombocytosis, polycythemia vera)
- Myelodysplastic disorders and acute myelomonocytic leukemia

Chemicals
- Mercury poisoning
- Venoms (reptiles, insects, jellyfish)
- Ethylene glycol
- Histamine

Trauma
- Thermal injury
- Hypothermia
- Crush injuries
- Electric shock

Endocrine and Metabolic Disorders
- Ketoacidosis
- Lactic acidosis
- Thyrotoxicosis

Hematologic Disorders (non-neoplastic)
- Acute hemolytic anemias and transfusion reactions
- Postsplenectomy
- Recovery from marrow failure

Other Disorders
- Tissue necrosis
- Pregnancy
- Eclampsia
- Exfoliative dermatitis
- Severe hypoxia
- Drugs: Corticosteroids, lithium chloride, and epinephrine

low LAP in a patient with neutrophilia should therefore lead to a diagnostic evaluation designed to rule out CML (Table 151–3 and Fig. 151–3).

Differential Diagnosis of Neutrophilic Leukemoid Reactions. Neutrophilic leukemoid reactions generally occur in patients who are obviously systemically ill. When the neutrophil count exceeds 80 × 10^9 per liter, or when the mildness of the systemic illness seems discordant with the extremely high level of neutrophils in the peripheral blood, the diagnosis most often considered is CML. A number of additional features distinguish leukemoid reactions from CML (Table 151–3). In the past the most definitive test for CML has been a marrow chromosome analysis for the Philadelphia chromosome (see Ch. 155). In the near future even more sensitive tests may be direct DNA analyses to detect structural changes in the bcr (breakpoint cluster region) locus on chromosome 22 or immunoassay for the abnormal c-abl gene product p210 (Table 151–3).

MONOCYTOSIS

Monocytosis is defined as absolute peripheral blood monocyte counts greater than 0.80 × 10^9 per liter in children and greater than 0.50 × 10^9 per liter in adults. The monocyte-macrophage is the most evolutionarily conserved blood cell. In fact, its ancestors, found in the circulation or coelomic cavity of marine invertebrates, produce monokines with high degrees of structural and biologic homology to those produced by monocytes of humans. The mononuclear phagocyte plays such an essential role in so many components of biologic life that it seems unlikely that absolute monocyte and macrophage deficiency would be compatible with life. Macrophage function is also described in Ch. 148.

Monocytes present antigen to lymphocytes, mediate cellular cytotoxicity, release procoagulants, participate in bone remodeling and wound repair, dispose of damaged cells, and regulate immune and hematopoietic responses by producing interleukin-1 (IL-1), tumor necrosis factor (TNF)-alpha, G-CSF, and certain alpha-interferons. Two factors stimulate the growth and differentiation of mononuclear phagocytes: M-CSF and GM-CSF (Fig. 151–3). Stromal cells, including endothelial cells and fibroblasts, constitutively produce M-CSF, a protein that acts only on cells of the monocyte lineage to stimulate their production, differentiation, and survival. Steady-state monocyte production probably depends upon M-CSF production. M-CSF production is not yet known to be inducible by factors released during the inflammatory response, but GM-CSF production is induced during inflammation (Fig. 151–2). Consequently, reactive monocytosis appears to reflect an increase of GM-CSF and possibly also of other factors that act synergistically.

The mononuclear phagocyte is more sluggish than the neutrophil in moving toward and killing bacteria, but is as effective, if not more so, in killing obligate intracellular parasites such as fungi, yeast, and viruses. In addition, it participates substantially in all types of granulomatous inflammation. Accordingly, monocytosis is often seen in patients with tuberculosis, syphilis, fungal infections, ulcerative and granulomatous colitis, and sarcoidosis (Table 151–4). Mild monocytosis is common in patients with Hodgkin's disease and a variety of cancers. High levels of monocytes in the blood are most often seen in patients with myeloid malignant diseases, including acute and chronic myelomonocytic leukemia, acute monocytic leukemia, and chronic myelogenous leukemia of the juvenile type.

EOSINOPHILIA

Eosinophilic leukocytosis (eosinophilia) exists when the esinophil count in the peripheral blood exceeds 0.4 × 10^9 per

TABLE 151–3. DISTINCTIONS BETWEEN NEUTROPHILIC LEUKEMOID REACTIONS AND CHRONIC MYELOGENOUS LEUKEMIA

Finding/Result	Leukemoid Reaction	CML
Presence of fever or other manifestations of acute or subacute illness	Usual*	Infrequent†
Splenomegaly	Rare	Frequent
Natural course of neutrophilia	Resolution linked temporally with abatement of underlying disease	Progressive slow increase over time
Peripheral blood:		
Basophilia	Rare‡	Common
Leukocyte alkaline phosphatase score	High	Low§
Philadelphia chromosome	Never	Frequent (85%)
Abnormal DNA: Rearrangement of breakpoint cluster region in DNA (chromosome 22)	Absent‖	Frequent (>85%)

*Regular exceptions to this rule are patients with leukemoid reactions associated with certain carcinomas (Table 151–1).

†Patients with CML are not exempt from developing infections. Some patients with infectious processes may be found to have CML. The ideal time to evaluate them diagnostically is after the inflammatory process resolves.

‡Patients with acute allergic reactions and patients with widespread parasitic diseases are frequently exceptions to this rule.

§Leukocyte alkaline phosphatase scores are sometimes normal in CML patients after splenectomy.

‖As described in Ch. 155, the Philadelphia chromosome forms when chromosome 22 breaks in a region called the breakpoint-cluster region (bcr). There are some patients with CML who have no Philadelphia chromosome on karyotypic analysis, yet do have bcr rearrangement on DNA analysis.

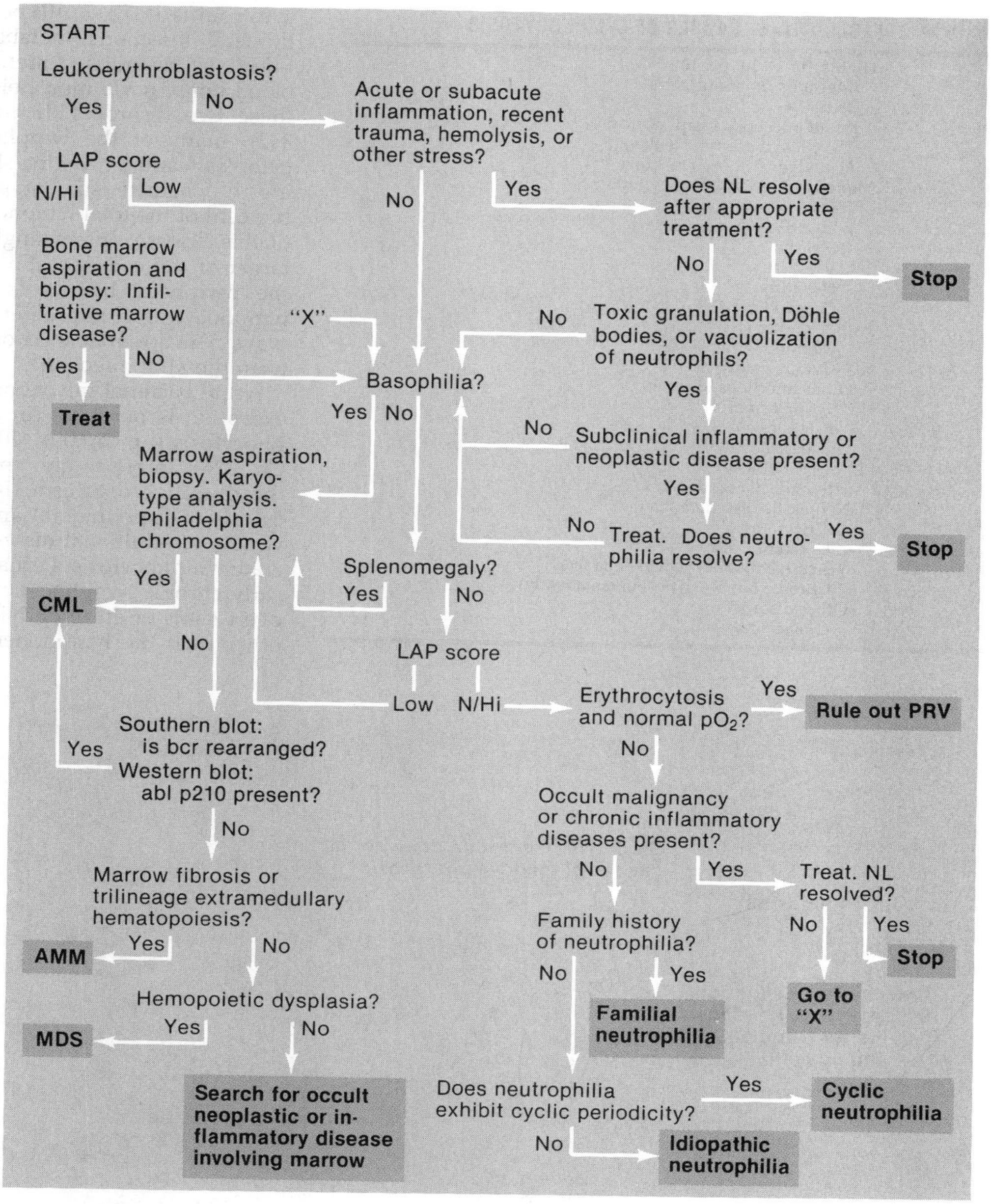

FIGURE 151–3. An algorithm for the evaluation of patients with neutrophilic leukocytosis (NL). LAP = Leukocyte alkaline phosphatase; N/Hi = normal or high; CML = chronic myelogenous leukemia; AMM = agnogenic myeloid metaplasia; PRV = polycythemia vera; MDS = myelodysplastic syndromes; abl p210 = the abnormally large protein that represents the product of the two fused genes, bcr and c-abl. Branch termini are enclosed in boxes.

TABLE 151–4. CAUSES OF MONOCYTOSIS

Infections
Tuberculosis
Brucellosis
Bacterial endocarditis
Typhoid and paratyphoid fevers
Listeriosis
Syphilis
Fungal infections
Recovery from acute infections
Protozoal infections
Neoplastic Disorders
Hodgkin's disease
Carcinoma (many)
Acute and chronic myelomonocytic leukemia, myelodysplastic syndromes, and chronic myelogenous leukemia of the juvenile type
Gastrointestinal Disorders
Ulcerative colitis
Granulomatous colitis
Cirrhosis
Sarcoidosis
Drug Reactions
Recovery from Marrow Suppression
Congenital Neutropenia

liter. Eosinophils are produced by progenitor cells in the marrow under the influence of at least two factors: GM-CSF and another protein that also stimulates the growth and differentiation of B-lymphocytes. Eosinophils function not only as phagocytes, but play an extraordinarily important role in modulating the potentially toxic effects of mast cell degranulation in hypersensitivity reactions.

The eosinophilic syndromes and the causes of eosinophilia are described in Ch. 162.

LYMPHOCYTOSIS

Lymphocytosis is defined as any lymphocyte count in excess of 5.0×10^9 per liter. Atypical lymphocytosis is present when atypical lymphocytes account for more than 20 per cent of the total peripheral blood lymphocyte population (see Ch. 342). The production and traffic of lymphocytes are clearly under tight control. A number of factors induce growth of T lymphocytes (IL-2 and IL-3), natural killer cells (IL-2), and B lymphocytes (IL-2, B cell stimulatory factor [BSF]-1, BSF-2, and B cell growth factor-II).

DIAGNOSIS. Mild to moderate lymphocytosis (lympho-

TABLE 151–5. CAUSES OF LYMPHOCYTOSIS

- **High (>15 × 10^9 per liter)**
  - Infectious mononucleosis
  - Pertussis
  - Acute infectious lymphocytosis
  - Chronic lymphocytic leukemia
  - Acute lymphocytic leukemia
- **Moderate (<15 × 10^9 per liter)**
  - Many viral infections
    - Infectious mononucleosis
    - Measles
    - Varicella
    - Hepatitis
    - Coxsackie
    - Adenovirus
    - Mumps
    - Cytomegalovirus
  - Other infectious diseases
    - Toxoplasmosis
    - Brucellosis
    - Tuberculosis
    - Typhoid fever
    - Syphilis (secondary)
  - Neoplastic disorders
    - Carcinoma
    - Hodgkin's disease
    - Acute lymphocytic leukemia (early)
    - Chronic lymphocytic leukemia (early)
  - Other disorders
    - Graves' disease

cyte counts < 12 × 10^9 per liter) is most commonly caused by viral infections, notably infectious mononucleosis and infectious hepatitis. Careful examination of the peripheral blood lymphocyte morphology can help distinguish between these two disorders. In infectious mononucleosis (see Ch. 342), many of the lymphocytes are large, with abundant cytoplasm and a ballerina-skirt-like cytoplasmic border. These are the characteristic "atypical" lymphocytes that exceed 20 per cent of the total lymphocyte population during the course of this disease. Interestingly, while the B lymphocyte is the target of the causative EB virus, the majority of the cells in the peripheral blood of patients with this disease are T lymphocytes. This proliferative response of T cells probably plays a major role in coordinating the process of recovery from the viral infection.

Acute bacterial infections rarely cause lymphocytosis. One exception is pertussis (in children) in which profound lymphocytosis (up to 60 × 10^9 per liter) is sometimes seen (see Ch. 276). Interestingly, specific soluble factors derived from the causative organism, *Bordetella pertussis*, induce lymphocytosis in experimental animals. In Table 151–5 are listed a variety of additional disorders associated with mild to moderate lymphocytosis. Perhaps with the exception of those with early chronic lymphocytic leukemia, most patients will have overt signs of an underlying illness involving anatomic sites other than the lymphohematopoietic system. This rule also

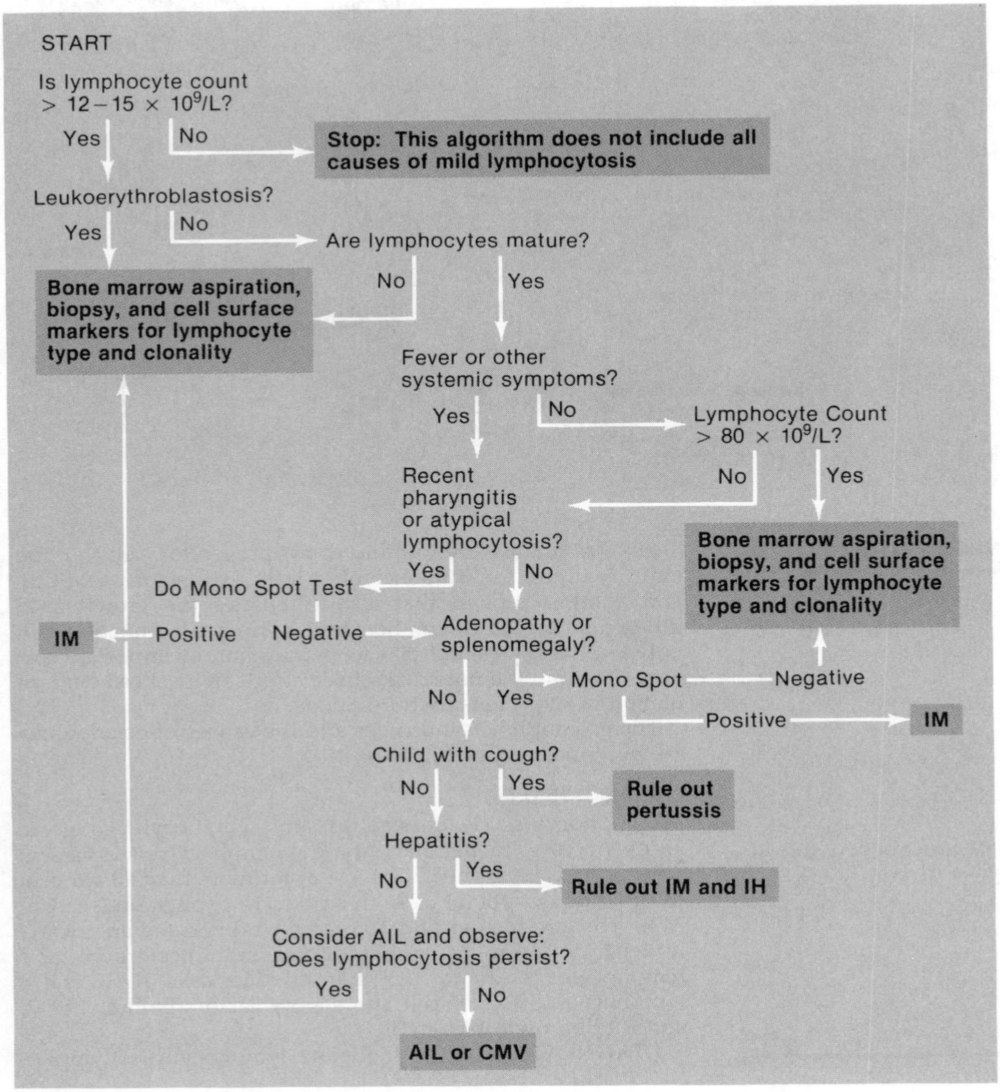

FIGURE 151–4. An algorithm for the evaluation of patients with lymphocytosis in excess of 12 × 10^9 per liter. IM = Infectious mononucleosis; CMV = cytomegalovirus infection; AIL = acute infectious lymphocytosis; IH = infectious hepatitis. Branch termini are enclosed in boxes.

holds true for patients with substantial lymphocytosis (> 12 to 15 × 10^9 per liter), the differential diagnosis of which is limited (Table 151–5). The diagnostic approach presented as an algorithm in Figure 151–4 depends simply upon establishing a tissue diagnosis to rule out malignant disease in patients who do not have clear-cut evidence of one of the benign disorders.

An important adjunct to histologic diagnosis is immunophenotypic analysis of the lymphocyte surface. Not only will such studies provide evidence for or against dominance of one lymphocyte type, but they are also capable of determining whether B lymphocytes in the circulation are all members of a single (therefore, likely neoplastic) clone.

Bagby GC, Dinarello CA, Wallace P, et al.: Interleukin 1 stimulates granulocyte macrophage colony-stimulating activity release by vascular endothelial cells. J Clin Invest 78:1316, 1986.

Broudy VC, Kaushansky K, Segal G, et al.: Tumor necrosis factor type alpha stimulates human endothelial cells to produce granulocyte/macrophage colony-stimulating factor. Proc Natl Acad Sci USA, 83:7467, 1986. Zucali J, Dinarello C, Oblon D, et al.: Interleukin 1 stimulates fibroblasts to produce granulocyte-macrophage colony-stimulating activity and prostaglandin E_2. J Clin Invest 77:1857, 1986. *These three papers provide important evidence that the production of granulopoietic factors by stromal cells can be stimulated by the monokines interleukin-1 and tumor necrosis factor-alpha. These in vitro observations provide insight into the importance of mononuclear phagocytes, the producers of monokines, as regulators of phagocyte production and function in inflammatory states. The reader is also referred to Figure 151–2.*

Cory S: Activation of cellular oncogenes in hemopoietic cells by chromosome translocation. Adv Cancer Res 47:189, 1986. *This review reports the pathophysiological significance of bcr gene rearrangement in cells from patients with chronic myelogenous leukemia.*

Donahue RE, Wang EA, Stone DK, et al.: Stimulation of haematopoiesis in primates by continuous infusion of recombinant human GM-CSF. Nature 321:872, 1986.

Fauci AS, Lane HC, Volkman DJ: Activation and regulation of human immune responses: Implications in normal disease states. Ann Intern Med 99:61, 1983. *This is an excellent review of lymphocyte function in health and disease. It covers B cell function and the linkage of T cell function with the function of B cells in a variety of disease states. The references are comprehensive.*

Metcalf D: The molecular biology of the granulocyte-macrophage colony stimulating factors. Blood 67:257, 1986. *This important paper describes the expanding knowledge of the granulocyte-macrophage colony-stimulating factors.*

Williams WJ, Beutler E, Erslev AJ, et al.: Hematology. 3rd ed. New York, McGraw-Hill Book Company, 1983. Wintrobe MM, Lee RE, Boggs DR, et al.: Clinical Hematology. 8th ed. Philadelphia, Lea & Febiger, 1981. *These textbooks of hematology include a number of chapters on phagocyte and lymphocyte production, traffic, distribution, and function. The reviews of neutrophilia, monocytosis, eosinophilia, and lymphocytosis are comprehensive and clinically relevant. Reference lists are encyclopedic and informative.*

152 CLONAL DEVELOPMENT AND STEM CELL ORIGIN OF PROLIFERATIVE DISORDERS

Philip J. Fialkow

Determination of whether a tumor arises from one or many cells can provide important clues about how it develops. For example, a neoplasm resulting from a rare event like mutation in a single somatic cell would by definition have a unicellular (clonal) origin. On the other hand, multicellular origin might be represented by a proliferative process caused by the presence of an abnormal growth factor.

The number of cells from which tumors arise can be conveniently investigated in a person who has at least two genetically distinct types of cells. The normal tissues contain cells of both types, but if the tumor is of clonal origin, it contains only one cell type.

One example of such a model system is the cellular mosaicism present in females heterozygous for the gene on the X chromosome that determines glucose-6-phosphate dehydrogenase (G6PD). In accordance with X chromosome inactivation, only one of the two G6PD genes is active in a given somatic cell. Thus, women who carry a gene for the usual type of G6PD (Gd^B) on one X chromosome and the common variant Gd^A on the other have two cell populations, one producing A type and the other B type G6PD. Since the two enzymes have different electrophoretic mobility, they are easily distinguishable. Cell proliferations with a clonal origin should exhibit only one type of enzyme (A *or* B), whereas those arising from many cells would usually have both A *and* B types. Once it has been determined that a proliferation is clonal, hierarchical relationships of stem cells can be investigated. For example, if both the granulocytes and erythrocytes of a heterozygous female with leukemia have only one and the same G6PD type, it can be inferred that the disease involves a stem cell multipotent for granulocytes and erythrocytes.

MYELOPROLIFERATIVE DISORDERS

Included in this group of diseases are chronic myelogenous leukemia, agnogenic myeloid metaplasia, polycythemia vera, and "essential" thrombocythemia. Although each disorder is characterized by predominance of one cell type (i.e., white cells, red cells, or platelets), there is often evidence of proliferation of other marrow cell types (e.g., in polycythemia vera erythrocytes predominate, but granulocytes and megakaryocytes also often are increased).

CHRONIC MYELOGENOUS LEUKEMIA. This disorder is of particular interest, since about 90 per cent of patients have a very specific and characteristic cytogenetic abnormality, the Philadelphia chromosome rearrangement (Ph) (see Ch. 155). Because Ph is so specific and when present is generally found in over 90 per cent of dividing marrow cells, it is most easily inferred that the disease develops from a single cell containing Ph.

Strong support for the clonal theory of Ph-positive chronic myelogenous leukemia was provided by the finding of only A *or* B G6PD in granulocytes from 32 patients with the disease, whereas both enzyme types were detected in the patients' normal tissues. Conversely, in Gd^B/Gd^A heterozygotes without blood cell abnormalities, with rare exceptions, the granulocytes show both B and A enzymes. The conclusion based on these and other observations that chronic myelogenous leukemia is a clonal disease obviously applies only to the stage at which the disorder is studied. Conceivably, many cells could be affected at an early phase, but when leukemia is clinically evident, only one clone is detected.

Ph has been found in erythroid precursors, suggesting that chronic myelogenous leukemia involves pluripotent stem cells. This postulate has been confirmed with G6PD: The same single-enzyme type found in the leukemic granulocytes was found in erythrocytes, eosinophils, monocytes, platelets, and B lymphocytes. These marker studies in chronic myelogenous leukemia provide definitive evidence for the existence in man of a stem cell pluripotent for lymphoid as well as myeloid cells.

OTHER MYELOPROLIFERATIVE DISORDERS. Although only a few patients have been evaluated with G6PD, the results suggest that the other chronic marrow cell proliferations—agnogenic myeloid metaplasia, polycythemia vera, essential thrombocythemia, and Ph-negative chronic myelogenous leukemia—are also clonal. Furthermore, in each instance, circulating red cells, granulocytes, and platelets displayed only one G6PD type, indicating that pluripotent stem cells were involved.

PATHOGENETIC IMPLICATIONS. The defect in chronic myelogenous leukemia seems to be intrinsic to the leukemic cells. Some workers have proposed that other myeloproliferations such as polycythemia vera or myeloid metaplasia result from proliferation of normal stem cells in response to abnormal stimuli. The G6PD studies suggest that the proliferating hemopoietic cells are very probably clonal and by inference that they are neoplastic in origin. Other points that have emerged from these studies are as follows:

Chromosomal Abnormalities. Specific cytogenetic abnormalities have been described in some patients with polycythemia vera (see Ch. 153). However, in the two studied Gd^B/Gd^A women with this disease, no chromosomal abnormalities were detected, indicating that at least in some patients these aberrations are not a prerequisite for the characteristic clonal proliferation of marrow stem cells. Accordingly, when a chromosomal abnormality occurs, it probably represents emergence of a subclone not required for the initial development of the disease.

G6PD studies of patients with chronic myelogenous leukemia suggest that there are clonally proliferating stem cells that lack Ph. Possibly at least two steps are involved in the pathogenesis of this leukemia—an early event leading to clonal proliferation of hemopoietic stem cells and a later event(s) resulting in the Ph and overt leukemia. The abnormal proliferation of Ph-positive cells is probably related to oncogene expression (see Ch. 169).

Myelofibrosis. Ph has not been detected in most studies of cultured marrow fibroblasts from patients with chronic myelogenous leukemia. It could be argued that the chromosomal abnormality arose in myeloid but not fibroblastic cells after the inception of the disease; however, the finding of normal double-enzyme G6PD types in the cultured fibroblasts indicates that they are not part of the neoplastic process. Similar observations suggest that the myelofibrosis that occurs in polycythemia vera and myeloid metaplasia is secondary. This is especially noteworthy for agnogenic myeloid metaplasia in which myelofibrosis is often the predominant clinical manifestation.

Remission. In clinical remission of chronic myelogenous leukemia or polycythemia vera achieved with conventional therapy, there is persistence of abnormal single-enzyme G6PD types in blood cells, and the percentage of Ph-positive marrow cells generally does not decline. Thus, even though these remissions may be prolonged, they are not accompanied by repopulation of the marrow with normal stem cells.

Residual Normal Stem Cells. In contrast to the results achieved with conventional therapy, about a third of patients with chronic myelogenous leukemia treated with intensive combination chemotherapy have reappearance in their marrows of large populations of Ph-negative cells. Studies of G6PD in one such patient indicated that the Ph-negative cells arose from nonclonal, presumably normal, stem cells. Studies of patients with polycythemia vera also suggest the presence of residual normal stem cells, but with their expression suppressed in vivo.

Summary. The myeloproliferative disorders appear to be clonal proliferations of pluripotent marrow stem cells, i.e., they are neoplasms with varying rates of progression. Myelofibrosis occurs in all of the disorders, but is apparently "reactive" and not part of the abnormal clone. Normal stem cells are present in these patients, and in some cases their expression is suppressed in vivo. Finally, since the clinical manifestations in each disorder are different despite the fact that the diseases all arise in pluripotent stem cells, the clinical variability presumably reflects differences in the responses of cells in the abnormal clones to certain regulatory factors. Determining the nature of these regulatory interactions may permit development of more efficient therapeutic modalities than are currently available.

ACUTE NONLYMPHOCYTIC LEUKEMIA

Many patients with acute nonlymphocytic leukemia have chromosomal abnormalities in marrow cells (see Ch. 156). The data suggest that within a given patient the chromosomally abnormal cells are members of a single clone. Findings of single-enzyme G6PD types in 26 heterozygotes with acute nonlymphocytic leukemia indicate that their diseases were clonal.

This leukemia has also been studied with an X chromosome inactivation marker system that has as its basis variations in noncoding intergenic DNA sequences termed restriction fragment length polymorphisms (RFLP's). Studies with RFLP's provide further support for the conclusion that acute nonlymphocytic leukemia develops clonally.

Stem cell relationships have been evaluated with G6PD in 18 patients with this leukemia. The observations in 13 relatively young patients that erythroid cells did not arise from the leukemic clone indicate that the clone did not prevent erythroid differentiation from normal progenitors. Conversely, in five elderly patients the leukemia involved stem cells pluripotent for at least granulocytes, erythrocytes, and platelets. Acute nonlymphocytic leukemia is therefore heterogeneous. In some patients it is expressed in cells with restricted differentiative expression; in others it involves stem cells with multipotent differentiative expression. Perhaps these differences underlie variations in cause and clinical features, including prognosis.

During some clinical remissions of this malignant disease the marrow seems to be repopulated by normal stem cells. For example, normal double-enzyme blood cell G6PD types were observed during remission in nine patients whose leukemia showed restricted differentiative expression. Thus, normal stem cells must have been present, but their proliferation was suppressed during the acute phase of the disease.

Another type of clinical remission, one that was associated with persistence of clonally derived stem cells, was found in two patients whose leukemia involved multipotent stem cells. Evidence that remission granulocytes were clonal was also found in 3 of 13 patients heterozygous for an RFLP.

The demonstration that clonal remissions are not uncommon suggests that this leukemia often has a multistep pathogenesis. Presumably an early event results in clonal proliferation of preleukemic stem cells that can differentiate to normal granulocytes. Overt leukemia evolves after a second step(s) occurs.

LYMPHOPROLIFERATIVE DISORDERS

IMMUNOGLOBULIN MOSAICISM. Immunoglobulin (Ig), as well as G6PD, is a useful marker in lymphoproliferative neoplasms. Since each Ig-synthesizing cell is committed to producing antibody molecules having only one variable region (idiotypic specificity) and only one light chain (κ or λ) and there are thousands of different antibodies, the immune system has extensive cellular mosaicism. The finding that a population of cells synthesizes only one type of Ig suggests that it is clonal. B lymphocytes, the precursors of plasma cells that secrete antibody, synthesize Ig that can be detected in the cytoplasm or on the cell's surface.

CHRONIC LYMPHOCYTIC LEUKEMIA. The proliferating cells in about 95 per cent of patients with this leukemia are B lymphocytes. The supposition that the disease is clonal based on Ig markers has been confirmed with G6PD. The G6PD studies also indicate that chronic lymphocytic leukemia is expressed in progenitors with differentiative expression restricted to the B-lymphocyte pathway and not to myeloid cells or at least to most blood T lymphocytes.

MULTIPLE MYELOMA. With rare exceptions, all the plasma cells in a given myeloma patient secrete Ig with the same light chain and idiotype, indicating clonal development. The total blood lymphocyte count is usually not increased in this disease. However, the fact that the surfaces of many circulating B lymphocytes and the cytoplasm of some pre-B cells have the same Ig molecules as those in the plasma indicates proliferation of a clone of early lymphocytes that ultimately differentiates into Ig-secreting plasma cells. This situation differs from that in chronic lymphocytic leukemia, in which maturation of the clone is restricted, i.e., most such patients do not have high levels of monospecific Ig in their serum.

WALDENSTRÖM'S MACROGLOBULINEMIA. This disease has features in common with chronic lymphocytic leukemia and multiple myeloma (see Ch. 163). As in myeloma, the same monospecific Ig found in the plasma is present on many marrow and circulating lymphocytes. In this sense Waldenström's macroglobulinemia and multiple myeloma might be regarded as forms of chronic lymphocytic leukemia in which the lymphocyte clone continues to mature from the small B cell to the mature plasma cell.

ACUTE LYMPHOCYTIC LEUKEMIA. In those few studied patients whose acute leukemia cells synthesize Ig, the data suggest clonal development. Studies with G6PD in untreated patients with the common form of this leukemia indicate that the disease is clonal and involves progenitors with differentiative expression limited to the lymphoid pathway. Cells in this type of acute lymphocytic leukemia do not have T cell surface markers or Ig synthesis. However, they do have rearranged Ig genes, indicating that they have B cell lineage differentiation potential. In many patients the Ig gene rearrangements are of a single type in all of the blast cells, providing more evidence that the common type of acute lymphocytic leukemia develops clonally. The presence of multiple Ig rearrangements found in some patients with B lymphoid malignant diseases probably results from the origin of the diseases in immature cells that continue to undergo Ig rearrangements as the neoplasms evolve. As differentiation proceeds within this clone, two or more subclones with different Ig gene rearrangements develop.

In 17 patients heterozygous for G6PD tested during remission, there was a return to nonclonal lymphopoiesis, indicating that the marrow was predominantly repopulated by normal cells. However, with a more sensitive Ig gene rearrangement marker technique, residual leukemic cells were found in remission stages of three of seven studied patients. This finding and the fact that the same monomorphic G6PD type found at diagnosis is present in relapse indicates that small numbers of leukemic cells persist during remission.

NON-HODGKIN'S LYMPHOMA. Ig markers in studies of B cell lymphomas indicate clonal development. Burkitt's lymphoma, a disease for which there is much circumstantial evidence of a viral cause, has been evaluated extensively with G6PD and Ig. The results indicate clonal development. Thus, if a virus causes the lymphoma, it either does so by inducing a rare change or constitutes but one of several factors necessary for tumorigenesis.

Burkitt's Tumor Relapses. Although the majority of patients with Burkitt's lymphoma have therapeutically induced clinical remissions, tumors reappear in over half the cases. Clinical and cell marker studies indicate that there are important biologic differences between early and late relapses. Thus, the G6PD and Ig types of early (<5 months) recurrent tumors were the same as those detected in the tumors on initial presentation, indicating re-emergence of the malignant clones. In contrast, the markers in some late (>5 months) Burkitt's tumor relapses were discordant with those originally found, indicating emergence of newly malignant cells or of neoplastic cells present but undetected when the patients were initially studied.

T CELL NEOPLASMS. T lymphocytes have on their surfaces receptors for antibody-bound antigen. In a process analogous to what occurs in B cell differentiation, as T lymphoid cells mature the T cell receptor genes undergo rearrangements. The finding in a neoplasm of such recombinations in the absence of Ig gene rearrangements indicates that the tumor is of T cell origin. The finding of one and the same T cell receptor gene rearrangement in all of the neoplastic cells indicates that the tumor developed clonally. With this system it has been shown, for example, that mycosis fungoides is a clonal neoplasm of T cell origin.

Korsmeyer AJ, Arnold A, Bakhsi A, et al: Immunoglobulin gene rearrangement and cell surface antigen expression in acute lymphocytic leukemias of T cell and B cell precursor origins. J Clin Invest 71:301, 1983.

Raskind WH, Fialkow PJ: The use of cell markers in the study of human hematopoietic neoplasia. In Weinhouse S, Klein G (eds.): Advances in Cancer Research. New York, Academic Press (in press). *A detailed review of studies of blood cell neoplasms with glucose-6-phosphate dehydrogenase, immunoglobulin, and T cell receptor markers; 209 references.*

153 ERYTHROCYTOSIS AND POLYCYTHEMIA

Paul D. Berk

Erythrocytosis, manifested by elevations of the red blood cell count, hematocrit, and hemoglobin concentration, represents a complex problem in differential diagnosis. Accurate diagnosis is crucial to appropriate management, particularly because therapy for certain diagnostic categories would be contraindicated in others.

Early in the evaluation of erythrocytosis it is important to differentiate an increase in the total red cell mass (absolute erythrocytosis) from a decrease in plasma volume (relative erythrocytosis). Patients with absolute erythrocytosis must be further categorized into those in whom excessive production of red cells results from a disorder intrinsic to the erythroid progenitor cells of the bone marrow (primary) or from excessive stimulation of an otherwise normal marrow by substances such as erythropoietin (secondary).

RELATIVE POLYCYTHEMIA

The hemoglobin concentration, hematocrit, and red blood cell count are usually interpreted as indicators of the circulating red blood cell or hemoglobin masses. In fact, these variables are merely measures of the extent to which the red cell mass is diluted in the plasma volume. Both the red cell mass and the plasma volume are regulated by separate and to a considerable extent independent physiologic controls. Hence, a patient with an elevated hemoglobin concentration, hematocrit, or red cell count may have (1) an increase in the red cell mass, i.e., an absolute erythrocytosis; (2) a reduction in the plasma volume; or (3) a combination of a red cell mass at the upper end of the normal range and plasma volume at the lower end of the normal range. These latter two situations have been termed relative or spurious polycythemia, since the elevated hemoglobin concentration, hematocrit, and red cell count do not reflect an absolute increase in the mass of circulating erythrocytes. Strictly speaking, the designation polycythemia should be reserved for conditions involving increased levels of other formed elements (granulocytes, platelets) in addition to erythrocytes; in fact, the term *polycythemia* is also widely applied to disorders characterized solely by abnormalities in erythroid parameters and will therefore be employed in this chapter.

The most frequent cause of relative polycythemia is dehydration. In settings in which dehydration is likely, fluid balance should be corrected before a hematologic evaluation of an elevated hematocrit is done. As an important first step, after dehydration is ruled out, patients with absolute polycythemia can be accurately distinguished from those with relative polycythemia by measurement of both the red cell mass and plasma volume, using ^{51}Cr-labeled erythrocytes and ^{125}I-albumin, respectively. This is especially important because, in the absence of conditions associated with arterial hypoxemia (cyanotic congenital heart disease, chronic pulmonary disease), cases of relative polycythemia are at least as common as cases of absolute polycythemia but need not be subjected to the extensive and expensive investigations that may be required to determine the cause of an absolute increase in the circulating red cell mass.

The normal red cell mass averages 30 ± 3 (SD) ml per kilogram in men and 27 ± 2 ml per kilogram in women. Although some studies indicate that hematocrits as high as 54 per cent in men or 48 per cent in women may be normal, increased red cell masses will be found in a small proportion of individuals of either sex with hematocrits in the upper 40's. As the hematocrit increases into the 50's, the proportion of patients with an increased red cell mass also increases but does not reach 100 per cent until the hematocrit is in excess of 60. Since approximately half of patients with polycythemia vera and other forms of true erythrocytosis and a large majority of those with spurious erythrocytosis present with hematocrits between 50 and 60, the need for direct measurement of the red cell mass to distinguish true polycythemia from spurious erythrocytosis is apparent.

Relative erythrocytosis, also called spurious polycythemia, stress polycythemia, and Gaisböck's syndrome, typically occurs in hypertensive obese middle-aged men, and especially in those who are heavy smokers. The male-female ratio is at least 5:1. Its underlying pathophysiology remains obscure. Both hypertension and its frequent therapy with diuretics may lead to reduction in the plasma volume. Smoking may contribute by two mechanisms. Both nicotine and carboxyhemoglobin, which circulates in smokers because of inhalation of carbon monoxide, may have mild diuretic effects. In addition, the presence of carboxyhemoglobin causes a shift to the left in the oxygen dissociation curve of the remaining hemoglobin, leading to mildly impaired tissue oxygenation. Normal compensatory mechanisms, in turn, lead to a modest increase in the red cell mass that may not always exceed the normal range, particularly when expressed per kilogram of body weight in an obese patient. In some smokers discontinuation of smoking results in cure of the erythrocytosis.

Relative erythrocytosis is not always a benign condition, the incidence of thromboembolic events reaching almost 30 per cent in some series, especially in patients with an absolute reduction in plasma volume. Treatment remains controversial, but maintenance of the hematocrit at no more than 50 per cent by a judicious phlebotomy regimen is often recommended and may be beneficial.

Burge PS, Johnson WS, Prankard TAJ: Morbidity and mortality in pseudo polycythemia. Lancet 1:1266, 1975. *Follow-up study documenting excess morbidity and mortality in patients with relative erythrocytosis.*

Humphrey PRD, Michael J, Pearson TC: Red cell mass, plasma volume and blood volume before and after venesection in relative polycythemia. Br J Haematol 46:435, 1980. *Documents that phlebotomy in relative polycythemia is followed by expansion of the plasma volume, so that hypovolemia does not occur.*

Smith JR, Landaw SA: Smokers' polycythemia. N Engl J Med 293:6, 1978. *A report convincingly linking smoking to polycythemia and suggesting that chain smoking is the link that ties stress to polycythemia.*

ABSOLUTE POLYCYTHEMIA: PATHOPHYSIOLOGY AND CLINICAL EVALUATION

Regulation of the Red Cell Mass

The circulating red cell mass is determined by a balance between the rate at which new erythrocytes are produced and released from the bone marrow and the rate of peripheral red cell destruction. The latter, as measured by studies of the red cell lifespan, is ordinarily fixed, with a normal mean value of about 100 days. While red cell lifespan may be reduced in pathologic states, there are no mechanisms by which it may be increased. Hence, physiologic regulation of the red cell mass occurs entirely by changes in the rate of red cell production.

Alterations in the red cell mass are effected so as to provide for a critical level of tissue oxygenation (Fig. 153–1). The principal sensors of the state of tissue oxygenation in adults are probably located in the kidney, although the existence of extrarenal oxygen sensors has also been proposed. The kidney responds to the perceived adequacy of oxygen delivery by modulating the output of the hormone erythropoietin. The gene for this carbohydrate-rich glycoprotein has been successfully cloned, and its biologic activity has been found to reside in a 166-amino acid polypeptide chain.

The initial commitment of pluripotent bone marrow stem cells to differentiate to the earliest erythroid-committed progenitors, the *erythroid burst-forming units* (BFU_E), depends principally on a T cell–derived growth regulator called *burst-promoting activity*. By contrast, erythropoietin, the principal regulator of the subsequent stages of erythropoiesis, appears to stimulate proliferation of the *erythroid colony–forming units* (CFU_E), the more differentiated but still morphologically unrecognizable progeny of the BFU_E. Since further differentiation of the CFU_E to early, recognizable proerythroblasts is a stochastic process, expansion of the pool of CFU_E results in an increase in the production of recognizable erythroid precursors in the marrow. Erythropoietin also shortens the overall maturation time of developing erythroid precursors and accelerates the release of reticulocytes into the circulation. Hence its net effect is to increase the output of red cells from the marrow and ultimately to expand the circulating red cell mass.

Mechanisms Producing Erythrocytosis

Erythrocytosis or "polycythemia" reflects an increase in marrow red cell production caused by increased proliferation of erythroid progenitors. This proliferation could be either "autonomous" as a result of an intrinsic cellular defect permitting escape from normal regulatory mechanisms or secondary to an external stimulus.

AUTONOMOUS PROLIFERATION. The increased erythroid activity in the primary polycythemias, including polycythemia rubra vera and the more recently described entity of

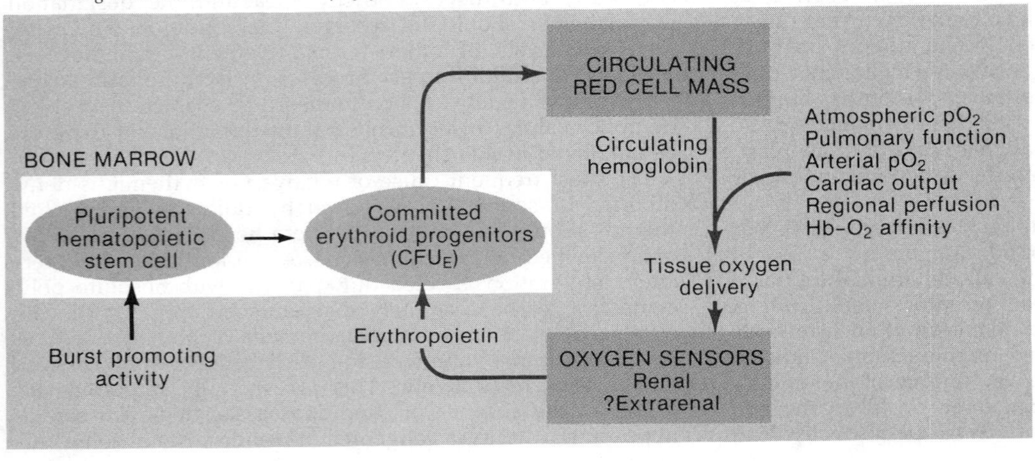

FIGURE 153–1. Relationship between tissue oxygen delivery, erythropoietin output, and the circulating red cell mass.

primary erythrocytosis, is seemingly autonomous in that increased red cell production occurs despite low or undetectable levels of erythropoietin as measured by in vivo bioassay techniques. Moreover, "endogenous colonies" of erythroid progenitors from such patients may be successfully grown in various in vitro tissue culture systems without added erythropoietin, which is otherwise essential for erythroid progenitor growth in vitro. Finally, phlebotomy to low normal or anemic levels produces an increase in erythropoietin production, indicating that the "servomechanism" relating erythropoietin output to tissue oxygen delivery is intact. The apparent erythropoietin independence of erythropoiesis in the primary polycythemias is now recognized to reflect a markedly increased sensitivity of erythroid progenitors to minute amounts of the hormone, rather than total erythropoietin independence.

SECONDARY PROLIFERATION. Alternatively, the proliferation could result from abnormalities in the erythropoietic regulatory mechanism extrinsic to the erythroid progenitors themselves. The increased red cell production in these circumstances is driven by increased levels of erythropoietin or other erythroid stimulatory substances, and erythroid progenitors require exogenous erythropoietin to grow successfully in vitro. These features characterize the various secondary polycythemias.

The secondary polycythemias can be further subdivided into three categories. The *first* is disorders in which the signal resulting in erythrocytosis, most often an increase in erythropoietin production, represents a physiologically appropriate response to poor tissue oxygenation caused by arterial hypoxemia, genetically determined or "acquired" high affinity hemoglobins that release oxygen to tissue inadequately, or reduced tissue perfusion. For these conditions, reduction of the red cell mass by phlebotomy, even to values still substantially greater than normal, may reduce tissue oxygen delivery and result in a further increase in erythropoietin output. The *second* category is disorders characterized by excessive autonomous production of erythropoietic stimulatory substances (erythropoietin, androgens, adrenal corticosteroids). Increased, autonomous erythropoietin production may occur in certain neoplasms, as a result of non-neoplastic lesions in the kidney (hydronephrosis, cysts, tumors, vascular lesions) that produce local ischemia involving the renal oxygen-sensing mechanism, or in certain rare, familial syndromes, without a demonstrable anatomic lesion. For the disorders in this category, erythropoietin production is not influenced by phlebotomy-induced changes in the red cell mass. The *third* category is the entity in which erythropoietin secretion remains under physiologic control in that it responds to phlebotomy, but at a level of production inappropriately high for the level of tissue oxygenation. A classification of the various absolute erythrocytoses, based on underlying mechanisms, is presented in Table 153–1.

TABLE 153–1. CAUSES OF ERYTHROCYTOSIS

I. Relative erythrocytosis (stress, spurious, or pseudopolycythemia; Gaisböck's syndrome)
II. Absolute erythrocytosis
   A. Primary (proliferative bone marrow disorder)
      1. Polycythemia vera
      2. Primary erythrocytosis
   B. Secondary (increased marrow stimulation by erythropoietin, etc.)
      1. Physiologically appropriate increased erythropoietin production
         a. Arterial hypoxemia
            i. High altitude
            ii. Chronic pulmonary disease
            iii. Cardiovascular shunt (right-to-left)
            iv. Massive obesity (pickwickian syndrome)
            v. Postural hypoxemia
         b. Abnormal release of oxygen from hemoglobin
            i. Hereditary high oxygen affinity hemoglobin
            ii. Congenitally decreased red cell 2,3-DPG
            iii. Smoker's polycythemia (carboxyhemoglobinemia)
         c. Interference with tissue oxygen metabolism
            i. Cobalt
      2. Physiologically inappropriate erythropoietin production
         a. Neoplasms
            i. Renal, adrenal, hepatocellular, and ovarian carcinomas
            ii. Cerebellar hemangioblastomas (e.g., von Hippel-Lindau syndrome)
            iii. Adrenal cortical adenoma and/or hyperplasia
            iv. Pheochromocytoma
            v. Large uterine fibroids (rare)
         b. Non-neoplastic renal diseases
            i. Cysts, hydronephrosis
            ii. Bartter's syndrome
            iii. Post-transplantation
         c. Autonomous, fixed increased erythropoietin production without demonstrable anatomic lesion (familial)
         d. Excessive basal erythropoietin output with further augmentation following phlebotomy (familial)
      3. Therapeutic administration or excess production of androgens or certain other corticosteroids

Pathophysiology of Absolute Erythrocytosis

Irrespective of underlying etiology, all disorders characterized by an absolute erythrocytosis share certain common clinical manifestations resulting from the expanded blood volume and increased blood viscosity. The increased blood volume leads to generalized vascular expansion and venous engorgement, which are reflected by the characteristic ruddy cyanosis of the skin and mucous membranes. These factors are magnified by the marked decrease in cerebral blood flow that accompanies elevation of the hematocrit and in turn contributes to headaches, tinnitus, a frequently described feeling of fullness in the head and neck, and light-headedness. There appears to be an increase in thrombotic complications, particularly involving the cerebrovascular circulation, in patients with markedly elevated hematocrit and expanded blood volume. Epistaxis and upper gastrointestinal hemorrhage are also more frequent in the hypervolemic patient. The increase in viscosity accompanying hypervolemia and erythrocytosis may result in a decrease in cardiac output, reduction in regional blood flow, and ultimately in an impairment of tissue oxygenation, even in cases in which the underlying initial stimulus was poor oxygen delivery.

In contrast to the consequences of expanded blood volume and blood viscosity, the consequences of bone marrow hyperactivity and of increased red cell destruction are minimal. Because expansion of the red cell mass often occurs very slowly, increases in bone marrow volume, alterations in the myeloid:erythroid ratio, and changes in reticulocyte count or plasma iron turnover may be difficult to appreciate. Similarly, although a doubling of the red cell mass results in a doubling of bilirubin production, this may be insufficient to drive the plasma unconjugated bilirubin concentration outside of its relatively wide normal range.

Clinical Evaluation of the Patient with Erythrocytosis

ROLE OF CONVENTIONAL DIAGNOSTIC METHODS. A systematic approach to the evaluation of the patient with erythrocytosis is illustrated in Figure 153–2. This algorithm ensures the correct classification of patients with relative as opposed to absolute erythrocytosis. In the majority of instances, patients with absolute erythrocytosis can also be appropriately classified as having primary or secondary erythrocytosis, and in the latter case, the specific underlying cause can be identified on the basis of conventional, widely available diagnostic studies. The diagnosis of polycythemia vera is discussed later in this chapter.

SPECIAL STUDIES: ASSAY OF ERYTHROPOIETIN AND ENDOGENOUS COLONY FORMATION. Erythropoietin is most commonly estimated by an in vivo bioassay in polycythemic mice. Injection of patient plasma or urine preparations into such animals stimulates the incorporation of ^{59}Fe into newly produced erythrocytes, to a degree proportional to the erythropoietin content of the injected material. When this assay is applied to urine samples, normal individuals have

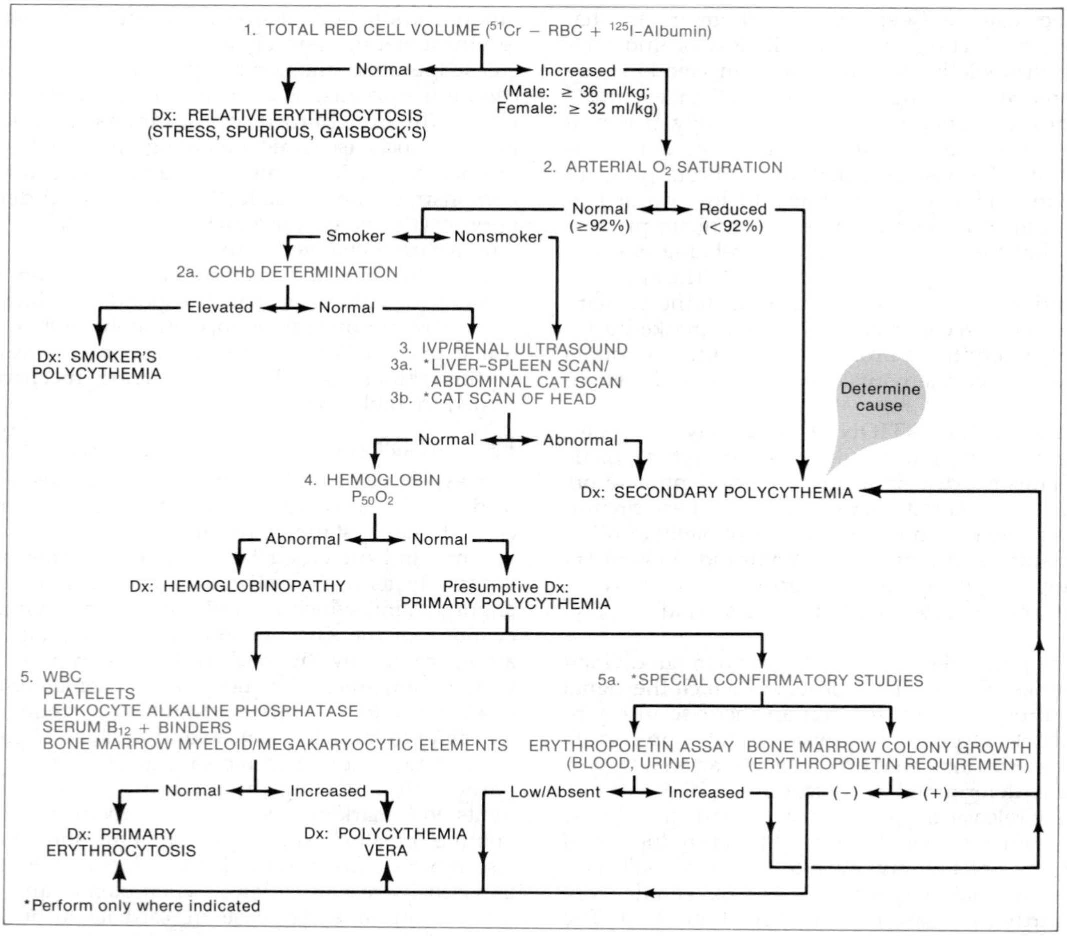

FIGURE 153–2. Algorithm for evaluation of an elevated hematocrit. Laboratory features suggestive of a myeloproliferative disease include elevated platelet and white blood cell counts and increased reticulin and clustered atypical megakaryocytes in a bone marrow biopsy. A careful history (e.g., ? family history of elevated hematocrit, ? heavy smoking) and physical examination (? splenomegaly, evidence of cardiac or pulmonary disease) provide indispensable information.

basal levels of erythropoietin excretion within a well-defined normal range. After phlebotomy urinary erythropoietin excretion increases, and an inverse logarithmic relationship is observed between the hematocrit and the erythropoietin excretion rate. Patients with hypoxic secondary erythrocytosis have variable basal values ranging from normal to increased, but all have increased values following reduction of hematocrit to normal by means of phlebotomy. In contrast, basal urinary erythropoietin excretion is very low in patients with polycythemia vera. Normal human plasma appears to contain 10 to 20 mU of erythropoietin per milliliter. The lower limit of sensitivity of the polycythemic mouse assay is approximately 50 mU per milliliter. Hence, when applied to plasma, this assay cannot distinguish normal subjects from those with polycythemia vera, since both groups fall below this sensitivity limit. The assay can detect the elevated levels seen in some cases of secondary polycythemia. Procedures to concentrate the plasma 40-fold may increase the sensitivity of this technique to approximately 5 mU per milliliter. Using this procedure, patients with polycythemia vera still had undetectable plasma levels of erythropoietin by bioassay, whereas most (but not all) normal subjects had detectable values averaging 7.8 ± 1.1 (SD) mU per milliliter, and the majority of patients with a clinical diagnosis of secondary polycythemia had elevated levels. Unfortunately, the concentration procedure is cumbersome and may introduce artifacts into the in vivo bioassay. Of alternative techniques for measuring erythropoietin, only a hemagglutination inhibition assay is commercially available, but its reliability has been questioned. Similarly, radioimmunoassay procedures report elevated erythropoietin levels in many cases of secondary polycythemia but equivalent levels in normal subjects and patients with polycythemia vera, possibly reflecting immunoreactive but biologically inert erythropoietin fractions or other materials. Only one experimental assay procedure purports to separate normal serum erythropoietin levels from reduced values in polycythemia vera.

The ability to grow erythroid progenitors from bone marrow or peripheral blood in vitro without added erythropoietin strongly supports the diagnosis of a primary bone marrow disorder of erythroid regulation.

As indicated in the foregoing discussion and in Figure 153–2, when erythropoietin assays and/or studies of in vitro endogenous colony formation are available, they may help to distinguish patients with primary polycythemias from those with secondary polycythemias. In addition, the influence of phlebotomy on erythropoietin output may separate the physiologically appropriate secondary polycythemias from those in which erythropoietin output is autonomous. In the majority of cases, these distinctions can be made on the basis of conventional diagnostic investigations.

Erslev AJ, Caro J: Pure erythrocytosis classified according to erythropoietin titers. Am J Med 76:57, 1984. *Clear demonstration of both the uses and limitations of erythropoietin bioassays in diagnosis of polycythemic states.*

Garcia JF, Ebbe SN, Hollander L, et al.: Radioimmunoassay of erythropoietin: Circulating levels in normal and polycythemic human beings. J Lab Clin

Med 99:624, 1982. *Report on the only erythropoietin radioimmunoassay that distinguishes the reduced values in polycythemia vera from normal levels.*
Golde DW, Hocking WG, Koeffler HP, et al.: Polycythemia: Mechanisms and management. Ann Intern Med 95:71, 1981. *An outstanding review of the pathophysiology, diagnosis, and management of the various polycythemias, with a comprehensive bibliography.*

SECONDARY POLYCYTHEMIAS

In the secondary polycythemias a normal bone marrow is stimulated to produce increased numbers of red blood cells, leading to an increase in the circulating red cell mass, as a result of increased production of erythropoietin or of other erythrostimulatory substances. These disorders all have in common the diverse symptomatic consequences of hypervolemia and increased blood viscosity described earlier. The secondary polycythemias may be classified into those in which the polycythemia is an appropriate physiologic response to inadequate tissue oxygenation and those in which the development of erythrocytosis is inappropriate to the oxygen balance of the patient (Table 153–1).

Physiologically Appropriate Polycythemias

HIGH ALTITUDE. In the presence of normal hemoglobin A and appropriate intraerythrocytic levels of 2,3-diphosphoglyceric acid (DPG), the partial pressure of oxygen in capillaries must be maintained close to 40 mm Hg to ensure adequate off-loading of oxygen to tissues. At sea level, where the atmospheric partial pressure of oxygen is approximately 160 mm Hg, oxygen is readily loaded onto the hemoglobin molecule, and the steep oxygen pressure gradient from the alveoli to the tissue capillaries ensures an adequate driving force for tissue oxygenation. In contrast, at elevated altitudes the atmospheric oxygen tension diminishes, and at approximately 5400 meters, the altitude of the highest permanent human settlement, atmospheric oxygen pressure is only 80 mm Hg, providing a much smaller alveolar–capillary oxygen pressure gradient. To provide adequate tissue oxygenation in the face of this reduced driving force, individuals constantly exposed to high altitude are acclimatized by two principal mechanisms, hyperventilation and the development of erythrocytosis. Hyperventilation causes a reduction in the pulmonary dead space and an increase in the surface area of adequately perfused alveoli. Erythrocytosis increases the oxygen-carrying capacity of circulating blood. Together, these two alterations permit acclimatization to occur without the need for a significant increase in cardiac output. In general, although a shift in the oxygen-hemoglobin dissociation curve to the right would also increase tissue oxygenation at a given capillary oxygen tension, such a change would also impair the on-loading of oxygen in the lungs at high altitudes. The latter appears to take precedence in that direct measurement of oxygen dissociation curves among individuals who live at higher altitudes generally reveals patterns within the normal range.

Approximately 25,000,000 people live at altitudes between 3000 and 5400 meters. The latter, with an atmospheric pressure of approximately one half normal, appears to represent the extreme limit of human long-term physiologic adaptation. Transient adaptation to higher levels is possible, as demonstrated by the successful 1978 scaling of Mount Everest (8848 meters), where atmospheric pressure is approximately one third of normal, without the use of administered oxygen.

Those who dwell for long periods at high altitudes typically develop an increased anteroposterior thoracic diameter, and a ruddy cyanosis secondary to hypervolemia. The increased blood volume is manifested in the engorged capillaries of the conjunctivae, skin, and mucous membranes, and may contribute to all of the classic symptoms of hypervolemia. The hematocrit is elevated, reflecting an increased red cell mass in the presence of a normal plasma volume. White blood cells and platelets are normal, and bone marrow aspirates may appear to be normal or to show modest erythroid hyperplasia. The acute and chronic effects of living at high altitude are further described in Ch. 537.

CARDIOPULMONARY DISEASE. Arterial hypoxemia, resulting from right-to-left shunts in congenital heart disease (see Ch. 49) or from chronic obstructive pulmonary disease (see Ch. 61), results in expansion of the red cell mass. This may be masked in part in both settings by a concomitant increase in plasma volume.

ALVEOLAR HYPOVENTILATION. Arterial hypoxemia, cyanosis, and secondary erythrocytosis may also result from either centrally mediated or peripheral impairment of alveolar ventilation. One of the settings in which this occurs, Monge's disease (chronic mountain sickness), is described in Ch. 537. Another is the so-called pickwickian syndrome, in which the work load of ventilation in a severely obese individual is aggravated by central hyporesponsiveness to hypoxemia and hypercapnia. In a third group of patients postural hypoxemia occurs during sleep. All of these conditions may be associated with increased erythropoietin production and secondary erythrocytosis.

ABNORMALITIES OF THE OXYGEN-HEMOGLOBIN DISSOCIATION CURVE. Abnormalities in the ability of hemoglobin to release oxygen to tissues, manifested by a shift in the oxyhemoglobin dissociation curve to the left, may occur on either a congenital or an acquired basis. At least 42 such hemoglobins have been described in association with erythrocytosis (Ch. 144). In most an amino acid substitution occurring in the contact area between the α and β chains interferes with the normal conformational changes that facilitate oxygen release from the molecule. The resulting high oxygen affinity hemoglobin results in noncyanotic tissue hypo-oxygenation and ultimately in secondary erythrocytosis. High affinity variants involving both α-chain substitutions (hemoglobin Capetown, hemoglobin Chesapeake) and β-chain substitutions (hemoglobin Ranier, hemoglobin Yakima) have been described. Most of these high affinity mutations are electrophoretically silent because there is no charge difference between the normal and variant hemoglobin. Hence, determination of an oxygen-hemoglobin dissociation curve or determination of the P_{50} is essential in the evaluation of patients suspected of having a high oxygen affinity hemoglobin. This suspicion particularly should be directed toward individuals in whom familial erythrocytosis is observed.

Secondary erythrocytosis may also occur in the presence of certain hereditary methemoglobinemias, disorders in which amino acid substitutions occur in the regions of the heme pockets. Most of these conditions are associated with hemolysis, but, in the few in which the rate of red cell destruction is near normal, compensatory mechanisms may result in a secondary erythrocytosis. Several different congenital disorders involving a decreased ability to synthesize 2,3-DPG have been described. Since reductions in red cell 2,3-DPG content are associated with an increased oxygen affinity for hemoglobin, such patients may behave clinically as if they had a high affinity hemoglobin disorder with resulting secondary erythrocytosis, even though they in fact have hemoglobin A. Finally, prolonged exposure to carbon monoxide, occasionally on an industrial basis but more frequently in chain smokers, results in erythrocytosis because carboxyhemoglobin has the effect of increasing the oxygen affinity of the remaining heme prosthetic groups. The hematocrit is often increased out of proportion to the red cell mass because of secondary effects of carboxyhemoglobin or nicotine or both in reducing the plasma volume.

Physiologically Inappropriate Erythrocytosis

NEOPLASMS AND NON-NEOPLASTIC RENAL DISEASES. Physiologically inappropriate erythrocytosis is seen in a variety of neoplasms, including renal and adrenal carcinoma, cerebellar hemangioblastoma, hepatocellular carcinoma, ovarian carcinoma, pheochromocytoma, and massive uterine fibroids (Ch. 173). The proportion of each of these tumors in which erythrocytosis develops is highly variable. It seems to be particularly high in cases of hepatocellular carcinoma. In most instances, increased erythropoietin production by the tumor is believed to be the underlying mechanism leading to erythrocytosis.

Secondary erythrocytosis also occurs in a variety of nonmalignant disorders of the kidney, including cystic disease and hydronephrosis, and following renal transplantation. Production of increased erythropoietin levels in the presence of renal cystic disease appears likely in view of the frequent documentation of high titers of the hormone in aspirated cyst fluid. Local intrarenal ischemia resulting from various types of renal pathology is believed to mediate an increased erythropoietin output in these disorders. Familial syndromes occur in which autonomous production of increased quantities of erythropoietin has been observed without a demonstrable anatomic lesion. Erythropoietin output in these syndromes does not vary in response to phlebotomy. A single report also describes an inappropriately high level of basal erythropoietin output in an individual in whom phlebotomy resulted in a further increase in hormone production. The nature of the underlying defect in these two syndromes is unclear.

DRUG INDUCED. Testosterone and its various derivatives, and a variety of adrenal corticosteroids, may stimulate red cell production. Testosterone-like compounds are often used therapeutically for this purpose in patients with renal failure who are undergoing dialysis or in patients with aregenerative anemia. In some instances, androgens will also stimulate granulocyte and platelet production. Occasionally, increased levels of steroid hormones, whether administered therapeutically or produced in the course of adrenal disorders, may result in secondary erythrocytosis.

Treatment of the Secondary Polycythemias

Hypervolemia and increased blood viscosity accompany the development of erythrocytosis. Accordingly, when a secondary erythrocytosis is not in response to an appropriate physiologic stimulus, reduction of hematocrit to less than 50 per cent by means of phlebotomy is an appropriate part of the treatment regimen, which should also address itself to the underlying disorder.

The issue is more complex in those secondary erythrocytoses that represent a physiologic response to poor tissue oxygenation. The beneficial effect of expansion of the red cell mass may ultimately be offset by the detrimental effect of increasing blood viscosity on cardiac output, systemic oxygen transport, and local tissue oxygen delivery. In a normovolemic state, oxygen transport is optimal at a hematocrit of 40 to 45 per cent. In the presence of hypervolemia, optimal oxygen delivery may occur at hematocrits close to 60 per cent. However, hematocrits higher than this inevitably impair oxygen delivery. Nevertheless, in a given patient, if an increase in the hematocrit to the region of 60 per cent does not achieve normal tissue oxygenation, a continued increase in erythropoietin output may result in overcompensation. This overcompensation may not only decrease net tissue oxygen delivery but may also impair regional blood flow in a number of organs, particularly within the cerebral circulation. In summary, in the physiologic secondary polycythemias, there is a balance between the beneficial effects of an increasing hematocrit and the negative consequences of an excessive increase in blood viscosity. In general, hematocrits in excess of 60 per cent are detrimental and should be reduced by phlebotomy. In patients with arterial hypoxemia resulting from pulmonary disease or right-to-left cardiac shunts, the optimal level of hemoglobin and hematocrit may be difficult to determine except by trial and error. In some cases, improvement in cerebral function and decrease in congestive heart failure may follow a reduction in blood volume to hematocrits in the mid 50's or even lower.

Bunn HF, Forget B: Hemoglobin: Molecular, Genetic and Clinical Aspects. Philadelphia, W. B. Saunders Company, 1986, pp 595–622. *This chapter presents an outstanding review of hemoglobin variants with abnormal oxygen binding and their clinical consequences, as well as a comprehensive bibliography.*

Chetty KG, Brown SE, Light RW: Improved exercise tolerance of the polycythemic lung patient following phlebotomy. Am J Med 74:415, 1983. *A detailed clinicophysiologic study documenting that patients with polycythemia due to chronic obstructive pulmonary disease benefit from reduction of hematocrit to the mid 50's by phlebotomy.*

Distelhorst CW, Wagner DS, Goldwasser E, et al.: Autosomal dominant familial erythrocytosis due to autonomous erythropoietin production. Blood 58:1155, 1981. *A well-described family with this rare syndrome. Bibliography includes references to cases with the slightly more common recessive variant.*

Erslev AJ: Blood and mountains. In Wintrobe MM (ed.): Blood, Pure and Eloquent. New York, McGraw-Hill Book Company, 1980, pp 257–280. *A lucid and fascinating review of the evolution of current concepts of human adaptation to the hypoxemia of high altitudes. Excellent bibliography.*

Whitcomb WH, Peschle C, Moore M, et al.: Congenital erythrocytosis: A new form associated with an erythropoietin-dependent mechanism. Br J Haematol 44:17, 1980. *An unusual syndrome characterized by inappropriately high basal erythropoietin output that increased further after phlebotomy.*

POLYCYTHEMIA VERA: A CLONAL STEM CELL DISORDER

Nature of the Defect in Polycythemia Vera

Polycythemia vera is a hematologic malignant disorder characterized by excessive proliferation of erythroid, myeloid, and megakaryocytic elements within the bone marrow, resulting in an increased red blood cell mass and, frequently, elevated peripheral granulocyte and platelet counts. Several lines of evidence, including cytogenetic observations and isoenzyme marker studies in G6PD heterozygotes, indicate that the increased proliferation of all three hematopoietic cell lines can trace its origin to a single abnormal clone, which has presumably developed at the level of the pluripotent stem cell (Ch. 152). B lymphocytes are also derived from the abnormal stem cell clone. Studies of the growth of both erythroid progenitors and granulocyte-macrophage progenitors (CFU-GM) in vitro have demonstrated the presence of residual normal stem cells in the marrow early in the disease, but a steady decline in the proportion of the normal elements as the duration of the illness lengthens.

Thrombotic episodes that are usually attributed to increased blood viscosity and/or thrombocytosis; hemorrhagic episodes associated with thrombopathy and/or the elevated platelet and erythrocyte counts; the development of a "spent" phase characterized by cytopenias, myelofibrosis, and myeloid metaplasia; and the transformation to acute leukemia are among the principal complications of this disorder. Polycythemia vera shares several clinical, pathophysiologic, and histologic features with agnogenic myeloid metaplasia, chronic myelogenous leukemia, and primary (essential) thrombocythemia, which are collectively classified as the myeloproliferative disorders (Ch. 154).

The excessive rate of erythropoiesis in polycythemia vera occurs despite bioassayable erythropoietin levels that are low or absent; endogenous erythroid colonies in this disorder can grow in vitro without added erythropoietin. These observations led to the concept that erythropoiesis in polycythemia vera was "autonomous." The growth of endogenous colonies from patients with polycythemia vera can be markedly reduced or eliminated by adding antierythropoietin antibody to the culture, however, and can be restored by the re-addition of minute quantities of the hormone. This suggests that erythroid progenitors in polycythemia vera, rather than being independent of the hormone, may be uniquely sensitive to trace levels of erythropoietin. In blood and bone marrow of patients with polycythemia vera, increased numbers of pluripotent colony-forming stem cells give rise to mixed colonies of granulocytic, erythroid, macrophage, and megakaryocytic elements (CFU-GEMM). These CFU-GEMM undergo erythroid differentiation without added erythropoietin and, compared to normal CFU-GEMM, exhibit increased megakaryocyte formation. The "endogenous" erythroid differentiation is abolished with antibodies to erythropoietin. Hence, both the increased "erythropoietin-independent" erythropoiesis and increased megakaryopoiesis characteristic of polycythemia vera reflect functional features of an identifiable abnormal pluripotent stem cell population.

The mechanism of malignant transformation in polycythemia vera is unknown. The rare occurrence of documented polycythemia vera in monozygotic twins and the only marginally increased incidence in first-degree relatives of affected patients suggest a minimal genetic role in most cases, and neither toxic chemicals nor exposure to radiation is established as an etiologic factor. Although two documented cases occurred among exposed observers of a 1957 nuclear test explosion, the incidence of polycythemia vera has not been appreciably increased in survivors of the Hiroshima and Nagasaki atomic bomb explosions. The disease is typically one of later life, with the median age at presentation being close to 60 years. Nevertheless, patients in their second through fourth decades are not rare. The disorder is characterized by a slight preponderance in males and a propensity to occur with somewhat increased frequency in patients of Jewish ancestry.

Clinical Manifestations

Multiphasic screening is currently resulting in an increasing percentage of cases being detected prior to the development of symptoms. Alternatively, a routine blood count may demonstrate increased hematocrit and other abnormalities in patients who present with only mild headaches and plethoric facies. Further symptoms as they develop usually will be referable to the combination of hypervolemia and hyperviscosity resulting from the increased red cell mass and blood volume, frequently aggravated by thrombocytosis and platelet dysfunction; to the local consequences of panhyperplasia of the bone marrow; or to the metabolic consequences of increased cell turnover.

SYMPTOMS. Headaches, tinnitus, light-headedness and vertigo, and blurred vision appear to result principally from increased blood viscosity and hypervolemia. Thrombotic complications, which may involve both arterial and venous occlusive events, are usually attributed to a combination of hyperviscosity, thrombocytosis, and platelet dysfunction. An increased incidence of epistaxis, spontaneous bruising, and upper gastrointestinal hemorrhage is also ascribed to the effects of hypervolemia and platelet dysfunction. Peptic ulcer disease seems to occur with increased frequency in patients with polycythemia vera as does pruritus, sometimes aggravated after a hot bath or shower, and occasionally so severe as to be disabling. The increased frequency of both peptic ulcer and pruritus may be related to the increased histamine release caused by excessive turnover of granulocytes and, more specifically, basophils. Approximately one third of patients complain of sweating and weight loss, presumed to be on the basis of a hypermetabolic state. Patients with polycythemia vera often complain of severe pain in their feet, which is characteristically relieved by very low doses of aspirin or nonsteroidal anti-inflammatory agents.

PHYSICAL FINDINGS. In established cases, physical examination typically reveals plethora or dusky cyanosis of the face, hands, feet, and mucous membranes. Engorgement of the conjunctivae and retinal veins is frequently present and, in patients with markedly increased hematocrit, retinal hemorrhages are occasionally seen. Mild hypertension is noted in approximately one third of patients. Ecchymoses are not infrequently observed. The most useful physical finding in terms of differential diagnosis is splenomegaly, which is present in approximately 75 per cent of patients with polycythemia vera and tends to exclude the diagnosis of most of the secondary polycythemias. Procedures such as abdominal computed tomography will demonstrate splenomegaly in a percentage of those patients in whom the spleen is not palpably enlarged. Splenic enlargement appears to reflect principally the development of extramedullary hematopoiesis. Hepatomegaly is present in approximately 40 per cent of patients.

Symptomatic bone pain and tenderness on physical examination, particularly in the ribs and sternum, are occasionally severe and reflect intense panhyperplasia of the bone marrow. In addition to hyperhistaminemia, the cellular proliferation of polycythemia vera results in overproduction of uric acid leading, not infrequently, to either uric acid stone diathesis or overt secondary gout.

Laboratory Data

The characteristic laboratory findings in polycythemia vera reflect the various consequences of increased bone marrow activity.

ERYTHROCYTES. Patients with this disorder typically present with an elevation of the hemoglobin concentration, hematocrit, and red blood cell count. Red blood cell morphology usually reveals hypochromic microcytic cells with a reduced mean corpuscular volume, suggestive of iron deficient erythropoiesis. This suggestion is frequently confirmed by a low serum iron level and absence of bone marrow iron stores. These features may occur prior to the onset of therapeutic phlebotomy and without any history of gastrointestinal blood loss and result from the shift of iron from various body storage pools into the circulating erythron as the red cell mass is expanded. This phenomenon may of course be exaggerated in patients who have gastrointestinal bleeding or in whom therapeutic phlebotomies have been initiated. Of the three conventional parameters reflecting the red cell mass, the red blood count is often most strikingly elevated, and red cell counts of 10×10^6 per microliter may be seen in the newly diagnosed case. In contrast, the hematocrit probably provides the best, although imperfect, simple guide to the size of the circulating red cell mass and to blood viscosity. It is difficult to define the precise upper limit for the normal hematocrit. As noted earlier, increased red cell masses may be found in a small percentage of patients with hematocrits of 48 per cent or above, and an increase in the hematocrit to greater than 60 per cent is required before the hematocrit alone can be taken positively as evidence for an absolute erythrocytosis. The plasma volume in polycythemia vera has variously been reported to be normal, reduced, or increased, and thus has no direct correlation with the red cell mass. The red cell lifespan is normal in the early phases of polycythemia vera, even in the presence of moderate splenomegaly. As the disease evolves, the development of increasingly ineffective erythropoiesis, and a larger element of extramedullary hematopoiesis with hepatomegaly and splenomegaly, results in progressive shortening of the red cell lifespan in some patients. This development is usually associated with the appearance of anisocytosis and poikilocytosis, nucleated red blood cells, and teardrop cells in the peripheral blood. When such studies are available, patients with untreated polycythemia vera will invariably demonstrate very low levels of plasma and urine erythropoietin and the ability to grow endogenous, erythropoietin-independent colonies of erythroid progenitors in vitro from either peripheral blood or bone marrow samples.

LEUKOCYTES. Sixty per cent of patients with polycythemia vera will have an increased granulocyte count in the peripheral blood at the time of diagnosis. Early in the disease, elevations are usually modest and involve the presence of only normal granulocytes and bands. Subsequently, striking elevations in total white count may achieve leukemoid proportions, associated with the appearance of early myeloid forms, particularly myelocytes and metamyelocytes. When the appearance of these cells is accompanied by increasing splenomegaly and the appearance of abnormal erythroid elements in the periphery, a significant element of myeloid metaplasia is likely. The alkaline phosphatase activity of circulating granulocytes is increased in polycythemia vera, in contrast to the reduction observed in chronic granulocytic leukemia. Increased granulocyte turnover is reflected by high serum and urine muramidase (lysozyme) levels, and by an increase in serum B_{12} and unbound B_{12} binding capacity that results from high levels of transcobalamins 1 and 3. The basophil count and, to a lesser extent, the eosinophil count may also be increased in polycythemia vera. Increased excretion of histamine metabolites reflects increased turnover of the former cell line.

PLATELETS. At diagnosis, the platelet count exceeds 500,000 per microliter in approximately half of patients with polycythemia vera, and striking elevations into the millions have been recorded. There is a tendency for the platelet count to increase with time, particularly in patients who are treated principally with phlebotomy. The platelets in polycythemia vera frequently appear morphologically abnormal, with megathrombocytes and megakaryocytic fragments being observed in the peripheral blood smear. An appreciable fraction of patients with polycythemia vera also have abnormalities of conventional studies of platelet function, including aggregation; a prolonged bleeding time may be present. Studies of prostaglandin metabolism also demonstrate decreased lipoxygenase activity and increased thromboxane A_2 production by the platelets of patients with polycythemia vera and other myeloproliferative diseases. However, it has not been possible to correlate either the height of the platelet count or the presence of platelet functional abnormalities with the propensity to thrombosis in these patients. In contrast, there seems to be a crude association between the extent of the elevation of the platelet count and the propensity to hemorrhagic complications.

BONE MARROW. The bone marrow in polycythemia vera is typically hyperplastic and reveals a panmyelosis. Because of the parallel increase in all three cell lines, the myeloid: erythroid ratio may be normal. Megakaryocytes are not merely increased but typically are seen in sheets or clumps, a finding strongly supportive of the diagnosis of a myeloproliferative disease. Bone marrow biopsy as well as aspirate is useful in the assessment of polycythemia vera, both because it gives a better indication of the extent of hypercellularity and because connective tissue staining will illustrate the extent of myelofibrosis. Serum levels of the procollagen III amino terminal peptide, now measurable by commercially available radioimmunoassay, also reflect the extent of myelofibrosis. Cytogenetic studies reveal various abnormalities in as many as 50 per cent of patients with polycythemia vera. Trisomy of chromosomes 8 and 9 or loss of chromosome 7 or its long arm (7q−) is the abnormality most frequently observed in untreated patients; loss of chromosome 5 or of the long arms of chromosome 5 (5q−) or 20 (20q−) has been observed in some patients, especially those treated with myelosuppressives. However, no abnormality is either specific for or diagnostic of polycythemia vera. Interestingly, the presence of cytogenetic abnormalities at the time of diagnosis appears to be of no prognostic significance.

MISCELLANEOUS. Low serum cholesterol concentrations are frequently observed in patients with polycythemia vera; these reflect accelerated catabolism of low density lipoproteins, presumably by the spleen. Hyperuricemia, reflecting a general increase in cell turnover, and an increase in lactic dehydrogenase and the indirect serum bilirubin concentration, reflecting accelerated erythroid turnover, are other commonly found abnormalities.

Diagnosis and Differential Diagnosis

Diagnosis of polycythemia vera is based on the demonstration of an increased red cell mass that is not associated with excessive erythropoietin production, as well as evidence of a concomitant increase in bone marrow production of granulocytes and thrombocytes. Polycythemia is one of two disorders characterized by "autonomous" erythropoiesis. It differs from the entity designated *primary erythrocytosis* in its associated increase in granulocyte and megakaryocytic proliferation and the presence of related abnormalities such as elevated levels of leukocyte alkaline phosphatase and serum B_{12}–binding proteins. The abnormalities in primary erythrocytosis are limited to the erythroid series, but within this sphere the low bioassayable erythropoietin levels and the presence of endogenous colonies are similar to those seen in polycythemia vera. Some argue that primary erythrocytosis represents a disorder arising in the committed erythroid stem cell compartment, i.e., at a later stage than the pluripotent stem cell affected in polycythemia vera, but primary erythrocytosis has not yet been demonstrated to be a clonal disorder. Others believe that these patients represent a forme fruste of typical polycythemia vera and that granulocytic or thrombocytic abnormalities will be revealed if patients are observed for sufficient periods.

The diagnosis of a primary bone marrow disorder with autonomous erythropoiesis may be made in accordance with the algorithm illustrated in Figure 153–2 by systematically excluding the various secondary causes of an absolute erythrocytosis. Patients appearing to have increased erythroid proliferation due to a primary bone marrow defect would be classified as having polycythemia vera if they have concomitant granulocytic or platelet abnormalities in the peripheral blood, evidence of a panmyelosis in the bone marrow, or splenomegaly. In the absence of these features, when abnormalities are restricted solely to the erythroid series, the diagnosis of primary erythrocytosis would be made.

The Polycythemia Vera Study Group has developed a set of empiric criteria that permit the diagnosis of polycythemia vera to be established in many patients within one to two office visits (Table 153–2). In patients who meet these criteria, the diagnosis of polycythemia vera is highly likely, the false-positive rate having been found to be less than 0.5 per cent. False-positive results are most likely in patients who are excessive users of both alcohol and tobacco. In this setting, excessive erythroid proliferation associated with carboxyhemoglobinemia and splenomegaly, leukocytosis, and increased leukocyte alkaline phosphatase activity and serum B_{12} associated with alcoholic liver disease may confound the diagnosis. The false-negative rate for the Polycythemia Vera Study Group criteria is unknown. Patients with early disease who do not yet meet these criteria may ultimately prove to have polycythemia vera, or at least a form of primary erythrocytosis, when more extensive evaluation is carried out in accordance with the criteria of Figure 153–2.

TABLE 153–2. PARAMETERS FOR THE DIAGNOSIS OF POLYCYTHEMIA VERA

A1 ↑ Red cell mass	B1 Thrombocytosis
Male: ≥ 36 ml/kg	Platelet count > 400,000/μl
Female: ≥ 32 ml/kg	B2 Leukocytosis: > 12,000/μl (no fever or infection)
A2 Normal art. O_2 sat. (≥ 92%)	B3 ↑ Leuk. alk. p'tase (LAP) (> 100)
A3 Splenomegaly	B4 ↑ Serum B_{12} (> 900 pg/ml) or ↑ $UB_{12}BC$ (> 2200 pg/ml)*

Dx. acceptable if following combinations are present:
A1 + A2 + A3
A1 + A2 + any two from category B
*$UB_{12}BC$ = unbound serum B_{12} binding capacity

Course

In the absence of treatment, polycythemia vera is a serious disease in which a high incidence of fatal thrombotic or hemorrhagic complications historically has led to a median survival of 6 to 18 months from diagnosis. Current treatment programs designed to maintain peripheral blood counts and the red cell mass at close to normal levels have achieved median survivals approximating 10 years, during the course of which aspects of the natural history of the disease have become more evident. In many patients, polycythemia vera is a readily managed disorder that remains asymptomatic for long periods. However, inadequate control of the red cell mass predisposes to both thrombotic and hemorrhagic complications, of which cerebrovascular, coronary, and abdominal vascular occlusions involving both arterial (e.g., mesenteric artery) and venous (Budd-Chiari syndrome) thromboses are most frequent. Thrombosis is the major cause of death in polycythemia vera, accounting for approximately one third of all fatalities. Transformation to acute leukemia, the development of other neoplasms, hemorrhage, and myelofibrosis are other major causes of fatality and collectively, along with thrombosis, account for 75 per cent of all deaths. Acute leukemia is clearly a part of the natural history of polycythemia vera, occurring with an incidence of up to 2 to 4 per cent even in patients who have not been exposed either to radiotherapy or to radiomimetic drugs.

Upper gastrointestinal hemorrhage, particularly from bleeding peptic ulcers, occurs with an increased incidence in patients with polycythemia vera. Underlying etiologic factors are believed to be increased acid secretion stimulated by hyperhistaminemia and vascular mucosal ischemia caused by increased blood viscosity and poor regional perfusion.

The complete natural history of polycythemia vera involves the ultimate transition from the proliferative phase, during which therapy is aimed at reducing peripheral blood counts, to a stable phase in which relatively normal blood counts may be maintained without therapy, to the so-called *burned out* or *spent phase.* Transition results predominantly from the gradual development of progressive myelofibrosis and, possibly, from a gradual reduction in the proliferative capacity of the abnormal hematopoietic clone. That myelofibrosis is a complication of polycythemia vera has long been recognized, but the nature of the association has been uncertain. The bulk of current evidence suggests that bone marrow fibroblasts in this setting are not part of the hematopoietic malignant clone. Similar conclusions have been reached in studies of the bone marrow fibroblast following transplantation. Hence, the increasing proliferation of fibroblasts and increased collagen deposition leading to myelofibrosis appear to be reactive phenomena rather than an intrinsic component of the neoplastic process. The clinical features and the management of postpolycythemic myelofibrosis do not differ appreciably from those of idiopathic myelofibrosis with myeloid metaplasia except that the incidence of acute leukemic transformation is markedly increased in the postpolycythemic setting, especially if the myelofibrosis follows treatment with radioactive phosphorus or chlorambucil (see Ch. 154).

Treatment

The initial treatment in any newly diagnosed case of polycythemia vera is phlebotomy. Efforts should be made to reduce the hematocrit to approximately 45 per cent, a level at which the complications of hypervolemia and hyperviscosity will be minimized. In patients with appreciable splenomegaly, the hematocrit no longer reliably reflects the red cell mass, which may continue to be significantly increased despite hematocrits in the upper 40's. The initial phlebotomy regimen may involve removal of 500 ml aliquots of whole blood as often as every two to three days until a normal hematocrit is achieved. Subsequent phlebotomies should be carried out as frequently as necessary to maintain the hematocrit at or below 45 per cent. As iron deficiency supervenes, red cell production will be retarded such that patients managed by phlebotomy alone may require as few as two or three phlebotomies per year.

Some investigators believe that phlebotomy alone, at rates sufficient to maintain a normal hematocrit and blood viscosity, is adequate to prevent the thrombotic complications of the disease and provides a minimal incidence of leukemic transformation. Others argue that some form of myelosuppression is preferable, in part because this offers an approach to the control of the thrombocytosis that is often a major clinical feature of the illness. Myelosuppression in this disorder has most often been carried out with radioactive phosphorus (^{32}P), with alkylating agents such as chlorambucil or busulfan, and more recently, with the nonalkylating myelosuppressive agent hydroxyurea.

In an ongoing randomized, controlled study in 431 patients, median survivals of 13.9 years with phlebotomy or 11.8 years with radioactive phosphorus therapy were significantly better than those achieved with chlorambucil (8.9 years), although the difference achieved statistical significance only after more than 10 years of treatment. Causes of death varied appreciably as a function of the treatment administered. Patients managed with phlebotomy alone had a significant excess incidence of severe and often fatal thrombotic complications, particularly in the first two to four years of treatment. Thrombotic complications were particularly frequent in more elderly patients (e.g., older than 70 years), in those with a high phlebotomy requirement (more than four to six per year), and in those who had had a prior history of a thrombotic event. Beyond three years the incidence of thrombotic complications became the same in patients treated with phlebotomy alone as in those treated with myelosuppression, suggesting that a subset of patients particularly susceptible to thrombosis had been selected out by this time. By contrast, myelosuppression with either ^{32}P or alkylating agents effectively decreased the risk of thrombotic complications in thrombosis-prone patients early in the disease. However, both chlorambucil and ^{32}P were associated with a statistically significant increased risk of acute leukemia, which became particularly prominent after five to seven years of treatment, and a somewhat later increased incidence of carcinomas of the skin and gastrointestinal tract. Thus, long-term myelosuppression with either of these agents is associated with an increased propensity for malignant transformation of the three rapidly proliferating tissues of the body: bone marrow, skin, and gastrointestinal mucosa. In addition, an increased incidence of intra-abdominal lymphocytic lymphoma has followed long-term treatment of polycythemia vera with chlorambucil.

Radioactive phosphorus, preferably given as an intravenous dose of 3 to 5 mCi, reliably produces a reduction in bone marrow proliferation with few immediate side effects. Chlorambucil or busulfan, administered either continuously or intermittently, also successfully controls peripheral counts in a high proportion of patients. In contrast to ^{32}P, myelosuppression with alkylating agents results in an appreciable incidence of cytopenias, which in the case of busulfan may be prolonged and troublesome. Because of these drug-related cytopenias and the fact that malignant complications occur both earlier and more frequently with chlorambucil than with ^{32}P, long-term treatment of polycythemia vera with alkylating agents can no longer be recommended. Although some argue that complications observed with chlorambucil should not preclude use of other alkylating agents, especially busulfan, there are sufficient anecdotal cases of leukemic transformation with all of the alkylating drugs that the burden of proof must be on those who argue for the safety of any such agent.

Hydroxyurea,* administered at a dose of 0.5 to 1.5 grams

*This use is not listed in the manufacturer's directive.

per day, has recently been shown to be an effective nonalkylating chemotherapeutic agent in the management of polycythemia vera. To date, this regimen has not been associated with an increased incidence of malignant transformation. However, the maximal follow-up with this agent, now approximately seven years, is too short for its full mutagenic potential to have been realized.

Since no form of treatment for polycythemia vera is without some risks, the following recommendations would appear to provide the best control of the disease with the fewest treatment-related complications. Because of the increased risk of thrombosis associated with age, patients over 70 are most effectively treated with a combination of ^{32}P and supplemental phlebotomy. Patients below the age of 50, and particularly those in the childbearing years, should be treated with phlebotomy alone whenever possible. Myelosuppression with hydroxyrurea would seem advisable in such younger patients if they are particularly at risk for thrombotic complications because of a high phlebotomy requirement or a history of prior thrombotic events. The role of myelosuppression is most uncertain in the age-group between 50 and 70. In the absence of thrombosis-associated risk factors, it is probably preferable to attempt to manage such patients by phlebotomy alone. If chemotherapy is deemed advisable, hydroxyurea would appear to be the agent of choice. Chlorambucil would now seem to be contraindicated for long-term therapy of polycythemia vera in view of its unacceptably high risk of leukemic and carcinogenic transformation, which may apply as well to other alkylating agents.

Although conclusive data are lacking, many physicians believe that a substantial increase in platelet count (i.e., in excess of 10^6 per microliter) is an indication for myelosuppressive therapy. Excessive splenic enlargement with local symptoms, bone tenderness, intractable pruritus, and poor veins may be other indications for the addition of myelosuppression to the treatment regimen. H_1 (cyproheptadine, 4 mg by mouth three times daily) and H_2 blockers (cimetidine, 300 mg by mouth three times daily), alone or in combination, provide relief from pruritus in some patients.

Attempts to reduce the incidence of thrombotic complications with the prophylactic use of platelet-antiaggregating agents, including aspirin and dipyridamole, have been unsuccessful. Indeed, not only has no significant benefit been achieved in terms of reduction in thrombosis, but these agents have been associated with a statistically significant increase in the incidence of gastrointestinal hemorrhage, particularly with prolonged administration to patients with platelet counts greater than 1 million. Hence, long-term prophylactic use of this group of agents cannot be recommended at this time. Short-term use of platelet-antiaggregating agents may be helpful during transient attacks of digital or cerebral ischemia, but such episodes are an indication for, and often respond to, myelosuppression.

Treatment of the burned-out myelofibrotic stage of polycythemia vera can be extremely difficult but does not differ from that described for idiopathic myelofibrosis. The acute leukemias that develop in polycythemia vera, either spontaneously or following myelosuppressive therapy, may be myeloid, myelomonocytic, lymphoid, or biphenotypic in morphology. In those patients with lymphoid morphology and/or increased levels of terminal deoxyribonucleotidyl transferase (TdT), a trial of vincristine and prednisone is indicated. Nevertheless, response to any form of treatment in these patients is infrequent, and median survival in a relatively recent series of postpolycythemic acute leukemias was approximately 30 days.

Meticulous control of blood volume and viscosity with the use of phlebotomy, supplemented when specifically indicated by judicious use of myelosuppression, can ensure most patients with polycythemia vera a prolonged period of relatively symptom-free survival. Median survival in recent series has exceeded 10 years, and symptom-free survival of 15 to 20 years is no longer uncommon. The longest documented survival following a well-founded diagnosis is 34 years.

Berk PD, Goldberg JD, Donovan PB, et al.: Therapeutic recommendations in polycythemia vera based on Polycythemia Vera Study Group protocols. Semin Hematol 23:132, 1986. *A detailed report on a continuous 19-year randomized control study of a large cohort of patients with polycythemia vera and the therapeutic recommendations derived from it. Part of a useful eight-article symposium on polycythemia vera.*

Caldwell GG, Kelley DB, Heath CW Jr, et al.: Polycythemia vera among participants of a nuclear weapons test. JAMA 252:662, 1984. *A provocative report that illustrates some of the difficulties in conclusively linking relatively uncommon disorders to radiation exposure.*

Conley CL: Polycythemia vera, diagnosis and treatment. Hosp Practice 22:107, 1987. *An excellent overview by a senior hematologist with great experience.*

Ellis JT, Peterson P, Geller SA, et al.: Studies of the bone marrow in polycythemia vera and the evolution of myelofibrosis and second hematologic malignancies. Semin Hematol 23:144, 1986. *An important review of bone marrow findings in polycythemia vera, exploring such issues as the evolution of fibrosis and second malignant disorders.*

Raskind WH, Jacobson R, Murphy S, et al.: Evidence for the involvement of B lymphoid cells in polycythemia vera and essential thrombocythemia. J Clin Invest 75:1388, 1985. *A concise paper illustrating how G6PD–isoenzyme analysis can be used to document that a particular cell line, in this case B lymphocytes, has a clonal origin.*

154 MYELOPROLIFERATIVE DISORDERS

Paul D. Berk

The normal bone marrow contains self-replicating pools of morphologically undifferentiated stem cells, recognizable hematopoietic cells undergoing differentiation and maturation, and connective tissue stromal elements. There is a hierarchy of stem cell populations: (1) a pluripotent stem cell capable under appropriate conditions of producing erythroid, myeloid, megakaryocytic, macrophage, and B lymphocyte progeny; (2) intermediate stem cells capable of producing several but not all of these lineages; and (3) committed, unipotent stem cells giving rise exclusively to erythroid, myeloid, or megakaryocytic offspring. The rate of proliferation, pool size, and rate of transition from less restricted to more restricted potential are carefully regulated so that the bone marrow can respond to the body's need for blood elements in a manner that is both selective in terms of the cell types produced and restricted or self-limited in duration (see Fig. 131–2). Thus in hemolysis, pyogenic infection, and immune platelet destruction, specific needs for increased production of erythrocytes, granulocytes, and platelets, respectively, are met ordinarily by selective erythroid, myeloid, or megakaryocytic hyperplasia of the marrow. Stromal cells such as fibroblasts do not appear to play a significant role in these responses.

In the myeloproliferative disorders, in contrast, each of the three major marrow cell lines proliferates in an unregulated, essentially autonomous and self-perpetuating manner. Four disorders—polycythemia vera, agnogenic myeloid metaplasia, chronic myelogenous leukemia, and essential thrombocythemia—can usefully be classified under this heading. Although the proliferation of one particular cell line may dominate the clinical picture, each of these is a clonal hematopoietic malignant disorder arising at the level of the pluripotent stem cell (Ch. 152). In each disorder erythroid, myeloid, and megakaryocytic elements proliferate excessively, but to varying degrees, in the bone marrow and in sites of extramedullary hematopoiesis (often resulting in splenomegaly). In each disorder there is a variable tendency for reactive proliferation of the otherwise normal bone marrow fibroblast—which is not a part of the malignant clone—with the development of myelofibrosis, and for termination in an acute blastic leukemia. Despite differences in the predominant cell line released into the periphery, bone marrows at the time of presentation show many similarities and may be indistinguishable, with clumps or sheets of abnormal megakaryocytes being common to all. Hyperuricemia secondary to increased cell turnover and abnormal levels of serum B_{12} and its binding proteins and of leukocyte alkaline phosphatase activity are also common to this group. Some investigators include acute leukemias of various types (notably erythroleukemia) and paroxysmal nocturnal hemoglobinuria within the myeloproliferative syndromes; others consider these disorders sufficiently different from the basic four to warrant their exclusion.

The myeloproliferative syndromes have long been considered to exhibit transitions between the various entities. The evolution of polycythemia vera into a disorder characterized by myelofibrosis with myeloid metaplasia is well documented, as is the transition of all entities—albeit with varying frequency—to acute leukemia. Other transitions have been harder to document. Thus, Philadelphia chromosome-positive chronic myelogenous leukemia may present transiently with elevated red cell and platelet counts but does not at this stage represent polycythemia vera. Similarly, a patient with polycythemia vera who has suffered a gastrointestinal hemorrhage may at initial examination have only an elevated platelet count, resembling essential thrombocythemia. Repletion of iron stores with resulting erythrocytosis does not represent a true transition from essential thrombocythemia to polycythemia vera.

Despite the failure to confirm true transitions among several of these disorders, the concept of a myeloproliferative syndrome involving the four basic entities just listed is now firmly supported by their clonal, morphologic, pathophysiologic, and clinical similarities. Various nonspecific cytogenetic abnormalities are also observed in each of these entities. The appearance of the Philadelphia (Ph^1) chromosome, characteristic of chronic myelogenous leukemia, is a late event in the pathogenetic evolution of the disorder and follows the initial development of the malignant clone of pluripotent stem cells.

Adamson JW, Fialkow PJ: The pathogenesis of myeloproliferative syndromes. Br J Haematol 38:299, 1978. *A concise review of cell biologic, cytogenetic, and enzymatic evidence for an analogous clonal origin of the major myeloproliferative disorders.*

Gilbert HS: Myeloproliferative disorders. Clin Geriatr Med 1:773, 1985. *A reassessment of the myeloproliferative disorder concept after 20 years of critical clinical experience.*

MYELOFIBROSIS WITH MYELOID METAPLASIA

Definition and Pathogenesis

Myelofibrosis with myeloid metaplasia is a syndrome in which morphologic evidence of excessive fibroblast proliferation and collagen deposition in the bone marrow is accompanied by myeloid metaplasia of organs such as the liver, spleen, and lymph nodes. These organs, involved normally in fetal but not adult erythropoiesis, become active sites of extramedullary hematopoiesis. Similar clinical syndromes may be seen in three distinct settings. The first of these is progressive hepatosplenomegaly and the evolution of a leukoerythroblastic peripheral blood picture indicative of myeloid metaplasia occurring in the absence of an apparent inciting cause. This disorder, termed *agnogenic myeloid metaplasia*, is a clonal stem cell hemopathy constituting one of the primary myeloproliferative syndromes. Second, a similar picture of myelofibrosis with myeloid metaplasia may evolve in the course of polycythemia vera or chronic granulocytic leukemia, either as a part of the natural history of the illness or as a consequence of the myelosuppressive therapies administered. The third setting is myeloid metaplasia with varying degrees of reactive myelofibrosis that may occur secondary to a wide spectrum of clinical disorders including, among others, severe hemolytic anemia, Hodgkin's disease, various nonhematopoietic neoplasms metastatic to the bone marrow, infections such as tuberculosis, or following bone marrow injury caused by radiation, benzol, fluorine, phosphorus, or strontium.

In myelofibrosis with myeloid metaplasia, the extent of extramedullary hematopoiesis tends to parallel the extent of bone marrow fibrosis. Indeed, it was previously believed that the mesenchymal cells in the liver, spleen, and lymph nodes resumed their embryonic potential for hematopoiesis in an attempt to compensate for myelophthisis. However, in some cases there is a dissociation between the degree of marrow fibrosis and extramedullary hematopoiesis resulting in (1) marrow fibrosis without evidence of significant myeloid metaplasia, or (2) progressive hepatosplenomegaly with a leukoerythroblastic peripheral blood picture in the absence of significant fibrosis. Pluripotent hematopoietic stem cells, presumably of bone marrow origin, are constantly present in the circulation of normal individuals and appear in increased numbers in the peripheral blood of patients with myelofibrosis. It is more likely that these circulating stem cells take up residence in organs such as the liver and spleen to produce extramedullary hematopoiesis than that this represents the reactivation of hematopoietic capabilities in local mesenchymal cells. Except in the secondary setting noted above, the primary pathogenetic event is believed to be a mutation leading to a malignant hematopoietic clone at the level of a pluripotent stem cell. The development of myelofibrosis appears to be a reaction to the presence of this proliferating clone. The release of increased megakaryocyte- and platelet-derived growth factor from the markedly expanded bone marrow megakaryocyte pool of the myeloproliferative syndromes may be in part responsible for the secondary fibroblast proliferation and collagen deposition. Colonization of the liver, spleen, and lymph nodes may, in this setting, represent a form of metastasis of abnormal stem cells to organs that retain an intrinsic potential to support erythropoiesis.

Clinical Features

Myelofibrosis with myeloid metaplasia, whether agnogenic or secondary to another myeloproliferative syndrome, is primarily a disorder of the middle-aged or older adult. At least 60 per cent of cases occur between the ages of 50 and 70, with no predilection for either sex. The onset of symptoms is usually insidious over several years and in most cases disease progression is slow. Most commonly presenting symptoms are referable to anemia with its consequent cardiovascular consequences, or to increased abdominal girth or discomfort resulting from splenic and hepatic enlargement. Bone pain, often migratory, and gouty arthritis occasionally bring the patient to medical attention. Deafness resulting from otosclerosis occurs in a small minority of cases. Increasing numbers of asymptomatic patients are being detected today in the course of routine screening laboratory or physical examinations.

On physical examination, splenomegaly is an almost universal finding. In approximately 85 per cent of cases, the spleen extends 8 cm or more below the left costal margin, and in one third of cases is enlarged more than 16 cm. Occasional patients without palpable splenomegaly will be demonstrated to have splenic enlargement by means of an isotopic or computerized tomographic imaging study. Rarely, significant myelofibrosis with cytopenia occurs, at least initially, without myeloid metaplasia and with no evidence of splenic enlargement. Hepatomegaly occurs in approximately 50 per cent of cases, frequently with mild abnormalities of liver function tests—especially elevation of alkaline phosphatase. Hepatomegaly in the absence of splenomegaly is extremely rare in agnogenic myeloid metaplasia or when the syndrome occurs secondary to another myeloproliferative disease, and points to a diagnosis of secondary myeloid metaplasia. Extramedullary hematopoiesis is frequently demonstrable histologically in lymph nodes, but clinically significant lymph node enlargement occurs in only 10 per cent of cases. Petechiae, caused by both thrombocytopenia and platelet dysfunction, have been reported in up to 25 per cent of patients, and jaundice, edema, and ascites are found in 10 to 20 per cent of cases.

Laboratory Data

At diagnosis, a mild to moderate degree of anemia is typical with the hemoglobin ranging between 9 and 13 grams per 100 ml. Red cells are initially normocytic and normochromic with mild poikilocytosis. Polychromatophilia, a modest reticulocytosis of 2 to 5 per cent, and occasional teardrop erythrocytes are seen (Color plate 3*D*). The presence of at least a few normoblasts and occasionally even earlier erythroid precursors is extremely common. As the disease progresses and the spleen enlarges, more severe anisocytosis, poikilocytosis, polychromasia, basophilic stippling, and normoblastosis may be sufficiently characteristic to indicate the diagnosis. The white blood cell count is initially normal in about one third of patients, elevated in approximately one half, and low in the remaining 15 per cent. Most typically, the count is in the range of 15,000 to 30,000 per cubic millimeter but counts as high as 70,000 per cubic millimeter are observed. The white count tends to fluctuate with time and often does not show the downward trend observed for the hemoglobin concentration and platelet count. A degree of granulocyte immaturity in the peripheral blood is typical, including the presence of as many as 10 per cent blasts. This does not necessarily suggest the evolution of acute leukemia, particularly when there are proportionate numbers of promyelocytes, myelocytes, and metamyelocytes as well. Basophilia and an acquired Pelger-Hüet anomaly are other typical features of the peripheral blood smear. The leukocyte alkaline phosphatase score is variable but is most often normal or increased. The platelet count initially is most often normal, although reduced or elevated counts are not uncommon. Exceedingly high counts in excess of 10^6 per microliter may cause this condition to be confused with the entity of primary thrombocytosis. Morphologically, megathrombocytes and megakaryocytic fragments are extremely common. Over time, the platelet count gradually tends to decrease, and thrombocytopenia is common late in the disorder. Overall, a peripheral blood smear demonstrating striking teardrop poikilocytosis, leukoerythroblastic nucleated cells, and megathrombocytes and megakaryocytic fragments is highly suggestive of the syndrome of myelofibrosis with myeloid metaplasia. Erythrocyte survival is almost invariably reduced and splenic sequestration often is present. Platelet production is usually increased even in patients with thrombocytopenia, associated with a marked increase in splenic pooling

Normal or slightly elevated serum levels of vitamin B_{12} and B_{12} binding proteins occur both in agnogenic myeloid metaplasia and postpolycythemia myelofibrosis, but the values are not as striking in those seen in chronic granulocytic leukemia. Hyperuricemia, due to increased uric acid production, is common. Miscellaneous laboratory abnormalities include high levels of LDH, modest elevations of serum transaminase and bilirubin levels, increased serum alkaline phosphatase activity caused by both hepatic and bone isoenzyme fractions, and modest increases in muramidase (lysozyme).

Cytogenetic abnormalities occur in up to 50 per cent of patients with agnogenic myeloid metaplasia, with trisomy for a C group chromosome being probably the most common consistent alteration. The Ph^1 chromosome is not present.

Osteosclerosis distributed primarily in the flat bones of the axial skeleton and in the metaphyseal ends of the femur and humerus may be recognized radiographically in up to 70 per cent of patients. Osteosclerosis involving the ear ossicles may result in deafness. The typical radiographic finding is the loss of definition of individual bony trabeculae, leading to a ground glass appearance.

Attempts to aspirate bone marrow almost invariably lead to a dry tap, even when the marrow is very cellular. Accordingly, bone marrow biopsy, either percutaneous or surgical, is usually required for diagnosis. Demonstration of bone marrow fibrosis, often with accompanying osteosclerosis, is the sine qua non. The bone marrow may sometimes be hypercellular, frequently demonstrating a panhyperplasia, in residual focal areas. Even in these areas, in which mature collagen may not be evident, an increase in reticulin fibers can usually be demonstrated by silver impregnation. Extramedullary hematopoiesis is demonstrable in both liver and spleen, but because of the risks involved in percutaneous biopsy of these organs, its diagnosis usually is based on the typical leukoerythroblastic blood picture and occasionally on isotopic erythrokinetic studies. The increase of bone marrow collagen content in myelofibrosis is principally the result of excessive collagen deposition and is reflected in an increase in the serum level of procollagen III amino terminal peptide.

Course of the Disease

The course of both agnogenic and postpolycythemic myelofibrosis is characterized by progressive splenic enlargement and, typically, by slightly less striking enlargement of the liver. The spleen will often fill the entire left side of the abdomen, extending beyond the midline to the right and down into the pelvis. The resulting early satiety, associated with a hypermetabolic state from increased cell turnover, may result in appreciable weight loss. Painful splenic infarcts may also complicate the disease. The marked splenic enlargement and consequent increase in splenic blood flow, coupled with increased resistance to flow within the liver caused by extramedullary hematopoiesis, lead to portal hypertension and its various complications including ascites, edema, and variceal hemorrhage in a small proportion of patients. Hepatic vein thrombosis with Budd-Chiari syndrome is another recognized complication. The progressive splenomegaly is accompanied almost inevitably by progressive anemia and thrombocytopenia, the former occasionally complicated by iron deficiency of blood loss or, less frequently, by folic acid deficiency. Although granulocyte counts are usually better maintained than those of other blood cellular elements, eventually granulocytopenia may develop. In this setting bacterial infections occur with increased frequency and may be a major factor leading to death. The association of myelofibrosis with tuberculosis is well documented, and this infection should be excluded by histologc and bacteriologic examination. When the two disorders coincide it is not clear whether myelofibrosis is always secondary to tuberculous infection of the marrow, or whether, conversely, tuberculosis has supervened in a patient with an underlying clonal hemopathy. Because of the almost inevitable hyperuricemia, attacks of gouty arthritis may develop in untreated patients.

Acute leukemic transformation is an occasional terminal event in agnogenic myeloid metaplasia. About 10 per cent of patients with polycythemia vera will develop a spent phase with advanced myelofibrosis. The likelihood of developing postpolycythemic myelofibrosis does not seem to be influenced by the type of therapy given for the underlying polycythemia, but evolution to the spent phase is a risk factor for subsequent development of acute leukemia. Once myelofibrosis has developed in this setting, the incidence of subsequent leukemic transformation (6 per cent in phlebotomy-treated patients, 45 per cent with chlorambucil, and 25 per cent with ^{32}P) is two and one half to four times greater than in similarly treated polycythemic patients who have not developed myelofibrosis.

Treatment and Prognosis

No agreement has been reached as to the optimal treatment of agnogenic myeloid metaplasia or of postpolycythemic myelofibrosis. There is thus far no effective treatment that inhibits the fibrotic process. Moreover, none of the conventional forms of treatment, including androgen therapy to stimulate erythropoiesis, chemotherapy, or splenectomy, has been shown to prolong life. Because of the relatively indolent progression of the disorder in most patients, a majority of hematologists undertake no specific treatment in the asymptomatic patient except for the administration of allopurinol at doses of 200 to 400 mg per day to avoid the complications of hyperuricemia.

In the presence of symptomatic anemia, androgens may be employed: testosterone enanthate, 200 to 600 mg weekly intramuscularly, or oxymetholone, 50 to 150 mg daily by mouth. Treatment must be continued for at least three months to establish whether a particular preparation is effective, and some hematologists argue that patients who fail to respond to one androgen preparation may ultimately respond to another. Androgens seem most effective in women who have been splenectomized previously or who have never had massive splenomegaly. The doses employed inevitably lead to excessive fluid accumulation and, in female patients, to significant masculinization. The hemolytic anemia almost never responds to corticosteroids; these drugs may, however, increase the risk of infection in granulocytopenic patients. In patients with marked thrombocytosis, busulfan, in an initial dose of 4 mg per day followed by lower doses as the platelet count normalizes, or hydroxyurea, at a dose of 500 to 1500 mg per day, is often effective in obtaining control of the platelet count. Although busulfan is widely used in this setting, its potential mutagenic risks are a cause for concern. These agents may occasionally produce a beneficial reduction in spleen size and/or increase the hemoglobin concentration, but equally frequently will result in suppression of erythropoiesis and thrombopoiesis. Radiation therapy to the spleen has largely been abandoned because the doses required to produce a meaningful reduction in spleen size often cause severe leukopenia and thrombocytopenia.

The role of splenectomy in patients with agnogenic myeloid metaplasia or postpolycythemic myelofibrosis is highly controversial. As a high risk procedure, it should probably be reserved for patients with severe hemolytic anemia, thrombocytopenia sufficient to produce bleeding, portal hypertension, or severe discomfort secondary to pressure symptoms or infarction. Striking thrombocytosis with thrombosis or hemorrhage or both may develop postoperatively and may require aggressive myelosuppression. In some patients splenectomy is followed by progressive enlargement of the liver, with recurrent hemolysis and thrombocytopenia. The diagnosis of acute leukemia is often difficult to make in these patients in whom the percentage of blasts in the peripheral blood may increase slowly and progressively for years.

Survival in agnogenic myeloid metaplasia and in postpolycythemic myelofibrosis is difficult to define with certainty. Several authors suggest that median survival in agnogenic myeloid metaplasia is approximately ten years from the onset of the disease and five years from the time of diagnosis. However, there is considerable heterogeneity, with both shorter and longer survival frequently observed.

Bone marrow transplantation has been attempted both by conventional techniques and after surgical manipulation of bone marrow cavity spaces in attempts to provide an improved microenvironment for the transplanted marrow. Only occasional successes have been reported, and this procedure must be considered highly experimental.

The syndrome of acute myelofibrosis, which is a rapidly progressive and fatal variant, has been shown by various cytologic marker studies to represent a form of acute megakaryocytic leukemia. It is believed that the release of platelet-megakaryocyte–derived growth factor from the malignant megakaryoblasts is responsible for the rapidly progressive marrow fibrosis. Induction chemotherapy may produce temporary hematologic remission, but only partial reversal of marrow fibrosis.

Berk PD, Castro-Malaspina H, Wasserman LR (eds.): Myelofibrosis and the Biology of Connective Tissue. New York, Alan R. Liss, Inc., 1984. *This book contains 29 concise chapters by multiple authors who review the available information about the regulation of fibroblast proliferation, collagen biosynthesis, cell biology of marrow stromal cells, and other aspects of basic biologic science believed to be relevant to the pathogenesis of myelofibrosis.*

Kroopman JE: The pathogenesis of myelofibrosis in myeloproliferative disorders. Ann Intern Med 92:858, 1980. *Excellent brief summary of speculations on the pathogenesis of myelofibrosis.*

Ruiz-Arguelles GJ, Marin-Lopez A, Lobato-Mendizabal E, et al.: Acute megakaryoblastic leukaemia: A prospective study of its identification and treatment. Br J Haematol 62:55, 1986. *An interesting study of diagnostic characterization and response to therapy of acute megakaryoblastic leukemia with myelofibrosis.*

Varki A, Lottenberg R, Griffith R, et al.: The syndrome of idiopathic myelofibrosis. Clinicopathologic review with emphasis on the prognostic variables predicting survival. Medicine 62:53, 1983. *This is a useful review of 88 consecutive patients with bone marrow fibrosis seen at Barnes Hospital. As noted in the title, there is considerable emphasis on prognostic features.*

ESSENTIAL THROMBOCYTHEMIA

Essential thrombocythemia, also known as a hemorrhagic thrombocythemia or essential thrombocytosis, is a primary myeloproliferative disorder in which the predominant laboratory feature is a persistent, striking elevation of the platelet count to values in excess of 1×10^6 per microliter. The disorder shows many features of polycythemia vera including an almost identical distribution of patient ages at the time of diagnosis, similar degrees of leukocytosis, and morphologically similar bone marrow abnormalities. Splenomegaly has been reported to occur in 30 to 75 per cent of cases. The criteria outlined in the following paragraph would restrict the diagnosis to patients who have either normal or reduced hemoglobin concentrations, those with concomitant erythrocytosis being classified as having polycythemia vera.

The Polycythemia Vera Study Group has proposed the following diagnostic criteria for essential thrombocythemia: (1) platelet count persistently greater than 1×10^6 per microliter in the absence of an identifiable cause such as malignant disease, infection, chronic inflammatory disease, or previous splenectomy; (2) normal total red cell volume, the measurement of which may be omitted if the hemoglobin concentration is less than 13 grams per 100 ml; (3) presence of iron in the bone marrow; if iron is absent, failure of the hemoglobin concentration to increase by more than 1 gram per 100 ml after a one-month trial of oral iron therapy; (4) absence of collagen fibrosis in bone marrow biopsy; and (5) absence of the Philadelphia chromosome from unstimulated metaphases obtained from a bone marrow aspirate. Because of both morphologic and clinical similarities, criteria 2 and 3 are necessary to exclude a diagnosis of polycythemia vera, whereas criteria 4 and 5 distinguish the disorder from agnogenic myeloid metaplasia and chronic myelogenous leukemia, respectively.

Clinical Features

The predominant clinical manifestations of essential thrombocythemia result from hemorrhagic and/or thrombotic events. Some patients have easy bruising, epistaxis, unexplained gastrointestinal bleeding, and an excessive tendency to postoperative hemorrhage. Conversely, other patients present evidence for microvascular occlusion in sites such as the extremities, the central nervous system, and the coronary circulation. The commonest manifestation of microvascular occlusion is burning pain in the feet, hands, and digits, which may progress to frank gangrene. Although these symptoms are striking when they occur, large numbers of patients, particularly younger patients, may be asymptomatic for long periods. Hence, the precise incidence of these complications is unknown. Similarly,transition to acute leukemia has been clearly documented, but there is no accurate estimate of its frequency, particularly in patients not previously exposed to mutagenic agents.

Course and Prognosis

The natural history of this disease is poorly appreciated, and most reports in the literature describe very small series of patients with a focus on a particular complication. Descriptions emphasizing hemorrhagic, thrombotic, and embolic episodes and a high fatality rate are directly contradicted by others emphasizing prolonged periods without complications. The largest series suggest a life expectancy perhaps analogous to that of polycythemia vera.

Therapy

Because of uncertainties about its natural history, there is a substantial lack of agreement about appropriate therapy for essential thrombocythemia. Despite strikingly high platelet counts, many hematologists recommend expectant management in asymptomatic patients under the age of 60, while others recommend the use only of platelet-antiaggregating agents (e.g., aspirin 300 mg per day with or without dipyridamole 50 mg three times daily).* However, the experience in polycythemia vera suggests that prolonged administration of platelet-antiaggregating agents may increase the risk of gastrointestinal hemorrhage. Chronic myelosuppression should be attempted in older patients and those who have a history of significant thrombotic episodes. In these cases, prevention of neurologic damage takes precedence over concern about long-term mutagenic effects of myelosuppression. Control of the thrombocytosis can be achieved with melphalan* 6 to 10 mg per day by mouth for one week followed by 4 to 6 mg per day until the platelet count is in the normal range. Subsequent maintenance with 2 to 6 mg per week is continued indefinitely, the appropriate dose depending on the platelet count. Alternatively, hydroxyurea* at an initial dose of 500 to 1500 mg per day, tapered to an individualized maintenance dose as the platelet count falls, or radioactive phosphorus 2.9 mCi per square meter of body surface area intravenously, repeated as necessary at intervals of not less than three months, is highly effective in achieving normalization of the platelet count. Patients presenting with serious thrombotic or hemorrhagic manifestations and uncontrolled thrombocytosis should be treated with platelet-antiaggregating agents, urgent plateletpheresis, and the initiation of a myelosuppressive regimen. Every effort should be made to avoid splenectomy in patients with essential thrombocythemia because of the extreme thrombocytosis and serious complications that often follow this procedure.

*This use is not listed in the manufacturer's directive.

Jabaily J, Iland HJ, Laszlo J, et al.: Neurologic manifestations of essential thrombocythemia. Ann Intern Med 99:513, 1983. *A contrary report on the largest series of patients with essential thrombocythemia yet assembled suggesting that approximately two thirds have evidence of at least transient neurologic dysfunction.*

Kessler CM, Klein HG, Havlik RJ: Uncontrolled thrombocytosis in chronic myeloproliferative disorders. Br J Haematol 50:157, 1982. *A retrospective study suggesting that, at least in the younger patient, severe thrombocytosis in myeloproliferative disease may have fewer complications than previously believed.*

Murphy S: Thrombocytosis and thrombocythaemia. Clin Hematol 12:89, 1983. *A detailed review of the pathogenesis, pathophysiology, and management of this puzzling disorder. Excellent bibliography.*

Murphy S, Iland H, Rosenthal D, et al.: Essential thrombocythemia: An interim report from the Polycythemia Vera Study Group. Semin Hematol 23:177, 1986. *A brief but useful update of Murphy's 1983 review.*

155 THE CHRONIC LEUKEMIAS

Bayard Clarkson

CHRONIC MYELOGENOUS LEUKEMIA (Chronic Myeloid Leukemia, Chronic Myelocytic Leukemia, Chronic Granulocytic Leukemia)

DEFINITION. Chronic myelogenous leukemia (CML) is a chronic form of leukemia originating in a primitive myeloid stem cell in which the leukemic cells retain the capacity for differentiation and are able to perform the essential functions of normal hematopoietic cells that they replace in the marrow. The leukemic cells have a pronounced tendency to undergo further malignant transformation with loss of ability to differentiate in later stages of the disease. Although commonly included among other myeloproliferative disorders (see Ch. 154), CML is a distinct entity that is easily recognized because the leukemic cells have a distinctive cytogenetic abnormality, the Philadelphia (Ph^1) chromosome.

ETIOLOGY. The etiology is unknown. The majority of patients with CML have no history of excessive exposure to ionizing radiation or chemical leukemogens, but the incidence increases greatly with exposure to high doses of radiation. This may occur following chronic exposure in radiologists who practice without adequate shielding, in patients who have received radiation treatments for ankylosing spondylitis or other chronic diseases, and in subjects exposed to a single massive dose of radiation as in the atomic bomb explosions in Japan in 1945. After subacute or acute exposure to large radiation doses there is a latent period of several years, after which the incidence of both acute myeloid leukemia and CML increases in an approximately linear relationship to the radiation dose. In the atomic bomb survivors the peak incidence occurred about seven years after the explosion and was about 50 times that of nonexposed subjects. The rate then declined, but still exceeded the national average 15 years later. Radiation hazards are more extensively discussed in Ch. 539.

The contribution of chemicals to the causation of CML is hard to assess. Any chemical capable of causing myelotoxicity or chromosome damage is suspect. However, persons in industrialized societies are exposed to such a wide variety of chemicals with these properties, including solvents, insecticides, hair dyes, and various drugs, that their very prevalence makes it difficult to incriminate specific candidates. Cytotoxic drugs, especially alkylating agents and those used in combination with radiation in the treatment of other neoplastic diseases (such as Hodgkin's disease), are known to increase the incidence of leukemia, usually after a latent period of several years.The most common type of leukemia is one of the variants of acute myeloid leukemia, but CML may also occur rarely. The minimal leukemogenic dose has not been established for any chemical or drug in humans, but it is only prudent to try to minimize unnecessary exposure to any potential leukemogens.

INCIDENCE AND PREVALENCE. The incidence of CML in the United States and most Western countries is about 1.5 per 100,000 population per year and accounts for about 15 per cent of all cases of leukemia. CML is slightly more frequent in men than women, but the course of the disease is the same. The median age is about 45 and the disease is uncommon below the age of 20. In children with CML in whom the Ph[1] chromosome is present, the course of the disease is similar to that of adults. A juvenile form of CML, described in very young children, has a more rapidly progressive course and the leukemic cells lack the (Ph[1]) chromosome.

Although a few instances have been noted of CML occurring in multiple family members, familial occurrence is uncommon, and children born to mothers who have the disease are normal.

PATHOGENESIS AND MECHANISMS. In over 90 per cent of cases the leukemic cells have a unique chromosomal abnormality, the Ph[1] chromosome. The Ph[1] anomaly results from a reciprocal translocation of a portion of the long arm of chromosome 22 to another chromosome, usually the long arm of chromosome 9, although sometimes to another chromosome. Both deletion of the long arm of number 22 and translocation to another chromosome must be demonstrated by appropriate banding studies to confirm Ph[1] positivity.

In Ph[1]-positive CML, the cellular oncogene c-abl, which is normally located on the long arm of chromosome 9 at band q34, is translocated to a small 6 kilobase (kb) region of chromosome 22 designated the breakpoint cluster region or bcr. This translocation results in the transcription of a novel hybrid bcr/c-abl 8.5 kb messenger RNA (mRNA) and its fusion protein product, a 210-kD phosphoprotein (P210). These novel products are larger than the corresponding normal c-abl mRNA (6 and 7 kg) and its protein (145 kD), and the P210 protein has altered tyrosine kinase activity. It is not yet known how these alterations relate to the CML cells' abnormal proliferative behavior. It is strongly suspected, however, that the hybrid bcr/abl gene has a key role in the pathogenesis of the disease because it is such a consistent finding. It is also analogous to a similar fusion protein in mouse cells transformed by the Abelson murine leukemia virus. Some patients present with many clinical features of CML, but do not have the Ph[1] chromosome in their marrow cells. The course of the disease is atypical in these patients, and they generally have a poor response to treatment and shorter survival than Ph[1]-positive patients. It appears that most of them are misdiagnosed as having Ph[1]-negative CML and have other myelodysplastic disorders, most commonly chronic myelomonocytic leukemia (CMMoL).

There is good evidence, based on the occurrence of CML in patients with chromosome mosaicism and in those heterozygous for the enzyme glucose-6-phosphate dehydrogenase, that the leukemic population arises from a single cell because the Ph[1] anomaly has been found to be restricted to just one of their dual cell lines (Ch. 152). The defect is an acquired one, since the Ph[1] marker is not present in nonhematopoietic cells, and monozygous twins of patients with CML do not have the Ph[1] chromosome in their myeloid cells. The presence of the Ph[1] genetic marker in erythrocyte, granulocyte, monocyte, and megakaryocyte precursors indicates that the original transformation occurred in an ancestral cell common to these myeloid cell types, but the exact location of the transforming event within the progenitor cell lineages is still uncertain.

The Ph[1] chromosome is absent in the majority of mature lymphocytes, although in about 20 per cent of patients some of the B cells contain the Ph[1] marker. T lymphocytes are rarely involved, although a few reports indicate some T cell precursors are Ph[1] positive. When one or more of the chronic phase leukemic cells undergo blastic transformation, in about 25 per cent of such cases the blasts have been found to have phenotypic properties associated with lymphocyte precursors, including high levels of terminal deoxynucleotidyl transferase and reactivity with specific antisera prepared against an antigen (cALLA) present on the common type of acute lymphoblastic leukemic cells. Some cases of CML blastic transformation have been reported in which the blasts contain intracellular IgM, a characteristic of pre-B cells. While in most cases of lymphoid blastic transformation detectable cytoplasmic and surface immunoglobulin are lacking, in the majority of cases there is rearrangement of the immunoglobulin heavy chain genes, and in some there is also progression to light chain–gene rearrangements. Since these gene rearrangements are a mandatory early step in B cell development and rarely occur within other human hematopoietic lineages, the findings provide strong evidence that the lymphoid blasts are early B cell precursors.

On the basis of serial hematologic examinations of atomic bomb survivors who developed CML, it has been estimated that about eight years elapse between the original mutational event that results in the first Ph[1]-positive leukemic cell in the marrow and the development of clinical symptoms when the diagnosis is ordinarily made. Since the average survival after diagnosis is three years, the total course of the disease is thus about 11 years. At the time of diagnosis 85 to 100 per cent of the dividing marrow cells contain the Ph[1] marker in the majority of patients. A few patients have lesser degrees of replacement of normal marrow cells by leukemic cells at diagnosis, and in such cases the leukemic and normal populations may coexist in nearly equal balance for a year or more before the leukemic cells eventually replace the normal cells. Cells containing the Ph[1] chromosome have not been found in normal subjects.

Why the leukemic cells have a proliferative advantage is not known. In the chronic stage of the disease the leukemic cells retain the capacity to differentiate almost normally, and the enzymatic and functional defects exhibited by the leukemic cells are not of sufficient severity to prevent them from carrying out their essential functions in supporting life in the absence of normal cells. Many of the defects somehow appear to be related to the increased mass of the leukemic population because such abnormalities as deficient neutrophil alkaline phosphatase, impaired phagocytic capacity of neutrophils, and various platelet and red cell abnormalities return toward normal after the cell density has been reduced by treatment.

There is characteristically a marked shift toward granulocyte differentiation at the expense of erythroid differentiation in untreated CML, but the myeloid-erythroid ratio usually returns toward normal after treatment. In most cases, neutrophilic granulocytes predominate, but eosinophilia and/or basophilia and monocytosis also occur frequently. Increased numbers of megakaryocytes and thrombocytosis frequently accompany the increased granulocyte production, but thrombocytopenia may also be observed. Some degree of anemia is common, and rarely erythrocytosis may occur.

The mass of myeloid tissue is usually greatly increased in CML at the time of diagnosis, sometimes tenfold or more. The leukemic granulocytic precursors in the marrow and spleen divide less rapidly than the corresponding cells in normal marrow, although their rate of proliferation may be nearly normal very early in the disease or after the myeloid mass has been reduced by treatment. In the chronic phase the percentage of myeloblasts is usually not increased compared to that in normal marrow, but their absolute number is greatly increased because of the expanded mass of myeloid tissue in the marrow, spleen, blood, and sometimes other extramedullary sites. There is also a greatly increased incidence of earlier committed granulocyte-monocyte precursors that form colonies and clusters in semisolid culture systems and that show nearly normal in vitro maturation and growth. The primary reason for the expanded myeloid mass is that the leukemic stem cells continue to proliferate after exceeding the cell density limit in the marrow at which normal stem cells arrest cell production. The specific biochemical abnormalities responsible for the failure of the multipotent leukemic stem cells to respond normally to feedback regulation are not yet understood, nor is it known how they may be related to the bcr/abl gene rearrangement.

The leukemic cells in chronic-phase CML have a striking

propensity for further malignant transformation. After a variable duration of the chronic phase, averaging about three years, the disease enters an accelerated or blastic phase. Such malignant progression occurs in about 80 per cent of patients and probably would eventually occur in all of them if they did not die of other complications of the disease or of unrelated causes. The Ph^1 chromosome is preserved, but the transformed cells may acquire additional chromosomal abnormalities such as an additional Ph^1 chromosome, trisomy of chromosome 8 or 17, or trisomy of the long arm of 17. The rapidity with which the transition occurs depends on the degree of further transformation and on the comparative proliferative properties of the chronic and acute phase stem cells. In the accelerated phase the cells retain their capacity for partial differentiation, whereas in the blastic phase they are arrested at the blastic level of differentiation. The direction of differentiation in the accelerated phase is variable as in the chronic phase. Transitional forms may occur among the chronic, accelerated, and blastic phases.

CLINICAL MANIFESTATIONS. Occasionally CML is diagnosed in an asymptomatic patient after incidental detection of splenomegaly or unexplained leukocytosis, basophilia, or thrombocytosis. Common early symptoms are *fatigue* and reduced exercise tolerance resulting from anemia, anorexia, reduction in food capacity, weight loss, and a sense of fullness in the left upper quadrant as a result of progressive splenic enlargement. Headaches, sweating, fever, and bone pain or tenderness may also occur, especially if the leukocyte count is very elevated. *Hemorrhagic manifestations* such as ecchymoses after minor trauma, petechiae, retinal hemorrhages, or hematuria may occur in patients in whom there is severe thrombocytopenia or in those with thrombocytosis with abnormal platelets. *Thrombotic episodes* such as splenic or myocardial infarction and thrombophlebitis are common, and priapism or severe headaches may result from leukostasis in patients with extreme leukocytosis. Acute *gouty arthritis* or *nephrolithiasis* is sometimes associated with elevated uric acid levels. Infections are uncommon in the chronic phase, but occasional patients may have unusual and persistent infections that are difficult to diagnose. Low-grade *fever* in the absence of infection is not unusual in the chronic phase when there is extreme leukocytosis, and the temperature returns to normal when the WBC is lowered by treatment.

PHYSICAL EXAMINATION. The most common finding on physical examination at diagnosis is *splenomegaly*. The spleen may be enormous and fill most of the abdomen, or only minimally enlarged; in less than 10 per cent of cases the spleen is not palpable or enlarged on splenic scan. Slight hepatomegaly is common, but when extreme liver enlargement occurs as a result of leukemic infiltration or there is infiltration of lymph nodes, skin, or other tissues, these are usually indications that the disease will have a rapidly progressive course. Patients who present with the disease already in blastic transformation or in whom this event occurs later in the course of the disease may exhibit any of the clinical findings associated with acute leukemia. Unlike acute leukemia, persistent fever unrelated to infection is common in the blastic phase of CML.

LABORATORY ABNORMALITIES. The most consistent laboratory abnormality at diagnosis is *leukocytosis* (Color plate 3C). The WBC count may range from a minimal elevation to over a million leukocytes per cubic millimeter. The marrow is hypercellular, and differential counts of both marrow and blood show a spectrum of mature and immature granulocytes similar to that found in normal marrow. Increased numbers of eosinophils and/or basophils are often present, and sometimes monocytosis is seen. Increased megakaryocytes are often found in the marrow, and sometimes fragments of megakaryocyte nuclei are present in the blood, especially when the platelet count is very high. The percentage of lymphocytes is reduced in both the marrow and blood in comparison to normal subjects, but the absolute lymphocyte count is usually normal or increased with normal proportions of B and T cells. The myeloid-erythroid ratio in the marrow is usually greatly elevated. The percentage of blasts in the marrow and blood is usually less than 3 per cent in the chronic phase at diagnosis and less than 1 per cent after the WBC count has been reduced by treatment; a persistent elevation of greater than 10 per cent usually indicates impending transformation. About half of patients present with some degree of *thrombocytosis* at diagnosis; thrombocytopenia is much less frequent. Extreme degrees of thrombocytopenia or thrombocytosis may develop as the disease progresses. In some patients, cyclic fluctuations of the leukocytes and platelets have been observed that are unrelated to treatment.

There may be no anemia at presentation, but variable degrees of *anemia* are common when the WBC count exceeds 50,000 per cubic millimeter. The anemia is normocytic and normochromic, unless complications such as bleeding occur, resulting in iron deficiency. Some patients, especially those with greatly enlarged spleens, have circulating nucleated erythrocyte precursors, but this finding is not usually prominent. There may be shortened red cell survival in patients with severe splenomegaly and/or hepatomegaly, but autoimmune hemolysis is not seen in uncomplicated CML. The reticulocyte count is normal or only slightly increased.

The mature granulocytes in CML usually have markedly diminished neutrophil alkaline phosphatase activity and their content of myeloperoxidase and lactoferrin may also be decreased. Plasma and leukocyte levels of histamine and histamine metabolites are usually elevated. Other common laboratory abnormalities in CML that are associated with the increased rates of cell production and turnover are elevated levels of serum uric acid, lactic dehydrogenase, vitamin B_{12}, the B_{12}-binding protein transcobalamin I, and serum urinary lysozyme. Hyperkalemia resulting from leakage of potassium from leukocytes occurs rarely. Hypercalcemia may also occur, usually in patients with blastic transformation or in those who are entering an accelerated phase and have lytic bone lesions.

Myelofibrosis, demonstrated by special stains of marrow biopsy specimens, may develop in the course of CML. Significant myelofibrosis is more often seen late in the course of disease, but rarely severe acute myelofibrosis is seen prior to treatment in patients with prominent megakaryocytic proliferation. The marrow histiocytes sometimes display prominent phagocytic activity and become engorged with glycolipids, resembling Gaucher cells.

Transition from the chronic phase to the accelerated or blastic phase may occur gradually over a year or longer or abruptly (blast crisis). The disease becomes progressively less responsive to previously effective treatment. Common signs and symptoms heralding such a change are progressive leukocytosis, thrombocytosis, or thrombocytopenia, anemia, increasing and painful splenomegaly, lymphadenopathy, hepatomegaly, or infiltration of other organs, fever, bone pain, development of destructive bone lesions, and thrombotic or bleeding complications. In the accelerated phase, the cells are still completely or partially differentiated, although they usually show increasing morphologic abnormalities. There are no standardized criteria for distinguishing between the accelerated and blastic phases, but most authorities use a persistent elevation of greater than 20 or 30 per cent blasts in the blood and/or marrow or of blasts plus promyelocytes of 30 per cent in blood or 50 per cent in marrow to define the blastic phase. When the spleen is the primary source of the transformed cells, the percentage of blasts in the blood may be higher than in the marrow. The blasts have the morphologic appearance of lymphoblasts in about 25 per cent of cases and contain terminal deoxynucleotidyl transferase, whereas in the remainder they are recognized as primitive myeloid precursors.

DIAGNOSIS. Persistent unexplained leukocytosis with circulating immature granulocytes and an enlarged spleen suggests the diagnosis of CML; some degree of splenomegaly is present at diagnosis in over 90 per cent of patients. A bone marrow aspiration and biopsy should always be done if the diagnosis of CML is suspected. Demonstration of the Ph^1 chromosome in dividing marrow cells provides confirmation of the diagnosis in Ph^1-positive CML. Occasional patients with complex variant translocations lack a morphologically apparent Ph^1 chromosome, but involvement of chromosomes 9 and 22 can be detected using appropriate molecular techniques.

Leukemoid reactions associated with infections are usually distinguishable in most cases because prominent splenomegaly is absent, neutrophil alkaline phosphatase activity is increased instead of low, and the Ph^1 chromosome is not present (see Ch. 151). Leukemoid or leukoerythroblastic reactions also occur with certain neoplasms, especially when there is involvement of the bone marrow, but sometimes even in the absence of marrow metastases. By appropriate cytochemical tests and analyses of surface antigens it is usually possible to distinguish metastatic tumor cells from immature hematopoietic cells. Leukoerythroblastic reactions may also be associated with hemorrhagic shock or hemolysis or as a rebound phenomenon following cytotoxic or infectious depression of the marrow, but a careful history, appropriate diagnostic tests, and a short period of observation should avoid confusion with CML.

Myelofibrosis, polycythemia vera, and other myeloproliferative variants may present with splenomegaly, leukocytosis, and immature granulocytes in the blood, but the neutrophil alkaline phosphatase activity is usually high in these disorders, and the Ph^1 chromosome is absent. The hematocrit is elevated in polycythemia vera (unless bleeding occurs), whereas it is normal or decreased in CML. Bone marrow biopsy and appropriate stains may reveal some increase in reticulin fibers or fibrosis in CML, but these findings are less prominent than in myelofibrosis. Patients who have the clinical manifestations of CML but without the Ph^1 chromosome may have mixed features of CML and other myeloproliferative disorders. Chronic monocytic or chronic myelomonocytic leukemia (CMMoL) and the chronic form of erythroleukemia are more properly regarded as variants of acute leukemia. Splenomegaly occurs frequently in CMMoL, but the leukocyte count is normal or only moderately elevated, the absolute monocyte count is usually increased, and the serum and urinary lysozyme levels are increased. The Ph^1 chromosome is not present, although other chromosomal abnormalities may occur.

Basophilic leukemia and eosinophilic leukemia may rarely occur as variants of CML or other myeloproliferative diseases and are usually associated with a poor prognosis. Basophilic leukemia should be distinguished from mast cell leukemia, in which urticaria pigmentosa is usually seen concomitantly. Thrombocythemia and megakaryocytic leukemia occur fairly commonly as variants of CML or other myeloproliferative disorders. Infrequently unexplained "essential" thrombocythemia and megakaryocytic hyperplasia are observed as isolated findings without Ph^1-positive cells in the marrow or other abnormalities of the myeloid elements. Such patients may later develop other manifestations of one of the myeloproliferative diseases.

Chronic neutrophilic leukemia is a rare disease, occurring mostly in older patients, which is characterized by marked splenomegaly, leukocytosis with 90 per cent or more mature neutrophils in the blood, elevated neutrophil alkaline phosphatase, and a chronic course. The absence of immature granulocytes in the blood and of the Ph^1 chromosome in the marrow distinguishes this type of leukemia from CML.

The first clinical manifestations of blastic transformation may occur in extramedullary sites such as the spleen, lymph nodes, meninges, or other tissues, while the marrow and blood are still filled with chronic-phase leukemic cells. If immature granulocytes are the predominant cell type, the extramedullary tumors may have a green hue owing to myeloperoxidase and are sometimes diagnosed as chloromas or granulocytic sarcomas. If the transformed cells resemble lymphoblasts, an erroneous diagnosis of lymphoma is sometimes made. Demonstration of the Ph^1 chromosome in the blasts will lead to the correct diagnosis. Since localized blastic lesions invariably become disseminated, usually within several months, systemic treatment, sometimes in addition to local irradiation, is justified once the diagnosis is made.

The leukemic cells in CML sometimes undergo early blastic transformation without recognition of the chronic phase, and patients may present with what appears to be acute leukemia, either lymphoblastic or one of the myeloid variants. A very large spleen, extreme leukocytosis (>400,000 per cubic millimeter), prominent eosinophilia and/or basophilia, and a normal or elevated platelet count should alert the physician to this possible diagnostic dilemma. However, all of these features may be absent in patients with CML presenting in blastic crisis de novo, and cytogenetic examination of the marrow is necessary to confirm the presence or absence of the Ph^1 chromosome.

All patients with a clinical diagnosis of acute lymphoblastic leukemia (ALL) should have cytogenetic analyses performed prior to treatment because Ph^1-positive ALL has a worse prognosis than the more common types of ALL. The incidence of Ph^1 + ALL is about 20 per cent and 2 per cent in adults and children, respectively, in patients with a suspected diagnosis of ALL. Ph^1 + ALL has recently been shown to include heterogeneous subtypes: some cases have similar bcr rearrangements as observed in classic CML, whereas in others the leukemic cells express unique abl-derived tyrosine kinases that are distinct from the bcr-abl–derived p210 protein of CML.

TREATMENT. Asymptomatic patients in the chronic phase in whom the WBC count is below 50,000 per cubic millimeter can be observed without treatment until the disease progresses and symptoms develop. When clinical manifestations appear they can usually be controlled with cytotoxic drugs or splenic irradiation, but unlike acute leukemia, true remissions are very rare and the marrow remains largely populated with leukemic cells containing the Ph^1 marker.

Chemotherapy. The most common conventional drug used is *busulfan*, but other alkylating agents such as cyclophosphamide and antimetabolites are also effective. One must be careful to avoid overtreatment of CML, as severe myelosuppression can occur. The usual starting oral dose of busulfan is 4 to 8 mg per day, but doses of 12 to 16 mg or higher may be required initially if the blood leukocyte and/or platelet counts are very high and rapid reduction is necessary. The dose should be reduced as the WBC count falls and the spleen shrinks during the first several weeks, roughly in proportion to halving of the WBC count. For example, if the initial WBC count is 100,000 per cubic millimeter and the initial dose of busulfan is 8 mg per day, when the WBC count reaches 50,000 per cubic millimeter the dose should be lowered to 4 mg per day. The drug should be stopped when the WBC count reaches about 25,000 per cubic millimeter, as it may continue to fall after stopping, and overtreatment can cause prolonged marrow hypoplasia. Other manifestations of chronic busulfan toxicity include sterility, dryness of skin and mucous membrane, hyperpigmentation, and rarely adrenal insufficiency and pulmonary fibrosis. In some patients the WBC count and spleen size may remain nearly normal without further treatment for months after initial control has been achieved, whereas others require continuous treatment. There is considerable variability in responsiveness, and the exact dose must be titrated individually. The dose of busulfan required to maintain control of the chronic phase is usually between 2 mg every other day and 4 mg per day. Some authorities prefer intermittent therapy rather than continuous treatment.

The amount of drug needed for control does not appear to be related to prognosis.

Purine and pyrimidine antagonists and hydroxyurea, a ribonucleotide reductase inhibitor, are also effective in controlling chronic-phase CML. The usual initial oral dose of *hydroxyurea* is between 1 and 3 grams per day, depending on the height of the WBC count and the body surface area. Hydroxyurea should be taken as a single dose at least an hour before eating. After the WBC count and spleen size are reduced to normal, the dose required for maintenance is usually between 0.5 gram every other day and 2.0 grams per day and must be titrated individually. Continuous treatment and close monitoring of the WBC count are necessary with hydroxyurea, as its inhibitory effects on myeloproliferation are much more transient than with busulfan and the WBC count may rise rapidly when it is discontinued. Hydroxyurea is generally well tolerated, but it may cause nausea, vomiting, diarrhea, stomatitis, dermatitis, and megaloblastosis.

Treatment of Acute Leukostatic or Thrombotic Complications. Some patients with CML may present with acute leukostatic or thrombotic complications (e.g., priapism, thrombophlebitis, infarctions of the spleen or other organs, sagittal sinus thrombosis, or other complications affecting the central nervous system), and in such cases it is mandatory to lower the WBC and/or platelet count rapidly with cytotoxic drugs. A continuous intravenous infusion of cytosine arabinoside, 200 mg per square meter of body surface area per 24 hours, or of hydroxyurea, 2 to 3 grams per square meter per day for four or five days, will usually lower the WBC and platelet counts rapidly, relieve the acute symptoms, and prevent additional complications. Leukapheresis and/or plateletpheresis is also effective in rapidly reducing the counts if a continuous flow centrifuge is available. The reduction is usually very transient, however, and chemotherapy should also be begun immediately for sustained control. Thrombocytosis sometimes persists after the WBC has been reduced by chemotherapy, and in such cases melphalan and/or thiotepa may be useful in controlling the platelets.

Tumor Lysis Syndrome. The patient should be well hydrated and allopurinol administered before beginning cytotoxic therapy when rapid cell lysis is anticipated in order to prevent exacerbation of hyperuricemia and development of uric acid nephropathy or acute arthritis. Hyperkalemia, hyperphosphatemia, increase of lactic dehydrogenase, and other biochemical abnormalities may also occur during sudden massive leukemic cell destruction (tumor lysis syndrome), but with adequate hydration to maintain a good urinary output and close monitoring, serious complications resulting from these biochemical alterations can usually be avoided.

Splenic Radiation. Splenic radiation is also effective in reducing the size of the spleen and WBC count. The radiation treatments should be given cautiously in fractionated doses over several weeks because the WBC count may continue to fall after stopping, and, as with busulfan, overtreatment can cause prolonged marrow hypoplasia. The total splenic dose needed for control is usually between 300 and 1200 rads, depending on the size of the spleen and radiation port, but the splenomegaly in some patients may be refractory to even larger doses. Splenectomy performed early in the chronic phase does not significantly affect survival, although in patients who are prone to develop massive splenomegaly it prevents later complications, which become difficult to manage (e.g., hypersplenism, inanition, repeated infarctions).

Aggressive Combination Chemotherapy. Some centers have taken a more aggressive therapeutic approach in chronic-phase CML with the use of combination chemotherapeutic regimens effective in acute myeloid leukemia. Complete remissions with marked reduction or disappearance of Ph^1-positive leukemic cells in the marrow have been obtained in 20 to 50 per cent of patients, but most of the remissions have been of short duration. Patients having remissions live longer than nonresponders, but overall survival does not appear to be significantly prolonged by the intensive treatment regimens employed to date.

Interferon Therapy. Both partially purified and recombinant human alfa-interferon have produced hematologic remissions in CML with partial or complete disappearance of Ph^1-positive metaphases from the marrow, but it is too soon to evaluate the effects of this treatment on survival. Trials of recombinant gamma-interferon have recently been started to determine if this will be equally or more effective, but the eventual role of the interferons and other biologic agents in the treatment of CML is not yet clear.

Marrow Transplantation (see Ch. 165). It has been possible to eradicate the leukemic clone only by administering very high doses of alkylating agents in combination with a supralethal dose of total body irradiation, followed by rescue with transplantation of marrow from a histocompatible donor. More than a dozen patients with CML with identical twins have been so treated, of whom the majority remain free of disease without further treatment with no detectable Ph^1-positive cells in the marrow for periods of up to ten years. The hazards associated with allogeneic marrow transplantation using histocompatible nonidentical sibling donors are still formidable, especially in older patients, but in the last six years several hundred patients with chronic-phase CML, mostly under the age of 50 years, have received allogeneic transplants at different centers throughout the world. The results are best if performed during the chronic phase, especially within the first year after diagnosis.

The probability of long disease-free survival is 50 to 70 per cent in different series if the transplant is done during the chronic phase; the remaining patients usually die within the first two years of complications related to the procedure, most often of interstitial pneumonia or graft-versus-host disease (GVHD). Depletion of T cells from the donor marrow with lectins or monoclonal antibodies has greatly reduced the incidence of GVHD, but it is not yet clear if overall survival will be improved; in some trials T cell depletion has been associated with an increased incidence of engraftment failure and leukemia relapse. The incidence of leukemic relapse reported so far in different series has varied from 0 to 20 per cent or higher, but because the disease may have a slow evolution, a longer period of observation will be necessary to determine the true incidence. Some patients have evidence of persistent Ph^1-positive cells in the marrow by karyotype analysis or bcr rearrangement but have not progressed to hematologic relapse.

Treatment of the Accelerated or Blastic Phase. When CML enters an accelerated phase it becomes increasingly refractory to therapy that was previously effective. Increasing doses of busulfan or hydroxyurea are required to control the WBC and spleen size and, in some cases, progressive thrombocytosis. In some cases, severe anemia and/or thrombocytopenia develops, either because of the disease or as a result of drug toxicity.

Therapy of the blastic phase is generally unsatisfactory, and most patients die within a few months after blastic transformation occurs. Hydroxyurea is most commonly used to control myeloid blastic transformation, but multidrug regimens designed for acute nonlymphoblastic leukemia are also used. In the 25 per cent of patients with lymphoblastic transformation, remission can often be achieved with prednisone and vincristine with reversion to the chronic phase, but these are usually of short duration and the average survival in different series was three to eight months. Complete remissions with disappearance of the Ph^1-positive cells in the marrow have rarely been achieved with intensive combinations of regimens designed for acute lymphoblastic leukemia, but these have all been only temporary and no cures have resulted. The average survival of patients with lymphoblastic transformation who are treated with modern intensive programs designed for ALL

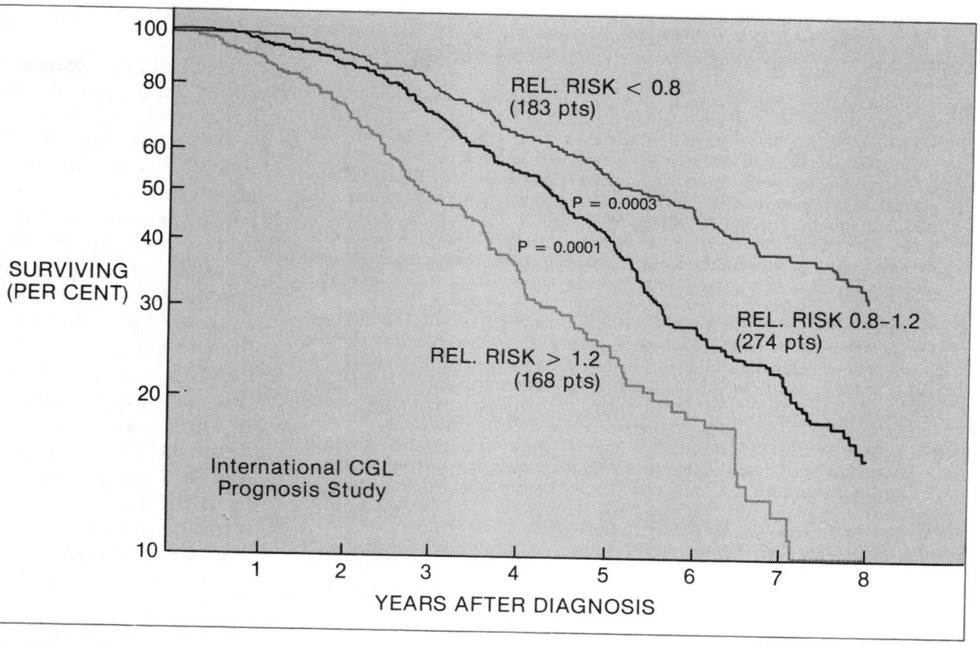

FIGURE 155–1. Actuarial survival of 625 patients with nonblastic Ph[1] chromosome–positive CML, 5 to 45 years old at the time of diagnosis, divided into low-, high-, and intermediate-risk groups, according to a Cox model with five variables, representing sex, spleen size, platelet count, hematocrit, and percentage of circulating blasts. The median survival of the 625 patients was 50.5 months. (From Sokal JE, et al.: Prognostic discrimination among younger patients with chronic granulocytic leukemia: Relevance to bone marrow transplantation. Blood 66:1352–1357, 1985.)

is about a year. The response is not significantly different in patients who initially present in blastic phase (Ph[1] + ALL) compared with those who develop lymphoblastic transformation after a recognized chronic phase. Any of the myriad complications seen in acute leukemia can be encountered during the blastic phase of CML. Meningeal leukemia should be treated with intrathecal methotrexate or arabinosylcytosine and/or cranial irradiation as in acute leukemia.

Since few patients respond satisfactorily to any treatment after myeloid blastic transformation is fully developed, there have been recent attempts to treat such patients aggressively with combination regimens designed for acute myeloid leukemia as soon as early evidence of impending blastic transformation can be detected, such as by appearance of additional chromosomal abnormalities or by a change in the growth pattern of the marrow colony forming cells in vitro. Although this approach may delay overt blastic transformation, it is not clear that survival is significantly affected. The results of aggressive treatment followed by allogeneic marrow transplantation in the accelerated or blastic phases are less favorable than in the chronic phase, with more early deaths due to complications, higher relapse rates, and only 10 to 25 per cent survivors after four years. Intensive treatment of the blastic phase followed by transplantation of stored autologous stem cells obtained from the marrow or blood during the chronic phase has been successful in temporarily restoring the disease to the chronic phase in some patients, but the mortality has been high, and it has not been demonstrated that overall survival is increased. No satisfactory methods have yet been found to selectively purge the marrow ex vivo of Ph[1]-positive leukemic progenitors while sparing normal stem cells.

PROGNOSIS. The median survival of patients with Ph[1]-positive CML from diagnosis is about three years, with a range of less than a year to over ten years. Although the clinical manifestations of the chronic phase can usually be readily controlled by appropriate treatment and most patients are able to lead normal lives, treatment has not substantially improved survival. Survival after development of an accelerated phase is usually less than a year and after blastic transformation only a few months, although patients with lymphoblastic transformation may live longer with appropriate treatment.

In a multi-institutional study of disease features at diagnosis in more than 800 patients with Ph[1]-positive nonblastic CML, the most important characteristics associated with shortened survival were older age, male sex (in patients under 45), large spleen, high platelet count, high percentages of blasts in blood and marrow, high percentages of eosinophils and basophils, presence of nucleated red cells in the blood, a high serum lactic dehydrogenase (LDH) level, and a low hematocrit. Using a Cox model generated with variables representing disease features found on regression analysis to have prognostic significance, the patients could be segregated into three groups with significantly different survival patterns, both for the total population of CML patients studied and for younger patients (aged 5 to 45 years) who might be candidates for bone marrow transplantation. Based on a Cox model using five variables: sex, spleen size, platelet count, hematocrit, and percentage of circulating blasts, the patients could be segregated into a high-risk group who had an actuarial mortality of 30 per cent during the first two years after diagnosis and an annual risk of 30 per cent thereafter, while the most favorable group had a two-year actuarial mortality of 9 per cent, an average annual risk thereafter of 17 per cent, and a median survival of five and one-half years (Fig. 155–1). Additional factors that have been reported to be associated with an unfavorable prognosis in other series are black race, cytogenetic abnormalities in addition to the Ph[1] chromosome, liver enlargement, and myelofibrosis. The predictive models are still undergoing refinement with inclusion of additional features of prognostic values, and they should prove useful in advising patients when to consider alternative forms of treatment, such as bone marrow transplantation.

Ben-Neriah Y, Daley GQ, Mes-Masson A-M, et al.: The chronic myelogenous leukemia-specific P210 protein is the product of the bcr/abl hybrid gene. Science 233:212, 1986. *A report of molecular biology studies demonstrating that the p210 kilodalton phosphoprotein in CML cells is the protein product of the novel 8.5-kilobase bcr/abl fusion transcript.*

Champlin R, Gale RP, Foon KA, et al.: Chronic leukemias: Oncogenes, chromosomes and advances in therapy. Ann Intern Med 104:671, 1986. *An excellent review describing recent developments in understanding the role of oncogenes and chromosomal rearrangements in the chronic leukemias, and including discussion of treatment with biologic agents and bone marrow transplantation.*

Clark SS, McLaughlin J, Crist WM, et al.: Unique forms of the *abl* tyrosine kinase distinguish Ph[1]-positive CML from Ph[1]-positive ALL. Science 235:85, 1987. *Some Ph[1]-positive ALL cells express unique* abl-*derived tyrosine kinases of 185 to 180 kilodaltons that are distinct from the* bcr-abl–*derived p210 protein of CML.*

De Klein A, Hagemeijer A, Bartram CR, et al.: *bcr* Rearrangement and translocation of the c-*abl* oncogene in Philadelphia positive acute lymphoblastic leukemia. Blood 68:1369, 1986. *The pH[1] chromosomes of patients with CML and Ph[1]-positive ALL are indistinguishable cytogenetically. However, whereas some of the latter have the same* bcr *rearrangement as in CML, others do not; Ph[1]-positive ALL thus includes several heterogeneous subtypes of leukemia.*

Erikson J, Griffin CA, Ar-Rushdi A, et al.: Heterogeneity of chromosome 22 breakpoint in Philadelphia-positive (Ph+) acute lymphocytic leukemia. Proc Natl Acad Sci USA 83:1807, 1986. *A recent report of molecular biology studies demonstrating heterogeneity in the breakpoints on chromosome 22 in Ph[1]-positive ALL.*

Goldman JM, Apperley JF, Jones L, et al.: Bone marrow transplantation for patients with chronic myeloid leukemia. N Engl J Med 314:202, 1986. *The results of allogeneic bone marrow transplantation are described in 52 patients with CML in the chronic phase and 18 patients with more advanced disease.*

Goto T, Nishikori M, Arlin Z, et al.: Growth characteristics of leukemic and normal hematopoietic cells in Ph[1]+ chronic myelogenous leukemia and effects of intensive treatment. Blood 59:793, 1982. *Report of a clinical trial in which patients in the chronic phase of CML were treated with a moderately intensive regimen consisting of splenectomy and combination chemotherapy. Although some complete remissions were achieved, these were usually of short duration. The results of other trials of splenectomy and intensive treatment are reviewed.*

Jain K, Arlin Z, Mertelsmann R, et al.: Philadelphia chromosome and terminal transferase positive acute leukemia: Similarity of terminal phase of chronic myelogenous leukemia and de novo acute presentation. J Clin Oncol 1:669, 1983. *A review of the clinical and laboratory features and results of intensive treatment of patients with CML with lymphoblastic transformation either presenting de novo as "Ph[1] + ALL" or as the terminal event after a chronic phase.*

Kantarjian HM, Smith TL, McCredie KB, et al.: Chronic myelogenous leukemia: A multivariate analysis of the associations of patient characteristics and therapy with survival. Blood 66:1326, 1985. *An analysis of pretreatment clinical and laboratory features in 303 patients with Ph[1]-positive chronic-phase CML to identify the factors of greatest prognostic significance.*

Koeffler HP, Golde DW: Chronic myelogenous leukemia: New concepts. N Engl J Med 304:1201, 1269, 1981. *Authoritative review that summarizes current knowledge of CML, with emphasis on pathogenesis and treatment. 204 references.*

Nitta M, Kato Y, Strife A, et al.: Incidence of involvement of the B and T lymphocytic lineages in chronic myelogenous leukemia. Blood 66:1053, 1985. *Peripheral blood lymphocytes were examined after stimulation in 32 patients with Ph[1]-positive CML. Most B cells and T cells were found to be Ph[1]-negative in the majority of patients, but about 20 per cent of patients had predominantly Ph[1]-positive B cells or a mixture of Ph[1]-positive and Ph[1]-negative cells that grew as established cell lines after transformation with Epstein-Barr virus.*

Pugh WC, Pearson M, Vardiman JW, et al.: Philadelphia chromosome–negative chronic myelogenous leukemia: A morphological reassessment. Br J Haematol 60:457, 1985. *Twenty-five cases originally classified as Ph[1]-negative CML were reexamined, and it was concluded that only one of the 25 was morphologically and clinically indistinguishable from Ph[1]-positive CML. The remainder consisted of a heterogeneous group of patients with other myelodysplastic disorders, particularly chronic myelomonocytic leukemia.*

Sokal JE, Baccarani M, Tura S, et al.: Prognostic discrimination among younger patients with chronic granulocytic leukemia: Relevance to bone marrow transplantation. Blood 66:1352, 1985. *A similar regression analysis was conducted in nonblastic CML patients aged 5 to 45 to permit identification of patients at high, intermediate, and low risk for survival. This is the age group usually considered for bone marrow transplantation, and the study may help in deciding when to recommend that the procedure be performed.*

Sokal JE, Cox EB, Baccarani M, et al.: The Italian Cooperative CML Study Group: Prognostic discrimination in "good-risk" chronic granulocytic leukemia. Blood April, 1984. *A multivariate regression analysis of the prognostic significance of disease features at the time of diagnosis in 813 patients with Ph[1] + nonblastic CML collected from six American and European series. With use of the Cox model, four key variables were found that enabled identification of low-, intermediate-, and high-risk groups of patients.*

Talpaz M, Kantarjian HM, McCredie KB, et al.: Hematologic remission and cytogenetic improvement induced by recombinant human interferon alpha in chronic myelogenous leukemia. N Engl J Med 314:1065, 1986. *A preliminary report describing the effects of recombinant human alfa-interferon in 17 patients with Ph[1]-positive CML. Fourteen patients responded of whom 13 had a hematologic remission and one a partial remission.*

Thomas ED, Clift RA, Fefer A, et al.: Marrow transplantation for the treatment of chronic myelogenous leukemia. Ann Intern Med 104:155, 1986. *This paper reports the results of the experience of the Seattle group in treating 198 patients with CML using bone marrow transplantation. The probability of long-term survival for allogeneic graft recipients was 49 per cent in the first chronic phase, 58 per cent in the second chronic phase, 15 per cent in the accelerated phase, and 14 per cent in the blastic phase.*

CHRONIC LYMPHOCYTIC LEUKEMIA

DEFINITION. Chronic lymphocytic leukemia (CLL) is a monoclonal neoplasm of slowly proliferating long-lived lymphocytes, usually B lymphocytes, which are immunologically defective.

ETIOLOGY. The etiology is unknown. Unlike the situation in acute and chronic myelogenous leukemia, exposure to ionizing radiation and cytotoxic drugs or chemicals does not result in an increased incidence of CLL. There does appear to be some genetic predisposition, since CLL is the most frequent type of leukemia occurring in multiple family members. There is no clear inheritance pattern, but siblings, especially brothers, appear to have the highest concordance of CLL. Except in rare high-incidence families, the incidence of CLL among close relatives is probably about three times that in the general population.

INCIDENCE. The incidence of CLL in the United States is about 3 per 100,000 population, or about 25 per cent of all leukemias. The incidence in most Western countries is similar, with CLL being slightly more common than CML. CLL is twice as common in males as in females. The mean age is about 60, and the incidence increases with age. It is rare before age 30 and almost never occurs in children. In Japan and several other Asian countries where reliable statistics exist, B cell CLL is very uncommon. This may be due to genetic factors; Japanese living in the United States have a slightly higher incidence than native Japanese, but still lower than the rest of the United States population. On the other hand, T cell variants of CLL and related lymphoproliferative diseases are not uncommon and appear to be endemic in certain areas of Japan. A human T cell leukemia-lymphoma virus (HTLV1) is strongly suspected of having an etiologic role in these T cell neoplasms in Japan, as well as in patients from the Caribbean and less often in the United States and other countries.

PATHOGENESIS AND MECHANISMS. In the great majority of cases, CLL results from a monoclonal proliferation of B lymphocytes, although a slight percentage of cases is derived from T cells. The leukemic B cells have monoclonal surface immunoglobulin (although in lower density than normal B lymphocytes), exhibit Ia-like cell surface antigens, carry receptors for the Fc fragment of IgG (as recognized by the binding of heat-aggregated IgG and several rosetting techniques) and for the C3d and occasionally the C3b complement components, and form spontaneous rosettes with mouse red blood cells. Intracellular crystalline inclusions containing IgM and λ light chains have been observed in the leukemic cells of some patients. A murine monoclonal antibody recognizes a 65,000- to 67,000-dalton antigen (Leu-1) present on B-CLL cells, but not on cells from other types of B cell leukemias or lymphomas. This surface antigen is also expressed by human thymocytes and peripheral T cells, but is absent on normal B cells. Other T cell antigens and the terminal deoxynucleotidyltransferase enzyme are absent on B-CLL cells.

The leukemic lymphocytes in CLL proliferate very slowly, as is also true of normal B lymphocytes and several other low-growth fraction B cell neoplasms such as multiple myeloma and most nodular lymphomas. The great majority of CLL lymphocytes are small cells that are in a quiescent state (G_0). In most cases, only a small fraction of the population consists of intermediate-sized or large lymphocytes, of which some are in various stages of the cell cycle preparing to divide; proliferation may be increased in lymph nodes compared to marrow or blood. Although only a small fraction of the total leukemic population is proliferating at any time, because the leukemic cells have a very long lifespan, they accumulate and continue to recirculate through the body.

The leukemic lymphocytes in CLL appear to be "frozen" in an intermediate stage of the B cell differentiation pathway, but can be induced in vitro with phorbol esters or B cell mitogens to differentiate into more mature B cells, including prolymphocytes, hairy cells, and plasma cells. CLL cells are immunologically defective, and they respond sluggishly to mitogens or immunologic stimuli. CLL cells produce an excess of free light chains, either kappa or lambda, but never both. Only a small percentage of patients secrete sufficient IgM to be detectable as a spike on electrophoresis.

In the early stages of CLL, T lymphocytes are present in the blood in normal or increased absolute numbers, although in reduced proportions. Purified T cells from CLL patients respond normally to mitogens, but form fewer T cell colonies in vitro compared to T cells from normal subjects and are defective in natural killer and antibody-dependent cell-mediated cytotoxicity. Normal T cells can be divided into sub-

TABLE 155–1. RAI'S STAGING SYSTEM FOR CLL*

Stage 0	Absolute lymphocytosis in blood of >15,000 per cubic millimeter
Stage I	Absolute lymphocytosis plus enlarged lymph nodes
Stage II	Absolute lymphocytosis plus enlarged liver and/or spleen (with or without lymph node enlargement)
Stage III†	Absolute lymphocytosis plus anemia (hemoglobin <11 grams per deciliter in males and <10 grams per deciliter in females)
Stage IV†	Absolute lymphocytosis plus thrombocytopenia (platelets <100,000 per cubic millimeter)

*From Rai KR, et al.: Clinical staging of chronic lymphocytic leukemia. Blood 46:219, 1975.

†In stages III and IV, patients may or may not have enlarged lymph nodes, liver, and/or spleen.

populations according to their type of Fc receptor for immunoglobulin: Tμ (IgM), Tα (IgA), and Tγ (IgG), or their reactivities with monoclonal antibodies. In CLL, the proportion of T cells with receptors for IgG (Tγ) is markedly increased, resulting in a decreased T helper cell (Tμ or T4/Leu-3) to T suppressor cell (Tγ or T8/Leu-2) ratio. The decreased T helper function and other immunologic abnormalities that have been described appear to be more pronounced in later stages of CLL.

CLINICAL MANIFESTATIONS. ***Staging.*** About 25 per cent of patients with CLL are asymptomatic when first seen, and the diagnosis is made following detection of lymphocytosis on an incidental blood count or in the course of investigating the cause of enlarged lymph nodes or splenomegaly. Some cases may have a very benign course, and the patient may remain asymptomatic for many years, whereas in others the disease can progress rapidly. The average survival in CLL is about four to five years. A simple clinical staging system for CLL (see Table 155–1) has proved of prognostic value in several large series. Median survival decreases with advancing stage: stage 0 = 14 (range 12 to 15) years; stage I = 8 (5 to 11) years; stage II = 6 (4 to 9) years; and stages III and IV = 2 (1 to 3½) years. A diagnosis of CLL may be made in some patients with a lesser degree of absolute lymphocytosis than 15,000 per cubic millimeter (i.e., earlier than stage 0) if cell marker studies demonstrate a monoclonal B cell population characteristic of CLL in the blood and marrow. The rate at which the disease progresses from early to late stages is quite variable in individual patients; stage II appears to be especially heterogeneous, and cases tend to diverge into low- or high-risk groups. Other investigators have reported that patients in the intermediate-risk group who had lymphocyte counts over 40,000 per cubic millimeter or diffuse instead of a nodular pattern of marrow involvement had shorter survival. A revised prognostic staging system was proposed by an international workshop on CLL that is based on the number of lymphoid areas involved and the degree of bone marrow failure (Table 155–2). Clinical enlargement of the spleen, of liver, and of lymph nodes in the cervical, axillary, and inguinal regions constitute five separate areas of involvement, each of which is considered one area irrespective of whether the lymphadenopathy is unilateral or bilateral. The advantages of

TABLE 155–2. INTERNATIONAL STAGING SYSTEM FOR CLL*

Clinical Stage†		
A A(0), A(I), or A(II)	No anemia or thrombocytopenia	Less than three areas of lymphoid enlargement
B B(I) or B(II)	No anemia or thrombocytopenia	Three or more involved areas
C C(III) or C(IV)	Anemia and/or thrombocytopenia	Regardless of the number of areas of lymphoid enlargement

*From Binet JL, et al.: A new prognostic classification of chronic lymphocytic leukemia derived from a multivariate survival analysis. Br J Haematol 48:356, 1981.

†It was recommended that the revised classification be integrated with the Rai system by using Roman numerals in parenthesis to represent the latter.

the revised system are that it has fewer stages (which should simplify design and evaluation of comparative therapeutic trials), it recognizes that anemia and thrombocytopenia have a similar prognosis and do not require separate stages, and it recognizes a predominantly splenic form of the disease that may have a relatively favorable prognosis. Survival curves have so far shown distinct differences among the three groups: the median survivals for groups A, B, and C were >10, 7, and 2 years, respectively.

Symptoms. Patients with early-stage disease are often asymptomatic, but increasing symptoms develop with advancing stage and include malaise, easy fatigability, anorexia, weight loss, low-grade fever, and night sweats. Bacterial infections, such as sinusitis, pneumonia, or cutaneous infections, are common and should be treated promptly with appropriate antibiotics. Patients in advanced stages become progressively more immunodeficient, anemic, and neutropenic and are unable to mobilize a normal response to infections. Viral infections such as herpes zoster are also common. Vaccinations for smallpox and other viral illnesses should be avoided because of the danger of generalized vaccinia or other severe reactions. Hyperreactivity to insect bites is common.

Physical Findings. Physical examination in stage 0 CLL (Rai classification) reveals no abnormalities, but in later stages the lymph nodes, spleen, and liver may become progressively enlarged, and there may also be extensive leukemic infiltration of other tissues, including the skin, orbit, conjunctivae, pharynx, lungs, pleura, heart, and gastrointestinal tract. Obstructive jaundice may occur from periportal infiltration or from nodes compressing the bile duct, and venous compression by enlarged nodes may cause edema and/or thrombophlebitis. Pronounced inanition is common late in the disease, and ascites and/or anasarca may develop in association with severe hypoalbuminemia. Leukostasis may cause priapism or infarctions of various organs. Bleeding manifestations such as bruising and epistaxis are common in advanced stages with severe thrombocytopenia. Leukemic involvement of the meninges is rare, but leukoencephalopathy may occur, probably owing to a viral infection.

LABORATORY ABNORMALITIES. The WBC count may range from a slight elevation to over a million per cubic millimeter. The *percentage of lymphocytes is always increased* and may be over 98 per cent (Color plate 3*F* and *G*). *Anemia, thrombocytopenia*, and *neutropenia* develop in advanced stages owing to impairment of normal hematopoiesis. The anemia is usually normochromic and normocytic, and the reticulocyte count is normal or reduced. Patients also frequently develop shortened red cell and/or platelet survival resulting from hypersplenism in advanced disease. Autoimmune hemolytic anemia, usually caused by warm reacting IgG antibodies, is common and may be accompanied by reticulocytosis, erythroid hyperplasia in the marrow, a positive direct Coombs antiglobulin test, and hyperbilirubinemia. Autoimmune thrombocytopenia or cold hemagglutinin disease may also occur, and occasionally such autoimmune phenomena may precede other clinical manifestations of CLL or develop shortly after beginning treatment.

Hypogammaglobulinemia is present at diagnosis in about half of patients and eventually develops in almost all of them as the disease advances. Any or all classes of immunoglobulins may be reduced. A small percentage of patients have monoclonal immunoglobulins or light chains demonstrable on electrophoresis or immunoelectrophoresis of the blood or urine. Rarely the abnormal proteins may cause hyperviscosity or cryoprecipitation. Angioneurotic edema may also occur rarely owing to formation of immune complexes.

Unlike CML, until recently no characteristic cytogenetic abnormality was described in CLL, and most studies showed normal karyotypes. Because CLL cells proliferate very slowly, in these earlier studies most of the metaphases analyzed were in normal dividing cells present in the specimen. Using B cell mitogens (e.g., pokeweed mitogen, protein A, or Epstein-Barr virus), chromosome abnormalities have been found in about half of patients with CLL. Trisomy 12 is the most common abnormality, being present in about one third of patients; in advanced disease additional chromosomal abnormalities may develop, probably because of clonal evolution. Abnormalities of chromosome 14 are also common, and several cases of CLL have been reported with translocations between chromosomes 11 and 14 t(11;14) (q13; q32). The heavy-chain immunoglobulin gene is located on chromosome 14, and the oncogenes c-ras-Kirsten and c-ras-Harvey, on chromosomes 11 and 12, respectively, but it is not known how these or other genes might be related to the causation of CLL.

Transformation of CLL cells to a more malignant phenotype is much less common than in CML. The most frequently described transformation is to a large-cell diffuse lymphoma (Richter's syndrome), but other types of transformations may also occur to "prolymphocytoid" leukemia, acute lymphoblastic leukemia (blast crisis), and multiple myeloma. The earlier reports are not informative as to whether the transformed cells arose by malignant evolution of the original CLL clone or were separate neoplasms, but both may occur, with malignant evolution probably being more common.

DIAGNOSIS. The diagnosis of CLL depends on the demonstration of a persistent absolute lymphocytosis in the blood and an increased percentage (usually >50 per cent) of small lymphocytes with round nuclei in the marrow. Pertussis and infectious lymphocytosis and other viral infections can sometimes cause striking lymphocytosis, but these illnesses usually occur in children or young adults, are usually accompanied by fever and other acute symptoms, and are of transient duration. Chronic infections such as tuberculosis may be accompanied by lymphocytosis, but this is usually less prominent than in CLL and appropriate workup should lead to the correct diagnosis. If there is any question about the diagnosis, appropriate cell marker studies should be performed to establish the monoclonality of the lymphocytic population and to distinguish CLL from other lymphoproliferative diseases. A schematic representation of normal B cell differentiation and related B cell neoplasms is shown in Figure 155–2.

If the lymph nodes are involved in CLL, the histologic pattern and immunologic markers characteristic of the cells are identical to those of diffuse well-differentiated lymphocytic lymphoma (DWDL), and these two diagnostic entities appear to be merely different variants of the same type of B cell neoplasia. DWDL may initially be localized in lymph nodes without involvement of the blood or marrow, but in more advanced stages it may be indistinguishable from CLL. Other types of disseminated lymphomas such as diffuse poorly differentiated lymphocytic lymphoma (DPDL), which may involve the blood and marrow, can be distinguished from CLL by differences in morphologic appearance of the tumor cells and appropriate cell marker analysis.

Waldenström's macroglobulinemia may be confused with

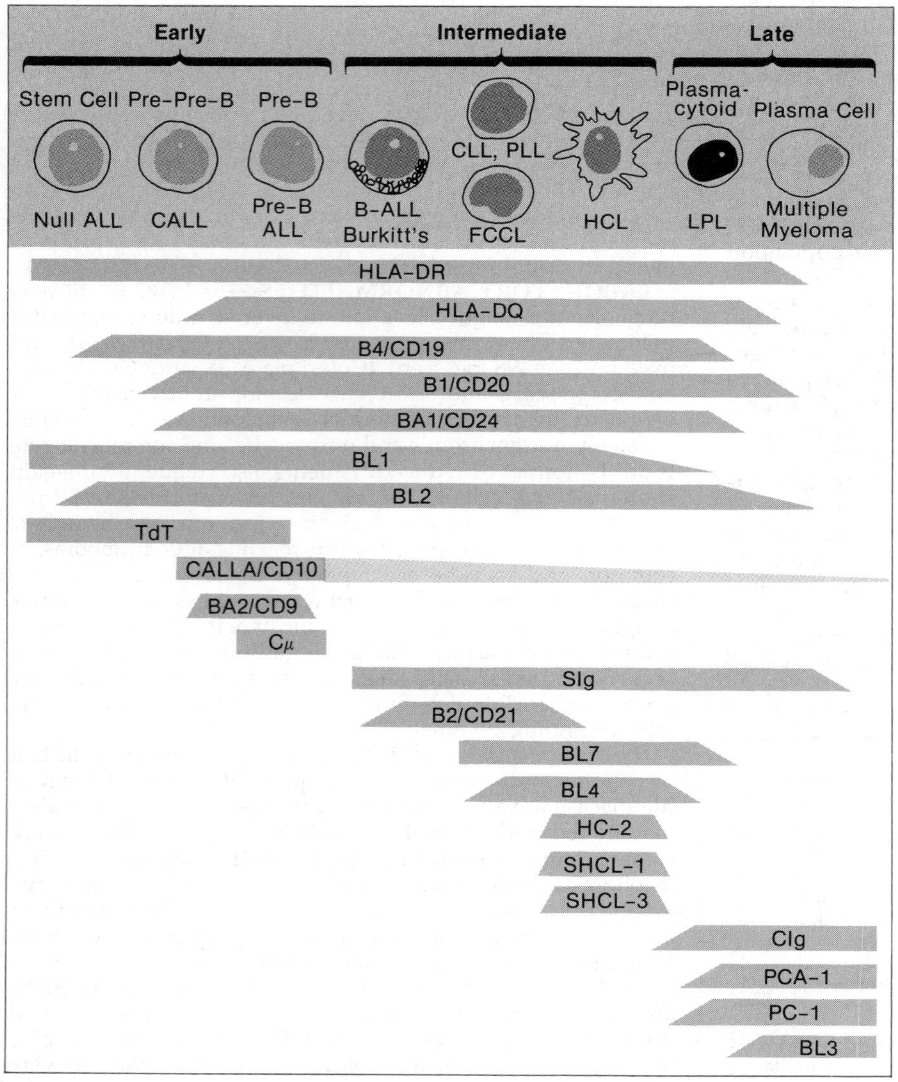

FIGURE 155–2. Schema of B cell differentiation and related B cell lymphoid neoplasms and the ranges of their reactivities with commonly used monoclonal antibodies recognizing B-cell associated antigens. (Prepared by Dr. Benjamin Koziner, Memorial Sloan-Kettering Cancer Center, New York, NY.)

Null ALL = Null acute lymphoblastic leukemia; CALL = common ALL; Pre-B ALL = common ALL with intracytoplasmic immunoglobulin μ heavy chain (Cμ); B-ALL = B cell ALL or Burkitt's lymphoma; CLL = chronic lymphocytic leukemia; PLL = prolymphocytic leukemia; FCCL = follicular center cell lymphoma; HCL = hairy cell leukemia; LPL = lymphoplasmacytoid lymphoma (Waldenström's macroglobulinemia); HLA-DR (Ia) = Dr-related locus of human leukocyte antigens; HLA-DQ = DQ-related locus of human leukocyte antigens; TdT = terminal deoxynucleotidyl transferase; Cμ = intracytoplasmic heavy chain (μ); SIg = surface immunoglobulin; CIg = intracytoplasmic immunoglobulin.

Commonly used monoclonal antibodies recognizing B-cell associated antigens include: anti-B1, B2, B4, CALLA (J-5), PCA-1, and PC-1, available from Coulter Immunology, Hialeah, FL; anti-BA1 and BA2 from Hibertech Inc., San Diego, CA; anti-BL1, BL2, BL3, BL4, and BL7 (Wang CY, et al.: J Immunol 133:684, 1984, and Knowles DM, et al.: Blood 62:191, 1983); anti-HC-2 (Posnett DN, et al.: J Immunol 133:1635, 1984); anti-SHCL-1 (Leu-14) and SHCL-3 (Leu-M5), available from Bectin-Dickinson, Mountain View, CA.

CD refers to antibody/antigen cluster designation defined by the Second International Workshop on Human Leukocyte Differentiation Antigens (Nadler LM: B cell/leukemia panel workshop: Summary and comments. In Reinherz EL, et al. (eds): Leukocyte Typing II. Vol. 2, New York, Springer-Verlag, 1986, p 1).

CLL, but the neoplastic lymphocytes in the former usually have a plasmacytoid appearance, more prominent surface, as well as cytoplasmic immunoglobulin, and they usually do not invade the blood to the same extent as CLL lymphocytes. There is invariably a prominent monoclonal IgM spike in the serum, whereas this is rare in CLL. A few cases may exhibit mixed features of the two entities.

Prolymphocytic leukemia is a rare disease occurring mostly in males in the sixth or seventh decade characterized by prominent splenomegaly, minimal adenopathy, and a poor prognosis. The prolymphocytes differ from CLL lymphocytes in that they are larger and have more cytoplasm, a more prominent nucleolus, and a greater density of surface immunoglobulin, which, again in contrast to CLL cells, exhibits polar migration (capping) after incubation at 37°C.

Hairy cell leukemia is sometimes misdiagnosed as CLL. In the former, the leukocyte count is usually low rather than elevated, and although hairy cells may resemble CLL lymphocytes on Romanowsky-stained smears, close scrutiny will reveal hair-like projections. If there is any doubt, special morphologic and cell marker studies should be performed, as described earlier.

Sézary's syndrome, a cutaneous lymphoma of helper T cell origin closely related to mycosis fungoides, is characterized by a chronic exfoliative erythrodermatitis and circulating atypical lymphocytes with cerebriform nuclei and acid phosphatase activity limited to the cytoplasmic granules instead of the Golgi zone. The prominent skin manifestations and the lesser degree of involvement of the marrow and lymph nodes usually suffice to differentiate Sézary's syndrome from T cell CLL.

Other T cell neoplasms that may be confused with CLL are adult T cell leukemia-lymphoma, T prolymphocytic leukemia, chronic T gamma-lymphoproliferative disease, and T hairy cell leukemia. In contrast to B cell CLL, skin involvement, lytic bone lesions, and hypercalcemia are common in adult T cell leukemia-lymphoma; some patients have been found to be infected with a retrovirus, termed human T cell leukemia-lymphoma virus 1 (HTLV1), which is suspected of causing the disease. The neoplastic cells in T gamma-lymphoproliferative disease are large granular lymphocytes, the WBC count is low with neutropenia, and lymphadenopathy and skin involvement are absent. Appropriate cell marker studies should always be performed to establish the correct diagnosis in CLL and related diseases as it is not always possible to distinguish between the different types on clinical or morphologic grounds.

TREATMENT. Since B cell CLL is a disease mainly affecting older persons, many of whom have a remarkably benign and prolonged course, and since there is no good evidence that early treatment will cure the disease or improve survival, most authorities recommend merely observing asymptomatic patients with early-stage disease until the disease progresses and symptoms develop. Indications for treatment include development of symptomatic or cosmetically disfiguring lymphadenopathy, progressive splenomegaly and/or hepatomegaly, recurrent infections, persistent unexplained fever, weight loss, and development of significant anemia, thrombocytopenia, and/or neutropenia resulting from progressive marrow infiltration, hypersplenism, or autoimmune complications. The rate at which the disease progresses from an early asymptomatic stage to an advanced stage requiring treatment is quite variable, and patients should be observed closely every few months until it can be determined whether their disease is going to remain indolent or become symptomatic. Some patients remain asymptomatic for many years without treatment.

Treatment should be begun when troublesome symptoms develop. *Chlorambucil* (Leukeran) is the most commonly employed drug, but other alkylating agents such as cyclophosphamide are also effective. Because of the slow proliferative rate of the neoplastic cells, antimetabolites are generally less effective, although arabinosyl cytosine has been reported to control the disease in some patients. The usual starting dose of chlorambucil is 6 to 12 mg (0.1 to 0.2 mg per kilogram of body weight) daily for three to six weeks, followed by a maintenance dose of 2 to 6 mg daily, the exact dose depending on the extent of disease, the severity of symptoms, and the patient's weight. The dose should be titrated individually according to the therapeutic response. The drug should be taken at least one hour prior to eating so as not to interfere with its absorption. About 70 per cent of previously untreated patients will show a satisfactory response to chlorambucil with reduction in the WBC count and shrinkage of the enlarged lymph nodes and organomegaly when present. Maintenance treatment is usually continued for six months to a year until a maximal response has been achieved. In some patients the disease may then remain asymptomatic for many months without further treatment, whereas others require continuous treatment for control.

Intermittent administration of chlorambucil has been recommended by some investigators and is probably slightly more effective and convenient than daily therapy. Various dosage schedules have been employed, usually 0.4 to 0.8 mg per kilogram as a single dose every two weeks or 0.4 to 2.0 mg per kilogram once a month. These high intermittent doses sometimes cause gastrointestinal toxicity, which may be partly alleviated by antiemetics. Myelosuppression is the usual dose-limiting toxicity, but immunosuppression, sterility, alveolar dysplasia, pulmonary fibrosis, chromosomal damage, and secondary acute myeloid leukemia may occur following chronic chlorambucil administration.

Corticosteroids are effective in controlling acute symptoms, especially autoimmune complications such as hemolytic anemia or thrombocytopenia. Corticosteroids may also have a pronounced cytolytic effect on the leukemic cells; the WBC count may fall rapidly, or it may rise temporarily concomitantly with regression of the enlarged lymph nodes and spleen. Prednisone is the corticosteroid most commonly prescribed, usually in doses of 10 to 20 mg daily, but larger doses of 50 to 100 mg may be necessary to control hemolytic anemia. Large doses of corticosteroids given over a prolonged period are inadvisable because they may cause severe cushingoid symptoms and increase the risk of infections. Most authorities now recommend that short courses of prednisone in relatively high doses (e.g., 80 mg daily for five days) be given as adjuvant therapy with intermittent chlorambucil, since intermittent steroid therapy produces the desired lymphocytolytic effect and improves the therapeutic response compared to chlorambucil alone while reducing the toxicity associated with continuous steroid administration. Long-term control of autoimmune complications associated with CLL such as hemolytic anemia, thrombocytopenia, or angioneurotic edema is dependent on adequate control of the leukemia. When the leukemic mass has been reduced sufficiently, the autoimmune manifestations usually subside. However, splenectomy is sometimes indicated to control hemolytic anemia, thrombocytopenia, or progressive splenomegaly refractory to drug treatment.

Local radiotherapy is often useful in the treatment of splenomegaly or greatly enlarged lymph nodes resistant to chemotherapy. Whole-body external radiation given cautiously in fractionated doses over several months has been reported to increase the incidence of remissions and prolong survival, and thymic radiation has also been reported to have a good therapeutic effect. However, both thymic and whole-body irradiation have also caused prolonged myelosuppression and fatalities in CLL and must be regarded as experimental forms of treatment that cannot be generally recommended.

Extracorporeal irradiation of the blood has also been shown to be effective in reducing the WBC count and organomegaly, but facilities for this procedure are not available in most centers and leukapheresis is more commonly employed. Leukapheresis is particularly useful in reducing very high lymphocyte counts and organomegaly in advanced disease in the presence of severe thrombocytopenia that limits additional cytotoxic drug therapy. Repeated leukapheresis may reduce the extent of leukemic infiltration of the marrow sufficiently to allow the platelet count to rise and permit resumption of chemotherapy.

In several clinical trials, patients with CLL have been treated more aggressively with various combinations of alkylating agents and other cytotoxic drugs in an attempt to increase the incidence of complete remissions and improve survival. With conventional doses of chlorambucil either alone or with prednisone, complete remissions are rare (0 to 20 per cent in different series), whereas with more intensive treatment higher remission rates have been reported (18 to 45 per cent). The relative effectiveness of the different regimens is difficult to compare, however, because of different patient populations and differing criteria for completeness of remission and durations of observations. Eradication of the leukemic clone has not been possible with any regimen. Patients having remissions live longer than nonresponders, but there is as yet no convincing evidence that overall survival is significantly improved. It is not yet known whether the more intensive regimens will result in a higher incidence of myeloid leukemia or other secondary malignant diseases in CLL.

Hypogammaglobulinemia when present usually persists even after the leukemic mass has been reduced by treatment. Administration of gamma globulin intramuscularly is of little value; clinical trials of various preparations of gamma globulin for intravenous use are currently under way to determine if it is possible to significantly correct the deficiency and reduce the incidence of infections and autoimmune cytopenias. In the rare patient who develops hyperviscosity or circulating autoantibodies, plasmapheresis with replacement by normal plasma is effective in temporarily lowering the abnormal proteins and relieving symptoms. When infections occur, every effort should be made to identify the offending organism and to begin specific antimicrobial treatment promptly.

Various monoclonal antibodies (MoAbs) to the neoplastic cells in B cell or T cell CLL have been investigated to determine their therapeutic efficacy. While some responses have been observed, they have usually been only partial and transient. Additional trials are in progress or planned with new, more specific MoAbs or those coupled with drugs, isotopes, or toxins, cocktails of several MoAbs, and MoAbs in combination with cytotoxic drugs. In contrast to hairy cell leukemia, the clinical trials of alfa-interferon in B cell CLL have shown it to be relatively ineffective, although about half of the patients with cutaneous T cell lymphomas have shown a partial or complete response to this interferon. Investigations of new methods of biologic therapy for CLL are continuing, and it is hoped that these investigations will lead to more selective and effective treatment.

PROGNOSIS. Median survival times of four to five years from diagnosis of CLL have been reported in most series. Since CLL has an extremely variable course, ranging from less than a year to more than 20 years, differences among series are probably due to inclusion of differing proportions of patients with early or advanced disease rather than to differences in treatment. The utility of the proposed clinical staging systems in predicting prognosis was mentioned earlier. There have also been attempts to correlate prognosis with various morphologic, immunologic, or proliferative characteristics of the leukemic cells, but these studies require extension and confirmation before their prognostic value can be accepted. Attempts to eradicate the disease with aggressive treatment have so far been unsuccessful, and there is as yet no convincing evidence that intensive treatment is preferable to more conservative treatment in prolonging overall survival.

Common causes of death in CLL are intercurrent infections, uncontrollable progressive leukemic infiltration of vital organs, extreme inanition, and bleeding. Since CLL occurs mainly in older persons, some patients also die as a result of unrelated diseases. Patients with CLL have a high incidence of second malignant tumors (3 to 34 per cent in different series), both cutaneous and nondermatologic. Many of the tumors were diagnosed prior to treatment of CLL and cannot be causally related to treatment. The incidence of acute myeloid leukemia is higher than expected in CLL following treatment and is probably related to administration of alkylating agents and/or radiation therapy, as has been reported in Hodgkin's disease and other neoplastic diseases.

Binet JL, Auguier A, Dighiero G: A new prognostic classification of chronic lymphocytic leukemia derived from a multivariate survival analysis. Cancer 48:198, 1981. *A report describing the proposed international prognostic staging system for CLL.*

Byhardt RW, Brace KC, Wiernik PH: The role of splenic irradiation in chronic lymphocytic leukemia. Cancer 35:1621, 1975. *A good review of the indications for splenic irradiation in control of CLL.*

Dillman RO, Shawler DL, Dillman JB, et al.: Therapy of chronic lymphocytic leukemia and cutaneous T-cell lymphoma with T101 monoclonal antibody. J Clin Oncol 8:881, 1984. *Report and brief review of investigational trials of monoclonal antibodies in CLL and cutaneous T cell lymphoma.*

Foon KA, Bottino GC, Abrams PG, et al.: Phase II trial of recombinant leukocyte A interferon in patients with advanced chronic lymphocytic leukemia. Am J Med 78:216, 1985. *Report of a phase II trial of recombinant alfa-interferon in CLL that demonstrated significant dose-dependent toxicity and only a few partial therapeutic responses. It was concluded that alfa-interferon is ineffective, at least in previously treated patients with advanced CLL.*

Foon KA, Todd RF: Immunologic classification of leukemia and lymphoma. Blood 68:1, 1986. *A comprehensive review of advances in the classification of leukemias and lymphomas, using batteries of monoclonal antibodies to define surface antigens, molecular probes to identify immunoglobulin and T cell receptor genes, cytochemical stains, and various other biochemical markers.*

Gale RP, Foon KA: Chronic lymphocytic leukemia. Recent advances in biology and treatment (review). Ann Intern Med 103:101, 1985. *Comprehensive, up-to-date review of developments in investigations of the biology and immunologic defects in CLL and also a good review of the differential diagnosis and conventional and investigational forms of treatment.*

Han T, Ozer H, Sadamore N, et al.: Prognostic importance of cytogenetic abnormalities in patients with chronic lymphocytic leukemia. N Engl J Med 310:288, 1984. *A good review of the cytogenetic abnormalities found in CLL with discussion of their clinical and immunologic significance.*

Juliusson G, Robert H-H, Ost A, et al.: Prognostic information from cytogenetic analysis in chronic B-lymphocytic leukemia and leukemic immunocytoma. Blood 65:134, 1985. *Another review of the cytogenetic abnormalities occurring in CLL with discussion of their prognostic importance.*

HAIRY CELL LEUKEMIA (Leukemic Reticuloendotheliosis)

DEFINITION. Hairy cell leukemia (HCL) is a chronic form of leukemia usually due to clonal proliferation of an unusual type of B lymphocyte. HCL accounts for approximately 2 per cent of all the leukemias. The etiology is unknown.

PATHOGENESIS AND MECHANISMS. Hairy cells are of B cell origin, as they have immunoglobulin gene rearrangements and are capable of monoclonal synthesis of immunoglobulin. Although their level of maturity within the B cell lineage varies, in most patients the neoplastic hairy cells appear to be preplasma cells. A few cases of T cell hairy cell leukemia have been reported.

The hairy cell appears on Wright-Giemsa–stained smears as an intermediate-sized or large lymphocyte (10 to 18 μ in diameter), with fine cytoplasmic projections that give the cell its name. The nucleus may be round, oval, horseshoe shaped, or slightly folded, and it is often eccentrically located. The chromatin can be evenly distributed, moderately coarse, or stippled, and one or more small nucleoli may be present. The cells usually have moderate amounts of pale blue-gray cytoplasm with irregular serrated edges and sometimes pseudopodial extensions (Color plate 3*H*). The cytoplasmic surface projections are best recognized under the phase-contrast microscope or the scanning electron microscope (Fig. 155–3). The latter reveals a characteristic surface pattern with prominent folds or ruffles that are similar to those present on monocytes but more conspicuous.

Cytochemical reactions are helpful in identifying hairy cells,

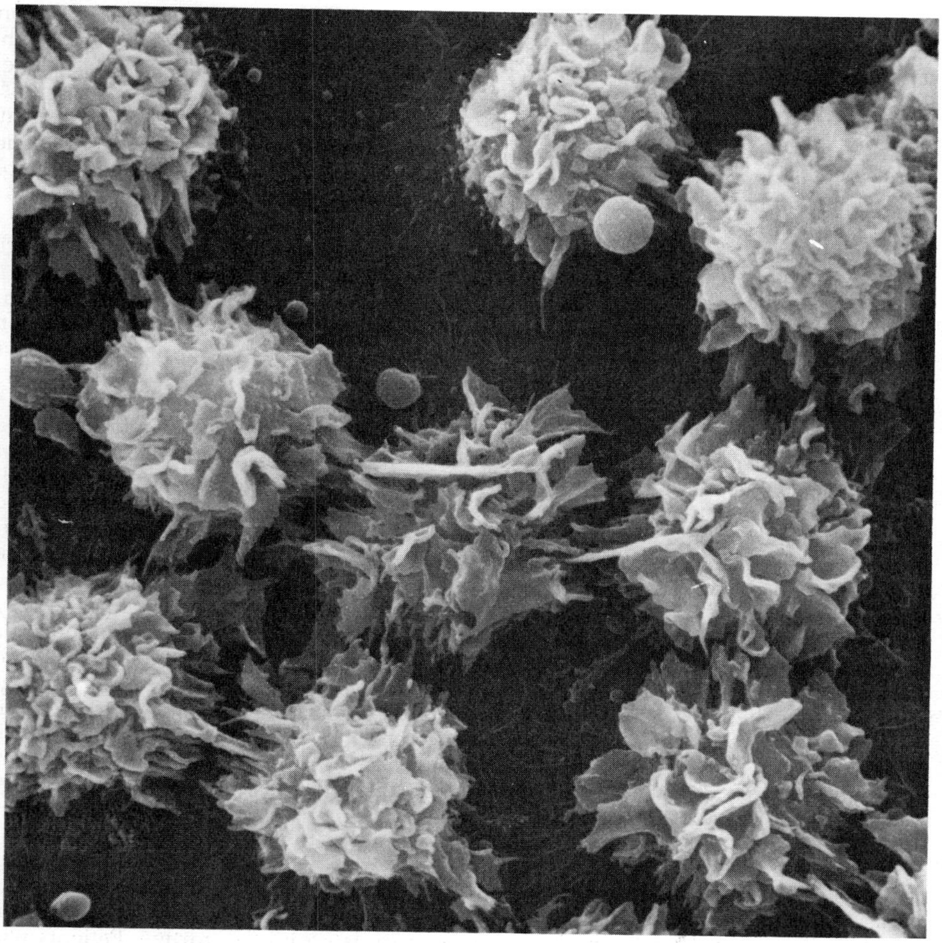

FIGURE 155–3. Hairy cells from the bone marrow as seen in the scanning electron microscope showing characteristic prominent surface ruffles. Magnification × 8750. (Courtesy of Dr. Etienne deHarven and Nina Lampen.)

but show variability in different cases and within the cells of any one population. Hairy cells are almost always positive for *acid phosphatase,* which is commonly, but not invariably, completely or partially resistant to addition of tartaric acid. However, a negative reaction does not exclude the diagnosis of HCL, and a positive reaction is not necessarily diagnostic. Hairy cells in the great majority of patients show varying degrees of positivity for alpha naphthyl acetate or butyrate esterase, and this reaction is usually completely inhibited by sodium fluoride. Cytochemical reactions associated with the granulocytic differentiation pathway (e.g., myeloperoxidase) are invariably negative in hairy cells. Lysozyme activity is absent in hairy cells, which helps to distinguish them from normal or leukemic monocytes.

Surface immunoglobulin (Ig) is present on hairy cells in the great majority of cases. The Ig is usually monoclonal, although in a few cases two different immunoglobulins have been reported. Hairy cells generally lack receptors for the third component of complement (C3), thus providing a helpful diagnostic distinction from monocytes and CLL cells, which carry the C3 receptor. Hairy cells may also frequently exhibit properties characteristic of monocytes (phagocytosis) and T lymphocytes (Tac antigen or interleukin-2 receptor). Several monoclonal antibodies with specificity for hairy cells are now available for confirmation of the diagnosis in difficult cases (see Fig. 155–2).

Hairy cells usually have very low proliferative activity; the percentage of hairy cells in the marrow or blood in DNA synthesis is almost invariably less than 1 per cent. Hairy cells also usually respond poorly in vitro to stimulation with mitogens. Chromosome abnormalities have been difficult to demonstrate because of the low incidence of mitoses, but trisomy of chromosome 12 (similar to CLL) has been reported in a few cases of HCL, as have abnormalities of the Y chromosome and of chromosomes 3, 6, and especially 14.

CLINICAL MANIFESTATIONS AND DIAGNOSIS. HCL occurs almost exclusively in adults and the median age at diagnosis is about 50 years. Males are affected about four times more frequently than females. Clinical manifestations are usually attributable to hairy cell infiltration of the bone marrow, which can cause suppression of normal hematopoiesis, and of the red pulp of the spleen, which can result in hypersplenism. The onset is usually insidious, and the most common symptoms are weakness caused by *anemia,* development of infections as a result of *neutropenia,* and pain or discomfort in the left hypochondrium owing to *progressive splenic enlargement.*

The liver is enlarged owing to hairy cell infiltration in about 40 per cent of cases, but prominent involvement of the lymph nodes is infrequent. Systemic vasculitis and lytic bone lesions associated with pain and sometimes pathologic fractures may occur. Infiltration of the skin or lungs occurs only rarely, and meningeal involvement is almost never seen.

The majority of patients have *pancytopenia,* but sometimes only one or two of the myeloid cell lines are depressed, most commonly the platelets and neutrophils. Monocytopenia is also frequent and may contribute to the increased susceptibility to infections. In most cases, hairy cells can be identified in smears of the blood or buffy coat, but in some patients they are very rare in the blood. Occasional patients have leukocytosis with numerous circulating hairy cells instead of leukopenia. The bone marrow is always diffusely infiltrated by hairy cells, but it may be difficult to aspirate the marrow in about half of the patients (i.e., "dry tap"). If the diagnosis of HCL is suspected but hairy cells cannot be demonstrated in the blood and bone marrow aspiration is unsuccessful, a marrow biopsy should be performed and imprint preparations made of the freshly obtained biopsy specimen so that the appropriate confirmatory cytologic and cytochemical tests can be done. Reticulin fibers are often increased in the marrow as well as in the spleen, and the marrow may also contain increased numbers of plasma cells. If a splenectomy is performed, experienced pathologists can usually make a definitive diagnosis because involvement of the red pulp by hairy cells and the presence of pseudosinuses are uniquely characteristic of HCL. Sections of liver biopsies show hairy cell infiltration largely confined to the portal areas without destruction of parenchymal hepatic cells. Liver function tests are often normal; the most common abnormality is an elevated serum alkaline phosphatase level that is related to the degree of periportal infiltration.

Other disease entities with which HCL may be confused are CLL, Waldenström's macroglobulinemia, some of the diffuse varieties of non-Hodgkin's lymphomas, histiocytic medullary reticulosis, and monocytic leukemia. The leukocyte count in HCL is usually low instead of elevated as in CLL. The serum immunoglobulins are usually normal or show a polyclonal increase in HCL in contrast to CLL, in which they are often depressed, or to Waldenström's macroglobulinemia, in which there is a monoclonal IgM spike. Histiocytic medullary reticulosis (HMR, malignant histiocytosis, histiocytic leukemia) is a rare, rapidly progressive fatal disease characterized by fever, wasting, jaundice, generalized lymphadenopathy, and hepatosplenomegaly. The involved organs are infiltrated with abnormal histiocytes that commonly show intense erythrophagocytosis, a functional characteristic rarely exhibited by hairy cells. Acute or chronic monocytic leukemia can also be confused with HCL, but the serum or urinary lysozyme levels in HCL are normal or low in contrast to the high levels found in monocytic leukemia.

Although the aforementioned clinical and laboratory features are useful in distinguishing HCL from other disease entities, the essential requirement for the diagnosis is positive identification of the characteristic hairy cells. Their unique features can readily be demonstrated by appropriate morphologic, cytochemical, and immunologic tests, as described under Pathogenesis. Although occasional cells closely resembling or identical to hairy cells have been observed in some varieties of non-Hodgkin's lymphomas, in none of these conditions or in any of the other lymphoproliferative or histiocytic-monocytic neoplasias mentioned earlier is the marrow diffusely infiltrated by characteristic hairy cells.

The diagnosis of HCL is not suspected prior to performing a splenectomy for some ill-defined condition such as "chronic anemia," "primary splenic lymphoma," or "myeloid metaplasia." However, experienced hematopathologists can usually readily diagnose HCL on examination of histologic sections of the spleen and distinguish this entity from lymphomas and other conditions causing splenic enlargement.

PROGNOSIS AND TREATMENT. HCL generally has a chronic course, with a median survival of three to five years and with some patients surviving many years. Rarely the disease is rapidly progressive and may be accompanied by massive infiltration of the skin and multiple internal organs, leading to death within a year. However, early death is most commonly due to infection as a consequence of neutropenia. A large variety of bacteria, fungi, viruses, and mycobacteria have been reported to cause terminal infections.

Patients who are relatively asymptomatic at the time of diagnosis should merely be observed, since the disease may progress very slowly and not require treatment for long periods.

Splenectomy. If there is progressive worsening of the anemia, thrombocytopenia, or neutropenia, splenectomy should be considered, as this has proved to be beneficial in about two thirds of cases and to improve survival in patients who respond favorably. A good response to splenectomy with improvement in one or more of the blood elements is not well correlated with spleen size, but patients with only patchy marrow involvement are more likely to have a favorable response than those whose marrows are densely infiltrated with hairy cells. Improvements in surgical techniques and in prevention of serious infections have greatly reduced the complications of splenectomy in recent years. The majority of patients with HCL will have some hematologic improvement after splenectomy, but the degree and duration of improvement are quite variable. In most cases the improvement will be noted within a few weeks after the operation. About 40 per cent of patients have no response or only a partial response, and in the latter relapse usually occurs within a few months. Forty to 60 per cent of patients in different series have a significant rise in the blood cell counts following splenectomy, with an average duration of response of over a year and with some patients remaining well for several years.

Chemotherapy and Biologic Therapy. Patients in whom the disease progressed after splenectomy heretofore presented a difficult therapeutic problem, but during the last several years two new therapeutic agents, alfa-interferon and pentostatin (2′-deoxycoformycin), have been shown to be highly effective forms of treatment.

In the past, many chemotherapeutic agents have been tried, but most were found to have limited usefulness or even to be deleterious. Glucocorticoids, alkylating agents in low doses, and androgens were employed most frequently. Glucocorticoids sometimes resulted in hematologic improvement and reduction in the size of the spleen, but even in patients who responded, the effect was usually short lived, and glucocorticoids significantly increased the risk of infection, especially fungal infections.

Antimetabolites and other cytotoxic drugs that affect only actively proliferating cells are ineffective and may be harmful in HCL, because the slowly proliferating hairy cells are less sensitive than the residual normal hematopoietic cells to such drugs. Patients with progressive disease who fail to respond to splenectomy or in whom relapse later occurs frequently benefit from treatment with low doses of alkylating agents (e.g., chlorambucil or cyclophosphamide) with a decrease in hairy cell infiltration of the marrow and improvement in the platelet and erythrocyte counts; however, the monocytopenia and granulocytopenia usually persist or may be worsened. Since alkylating agents may cause further myelosuppression, such therapy should be limited to patients whose disease is clearly progressing following splenectomy. Some cases that fail to respond to chlorambucil or that have relapsed show significant hematologic improvement with androgens (e.g., Halotestin* 10 mg three times a day or oxymetholone* 150 mg four times a day), and sometimes the responses are prolonged. However, it is not yet clear what proportion of patients can be expected to have a significant response to androgens, and further trials are indicated. Patients with leukocytosis and large numbers of circulating hairy cells may benefit from intensive leukapheresis, but no significant improvement can be expected in the majority of patients who are leukopenic. A few patients with refractory disease and severe neutropenia and thrombocytopenia secondary to bone marrow replacement by hairy cells have had durable remissions following intensive chemotherapy. However, such aggressive therapy is extremely hazardous and requires intensive supportive treatment, including repeated granulocyte and platelet transfusions during the period of prolonged marrow aplasia; it cannot be recommended except as experimental treatment of patients refractory to conventional treatment in centers specially equipped to provide adequate supportive therapy.

Alfa-interferon is highly effective in the treatment of HCL. The majority of patients show a beneficial response to either

*This use is not listed in the manufacturer's directive.

natural or biosynthetic (recombinant) alfa-interferons. The responses are often observed within a month after beginning treatment and may lead to a substantial reduction in hairy cell infiltration of the marrow and normalization of hematopoiesis, including recovery of the monocyte and granulocyte counts, which does not usually occur during treatment with low-dose chlorambucil. Complete remissions with disappearance of all hairy cells from the marrow almost never occur, and there is no evidence that alfa-interferon is curative.

The doses of alfa-interferon have varied in the different clinical trials, but relatively low doses were found to be effective (i.e., 2 million U per square meter of body surface area three times weekly by self-administered subcutaneous injection). Some toxicity was observed in most patients, including fever, fatigue, myalgias, dryness of mucous membranes, myelosuppression, liver function abnormalities, paresthesias, and alopecia, but toxic effects were usually considered acceptable when weighed against the favorable hematologic responses.

Alfa-interferon is already generally considered the treatment of choice in patients with progressive disease after splenectomy, and it is currently being evaluated as first-line treatment, especially in patients whose marrow is densely infiltrated with hairy cells and in whom splectomy is relatively ineffective.

Pentostatin (2′-deoxycoformycin) is also effective in HCL. This drug was originally used clinically in relatively high doses for treatment of T cell neoplasias and various other tumors, but it was largely abandoned because of severe toxicity and the relative lack of antitumor effect. Given in low doses, however, deoxycoformycin is very effective in treating HCL. Some patients have even had complete remission with complete clearing of hairy cells from the marrow. Deoxycoformycin is still considered an investigational agent, and the optimal dosage schedule and response and toxicity patterns are currently being determined in multi-institutional clinical trials.

Bouroncle BA: Leukemic reticuloendotheliosis (hairy cell leukemia). Blood 53:412, 1979. *A review of the manifestations of hairy cell leukemia by the physician who first recognized this disease as a clinical entity.*

Cheson BD, Martin A: Clinical trials in hairy cell leukemia. Ann Intern Med 106:871, 1987. *An excellent review of current therapy for hairy cell leukemia. 71 references.*

Golomb HM: Hairy cell leukemia: Lessons learned in 25 years. J Clin Oncol 1:652, 1983. *Good review of the clinical features, therapeutic options, and biology of HCL with list of pertinent references.*

Jacobs AD, Champlin RE, Golde DW: Recombinant α-2-interferon for hairy cell leukemia. Blood 65:1017, 1985. *The results of a clinical trial of recombinant alfa-interferon are reported that confirm the beneficial therapeutic effects of this agent in HCL as originally reported by Quesada, et al. (see reference below).*

Jansen J, LeBien TW, Kersey JH: The phenotype of the neoplastic cells of hairy cell leukemia studied with monoclonal antibodies. Blood 59:609, 1982. *Eighteen cases of hairy cell leukemia were studied with a battery of polyclonal anti-Ig and monoclonal antibodies. The results support the B cell origin of HCL and suggest that the maturation arrest in HCL is at a more mature stage than in CLL.*

Spiers ASD, Moore D, Cassileth PA, et al.: Remissions in hairy-cell leukemia with pentostatin (2′-deoxycoformycin). N Engl J Med 316:825, 1987.

Westbrook CA, Golde DW: Clinical problems in hairy cell leukemia: Diagnosis and management. Semin Oncol 11 (4 Suppl. 2):514, 1984. *A good general review of the clinical aspects of HCL.*

156 THE ACUTE LEUKEMIAS

Howard J. Weinstein

DEFINITION. The acute leukemias are primary malignant diseases of the blood-forming organs characterized by a predominance of immature myeloid or lymphoid precursors (blasts). The blasts progressively replace normal bone marrow, migrate, and invade other tissues. There is diminished production of normal erythrocytes, granulocytes, and platelets in acute leukemia, and this leads to the most important complications of this disease—anemia, infection, and hemorrhage.

The acute leukemias are classified morphologically by reference to the predominant cell line involved as lymphoblastic (ALL) and myelogenous (AML) forms. If untreated, both forms are universally fatal within a period of months to one year. Therapy has markedly altered prognosis, and many patients with acute leukemia remain free of disease for prolonged periods.

ETIOLOGY. The mechanism of leukemogenesis in humans is unknown, but inciting agents are well established.

Ionizing Radiation. Physicians and scientists exposed to excessive amounts of radiation during the early years of research on medical application of x-rays, patients given low-dose radiation for rheumatoid spondylitis, and persons exposed acutely to radiation during the nuclear attacks on Hiroshima and Nagasaki in 1945 have all been found to have an increased incidence of leukemia. This increase involved chronic myelocytic leukemia (CML), ALL, and AML in survivors of the atomic bombings and has been dose related. The first cases of leukemia were noted two years after irradiation. A peak was reached after five to seven years and diminished to baseline levels by about 1970. Studies of the effects of diagnostic x-ray exposure, including fetal exposure, have not consistently shown an increased incidence of leukemia.

Oncogenic Viruses (see also Ch. 169). Horizontally transmissible RNA viruses (retroviruses) are clearly capable of inducing acute leukemia in mice, domestic cats, cattle, chickens, and gibbon apes. Unequivocal evidence for either an endogenous or a horizontally transmitted human leukemia virus is still lacking. A naturally occurring human type C retrovirus, human T cell leukemia virus (HTLV1), has recently been isolated from malignant lymphocytes of adults with a rare T cell leukemia-lymphoma. HTLV-associated leukemia is prevalent in certain geographic regions such as Southwestern Japan, the Caribbean, and areas of South America. In areas where clustering of adult T cell leukemia-lymphoma occurs, most patients and 10 per cent of healthy individuals have natural antibodies to HTLV, suggesting that HTLV is a common infection. The molecular mechanism of neoplastic transformation of human T cells by HTLV is currently not known.

Genetic and Congenital Factors. The strongest evidence for a genetic predisposition to acute leukemia is the occurrence of this disease in identical twins. If one of a set of identical twins develops leukemia before six years of age, the risk of disease in the other twin is 20 per cent. Leukemia usually develops in a co-twin within months of the first case. Concordant leukemia in monozygotic infant twins may reflect a common prezygotic determinant, shared intrauterine insult, or blood-borne metastases from one twin to the other. For fraternal twins and siblings the risk of developing leukemia is between twofold and fourfold higher than for children in the general population.

Congenital conditions associated with chromosomal instability and a predisposition to acute leukemia include three autosomal recessive disorders: Bloom's syndrome, Fanconi's anemia, and ataxia-telangiectasia. Ataxia-telangiectasia is commonly accompanied by rearrangement of the long arm of chromosome 14 and is one of the inborn immunodeficiency syndromes that predispose to lymphoreticular neoplasms, including acute lymphoblastic leukemia.

Down's syndrome (trisomy 21) is associated with a 10- to 20-fold increased risk of leukemia during the first decade of life. The cell types of leukemia follow the usual distribution, but the age peak is nearly three years earlier than expected. Newborns with Down's syndrome may show a transient proliferation of blast cells (usually myeloblasts) that is often clinically and hematologically indistinguishable from congenital leukemia. In contrast to congenital leukemia, complete permanent recovery occurs within weeks to months without specific antileukemia therapy.

Chemical Agents. Many chemicals have been associated with leukemia. Benzene exposure increases the risk of AML, with bone marrow hypoplasia and/or pancytopenia often preceding the diagnosis of leukemia. Less convincing reports have implicated chloramphenicol and phenylbutazone as leukemogenic agents.

An increased risk for AML and myelodysplastic syndromes has been documented in patients treated with alkylating agents for neoplastic and non-neoplastic diseases. The ten-year cumulative risk ranges from 2 to 10 per cent and has been related to cumulative dose and type of alkylating agent. Many of these secondary leukemias have developed in the absence of radiation or underlying diseases that produce immunologic deficiency.

INCIDENCE. The leukemias account for approximately 3 per cent of all cancer in the United States. The overall frequency of leukemia, as reflected in mortality statistics, increased steadily in developed countries over the first half of the twentieth century and has remained stable during the past three decades. It is believed that this pattern reflected improving ability to diagnose leukemia and increasing accuracy of death records.

The age-adjusted incidence of leukemia is about 8 to 10 per 100,000 persons per year. Acute leukemia accounts for nearly half of all leukemias. The peak incidence of ALL occurs between the ages of two and four years, whereas the incidence of AML progressively increases with advancing age. The ratio of ALL to AML is 4:1 in persons under the age of 15, but this ratio is reversed in adults. Acute leukemia is more common in males than in females and in whites than in blacks.

PATHOPHYSIOLOGY. The molecular basis of leukemic transformation in man is unknown. The fundamental defect in acute leukemia appears to be unregulated proliferation of early precursor cells that have lost their capacity to differentiate in response to normal hormonal signals and cellular interactions. Previously the accumulation of the leukemic cell population was attributed only to rapid and uncontrolled proliferation.

A leukemic transformation may arise at any point during the differentiation of the hematopoietic pluripotential stem cell. Chromosome and glucose-6-phosphate dehydrogenase isozyme studies show that both ALL and AML are of unicellular (clonal) origin (see Ch. 152) and that the cellular level of origin of AML is heterogeneous. In some patients with AML the leukemia is expressed in the erythrocytic and granulocytic pathways, suggesting involvement of the CFU-S (myeloid stem cell). In other patients, the leukemia is expressed in cells restricted to granulocytic and macrophage lineage, suggesting involvement of CFU-GM (committed granulocyte-macrophage progenitor). Acute lymphoblastic leukemia is superimposed on normal hematopoietic cells that are products of normal CFU-S because committed myeloid progenitors in ALL do not contain chromosomal markers that are found in the leukemic lymphoblasts.

In acute leukemia, both normal and malignant cells coexist and compete for ascendancy within the bone marrow. Antileukemic therapy destroys the leukemic clone and allows for return of normal hematopoiesis. This is in contrast to chronic myelogeneous leukemia, in which few normal myeloid stem cells are detectable at any time during the course of the disease.

Certain in vitro investigations and clinical studies provide some evidence that acute leukemia, although clonal, can be influenced by extracellular leukemogenic factors or deficiencies of differentiation factors. Acute leukemia has appeared in the engrafted cells of several leukemic patients who received marrow transplants from histocompatible siblings, for example, suggesting that leukemogenesis may result from unidentified factors that persist in certain susceptible hosts.

CLASSIFICATION. The acute leukemias are extraordinarily heterogeneous, reflecting the complexities of hematopoietic differentiation. The various types of acute leukemia are characterized by multiple methods that include morphology, histochemistry, cell surface and cytoplasmic markers, and cytogenetic and molecular genetic changes.

Morphology and Histochemistry. Blast cells are immature precursors, lacking many of the features for differentiating a lymphoid from a myeloid origin. The capacity to distinguish these blasts is of marked therapeutic and prognostic importance; various cytologic criteria have been established to differentiate between them.

Using the French-American-British (FAB) international morphologic classification, ALL has been divided into subgroups L1 to L3 and AML into subgroups M1 to M7. In L1 the lymphoblasts treated with Wright's stain are small and uniform in size, have smooth, homogeneous nuclear chromatin with indistinct nucleoli, and only a small rim of pale blue staining cytoplasm. L2 blasts are larger and nonuniform in size, have more prominent nucleoli, and a variable amount of cytoplasm. L3 blasts have deeply basophilic, vacuolated cytoplasm and are indistinguishable from Burkitt's lymphoma cells. The majority of L1 and L2 types of lymphoblasts are reactive with periodic acid–Schiff (PAS), and nonreactive with myeloperoxidase. The vacuoles in the L3 blasts are PAS negative, but stain positively for neutral fat (oil red O).

A summary of the AML subtypes and their histochemical reactivity is listed in Table 156–1. Auer rods, which are azurophilic granular cytoplasmic inclusion bodies, are thought to be pathognomonic of AML and are most commonly seen in the M2 and M3 subtypes. Acute leukemias derived from eosinophilic and basophilic precursors, although uncommon, display unique characteristics as well as many features in common with other AML's. Acute megakaryocytic leukemia represents the M7 subtype of AML.

Surface Markers. Four broad subclasses of ALL are defined by leukemic cell surface markers and have prognostic and therapeutic significance. This classification of ALL and the approximate percentage of patients in each subclass is shown in Table 156–2.

The common ALL antigen, or CALLA, is a glycosylated polypeptide that is expressed on the cell surface in approximately 60 and 50 per cent of cases of childhood and adult ALL, respectively. CALLA is also detected in some of the non-Hodgkin's lymphomas, in one third of cases of blast crisis of Ph^1 chromosome–positive CML, on a small percentage of normal bone marrow cells, and on some nonhematopoietic tissues. The early precursor B ALL blasts have undergone immunoglobulin gene rearrangements, indicating a commitment to B cell differentiation.

Patients with T cell ALL have a characteristic clinical presentation—that is, adolescent males with a high white blood cell count and a mediastinal mass. The T lymphoblasts from these patients display markers that characterize their phenotype as early, mid, or late thymocyte.

Blast cells from patients with AML react with many monoclonal antibodies that define antigens at various stages of erythroid, granulocytic, monocytic, and megakaryocytic differentiation. Myeloid leukemic blasts in most instances have Ia antigens, but lack T cell, B cell, and CALLA antigens. A small percentage of cases of ALL and AML express lineage nonspecific markers (e.g., rearranged immunoglobulin genes in a myeloblast) and are referred to as mixed lineage leukemias. It is not clear if these mixed phenotypes represent aberrant differentiation or transformation of an early bipotent stem cell.

Cytoplasmic Markers. At least five cytoplasmic marker enzymes have been used in the classification of acute leukemias: terminal deoxynucleotidyl transferase, hexosaminidase, *N*-alkaline phosphatase, 5′-nucleotidase, and adenosine deaminase. T lymphoblasts have diminished 5′-nucleotidase and

TABLE 156–1. FAB CLASSIFICATION OF ACUTE MYELOGENOUS LEUKEMIA

FAB Class	Common Name	Morphology	Histochemistry	Unique Clinical or Laboratory Features
M1	Acute myelocytic leukemia without differentiation	Myeloblasts predominate; distinct nucleoli; few granules	MP+	−7/del 7q, +8
M2	Acute myelocytic leukemia with differentiation	Myeloblasts and promyelocytes predominate; further maturation abnormal	MP+	Myeloblastomas, t(8;21)
M3	Acute promyelocytic leukemia	Promyelocytes predominate; hypergranular; may have reniform or bilobed nuclei with small granules	MP+	DIC, t(15;17)
M4	Acute myelomonocytic leukemia	Myelocytic and monocytic maturation evident; peripheral monocytosis	MP+ NSE+	inv 16, +8, eosinophilia, extramedullary leukemia (skin, gums, CNS)
M5	Acute monocytic leukemia with differentiation	Promonocytes or undifferentiated blasts, cerebriform nuclei, cytoplasmic pseudopods	NSE+	t (——,11), infants, extramedullary leukemia
M6	Erythroleukemia	Bizarre, multinucleated, megaloblastoid erythroblasts predominate; myeloblasts also present	MP+ (myeloblast), PAS+ (erythroblasts)	Complex chromosomal abnormalities
M7	Megakaryocytic leukemia	Pleomorphic, undifferentiated, cytoplasmic blebs	Platelet peroxidase by electron microscopy	Myelofibrosis or increased bone marrow reticulin

FAB = French-American-British classification; MP = myeloperoxidase; NSE = nonspecific esterase; PAS = periodic acid–schiff; t = translocation; S = deletion (loss of entire chromosome or part of the long arm); DIC = disseminated intravascular coagulation; inv = inversion; t (——,11) = translocations with band 11q23 and one of several reciprocating chromosomes (6, 9, 10, 17, 19); t = trisomy.

increased adenosine deaminase activity as useful distinguishing characteristics. For example, deoxycoformycin, an inhibitor of adenosine deaminase, has induced remission in T cell ALL. Terminal deoxynucleotidyl transferase activity provides excellent diagnostic differentiation between ALL and AML, as it is present in 95 per cent of cases of ALL and is mostly absent in AML. It has also correctly defined the lymphoblastic crisis in CML and predicted the efficacy of ALL therapy in its management.

Chromosomal Changes. A detectable nonrandom chromosomal change is usually present in the leukemic cells in over 80 per cent of patients with ALL and AML. A normal karyotype appears with remission, and the original chromosome aberration reappears at the time of relapse. Moreover, specific chromosomal abnormalities correlate with particular FAB subtypes of AML (Table 156–2). Loss of chromosomes 5 or 7 or trisomy 8 has been most consistently observed in patients with myelodysplastic syndromes (preleukemia) or secondary AML (previous history of radiation, cytotoxic drugs, or exposure to strong mutagenic agents).

In ALL the modal chromosome numbers appear to be much higher than in AML. Consistent chromosome translocations have been correlated with various immunophenotypes of ALL (e.g., t(11;14) with T cell, t(8;14) with B cell, and t(1;19) with pre-B cell). An interesting subgroup of patients with ALL include those with a Ph^1 chromosome. It is unclear if Ph^1-positive ALL represents the lymphoblastic crisis of chronic myelogenous leukemia or a different leukemia.

TABLE 156–2. IMMUNOLOGIC CLASSIFICATION OF ACUTE LYMPHOBLASTIC LEUKEMIA

	Early Precursor B	Pre-B	B	T	Unc
Frequency (per cent)	15	60	<5	15	5
Immune phenotype					
Ia	+	+	+	–	–
B4	+	+	+	–	–
CALLA	–	most	rare	rare	–
cIg	–	20–30%	–	–	–
sIg	–	–	+	–	–
Sheep RBC rosettes	–	–	–	most	–
Thymocyte antigens	–	–	–	+	–

Ia = Class II histocompatibility antigen; B4 = early B cell antigen; CALLA = common acute lymphoblastic leukemia antigen; cIg = cytoplasmic immunoglobulin (u heavy chain); sIg = surface immunoglobulin; Sheep RBC rosettes = receptor on T lymphocytes that spontaneously binds sheep erythrocytes; Thymocyte antigens = early to late thymocyte antigens recognized by a series of anti-T monoclonal antibodies; Unc = unclassified.

The mechanism by which cells carrying chromosomal abnormalities gain selective advantage is beginning to be understood. The chromosome position of several cellular oncogenes is now known. The cellular oncogenes are homologous to recognized transforming genes of the acute retroviruses. Little is known about their function in the human genome, but they may be in part responsible for control of cellular proliferation and differentiation. These cellular oncogenes may be perturbed or activated by several mechanisms, including chromosome rearrangement, alteration in gene dosage (gain or loss of a chromosome), or small mutations. Activation or altered expression of cellular oncogenes may turn out to be one of several key steps in neoplastic transformation (see Ch. 169 for a more detailed discussion).

CLINICAL MANIFESTATIONS. The signs and symptoms of acute leukemia relate to decreased numbers of normal hematopoietic cells and invasion of other organs by leukemic cells. Why normal hematopoiesis is suppressed in leukemia is not known. It may result in part from the release of suppressor substances by leukemic blasts.

Anemia. Asthenia, pallor, headache, tinnitus, dyspnea, angina, edema, and congestive heart failure may all indicate anemia. The anemia generally results from decreased erythropoiesis and blood loss. Evidence of specific antibody-mediated hemolysis is uncommon.

Hemorrhage. Hemorrhagic manifestations in newly diagnosed acute leukemia are usually caused by thrombocytopenia. Oozing gums, epistaxis, petechiae, ecchymoses, menorrhagia, melena, and excessive bleeding after tooth extraction are common initial manifestations. Retinal hemorrhages and subarachnoid bleeding are rare. Most thrombocytopenic bleeding occurs when the platelet count is less than 20,000 per microliter.

Intracranial hemorrhages may result from leukostasis, i.e., intravascular clumping of blasts, especially within small vessels of the brain, leading to infarction and hemorrhage. Leukostasis occurs most frequently in acute myelogenous leukemia when the peripheral leukocyte count is in excess of 150,000 per microliter.

In acute promyelocytic leukemia, the abnormal granules in the blast appear to contain tissue thromboplastin activity or fibrinolysins that initiate disseminated intravascular coagulation or fibrinolysis. Massive hemorrhage can occur in this setting (see Ch. 167).

Infection. Most early infections in acute leukemia are presumably bacterial, but specific etiologic agents are often not found. Leukemia may first be recognized by the occurrence of an infection (respiratory, dental, sinus, perirectal abscess, urinary tract, and skin) that never fully clears. These early infections appear to be attributable to granulocytopenia, with the risk of infection being greatest when the absolute granulocyte count is less than 200 cells per microliter. Repeated search for an infectious source of fever is required in all patients, because "leukemic fever" is extremely rare.

Leukemic Infiltration. Although leukemia is primarily a disease of bone marrow and peripheral blood, other tissues may also become infiltrated by the blast cells. The organs most commonly showing initial clinical involvement are the liver, spleen, and superficial lymph nodes. Bone pain is one of the initial symptoms in 25 per cent of patients with acute leukemia, and children with ALL may present with migratory joint pain accompanied by swelling and tenderness that may be confused with juvenile rheumatoid arthritis. These symptoms may be the result of direct leukemic infiltration of the periosteum, periosteal elevation by underlying cortical disease, bone infarction, or expansion of the marrow cavity by leukemic cells.

Central nervous system leukemia (leptomeningeal involvement) is clinically present at the time of diagnosis in about 2 per cent of patients. The most common signs and symptoms include vomiting, headache, papilledema, nuchal rigidity, and cranial nerve palsies. Pleocytosis with the presence of blasts usually makes the diagnosis a simple one, but even with cytocentrifugation techniques, between 5 and 15 per cent of patients with arachnoid infiltration will not have identifiable leukemic cells in the spinal fluid.

Thymic or mediastinal infiltration, most commonly seen in T cell ALL, may cause life-threatening airway or vascular compression. Patients with the monocytic variants of AML frequently have skin and gum infiltration.

Chloromas or myeloblastomas are localized tumors seen in patients with AML that often appear green on the cut surface because of the presence of large amounts of the enzyme myeloperoxidase. These tumors may arise in bones or soft tissues and are frequently seen in the epidural area and around the orbits. Chloromas may appear before the onset of detectable bone marrow disease, or they may herald relapse.

LABORATORY MANIFESTATIONS. Clinical laboratory data often provide a broad spectrum of abnormal findings in the patient with newly diagnosed acute leukemia. Anemia, abnormal white cell and differential blood counts, and thrombocytopenia are common, but as many as 10 per cent of patients may have normal routine blood counts at the time of diagnosis even when the bone marrow is replaced by leukemic cells. Pancytopenia without recognizably abnormal leukocytes is found in a small percentage of patients and has been called aleukemic leukemia.

Blast cells are usually easily detectable in the peripheral blood when the white count exceeds 5000 per microliter (Color plate 3*I* and *J*). The morphology of peripheral blasts may not accurately reflect the status of the bone marrow. For example, normal myeloblasts may be detected in the circulation when lymphoblasts invade the marrow as part of the so-called leukoerythroblastic response to marrow invasion. The definitive diagnosis of leukemia should be made only from a bone marrow aspiration. The marrow specimen is usually hypercellular and contains from 30 to 100 per cent blast cells (Color plate 3*K*). Occasionally bone marrow aspiration results in a "dry tap." This may be attributed to a very packed marrow, reticulum fibrosis, or bone marrow necrosis within the marrow cavity. Marrow needle biopsy will usually produce an adequate specimen. The sample obtained by this technique should be touched to glass slides before it is placed in a fixative, because such touch preparations are very useful in assessing morphology.

Muramidase, or lysozyme, is a hydrolytic enzyme that is present in the primary granules of primitive granulocyte and monocyte precursor cells. Elevated serum and urine levels of this enzyme may be present in AML, with the highest levels in the monocytic and myelomonocytic subtypes. Renal tubular dysfunction and hypokalemia have been reported with increased blood and urine lysozyme. Hyperkalemia, hypocalcemia, and hyperphosphatemia have been associated with hyperleukocytosis and tumor lysis.

DIFFERENTIAL DIAGNOSIS. The diagnosis of acute leukemia is seldom difficult. Infections, neoplasms, and other marrow infiltrations may lead to leukocytosis and to immature cells in the peripheral blood. These leukemoid reactions generally mimic chronic myelogenous leukemia (see Ch. 155). Neutropenia induced by drugs, toxins, or infection may result in bone marrow that is left shifted (filled with myeloblasts and promyelocytes). This normal, early myeloid population can be confused with AML, but it will mature in a few days, thus establishing the diagnosis.

Infectious mononucleosis and other viral illnesses can masquerade as ALL. This differential diagnosis is particularly difficult in the rare patient whose viral illness is complicated by thrombocytopenic purpura or immunohemolytic anemia. Patients with both acute leukemia and aplastic anemia may present with pancytopenia. The bone marrow aspirate in aplastic anemia will be hypocellular, but rarely the two diseases cannot be differentiated initially because a small number of patients with acute leukemia have hypocellular bone marrow.

THERAPY. The possibility of cure for both ALL and AML has become realistic. Complete remission is required to provide a significant prolongation of survival. Such a remission is commonly defined as the reduction of leukemic cells to undetectable levels and the restoration of normal bone marrow function. This includes a return to less than 5 per cent blasts in the bone marrow; normalization of hemoglobin, granulocyte, and platelet counts; resolution of organomegaly; and return of the patient to normal lifestyle.

Initial treatment is directed toward correcting metabolic abnormalities, anemia, and thrombocytopenia and toward controlling infection and preventing hyperuricemia. This may require up to 48 hours, but can usually be achieved in 24 hours. Immediate administration of chemotherapy is necessary to prevent leukostasis in patients with AML and high white cell counts (>200,000 per microliter). Allopurinol is started at diagnosis to decrease the formation of relatively insoluble uric acid from the catabolic products of leukemia cells. Hyperuricemia may occur prior to antileukemic treatment and occasionally may be severe enough to produce impaired renal function before therapy can be started. In this setting, alkalinization and high urine flow should be established before cytotoxic therapy is initiated.

Acute Lymphoblastic Leukemia. Once the patient's condition is stabilized, antileukemic chemotherapy should begin without delay. Therapy is divided into three phases: remission induction, central nervous system prophylaxis, and treatment in remission (maintenance or continuation therapy).

REMISSION INDUCTION. Combinations of two agents have been consistently superior to single agents for inducing complete remission of patients with ALL. The most effective combination has been vincristine and prednisone, which produces complete remission in more than 90 per cent of pediatric patients and 50 per cent of adults with ALL. For patients over 15 years of age, the addition of a third drug (L-asparaginase, doxorubicin, or daunorubicin) increases the remission rate to over 80 per cent. In several studies the remission rates fell to 60 to 70 per cent in patients over 30 years of age.

CENTRAL NERVOUS SYSTEM PROPHYLAXIS. An important advance in the treatment of childhood ALL was CNS prophylaxis. As more children experienced longer bone marrow remission, the CNS became the first site of relapse in over 50 per cent of patients. The risk of relapse in the CNS can be markedly reduced by treatment with irradiation, 2400 rads to the cranial-spinal axis or 2400 rads to the cranium, combined with four doses of methotrexate given intrathecally. Intrathecal methotrexate alone is effective CNS prophylaxis in selected patients with ALL. Treatment of the CNS sanctuary reduces the frequency of subsequent bone marrow relapse and increases the percentage of children whose disease remains in continuous complete remission. CNS prophylaxis is usually administered following completion of the induction regimen and is now routinely used in all childhood and most adult ALL treatment programs. In the adult age group, CNS leukemia is significantly reduced by similar prophylaxis, but this has not resulted in longer bone marrow remission.

Cranial irradiation combined with intrathecal methotrexate is very effective CNS prophylaxis, but carries some risk of CNS damage. For example, irradiation alters vascular permeability to methotrexate, such that subsequent administration of parenteral methotrexate in large doses may result in a demyelinating leukoencephalopathy.

Maintenance or Continuation Therapy. After remission induction and CNS prophylaxis, continued therapy is necessary to prevent bone marrow relapse. Standard maintenance regimens have included 6-mercaptopurine, methotrexate, and periodic pulses of the remission-induction drugs. The above type of therapy is of relatively limited value for adults and high-risk children with ALL. Multiple cell cycle–specific and nonspecific agents have been intensively used before maintenance therapy to prevent the emergence of drug-resistant leukemic cells. These newer drug regimens appear to have improved durations of remission for high-risk patients.

How long maintenance therapy should be continued is unclear, in part because of the inability to assess minimal residual disease (less than 10^9 leukemic cells). In the absence of objective evidence, patients have been treated for two and one-half to five years.

Relapse. The most common site of relapse is in the bone marrow, with the highest risk during the first two years after diagnosis. CNS relapse has dramatically declined with the routine use of CNS prophylactic therapy; however, the testes are an important extramedullary site of relapse. If testicular relapse occurs during or following cessation of therapy, irradiation in a dose of 2400 rads should be given to both testes. As when CNS relapse occurs, systemic spread must be assumed, and therefore systemic as well as local therapy should be given. The prognosis for males with late testicular relapse appears to be favorable (data apply to children).

Approximately 80 per cent of children and 50 per cent of adults who have relapse will achieve second remissions with the original induction chemotherapy, but these are short lived. A second course of chemotherapy may be curative for a small percentage of patients whose initial remission was greater than two to three years. Bone marrow transplantation, however, is potentially useful therapy for these patients.

Bone Marrow Transplantation (see Ch. 165). The initial trials of bone marrow transplantation in ALL involved patients with advanced resistant disease and resulted in long-term survival in 10 per cent. Earlier application of transplantation in patients with ALL has been more successful. Several centers have reported survival of 30 per cent in patients with ALL who underwent transplantation in second or subsequent remission. Marrow transplantation in first remission is now being considered for very high risk patients. Autologous bone marrow transplantation is an interesting approach for patients who lack HLA-identical donors. Bone marrow is obtained in second remission, is treated in vitro by physical, immunologic (e.g., anti-CALLA antibody), or pharmacologic techniques to remove residual leukemia cells, and is cryopreserved. The patient receives supralethal chemoradiotherapy and reinfusion of autologous "treated" bone marrow. The survival rate has been 20 to 30 per cent after autologous transplantation. Recurrent leukemia remains a major problem after allogeneic or autologous transplantation for ALL.

Prognosis. The cure rate for children with ALL now routinely approaches 60 to 70 per cent, but is no more than 30 per cent for adults. In childhood studies, relatively favorable prognostic factors include age of two to ten years, white race, female sex, a white blood count less than 20,000 per microliter, and CALLA positivity. Over 70 per cent of patients in this group remain in continuous complete remission for five or more years after diagnosis. Less favorable prognostic factors include age less than two or greater than ten years, male sex, a mediastinal mass, L3 or Burkitt-type leukemia, Ph^1 chromosome, and an extremely elevated white blood cell count. The presence of T cell disease has a strong correlation with some high-risk clinical features, but is not an independent prognostic variable. The poorer prognosis observed in the older age group may in part be due to a different distribution of biologic subsets of ALL between adults and children.

Acute Myelogenous Leukemia. Progress in the treatment of AML has not equaled that in the management of ALL. More effective antileukemic chemotherapy and more sophisticated supportive care have recently increased the complete remission rate and the duration of remission, however.

Remission Induction. Remission induction is now successful in 50 to 85 per cent of patients (adults and children) with AML. The drug dosages necessary to kill myeloblasts come dangerously close to destroying normal marrow cells and cause prolonged bone marrow aplasia until normal hematopoietic progenitors can repopulate the marrow. Therefore, effective remission induction programs are associated with considerable morbidity and mortality. The introduction of cytosine arabinoside (ara-C) and the anthracyclines (daunorubicin and doxorubicin) represented a major advance in the therapy of AML. Remission can be achieved in the majority of patients under 60 years of age with a single course of seven days of cytosine arabinoside and three days of daunorubicin or doxorubicin. In the past, only about one third of patients over age 60 achieved complete remission, but recent results are more encouraging.

Consolidation and Intensification Chemotherapy. As in ALL, remission induction therapy reduces but does not eradicate the leukemic clone of cells. Therefore, additional therapy is necessary to achieve prolonged remissions in patients with AML. With most chemotherapy treatment programs, median durations of remission have been 12 to 18 months, but with only 10 to 20 per cent of patients who achieved remission remaining as leukemia-free survivors at five or more years.

In an effort to increase leukemic cell kill during remission, patients have been treated with intensification or consolidation chemotherapy for periods of a few months to one year after induction of remission. This has been based on the steep dose response curve for most chemotherapeutic agents. In some studies, sequential "non-cross-resistant" drug combinations have been administered to circumvent the problem of acquired drug resistance. The chemotherapeutic strategies used have resulted in marked improvements in durations of remission for patients of less than 18 years with AML (life table estimates of 45 per cent leukemia-free survival at five years). For similarly treated adults (18 to 60 years), median durations were longer compared to standard maintenance chemotherapy regimens, but a higher plateau of five-year leukemia-free survival was not achieved. It does not appear that maintenance chemotherapy after consolidation or intensification treatment is of additional therapeutic benefit.

Bone Marrow Transplantation (see Ch. 165). Over the past 10 years bone marrow transplantation has become an important therapeutic method in AML. Marrow grafting has been generally limited to persons less than 45 years of age with AML who have HLA-identical donors. Transplantation is ideally performed as soon as the patient enters complete remission. The outcome of bone marrow transplantation for patients with AML with first remission is promising. Leukemia-free survival estimates are as high as 50 to 60 per cent for young patients (<20 years), but decrease in older adults (>35 years). Relapse of leukemia after marrow transplantation has not been a major obstacle to success. Graft-versus-host disease and interstitial pneumonitis account for the major mortality and morbidity in these patients. For children and young adults (<35 years) there is a trend toward improved survival for those receiving a bone marrow transplant compared to chemotherapy in first remission. Bone marrow transplantation is the current treatment of choice for the patient with AML who has had relapse after an initial course of chemotherapy.

Central Nervous System Leukemia. CNS relapse is substantially less common (5 to 20 per cent) than in ALL, in part because of earlier death from systemic disease. Patients with myelomonocytic or monocytic leukemia are at increased risk for CNS disease. CNS prophylaxis is not routinely used for adults with AML. It is frequently employed in pediatric patients with AML, but it has not impacted upon overall survival.

Prognosis. The cure rate for children with AML (greater than five years of continuous remission) approaches 30 to 40 per cent, but is no more than 20 per cent for adults. Correlations among age, sex, performance status, morphologic classification, blast cytokinetics, platelet count, splenomegaly, and the response to therapy have been described but are controversial. There is a correlation between the karyotypic abnormality in pretreatment bone marrow samples and response to therapy. Patients with deletions of chromosome 5 or 7 represent a group of patients who are likely to have short survival times.

The terms "myelodysplastic syndromes" or "preleukemia" and "smoldering leukemia" have been applied to a spectrum of abnormalities of bone marrow function characterized by normal to increased marrow cellularity and ineffective hematopoiesis. These patients often have a panmyelopathy, and chromosomal abnormalities are present in up to 75 per cent of cases. Many of these patients will develop AML within 6 to 18 months after diagnosis. The response to chemotherapy is poor, and bone marrow transplantation should be considered for the child or young adult with these diseases.

AML has been reported in patients who received chemotherapy (alkylating agents and nitrosoureas) for neoplastic diseases, including malignant lymphoma, ovarian carcinoma, and gastrointestinal carcinoma. The response of these patients to chemotherapy is also poor, with remission rates of less than 50 per cent in most series.

Immunotherapy. Most studies find immunotherapy to be effective against only relatively small numbers of tumor cells, usually less than 10^5. Because of this limitation the majority of immunotherapy trials have been performed in patients whose disease is in remission. A variety of immunotherapeutic agents have been examined, including BCG, *Corynebacterium parvum*, levamisole, and irradiated allogeneic leukemic blast cells with BCG. In most trials, patients have been randomized to receive chemotherapy alone, immunotherapy alone, or both chemotherapy and immunotherapy. Immunotherapy has almost always failed to increase remission durations in AML and ALL. Recent studies have focused on conjugating monoclonal antibodies to drugs or toxins that can target specific cells, and the use of biologic response modifiers such as the interferons and interleukins.

Supportive Care. Advances in the treatment of acute leukemia, especially AML, have depended on progress in the control of infection and bleeding. Infection is a major complication of induction chemotherapy for AML, with mortality of 20 to 30 per cent. Neutropenia, impaired immunity, central venous catheters, and drug toxicity to nonhematopoietic tissues (gastrointestinal tract) are predisposing factors. Virtually all patients with AML become febrile while receiving induction chemotherapy. Although infection is usually suspected, it is documented in only 50 to 70 per cent of cases. Nevertheless, febrile, neutropenic (less than 500 granulocytes per cubic millimeter) patients should receive broad-spectrum antibiotics immediately after appropriate cultures have been obtained. A semisynthetic penicillin and an aminoglycoside are generally included. Enteric gram-negative bacilli colonizing the gastrointestinal tract and gram-positive bacteria (e.g., *Staphylococcus epidermidis*) are responsible for the majority of infections.

Oral nonabsorbable antibiotics, protected environments (laminar airflow), and granulocyte transfusions during induction of remission in patients with AML are not of proven benefit. Oral nonabsorbable antibiotics reduce enteric colonization and have been shown to reduce systemic infection. Several studies indicate a decreased incidence of infections in protected environments, but overall remission rates remain unchanged. Therapeutic granulocyte transfusions in some studies have improved survival in patients with gram-negative bacteremia, but in general they have a limited role because of newer and more potent antibiotics.

In addition to bacteria, a variety of opportunistic organisms invade the immunosuppressed host. Patients receiving "broad-spectrum" antibiotics who remain febrile and granulocytopenic for approximately one week should be carefully observed for fungal infections, and empiric treatment with amphotericin B should be begun. *Pneumocystis carinii* threatens the immunosuppressed host and causes severe interstitial pneumonitis. Infection with this organism can be prevented by prophylactic therapy with trimethoprim-sulfamethoxazole. The severity of chickenpox can be reduced by the prophylactic administration (within 96 hours of exposure) of zoster immune globulin in patients in whom serologic examination indicates lack of varicella-zoster antibody and who are exposed to chickenpox or zoster. Acyclovir is useful for the treatment of varicella-zoster infection.

Platelet transfusions from HLA-mismatched donors are successful in restoring hemostasis in thrombocytopenic patients, but result in alloimmunization in 30 to 50 per cent of patients (see Ch. 166). The alloimmunized patient may be managed by the use of HLA-matched platelets, single-donor platelets obtained by plateletpheresis, or autologous cryopreserved platelets. There is controversy whether platelets should be transfused prophylactically (i.e., when platelet count is less than 20,000 per microliter) or whether they should be used only for active bleeding. The patient's overall clinical status and platelet responsiveness are factors to be taken into consideration in making this decision. The hemorrhagic complications of acute promyelocytic leukemia can be prevented and controlled by administration of heparin.

Transfusion of blood products from normal donors has been associated with graft-versus-host disease in the immunosuppressed and myelosuppressed patient with acute leukemia. Irradiation of blood products at dosages sufficient to destroy T lymphocytes prevents the development of graft-versus-host disease.

Applebaum FR, Dahlberg S, Thomas ED, et al.: Bone marrow transplantation or chemotherapy after remission induction for adults with acute nonlymphoblastic leukemia. Ann Intern Med 101:581, 1984. *One of several studies comparing the outcome of marrow transplantation with that of continued chemotherapy for adults with AML.*

Bennett JM, Catovsky D, Daniel MT, et al.: Proposals for the classification of the acute leukemias. Br J Haematol 33:451, 1976. *Detailed description of the French-American-British (FAB) classification of acute leukemia.*

Casciato DA, Scott JL: Acute leukemia following prolonged cytotoxic agent therapy. Medicine 58:32, 1979. *Includes a complete review of drug-induced leukemia and a complete bibliography.*

Foon KA, Todd RF: Immunologic classification of leukemia and lymphoma. Blood 68:1, 1986. *Detailed review of the cell surface phenotypes in the leukemias and lymphomas.*

Gale RP: Advances in the treatment of acute myelogenous leukemia. N Engl J Med 300:1189, 1979. *Excellent clinical review of current therapies and supportive care for patients with AML. Includes a complete bibliography.*

Gallo RC, Wong-Staal F: Retroviruses as etiologic agents of some animal and human leukemias and lymphomas and as tools for elucidating the molecular mechanism of leukemogenesis. Blood 60:545, 1982. *Review of viral etiology of leukemias including the HTLV retrovirus.*

McCulloch EA: Stem cells in normal and leukemic hemopoiesis. Blood 62:1, 1983. *Good review and bibliography of the nature of differentiation in normal and leukemic process.*

Murphy SB (ed.): Acute Lymphoblastic Leukemia. Semin Oncol 12:79, 1985. *Excellent chapters on the biology and treatment of ALL in both children and adults.*

Prentice HG (ed.): Infections in Haematology. Clin Haematol 13:523, 1984. *Includes chapters on infection prophylaxis and treatment of bacterial, viral, and fungal infections of the immunocompromised host.*

Rowley JD: Biological implications of consistent chromosome rearrangements in leukemia and lymphoma. Cancer Res 44:3159, 1984. *Complete review of consistent chromosomal lesions in the leukemias and oncogene mapping.*

Thomas ED: Bone marrow transplantation in hematologic malignancies. Hosp Pract 22:77, 1987. *Overview of marrow transplantation for acute leukemia.*

157 INTRODUCTION TO NEOPLASMS OF THE IMMUNE SYSTEM

Carol S. Portlock

Neoplasms of the immune system are a heterogeneous group of tumors whose cells of origin may be the lymphocyte, the histiocyte, or other cell components of the immune system. Each neoplasm is thought to be a monoclonal expansion of malignant cells, although this has only been conclusively demonstrated for lymphocytic tumors. Interestingly, these neoplasms often retain many morphologic, functional, and migratory characteristics common to their normal cell counterparts.

With increasing understanding of the normal immune system, it has become possible to classify malignant immune disorders according to their cell of origin. Table 157–1 lists these neoplasms, utilizing current immunologic concepts. Tumors of B lymphocyte lineage are identified by the presence of cell surface immunoglobulin, utilizing fluorescent anti-immunoglobulin antibodies. Each B lymphocytic neoplasm can be immunotyped according to its heavy chain and light chain classes and can be shown to be a monoclonal process. Such immunologic phenotyping may identify distinct groups of patients with different clinical presentations and prognoses. In addition to membrane-bound immunoglobulin, malignant B lymphocytes may have Ia antigen and Fc receptors, as well as receptors for complement.

Tumors of T lymphocyte lineage are identified in vitro by the formation of E rosettes after incubation with sheep erythrocytes. Moreover, monoclonal antibodies that react with normal T cell differentiation antigens can be used to detect distinct malignant T cell subsets. Enzyme determination of terminal deoxynucleotidyl transferase (TdT) may also identify a T cell lineage, as well as pre-B and lymphoid stem cells.

TABLE 157–1. LYMPHOMAS AS NEOPLASMS OF THE IMMUNE SYSTEM

Cell of Origin	Neoplasm
I. B cell	
Medullary B cell	Chronic lymphocytic leukemia, diffuse small lymphocytic lymphoma
Follicular B cell	Follicular lymphomas, diffuse mixed lymphoma, diffuse large cell lymphoma, Burkitt's lymphoma
Immunoblastic B cell	Diffuse immunoblastic lymphoma
II. T cell	
Thymic T cell	Lymphoblastic lymphoma
Mature T cell	Peripheral T cell lymphomas, chronic lymphocytic leukemia (rare), HTLV-I–associated lymphoma, mycosis fungoides, Sézary's syndrome
Immunoblastic T cell	Diffuse immunoblastic lymphoma
III. Histiocytic	
Histiocyte	Malignant histiocytosis, true histiocytic lymphoma (rare)
IV. Unknown	Hodgkin's disease

Modified from Strauchen JA: West J Med 135:276, 1981.

With utilization of these immunologic techniques, however, some tumors that are of lymphocyte origin morphologically cannot be shown to contain B or T cell surface markers and consequently are termed null cell. Nevertheless, immunoglobulin gene rearrangements may be detected in such null cells, suggesting a pre-B cell origin. Moreover, specific rearrangements of the T cell receptor gene loci identify tumors of T cell origin. Tumors of histiocytic lineage have not yet been identified by monoclonal antibody techniques. These cells lack endogenous immunoglobulin, but may acquire exogenous immunoglobulin on their cell surface. They may be rich in lysozyme or muramidase, and as phagocytic cells, they can be shown to ingest latex particles or sensitized erythrocytes. The cell lineage of the Reed-Sternberg cell in Hodgkin's disease is not known with certainty. It has in vitro characteristics in common with both histiocytes and lymphocytes. It may derive from a dendritic cell or lymphocyte.

In addition to a specific immunologic phenotype, chromosomal abnormalities can be detected in the majority of immune system neoplasms. In many the karyotype appears to be specific (follicular lymphomas, Burkitt's lymphoma, mycosis fungoides). Another marker that appears to be specific is the presence of antibodies to the human retrovirus HTLV-1 (human T cell lymphoma virus) found in patients with mature T cell lymphoma. These and other in vitro methods may provide additional information for defining prognostically important patient subsets.

Each neoplasm of the immune system is a distinct clinicopathologic entity. However, these disorders tend to share some common clinical features. For example, systemic symptoms of fever, night sweats, and weight loss may be present and tend to correlate with advanced stage of disease. The neoplasm usually arises in one or more organs of the hematopoietic system (lymph nodes, spleen, liver, bone marrow) and if untreated or ineffectively treated, it tends to disseminate to all those organs, as well as to other sites. Bone marrow involvement with or without peripheral blood manifestation is common in certain disorders and may be the predominant feature. Meningeal infiltration is often present when aggressive neoplasms involve the bone marrow.

PATHOLOGY AND CLASSIFICATION

Neoplasms of B or T lymphocytic lineage are termed non-Hodgkin's lymphomas. They are a diverse group of diseases with varying clinical presentations, responses to therapy, and prognoses. The Rappaport histopathologic classification of the non-Hodgkin's lymphomas (Table 157–2) has been used successfully in clinical trials and practice. It has permitted the identification of specific clinicopathologic entities and of favorable and unfavorable prognostic groups since 1966. Nevertheless, the Rappaport classification, based exclusively upon morphologic concepts, does not take into account recent information regarding the immune system. For example, the term "histiocytic" lymphoma is generally incorrect because virtually all of the non-Hodgkin's lymphomas are of lymphocytic origin.

Table 157–2 juxtaposes a more recent National Cancer Institute working formulation with the Rappaport classification. Tumor architecture is an important feature in both: Rappaport's "nodular" is replaced by the more immunologically accurate term "follicular." Cell morphology is more descriptive in the working formulation and "histiocytic" is replaced by "large cell." Prognostically favorable and unfavorable groups are termed low, intermediate, and high grade. The low-grade category includes small lymphocytic consistent with chronic lymphocytic leukemia; a miscellaneous category includes mycosis fungoides and true histiocytic lymphoma.

Many non-Hodgkin's lymphomas may exhibit two distinct histologic subtypes. Both the architecture and the cell type

TABLE 157–2. CLASSIFICATION OF THE NON-HODGKIN'S LYMPHOMAS

NCI Working Formulation (1982)	Rappaport Classification (1966)
Low grade	
Small lymphocytic (SLL)	Diffuse lymphocytic, well differentiated (DLWD)
Follicular, small cleaved cell (FSCL)	Nodular lymphocytic, poorly differentiated (NLPD)
Follicular, mixed small cleaved and large cell (FML)	Nodular mixed lymphocytic-histiocytic (NML)
Intermediate grade	
Follicular, large cell (FLCL)	Nodular histiocytic (NHL)
Diffuse, small cleaved cell (DSCL)	Diffuse lymphocytic, poorly differentiated (DLPD)
Diffuse, mixed small cleaved and large cell (DML)	Diffuse mixed lymphocytic-histiocytic (DML)
Diffuse, large cell (cleaved and noncleaved) (DLCL)	Diffuse histiocytic (DHL)
High grade	
Large cell immunoblastic (IBL)	Diffuse histiocytic (DHL)
Lymphoblastic (convoluted and nonconvoluted) (LL)	
Small noncleaved cell (Burkitt and non-Burkitt) (SNCL)	Diffuse undifferentiated (DUL)

may change, usually evolving from a low-grade lymphoma to an intermediate or high-grade lymphoma. Rarely, two histologic subtypes may be present at diagnosis in the same lymph node (composite lymphoma). More often, two histologic subtypes may be seen at diagnosis in two separate biopsy specimens; most frequently, one is seen at diagnosis and a second at relapse or autopsy. It is thought that such "transformation" represents clonal expansion of a more aggressive cell line. Its clinical importance is that both therapy and prognosis may be dramatically altered by its emergence.

DIAGNOSIS AND STAGING

The diagnosis of a neoplasm of the immune system is based upon pathologic classification of biopsy material. This requires adequate tissue (preferably lymph node, so that both architecture and cell type may be assessed), proper handling, and excellent hematopathologic interpretation. Special studies such as imprints, immunotyping, gene rearrangement, karyotyping, TdT determination, and electron microscopy may provide additional information for classification. Since these latter studies require fresh tissue and special handling, it is important that the pathologist be involved *before* biopsy. Likewise, it is important that each case be evaluated jointly by a medical oncologist, radiation therapist, surgeon, and radiologist from the outset.

With the diagnosis established, the extent of disease should be completely defined. Since each neoplasm has distinct clinicopathologic features, the choice of staging studies will be based on that information. All patients should have a complete history, particularly assessing the presence or absence of systemic symptoms, and physical examination. All nodal areas should be examined, including Waldeyer's ring and preauricular, epitrochlear, and popliteal lymph nodes. In addition to liver and spleen, epigastric or other abdominal masses may be found. The lungs, skin, breasts, testicles, and central nervous system should be carefully examined for extranodal involvement. Blood counts and liver and renal function tests are necessary in all patients. In addition to chest radiography, tomography or computed tomography may be indicated in an abnormal chest. Abdominal CT and lymphography are often complementary and not mutally exclusive. Gallium 67 scanning may be useful, but is not a diagnostic method. Liver and spleen scans are of minimal value. Studies of bone or gastrointestinal tract should be performed only when symptoms are present. Bone marrow biopsy is often indicated, particularly if advanced clinical disease is present or the patient has a low-grade lymphoma. CSF cytology should be determined in all patients with intermediate and high-grade lymphomas who have bone marrow involvement and in all patients with Burkitt's lymphoma, lymphoblastic lymphoma, or malignant histiocytosis.

Several different staging systems are applied to neoplasms of the immune system. Their purpose is to define disease extent, to assist in treatment strategies, to evaluate therapeutic results, and to determine prognosis. In Hodgkin's disease the utility of staging has been elegantly demonstrated, and excellent clinical care demands careful clinical and pathologic staging. Staging laparotomy with splenectomy and biopsy of liver, lymph nodes, and bone marrow was developed for adequate intra-abdominal assessment of Hodgkin's disease. It accurately identifies pathologic stage and its results often dictate treatment strategy. The Ann Arbor staging system for Hodgkin's disease has also been applied to the non-Hodgkin's lymphomas. In this setting it has less value in determining therapy but remains an important prognostic variable. Modified staging systems are used in pediatric lymphomas, chronic lymphocytic leukemia, Burkitt's and lymphoblastic lymphomas, and mycosis fungoides. Since pathologic intra-abdominal assessment is rarely needed to determine treatment in the non-Hodgkin's lymphomas, staging laparotomy is usually unnecessary. Nonetheless, careful clinical staging is imperative in all cases.

DIFFERENTIAL DIAGNOSIS

The differential diagnosis of neoplasms of the immune system is usually that of lymphadenopathy. Reactive processes, infections, other malignant tumors, and collagen-vascular disorders may all cause enlarged lymph nodes or hepatosplenomegaly or both. The location(s) of the lymph nodes, their size, shape, consistency, rapidity of onset, and other characteristics may aid in determining etiology.

Regional lymph node hyperplasia may be seen with acute or chronic infections of the extremities and with vaccinations or insect bites. Diffuse lymphadenopathy may occur following ingestion of phenytoin. Other diffuse reactive processes such as acquired immunodeficiency syndrome, angioimmunoblastic lymphadenopathy, and collagen-vascular disorders may be associated with an increased likelihood of developing lymphoma. Consequently, a single lymph node biopsy may not solve the diagnostic dilemma. That is why pathologic consultation before biopsy is recommended.

Among infectious etiologic factors, viral illnesses predominate and often produce bizarre pathologic material. Infectious mononucleosis may present with features common to Hodgkin's disease. Cytomegalovirus, cat scratch disease, toxoplasmosis, tuberculosis, and syphilis are other considerations. Other malignant neoplasms usually involve lymph nodes by regional spread. For example, cervical lymphadenopathy may be the first symptom of a malignant tumor involving the oropharynx or nasopharynx. Likewise, breast cancer may present with axillary adenopathy and a microscopic primary tumor.

In virtually all instances, the only way to determine conclusively the cause of lymphadenopathy is by pathologic tissue examination. Low cervical and supraclavicular lymph nodes are more likely to yield diagnostic material than axillary and inguinal nodes. When only intrathoracic or abdominal disease is present, bone marrow biopsy may provide diagnostic information and obviate the need for surgery. Fine needle aspiration is of lesser value in neoplasms of the immune system than in solid tumors, because cell morphology and architecture are both important diagnostic parameters.

Berard CW: A multidisciplinary approach to non-Hodgkin's lymphomas. Ann Intern Med 94:218, 1980. *A discussion moderated by Berard of the immunologic concepts pertinent to an understanding of the non-Hodgkin's lymphomas.*

Foon KA, Todd RF III: Immunologic classification of leukemia and lymphoma.

Blood 6:1, 1986. *A comprehensive review of monoclonal antibody and molecular methods of classifying the leukemias and lymphomas.*
Non-Hodgkin's lymphoma pathologic classification project. National Cancer Institute sponsored study of classifications of non-Hodgkin's lymphomas: Summary and description of a working formulation for clinical usage. Cancer 49:2112, 1982. *The working formulation is presented and six pathologic classifications are compared.*

158 THE NON-HODGKIN'S LYMPHOMAS

Carol S. Portlock

The non-Hodgkin's lymphomas are the single largest group of neoplasms of the immune system. Composed of more than ten distinct disease entities, the non-Hodgkin's lymphomas are best understood as a heterogeneous group of malignant diseases whose common link is a characteristic monoclonal expansion of malignant B or T lymphocytes.

EPIDEMIOLOGY

The non-Hodgkin's lymphomas may occur at any age, although they are rarely diagnosed during the first year of life. They occur with increasing frequency throughout adulthood. The incidence is estimated to be approximately 27,000 cases per year in the United States (1986) with males affected more often than females. Moreover, male predominance is most evident among young patients in association with the aggressive histologic subtypes of lymphoblastic and Burkitt's lymphomas.

Geographic clustering is characteristic of some non-Hodgkin's lymphomas: Burkitt's lymphoma in central Africa; adult T cell leukemia/lymphoma in southwestern Japan and the Caribbean; and small intestinal lymphoma with associated immunoglobulin disorders in the Middle East.

Preceding immune dysfunction has been associated with the development of aggressive non-Hodgkin's lymphomas. Congenital immunodeficiency states associated with lymphoma include severe combined immunodeficiency, ataxia-telangiectasia, Wiskott-Aldrich syndrome, X-linked lymphoproliferative syndrome, and common variable immunodeficiency (Ch. 419). Transplant recipients, patients with autoimmune states, and patients with AIDS (acquired immunodeficiency syndrome) also have increased risk of developing lymphoma.

ETIOLOGY AND PATHOGENESIS

The etiology of the non-Hodgkin's lymphomas is unclear. Perhaps the best studied lymphoma is Burkitt's (Ch. 159), with which the Epstein-Barr virus (EBV) has been associated and for which specific chromosomal and oncogene translocations have been implicated in its pathogenesis.

Adult T cell leukemia/lymphoma (ATL), a rare and recently discovered disorder, is associated with a unique human retrovirus, HTLV-I. ATL is endemic in southwestern Japan where 12 to 15 per cent of normal persons have HTLV-I antibodies; it is also found in the Caribbean basin.

The specific chromosomal translocations seen in Burkitt's lymphoma have uniformly involved the *c-myc* oncogene on chromosome 8 and the immunoglobulin heavy- or light-chain genes on chromosomes 14, 2, or 22. Specific chromosomal translocations have also been reported in follicular lymphomas, involving chromosomes 11 and 14 or 18 and 14. The translocation site on chromosome 14 is identical to that in Burkitt's lymphoma, and by analogy, suggests that a transforming gene on chromosome 11 or 18 is activated when brought into proximity with the immunoglobulin heavy-chain locus. These oncogenes, *bcl-1* (on chromosome 11) and *bcl-2* (on chromosome 18), have been identified and cloned.

In addition to the etiologic considerations of oncogenic viruses and oncogene transformation, other factors that have been associated with an increased incidence of lymphoma include ionizing radiation (whole-body dose greater than 100 rads), hereditary predisposition, and congenital or acquired immunodeficiency.

PATHOLOGY AND CLINICAL FEATURES

Many different pathologic classifications have been proposed for the non-Hodgkin's lymphomas (Ch. 157). Rappaport's classification (Table 157–2) has been the most successfully utilized and applied in clinical trials, while that of Lukes and Collins is more immunologically correct, classifying diseases based on their cell of origin. The National Cancer Institute Working Formulation (1982) is being increasingly accepted, since it is proving both clinically useful and immunologically correct.

Pathologic interpretation of the non-Hodgkin's lymphomas can be supplemented with a variety of complementary studies. Immunophenotyping may identify the cell of origin by demonstrating B cell monoclonal surface immunoglobulin, T cell sheep erythrocyte rosettes (E rosettes), and B or T cell differentiation antigens. Clonality may also be ascertained by detection of the rearrangement of the B cell immunoglobulin genes or of the T cell receptor gene loci. Moreover, the karyotype may reveal a specific chromosomal translocation. The presence of antibody against HTLV-I suggests a T cell lymphoma, whereas HTLV-III antibody suggests an aggressive B cell neoplasm.

Each disease entity of the Working Formulation has a distinct clinical presentation and prognosis, as noted below. The pathologic appearance and some of the clinical characteristics of each category, as outlined in the Working Formulation, are listed in Tables 158-1 and 158-2.

LOW GRADE. The low-grade lymphomas (small lymphocytic [SLL]; follicular, predominantly small cleaved cell [FSCL]; and follicular, mixed, small cleaved and large cell [FML]) have several clinical characteristics in common: (1) Each has a history of waxing and waning or slowly progressive adenopathy. (2) These are rubbery, mobile lymph nodes that are rarely fixed and have no overlying skin infiltration; lymph nodes may be very bulky but are rarely painful. (3) Liver and

TABLE 158–1. PATHOLOGIC CHARACTERISTICS OF THE NON-HODGKIN'S LYMPHOMAS

Subtype	Architectural Pattern	Malignant Lymphocyte Cytology	Immunophenotype/ Immunogenotype
SLL	Diffuse	Small round cells	B cell; rarely T-cell
FSCL	Follicular	Small cleaved cells	B cell
FML	Follicular	Small cleaved cells admixed with large cells, cleaved or noncleaved	B cell
FLCL	Follicular	Large cells cleaved or noncleaved	B cell
DSCL	Diffuse	Small cleaved cells	B cell; occasionally T cell
DML	Diffuse	Admixture of small and large cells cleaved or noncleaved	B cell; T cell
DLCL	Diffuse	Large cells cleaved or noncleaved	B cell; T cell
IBL	Diffuse	Large cells; plasmacytoid, clear, or polymorphic cell variants	B cell; T cell
LBL	Diffuse "starry sky"	Lymphoblasts, convoluted or nonconvoluted nuclei	Thymic T cell
SNCL	Diffuse "starry sky"	Noncleaved cells, round nuclei with prominent nucleoli	B cell

TABLE 158–2. CLINICAL CHARACTERISTICS OF THE NON-HODGKIN'S LYMPHOMAS

Subtype	% of all Lymphomas	Median Age, yr	Sex Ratio M:F	% PS I, II	% PS III, IV	% Bone Marrow Involvement
SLL	3.6	61	1.2:1	11	89	71
FSCL	22.5	54	1.3:1	18	82	51
FML	7.7	56	0.8:1	27	73	30
FLCL	3.8	55	1.8:1	27	73	34
DSCL	6.9	58	2:1	28	72	32
DML	6.7	58	1.1:1	45	55	14
DLCL	19.7	57	1:1	46	54	10
IBL	7.9	51	1.5:1	52	49	12
LBL	4.2	17	1.9:1	27	74	50
SNCL	0.5	30	2.6:1	34	66	14

spleen are frequently involved pathologically and may be enlarged; liver function tests are usually normal, although the alkaline phosphatase may be mildly increased. (4) Bone marrow involvement is common; circulating lymphoma cells may be identified on smear or by cell-sorting techniques. (5) Blood counts are usually normal at diagnosis. Elevation of the white blood cell count with circulating cells, anemia with autoimmune hemolytic anemia, and cytopenias secondary to hypersplenism or bone marrow replacement are uncommon complications. (6) Other extranodal disease sites may include pleura, lung, skin, breast, and gastrointestinal tract. (7) Enlarged lymph nodes may cause lymphedema, ureteral obstruction, or epidural cord compression. (8) Central nervous system (meningeal or parenchymal), renal, or testicular infiltration does not occur.

INTERMEDIATE GRADE AND HIGH GRADE. As a group, the intermediate (follicular, predominantly large cell [FLCL]; diffuse, small cleaved cell [DSCL]; diffuse, mixed small and large cell [DML]; and diffuse, large cell [DLCL]) and high-grade lymphomas (large cell immunoblastic [IBL]; lymphoblastic [LBL]; and small noncleaved cell, including Burkitt's lymphoma and diffuse and undifferentiated lymphoma, non-Burkitt's type [SNCL]) have several general clinical features in common: (1) There is a history of abrupt onset with rapidly enlarging lymph node masses. (2) Lymph nodes may be rubbery and mobile but may also be hard, fixed, and with overlying skin infiltration. Masses may be warm, erythematous, and painful. (3) Bulky lymph node masses (>10 cm) may be present in the mediastinum, retroperitoneum, and/or mesentery. (4) Waldeyer's ring may be involved and is often associated with extranodal disease of the stomach or small bowel or both. (5) Hepatosplenomegaly may be present, and liver function tests may be abnormal. Porta hepatis or even intrahepatic obstructive patterns may be seen. (6) Extranodal involvement is common: stomach, small bowel, lung, skin, bone, and central nervous system (particularly meningeal disease in association with bone marrow involvement). Rarely ovarian, testicular, or renal disease may be present. (7) Bone marrow involvement and circulating cells are less commonly seen at diagnosis than in low-grade lymphomas. A leukemic picture may emerge, however, when progressive disease develops. (8) Lymph node masses may cause lymphedema, ureteral obstruction, vascular obstruction (superior vena cava syndrome, thrombophlebitis), and epidural cord compression.

MISCELLANEOUS. A miscellaneous category of the Working Formulation includes mycosis fungoides—a rare helper T cell lymphoma of the skin; composite lymphoma—multiple histologic subtypes (e.g., FSCL and IBL) occurring simultaneously; and true histiocytic lymphoma.

Since the Formulation's publication in 1982, additional mature T cell lymphomas have been recognized. The peripheral T cell lymphomas are a diverse group of "post-thymic" neoplasms, whose cell of origin is the differentiated T cell. Their morphology includes diffuse small-cell, mixed-cell, large-cell, or immunoblastic lymphoma, as well as subgroups with histologic features of angioimmunoblastic lymphadenopathy, lymphomatoid granulomatosis, Hodgkin's-like disease, or Lennert's lymphoma. Clinical features include a 2:1 male predominance, prominent extranodal disease (particularly lung involvement) in the majority, systemic symptoms, and skin rash. In general, response to treatment and survival appear to parallel their counterparts in the Working Formulation.

HTLV-I associated adult T cell leukemia/lymphoma is characterized by geographic clustering, the presence of antibody to HTLV-I, and a rapidly fatal clinical course. Clinical features include abrupt onset of generalized lymphadenopathy, hepatosplenomegaly, skin infiltration, lytic bone disease, bone marrow involvement with circulating cells, and hypercalcemia. In spite of intensive chemotherapy, median survival is less than one year. Although clinically distinct, this rare T cell lymphoma is not easily distinguishable pathologically from other T cell lymphomas. Diffuse small-cell, mixed-cell, large-cell, and undifferentiated cell types have all been described. Therefore, clinical suspicion and the presence of HTLV-I antibody are necessary to confirm the diagnosis.

DIAGNOSIS AND STAGING

As discussed in Ch. 157, the diagnosis of a non-Hodgkin's lymphoma requires skilled interpretation of adequate tumor tissue, preferably from an involved lymph node, so that tumor architecture as well as cell type may be assessed. B cell and T cell typing studies may complement the pathologic interpretation, but do not supplant it. The clinical history and ancillary studies, e.g., HTLV-I or -III antibody, may also contribute. Once a diagnosis has been established, then it is useful to determine the extent of disease through staging.

The Ann Arbor staging system utilized for Hodgkin's disease (see Ch. 160) is also used in the management of non-Hodgkin's lymphomas. Although of clinical value, this staging system has several shortcomings when applied to non-Hodgkin's lymphomas: Factors such as disease site, disease bulk, and extent of extranodal involvement are not considered. In addition, the presence of systemic symptoms plays a lesser role in influencing treatment planning and prognosis in non-Hodgkin's lymphoma. Nevertheless, thorough pretreatment staging is necessary in all patients.

Noninvasive studies, which should be obtained in all patients, are listed in Table 158–3.

Based on this information, clinical stage of the lymphoma can be determined. Since bone marrow involvement is so common, particularly in low-grade lymphoma, bilateral percutaneous bone marrow biopsies are often the simplest way to establish pathologic stage IV disease.

Pathologic confirmation of other extranodal sites may be appropriate, as when gastroscopic biopsy, pleural cytology, or skin biopsy is obtained. Laparotomy or thoracotomy is indicated only in those patients with no other evident disease or when a gastrointestinal tumor is removed prior to treatment. Staging laparotomy as performed for Hodgkin's disease is rarely if ever indicated.

TABLE 158–3. NONINVASIVE STUDIES IN NON-HODGKIN'S LYMPHOMA

History with assessment of systemic symptoms, predisposing epidemiologic factors
Physical examination
CBC and platelet count; Coombs' test if anemic
Liver and renal function tests
Serum immunoglobulins in low-grade lymphomas
Antibody for HTLV-I or HTLV-III, if indicated
Chest radiograph, PA and lateral
Chest computed tomography, if indicated
Abdominal and pelvic computed tomography
If unavailable, abdominal ultrasound study
If normal, lymphography possibly indicated
Bone scan and bone radiographs if clinical involvement suspected
Upper gastrointestinal series, if clinical involvement suspected or if Waldeyer's ring involved
Gallium scan (in SNCL)
CSF cytology (in all patients with intermediate or high-grade lymphomas and known bone marrow disease)

TREATMENT

In defining a treatment approach for the patient with non-Hodgkin's lymphoma, it is necessary to consider such factors as histologic subtype, stage, sites of disease, tumor bulk, thoroughness of initial staging, general medical condition, and age, as well as the goals and effectiveness of therapy. In practical terms the non-Hodgkin's lymphomas can be considered in two broad categories: those diseases that progress slowly and have an indolent natural history (the low-grade lymphomas) and those diseases that present aggressively, progress rapidly, and if unsuccessfully treated are soon fatal (the intermediate and high-grade lymphomas).

LOW-GRADE LYMPHOMAS. As outlined above, low-grade lymphomas infrequently present with truly localized disease (pathologic stage I or II). Only 11 to 27 per cent, depending upon histologic subtype, are therefore eligible for regional treatment with radiation therapy. Although uncommon, this disease presentation appears to be highly favorable, with more than 75 per cent of patients remaining free of disease for ten years or longer after irradiation alone (3500 to 4400 rads to the region).

Many more patients appear to have clinically localized disease after noninvasive staging and bone marrow biopsy, but have not undergone complete laparotomy staging. Under these circumstances, radiation therapy may still accomplish good local control. Many patients, however, will have undetected microscopic disease outside the treatment portal that will slowly progress and lead to disease recurrence several years after initial therapy. Nevertheless, irradiation may still be a reasonable choice, since relapse may occur years later, and salvage treatment at relapse may be effective. Patients eligible for this approach are those with peripheral lymph node presentations (stage I and II) involving cervical, supraclavicular, axillary, or inguinal regions. Abdominal masses usually require whole-abdominal irradiation in which this approach may not be justified. Thoracic presentations are rare.

The majority (74 to 89 per cent) of patients with low-grade lymphomas have advanced stage (III or IV) disease and are therefore ineligible for localized treatment approaches. Optimal management of such patients remains controversial. Complete disappearance of all known tumor (including bone marrow biopsy) may be induced in more than 80 per cent of patients with single or multiagent chemotherapy, with whole-body irradiation, or with combined chemotherapy-irradiation. Unfortunately, remissions are usually limited to two and one half to five years. These seemingly complete responders actually have persistent circulating lymphoma cells in their peripheral blood. The presence of such cells correlates with subsequent relapse.

The most successful current chemotherapy program is C-MOPP (cyclophosphamide, vincristine (Oncovin), procarbazine, and prednisone). Initially employed in advanced stage FML, ten-year results reveal six of twelve complete responders still in remission. Although a larger prospective study did not confirm the remission durability of C-MOPP in FML, it did show a significant remission advantage in FSCL. Current investigative programs are designed to intensify the chemotherapy-radiation therapy regimens in an attempt to eradicate the malignant clone.

In summary, a standard treatment regimen in advanced low-grade lymphoma has not been established. Daily single-agent cyclophosphamide; daily or pulse chlorambucil; combinations of cyclophosphamide, vincristine, prednisone with or without procarbazine or Adriamycin are reasonable choices depending upon the clinical circumstances. Enrollment in a protocol regimen is encouraged whenever possible, since an optimal treatment regimen has not been identified.

Another management approach in patients with advanced stage low-grade non-Hodgkin's lymphomas is initial treatment deferral with institution of therapy when there is disease progression. This approach is based on the premise that treatment at diagnosis does not appear curative. Many patients have indolent, slowly progressive disease, and treatment deferral does not appear to compromise therapeutic outcome. Approximately one half of all patients may be eligible for observation at diagnosis; the median treatment-free period correlates with histology: more than eight years for SLL, five years for FSCL, and ten months for FML.

Biologic therapies have also been investigated in low-grade lymphomas and appear to have transient efficacy. These include monoclonal antibody therapy directed specifically against the malignant B cell immunoglobulin idiotype, antibody against B cell differentiation antigens, and alpha-interferon.

In up to 50 per cent of patients low-grade lymphomas may change with or without treatment from an indolent to an aggressive form by the eighth year following diagnosis. Most often the transformation presents as rapidly growing disease in one or more sites, while the low-grade component remains stable or progresses slowly. Pathologic study reveals DLCL, IBL, or other aggressive subtypes, and studies of clonality are consistent with the low-grade histology (B cell primarily). Most transformations represent emergence of an aggressive subclone from the original indolent disease, but some cases appear to represent the emergence of a completely new second neoplasm that is a clonally distinct, aggressive lymphoma in the setting of indolent lymphoma.

Histologic transformation is important to recognize, since it has prognostic and therapeutic implications. Median survival is less than one year following its emergence, and intensive treatment programs are necessary to gain disease control. Some patients appear to have the aggressive component eradicated by such measures, often with persistence or later relapse of the indolent histology.

INTERMEDIATE AND HIGH-GRADE LYMPHOMAS. Intensive combination chemotherapy is the mainstay of curative treatment in the aggressive non-Hodgkin's lymphomas. Of the half of all patients who may present with regional disease alone, only that small subset with pathologic stage I presentation may be eligible for radiation therapy alone. This is because the intent and realistic goal of treatment in the aggressive lymphomas is always cure, and relapse must be avoided whenever possible.

The expectation of cure in the vast majority of patients with aggressive lymphomas, regardless of stage, is based upon the following observations in advanced disease: (1) Tumors are rapidly proliferating and initially very sensitive to combination chemotherapy. (2) Survival curves in advanced disease are biphasic, revealing a rapid death rate during the two years (composed of partial and nonresponding patients) and then a plateau of cured cases (composed of complete responders). (3) With intensifying drug regimens the proportion of com-

TABLE 158–4. REPRESENTATIVE DRUG COMBINATIONS FOR INTERMEDIATE AND HIGH-GRADE NON-HODGKIN'S LYMPHOMAS

MACOP-B		
Methotrexate	400 mg/m² IV	Weeks 2, 6, 10 with leucovorin
Adriamycin	50 mg/m² IV	Weeks 1, 3, 5, 7, 9, 11
Cyclophosphamide	350 mg/m² IV	Weeks 1, 3, 5, 7, 9, 11
Oncovin	1.4 mg/m² IV	Weeks 2, 4, 6, 8, 10, 12
Prednisone	75 mg PO	Daily, dose tapered over the last 15 days
Bleomycin	10 U/m² IV	Weeks 4, 8, 12
Co-trimoxazole	2 tab PO	Twice daily throughout
ProMACE-MOPP		
Prednisone	60 mg/m² PO	Days 1–14
Methotrexate	500 mg/m² IV	Day 15 with leucovorin
Adriamycin	25 mg/m² IV	Days 1 and 8
Cyclophosphamide	650 mg/m² IV	Day 1
Etoposide (VP–16)	120 mg/m² IV	Day 1
Mechlorethamine	6 mg/m² IV	Day 8
Oncovin	1.4 mg/m² IV	Day 8
Procarbazine	100 mg/m² PO	Days 8–14
Prednisone	60 mg/m² PO	Days 8–14
m-BACOD		
Methotrexate	200 mg/m² IV	Days 8 and 15 with leucovorin
Bleomycin	4 mg/m² IV	Day 1
Adriamycin	45 mg/m² IV	Day 1
Cyclophosphamide	600 mg/m² IV	Day 1
Oncovin	1 mg/m² IV	Day 1
Dexamethasone	6 mg/m² PO	Days 1–5
CHOP-B		
Cyclophosphamide	1 gram/m² IV	Day 1
Hydroxydaunomycin/ Adriamycin	40 mg/m² IV	Day 1
Oncovin	2 mg IV	
Prednisone	100 mg PO	Days 1–5
Bleomycin	15 U IV	Days 1 and 5

plete responders may be increased and, likewise, the proportion cured. (4) Increasing tumor bulk correlates with decreased complete response, the emergence of drug resistance, and poor survival. (5) The highest complete response rates to combination chemotherapy are achieved in patients with regional or disseminated nonbulky disease.

Commonly used agents in combination regimens include: cyclophosphamide, Adriamycin, vincristine, prednisone, methotrexate, bleomycin, etoposide, and cytosine arabinoside. Representative regimens are listed in Table 158–4. Treatment should be initiated promptly after diagnosis and appropriate noninvasive staging; the regimen must be intensive (leading to at least moderate toxicity), administered in high and often escalating doses, on a rigorous schedule; attention must be paid to rapidity of response and any evidence of early drug resistance; and after a defined treatment course, complete restaging is undertaken. Utilizing these guidelines, at least 60 per cent of patients with advanced disease and more than 80 per cent with localized disease will achieve complete response. The majority of complete responses (>70 per cent) are durable, and maintenance chemotherapy is unnecessary.

Intensification of drug treatment has led to further improvement in the results of combination chemotherapy. The MACOP:B drug regimen, for example, delivers high-dose, weekly alternating therapy for 12 weeks followed by no maintenance chemotherapy. Preliminary results reveal 51 of 61 patients (83 per cent) with DLCL achieving complete response and 90 per cent disease free at two years. Another investigative approach has been the use of potentially lethal doses of chemotherapeutic agents with autologous bone marrow rescue in high-risk patients. Preliminary reports suggest that this approach is superior to standard combination chemotherapy.

SPECIAL CONSIDERATIONS. ***Histopathologic Subtype.*** Lymphoblastic lymphoma and SNCL are often treated with modified intensive drug programs, and all patients require central nervous system prophylaxis.

Mediastinal Disease. Superior vena cava syndrome may be present and is effectively managed with irradiation and/or chemotherapy. Biopsy of undetermined mediastinal masses must be accomplished with less than 750 to 1000 rads (200 to 250 rad fractions) prophylactic irradiation before biopsy.

Gastrointestinal Disease. Perforation or bleeding or both are frequent complications prior to or following treatment. To avoid this, surgical resection of the involved region is often recommended prior to therapy.

Central Nervous System. All patients with lymphoblastic lymphoma and SNCL, as well as those with other aggressive histologic types and bone marrow involvement, are at risk for meningeal disease. CSF cytology is determined before therapy, and meningeal prophylaxis is given.

Primary brain lymphoma, as often identified in immunodeficient patients, requires high-dose whole-brain irradiation with or without chemotherapy.

Tumor Masses Larger than 10 Cm. Supplementary irradiation is often administered concurrently with or following chemotherapy. Residual fibrosis may occasionally persist after therapy.

Tumor Lysis Syndrome. Rapid tumor shrinkage with excess urate production should be anticipated in all patients and allopurinol administered. With bulky or disseminated tumor or both, rapid cell lysis may lead to hyperkalemia, hypocalcemia, hyperphosphatemia, hyperuricemia, and acute renal failure. Patients with SNCL and lymphoblastic lymphoma are most often affected (see Ch. 159).

PROGNOSIS

The Working Formulation identifies more than ten distinct disease entities and groups them according to prognosis. The survival curves upon which these prognostic groups were initially based are no longer entirely valid because of improved treatment methods. Nevertheless, it is still important to recognize a low-grade category in which the lymphoma progresses slowly and has an indolent natural history, as well as intermediate and high-grade categories in which the disease

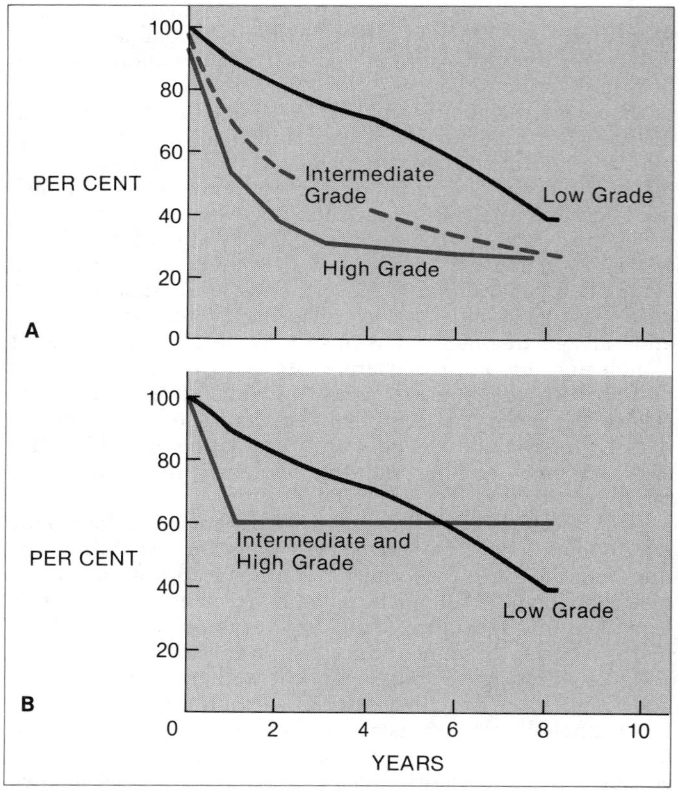

FIGURE 158–1. *A*, Actuarial survival according to histologic grade, based on 1975 data, as reported in the Working Formulation (1982). *B*, Hypothetical actuarial survival according to histologic grade, based on 1985 data (see text).

presents aggressively, progresses rapidly and, if unsuccessfully treated, is soon fatal.

In Figure 158–1*A* are the overall survival curves of the original Working Formulation (based on 1975 data) according to prognostic category. The median survivals are approximately six and one half years for the low-grade, two and one half years for the intermediate-grade, and one and one half years for the high-grade categories. Figure 158–1*B* illustrates representative overall survival curves based on 1985 data, according to prognostic category. The median survival in the low-grade category is six and one half years, unchanged from the original Working Formulation; whereas the median survival for the intermediate and high-grade categories has not yet been reached, and at least 60 per cent of all patients remain alive and disease free at five years. Followed to eight years, the curves overlap as patients in the low-grade category succumb to progressive lymphoma, while patients in the intermediate and high-grade categories continue disease free.

This, then, is the prognostic paradox of the non-Hodgkin's lymphomas: Initially favorable and indolent, the low-grade histologic types are, in fact, the unfavorable category with longer observation; and initially unfavorable and aggressive intermediate and high-grade histologic types are, in fact, the favorable categories, since cure may be regularly achieved.

Broder S: T-cell lymphoproliferative syndrome associated with human T-cell leukemia/lymphoma virus. Ann Intern Med 100:543, 1984. *HTLV-I–associated adult T cell leukemia-lymphoma is discussed in detail in this NIH symposium: clinical features, pathology, epidemiology, and molecular biology.*

Klimo P, Connors JM: MACOP-B chemotherapy for the treatment of diffuse large-cell lymphoma. Ann Intern Med 102:596, 1985. *An intensive weekly combination chemotherapy program completed in three months, yielding complete responses in 51 of 61 patients. Relapse-free survival for complete responders was 90 per cent at two years post-therapy.*

Matis LA, Young RC, Longo DL: Nodular lymphomas: Current concepts. CRC Crit Rev Oncol Hematol 5:171, 1986. *A thorough review of low-grade lymphomas: Clinical management, immunobiology, and molecular biology.*

Skarin AT (ed.): Update on treatment for diffuse large-cell lymphoma. In Advances in Cancer Chemotherapy. Park Row Publishers, Inc., 1986. *Proceedings of a symposium updating combination chemotherapy regimens for diffuse large cell lymphoma.*

Sweet DL, Kinzie J, Gaeke ME, et al.: Survival of patients with localized diffuse histiocytic lymphoma. Blood 58:1218, 1981. *Results of radiation therapy alone in pathologic stage I and II patients. At 11 years, disease-free survival was 93 per cent for stages I and IE; 33 per cent for stages II and IIE.*

The Non-Hodgkin's Lymphoma Pathologic Classification Project: National Cancer Institute sponsored study of classifications of non-Hodgkin's lymphomas: Summary and description of a working formulation for clinical usage. Cancer 49:2112, 1982. *The Working Formulation is presented in detail with pathologic and clinical analyses.*

Waldmann TA, Korsmeyer SJ, Bakhshi A, et al.: Molecular genetic analysis of human lymphoid neoplasms: Immunoglobulin genes and the *c-myc* oncogene. Ann Intern Med 102:497, 1985. *Immunoglobulin gene rearrangement is reviewed and its clinical utility assessed; translocations in Burkitt's lymphomas are also discussed.*

Weis JW, Winter MW, Phylikey RL, et al.: Peripheral T-cell lymphomas: Histologic, immunohistologic, and clinical characterization. Mayo Clin Proc 61:411, 1986. *A review of 40 cases of peripheral T-cell lymphomas emphasizing their histologic and clinical diversity as well as the importance of immunophenotyping.*

Ziegler JL, Beckstead JA, Volberding PA, et al.: Non-Hodgkin's lymphoma in 90 homosexual men: Relation to generalized lymphadenopathy and the acquired immunodeficiency syndrome. N Engl J Med 311:565, 1984. *Aggressive histology of non-Hodgkin's lymphomas involving central nervous system, gastrointestinal tract, and other unusual extranodal sites are described in high-risk homosexual males.*

159 BURKITT'S LYMPHOMA

Carol S. Portlock

Burkitt's lymphoma is a rare monoclonal B cell neoplasm of great biologic importance. It was first described in 1958 by Dr. Denis Burkitt, who reported rapidly growing jaw tumors and abdominal masses in Ugandan children. Over the next 25 years, the elucidation of its unique epidemiologic, pathologic, clinical, and laboratory features has pioneered research into the etiology, pathogenesis, and therapy of lymphoma.

EPIDEMIOLOGY

Burkitt's lymphoma is the most common childhood malignant disorder in Uganda. The disease is found along a "lymphoma belt" lying approximately 10 degrees north and 10 degrees south of the African equator. Within the belt there are altitude, temperature, and rainfall restrictions; these climatic conditions are similar to those of Papua, New Guinea, where Burkitt's lymphoma is also commonly identified. Holoendemic or hyperendemic malaria follows the geographic distribution of the lymphoma belt and originally suggested to Burkitt a mosquito-borne vector and/or associated host immune dysfunction.

In addition to its geographic restrictions, endemic Burkitt's lymphoma is associated with time-space clustering. Nonendemic Burkitt's lymphoma, a similar disease occurring rarely and sporadically in other areas of the world (less than one case per million annually in the United States), has also been reported to occur in time-space clusters. Moreover, nonendemic Burkitt's lymphomas may be associated with preceding immune dysfunction (e.g., organ transplantation and acquired immune deficiency syndrome).

ETIOLOGY AND PATHOGENESIS

The Epstein-Barr virus (EBV) is present in almost 90 per cent of African Burkitt's lymphoma but less than half of nonendemic cases. Whether the virus plays an etiologic role or is merely a passenger in Burkitt's lymphoma remains controversial. Typically, primary EBV infection precedes the development of Burkitt's lymphoma by at least seven or more months. Ugandan children with high EBV capsid antigen titers have a 30-fold greater risk of developing Burkitt's lymphoma as compared with controls. Elevated EBV/VCA titers are also associated with a favorable prognosis in both African and nonendemic tumors.

Specific chromosomal translocations have been identified in Burkitt's lymphoma (with or without the concurrent detection of EBV) and involve chromosomes 2, 8, 14, and 22. The most frequent translocation is t(8;14) (q24;q32) and less commonly t(2;8) (p12;q24) and t(8;22) (q24;q11). The immunoglobulin heavy chain maps to chromosome 14, κ light chain to chromosome 2, and λ light chain to 22. In cell culture, there is a direct correlation between the kind of light chain expressed and the type of chromosomal translocation. Moreover, the cellular oncogene *c-myc* maps to chromosome 8 and is involved in each of the three translocations specific to Burkitt's lymphoma. When *c-myc* is translocated to chromosome 14 within the immunoglobulin heavy-chain gene, the break may occur at different nucleotide sequences, e.g., the variable or switch regions, in different Burkitt's cell lines. It is proposed that this transposition of the oncogene to a transcriptionally active site may thus lead to oncogene activation and ultimately, lymphomagenesis. The delineation of the role of *c-myc* and/or other oncogenes in the etiology of Burkitt's lymphoma and the inter-relationship of *c-myc* (if any) with EBV awaits future research.

PATHOLOGY

Burkitt's lymphoma is classified as a high-grade small noncleaved cell malignant lymphoma. It is composed of intermediate-size lymphoid cells containing round nuclei of uniform size and shape, with coarse chromatin and one or more distinct nucleoli. A rim of basophilic cytoplasm is usually present. Large numbers of mitotic figures are invariably seen and a "starry sky" pattern is characteristic. The cells are of monoclonal B cell lineage, expressing IgM of a single light-chain class on their cell surface.

CLINICAL FEATURES

Although similar histologically, African and nonendemic Burkitt's lymphomas are clinically distinct. The African disease affects children aged 2 to 16, average 7 years, with a 2:1 male predominance. Bulky extranodal tumors of the jaw (70 per cent), abdominal viscera (50 per cent), particularly kidneys, ovaries, and retroperitoneum, and meninges (30 per cent) predominate. Nonendemic Burkitt's affects children primarily, average 11 years, but has been documented in adults as old as 70 years. Male predominance is only evident in patients younger than 15 years. Jaw tumors are rare, abdominal disease involves mesenteric lymph nodes rather than viscera, and bone marrow involvement is frequent.

Burkitt's lymphoma has a growth fraction approaching 100 per cent and a tumor doubling time in vivo of less than three days. Patients present with dramatic enlargement of tumors, and these rapidly enlarging masses may obstruct the gastrointestinal tract or ureters or compress nerve roots or spinal cord. Metabolic consequences of rapid tumor growth include excess urate and lactic acid production as well as acute renal failure.

DIAGNOSIS AND STAGING

The diagnosis must be established by biopsy, since the clinical features are not specific. Diseases that may present similarly include other non-Hodgkin's lymphomas, acute myelogenous leukemia with chloromas, plasmacytoma, fibrous dysplasia of bone, disseminated fungal infection, and several pediatric solid tumors (rhabdomyosarcoma, neuroblastoma, retinoblastoma, and Wilms' tumor). In addition to pathologic sections, touch imprints, immunotyping, and tumor karyotype may be of value.

Rigorous staging is of less therapeutic and prognostic importance in Burkitt's lymphoma than in other lymphomas because all patients receive chemotherapy and the rapidity of disease progression demands treatment within 48 hours of presentation. Nevertheless, it is important to document disease extent to evaluate therapeutic efficacy. Studies should include a careful history and physical examination, blood counts, chemistries (including lactate dehydrogenase), chest radiograph, abdominal computed tomography, gallium 67 scan, bone marrow biopsy or aspirate, and CSF cytology.

MANAGEMENT AND PROGNOSIS

The most important prognostic variable in Burkitt's lymphoma is total tumor volume at initiation of chemotherapy. Surgical debulking prior to chemotherapy is clearly of value in those patients with localized disease. On the other hand, radiation therapy does not offer the same benefit. Combination chemotherapy is used in all patients and may be highly effective. High dose cyclophosphamide may be curative as a single agent; however, the complete response rates and remission durability of combination regimens are superior.

Prior to initiation of chemotherapy it is mandatory to carry out anticipatory therapy of uric acid nephropathy and acute tumor-lysis syndrome (rapid rises in serum potassium, phosphate, uric acid, xanthine, and LDH with reciprocal fall in serum calcium).

With current combination chemotherapy programs (which include cyclophosphamide, Adriamycin, vincristine, and methotrexate) virtually all patients achieve complete remission, while approximately half will have relapse. In spite of CNS prophylaxis, meningeal relapse is common. Nevertheless, aggressive second-line approaches, including high dose regimens with bone marrow transplantation, may be curative. Most relapses after discontinuing initial treatment occur during the first three to six months and are unaffected by maintenance therapy. However, in African Burkitt's lymphoma, very late relapses (occurring 12 to 79 months after discontinuation of treatment) have been reported. Whether some of these relapses represent second neoplasms is not known.

Burkitt DP: The discovery of Burkitt's lymphoma. Cancer 51:1777, 1983. *A personal account.*

Magrath IT, Janus C, Edwards BK, et al.: An effective therapy for both undifferentiated (including Burkitt's) lymphomas and lymphoblastic lymphomas in children and young adults. Blood 63:1102, 1084. *Results of a multiagent intensive drug combination program with intrathecal chemotherapy are described.*

Ziegler JL: Burkitt's lymphoma. N Engl J Med 305:735, 1981. *A complete review of laboratory and clinical data, as well as recommendations for management.*

160 HODGKIN'S DISEASE

John H. Glick

DEFINITION. Hodgkin's disease is a unique malignant disorder, usually arising in lymph nodes, with a characteristic histopathologic appearance. It is defined by the presence of the virtually pathognomonic Reed-Sternberg giant cell in an appropriate cellular background. The disease was first recognized as a distinct clinicopathologic entity in 1832 by Thomas Hodgkin, who described seven patients with a fatal illness involving "hypertrophy of the lymphatic system." Although the etiology is unknown, definitive evidence has emerged that Hodgkin's disease is indeed a malignant neoplasm and not a granulomatous infection or a chronic immunologic disorder. Advances in the pathology, staging, and treatment of Hodgkin's disease during the past two decades have provided a dramatic improvement in the prognosis and potential for cure of all patients with this disease.

ETIOLOGY AND PATHOGENESIS. The cause of Hodgkin's disease is unknown, and the nature of the Reed-Sternberg cell remains an enigma. The Reed-Sternberg giant cell as well as its mononuclear variants is malignant, as established by sustained proliferation in vitro, aneuploidy, and heterotransplantability when inoculated intracerebrally into nude mice. Spleen cells taken from Hodgkin's patients have been grown in tissue culture, with the demonstration of macrophage characteristics, including phagocytic activity and surface receptors for the Fc fragment of immunoglobulins and for the C3b component of complement. Reed-Sternberg cells closely resemble interdigitating reticulum cells found in the interfollicular or T cell region of lymph nodes. Both demonstrate strong expression of human Ia-like antigens, a close physical association with helper/inducer T cells, and a lack of at least two common macrophage antigens. Malignant transformation of the interdigitating reticulum cell to a Reed-Sternberg cell could result in diminished antigen-presenting capacity and could contribute to the known defect in T cell–mediated immunity commonly observed in Hodgkin's disease patients.

The controversy pertaining to the cell of origin is far from resolved. A mouse monoclonal antibody against the Hodgkin cell line L428 has been noted to be specific for both Reed-Sternberg cells and their mononuclear variants, and for a minute and distinct new cell population in normal tonsils and lymph nodes. This observation suggests that a previously unrecognized early myeloid-monocytoid cell may be the progenitor of the Reed-Sternberg cell.

No confirmation of a suggested bacterial, viral, or fungal cause has been obtained. The problem of frequent secondary infections in the immunocompromised patient with advanced Hodgkin's disease continues to thwart investigators searching for an infectious origin. Any theory of the cause of Hodgkin's disease must account for the wide panorama of histopathologic and clinical presentations, the variety of neoplastic giant cells, the signs of an inflammatory reaction and infectious-like symptoms, the characteristic immunologic defects, and the specific epidemiologic patterns.

EPIDEMIOLOGY. Only 7100 new cases of Hodgkin's disease are diagnosed each year in the United States, with approximately 1600 deaths. These patients average 32 years of age and are more commonly male than female. The age-specific distribution curve is an unusual bimodal pattern for both sexes, with the first peak at ages 15 to 35 and the second after age 50. Hodgkin's disease is distributed throughout the world, but the age-specific rates differ markedly in different countries. The developed areas of the United States and Northern Europe have a prominent young adult peak, which is lower in less developed countries and absent in Japan.

There is an inverse risk with family size, with a rate 2.5 times greater among persons without siblings than those with four or more siblings. There is up to a seven-fold increased risk among siblings of young adults with Hodgkin's disease. Increased risk also occurs with early birth order position and improved living conditions. All these factors tend to decrease and delay exposure to infectious agents. It has been suggested that Hodgkin's disease may be an age-dependent host response to a common infection. Population-based studies have failed to document significant "clustering" of cases. No increased risk in medical personnel exposed to large numbers of Hodgkin's patients has been observed. Thus, at the present time, there is no firm evidence for a contagious etiology.

PATHOLOGY. Histologic diagnosis of Hodgkin's disease requires the presence of characteristic Reed-Sternberg giant cells in association with an appropriate stromal background or cellular milieu. The classic Reed-Sternberg cell (Fig. 160–1*A*) is a large, bilobed cell with prominent eosinophilic nucleoli, perinucleolar clearing, thick nuclear membrane, and relatively abundant cytoplasm. Distinctive multinuclear giant cells in lacunar-like spaces (Fig. 160–1*B*) are associated with the nodular sclerosis subtype and are considered Reed-Sternberg variants. Mononuclear variants are also found on biopsy but cannot be considered as reliably diagnostic. Although the diagnosis of Hodgkin's disease is rarely made in the absence of Reed-Sternberg cells, the presence of such a cell is not pathognomonic of the disease. Cells indistinguishable from or closely resembling Reed-Sternberg cells may be found in reactive conditions such as infectious mononucleosis in which immunoblasts, or transformed lymphocytes, may mimic Reed-Sternberg cells. The character of the stromal background is as important for the diagnosis of Hodgkin's disease as is the Reed-Sternberg cell. This background consists of a mixed population of cytologically benign cells, including reactive lymphocytes, benign histiocytes, plasma cells, and eosinophils.

Frozen section material should not be used to make a definitive diagnosis when Hodgkin's disease is suspected because of the presence of artifacts. Formalin-fixed tissue is required for careful histologic review. If any uncertainty of diagnosis exists, consultation with an experienced hematopathologist is required. The monoclonal antibody Leu-M1, which reacts with granulocytes, stains Reed-Sternberg cells and their mononuclear variants. This immunodiagnostic marker may be particularly useful in distinguishing Hodgkin's disease from other lymphoproliferative disorders such as peripheral T cell lymphomas. Needle aspiration of lymph nodes for diagnostic purposes is generally not reliable because insufficient tissue is obtained for accurate evaluation.

Hodgkin's disease is subclassified histopathologically into four subtypes according to the Rye classification (Table 160–1). The relative frequency of the four groups is variable in different series, depending on epidemiologic and patient referral factors. The natural history of Hodgkin's disease correlates well with the histopathologic groups. The *lymphocyte predominance type* is the most favorable and is associated with early stage disease in asymptomatic patients with nodal presentations. The *nodular sclerosis variety* has a relatively favorable prognosis, usually occurs in young women with multiple node groups, and frequently involves the mediastinum. The *mixed cellularity pattern* tends to occur in middle-aged patients with systemic symptoms and more extensive disease than is first evident on initial presentation. The *lymphocyte depletion subtype* has the least favorable prognosis, as it generally occurs in patients with advanced stage disease, systemic symptoms, and frequently involves the bone marrow. Advances in aggressive therapy, after precise staging, have obscured the prognostic value of histopathologic classification.

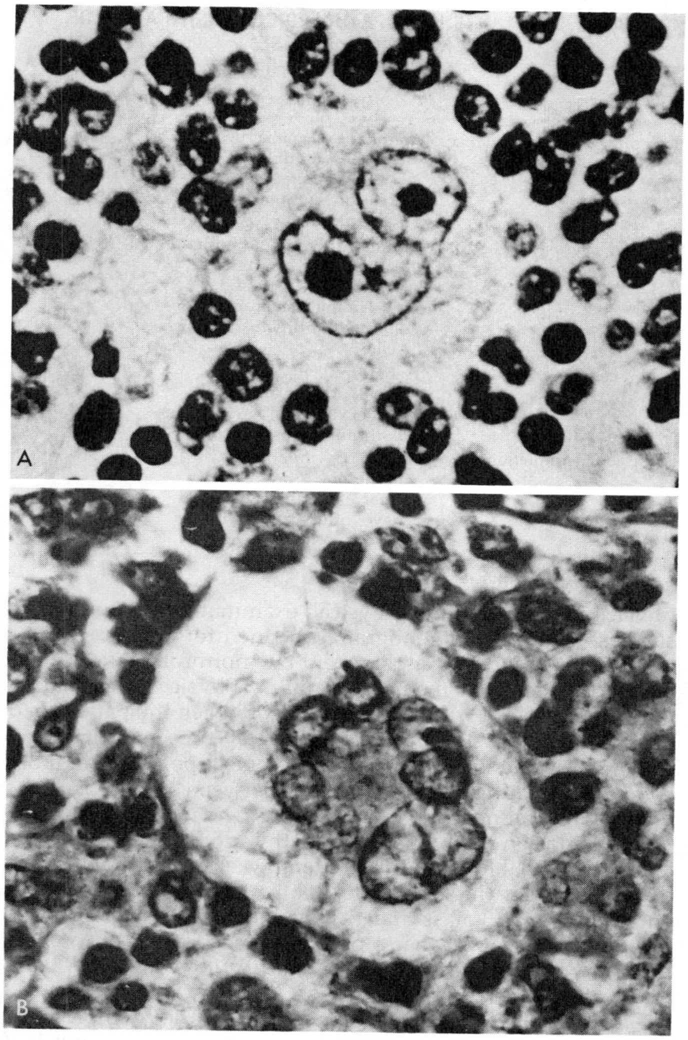

FIGURE 160–1. Pathologic diagnosis. *A*, Diagnostic Reed-Sternberg cell with large inclusion-like nucleoli, high power. *B*, Reed-Sternberg cell variant, lacunar cell type, high power. (Reprinted by permission from Tindle BH: Pathology of Lymphomas. In Bennett JM [ed.]: Lymphomas I. The Hague, Martinus Nijhoff, 1981, p 70.)

CLINICAL MANIFESTATIONS. The initial presentation and subsequent clinical course of patients with Hodgkin's disease can be extremely variable, depending on when in the natural history the patient first seeks medical attention.

Adenopathy. The majority of patients present with a painless and enlarging mass, most commonly in the neck, but occasionally in the axilla or inguinal-femoral region. This lymphadenopathy is usually discovered accidentally by the patient and is often the only manifestation of the disease at the time of diagnosis. Upon examination, this mass is found to be a discrete rubbery usually nontender lymph node or group of surrounding enlarged and matted lymph nodes. Asymptomatic lymphadenopathy also may be noted by the

TABLE 160–1. RYE HISTOPATHOLOGIC CLASSIFICATION OF HODGKIN'S DISEASE*

Subgroup	Major Histologic Features	Relative Frequency
Lymphocyte predominance	Abundant normal-appearing lymphocyte infiltrate with or without benign histiocytes; occasionally nodular; rare Reed-Sternberg (R-S) cells	5–15%
Nodular sclerosis	Nodules of lymphoid infiltrate of varying size, separated by bands of collagen and containing numerous "lacunar" cell variants of R-S cells	40–75%
Mixed cellularity	Pleomorphic infiltrate of eosinophils, plasma cells, histiocytes, and lymphocytes with numerous R-S cells	20–40%
Lymphocyte depletion	Paucity of lymphocytes with numerous R-S cells, often bizarre in appearance; may have diffuse fibrosis or reticulum fibers	5–15%

*Modified from Lukes and Butler.

physician on a routine physical examination. In other instances, a chest roentgenogram, obtained for either a routine purpose or because of a persistent dry nonproductive cough, may demonstrate a mediastinal mass. Physical examination may then disclose lymphadenopathy of which the patient had been unaware. Although these typical presentations may occur at any age with any histopathologic type, they are more common in young patients, usually between 15 and 35 years of age with the nodular sclerosis histologic pattern.

The duration of lymphadenopathy prior to diagnosis is extremely variable. Typically, several weeks to several months elapse between the time of the patient's first observation of an asymptomatic mass and the diagnostic biopsy. However, some patients report that a particular mass has been present for many months to several years, with intermittent waxing and waning in size.

Fever and Systemic Symptoms. Although the asymptomatic presentation is most common, one quarter to one third of patients will present with unexplained and persistent fever and/or night sweats as initial symptoms. Fatigue and weight loss may be associated complaints. Patients with these symptoms tend to be in the older age group, are more often men than women, and are generally discovered to have more widespread disease than the usual patient presenting without symptoms. Although superficial lymphadenopathy is present in most such patients, occasionally palpable lymphadenopathy is absent in the patient past the age of 40 with severe systemic symptoms. These patients present with fever of undetermined origin. Extensive diagnostic efforts may be required to discover the presence of Hodgkin's disease, including lymphangiography, abdominal CT scanning, bone marrow biopsies, or even exploratory laparotomy.

The presence of fever, drenching night sweats requiring the changing of bed clothing, or weight loss exceeding 10 per cent of baseline body weight during the six months preceding diagnosis constitute systemic or B symptoms for staging purposes, and confer an adverse prognosis.

Although fever secondary to Hodgkin's disease is usually low grade, occasional patients have intermittent evening fever lasting several days, alternating with afebrile periods lasting days or weeks. This cyclic fever has been labeled the *Pel-Ebstein type* but is rarely the presenting manifestation of the disease.

Pruritus. Pruritus is another characteristic systemic symptom of Hodgkin's disease. It may be mild and localized, but usually progresses and becomes generalized. Severe pruritus may result in extensive excoriations and inability to sleep. It is rarely relieved by topical medications or antihistamines. The prognostic significance of pruritus itself is unclear. It rarely occurs in the absence of fever and/or night sweats but is no longer considered as a B symptom because its presence does not correlate with an adverse prognosis. Generalized severe pruritus may occur in patients with non-Hodgkin's lymphomas and in other medical and dermatologic conditions, but its presence should always suggest Hodgkin's disease. Its cause is unknown.

SELECTED CLINICAL PROBLEMS. A wide variety of other symptoms may initially call the attention of patients and their physicians to the disease. These same problems occur more commonly as the course of Hodgkin's disease progresses. In addition, almost all patients receive treatment that profoundly affects the natural history of their illness, resulting in either apparent cure or persistent relapsing Hodgkin's disease, or frequently in complications that become difficult to separate from the manifestations of the disease itself.

Pulmonary involvement occurs in only 10 to 20 per cent of patients at presentation. It appears to arise by spread along lymphatics from ipsilateral hilar lymph nodes. Hodgkin's disease frequently involves the lungs with a patchy pulmonary infiltrate without circumscribed borders. Its appearance is variable, and it must be distinguished from radiation effects, drug reactions, and the wide variety of pulmonary infections that occur in these immunocompromised patients. In a severely ill patient in whom the diagnosis is uncertain, the therapeutic significance of these lesions is so great that bronchoscopy with transbronchial biopsy or diagnostic thoracotomy may be justified. Pleural effusions—transudates, exudates, or chylous—are most frequently caused by central lymphatic and venous obstruction resulting from Hodgkin's disease in the mediastinum or obstruction of the thoracic duct. These effusions are rarely caused by direct pleural involvement, and cytologic examination of the fluid or pleural biopsy infrequently reveals diagnostic Reed-Sternberg cells.

Superior vena caval obstruction or compression of the upper airway by mediastinal Hodgkin's disease may be the initial presentation or a complication in the course of the disease. Myocardial involvement is extremely unusual, but pericardial effusions may occur from direct invasion by adjacent mediastinal Hodgkin's disease. Effusions rarely produce cardiac tamponade, and this complication is more often a consequence of radiation-induced pericarditis.

Spinal cord compression, usually caused by epidural spread of tumor from paravertebral lymph nodes through intervertebral foramina in the thoracic or lumbar regions, may be a devastating acute complication. This syndrome may be seen in patients with an otherwise favorable prognosis, although it usually occurs in patients with progressive tumor in whom primary treatment has failed. Back or neck pain, either directly over the vertebral body or occurring in a radicular pattern, should promptly raise the suspicion of cord compression. Symptoms suggestive of more advanced cord compression include numbness, tingling or weakness of an extremity, motor weakness, and bladder or bowel dysfunction. Prompt diagnostic evaluation, including myelography and/or CT scanning, are mandatory, as is prompt therapeutic intervention with immediate radiotherapy to prevent permanent neurologic damage. Surgical decompression is rarely indicated.

Bone involvement may occur from hematogenous spread in advanced disease or by local nodal spread to adjacent bone. Bone involvement often produces pain but rarely fracture, since the bone lesion is generally osteoblastic or mixed osteoblastic and osteolytic.

Hepatic involvement is present in less than 5 per cent of patients at the time of diagnosis and is generally focal in nature. Liver involvement in Hodgkin's disease is almost always associated with splenic involvement. Massive hepatomegaly or jaundice is rarely seen at the time of initial presentation. However, as the liver becomes progressively involved, diffuse infiltration of the portal spaces may be associated with serious hepatic dysfunction and laboratory features of intrahepatic biliary obstruction. Rarely, enlarged lymph nodes in the porta hepatis may produce extrahepatic biliary obstruction. Direct *renal involvement* is rarely a clinically significant problem, but ureteral obstruction and hydronephrosis, secondary to massive retroperitoneal lymphadenopathy, may be seen in far-advanced disease. The nephrotic syndrome, presenting as lipoid nephrosis, is a rare manifestation of Hodgkin's disease and is occasionally accompanied by evidence of glomerular immune complex deposition.

Infectious complications are common in patients with Hodgkin's disease and may or may not be temporarily related to concurrent treatment. Virtually all patients with uncontrolled Hodgkin's disease who succumb to this disorder will have episodes of serious infections at some point in the course of their disease. Localized or disseminated herpes zoster is the most frequently diagnosed serious viral infection, while cryptococcosis, especially of the lungs and meninges, is the most virulent of the fungal complications. *Pneumocystis carinii* pneumonia causes diffuse pulmonary infiltrates and may appear in patients whose disease is in remission between cycles of chemotherapy, as well as in patients in whom relapse occurs. Toxoplasmosis is being recognized with increasing frequency, while tuberculosis has become distinctly uncommon in this population. Children who have undergone splenectomy are particularly predisposed to overwhelming pneumococcal infections unless prophylactic antibiotics or pneumococcal vaccine is administered.

Immunologic abnormalities are common in patients with Hodgkin's disease even at the time of initial diagnosis and prior to initiation of any treatment. A significantly higher frequency of cutaneous anergy is observed than in a control population. The presence or absence of anergy, however, has been shown to have no influence on the prognosis within a specific stage, given the effectiveness of modern therapy. Thus, there is no role for the routine anergy panel. With refined immunologic techniques, a defect in delayed hypersensitivity and T lymphocyte transformation can be detected even in early stage I disease. These deficits are aggravated by therapy and persist for many years even after successful curative treatment. A serum factor, probably an immune complex, has been identified that interferes with T cell function. This factor can be removed in vitro, can block the usual T cell reactions of normal cells, and is probably different from prostaglandins, which are also increased in the serum of some patients. Therapy for Hodgkin's disease undoubtedly accentuates the T cell abnormality. However, it is still unknown whether the observed immunologic abnormalities contribute to the pathogenesis of the disease or are merely secondary phenomena.

STAGING. The progress achieved in the treatment of Hodgkin's disease has paralleled the improvement in techniques for identifying the extent or stage of disease in the untreated patient. In view of the current choices of therapy, it is essential that all cases of Hodgkin's disease be completely evaluated before therapeutic decisions are made. The primary goals of staging are to assess the extent of disease, facilitate the selection of an appropriate treatment program, provide an accurate determination of prognosis, and establish a baseline for re-evaluation following completion of therapy.

The staging classification in current use is outlined in Table 160–2. Patients are assigned a *clinical stage* (CS) on the basis of their initial biopsy, systemic symptoms, physical examination, laboratory results, and radiologic procedures. However, treatment decisions are generally based on a *pathologic stage* (PS), after the extent of involvement has been documented with appropriate biopsies. The basic staging classification is modified by the adverse prognostic significance of systemic symptoms (B disease) and by the realization that localized contiguous extranodal extension (E disease) generally does not carry the same poor prognosis as hematogenous extranodal involvement (stage IV disease).

TABLE 160–2. MODIFIED ANN ARBOR STAGING CLASSIFICATION

Stage	
I	Involvement of a single lymph node region (I) or of a single extralymphatic organ or site (I_E)
II	Involvement of two or more lymph node regions on the same side of the diaphragm (II) or localized involvement of an extralymphatic organ or site and of one or more lymph node regions on the same side of the diaphragm (II_E)
III	Involvement of lymph node regions on both sides of the diaphragm (III), which may also be accompanied by involvement of the spleen (III_S) or by localized involvement of an extralymphatic organ or site (III_E) or both (III_{SE})
III_1	Involvement limited to the lymphatic structures in the upper abdomen; that is, spleen, or splenic, celiac, or hepatic portal nodes, or any combination of these
III_2	Involvement of lower abdominal nodes; that is, para-aortic, iliac, inguinal or mesenteric nodes, with or without involvement of the splenic, celiac, or hepatic portal nodes
IV	Diffuse or disseminated involvement of one or more extralymphatic organs or tissues, with or without associated lymph node involvement

E = extralymphatic site; S = splenic involvement.
Note: The presence of fever, night sweats, and/or unexplained loss of 10 per cent or more of body weight in the 6 months preceding diagnosis is denoted by the suffix letter B. The letter A indicates the absence of these symptoms. Each patient is assigned a clinical stage (CS) on the basis of the initial biopsy, physical examination, laboratory and radiologic results, and a pathologic stage (PS) on the basis of subsequent biopsy results, whether normal or abnormal.

Within each stage of Hodgkin's disease there is a spectrum of patients who have a more or less favorable prognosis, depending on the site or sites of disease, size of the tumor masses, and degree of symptoms. The importance of these prognostic factors and substages within the Ann Arbor classification has become increasingly recognized, because treatment methods are now tailored to individual clinical situations. Controversy exists about the prognostic and therapeutic significance of the E lesion, the size of a mediastinal mass, and the substaging of IIIA patients. PS IIIA disease, for example, may be subdivided into a prognostically favorable III_1 group, in which abdominal disease is confined to the upper abdominal nodes and/or the spleen, and a less favorable III_2 group with disease extending to the lower abdomen, including the para-aortic, iliac, or inguinal lymph nodes. A complete knowledge of staging is vital to guide an efficient but thorough diagnostic evaluation. The tests performed as part of a staging evaluation must be individualized rather than obtained automatically.

DIAGNOSTIC EVALUATION. Recommended staging procedures are outlined in Table 160–3. This evaluation should

TABLE 160–3. DIAGNOSTIC EVALUATION

A. Required procedures
   1. Histologic confirmation by biopsy
   2. Detailed history for unexplained fever, weight loss, night sweats, and pruritus
   3. Physical examination to document all areas of lymphadenopathy, including Waldeyer's ring; size of liver and spleen; bony tenderness. Neurologic evaluation
   4. Laboratory studies
      a. CBC and platelet count, ESR
      b. Serum alkaline phosphatase, LDH
      c. Renal function, including uric acid
      d. Liver function
   5. Radiologic studies
      a. Chest roentgenogram
      b. Bipedal lymphangiogram
      c. CT of the chest and whole abdomen including the pelvis
B. Frequently performed procedures under specific clinical conditions
   1. Bone marrow biopsy (needle or open surgical technique)
   2. Bone roentgenography and scanning for areas of bone pain or tenderness
   3. Gallium whole-body scanning
   4. Staging laparotomy and splenectomy, if therapeutic decisions will depend on the identification of subdiaphragmatic disease

commence promptly after the initial biopsy establishes the diagnosis.

History and Physical Examination. A careful history and physical examination are essential to discover characteristic systemic symptoms and to describe all the lymph node areas of the body. Enlarged lymph nodes are not necessarily involved by disease; reactive lymphoid hyperplasia occasionally occurs in some patients with Hodgkin's disease. If confirmation of Hodgkin's disease in suspicious lymph nodes will change the therapeutic approach, then additional biopsies should be obtained. Although Waldeyer's ring involvement is uncommon in Hodgkin's disease, the lymphoid tissues in this region should be evaluated by physical examination. The size of the liver and spleen should be carefully determined, although mild enlargement of either organ may merely be a sign of nonspecific hypertrophy rather than involvement by Hodgkin's disease. A palpable abdominal mass caused by enlarged mesenteric or para-aortic lymph nodes is a rare initial finding. The bones should be examined for areas of tenderness, and a careful baseline neurologic examination performed.

Laboratory Studies. Routine laboratory tests include a complete blood count, erythrocyte sedimentation rate (ESR), urine analysis, renal and liver function tests, and serum alkaline phosphatase. Mild to moderate anemia may be found in patients with widespread disease and is often associated with normal indices, normal or low reticulocyte count, and a negative Coombs' test. Anemia in a patient with Hodgkin's disease is usually caused by the typical chronic anemia of malignancy, and rarely is secondary to hypersplenism, marrow involvement, or a Coombs'-positive hemolytic anemia. A moderate to marked neutrophilic leukocytosis and thrombocytosis are characteristic of active, symptomatic Hodgkin's disease. Occasionally, the granulocytosis may be so marked as to suggest chronic granulocytic leukemia, but more careful evaluation usually demonstrates that this represents a "leukemoid" reaction. Eosinophilia of a mild degree is common. In patients with severe and longstanding pruritus, moderate or marked eosinophilia frequently occurs. Absolute lymphopenia (<1000 per cubic millimeter) may be seen in a small percentage of patients with more advanced disease, and is usually a poor prognostic sign.

The ESR is commonly elevated in patients with active disease, but has limited sensitivity. Other nonspecific laboratory abnormalities include increased levels of serum alpha$_2$-globulin, fibrinogen, haptoglobin, copper, and zinc; depression of serum iron and iron-binding capacity; and increase of leukocyte alkaline phosphatase. An elevated serum alkaline phosphatase level may be a nonspecific finding or secondary to involvement of bone, bone marrow, or liver with Hodgkin's disease. Elevation of the serum uric acid level is rare at the time of initial presentation, except in advanced stages of disease with massive nodal or bone marrow involvement.

Radiologic Studies. Radiologic examinations should include routine chest roentgenograms, which will demonstrate mediastinal involvement in 50 to 60 per cent of patients. In contrast, hilar disease is seen at presentation in less than 20 per cent of cases. In the absence of mediastinal involvement, hilar disease is unusual. Whole lung tomography is of marginal value and has been replaced by computed tomography (CT) of the chest. CT allows better definition of mediastinal, hilar, and paravertebral adenopathy, and pulmonary involvement. CT of the chest is indicated for all patients. Its role is to define more precisely the extent of disease, including possible localized extension into the pulmonary parenchyma, as well as to assist in radiation treatment planning. The presence of a small pleural effusion in the patient with a mediastinal mass does not necessarily indicate malignant involvement of the pleura. Thoracentesis or pleural biopsy is rarely diagnostic of Hodgkin's disease in these situations.

Subdiaphragmatic sites are best evaluated by performing both bipedal lymphangiography and abdominal-pelvic CT. These examinations are complementary, and neither procedure should replace the other. The lymphangiogram is the most reliable means of assessing involvement of retroperitoneal or pelvic lymph nodes, in that abnormalities of intranodal architecture can be demonstrated in up to 25 per cent of cases at presentation (Fig. 160–2). The overall accuracy of this procedure is 80 to 90 per cent. Lymphangiography is also valuable in preparation for exploratory laparotomy, in that it directs the surgeon to potentially abnormal areas for lymph node biopsy. Lymphangiography is also helpful for planning radiotherapy fields, and especially for assessing the degree of response to therapy during serial follow-up evaluation of the involved retroperitoneal lymph nodes.

Abdominal CT can complement lymphangiography by demonstrating lymphadenopathy in the mesentery, porta hepatis, celiac nodes, and para-aortic nodes above the level of those opacified by the lymphangiogram. CT can only assess nodal involvement when there is an increase in lymph node size. In contrast, lymphangiography provides information on abnormal architecture even in unenlarged nodes. Thus, reliance on CT alone may lead to understaging.

Routine bone scans or skeletal x-ray examinations are not indicated in the asymptomatic patient with a normal alkaline phosphatase. However, in those patients with areas of bone pain or tenderness, bone scans complemented by selective x-ray examinations are indicated to detect osseous lesions.

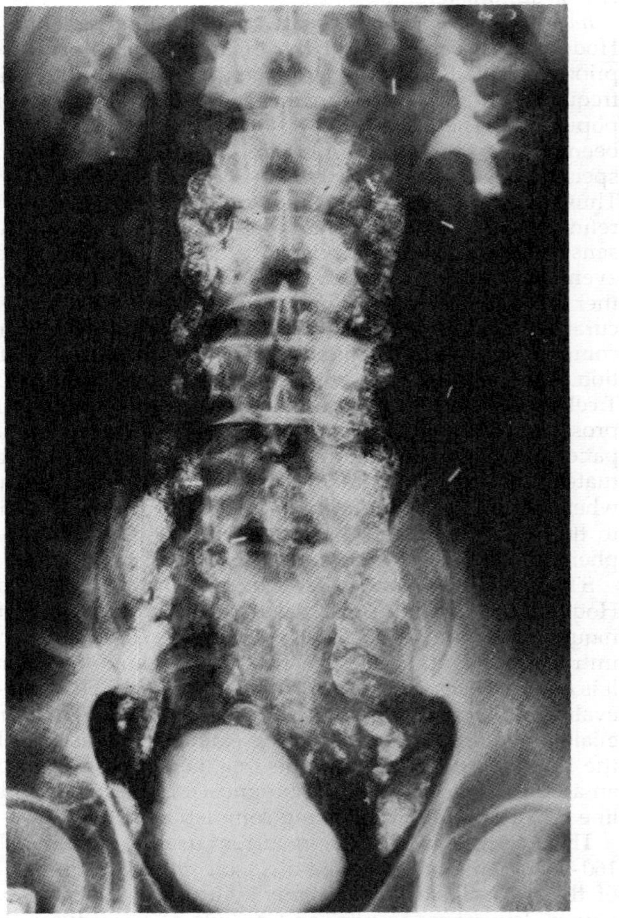

FIGURE 160–2. Abnormal lymphangiogram with enlargement and distortion of the internal architecture in the pelvic, iliac, and paraaortic lymph nodes. Despite the extensive lymphadenopathy, little displacement of the ureters and no obstruction of the upper urinary tracts were seen. (Reprinted by permission from Kaplan HS: Hodgkin's Disease. 2nd ed. Cambridge, Harvard University Press, 1980, p 194.)

Unless the patient has significant hepatomegaly or marked elevations of the liver function tests, liver-spleen scan is not indicated. CT of the liver is more useful in this situation. A single percutaneous needle biopsy of the liver is rarely diagnostic, because of the focal nature of hepatic involvement. Gallium whole-body scans can be helpful in evaluating initial disease as well as potential sites of recurrence, especially in the mediastinum, but cannot be used as evidence of Hodgkin's disease without biopsy confirmation.

Bone Marrow Biopsy. This procedure should be performed in all patients with systemic symptoms or clinical stage III disease or both. It is also useful in patients with significant peripheral blood count abnormalities, increased serum alkaline phosphatase of bony origin, and in those patients with abnormal bone roentgenograms or scans. Hodgkin's disease in the bone marrow is rarely demonstrable by simple marrow aspiration. Involvement is usually focal, often associated with fibrosis, and is diagnosed more readily by either a unilateral or bilateral bone marrow biopsy.

Staging Laparotomy. In the absence of medical contraindications, an exploratory laparotomy with splenectomy is widely employed as part of the routine staging evaluation to identify and confirm the presence of Hodgkin's disease below the diaphragm. The purpose of the laparotomy is diagnostic, the results of which may alter treatment selection significantly. Laparotomy findings that frequently influence both the staging and subsequent treatment include detection of Hodgkin's disease in the spleen, detection of the extent of splenic involvement, and detection of presence of disease in the celiac or retroperitoneal lymph nodes. Secondary benefits from the laparotomy include attempting to preserve ovarian function by means of an oophoropexy when pelvic irradiation is to be utilized in young women, reducing required irradiation fields when the spleen is treated, and improving the peripheral blood counts in the occasional patient with hypersplenism. In one quarter of patients with normal-sized spleens on physical examination, Hodgkin's disease will be found in the spleen removed at surgery. Conversely, approximately 50 per cent of patients with clinical or radiologic enlargement of the spleen do not have histologic involvement. The identification of Hodgkin's disease in the liver is especially difficult. Physical examination, routine liver function tests, and liver scans correlate poorly, if at all, with histologic verification. Liver involvement can be demonstrated at laparotomy on wedge or needle biopsy and is more often found in patients with significant splenomegaly and/or abnormal lymphangiograms.

Staging laparotomy is not a routine diagnostic procedure and should be performed only in those patients in whom the results will potentially modify treatment selection. Discussion of potential treatment options with the radiotherapist or medical oncologist for each stage of Hodgkin's disease should be held prior to the decision to perform a laparotomy. Thus, staging laparotomy with splenectomy is generally recommended for patients with clinical stage I to IIA/B or IIIA disease. Patients with stage IIIB or IV disease are not candidates for laparotomy because combination chemotherapy will be used as their primary method of treatment.

In some cases, staging laparotomy must be deferred or omitted. The patient who presents with massive mediastinal lymphadenopathy should not undergo laparotomy because of the dangers of anesthesia in these patients. In addition, combination chemotherapy is frequently employed in patients with large mediastinal masses, thus eliminating the need for precise staging below the diaphragm.

As a result of staging laparotomy and splenectomy, approximately one third of patients with clinical stages I and II are found to have either subdiaphragmatic lymph node disease or splenic involvement, necessitating extension of the subdiaphragmatic radiation portals. If extensive splenic involvement (> four nodules) is documented, either combination chemotherapy alone or a combined modality program is required. Approximately one quarter of clinical stage IIIA patients (i.e., those with suspicious lymphangiograms or abdominal CT scans) have a negative staging laparotomy that allows their pathologic stage to be downgraded to I or II. Although the results of the laparotomy allow change in the stage in as many as 35 per cent of patients, this change modifies the treatment plan in only approximately 20 per cent, depending on the extent of disease found below the diaphragm. Even in the hands of experienced surgeons, staging laparotomy is associated with a small risk of perioperative morbidity, including infection, fever, and phlebitis, Rare fatalities have been reported. Because of occasional severe bacterial infections occurring after splenectomy, pneumococcal vaccine should be administered preoperatively.

MODE OF SPREAD. Careful mapping of initial sites of involvement of Hodgkin's disease and the use of lymphangiography, staging laparotomy, and splenectomy provide evidence that involvement of various lymph node groups is distinctly nonrandom. Two different theories have been proposed to account for the nonrandom patterns of spread: (1) The *contiguity theory* (Rosenberg and Kaplan) postulates that the disease is unifocal in origin, beginning in an initial focus within the lymphatic system and spreading via lymphatic channels to contiguous lymphatic structures. The contiguity theory has been challenged because of the frequency of cervical, supraclavicular, and retroperitoneal lymph node involvement without intervening mediastinal disease, as well as the common involvement of the spleen, which has no afferent lymphatics. (2) The *susceptibility theory* (Smithers) postulates that the disease is multifocal in origin. The giant cells of Hodgkin's disease are thought to migrate in and out of lymph nodes from the bloodstream but are thought to grow only in preferential sites, presenting an appearance of contiguous spread. Noncontiguous spread is more common in the mixed cellularity and lymphocyte depletion subtypes, when multiple sites are present and when vascular invasion is present. However, the role of vascular invasion in the spread of Hodgkin's disease is not fully understood. Vascular invasion in the spleen may lead to hematogenous dissemination, since the spleen is almost invariably involved when Hodgkin's disease is present in the liver or bone marrow.

TREATMENT. The prognosis for patients with Hodgkin's disease has improved dramatically during the past three decades because of (1) the advances in precise staging and an awareness of the important prognostic factors previously described, (2) the development of supervoltage radiotherapeutic techniques, and (3) the use of effective combination chemotherapy programs.

Radiotherapy. Important factors in determining the success of radiation therapy include the radiation dose per field, the extent of the fields employed, the beam energy, and precision of treatment planning. A tumoricidal dose of 3600 to 4400 rads is required to eradicate the lesions of Hodgkin's disease. Lymphoid regions adjacent to areas of known disease or those that are contiguous via lymphatic channels are usually treated to full dose. Apparently uninvolved areas are treated prophylactically for subclinical disease with dosages of 3600 rads. Large fields, shaped to conform to the patient's anatomy, are designed to treat multiple contiguous lymph node regions. A *mantle* port covers the cervical, supraclavicular, infraclavicular, axillary, mediastinal, and hilar lymph nodes. The *para-aortic* field includes the para-aortic lymph nodes from the level of the diaphragm down to the aortic bifurcation but omits the pelvis and treats the splenic hilar lymph nodes in a patient with a prior splenectomy. An *inverted Y* port includes in one field not only the para-aortic and splenic hilar lymph nodes but also extends into the pelvis to encompass the iliac and inguinal-femoral lymph nodes. The combination of a mantle and para-aortic field is also referred to as subtotal nodal or extended field irradiation. *Total lymphoid irradiation* implies sequential treatment to both a mantle and an inverted Y field.

The use of sequential large field irradiation minimizes the risk of either overlap or underdosage, which could result in either undue normal tissue toxicity or inadequate therapy. Treatment of these large fields requires supervoltage radiation. This capability is available primarily with contemporary linear accelerators, which have the advantages over cobalt of skin sparing, increased depth dose, and sharp beam edges with reduced lateral scatter. The use of a treatment simulator to plan the radiotherapy fields and proper field verification (portal films) during the treatment process is essential.

Definitive radiation therapy alone is appropriate initial management for the majority of patients with pathologic stage I and II Hodgkin's disease. Mantle and para-aortic radiation is the treatment of choice for stages IA and IIA disease, providing an 85- to 90-per cent chance of cure with irradiation alone. Patients with stage IB and IIB disease are treated with mantle and para-aortic or total lymphoid irradiation and have a 70 to 75 per cent chance of cure with such treatment. Controversy exists about the indications for using both radiotherapy and chemotherapy in stage I or II patients who present with large mediastinal masses, limited contiguous extranodal disease (the E lesion of the Ann Arbor system), or systemic symptoms. In each of these disease settings, the use of radiation alone results in a lower disease-free survival rate than when a combined modality program is employed as the initial treatment, although the use of chemotherapy at relapse may provide an equivalent chance of cure. Patients with III_SA or III_1A Hodgkin's disease and minimal splenic involvement are usually treated with total lymphoid irradiation alone. Controversy exists whether prophylactic hepatic radiation should be delivered to those patients with splenic involvement.

Complications of radiation are related to the technique employed, dosage administered, and irradiated volume. Acute side effects of radiotherapy include transient nausea and vomiting, dysphagia, and marrow suppression. These effects subside shortly after radiation therapy is completed. Late potential side effects of radiation include hypothyroidism, pneumonitis, transient myelitis (generally manifested as electric-like shocks in limbs on neck flexion known as *Lhermitte's sign*), and rarely pericarditis. Persistent myelosuppression is a rare late complication. Radiation-induced decreased bone growth has been noted in children.

Chemotherapy. The major advance in the treatment of stage IIIB and IV Hodgkin's disease was the development of curative combination chemotherapy. The initial studies from the National Cancer Institute demonstrated that a four-drug combination known as MOPP (nitrogen mustard, vincristine, procarbazine, and prednisone) was capable of producing documented complete remissions in 70 to 80 per cent of patients with advanced Hodgkin's disease. At least one half to two thirds of the patients who achieved complete remission with MOPP have not had recurrence after more than 10 to 20 years of observation. Thus, 50 per cent of all patients with stage IIIB and IV who underwent treatment were cured with MOPP chemotherapy alone.

The potential for clinical cure of Hodgkin's disease with chemotherapy exists for all histologic subtypes, stages, and extranodal sites of disease. Patients who have received prior radiotherapy in whom relapse subsequently occurs have an equivalent chance of being cured with "salvage" chemotherapy. Older patients and those with bone marrow involvement, systemic symptoms, bulky disease, and poor performance status have a less favorable long-term response with chemotherapy. The best results have been reported for asymptomatic patients with disease limited to the lymph nodes and/or lung.

It is essential to administer the drugs in the MOPP regimen at full doses and in a timely fashion. Therapy is repeated every four weeks for a minimum of six cycles. An additional two cycles are administered after a complete clinical remission is obtained. At that time, chemotherapy is discontinued only when repeat restaging studies document that a true complete remission has been obtained. The restaging diagnostic evaluation includes repeat radiologic procedures and biopsies as indicated to verify the complete response status. Maintenance chemotherapy beyond the documentation of a restaged complete remission is of no advantage in improving either disease-free or overall survival.

No alternative four- or five-drug combinations have been demonstrated conclusively to be superior to MOPP, considering differences in patient selection, prognostic factors, restaging evaluation, and adequate follow-up. However, comparable results to MOPP have been achieved with a variety of alternative chemotherapy programs that offer significantly less toxicity than MOPP. Combinations that contain cyclophosphamide or chlorambucil instead of nitrogen mustard, vinblastine in place of vincristine, and/or the addition of a nitrosourea appear to be as efficacious as MOPP in producing durable complete responses but have substantially fewer side effects. The BCVPP (BCNU, cyclophosphamide, vinblastine, procarbazine, and prednisone) regimen is one example of an equally effective and less toxic alternative to MOPP.

Patients who have relapsed after definitive irradiation for early stage disease are often salvaged and cured with chemotherapy. Patients who have relapsed after initial chemotherapy have a poorer but not hopeless outlook. Patients who have recurrence after a MOPP-induced complete remission of at least one year may benefit from a second course of the same therapy and achieve a second long-term complete remission, but cure is unlikely. Patients who are definitely MOPP resistant should be treated with chemotherapy regimens that contain different or non-cross-resistant drugs. The ABVD program (Adriamycin, bleomycin, vinblastine, and DTIC) is a widely used second-line regimen that results in complete remission in 30 to 60 per cent of patients. However, the follow-up is still too limited to place confidence in the curative potential of these second-line chemotherapy programs.

The identification of an active non-cross-resistant combination in the patient who has had a relapse led to the investigation of sequential alternating chemotherapy regimens (i.e., MOPP alternating monthly with ABVD or a hybrid of seven drugs MOPP/ABV in one monthly cycle) as primary induction therapy. By exposing tumor cells to more drugs early in the course of disease, drug-resistant clones might be eradicated before growing too large to be cured. The objective is to increase the complete remission rates over that which has been demonstrated with MOPP and, more importantly, to improve relapse-free and overall survival. This approach shows considerable promise, especially for patients with stage IV disease, but longer follow-up will be required before this strategy can be adopted as standard practice for advanced Hodgkin's disease.

The major complication of chemotherapy is bone marrow suppression with increased risk of infection and, rarely, hemorrhage. The peripheral blood counts are monitored carefully during chemotherapy and drug doses are adjusted depending on the degree of myelosuppression. However, drug dose reductions made simply for the purpose of decreasing subjective toxicity are inappropriate because the opportunity for cure is also reduced. Sterility, more commonly seen in males, is a permanent side effect of chemotherapy. Significant nausea and vomiting are seen with the MOPP and ABVD regimens. These drug programs often produce serious psychologic problems that require effective counseling, as well as antiemetic agents. Mild peripheral neuropathy is commonly seen with vincristine, but paresthesias are not an indication to reduce drug dosage. Acute leukemia as a late effect of chemotherapy alone is a recognized but unusual complication.

Combined Modality Therapy. Combinations of irradiation and chemotherapy in the treatment of Hodgkin's disease have been utilized during the past 15 years with the goal of increasing the cure rate. It is logical to assume that combination chemotherapy, effective in curing a significant percentage of patients with advanced disease, should be even more effective for occult disease that might be present after radiation therapy. Patients who have recurrence after receiving MOPP chemotherapy frequently have relapse in sites of major pretreatment involvement, including bulky lymph node areas. An additional rationale for combined modality therapy includes improved management of childhood Hodgkin's disease by reduction of radiation fields that may cause bone growth retardation, decreased requirement for staging laparotomy, and reduced complications from newer radiotherapy techniques involving larger treatment fields.

Adjuvant chemotherapy can substitute effectively for prophylactic irradiation of apparently uninvolved sites, but to date there is no clear justification for the routine use of a combined-modality approach for the overwhelming majority of patients with pathologic stage I or II disease. However, there are certain subsets of patients with early stage Hodgkin's disease for whom combined modality treatment is indicated because of an unacceptably high relapse rate; that is, patients with large mediastinal masses or contiguous extranodal involvement.

The treatment of pathologic stage IIIA Hodgkin's disease remains controversial. Retrospective studies have concentrated on identifying prognostic subgroups in which there is an unacceptably low disease-free survival with radiotherapy alone. At the present time, it would be premature for radiation therapists to abandon total nodal irradiation in III_1A patients in whom the prognosis is favorable and who at laparotomy are found to have minimal involvement of the spleen or upper abdominal nodes. In this subgroup, only those who relapse after primary radiotherapy should receive combination chemotherapy. For patients with clinical stage IIIA/pathologic III_2A disease, and for those with extensive splenic involvement, no one management strategy has been proved superior. Acceptable treatment alternatives for this subgroup include combined modality therapy with total nodal or subtotal nodal radiotherapy plus MOPP, initial chemotherapy followed by irradiation to sites of pretreatment involvement, and chemotherapy alone. Although combination chemotherapy remains the mainstay for stage IIIB disease, both improved disease-free and overall survival may be obtained for these patients in whom initial MOPP chemotherapy followed by or sequenced with total nodal irradiation is utilized.

Significant improvement in survival rates as a result of combined modality programs has not been clearly demonstrated for certain subsets of patients. In part, this is because of the long time (ten or more years) required to establish an overall survival benefit. Combined modality programs generally demonstrate improved disease-free survival, but interpretation of current clinical trials must be tempered by the observation that patients who relapse after radiation alone are frequently salvaged or cured with chemotherapy administered only at the time of relapse. It may be more acceptable to treat patients conservatively at the onset of their disease with one method, reserving the more complicated combined modality programs for those patients with poor prognostic factors and an unacceptably high relapse rate after primary irradiation alone.

The complications and morbidity of combined modality programs are significant. The potential risk of acute complications, including profound and prolonged myelosuppression, sterility of both men and women, and demonstrated risk of second malignant tumors, has modified the enthusiasm for a combined modality approach. The incidence of acute myelomonocytic leukemia is approximately 5 to 7 per cent for patients at risk for seven to ten years following combined modality treatment. Paradoxically, this incidence is greatest in patients over the age of 40 years, the group most likely to have an unfavorable prognosis.

Recommended Therapy. The recommended therapy for a patient with Hodgkin's disease must be individualized. Important management considerations include stage and bulk of disease, age, prior therapy, medical complications, and availability of modern skills in radiotherapy and chemotherapy. The improved results of aggressive therapy after accurate clinical evaluation and pathologic staging are achievable only by experienced teams of physicians working closely together to achieve the excellent cure rates now possible while avoiding the risks of excesses in treatment. The recommended therapeutic approaches for the previously untreated adult patient with various stages of Hodgkin's disease are listed in Table 160–4. Estimated results are expressed as the percentage of patients likely to achieve a disease-free interval of five years. Careful evaluation of their condition and observation of a high proportion of patients, perhaps 90 or 95 per cent, who have survived free from relapse for five years demonstrate that they are cured of their disease.

An early stage patient who has relapsed after radiation therapy alone may be cured with salvage chemotherapy. Thus, freedom from first or even second relapse must be considered in the evaluation of both disease-free and overall survival when the results of current clinical trials are analyzed. With dramatically improved treatment results, the challenge

TABLE 160–4. THE TREATMENT OF HODGKIN'S DISEASE IN ADULTS

Ann Arbor Pathologic Stage	Recommended Therapy	Estimated 5-Year Disease-Free Survival (%)	Investigational Therapy
IA, I_EA, IIA, II_EA*	Mantle and para-aortic radiotherapy	85–90	Limited-field radiotherapy ± combination chemotherapy
IB, I_EB, IIB, II_EB*	Mantle and para-aortic or total lymphoid radiotherapy	70–75	Limited-field or subtotal lymphoid radiotherapy + combination chemotherapy; chemotherapy alone
III_1A, III_SA, III_EA*†	Total lymphoid radiotherapy ± chemotherapy	70–80	Total lymphoid radiotherapy, including hepatic irradiation; combination chemotherapy
III_2A	Combination chemotherapy (i.e., MOPP) ± total lymphoid radiotherapy	65–75	Combination chemotherapy + limited-field radiotherapy to areas of pretreatment involvement
IIIB, III_SB, III_EB	Combination chemotherapy (i.e., MOPP)	60	Combination chemotherapy + either total lymphoid radiotherapy or limited-field radiotherapy to areas of pretreatment involvement
IVA, IVB	Combination chemotherapy (i.e., MOPP)	50	Alternating non-cross-resistant chemotherapy (i.e., MOPP-ABVD); combination chemotherapy followed by limited-field radiotherapy to areas of pretreatment involvement

*Patients with large mediastinal masses (>0.33 of the transverse diameter of the chest) will be controlled by irradiation alone in approximately 40 to 50 per cent of cases and should receive combined modality therapy (chemotherapy and irradiation) as primary management.

†Patients with extensive involvement of the spleen (>4 nodules) will be controlled by irradiation alone in approximately 40 per cent of cases and should receive combined modality therapy (chemotherapy and irradiation), or chemotherapy alone as primary management.

facing physicians and investigators caring for patients with all stages of Hodgkin's disease is to weigh carefully the toxicity-benefit ratio for each new recommended regimen.

PROGNOSIS. Hodgkin's disease is a curable malignant condition. Advances in histopathologic classification, precise diagnostic evaluation, and selection of appropriate aggressive therapy have led to continuous improvement in both disease-free and overall survival. Survival figures and prognostic factors that were acceptable 10 or even 20 years ago are not acceptable today. The five-year survival rate has increased from approximately 25 to 50 per cent 20 years ago to at least 75 per cent today.

The success of modern radiotherapy, chemotherapy, or combined modality programs has obscured the significance of such important prognostic factors as histologic subtype, stage of disease, and the presence of systemic symptoms. In recent years, newer prognostic factors have been identified, including anatomic substage III_2A, five or more sites of lymph node involvement, extensive splenic disease, bulky mediastinal lymphadenopathy, and contiguous extranodal extension. Combined modality treatment programs or chemotherapy alone is recommended for patients with these unfavorable prognostic factors. However, any potential disease-free survival advantage seen after combined modality therapy must be balanced by the potential risk of late complications, particularly second malignant conditions, and must be translated into an overall survival benefit before general acceptance.

Table 160–4 presents a reasonable estimate of prognosis, recommended therapy, and current appropriate investigative approaches for the various stages of Hodgkin's disease. These treatment recommendations provide only the broadest of guidelines. Therapy must be individualized, depending on the specific clinical situation and the skill and experience of physicians treating the patient. Any treatment recommendations and estimates of cure must be viewed with the understanding that the management of Hodgkin's disease is dynamic, constantly undergoing change and refinement, and is designed to provide each patient with the best probability of cure and the least possibility of long-term toxicity.

Bakemeier R, Anderson J, Costello N, et al.: BCVPP chemotherapy for advanced Hodgkin's disease: Evidence for greater duration of complete remission, greater survival, and less toxicity than with a MOPP regimen. Ann Intern Med 101:447, 1984. *A large randomized trial that demonstrates that BCVPP is at least as effective as MOPP, but produces significantly less toxicity.*

Bonadonna G, Valagussa P, Santoro A: Alternating non-cross-resistant combination or MOPP in stage IV Hodgkin's disease: A report of 8-year results. Ann Intern Med 104:739, 1986. *An updated report of alternating monthly MOPP-ABVD for stage IV. The patient numbers are small, and the results have not yet been confirmed.*

Canellos G, Come S, Skarin A: Chemotherapy in the treatment of Hodgkin's disease. Semin Hematol 20:1, 1983. *A thorough review of the status of chemotherapy for both early and advanced stages of disease.*

Glick J, Tsiatis A: MOPP/ABVD chemotherapy for advanced Hodgkin's disease. Ann Intern Med 104:876, 1986. *A concise editorial summarizing current results and investigational approaches in advanced Hodgkin's disease. An analysis of the statistical pitfalls of these clinical trials is presented.*

Kaplan H: Hodgkin's disease. 2nd ed. Cambridge, Harvard University Press, 1980. *A detailed, extensively illustrated and referenced volume covering every aspect of the disease as seen by one of the acknowledged experts and pioneers in the field.*

Klimo P, Connors J: MOPP/ABV Hybrid Program: Combination chemotherapy based on early introduction of seven effective drugs for advanced Hodgkin's disease. J Clin Oncol 3:1174, 1985. *A preliminary report of the MOPP/ABV hybrid regimen. Although their results are encouraging, the patient numbers are small and the follow-up too short to allow any conclusions to be drawn as to its superiority over conventionally accepted regimens.*

Leslie N, Mauch P, Hellman S: Stage IA to IIB supra-diaphragmatic Hodgkin's disease. Cancer 55:2072, 1985. *A thoughtful review of the treatment of early stage Hodgkin's disease, emphasizing the experience of the Harvard Joint Center for Radiation Therapy.*

Longo D, Young R, Wesley M, et al.: Twenty years of MOPP therapy for Hodgkin's disease. J Clin Oncol 4:1295, 1986. *A classic and important long-term follow-up report of MOPP-treated patients by the National Cancer Institute group.*

Proceedings of the Symposium on Contemporary Issues in Hodgkin's Disease: Biology, Staging, and Treatment. Cancer Treat Rep 66:601, 1982. *A collection of important papers covering all aspects of Hodgkin's disease. The papers on biology, staging, treatment, and complications are especially worthwhile.*

Rosenberg S, Kaplan H: The evolution and summary results of the Stanford randomized clinical trials of the management of Hodgkin's disease. Int J Radiat Oncol Biol Phys. 11:5, 1985. *An update with long-term follow-up on the important Stanford controlled trials of the use of radiotherapy with or without adjuvant chemotherapy.*

161 LANGERHANS CELL (EOSINOPHILIC) GRANULOMATOSIS

Jerome E. Groopman

The numerous and sometimes confusing classifications of clinical disorders associated with Langerhans cell proliferation reflect our ignorance of both the cause and pathophysiology of many of these diseases. The Langerhans cell belongs to the larger family of cells termed *histiocytes.* Histiocytes are tissue macrophages and include the hepatic Kupffer cell, the alveolar macrophage of the lung, the giant cell of granulomas and the osteoclast in addition to the dermal Langerhans cell. The microglial cell of the brain is probably of macrophage origin as well. All of these tissue macrophages derive from precursor cells that normally reside in bone marrow, mature into circulating blood monocytes, and then egress into tissues and differentiate into a particular type of histiocyte.

A number of benign disorders are associated with proliferation of histiocytes and their fusion into multinucleated giant cells that form granulomas. Langerhans cell (eosinophilic) granulomatosis is an idiopathic benign disease characterized by proliferation and infiltration of tissue by histiocytes and eosinophils. Although this disorder was previously termed eosinophilic granuloma, the proliferating cell that appears primarily responsible for the clinical manifestations of the disorder is the Langerhans cell. The eosinophils may take residence in the lesion because of potent eosinophilic chemotactic factors released secondarily by the histiocytes. Langerhans cell granulomatosis is a distinct disorder unrelated to the eosinophilic syndromes (Ch. 162).

The interaction of "activated macrophages" with surrounding normal tissues may form the pathophysiologic substructure of many of the clinical features of Langerhans cell granulomatosis.

Clinical conditions of unknown cause characterized pathologically by proliferation of tissue macrophages in sheetlike masses with interspersed eosinophils have been difficult to define as specific disease entities. There is great histologic variability within these disorders, and lesions taken from different sites in the same patient may differ pathologically. The clinical course and prognosis do not correlate with histopathologic findings. The concept of Langerhans cell granulomatosis, Hand-Schüller-Christian disease (the classic triad of exophthalmos, diabetes insipidus, and bone destruction) and Letterer-Siwe disease as elements of a continuum termed *histiocytosis X* fails to recognize important differences in clinical course, organ involvement, and therapeutic response. This chapter will discuss unifocal Langerhans cell granulomatosis, multifocal Langerhans cell granulomatosis, and Letterer-Siwe disease. These are the best characterized idiopathic histiocytoses, yet in clinical practice many cases do not readily fit into these categories.

UNIFOCAL LANGERHANS CELL (EOSINOPHILIC) GRANULOMATOSIS

Unifocal Langerhans cell granulomatosis is a benign disorder generally occurring in males during childhood or early adult life. It may occur as late as the sixth or seventh decade of life.

CLINICAL MANIFESTATIONS. The most common presentation of the disorder is a single osteolytic lesion in a long or flat bone, most frequently in the calvarium or femur in children and in a rib in adults. The predilection for skull, femur, rib, pelvis, vertebra, and mandible is not understood. The small bones of the distal extremities are not generally involved. Although the lesions are usually purely lytic, mixed blastic and lytic lesions occur. Pain and swelling over the affected area are common presenting symptoms, although disruption of teeth with mandibular disease, fracture, and otitis media due to mastoid involvement are not infrequent. Many lesions are asymptomatic and diagnosed serendipitously during radiologic evaluation for unrelated problems. Unifocal Langerhans cell granulomatosis of lymph nodes, thymus, or salivary glands is very rare and has the same benign course as that of the more frequent bony lesions. Unifocal Langerhans cell granulomatosis is rarely associated with systemic symptoms and there are no characteristic laboratory findings. Diagnosis is established by biopsy.

DIAGNOSIS. The bone scan is very useful in determining that the lesion is indeed unifocal and in following patients over time for development of new osteolytic lesions. An open biopsy should be performed for diagnosis. Pathologically, an infiltrate with foamy macrophages and admixed eosinophils favors the diagnosis of Langerhans cell granulomatosis. Langerhans' histiocytes contain a cytoplasmic inclusion of unknown composition but with constant thickness and striation termed an *X body.* They also stain by immunoperoxidase for a cytoplasmic protein termed S-100; detection of S-100 assists the histopathologic diagnosis of Langerhans cell granulomatosis.

TREATMENT. At the time of biopsy, curettage, with or without bone chip packing, should be carried out. This simple surgical approach is almost uniformly successful as definitive therapy for an individual lesion. Lesions in anatomic sites that are difficult to approach surgically, such as weight-bearing bones or cervical vertebrae, are best treated by low-dose (300 to 600 rads fractioned total dose) local supervoltage irradiation. This low-dose radiotherapy generally eradicates the proliferating histiocytes and allows for normal bone repair, while high-dose radiotherapy leads to tissue damage and resultant poor healing. Surgical decompression followed by low-dose irradiation is sometimes indicated for lesions requiring emergency intervention, such as those compressing the spinal cord. Patients should be carefully followed after therapy for the development of new lesions, which generally arise within the first year after diagnosis. Individuals with a lesion in the bones of the head, neck, or pelvis are more likely to have subsequent disease. Bone scans to detect new lesions and plain films to follow the known site of involvement should be obtained every six months for one to two years after therapy. Extraosseous Langerhans cell granulomatosis involving soft tissue is generally successfully managed by complete surgical excision if possible, or by low-dose irradiation.

MULTIFOCAL LANGERHANS CELL (EOSINOPHILIC) GRANULOMATOSIS

CLINICAL MANIFESTATIONS. Similar to the unifocal form, multifocal Langerhans cell granulomatosis generally presents in children, predominantly in males, and often with *bone lesions.* In addition to the calvarium, the sphenoid bone, sella turcica, mandible, and long bones of the upper extremities may be involved. This tropism for the head is unexplained but may indicate local reaction to an inciting agent that enters via the nasopharynx or oropharynx. Complications of this disorder include chronic otitis media caused by destruction of temporal and mastoid bones, proptosis with orbital masses, loose teeth with infiltration of maxilla or mandible, and both anterior and posterior pituitary dysfunction with involvement of the sella turcica. This last complication may occur with focal disease of hypothalamus or pituitary without bone involvement, and growth retardation of the patient may occur. Diabetes insipidus is caused by granulomatous involvement of the hypothalamus or pituitary and may be either transient or permanent. The classic triad of lytic skull lesions, exophthalmos, and diabetes insipidus called *Hand-Schüller-Christian disease* is best viewed as a subset of multifocal Langerhans cell (eosinophilic) granulomatosis. Dermal lesions may appear papulosquamous, seborrheic, eczematous, and rarely xanthomatous. Vulvar lesions with ulceration are not uncommon. Hepatosplenomegaly and lymphadenopathy are unusual in multifocal Langerhans cell granulomatosis.

In *Langerhans cell granulomatosis* the lung is an important extraosseous site of involvement. The disorder mainly affects young adult men and often presents with a chronic cough, pneumothorax, and constitutional symptoms. The chest radiograph usually shows a diffuse micronodular and interstitial infiltrate involving the mid-zones and bases of the lungs with relative sparing of the costophrenic angles. Ultimately a honeycomb appearance may occur; it is caused by coalescence of small parenchymal pulmonary cysts. Fibrosis is a late finding that may lead to chronic cor pulmonale. Pulmonary function tests may show restrictive impairment. Diagnosis is best made by biopsy that shows the mixed histiocytic-eosinophilic infiltrate with a variable degree of fibrosis. Pulmonary Langerhans cell granulomatosis has a highly variable natural history. Spontaneous remissions are not infrequent, but prognosis is poorer at the extremes of age and with involvement of extrapulmonary organs.

DIAGNOSIS. There are no distinctive laboratory abnormalities in multifocal Langerhans cell granulomatosis. The leukocyte count is generally normal and eosinophilia is not present unless it is from another cause. Hypercalcemia generally does not result from bone lesions.

The diagnosis of multifocal Langerhans cell granulomatosis is definitively made by biopsy, usually of a bone lesion. Again, S-100 detected by the immunoperoxidase method may be useful in confirming the diagnosis. The extent of multifocal involvement is established by physical examination, chest radiography, bone scanning, and if indicated, computed tomography of the brain. This last test is useful for hypothalamic or pituitary lesions associated with diabetes insipidus.

TREATMENT. The natural history of multifocal Langerhans cell granulomatosis is relatively favorable when cases best diagnosed as Letterer-Siwe disease (see below) are excluded. Destructive lesions of bone when present early in the clinical course may predict a better outcome. The therapy is guided by the particular organs involved. Diabetes insipidus and growth retardation should be treated by hormonal replacement with vasopressin (Ch. 226) and human growth hormone, respectively. Low-dose irradiation to the suprasellar area may restore endocrine function in certain individuals. The seborrheic dermal eruption is responsive to tar treatments. X-irradiation using doses generally below 600 rads to symptomatic bony lesions is nearly always effective. Surgery may be necessary to relieve spinal cord compression and mastoid problems and to excise skull lesions eroding through skin. Oral granulomatosis can be treated with dexamethasone elixir used as a mouth rinse three times a day. Similarly, topical steroid creams may accelerate the healing of vulvar lesions.

Systemic therapy is indicated when either radiation fails or multiple sites demand treatment. Corticosteroids alone may achieve dramatic results. Prednisone at a single dose of 0.5 to 1.0 mg per kilogram can be used in the acute phase. Alternate day corticosteroid therapy can be initiated after remission is achieved. Use of cytotoxic agents, such as vinblastine or methotrexate, is generally reserved for aggressive and refractory disease.

There is insufficient experience to recommend a single first-line chemotherapeutic regimen. Addition of vinblastine at a dose of 0.1 mg per kilogram intravenously every week for four to eight weeks is generally successful in achieving remission. It is unclear whether maintenance chemotherapy with weekly vinblastine or prednisone is required to sustain remission. Should disease recur within several months after discontinuation of therapy for the acute phase, the patient should be re-treated with the initially successful regimen and receive maintenance therapy. The striking variability in clinical course makes it difficult to generalize with regard to therapeutic guidelines.

LETTERER-SIWE SYNDROME

In 1924 Letterer described a six-month-old child with diffuse purpura, fever, otitis media, lymphadenopathy, and hepatosplenomegaly. Nine years later, Siwe included this case in a series of six similar cases. In all instances, there was diffuse tissue infiltration by histiocytes. The histiocytes of Letterer-Siwe disease have abundant acidophilic cytoplasm and are often vacuolated. There may be prominent hemophagocytosis. Generally there is a relative paucity of eosinophils in the histiocytic infiltrates.

CLINICAL MANIFESTATIONS. Children are usually affected in the first years of life, although an adult form of the syndrome may exist. Liver, spleen, lymph nodes, lung, and bone are the most commonly affected areas. Laboratory evaluation often demonstrates leukocytosis, although pancytopenia caused by hypersplenism or bone marrow infiltration may be seen. The dermal lesion of Letterer-Siwe disease is generally a brown-red, scaly eczematoid or seborrheic eruption, and purpura secondary to thrombocytopenia may be present. Hepatosplenomegaly may occur with or without jaundice or elevated levels of hepatic parenchymal enzymes. There is no familial or hereditary predisposition, and that distinguishes Letterer-Siwe disease from another histiocytic disorder of infants, familial erythrophagocytic lymphohistiocytosis. A clinical pathologic syndrome nearly identical to Letterer-Siwe disease has been described in immunologically compromised children infected with a variety of viruses. In addition, certain cases termed Letterer-Siwe disease may actually be unusual forms of malignant lymphoma.

TREATMENT. The course of Letterer-Siwe disease is commonly fulminant and fatal. Spontaneous remissions are rare. It is important to distinguish Letterer-Siwe disease from disorders of infectious or clearly neoplastic origin before initiating therapy. Systemic symptoms of Letterer-Siwe disease often improve with corticosteroids and focal lesions may be palliated with radiotherapy. Occasionally, clinical remission has been achieved with chemotherapy, particularly vinblastine and prednisone. If this regimen fails, methotrexate and 6-mercaptopurine may be used. Successful allogeneic bone marrow transplantation has been reported in a single case.

Chu T, D'Angio GJ, Favara B, et al.: Histiocytosis syndromes in children. Lancet 1:208, 1987. *This brief article offers an up-to-date classification of this group of disorders "not only as a standard for diagnosis and patient management but also for research and for use in publications on the subject."*

Elema JD, Atmosoerodjo-Briggs JE: Langerhans' cells and macrophages in eosinophilic granuloma: An enzyme-histochemical, enzyme-cytochemical, and ultrastructural study. Cancer 54:2174, 1984. *An excellent description of histopathology of histocytic disorders with emphasis on diagnostic markers such as the S-100 protein.*

Greenberger JS, Crocker AC, Vawter G, et al.: Results of treatment of 27 patients with systemic histiocytosis (Letterer-Siwe syndrome, Schuller-Christian syndrome and multifocal eosinophilic granuloma). Medicine 60:311, 1981. *A detailed analysis of therapy of histiocytic disorders at a single academic medical center.*

Groopman JE, Golde DW: The histiocytic disorder: A pathophysiologic analysis. Ann Intern Med 94:95, 1981. *Comprehensive review of the histiocytic disorders with emphasis on pathophysiologic mechanisms; extensive bibliography.*

Komp DM: Langerhans cell histiocytosis. N Engl J Med 316:747, 1987. *An informative editorial with an excellent bibliography.*

Risdall RJ, McKenna RW, Nesbit ME, et al.: Virus-associated hemophagocytic syndrome. A benign histiocytic proliferation distinct from malignant histiocytosis. Cancer 44:993, 1979. *Importance of considering infectious causes of clinicopathologic syndromes easily misdiagnosed as histiocytic disorders.*

Sims DG: Histiocytosis X: Follow-up of 43 cases. Arch Dis Child 52:433, 1977. *A large series followed over a long period; illustrates the striking variability in clinical course.*

Zinkham WH: Multifocal eosinophilic granuloma: Natural history, etiology and management. Am J Med 60:457, 1976. *A comprehensive and well-written clinical paper; of great assistance in clinical management.*

162 EOSINOPHILIC SYNDROMES

David A. Bass

Many diseases that cause eosinophilia, such as parasitic infestations, allergies, and drug reactions, are discussed elsewhere in this book. This chapter provides a brief summary of the distinctive qualities of eosinophils and the types of disease that may be associated with eosinophilia in the peripheral blood.

Eosinophils are granulocytic leukocytes and share with neutrophils similar life cycles, morphology, lysosomal enzymes, potent oxidative metabolism, and phagocytic ability. The distinctive qualities of eosinophils become apparent in their responses during specific immunologic and inflammatory processes. Acute inflammation causes stimulation of neutrophil production, inhibition of eosinophil production, and eosinopenia in the peripheral blood. Administration of glucocorticosteroids causes eosinopenia and neutrophilia. Moreover, unlike neutrophils, eosinophils appear closely linked to the immune system. Eosinophil stimulation most commonly follows repeated or prolonged antigenic exposure, especially when the antigens are deposited in tissues and elicit hypersensitivity reactions. Stimulation of eosinophilia in delayed hypersensitivity reactions is T lymphocyte dependent. During immune responses to metazoan parasites, lymphocytes release substances that stimulate eosinopoiesis.

The functions of eosinophils remain a subject of debate. The two currently favored hypotheses appear contrasting, if not contradictory. One hypothesis views the eosinophil as a protective killer cell, similar to the neutrophil, but specifically involved in defense against metazoan parasites. The alternative theory views the eosinophil as an anti-inflammatory modulator of hypersensitivity reactions, serving to constrain the immune response and minimize its unnecessary spread.

Eosinophils may on occasion be harmful rather than beneficial. Prolonged, marked eosinophilia may be associated with Löffler's endomyocardial disease, discussed below. Eosinophils may also contribute to localized tissue damage in specific syndromes. For example, a component of eosinophil granules, the major basic protein, causes cytopathic changes in tracheal epithelium in vitro that are similar to the changes observed in patients with asthma.

EOSINOPHILIC SYNDROMES AFFECTING ORGAN SYSTEMS

HYPEREOSINOPHILIC SYNDROME. This is a myeloproliferative syndrome with persistent, marked eosinophilia (above 1500 per cubic millimeter) and evidence of organ involvement. Eosinophilic infiltrates may cause dysfunction of diverse tissues, including the following: The heart may reveal the changes of Löffler's endomyocardial disease. Most patients have hepatosplenomegaly, although laboratory studies of hepatic functions demonstrate minimal abnormalities, usually limited to a modest elevation of serum alkaline phosphatase. Central nervous system complications may present as diffuse changes (confusion, delusion, psychosis, coma) or localized problems, including peripheral neuropathies or hemiparesis. Gastrointestinal involvement may cause diarrhea, nonspecific abdominal pains, and occasionally malabsorption syndromes. Pulmonary involvement may present as interstitial infiltrates that contain large numbers of eosinophils on biopsy. Pleural effusions may occur. Rashes occur in 25 to 50 per cent of the patients and are usually nonspecific, urticarial, or maculopapular. The presence of angioedema has been suggested to be a favorable indicator of therapeutic responses. Patients often have a mild normochromic normocytic anemia, but severe anemia or thrombocytopenia is rare. Once organ involvement is demonstrated, the prognosis without treatment is poor, with about half dying by nine months.

However, about one third of the patients with this syndrome may respond to corticosteroid therapy; moreover, the majority of the remainder may have a favorable response to hydroxyurea. Death is often due to cardiac involvement with endomyocarditis and congestive failure. Death caused by infections or thrombocytopenia with bleeding is unusual. Rare cases have terminated in a blastic crisis, even following "successful" treatment with hydroxyurea.

EOSINOPHILIC LEUKEMIA. Eosinophilic leukemia is rare. A number of patients have been described with immature eosinophils in the peripheral blood, thrombocytopenia, and severe anemia. In some patients chromosomal aberrations, including the Philadelphia chromosome, have been described.

LÖFFLER'S ENDOMYOCARDIAL DISEASE. This involves a thickening of the endocardium with subendocardial myocardial degeneration and infiltration by eosinophils. Either or both ventricles may be involved; atria are usually minimally affected. It may present as a restrictive cardiomyopathy and/or valvular dysfunction, usually mitral regurgitation, leading to right- or left-sided congestive heart failure. Mural thrombi may further compromise cardiac function or cause embolic events. Over 90 per cent of the patients are males. This disease may be due to the release of some component of eosinophil leukocytes, since it has been observed during diverse illnesses characterized by great and prolonged blood eosinophilia, i.e., an eosinophil count higher than 2000 per cubic millimeter for longer than 12 months, including solid tumors, metazoan parasites, hypersensitivity vasculitis, the hypereosinophilic syndrome, and eosinophilic leukemia.

DISEASES ASSOCIATED WITH EOSINOPHILIA

(Table 162–1)

ALLERGIES AND DRUG REACTIONS. These are discussed in other chapters. Although acute allergic reactions may cause leukemoid eosinophilic responses (eosinophils above 20,000 per cubic millimeter), chronic allergy is rarely associated with eosinophil counts above 2000 per cubic millimeter.

INFECTIONS. Infestations by *invasive metazoan parasites* almost always cause eosinophilia. Noninvasive helminths (e.g., pinworm, whipworm) or encysted parasites (e.g., echinococcus) are less regularly associated with peripheral eosinophilia. Protozoa do not usually cause eosinophilia. Mycobacterial and fungal infections are not usually associated with eosinophilia; however, about 10 per cent of patients with afebrile *tuberculosis* may have a modest increase in blood eosinophils. Acute *coccidioidomycosis* often causes immunologic manifestations, including erythema nodosum, erythema multiforme, urticaria, polyarthritis, and eosinophilia. Acute bacterial and viral infections are usually associated with eosinopenia in the peripheral blood. Exceptions to this rule include the eosinophilias of *chlamydial pneumonia of infancy, cat scratch disease, infectious lymphocytosis,* and occasional cases of *infectious mononucleosis.* During the convalescent phase of acute infections, occasional patients will develop a transient, usually mild eosinophilia. In scarlet fever, eosinophilia regularly appears coincidentally with the characteristic rash.

SKIN DISEASES. Diverse skin diseases may be associated with eosinophilia. Best documented are the eosinophilias of *atopic dermatitis, eczema, acute urticaria* (but not chronic urticaria or angioneurotic edema), *pemphigus, bullous pemphigoid, herpes gestationis,* and *Wells' syndrome.* Eosinophil counts may be useful in the evaluation of *toxic epidermal necrolysis.* Eosinophil counts are usually elevated when this entity is due to a drug reaction but are usually reduced when staphylococci are the cause.

PULMONARY EOSINOPHILIAS. See Ch. 63.

EOSINOPHILIC GASTROENTERITIS. See Ch. 162.

NEOPLASTIC DISORDERS. A small proportion, about 5 per cent, of patients with *carcinomas* and *sarcomas* may have eosinophilia. Eosinophilia with solid tumors may be indicative of metastatic dissemination. A mild eosinophilia accompanies *Hodgkin's disease* in roughly one fifth of patients; however, in occasional cases, marked eosinophilia (up to 98 per cent) has occurred. *Immunoblastic lymphadenopathy* is associated with eosinophilia in about one third of cases. Cutaneous involvement with neoplastic disorders, including histiocytic medullary reticulosis, mycosis fungoides, and Sézary's syndrome, may have an associated eosinophilia.

TABLE 162–1. DISORDERS ASSOCIATED WITH EOSINOPHILIA

- **I. Allergy**
  - A. Allergic rhinitis
  - B. Asthma
  - C. Atopic dermatitis
  - D. Acute urticaria
  - E. Drug reactions
- **II. Infectious diseases**
  - A. Tissue-invasive helminths
    - 1. Major tropical
      - a. Filariasis
      - b. Schistosomiasis
    - 2. North America
      - a. Strongyloidiasis
      - b. Trichinosis
      - c. Toxocariasis
      - d. Ascariasis
      - e. Occasional in hookworm disease, echinococcosis, cysticercosis
  - B. Other infections
    - 1. Acute coccidioidomycosis
    - 2. Afebrile tuberculosis
    - 3. Cat scratch disease
    - 4. Chlamydial pneumonia of infancy
    - 5. Convalescent phase of many infections, especially scarlet fever
- **III. Other cutaneous diseases**
  - A. Bullous pemphigoid
  - B. Herpes gestationis
  - C. Recurrent granulomatous dermatitis
  - D. Scabies
- **IV. Other pulmonary diseases**
  - A. Transient pulmonary eosinophilic infiltrates (Löffler's syndrome)
  - B. Hypersensitivity pneumonitis
  - C. Allergic bronchopulmonary aspergillosis
  - D. Tropical eosinophilia
  - E. Chronic eosinophilic pneumonia
- **V. Connective tissue diseases**
  - A. Polyarteritis group
    - 1. Allergic granulomatosis (Churg-Strauss type)
    - 2. Angiitis with hepatitis B antigenemia
  - B. Rheumatoid arthritis (severe)
  - C. Eosinophilic fasciitis
  - D. Sjögren's syndrome
- **VI. Neoplastic and myeloproliferative diseases**
  - A. Solid tumors, especially mucin secreting, epithelial cell origin especially when metastatic to serosa or bone
  - B. Lymphoid
    - 1. Lymphomas, especially T cell type and Hodgkin's disease
    - 2. T cell and acute lymphoblastic leukemias
    - 3. Occasional with myeloma (heavy chain disease)
  - C. Hypereosinophilic syndrome
  - D. Other
    - 1. Histiocytosis with cutaneous involvement
    - 2. Angiolymphoid hyperplasia (Kimura's disease)
- **VII. Immunodeficiency diseases**
  - A. Selective IgA deficiency
  - B. Swiss-type and sex-linked combined immunodeficiency
  - C. Nezelof syndrome
  - D. Wiskott-Aldrich syndrome
  - E. Hyper-IgE syndrome
  - F. Graft versus host reactions
- **VIII. Occasional causes of eosinophilia**
  - A. Eosinophilic gastroenteritis
  - B. Inflammatory bowel disease
  - C. Chronic active hepatitis
  - D. Long-term dialysis
  - E. Acute pancreatitis
  - F. Postirradiation
  - G. Hypopituitarism
  - H. Other localized disorders with occasional blood eosinophilia
    - 1. Eosinophilic lymphadenitis
    - 2. Eosinophilic cystitis
    - 3. Eosinophilic cholecystitis
    - 4. Eosinophilic meningitis

IMMUNE DISEASES. In the absence of pulmonary involvement, polyarteritis is rarely associated with eosinophilia. By contrast, *polyarteritis with pulmonary involvement* (asthma) and the *allergic granulomatosis of Churg and Strauss* are associated with eosinophilia in a great majority of cases. The syndrome of *polyarteritis in association with hepatitis antigenemia* may also be accompanied by eosinophilia. Mild eosinophilia occurs in about 10 per cent of patients with *rheumatoid arthritis* at some time during their disease. Occasional cases, usually those of long standing with nodules and pleuropulmonary involvement, may have marked peripheral blood eosinophilia. The syndrome of *eosinophilic fasciitis* is discussed in Ch. 437. In one large series, about two thirds of patients with *Sjögren's syndrome* had eosinophilia. Mild eosinophilia is often noted in *immune deficiency syndromes,* whether involving the T or B lymphocyte series, and in certain defects of neutrophil production or function. Such patients may respond to pulmonary infection by *Pneumocystis carinii* with marked eosinophilia. The syndrome of *eosinophilic lymphadenitis* is characterized by peripheral blood eosinophilia associated with localized, usually inguinal or axillary, lymphadenopathy. The response appears to follow repeated local exposures to an antigen, such as an insect sting, on a peripheral extremity. Involved lymph nodes may be densely infiltrated with eosinophils.

Many other diseases of presumed immunologic etiology are not associated with eosinophilia; these include systemic lupus erythematosus, systemic sclerosis, glomerulonephritis, acute rheumatic fever, serum sickness, autoimmune hemolytic anemia, thrombocytopenic purpura, Hashimoto's thyroiditis, pernicious anemia, and myasthenia gravis.

RADIATION-RELATED EOSINOPHILIA. About 40 per cent of patients with an intra-abdominal neoplasm exhibit eosinophilia during the first few weeks of radiation therapy. Such patients may also develop proctitis with a marked local infiltration of eosinophils.

INFLAMMATORY BOWEL DISEASE. Local inflammatory lesions of *ulcerative colitis* may be rich in eosinophils, and a slight elevation of blood eosinophils may occur in this disease. Some observers have also reported modest eosinophilia during symptomatic phases of *Crohn's disease,* and this may be a helpful guide in differentiating Crohn's disease from acute appendicitis.

CHRONIC ACTIVE HEPATITIS. About one third of patients with chronic hepatitis have eosinophils in excess of 5 per cent.

DRESSLER'S SYNDROME. Although not mentioned in recent reviews, 20 per cent of the patients in Dressler's original series had eosinophilia.

PANCREATIC DISEASES. A distinctive clinical syndrome associated with acinar cell carcinoma of the pancreas includes polyarthritis, subcutaneous panniculitis, and blood eosinophilia. Similar symptoms and signs may be observed two to six weeks following acute pancreatitis.

DIALYSIS. About one third of patients undergoing long-term hemodialysis develop blood and bone marrow eosinophilia without apparent cause. Similarly, long-term peritoneal dialysis may evoke an eosinophilic peritoneal effusion and occasionally elevated numbers of eosinophils in the blood. This eosinophilic peritonitis may be associated with abdominal pain and fever, and may be mistaken for a bacterial infection unless a differential count of the exudate is obtained.

ADDISON'S DISEASE. Although occasional patients with Addison's disease and eosinophilia have been observed, this is not typical. In one series, the only patients with eosinophilia had hypopituitarism.

Fauci AS, Harley JB, Roberts WC, et al: The idiopathic hypereosinophilic syndrome: Clinical, pathophysiologic, and therapeutic considerations. Ann Intern Med 97:78, 1982. *An excellent up-to-date summary of the eosinophil and hypereosinophilia from the National Institutes of Health.*

Weller PF, Goetzl EJ: Dermatological conditions associated with eosinophilia and eosinophilic diseases. In Kay AB, Goetzl EJ (eds.): Contemporary Issues in Clinical Immunology and Allergy: Immunodermatology. Edinburgh, Churchill Livingstone, 1984. *A general review of the disorders associated with eosinophilia and how they should be approached clinically.*

163 PLASMA CELL DISORDERS

Sydney E. Salmon

GENERAL CONSIDERATIONS

The plasma cell disorders are a group of related neoplastic diseases associated with proliferation of a single clone of immunoglobulin-secreting plasma cells derived from the B cell series of immunocytes. This group of disorders has variously been referred to with a series of synonymous terms: monoclonal gammopathies, plasma cell dyscrasias, gammopathies, immunoglobulinopathies, paraproteinemias, and dysproteinemias.

The plasma cell disorders to be discussed here are monoclonal neoplasms; their secreted immunoglobulin products are electrophoretically and immunologically homogeneous and therefore readily distinguished from the heterogeneous populations of immunoglobulin-antibody molecules secreted by the numerous clones of normal B cells. There are five major classes of immunoglobulins synthesized by B lymphocytes and plasma cells: IgG, IgA, IgM, IgD, and IgE (see Ch. 417). Immunoglobulins are antibody protein molecules that all have a basic monomeric unit structure of two heavy (H) chains and two light (L) chains, which each have "constant" and "variable" regions with respect to amino acid sequence. IgG, IgA, IgD, and IgE are synthesized and secreted as monomers with molecular weights in the range of 150,000 to 190,000; IgM is secreted as a pentameric structure with a molecular weight of 900,000. Class specificity of each immunoglobulin is defined in terms of a series of antigenic determinants on the constant regions of the H chains (γ, α, μ, δ, ϵ). There are also two major types of L chains (κ and λ) defined by antigenic determinants on the constant regions of the L chains. The amino sequence in the variable regions of immunoglobulin molecules corresponds to the zone of the active antigen-combining site of the antibody, whereas the constant regions convey other biologic properties. (Structural and functional properties of immunoglobulins are summarized in Table 417–1 and Figure 417–1).

A homogeneous immunoglobulin, as a sharp peak or "spike" in the beta or gamma globulin zone on electrophoresis, is referred to as an M-component. Electrophoresis and immuno-electrophoresis, respectively, are used to quantitate and qualitatively identify M-components. Definition of an M-component as monoclonal (having a single H chain and a single L chain type) requires immunoelectrophoretic or immunofixation studies or both.

Plasma cells represent the most well-differentiated progeny in the B cell series of immunocytes. They contain substantial quantities of rough-surfaced endoplasmic reticulum that is rich in RNA, and are specialized for production of antibody molecules at a rapid rate. In the normal immune response, individual plasma cells can synthesize and secrete immunoglobulin at rates up to 100,000 molecules per minute. Immunoglobulin secretion rates of neoplastic plasma cells are generally somewhat lower than those for normal plasma cells. Additionally, in neoplastic clones, H and L chain biosynthesis is sometimes "unbalanced" with excessive synthesis of free L chains, which are usually secreted by the cell as L chain dimers of molecular weight 60,000. The relatively low molecular weight of secreted L chains permits them to undergo renal glomerular filtration. While limited amounts of free L chains can be reabsorbed and catabolized by the renal tubule, excessive amounts are excreted in the urine. Monoclonal L chains in the urine in association with B cell neoplasms are referred to as *Bence Jones proteins*, in tribute to the clinical chemist who discovered their differential solubilization on boiling and precipitation on cooling. Electrophoretic and immunologic techniques are now used to assess urinary L chain excretion. The B lymphoid cell precursors of plasma cells have somewhat more limited capability for immunoglobulin synthesis; the immunoglobulin they produce is more frequently displayed on the cell membrane than secreted by the cell. In some instances, individual lymphoid cells may display more than one immunoglobulin on their surfaces (particularly IgD plus IgM). In such instances, both molecules express the identical L chain type and apparent antibody specificity, and the immunoglobulin class expressed is in the course of being "switched" in association with clonal proliferation and differentiation. A number of the B cell neoplasms discussed in this text are manifest as if frozen at various points along this differentiation pathway. Most cases of chronic lymphocytic leukemia, non-Hodgkin's lymphoma, multiple myeloma, macroglobulinemia, and related disorders appear to originate from monoclonal B cell progenitors and are expressed as immunoglobulin-synthesizing neoplasms with either surface membrane or secreted monoclonal immunoglobulin (see Ch. 152). Despite the apparently common origin of these neoplasms, the clinical manifestations, response to treatment, and prognosis of these neoplasms differ substantially. In most instances, the tumor stem cells for one of these neoplasms (those progenitor cells responsible for the metastatic spread and self-renewal of the tumor) give rise to cells that express

TABLE 163–1. CLASSIFICATION OF DISORDERS ASSOCIATED WITH MONOCLONAL IMMUNOGLOBULIN (M-COMPONENT SECRETION)

Disorder	M-Component	
1. Plasma cell neoplasms		
A. Multiple myeloma	IgG>IgA>IgD>IgE ± free L chain or L chain alone (κ>λ) rarely biclonal or without detectable Ig abnormality	
B. Macroglobulinemia	IgM ± free L chain (κ>λ)	
C. H chain diseases	γ, α, or μ chain or fragment; ?, δ, or ε	
D. Primary amyloidosis	Free L chain (κ>λ) or L chain fragment alone or plus IgG, IgA, IgM, or IgD	
E. Monoclonal gammopathy of unknown significance	IgG, IgM, IgA, or IgD usually without L chain secretion	
2. Other B cell neoplasms	*M-component* (occasionally secreted)	
A. Chronic lymphocytic leukemia	IgM>IgG	
B. B cell non-Hodgkin's lymphomas (any morphologic pattern or lymphoid cell types)		
3. Nonlymphoid neoplasms—Chronic myelogenous leukemia; carcinoma of colon, breast, prostate, or other sites	No consistent patterns	
4. "Autoimmune" or autoreactive disorders	*M-component*	*Antibody activity of M-component*
A. Cold agglutinin disease (some characteristics of Waldenström's macroglobulinemia)	IgMκ most common	Anti-I antigen of RBC membrane
B. Mixed cryoglobulinemia	IgM	Anti-IgG
C. Hypergammaglobulinemia	IgG	Anti-IgG
D. Sjögren's syndrome	IgM	?
5. Miscellaneous inflammatory, storage, or infectious disorders		
Lichen myxedematous	IgGλ	
Gaucher's disease	IgG	
Cirrhosis, sarcoidosis, parasitic diseases, renal acidosis	No consistent pattern	

the original differentiation state and clinical features of the particular neoplasm (e.g., multiple myeloma). In occasional instances of plasma cell neoplasia (and chronic lymphocytic leukemia and follicular lymphoma) apparent "subcloning" occurs during the patient's clinical course, and the pattern of histology and tumor growth takes on a less differentiated form—e.g., as a poorly differentiated large cell lymphoma. Such transformations are often associated with some change in immunoglobulin synthesis or secretion. Immunologic commonality with the original clone can usually be found, however, by the use of sophisticated techniques. A classification of B cell disorders associated with secretion of an M-component appears in Table 163–1.

Stites DP, Stobo JD, Wells JV: Basic and Clinical Immunology. 6th ed. Los Altos, Lange Medical Publications, 1987. *An excellent and reasonably priced text on immunology for students, house staff, and physicians.*

MULTIPLE MYELOMA

DEFINITION. Multiple myeloma (plasma cell myeloma, myelomatosis) is a disseminated malignant disease in which a clone of transformed plasma cells proliferates in the bone marrow, disrupting its normal functions as well as invading the adjacent bone. The disease is frequently associated with extensive skeletal destruction, hypercalcemia, anemia, impaired renal function, immunodeficiency, and increased susceptibility to infection. Amyloidosis, clotting disorders, and other protein abnormalities are occasional associations. The neoplastic plasma cells usually produce and secrete M-component immunoglobulin, the amount of which in any given case varies proportionally with the total body tumor burden.

ETIOLOGY. The etiology of human myeloma is unknown; however, genetic predisposition, oncogenic viruses, inflammatory stimuli, and chronic antigenic stimulation have all been implicated.

A mouse model of myeloma has provided some basis for the aforementioned hypotheses. Myeloma can be readily induced in the inbred BALB-C strain of mice by intraperitoneal injection of mineral oil. Such mice are known to harbor oncogenic type C RNA viruses. Of interest, BALB-C mice raised in a germ-free environment fail to develop myeloma after oil injection (although other lymphoid neoplasms may arise). This suggests that bacterial antigenic exposure may be required to increase sufficiently the proliferation of populations of immunoglobulin-producing B cells to render them susceptible to myeloma induction. Myeloma appears to be epizootic, having been reported in rats, dogs, cats, horses, and other mammalian species.

INCIDENCE AND PREVALENCE. Multiple myeloma is a disease most frequently observed in the middle-aged and elderly (median age 60), with an incidence that increases with age. Rare cases have been reported in younger persons, including a few teenagers. The annual incidence of myeloma is 3 per 100,000 population (about as common as Hodgkin's disease). It is slightly more common in males than females, and has been reported in all racial groups. Myeloma accounts for about 10 per cent of hematologic malignant tumors and 1 per cent of all forms of cancer.

PATHOPHYSIOLOGY. The symptoms and signs of multiple myeloma and its consequences on the patient are related primarily to (1) the growth kinetics of the neoplastic plasma cells and the total body tumor burden and (2) secreted products of the tumor cells which have physiochemical, immunologic, or humoral effects. The various secreted products can induce a wide variety of clinical syndromes in patients with myeloma.

MYELOMA CELL MASS. Once transformed plasma cells begin to proliferate in a malignant fashion, the clone appears to grow relatively rapidly with a tumor stem cell doubling time of 24 to 48 hours. Although the neoplasm appears to originate from a single transformed cell (10^0 cells) at a single location, progressive myeloma growth is associated with hem-

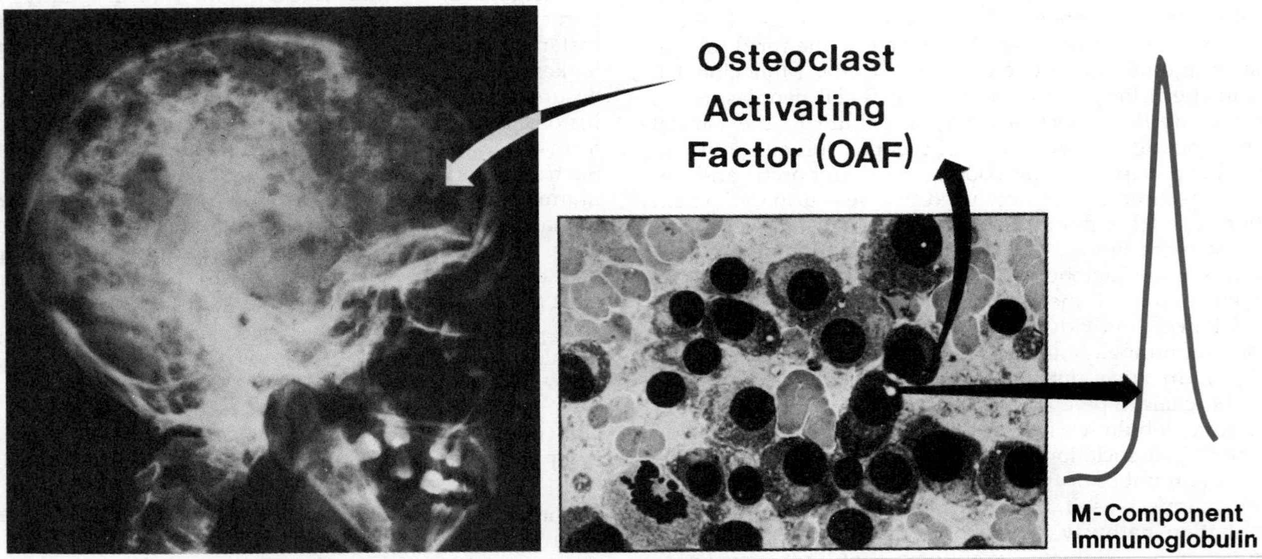

FIGURE 163–1. Clinicopathologic features of multiple myeloma. The type of extensive skeletal destruction ("Swiss cheese"-like lesions) observed in Stage III myeloma patients is represented by the skull at the left of the figure. The patient's bone marrow (center) contains an infiltrate of neoplastic plasma cells which can synthesize and secrete both an osteoclast activating factor (OAF), and a monoclonal immunoglobulin, which appears as a "spike" on protein electrophoresis. Serial measurements of the M-component provide a useful quantitative marker for growth or regression of the neoplasm, as the M-component production rate per myeloma cell remains relatively constant in most cases.

atogenous spread of the neoplastic cells to various skeletal sites, leading to widespread involvement of the bone marrow with nodules or sheets of plasma cells (Fig. 163–1). Marrow involvement leads to development of a normochromic normocytic anemia that is apparent in virtually all patients with myeloma. This appears to be the consequence of tumor-related inhibition of erythropoiesis as well as the disturbance of marrow architecture. A slight shortening of red cell survival, iron deficiency, and blood loss may also contribute to the anemia. High concentrations of a serum M-component may lead to blood sludging and hyperviscosity. Rouleaux formation observed on the peripheral blood smear and an increase in the sedimentation rate are also due to high concentrations of myeloma globulins in the plasma. In addition to monoclonal immunoglobulin, myeloma cells also secrete calcium-mobilizing substances, osteoclast activating factors (OAF's), which stimulate local bone resorption by osteoclasts in the vicinity of foci of myeloma in the bone marrow. Simultaneously, local osteoblastic activity is inhibited. Radiographically, this may result in osteopenia resembling osteoporosis and in discrete osteolytic bone lesions as well as hypercalcemia and hypercalciuria (Fig. 163–2). Several peptides with OAF activity have been isolated. Tumor growth factor alpha (TGF-α) is one of the major growth factors that mobilizes calcium from bone. Secretion of the M-component immunoglobulin appears to occur at a relatively constant rate per myeloma cell in approximately 90 per cent of myeloma patients. Availability of this tumor marker permits quantitation of the total body tumor burden because both the cellular synthetic rate of the M-component and its total body synthetic rate can be determined. "Early myeloma" is associated with a substantial tumor burden $\approx 5 \times 10^{12}$ myeloma cells (about 0.5 kg). As the total body tumor mass reaches the clinical level of detection, its growth rate slows substantially (to a doubling time of two to six months) following a typical gompertzian growth curve (see Ch. 168). Cytokinetically, this slowing of growth is associated with a fall in the fraction of tumor cells traversing the cell cycle, as determined with tritiated thymidine autoradiography. Patients with extensive myeloma who are close to death generally have $>3 \times 10^{12}$ myeloma cells in the body (3.0 kg) as well as extensive lytic bone lesions and fractures and other findings characteristic of myeloma.

M-Components in Myeloma. The monoclonal immunoglobulin types that are secreted as M-component are usually IgG, IgA, or free L chains of Ig. Occasionally, the M-component will be IgD and extremely rarely, IgE. (IgM secretion is characteristically associated with macroglobulinemia.) The frequency of these different immunologic types of plasma cell disorders is roughly proportional to the serum concentration (see Table 417–1) and total body synthetic rate for the various immunoglobulins. When L chains are secreted (as dimers) into the plasma, they are rapidly extracted and metabolized by the kidney and thus are not usually detected on serum electrophoresis. When the renal threshold is exceeded, L chains appear in the urine (Bence Jones proteins). If the patient has renal failure (sometimes induced by L dimers), a serum M-component composed only of L chains may appear. L chains or L chain fragments with high tissue affinity are sometimes deposited as a characteristic infiltrative deposit ("amyloid") in certain tissues (see Immunocytic [Primary] Amyloidosis below).

If an IgG or IgA M-component has a high intrinsic viscosity (related to molecular aggregation or asymmetry) and is present in high concentrations, hyperviscosity and bleeding disorders may develop. These complications are less common in myeloma than in macroglobulinemia. Serum M-components can induce bleeding disorders by complexing or binding immunologically with coagulation factors I, II, V, VII, or VIII. Occasionally, M-components will have narrow thermal amplitude and form cryoglobulins (including mixed cryoglobulin) and lead to Raynaud's phenomenon, impaired circulation, and potential gangrene after cold exposure. Some of these bleeding and circulatory syndromes and other immunologically predicated syndromes (e.g., hemolytic anemia, hyperlipidemia) can now be defined as being due to the M-component's having specific antibody function. These antibodies may have a low binding affinity for a normal antigenic determinant in blood or other tissue, but this may suffice for an interaction in the presence of the large amount of M-component present. Virtually all myeloma immunoglobulins are thought to have some antigen-binding specificity (as the

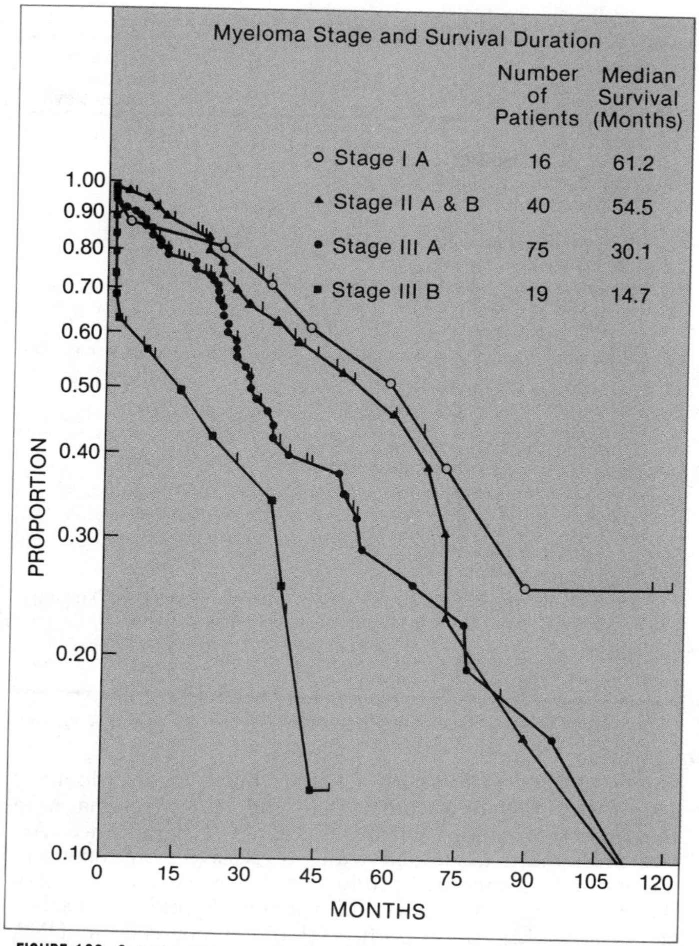

FIGURE 163–2. Life table survival curves for 150 patients with multiple myeloma categorized by stage. (○) Stage IA, (▲) Stages IIA and B, (●) Stage IIIA, and (■) Stage IIIB. Stage IA survival is significantly better than that of Stages IIIA and IIIB. Stages IIA and B are significantly better than Stages IIIA and IIIB. Stages IIIA and IIIB are significantly different from one another. (From Durie BGM, Salmon SE, Moon TE: Blood 55:364, 1980. With permission of the authors and publisher.)

neoplasm arises from a normal committed antibody-producing clone), but in most instances the antibody specificity of any given patient's M-protein remains unknown. Only in the exceptional clinical syndromes (such as those mentioned above) is it likely to be discovered or characterized.

Renal Failure. Renal failure is observed in at least 20 per cent of patients with myeloma and is frequently of mixed pathogenesis. Hypercalcemia leads to calcium nephropathy and is the most common cause of renal failure in myeloma. Second in importance is the presence of heavy Bence Jones proteinuria, which also leads to tubular injury. Additional factors that may also contribute to renal failure in myeloma include hyperuricemia (in association with increased tumor cell DNA turnover), pyelonephritis, and amyloidosis. Functional abnormalities of the kidney in myeloma include acute and chronic renal failure, defects in urine concentration and acidification, and acquired Fanconi syndrome. Histologically the kidneys are usually enlarged; the glomeruli are usually normal. A characteristic "blocked pipe" appearance with eosinophilic casts surrounded by an epithelial syncytium in distal tubules and collecting ducts is the hallmark of "myeloma kidney." This is somewhat more common in patients with lambda L chain excretion.

Immunodeficiency. Patients with myeloma usually have severely depressed serum levels of normal immunoglobulins and a compromised ability to manifest a normal humoral immune response after antigenic stimulation. Consequently, they are highly susceptible to infection from common encapsulated organisms (e.g., pneumococcus), and pneumonia and other septic episodes are quite common in patients at the time of diagnosis or when the disease has relapsed. A series of mechanisms appears to be responsible for this immunodeficiency syndrome. In the BALB-C mouse model (and presumably in man), myeloma cells secrete an inhibitory substance (not immunoglobulin) that activates macrophage-mediated suppression of proliferation of normal antibody producing B-cell clones. Such macrophage-induced suppression of normal immunoglobulin synthesis has been observed in patients with myeloma. Additionally, in IgG myeloma the secreted IgG M-component accelerates the catabolism of the patient's normal IgG. This is because the IgG fractional catabolic rate increases as the total serum IgG concentration rises, resulting in a shorter half-life for both myeloma and normal IgG. These defects in humoral immunity are often compounded by faulty granulocyte function wherein opsonization and phagocytosis of bacteria may be impaired by the large quantities of M-protein. Finally, the number of available circulating granulocytes may be significantly reduced as a consequence of the disease or myelosuppression secondary to chemotherapy.

CLINICAL MANIFESTATIONS (Table 163–2). Presenting symptoms and signs of myeloma include bone pain (often associated with pathologic fractures of the spine or ribs), weakness resulting from anemia, recurrent infection, hypercalcemia (associated with confusion, polyuria, and constipation), and azotemia, occasionally with paralysis secondary to spinal cord compression or with bleeding disorders. Asymptomatic patients are sometimes identified by the presence of proteinuria in the absence of hypertension, or the presence of increased total serum protein on a multichemistry profile. Not infrequently the presentation is that of back pain, anemia, and a very high sedimentation rate in an older patient. Some patients present with acute renal failure with oliguria, especially following dehydration.

DIAGNOSIS. Patients with one or more of the aforementioned symptoms and signs require laboratory confirmation of the diagnosis of multiple myeloma. Patients may have pallor or focal bone tenderness on examination, but there are no characteristic physical findings. In advanced stages of myeloma, soft tissue plasmacytomas (usually as direct extensions from underlying ribs or other bones) may develop. Lymphadenopathy or splenomegaly is only an occasional finding. The laboratory diagnosis of myeloma includes serum electrophoresis, electrophoresis of a 24-hour urine specimen (with immunologic typing of any serum and/or urine M-components found), and bone marrow aspiration. A complete skeletal x-ray survey should be carried out. Radionuclide bone scans are of little or no value because the suppression of osteoblastic activity associated with myeloma inhibits radionuclide uptake into the lesions. This is also the presumed explanation of the fact that the serum alkaline phosphatase level is usually normal despite severe bony involvement. Typical skeletal x-ray findings appear in Figure 163–1.

TABLE 163–2. CLINICAL MANIFESTATIONS OF MULTIPLE MYELOMA

Bone involvement—osteolysis due to OAF; pain; pathologic fractures; hypercalcemia
Anemia—decreased RBC production plus mild hemolysis
Renal failure—due to calcium nephropathy, L chains, uric acid, amyloid, infection, proteinuria (hypertension is rare), uremia; occasionally acute, oliguric renal failure
Recurrent infections—especially respiratory
Amyloidosis (develops in about 15 per cent)
Plasmacytomas
Rare paraprotein-associated syndromes—hyperviscosity syndrome, cryoglobulinemia, hyperlipoproteinemia
Hemorrhagic diatheses
Very high erythrocyte sedimentation rate and rouleaux formation on blood smear (with serum M-component)

A complete blood count with differential, serum calcium and albumin determinations, one or more tests of renal function, and measurement of serum immunoglobulin and serum beta$_2$ microglobulin levels are also useful. These tests aid in staging of the disease and distinguishing myeloma from other disorders. Patients suspected of having myeloma on the basis of skeletal and/or bone marrow involvement but lacking a serum M-component generally have L chain myeloma. This is usually identifiable on protein electrophoresis of a 24-hour urine concentrate. Dipsticks for detecting proteinuria are unreliable for detection of urinary L chains, and the heat test for Bence Jones proteins is positive in only about one half of cases of L chain myeloma. Urinary L chains also occur in some patients with primary amyloidosis and about 20 per cent of patients with macroglobulinemia. The rare patients with H chain disease also have urinary or serum M-components on electrophoresis. However, the clinical presentation and immunologic findings are otherwise quite different in those entities.

The definitive diagnosis of multiple myeloma requires the demonstration of plasmacytosis in the marrow (Color plate 3*L*) or a soft tissue lesion and the presence of significant M-component production plus some evidence of invasiveness. The presence of lytic bone lesions is the best sign of invasiveness. The suppression of normal immunoglobulins, as well as anemia, hypercalcemia, azotemia, bone demineralization, compression fractures, and disease progression, is supportive in making the diagnosis when the major criteria are not all present. Other disorders that must be distinguished from myeloma include monoclonal gammopathy of unknown significance (see under Monoclonal Gammopathies of Undetermined Significance) and metastatic carcinomas. Additionally, indolent myeloma and the occasional case of solitary plasmacytoma (soft tissue) must be distinguished from myeloma because these patients do not require systemic chemotherapy. In patients with myeloma approximately 53 per cent of M-components are IgG, 25 per cent IgA, and 1 per cent IgD. About 20 per cent have apparent pure Bence Jones (L chain) myeloma, with only urinary L chain excretion. Two thirds of patients who have a serum M-component (IgG or IgA) also have concomitant Bence Jones proteinuria. Fewer than 1 per cent of patients have no definable M-component in the serum or urine. Such patients usually have L chain myeloma also, but this is masked by the ability of the kidney to completely catabolize the presented L chains. Immunofluorescent studies of the bone marrow plasma cells with anti-L chain antisera generally identify such patients. One relatively uncommon presentation of myeloma is with plasma cell leukemia. Such patients often have hepatosplenomegaly and occasionally lymphadenopathy as well as an M-component, bone lesions, and a circulating plasma cell count of greater than 2000 per cubic millimeter.

CLINICAL STAGING. As is the case in other neoplasms, quantitative staging information is useful in projecting the prognosis for individual patients and for deciding on the approach and intensity of treatment. A prognostically useful staging system has been developed for myeloma by correlating various pretreatment prognostic factors (hemoglobin, calcium, quantity of M-component secretion, and degree of skeletal involvement on roentgenograms) with the total body tumor cell number as measured immunologically (Table 163–3). Thus, myeloma patients can be categorized as having Stage I (low), II (intermediate), or III (high) disease with respect to tumor burden.

Impairment of renal function has an adverse effect on survival. Cases in which the serum creatinine level is greater than 2.0 mg per deciliter are thus staged with the additional designation B, whereas those with more normal renal function are classed as A. The effect of stage on prognosis is depicted in Figure 163–2. Patients with Stage IA disease sometimes require observation without treatment or, if available, cell kinetic studies to establish whether they actually do have progressive myeloma rather than indolent myeloma or a monoclonal gammopathy of undetermined significance. Active myeloma is associated with progressive symptoms and increasing M-component production. In vitro flash labeling of the marrow myeloma cells with tritiated thymidine reveals a significantly higher proportion of the tumor cells in DNA synthesis in myeloma than in either indolent myeloma or monoclonal gammopathy of unknown significance. Urinary L chain excretion also serves as a signal of an aggressive tumor.

TABLE 163–3. MYELOMA STAGING SYSTEM

Stage	Criteria	Measured Myeloma Cell Mass (Cells × 10^{12} per Square Meter)
I.	*All* of the following:	<0.6 (low)
	1. Hemoglobin value >10 grams/dl	
	2. Serum calcium value (≤12 mg/dl)	
	3. On x-ray, normal bone structure (scale 0) or solitary bone plasmacytoma only	
	4. Low M-component production rates	
	a. IgG value <5 grams/dl	
	b. IgA value <3 grams/dl	
	c. Urine L chain M-component on electrophoresis <4 grams/24 hours	
II.	Fitting neither Stage I nor Stage III	0.6–1.20 (intermediate)
III.	One or more of the following:	>1.20 (high)
	1. Hemoglobin value <8.5 grams/dl	
	2. Serum calcium value >12 mg/dl	
	3. Advanced lytic bone lesions (scale 3)	
	4. High M-component production rates	
	a. IgG value >7 grams/dl	
	b. IgA value >5 grams/dl	
	c. Urine L chain M-component on electrophoresis >12 grams/24 hours	

Subclassification:
A = Relatively normal renal function (serum creatinine value <2.0 mg/dl)
B = Abnormal renal function (serum creatinine value ≥2.0 mg/dl)
Examples:
Stage IA = Low cell mass with normal renal function
Stage IIIB = High cell mass with abnormal renal function

From Durie BGM, Salmon SE: Cancer 36:842, 1975.

Measurement of serum beta$_2$-microglobulin can be used as an additional prognostic factor, as its serum concentration appears to reflect myeloma cell burden as well as renal functional impairment. Serum beta$_2$ microglobulin levels of greater than 6 μg per milliliter are associated with a poor prognosis. However, beta$_2$-microglobulin does not distinguish between low cell mass myeloma and "monoclonal gammopathies of unknown significance."

TREATMENT AND PROGNOSIS. Some patients with myeloma have relatively indolent disease that, in Stage I cases, is sometimes confused with monoclonal gammopathies of unknown significance. The overwhelming majority of patients have more advanced disease and require active systemic treatment. Two areas of treatment are important: (1) systemic chemotherapy for multiple myeloma, and (2) supportive care for treatment of complications of the disorder (e.g., spinal cord compression, bone pain, hypercalcemia, sepsis, anemia, and renal failure).

Systemic Chemotherapy. Improvements in systemic chemotherapy for multiple myeloma (in the 1960's) resulted in an increased life expectancy for these patients. Prior to this era, the median life expectancy of untreated myeloma patients was less than one year (3.5 to 8.5 months), whereas at present, with optimal chemotherapy, it is about three years on average, and up to five years or more for patients who respond to chemotherapy. Survival is also influenced by the presenting clinical stage and renal function.

Cell cycle nonspecific cytotoxic drugs (alkylating agents, nitrosoureas, and anthracycline antibiotics) have proved to be the most useful agents in the chemotherapy of myeloma. Vinca alkaloids and corticosteroids appear to potentiate the efficacy of the other cytotoxic drugs. Human leukocyte interferons, including the recombinant alfa interferons, are also useful agents in the treatment of myeloma and are currently being evaluated to define their role in combination with other drugs.

Systemic chemotherapy for myeloma traditionally has employed single-agent chemotherapy with an oral alkylating agent plus prednisone. To prevent complications such as hypercalcemia, hyperuricemia, and azotemic patients should be well hydrated before treatment is initiated and ambulated if at all possible. Prevention of treatment-associated hyperuricemia with allopurinol is also of value during the first few months of treatment. (Management of other complications of myeloma is described under Supportive Care.)

The single agents most widely used for the treatment of myeloma are melphalan (Alkeran, L-phenylalanine mustard) and cyclophosphamide (Cytoxan). Either can be given on a chronic low dose daily basis or in intermittent pulsed courses of therapy. Although equivalent therapeutic results appear to be obtained with either of these schedules, the intermittent course necessitates fewer physician visits and may be associated with less late failure of hematopoietic stem cells. For the intermittent pulse schedules, melphalan is generally administered in a total dose of 8 mg per square meter per day orally for four days and repeated every three to four weeks. Alternatively, higher doses may be given with longer intervals between treatments. Cyclophosphamide is given in a dose of 0.8 gram per square meter either intravenously as a single dose or in divided daily oral doses over four days, every three to four weeks. Both of these alkylating agent schedules usually incorporate a course of 60 mg per square meter of prednisone per day for four days. The amounts given of both of the alkylating agents must be monitored closely with regard to the magnitude and duration of toxic side effects, particularly myelosuppression. Oral melphalan seems to vary significantly in bioavailability from patient to patient. In lieu of an assay for its plasma level, it is important to use a sufficient dose to induce some myelosuppression. Both melphalan and cyclophosphamide dosages are generally reduced if the total white blood count at the time of the next treatment is less than 3000 and the granulocyte count less than 2000 or the platelet count less than 100,000. Melphalan, cyclophosphamide, and the nitrosourea carmustine (BCNU) have been combined in various ways, often with the addition of vincristine (Oncovin) and sometimes doxorubicin (Adriamycin). Results with these more intensive regimens, including alternations of a number of active agents, appear better in high tumor burden patients (Stage III) than simple combinations of an alkylating agent and prednisone. Very high intravenous doses of melphalan have been administered to myeloma patients along with aggressive supportive care. While this approach has induced excellent remissions in some patients, it remains quite toxic and experimental. Whether therapy is warranted for Stage I patients remains to be defined, as the treatment often causes toxicity, and therapy can be delayed until clearer evidence of invasiveness is present.

After systemic chemotherapy is initiated, patients with responsive myeloma generally have prompt relief of bone pain and reversal of symptoms and signs of hypercalcemia, anemia, and recurrent infection. Other symptoms frequently improve, and there is often a feeling of general well-being. However, major healing of osteolytic lesions or improvement in the depressed levels of normal immunoglobulins is distinctly uncommon, suggesting some persisting cellular or humoral defect in the recovery from these two myeloma-induced abnormalities. Associated with such symptomatic and general improvement, the quantity of the M-component produced falls progressively as the myeloma cells responsible for its synthesis are killed by the cytotoxic agents. The rate of fall of the serum M-component concentration or of urinary L chain excretion depends both upon the rate of kill of the myeloma cells and upon the fractional catabolic rate of the immunoglobulin. Inasmuch as L chains have a fractional catabolic rate of about six hours, their excretion can be substantially reduced within three to four days after effective lysis of tumor cells. However, the various serum M-components are metabolized more slowly; reduction in the IgG M-component marker of tumor burden may lag four to six weeks behind symptomatic improvement with chemotherapy. With currently available treatment some 60 to 75 per cent of myeloma patients achieve at least 75 per cent reduction in the total body myeloma cell mass (as calculated from reductions in M-component synthesis). In general, at least this degree of reduction in tumor burden is required to observe significant improvement in survival with chemotherapy. Lesser degrees of tumor regression are observed in the remainder of patients. Although classed as "nonresponders," most achieve some symptomatic benefit. Patients who achieve objective response generally have a persistent and stable low level of monoclonal plasma cells in the bone marrow and M-component secretion despite continued cytotoxic therapy. Cell kinetic studies in remission indicate that the residual tumor cells are hypoproliferative. In some instances, patients can be followed in a remission without continued administration of chemotherapy. However, this is a difficult course to follow in patients who present with Stage III disease or who have Bence Jones myeloma, as these patients tend to relapse quickly (within less than six months) when treatment is discontinued. Most myeloma patients who achieve remission have less than one log of tumor regression (90 per cent) with treatment, and only about 10 per cent of patients have as much as a two log regression (99 per cent). Thus, even in remission, there is a large subclinical residue of tumor cells (greater than 10^{10} tumor cells). Even though many of these cells may not be in the tumor stem cell compartment, there is still a sufficient number of malignant cells present to lead to eventual relapse in virtually all patients with multiple myeloma. Cures will require development of more effective therapy in the future. Patients who present with renal failure and those whose tumor clones produce only L chains (particularly of the λ type) tend to have a poorer response to treatment with more frequent early relapse and shorter survival than those who present with a serum M-component. Outcome in IgG cases also tends to be somewhat better than that in IgA cases. Among Stage III cases, the fraction of the tumor cells in DNA synthesis (growth fraction) also affects prognosis, with the patients with a high growth fraction having relatively brief responses to treatment and short survival. Patients presenting with plasma cell leukemia also have a high growth fraction, poor response to treatment, and short survival.

Patients with tumors exhibiting a high growth fraction tend to respond very quickly to chemotherapy, with a rapid fall in the M-component to remission levels (e.g., within six weeks), but then relapse occurs quickly. More durable responses require three to eight months to achieve. For patients who achieve objective remission, serial monitoring of the quantity of serum and/or urinary M-component on electrophoresis or with nephelometry provides an excellent means for assessing the stability of the remission and for detecting relapse at its earliest stages, often before the patient develops recurrent hypercalcemia or new lytic lesions.

In most patients with myeloma who achieve 75 per cent tumor regression, remission remains for at least three years before relapse occurs, as manifested by a rising M-component or new symptoms. In only occasional Stage III patients is the disease still in remission beyond six years after the diagnosis (Fig. 163–2). Some useful approaches to secondary chemotherapy have been devised that are beneficial to patients in whom relapse results from primary treatment. For example, there is not complete cross-resistance between melphalan and cyclophosphamide, and disease relapsing after treatment with one of these agents will occasionally respond to the other. A more useful approach has been that of the intravenous combination of carmustine (BCNU) and doxorubicin (Adriamycin) with each drug administered at a dosage of 30 mg per square meter every three weeks. Vincristine (Oncovin) and prednisone can be administered along with these drugs in an attempt to potentiate their effect. About one half of patients who initially respond to alkylating agents can achieve second remissions with these agents. Alfa interferons have also been useful for inducing secondary remissions. Second remissions rarely last longer than one year. The terminal phase of myeloma is characterized by symptoms and signs of progressive growth of the drug-resistant tumor (e.g., bone pain, hypercalcemia, fractures, rising M-component, anemia, and renal failure). A late complication of treatment of myeloma (particularly with melphalan) is injury of normal bone marrow stem cells. This injury can result in development of a chronic refractory sideroblastic anemia or acute myelogenous leukemia. It has been projected that well over 5 per cent of myeloma patients may eventually develop leukemia as a result of treatment. However, the risk-benefit ratio for myeloma patients still favors use of systemic chemotherapy. The immediate cause of death is frequently sepsis or renal failure. Recent advances in chemotherapy have resulted in some improvement in the prognosis for patients with myeloma. Better results will require the identification of new drugs with significant antimyeloma activity.

Supportive Care. Patients with newly diagnosed myeloma and those whose disease has relapsed often have problems that require immediate or emergency management that may have to be carried out concomitantly with initiation of chemotherapy.

HYPERCALCEMIA AND OSTEOLYSIS. Hypercalcemia as a metabolic complication of osteolysis is common in myeloma; the serum calcium should be determined initially even in patients lacking the characteristic symptoms of confusion, irritability, and constipation. The effects of hypercalcemia relate to the ionized fraction, which is greater when the serum albumin level is low. When serum calcium is only modestly increased (e.g., 11.5 to 12 mg per deciliter), hydration with several liters of intravenous saline, alone or with furosemide, will often suffice until the effect of systemic chemotherapy can induce a more sustained reduction in the calcium. Ambulation should be encouraged, as it also reduces bone resorption. Oral phosphate solutions (Fleet's phosphosoda enemas) may also prove useful for mild hypercalcemia if renal function is not impaired and the serum phosphate is not increased. Greater degrees of hypercalcemia (serum calcium $>$12 mg per deciliter) represent a medical emergency because of both cardiac and renal effects, and often require the addition of more aggressive measures, including large doses of corticosteroids. Injections of calcitonin or mithramycin are also indicated if the level of serum calcium is very high (e.g., $>$ 14 mg per deciliter) or if the response to steroids is not rapid. Mithramycin (25 μg per kilogram of body weight) can often normalize the serum calcium in less than 24 hours, but frequently repeated injections are undesirable, as they can induce thrombocytopenia, which may compromise the ability to administer systemic chemotherapy for myeloma. (See Ch. 247 for a further discussion of the treatment of hypercalcemia.)

SPINAL CORD COMPRESSION. Developing neurologic symptoms in the lower extremities plus focal back pain in a patient with myeloma should lead to an emergency evaluation for the possibility of cord compression secondary to an extradural plasmacytoma. Consultations involving neurology, radiation therapy, and neurosurgery should be obtained promptly. If the diagnosis is established with magnetic resonance imaging or myelography before paralysis develops, the chance for recovery of neurologic function with high dose steroids and emergency radiotherapy (with or without laminectomy) is excellent. Delays in diagnosis or therapy (even 12 hours) can leave the patient with irreversible paraplegia.

BONE PAIN. Bone pain caused by expanding plasmacytomas can usually be managed with analgesics and systemic chemotherapy. In some instances a single bony lesion will be responsible for the patient's pain. Such focal lesions can usually be palliated effectively and quickly with moderate doses of local radiotherapy (2000 to 3000 rads). Radiotherapy generally should be used only if pain is not relieved promptly with chemotherapy, and it should be limited to a relatively small field, as it impairs normal bone marrow function. Long delays in systemic chemotherapy for administration of radiotherapy should be avoided, as new bony lesions often develop during such intervals.

ANEMIA. Transfusion of packed red blood cells is often required in the initial management of Stage III myeloma patients. Occasionally, normal hematopoiesis can be stimulated with androgens. Other hematinics (iron, folic acid, vitamin B_{12}) are not of value. Patients experiencing an objective response to myeloma chemotherapy generally have a rise in hemoglobin of several grams during the first year after initiation of treatment.

INFECTION. Because of the known increased incidence of bacterial infection in myeloma (particularly pneumococcal), various efforts have been made to prevent infection. Immunization with polyvalent pneumococcal vaccine is of limited utility because of the profound defect that myeloma patients have in responding to carbohydrate antigens. Prophylactic administration of large doses of gamma globulin has proved ineffective, in part because of the hypercatabolism of all IgG in patients with IgG myeloma. Prophylactic use of antibiotics (penicillin, ampicillin) is of some benefit in infection-prone patients. If the patient can be depended upon to recognize the earliest signs of infection, prompt treatment at the time of fever or sputum production will usually suffice. When a patient with myeloma has a major septic episode, bactericidal antibiotics must be administered in adequate dosage. Nephrotoxic antibiotics (e.g., aminoglycosides) should be avoided in view of the frequency of overt or subclinical renal impairment in myeloma.

RENAL INSUFFICIENCY. Renal failure is a major cause of death in multiple myeloma. The major causes of renal failure are hypercalcemia and Bence Jones proteinuria. Both are potentially treatable. The patient should be kept well hydrated, and treated promptly for hypercalcemia when it is present. Allopurinol should also be used to prevent hyperuricemia and hyperuricosuria. Intravenous pyelography can precipitate renal failure in myeloma patients (perhaps because of dehydration) and should be approached with caution and with maintenance of hydration. Acute renal failure should be treated aggressively with standard measures, including hemodialysis, with the understanding that it may no longer be required if the injury is not too severe and if a good response is seen to chemotherapy. When the disease is in remission some patients have been supported with long-term hemodialysis. Long-term dialysis is clearly not indicated if the patient fails to achieve clinical remission with systemic chemotherapy.

VARIANT FORMS OF MYELOMA. ***Indolent Myeloma.*** About 5 per cent of patients under evaluation for multiple myeloma have a more indolent form of the disease with a life expectancy of up to ten years. Such patients are currently difficult to identify prospectively without specialized testing or a period of observation without treatment. Some are asymptomatic patients in whom the diagnosis is made after routine biochemical studies. One or two lytic bony lesions may be present. Most such patients have Stage I myeloma, and significant bone pain, hypercalcemia, azotemia, and Bence Jones proteinuria are absent. The tumor cells in indolent myeloma are hypoproliferative with a tumor cell tritiated thymidine labeling index of less than 0.5 per cent. Patients with indolent myeloma can be followed symptomatically without initiation of systemic chemotherapy. This group is relatively rare, however, and it is probably better to err on the side of treatment if the evidence for indolence is equivocal.

Solitary Myeloma. Occasional patients present with an apparently solitary myeloma. Bilateral core bone marrow biopsies from the iliac spine and a sternal aspirate, as well as electrophoretic studies of the blood and urine, should be performed in all cases thought to involve a solitary lesion. Only about half of patients with solitary myeloma have a demonstrable M-component, and even then a relatively small one. The normal immunoglobulins should also not be depressed in patients with a solitary lesion. Those involving soft tissues (particularly in the head and neck region) have a relatively high probability of being solitary and can often be managed with local surgery and radiation therapy. After effective local treatment of a soft tissue plasmacytoma, myeloma proteins in the blood or urine should disappear promptly. If they do not, occult dissemination can be predicted. In general, patients with a solitary soft tissue plasmacytoma will not require chemotherapy.

In contrast, patients with apparently solitary myeloma of bone generally do have additional occult disease. They also frequently respond unusually well to systemic chemotherapy after the original local lesion is treated with about 4000 rads of radiation. Patients with apparently solitary myeloma of bone can often be followed in unmaintained remission after the initial year of treatment with radiation and chemotherapy.

Barlogie B, Smith L, Alexanian R: Effective treatment of advanced multiple myeloma refractory to alkylating agents. N Engl J Med 310:1353, 1984. *Describes a useful vincristine-doxorubicin-dexamethasone combination treatment of patients with myeloma in relapse.*

Bataille R, Durie BGM, Grenier J: Prognostic factors and staging in multiple myeloma: A reappraisal evaluating new parameters. Blood 64(Suppl 5):152a, 1984. *An assessment of several staging systems for myeloma as well as of serum beta$_2$-microglobulin as a prognostic factor.*

Durie BGM, Dixon DO, Carter S, et al.: Improved survival duration with combination chemotherapy induction for multiple myeloma: A Southwest Oncology Group Study. J Clin Oncol 4:1227, 1986. *Describes an excellent treatment option for remission induction in patients with active myeloma.*

Durie BGM, Salmon SE, Moon TE: Pretreatment tumor mass, cell kinetics and prognosis in multiple myeloma. Blood 55:364, 1980. *A detailed analysis of tumor cell burden, thymidine labeling, response to treatment, and survival in myeloma which identifies kinetically unfavorable patient groups.*

Quesada JR, Alexanian R, Hawkins M, et al.: Treatment of multiple myeloma with recombinant alfa interferon. Blood 67:275, 1986. *A report summarizing the usefulness of interferon in myeloma therapy. Patients receiving this therapy often had improvement in normal immunoglobulin synthesis.*

Salmon SE (ed.): Myeloma and Related Disorders. Clin Haematol Vol 2, 1982. *A review by leading clinical investigators of major clinical and research advances that pertain to multiple myeloma and related entities.*

Salmon SE, Haut A, Bonnet JD, et al.: Alternating combination chemotherapy improves survival in multiple myeloma: A Southwest Oncology Group Study. J Clin Oncol 1:453, 1983. *Evidence supporting the use of aggressive combination chemotherapy for advanced stage myeloma patients.*

MACROGLOBULINEMIA OF WALDENSTRÖM

DEFINITION. Waldenström's macroglobulinemia is characterized by the proliferation and accumulation of malignant cells with lymphoplasmacytic morphology that secrete IgM M-components. Sites of B cell development, including the bone marrow, lymph nodes, and spleen, are usually involved. Major clinical manifestations of the disorder are related to hyperviscosity of the circulating intravascular macroglobulin. The disease has some similarities with myeloma, lymphoma, and chronic lymphocytic leukemia.

ETIOLOGY AND PATHOPHYSIOLOGY. Waldenström's macroglobulinemia is of unknown etiology, but appears to have a slightly increased familial incidence. It has a slight male predominance and increases in incidence with age, usually beginning in the fifth or sixth decade. The neoplasm appears to originate in a plasmacytic lymphocyte in the B cell series, which proliferates in the bone marrow and/or lymph nodes and spleen. Cytogenetic markers are sometimes found but are nonspecific. IgM M-components frequently have physiochemical properties that lead to hyperviscosity, cryoprecipitation, or bleeding phenomena. In contrast to myeloma, osteolysis, renal impairment, and amyloidosis are quite rare in macroglobulinemia.

CLINICAL FEATURES. The clinical onset of macroglobulinemia is often gradual and associated with increasing weakness, fatigue, epistaxis, or other bleeding manifestations. Recurrent infection, visual difficulties, weight loss, or neurologic symptoms are also common. Bone pain is not a symptom of macroglobulinemia, and skeletal x-rays are usually unremarkable. On physical examination, patients often exhibit pallor, lymphadenopathy, and hepatosplenomegaly. Ophthalmoscopic examination usually reveals marked dilatation and vascular segmentation of the retinal veins ("sausage links") secondary to hyperviscosity, and occasional retinal hemorrhages and exudates. About one fourth of macroglobulinemic patients present with neurologic signs secondary to slow blood flow or sludging, including peripheral neuropathy, transient paresis, abnormal reflexes, headache, dizziness, deafness, and/or impaired state of consciousness or coma. Hyperviscosity also leads to bleeding and oozing from mucous membranes. Such symptoms and signs of hyperviscosity are uncommon when the serum viscosity is less than 4 units (normal, 1.4 to 1.8) and increase dramatically in frequency with values above 6 units.

Laboratory findings include a normochromic normocytic anemia, which is partially due to a reduced red cell mass and partially to an expanded plasma volume as a result of hyperviscosity. Rouleaux formation is quite prominent, and the sedimentation rate is increased markedly unless plasma gelation occurs. Plasmacytic lymphocytes are often present on the blood smear and are sometimes present in leukemic proportions. Coombs-positive hemolytic anemia or cold hemagglutinins are occasional findings. (The cold hemagglutinin syndrome is a variant of macroglobulinemia.) An M-component is present on serum electrophoresis in macroglobulinemia and can be shown to be monoclonal IgM with immunoelectrophoresis. Eighty per cent of IgM M-components have κ L chains, and the remaining 20 per cent are λ. Most macroglobulins will precipitate in distilled water (Sia test); however, this test is nonspecific. About 10 per cent of macroglobulins have cryoglobulin properties; some will form gels as the patient's blood is drawn unless a prewarmed syringe is used and subsequent separative procedures are carried out at 37° C. Bence Jones (L chain) proteinuria is also present in 10 per cent of patients with macroglobulinemia. The serum viscosity is usually increased. Normal immunoglobulins (IgG or IgA) are commonly reduced. The bone marrow aspirate usually reveals a substantial infiltrate with plasmacytic lymphocytes and plasma cells.

DIAGNOSIS. The diagnosis of Waldenström's macroglobulinemia requires the presence of typical symptoms and signs, the presence of an IgM M-component of greater than 3 grams per deciliter, and histologic evidence on bone marrow aspirate or biopsy. The differential diagnosis from chronic lymphocytic leukemia, lymphoma, multiple myeloma, and monoclonal gammopathies of undetermined significance depends upon the presence of characteristic immunologic and clinical features. Intermediate forms with characteristics of several of these related B cell disorders occasionally occur. IgM elevations of smaller magnitude are also seen in a variety of infectious and inflammatory disease, including those listed in Table 163–1.

TREATMENT AND PROGNOSIS. Patients with macroglobulinemia who present with a severe hyperviscosity syndrome and marked neurologic findings (e.g., impending coma or paresis) or serious bleeding should be treated by intensive emergency plasmapheresis. This is best accomplished with an intermittent or continuous flow blood cell separator. Red cell transfusion and/or volume replacement is generally required, as 6 to 8 liters of plasma may have to be removed during the first two to four days. Plasmapheresis is quite effective in macroglobulinemia because 90 per cent of the M-component remains in the intravascular compartment as a result of its high molecular weight.

Inasmuch as plasmapheresis removes only a troublesome tumor product and does not alter the underlying tumor, specific therapy requires the suppression of the neoplasm with systemic chemotherapy.

Chlorambucil (Leukeran) is usually administered orally at a dosage of 6 to 8 mg per day, with dosage adjustments made in accord with the WBC and platelet count. Although chlorambucil is well tolerated, the various drug regimens used in the treatment of multiple myeloma are useful in macroglobulinemia and are quite acceptable alternatives. Once patients achieve remission with chemotherapy (at least 80 per cent of cases), intermittent plasmapheresis can usually be discontinued. Systemic treatment is usually continued indefinitely in macroglobulinemia, since treatment, although suppressive, does not eradicate the IgM producing clone. Alfa interferon may be of some use for patients with macroglobulinemia that becomes refractory to alkylating agents.

The median survival in macroglobulinemia is about three years; however, many patients may have an indolent disease and may survive for ten years or more.

MacKenzie MR, Fudenberg HH: Macroglobulinemia: An analysis of 40 patients. Blood 39:874, 1972. *Useful review of clinical and laboratory features of macroglobulinemia of Waldenström.*

Waldenström J: Studies on conditions associated with disturbed gamma globulin formation (gammopathies). Harvey Lect 56:211, 1961. *A lengthy and stimulating discussion of macroglobulinemia and related plasma cell disorders by the clinical investigator who first described macroglobulinemia.*

HEAVY CHAIN DISEASES

The heavy chain diseases are a group of rare lymphoplasmacytic neoplasms associated with secretion of a monoclonal heavy chain or heavy chain fragment by the neoplastic cells. Thus far, H chain diseases related to the three major immunoglobulin classes have been reported (γ, α, μ). The clinical syndromes vary with H chain type but have some similarities with other B cell neoplasms.

GAMMA (γ) CHAIN DISEASE. This syndrome was the first heavy chain disease to be recognized. More than 50 cases have been reported. The symptoms and clinical presentation are similar to those of malignant lymphomas; the patients frequently have recurrent infections, lymphadenopathy, and hepatosplenomegaly. Characteristically, edema of the soft palate and uvula associated with Waldeyer's ring involvement occurs in γ heavy chain diseases. Normochromic normocytic anemia is typical, and many patients are pancytopenic save for an eosinophilia. Several patients have also manifested plasma cell leukemia, but skeletal lesions are uncommon.

Histologic studies of the lymph nodes and bone marrow usually reveal a pleomorphic infiltrate of lymphoplasmacytic and large lymphoid cells and eosinophils, abnormalities reminiscent of Hodgkin's disease.

All patients have free γ heavy chains present in the serum and urine determined by immunologic and electrophoretic techniques. The urinary protein lacks the heat properties of L chains. Immunoelectrophoresis shows the monoclonal peak to have γ chain determinants but to lack κ or λ L chains. Of interest, there is a large deletion (200 amino acids) in the variable region of the γ chain. As in myeloma and macroglobulinemia, normal immunoglobulins are reduced. Although in some patients there has been a rapid downhill course, use of intensive combination chemotherapy (as in diffuse lymphomas) has resulted in long survival in some patients.

ALPHA (α) CHAIN DISEASE. This rare and interesting syndrome has a characteristic genetic and geographic distribution and is about twice as common as γ chain disease. It has been observed predominantly in young Arabs and non-Ashkenazic Jews living in the Middle East ("Mediterranean lymphoma"). However, the disease does occur in patients of other ethnic backgrounds. Patients usually present with abdominal discomfort and weight loss owing to malabsorption and diarrhea and have extensive mesenteric and small-intestinal lymphatic involvement with lymphoma (see Ch. 104). The lamina propria is extensively infiltrated with neoplastic plasma cells. Cellular morphology is similar to that in γ chain disease; however, marrow involvement is rare. Pulmonary involvement has been observed in two children with α chain disease.

Immunodiagnosis of α chain disease is relatively difficult, as a sharp M-component spike is usually not observed in the serum or urine, and the entity must be thought of in patients with intestinal lymphoma. Alpha chains have a tendency to polymerize and thereby become heterodisperse on electrophoresis, giving the appearance of either a normal serum electrophoresis or diffuse hypergammaglobulinemia. Immunoelectrophoresis, however, demonstrates that only the α chain is present and that L chains are absent. The α chains are monoclonal. Only about half of the patients have free α chain in the urine, presumably because of the tendency for formation of large complexes which do not pass the glomerulus. Although most cases of α chain disease have been fatal, some patients have achieved remissions with chemotherapy. A few patients have achieved remission with antimicrobial therapy, suggesting that an infectious agent may underlie this unusual monoclonal B cell proliferation.

MU (μ) CHAIN DISEASE. Secretion of free μ heavy chains into the plasma is a rare occurrence in chronic lymphocytic leukemia. The seven patients reported have had longstanding disease with retroperitoneal adenopathy and hepatosplenomegaly. Bone marrow aspiration has shown vacuolated lymphoplasmacytic cells. Hypogammaglobulinemia was seen on serum electrophoresis, and immunoelectrophoresis was required to detect the small amount of free μ chains. Most of the patients also had substantial amounts of κ L chain in the urine. The monoclonal lymphoid cells of the neoplasm appear to have a defect in H-L chain assembly, as intracellular L chains are detectable but do not assemble normally into IgM prior to secretion.

Franklin EC: μ-Chain disease. Arch Intern Med 135:71, 1975. *The major clinical features of μ-chain disease are summarized.*

Seligman M: Immunochemical, clinical and pathological features of α chain disease. Arch Intern Med 135:71, 1975. *A clinically relevant immunologic description of α-chain disease.*

IMMUNOCYTIC (PRIMARY) AMYLOIDOSIS

(see also Ch. 210)

DEFINITION. Amyloidosis is not a single disease entity but a term applied to a complex of disorders associated with deposition of insoluble fibrillar proteins in virtually pure form in various tissues of the body. The disease complex was first designated "amyloid" in the 1850's by Virchow, who considered the "waxy, eosinophilic" homogeneous and amorphous tissue deposits to be composed of polysaccharide or starch-like substances. Amyloid stains pink with hematoxylin and eosin and metachromatically with methyl or crystal violet. Congo red stain produces green birefringence under polarized light and is the most specific light microscopic stain for amyloid. Under the electron microscope, amyloid has a characteristic fibrillar B-pleated sheet structure. This structure is not found in normal mammalian tissues.

A complete description of the various forms of amyloidosis is contained in Chapter 210 and a classification based on the chemistry of the amyloid fibrils is presented in Table 210–1. Since immunocytic (primary or AL) amyloidosis may shade into the plasma cell disorders, a further brief summary is given here.

PATHOPHYSIOLOGY (Table 163–4). Amyloid fibrils from primary amyloidosis are homogeneous and homologous to the variable region fragment of either κ or λ L chains (Ig-V_L) and thus have been defined as immunoglobulin amyloid-fibril

TABLE 163–4. CLASSIFICATION OF THE ACQUIRED SYSTEMIC AMYLOIDOSES (β-Fibrilloses)

Classification	Major Protein Component
A. Immunocytic amyloidosis	
1. No evidence of coexisting disease	AL
2. Multiple myeloma	AL
3. Other monoclonal gammopathy	AL
4. Agammaglobulinemia	AL
B. Reactive systemic amyloidosis	AA
1. Acute recurrent and chronic infections	AA
2. Chronic inflammatory conditions (e.g., rheumatoid arthritis)	AA
C. Localized amyloid (involvement of a single organ without generalized involvement)	AL
D. Familial amyloidosis	AA, PA

AL = Amyloid light chain; AA = Amyloid A (protein A); PA = Prealbumin amyloid.

proteins (AL). There is a clear relationship between amyloid-fibril deposits and Bence Jones proteins, which are related to multiple myeloma and related plasma cell disorders. Furthermore, AL appear to be produced in these disorders through a proteolytic mechanism to which only certain free L chains (and not intact Ig components) are susceptible. Such "amyloidogenic" L chains are more frequently of λ than κ L chain type. The characteristic "B-pleated sheet" amyloid fibrils can be produced in vitro by treating certain Bence Jones proteins with proteolytic enzymes. As a result of these studies and the finding of AL type amyloid fibrils in association with virtually all monoclonal gammopathies (including myeloma, macroglobulinemia, H chain diseases, B cell lymphoid neoplasms, and gammopathies of unknown significance) as well as agammaglobulinemia, Glenner proposed that primary amyloidosis be designated *immunocytic amyloid*. This designation clearly has a recognizable relationship to the pathophysiology of amyloid formation in monoclonal B cell disorders.

CLINICAL FEATURES. Patients with immunocytic amyloid present with complaints of weakness, weight loss, ankle swelling, paresthesias, and lightheadedness. Symptoms of multiple myeloma may also be present when the amyloid is associated with that disorder (about 15 per cent of myeloma cases). Major physical findings of immunocytic amyloid include enlargement of the tongue, purpura, hepatomegaly, and occasional splenomegaly. Skin manifestations can include plaques, papules, or nodules. Involvement of periarticular regions can give an appearance similar to that of rheumatoid arthritis. Involvement of the glenohumoral joint leads to a characteristic "shoulder pad sign." Periorbital purpura may appear spontaneously or after straining ("raccoon eyes"). Purpuric bleeding is sometimes associated with an acquired deficiency of factor X. Ankle edema in amyloidosis is often associated with congestive heart failure or the nephrotic syndrome. Heart failure occurs in about 30 per cent of patients, and renal involvement is a leading cause of death. The carpal tunnel syndrome, peripheral neuropathy, and orthostatic hypotension are additional associations with amyloid infiltration.

Laboratory findings include evidence of anemia and/or renal failure in about half of the patients. Ninety per cent have proteinuria. Serum immunoelectrophoresis reveals an M-component in about half of the patients with amyloidosis and in three quarters of those with amyloid associated with myeloma. Addition of urinary immunoelectrophoresis permits detection of an M-component in almost 90 per cent of cases. λ L chain excretion is more common than κ (2 to 1) in amyloidosis. Some increase in marrow plasma cells is common.

Diagnosis of amyloidosis requires tissue biopsy and demonstration of amyloid deposition by the green birefringence of the Congo red stain by polarization microscopy. If easily obtained, the initial biopsy should be of the organ suspected of being infiltrated with amyloid. Alternatively, the first biopsy may be taken from the rectal mucosa, as it is relatively safe and easy to obtain, and with adequate tissue is positive in more than 75 per cent of cases. Other useful biopsy sites include the gingiva, skin, kidney, and carpal ligament (in patients with the carpal tunnel syndrome). Endomyocardial biopsy via catheter has led to the detection of amyloid in unexplained cases of cardiac failure.

TREATMENT. Because of the relationship of AL amyloid to monoclonal plasma cell proliferation, systemic chemotherapy with alkylating agent-prednisone combinations has been tried with some evidence of improvement or halting in progression of amyloid deposition. Therefore, a trial of therapy similar to that used for myeloma is warranted. Unfortunately, treatment has not yet significantly improved survival. Colchicine has been tried in AL amyloid without proven success. Supportive measures in systemic amyloidosis include management of cardiac and renal failure. Congestive heart failure caused by amyloid does not usually respond to cardiac glycosides, and sudden deaths from arrhythmia have been reported. Diuretics have been useful for relief of edema.

The prognosis in systemic immunocytic amyloidosis is poor. In one review of 236 cases, the average survival was 14.7 months for patients without underlying myeloma (about 50 to 60 per cent of cases) and four months for those with amyloidosis and myeloma (about 20 per cent of cases).

Buxbaum JN, Hurley ME, Chuba J, et al.: Amyloidosis of the AL type: Clinical, morphologic, and biochemical aspects of the response to therapy with alkylating agents and prednisone. Am J Med 67:867, 1979.

Durie BGM, Persky B, Soehnlen BJ, et al.: Amyloid production in human myeloma stem-cell culture, with morphologic evidence of amyloid secretion by associated macrophages. N Engl J Med 307:1689, 1982.

Kyle RA, Greipp PR: Amyloidosis (AL), clinical and laboratory features in 229 cases. Mayo Clin Proc 58:665, 1983. *The best current review of this entity drawing upon the extensive Mayo experience.*

MONOCLONAL GAMMOPATHIES OF UNDETERMINED SIGNIFICANCE

If a patient has an M-component in the serum but lacks other diagnostic findings for myeloma, macroglobulinemia, or one of the other plasma cell neoplasms, the disorder is best classified as monoclonal gammopathy of unknown significance (MGUS). Formerly, the term "benign monoclonal gammopathy" was applied; however, this term is misleading, as some patients in this category do, in fact, develop myeloma or macroglobulinemia after a period of follow-up. Serum M-components without other signs of myeloma or macroglobulinemia occur in about 1 per cent of the population above age 50 and 3 per cent above age 70. Most of these persons never develop signs of a malignant plasma cell disorder. A number of patients have been followed for 15 years or more without developing myeloma.

Patients with monoclonal gammopathy of unknown significance have relatively small M-components present in the serum (usually less than 2 grams per deciliter) and do not excrete urinary L chains (Bence Jones protein). The bone marrow plasma cell percentage is generally less than 5 per cent. Marrow plasma cells from patients with MGUS have an extremely low tritiated thymidine labeling index (less than 0.5 per cent). When anemia, osteolytic lesions, hypercalcemia, Bence Jones proteinuria, or renal failure is present, the patient does not fall in the category of having a monoclonal gammopathy of undetermined significance and should be considered to have a malignant disorder. The levels of nonmonoclonal immunoglobulins are sometimes normal in monoclonal gammopathy of unknown significance, but this does not provide significant differentiation between benign and malignant plasma cell disorders. If there is only a serum M-component and no clear associated disease demonstrable by baseline observations, the patient should be followed without any treatment for the monoclonal gammopathy. In general, the patient should be seen at least every three months during the first year and at intervals of six months thereafter. If the monoclonal protein increases by 50 per cent on repeated serum electrophoresis, then a complete re-evaluation is warranted. In a five-year study of the natural history of 241 cases of monoclonal gammopathy of unknown significance, 57 per cent of patients retained stable protein levels; 9 per cent had a 50 per cent increase in the serum M-component or developed Bence Jones proteinuria; 23 per cent died without five-year serum studies; and 11 per cent developed myeloma, macroglobulinemia, or amyloidosis.

OTHER DISEASES ASSOCIATED WITH MONOCLONAL GAMMOPATHY. Patients with a variety of diseases have a monoclonal gammopathy of unknown significance. Among neoplastic diseases, monoclonal gammopathy has been observed in association with colonic cancer and certain other carcinomas, as well as with several B cell neoplasms (chronic lymphocytic leukemia and various lymphomas). M-components in lymphoid neoplasia may relate to their B cell origin and function. The explanation for an association with nonlymphoid neoplasms remains obscure, and could be coincidental. The incidence of monoclonal gammopathy in this latter group may be no greater than in the general population of that age range.

Among non-neoplastic disorders, a monoclonal gammopathy is regularly associated with the rare skin disorder lichen myxedematosus (papular mucinosis). Patients with this disorder have diffuse progressive deposition of protein in the dermis in association with the presence of a highly cationic IgG M-component, which usually has λ L chains. Monoclonal gammopathies are occasionally associated with other disorders, including Gaucher's disease, hepatitis and other liver diseases, collagen vascular diseases, and myasthenia gravis. Transient monoclonal gammopathies are sometimes observed after bone marrow transplantation, particularly in children with immunodeficiency syndrome.

Kyle RA: Monoclonal gammopathy of undetermined significance. Natural history in 241 cases. Am J Med 64:814, 1978. *An excellent and detailed analysis of the Mayo Clinic experience.*

Miglione PJ, Alexanian R: Monoclonal gammopathy in human neoplasia. Cancer 21:1127, 1968. *These authors analyze the experience at M.D. Anderson Hospital in Houston and suggest that monoclonal gammopathy associated with neoplasms other than myeloma or macroglobulinemia is only coincidental.*

Talerman A, Haije WG: The frequency of M-components in sera of patients with solid malignant neoplasms. Br J Cancer 27:276, 1973.

164 DISEASES OF THE SPLEEN

Douglas V. Faller

PHYSIOLOGY AND FUNCTIONS

The spleen, the largest lymphoid organ in the body, plays a major role in the cellular and humoral immune response to infection and inflammation. In addition, with its unique architecture and network of fixed phagocytic cells, the spleen is the primary filter for circulating senescent cells, antigens, and microorganisms. A spleen of average size (135 grams) receives a blood flow of 300 ml per minute. Splenic vessels from the hilus penetrate into trabeculations formed by invaginations of the splenic capsule (Fig. 164–1). The central arterioles, surrounded by sheaths of lymphoid tissue, have branches (follicular arterioles) that take off at right angles, effectively skimming plasma and circulating antigens from the blood and delivering them directly to the splenic immune system. The terminal arterioles are open ended and dump the remaining concentrated blood cells into the splenic cords. Some cells are shunted rapidly into the venous collection system, but many percolate slowly through the open splenic cords for several minutes before squeezing through 0.5 to 2.5 μm slits between the endothelial cells and the discontinuous basement membrane of the venous sinusoids and re-entering the splenic venous system. The cut surface of the spleen displays a prominent red pulp, dotted with islands of white pulp, which serve to compartmentalize the filtrative and immunologic functions of the spleen, respectively.

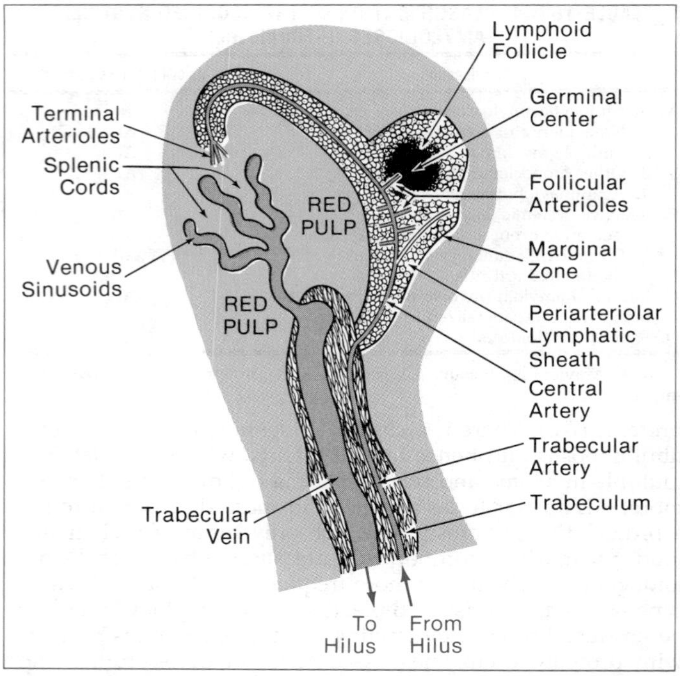

FIGURE 164–1. Diagrammatic representation of the structure of the spleen.

THE WHITE PULP. The white pulp consists of periarteriolar lymphatic sheaths, with a mantle layer of small lymphocytes (predominantly T lymphocytes) surrounding lymphoid germinal centers, which contain B cells and plasmablasts. Blood-borne antigens and pathogens are concentrated and contact immune responder cells in the white pulp. Circulating particulate antigens and opsonized microorganisms are rapidly phagocytized by macrophages in both the white and red pulp and are presented to the lymphocytes surrounding the germinal centers in the white pulp. Reactive plasmablasts secreting IgM appear, and the germinal centers enlarge within 24 hours. Consequently the white pulp component of the spleen hypertrophies in response to infection and antigenic stimulation. The spleen is therefore important in mounting a response to new immune challenges and serves as the major source of IgM production in the body. The marginal zone of the spleen surrounds these periarteriolar lymphatic sheaths of the white pulp with a dense reticulum in which the terminal arterioles end. This marginal zone blends into the red pulp.

THE RED PULP. The splenic cords (of Billroth) make up the red pulp. Erythrocytes slowly traverse these nonendothelialized cords and are subjected to metabolic conditions (including hypoxia, glucose deprivation, and low pH) that stress senescent or even mildly damaged cells. Defective erythrocytes with abnormally stiff cytoplasm (as in the sickle cell hemoglobinopathies), deficient cellular membrane (as in the spherocytic hemolytic diseases), or excessive rigidity of membrane proteins (as in the thalassemia syndromes) are then *culled* from this delayed microcirculation by the avidly phagocytic macrophages, reticular cells, and littoral cells that line the cords. *Pitting* of inclusions from erythrocytes is also performed by these phagocytes as the red cells attempt to squeeze through narrow fenestrations into the venous sinuses. This pitting function removes Howell-Jolly bodies (nuclear remnants), Heinz bodies (denatured hemoglobin), and intraerythrocytic parasites, such as malaria and *Bartonella*. New reticulocytes are *conditioned* in this environment, losing up to 30 per cent of their cell membrane and any remaining mitochondria. Iron from ingested red blood cells is stored by the splenic phagocytes and released to the plasma for *reutilization of iron.* In states of abnormal hemolysis, a buildup of hemosiderin occurs in these cells.

The spleen serves as a *reservoir* for platelets, with up to a third of the total platelet mass being sequestered there at any one time in a freely exchangeable pool. In certain disease states this reservoir function can be exaggerated. Acute entrapment of erythrocytes in the splenomegalic crisis of hemoglobin SC disease or the blackwater fever crisis of falciparum malaria can result in profound shock. Although the spleen is a blood-forming organ until five months of gestation, *hematopoiesis* in the adult spleen occurs only as a result of pathologic, usually neoplastic, conditions. Evidence exists for involvement of the spleen in the *regulation of blood volume* and in the *catabolism of low-density lipoproteins.*

EVALUATION OF THE SPLEEN

The spleen lies against the posterior abdominal wall and the diaphragm. When the spleen enlarges its lower pole moves down, anteriorly and to the right. It is best identified by detection of its movement during respiration. A palpable spleen is nearly always significantly enlarged, except in the very young. Imaging of the spleen and liver can be performed after injection of radiolabeled colloid. To visualize the spleen alone, or to identify accessory spleens, heat- or chemically damaged red blood cells tagged with ^{51}Cr or ^{99m}Tc are used. This test can also be used as an indicator of splenic function.

SPLENOMEGALY

Five general mechanisms may enlarge the spleen: (1) reactive proliferation of lymphoid cells; (2) infiltration by neoplastic cells or lipid-laden macrophages; (3) extramedullary hematopoiesis; (4) proliferation of phagocytic cells; and (5) vascular congestion. Diseases may cause splenomegaly by one or by a combination of these mechanisms (Table 164–1). The causes of massive splenomegaly (greater than 3000 grams) are somewhat more limited (Table 164–2). The myelodysplastic disorders and malignant lymphoid disorders are the most common causes of chronic massive splenomegaly in nontropical countries. Splenomegaly can present as an isolated finding on physical examination, in association with a systemic disorder, or be discovered as a consequence of the secondary hematologic effects of splenic enlargement—the hypersplenism syndrome.

Evaluation of splenomegaly should include examination of the peripheral blood. A spleen scan is recommended to determine the size and shape of the spleen and to look for defects suggestive of tumors, cysts, or nonsplenic masses displacing the spleen. In general, diagnostic tests are not performed on the spleen itself; they are oriented toward the diagnosis of disease states producing splenomegaly. If lymphadenopathy is present, lymph node biopsy may yield a diagnosis. When systemic symptoms accompany splenomegaly but no lymphadenopathy is appreciated, a laparotomy with biopsies of liver, spleen, and lymph nodes is sometimes indicated. Such a study will produce a diagnosis of lymphoma in one third of cases, congestive splenomegaly in one quarter, and an inflammatory state in one fifth.

TABLE 164–1. CAUSES OF SPLENOMEGALY

Infection (lymphoid hyperplasia)
Viral, parasitic, bacterial, fungal
Inflammation (lymphoid hyperplasia)
Rheumatoid arthritis, sarcoidosis, systemic lupus erythematosus, renal dialysis, beryllium
Neoplasms (infiltrative or myeloproliferative)
Leukemia, lymphoma, polycythemia vera, myeloid metaplasia, cysts, metastatic tumors, primary tumors
Hemolytic Disease (phagocytic hyperplasia)
Spherocytosis, thalassemia major, pyruvate kinase deficiency
Deficiency Diseases
Iron deficiency, pernicious anemia
Infiltration
Gaucher's disease, Neimann-Pick disease, amyloidosis, extramedullary hematopoiesis
Splenic Vein Hypertension (vascular congestion)
Cirrhosis, splenic or portal vein thrombosis, hepatic schistosomiasis
Endocrine
Graves' disease, Hashimoto's thyroiditis
Hemophilia (subsequent to intensive therapy with clotting-factor concentrate)

TABLE 164–2. CAUSES OF MASSIVE SPLENOMEGALY

Acute
Malaria (falciparum) with splenic sequestration crisis
Sickle cell anemia with splenic sequestration crisis
Chronic
Myelodysplastic
Chronic myelogenous leukemia
Myeloid metaplasia
Polycythemia vera (end-stage)
Primary thrombocythemia
Neoplastic
Lymphoma
Malignant reticuloendotheliosis
Hodgkins' disease
Hairy-cell leukemia
Hematologic
Thalassemia major
Sickle cell anemia (rare)
Inflammatory-infiltrative
Gaucher's disease
Sarcoidosis
Felty's syndrome
Infectious
Malaria
Kala-azar

INFECTION. Systemic infections are the most common causes of moderate and transient splenomegaly. Splenic enlargement is the rule in mononucleosis due to Epstein-Barr virus infection, but is less frequent in the heterophil-negative mononucleosis syndromes associated with cytomegalovirus, adenovirus, or acquired toxoplasmosis. Splenomegaly can be massive, however, in congenital toxoplasmosis or other infectious causes of the TORCH syndrome. A palpable spleen is often detected in the course of viral hepatitis and influenza and less often in association with infectious lymphocytosis, pertussis, and roseola infantum. Bacterial infections causing splenomegaly include secondary syphilis and acute brucellosis. Hematogenous spread of tuberculosis or histoplasmosis can involve the spleen. Splenomegaly is common in tropical populations and is due to malaria, schistosomiasis, leishmaniasis (kala-azar), chronic worm infestation, and other disorders. Rickettsial infection can produce splenic enlargement, a palpable spleen being noted in up to 40 per cent of patients with Rocky Mountain spotted fever. Modest splenomegaly is appreciated in 30 to 80 per cent of patients with the lymphadenopathy accompanying the acquired immunodeficiency disease–related complex (ARC).

INFLAMMATION. Splenomegaly is found in systemic lupus erythematosus (20 per cent), rheumatoid arthritis (5 to 10 per cent), and Behçet's disease and frequently results in production of cytopenias by hypersplenism. Angioimmunoblastic lymphadenopathy, sometimes associated with anticonvulsant administration, is characterized by splenomegaly, autoimmune hemolytic anemia, and dysproteinemia. Regional ileitis is occasionally accompanied by a histiocytic infiltration of the spleen.

NEOPLASMS. The myelodysplastic disorders and leukemias commonly infiltrate the spleen, causing modest to massive enlargement. Splenic involvement is noted in 30 to 40 per cent of adult non-Hodgkin's lymphoma at presentation. Primary malignant tumors of the spleen are rare and include lymphangiosarcomas, hemangiosarcomas, fibrosarcomas, and leiomyosarcomas. They may present with local or systemic problems and are diagnosed by spleen scan and angiography. Metastatic tumor is a rare cause of splenomegaly.

STORAGE DISEASES. Previously undiagnosed Gaucher's disease is a cause of asymptomatic splenomegaly. Niemann-

Pick disease and the sea-blue histiocyte syndrome can also present in this way. Diagnosis can often be made by bone marrow biopsy.

CHRONIC CONGESTIVE SPLENOMEGALY (BANTI'S SYNDROME). This complex is characterized by splenomegaly, pancytopenia as a consequence of hypersplenism, and gastrointestinal bleeding secondary to portal hypertension. The splenic vein hypertension is due to either intrahepatic disease (e.g., cirrhosis or schistosomiasis) or extrahepatic disease (such as portal or splenic vein thrombosis). Splenic vein thrombosis is most commonly caused by compression of the splenic vein by tumor or fibrosis. Pregnancy, trauma, or intravascular coagulation can predispose to portal vein thrombosis. The spleen is markedly enlarged and congested, with distended veins and venous sinuses. Periarteriolar hemorrhage, siderotic nodules, hyperplasia of the red pulp, and progressive fibrosis occur. Symptoms can range from vague gastrointestinal complaints to catastrophic bleeding from esophageal or gastric varices. Hematologic cytopenias may be severe, but are rarely the major medical concern. Etiologic studies of congestive splenomegaly should include evaluation for alcoholism, liver function tests, liver-spleen scan, liver biopsy, and a search for varices. If no liver disease is found, venous obstruction should be considered and splenoportal venography performed. Splenic or hepatic vein thrombosis may be the initial presentation in an occult myeloproliferative disease, particularly polycythemia vera.

HYPERSPLENISM

Hypersplenism is an exaggeration of normal splenic function, with enhanced filtration and phagocytosis of the cellular elements of the blood. The hyperplastic spleen can sequester as much as 90 per cent of the total platelet pool or 45 per cent of the red cell mass. Four criteria support the diagnosis of hypersplenism: (1) cytopenia of one or more hematologic cell lines; (2) compensatory reactive marrow hyperplasia; (3) splenomegaly; (4) correction of abnormalities by splenectomy.

Hypersplenism is frequently secondary to splenic enlargement. Splenomegaly due to infiltrative diseases (lymphoma, chronic leukemia, Gaucher's disease, amyloidosis) is not usually associated with the severe cytopenias of hypersplenism. Enlargement of the spleen due to hypertrophy of the phagocytic elements (inflammatory diseases) or secondary to congestive splenomegaly with slowing of the cellular transit time through the spleen, however, is frequently accompanied by anemia, thrombocytopenia, or granulocytopenia of varying degrees. The erythrostatic environment of hypersplenism is especially threatening to red blood cells with mild intrinsic abnormalities. The patient with well-compensated hereditary spherocytosis or elliptocytosis may experience acute, severe hemolysis from the transient splenic enlargement accompanying mononucleosis. Similarly the anemia of chronic liver disease may worsen as the increasing pressure in the portal system causes stasis and destruction of acanthocytes in the spleen. The harsh metabolic environment of the splenic cords (hypoxia, low glucose levels, and low pH) is exaggerated in the enlarged and congested spleen. In addition, phagocytosis of red cells or platelets stimulates more reactive hyperplasia of splenic histiocytes, begetting more hypersplenism. This is the mechanism underlying *primary hypersplenism*, in which the spleen hypertrophies because of phagocytosis of defective red cells (hereditary spherocytosis), antibody-coated red cells (autoimmune hemolytic anemia), or antibody-coated platelets (autoimmune thrombocytopenia). Hypersplenism can be documented and quantified by demonstrating a decrease in the circulating half-life of labeled erythrocytes along with an increase in the spleen-liver uptake ratio.

INDICATIONS FOR SPLENECTOMY

Splenectomy may be indicated for either of two medical conditions: (1) to stage or control a basic disease process (Hodgkin's disease, hereditary spherocytosis, autoimmune cytopenias) or (2) to alleviate the consequences of hypersplenism secondary to other disease processes. In addition, the spleen may have to be removed because of traumatic or, rarely, spontaneous rupture causing intra-abdominal hemorrhage.

THROMBOCYTOPENIA. *Chronic autoimmune thrombocytopenia* (ITP) refractory to corticosteroid therapy will usually improve (70 to 90 per cent) after splenectomy, with the platelet count becoming normal in 60 per cent. Those who do not respond completely can often be maintained on a lower corticosteroid dose. The thrombocytopenia accompanying *systemic* or *discoid lupus* responds only poorly to splenectomy. *Thrombotic thrombocytopenic purpura* has been treated in the past with splenectomy and steroid therapy, but newer multimodal treatments, including plasmapheresis or plasma exchange, appear more promising (Ch. 166).

HEMOLYTIC ANEMIAS. *Autoimmune hemolytic anemia* caused by warm-reacting antibodies that does not resolve after two months of corticosteroid therapy may be treated by splenectomy. Two thirds of such patients will have complete or partial remission, but the relapse rate is high. Splenectomy is a uniformly effective treatment for the anemia of *hereditary spherocytosis* (Ch. 138). Surgery should be delayed until the age of five years, if possible, to decrease the risk of overwhelming sepsis. Other congenital hemolytic anemias do not respond as consistently to splenectomy, and the decision to remove the spleen should be based on the severity of the anemia and lack of response to alternative treatments.

LEUKEMIAS. Splenectomy is routinely performed for symptomatic cytopenias or splenomegaly in *hairy-cell leukemia* (leukemic reticuloendotheliosis). Improvement occurs in up to 85 per cent of patients, but recurrence of cytopenias is common. Early splenectomy is no longer recommended, and the advent of alpha-interferon therapy for this disease may relegate splenectomy to a secondary role (Ch. 155). In the past, splenectomy was commonly carried out in patients with *chronic myelogenous leukemia* for relief of symptoms or prior to bone marrow transplantation. Any benefit is transient, however; survival is not affected, and the operation in this setting is associated with a high mortality. Splenectomy can provide useful palliation in patients with *chronic lymphocytic leukemia* who have symptomatic splenomegaly or autoimmune hemolytic anemia. Splenectomy improves the hematologic status and the quality of life in cases of severe agnogenic myeloid metaplasia (Ch. 154).

STORAGE DISEASES. Splenectomy can be performed in *Gaucher's disease* when splenomegaly produces mechanical or cytopenic problems. The spleen serves as a storage area for undigested cerebroside, so it is possible that splenectomy might accelerate the disease (Ch. 185).

FELTY'S SYNDROME. Neutropenia of variable degrees and splenomegaly, occasionally accompanied by thrombocytopenia or anemia, occurs in about 1 per cent of patients with rheumatoid arthritis. The spleen appears to be both the source of the antibody coating the neutrophils and the means of their destruction. If the neutropenia is severe enough to cause frequent infections or skin ulcerations, splenectomy is beneficial in 60 to 80 per cent of patients.

THALASSEMIA MAJOR. In the setting of longstanding thalassemia, therapeutic splenectomy is often required. It appears, however, that aggressive transfusion regimens combined with iron chelation therapy may reduce the incidence of severe hypersplenism.

RENAL DIALYSIS HYPERSPLENISM. Up to 10 per cent of uremic patients undergoing long-term dialysis develop signs of hypersplenism. Splenectomy may decrease bleeding tendencies and transfusion requirements in this setting.

ALTERNATIVES TO SPLENECTOMY. Therapy with glucocorticoids inhibits phagocytosis and can provide a useful "chemical splenectomy" in short-term situations. Partial splenectomy is sometimes advocated in children to reduce the risk of postsplenectomy complications. Partial or complete embolization of the spleen using percutaneous catheterization is a relatively safe, effective, and noninvasive approach when surgery is contraindicated. Splenic irradiation (100 to 500 rads) can provide transient therapy for hypersplenism or splenomegaly due to infiltrative diseases.

POSTSPLENECTOMY SYNDROMES AND HYPOSPLENISM

HEMATOLOGIC SEQUELAE. The hyposplenic or postsplenectomy state can often be diagnosed by examination of the peripheral blood smear. In the absence of splenic culling and pitting functions, nucleated red blood cells, Howell-Jolly and Heinz body inclusions, siderocytes, and acanthocytes are found in the circulation. Reticulocytes are no longer conditioned, and their redundant cell membrane produces target cells upon drying and staining.

A transient and modest increase in the leukocyte count occurs after splenectomy and lasts one to two weeks. The bulk of this *leukocytosis* is accounted for by early *neutrophilia*. Later, *lymphocytosis* and *monocytosis* become more prominent.

Splenectomy routinely results in prominent postoperative *thrombocytosis*, often producing platelet counts of 1 million or more per cubic millimeter for weeks to months following surgery. This elevation may persist in 40 per cent of patients. The risk of consequent thromboembolic phenomena is high only after splenectomy in the setting of myeloproliferative disease or paroxysmal nocturnal hemoglobinuria. Attempts should be made to decrease the platelet count with chemotherapy before surgery in such cases. Following surgery, therapy with anticoagulants and antiplatelet agents should be considered, especially if the patient is bedridden.

INFECTION. In the absence of the spleen, or in the setting of functional asplenia, certain inadequacies of immune function can be demonstrated. IgM levels fall, and complement-mediated opsonization is decreased. This is in part due to a fall in the levels of tuftsin and properdin, two opsonic proteins produced by the spleen. The ability to phagocytose circulating antigens is compromised, as is cell-mediated immunity.

The risk of *overwhelming sepsis* following splenectomy or in functional asplenia is especially high in children, being as high as 10 per cent in debilitated infants. The incidence falls in older children (1 per cent) and is rare, but reported, in adults. The etiologic organisms are encapsulated bacteria, predominantly pneumococcus and less commonly meningococcus or *Hemophilus influenzae*. These are poorly opsonized in the body, and the intact spleen, with its slow, tortuous blood flow past avid phagocytes, appears to be the primary site for clearance of these pathogens. All patients with decreased splenic function, whether due to functional hyposplenism or to splenectomy (traumatic or therapeutic) must be warned to take any febrile illness seriously. Prophylaxis with penicillin is recommended for all children with asplenia or splenic hypofunction (e.g., sickle cell anemia). Immunization with polyvalent vaccines to pneumococci, meningococci, and *H. influenzae* is advised for patients over the age of three years. Serologic response to these vaccines is not always normal in hyposplenia or asplenia. The timing of vaccine administration (before or after splenectomy) is not important, but vaccination should precede any chemotherapy, if possible. Serious infections with unusual organisms like *Babesia* or *Bartonella* also occur in asplenic individuals. A concurrent viral infection may predispose hyposplenic patients to fulminant bacteremias.

FUNCTIONAL HYPOSPLENISM. Repeated symptomatic or silent infarction of the spleen in the course of veno-occlusive diseases, like the sickle cell syndromes, results in substantial or total loss of splenic tissue *(autosplenectomy)*. The spleen is shrunken and fibrosed. Circulating erythrocytes reflect the loss of the splenic filtration function and are found to contain mitochrondrial remnants and inclusions of nuclear fragments (Howell-Jolly bodies) and denatured hemoglobin (Heinz bodies). Bizarrely shaped red cells, target cells, and large platelets are observed. Hyposplenism can occur even with a large or normal-sized spleen if splenic tissue has been replaced by sarcoid granulomas, amyloid, or multiple myeloma or if splenic phagocytes have been paralyzed by high-dose corticosteroid therapy. Other diseases linked with hyposplenism include ulcerative colitis, celiac disease, dermatitis herpetiformis, systemic lupus erythematosus, primary thrombocythemia, and Graves' disease. Such patients run the same risk of fulminant bacteremia as do those who have had their spleen surgically removed.

CONGENITAL ASPLENIA. This uncommon condition is associated with symmetric development of normally asymmetric organs or pairs of organs. Complex and multiple cardiovascular anomalies are the rule.

OTHER DISEASES OF THE SPLEEN

SPLENIC RUPTURE. Rupture of the capsule may be precipitated by trauma, overly zealous palpation of an enlarged spleen (secondary to mononucleosis, sepsis, or leukemia), or rarely by dissection of a pancreatic pseudocyst into the spleen. The patient presents with left upper-quadrant pain, sometimes radiating to the left scapular region, and abdominal guarding and rigidity and progresses to hypovolemic shock. Usually emergency splenectomy is indicated. In selected cases, nonoperative management or splenorraphy, including wrapping of the ruptured capsule ("hair netting"), is a treatment option to splenectomy.

SPLENIC INFARCTION. Infarction usually occurs in the setting of splenic enlargement secondary to myeloproliferative disease or vascular occlusive phenomena (sickle hemoglobinopathies, including SS, SA, S thal, and SC diseases). These may be silent infarctions or present with severe left upper-quadrant pain.

ARTERIAL ANEURYSMS. These lesions are most common in women beyond middle age. They may be asymptomatic or cause left upper-quadrant pain or vague gastrointestinal complaints. The aneurysm or the spleen is sometimes palpable, and a bruit may be appreciated. Radiologic studies can reveal a calcified aneurysmal wall, and the diagnosis is made by sonography or angiography. Embolization of such aneurysms has been successful in situations in which surgery is contraindicated.

SPLENIC HEMANGIOMATOSIS. Diffuse cavernous hemangiomatosis of the spleen is rare, but the cavernous hemangioma is the most common benign tumor involving the spleen. The patient can present with splenic infarctions, splenomegaly, or thrombocytopenia secondary to platelet destruction within the hemangiomas, or the finding of hemangiomatosis may be incidental. The diagnosis can usually be made by computed tomography or sonography.

SPLENIC CYSTS. Echinococcal infection should be suspected in a patient with an appropriate travel history, single or multiple splenic cysts with calcified walls, and eosinophilia. Serologic studies may be helpful in establishing the diagnosis. True splenic cysts (dermoids and mesenchymal inclusion cysts) are embryonic rests and may be diagnosed by scan and angiography.

SPLENIC ABSCESS. An occult, deep-seated infection, splenic abscess usually follows a bacteremic episode. The source of the septicemia can be infected endocardium; lung (pneumonia, lung abscess, empyema); skin or soft tissue; pelvis (pelvic inflammatory disease or septic abortion); nasopharynx; or ear. Predisposing factors include previous splenic damage by infarction (secondary to sickle cell disease or leukemia), trauma, and infection (malaria, typhoid, amoeba, cysts). Extension of an abscess into the spleen from adjacent perforated abdominal organs (stomach, transverse colon, tail of pancreas) can occur. In most series, streptococci are the most common etiologic agents, followed by staphylococci and, with increasing frequency, by gram-negative organisms (*Salmonella, Enterobacteriaceae, Pseudomonas, Serratia, Bacteroides*) and anaerobes. Presenting symptoms include fever, chills, and left upper-quadrant pain, often accompanied by tenderness, muscle spasm, and subcutaneous edema over the spleen. Infection localized to the upper pole of the spleen can produce pleuritic pain and even left pleural effusion. An abscess in the lower pole may result in signs of peritoneal inflammation. A splenic friction rub may be appreciated. Splenic scan, sonography, and computed tomography aid in the diagnosis. The differential diagnosis must include subphrenic abscess, pulmonary empyema, splenic infarction, perinephric abscess, neoplasms, and pancreatic pseudocyst. A combination of antibiotics and surgical intervention, usually splenectomy, is indicated. Single abscesses respond well, but multiple abscesses, often the result of generalized sepsis in a debilitated or immunocompromised patient, are associated with a high mortality.

Chaikof EL, McCabe CT: Fatal overwhelming postsplenectomy infection. Am J Surg 149:534, 1985. *A review of infection patterns in 776 splenectomized adults and children.*

Chun CH, Raff MJ, Contreras L, et al.: Splenic abscess. Medicine, 59:50, 1980. *Comprehensive review of this often fatal disease, discussing etiology, predisposing factors, diagnosis, and treatment.*

Crosby WH: The spleen. In Wintrobe MM (ed.): Blood, Pure and Eloquent. New York, McGraw-Hill Book Company, 1980, p 96. *Historical review of our understanding of splenic function and hypersplenism.*

Eichner ER: Splenic function: Normal, too much and too little. Am J Med 66:311, 1979. *Useful summary of hypersplenic and hyposplenic states, with recommendations for management.*

Mucha P Jr: Changing attitudes toward the management of blunt splenic trauma in adults. Mayo Clin Proc 61:472, 1986. *Discusses splenic preservation and alternatives to splenectomy.*

165 BONE MARROW TRANSPLANTATION

Rainer Storb

MARROW TRANSPLANT PRINCIPLES. Transplantation of marrow from a donor identical with the recipient at the major histocompatibility complex reduces graft-versus-host disease (GVHD) and improves survival of the recipient. Successful human transplantation using allogeneic, HLA-identical sib donors was carried out first in children with immunodeficiency diseases (reviewed in Ch. 419) and subsequently in patients with severe aplastic anemia and leukemia.

Marrow transplantation differs in several aspects from transplantation of solid organs, in particular kidney (see Ch. 80): (1) the host-versus-graft reaction can generally be abrogated by a single short course of high-dose immunosuppressive therapy given immediately before transplantation; (2) preceding blood transfusions are not beneficial but rather can interfere with subsequent marrow engraftment, particularly in patients with aplastic anemia; (3) donors have mostly been HLA-identical family members; (4) donors do not suffer a permanent organ loss, since the removed marrow is replaced within weeks; and (5) post-grafting immunosuppression of recipients can generally be terminated after 3 to 12 months.

To prepare for marrow transplantation the recipient's immune system must first be destroyed. This is effectively accomplished by use of cyclophosphamide (CY), at 50 mg per kilogram per day for four days, or total body irradiation (TBI), at 800 to 1500 rad midline tissue doses (4 to 25 rad per minute) either alone or combined with CY or other chemotherapeutic agents. This program not only sets the stage for establishment of the allogeneic graft but also serves to kill leukemic cells, if that is the patient's basic disease.

After the conditioning regimen, 2 to 6 $\times$ 10^8 donor marrow cells per kilogram are infused intravenously. Most grafts are initially successful such that within two to four weeks marrow cellularity increases and peripheral blood counts of donor origin rise. Over time, all hematopoietic and immune cells of the recipient are replaced by those from the marrow donor, including plasma cells and tissue macrophages.

COMPLICATIONS. *Graft-versus-host disease* may occur when genetically foreign, immunologically active lymphocytes are transferred into an immunosuppressed recipient incapable of rejecting the lymphocytes. This condition is met within all allogeneic marrow transplant recipients (donors are other than monozygous twins). Donor T lymphocytes present in the marrow inoculum recognize histocompatibility antigens of the host as foreign, become sensitized, proliferate, and attack recipient tissue, thereby producing the clinical syndrome of GVHD. The main targets of GVHD are skin, gastrointestinal tract, and liver. Methotrexate or cyclosporine is given within the first 3 to 12 months after grafting as perhaps the most effective immunosuppressive agent to prevent GVHD. Best results seem to be achieved when both drugs are combined. Once the drugs are discontinued, many patients do well with persisting graft-host tolerance. However, acute GVHD occurs in approximately 35 to 60 per cent of the patients, and as many as 40 per cent of afflicted patients die from associated infections. Xenogeneic antihuman thymocyte globulin (ATG), prednisone, or cyclosporine has been used to treat acute GVHD with some success. Better approaches to prevent or treat acute GVHD are necessary, such as the more imaginative use of known immunosuppressive agents, the use of "germ-free" isolation, or the removal of T cells from the marrow inoculum by antibodies to human T lymphocytes.

Chronic GVHD affects approximately 25 to 45 per cent of patients surviving more than 180 days. It is most frequent in older patients and those who had acute GVHD. It may affect the same organs that are involved in acute GVHD and, additionally, mucous membranes. It resembles collagen vascular diseases and is characterized by severe immune deficiency, impaired granulocyte chemotaxis, and recurrent, sometimes life-threatening bacterial infections. Combination therapy with prednisone and azathioprine, CY, or procarbazine is effective in most patients with chronic GVHD.

Interstitial pneumonias, either of unknown etiology or associated with infectious agents such as cytomegalovirus, are a cause of morbidity and fatality during the first four months after grafting. They are a major problem in patients treated with TBI and then receiving transplants for leukemia and a minor problem in CY-treated patients receiving transplants for aplastic anemia. Probably these infections are the result of deficient immune reactivity of the compromised host (see Ch. 258) although radiation effects may also play a role. Effective methods of accelerating the immune reconstitution and/or the use of antiviral agents or hyperimmune globulin might be of value in obviating the problem of interstitial pneumonia.

CLINICAL RESULTS

SEVERE APLASTIC ANEMIA. Aplastic anemia is most frequently attributable to a stem cell defect (see Ch. 133). In many cases infusion of marrow from a monozygotic twin (syngeneic transplant) has been successful in reconstituting the marrow without immunosuppression of the recipient. Some syngeneic grafts have been successful only after preparation with CY and a second transplant, suggesting that these cases may involve other mechanisms, perhaps of autoimmune etiology, which can be overcome by CY.

Allogeneic marrow transplantation (donors are HLA-identical family members) is often effective therapy for severe aplastic anemia, with significantly better survival.

Marrow graft rejection has been a major problem in aplastic anemia. Two factors have predicted graft rejection: (1) positive in vitro tests of cell-mediated immunity, indicating reaction

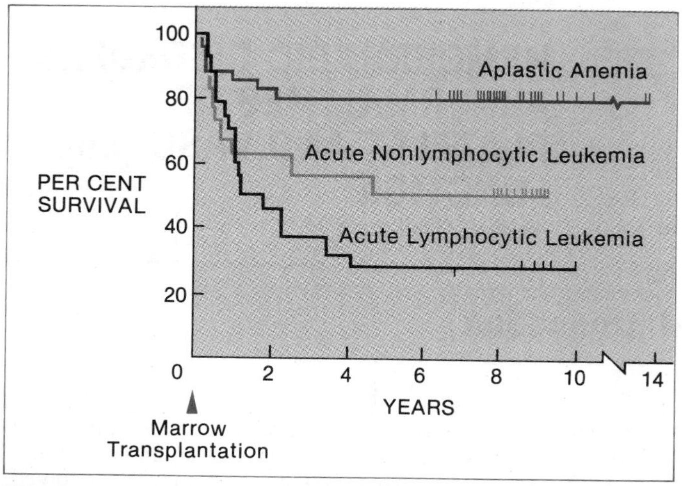

FIGURE 165–1. The survival of 43 untransfused patients with aplastic anemia, 22 patients with acute nonlymphoblastic leukemia having transplants in first remission, and 22 patients with acute lymphoblastic leukemia having transplants in second or subsequent remission after marrow grafts from HLA-identical family members. The surviving patients with leukemia remain in unmaintained remission. Day "0" is the day of marrow transplantation. The tick marks indicate living patients. Survival is as of May 1986.

of recipient lymphocytes against donor cells before transplantation; and (2) a low number of transplanted marrow cells ($<3 \times 10^8$ per kilogram). Transfusion-induced sensitization is the major cause of graft rejection. In our experience when transplantation is carried out in patients who have not received transfusions before transplantation, graft failure is the exception. Eighty-three per cent of our 43 patients are alive between 4 and 14½ (median 7) years after grafting (Fig. 165–1). We believe that the immunologic mechanisms involved in graft failure are, for the most part, iatrogenic (i.e., induced by previous blood transfusion).

Many programs are being carried out to avoid rejection in multiply transfused patients by using more intensive immunosuppressive conditioning regimens. In all programs CY is used, but other features of the conditioning regimens vary. In Seattle methotrexate and cyclosporine are used after grafting, and viable donor buffy-coat cells are infused together with the marrow inoculum. The donor's peripheral blood is a potential source of additional pluripotent hematopoietic stem cells and/or lymphoid cells capable of overcoming rejection. As a rule, the rejection rates have decreased and survival has increased. Of the last 65 Seattle patients with aplastic anemia who received marrow grafts from HLA-identical siblings following multiple transfusions, 70 per cent are alive after follow-up periods of 4 to 10½ years.

Most of the regimens have associated risks. The addition of buffy-coat cells may lead to an increased risk of chronic GVHD. Radiation regimens carry the potential risk for late malignant disease. Because of these problems and the still existing mortality from rejection, emphasis should be placed on measures to prevent rather than overcome sensitization by blood transfusions. For this the physician should be aware of the possibility of marrow transplantation when aplastic anemia is first diagnosed. If an HLA-identical family member is available, early transplantation before transfusions is the therapy of choice.

LEUKEMIA. Marrow grafting for leukemia presents the same general transplantation problems encountered for aplastic anemia. However, graft rejection is rare. The unique problem is recurrence of leukemia. Formerly marrow transplantation was carried out only after failure of all other therapy when patients were undergoing advanced relapse. Of the first 100 patients with acute leukemia receiving grafts in Seattle after CY and TBI, 12 per cent are alive with the disease in remission between 11 and 16 years without any maintenance therapy. Approximately 75 per cent of all patients could be expected to have recurrent leukemia unless they died of other causes. Leukemic recurrence usually originated from host-type cells, indicating that it is difficult to kill every leukemic cell once the patient has reached the end-stage of the disease. Current attempts to reduce the rate of leukemic relapse and increase long-term survival in patients with leukemia receiving transplants in the end-stage of their disease involve the use of higher doses of TBI by means of fractionating the radiation and the use of additional chemotherapeutic agents. Perhaps these attempts are doomed to failure since, in an exponential cell kill process, it is difficult to kill the last leukemic cell. Some of the apparent cures may have occurred because of leukemic cell kill by immune mechanisms directed at non-HLA antigens expressed on leukemic cells. This is suggested by the observation of a graft-versus-leukemia effect in man.

It is attractive to carry out marrow transplantation earlier in the course of the disease while the disease is in remission. The advantages of this approach include treatment when the number of leukemic cells in the body is small and before the cells become resistant to therapy, and while the patient is in good clinical condition and therefore better able to tolerate the therapy. Accordingly, we began in 1976 to treat patients with acute nonlymphoblastic leukemia by marrow grafting when the disease was in first or subsequent remission and those with acute lymphoblastic leukemia when it was in second or subsequent remission after conditioning with CY and TBI.

Patients with acute nonlymphoblastic leukemia who received chemotherapy have an approximate median duration of survival of 2 years (see Ch. 156). Only 15 to 20 per cent of patients who received chemotherapy are alive at five years. Of the first 22 patients with *acute nonlymphoblastic leukemia* treated by marrow transplantation during *first remission,* 12 are alive with the disease in unmaintained remission between eight and ten years after transplantation (Fig. 165–1). The survival curve shows a plateau at 55 per cent.

Approximately 50 per cent of patients with acute lymphoblastic leukemia, especially children, can be cured by chemotherapy (see Ch. 156). Once relapse has occurred, another remission can often be induced with chemotherapy, but long-term survival is poor, with very few of the patients alive at two years. Treatment of patients with acute lymphoblastic leukemia during second or subsequent remission by marrow transplantation seems justified in an attempt to change the otherwise grim outlook and perhaps "cure" some of these patients of their disease.

The survival curve of the first 22 patients with *acute lymphoblastic leukemia in second or subsequent remission* receiving marrow grafts in Seattle shows a plateau at 27 per cent 8½ to 10 years after transplantation (Fig. 165–1).

The results of marrow transplantation for the treatment of patients with *chronic granulocytic leukemia* in blast crisis have been similar to those in patients with leukemia in relapse. The projected survival is approximately 15 per cent (Fig. 165–2). The patients' marrows show absence of the Philadelphia chromosome, a unique result.

Transplantation during the *chronic phase of chronic granulocytic leukemia* promises to improve these results. Although follow-up is still short, it appears that long-term disease-free survival will be on the order of 50 per cent (Fig. 165–2).

Marrow transplantation has now also been successfully applied to the treatment of patients with non-Hodgkin's lymphoma, myelofibrosis, multiple myeloma, preleukemia, and hairy cell leukemia.

Common to all results of marrow grafting for leukemia and lymphoma is the problem of recurrence of disease due to host cells that have survived the high-dose chemoradiation therapy. New treatment programs being explored in a number of

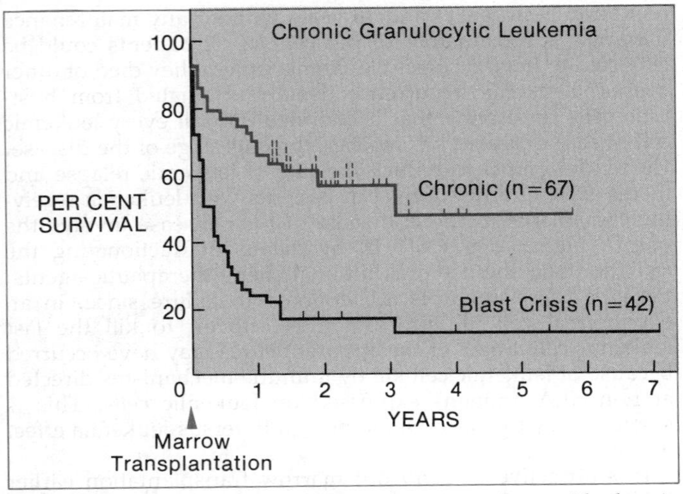

FIGURE 165–2. Survival after marrow grafting in patients with chronic granulocytic leukemia having transplants either in blast crisis or in chronic phase. The tick marks indicate living patients. Survival is as of March 1985.

centers are aimed at more effectively destroying the malignant cells, thereby increasing the success of marrow transplantation.

CONCLUSIONS

Marrow transplantation, once considered a desperate form of therapy in patients with end-stage disease, has now become increasingly successful when used early in the course of aplastic anemia or leukemia. The current success now obliges the physician to identify, soon after diagnosis, those patients who have suitable donors and who may be candidates for transplantation. Marrow grafting has now been extended to the therapy of patients with other hematologic malignant diseases and genetic disorders of hematopoiesis. In the longest survivor with malignant non-Hodgkin's lymphoma, the disease is now in unmaintained remission 16 years after marrow grafting. Cures of congenital Fanconi's anemia, paroxysmal nocturnal hemoglobinuria, thalassemia major, osteopetrosis, and certain genetic storage diseases have been achieved by marrow transplantation.

Many patients do not have HLA-identical sibs, and very few have monozygotic twins. To extend marrow transplantation to a larger number of patients, the use of less well matched family members has been explored with success. Successful human transplants from unrelated donors for the treatment of patients with acute leukemia and aplastic anemia have been carried out.

With the establishment of techniques to "purge" marrow from unwanted malignant cells and to cryopreserve marrow for indefinite periods, in recent years we have seen a renaissance of autologous marrow transplantation for the treatment of malignant diseases. Autologous marrow is attractive, since it avoids the problem of GVHD.

Moller G (ed.): Graft-versus-host reaction. Immunol Rev, Vol 88, 1985. *Reviews by multiple authors of the pathophysiology, immunology, treatment, and prevention of acute and chronic graft-versus-host disease in experimental animals and in man.*

Storb R, Thomas ED: Current state of marrow transplantation. In Silker, R, Gordon AS, Lobue J (eds.): Contemporary Hematology/Oncology, Vol. 3. New York, Plenum Medical, 1984, pp 235–266. *General review with emphasis on GVHD, immunological aspects, opportunistic infections, and recurrence of leukemia.*

Van Bekkum DW, Lowenberg B (eds.): Bone Marrow Transplantation: Biological Mechanisms and Clinical Practice. Vol 3. New York, Marcel Dekker, 1985. *Current state of experimental research and clinical applications in the area of bone marrow grafting. Written by multiple authors.*

Van Rood J, Zwaan F (eds.): Bone Marrow Transplantation. Semin Hematol, Vol 21, 1984. *Multiple-author reviews of marrow transplantation for malignant and nonmalignant hematologic diseases, including late complications and immune reconstitution.*

166 HEMORRHAGIC DISORDERS: ABNORMALITIES OF PLATELET AND VASCULAR FUNCTION

Aaron J. Marcus

Introduction

MECHANISMS OF NORMAL HEMOSTASIS

In hemostasis a sequence of local events culminates in spontaneous arrest of bleeding from a traumatized blood vessel. Three closely linked biologic systems are involved: *blood vessels, platelets,* and *coagulation proteins.* The initial response to interruption of vascular continuity is known as *primary hemostasis* and involves platelets and the vessel surface. Coagulation proteins do not play a role at this juncture. Vascular injury is immediately followed by vessel contraction and platelet adhesion to exposed subendothelial collagen. This adhesive process involves platelet membrane glycoprotein Ib (GPIb) and is mediated by Factor VIII–related von Willebrand factor (Factor VIII: vWF) polymers that adsorb to exposed subendothelial collagen and to platelets. Collagen is an agonist for adherent platelets and induces configurational and biochemical alterations therein. These include (1) secretion of biologically active substances stored in intracellular platelet granules (release reaction); (2) enzymatic liberation of arachidonic acid (by phospholipase[s]) and its oxygenation, mainly to thromboxane A_2 (TXA_2) and 12-hydroxyeicosatetraenoic acid (12-HETE); (3) a rearrangement of platelet surface phospholipoprotein, such that it develops procoagulant properties. These include ability to bind and catalyze activation of Factor X and conversion of prothrombin to thrombin. The proteolytic enzyme thrombin is a strong stimulus for further platelet aggregation, TXA_2 formation, the release reaction, and further catalysis of fibrin formation.

Platelet secretion can be induced not only by collagen and thrombin, but also by adenosine diphosphate (ADP) and epinephrine. Released platelet products are classified according to their intracellular granule of origin. Thus ADP, serotonin (5-hydroxytryptamine, 5-HT, a powerful vasoconstrictor substance), and calcium originate from dense granules and serve to recruit additional platelets into the hemostatic plug. Alpha-granule components include platelet factor 4 (a heparin-neutralizing protein); beta-thromboglobulin (a platelet-specific protein of unknown function); platelet-derived growth factor (PDGF), which stimulates proliferation of smooth muscle and fibroblasts; Factor VIII: vWF; Factor V; thrombospondin; fibrinogen; albumin; and fibronectin. The threshold for release of alpha-granule components by stimuli is lower than that required for dense body release.

Platelet recruitment, as initiated by released ADP and TXA_2, results in further stimulation, aggregation, and augmentation of hemostatic plug formation (Fig. 166–1). In addition, released ADP induces exposure of platelet fibrinogen-binding sites. Exposure of the platelet fibrinogen receptor results from structural transformation of platelet glycoproteins IIb and IIIa during platelet activation. These proteins form a heterodimer complex that expresses fibrinogen receptor activity.

As mentioned, platelet-collagen contact results in liberation of the essential fatty acid, arachidonate, which is oxygenated by two enzymes: a particulate cyclo-oxygenase and a cytoplasmic lipoxygenase. Cyclo-oxygenation of arachidonate (which is inhibited by aspirin acetylation) results in formation of endoperoxides (PGG_2 and PGH_2), which are transient

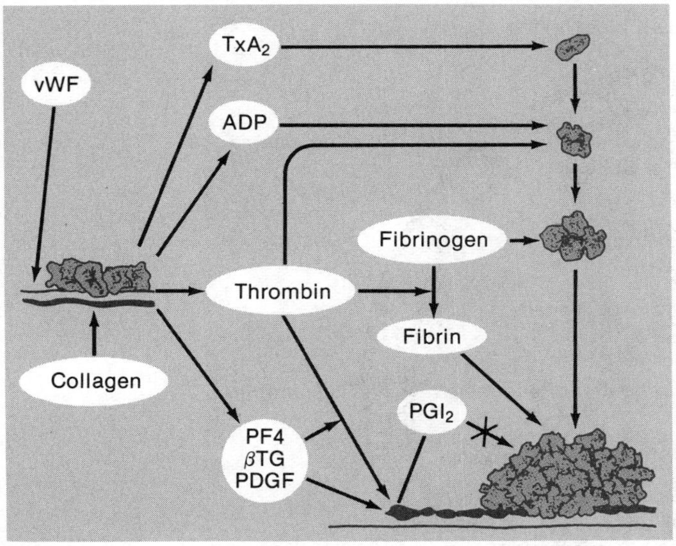

FIGURE 166–1. Reactions of primary (*left*) and secondary (*right*) hemostasis. Following injury of intact vascular endothelium, collagen exposure in the presence of Factor VIII:vWF results in platelet adhesion and activation. These activated platelets release ADP and 5-HT from dense granules and proteins from alpha granules (platelet factor 4, beta-thromboglobulin, and platelet-derived growth factor). Thromboxane is formed from free arachidonic acid and the stimulated platelet phospholipoprotein surface catalyzes activation of Factor X in the formation of thrombin. TxA_2, ADP, and thrombin "synergize" to induce shape change, aggregation, and release in platelets arriving at the injury site. Thrombin formation with consequent conversion of fibrinogen to fibrin comprises secondary hemostasis. Prostacyclin (PGI_2) and other eicosanoids are synthesized by endothelial cells from arachidonate in response to injury, collagen, thrombin, and released platelet endoperoxides. Endothelial cell eicosanoids may regulate the size and extent of platelet deposition in the hemostatic plug (or under pathologic conditions—the thrombus). (Modified from Thompson AR, Harker LA: Manual of Hemostasis and Thrombosis. 3rd ed. Philadelphia, FA Davis Company, 1983.)

intermediates in TXA_2 formation (Fig. 166–2). TXA_2 is rapidly released into the surrounding medium where it induces further platelet aggregation and vasoconstriction. TXA_2 inhibits platelet adenylate cyclase, thereby inducing a fall in cyclic AMP, which in turn increases calcium mobilization. The level of free intracellular calcium is the final determinant of platelet responsiveness. Thrombin and collagen also promote intracellular platelet calcium mobilization independent of, but by comparable mechanisms to, TXA_2. Ionized platelet calcium induces: (1) complex formation with its binding protein, calmodulin, (2) activation of kinases that phosphorylate platelet myosin, (3) activation of phospholipases, and (4) initiation of secretion. In sharp contrast, endothelial cell endoperoxides are converted to prostacyclin (PGI_2) and other eicosanoids. PGI_2 inhibits platelet aggregation and release by increasing platelet cyclic AMP levels, thereby blocking calcium mobilization (Fig. 166–2).

Although primary hemostasis represents a complex sequence of events, its clinical assessment is relatively simple. The bleeding time is a sensitive and reliable index of primary hemostasis. If the bleeding time is prolonged and the platelet count over 100,000 per microliter, primary hemostasis is impaired because of a platelet defect. The qualitative defect can be caused by poor adhesion to the vessel wall or poor platelet cohesion (aggregation). Alternatively, impairment of platelet plug formation as manifested by prolonged bleeding time can be due to thrombocytopenia (platelet count $< 100,000$ per microliter).

In *secondary hemostasis*, platelets have already aggregated at the site of injury, and the exposed surface membrane phospholipoprotein on activated platelets has catalyzed Factor X activation and prothrombin conversion to thrombin. Thrombin formation is a critical step that amplifies the reactions of primary hemostasis as well as those leading to fibrin formation and stabilization of the platelet plug (or under pathologic conditions, the thrombus). The actions of thrombin in hemostasis are (1) direct irreversible platelet aggregation with release of ADP, 5-HT, and proteins from alpha-granules; (2) initiation of phospholipase activity culminating in production of TXA_2, thereby indirectly augmenting vasoconstriction, aggregation, and release; (3) conversion of fibrinogen to fibrin strands that consolidate the platelet mass; (4) exposure of platelet receptors for Factor Va to which Factor Xa binds, and enhancement of further thrombin formation; (5) activation of Factor XIII, which catalyzes formation of covalent amide bonds between fibrin polymers, resulting in clot stabilization and completion of the hemostatic process.

Thompson AR, Harker LA: Manual of Hemostasis and Thrombosis. 3rd ed. Philadelphia, F. A. Davis Company, 1983. *This is a compact but very thorough manual that details a pathophysiologic approach to the diagnosis and management of patients with hemostatic and thrombotic disorders. The sequential organization, tables, and figures are presented in a comprehensive manner.*

BLOOD PLATELETS

Platelets are anucleate cytoplasmic fragments derived from marrow megakaryocytes by extension of cytoplasmic processes that undergo attenuation, develop constrictions at their distal ends, and then rupture in the form of free platelets. Production and release of platelets from the marrow may be controlled by two "thrombopoietins"—one regulating the quantity of megakaryocyte-committed stem cells and another modulating megakaryocyte maturation. The presence of large platelets (megathrombocytes) in the circulation may be directly related to the degree of thrombopoietic stimulation. Platelets, which normally circulate for about ten days, are 3.6 ± 0.7 μm in diameter. The normal platelet count is 150,000 to 400,000 per microliter. On a stained blood smear one can visualize about three to ten platelets per oil-immersion field. Approximately 70 per cent of platelets are circulating, and 30 per cent are in the spleen.

Despite its comparatively simple structure the platelet is functionally complex. Stimulated platelets adhere to damaged vessel surfaces (adhesion) as well as to each other (cohesion or aggregation). Stimulation is also a prerequisite for the release reaction and transformation of arachidonic acid to TXA_2, which reinforces hemostatic function. Platelets maintain "vascular integrity" through obscure mechanisms. Rapid onset of thrombocytopenia is often associated with spontaneous hemorrhage into the skin and mucous membranes, whereas in chronic thrombocytopenias there is an ill-defined compensatory mechanism for missing "vascular integrity factor(s)" and hemorrhage is less frequent. Platelets function in the intrinsic coagulation system. The phospholipoprotein surface of stimulated platelets binds and catalyzes interactions between activated coagulation factors culminating in thrombin formation, a property formerly termed platelet factor 3.

Platelets mediate clot retraction, probably via the contractile protein actomyosin. This may play a role in vivo during consolidation of hemostatic plug formation and can be studied in vitro as a well-defined metabolic process.

Platelets, therefore, intrinsically possess multiple mechanisms for responding to and repairing effects of vascular damage. These include a factor(s) for maintaining vascular integrity, the capacity to spontaneously arrest bleeding through plug formation, the ability to catalyze fibrinogen polymerization—thereby stabilizing the plug, and mechanisms for release of growth factors to enhance repair and healing. These processes occur in varying degrees, depending upon strength and concentration of the stimuli. Failure of one mechanism (as in the case of TXA_2 inhibition by aspirin ingestion) results in a minor hemostatic defect, since others such as thrombin responsiveness remain intact. Figure 166–3

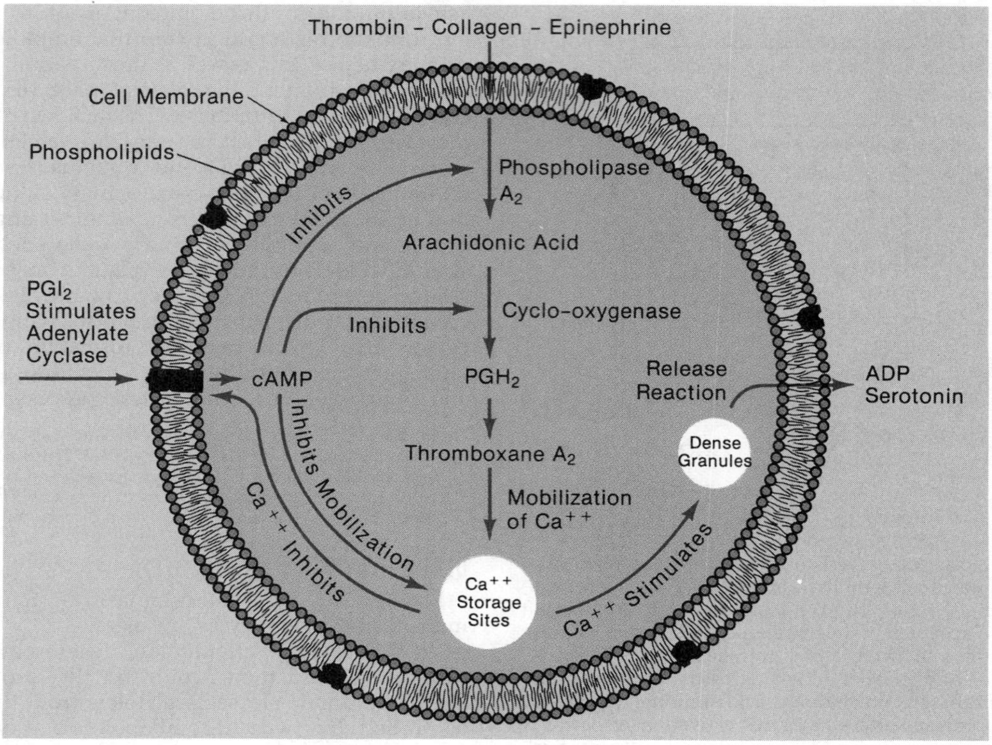

FIGURE 166–2. Diagram of events associated with activation of the platelet arachidonic acid cyclooxygenase pathway. The end product, thromboxane A_2, induces intracellular calcium mobilization and is also released into the microenvironment where it acts as a direct agonist for additional platelet aggregation and vasoconstriction. Mobilized calcium is the major stimulus for initiation of dense granule secretion. ADP and serotonin are among the most important products of the platelet release reaction. The increase in intracellular calcium also inhibits adenylate cyclase, thus lowering cyclic AMP levels, which further promotes aggregation and release. In contrast, PGI_2, the major cyclooxygenase product of endothelial cells, stimulates adenylate cyclase, thus elevating platelet cyclic AMP and blocking calcium mobilization and its consequences. In this manner PGI_2 attenuates platelet responsiveness. Platelets also contain a lipoxygenase pathway of arachidonate metabolism, of which the end product is the chemotactic monohydroxy fatty acid, 12-HETE. In contrast to the cyclooxygenase pathway shown here, the lipoxygenase reactions are not inhibited by aspirin. (From Gorman RR, Marcus AJ: Prostaglandins and cardiovascular disease. Current concepts. A Scope publication. Upjohn Company, 1981.)

depicts platelet ultrastructure with emphasis on functional correlations associated with specific organelles.

Colman RW, Hirsh J, Marder V, et al. (eds.): Hemostasis and Thrombosis: Basic Principles and Clinical Practice. Philadelphia, JB Lippincott Company, 1982. *This book presents the biochemistry and physiology of hemostasis and the pathophysiology of thrombosis in detail. Emphasis is on diagnosis and treatment of hemorrhagic diseases and thrombotic diatheses.*

Marcus AJ: The eicosanoids in biology and medicine. J Lipid Res 25:1511, 1984. *A review and discussion of how eicosanoids and their precursors from multiple cell types exert biologic effects in the microenvironment.*

CLINICAL ASSESSMENT OF PATIENTS WITH POSSIBLE BLEEDING DISORDERS

The physician is required to evaluate the condition of a patient in two clinical settings to determine if a bleeding tendency is present. (1) A screening evaluation is required before the patient undergoes a surgical procedure. (2) The patient has previously experienced an episode(s) of hemorrhage—either spontaneous or following trauma.

In both instances a meticulous personal and family history, in addition to a physical examination, together with sequentially selected laboratory screening tests, will establish that (1) a hemorrhagic tendency is or is not present; (2) the bleeding diathesis is due to a coagulation abnormality, a vascular defect, or a platelet disorder; (3) the disorder is congenital or acquired (Table 166–1).

MEDICAL, FAMILY, AND DRUG HISTORY. A history of excessive bleeding or bruising occurring spontaneously or following minor trauma is of significance. This is especially true if the bruise is 3 cm or larger. Although such episodes are usually associated with a vascular abnormality, they also occur in coagulation and platelet disorders. The patient should be questioned concerning unusual bleeding following dental extraction or surgery. Characteristically, bleeding in platelet

TABLE 166–1. DIFFERENTIAL CLINICAL DIAGNOSIS OF COAGULATION, PLATELET, AND VASCULAR DISORDERS

	Coagulation Defect	Platelet Disorder	Vascular Abnormality
Family history	Usually positive	Negative	Usually negative
Sex predominance	Males	Frequently females	Mainly females
Nature of symptoms and signs	Visceral, intramuscular and joint hemorrhage; spontaneous and post-mild trauma	Cutaneous, mucous membrane, and CNS hemorrhage; petechiae, purpura, hematuria; hemarthroses rare	Ecchymoses, purpura, frequently spontaneous; melena; no hemarthroses
Time sequence of hemorrhage	Post-traumatic delay followed by persistent oozing	Concomitant with and immediately following trauma; usually of short duration	Post-traumatic or spontaneous localized ecchymoses; generalized bleeding rare
Response to local pressure	Usually ineffective	Usually effective	Effective

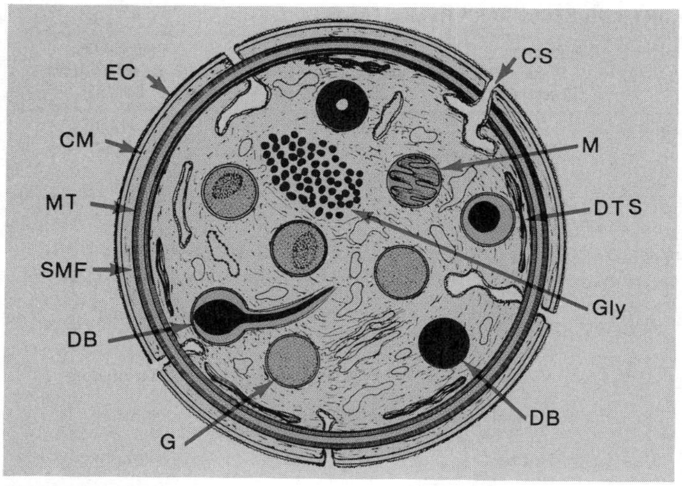

FIGURE 166–3. Diagrammatic representation of platelet ultrastructure. The glycoprotein-rich exterior coat (EC) contains receptors for platelet agonists and inhibitors. Signal transduction also occurs at this site. The cell membrane (CM) consists of the classic lipid bilayer and is rich in arachidonic acid, which is esterified to phospholipid. In activated platelets the CM undergoes a rearrangement to form a catalytic lipoprotein surface for acceleration of coagulation. Concomitantly, membrane calcium release promotes activation of phospholipases for initiation of eicosanoid formation. The submembrane filaments (SMF), now recognized as actin, form parallel structures that induce pseudopod formation upon platelet stimulation. These filaments also line channels of the surface-connected canalicular system (CS). The circumferential microtubule system (MT) constitutes the cytoskeleton, which maintains the disc shape of unstimulated circulating platelets. Platelets also contain mitochondria (M), glycogen (Gly), and dense bodies (DB), which represent sites of storage for ADP, 5-HT, and calcium. Platelet granules (G) are of two types: some are lysosomal, and others contain secretable proteins of the "adhesive" type (fibrinogen, von Willebrand factor, thrombospondin, and fibronectin), as well as PF_4, beta-thromboglobulin, and PDGF. The dense tubular system (DTS) and the surface-connected canalicular system are membrane systems in the platelet, which are counterparts of sarcoplasmic reticulum as defined in other cells. (Courtesy of Dr. James G. White: CRC Critical Reviews in Oncology/Hematology, 4:337, 1986. Copyright CRC Press, Inc., Boca Raton, FL.)

diseases is immediate and transient, and blood loss is minimal to moderate. In coagulation disorders, postoperative or posttraumatic hemorrhage is delayed, prolonged, and moderate to severe. Mucous membrane bleeding such as epistaxis is a common presenting symptom in platelet diseases. Family history is critical, especially in males, since deficiencies of Factors VIII and IX are linked to the X chromosome. Factor VIII deficiency (hemophilia A) accounts for approximately 85 per cent of congenital coagulation disorders. An additional 10 per cent are due to Factor IX deficiency. The other coagulation defects (autosomal recessive) comprise the remaining 5 per cent. In 30 per cent of patients with hemophilia, a family history cannot be elicited.

Acquired abnormalities of platelets, blood vessels, and coagulation factors or a combination of these (including circulating anticoagulants) occur as complications of systemic disorders such as liver disease, malignant disease, systemic lupus erythematosus (SLE), and uremia. A major facet of the history concerns medication. *Aspirin ingestion* during the previous week will interfere with platelet function and will also increase the severity of a hemostatic disorder already present. Drugs known to interfere with platelet function are listed in Table 166–2. Patients taking coumarin anticoagulants or heparin (including those surreptitiously using these drugs) must be identified.

PHYSICAL EXAMINATION. Information from the history is confirmed and extended by physical examination. Presence and distribution of petechiae, purpuric spots, or ecchymoses should be noted. *Petechiae* are pinpoint lesions resulting from breakage or increased permeability of arterioles, capillaries, or venules. They appear at pressure points and mucosal surfaces. Petechiae are characteristically observed in symptomatic patients with thrombocytopenia. A *purpuric lesion* represents confluent petechiae, also associated with thrombocytopenia. An *ecchymosis* is an extension of the purpuric lesion, indicating that extravasated blood has traversed fascial planes. A *dissecting hematoma* is the most serious form of an ecchymosis. Spontaneous ecchymoses occur in defects in coagulation. *Hemarthroses* or ankylosed joints strongly suggest Factor VIII or Factor IX deficiency. Lesions of Osler-Weber-Rendu disease (hereditary telangiectasia) and spider telangiectasia may resemble petechiae, but blanch on pressure. Cherry hemangioma and angiokeratomas (Fabry's disease) usually do not blanch.

Triplett DA: Hemostasis: A Case Oriented Approach. New York, Igaku-Shoin, 1985. *This text emphasizes prerequisites for diagnosis and care of patients with hemorrhagic or thrombotic disorders. Authentic cases from hospital archives have been utilized for presentation and discussion.*

SEQUENCE OF LABORATORY STUDIES OF HEMOSTATIC FUNCTION

Although a tentative diagnosis of a hemorrhagic diathesis can be made from the history and physical examination, precise characterization requires laboratory studies. Basic screening tests are carried out first. These procedures examine the integrity of platelet, vascular, and coagulation components of hemostasis: (1) microscopic examination of the peripheral blood smear, (2) platelet count, (3) bleeding time, (4) prothrombin time (PT), (5) activated partial thromboplastin time (APTT or PTT), and (6) thrombin time (TT). More sophisticated and expensive assays should not be done unless indicated by abnormal results of screening tests (Table 166–3 and Fig. 166–4).

Platelet numbers and gross morphology can be evaluated from inspection of the peripheral blood smear. In addition, visualization of other formed elements is helpful in patient evaluation. Schistocytes suggest microangiopathic hemolytic anemia as occurs in disseminated intravascular coagulation (DIC). The presence of large platelets indicates increased platelet turnover as seen in immune thrombocytopenia or platelet destruction by artificial cardiac prostheses.

Platelet counts below 100,000 per microliter are the most common cause of serious bleeding. There is an inverse relationship between platelet count and bleeding time. Platelet counts below 50,000 per microliter require phase microscopy for accurate enumeration.

The *bleeding time* is usually determined by a modified Ivy method in which an incision 1 cm long and 1 mm deep is made on the volar surface of the forearm while 40 mm Hg of pressure is maintained on the upper arm with a blood pressure cuff. The bleeding time usually exceeds nine minutes under the following conditions: (1) thrombocytopenia (platelet counts $<$ 100,000 per microliter), (2) qualitative platelet defects, (3) von Willebrand's disease, and (4) vascular defects.

Following aspirin ingestion, the bleeding time may be prolonged from the normal range of two to six minutes to a mean value of nine and one-half minutes. Alcohol and aspirin are synergistic in extending the bleeding time. A prolonged

TABLE 166–2. DRUGS ASSOCIATED WITH ABNORMALITIES IN PLATELET FUNCTION

Aspirin	Low molecular weight dextran
Chlorpromazine	Meclofenamic acid
Clofibrate	Nitrofurantoin
Dipyridamole	Penicillins
Ethanol	Phenylbutazone
Glyceryl guaiacolate (Guaifenesin)	Sulfinpyrazone
Hydroxychloroquine	Tricyclic antidepressants
Indomethacin	*Vinca* alkaloids

TABLE 166–3. SCREENING TESTS FOR PRIMARY AND SECONDARY HEMOSTASIS

Disorder	Platelet Count (~300 × 10^3/cu mm)	Bleeding time (<9 minutes)	Clot Retraction	Prothrombin Time (12 seconds)	Activated Partial Thromboplastin Time (33–45 Seconds)	Thrombin Time (3–5 Seconds Above Control)
Thrombocytopenia	Low	Prolonged	Poor to absent	Normal	Normal	Normal
Vascular defects	Normal	Prolonged (tourniquet test positive)	Normal	Normal	Normal	Normal
Qualitative platelet defect	Normal	Prolonged	Normal (poor to absent in thrombasthenia)	Normal	Normal	Normal
Extrinsic coagulation system						
Factor VII deficiency	Normal	Normal	Normal	Prolonged	Normal	Normal
Factor II, V, or X deficiency	Normal	Normal	Normal	Prolonged	Prolonged	Normal
Intrinsic coagulation system						
Factor VIII and IX deficiency	Normal	Normal	Normal	Normal	Prolonged	Normal
von Willebrand's disease	Normal	Prolonged	Normal	Normal	Variable—usually prolonged	Normal
Afibrinogenemia, dysfibrinogenemia	Normal	Variable	Normal	Normal	Normal	Prolonged
DIC, liver failure	Usually low	Variable, often prolonged	Sometimes poor	Prolonged	Prolonged	Prolonged

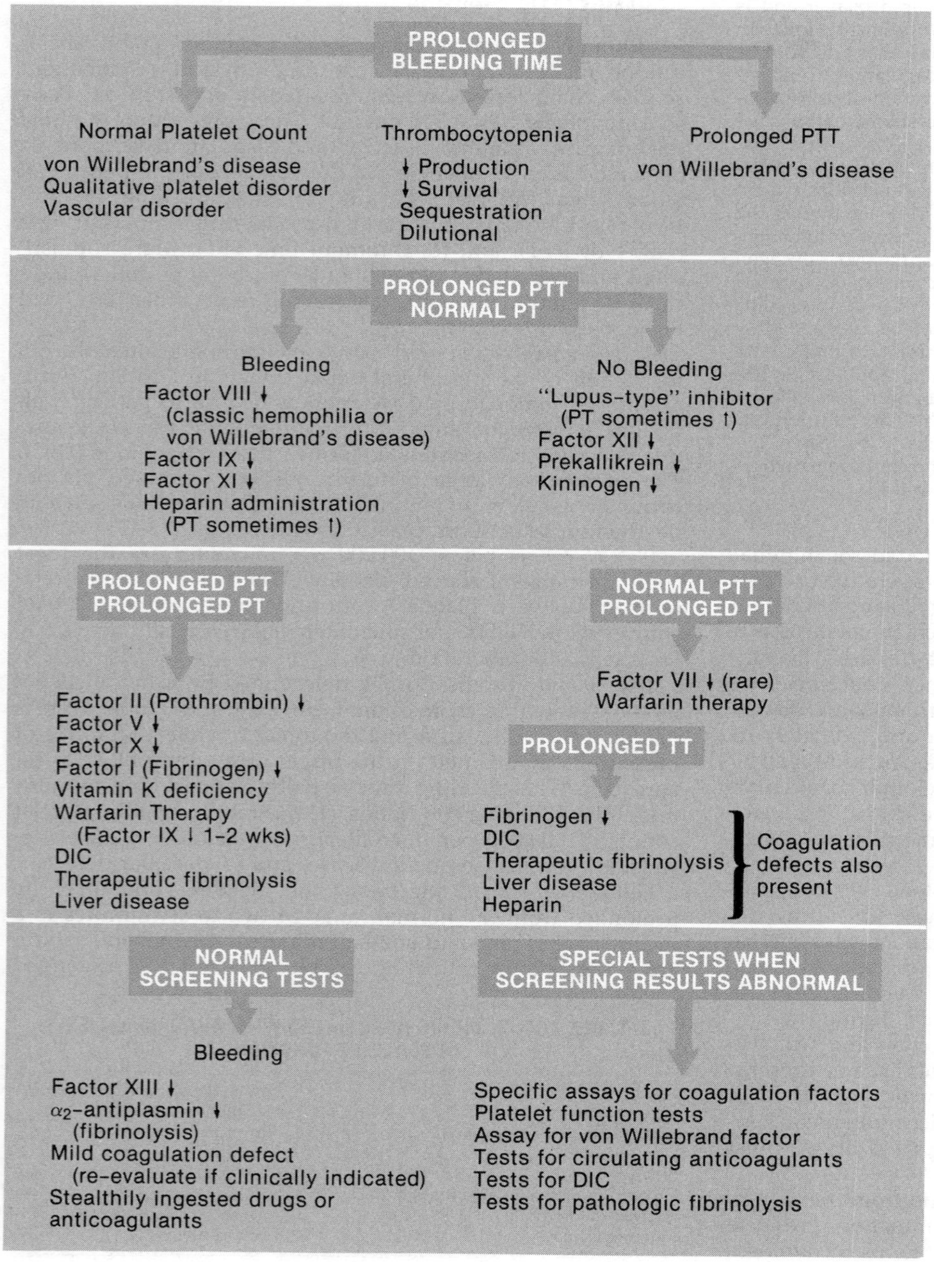

FIGURE 166–4. Sequential interpretation of screening tests in Table 166–3.

bleeding time in the setting of a normal platelet count defines a vascular abnormality or a qualitative platelet disorder. Approximately 43 per cent of such patients have von Willebrand's disease; 27 per cent will be diagnosed as having vascular purpura (platelets and coagulation normal), 16 per cent have thrombasthenia, 7 per cent have thrombocytopathy with normal-appearing platelets, and 7 per cent have thrombocytopathy with abnormal platelet morphology.

The *prothrombin time* provides an overall assessment of the extrinsic coagulation system. Since factor VII is the first coagulation protein to be depleted by oral anticoagulants, the PT is important for monitoring such patients. In congenital and acquired deficiencies of factors VII, X, V, II, and fibrinogen, the PT will be prolonged.

The *activated partial thromboplastin time* is an excellent screening procedure for the intrinsic coagulation system. The "contact" components of the intrinsic system (Factor XII and cofactors) are activated by particulate ingredients of a reagent such as kaolin or celite. The remaining coagulation proteins are activated by phospholipid in the reagent. If the patient has a normal PT but prolonged PTT, a deficiency of the intrinsic system (Factors XII, XI, VIII, IX, Fletcher factor, and Fitzgerald factor) exists or a circulating anticoagulant is present. Patients with the lupus anticoagulant frequently have a normal PT and prolonged PTT. The PTT is also utilized in monitoring heparin therapy.

The *thrombin time* provides information concerning quantitative and qualitative aspects of plasma fibrinogen and is also influenced by inhibitors. Thus the thrombin time will be prolonged in hypofibrinogenemia, dysfibrinogenemias, during heparin therapy, by the presence of fibrinogen-fibrin split products, and paraproteins. The thrombin time is usually prolonged if the fibrinogen level is below 100 mg per deciliter (Fig. 166–4).

Confirmatory screening tests include procedures for identification of fibrinogen-fibrin degradation products as occur in DIC. When a circulating anticoagulant is suspected on the basis of a prolonged PTT, the patient's plasma is diluted 1:1 with normal pooled plasma. If the PTT is not corrected by this maneuver, a circulating anticoagulant is probably present. Evaluation of clot retraction is simple and inexpensive. If clot retraction is normal, it indicates that platelet numbers, platelet function, the quantity of fibrinogen, and packed cell volume are satisfactory. Clot retraction is defective to absent in thrombasthenia and thrombocytopenia.

An occasional result in routine screening procedures is the combination of normal coagulation tests, normal platelet count and morphology, but a slightly prolonged bleeding time. This mild qualitative platelet defect is most commonly due to ingestion of aspirin or a medication containing aspirin. Another offender is guaifenesin (glyceryl guaiacolate), a component of cough remedies (Table 166–2).

Platelet aggregometry can provide additional information concerning a possible platelet qualitative defect. Aggregation is measured as an increase in light transmission through stirred platelet-rich plasma while a specific agonist is added. Test substances include ADP, collagen, epinephrine, sodium arachidonate, and the agglutinating agent ristocetin. A ristocetin agglutination study for von Willebrand's disease is mandatory if the PTT is prolonged, the bleeding time excessive, and the platelet count normal. In von Willebrand's disease the platelets are unresponsive to ristocetin. In contrast, platelets from patients with thrombasthenia will *agglutinate* upon addition of ristocetin, but will not *aggregate* in the presence of standard stimuli.

Patients with acquired defects in the platelet release reaction (drugs, following cardiopulmonary bypass, uremia) and those with congenital release abnormalities demonstrate a single, reversible wave of platelet aggregation. Platelets from patients who have recently ingested aspirin are unresponsive to arachidonate, and those from patients with myeloproliferative disorders are unreactive to epinephrine. Correlations between results of in vitro platelet aggregometry may not always be in direct relationship to the hemostatic defect observed clinically. Therefore, aggregometry information should be regarded as largely supportive and correlated with the value obtained for the bleeding time. Further evaluation usually is not required in the patient whose coagulation- and platelet-screening tests are normal. There are instances, however, in which mild clinical and laboratory coagulation or platelet disturbances require further elucidation. This is done by performance of specific assays for coagulation factors or platelet aggregometry or both with an extended group of stimuli at varying concentrations.

Harker LA, Zimmerman TS (eds.): Measurements of Platelet Function. Methods in Hematology Series. Vol. 8. New York, Churchill Livingstone, 1983. *This book is a compilation of recommended methods for evaluating platelet function.*

Sirridge MS, Shannon R: Laboratory Evaluation of Hemostasis and Thrombosis. 3rd ed. Philadelphia, Lea & Febiger, 1983. *This volume covers basic aspects of hemostasis and thrombosis and features detailed descriptions of diagnostic procedures, reagents employed, and interpretations of laboratory tests.*

Quantitative Platelet Disorders

THROMBOCYTOPENIA

Thrombocytopenia is defined as a platelet count below 100,000 per microliter. Except for chronic, longstanding thrombocytopenia, hemorrhage is inversely proportional to the platelet count (especially in disorders of platelet production). Platelet counts in the range of 40,000 to 60,000 per microliter may lead to post-traumatic bleeding, and at 20,000 per microliter, spontaneous hemorrhage can occur. Particularly hazardous are central nervous system and gastrointestinal hemorrhage. Fever, anemia, and chronic inflammation in thrombocytopenic patients render them more susceptible to bleeding and less responsive to platelet transfusions.

There are four basic mechanisms of thrombocytopenia (Table 166–4): (1) decreased or ineffective platelet production, (2) shortened platelet survival time in the circulation due to

TABLE 166–4. CAUSES OF THROMBOCYTOPENIA

I. Decreased platelet production
- Reduced megakaryocytes in marrow
  - Marrow infiltration—malignant disease, myelofibrosis, chemicals, and drugs
  - Marrow hypoplasia—radiation, chemicals, insecticides, drugs, viruses, idiopathic, alcohol
  - Congenital—Fanconi's pancytopenia, thrombocytopenia with absence of radius, autosomal recessive thrombocytopenia, cyclic thrombocytopenia, infection (congenital rubella)
- Ineffective thrombocytopoiesis (normal or increased marrow megakaryocytes)
  - Hereditary
    - Autosomal dominant thrombocytopenia
    - May-Hegglin anomaly
    - Wiskott-Aldrich syndrome
  - Megaloblastic anemias
    - Di Guglielmo's syndrome
    - Preleukemia

II. Decreased platelet survival
- Increased destruction
  - Drug-induced thrombocytopenic purpura
  - Idiopathic thrombocytopenic purpura
  - Post-transfusion purpura
  - Isoimmune neonatal purpura
  - Secondary immunologic purpura
  - HIV infection (AIDS)
- Increased consumption
  - Thrombotic thrombocytopenic purpura
  - Disseminated intravascular coagulation
  - Cavernous hemangioma
  - Hemolytic-uremic syndrome
  - Acute infections
  - Cardiopulmonary bypass

III. Sequestration (hypersplenism)

IV. Dilutional thrombocytopenia

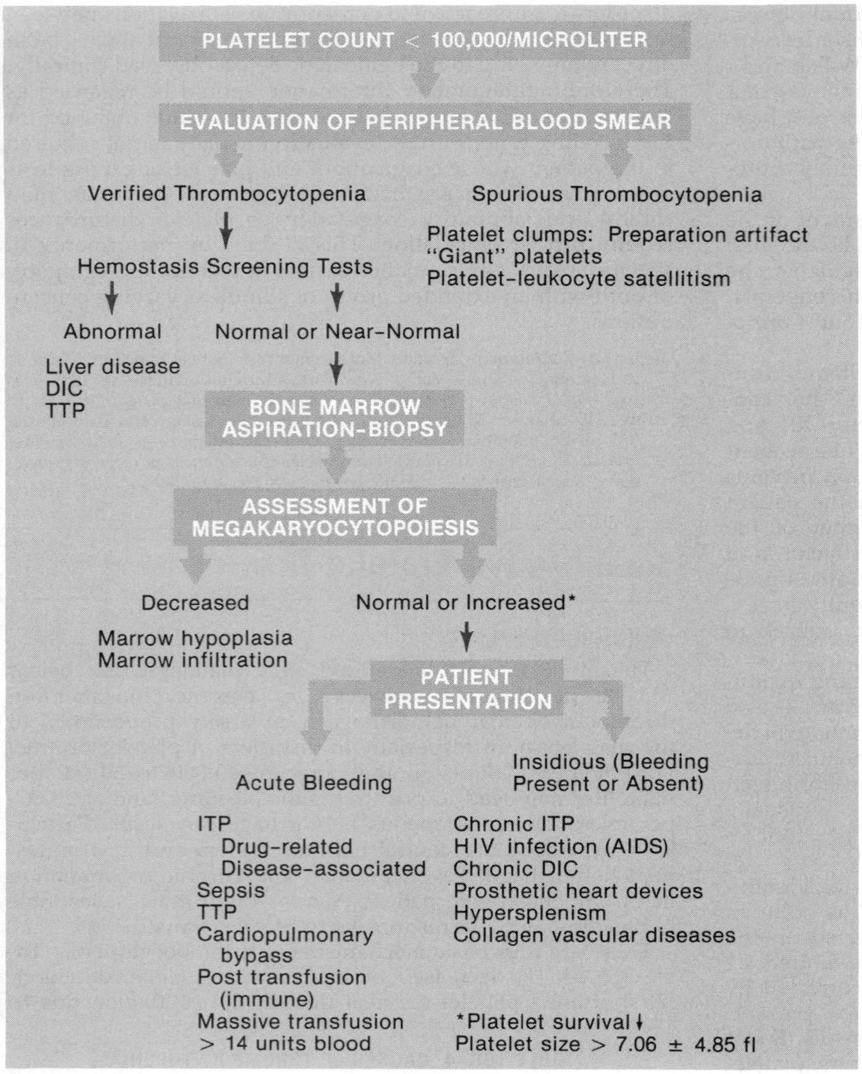

FIGURE 166–5. Evaluation of the thrombocytopenic patient. (Modified from Nathan DG, Oski FA: Hematology of Infancy and Childhood. Philadelphia, WB Saunders Company, 1981.)

increased destruction or consumption or both, (3) splenic sequestration, (4) intravascular dilution of circulating platelets. A diagnostic approach to thrombocytopenic patients is outlined in Figure 166–5.

Decreased Platelet Production

REDUCED MEGAKARYOCYTES. Reduced platelet production by megakaryocytes may result from marrow replacement, chemical injury, or congenital disorders. Compromise of erythroid or myeloid elements may also occur. Since the basic defect is the rate at which platelets enter the circulation, platelet survival is normal or slightly decreased. Mechanical displacement of megakaryocytes in the marrow may be due to metastatic carcinoma, myeloma, leukemias or lymphomas, xanthomatoses, myelofibrosis, and granulomas. Radiation, drugs, or infectious agents may also be responsible for decreased megakaryocytopoiesis. Cancer chemotherapeutic agents predictably induce megakaryocyte damage. Other offending substances include alcohol, anticonvulsants, tranquilizers, thiazides, solvents, and insecticides. Megakaryocytic hypoplasia may occur in congenital diseases such as pancytopenias associated with Fanconi's syndrome—a fatal childhood illness characterized by multiple congenital and skeletal abnormalities. Another autosomal recessive disorder, congenital hypoplastic thrombocytopenia, associated with absent radii (TAR syndrome) is characterized by an early hemorrhagic diathesis. Megakaryocytic hypoplasia also occurs as an autosomal recessive trait in the absence of other somatic abnormalities and as a result of congenital intrauterine rubella infection.

INEFFECTIVE THROMBOCYTOPOIESIS. Ineffective thrombocytopoiesis is characterized by increased marrow megakaryocytes but a decrease in circulating platelets. The defect may involve (1) defective platelet formation, (2) abnormal release of platelets from the marrow, and (3) destruction of platelets in the marrow. An autosomal dominant form of this ineffective thrombocytopoiesis, sometimes in association with increased serum IgA, nephritis, deafness, and "giant" platelets, has been reported. Ineffective platelet production also occurs in the May-Hegglin anomaly (autosomal dominant), the Wiskott-Aldrich syndrome (sex-linked recessive), and DiGuglielmo's disease. Vitamin B_{12} and folate deficiencies are characterized by an increase in megakaryocyte cytoplasmic mass but relatively ineffective platelet production. Thrombocytopenia associated with excessive alcohol ingestion is complex and due to several factors such as megakaryocytic hypoplasia, splenic platelet pooling, shortened platelet survival time, and folate deficiency.

Decreased Platelet Survival Due to Increased Destruction

Drug-Induced Thrombocytopenic Purpura

At least 70 drugs have been implicated in or proven to induce thrombocytopenic purpura (Table 166–5). In these thrombocytopenias, marrow megakaryocytes are increased and platelets are destroyed peripherally. In adults with thrombocytopenic purpura, a drug etiology should be considered

TABLE 166–5. THERAPEUTIC AND CHEMICAL AGENTS THAT MAY PRODUCE THROMBOCYTOPENIC PURPURA

I. Direct marrow suppressants	
Generalized marrow hypoplasia or aplasia	
Antimetabolites	
Antimitotic agents	
Anti-tumor antibiotics	
Benzene and derivatives	
Ionizing radiation	
Nitrogen mustard and congeners	
Occasional association with marrow hypoplasia or aplasia	
Chloramphenicol	
Gold compounds	
Methylphenylethyl hydantoin (Mesantoin), trimethadione (Tridione)	
Phenylbutazone	
Quinacrine	
Selective suppression of megakaryocytes	
Chlorothiazides	
Estrogenic hormones	
Ethanol	
Tolbutamide	
II. Production of thrombocytopenia by an immunologic mechanism	
Acetazolamide (Diamox)	p-Aminosalicylic acid (PAS)
Carbamazepine	Phenytoin (Dilantin)
Chlorothiazides	Quinidine
Chlorpropamide	Quinine
Desipramine	Rifampin
Digitoxin	Stibophen (Fuadin)
Gold salts	Sulfamethazine
Hydroxychloroquine	Sulfathiazole
Methyldopa	
III. Direct damage to circulating platelets	
Heparin	
Ristocetin	
IV. Probable immunologic mechanism; antibodies not always demonstrated	
Acetaminophen	Organic hair dyes
Aminopyrine	Nitroglycerin
Aspirin and sodium salicylate	Paramethadione
Barbiturates	Penicillin
Bismuth	Phenacetin
Carbutamide	Phenylbutazone
Cephalothin	Potassium iodide
Chloroquine	Prednisone
Chlorpheniramine maleate	Prochlorperazine
Chlorpromazine	Promethazine
Codeine	Propylthiouracil
Dextroamphetamine sulfate	Pyrazinamide
Diazoxide	Reserpine
Digitalis and digoxin	Spironolactone
Disulfiram (Antabuse)	Streptomycin
Ergot	Sulfonamides (sulfadiazine, sulfadimetine, sulfamerazine, sulfamethoxazole, sulfisoxazole)
Erythromycin	Tetracycline
Insecticides	Tetraethylammonium (TEA)
Iopanoic acid (Telepaque)	Thiourea
Isoniazid	Trimethadione
Meperidine	Trimethoprim-sulfamethoxazole
Meprobamate	Turpentine
Mercurial diuretics	

first. This is true even if a medication has been used without previous ill effects.

Typically the patient may become symptomatic with flushing and chills within a few minutes after ingestion of the offending agent. Hemorrhage from the gastrointestinal and urinary tracts may occur 1 to 12 hours later. This is followed or accompanied by petechiae and purpuric lesions in dependent areas, although the palms and soles are usually spared. Hemorrhagic bullae may appear on the oral mucosa, which is pathognomonic of thrombocytopenic purpura. The petechiae are nontender and nonpruritic and do not have an erythematous border—which distinguishes them from allergic skin reactions.

PATHOGENESIS OF DRUG-RELATED THROMBOCYTOPENIAS. A drug rarely induces thrombocytopenia by direct action on circulating platelets. This occurred with the antibiotic ristocetin, which is no longer in clinical use. Many drugs have been suspected, and in some cases they have proven to induce thrombocytopenia by an antibody-mediated immune mechanism.

Heparin, whether administered intravenously or subcutaneously, can induce thrombocytopenia with little or no consequences or a thrombocytopenia that is complicated by a thrombotic diathesis. In the mild form, platelet counts are in the range of 100,000 per microliter, and spontaneous bleeding seldom occurs. Patients do not necessarily give a history of receiving heparin in the past. The thrombocytopenic effect may be related to the use of heparin subfractions with a lesser affinity for antithrombin III. This mild syndrome may eventually be eliminated when purified heparin preparations are developed with near-total affinity for antithrombin III. The mild thrombocytopenia occurs within 15 days of heparin administration and is completely reversible upon cessation of heparin therapy. Since the patients are usually asymptomatic, future use of heparin, if required, may be considered. The severe symptomatic heparin-induced thrombocytopenia is slow in onset and increases in severity within a two-week period. The chronology of the event suggests an immune mechanism, and antibodies to the platelet-heparin complex have been identified. The in vivo aggregation of platelets that ensues can result in occlusive vascular lesions in multiple locations. Embolic complications also occur, but hemorrhage is rare. Future therapy with heparin is contraindicated.

Among the most widely studied drug-induced thrombocytopenias is that due to *quinidine*. It serves as a model for chemically related compounds as well as other agents that induce thrombocytopenia.

The immunologic reaction that terminates in platelet destruction occurs in the following manner: (1) The drug (or one of its derivatives or metabolites) acts as a hapten and forms a complex with a plasma protein ("carrier"). (2) The complex formed is antigenic and induces production of high-affinity antibodies. When the drug is reingested the antibody can bind to the drug (hapten) itself. (3) The antigen-antibody complex then adsorbs to platelets via their Fc receptor. (4) Adsorption of the antigen-antibody complex by platelets is nonspecific, i.e., the platelets are "innocent bystanders." (5) Antibody-coated platelets are rapidly and efficiently "recognized" by the reticuloendothelial system and removed from the circulation prematurely, giving rise to thrombocytopenia when bone marrow reserve decompensates.

DIAGNOSIS OF DRUG-INDUCED THROMBOCYTOPENIA. A detailed history concerning drug ingestion or unusual environmental exposure is mandatory. Intake of beverages such as tonic water should also be checked, since it contains quinine, which can induce thrombocytopenia ("cocktail purpura"). If possible, all medications should be withdrawn until a diagnosis has been established. This also serves as a diagnostic test, since the purpura may resolve following removal of an offending drug.

In vitro assays for detection of possible circulating drug-induced antibodies are difficult to perform in most laboratories. No single test (complement fixation, "immunoinjury tests," ^{51}Cr release) will detect all antibodies. Direct binding assays for IgG or complement on the platelet surface are useful but cumbersome and produce variable results. Readministration of the drug, even in smaller doses for confirmation of an etiologic diagnosis, is not recommended. If other hematologic parameters are normal, a bone marrow examination is not necessary. However, if thrombocytopenia persists for more than two weeks after abstinence from the drug, another diagnosis should be considered, and a bone marrow examination is indicated. Exceptions include gold salts and arsenicals, which are excreted slowly.

TREATMENT OF DRUG-INDUCED, ANTIBODY-MEDIATED THROMBOCYTOPENIA. Usually no treatment is necessary, since withdrawal of the offending agent results in recovery. If purpura increases in severity or spontaneous bleeding occurs from mucous membranes, corticosteroid therapy is recommended because it will inhibit phagocytosis of antibody- or complement-coated platelets by macrophages in the spleen. Also, steroids have a beneficial effect on vascular integrity. If the platelet count is below 30,000 per microliter initially, corticosteroids should be administered. Rare instances of life-threatening hemorrhage must be managed with platelet transfusions or, as a last resort, exchange transfusions, on the presumption that the latter would lower plasma concentrations of drug and antibody. Since antibodies in drug-induced thrombocytopenia are specific, alternative pharmacologically equivalent compounds can be substituted. Future use of the offending drug is contraindicated.

King DJ, Kelton JG: Heparin-associated thrombocytopenia. Ann Intern Med 100:535, 1984. *This review discusses the diagnosis and treatment of heparin-induced thrombocytopenia as a laboratory finding in the absence of symptomatology and the syndrome of heparin-associated thrombocytopenia plus arterial thrombosis. The latter can result in stroke, myocardial infarction, and death.*

Idiopathic Thrombocytopenic Purpura

DEFINITION. Idiopathic thrombocytopenic purpura (ITP) refers to thrombocytopenia occurring in the absence of toxic exposure or a disease associated with decreased platelets. In at least 85 per cent of patients with ITP an immunologic mechanism involving IgG-type antibodies can be demonstrated. Since platelet destruction is immune mediated in most cases, the term *autoimmune thrombocytopenic purpura* (ATP) has been suggested. There are two forms of ITP, acute and chronic. Both are characterized by normal or increased marrow megakaryocytes (number and volume), shortened platelet survival, and absence of splenomegaly.

ACUTE ITP. Acute ITP occurs most frequently in childhood (ages two to six) and affects both sexes equally. A history of antecedent upper respiratory viral infection one to three weeks prior to onset can be elicited in 80 per cent of cases. There is a peak seasonal incidence in fall and winter, which may parallel prevalence of viral respiratory infections. Symptomatic patients abruptly develop petechial hemorrhages and purpura. Hemorrhagic bullae in the oral cavity may occur along with epistaxis and gastrointestinal and genitourinary bleeding. Platelet counts of 20,000 per microliter or less are commonly observed. Although the patient is at risk for intracranial hemorrhage, this rarely occurs. If splenomegaly is present it usually reflects the previous viral illness. Peripheral blood smears demonstrate eosinophilia and lymphocytosis. Since 80 per cent of patients recover spontaneously in two weeks to six months, the prognosis of acute ITP in children is excellent. Recurrence after complete recovery is rare, and mortality is less than 1 per cent. In adults, however, spontaneous remission will not occur in 90 per cent of patients with acute ITP.

Therapy is not required unless atraumatic mucous membrane hemorrhage continues and new crops of ecchymoses appear. Some physicians treat all patients with short-term prednisone therapy (1 to 2 mg per kilogram body weight daily) for four weeks when the risk of hemorrhage is maximal. Since spontaneous remission occurs in most children, objective evaluation of corticosteroid therapy is difficult. In rare situations in which life-threatening hemorrhage occurs, platelet transfusions are indicated. Intravenous infusion of high-dose gamma globulin (1.0 to 2.0 grams per kilogram body weight) may induce an increase in platelet counts of patients with ITP. This is due to blockade of Fc receptors on macrophages in the reticuloendothelial system by the immunoglobulin. Thus antibody-coated platelets remain in the circulation. Responses are frequently transient, and a five-day course of treatment costs $6000. However, a single transfusion of gamma globulin (400 mg per kilogram) may be effective in preparation for platelet transfusion or splenectomy in uncontrolled life-threatening acute ITP.

Approximately 10 to 15 per cent of adult patients with acute ITP will not fully recover in six months. If the patient is symptomatic, or if platelet counts are below 100,000 per microliter, treatment with corticosteroids is required. Children who do not respond to a course of prednisone (80 to 100 mg per day) within 6 to 12 months should be considered for splenectomy. Permanent remission occurs following splenectomy in 85 per cent of patients.

CHRONIC ITP. Chronic ITP in adults can begin insidiously or result from an episode of acute ITP, from which 90 per cent of adults do not undergo spontaneous remission. Although it occurs at any age, chronic ITP is observed most frequently between 20 and 40 years, with women affected more frequently than men (ratio 3:1). In the insidious form there is gradual onset of mucosal petechiae, ecchymoses, epistaxis, and menorrhagia. Cutaneous hemorrhage is more common in distal portions of the extremities. Palpable splenomegaly is not a characteristic of chronic ITP. If present, the diagnosis should be questioned. Platelet counts are in the range of 30,000 to 80,000 per microliter, and bone marrow megakaryocytes are normal or increased in number and volume (Fig. 166–5).

Clinically, chronic ITP undergoes remissions and relapses alternating over long periods. Exacerbations are sometimes cyclic and can be correlated with phenomena such as menstruation. Thus evaluation of treatment is difficult. Although acute ITP in children is not accompanied by immune-type disorders, in adults with chronic ITP periodic evaluation is required for coexistence of diseases such as systemic lupus erythematosus, lymphoproliferative disorders, and autoimmune hemolytic anemia (Evans' syndrome).

THROMBOCYTOPENIA IN THE ACQUIRED IMMUNODEFICIENCY SYNDROME (AIDS). One of the most common hematologic complications of infection with HIV is thrombocytopenia. These patients do not have splenomegaly, and marrow megakaryocytes are normal. The thrombocytopenia is associated with deposition of immune complexes and complement on the platelet surface. This is in contrast to classical ITP (ATP) in which antiplatelet IgG antibody is bound to the platelet surface. Superimposed on this cause of thrombocytopenia, decreased production of platelets may also result from marrow replacement with tumor or infiltration by fungi or mycobacteria (Fig. 166–5).

Thrombocytopenia in patients with AIDS or AIDS-related complex (ARC) may occur early in the course of HIV infections. The use of corticosteroids has resulted in transient improvement in circulating platelet counts, but long-term therapy with steroids in these patients is hazardous. Vincristine or vinblastine has induced temporary improvement, and danazol has been of minimal usefulness. Most patients have been managed conservatively, with splenectomy considered as a last resort. High-dose intravenous gamma globulin has provided benefit over a period of several months.

PATHOGENESIS OF ITP. The pathophysiology and clinical manifestations in 85 to 95 per cent of patients with chronic ITP are due to production of an antiplatelet IgG antibody that binds to platelets and results in premature splenic removal of these platelets. Hepatic removal occurs in highly sensitized patients. Splenic destruction of antibody-damaged platelets occurs because splenic macrophages contain receptors for the Fc portion of the IgG molecule. Platelet-bound IgG has also been identified in patients with malignant tumors, leukemias, thrombotic thrombocytopenic purpura, aplastic anemia, and sepsis. Platelet antigens also fix complement. In ITP, platelets may also contain surface-bound IgM (up to 20 per cent of cases). These platelets are removed by the liver. Hepatic removal of antibody-coated platelets may account for failure of splenectomy to induce complete long-term remissions in about 50 per cent of patients with ITP.

DIAGNOSIS OF CHRONIC ITP. Criteria for diagnosis include (1) evidence of increased platelet destruction as demonstrated by a shortened survival time (in "compensated thrombocytolytic states" the platelet count may be normal or near normal). (2) Increased megakaryocyte size and number in the marrow. (3) Demonstration of antibody bound to platelets by a reliable technique. (4) Other clinical disorders that might meet criteria 1 to 3 should be ruled out. (Drug-induced immunologic thrombocytopenia may be difficult to differentiate from ITP. Platelet counts should return to normal 7 to 14 days following discontinuation of the drug.) (5) Presence of splenomegaly virtually excludes the diagnosis of ITP.

If the patient's platelets *do not contain demonstrable antiplatelet antibody* by available techniques and the other criteria cited above can be met, the term *ITP* should be used (5 to 10 per cent of cases). Patients in whom *platelet antibody can be demonstrated* are classified as *ATP*. Other clinical disorders considered in the differential diagnosis include the thrombocytopenia associated with HIV infection, SLE, lymphomas, and hypersplenism (Fig. 166–5).

TREATMENT. Major therapeutic methods for chronic ITP are: corticosteroids, splenectomy, immunosuppressive agents, and high-dose intravenous gamma globulin. The clinical course of chronic ITP is variable. Spontaneous recovery occurs in less than 10 per cent of cases. Patients whose platelet counts are in the range of 100,000 per microliter and whose hemorrhagic manifestations are minimal may be observed at bimonthly intervals. Maintenance of normal to near-normal hemostasis (occasional cutaneous petechiae or bruising) is more important than the platelet count per se. Hemostasis can be achieved with platelet counts of 40,000 to 60,000 per microliter.

Corticosteroids. If platelet counts remain below 40,000 per microliter and spontaneous bleeding persists, therapy with prednisone is indicated (1 mg per kilogram daily); 70 to 90 per cent of patients respond with an increase in platelets and decrease in hemorrhagic diathesis. The hemorrhagic disorder frequently improves prior to the rise in platelet count. This may be due to a direct effect of corticosteroids on capillaries in improving their physical integrity. Although a clinical response to corticosteroids may occur in 48 hours, beneficial effects become fully evaluable in 1 to 3 weeks. After four to six weeks the corticosteroid dose is gradually tapered and discontinued, especially if no bleeding is present. About 20 per cent of patients have a long-term beneficial response to corticosteroids. If subsequent relapse occurs, readministration of corticosteroids should induce another remission. Over many months only 10 to 15 per cent of patients treated with corticosteroids remain in permanent remission. The subsequent course may become unfortunate, characterized by corticosteroid refractoriness and prohibitive toxicity. The next consideration is splenectomy.

The beneficial effect of corticosteroids in ITP is due to prevention of sequestration of antibody-coated platelets by splenic phagocytic cells. Mononuclear cell phagocytic capacity, chemotaxis, and adherence properties of antibody-coated platelets are all reduced by corticosteroids. Other corticosteroid effects include an increase in platelet production, impairment of immunoglobulin synthesis, and inhibition of antibody-platelet interaction.

Splenectomy. When patients become unresponsive to corticosteroids or require toxic levels to maintain hemostatic balance, splenectomy is indicated. This results in removal of the major site of platelet destruction and a significant source of antiplatelet antibody production. About 70 to 80 per cent of patients improve after splenectomy, and in 60 per cent platelet counts return to normal. In those who respond, there is normalization of platelet survival and decrease in platelet-bound IgG. Interestingly, antiplatelet antibody is still detectable in the plasma and platelets of some patients with ITP in remission. ITP remains in permanent remission in two thirds of splenectomized patients, and in the one third whose platelet counts remain below 100,000 per microliter, bleeding symptoms no longer occur. Over a five-year period, relapse occurs after splenectomy in about 10 to 12 per cent of patients. Many of these patients can be maintained on low-dose prednisone (10 mg or less daily). The presence of an accessory spleen should always be considered in patients who do not respond completely to splenectomy or in whom relapse occurs soon after a successful splenectomy-induced remission.

Although patients tolerate splenectomy rather well in the setting of severe thrombocytopenia, those with life-threatening bleeding may be prepared for surgery with a single (400 mg per kilogram) intravenous dose of gamma globulin, followed by platelet transfusions preoperatively.

Some observers recommend splenectomy in all patients with ITP of more than 6 months' duration who cannot be maintained therapeutically with 5 to 10 mg prednisone daily. With regard to pneumococcal infection in the postsplenectomy state, prophylactic administration of Pneumovax is recommended 1 to 2 weeks prior to splenectomy in both adults and children.

Management of Patients No Longer Responsive to Corticosteroids and Splenectomy (Refractory ITP). Over a period of years, relapse occurs in the postsplenectomy state in 10 to 12 per cent of patients with chronic ITP. It cannot be managed with corticosteroids, and hemorrhagic manifestations continue to develop. Immunosuppressive drug therapy has been moderately successful in some instances, but the disorder does not lend itself to controlled therapeutic studies. Azathioprine and cyclophosphamide have been useful, and in some cases prolonged remissions have been reported. It may require up to two months to observe a beneficial effect. Vincristine has also been effective, either alone or followed by maintenance therapy with cyclophosphamide. The long-term effects and toxicity of immunosuppressive therapy are not known, so these agents should be used with caution.

High-dose intravenous gamma globulin is an important method for treatment of ITP in children and adults. The induction of temporary reticuloendothelial blockade (Fc receptor) and other, unknown, mechanisms are thought to be responsible for the rise in platelet count. Danazol,* a modified androgen preparation devoid of masculinizing effects, has been used in doses of 200 to 400 mg per day as a substitute for corticosteroids. Partial success in restoration of platelet counts has been reported, as has synergy with corticosteroids.

Platelet transfusions for life-threatening bleeding in ITP were previously ineffective and used only as a last resort. Pretreatment with gamma globulin may facilitate such therapy when required.

In *neonatal ITP*, IgG antibody is passively transferred across the placenta. The disorder can occur whether the mother's disease is in remission or whether she is thrombocytopenic. The infant's platelet count may be normal at birth, but decreases in 12 to 24 hours. Treatment of the mother with prednisone (10 to 20 mg per day) for 10 to 14 days prior to term is recommended, which also permits vaginal delivery.

*Four patients receiving danazol therapy for endometriosis developed a reversible ITP-like syndrome. Thus, platelet counts should be closely monitored in patients with ITP receiving danazol therapy (Arrowsmith JB, Dreis M: N Engl J Med 315:585, 1986).

Baumann MA, Menitove JE, Aster RH, et al.: Urgent treatment of idiopathic thrombocytopenic purpura with single-dose gammaglobulin infusion followed by platelet transfusion. Ann Intern Med 104:808, 1986. *Work described here represents an extension of the use of intravenous high-dose gamma globulin for therapy of ITP. Use of a large single dose followed by allogeneic platelet transfusion allows for control of bleeding and preparation for emergency surgery in ITP.*

Harrington WJ: Are platelet-antibody tests worthwhile? N Engl J Med 316:211, 1987. *The author discusses the important role of serologic testing for platelet antibodies in the diagnosis of ITP. Antibody measurements have been less valuable as guides for therapy. Patients with ITP who have normal to increased megakaryocytes in the bone marrow and have not responded to standard conservative therapeutic modalities are candidates for splenectomy.*

Karpatkin S: Autoimmune thrombocytopenic purpura. Semin Hematol 22:260, 1985. *A scholarly monograph that discusses and evaluates all recent clinical and research aspects of autoimmune and idiopathic thrombocytopenia. The concept of "ATP" is developed.*

McMillan R: Chronic idiopathic thrombocytopenic purpura. N Engl J Med 304:1135, 1981. *This review thoroughly encompasses current clinical, laboratory, and therapeutic aspects of ITP.*

Picozzi VJ, Roeske WR, Creger WP: Fate of therapy failures in adult idiopathic thrombocytopenic purpura. Am J Med 69:690, 1980. *An interesting retrospective study in which spontaneous recovery in patients with ITP was surprisingly frequent.*

Post-transfusion Purpura

Post-transfusion purpura is a very rare disorder (approximately 40 cases reported), clinically indistinguishable from fulminant ITP or drug-induced thrombocytopenia. Most cases have occurred in women who had previous pregnancies. The purpuric episode occurs five to eight days following blood transfusion. The patients are thought to have developed an antibody to a genetically determined platelet antigen known as Pl^{A1}, which is present in 98 per cent of the population. It is assumed that the patient became sensitized during pregnancy when fetal platelets (containing Pl^{A1} antigen inherited from the father) became accessible to the maternal circulation. The antigen may then have eluted from the Pl^{A1}-positive fetal platelets and adsorbed to the patient's platelets in a passive manner. Although 1 in 50 recipients is mismatched with respect to the Pl^{A1} antigen, post-transfusion purpura is very rare and production of the antibody is transient. Platelet counts are less than 10,000 per microliter, and thrombocytopenia may persist up to seven weeks. Corticosteroids have been employed for treatment, but frequently the severity of thrombocytopenia and hemorrhagic diathesis has prompted use of exchange transfusions and plasmapheresis. Platelet transfusions are ineffective. Definitive diagnosis is made by detection of the anti-Pl^{A1} antibody by agglutination and complement fixation techniques. Post-transfusion purpura as a syndrome may be heterogeneous and not limited to females or Pl^{A1}-negative individuals.

Isoimmune Neonatal Purpura

If the fetus has inherited a paternal platelet-specific antigen that induces IgG antibody formation by the mother, these antibodies cross the placenta and adsorb to fetal platelets. Frequently the Pl^{A1} system has been implicated (about 50 per cent of cases). Hemorrhage may not be present at birth, but several hours later, petechiae, ecchymoses, and hematomas develop. The most urgent complication is intracranial hemorrhage (mortality 10 to 15 per cent). Therapy has included corticosteroids and, when necessary, platelet transfusions or exchange transfusions. Recovery is usually uneventful, and platelets return to normal within 14 to 21 days. An important differential is that between neonatal ITP and isoimmune neonatal purpura. Thus platelet counts and morphology should be part of prenatal care.

Secondary Autoimmune Thrombocytopenia

Immune-mediated thrombocytopenia, including the presence of platelet-associated IgG (which may not be specific), occurs as a complication of systemic diseases. Most frequent are SLE and lymphoproliferative disorders. About 10 to 15 per cent of patients with SLE develop an ITP-like syndrome in the course of their disease or even have it at initial presentation. The higher incidence of SLE in females and in chronic ITP parallels the increase in frequency of the HLA-DRw2 system in these disorders. Of patients initially presenting with chronic ITP, 25 to 30 per cent may eventually be found to have SLE. Immunologic tests for SLE should be carried out in all new cases of ITP. An ITP-like syndrome may develop in patients with Hodgkin's disease, lymphomas, chronic lymphocytic leukemia, and sarcoidosis. Other reports of this ITP-like illness have appeared in association with thyrotoxicosis, tuberculosis, Hashimoto's thyroiditis, scleroderma, rheumatoid arthritis, and malignancies.

In allergic reactions to insect bites, tetanus toxoid, foods, or vaccines or recovery from viral infections such as rubella or infectious mononucleosis, platelets may be damaged by antigen-antibody complexes and then sequestered in the reticuloendothelial system, rendering the patient thrombocytopenic. In Evans's syndrome, chronic ITP is associated with a Coombs-positive autoimmune hemolytic anemia.

Decreased Platelet Survival Due to Increased Consumption

Thrombotic Thrombocytopenic Purpura (Moschcowitz's Syndrome)

Thrombotic thrombocytopenic purpura (TTP) is a generalized disorder of the microcirculation characterized by thrombocytopenic purpura, microangiopathic hemolytic anemia, transient and fluctuating neurologic signs, renal dysfunction, and a febrile course. More than 400 cases have been reported, of which two thirds have been in women with a mean age of 39. The bleeding is widespread and includes petechiae, ecchymoses, gastrointestinal hemorrhage, retinal bleeding, and hematuria. The neurologic findings are variable and may include an organic mental syndrome, paresis, aphasia, slurred speech, headache, vertigo, and seizures. The renal disease is usually progressive and characterized by hematuria, proteinuria, and an elevated blood urea nitrogen level.

All patients present with thrombocytopenia (platelets less than 50,000 per microliter). The peripheral blood smear demonstrates characteristic abnormalities of microangiopathic hemolytic anemia—fragmented red cells (schistocytes), burr cells, helmet-shaped erythrocytes, and normoblasts. The Coombs test is negative, and there is marked reticulocytosis. In early stages of the disease, laboratory tests do not indicate the presence of disseminated intravascular coagulation (DIC). However, as the illness progresses to hepatic and renal decompensation or onset of sepsis, frank DIC occurs.

The pathologic lesion of TTP is characteristic. Hyaline thrombi occlude arterioles and capillaries of virtually every tissue. Although endothelial cell proliferation may be observed in proximity to the lesions, inflammatory reactions and vasculitis are not observed. The hyaline material is thought to consist of dense platelet aggregates surrounded by thin layers of fibrin.

The etiology of these diffuse occlusive lesions in the microcirculation is unknown. In one third of patients a history of antecedent upper respiratory tract infection can be elicited. TTP has been linked with oral contraceptives, antibiotics, surgery, pregnancy, meningococcal infections, coxsackievirus B, vaccines, and mycoplasmas. An immune mechanism might be involved in the pathogenesis of TTP, since it has been associated with SLE, low levels of serum complement, and identification of complement components in vascular lesions. Successful therapeutic use of plasma, exchange transfusions, and plasmapheresis supports the concept that vascular injury, platelet sequestration, and microvascular thrombosis in TTP could result from deposition of immune complexes in arterioles and capillaries. However, circulating immune complexes in TTP have yet to be identified.

In a typical case the presence of thrombocytopenia, hemolytic anemia, neurologic abnormalities, fever, and renal dysfunction confirm the diagnosis. If the patient is seen late in the course, laboratory tests will indicate DIC. The hemolysis and symptomatology in DIC accompanying other diseases is not as severe, however, as that in TTP. The hemolytic-uremic syndrome (HUS) observed in infants and children may resemble TTP, but neurologic symptoms are rare. TTP involves more organ systems, and HUS is characterized by more serious renal involvement, frequently complicated by severe hypertension. A TTP-like syndrome can occur in patients with malignant disease in association with or following chemotherapy.

Biopsies of marrow, skin, muscle, gingivae, and lymph nodes in TTP have yielded variable results (positive in up to two thirds of cases). Biopsy of petechial sites has been reported to be diagnostic. Hyaline thrombi can be demonstrated in dermal capillaries.

In the past TTP was fatal in 50 to 80 per cent of cases. Therapy has always been difficult to evaluate. It included splenectomy, massive corticosteroids, and inhibitors of platelet function (dipyridamole, aspirin, and dextran)—all with varying degrees of success. Newer therapeutic advances have markedly improved the previously unfavorable prognosis in TTP. Plasma infusions, exchange transfusions, and plasmapheresis have all been utilized with highly encouraging results. Many patients have undergone complete remissions of long duration, and others have been successfully maintained with intermittent plasma infusions. Thus, plasma infusions, plasmapheresis, or both are currently regarded as the treatment of choice. Corticosteroids, aspirin, and dipyridamole may be employed initially, but in the absence of a rapid response, plasma therapy should be initiated. The most adequate trial is 2 to 7 plasma volume exchanges over a two-week interval.

Lian EC-Y, Mui PTK, Siddiqui FA, et al.: Inhibition of platelet-aggregating activity in thrombotic thrombocytopenic purpura plasma by normal adult immunoglobulin G. J Clin Invest 73:548, 1984. *Normal IgG inhibits platelet-aggregating activity present in TTP plasma.*

Marcus AJ: Moschcowitz revisited. N Engl J Med 307:1447, 1982. *Discussion of a new approach to the pathogenesis and treatment of chronic TTP.*

Disseminated Intravascular Coagulation

Disseminated intravascular coagulation (DIC), also known as defibrination syndrome or consumption coagulopathy, represents a complication of medical, surgical, and obstetric situations in which the intrinsic and extrinsic coagulation systems are activated with resulting local and general escape of thrombin into the circulatory system. In DIC fibrinogen is depleted, and platelets are activated and deposited in the microcirculation, leading to thrombocytopenia. The initial thrombotic phase is followed by a hemorrhagic disorder due to depletion of platelet and coagulation factors. Hemorrhage into skin and mucous membranes is followed by bleeding in other tissues and organs. Fibrinolysis ensues, and degradation products formed by the action of plasmin appear as a secondary complication. Thrombocytopenia is usually out of proportion to the coagulation abnormality (platelet counts are well below 100,000 per microliter). The accumulation of fibrinogen-fibrin degradation products due to secondary fibrinolysis further inhibits platelet function. Systemic diseases in which there is tissue damage with release of procoagulant substances and proteases, circulatory stasis, and shock all contribute initiating mechanisms for DIC. The underlying condition should be managed first, and if necessary, plasma, cryoprecipitate, and platelet transfusions are utilized. Heparin should be avoided, except in DIC occurring as a complication of progranulocytic leukemia in which there is intravascular release of tissue factor. Additional features of DIC are discussed in Ch. 167.

Cavernous ("Giant") Hemangioma (Kasabach-Merritt Syndrome)

Approximately 3 per cent of infants with hemangiomas, either subcutaneous or visceral, have thrombocytopenia. Bleeding may occur during the first few days of life or be delayed for several years. The hemangiomas occur subcutaneously or in viscera, but both types of lesions rarely coexist. Although the term *giant* has been used to describe the lesions, size is not correlated with thrombocytopenia. Low platelet counts can be associated with hemangiomas 5 to 6 cm in diameter. Concomitant with development of bleeding complications, the hemangioma may change in size and consistency. Purpura and ecchymoses develop around the lesion per se, followed by DIC. The lesions may regress within five years. Mild thrombocytopenia in the absence of significant bleeding is treated with corticosteroids. Heparin therapy has been used with transient results and is not recommended. Symptomatic patients should be managed with surgical removal of the primary lesion. In vital areas such as the neck and thorax radiotherapy may be required.

Hemolytic-Uremic Syndrome (Gasser's Syndrome)

The hemolytic-uremic syndrome (HUS) occurs mainly in infants and young children and is characterized by a Coombs-negative microangiopathic hemolytic anemia, thrombocytopenia, and acute renal failure. Occasional cases occur in adolescents and young adults. Rarely, HUS complicates immunization procedures or penicillin therapy. A typical episode is preceded by abdominal pain, vomiting, and diarrhea. Anemia, hemorrhage, renal insufficiency, and cardiac decompensation ensue. In contrast to TTP, neurologic signs and symptoms are rare. The thrombocytopenia (85 per cent of cases) is an example of selective platelet consumption without an increase in fibrinogen turnover. Although laboratory features of DIC may be observed early in the course, coagulation factor levels subsequently increase as a "rebound" phenomenon. Thus HUS is not actually an example of DIC.

A syndrome similar to HUS has been reported in women in association with pregnancy, the postpartum period, and ingestion of oral contraceptives. This may be a variant of HUS and is later complicated by nephrosclerosis.

The pathologic lesion of HUS consists of occlusive hyaline deposits closely associated with endothelial cells in the renal microcirculation. Fibrinogen and platelets have also been identified in small blood vessels. HUS may result from an incomplete response to a primary antigenic stimulus with subsequent formation of circulating immune complexes and fibrin deposition in the renal microvasculature.

Therapy in HUS is primarily directed toward management of renal failure with peritoneal dialysis. The combination of packed erythrocyte transfusions, dialysis, and other vigorous supportive measures has reduced the overall mortality from 35 per cent to 5 per cent. Corticosteroids, heparin, fibrinolytic agents, and inhibitors of platelet aggregation have not been consistently beneficial. In analogy with therapy for TTP, plasma infusion, plasmapheresis, and exchange transfusion may be of value.

Kaplan BS, Drummond KN: The hemolytic-uremic syndrome is a syndrome. N Engl J Med 298:964, 1978. *This discussion considers the definition and pathogenesis of the hemolytic-uremic syndrome. The central feature is damage to the vascular endothelium in glomerular capillaries and renal arterioles. Differentiation of this disorder from TTP is discussed.*

Thrombocytopenia in Acute Infections

Bacterial, viral, fungal, rickettsial, and protozoan infections can be associated with thrombocytopenia. In febrile patients with platelet counts below 150,000 per microliter the possibility of gram-negative sepsis or, less commonly, gram-positive sepsis should be evaluated. In some cases platelet production may be suppressed, and in others direct platelet destruction by viruses and bacteria has been demonstrated in vitro. Development of DIC as a complication of infection would further contribute to thrombocytopenia. Toxins produced by microorganisms can bind to platelets and induce aggregation and release. Circulating immune complexes may adsorb to platelets, resulting in their premature removal from the circulation. Only a small percentage of patients with infections develop a hemorrhagic diathesis on the basis of thrombocytopenia. Platelet levels return to normal during recovery.

Thrombocytopenia in Cardiopulmonary Bypass

Thrombocytopenia is one of several hemostatic complications occurring during cardiopulmonary bypass. In some instances it is part of the consumption coagulopathy, but in others it is due to platelet contact with surfaces of oxygenators. This contact may induce platelet activation. Traces of thrombin, which form in the pump or at surgical sites, further stimulate platelets. Currently, platelet transfusions are used to restore hemostasis, but controlled studies to verify their effectiveness have not been carried out. Therapeutic use of platelets may be excessive. Prostacyclin or stable derivatives thereof are currently under study, since they increase platelet cyclic AMP and could block platelet aggregation and release in the extracorporeal circulatory apparatus.

Thrombocytopenia Due to Splenic Sequestration

Splenomegaly accompanying any disease may result in platelet counts of 50,000 to 100,000 per microliter (see Ch. 164). A hemorrhagic diathesis in this setting alone is rare, but trauma or surgery in such patients may be complicated by excessive bleeding. Bone marrow megakaryocytes are normal to increased, and anemia and thrombocytopenia may also occur. In normal subjects 30 per cent of the platelet mass is present in the spleen, but in hypersplenic patients, this may approach 90 per cent. Platelet pooling in the hypersplenic state should be distinguished from actual platelet destruction, as occurs in the immune thrombocytopenias. In chronic ITP the reticuloendothelial system in the spleen prematurely destroys the antibody-coated platelets. In hypersplenism the platelets are essentially normal, but their transit time through the spleen is delayed. This has been verified by studies of platelet survival curves in hypersplenism, in which recovery in the peripheral blood is low but platelet lifespan is normal. The splenic pooling defect does not require therapy unless accompanying anemia mandates splenectomy to decrease transfusion requirements. Splenectomy, if carried out for that reason, will also result in restoration of normal platelet counts. During *hypothermia* there is a reversible thrombocytopenia that is thought to be due to transient sequestration in the spleen and liver.

Thrombocytopenia in the Massively Transfused Patient

In addition to effects of dilution, at least three hemostatic defects occur in patients receiving massive transfusions (10 to 20 units of whole blood or equivalent): (1) thrombocytopenia, (2) platelet dysfunction, and (3) a coagulation defect. If there is concomitant DIC, Factor VIII levels may fall below 25 per cent, necessitating use of cryoprecipitate, which will also provide fibrinogen. Platelet counts fall to 50,000 per microliter, but rarely below this level. Platelet transfusions may be required, but this should be governed by clinical evaluation rather than the platelet count per se. Screening tests for DIC, including thrombin times and measurement of fibrinogen-fibrin degradation products, should be carried out (Table 166–3 and Fig. 166–4). The thrombocytopenia is usually reversible within three to five days.

THROMBOCYTOSIS AND THROMBOCYTHEMIA

Thrombocytosis represents an elevation in platelet count beyond 400,000 per microliter and occurs in three forms: (1) transitory or "physiologic," (2) reactive or "secondary," and (3) autonomous or "primary" (thrombocythemia).

TRANSITORY THROMBOCYTOSIS. This occurs following exercise and physical stress. It may reflect platelet release from the lung, since it occurs in splenectomized individuals. Epinephrine administration produces a 20- to 50- per cent rise in platelet count, which originates from the splenic pool since it does not occur in asplenic persons. Transitory thrombocytosis results from mobilization of preformed platelets rather than from accelerated platelet production, as occurs in the other two forms of thrombocytosis.

SECONDARY OR REACTIVE THROMBOCYTOSIS. This results from accelerated platelet production, via an unknown stimulus. Reactive thrombocytosis occurs in response to hemorrhage, acute and chronic inflammatory disorders, malignant diseases, hemolysis, and the postsplenectomy state. Successful treatment of the underlying disorder reverses the thrombocytosis. It is rarely necessary to employ therapeutic methods to lower platelet counts. Reactive thrombocytosis following splenectomy is observed during the early postoperative period, and platelet levels may reach 1,000,000 per microliter during the ensuing months. Thrombotic or hemorrhagic complications rarely occur, however, and therapy is not required. Reactive thrombocytosis also occurs as a "rebound" phenomenon following a thrombocytopenic state, as in withdrawal of myelosuppressive drugs, recovery from acute alcoholism, and therapy for vitamin B_{12} deficiency. Thrombocytosis also occurs in association with iron deficiency, but may be secondary to blood loss. Iron may in some way regulate thrombocytopoiesis.

PRIMARY THROMBOCYTHEMIA. In primary thrombocythemia increased platelet production is sustained and *independent of normal regulatory processes*. Marrow megakaryocyte mass is markedly increased, and platelet production is correspondingly elevated as much as 15-fold. Platelet counts occur in the range of one to two million per microliter and may be associated with either hemorrhage or thrombosis. The Philadelphia chromosome is absent, and red cell mass is not increased. Importantly, an underlying disorder associated with secondary (reactive) thrombocytosis must be ruled out.

When hemorrhage occurs, it is usually from mucosal surfaces and related to a functional platelet abnormality. Platelets from patients with primary thrombocythemia do not respond normally to epinephrine stimulation in vitro. The thrombotic diathesis could be due to an increased circulating platelet mass per se and excessive TXA_2 production. This is because platelets utilize endoperoxides released from those in proximity for production of additional thromboxane—thereby resulting in enhanced platelet aggregation and vasoconstriction. Along with polycythemia vera, chronic myelogenous leukemia, and agnogenic myeloid metaplasia, primary polycythemia is considered a chronic myeloproliferative disease (see Ch. 154 for a more detailed description of this entity). Primary thrombocythemia also accompanies or evolves into chronic myelogenous leukemia, polycythemia vera, and agnogenic myeloid metaplasia. In common with the latter diseases, primary thrombocythemia is a clonal disorder, originating from a multipotential stem cell. Palpable splenomegaly is present in 80 per cent of cases. Most patients are over 55 years of age, and in this group cardiovascular disease frequently complicates the bleeding or thrombotic diathesis. Splenic infarction and atrophy as a complication of thrombosis occur in 20 per cent of patients. Splenic atrophy is associated with earlier mortality.

In addition to gastrointestinal bleeding, hemorrhage also occurs in skin and mucous membranes. Although episodes of hemorrhage and thrombosis occur in alternating fashion, thromboembolic phenomena, observed in 30 per cent of cases, are the most common cause of death.

Blood smears demonstrate platelet aggregates, giant forms, and fragments of megakaryocytic cytoplasm. Microscopic bone marrow specimens are markedly hypercellular with a background of platelet aggregates. In contrast to polycythemia vera, marrow iron content is normal or increased.

The thrombocytosis gives rise to spurious laboratory values for substances that are normal platelet constituents released into serum upon clotting. Thus there is pseudohyperkalemia and increases in serum acid phosphatase, lactic dehydrogenase, and zinc. These values are normal if the patient's cell-free plasma is retested as a control. Automated laboratory counting devices may estimate large platelets as erythrocytes, rendering the platelet count falsely low. *This emphasizes the importance of monitoring peripheral blood smears.*

The incidence of clinical bleeding or thrombosis does not correlate with laboratory values or in vitro tests of platelet function. However, reducing platelet production (and erythropoiesis, if excessive) is beneficial, especially in symptomatic patients. Some observers believe that patients over 50 years of age with platelet counts greater than 1,000,000 per microliter should be treated with cytoreduction, even if asymptomatic. Alkylating agents are useful for this purpose. These include ^{32}P(2.3 mCi/m^2), phenylalanine mustard, 1 to 4 mg daily by mouth, or hydroxyurea, 15 to 30 mg per kilogram.

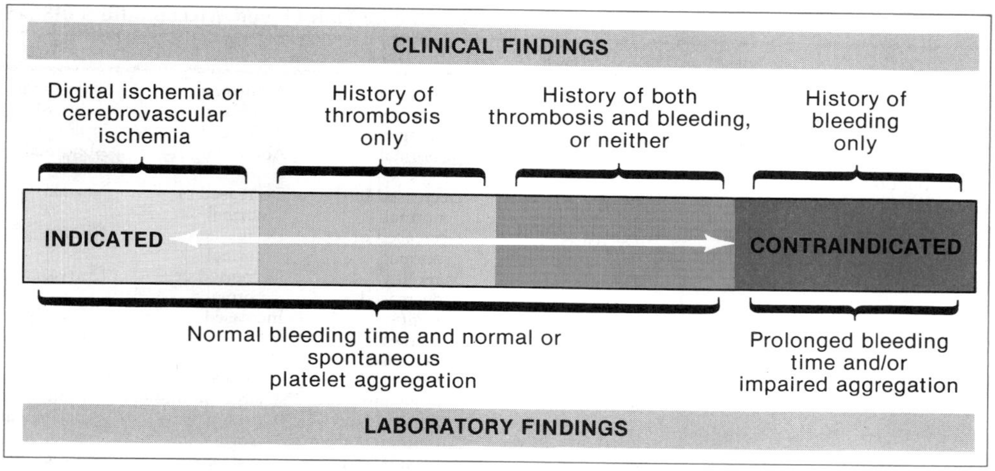

FIGURE 166–6. Correlations between clinical and laboratory results and indications for platelet cyclooxygenase inhibition with aspirin in autonomous thrombocythemia. Inhibition of platelet function may not reduce incidence of thromboembolic complications but may lower the degree of platelet responsiveness. Suggested aspirin dose: 325 mg per day. (Adapted from Schafer AI: Bleeding and thrombosis in the myeloproliferative disorders. Blood 64:1, 1984.)

Re-treatment in 3 to 6 months may be necessary. Platelet counts should be maintained at 600,000 per microliter. In emergency situations involving massive hemorrhage, plateletpheresis is recommended for an immediate (although transient) therapeutic effect.

About 40 per cent of patients with myeloproliferative disorders have a deficiency in platelet arachidonic acid lipoxygenase. This allows for shunting of free arachidonate through the cyclo-oxygenase pathway and production of excessive TXA_2. Paradoxically, such patients with enhanced TXA_2 production may have a bleeding tendency.

Since the thrombotic diathesis may be a complication of excessive quantities of activated platelets in the circulation, therapy with aspirin (325 mg daily) and dipyridamole* (75 mg three times daily) is recommended as prophylaxis. Since aspirin may also induce bleeding, criteria for its use can be summarized as follows: (1) Aspirin is contraindicated in patients with a previous history of hemorrhage, especially if the bleeding time is prolonged and if in vitro platelet aggregation tests indicate a defect. (2) Patients with no history of previous bleeding who have evidence of thrombosis in the extremities or in the cerebral or myocardial circulation should be treated with aspirin and dipyridamole (in conjunction with cytoreduction). Treatment for patients with a mixed history of bleeding and thrombosis must be individualized. If they have symptoms of thrombosis and the platelet count is between 750,000 and 1,000,000 per microliter, aspirin and dipyridamole are administered with caution, i.e., the patient is observed at monthly intervals and appropriately instructed. These criteria are summarized in Figure 166–6.

Schafer AI: Bleeding and thrombosis in the myeloproliferative disorders. Blood 64:1, 1984. *This review discusses the pathogenesis of autonomous thrombocytosis that occurs in myeloproliferative disorders. Therapeutic efficacy of cytoreduction and inhibition of platelet function are thoughtfully considered.*

*This use is not listed in the manufacturer's directive.

Qualitative Platelet Disorders

Patients with a prolonged bleeding time and normal platelet count have a qualitative platelet defect (Fig. 166–4). The abnormality may be intrinsic to the platelet or be due to a deficiency and/or a structural defect of plasma proteins that modulates platelet adhesion to subendothelium or platelet aggregation. One of three aspects of platelet function is abnormal in congenital or acquired qualitative platelet disorders: adhesion, aggregation, or the release reaction.

Coller BS: Disorders of platelets. In Ratnoff OD, Forbes CD (eds.): Disorders of Hemostasis. Orlando, Grune & Stratton, 1984, pp 73-176. *This is an excellent monograph, describing in great detail currently important aspects of platelets in hemostasis, coagulation, and thrombosis. Discussions of each topic, tables, illustrations, and references are excellent.*

BERNARD-SOULIER SYNDROME (Giant Platelet Syndrome)

This very rare congenital bleeding disorder, transmitted as an autosomal recessive trait, is characterized by platelets that vary in size and morphology. Cutaneous, mucous membrane, and visceral hemorrhages occur, and fatalities have been reported. The bleeding time is markedly prolonged because of failure of platelets to adhere to subendothelium. Prothrombin consumption is abnormal, reflecting poor clot-promoting properties of the platelets. This may be due to impaired binding of coagulation proteins to the platelet surface. Platelet aggregation in response to collagen, epinephrine, and ADP is normal, since these are cohesive functions and not related to surface adhesion. There is no agglutination in response to ristocetin, however, because GPIb (missing in the Bernard-Soulier syndrome) is the receptor for von Willebrand factor when platelets are exposed to ristocetin. GPIb-deficient platelets from patients with Bernard-Soulier syndrome cannot bind von Willebrand factor. This is in contrast to patients with von Willebrand's disease in which vWF is deficient or abnormal. In this case ristocetin agglutination is corrected by addition of normal plasma or purified von Willebrand factor, which does bind to their platelets. Platelet transfusions are effective, but may be complicated by development of alloantibodies to GPIb (missing from the patient's platelets), and should be utilized only in urgent clinical situations.

VON WILLEBRAND'S DISEASE (see also Ch. 167)

Von Willebrand factor (vWF) mediates adhesion (via GPIb) between platelets and the vessel wall (Fig. 166–1). vWF is a glycoprotein synthesized in endothelial cells and megakaryocytes and then released into plasma. It circulates as a heterogeneous group of disulfide-linked multimers ranging in molecular weight from 800,000 to 12,000,000 with subunits in the range of 200,000. The pathogenesis of bleeding in von Willebrand's disease (vWD) relates to the absence of platelet adhesion to subendothelium as mediated by vWF. The patient's plasma is also deficient in Factor VIII coagulant activity.

Von Willebrand's disease has been classified into several types and subtypes, all related to defects involving the vWF protein (Table 166–6). *Type IA vWD* (autosomal dominant), the most common form, is associated with a moderate bleeding diathesis. Circulating levels of all vWF multimers are decreased, but their structure is normal. Factor VIII coagulant activity is low, and ristocetin agglutination is absent. *Type IB vWD* is a slight variant of Type IA. All multimers are present, but the large ones are decreased relative to the smaller multimers. *Type IIA vWD* is less common. Multimer assembly from normal subunits is defective, and large and intermediate multimers are missing from plasma and platelets. Congenital inability to assemble intermediate and high-molecular weight multimers is inherited as an autosomal dominant. Ristocetin-induced agglutination activity is markedly decreased, and

TABLE 166–6. CLASSIFICATION OF VON WILLEBRAND'S DISEASE

	Type IA	Type IB	Type IIA	Type IIB	Type IIC	Type IID	Type III
Genetic transmission	Autosomal dominant	Autosomal dominant	Autosomal dominant	Autosomal dominant	Autosomal recessive	Autosomal dominant	Autosomal recessive
Bleeding time	Prolonged	Prolonged	Prolonged	Prolonged	Prolonged	Prolonged	Prolonged
Crossed immuno-electrophoresis	Normal	Normal	Abnormal	Abnormal	Abnormal	Abnormal	Variable (mostly abnormal)
VIIIC	Decreased	Decreased	Decreased or normal	Decreased or normal	Normal	Normal	Markedly decreased
vWF*	Decreased	Decreased	Decreased or normal	Decreased or normal	Normal	Normal	Minute amounts or absent
Ristocetin cofactor	Decreased	Decreased	Markedly decreased	Decreased or normal	Decreased	Decreased	Absent
RIPA†	Decreased or normal	Decreased or normal	Absent or markedly decreased	Increased	Markedly decreased	Decreased	Absent
Multimeric structure	Normal in plasma and platelets	Large multimers are present but are decreased relative to small multimers	Absence of large and intermediate multimers from plasma and platelets	Absence of only larger multimers from plasma. Normal in platelets	Absence of large multimers from plasma and platelets. Triplet structure is aberrant	Absence of large multimers from plasma. Triplet structure is aberrant but different from IIC	Variable

From Ruggeri ZM, Zimmerman TS: Platelets and von Willebrand disease. Semin Hematol 22:203, 1985.
*Measured as antigen by reaction with specific antibodies.
†RIPA = ristocetin-induced platelet aggregation in platelet-rich plasma.

Factor VIII procoagulant activity can be low. In *type IIB vWD* the very largest multimers are absent from plasma, but these multimers have an abnormal affinity for and are present on the patient's platelets and endothelial cells. Platelets that have adsorbed the vWF multimers in type IIB may agglutinate and be cleared from the circulation—thus causing thrombocytopenia. This may also account for the rapid disappearance of large multimers from the plasma and also the prolonged bleeding time. In vitro platelets from patients with type IIB vWD are highly sensitive to ristocetin because of the adsorbed vWF.

Clinically, *type III vWD* patients are the most severely affected. Fortunately this variant is rare, since it represents the homozygotic or double heterozygotic state. Levels of vWF in the circulation, platelets, endothelial cells, and subendothelium are virtually undetectable. Factor VIII:C is also deficient. These patients clinically represent an extreme form of type I vWD.

PSEUDO-VON WILLEBRAND'S DISEASE OR PLATELET-TYPE vWD. Platelets from these patients have an unexplained increased affinity for binding the larger vWF multimers, which are structurally normal. The plasma is almost devoid of large multimers although low molecular weight multimers remain. The bleeding disorder is similar to vWD, but the *abnormality is platelet mediated*. Ristocetin-induced agglutination is enhanced and occurs at low concentrations. Thrombocytopenia and abnormalities of platelet morphology have been reported. In vitro, cryoprecipitate will agglutinate platelets from these patients in the absence of any other agonist, attesting to their sensitivity. This is in contrast to type IIB vWF, in which ristocetin is necessary, albeit at low levels.

Treatment of vWD is directed toward correction of the plasma defect in vWF and Factor VIII, and it differs among the subtypes. For type I vWD the treatment of choice is cryoprecipitate, since this contains high concentrations of vWF, especially the high molecular weight multimers. Fresh or fresh-frozen plasma may be used if cryoprecipitate is not available, and the fluid burden can be tolerated. Cryoprecipitate will shorten the bleeding time to a varying degree for about a 12-hour period. For severe bleeding episodes, as much as 30 to 50 units of cryoprecipitate per kilogram may be required to normalize the Factor VIII level and correct the bleeding time. Epsilon-aminocaproic acid (EACA), which blocks fibrinolysis and stabilizes clot formation, is recommended for prophylactic use prior to dental extraction or minor surgery (50 to 100 mg per kilogram orally or intravenously).

The synthetic analogue of antidiuretic hormone, 1 deamino 8-d-arginine vasopressin (DDAVP), induces a threefold increase in vWF in patients with type I vWD (also Factor VIII). Peak response occurs 30 to 60 minutes after infusion. Prophylactic use of DDAVP and its therapeutic use for mild to moderate bleeding in type I vWD is a major advance, since it can replace therapy with blood components.

Cryoprecipitate should be used for treatment of hemorrhage in type IIA vWD, in which large vWF multimers are absent from plasma and platelets. DDAVP may be tried, since it will increase the low molecular weight vWF components, but it may not improve ristocetin cofactor activity or the bleeding time.

In type IIB vWD, in which there is vWF on the platelets and in endothelial cells, DDAVP infusion may induce release of the abnormal vWF multimers from these tissues with ensuing platelet agglutination in vivo and thrombocytopenia. Thus, DDAVP should not be used in type IIB vWD. For type IIB vWD, cryoprecipitate is recommended. In pseudo-vWD or platelet type vWD there is also platelet-bound normal vWF. In this instance, both DDAVP and cryoprecipitate will elevate plasma levels of large multimers of vWF, but may lead to in vivo agglutination and thrombocytopenia. Thus they should be used with caution. Cryoprecipitate is useful in type III vWD (which clinically resembles severe type I). Use of Factor VIII concentrates is not indicated for treatment of vWD because only low levels of vWF are present and mucosal bleeding is not controlled.

Moroose R, Hoyer LW: Von Willebrand factor and platelet function. Ann Rev Med 37:157, 1986. *This article contains a clear summary of current concepts of vWF-platelet interactions, reviews current research, and presents an update of therapy of von Willebrand's disease.*

Ruggeri ZM, Zimmerman TS: Platelets and von Willebrand disease. Semin Hematol 22:203, 1985. *This review considers recent information on structure-function relationships of von Willebrand factor. Interactions among vWF, platelets, and subendothelium are discussed. Subtypes of vWD are classified in detail.*

THROMBASTHENIA (Glanzmann's Disease)

Thrombasthenia, inherited as an autosomal recessive defect in platelet function, results in a lifelong mild to severe hemorrhagic tendency. Bleeding is of the mucosal type: epistaxis, gastrointestinal hemorrhage, and menorrhagia. Thrombasthenia is characterized by (1) normal platelet count, (2) prolonged bleeding time, (3) clot retraction that is poor or absent, (4) normal agglutination with ristocetin (GPIb, the platelet receptor for vWF is intact), (5) no aggregation in response to ADP, collagen, thrombin, epinephrine, arachidonate, or endoperoxide PGH_2 (although TXA_2 synthesis is normal). In in vitro systems thrombasthenic platelets undergo normal shape change and adhere normally in a single layer to subendothelium. However, "recruitment" of additional platelets to form a normal hemostatic plug is absent. This is in direct contrast to platelets of the Bernard-Soulier syndrome in which there is no adherence to subendothelium because of the absence of GPIb.

PATHOPHYSIOLOGY OF THROMBASTHENIA. Platelet-platelet interactions (cohesion) are grossly defective. The essential modulator of the platelet cohesion reaction is fibrinogen. Whereas unstimulated normal platelets do not bind fibrinogen, platelet activation by agonists such as ADP, thrombin, or epinephrine induces rapid expression of fibrinogen receptors. Platelets in thrombasthenia are incapable of binding fibrinogen, even in the presence of agonists. Solubilized membrane glycoproteins from normal platelets contain approximately 18 per cent of the total protein content as a complex of glycoproteins IIb and IIIa, which forms in the presence of calcium. This complex is diminished to absent in thrombasthenia. The two abnormalities mentioned above, i.e., absence of fibrinogen binding and quantitative deficiency of glycoproteins IIb and IIIa, explain the defect in thrombasthenia. Normally when platelets are stimulated, surface glycoproteins IIb and IIIa change structurally to become the fibrinogen receptor. In thrombasthenia the near-absence of the GPIIb-IIIa complex does not allow for fibrinogen binding. This is presumed to be the cause of the platelet abnormality. In a variant of thrombasthenia the GPIIb-IIIa complex is structurally abnormal so that fibrinogen is not bound. This further verifies the necessity for fibrinogen binding for platelet aggregation. Platelet fibrinogen itself is reduced or absent in thrombasthenia, as are the platelet surface antigens Pl^{A1} and Pl^{A2}.

For treatment of clinically significant hemorrhage, platelet transfusions are indicated. They should be reserved for severe bleeding, however, because of possible development of antibodies to glycoproteins IIb and IIIa. The antibody will interfere with functional integrity of platelets transfused at a later date.

George JN, Nurden AT, Phillips DR: Molecular defects in interactions of platelets with the vessel wall. N Engl J Med 311:1084, 1984. *This Medical Progress article classifies and discusses the pathogenesis and molecular defects of congenital disorders of platelet-vessel wall interactions that result in hemorrhagic disease. Glycoproteins of platelets and plasma are considered in relation to their involvement in primary hemostasis.*

Leung L, Nachman R: Molecular mechanisms of platelet aggregation. Ann Rev Med 37:179, 1986. *A concise analysis of molecular events accompanying platelet stimulation, including assembly of adhesive proteins on the platelet surface.*

ABNORMALITIES OF THE PLATELET RELEASE REACTION

When platelets are stimulated, the initial response results from the direct action of the agonist at its receptor site. The response is recorded in vitro as an initial wave of aggregation. This is normally followed by a "second wave" of aggregation, which is irreversible (in contrast to the first wave). The second wave is fibrinogen dependent, requires release of dense granule constituents such as ADP and 5-HT, and is accompanied by synthesis of TXA_2. Defects in the above processes result in a single reversible wave of aggregation, which is abnormal. Clinically, defects in the release reaction result in a syndrome characterized by mild mucocutaneous, postpartum, and postoperative bleeding and menorrhagia. The bleeding time is slightly prolonged, platelet counts and coagulation profiles are normal. Release reaction disorders can be subdivided as follows: (1) "storage pool" deficiency in which the release defect is due to a paucity of dense granules or alpha-granules within the platelet (a hereditary disorder in which alpha-granules are deficient is known as the gray platelet syndrome); (2) defects due to an abnormality in the release mechanism itself in the setting of a normal granule population (this is also known as the aspirin-like syndrome); (3) disorders of nucleotide metabolism.

Hereditary deficiency of dense granules, as expected, results in a defect in platelet hemostatic function. This includes the Hermansky-Pudlak syndrome, which is also associated with albinism and the presence of ceroid-like pigment in macrophages. Another example of hereditary dense granule deficiency is the Chédiak-Higashi syndrome (oculocutaneous albinism, infections, and bleeding). In the Wiskott-Aldrich syndrome (thrombocytopenia, infections, and eczema) hemorrhage is disproportionate to the bleeding time. Platelet granule abnormalities have also been reported.

Patients whose platelets appear to have normal dense granule content but deficient release have been classified as having an aspirin-like disorder because of its clinical resemblance to the effects of aspirin ingestion. This disorder must be differentiated from situations in which patients have surreptitiously ingested aspirin or aspirin-containing medications. Reports of cyclo-oxygenase deficiency and TXA_2 insensitivity have appeared, but these are apparently quite rare.

Patients with glycogen storage disease, type I (glucose 6-phosphatase deficiency), can develop a mild hemorrhagic tendency with a long bleeding time. The disorder of nucleotide metabolism resulting from the glucose 6-phosphatase deficiency induces a defect in platelet ADP release, which is more accentuated during periods of hypoglycemia. The syndrome is correctable by intravenous administration of glucose.

In general, patients with abnormalities of the platelet release reaction experience mild to moderate defects in hemostasis. Major surgical procedures and trauma may result in more serious hemorrhage, requiring vigorous therapeutic measures. This emphasizes the importance of preoperative screening as described in Table 166–3 and Figure 166–4. These patients should avoid aspirin or medications containing acetylsalicylic acid, since they will worsen the hemostatic defect.

ACQUIRED DISORDERS OF PLATELET FUNCTION—SYSTEMIC DISEASES

UREMIA. In uremia, patients may develop a hemorrhagic disorder secondary to a defect in platelet function. Abnormalities of adhesion and release as manifested by prolonged bleeding times are observed. Reversal of the clinical and laboratory platelet defects occurs following dialysis. This suggests that platelet dysfunction in uremia is induced by a dialyzable substance(s). Guanidinosuccinic acid, phenols, and urea are compounds implicated in the "uremic platelet defect."

AUTOIMMUNE AND LYMPHOPROLIFERATIVE DISEASES. Acquired von Willebrand's disease has been reported in association with these syndromes. Clinically the bleeding resembles that encountered in mild to moderate vWD. There may be an antibody to the Factor VIII:vWF complex, or the larger vWF multimers may be cleared. Acquired vWD has also been reported in association with SLE, monoclonal gammopathy, hypernephroma, and myeloproliferative disorders.

DYSPROTEINEMIAS. The hemorrhagic diathesis complicating these disorders is multifactorial. The final common denominator is interference with platelet surface-related function. Contributory factors include absorption of paraproteins to platelet and vessel surfaces, plasma hyperviscosity, thrombocytopenia, and coagulation abnormalities. Macroglobulinemia and IgA and IgG myeloma are most frequently associated with these functional disorders. The plasma expander *dextran* can induce defects in platelet function comparable to those seen in the dysproteinemias.

OTHER SYSTEMIC DISEASES. Prolonged bleeding times and platelet functional abnormalities have been reported in many systemic diseases and in association with their treatment. These include acute and chronic leukemias, SLE, pernicious anemia, scurvy, amyloidosis (Factor X deficiency has also been described), homocystinuria, and cirrhosis. Patients with diseases complicated by sepsis and treated with carbenicillin develop a hemostatic defect, as demonstrated by prolonged bleeding time and purpura. The DIC associated with systemic diseases results in platelet dysfunction, which compounds the other coagulation defects. Proteolytic degradation products of fibrinogen-fibrin digestion absorb to platelets and inhibit hemostatic plug formation.

Platelet Transfusions

Platelet transfusions are utilized to control serious hemorrhage in thrombocytopenic patients or in individuals with severe qualitative platelet defects. Major bleeding can be anticipated in patients with platelet counts below 25,000 per microliter; platelet numbers less than 10,000 per microliter are associated with increased morbidity from spontaneous or traumatic bleeding. In the absence of complicating factors such as fever, sepsis, mucosal ulceration, and hypersplenism, patients with megakaryocytic aplasia do not hemorrhage if the platelet count is 5000 per microliter or greater. In the immune thrombocytopenias, platelet counts of 1000 per microliter can be hemostatically sufficient. Patients with thrombocytopenia complicated by platelet dysfunction (neoplasia, drugs, uremia) require platelet counts of 20,000 per microliter or more for prevention of spontaneous hemorrhage. Bleeding time determinations are valuable in the management of individual patients, since it may correlate with the platelet concentration required for adequate hemostasis. As shown in Figures 166–4 and 166–5, coagulation parameters in thrombocytopenic patients are important, since they may contribute to the bleeding diathesis, and obviously coagulation defects do not respond to platelet administration.

If possible, platelets should be transfused approximately 90 minutes following decision and requisition. The usual dose is one unit of platelet concentrate (platelets suspended in 50 ml of plasma) per 10 kilograms of body weight. Clinical and laboratory evaluation is mandatory for judging the effectiveness of a given platelet transfusion and constitutes the major determinant of expected effectiveness of future transfusions. A platelet count should be obtained immediately preceding transfusion and one hour post-transfusion, and a final count should be made approximately 24 hours later. If a concentrate of random donor platelets did not increase the platelet count by 25,000 per microliter, the transfusion was of minimal value, and future transfusions will require quantitatively more platelets or platelets from an HLA-matched donor. After exposure to platelets from approximately 20 separate donors, patients become alloimmunized, and such transfusions are no longer useful therapeutically. This is evidenced by a lack of platelet increment at the one-hour period following transfusion. Thereafter platelets from histocompatible siblings or HLA-matched platelets are required for hemostasis. Thus, platelets are most useful as short-term therapy in hypoproliferative thrombocytopenia and in patients receiving chemotherapy with agents having a temporary marrow-suppressive effect.

Isoimmunization occurs less rapidly in leukemic patients than in patients with aplastic anemia, probably because chemotherapeutic agents are immunosuppressive. Routine use of prophylactic platelet transfusions is controversial, but many oncology centers utilize such treatment in patients whose platelet counts fall below 20,000 per microliter (4- to 6-unit transfusions are recommended).

Although reduction in platelet count and a platelet functional defect associated with cardiopulmonary bypass are documented, the effectiveness of platelet transfusions in this situation is difficult to evaluate. Current consensus is that routine administration of platelets during cardiovascular bypass procedures is probably not indicated.

Possible complications of platelet transfusions should temper decisions to initiate them. Patients receiving platelet concentrates from multiple donors undergo a risk as high as 40 per cent for post-transfusion hepatitis. Evidence of chronic hepatitis will develop in 50 per cent of recipients. Other complications include allergic and febrile reactions, AIDS, malaria, Chagas' disease, several viral infections, and graft-vs.-host (GVH) disease.

When thrombocytopenic bleeding complicates disorders characterized by increased platelet destruction or consumption, platelet transfusions in the past have been rather ineffective, mainly because transfused platelets were rapidly destroyed. High-dose intravenous gamma globulin may improve platelet counts rapidly in disorders such as acute ITP and preoperatively in patients with severe thrombocytopenia requiring splenectomy.

Eisenstaedt R: Blood component therapy in the treatment of platelet disorders. Semin Hematol 23:1, 1986. *This review discusses the therapeutic use of platelet transfusions in quantitative and qualitative platelet diseases. There is also detailed consideration of the ever increasing group of complications associated with platelet administration.*

Vascular Purpuras

As part of the hemostatic response, blood vessels constrict when severed or traumatized. Tests of hemostasis in current use mainly evaluate coagulation mechanisms and platelet function. Aside from the Rumpel-Leede tourniquet test and bleeding time, there are no specific methods to assess a vascular contribution to a hemostatic defect. Thus the diagnosis of vascular purpura is one of exclusion after qualitative and quantitative platelet disorders, coagulation defects, and fibrinolytic disorders have been ruled out. Patients usually present with easy bruisability and spontaneous bleeding from small blood vessels in the form of petechiae, ecchymoses, or both. In addition to a positive Rumpel-Leede vascular fragility test, the bleeding time is prolonged (Tables 166–3 and 166–7 and Figure 166–4).

ALLERGIC PURPURA (HENOCH-SCHÖNLEIN SYNDROME OR "ANAPHYLACTOID PURPURA"). Allergic purpura occurs mainly in children two to seven years of age with male predominance. Onset is sudden with an urticarial lesion, which fades and is replaced by red maculopapular rashes. The latter coalesce to form symmetric ecchymoses, especially over the extensor aspects of the lower extremities and buttocks. Two thirds of children have periarticular joint involvement, characterized by nonmigratory polyarthralgias in the ankles and knees. Abdominal pain with colic, accompanied by melena, occurs as a result of hemorrhage and edema in the small intestine. Occasionally this is complicated by intussusception. Acute glomerulonephritis with hematuria,

TABLE 166–7. VASCULAR PURPURAS

- Allergic purpura (Henoch-Schönlein)
- Dysproteinemias
  - Macroglobulinemia
  - Cryoglobulinemia
  - Primary hyperglobulinemic (benign) purpura
  - Multiple myeloma
  - Amyloidosis
- Purpura simplex
- Drug-induced vascular purpura
- Senile purpura
- Hereditary disorders of connective tissue
  - Ehlers-Danlos syndrome
  - Pseudoxanthoma elasticum
  - Marfan's syndrome
  - Osteogenesis imperfecta
- Cushing's syndrome
- Scurvy
- Autoerythrocyte and DNA sensitivity

proteinuria, and edema can occur during the second or third week. Renal involvement may be accompanied by hypertension with a transient decrease in renal function, which rarely progresses to chronic renal failure (less than 15 per cent). Skin biopsies during the acute episode reveal aseptic vasculitis with perivascular cuffing, fibrinoid necrosis, platelet plugging, and interstitial edema. Substances identified at the site of the inflammatory lesions include IgA, IgM, C3 to C5, and properdin. Similar lesions have been identified in the bowel, and renal biopsies have demonstrated segmental or (rarely) diffuse glomerular proliferation with occlusion of capillaries by fibrinoid material. A possible relationship between Henoch-Schönlein purpura, Buerger's disease, and other forms of IgA nephropathy is discussed in Ch. 81. Although the histopathologic lesions resemble those experimentally induced in immune complex disease, no antigen has been identified in association in Henoch-Schönlein purpura.

Patients with abdominal and joint involvement have been managed with prednisone to reduce the edema and inflammatory response. Corticosteroids, however, have no effect on the renal lesion and do not modify the skin manifestations. The long-term prognosis is good in the absence of chronic renal disease, although a 50 per cent recurrence rate during the initial weeks of recovery has been reported.

PARAPROTEINEMIAS. Vascular-type purpura occurs in paraproteinemias. The hemostatic defect is also attributable to complications of the primary disease such as bone marrow replacement, liver dysfunction, and uremia. Acquired deficiencies of coagulation factors and thrombocytopenia are common. This includes absorption of Factor X to amyloid and coating of the platelet surface and canalicular system with paraprotein. Hyperviscosity and "sludging" of erythrocytes and granulocytes in capillaries, leading to direct endothelial damage inflicted by precipitated paraproteins, also contribute to the vascular purpura.

In *cryoglobulinemia* (and cryofibrinogenemia), exposure of extremities to low temperature can induce purpuric lesions with subsequent ulceration. This is due to cryoglobulin precipitated on the vascular surface, which then interferes with vessel integrity. Complexes among fibrinogen, fibrin, and fibronectin have been identified as cryofibrinogens. These patients fare better in warm climates.

In *macroglobulinemia*, mucosal bleeding is more common than cutaneous hemorrhage. Patients with *primary hyperglobulinemic purpura* develop recurrent episodes of purpura, especially following exertion or physical trauma. The lower extremities are affected more commonly, and the purpuric episodes are preceded by a prodrome of itching and erythema. Progressive pigment deposition with discoloration at the site of the lesion is common. The hyperglobulinemia is monoclonal and of the IgM type. Epistaxis, purpura, and spontaneous bruisability are frequent. *Benign hyperglobulinemic purpura* occurs in systemic diseases such as Sjögren's syndrome, SLE, and rheumatoid arthritis.

In *myeloma*, the most common cause of hemorrhage is thrombocytopenia. Coagulation disorders, a qualitative platelet abnormality, and vascular purpura are also observed (see Ch. 163). Patients with IgA and IgG myeloma are at higher risk for qualitative platelet defects, which are reversible if the immunoglobulin level is reduced following successful therapy. In *amyloidosis* the protein is deposited in skin and subcutaneous tissues. This results in increased vascular fragility, manifested by purpura and subcutaneous hemorrhage (also due to Factor X absorption). Periorbital purpura ("raccoon eyes") is particularly diagnostic in amyloidosis (see Ch. 163).

PURPURA SIMPLEX (SIMPLE BRUISING). The lesions of this disorder are mild, occurring most frequently in women of childbearing age. Hemorrhage is limited to the skin in the form of circumscribed purpura, especially on the lower extremities and trunk. Occurrence during or preceding menstrual periods is frequent. The syndrome, also referred to as devil's pinches, is mainly of cosmetic import and does not require treatment. However, patients should be encouraged to avoid aspirin or aspirin-containing medications.

KAPOSI'S HEMORRHAGIC SARCOMA. Previously observed on the lower extremities of males over 50 years of age, these lesions more recently have been reported in association with immunosuppressive therapy and in patients with HIV infections. The hemorrhagic nodules result from proliferation of vascular elements. Local hemorrhage, followed by hemosiderin deposition, results in the characteristic violaceous or dark brown lesions. In about 10 per cent of cases, lesions are not limited to lower extremities, but appear in the gastrointestinal tract, liver, and lungs.

DRUG-INDUCED VASCULAR PURPURA. Many drugs produce generalized purpura in the absence of thrombocytopenia or a qualitative platelet defect. Examples include iodides, quinine, penicillins, chlorothiazides, sulfa drugs, and coumarin anticoagulants. Upon discontinuance of the offending drug, the purpura subsides. Screening procedures for diagnosis of this entity in contrast to other forms of purpura are outlined in Tables 166–3 and Figure 166–4.

SENILE PURPURA. This disorder should more appropriately be referred to as purpura in the elderly. It results from degeneration and loss of collagen, elastin, and subcutaneous fat in dermal tissues. The purpura most commonly occurs on extensor aspects of the forearms and hands. Anatomic locations that received exposure to actinic radiation are also affected. Lesions consist of red to purple ecchymoses that occur spontaneously. They persist for weeks and may result in residual hemosiderin pigmentation, probably reflecting poor phagocytic function in those anatomic locations. There is no therapy of proven value.

HEREDITARY DISORDERS OF CONNECTIVE TISSUE. Hereditary connective tissue disorders are mesenchymal dysplasias in which connective tissue and perivascular supporting structures of blood vessels are abnormal. This is also manifested by structural defects in larger blood vessels, resulting in increased vascular fragility and abnormal platelet adhesiveness. The hemorrhagic disorder can vary from benign bruisability to serious hemorrhage from viscera or large blood vessels.

CUSHING'S SYNDROME. Vascular purpura on the trunk and extremities occurs as a complication of chronic administration of high-dose corticosteroids or as a feature of Cushing's syndrome (Ch. 230). Bruising occurs spontaneously or following minor trauma. Pathogenesis of the vascular purpura may be related to a catabolic effect of steroids on perivascular supporting tissues. The purpura disappears upon cessation of corticosteroid administration or successful treatment of Cushing's syndrome.

SCURVY. In vitamin C deficiency, collagen synthesis is defective, as is deposition of "intercellular cement" along endothelial linings and perivascular supporting tissues of small vessels. Gingival bleeding and hemorrhage into subcutaneous tissues and muscle occur. Dermal bleeding is conspicuous around hair follicles. Subperiosteal hemorrhage is common in children but rare in adults, who more frequently develop intramuscular hematomas. Other vitamin and nutritional deficiencies usually coexist and complicate the clinical presentation. In adults 1 gram of ascorbic acid daily will terminate the scurvy and its associated hemorrhagic disorder.

AUTOERYTHROCYTE AND DNA SENSITIVITY. Autoerythrocyte sensitivity is characterized by formation of painful ecchymoses on the extremities, preceded by sensations of itching or burning, frequently coincident with emotional stress. The lesions may progressively enlarge and have an erythematous border. Headache, nausea, and vomiting with gastrointestinal, genitourinary, or intracranial bleeding may occur. About 100 patients have been described, of whom 95 per cent are women. Intradermal injection of autologous erythrocytes or erythrocyte stroma results in appearance of similar ecchymoses at the injection site. Thus the purpura may be due to autosensitization to an erythrocyte membrane component. Characteristically there are remissions and exacerbations over long periods.

The syndrome of DNA autosensitivity resembles autoerythrocyte sensitization. The lesions begin as painful nodules on the extremities, which enlarge and become indurated. Ecchymoses occur 24 hours later and may become bullous. Resolution occurs spontaneously. Intradermal injection of the patient's leukocytes or a solution of DNA into the skin will induce an ecchymosis. In some instances chloroquine therapy has been successful.

Ratnoff OD: The psychogenic purpuras: A review of autoerythrocyte sensitization, autosensitization to DNA, "hysterical" and factitial bleeding, and the religious stigmata. Semin Hematol 17:192, 1980. *This is a scholarly summary of the latest information concerning autoerythrocyte sensitization and sensitization to DNA. It also discusses the controversial relationship between emotional stress and the development of a hemorrhagic diathesis.*

Hereditary Hemorrhagic Telangiectasia (Osler-Weber-Rendu Disease)

Hereditary hemorrhagic telangiectasia is a bleeding disorder resulting from a vascular developmental abnormality. It is transmitted as an autosomal dominant trait—thus a family history of bleeding in both sexes is verifiable. The telangiectases result from dilatation and convolution of venules and capillaries in the skin and mucous membranes. Vessel walls are thinned to the level of a single layer of endothelium that has neither anatomic support nor contractile properties. These fragile, angiomatous masses of vascular components bleed spontaneously or following minor trauma. This disease is the most common hereditary vascular disorder associated with a hemorrhagic diathesis. Visible lesions, approximately 3 mm in diameter, occur on nasal mucous membranes, lips, gingiva, buccal mucosa, palate, both sides of the tongue, face, trunk, and palmar and plantar surfaces. The telangiectases are violaceous and flat, blanch on pressure exerted by a glass slide, and are variable in shape from pinpoint to nodular to spider-like. The telangiectases can be seen in children, but their appearance increases with age, peaking between the fourth and fifth decades. This correlates with an increase in the frequency and severity of hemorrhagic episodes. Bleeding is less severe in females. Visceral telangiectases occur in the gastrointestinal, respiratory, and genitourinary tracts.

Mucous membrane bleeding, especially epistaxis, is the most common clinical problem. In any given patient, however, telangiectases in other locations may become the source of chronic, recurrent hemorrhage. Fortunately hemostatic and coagulation values are normal, allowing patients to tolerate surgical procedures when required. Iron deficiency anemia is a common complication.

Vascular malformations in the lung result in pulmonary arteriovenous fistulas in 20 per cent of patients. These malformations, which increase in size and frequency with age, are usually multiple and constitute a source of hemoptysis as well as foci of infection. Shunting of blood through the pulmonary arteriovenous fistulas may induce hypoxemia, digital clubbing, and polycythemia. Recurrent brain abscesses and cerebral embolism have resulted from this pulmonary shunting abnormality. Arteriovenous fistulas also occur in the cerebral, hepatic, and splenic circulation, in addition to hemangiomas in the liver and polycystic kidneys.

The diagnosis is readily made in the setting of repeated episodes of hemorrhage, the presence of multiple telangiectases, and a characteristic family history. The diagnosis may be more difficult when bleeding is mild, telangiectases are absent from the skin or not readily visible, and the family history is unclear. Fiberoptic endoscopy has been helpful in diagnosis. Pulmonary arteriovenous fistulas are demonstrable by pulmonary angiography.

Treatment is mainly supportive and symptomatic. Iron deficiency should be treated by replacement therapy, used parenterally if necessary to maintain the storage pool. The latter is preferable to repeated transfusions. Whenever possible, hemorrhage should be controlled locally. Topical hemostatic agents are useful if the site is accessible. Cautery of bleeding sites not readily accessible is useful mainly as a temporary measure. Estrogens have been utilized to induce squamous metaplasia of the nasal mucosa, but this therapy is controversial. Surgical intervention for uncontrollable bleeding or for removal of arteriovenous fistulas should be considered on an individual basis. Use of oral contraceptives by females is debatable, since it is not known whether the low quantities of estrogen in these agents enhance or reduce the tendency to bleed. Despite the lack of specific therapeutic measures and the potential hazard of spontaneous hemorrhage, the prognosis in hereditary hemorrhagic telangiectasia is relatively good.

167 DISORDERS OF BLOOD COAGULATION

Deane F. Mosher

Normal hemostasis requires interactions among blood vessels, the formed elements of blood, especially platelets and monocytes, and blood coagulation proteins. The general biology of hemostasis and the approach to a patient suspected of having a hemorrhagic diathesis have been discussed in Ch. 166, Hemorrhagic Disorders: Abnormalities of Platelet and Vascular Function. In the present chapter, attention is focused on hemorrhagic and thrombotic disorders that occur as a consequence of abnormalities of blood coagulation proteins.

REVIEW OF BLOOD COAGULATION

Blood coagulation, initiated by substances in injured tissues, is propagated by an interlocking network of enzymic events, the so-called coagulation cascade. These controlled reactions insure that blood coagulation happens quickly and yet remains localized. Blood coagulation results in the formation of a protein scaffolding, the fibrin clot, that controls bleeding and serves as a nidus for subsequent cellular ingrowth and tissue repair. After several days the fibrin clot is lysed and replaced by a more permanent scaffolding of connective tissue matrix molecules. Abnormalities that result in delay of clot formation or in premature lysis of clots are associated with a bleeding tendency. Abnormalities that result in inappropriate activation or localization of blood coagulation are associated with thrombosis.

COAGULATION PROTEINS. Coagulation and fibrinolysis involve many proteins (Table 167–1). This list grows larger as blood coagulation mechanisms are studied in greater depth. Structural and functional similarities allow one to put the proteins into one of several groups. Some are zymogens of serine proteinases and hence members of the serine proteinase family of proteins. Among the serine proteinase family are five proteins (factors II, VII, IX, and X and protein C) that are modified by vitamin K–dependent post-translational carboxylation of glutamic acid residues. A sixth plasma protein, protein S, is also modified by this reaction. The modification allows the six proteins to bind Ca^{++} and phospholipids and thereby participate efficiently in blood coagulation. Factors V and VIII function as helper proteins during blood coagulation

TABLE 167–1. PROTEINS INVOLVED IN BLOOD COAGULATION AND FIBRINOLYSIS

Proteins	Synonym	Size in Kilodaltons*	Plasma Concentrations in mg/dl (μm)*	Kind of Protein	Function†
Fibrinogen	Factor I	340	300(9)	Structural protein, unique	Gels to form clot
Factor II	Prothrombin	72	15(2)	Vit. K–dependent zymogen of serine proteinase	Activates I, V, VIII, XIII, protein C, and platelets
Factor V	Proaccelerin	350	2(0.05)	Ceruloplasmin-like binding protein	Supports X_a activation of II
Factor VII	Stable factor	50	0.1(0.02)	Vit. K–dependent zymogen of serine proteinase	Activates IX and X
Factor VIII	Antihemophilic factor	350	0.1(0.003)	Ceruloplasmin-like binding protein	Supports IX_a activation of X
Factor IX	Christmas factor	57	1(0.2)	Vit. K–dependent zymogen of serine proteinase	Activates X
Factor X	Stuart-Prower factor	59	1(0.2)	Vit. K–dependent zymogen of serine proteinase	Activates II
Factor XI	Plasma thromboplastin antecedent	160	0.5(0.03)	Zymogen of serine proteinase	Activates XII and prekallikrein
Factor XII	Hageman factor	75	2(0.2)	Zymogen of serine proteinase	Activates XI and prekallikrein
Factor XIII	Fibrin-stabilizing factor	320	3(0.08)	Zymogen of transglutaminase	Cross-links fibrin and other proteins
von Willebrand factor	Factor VIII–related antigen	800–20,000	2(0.05)	Structural protein, unique	Binds VIII, mediates platelet adhesion
Prekallikrein	—	88	2(0.3)	Zymogen of serine proteinase	Activates XII and prekallikrein, cleaves HMWK
High molecular weight, kininogen (HMWK)	—	150	2(0.2)	Binding protein, unique	Supports reciprocal activation of XII, XI, and prekallikrein
Fibronectin	—	450	40(1)	Structural protein, unique	Mediates cell adhesion
Major antithrombin	Antithrombin III	60	20(2.5)	Serpin	Inhibits II_a, X_a, and other proteases; cofactor for heparin
Minor antithrombin	Heparin cofactor II	55	5(0.6)	Serpin	Inhibits II_a, cofactor for heparin and dermatan sulfate
Protein C	—	62	0.4(0.06)	Vit. K–dependent zymogen of serine proteinase	Inactivates V and VIII
Protein S	—	69	3(0.4)	Vit. K–dependent binding protein	Cofactor for protein Ca, binds C4b-binding protein
Plasminogen	—	86	10(1.2)	Zymogen of serine proteinase	Lyses fibrin and other proteins
Alpha-2-antiplasmin	—	60	3(0.5)	Serpin	Inhibits plasmin
Prourokinase	—	50	—	Zymogen of serine proteinase	Activates plasminogen
Tissue plasminogen activator	TPA	55	—	Serine proteinase	Activates plasminogen
Plasminogen activator inhibitor I	—	52	—	Serpin	Inactivates TPA
Plasminogen activator inhibitor II	—	55	—	Serpin	Inactivates urokinase

*For comparison, the size of albumin is 68 kilodaltons, and the plasma concentration of albumin is 3500 mg/dl (510 μm).
†For zymogens, the function after activation is given.

and are homologous to one another and to ceruloplasmin, a Cu^{++}-binding plasmin protein. Other proteins are *ser*ine *pro*teinase *in*hibitors and hence members of the "serpin" family of proteins. Most of the proteins listed in Table 167–1, including the vitamin K–dependent factors, are synthesized by hepatocytes. A number of the proteins, however, can also be synthesized by other cell types such as megakaryocytes, monocyte-macrophages, and endothelial cells.

GENERAL MECHANISMS. Blood coagulation is activated, propagated, and controlled by mechanisms found in other proteolytic effector systems (e.g., complement). These mechanisms include:

1. Sequential activation by limited proteolytic cleavage
2. Amplification of the response by feedback activation loops
3. Use of binding or helper proteins to bring reactants together
4. Destruction of activated proteins by further proteolytic cleavage
5. Inhibition of activated proteinases by stoichiometric complex formation with specific inhibitor proteins, *i.e.*, the serpins

In addition, there is a mechanism that is so far unique to blood coagulation:

6. Formation of a five-part complex of an activated vitamin K–dependent factor, to-be-activated vitamin K–dependent zymogen, helper protein, Ca^{++}, and phospholipid surface (Fig. 167–1*C*).

EXTRINSIC AND INTRINSIC PATHWAYS. Blood coagulation can be initiated by exposure of blood to a specific cellular lipoprotein called tissue factor (the "extrinsic system") or by activation of contact factors of plasma (the "intrinsic system"). Both of these initiation pathways lead to a common pathway, which results in the elaboration of thrombin, the master coagulation enzyme. As shown in Figure 167–1*A*, the concept of the two initiation pathways and the common pathway is useful in understanding two major coagulation tests, the activated partial thromboplastin time (APTT), in which blood plasma is activated by the intrinsic pathway, and the prothrombin time, in which tissue factor is added to plasma so that activation proceeds by the intrinsic pathway. It is unlikely that the two initiation pathways are so clearly delineated in vivo. Activation of factor IX, an intrinsic factor, by factor VII, an extrinsic factor, must be of considerable

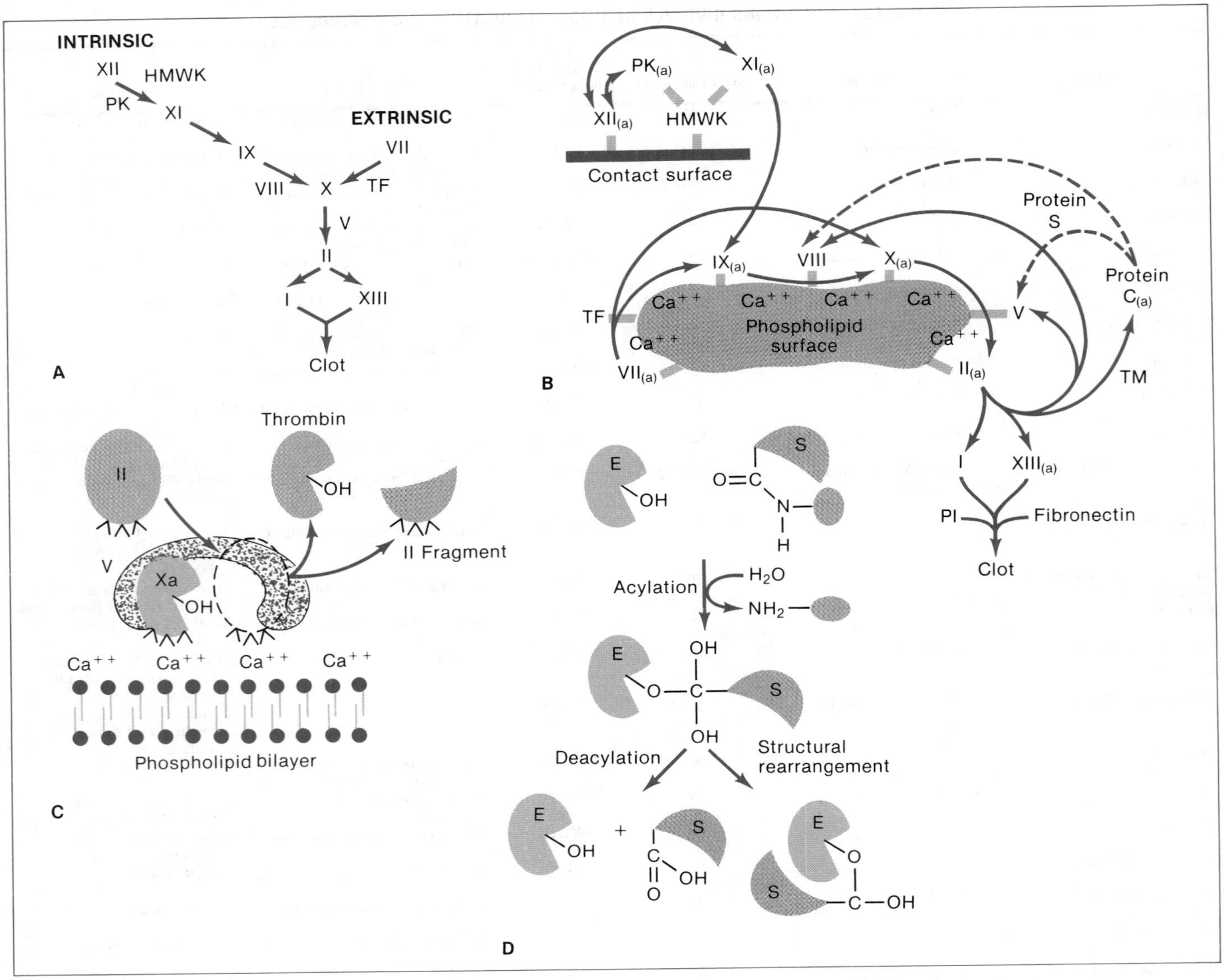

FIGURE 167–1. Diagrams of interactions among coagulation factors. PK = prekallikrein; HMWK = high molecular weight kininogen; TF = tissue factors; PI = alpha-2-antiplasmin; TM = thrombomodulin. *A* (the so-called Y diagram) depicts the intrinsic and extrinsic pathways in their simplest forms. *B* is organized around the contact surface and the phospholipid surface. Solid lines indicate activation. Broken lines indicate inactivation. The stippled patches indicate binding of proteins to surfaces or to one another. The subscript (a) indicates proteins that are zymogens and can be converted to active enzymes. *C* is a close-up of activation of prothrombin (factor II) on a phospholipid surface to which factors X_a and V are also bound. Prothrombin is cleaved, generating thrombin and a large fragment. *D* depicts the reaction of a serine proteinase (E) with a substrate or serpin(s). The proteinase attacks a peptide bond in the substrate or serpin, forming an acylenzyme intermediate. If the attack is on a serpin, it stays bound to the proteinase, and the proteinase is inhibited. With a substrate, the intermediate is deacylated, completing cleavage of the peptide bond and regenerating the proteinase.

importance because deficiencies of factors VII and IX, as well as the factors that follow factor IX in the intrinsic and common pathways, *i.e.*, factors VIII, X, V, II, and I, all are associated with a bleeding tendency. In contrast, deficiency of factor XII, prekallikrein, or high-molecular-weight kininogen does not cause a bleeding problem, and factor XI deficiency is associated with a bleeding tendency in only a minority of cases.

Tissue Factor and the Extrinsic Pathway. Factor VII is unique among coagulation factors because it circulates in an active configuration. To initiate coagulation, however, factor VII requires tissue factor. A major initiating stimulus to coagulation, therefore, is exposure of blood to tissue factor. Tissue factor is present in many types of cells, including fibroblasts, endothelial cells, and monocytes. Normally, tissue factor is cryptic. In response to a variety of stimuli, such as mechanical disruption in the case of fibroblasts or exposure to lymphokines or monokines in the case of monocytes or endothelial cells, tissue factor becomes expressed on cell surfaces.

In the presence of tissue factor, phospholipid, and Ca^{++}, factor VII can activate factors IX and X (Fig. 167–1*B*). Factor X_a then activates factor II, and factor II_a (thrombin) cleaves fibrinogen to fibrin. The time to clot formation after addition of tissue factor, phospholipid, and Ca^{++} to citrated platelet-poor plasma is called the prothrombin time. When determined with an excess of tissue factor (as is generally done), the prothrombin time measures only factors of the extrinsic and common pathways and does not measure factor IX. When the concentration of tissue factor is low, presumably the more common situation in the body, a considerable portion of the

X-activating capability of factor VII is generated through factor IX, because there is ten times more factor IX than factor VII.

Contact Factors and the Intrinsic System. Activation of contact factors constitutes a second pathway for activating factor X. Negatively charged surfaces, such as sulfatide micelles, glass, kaolin, and celite, bind factor XII and high molecular weight kininogen (HMWK). HMWK, in turn, binds prekallikrein and factor XI. Binding to surfaces initiates a series of reciprocal cleavages of factor XI and prekallikrein by activated factor XII and of factor XII by activated factor XI and kallikrein (Fig. 167–1*B*). Activated factor XI activates factor IX in a reaction that requires Ca^{++}. Kallikrein also releases bradykinin, a vasoactive and pain-causing octapeptide, from HMWK and low molecular weight kininogen. In the APTT, platelet-poor citrated plasma is allowed to incubate for three to five minutes with kaolin or ellagic acid to optimally activate factor XI. Ca^{++} and phospholipid are then added so that activated factor XI (XI_a) can activate factor IX, factor IX_a can activate factor X, and so on.

Amplification of Activation Pathways. Three analogous five-part propagating reactions take place: (1) factor VII activates factor X or IX in the presence of tissue factor, Ca^{++}, and phospholipid; (2) factor IX_a activates factor X in the presence of factor VIII, Ca^{++}, and phospholipid; and (3) factor X_a activates factor II in the presence of factor V, Ca^{++}, and phospholipid. The phospholipid requirement for reaction (1) is satisfied by the surface of the tissue factor–containing cell. For the reactions involving factor VIII or V, the phospholipid requirement is satisfied by platelet phospholipid.

Factor VIII is a trace protein of plasma, and large amounts have become available only recently. The five-part reaction we know most about, therefore, is the one that involves factor V (Fig. 167–1*C*). Factors X_a and II bind to the phospholipid surface in interactions that require gamma-carboxyl glutamic acid residues; the binding is Ca^{++} dependent. Factor V contains domains for binding factors X_a and II, Ca^{++}, and the phospholipid surface. Stimulated platelets contain discrete binding sites for factor V. The accelerating role of platelets in the X_a-V-II reaction is called platelet factor 3 activity. Formation of the five-part complex dramatically increases the rate constant (K_{cat}) for activation of factor II by factor X_a. In the five-part complex, factor V is most effective after it has been cleaved by factor II_a (thrombin). Thus, thrombin is initially generated at a sluggish rate, but once a small amount of thrombin is generated so that it can cleave factor V to a more active form, subsequent thrombin generation is rapid and efficient, consuming almost all of the factor II in plasma.

LOCALIZATION AND INHIBITION OF BLOOD COAGULATION. Blood coagulation is efficiently activated only on a phospholipid surface (Fig. 167–1), and thus activation is localized to the area of injury. Several mechanisms dampen activation and insure that activated factors do not escape and cause thrombosis at a distant site.

Thrombin exhibits acquired altered specificity when complexed to thrombomodulin, a protein on the luminal surface of endothelial cells. Rather than acting upon fibrinogen or factors V and VIII, thrombin cleaves and activates protein C (Fig. 167–1*B*). Activated protein C, in turn, cleaves thrombin-activated factors V and VIII further so that V and VIII are no longer active. In addition, activated protein C enhances fibrinolysis, probably by neutralizing the major inhibitor of tissue plasminogen activator (see below). Activation of protein C by thrombin-thrombomodulin complex, therefore, is a powerful anticoagulant event, just as the activation of factors V and VIII by thrombin is a powerful procoagulant event. The cleavage of factors V and VIII by activated protein C requires the sixth vitamin K–dependent protein of plasma, protein S. Protein S serves as a cofactor for activated protein C rather than acting as a proteinase.

Two antithrombins in plasma inhibit thrombin and other serine proteinases that are generated during blood coagulation. The antithrombins, members of the serpin family, are substrates for the proteinases. Upon cleavage the antithrombins undergo a structural rearrangement that allows them to form tight one-to-one complexes with the proteinases (Fig. 167–1). As a result, the proteinases are irreversibly inhibited. The major and minor antithrombins, also called antithrombin III and heparin cofactor II, account for approximately 80 per cent and 20 per cent, respectively, of the inhibitory activity in plasma toward thrombin. The rates at which both antithrombins combine with coagulation proteinases are accelerated manyfold by heparin and by heparan sulfate proteoglycan on the luminal surface of endothelial cells. The acceleration explains the anticoagulant action of heparin. The rate at which the minor antithrombin combines with thrombin is accelerated by dermatan sulfate, a glycosaminoglycan found in the vessel wall.

As described in more detail below, inherited deficiency states of protein C, protein S, the major antithrombin, and the minor antithrombin have all been associated with thrombotic diatheses.

STRUCTURE OF FIBRINOGEN AND FIBRIN. Fibrinogen and fibrin monomer are extended trinodular molecules made up of pairs of three polypeptide chains: alpha, beta, and gamma (Fig. 167–2*A*). The three chains run through half of the molecule, that is, through half of the central E nodule and the whole of one of the two peripheral D nodules. The chains are thought to adopt a coiled-spring structure between the E and D nodules. This portion of the molecule is particularly susceptible to degradation by the principal fibrinolytic enzyme, plasmin. The nodules resist degradation by plasmin. Thus the products of complete lysis of a clot by plasmin are one E nodule, two D nodules, and small fragments (Fig. 167–2*B*).

Thrombin cleaves negatively charged small peptides, called fibrinopeptides A and B, from the amino terminals of the alpha and beta chains in the E nodule of fibrinogen. Release of these peptides, which account for less than 3 per cent of the mass of fibrinogen, converts fibrinogen to a clottable derivative called fibrin monomer. At concentrations 1000-fold lower than physiologic, fibrin monomer will assemble to form an infinite branching network of fibrils (Fig. 167–2*B*). At physiologic fibrin concentrations, this network constitutes a strong gel and immobilizes blood. Fibrinogen is usually completely converted to fibrin during blood coagulation. Thus the concentration of fibrinogen antigen in serum is about 0.02 mg per deciliter, as compared to 200 mg per deciliter in plasma. Fibrinogen, however, forms soluble complexes with fibrin monomer when the concentration of thrombin is low. The soluble complexes can escape from areas of active coagulation and be detected in the circulation.

The fibrin gel is modified by thrombin-activated factor XIII. This enzyme, a transglutaminase, acts upon selected glutaminyl residues in fibrin and other proteins, including fibronectin and alpha-2-antitrypsin, to cause covalent protein-protein cross-linking (Fig. 167–2*C*). Cross-links are introduced between gamma chains of adjacent D domains, thus ligating the fibrin fibril end to end (Fig. 167–2*B*). Cross-linking of gamma chains renders the clot insoluble in protein denaturants such as 6 M urea. The alpha chains can ligate side to side among themselves or be cross-linked to fibronectin or alpha-2-antiplasmin. Both the "hardening" of the fibrin clot by cross-linking and the incorporation of other proteins into the clot are probably important. Many cell types have specific receptors for fibronectin that they use to migrate into fibronectin-containing clots. Alpha-2-antiplasmin is a serpin that rapidly forms a one-to-one complex with plasmin. Cross-linked alpha-2-antiplasmin serves to protect the clot from low levels of fibrinolysis. Deficiency of factor XIII or of alpha-2-antiplasmin is associated with a bleeding tendency, and some patients with factor XIII deficiency suffer from poor wound healing.

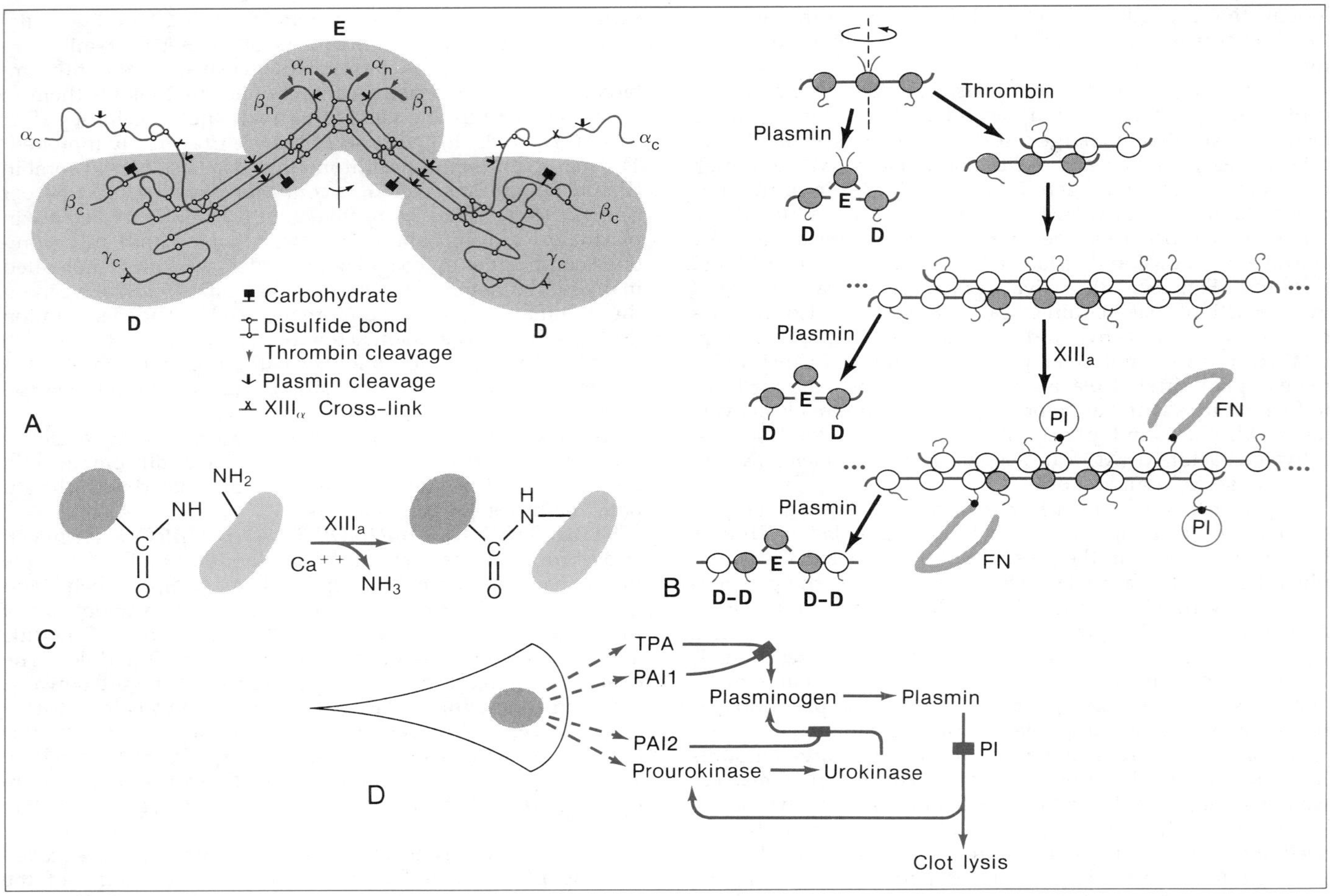

FIGURE 167–2. *A,* Disposition of the six chains of fibrinogen. Fibrinogen is composed of a central E nodule and two peripheral D nodules. One set of three nonidentical chains—alpha, beta, and gamma—runs through half the molecule and is bound to the other set by disulfide linkages in the E domain, where the amino termini of all six chains come together. The strands connecting the peripheral nodules to the central nodule contain all three chains. The carboxyl terminal regions of the three chains constitute the globular D domain. In addition, the extreme carboxyl terminal region of the alpha chain extends out from the D domain. Thrombin releases acidic fibrinopeptides A and B from the E domain to yield fibrin; plasmin cleaves the molecule between E and D. *B,* Activation, assembly, cross-linking, and lysis of fibrinogen and fibrin. Fibrinogen and fibrin are both trinodular proteins. Clotting is initiated by release of the negatively charged fibrinopeptides from the E nodule. Assembly is driven by noncovalent E nodule–D nodule interaction. End-to-end covalent cross-linking occurs between gamma chains. Alpha-2-antiplasmin (PI) and fibronectin (FN) cross-link to the extended carboxyl terminal portion of the alpha chain. Plasmin cleaves this portion of the alpha chain and separates the D and E nodules. *C* diagrams the cross-linking reaction catalyzed by factor XIII. *D* depicts the activation of plasminogen by its physiologic activators, urokinase and tissue plasminogen activator (TPA), and the control of the activation by plasminogen activator inhibitors (PAI1 and PAI2). These four molecules are secreted by cells. Plasmin is inhibited by alpha-2-antiplasmin (PI).

FIBRINOLYSIS. Cleavage of plasminogen to the active proteinase plasmin is carried out by two plasminogen activators: tissue plasminogen activator (TPA) and urokinase (Fig. 167–2*D*). TPA is secreted as an active serine proteinase, whereas urokinase can be activated from a somewhat active precursor, prourokinase. Among the activators of prourokinase is plasmin. TPA, plasminogen, and plasmin all bind to fibrin, and it is in a fibrin clot that TPA can activate plasminogen to plasmin most efficiently. Prourokinase does not bind to fibrin. However, small amounts of plasmin already bound to fibrin can activate prourokinase to urokinase, which then can activate more plasminogen to plasmin.

Localization of fibrinolysis to the fibrin clot is further insured by an efficient array of inhibitors. Cells secrete specific inhibitors of TPA and urokinase, presumably to regulate fibrinolysis in their local environment. Indeed, tightly controlled secretion of activator and inhibitor may allow a cell to localize plasminogen activation to volumes that are only nanometers across. Anti-TPA is present in the circulation in low concentrations. Also in the circulation is alpha-2-antiplasmin, which inhibits plasmin extremely rapidly and efficiently.

Plasmin degrades a variety of proteins in addition to fibrin, especially connective tissue proteins, and undoubtedly has other physiologic functions besides lysis of fibrin clots. For instance, ovarian follicular cells secrete plasminogen activator in response to hormonal stimulation just prior to ovulation and thereby initiate degradation of the follicular wall.

Epsilon-aminocaproic acid (EACA) and its cyclic analogue, tranexamic acid, bind to a single site on plasminogen and plasmin and inhibit binding of these molecules to fibrin. As a result, the molecules are good inhibitors of plasminogen activation.

Streptokinase, a bacterial protein, forms a complex with plasminogen and causes a conformational change that opens up the active site of plasminogen. The streptokinase-plasminogen complex can degrade fibrin and activate free plasminogen to plasmin. The complex is not inhibited by alpha-2-antiplasmin.

Colman RW, Hirsh J, Marder VJ, Salzman EW (eds.): Hemostasis and Thrombosis: Basic Principles and Clinical Practice. 2nd ed. Philadelphia, J. B. Lippincott Company, 1987. *Extensive information about the structure and function of blood coagulation proteins with earnest attempts to relate biochemical facts to clinical problems.*

APPROACH TO PATIENTS WITH COAGULATION DISORDERS

HISTORY AND PHYSICAL EXAMINATION. There are three components to effective hemostasis: the blood vessel, platelets, and the network of soluble factors. Abnormal bleeding occurs with much greater frequency when two of the three components are compromised as, for example, in a hemophilic patient who suffers trauma or takes aspirin, or in a patient with peptic ulcer and thrombocytopenia. Disorders of platelets or blood vessels often cause mucosal or superficial bleeding; deficiency of a coagulation factor results in a tendency to form soft tissue hematomas or to suffer from repeated hemarthroses. Thrombosis tends to occur when there is inflammation, abnormalities of the luminal surface of a large blood vessel, or stasis.

A personal history, family history, and physical examination are important parts of the evaluation of a possible coagulation problem. In taking a history, it is not enough simply to ask: "Do you or your close relatives bleed or clot abnormally?" One must also determine how the hemostatic system has been stressed: "Have you had any operations or tooth extractions? If so, did you bleed abnormally or require blood transfusions afterward? Are your menstrual periods heavy? Do you bruise easily? Do you take iron tablets? Have you ever had a limb immobilized?" And so on. A formal family tree indicating how many family members are at risk and which ones have symptoms or laboratory evidence of a coagulation disorder should be constructed.

LABORATORY SCREENING TESTS. When a bleeding disorder is suspected a group of reproducible and fairly inexpensive laboratory tests should detect most clinically significant abnormalities of platelets, blood vessels, and the coagulation factor network:

1. A complete blood count and examination of the blood smear screen for abnormalities in bone marrow function or platelet number and morphologic changes in red cells caused by intravascular thrombosis or microangiopathy.
2. A quantitative platelet count provides more definitive information about platelet number.
3. A template bleeding time screens for abnormalities of blood vessels and platelets.
4. The prothrombin time and APTT screen for abnormalities of the extrinsic and intrinsic coagulation pathways, respectively. Both tests are sensitive to abnormalities of the common pathway. The prothrombin time or APTT should be abnormally long if a single factor is below 20 to 40 per cent of its normal plasma concentration.
5. The solubility of the fibrin clot in concentrated (6 M) urea will detect clinically significant deficiency of factor XIII. In the absence of factor XIII the clot will not be covalently cross-linked and therefore will be soluble.

Evaluation of a Prolonged Prothrombin Time or APTT. The first step is to perform mixing experiments of normal plasma and the abnormal plasma to decide whether the abnormal plasma is deficient in a coagulation factor or contains an inhibitor of coagulation. If the screening test of the mixture is normal, it is likely that the abnormal plasma is deficient in one or more factors, and specific factor assays can be done to identify the deficiency. If the screening test of the mixture is abnormal, it is likely that the abnormal plasma contains an inhibitor. Inhibitors may be of the so-called lupus type and directed against the phospholipid used in the assays or more rarely may be directed against a single coagulation factor. Lupus-type inhibitors rarely cause clinical bleeding. Indeed, as described below, some patients with lupus-type inhibitors suffer from repeated episodes of venous and arterial thrombosis. Inhibitors directed against single factors, especially VIII and IX, may cause serious bleeding.

SPECIFIC TESTS OF INDIVIDUAL PROTEINS. A plasma protein can be measured as the protein per se, usually with an immunoassay, or for protein activity. Plasma contains many different proteins, some of which will influence the activity of the coagulation factor of interest and others of which may influence the end point of the assay. Activity assays for coagulation proteins are therefore less straightforward than many laboratory measurements. In general, there are two approaches for such activity assays: use of factor-deficient plasmas and use of chromogenic substrates.

Use of Factor-Deficient Plasmas. Normal and patient's plasma are compared for their ability to correct the prothrombin time or APTT of plasma from an individual severely deficient in the factor of interest. Thus factor VIII can be measured, using plasma from an individual with severe classic hemophilia. If the patient has a factor VIII deficiency, the patient's plasma should correct the APTT of the hemophilic patient's plasma less well than does normal plasma. By convention, the normal plasma is said to have 100 per cent or 1 unit per milliliter of activity. If a 1/10 dilution of the patient's plasma has the correcting power of a 1/100 dilution of normal plasma, the patient will be said to have a factor VIII activity of 10 per cent or 0.1 unit per milliliter. Such an assay should be accurate to within 10 to 20 per cent of the reported value.

Use of Chromogenic Substrates. A chromogenic substrate is a small peptide that is cleaved rapidly and relatively specifically by an activated proteinase to yield a colored product. The rate of cleavage can be measured with high precision in a spectrophotometer, using dilute solutions of plasma. As an example, plasminogen can be assayed by addition of streptokinase to diluted plasma and quantification of cleavage of a chromogenic substrate by streptokinase-plasminogen complexes. Alternatively, antiplasmin can be assayed by addition of plasmin to diluted plasma and quantification of the loss of the ability of plasmin to cleave the same substrate due to formation of plasmin-inhibitor complexes. Such assays should be accurate to within 3 to 5 per cent of the reported value, but may be subject to artifact. For instance, a patient with a recent streptococcal infection could have artifactually low apparent plasminogen activity due to neutralizing antibodies to streptokinase.

Indications for Specific Tests. When there is a suspicious bleeding history but normal screening tests, several specific assays should be considered. Mild factor VIII or IX deficiency (10 to 40 per cent of normal) is clinically significant, but may result in a screening APTT that is at the upper limits of normal but still within the normal range. Deficiency of plasma alpha-2-antiplasmin can be diagnosed only with a specific assay.

Evaluation of a possible thrombotic diathesis, at present, can be done only with specific assays for proteins C and S, the two antithrombins, plasminogen, and perhaps other components of the fibrinolytic system.

Diagnosis of a 50 Per Cent Deficiency State. Laboratory studies of family members are often crucial to the evaluation, especially when the diagnosis centers around a heterozygous (50 per cent of normal) deficiency. The normal level (i.e., the value in 99 per cent of normal individuals) of a coagulation factor is typically 70 to 140 per cent; the level of the factor in individuals with heterozygous deficiency is typically 35 to 70 per cent; and the assay for the factor is accurate to within only 5 to 10 per cent of the reported value. The problem of distinguishing the 50 per cent deficiency state from normal is therefore a formidable one. If the apparent deficiency is found in other family members at risk, one can be much more confident that a true deficiency state exists. For example, a random woman with a 50 per cent factor VIII level is probably not a carrier of classic hemophilia. If the sister of a hemophilic patient has a 50 per cent factor VIII level, however, the sister has a 95 per cent chance of being a carrier. Heterozygous deficiency states associated with thrombosis (i.e., deficiency of the major antithrombin, the minor antithrombin, protein C, or protein S) present a similar problem. The most important facet of the care of a patient with heterozygote deficiency is appropriate counseling. Therefore a physician should not be reluctant to arrange extensive family studies. To give an example, it would be much more efficient (and cost-effective) to identify a patient with antithrombin deficiency as part of a family study and counsel that patient that he or she is at risk for thrombosis after surgery than to screen all patients prior to surgery with a specific assay for antithrombin. In the future it is likely that informative protein or restriction fragment length polymorphisms will be identified that will allow most deficiency states to be traced in families with more than 99 per cent confidence.

Suchman AL, Griner PF: Diagnostic uses of the activated partial thromboplastin time and prothrombin time. Ann Intern Med 104:810, 1986. *Critical evaluation of when these tests should be ordered and how the tests should be interpreted.*

INHERITED DISORDERS OF BLOOD COAGULATION

General Comments

The plasma protein coagulation factors that are named with Roman numerals, with the exception of factor XII, were identified as a consequence of patients presenting with bleeding disorders, eventually recognized as unique and familial. Bleeding may be due to a structural defect in a coagulation factor or to a lack of its synthesis. In the former situation there will be immunologically cross-reacting material (CRM) present in the patient's plasma, and the patient is said to be CRM+. In the latter situation the patient is said to be CRM−. Genetic material for most of the coagulation factors has been cloned, and considerable information about the exact genetic defects that underlie inherited bleeding disorders is being generated. It is likely that a number of different genetic defects will be demonstrated for each coagulation factor, in analogy to the many defects in the β globin gene in patients with hemoglobinopathy or thalassemia. In other words, Murphy's law of genetic disease—"Whatever can go wrong with a gene will go wrong"—will be proven again and again. Future studies of genetic defects of coagulation proteins will undoubtedly give important new insights into the functions of these proteins, will allow deficient patients to be separated into subgroups in ways that are clinically relevant, and, as described above, will allow more definitive diagnosis of heterozygous deficiency states.

GENETICS. Deficiencies of factors VIII and IX are inherited as X-linked traits with bleeding occurring in the male hemizygotes. Von Willebrand disease is usually an autosomal dominant disorder, although rare patients have severe autosomal recessive disease. Deficiencies of all of the other coagulation factors are transmitted as autosomal recessive traits, with clinically significant bleeding usually manifested only in patients with homozygous deficiency. Heterozygous carriers may have reduced plasma levels of a coagulation factor activity, but the deficiency seldom affects hemostasis. In the case of protein deficiencies associated with familial tendency to thrombosis, however, heterozygotes with 50 per cent of the normal level of the protein are at risk. Inherited deficiencies may be combined. Most frequently cited are patients with combined factor V and factor VIII deficiencies that appear to be familial. The reason for the association is not known, although it is intriguing that factors V and VIII are homologous to one another and perform analogous functions (Fig. 167–1). Combined deficiencies in the functions of factors II, VII, IX, and X have been observed in patients with congenitally defective vitamin K–dependent gamma-carboxylation.

TREATMENT STRATEGIES. The most obvious treatment is replacement of the missing factor. Concentrates of factors VIII and IX are readily available at a cost of 12 to 20 cents per unit. Because of its large size, factor VIII distributes mainly in the blood plasma. There is approximately 40 ml of plasma per kilogram of body weight. Thus it would take 1400 units of factor VIII (at a cost of $168 to $280) to raise the plasma factor VIII level of a 70-kg patient with severe classic hemophilia from less than 1 per cent (<0.01 unit per milliliter) to 50 per cent (0.5 unit per milliliter) as calculated by the following formula:

$$0.5 \text{ unit/ml} \times 40 \text{ ml/kg} \times 70 \text{ kg} = 1400 \text{ units}$$

Because of its smaller size, factor IX distributes in a volume 1½-fold to 2-fold greater than the plasma volume. Thus, proportionately more factor IX than factor VIII must be infused to achieve a similar response in a patient with hemophilia B. Because of its longer half-life in the body, however, factor IX needs to be given less often than factor VIII to maintain a therapeutic level.

The above calculation points out one of the drawbacks of replacement therapy: cost. A shortage of concentrates is a potential problem, but at present there is enough source plasma to supply the needs of hemophilic patients. The most important, indeed overriding, problem with purified factor concentrates is with contaminating viruses. Each batch of concentrate is made from thousands of units of plasma, some of which come from commercial plasmapheresis centers. There is a high likelihood that recipients will be infected with hepatitis B, non-A, non-B hepatitis, and/or human immunodeficiency virus (HIV). This likelihood can be minimized by use of source plasma that does not contain antibodies to the viruses and has a normal level of transaminase. The infectivity of concentrates can be further decreased and perhaps eliminated by subjecting the concentrates to treatment (e.g., heating or extraction with an organic solvent) that will inactivate the viruses but preserve the activity of the factor of interest. It will be some time before efficacies of the attenuation processes are completely known or before products made by recombinant DNA techniques are available. In the meantime the clinician and patient must weigh the convenience and effectiveness of potentially infective factor concentrates against treatments that are more cumbersome but minimize exposure to multiple donors (e.g., use of cryoprecipitate rather than factor VIII concentrate) or do not require exposure to blood products at all (e.g., use of desmopressin to transiently raise the level of factor VIII and EACA to minimize mucosal bleeding).

When elective procedures are contemplated that require prophylactic therapy to raise factor levels, it is wise to test the proposed therapy prior to the procedure to be sure that target levels can be achieved.

HEMOPHILIA A (FACTOR VIII DEFICIENCY)

Hemophilia A, the most frequently encountered serious inherited disorder of blood coagulation, occurs in 1 of 10,000 males. Some patients lack plasma factor VIII, whereas others have a nonfunctional factor VIII molecule present in normal concentrations. The majority of hemophilic patients give a positive family history with an X-linked inheritance pattern. In the remainder the mutation of the factor VIII gene may be new. A hemophilic patient's daughters will all be carriers, but all his sons will be normal. A carrier woman has a 50 per cent chance of producing a hemophilic male or a female carrier. Because of random inactivation (lyonization) of the X chromosome, the carrier is a genetic mosaic with two populations of cells containing either a normal X chromosome or an abnormal X chromosome (bearing the hemophilic gene). Therefore, a carrier should have about 50 per cent of the normal level of factor VIII activity. The range of factor VIII levels in carriers is broad, probably because inactivation of one of the X chromosomes is often disproportionate. If extreme lyonization occurs so that the preponderance of cells in the carrier female contains the X chromosome with the hemophilic gene and the factor VIII level is less than 40 per cent of normal, the woman may have clinical features of mild hemophilia.

CLINICAL MANIFESTATIONS. In general, the degree of factor VIII deficiency correlates with the frequency of clinically significant bleeding. Furthermore, the degree of deficiency and bleeding severity tend to be similar in affected members of a given family. Hemophilia, therefore, is often classified as severe (<1 per cent normal activity), moderate (1 to 5 per cent normal activity), or mild (5 to 25 per cent normal activity). Bleeding from the umbilical cord is rare at birth, presumably because the extrinsic limb of the coagulation system functions normally in the presence of high concentrations of tissue factor.

Hematomas and Internal Hemorrhage. Depending on the severity of the deficiency, soft tissue hematomas may develop in early infancy. More difficulties begin when the child becomes physically active, and these continue throughout life. Hematomas often occur in muscles and soft tissues. Considerable blood loss can occur into thigh muscles or the retroperitoneum; extent of blood loss in these areas may be difficult to discern clinically and is frequently underestimated. The bleeding of hemophilia can involve virtually any anatomic area and give rise to secondary symptoms and signs caused by compression. If bleeding occurs in the pharynx or neck, airway obstruction can result. Severe bleeding may occur from peptic ulcerations. Partial intestinal obstruction may result from hemorrhage into the bowel wall. Mesenteric bleeding can lead to the development of bowel ischemia and necrosis. Hematuria can be painless or may present as ureteral colic due to formation of clots that obstruct the ureter. Subdural hematomas and other central nervous system hemorrhages are uncommon, but represent a major cause of death and disability. Many bleeding episodes appear to develop spontaneously without a history of trauma or other provoking causes. Such spontaneous bleeding may occur during periods of stress, as before school examinations or following family dissension. When bleeding follows trauma, it may be delayed, since the primary hemostasis furnished by vessels and platelets is intact (see Ch. 166).

Hemarthroses. Bleeding occurs in joints, usually in the elbows, knees, and ankles and less often in the wrist and hand. In about half of hemophilic patients, repeated hemarthroses result in eventual deformity and crippling. These patients have factor VIII activity levels well below 5 per cent of normal and usually less than 1 per cent of normal. The patient experiences considerable pain with bleeding into joints due to distension of the joint capsule. Movement is severely limited, causing disuse atrophy of the muscles about the joint. Pressure erodes the ends of long bones, causing periosteal pain, eventual necrosis, and pseudocyst formation. Hemarthrosis causes proliferation of the synovium. Thus a vicious cycle is set in play in which a joint, once weakened, may experience hemorrhage again and again in a seemingly spontaneous manner.

Bleeding after Surgery. Major or minor surgery, including dental extractions, can result in marked blood loss in a hemophilic patient and therefore must be carried out in conjunction with factor VIII replacement therapy to assure adequate hemostasis. Even those patients with mild hemophilia, factor VIII levels of 5 to 25 per cent of normal, may develop clinically significant bleeding with surgery or trauma and require replacement therapy.

DIAGNOSIS. A history of joint and soft tissue bleeding, a family history compatible with X-linked inheritance, and the presence of arthropathy on physical examination would all point to the diagnosis of sex-linked hemophilia. Factor VIII deficiency is most likely, although IX deficiency (hemophilia B) must also be considered. Laboratory screening tests should show a normal prothrombin time and prolonged APTT. The abnormal APTT should be corrected by all deficient plasmas except those from individuals with known factor VIII deficiency. In particular, the abnormal APTT should be corrected by plasma from a patient with factor IX deficiency. If plasmas from patients with known deficiencies are not available, correction can be attempted with normal plasma absorbed with barium salts (which will remove factor IX but not factor VIII) and serum (which contains factor IX but not active factor VIII). Absorbed plasma, but not serum, will correct the abnormal APTT of a patient with factor VIII deficiency. As described above, a quantitative assay for factor VIII can be done by testing the ability of dilutions of the patient's plasma to correct the defect in factor VIII–deficient plasma.

Von Willebrand factor (see below) stabilizes factor VIII in the circulation; severe deficiency of von Willebrand factor is therefore accompanied by severe deficiency of factor VIII, and hemophilia A can be confused with von Willebrand disease. Unlike hemophilia, however, von Willebrand disease is inherited as an autosomal dominant trait and may present with a history of vascular type bleeding. Upon screening, the bleeding time should be grossly prolonged in von Willebrand disease, whereas the bleeding time is usually at the upper limit of normal or only slightly prolonged in hemophilia. Further investigation should demonstrate deficiency or abnormality of von Willebrand factor and defective platelet aggregation mediated by the antibiotic ristocetin in von Willebrand disease but not in hemophilia. If the diagnosis remains in doubt, it may be helpful to perform laboratory tests on family members to determine the inheritance pattern of the deficiency.

TREATMENT. The patient and family must learn about the nature of hemophilia, the anticipated severity of the patient's disease, the recognition and management of various types of bleeding episodes, the difference the disorder may make in the patient's future life style, and the genetics of its transmission.

General Considerations. A major goal of patient, family, and physician is to have the patient lead as normal a life as possible. This will entail some restrictions of activities as a child and limitations on career choices. The physician, guided by the medical history, the degree of physical impairment, the severity of bleeding in affected family members, and the plasma level of factor VIII, should advise the patient to participate in activities commensurate with the severity of his disease. A hemophilic child should be reared in a protective environment until he understands the consequences of hemophilia and can take responsibility for his actions. The physician should be alert for denial mechanisms sometimes constructed by patient and parents about the disease. For example, the patient may develop a willingness and receive unconscious encouragement from the parents to participate in dangerous activities or to forgo needed treatments. With maturity, the patient usually accepts the constraints imposed by his disease. He should be encouraged to develop his education and interests as fully as possible and counseled to adopt a career that does not expose him to undue hazards, is compatible with his physical capabilities, and allows him access to adequate health insurance coverage.

To be free to develop as normal a life as possible, the patient must participate in a major way in his medical care. This has led to the widespread adoption of home care programs in which the patient treats himself at home with the backup of a primary physician, a nurse coordinator, and a multidisciplinary team of a hematologist, orthopedic surgeon, dentist, social worker, financial counselor, and so on. It is reasonable to expect a responsible patient in a home care program to work or go to school full time, to require a minimum of emergency room visits, and to be hospitalized only for major trauma, medical illness, or elective surgery. The major cost of such a program is replacement therapy: A 70-kg patient who has severe hemophilia and needs to give himself an infusion every other week would consume approximately \$6000 (25 × \$250) in blood products per year. Home care programs, however, are cost effective because bleeding episodes are treated when first symptomatic and do not proceed to the point at which hospitalization is required for aggressive replacement therapy and pain management. About 50 per cent of patients with hemophilia A have enough problems to make home care worthwhile.

Patients receiving long-term replacement therapy need regular evaluation at 6- to 12-month intervals. The clinic visit should include a physical examination with special attention paid to joints, an inhibitor screen, a chemistry panel with special attention paid to liver function, and tests for antibodies to hepatitis viruses and HIV.

Factor VIII Preparations. Bleeding episodes are managed primarily by administration of factor VIII, either in the form of cryoprecipitate or as a commercially prepared lyophilized concentrate. The use of cryoprecipitate or factor VIII concentrate avoids the complication of volume overload that would occur with the large amount of plasma that would be necessary to attain acceptable levels of factor VIII activity.

Blood banks prepare cryoprecipitate by freezing individual bags of fresh normal plasma, each containing approximately 200 units of factor VIII activity in 200 ml of plasma, at −90°C and then thawing at 4°C. Approximately 50 per cent of the factor VIII contained in the plasma remains as a precipitate, which is separated from the bulk of the plasma and stored frozen in individual bags containing approximately 100 units of factor VIII activity in 20 to 40 ml of residual plasma. When needed, the appropriate number of bags is thawed at 37°C, and the contents are pooled and administered intravenously to the patient.

Lyophilized factor VIII concentrate has been taken through several purification steps and is available in vials containing different amounts of factor VIII activity (exact amounts stated on the labels). The concentrates are readily soluble upon addition of diluent and thus can be prepared and administered intravenously within 30 minutes.

The major advantage of cryoprecipitate, especially for the patient who needs only occasional infusions of factor VIII, is that it exposes the recipient to fewer donors and thus minimizes the chance of blood-transmitted viral infection. Indeed, individuals have been supported from infancy to young adulthood with cryoprecipitate prepared from plasma donated sequentially by the same donor. The major disadvantages of cryoprecipitate are the inconvenience of thawing and pooling bags prior to administration and the need for the bags to stay frozen at −20°C until the time of administration in a home freezer that does not have a frost-free cycle and preferably has a device that graphs temperature over time.

The major advantages of lyophilized concentrates are stability on storage and convenience of administration. Another major advantage of concentrates in the future will be the knowledge that the concentrates have been processed to totally inactivate HIV and possibly also hepatitis B and the agent(s) of non-A, non-B hepatitis.

Patients should be vaccinated against hepatitis B at the time of diagnosis and will be prime candidates for vaccines that may be developed in the future for non-A, non-B hepatitis viruses and HIV.

Replacement Therapy. Intensity of replacement therapy depends on the estimated plasma level of factor VIII required to halt the bleeding and the disappearance rate of the infused factor VIII. Very early hemarthrosis can be managed with a single infusion to attain a peak factor VIII level of 25 to 50 per cent of normal. For more extensive hemorrhage, factor VIII infusions are usually continued for two days after cessation of symptoms or signs of bleeding. Early hemarthrosis or hematuria can be managed by maintenance of the plasma factor VIII level at 25 to 50 per cent of normal for two to three days. Muscle hematomas require a longer period of sustained factor VIII levels, in the range of 40 to 60 per cent of normal for four to six days. Major trauma or surgery requires that the factor VIII level be maintained at more than 70 per cent of normal until hemostasis is achieved and then in the range of 25 to 50 per cent of normal for 10 to 14 days. Plasma factor VIII can be measured after administration of the calculated dose to document that the desired peak level has been achieved and prior to subsequent scheduled doses to determine whether desired levels have been sustained. If a low factor VIII level persists despite replacement therapy, it may be that simply not enough factor VIII is being given, that the factor VIII concentrates contain less than their stated activity, or that the patient has developed an inhibitor that neutralizes infused factor VIII.

The amount of concentrate needed to achieve and maintain a desired level of factor VIII activity can be estimated by knowing (1) that the patient's plasma volume is about 40 ml per kilogram of body weight, (2) the amount of factor VIII activity in the average bag of cryoprecipitate (usually about 100 units) or in available vials of lyophilized concentrate factor VIII activity, and (3) that factor VIII has a half-life of about 10 to 12 hours in the circulation. Therefore replacement therapy is ordinarily given three times a day when tight control of the level is needed and twice a day when deeper troughs in the level can be tolerated.

Treatment of Hemarthroses. In addition to replacement therapy, joint bleeding is initially managed by immobilization of the affected limb and application of ice packs to diminish swelling and discomfort of the joint. Because of the risk of introducing infection or of causing additional bleeding, hemarthroses should not be aspirated unless such acute pain and tension are present that pressure necrosis is a major possibility. Aspiration should be performed only after administration of replacement factor VIII. Splinting or using elastic bandages over a hemarthrosis may make the patient more comfortable and insure that a position of joint function is maintained during the acute stage. When pain and swelling have subsided, the patient should begin rehabilitation to regain motion and strength in conjunction with prophylactic replacement therapy. Patients with joint disease may benefit from periodic assessment by an orthopedic surgeon. In properly selected patients, synovectomy and artificial joint replacement have been very successful in improving the usefulness of severe chronic joint deformity.

Dental Care. The patient should be instructed about the importance of dental hygiene and should have frequent dental examinations. Bleeding in deep tissues of the oropharynx can be life threatening. Therefore, a local anesthetic should be administered by needle puncture only after prophylactic administration of factor VIII concentrate. Extraction also requires prior administration of factor VIII concentrate. For patients with mild or moderate hemophilia, it is likely that adequate levels of factor VIII can be achieved with use of desmopressin, as described below for patients with von Willebrand disease. Administration of EACA by mouth, also described below, is useful in prevention of rebleeding after tooth extraction.

Use of Analgesics. Bleeding can cause extraordinary pain, especially in joints. Injudicious use of narcotics can lead to addiction in hemophilic patients. Aspirin must be avoided by the hemophilic because it decreases platelet aggregation and accentuates bleeding. Acetaminophen and codeine are recommended as the first choices of analgesics. In selected cases, ibuprofen can be given for chronic joint pain. The likelihood that ibuprofen will cause increased bleeding can be assessed by a template bleeding time after the patient has received the drug for several days. If the bleeding time is prolonged compared to the bleeding time before therapy, the drug should be discontinued.

Factor VIII Inhibitors. The possibility that the patient has acquired neutralizing antibodies to factor VIII (factor VIII inhibitor) should be of constant concern. An inhibitor may initially appear at almost any time in the life of a hemophilic patient and need not be associated with any obvious change in the clinical severity of the disorder. Patients with inhibitors present special problems. Much depends on the titer of the inhibitor, which is commonly expressed in Bethesda units: 1 Bethesda unit, by definition, inhibits 1 unit of factor VIII, i.e., the factor VIII in 1 ml of normal plasma. If one calculates the amount of factor VIII required to neutralize the inhibitor and achieve a 50 per cent normal level of circulating factor VIII in a patient who weighs 70 kg and has a plasma volume of 2,800 ml and an inhibitor titer of 10 Bethesda units per milliliter, the amount (and cost) is immense:

$$2800 \text{ ml} \times 10.5 \text{ units/ml} = 29{,}400 \text{ units (cost} = \$3528 \text{ to } \$5880)$$

Several strategies are available, all expensive and none totally adequate. Because some inhibitors take up to several hours to complex with and inhibit factor VIII, it may be possible to maintain factor VIII levels at a therapeutic level by constant infusion. If the inhibitor is of modest titer (1 to 10 Bethesda units per milliliter), it may be possible to remove enough inhibitor by plasmapheresis to make therapy feasible with lower amounts of factor VIII. A patient receiving factor VIII concentrate may have an anamestic immune response with an increase in the titer and avidity of his inhibitor. Therefore, everything possible should be done to achieve permanent hemostasis in the four- to six-day "golden period" during which replacement therapy is possible. Patients with high titers of rapidly acting inhibitor can be given activated factor IX concentrate that also contains activated factor X and therefore "bypasses" factor VIII in the coagulation cascade. Such a concentrate, unfortunately, is expensive and has considerable thrombogenic potential.

AIDS. Regardless of whether they have antibodies to HIV, patients who have used significant quantities of blood products must take proper precautions to protect their close contacts and loved ones. They can be assured that the virus is not transmitted by casual household contact. They must be taught safe disposal procedures for needles and other injection paraphernalia. It should be strongly recommended that condoms be used during all sexual intercourse. This raises an irreconcilable conflict for couples considering pregnancy. There is a high likelihood of transmission of HIV to the newborn of a virus-positive mother. Thus, wives of men with hemophilia who are considering pregnancy should receive specific education and counseling and be tested for antibodies to HIV before pregnancy occurs.

PROGNOSIS. Factor VIII concentrate is a two-edged sword. The major long-term complications of moderate and severe hemophilia are (1) progressive joint deformity and crippling, (2) development of inhibitors to factor VIII activity, (3) hepatitis and cirrhosis, and (4) acquired immune deficiency syndrome.

Despite the availability of replacement therapy, many hemophiliacs, for a variety of reasons, are treated inadequately or haphazardly and become severely crippled and, ultimately, chronic invalids. The last three of the four complications listed above are seen more often in patients who receive frequent replacement therapy. Up to 15 per cent of hemophilic patients develop inhibitory antibodies to factor VIII activity, usually in childhood. The tendency to develop antibodies may be genetic. If so, the accumulating information about lesions in hemophilic factor VIII genes should lead to knowledge that will allow identification of patients at high risk for development of inhibitors. Most patients who have received factor VIII concentrate in the past have been exposed to hepatitis viruses and HIV. The risks of chronic hepatitis and AIDS in exposed individuals are both probably greater than 10 per cent. On the whole, the availability of concentrates has been beneficial and has improved the prognosis of all forms of hemophilia A—mild, moderate, and severe. With the elimination of viruses in concentrates and a better understanding of inhibitor formation, it is reasonable to hope that future cohorts of hemophiliacs will enjoy the benefits of replacement therapy without the complications. Patients who have been treated in the past, however, are at risk for these complications, especially AIDS, and thus their prognosis is guarded.

CARRIER DETECTION. Women who have relatives with hemophilia frequently seek help to determine whether they may pass the disorder to their children. Daughters of men with the disorder, mothers of more than one hemophilic son, and mothers who have a hemophilic son and another hemophilic male relative in their pedigree are obligate carriers of the hemophilic gene. Only about 15 per cent of the instances of hemophilia arise because of spontaneous mutation. Determination of factor VIII procoagulant activity is of limited usefulness in the identification of carrier women, because low-normal levels overlap with factor VIII levels found in obligate heterozygotes. A major reason for scatter in factor VIII levels is scatter in the levels of von Willebrand factor, which functions as a carrier protein for factor VIII. Therefore the overlap between normal persons and obligate carriers is decreased considerably if the factor VIII level is corrected for the level of immunoreactive von Willebrand factor (sometimes called factor VIII–related antigen). When the ratios of these two proteins are analyzed by logarithmic discriminant analysis, greater than 95 per cent of carriers can be identified. Such an analysis is best done by a laboratory that is highly experienced with the assays and has proven the validity of the analysis in an adequate number of obligate carriers.

Several restriction fragment length polymorphisms close to the gene for factor VIII have been shown to be useful in tracing hemophilia A in families. In families in which the polymorphisms segregate with hemophilia, the polymorphisms can identify carriers with greater than 99 per cent confidence. The polymorphisms also can be used to diagnose hemophilia in fetuses in the first trimester, whereas assays of factor VIII per se can only be done in the second trimester when the fetal circulation is accessible for blood sampling by fetoscopy.

Graham JB, Green PP, McGraw RA, et al.: Application of molecular genetics in prenatal diagnosis and carrier detection in the hemophilias: Some limitations. Blood 66:759, 1985. *Summarizes the initial cloning literature on factor VIII and the potential application to patients.*

Levine PH: The clinical manifestations and therapy of hemophilias A and B. In Colman RW, Hirsh J, Marder VJ, et al. (eds.): Hemostasis and Thrombosis: Basic Principles and Clinical Practice. 2nd ed. Philadelphia, J. B. Lippincott Company, 1987, pp 97–111.

VON WILLEBRAND DISEASE

This disorder, named for the Finnish physician who described it in 1926, is due to a deficiency or abnormality of a plasma protein, von Willebrand factor, that is required for the stabilization of factor VIII in the circulation and for the normal adherence of platelets to sites of vascular injury. The gene for von Willebrand factor is on chromosome 12. The hallmarks of von Willebrand disease historically have been a low factor VIII level, a long bleeding time, and autosomal inheritance. The last two characteristics distinguish von Willebrand disease from hemophilia A. With extensive characterization of von Willebrand factor over the last decade has come a broadening of the definition of von Willebrand disease so that the name now encompasses a heterogeneous group of defects of von Willebrand factor.

FUNCTION OF VON WILLEBRAND FACTOR. Factor VIII and von Willebrand factor circulate in normal plasma as a complex. Endothelial cells and megakaryocytes-platelets synthesize, store, and secrete von Willebrand factor. Secretion increases when endothelial cells are stimulated or injured. Therefore the concentration of plasma von Willebrand factor is labile and can be increased by stimuli as innocuous as a vigorous Valsalva maneuver, and it is common to find levels of von Willebrand factor elevated twofold to tenfold in ill patients. Von Willebrand factor exists as a series of multimers ranging in size from 850,000 to 12,000,000 daltons. The largest multimers, which have a half-life in the circulation of only several hours, are most active in mediation of platelet adhesion. Both large and small multimers complex with factor VIII. Von Willebrand factor can interact with platelets in two different ways. It binds to platelet glycoprotein Ib in a reaction that is greatly enhanced by ristocetin (an antibiotic that cannot be used because it causes thrombocytopenia). It also binds to platelet glycoprotein IIb-IIIa complex, but only when platelets are activated. Von Willebrand factor binds to collagen and other components of the vessel wall and thus mediates attachment and spreading of platelets to the subendothelium of damaged vessels. The role of von Willebrand factor in platelet adhesion is especially important when blood passes through the blood vessel at high shear rate and the red blood cell count is normal or increased.

PATHOGENESIS OF VON WILLEBRAND DISEASE. In classic (type I) von Willebrand disease, patients have prolonged bleeding time, abnormal platelet aggregation in response to ristocetin, and parallel decreases in plasma factor VIII activity, immunoreactive von Willebrand factor, and ristocetin cofactor activity. Patients with severe, usually homozygous, disease can have less than 1 per cent of normal von Willebrand factor in plasma and platelets and no detectable von Willebrand antigen in endothelial cells. Their factor VIII levels may be less than 5 per cent of normal. Intravenous infusion of small amounts of normal plasma, hemophilic plasma, or normal serum into patients with severe von Willebrand disease results in a prolonged increase in factor VIII that is out of proportion to the factor VIII content of the transfused plasma or serum. This probably results from stabilization of the patients' endogenously produced factor VIII by infused von Willebrand factor.

A number of qualitative abnormalities of von Willebrand factor result in variant diseases called type IIA, type IIB, and so on. In type IIA disease the large and intermediate-sized multimers are not present in plasma or platelets. Von Willebrand factor function (e.g., ristocetin cofactor activity) is decreased more than von Willebrand factor antigen. These patients have abnormal platelet adhesion and long bleeding times, but normal factor VIII activity. Abnormal multimer patterns can be ascertained by probing separated plasma proteins with antibodies to von Willebrand factors after agarose gel electrophoresis. Subtypes IIC, IID, etc., of von Willebrand disease have been identified, based on additional subtle abnormalities in the electrophoretic pattern of the multimers. In type IIB disease the largest multimers are missing from plasma but not from platelets, and the abnormal von Willebrand factor causes platelet aggregation at lower than usual ristocetin concentration. It is thought that the largest multimers are missing from plasma because the multimers bind spontaneously to platelets. In principle, such a spontaneous interaction could be due to defects in the patient's von Willebrand factor or in the patient's platelets ("platelet von Willebrand disease"), and indeed patients have been identified in whom the defect is in the platelets.

CLINICAL MANIFESTATIONS. Von Willebrand disease has a broad spectrum of clinical and laboratory features. It can range from a severe hemorrhagic disorder, in which the level of factor VIII is low enough and the bleeding problems severe enough that the disease must be differentiated from classic hemophilia, to an asymptomatic condition that is a laboratory curiosity. The severity of symptoms due to von Willebrand disease can vary considerably even among afflicted family members, probably because there are a number of factors that control the synthesis and secretion of von Willebrand factor.

Patients with severe disease usually have inherited it from both parents, as either a true homozygous or as a double heterozygous disease. The principal bleeding problems are of the superficial type. Epistaxis is a frequent complaint, especially early in life, as is easy bruising. Hematuria and gastrointestinal bleeding occur less frequently, and hemarthroses are quite rare. Without adequate replacement therapy, postoperative bleeding is a major hazard. In patients with heterozygous type I or II disease, the hemorrhagic tendency usually becomes evident or troublesome only with trauma, surgery, or dental extractions. Women with the disorder commonly experience excessive menses and postpartum bleeding. In all forms of the disease, the frequency and severity of bleeding tend to lessen with age.

DIAGNOSIS. The classic findings in type I von Willebrand disease are prolonged bleeding time and a low level of factor VIII. Confirmatory testing should reveal a low level of immunoreactive von Willebrand factor and absence or diminished platelet aggregation when ristocetin is added to the patient's platelet-rich plasma. The analysis using ristocetin can be made more sensitive and quantitative by testing the ability of dilutions of the patient's plasma to support agglutination of washed platelets; this is often called the ristocetin cofactor titer. Patients with severe type I disease lack von Willebrand factor antigen when endothelial cells of skin biopsies are stained by immunofluorescence or platelets are lysed and subjected to immunoassay.

Electrophoretic analysis of the site distribution of von Willebrand factor multimers should be done in patients who are suspected of having type II von Willebrand disease on the basis of bleeding problems, prolonged bleeding time, and abnormal ristocetin-induced platelet aggregation but normal or only slightly decreased levels of von Willebrand factor and factor VIII. In type IIA disease the larger multimers are missing in both plasma and platelets. In type IIB disease (hypersensitivity to ristocetin) the larger multimers are missing in plasma but not in platelets.

It may be very difficult to know for sure whether someone with mild decreases in von Willebrand factor and factor VIII, say to 50 per cent of normal, has von Willebrand disease. A number of factors influence the plasma concentration of von Willebrand factor. For instance, people with type O blood have lower levels than people with types A and B. As another example, hypothyroidism causes the level of von Willebrand factor to fall. As mentioned above, endothelial cells can be stimulated to release von Willebrand factor. Thus, one must worry about both overdiagnosis and underdiagnosis. Serial studies of the same patient and studies of other family members can be helpful. Because symptoms in such patients are mild and tend to decrease with age, however, it may suffice to be honest with such patients about the ambiguities of the laboratory tests and counsel them to alert their physician about the possibility of von Willebrand disease in the event of trauma or major surgery.

TREATMENT. Indications for therapy in von Willebrand disease include surgery, severe epistaxis, severe menorrhagia, and recurrent gastrointestinal bleeding.

Replacement Therapy. Cryoprecipitate is equally rich in factor VIII and von Willebrand factor and therefore will correct both the deficiency of factor VIII and the long bleeding time of type I von Willebrand disease. Factor VIII concentrates are poor in von Willebrand factor and will not correct the bleeding time defect. Hence, replacement therapy in von Willebrand disease should be with cryoprecipitate rather than factor VIII concentrate. Because the largest multimers of von Willebrand factor are cleared rapidly after infusion, the bleeding time is usually corrected only transiently. The smaller multimers allow the patient's own factor VIII to circulate, and the factor VIII level may remain elevated for considerably longer than would be predicted, based on the amount of infused factor VIII. In the case of ongoing hemorrhage or major surgery, cryoprecipitate should be given, using the guidelines described above for factor VIII replacement in hemophilia A. The infusion should be given immediately prior to maneuvers designed to achieve hemostasis. This will insure that the bleeding time as well as the factor VIII level is maximally corrected. It is not practical to give cryoprecipitate often enough to keep the bleeding time continuously corrected or to quantify the correction with serial bleeding times. Therefore, once hemostasis is achieved, therapy should be directed toward keeping the level of factor VIII in the appropriate therapeutic ranges as described above for hemophilia A. This probably will require less cryoprecipitate than if one were treating a hemophiliac.

Desmopressin. There are difficulties in obtaining an effective virus-free purified concentrate of von Willebrand factor. The largest multimers are hard to purify, and the potential market is small enough that there is no economic incentive to develop such a product by recombinant DNA techniques. Therefore, considerable attention has been devoted to the therapeutic potential of desmopressin (1-desamino-8-D arginine vasopressin, DDAVP), especially in patients with mild von Willebrand disease. Desmopressin causes release of von Willebrand factor and plasminogen activator from endothelial cells. EACA suppresses baseline and desmopressin-stimulated fibrinolysis and may be useful as an adjunctive therapy. Desmopressin, 0.3 μg per kilogram of body weight in 50 ml of saline, is given over 15 minutes. In type I disease, severalfold increases of both factor VIII and von Willebrand protein occur 15 to 30 minutes after infusion, with a concomitant decrease in the bleeding time. The effect may last for several hours. The magnitude and duration of the response vary among individual patients, especially among those with type IIA disease. Desmopressin is contraindicated in type IIB disease because appearance of the large multimers in the circulation can cause thrombocytopenia.

To learn if the treatment is feasible in a given patient, one should quantify the response to a test dose of desmopressin at the time of diagnosis or five to seven days prior to a planned procedure. For oral surgical procedures, EACA is given orally in a dosage of 75 mg per kilogram every six hours for seven to ten days beginning the evening before the procedure. It is controversial whether an antifibrinolytic agent should be given with major surgery.

Menstruation and Pregnancy. Excessive menstrual blood loss can be managed with hormonal suppression. Levels of factor VIII, von Willebrand factor, and ristocetin cofactor activity may become normal during pregnancy. Therefore, these tests, along with determination of the bleeding time, should be repeated during the third trimester to plan for replacement therapy during delivery. Cryoprecipitate should be given if the factor VIII level remains low. If the factor VIII level is greater than 50 per cent, but the bleeding time remains long, cryoprecipitate should be on call, because postpartum blood loss is frequently severe enough to require replacement infusion.

Complications of Therapy. Chronic arthropathy is less common in von Willebrand disease than in hemophilia A. The complications of replacement therapy for severe von Willebrand disease are the same as those described above for hemophilia A. Rarely, antibodies that inhibit the activity of von Willebrand protein develop. Patients receiving blood products should be vaccinated against hepatitis B and monitored for the acquisition of hepatitis viruses and HIV.

Moroose R, Hoyer LW: Von Willebrand factor and platelet function. Ann Rev Med 37:157, 1986. *Review of recent advances in knowledge of von Willebrand factor.*

Richardson DW, Robinson AG: Desmopressin. Ann Intern Med 103:228, 1985. *Review of the effectiveness of this drug in a variety of situations, including mild hemophilia, von Willebrand disease, liver disease, and uremia.*

HEMOPHILIA B (FACTOR IX DEFICIENCY)

Factor IX deficiency is inherited as an X-linked disorder that presents with the historical and clinical features of classic hemophilia (hemophilia A). The deficiency is most often quantitative, but can be due to qualitative defects of factor IX structure. The severity of bleeding is usually similar in members of a single family. In general, for a given degree of deficiency, factor IX–deficient patients have fewer symptoms than do patients with factor VIII deficiency, e.g., patients with severe (<1 per cent of normal) factor IX deficiency have the symptoms of patients with mild (1 to 5 per cent of normal) factor VIII deficiency. Nevertheless, factor IX deficiency causes serious bleeding problems. Patients with factor IX deficiency can be more cavalier about their disease than can patients with factor VIII deficiency, and therefore they are not as quick to seek medical attention when they need it—sometimes to their detriment.

CLINICAL MANIFESTATIONS. Many patients with low levels of factor IX are asymptomatic until the hemostatic system is stressed by surgery or trauma. Patients with the most severe disease may develop muscle hematomas, gastrointestinal hemorrhage, and bleeding into large joints with progression to crippling joint deformities.

DIAGNOSIS. This disorder is suspected with the finding of a normal prothrombin time and prolonged APTT that can be corrected by normal serum but not by barium sulfate–adsorbed plasma. The inability of the patient's plasma to correct the prolonged APTT of plasma from a patient with known factor IX deficiency establishes the diagnosis.

TREATMENT. The care and long-term goals of therapy for the patient with factor IX deficiency are similar to those described above for the patient with hemophilia A. Most patients will need less care than if they had hemophilia A, but they require the same intensity of education and counseling.

Replacement Therapy. Fresh frozen plasma is used to treat mild to moderate bleeding, especially in those patients who have hemorrhagic episodes infrequently. Ordinarily, transfusion of 500 ml of plasma twice daily is sufficient to maintain a level of factor IX activity 10 to 12 per cent above baseline. EACA can be used as an adjunct to transfusions of plasma in patients with mucosal bleeding or dental work.

Patients with moderate to severe hemorrhage, such as large hemarthroses or muscle hematomas, and patients being prepared for surgery can be treated with commercially prepared factor IX concentrate, aiming for levels that are approximately two-thirds as high as those described above for factor VIII replacement therapy. Because the volume of distribution and the half-life of factor IX are both greater than for factor VIII, a greater loading dose of factor IX must be given than for factor VIII, but subsequent doses can be given less frequently. The length of therapy is dependent on the severity of the hemorrhage and the patient's response. Therapy is generally continued for two days after bleeding and related symptoms have subsided.

Complications of Therapy. Presently available factor IX concentrates are a mixture of all of the vitamin K–dependent factors—factors II, VII, IX, and X and proteins C and S—and are heat treated. Factor IX stands up to heat treatment better than factor VIII, and therefore the concentrates are heated more vigorously and should be freer of infectious HIV than are factor VIII concentrates. However, the concentrates are not free of infectious hepatitis viruses. Patients therefore should be immunized against hepatitis B.

Factor IX concentrates contain trace amounts of activated vitamin K–dependent factors and therefore are thrombogenic and carry a risk for thromboembolism, especially when used in high dosage in patients who have liver disease or are immobilized after surgery. EACA greatly enhances the risk of thromboembolism and should never be used as an adjunct to factor IX concentrates. Indeed, some advocate that low-dosage heparin (5000 units every 12 hours) and plasma (as a source of antithrombins) be given to surgical patients receiving factor IX concentrate. Because of these potential complications, it is advisable to reserve the use of factor IX concentrates for patients who have acquired antibody to hepatitis B surface antigen as a result of prior exposure or immunization and for whom the benefits of treatment outweigh the risks of thromboembolism. In a situation in which levels greater than 10 to 15 per cent above baseline are desired but use of factor IX concentrate is contraindicated, plasmapheresis can be used to prevent volume overload.

Antibody inhibitors to factor IX occur in 5 to 10 per cent of treated patients.

CARRIER DETECTION. The normal range for factor IX is narrower than the normal range for factor VIII, and therefore carrier testing based on coagulation assays is better for hemophilia B than for hemophilia A. Nevertheless, laboratory definition of the carrier state is still an exercise in probabilities and is best done with genetic markers. The factor IX gene is more polymorphic than the factor VIII gene, and it seems likely that informative genetic markers will be found in most families. However, it is worthwhile doing factor IX activity assays in known and potential carriers, because women who are carriers may have factor IX levels that are sufficiently low to cause mild bleeding, especially after trauma or surgery.

Thompson AR: Structure, function, and molecular defects of factor IX. Blood 67:565, 1986. *Comprehensive summary of information about factor IX and hemophilia B.*

DEFICIENCIES OF CONTACT FACTORS

Deficiencies of factor XII, prekallikrein, or high molecular weight kininogen are clinically benign, and deficiency of factor XI may sometimes be benign. Patients with these abnormalities, however, have APTT's that are as prolonged as are those of patients with factor VIII or IX deficiency. Therefore it is important to establish the correct diagnosis and to counsel the patient that he or she has a laboratory abnormality that carries no risk for bleeding.

Deficiency of Factor XII, Prekallikrein, or High Molecular Weight Kininogen

These autosomal recessive disorders are almost always asymptomatic and are usually identified as a result of delayed coagulation times in routine laboratory assays. The deficiencies should be suspected when the APTT is prolonged in a patient who does not have a history of any bleeding tendency. The APTT of a mixture of patient's plasma and normal plasma should be normal, i.e., with no inhibitor demonstrable. The plasma concentrations of factors VIII and IX should be normal. The coagulation defect can be identified by the inability of the patient's plasma to correct the APTT of plasma from a patient known to have a deficiency of factor XII, prekallikrein, or high molecular weight kininogen.

Deficiency of Factor XI

Factor XI deficiency is fairly common among Ashkenazi Jews, and the prevalence of homozygous factor XI deficiency in cities with a sizable Jewish population is comparable to the prevalence of hemophilia A. The defect is usually asymptomatic, but it does occasionally cause spontaneous bleeding. Major bleeding into muscles or joints is rare. The inheritance pattern is autosomal recessive so that the deficiency is found with equal frequency in men and women. The APTT is prolonged. The prothrombin time and bleeding time are normal. Normal serum or barium sulfate–adsorbed plasma will both correct the APTT. Specific assays for factors VIII and IX are normal. The diagnosis is established by demonstrating that the patient's plasma does not correct the APTT of plasma known to be deficient in factor XI.

Clinically significant bleeding usually occurs in association with trauma, surgery, or dental extractions. Fresh frozen plasma, 10 to 20 ml per kilogram, should be given as treatment of bleeding or as prophylaxis for surgery. One infusion should suffice, because factor XI has a half-life of about 72 hours.

Silverberg M, Kaplan AP, Colman RW: Contact activation and its abnormalities. In Colman RW, Hirsh J, Marder VJ, et al. (eds.): Hemostasis and Thrombosis: Basic Principles and Clinical Practice. 2nd ed. Philadelphia, J. B. Lippincott Company, 1987, pp 18–38. *Well-referenced description of the biochemistry of factor XI and the deficiency state.*

DEFICIENCIES OF THE EXTRINSIC AND COMMON PATHWAYS

Deficiencies of factors VII, X, V, and II are all associated with clinically significant bleeding. The hemorrhagic diathesis is not as predictable or severe as in hemophilia A, but replacement therapy probably will be required at some point in a patient's lifetime, especially to control bleeding from mucous membranes, after dental extractions, or during menses.

Deficiency of Factor VII

This is a rare autosomal recessive defect, having been reported in fewer than 100 patients. Both qualitative and quantitative abnormalities of factor VII occur, and patients can be either mixed heterozygotes or true homozygotes.

CLINICAL MANIFESTATIONS. Patients have a history of bleeding, usually beginning in infancy or early childhood. Bleeding, however, is frequently mild, even in patients with severe deficiency. Heterozygous relatives have no bleeding tendency. Mucous membrane bleeding, epistaxis, intramuscular hemorrhage, hemarthroses, and menorrhagia are the most common problems; gastrointestinal bleeding is less common, hematuria occurs only occasionally, and central nervous system bleeding is rare. Bleeding after dental extractions is predictable, and such extractions should be done with prophylactic replacement therapy. Clinical manifestations of bleeding can vary from mild to severe in the same patient. In fact, patients with impressive bleeding histories have undergone major surgery without accompanying hemorrhage. This phenomenon is unexplained and not consistent with the central role assigned to factor VII in the physiologic initiation of blood coagulation. Also incongruent are observations of thromboembolism in factor VII–deficient patients.

DIAGNOSIS. A diagnosis of factor VII deficiency should be considered if the prothrombin time is prolonged whereas the APTT is normal. The coagulation time of the patient's plasma in response to Russell's viper venom, which directly activates factor X, is normal. The diagnosis is established by the inability to correct the patient's prothrombin time with plasma from a person known to have factor VII deficiency.

TREATMENT. Bleeding is treated with plasma, not necessarily fresh frozen because factor VII is very stable. The half-life of factor VII is two to six hours, and therefore frequent treatment is needed during a bleeding episode. Levels of 15 to 20 per cent of normal can be obtained with a loading dose of plasma of 10 to 20 ml per kilogram followed by 3 to 6 ml per kilogram every 12 hours and should suffice to stop bleeding or as prophylaxis for surgery. Commercially available factor IX concentrates, which contain factors VII, IX, X, and II, can be used if it is essential to avoid any possibility of intravascular volume overload; such concentrates carry the risk of thromboembolism and hepatitis. Menorrhagia may require treatment with oral contraceptive agents.

Deficiency of Factor X

This is also a rare autosomal recessive disorder secondary to absence of or reduced synthesis of a normal molecule and/or production of a normal amount of antigen that has little or no function. Clinical symptoms include epistaxis, occasional mucous membrane, joint, and muscle hemorrhages, and gastrointestinal bleeding. Women may have severe, life-threatening menses and postpartum hemorrhage. The diagnosis is suspected when both the prothrombin time and APTT are prolonged. The abnormal tests correct with normal serum, but not with barium sulfate–adsorbed plasma.

The clotting time of plasma in response to Russell's viper venom is usually prolonged, although an abnormal factor X has been described that is activated normally by Russell's viper venom but not by the intrinsic or extrinsic systems of blood coagulation. The diagnosis is established by demonstration that the abnormal plasma does not correct plasma known to be specifically deficient in factor X. Bleeding episodes are treated with plasma as described above for factor VII deficiency; plasma needs to be given less often because the plasma half-life of factor X is 24 to 48 hours.

Deficiency of Factor II (Prothrombin)

Like deficiency of factors VII and X, factor II deficiency (hypoprothrombinemia) is a rare recessive disorder due to decreased synthesis of factor II and/or synthesis of a dysfunctional molecule. Bleeding ranges from mild to severe and generally occurs only if the factor II activity level is less than 20 per cent of normal. Symptoms include umbilical bleeding at birth, epistaxis, menorrhagia, postpartum hemorrhage, and bleeding after trauma or minor surgical procedures. The diagnosis is suspected if the prothrombin time and APTT are prolonged and the thrombin time is normal. Neither serum nor barium sulfate–adsorbed plasma will correct the abnormalities. A specific assay can be done based on the relative ability of the unknown to correct the prothrombin time of known factor II–deficient plasma. Alternatively, a test can be done in which clotting of plasma is initiated with Taipan venom, a specific activator of factor II. Bleeding is treated with infusions of fresh frozen plasma as described above for factor VII deficiency. Infusions are necessary only every two days, since the half-life of factor II is about 72 hours.

Global Deficiency of Vitamin K–Dependent Factors

Several patients have been described who presented as infants with bleeding, grossly prolonged prothrombin time and APTT, and low levels (<5 per cent of normal) of factors II, VII, IX, and X even though there was no evidence of liver disease, malabsorption, or ingestion of coumarin drugs. The levels of the vitamin K–dependent factors increased to 30 to 40 per cent of normal when the patients were given pharmacologic doses (10 mg per day) of vitamin K, and the patients did well with minimal symptoms. This syndrome is probably due to some abnormality of vitamin K metabolism, such as an abnormality of vitamin K epoxide reductase.

Deficiency of Factor V

This disorder usually is inherited as an autosomal recessive trait, although families in which there is dominant transmission have been identified. Most patients lack factor V antigen.

CLINICAL MANIFESTATIONS. As with deficiencies of the other common pathway components, severity of bleeding symptoms is variable, and hemorrhage most often involves the mucous membranes of the nose and oral cavity. Hemarthroses are unusual. Menorrhagia may be so severe as to be life threatening. Some women with factor V deficiency, however, have normal menses or only mild menorrhagia. Obstetric deliveries may occur with little or no bleeding, but postpartum hemorrhage is frequent and requires replacement therapy.

DIAGNOSIS. Both the APTT and prothrombin time are prolonged. The prothrombin time can be corrected by barium sulfate–adsorbed fresh plasma, but not by serum. Definitive diagnosis is established if the patient's plasma does not correct the deficiency of a patient known to lack factor V activity. For unknown reasons, the bleeding time is prolonged in about one third of factor V–deficient patients.

THERAPY. Factor V is an extremely labile protein. Treatment, therefore, should be with plasma that is either fresh or was frozen while fresh and has not been stored for more than several months. The therapeutic goal should be a factor V activity level greater than 25 per cent of normal. Because factor V is larger than the vitamin K–dependent factors, it should be possible to achieve such a level with the doses of plasma described above for factor VII deficiency. The plasma half-life of factor V activity is 12 to 36 hours. Cryoprecipitate and factor VIII concentrate are not enriched in factor V. Surgery should be done under the "cover" of prophylactic replacement therapy.

Platelets contain 10 to 20 per cent of the factor V in blood, and therefore platelet concentrates are a good source of factor V. Several patients have responded well to platelet transfusion after developing neutralizing antibodies to factor V.

Combined Deficiencies of Factors V and VIII

A number of patients have mild deficiencies of both factors V and VIII inherited as an autosomal recessive trait. The basis of the syndrome is unknown, but it probably is related to some post-translational modification of the two homologous proteins which is necessary for their function. Therapy should be directed toward replacement of both proteins.

Roberts HR, Foster PA: Inherited disorders of prothrombin conversion. In Colman RW, Hirsh J, Marder VJ, et al. (eds.): Hemostasis and Thrombosis: Basic Principles and Clinical Practice. 2nd ed. Philadelphia, J. B. Lippincott Company, 1987, pp 162–181. *Thoroughly referenced, and an excellent source of more detailed information about the diagnosis and management of patients with rare but clinically important factor deficiencies.*

ABNORMALITIES IN CONVERSION OF FIBRINOGEN TO FIBRIN

Disorders of Fibrinogen

These fall into two categories: absence (afibrinogenemia) or a low content (hypofibrinogenemia) of plasma fibrinogen and abnormally functioning plasma fibrinogen (dysfibrinogenemia). Afibrinogenemia and hypofibrinogenemia are autosomally recessive traits. Dysfibrinogenemia can be autosomally dominant or recessive.

AFIBRINOGENEMIA. In patients with absence of or low content of fibrinogen, the bleeding tendency may be noted at birth as continued oozing from the umbilical stump. The intensity and frequency of bleeding after trauma or surgery vary from mild to severe. Death from intracranial hemorrhage may occur in infancy or early childhood. It is not understood why some patients have a minimal bleeding tendency whereas others are very symptomatic. All assays that require formation of fibrin as an endpoint are abnormal. Plasma fibrinogen cannot be detected by immunologic or chemical (salting out) methods. The bleeding time may be markedly prolonged. Bleeding episodes should be treated with cryoprecipitate, which contains eightfold to tenfold more fibrinogen than does an equivalent amount of plasma. Plasma fibrinogen concentrations greater than 100 mg per deciliter are generally adequate and can be achieved by administration of one bag of cryoprecipitate for each 10 kg of body weight.

DYSFIBRINOGENEMIA. Dysfibrinogenemias are usually named after the cities in which they were discovered. The clinical features are very variable. Most individuals are asymptomatic. Some have mild to moderate bleeding tendencies, usually manifest only after surgery or trauma. Wound dehiscence is a problem in some. Some have a tendency for thrombosis. The abnormal proteins have a fascinating array of defects. For instance, several of the abnormal fibrinogens are poor substrates for thrombin, so that the fibrinopeptides are released slowly. Other abnormal fibrinogens, once converted to fibrin monomer by thrombin, display impaired aggregation into a fibrin gel. The diagnosis of these disorders should be suspected when delayed or poorly formed fibrin endpoints are observed in the prothrombin time, APTT, and thrombin time assays. The fibrinogen level, measured immunologically or chemically, is normal to low-normal. The majority of patients do not require treatment. In instances of bleeding or before surgical procedures on a patient known to have a propensity to bleed, replacement therapy in the form of cryoprecipitate should be given to attain a functioning plasma fibrinogen level of 100 to 150 mg per deciliter. Because the half-life of fibrinogen is four days, such infusions need to be given only once every several days. There are no absolute guidelines for how long therapy must be continued, but infusions of cryoprecipitate should be administered for two days after bleeding stops.

Deficiency of Factor XIII

Bleeding symptoms in factor XIII deficiency occur in individuals with less than 1 to 2 per cent of normal plasma factor XIII activity. The symptomatic deficiency state is an autosomal recessive trait. The bleeding diathesis is commonly apparent at birth as umbilical stump hemorrhage and continues throughout life. Wounds ooze slowly for days and heal poorly with scar formation. Intracranial hemorrhage after inapparent or only minor trauma is common. Males tend to be sterile, and women with the disorder have a high incidence of fetal loss unless they receive replacement therapy during pregnancy. Thrombin formation or conversion of fibrinogen to fibrin is not impaired. Consequently the prothrombin and APTT are normal. Platelet function tests are also normal. The laboratory diagnosis consists of demonstrating that a fibrin clot, made by recalcification of the patient's plasma, dissolves overnight at room temperature in 5 M urea or 1 per cent monochloroacetic acid. Fibrin clots formed in the presence of greater than 1 to 2 per cent of the normal concentration of factor XIII remain intact indefinitely in these solvents.

Treatment consists of giving fresh frozen plasma. Correction of the plasma concentration of factor XIII to 5 to 10 per cent of normal will provide normal hemostasis. The half-life of factor XIII is approximately 12 days, and thus prophylactic replacement therapy is feasible. Because central nervous system hemorrhage is a major risk, factor XIII–deficient patients are commonly given 5 to 10 ml per kilogram of fresh frozen plasma every three weeks. Extra plasma should be given in preparation for surgery or other head trauma. Development of inhibitory antibody to factor XIII as a consequence of transfusion therapy is apparently rare.

Deficiency of Alpha-2-Antiplasmin

Congenital homozygous deficiency of alpha-2-antiplasmin is associated with a severe, hemophilia-like, bleeding tendency. Heterozygous family members with plasma concentrations of the inhibitor 50 per cent of normal have a mild bleeding tendency characterized by postoperative bleeding, excessive bleeding after tooth extraction, and easy bruising after trauma. Levels of alpha-2-antiplasmin can be quantified with an activity assay. Patients with severe homozygous deficiency have fewer bleeding episodes when they receive long-term treatment with tranexamic acid. Heterozygotes would probably also benefit from treatment with tranexamic acid or EACA when symptomatic or when their antiplasmin level is depleted by stresses such as major surgery.

Gralnick HR: Congenital disorders of fibrinogen. In Williams WJ, Beutler E, Ersley AJ, et al. (eds.): Hematology. New York, McGraw-Hill Book Company, 1983, pp 1399–1410. *Detailed information about inherited fibrinogen abnormalities.*

Kitchens CS, Newcomb TF: Factor XIII. Medicine 58:413, 1979. *A comprehensive review.*

Kluft C, Vellenga E, Brommer JP, et al.: A familial hemorrhagic diathesis in a Dutch family: An inherited deficiency of alpha-2-antiplasmin. Blood 59:1169, 1982. *Description of a fairly large kindred.*

INHERITED TENDENCIES TOWARD THROMBOSIS

There has been considerable progress in the biochemical definition of hypercoagulability. Quantitative or functional deficiencies of four plasma proteins—protein C, protein S, the major antithrombin, and the minor antithrombin—have been reported to be associated with a tendency toward thrombosis in affected families. Abnormalities of homocysteine metabolism have been shown to be associated with arterial thrombosis (Ch. 194). As more is learned about fibrinolysis, it is likely that genetic abnormalities of plasminogen, plasminogen activators, and plasminogen activator inhibitors will be identified that are associated with a thrombotic diathesis.

APPROACH TO THE PATIENT WITH A SUSPECTED THROMBOTIC TENDENCY. Patients with the recently described deficiency syndromes are fairly rare. It is therefore difficult to make firm guidelines about when or how to search for deficiency states and how to treat or counsel affected individuals. In general, it is worthwhile to evaluate the status of patients with family histories of thrombosis, young (<40 years old) patients, and patients with rare types of thrombosis (e.g., dural sinus or mesenteric vein thrombosis). Patients should be questioned and their status evaluated to ascertain whether they or family members have or have had conditions that would put them at risk for thrombosis (obesity, prolonged immobilization, injury to or abnormalities of vessels) or causes for secondary hypercoagulability (myeloproliferative syndrome, paroxysmal nocturnal hemoglobinuria, malignant disease, lupus anticoagulant). It has been estimated that of patients with "unexpected thrombosis," 1 to 2 per cent will have deficiency of the major antithrombin, 5 per cent will have deficiency of protein C, and 5 per cent will have deficiency of protein S. In my practice the laboratory evaluation in individuals with a possible thrombotic diathesis includes activity assays of total antithrombin and plasminogen (readily available) and immunoassays of proteins C and S (available in coagulation reference laboratories). Plasma is also frozen at −70°C with the anticipation that new tests may become available in the future. For especially suspicious cases, plasma can be sent to reference or research laboratories for functional assays of proteins C and S and immunoassay and functional assay of the minor antithrombin. Patients with premature peripheral or cerebral occlusive arterial disease should be screened for excessive homocysteine accumulation after a standardized methionine-loading test.

The number of assays that could be done on a patient with a probable thrombotic diathesis is seemingly endless. Consider just the example of protein C. If protein C antigen is normal, protein C function could be impaired. Functional activities of protein C that could be impaired include: ability to generate an active site; ability to become activated by thrombin-thrombomodulin complex; ability once activated to cleave its physiologic substrates, factors V and VIII; ability to interact with protein S; and so on. In the future it is likely that screening assays will be developed to evaluate the protein C–protein S system, the antithrombins, and the fibrinolytic system. These screening assays, unfortunately, are unlikely to be as simple, inexpensive, and comprehensive as are the screening assays that we have for the coagulation cascade. And until the assays are developed, we must make do with the present laboratory tests, which, although not totally satisfactory, are extremely useful in selected situations.

Deficiency of Protein C

Two syndromes of hereditary protein C deficiency have been described: (1) heterozygous deficiency in which half-normal concentrations of protein C are associated with an increased risk of venous thromboembolism and (2) homozygous deficiency in which total lack (<1 per cent of normal) of protein C is associated with neonatal purpura fulminans (ischemic necrosis of skin and digits) and massive venous thrombosis. Not all individuals with heterozygous deficiency have thrombosis. In families in which there is thrombosis, some family members with 50 per cent levels are asymptomatic, i.e., the phenotype displays autosomal dominance with incomplete penetrance. In several large kindreds ascertained because of infants with homozygous deficiency, none of more than 30 individuals with heterozygous deficiency had a history of venous thrombosis, i.e., in some families heterozygous deficiency apparently does not increase the risk for thrombosis. It is likely, however, that homozygous deficiency is invariably associated with problems. Indeed, the syndrome of coumarin-induced skin necrosis recapitulates the syndrome of homozygous deficiency. Upon initiation of warfarin therapy, the plasma concentration of protein C, which has a half-life of six hours, falls more quickly than the concentrations of factors II, IX, and X, thus causing a hypercoagulable state.

The diagnosis of protein C deficiency is usually based on decreased amounts of antigen in plasma. For patients receiving long-term therapy with warfarin, other vitamin K–dependent proteins, e.g., factors X and II, are also measured with an immunoassay to correct for the 35 to 50 per cent drop in the level of circulating vitamin K–dependent proteins due to undercarboxylation. As discussed above, the antigenic measurements will not detect individuals with dysfunctional protein C.

Because not everyone with heterozygous protein C deficiency has thrombosis, long-term anticoagulation should be reserved for individuals who have had a thrombotic episode unless the family history is so striking that the physicians and affected members agree that prophylactic treatment is warranted. Asymptomatic family members should be counseled that they are at greater risk for thrombosis and advised about the dangers of prolonged immobilization of limbs, obesity, and smoking. When warfarin therapy is started in a patient with heterozygous deficiency, the anticoagulant effect should be achieved at a leisurely pace by daily administration of the predicted maintenance dose rather than by administration of a loading dose of drug. It is preferable to begin warfarin therapy while the patient is being treated with heparin. However, one should be aware that heparin induces thrombocytopenia and thrombosis in some patients, especially those who have received heparin for more than ten days.

Infants with homozygous protein C deficiency respond acutely to administration of plasma or factor IX concentrate, which is rich in protein C. Oral anticoagulants can be used to decrease the frequency of thrombotic events.

Deficiency of Protein S

In a number of families, decreased levels of plasma protein S antigen or activity are associated with venous thrombosis. Correlation between antigen and activity is poor, probably because a fraction of protein S in plasma is complexed with C4b-binding protein, and only the fraction of protein S that is free has anticoagulant activity. The tendency toward thrombosis is inherited as an autosomal dominant trait with incomplete penetrance. Affected individuals tend to have levels of protein S that are 50 per cent of normal, i.e., they are heterozygous for the deficiency. The incidence of symptomatic heterozygous protein S deficiency is probably the same as the incidence of symptomatic protein C deficiency. Pending further information about this recently described syndrome, it seems reasonable to approach and treat heterozygous protein S deficiency using the guidelines described above for heterozygous protein C deficiency.

Deficiency of the Major Antithrombin (Antithrombin III)

The average concentration of the major antithrombin in deficient patients is approximately 50 per cent of normal. The most frequent manifestation of thromboembolism is lower extremity thrombophlebitis, often bilateral and recurrent and often with pulmonary embolism. Patients may develop venous insufficiency and chronic leg ulcers. Upper extremity thrombophlebitis and mesenteric vein thrombosis are less common. Rare patients may develop retinal or cerebral vein thrombosis, thrombosis of the renal vein or inferior vena cava, Budd-Chiari syndrome, priapism, or widespread clotting and defibrination syndrome. The cumulative incidences of thromboembolism are estimated to be 15 per cent by age 19, 50 per cent by age 29, and 85 per cent in individuals over 40 years. Complete, i.e., homozygous, lack of the major antithrombin has not been described. Patients homozygous for a dysfunctional antithrombin, however, have been reported.

Antithrombin deficiency can be ascertained by an activity assay in which diluted plasma and heparin are mixed with a known concentration of thrombin, and the amount of uninhibited thrombin is quantified with a chromogenic substrate. Ongoing thrombosis and heparin therapy both lower the concentration of plasma antithrombin. Therefore the diagnosis of antithrombin deficiency is best made after the patient has recovered from a thrombotic event.

A patient with acute thrombosis should be treated with heparin. Because of depletion of the major antithrombin, the level of antithrombin may become so low that the patient is resistant to heparin. In this case, a source of antithrombin should be infused, in the form of either fresh frozen plasma or, if available, antithrombin concentrate. The half-life of antithrombin is 16 to 24 hours. Administration of warfarin should be started promptly, and the patient probably should receive warfarin indefinitely.

Prophylactic use of anticoagulants should be considered in view of the spontaneous and unpredictable occurrence of thromboembolism with the potential for a fatal outcome. At the very least, affected individuals should be counseled about the risks of the disorder. Pregnancies should be managed in high-risk clinics prepared to cope with the difficult questions of how, when, or whether anticoagulants should be administered during the pregnancy.

Deficiency of the Minor Antithrombin (Heparin Cofactor II)

Two families have been reported in which half-normal plasma concentrations of the minor antithrombin were associated with venous and arterial thrombosis. The number of family members studied was not large enough to prove formally that the deficiency state segregates with the thrombotic deficiency, but the reports certainly are suggestive. If the association is confirmed in larger kindreds, low concentrations of minor antithrombin in a patient who has had a thrombotic event would be an indication for long-term warfarin therapy.

Boers GHJ, Smals AGH, Trijbels FJM, et al.: Heterozygosity for homocystinuria in premature peripheral and cerebral occlusive arterial disease. N Engl J Med 313:709, 1985. Mudd SH: Vascular disease and homocysteine metabolism. N Engl J Med 313:751, 1985. *Descriptions and discussions of homocystinuria as a cause of premature arterial disease.*

Clouse LH, Comp PC: The regulation of hemostasis: The protein C system. N Engl J Med 314:1298, 1986. *Summary of the biochemical and clinical evidence for the importance of proteins C and S, especially protein C, in prevention of thrombosis.*

Cosgriff TM, Bishop DT, Hershgold EJ, et al.: Familial antithrombin III deficiency: Its natural history, genetics, diagnosis and treatment. Medicine 62:209, 1983. *Comprehensive review of deficiency of the major antithrombin.*

Kamiya T, Sugihara T, Ogata K, et al.: Inherited deficiency of protein S in a Japanese family with recurrent venous thrombosis: A study of three generations. Blood 67:406, 1986. Comp PC, Doray D, Patton D, et al.: An abnormal plasma distribution of protein S occurs in functional protein S deficiency. Blood 67:504, 1986. *Studies of two large kindreds that point out some of the clinical and laboratory features of protein S deficiency.*

Rodgers GM, Shuman MA: Congenital thrombotic disorders. Am J Hematol 21:419, 1986. *Particularly good for its summary of the literature concerning the fibrinolytic system.*

Schafer AI: The hypercoagulable states. Ann Intern Med 102:814, 1985. *Balanced and well-referenced overview of primary and secondary causes of thrombosis.*

Tran TH, Marbet GA, Duckert F: Association of hereditary heparin co-factor II deficiency with thrombosis. Lancet 2:413, 1986. Sie P, Dupouy D, Pichon J, et al.: Constitutional heparin co-factor II deficiency associated with thrombosis. Lance 2:414, 1986. *Initial reports that deficiency of the minor antithrombin in plasma may predispose individuals to thrombosis. Representative of the tenuous but provocative arguments found in papers describing new deficiency syndromes associated with thrombosis.*

ACQUIRED DISORDERS OF BLOOD COAGULATION

GENERAL COMMENTS. In a number of clinical situations, the APTT and/or prothrombin time are prolonged because of acquired deficiencies: vitamin K deficiency secondary to malabsorption or dietary deficiency, severe liver disease, use of coumarin anticoagulants to lower the activity of vitamin K–dependent factors, and consumption coagulopathy associated with severe illness. Rarer causes of acquired deficiencies include selective urinary loss of a coagulation factor in nephrotic syndrome, selective adsorption of a coagulation factor, especially factor X, to amyloid, and selective depletion of a clotting factor due to development of a non-neutralizing antibody to the factor.

Vitamin K Deficiency

METABOLISM AND FUNCTION OF VITAMIN K. Vitamin K is required for the post-translational gamma-carboxylation of specific glutamyl residues in factors VII, IX, X, and II and of proteins C and S and certain other proteins, e.g., osteocalcin, which constitutes 1 per cent of the protein in bone. In vitamin K–deficient states, levels of the vitamin K–dependent plasma proteins are near normal; however, the functions of these proteins in reactions and assays (e.g., the prothrombin time) that require a phospholipid surface are severely impaired. As vitamin K deficiency develops, the activities of factor VII and protein C decrease rapidly, followed by diminished activities of factors IX, X, and II.

There are limited body stores of vitamin K. A normal diet containing green leafy vegetables provides 300 to 500 μg of vitamin K, more than enough to meet the adult daily requirement of 1 μg per kilogram of body weight. In addition, vitamin K synthesized by normal gastrointestinal bacterial flora contributes to the daily requirement. Vitamin K is a fat-soluble vitamin, and solubilization of fat must occur before vitamin K can be absorbed (Ch. 104). Hence, vitamin K deficiency may occur in bile salt–deficient states, in all malabsorptive disorders, or with an inadequate dietary intake combined with gastrointestinal sterilization by orally administered antibiotics. Vitamin K occurs naturally in two forms, vitamin K_1 (phylloquinone) and vitamin K_2 (menaquinones), both of which require lipid for absorption. A synthetic water-soluble form, vitamin K_3 (menadione), is commercially available. Despite its ready absorption from intestine, menadione must be converted to vitamin K_2 by the liver and therefore is not as rapidly effective as vitamin K_1 in promoting the gamma-carboxylation reaction.

VITAMIN K DEFICIENCY OF THE NEWBORN. At birth, vitamin K levels are low, and production of vitamin K by intestinal bacteria is insufficient to meet an infant's requirements for production of normally functioning coagulation factors. The vitamin K–deficient state lasts for three to five days and may be the reason Israelites did not circumcise their babies until the eighth day (Leviticus 12:3). Cow's milk contains some vitamin K, but human milk contains essentially none (1 to 2 μg per liter). Unless vitamin K is given, the physiologic state of neonatal hypoprothrombinemia can lead to hemorrhagic disease of the newborn in the following high-risk groups: premature infants; breast-fed infants; infants of mothers who are receiving vitamin K antagonists, especially hydantoin anticonvulsants; and infants with malabsorption. If the prothrombin time is prolonged to greater than twice normal, it is common to encounter bleeding from the umbilicus, ecchymoses and hematomas, hematuria, and, most importantly, intracranial hemorrhage. Prophylactic intramuscular administration of a 1-mg dose of vitamin K_1 at delivery virtually eliminates the risk of subsequent hemorrhage. Excessive administration (5 mg or more) of vitamin K_3 may cause hemolytic anemia and kernicterus in the newborn and should be avoided.

MALABSORPTION SYNDROMES. Malabsorptive states (Ch. 104) with impaired absorption of fat, such as adult celiac disease, regional enteritis, use of cholestyramine or neomycin, or deficient intraluminal bile salts (obstruction of biliary ducts, cholestatic liver disease), are often associated with vitamin K deficiency. Similarly, various chronic diarrheas can cause vitamin K deficiency, presumably because of decreased transit time and relative malabsorption of fats. The hallmark of vitamin K deficiency is prolonged prothrombin time. If the prothrombin time is longer than twice normal, the patient likely will have ecchymoses, gingival bleeding, hematomas, hematuria, and/or melena. Daily oral administration of vitamin K_1 in supraphysiologic doses (2 to 10 mg) prevents the deficiency and should be routine in patients with malabsorption of fat. The bleeding tendency, once developed, is easily corrected by giving 10 to 25 mg of vitamin K_1 intramuscularly. In cases in which the bleeding diathesis is so severe that intramuscular injections are contraindicated, 20 to 40 mg of vitamin K_1 may be infused intravenously. It should be infused slowly at a rate of 1 mg per minute because the vehicle in which the vitamin is dissolved can cause an adverse reaction. If this does not correct the prothrombin time, it is unlikely that additional vitamin K will have any effect.

DEBILITATED PATIENTS WHO MAY BE RECEIVING ANTIBIOTICS. Patients who are without oral intake for more than several days and receiving antibiotics should be given parenteral vitamin K_1 at a dosage of 150 μg per day because they are likely to become vitamin K deficient. Patients with uremia or malignant disease are at special risk and may become vitamin K deficient on the basis of poor oral intake alone.

Some third-generation cephalosporins have a hypothrombinemic effect that is greater than would be expected from elimination of bowel flora. It has been suggested that the N-methylthiotetrazole side chain shared by cefamandole, moxalactam, and cefoperazone is cleaved from the antibiotic and interferes with the action of vitamin K, especially in patients who are borderline deficient in vitamin K.

COUMARIN ANTICOAGULANTS. Warfarin and other coumarin anticoagulants competitively inhibit the effects of vitamin K in the post-translational gamma-carboxylation of vitamin K–dependent plasma proteins. Upon initiation of therapy, the activities of the proteins with the most rapid half-lives will be lost first. Thus the activities of the vitamin K–dependent proteins become depressed in the following order: factor VII and protein C, factor IX, factor X, and factor II. Coumarin anticoagulants are administered for a long time for the prevention of recurrent thromboembolism in patients who have experienced deep vein thrombosis and pulmonary embolism or myocardial infarction. Patients should be reliable, able to be supervised, and without known potential sources of hemorrhage in the central nervous, gastrointestinal, or genitourinary systems. The art of administration of warfarin involves balancing drug intake against vitamin K intake so as to prolong the prothrombin time about one and one-half times as compared to a normal control, e.g., 17 to 19 seconds as compared to a control of 12 seconds. Ratios below this value are less effective in preventing thrombosis, whereas values twice normal or greater carry a high risk for hemorrhage. An adult receiving a normal diet will usually need 5 to 10 mg of warfarin per day to achieve the desired ratio. After initiation of therapy, it will take three to four days before the chosen dose of warfarin will cause its maximal effect on the prothrombin time. The dose can then be altered to maintain the prothrombin time in the therapeutic range.

Once the prothrombin time is stabilized, it needs to be checked only every three to four weeks if the patient is on a stable diet and in usual health. The therapeutic dose of warfarin may change dramatically if the diet is changed or if changes are made in the intake of one of the many drugs that enhance or depress the effect of warfarin (Table 167–2). Patients should wear a bracelet or neck tag stating that they are receiving an oral anticoagulant. They should not take aspirin in any of its forms.

It is not uncommon for patients to experience slight gingival bleeding, purpura with minimal trauma, or trace hematuria

TABLE 167–2. DRUGS AND CONDITIONS THAT INFLUENCE RESPONSE TO WARFARIN

Increased Resistance to Warfarin	
Hereditary warfarin resistance	Increased warfarin metabolism
Increase in vitamin K	Barbiturates
Reduced drug absorption	Primidone
Malabsorption syndrome	Carbamazepine
Liquid paraffin laxatives	Ethchlorvynol (Placidyl)
Cholestyramine resin	Glutethimide (Doriden)
Magnesium trisilicate	Meprobamate
	Griseofulvin
	Rifampin
	Nafcillin
Increased Sensitivity to Warfarin	
Vitamin K deficiency	Synergism with warfarin
Malabsorption syndrome	Vitamin E
Wide-spectrum antibiotics	Anabolic steroids
Liquid paraffin	Danazol
Clofibrate	Blocking of warfarin metabolism
Displacement of albumin binding	Phenytoin sodium (Dilantin)
Phenylbutazone	Chloramphenicol
Aspirin	Clofibrate
Indomethacin	Tricyclic antidepressants
Sulindac	Erythromycin
Mefenamic acid	Cimetidine
Tolmetin	Sulfamethoxazole-trimethoprim
Ibuprofen	Sulfinpyrazone
Naproxen	Unknown mechanism
Fenoprofen	Quinine
Phenytoin sodium (Dilantin)	Quinidine
Oral hypoglycemic agents	Phenothiazine
Nalidixic acid	Disulfiram (Antabuse)
Estrogen	Sulfisoxazole
Miconazole	Amiodarone

From Peterson CE, Kwaan HC: Current concepts of warfarin therapy. Arch Intern Med 146:581, 1986.

while receiving anticoagulants in the therapeutic range. These symptoms become more marked when there is overanticoagulation, and the patient is at risk for severe gastrointestinal or genitourinary hemorrhage, bleeding or hematoma formation after trauma, and intracranial bleeding. If the prothrombin time is prolonged and increased bleeding is not a clinical problem, warfarin, which has a half-life of 35 hours, can be omitted until the desired prothrombin time is obtained. When overanticoagulation results in clinically significant bleeding, the physician can give fresh frozen plasma, 10 to 20 ml per kilogram, as a source of normal vitamin K–dependent proteins, and/or give vitamin K, depending on the immediacy of the problem and whether continuation of warfarin is necessary. The effect of plasma on the prothrombin time is immediate but temporary. The use of factor IX concentrates to treat warfarin overdose should be avoided because of occasional thrombotic complications and the risk of hepatitis. Oral or intramuscular vitamin K_1, 5 to 25 mg, should correct the prothrombin time within 8 to 24 hours. Slow intravenous infusion of vitamin K, 20 to 40 mg, should correct the prothrombin time in four to six hours. Administration of more than 5 mg of vitamin K will make the patient warfarin resistant and necessitate a round of re-anticoagulation. Therefore the best strategy for the patient who needs continued anticoagulation is to give plasma and small doses (1 to 2 mg) of vitamin K while closely monitoring the prothrombin time and clinical state.

Patients occasionally present with bleeding complications after ingestion of a coumarin compound, either surreptitiously or as a suicide attempt. Patients who take coumarins surreptitiously are usually depressed and receive gain from medical attention. They often belong to a health profession. The coumarin compounds in rat poisons are much more powerful than warfarin and can cause extreme resistance to vitamin K for weeks and even months.

Coumarin anticoagulants should not be given from the 6th to the 12th week of gestation because of the high likelihood that characteristic facial and skeletal malformations, the so-called coumarin embryopathy, will be induced. Use of coumarin drugs in the second and third trimesters is associated with an increased incidence of CNS malformations presumed to be due to sporadic intracranial hemorrhages. If anticoagulation is needed during pregnancy, one approach is to switch to subcutaneous heparin between the 6th and 12th week and after the 38th week.

Barza M, Furie B, Brown AE, et al.: Defects in vitamin K–dependent carboxylation associated with moxalactam treatment. J Infect Dis 153:1166, 1986. *Interim summary of the moxalactam story.*

Hull R, Hirsh J, Ray R, et al.: Different intensities of oral anticoagulant therapy in the treatment of proximal-vein thrombosis. N Engl J Med 307:1676, 1982. *Good data in support of less intensive therapy.*

Iturbe-Alessio I, Fonseca MdC, Mutchinik O, et al.: Risks of anticoagulant therapy in pregnant women with artificial heart valves. N Engl J Med 315:1390, 1986. *One group's approach to a difficult subject.*

Lipton RA, Klass EM: Human ingestion of a "superwarfarin" rodenticide resulting in a prolonged anticoagulant effect. JAMA 252:3004, 1984. Jones EC, Growe GH, Naiman SC: Prolonged anticoagulation in rat poisoning. JAMA 252:3005, 1984. *Illustrative case reports.*

O'Reilly RA: Vitamin K antagonists. In Colman RW, Hirsh J, Marder VJ, et al. (eds.): Hemostasis and Thrombosis: Basic Principles and Clinical Practice. 2nd ed. Philadelphia, J. B. Lippincott Company, 1987, pp. 1367–1372.

Peterson CE, Kwaan HC: Current concepts of warfarin therapy. Arch Intern Med 146:581, 1986. *A concise review.*

Suttie JW: Vitamin K–dependent carboxylase. Ann Rev Biochem 54:459, 1985. *Update on the biochemistry of vitamin K action and the opposing effect of the coumarin.*

Liver Disease

The liver is the major site of synthesis of fibrinogen, plasminogen, the vitamin K–dependent proteins, the antithrombins, and many other plasma proteins. The mechanisms by which steady state concentrations of these proteins in plasma are regulated are obscure. As part of the "acute phase reaction" in response to interleukin-1 and tumor necrosis factor, the synthesis of many plasma proteins, especially fibrinogen, increases at the expense of albumin synthesis. The normal liver seems to have a considerable reserve for production of fibrinogen but to be working at near maximal capacity in the synthesis of vitamin K–dependent proteins.

Patients with liver disease occasionally develop petechiae, ecchymoses, prolonged bleeding from venipunctures, and/or gastrointestinal hemorrhage. Clinically significant bleeding may occur with biopsies and surgery. The causes of these problems are diverse.

In patients with alcoholic liver disease, bleeding can be secondary to dietary *vitamin K deficiency* and will respond promptly to oral vitamin K. With more advanced disease, patients may become vitamin K deficient on the basis of fat malabsorption as well as poor nutrition, and parenteral vitamin K must be given. The synthesis of vitamin K–dependent factors becomes impaired as hepatocytes are lost, rendering the patient resistant to parenteral vitamin K. A poor prognosis is associated with a prolonged prothrombin time (greater than 1½ times normal) that does not become corrected after intravenous vitamin K. If the patient no longer responds to parenteral vitamin K, abnormal bleeding or correction of the prothrombin time prior to invasive procedures will require transfusions of fresh frozen plasma. In fulminant hepatocellular disease, *hypofibrinogenemia* can be profound enough to be considered the cause of bleeding; in such cases, both fresh frozen plasma and cryoprecipitate should be given.

Acquired dysfibrinogenemia, manifested by abnormal fibrin polymerization, has been observed in a number of patients having hepatic diseases such as alcoholic cirrhosis, postnecrotic cirrhosis of unknown cause, drug-induced hepatic failure, and hepatoma. The fibrinogen in these patients has about twice the normal content of sialic acid, indicating an overall increase in the amount of attached carbohydrate. The clotting of these fibrinogens by thrombin is delayed in proportion to the increase of sialic acid. If the liver disease improves, the defect may disappear.

Patients with liver disease commonly have *increased fibrinolysis,* because of an inability to maintain normal levels of alpha-2-antiplasmin and/or decreased hepatic clearance of plasminogen activators. Enhanced fibrinolysis, however, is rarely the primary cause of bleeding. Occasionally, chronic, smoldering *disseminated intravascular coagulation* may develop, in which case the platelet count is decreased and levels of several coagulation factors fall because of consumption. These patients do not require therapy unless they exhibit clinically significant bleeding, in which case the approach should be the same as for patients with other causes of diffuse intravascular coagulation (see below). Patients in whom LeVeen peritoneovenous shunts have been placed and women with acute fatty liver of pregnancy and marked deficiency of the major antithrombin (<25 per cent of normal) are at particular risk to develop disseminated intravascular coagulation.

Efforts should be made to normalize the prothrombin time, fibrinogen concentration, and platelet count in patients with liver disease prior to surgery, biopsy, or other invasive procedures. Factor IX concentrates are not recommended for prophylaxis in patients in whom the prothrombin time will not correct with parenteral vitamin K because such patients are likely to be deficient in plasma antithrombin, to have decreased hepatic clearance of activated clotting factors, and therefore to be at risk for thromboembolism. Platelet concentrates should be given if the platelet count is less than 75,000 per microliter. If hypersplenism is the cause of thrombocytopenia, however, it may be difficult to achieve a satisfactory platelet count.

Blanchard RA, Furie BC, Jorgensen W, et al.: Acquired vitamin K–dependent carboxylation deficiency in liver disease. N Engl J Med 305:242, 1981. *Interesting clinical study of circulating levels of normal and abnormal factor II.*

Liebman HA, McGehee WG, Patch MJ, et al.: Severe depression of antithrombin III associated with disseminated intravascular coagulation in women with fatty liver of pregnancy. Ann Intern Med 98:330, 1983. *Presents argument that acquired deficiency of the major antithrombin can cause widespread thrombosis.*

Mannucci PM, Forman SP: Hemostasis and liver disease. In Colman RW, Marder VJ, Salzman EW (eds.): Hemostasis and Thrombosis: Basic Principles and Clinical Practice. Philadelphia, J. B. Lippincott Company, 1982, pp 595–601. *Review with good references.*

Renal Disease

Patients with uremia occasionally develop purpura, mucous membrane bleeding, gastrointestinal hemorrhage, and prolonged bleeding from venous and arterial needle puncture sites. Such patients usually have a prolonged bleeding time. The pathogenesis of the bleeding tendency is complex. The platelet count may be low. More importantly, platelet function is abnormal because of accumulation of a dialyzable substance in the circulation (Ch. 166). Anemia contributes to platelet dysfunction in vivo, because the stirring action of red cells causes a large increase in the diffusivity of platelets and allows platelets to be transported efficiently to areas where the vessel wall is injured. Daily infusion of cryoprecipitate has been useful in correcting the bleeding tendency in uremia. Although uncertain, the correction may be related to the high molecular weight von Willebrand factor multimers contained in cryoprecipitate. Desmopressin, which is effective in raising the plasma level of von Willebrand factor in patients with von Willebrand disease (see above), temporarily corrects the bleeding time in patients with uremia. Daily intravenous administration of conjugated estrogens may also correct the bleeding time over a period of days. Thus a number of therapeutic maneuvers can be tried in a symptomatic uremic patient: dialysis to restore platelet function; transfusion to normalize red cell and platelet number; and administration of cryoprecipitate, desmopressin, or conjugated estrogen.

Coagulation factors, especially vitamin K–dependent factors and factor V, tend to be at low concentration in chronic renal disease, although not to levels that should cause bleeding. Some of these deficiencies probably result from hepatic insufficiency or from vitamin K deficiency secondary to oral antibiotic therapy, malabsorption caused by uremic enteritis, and diminished dietary intake. Very low plasma factor IX levels (10 per cent of normal) have been observed in patients with severe nephrotic syndrome and preferential loss of factor IX into the urine. Subclinical disseminated intravascular coagulation occasionally occurs in patients with chronic renal disease, as evidenced by elevated amounts of fibrin degradation products in serum and urine. It has been suggested that loss of the major antithrombin in nephrotic syndrome may cause renal vein thrombosis. There are no clear guidelines as to when and how to treat such deficiencies. If the prothrombin time is long or the factor IX level is low in a patient who is bleeding, fresh frozen plasma is the replacement product of choice, although it may be difficult to give enough to someone who cannot compensate for the large volume.

di Minno G, Martinez J, McKean, M-L, et al.: Platelet dysfunction in uremia: Multifaceted defect partially corrected by dialysis. Am J Med 79:552, 1985. Castillo R, Lozano T, Escolar G, et al.: Defective platelet adhesion on vessel subendothelium in uremic patients. Blood 68:337, 1986. *Two studies of platelet function in uremic patients.*

Janson PA, Jubelirer SJ, Weinstein MJ, et al.: Treatment of the bleeding tendency in uremia with cryoprecipitate. N Engl J Med 303:1318, 1980. Mannucci PM, Remuzzi G, Pusineri F, et al.: Deamino-8-D-arginine vasopressin shortens the bleeding time in uremia. N Engl J Med 308:8, 1983. Livio M, Mannucci PM, Vigano G, et al.: Conjugated estrogens for the management of bleeding associated with renal failure. N Engl J Med 315:731, 1985. *Contain results of three different but possibly related approaches to improvement of the bleeding time in uremic patients. The mechanisms of the favorable clinical effects are enigmas.*

Livio M, Gotti E, Marchesi D, et al.: Uraemic bleeding: Role of anaemia and beneficial effect of red cell transfusions. Lancet 2:1013, 1982. *Evidence that patients with higher hematocrits have more normal bleeding times.*

Sporadic Acquired Factor Deficiency

A number of patients with amyloidosis have factor X deficiency because of its removal from the circulation through binding of zymogen factor X to the amyloid deposits. Patients present with mild to severe bleeding just as do individuals with the inherited form of factor X deficiency. Replacement therapy can be given with plasma or factor concentrates. However, the in vivo half-life of factor X is shortened.

Occasionally a patient is seen with isolated factor deficiency but no evidence of a neutralizing antibody, e.g., when the patient's plasma is mixed 1:1 with normal plasma, the factor level in the mixture is 50 per cent. Such a patient with factor II deficiency was recently studied in depth and shown to have a non-neutralizing antibody to factor II. Administration of corticosteroids was associated with a rise in factor II activity and cessation of bleeding, but circulating factor II was bound to antibody. These observations suggested that non-neutralizing antibodies to factor II cause plasma factor II deficiency because of rapid clearance of the antigen-antibody complexes, which is slowed by corticosteroids. Demonstration of non-neutralizing antibodies requires special techniques and takes some time. Therefore, in a patient who is bleeding seriously, one may need to begin administration of corticosteroids, possibly supplemented with fresh frozen plasma, before the diagnosis is established.

Bajaj SP, Rapaport SI, Barclay S, et al.: Acquired hypoprothrombinemia due to nonneutralizing antibodies to prothrombin: Mechanism and management. Blood 65:1538, 1985. *Although this paper describes only one patient, it illustrates what may be a fairly common happening.*

Greipp PR, Kyle RA, Bowie EJ: Factor X deficiency in amyloidosis: A critical review. Am J Hematol 11:443, 1981. *Well-documented description of the cause of this deficiency.*

Syndromes of Disseminated Intravascular Coagulation (DIC)

GENERAL COMMENTS. In the following discussion, DIC is divided into four clinical syndromes: (1) *compensated DIC,* which may be associated with thrombosis but does not result in bleeding; (2) *defibrination syndrome,* in which the mechanisms that localize blood coagulation are overwhelmed by release of tissue factor, leading to massive utilization and depletion of fibrinogen, other clotting factors, and platelets and resultant thrombosis and/or bleeding; (3) *primary fibrin-*

olysis, in which the mechanisms that localize fibrinolysis are overwhelmed by release of plasminogen activators, leading to bleeding; and (4) *microangiopathic thrombocytopenia*, in which platelet microthrombi are widespread, leading to depletion of platelets, ischemic necrosis of tissues, and microangiopathic changes in red cells. The causes of DIC syndromes are many, and there is considerable overlap among syndromes. Patients with DIC often have multiple medical problems, including bone marrow failure, liver failure, renal failure, vitamin K deficiency, and the like, which may complicate the clinical and laboratory analysis in a given patient. Much of the controversy that surrounds DIC undoubtedly stems from attempts to lump diverse conditions and patients together. Despite its oversimplicity, the following scheme is useful because the treatments of the four paradigm syndromes are quite different. For many of the diseases associated with DIC, specific descriptions of the DIC and recommendations for treatment can be found under individual diseases elsewhere in this textbook.

COMPENSATED DIC. Patients with serious underlying diseases (trauma, infection, malignant tumor, etc.) usually have increased production and consumption of platelets, fibrinogen, and other coagulation proteins. Patients with traumatized or inflamed tissues manifest an "acute phase reaction" mediated by interleukin-1 and tumor necrosis factor in which hepatic plasma protein synthesis is altered. A number of plasma alpha-1, alpha-2, and beta globulins, including alpha-2-antiplasmin and fibrinogen, increase in concentration, whereas other plasma proteins, including transferrin and albumin, decrease in concentration. In areas of trauma or inflammation, there is ongoing coagulation and fibrinolysis. Under such conditions, unclottable fibrin degradation products can be detected by immunoassay in serum. However, the prothrombin time is normal, the platelet count is normal or only minimally decreased, and plasma fibrinogen concentration is elevated. There is speculation that low-grade DIC is associated with microemboli and microthrombi that contribute to the organ failure commonly found in patients with severe illnesses. At this point, however, the only indication to use heparin or other anticoagulants in such patients is as prophylaxis or treatment of thrombosis in large vessels. An outstanding example of the need for anticoagulation is in the Trousseau syndrome of "migratory" venous thrombosis in patients with malignant disease (Ch. 171). Warfarin therapy is often ineffective in such patients, and they must instead be started on a long-term regimen of heparin therapy.

DEFIBRINATION SYNDROME. The prototype of defibrination syndrome is the rapid onset of generalized bleeding that occurs when tissue factor is released into the circulation after massive brain trauma or during amniotic fluid embolization. Laboratory tests in such patients demonstrate gross depletion of platelets and fibrinogen, increase in fibrin degradation products, prolongation of prothrombin time, and variable decreases in factors V and VIII, factor II and the other vitamin K–dependent factors, the antithrombins, and plasminogen. Defibrination syndrome occurs most frequently with shock, sepsis, cancer, burns, and obstetric complications. Patients with sepsis, especially due to meningococcus, may develop purpura fulminans or the Waterhouse-Friderichsen syndrome (hemorrhagic necrosis of vital organs, including the adrenals). The patient's hemostatic system must be supported while the patient is resuscitated and the underlying cause is treated. Thus the patient should receive platelet concentrates, cryoprecipitate as a source of fibrinogen, and fresh frozen plasma as a source of other plasma proteins, especially the antithrombins. An appropriate mix is 10 bags of cryoprecipitate for every 2 to 3 units of plasma. One's goals should be a platelet count of more than 50,000 per microliter, a fibrinogen concentration greater than 100 mg per deciliter, a prothrombin time that is within 2 to 3 seconds of normal, and a concentration of antithrombins that is greater than 40 per cent of normal. The role of heparin is controversial. It is my view that, unless the patient improves quickly or active bleeding cannot be controlled, heparin should be infused in low dosages (10 to 15 units per kilogram per hour after a loading dose of 30 to 40 units per kilogram) with the goal of dampening further defibrination as the patient's clotting components are replenished with cryoprecipitate and plasma. If the patient has overt thrombosis, the dose of heparin can be increased. The low dose of heparin should not cause lengthening of the prothrombin time or APTT or exacerbate the bleeding diathesis. Patients who are severely ill and have defibrination syndrome are at high risk of becoming vitamin K deficient and therefore should receive parenteral vitamin K.

PRIMARY FIBRINOLYSIS. Primary fibrinolysis, in its pure form, is rare and results from massive release of plasminogen activator. Conditions associated with DIC that cause "primarily" fibrinolysis, if not primary fibrinolysis, include carcinoma of the prostate, acute promyelocytic leukemia, hemangiomas, and sustained release of plasminogen activator by endothelial cells due to injection of venoms. A critical point is reached when enough plasmin is activated to deplete the circulation of alpha-2-antiplasmin. This allows plasmin to work unopposed on a variety of substrates in blood. Fibrinogen is lysed to fibrinogen degradation products. Because of the lack of fibrinogen and the inhibitory effect of degradation products on fibrin polymerization, the prothrombin time is prolonged. The platelet count, however, is appropriate for the state of the bone marrow, and antithrombin levels are normal. Ecchymoses, mucosal bleeding, and bleeding from needle puncture sites can be extensive. It is usually possible to give enough cryoprecipitate to keep plasma fibrinogen at a concentration greater than 100 mg per deciliter. There is, however, no concentrated source of alpha-2-antiplasmin. EACA, 1 gram per hour in an adult, may be effective in minimization of bleeding, and in my view it should be given a therapeutic trial in a symptomatic patient if the activity of alpha-2-antiplasmin in plasma is less than 35 to 40 per cent of normal. If there is a worry about induction of thrombosis with EACA, heparin in a low dose can be infused simultaneously as described above.

THERAPEUTIC FIBRINOLYSIS (THROMBOLYSIS). Intravenous administration of streptokinase, urokinase, or tissue plasminogen activator is accepted useful therapy for deep vein thrombosis, pulmonary embolism, acute myocardial infarction, and peripheral arterial thromboembolism. These agents re-establish patency of vessels more quickly than does heparin. The dosage and method of administration of the agents are specific for the different conditions, and in some instances the agent is administered by selective catheterization of the involved vessel.

In the case of streptokinase or urokinase administered systemically, therapeutic effectiveness requires that systemic fibrinolysis be achieved, i.e., that the patients develop iatrogenic primary fibrinolysis. Prolongation of the thrombin time to twice normal is often taken as evidence that the desired effect has been achieved. Such patients also have decreased plasma fibrinogen, plasminogen, and alpha-2-antiplasmin. In the case of streptokinase administered locally or TPA administered systemically or locally, thrombi can be lysed with variable and sometimes minimal evidence of systemic fibrinolysis.

If the level of plasminogen falls to zero, the patient will be relatively resistant to further infusion of fibrinolytic agents. At that point, or at the end of the planned infusion, there is hypercoagulability, and anticoagulation with heparin should be carried out.

The main complication of fibrinolytic therapy is hemorrhage, usually in the form of continuous, slow oozing at sites of invasive procedures. If a pressure dressing does not control this bleeding, administration of the agent can be discontinued with the anticipation that fibrinolytic activity will subside within a few hours. Fresh frozen plasma can be given if the bleeding is severe.

MICROANGIOPATHIC THROMBOCYTOPENIA. The hallmarks of microangiopathic thrombocytopenia are a low platelet count and fragmented red cells on blood smear. Although the serum may contain fibrin degradation products, the prothrombin time is generally not elevated, and the fibrinogen concentration is normal or increased. Microangiopathic thrombocytopenia can be seen in patients with sepsis, malignant disease, immune complex disease, vasculitis, malignant hypertension, eclampsia, vascular malformations, and intravascular aspergillosis. The prototype conditions, however, are hemolytic uremic syndrome (HUS) and thrombotic thrombocytopenic purpura (TTP) (Ch. 81). HUS involves mainly the vessels of the kidney, usually occurs in children, and usually is self-limited. TTP involves many organs, including the brain, usually occurs in adults, and usually causes death unless aggressively treated. Acute neurologic symptoms are the most striking feature of full-blown TTP. The pathogenesis of HUS and TTP is obscure. It has been suggested that patients lack prostacyclin; have von Willebrand factor multimers that are extra large and cause spontaneous platelet aggregation; have autoantibodies that damage endothelial cells; or have a circulating substance, possibly of microbial origin, that causes spontaneous platelet aggregation and that is neutralized by immunoglobulin present in normal plasma. There are intriguing instances in which HUS or TTP occurs in small clusters, is recurrent, or is familial. Whatever the cause(s), both HUS and TTP respond in the majority of cases to infusion of fresh frozen plasma. In some cases the requirement for plasma is so great that plasma exchange is necessary. In other cases, occasional infusion of 1 to 2 units of plasma will suffice. If extensive plasmapheresis fails, therapeutic options include use of drugs that inhibit platelet aggregation, splenectomy, and use of vincristine.

SNAKE BITES. Venoms from various snakes, especially the vipers and rattlesnakes, contain proteins that can, depending on the species, clot fibrinogen, activate factor II, factor X, protein C, or platelets; or cause release of plasminogen activator from endothelial cells. Fortunately the clinical problems associated with DIC's from venoms are not as striking as the laboratory abnormalities displayed by the victims. Treatment in most instances can be conservative: administration of antivenoms, transfusion of platelets and/or plasma, and general supportive therapy. In some instances, hypofibrinogenemia and thrombocytopenia persist for weeks.

Aster RH: Plasma therapy for thrombotic thrombocytopenic purpura: Sometimes it works, but why? N Engl J Med 312:985, 1985. *Interim analysis of a perplexing question.*

Marder VJ, Martin SE, Colman RW: Clinical aspects of consumptive thrombohemorrhagic disorders. In Colman RW, Marder VJ, Salzman EW (eds.): Hemostasis and Thrombosis: Basic Principles and Clinical Practice. Philadelphia, J. B. Lippincott Company, 1982, pp 664–693. *Richly referenced, well-organized discussion of DIC in its many guises.*

Schwartz BS, Williams EC, Conlan MG, et al.: Use of epsilon aminocaproic acid (EACA) in treatment of patients with acute promyelocytic leukemia and acquired alpha-2-antiplasmin deficiency. Ann Intern Med 105:873, 1986. *Emphasizes the importance of plasma alpha-2-antiplasmin concentration in the evaluation of fibrinolytic states.*

Verstraete M, Collen D: Thrombolytic therapy in the eighties. Blood 67:1529, 1986. *A review of a rapidly evolving field.*

ANTICOAGULANTS

GENERAL COMMENTS. An anticoagulant is any substance that, when added to blood, decreases the ability of the blood to clot. By this definition the coumarin antagonists of vitamin K are not anticoagulants, because their effect is to interfere with the hepatic synthesis of normal clotting factors. The four general categories of anticoagulation important to human clinical disease are (1) heparin and heparin-like substances, (2) factor VIII inhibitors, (3) anticoagulants associated with lupus erythematosus (so-called lupus anticoagulant), and (4) miscellaneous rare inhibitors of other clotting factors.

Heparin

Heparin is used commonly for its anticoagulant properties in the prevention of and therapy for thromboembolism and to keep blood fluid during extracorporeal circulation. By definition, 1 unit of heparin will render 1 ml of sheep blood incoagulable. The therapeutic concentration in a human (i.e., a patient with an APTT 1½ times longer than normal) is 0.1 to 0.3 units per milliliter.

Bleeding is the most common complication of heparin therapy. This can be minimized by (1) administration of the drug by continuous infusion rather than in boluses; (2) quantification of the anticoagulant effect at regular intervals by whole blood clotting times or APTT; (3) selection of patients who do not have an occult bleeding site or underlying bleeding diathesis; and (4) prohibition of aspirin and intramuscular injections. Despite this, purpura, ecchymoses, hematomas, gastrointestinal hemorrhage, hematuria, retroperitoneal bleeding, or bleeding at sites of invasive procedures may occur. Heparin is cleared from the circulation within two to four hours. Therefore if bleeding is minimal and can be controlled by local measures, discontinuation of heparin may be all that is necessary. If bleeding is severe, the effects of heparin can be counteracted by giving 1 mg of protamine sulfate for each 100 units of heparin estimated to be in the patient's circulation.

After seven to ten days of heparin therapy, thrombocytopenia sometimes occurs, subsiding when heparin is discontinued. Mild thrombocytopenia is likely due to a direct effect of heparin on platelets. In some patients the thrombocytopenia can be severe and associated with venous and/or arterial thrombosis and DIC. In these patients the thrombocytopenia is probably immunologically mediated. It is important to be alert for such a patient, because one's tendency is to treat the thrombosis by increasing the dose of heparin, only to make the situation worse. Heparin therefore should be discontinued if the platelet count drops precipitously. Low-molecular-weight heparin holds the promise of providing anticoagulant activity without undesirable reactions with platelets and may be a therapeutic option in the future for patients with heparin-induced thrombocytopenia. For the present, however, the best defense is prophylactic, i.e., to initiate warfarin therapy early so that a stable anticoagulant effect is achieved during the first week of heparin therapy.

Several patients with neoplastic plasma cell disorders have had clinical bleeding due to a circulating heparin-like proteoglycan that required the major antithrombin for its function and could be neutralized by protamine sulfate.

Turpie AGG, Levine MN, Hirsh J, et al.: A randomized controlled trial of a low-molecular-weight heparin (enoxaparin) to prevent deep-vein thrombosis in patients undergoing elective hip surgery. N Engl J Med 315:925, 1986. Salzman EW: Low-molecular-weight heparin: Is small beautiful? N Engl J Med 315:957, 1986. *Good update and review of trends in heparin therapy.*

Factor VIII Inhibitors

An endogenously produced anticoagulant, usually referred to as a circulating anticoagulant or a circulating inhibitor, is an antibody that interacts with a clotting factor in a manner that neutralizes the functional activity of the factor. Production of such an antibody is pathologic and often results in hemorrhage. Factor VIII inhibitors are commonly observed in hemophilia A (factor VIII deficiency), but are rare in nonhemophilic patients. Conditions in which sporadic factor VIII inhibitors occur include the postpartum state, diseases of immunologic dysfunction, and old age. The sporadic inhibitors induce a hemophilia-like state, i.e., a significant bleeding diathesis, but are unlike the inhibitors of hemophilic patients in several ways. They tend to be of low titer (<1 to 20 Bethesda units) and to bind factor VIII weakly. Titers often drop when patients are treated with cytoxan, 1 gram intravenously, and prednisone, 80 mg per day to be tapered once an effect is seen. Such a therapeutic response is rare in patients with hemophilia and an inhibitor. Acute bleeding episodes can be managed with variable success by continuous infusion of factor VIII concentrate or cryoprecipitate.

When a factor VIII inhibitor is present, the prothrombin time is normal but the APTT is prolonged. If the patient's plasma is incubated for several hours with an equal quantity of normal plasma, the APTT of the mixture should be prolonged. The factor VIII level in the patient's plasma and in the mixture of patient's plasma and normal plasma should be low no matter what dilutions are tested, whereas the factor IX level should be normal. These characteristics distinguish factor VIII inhibitors from the antiphospholipid inhibitors associated with lupus erythematosus (lupus-type inhibitors). A lupus-type inhibitor may cause prolongation of the prothrombin time, especially when the test is done with diluted thromboplastin; does not require an incubation period to express inhibitory activity in mixtures of patient's and normal plasma; and may interfere with the assays for both factors VIII and IX when the patient's plasma is tested at a 1:10 dilution but not when the patient's plasma is tested at a 1:200 or 1:500 dilution. The implications of having a factor VIII inhibitor versus a lupus-type inhibitor are very different, and the physician and laboratory must be sure that the correct diagnosis is made, even though there is no single test with which to make the distinction.

Herbst KD, Rapaport SI, Kenoyer DG, et al.: Syndrome of an acquired inhibitor of factor VIII responsive to cyclophosphamide and prednisone. Ann Intern Med 95:575, 1981. *Good description of six nonhemophilic patients with inhibitors.*

Lupus-Type Inhibitors

Patients with systemic lupus erythematosus sometimes develop a circulating anticoagulant unrelated to the severity or duration of disease. A similar inhibitor sometimes occurs in patients who do not have lupus. Patients who have the lupus-type inhibitor also may have anticardiolipin antibodies and thrombocytopenia. Only rarely is the inhibitor associated with clinically significant bleeding. When patients with the inhibitor do bleed, it is due to thrombocytopenia, platelet dysfunction, and/or acquired factor II deficiency. Instead, patients with the lupus-type inhibitor are at increased risk of having recurrent thromboembolic events. Thrombosis can involve both veins and arteries. There is probably accelerated atherosclerosis. Women with the inhibitor have a greatly increased incidence of spontaneous abortion. Some patients have neurologic abnormalities that may be due to cerebral thrombosis or myelitis or both. In short, the problems associated with a lupus-like inhibitor can be devastating.

Inhibition of clotting tests is thought to be a consequence of binding of the inhibitor to the acidic phospholipids used in the prothrombin time and APTT. The prolongations of both assays can be very impressive. Presumably, platelet membranes, rather than phospholipid micelles, provide the surface for activation of factors X and II, thus accounting for the fact that clinically significant bleeding does not occur. The pathogenesis of the thrombotic diathesis associated with lupus-type inhibitors is unknown. A reasonable hypothesis is that the lupus-type inhibitor and the anticardiolipin are members of a cross-reacting family of antiphospholipid antibodies, and within the family are antibodies that react in a noxious fashion with endothelial cells, e.g., to block prostacyclin production or to inhibit the cofactor activity of thrombomodulin in the protein C–protein S pathway.

Without knowledge of the pathogenesis of the thromboembolism there is no rational approach to treatment. Anticoagulants should be given, but may not be effective. It also is reasonable to try immunosuppressive therapy or plasmapheresis. Administration of corticosteroids and low-dose aspirin during pregnancy had favorable laboratory and clinical effects in a group of women with the inhibitor and impressive histories of spontaneous abortion.

Branch DW, Scott JR, Kochenour NK, et al.: Obstetric complications associated with the lupus anticoagulant. N Engl J Med 313:1322, 1985. Feinstein DI: Lupus anticoagulant, thrombosis, and fetal loss. N Engl J Med 313:1348, 1985. *Article and accompanying editorial that illustrate well the dilemmas of lupus-type inhibitors.*

Miscellaneous Inhibitors of Clotting Factors

Approximately 5 per cent of patients with factor IX deficiency (hemophilia B) develop inhibitors to factor IX after repeated transfusion. Inhibitors to factor V have been reported in about eight patients, only one of these being a factor V–deficient patient. Acquired inhibitors to von Willebrand factor activity have developed in a very few patients. An IgG inhibitor was found in a factor XIII–deficient patient following transfusion. A few patients receiving isoniazid have developed an inhibitor directed toward the fibrin cross-linking sites; this results in defective fibrin polymerization.

Myeloma or macroglobulinemia may give rise to defective fibrin polymerization as a result of interference by high concentrations of gamma globulin. If overt bleeding occurs, plasmapheresis may restore adequate hemostasis by reducing serum protein concentration.

A very interesting inborn error of alpha-1-antiproteinase (alpha-1-antitrypsin) has been reported in which the mutant serpin is a rapid, specific inhibitor of thrombin, thus causing a severe hemorrhagic diathesis.

PART XIII

ONCOLOGY

168 INTRODUCTION

John Laszlo

HISTORICAL BACKGROUND AND DEFINITIONS

Cancer is an English term derived from the Greek word for crab, *Karkinos*, which was believed to be first used by Hippocrates, who attributed this affliction to an excess of black bile. Cancer was known in antiquity, being described in the early writings of Greeks and Romans. Tumors in Egyptian mummies dating back 5000 years represent the first known human malignant growths, although there is pathologic evidence of bone tumors occurring in dinosaurs and other prehistoric animals.

Peyton Rous, a Nobel laureate for his pioneering work on viral causes of animal tumors, wrote: "Tumors destroy man in an unique and appalling way, as flesh of his own flesh, which had somehow been rendered proliferative, rampant, predatory and ungovernable."

Cancer is a prevalent group of diseases, with more than 900,000 new cases diagnosed annually in the United States and more than 600,000 deaths. Trends in the cancer death rates for males and females are shown in Figures 168–1 and 168–2. More than five million Americans have survived cancer; in more than three million of these the diagnosis was established five or more years ago.

Any definition of cancer must consider (1) the property of an uncontrollable growth of cells originating from normal tissues and (2) the property of killing the host by means of local extension or distant spread (metastasis). Cancer has been defined in terms of an autonomous growth that is unresponsive to normal regulatory factors; in terms of the irreversibility with which cancer cells progressively lose the differentiated characteristics and functions of the normal tissue of origin; on the basis of morphologic or cytogenetic features; and on the basis of reversion to growth and antigenic properties characteristic of fetal cells. All of these qualities are typical of most cancer cells, but they are not universally characteristic. The exceptions make any single definition suspect. Some endocrine-related tumors, for example, not only closely resemble the morphologic features of the tissue of origin but also mimic its functions. They may even be at least partially responsive to hormonal control.

Certain animal and human tumors are capable of differentiation and even spontaneous remission. The embryonal cell carcinoma, for example, may begin with a single type of undifferentiated cell and give rise to highly differentiated teratoid tumors containing tissues such as cartilage and hair. Human leukemic cells can be stimulated to undergo terminal differentiation in vitro, and there is the potential to accomplish this by pharmacologic means in patients. Even the property of rapid growth is not characteristic of most tumors, nor does it distinguish a tumor from rapidly growing fetal tissues or certain normal adult tissues such as bone marrow cells or gastrointestinal epithelium. For example, chronic lymphocytic leukemia results from the accumulation of a slowly proliferating clone of small (B) lymphocytes that are identifiable because they share characteristic enzymatic and cell membrane properties. Etiology is not useful as a means of separating cancers from normal tissues, since the etiology is usually unknown. Indeed, different causes of a single type of malignant tumor may give rise to varying behavior. For example, acute myelogenous leukemia arising de novo differs in its behavior from a morphologically similar leukemia caused by exposure to ionizing radiation.

Shimkin MB: Contrary to Nature. Washington, D.C., US Department of Health, Education and Welfare, 1977. *An outstanding and eminently readable work on the development of knowledge about cancer from earliest records to modern times. This well-illustrated book traces the impact of the scientists and institutions that have contributed to cancer research throughout the world.*

ETIOLOGY

Many chemicals (benzpyrene, aflatoxin, arsenicals, asbestos), viruses, and physical agents (ionizing radiation, ultraviolet light) can serve as carcinogenic stimuli capable of inducing malignant transformation in animals or humans (Ch. 170). Some cancers are iatrogenic in origin, as in patients who develop acute leukemia or other cancers years after being cured of systemic cancer by the use of cytotoxic chemotherapeutic drugs, or in patients who receive prolonged immunosuppressive therapy as part of their renal transplantation program.

Substances that are not themselves carcinogens may serve as co-carcinogens in that they promote tumor formation when given in conjunction with or following exposure to specific carcinogens. The major public health hazard relating to cancer in the United States is from the use of *tobacco products. The incidence, time to occurrence, and site of cancer depends upon the frequency and mode of use (smoking, chewing), as well as on exposure to potentiating factors such as alcohol or asbestos.* About one third of cancers in the United States and Europe are related to the use of tobacco products. Additionally, *host susceptibility* is a critical determinant in the carcinogenic process, for a known carcinogen may cause cancer, premalignant changes, or no detectable effect in a given person. This is partly explained by genetic (or acquired) differences in the metabolism of a precursor to the proximate carcinogen and by differences in hormonal milieu and immunologic resistance.

In addition to the use of tobacco, other aspects of lifestyle appear to be important contributors to human carcinogenesis. A high intake of dietary fat increases susceptibility of numerous forms of cancer. Low fiber and low calcium intake appear to increase the risk for colon cancer. High alcohol intake increases oral cancer. All of these are common in most industrialized nations of the Western world. Sexual lifestyle also can be etiologic, as with the high incidence of cervical cancer among women who have many sexual partners (presumably due to papilloma virus) and the high incidence of Kaposi's sarcoma among male homosexuals with AIDS.

Fundamental mechanisms that govern the etiology of human cancer, a subject devoid of new ideas for many years, have recently become enormously exciting as new information

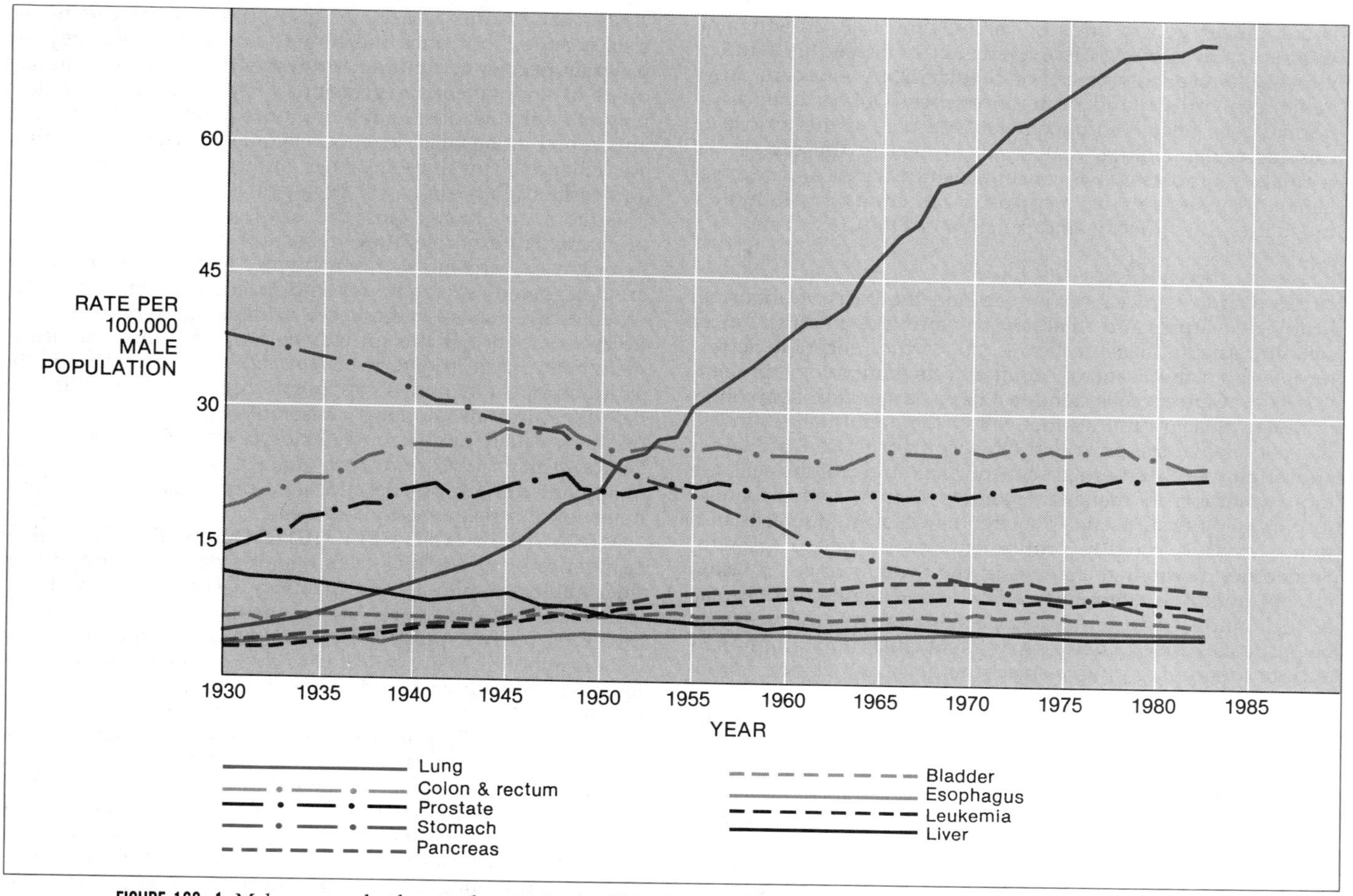

FIGURE 168–1. Male cancer death rates by site in the United States, 1930 to 1983. The rate for the male population is standardized for age on the 1970 United States population. Sources for statistics are the National Vital Statistics Division and Bureau of the Census, United States. (Courtesy of the Epidemiology and Statistics Department, American Cancer Society.)

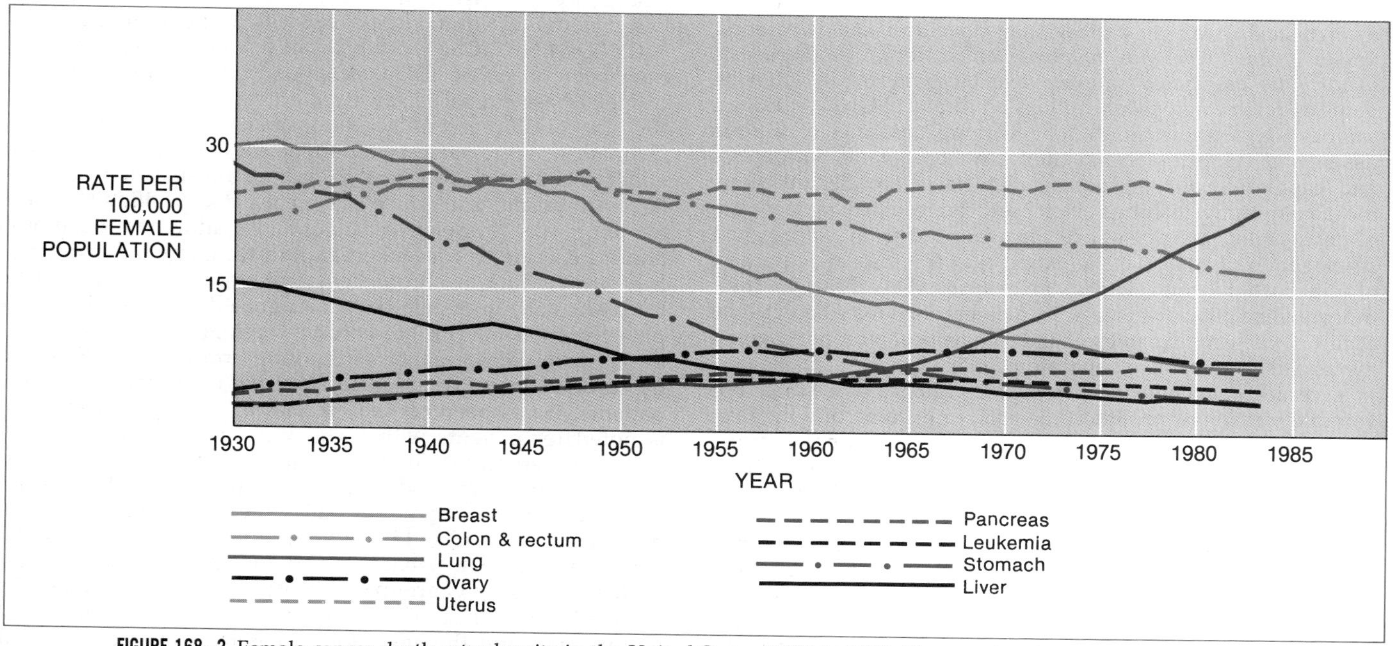

FIGURE 168–2. Female cancer death rates by site in the United States, 1930 to 1983. The rate for the female population is standardized for age on the 1970 United States population. Sources for statistics are the National Vital Statistics Division and Bureau of the Census, United States. (Courtesy of the Epidemiology and Statistics Department, American Cancer Society.)

about cancer genes, viruses, carcinogens, cell growth, and differentation is being discovered. Retroviruses (RNA tumor viruses), oncogenes (pieces of cellular DNA found in oncogenic retroviruses) and proto-oncogenes (DNA sequences in normal cells related to oncogenes) are part of the lexicon of this molecular biology that seeks to explain these essential regulatory processes. For cancer-causing viruses and carcinogens to cause heritable neoplastic cell transformation they must alter the structure and function of DNA (Ch. 169).

HISTOLOGY, METASTASIS, AND GROWTH

The diagnosis of cancer is made on the basis of abnormal histologic features and an abnormal pattern of growth. Cancer cells in variable measure bear some of the morphologic features of both the tissue of origin and its embryologic progenitor cell. Cancer cells tend to have large and sometimes irregular nuclear outlines that reflect the abnormalities in cell division and in the polyploid DNA content. Nuclei are larger and often more numerous than normal, and mitotic cells are more common in malignant tumors than in either benign tumors or normal tissue. The frequency of mitotic cells in a tumor mass is roughly proportional to its rate of growth. Sometimes qualitative changes in the process of cell division lead to multinucleated and variably sized giant cells. Special histochemical and immunologic stains and procedures may be particularly useful in classifying leukemias and lymphomas and for identifying unique structures such as melanin, myofibrils, and immunoglobulin markers.

The growth pattern of tumor cells is always abnormal compared to the tissue of origin. In benign tumors, cells resemble normal tissue; their pattern of growth is usually circumferential and rounded in gross appearance, and often the tumor is encapsulated by surrounding fibrous tissue. These slow-growing tumors do not become necrotic and hemorrhagic, in contrast to malignant tumors, which more readily outgrow their vascular supply. Benign tumors may show a spectrum of variation from normal, and on occasion the distinction between a benign and a malignant lesion on the basis of histology alone may be subtle. Malignant tumors are more deviant in their cellular and organizational characteristics, and the cells adhere less to one another. Aided by the elaboration of proteases, they thus tend to spread locally and replace normal stromal and parenchymal cells and also to metastasize. As they grow they develop their own blood vessels, presumably in response to a tumor angiogenesis factor. The associated unique vascular pattern can often be demonstrated angiographically as a "tumor blush." Although tumors may be surrounded by varying amounts of fibrous tissue and lymphoid cells, they tend to invade lymphatics and capillaries. When tumors metastasize to distant sites, most commonly to lungs, liver, and bone marrow, they are often rounded in appearance, growing out from a presumed single clone of cells. To the extent that the histologic pattern of the parent tumor varies, metastases may differ in their morphologic characteristics. This divergence may be extreme at times, causing the pathologist to question whether a given metastasis represents a separate primary tumor.

A clinically recognizable tumor includes (1) a small but variable fraction of proliferating cells, only some of which are clonogenic in that they can give rise to additional tumors, and (2) nonproliferating cells, some of which are potentially clonogenic if properly stimulated and the remainder of which lack the capacity for cell division and are themselves programmed for death. A spectrum of morphologic findings may reflect stages in neoplastic transformation. Dysplastic changes of bronchial epithelium or of the cervix are considered to be premalignant, although not necessarily destined to become cancerous, particularly if the inciting stimulus is removed. As cells become more anaplastic in appearance, they may begin to show microscopic invasion, progressing from carcinoma in situ to microscopic invasion to overt invasive disease. *Dysplastic* changes in other organs also precede frank carcinomatous changes, but once the tumors are established they are programmed for continuing survival and growth, save in rare cases of spontaneous regression. Malignant transformation may possibly be considerably more frequent than is clinically apparent but be held in check by mechanisms of immune surveillance. This hypothesis is attractive but controversial and certainly has not as yet been proved.

Tumors are named for the cell type from which they originate. For example, they are termed carcinoma if epithelial in origin or sarcoma if mesenchymal in origin. Carcinomas are designated as squamous cell or adeno in type, depending whether they show microscopic evidence of keratin or glandular formation. If the growth pattern of tumors is clearly malignant, then the term *carcinoma* or *sarcoma* should be included in the name. A carcinoma that has lost its differentiated features and no longer resembles a recognizable cell of origin is called undifferentiated or poorly differentiated, as the case may be. Careful morphologic classification of some malignant tumors can be critical in predicting their biologic behavior and response to treatment.

METASTASIS AND CELL HETEROGENEITY. The lack of adherence of tumor cells to one another accounts in part for their ability to migrate and invade adjacent tissues and also to spread to distant sites. Tumor masses are not homogeneous; their biologic properties vary from one subpopulation of cells to another. Many cancer cells may be shed from a tumor; fewer may invade and erode a blood vessel to be disseminated by the circulation; and only a rare cell may have the capacity to lodge successfully in a supportive site and begin to grow into a discrete metastasis. One subpopulation of cancer cells may be more successful in growing in lung, whereas another may grow better in liver or bone marrow, for reasons that are not currently understood. Curiously, extensive selective pressures make metastasis an unlikely event for any given cell. The mere presence of tumor cells in the venous drainage of a tumor specimen does not necessarily presage the development of a metastasis. Metastases, like the primary tumor, may cause pressure symptoms or replace normal tissues to damage the host further. The phenotypic heterogeneity of tumors may explain the emergence of resistant lines following chemotherapy, radiation therapy, or hormonal therapy. The emergence of resistant lines is based on chromosomal instability, clonal selection, and the capacity for gene amplification.

CYTOGENETICS. Many types of cytogenetic abnormalities have been observed in leukemias and other cancers by study of metaphase preparations, by high resolution banding with the use of fluorescent acridine stains, and by other new techniques. The most common of the recurring defects is either a band deletion or a reciprocal translocation between two chromosomes in which one breaks at a specific site. There has long been evidence of aneuploidy, additions, deletions, and translocations for leukemias and for many other tumors. Increasingly unique chromosomal abnormalities characteristic for particular tumors are being recognized, e.g., the Philadelphia chromosome (Ph^1) in chronic myelogeneous leukemia, a translocation abnormality of the long arm of the G22 to the C9 chromosome. Present in some 85 per cent or more of CML patients, it has been correlated with a better prognosis than is noted for patients with CML who lack this marker chromosome (see Ch. 155). Clonal abnormalities also occur in myeloid, erythroid, and megakaryocytic cells, indicating an earlier common progenitor cell as the source of this clonal malignancy (see Ch. 152). Other interesting chromosomal abnormalities have been reported for specific tumor types, such as a missing G group chromosome in meningiomas, the frequent occurrence of a 14 q^+ translocation in malignant lymphomas, and the aneuploid cytogenetic characteristics of adult leukemia. A series of chromosomal abnormalities are found in Burkitt's lymphoma, Wilms' tumor, neuroblastoma, and small cell lung cancer.

Pierce GB, Fennell RH: Pathogenesis of cancer: In Holland JF, Frei E III (eds.): Cancer Medicine. Philadelphia, Lea & Febiger, 1982, p 149. *A lively discussion of the properties of cancer cells and how they relate in histology and growth to the normal cells of origin. Subsequent chapters on tumor invasion, metastases, cell kinetics, and cytogenetics also give details to supplement this introductory chapter.*

Yunis JJ: The chromosomal basis of human neoplasia. Science 221:227, 1983. *Summarizes evidence obtained by newer techniques that chromosomal abnormalities exist in most malignant neoplasms. It integrates the emerging oncogene story with findings of consistent morphologic evidence of chromosomal deletion, translocation, and so on.*

GROWTH KINETICS. Oncologists endeavor to quantify the growth rate of tumors as objectively as possible, using such parameters as the growth fraction of tumors, the duration of the cell cycle, the number of cells in the resting (G_0) phase, and the rate of cell death and removal (Fig. 168–3). The kinetics of tumor growth are crucial in determining prognosis and are also factors in determining response to chemotherapy. "Doubling time" tends to be characteristic of particular tumors. *A tumor that has reached the size of clinical detectability (ca. 1 cm) has already undergone approximately 30 doublings to reach 10^9 cells. Only 10 further doubling cycles are required to produce a tumor burden of approximately 1 kg, which is usually lethal.*

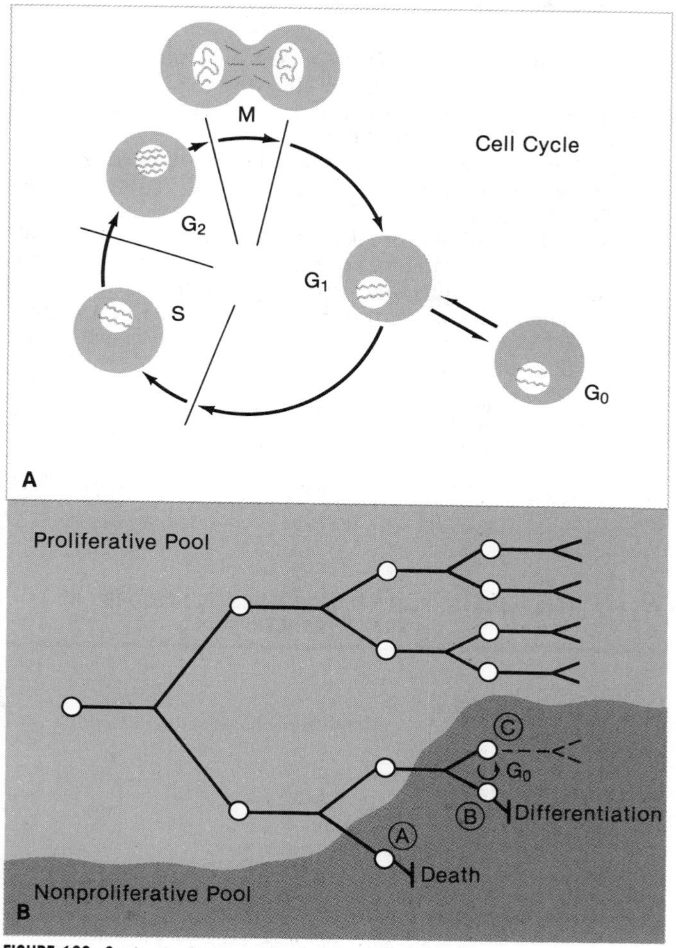

FIGURE 168–3. *A*, A diagrammatic representation of the events during the cell cycle. M is the period of mitosis—approximately one hour from prophase to cell division. G_1 reflects normal cell metabolism prior to DNA synthesis and usually constitutes more than half of the total cell generation time. Cells not actively undergoing replication are described as being G_0; here they may remain indefinitely or be recruited back into the cycle. The DNA synthetic (S) phase is generally 6 to 24 hours. *B*, A schematic representation of tumor growth. As the cell population expands, a progressively higher percentage of cells leave the proliferative pool by death (A), by differentiation (B), or by entering resting phase G_0 (C) from which they may be recruited back into the proliferative pool if the population site is reduced.

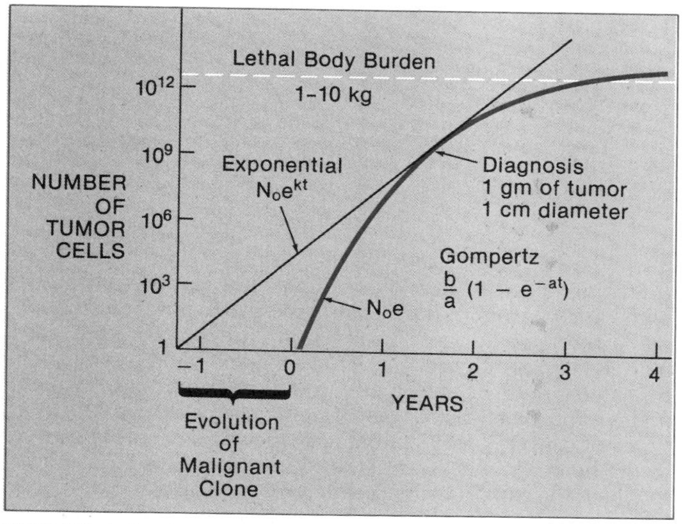

FIGURE 168–4. A schematic log-linear plot to describe models of exponential and gompertzian growth curves. Over any short span of observation it is not possible to distinguish between the two, but conclusions drawn about the latent period, prognosis, and susceptibility to treatment may be quite different between the two models. (Courtesy of Dr. Edwin Cox.)

The simple exponential growth curve is a useful first approximation to the growth of tumors (Fig. 168–4). Deviation of the growth rate from a simple exponential expression has important implications for early diagnosis and for explaining difficulties in curing bulky tumors. As most tumors grow, the generation time of dividing cells remains fairly constant, but an ever increasing percentage of daughter cells enters a nonproliferating state, G_0, from which they may (potentially) be recruited back into cell cycle if the tumor cell population is reduced (Fig. 168–3). In many instances, less than 10 per cent of the cells constituting the tumor mass are actively proliferating by the time the tumor is detected; thus the remaining 90 per cent of cells are not susceptible to most antimetabolites because they are not engaged in DNA synthesis. The progressive movement of cells into G_0 and the increasing relative death rate of cells as the tumor grows larger combine to produce a slowing of the relative growth rate, reflected in a deviation of the growth curve away from a simple exponential function.

Tumor growth curves are often better described by the Gompertz equation, which has also been found useful to describe biologic growth, such as the growth of the human fetus, of individual organs, and of transplantable tumors. Tumors described by the Gompertz curve appear to be growing exponentially over any short span of observation, up to three or four doublings. Observation over a longer time span reveals the gradual slowing of relative growth rate (Fig. 168–4), to an eventual plateau level at which the rate of new cell production just equals the rate of cell loss. Fitting an exponential curve to tumors that show a Gompertz growth characteristic is somewhat misleading in that it underestimates the underlying growth rate, overestimates the latent cell line, and predicts more rapid progression and death than are observed.

A number of concepts for cancer treatment based on this kinetic model have been suggested (see Ch. 176). One of these is surgical "debulking" of tumors to reduce them to a small size at which their growth rate increases and the cells are more susceptible to chemotherapy as a function of increased cell division. The availability of more potent and potentially curative chemotherapy programs has given this added importance. A second and related notion is that of deriving comparable equations for expressing cell killing by drugs, in order to predict how many courses of treatment would be required to achieve a total cell kill.

Lloyd HH: Estimation of tumor cell kill from Gompertz growth curves. Cancer Chemother Rep 59:267, 1975. *Illustrates Gompertz growth curves for experimental tumors and applies theories on tumor growth rates to estimate tumor cell killing due to treatment.*

Rai KR, Sawitsky A, Cronkite DP, et al.: Clinical staging of chronic lymphocytic leukemia. Blood 46:219, 1975. *Tumor burden and prognosis can be predicted for some malignant growths by statistical analysis of simple descriptors. More complex and sophisticated systems for multiple myeloma have also been developed that depend upon estimating the mass of malignant cells by its immunoglobulin products* (e.g., Durie et al.: Blood 55:364, 1980).

STAGING, CLASSIFICATION, MARKERS, AND PROGNOSIS

Staging and classification of the clinical features of patients with cancer are important to provide prognostic information, guide therapy, design clinical trials, and communicate information among physicians. The complex TNM system, the three elements of which are the primary *t*umor, regional *n*odes, and *m*etastasis, was designed to be applicable to all types of cancer. TNM staging is particularly useful in cancers of the head and neck, breast, and most types of lung cancer, in which the clinical course is often reproducible and described by progression of disease as a local growth, followed by increasing regional node involvement, and finally by distant metastasis (Table 168–1). By contrast, it is less useful for tumors such as small cell lung cancer, which tend to metastasize early. The size of the primary tumor ranges up to 2 cm for T_1 lesions, 2 to 4 cm for T_2, and larger than 4 cm for T_3 (these criteria vary slightly for some other tumors). Progressive involvement of regional nodes is clinically assessed from the nondemonstrable N_0 to the large and fixed nodes of an N_3 lesion. Metastases are either clinically unsuspected, M_0, or are present beyond the cervical lymph nodes, M_1, in the case of head and neck cancer. Related staging systems based on anatomic extent of disease are also useful for tumors such as cervical cancer and Hodgkin's disease. Indeed, the combined contribution of careful morphologic classification, clinical staging, and substaging together with systematic treatment is best demonstrated in Hodgkin's disease, in which these concerted studies have raised the overall curability from 10 per cent to over 80 per cent during the past 25 years.

The use of the TNM system by practicing physicians is still the exception rather than the rule. In addition to anatomic extent of disease, other determinants affect prognosis, response to treatment, and quality of life (Table 168–2). Table 168–3 relates the general factors listed in Table 168–2 to specific prognostic factors in breast cancer, and is designed to include almost all factors potentially relevant to outcome. Not all of these are equally important, or even comparable for different tumors. In breast cancer the most commonly used information includes the characteristics of the local lesion (size, location, fixation, skin or nipple involvement), extent of regional node involvement, presence of metastases, and type of hormonal receptors on the tumor. The Karnofsky scale (Table 168–4) is the most widely used shorthand measure of a patient's performance status.

Other types of tumor markers may be useful in diagnosing or in following the response to treatment of various cancers (see Ch. 172). Some of these are relatively specific markers such as the beta subunit of HCG, alpha-fetoprotein, thyrocalcitonin, breast cyst antigen, serum acid phosphatase, monoclonal immunoglobulins, and urinary lysozyme. Others such as carcinoembryonic antigen (CEA) and serum LDH are quite nonspecific, but may nevertheless be useful in charting the progress of treatment.

American Joint Committee for Cancer Staging and End-Results Reporting: Manual for Staging of Cancer. Chicago, American Joint Committee, 1978. *This manual is available free of charge from the American Joint Committee, 55 East Erie St., Chicago, Ill. 60611*

Cox EB, Laszlo J, Freiman A: Classification of cancer patients: Beyond TNM. JAMA 242:2691, 1979. *A critical review of the elements of classification systems, with a discussion of how computers can help to expand clinicians' ability to assess individual patients.*

TABLE 168–1. THE TNM SYSTEM

Primary Tumor (T)	
T_0	No evidence of primary tumor
T_{1b}	Carcinoma in situ
T_1, T_2, T_3, T_4	Progressive increase in tumor size and involvement, e.g., for breast cancer, 0–2 cm, 2–5, >5, any size plus skin or chest wall
Regional Lymph Nodes (N)	
N_0	Regional nodes not demonstrable
N_{1a}, N_{1b}	Homolateral regional nodes (breast): metastases not suspected (a), suspected (b)
N_2, N_3	Homolateral regional nodes: fixed axillary (N_2), homolateral supraclavicular (N_3), or edema of arm; metastases suspected
N_x	Regional lymph nodes cannot be assessed clinically
Distant metastasis (M)	
M_0	No known distant metastasis
M_1	Distant metastasis present
Specific site ________	

The Manual for Staging of Cancer may be obtained free of charge from the American Joint Committee, 55 East Erie Street, Chicago, Ill. 60611.

TABLE 168–2. POSSIBLE DETERMINANTS OF RESPONSE TO TREATMENT AND LENGTH AND QUALITY OF SURVIVAL

I. Biologic characteristics of tumor
   a. Growth fraction
   b. Generation time
   c. Rate of spontaneous cell loss
   d. Degree of differentiation, cell-cell interaction
   e. Propensity to metastasis
II. Host resistance
   a. Status of immune competency
   b. Nutrition
   c. Co-morbid medical conditions
III. Host-tumor interaction
   a. Microenvironment, invasiveness
   b. Location of tumor
      (1) Interference with function of vital organs
      (2) Extirpation without harm to vital functions
   c. Systemic effects of tumor, paraneoplastic syndromes
   d. Occurrence of metastasis (regional node involvement)
   e. Site of metastasis, multiple versus single
   f. Endocrine and other metabolic modulation of tumor growth
IV. Effect of treatment on the tumor versus effect on host
   a. Completeness of extirpation of primary tumor
   b. Timing of primary extirpation with respect to occurrence of metastasis
   c. Dose-response relationship to tumor cell killing
   d. Toxicity, therapeutic ratio
   e. Reinforcement of normal host defense mechanisms (immunostimulation, fibrosis in irradiated area)

TABLE 168–3. POTENTIAL PROGNOSTIC FACTORS IN BREAST CANCER*

Primary disease
- Epidemiology
  - Familial occurrence (I, II, III)
  - Endocrine milieu (menstrual history, hormone administration) (IIIf)
- Primary lesion
  - Size (IVb)
  - Location (IIIb, IIId, IVa)
  - Histologic type and grade (Ia, Id, IIIa)
  - Ulceration, invasion, fixation (IIIa, IIIb)
  - Kinetic analysis, thymidine labeling (Ia, Ib, Ic)
  - Pathology description of surgical specimen (IVa)
- Extraprimary
  - Involvement of regional lymph nodes (Ie, IIId, IIIe, IVb)
  - Metastatic involvement—history and physical examination, screening and selected special studies (Ie, IIId, IIIe, IVb)

Recurrent disease
- Time to first recurrence (Ia, Ib, Ic, IIIf, IVa)
- Site(s) of metastasis (Ie, IIIa, IIIb, IIIf)
- Hormone receptors and hormonal responsiveness (IIIf, IVd)
- Doubling time, kinetic studies (Ia, Ib, Ic)
- Response to chemotherapy (IVc, IVd)
- Response to radiation therapy (IVc, IVd, IVe)
- Serum calcium (IIIc)

General
- Skin testing, immunoglobulin levels, macrophage chemotaxis (IIa)
- General medical history and physical (IIb, IIc)

*Numerals refer to Table 168–2.

TABLE 168–4. "PERFORMANCE STATUS" (KARNOFSKY SCALE)

Criteria of Performance Status (PS)		
Able to carry on normal activity; no special care is needed	100	Normal; no complaints; no evidence of disease
	90	Able to carry on normal activity; minor signs or symptoms of disease
	80	Normal activity with effort; some signs or symptoms of disease
Unable to work; able to live at home and care for most personal needs; a varying amount of assistance is needed	70	Cares for self; unable to carry on normal activity or to do active work
	60	Requires occasional assistance but is able to care for most needs
	50	Requires considerable assistance and frequent medical care
Unable to care for self; requires equivalent of institutional or hospital care; disease may be progressing rapidly	40	Disabled; requires special care and assistance
	30	Severely disabled; hospitalization is indicated although death not imminent
	20	Very sick; hospitalization necessary; active supportive treatment is necessary
	10	Moribund, fatal processes progressing rapidly
	0	Dead

DIAGNOSIS OF CANCER AND ITS COMPLICATIONS

GENERAL EVALUATION. The diagnosis of cancer can be simple or it can tax all of the skills of clinical investigation, depending on the site and extent of the disease The challenge is to detect cancer as early as possible, when it is most likely to be curable. In large cancer centers one third of new patients are found to have in situ or localized cancer, one quarter to have regional disease, and one third to have distant disease. The rest of the cancers are unknown or unstaged. Early detection of localized, malignant disease is aided by an awareness of risk factors in the family history, personal habits (tobacco, alcohol, sun exposure) and occupational exposure (e.g., asbestos, chromium, plastic factory). It also requires attention to subtle and nonspecific symptoms of fatigue, weakness, weight loss, depression, headache, pain, changes in bowel habits, persistent cough or hoarseness, and other clues from the history. The frequency with which the diagnosis of cancer results from attention to such nonspecific manifestations is obviously much less than if the patient presents with physical evidence such as masses in the skin or abdomen, enlargement of nodes or organs, evidence of lymphatic or venous obstruction, or pleural or ascitic effusions.

The physician should carefully examine the nose, oral cavity, pelvis, and rectum for masses or ulcerated lesions as part of any complete evaluation, and these should not be "deferred." More subtle clues may be seen in the skin with petechiae, with hyperpigmentation of skin folds (acanthosis nigricans), rarely with herpes zoster that can antedate the finding of certain cancers such as lymphoproliferative cancers, or with peculiar types of neuromyopathies (see Ch. 174 and 175). Leads from laboratory testing may be found in unexplained anemia, thrombocytopenia, hypercalcemia, or elevation of serum LDH and alkaline phosphatase, or by specific search for tumor markers.

INITIAL DIAGNOSIS. There are two major categories of diagnostic problems: obtaining the original diagnosis, and correctly identifying the many types of complications or intercurrent illnesses which may arise during the course of the disease. The former is usually the simpler of the two, requiring a tissue diagnosis, for example, in a patient who has a signal lesion in the lung, an enlarging lymph node, or a skin lesion. Intra-abdominal disease is more difficult to find—for example, in the patient with anorexia and extensive weight loss who has a pancreatic neoplasm. Fortunately, advances in imaging techniques (ultrasound, CT scanning, liver and spleen scanning) frequently help to demonstrate pancreatic tumor tissue when it exists (see Ch. 109). Radionuclide bone scanning is a powerful tool for detecting metastases that are not yet visible on standard bone radiographs, although bone scans may also be abnormal owing to arthritis or previous trauma. *Indirect diagnostic techniques are not a substitute for a histologic or cytologic diagnosis of cancer.* Occasionally it may not be possible to obtain tissue for histologic diagnosis, e.g., when there is a deep-seated brain tumor.

Physicians often face the diagnostic dilemma posed by the discovery of a metastatic lesion when the primary site of tumor is unknown. For example, a mass on the arm is excised and found to be an adenocarcinoma, but radiographic studies of lung, bowel, and kidneys are normal. The most common sources of such lesions are tumors of the lung and pancreas. Even so, the majority of primary sites are never found. It is of dubious value to perform blind and invasive diagnostic procedures in the absence of some directive clues. One constructive action that can be taken is to consider the possibility of extragonadal germ cell tumors in patients under 50 years of age. The finding of mediastinal, retroperitoneal, or lymph node involvement and high HCG or alpha-beta protein levels may be indicative of germ cell tumors. These may respond dramatically to cisplatin-based chemotherapy programs.

DETECTION AND SCREENING. How can the presence of cancer be detected at a curable stage in asymptomatic people? It is not sufficient to make an earlier diagnosis unless that knowledge prolongs life. Detailed discussion of the cost-benefit factors of various screening techniques is beyond the scope of this chapter. It is almost impossible to prove that a detection test decreases mortality. Simple and inexpensive measures such as self-examination of the breasts or testes, routine cervical cytology, and examination of stools for occult blood seem more likely to be of value, particularly in high risk groups, than frequent chest x-ray examinations, routine proctoscopy, and widespread mammography. The latter procedures are better advised for specific high-risk groups, but even some of these points are highly debatable. For example, mammography is the most effective means of detecting small (<0.5 cm) cancers, and the cost of this procedure is falling, which improves the risk-benefit ratio. The routine use of mammography leads to additional biopsies, however, which are costly, and usually the results show the lesion is benign. This creates a dilemma of some magnitude, as does screening stool specimens for occult blood. (The American Cancer Society is a good source of guidelines for various screening procedures.)

Diagnostic approaches taken for the *symptomatic patient* are relatively direct compared to the question of cost-effectiveness of mass screening, which is more difficult and controversial. How much testing is advisable for a concerned asymptomatic patient who can afford noninvasive procedures even if they have a lower yield than would seem appropriate for mass screening? There are no good sources or valid generalizations about this subject, and the answer will depend on the information and attitude of the doctor and relationship with the patient. It comes down to the doctor recommending what would be optimal and the patient selecting on the basis of all information.

DIAGNOSTIC PROBLEMS DURING CONTINUING CARE OF THE PATIENT WITH CANCER. The physician who undertakes the continuing care of a patient with cancer must be vigilant in promptly identifying complications arising from the progression of tumor, and in detecting curable intercurrent illness which may be mistaken for manifestations of cancer itself. The patient with a known tumor who develops anorexia, weight loss, and jaundice may have cholecystitis and biliary obstruction, rather than metastatic cancer, and may die from that disorder unless the correct diagnosis is established. Furthermore, some potentially treatable conditions are actually caused by the cancer therapy—as in postoperative adhesions or radiation-induced strictures leading to bowel obstruction, or chemotherapy-induced immunosuppression leading to an opportunistic fungal infection. Certain drugs may even produce complications that simulate paraneoplastic syndromes, such as inappropriate secretion of ADH, neuromyopathy, or cerebellar degeneration. Although errors in diagnosis of intercurrent medical and surgical illness sometimes seem almost inevitable, the best way to minimize these problems is to *assume that each new condition is due to a nonmalignant process, until it is proven otherwise.*

Eddy DM: Finding cancer in asymptomatic people. Cancer 51:2440, 1983. *The author reviews the degrees of evidence that early detection tests are effective in reducing mortality, with emphasis on the two areas (breast, lung) in which randomized controlled studies exist.*

Greco FA, Vaughn WK, Hainsworth JD: Advanced poorly differentiated carcinoma of unknown primary site: Recognition of a treatable syndrome. Arch Intern Med 104:547, 1986. *A positive approach to treatment of patients who have cancer of unknown origin.*

PRINCIPLES OF MANAGEMENT OF THE PATIENT WITH CANCER

APPROACHES TO TREATMENTS. A therapeutic strategy should be clearly defined for each patient with cancer, once the diagnosis has been firmly established, staging of the tumor has been carried out, and careful assessment has been made of the patient's overall physical, physiologic, and social situation. Such a strategy is often best devised by a multidisciplinary team, including medical, surgical, and radiation oncologists who will weigh the possibilities of cure or significant palliation, consider the various treatment options and their expected untoward effects, and then embark on a therapeutic trial. Fortunately the therapeutic horizons are constantly changing. For example, patients with disseminated testicular cancer, acute lymphocytic leukemia, Ewing's sarcoma, Wilms' tumor, ovarian carcinoma, Hodgkin's disease, and histiocytic lymphoma now have an excellent chance for a cure, whereas this would have been impossible even in the recent past. Since the outcome for an individual patient cannot be precisely predicted, the initial treatment plan must often be updated on the basis of changing circumstances or after restaging procedures, in order to provide the broadest chance of response to therapy. Obviously surgery or localized radiation therapy with the aim of cure is a desirable option if the clinical circumstances are appropriate. Surgery is used as the sole initial treatment for over 50 per cent of patients with *all* types of localized cancer, the remainder being treated either with radiation alone or in various combinations with or without chemotherapy. Local or regional recurrences may still permit localized radiotherapy with the intent of cure, but systemic disease requires chemotherapy if all tumor cells are to be reached. The difficulty of attempting to predict tumor response to chemotherapy may one day be overcome through in vitro sensitivity tests, but for the present the selection process depends upon prior reports of clinical trials for particular types of cancer.

Forty to fifty per cent of all patients with cancer are potentially curable at the time of diagnosis. It is more important to understand the principles underlying the various types of treatment, the order in which they are used, and how aggressively they are to be applied than to remember their dosage schedules. The risk of serious side effects may be much more acceptable to a patient who stands a good chance for a cure than to one who does not. A limited trial of therapy in patients who have tumors that are unlikely to respond is usually warranted, with a careful look for changes in tumor size or tumor markers. At least such an approach gives patients an opportunity for palliation, without committing them to many months of ineffective treatment. These judgmental decisions must bridge the gap between careful assessment of the individual patient and knowledge concerning current therapeutic methods. After careful explanation by the physician of all options, it is the competent patient who must make the ultimate decisions about treatment. Therefore, it is essential to develop a meaningful therapeutic alliance in dealing with such choices.

SUPPORTIVE CARE. In its broadest sense, "supportive care" refers to all types of medical care required to provide for the needs of the patient with cancer. Certain specific supportive care programs for patients receiving aggressive chemotherapy for leukemia and other conditions have led to gratifying improvements in cure rates by anticipating and/or counteracting potentially fatal complications such as *infection and bleeding.* Early detection and vigorous treatment with newer antibiotics can be lifesaving for infected patients during periods of severe granulocytopenia. It has become unusual to see a fatal infection during the first few such episodes in the treatment of cancer. Similarly, platelet transfusions can minimize the risk of hemorrhage during periods of profound thrombocytopenia. These two advances, together with aggressive systemic and intrathecal chemotherapy, are responsible for the 50 per cent cure rate that can now be achieved in childhood leukemia, for example.

Severe *nausea and vomiting* induced by combination chemotherapy may be major, even limiting, factors in patient compliance because of the serious deterioration in the quality of life induced by these potent drugs. The woman receiving adjuvant chemotherapy for breast cancer or the man being treated for testicular cancer may endure a year of these exhausting side effects unless an effective antiemetic program is administered. Many patients fail to respond to conventional antiemetics, such as large doses of phenothiazines, but may respond very well to high dose metoclopramide and steroids, haloperidol, delta-9-tetrahydrocannabinol (THC) and other antiemetics. The effectiveness of antiemetic drugs varies, depending on the type of chemotherapy, with high dose cisplatinum therapy being the most potent and difficult emetic stimulus to control. Anxiety is a very important part of the whole symptom complex. It frequently leads to anticipatory nausea and vomiting. The anxiety portion can be alleviated by benzodiazepines such as lorazepam.

General supportive care also involves meeting nutritional, rehabilitative, psychosocial, and analgesic requirements (see below). Anorexia and weight loss are almost invariably associated with advanced cancer; occasionally profound *cachexia* may occur in a patient with only a small and apparently localized lesion such as lung cancer. There are several potential explanations for the varying *nutritional problems*—anatomic causes such as abdominal pressure or head and neck surgery, liver disease, paraneoplastic syndromes, effects of chemotherapy, depression, or the release of peptides such as cachectin. In the individual patient it is often difficult to sort out the factors that contribute to anorexia and hypercatabolism, and frequently they occur together. Regardless of etiology it is important to reverse this catabolic trend, since malnourished patients tolerate the usual courses of chemotherapy or radiation therapy very poorly and may die prematurely of complications related to treatment toxicity. Thus, in the case of a patient with recurrent cancer of the head and neck, improvement in nutrition is often a necessary prerequisite to the use of chemotherapeutic drugs. Increasingly, oncologists are using parenteral or tube feedings prior to major cancer surgery, radiation therapy, or chemotherapy. The dietitian familiar with the practical problems faced by these patients is an essential member of the team working with the patient and family.

Hyperuricemia and *hyperuricosuria* have the potential of producing acute urate nephropathy in patients in whom tumors are rapidly destroyed by chemotherapy. This complication can be effectively prevented by the use of allopurinol to block urate synthesis and by vigorous hydration prior to and during administration of cytotoxic therapy for lymphocytic leukemia or lymphoma, for example.

Every physician caring for patients with cancer must appreciate the cumulative debilitating effects of bed rest, continuous intravenous infusions, weight loss, and cytotoxic chemotherapy. Losses of muscle mass and bone structure are predictable in patients with advanced cancer, and they predispose to further immobility, hypercalcemia, and fractures. A simple and useful exercise program developed by Rosenbaum and associates can be done at home or in the hospital. The program also contributes to a feeling of well-being and preservation of body image.

The *psychosocial problems* that may be encountered by patients with cancer are profound and varied. Many of these are not unique to cancer and occur in age-matched patients with other types of chronic illness and shortened life expectancy. Shock, bereavement, anger, denial, withdrawal, and depression are common responses of people faced with such overwhelming problems. Disfigurement, feelings of shame and disgrace, loss of sexual activity, and job discrimination are problems that are more prevalent in patients with cancer than in those with many other illnesses. *The attitude of the physician and staff* is of key importance in helping the patient make the best possible adjustment, given all of the premorbid factors and limitations imposed by the illness. The physician who (verbally or nonverbally) conveys the impression that "There is nothing further that I can do" is sentencing his patient to untold misery or forcing him into the waiting arms of enthusiastic cancer quacks. All patients need help. Most patients respond positively to it, and they appreciate a gently supportive role that stresses honesty, trust, and a willingness simply to be available to help both patient and family with their fears and needs.

The *care of the patient who is dying of cancer* is the most sensitive issue for both patient and family. This is also commonly the period in which patients feel abandoned by physicians who themselves are frustrated by their inability to cure or cause remission of the illness and by the tragic human circumstances that often accompany such illnesses. Indeed, these take their toll on doctors and nurses as well as on relatives and friends, and busy cancer clinics recognize the need for support groups for their staff. (Indeed, unless there is an active self-renewing effort, oncology workers are subject to "burnout," an insidious syndrome difficult to recognize.) The physician must always prepare a reassuring setting so that when specific therapy is no longer warranted, patient comfort will be attended to in a considerate and thoughtful manner. In the final weeks of the illness, family members may require even more attention than the patient, and the team of doctor, nurse, social worker, and chaplain should provide the necessary support for all concerned including staff.

Patients fear *pain* perhaps more than any other aspect of cancer, and there are many misconceptions about this subject by the public. Yet adequate techniques are available to control pain in most patients, if these are used in a timely and appropriate fashion. Here again a carefully obtained history is an important initial step in diagnosis, for a patient with pain may have anything from cord compression or bone metastasis to a benign condition such as arthritis. The complaint of pain may even reflect the fear of abandonment. Relatively simple radiotherapy or neurosurgical procedures employed sufficiently early for localized pain and the *liberal use of narcotics for severe generalized pain* are usually successful in alleviating cancer-related pain. One need not be concerned with potential narcotic addiction in dying patients. Patients themselves are often reluctant to take adequate doses of analgesics and should be encouraged to take them with sufficient frequency to alleviate pain *before* it becomes very severe.

Depending on the wishes of the family, it is often preferable to provide for the care of the dying patient in his or her own home. This can be done with a home care program supplemented by visiting nurses and volunteers. *Hospice programs* are rapidly developing in the United States, and these can provide the supportive ingredients for both the patient and family that others cannot supply. The patient is often much more comfortable in familiar surroundings and near to loved ones. Family and friends usually respond willingly to their duties when properly directed. Finally, the savings in costly hospitalizations can conserve already depleted financial resources. Indeed, careful curbing of unnecessary costly tests and interventions can make an enormous financial difference over the course of the illness.

DeVita VT, Hellman S, Rosenberg SA (eds.): The Principles and Practice of Oncology. Philadelphia, J. B. Lippincott Company, 1985. *A major text of oncology that is particularly useful for looking up specific tumors and treatment.*

Holland JF, Frei E III (eds.): Cancer Medicine. Philadelphia, Lea & Febiger, 1982. *Excellent textbook with resource materials for all levels of study. It is an oncology textbook with general articles on diagnostic procedures and principles of treatment, as well as hard-to-find highly technical and basic articles related to various aspects of cancer research.*

Laszlo J: Antiemetics and Cancer Chemotherapy. Baltimore, Williams & Wilkins Company, 1983. *The first detailed study of the neurophysiology, fluid balance, drug therapies, and behavioral therapy of the nausea and vomiting produced by chemotherapeutic drugs.*

Laszlo J: Physician's Guide to Cancer Care Complications: Prevention and Management. New York, Marcel Dekker, 1986. *Careful review of the complications of surgery, radiation therapy, and chemotherapy from experts who have special interests in minimizing predictable problems in management of patients with cancer.*

Rosenbaum EH, Rosenbaum IR: A Comprehensive Guide for Cancer Patients and Their Families. Palo Alto, CA, Bull Publishing Co., 1980. *A sensitive and practical manual describing the attitudes, stresses, and losses of the patient who has cancer, and a helpful guide to rehabilitative services, nutrition, and bed care management. Encompasses the range of personal support services to patients in a book that is suitable for the entire health team.*

169 ONCOGENES

J. Michael Bishop

CANCER AS A GENETIC DISEASE

Astute observers have long nurtured the thought that cancer might be at its heart a genetic disease. The thought was at first vague and arose from seemingly disparate discoveries that included the existence of heritable diatheses to cancer, the presence of abnormal chromosomes in cancer cells, and the likelihood that many carcinogens act by inducing mutations in cellular DNA. Medical geneticists and epidemiologists first conceived the possibility of "cancer genes," prompted by occasional examples of human tumors whose occurrence seemed dictated by recessive or dominant inherited traits. Now the long-imagined cancer genes have been brought to view, unearthed by two experimental strategies; the use of viruses that cause tumors in animals and the search for tumorigenic genes in the DNA of cancer cells. From these studies we have learned that the human genome contains a set of genes (more than 20 loci but perhaps less than 100) that may lie at the heart of every cancer. These genes are called *proto-oncogenes* (to designate them as precursors to oncogenic determinants) or *cellular oncogenes* (to designate them as potentially oncogenic determinants that are part of the genetic dowry of all normal cells), and their value to cancer research is beyond measure. They are our present best hope of achieving an understanding of the molecular mechanisms by which cancer arises, a keyboard on which many different carcinogens may play, the possible components of a final common pathway to neoplastic growth.

FIRST DESCRIPTIONS: VIRAL ONCOGENES

Documentation that specific genes can elicit cancerous growth emerged first from the study of viruses that cause tumors in animals. By the use of formal genetic analyses, and

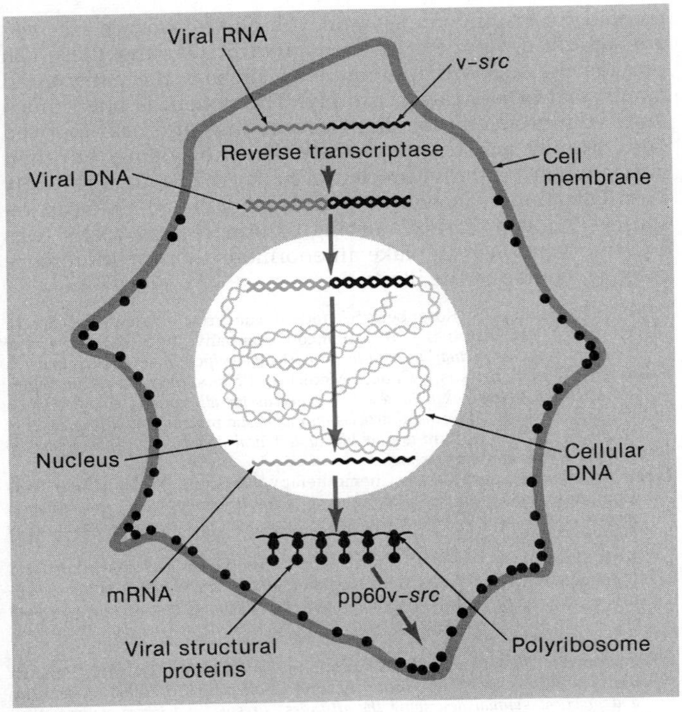

FIGURE 169–1. The molecular life cycle of retroviruses leads to insertion of viral genes into the chromosome of the host cell and the subsequent production of viral proteins that can transform the cell to neoplastic growth. In the example illustrated, the protein encoded by the *src* oncogene of the Rous sarcoma virus attaches to the inner surface of the plasma membrane and catalyzes phosphorylation of tyrosine residues in cellular proteins. (Modified from Bishop JM: Oncogenes and proto-oncogenes. Hosp Pract 18:68, 1983, with permission from HP Publishing Co., Inc.)

later of recombinant DNA, investigators were able to show that the tumorigenicity of many viruses can be attributed to domains within the genomes of the viruses. In time, these domains became known as oncogenes because they are oncogenic and are coincident with active viral genes that encode proteins produced in infected cells.

The most decisive paradigm for the genetic origins of cancer emerged from the study of retroviruses, whose genes are carried in RNA but are copied into DNA by reverse transcriptase early in viral replication. The life cycle of retroviruses provides a microcosm of carcinogenesis (Fig. 169–1). The viral DNA produced by reverse transcriptase is inserted (or "integrated") into the chromosomal DNA of the host cell. Thereafter, the cell uses its own machinery to express the integrated viral genes. These events hold two possibilities for carcinogenesis. First, the integration of viral DNA is potentially mutagenic: It can damage vital cellular genes, and it can influence their expression by bringing them under the sway of powerful viral signals. Virologists call this *insertional mutagenesis*; it may indeed be tumorigenic (see below), and the cellular genes perverted by viral DNA are candidate "proto-oncogenes." Second, some (but not all) retroviruses carry oncogenes whose expression is sufficient to give rise to cancerous growth. The oncogenes of retroviruses make no apparent contribution to viral replication; therefore, their presence in viral genomes posed a puzzle. The puzzle was solved with the discovery that retroviral oncogenes are not viral genes at all, but wayward copies of cellular genes acquired during the course of viral replication by a process known formally as transduction, and carried as mere passengers in the viral genome. It is likely that transduction by retroviruses is a rare accident of nature, without design for the virus, and attributable to details of the curious means by which retroviruses replicate. There is no reason to believe that the transduction is limited to genes with tumorigenic potential. However, transduction by retroviruses is of profound consequence because it has brought to view cellular genes whose activities may be central to all forms of carcinogenesis. Many decades might have been necessary to find these genes in the morass of the mammalian genome; instead, the genes were manifested in viruses, excerpted, and made available for close scrutiny.

THE PATHOGENIC MECHANISMS OF RETROVIRAL ONCOGENES

The study of viral oncogenes began with the hope that the mechanisms by which these genes act might help to reveal the inner workings of the cancer cell, to elucidate the biochemical abnormalities that prompt cancerous growth. This is now a burgeoning prospect because the number of retroviral oncogenes has grown to at least 20, each inducing specific forms of malignancy, each encoding a protein whose action apparently causes harm (Table 169–1). The first hint of how informative these genes might be came with the discovery that several retroviral oncogenes encode protein kinases, located on the plasma membrane of the cell and possessing a previously unencountered substrate specificity for tyrosine. It would be difficult to envision a better explanation for neoplastic transformation: By phosphorylating numerous cellular proteins, a single enzyme could rapidly change myriad aspects of cellular structure and function. If the phosphorylated

TABLE 169–1. THE PROTEINS ENCODED BY RETROVIRAL ONCOGENES

Oncogenes	Tumorigenicity	Biochemical Properties	Subcellular Location	Cellular Homologue
abl	Lymphoma	Protein kinase	Plasma membrane	
*erb-A**	?	?	?	
erb-B	Erythroleukemia	Glycosylated	Intracellular and plasma membranes	Receptor for EGF
*ets**	?	?	?	
fgr	Sarcoma	Protein kinase	Plasma membrane	
fms	Sarcoma	Glycosylated	Plasma membrane	Receptor for CSF-I
fos	Osteosarcoma	?	Nucleus	
fps/fes†	Sarcoma	Protein kinase	Plasma membrane	
kit	Sarcoma	Protein kinase	Plasma membrane	
mos	Sarcoma	?	Cytoplasm	
myb	Myelomonocytic leukemia	?	Nucleus	
myc	Carcinomas, leukemia and sarcoma	Binds to DNA	Nucleus	
raf/mht/mil†	Sarcoma	Glycosylated	Membranes	
ras	Sarcoma and erythroleukemia	Binds and hydrolyzes GTP	Plasma membrane	G/N regulatory proteins
rel	Lymphoma	?	?	
ros	Sarcoma	Protein kinase	Plasma membrane	
sis	Sarcoma	Growth factor	Cytoplasmic	Subunit 2 of PDGF
ski	Sarcoma	?	Nucleus	
src	Sarcoma	Protein kinase	Plasma membrane	
yes	Sarcoma	Protein kinase	Plasma membrane	

*The exact contribution of *erb-A* and *ets* to tumorigenesis by the viruses in which they occur is not yet apparent.
†Multiple names denote genes isolated from different species but later proved to be homologous.

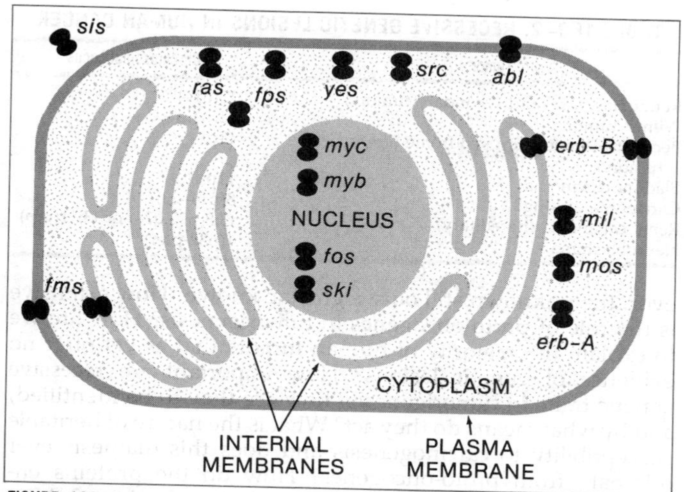

FIGURE 169–2. The products of oncogenes assume diverse locations within the cell, where they perform functions involved in the regulation of cellular growth and differentiation. (Modified with permission from Hunter T: The proteins of oncogenes. Sci Am 251:78, 1984.)

proteins can be found (only a few have been, to date), a door will be opened to the secrets of neoplastic growth.

Protein phosphorylation is not the only means by which retroviral oncogenes may act (Table 169–1). As more and more of the proteins encoded by oncogenes came into view, a provocative diversity emerged: Some of the proteins are protein kinases, others are not (one is a component of the growth factor normally released by platelets); some attack in the nucleus of the cell, some in the cytoplasm, some at the plasma membrane (Fig. 169–2); and there is little correlation between what we now know of how oncogenes function and the character of their tumorigenicities. What does this diversity signify? The growth of cells is regulated by an interdigitating network that spans from the surface of the plasma membrane to the depths of the nucleus. If that network were to be touched at any point by an adverse influence and tilted out of balance, cancerous growth might ensue. Perhaps the diverse means by which different oncogenes act may mirror various components of the regulatory network, revealing how the network performs its task. By studying oncogenes, we are likely to be learning of both cancerous and normal growth at one and the same time. It is an old adage of medical science that study of the abnormal can reveal the normal.

PROTO-ONCOGENES AND ONCOGENES

The cellular genes whose transduction engenders retroviral oncogenes provided the first glimpse and the first definition of proto-oncogenes. By all available criteria, these are cellular genes, not viral genes in disguise. They can be found in every member of every vertebrate species examined, probably in all metazoan organisms. Evolutionary conservation of this magnitude signifies that the proto-oncogenes serve essential functions for the species in which they are harbored. Proto-oncogenes are expressed in normal cells and tissues, and their expression can vary from one tissue to another, from one embryologic lineage to another, from one time in embryogenesis to another. It is widely assumed that, in their normal guise, proto-oncogenes help to control the growth and development of cells and organisms. This assumption has been strengthened by the discovery that several of the proto-oncogenes encode proteins known to participate in the regulation of cellular proliferation, including platelet-derived growth factor (PDGF) and the receptors for epidermal growth factor (EGF) and colony-stimulating factor I (CSF-I) (Table 169–1).

Why are the transduced forms of proto-oncogenes tumorigenic? What converts a proto-oncogene, a compliant member of the cellular citizenry, to an oncogene—an unruly and potentially lethal enemy? The possible answers to these questions have taken two general forms: Transduction may have unleashed the genes from their usual controls and outlandish or inappropriate expression of otherwise normal genes might be the fatal flaw; alternatively, mutation during or after transduction could change the structure of the genes and the proteins they encode, giving rise to abnormal function. For the moment, it appears that either explanation may on occasion apply. There is no question but that transduction by retroviruses mandates relatively vigorous gene expression. Comparisons of retroviral oncogenes to their cellular progenitors have revealed a variety of structural changes sufficient to evoke anomalous function. These issues are not arcane: they prefigure the debate over whether, and if so how, proto-oncogenes might be the intrinsic "cancer genes" of human cells.

PROTO-ONCOGENES AS CANCER GENES

Do proto-oncogenes participate in many or all forms of tumorigenesis? Are they a common keyboard for all the players in carcinogenesis? Since these questions were first raised, the pertinent evidence has grown from a thin thread to a rich and provocative fabric of experimental observation.

1. Direct manipulation of proto-oncogenes isolated by molecular cloning has revealed that some (but not all) of these ostensibly normal genes can elicit neoplastic growth if they are first attached to viral signals that command vigorous gene expression and then inserted into cells in culture.

2. There is evidence that retroviruses without oncogenes of their own initiate tumorigenesis by the mutation of proto-oncogenes. The mutations may be of two sorts: those that enhance expression of a gene and those that change the structure of the protein(s) encoded by a gene.

3. Some human tumors (the exact number is not yet clear) display karyotypic evidence of gene amplification (double-minute chromosomes and homogeneously staining regions in marker chromosomes) and contain one or another proto-oncogene whose number has been multiplied as much as 200-fold over normal. As a consequence of amplification, the proto-oncogene is expressed in inordinately large amounts. Amplification of proto-oncogenes has been found in two patterns: as sporadic and occasional features of diverse tumors and as a common feature of particular tumors. The latter pattern gives promise of being clinically useful. For example, amplification of a proto-oncogene known as N-*myc* is a frequent feature of human neuroblastomas and appears to connote an ominous prognosis that will justify attempts at new therapeutic regimens.

4. At least several of the chromosomal translocations that typify a substantial variety of human tumors move a proto-oncogene from one chromosome to another. As a consequence, expression of the proto-oncogene may be altered, or the gene may sustain mutations within the domain that encodes a protein. Present examples include Burkitt's lymphoma (translocation of the proto-oncogene c-*myc*) and chronic myelogenous leukemia (translocation of c-*abl*), in which the Philadelphia chromosome (Ph^1) raised the possibility many years ago that consistent forms of chromosomal damage might figure in tumorigenesis.

BIOLOGICALLY ACTIVE ONCOGENES IN THE DNA OF HUMAN TUMORS

The frequency with which proto-oncogenes first identified through the use of retroviruses have been implicated in the genesis of human tumors is not easy to dismiss as coincidence. The incriminating evidence remained entirely circumstantial, however, until a direct assault revealed biologically active oncogenes in human tumors. Application of DNA from a variety of human tumors to cells in culture can elicit neoplastic growth, as if the DNA contained oncogenes of the sort once found only in viruses. Approximately 20 per cent of all human tumors demonstrate activity of this type, no matter what their histopathology. The responsible genes have now been identified for a substantial variety of tumors. With remarkable frequency, they have proved to be one or another member of a family of proto-oncogenes known as *ras* genes and already familiar to us from the study of retroviruses. But other genes have been found as well—some that were known to us before from the study of retroviruses, others that are entirely new to us. Many of the oncogenes appear to be active because they have suffered mutations that change single amino acids in the protein products of the genes.

ONCOGENES AND THE MULTIPLE STEPS IN CARCINOGENESIS

The attribution of tumorigenesis to oncogenes seemed at first glance simplistic, since the genesis of tumors has long been described as a protracted and complex sequence of events. However, the identification of oncogenes and the proto-oncogenes from which they are derived has given us a tool with which to recognize several separate steps in tumorigenesis. In at least some human and animal tumors, it is possible to point to at least two coexistent genetic lesions afflicting proto-oncogenes in various ways. For example, two oncogenes have been incriminated in the genesis of Burkitt's lymphoma: a proto-oncogene that has been relocated and possibly activated by chromosomal translocation, and another gene whose action transforms rodent cells in culture, perhaps because a mutation has altered the protein encoded by the gene.

The manner in which such pairings might exemplify distinct steps in carcinogenesis has been demonstrated by experiment. Two oncogenes can be combined to elicit a tumorigenic phenotype in cultures of embryonic rodent cells that could not be rendered tumorigenic by either of the oncogenes alone. Medical geneticists have in the past suggested that at least some tumors may owe their origins to no more than two genetic lesions. These suggestions now appear more credible than ever before.

RECESSIVE GENETIC DAMAGE IN TUMORS

The oncogenes considered so far are thought to be genetically dominant: Their abnormalities have an impact even when a normal allele of the same gene is also present in the cell. But at least some human tumors (and perhaps all) also bear lesions that are recessive, that make their presence known only when no normal counterpart is present. By inference from karyotypes and by the use of restriction endonucleases, substantial evidence has been obtained for the presence of recessive mutations in a variety of tumors. The examples of retinoblastoma and Wilms' tumor are presently the most celebrated, but other (and more common) examples are now emerging as well (Table 169–2). In each instance, the faulty chromosome—and sometimes the responsible region of that chromosome—is known. But no particular gene has yet been incriminated, nor do we know how recessive mutations might interact with dominant oncogenes.

Recessive mutations explain hereditary diatheses to several forms of neoplasm (again, retinoblastoma and Wilms' tumor are the seminal examples). By contrast, there is as yet no evidence to implicate any of the dominant oncogenes in the inheritance of cancer.

THE FUTURE

By one means or another, at least 11 proto-oncogenes have been implicated in different types of tumorigenesis. In some instances, expression of the gene is enhanced; in other instances, the structure of the protein encoded by the gene has been changed. In a few instances, both of these events may have occurred. These are remarkable conclusions, reached within a decade of the discovery of proto-oncogenes. However, the unknown still outweighs the known. How extensive is the role of proto-oncogenes in tumorigenesis? How are we to explain the majority of human tumors that as yet offer no evidence of genetic lesions? How important are recessive genetic traits in tumorigenesis, how are they to be identified, and by what means do they act? What is the nature of heritable susceptibility to carcinogenesis and does this diathesis ever originate from proto-oncogenes? How do the proteins encoded by oncogenes conduct their nefarious business? After all, will we be able to parlay the growing information about oncogenes into devices for the prevention, diagnosis, and treatment of human cancer? It is too early to foretell how quickly the answers to these questions may come, but there now seems little reason to doubt that we have laid hold of cancer with a grip that should eventually extract the deadly secrets of the disease.

TABLE 169–2. RECESSIVE GENETIC LESIONS IN HUMAN CANCER

Tumor	Chromosomal Locus
Retinoblastoma (and secondary tumors)	13(q14)
Wilms' tumor	11(p13)
Beckwith-Wiedemann syndrome (embryonal tumors)	11p
Bladder carcinoma	11p
Carcinoma of lung	3(p14–23)
Renal carcinoma (hereditary)	t3;8(p12;q24) or t3;11(p;p)
Neuroblastoma	1(p32-pter)

Bishop JM: The molecular biology of RNA tumor viruses: A physician's guide. N Engl J Med 303:675, 1980.
Bishop JM: Oncogenes. Sci Am 246(3):80, 1982.
Bishop JM: Cellular oncogenes and retroviruses. Ann Rev Biochem 52:301, 1983.
Bishop JM: Oncogenes and proto-oncogenes. Hosp Pract 18:67, 1983.
Bishop JM: Trends in oncogenes. Trends Genet 1:245, 1985.
Hunter T: The proteins of oncogenes. Sci Am 251(2):70, 1984.
Varmus HE: The molecular genetics of cellular oncogenes. Ann Rev Genet 18:553, 1984.
Weinberg RA: A molecular basis of cancer. Sci Am 249(5):126, 1983.
Weinberg RA: The action of oncogenes in the cytoplasm and nucleus. Science 230:770, 1985.
All of these references offer general reviews of this rapidly expanding area of medical research.

170 EPIDEMIOLOGY OF CANCER

Joseph F. Fraumeni, Jr.

Epidemiology has contributed substantially to knowledge about the origins of human cancer, and provides the foundation for measures designed to prevent cancer. The approach dates from the eighteenth century, when the occupational physician Bernardino Ramazzini reported that nuns were at high risk of breast cancer, and the surgeon Percivall Pott observed that chimney sweeps exposed to soot were prone to scrotal cancer. The initial leads to epidemiologic investigation have often come from astute clinicians who noted an excessive number of patients with the same tumor and traced the "cluster" to a particular cultural, occupational, or iatrogenic exposure. Major insights into cancer etiology are provided also by experimental approaches to detect carcinogens in laboratory animals or mutagens in short-term test assays, and to clarify basic mechanisms of carcinogenesis. In recent years the pace of epidemiologic and experimental research in cancer etiology has accelerated, including efforts to identify environmental factors, which are generally held responsible for a large proportion of cancers in the general population.

PATTERNS OF CANCER OCCURRENCE

Cancer is second only to heart disease as a cause of death in the United States, and accounts for 22 per cent of all deaths.

It is estimated that in 1986 about 930,000 Americans developed cancer, excluding in situ carcinomas and nonmelanoma skin cancer, and that about 472,000 died from the disease. The most common cancers occur in the lung in males, the breast in females, and the colon and rectum in each sex.

It has been widely claimed that 80 to 90 per cent of all cancer is related to environmental influences, particularly those related to life style practices. These estimates are derived from the substantial international variation in cancer incidence, in which rates for the lowest-risk countries are subtracted from the rates prevailing in the United States. The resulting difference is attributed to environmental causes, and the lowest risk is assumed to represent the baseline level for tumors that develop "spontaneously" and cannot be prevented. Around the world the reported age-adjusted incidence rates for total cancer vary by a factor of about three, whereas the rates for certain anatomic sites, particularly the esophagus and liver, vary by more than 100-fold. Even the risks for the more common tumors in Western countries differ by factors of about 8 to 40. Although some of this variation may have a genetic basis, evidence supporting a major role for environmental factors can be found in the experience of migrant populations, such as the Japanese who moved to Hawaii and California. Generally, as migrant groups adopt customs of the new land, their risk of various cancers shifts away from the rate prevailing in the country of origin to approximate that of the host country. The change in incidence for some cancers, notably cancer of the colon, is often evident within two to three decades of migration, whereas the change for other cancers, notably cancer of the breast, requires more than one generation. Although variations within countries are not as great as those seen internationally, the mapping of cancer death rates in the United States at the county level has revealed geographic clustering that provides leads to the investigation of environmental exposures.

Variations in cancer incidence and mortality over time may also reflect environmental factors, although some fluctuations can be explained by changing medical practices and reporting procedures. Most dramatic has been the increase in lung cancer rates in the United States and other countries; in the 1950's cigarette smoking was determined to be responsible. Upward trends have been noted also for thyroid cancer resulting from x-ray therapy to the head and neck during childhood, malignant melanoma from changing clothing styles and recreational exposures to sunlight, and endometrial cancer from the use of menopausal estrogens. The increases in prostatic cancer and multiple myeloma, however, are at least partly due to improvements in diagnostic measures. In the black population of the United States, sharp increases over time have been reported for cancers of the lung, esophagus, prostate, and pancreas and multiple myeloma, and these tumors are now more common in blacks than whites. Several cancers have shown little change, while a few have displayed downward trends, including cancers of the stomach, cervix, and liver.

THE CAUSES OF CANCER

Although much remains to be learned about the factors responsible for variations of cancer in the general population, several environmental exposures have been identified as causes of cancer (Table 170–1). The evidence is based primarily on case-control studies (comparing the past experience of persons with and without a particular cancer) or cohort studies (following-up individuals whose experiences and characteristics are already defined). There is a growing recognition, however, that most cancers result from the combined effects of multiple exposures and susceptibility states. This is consistent with multistage models in which different risk factors accelerate the transition rates at various stages of carcinogenesis. Some affect early stages as initiators, others act at late stages as promoters, and still others influence both early and late stages. It is generally thought that cumulative environmental exposures, long latency periods, and multistage processes account for the increasing risk of most cancers with advancing age.

TABLE 170–1. ENVIRONMENTAL CAUSES OF HUMAN CANCER

Agent	Type of Exposure	Site of Cancer
Alcoholic beverages	Drinking	Mouth, pharynx, esophagus, larynx, liver, breast
Alkylating agents (melphalan, cyclophosphamide, chlorambucil, semustine)	Medication	Leukemia
Androgen-anabolic steroids	Medication	Liver
Aromatic amines (benzidine, 2-naphthylamine, 4-aminobiphenyl)	Manufacture of chemicals	Bladder
Arsenic (inorganic)	Mining and smelting of certain ores, pesticide manufacturing and application, medication and contaminated drinking water	Lung, skin, liver (angiosarcoma)
Asbestos	Manufacturing and application	Lung, pleura, peritoneum, gastrointestinal tract
Benzene	Leather, petroleum, and other industries	Leukemia
Bis(chloromethyl)ether	Manufacture of ion exchange resins	Lung
Chlornaphazine	Medication	Bladder
Chromium compounds	Manufacturing	Lung
Estrogens	Medication	
Synthetic (DES)		Vagina, cervix (adenocarcinoma)
Conjugated (Premarin)		Endometrium
Steroid contraceptives		Liver (benign)
Immunosuppressants (azathioprine, cyclosporin)	Medication	Lymphoma (histiocytic), skin (squamous carcinoma), soft tissue sarcoma
Ionizing radiation	Atomic blasts, medical use, radium dial painting, uranium and metal mining	Nearly all sites
Isopropyl alcohol production	Manufacturing by strong acid process	Nasal sinuses
Mustard gas	Manufacturing in wartime	Lung, larynx, nasal sinuses
Nickel dust	Refining	Lung, nasal sinuses
Phenacetin-containing analgesics	Medication	Renal pelvis
Polycyclic hydrocarbons	Coal carbonization products and some mineral oils	Lung, skin (squamous carcinoma)
Tobacco chews and powder	Snuff dipping and chewing of tobacco, betel, lime	Mouth
Tobacco smoke	Smoking, especially cigarettes	Lung, larynx, mouth, pharynx, esophagus, bladder, pancreas, kidney
Ultraviolet radiation	Sunlight	Skin, including melanoma
Vinyl chloride	Manufacture of polyvinyl chloride	Liver (angiosarcoma)
Wood dusts	Furniture manufacturing	Nasal sinuses

TOBACCO. The principal carcinogenic hazard in western countries is tobacco smoking, which produces cancers of the lung, larynx, mouth, pharynx, esophagus, bladder, pancreas, kidney, and possibly cervix. It is estimated that smoking, especially cigarettes, contributes to about 30 per cent of all cancer in men and women combined. The greatest impact is on lung cancer, with the risk for male smokers of two or more packs per day being about 20 times that of nonsmokers. However, the rates for lung cancer are now rising more sharply in women than in men, reflecting the growing popularity of cigarettes among women in the past 20 to 30 years. Smokers of filter-tipped cigarettes with reduced tar and nicotine have a lower risk of lung cancer than do smokers of nonfilter cigarettes, but still a much higher risk than do nonsmokers. Smokeless tobacco products are also of concern, since oral cancer has been linked with snuff dipping, a common practice in rural southern areas of the United States. In parts of Asia, oral cancer is very common in people exposed to various tobacco chews, which are often mixed with betel, lime, and other agents that may enhance the risks.

ALCOHOL. Consumption of alcoholic beverages has been shown to multiply the effects of tobacco smoking on cancers of the mouth, pharynx, esophagus, and larynx. Heavy drinking also increases the risk of liver cancer, particularly among cirrhotic patients. Ethanol is not carcinogenic in laboratory animals, so the mechanism by which alcohol promotes carcinogenesis is not clear. Under suspicion are nutritional deficiencies associated with heavy drinking, the effects of congeners or contaminants (e.g., nitrosamines, hydrocarbons) in alcoholic beverages, and the capacity of alcohol to solubilize carcinogens or enhance their penetration into tissue.

SOLAR RADIATION. The dominant risk factor for nonmelanoma skin cancer (squamous and basal cell carcinomas) and for malignant melanoma is ultraviolet (UV) radiation from the sun. The evidence is based on the tendency for skin cancers to arise on sun-exposed surfaces, the high rates among outdoor workers, the inverse correlation between skin cancer incidence and distance from the equator, the predisposition of light-skinned and especially fair-complexioned populations who sunburn easily, the resistance of dark-skinned populations with protective melanin pigment, the exceptional risks of skin cancer among persons with genetic diseases exacerbated by sunlight (e.g., xeroderma pigmentosum, albinism), and the capacity of UV radiation in repeated doses to induce skin cancer in experimental animals.

IONIZING RADIATION. Although ionizing radiation probably accounts for less than 3 per cent of all cancer, it appears that virtually no site of the body is spared from its carcinogenic effects. It is difficult to measure directly the effects of low doses of sparsely ionizing radiation, such as x- or gamma rays, but extrapolations are possible by studying populations who have been exposed to high and moderate doses for medical, occupational, or military reasons. In general, the breast, thyroid, and bone marrow are the most radiosensitive organs. Radiogenic leukemia shows a wavelike pattern with the excess risks starting about two to four years after exposure, peaking at six to eight years, and declining to normal within 25 years. In contrast, radiogenic carcinomas have a minimal latent period of five to ten years and a temporal distribution that resembles the natural incidence curve, suggesting that age-dependent factors influence tumor expression. Surveys of medically irradiated populations have revealed an excess risk of leukemia and other cancers among patients treated for ankylosing spondylitis, benign gynecologic diseases, and various neoplasms; breast cancer among women treated for postpartum mastitis or who received fluoroscopies to monitor pneumothorax treatment of tuberculosis; thyroid cancer among children treated for thymus enlargement, benign head and neck disease, or tinea capitis; leukemia and other childhood cancers following prenatal x-ray exposure; and various cancers following use of radioactive compounds (osteosarcoma with radium-224, leukemia with phosphorus-32, and leukemia and liver angiosarcoma with Thorotrast).

OCCUPATIONAL HAZARDS. Occupational exposures are usually reported to account for less than 5 per cent of all cancer in men, but the percentage is higher for certain tumors, such as the bladder. Most occupational carcinogens have been first detected through clinical and epidemiologic observations with subsequent confirmation by laboratory studies. However, inorganic arsenic has not been shown to be carcinogenic in laboratory animals. In the case of mustard gas and vinyl chloride, the risks were detected in humans after the substances had been shown to induce tumors in laboratory animals, although little attention was given to the experimental studies when first reported. The effects of some agents, particularly asbestos and radon, are greatly potentiated by cigarette smoking, so that programs to reduce either the workplace exposure or smoking would significantly lower but not eliminate the occupational risk. A number of manufacturing industries (e.g., furniture, leather, rubber) are associated with cancer risk, although the specific carcinogens have not been identified. Industrial hazards and their detection have important implications beyond the work force, since most agents are not confined to the plant but ultimately become part of the general environment to which large segments of the population may be inadvertently exposed.

ENVIRONMENTAL POLLUTION. Pollutants in the urban air have long been suspected in the etiology of lung cancer, with fossil fuel combustion products, especially polycyclic hydrocarbons, being of special concern. In several studies the rates for lung cancer have shown correlations with measurement of benzo(*a*)pyrene in the ambient air, yet the available evidence suggests that the urban excess of lung cancer is mainly due to cigarette smoking and partly to occupational exposures. In the large-scale survey of the American Cancer Society, age- and smoking-standardized rates for lung cancer were computed among men not occupationally exposed to dust, fumes, or vapors. No major differences in mortality were seen between urban and rural areas, or between cities characterized by indices of pollution. Another approach has been to extrapolate from studies of workers heavily exposed to hydrocarbons, with the results suggesting only small effects from urban air pollutants. In some studies the effects of smoking a particular amount were greater in urban than rural areas, suggesting that tobacco smoke may interact with carcinogens in the ambient atmosphere.

Asbestos bodies and calcified pleural plaques have been reported in large segments of the urban population, but the carcinogenic effects following nonoccupational exposures are uncertain. It is clear, however, that mesotheliomas may result from neighborhood exposures to asbestos industries and from household contact with asbestos dust, particularly through laundering of work clothing. Another hazard may result from airborne levels of arsenic, since high mortality from lung cancer has been reported among male and female residents in communities with arsenic-emitting smelters.

Recent interest has centered on contaminants in drinking water, since several halogenated organic compounds produced during chlorination are carcinogenic and mutagenic in laboratory tests. Levels of these compounds in drinking water have shown correlations with the rates for cancers of the bladder, colon, and rectum in the same area.

MEDICATIONS. Several carcinogens have been detected by studies of patients exposed to medicinal agents. Some drugs have been withdrawn from clinical practice, while others are retained since risk-benefit considerations may warrant their use in certain conditions. A major discovery in this area was that synthetic estrogens given during pregnancy produce adenocarcinomas of the vagina and cervix several years later in daughters exposed in utero. This was the first demonstration of transplacental carcinogenesis in humans. Endometrial cancer was then firmly linked to the use of conjugated estrogens for menopausal symptoms, and further studies suggested that the occurrence of breast cancer might also be excessive in long-term users. Oral contraceptives have been related to benign liver tumors, to endometrial cancer among users of the sequential type of contraceptives, and possibly to cervical cancer and to breast cancer among some high-risk women (e.g., with benign breast disease). A reduced risk of endometrial and ovarian cancers has been reported with the use of combined oral contraceptives.

An excess risk of acute nonlymphocytic leukemia, and perhaps other cancers, has been seen among patients receiving certain alkylating agents. These risks may be acceptable when treating conditions with a poor prognosis such as metastatic cancer, but for conditions with a favorable long-term prognosis the benefits of treatments should be carefully weighed against the risks. These drugs may exert their action in part by breaking chromosomes, since other leukemogens (radiation, benzene) have a similar effect.

Immunosuppressive agents have been assessed primarily by studies of renal transplant recipients, most of whom have had azathioprine and corticosteroids. The risk of histiocytic lymphoma is very high, and first appears within months of transplantation. This explosive onset has suggested that a latent oncogenic virus may be activated by immunologic mechanisms. For all other cancers combined, the excess risk is about two-fold and first becomes evident about two years after transplantation. It has not affected all forms of cancer, as might be predicted by the hypothesis of "immunologic surveillance," but increased risks have been noted for cancers of the liver, biliary system, and bladder, and for soft-tissue sarcomas, adenocarcinoma of the lung, squamous carcinoma of the skin, and malignant melanoma. Recently, other groups of patients receiving immunosuppressants have shown an excess of lymphomas, squamous carcinoma of the skin, and soft-tissue sarcomas, but at lower rates than those seen in transplant patients. It is noteworthy that the predominance of lymphomas with drug-induced immunosuppression is seen also among patients with primary immunodeficiency syndromes.

INFECTIOUS AGENTS (see also Ch. 169). Evidence is increasing that both DNA and RNA viruses are causally related to certain forms of human cancer. The epidemiologic patterns of cervical cancer have long suggested venereal transmission of an infectious agent, with human papillomaviruses and herpes simplex virus type 2 being chief suspects. The Epstein-Barr virus (EBV) is linked to nasopharyngeal cancer and Burkitt's lymphoma, particularly in areas of the world where these tumors are highly prevalent. Hepatitis B infection is related to hepatocellular carcinoma, especially in endemic regions of Africa and Asia. Outbreaks of adult T cell leukemia in certain areas, especially in Japan and the Caribbean, have been linked to infection with the human T-lymphotropic virus type I (HTLV-I). Another human retrovirus (HTLV-III), also known as lymphadenopathy-associated virus (LAV) or human immunodeficiency virus (HIV), has been shown to cause the acquired immunodeficiency syndrome (AIDS). Recognized in epidemic form since 1981, AIDS affects mainly homosexual men, hemophiliacs, and intravenous drug abusers and is often accompanied by Kaposi's sarcoma and non-Hodgkin's lymphoma (Ch. 158).

If viruses are oncogenic in humans, it seems likely that predisposing factors are operating. Thus, EBV may interact with certain histocompatibility antigens to produce the high rate of nasopharyngeal cancer in Chinese populations, with persistent malarial infections to induce African Burkitt's lymphoma, or with a genetic immunodeficiency trait to cause family clusters of lymphoma. Hepatitis B infection may combine with dietary aflatoxin to produce liver cancer in endemic regions. In animal models the production of immunodeficiency enhances viral carcinogenesis, so that the narrow range of tumors complicating immunodeficiency states of humans suggests that viruses play only a limited role in human cancer.

Parasitic infections affect the risk of cancer in certain areas of the world. In Africa and Papua New Guinea, the geographic patterns of malaria and Burkitt's lymphoma are closely correlated; in the Middle East and North Africa schistosomiasis produces squamous carcinoma of the bladder; and in Asia infestation with liver flukes (clonorchiasis and opisthorchiasis) predisposes to cholangiocarcinoma.

NUTRITION. International correlations and migrant studies have suggested that certain features of the affluent Western diet contribute to a sizable proportion of all cancers. Various nutritional hypotheses are under study, although the mechanisms appear complex and difficult to unravel. For example, high dietary fat may affect the risk of colonic cancer by increasing the concentration of bile acids in the bowel, which are then metabolized by bacterial flora into carcinogens or co-carcinogens, and it may promote the development of breast cancer by increasing estrogen production and prolactin release. Dietary fat and caloric excess may also contribute to endometrial cancer and the associated manifestations of obesity, diabetes, and hypertension.

It appears also that a low intake of certain food classes may predispose to cancer. In several studies, the risk of colonic cancer has been inversely related to the consumption of fiber, which may protect against intestinal carcinogens or precursors by dilutional or other effects. Micronutrients and trace metals may also have a protective influence, since cancers of the lung and other sites have been associated with a low intake of vitamin A, beta-carotene, and selenium. The risk of stomach cancer has been related to a deficiency of fruits and vegetables containing vitamin C, which may act by inhibiting the formation of carcinogenic nitrosamines in the stomach. In a study of colonic cancer, patients ingested smaller than usual amounts of cruciferous vegetables (e.g., broccoli, cabbage, Brussels sprouts, cauliflower), containing indole compounds, which can inhibit carcinogenesis in laboratory animals. In esophageal cancer, the high rate among black males has been attributed to heavy alcohol consumption and generalized poor nutrition.

A variety of other dietary factors, including additives and contaminants, have fallen under suspicion. The consumption of aflatoxin, a carcinogenic metabolite of the fungus *Aspergillus flavus*, correlates closely with the distribution of liver cancer

TABLE 170–2. HEREDITARY NEOPLASMS

	Inheritance*	Features
Retinoblastoma	AD	Susceptibility to second primary tumors, including osteosarcoma of leg and radiogenic sarcoma of orbit; chromosome deletion (13q14) in some cases
Nevoid basal cell carcinoma syndrome	AD	Basal cell cancers of skin increased by UV and ionizing radiation; medulloblastoma, ovarian fibromas, and developmental defects in some cases
Multiple endocrine neoplasia I (Wermer's syndrome)	AD	Adenomas of anterior pituitary, parathyroid, pancreatic islet cells, thyroid, and adrenal cortex; carcinoid tumors of intestine and bronchus in some cases
Multiple endocrine neoplasia II (Sipple's syndrome)	AD	Pheochromocytoma and medullary thyroid carcinoma; parathyroid tumors and neurofibromas in some cases
Chemodectomas	AD	Paragangliomas from chemoreceptor system
Polyposis coli	AD	Multiple adenomatous polyps and adenocarcinomas of large bowel; some families feature osteomas, fibromas, lipomas, and epidermal cysts (Gardner's syndrome)
Tylosis with esophageal carcinoma	AD	Squamous cell carcinoma of esophagus with keratoses of palms and soles
Dysplastic nevus syndrome	AD	Hereditary melanomas derived from nevi, especially after sun exposure

*AD = autosomal dominant.

TABLE 170–3. HEREDITARY PRENEOPLASTIC SYNDROMES

	Inheritance*	Neoplasms
Phacomatoses		
Neurofibromatosis	AD	Sarcomatous change in 10% of cases; gliomas of brain and optic nerve, acoustic neuromas, meningiomas, and acute leukemia
Tuberous sclerosis	AD	Hamartomatous growths in several organs; brain tumors, chiefly giant-cell astrocytoma, in 1–3% of patients
von Hippel-Lindau syndrome	AD	Angiomatosis of retina and cerebellum; renal adenocarcinoma, pheochromocytoma, and ependymoma in some cases
Multiple exostoses (diaphyseal aclasis)	AD	Chondrosarcoma in 5–11% of patients
Peutz-Jeghers syndrome	AD	Rare malignant change in hamartomatous polyps of gastrointestinal tract; ovarian neoplasms in 5% of female patients
Cowden's multiple hamartoma syndrome	AD	Oral papillomas, cystic mastopathy and breast cancer, thyroid and colonic neoplasms
Genodermatoses		
Xeroderma pigmentosum	AR	Various skin cancers in all patients exposed to sunlight; defective cellular repair of DNA damage induced by UV light
Albinism	AR	Skin cancers, chiefly squamous, in sun-exposed areas
Epidermodysplasia verruciformis	AR	Skin cancers, chiefly squamous, in multiple warts induced by papillomavirus
Polydysplastic epidermolysis bullosa	AR	Skin cancers, chiefly squamous, in scars
Dyskeratosis congenita	AR	Squamous carcinomas of skin and mucous membranes; features of Fanconi's anemia in several cases
Werner's syndrome (adult progeria)	AR	Soft tissue sarcoma, other tumors
Chromosome instability		
Bloom's syndrome	AR	Acute leukemia, lymphoma, other cancers
Fanconi's anemia	AR	Acute myelomonocytic leukemia and squamous carcinoma of mucous membranes; hepatoma reported after androgen-anabolic steroids
Immune deficiency		
Ataxia telangiectasia	AR	Lymphoma, lymphocytic leukemia, stomach cancer, other tumors; chromosome fragility and ineffective DNA repair reported; heterozygous carriers prone to leukemia, lymphoma, and carcinomas of biliary tract, stomach and ovary
Common variable immunodeficiency	?AR	Lymphoma, stomach cancer
Wiskott-Aldrich syndrome	XR	Lymphoma, acute leukemia
X-linked (Bruton's) agammaglobulinemia	XR	Lymphoma, acute leukemia
X-linked lymphoproliferative syndrome	XR	Abnormal response to infection by Epstein-Barr virus, resulting in severe infectious mononucleosis, immunoblastic sarcoma, B cell lymphoma, or plasmacytoma

*AD = autosomal dominant; AR = autosomal recessive; XR = X-linked recessive.

in Africa. Coffee intake has been associated with bladder and pancreatic cancers in some studies, but causal relationships have not been established. The artificial sweeteners saccharin and cyclamate are weak bladder carcinogens or co-carcinogens in laboratory animals, but a recent large-scale study of bladder cancer indicated that the risk in humans is very small if present at all. Cooking practices may generate hydrocarbons or other carcinogens at high temperatures, although no epidemiologic observations are available.

GENETIC SUSCEPTIBILITY. Compared to environmental factors in cancer, genetic determinants are less conspicuous and more difficult to identify by clinical and epidemiologic means. Although racial and ethnic differentials for most cancers appear largely modulated by environmental influences, genetic factors may contribute to some high rates (e.g., nasopharyngeal cancer among Chinese and gallbladder cancer among American Indians and certain Hispanic groups) and some low rates (e.g., testicular cancer and Ewing's sarcoma among blacks in Africa and the United States). Genetic susceptibility is most evident for skin cancer, since ethnic variations correspond to the degree of protective skin pigmentation.

Although only a small percentage of cancer is inherited in a mendelian fashion, over 200 single-gene disorders have been linked to neoplasia. Table 170–2 lists some cancers that occur as an inherited trait (hereditary neoplasms), and Table 170–3 presents those arising as a complication of inherited precursor lesions (preneoplastic states). In some syndromes environmental factors contribute to the development of cancer. Neoplasms of a hereditary nature tend to occur earlier in life than do nonfamilial occurrences of the same tumor, and usually arise from multiple foci within the affected organ.

In contrast to the hereditary syndromes, the common human cancers show small familial risks, on the order of two- to three-fold. However, the familial risks for breast and colonic cancers are as high as 20- to 30-fold among subgroups of patients with early onset and bilateral or multifocal origin. Familial susceptibility also appears to enhance the effects of environmental exposures, such as smoking in lung cancer, and sunlight exposure in melanomas derived from dysplastic nevi. In some families there are remarkable aggregations of cancer consistent with an autosomal dominant mode of inheritance. These "cancer families" may display either a single type of cancer or a constellation of multiple cancers, especially adenocarcinomas of the colon and endometrium, or the breast and ovary. Other families are prone to diverse cell types of childhood and adult cancers, particularly soft-tissue and bone sarcomas, breast carcinoma, brain tumors, adrenocortical neoplasms, and leukemia. The delineation of genetic and familial syndromes is helpful in applying laboratory probes to clarify the heritable component and basic mechanisms of carcinogenesis, and in targeting screening and prevention programs designed to protect high risk individuals.

Chaganti RSK, German JL (eds.): Genetics in Clinical Oncology. New York, Oxford University Press, 1985. *A concise guide to the heritable aspects of cancer and the application of cancer genetics to clinical medicine.*

Doll R, Peto R: The causes of cancer: Quantitative estimates of avoidable risks of cancer in the United States today. J Natl Cancer Inst 66:1191, 1981. *A critical review of carcinogenic hazards with emphasis on quantitative risk assessment and the preventable nature of most forms of cancer.*

Schottenfeld D, Fraumeni JF Jr (eds.): Cancer Epidemiology and Prevention. Philadelphia, W. B. Saunders Company, 1982. *A detailed survey of cancer epidemiology, with 70 chapters covering virtually all aspects of the field. The contribution of epidemiology to the development and evaluation of preventive measures is emphasized.*

Vessey MP, Gray M (eds.): Cancer Risks and Prevention. New York, Oxford University Press, 1985. *A review of cancer risk factors and the methods used to apply this information to cancer prevention.*

171 PARANEOPLASTIC SYNDROMES

Paul A. Bunn, Jr.

The paraneoplastic syndromes are a heterogenous group of signs and symptoms indirectly caused by cancers at a distance from the primary tumor or its metastases. These "remote" or "biologic" effects of malignancy are not a direct effect of the primary or metastatic cancer. Distinguishing between the tumor and the paraneoplastic syndrome is the most important step in the differential diagnosis. The majority of paraneoplastic syndromes are caused by proteins secreted by these tumors. In some instances (e. g., endocrine paraneoplastic syndromes), the proteins (hormones) are well characterized, and the pathophysiology is well understood. These paraneoplastic syndromes invariably improve with effective antineoplastic therapy. In addition, drugs that interfere with the hormone action may be useful in severe cases or when the tumor fails to respond to therapy. In other instances the etiology of the syndrome is not clear, and the syndrome may not improve even with effective antitumor therapy. This is often true of the neurologic syndromes, perhaps because the nervous system cannot regenerate and damage is often permanent. Some of these syndromes may be caused by an immunologic reaction to tumor antigens that are shared with normal cells.

Recognizable paraneoplastic syndromes, other than wasting of the host or tumor cachexia, occur in a minority of cancer patients. They may be extremely important, however, in the early detection of the original cancer or may be the first sign of recurrence. They may also simulate metastatic disease and thus prevent patients from receiving curative therapy. Conversely, signs and symptoms of metastatic disease may be falsely ascribed to a paraneoplastic syndrome and thus lead to the withholding of appropriate therapy. Paraneoplastic syndromes may be disabling but treatable with proper recognition. Thus, establishing a diagnosis is extremely important. True paraneoplastic syndromes must be distinguished from those caused by the primary tumor or its metastases, infections, toxicities of therapy, vascular abnormalities, obstruction caused by a tumor or its products, and fluid and electrolyte abnormalities. It is also important to understand which paraneoplastic syndromes respond to primary antitumor therapy. Alternative forms of therapy aimed at symptomatic control should be considered in those syndromes in which response to primary antitumor therapy is unlikely.

WASTING OF THE HOST. Wasting of the host, sometimes called tumor cachexia or the cachexia of malignant disease, is the most common of the paraneoplastic syndromes. The catabolic phase that usually accompanies malignant disease may be out of keeping with the size of the tumor and may be complex in its pathogenesis—decreased caloric intake (there is often a perverted sense of taste and smell with aversion to specific foods), malabsorption, loss of protein (e.g., hemorrhage or effusions), fever, and possibly a change in metabolic pathways. For example, increased anaerobic glycolysis with enhanced gluconeogenesis from amino acids and partial insulin resistance have been described. Possibly factors capable of distorting metabolism are secreted by the tumor, for example, cachectin, a macrophage-derived factor that is capable of inhibiting the activity of certain lipogenic enzymes. Certainly the caloric expenditure tends to remain high, and the basal metabolic rate is increased, despite the reduced intake of calories, suggesting a deranged metabolism.

Treatment of the underlying tumor is the major approach to therapy. Replacement alimentation is reserved for patients undergoing surgical treatment or for patients with severe nutritional deficiency but for whom there is hope for significant remission or cure.

ENDOCRINE PARANEOPLASTIC SYNDROMES. The original description of a paraneoplastic syndrome was that of ectopic Cushing's syndrome, as reported by Brown in 1928. The endocrine neoplastic syndromes are listed in Table 173–1 and are described in detail in Ch. 173, to which the reader is referred.

NEUROLOGIC PARANEOPLASTIC SYNDROMES (Table 171–1). Neurologic signs and symptoms appear frequently in cancer patients and are most often directly related to metastases, fluid and electrolyte abnormalities, vascular abnormalities, infections, or toxicity of therapy. True paraneoplastic syndromes are generally diagnosed by exclusion of these other conditions (Ch. 174). Subacute cerebellar degeneration, subacute motor neuropathy, sensory neuropathy, Eaton-Lambert syndrome, and dermatomyositis in older males are so strongly associated with cancer that their presence should lead to a search for a primary tumor when none is evident.

HEMATOLOGIC PARANEOPLASTIC SYNDROMES. Cancers may indirectly affect any of the hematopoietic cell lines, producing increases or decreases in either individual cell lineages or multiple lineages. Increased cell numbers are generally produced when the tumor secretes a stimulatory hormone/growth factor.

Erythrocytosis most often results from erythropoietin production by renal or liver tumors. In a large review, paraneoplastic erythrocytosis when found was most often associated with hypernephromas (35 per cent), benign renal abnormalities (14 per cent), hepatomas (19 per cent), cerebellar hemangioblastomas (15 per cent), uterine tumors (7 per cent), adrenal tumors and pheochromocytomas (3 per cent), and miscellaneous tumors (3 per cent). In rare cases, induction of local kidney or systemic hypoxia by tumors may also result in erythrocytosis.

Leukemoid reactions, granulocytosis, eosinophilia, and/or basophilia are most often produced when the tumor secretes a colony-stimulating factor (CSF) and thus are corrected by effective treatment of the primary tumor. Granulocytosis is most often associated with lung, gastric, pancreatic, and brain cancers; melanomas; and Hodgkin's and non-Hodgkin's lymphomas. Eosinophilia is most often associated with lymphomas, especially Hodgkin's disease, and gastrointestinal carci-

TABLE 171–1. PARANEOPLASTIC SYNDROMES

1. Wasting of the host—"tumor cachexia"
2. Endocrine/hormone—see Table 173–1
3. Neuromyopathies—see Table 174–1
4. Hematologic
   - Erythrocytosis, granulocytosis, thrombocytosis
   - Anemia (chronic disease, pure red cell aplasia, hypersplenic, autoimmune hemolytic anemia, microangiopathic hemolytic anemia)
   - Granulocytopenia, thrombocytopenia
5. Thromboembolic
   - Venous thrombosis (Trousseau's syndrome)
   - Disseminated intravascular coagulation
   - Nonbacterial thrombotic endocarditis (murantic endocarditis)
6. Renal
   - Secondary to hormonal or metabolic effects
   - Glomerulopathies—including the nephrotic syndrome
   - Miscellaneous—myeloma kidney, amyloidosis, uric acid nephropathy, etc.
7. Dermatologic—see Table 175–4
8. Gastrointestinal
   - Anorexia, nausea, vomiting
   - Protein-losing enteropathy
   - Malignant hepatopathy
9. Miscellaneous
   - Lactic acidosis
   - Clubbing/hypertrophic pulmonary osteoarthropathy
   - Hyperlipidemia
   - Hypertension—hypotension
   - Hyperamylasemia
   - Amyloidosis
   - Arthritis

nomas. These syndromes must be differentiated from chronic myelogenous leukemia and other causes of leukemoid reactions such as infection, inflammatory diseases, metabolic diseases, and certain drugs (Ch. 151).

Anemia is frequently associated with malignant disease, and granulocytopenia and thrombocytopenia may also be paraneoplastic in nature. *Autoimmune hemolytic anemia* is most often associated with B cell lymphoproliferative neoplasms and less often with ovarian and lung cancers (Ch. 139). Successful treatment of the primary tumor often leads to improvement; corticosteroids are usually unsuccessful. *Pure red cell aplasia* is found in association with thymomas (50 per cent) and a variety of other cancers.

Microangiopathic hemolytic anemia, a rare cause of anemia in patients with cancer, is diagnosed by the presence of severe hemolytic anemia with fragmented erythrocytes seen in the blood smear and a negative Coombs test. Most often this syndrome is associated with mucin-producing adenocarcinomas, especially those from the stomach (55 per cent), breast (13 per cent), lung (7 per cent), and unknown primary site (10 per cent). It is often abrupt in onset and associated with thrombocytopenia and disseminated intravascular coagulation.

Granulocytopenia is usually the result of chemotherapy, radiation therapy, severe infection, or marrow involvement, but has been reported rarely in association with thymoma. A syndrome resembling *idiopathic thrombocytopenic purpura (ITP)* may occur in association with lymphomas (especially chronic lymphocytic leukemia, Hodgkin's disease, and immunoblastic lymphadenopathy) and less frequently with other malignant disorders.

THROMBOEMBOLIC PARANEOPLASTIC SYNDROMES. A *hypercoagulable* state is frequent in cancer patients and may manifest as: (1) *migratory thrombophlebitis* (Trousseau's syndrome); (2) subacute or overt *disseminated intravascular coagulation* (DIC); and (3) *nonbacterial thrombotic endocarditis* (NBTE, murantic endocarditis); or (4) a combination of these three.

Thrombophlebitis occurs in as many as 1 to 11 per cent of cancer patients and is most often associated with mucin-producing adenocarcinomas of the gastrointestinal tract. It may also be seen with lung, breast, ovarian, and prostate cancers. The treatment of migratory thrombophlebitis is difficult; acute episodes require heparin. Long-term therapy with warfarin is generally unsuccessful, but long-term administration of subcutaneous heparin has had some limited success.

DIC may present as an acute hemorrhagic diathesis or be discovered incidentally as chronic laboratory abnormalities. Coagulation abnormalities by laboratory test may be seen in as many as 90 per cent of patients with cancer, but most of these never develop overt bleeding episodes. Acute episodes are most frequently associated with acute promyelocytic leukemia (APL) and adenocarcinomas (especially prostatic). Identification and treatment of all precipitating factors are the keystones to the management of DIC. This includes therapy for the primary tumor as well as for infection, acidosis, and other factors. Heparin is often used prophylactically in APL although this is not mandatory if all coagulation parameters are normal and are monitored closely. For overt DIC, heparin appears to be superior to warfarin; spontaneous remission of DIC may occur in adenocarcinomas without any therapy.

NBTE is characterized by sterile verrucous lesions on the left-sided heart valves; these thrombi may embolize to the brain and other vital organs. These occur most often with mucin-producing adenocarcinomas. Therapy is directed to the primary tumor. The therapeutic role of heparin and warfarin is uncertain.

RENAL PARANEOPLASTIC SYNDROMES. Most renal abnormalities that occur in patients with cancer are due to metatases, obstruction, electrolyte and fluid imbalances, toxicity of therapy, or infection. The most common renal paraneoplastic syndrome, other than those linked to hormones (e.g., SIADH), is the nephrotic syndrome. In one report 10 per cent of patients with nephrotic syndrome had underlying malignant disease, with Hodgkin's disease being the most frequently associated disorder. Most of these patients have lipoid nephrosis (minimal change glomerulopathy). In contrast, patients with non-Hodgkin's lymphomas often have immunoglobulin deposits suggesting an immune complex etiology. In both instances the nephrotic syndrome resolves if there is a response to antitumor therapy. Patients with carcinomas most often have membranous glomerulonephritis with subepithelial electron-dense deposits. Other renal abnormalities associated with cancer include (1) the host of abnormalities associated with multiple myeloma and amyloidosis (Ch. 163); (2) the potassium wasting and hypokalemia syndrome caused by lysozyme secreted by patients with acute myelogenous leukemia (M4 or M5); (3) the syndrome of intrarenal obstruction preceded by mucoprotein secreted by patients with pancreatic carcinoma; and (4) the syndrome of nephrogenic diabetes insipidus found in some patients with leiomyosarcoma.

DERMATOLOGIC PARANEOPLASTIC SYNDROMES. This group of syndromes is summarized in Ch. 175. The strongest dermatologic associations with malignant disease are with acanthosis nigricans, erythema gyratum repens, tylosis, dermatomyositis in older males, flushing in the carcinoid syndrome and with the hereditary syndromes (Gardner's syndrome, Peutz-Jegher's syndrome, etc).

GASTROINTESTINAL PARANEOPLASTIC SYNDROMES. *Protein-losing enteropathy* may be produced by inflammation and ulceration of the mucosa, obstruction of intestinal lymphatics (lymphomas), congestive heart failure (carcinoid, pericardial constriction), and by undefined mechanisms. While hypoalbuminemia is common in cancer patients, true protein-losing enteropathy is rare.

Malignant *hepatopathy* (Stauffer's syndrome) is characterized by biochemical abnormalities (increased alkaline phosphatase, hypercholesterolemia, prolonged prothrombin time) and hepatosplenomegaly in association with hypernephroma or malignant schwannoma without liver metastases. These abnormalities improve following resection of the primary tumor.

MISCELLANEOUS PARANEOPLASTIC SYNDROMES. *Fever* is a common finding in cancer patients and is often idiopathic. This is most common in lymphomas (where it is associated with a poor prognosis), hypernephromas, osteogenic sarcomas, and myxomas, although it may be found with other tumors. It almost always disappears with successful antitumor therapy. *Lactic acidosis* may be associated with acute leukemias and lymphomas and responds to successful antitumor therapy. *Hyperlipidemias* have been reported in association with multiple myeloma, hepatoma, and colon cancer.

Hypokalemia and hypertension with tumor production of renin have been reported with lung cancer, hypernephroma, and Wilms' tumor. *Hypotension* has been reported in association with a prostaglandin A–secreting hypernephroma and with intrathoracic tumors secondary to abnormal baroreceptor responses. *Hyperamylasemia* may be caused by lung cancers, especially adenocarcinomas, and is generally not associated with symptoms.

Hypertrophic pulmonary osteoarthropathy is characterized by clubbing, periostitis of the long bones, and occasionally polyarthritis. Involved bones include the distal ends of the tibia, fibula, humerus, radius, or ulna. It is associated most frequently with lung cancer (except small-cell), mesothelioma (especially the benign form), and other cancers when they metastasize to the lungs or mediastinum. The abnormalities improve with successful treatment of the primary tumor. The etiology is unknown.

Amyloidosis occurs in association with multiple myeloma, lymphoma, or carcinomas (especially hypernephroma) in about 15 per cent of cases. The amyloidogenic protein is monoclonal light-chain (AL) in the case of B cell tumors; other proteins (AA) are associated with other tumors (Ch. 210). Amyloidosis causes signs and symptoms by deposition in nerves, heart, kidney, and joints. Prognosis is poor, and there is no specific therapy. *Polyarthritis* has been reported in association with breast and other cancers. *Polymyalgia rheumatica* may precede development of several forms of cancer, and *systemic lupus erythematosus* (SLE) is associated with lymphomas, leukemias, thymomas, and testicular, lung, and ovarian cancers. Remission of SLE may occur with successful antitumor therapy.

Antman KH, Skarin AT, Mayer RJ, et al.: Microangiopathic hemolytic anemia and cancer: A review. Medicine 58:377, 1979. *Reviews the clinical manifestations and etiology of this syndrome.*

Barnes BE: Dermatomyositis and malignancy. A review of the literature. Ann Intern Med 84:68, 1976. *This review evaluates the association of dermatomyositis and malignant disease and shows the strong association in older males.*

Bunn PA Jr, Minna JD: Paraneoplastic syndromes. In DeVita VT, Hellman S, Rosenberg SA (eds.): The Principles and Practice of Oncology. Philadelphia, JB Lippincott Company, 1985, pp 1797–1842. *This chapter is an extensive review of all types of paraneoplastic syndromes with a complete bibliography*

Crowthers D, Bateman CJT: Hematologic aspects of systemic disease—malignant disease. Clin Hematol 1:447, 1972. *This review discusses the various hematologic paraneoplastic syndromes in more detail.*

Markham M: Response of paraneoplastic syndromes to antineoplastic therapy. West J Med 144:5, 1986. *A thorough review of the paraneoplastic syndromes that improve or disappear in response to effective antitumor therapy*

McKinney TD (ed.): Renal Complications of Neoplasia. New York, Praeger, 1986. *A thorough review of all of the renal paraneoplastic syndromes.*

Rickles FR, Edwards RL: Activation of blood coagulation in cancer: Trousseau's syndrome revisited. Blood 63:14, 1983. *Reviews the possible causes of the hypercoagulable state in cancer.*

Sack GH, Levin J, Bell WR: Trousseau's syndrome and other manifestations of chronic disseminated coagulopathy in patients with neoplasms. Medicine 56:1, 1977. *A thorough review of the various manifestations of the hypercoagulable state associated with cancer.*

Torti FM, Dieckmann B, Beutler B, et al.: A macrophage factor inhibits adipocyte gene expression: An in vitro model of cachexia. Science 229:867, 1985. Theologides A: Anorexins, asthenins, and cachectins in cancer. Am J Med 81:696, 1986. *These two articles suggest that "cachectin"–"tumor necrosis factor" and/or other monokines may play a role in the cachexia of malignant disease.*

172 TUMOR MARKERS

Paul A. Bunn, Jr.

In malignant disease there is aberrant expression of a number of genes. Many of the products of these genes, including hormones, enzymes, immunoglobulins, and a variety of other proteins, may be secreted by the tumor cell. If there is sufficient secretion (dependent on the tumor burden and the secretory capacity of each cell) without rapid metabolic degradation, the secreted protein may be detectable in the serum. These proteins or biomarkers are potentially useful for (1) screening populations, (2) early detection of patients with suspected disease, (3) assessing tumor burden and prognosis, (4) assessing response to therapy, and (5) evaluating early recurrence. Currently available radioimmunoassays can often detect minute amounts (nanograms) of the marker substance. All of the marker proteins, however, are products of normal cells and may be present in small amounts in normal serum. Furthermore, the levels of some marker proteins may also increase with inflammation. Thus the specificity of each marker must be well defined. Very few tumor markers are sufficiently sensitive and specific to be useful for each of these above purposes. The most established tumor markers include the beta subunit of human chorionic gonadotropin (beta-HCG), alpha fetoprotein (AFP), idiotypic immunoglobulins, and carcinoembryonic antigen (CEA). A list of currently used markers is shown in Table 172–1.

HORMONES. Human chorionic gonadotropin *HCG* is a two-chain (alpha and beta subunits) glycoprotein hormone secreted by the trophoblastic epithelium of the placenta. The beta subunit is normally present in maternal serum during pregnancy, but its presence in males and nonpregnant females is indicative of cancer. Measurement of HCG has been used

TABLE 172–1. TUMOR CELL MARKERS

Marker	Tumor Types
Hormones	
Beta subunit of chorionic gonadotropin	Testicular cancers, choriocarcinoma, hydatidiform mole
AVP, ACTH	Small-cell lung; APUD tumors
Calcitonin	Medullary thyroid carcinoma, small-cell lung and APUD tumors
Gastrin-releasing peptide (bombesin)	Small-cell lung cancer
Placental lactogen	Trophoblastic tumors, various carcinomas
Oncofetal Proteins	
Alpha-fetoprotein	Hepatoma, testicular cancers
Carcinoembryonic antigen (CEA)	Gastrointestinal tract, breast, lung, ovarian cancers
Enzymes	
L-dopa decarboxylase	Small-cell lung cancer
Creatine phosphokinase (BB)	Prostate cancer, small-cell lung cancer
Neuron-specific enolase	Prostate cancer, small-cell lung cancer, others
Acid phosphatase (prostate specific)	Prostate cancer
Placental alkaline phosphatase	Uterus, ovary, breast, lung cancers
Lysozyme	Acute nonlymphatic leukemia (myelomonocytic and monocytic types)
Serum galactosyltransferase	Gastrointestinal carcinomas, breast and prostate cancers
Lactic dehydrogenase (LDH)	Lymphomas, Ewing's sarcoma, various carcinomas
Secreted Tumor Antigens	
CA 125	Ovarian cancer, other epithelial cancers
CA 19-9	Various carcinomas
Other glycosphingolipids	Various carcinomas
β_2 microglobulin	Multiple myeloma
Miscellaneous	
Vitamin B_{12}–binding proteins	Acute or chronic myelogenous leukemia, myeloproliferative disease
Immunoglobin	B cell lymphoproliferative diseases
Polyamines	Various carcinomas
Chromogranin A	Small-cell lung cancer
Proton NMR spectroscopy	All malignant tumors

for the diagnosis and management of trophoblastic tumors (choriocarcinoma, hydatidiform mole), and certain germ cell tumors of the testes. Its level has prognostic importance. The rate of decline may be used to assess the effectiveness of therapy, and its reappearance is direct evidence of tumor recurrence. Extragonadal germ cell tumors often secrete beta-HCG and it can be used to help confirm the origin of undifferentiated mediastinal or retroperitoneal tumors. Beta-HCG may also be secreted by adenocarcinomas of the ovary, pancreas, stomach, and lung and by hepatomas.

A variety of other hormones may be useful tumor markers. Human placental lactogen is secreted by the majority of trophoblastic tumors and a minority of lung cancers, hepatomas, endocrine tumors, leukemias, and lymphomas.

Polypeptide hormones such as adrenocorticotropic hormone (*ACTH*) and arginine vasopressin (*AVP*) may be useful markers when produced by small-cell lung cancer or other tumors with properties of amine precursor uptake and decarboxylation (APUD tumors). Similarly, *calcitonin* is used to predict medullary carcinoma of the thyroid in families or it can be used as a marker in APUD tumors that secrete it. *Gastrin-releasing peptide* (bombesin-like protein) is produced by the majority of small-cell lung cancers. It is not an ideal tumor marker, however, because it is rapidly degraded in plasma. Elevated levels in the cerebrospinal fluid (CSF) may be useful for predicting leptomeningeal metastases.

ONCOFETAL PROTEINS. *Alpha-fetoprotein* (AFP) is normally secreted in large amounts during the twelfth through fifteenth weeks of gestation and then declines to low levels (<40 ng per milliliter) by the age of one year. Elevated levels occur in the majority (75 per cent) of patients with embryonal and teratocarcinomas of the testes and ovary, as well as in those with extragonadal germ cell tumors. Like beta-HCG, the level has prognostic implications; the rate of decline predicts the effectiveness of therapy, and a rising titer is direct evidence of tumor progression. Elevated AFP levels are present in 70 to 95 per cent of hepatomas. The incidence is highest in areas where hepatoma is endemic. AFP is increased in a minority of patients with cancers of the pancreas, stomach, colon, and lung. Since AFP is produced by normal cells, there are instances of "false positives." AFP may be produced by benign liver tumors, by cirrhotic livers, or during hepatitis, although these entities usually produce levels less than 500 ng per milliliter. AFP may be increased in patients with ataxia-telangiectasia.

Carcinoembryonic antigen (CEA) is normally secreted during the second to sixth months of gestation. In nonsmoking adults, serum levels are less than 2.5 ng per milliliter, whereas smokers have normal levels up to 5 ng per milliliter. Serum levels of CEA may increase in a variety of inflammatory conditions (e.g., cirrhosis, pancreatitis, inflammatory bowel disease, and rectal polyps) as well as in a variety of human cancers.

Elevated levels of CEA are reported in patients with colon cancer (60 to 90 per cent), pancreatic cancer (80 per cent), gastric cancer (60 per cent), lung cancer (75 per cent), breast cancer (50 per cent), and many other malignant tumors in lower frequency. The frequency with which the level of CEA is elevated and the level attained are dependent on the extent of disease, the degree of differentiation (well-differentiated tumors produce more), and the presence of liver metastases. Because of the high false positive rate in inflammatory diseases, the principal use of CEA is in monitoring response to therapy and disease progression, especially for carcinoma of the colon (Ch. 107). Elevated levels should return to normal following complete resection of the primary tumor. A persistent elevation or an increasing concentration is highly suggestive of residual or recurrent tumor. Surgical reexploration in the face of increasing CEA without clinical evidence of disease may lead to discovery of surgically resectable recurrences. These patients may then have a long disease-free survival.

Radiolabeled antibodies to CEA and AFP are being evaluated for their ability to detect metastatic disease and for therapy. Preliminary studies show sensitivities in the range of 60 to 80 per cent.

ENZYMES. A variety of enzymes are also useful tumor markers in some settings. The key APUD enzyme, L-dopa decarboxylase, is often increased in patients with small-cell lung cancer and other APUD tumors. The serum level of the BB isoenzyme of creatine phosphokinase is elevated in the majority of patients with small-cell lung cancer or cancer of the prostate. Serum levels of neuron-specific enolase are often elevated in patients with these same tumors.

Prostatic epithelium also produces a specific *acid phosphatase* (*prostatic acid phosphatase*) whose serum level is elevated in about one third of patients with occult prostatic cancer and in 75 per cent of patients with more advanced prostatic cancers. *Placental alkaline phosphatase* is secreted by a minority of cancers of the female reproductive organs and breast and lung cancers. *Lysozyme*, a monocyte-derived enzyme, is frequently increased in patients with acute monocytic and myelomonocytic leukemia. An isoenzyme of *serum galactosyltransferase* is present in the serum of patients with gastrointestinal carcinomas (75 per cent), and breast cancer (78 per cent), as well as in a minority of patients with prostatic cancer and lymphoproliferative cancers. Serum lactic dehydrogenase (LDH) levels are elevated in a variety of malignant diseases, including lymphomas (especially Burkitt's), Ewing's sarcomas, and a variety of carcinomas. The extent of elevation may provide prognostic information as well as a useful measure of antitumor response.

SECRETED TUMOR ANTIGENS. The development of monoclonal antibody technology has led to recognition of many new glycoprotein and glycolipid antigens on tumor cells that may be secreted into the plasma. The antigen recognized by the monoclonal antibody *CA 125* is a useful marker for the majority of patients with ovarian cancer. *CA 19-9* recognizes an antigen secreted by many epithelial carcinomas, including colon cancer, but this marker is probably less useful than CEA. Many epithelial carcinomas, especially adenocarcinomas, secrete glycosphingolipids such as Lewis blood group antigens and human milk fat globule antigens. The value of these markers remains to be established. β_2 microglobulin, an HLA class I antigen, is present on the cell surface of most nucleated cells. It is secreted into the plasma in excess amounts in patients with multiple myeloma, where its level has prognostic value and may be useful in assessing response to therapy.

MISCELLANEOUS. *Vitamin B_{12}*–binding proteins are frequently increased in myeloproliferative disorders and occasionally in acute or chronic myelogenous leukemias. The idiotypic *immunoglobulins* produced by B cell lymphoproliferative malignant disorders are excellent tumor markers and may be used to assess tumor burden as well as to follow response to therapy. More than 99 per cent of patients with multiple myelomas and Waldenstrom's macroglobulinemia secrete a heavy chain or a light chain (Ch. 163). Occasionally these tumors secrete globulins of more than one idiotype. Monoclonal antibodies to the idiotypic immunoglobulin are being evaluated as therapeutic agents. *Polyamines* are generally secreted in direct relation to the rate of proliferation. In many malignant diseases their quantitation has proven to be useful for prognosis and in assessing response. They are not sufficiently sensitive or specific for widespread use. *Chromogranin A* is a 68,000-dalton protein found in the neurosecretory granules of normal and malignant APUD cells. Serum measurement by radioimmunoassay may be a useful marker of small-cell lung cancer disease activity. *Water-suppressed proton nuclear magnetic resonance spectrum* of plasma is dominated by the resonances of plasma lipoprotein lipids. This spectrum narrows in patients with all types of cancer evaluated and is thus a potentially valuable approach to the early detection of cancer and the monitoring of therapy.

Aroney RS, Dermody WC, Aldernderfer P, et al.: Multiple sequential biomarkers in monitoring patients with carcinoma of the lung. Cancer Treat Rep 68:859, 1984. *Reviews the variety of proteins secreted by small-cell lung cancers that can be used as tumor markers.*

Fossel ET, Carr JM, McDonagh J: Detection of malignant tumors. Water suppressed proton nuclear magnetic resonance spectroscopy of plasma. N Engl J Med 315:1369, 1986. *This stimulating novel technique was valuable in the early diagnosis and follow-up of a variety of malignant tumors.*

Hakomori S: Glycosphingolipids. Sci Am 254(5):44, 1986. *This article reviews the various glycosphingolipid antigens present on cancer cells.*

Novis BH, Gluck E, Thomas P, et al.: Serial levels of CA 19-9 and CEA in colonic cancer. J Clin Oncol 4:987, 1986. *An article comparing the utility of these markers.*

Rosen SW, Weintraub BD, Vaitukaitus JL, et al.: Placental proteins and their subunits as tumor markers. Ann Intern Med 82:71, 1975. *A review of the value of placental proteins as tumor markers.*

Sobol RE, O'Connor DT, Addison J, et al.: Elevated serum chromogranin A concentrations in small cell lung cancer. Ann Intern Med 105:698, 1986. *This article is an example of one of several markers of neuroendocrine cells that are useful in following the course of small-cell lung cancer patients.*

Wanebo HJ, Rao B, Pinsky CM, et al.: Preoperative carcinoembryonic antigen level as a prognostic indicator in colorectal cancer. N Engl J Med 299:448, 1978. *This article shows the value of oncofetal markers as prognostic indicators.*

173 ENDOCRINE MANIFESTATIONS OF TUMORS: "ECTOPIC" HORMONE PRODUCTION

William D. Odell

Cancers often produce symptoms by means of the elaboration of humoral or hormonal substances in addition to those symptoms produced directly by tumor mass or invasion.

Although several chemical classes of hormones exist, these cancer humoral or hormonal substances are usually protein or peptide in nature. These protein substances are so ubiquitously distributed in noncancerous tissues that it is difficult to determine whether they are ectopic or eutopic. Furthermore, all cancers appear to be associated with production of such proteins, usually in markedly increased amounts over normal tissues. These proteins are usually biologically inactive or weakly bioactive and produce no recognizable clinical symptoms. When biologically active substances are produced, clinical symptoms result. A very large number of proteins are produced by cancers; those that are hormones or hormone precursors are listed in Table 173–1. Steroids or thyronines seem not to be secreted as part of ectopic endocrine syndromes, although rarely a cancer may convert a bioinactive steroid such as dehydroepiandrosterone to a bioactive one. As discussed under hypercalcemia, some malignant tumors may convert 25-hydroxyvitamin D to 1,25-dihydroxyvitamin D.

ECTOPIC ACTH PRODUCTION. The association of Cushing's syndrome with carcinoma is the most common ectopic endocrine syndrome. Fifty per cent of reported patients have carcinoma of the lung (predominantly oat cell or small round cell), 10 per cent have carcinoma of the thymus, 10 per cent have carcinoma of the pancreas (including carcinoids and islet cell tumors), 5 per cent have medullary carcinoma of the thyroid (which also produces calcitonin), and 5 per cent have neoplasms derived from the neural crest (pheochromocytoma, neuroblastoma, paraganglioma, and ganglioma). Considered conversely, about 3 per cent of patients with oat cell carcinoma of the lung have clinical or laboratory evidence of Cushing's syndrome—often extremely subtly manifested. Although other carcinomas are associated with Cushing's syndrome less frequently, numerous isolated case reports suggest that any carcinoma may show this association.

Immunoactive ACTH can be detected universally in extracts prepared from carcinomas of the lung, colon, stomach, pancreas, or esophagus. In fact, a large glycoprotein containing immunoactivities of both ACTH and beta-melanocyte-stimulating hormone may be extracted from all normal nonendocrine tissues. This material, present in small quantities in normal tissues, is present in large quantities in extracts of carcinomas, regardless of histologic type. It has no biologic activity in sensitive dispersed adrenal cell assays in vitro, but is converted to a 4500 MW bioactive ACTH by exposure to trypsin. Presumably this material in both normal tissue extracts and carcinomas is *proopiomelanocortin* (POMC). An identical material is detectable in the blood of 70 per cent of patients with carcinoma of the lung, regardless of histologic type, using immunoassays. However, only some carcinomas enzymatically convert this biologically inactive POMC to biologically active ACTH. This conversion process is preferentially associated with the histologic types of neoplasms previously listed as being associated with clinical Cushing's syndrome.

POMC, in addition to the ACTH sequence, also contains the sequence of the endorphins, lipotropin, and beta-melanocyte-stimulating hormone. Previous reports of MSH and lipotropin production by cancers are best explained by detection of circulating POMC per se or its cleavage products, lipotropin and/or MSH.

The symptoms produced by the ectopic production of *bioactive* ACTH are varied, ranging from none—simply the laboratory data of increased cortisol—to full features of Cushing's syndrome. Often they are subtle, consisting only of mild weakness or the laboratory finding of hypokalemia without physical abnormalities. Hypokalemia is uncommon in Cushing's disease of pituitary origin. The classic Cushing's syndrome is not commonly associated with cancer, for such physical changes usually require from months to years to be produced and often the neoplasm is present but a short while.

TABLE 173–1. HORMONES REPORTED TO BE SECRETED BY CANCERS

Proopiomelanocortin	Calcitonin
ACTH	Growth hormone
Chorionic gonadotropin	Prolactin
Alpha peptide chain	Gastrin
Beta peptide chain	Secretin
Vasopressin	Glucagon
Somatomedins	Corticotropin releasing hormone
Hypoglycemia-producing factor	Growth hormone releasing hormone
Growth factors	Gastrin-releasing peptide
Osteoclast-activating factor	Somatostatin
1,25-Dihydroxyvitamin D	Chorionic somatotropin
Parathormone-like-factors	Neurophysins
Erythropoietin	Eosinophilopoietin
Hypophosphatemia-producing factor	

The occurrence of psychosis, weakness, hypokalemia, or an abnormal glucose tolerance curve in a patient with known cancer suggest ectopic bioactive ACTH production. Plasma ACTH concentrations are often extremely high, unlike those in Cushing's disease, which are usually "normal" but in association with an elevated cortisol concentration. In addition, suppression with high doses of oral dexamethasone (8 mg per day) usually does not occur in ectopic ACTH syndrome, but does occur in Cushing's disease (of pituitary origin). Adrenal carcinomas or adenomas producing excess cortisol are associated with undetectable or very low levels of plasma ACTH in conjunction with elevated plasma cortisols (see Ch. 230).

Approximately 50 to 60 per cent of patients with bronchial adenoma and ectopic Cushing's syndrome show cortisol or ACTH suppression with administration of large doses of dexamethasone. The most likely explanation is that these neoplasms produce corticotropin-releasing hormone (CRH) (a 41-amino acid peptide normally produced by the hypothalamus to control pituitary ACTH secretion). The tumor CRH stimulates secretion of ACTH by the normal pituitary. In such patients dexamethasone inhibits CRH action directly at the pituitary gland. Although this hypothesis is untested with respect to bronchial adenoma–ACTH syndrome, the production of CRH-like material by tumors has been described.

Treatment of Cushing's syndrome caused by cancer depends upon resection of the tumor or effective chemotherapy. If this is not possible, treatment with drugs that interfere with adrenal steroid synthesis prevents the continued ACTH production from stimulating excess adrenal secretion of cortisol—e.g., metyrapone, aminoglutethimide, or ketoconazole.

In summary, POMC is probably produced in small quantities by all normal nonendocrine tissues. It may be an autocrine or paracrine substance. Cancers produce increased quantities of POMC that can often be detected by immunoassay in increased quantities in the blood of patients with cancer. Selected carcinomas, related to histologic type, metabolize POMC to biologically active ACTH and occasionally MSH or lipotropin, producing the so-called ectopic ACTH-MSH syndrome. These and similar data concerning chorionic gonadotropin (CG) have led to the belief that ectopic humoral syndromes are not ectopic. Why some cancers metabolize POMC and most do not remains an important unanswered question.

HYPERCALCEMIA AND CANCER. Hypercalcemia is a common finding in patients with cancer. In a large series of patients with bronchogenic carcinoma, 12.5 per cent were hypercalcemic. The frequency of hypercalcemia varied with histologic type: 23 per cent with epidermoid carcinoma, 12.5 per cent with anaplastic carcinoma, and 2.5 per cent with adenocarcinoma. When carcinoma-associated hypercalcemia occurs, the tumors most frequently found are carcinoma of the lung (approximately 35 per cent), carcinoma of the kidney (24 per cent), and carcinoma of the ovary (8 per cent). However, any carcinoma may produce hypercalcemia. The cause of hypercalcemia in the majority of patients remains controversial. Multiple substances appear to be involved. Most of these factors appear to stimulate osteoclast activity with resultant increased bone resorption. This increased resorption is not associated with increased bone formation. Such "uncoupling" of resorption and formation is characteristic of cancer hypercalcemia.

The mechanisms of hypercalcemic caused by solid tumors are different from those caused by malignant hematologic disease. The malignant hematologic diseases appear to produce one or more factors that act locally (paracrine effects) to stimulate bone resorption. In contrast, solid tumors causing hypercalcemia act by producing factors that circulate as a hormone and stimulate osteoclastic activity. In addition, the hypercalcemia caused by both solid tumors and hematologic malignant disease is commonly associated with decreased renal clearance of calcium.

Hematologic Malignant Disease and Hypercalcemia. Most patients with multiple myeloma have extensive bone destruction, and 20 to 40 per cent develop hypercalcemia. This hypercalcemia is produced by increased osteoclast activity caused by locally acting factors produced by the myeloma cells. These factors probably include (1) osteoclast-activating factor (OAF), a bone-resorbing protein produced by activated normal lymphocytes; (2) lymphotoxin (produced by lymphocytes); and (3) tumor necrosis factor, also called cachectin (produced by monocytes). All of these proteins stimulate bone resorption in vitro. Decreased renal excretion of calcium is also important in the development of hypercalcemia in these patients.

Many patients with adult T cell lymphoma develop hypercalcemia. Most of the hypercalcemic patients have lymphoma caused by a type C retrovirus, HTLV-I. These cells produce several factors that increase osteoclast activity, including OAF, colony-stimulating factors, and gamma interferon. These tumor cells also produce lymphokines, and thus additional possibilities include lymphotoxin and/or tumor necrosis factor. In addition, these tumor cells hydroxylate 25-hydroxyvitamin D to 1,25-dihydroxyvitamin D, which may also contribute to hypercalcemia by increasing bone resorption in patients with HTLV-I lymphoma.

Solid Tumors and Hypercalcemia. Solid tumors produce a humoral substance or substances that stimulate osteoclast activity. This syndrome of solid-tumor hypercalcemia is usually associated with increased renal cyclic AMP production, inhibition of renal tubule phosphate reabsorption, and increased renal calcium reabsorption, all consistent with the effects of parathormone (PTH). There is no renal bicarbonate wasting, however, as is observed in primary hyperparathyroidism.

Contrary to previous concepts, the hypercalcemia is not due to the ectopic production of PTH: (1) With current assays, PTH is either suppressed or undetectable in this syndrome. (2) PTH messenger RNA is not detectable in such tumors. (3) Anti-PTH antibodies do not inhibit the biologic action of the hypercalcemic factor(s) in in vitro assays of tumor and blood extracts of patients with solid tumors and hypercalcemia. This PTH-like factor does bind to PTH receptors in in vitro cell systems, and its binding is abolished by specific PTH antagonists acting at the receptor level. Purification and characterization of this PTH-like factor are being actively pursued.

Several other proteins that stimulate osteoclastic activity in in vitro assays are also produced: transforming growth factor alpha (TGF-alpha), platelet derived growth factor (PDGF), transforming growth factor beta (TGF-beta). The *sis* oncogene codes for a peptide with homology to PDGF. In vitro PDGF enhances the osteoclast-stimulating potency of TGF-beta and -alpha.

Prostaglandins. Several reports describe hypercalcemia produced by carcinomas that were associated with increased prostaglandin excretion or production. In a few patients, treatment with indomethacin returned elevated serum calcium levels to normal. However, as large numbers of patients were studied, no investigators have reported success with routine use of indomethacin as treatment for hypercalcemia caused by cancer. Production of prostaglandins by cancer with release systemically is probably not a common cause of hypercalcemia in patients.

Concurrent Primary Hyperparathyroidism. Hyperparathyroidism per se is a common disorder and has repeatedly been described in patients with known cancers. The presence of hyperparathyroidism in a patient with cancer may be suggested by a high plasma PTH level (which is very rare in cancer), using amino terminal PTH immunoassays.

Summary. Hypercalcemia is a common abnormality produced by cancer. Since hypercalcemia may itself produce considerable morbidity or even death, recognition and prompt treatment are essential, and the diagnosis should be considered in any patient with cancer who develops polyuria, constipation, lethargy, or personality change. Patients with known carcinomas may be eucalcemic when active and ambulatory, but may rapidly develop dangerous hypercalcemia when immobilized. The nonspecific treatment of severe hypercalcemia is described in Ch. 247. It generally depends on infusions of saline, diuresis with furosemide, and ambulation. If this does not suffice, treatment with mithramycin, which inhibits bone resorption, may be necessary as an emergency procedure. The administration of calcitonin and glucocorticoids has been used for short-term treatment. Diphosphonate or phosphate, given orally, has been used for long-term treatment. Obviously therapy directed toward the tumor itself should be concomitantly employed, but this is much more slowly effective, if at all.

HYPOPHOSPHATEMIA. A rare syndrome of profound hypophosphatemia, with normal serum calcium, in association with an unusual variety of neoplasms, has been described in perhaps 20 patients. The neoplasms producing this syndrome include pleomorphic sarcomas, hemangiomas, giant cell tumors of bone, or benign osteoblastomas. This syndrome may be more common than previously recognized, being sometimes erroneously reported as adult-onset vitamin D–resistant rickets. Recently, patients with prostatic carcinoma were reported to have hypophosphatemia. The syndrome is associated with dramatic phosphaturia, normal or undetectable plasma PTH, normal serum calcium, and, often, severe muscle spasms. There is severe osteomalacia with bone pain and fractures that occur with minimal trauma. In some (perhaps all) patients, the profound phosphaturia is also associated with aminoaciduria and glucosuria. Blood concentrations of 25-hydroxyvitamin D are normal; 1,25-dihydroxyvitamin D concentrations are low. The serum phosphorus returns to normal following resection of the tumor or following treatment with 1,25-dihydroxyvitamin D. These tumors apparently elaborate a material that inhibits 1-hydroxylation of vitamin D by the kidney.

CHORIONIC GONADOTROPIN. A substance similar but probably not identical to normal chorionic gonadotropin (CG) is elaborated by all normal human tissues and is extractable from all carcinomas. In about 5 to 15 per cent of patients with carcinomas of all kinds, this gonadotropin is detectable in blood. The difference between CG secreted by the trophoblast and that contained in normal tissues lies in the carbohydrate composition. Carbohydrate constitutes about a third of the molecular weight of trophoblast CG. Normal tissue CG contains little or no carbohydrate. The degradation rate or metabolic clearance rate of CG from plasma is inversely related to its carbohydrate content. Thus, presumably, carbohydrate-free CG has extremely little biologic activity in vivo and is cleared from plasma with a half-life of minutes. Carbohydrate-rich CG is cleared slowly with a half-life of hours. All carcinomas also secrete CG. However, those associated with detectable blood concentrations also glycosylate this material, increasing biologic activity and slowing metabolic clearance sufficiently to reach detectable blood concentrations. Approximately 10 per cent of patients with a wide variety of carcinomas have elevated blood CG (e.g., carcinoma of the lung, stomach, pancreas, colon). Men with such tumors often have mild gynecomastia. A rare syndrome produced by CG is precocious puberty in boys with hepatoblastoma.

HYPOGLYCEMIA AND CANCER. Tumor-associated hypoglycemia occurs most frequently with neoplasms that can be loosely termed mesotheliomas. They include more specifically fibrosarcomas, neurofibromas, neurofibrosarcomas, spindle cell carcinomas, rhabdomyosarcomas, and leiomyosarcomas. Such tumors are usually large when hypoglycemia is noted, ranging in size from 800 to 10,000 grams, and are found mainly in the abdomen. They may also develop within the thorax. In the remaining one third, the most frequent tumors are hepatic carcinomas (21 per cent), adrenal cortical carcinomas (6 per cent) and a variety of anaplastic adenocarcinomas, pseudomyxomas, and cholangiomas. Studies utilizing both tumor extracts and blood samples can be summarized as follows: (1) A hypoglycemic factor that mimics insulin activity by in vitro bioassay is often demonstrable; (2) insulin itself is usually not demonstrable by insulin radioimmunoassay; and (3) a substance is often detectable in increased concentrations as measured by radioreceptor assays that quantify somatomedins and so-called nonsuppressible insulin-like activity or insulin-like growth factors (IGF-I and IGF-II). Thus, hypoglycemia associated with cancer may be caused by one or more of the somatomedins, a family of protein substances normally elaborated by the liver that differ structurally from insulin but that have many of its biologic properties. Current assay systems indicate that such substances are increased in blood and tumor extracts from some (perhaps 50 per cent), but not all, of the patients with this syndrome.

GROWTH HORMONE AND GROWTH HORMONE RELEASING HORMONE. Acromegaly associated with bronchial carcinoid or pancreatic islet cell tumor occurs in a small number of patients. In at least five of these patients, growth hormone (GH) secretion was restored to normal or the clinical signs of acromegaly subsided after the extrapituitary tumor was removed without any therapy being directed toward the pituitary gland. Extracts from such an adenoma were found to contain a potent substance capable of releasing GH from dispersed pituitary cells in culture. This GH releasing hormone (GHRH) has been shown to be probably identical to that produced by the hypothalamus normally to control secretion of GH. Elaboration of GHRH by a peripheral tumor may therefore have the potential of leading to a pituitary tumor. The presence of an extrapituitary tumor should be excluded in any patient with acromegaly.

In addition to elaboration of GHRH, tumors could elaborate GH per se. High concentrations of GH have been found in extracts of ovarian carcinomas in patients without acromegaly.

CALCITONIN. Calcitonin is normally secreted by the parafollicular cells of the thyroid gland and serves as an excellent hormonal marker of tumors developing from these cells—medullary carcinomas (Ch. 248). Calcitonin is also secreted ectopically by a variety of carcinomas, but since this hormone has little or no biologic effect in normal adults, no symptoms are produced. Elevated plasma concentrations of calcitonin have been described in patients with carcinomas of the lung (regardless of histologic type), colon, breast, and pancreas. Direct synthesis of calcitonin by the tumor or an arteriovenous gradient of the hormone across a tumor has not been reported.

VASOPRESSIN. Schwartz and Bartter first described the syndrome of cancer associated with hyponatremia, hypervolemia, renal sodium loss, and inappropriately high urine osmolality to which their name is sometimes attached (see Ch. 77). The associated symptoms are those of decrease in mental acuity, confusion, or even seizures. This syndrome has been attributed to secretion of arginine vasopressin (AVP) by the tumor; vasopressin has been demonstrated by bioassay and radioimmunoassay in extracts of such neoplasms, and synthesis of AVP (incorporation of tritiated amino acids) by extracts of lung cancer has been found in vitro. Ectopic production of vasopressin is very common in patients with carcinoma of the lung (found in 42 per cent in one series). Excess vasopressin produces no symptoms unless the patient continues to drink "excess" water. In normal persons thirst is suppressed by a fall in plasma osmolality. Possibly the smaller percentage of patients with excess vasopressin who develop symptoms of water intoxication and hyponatremia have both a sustained hypersecretion of vasopressin and a defect in thirst control. The treatment of the syndrome of inappropriate secretion of antidiuretic hormone, sometimes called SIADH, is considered in Ch. 77.

A single larger precursor molecule contains the amino acid sequence of both neurophysin II and arginine vasopressin (see Ch. 227). Normally enzymatic cleavage releases neurophysin II and vasopressin on a mole-for-mole basis. Elevation of plasma neurophysin has been found in approximately 40 per cent of unselected patients with lung carcinoma, a value similar to that found for vasopressin.

ERYTHROPOIETIN. This glycoprotein hormone is normally secreted by the kidney and stimulates differentiation of early red cell stages, resulting in increased red cell production (see Ch. 153). A variety of benign and malignant conditions involving the kidney are associated with erythrocytosis. About two thirds of patients with erythropoietin-induced erythrocytosis have hypernephroma, renal cysts, or hydronephrosis. These are not examples of ectopic hormonal syndromes, but represent retained properties of a neoplasm derived from the tissue normally producing the hormone. About one third of patients have neoplasms derived from tissues not known to produce erythropoietin normally. These include hemangioblastomas (21 per cent), uterine fibromas (6 per cent), adrenal cortical neoplasms (3 per cent), ovarian neoplasms (3 per cent), hepatomas (3 per cent), and pheochromocytomas (1 per cent). The biochemical characteristics of the tumor-produced erythropoietin are indistinguishable from erythropoietin produced by the normal kidney.

EOSINOPHILOPOIETIN. Eosinophilia occurs in an occasional patient with malignant disease. Eosinophilia, irrespective of cause, is in turn often associated with endocardial fibrosis, mural thrombus development, and embolic phenomena. An undifferentiated lung carcinoma that produced this syndrome was found to contain large amounts of an eosinophilopoietin-like material, measured by an in vitro eosinophil colony growth assay. In proximity to fibrotic cardiac endothelium were masses of aggregated eosinophils. These eosinophils were shown to generate large amounts of toxic oxygen species, demonstrated to be toxic to cultured endothelial cells in vitro.

SUMMARY. A large variety of protein hormones or protein hormone-like materials are produced by cancers. Most are biologically inert or weakly bioactive. Similar or identical substances are often produced by most or all normal tissues (e.g., POMC, CG) or by a selected group of normal tissues (e.g., erythropoietin, IGF-I and II). Selected carcinomas, correlated with histologic type, metabolize some of these substances into bioactive forms, producing humoral syndromes. It may presently be hypothesized that ectopic hormone production is not ectopic. Detection and quantification of the biologically inactive or weakly bioactive proteins have been useful in early tumor diagnosis and in following response to therapy.

GENERAL REFERENCES

Frohman LA: Ectopic hormone production. Am J Med 70:995, 1981. *An editorial overview of current concepts concerning production of hormones by tumors. There is a short but useful list of references.*

Mundy GR: Ectopic hormonal syndromes in neoplastic diseases. Hosp Prac 22:113, 1987. *A recent useful review.*

Odell WD: Humoral manifestations of cancer. *In* Williams RH (ed.): Textbook of Endocrinology, 7th ed. Philadelphia, W.B. Saunders Company, 1984, Chapter 31. *A more detailed review of humoral syndromes produced by cancer.*

PROOPIOMELANOCORTIN, LIPOTROPIN, MSH

Saito E, Iwasa S, Odell WD: Widespread presence of large molecular weight adrenocorticotropin-like substances in normal rat extrapituitary tissues. Endocrinology 113:1010, 1983. *This paper shows for the first time that proopiomelanocortin is extractable from all normal nonendocrine tissues.*

HYPERCALCEMIA

Bender RA, Hansen H: Hypercalcemia in bronchogenic carcinoma. A prospective study of 200 patients. Ann Intern Med 80:205, 1974. *An analysis of the frequency of hypercalcemia in patients with various histologic types of lung cancer.*

Breslau NA, McGuire JL, Zerwekh JE, et al.: Hypercalcemia associated with increased serum calcitriol levels in three patients with lymphoma. Ann Intern Med 100:1, 1984. *Evidence for another interesting mechanism for tumor-associated hypercalcemia—that of production of the most active form of vitamin D.*

Goltzman D, Stewart AF, Broadus AE: Malignancy-associated hypercalcemia: Evaluation with a cytochemical bioassay for parathyroid hormone. J Clin Endocrinol Metab 53:899, 1981.

Merendino JJ Jr, Insogna KL, Milstone LM, et al.: A parathyroid hormone-like protein from cultured human keratinocytes. Science 231:388, 1986.

Mundy GR: Pathogenesis of hypercalcemia of malignancy. Clin Endocrinol 23:705, 1985. *This is an outstanding review of hypercalcemia caused by cancer.*

Simpson EL, Mundy GR, D'Souza SM, et al: Absence of parathyroid hormone messenger RNA in nonparathyroid tumors associated with hypercalcemia. N Engl J Med 309:325, 1983.

HYPOPHOSPHATEMIA

Weidner N, Cruz DS: Phosphaturic mesenchymal tumors: A polymorphous group causing osteomalacia or rickets. Cancer 59:1442, 1987. *This is an excellent review of this intriguing topic of the production of reversible metabolic bone disease by tumors.*

CHORIONIC GONADOTROPIN

Yoshimoto Y, Wolfsen AR, Odell WD: Glycosylation, a variable in the production of hCG by cancers. Am J Med 67:414, 1979. *This study demonstrates that hCG-like material is present in extracts of all carcinomas and of all normal human tissues. The hCG in most carcinomas and in all normal tissues except the placenta is very low in or free of carbohydrate. The hCG extracted from placenta or present in cancers or blood of patients with cancer associated with detectable hCG is carbohydrate rich.*

HYPOGLYCEMIA

Gordon P, Hendricks CM, Kahn CR, et al.: Hypoglycemia associated with non-islet-cell tumor and insulin-like growth factors. N Engl J Med 305:1452, 1981.

GROWTH HORMONE AND GROWTH HORMONE RELEASING HORMONE (GHRH)

Frohman LA, Szabo M, Berelowitz M, et al.: Partial purification and characterization of a peptide with growth hormone-releasing activity from extrapituitary tumors in patients with acromegaly. J Clin Invest 65:43, 1980. *This manuscript is a good source of reference for this syndrome. In addition, this offers the first chemical characterization of GHRH extracted from extrapituitary tumors causing pituitary tumors and acromegaly.*

CALCITONIN

Schwartz KE, Wolfsen AR, Forster B, et al.: Calcitonin in the nonthyroidal cancer. J Clin Endocrinol Metab 49:438, 1979. *This report offers a good review of earlier publications and itself indicates the frequency of elevated blood calcitonin in patients with a wide variety of carcinomas. Fluctuations in calcitonin in parallel with removal and relapse of the tumor are shown.*

VASOPRESSIN

Robertson GL, Berl T.: Water metabolism. In Brenner BM, Rector FC Jr (eds.): The Kidney, 3rd ed. W.B. Saunders Co., Philadelphia, 1986, pp. 385–432. *This is an excellent and up-to-date review of the SIADH in the context of a more general discussion of the control of water metabolism.*

EOSINOPHILOPOIETIN

Slungaard A, Ascensao J, Zanjani E, et al.: Pulmonary carcinoma with eosinophilia: Demonstration of a tumor-derived eosinophilopoietic factor. N Engl J Med 309:778, 1983.

174 NONMETASTATIC EFFECTS OF CANCER ON THE NERVOUS SYSTEM

Jerome B. Posner

When patients with systemic cancer develop nervous system dysfunction, metastasis is usually the cause. However, cancer exerts deleterious effects on the nervous system by mechanisms other than metastases. Recognition of these nonmetastatic neurologic complications can prevent inappropriate and perhaps harmful therapy directed at a nonexistent metastasis. Since at times the nervous system symptoms precede the discovery of the cancer, they can also lead the physician to the diagnosis of an otherwise occult neoplasm.

An almost bewildering variety of neurologic disorders have been ascribed to effects of systemic cancer (Table 174–1). Most patients with nervous system dysfunction not caused by metastases are eventually found to be suffering from infection, vascular or metabolic disorders, or from unwanted side effects of chemotherapy. This chapter discusses two other types of nervous system damage related to cancer not described elsewhere in this book: "remote effects" or paraneoplastic syndromes (Table 174–2), and radiation injury.

REMOTE EFFECTS

Remote effects of cancer on the nervous system, paraneoplastic syndromes, are terms that refer to nervous system dysfunction of unknown cause occurring almost exclusively or at higher frequency in patients with cancer. These syndromes are not common. In a series of 1465 patients with cancer, about 7 per cent were found to have unexplained neurologic dysfunction, usually weakness and wasting of proximal muscles associated with absence of or diminished deep tendon reflexes. The more classic paraneoplastic syndromes, cerebellar degeneration and myelopathy, occurred three times each; there was no instance of sensory neuronopathy. Therefore, excluding patients with mild peripheral neuropathy or myopathy possibly associated with cachexia, remote effects probably occur in less than 1 per cent of unselected patients with cancer. Lung cancer, particularly small cell cancer, accounts for more than 50 per cent of cases; the incidence is greatest among patients with ovarian and small cell lung cancer. Because of its rarity, the diagnosis of remote effects should never be

TABLE 174–1. NONMETASTATIC EFFECTS OF CANCER ON THE NERVOUS SYSTEM

Remote Effects or Paraneoplastic Syndromes (see Table 174–2)
Side Effects of Therapy
Chemotherapy
Radiation therapy (see Table 174–3)
Metabolic and Nutritional Abnormalities
Destruction of vital organs (e.g., liver)
Elaboration of hormonal substances by tumor
Competition between tumor and brain for essential substrates (e.g., glucose)
Malnutrition
Infections (usually associated with lymphomas)
Parasites (e.g., toxoplasmosis)
Fungi (e.g., cryptococcosis, aspergillosis, mucormycosis)
Bacteria (e.g., *Listeria monocytogenes* infection)
Viruses (e.g., herpes zoster)
Vascular Disease
Intracranial hemorrhage
Cerebral infarction

TABLE 174–2. REMOTE EFFECTS OF CANCER ON THE NERVOUS SYSTEM (PARANEOPLASTIC SYNDROMES)

Brain and Cranial Nerves
Subacute cerebellar degeneration
Opsoclonus-myoclonus
Limbic encephalitis
Brain stem encephalitis
Optic neuritis
Retinal degeneration
Spinal Cord
Necrotizing myelopathy
Subacute motor neuronopathy
Motor neuron disease
Myelitis
Dorsal Root Ganglia
Subacute sensory neuronopathy
Peripheral Nerve
Subacute or chronic sensorimotor peripheral neuropathy
Acute polyradiculoneuropathy (Guillain-Barré syndrome)
Remitting and relapsing peripheral neuropathy
Mononeuropathies
Mononeuritis multiplex
Brachial neuritis
Autonomic neuropathy
Peripheral neuropathy associated with paraproteinemia
Neuromuscular Junction and Muscle
Lambert-Eaton myasthenic syndrome
Myasthenia gravis
Dermatomyositis, polymyositis
Acute necrotizing myopathy
Carcinoid myopathies
Myotonia
Cachectic myopathy
"Neuromyopathy"

accepted until a thorough evaluation has excluded metastatic or other nonmetastatic causes of neurologic dysfunction. In particular, infiltration of nerve roots by tumor in the leptomeninges may mimic paraneoplastic peripheral neuropathy.

The etiology of remote effects is unknown. Hypotheses have included opportunistic viral infections, competition between tumor and nervous system for essential metabolites, and secretion by tumor of a neurotoxin. The hypothesis for which there is most evidence is that remote effects are autoimmune responses. The evidence includes the demonstration of autoantibodies reactive with specific neurons in the serum of patients with paraneoplastic cerebellar degeneration (see below), subacute sensory neuronopathy (see below), and some other paraneoplastic disorders. Plasma and IgG from patients suffering from Lambert-Eaton myasthenic syndrome (see below) passively transfer that neuromuscular defect to experimental animals. It seems likely that remote effects of cancer are a heterogeneous group of disorders in which different pathogenetic mechanisms play a role. Furthermore, although the disorders described in this chapter are separated by their clinical signs into anatomic categories, more than one clinical syndrome may be present in a given patient. This is particularly true of the dementias, which are often lumped together with brain stem, cerebellar, and spinal cord lesions as carcinomatous encephalomyelitis, and also of myopathy and peripheral neuropathy associated with cancer, often called carcinomatous neuromyopathy.

Brain and Cranial Nerves

CEREBRUM. Cerebral remote effects are usually characterized by dementia with or without other neurologic findings. Dementia usually begins insidiously and progresses. Loss of recent memory and affective alterations, either anxiety or depression, characterize the disorder. Seizures are prominent in some patients, and others have a fluctuating confusional state. When other abnormal neurologic signs are present, they usually point to brain stem, cerebellar, or peripheral nerve involvement. The electroencephalogram is diffusely slow, and the cerebrospinal fluid sometimes contains 10 to 40 lymphocytes per cubic milliliter and a slight elevation of the protein concentration.

Pathologically, there are two main groups. In some patients, no significant pathologic changes are found in the cerebrum despite unequivocal clinical dementia. Other patients demonstrate widespread cerebral neuronal loss and perivascular collections of lymphocytes, particularly in the medial temporal lobes (limbic encephalitis) or the thalamus. The differential diagnosis includes brain or leptomeningeal metastases, fungal or parasitic infections (including multifocal leukoencephalopathy), and metabolic encephalopathy. Focal cerebral signs other than dementia, CT and MRI (Ch. 456), and cerebrospinal fluid studies support the diagnosis of infection or metastatic disease. Metabolic encephalopathy can usually be diagnosed by appropriate laboratory tests, as indicated in Ch. 457. Progressive dementia in middle age accompanied by cerebellar, brain stem, or peripheral nerve dysfunction but no other focal cerebral signs suggests dementia as a remote effect of cancer. There is no specific treatment for these dementias, but they may improve with successful therapy of the cancer.

BULBAR ENCEPHALITIS. Brain stem dysfunction associated with dementia, which develops insidiously or subacutely and is progressive, may be a remote effect of the cancer. The brain stem signs include vertigo, nystagmus, dysphagia, ophthalmoplegia, and at times ataxia and extensor plantar reflexes. The pathologic changes, predominantly in the lower pons and medulla, are those of neuronal loss and perivascular lymphocytic cuffing. The lymphocytic infiltration is responsible for the term *encephalitis*. The cause is unknown, and there is no effective treatment.

CEREBELLUM. Paraneoplastic cerebellar degeneration is clinically sufficiently characteristic to suggest cancer even when neurologic symptoms predate diagnosis of the tumor. Symptoms usually evolve over weeks, with bilateral and symmetric cerebellar dysfunction, the patient being equally ataxic in arms and legs. Severe dysarthria is usually present, and vertigo and diplopia are common, but nystagmus may be absent. Many patients have neurologic signs pointing to disease outside the cerebellum: extensor plantar responses are common; tendon reflexes may be either diminished or exaggerated; and dementia occurs in about half. The cerebrospinal fluid is usually normal, but there may be as many as 40 lymphocytes per cubic milliliter and an elevated protein content. The disease, which may be associated with any cancer, precedes the discovery of the neoplasm by periods of from weeks to three years in more than half the patients. Cerebellar atrophy may be seen on a CT scan, particularly if done late in the course of the illness. Characteristic pathologic changes consist of diffuse or patchy loss of Purkinje cells in all areas of the cerebellum. There may be lymphocytic cuffs around blood vessels, particularly in the deep nuclei. This illness can be distinguished from cerebellar metastases by the symmetry of its signs and the absence of increased intracranial pressure, and from alcoholic-nutritional cerebellar degeneration because dysarthia and ataxia in the upper extremities are prominent in the carcinomatous cerebellar degenerations, and are usually mild or absent in the alcoholic variety. The hereditary cerebellar degenerations rarely run so rapid a course. At times the disorder stabilizes or improves with successful treatment of the tumor. Autoantibodies that react to cytoplasm of Purkinje cells have been identified in the serum of women with paraneoplastic cerebellar degeneration and breast or ovarian cancer. The antigen identified by the antibody has been identified in the tumor of at least one patient suffering cerebellar degeneration. The role of the autoantibody in the pathogenesis of the disease is not established.

Another, less common, cerebellar syndrome is that of opsoclonus (spontaneous, conjugate, chaotic eye movements most severe when voluntary eye movements are attempted). Opsoclonus is frequently associated with cerebellar ataxia and myoclonus of the trunk and extremities. It is most common in children as a remote effect of neuroblastoma. In children, the neurologic symptoms may respond to adrenocorticosteroids or to treatment of the tumor.

Spinal Cord

Two rare but distinct myelopathies complicate cancer: The first, *subacute motor neuronopathy,* affects anterior horn cells, usually in patients with Hodgkin's disease or other lymphomas. The course is subacute, with progressive painless asymmetric lower motor neuron weakness of legs and arms. Some patients complain of sensory symptoms, but sensory loss is mild or absent despite profound weakness. The major pathologic finding is neuronal degeneration of anterior horn cells. Sometimes there is inflammation in the anterior horns and demyelination in the white matter of the spinal cord. The clinical course is different from most remote effects in that many patients improve spontaneously, independent of the course of the underlying lymphoma. The etiology is unknown, but a similar disorder in mice harboring lymphomas appears to be caused by a virus. Rarely, gray matter myelopathies with clinical courses resembling syringomyelia or autonomic insufficiency (q.v.) complicate systemic cancer.

The second complicating condition is *subacute necrotic destruction of the spinal cord,* a myelopathy in which both gray and white matter are affected equally. Clinically, there is rapidly ascending sensory and motor loss, usually to midthoracic levels, the patient becoming paraplegic and incontinent within hours or days. The neurologic symptoms often precede the discovery of the neoplasm, and the illness is clinically and pathologically indistinguishable from idiopathic subacute necrotic myelopathy. Since epidural spinal cord compression from metastatic tumor or arteriovenous spinal cord anomalies may present similar clinical signs, a myelogram is essential. In addition to the two aforementioned entities, many patients with paraneoplastic cerebellar degeneration develop extensor plantar responses, mild sensory changes, and reflex asymmetries and weakness associated with degenerations of long tracts and anterior horn cells of the spinal cord. However, spinal cord symptoms do not predominate in these patients. Amyotrophic lateral sclerosis has been reported as a remote effect of cancer, but it is doubtful that it occurs in patients with cancer more often than in the general population.

Peripheral Nerves and Dorsal Root Ganglia

Four clinical peripheral nerve disorders occur in association with cancer. Characteristic of carcinoma is a *subacute sensory neuronopathy* marked by loss of sensation with relative preservation of motor power. The illness sometimes precedes the appearance of the carcinoma and progresses over a few months, leaving the patient with moderate or severe disability. The cerebrospinal fluid protein is usually elevated. Pathologically, there is destruction of posterior root ganglia with perivascular lymphocytic cuffing and wallerian degeneration of sensory nerves. Many of the patients have inflammatory and degenerative changes in brain and spinal cord as well. The disorder is usually associated with small cell carcinoma, and in some such patients serum autoantibodies reacting against the nuclei of neurons but not other cells have been identified. The antibody is specific for the disorder, but its role in pathogenesis is not known. There is no treatment.

More common than sensory neuropathy is a *distal sensorimotor polyneuropathy* characterized by motor weakness, sensory loss, and absence of distal reflexes in the extremities. The illness is pathologically characterized by either segmental demyelination or wallerian degeneration (or both) of sensory and motor peripheral nerves. Pathologically and clinically, the sensorimotor neuropathy is indistinguishable from polyneuropathies not associated with cancer. Indeed, some have suggested that the late or terminal polyneuropathy may be due to nutritional deprivation associated with cancer. Its etiology, however, is not clear, and it does not respond to treatment with vitamins and other nutritional supplements.

A *polyneuritis* clinically and pathologically indistinguishable from acute postinfectious polyneuropathy (Guillain-Barré syndrome) also complicates cancer, particularly Hodgkin's disease, with impaired immunity. A few patients with *neuropathy limited to the autonomic nervous system* have been reported.

Neuromuscular Junction and Muscles

NEUROMUSCULAR JUNCTION. *Myasthenia gravis* is associated with thymomas, but usually not other systemic tumors. The Lambert-Eaton myasthenic syndrome is characterized by weakness and fatigability of proximal muscles, particularly of the pelvic girdle and thighs. The cranial nerves and respiratory muscles are usually spared. Patients often complain of dryness of the mouth, impotence, pain in the thighs, and peripheral paresthesias. On examination there is weakness of the proximal muscles, but strength increases over several seconds of a sustained contraction. The deep tendon reflexes are diminished or absent. The diagnosis is made by electromyographic studies in which repeated nerve stimulations at rates above ten per second cause a progressive *increase* in the size of the muscle action potential (the opposite of myasthenia gravis). About two thirds of patients with this syndrome either have or will develop cancer, usually small cell carcinoma of the lung. The neuromuscular defect in this illness is believed to be deficient release of acetylcholine. Similar findings have been produced in experimental animals by injection of either serum IgG or extract of tumor in patients with the disorder, suggesting an autoimmune etiology. Plasmapheresis and immune-suppressant drugs may relieve symptoms. The illness responds poorly to anticholinesterase drugs, but does respond to guanidine hydrochloride given in doses of 15 to 40 mg* per kilogram per day.

MUSCLE. Typical *dermatomyositis* or *polymyositis* may occur as a remote effect of cancer (Ch. 443). Fewer than 10 per cent of patients with this disorder have cancer, but the figure is higher in older patients. The clinical picture of polymyositis associated with cancer (i.e., subacute development of weakness, particularly involving proximal muscles and sometimes bulbar muscles) is indistinguishable from that of dermatomyositis or polymyositis not associated with cancer. Pathologically, there may be two groups: one with the typical inflammatory lesions of polymyositis and one with little inflammation but severe muscle necrosis. The latter group may suffer an explosive clinical course. The patients respond somewhat less well to corticosteroid therapy than do those with dermatomyositis unaccompanied by cancer, although substantial improvement with steroid treatment does occur in some.

Muscle Weakness. Some patients with cancer complain of *weakness* and *fatigability* that seem worse than can be accounted for by their cancer alone. Cachexia and weight loss alone do not usually cause measurable muscle weakness. The weakness is usually proximal and produces particular difficulty climbing stairs or getting out of low chairs. Ankle reflexes may be diminished or absent. Further neurologic evaluation does not yield findings diagnostic of one of the remote effects of cancer described above. Brain and his colleagues have labeled this entity a neuromyopathy because its exact anatomic locus is unclear, but others have suggested that it is a nonspecific accompaniment of cachexia and systemic illness. Specific (type II) muscle fiber atrophy develops early in patients with systemic cancer. The cause and treatment of the weakness are unknown.

Anderson NE, Cunningham JM, Posner JB: Autoimmune pathogenesis of paraneoplastic neurological syndromes. CRC Crit Rev Clin Neurobiol. (in

*May exceed manufacturer's recommended maximum dosage.

press) *A comprehensive review of paraneoplastic syndromes, with emphasis on the evidence for autoimmune pathogenesis.*
Henson RA, Urich H: Cancer and the Nervous System. Oxford, Blackwell Scientific Publications, Ltd., 1982. *Comprehensive descriptions of all of the paraneoplastic disorders affecting the nervous system.*

NERVOUS SYSTEM INJURY FROM THERAPEUTIC RADIATION

Adverse effects of ionizing radiation on the nervous system (Table 174–3) are related to the total dose of radiation, the size of each fraction, the total duration over which the dose is received, and the volume of nervous system tissue irradiated. Other factors, such as underlying nervous system disease (e.g., brain tumor, cerebral edema), previous surgery, concomitant use of chemotherapeutic agents, and individual susceptibility make it impossible to define precisely a safe dose of radiation therapy for a given individual. However, guidelines allow the radiation therapist to calculate generally safe nervous system doses. Adverse effects may involve any portion of the central or peripheral nervous system and may occur acutely or be delayed weeks to years following irradiation.

CLINICAL MANIFESTATIONS. *Acute encephalopathy* may follow large radiation doses to the brains of patients with increased intracranial pressure, particularly in the absence of corticosteroid prophylaxis. Immediately following treatment, susceptible patients develop headache, nausea and vomiting, somnolence, fever, and occasionally worsening of neurologic signs, rarely culminating in cerebral herniation and death. Acute encephalopathy usually follows the first radiation fraction and becomes progressively less severe with each ensuing fraction. This disorder is believed to result from increased intracranial pressure and/or brain edema from radiation-induced alteration of the blood-brain barrier. It responds to corticosteroids. Acute worsening of neurologic symptoms does not occur after spinal cord irradiation.

Early delayed reactions appear 6 to 16 weeks after therapy and persist for days to weeks. A transient, diffuse encephalopathy commonly follows prophylactic irradiation of the brain for leukemia in children and for small cell lung cancer in adults. The disorder is characterized by somnolence, often associated with headache, nausea, vomiting, and sometimes fever. The electroencephalogram may be slow, but there are no focal signs. Whole-brain irradiation for brain tumor sometimes causes lethargy and worsening of focal neurologic signs, simulating progression of the brain tumor. CT may also indicate worsening. Both disorders usually respond to steroids, but if untreated will resolve spontaneously. A brain stem disorder characterized by diplopia, ataxia, dysarthria and dysphagia, and associated with foci of demyelination resembling acute multiple sclerosis, rarely follows irradiation to the brain stem. *Early delayed myelopathy* follows radiation therapy to the neck or upper thorax and is characterized by Lhermitte's sign (an electric shock–like sensation radiating into various parts of the body when the neck is flexed). The symptoms resolve spontaneously. Early delayed radiation syndromes are believed to result from demyelination, possibly due to radiation-induced damage to oligodendroglia.

TABLE 174–3. RADIATION INJURY TO THE NERVOUS SYSTEM

Time After RT	Organ Affected	Clinical Findings
Primary injury		
Immediate (min to hrs)	Brain	Acute encephalopathy
Early delayed (6–16 wks)	Brain	Somnolence, focal signs
	Spinal cord	Lhermitte's sign
Late delayed (mos to yrs)	Brain	Dementia, focal signs
	Spinal cord	Transverse myelopathy
	Peripheral nerves	Paralysis, sensory loss
Secondary injury (years)	Several	Brain, cranial and/or peripheral nerve sheath tumors
	Arteries (atherosclerosis)	Cerebral infarction
	Endocrine organs	Metabolic encephalopathy

Late delayed radiation injury appears after months to years and may affect any part of the nervous system. In the brain, there are two clinical syndromes. The first follows whole-brain irradiation either prophylactically or in some patients with primary and metastatic brain tumors. The disorder is characterized by dementia without focal signs. There is cerebral atrophy on CT scan, pathologic changes are nonspecific, and there is no treatment. The second disorder affects patients who receive either focal brain irradiation during therapy of extracranial neoplasms or whole-brain irradiation for intracranial neoplasms. Neurologic signs suggest a mass and include headache, focal or generalized seizures, and hemiparesis. Brain CT scans reveal a hypodense mass, sometimes with contrast enhancement. Neuropathologic features include coagulative necrosis of white matter, telangiectasia, fibrinoid necrosis and thrombus formation, and glial proliferation and bizarre multinucleated astrocytes. The clinical and CT findings cannot be distinguished from brain tumor, and the diagnosis can be made only by biopsy. Corticosteroids sometimes ameliorate symptoms. The treatment, if the disorder is focal, is surgical removal. *Late delayed myelopathy* is characterized by progressive paralysis, sensory changes, and sometimes pain. A Brown-Sequard syndrome (weakness and loss of proprioception in the extremities of one side with loss of pain and temperature sensation on the other) is often present at onset. Patients occasionally respond transiently to steroids, and the disorder may stop progressing, but generally patients become paraplegic or quadriplegic. Pathologic changes include necrosis of the spinal cord. *Late delayed neuropathy* may affect any cranial or peripheral nerve. Common disorders are blindness from optic neuropathy and paralysis of an upper extremity from brachial plexopathy after therapy for lung or breast cancer. The pathogenesis is probably fibrosis and ischemia of the plexus. There is no treatment.

Radiation-induced tumors, including meningiomas, sarcomas, or, less commonly, gliomas, may appear years to decades after cranial irradiation and may follow even low doses. Malignant or atypical nerve sheath tumors may follow irradiation of the brachial, cervical, and lumbar plexuses. The central nervous system may also be damaged when radiation alters extraneural structures. Radiation therapy accelerates *atherosclerosis*, and cerebral infarction associated with carotid artery occlusion in the neck may occur many years after neck irradiation. *Endocrine* (pituitary, thyroid, parathyroid) dysfunction from radiation may be associated with neurologic signs. Hypothyroidism often presents as a neurologic disorder, and hyperthyroidism or hyperparathyroidism from radiation may also cause an encephalopathy.

Gilbert HA, Kagan AR (eds.): Radiation Damage to the Nervous System. A Delayed Therapeutic Hazard. New York, Raven Press, 1980. *A comprehensive description of all of the nervous system side effects of therapeutic irradiation.*

175 CUTANEOUS MANIFESTATIONS OF INTERNAL MALIGNANCY

Frank Parker

Cutaneous changes associated with internal malignant disease are diverse. Some skin alterations are clear indicators of underlying malignant disease. Others, less specific, arise in either the presence or absence of malignancy, but occur with sufficient frequency to arouse suspicion and the need to search for underlying carcinoma or lymphoma. These various skin findings may precede any signs associated with the internal malignant disease; they are therefore of crucial importance in early identification and cure of internal neoplasms.

Skin manifestations of internal malignant disease can be classified into two major groups: (1) those in which malignant cells can be found in the skin on biopsy (specific skin lesions) and (2) those in which malignant cells cannot be identified on a skin biopsy (nonspecific skin lesions). The specific lesions are diagnostic of the internal malignant disease, while the nonspecific skin alterations may or may not be associated with an internal neoplasm. Some of the nonspecific skin changes are clear indicators of underlying tumor; others merely arouse concern.

SPECIFIC SKIN LESIONS ASSOCIATED WITH INTERNAL MALIGNANT DISEASE

Carcinomas, leukemia, lymphoma, plasma cell dyscrasias, and sarcomas can all affect the skin specifically in clinically identifiable patterns. A biopsy of a suspicious skin lesion is helpful because the tissue of origin (primary underlying neoplasm) can often be identified.

Skin Metastases (Table 175–1 and Color plate *6A*)

Metastases to the skin are comparatively rare (approximately 1 to 5 per cent of internal malignancies), but when present are readily diagnosed by biopsy. Cutaneous metastases usually appear as flesh-colored to red-purple or brownish solitary papules or nodules, stony-hard to the touch, and often innocent in appearance. There is no relationship between site of origin and size, color, and consistency of the metastatic deposit. Lung cancer in men and breast cancer in women most commonly involve the skin; other sources include malignant tumors of the gastrointestinal tract, kidney, ovary, uterus, and urinary bladder and oral cavity carcinomas.

Clinical patterns of metastatic spread to skin depend on several factors such as the organ of origin and whether tumor is disseminated by lymphatics or blood. In general, those neoplasms that spread via lymphatics, such as breast and oral cavity carcinoma, localize in the skin late in the clinical course. Tumors that often embolize through venous channels, such as those arising in the lung, kidney, and ovary, can appear early in the skin and thus may be the first indication of the internal malignant disease.

Certain areas of the skin are predisposed to metastases, localizing near the site of the primary cancer (Table 175–1). Thus, abdominal wall metastases, especially around the umbilicus (Sister Mary Joseph's nodules), arise from neoplasms of the stomach, kidney, and ovary. The lower abdominal wall and external genitalia metastases arise from cancers of the genitourinary systems; face and neck skin metastases, from carcinomas of the oropharynx; and the scalp is a favorite site for metastases from breast, lung, and the genitourinary system.

TABLE 175–1. INTERNAL MALIGNANCIES METASTATIC TO SKIN CLINICAL FEATURES AND AREAS OF DISTRIBUTION

Primary Internal Malignancy	Cutaneous Clinical Features	Areas of Distribution
Breast	Papules, nodules—rock hard En cuirasse—scirrhous form Erysipelatoides—cellulitis form Alopecia neoplastica	Chest wall Trunk Scalp
Lung	Papules, nodules Scirrhous—morpheic form Erysipeloides—cellulitis form Alopecia neoplastica	Chest wall Scalp Face
Kidney	Angiomatous, pulsatile nodules Scirrhous—en cuirasse form Alopecia neoplastica	Abdominal wall, trunk Scalp Face External genitalia
Stomach, bowel, pancreas	Nodules Scirrhous—en cuirasse form Cellulitis—erysipelatoides	Anterior abdomen Periumbilical
Ovary, uterus	Nodules Cellulitis form—erysipelatoides	Umbilicus, abdomen
Oral cavity	Nodules	Face and neck
Thyroid	Pulsatile angiomatous nodules	Anywhere

Some patterns of metastatic disease are characteristic. For example, metastases to the scalp simulate wens or turban (pilar) tumors that may ulcerate. More distinctive is "alopecia neoplastica"—that is, areas of scarring alopecia in the scalp with induration and atrophy that simulate alopecia areata. Metastases from the breast and, less commonly, from the stomach, prostate, lung, uterus, and pancreas can produce dramatic changes in the chest wall: carcinoma en cuirasse. This scirrhous form of cutaneous metastatic spread produces extensive fibrosis of the dermis as a result of lymphatic involvement and obstruction by the cancer cells so that large areas of the chest are girdled by a thick, rigid encasement to which pink to flesh-colored papules and nodules evolve to form morphea-like plaques. The distinctive skin lesion of inflammatory carcinoma, or "carcinoma erysipeloides," is usually caused by breast cancer (less frequently by malignant tumors of the uterus, lung, and gastrointestinal tract) and simulates cellulitis over the ipsilateral chest wall anteriorly. Renal cell carcinoma and medullary and anaplastic forms of thyroid cancer, which are highly vascularized tumors, may simulate hemangiomatous nodules that pulsate on palpation when deposited in the skin. *Inflammatory oncotaxis* is a term describing the attraction of cancer cells to an area of tissue trauma resulting presumably because trauma (surgery and radiation) causes inflammation and capillary disruption, thus predisposing cancer cells to settle in these areas. For example, cutaneous metastases from colon, kidney, and cervix have been known to localize in abdominal wall surgical incisions.

Prognosis among patients with cutaneous metastases is poor, as they imply metastases elsewhere internally. If a cutaneous metastatic lesion is discovered years after the primary cancer is diagnosed, a second internal cancer should be ruled out, since only 10 per cent of internal cancers (mostly breast carcinoma) spread to the skin after five years' time. Clearly any skin nodule or papule of obscure origin and uncertain diagnosis should undergo biopsy, especially if there are reasons to suspect malignancy.

Lymphomas

Specific cutaneous involvement (neoplastic cellular proliferation in the skin) is seen less frequently in the lymphoma-leukemia group of neoplasms when compared with carcinomas. Rather, cutaneous manifestations are more often nonspecific (i.e., pruritus, petechiae, purpura, infections) in patients with leukemias and lymphomas, occurring in 25 to 40 per cent of such patients (see below, Nonspecific Skin Lesions Associated with Internal Malignant Disease). The specific skin lesions that are seen are similar in patients with lymphoma and leukemia, regardless of the various types of these neoplasms. Thus, skin lesions in all forms of lymphomas and leukemias appear as red, blue, and violaceous asymptomatic macules, nodules, and plaques that may ulcerate. Particularly suggestive are thickened, beefy-red arcuate lesions as well as poikilodermatous plaques (hyperpigmentation and hypopigmentation with telangiectasis throughout the thickened patches).

Cutaneous T Cell Lymphomas (Table 175–2)

These lymphomas are lymphoproliferative disorders of helper T lymphocytes with an affinity for skin (epidermotropism) in which atypical lymphocytes accumulate in clusters in the epidermis to form so-called Pautrier's abscesses. They represent at least three types of lymphoma: mycosis fungoides, Sézary syndrome, and adult T cell lymphoma, each

TABLE 175–2. CUTANEOUS T CELL LYMPHOMAS

Lymphoma	Skin Lesions	Other Features
Mycosis fungoides	Erythematous patches, plaques, tumors, erythroderma	Late involvement of lymph nodes, internal organs
Sézary syndrome	Erythroderma with ectropion and leonine facies; often spares body folds	Sézary cells in blood with high WBC, hepatosplenomegaly, lymphadenopathy
Adult T cell lymphoma	Erythroderma, papules, nodules	HTLV 1 virus antibodies, hepatosplenomegaly, osteolytic bone lesions, hypercalcemia
T immunoblastic lymphoma	Plaques, tumors	Arise from pre-existing mycosis fungoides or Sézary syndrome
Chronic lymphoblastic leukemia, T cell type	Erythroderma, plaques, nodules	Prolonged course
T lymphoblastic lymphoma	Tumors of skin	Rapidly fatal with bone marrow and mediastinal involvement

of which presents with variable clinical characteristics and biologic behavior.

Mycosis fungoides (Color plate 6B) usually follows a prolonged course, beginning with nonspecific skin lesions (so-called premycotic stage) that, after a variable number of years, evolve into histologically specific skin lesions (cutaneous patches, plaques—the mycotic stage) and then into ulcerative nodules and tumors (tumor stage).

Extracutaneous disseminated disease involves first lymph nodes and then, in advanced stages, liver and spleen and other internal organs. Less commonly the disease may begin with cutaneous nodules and tumors without evolving from patches and plaques. Several types of clinical lesions (patches, plaques, and tumors) may coexist in any one patient. The premycotic stage (biopsy of lesions is nonspecific) can persist from a few months to more than 40 years, the morphology of the skin lesions resembling a number of banal dermatoses: psoriasis or eczema or poikilodermatous telangiectatic, stippled pigmented patches. In the plaque stage the premycotic lesions become infiltrated, although indurated, red-purple plaques also arise from previously uninvolved skin. The lesions usually are oval to round, but they may also be arciform or annular or assume a horseshoe shape, or the entire integument may be infiltrated, producing a thickened, red hide (erythroderma). In the final stage, tumors develop from pre-existing plaques, erythroderma, or previously uninvolved skin. Tumors may be a few centimeters to 10 cm in size and often ulcerate. It is difficult to diagnose mycosis fungoides in the premycotic stage; it requires multiple skin biopsies over extended periods.

The *Sézary syndrome* (Color plate 6C), the leukemic variant of mycosis fungoides, consists of generalized exfoliative dermatitis with edema, redness, and thickening of the skin associated with ectropion, leonine facies, keratoderma of the palms and soles, hepatosplenomegaly, and lymphadenopathy associated with large numbers of atypical T lymphocytes in the circulation. The latter, so-called Sézary cells, represent T cells with highly convoluted nuclei identical to the cells infiltrating the skin in mycosis fungoides. The immediate source of the circulating Sézary cells appears to be the skin, as the bone marrow is rarely involved. In many patients mycosis fungoides pursues a chronic course, and the patients die of unrelated causes; some experience rapid progression to cutaneous tumors and ulcerative lesions and disseminated disease (visceral involvement is frequently diffuse and resembles leukemic infiltrates). Sézary syndrome has a particularly poor prognosis. Staphylococcal or *Pseudomonas* septicemia is the most common terminal event, accounting for half of the deaths.

Adult T cell lymphoma, which is associated with a retrovirus, human T cell lymphoma virus (HTLV), occurs mainly in blacks in the United States. Cutaneous findings are prominent in 70 per cent of patients and may be the presenting feature. Flesh-colored papules, nodules, and tumors as well as generalized erythroderma may be present. The papules are diffusely disseminated over the trunk and coalesce to form plaques. Patients also display peripheral and mediastinal lymphadenopathy, and hepatosplenomegaly is found in half of the patients. A unique feature of this lymphoma is trabecular and bone marrow involvement with multiple "punched-out" osteolytic lesions in the axial skeleton and long bones associated with extreme hypercalcemia.

Several other forms of T cell lymphomas occur with skin involvement and are outlined in Table 175–2.

Non-Hodgkin's Lymphomas and Cutaneous B Cell Lymphomas (see Ch. 158)

Red, blue, or violaceous skin lesions occur in all forms of non-Hodgkin's lymphoma. They appear as papules, nodules, and plaques with occasional large, ulcerated tumors that evolve in the skin after lymph node involvement. Skin involvement can be seen as the initial presentation, or it may occur late in the course of the disease. It appears to have no impact on prognosis.

Hodgkin's Disease (see Ch. 160)

The skin is not commonly involved in a specific way, but when it is, the erythematous papules, nodules, and plaques that often ulcerate are indistinguishable from the skin lesions found in non-Hodgkin's lymphoma. The site of predilection is the thoracic wall, spread being via retrograde lymphatic drainage pathways from massively enlarged axillary and cervical lymph nodes. Specific cutaneous involvement is seen in those patients with extensive and highly aggressive Hodgkin's disease.

Leukemias

Leukemia cutis usually develops months after the diagnosis of leukemia (55 per cent of patients) or at the time of diagnosis (38 per cent), but it can occasionally precede systemic disease and be the first sign of the underlying condition. Red to violaceous papules, nodules, and thickened plaques are the usual forms that leukemic infiltrates take, but rarely is erythroderma found. When chronic myelogenous leukemia (CML) enters the blast phase, greenish tumors may develop in the skin, forming chloromas or granulocytic sarcomas (see Ch. 155). Skin lesions in acute leukemias and chronic lymphocytic leukemia (CLL) are found on the face and extremities, while those associated with CML are more commonly seen on the trunk. In monocytic leukemia, widespread leukemia skin infiltrates occur, and oral mucosal involvement (gingival hyperplasia) is commonplace. In general, the histology of leukemic cells in skin for various forms of leukemia mimics that seen in the blood and bone marrow, but it is difficult to diagnose the type of leukemia from skin biopsies.

Plasma Cell Dyscrasias

Specific skin manifestations of multiple myeloma, extramedullary plasmacytoma, and Waldenström's macroglobulinemia consist of lymphoplasmacytoid cell infiltrates or deposition of monoclonal paraprotein immunoglobulins (see Ch. 163). Bluish-red and flesh colored nonulcerated nodules and plaques on the trunk are observed in 4 per cent of patients with multiple myeloma, representing in most instances extensions from underlying medullary plasma cell proliferation.

Cutaneous Histiocytic Malignant Tumors

Malignant tumors of histiocytes may be solitary or present as disseminated disease. *Malignant histiocytosis* (histiocytic medullary reticulosis), a systemic, progressive proliferation of atypical histiocytes, produces wasting, fever, lymphadenopathy, hepatosplenomegaly, pancytopenia, and skin lesions. Children and adults are affected, and skin lesions are an integral part of the disease, especially in children (up to 90 per cent have cutaneous changes). The reddish-purple papulonodular and ulcerative plaques occur over the trunk and face early in the clinical course. Malignant histiocytosis is fatal in adults, but is somewhat less aggressive in children.

Angioblastic Lymphadenopathy

Immunologically mediated, this often fatal disorder is characterized by proliferation of plasmacytoid immunoblasts and plasma cells. Fever, malaise, weight loss, hepatosplenomegaly, and generalized lymphadenopathy are accompanied in 40 per cent of cases by generalized, maculopapular, purpuric, and, at times, exfoliative erythroderma. Biopsy findings of involved lymph nodes are diagnostic (proliferation of plasma cells, arborizing vessels, and deposition of amorphous material), while skin biopsy reveals a lymphohistiocytic vasculitis composed of plasma and immunoblast-like cells.

Neuroblastoma

Neuroblastoma, a poorly differentiated tumor derived from primordial neural crest cells, arises within the sympathetic ganglion (cervical, thoracic, and pelvic tumors) and adrenal glands of children. It frequently metastasizes to bone, lymph nodes, liver, and skin. Bluish nodules appear over a wide area (causing these children to be called blueberry-muffin children). A helpful clinical sign occurs after rubbing these lesions: They blanch with a halo of surrounding erythema, probably related to the release of catechols contained in the cells of the tumors. Even though patients with neuroblastoma are not hypertensive, 85 per cent have increased urinary catecholamine metabolites.

Kaposi's Sarcoma (Color Plate 6*D–F*)

Kaposi's sarcoma, a multifocal, vascular malignant tumor, can occur in four major clinical settings: African Kaposi's, classic Kaposi's in elderly Jewish or Mediterranean males, Kaposi's secondary to immunodeficiency conditions, and Kaposi's sarcoma occurring as a complication of acquired immunodeficiency syndrome (AIDS). In each instance the skin lesions are identical histologically and clinically; they present as purplish-brown macules, plaques, papules or nodules. The distribution and course of these sarcomatous lesions, however, vary according to the clinical setting (Table 175–3). Thus, classic Kaposi's sarcoma occurs in elderly males of Mediterranean background as purplish macules that may progress to infiltrative plaques and nodules on the distal extremities, following an indolent course. The Kaposi's sarcoma occurring in young homosexuals and others with AIDS is characterized by widely distributed, red-brown macules, papules, nodules over the upper body and progresses in a fulminant course. The Kaposi's lesions in AIDS often follows skin cleavage lines and frequently involve the oropharyngeal mucosa, appearing as purple hemorrhagic plaques. The importance of the immune status in the evolution of Kaposi's sarcoma is dramatically illustrated in renal transplant patients who are immunosuppressed. Kaposi's sarcoma develops after 9 to 16 months following transplantation and initiation of immunosuppressive drugs. Rapidly progressive, widespread, red to purple papules ensue, but they may regress when immunosuppressive therapy is withdrawn.

NONSPECIFIC SKIN LESIONS ASSOCIATED WITH INTERNAL MALIGNANT DISEASE (Table 175–4)

Malignant cells cannot be identified in the skin in a wide variety of cutaneous manifestations of internal malignant disease. The pathogenesis of these disparate skin reactions is obscure. Often the only evidence that malignancy and cutaneous changes are related is the observation that following removal of the tumor or treatment of the neoplasm the skin change subsides or disappears and may subsequently exacerbate if the neoplasm recurs. Skin manifestations may coincide with, antedate, or follow the clinical diagnosis of internal malignant disease.

Although nonspecific manifestations are often highly suggestive of underlying malignant disease, they are more frequently seen with other nonmalignant conditions. When these skin changes are observed, therefore, an internal neoplasm is only one of several possibilities in the differential diagnosis.

Nonspecific skin manifestations can be considered under two major headings: (1) skin changes common to many skin diseases, including internal malignancy and (2) syndromes and entities commonly associated with internal neoplasia.

Skin Changes Common to Many Skin Conditions, Including Internal Malignancy

Pruritus, unassociated with detectable abnormalities of the skin except for secondary lesions such as excoriations or prurigo-like papules, may be an important manifestation of various internal malignant diseases, including Hodgkin's disease, lymphocytic leukemia, carcinoid, polycythemia vera (in

TABLE 175–3. KAPOSI'S SARCOMA: COMPARISON OF VARIOUS FORMS

	Classic Form	African Form	Immunologic Deficiency State	AIDS Associated
Age	40–70 years	Middle age	Any age	20–50 years
Sex	M:F, 10–15:1	—	M or F	Mostly males
Social characteristics	Mediterranean or Jewish ancestry	Blacks in equatorial Africa	Patients taking immunosuppressive drugs—renal transplant, etc.	Homosexuals, drug addicts, hemophiliacs
Occurrence	0.2% cancers in USA	10% of all malignant tumors in Africa	400% greater incidence than population at large	Increasing; 35% of AIDS patients
Clinical appearance of skin lesion	Multiple purple-brown macules, papules, plaques, nodules	Nodules, exophytic lesions, infiltrative, burrowing plaques	Papules, nodules	Multiple purple-brown macules, papules, nodules; follow cleavage lines of skin
Cutaneous location	Lower legs most often, occasionally arms	Extremities	Trunk, neck—widespread lesions	Widespread—upper body, face, neck
Mucosal involvement	Rare	Rare	—	Common
Node and systemic involvement	Rare—occasionally nodes, GI tract, liver in 10% of patients	Uncommon	—	Frequent; 75% with visceral involvement; 5% visceral lesions only
Course and prognosis	Indolent course, 15% mortality within 10 years	Indolent course	Good; may regress if immunosuppressive drugs can be stopped	Fulminant condition, poor prognosis
Response to therapy	Excellent	—	Good	Poor

TABLE 175–4. NONSPECIFIC SKIN LESIONS ASSOCIATED WITH INTERNAL MALIGNANCIES

I. Skin lesions common to many skin conditions, including internal malignancy
II. Syndromes and entities commonly associated with internal malignancy
  A. Nongenetic syndromes
    1. High incidence of association with internal malignancy
      Paget's disease
      Stewart-Treves syndrome
      Acanthosis nigricans
      Dermatomyositis
      Leser-Trélat syndrome
      Glucagonoma syndrome
      Bazex syndrome
      Pulmonary osteoarthropathy
      Carcinoid syndrome
    2. Low incidence of association with malignancy
      Sweet's syndrome
      Amyloid
      Urticaria pigmentosa and mastocytosis syndrome
      Bowen's disease
  B. Genetic syndromes
    1. High incidence of association with malignancy
      Torre's syndrome
      Gardner's syndrome
      Cowden's syndrome
      Multiple endocrine neoplasia III
      Ataxia-telangiectasia
    2. Low incidence of association with malignancy
      Neurofibroma
      Peutz-Jeghers
      Basal cell carcinoma nevus syndrome
      Bloom's syndrome

which pruritus often occurs after exposure to heat), and, less commonly, carcinoma. The itching may be mild or severe, localized or generalized, intermittent or constant. In Hodgkin's disease, itching is usually continuous and may be localized to the feet and lower part of the body, only later to become generalized. Up to 30 per cent of patients with Hodgkin's disease may itch. Pruritus of leukemia has a greater tendency to be generalized and may evolve into generalized erythroderma. Carcinomas of the gastrointestinal tract, lung, ovary, and prostate may also be associated with itching, which may precede recognition of these cancers by a year. Although dry skin (xerosis) is the most common cause of pruritus, other systemic causes of this bothersome symptom should be sought in addition to malignant disease, including drug reactions, cholestatic liver disease, uremia, diabetes, and thyroid disease.

Erythroderma, or exfoliative dermatitis, is a cutaneous reaction pattern with various causes. In 10 per cent of patients, total-body cutaneous redness, edema, scaling, and lichenification are associated with malignancy. In clinical practice the usual cause of exfoliative dermatitis is either a drug reaction or a generalized exacerbation of a pre-existing dermatosis such as atopic dermatitis, psoriasis, or contact dermatitis. When it is due to malignant disease, erythroderma is most pathognomonic of Hodgkin's disease, less frequently seen in lymphocytic leukemia, or rarely associated with underlying carcinoma. Erythroderma may be the first sign of Hodgkin's disease or leukemia. Skin biopsies do not reveal lymphomatous or leukemic infiltrates, although the patients clinically look similar to those with Sézary's syndrome (in which skin biopsies display diagnostic Sézary cells).

Figurate erythemas are red, gyrate, serpiginous, and annular bands that take on a pattern reminiscent of a wood grain and have been given descriptive names such as erythema gyratum repens and erythema annular centrifugum. These lesions are occasionally associated with neoplasia, especially breast and lung cancer.

Urticaria-like lesions, flesh-colored to red pruritic papules, nodules, and plaques, at times accompany leukemia, so-called leukemids. They may precede the development of leukemia by many months, and biopsy of the lesions does not show malignant cells. Treatment and control of leukemia often result in clearing.

Acquired hypertrichosis lanuginosa (malignant down), the sudden onset of excessive growth of fine, long, unpigmented fetal hair (lanugo) over the face, trunk, and limbs, has been associated with breast, uterine, pancreatic, pulmonary, and gastrointestinal carcinomas as well as lymphomas.

Herpes zoster is increased in incidence in patients with Hodgkin's disease and chronic lymphocytic leukemia as well as with a variety of neoplasms that are being managed with chemotherapy. This is evidence of the important role that impaired cellular immunity plays in activating viral replication. The painful, unilateral, grouped, clear, and often hemorrhagic umbilicated vesicles in a dermatomal distribution are readily recognized (see Ch. 343).

A number of miscellaneous dermatoses have occasionally been associated with internal malignant disease, but it is not entirely clear whether these associations are real or fortuitous. Table 175–5 lists some of these.

Syndromes and Entities Associated with Internal Neoplasia

A number of unique cutaneous syndromes, both genetic and nongenetic, are associated with internal neoplasms with sufficient frequency to alert the clinician to look for these potentially curable neoplasms early in their evolution. In some instances there is a high incidence of associated neoplasms, while in others this association is less clear.

Nongenetic Syndromes and Entities Associated with Internal Malignant Disease

HIGH INCIDENCE OF CUTANEOUS LESIONS ASSOCIATED WITH MALIGNANCY. *Paget's disease* of the breast is invariably found with an underlying intraductal mammary carcinoma. Erythematous scaling or weeping, sharply marginated patches on the nipple and areola of one breast should alert the clinician to examine the breast carefully. A breast mass may not be palpable or may not be definitely found with mammography, but in virtually every case an underlying carcinoma is present. Paget's disease can also occur in the anogenital region (extramammary Paget's disease). In this disorder, eczematous, pruritic, crusted, lichenified, well-demarcated patches may involve the lower abdominal wall, inguinal regions, genitalia, or perianal area. In up to 50 per cent of such patients, an underlying carcinoma of the rectum, prostate, urethra, other parts of the genitourinary tract, or apocrine gland is found. Biopsies taken from mammary and extramammary Paget's disease show the same diagnostic features, namely, large, round cells with clear cytoplasm in the epidermis (Paget's cells).

Stewart-Treves syndrome is the occasional occurrence of lymphoangiosarcoma as a complication of chronic lymphedema of the arm after radical mastectomy for carcinoma of the breast. Angiomatous, livid, or dusky red blebs and nodules exuding fluid may evolve from 2 to 20 years following mastectomy and the onset of the lymphedema. Angiosarcoma has also developed in congenital lymphedema as well as in lymphedema of the legs following surgery for cervical cancer.

TABLE 175–5. DERMATOSES ASSOCIATED WITH INTERNAL MALIGNANT DISEASE

Dermatosis	Associated Cancer
Bullous lesions: pemphigoid, pemphigus, dermatitis herpetiformis	Rectal, breast, larynx, lymphoma
Tylosis: palmar hyperkeratosis	Esophagus
Acquired ichthyosis	GI leiomyosarcoma, lymphoma, multiple myeloma, lung, breast
Palmar fasciitis and polyarthritis: palmar fascial thickening with erythema, swelling of palms and dorsum of hands	Ovary

Acanthosis nigricans (Color plate 6G) presents as soft, velvety, verrucous, brown hyperpigmentation of the body folds, especially those of the neck, axillae, and groin. When it occurs in patients over the age of 40 years, it is often a sign of an underlying malignant tumor, usually adenocarcinoma (most often stomach, gastrointestinal tract, and uterus; less commonly, ovary, prostate, breast, and lung) and rarely lymphoma. Acanthosis nigricans involving the tongue and oral mucosa is highly suggestive of underlying malignancy. Acanthosis nigricans may appear before the malignant neoplasm 20 per cent of the time. Regression of the skin sign following therapy for the tumor and reappearance with reactivation of the tumor have been observed, suggesting that the underlying tumor secretes an as yet unidentified substance that is responsible for the verrucoid skin lesions. Acanthosis nigricans is more commonly found in individuals under 40 years of age, and then it is not usually associated with malignancy but rather with obesity or a variety of endocrinopathies (Cushing's disease, acromegaly, polycystic ovaries, hypothyroidism and hyperthyroidism, insulin-resistant diabetes). It also occurs on a familial basis. Special concern must be given to nonobese adults who have recently developed the verrucous areas in body folds. In 80 to 90 per cent of all instances the cancer arises in the stomach.

Dermatomyositis (Color plate 6*H*) developing in individuals over 40 years of age also calls for a careful search for underlying carcinoma (see Ch. 443). Although there is disagreement whether the incidence of internal malignant disease is increased in dermatomyositis, numerous cases have been reported with this association. Not uncommonly the dermatomyositis resolves upon removal of the carcinoma, but the syndrome recurs if the tumor reappears. In some instances the dermatomyositis precedes the cancer by several years. The search for neoplasm should be continued, therefore, even if the initial evaluation fails to find it, especially with (1) failure of the dermatomyositis to respond to conventional therapy (i.e., after systemic steroids), (2) a history of previous malignant disease, or (3) presence of atypical symptoms of the dermatomyositis. Malignant tumors of the breast and lung are those most commonly associated with dermatomyositis. Dermatomyositis is recognized by proximal muscle pain and weakness and a characteristic dermatitis that includes heliotrope rash (edematous, dusky, violaceous discoloration of the eyelids) along with a brilliant violaceous, erythematous telangiectatic scaling rash over the cheeks, forehead, V of the neck, elbows, and knees. Gottron's papules, slightly elevated red to violaceous papules or small plaques over the knuckles, are also an important finding in dermatomyositis.

The *Leser-Trélet sign,* the sudden appearance and growth of multiple seborrheic keratoses, occurs with underlying cancer in the elderly. This sign has been the subject of controversy, since seborrheic keratoses of the same histologic type are common in the elderly. Nevertheless, several case reports have described new and enlarging keratoses in association with cancer of the lung, adenocarcinoma of the bowel, mycosis fungoides, and Sézary's syndrome and, in some of these patients, the keratoses regressed when the malignant tumor was treated.

Necrolytic migratory erythema, associated with alpha-cell tumors of the pancreas and elevated glucagon levels, evolves as gradually enlarging erythematous patches with central, superficial blister formation progressing to central crusting and healing. Annular and figurate lesions result, with exudative, erosive, and crusting areas most pronounced in the perineum, groin, and perioral areas. Painful glossitis may be another prominent sign of the glucagonoma syndrome. The skin rash and stomatitis often resolve within a week after the tumor is removed. The pathogenesis of the skin and mucous membrane lesions is unclear. The glucagonoma syndrome is discussed more completely in Ch. 233. Similar skin lesions may be seen in association with severe zinc deficiency.

Bazex syndrome, or acrokeratosis paraneoplastica, is a unique cutaneous marker of carcinomas of the upper respiratory tract, especially seen with squamous cell carcinomas of the oral, pharyngeal, laryngeal, esophageal, and bronchial areas, primarily in males. When the tumor is asymptomatic, red to violaceous, scaling, psoriasis-like patches are found confined to the bridge of the nose, the fingers, toes, and margins of the ear helices. The nail folds are often red, scaling, and tender with grooving of the nails and onycholysis. Later the eruption on the acral areas becomes more extensive, spreading from the fingers to the palms and soles, which, in turn, become red and scaling and form a honeycomb-like thickening. The fingers and toes become violaceous and bulbous, and the rash evolves on the nose. In the last stage, if the tumor has not been treated and has progressed, new scaling lesions resembling psoriasis spread over the face, trunk, knees, arms, and scalp. Nail dystrophy (ridged, brittle, crumbling nails) is extensive.

Clubbing of the fingers is a well-known manifestation of bronchogenic carcinoma, mesothelioma, metastatic carcinoma to the thorax (from the colon, larynx, breast, or ovary) and occasionally Hodgkin's disease. *Hypertrophic pulmonary osteoarthropathy* is the term used when clubbing is accompanied by subperiosteal new bone formation along the shafts of the long bones of the extremities and digits. Joints of the ankle, knees, wrists, and hand may be painful and swollen. In some patients cutaneous thickening of the forearms and legs produces cylindric enlargement of the limbs, and the facial features become coarse with deep facial furrows simulating acromegaly. At times, deep confluent skin wrinkles evolve over the forehead and scalp, a condition termed *pachydermoperiostosis* when the skin changes accompany acromegaloid features.

Carcinoid, malignant tumor of the chromaffin cells of the gastrointestinal tract and, less frequently, the bronchus, may be associated with intermittent scarlet to violet red flushing of the head, neck, and upper part of the trunk. Eventually the erythema becomes permanent, and telangiectasis and tortuous veins evolve in the flushed areas. This syndrome and its cutaneous manifestations are described more fully in Ch. 243.

LOW INCIDENCE OF CUTANEOUS LESIONS ASSOCIATED WITH MALIGNANCY. *Amyloid deposits* in the skin may occur without obvious cause (cutaneous amyloidosis) as part of an inherited syndrome or secondary to plasma cell dyscrasias—either primary systemic amyloidosis or multiple myeloma. In the case of plasma cell dyscrasias, shiny, translucent, waxy, firm purpuric papules and plaques occur on the mucocutaneous junctions of the eyes, nose, and mouth along with macroglossia. Occasionally, infiltrated papules are not apparent, and only purpuric lesions evolve around the eyes ("raccoon eyes").

Urticaria pigmentosa consists of skin lesions that appear as numerous red-brown macules and papules on the trunk and extremities. Light stroking of the skin lesions causes urtication with edema and a red flare due to the release of histamine from the mast cells infiltrating the skin (Darier's sign). These skin lesions are sometimes associated with systemic mastocytosis (see Ch. 427) or, more rarely, with mast cell leukemia or myeloproliferative disorders (myelofibrosis, myeloid metaplasia, polycythemia, and granulocytic leukemia) with extensive infiltration of mature mast cells in the marrow and mast cells or basophils in the peripheral blood.

Bowen's disease of the skin consists of multiple superficial squamous cell cancers occurring in non–sun-exposed areas of the body, particularly in individuals with a history of long-term ingestion or exposure to arsenicals (drinking of well water, exposure to insecticides or industrial arsenicals). Bowen's skin lesions appear as discrete, red, scaling, flat to slightly raised patches that mimic eczematous or psoriatic patches. These skin lesions should be removed to prevent progression to invasive squamous cell carcinoma. The relationship of these lesions to internal malignancy is controversial, but a careful search for cancers of the larynx, lung, esophagus, liver, and bladder is warranted.

Sweet's syndrome (acute febrile neutrophilic dermatosis) is associated rarely with underlying chronic myelogenous leukemia. Red, tender, infiltrated plaques and annular lesions are distributed asymmetrically on the face, neck, and upper arms. The skin lesions consist of massive polymorphonuclear infiltration of the dermis, of unknown cause. Patients with Sweet's syndrome also suffer from fever, malaise, peripheral leukocytosis, arthralgias and arthritis, and conjunctivitis and episcleritis. Peripheral leukocyte counts generally range from 15,000 to 20,000 with 80 to 90 per cent mature polymorphonuclear leukocytes. Careful evaluation of the peripheral cells and occasionally of the bone marrow is indicated because of the possibility of coincident myelogenous leukemia.

Genetic Syndromes Associated with Internal Malignant Disease

HIGH INCIDENCE OF ASSOCIATION WITH INTERNAL MALIGNANCY. *Gardner's syndrome* consists of multiple epidermoid and sebaceous cysts of the face and scalp, fibrous tissue tumors of the skin (desmoid tumors, fibromas and fibrosarcomas), osteomas of the membranous bones of the face and head, and polyps of the colon and rectum (Ch. 107). No patients with this syndrome live beyond the seventh decade without developing adenocarcinoma of the bowel.

Cowden's disease, a condition in which there are numerous hamartomas of the skin, mucous membranes, and internal organs, is associated with malignant neoplasms of the breast and thyroid in a high percentage of patients. The hamartomas present on the skin as keratotic, warty papules and nodules on the central area of the face and on the hands and arms. Papular, cobblestone lesions may appear on the gingiva, palate, tongue, and larynx.

Torre's syndrome, another autosomal dominant condition, consists of multiple sebaceous gland tumors, sebaceous adenomas, sebaceous hyperplasia, and basal cell cancers with sebaceous differentiation. It is associated with cancers of the colon, duodenum, ampulla of Vater, uterus, and genitourinary tract. The skin tumors in this condition are yellowish or red papules and nodules.

Multiple Endocrine Neoplasia Type III (see Ch. 241). Medullary carcinoma of the thyroid and pheochromocytoma are found in association with a marfanoid habitus and multiple whitish to pink papular mucosal neuromas studding the lips, tip of the tongue, and, less often, the buccal mucosa, gingivae, palate, and pharynx. Neuromas also develop on the conjunctivae and corneas, and thickened corneal nerves may be found with slit lamp examination.

Ataxia-telangiectasia, an autosomal recessive disorder associated with lymphomas, is recognized by telangiectasias over the ears, eyelids, nose, butterfly area of the face, and conjunctivae in association with progressive cerebellar ataxia, profound immunologic deficiency, and sinopulmonary infections (see Ch. 419). Hodgkin's disease, non-Hodgkin's lymphoma, or leukemia develops in 10 per cent of patients, with other malignant neoplasms such as ovarian dysgerminomas, gliomas, cerebellar medulloblastomas, and gastric adenocarcinomas occurring less frequently. Persons with *Wiskott-Aldrich syndrome* also display a propensity to malignant lymphomas (79 per cent) or leukemias (13 per cent) by the age of ten years, probably related to widespread immunologic abnormalities of both the humoral and cell-mediated systems found in this condition. The skin changes are similar to atopic dermatitis (and are associated with petechiae due to thrombocytopenia).

LOW INCIDENCE OF ASSOCIATION WITH INTERNAL MALIGNANCY. Some dominant inherited conditions are associated with internal malignancy, but the relationship is not frequently found. Thus, patients with *neurofibromatosis* have café au lait spots, axillary freckles, and multiple neurofibromas. They are prone to develop pheochromocytomas (10 per cent of patients by the age of 60 years), acoustic neuromas, and neurofibrosarcomas.

Patients with the *Peutz-Jeghers syndrome* have numerous brown-black macules on the lips, perioral regions, hands, and feet in association with hamartomatous polyps of the small bowel, stomach and, less commonly, colon (see Ch. 107). Malignancy occasionally develops in the polyps. *Nevoid basal cell carcinoma syndrome* is occasionally associated with the development of medulloblastoma or fibrosarcoma of the jaw.

Bloom's syndrome (telangiectatic redness of the skin in photoexposed areas and stunted growth) and the *Chédiak-Higashi syndrome* (light coloration of skin and hair) are autosomal recessive conditions associated with a propensity to develop leukemias and lymphomas.

Braverman IM: Skin Signs of Systemic Disease. Philadelphia, W. B. Saunders Company, 1981. *This classic book, on all skin signs associated with systemic disease, has many useful pictures of the cutaneous lesions related to internal malignant disease.*

Callen JP: Cutaneous Aspects of Internal Disease. Chicago, Year Book Medical Publishers, 1981. *This book, written by a number of authoritative authors, reviews in detail the varied manifestations of cutaneous signs of internal malignancy. Part 3 is especially useful in covering the hematologic and oncologic cutaneous signs of systemic lymphomas and carcinomas.*

Thiers BH, Maize C (eds.): Symposium on Cutaneous T Cell Lymphoma and Related Disorders. Dermatol Clin Vol. 3, No. 4, 1985. *A series of articles relating to the basic scientific and clinical features of cutaneous lymphomas by a number of authorities in the field.*

176 PRINCIPLES OF CANCER THERAPY

Bruce A. Chabner

During the past two decades, fundamental changes have taken place in the treatment of cancer. Once an undertaking with limited expectations, the treatment of cancer is now increasingly effective because of the development of new drugs and more effective radiotherapy and surgery. Many advanced malignant diseases affecting younger age groups, such as the lymphomas, choriocarcinoma, testicular cancer, and childhood leukemia, can often be cured by drug therapy with or without irradiation. The solid neoplasms of later life, particularly adenocarcinomas originating in the gastrointestinal tract and lung, remain a formidable therapeutic challenge in which the potent toxicities and risks of aggressive therapy must be carefully weighed against the limited benefits likely to result. Here the major hope is for the cure of patients at initial presentation through aggressive use of all methods of treatment, including drugs. This chapter will consider the basic biologic and pharmacologic principles that govern the selection of a therapeutic plan for cancer patients. The treatment of specific tumors will be discussed elsewhere.

The objectives of cancer treatment are not the same for all patients and all diseases. They are conditioned by an appreciation of the potential for cure or palliation and an assessment of the patient's tolerance to the side effects of possible treatments. For potentially curable patients, it is imperative that an optimal regimen be selected and pursued without compromise or dosage reduction. On the other hand, curative regimens may not be appropriate for some patients. For example, although curative chemotherapy exists for the majority of patients with diffuse histiocytic lymphoma, not all patients with this diagnosis are appropriate candidates for intensive therapy. Older patients, for example, may have serious medical problems, such as cardiac or pulmonary disease, that preclude aggressive treatment. In such cases, the physician must weigh the chances of successful treatment against the probability of life-threatening side effects and must discuss these conditions frankly with the patient and family. At times, less intensive treatment or only supportive care with pain control and psychologic support may be the wisest therapeutic choice.

Palliation of symptoms and attention to the details of good medical care are often neglected in patients who have reached an incurable phase of their illness. Detection and treatment of complications such as intestinal obstruction, brain metastases, and hypercalcemia, although not affecting the ultimate outcome of disease, may allow the patient extended periods of functional and pain-free life. Thus, it is vital for the physician to listen to the patient's complaints, to conduct periodic physical examinations, and to maintain a concerned and supportive relationship, despite knowledge of the likely eventual outcome.

DETERMINANTS OF TREATMENT PLAN

The primary determinants in the choice of treatment are (1) the histologic diagnosis of the malignant tumor, (2) the stage or extent of disease (including specific sites of organ involvement), and (3) an assessment of the biologic features or specific growth characteristics of the individual tumor.

DIAGNOSIS AND CLASSIFICATION. Accurate pathologic diagnosis and classification of a tumor are obviously crucial. Correct subtyping of tumors is important for many tumors, such as the lymphomas, carcinoma of the lung, and ovarian carcinoma. These general categories encompass disease types with variant patterns of clinical progression and response to treatment. *Histologic grading* is also required for an accurate prognosis and as a guide to therapy in some tumors. Biochemical characterization may be required to identify tumors, e.g., mediastinal malignant teratomas that contain marker proteins (beta-subunits of human chorionic gonadotropin or alpha-fetoprotein); these features assist in distinguishing these from other undifferentiated carcinomas. Similarly, histiocytic lymphoma may be difficult to distinguish from an unusual primary occurrence of acute myeloid leukemia arising in lymph node or bone or from undifferentiated carcinomas unless appropriate touch preparations, histochemical stains, and patterns of reactivity with monoclonal antibodies are examined. The subclassification of lymphoid leukemias, such as B and T cell chronic lymphocytic leukemia (CLL) and childhood acute lymphocytic leukemia, may require the use of cell-surface immunologic typing, in addition to the usual histologic evaluation. The prognosis and treatment of each of these disorders are distinct and different. Genetic techniques, such as chromosomal or oncogene analysis, may be required to distinguish neuroblastoma from neuroepithelioma (Table 176–1). *The internist must always consider the possibility of an alternative, treatable diagnosis, and must seek expert pathologic clarification before committing the patient to a plan of treatment.*

STAGING. In general, knowledge of the extent of a malignant disease (*staging*) is essential to plan effective treatment. In selected cases, staging procedures may pose inappropriate risks to the patient and should never take precedence over necessary therapeutic intervention. For patients with life-threatening local complications of disease, such as upper airway obstruction, superior vena cava obstruction, or biliary obstruction, definitive staging should be delayed to administer surgical or local radiation therapy or chemotherapy.

Staging strategies are based on a knowledge of the natural history of disease, specifically its likely patterns of dissemination to regional and distant sites. In development of a staging plan, the morbidity of a given procedure must be balanced against its probable yield of positive information (the risk-benefit ratio). The procedure should be performed only if the results obtained would affect the treatment decision. For example, a procedure such as lymphangiography, which has low morbidity in the absence of compromised pulmonary function, has great usefulness in lymphomas because of its high yield of positive results and the major impact of these results on treatment choice. In contrast, the staging laparotomy frequently employed to define intra-abdominal disease in Hodgkin's disease has only limited utility in non-Hodgkin's lymphomas. The latter diseases are usually disseminated at presentation and in advanced stages are not approriately treated for cure with local therapeutic measures such as radiation therapy. For patients with solid tumors of epithelial origin (carcinomas), an orderly progression of disease occurs, first with involvement of local lymph nodes, and then dissemination to distant sites such as lung, bone, and liver. In such patients, the initial diagnostic workup usually includes bone and liver scans and chest x-ray; if these sites are free of tumor, a definitive surgical procedure is undertaken, with removal of the primary mass and adjacent lymph nodes. In general, the physician should resist the temptation to order batteries of duplicative tests, such as CT and ultrasound evaluations, or tests that have low yield in the absence of localizing symptoms, such as bone scans in asymptomatic patients with clinically localized breast cancer.

BIOLOGIC CHARACTERISTICS OF THE TUMOR. In planning a treatment program, the physician must also take into account the biologic characteristics of the tumor, and in particular its growth rate. Aggressive treatment is likely to be least beneficial and effective in tumors that contain a small fraction of actively dividing cells. Thus, certain patients with chronic lymphocytic leukemia may give a clinical history indicating extremely indolent clinical behavior of the tumor over a period of several years. These patients are unlikely to be cured by aggressive treatment, and many can be safely observed without treatment. In contrast, other patients with the same diagnosis but with the prolymphocytic leukemia variant may have a more aggressive clinical course indicating a need for early aggressive combination chemotherapy. In summary, although the clinical impression of tumor growth rate is not frequently used as a determinant of a therapeutic choice, it may be an important criterion in determining when to begin chemotherapy in patients with chronic lymphocytic leukemia, multiple myeloma, and other "indolent" types of malignant disease.

The foregoing information concerning pathology, stage, and clinical progression must then be synthesized to yield a clear understanding of the clinical circumstances at the time of making a decision about treatment. At this point, certain questions must be faced: (1) Is cure possible and, if so, by what therapies? What are the possible short-term and long-term side effects of the various alternative therapies? (2) If cure is impossible, is significant prolongation of survival possible and, if so, at what cost to the patient's sense of well-being and his or her ability to derive satisfaction from daily life? (3) Is palliation of symptoms a more reasonable objective than undertaking life-threatening treatment? In no other specialty of medicine is the treatment decision more influenced by the personal philosophies of physician and patient and

TABLE 176–1. ANALYSIS OF ONCOGENE EXPRESSION, KARYOTYPE, AND NEURAL ENZYMES ALLOWING SUBCLASSIFICATION OF HISTOLOGICALLY INDISTINGUISHABLE FORMS OF PERIPHERAL NERVOUS SYSTEM TUMORS*

Genetic Alterations	Neuroblastoma	Peripheral Neuroepithelioma
Cytogenetic		
Double-minute chromosomes or homogeneously staining regions	+	−
Reciprocal translocation involving chromosomes 11 and 22	−	+
Molecular Genetic		
Amplified N-*myc* oncogene	+	−
High-level N-*myc* expression (RNA)	+	−
Neurotransmitter-associated Enzymes		
Dopamine hydroxylase } Tyrosine hydroxylase }	+	−
Choline acetyltransferase	−	+

*Peripheral neuroepithelioma is highly responsive to combined-method therapy, whereas neuroblastoma is more refractory to treatment. (See Israel MA: The evolution of clinical molecular genetics. Am J Pediatr Hematol/Oncol 8:163, 1986.)

TABLE 176–2. COMBINED-METHOD THERAPY OF PRIMARY BREAST CANCER

Aim	Therapeutic Procedure	Rationale
Control of primary tumor	1. Local excision	Removal of bulk tumor and preservation of breast
	2. High-dose local irradiation	Sterilization of residual microscopic tumor implants of radiosensitive tumor
Prevention of distant recurrence	Adjuvant chemotherapy with 5-fluorouracil, cyclophosphamide, methotrexate	Treatment for occult metastases in patients with positive lymph nodes

their assessment of potential risks and benefits. Increasingly, conclusions from prospective clinical trials are providing a rational basis for making these decisions. While there is no single simple answer for all patients with the same diagnosis, no patient should be discouraged from aggressive therapy if there exists a reasonable chance for cure.

MANAGEMENT OF LOCAL-REGIONAL DISEASE

CANCER SURGERY. Prior to the advent of radiotherapy in the 1920's and chemotherapy in the 1950's, cancer treatment was the exclusive province of the surgeon. Cancer surgery for localized tumors is based on the principle of first establishing a diagnosis, secondly determining the extent of local disease, and thirdly establishing tumor-free surgical margins whenever possible. Current treatment often calls for integration of surgery with radiotherapy or chemotherapy to preserve bodily function and to prevent distant metastases. As examples, limited, limb-sparing surgery with high-dose irradiation may be used for soft tissue sarcomas of the extremities (Table 176–2) and surgical biopsy followed by local irradiation for primary breast cancer less than 5 cm diameter (see Ch. 240). The medical oncologist and radiotherapist should participate in treatment planning before definitive surgical procedures are undertaken.

Surgical resection of regional lymph nodes is performed for both diagnostic and, less frequently, therapeutic reasons. In some instances—e.g., testicular carcinoma with occult retroperitoneal lymph node metastases and in carcinomas of the head and neck—radical lymphadenectomy may be curative. In most other carcinomas (breast carcinoma, malignant melanoma, and colon carcinoma), lymph node dissection provides important staging information, but, if lymph nodes are positive, the operation is usually not curative because of the strong association between nodal metastases and later relapse in distant sites. This prognostic information is of particular benefit for diseases in which effective adjuvant therapy is available. In breast cancer, gastric carcinoma, and rectal carcinoma, lymph node dissection has become a staging, rather than a purely therapeutic, procedure. Its findings are critical in making the decision whether to use adjuvant chemotherapy.

While the role of surgery for treatment of local and regional disease has been modified to accommodate multimethod strategies, its employment in patients with disseminated disease has expanded. Early and aggressive resection of pulmonary metastases in patients with osteogenic sarcoma or soft tissue sarcoma has led to improved survival rates and occasional cures. Surgical resection of solitary intracranial metastases is clearly indicated for patients with breast cancer or malignant melanoma if this lesion is the sole site of metastatic disease. Reduction of tumor bulk by surgery, while not curative in its own right, may increase recruitment of previously dormant cells into active DNA synthesis and thereby render the residual tumor more susceptible to chemotherapy or radiotherapy.

In summary, the specific indications for surgery vary with clinical diagnosis and circumstances and need not be restricted to primary curative treatment of nonmetastatic disease.

RADIATION THERAPY. As an alternative to surgery, radiation therapy possesses significant advantages for locoregional treatment of malignant disease, because it produces less acute morbidity and loss of function of the affected body part. Radiotherapy exerts its biologic effect through the formation of ion pairs or reactive oxygen metabolites such as superoxide, H_2O_2, or hydroxyl radicals. These products cause breaks in DNA, which, if not repaired, may lead to cell death. Mutagenesis and carcinogenesis, resulting from sublethal effects of radiation on DNA, are other recognized late effects of radiation therapy. Radiation therapy may be delivered in the form of electromagnetic waves, such as x-rays or gamma rays, or as particle streams, such as heavy ions, protons, neutrons, pi mesons, or electrons. The characteristics of these forms of radiation have important implications for their clinical use. Electron-beam irradiation deposits its energy at the skin. Low energy x-rays, or *kilovoltage* x-rays, yield their energy readily as they pass through tissue, and consequently cause considerable damage to skin and normal tissues overlying deep-seated tumors. Higher energy x-rays, generated by linear accelerators, and gamma radiation generated by a ^{60}Co-machine, cause less skin damage, a significant advantage in the treatment of visceral tumors such as gastrointestinal carcinomas, brain tumors, or carcinoma of the lung. Charged particle beams, particularly protons, heavy ions, and pi mesons, have the further advantage of depositing their energy in a sharply focused peak below the skin surface (Fig. 176–1).

The biologic effects of conventional x-ray therapy in both the kilovoltage and megavoltage energy range are greatly enhanced by the presence of oxygen. Hypoxic cells, as found in the poorly vascularized centers of large tumors, are relatively insensitive to x-rays. In contrast, high-energy particle beams, such as neutrons, heavy ions, and protons, are less dependent on oxygen in their cytotoxic action. Thus, with respect to biologic action and dose-distribution characteristics,

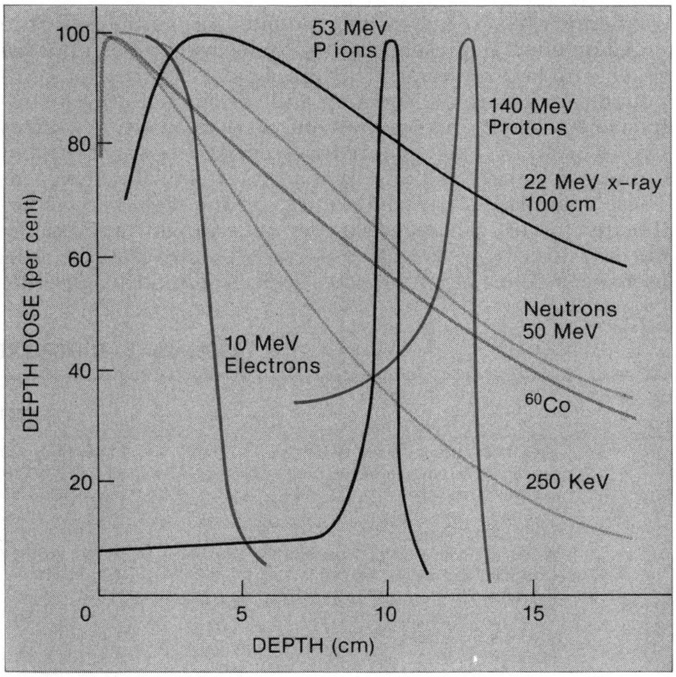

FIGURE 176–1. Penetration of various types of x-rays. Percentage of radiation dose absorbed at indicated depth below skin surface. MeV = Million electron volts; KeV = thousand electron volts. (From Becker FF [ed.]: Cancer, A Comprehensive Treatise. Vol VI. New York, Plenum Press, 1977.)

TABLE 176–3. NORMAL TISSUE TOLERANCE TO RADIOTHERAPY

Tissue	Toxic Effect	Dose Limit (Rads)*
Bone marrow	Aplasia	250
Liver	Hepatitis	2500
Intestine	Ulceration, perforation, fibrosis	4500
Brain	Infarction, necrosis	5000
Spinal cord	Infarction, necrosis	4500
Heart	Pericarditis	4500
Lung	Pneumonitis, fibrosis	1500
Kidney	Nephrosclerosis	2000
Skin	Sclerosis, dermatitis	5500

*Radiation delivered in 200-rad fractions, to whole organ, five days per week, will produce a 5 per cent incidence of toxicity.

particle therapy has significant theoretic advantages for treating large, poorly vascularized visceral tumors.

Radiotherapy is typically administered in fractionated doses of 150 to 250 rads per day, four or five days per week, for four to seven weeks. Fractionation produces an improved therapeutic index as compared with single large doses, possibly because of the greater capacity of normal cells to repair radiation-induced damage as compared to tumors. For single doses of radiation, a shoulder is observed in the curve that relates dose to cell kill. The width of this shoulder is believed to reflect the ability of the cell to repair DNA breaks. In general, normal cells have a broader radiation dose-response shoulder and therefore tolerate individual doses of radiation with less damage than do malignant cells. Fractionation of doses has the further advantage of allowing time for death of tumor cells in the interval between fractions; the reduction in tumor size is associated with improved oxygenation of formerly hypoxic tumor cells, rendering them more sensitive to subsequent radiation. The choice of fraction size and total dose is determined by the relative radiosensitivity of the tumor and the tolerance of normal tissue in the irradiated field (Table 176–3). Less sensitive tumors, such as malignant melanoma or sarcomas, are usually treated with larger individual fractions. Fraction size may be increased if a more rapid therapeutic effect is required.

Attempts have been made to identify drugs that enhance radiation effect (radiosensitizers) or selectively protect normal tissues (radioprotectors). The nitroimidazole class of compounds, including the common antitrichomonal drug metronidazole (Flagyl) and less neurotoxic derivatives, sensitizes hypoxic cells in tissue culture by accepting free electrons and forming toxic free-radicals in a manner similar to oxygen. These compounds have little effect on the toxicity of radiotherapy for oxygenated cells and thus do not appreciably increase toxicity to normal tissues. A second class of radiosensitizers, the halopyrimidines such as bromodeoxyuridine, is incorporated into DNA, which sensitizes the nucleic acid to strand breakage by irradiation. Clinical trials of such compounds have not been completed at this writing. An alternative approach is the use of protective compounds such as sulfhydryl compounds that interact with and detoxify the free-radicals produced by irradiation. These compounds would have to be selectively taken up by normal tissues to create a therapeutic advantage. Their use is still experimental.

Nonpharmacologic measures may also enhance radiation effects; these measures include hyperbaric oxygenation, which decreases the proportion of anoxic, and thus radioresistant, cells, and hyperthermia, which enhances toxicity to both normal and malignant cells. Neither of these ancillary measures has received thorough clinical trial.

THE MANAGEMENT OF METASTATIC CANCER. Approximately 40 per cent of patients with cancer are cured by local or regional forms of treatment. For the remainder, systemic therapy is used at some time during their illness, and in selected diseases and selected clinical situations this therapy may be curative (Table 176–4). In other diseases (Table 176–5), drug therapy produces partial or complete regression in the majority of patients, and treatment is associated with prolongation of survival for some patients. However, few of these patients are cured by chemotherapy, and relapse eventually leads to death. It has been estimated that approximately 40,000 cancer patients each year are cured by chemotherapy, either by treatment of clinically apparent metastatic disease

TABLE 176–4. TUMORS CURABLE WITH CHEMOTHERAPY

	Agent(s)	Long-Term Disease-Free Survival (%)
Curable with Single-Agent Chemotherapy		
Choriocarcinoma (low-risk patients)	MTX	90
Burkitt's lymphoma (Stage I)	Alk	90
Curable with Combination Chemotherapy		
Acute lymphocytic leukemia	Vin, Pred, Anth, MTX, 6-MP	60
Hodgkin's disease (stages III and IV)	Alk, Vin, Pro, Pred	60
Diffuse histiocytic lymphoma (stage II–IV)	Alk, Vin, Pro, Pred, MTX, Anth	70
Nodular mixed lymphoma (stage II–IV)	Alk, Vin, Pro, Pred	75
Testicular carcinoma (stage II–III)	Vel, Plat, Bl, VP-16	70–90
Childhood sarcomas (with radiation and surgery)	Act-D, Alk, Vin	70–90
Childhood lymphomas	Alk, Vin, Pred, Anth	75

Act-D = actinomycin D; Alk = alkylating agent; Anth = anthracycline; Bl = bleomycin; 6-MP = 6-mercaptopurine; MTX = methotrexate; Plat = *cis*-platinum; Pred = prednisone; Pro = procarbazine; Vel = vinblastine (Velban); Vin = vincristine.

TABLE 176–5. TUMORS RESPONSIVE TO CHEMOTHERAPY

	Agents*	Partial or Complete Response (%)	Long-Term Disease-Free Survival (%)
Breast carcinoma (Stage III–IV)	MTX, FU, Alk, Anth	75	rare
Small cell carcinoma of the lung	Alk, MTX, Pro, Anth, VP-16	90	10
Gastric carcinoma	FU, Anth, Mit	50	rare
Ovarian carcinoma	MTX, FU, Alk, Plat, Hex	75	10–20
Multiple myeloma	Alk, Pred, Vin, Anth	75	rare
Acute nonlymphocytic leukemia	Ara-C, Anth, Alk	75	20
Chronic lymphocytic leukemia	Alk, Pred	75	rare
Prostate cancer	H T	75	rare
Head and neck cancer	Bl, MTX, Plat	75	rare
Mycosis fungoides	Alk, MTX	75	rare
Bladder cancer	Alk, MTX, Plat, Vel	60	rare

*Combination therapy yields responses in majority of patients, but less than 25% have long-term disease-free survival. Median survival of treated patients is prolonged.

Act-D = actinomycin D; Alk = alkylating agents; Anth = anthracycline (Adriamycin or daunomycin); Ara-C = cytosine arabinoside; Bl = bleomycin; FU = 5-fluorouracil; Hex = hexamethylmelamine (investigational drug available from National Cancer Institute); H T = hormonal therapy; Mit = mitomycin C; MTX = methotrexate; Plat = *cis*-platinum; Pred = prednisone; Pro = procarbazine; Vel = vinblastine (Velban); Vin = vincristine.

or by adjuvant chemotherapy. The therapeutic index, or margin of safety between therapeutic and toxic drug doses, is extremely narrow for many of the effective compounds; thus, small changes in pharmacokinetics or increased patient sensitivity to drug action may lead to unacceptable toxicity. In this setting, the clinician requires as much information as possible concerning the determinants of tumor cell kill, prediction of antitumor effects, pharmacokinetics, and drug interactions to maximize the effectiveness of therapy and to avoid needless toxicity.

The Kinetic Basis of Drug Therapy

FRACTIONAL KILL HYPOTHESIS. The kinetics, or growth cycle, of mammalian cells have been summarized in Ch. 168. In treating experimental tumors, a constant fraction of the total cell population is killed by a given dose of drug. Since each treatment cycle kills a specific fraction of the remaining cells, the results of treatment are a direct function of the dose of drug administered and the frequency with which treatment is repeated. However, because tumors in humans are large and are composed of heterogeneous cell populations, the "fractional kill" hypothesis does not apply as well in this situation. Treatment will eliminate sensitive cells, leaving behind the more drug-resistant population. In addition to the problem of drug resistance, most human neoplasms contain a large fraction of slowly dividing or nondividing cells (termed G_0 cells) (Fig. 176–2). Since many antineoplastic agents are most effective against rapidly dividing cells, the initial kinetic stage is unfavorable for drug treatment. However, if the number of tumor cells can be reduced by surgical treatment or radiotherapy, the remaining cells are recruited into active proliferation and become increasingly susceptible to therapy with drugs. Through this mechanism, an initially slowly responding tumor may actually become more responsive to therapy as its size is reduced by treatment.

HETEROGENEITY OF HUMAN TUMORS. The fractional kill hypothesis assumes that tumors are composed of a uniformly sensitive population of cells. Most human tumors do evolve from a single clone of malignant cells, as judged by the presence of unique chromosomal markers or by G6PD typing (see Ch. 152). However, as tumors grow, significant mutation takes place, and advanced tumors are composed of multiple cell types that differ in their biochemical and morphologic characteristics and, most importantly, in their sensitivity to treatment. Drug-resistant cells are believed to arise from a parent-sensitive population by random mutation. The probability that a drug-resistant cell exists in a tumor is a function of the mutation rate for the drug-resistance gene and the absolute number of tumor cells. Thus, the chances for cure are greatest when the tumor population is smallest and least likely to contain treatment-resistant mutants. Also, combination therapies employing drugs with differing mechanisms of action are more likely to eradicate a tumor population than single-agent treatment, since a given cell is less likely to be simultaneously resistant to more than one agent.

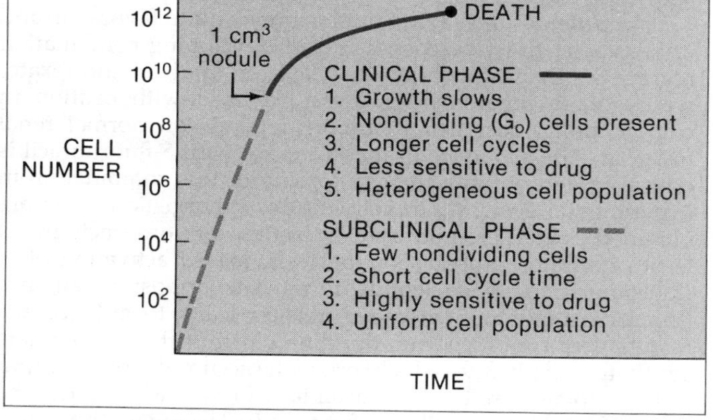

FIGURE 176–2. Kinetic phases of tumor growth.

PREDICTION OF DRUG RESPONSE. The selection of drugs for treating individual patients is primarily based on past experience in treating patients with the same histologic diagnosis and the same stage of disease. It would be highly desirable to be able to predict the sensitivity of individual tumors to treatment, and thus avoid needless toxicity of ineffective agents. The most successful laboratory aid for predicting response is the measurement of hormone receptors as a guide for hormonal therapy of breast cancer. This topic will be considered in detail later in this chapter. Biochemical tests based on the mechanism of drug action or mechanisms of tumor resistance are able to predict response in animal tumors, but have not been used extensively in clinical trials. A notable exception is the treatment of acute myeloblastic leukemia with cytosine arabinoside. The duration of complete remission in this disease may be predicted prior to treatment by the ability of leukemic cells to activate this drug and retain its triphosphate form. Attempts to develop drug sensitivity testing based on in vitro cultures of primary human tumors have met with mixed success; in general, these assay systems are too unreliable and too labor-intensive to be useful for routine clinical use.

PHARMACOKINETIC DETERMINANTS OF RESPONSE

The outcome of cancer chemotherapy depends in large part on the inherent sensitivity of the tumor under treatment to the agents being used. However, pharmacokinetic factors such as drug absorption, metabolism, and elimination also influence response and are extremely variable from one patient to the next. The oral route of drug administration is sparingly used in cancer chemotherapy. Up to tenfold variability in the bioavailability of orally administered 6-mercaptopurine, methotrexate, hexamethylmelamine,* 5-fluorouracil, and melphalan has been reported.

Most agents are given intravenously to assure adequate drug entry into the bloodstream. A few agents can be administered by other routes. Cytosine arabinoside, an antileukemic drug, may be given subcutaneously, a route that produces slow absorption and more prolonged drug concentrations in plasma than observed by the intravenous route. Methotrexate or cytosine arabinoside may be administered into the lumbar space for treatment of meningeal leukemia, lymphoma, or carcinoma, although neurotoxic side effects (coma, seizures, meningeal irritation) are observed with methotrexate, particularly at doses above 12 mg.

Several drugs have been administered by the intraperitoneal route, including methotrexate, 5-fluorouracil, and *cis*-platinum, for treatment of malignant disease confined to the peritoneal surfaces, such as ovarian cancer. The advantage of this route is that drug, instilled in a volume of 2 liters of dialysate, exits slowly from the peritoneal space, producing a marked concentration gradient of 100- to 1000-fold between the peritoneal fluid and plasma. Metabolism of drug in the liver as it exits from the peritoneum through the portal circulation further reduces drug concentrations reaching the systemic circulation. This type of therapy has produced documented remissions in ovarian cancer resistant to conventional regimens, but it is complex to administer, does not effectively treat disease outside the peritoneum, and thus has uncertain value in the general management of this disease.

For metastatic tumor confined to the liver, as often occurs in patients with previously resected colon cancer, hepatic arterial perfusion with 5-fluorouracil or 5-fluorodeoxyuridine appears to produce a higher response rate than intravenous therapy with the same agents; continuous infusions of two

*Investigational drug available from National Cancer Institute.

TABLE 176–6. DOSE ADJUSTMENTS FOR ALTERED RENAL OR HEPATIC FUNCTION

Condition	Agent	Dose Adjustment*
Altered renal function	Methotrexate *cis*-Platinum VP-16 Hydroxyurea Bleomycin	Decrease dose in proportion to decrease in creatinine clearance
Altered hepatic function	Adriamycin Vincristine Velban Vindesine	Decrease dose by 50% in patients with serum bilirubin >3.0 mg/dl

*Guidelines are approximations. Doses should be further adjusted on the basis of toxicity resulting from the initial dose.

weeks' duration, or longer, are well tolerated, since the drugs are degraded in their flow through the liver before they can enter the systemic circulation. Disadvantages of this therapy are local catheter complications, the need for a constant infusion device, and the failure to treat disease outside the liver. Biliary sclerosis is a known complication. Intra-arterial perfusion of extremity sarcomas and melanomas has been performed in experimental studies but has uncertain efficacy.

Elimination rates for commonly used drugs vary considerably and are not always predictable on the basis of renal or hepatic function. Alterations in drug dosage are necessary for patients with compromised ability to excrete or metabolize specific drugs (Table 176–6). For agents not listed in the table, reductions in drug dosage should not be made unless mandated by leukopenia, thrombocytopenia, serious infection, or other life-threatening complications, as dose reduction can only compromise the chances for response.

Drug-level monitoring has not been used as a standard guide to dose adjustment, except for the monitoring of high-dose methotrexate therapy (see below). The high reactivity, complex metabolism, and low plasma concentrations of anticancer drugs in general have made such monitoring difficult for other agents, except in investigative settings.

ASSESSMENT OF RESPONSE

An objective assessment of the response of a tumor to treatment is of central importance. Too often subjective impressions of improvement based on a patient's sense of well-being or performance status are not borne out by objective criteria. The standard criterion for partial response is a 50 per cent or greater reduction in the sum of the product of perpendicular diameters of all lesions measurable by physical examination or by radiologic techniques. A complete response denotes complete disappearance of disease, and in most diseases *should be documented by pathologic restaging if possible*. Pathologic restaging requires rebiopsy of previously involved organ sites. For tumors that secrete quantifiable marker proteins, such as gestational choriocarcinoma or germ cell tumors of the testis, a fall of these markers to normal levels and a persistence at this level for two to three months is necessary for a judgment of complete remission. Even in the presence of normal markers, persistent abnormalities on chest film or computed scanning may still require biopsy. For example, in patients with testicular carcinoma who present with intra-abdominal tumor, the induction of remission must be verified by repeat biopsy of retroperitoneal lymph nodes, even if radiographs and markers are negative. Partial responses rarely lead to significantly improved survival.

STRATEGIES OF CLINICAL CHEMOTHERAPY

COMBINATION CHEMOTHERAPY. ***Background.*** The first effective drugs for treating cancer were introduced in the mid and late 1940's, but initial therapeutic results were disappointing. Although impressive regressions of acute lymphocytic leukemia and adult lymphomas were obtained with nitrogen mustard, antifolates, corticosteroids, and the vinca alkaloids, responses were only partial in degree and of short duration. Attempts at retreatment usually met with a diminished response or frank resistance to further therapy. Increased doses could not be given because of prohibitive bone marrow toxicity or neurotoxicity, and few patients derived lasting benefit. The single exception was the cure of choriocarcinoma by methotrexate. The introduction of combination chemotherapy for acute lymphocytic leukemia of childhood in the early 1960's marked a turning point in the effective treatment of neoplastic disease. Such combinations of chemotherapeutic agents are now the standard for the treatment of most advanced cancers.

Rationale. The principal rationale for combination chemotherapy derives from an appreciation of the reasons for failure of single-agent treatment: (1) De novo resistance to any given single agent is frequent, even in the most responsive tumors. (2) Initially responsive tumors rapidly acquire resistance after drug exposure. Drugs either induce resistance or select resistant mutants from an initially heterogeneous tumor cell population. However, since the various anticancer drugs have diverse mechanisms of action, cells resistant to one agent might still be sensitive to the several other drugs in the regimen. If drugs have different, nonoverlapping toxicities, each can be used in full dosage in a combination regimen. For example, drugs such as vincristine, prednisone, bleomycin, and hexamethylmelamine, which lack bone marrow toxicity, are particularly valuable for combination with myelosuppressive agents. On the basis of these principles, curative combinations have been devised for acute lymphocytic leukemia (vincristine-prednisone ± Adriamycin and L-asparaginase), Hodgkin's disease (nitrogen *m*ustard-vincristine [*O*ncovin]-*p*rednisone-*p*rocarbazine; called MOPP), histiocytic lymphoma (C-MOPP), and testicular carcinoma (bleomycin-vinblastine-*cis*-platinum). The cure of advanced malignancy, when possible, is primarily achieved with combination regimens (Table 176–5).

Scheduling. The scheduling of drugs in combinations was initially based on convenience and empirical experience. Intermittent cycles of therapy allow for periods of recovery of host bone marrow and immune function. More recent combinations have incorporated nonmyelosuppressive agents in the "off period" between doses of myelotoxic drugs. High-dose methotrexate with leucovorin rescue has proved to be particularly useful in this capacity in the off period because of its minimal effect on white blood cell and platelet counts. Logic dictates the initial use of drugs that kill in all phases of the tumor cell growth cycle, such as the alkylating agents or nitrosoureas (if active against the disease in question), to reduce tumor bulk and thereby recruit slowly dividing cells into active DNA synthesis, then to be followed by cell cycle–dependent agents (such as methotrexate or the fluoropyrimidines) that kill preferentially in the DNA synthetic phase. An example of such a regimen in which the cycle-nonspecific drugs are followed by cycle-specific agents is shown in Table 176–7.

Drug Interactions. Drug interactions, both favorable and unfavorable, must be considered in developing combination regimens. Drugs such as *cis*-platinum and methotrexate, which cause renal toxicity, must be used with caution in combination since their excretion depends on normal renal function. The sequence of methotrexate with 5-fluorouracil is critical in determining the cytotoxicity of this combination in experimental systems. In cell culture, synergistic results are obtained when methotrexate precedes 5-fluorouracil by at least one hour, probably owing to increased activation of 5-fluorouracil to its nucleotide form. The opposite sequence (fluoropyrimidine, then methotrexate) leads to antagonistic results because of fluoropyrimidine block of the thymidylate synthetase pathway, which prevents accumulation of intracellular folates in the dihydrofolate form and negates the effect of inhibition of dihydrofolate reductase by methotrexate

TABLE 176–7. STRATEGIES FOR COMBINATION CHEMOTHERAPY: USE OF NON–CROSS-RESISTANT DRUGS IN SEQUENCE IN MACOP-B REGIMEN

	Week 1	2	3	4	5	6	7	8	9	10	11	12
Doxorubicin 50 mg/m²	x		x		x		x		x		x	
Cyclophosphamide 350 mg/m²	x		x		x		x		x		x	
Methotrexate 400 mg/m²		x				x				x		
Vincristine 1.4 mg/m²		x		x		x		x		x		x
Bleomycin 10 U/m²				x				x				x
Prednisone 75 mg daily	→ (continuous, weeks 1–12)											
Leucovorin, 15 mg every 6 hr for 6 doses, beginning 24 hr after methotrexate												

Adapted from Ann Intern Med 102:596, 1985.

Notable features:

1. Early use of all six agents discourages outgrowth of resistant tumor cells.
2. Therapy begun with drugs that are not cell cycle–specific, followed by cycle-specific agents in week 2.
3. Nonmyelosuppressive drugs in weeks 2, 4, 6, 8, 10, and 12 allow recovery from drugs in odd-numbered cycles.

(Fig. 176–3). Similarly, L-asparaginase prior to methotrexate aborts the toxic effect of the antifolate, and is therefore avoided in clinical scheduling. *cis*-Platinum, a drug that covalently binds to DNA, markedly enhances the toxicity of antimetabolites, such as 5-fluorouracil and cytosine arabinoside. Methotrexate and 6-mercaptopurine are highly synergistic; methotrexate blocks de novo purine biosynthesis, thus augmenting the uptake and utilization of preformed purines such as 6-mercaptopurine.

Adjustments Within Combinations. All drug combination regimens require dose adjustment scales to allow increases or decreases of dose according to toxicity. It becomes difficult to determine which of the several agents is responsible if overlapping toxicity patterns are present. In this setting, arbitrary scales of dose adjustment according to bone marrow toxicity or other readily identifiable and quantifiable toxicity are usually provided with protocols.

New Strategies. In the first combination chemotherapy trials, such as MOPP chemotherapy of Hodgkin's disease, the overall strategy was to deliver intensive therapy over a finite time period and then to restage the condition to rule out the presence of occult residual disease. Treatment was discontinued in those patients having complete remission. The duration of unmaintained complete remission then served as an index of the completeness of response. In an effort to improve the long-term disease-free survival rate associated with cyclic chemotherapy, this basic strategy has been modified in the following ways:

1. Alternative combinations to the primary regimen have been identified by trials in patients resistant to the primary treatment. An example is the ABVD regimen for Hodgkin's disease, which incorporates four agents (Adriamycin, bleomycin, vinblastine, and DTIC) that are non–cross-resistant with the MOPP drugs. The second regimen can then be used in alternating cycles of treatment with the primary combination, or one set of drugs can be used on day 1 and a second set on day 8 of a 28-day cycle. The day 1–day 8 alternation has the better chance of discouraging the development of drug-resistant cells (see Table 176–7).

2. An alternative is to use non–cross-resistant agents for maintenance therapy, after induction of complete remission with the standard combinations, as is standard practice in childhood leukemia.

COMBINED RADIATION AND CHEMOTHERAPY. Chemotherapy can often be usefully combined with other forms of treatment, such as irradiation or surgery. As an example, surgical resection of residual testicular carcinoma following chemotherapy leads to cure of a fraction of patients who would otherwise be only partial responders. There is evidence that the combination of irradiation and chemotherapy may improve the complete response rate and survival in children with Wilms' tumor and embryonal rhabdomyosarcoma.

Unfortunately, chemotherapy and radiotherapy have synergistic actions on *both* normal and malignant tissue, and this may lead to problems in their integrated use. The normal tissue of greatest concern is the bone marrow. Radiation given to the pelvic or midline abdominal areas produces a decline in blood counts and a decrease in bone marrow reserve. Appropriate shielding of the pelvic structures and the use of megavoltage radiation with limited scatter can preserve a significant portion of this marrow-bearing tissue. The sequence of administration may be of crucial importance. For example, chemotherapy followed by total nodal irradiation is less well tolerated because of severe myelosuppression in the radiation phase of treatment. One must anticipate cumulative effects of both chemotherapy and irradiation on bone marrow reserve.

High-dose chemotherapy (usually cyclophosphamide) and total-body irradiation have been used to eradicate residual acute myelocytic leukemia in children and young adults. These patients are rescued from lethal toxicity by allogeneic bone marrow transplantation (see Ch. 165). Similar therapy for solid tumors, using BCNU, alkylating agents, or combinations of drugs with autologous bone marrow reconstitution, has been successful in selected cases of lymphoma, but remains experimental because of its extreme toxicity to bone marrow, liver, and lung, and the high rate of tumor recurrence.

Other examples of interactions between chemotherapeutic agents and irradiation are as follows: (1) Adriamycin and concurrent mediastinal irradiation enhance toxicity for the heart, esophagus, and lung. (2) Bleomycin enhances x-ray damage to pulmonary tissue. (3) Methotrexate may produce recall reactions in previously irradiated skin. (4) Prednisone suppresses the immediate reaction to pulmonary irradiation, but withdrawal of steroids may be associated with a serious flare in radiation-induced pneumonitis. Reduction of radiation dose or an alteration in drug dose or schedule may be necessary to avoid untoward effects.

The *carcinogenicity* of both radiotherapy and chemotherapy is another negative consideration in their combined use. Agents listed in Table 176–8 are strongly suspected of being carcinogenic, based on (1) association with a high incidence of second malignant tumors in humans, (2) proven carcinogenicity in animals, or (3) strongly positive mutagenicity in bacterial assays. Irradiation is also strongly mutagenic and carcinogenic. The combination of alkylating agents and procarbazine with irradiation has led to an estimated 5 per cent incidence of second malignant disease (most frequently acute myelocytic leukemia) in patients with Hodgkin's disease. The carcinogenic potential of specific regimens is difficult to quantitate because of the brief survival of many patients undergoing such treatment and uncertainty as to the number of patients at risk in retrospective studies. Nonetheless, there is sufficient evidence of irradiation-drug synergy to warrant caution in accepting combinations of irradiation and carcinogenic drugs, particularly for patients who have an excellent chance of cure or long-term survival by single-method treatment.

Both irradiation and chemotherapy are capable of producing *infertility*. Cyclophosphamide, chlorambucil, busulfan, mel-

TABLE 176–8. CARCINOGENICITY OF ANTINEOPLASTIC AGENTS

	Second Tumors in Humans	Carcinogen in Animals	Mutagen*
High risk			
Cyclophosphamide	+	+	+
Melphalan	+	+	+
Chlorambucil	+	+	NR
Procarbazine	+	+	–
Methyl CCNU	+	+	NR
6-Mercaptopurine	+	+	+
Adriamycin	NR	+	+
Low risk			
Methotrexate	–	–	–
Cytosine arabinoside	–	–	–
5-Fluorouracil	–	NR	–
Risk unknown			
Bleomycin	NR	–	–
Cis-platinum	NR	NR	+
Actinomycin D	NR	–	+
Vincristine	NR	–	–
Vinblastine	NR	+	–

*Mutagen in Ames assay using *Salmonella typhimurium* testor strain and rat liver microsomes.

NR = not reported.

phalan, and procarbazine, as well as combination regimens, cause infertility in both males and females, often with permanent sterility in males and in women over 40 years. Adriamycin, *cis*-platinum, the vinca alkaloids, the antimetabolites, and the nitrosoureas have not been carefully studied in this respect. In men, the development of azoospermia is usually but not always irreversible.

ADJUVANT THERAPY. Adjuvant therapy is treatment given after surgical resection of a primary tumor in an effort to prevent recurrence at distant sites. The need for adjuvant therapy arises from two sources: (1) the high recurrence rate of certain tumors following surgery for apparently localized disease (e.g., breast cancer, soft tissue sarcoma, osteogenic sarcoma, Dukes' B and C colon and rectal cancer, and various solid neoplasms of childhood), and (2) the failure of chemotherapy or combined-method treatment to cure patients after recurrence of disease. Tumors are generally most susceptible to chemotherapy at their earliest stages of growth. This increased sensitivity of small tumors is based on a higher growth fraction, a shorter cell cycle time, and a decreased probability of there being drug-resistant cells in the population; these factors allow for a greater fractional cell kill for a given drug dose. As a tumor enlarges, its growth fraction decreases, the cell cycle time lengthens, and the probability of drug-resistant mutations arising increases. In addition, patients are able to accept chemotherapy best when they are not debilitated by metastatic disease.

There are disadvantages of adjuvant therapy related to both short-term and long-term risks. An unidentifiable fraction of patients receiving adjuvant treatment will have been cured by the primary surgical procedure and therefore will be experiencing needless risks and toxicity. In considering adjuvant therapy, late complications such as carcinogenicity (Table 176–8) and sterility assume greater importance. Nonetheless, intensive treatment in the adjuvant setting offers a higher probability of cure than treatment at later stages of disease.

ANTINEOPLASTIC DRUGS

The effective and safe use of cancer chemotherapeutic agents requires a fundamental understanding of their action, interactions, pharmacokinetics, and toxicity in man. Primary reviews of antineoplastic drugs should be consulted for more detailed information.

ANTIMETABOLITES. ***Antifolates.*** Antimetabolites act as fraudulent substrates for vital biochemical reactions. Most of the effective antimetabolites used in cancer treatment inhibit the synthesis of DNA or its precursors. The first antimetabolite to be used clinically was aminopterin. It has since been replaced by another folate analogue, *methotrexate,* which has more predictable clinical toxicity and at least equal clinical activity. Tetrahydrofolates, among other functions, provide one-carbon groups used in the synthesis of the purine nucleotides and thymidylate, which are precursors of DNA (Fig. 176–3). In the synthesis of thymidylate, N^{5-10} methylenetetrahydrofolate donates its one-carbon methylene group and at the same time is oxidized to dihydrofolate, an inactive form of folic acid. Methotrexate and its polyglutamate metabolites inhibit dihydrofolate reductase (DHFR) (Fig. 176–3), the enzyme responsible for reducing inactive dihydrofolate back to the active tetrahydrofolate form. The block in DHFR depletes folate cofactor pools, leads to a buildup of toxic dihydrofolate, and shuts down the synthesis of purine nucleotides and thymidylate. The polyglutamate forms of methotrexate, particularly those with three or four additional glutamates, are preferentially retained within tumor cells and are potent inhibitors of a number of folate-dependent enzymes in addition to dihydrofolate reductase.

The biochemical effects of methotrexate can be reversed by administration of the reduced folate leucovorin. This leucovorin "rescue" prevents methotrexate toxicity to bone marrow and gastrointestinal epithelium if administered in sufficient doses within 36 hours after infusions of high doses of methotrexate. Methotrexate infusion of 6 to 36 hours in duration, and in total doses of 1500 mg per square meter* or greater, can be given safely if followed by leucovorin rescue. The dose of leucovorin required (usually 15 to 50 mg per square meter every 6 hours for 48 hours) depends on the methotrexate

*Exceeds manufacturer's recommended maximum dose.

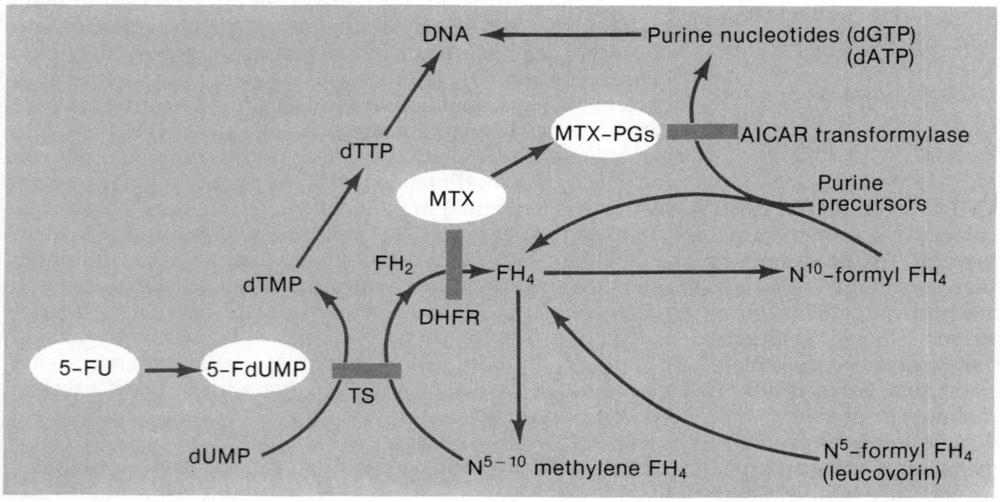

FIGURE 176–3. Sites of action of methotrexate (MTX) and 5-fluorodeoxyuridylate (5-FdUMP). DHFR = Dihydrofolate reductase; TS = thymidylate synthase; AICAR transformylase = aminoimidazolecarboxamide ribonucleotide transformylase; FH_2 = dihydrofolic acid; FH_4 = tetrahydrofolic acid. Note that MTX-PG's (MTX polyglutamates) directly inhibit AICAR transformylase and TS (not shown), in addition to inhibition of DHFR.

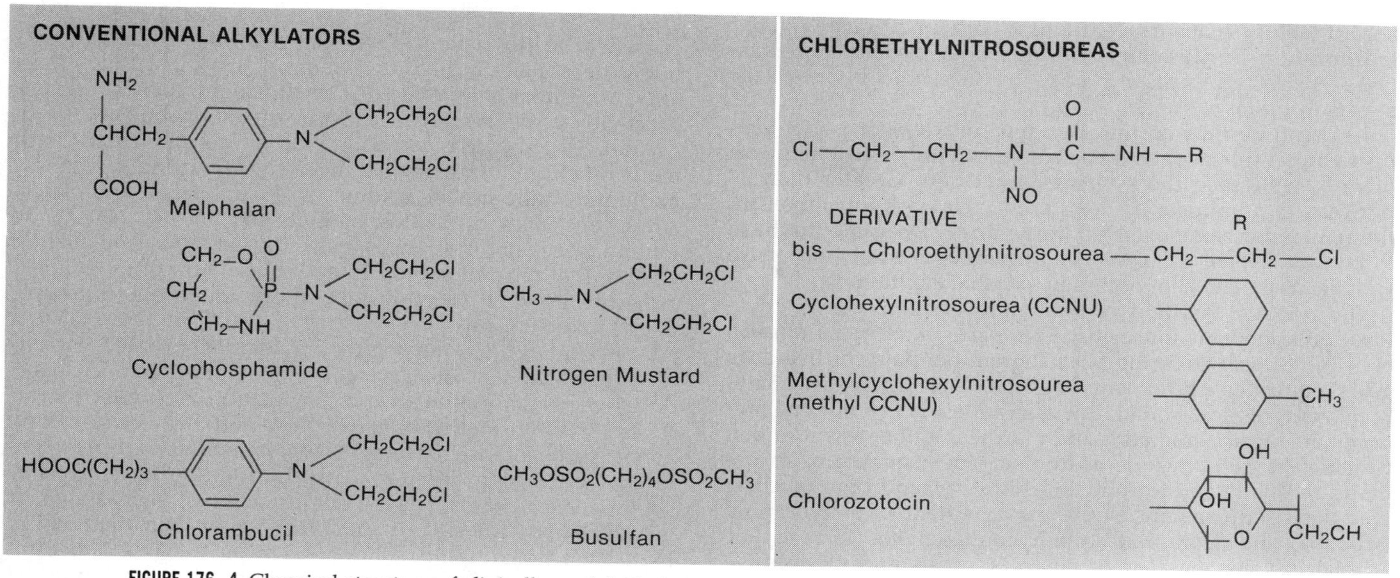

FIGURE 176–4. Chemical structure of clinically useful alkylating agents and the related class of nitrosourea compounds.

concentration at the time of rescue and may have to be increased in patients with inadequate renal function and delayed drug elimination.

Tumor cells acquire resistance to antifolates by several different biochemical mechanisms: (1) deletion of a high-affinity, carrier-mediated transport system for reduced folates, shared by methotrexate; (2) an increase in the concentration of DHFR; (3) an altered reductase that fails to bind methotrexate; and (4) decreased thymidylate synthesis activity. An increase in enzyme concentration owing to amplification of the reductase gene is readily induced by exposure of cells to gradually increasing drug concentration in tissue culture and has been documented to occur in the clinical setting. In attempts to overcome resistance, high doses of methotrexate (1500 mg per square meter* or greater) are given in 6- to 36-hour infusions, followed by repeat doses of the rescue agent leucovorin. This therapy is designed to provide sufficiently high drug concentrations to penetrate the cell membrane by passive diffusion and to saturate increased concentrations of enzyme. Methotrexate may be administered intravenously in doses ranging from 25 to 7500 mg per square meter.* Its primary plasma half-life is approximately two to three hours with excretion largely by the kidney (90 per cent). In patients with abnormal renal function or in those receiving doses above 1000 mg per square meter, monitoring of drug concentration in plasma is recommended to avoid serious toxicity. Methotrexate concentrations in plasma can be measured accurately with a competitive binding assay or radioimmunoassay and are useful for detecting patients at high risk of toxicity, who should then receive leucovorin rescue doses.

Methotrexate distributes slowly into "third spaces" such as ascites, pleural effusions, or cerebrospinal fluid. In patients with effusions or ascites the slow reentry of drug into the systemic circulation has been associated with a prolonged terminal half-life and unexpected toxicity. Systemic methotrexate enters spinal fluid poorly with concentrations only 3 per cent of those simultaneously in plasma. Only with high-dose methotrexate therapy are cytotoxic concentrations achieved in the spinal fluid. Alternatively, methotrexate may be injected directly into the lumbar intrathecal space or directly into the ventricle through an indwelling reservoir.

Acute methotrexate toxicity results from its effects on rapidly proliferating tissues (bone marrow and intestinal and oral epithelium). Drug concentrations of 1×10^{-8} M or greater in plasma produce myelosuppression and mucositis, which peak 5 to 14 days following a bolus dose or short-term infusion, with rapid recovery. More prolonged toxicity may be observed in patients who fail to eliminate the drug normally. High-dose therapy with methotrexate may lead to acute renal injury, believed to result from intrarenal precipitation of methotrexate or methotrexate-derived material. This can be prevented by vigorous pretreatment hydration, urine alkalinization (pH≥7), and, in patients with underlying renal disease, dose reduction proportional to the decrease in renal function. Renal toxicity and delayed drug excretion are aggravated by concomitant use of nonsteroidal anti-inflammatory drugs. Both acute and chronic hepatotoxicity may be caused by methotrexate with acute increase of serum levels of hepatic enzymes and, in patients receiving long-term oral treatment, hepatic fibrosis and cirrhosis. An acute pneumonitis, possibly of hypersensitivity origin, and rare episodes of anaphylaxis have been described.

Various manifestations of neurotoxicity are observed in up to 30 per cent of patients receiving intrathecal methotrexate, including motor dysfunction, cranial nerve palsies, coma, or seizures. Symptoms are accompanied by increased spinal fluid pressure and protein concentration and a reactive pleocytosis. Continued methotrexate treatment in this setting may be fatal.

Fluoropyrimidines. 5-Fluorouracil (5-FU), an analogue of thymine, inhibits thymidylate synthesis (Fig. 176–4). 5-FU has activity against many solid tumors, including breast, colon, head and neck, and ovarian carcinoma, and is now commonly used in combination therapy. Two biochemical actions may account for its cytotoxicity. 5-FU is converted to its corresponding ribose-triphosphate (5-FUTP) which, in turn, is incorporated in RNA and inhibits RNA processing and function. A second metabolite, 5-FdUMP, binds tightly to thymidylate synthase and inhibits the eventual formation of dTTP, one of the four necessary precursors of DNA. Resistance to 5-FU develops through deletion of one of the several key enzymes required for its activation (uridine kinase, nucleoside phosphorylase, and orotic acid phosphoribosyl transferase) or through amplification of thymidylate synthetase.

5-FU is usually given intravenously or intra-arterially because of erratic oral absorption and rapid first-pass metabolism in the liver. It may be given with leucovorin to enhance its binding to thymidylate synthase. Leucovorin increases 5-FU gastrointestinal toxicity and may enhance its therapeutic activity in breast and colon cancer. After intravenous administration of 10 to 15 mg per kilogram, peak plasma concentrations reach 0.1 to 1 mM, but rapid metabolism to dihydrofluorouracil in the liver and other tissues leads to an

*Exceeds manufacturer's recommended maximum dose.

abrupt fall in plasma concentrations with a half-time of about ten minutes. By six hours after injection, plasma concentrations of 5-FU are below 1 μM, the threshold for cytotoxic effects in tissue culture.

5-FU can be infused into the hepatic artery or portal vein for treatment of hepatic metastases, and only small amounts of drug will reach the systemic circulation. Greater than 80 per cent of administered 5-FU is inactivated by metabolism, the remainder being excreted in the urine. Doses do not have to be modified in the presence of hepatic dysfunction, since significant metabolism occurs in extrahepatic tissues.

The primary toxicities of *bolus* intravenous 5-FU are myelosuppression and mucositis. *Continuous intravenous infusion* of 5-FU at doses of 30 mg per kilogram per day* for five days gives equivalent therapeutic results, but different toxicity. Myelosuppression is mild, but gastrointestinal symptoms predominate (again, stomatitis and diarrhea). Other less common toxicities of 5-FU include acute neurologic symptoms in patients receiving intracarotid infusions, a syndrome of chest pain and serum enzyme elevations consistent with myocardial ischemia, and acute and chronic conjunctivitis. Intrahepatic arterial infusion has led to biliary sclerosis and progressive jaundice.

Cytosine Arabinoside. Cytosine arabinoside (ara-C, cytarabine) is an analogue of deoxycytidine, differing only in the substitution of the sugar arabinose for deoxyribose. Ara-C readily penetrates cells by a carrier-mediated process and then is converted to its active form, ara-CTP. Ara-C is incorporated into DNA and causes premature termination of the growing strand of newly synthesized DNA. Two inactivating enzymes, cytidine deaminase and dCMP deaminase (which degrade ara-C and ara-CMP, respectively), are present in high concentration in some tumors and are thought to exert an important negative influence on drug action. Ara-C kills cells selectively during the S phase of the cell cycle and has little activity against slowly growing solid tumors.

Resistance to ara-C is not well understood, but may relate to (1) deletion of deoxycytidine kinase, a necessary enzyme for activation, (2) an increased intracellular pool of dCTP (the nucleotide that competes with ara-CTP), (3) increased cytidine deaminase, or (4) a deficiency of the membrane transport process. In patients with leukemia, clinical response to ara-C may be predicted by the ability of leukemic cells to form and to retain ara-CTP after exposure to ara-C in vitro.

Ara-C is administered intravenously and is distributed rapidly into total body water, including cerebrospinal fluid. Owing to rapid inactivation (half-time of seven to twenty minutes) and its S-phase specificity, ara-C is given by continuous infusion in dosages of 100 mg per square meter per day or in a bolus of 50 to 100 mg every eight to twelve hours, for five to ten days. More than 70 per cent of administered ara-C is excreted in the urine as its inactive metabolite ara-U, which is formed in liver, plasma, granulocytes, and other sites. Alternatively, ara-C has been given in very high doses (up to 3 grams per square meter*) every 12 hours for six days, a regimen that appears to improve the response rate in refractory types of acute myelocytic leukemia. Alternatively in patients with preleukemic syndromes or in elderly patients, ara-C has been administered in low doses of 10 to 20 mg per square meter per day subcutaneously. Responses in preleukemic patients have been ascribed to an induction of tumor differentiation by low levels of ara-C.

Ara-C may also be administered intrathecally for treatment of meningeal leukemia or carcinomatosis. Because spinal fluid contains little cytidine deaminase, intrathecal doses of 50 mg per square meter yield high peak levels (1 mM), which decline with a half-time of two hours.

The primary side effects of ara-C are myelosuppression and gastrointestinal epithelial injury (nausea, vomiting, diarrhea). Patients frequently develop mild serum enzyme elevations consistent with hepatocellular damage, but these changes rarely necessitate a discontinuation of treatment. High-dose ara-C treatment causes cerebral dysfunction, ataxia, and conjunctivitis, toxicities not seen with conventional doses.

Ara-C has shown synergistic biochemical interaction with many other antitumor agents, including alkylating agents, *cis*-platinum, thiopurines, uridine analogues, and antifolates. Ara-C enhances cyclophosphamide and BCNU activity by inhibiting repair of strand breaks caused by the alkylating agents. Methotrexate given three to six hours prior to ara-C enhances ara-CTP formation in experimental tumors by undefined mechanisms.

A second cytidine analogue, *5-azacytidine* (*5-azaC*), is activated to 5-azaCTP, which is incorporated into RNA and causes defective protein synthesis and degradation of polyribosomes. It also inhibits methylation of DNA and thus can activate genes, such as those for fetal hemoglobin, which are normally inactivated during differentiation. In addition to its antileukemic activity, 5-azaC has the unique action of increasing fetal hemoglobin synthesis in patients with beta-thalassemia (Ch. 142). The rapid decomposition of 5-azaC in alkaline or neutral solution necessitates either fresh mixing prior to administration or formulation at a slightly acid pH in Ringer's lactate (pH 6.2). The drug undergoes rapid removal from the plasma, either through metabolism or chemical decomposition. Less than 2 per cent of an administered dose remains in plasma as parent compound 30 minutes after administration. The primary toxicities of 5-azaC are myelosuppression and severe and prolonged nausea and vomiting. The latter symptoms are lessened by a prolonged or continuous infusion, with no apparent change in its therapeutic efficacy.

Purine Analogues. 6-Mercaptopurine (6-MP) and 6-thioguanine (6-TG) have the single substitution of a thiol group in place of the 6-hydroxyl group found in the basic purine nucleus. Both require activation to the nucleotide level by hypoxanthine-guanine phosphoribosyltransferase (HGPRT'ase) to inhibit de novo purine biosynthesis and block the conversion of the purine precursor inosinic acid to adenylic acid or to guanylic acid. The triphosphate nucleotides of 6-TG and 6-MP are incorporated into DNA and produce delayed toxicity after several cell divisions. Biochemical resistance to these agents in human leukemic cells is commonly associated with increased concentrations of a degrading enzyme, a membrane-bound alkaline phosphatase, or decreased concentrations of the activating enzyme HGPRT'ase. 6-MP is not reliably absorbed orally; 6-TG is erratically absorbed, and is thus administered by intravenous infusion. 6-MP is rapidly eliminated (plasma half-time 20 to 45 minutes) by oxidation to 6-thiouric acid catalyzed by xanthine oxidase. This reaction is inhibited by allopurinol; thus the dose of orally administered 6-MP must be reduced 75 per cent in the presence of the xanthine oxidase inhibitor. 6-TG is degraded by desulfuration and by oxidation with a plasma half-time of 80 to 90 minutes. No reduction in 6-TG dosage is required for patients who are also receiving allopurinol. Both agents are well tolerated in doses of approximately 100 mg per square meter for at least five days. 6-MP is used at reduced doses for maintenance of remission.

The primary toxicity of both thiopurines is myelosuppression and epithelial injury. Myelosuppression is maximal within seven days of drug administration, and recovery occurs in one to two weeks. Both drugs produce reversible hepatotoxicity with enzyme and bilirubin increases in a pattern suggesting cholestatic jaundice. Mucositis, esophagitis, and gastrointestinal complaints are usually mild.

The 6-thiopurines and the related compound azathioprine, which is metabolized to 6-mercaptopurine by the liver, are potent suppressors of cell-mediated immunity and thus find numerous applications for treating autoimmune diseases and preventing transplant rejection. Immunosuppression with

*Exceeds manufacturer's recommended maximum dose.

these agents can be achieved at doses that produce little decrease in the white blood cell count. Long-term immunosuppressive therapy with azathioprine, prednisone, and other immunosuppressive agents in renal transplantation is associated with an increased risk of squamous carcinomas of skin and histiocytic lymphoma and predisposes patients to bacterial and opportunistic infections.

An unusual purine analogue, deoxycoformycin, has the ability to induce remissions in hairy cell leukemia (see Ch. 155) and chronic lymphocytic leukemia. When used in low dosages of 4 mg per square meter every two weeks, this drug effectively blocks adenosine deaminase activity leading to dATP accumulation and cell death. In high-dose regimens, it causes somewhat unpredictable, but occasionally severe, neurotoxicity or renal failure.

ALKYLATING AGENTS. Alkylating agents kill tumor cells and normal dividing tissues by forming covalent bonds with nucleic acids. The alkyl groups attach to DNA, interfere with its integrity, and thereby produce significant cytotoxic, mutagenic, and carcinogenic effects.

Alkylating agents spontaneously form positively charged carbonium ions in aqueous solution. In the case of chloroethyl derivatives, the alkylating intermediate is $R\text{-}CH_2CH_2^+$, which attacks nucleophilic (electron-rich) sites on nucleic acids, proteins, sulfhydryls (glutathione), and amino acids. It is likely that the primary cytotoxic and mutagenic effects of alkylating agents result from binding to guanine (which accounts for about 90 per cent of alkylated sites), adenine, and cytosine. Based alkylation leads to misreading of the DNA code, but also single-strand breakage. Cross-linkage of DNA occurs when bifunctional alkylating agents are employed. These agents, such as nitrogen mustard, possess two chloroethyl groups, each capable of forming a reactive carbonium ion. The formation of cross-links correlates closely with the lethality of alkylating agents and nitrosourea derivatives in cell culture. Alkylating agents such as nitrogen mustard and cyclophosphamide kill cells in all phases of the cell cycle, but have quantitatively greater activity against rapidly dividing cells.

Alkylating agents share a common mechanism of action, but they differ in their pharmacokinetic features, lipid solubility, chemical reactivity, metabolism, and membrane transport properties (Table 176–9). Tumors may therefore differ in their response or resistance to agents in this class. For example, nitrosoureas and *cis*-platinum may be effective against tumors resistant to cyclophosphamide. The structures of commonly used alkylating agents are shown in Figure 176–4.

Nitrogen mustard (mechlorethamine), the first alkylating agent to receive clinical trial, is used primarily for treatment of malignant lymphomas and as a topical solution for treatment of mycosis fungoides. Nitrogen mustard enters cells through an active transport mechanism shared with the physiologic amine choline. Resistance is believed to result from enhanced repair of DNA alkylation or inactivation by cellular thiols. The primary clinical toxicities of nitrogen mustard consist of myelosuppression and gastrointestinal symptoms (nausea and vomiting). Minor cholinergic side effects occur at high doses and include lacrimation, diarrhea, and diaphoresis. The high chemical reactivity of this compound causes severe local tissue injury when infiltrated into the skin. It is used to ablate the pleural space in patients with chronic pleural effusion (0.2 to 0.4 mg per kilogram into the pleural space after draining the effusion).

TABLE 176–9. ALKYLATING AGENTS

Agent	Route (IV/PO)	Schedule	Dose (mg/m²)	Plasma t½ (hr)
Cyclophosphamide	IV	q.d. × 5	400	6–12
	PO	q.d.	50–100	
Chlorambucil	PO	q.d.	1–2	1.5
Melphalan	IV	q.d. × 5	4	1.8
	IV	q. 4 w.	8	
	PO	q.d. × 5	8	
Nitrosoureas				
BCNU	IV	q. 6 w.	150–225	RCD
CCNU	PO	q. 6 w.	100–150	RCD
Methyl CCNU	PO	q. 6 w.	150–200	RCD

RCD = rapid chemical degradation.

Cyclophosphamide (Cytoxan) has largely replaced nitrogen mustard in clinical use. The drug requires hepatic activation in a multistep process to yield the active compound, phosphoramide mustard, and a side product, acrolein. Acrolein may be responsible for the common side effect of hemorrhagic cystitis, a complication that can be reduced by orally administered thiols. Cyclophosphamide is well absorbed orally, but is usually given by intravenous infusion. It produces only mild thrombocytopenia in comparison with leukopenia. Nausea, vomiting, and alopecia are common side effects. Attempts to prevent cystitis by vigorous hydration of patients carry the risk of inducing symptomatic hyponatremia, since in high-dose infusion regimens (doses of 50 mg per kilogram) cyclophosphamide causes inappropriate water retention owing to direct effects on the renal tubule. Hyponatremia, seizures, and death have occurred as a consequence of water retention. Other toxicities associated with cyclophosphamide treatment include suppression of humoral and delayed immunity, acute myocardial necrosis (after high-dose administration associated with bone marrow transplantation), and, after prolonged courses of treatment, acute myeloblastic leukemia and pulmonary fibrosis.

Melphalan (L-phenylalanine mustard, Alkeran) has activity similar to that of cyclophosphamide (lymphomas, breast and ovarian cancer, multiple myeloma) but does not cause hemorrhagic cystitis. The drug has variable bioavailability by the oral route; thus, the average dose of 0.1 to 0.2 mg per kilogram must be adjusted according to bone marrow tolerance. Melphalan enters cells by active transport, utilizing amino acid transport systems. After intravenous administration, the parent compound disappears from plasma with a half-life of approximately two hours. Less than 15 per cent of the drug is excreted in the urine intact.

Chlorambucil (Leukeran), a close structural congener of melphalan, is also stable in aqueous solution and is given orally. Thus, it is a convenient alkylating agent for treating chronic lymphocytic leukemia, nodular lymphomas, or multiple myeloma, which require long-term management. It has suppressive effects on both granulocytes and platelets, but few other side effects. Like cyclophosphamide and melphalan, chlorambucil therapy has been linked to late occurrences of acute myeloblastic leukemia.

Busulfan (Myleran) consists of two labile methane-sulfonate groups attached at opposite ends of a four-carbon alkyl chain. This compound is sufficiently stable for oral administration, but it rapidly forms carbonium ions leading to alkylation of DNA. It is primarily used for the treatment of chronic granulocytic leukemia, in which its myelosuppressive action provides effective, long-term regulation of the white blood cell count. Myelosuppression is not quickly reversible and may be permanent if excessive doses are used. In addition to myelosuppression, busulfan causes diffuse pulmonary fibrosis and an addisonian-like state characterized by cutaneous hyperpigmentation and weakness, but without abnormal adrenal function.

The *chloroethylnitrosoureas* form a structurally distinct group of alkylating agents. These highly lipid-soluble, chemically reactive compounds have clinical activity against the lymphomas, malignant melanoma, brain neoplasms, and gastrointestinal carcinomas. A new glycosylated nitrosourea, chlorozotocin,* has a similar spectrum of activity but less bone marrow toxicity. Chemical decomposition of these agents yields a reactive chloroethyl carbonium ion ($ClCH_2CH_2^+$) that alkylates DNA. Decomposition of nitrosoureas also yields isocyanates

*Investigational drug.

of differing reactivity that may attack NH_2 groups in a carbamylation reaction and are believed to inhibit DNA repair and to alter maturation of RNA. Because of the extreme clinical reactivity of these compounds in aqueous solution, intact parent compounds (BCNU, CCNU, or methylCCNU) have not been detected in plasma, and little is known about their disposition in man. The high lipid solubility of the nitrosoureas may account for their activity against intracranial tumors, in which the chloroethyl portion of CCNU reaches concentrations 30 per cent of those found simultaneously in plasma. The primary toxicity of the nitrosoureas is delayed and cumulative myelosuppression. Nadir leukopenia and thrombocytopenia occur six to eight weeks after dosage. These compounds are strongly carcinogenic in animal test systems, and methylCCNU has been associated with acute myeloblastic leukemia in humans. Pulmonary fibrosis and renal failure are observed in patients after prolonged courses of treatment (greater than 1500 mg per square meter of BCNU or its congeners). High doses of BCNU (above 500 mg per square meter*) have been used to eradicate tumors such as malignant melanoma or lymphoma, followed by autologous bone marrow transplantation, and are associated with severe, and at times fatal, hepatic and pulmonary toxicity.

***CIS*-PLATINUM.** *Cis* (II) platinum diamminedichloride (cisDDP), the only heavy metal compound used as a cancer chemotherapeutic agent, has a unique mechanism of action and spectrum of biologic effects. It possesses important therapeutic activity against testicular tumors, ovarian carcinoma, bladder cancer, and head and neck cancer. The cis-dichloro structure has cytotoxic activity by virtue of its ability to form covalent bonds and cross-links with DNA. The chloride ions of the coordinate complex are readily displaced by water, generating two positively charged sites. This activated complex then interacts with a nucleophilic site on DNA, RNA, or protein to form covalent cross-links in a manner similar to alkylating reactions. The formation of cross-links continues for hours after drug exposure, and is opposed by repair processes that excise and rebuild damaged segments of DNA. It is likely that the ability to repair DNA is an important determinant of sensitivity to this drug. *cis*-Platinum causes profound cumulative nephrotoxicity due to the reactivity of the parent compound excreted in glomerular filtrate. This toxicity can be prevented by maintaining a high urine flow and a high chloride concentration in urine.

Cis-platinum is usually administered after a four- to six-hour period of hydration and diuresis with 1 liter of a sodium chloride solution. The intravenous dose administered is 40 to 75 mg per square meter and varies according to frequency of administration and individual patient tolerance. An alternative schedule is 20 mg per square meter per day for five days, a regimen that causes less nephrotoxicity and nausea. The renal toxicity of high doses of *cis*-platinum (up to 120 mg per square meter) can be prevented by chloride diuresis with 250 ml of hypertonic saline, given over a one-hour period. The clearance of total platinum from plasma proceeds rapidly during the first few hours after injection (half-time 20 to 60 minutes), but slowly thereafter, owing to covalent binding of drug to serum proteins. The drug bound to protein is inactive. Between 20 and 75 per cent of administered drug is excreted in the urine in the 24 hours after administration. The remainder is probably bound to tissues or plasma protein. *Cis*-platinum penetrates poorly into the central nervous system, the plasma-cerebrospinal fluid ratio being 21:1 or greater. There is considerable interest in the use of *cis*-platinum by intraperitoneal instillation, 90 mg per square meter in 2 liters of dialysate, for treatment of ovarian cancer.

Cis-platinum causes nephrotoxicity in 30 per cent of patients treated with 50 to 75 mg per square meter per course unless preventive pretreatment hydration is undertaken. The primary pathologic findings are coagulative necrosis of the distal tubular epithelium and collecting ducts. In patients with platinum nephrotoxicity, changes in tubular function include magnesium wasting and the excretion of high molecular weight proteins. Hypomagnesemia, a common finding in patients treated with *cis*-platinum, is usually asymptomatic but may lead to tetany. Nausea and vomiting are distressing symptoms in patients taking *cis*-platinum and are poorly relieved by standard antiemetics. These symptoms may be lessened by giving smaller doses once daily for five days. *Cis*-platinum causes only moderate myelosuppression. Leukopenia, thrombocytopenia, and anemia may develop in patients after extended treatment or during high-dose therapy. Other toxicities include a distal, sensory neuropathy after prolonged treatment; hypersensitivity reactions such as urticaria, wheezing, and hypotension (which can be prevented in some patients by pretreatment with antihistamines and corticosteroids); and a progressive loss of high frequency hearing, particularly in older patients.

Analogues of *cis*-platinum, such as CBDCA [carboplatin], appear to cause less nephrotoxicity and ototoxicity and are undergoing clinical evaluation at this time. CBDCA causes greater myelosuppression than *cis*-platinum, perhaps because higher doses are tolerated without renal toxicity.

ANTITUMOR ANTIBIOTICS. ***Bleomycin.*** Bleomycin, a mixture of antibiotic peptides, is widely used for treating lymphomas, testicular cancer, and head and neck cancer. Bleomycin produces single- and double-strand breaks in DNA through a complex sequence of reactions, beginning with its binding to DNA. Ferrous ion (Fe^{2+}), which is intimately bound to bleomycin, then undergoes spontaneous oxidation to the Fe^{3+} state, liberating an electron that is accepted by oxygen to form reactive oxygen species such as the superoxide or hydroxyl radicals, which in turn attack the deoxyribose backbone of DNA, releasing free bases and leading to strand breaks.

Bleomycin kills cells preferentially during the premitotic, or G_2, phase or in the mitotic phase of the cell cycle. The possibility of increasing cell kill by exposing cells during the G_2 phase or mitosis has led to continuous infusion of bleomycin. The determinants of bleomycin sensitivity are poorly understood. There is indirect evidence that the same processes required to repair radiation damage to DNA also repair bleomycin-induced lesions.

Bleomycin is administered by subcutaneous, intramuscular, or intravenous injection with no obvious difference in clinical response rates. Following an intravenous bolus injection of 15 units per square meter, bleomycin has a biphasic plasma disappearance with half-times of 24 minutes and two to four hours. The drug is primarily excreted unchanged in the urine. Bleomycin pharmacokinetics are therefore markedly altered in patients with abnormal renal function. A half-time of 21 hours has been reported in a patient with a creatinine clearance of 11 ml per minute; a decreased dosage of bleomycin (25 to 50 per cent of normal) is indicated for patients with compromised renal function.

Bleomycin has myelosuppressive toxicity only at high doses (above 25 units per square meter*) or in patients with hypoplastic bone marrow. The most important toxicity of bleomycin is progressive interstitial pulmonary fibrosis, manifested first by cough, dyspnea, and bibasilar pulmonary infiltrates on a chest radiograph. The diffusion capacity of the lung progressively decreases with increased total doses of the drug. The decline becomes more rapid above doses of 250 units, and the incidence of significant pulmonary toxicity is 10 per cent at total doses above 450 units. Toxicity is more likely to occur in patients over 70 years of age, in patients with underlying lung disease, in patients receiving high concentrations of oxygen during anesthesia subsequent to bleomycin therapy, and in those previously treated with pulmonary irradiation. Anti-inflammatory agents such as corticosteroids have not been proved to prevent or effectively treat this

*This exceeds the manufacturer's recommended dosage.

*This exceeds the manufacturer's recommended dosage.

fibrosis. The clinical symptoms and x-ray findings of bleomycin pulmonary toxicity are difficult to distinguish from other pulmonary syndromes observed in cancer patients, such as progressive tumor, infectious processes such as *Pneumocystis carinii* or cytomegalovirus, or radiation pneumonitis. Open lung biopsy, often required to rule out these other processes, reveals an acute inflammatory infiltrate, interstitial and intra-alveolar edema, pulmonary hyaline membrane formation, and interstitial fibrosis.

Bleomycin also causes cutaneous toxicity with erythema, induration, thickening, and eventual peeling of skin over the fingers, palms, and extremity joints. Many patients develop hyperpigmentation of skin creases and a general skin darkening. Raynaud's phenomenon has also been reported during bleomycin therapy. Other less frequent toxicities include acute hypertension (at doses greater than 25 units per day), hyperbilirubinemia, fever, and hypersensitivity reactions with urticaria and bronchospasm.

Anthracyclines. Daunomycin and doxorubicin (Adriamycin) belong to the anthracycline class of antibiotics produced by *Streptomyces* species. Anthracyclines have a wide spectrum of clinical activity, including breast cancer, leukemia, and sarcomas. Anthracyclines have many biologic and biochemical effects, including (1) chelation of divalent cations, especially Fe^{2+}, with production of oxygen radicals and superoxide, (2) cyclic oxidation-reduction of the quinone-hydroquinone functional group; and (3) intercalation between strands of the DNA double helix. Intercalation results in inhibition of DNA, RNA, and ultimately protein synthesis. The generation of free radicals of either the drug itself or oxygen is responsible for cytotoxicity.

The anthracyclines induce single-stranded DNA breaks. These breaks are believed to result either from drug-induced cleavage mediated by the enzyme topoisomerase II or from free radicals initiated by reduction of the anthracyclines. Tocopherol (vitamin E), a known free-radical scavenger, lessens oxygen radical generation by doxorubicin in vitro and in animals lessens the cardiac toxicity of Adriamycin without diminishing its antitumor activity. The reason for the particular susceptibility of the heart to doxorubicin action is not clear, but may be due to the lack of free-radical detoxifying enzymes, particularly glutathione peroxidase in that organ.

Assay methods for the anthracyclines have been developed but are not routinely available. The pharmacokinetics of the parent drug include half-lives of 11 minutes, 3 hours, and 25 to 28 hours. The liver is the main site of metabolism of both doxorubicin and daunorubicin. As a result, drug dosages are often modified in the face of abnormal liver function, but precise guidelines based on pharmacokinetics are not available.

Myelosuppression and mucositis are the dose-limiting acute toxicities of the anthracyclines. Alopecia is also common. Extravasation of these agents leads to severe local reaction, beginning as erythema and pain that progress over weeks to deep ulcerative lesions requiring surgical debridement and grafting.

Cardiac damage is the most serious toxicity caused by these agents. In rare instances, an acute syndrome develops hours to days after a dose of doxorubicin or daunorubicin and consists of arrhythmias or pump failure, but clinically significant acute effects are unusual (supraventricular arrhythmias, heart block, and ventricular tachycardia). A more serious toxicity is cumulative, dose-dependent cardiomyopathy, which leads to congestive heart failure in 1 to 10 per cent of the patients who receive more than 550 mg per square meter of doxorubicin or daunomycin. A progressive decrease in cardiac contractility is observed with increasing total dose and is associated with progressive pathologic changes on endocardial biopsy. Congestive heart failure may not appear until up to nine months after cessation of anthracycline therapy. There are no proven methods for preventing acute or chronic anthracycline-induced cardiac damage. Various doxorubicin analogues, many of which have less cardiac toxicity than the parent compound in animals, are undergoing evaluation in humans. The most promising appear to be 4^1-epidoxorubicin and mitoxantrone, the latter a related anthracenedione. Both of these agents have activity in lymphomas and breast cancer.

Mitomycin. Mitomycin C is an antibiotic with clinical activity in gastrointestinal tumors, breast cancer, and ovarian cancer. Its mechanism of action is unclear, but may be the result of free radical generation or alkylation. Only when metabolically activated does the drug alkylate DNA, producing intrastrand and interstrand cross-links, inhibition of DNA synthesis, and cell death.

There is little information on the pharmacokinetics and disposition of this agent. Bolus intravenous doses of 22.5 to 45 mg per square meter* produce peak plasma levels of 0.4 μg per milliliter. Metabolic activation occurs in many tissues and may account for its rapid clearance from the plasma. The liver does not play a necessary role in metabolic activation, and dose modification is not indicated in the presence of liver disease.

The major dose-limiting toxicity of mitomycin C is myelosuppression, which is delayed in onset and cumulative with successive cycles of therapy. Leukocyte and platelet counts usually reach a nadir four to six weeks after treatment. Doses often require modification by the third course of treatment. This drug has been implicated in unusual instances of interstitial pneumonitis, nephrotoxicity, and a syndrome characterized by intravascular hemolysis and renal failure (the hemolytic-uremic syndrome). Mitomycin C may accelerate the development of anthracycline-induced cardiomyopathy.

Actinomycin D. Actinomycin D has activity in the treatment of Wilms' tumor, Ewing's sarcoma, embryonal rhabdomyosarcoma, and gestational choriocarcinoma. This antibiotic intercalates with DNA by virtue of a specific interaction between its cyclic polypeptide chains and deoxyguanosine, causing inhibition of DNA-directed RNA synthesis. Actinomycin D also causes single-stranded DNA breaks.

Actinomycin D is primarily excreted unchanged in bile and urine. Clearance of the drug from plasma is rapid initially, but a slow phase (half-time of 36 hours) of drug disappearance predominates, corresponding to slow release of drug from tissues. Human pharmacologic data are inadequate to allow rational dose modification in the face of liver or renal failure. The dose-limiting toxicity of this agent is myelosuppression, but gastrointestinal side effects are also prominent, and include abdominal pain, cramps, diarrhea, and mucositis. Actinomycin D also enhances x-irradiation toxicity to skin, the gastrointestinal tract, and other sites. A cutaneous recall reaction may occur in patients treated with actinomycin D several months after x-irradiation.

PLANT PRODUCTS. The Vinca alkaloids vincristine and vinblastine, derived from the ornamental shrub *Vinca rosea* (periwinkle), and the epipodophyllotoxins VM-26† and VP-16, derived by modification of a product of the mandrake plant, are among the few plant products with clinically useful cytotoxic activity. Resistance to these agents, as well as to the anthracyclines and actinomycin D, may develop through amplification of a drug-binding glycoprotein, the P-170 glycoprotein, a change that confers multidrug resistance to natural product agents of diverse structure. This pattern of multidrug resistance is believed to result from increased efflux of the anticancer drugs from the tumor cell.

Vinca Alkaloids. The vinca alkaloids bind to tubulin, an intracellular protein that polymerizes to form the microtubular apparatus. Microtubules are components of the mitotic spindle, but also play an important role in maintaining cell

*This exceeds the manufacturer's recommended dosage.

†Investigational drug that has been recommended for approval by FDA Oncologic Drug Advisory Committee.

structure and in providing channels for movement of cellular secretions and neurotransmitters. The vinca alkaloids inhibit the assembly of microtubules and cause dissolution of the mitotic spindle. Vincristine and vinblastine are given intravenously in dosages of 1.0 to 1.4 mg per square meter and 2 to 4 mg per square meter, respectively, at weekly intervals. Only minute concentrations of these alkaloids (less than 0.01 μM) are required to kill sensitive cells. Both alkaloids undergo hepatic metabolism and biliary excretion. Very little parent drug is excreted in the urine. A 50 per cent reduction in dose of either vinca alkaloid is recommended for patients with hepatic dysfunction and a serum bilirubin above 3 mg per deciliter; no dose adjustment is necessary for patients with altered renal function.

Total doses of vincristine greater than 2 mg often cause a progressive neurotoxicity, particularly in older patients and in those receiving weekly treatment. Patients experience a decrease in deep tendon reflexes, paresthesias of the fingers and lower extremities, and, at more advanced stages, cranial nerve palsies, and profound weakness of the dorsiflexors of the foot and extensors of the wrist. The sensory changes may improve with discontinuation of vincristine, but motor deficits usually show little improvement. Vincristine causes little myelosuppression. The platelet count may actually rise during treatment as a result of endoreduplication of megakaryocytes. In contrast, vinblastine is highly toxic to bone marrow, producing leukopenia and thrombocytopenia. Mucositis is also a frequent side effect, but neurotoxicity is rare. Vindesine,* another vinca alkaloid, causes both myelosuppression and moderately severe neurotoxicity. Vincristine promotes release of antidiuretic hormone and may rarely cause symptomatic dilutional hyponatremia. This syndrome is easily treated by fluid restriction.

Podophyllotoxins. Two glycosidic derivatives of podophyllotoxin, VP-16 and VM-26, have important clinical activity in the treatment of lymphomas, small-cell carcinoma of the lung, leukemia, and testicular cancer. They promote DNA strand breaks mediated by the enzyme topoisomerase II. VP-16 and VM-26 have no effect on microtubular assembly and arrest cells in G_2 rather than in mitosis. VP-16 and VM-26 are given intravenously. VP-16 has a shorter terminal half-life, less metabolic alteration, and greater renal excretion (30 per cent unchanged in urine) than VM-26. VP-16 dosage should be reduced by at least 50 per cent in patients with serum creatinine of 2 mg per deciliter or higher. Both drugs penetrate poorly into the cerebrospinal fluid despite their high lipid solubility. The primary route of elimination for VM-26 is metabolic.

Typical well-tolerated intravenous dosages of VP-16 are 45 mg per square meter per day for seven days, 86 mg per square meter per day twice weekly, and 290 mg per square meter once weekly. VM-26 is usually given in weekly dosages of 67 mg per square meter. The dose-limiting toxicity for both drugs is leukopenia. Nausea, vomiting, and neurotoxicity (paresthesias or tendon reflex depression) occasionally occur in patients receiving these drugs.

OTHER AGENTS. ***Hexamethylmelamine.*** Hexamethylmelamine (HMM) exhibits significant activity against ovarian cancer, breast cancer, the lymphomas, and small-cell carcinoma of the lung. The methylamines can be converted by enzymatic hydroxylation to methylol ($R\text{-}CH_2OH$) analogues, which are cytotoxic in tissue culture and may be the active alkylating form of the drug. Because of its limited aqueous solubility, HMM can be given only by the oral route. Usual dosages of 4 to 12 mg per kilogram per day are given for courses of 14 to 21 days. However, the bioavailability of HMM by this route is highly variable. The parent compound has a half-time of 4.7 to 10.2 hours in plasma. HMM produces nausea and vomiting as its dose-limiting toxicity. HMM also produces neurotoxic symptoms, such as mood alterations, hallucinations, and peripheral neuropathy. These effects gradually increase in severity during a protracted course of treatment and disappear upon drug withdrawal.

Dacarbazine (DTIC). DTIC, an imidazole-4-carboxamide derivative, was first synthesized as an inhibitor of purine biosynthesis but, in fact, functions as an alkylating agent. It is active against Hodgkin's disease, malignant melanoma, and soft tissue sarcomas. The metabolic activation of this agent by hepatic microsomes leads to production of an active methyl cation (CH_3^+), which binds to nucleic acid bases. This alkylation is believed to be responsible for the cytotoxic action of DTIC. Schedules of intravenous administration vary from 150 to 300 mg per square meter per day for five to ten days, depending on prior treatment history, concurrent therapy, and patient tolerance. There is no accurate information on its pharmacokinetics or metabolism in man. Severe nausea and vomiting occur during the first days of treatment but may be lessened by reducing the initial dose and gradually increasing the dose during the course of treatment. Mild myelosuppression may occur two to three weeks following treatment. Other toxicities include a flu-like syndrome and a possible enhancement of doxorubicin cardiac toxicity.

Procarbazine. Procarbazine has become an important agent in the treatment of Hodgkin's disease, brain tumors, and lung cancer. It undergoes metabolic activation, yielding a methyldiazonium ion ($^+CH_2{-}N{=}NH$), which becomes bound to nucleic acids, phospholipids, and protein. The pharmacokinetics of procarbazine in humans have been incompletely characterized. The parent drug disappears from plasma with a rapid half-time of seven minutes following intravenous administration. Procarbazine is usually administered orally in daily doses of 100 mg per square meter per day for 10 to 14 days.

Procarbazine may produce a number of adverse reactions. It causes moderate nausea and decreased appetite, mild to moderate leukopenia and thrombocytopenia, and, less frequently, neurotoxicity (paresthesias of the extremities, drowsiness, or depression). The mental status changes may be related to inhibition of monoamine oxidase; therefore, patients taking procarbazine should avoid foods containing tyramine, such as wine, bananas, yogurt, and ripe cheese, since these may provoke a hypertensive crisis. Other monoamine oxidase inhibitors should not be used with this drug. Procarbazine has an Antabuse-like action, which may lead to sweating, flushing, and headache upon ingestion of alcohol. It also causes hypersensitivity reactions, most prominently a maculopapular rash or pulmonary infiltrates. In addition to its cytotoxic action, procarbazine is a potent immunosuppressant, teratogen, and carcinogen. The compound is highly mutagenic in bacterial assays and produces both carcinomas and acute myelocytic leukemia in rodents and monkeys. An increased incidence of second tumors, most prominently acute leukemia, has been observed in patients receiving MOPP combination chemotherapy with irradiation for Hodgkin's disease, and procarbazine is suspected of being the responsible carcinogen in this combination. Thus, its use for non-neoplastic diseases should be carefully weighed with these late toxicities in mind.

L-Asparaginase. L-Asparagine is a nonessential amino acid synthesized by transfer of an amine group to L-aspartic acid. The synthetic reaction is catalyzed by the enzyme L-asparagine synthetase, which is found in many tissues but is lacking in certain human malignant diseases, particularly lymphoid tumors. In tumor cells lacking L-asparagine synthetase, the amino acid can be obtained only from the plasma pool of amino acids. The enzyme L-asparaginase, obtained from *Escherichia coli* or *Erwina carotovora*, degrades asparagine and has potent activity against childhood acute lymphocytic leukemia.

*Investigational drug that has been recommended for approval by FDA Oncologic Drug Advisory Committee.

Resistance to L-asparaginase arises through an increase in L-asparagine synthetase activity in tumor cells. Preparations of L-asparaginase from different bacterial strains have slightly different properties and are not cross-reactive in immunologically sensitized patients. Thus, preparations from *Erwinia* may be used in patients who are hypersensitive to the *E. coli* L-asparaginase. Most L-asparaginase preparations contain L-glutaminase activity, which is 3 to 5 per cent of the L-asparaginase activity. The usual doses are 6000 IU per square meter every other day for three to four weeks, or 1000 to 2000 IU per square meter daily for ten to twenty days.

The half-life of L-asparaginase in plasma is 14 to 22 hours, but there is considerable variation among different preparations. Plasma clearance is greatly accelerated in hypersensitive patients, and enzyme activity may disappear from plasma within four hours. The enzyme distributes primarily within the intravascular space. However, the cerebrospinal fluid concentration of asparagine falls rapidly, and an antileukemic effect is exerted in this sanctuary. The primary toxicities of L-asparaginase are related to immunologic sensitization or result from decreased protein synthesis. Positive skin tests to L-asparaginase are rarely observed in untreated persons, but anaphylaxis may occur with the first dose of drug. Allergic reactions, such as urticaria, laryngeal edema, bronchospasm, or hypotension, occur following multiple courses of the enzyme. Passive hemagglutinating antibodies are observed in patients who subsequently develop anaphylaxis, and complement-fixing antibodies are found in serum after an anaphylactic episode. Toxic effects resulting from inhibition of protein synthesis include hypoalbuminemia and decreased serum fibrinogen, prothrombin, antithrombin III, and other clotting factors, leading to either hemorrhagic or thrombotic episodes; decreased serum insulin with hyperglycemia; decreased serum lipoproteins; and, in 25 per cent of patients, cerebral dysfunction with confusion, stupor, or frank coma. Other toxicities not explained by inhibition of protein synthesis include acute pancreatitis and abnormal liver function tests (increased serum bilirubin, SGOT, and alkaline phosphatase). Approximately 65 per cent of patients receiving L-asparaginase experience nausea, vomiting, and chills as an immediate reaction, but these side effects are controlled by antiemetics, antihistamines, or corticosteroids. L-Asparaginase has no known toxicity to gastrointestinal mucosa or bone marrow and thus is easily used in combination chemotherapy. The only well-established drug interactions are its ability to terminate methotrexate action and its enhancement of ara-C cytotoxicity. Large doses of the antifolate are well tolerated if followed at 24 hours by L-asparaginase rescue because the duration of effective exposure of the bone marrow and gastrointestinal mucosa to methotrexate is limited. The combination of methotrexate and L-asparaginase may have value in the treatment of acute lymphocytic leukemia.

HORMONAL THERAPY

Steroid hormones, like the polypeptide hormones, initiate their action at the cellular level by their binding to discrete receptors. These receptors are present in tumors derived from steroid-responsive normal tissues, such as endometrium, prostate, or breast, and can be assayed in tumor homogenates by competitive binding methods. The correlations between estrogen steroid receptor content and clinical response is strong. For example, the response rate to hormonal manipulation in estrogen receptor–positive (ER^+) patients with breast cancer is approximately 65 per cent, whereas it is less than 10 per cent in ER^- patients. Thus ER^- patients can safely be excluded from consideration for endocrine therapy on the basis of the assay. At least three factors must be kept in mind in assessing the value of the steroid receptor assay: (1) The laboratory performing the test should conform in its methods to nationally established standards. (2) Repeat evaluation of receptor status should be undertaken with each change in therapy, if possible, since receptor status may evolve with time and with intervening treatment. For example, changes from ER^+ to ER^- status clearly occur in approximately 20 per cent of patients having sequential analyses of metastatic breast cancer. (3) Multiple sites should be evaluated if accessible, since biopsy results will differ in receptor content in 10 to 20 per cent of patients with metastatic breast cancer.

The general mechanism of action of steroid hormones is described in Ch. 221. In brief, this action is initiated by binding of the hormone to cytoplasmic receptor, followed by transformation of the steroid-receptor complex to an "active" form, translocation of the receptor-steroid complex to the nucleus, and binding of the complex to an acceptor site on chromatin. Nuclear binding then affects the transcription of messenger RNA coding for specific protein, such as growth-promoting or growth-inhibiting factors, leading ultimately to cell death. In experimental systems, many possible mechanisms of steroid resistance, in addition to absence of the receptor protein, have been identified involving defects in receptor binding, complex transformation and translocation, and nuclear binding. Steroid antagonists, such as the anti-estrogen tamoxifen, bind to receptor and undergo translocation but fail to initiate the transcriptional changes produced by the native steroids or elicit growth-inhibiting proteins. A list of commonly used steroid hormones and antagonists, as well as their major pharmacologic properties, is provided in Table 176–10.

Surgical or radiotherapeutic ablation of an endocrine gland presents an alternative to hormonal therapy in some cases, but has the obvious disadvantage of the ablative procedures itself, and produces in some cases undesirable hormonal deficiencies. For example, adrenalectomy for metastatic breast cancer leads to glucocorticoid and mineralocorticoid deficiency which necessitates replacement therapy. Ablative procedures currently represent first-line therapy only in prostatic cancer, male breast cancer, and premenopausal female breast cancer. As an alternative to adrenalectomy, the production of estrogenic steroids by the adrenal may be inhibited by aminoglutethimide, plus a glucocorticoid (added to suppress pituitary ACTH production).

Analogues of luteinizing hormone releasing hormone (LHRH) are capable of inducing a fall in plasma testosterone levels to castration values. These analogues are effective in producing remission in patients with prostatic cancer, and are an effective alternator to orchiectomy or estrogens.

BIOLOGIC THERAPIES

Surgery, irradiation, and cytotoxic chemotherapy are the principal methods of cancer treatment, but they have the inherent disadvantage of damaging normal tissues. As the result of advances in understanding cancer biology and immunologic defenses against cancer, attention has turned to biologic substances that modify or augment the host response. These biologic response modifiers (BRMs) offer the promise of greater specificity and fewer side effects and are depicted in Figure 176–5.

The basis for immunologic approaches to cancer treatment arises from the knowledge that both cellular and humoral defenses exist against cancer. The cellular defenses include at least three classes of naturally occurring cytotoxic lymphocytes (natural killer cells, lymphokine-activated killer [LAK] cells, and natural cytotoxic cells) that are capable of recognizing and killing tumor cells. These cells can be stimulated to proliferate, and their antitumor activity can be enhanced by administration of biologic substances such as the interferons and interleukins. In addition, humoral substances secreted by

TABLE 176–10. HORMONES AND HORMONE ANTAGONISTS IN CANCER TREATMENT

Agent	Route	Dose and Schedule	Acute Toxicity	Late Complications	Uses
Estrogen					
Diethylstilbestrol	PO	5 mg t.i.d. (breast) 1–3 mg q.d. (prostate)	Nausea, vomiting, sodium and fluid retention, uterine bleeding, hypercalcemia (in patients with bone metastases)	Feminization, risk of death from cardiovascular disease	Prostate cancer, postmenopausal breast cancer
Estrogen antagonist					
Tamoxifen	PO	10 mg b.i.d.	Hypercalcemia, nausea, thrombocytopenia (transient), mild estrogenic action, hot flashes	Retinal degeneration, cataracts in high doses (above 40 mg/day)	Breast cancer
Progestins					
Hydroxyprogesterone	IM	1 gram b.i.w.	Fluid retention, hypercalcemia, cholestatic jaundice		Breast, endometrial, renal cancer
6-Methyl hydroxyprogesterone	IM PO	200–600 mg b.i.w. 100–200 mg q.d.			
Megestrolacetate	PO	160 mg q.d.			
Androgens					
Fluoxymesterone	PO	10–20 mg q.d.	Cholestatic jaundice (fluoxymesterone), virilization, fluid retention, ureteral obstruction (males), hypercalcemia (in patients with bone metastases)	Hepatic adenomas, hepatoma	Breast carcinoma in ER^+ patients who have prior response to estrogen or anti-estrogen therapy
Glucocorticoids					
Prednisone	PO	40 mg/m^2 q.d.	Fluid retention, hyperglycemia, euphoric state, hypokalemia	Osteoporosis, immunosuppression, cushingoid habitus, gastrointestinal ulcers, hypertension, suppression of pituitary-adrenal axis	Lymphomas, leukemia, multiple myeloma, breast cancer
Hydroxycortisone hemisuccinate	IV	200 mg/m^2 q.d.			
Dexamethasone	PO	2–10 mg/m^2 q.d. in divided doses		Same as above	Cerebral edema

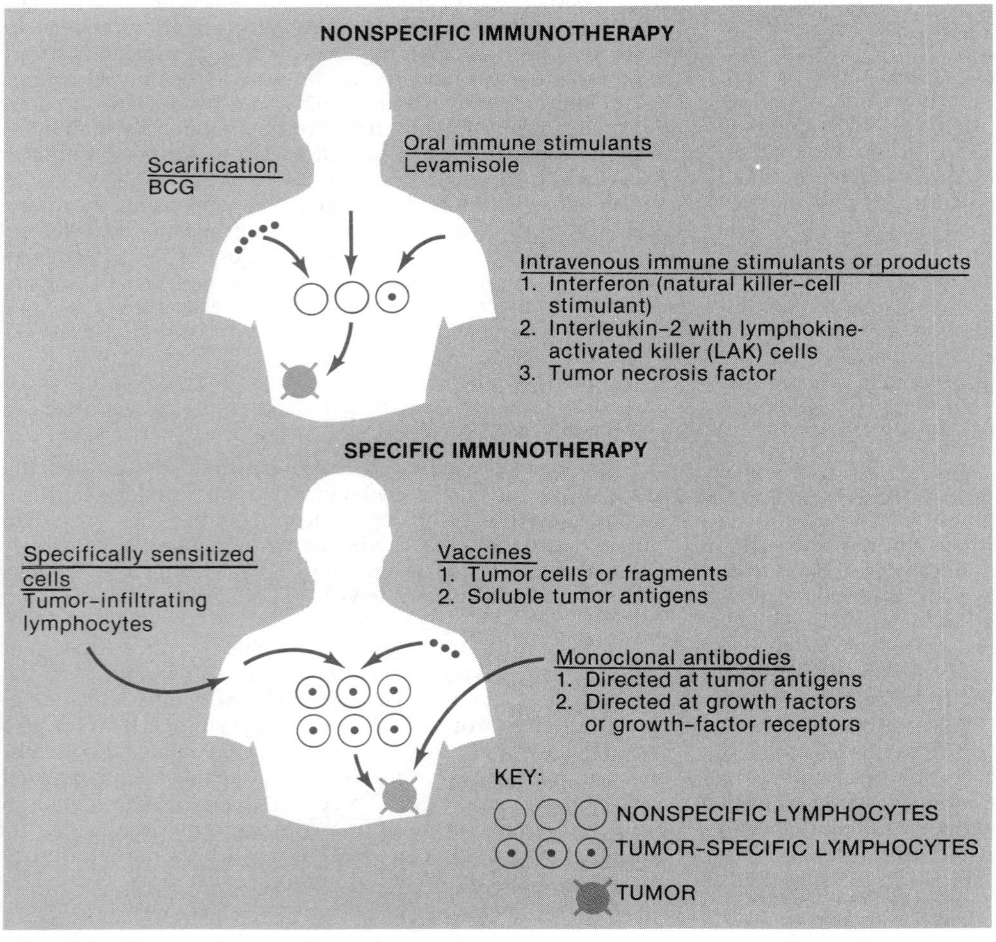

FIGURE 176–5. Concepts of tumor immunotherapy. Nonspecific therapies cause proliferation of a broad range of immune cells, some of which have inherent antitumor activity, such as natural killer cells or LAK cells. Specific immunotherapies employ products that have specificity for a particular tumor based on the tumor's surface antigens or based on its growth factor requirements. These antigens, or growth-factor requirements, may be shared by normal cells derived from the same tissue.

TABLE 176–11. PROMISING BIOLOGIC APPROACHES FOR CANCER THERAPY

Target	Role in Cancer Progression	Therapeutic Concept
Epidermal growth factor (EGF)	Stimulates cancer cell proliferation of epithelial–derived cancers	Employ monoclonal antibody to EGF receptor
Bombesin	Stimulates proliferation of small-cell carcinoma of the lung	Employ monoclonal antibody to bombesin
Laminin	Basement membrane protein to which cancer cells attach during invasion and metastasis	Prevent attachment with administration of soluble laminin fragments
Interleukin-2 (IL-2)	Stimulates proliferation of neoplastic T cells	Employ monoclonal antibody to IL-2 receptor

lymphocytes, such as the interferons and tumor necrosis factor, have direct antitumor activity. The most successful use of biologic substances has been in the treatment of hairy cell leukemia, chronic granulocytic leukemia, and non-Hodgkin's lymphoma with alfa-interferon. An early trial of LAK-cell therapy—using cells taken from the host, expanded in vitro in the presence of IL-2, and reinfused in the presence of IL-2—has produced responses in patients with renal carcinoma, malignant melanoma, and colon cancer, but this treatment is compromised by significant host toxicity related to IL-2, including marked fluid retention.

An alternative approach is to develop antibodies that recognize antigens specific for a malignant tissue, such as the anti–B-cell antibodies used to clear bone marrow cells of B cell lymphomas in bone marrow autotransplantation. While tumor-specific antigens have been identified in experimental neoplasms, such antigens have been difficult to isolate in human tumors. However, in at least one setting, a tumor-specific antigen has been used as the target for monoclonal antibody therapy in man; the idiotypic immunoglobulin found on the surface of lymphoma cells has been used as the antigen to elicit antibody specific for that tumor. While patients with lymphoma have shown consistent tumor regression with such therapy, preparation of such anti-idiotypic antibody is arduous, and most responses have been only temporary. Radiolabeled monoclonal antibodies have proven capable of localizing to tumor deposits, but in early clinical trials these antibodies have little cytotoxic effect. Attempts to arm antibodies with alpha- or beta-particle emittors, or with toxins such as the ricin-A chain, are in progress.

Other, less-well-understood immunotherapies have been tested, including tumor vaccines, nonspecific immunostimulants such as BCG (bacillus Calmette-Guerin), and macrophage stimulators such as muramyl dipeptide. None has an established place in cancer therapy, with perhaps the exception of intravesicular instillation of BCG in patients with bladder carcinoma is situ.

Biologic properties of tumor, including dependence on specific factors for growth and metastasis, are also being examined as targets for biologic therapies; promising ideas are listed in Table 176–11.

CONCLUSIONS

In perhaps no other specialty of internal medicine is the physician faced with more crucial choices and a smaller margin for error than in the treatment of a patient with cancer. Because of the potency of the drugs used and the fact that vital-organ function may be compromised by the malignant process, the physician must take into account physiologic and pharmacologic factors in choosing regimens, doses, and duration of therapy. In addition, the physician must never lose sight of the reality that poorly conceived or inadequately administered treatment carries with it the certainty of a fatal outcome.

Chabner BA: The Pharmacologic Basis of Cancer Treatment. Philadelphia, W. B. Saunders Company, 1982. *A text covering both the clinical and experimental pharmacology of anticancer drugs, with particular emphasis on clinical pharmacokinetics, cell kinetics, and drug interactions.*

De Vita VT Jr, Hellman S, Rosenberg SA: Cancer: Principles and Practice of Oncology. 2nd ed. Philadelphia, J. B. Lippincott Company, 1986. *A detailed consideration of three treatment methods of cancer: surgery, irradiation, and chemotherapy.*

Goldie JH, Goldman AJ: A mathematic model for relating the drug sensitivity of tumors to their spontaneous mutation rate. Cancer Treat Rep 63:1727, 1979. *The most useful and illuminating analysis of the relationship of spontaneous mutation rate to drug resistance.*

Pinedo HM, Chabner BA: Cancer Chemotherapy. Amsterdam, Elsevier-North Holland, 1986. *A yearly update of drug research and clinical chemotherapy, with detailed and critical evaluation of important new papers.*

Rosenberg SA, Lotze MT, Muul LM, et al.: Observations on the systemic administration of autologous lymphokine—activated killer cells and recombinant interleukin-2 to patients with metastatic cancer. N Engl J Med 313:1485, 1985. *A landmark study describing the response of patients with various solid tumors to LAK cells with a recombinant growth factor, interleukin-2. This is the first positive trial of an anticancer therapy based on cell-mediated immunity.*

Tannock I: A presentation of classical cell kinetics and its application to cancer chemotherapy: A critical review. Cancer Treat Rep 62:1117, 1978. *A lucid discussion of the basic principles of cellular kinetics and their application, or lack thereof, in the design of current clinical chemotherapy regimens.*

PART XIV

METABOLIC DISEASES

177 INTRODUCTION

James B. Wyngaarden

The term *metabolism* encompasses the numerous chemical transformations that occur within living organisms. These are often divided into two large categories. Those reactions or processes that are synthetic, and in general result in a larger molecule than any of the reactants, are called *anabolic*. Such reactions are usually energy requiring. Those reactions that are degradative and involve the breakdown of large molecules into smaller products are termed *catabolic*. Such processes are essentially energy yielding. The term *intermediary metabolism* refers to all changes that take place between the moment of entry of a nutrient into the organism and the discharge of all of the chemical products into the environment. It is customary to consider separately the intermediary metabolism of carbohydrates, lipids, and proteins, although no sharp lines can be drawn among these three areas of knowledge. The term *basal metabolism* refers to energy requirements for maintenance and conduct of cellular and tissue processes under conditions in which the effects of muscular activity and the work of digestion and metabolism of foodstuffs are minimal.

Part XIV of this textbook is concerned with Metabolic Diseases. A disorder is classified as a metabolic disease when the fundamental pathogenetic mechanism involves a chemical transformation or process. Many diseases of metabolism involve specific enzyme or other protein abnormalities. When these can be attributed to an underlying genetic abnormality, they are termed *inborn errors of metabolism* (see Ch. 34). Disorders associated with specific enzyme defects have been described for more than 100 individual enzymes. Most of these are described somewhere in this textbook, but not all have been collected into Part XIV. For example, hemolytic anemias attributable to specific enzyme defects are included with the other hemolytic anemias in Part XII, Hematologic Diseases, and adrenal hyperplasia attributable to specific enzyme defects is discussed in Part XVI, Endocrine and Reproductive Diseases. The disorders included in this Part are chiefly those whose manifestations are multisystemic or in which the biochemical and genetic factors dominate the description.

PATHOGENESIS OF HEREDITARY METABOLIC DISEASES. The etiology of an inborn error of metabolism is a mutant gene. The alteration in DNA structure produces a disturbance in protein structure and function, which in turn affects cell and organ function. Hereditary metabolic diseases can be considered in terms of these three sequential levels.

Altered DNA Structure. The nature of mutations can be deduced from changes in amino acid sequences in the mutant proteins and the genetic codes (see Ch. 33). This approach has been applied most extensively in studies of variant hemoglobins and glucose-6-phosphate dehydrogenases. DNA restriction enzyme analyses and DNA sequencing techniques now permit direct analysis of alterations in DNA structure. By these methods, point mutations, deletions, and insertions are now readily identified, and hybrid proteins or prematurely terminated or aberrantly extended proteins or totally deleted proteins explained in terms of genetic mechanisms. Restriction endonucleases identify variations in gene structure as fragment-length polymorphisms. The latter approach has provided first clues to the genetic abnormality in Huntington's disease and cystic fibrosis. With the availability of DNA cloning techniques it is now possible to study directly the altered DNA sequence in many human mutations, even those that involve genes that code for quantitatively minor proteins such as enzymes. These techniques also disclose mutations in noncoding regions of DNA that affect rate of synthesis, processing, or stability of specific messenger RNAs.

Altered Protein Function. Abnormalities in the synthesis or structure of a specific enzyme protein result in absence of or reduced or (occasionally) enhanced rates of a specific enzyme-catalyzed reaction. In most genetic enzyme deficiency states, a reduced but detectable level of enzymatic activity can be measured by sensitive assays. The residual enzyme activity can frequently be attributed to a catalytically abnormal enzyme, which may exhibit decreased affinity for substrates, cofactors, or inhibitors. In the most extensively studied series of enzyme defects, those involving glucose-6-phosphate dehydrogenase, most of the enzyme deficiencies reflect unstable enzymes whose activities decay as the erythrocyte ages. This is a common mechanism of enzyme deficiency in the anucleated red blood cell, but has not been demonstrated to be an important cause of enzyme deficiency in disorders that affect primarily nucleated cells. The most interesting example of mutations leading to increased enzyme activities involves phosphoribosylpyrophosphate synthetase. Different mutations in an X-linked structural gene lead to four discrete subtypes exhibiting (1) reduced sensitivity to nucleotide regulators, (2) increased affinity for substrate, (3) increased specific activity per enzyme molecule, or (4) a combination of (1) and (3). Relatively few lesions, other than hemoglobinopathies, have been attributed to mutations in genes coding for nonenzymic proteins. One example is the ZZ variant of alpha$_1$-antitrypsin deficiency, in which an altered protein is not susceptible to normal post-translational processing (glycosylation), with the result that the defective glycoprotein cannot be secreted by the liver. In some nonenzymic proteins, a structural abnormality leads to aggregation (e.g., sickle cell hemoglobin). In others, the mutation affects the affinity of a receptor for a specific ligand (e.g., the low-density lipoprotein [LDL] receptor in familial hypercholesterolemia and the cytoplasmic androgen receptor in complete testicular feminization).

Disrupted Cell and Organ Function. Most genetic diseases first come to clinical attention because of disturbances at the level of cell and organ function. Several types of derangements occur:

1. Altered flux through metabolic pathways. This is the most frequent basis of recognition of an inborn error of metabolism. The product may be missing (albinism), or a

precursor may accumulate (mucopolysaccharidoses) or be shunted into a toxic metabolite (phenylketonuria).

2. Disordered feedback regulation of synthetic pathways. Decreased synthesis of a regulatory end-product may result in faulty control of an early step of the pathway with excessive production of intermediates. The classic example is acute intermittent porphyria, in which a deficiency of uroporphyrinogen synthetase leads to diminished production of heme, a normal feedback inhibitor of porphyrin synthesis. Decreased production of heme leads to overactivity of δ-aminolevulinic acid synthetase, overproduction of nonheme porphyrins, and acute intermittent porphyria.

3. Disordered membrane function. This is the basis for a large group of genetic diseases in which there is impairment of a specific function of a plasma membrane protein. In one type, transmembrane transport of specific small molecules is defective, apparently because a membrane carrier protein is nonfunctional. The affected substrates can be amino acids (cystinuria), carbohydrates (renal glycosuria), or ions (renal tubular acidosis). In another type, receptor-mediated endocytosis of a macromolecule is defective. In familial hypercholesterolemia a mutation in the gene that codes for a receptor results in defective uptake and degradation of LDL by body cells, resulting in accumulation of LDL and its cholesterol in plasma and arterial walls. Still another type involves a defect in a plasma membrane protein whose action is required for hormone action. In pseudohypoparathyroidism, the guanosine triphosphate (GTP)–sensitive N protein is defective, and parathyroid hormone cannot stimulate adenylate cyclase in the target cell. The latter two types of defects are inherited as dominant traits, in contrast to those that involve transmembrane transport of small molecules which behave as recessive traits.

4. Disordered intracellular compartmentation. A few examples of primary genetic defects in cell compartmentation are known. The ZZ variant of alpha$_1$-antitrypsin deficiency, discussed above, is one. Another is I-cell disease, in which there is a deficiency of a processing enzyme that is normally responsible for the occurrence of mannose-6-phosphate residues in lysosomal enzymes. In the absence of mannose-6-phosphate residues, enzymes do not bind to a specific receptor that directs them to the lysosome, and these enzymes pass through the cell into the plasma like a secretory protein. An additional example is a rare form of familial hypercholesterolemia in which there is an abnormal cell surface receptor that can bind LDL but cannot transport it into the cell.

5. Distorted cell or tissue architecture. The distorted shapes of erythrocytes in sickle cell diseases and in hereditary spherocytosis are examples of this type. Another example is illustrated by the immotile cilia syndrome (Kartagener's syndrome), in which a structural protein of cilia, dynein, is defective. In consequence the "dynein arms" that cross-link microtubules are missing, they cannot slide properly, and cilia cannot undulate. Still another type is exemplified by Type VI Ehlers-Danlos syndrome, in which collagen is deficient in hydroxylsine and does not cross-link normally.

ACQUIRED METABOLIC DISEASES. There are many examples of metabolic diseases that are acquired rather than hereditary. Gout exists in primary and secondary varieties. The secondary types occur because of excessive nucleic acid turnover in myeloproliferative diseases or chronic hemolytic anemias, or because of impaired renal excretion of uric acid resulting from drug effects upon the kidney or acquired renal disease. Certain varieties of porphyria can be attributed to acquired intoxications. Hyperlipoproteinurias are common accompaniments of other diseases: hypothyroidism, the nephrotic syndrome, acute and chronic alcoholism, biliary obstruction. In many conditions there is a prominent interaction between hereditary and environmental factors: obesity and diabetes mellitus, ingestion of phenylalanine-containing proteins in phenylketonuria, ingestion of milk in galactosemia. Without the environmental stress these conditions would remain silent.

Some of the diseases of metabolism are very common, such as diabetes, with a prevalence in the United States of about 2.5 per cent, and the hyperlipidemias. Others are quite rare, and a few are perhaps more properly regarded as biochemical anomalies rather than diseases—pentosuria, for example. The study of rare metabolic disorders has provided a better understanding of normal metabolic processes, and in some instances has allowed early recognition of a disorder whose manifestations are preventable simply by adjustment of diet (galactosemia, phenylketonuria). The identification of specific enzyme defects has led to attempts at replacement therapy with inklings of success following enzyme infusion (Gaucher's disease, Fabry's disease) or organ transplantation (bone marrow in immunologic deficiency states; kidney in cystinosis, Fabry's disease, Gaucher's disease).

Bondy PK, Rosenberg LE (eds.): Metabolic Control and Disease. 8th ed. Philadelphia, W. B. Saunders Company, 1980. *An excellent general text.*

Stanbury JB, Wyngaarden JB, Fredrickson DC, et al. (eds.): The Metabolic Basis of Inherited Disease. 5th ed. New York, McGraw-Hill Book Company, 1983. *An authoritative text that presents detailed discussions of various hereditary diseases of metabolism by recognized experts on each topic.*

Disorders of Carbohydrate Metabolism

178 GALACTOSEMIA

Stanton Segal

The galactosemias are toxicity syndromes exhibited by patients with an inherited inability to metabolize the sugar, galactose, which is a constituent of the disaccharide lactose found in milk and milk products. There are three disorders, each of which results from a deficiency of one of the enzymes that catalyze the normal conversion of galactose to glucose: galactokinase, galactose-1-phosphate uridyltransferase, and uridine diphosphate-4-epimerase. A defect in galactokinase is manifested primarily by cataract formation early in life. Uridyltransferase deficiency, which is the most prevalent and commonly referred to as classic galactosemia, results in a syndrome of nutritional failure, liver disease, abnormal renal tubule function, cataracts, mental retardation, and ovarian abnormalities in affected females. A deficiency of epimerase activity clinically resembles transferase deficiency, but may exist in a more benign form when the enzyme defect is limited to red blood cells. For all three disorders, the elevations of the level of galactose and its metabolites in blood, urine, and tissues can be corrected and the clinical manifestations alleviated by omission of dietary galactose.

ETIOLOGY. Galactokinase, galactose-1-phosphate uridyltransferase, and uridine diphosphate-4-epimerase deficiencies are all autosomal recessive genetic disorders. The individual human genes have been located on chromosomes 17, 9, and 1 respectively. The tissues of obligate heterozygotes contain about 50 per cent of the normal enzyme activity, while homozygotes exhibit absence of or very little activity. Immunoelectrophoretic analysis has shown that patients with transferase deficiency produce a protein similar to the normal, but with severely reduced enzyme activity or reduced stability, suggesting single amino acid substitution defects in the majority rather than deletion mutations.

PREVALENCE. Uridyltransferase deficiency has a prevalence of 1 per 40,000 births and a carrier rate of about 1 per cent in the U.S. population. A gene known as the Duarte variant is allelic to the normal transferase and codes for a protein that is electrophoretically different and enzymatically less active. The gene frequency of the Duarte variant is about 0.05 per cent, and homozyotes for the Duarte variant have about 50 per cent of normal transferase activity in their red blood cells. With widespread neonatal screening a number of babies have been detected with low red cell transferase activity who are compound heterozygotes with one gene for defective transferase and another for the Duarte variant. Such infants have only 10 to 25 per cent of red cell enzyme activity, but rarely have impaired galatose utilization that requires treatment.

Galactokinase deficiency is quite rare, having a prevalence of one in 500,000 to one in one million births. Epimerase deficiency is also rare. The benign type has mainly been described in Swiss and Japanese populations, while only a few cases of symptomatic epimerase deficiency have been detected.

PATHOGENESIS. Galactose is converted to glucose by a unique series of three enzyme reactions. The first enzyme in the pathway, galactokinase, causes galactose to react with ATP to form galactose-1-phosphate:

$$\text{Galactose} + \text{ATP} \rightarrow \text{Galactose-1-P}$$

Next, galactose-1-P reacts with UDP-glucose to form UDP-galactose in a reaction catalyzed by uridyltransferase:

$$\text{Galactose-1-P} + \text{UDP-glucose} \rightleftharpoons \text{Glucose-1-P} + \text{UDP-galactose}$$

The third enzyme, epimerase, performs the spatial change of the hydroxyl group about the fourth carbon to convert galactose to glucose:

$$\text{UDP-galactose} \rightleftharpoons \text{UDP-glucose}$$

In the presence of pyrophosphate, UDP-glucose pyrophosphorylase cleaves UDP-glucose to glucose-1-phosphate, which is converted to glucose-6-phosphate by phosphoglucomutase and then enters various other pathways of glucose metabolism. Normally this pathway functions efficiently. Galactose rapidly disappears from blood after intravenous infusion, even faster than a comparable amount of glucose. In normal individuals liver extraction of galactose results in a rise in the level of blood glucose.

In each of the three forms of galactosemia, diminished enzyme activity produces an accumulation of the substrates proximal to the metabolic block: galactose in galactokinase deficiency, galactose and galactose-1-phosphate in transferase deficiency, and galactose, galactose-1-phosphate plus UDP-galactose in epimerase deficiency. When galactose is increased, alternative pathways form large amounts of otherwise trace metabolites. In one reaction galactose is reduced to form the sugar alcohol, galactitol, while in another galactose is oxidized to galactonic acid. These metabolites accumulate in tissues and are excreted in considerable amounts in the urine.

Identification of accumulated metabolites and the elucidation of alternative pathways have provided insights into the relationship of biochemical toxicity and clinical manifestations of the disorders. In galactokinase deficiency, in which galactose and metabolites of alternative pathways are increased, the principal clinical finding is cataracts, without multiple organ involvement. These findings implicate galactose-1-phosphate as causing the severe multisystem disease of transferase deficiency and systemic epimerase deficiency. Cataract formation appears to be due to the formation of galactitol by lens aldose reductase. Galactitol, which cannot be further metabolized, accumulates in the lens and produces osmotic changes with imbibition of fluid, lens swelling, and protein precipitation. The exact biochemical alterations in target organs affected by transferase deficiency have not been defined. There are no structural alterations of the brain associated with mental retardation in cases of transferase deficiency, but liver dysfunction is accompanied by altered architecture of liver characterized by pseudoacinar formation of hepatic cells. The ovaries of females afflicted with hypogonadism may be small, fibrotic, or streaked.

The fact that galactose-1-phosphate can be increased in red cells of transferase-deficient patients and that mental retardation and ovarian abnormalities can occur in patients with no exposure to galactose has fostered the concept that there is continuous self-intoxication in this disorder. This could occur as a result of the formation of UDP-galactose from UDP-glucose via epimerase activity and subsequent pyrophosphorolysis of UDP-galactose to liberate galactose-1-phosphate. The pyrophosphorylase plays a dual role in the process, since it is also responsible for the formation of UDP-glucose from uridine triphosphate and glucose-1-phosphate.

CLINICAL MANIFESTATIONS. Cataracts are the principal finding in patients with galactokinase deficiency, who otherwise are healthy. The cataracts are usually discovered in infants and children examined for other medical reasons. Pseudotumor cerebri has been described in some galactokinase-deficient patients as well as those with transferase deficiency. Cataracts have been observed in some heterozygous carriers, and patients under 40 years with cataracts frequently have lower than normal red cell galactokinase levels.

Uridyltransferase deficiency usually manifests itself shortly after birth or within the first few weeks of life with growth failure, vomiting, diarrhea, hepatomegaly, ascites, jaundice, hemolytic anemia, hypoglycemia, proteinuria, and a renal Fanconi syndrome. Cataracts may not be easily observed with an ophthalmoscope in young infants, but are found on slit lamp examination. Infants with this disease may die in the first few days of life from overwhelming *Escherichia coli* sepsis before other manifestations are evident. Without elimination of galactose from the diet, severely affected infants will die of inanition and liver failure. Occasionally, because of vomiting, the infant's formula will be changed to one that is galactose free, with subsequent cessation of the toxicity syndrome. Later in childhood these patients have severe mental retardation and cataracts after milk is reintroduced into the diet. Mental retardation is frequent if therapy is not initiated within the first two to three months of life. Postpubertal females have a high incidence of hypergonadotropic hypogonadism expressed as either primary or secondary amenorrhea, but the testes of male patients are normal. There is no correlation of the clinical course with ovarian function, but the frequency of hypogonadism appears to be higher where diet therapy was delayed.

Black patients with transferase deficiency may have a milder toxicity syndrome and in some cases have no symptoms. This has been called the Negro variant. Such patients have been found to metabolize some galactose because of the presence of 10 per cent of normal transferase activity in liver and intestinal mucosa. A toxicity syndrome resembling transferase deficiency occurs in cases of systemic epimerase deficiency.

DIAGNOSIS. Galactokinase deficiency should be suspected in any infant or child with cataracts and the diagnosis confirmed by assay of red blood cell or cultured fibroblast galactokinase. A presumptive diagnosis is possible by detection of reducing sugar in urine that is glucose oxidase negative (galactose) or by chromatographic analysis for galactitol in the urine. These urinary findings also obtain in transferase deficiency, whose definitive diagnosis require the assay of red cell transferase activity. Since severely affected babies may be given blood transfusions before a diagnosis of galactosemia is considered, red cell transferase assay should be delayed until transfused blood has been replaced by the infant's own cells. However, assay of transferase in parents' red cells and the findings of 50 per cent of normal activity in both may be helpful in making a presumptive diagnosis in such infants or in those who may have died before specimens for assay were obtained.

In the differential diagnosis, hereditary fructose intolerance with hepatomegaly, liver dysfunction, hypoglycemia, renal Fanconi syndrome, and nonglucose reducing substance in the urine should be considered. Lactosuria, a common finding in a variety of gastrointestinal disorders, also causes a positive test result for reducing substance. However, many laboratories use glucose oxidase-based tests for blood and urinary sugar determination, and in such instances, galactosemia and galactosuria would go undetected. The greatest confusion in differential diagnosis is the distinction between transferase deficiency and primary liver disease. Because the liver is the major organ metabolizing galactose, any disruption of hepatocellular function may result in galactosemia and galactosuria. Red cell transferase assay should be employed to make the distinction. Patients with clinical findings resembling classic transferase deficiency galactosemia who have normal red cell transferase activity should also be tested for red cell epimerase activity.

Besides the quantitative assay of red cell transferase, the performance of starch gel electrophoresis or isoelectric focusing to determine isoenzyme banding may be useful in distinguishing the carrier for classic galactosemia, the homozygous Duarte variant whose red cell enzyme activity is comparable to carriers for the classic disease, and mixed Duarte–classic galactosemia carriers who have 10 to 25 per cent of normal activity, as well as the Rennes and Chicago variants of transferase deficiency. In addition to these variants with diminished red cell activity and electrophoretic abnormalities, there are other variant forms. The Indiana variant has typical symptoms of transferase deficiency galactosemia and unstable red cell activity, while clinical disease in the Munich variant is caused by abnormal inhibition of transferase by glucose-1-phosphate, the product of the reaction.

Many cases are presently diagnosed as a result of neonatal screening. More than one half of the states in the United States and several foreign countries test all newborns by analysis of heel-stick-blood spots on filter paper. All of the procedures used will detect transferase deficiency. Some will also detect galactokinase or epimerase deficiency. All positive test results require confirmation by quantitative assay of the individual enzymes. Such screening has resulted in delineation of the benign form of epimerase deficiency in which galactose-1-phosphate appears to accumulate only in red blood cells. Subsequent studies have indicated the epimerase in such cases is unstable because of increased requirement for cofactor NAD, which can be supplied by other cells but not red blood cells.

TREATMENT. The institution of a galactose-free diet is the cornerstone of treatment. With galactose elimination, early cataracts may regress. Liver dysfunction and renal tubule abnormalities disappear, and growth and development are normal. Besides the banning of milk and all milk products, care should be taken to eliminate foods in which milk is used in cooking and baking or lactose has been added. There is no indication that the ability to metabolize galactose increases with age, so that dietary restrictions should not be relaxed in older children.

PROGNOSIS. Untreated patients with transferase deficiency may not survive. Those who do will be severely retarded mentally. The best prognosis for normal mentation occurs in those treated at birth or shortly thereafter. Those treated after three months of age have a poorer outcome. Despite excellent treatment from birth, patients with a normal IQ may not do well in school and may have diminished attention span and visual-perceptual difficulties. A significant number may have abnormal EEG patterns. The possibility exists that continuous self-intoxication with endogenous galactose-1-phosphate formation underlies the less than perfect mental outcome and ovarian atrophy in transferase deficiency, even with excellent dietary treatment.

PREVENTION. The best outcome results from the earliest dietary treatment. Heterozygote mothers of known galactosemic patients should receive a galactose-free diet to prevent any intrauterine exposure of a fetus who may be affected. Prenatal diagnosis can be performed by enzyme assay of cultured amniotic cells.

Fishler, Koch R, Donnell GN, et al.: Developmental aspects of galactosemia from infancy to childhood. Clin Pediatr 19:38, 1980. *Data describing outcome of dietary treatment of uridyltransferase-deficient patients in relation to age of diagnosis reveals normal IQ but abnormal visual-perceptual status and EEG in patients well treated before three months of age.*

Kaufman FR, Kogut MD, Donnell GN, et al.: Hypergonadotropic hypogonadism in female patients with galactosemia. N Engl J Med 304:944, 1981. *Describes amenorrhea and ovarian abnormalities in patients with uridyltransferase deficiency.*

Levy HL, Hammersen G: Newborn screening for galactosemia and other galactose metabolic defects. J Pediatr 92:871, 1978. *Details of methods and results of worldwide screening of about six million infants.*

Segal S: Disorders of galactose metabolism. In Stanbury JB, Wyngaarden JB, Fredrickson DS, et al. (eds.): The Metabolic Basis of Inherited Disease. 5th ed. New York, McGraw-Hill Book Company, 1983, pp. 167–192. *A comprehensive treatise of the enzymology and metabolism of galactose, the biochemical basis of galactose toxicity, and the clinical aspects of inherited disorders.*

179 THE GLYCOGEN STORAGE DISEASES

R. Rodney Howell

Glycogen is the principal storage form of carbohydrate in man and is found in varying concentrations in virtually all cells. Glycogen is composed exclusively of glucose molecules, and differs from starch in having a highly branched structure that greatly enhances its solubility.

In the glycogen storage diseases the tissue concentration of glycogen is most commonly elevated, but in certain of these disorders the significant abnormality is in the structure of glycogen. Although liver glycogen content reflects to some extent the nutritional status of the subject, excessive alimentation does not lead to abnormal accumulation of hepatic glycogen in the normal subject in the absence of corticosteroid treatment.

The glycogen storage diseases are of historic importance in that the first direct demonstration of a liver enzyme deficiency in man was made in glycogen storage disease by the Coris over 35 years ago.

As new specific enzyme defects were recognized, the Coris began a numbering system for the glycogen storage diseases that has been in wide use. However, we will not refer to the numbering system here; its use is to be discouraged, because the numbers beyond VI vary considerably from author to author and the existence of some of the conditions defined by recent numbers is in doubt.

Although most of the glycogen storage diseases produce fairly widespread accumulation of glycogen, in large part the diseases present clinically as either hepatic or muscular forms.

THE HEPATIC FORMS OF GLYCOGEN STORAGE DISEASE. Hepatorenal glycogen storage disease (von Gierke's disease) is the prototype of the hepatic forms of glycogen storage disease. Glucose-6-phosphatase deficiency is the basic defect. Children with this disorder have proportionately short stature with a very prominent abdomen and massive enlargement of the liver. The hepatic enlargement is due to both glycogen and lipid accumulation. Although the kidneys are enlarged because of the deposition of glycogen, this cannot be appreciated clinically except by radiographic examination. The eyes reveal multiple bilateral, symmetric, yellowish, discrete, paramacular lesions, which are specific for this form of glycogen storage disease. Xanthomas are common over the extensor surfaces of the arms and legs; bleeding may present major clinical problems.

Prominent hypoglycemia on fasting and a reduced rise in blood sugar after subcutaneous injection of epinephrine or glucagon are typical. The response to glucagon and epinephrine is rarely "flat," because the degradation of branch points of glycogen leads to glucose release even in the absence of glucose-6-phosphatase. Dramatic increases of blood lactate, pyruvate, triglycerides, cholesterol, and uric acid are usual.

After puberty the hyperuricemia with complicating clinical gouty arthritis (see Ch. 195) and the occurrence of multiple benign hepatic adenomas (and very rarely hepatic carcinoma) become the main clinical problems. Death from renal disease, possibly related to uric acid, has occurred in several adult patients.

The precise diagnosis must be routinely established by a liver biopsy and the demonstration of deficient activity of the enzyme glucose-6-phosphatase. Patients are recognized in whom no glucose-6-phosphatase activity is demonstrated on a fresh biopsy sample, but completely normal activity is demonstrated on the frozen sample. This condition represents a defect in glucose-6-phosphate translocase, a specific protein that shuttles glucose-6-phosphate across the membrane.

Other prominent forms of hepatic glycogen storage disease appear clinically similar to glucose-6-phosphatase deficiency glycogen storage disease except that they are milder. In the deficiency of the debrancher enzyme there is excessive accumulation of glycogen of abnormal structure. The stored glycogen has short outer branches. These patients generally have much milder hypoglycemia and much milder growth retardation and do not present with hyperuricemia or the severe lipid problems that are seen in glucose-6-phosphatase deficiency glycogen storage disease. Hepatic adenomas are not known to occur.

The typical patient with debrancher deficiency glycogen storage disease tends to achieve more normal height, and following puberty the liver will frequently appear normal in size. Because of the generalized nature of the enzyme defect in these patients (including liver as well as muscle), some of these patients have had significant myopathy in adulthood related to storage of abnormally structured glycogen. Muscle weakness and wasting can be the predominant findings in the older patient. The diagnosis is usually established by assaying liver, muscle, white cells, or red cells for the specific debranching enzyme. Direct liver assay is often required.

A genetic deficiency of the branching enzyme presents as liver failure in early infancy. These children display the usual hallmarks of liver failure (jaundice, ascites), usually by age two years. Muscle weakness can be prominent. A deficiency of the branching enzyme can be demonstrated in leukocytes and in fibroblasts as well as in liver tissue. The glycogen content of the liver is usually within or below normal range, but the structure demonstrates very long outer branches secondary to deficiency of the branching enzyme.

A group of patients has been recognized with very mild clinical symptoms of hypoglycemia and growth retardation but with substantial hepatomegaly. Some lack clinical symptoms. On biochemical examination they have a significant increase of normally structured liver glycogen and a deficiency of the enzyme phosphorylase. The deficiency in all instances has been partial (perhaps total deficiency would be lethal). The outlook in phosphorylase-deficient patients is good, and ordinarily no specific treatment is required.

Further study of patients with defects in the phosphorylase system has demonstrated a substantial number of males who are genetically deficient in the enzyme phosphorylase b kinase. This glycogen storage disease is different from all others (which are inherited as autosomal recessive traits), in that phosphorylase b kinase activity is inherited in an X-linked recessive manner. Females who carry this gene (heterozygotes) may have modest hepatomegaly, whereas affected males (hemizygotes) have substantial hepatomegaly without the other major symptoms of hypoglycemia or hyperlipidemia. Their response to epinephrine and glucagon is variable, but they routinely have significant plasma elevations of liver enzymes such as SGOT and SGPT. Leukocyte phosphorylase b kinase assays can usually establish the diagnosis.

Treatment of the Hepatic Forms of Glycogen Storage Disease. A variety of hormonal treatments, such as thyroxine and glucagon administration, have been ineffective in the hepatic forms of glycogen storage disease. Some patients have benefited from portacaval shunting, most specifically in restoration of growth. Because of substantial morbidity this treatment is no longer recommended.

At present, the most appropriate treatment for the symptomatic forms of hepatic glycogen storage disease is nasogastric infusion of a high carbohydrate diet. Continuous nasogastric feeding overnight with either carbohydrate alone or carbohydrate plus protein is of great benefit not only in restoring growth toward normal but also, importantly, in restoring the lipid and carbohydrate abnormalities toward normal. Oral cornstarch during the day is helpful. These treatments, currently in wide use, are safe and their clearest benefit is on growth.

The adult patient with hyperuricemia and gout is effectively treated with allopurinol and is usually not responsive to uricosuric drugs. Liver transplantation has been performed in patients with glucose-6-phosphatase, debrancher, and brancher enzyme deficiency. This treatment is likely to be of increasing importance in seriously affected persons.

THE MUSCULAR FORMS OF GLYCOGEN STORAGE DISEASE. The most dramatic of the muscular forms of the glycogen storage diseases is generalized glycogen storage disease (Pompe's disease). There is prominent deposition of glycogen in all muscular tissues and a genetic deficiency of the lysosomal enzyme alpha-1,4-glucosidase.

This condition was originally described in infants, with the typical child dying of cardiorespiratory disease in the first two years of life. In recent years, additional patients with muscular glycogen storage disease, secondary to deficiency of alpha-1,4-glucosidase, have presented with muscular weakness in late childhood or in adulthood. Patients presenting as young adults have commonly been diagnosed as having muscular dystrophy. Respiratory failure has been the presenting symptom in certain adults. Cardiac involvement has been either minimal or absent in the older patients.

The diagnosis of this form of glycogen storage disease depends on a muscle biopsy that demonstrates an increased concentration of glycogen, which on electron microscopy is seen within the lysosome. Alpha-1,4-glucosidase deficiency is transmitted in an autosomal recessive manner. Specific enzyme analyses of leukocytes may demonstrate an absence of an acid alpha-1,4-glucosidase, but such studies are not always reliable. The presence in white cells of a neutral maltase that has considerable activity in the range of pH 4 can lead to relatively normal white cell activities for alpha-1,4-glucosidase, although the acid maltase characteristic of the lysosome is deficient. There is a consistent deficiency of alpha-1,4-glucosidase activity in cultured skin fibroblasts. Patients with myopathy appearing in late adulthood must be considered as potential candidates for alpha-1,4 glucosedase deficiency glycogen storage disease, as well as for debrancher deficiency glycogen storage disease, as mentioned above.

Muscle phosphorylase deficiency or McArdle's disease is perhaps the rarest of the glycogen storage diseases. Patients with this disorder are probably under-recognized, for their symptoms appear functional. Patients are usually asymptomatic until adolescence or early adulthood when they develop painful muscle cramps after exercise. If exercise is continued, myoglobinuria and renal failure may ensue.

These patients demonstrate absence of the increase in venous lactate that follows anaerobic exercise. The condition should be suspected in healthy, well-developed adults with painful muscle cramps after exercise who demonstrate no increase in lactate after exercise. A specific diagnosis is made on muscle biopsy, which demonstrates an increased concentration of structurally normal glycogen and a deficiency of phosphorylase activity. This condition is inherited as an autosomal recessive trait.

Patients with a genetic deficiency of muscle phosphofructokinase activity appear clinically identical to patients with an absence of muscle phosphorylase activity. The diagnosis is established in a similar fashion; they have painful muscle cramps after exercise, demonstrate no increase in venous lactate after anaerobic exercise, and show increased concentration of glycogen in the muscle, but absence of muscle phosphofructokinase activity.

Isolated patients have been reported in whom activities of phosphohexoisomerase, phosphoglucomutase, or cyclic 3′,5′-AMP-dependent kinase have been deficient, but these conditions need further clarification. Reported deficiencies of UDP-8-glycogen transferase activity probably represent defects in gluconeogenesis; the low enzyme activity is likely a reflection of the well-known instability of the enzyme when tissue glycogen content is low.

Treatment of the Muscular Glycogen Storage Diseases. Patients with deficiencies of phosphofructokinase or of phosphorylase in muscle can be benefited by avoiding strenuous exercise. There is some suggestion that isoproterenol (which increases blood flow to the muscle) may be helpful by making more glucose available for direct utilization by muscle.

At present there is no specific treatment for Pompe's disease (alpha-1,4-glucosidase deficiency glycogen storage disease). A strain of cattle in Australia affected with a condition identical to Pompe's disease in man is proving valuable as an experimental model. Bone marrow transplants have been tried; they are not likely to be effective in man.

PRENATAL DIAGNOSIS OF THE GLYCOGEN STORAGE DISEASES. Glucose-6-phosphatase deficiency glycogen storage disease cannot be diagnosed by amniocentesis because the enzyme deficient in this condition (glucose-6-phosphatase) is not present in normal cultured human fibroblasts. New techniques of molecular genetics (e.g., restriction mapping) should permit prenatal diagnosis in the near future. However, the enzyme alpha-1,4-glucosidase is active in normal cultured skin fibroblasts, and Pompe's disease can be reliably diagnosed in utero. Debrancher deficiency glycogen storage disease is difficult to establish in utero. Although the debranching enzyme is present in normal fibroblasts, widespread tissue variability of the inherited deficiency makes the prenatal diagnosis of this disorder difficult. Brancher deficiency glycogen storage disease can be diagnosed in utero.

Phosphorylase b kinase deficiency can be diagnosed in cultured human fibroblasts. The mildness of this condition, however, makes prenatal diagnosis inappropriate.

Beratis NG, LaBadie GU, Hirschhorn K: Genetic heterogeneity in acid alpha-glucosidase deficiency. Am J Hum Genet 35:21, 1983. *Study examines differences at the molecular level among the several clinical forms of acid alpha-glucosidase deficiency.*

Chen YT, Cornblath M, Sidbury JB: Cornstarch therapy in Type I glycogen storage disease. N Engl J Med 310:171, 1984. *The usefulness of oral cornstarch to maintain blood sugar concentrations is demonstrated.*

Folk CC, Greene HL: Dietary management of Type I glycogen storage disease. J Am Diet Assoc 84:293, 1984. *A detailed approach to the nutritional treatment of the hepatic glycogen storage diseases.*

Howell RR, Williams JC: The glycogen storage diseases. In Stanbury JB, Wyngaarden JB, Fredrickson DS, Goldstein JL, Brown MS et al. (eds.): The Metabolic Basis of Inherited Disease. 5th ed. New York, McGraw-Hill Book Company, 1983. *This is a thorough coverage of the clinical and biochemical aspects of the glycogen storage diseases. This article is extensively referenced.*

Narisawa K, Otomo H, Igarashi Y, et al.: Glycogen storage disease type Ib: Microsomal glucose-6-phosphatase system in two patients with different clinical findings. Pediatr Res 17:545, 1983. *This article summarizes current information about the microsomal glucose-6-phosphatase system and the glucose-6-phosphate translocase.*

Starzl TE, Iwatsuki S, Shaw BW Jr, et al.: Analysis of liver transplantation. Hepatology 4:47S, 1984. *A review of liver transplantation in genetic as well as other diseases.*

180 PENTOSURIA (Essential Pentosuria)

R. Rodney Howell

Pentosuria is an innocuous, rather common heritable abnormality of carbohydrate metabolism that occurs almost exclusively in Jews and Lebanese. It is transmitted in an autosomal recessive fashion with an estimated prevalence of 1:2000 to 1:5000 in these populations. Affected persons excrete between 1 and 4 grams of the pentose L-xylulose in the urine daily. Loading of the glucuronic acid cycle by the oral administration of glucuronolactone will cause an increase in urinary L-xylulose excretion in the homozygote and a lesser response in the heterozygote. Red blood cells of normal persons contain two L-xylulose reductases: a major and a minor isozyme. The residual enzyme activity in red cells of pentosuric persons and the normal minor isozyme have similar Michaelis constants for L-xylulose and xylitol and also possess other similar biochemical properties. Homozygosity for the pentosuria allele results in absence of the major isozyme and in a residual isozyme that is identical to the minor isozyme of normal persons. The presence in the urine of L-xylulose, a reducing sugar, has in the past led to false diagnoses of diabetes. The sugar can easily be distinguished from others by paper or thin-layer chromatography. Glucose oxidase, which is the reagent in the commonly used dipstick type of urine test, does not react with this sugar, whereas reducing agents will.

Hiatt HH: Pentosuria. In Stanbury JB, Wyngaarden JB, Fredrickson DS (eds.): The Metabolic Basis of Inherited Disease. 4th ed. New York, McGraw-Hill Book Company, 1978, p 110. *This is a detailed review of the history and biochemistry of essential pentosuria.*

Lane AB: On the nature of L-xylulose reductase deficiency in essential pentosuria. Biochem Genet 23:61, 1985. *This reference summarizes our current understanding of the L-xylulose reductases and their deficiency in pentosuria.*

181 ESSENTIAL FRUCTOSURIA AND HEREDITARY FRUCTOSE INTOLERANCE

R. Rodney Howell

ESSENTIAL FRUCTOSURIA (FRUCTOSURIA). Fructosuria is a rare asymptomatic condition caused by a deficiency of the enzyme fructokinase. It is inherited in an autosomal recessive manner and has a recognized prevalence of 1:130,000. Fructokinase activity is normally present only in liver, kidney, and intestinal mucosa and catalyzes the first reaction in the major pathway of fructose utilization in man.

The diagnosis of fructosuria is established indirectly by a fructose loading test. Following such a load, an excessive rise in fructose concentration in the blood and the chromatographic identification of significant amounts of fructose in the urine are diagnostic. In normal persons after fructose loading the blood fructose concentration will peak at one hour and does not exceed 25 mg per deciliter, with no significant concentration of fructose in the urine. Hepatic fructokinase activity is undetectable in tissue from patients with essential fructosuria. Fructose is a reducing sugar and reacts with Clinitest tablets and other reducing agents, so confusion with diabetes must be avoided. Since fructose does not react with glucose oxidase in the urine dipstick utilized in most clinical laboratories, the confusion of this benign condition with diabetes is less of a problem now than in the past.

HEREDITARY FRUCTOSE INTOLERANCE. Hereditary fructose intolerance is a potentially life-threatening disorder and can be suspected from a detailed nutritional history. This condition is due to a structural mutation of the liver enzyme fructose-1-phosphate aldolase (aldolase B) and is transmitted in an autosomal recessive fashion. In humans there are three types of aldolases (A, B, and C) that are tetrameric molecules that may form hybrids. They differ in their tissue distribution and in their activity ratios toward their two substrates fructose-1,6-diphosphate (FDP) and fructose-1-phosphate (F1P). Aldolase B is characterized by an activity ratio of 1 and is present in large amounts in liver, renal cortex, and small intestine. Tissue from patients with hereditary fructose intolerance exhibits profound deficiency of activity against fructose-1-phosphate and modest reduction in activity against fructose-1,6-diphosphate.

Symptoms are present only after the ingestion of fructose. Immediately after fructose ingestion there is a brisk reduction in blood glucose and serum phosphorus concentrations and a marked increase in serum uric acid concentration. There is a striking deterioration of renal tubular function as manifested by the inability to acidify the urine, bicarbonaturia, aminoaciduria, and phosphaturia in the presence of a falling serum phosphorus concentration. Hypokalemia may occur. The infant who continues to ingest fructose will exhibit vomiting, failure to thrive, hypotonia, jaundice, hepatosplenomegaly, ascites, bleeding disorders, abnormal liver function test results, hypoglycemia, acidosis, proteinuria, and fructosuria. The differential diagnosis includes galactosemia and tyrosinemia, and diagnosis can be difficult.

The acidosis is due primarily to excess lactic acid and to a lesser extent to proximal renal tubular dysfunction. The fructosemia and fructosuria are secondary to the inhibition of fructokinase by its accumulated reaction product fructose-1-phosphate. The hypoglycemia following ingestion of fructose results from a defect in the phosphorolysis of glycogen to glucose-1-phosphate.

Liver biopsies show early stages of cirrhosis. The brain may show diminished neurons. In spite of the recurrent hypoglycemia in infancy, affected adults have normal intelligence.

The dose-dependent reduction of ATP and the accumulation of fructose-1-phosphate within the renal cortex have been thought to explain the Fanconi-like syndrome observed in these patients. The reduction of phosphate is, however, of greatest importance. The hyperuricemia results from the increased conversion of adenine nucleotides to urate induced by fructose and from decreased renal clearance of urate in the presence of elevated blood lactate concentrations.

In patients with hereditary fructose intolerance, clinically important chronic fructose intoxication can occur after infancy without causing symptoms of acute fructose intoxication. This is expressed as isolated, reversible retardation of somatic growth. Older affected children and adults are protected by the development of an aversion to sweets and a self-imposed fructose-free diet.

If the diagnosis of hereditary fructose intolerance is suspected the immediate elimination of fructose from the diet is recommended. The diagnosis is established by the intravenous fructose tolerance test after several weeks of fructose withdrawal; should the diagnosis still be uncertain, liver biopsy is advised for assay of aldolase and reference enzymes and for histologic study.

The treatment is the exclusion of fructose from the diet. With a fructose-free diet the patient's outlook is favorable.

Cox TM, O'Donnell MW, Camilleri M: Allelic heterogeneity in adult hereditary fructose intolerance. Detection of structural mutations in the aldolase B molecule. Mol Biol Med 1:393, 1983. *Molecular studies in aldolase B in hereditary fructose intolerance; structural defects are shown.*

Gregori C, Besmond C, Odievre M, et al.: DNA analysis in patients with hereditary fructose intolerance. Ann Hum Genet 48:291, 1984. *Molecular genetic studies in 11 patients with hereditary fructose intolerance; major deletion of the gene was not observed.*

Gitzelmann R, Steinmann B, van den Berghe G: Essential fructosuria, hereditary fructose intolerance, and fructose-1,6-diphosphate deficiency. In Stanbury JB, Wyngaarden JB, Fredrickson DS, et al. (eds.): The Metabolic Basis of Inherited Disease. 5th ed. New York, McGraw-Hill Book Company, 1983. *This review covers in detail the clinical and biochemical aspects of hereditary fructose intolerance and essential fructosuria.*

Mock DM, Perman JA, Thaler M, et al.: Chronic fructose intoxication after infancy in children with hereditary fructose intolerance. A cause of growth retardation. N Engl J Med 309:764, 1983. *Reviews and focuses on growth retardation as a feature of chronic, rather than acute, fructose intoxication.*

Morris, RC, McInnes RR, Epstein CJ, et al.: Genetic and metabolic injury of the kidney. In Brenner BM, Rector FC (eds.): The Kidney. Philadelphia, W. B. Saunders Company, 1976, pp 1214–1218. *This chapter details the mechanism of renal injury in hereditary fructose intolerance.*

Steinmann B, Gitzelmann, R: The diagnosis of hereditary fructose intolerance. Helv Paediatr Acta 36:297, 1981. *Excellent review of diagnostic tests for hereditary fructose intolerance.*

182 PRIMARY HYPEROXALURIA

Lloyd H. Smith, Jr.

Primary hyperoxaluria is a general term for two rare genetic disorders of glyoxylate metabolism productive of excessive synthesis and urinary excretion of oxalic acid. Both disorders are transmitted as autosomal recessive traits. The diseases are characterized by the onset in childhood of recurrent calcium oxalate nephrolithiasis or nephrocalcinosis, or both, usually leading to early death secondary to renal failure. In addition to the usual clinical features of uremia, severe peripheral vascular insufficiency may complicate the course of the disease. At postmortem examination calcium oxalate may be found widely deposited in extrarenal sites, a condition known as *oxalosis.* More rarely, milder forms of the disease may be found in adults. Although oxalate is an important constituent in approximately two thirds of all kidney stones, most adult patients with calcium oxalate nephrolithiasis excrete normal amounts of urinary oxalate (Ch. 90).

Primary hyperoxaluria Type I (glycolic aciduria) represents a genetic defect in the activity of peroxisomal alanine: glyoxylate aminotransferase. The resulting accumulation of glyoxylate leads to its excessive oxidation to oxalate and its reduction to glycolate, both of which are excreted in increased amounts in the urine (more than 60 mg per 1.73 square meters per 24 hours each). In *primary hyperoxaluria Type II* (L-glyceric aciduria) there is a defect in the enzyme D-glyceric dehydrogenase. Hydroxypyruvate accumulates and is reduced by lactic dehydrogenase (LDH) to L-glyceric acid, a compound that is undetectable in normal urine. The reduction of hydroxypyruvate to L-glycerate is probably coupled to the oxidation of glyoxylate to oxalate, both catalyzed by LDH. Each disease can be diagnosed by the characteristic pattern of metabolites in urine: Type I, oxalate and glycolate; Type II, oxalate and L-glycerate. Pyridoxine deficiency in laboratory animals and man also leads to hyperoxaluria and even oxalosis with a urinary pattern similar to that of the genetic disease Type I. With the onset of renal failure the clearance of oxalate is reduced (its clearance is normally about 1.2 times that of creatinine) so that its urinary excretion may return to normal. The diagnosis may then be difficult to establish because of the unreliability of currently available methods for measuring serum oxalate.

No specific methods of treatment are now available. Efforts are directed toward reducing the amount of oxalate excreted and increasing its solubility. Large amounts of pyridoxine (200 to 400 mg per 24 hours) may decrease oxalate excretion in the Type I disease. More physiologic doses of pyridoxine (2 to 10 mg) may be effective in some patients. Dilute urine should be maintained by forcing fluids, and a phosphate or magnesium oxide supplement may offer partial protection against stone formation. Renal homotransplantation has been disappointing because of rapid deposition of calcium oxalate in the transplanted kidney, but there have been some reports of success. Long-term dialysis and pyridoxine are therefore indicated when renal failure is severe. Nitroglycerin has been reported to be effective in treatment of the peripheral vascular insufficiency associated with oxalosis. A search for an inhibitor of oxalate synthesis is highly indicated.

Increased urinary excretion of oxalate and stone diathesis (in the absence of glycolic aciduria or L-glyceric aciduria) occur in many patients who have small bowel disease and malabsorption. Normally oxalate and fatty acids of the small intestine compete for available calcium ion, and calcium oxalate is poorly absorbed. This important form of acquired hyperoxaluria results from excessive absorption of dietary oxalate in the presence of significant steatorrhea. It can be controlled by a low oxalate diet.

Danpure CJ, Jennings PR, Watts RWE: Enzymological diagnosis of primary hyperoxaluria type I by measurement of hepatic alanine: Glyoxylate aminotransferase activity. Lancet 1:289, 1987. *In contrast to the previous suggestion of a carboligase defect, this new study seems to establish this disorder as a specific transaminase defect. This is more consistent with the therapeutic response to pyridoxine.*

Earnest DL: Enteric hyperoxaluria. Adv Intern Med 24:407, 1979. *An excellent general review of the clinical features, pathogenesis, and treatment of the most frequent cause of hyperoxaluria, that associated with its excessive absorption from dietary sources.*

Yendt ER, Cohanim M: Response to a physiological dose of pyridoxine in Type I primary hyperoxaluria. N Engl J Med 312:953, 1985. *This article describes varying degrees of sensitivity in the reduction in oxalate excretion during pyridoxine therapy and raises the intriguing possibility that in some patients the diagnosis may be obscured by small amounts of the vitamin.*

Disorders of Lipoprotein Metabolism

183 THE HYPERLIPOPROTEINEMIAS

John D. Brunzell

Disorders of lipoprotein metabolism are related to abnormalities in the synthesis and degradation of plasma lipoproteins. These abnormalities may result from primary inborn errors of metabolism or may be secondary to a variety of other disease states. Hyperlipidemia, the elevation of plasma cholesterol and/or triglyceride concentrations, is the hallmark of the lipoprotein disorders. Clinical delineation of these disorders is important because of the association of some with premature coronary artery disease and others with recurrent pancreatitis.

The classification of disorders of lipoprotein metabolism was first based on the varieties of xanthomas that occur and the appearance of plasma turbidity due to the accumulation of large, light-scattering lipoprotein particles in plasma. With the discovery of relatively discrete lipoprotein species, classification of these disorders was based on separation of lipoproteins by ultracentrifugation or by electrophoresis. Understanding of lipoprotein physiology has allowed classification of lipoprotein disorders according to pathophysiologic defects, with specific discrete apoprotein, enzyme, or receptor abnormalities identified in some disorders.

PHYSIOLOGY OF LIPOPROTEIN TRANSPORT

Structure and Function of Lipoproteins

The structure of the lipoprotein macromolecule is well suited for the solubilization of lipids in plasma. The nonpolar lipids—cholesteryl ester and triglyceride—are present in the lipoprotein core surrounded by a monolayer composed of specific proteins and the polar lipids, unesterified cholesterol and phospholipid. This monolayer allows the lipoprotein to remain miscible in plasma.

The lipoproteins function as an efficient vehicle for site-to-site transport of triglyceride and cholesterol of both exogenous and endogenous origin. Although caloric need is fairly constant throughout the day, food is ingested only periodically. The excess calories that enter the circulation with each meal are transported mainly as triglyceride to be stored in adipose tissue for future utilization between meals as free fatty acids. Ingested and synthesized cholesterol also needs to be transported to extrahepatic tissues to serve as a source of membrane cholesterol and as substrate for steroid hormone synthesis. The transport of triglyceride and cholesterol is accomplished by a spectrum of lipoproteins that have been classified by arbitrary operational boundaries according to either their density by ultracentrifugation or mobility by electrophoresis (Fig. 183–1). Fortunately the lipoproteins, as separated by ultracentrifugation or electrophoresis, are so similar that the synonyms based on each of these methods of separation are essentially interchangeable.

The triglyceride-rich lipoproteins can enter the plasma as chylomicrons derived from dietary fat adsorbed from the gut or endogenously as triglyceride-rich very low density lipoprotein (VLDL) synthesized from glucose or circulating free fatty acids in the liver. After removal of some of their triglycerides and surface components, the remaining lipoprotein remnant of the chylomicron is taken up by the liver and degraded. The remnant of endogenous triglyceride-rich lipoprotein probably also requires the liver for further processing. In contrast to the chylomicron, however, only some components of VLDL are removed, resulting in formation of the low-density cholesterol-rich lipoprotein.

This is likely to be an oversimplification, as there is a continuous spectrum of particles, and lipoproteins enter and exit at many sites along this spectrum of varying lipoprotein sizes. High-density lipoproteins interact with this system for transport of triglyceride and cholesteryl ester, as will be noted later.

Both the physiology and the pathophysiology of lipoproteins can be evaluated by examining the sites of lipoprotein production and the multiple steps in lipoprotein catabolism. Most pathophysiologic abnormalities leading to hyperlipi-

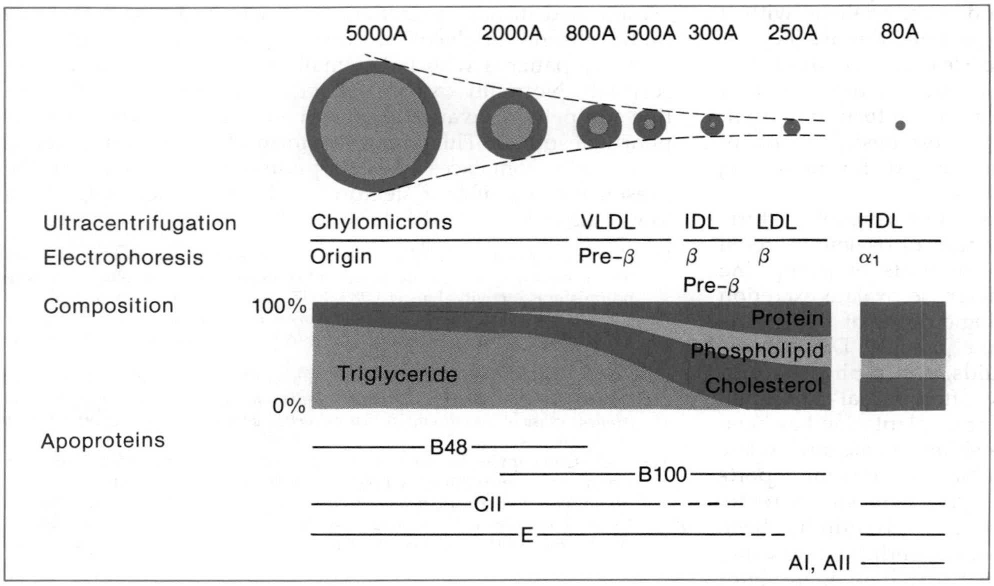

FIGURE 183–1. Classification of plasma lipoproteins by physical and chemical properties. (Modified from Bierman EL: Current Concepts: Hyperlipoproteinemia. The Upjohn Company, 1984.)

demic states can be understood by examining four sites of regulation of plasma lipoprotein transport: (1) triglyceride-rich lipoprotein input, (2) lipoprotein lipase–mediated triglyceride catabolism, (3) remnant catabolism, and (4) cholesterol-rich lipoprotein catabolism (Fig. 183–2).

Production of Triglyceride-Rich Lipoproteins

After hydrolysis of dietary triglycerides in the small intestine, the resulting fatty acids and monoglycerides are taken up by the absorptive cells of the small intestine and incorporated into large triglyceride-rich lipoproteins with a specific form of apoprotein B (apo B-48), phospholipid, and a small amount of cholesterol. These chylomicrons are secreted from the absorptive cells into the lymphatics and subsequently enter the plasma via the thoracic duct. Chylomicron secretion and transport represent a system of high-capacity energy transport, allowing calories ingested at one time, over and above immediate needs, to be transferred to sites of storage for use between meals. The chylomicron remnant taken up and degraded by the liver suppresses synthesis of components of endogenous triglyceride-rich lipoproteins.

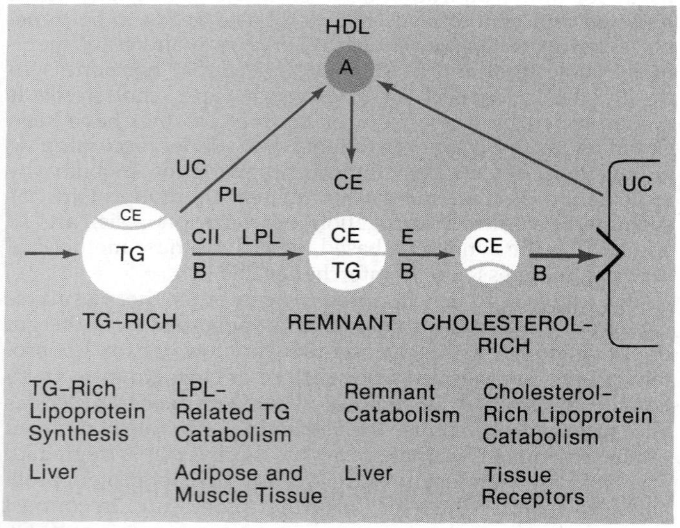

FIGURE 183–2. The triglyceride-rich lipoprotein (VLDL) is synthesized in the liver and contains apo-B, which remains with the particle through its subsequent catabolism. The triglyceride-rich lipoprotein core contains triglyceride (TG) and cholesteryl ester (CE) and surface unesterified cholesterol (UC) and phospholipid (PL). Upon entering plasma, acquired apo CII activates lipoprotein lipase (LPL) to catabolize TG core. The resulting remnant acquires apo-E, which interacts with hepatic receptors to catabolize remnant to cholesterol-rich low density lipoprotein (LDL). The LDL binds to high-affinity receptor, with subsequent intracellular degradation of the lipoprotein. High density lipoproteins with apoproteins AI and AII (A) acquire surface components of lipoproteins and plasma membranes of cells and form cholesteryl esters. These cholesteryl esters exchange with other lipoproteins or are delivered directly to the liver and may be the primary source of biliary cholesterol and bile acids.

Input into plasma of triglyceride-rich lipoproteins also occurs from endogenous sources. During meals, plasma free fatty acids enter the liver, where they may be esterified with glycerole to form triglyceride. Between meals, free fatty acids are mobilized from adipose tissue triglyceride stores. These serve as a potential source for hepatic triglyceride synthesis. Lipogenesis, synthesis of fatty acids de novo from carbohydrate, also occurs in the liver. Fatty acids in the cytosol of the hepatocyte can either enter mitochondria, when oxidation occurs, or can remain in the cytosol, where they are esterified to form triglyceride. These processes appear to be regulated by changes in insulin and glucagon levels that occur with feeding: glucagon enhances and insulin prevents mitochondrial fatty acid uptake by regulating long-chain acyl carnitine transferase. Insulin also induces lipogenic enzymes in the hepatocytes that regulate the synthesis of fatty acids.

Triglyceride synthesized in the liver, together with cholesteryl ester, is combined with the lipoprotein monolayer composed of phospholipid, unesterified cholesterol, and apoprotein B, and secreted into the hepatic venous outflow as triglyceride-rich VLDL. Hepatic apoprotein B (apo B-100) in VLDL has a larger molecular weight than intestinal apoprotein B (apo B-48) found in chylomicrons.

In normal individuals, the majority of triglyceride input into the plasma is of dietary origin. While the average American diet contains about 100 grams of triglyceride per day, less than 30 grams of triglyceride are secreted endogenously.

Lipoprotein Lipase-Mediated Triglyceride Catabolism

The triglyceride that enters the plasma in chylomicrons and endogenously synthesized triglyceride-rich lipoproteins is transported to adipose tissue for storage or to muscle for utilization. The enzyme in adipose tissue and muscle that catalyzes this triglyceride uptake is lipoprotein lipase. In adipose tissue the enzyme is synthesized in the fat cell, and following secretion and transport to the capillary endothelial cell, hydrolyzes the triglyceride in these lipoproteins at the endothelial surface. At least two of the three fatty acids potentially releasable from triglyceride hydrolysis are then transported to the fat cell where they are re-esterified with glycerol and stored as intracellular adipocyte triglyceride. The vast majority of the triglyceride in the adipocyte enters by this mechanism; little lipogenesis de novo from glucose occurs in adipose tissue in humans. The functional activity of lipoprotein lipase in adipose tissue is increased during and after meals. In humans, most of this increase in function is due to the increase in triglyceride-rich lipoproteins that serve as enzyme substrate. Although insulin is required to maintain lipoprotein lipase levels in adipose tissue, little change in enzyme levels occurs with normal meals. Between meals, calories stored as triglyceride are released from the adipocyte as free fatty acids. This hydrolysis of intracellular adipocyte triglyceride is mediated by "hormone-sensitive" lipase of the fat cells. Between meals, when insulin levels are low and glucagon is increasing, hormone-sensitive lipase activity increases, and free fatty acids are released to be used for energy utilization by most tissues of the body.

The interaction of lipoprotein lipase with triglyceride in triglyceride-rich lipoproteins requires a cofactor, apoprotein CII. When secreted from the absorptive cell of the gut and from the liver, chylomicrons and VLDL do not contain this activator. Shortly after entering plasma these lipoproteins pick up apoprotein CII from a reservoir in circulating high-density lipoprotein (HDL). Thus the triglyceride-rich lipoproteins contain both substrate and activator for their hydrolysis by lipoprotein lipase. Following hydrolysis of the triglyceride in these lipoproteins, the apoprotein CII is released and again picked up by HDL. Thus, HDL appears to serve as a shuttle for apoprotein CII (as well as other lipoprotein components) (see below). Other apoproteins (CI and CIII) are transferred bidirectionally between triglyceride-rich lipoproteins and HDL and may play a role in lipoprotein lipase triglyceride hydrolysis, as well as other lipoprotein interactions.

Remnant Lipoprotein Catabolism

Following hydrolysis of the triglyceride in triglyceride-rich lipoproteins and the simultaneous removal of surface components, "remnant" lipoproteins are formed from chylomicrons and endogenous triglyceride-rich lipoproteins. The intermediate-density lipoprotein fraction isolated by ultracentrifugation consists largely of remnant particles of VLDL. Those remnants formed from chylomicrons and large endogenous VLDL often distribute, however, in the density range of small VLDL. Thus, remnants and endogenously synthesized triglyceride-rich lipoproteins cannot be separated completely by ultracentrifugation. Once formed, the remnant has a short half-life in plasma and appears to be taken up by the liver (Fig. 183–3). The endogenous triglyceride-rich lipoprotein remnant is further processed into the cholesterol-rich low-density lipoprotein (LDL). During this catabolic process, further triglyceride and cholesterol as well as some surface proteins are removed. The remnant lipoprotein contains apoprotein B, and several forms of apoprotein C and apoprotein E. The apoprotein E that accumulates as the remnant lipoproteins are formed appears to be important for hepatic uptake of those remnants. There is a complex interaction of hepatic receptors specific for apoprotein E and other receptors that bind both apoprotein B and apoprotein E, with the apoproteins in the remnant lipoproteins regulating their hepatic uptake. By the time the cholesterol-rich LDL has been formed, apoprotein B is the only apoprotein of the triglyceride-rich lipoproteins remaining.

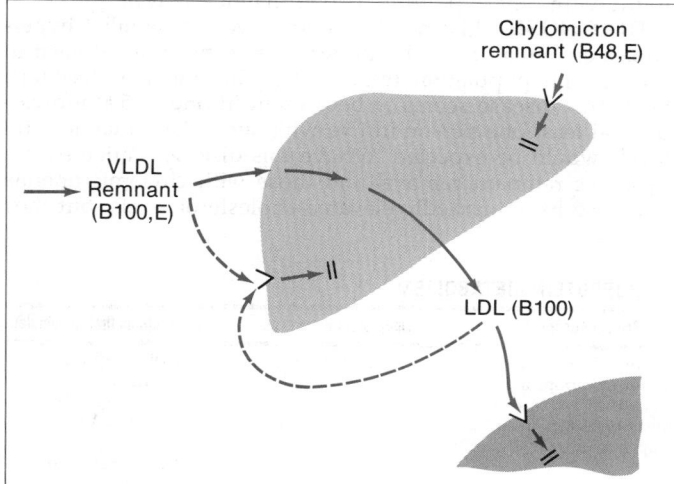

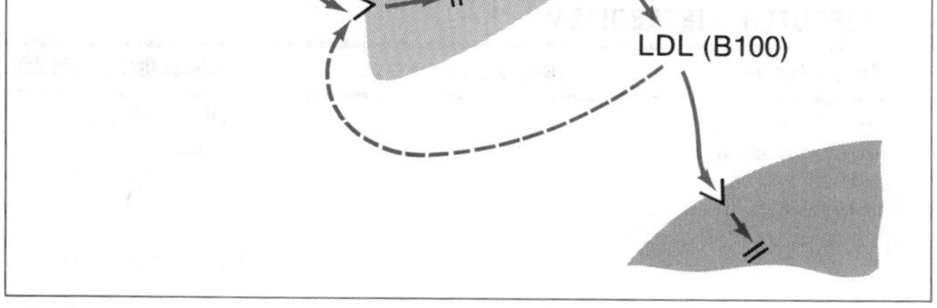

FIGURE 183–3. The liver is involved in the conversion of VLDL remnants containing apo B-100 and apo E to LDL, which are terminally catabolized via the LDL receptor in peripheral or hepatic tissue. The chylomicron remnant containing apo B-48 and apo E is processed completely in the liver via the apo E or chylomicron receptor.

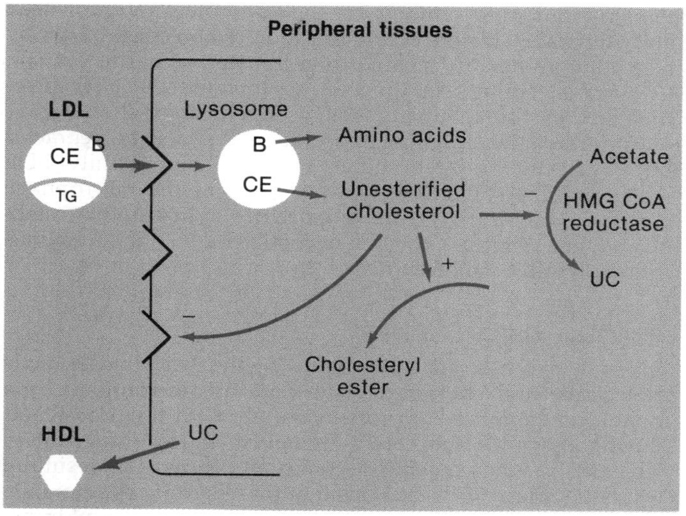

FIGURE 183–4. LDL containing apo B are removed from plasma by a high-affinity receptor and are processed in the lysosome. The resulting unesterified cholesterol regulates the cellular homeostatic mechanisms.

Cholesterol-Rich Low-Density Lipoprotein Catabolism

As the cholesterol-rich LDL normally arises from the remnant lipoprotein of VLDL, it contains the same amount of apoprotein B per lipoprotein particle as endogenous triglyceride-rich VLDL, while other apoproteins have been almost entirely removed, together with much of the phospholipid and some cholesterol. The cholesterol-rich lipoprotein can be removed from plasma by extrahepatic tissues where it functions as the chief source of cholesterol for membrane synthesis or steroid hormone synthesis by these tissues. Alternatively the lipoprotein may be taken up by the liver and degraded if not utilized peripherally. Apoprotein B in the cholesterol-rich lipoprotein appears to be recognized by a specific, high-affinity binding site in tissues (Fig. 183–4). Once bound, the lipoprotein is internalized by the cell in an endocytotic vesicle that fuses with a primary or pre-existing secondary lysosome. The protein moiety is degraded and the cholesteryl ester hydrolyzed to unesterified cholesterol by a lysosomal acid cholesteryl ester hydrolase. Hydrolysis of the triglyceride and phospholipid may also occur in the lysosome. The cell is able to regulate its own cholesterol content through a feedback control system in which intracellular free cholesterol suppresses endogenous cholesterol production by inhibiting the rate-limiting enzyme in cholesterol synthesis (HMG-CoA reductase). Furthermore, accumulation of intracellular free cholesterol limits the further uptake of cholesterol-rich lipoproteins by inhibiting synthesis of the lipoprotein receptor itself and stimulates its own re-esterification to cholesteryl ester by activating an acyl CoA:cholesterol transferase in the cytosol. Cholesterol content in the cell is regulated by a receptor-mediated system involving HDL as a vehicle for cholesterol.

Apoprotein B containing lipoproteins may also be degraded by a scavenger system other than the high-affinity LDL receptor. This scavenger pathway involves the macrophage system and assumes greater importance in lipoprotein catabolism when defects in the LDL receptor or other abnormalities in lipoprotein catabolism exist.

Lipoprotein Surface Catabolism

Newly synthesized lipoproteins with their hydrophobic triglyceride and cholesteryl ester core are surrounded by a monolayer composed of protein, unesterified cholesterol, and phospholipid. As the core is removed and the lipoprotein decreases in size, several mechanisms process the resulting "excess" surface. The catabolism of these surface components involves HDL and the enzyme lecithin-cholesterol-acyl-transferase (LCAT). HDL synthesized by the liver and the intestine, is composed of phospholipid and two major structural apoproteins, apoprotein AI and apoprotein AII. This HDL serves as an acceptor for the phospholipid (mainly lecithin) and unesterified cholesterol from the triglyceride-rich lipoprotein surface. LCAT associated with HDL then removes a fatty acid from lecithin and transfers it to cholesterol, producing cholesteryl ester and lysolecithin. The cholesteryl ester is transferred from HDL to the liver directly or after transfer to other lipoproteins via lipid transfer protein, making the HDL apoproteins available to shuttle more lipoprotein surface components. HDL, LCAT, and transfer proteins may also play a role in the regulation of intracellular cholesterol content by enhancing the efflux of free cholesterol from extrahepatic tissues. Thus, HDL may play a role in the transport of cholesterol from cells to liver where it is ultimately excreted. In addition, HDL serves as the shuttle for apoprotein CII and apoprotein E to and from triglyceride-rich lipoproteins as part of their catabolism.

Cholesterol Excretion

Cholesterol and phospholipids are excreted as such in the bile, or after conversion of cholesterol into bile acid. A large proportion of the secreted bile acids is reabsorbed in the enterohepatic circulation and recycled. However, a net loss of bile acid, cholesterol, and phospholipid in the stool occurs by this pathway.

The definitive source of the cholesterol for output in the bile and for bile acid formation has not been determined. Cholesterol excreted into the bile may be synthesized directly in the liver. Alternatively, cholesterol may be secreted from the liver and gut in triglyceride-rich lipoproteins and may be esterified by the LCAT-HDL system, and may reenter the liver directly with HDL or via remnant lipoproteins.

INBORN ERRORS OF LIPOPROTEIN METABOLISM

The primary, or inborn, errors of lipoprotein metabolism leading to hyperlipidemia generally can be grouped into disorders associated with overproduction of triglyceride-rich lipoproteins or disorders due to defects in one of three catabolic steps in lipoprotein degradation (see Fig. 183–2). Much more is known about defects in lipoprotein catabolism than about defects leading to lipoprotein overproduction (Table 183–1).

Defective Low-Density Lipoprotein Catabolism: Familial Hypercholesterolemia

DEFINITION. Familial hypercholesterolemia is an autosomal dominant trait with defective receptors for plasma LDL. An increase in LDL cholesterol is associated with characteristic xanthomas in the Achilles tendons, the patellar tendons, the extensor tendons of the hands, and with early coronary artery disease.

ETIOLOGY AND PATHOGENESIS. This disorder in LDL catabolism is caused by one of several alleles producing an abnormal LDL receptor. One of these alleles is associated with absence of LDL receptor synthesis and the others with the production of receptors of abnormal composition. These nonfunctional receptors are associated with decreased LDL catabolism and, in the heterozygote, with an approximate twofold increase in LDL levels. In the very rare homozygote, no receptor degradation occurs, and LDL is removed by a lower-affinity "scavenger" pathway with a sixfold or greater increase of cholesterol-rich lipoproteins in plasma.

CLINICAL MANIFESTATIONS. This disorder often manifests as coronary artery disease in a young male, who then is noted to have elevated cholesterol levels. The mean age of the first myocardial infarction in males with familial hypercholesterolemia who develop atherosclerosis is about 41 years. Affected women without additional risk factors often go through life without clinical manifestations of atherosclerosis. Low HDL cholesterol levels and cigarette smoking have marked effects on accelerating coronary artery disease and may be the major determinants of clinical disease in females. Peripheral vascular disease and cerebrovascular disease do not seem to be increased as much as coronary artery disease in this disorder. Lipid deposits in tendons are pathognomonic for this disorder. These xanthomas, usually bilateral, may be nodular irregularities in the Achilles tendons or extensor tendons of the hands, but can extend to diffuse, generalized thickening. Corneal arcus and xanthalasma may occur but are found with other lipoprotein abnormalities as well.

DIAGNOSIS. Plasma cholesterol levels in familial hypercholesterolemia are in the upper 1 per cent of levels seen in the general population (e.g., 300 to 500 mg per deciliter). Since this disease seems to be present in one in 500 individuals, at least one person in five with such plasma cholesterol levels would be expected to have this disease. Patients with defective remnant removal and those with chylomicronemia may also have markedly elevated cholesterol levels, but they

TABLE 183–1. INBORN ERRORS OF LIPOPROTEIN METABOLISM

Name	Prevalence	Physiologic Abnormality	Protein Abnormality	Lipoprotein Phenotype	Lipoproteins that Accumulate
Familial hypercholesterolemia	1/500	↓ LDL catabolism	Abnormal LDL receptor	IIA (IIB)	LDL ± VLDL
Familial dysbetalipoproteinemia	1/10,000	↓ Remnant catabolism	Abnormal apoprotein E	III	β VLDL
Lipoprotein lipase or Apo CII deficiency	Very Rare	↓ TG catabolism	Absence of LPL or apoprotein CII	I (V)	Chylo ± VLDL
Familial hypertriglyceridemia	? 1/200	↑ VLDL-TG and bile acid synthesis	?	IV (V)	VLDL ± Chylo
Familial combined hyperlipidemia	? 1/100	↑ Apoprotein B synthesis	? Apoprotein B	IIA, IIB, IV	LDL and/or VLDL

Phenotypes based on World Health Organization recommendations.
Chylo = chylomicron.

can be distinguished by the degree of coincident hypertriglyceridemia. Hypothyroidism and the nephrotic syndrome are also associated with elevated cholesterol levels. The increase in LDL in familial hypercholesterolemia uniquely is persistent, is almost always present in a parent, and is detectable at birth. The coexistence of tendon xanthomas and hypercholesterolemia is diagnostic of this disorder. Unilateral Achilles tendon thickening may be the result of injury.

TREATMENT. Discontinuation of smoking should be the first consideration for those who smoke. A low saturated fat, low cholesterol diet should be initiated in all affected individuals with this disorder, even though only a 5 to 15 per cent reduction in LDL levels occurs. Normalization of LDL levels occurs with the combination of a bile acid-binding resin (15 to 30 grams per day in divided doses with meals) and very high dose nicotinic acid with meals and at bedtime (2 to 7.5 grams per day). Compliance with each drug regimen has been poor. Fat-soluble vitamins should be given at bedtime, since the resins (colestipol or cholestyramine) prevent their absorption. Some recommend therapy with nicotinic acid and resins for all affected individuals. More conservatively, treatment can be restricted to postadolescent males and women with additional risk factors for coronary artery disease. Drugs that suppress hepatic HMG-CoA reductase and hepatic cholesterol synthesis may be available soon and should simplify the treatment of this disorder.

Remnant Removal Disease: Dysbetalipoproteinemia

DEFINITION. This disorder is due to the interaction between (1) an autosomal recessive defect in apoprotein E with abnormal remnant catabolism and (2) independent overproduction of triglyceride-rich lipoproteins. This results in the accumulation of postlipoprotein lipase remnants from both chylomicrons and endogenously synthesized VLDL that cause xanthomas and coronary artery and peripheral vascular disease.

ETIOLOGY AND PATHOGENESIS. About 1 per cent of individuals have two genes leading to an abnormal apoprotein E. Multiple alleles exist for apoprotein E; those producing amino acid substitutions in a critical region of the apoprotein have abnormal apoprotein E binding to hepatic membranes. Affected individuals either have two identical abnormal genes or are compound heterozygotes with two different abnormal genes. Most of these individuals do not have hyperlipidemia but rather have low plasma cholesterol and LDL levels, presumably because of defective conversion of VLDL remnants to LDL. VLDL remnants that are cholesteryl ester enriched are present, but plasma triglyceride levels are usually normal. About one in 100 individuals with this abnormal apoprotein E has hyperlipidemia with remnant removal disease. These individuals appear to have an independent abnormality leading to hypertriglyceridemia in addition to the defect in apoprotein E, and accumulate significant levels of chylomicron and VLDL remnants. Much rarer forms of remnant removal disease are caused by total absence of apoprotein E or an absence of postheparin plasma hepatic triglyceride lipase.

CLINICAL MANIFESTATIONS. This disorder may present initially as premature clinical atherosclerosis or as planar or tuberous xanthomas, or it may be detected as hyperlipidemia on routine laboratory screen. This disorder is usually not manifested as an abnormality in triglyceride or cholesterol levels in men until the third or fourth decade or in women until after menopause. The coexistent apoprotein E abnormality can be detected at birth. The onset of the xanthomas also is late. Planar xanthomas of the palmar crease and tuberous or tuberoeruptive xanthomas are highly suggestive of this disorder, although both can occur in severe, chronic obstructive liver disease with residual hepatocellular function. Atherosclerosis often is first noted in men around age 50 years. Peripheral vascular disease often predominates, but coronary artery disease is increased as well. In females, development of peripheral vascular and coronary artery disease after menopause is rapid as compared with nonaffected females. The presence of estrogen in the premenopausal state seems to minimize the defect in remnant catabolism.

DIAGNOSIS. The presence of palmar or tuberous xanthomas in the absence of liver disease is diagnostic. Plasma cholesterol and triglyceride are increased to similar levels. A method for separation of VLDL from the remainder of the more dense lipoproteins is necessary to demonstrate that these VLDL are cholesteryl ester enriched and have beta mobility on electrophoresis ("beta VLDL") rather than the typical pre-beta mobility of VLDL. An abnormal apoprotein E can usually be demonstrated by isoelectric focusing. The concentration of LDL is typically low, and HDL is often normal or slightly depressed. Hypothyroidism can aggravate this disorder or rarely can lead to remnant accumulation by itself.

TREATMENT. In obese individuals with this disorder, weight loss should be considered in lowering triglyceride and cholesterol levels. In postmenopausal females, low-dose ethinyl estradiol seems to normalize the defect in remnant removal and to correct the hypercholesterolemia. Clofibrate (1 gram twice a day) or gemfibrozil (0.8 gram* twice a day) also is effective in decreasing lipid levels. Alternatively, high-dose nicotinic acid is considered by some investigators as the drug of choice for treatment of this disorder. There is evidence that the form of atherosclerosis occurring with this disorder may be partially reversible with treatment.

Defective Lipoprotein Lipase–Related Triglyceride Catabolism

DEFINITION. Familial lipoprotein lipase (LPL) deficiency is a rare autosomal recessive trait characterized by complete absence of active enzyme protein in all tissues leading to massive hypertriglyceridemia from birth and recurrent episodes of pancreatitis. Similar syndromes also are caused by inborn defects in other aspects of the LPL system.

ETIOLOGY AND PATHOGENESIS. Hydrolysis of triglyceride from chylomicrons and endogenous VLDL in vivo requires both lipoprotein lipase and its activator apo CII. A defect of either of these proteins is associated with severely decreased triglyceride removal and massive hypertriglyceridemia. In infants and young children the triglyceride accumulates primarily as chylomicron triglyceride of dietary origin. As the patient gets older, a defect in VLDL triglyceride removal becomes more apparent as well. Both LPL and apoprotein CII deficiency are autosomal recessive disorders; often consanguinity can be documented. Individuals also exist who have LPL activity missing from only selected tissues or have a familial inhibitor of LPL activity. These latter groups usually have less severe hypertriglyceridemia and become symptomatic later in life than in the classic form of LPL deficiency.

CLINICAL MANIFESTATIONS. Infants with LPL deficiency rapidly manifest intolerance to fatty foods. As these children grow, they learn to avoid certain high fat foods such as whole milk. Abdominal pain, often with pancreatitis, occurs in association with the high levels of chylomicron triglyceride. Eruptive xanthomas occur on extensor surfaces, notably the elbows, knees, and the buttocks, and are pathognomonic for chronic chylomicronemia. Hepatomegaly and occasionally splenomegaly occur because of the accumulation of lipid-laden foam cells. The hepatosplenomegaly rapidly diminishes on a fat-free diet, which clears the chylomicronemia. Eruptive xanthomas also disappear with time after lowering of chylomicron levels. Other signs and symptoms seen with chronic chylomicronemia may also occur (see below).

*This dose exceeds the manufacturer's recommended dosage.

DIAGNOSIS. A young child with abdominal pain and milky, lactescent plasma should be studied for a genetic abnormality in LPL. Other causes of chylomicronemia before adulthood relate to the occurrence of a common form of hypertriglyceridemia with diabetes or glucocorticoid therapy. Absent or diminished activity of lipoprotein lipase can be demonstrated in adipose tissue or muscle tissue, or in plasma after intravenous heparin. Apoprotein CII deficiency can be detected by radioimmunoassay or by gel electrophoresis of the protein components of lipoproteins.

TREATMENT. In all the inborn errors of the LPL-related triglyceride removal system associated with chylomicronemia, a decrease in total dietary fat is absolutely indicated. A total of polyunsaturated and saturated fat as low as 10 to 20 per cent of calories is often required. Medium-chain triglycerides can be used to prepare some foods, since their fatty acids leave the gut unesterified via the portal vein rather than via the thoracic duct as chylomicron triglyceride. The goal is to decrease the amount of dietary fat to a level low enough to eliminate the occurrence of abdominal pain. These individuals can also be sensitive to agents that raise endogenous VLDL levels, such as alcohol or glucocorticoids, and to the effects of pregnancy.

Other Genetic Disorders with Mild to Moderate Hypertriglyceridemia

A number of less well characterized disorders associated with persistent or intermittent elevated VLDL levels exist. Some may be associated with increased hepatic secretion of VLDL, others with defective VLDL catabolism. It has been useful to classify those conditions into several relatively homogenous groups on the basis of the existence of large, well-characterized families for each.

FAMILIAL HYPERTRIGLYCERIDEMIA. This apparently autosomal dominant trait may be quite common. Individuals with familial hypertriglyceridemia appear to have a defect leading to enhanced hepatic triglyceride synthesis with subsequent secretion of triglyceride-enriched, large VLDL. These individuals may also have increased cholesterol and cholic acid synthesis. LPL-related triglyceride removal and remnant lipoprotein catabolism appear to be normal. LDL levels are normal, while HDL is triglyceride-enriched with depletion of HDL cholesterol.

Most individuals with this disorder do not have an increased predisposition for coronary artery disease, remain asymptomatic, and are detected by routine lipid screen. Occasionally with the onset of another disorder associated with elevated triglyceride levels, they will develop the chylomicronemia syndrome (see below). These individuals develop no characteristic xanthomas. There is no increase in obesity in this disorder, and no increase in the frequency of diabetes.

Individuals with this disorder have persistent hypertriglyceridemia once they become adults. Below the age of 20, the abnormality is not manifest. Some of the increase in VLDL may persist after weight loss. Increased levels of LDL do not occur. One parent is characteristically affected, as are half of the siblings. These individuals appear to be quite sensitive to other factors that cause only mild hypertriglyceridemia in normal adults: obesity and alcohol, and estrogen, diuretic, beta-adrenergic blocker, and glucocorticoid therapy.

Treatment with clofibrate or gemfibrozil usually leads to significant decreases in VLDL levels. In families without evidence of increased atherosclerosis, no known benefit accrues from this therapy, and it should be discouraged. Drugs causing elevation of triglyceride levels should be avoided because they may precipitate massive chylomicronemia and pancreatitis.

FAMILIAL COMBINED HYPERLIPIDEMIA. This disorder was first suggested in 1973 to be very common in those with premature coronary heart disease, to be inherited as an autosomal dominant trait, and to be characterized by different "combinations" of hyperlipidemia: elevated cholesterol level alone, elevated triglyceride level alone, or elevations in levels of both lipids (familial multiple lipoprotein-type hyperlipidemia). It now appears that this disorder is better characterized as one with elevated plasma apoprotein B levels with variable lipid phenotype even in the same individual at different times, in contrast with familial hypercholesterolemia. The increase in apoprotein B, whether in VLDL or in LDL, appears to be caused by increased hepatic synthesis of the apoprotein. These individuals also have abnormalities in HDL with a mild decrease in HDL cholesterol and apoprotein AI.

Males with this disorder have premature coronary artery disease with mean age of infarct at about 40 years. Smoking has a marked effect on the prevalence of clinical heart disease. Individuals with this disorder are slightly more obese and may have more systemic hypertension. They have no characteristic xanthomas, but occasionally have nonspecific xanthalasma.

OTHER FORMS OF HYPERTRIGLYCERIDEMIA. Individuals with chylomicronemia and triglyceride levels between 1000 and 2000 mg per deciliter are said to aggregate in families. In addition, there are individuals with primary hypertriglyceridemia noted to have a defect in VLDL removal not characterized by one of the above defects in the lipoprotein lipase system.

APPROACH TO THE PATIENT WITH MILD TO MODERATE HYPERTRIGLYCERIDEMIA. The major concern for the individual with hypertriglyceridemia relates to a possible increase in risk for atherosclerosis. When an individual is identified with elevated plasma triglyceride levels, acquired forms of hyperlipidemia should be identified and treated, and the primary forms of hypertriglyceridemia associated with defective remnant catabolism or LPL deficiency should be ruled out.

Elevations in plasma triglyceride levels often serve as a marker for associated abnormalities potentially related to atherosclerosis. A strong family history of early coronary artery disease in the father or mother's male relatives helps to identify such a hypertriglyceridemic individual at risk for early atherosclerosis.

The hypertriglyceridemic individuals who intermittently develop hypercholesterolemia caused by increased LDL levels as well as those who have elevated LDL apoprotein B levels with normal LDL cholesterol also seem to be ones with increased risk for atherosclerosis.

The level of HDL cholesterol is often low in the presence of hypertriglyceridemia. This can occur with familial LPL deficiency and with familial hypertriglyceridemia and does not seem to be associated with the increase in coronary risk seen with a low HDL cholesterol level in the absence of hypertriglyceridemia. However, a decrease in the level of the major apoprotein of HDL, apoprotein AI, seems to be a good predictor of risk, even in the presence of hypertriglyceridemia.

The aforementioned abnormalities characteristic of the hypertriglyceridemic subject at risk for atherosclerosis are similar to those in familial combined hyperlipidemia, which may account for a significant portion of this group.

While weight loss and clofibrate (or gemfibrozil) therapy lower VLDL levels, those at risk for early coronary disease may respond with an increase in LDL levels. Preferred therapy for the hypertriglyceridemic individual at risk, in particular the one with familial combined hyperlipidemia, may be like that used to treat elevated LDL levels in familial hypercholesterolemia: combined bile acid resin and high-dose nicotinic acid therapy, in addition to a diet low in saturated fat and cholesterol. Because of the uncertainty of the significance of elevated triglyceride levels and the unknown risks of lifelong drug therapy, many authorities have recommended diet therapy alone for hypertriglyceridemia.

TABLE 183–2. ACQUIRED DISORDERS OF LIPOPROTEIN METABOLISM

A. Hypertriglyceridemia
   1. Mild to moderate hypertriglyceridemia
      a. Diabetes mellitus*
      b. Uremia and/or dialysis*
   2. Minimal hypertriglyceridemia alone
      a. Obesity
      b. Estrogen*
      c. Alcohol*
      d. Beta-adrenergic blocking agents*
   3. Rare forms of moderate to marked hypertriglyceridemia
      a. Systemic lupus erythematosus
      b. Dysgammaglobulinemias
      c. Glycogenosis type I
      d. Lipodystrophy
B. Combined hyperlipidemia
   1. Hypothyroidism*
   2. Nephrotic syndrome
   3. Glucocorticoid excess*
   4. Diuretics*
C. Hypercholesterolemia
   1. Acute intermittent porphyria
   2. Anorexia nervosa

*Can be associated with chylomicronemia syndrome when it occurs with the familial forms of hypertriglyceridemia.

ACQUIRED DISORDERS OF LIPOPROTEIN METABOLISM

Some disease states are associated with mild to moderate hyperlipidemia in the absence of primary forms of hyperlipidemia, while others seem to have a significant effect only in the presence of a familial form of hyperlipidemia. In general, these can be divided into conditions associated with increased levels of triglyceride-rich lipoproteins and those associated with multiple lipoprotein-type expression (acquired combined hyperlipidemia) (Table 183–2).

Hypertriglyceridemia

DIABETES MELLITUS. Persons with untreated insulin-dependent diabetes and untreated symptomatic non-insulin-dependent diabetes have low adipose tissue or muscle lipoprotein lipase activity with a mild to moderate increase in triglyceride levels and decreased HDL cholesterol levels. With insulin resistance and milder degrees of insulin deficiency, hypertriglyceridemia is caused by excess free fatty acids mobilized from adipose tissue that are re-esterified in the liver and secreted as endogenous VLDL. Treatment with insulin or oral sulfonylurea agents will correct the abnormality in LPL over a period of weeks. In the treated diabetic, variability in free fatty acid mobilization and hepatic triglyceride synthesis, related to the degree of diabetic control, accounts for most of the variation in triglyceride levels.

CHRONIC UREMIA AND DIALYSIS. Many individuals with chronic uremia have elevated VLDL levels with hypertriglyceridemia and low HDL cholesterol levels. This persists after initiation of maintenance hemodialysis or peritoneal dialysis. These lipoprotein abnormalities appear to be related to defects in LPL-mediated triglyceride removal and, with smoking and hypertension, account for the marked atherosclerosis in the dialysis population.

OTHER. Obesity, estrogen use, and alcohol are associated with minimal to mild increases in triglyceride levels, usually not to levels considered abnormal, which appear to be caused by modest increases in hepatic VLDL secretion. Diuretic agents and beta-adrenergic blocking agents are also associated with small increases in triglyceride levels. The diuretics often raise LDL levels, while the beta-blocking agents decrease HDL.

Moderate to marked hypertriglyceridemia occurs extremely rarely in systemic lupus erythematosus or dysgammaglobulinemia caused by an immunoglobulin lipoprotein interaction. Moderate hypertriglyceridemia can also occur in rare disorders such as glycogenosis (type I), lipodystrophy, and carnitine-palmitoyl transferase deficiency.

Combined Hyperlipidemia

HYPOTHYROIDISM. Thyroid hormone appears to be necessary for proper functioning of most steps in lipoprotein metabolism. Thyroxine is necessary for maintenance of the LDL receptor; in hypothyroidism LDL levels are elevated because of defective catabolism. Remnant removal is impaired, resulting in the accumulation of chylomicron with VLDL remnants, and finally the LPL level is low, resulting in hypertriglyceridemia. Thyroxin replacement corrects all of these defects.

NEPHROTIC SYNDROME. With urinary loss of albumin and the development of hypoalbuminemia, increases in levels of VLDL or LDL or both occur. These lipoprotein abnormalities are associated with increased hepatic lipid synthesis and defective catabolism of triglyceride-rich lipoproteins. The latter defect may be related to the loss in the urine of cofactors required for LPL function.

GLUCOCORTICOID EXCESS. Excess glucocorticoid levels caused by Cushing's syndrome or exogenous steroid therapy are associated with elevated VLDL and/or LDL levels. The best studied situation is in the glucocorticoid-treated renal transplant subject, who in the absence of uremia or proteinuria has combined hyperlipidemia.

Hypercholesterolemia

Elevated LDL levels may occur in occasional individuals in response to high saturated fat and cholesterol feeding. Much of the hypercholesterolemia in the population has remained unexplained and has been termed multifactorial, suggesting that it is due to interaction of multiple genes (polygenic) with the environment. Elevated LDL levels occur in acute intermittent porphyria and have been reported with hepatomas and in anorexia nervosa.

CHYLOMICRONEMIA SYNDROME

DEFINITION. Marked chylomicronemia with plasma triglyceride levels in excess of 2000 mg per deciliter is associated with a constellation of signs and symptoms called the chylomicronemia syndrome.

ETIOLOGY AND PATHOGENESIS. This syndrome can occur because of one of several inborn errors in the lipoprotein lipase system for plasma triglyceride removal as noted earlier. Much more commonly, the marked hypertriglyceridemia occurs as a result of the interaction of two common forms of hypertriglyceridemia, usually one genetic and one acquired. Untreated symptomatic diabetes mellitus in the presence of familial hypertriglyceridemia, familial combined hyperlipidemia, or, less commonly, remnant removal disease is a frequent cause of chylomicronemia. Commonly used drugs that interact with these inborn errors are the estrogens, diuretics, beta-adrenergic blocking agents, alcohol, and glucocorticoids. The effects of these drugs are often markedly exaggerated in patients with pre-existing hyperlipidemia. Hypothyroidism and uremia may also occasionally contribute.

CLINICAL MANIFESTATIONS. For unexplained reasons, some individuals are asymptomatic with plasma triglyceride levels as high as 29,000 mg per deciliter. More commonly, abdominal pain and/or pancreatitis or even chest pain is present. Impairment of recent memory can often be detected and the patient may complain of paresthesias of the extremities, similar to the carpal tunnel syndrome. Lipemia retinalis can often be observed, hepatomegaly is common, splenomegaly can occur, and eruptive xanthomas are evidence of chronic chylomicronemia. All of these symptoms and signs clear when triglyceride levels are decreased below 1000 or 2000 mg per deciliter. Marked hypertriglyceridemia may cause insulin resistance and impair control of diabetes. Also, many routine laboratory tests are invalid in the presence of milky plasma. Simple removal of chylomicrons from plasma by short-term ultracentrifugation helps to avoid this problem.

DIAGNOSIS. It is very simple to make a presumptive diagnosis of chylomicronemia syndrome by visual examination of the patient's plasma. Milky plasma always indicates the presence of chylomicrons, as does a plasma triglyceride level above 1000 mg per deciliter. In the presence of symptoms and signs of the chylomicron syndrome, a definitive diagnosis is made if these clear when the triglyceride level is lowered.

TREATMENT. With pancreatitis, the discontinuation of oral intake will rapidly decrease triglyceride levels. With refeeding, fat must be avoided initially and replaced slowly. Often, mild to moderate abdominal pain can be treated by lowering dietary fat content and avoiding alcohol. The mainstay of treatment is to identify the causes of the elevation in triglyceride levels. A genetic form of hypertriglyceridemia is invariably present and may need to be treated with clofibrate, gemfibrozil, or nicotinic acid. The last drug is difficult to use in diabetic patients because it impairs insulin sensitivity. The acquired disease or agent contributing to the hypertriglyceridemia should be treated or removed. Slowly, the patient can be refed while the plasma is watched for turbidity and the patient's symptoms and signs are observed. With appropriate therapy, the chylomicronemia syndrome should rarely recur.

HYPERLIPIDEMIA AND ATHEROSCLEROTIC VASCULAR DISEASE

Although the etiology of atherosclerosis is multifactorial, the development of premature coronary artery disease and peripheral vascular disease is strongly dependent on abnormalities in plasma lipoprotein metabolism. Thus, coronary artery disease in men under the age of 50 years and in women of any age is more likely to occur in the presence of one of the inborn errors or acquired forms of hyperlipidemia. Independently, HDL may protect against atherosclerosis. Differences in HDL cholesterol levels between men and women may explain a large part of the sex difference in development of atherosclerosis.

Familial hypercholesterolemia unequivocally is associated with premature coronary artery disease and aggravated by cigarette smoking and low HDL cholesterol levels. Remnant removal disease is also associated with peripheral vascular disease and coronary artery disease. Familial hypertriglyceridemia may impose some increased risk for atherosclerosis in a few families, but atherosclerosis is generally not increased in this form in hypertriglyceridemia. The increased atherosclerosis seen in diabetics and in patients undergoing long-term hemodialysis may also be related in part to abnormalities in lipoprotein metabolism. One must be concerned that the lipoprotein changes seen with diuretic and beta-adrenergic blocking therapy for elevated blood pressure may contribute to coronary artery disease.

Nonetheless, all of these factors still account for only a minor part of premature atherosclerosis. Mildly elevated levels of LDL, apoprotein B, or triglyceride and low levels of HDL cholesterol and apoprotein AI have been suggested to be present in the majority of patients with premature coronary artery disease. The frequency of familial combined hyperlipidemia in this undefined heterogeneous group of individuals has yet to be determined.

The goal of therapy aimed at correcting hyperlipidemia is to prevent the progression of atherosclerosis. Direct evidence now suggests this may be possible in some individuals with specific lipoprotein abnormalities. Young individuals at risk can be identified as those with a family history of premature coronary artery disease or known acquired causes of hyperlipidemia (Table 183–2). After consideration of the acquired causes of hyperlipidemia, individuals with plasma cholesterol levels in the upper 25th percentile of the normal distribution should be treated with a low-saturated fat, low-cholesterol diet. Young and middle-aged men whose LDL cholesterol remains in the upper fifth to tenth percentile should be considered for therapy with a bile acid–binding resin, high-dose nicotinic acid, or neomycin. Combinations of a resin with nicotinic acid or with a fibric acid derivative (clofibrate or gemfibrozil) may be of further benefit. The use of the fibric acid drugs alone does not seem warranted because of the tendency for LDL to increase in those with hyperlipidemia who are at risk for premature coronary disease.

RARE DISORDERS OF LIPOPROTEIN METABOLISM

Several rare inherited disorders of lipoprotein metabolism are of considerable theoretical importance because they assist in understanding normal lipoprotein physiology. Each of these disorders is an autosomal recessive trait.

Abetalipoproteinemia presents in early childhood and is associated with absence of apoprotein B–containing lipoproteins due to defective synthesis. Intestinal fat malabsorption, ataxia, neuropathy, retinitis pigmentosa, and acanthocytosis result. *Tangier disease* presents in childhood with absence of HDL and extremely low levels of apoproteins AI and AII. Cholesteryl esters deposit in tonsils and other lymphoid tissues and corneal opacities develop. *Lecithin-cholesterol acyltransferase deficiency* presents in the young adult as hemolytic anemia and renal failure. Although the free cholesterol level in plasma is variable, the cholesteryl ester level is very low. Other even rarer disorders are described in recent reviews.

Disorders of lipoprotein and lipid metabolism. In Stanbury JB, Wyngaarden JB, Fredrickson DS, et al. (eds.): The Metabolic Basis of Inherited Disease. 5th ed. New York, McGraw-Hill Book Company, 1983, pp 589–747. *Seven extensive reviews in great detail about the inborn errors leading to abnormalities in plasma lipoproteins.*

Havel RJ: Symposium on lipid disorders. Med Clin North Am 66:317, 1982. *Contains 12 review articles by experts in the field concerning basic biochemistry and physiology of lipoproteins, pathophysiology of specific diseases, and therapy of these disorders.*

Journal of Lipid Research 25:1425–1634, 1984. *Series of articles ranging from basic biochemistry of lipids to clinical lipoprotein disorders.*

184 FABRY'S DISEASE (Glycosphingolipidosis)

James B. Wyngaarden

DEFINITION. Fabry's disease is an inborn error of glycosphingolipid metabolism characterized by telangiectatic skin lesions, hypohidrosis, corneal opacities, acral pain and paresthesias, intermittent fevers, renal failure, and cardiovascular, gastrointestinal, and central nervous system disturbances.

PREVALENCE. The disease has an estimated prevalence of 1:40,000 births.

ETIOLOGY AND PATHOGENESIS. Fabry's disease is an X-linked condition, fully manifest in the hemizygous male. Heterozygous females may exhibit the disease in an attenuated form, and usually show corneal clouding; occasionally a female may have most of the features of the full syndrome, including renal failure.

The biochemical defect is a deficiency of the lysosomal enzyme, alpha-galactosidase-A. The enzymatic defect leads to a progressive deposition of neutral glycosphingolipids with terminal alpha-galactosyl moieties in most visceral tissues and fluids of the body. The most prominent of these is a trihexosylceramide called globotriaosylceramide, a degradation product of a constituent of membrane called globoside. The majority of anatomic and physiologic abnormalities observed in Fabry's disease can be related to the cumulative deposition of glycosphingolipid, particularly in the lysosomes of the cardiovascular-renal system.

PATHOLOGY. Morphologically, Fabry's disease is characterized by widespread tissue deposits of a crystalline glycosphingolipid that shows birefringence under polarized light. The glycosphingolipid is deposited in all areas of the body, predominantly in the lysosomes of endothelial, perithelial, and smooth muscle cells of blood vessels. Lipid deposits are also prominent in epithelial cells of the cornea, in glomeruli and tubules of the kidney, in muscle fibers of the heart, and in ganglion cells of the dorsal roots and autonomic nervous system. The skin lesions are telangiectases or small superficial angiomas. Capillaries, venules, and arterioles show pathologic lipid storage, and there is marked dilatation of the capillaries of the dermal papillae just below the epidermis. The larger lesions are usually located in the upper dermis, where they may produce elevation, flattening, or hypertrophy of the epithelium, with keratosis; hence the term *angiokeratoma*. On electron microscopy lipid inclusions show a concentrically arranged lamellar structure with alternating light- and dark-staining bands. Peripheral nerves show densely stained inclusions in the cytoplasm of perineurial fibroblasts and the endothelial cells of the endoneurial blood vessels. There is loss of unmyelinated neurons but not of myelinated neurons. Some neurons contain ceramide trihexoside.

CLINICAL MANIFESTATIONS. *Telangiectases* may occur in childhood and lead to early diagnosis. They increase in size and number with age, and range from barely visible to several millimeters in diameter. The lesions are punctate, dark red to blue-black, and flat or slightly raised. They do not blanch with pressure, and the larger ones may show slight hyperkeratosis. The lesions tend to occur in the "bathing trunk area," but may occur anywhere, including the oral mucosa. The hips, thighs, buttocks, umbilicus, lower abdomen, scrotum, and glans penis are common sites, and there is a tendency toward bilateral symmetry. In some patients skin lesions are absent and lesions are entirely visceral. Sweating is often decreased, and hair may be sparse; shaving may be required only infrequently. Ocular lesions may be present in all elements of the eye. The most prominent are in the cornea, conjunctiva, and retina. Corneal opacities, observed by slit lamp examination, are present in most heterozygotes. The conjunctival and retinal vessels may show mild to marked tortuosity, with aneurysmal dilatations of thin-walled venules, as well as angulation and segmental, sausage-like dilatation of veins.

Pain is the most debilitating symptom. Fabry's crises, lasting from minutes to several days, consist of agonizing, burning pain in palms, soles, and proximal extremities, associated with fever. The pain may become more severe with age, or may disappear. Attacks of abdominal or flank pain may simulate appendicitis or renal colic. In addition, there may be chronic troublesome paresthesias of hands and feet.

With increasing age progressive infiltration of the cardiovascular-renal system with glycosphingolipid gives rise to anginal chest pain, myocardial infarction, cardiomegaly, or congestive heart failure. Involvement of renal parenchymal vessels leads to hypertension. During childhood and adolescence protein, red cells, casts, and desquamated kidney and urinary tract cells appear in the urine. Azotemia is common in the second to fourth decade. Birefringent lipid globules with characteristic Maltese crosses within and without cells can be observed in the urine sediment by polarized light microscopy. Other features may include chronic bronchitis and dyspnea, lymphedema of the legs without hypoproteinemia, episodic diarrhea, osteoporosis, retarded growth, and delayed puberty. The mean age at death is 41 years, but survival may extend into the sixties.

DIAGNOSIS AND DIFFERENTIAL DIAGNOSIS. The diagnosis in hemizygous males is most readily made from the history of painful paresthesias and episodic crises with fever, and the observation of characteristic skin lesions, corneal opacities, and conjunctival lesions. The disorder is often misdiagnosed as rheumatic fever, erythromelalgia, or neurosis. The skin lesions must be differentiated from the benign angiokeratomas of the scrotum of older men (Fordyce's disease) or from angiokeratoma circumscripta. Angiokeratomas identical to those of Fabry's disease have been reported in fucosidosis and sialidosis. The diagnosis is confirmed biochemically by demonstration of markedly alpha-galactosidase-A activity in plasma or serum, leukocytes, tears, biopsied tissue, or cultured skin fibroblasts. Increased levels of globotriaosylceramide are found in urinary sediment, plasma, or cultured fibroblasts.

Suspect heterozygotes may show corneal opacities, isolated skin lesions, and lipid-laden cells in skin or other tissues or in urinary sediment. Intermediate activities of alpha-galactosidase-A can usually be demonstrated.

Prenatal diagnosis of Fabry's disease may be made by amniocentesis at approximately 14 weeks of gestation and demonstration of deficient alpha-galactosidase-A activity and XY karyotype in cultured amniotic cells, and accumulated trihexosylceramide in amniotic acid.

TREATMENT. Pain may be relieved with phenytoin or carbamazepine in some patients. Maintenance administration of phenytoin, carbamazepine, or both, or corticosteroid therapy has also provided symptomatic relief. Renal insufficiency is treated with long-term hemodialysis or renal transplantation. In some recipients biochemical and clinical regression, with relief of pain, has followed placement of renal allografts. Alpha-galactosidase-A purified from human placenta has been administered to several hemizygotes. The enzyme was rapidly cleared from plasma and taken up by liver. There was a reduction in level of circulating trihexosylceramide. Current research centers on target delivery of enzyme and methods of protecting it from rapid inactivation.

Case Records of the Massachusetts General Hospital: Case 2–1984 (Fabry's Disease). N Engl J Med 310:106, 1984. *Excellent presentation of nervous system involvement in Fabry's disease.*

Desnick RJ, Klionsky B, Sweeley CC: Fabry's disease (α-galactosidase A deficiency). In Stanbury JB, Wyngaarden JB, Fredrickson DS, et al. (eds.): The Metabolic Basis of Inherited Disease. 5th ed. New York, McGraw-Hill Book Company, 1983. *A definitive chapter describing clinical, pathologic, and biochemical manifestations of Fabry's disease; 400 references.*

Goldman ME, Cantor R, Schwartz MF, et al.: Echocardiographic abnormalities and disease severity in Fabry's disease. J Am Coll Cardiol 7:1157, 1986. *Echocardiographic evidence of Fabry's disease appears to correlate with age-related severity of disease.*

185 GAUCHER'S DISEASE

Edwin H. Kolodny

DEFINITION. This relatively common familial disorder results from progressive accumulation of glucocerebroside within phagocytic cells of the monocyte-macrophage system involving principally the liver, spleen, bone marrow, and lymph nodes. Three genetically distinct clinical types have been differentiated: type 1, a chronic non-neuronopathic or "adult" form that may appear at any age and is associated with hypersplenism and bone lesions; type 2, an acute neuronopathic or "infantile" form that presents in infancy with multiple brain stem signs; and type 3, a "juvenile" subacute neuronopathic form that presents in childhood and causes seizures and mental deterioration. The activity of glucocerebrosidase is deficient in all three types, but each is due to a different mutation.

PATHOLOGIC PHYSIOLOGY AND PATHOGENESIS. Glucocerebroside contains equimolar amounts of spingosine, fatty acid, and glucose. Considerable quantities of this compound are generated daily by the turnover of senescent red and white blood cells. In the central nervous system, glucocerebroside is produced in the course of ganglioside metabolism. A deacylated derivative, glucosylsphingosine, also accumulates in Gaucher's disease. This highly cytotoxic compound is probably responsible for the nerve cell destruction that occurs in the neuropathic forms of the disease. Both of these glycolipids are degraded by acidic glucosylceramide-β-D-glucosidase (glucocerebrosidase; E.C. 3.5.1.2.1), a lysosomal enzyme with multiple molecular forms. Its catalytic efficiency is increased by a low molecular weight, heat-stable protein that combines with the enzyme-lipid complex. The gene for glucocerebrosidase has been mapped to the q21 region of chromosome 1, and its cloned cDNA has been used as a molecular probe to identify the catalytic site of the enzyme and variations in restriction pattern of genomic DNA from Gaucher patients.

A distinctive morphologic feature is the *Gaucher cell*, a large round or polyhedral phagocyte, 20 to 100 μ in diameter, containing one or more small eccentrically placed nuclei and a pale, striated cytoplasm resembling wrinkled tissue paper or crumpled silk (Fig. 185–1*A*). Under the electron microscope, this fibrillary network consists of numerous dilated saclike structures resembling lysosomes containing tubules; these are similar to the twisted bilayers characteristic of glucocerebroside deposits. The reaction of the Gaucher cell cytoplasm with the periodic acid–Schiff stain is strongly positive. Stains for iron and acid phosphatase are also positive, but the reaction with lipid stains is weak. The bone marrow of patients with chronic myelogenous leukemia often contains cells with a similar appearance; the deposits in these "pseudo-Gaucher" cells are linear rather than twisted.

Glucosylceramide is increased two- to three-fold in plasma and more than 200-fold in the spleen and liver. Gaucher cells are present in virtually all organs surrounding small blood vessels and as sheets infiltrating their parenchyma. The spleen

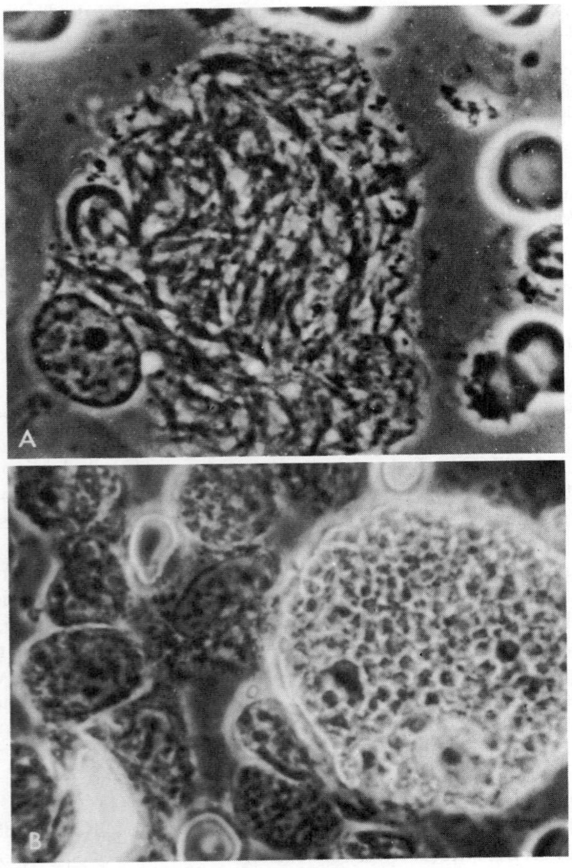

FIGURE 185–1. Appearance of the typical Gaucher cell (*A*) and a foam cell seen in Niemann-Pick disease (*B*). Both are viewed under phase microscopy in unstained smears of aspirated bone marrow. Magnification can be estimated from adjacent red cells.

may become massively enlarged and develop multiple infarcts and fibrosis. The red pulp of the spleen appears white because of lipid infiltration by Gaucher cells; foci of extramedullary hematopoiesis can occur. In most patients the liver is also enlarged, the Kupffer cells of their sinusoids transformed into Gaucher cells. Fibrosis is present, but there is no proliferation of the bile ducts and liver failure is rare. Excretion of glucosylceramide into the bile probably prevents more massive accumulation within the liver. In some cases, portal hypertension develops.

Gaucher cells may completely fill the medullary cavity of bone, cause thinning of the cortex, loss of its normal trabeculation, patchy myelosclerosis, bone infarcts, and osteonecrosis. The metaphyseal plate in the long bones is especially prone to damage. An *Erlenmeyer flask deformity* of the distal femur is an early radiographic sign of bone involvement. With progression of the disease, spontaneous fractures and painful lytic lesions are found. Diffuse pulmonary infiltration can occur with direct involvement of the alveoli, pleura, and interstitium resulting in dyspnea and cor pulmonale. Renal involvement with severe proteinuric nephropathy and glomerulonephritis occurs in a few cases.

Central nervous system pathology has been found in all three types. Perivascular collections of Gaucher cells, nerve cell loss, neuronophagia, and infiltration of microglia are the principal changes observed. The most affected area in type 2 are the deeper layers of the frontal cortex and the nuclei of the basal ganglia, midbrain, and brain stem. The high concentrations of glucosylsphingosine, a cytotoxic compound, present in the brain, liver, and spleen of type 2 patients probably contribute to the necrosis that occurs in these tissues.

The activity of tartrate-resistant acid phosphatase and angiotensin converting enzyme and concentrations of several serum proteins, including the immunoglobulins, are increased, especially in type 1 patients. The increased acid phosphatase is the type 5 isozyme and therefore of osteoclastic origin and indicative of bone involvement. Some older patients develop a monoclonal gammopathy with multiple myeloma. Leukemias and other forms of malignant neoplasms are also more frequent in elderly patients with type 1 disease.

CLINICAL MANIFESTATIONS. ***Chronic Non-neuropathic Type.*** This disease is transmitted as an autosomal recessive trait and affects both sexes equally. It has been observed in whites, blacks, and Asians, but more than one half of cases are found in Ashkenazic Jews. Since one in 20 of this population is a carrier, it is not unusual for the disease to appear in two successive generations of the same family. Clinical symptoms in this so-called adult form may appear at any age, from the first year of life to the ninth decade. One third of all cases are diagnosed in the first decade. The majority of these children are not of Jewish ancestry. They develop massive enlargement of the spleen and evidence a delay in somatic growth that may severely hamper their intellectual and social development. The condition in another 25 per cent of patients is not diagnosed until after age 30. These patients have a much more benign course. Only rarely do these individuals have serious hematologic or osseous complications.

The most common presenting symptom is excessive fatigue associated with a hypochromic anemia and splenomegaly. Frequently there is a long history of bleeding tendency such as repeated epistaxis and ecchymoses, but this rarely attracts medical attention unless it is associated with a major hemorrhage such as splenic rupture, bleeding from esophageal varices, subdural hematoma, or hemopericardium. The first indication in some patients may be the appearance of bone or joint pain or a pathologic fracture. Lytic lesions develop in the shafts of the long bones, vertebrae, ribs, and pelvis. This produces osteosclerosis and, in the most virulent cases, osteonecrosis and eventually collapse of bone. In the acute crises affecting bone or joints there is severe incapacitating pain, erythema, swelling, tenderness, and occasionally joint effusion. While only 20 per cent of all type 1 patients have significant clinical involvement of bone, more than one half have radiologic evidence of the Erlenmeyer flask deformity with tapering of the midshaft of the femur and failure of normal trabeculation causing a widening of the distal end.

The clinical course is variable. In response to an acute infection, the size of the spleen may increase dramatically and then regress, but slowly progressive splenomegaly is the usual pattern. Anemia, thrombocytopenia, and leukemia are frequent but rarely cause significant morbidity. Bleeding may occur if the platelet count falls below 50,000 to 70,000 per cubic millimeter; however, the count usually rises again spontaneously within a few weeks. Hepatomegaly with a firm liver edge is common, and in a few severe cases liver failure and portal hypertension occur.

Acute Neuronopathic Type. This form of the disease is much rarer than the adult type 1 variety. It is observed in infants of different ethnic groups and does not show any predilection for Jews. The disease usually presents a few months after birth with retroflexion of the head, strabismus, increasing muscular hypertoncity, and marked increase in the size of the liver and spleen. In some cases, developmental milestones are normal until the second or third year. The major central nervous system signs reflect brain stem and and cranial nerve involvement. There are extreme arching of the neck, retraction of the lips, trismus, laryngeal spasm with a chronic cough and stridor, and spastic rigidity of the extremities. Seizures and psychomotor retardation also occur. Death results from respiratory infection within a few months to two years after signs appear.

Juvenile Type. This includes a heterogeneous group of patients with signs of the chronic adult type combined with progressive neurologic disease that begins in childhood or adolescence. A subtype of this disease that occurs in Swedish youngsters is referred to as the Norrbottnian variant. Their growth is retarded, and there are hypersplenism and skeletal changes of the type that occurs in the chronic non-neuropathic form. In addition, they develop oculomotor apraxia, convergent squint, seizures, and a delay in motor development. In splenectomized patients, white retinal infiltrates may appear, the infiltration of glucosylceramide into the central nervous system is accelerated, and the pace of mental deterioration is faster than in nonsplenectomized patients. In other patients with the juvenile type, the principal manifestations are medication-resistant myoclonic seizures and slow intellectual decline.

DIAGNOSIS. Gaucher's disease should be suspected in any patient with unexplained splenomegaly and a bleeding tendency, bone or joint pains, or pathologic fractures. A radioisotope scan of the liver and spleen will reveal the extent of the hepatosplenomegaly and the presence of infarcts. Radionuclide scintigraphy or magnetic resonance imaging is useful for locating lytic changes in bone. The bone marrow may demonstrate Gaucher cells. The diagnosis is established by assaying the activity of glucosylceramide-β-D-glucosidase in leukocytes or cultured fibroblasts. The artificial fluorogenic substrate, 4-methylumbelliferyl-β-glucoside, is commonly employed as a substitute for the natural lipid substrate. The degree of enzyme deficiency is similar in all three clinical subtypes of Gaucher's disease. Within the same family, expression of the disease may vary considerably so that enzyme assays should be done on all close relatives of the patient, whether or not they are symptomatic. Heterozygotes have approximately one half the normal enzyme activity; however, with current methods the range of values overlaps with the normal range. Therefore, carrier detection cannot be done with 100 per cent certainty. Prenatal diagnosis is possible using cultured amniotic cells.

TREATMENT AND PROGNOSIS. Iron therapy may partially correct the anemia, but the persistent use of iron in the presence of adequate iron stores increases the risk of hemochromatosis. Splenectomy is performed for severe and persistent thrombocytopenia or when mechanical factors cause massive swelling, abdominal pain, or gastrointestinal dysfunction. Correction of the thrombocytopenia occurs immediately after the operation with a less dramatic improvement noted in the anemia. In children, the growth curve usually improves. However, splenectomy may hasten the pace of lipid deposition into the liver and bones, and osteolytic lesions may appear within a few months after the operation. Therefore, the surgeon may elect to leave in place any accessory spleen tissue that is present or to perform a partial splenectomy. Acute lesions in bone and joints are initially treated with immobilization and the prevention of weight bearing. However, as soon as possible a graduated program of exercises is introduced to maintain joint mobility and prevent further loss of bone. Fractures of the head and neck of the femur are usually treated by prosthetic hip replacement. Enzyme replacement therapy and bone marrow transplantation have been tried in a few patients without long-term benefit. The prognosis in children with the early onset form of the type 1 disease is poor because of the severe lung, liver, and bone involvement in these cases. In milder cases of later onset, longevity is normal. Children with the infantile neuronopathic form do not survive beyond age two to three years, whereas those with the juvenile subacute neuronopathic variant may live into their third decade.

Brady RO, Barranger JA: Glucosylceramide lipidosis: Gaucher's disease. In Stanbury JB, Wyngaarden JB, Fredrickson DS, et al. (eds.): The Metabolic Basis of Inherited Disease. 5th ed. New York, McGraw-Hill Book Company, 1983. *A review of the clinical and metabolic abnormalities in Gaucher's disease.*

Desnick RJ, Gatt S, Grabowski GA (eds.): Gaucher Disease: A Century of Delineation and Research. New York, Alan R. Liss, 1982. *A complete review of all aspects of Gaucher's disease based on reports presented at the First International Symposium on Gaucher Disease held in July, 1981.*

Ginns EI, Choudary V, Tsuji S, et al.: Gene mapping and leader polypeptide sequence of human glucocerebrosidase: Implications for Gaucher disease. Proc Natl Acad Sci USA 82:7101, 1985. *This report describes the mapping of the structural gene for glucocerebrosidase to chromosome 1 band q21 using radiolabeled human glucocerebrosidase cDNA. For other reports describing the cDNA see Proc Natl Acad Sci USA 82:5442 and 7289, 1985, and J Biol Chem 261:50, 1986.*

Rosenthal DI, Scott JA, Barranger J, et al.: Evaluation of Gaucher disease using magnetic resonance imaging. J Bone Joint Surg 68:802, 1986. *The sensitivity of MRI in detecting bone lesions is documented in this study of 24 patients.*

Rubin M, Yampolski I, Lambrozo R, et al.: Partial splenectomy in Gaucher's disease. J Pediatr Surg 21:125, 1986. *A review of the surgical outcome in 11 children with type 1 Gaucher's disease.*

Stowers DW, Teitelbaum SL, Kahn AJ, et al.: Skeletal complications of Gaucher disease. Medicine 64:310, 1985. *Description of bone findings in 327 patients with Gaucher's disease.*

186 NIEMANN-PICK DISEASE

Edwin H. Kolodny

DEFINITION. The eponym Neimannn-Pick disease originally referred to the classic infantile form of lipid storage disease described more than a half century ago. The lysosomal enzyme sphingomyelinase is absent in this disease; this causes widespread deposition of sphingomyelin, a ceramide phospholipid. Foam cells proliferate within the liver, spleen, and bone marrow, and there is nerve cell loss within the central nervous system. This acute neuronopathic form was subsequently designated as type A to distinguish it from other variants of sphingomyelin lipidosis which have since been described. These variants are distinguished by their age of onset, degree of central nervous system involvement, and sphingomyelinase activity (Table 186–1).

PATHOLOGY. *Foam Cell.* The cytoplasm of this large histiocyte contains numerous uniform-sized lipid-staining droplets that create a fine reticulated web resembling a hon-

TABLE 186–1. THE SPHINGOMYELIN LIPIDOSES

Type	Descriptive Name	Racial and/or Geographic Predilection	Affects Brain	Deficiency
A	Acute neuronopathic	Ashkenazic Jewish	Yes	Sphingomyelinase
B	Chronic non-neuronopathic	No	No	Sphingomyelinase
C	Subacute neuronopathic or juvenile dystonic lipidosis	No	Yes	Cholesterol esterification
D	Nova Scotian	Yarmouth County, Nova Scotia	Yes	Unknown
E	Adult non-neuronopathic	No	No	Unknown

eycomb or mulberry (see Fig. 185–1*B*). Under the electron microscope these cytosomes consist of both concentrically laminated membranous arrays and dense homogeneous bodies. Foam cells are present in the tissues of the reticuloendothelial system.

Sphingomyelin. The ceramide and phosphorylcholine portions of this lipid are linked by a phosphodiester bond that under normal circumstances is cleaved by sphingomyelinase. Sphingomyelin is increased 15- to 45-fold in the liver and spleen of patients with type A Niemann-Pick disease, and about half as much in type B patients. The organs of type C patients exhibit a three- to six-fold increase in sphingomyelin, but it is not the major accumulating lipid in this variant. Sphingomyelin storage occurs in the brain of type A but not type B patients. Patients with every variety of Niemann-Pick disease also accumulate bis (monoacylglycero) phosphate, unesterified cholesterol, glucosylceramide, and other neutral glycolipids.

Sphingomyelinase. Patients with type A and type B Niemann-Pick disease are totally deficient in sphingomyelinase, the acid hydrolase that removes the phosphorylcholine moiety from sphingomyelin. The absence of this phosphodiesterase probaby explains the simultaneous increase of bis (monoacylglycero) phospate. In type C patients, sphingomyelinase may be normal or partially deficient, but the principal finding is a defect in esterification of nonlipoprotein cholesterol. A low molecular weight protein, SAP-2, stimulates spingomyelinase by binding to the enzyme. The gene for this activator has been mapped to chromosome 10, but no cases of SAP-2 deficiency associated with Niemann-Pick disease have been reported.

CLINICAL MANIFESTATIONS. ***Type A.*** Hepatosplenomegaly, diffuse pulmonary infiltration, and developmental delay are noticeable as early as one to two months of age. Weight gain is poor partly because of vomiting associated with feedings. Lymphadenopathy, opisthotonic posturing, and seizures develop. Eye signs include periorbital puffiness, clouding of the corneas, yellowish discoloration of the lens, and cherry-red maculae. The skin becomes brownish-yellow, and xanthomas may appear. The affected child becomes emaciated with very thin extremities, a protuberant abdomen, and ascites. Developmental milestones normal for a one-year-old are never attained, and after the child lingers in a vegetative state for many months, death occurs, usually before the fourth year. Postmortem studies reveal a large yellow liver and atrophic brain with widespread nerve cell loss and gliosis. The cytoplasm of remaining neurons and of the glial cells is ballooned with lipid inclusions. A high percentage of patients with this rare autosomal recessive disorder are of Ashkenazic Jewish ancestry.

Type B. Severe early involvement of the lungs, liver, and spleen also characterizes type B Niemann-Pick disease, but mental development in this variant is normal. The chest radiograph reveals nodular densities throughout the lung fields and thickening of the interlobar fissures. Signs of hypersplenism such as mild anemia, leukopenia, and thrombocytopenia with easy bruising often occur. A few patients have been described with a brownish-red spot in the macula, and sea-blue histiocytes are sometimes found in the bone marrow. These cells contain ceroid that confers on them a bluish cast when stained with Giemsa. Normal longevity is possible but may be limited by chronic pulmonary insufficiency and the mechanical effects of the enlarged spleen and liver on other abdominal organs.

Type C. This diagnosis has been applied to a heterogeneous group of patients with a variable age of onset. In some cases, jaundice is present during the first three months, but this subsides despite the progression of the disease. A liver biopsy in these instances may show chronic hepatitis with giant cells. One group of type C patients, between one and one-half and three years of age, exhibits slowing of speech and motor development and then develops blindness and spasticity. The condition of these children deteriorates rapidly over a two-year period and they die at age five to six years. Other type C patients may not develop overt neurologic symptoms until after age five years. These consist of a decline in intellect, progressive impairment of vertical gaze, dysarthria, dysphagia, incoordination, seizures, and involuntary movements. A few have also developed cataplexy. These patients usually survive into adult life.

Type D. This designation is used for cases similar to type C occurring in descendents of an Acadian couple born in Yarmouth, Nova Scotia, in the 1600's. No sphingomyelinase deficiency has been reported in these cases.

DIAGNOSIS. Niemann-Pick disease should be suspected whenever foam cells are present in the bone marrow of a patient with hepatosplenomegaly. The infant of Ashkenazic Jewish heritage who develops slowly would suggest the type A variant. Early jaundice and a subsequent period of normal development might stimulate a work-up for type C Neimann-Pick disease. The foam cell, a lipid-laden histiocyte, should not be confused with the Gaucher cell, which also contains lipid, but of a different morphologic appearance. Foam cells also occur in hypertriglyceridemia and certain other lysosomal storage diseases such as fucosidosis, mannosidosis, GM_1 gangliosidosis, Sandhoff's disease, Wolman's disease, and I-cell disease. In long-standing cases of type B disease, sea-blue histiocytes containing a ceroid-like material are also observed in the bone marrow. The definitive diagnosis of Niemann-Pick disease types A and B is based upon the assay of sphingomyelinase activity. Homogenates of cultured skin fibroblasts or leukocytes from these patients, when incubated with sphingomyelin labeled with ^{14}C in the choline portion of the molecule, have less than 5 per cent of control activity. Intermediate values are obtained for type A and type B heterozygotes. Type C homozygotes may exhibit a partial deficiency, but type C heterozygotes cannot be determined enzymatically. The defect in cholesterol esterification present in type C patients can be demonstrated in fibroblast culture by incubating the cells with LDL protein and ^3H-labeled oleate and then analyzing their content of unesterified and esterified cholesterol. Prenatal diagnosis of type A and type B Neimann-Pick disease is accomplished by determining the enzyme activity of cultured amniotic fluid cells.

TREATMENT. There is no specific treatment available for any of the sphingomyelin storage diseases. In type B patients splenectomy may be done to relieve mechanical pressure within the abdomen or to correct a thrombocytopenia with hemorrhagic diathesis. Neither replacement with exogenous enzyme nor organ transplants have been successful, but it is possible that bone marrow transplantation will in the future prove beneficial to patients without central nervous system involvement. Animal models of Niemann-Pick disease are available for laboratory trials of potential new therapies.

Besley GTN, Moss SE: Studies on sphingomyelinase and β-glucosidase activities in Niemann-Pick disease variants. Phosphodiesterase activities measured with natural and artificial substrates. Biochim Biophys Acta 752:54, 1983. *Sphingomyelinase activity in cultured skin fibroblasts and liver is characterized and the deficiency in types A, B, and C Neimann-Pick disease described.*

Brady RO: Sphingomyelin lipidosis: Neimann-Pick disease. In Stanbury JB, Wyngaarden JB, Fredrickson DS, et al. (eds.): The Metabolic Basis of Inherited Disease. 5th ed. New York, McGraw-Hill Book Company, 1983. *A comprehensive review of the different clinical forms of sphingomyelin lipidoses. Details of their pathology, metabolic disturbance, and enzymatic aspects are provided, as well as a complete bibliography.*

Breen L, Morris HH, Alperin JB, et al.: Juvenile Niemann-Pick disease with vertical supranuclear ophthalmoplegia. Arch Neurol 38:388, 1981. *A comprehensive review of the clinical features in the later-onset form of type C. References to the sea-blue histiocyte syndrome are included.*

Pentchev PG, Comly ME, Kruth HS, et al.: A defect in cholesterol esterification in certain patients designated as Niemann-Pick disease type C. Proc Natl Acad Sci USA 82:8247, 1985. *Description of the enzyme defect in type C Niemann-Pick disease.*

Winsor EJ, Welch JP: Genetic and demographic aspects of Nova Scotia Niemann-Pick disease. Am J Hum Genet 30:530,1978. *A useful source of references to type D Niemann-Pick disease.*

Inborn Errors of Amino Acid Metabolism

187 HYPERAMINOACIDURIA (With a Classification of the Inborn and Developmental Errors of Amino Acid Metabolism)

Charles R. Scriver

Study of the inborn errors of amino acid metabolism has improved our knowledge of metabolism, and in several instances has improved diagnosis and treatment of specific diseases. The inborn errors of renal transport are important "probes" of the mechanisms dedicated to amino acid reabsorption. They identify either the carriers or the metabolic processes that are coupled to the transcellular flux that achieves net reabsorption.

A certain amount of L-aminoaciduria, representing less than 2 to 3 per cent of the total urinary nitrogen, is a normal phenomenon. A small fraction, usually less than 5 per cent, of the filtered load of the amino acids in plasma is not reabsorbed completely by the proximal portion of the renal tubule and is excreted in the urine. In the healthy person, the efficiency of renal tubular transport of the individual amino acids is related to their chemical and steric structure, the amount in the glomerular filtrate, and the sex, age, and physiologic state of the subject.

Abnormal aminoaciduria will result when there is an acquired or hereditary disturbance of cellular metabolism or transport of amino acids. The known hyperaminoacidurias (see Table 187–1, which also includes several inborn errors of amino acid metabolism not necessarily associated with hyperaminoaciduria per se, but identified by organic acid and fatty acid derivatives) can be classified according to four basic mechanisms (Fig. 187–1):

1. *Saturation*: Amino acid is at elevated concentration and approaches or exceeds the capacity of the system to reabsorb it ("overflow" aminoaciduria).
2. *Competition*: One amino acid at elevated concentration competes with others sharing access to a transport system ("combined" aminoaciduria).
3. *Modification of reactive site(s)*: Amino acid(s) is (are) not transported efficiently because access to the system is impaired ("renal" aminoaciduria).
4. *Inhibition of substrate transfer*: Energy-dependent processes coupled to the carrier and transfer of substrates across membranes are impaired ("renal" aminoaciduria).

The individual mechanisms required for transport of each amino acid can be grouped into at least five major gene-controlled and non-overlapping systems, each having a preference for a particular group of amino acids normally found in plasma and revealed by a mendelian phenotype (see Table 187–1, Group III). Another series of carriers appears able to recognize individual free amino acids, with perhaps one site for each of the protein amino acids. (Yet another series permits transepithelial absorption of oligopeptides, with hydrolysis following uptake of the peptides.)

Text continued on page 1155

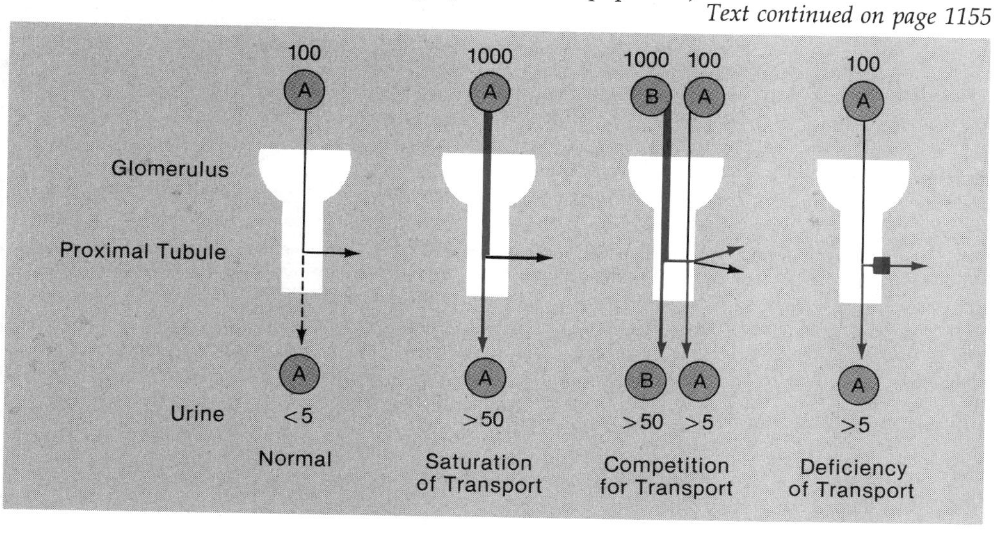

FIGURE 187–1. Mechanisms of hyperaminoaciduria. *Panel 1*: Normal reabsorption reclaims > 95 per cent of filtered amino acid molecules. Hyperaminoaciduria can occur if (*Panel 2*) filtered load increases (10× increase shown) and transport mechanism is saturated, or (*Panel 3*) amino acid in excess competes with another on a shared carrier, or (*Panel 4*) carrier is modified (mutant) or coupling of energy to carrier is impaired.

TABLE 187–1. HEREDITARY AND ACQUIRED AMINOACIDOPATHIES

The aminoacidurias presented in this table are divided into acquired and inherited types. Disturbances related to perinatal adaptive phenomena of multifactorial origin are included. The classification recognizes physiologic factors affecting amino acid distribution between plasma and urine, and whether the disorder primarily affects catabolism or membrane transport of the amino acid(s). Thus the disorders are grouped according to mechanism and preferred fluid for detection. The data refer to those conditions associated with perturbation of the normal content of ninhydrin-reactive metabolites in plasma or urine; some exceptions have been made to include ninhydrin-negative metabolites.

GROUP IA

The primary defect is in catabolism. There is a low renal clearance of amino acid but a hyperaminoaciduria by saturation of transepithelial transport. Detection in the plasma is preferable unless otherwise indicated, but the use of urine for screening (or diagnosis) is not precluded; assignment to this group implies primarily that diagnosis (or screening) of the condition is feasible by virtue of significant metabolite accumulation in blood (or plasma).

Amino Acid Affected: ↓ = decreased; ↑ = increased. Source of enzyme number is *Enzyme Commission*. IP = apparent inheritance pattern; AR = autosomal recessive; AD = autosomal dominant; (AR) = probably autosomal recessive; XL = X-linked. *Remarks:* CNS = central nervous system; CoA = coenzyme A; CSF = cerebrospinal fluid.

Condition or Disease	Amino Acid Affected	Enzyme Affected (Synonym) *In Group A*	IP	Remarks
		Common Perinatal (Adaptive) Traits*		
Neonatal hyperphenylalaninemia	Phenylalanine	Phenylalanine 4-monooxygenase (phenylalanine-hydroxylating system) [1.14.16.1]	—	Benign; may respond to folic acid; often occurs with tyrosinemia
Neonatal tyrosinemia	Tyrosine	4-Hydroxyphenylpyruvate dioxygenase (*p*-hydroxyphenyl pyruvic acid hydroxylase) [1.13.11.27]	—	Benign; responds to ascorbic acid and reduced protein intake
Hypermethioninemia	Methionine	? Methionine adenosyltransferase (ATP:L-methionine *S*-adenosyltransferase) [2.5.1.6]	—	Benign; usually found with high protein intake
Hyperhistidinemia	Histidine	? L-Histidine ammonia-lyase [4.3.1.3]	—	Benign; related to high protein intake
		Inherited Traits		
Hyperphenylalaninemia				
Classic phenylketonuria	Phenylalanine	Phenylalanine 4-monooxygenase (L-phenylalanine, tetrahydropteridine:oxygen oxidoreductase [4-hydroxylating]) [1.14.16.1]	AR	Plasma phenylalanine > 16 mg/100 ml; causes mental retardation; when untreated, L-phenylalanine tolerance in diet is 250–500 mg/day
Atypical phenylketonuria	Phenylalanine	Same	(AR)	Plasma phenylalanine > 16 mg/100 ml; similar to entry above, but dietary tolerance for L-phenylalanine is > 500 mg/day
Transient phenylketonuria	Phenylalanine	Same	(AR)	Plasma phenylalanine > 16 mg/100 ml; change in status to that of next entry or normal, several months or years after birth
Benign hyperphenylalaninemia	Phenylalanine	Same	AR	Plasma phenylalanine < 16 mg/100 ml on normal diet; benign trait
Dihydropteridine reductase deficiency	Phenylalanine	Dihydropteridine reductase [1.6.99.7]	AR	Deficient tetrahydrobiopterin cofactor also impairs biosynthesis of L-DOPA and 5-HT in CNS; low phenylalanine diet does not correct this
Biopterin synthesis defect	Phenylalanine	Various enzymes in synthesis pathway	AR	See preceding entry
Hypertyrosinemias				
Tyrosinosis (Medes)	Tyrosine	? Tyrosine aminotransferase (L-tyrosine:α-ketoglutarate aminotransferase) [2.6.1.5]	(AR)	One case known; myasthenia gravis probably incidental finding
Hypertyrosinemia I	Tyrosine (and methionine in acute stage)	Fumarylacetoacetate hydrolase [3.7.1.2]	AR	Hepatic cirrhosis and renal tubular failure; usually fatal in absence of tyrosine restriction
Hypertyrosinemia II	Tyrosine	Soluble (cytosol) tyrosine aminotransferase [2.6.1.5]	AR	Associated with developmental retardation; Richner-Hanhart syndrome in some patients
Hawkinsinuria	Tyrosine	4-Hydroxyphenyl pyruvate dioxygenase [1.13.11.27]	AD	Disease signs are variable and include failure to thrive; reflect formation of epoxides and adducts of glutathione
Hyperhistidnemia†				
Classic form	Histidine (alanine in some cases)	L-Histidine ammonia-lyase [4.3.1.3]; liver, epidermis	AR	Harmless condition in majority
Branched-chain hyperaminoacidemia‡				
Classic maple syrup urine disease	Leucine, isoleucine, valine, alloisoleucine	Branched-chain α-ketoacid lipoate oxidoreductase (probably decarboxylase component) [1.2.4.3(4)]	AR	Postnatal collapse; mental retardation in survivors; diet therapy can be effective
Intermittent form	Leucine, isoleucine, valine, alloisoleucine	Branched-chain α-ketoacid oxidase(s)§ [1.2.4.3(4)]	(AR)	Intermittent symptoms; development may be otherwise normal
Mild form	Same	Same	(AR)	Unremittent; milder than classic form
Thiamine-responsive form	Same	Same	(AR)	Mild form; responsive to thiamine (vitamin B_1)

TABLE 187–1. HEREDITARY AND ACQUIRED AMINO ACIDOPATHIES *Continued*

Condition or Disease	Amino Acid Affected	Enzyme Affected (Synonym) *In Group A*	IP	Remarks
		Inherited Traits (Continued)		
Multiple dehydrogenase form	Same (plus pyruvate and α-ketoglutarate)	Dihydrolipoamide dehydrogenase [1.8.1.4]	(AR)	Congenital lactic acidosis plus branched-chain amino-keto acid disorder
Hypervalinemia	Valine	Branched-chain amino-acid aminotransferase (valine aminotransferase) [2.6.1.66]	AR	Retarded development and vomiting; responds to diet
Type I hyperlysinemia	Lysine	Deficient "aminoadipic semialdehyde synthase" (bifunctional enzyme with lysine-ketoglutarate reductase [1.5.1.8] + saccharopine reductase [1.5.1.9] activities)	AR	Associated with mental retardation, hypotonia
Type 2 hyperlysinemia	Lysine, methionine and homocyst(e)ine	Only saccharopine reductase activity of bifunctional enzyme is deficient	AR	Same as above
Homocyst(e)inuria (methylene THF reductase deficiency)	Methionine (low) and homocyst(e)ine (high)	5,10-Methylenetetrahydrofolate reductase [1.7.99.5]	AR	Defective remethylation of homocysteine to methionine; neurologic and behavioral symptoms associated
Homocyst(e)inuria (with methylmalonic aciduria)	Homocyst(e)ine (high), methionine (low); plus methylmalonate	a. Defective cobalamin coenzyme biosynthesis b. Defective cobalamin transport (lysosomal)	AR (AR)	Defective remethylation of homocysteine and methylmalonyl-CoA mutase (MMA mutase) activity; severe neurologic signs and acidosis after birth
Cystathioninuria†	Cystathionine	Cystathionine γ-lyase [4.4.1.1]	AR	Probably benign trait; vitamin B_6 corrects biochemical trait in most patients
Hyperglycinemias				
Ketotic form	Glycine and other glucogenic amino acids	Propionyl-CoA carboxylase (ATP-hydrolyzing) propanoyl-CoA:carbon-dioxide ligase [ADP-forming]) [6.4.1.3]	AR	Ketosis, neutropenia, mental retardation; often fatal; detectable in skin fibroblasts
Ibid.	Ibid.	Methylmalonyl-CoA mutase [5.4.99.2]	AR	Symptoms are those of methylmalonic aciduria with acidosis (some mutase-affected patients are responsive to vitamin B_{12})
Ibid.	Ibid.	Acetyl-CoA acyltransferase (β-ketothiolase) [2.3.1.16] deficiency¶	AR	Signs are those of α-methyl-β-hydroxybutyric aciduria (with or without tiglic aciduria) and acidosis
Nonketotic form	Glycine	Glycine cleavage reaction (CO_2, NH_3, and hydroxymethyltetrahydrofolate formed) [1.4.4.2, 2.1.2.10]	AR	Severe CNS depression soon after birth; high CSF:plasma glycine ratio; benzoate decreases plasma glycine; no effect on CNS prognosis; strychnine improves seizures
Sarcosinemia†	Sarcosine	Sarcosine oxidase (sarcosine:oxygen oxidoreductase [demethylating]) [1.5.3.1]	AR	Benign trait (probably)
"Sarcosinemia" (glutaric aciduria, type II)	Sarcosine (glutaric acid and multiple fatty acids)	? Electron transfer flavoprotein (affecting multiple aryl-CoA dehydrogenases) [1.3.99.2-3]	AR	Postnatal lethargy, vomiting, coma, and acidosis; odor; multiple abnormalities of fatty acid oxidation
Hyperprolinemias				
Type I	Proline	L-Proline dehydrogenase (oxidase) [1.5.99.8]	AR	Benign trait
Type II	Proline	1-Pyrroline dehydrogenase (Δ^1-pyrroline-5-carboxylate:NAD^+ oxidoreductase) [1.5.1.12]	AR	Benign trait; Δ^1-pyrroline-5-carboxylate and 3-hydroxy-1-pyrroline-5-carboxylate excreted in urine
Hyperhydroxyprolinemia	Hydroxyproline	4-Hydroxy-L-proline dehydrogenase (oxidase) [1.1.1.104]	AR	Benign trait
Hyperlysinemias, Hypertryptophanemias, and Related Diseases				
Type I	Lysine (and glutamine)	Saccharopine dehydrogenase ($NADP^+$, lysine-forming) [1.5.1.8]	AR	Associated with mental retardation and hypotonia
Saccharopinuria†	Lysine, saccharopine, citruline	? Saccharopine dehydrogenase ($NADP^+$, L-glutamate-forming) (saccharopine dehydrogenase) [1.5.1.10]	AR	Associated with mental retardation
Pipecolic acidemia†	Pipecolic acid	L-Pipecolate dehydrogenase (pipecolate oxidase) [1.5.99.3]	AR	Hepatomegaly and mental retardation (peroxisomal dis.)
α-Aminoadipic aciduria	α-Aminoadipic acid	? Mitochondrial α-aminoadipate amino transferase [2.6.1.39]	(AR)	Variable clinical features
α-Ketoadipic aciduria	α-Aminoadipic and α-ketoadipic acids	? α-Ketoadipic decarboxylase	(AR)	Mental retardation
Glutaric aciduria type I	Glutaric acid	? Glutaryl-CoA dehydrogenase [1.3.99.7]	(AR)	Mental retardation
Glutaric aciduria type II (multiple acyl-CoA dehydrogenase deficiency)	Glutaric acid, complex organic aciduria, sarcosine	Electron transport flavoprotein [1.3.99.2-3]	AR	Severe form, neonatal metabolic disease; adult form, recurrent hypoglycemia
Hydroxylysinemia	Free hydroxylysine	? Hydroxylysine kinase [2.7.1.81]	(AR)	Mental retardation
Tryptophanemia	Tryptophan (with indoleketonuria)	? Formamidase [3.5.1.9]	(AR)	Variable, probably benign

Table continues on following page. See page 1154 for footnotes.

TABLE 187–1. HEREDITARY AND ACQUIRED AMINOACIDOPATHIES *Continued*

Condition or Disease	Amino Acid Affected	Enzyme Affected (Synonym) *In Group A*	IP	Remarks
		Inherited Traits (Continued)		
Hyperammonemias				
Carbamyl phosphate synthetase (CPS) deficiency	Glycine, glutamine	Carbamate kinase (ATP:carbamate phosphotransferase) [2.7.2.2]	AR	Group of diseases with ammonia intoxication, protein intolerance, hepatomegaly, vomiting, etc.; argininosuccinic aciduria also has trichorrhexis nodosa
Ornithine transcarbamylase (OTC) deficiency	Glutamine	Ornithine carbamoyltransferase (carbamoylphosphate:L-ornithine carbamoyltransferase [2.1.3.3]	XL	Same as above
Citrullinemia	Citrulline	Argininosuccinate synthetase (L-citrulline:L-aspartate ligase [AMP-forming]) [6.3.4.5]	AR	Same as above
Argininosuccinicaciduria†	Argininosuccinic acid	Argininosuccinate lyase (L-argininosuccinate arginine-lyase) [4.3.2.1]	AR	Same as above
Hyperargininemia	Arginine	Arginase (L-arginine amidinohydrolase) [3.5.3.1]	AR	Deterioration of CNS function and IQ in childhood; hyperammonemia (inconstant) aggravated by protein
Hyperornithinemia	Ornithine	Unknown (mitochondrial ornithine transport system?)	AR	Associated with hyperammonemia and homocitrullinemia (HHH syndrome)
Hyperornithinemia (without hyperammonemia)	Ornithine	L-Ornithine; 2-oxoacid aminotransferase [2.6.1.13]	AR	Associated with gyrate atrophy of choroid and retina but no hyperammonemia
Hyperalaninemia	Alanine	Pyruvate dehydrogenase (lipoate) (pyruvate dehydrogenase) [1.2.4.1] deficiency, pyruvate carboxylase [6.4.1.1] deficiency, and other defects	AR	Lactic acidosis, intermittent ataxia, mental retardation
			AR	Intermittent lactic acidosis, intermittent hypoglycemia
Aspartylglucosaminuria	Glycoasparagines	Aspartylglucosylaminase (2-acetamido-1[β^1-L-aspartamido]-1,2-dideoxyglucose amidohydrolase) [3.5.1.26]	AR	Lysosomal disease; mental retardation
Glutathionemia†	Glutathione or related peptides	γ-Glutamyltransferase (γ-glutamyltranspeptidase) [2.3.2.2]	AR	Mental retardation associated with finding
Hyperthreoninemia	Threonine	Unknown	(AR)	Seizures
		Other Conditions Which May Affect Amino Acids in Plasma		
Protein-calorie malnutrition	Tryptophan/leucine/isoleucine/valine ↓; tyrosine/glycine/proline ↑	—	—	Severity of change related to severity of malnutrition
Prolonged fasting	Alanine ↓; threonine, glycine ↑	—	—	Early fasting does not show same pattern
Obesity	Leucine/isoleucine/valine/phenylalanine/tyrosine ↑; glycine ↓	—	—	Reflects insulin insensitivity
Hepatitis	Methionine/tyrosine ↑	—	—	Reflects severity of liver disease

*These conditions have been detected by screening methods applied in the newborn period of life. They should not be misdiagnosed as permanent disorders of amino acid metabolism also identifiable by screening.

†Urine screening is as efficient as, or even more reliable than, blood screening in these conditions.

‡A number of disorders of branched-chain amino acid catabolism cause accumulation of substances that are ninhydrin negative. These compounds can usually be detected by gas-liquid chromatographic methods (see Goodman SI: Am J Hum Genet 32:781, 1980).

§Partial activity; more than 2 per cent of normal.

¶Hyperglycemia observed only in some patients with this enzyme deficiency.

GROUP IB

The primary defect is in catabolism. There is a high renal clearance of amino acid and a hyperaminoaciduria by saturation of transepithelial transport. Detection in the urine is preferable.

Source of enzyme number is *Enzyme Commission*. IP = apparent inheritance pattern; AR = autosomal recessive; (AR) = probably autosomal recessive; AD = autosomal dominant.

Condition or Disease	Substance Affected (Synonym)	Enzyme Affected (Synonym) [Enzyme Commission No.]	IP	Remarks
Hypophosphatasia	Phosphoethanolamine	? Deficiency of ethanolaminephosphate phospho-lyase (*O*-phosphorylethanolamine phospho-lyase) [4.2.99.7]	AR	"Rickets" unresponsive to vitamin D; craniosynostosis; hypercalcemia
Pseudohypophosphatasia	Phosphoethanolamine	? Same as above; activity present but altered	(AR)	Same as above
β-Aminoisobutyric-aciduria	β-Aminoisobutyric acid	?	AD/AR	Benign polymorphic trait

TABLE 187–1. HEREDITARY AND ACQUIRED AMINOACIDOPATHIES *Continued*

Condition or Disease	Substance Affected (Synonym)	Enzyme Affected (Synonym) *In Group A*	IP	• Remarks
4-Hydroxybutyric aciduria (γ-amino butyrate pathway)	γ-OH butyrate	Succinic semialdehyde dehydrogenase [1.2.1.24]	AR	Mental retardation, hypotonia. Detectable by GC/MS analysis of urine, plasma, CSF
Hyper-β-alaninemia	β-Alanine	? β-Alanine-pyruvate aminotransferase (β-alanine transaminase) [2.6.1.18]		Seizures; somnolence; mental retardation
Carnosinemia	Carnosine	Aminoacyl-histidine dipeptidase (carnosinase) [3.4.13.3]	AR	Seizure and mental retardation; or benign possibly
Pyroglutamic aciduria*	L-Pyroglutamic acid (5-oxo-L-proline; pyrrolidone-2-carboxylic acid)	Glutathione synthetase [6.3.2.3]	AR	L-Pyroglutamic acid (5-oxo-L-proline) results from overproduction via modified γ-glutamyl cycle

*Urine screening is as efficient as, or even more reliable than, blood screening in these conditions

GROUP II

There is a primary defect in catabolism and a secondary defect in transport. Hyperaminoaciduria is of combined origin—saturation and competition. Detection is possible in both plasma and urine.

Disease	Amino Acids *Affected in Plasma*	Amino Acids *Present in Urine*	Remarks
Hyperprolinemia, types I and II	Proline	Proline, + hydroxyproline and glycine	See entries in Group IA; competition occurs on iminoglycine transport system (see Group III)
Hyper-β-alaninemia	β-Alanine	β-Alanine, + β-aminoisobutyric acid and taurine	See Hyper-β-alaninemia in Group IB; competition occurs on β-amino transport system
Hyperlysinemia	Lysine	Lysine, + ornithine and arginine	See entries in Group IA; competition occurs on "dibasic" transport system (see Group III)
Hyperargininemia	Arginine	Ornithine and lysine, and sometimes generalized hyperaminoaciduria	See entry Hyperargininemia in Group IA; competition occurs on "dibasic" transport system (see Group III); pathogenesis of generalized aminoaciduria unknown

GROUP III

The primary defect is in the renal membrane transport site. There is a high renal clearance of amino acid, and detection is possible only in the urine. *Activity Affected:* Presumed gene product activity affected by mutant gene. IP = apparent inheritance pattern; AD = autosomal dominant; (AD) = probably autosomal dominant; AR = autosomal recessive; (AR) = probably autosomal recessive; XL = X-linked. *Remarks:* PTH = parathyroid hormone.

Trait	Substance Affected	Activity Affected	Other Tissues Affected	IP	Remarks
		Common Perinatal (Adaptive) Trait			
Neonatal iminoglycinuria	Proline, hydroxyproline, glycine	Specific proline and specific glycine transport (probably)	—	—	Benign adaptive trait; prolinuria subsides at ~ 100 days, glycinuria at ~ 200 days after full-term birth
Neonatal cystine-lysinuria	Cystine and dibasic amino acids (lysine, ornithine, and arginine)	Specific dibasic transport system	—	—	Transient; evident in newborn period in some but not all infants
		Inherited Hyperaminoacidurias			
Selective					
Hyperdibasic aminoaciduria type 2 (Lysinuric-protein intolerance)	Lysine, ornithine, arginine ("dibasic" group)	Shared "dibasic" amino acid transport system in basolateral membrane	Intestine (basolateral membrane, efflux defect). Fibroblasts (plasma membrane; efflux defect on γ^+ system)	AR	Associated with protein intolerance, failure to thrive, hyperammonemia basolateral membrane defect; silent carrier
Hyperdibasic aminoaciduria type I	Lysine, ornithine, arginine	Shared "dibasic" amino acid transport system (brush-border membrane)	Intestine	AR/AD	Associated with mental retardation in one reported patient; carriers have hyper dibasic aminoaciduria
Isolated hyperlysinuria	Lysine	Lysine-specific system (brush border)	Intestine	AR	One proband reported
Classic cystinuria	Lysine, ornithine, arginine, and cystine	Shared membrane system in brush-border membrane	Intestine	AR	"Negative" reabsorption of affected amino acid can occur; three alleles (? same locus), each causing different phenotypes: in type I carrier (vs. types II and III) no excess of amino acids in urine ("silent"); in type III patient, intestinal transport intact (or partial defect)
Hypercystinuria	Cyst(e)ine	Specific system for cyst(e)ine	?	(AR)	One pedigree only
Iminoglycinuria	Proline; hydroxyproline; glycine	Shared system for imino acids, glycine (and sarcosine)	Intestine	AR	Four alleles (? same locus); I and II are silent carriers; III and IV are hyperglycinuric carriers; I associated with intestinal defect; IV with K_m mutant

Table continues on following page. See page 1154 for footnotes.

TABLE 187–1. HEREDITARY AND ACQUIRED AMINOACIDOPATHIES *Continued*

Trait	Substance Affected	Activity Affected	Other Tissues Affected	IP	Remarks
		Inherited Hyperaminoacidurias (Continued)			
Hartnup disorder	Neutral amino acids (excluding imino acids, glycine, cyst(e)ine and β-amino acids	Shared system for large neutral amino acid group (luminal membrane)	Intestine	AR	Three alleles (? same locus); I, intestine affected; II, intestine normal; III, kidney normal; carrier "silent" in all
Hyperhistidinuria	Histidine		Intestine	AR	Associated with mental retardation in siblings
Hyperdicarboxylic aminoaciduria (glutamate-aspartate transport defect)	Glutamic acid, aspartic acid	Shared dicarboxylic acid transport system (brush-border membrane)	Intestine ±	AR	Benign
Idiopathic (primary genetic) Fanconi syndrome	Generalized effect on all solutes and water	? Coupling of energy; ? tight junction integrity	Secondary to renal phenotype	AR (and AD)	Adult onset and infantile-childhood forms are differentiated; basic defect unknown; probably several alleles
Secondary genetic forms of Fanconi syndrome					
Cystinosis; type I, type II	Same as above (secondary response)	Cystine storage (lysosomal defect), with secondary damage to tubule and glomerulus (later)	Secondary to renal phenotype	AR*	Several alleles; infantile (type I) and adolescent (type II) forms have differing rates for onset of nephropathy; "adult" form (type III) has no nephropathy
Hereditary fructose intolerance	Same as above, + fructose	Fructose-1-phosphate aldolase (fructose bisphosphate aldolase) (with secondary effects on cellular ATP)	Secondary to renal phenotype (hepatic cirrhosis)	AR	Nephropathy dependent on intact PTH-cAMP axis in kidney; responds to fructose withdrawal
Galactosemia	Same as above, + galactose	Galactose-1-phosphate uridylytransferase (with secondary effects on cellular ATP)	Secondary to renal phenotype (cataracts, CNS effects)	AR	Fanconi's syndrome responds to galactose withdrawal; "Galactosemia" due to galactokinase deficiency does *not* have Fanconi's syndrome
Hereditary tyrosinemia	Same as above, + tyrosine metabolites	Unknown (with secondary effects on cellular ATP)	Secondary to renal phenotype (hepatic cirrhosis)	AR	Fanconi's syndrome responds to tyrosine restriction
Wilson's disease	Same as above, with proximal and distal renal tubular acidosis	Unknown (? secondary effects on cytochrome oxidase system)	Hepatolenticular degeneration	AR	Fanconi's syndrome responds to depletion of copper storage
Lowe's oculocerebrorenal syndrome	Generalized dysfunction with defective urinary NH_3 production	Unknown	An oculocerebro-intestinal-renal syndrome (? involving tissues with high γ-glutamyl cycle activity)	XL†	Basic defect still unknown: treatment for tubular reclamation defects does not improve mental retardation or the cataracts and hydrophthalmia
Vitamin D dependency (pseudodeficiency rickets)	Generalized defect (secondary response)	Type I: 25-Hydroxyvitamin D-1-α-hydroxylase Type II: Defective binding of hormone	Deficiency of synthesis or binding affects intestinal absorption of calcium and initiates PTH response	AR	Nephropathy dependent on PTH excess and hypocalcemia (phenocopy occurs in vitamin D deficiency)
Miscellaneous					
Glycoglycinuria	Glucose and glycine	Unknown (the two solutes do *not* share a common carrier)	—	(AD)	Asymptomatic; normal-Tm (type B) glucosuria; possibility that there is a heterozygous manifestation of a Fanconi-like tubulopathy merits consideration
Luder-Sheldon syndrome	Generalized amino acids, glucose, and phosphate	Unknown	—	AD	Symptoms of Fanconi's syndrome have occurred in probands
Rowley-Rosenberg syndrome	Generalized aminoaciduria	Unknown	—	(AR)	Associated components of syndrome; growth retardation, muscular hypoplasia, pulmonary involvement, and right ventricular hypertrophy

*For each type

†Recessive.

Benson PF, Fensom AH: Genetic Biochemical Disorders. Oxford Monographs on the Medical Genetics No. 12. Oxford, Oxford University Press, 1985. *A "handbook," leaner than* The Metabolic Basis of Inherited Disease *(the standard "encyclopedia"), that covers, in short essays, nearly all entries in Table 187–1.*

Scriver CR, and Tenenhouse HS: Mendelian phenotypes as "probes" of renal transport systems for amino acids and phosphate. Handbook of Physiology (Renal Section, 1987). *A review of the amino acid transport systems (in kidney and other tissues) delineated by mutations in man and of their relative importance in metabolic homeostasis.*

Wellner D, Meister A: A survey of inborn errors of amino acid metabolism and transport in man. Annu Rev Biochem 50:911, 1981. *A crisp review of events in a field that now moves more slowly than it once did.*

The *group-specific sites* are classified into the β-amino system and the α-amino systems. Within the following list, the representative inborn error of amino acid metabolism that reveals the system is also indicated.

1. *The β-amino system*: β-alanine, β-aminoisobutyric acid, and taurine (viz., hyper-β-alaninemia)
2. *The α-amino systems*:
   a. "Dibasic" systems
      i. System I: lysine, arginine, ornithine, and cystine in brush border membrane (viz., cystinuria)
      ii. System II: lysine, arginine, ornithine in basal-lateral membrane (viz., lysinuric-protein intolerance)
   b. "Acidic" system: aspartic, glutamic (viz., dicarboxylic aminoaciduria)
   c. "Neutral" systems
      i. System I: proline, hydroxyproline, and glycine (viz., hyperprolinemia and renal iminoglycinuria)
      ii. System II: the remaining neutral α-amino acids (viz., Hartnup disorder)

It is usually possible to classify the aminoaciduria and its pathogenesis by analyzing the amino acid content of plasma and urine collected conjointly (see Table 187–1 and Fig. 187–1). Elution chromatography and gas chromatography–mass spectrometry will reveal the details of hyperaminoaciduria and any related organic aciduria. The recognition of a specific disorder of amino acid metabolism may provide an opportunity for treatment and, by genetic counseling, could prevent disease in relatives.

Rosenberg LE, Scriver CR: Disorders of amino acid metabolism In Bondy PK, Rosenberg LE (eds.): Metabolic Control and Disease. Philadelphia, W. B. Saunders Company, 1980, pp 583–776.
Scriver CR, Rosenberg LE: Amino Acid Metabolism and Its Disorders. Philadelphia, W. B. Saunders Company, 1973.
Wellner D, Meister A: A survey of inborn errors of amino acid metabolism and transport in man. Annu Rev Biochem 50:911. 1981

188 THE HYPERPHENYLALANINEMIAS

Lloyd H. Smith, Jr.

Phenylalanine is an essential amino acid. In its main metabolic pathway phenylalanine is irreversibly hydroxylated in the 4 position of its phenyl ring to form tyrosine, a reaction catalyzed by phenylalanine hydroxylase (Fig. 188–1). In addition to its role in protein synthesis, tyrosine is necessary as a precursor of the biogenic amines dopamine and norepinephrine in the central nervous system, of thyroxine and triiodothyronine in the thyroid gland, and of melanin in melanocytes. The hydroxylation of phenylalanine to form tyrosine is a complex reaction that requires the apoenzyme phenylalanine hydroxylase, oxygen, and a specific cofactor, tetrahydrobiopterin, as an electron donor. In the process of the reaction tetrahydrobiopterin is oxidized to dihydroquinone and must be regenerated by dihydropteridine reductase (and NADH) before it is again functional in phenylalanine metabolism (Fig. 188–1). In this system there are several sites for possible metabolic errors, and in fact a number of disorders have been described characterized by hyperphenylalaninemia (greater than 1.2 mg per deciliter of plasma). When phenylalanine accumulates there is increased shunting into its minor metabolites: phenylpyruvate, phenyllactate, phenylacetate, and phenylacetylglutamine.

CLASSIC PHENYLKETONURIA

Phenylketonuria was one of the first metabolic abnormalities to be established as a cause of mental deficiency, being discovered in 1934 by Følling with the use of the ferric chloride test (for phenylpyruvate). Phenylketonuria is an autosomal recessive disorder, which in the homozygote results in a severe deficiency of phenylalanine hydroxylase activity secondary to an abnormality of the apoenzyme. Heterozygotes have partial activity, which is sufficient to maintain normal plasma levels of phenylalanine in most circumstances. Phenylketonuria occurs with a prevalence of approximately 1 in each 10,000 to 12,000 births in whites and Orientals with a carrier rate of 2 per 100, but it occurs much less frequently in blacks.

CLINICAL MANIFESTATIONS. Patients with phenylketonuria are usually normal at birth. If the disease is unrecognized and untreated, however, the infant during the first year of life gradually develops mental retardation, delayed psychomotor maturation, tremors, seizures, eczema, a tendency to hypopigmentation, and hyperactivity. Impairment of mental function is usually severe, with I.Q. scores less than 50, and this taken with the other neurologic problems leads to the need for the majority of untreated patients to be institutionalized. There may be a "mousy odor" to the patient, and especially to the urine, which has been attributed to phenylacetic acid. Early diagnosis and treatment of phenylketonuria, within the first month of life, will prevent the development of these clinical complications.

PATHOGENESIS. The marked reduction in phenylalanine hydroxylase activity in classic phenylketonuria results in hyperphenylalaninemia with concentrations usually exceeding 16 mg per deciliter of plasma (approximately 1 mM). In addition, the shunting of phenylalanine into its transamination pathway leads to the excessive production and urinary excretion of phenylpyruvate and the other metabolites listed earlier. The mechanism of the neurologic deficit in phenylketonuria has not been established, but it is clearly related to the accumulation of phenylalanine (or its metabolites) rather than to a deficiency of tyrosine or its metabolites, since control of the hyperphenylalaninemia by diet prevents complications. Phenylalanine may inhibit the transport and therefore the availability of other amino acids to the brain during a critical time in its growth and maturation. Phenylalanine has been shown to be a competitive inhibitor of tyrosinase in the pathway of melanin synthesis, which is the probable explanation for the pigment dilution seen in untreated patients. In phenylketonuria tyrosine becomes an essential amino acid, but this requirement for tyrosine is usually adequately met from dietary sources.

DIAGNOSIS. The diagnosis of phenylketonuria is now usually made by screening techniques during the neonatal period. These techniques depend upon the demonstration of hyperphenylalaninemia rather than urinary phenylketonuria, since the transaminase necessary for the formation of phenylpyruvate may not be fully active in the neonatal period. The most widely used test is the Guthrie bacterial inhibition assay, which can detect excess levels of phenylalanine from a single drop of capillary blood collected from a heel prick onto a special type of filter paper. An abnormal result must be followed up with more specific determinations of plasma phenylalanine, which is usually found to be more than 16 mg per deciliter when there is normal protein ingestion after the first few days of life. The differentiation of phenylketonuria from the other forms of the hyperphenylalaninemias depends upon the level of amino acid measured, whether it is sustained with time, and the biochemical and clinical response to dietary therapy. The recent cloning of the human phenylalanine hydroxylase gene now allows for the prenatal detection of about 87 per cent of either the carrier state or the homozygous disease in white families based on locus-specific DNA polymorphisms. The involved gene is on chromosome 12.

TREATMENT. In the absence of any method to replace the missing phenylalanine hydroxylase apoenzyme, treatment is dependent upon dietary restriction of phenylalanine. By the

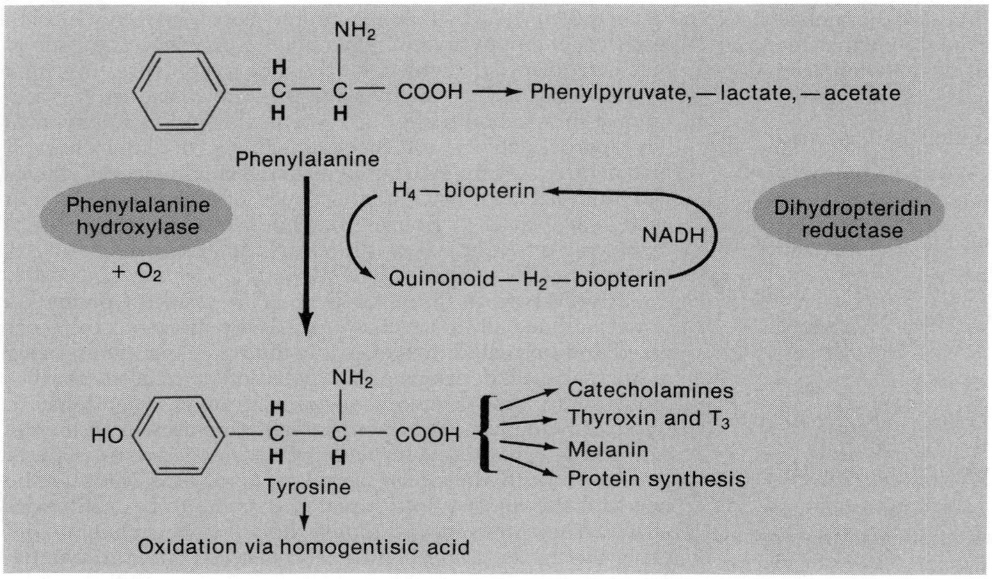

FIGURE 188–1. Pathways of phenylalanine and tyrosine metabolism.

use of special semisynthetic diets, such as Lofenalac or PKUaid in the United States, it is possible to reduce phenylalanine intake to 250 to 500 mg per day while maintaining good nutrition for all other dietary requirements. Phenylalanine ingestion is monitored to maintain its plasma level in the range of 3 to 12 mg per deciliter. This regimen has been found to be highly successful in preventing the clinical manifestations of the disease. Scrupulous adherence to such a dietary regimen is of particular importance during the early months of life. In the absence of clearly established guidelines, it is probably wise to continue dietary therapy at least through the first decade and perhaps indefinitely. It is particularly important that a woman with phenylketonuria maintain careful dietary control of her plasma levels of phenylalanine during pregnancy in order that the developing central nervous system of the fetus may not be damaged during intrauterine life.

HYPERPHENYLALANINEMIC VARIANTS

A number of variants from classic phenylketonuria may also be associated with increased concentrations of plasma phenylalanine in newborns. This is not surprising in view of the usual heterogeneity of genetic disorders and also the number of factors in the complex reaction catalyzed by phenylalanine hydroxylase (Fig. 188–1). It is important to distinguish these variants from classic phenylketonuria because they may have different prognoses and require different treatment programs. The benign disorders must also be carefully distinguished from "malignant hyperphenylalaninemia," as noted below.

TRANSIENT PHENYLKETONURIA. A number of patients exhibit the chemical findings of phenylketonuria at birth but have disappearance of these abnormalities over the following few weeks. It has been assumed that this syndrome represents a maturational delay in the development of some component of the phenylalanine hydroxylase system, although this has not been established. Dietary control of hyperphenylalaninemia is indicated during the initial phases of this syndrome (when it may not be distinguishable from classic phenylketonuria), but can later be discontinued.

PERSISTENT HYPERPHENYLALANINEMIA. Some patients exhibit milder forms of phenylketonuria and probably represent variants with higher residual activities of phenylalanine hydroxylase. Even in the absence of dietary control, their plasma levels of phenylalanine may be in the range of 4 to 16 mg per deciliter, levels not ordinarily associated with mental deficiency. Many of these patients do not require therapy and would never have come to attention were it not for mass screening programs for newborns. This is a heterogeneous group of patients with varying degrees of impairment in the metabolism of phenylalanine.

MALIGNANT HYPERPHENYLALANINEMIA. A small number of patients in whom phenylketonuria is diagnosed by the criteria just outlined fail to respond clinically to dietary restriction of phenylalanine. The hyperphenylalaninemia responds to diet as anticipated, but despite this chemical response they develop progressive neurologic deficits and seizures and usually die in the first few years of life. These patients, who represent between 1 and 3 per cent of all infants with a positive Guthrie test, are missing dihydropteridine reductase, necessary for the regeneration of the tetrahydrobiopterin cofactor of phenylalanine hydroxylase (Fig. 188–1). Activity of dihydropteridine reductase can be assayed in skin fibroblasts and in peripheral blood cells (lymphocytes, granulocytes, and platelets). More rarely they may retain the reductase but exhibit a block in the biosynthesis of the cofactor. Although the adverse effects of the resulting defect in phenylalanine metabolism can be largely circumvented by diet, tetrahydrobiopterin is also a cofactor for at least two other hydroxylations important in the production of neurotransmitters in the central nervous system: the hydroxylation of tryptophan to 5-hydroxytryptophan and of tyrosine to L-dopa. It is assumed that these deficits, or deficits of other reactions not yet demonstrated that require the cofactor, explain the progressive neurologic abnormalities. A rapid test for malignant hyperphenylalaninemia is available in that a single oral dose of tetrahydrobiopterin* (2 mg per kilogram) will reduce the plasma phenylalanine to normal in six hours in these patients. Classic phenylketonuria, as expected, shows no response. Treatment of these patients is being attempted with 5-hydroxytryptophan and L-dopa as well as with a low phenylalanine diet. These patients can be treated with tetrahydrobiopterin and neurotransmitters without dietary restriction of phenylalanine. Tetrahydrobiopterin is not transported in significant amounts into the brain, so treatment with it alone does not suffice as replacement in malignant hyperphenylalaninemia.

*Investigational drug.

Daiger SP, Lidsky AS, Chakroborty R, et al.: Polymorphic DNA haplotypes at the phenylalanine hydroxylase locus in prenatal diagnosis of phenylketonuria. Lancet 1:229, 1986. *Description of the current status of using restriction fragment length polymorphisms for this purpose, with accuracy of diagnosis of approximately 87 per cent for siblings at risk.*

Danks DM, Schlesinger P, Firgaira F, et al.: Malignant hyperphenylalaninemia—clinical features, biochemical findings and experience with administration of biopterins. Pediatr Res 13:1150, 1979. *This report presents four patients with this most recently described variant of hyperphenylalaninemia and summarizes current clinical and biochemical knowledge concerning the effects of biopterin deficiency.*

Kaufman S, Woo S, Scriver CR: Disorders of phenylalanine metabolism. In Scriver CR, Beaudet A, Sly W, et al. (eds.): The Metabolic Basis of Inherited Disease. 6th ed. New York, McGraw-Hill Book Company, 1988, in press. *Although the emphasis in this review is on the pathogenesis of the various forms of the hyperphenylalaninemias, there is a reasonable clinical description and an extensive and useful bibliography.*

Ledley FD, Levy HL, Woo SL: Molecular analysis of the inheritance of phenylketonuria and mild hyperphenylalaninemia in families with both disorders. N Engl J Med 314:1276, 1986. *Demonstration of multiple and distinct mutations in the phenylalanemia hydroxylase gene.*

189 ALCAPTONURIA

James B. Wyngaarden

DEFINITION. Alcaptonuria is a rare hereditary disease in which homogentisic acid oxidase activity is missing. Homogentisic acid produced during the metabolism of phenylalanine and tyrosine accumulates and is excreted in the urine. It causes pigmentation of cartilage and other connective tissue (ochronosis) and in later years a degenerative arthritis of the spine and the larger peripheral joints. The disease has historic significance, for it was chiefly on the basis of study of families with alcaptonuria that Sir Archibald Garrod developed the concept of inborn errors of metabolism. The disease is inherited as an autosomal recessive trait. No method of detection of heterozygotes has been found.

INCIDENCE AND PREVALENCE. At least 600 cases have been reported, including one in an Egyptian mummy 3500 years old. A prevalence of three to five per million individuals was found in Northern Ireland.

PATHOGENESIS. The activity of homogentisic acid oxidase in the normal adult human liver is sufficient to metabolize over 1600 grams of homogentisic acid per day. Normally, no homogentisic acid can be detected in plasma or urine. In alcaptonuric individuals there is no detectable activity of this enzyme in liver or kidney tissue. Plasma levels of homogentisic acid rise to about 3 mg per deciliter, and the urinary excretion ranges from 4 to 8 grams per day. Mammalian tissue contains an enzyme called homogentisic acid polyphenoloxidase that catalyzes the oxidation of homogentisic acid to an ochronotic pigment, but pigment can also be produced nonenzymatically in the presence of oxygen and alkali, as for example in urine. The homogentisic acid polymer has a high affinity for cartilage and connective tissue macromolecules. The stained tissue is fragile and eventually may break down, leading to degenerative intervertebral disc or joint disease. Homogentisic acid may also have a direct effect upon collagen synthesis through inhibition of lysyl hydroxylase.

PATHOLOGY. In an adult alcaptonuric patient cartilage in many areas, particularly the costal, laryngeal, and tracheal cartilage, is densely pigmented, sometimes being coal-black in appearance. Pigmentation is also present throughout the body in fibrous tissue, fibrocartilage, tendons, and ligaments. To a lesser degree it is also found in the endocardium, in the intima of larger vessels, in various organs such as kidney and lung, and in the epidermis.

CLINICAL MANIFESTATIONS. Homogentisic acid is present in urine from birth, but urine is colorless when passed. Before the days of disposable diapers the diagnosis was sometimes made when diapers turned brown in alkaline soaps. Pigment may appear in perspiration and stain clothing in the axillary and genital regions. Generally, the earliest change that can be detected externally is a slight pigmentation of the sclerae or the ears, beginning at 20 or 30 years of age. The cartilage of the ears may be slate blue or gray and feel irregular and thickened. Sometimes dusky discolorations of underlying tendons can be seen through the skin over the hands. In many patients, however, pigment is scarcely evident. The arthritis usually presents with limitation of motion of the hips, knee joints, or shoulders. There may be periods of acute inflammation, and later there is usually rather marked limitation of motion and ankylosis in the lumbosacral region. The arthritic complications are often severe and painful and may lead to extensive crippling. In addition, alcaptonuric patients appear to have a high incidence of cardiovascular disease, including generalized arteriosclerosis and chronic mitral and aortic valvulitis, with calcification of valves and annulus. At least one degenerated pigmented aortic valve has been replaced with a prosthesis. Myocardial infarction is a common cause of death. Other reported complications include ruptured intervertebral discs, prostatitis, and renal stones.

X-RAY CHANGES. These may be almost pathognomonic of alcaptonuria. The vertebral bodies of the lumbar spine show degeneration of the intervertebral discs with narrowing of the space and dense calcification of remaining disc material. There is variable fusion of vertebral bodies, but little osteophyte formation and minimal calcification of intervertebral ligaments. The degenerative changes of ochronotic arthritis are most severe in the hip, shoulder, and knee, and there may be calcific deposits in the tendons. The sacroiliac joints and smaller joints of the extremities usually show little or no abnormality. Ear cartilage may be calcified.

DIAGNOSIS AND DIFFERENTIAL DIAGNOSIS. The diagnosis is suggested by the history of pigmentary changes of urine, the presence of non-glucose reducing substance, the pigmentation of sclerae or cartilage, the arthritic episodes, and especially the typical x-ray changes of the lumbar spine. Specific identification of homogentisic acid in urine can be accomplished by chromatographic or enzymatic assays.

The ochronotic changes of skin and cartilage may be confused with pigmentary changes resulting from prolonged use of Atabrine, or use of carbolic acid dressings for chronic cutaneous ulcers. The arthritis must be differentiated chiefly from rheumatoid arthritis, osteoarthritis, and gout.

TREATMENT. There is no effective treatment. Dietary restriction of phenylalanine and tyrosine of the degree necessary to reduce homogentisic aciduria is impractical and potentially deleterious. Large amounts of ascorbic acid have been given in an effort to reduce pigment formation. Ascorbic acid protects lysyl hydroxylase from inhibition by homogentisic acid in vitro. It does not alter the metabolic defect.

Justesen P, Anderson PE Jr: Radiologic manifestations in alcaptonuria. Skeletal Radiol 11:204, 1984. *Characteristic radiologic findings are demonstrated.*

La Du BN: Alcaptonuria. In Stanbury JB, Wyngaarden JB, Fredrickson DS (eds.): The Metabolic Basis of Inherited Disease. 4th ed. New York, McGraw-Hill Book Company, 1978, p 268. *A detailed discussion of the history, clinical features, and biochemical derangements of alcaptonuria and ochronosis.*

190 HISTIDINEMIA

Lloyd H. Smith, Jr.

Histidinemia is a rare genetic disorder, probably transmitted as an autosomal recessive trait, in which the activity of histidase is markedly diminished. As a result there is a block in the conversion of histidine to urocanic acid. Histidine accumulates in the blood and is transaminated in increased amounts to imidazolepyruvic acid. In a screening program of urine specimens from newborns in Massachusetts, a prevalence of 1 in 14,190 was found for histidinemia. The diagnosis is established by demonstrating fasting hyperhistidinemia (four to ten times increased over the normal of approximately

1 mg per deciliter), histidinuria, and urinary imidazolepyruvic acid (which will give a positive ferric chloride test or Phenistix test for phenylketonuria). The enzyme defect can be demonstrated in biopsy specimens from skin and liver. In several patients low levels of platelet serotonin have been noted. In the past, varying degrees of mental retardation and of speech defects have been attributed to this genetic disorder. More recent evidence suggests that these represented the bias of ascertainment and that histidinemia has no demonstrated biologic disadvantage.

191 THE HYPERPROLINEMIAS AND HYDROXYPROLINEMIA

Lloyd H. Smith, Jr.

The imino acids proline and hydroxyproline are nonessential; proline is readily synthesized in the body from glutamate and ornithine and hydroxyproline from proline. The synthesis of hydroxyproline occurs uniquely in peptide linkage largely as a constituent of collagen. Three rare genetic disorders of the degradative pathways of the acids have been described.

HYPERPROLINEMIAS. Two distinct disorders of proline metabolism, both transmitted as autosomal recessive traits, are associated with hyperprolinemia. In Type I hyperprolinemia there is a block in the metabolism of proline to Δ'-pyrroline-5-carboxylate because of decreased activity of the enzyme proline oxidase. In Type II hyperprolinemia there is a block at the second step in the degradative pathway, the conversion of Δ'-pyrroline-5-carboxylate to L-glutamate, because of decreased activity of Δ'-pyrroline-5-carboxylate dehydrogenase. In both disorders the accumulation of proline in the blood leads to prolinuria and, through competition for a common renal tubular transport mechanism, to hydroxyprolinuria and glycinuria as well. In the Type II disorder there is also excessive urinary Δ'-pyrroline-5-carboxylate. The disorders can be diagnosed by finding the characteristic changes of hyperprolinemia and iminoaciduria as noted above. Although various forms of renal disease have been described with the Type I disorder and neurologic abnormalities and seizures in some patients with either Type I or Type II hyperprolinemia, these may represent the bias of ascertainment. Since no clinical entity has been clearly established, there is no indicated therapy for either form of hyperprolinemia.

HYDROXYPROLINEMIA. An increased plasma level of free hydroxyproline associated with hydroxyprolinuria has been described in members of several families, but this disorder has not resulted in prolinuria or glycinuria. The disorder is assumed to be an autosomal recessive trait in which the homozygote has deficient activity of hydroxyproline oxidase. There is no associated abnormality of collagen metabolism, and the urinary excretion of peptide-bound hydroxyproline is normal. As in the case of the hyperprolinemias, no clinical entity has been demonstrated and no treatment is indicated.

192 DISEASES OF THE UREA CYCLE

Lloyd H. Smith, Jr.

Humans are ureotelic; they are dependent upon the synthesis of urea for nitrogen excretion. The only source of net urea formation is through the urea cycle (Fig. 192–1), which consists of five enzymes necessary for the sequential synthesis of carbamyl phosphate, citrulline, argininosuccinate, arginine, and urea. When the function of this pathway is impaired, ammonia tends to accumulate. The associated clinical abnormalities show certain common features such as mental retardation and severe neurologic dysfunction. Genetic diseases associated with blocks at each of these five steps have been discovered and will be described briefly below. In addition, one patient has been described with deficiency of N-acetylglutamate synthetase, which catalyzes the formation of acetylglutamate, which is required for the activation of carbamyl phosphate synthetase in step 1, as shown in Figure 192–1.

CARBAMYL PHOSPHATE SYNTHETASE (CPS) DEFICIENCY. Carbamyl phosphate (CAP) channeled for urea synthesis, in contrast to pyrimidine-channeled CAP, is synthesized in mitochondria from ammonia, bicarbonate, and ATP in a reaction catalyzed by CPS in the presence of N-acetylglutamate as an enzyme activator. Approximately 19 patients with deficiency of CPS have been discovered, usually presenting with hyperammonemia, protein intolerance, and neurologic symptoms during the neonatal period. The diagnosis is established by measuring carbamyl phosphate synthetase in a liver biopsy or in peripheral leukocytes. There are no characteristic changes in amino acids in blood or urine.

ORNITHINE CARBAMYL TRANSFERASE (OCT) DEFICIENCY. OCT catalyzes the mitochondrial carbamylation of ornithine by CAP to form citrulline. Approximately 40 to 50 patients have been described with hyperammonemia and neurologic abnormalities secondary to deficient activity of OCT. The disorder seems to be transmitted as a sex-linked dominant trait with hemizygous males rarely surviving the neonatal period; females manifest varying degrees of protein intolerance. As in the case of CPS deficiency, there are no detectable abnormalities of amino acid metabolism. Mitochondrial CAP accumulates, however, and spills over into the cytosol to drive pyrimidine synthesis (Fig. 192–1). This results in orotic aciduria as a constant finding. The enzyme defect can be shown in biopsy specimens from liver or intestinal mucosa or in leukocytes. Prenatal diagnosis of the disease is now possible using a gene-specific probe.

ARGININOSUCCINATE (ASA) SYNTHETASE DEFICIENCY (CITRULLINEMIA). Citrulline synthesized in mitochondria normally diffuses into the cytosol, where it is condensed with L-aspartic acid in the presence of ATP to form argininosuccinic acid. This reaction is catalyzed by ASA synthetase. Approximately 20 patients who have been documented as having neonatal citrullinemia have exhibited marked heterogeneity in the severity of their clinical and

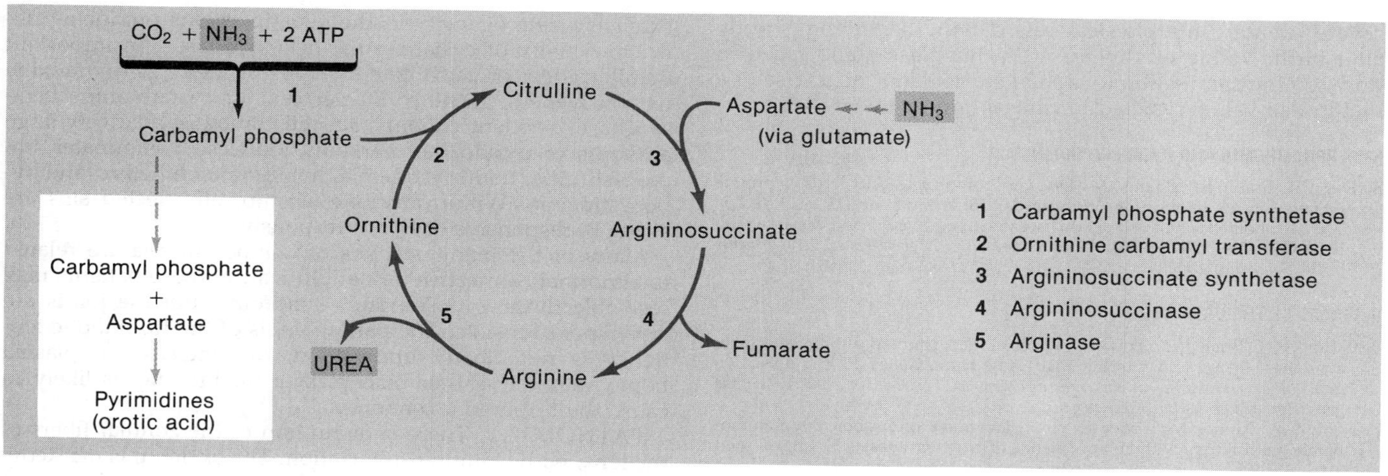

FIGURE 192–1. The urea cycle.

chemical manifestations. The associated hyperammonemia is in general less severe than in deficiency of CPS or OCT, but does occur after protein ingestion. Citrulline is increased in blood and urine, and secondary orotic aciduria has been noted, presumably reflecting excess CAP. Patients with a late onset form of presentation have been described, especially from Japan.

ARGININOSUCCINASE (ASase) DEFICIENCY (ARGININOSUCCINIC ACIDURIA). Cytosolic argininosuccinic acid undergoes reversible cleavage to arginine and fumarate catalyzed by ASase. Approximately 60 patients have been described with argininosuccinic aciduria. Clinical findings, which vary widely in severity, have included mental retardation, seizures, ataxia, hepatomegaly and hepatic fibrosis, and friable hair (trichorrhexis nodosa). In addition to large amounts of ASA in blood, urine, and cerebrospinal fluid (readily demonstrable by chromatography), patients with ASase deficiency may have citrullinemia.

ARGINASE DEFICIENCY (HYPERARGININEMIA). Arginine is hydrolyzed to urea and ornithine, catalyzed by arginase, in the last step of the urea cycle. Only 13 patients have been described with deficiency of arginase, which has been associated with mental retardation and spasticity. Arginine is increased in blood and urine and may occasionally cause secondary cystinuria owing to competitive inhibition of the renal tubular transport of dibasic amino acids. Hyperammonemia may be found after protein ingestion. The absence of arginase can be conveniently demonstrated in circulating erythrocytes.

193 BRANCHED-CHAIN AMINOACIDURIA

Lloyd H. Smith, Jr.

Leucine, isoleucine, and valine are essential, so-called branched-chain amino acids, which have certain structural resemblances and share some common metabolic pathways. Three rare genetic disorders in the degradative pathways of the branched-chain amino acids will be described briefly.

MAPLE SYRUP URINE DISEASE. This disorder, also called *branched-chain ketonuria*, derives its name from the characteristic odor of the urine of affected infants. The disease is transmitted as a rare (1 in 120,000 to 290,000 births) autosomal recessive trait in which the affected homozygote exhibits deficient activity in the complex oxidative decarboxylation pathway of the keto acids of leucine, isoleucine, and valine. As a consequence these three amino acids and their corresponding keto acids accumulate in excess in blood and urine and presumably throughout the body. A few patients have a variant disorder that responds to treatment with large amounts of thiamine (20 times the normal daily requirement). These patients have a dehydrogenase enzyme with a decreased affinity for alpha-ketoisovalerate and thiamine pyrophosphate. The pathogenesis of the deleterious effects in maple syrup urine disease has not been firmly established and may be complex, but probably relates mostly to the accumulation of leucine.

Severe hypotonia, lethargy, feeding difficulties, and hypoglycemia develop in the first week in an infant who seemed normal at birth. Convulsions and decorticate rigidity may develop, and most patients die, often of intercurrent infection, within the first year of life (often within the first few weeks). The diagnosis can usually be suspected from the characteristic odor of the urine and is confirmed by the abnormal pattern of amino acids and keto acids in blood and urine. The enzyme defect is demonstrable in leukocytes and fibroblasts. Treatment—by careful dietary control of leucine, isoleucine, and valine—is simple in theory but difficult in practice because of the necessity to balance three individual essential amino acids that are not easily analyzed. In those few cases in which rigid dietary control with careful monitoring of plasma levels has been instituted early, the results have been gratifying. A few patients have been described with milder variants of maple syrup urine disease. Thiamine therapy should be tried, as noted.

ISOVALERIC ACIDEMIA. This rare genetic disorder in the degradative pathway of leucine is due to a block in the conversion of isovaleric acid to beta-methylcrotonic acid, which is catalyzed by isovaleryl-CoA dehydrogenase. Isovaleric acid accumulates in blood and urine and gives rise to an odor that has been described as like sweaty feet. The pathogenesis of the associated clinical features has not been established. Symptoms, which usually begin in the first week of life, consist of attacks of vomiting, acidosis, tremors, lethargy, or even coma. Leukopenia, anemia, and thrombocytopenia have been observed during acute attacks. Patients who survive have generally exhibited mental retardation. As in the case of maple syrup urine disease, which it may clinically resemble, isovaleric acidemia may be suspected from the associated odor. The diagnosis is established by the demonstration of excess isovaleric acid in the serum by gas-liquid chromatography or of isovalerylglycine in the urine. Treatment is by strict control of dietary leucine.

HYPERVALINEMIA. This disorder has been described only in one Japanese infant who exhibited vomiting and severe mental and physical retardation, beginning shortly after birth. Valine was increased in his plasma and failed to undergo transamination to alpha-ketoisovaleric acid. Use of a diet low in valine resulted in clinical improvement.

HYPERPROLINEMIA AND HYDROXYPROLINEMIA

Scriver CR, Smith RJ, Phang JM: Disorders of proline and hydroxyproline metabolism. In Stanbury JB, Wyngaarden JB, Fredrickson DS, et al. (eds.): The Metabolic Basis of Inherited Disease. 5th ed. New York, McGraw-Hill Book Company, 1983, p 360. *An extensive analysis of the chemical derangements in these rare disorders.*

DISEASES OF THE UREA CYCLE

Beaudet AL, O'Brien WE, Bock H-GO, et al.: The human argininosuccinate synthetase locus and citrullinemia. Adv Hum Genet 15:161, 1986. *An excellent general review of this rare disorder, with particular emphasis on the molecular analysis of the defective gene.*

Brusilow SW, Danney M, Waber LJ, et al.: Treatment of episodic hyperammonemia in children with inborn errors of urea synthesis. N Engl J Med 310:1630, 1984. *A review of interesting new therapeutic approaches.*

Brusilow SW, Horwich AL: Disorders of the urea cycle. In Scriver CR, Beaudet A, Sly W, et al. (eds.): The Metabolic Basis of Inherited Disease. 6th ed. New York, McGraw-Hill Book Company, 1988, in press. *A large number of disorders are associated with derangements in urea synthesis. This chapter gives a lucid summary of the biochemistry of urea synthesis and the pathogenesis of the various disorders associated with that pathway. As always in* The Metabolic Basis of Inherited Disease, *there is a large and useful bibliography.*

Rowe PC, Newman SL, Brusilow SW: Natural history of symptomatic partial ornithine transcarbamylase deficiency. N Engl J Med 314:541, 1986. *Studies of the disease in a series of symptomatic female heterozygotes with a description of clinical manifestations, therapy, and outcome.*

BRANCHED-CHAIN AMINOACIDURIA

Danner DJ, Armstrong N, Heffelfinger SC, et al.: Absence of branched-chain acyl-transferase as a cause of maple syrup urine disease. J Clin Invest 75:858, 1985. *The demonstration of a specific enzyme defect in the 4-enzyme complex that normally decarboxylates these keto acids.*

Elsas LJ: Disorders of branched chain amino acid metabolism. In Scriver CR, Beaudet A, Sly W, et al. (eds.): The Metabolic Basis of Inherited Disease. 6th ed. New York, McGraw-Hill Book Company, 1988, in press. *This is the most sophisticated general presentation of the pathogenesis of this group of disorders. Although the emphasis is on the biochemical basis, there is a useful clinical discussion and an extensive bibliography.*

194 HOMOCYSTINURIA

S. Harvey Mudd

DEFINITION. The term *homocystinuria* designates a biochemical abnormality, not a disease entity. Several known genetic disorders lead to homocystinuria. Most common is cystathionine beta-synthase deficiency. In this condition ectopia lentis, mental retardation, bony abnormalities, osteoporosis, and thromboembolic phenomena are frequent.

PREVALENCE. More than 600 adequately documented cases of cystathionine beta-synthase deficiency have been reported. Screening of newborn infants indicates a *minimal* prevalence of 1 in 200,000 worldwide.

ETIOLOGY AND PATHOGENESIS. Cystathionine beta-synthase deficiency is inherited as an autosomal recessive trait. Deficient activity of this enzyme has been demonstrated in liver extracts, in brain, and in cultured skin fibroblasts and lymphocytes. The enzyme deficiency results in failure of homocysteine to react with serine to form cystathionine on the pathway to cysteine. Homocystine is the disulfide oxidation product formed from two molecules of homocysteine. Normally homocystine is not detected in human plasma by methods of the usual sensitivity. In cystathionine beta-synthase-deficient patients fasting plasma concentrations up to 0.2 μmol per milliliter of homocystine have been reported. The urine may contain up to 1 mmol of homocystine per day. Plasma methionine levels are also raised, and plasma cystine is low. Detailed studies, chiefly of cultured fibroblasts, suggest extensive heterogeneity in the genetic lesions producing deficient activity of cystathionine beta-synthase. An important manifestation of such genetic heterogeneity is pyridoxine responsiveness. In 40 to 50 per cent of cystathionine beta-synthase–deficient patients, administration of relatively large amounts of pyridoxine markedly reduces or eliminates homocystinuria, homocystinemia, hypermethioninemia, and hypocystinemia. Within any one sibship, all affected sibs are either B_6 responsive or B_6 nonresponsive.

Many of the manifestations of homocystinuria are related to abnormal connective tissue. Outwardly these patients may resemble those with Marfan's syndrome, but the joints are not hyperextensible. The pathogenesis of the thrombotic tendency is not clearly understood, but increase of plasma homocyst(e)ine, rather than plasma methionine, is likely to cause the thrombotic tendency.

PATHOLOGY. There is disruption of the zonular fibers of the lens, with resulting subluxation. The skeleton is markedly osteoporotic, and the vertebrae show rarefaction with biconcave compression. Thrombi and emboli have been reported in almost every artery or vein. These result in brain infarcts, coronary occlusion, and myocardial infarction, pulmonary infarcts, renal infarcts, and thrombophlebitis with pulmonary emboli.

CLINICAL MANIFESTATIONS. Among individuals with cystathionine beta-synthase deficiency there is marked variation with regard to the major clinical features of this condition, their time of onset, and severity. Clinical manifestations tend to be less prevalent, slower in onset, or less marked among B_6-responsive patients than among nonresponsive ones. A survey of 629 patients showed that mental capabilities ranged from severely retarded to IQ's as high as 130. Median IQ for B_6-responsive patients was 78; for B_6-nonresponsive patients, 56. Mental retardation, when present, most commonly becomes manifest during the first few years of life.

The incidence of dislocated optic lenses increases with age. By the age of 10 years, 55 per cent of B_6-responsive patients have dislocated lenses; 82 per cent of B_6-nonresponsive patients. Acute glaucoma and reduced visual acuity may result.

Thromboembolism is the life-threatening complication of cystathionine beta-synthase deficiency. By age 15, chances of having had a clinically detected thromboembolic event are 12 per cent among B_6-responders and 27 per cent among B_6-nonresponders. Large and small arteries and veins may be affected. Major cerebral vascular thrombosis may occur. Venous thrombosis with pulmonary emboli is common. By age 30 years, 4 per cent of B_6-responsive patients had died and 23 per cent of B_6-nonresponsive patients.

The spine is the most common site of osteoporosis, followed by the long bones. By age 15, chances of having radiologically detected spinal osteoporosis are 36 per cent among B_6-responders and 65 per cent among B_6-nonresponders. Scoliosis occurs in many individuals, although kyphosis is infrequent. Vertebral collapse and pathologic fractures of long bones may occur. The long bones are generally thin and excessively lengthened. Pectus carinatum or excavatum is common.

DIAGNOSIS AND DIFFERENTIAL DIAGNOSIS. The diagnosis is suggested by ectopia lentis and thromboembolic phenomena, together with other aforementioned features. The urinary cyanide-nitroprusside reaction is positive. Other disulfidurias, for example, cystinuria, also produce a positive cyanide-nitroprusside reaction, so homocystinemia and homocystinuria distinguish cystathionine beta-synthase deficiency from alternative forms of disulfiduria. Cystathionine beta-synthase deficiency is confirmed by demonstration of markedly reduced enzyme activity with cultured skin fibroblasts or phytohemagglutinin-stimulated lymphocytes or in a liver biopsy specimen.

Heterozygotes may be identified by assay of cystathionine beta-synthase activity in liver biopsy tissue. Cystathionine beta-synthase activities in cultured fibroblasts or phytohemagglutinin-stimulated lymphocytes from most heterozygotes are below the control range, but there is some overlap. For unequivocal identification such studies are best accompanied by methionine loading tests. In some young adults premature peripheral or cerebral occlusive arterial disease may be due to heterozygosity for cystathionine beta-synthase deficiency.

Rarer forms of homocystinuria are caused by decreased 5-methyltetrahydrofolate-dependent homocysteine methylation, owing either to decreased 5,10-methylenetetrahydrofolate reductase activity or to a variety of lesions that interfere with the ability to produce methylcobalamin. In all of these, plasma methionine levels are low. The condition is first noted in childhood. Homocystinuria also occurs following 6-azauridine triacetate administration.

TREATMENT. Management is directed toward the biochemical abnormality with the aim of preventing or ameliorating clinical manifestations, and toward the clinical treatment of complications.

Newborns known to have the abnormality have almost always been treated with a low-methionine diet (usually accompanied by cystine supplementation). Such therapy prevents mental retardation and may decrease the rate of lens dislocations and reduce the incidence of seizures. It is too early to assess the effects on thromboembolic events, osteoporosis, or mortality. When the condition is diagnosed at later ages in B_6-responsive patients, pyridoxine treatment (doses up to 500 to 1000 mg per day) accompanied by folate repletion has been shown to produce a statistically significant reduction in the rate of initial thromboembolic events. When diagnosis is made at later ages in B_6-nonresponsive patients, strict methionine limitation, if accepted and carefully adhered to, may be beneficial in preventing thromboembolic events. Recently, in early studies of such patients, betaine, which lowers homocysteine by accelerating its methylation, has appeared useful. Antithrombotic therapy with aspirin and dipyridamole has also been advocated.

Boers GHJ, Fowler B,. Smals AGH, et al.: Improved identification of heterozygotes for homocystinuria due to cystathionine synthase deficiency by the combination of methionine loading and enzyme determination in cultured fibroblasts. Hum Genet 69:164, 1985. *When liver tissue is not available.*

Boers GHJ, Smals AGH, Trijbels FJM, et al.: Heterozygosity for homocystinuria in premature peripheral and cerebral occlusive arterial disease. N Engl J Med 313:709, 1985. *A possible cause of early, otherwise unexplained, thromboembolic events.*

Carson NAJ: Homocystinuria: Clinical and biochemical heterogeneity. In Cockburn F, Gitzelmann R (eds.): Inborn Errors of Metabolism in Humans. Lancaster, Eng., MTP Press, 1982. *Successful treatment of late-diagnosed B_6-nonresponsive patients by methionine restriction.*

Mitchell GA, Watkins D, Melancon SB, et al.: Clinical heterogeneity in cobalamin C variant of combined homocystinuria and methylmalonic aciduria. J Pediatr 108:410, 1986. *Contains a useful brief summary of other causes of homocystinuria.*

Mudd SH, Skovby F, Levy HL, et al.: The natural history of homocystinuria due to cystathionine-β-synthase deficiency. Am J Hum Genet 37:1, 1985. *An international questionnaire study covering 629 patients. The natural history of the untreated disease is defined for the major clinical manifestations and the effects of therapies evaluated statistically.*

Mudd SH, Levy HL: Disorders of transsulfuration. In Stanbury JB, Wyngaarden JB, Fredrickson DS, et al. (eds.): The Metabolic Basis of Inherited Disease. 5th ed. New York, McGraw-Hill Book Company, 1983. *A detailed review of the clinical features of 350 confirmed cases of cystathionine β-synthase deficiency, with a discussion of metabolic factors in homocystinuria.*

Wilcken DEL, Wilcken B, Dudman NPB, et al.: Homocystinuria—the effects of betaine in the treatment of patients not responsive to pyridoxine. N Engl J Med 309:448, 1983. *Eleven patients responded with a substantial decrease in plasma homocysteine levels and an increase in total cysteine levels. In six there was prompt clinical improvement, such as darkening of new hair and improvement in behavior.*

Disorders of Purine and Pyrimidine Metabolism

195 GOUT

James B. Wyngaarden

Gout is a term representing a heterogeneous group of genetic and acquired diseases manifested by *hyperuricemia* and a characteristic *acute inflammatory arthritis* induced by *crystals* of monosodium urate monohydrate. Some patients develop aggregated deposits of these crystals (*tophi*) in and around the joints of the extremities that can lead to severe crippling. Many patients develop a *chronic interstitial nephropathy*. In addition, uric acid *urolithiasis* is common in gout.

Some patients develop all of the features of the disease described above, but these manifestations can occur in different combinations. However, essential hyperuricemia alone, even when complicated by uric acid lithiasis, should not be called gout; gout signifies inflammatory arthritis or tophaceous disease.

A classification emphasizing the heterogeneity of gout is presented in Table 195–1.

PREVALENCE AND INCIDENCE. The prevalence of gout varies from about 0.13 to 0.37 per cent in Europe and the United States to 10 per cent in adult male Maori of New Zealand. Exceptionally high prevalences are also found in Filipinos (in the United States, but not in the Philippines) and in the natives of the Mariana Islands. During World Wars I and II acute gouty arthritis was uncommon in Europe. When dietary protein again became plentiful, its frequency returned to prewar levels. Although formerly rare in Japan, gout has now become common in parallel with the increase in protein consumption in that country.

Primary gout is chiefly a disease of adult men; only about 5 per cent of cases are found in women, largely in the postmenopausal group. The frequency of gout is increased in patients taking diuretics, especially of the thiazide group; in certain nephropathies; and in polycythemia vera, myeloid metaplasia, or chronic hemolysis. Gout in all of its forms makes up about 5 per cent of arthritis cases.

GENETICS OF GOUT. A family history of clinical gout is generally found in 6 to 18 per cent of patients in the United States and Denmark. Figures of 40 to 80 per cent have been reported from England, and also from the United States following tenacious family studies. About 25 per cent of first-degree relatives of gouty subjects are hyperuricemic, and about 20 per cent of these have symptomatic gout. Familial hyperuricemia is polygenic and multifactorial. Hyperuricemia is correlated with maleness, surface area, obesity, ponderal index, protein intake, social status, and educational level. Thus many variables affect the phenotypic expression of hyperuricemia. In primary gout associated with hypoxanthine-guanine phosphoribosyltransferase (HGPRT) deficiency and phosphoribosylpyrophosphate (PP-ribose-P) synthetase variants, the genetic transmissions are X linked. Glycogen storage disease type I, which is associated with a specific form of secondary gout, is an autosomal recessive trait.

PATHOGENESIS AND PATHOLOGY. The hallmark of gout is hyperuricemia. The risk of gout increases with the

TABLE 195–1. CLASSIFICATION OF HYPERURICEMIA AND GOUT

Type	Disturbance in Uric Acid Metabolism	Inheritance
Primary		
I. Idiopathic (>99% of primary gout)		
A. Normal urinary excretion (80–90% of primary gout)	Decreased renal clearance ± overproduction	Polygenic
B. Increased urinary excretion (10–20% of primary gout)	Overproduction ± decreased renal clearance	Polygenic
II. Associated with specific enzyme or metabolic defects (<1% of primary gout)		
A. Increased activity of PP-ribose-P synthetase	Overproduction; increased synthesis of PP-ribose-P	X-linked
B. "Partial" deficiency of hypoxanthine-guanine phosphoribosyltransferase	Overproduction; increased PP-ribose-P concentration	X-linked
Secondary		
I. Associated with increased purine biosynthesis de novo		
A. "Complete" deficiency of hypoxanthine-guanine phosphoribosyltransferase	Overproduction; Lesch-Nyhan syndrome	X-linked
B. Glucose-6-phosphatase deficiency	Overproduction and decreased renal clearance; glycogen storage disease, type I (von Gierke)	Autosomal recessive
II. Associated with increased nucleic acid turnover	Overproduction, e.g., chronic hemolysis; polycythemia; myeloid metaplasia	—
III. Associated with decreased renal clearance of uric acid	Reduced renal functional mass; inhibition of secretion and/or enhanced reabsorption by drugs, toxins, or endogenous metabolic products	—

degree of hyperuricemia and also with age (Table 195–2). Virtually all patients with gout have serum urate values above 7.0 mg per deciliter. An occasional patient will have a lower value at the time of attack, perhaps attributable to the urate diuresis that sometimes accompanies the inflammatory response. Repeat analyses will almost always show hyperuricemia during quiescent periods.

In normal prepubertal children, serum urate values average 3.6 mg per deciliter in both sexes. At puberty these levels increase, and thereafter mean values are 5.1 mg per deciliter in males and 4.1 mg per deciliter in females. After the menopause, mean values in females increase to approximate levels in males. In the United States the central 95 per cent segment of the distributions encompasses values of 2.2 to 7.5 mg per deciliter in adult males and 2.1 to 6.6 mg per deciliter in adult premenopausal females. Definitions of hyperuricemia based on distributions of serum urate are useful for epidemiologic studies. But statistical expressions are not adequate definitions of the pathophysiologic significance of hyperuricemia, for it is the *solubility* of urate in plasma and body fluids that is important. There is no evidence that urate in solution is toxic; all of the features of gout derive from responses to the urate crystal.

TABLE 195–2. PREVALENCE OF GOUTY ARTHRITIS IN MEN IN RELATION TO SERUM URATE CONCENTRATION AND AGE

Serum Urate Level (mg/dl)	Mean Age 49 Years* (%)	Mean Age 58 Years† (%)
6.0–6.9	2	2
7.0–7.9	4	17
8.0–8.9	11	25
9.0–9.9	30	90
10 +	48	90

*Zalokar et al.: Chron Dis 25:305, 1972.
†Hall et al.: Am J Med 42:27, 1967.

TABLE 195–3. SOLUBILITY OF URATE ION AS A FUNCTION OF TEMPERATURE IN THE PRESENCE OF 140 mM Na⁺*

Temperature (° C)	Maximal Equilibrium Concentration of Urate in the Presence of 140 mM Na^+ (mg/dl)
37	6.8
35	6.0
30	4.5
25	3.3
20	2.5
15	1.8
10	1.2

*From Loeb: Arthritis Rheum 15:189, 1972.

The solubility of urate in body fluids is strongly influenced by pH and temperature (Table 195–3). At pH 7.4 and 37°C, the solubility of urate in fluid having the sodium composition of plasma is 6.4 to 6.8 mg per deciliter. An additional 0.4 mg per deciliter is protein bound, chiefly to an alpha$_1$-alpha$_2$-globulin. Thus 7.0 mg per deciliter is about the solubility limit of urate in plasma at normal central body temperature. But solubility is considerably less at the temperature of peripheral joints, which may be 32°C in the knee, and 29°C in the ankle (Hollander, 1949). Concentrations of plasma urate above 7 mg per deciliter at 37°C define hyperuricemia in a physicochemical sense. Urate forms stable supersaturated solutions, but such solutions are poised for crystal formation when perturbed.

Mechanisms of Hyperuricemia. The concentration of urate in plasma is determined by the balance between absorption and production of purines on the one hand and destruction and excretion on the other. Exogenous purines contribute substantially to body uric acid stores. Purine restriction leads to a reduction of serum urate of 0.6 to 1.8 mg per deciliter in normal subjects. Similar regimens have little effect on hyperuricemia of gouty subjects who greatly overproduce purines, but exhibit comparable effects in patients with reduced renal urate clearance. Abnormalities of purine absorption have not been implicated as a cause of hyperuricemia.

Human beings lack uricase; therefore uric acid is the end-product of purine metabolism. In normal subjects approximately one third of the uric acid disposed of each day is degraded by bacteria in the gut, and two thirds is excreted unchanged by the kidney. Decreased uricolysis has been excluded as a mechanism for hyperuricemia. In fact, with high urate concentrations in body fluids, enteric uricolysis is enhanced; with the onset of renal insufficiency, intestinal uricolysis assumes increased importance and in extreme instances may account for 80 per cent of daily urate disposition. By contrast, both increased purine biosynthesis and decreased renal excretion of uric acid play important roles in the pathogenesis of primary hyperuricemia.

Random urine samples in normal men commonly contain 500 to 1000 mg per 24 hours. On a purine-restricted diet these values average 418 ± 70 mg per 24 hours. Gouty subjects show slightly higher average values, 497 mg per 24 hours, but the overlap with the normal range is extensive. From 10 to 20 per cent of gouty subjects show basal values above the upper limits of normal. Because of the insensitivity of urinary urate measurements in the assessment of purine production, isotopic tracer studies have been employed for this purpose. With labeled uric acid the miscible pool of uric acid in normal man averages 1200 mg, and the daily rate of production averages 750 mg. From one half to three fourths of the pool turns over each day. The difference between the rate of production and the rate of excretion of urate ranges from 100 to 365 mg per day and represents the amount of intestinal uricolysis.

A second method of study involves measurement of incorporation of an isotopically labeled purine precursor, usually glycine, into urinary uric acid. The incorporation can be corrected for extrarenal disposal to give total incorporation values. By use of these methods, evidence of some degree of excessive production of uric acid has been obtained in about two thirds of gouty patients studied. The most extreme values are found in subjects with HGPRT deficiency or PP-ribose-P synthetase variants, but these represent fewer than 1 per cent of gouty subjects. Many patients whose 24-hour urinary uric acid values fall within the normal range show modest increases in the rate of turnover of an enlarged uric acid pool and/or overincorporation of glycine into urate. Studies of the intramolecular distribution of ^{15}N in uric acid following administration of ^{15}N-glycine show excessive labeling of position 9, which is derived from the amide-N of glutamine and from ammonia. Thus many more gouty subjects show evidence for mild overproduction of purine than would have been deduced from urinary uric acid measurements alone.

The first unique reaction of purine biosynthesis and the site of metabolic regulation by purine ribonucleotide inhibitors is that which synthesizes phosphoribosylamine, catalyzed by amidophosphoribosyltransferase:

$$\text{Glutamine} + \text{PP-ribose-P} + H_2O \xrightarrow{Mg^{2+}} \text{phosphoribosylamine} + \text{glutamic acid} + \text{PPi}$$

There are several possible mechanisms for loss of regulation at this site and acceleration of purine biosynthesis. These include (1) excessive concentrations of the substrates PP-ribose-P, glutamine, or both; (2) a structural alteration or increased amount of the enzyme, rendering it more active or less sensitive to inhibition by purine ribonucleotides; or (3) a reduced concentration of one of the regulatory nucleotides (AMP or GMP) which exert cooperative allosteric inhibition of enzyme activity. Intracellular levels of PP-ribose-P are strikingly raised in HGPRT deficiency and also in PP-ribose-P synthetase overactivity. The increased concentration of PP-ribose-P drives purine biosynthesis both by furnishing more of the rate-limiting substrate and by allosteric activation of amidophosphoribosyltransferase. PP-ribose-P turnover is accelerated in gouty patients in whom uric acid is overproduced. However, erythrocyte PP-ribose-P levels are normal in gouty patients without specific enzyme defects. Plasma glutamate values are slightly raised in gouty subjects, both in the fasting state and after oral glutamate loads, but plasma glutamine levels are normal. Although reduced activities of glutaminase and of glutamic dehydrogenase have been postulated in gout, no direct evidence for such enzyme deficiencies exists. Any process that results in accelerated breakdown of intracellular adenyl nucleotides may lead to hyperuricemia by prompt degradation of daughter purine compounds to uric acid and to secondary acceleration of purine synthesis de novo through release of inhibition of amidophosphoribosyltransferase. This biphasic mechanism has been implicated in glycogen storage disease type I following fructose infusion, following alcohol ingestion, and in a gouty patient with a variant AMP deaminase that showed reduced sensitivity to GTP, its normal regulator. The last example has been proposed as a possible general mechanism in idiopathic gout. There are no examples of gout attributable to intrinsic alterations of the amidophosphoribosyltransferase itself.

In the normal turnover of nucleic acids and nucleotides some are degraded to free purine bases, chiefly hypoxanthine and guanine. Nucleotides synthesized de novo in excess of nucleotide and nucleic acid requirements are promptly degraded to hypoxanthine. Guanine is deaminated to xanthine by guanase. Hypoxanthine and xanthine are oxidized to uric acid by xanthine oxidase (Fig. 195–1). Hepatic xanthine oxidase activity is increased in gouty overproducers, but this appears to be an induced rather than a primary change. Nevertheless this is an additional factor contributing to accelerated uric acid synthesis in these patients.

In a substantial fraction of gouty subjects the immediate pathogenetic mechanism of hyperuricemia appears to be a decreased renal tubular clearance of urate. Renal excretion of urate is a complex function of glomerular filtration, tubular reabsorption, and tubular secretion. Filtration of plasma urate is assumed to be complete, on the basis of micropuncture studies in animals and ultrafiltration studies of human plasma in vitro. Less than 5 per cent of plasma urate is protein bound in man under physiologic conditions at 37°C. Filtered urate appears to be almost completely reabsorbed in the proximal tubule (presecretory reabsorption). Some of the secreted urate is also reabsorbed in the distal portion of the proximal tubule and to a lesser extent in the ascending portion of the loop of Henle and in the collecting ducts (postsecretory reabsorption). The urate that is excreted is thought to arise almost entirely by tubular secretion. These conclusions rest on clearance studies with and without inhibitors of reabsorption, such as probenecid, or of secretion, such as pyrazinamide, which have major limitations.

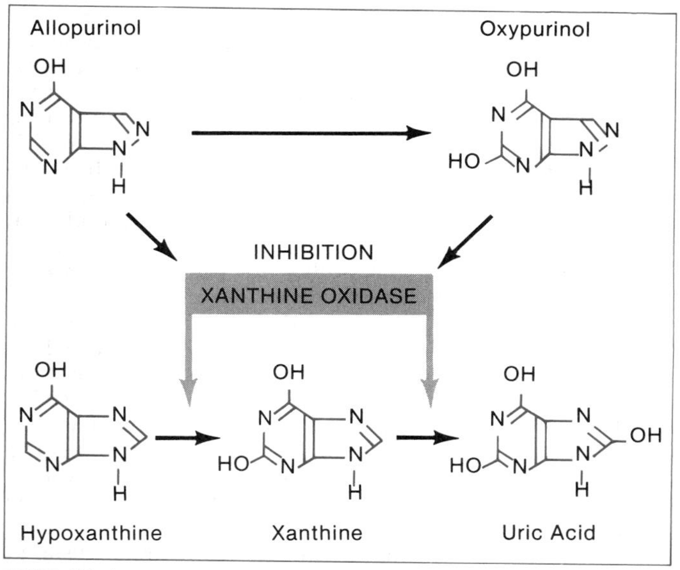

FIGURE 195–1. Pathway of uric acid synthesis catalyzed by xanthine oxidase and the site of action of allopurinol.

Studies in gouty patients have been interpreted as indicating reduced secretion of urate per nephron, but enhanced postsecretory reabsorption would also explain the data. The difference in renal tubular handling of urate in gout is small, and conclusions rest upon statistical analysis of clearance data on groups of patients. On this basis the renal contribution to hyperuricemia is most marked in patients with normal 24-hour excretion values of urate, normal turnover values of the uric acid pool, and normal values of glycine incorporation into uric acid. But reduced renal urate clearances per nephron are not restricted to this group. With the exception of patients with HGPRT deficiency or PP-ribose-P synthetase variants, overproducer gouty subjects as a group also show reduced renal urate clearance (Simkin). Thus, although some investigators have separated the large group of patients with an undefined biochemical lesion, *idiopathic gout*, into two discrete subgroups termed metabolic (overproducer) and renal gout, the evidence does not support such a categoric distinction, inasmuch as many subjects show both defects. Since chronic excessive alcohol consumption is common in gouty subjects and causes excessive turnover of adenine nucleotides and increased urate production and excretion, it is possible that some of the metabolic contributions to hyperuricemia in idiopathic gout are alcohol related.

The complexity of the pathogenesis of hyperuricemia is illustrated by two additional observations. The first is that asymptomatic hyperuricemia begins at puberty in the male as an exaggeration of the modest increase in serum urate concentration that normally occurs at that age and at the menopause in the female. Clearly hormonal factors influence serum urate levels. The second is that both pathogenetic mechanisms may be reversible. Subjects with primary (idiopathic) gout are on average 15 to 30 per cent overweight, and 75 per cent or more show fasting hypertriglyceridemia. (Hyperuricemia is present in more than 80 per cent of all patients with hypertriglyceridemia.) In some gouty patients, weight reduction and abstinence from alcohol reverse hypertriglyceridemia, hyperuricemia, excessive urate excretion, and evidence of overproduction by isotopic studies, as well as evidence of impaired renal urate clearance.

The Acute Gouty Attack. In 1859, A. B. Garrod, in the second and fourth of his ten propositions on the "The True Nature of Essence of Gout," wrote: "Investigations recently made in the morbid anatomy of gout, prove incontestably that true gouty inflammation is *always* accompanied with a deposition of urate of soda in the inflamed part. . . . The deposited urate of soda may be looked upon as the cause, and not the effect, of the gouty inflammation." In 1899 Freudweiler reproduced acute gouty attacks by injection of microcrystals of sodium urate. The role of the urate crystal in acute gout was rediscovered in 1961 by McCarty and Hollander. In laboratory animals experimental gouty arthritis requires the presence of leukocytes. However, synovitis can also be produced experimentally by other crystals of similar size and shape, and occurs in pseudogout caused by calcium pyrophosphate dihydrate crystals.

Although a number of cellular mechanisms are activated by the urate crystal, the exact sequence by which inflammation is initiated is uncertain. Hagemen factor, kallikrein, kinin-like peptides, and the complement system all participate in the response, but each has also been excluded as an obligatory factor in the inflammatory reaction. Urate crystals are leukotactic. Leukocytes and synovial lining cells ingest the urate crystals. Within minutes leukocytes release leukotriene B_4 (LTB_4) and a glycoprotein chemotactic factor (mw = 11,500). Production of these chemoattractants is blocked by colchicine. The acute inflammatory response to injected urate crystals is also blocked by prior treatment with colchicine, but the inflammatory response to purified crystal-induced chemotactic factor is not. Thus this factor and LTB_4 may be important mediators of the inflammatory reaction in gout. Monocytes are also stimulated by urate crystals in vitro, with release of interleukin-1. IL-1 may also contribute to initiation and amplification of gouty inflammation.

Crystal-cell interactions may be modulated by proteins adherent to the crystals. Crystals from patients with acute gout have surface coats of IgG, and to a lesser extent of IgM, IgA, C_3, and fibrinogen, but not of albumin. In studies in vitro, IgG coating enhances neutrophil responsiveness to urate crystals, whereas certain other proteins inhibit. Such modulating factors may account for the variable inflammatory responses to urate crystals in gouty subjects.

Phagocytosis of the crystal leads to rapid destruction of the phagolysosome membrane with release of hydrolytic enzymes into the cell. This results in cell necrosis and release of the crystal and lysosomal and cytoplasmic enzymes into the surrounding tissue. In a simulated system (liposomes) phospholipid membranes are susceptible to urate-induced lysis if they contain cholesterol or testosterone and refractory if they contain beta-estradiol. These observations suggest obvious interpretations, based upon the relative preference of gout for men and postmenopausal women.

The events leading to the putative burst of microcrystals of urate that initiates the acute attack are largely speculative. Three major theories have been advanced. The first postulates that trauma may result in shedding of crystals from preexisting cartilaginous tophi into the synovial fluid. The second emphasizes the ability of organized proteoglycans of cartilage to absorb (solubilize) urate. Disruption and increased turnover of proteoglycans are postulated to occur following trauma, with release of additional urate into the already supersaturated synovial fluid, and resulting crystallization. The third postulates a joint effusion with trauma, followed by a more rapid rate of reabsorption of water than of solute, resulting in further supersaturation of synovial fluid with urate, and precipitation of crystals. The first metatarsophalangeal joint is exposed to the greatest pressure per unit area of any joint in the body during walking, and it and other lower extremity joints, which are the joints predominantly involved in gout, are especially susceptible to trauma. In addition, the low temperature of peripheral leg joints will favor crystallization of urate from supersaturated synovial fluid. Thus each of these theories, which are not mutually exclusive, has merit.

Tophi. The pathognomonic lesion of gout is the *tophus*, a deposit of fine acicular crystals of monosodium urate monohydrate, surrounded by a mononuclear reaction and a foreign body granuloma of epithelial and giant cells, some of which may be multinucleate. Urate crystals are water soluble, but when tissues are treated with nonaqueous fixatives (e.g., absolute alcohol) the crystals are preserved and are brilliantly anisotropic and negatively birefringent in compensated polarized light. Tophi are commonly found in articular and other cartilage, synovia, tendon sheaths and other periarticular structures, epiphyseal bone, the subcutaneous layers of the skin, and the interstitial areas of the kidney. The articular cartilages are the most common and at times the exclusive sites of urate deposition. The deposits, although superficial, are actually embedded in the intercellular matrix. In the joint, cartilaginous degeneration, synovial proliferation and pannus, destruction of subchondral bone, proliferation of marginal bone, and sometimes fibrous or bony ankylosis develop. The punched-out lesions of bone commonly seen on roentgenograms represent marrow tophus deposits, which may communicate with the urate crust on the articular surface through defects in the cartilage. In vertebral bodies, urate deposits involve the marrow spaces adjacent to the intervertebral discs, as well as the discs themselves.

All of these sites of urate deposition are rich in proteoglycans, and the postulated role of these substances in attracting and solubilizing urate when organized, and of releasing urate during metabolic turnover, cited above, may serve to explain both localization and occurrence of tophi. Curiously, the process in the tissues evokes only a minimal inflammatory response in comparison with the violence of the acute gouty attack brought about by crystals within the synovial space. Urate crystals stimulate mesenchymal cells of joints to produce collagenase and prostaglandin E_2, both of which may play roles in articular destruction.

The Gouty Kidney. The only distinctive histologic feature of the gouty kidney is the presence of sodium urate crystals in the medulla or pyramids and surrounding round cell and giant cell reaction. These are found in a high percentage of gouty patients at autopsy and are associated with acute and chronic interstitial inflammatory changes, fibrosis, tubular atrophy, glomerular sclerosis, and arteriolar nephrosclerosis. The earliest change in the kidney is an interstitial reaction, maximal near the loops of Henle, associated with tubular damage. In kidneys without tophi the interstitial reaction tends to spare the medulla and juxtamedullary cortex. Although renal disease is common in gout, it is generally mild and only slowly progressive. The origin of the interstitial nephropathy is not known. It is not even certain that in the absence of crystalline deposits it is related to hyperuricemia. Other possibilities include nephrosclerosis, uric acid stone disease, urinary infection, aging, and lead poisoning. Crystalline deposits may occur within the distal tubules and collecting ducts and are probably composed of uric acid and related to the intratubular concentration of uric acid and the acid pH of the urine; they lead to dilatation and atrophy of the more proximal tubules. Deposits within the interstitium are composed of sodium urate and are believed to be related to the elevated urate concentration of plasma and interstitial fluid.

Uric Acid Urolithiasis. The overall incidence of renal stones in gout is about 20 per cent, about 200-fold higher than in the general population. In 84 per cent of gouty subjects, the stones are pure uric acid (not sodium urate); in 4 per cent, uric acid and calcium oxalate; and in 12 per cent, calcium oxalate or phosphate alone. The incidence of stones rises with the degree of hyperuricemia and approximates 50 per cent at serum urate values above 12 mg per deciliter. Marked hyperuricemia probably influences stone formation primarily by increasing uric acid *excretion*. The incidence of stones rises above 20 per cent in gouty subjects when the uric acid excretion exceeds 700 mg per 24 hours, and reaches 50 per cent at values above 1100 mg per 24 hours. Patients with increased uric aciduria also have an increased incidence of calcium oxalate stones. Urate (not uric acid) can participate in "heterogeneous nucleation" with calcium oxalate.

Other factors in the pathogenesis of uric acid stones include the *concentration of uric acid in urine*, the *acidity* of urine, and possibly the availability of stone *matrix* and the level of *solubilizing substances* in the urine. The solubility of urate decreases with fall of pH because of the shift to free uric acid. The pKa of uric acid is 5.75. In plasma at pH 7.4 more than 99 per cent is present in ionized form (urate), whereas in urine at pH 5.0 about 85 per cent is un-ionized (uric acid). At this pH only 15 mg of uric acid per deciliter of urine are soluble at 37°C, so supersaturation is required to excrete an average uric acid load in a normal urine volume. The solubility increases more than 10-fold at pH 7.0 and more than 100-fold at pH 8.0 over pH 5.0.

Both gouty and nongouty uric acid stone formers exhibit unusually low urinary pH values when fasting and throughout the day. The persistently acid urine has been attributed to subnormal ammonium production with a compensatory increase in titratable acidity. There is debate whether these data reflect occult or measurable renal damage (e.g., interstitial nephropathy), aging, or an intrinsic renal defect. Regardless of the explanation, the tendency toward persistently acid urine favors uric acid stone formation.

CLINICAL MANIFESTATIONS. The clinical manifestations of gout are conveniently described in four categories: acute gouty arthritis, tophaceous gout, gouty nephropathy, and uric acid urolithiasis.

Clinical gout is extraordinarily rare before puberty, when males at risk for primary idiopathic gout first develop hyperuricemia. Exceptions occur in the juvenile gout of the Lesch-Nyhan syndrome or glycogen storage disease type I, in which marked hyperuricemia is present from infancy. Only about 20 per cent of hyperuricemic subjects ever develop acute gout, although this figure rises as the degree of hyperuricemia increases (Table 195–2). The peak age of onset of gout is about 45 years in men. Thus the usual gouty male is exposed to 30 years of hyperuricemia before an attack occurs. In women gout usually occurs some years after the menopause, when serum urate values rise to hyperuricemic levels in those genetically at risk for gout.

Acute Gouty Arthritis. When acute gouty arthritis develops, it often appears as a fulminating arthritic attack of incapacitating severity. Acute gout is predominantly a disease of the lower extremity. Seventy-five to 90 per cent of initial attacks are monoarticular, and at least half of first attacks involve the metatarsophalangeal joint of the great toe (podagra). Next in order of frequency as sites of initial involvement are the instep, ankle, heel, knee, wrist, finger, and elbow. Later attacks are more often polyarticular and may include the shoulder or hip, or rarely such joints as the sacroiliac, sternoclavicular, mandibular, or even the spine. The more distal the site of involvement, the more typical are the attacks.

Some patients report short trivial episodes of "ankle sprains" or sore heels or twinges of pain in the great toe prior to the first attack, sometimes going back over several years. More often the first attack occurs with explosive suddenness during apparent excellent health, often at night. Within minutes to hours the affected joint becomes hot, dusky red, and exquisitely painful. Lymphangitis may be evident. Systemic signs of inflammation may include fever, leukocytosis, and elevation of the erythrocyte sedimentation rate. The inflammatory reaction may suggest a cellulitis or septic joint, and on occasion a joint is erroneously incised by an unwary physician.

Acute gouty arthritis often follows a precipitating event, such as trauma, surgery, alcohol or dietary overindulgence, starvation, or infection. Attacks may follow a long walk, golf, or hunting trip (e.g., "pheasant hunter's toe"). Postoperative gout usually occurs on the third to the fifth day and has been attributed to the subsidence of the adrenal alarm by analogy with the recrudescence of acute gout that may follow cessation of steroid therapy. Alcohol intoxication and starvation increase serum urate levels by inhibition of renal excretion by the accompanying lactic acidosis and ketosis, respectively. Regular ingestion of alcohol also increases urate production by stimulating purine nucleotide catabolism. Thus the legendary association of gout with imbibition has now acquired a sound metabolic explanation. Experimentally, urate crystals coated with endotoxins are particularly inflammatory; a subthreshold dose of injected uncoated crystals becomes violently inflammatory when endotoxin is given intravenously. Perhaps these observations bear upon the role of infection in precipitating attacks. It is postulated that uricosuric agents and allopurinol may induce acute attacks by lowering synovial fluid urate and favoring shedding of synovial crystals during dissolution.

The course of an untreated attack is highly variable. Initial attacks are usually self-limited. Mild attacks may subside in several hours or a few days. Severe attacks may last many days to several weeks. As the attack subsides, the inflamed skin may desquamate. Once the attack has broken, recovery is generally rapid and complete. The patient then re-enters an asymptomatic phase, often termed *intercritical* gout in recognition of the tendency of acute attacks to recur. The subsequent course of gout is difficult to predict. Some patients never have a second attack. Others never fully recover from the first episode and suffer a series of exacerbations leading directly to chronic gouty arthritis. More commonly a pattern of recurrences develops. In an extensive series, 62 per cent of patients had recurrences within the first year, 16 per cent in one to two years, 11 per cent in two to five years, and 4 per cent in five to ten years; 7 per cent had no recurrence during prolonged follow-up. In the untreated patient the frequency of attacks often increases, and they may become more severe, last longer, and eventually resolve less completely. The patient may reach a state in which he or she is rarely free of gouty inflammation, and in which residual swelling, stiffness, and joint pain give permanent disability not responsive to measures usually effective in acute attacks.

Tophaceous Gout. Before effective control of hyperuricemia became possible, more than one half of gouty patients developed visible tophi. The incidence now ranges from 13 to 25 per cent. In noncompliant patients it still exceeds 50 per cent. Development of tophi is correlated with the degree of hyperuricemia, severity of renal involvement, and duration of disease. The time from initial attack to visible tophaceous involvement ranged from 3 to 42 years in one large series, with an average of 11.6 years. In 0.5 per cent of patients, tophi are present at the time of the initial attack; virtually all such patients have gout secondary to a myeloproliferative disease.

Chronic gouty arthritis is a consequence of the progressive inability to dispose of urate as rapidly as it is produced. Crystalline deposits of urate appear in and around joints.

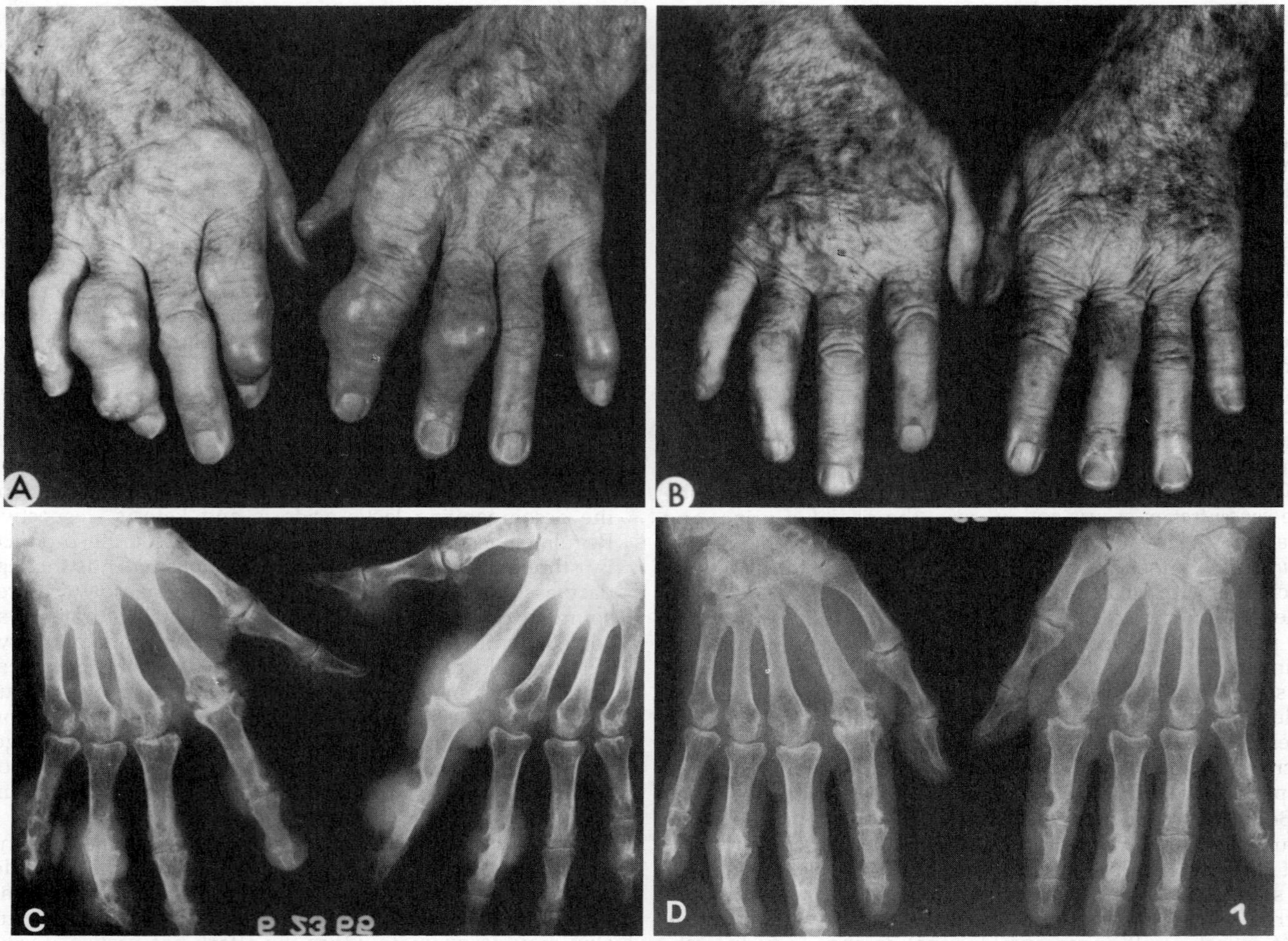

FIGURE 195–2. Chronic gouty arthritis (*A*) with tophaecous destruction of bone and joints (*C*), and improvement after three years of treatment with allopurinol, prophylactic colchicine, and a moderately low purine diet (*B* and *D*). (Courtesy of R. Wayne Rundles, Duke University Medical Center.)

Destruction of tissue is particularly evident in cartilage and bone, leading to radiolucent "punched-out" lesions, and to cortical erosions with characteristic "overhanging margins" (Fig. 195–2). A frequent site of tophaceous deposits is the external ear, especially in the helix and antihelix. Subcutaneous deposits, especially of fingertips, palms, and soles, may be visible as yellowish-white infiltrates. Tophaceous deposits may produce irregular asymmetric tumescences over joints. The classic gout shoe has a window cut to accommodate a tender prominent joint, usually the first metatarsophalangeal. At later stages, fusiform or nodular enlargements of Achilles tendons, or saccular distensions of olecranon bursae, are common and characteristic.

The process of tophaceous deposition advances insidiously, and although the tophi themselves are relatively painless, often progressive stiffness and persistent aching limit the use of affected joints. Eventually extensive destruction of joints and large subcutaneous tophi may lead to grotesque deformities and progressive crippling (Fig. 195–2). The tense, shiny, thin skin overlying the tophus may ulcerate and extrude white chalky or pasty material composed of myriads of fine, needle-like crystals. The olecranon bursa may be massively distended with "urate milk." Rarely tophi may involve the tongue, epiglottis, vocal cords, arytenoid cartilage, corpus cavernosum and prepuce of the penis, aorta, aortic or mitral valves, and cardiac conducting system, causing rhythm disturbances. They do not involve the liver, spleen, lungs, or central nervous system.

As chronic gouty changes and renal disease advance, acute attacks occur less frequently and are milder. No joint is exempt from chronic gouty involvement, although those of the lower extremity and hand are most commonly involved. The hip and spinal joints are rarely affected by tophaceous changes in the absence of extensive disease elsewhere. Radiographic changes of the sacroiliac joint and aseptic necrosis of the hip are sometimes attributable to gout.

Gouty Nephropathy. Renal disease is common in gout. One third of patients show isosthenuria and moderate proteinuria. The glomerular filtration rate is well preserved in many gouty subjects, but in others it gradually falls. Decline in renal function appears to be correlated with aging, renal vascular disease and hypertension, renal calculi, pyelonephritis, or independently occurring nephropathy, including that of lead poisoning. Only occasionally is it ascribable to gout alone. Hyperuricemia alone had no deleterious effect upon renal function during follow-up studies of gouty subjects ranging up to 12 years (Berger and Yu). Renal dysfunction does not shorten life expectancy in the average gouty subject, even though uremia is the eventual cause of death in 17 to 25 per cent of subjects. The majority of gouty patients die of cardiac or cerebral vascular disease (60 per cent) or malignant disease, which occur in about the same incidence and at about the same time of life as in nongouty American males.

Hypertension is present in one third to one half of patients and may be severe (diastolic pressure >130 mm Hg) in 10 per cent. Arterial and arteriolar nephrosclerosis are frequently prominent post mortem. There are no characteristic clinical or laboratory features to distinguish gouty kidney from other causes of chronic renal failure, except for the association of gout with the former. Renal failure from gouty nephropathy in the absence of gouty arthritis, tophi, or stones is extraordinarily rare; indeed, the entity is open to question.

Gouty nephropathy, sometimes referred to as *urate nephropathy* to emphasize the identity of the interstitial crystals, must be distinguished from *uric acid nephropathy*, an entirely different entity leading to acute renal failure from tubular obstruction by uric acid crystals.

Urolithiasis. The incidence of urolithiasis in gout is correlated with both the degree of hyperuricemia and the magnitude of the 24-hour uric acid excretion. Above serum levels of 12 to 13 mg per deciliter or excretion values of 1100 mg per 24 hours, the incidence is 50 per cent. Many of these subjects will have secondary gout, with a myeloproliferative disease such as polycythemia vera or myeloid metaplasia. The incidence of stones in such patients is 35 to 40 per cent. Of gouty subjects who pass stones, about one third have their first episode of urolithiasis before the onset of gouty arthritis, sometimes more than a decade earlier. Pure uric acid stones are radiolucent and are demonstrable in the body only by use of contrast media. Renal stones are reduced in frequency in gouty patients given allopurinol.

GOUT ASSOCIATED WITH SPECIFIC ENZYME DEFECTS. Gout occurring on the basis of specific enzyme defects has special clinical features. These forms of gout are rare, accounting for fewer than 1 per cent of cases.

Glycogen Storage Disease Type I (see Ch. 179). Over 50 cases of von Gierke's glycogen storage disease (glucose-6-phosphatase deficiency) and gout have been recorded. Gout does not complicate other forms of glycogen storage disease. Affected subjects may develop gouty arthritis by the end of the first decade of life. Chronic tophaceous gout and gouty nephropathy may account for a major portion of morbidity when these patients become adults. The sexes are involved equally. Avoidance of nocturnal hypoglycemia by a diet high in starch or by continuous intragastric feeding may markedly reduce or even correct hyperuricemia and ameliorate gout. The hyperuricemia also responds to allopurinol, less well to uricosuric agents because of renal disease.

Hypoxanthine-Guanine Phosphoribosyltransferase Deficiency. Deficiency of HGPRT gives rise to two different X-linked syndromes. A complete deficiency is associated with the Lesch-Nyhan syndrome (see Ch. 196). There is extreme exaggeration of uric acid production, and the greatly increased excretion leads to crystalluria, renal stones with ureteral colic, and sometimes uric acid nephropathy. Death from renal failure usually occurs by age ten; if allopurinol therapy is begun early, the patients may live into their 20's. A few of the more than 100 reported patients, all males, have had typical attacks of gouty arthritis.

An incomplete deficiency of HGPRT is associated with renal stones and recurrent acute gouty arthritis. Erythrocytes show from 0.2 to 50 per cent of normal HGPRT activity; the disorder is heterogeneous. Fifteen per cent of patients show minimal to moderate neurologic dysfunction resembling spinocerebellar ataxis or cerebral palsy. A few have survived neonatal episodes of uric acid nephropathy. Gout usually begins in the second or third decades; tophi develop early. Three quarters of patients have renal stones, half of these before age ten. These subjects have more marked hyperuricemia (usually >10 mg per deciliter) and uricaciduria (usually >1 gram per 24 hours) than most gouty subjects. Fewer than 100 cases—again, all males—have been described. HGPRT normally catalyzes a reaction between hypoxanthine or guanine and PP-ribose-P in reconstituting ribonucleotides, often called a "salvage" reaction. In HGPRT deficiency intracellular PP-ribose-P levels are raised and drive the first reaction of purine biosynthesis to excess. The female heterozygous carriers of complete HGPRT deficiency are not hyperuricemic, and their erythrocytes show normal HGPRT assay values. Carriers of the partial defect may be hyperuricemic and may show intermediate levels of HGPRT activity. Presumably, only cells possessing at least minimal HGPRT activity survive lyonization. Heterozygotes for the partial defect may develop uric acid stones or typical gout, which may occur before the menopause. Partial HGPRT deficiency should be considered in all females with gout or uric acid stones who exhibit raised urinary uric acid excretion values.

Phosphoribosylpyrophosphate Synthetase Variants. These patients resemble those with partial HGPRT deficiency in showing marked hyperuricemia and uricaciduria, and in developing uric acid stones or gout, and sometimes uric acid nephropathy, at an early age. They do not have neurologic abnormalities. Purine overproduction is prodigious. The enzyme abnormalities, of which there are four different types leading to increased activity, result in increased intracellular concentrations of PP-ribose-P and excessive purine biosynthesis. This, too, is an X-linked disorder, and all gouty patients are males. Fewer than 20 families have been identified with this disorder.

SECONDARY GOUT. Any acquired hyperuricemic state may be complicated by secondary gout. This disorder occurs in 5 to 10 per cent of patients with polycythemia vera or myeloid metaplasia, occasionally in secondary polycythemia complicating congenital heart disease or chronic pulmonary disease, in chronic myelogenous leukemia, in multiple myeloma, or in chronic hemolytic anemias. In such instances the mean age of onset is later (59 years), women are more commonly involved (16 per cent), and both serum and urinary uric acid values tend to be higher than in idiopathic primary gout. Acute gouty arthritis may occasionally antedate evidence of the myeloproliferative disorder by many months, or even by several years. A syndrome of coexisting sarcoidosis, psoriasis, and gout has been described but may represent fortuitous concurrence of common diseases.

In all the instances mentioned above, hyperuricemia appears to result from an increase in turnover of nucleic acid. Hyperuricemia may also result from reduced renal excretion of urate, either because of drug effects or because of parenchymal disease.

Hyperuricemia frequently follows the use of potent diuretic agents. Mean increases in serum urate concentrations are less than 2 mg per deciliter, but some subjects exhibit rises of 4 to 5 mg per deciliter. The hyperuricemic effect of diuretic agents results from salt and water loss, volume contraction, and avid solute reabsorption (including urate) in the proximal tubule. Typical gouty attacks may occur in patients receiving such drugs as hydrochlorothiazide, ethacrynic acid, or furosemide. In the 14-year study of the adult population of Framingham, Massachusetts, one half of the new cases of gout occurred in subjects taking potent diuretics. Three to five per cent of patients with gout have diabetes, but this incidence is not far from that of diabetes in the population of equivalent age. In markedly obese patients, total caloric restriction may result in extreme hyperuricemia, which is correlated with serum levels of beta-hydroxybutyric acid and may be associated with severe attacks of acute gouty arthritis, especially of knees and ankles.

Chronic renal disease is a frequent cause of hyperuricemia, but only about 1 patient per 1000 develops gout. Uremia appears to interfere in some way with the inflammatory response to urate crystals. Gout continues to be found in patients who survive lead exposure early in life and go on to develop slowly progressive lead nephropathy. In addition, saturnine gout is particularly prevalent in the southeastern United States, where it is attributed to the chronic ingestion of moonshine whiskey of high lead content with resulting renal tubular damage. Lead nephropathy and polycystic renal disease predispose to gout more often than do other forms of chronic renal disease.

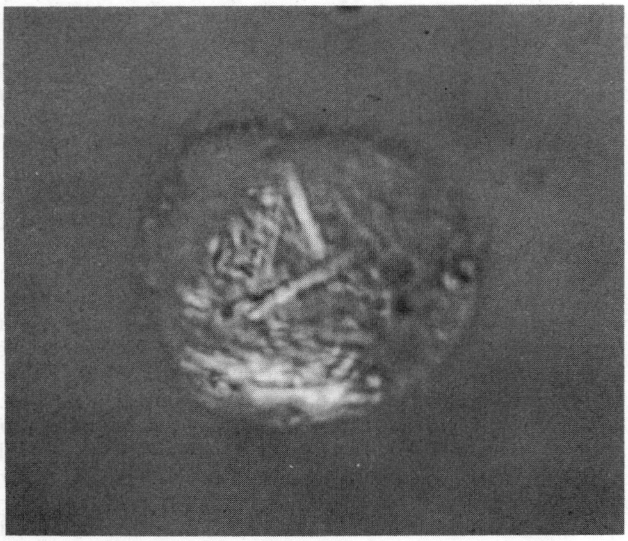

FIGURE 195–3. Sodium urate monohydrate crystals phagocytized by leukocyte in synovial fluid from acute gouty arthritis, examined by polarized light. (Courtesy of Edward W. Holmes, Duke University Medical Center.)

DIAGNOSIS. The diagnosis of acute gouty arthritis is not difficult when there is an explosive onset of a typical inflammatory attack of characteristic severity in a peripheral joint, especially of the lower extremity. The diagnosis is established by the demonstration of typical negatively birefringent needle-shaped crystals of sodium urate in the leukocytes of synovial fluid (Fig. 195–3). With proper technique, including the use of a polarizing microscope, intraleukocytic sodium urate crystals are found in over 95 per cent of aspirates from joints in acute gout. The leukocyte count may range from 1000 to more than 50,000, depending on the acuteness of the inflammation. A Gram stain should always be obtained to evaluate infection, which may coexist. In the rare event of failure to find crystals on the first attempt, a second aspirate obtained some hours later is usually positive. Urate crystals must be distinguished from calcium pyrophosphate dihydrate crystals of pseudogout. The latter are weakly positively birefringent under polarized light and usually more rectangular than urate crystals. Every patient suspected of having gout should have the diagnosis confirmed by crystal demonstration. It is not necessary to repeat the procedure in later attacks, unless they are atypical and other diagnoses (trauma, infection) are also under consideration. A rapid response of pain and inflammation to the administration of colchicine is so characteristic as also to be of diagnostic value. Responses of rheumatoid arthritis and sarcoid arthritis to colchicine are not so dramatic or complete as those in gout. The finding of hyperuricemia is anticipated and helpful, but since hyperuricemia is common (13 per cent of hospitalized male patients), it may coexist with other acute arthropathies. The presence of tophi or of typical roentgenographic findings of punched-out, destructive bony lesions will help establish the diagnosis of chronic tophaceous gout, but does not prove that the current event is acute gout. Only the demonstration of a large proportion of intraleukocytic crystals of sodium urate in the synovial fluid of the involved joint will do that. In 70 per cent of patients with crystal-proven gout, extracellular urate crystals are demonstrable in asymptomatic first metatarsophalangeal joints. Such crystals are rare (5 per cent) in hyperuricemic subjects who have never had clinical gout.

Each gouty patient should also have a determination of the 24-hour urinary excretion of uric acid. The sample should be collected after three days of moderate purine restriction, during an intercritical period. Values of greater than 600 mg per 1.72 square meters per day under these conditions probably indicate overproduction, and those of over 800 mg per day warrant additional studies for a specific subtype of primary gout, such as HGPRT deficiency of PP-ribose-P synthetase overactivity, or of secondary gout, such as a myeloproliferative disorder. Elevated urinary uric acid values also signify that the patient is at higher risk for renal stone and represent an indication for allopurinol rather than uricosuric drug therapy for gout.

Chronic gouty arthritis may be diagnosed by the presence of urate deposits in or near the affected joints or bursae or of soft-tissue deposits in the helix of the ear, the fingertips, the Achilles tendon, or other locations. The diagnosis may be confirmed by removal of the chalky contents of a tophus, by microscopic identification of sodium urate crystals by optical means, by chemical identification by the murexide test, or, preferably, by ultraviolet spectrophotometry and degradation by uricase.

DIFFERENTIAL DIAGNOSIS. Acute gout must be differentiated from acute rheumatic fever, rheumatoid arthritis, traumatic arthritis, osteoarthritis, pyogenic arthritis, sarcoid arthritis, cellulitis, bursitis, tendinitis, and thrombophlebitis. Podagra, the most common initial presentation of gout, can be mimicked by trauma, degenerative arthritis, acute sarcoidosis, psoriatic arthritis, pseudogout, palindromic rheumatism, Reiter's syndrome, or infection. Acute monoarticular arthritis of the great toe in the immediate postoperative period following parathyroidectomy can be caused by hydroxyapatite crystals. These various forms of "pseudopodagra" may be suggested by a negative examination of synovial fluid for urate crystals. Pseudogout (see Ch. 444), which is manifested by acute attacks of arthritis of knees and other joints, is usually accompanied by calcification of joint cartilage; the synovial fluid contains nonurate crystals of calcium pyrophosphate. However, gout and pseudogout may coexist, and both types of crystals will then be found in synovial fluid leukocytes.

Chronic gouty arthritis must chiefly be differentiated from rheumatoid arthritis, osteoarthritis, traumatic arthritis, and residua of pyogenic arthritis. The history of onset, progression, response to colchicine, and demonstration of hyperuricemia, asymmetric tumescences, typical roentgenographic changes, and tophi or crystals of urate in synovial fluid and leukocytes should establish the diagnosis.

TREATMENT. The therapeutic aims in gout are (1) to terminate the acute gouty attack as promptly and gently as possible, (2) to prevent recurrences of acute gouty arthritis, (3) to prevent or reverse complications of the disease resulting from deposition of sodium urate in joints and kidneys, and (4) to prevent formation of uric acid kidney stones. The therapeutic program differs according to the stage of the disease and the complications present. In the majority of patients it is possible to abort or prevent acute attacks, to control hyperuricemia, and to prevent chronic gouty arthritis, nephropathy, and stones.

Acute Attack. The affected joint should be placed at rest, and an anti-inflammatory agent administered promptly. Three types of agents are available: colchicine, nonsteroidal anti-inflammatory agents, and glucocorticoids (or ACTH). *Colchicine* is the only agent of specific diagnostic value in acute gout. It should be given as soon as the diagnosis is suspected. The initial dose of 0.6 to 1.2 mg of colchicine is followed by 0.6 mg every hour for eight hours and then every two hours until pain is relieved or until nausea, vomiting, cramping, or diarrhea develops. Maximum tolerated doses range from 4 to 8 mg. In many patients dramatic relief of pain and onset of gastrointestinal side effects occur simultaneously. The diarrhea may be treated with paregoric, 4 ml, or Kaopectate, 30 ml, after each loose stool. Colchicine should be discontinued until gastrointestinal symptoms subside. Since the effective dose of colchicine varies, each patient should learn his or her own tolerance dose and stop just short of this in treatment of subsequent attacks. If started promptly, colchicine affords relief over 90 per cent of the time; if treatment is delayed beyond 12 hours, only 75 per cent of patients will respond within 24 to 48 hours. Since colchicine is concentrated within cells and turns over with a half-life of about 30 hours, repeated courses of colchicine carry a higher risk of toxicity; treatment failures should be treated with a nonsteroidal anti-inflammatory drug (NSAID).

Colchicine may also be given intravenously (subcutaneous infiltration may result in tissue necrosis). The usual initial dose is 1 to 2 mg in 20 ml saline solution given slowly, and if a single dose is not effective, the injection may be repeated once in four to five hours (maximum intravenous dose, 3 to 5 mg). Gastrointestinal symptoms are uncommon with intravenous administration, although occasionally nausea will occur.

Dose-related toxic responses to colchicine include alopecia (reversible), bone marrow suppression (leukopenia, thrombocytopenia, anemia), and hepatocellular damage. The drug should not be used in patients with advanced hepatic or renal disease.

NSAID's are equally effective in acute gout, and are usually preferred over colchicine because they are so much milder for the patient. Indomethacin has been most widely used. It is given orally in initial doses of 50 mg three or four times a day. When pain is relieved, doses are tapered over another 48 to 72 hours. Larger doses may cause severe headache, gastric distress, or a transient depersonalization reaction in some patients, but these side effects have been noted only rarely in gouty patients receiving short courses of the drug. *Phenylbutazone* and *oxyphenbutazone* (Tandearil) are also effective in acute gouty arthritis and may be preferred when the gouty attack has proceeded for some time or when the attack does not abate completely with colchicine or indomethacin. The initial dose is 400 mg orally, followed by 100 mg every four to eight hours for two to three days. Bone marrow suppression may rarely occur, even after a short course of either drug. Other NSAID's, such as *naproxen* and *ibuprofen,* can also be used, especially in patients with a history of peptic ulcer. With all NSAID's, renal function should be monitored, especially in hypertensive patients.

If full doses of colchicine or NSAID's are contraindicated (e.g., in postoperative gout) or ineffective, *ACTH* may be employed by intravenous drip (40 units per day) or as intramuscular gel (40 to 80 units per day), or systemic glucocorticoids may be given for two to three days, rarely longer, following which the doses are reduced in stepwise fashion and discontinued. Unfortunately, rebound attacks of gout are rather common after such therapy. *Triamcinolone hexacetonide* in a dose of 5 to 20 mg injected intra-articularly into the involved joint is useful in treating acute gout limited to a single joint or bursa, particularly in patients in whom the standard drugs cannot be used, and relief from pain is usually prompt and complete within 24 to 36 hours. Steroid hormones are not recommended for parenteral use in acute gout, as the effects are inconsistent and rebound attacks frequent.

Uricosuric agents and allopurinol are of no value in treatment of the acute attack.

Interval Phase. The patient with gout should avoid high purine foods so as to lessen the burden of uric acid excretion. A severe limitation of purine-containing foods is rarely indicated, unless renal function is poor. Gradual weight reduction is indicated if the patient is overweight, and may of itself reduce hyperuricemia and the tendency to develop attacks of gout. Sudden weight reduction may precipitate gouty attacks and should be avoided. In general, diets of moderate protein content, somewhat low in fat, are preferred. Hypertension should be treated vigorously, even if antihypertensive agents worsen hyperuricemia; the result can be countered with appropriate antihyperuricemic drug therapy.

A high fluid intake is advisable to maintain a urinary output of 2000 ml per day. Uric acid excretion is thus promoted, and the dangers of crystal formation in the kidney or ureter are reduced. Beer, ale, and wine should be avoided, as they may precipitate attacks. Distilled alcoholic beverages in moderation generally have little influence on the gouty process. Illicit liquor (moonshine) should be prohibited. Excessive alcohol use in any form should be avoided, as it enhances purine production and also leads to hypertriglyceridemia.

Patients who recognize prodromal symptoms may abort acute attacks by prompt institution of colchicine, phenylbutazone, or indomethacin therapy; they frequently require only a few tablets to achieve success. The daily ingestion of 0.6 to 1.8 mg of colchicine is generally effective in reducing the number of acute gouty attacks in patients who are subject to frequent episodes. Toxicity is rare, but may include alopecia, bone marrow suppression, and hepatocellular damage. Maintenance colchicine therapy is particularly important during the first months or year after institution of uricosuric drugs or of allopurinol. Daily ingestion of indomethacin, 25 or 50 mg has also been employed for this purpose and appears to be effective. The risks of renal and gastrointestinal toxicity make use of indomethacin undesirable as a prophylactic agent or as therapy for chronic gouty arthritis.

Chronic Gouty Arthritis. Use of a drug to lower the serum level of uric acid to 6 mg per 100 ml or less is indicated in all gouty patients with visible tophi, with roentgenographic evidence of urate deposits, or with a history of two or more major attacks of acute gouty arthritis. Allopurinol is the drug of choice unless the patient is already well managed with a uricosuric agent. With either type of agent the number of acute gouty attacks may be increased during the first few months unless maintenance colchicine therapy is given, whereas after 12 to 18 months the number may be decidedly reduced.

Allopurinol controls serum urate levels by inhibiting xanthine oxidase and thereby regulating production of uric acid (Fig. 195–1). Allopurinol is converted to oxipurinol in the body, and the latter compound has a longer biologic half-life (28 hours), ultimately being largely excreted in the urine. Inhibition of conversion of hypoxanthine and xanthine to uric acid permits these precursors to be excreted instead. In gouty subjects other than those with HGPRT deficiency, the increment in hypoxanthine plus xanthine excretion is only about two thirds of the decrement in uric acid excretion, presumably because of enhanced feed-back inhibition of purine synthesis de novo by nucleotides reconstituted from hypoxanthine. The induced xanthinuria has not resulted in xanthine stone formation in the usual gouty subjects, but has done so in a rare patient with HGPRT deficiency and in patients being treated with antineoplastic agents. Use of allopurinol results in reduction of levels of uric acid in serum *and in urine.* The drug is effective even in the presence of renal failure, when uricosuric agents generally are not. Its action is not blocked by salicylates. The usual dose is 300 mg, given orally once a day. In the presence of moderate nitrogen retention the dose of allopurinol should be reduced by one half or more (see Ch. 24), as the biologic half-life of the active metabolite, oxipurinol, is prolonged. Allopurinol is usually well tolerated, but may cause gastric irritation, diarrhea, or skin rash or induce an attack of gout. Toxic hepatitis, epidermal necrolysis, and vasculitis may occasionally be severe, even fatal. Toxic effects are more frequent and more severe in the presence of renal failure. Intramuscular crystals of xanthine and oxipurinol have been described in patients receiving allopurinol, but their significance in terms of toxicity is not clear. Uricosuric agents may be used concurrently with allopurinol to hasten mobilization of urate deposits, but combined therapy may require larger doses of allopurinol because uricosuric drugs also enhance the excretion of oxipurinol. Since allopurinol decreases uric acid excretion, it is also very useful in controlling uric acid stone formation, especially in patients who are overproducers of uric acid. If the serum urate values can be controlled at levels below saturation of urate in body fluids, extensive resolution of soft tissue tophi and modest reduction in size of bony erosions may be achieved, together with some recalcification of bony lesions (Fig. 195–2). Joint mobility and comfort may be greatly improved.

Uricosuric drugs block tubular reabsorption of filtered urate. Those of use in gout are probenecid and sulfinpyrazone. These agents begin to lose effectiveness when the creatinine clearance falls below 80 ml per minute and are completely ineffective when the clearance falls below 30 ml per minute. *Probenecid* is given in doses of 0.5 gram to 3 grams daily in two or three evenly spaced doses (average dose, 1 to 1.5 grams). This drug may produce gastrointestinal upsets, headaches, or skin rash. *Sulfinpyrazone* may be given in doses of 100 to 600 mg daily in three or four divided doses (average dose, 300 mg). This drug is related to phenylbutazone and may cause untoward reactions, but is generally somewhat better tolerated than probenecid. *Salicylates* block the uricosuric action of both probenecid and sulfinpyrazone and must not be used concurrently. Salicylates are uricosuric when given in high doses (4 to 6 grams daily), but few patients can tolerate these quantities.

With all uricosuric agents the doses should be low initially, to avoid sudden excretion of large quantities of urate, and increased at weekly intervals to maintenance levels. Fluids should be forced to prevent formation of concentrated urine, especially during the late hours of the night. During the first days or weeks of therapy the urine should be kept at pH 6 or above, by administration of sodium bicarbonate or sodium citrate–citric acid (Shohl's solution); this may be difficult to achieve, as acid urine tends to be produced in gouty patients. In patients in whom urate is being mobilized, and especially those in whom uric acid gravel is formed, alkalinization during the night, when fluid intake is reduced, is important. A single 250-mg tablet of acetazolamide (Diamox) taken at bedtime will serve to keep the urine alkaline and dilute throughout the night.

In selected patients surgical removal of large extra-articular urate deposits, such as those in olecranon bursae, may be advisable. Occasionally amputation of irreparably damaged digits, especially those containing draining sinuses, is indicated. Physical therapy and appropriate self-help devices are valuable in patients who are partially disabled.

Asymptomatic Hyperuricemia. Asymptomatic hyperuricemia is frequent in family members of patients with gout and in the general population. It usually requires no therapy, as only about one fifth of patients will ever develop articular attacks, and adequate therapy can be instituted when these supervene. Exceptions may exist in patients with markedly elevated serum levels of uric acid, especially if urinary urate excretion is low and there is a family history of tophaceous disease. In such circumstances the asymptomatic subject should be treated with allopurinol before articular or renal complications develop. It is essential that the physician maintain frequent close observation of the patient.

Berger, L. Yu T-F: Renal function in gout: IV. An analysis of 524 gouty subjects including long-term follow-up studies. Am J Med 59:605, 1975. *An important study showing that deterioration of renal function in gout is largely associated with aging, renal vascular disease, hypertension, renal calculi with pyelonephritis, or independently occurring nephropathy. Hyperuricemia alone had no deleterious effect on renal function over periods up to 12 years.*

Cherian PV, Schumacher HR Jr: Immunochemical and ultrastructural characterization of serum proteins associated with monosodium urate crystals (MSU) in synovial fluid cells from patients with gout. Ultrastruct Pathol 10:209, 1986. *Various proteins associated with intracellular urate crystals, IgG > IgM or IgA > C3 or fibrinogen, may influence the inflammatory properties of those crystals.*

Reibman J, Haines KA, Rich AM, et al.: Colchicine inhibits ionophore-induced formation of leukotriene B_4 by human neutrophils: The role of microtubules. J Immunol 136:1027, 1986. *The mechanisms of colchicine action in inhibiting production of leukotriene B_4 by neutrophils appears to depend upon its effect upon the number and integrity of the microtubules.*

Simkin PS: Uric acid excretion in patients with gout. Arthritis Rheum 22:98, 1979. *An analysis of six published studies relating the rate of urate excretion to plasma urate levels in normal and gouty subjects. The kidneys of the average gouty person lag significantly behind the normal in their response to any concentration of plasma urate. The kidneys of overproducers (38 of 73 gouty subjects) were no less handicapped than those of other gouty subjects.*

Spillberg I, Mandell B, Mehta J, et al.: Mechanism of action of colchicine in acute urate crystal-induced arthritis. J Clin Invest 64:775, 1979. *Phagocytosis of urate crystals by neutrophils induces the synthesis and release of a glycoprotein that is chemotactic both in vitro and in vivo. Colchicine decreases production and release of this factor. Colchicine abrogates the acute arthritis produced by urate crystals in rabbits, but has no effect upon the arthritis induced by injection of purified cell-derived chemotactic factor.*

Wyngaarden JB, Kelley WN: Gout. In Stanbury JB, Wyngaarden JB, Fredrickson DS, et al. (eds): The Metabolic Basis of Inherited Disease. 5th ed. New York, McGraw-Hill Book Company, 1983. *A detailed account of purine metabolism and the pathogenesis of primary gout.*

Wyngaarden JB, Kelley WN: Gout and Hyperuricemia. New York, Grune & Stratton, 1976. *Everything you have always wanted to know about gout but never dared to ask, condensed into 500 pages.*

196 OTHER DISORDERS OF PURINE METABOLISM

Edward W. Holmes

XANTHINURIA

Classic xanthinuria, which is inherited as an autosomal recessive trait, is the consequence of an isolated deficiency of xanthine oxidase. As a result of this enzyme deficiency, uric acid is replaced by xanthine and hypoxanthine as the end products of purine metabolism. Serum urate concentrations in these patients range from 0 to 1.4 mg per deciliter and urinary uric acid excretion ranges from 0 to 8 mg per day; serum oxypurine (xanthine plus hypoxanthine) concentrations and urine oxypurine excretion are increased in this disorder.

More than 50 patients with classic xanthinuria have been described, and the prevalence of this disorder is estimated to be approximately 1 in 45,000. Over 50 per cent of individuals with classic xanthinuria are asymptomatic, the diagnosis being suspected by the incidental finding of a very low serum urate concentration during evaluation of presumably unrelated medical problems. The diagnosis is virtually established by the demonstration of low serum and urinary uric acid levels in association with increased urinary oxypurine excretion, and it is confirmed by assaying liver or intestinal mucosa for xanthine oxidase activity. One third of patients develop radiolucent renal calculi composed of xanthine. Four adult patients have had myopathic symptoms characterized by muscle cramps following exercise, and crystalline deposits of xanthine and hypoxanthine have been found in skeletal muscle. Recurrent polyarthritis has been described in three patients, and it has been suggested but not established that this symptom may represent crystal-induced synovitis.

A new subtype of xanthinuria has been described in which the deficiency of xanthine oxidase is associated with a deficiency of sulfite oxidase. Both of these enzymes require a molybdenum cofactor for catalytic activity, and absence of this cofactor has been demonstrated in the liver of a patient with this combined enzyme defect. Five patients have been reported with an inherited deficiency of these two enzymes, and all five presented in the first weeks of life with a severe neurologic disorder characteristic of isolated sulfite oxidase deficiency. Symptoms include feeding difficulties from birth, tonic-clonic seizures, nystagmus, enophthalmus, ocular lens dislocation, and Brushfield spots. As in isolated sulfite oxidase deficiency, urinary excretion of sulfate is low while that of sulfite, thiosulfate, S-sulfocysteine, and taurine is increased. Characteristic biochemical findings of xanthinuria are also present.

An acquired phenocopy of the combined defect has been

described in a 20-year-old male with short-bowel syndrome maintained for 18 months with total parenteral nutrition. In addition to hypouricemia and hypouricaciduria, urinary excretion of sulfite and thiosulfate was increased while excretion of sulfate was decreased. Following infusion of commercially available amino acid solutions the patient experienced headaches, night blindness, irritability, lethargy, and then coma.

The prognosis in classic xanthinuria is excellent, as shown by the high percentage of patients who are asymptomatic. Therapy for xanthine calculi includes high fluid intake, and on occasion allopurinol has been used in patients with residual xanthine oxidase activity to increase the excretion of hypoxanthine relative to xanthine, the former being more soluble than the latter. In patients with the inherited form of combined xanthine oxidase and sulfite oxidase deficiency, the neurologic symptoms have been refractory to therapy with a number of agents, including oral ammonium molybdate. With the acquired form of this combined disorder, treatment with ammonium molybdate reversed the biochemical abnormalities and the neurologic symptoms were markedly ameliorated.

Holmes EW, Wyngaarden JB: Hereditary xanthinuria. In Stanbury JB, Wyngaarden JB, Fredrickson DS, et al.: (eds.): The Metabolic Basis of Inherited Disease. 5th ed. New York, McGraw-Hill Book Company, 1983, pp 1192–1201. *A thorough coverage of the clinical and biochemical abnormalities found in classic xanthinuria, as well as the inherited and acquired forms of the combined deficiency of xanthine oxidase and sulfite oxidase.*

Wadman SK, Duran M, Beemer FA, et al.: Absence of hepatic molybdenum cofactor: An inborn error of metabolism leading to a combined deficiency of sulfite oxidase and xanthine dehydrogenase. J Inherited Metab Dis 6:78, 1983. *Metabolic and clinical observations on five patients with this disorder.*

THE LESCH-NYHAN SYNDROME AND PARTIAL DEFICIENCY OF HYPOXANTHINE-GUANINE PHOSPHORIBOSYLTRANSFERASE

The Lesch-Nyhan syndrome, caused by a virtually complete deficiency of hypoxanthine-guanine phosphoribosyltransferase (HGPRT) activity, is manifested clinically by hyperuricemia, excessive production of uric acid, and neurologic features including self-mutilation, choreoathetosis, spasticity, and mental retardation. Partial deficiency of HGPRT activity is associated with uric acid overproduction, severe gout, and occasionally neurologic abnormalities, but self-mutilation is absent. The Lesch-Nyhan syndrome occurs in about one in 100,000 births, and partial deficiency of HGPRT is noted in less than 1 per cent of the gouty population.

ETIOLOGY AND PATHOGENESIS. Studies have demonstrated a single but different amino acid substitution in 16 mutant forms of HGPRT documenting marked genetic heterogeneity in this disorder. Failure to reutilize hypoxanthine in the salvage pathway as a result of HGPRT deficiency leads to increased oxidation of this purine base to uric acid. An increase in the intracellular concentration of phosphoribosylpyrophosphate, which also results from reduction in hypoxanthine reutilization, leads to an increase in the rate of purine biosynthesis de novo. The combined effect of these abnormalities is increased uric acid production resulting in hyperuricaciduria, which predisposes to uric acid crystal and stone formation, and hyperuricemia, which leads to gouty arthritis and tophaceous deposits. The biochemical basis for the unusual and devastating neurologic abnormalities seen in the Lesch-Nyhan syndrome is not clearly understood, but abnormalities in dopamine neuron function have been described. Position emission tomography has demonstrated a selective decrease in glucose utilization in the caudate.

CLINICAL MANIFESTATIONS. The gene for HGPRT is located on the X chromosome, and consequently the deficiency of HGPRT activity is fully expressed only in affected males. Females heterozygous for HGPRT deficiency may have subtle abnormalities in purine metabolism, but they are generally asymptomatic.

Infants with the Lesch-Nyhan syndrome are normal at birth, and the earliest consistent abnormality is a delay in motor development noted at three to four months of age. Between eight and twelve months extrapyramidal signs develop leading to choreoathetosis, and at about one year of age signs of pyramidal tract involvement, such as hyper-reflexia, clonus, and scissoring of the legs, appear. Compulsive self-destructive behavior appears any time between early childhood and adolescence. This is the most distinctive neurologic feature of the syndrome, and is manifested by biting of the fingers, lips, and buccal mucosa. Repeated attempts at self-injury, such as placing extremities in dangerous areas and self-inflicted head trauma, are also common. Sensation is intact in these children. Mental retardation is noted in most cases, but it is unclear whether the enzyme deficiency per se causes this or whether it is the result of poor performance on formal testing in children with dysarthria and choreoathetosis. Growth retardation is also a prominent feature of the syndrome. Uric acid crystalluria may be noted as orange crystals on the diaper during the first weeks of life and in untreated patients progresses to uric acid nephrolithiasis, obstructive uropathy, and azotemia. Hyperuricemia is usually present and may attain levels of 18 mg per deciliter, but the serum urate concentration may be normal, especially before puberty. Gout is unusual in the Lesch-Nyhan syndrome before 12 to 15 years of age. Death usually occurs in the second or third decade from infection or renal failure.

Patients with partial deficiency of HGPRT develop uric acid crystalluria and renal calculi in childhood, and gouty arthritis often occurs before 20 years of age. Neurologic manifestations, including mental retardation, mild spastic quadriplegia, dysarthria, cerebellar ataxia, and seizures, are noted in 20 per cent of patients with partial HGPRT deficiency, but self-mutilation does not develop. Patients with partial HGPRT deficiency may seek medical attention with the only symptom being the passage of a renal calculus or an attack of gouty arthritis. Life expectancy is normal in these patients.

DIAGNOSIS. Self-destructive behavior is the most distinguishing clinical feature of the Lesch-Nyhan syndrome; whereas retarded children with other disorders will bite their fingers, mutilation to the point of tissue destruction is rare in any disorder other than the Lesch-Nyhan syndrome. Severe self-biting in other neurologic disorders is usually associated with a loss of pain sensation. As pointed out, hyperuricemia is usually present, but this is not an invariable finding. The diagnosis is established by demonstrating a virtual absence of HGPRT activity in readily accessible tissues such as erythrocytes. Analyses of erythrocyte lysates are not useful in identifying heterozygous female carriers, but this can be accomplished with cell culture of skin fibroblasts or through analysis of hair follicles.

Partial deficiency of HGPRT should be suspected in male patients with the onset of gouty arthritis before 20 years of age and in young males with uric acid crystalluria or uric acid nephrolithiasis. Uric acid overexcretion is found invariably in patients with normal renal function, and the diagnosis is confirmed by enzyme assay. Patients with partial HGPRT activity will have erythrocyte lysate values that are usually in the range of 0.1 to 5 per cent of control values, rarely up 30 to 50 per cent of control values, while Lesch-Nyhan patients will have values less than 0.01 per cent of control values.

TREATMENT. Uric acid stone formation, tophi, and gouty arthritis can be controlled in both the Lesch-Nyhan syndrome and partial deficiency of HGPRT with drugs that inhibit xanthine oxidase activity. However, a few patients have developed xanthine stones with this therapy. No drugs have been found that correct the neurologic deficits, but supportive measures such as restraints that reduce the tendency to self-mutilation are well accepted by the patient. Drugs such as diazepam help control the movement disorder. Given the devastating neurologic complications of the Lesch-Nyhan syndrome, therapeutic abortion has been used as a preventive measure following heterozygote identification and intrauterine diagnosis.

Edwards NL, Recker D, Fox IH: Overproduction of uric acid in hypoxanthine-guanine phosphoribosyltransferase deficiency. J Clin Invest 63:922, 1979. *A careful analysis of the basis for uric acid overproduction in patients with HGPRT deficiency.*

Kelley WN, Wyngaarden JB: Clinical syndromes associated with hypoxanthine-guanine phosphoribosyltransferase deficiency. In Stanbury JB, Wyngaarden JB, Fredrickson DS, et al. (eds.): The Metabolic Basis of Inherited Disease. 5th ed. New York, McGraw-Hill Book Company, 1983, pp 1115–1143. *A detailed description of the clinical and biochemical consequences of HGPRT deficiency.*

Wilson JM, Stout JT, Palella TD, et al.: A molecular survey of hypoxanthine-guanine phosphoribosyltransferase deficiency in man. J Clin Invest 77:188, 1986. *A description of specific mutations at the molecular level in patients with HGPRT deficiency.*

2,8-DIHYDROXYADENINE RENAL STONES

Deficiency of adenine phosphoribosyltransferase, an enzyme in the salvage pathway of purine nucleotide synthesis, leads to the accumulation and increased urinary excretion of 2,8-dihydroxyadenine, the product of adenine oxidation by xanthine oxidase. Because of the insolubility of this purine, patients with this autosomal recessive disorder are predisposed to development of renal calculi composed of 2,8-dihydroxyadenine. Six individuals homozygous for this enzyme deficiency have presented with acute renal failure, and three of these patients suffered permanent renal damage. Renal colic may occur within the first months of life, as late as 40 years of age, or individuals with this disorder may be asymptomatic. 2,8-Dihydroxyadenine stones are usually radiolucent. The diagnosis is confirmed by analysis of the stone with ultraviolet, infrared, or mass spectrometry or x-ray crystallography, or by demonstrating the absence of adenine phosphoribosyltransferase activity in erythrocyte lysates. Except for the excessive excretion of adenine and its metabolites with the consequent development of renal calculi, no other biochemical or clinical abnormalities have been reported in individuals homozygous for this enzyme deficiency.

The prevalence of the homozygous state is not documented, but it is calculated to occur once in 35,000 to 250,000 births, since the prevalence of heterozygosity for adenine phosphoribosyltransferase deficiency varies from 0.4 to 1.0 per 100. Individuals heterozygous for the enzyme deficiency have no recognized clinical abnormalities.

Prognosis depends on renal function at the time of diagnosis. Therapy with dietary purine restriction, high fluid intake, and allopurinol—to prevent oxidation of adenine to 2,8-dihydroxyadenine—is effective in reducing stone formation and preserving renal function.

Simmonds A, Van Acker KL: Adenine phosphoribosyltransferase deficiency. In Stanbury JB, Wyngaarden JB, Fredrickson DS, et al. (eds.): The Metabolic Basis of Inherited Disease. 5th ed. New York, McGraw-Hill Book Company, 1983. *A detailed review of all known cases of complete APRT deficiency and discussion of the metabolic defect.*

Van Acker KJ, Simmonds A, Potter C, et al.: Complete deficiency of adenine phosphoribosyltransferase. Report of a family. N Engl J Med 297:127, 1977. *Adenine, 8-hydroxyadenine and 2,8-dihydroxyadenine amounted to 25 per cent of urinary purines in two homozygous male children, one of whom had "pure uric acid stones" later correctly identified as 2,8-dihydroxyadenine.*

MYOPATHY ASSOCIATED WITH MYOADENYLATE DEAMINASE DEFICIENCY

Deficiency of myoadenylate deaminase has been noted in approximately 2 per cent of muscle biopsies submitted for routine investigation in some centers. This isozyme of adenosine monophosphate (AMP) deaminase is found only in skeletal muscle, and this is the only organ affected by this enzyme deficiency. In approximately half of the cases that have been carefully studied, AMP deaminase deficiency is not associated with other neuromuscular pathology, and in these individuals the enzyme deficiency is marked (<1 per cent of normal). In cases in which the residual enzyme activity is higher (1 to 10 per cent of normal) the patients have a broad spectrum of neuromuscular diseases. Three quarters of patients with primary myoadenylate deaminase deficiency report exercise-related symptoms of easy fatigability, cramps, and myalgias, usually beginning in childhood or young adulthood. Weakness without exercise is noted in less than one third of patients. Hypotonia has been described in two patients. Reduced AMP deaminase activity has occasionally been reported in patients with other neuromuscular disorders, but no definite association of this enzyme deficiency has been established with any symptom complex other than easy fatigability, cramps, and myalgias. Since a few individuals with myoadenylate deaminase deficiency have been reported to be asymptomatic, factors in addition to AMP deaminase deficiency may contribute to the exercise-related manifestations described above.

Serum creatine kinase activity is mildly and variably increased in about one half of patients with this disorder, and routine laboratory studies including electromyography and histochemistry of muscle are not diagnostic. In the patient with exercise-related symptoms the specific diagnosis of myoadenylate deaminase deficiency is suggested by the finding of reduced NH_3 production in a forearm ischemic exercise test. NH_3 is a product of AMP deamination, a normal consequence of ATP catabolism in skeletal muscle. However, not all patients with reduced NH_3 production following ischemic forearm exercise will have myoadenylate deaminase deficiency, and the diagnosis needs to be confirmed by direct assay of AMP deaminase activity in skeletal muscle.

AMP deaminase is one of the components of the purine nucleotide cycle, a series of reactions that is potentially important in energy production and utilization in skeletal muscle. Deficiency of myoadenylate deaminase activity may impair energy generation through diminished production of citric acid cycle intermediates, and it may adversely affect energy utilization through a reduction in the rate of adenosine triphosphate (ATP) hydrolysis by myofibrillar ATPase.

Prognosis in myoadenylate deaminase deficiency is generally good. Present experience suggests the symptoms are slowly progressive, and the disorder leads to mild disability in most cases, although there have been exceptions to these generalizations. No effective therapy is available at this time.

Fishbein WN: Myoadenylate deaminase deficiency: Inherited and acquired forms. Biochem Med 33:158, 1985. *Review of biochemical data supporting primary and secondary forms of AMP deaminase deficiency.*

Sabina RL, Swain JL, Olanow CW, et al.: Myoadenylate deaminase deficiency: Functional and metabolic abnormalities associated with disruption of the purine nucleotide cycle. J Clin Invest 73:720, 1984.

Swain JL, Sabina RL, Holmes EW: Myoadenylate Deaminase Deficiency. In Stanbury JB, Wyngaarden JK, Fredrickson DS, et al. (eds.): The Metabolic Basis of Inherited Disease. 5th ed. New York, McGraw-Hill Book Company, 1983, pp 1184–1191. *Discussion of the clinical and biochemical findings in 26 patients with myoadenylate deaminase deficiency, as well as a review of the role of the purine nucleotide cycle in skeletal muscle function.*

IMMUNE DYSFUNCTION ASSOCIATED WITH PURINE ENZYME DEFICIENCIES

Adenosine deaminase deficiency is an uncommon disorder, approximately 100 to 150 families having been identified, that leads to a clinical syndrome of severe combined immunodeficiency, i.e., a defect in both T cell and B cell function. About one fifth of patients with severe combined immunodeficiency, in which the disorder is inherited as an autosomal recessive condition, or more rarely as an X-linked recessive disorder, will have this enzyme deficiency. Approximately 85 per cent of patients with adenosine deaminase deficiency come to medical attention at one to two months of age with recurrent infections of the skin and the gastrointestinal and respiratory systems. Both ordinary and opportunistic pathogens are encountered, and candidiasis is almost invariably present. Diarrhea is common, as well as delayed physical growth and development. Physical findings are for the most part unremarkable except for the absence of lymph nodes and pharyngeal lymphoid tissue. A rachitic rosary, or prominence of the costochondrial junctions, has been noted in some patients. Laboratory tests show absence of a thymic shadow, lymphopenia, negative skin test results for delayed hypersensitivity, attenuated lymphocyte responses to lectins and antigens in vitro, and hypogammaglobulinemia. The diagnosis is established by documenting adenosine deaminase deficiency in erythrocyte lysates or other cell extracts. Approximately 15 per cent of individuals with this disorder have a milder disease with later age of onset and relative sparing of humoral immunity. In the severe form of this disorder, if untreated, overwhelming infection and sepsis lead to death before two years of age.

Current mechanisms favored to explain the immune defects observed in adenosine deaminase deficiency are deoxy-ATP accumulation leading to inhibition of ribonucleotide reductase with resultant decrease in DNA replication, and S-adenosylhomocysteine accumulation leading to inhibition of transmethylation reactions. Either or both of these proposed mechanisms could reduce lymphocyte proliferation and function.

Treatment of adenosine deaminase deficiency by bone marrow transplantation has resulted in virtually complete immune reconstitution in some patients, and at present this is the preferred therapy if compatible donors are available. Enzyme replacement with repeated transfusions of irradiated red blood cells (to prevent graft-versus-host disease) has improved immune function in some patients.

Purine nucleoside phosphorylase deficiency is less common than adenosine deaminase deficiency, approximately 15 to 20 patients having been recognized with this disorder. Purine nucleoside phosphorylase deficiency is also inherited as an autosomal recessive disorder, but it leads to a defect in cell-mediated immunity with little if any abnormality in humoral immunity. In patients with this disorder diagnosis has been made as early as four months and as late as nine years of age, with infections involving skin, lung, middle ear, mastoids, and urinary tract. Infections with nonbacterial agents have been most common, reflecting the primary defect in cellular immunity. Laboratory tests show lymphopenia, diminished number of circulating T cells, reduced lymphocyte response to antigens, and negative skin test results for delayed hypersensitivity. Immunoglobulin levels are normal, but several patients have exhibited signs of immunoregulatory abnormalities as shown by autoimmune hemolytic anemia, antinuclear antibodies, and rheumatoid factor. In addition, patients with purine nucleoside phosphorylase deficiency have hypouricemia, a finding of no clinical consequence in itself, but one that suggests the diagnosis of this enzyme deficiency in a child with recurrent infections.

Confirmation of the diagnosis is obtained by assay of erythrocyte lysate or other cell extracts for purine nucleoside phosphorylase activity. It has been proposed that accumulation of deoxyguanosine triphosphate in T lymphocytes with resultant inhibition of ribonucleotide reductase and DNA replication is responsible for the immune defect in this disorder. Prognosis in purine nucleoside phosphorylase deficiency is generally better than that for adenosine deaminase deficiency, but therapy with bone marrow transplantation and erythrocyte transfusion has been less successful.

Adenosine deaminase in disorders of purine metabolism and in immune deficiency. Ann NY Acad Sci vol. 451, 1985. *A collection of papers dealing with clinical, metabolic, and immunologic aspects of adenosine deaminase deficiency.*

Giblett ER: Adenosine deaminase and purine nucleoside phosphorylase deficiency: How they were discovered and what they may mean. In Elliot K, Whelan J (eds.): Enzyme Defects and Immune Dysfunction. Ciba Found Symp 68:3, 1979. *An interesting story about scientific serendipity and discovery of a new group of clinical disorders.*

Kredich N, Hershfield MS: Immunodeficiency diseases caused by adenosine deaminase deficiency and purine nucleoside phosphorylase deficiency. In Stanbury JB, Wyngaarden JB, Fredrickson DS, et al. (eds.): The Metabolic Basis of Inherited Disease. 5th ed. New York, McGraw-Hill Book Company, 1983, p 1157. *An authoritative review of the clinical, laboratory, and biochemical abnormalities in these disorders. This chapter also includes a detailed discussion of purine nucleoside metabolism in normal and pathological situations.*

197 DISORDERS OF PYRIMIDINE METABOLISM

Lloyd H. Smith, Jr.

Pyrimidine nucleotides share equally with purine nucleotides the chemical chore of transmitting genetic information for reproduction or for phenotypic expression within the cell. They also function in the intermediary metabolism of lipids and carbohydrates. Only a few disorders of pyrimidine metabolism have been recognized.

Hereditary orotic aciduria is a rare genetic disorder of pyrimidine metabolism characterized by megaloblastic anemia resistant to the usual hematinic agents, leukopenia, failure of normal growth and development, and the continued excessive urinary excretion of orotic acid. Patients also have impaired cellular immunity with intact humoral immunity. Orotic acid is highly insoluble and often forms a heavy sediment of urinary crystals that may on occasion result in ureteral or urethral obstruction. The disorder, which is transmitted as an autosomal recessive trait, is usually characterized by reduced activities of two consecutive enzymes in pyrimidine biosynthesis, orotate phosphoribosyltransferase (OPRT) and orotidine 5′-phosphate decarboxylase (ODC). Both enzymatic activities may reside in a single multifunctional protein for which the gene is located on the long arm of chromosome 3. A single patient has been described with isolated deficiency of ODC. There is a prompt and sustained hematologic and general clinical response to oral uridine (2 to 4 grams per day), which must be continued indefinitely as replacement therapy. The disease has attracted special attention because it represents a block in the de novo pathway of pyrimidine synthesis, is an example of a double enzyme defect, and produces a requirement for replacement of a normal metabolic intermediate, uridine.

Orotic aciduria, without the characteristic hematologic abnormalities, also occurs in *ornithine transcarbamylase deficiency*. It is presumed that this results from the overflow of carbamyl phosphate from urea synthesis (partially blocked in this disease) to pyrimidine synthesis. Orotic aciduria has also been found in purine nucleoside phosphorylase deficiency and in PP-ribose-P synthetase deficiency (see Ch. 419).

Excessive urinary excretion of orotic acid and orotidine occurs during treatment with *allopurinol* or *6-azauridine*.* Metabolic products of both compounds inhibit orotidine 5′-decarboxylase activity.

Beta-aminoisobutyric aciduria is a benign hereditary disorder of thymine catabolism that occurs in 5 to 10 per cent of Caucasians and in a much higher percentage of Asians. The defect presumably lies in the transamination of beta-aminoisobutyric acid to methylmalonic acid semialdehyde. The aminoaciduria that results, representing the only known disorder of pyrimidine catabolism, has no known biologic disadvantage.

Pyrimidine 5′-nucleotidase deficiency is a rare form of hereditary hemolytic anemia, transmitted as an autosomal recessive trait. The erythrocytes exhibit prominent basophilic stippling owing to aggregates of undegraded ribosomes and on analysis contain very high concentrations of cytidine and uridine nucleotides. The mechanism by which the nucleotidase deficiency leads to hemolysis is unclear. Lead inhibits pyrimidine 5′-nucleotidase activity and leads to a similar anemia with basophilic stippling, possibly through this mechanism.

Becoft DMO, Suttle DP, Webster DR: Orotic aciduria. In Scriver CR, Beaudet A, Sly W, et al. (eds.): The Metabolic Basis of Inherited Disease. 6th ed. New York, McGraw-Hill Book Company, 1988, in press. *This is the most*

*Investigational drug.

complete description of normal pyrimidine metabolism in man and the derangements that occur in hereditary orotic aciduria.

Girot R, Hamet M, Perignon J-L, et al.: Cellular immune deficiency in two siblings with hereditary orotic aciduria. N Engl J Med 308:700, 1983. *Two children with orotic aciduria exhibited impaired cellular immunity but normal humoral immunity, analogous to that seen with purine nucleoside phosphorylase deficiency.*

Smith LH Jr: Purine and pyrimidine metabolism in man. In Smith LH Jr, Thier SO (eds.): Pathophysiology: The Biological Principles of Disease. 2nd ed. International Textbook of Medicine, Vol 1. Philadelphia, W. B. Saunders Company, 1985. *This chapter in the companion textbook of pathophysiology gives a classification and general survey of the currently recognized diseases involving the synthesis or degradation of pyrimidines.*

Valentine WN, Fink K, Paglia DE, et al.: Hereditary hemolytic anemia with human erythrocyte pyrimidine 5′-nucleotidase deficiency. J Clin Invest 54:866, 1974. *This is the original and still the best description of the altered pyrimidine metabolism leading to hemolytic anemia in this rare but interesting genetic disease.*

Inherited Disorders of Connective Tissue

198 THE MUCOPOLYSACCHARIDOSES

William S. Sly

The mucopolysaccharidoses are a group of lysosomal storage diseases, each of which is produced by an inherited deficiency of an enzyme involved in degradation of acid mucopolysaccharides (now called glycosaminoglycans and abbreviated GAG's). They are clinically progressive and have many common features that result from accumulation of partially degraded GAG's in various tissues. They produce disability primarily from storage-related abnormalities of the connective tissue, the heart, the bony skeleton, and the central nervous system.

Delineation of this group of diseases on the basis of clinical features, radiologic findings, and biochemistry of the urinary GAG's led to the famous classification of McKusick into MPS I to VI in 1966. Over the next six years, an exciting series of investigations from the laboratories of Neufeld and co-workers led to the discoveries that fibroblasts from patients with these disorders show storage abnormalities in culture, that fibroblasts from genetically different patients could "cross-correct" each other in culture, and that this "cross-correction" was due to secretion and recapture of lysosomal enzymes by the complementing fibroblast cell lines, each of which could secrete the enzyme the other was missing and take up the "corrective factor" for which it was deficient. These complementation studies served for nearly a decade as means for clinical diagnosis, for segregation of the disease into complementation groups (e.g., segregation of Hurler's and Scheie's syndromes into one complementation group, and separation of Sanfilippo's syndrome into several complementing groups), and also guided the purification of the corrective factors, each of which was eventually identified as a specific GAG degradative enzyme. Although still useful in certain situations, the complementation assays have largely been replaced by direct assays for the enzymes listed in Table 198–1 as deficient for each of the disorders.

ETIOLOGY OF GLYCOSAMINOGLYCAN STORAGE. The GAG's are long linear polysaccharide molecules composed of repeating dimers, each of which contains a hexuronic acid (or galactose in the case of keratan sulfate) and an amino sugar. They are usually found in covalent linkage to a core protein on which they are synthesized and from which they branch like bristles from a brush. The individual GAG's differ from each other in the hexuronic acid-amino sugar combinations in the repeating dimers, in the linkages between these components, in the linkages between repeating dimers, and in the degree to which individual sugar components are N-acetylated or sulfated. The major GAG's and their respective repeating dimers are chondroitin sulfate (glucuronic acid β1-3 N-acetylgalactosamine-4/6-sulfate); dermatan sulfate (iduronic acid α1-3 N-acetylgalactosamine-4-sulfate); heparan sulfate, which has both glucuronic acid and iduronic acid linked β1-4 and α1-3, respectively, to either N-acetylglucosamine or glucosamine N-sulfate; and keratan sulfate (galactose β1-4 N-acetylglucosamine-6-sulfate). The large proteoglycan molecules made up of protein cores and their GAG branches are secreted by cells and make up a significant fraction of the extracellular matrix of connective tissue. Their turnover depends on their subsequent internalization by endocytosis, their delivery to lysosomes, and their digestion by lysosomal enzymes. Lysosomal proteases digest the core protein, endoglycosidases reduce the size of the GAG's to oligosaccharides of varying length, and many exoglycosidases act sequentially to degrade the GAG's to their monosaccharide components. Each lysosomal enzyme is specific for a specific linkage. An inherited deficiency for any enzyme involved will disrupt the sequential degradative process and lead to accumulation in lysosomes of partially degraded GAG. The accumulation is progressive and eventually disrupts cellular architecture and disturbs cell function. The tissues and organs most affected and the severity depend on the degree of enzyme deficiency, i.e., whether partial or complete. Severity also depends on which enzyme is missing, since individual GAG's vary in their tissue distribution and their rate of turnover.

The enzyme deficiencies, the major storage products, and the clinical features for the mucopolysaccharidoses are summarized in Table 198–1. There is marked genetic heterogeneity within this group of disorders, with many different clinical phenotypes resulting from the different enzyme deficiencies (see MPS I–VII, Table 198–1). It is now clear also that quite different phenotypes can result from the same enzyme deficiency, depending on whether it is partial or complete (see MPS I-H, MPS I-S, and MPS I-H/S in Table 198–1).

GENETICS OF THE MUCOPOLYSACCHARIDOSES. Except for Hunter's syndrome (MPS II), in which the missing enzyme is specified by a gene on the X chromosome and the inheritance is X linked, all of the mucopolysaccharidoses result from deficiencies of enzymes specified by autosomal genes. Thus the inheritance pattern is autosomal recessive. In most cases, affected offspring can be shown to be the products of heterozygous carrier parents, both of whom have about half normal levels of the enzyme for which the affected patient is deficient. Even though the enzymes can now be measured for most of these disorders, the disorders are too rare to make screening for carriers practical. However, carrier status can be determined by enzyme assays in high-risk individuals, and prenatal diagnosis for most of these disorders is available to high-risk mothers, such as mothers of an affected offspring, who face a 25 per cent chance of another affected offspring in a subsequent pregnancy.

CLINICAL AND PATHOLOGIC CONSEQUENCES OF GLYCOSAMINOGLYCAN STORAGE. Connective tissue storage produces connective tissue laxity in most of these disorders, manifest by inguinal and umbilical hernias. Connective tissue thickening also occurs, owing in part to GAG storage and in part to excessive collagen deposition. This combination leads to coarse facial features, peripheral nerve entrapments, thickened meninges that may lead to cord compression and hydrocephalus, and thickened joint capsules. Connective tissue deposition in valve leaflets, the endocardium, and the myocardium produces symptomatic heart disease, a common cause of death in these patients to which coronary vascular insufficiency also contributes. Most of these disorders produce short stature, partly because of impaired long bone growth and partly because of vertebral abnormalities. These and many other changes in the bony skeleton are collectively referred to as *dysostosis multiplex*. Central nervous system storage may produce progressive mental retardation, especially in disorders involving impaired degradation of heparan sulfate (MPS I, II, and III). Corneal clouding and visual handicap result from storage of the partially degraded GAG's in the corneal stroma, especially in disorders involving impaired degradation of dermatan sulfate and keratan sulfate (MPS I, IV, and VI). Hepatomegaly is common and may be massive, but rarely is important clinically. Excessive urinary excretion of incompletely degraded GAG's (mucopolysacchariduria) is a constant finding of considerable diagnostic significance (Table 198–1) but has little pathologic significance.

HURLER'S SYNDROME (MPS I-H). ***Pathology.*** The basic defect is a deficiency of alpha-L-iduronidase, an enzyme that participates in degradation of dermatan sulfate and heparan sulfate. Accumulation of membrane-bound storage material in parenchymal and mesenchymal cells is the chief pathologic finding. It affects every organ. Vacuolated cells distended with storage material distort normal cell and tissue architecture. In most cells this storage material is granular and composed of GAG's. In neurons, lipids are also present, presumably because stored GAG's inhibit sphingolipid degradation.

Clinical Features. Although patients are thought to be normal until six months of age, they develop persistent nasal discharge, noisy breathing, frequent upper respiratory infections, stiff joints, a thoracolumbar gibbus, and some degree of chest deformity in the last half of the first year of life. Over the second year, the classic syndrome develops with large head, coarse features, corneal clouding, hypertelorism, prominent eyebrows, thick lips, and broad flat nose with depressed nasal bridge. The hands are short and stubby, and joint limitation produces a clawhand deformity. Abdominal protuberance results from hepatosplenomegaly and lax abdominal musculature, often with inguinal and umbilical hernias. Dwarfism is obvious by the end of the second year, by which time cardiac murmurs are present.

Developmental delay is obvious before 18 months of age, and mental retardation progresses slowly. Limitation of joint movement leads to contractures of the hands, the elbows, and the knees. Death usually occurs by the age of 10 from pneumonia or heart failure, after about five years of steady regression and nearly total loss of acquired skills. Hearing loss is usually moderate to severe, and coronary insufficiency and peripheral vascular insufficiency are important late findings.

Radiologic abnormalities of dysostosis multiplex are striking. The skull is large and scaphocephalic, and the calvarium is thickened. The sinuses are poorly developed. The sella is enlarged anteriorly and referred to as J shaped. The ribs are oar shaped, being narrow posteriorly and greatly expanded anteriorly. The medial third of the clavicle is thickened. The vertebrae are initially rounded and appear ovoid. One or two lower thoracic and upper lumbar vertebrae are often hypoplastic and wedge shaped, producing the gibbus deformity. The pelvis shows flared iliac wings, a small body of the ilium, and shallow oblique acetabula. The hips show coxa valga deformities. The metatarsals and phalanges are short and wide; the proximal ends of the metacarpals taper sharply, a classic finding called proximal pointing. The long tubular bones have expanded diaphyses. There is loss of normal angulation of the humerus at the shoulder. The radiologic changes are progressive, but the changes vary considerably from patient to patient at a given age. The lower extremities are generally more mildly affected than the upper extremities, except for the hips, which often show changes resembling aseptic necrosis of the femoral heads that correlate with severe hip disability clinically.

Diagnosis. The diagnosis can be suspected on clinical and radiologic grounds, supported by demonstration of mucopolysacchariduria (DS>HS), and established definitively by demonstration of the enzyme deficiency, using the commercially available phenyl-L-iduronide substrate. Enzyme activity can be measured in extracts of leukocytes or cultured fibroblasts.

Treatment. Only supportive and symptomatic treatment can be offered to patients, as no effective treatment for the storage abnormality is available.

SCHEIE'S SYNDROME (MPS I-S). This rare disorder is also due to a deficiency of alpha-L-iduronidase and is characterized by severe corneal clouding, deformity of the hands, and aortic valve disease. Symptoms appear between the ages of 5 and 15. The height is normal, as is the intelligence. The striking joint stiffness of the hands is similar to that seen in Hurler's syndrome but is complicated by the carpal tunnel syndrome with median nerve entrapment. Aortic stenosis, regurgitation, or both are present but are usually not symptomatic in early life. Life expectancy may be nearly normal. Diagnosis depends on the same criteria as for Hurler's syndrome. Corneal transplant and aortic valve replacement are reasonable, since intelligence is normal.

THE HURLER-SCHEIE COMPOUND (MPS I-H/S). Some patients with a phenotype that is intermediate between that of Hurler's and Scheie's syndromes are thought to represent compound heterozygotes, having inherited one Hurler and one Scheie gene from each parent.

HUNTER'S SYNDROME (MPS II). Hunter's syndrome is distinguished from Hurler's syndrome by three features: (1) slower progression with longer survival, (2) lack of corneal clouding, and (3) X-linked rather than autosomal recessive inheritance. A severe and a mild form exist. The severe form has most of the features of Hurler's syndrome, but they are slightly milder except for hearing impairment, which is more severe. The patients usually die by age 15. A much milder form has been reported with near-normal intelligence and near-normal survival. Diagnosis is made on the basis of the clinical findings, radiologic evidence of dysostosis multiplex, increased urinary GAG's, and demonstration of sulfoiduronate sulfatase deficiency on serum or on extracts of leukocytes or cultured fibroblasts. Carrier detection is still imperfect, but prenatal diagnostic tests are reliable.

SANFILIPPO'S SYNDROME (MPS III). This syndrome can be produced by a deficiency of at least four different enzymes, all of which participate in degradation of heparan sulfate (Table 198–1). Early development is normal but slows or halts between the ages of two and six years, after which mental deterioration is often rapid. Gait becomes unsteady, muscles atrophy, and the patient becomes bedridden. Death usually occurs by puberty. The head is large, the hair coarse, and hirsutism common. Visceromegaly is mild to absent. Cardiac involvement is rare. Height may be normal through the first decade and then falls behind. Skeletal findings of dysostosis multiplex are mild and include thickened calvarium, ovoid vertebral bodies, mild dysplasia of the pelvis, and mild rib changes. The clinical diagnosis may be suspected from the severe mental retardation, which appears disproportionate with relatively mild somatic and radiologic abnor-

TABLE 198–1. THE MUCOPOLYSACCHARIDOSES (MPS STORAGE DISEASES I TO VII)

Abbreviation	Eponym	Enzyme Deficiency	Major Storage Product	Urinary GAG's	Clinical Features
MPS I-H	Hurler's	α-L-Iduronidase	DS + HS	↑ 5–25X DS > HS	Onset 6–12 months, coarse features, rhinorrhea, grunting respiration, corneal clouding, cardiac disease, visceromegaly, dwarfism, dysostosis multiplex, progressive mental retardation after the first year; death by 5–10 years
MPS I-S (formerly MPS V)	Scheie's	α-L-Iduronidase	DS + HS	↑ 5–25X DS > HS	Onset 5–15 years, corneal clouding, stiff joints, clawhand, genu valgum, dysostosis multiplex, aortic valve disease; however, normal height, normal intelligence, and long survival (difficult to distinguish clinically from mild MPS VI)
MPS I-H/S	Hurler-Scheie	α-L-Iduronidase	DS + HS	↑ 5–25X DS > HS	Onset 2–4 years, all findings of MPS-H but milder, slower progression, and survival into 20's
MPS II, severe	Hunter's severe form	L-Sulfoiduronate sulfatase	HS + DS	↑ 5–25X DS = HS	Onset 2–4 years, clear corneas, deafness, all other features of MPS I-H, but milder; mental retardation progresses to profound state; death by 10–15 years
MPS II, mild	Hunter's mild form	L-Sulfoiduronate sulfatase	HS + DS	↑ 5–25X DS = HS	Onset in first decade, short stature, clear corneas, joint stiffness, dysostosis multiplex, visceromegaly, cardiac disease, nerve entrapments, near-normal intelligence; survival to 30's–60's, depending on heart involvement
MPS III-A	Sanfilippo's, type A	Heparan sulfate sulfamidase	HS	↑ 5–20X 85% HS	Onset 2–6 years, large head, normal height; Hurler-like features, dysostosis multiplex, hepatomegaly are all mild; mental retardation is rapidly progressive and severe; death at end of puberty
MPS III-B	Sanfilippo's, type B	N-acetyl-α-D-glucosaminidase	HS	↑ 5–20X 85% HS	Clinically indistinguishable from MPS III, type A
MPS III-C	Sanfilippo's, type C	Acetyl CoA: α-glucosamide N-acetyltransferase	HS	↑ 5–20X 85% HS	Clinically indistinguishable from MPS III, type A
MPS III-D	Sanfilippo's, type D	N-acetyl-α-D-glucosamine-6-sulfatase	HS	↑ 5–20X 85% HS	Clinically indistinguishable from MPS III, type A
MPS IV-A	Morquio's, classic form	N-acetylgalactosamine-6-sulfatase (gal-6-sulfatase)	KS + Ch 6-S	↑ 3–5X KS + Ch-S	Characteristic facies, short-trunk dwarfism, deformed thorax, corneal clouding, hearing deficit, aortic valve disease, unstable neck, spinal cord transection; intelligence is normal; death usually in 20's from cardiorespiratory problems
MPS IV-B	Morquio-like syndrome	β-Galactosidase deficiency	KS + Ch 4-S	↑ 2–5X KS = Ch-S	Short stature, corneal clouding, mild dysostosis multiplex, prominence of lower face, pectus carinatum, hip deformity, normal intelligence
MPS VI	Maroteaux-Lamy, severe	N-acetylgalactosamine-4-sulfatase (arylsulfatase B)	DS + ?Ch 4-S	↑ 4–20X 70–90% DS	Onset age 2–4 years, growth failure from age 4 slowly progressive, joint stiffness, corneal clouding, aortic valve disease, and severe hip deformity; dysostosis multiplex, striking white cell inclusions; intelligence normal; death in 20's
	Maroteaux-Lamy, mild	N-acetylgalactosamine-4-sulfatase (arylsulfatase B)	DS + ?Ch 4-S	↑ 4–20X 70–90% DS	Onset 5–7 years, short stature, severe osseous changes, especially in the hips; nerve entrapment, corneal clouding, aortic valve disease; normal intelligence, long survival; difficult to distinguish from MPS I-S
MPS VII	Sly	β-Glucuronidase	HS, DS, Ch-S	↑ 6–8X HS, DS Ch 4/6-S	Onset 1–2 years, mild to moderate Hurler-like features, dysostosis multiplex, pectus carinatum, visceromegaly, cardiac murmurs, short stature, moderate mental retardation; slowly progressive after infancy; striking granulocyte inclusions; milder forms exist, as does a more severe form with neonatal ascites and death within two years.

DS = dermatan sulfate; HS = heparan sulfate; Ch-S = chondroitin sulfate; KS = keratan sulfate.

malities, supported by the presence of heparan sulfaturia, and established definitively by demonstration of the specific enzyme deficiency.

MORQUIO'S SYNDROME, CLASSIC FORM (MPS IV-A). The predominant clinical features relate to skeletal abnormalities and to symptoms of spinal cord compression resulting from instability of the neck. Intelligence is normal. By the age of two years, pigeon chest deformity, genu valgum, and gait disturbance appear. Knees and wrists enlarge. The neck appears short, and the head seems to sit on the deformed thorax. Universal platyspondylisis, evident on x-ray examination, kyphoscoliosis, and contractures at the knees and hips all contribute to dwarfism. The face is unusual because of mid-face hypoplasia, depressed nasal bridge, flared nares, and prominence of the lower third of the face on side view. The teeth are wide spaced and the dental enamel thin. Corneal clouding is mild but slowly progressive. Long survival is rare, with death between the ages of 20 and 40 from cardiopulmonary complications. The cardiac disease is valvular (aortic regurgitation). The respiratory problems arise from thoracic deformities and from neurotrophic myelopathy caused by atlantoaxial subluxation. Diagnosis depends on the clinical and radiologic features, which are characteristic; the finding of keratan sulfaturia (which may disappear in adolescence); and the deficiency for N-acetylgalactosamine-6-sulfatase, which is active on both GalNAc 6-S in chondroitin sulfate and Gal 6-S in keratan sulfate. The enzymatic assay is available in only a few laboratories. Treatment is symptomatic. Posterior cervical fusion should be done early in the disease to prevent spinal cord damage. Correction of the genu valgum requires a single operation at about six years.

THE MORQUIO-LIKE SYNDROME WITH BETA-GALACTOSIDASE DEFICIENCY (MPS IV-B). Short stature, mild pectus carinatum, corneal clouding, odontoid hypoplasia with cervical instability, mild dysostosis multiplex, moderate lumbar kyphosis, and mild genu valgum are all features that are found in this Morquio-like disease resulting from beta-galactosidase deficiency. Absent are hearing deficit, dental abnormalities, cardiac murmurs, hepatomegaly, and joint laxity. Keratan sulfaturia is present. The diagnosis is based on normal N-acetylgalactosamine-6-sulfatase levels and reduced beta-galactosidase levels. Presumably this disorder reflects a mutation that impairs the activity of the enzyme on galactose linkages in keratan sulfate but spares its activity on GM_1 ganglioside. Thus the findings of chondrodystrophy predominate, and the neurologic manifestations of GM_1 gangliosidosis are absent.

THE MAROTEAUX-LAMY SYNDROME, SEVERE AND MILD TYPES (MPS VI). Maroteaux and colleagues recognized a new form of mucopolysaccharidosis in 1963 that resembled Hurler's syndrome but differed in that intelligence of the dwarfed, deformed patients was spared; the urinary GAG was almost exclusively dermatan sulfate; and the leukocytes exhibited striking metachromatic inclusions. Affected patients often die in their 20's with cardiac failure. Many suffer cervical cord compression and hydrocephalus resulting from thickened meninges. Since specific enzymatic assays have become available both for arylsulfatase B, missing in MPS VI, and alpha-L-iduronidase, missing in MPS I, it has become clear that many patients with milder forms of MPS VI exist who might previously have been thought to have Scheie's syndrome. No specific treatment is available for the storage abnormality. However, shunting for hydrocephalus, spinal fusion for atlantoaxial subluxation, corneal transplants for visual handicap, and cardiac valve and hip replacement are all reasonable when required, because intelligence is preserved and patients with milder forms of the abnormality have the potential for long survival.

BETA-GLUCURONIDASE DEFICIENCY MUCOPOLYSACCHARIDOSIS (MPS VII). Most patients present by age three with a Hurler-like illness manifest by frequent upper respiratory infections, chest deformities, cardiac murmurs, hepatosplenomegaly, hernias, dysostosis multiplex, and mild to moderate mental retardation. Many develop corneal clouding. About 20 patients, showing a wide range of clinical severity, have been recognized. Most of the patients have shown slow progression in clinical abnormalities after the age of six. The natural history beyond the teens is yet to be determined. Urinary GAG's have been increased, and heparan sulfate, dermatan sulfate, and chondroitin sulfate have all been reported to be increased in urine. Striking inclusions in leukocytes are typical, as in MPS VI. The diagnosis depends on the demonstration of the enzyme deficiency. Carrier detection and prenatal diagnosis are available.

OTHER DISORDERS RELATED TO THE MUCOPOLYSACCHARIDOSES. Mucolipidosis II (also called I-cell disease) and mucolipidosis III (also called pseudo-Hurler polydystrophy) are severe and milder forms, respectively, of a Hurler-like disease with many features in common with the mucopolysaccharidoses. However, these patients do not have mucopolysacchariduria.

These disorders result, not from a deficiency for a single lysosomal enzyme like the mucopolysaccharidoses, but from a defect in the processing N-acetylglucosaminyl phosphotransferase that normally targets acid hydrolases to lysosomes. Failure to add the phosphomannosyl-recognition marker that normally directs their segregation into lysosomes allows acid hydrolases to be secreted instead. As a consequence, there is an intracellular deficiency of most of the enzymes involved in the degradation of GAG's (and an extracellular excess), which is part of a general pattern of deficiency involving nearly all lysosomal enzymes. The absence of mucopolysacchariduria, and the 10- to 50-fold elevations of levels of acid hydrolases in serum, distinguish these two disorders from the single-enzyme deficiency mucopolysaccharidoses.

Another group of disorders, not classified with the mucopolysaccharidoses, may produce a Hurler-like picture, including mental retardation, visceromegaly, and dysostosis multiplex. These disorders result from single-enzyme deficiencies for enzymes involved in the catabolism of the oligosaccharide components of glycoproteins. Included are mannosidosis, fucosidosis, and the more recently delineated group of sialidoses (one of which has been described under the name mucolipidosis I). The sialidoses result from a deficiency of oligosaccharide N-acetylneuraminidase. The primary storage products in these disorders are oligosaccharides derived from glycoproteins. However, there is some storage of keratan sulfate as well. It appears that these enzymes are required for degradation of some oligosaccharide side chains on keratan sulfate. Impaired degradation of keratan sulfate may explain the dysostosis multiplex that mimics the skeletal findings of the mucopolysaccharidoses in these disorders.

Kelly TE: The mucopolysaccharidoses and mucolipidoses. Clin Orthop 114:116, 1976. *A nice summary of clinically relevant information.*
McKusick VA, Neufeld EF, Kelly TE: The mucopolysaccharide storage diseases. In Stanbury JB, Wyngaarden JB, Fredrickson DS, et al. (eds.): The Metabolic Basis of Inherited Disease. 5th ed. New York, McGraw-Hill Book Company, 1983. *A comprehensive chapter with good historical perspective.*
Neufeld EF, Muenzer J: The mucopolysaccharide storage diseases. In Scriver CR, Beaudet AL, Sly WS, et al. (eds.): The Metabolic Basis of Inherited Disease. 6th ed. New York, McGraw-Hill Book Company, 1988. *A current, comprehensive treatment of biochemical and genetic information.*

199 THE MARFAN SYNDROME

Peter H. Byers

DEFINITION. The Marfan syndrome is a dominantly inherited connective tissue disorder characterized by musculoskeletal abnormalities (arachnodactyly, tall stature, scoliosis, pectus deformities, and ligamentous laxity), cardiovascular abnormalities (mitral valve prolapse and regurgitation, aortic valve insufficiency, and aortic dilatation, aneurysm, and dissection), lens dislocation, and myopia.

ETIOLOGY AND PATHOGENESIS. For most patients the molecular defect is not known. However, increased production of hyaluronic acid by cultured fibroblasts, the synthesis of an α2(I) chain of type I collagen that contains a small insertion, and alterations in the cross-linking of collagen and elastin in the aorta have each been identified in at least one patient.

PREVALENCE. The Marfan syndrome affects about 1 in 15,000 individuals without racial or ethnic predilection.

PATHOLOGY. The mitral and aortic valves are characterized by "myxomatous degeneration" or the appearance of large pools of nonfibrous material that separates the normal cells of the valves. The valves may be thickened. In the absence of dissection there is accumulation of metachromatic material in the aortic media and disruption of the normal elastic laminae. Aortic dissection characteristically begins in the ascending aorta and may proceed in both directions. Death frequently results from cardiac tamponade due to hemopericardium, coronary occlusion, occlusion of the arteries to the brain, internal hemorrhage, or loss of perfusion of multiple abdominal organs.

CLINICAL MANIFESTIONS. The Marfan syndrome is highly variable in its clinical manifestations, and affected members within the same family may differ in the degree to which they express the mutation; the differences between families may be explained, in part, by different mutations in connective tissue genes. The diagnosis can be made occasionally in newborns because of lens dislocation, mitral valve prolapse, scoliosis, and tall stature with arachnodactyly. More commonly, affected infants may be tall, but cardiac findings are minimal. Many have mild to moderate scoliosis with pectus deformities (excavatum or carinatum); progression of scoliosis or pectus deformities may be rapid during the adolescent growth spurt. About half the patients with the Marfan syndrome have ocular lens dislocation, usually in a superior and nasal direction and generally nonprogressive. Cataract formation and glaucoma are occasional complications of ectopia lentis. Mitral prolapse is seen in virtually all patients with the Marfan syndrome and in some progresses to symptomatic mitral regurgitation; associated rhythm disturbances may be symptomatic.

The major life-threatening complication of the Marfan syndrome is aortic dissection and rupture, and most deaths result from cardiovascular disease. The risk of dissection is well correlated with aortic diameter. In some children aortic root diameters, measured by echocardiography, are greater than normal but, more commonly, aortic diameters do not exceed the normal range (20 to 37 mm) until adulthood and usually enlarge gradually, although the rate may vary. Aortic dissection in the Marfan syndrome is occasionally asymptomatic, but usually there is prolonged, severe substernal chest pain of a tearing or searing quality, often with radiation into the neck, back, and arms. It is often accompanied by diaphoresis, hypotension, and shock. Blood pressure in the two arms may differ. Rarely, pregnancy may be complicated by dissection, even in the presence of a normal aortic diameter.

DIFFERENTIAL DIAGNOSIS. The Marfan syndrome is one of several disorders in which the characteristic habitus is seen. *Contractural arachnodactyly* is a dominantly inherited disorder characterized by arachnodactyly, joint contracture rather than joint laxity, small cup-shaped ears, pectus deformity, mild scoliosis, and mitral valve prolapse, but lens dislocation is absent, and aortic dilatation is not a complication. *Homocystinuria* (see Ch. 194) is characterized by autosomal recessive inheritance, tight joints, peripheral vascular disease, thrombosis of arterial vessels, and, often, mild mental retardation. The diagnosis is confirmed by detection of excessive homocystine in the urine. In the *nonasthenic form* of the Marfan syndrome, body habitus is normal, but lens dislocation and mitral prolapse are common, and death from aortic aneurysm and dissection often establishes the diagnosis. Aortic dissection generally occurs in the fifth to seventh decades; the disorder is inherited in an autosomal dominant fashion. The *mitral valve prolapse syndrome* is commonly mistaken for the Marfan syndrome because of the presence of mitral valve prolapse, tall stature, and some of the mild skeletal features of the Marfan syndrome. The disorder is inherited in an autosomal dominant fashion; the absence of lens dislocation and progressive aortic root dilatation distinguish it from the Marfan syndrome. Patients with the *Stickler syndrome* may have a marfanoid habitus, degenerative arthritis of multiple joints, cleft palate, and, generally, vitreal degeneration. The *marfanoid habitus* may be seen in some patients with sickle cell disease, the Klinefelter syndrome (the 47 XXY karyotype, see Ch. 36), and multiple endocrine adenomatosis type IIB (see Ch. 241).

TREATMENT. Treatment of the Marfan syndrome has several objectives: control of excessive height, prevention of glaucoma, regulation of blood pressure, and prevention of aortic dissection. Excessive height may be controlled by administration of testosterone (to boys) and estrogens (to girls) prior to puberty to hasten epiphyseal closure. Routine ophthalmologic examination is important to assure that dislocation of the lens into the anterior chamber does not occur and to treat any retinal detachment (the consequence of the high myopia that accompanies the syndrome). Rarely the lenses must be removed because of recurrent anterior chamber displacement or because the lens edge is in the center of the visual field and adequate correction cannot be achieved. Blood pressure should always be maintained in the normal range because hypertension is known to increase the risk of dissection, even in normal persons. There is some indication that treatment with agents that decrease cardiac contractility (beta-adrenergic blockers, for example) may delay the rate of aortic progression, but this is an area of controversy, and appropriate controlled studies have not yet been published; nonetheless, in some centers such treatment is routine.

Recently, the advances in surgical technique have made replacement of diseased portions of the aorta a routine treatment that appears to provide increased life expectancy. Replacement should be considered when aortic root diameter reaches approximately 55 mm and prior to decompensation of the left ventricle as a result of aortic valve insufficiency. A composite graft that includes an aortic valve is now used. In some patients, mitral valve function is compromised and the valve requires replacement. Techniques for replacement of large portions of the aorta have also helped to prolong survival.

PROGNOSIS. The prognosis in the Marfan syndrome depends largely on the vascular complications. In one major study the mean age of death for all affected individuals was in the early 40's, and virtually all died of the cardiovascular complications. The judicious use of surgical replacement of the ascending aorta and, if needed, of additional parts of the aorta appears to prolong survival. If the controlled studies of treatment with beta-adrenergic blockage demonstrate effectiveness, then another treatment of the cardiovascular complications will be available.

Patients with the Marfan syndrome should be observed yearly by an internist, a family physician, or a geneticist. Echocardiography should be performed yearly to follow aortic root diameter and the magnitude of mitral regurgitation and aortic insufficiency. Patients should see an ophthalmologist regularly and should consult with a cardiac surgeon as the aortic root diameter passes 50 to 55 mm.

Pregnancy usually is completed without complication, but women in whom the aortic diameter is greater than 40 mm (above the upper limits of normal) may be at greater risk for complications. All pregnancies should be followed in a high-risk center.

Prenatal diagnosis, the only form of prevention, is not currently available. Genetic counseling is important for all members of the proband's family to identify those who are affected.

Gott VL, Pyeritz RE, Magovern GJ Jr, et al.: Surgical treatment of aneurysms of the ascending aorta in the Marfan syndrome: Results of composite-graft repair in 50 patients. N Engl J Med 314:1070, 1986. *A review of the surgical approach to the patient with the Marfan syndrome; outcome, complications, criteria for selection, and longevity.*

Maumenee IH: The eye in the Marfan syndrome. Trans Am Ophthalmol Soc 79:684, 1981. *The most comprehensive review of the eye findings in the Marfan syndrome and their differential diagnosis.*

McKusick VA: Heritable Disorders of Connective Tissue. 4th ed. St. Louis, CV Mosby Company, 1972, pp 61–200. *Still the most comprehensive description of patients with the Marfan syndrome. Many case histories, easy and interesting to read; anecdotal.*

Pyeritz RE, McKusick VA: The Marfan syndrome: Diagnosis and management. N Engl J Med 300:772, 1979. *A more formal statistical compilation of the frequency of physical findings and complications in patients with the Marfan syndrome. Recommendations for management and follow-up.*

200 EHLERS-DANLOS SYNDROME

Peter H. Byers

DEFINITION. Ehlers-Danlos syndrome (EDS) is a group of more than ten inherited connective tissue disorders characterized by abnormalities of the skin, ligaments, and internal organs. The clinical manifestations include skin fragility, abnormal scar formation, excessive bruising, joint laxity, and, in one variety, rupture of viscera and arteries (Table 200–1).

ETIOLOGY. EDS results from mutations in the synthesis and processing of types I and III collagens, the major proteins of skin, ligaments, tendons, blood vessels, and viscera. The molecular bases of EDS types I, II, III, V, and VIII are not known. The known defects include mutations affecting the structure, synthesis, processing, or stability of type III collagen (EDS type IV); deficient hydroxylation of lysyl residues in type I and type III collagen (EDS type VI); defective conversion of type I procollagen to collagen (EDS type VII); defective collagen cross-linking and abnormal cellular utilization of copper (EDS type IX); and a functional defect in fibronectin (EDS type X).

PREVALENCE. The aggregate frequency of EDS is about one in 5000 births. EDS type III, benign familial hypermobility,

TABLE 200–1. CLINICAL FEATURES, MODE OF INHERITANCE, AND BIOCHEMICAL DISORDERS OF THE EHLERS-DANLOS SYNDROME

Type	Clinical Features	Inheritance	Biochemical Disorders
I. Gravis	Soft, velvety, hyperextensible skin; easy bruising; "cigarette-paper" scars; hypermobile joints; varicose veins; prematurity	AD	Not known
II. Mitis	Similar to type I, but less severe	AD	Not known
III. Familial hypermobility	Soft skin, no scarring, marked large and small joint hypermobility	AD	Not known
IV. Arterial	Thin, translucent skin with visible veins; marked bruising; skin and joints have normal extensibility; arterial, bowel and uterine rupture	AD (AR)	Abnormal type III collagen synthesis, secretion or structure
V. X linked	Similar to type II	XLR	Not known
VI. Ocular	Soft, velvety, hyperextensible skin; hypermobile joints, scoliosis; ocular fragility and keratoconus	AR	Lysyl hydroxylase deficiency
VII. Arthrochalasis multiplex congenita	Congenital hip dislocation, joint hypermobility; soft skin with normal scarring	AD	Abnormal structure of the aminoterminal cleavage site in pro $\alpha1(I)$ and pro $\alpha2(I)$
VIII. Periodontal	Generalized periodontitis; skin similar to type II	AD	Not known
IX. Cutis laxa, bladder diverticula	Soft, extensible, lax skin; bladder diverticula and rupture; short arms, limited pronation and supination; broad clavicles; occipital horns	XLR	Abnormal copper utilization with defect in lysyl oxidase
X. Fibronectin defect	Similar to type II	AR	Defect in fibronectin

accounts for most patients identified as having EDS; some forms are uncommon (EDS types IV, VI, VII, and VIII); others have been found in only a few families (EDS types IX and X). There is no racial or ethnic predisposition for any of the common types of EDS.

PATHOLOGY AND PATHOGENESIS. Dermal collagen fibrils in patients with EDS types I, II, and III are larger than normal and irregular in outline when viewed by electron microscopy. In EDS type IV, skin is thin and collagen fibril diameter is frequently smaller than normal. Arterial wall thickness is usually less than normal, and tensile strength is diminished. Fibroblastic cells in dermis frequently have marked dilatation of the rough endoplasmic reticulum as a result of defective secretion of type III procollagen. Death results from arterial rupture (with the presenting signs depending on the site of rupture), bowel rupture with sepsis, and rupture of the gravid uterus during late gestation or delivery. In EDS type VI the ultrastructural abnormalities of collagen fibrils are similar to those seen in EDS types I, II, and III. There are no specific pathologic features of the other types of EDS.

CLINICAL MANIFESTATIONS. The clinical manifestations of each type of EDS are different (Table 200–1); it is important to identify patients with EDS type IV because of the grave consequences of the disease and to identify those with EDS types VI, V, and IX because of the risk of recurrence in their families.

EDS types I and II are characterized by marked joint laxity, soft, velvety, and hyperextensible skin, easy bruising, and "cigarette-paper" scars in areas of trauma. They differ in severity. Prematurity is common in EDS type I but rare in EDS type II. The major complications of both are the recurrent joint dislocations, skin fragility, and a high frequency of early-onset osteoarthritis. Many of the manifestations are more severe in childhood and decrease following puberty. At present the diagnosis depends on recognition of the appropriate clinical findings; electron microscopic studies of dermis may be confirmatory but are not specific. Patients with EDS type III are commonly seen by rheumatologists because of the joint discomfort and early onset degenerative joint disease.

EDS type IV, the most severe form, usually results from heterozygous (dominant) mutations in the genes of type III collagen; autosomal recessive inheritance has been described but is rare. The diagnosis is confirmed by finding decreased amounts of type III collagen in skin or by identifying a defect in the structure, synthesis, or secretion of type III procollagen by cultured dermal fibroblasts. In the newborn period some infants already have bruising, but most affected infants are difficult to identify. By adolescence the veins are readily visible on the trunk and extremities, and bruising is common. Vascular or bowel rupture is rare during childhood. Arterial fragility may manifest as sudden death, stroke, shock from retroperitoneal or intra-abdominal bleeding, or compartmental syndromes, depending on the site of vessel rupture. Prompt surgical intervention may be lifesaving, although tissue friability may make repairs difficult. Pregnancy may be complicated by arterial or uterine rupture, either of which is often fatal. Recurrent abdominal pain may result from repeated mural hemorrhage in the small intestine. Survival beyond the fifth decade is rare.

EDS type VI is an autosomal recessive disorder characterized by a marfanoid habitus, skin and joint findings similar to those in EDS type II, ocular fragility, and scoliosis. The diagnosis is made by finding decreased amounts of hydroxylysine in skin and confirmed by low levels of lysyl hydroxylase measured in cultured dermal fibroblasts. Late complications may include vascular rupture, and blindness from retinal detachment or globe rupture.

The initial presentation of EDS type VII is often in the newborn period, the patient having bilateral hip dislocation and marked joint laxity. The hips are often difficult to stabilize, and recurrent dislocation may continue at the hips and other joints. When suspected clinically the diagnosis can be confirmed in some patients by identifying intermediates in the conversion of type I procollagen to collagen in skin and confirming the defect in cultured dermal fibroblasts.

EDS type VIII is characterized by the combination of noninflammatory gingival loss (often leading to loss of teeth) and the cutaneous and joint signs of the EDS type II phenotype.

EDS type IX is noted in childhood with skin hyperextensibility and laxity, drooping facies, and minor skeletal anomalies. Evidence of bladder dysfunction may be present by the age of six years, and diverticula of the bladder and hydronephrosis may be apparent by that age. Mild chronic diarrhea, orthostatic hypotension, short upper arms with limited pronation and supination, and the growth of occipital inferior horns become apparent during adolescence. Intelligence is usually in the normal range; inheritance is X-linked recessive. The diagnosis is made by the low serum copper and ceruloplasmin levels and confirmed by low lysyl oxidase levels in cultured dermal fibroblasts. Maintenance of normal urinary drainage is important to prevent renal failure, and continuing bladder drainage may be essential to prevent rupture. There is some variation in severity among families.

DIFFERENTIAL DIAGNOSIS. The differential diagnosis is generally limited to the varieties of EDS, although some patients with the Marfan syndrome have marked joint laxity and others with forms of osteogenesis imperfecta have joint laxity and easy bruising. Patients with EDS type IV and EDS types I and II are often investigated for a bleeding diathesis before the correct diagnosis is made. Because of joint instability and laxity many patients with EDS types I, II, III, VI, and VII are investigated for developmental delay before it is recognized that they have a form of EDS.

TREATMENT. The gaping skin wounds that occur in some forms of EDS should be approximated carefully, and the removable sutures should be left in place for twice the usual time. Recurrent dislocations can often be repaired surgically although further recurrence is more common than in unaffected individuals. Arterial rupture in patients with EDS type IV needs to be treated surgically unless bleeding is controlled by compartmental limitation (e.g., some retroperitoneal bleeding). The repair of affected arteries is often difficult because of extreme friability. If colon rupture recurs, the colon should be excised to prevent further episodes. Rupture of the small bowel is very rare. Some patients with EDS type VI respond to ascorbic acid (1 to 4 grams per day) with some symptomatic improvement and increased excretion of hydroxylysine in the urine. There is no metabolic treatment for other forms of EDS, and management is largely symptomatic.

PROGNOSIS. The prognosis in EDS depends on the specific type with which the patient is affected. Life expectancy is considerably shortened in EDS type IV because of organ and vessel rupture and may be decreased in EDS type VI; in all others, life expectancy is normal. With the exception of EDS type VI, no specific therapy is available that affects the natural history of the condition.

Prevention by prenatal diagnosis is feasible for some types of EDS. Heterozygosity for the EDS type VI mutation has been recognized by examination of amniotic fluid cells in a family at risk for recurrence. The structural mutations in EDS type VII and in EDS type IV should be recognizable by studies of collagens synthesized by chorionic villus cells in culture, but this approach has not yet been used. Analysis of copper uptake and distribution by amniotic fluid cells should facilitate prenatal diagnosis of EDS type IX. All families should have genetic counseling once a proband is identified.

Byers PH, Holbrook KA: Molecular basis of clinical heterogenity in the Ehlers-Danlos syndrome. Ann NY Acad Sci 460:298, 1985. *The most comprehensive and up-to-date review of the molecular lesions in EDS.*

Hollister DW, Byers PH, Holbrook KA: Genetic disorders of collagen metabolism. Adv Hum Gene 12:1, 1982. *Detailed biochemical and clinical description of the different forms of EDS.*

McKusick VA: Heritable Disorders of Connective Tissue. 4th ed. St Louis, C. V. Mosby Company, 1972, pp 292–371. *Although the classification is not up to date, the richness of clinical detail is unsurpassed. A delight to read because of the many case histories and the personal touch.*

201 OSTEOGENESIS IMPERFECTA

David W. Rowe

Osteogenesis imperfecta is a heritable disorder of connective tissue that results primarily in fragile bones that break with minimal trauma. The disease may be limited to a few fractures in childhood, cause 50 to 100 fractures by adulthood with severe long-bone deformity, or cause death in the newborn. The prevalence is 5 per 100,000 live births, and there is no known racial or ethnic predilection. Interest in this disease is increasing as advances in molecular biology are applied to defining the underlying abnormalities within the type I collagen genes. There is also the hope that understanding the mutations of mild osteogenesis imperfecta will give insight into certain forms of osteoporosis that have a familial or genetic component.

PATHOGENESIS. The tissues that are abnormal in osteogenesis imperfecta are composed primarily of type I collagen. This collagen type is a triple helical molecule formed by two genetically distinct but related polypeptide chains in a ratio of two alpha-1 (I) and one alpha-2 (I) chains. The mildest form of osteogenesis imperfecta (type I—see below) appears to result from underproduction of type I collagen owing to reduced accumulation of alpha-1 (I) collagen mRNA within the cytoplasm. In the more severe forms of osteogenesis imperfecta (types II, III, and IV), there are mutations within the helical regions of either the alpha-1 (I) or the alpha-2 (I) chain. These changes result from either a partial gene deletion or a nucleotide point mutation that alters an amino acid essential for the helical conformation of the alpha chains. Molecules containing a mutant alpha chain do not form normal triple helical molecules. A molecule containing a mutant chain can interfere with the interactions of adjacent molecules, thus weakening the entire structure. The severity of the clinical defect is probably related to the qualitative nature of the mutation and the extent to which the abnormal chains accumulate within specific tissues (Table 201–1).

TYPES AND CLINICAL MANIFESTATIONS. The terms *osteogenesis imperfecta tarda* or *congenita* have been replaced by a classification scheme based on relatively distinct syndromes that reflect *fundamentally different defects in type I collagen* biosynthesis. Osteogenesis imperfecta type I is the mildest form and is associated with nondeforming fractures during childhood which cease after puberty. Fractures can reappear with trauma and in postmenopausal women. In most cases a dominant family history can be elicited having the associated features of blue sclerae, joint laxity, and thin skin, findings that are less obvious in older affected individuals. More variable are hearing abnormalities, short stature, and dentinogenesis imperfecta. Sporadic cases occur and presumably reflect a new mutation. By contrast, the most severe form of osteogenesis imperfecta (type II) results in infants that do not survive the newborn period. Their bones have a crumpled appearance on roentgenography and are so weak that dismemberment may occur. The disorder is usually acquired as a sporadic new mutation, although cases have been observed that suggest a recessive mode of inheritance. In osteogenesis imperfecta type III, there are severe deformities of long bones, marked short stature, and moderate joint laxity. Gray sclerae, impaired hearing, and dentinogenesis imperfecta are frequently present. Fractures and deformity are usually present at birth such that ambulation is never possible. Severe scoliosis can progress to cause respiratory failure. The inheritance is recessive. Osteogenesis imperfecta type IV is less severe, but usually results in moderate long-bone deformity. Ambulation is possible but may require external bracing or internal fixation of the long bones. Blue sclerae, lax joints, and hearing impairment are less common, while dentinogenesis imperfecta is more frequently found. Both dominant and recessive modes of inheritance occur. This is the most heterogeneous group and any individual case may have features of either type I or type III.

DIAGNOSIS. The diagnosis of each form of osteogenesis imperfecta is based on the history, physical examination, family pedigree, and x-ray features. The bone biopsy is not usually of diagnostic aid. Only the milder forms of this disease should pose a diagnostic problem with other disorders that cause minimal bone deformity or fractures. The bowing and fractures associated with osteomalacia or rickets are differentiated by roentgenography and the biochemical measures of calcium, phosphorus, PTH, and vitamin D. Juvenile, disuse,

TABLE 201–1. CLINICAL CLASSIFICATION OF OSTEOGENESIS IMPERFECTA

Type	Description	Inheritance	Suspected Mutation
I	Mild, nondeforming	AD	Deficient amounts of alpha-1 (I) mRNA
II	Lethal	NM, AR	Mutation within helical domain of alpha-1 (I)
III	Severe long-bone deformity and scoliosis	NM, AR	Poorly defined
IV	Mild with long-bone deformity	AD	Mutation within helical domain of alpha-2 (I)

AD = autosomal dominant; AR = autosomal recessive; NM = new mutation.

and steroid-induced osteoporosis can be distinguished by history. Other rare diagnoses to be considered are infantile cortical hyperostosis (Caffey's disease) and hypophosphatasia. Studies of collagen synthesis and collagen mRNA in cultured fibroblasts plus analysis of restriction fragment length polymorphisms for the type I collagen genes are beginning to provide the means for a specific diagnosis for the various forms of the disease. However, most of these methods remain experimental, and one must rely primarily on ultrasonography for intrauterine diagnosis of the severe forms (type II and type III) of the disease.

TREATMENT. The use of supplemental calcium, vitamin D, fluoride, anabolic steroids, calcitonin, and pyrophosphate has not been shown to provide a satisfactory response. Since many of these drugs were used in heterogeneous groups of patients with osteogenesis imperfecta, there may be subgroups of patients who could benefit from certain medical regimens. At present, therapy is primarily orthopedic with external bracing, and surgical straightening with intramedullary splinting (rodding) of the long-bone deformities. Use of lightweight plastic bracing will assume a greater role in promoting ambulation. However, attempts to halt the progression of scoliosis in osteogenesis imperfecta have not been successful. In all forms of osteogenesis imperfecta maintenance of good muscle tone and range of motion is crucial for the optimal use of the extremities. Creative use of physical therapy, especially in the form of swimming, may be the most useful preventive measure in this disorder.

Akeson WH, Bornstein P, Glimcher MJ: Symposium on Heritable Disorders of Connective Tissue. St. Louis, C. V. Mosby Company, 1982. *See Chapters 20–23 for a general review of clinical, morphologic, and biochemical aspects of osteogenesis imperfecta.*

Albright JA, Millar EA: Osteogenesis imperfecta. Clin Orthop 159:2, 1981. *A collection of numerous articles on the pathology and treatment of this disease.*

Byers PH, Bonadio JF: The molecular basis of clinical heterogeneity in osteogenesis imperfecta: Mutations in type I collagen genes have different effects on collagen processing. In Lloyd JK, Scriver CR (eds.): Genetic and Metabolic Disease in Pediatrics. London, Butterworths International Medical Reviews, 1985. *Most current and best-written review of the molecular basis of osteogenesis imperfecta.*

Smith R, Francis MJO, Houghton GP: The Brittle Bone Syndrome. London, Butterworth Co., 1982. *A comprehensive review by one group of investigators having a large experience with osteogenesis imperfecta. Chapter 7 has a good differential diagnosis.*

202 PSEUDOXANTHOMA ELASTICUM

Jouni Uitto

Pseudoxanthoma elasticum (PXE) (synonyms: Grönblad-Strandberg syndrome, systemic elastorrhexis) is a generalized progressive connective tissue disorder primarily affecting the elastic fibers. Clinically, PXE manifests as characteristic cutaneous lesions, ocular changes, and widespread vascular abnormalities. The relative severity of these changes results in a variety of clinical pictures. The onset of the disease may be in early childhood, and in most cases the cutaneous changes are evident before the age of 30 years. The exact incidence of PXE is not known, although estimates are about 1 in 160,000 persons. The male-female ratio is probably 1:1.

CLINICAL MANIFESTATIONS. ***Skin.*** The primary cutaneous lesions are relatively small (1 to 3 mm) yellowish papules that give the affected area a pebbly, "plucked chicken skin" appearance. The primary lesions tend to coalesce into larger plaques, and the skin of the involved areas becomes thickened and leathery (Fig. 202–1). Gradually, the affected skin becomes redundant, lax, and inelastic. The predilection sites are the face, neck, axillary folds, lower abdomen, and thighs. The nasolabial folds and chin creases may be strikingly accentuated. Yellowish lesions similar to those noted on the skin can also be seen on the mucous membranes.

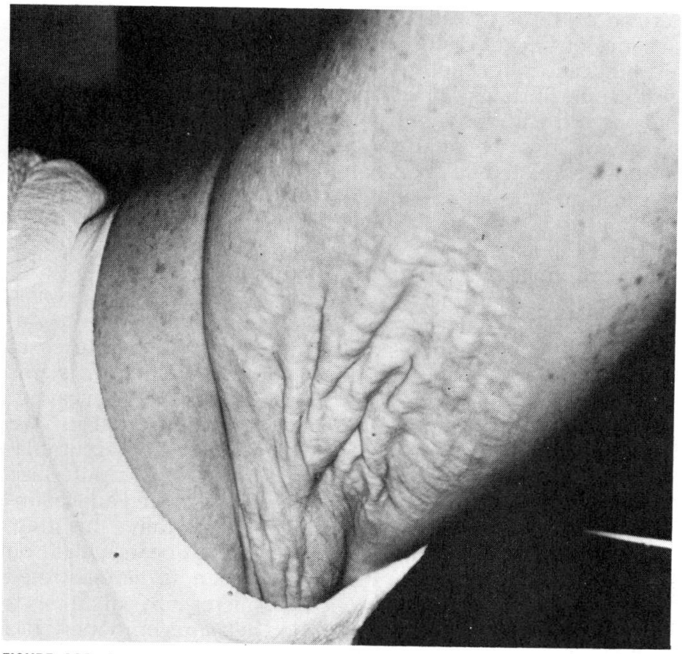

FIGURE 202–1. Typical cutaneous manifestations of pseudoxanthoma elasticum. The lesion demonstrates redundant and inelastic skin in the axillary fold.

Eye. The ocular changes are characterized by angioid streaks, i.e., grayish or brownish-red, poorly defined streaks radiating across the fundus of the eye. Their development usually starts later than that of the cutaneous lesions, often during the third or fourth decade. The ocular changes are commonly bilateral and include hemorrhages and exudates in Bruch's membrane, an elastin-rich structure located between the retina and the choroid. The degenerative changes of the eye frequently lead to impaired vision, and complete blindness, although rare, is one of the major complications of PXE. Angioid streaks may be present without noticeable cutaneous changes, but other accompanying observations, such as vascular changes, may lead to correct diagnosis of PXE. Angioid streaks can also be associated with other diseases—for example, Paget's disease of bone, sickle cell anemia, tumoral calcinosis, lead poisoning, and idiopathic thrombocytopenia.

Vascular Manifestations. The early manifestations of arterial involvement include hypertension, weak peripheral pulses, and, occasionally, intermittent claudication. The most devastating complications develop as a result of coronary occlusion or cerebral hemorrhage; the most frequent complication is recurrent bleeding from the gastrointestinal tract. A common site of the gastrointestinal bleeding is the gastric mucosa, where the elastic fibers of the arteries are particularly affected. Bleeding from the urinary tract can also occur.

INHERITANCE. Most cases of PXE are inherited as an autosomal recessive disease. However, autosomal dominant inheritance has been documented in a few families. The classification proposed by Pope divides the dominantly inherited form of PXE into two categories. The type I dominant form is characterized by classic cutaneous changes associated with severe vascular complications. The type II dominant form, which is more frequent than type I, is characterized by focal cutaneous involvement associated with hyperextensible skin, blue sclerae, high arched palate, and loose-jointedness. The type I recessively inherited form is the classic, most frequently encountered type of pseudoxanthoma elasticum, characterized by typical cutaneous, vascular, and ocular manifestations. The type II recessively inherited disease, characterized by generalized cutaneous involvement and by the absence of vascular and ocular manifestations, is very rare.

In addition to the inherited forms, several cases with cutaneous findings consistent with PXE but without family history and without vascular or ocular involvement have been reported. In some of these cases, the development of skin lesions is related to external trauma, such as exposure to Norwegian saltpeter. Patients with an unusual perforating variant of cutaneous PXE have been described. In these patients the lesions are confined to the abdomen, most often in a periumbilical distribution. Periumbilical perforating PXE appears to be a distinct acquired form of the disease.

PATHOLOGY. Histopathologic examination of the involved skin demonstrates an accumulation of structures in the middle or lower dermis that stain positively with stains specific for elastic fibers, e.g., Verhoeff stain. In contrast to the elastic fibers in normal skin, the elastic material in PXE appears irregularly clumped and fragmented. The accumulation of elastic fibers has also been quantitated by computerized morphometric analyses and by assay of desmosine, an elastin-specific cross-link compound. Characteristically the fragmented elastic fibers contain calcium that appears bluish on routine hematoxylin-eosin stain and that can be demonstrated by calcium-specific stains. Electron microscopy of affected skin demonstrates that the amorphous elastin component has been replaced by bundles of granular material with staining properties different from normal elastin. Also, foci containing calcium hydroxyapatite crystals can be detected in the elastic fibers. These morphologic findings thus provide evidence for derangement in the organization of the elastic structures in PXE. Biochemical proof of the exact molecular defect in the structure or metabolism of elastin is, however, lacking, and it is unclear whether the calcification of elastic fibers is a primary or secondary event.

THERAPY. No specific treatment is available, and the primary prevention entails genetic counseling. Although treatment with vitamin E, vitamin C, or a low calcium diet has been advocated in isolated case reports, no clinical proof of their efficacy is available in the form of controlled clinical trials. In selected cases, plastic surgery may be helpful in improving the cosmetic appearance of the skin.

Neldner KH, Martinez-Hernandez A: Localized acquired cutaneous pseudoxanthoma elasticum. J Am Acad Dermatol 1:523, 1979. *Clinical description of a distinct acquired form of pseudoxanthoma elasticum.*

Pope FM: Two types of autosomal recessive pseudoxanthoma elasticum. Arch Dermatol 110:219, 1974. *A clinical study establishing the genetic heterogeneity of this condition.*

Rosenbloom J: Elastin: Relation of protein and gene structure to disease. Lab Invest 51:605, 1984. *A comprehensive review on elastin structure and metabolism.*

Uitto J: Elastic fibers in cutaneous diseases. Curr Concepts Skin Dis 6:19, 1985. *A review of the molecular defects of elastin in heritable connective tissue diseases, including pseudoxanthoma elasticum.*

Uitto J, Paul JL, Brockley K, et al.: Elastic fibers in human skin: Quantitation of elastic fibers by computerized digital image analyses and determination of elastin by a radioimmunoassay of desmosine. Lab Invest 49:499, 1983. *Demonstration of increased elastin concentrations in the lesional skin in pseudoxanthoma elasticum.*

Disorders of Porphyrins or Metals

203 PORPHYRIA

D. Montgomery Bissell

Porphyrias are characterized clinically by neurologic and/or cutaneous manifestations and chemically by overproduction of porphyrins or the porphyrin precursors, delta-aminolevulinic acid (ALA) and porphobilinogen (PBG). The most important members of this group of diseases are hereditary, but acquired porphyria occurs also; in all instances, porphyria must be distinguished from simple porphyrinuria, which accompanies a variety of common conditions and is without clinical significance.

BIOSYNTHESIS OF HEME. Heme is a metalloporphyrin, a member of a group that includes chlorophyll and vitamin B_{12}. These have been termed the molecules of life, in view of their importance to aerobic metabolism. Heme is formed from succinyl CoA and glycine in a series of enzyme-catalyzed steps (Fig. 203–1). The initial enzyme of the pathway, ALA synthetase, is rate-determining for the overall synthesis. Its activity is regulated in a "feedback" manner, so that it responds rapidly to the changing needs of the tissue for heme. When a relative deficiency of heme occurs—from increased heme-protein formation or impaired heme synthesis or both—ALA synthetase is stimulated, and the flow of heme precursors into the pathway increases. With formation of the initial porphyrin-like intermediate uroporphyrinogen, a branch point occurs involving different porphyrin isomers. While there are four possible isomers of uroporphyrinogen, only I and III occur in nature, isomer III being the physiologic intermediate. The isomer I pathway is abortive, proceeding only as far as coproporphyrin I, and normally is inconsequential. Metabolism of uroporphyrinogen III involves modifications of porphyrin side chains that render the molecule progressively more lipophilic and redirect its excretion from the body. Whereas the water-soluble ALA, PBG, and uroporphyrin are excreted entirely or very largely in urine, coproporphyrin is excreted in both urine and feces and protoporphyrin solely in feces. The porphyrinogens constitute the true intermediates of heme synthesis. The porphyrins—with the exception of protoporphyrin—are side products of the pathway that are irreversibly oxidized and must be excreted. Although loss of heme precursors from the pathway occurs and is measurable in urine or stool, it normally represents less than 1 per cent of heme synthesis. Increased excretion of these compounds implies an underlying disturbance of heme formation, either hereditary or acquired.

TISSUE SITES OF PORPHYRIN PRODUCTION. Heme serves as the prosthetic group for mitochondrial cytochromes as well as for other heme proteins and therefore is required by all cells in the body; presumably each tissue provides its own heme by endogenous synthesis. This requirement, however, varies widely among individual tissues, reflecting large differences in the concentration and turnover of specific heme proteins. Relatively high rates of heme synthesis are characteristic of both bone marrow and liver. In bone marrow, heme synthesis is devoted very largely to formation of hemoglobin; in liver, heme is required for several relatively short-lived heme proteins, in particular a group of microsomal cytochromes known as P-450. In rat liver, turnover of these cytochromes appears to account for 60 to 70 per cent of heme utilization. Synthesis of hepatic cytochrome P-450 is inducible by numerous drugs and possibly also by endogenous lipophilic substances, and administration of an inducing drug results in stimulation of ALA synthetase and a consequent increase in the rate of heme formation. In extrahepatic tissues (including bone marrow), the regulatory role of ALA synthetase remains poorly defined, and inducing effects of administered drugs have not been documented.

CLASSIFICATION, GENETICS, AND PREVALENCE. In the hereditary porphyrias, the specific genetic defect presum-

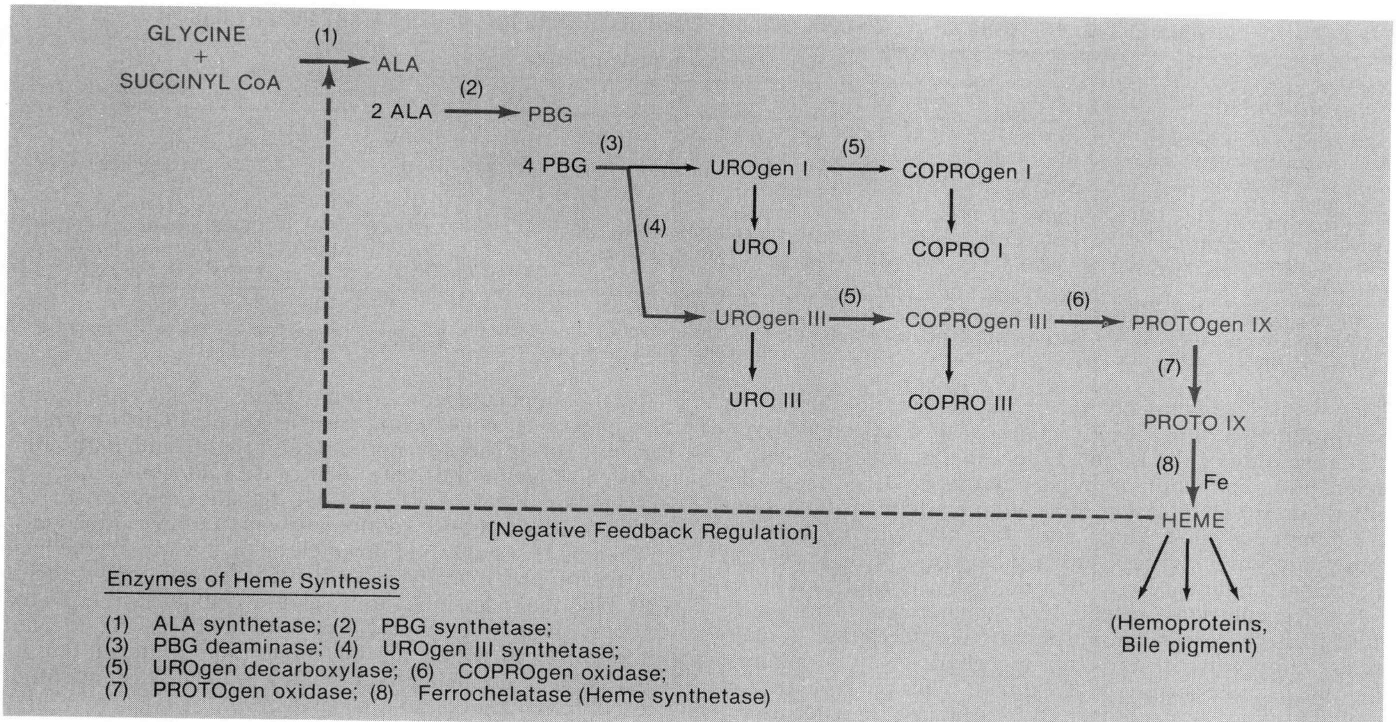

FIGURE 203–1. Pathway of heme biosynthesis (ALA = δ-aminolevulinic acid; PBG = porphobilinogen; URO = uroporphyrin; COPRO = coproporphyrin; PROTO = protoporphyrin).

ably is present in all cells of the body. However, for reasons as yet unclear, abnormal porphyrinogenesis is confined largely to either bone marrow or liver, with the possible exception of protoporphyria, which may involve both tissues. Accordingly, the classification presented in Table 203–1 separates the porphyrias into erythropoietic and hepatic types. Other tissues may be affected by the porphyria-producing lesion, but their contribution to total body production of heme precursors is small. Congenital erythropoietic porphyria and delta-aminolevulinic aciduria are rare autosomal recessive diseases; the other hereditary porphyrias are dominant disorders, and the sexes are equally affected. Although their distribution appears to be worldwide, accurate prevalence figures are not available because many carriers in the general population are asymptomatic. Clinically manifest hepatic porphyria appears to be much more common in whites than in blacks or Asians; whether this reflects differences in carrier rates or only variable clinical expression of the defect among these populations is unknown.

BIOCHEMICAL CHARACTERIZATION. While the porphyrias as a group represent disturbances of heme synthesis, they may be differentiated on the basis of the specific enzymatic defect in each type and the unique pattern of excretion of heme precursors (ALA, PBG, or porphyrins) associated with each defect (Table 203–2). This pattern is determined with quantitative tests; qualitative tests such as the Watson-Schwartz test for PBG are best reserved for urgent circumstances or when quantitative determinations are unavailable. With examination of the entire array of heme precursors in urine and feces, true porphyrias are readily differentiated from asymptomatic porphyrinuria, which may accompany acute liver disease, various tumors (hepatoma, Hodgkin's disease), and neurologic diseases. Porphyrinuria in these instances generally involves an isolated increase in urine coproporphyrin, with or without a modest increase in uroporphyrin. In lead poisoning, urine exhibits a significant increase in ALA with a lesser increase in coproporphyrin; PBG and fecal porphyrins are normal. None of these patterns resembles those associated with porphyria (Table 203–2).

Overproduction, with excess excretion, of ALA and PBG or porphyrins is associated with specific clinical manifestations. Increased circulating ALA and PBG are linked to a variety of neurologic problems that may include psychosis, seizures, and paresis. A neuropathic effect of ALA or PBG has been postulated. By contrast, overproduction of porphyrins is associated predominantly with cutaneous photosensitivity; no effect on neurologic function has been observed. The dermatologic effects of porphyrins are proportional to their approximate concentration in subcutaneous tissues and depend on excitation of porphyrins by visible light (peak effective wavelength, ca. 400 nm).

TABLE 203–1. CLASSIFICATION OF THE PORPHYRIAS

Erythropoietic
Congenital erythropoietic porphyria (Günther's disease)
Protoporphyria (erythropoietic or erythrohepatic protoporphyria)
Hepatic
Acute intermittent porphyria (pyrroloporphyria)
Hereditary coproporphyria
Variegate porphyria (South African porphyria)
Delta-aminolevulinic aciduria
Porphyria cutanea tarda (symptomatic porphyria)
Toxic porphyria

CONGENITAL ERYTHROPOIETIC PORPHYRIA

Fewer than 100 patients with this condition have been described. Pink urine and cutaneous photosensitivity are the principal manifestations and, classically, are present from early childhood. While the diagnosis usually is made at this time, a first presentation has been described also in adults, whose clinical state resembled that of relatively severe porphyria cutanea tarda (see below). Acute attacks of abdominal pain with neurologic manifestations do not occur. Cutaneous lesions consist of bullae, vesicles, and shallow ulcers on light-exposed skin. Repeated injuries are accompanied by hypertrichosis and, in patients surviving beyond childhood, may cause disfiguring scars with loss of portions of the nose, ears, eyelids, and digits. Erythrodontia, reflecting accumulation of porphyrins in teeth and bones, and splenomegaly also have been present in a high proportion of cases, associated with a compensated hemolytic anemia, which may be intermittent.

TABLE 203–2. PATTERNS OF OVERPRODUCTION OF HEME PRECURSORS IN THE HEREDITARY PORPHYRIAS

Type of Porphyria	Heme Precursors Present in Abnormal Amounts: *Urine*	*Feces*	*RBC*	*Plasma*	Enzyme Defect
Delta-aminolevulinic aciduria	**ALA*** > PBG > URO < COPRO	—	—	—	PBG synthetase (2)†
Acute intermittent porphyria	ALA < **PBG** > > URO	—	—	ALA, PBG	PBG deaminase (3)
Congenital erythropoietic porphyria	URO > > COPRO	URO > COPRO	**URO**	URO	?UROgen III synthetase (4)
Porphyria cutanea tarda	**URO** > > COPRO	URO	—	URO	UROgen decarboxylase (5)
Hereditary coproporphyria	ALA < PBG < URO < COPRO	**COPRO** > > PROTO	—	COPRO	COPROgen oxidase (6)
Variegate porphyria	ALA < PBG < URO < COPRO	COPRO < **PROTO**	—	COPRO, PROTO	PROTOgen oxidase (7)
Protoporphyria	—	PROTO	**PROTO**	PROTO	Ferrochelatase (8)

*The diagnostic abnormality for each type is in boldface type.
†Numbers in parentheses denote the position of the enzyme defect in the heme synthetic pathway (see Fig. 203–1).
ALA = δ-aminolevulinic acid; PBG = porphobilinogen; URO = uroporphyrin; COPRO = coproporphyrin; PROTO = protoporphyrin.

The chemical abnormality that characterizes this disease is overproduction of uroporphyrin and also of coproporphyrin, predominantly of the isomer I type; this is consistent with a defect in the formation of uroporphyrinogen III, although the inherited enzymatic lesion remains to be defined. Blood and urine both exhibit striking—and often massive—increases in these porphyrins, whereas urinary ALA and PBG are present in normal amounts. Circulating normoblasts and, to a lesser extent, reticulocytes, exhibit intense fluorescence owing to their high content of uroporphyrin. The feces also contain excess uroporphyrin and coproporphyrin with a minimal increase in protoporphyrin. Treatment relies on avoidance of sunlight; topical sunscreens and β-carotene (the latter useful in protoporphyria) are of no proven value. In patients with hemolysis, splenectomy may lead to prolongation of red cell lifespan and diminished porphyrin excretion.

PROTOPORPHYRIA

A relatively common condition, in most patients this is manifest solely as cutaneous photosensitivity. Within minutes of exposure, sunlight causes a burning, stinging sensation or pruritus of unprotected skin, followed by erythema and/or edema (solar urticaria). Attacks subside over a period of hours, often without sequelae; in some patients, repeated episodes lead to thickening of the skin (solar eczema). The cutaneous manifestations associated with other types of porphyria (bulla formation, mechanical fragility, or hypertrichosis) are absent in protoporphyria. The disease is characterized chemically by excess protoporphyrin IX in erythrocytes, plasma, and feces. Excretion of ALA, PBG, and uroporphyrin is normal, whereas fecal coproporphyrin may be moderately increased. Diffusion of protoporphyrin from red cells to plasma and cutaneous tissues appears to be responsible for the observed photosensitivity and distinguishes protoporphyria from other, acquired conditions with elevation of the level of red cell porphyrin. In iron deficiency, lead intoxication, and certain refractory chronic anemias, excess protoporphyrin is present in erythrocytes but is bound within the cell; plasma protoporphyrin levels invariably are normal, and cutaneous symptoms are absent.

The hereditary defect is a partial deficiency of ferrochelatase, which is the final enzyme of the heme synthetic pathway, catalyzing the conversion of protoporphyrin to heme. In some patients, the excess protoporphyrin appears to be derived entirely from the bone marrow, whereas in others the liver has been implicated as well. The clinically latent carrier state is frequent. About 10 per cent of patients form protoporphyrin-containing gallstones, and subclinical liver disease also appears to be relatively common, presumably because of deposition of protoporphyrin in the liver. In rare instances, the presenting manifestation is cholestasis, with inflammation, fibrosis, and crystalline protoporphyrin inclusions in bile canaliculi and liver cells. Progression to portal hypertension and death may be rapid. Fatal hepatic involvement has been associated with markedly elevated plasma protoporphyrin concentrations (>1000 μg per deciliter).

Treatment of cutaneous manifestations includes administration of beta-carotene, which increases the patient's tolerance for sunlight apparently by quenching light- and porphyrin-induced active intermediates that cause cutaneous injury. As a screening measure for possible hepatic involvement, all patients should receive routine evaluation of liver function.

There is no established prophylaxis or therapy for the liver disease of protoporphyria. Individual case reports suggest that blood transfusions, iron, cholestyramine, or activated charcoal may be beneficial, the latter two serving to bind protoporphyrin within the intestinal lumen, interrupting its enterohepatic circulation and thereby reducing the amount of protoporphyrin presented to the liver.

HEPATIC PORPHYRIA WITH NEUROLOGIC MANIFESTATIONS

DEFINITIONS. *Acute Intermittent Porphyria.* This disease is caused by a hereditary partial deficiency of PBG deaminase and is characterized by excretion of excess ALA and PBG in urine. Acute neurologic attacks occur; cutaneous symptoms are not a feature of this type of porphyria.

Hereditary Coproporphyria. A partial deficiency of coproporphyrinogen oxidase is present, leading to excretion of excess ALA, PBG, uroporphyrin, and coproporphyrin in urine and excess coproporphyrin in feces. In addition to acute neurologic attacks, approximately 30 per cent of patients experience cutaneous manifestations consistent with overproduction of porphyrins.

Variegate Porphyria. This type results from a partial deficiency of protoporphyrinogen oxidase and is characterized by excess excretion of the entire series of heme precursors; excretion of protoporphyrin in feces is characteristically high. Erythrocyte porphyrin levels are normal. Cutaneous photosensitivity or unusual fragility of sun-exposed skin is present in a majority of affected individuals and may be a chronic manifestation; the lesions are similar to those present in porphyria cutanea tarda (see below). However, as in the two preceding types, the occurrence of acute neurologic attacks is the most important clinical feature.

Delta-aminolevulinic Aciduria. There is profound deficiency of PBG synthetase in this condition, associated with excess ALA in the urine. Coproporphyrin also is increased, for reasons as yet unclear. The urinary findings are similar to those in persons with heavy metal intoxication, which must be excluded. The clinical presentation is identical to that of acute intermittent porphyria, except that symptoms occur only in homozygotes.

PATHOGENESIS. The individual genetic defect in each type appears to limit the flow of heme precursors and to be responsible for potential or actual heme deficiency in the liver. Circumstances that increase the demand for heme synthesis—the classic example being induction of cytochrome P-450 by barbiturates—cause the deficiency to be expressed, leading to derepression of ALA synthetase, overproduction of heme precursors preceding the genetic defect, and clinical symptoms. In addition to drugs, changes in endogenous factors have also been implicated in precipitating acute attacks. Involvement of steroid hormones is suggested by the fact that symptoms are rare prior to puberty, and disease is expressed clinically in women more often than in men. Estrogens (including oral contraceptives) are among the drugs that precipitate attacks, and cyclic premenstrual exacerbations occur in some women, resolving with onset of menstruation. The effect of pregnancy on disease activity is unpredictable. Infection or fasting (deliberate or as a result of concurrent illness) also predisposes carriers to acute attacks.

CLINICAL PRESENTATION. Acute neurologic attacks are common to all of the porphyrias cited above, and their identical presentations and management justify treating these types as a group. An acute attack consists of abdominal, back, or extremity pain, initially subacute but increasingly intense over a period of 24 to 48 hours until it may suggest acute cholecystitis, appendicitis, or other surgical diagnosis. Anorexia, nausea, and vomiting are frequent. Constipation typically is longstanding and worsens at the onset of an attack. In evaluating pain, the examiner may be impressed that the severity of the symptoms is out of proportion to the abdominal findings; rebound tenderness is seldom present. Tachycardia is a frequent finding and a useful parameter of disease activity. Fever is unusual and suggests a concurrent infectious process. X-ray examination of the abdomen may show dilated loops of small bowel consistent with paralytic ileus. In general, the abdominal manifestations are believed to represent a neurogenic motility disturbance of the bowel. They often occur in association with frank neurologic dysfunction: Generalized seizures or mental abnormalities that range from confusion to psychosis may be presenting features of an acute attack. With prolonged attacks, motor and sensory deficits appear and may progress to quadriplegia, respiratory paralysis, and death. The neuropathic changes are variable; patchy demyelination of peripheral nerves and focal degeneration of the autonomic nervous system have been described. Routine laboratory tests generally are unremarkable. Anemia is not a feature of the hepatic porphyrias, and blood loss does not precipitate acute attacks. Liver function test results similarly are normal, apart from slight increase of serum transaminase activity. Hyponatremia occurs in a minority of patients but occasionally is striking; it may reflect inappropriate secretion of antidiuretic hormone, complicated in some instances by aggressive intravenous fluid therapy with glucose and water.

Apart from acute episodes, in which the diagnosis is obvious, carriers of these genetic defects may complain of mood swings and bodily pains, which fail to suggest a specific diagnosis and may be without associated physical findings. The porphyric nature of such symptoms often is difficult to resolve. Although excretion of heme precursors is uniformly increased in acute attacks, it varies widely among asymptomatic carriers and thus does not provide a secure basis for differentiating porphyric from nonspecific manifestations. Treatment is empiric, with due regard for those drugs that may induce acute attacks (see below). There is no evidence that dietary manipulations (e.g., excess carbohydrate) are useful.

DIAGNOSIS. Urinary PBG is increased in these porphyrias during acute attacks (except in delta-aminolevulinic aciduria) and remains increased while symptoms persist. This may be documented by rapid qualitative methods (Watson-Schwartz or Hoesch tests) in which PBG reacts with Ehrlich's reagent (dimethylaminobenzaldehyde in HCl) to form a red complex that is not extractable with *n*-butanol. Positive test results should be confirmed by quantification of urinary PBG by ion-exchange column chromatography. With quantification of urinary and fecal porphyrins, the specific type of porphyria usually can be established. Uroporphyrin often is reported as increased in acute intermittent porphyria, despite the fact that its formation theoretically is compromised by the genetic defect of this type. This apparently reflects nonenzymatic conversion of PBG to a dark uroporphyrin-like compound (porphobilin), which may occur in the urinary bladder. The conversion is accelerated by exposure of urine to light, accounting for the visible darkening of voided urine from patients with acute intermittent porphyria. A "urine porphyrin screen" does not measure PBG and therefore could be misleading in the investigation of patients with acute abdominal pain.

In the absence of clinical symptoms, increase of urinary PBG is inconstant. In 20 to 30 per cent of asymptomatic carriers of acute intermittent porphyria, PBG in urine is within the normal range. In these cases, assay of erythrocyte PBG deaminase may be used to identify carriers. This activity is significantly reduced in affected persons and is abnormal regardless of the age or clinical state of the person. Many asymptomatic carriers with hereditary coproporphyria or variegate porphyria excrete PBG in normal amounts. Identification of carriers requires measurement of fecal coproporphyrin in the case of hereditary coproporphyria and fecal protoporphyrin for variegate porphyria. While the inherited defects in these types of porphyria are known, the enzymes are intramitochondrial; therefore, their assay requires nucleated cells (leukocytes or cultured skin fibroblasts) and at present is a research procedure.

MANAGEMENT. Emphasis is on the prevention of acute neurologic attacks. In families with a known case of porphyria, identification of carriers is mandatory, using the appropriate screening procedure for the type of porphyria involved (see above). Carriers should be instructed as to the hazards of fasting and of taking drugs that may precipitate acute attacks (Table 203–3). Carriers of hereditary coproporphyria or variegate porphyria who experience cutaneous manifestations in the absence of a porphyrogenic drug should minimize their exposure to sunlight and wear protective clothing.

The management of neurologic exacerbations includes immediate withdrawal of possible offending drugs, administration of carbohydrate, correction of electrolyte abnormalities, and general supportive care. Carbohydrate is given to reverse the fasting state, usually as intravenous dextrose because of nausea or vomiting, and in amounts approaching 400 grams per day. To avoid administration of a water load, hypertonic solutions may be infused by a central line. Seizures, when present, generally occur early in the course of an attack and respond to parenteral diazepam. For analgesia, chlorpromazine may be used, although the specificity of its action is uncertain; excessive sedation is a troublesome side effect. In many patients, meperidine will be required despite the danger of addiction. Propranolol counters the tachycardia of acute attacks; it should be introduced at very low doses (e.g., 10 mg twice daily).

If acute manifestations fail to respond to these measures within 48 hours, treatment with hematin (hydroxyheme) is

TABLE 203–3. HAZARDOUS AND SAFE DRUGS IN PORPHYRIA WITH NEUROLOGIC MANIFESTATIONS

May Precipitate Acute Attacks	Believed to Be Safe
Apronalid	Aspirin
Barbiturates	Bromides
Chlordiazepoxide	Chlorpromazine
Chloroquine	Corticosteroids
Chlorpropamide	Diazepam
Dichloralphenazone	Dicumarol
Ergot preparations	Digoxin
Estrogens	Diphenhydramine
Ethanol	Ether
Glutethimide	Guanethidine
Griseofulvin	Meperidine
Hydantoins	Morphine
Imipramine	Neostigmine
Meprobamate	Nitrous oxide
Methsuximide	Penicillins
Methyldopa	Propranolol
Methyprylon	Tetracyclines
Novonal	
Sulfonamides	

indicated with the rationale that it compensates for the genetic impairment of endogenous heme synthesis. The solution consists of pyrogen-free hemin (ferriprotoporphyrin IX chloride) dissolved in aqueous sodium carbonate (10 grams per liter), adjusted to pH 8.0 with HCl and sterilized by membrane filtration. It is infused slowly (over 10 to 15 minutes) into the largest available vein. A dose of 2 mg per kilogram body weight at 24-hour intervals usually is effective, as shown by a decline in urinary PBG to less than 10 per cent of the pretreatment level. If the response to this regimen is unsatisfactory, the frequency of the dose may be doubled. However, the total administered hematin should not exceed 6 mg per kilogram body weight per day. Subjective improvement parallels the chemical response and is evident 72 to 96 hours after the initial hematin infusion. Improvement in neurologic deficits depends on the underlying pathologic condition. Hematin may arrest a progressive neuropathy, but has no effect on established lesions involving demyelination. With cessation of hematin treatment, a rise in urinary PBG may occur, although the patient's condition usually remains stable (Fig. 203–2).

Hematin is available commercially as a powder (Panhematin), which is reconstituted for use with sterile water. The prepared solution is unstable and should be infused promptly. It may be stored at 4°C for up to 12 hours, but then should be discarded. Side effects of hematin administration include chemical phlebitis at the site of infusion (4 per cent of cases) and reduced clotting activity. Abnormal coagulation tests and reduced platelets have been observed in several patients receiving hematin. These effects are dose related and may be due to decay product(s) of dissolved hematin rather than to hematin itself. They are minimized by the use of freshly prepared material. When present, they are maximal 10 minutes after injection of hematin, diminished at 5 hours, and undetectable at 48 hours. Clinically significant bleeding has not occurred except in patients also receiving another anticoagulant. The findings suggest that hematin should not be used in patients with impaired coagulation or in those undergoing surgical procedures. At doses substantially in excess of the recommended maximum, hematin has caused renal toxicity, which was reversible. Similar problems have not been observed with the usual doses, despite the fact that

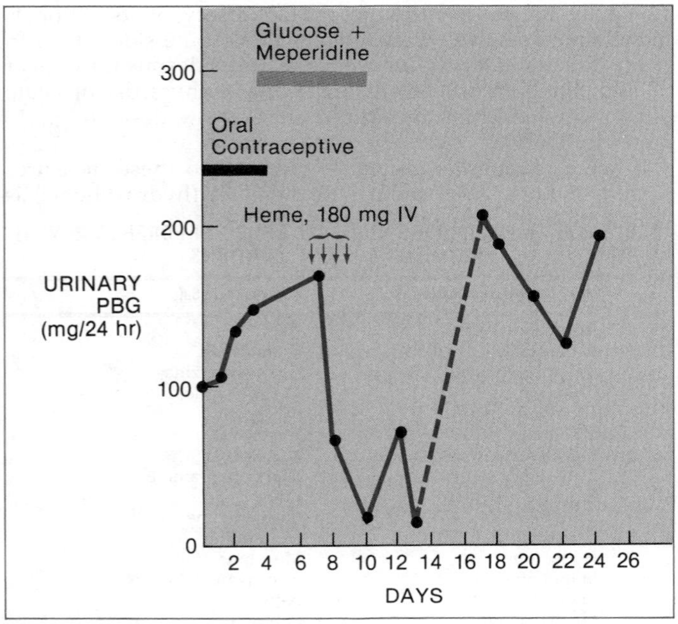

FIGURE 203–2. Acute intermittent porphyria in a patient taking oral contraceptive medication: response of urinary PBG (porphobilinogen) to administered heme (hematin). Normal PBG less than 2 mg per 24 hours.

patients with acute hepatic porphyria may exhibit reduced renal function.

For women with regular and disabling premenstrual porphyric symptoms, prophylactic hematin (administered one or two days prior to the expected onset of symptoms) and ovulatory suppression with oral contraceptives have been tried. From the limited experience to date, neither therapy can be considered established. Ovulatory suppression by means of peptide analogues of luteinizing hormone releasing hormone (LH-RH) is logical, because such analogues lack the porphyria-inducing properties of contraceptive steroids, and this approach is being evaluated at the present time.

PROGNOSIS. The vast majority of carriers remain asymptomatic, provided that they avoid drugs associated with exacerbations, and their longevity appears to be unaffected. Acute neurologic attacks formerly carried a substantial mortality. However, as a result of hematin therapy and modern intensive care for complications such as respiratory failure, the outlook for these patients is much improved. Neurologic deficits may require months or years to resolve, but complete recovery is observed in many instances. Although mental abnormalities occur in acute attacks, these are neither persistent nor progressive.

PORPHYRIA CUTANEA TARDA

This relatively common condition is characterized by mechanical fragility and blistering of light-exposed skin. Acute neurologic attacks do not occur. The onset of manifestations is insidious, patients often failing to associate cutaneous lesions with sun exposure. Seemingly trivial trauma to the dorsa of the hands, arms, face, or feet leads to vesicles that rupture to an open sore, eventually healing with scar formation. Sclerodermoid changes and hypertrichosis may occur. A history of ethanol abuse and/or chronic liver disease can be obtained from a majority of patients with this type of porphyria. The pathologic changes seen in liver biopsies are nonspecific and do not correlate with the severity of the porphyria. In a few patients, hepatomas containing a high concentration of porphyrin have been diagnosed and presumably were the cause of cutaneous manifestations. Almost all liver biopsy specimens exhibit an increase in stainable iron, and freshly obtained tissue is fluorescent under ultraviolet light because of its high content of uroporphyrin. Associations of this disease with systemic lupus erythematosus, diabetes mellitus, and hemochromatosis (heterozygous state) have been reported.

Urine from patients is red-orange or brown. Its uroporphyrin content (predominantly isomer I) is strikingly elevated; cutaneous manifestations are associated with levels greater than 800 μg per 24 hours (normal, <50 μg per 24 hours). Urinary coproporphyrin excretion is moderately increased, whereas fecal coproporphyrin and protoporphyrin are normal. This pattern clearly distinguishes patients with porphyria cutanea tarda from those with variegate porphyria and cutaneous manifestations (Table 203–2).

The *pathogenesis* of porphyria cutanea tarda is incompletely understood. The pattern of porphyrin excretion, with predominance of isomer I compounds, suggests a partial defect at the level of uroporphyrinogen III synthetase; on the other hand, excretion of uroporphyrin is greater than that of coproporphyrin, consistent with deficient activity of uroporphyrinogen decarboxylase. A partial deficiency of the latter activity appears to be present in the liver of all patients with porphyria cutanea tarda. Whether or not this represents a hereditary abnormality in all cases is controversial at present. In some patients the defect is expressed not only in liver but also in erythrocytes; first-degree relatives of these patients also exhibit the defect in a pattern consistent with autosomal dominant inheritance. On the other hand, in some patients the defect is detectable solely in liver tissue. The erythrocyte enzyme of the patient and family members is normal. The latter has been termed *sporadic* porphyria cutanea tarda. The available data are insufficient for determining whether this is an acquired disease or a hereditary variant of porphyria cutanea tarda. Because of the regular association of porphyria cutanea tarda with hepatic siderosis and moderately increased transferrin saturation (averaging 60 per cent), testing for the hemochromatosis gene has been carried out (see Ch. 206). Heterozygosity for hemochromatosis (by HLA testing) appears to occur frequently in persons with clinically evident porphyria cutanea tarda and may be required for its expression. Regardless of the genetic component, it is clear that environmental or purely acquired factors play a central role in the pathogenesis of symptoms. Dietary iron, ethanol ingestion, and certain drugs (notably, estrogens) all may provoke increased porphyrin production, apparently acting in concert with the underlying genetic defect to compromise heme synthesis at the level of uroporphyrinogen III formation. The cutaneous manifestations of porphyria cutanea tarda have been observed in a few patients with renal failure receiving hemodialysis, and increase of plasma uroporphyrin has been noted; the pathogenesis is obscure.

Management involves attention to possible aggravating factors: administered iron, estrogen, ethanol, or occupational exposure to noxious chemicals should be eliminated, and this alone may lead to a reduction in porphyrin excretion and remission of cutaneous manifestations. However, phlebotomy, to remove iron from the liver and accelerate resolution of the disease, usually is indicated. With monitoring of the patient's hemoglobin level, 500 to 1000 ml of blood may be removed once or twice monthly, until urine porphyrin levels begin to decline. The time-course of the response varies widely among patients, averaging six months. For patients with disabling cutaneous disease and unable to tolerate phlebotomy, chloroquine* at low doses may be introduced. However, this carries a definite risk of a hepatotoxic reaction, and close monitoring of liver function is required. Plasmapheresis also may be useful for directly reducing the concentration of circulating uroporphyrin. Topical sunscreens and beta-carotene offer little or no protection against light-induced damage in this disease. When pathogenic environmental factors have been eliminated, a clinical response is observed in virtually all patients treated with serial phlebotomies and usually is long lasting.

TOXIC PORPHYRIA

Cutaneous porphyria on a large scale occurred in Turkey in 1959, when several thousand persons consumed grain that had been treated with a fungicide (hexachlorobenzene). Other cases have resulted from accidental or industrial exposure to hepatotoxins, epidemiologic considerations indicating that the disease is acquired rather than hereditary. The clinical manifestations and laboratory abnormalities are indistinguishable from those of porphyria cutanea tarda.

Anderson KE, Spitz IM, Sassa S, et al.: Prevention of cyclical attacks of acute intermittent porphyria with a long-acting agonist of luteinizing hormone-releasing hormone. N Engl J Med 311:643, 1984. *Premenstrual porphyric attacks and a possible new treatment for them.*

Bissell DM: Haem metabolism and the porphyrias. In Wright R, Millward-Sadler GH, Alberti KGMM, Karran S (eds.): Liver and Biliary Disease. 2nd ed. London, Balliere, Tindall & Cox, 1985, pp 387–413. *The hepatic porphyrias, with emphasis on the clinical aspects.*

Goetsch CA, Bissell DM: Instability of hematin used in the treatment of acute hepatic porphyria. N Engl J Med 315: 235, 1986. *A discussion of hematin therapy, with evidence that some treatment failures and side effects of hematin result from the use of decayed material.*

Kappas A, Sassa S, Anderson KE: The porphyrias. In Stanbury JB, Wyngaarden JB, Fredrickson DS, et al. (eds.): The Metabolic Basis of Inherited Disease. 5th ed. New York, McGraw-Hill Book Company, 1983, pp 1301–1384. *A detailed review of genetic and biochemical aspects of the porphyrias.*

Kushner JP, Edwards CQ, Dadone MM, et al.: Heterozygosity for HLA-linked hemochromatosis as a likely cause of the hepatic siderosis associated with sporadic porphyria tarda. Gastroenterology 88:1232, 1985. *A discussion of familial and sporadic porphyria cutanea tarda and of the possible involvement of the hemochromatosis gene in the expression of this porphyria.*

Ridley A: The neuropathy of acute intermittent porphyria. Q J Med 38:307, 1969. *Neurologic manifestations in 25 patients.*

*This use is not listed in the manufacturer's directive.

204 ACATALASIA

James B. Wyngaarden

DEFINITION AND SYNONYMS. Acatalasia is a rare inherited deficiency of catalase in erythrocytes (acatalasemia) and other tissues. In some subjects acatalasia is associated with severe gangrenous lesions of the oral cavity and destruction of alveolar bone (Takahara's disease).

EPIDEMIOLOGY. Acatalasia was discovered in Japan in 1946. Takahara's disease occurs chiefly among Japanese and Koreans but has also occurred in Peru. Asymptomatic acatalasemia has been reported from Japan, Korea, Switzerland, Israel, Mexico, and Peru, and hypocatalasemia from several additional countries, including the United States.

ETIOLOGY AND PATHOGENESIS. Acatalasia is inherited as an autosomal recessive condition and is often associated with consanguinity. In Japan the estimated frequencies of homozygotes and heterozygotes are 4×10^{-6} and 1.7×10^{-3}, respectively. The distribution of blood catalase values among homozygous affected, heterozygous, and normal subjects is triphasic, without overlap. Residual catalase activity among Japanese with acatalasia is very low; the enzyme is electrophoretically normal, of normal stability, and low specific activity. Among Swiss homozygotes, residual catalase activity is higher, and the enzyme is electrophoretically abnormal and heat labile. Swiss heterozygotes have normal blood catalase levels.

Takahara's disease results from oral sepsis with hydrogen peroxide–producing bacteria and appears to be restricted to subjects with very low catalase activities. Acatalasemic Japanese with Takahara's disease have 0.23 per cent of normal catalase activity; those without have 0.57 per cent. Homozygotes from Switzerland, Israel, and Mexico have higher values and are clinically normal. Homozygotes have been classified into five subtypes by Aebi and Wyss, on the basis of genetic and clinical heterogeneity.

CLINICAL MANIFESTATIONS. About one half of acatalasemic subjects remain asymptomatic throughout life. Takahara's disease usually begins before age ten, sometimes during infancy. Over 50 cases have been reported. Mild disease consists of ulcers in the dental alveoli or in tonsillar crypts. In moderate disease (the most common) there is alveolar gangrene, recession of alveolar bone, and loss of teeth. In severe cases there is widespread destruction with gangrene of the maxilla and soft tissue, similar to noma. After healing, extensive scarring may limit opening of the mouth. Gangrenous lesions of the oral cavity are rare after puberty.

DIAGNOSIS. The disease should be suspected in any child with shaggy discolored ulcers of dental alveoli or gangrenous lesions of the mouth. A presumptive diagnostic test is easily performed as follows: When hydrogen peroxide is added to acatalasemic blood, it turns brown-black because of formation of methemoglobin, whereas normal blood bubbles vigorously and remains pink. Asymptomatic acatalasemic and hypocatalasemic subjects have been diagnosed in family studies or in population surveys by quantitative assays of blood catalase activity.

TREATMENT. Curettage and excision of granulating tissue, drainage, irrigation of septic areas, extraction of teeth, and antibiotic therapy have been employed. Reconstructive surgery and bone grafts have been required. Direct application of crystalline catalase suspensions and transfusions of normal catalase-rich whole blood have been suggested. Once healing has taken place the disease does not recur.

Aebi HE, Wyss SR: Acatalasemia. In Stanbury JB, Wyngaarden JB, Fredrickson DS, et al. (eds.): The Metabolic Basis of Inherited Disease. 5th ed. New York, McGraw-Hill Book Company, 1983. *An authoritative review of genetic, metabolic, and clinical features of acatalasia.*

Matsunaga T, Segar R, Höger P, et al.: Congenital acatalasemia: A study of neutrophil functions after provocation with hydrogen peroxide. Pediatr Res 19:1187, 1985. *Chemotaxis of neutrophils is depressed by H_2O_2 in vitro. This mechanism may contribute to the formation of mucosal ulcers in acatalasia.*

205 WILSON'S DISEASE

Andrew Deiss

DEFINITION. Wilson's disease (hepatolenticular degeneration) is a hereditary disorder characterized by the accumulation of copper in the body, especially in the liver, brain, kidneys, and corneas. The excess copper leads to tissue injury and ultimately, if effective treatment is not instituted, to death.

ETIOLOGY AND PREVALENCE. Wilson's disease is inherited as an autosomal recessive trait. The gene responsible for the disturbance in copper metabolism is closely linked to the locus for esterase D on the long arm of chromosome 13. The prevalence of the disease is approximately 30 per million.

PATHOGENESIS. Normally, loss of copper from the body occurs primarily through the bile. Much of biliary copper is secreted in a poorly absorbable form and thus is lost in the feces. Copper balance is normally maintained by this mechanism. In Wilson's disease biliary excretion of copper is impaired, and as a consequence total body copper is progressively increased. The specific nature of the metabolic abnormality that causes this defect is not known.

Positive copper balance begins in infancy in Wilson's disease and continues thereafter unless appropriate therapy is given. However, the distribution of copper changes as the disease progresses. Liver copper is actually greater in presymptomatic homozygotes than in symptomatic ones. Thus not only does net deposition of liver copper cease, but a portion of previously deposited copper is lost from the liver and deposited elsewhere. This copper redistribution probably takes place when liver injury occurs. If this injury occurs abruptly in many hepatocytes, liver disease may be clinically manifested and a large amount of copper may be released over a short period, creating the potential for acute erythrocyte injury and hemolytic anemia as well. However, if hepatocyte injury is more gradual, acute liver disease will not occur, and the patient will remain asymptomatic as the important site of copper deposition shifts to the brain. With the latter course, most patients will present at a later time with neurologic or psychiatric symptoms, usually with clinically inapparent cirrhosis.

The serum concentration of the copper-containing protein ceruloplasmin is low in 95 per cent of patients with Wilson's disease. The mechanism for the hypoceruloplasminemia is not known, but it is not believed to play a pathogenetic role in the disease.

PATHOLOGY. The diagnosis cannot be made on the basis of histologic sections of the liver. Fatty change and glycogen-filled nuclei are present early, followed later by piecemeal necrosis, lymphocytic infiltration, erosion of limiting plates, parenchymal collapse, and fibrosis. Ultimately these abnormalities evolve into postnecrotic cirrhosis. Stains for copper are unreliable, being negative most frequently during the early stages of the disease when diagnostic help is most needed.

In the brain abnormal astrocytes and neuronal necrosis are widely distributed, and there is atrophy or cavitation of the basal ganglia and occasionally the cerebral cortex.

CLINICAL MANIFESTATIONS. Wilson's disease is a disorder of young persons. Although the disease may occur at any time from the age of five years into the sixth decade, two thirds of patients seek medical attention between the ages of eight and twenty. The physician should suspect the disorder in children under the age of 15 years with signs of progressive hepatic dysfunction or in young people over that age with characteristic neurologic abnormalities.

The hepatic symptoms are quite diverse. Commonly a brief illness characterized by malaise, anorexia, jaundice, and increased aminotransferases is mistaken for viral hepatitis. Similar episodes may recur at intervals of months or years, or a latent period may occur during which the patient is asymptomatic until neurologic symptoms begin. If clinically overt hepatocyte injury persists over a longer period, a syndrome resembling chronic active hepatitis results. Occasionally liver injury occurs precipitously; without rapid institution of appropriate treatment, death is likely in these patients and the need for prompt diagnosis is urgent. More commonly, however, hepatocyte injury is gradual and is not accompanied by symptoms of liver disease; nevertheless cirrhosis develops ultimately in all patients. This liver injury may not be recognized until neurologic disease is evaluated.

Episodes of hemolytic anemia occur when massive release of copper from the liver takes place. Thus hemolysis is usually accompanied by overt liver disease; it occurs regularly in patients with fulminant hepatic failure. Hemolysis usually lasts only a short period and disappears spontaneously.

The neurologic signs at onset may take a variety of forms. Patients may start with a slightly dystonic facies in which the upper lip is drawn tightly over the teeth. Shortly afterwards they develop awkward, dystonic postures in the upper extremities and often an unsteady gait. Once recognized by prior experience, these particular neurologic manifestations are seldom mistaken. In other patients, tremor may be the initial sign, often a characteristic "wing-beating" rhythmic oscillating tremor of the upper extremities that in severe cases gradually extends to the trunk. Frequently loss of coordination of fine movements, such as those required for handwriting, is the earliest neurologic sign. As the disease progresses, patients may develop combinations of these abnormalities. Dysarthria, rigidity, drooling, and titubation are late features. Seizures are infrequent and sensory abnormalities absent. The Kayser-Fleischer (K-F) ring, described below, is definitively diagnostic in the neurologic variety and nearly so in the hepatic form of the disease.

Psychological symptoms of Wilson's disease are prominent and consist of early development of intellectual deterioration, personality changes, and unstable behavior. Children begin to fail at school, and young adults may show difficulty in performing jobs once considered routine. Schizophreniform symptoms and other forms of bizarre behavior may appear, but the mental status examination always shows signs of organic dementia. Effective removal of excess copper often improves but usually fails to eliminate these symptoms completely.

Kayser-Fleischer rings are golden brown or greenish rings or arcs in Descemet's membrane at the limbus of the cornea. They are composed of copper-containing granules and develop primarily after redistribution of liver copper. They may be visible with the unaided eye, but slit-lamp examination should always be obtained. K-F rings are present in all or nearly all patients in the neurologic or psychiatric stage of the disease, but are not present in about one third of those with hepatic symptoms.

Rare symptoms ascribable to Wilson's disease include cholelithiasis, sunflower cataracts, arthropathy, renal calculi, and the Fanconi syndrome.

DIAGNOSIS. The classic diagnostic features of K-F rings, low serum ceruloplasmin concentration (<20 mg per deciliter) and increased amounts of liver and urine copper (>250 μg per gram of dry weight and >100 μg per 24 hours, respectively) are present in nearly all patients with fully evolved neurologic Wilson's disease, but only in about two thirds of those presenting with liver disease. In these patients, K-F rings often have not yet formed, and the serum ceruloplasmin concentration may be difficult to interpret. Even in Wilson's disease, serum ceruloplasmin increases during inflammation, estrogen administration, and pregnancy and may decrease during liver failure. Measurement of the copper content of the liver should resolve the problem. Hepatic copper is often greater than normal (50 μg per gram of dry weight) in a variety of chronic liver diseases, but it seldom reaches the concentration seen in most patients with Wilson's disease (>250 μg per gram of dry weight). In a patient with a disease clinically suggestive of Wilson's disease, hepatic copper of this magnitude is essentially diagnostic. All measurements of copper metabolism should be entrusted only to laboratories experienced with their determination, and the normal values of that laboratory should be used.

In primary biliary cirrhosis and chronic cholestasis, diseases with acquired abnormalities of copper excretion, liver copper may be greatly increased and K-F rings occur rarely. The age, symptoms, and laboratory abnormalities of patients with these diseases help distinguish them from Wilson's disease.

Early during the hemolytic anemia the urinary copper excretion is very great. The Coombs test result is negative. When hemolysis and acute liver disease occur concurrently in a young person, Wilson's disease is the most probable cause.

Examination of all siblings of patients with Wilson's disease is mandatory to identify presymptomatic homozygotes. K-F rings will be absent. Serum ceruloplasmin concentration is reduced in 95 per cent of homozygotes and 10 per cent of heterozygotes. If it is low, liver copper content should be measured. Hepatic copper is slightly increased in most heterozygotes. If the copper is greater than 250 μg per gram of dry weight, Wilson's disease is present, and it should be treated as in symptomatic patients. Heterozygotes never become symptomatic and should not be treated. Some homozygotes will be missed by this evaluation, so continued follow-up is necessary.

TREATMENT. Without effective lifetime therapy, Wilson's disease is inevitably fatal. If treatment is begun early enough, symptomatic recovery usually is complete, and a life of normal length and quality can be expected. If treatment is begun too late, death may not be prevented, or recovery will be only partial.

Effective therapy depends upon establishing negative copper balance, thereby preventing deposition of more copper and mobilizing for excretion excess copper already deposited. The copper chelating agent, D-penicillamine, should be given to all patients initially. The usual dose is 1 to 1.5 grams per day, given in divided doses before meals and at bedtime. Response typically is quite slow, occurring over months, but it may occur more rapidly. A year or more is often required to obtain maximum improvement. About 10 per cent of patients experience a worsening of their neurologic symptoms during the first month or two of treatment, and this phenomenon should not suggest that the diagnosis is in error. Compliance and the effectiveness of therapy must be monitored at one- to two-month intervals with measurements of urine copper, serum ceruloplasmin, and serum non-ceruloplasmin copper (total serum copper minus ceruloplasmin copper). Non-ceruloplasmin copper should decrease early and ceruloplasmin more gradually if treatment is adequate. Urine copper will increase at once to 1 to 5 mg per 24 hours during the first few months, then gradually decrease as the excess of copper decreases.

Toxic effects are frequent. Rash, fever, adenopathy, neutropenia, or thrombocytopenia often occurs during the first two weeks of treatment. In such circumstances, penicillamine should be discontinued; when the symptoms have cleared, prednisone should be begun at a dose of 40 mg per day and penicillamine resumed at 250 mg per day and gradually increased to full dose over a period of a few weeks. The steroids can then be tapered and stopped. Side effects that occur later after initiation of penicillamine administration include proteinuria, nephrotic syndrome, systemic lupus erythematosus, Goodpasture's syndrome, and a variety of chronic skin diseases. These side effects can often be reversed by temporarily stopping penicillamine and resuming it after the symptoms have abated, sometimes with the addition of steroids. Suspension of treatment should never be permitted for more than a few months.

If penicillamine toxicity is intolerable, trientine (250 mg four times a day) is an effective alternative. Zinc acetate also produces a negative copper balance with tolerable side effects, but there is little experience with its use.

Some patients, especially those with fulminant hepatic failure, are so severely ill that the benefits of medical treatment cannot occur rapidly enough to prevent death. In these patients, liver transplantation, if successful, is curative.

Cartwright GE: Diagnosis of treatable Wilson's disease. N Engl J Med 298:1347, 1978. *An excellent description of the protean and often confusing clinical presentations of Wilson's disease and a few illustrations of what happens when the diagnosis is missed.*

Deiss A, Lynch RE, Lee GR, Cartwright GE: Long-term therapy of Wilson's disease. Ann Intern Med 75:57, 1971. *The natural history of Wilson's disease is related to the evolving pattern of copper deposition.*

Scheinberg IH, Sternlieb I: Wilson's Disease. Philadelphia, W. B. Saunders Company, 1984. *The authoritative monograph based on the author's vast experience with all aspects of Wilson's disease.*

Sternlieb I, Scheinberg IH: Prevention of Wilson's disease in asymptomatic patients. N Engl J Med 278:352, 1968. *An important report defining the criteria for identifying homozygotes and heterozygotes in families of patients with Wilson's disease.*

206 HEMOCHROMATOSIS (Iron Storage Disease)

Arno G. Motulsky

DEFINITION. The most common generalized iron storage disease in the United States and in persons of European origin is a genetic disorder known as primary or idiopathic hemochromatosis that is linked to the HLA locus. Massive iron deposits in parenchymal cells may develop after years of increased iron absorption, and functional organ impairment of the liver, heart, and other organs ensues. Secondary hemochromatosis with parenchymal cell involvement also occurs in a variety of anemias associated with both ineffective erythropoiesis and increased iron absorption—most commonly in homozygous beta-thalassemia. Blood transfusions contribute further to the pathologic iron overload. In these patients, clinical signs and symptoms of excessive iron storage develop in adolescence or even earlier.

Hemochromatosis affecting parenchymal tissues needs to be differentiated from iron loading of macrophages of the reticuloendothelial system that is relatively benign. If severe and generalized, the latter condition is known as hemosiderosis and typically occurs after multiple blood transfusions in patients with aplastic anemia in whom iron absorption is not increased. Iron overload of parenchymal liver cells is rarely observed under such conditions and occurs only with massive iron deposits after considerable time has elapsed to permit redistribution of iron.

ETIOLOGY, GENETICS, AND PATHOGENESIS. "Idiopathic" hemochromatosis is caused by an autosomal recessive gene that causes increased iron absorption in the gut. The nature of the metabolic abnormality remains unknown but may relate to failure of iron storage in gastrointestinal and reticuloendothelial cells. Thus, instead of being stored normally in such cells, iron enters the bloodstream to be deposited in parenchymal cells of the liver and other organs. Clinical signs and symptoms will develop after many years of excessive iron absorption when total body iron stores have reached levels of 15 to 40 grams as compared with normal iron stores of 0.2 to 2.0 grams.

The gene for hemochromatosis is located on the short arm of chromosome 6 and is linked to the HLA locus. The hemochromatosis gene is physically close to the HLA-A allele of the HLA complex. About 70 per cent of hemochromatosis patients carry the HLA-A_3 allele as compared to 25 to 30 per cent of the general population.

Recombination between the hemochromatosis gene and the HLA-A allele is very rare. Since these genes are separate, hemochromatosis is not likely to be a direct effect of HLA-A gene action. An increased frequency of HLA B_7 and HLA B_{14} is also observed and is caused by "hitchhiking" of each of these determinants on the chromosome carrying the hemochromatosis gene (linkage disequilibrium). The development of clinical hemochromatosis in the vast majority of cases requires the "double dose" of the mutant gene, and affected patients are homozygotes. Among sibships that include at least one affected homozygote with hemochromatosis, additional homozygotes as well as heterozygote carriers can often be defined by HLA testing using the principles of genetic linkage. Thus, the HLA status of the affected patient who has inherited a hemochromatosis gene from each parent is determined (Fig. 206–1). Sibs with both HLA haplotypes identical to that of the affected patient will carry the linked hemochromatosis allele on the maternal as well as the paternal chromosome 6. Such persons are homozygous, are at high risk to develop iron overload, or may already be affected. Sibs who share only one HLA haplotype are heterozygotes, and sibs who share none are normal, not having inherited any hemochromatosis gene. No test to detect heterozygotes in the general population exists. Detection of homozygotes in the population at large must utilize measures of iron status (transferrin saturation, serum ferritin) and nonspecific indices of liver damage (e.g., transaminase). HLA testing is not useful for detection in the population.

Homozygotes for hemochromatosis absorb increased iron. The actual amount of stored iron at a given time depends upon additional factors such as age, sex, iron content of food, caloric intake, degree of alcohol ingestion, and unknown factors. Not enough iron to produce clinical findings will have been absorbed in younger persons. Males generally eat larger quantities of food than females and therefore absorb more iron. Most importantly, females lose iron periodically during menstruation and occasionally during pregnancy. Therefore, while the prevalence of homozygotes for the hemochromatosis gene is identical in both sexes, *clinically* apparent hemochromatosis occurs about ten times more frequently in males. Excessive alcohol intake further contributes to liver damage, and many patients with the clinical disease give a history of excessive alcohol intake. Alcohol may stimulate iron absorption, and certain alcoholic beverages such as red wines contain increased amounts of iron. Ingestion of iron-containing medications—particularly over prolonged periods—would cause additional iron absorption.

Excessive iron in various parenchymal organs, particularly the liver and the heart, is required before clinical manifestations develop. There is a fairly good correlation between the quantity of iron stored and the development of clinical signs

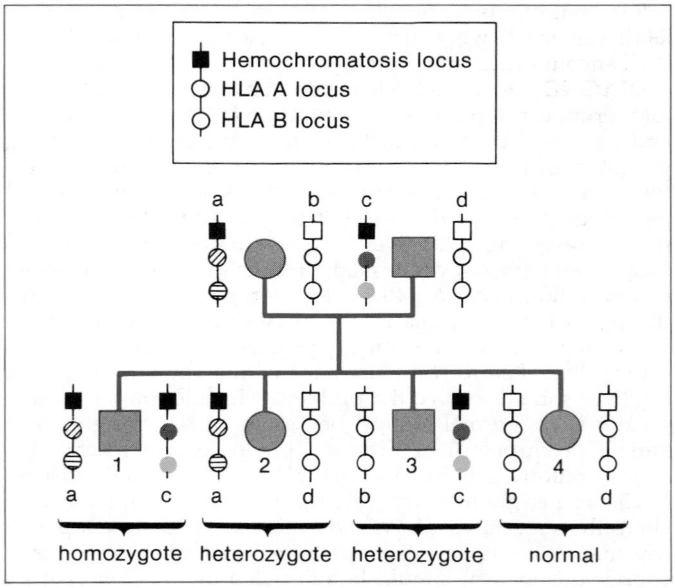

FIGURE 206–1. Hypothetical distribution of iron-loading alleles, each designated by an HLA haplotype, among family members of a patient (1) with fully developed idiopathic hemochromatosis. The "topographic" relationships between the gene (■) and the HLA loci (○) are diagrammatic approximations. The mother of the patient has two number 6 chromosomes, designated a and b, of which chromosome a carries the mutant allele of the hemochromatosis locus. In the father the mutant allele occurs on the sixth chromosome that is designated c. The patient inherited both mutant genes and is a homozygote. (From Bothwell TH, Charlton RW, Motulsky AG: Idiopathic hemochromatosis. In Stanbury JB, Wyngaarden JB, Fredrickson DS, Goldstein JL, Brown MS [eds.]: The Metabolic Basis of Inherited Disease. 5th ed. New York, McGraw-Hill Book Company, 1983.)

and symptoms. Heterozygotes for the hemochromatosis gene may absorb somewhat increased amounts of iron, and minor abnormalities of iron loading have sometimes been detected. Test results of iron status in heterozygotes are closer to those found in normals than to those in homozygotes for hemochromatosis; clinical manifestations rarely if ever occur. It is conceivable that heterozygotes are at higher risk to develop iron overload under conditions at which normal persons would not be affected. However, iron overload in alcoholic liver disease appears not to be associated with the heterozygote state for hemochromatosis. Not all homozygotes develop clinical disease. The fraction of those who do so depends upon the various circumstances affecting iron balance already discussed. It is clear that full-blown clinical findings are the "tip of the iceberg" and that many homozygotes may have no symptoms or exhibit only mild clinical findings that are not recognized as being related to the underlying iron storage disease.

PATHOLOGY. Although iron in reticuloendothelial cells is relatively harmless, parenchymal cell deposits are noxious to tissues. Iron in hemochromatosis is stored mostly in parenchymal cells as insoluble granular gold-brown aggregates known as *hemosiderin*. Normally, most iron is stored as ferritin, but with increasing iron overload the proportion of hemosiderin increases. With advancing hemosiderosis, fibrosis increases, and cirrhosis is frequent in fully developed cases. In such patients wide fibrotic bands characteristically separate liver lobules to cause monolobular cirrhosis.

Skin pigmentation is caused by melanin in the deeper epidermis while the slate-gray appearance in some cases is caused by hemosiderin. Pancreatic iron deposits are more marked in exocrine than in endocrine cells, and fibrosis is the rule. Iron pigment may be deposited in myocardial fibers. Synovial linings as well as various endocrine glands, including thyroid, parathyroid, and anterior pituitary, may be heavily infiltrated with hemosiderin. Testicular atrophy without hemosiderin deposits is frequent. These descriptions refer to fully developed cases. Early cases exhibit significantly fewer pathologic findings.

PREVALENCE. Studies in Utah, Brittany (France), and Sweden suggest homozygote frequencies varying between 1/200 and 1/600. This implies a high frequency of the heterozygote state for the disease, ranging from 8 to 13 per cent. Such frequencies make hemochromatosis one of the most common genetic diseases. Since only a certain portion of homozygotes will develop typical clinical findings, the frequency of the clinical disease will be lower and was estimated to be roughly 1/5000 in the Pacific Northwest of the United States and 1/500 and 1/1000 in autopsy series in Scotland and Southern Sweden, respectively. More prevalence studies are required.

CLINICAL MANIFESTATIONS IN THE FULL-BLOWN DISEASE. Because of the long time required to produce organ damage, the onset of clinical disease is usually, but not always, delayed to the age of 40 to 60. Males are more frequently and earlier affected than menstruating females. The most important clinical signs and symptoms in the fully developed disease include hepatomegaly, skin pigmentation, weakness and lethargy, chronic abdominal pain, diabetes, arthralgia, loss of libido, and impotence. However, more and more patients are being discovered in the early stages of the disease with few or no clinical findings.

The *skin pigmentation* causes browning of the skin that is most pronounced in exposed areas and scars. With increasing hemosiderin deposits, the skin takes on a slate-gray appearance.

Hepatomegaly is the most common physical finding and may occur without symptoms and with normal liver function test results. Portal hypertension and esophageal varices are seen less frequently than in Laennec's cirrhosis. Episodes of hepatic failure are rare, but may be precipitated by blood loss or surgical procedures. *Splenomegaly* occurs. Chronic aching *abdominal pain* is common once cirrhosis has developed and may be the presenting symptom. Carcinoma of the liver is a relatively frequent late complication. Unfortunately, *once cirrhosis has developed, the risk of a malignant hepatoma appears undiminished by iron removal and emphasizes the importance of early case detection and initiation of iron-removing therapy* (see below). Dysrhythmia and refractory cardiac failure may occur and may present clinically as *congestive cardiomyopathy*.

Insulin-dependent diabetes is often seen. A family history of diabetes unrelated to iron storage is more common among patients with hemochromatosis than among controls, suggesting expression of a genetic predisposition to diabetes in persons with liver and pancreatic injury. *Arthralgia* and *arthropathy* different from rheumatoid arthritis and osteoarthritis are common. The second and third metacarpophalangeal joints are usually first involved. Knees, hips, shoulders, and lower back may be affected and acute synovitis with pseudogout of the knees has been observed. Roentgenograms show chondrocalcinosis with small cysts characteristically affecting the second or third metacarpophalangeal joints. Osteoporosis is sometimes observed. *Loss of libido* and sexual impotence with testicular atrophy are common. Scanty body hair may be present long before significant hepatic impairment. Clinically manifest *hypogonadism* is usually of hypogonadotrophic origin. Marked lethargy, increased sleep requirements, and inability to think clearly are frequent complaints.

DIAGNOSIS. The clinical diagnosis of hemochromatosis requires a high index of suspicion and needs to be sought more frequently. Many patients are being detected fortuitously after discovery of abnormally saturated transferrin levels during general workups. Iron overload should be carefully considered among patients (particularly males) who present with any one or a combination of the following: hepatomegaly, weakness and lethargy, abnormal skin pigmentation, atypical arthritis, diabetes, impotence, unexplained chronic abdominal pain, or idiopathic cardiomyopathy. Excessive alcohol intake increases the diagnostic probability. A careful history of such illness among sibs should be obtained, and diagnostic suspicions should be particularly high when the family history is positive for the various clinical findings that might suggest this disease.

The diagnosis requires laboratory testing of iron status. The most practical screening test is the determination of serum iron and of transferrin saturation. Serum iron is characteristically elevated in patients with hemochromatosis, and there is increased iron saturation of transferrin, ranging between 60 and 100 per cent (normal, less than 50 per cent). However, abnormally high transferrin saturation can occur as a result of sample contamination, physiologic plasma iron fluctuation, iron therapy, liver disease, and red cell disorders. An abnormal value for transferrin saturation is seen early in the course of the disease and does not reflect the extent of iron storage. In contrast, a valuable noninvasive test to assess iron stores is the measurement of serum ferritin, which correlates reasonably well with the extent of iron storage in the absence of excessive alcohol consumption, inflammation, rheumatoid arthritis, neoplasia, and liver disease such as that induced by drugs or viral hepatitis. Without such complications, a level above 300 μm per liter in males and above 200 μg per liter in females indicates increased iron stores and requires further investigation. Patients with fully developed hemochromatosis have ferritin levels ranging between 700 and several thousand micrograms per liter. However, rare families with significant iron overload and normal ferritin values have been described. Various imaging techniques such as hepatic computerized tomography and nuclear magnetic resonance may become useful for the assessment of hepatic iron stores.

Because of problems with specificity and sensitivity with all laboratory and imaging tests, the definitive test for hemochromatosis is a *liver biopsy*. Parenchymal hemosiderin deposits can be demonstrated histochemically, and the actual concentration of iron should be estimated biochemically. The extent of liver damage and cirrhosis can be determined by histologic examination.

DIFFERENTIAL DIAGNOSIS. The most common differential diagnostic problem is raised by alcoholic liver disease not associated with HLA-linked hemochromatosis. Many such patients have an increased amount of stainable liver iron but no increased iron stores (usually less than 3 grams). Unlike genetic hemochromatosis, the iron in this disease is mostly located in reticuloendothelial cells. Liver function abnormalities are more severe than in hemochromatosis. Appropriate tests (including serum ferritin, liver biopsy, and even a trial of phlebotomies) can establish whether there is increased generalized iron storage. HLA testing and studies of iron status in family members may be helpful, since familial aggregation is not seen in patients with alcoholic liver disease. Iron overload due to chronic anemias (see below) such as beta-thalassemia major rarely raises diagnostic problems, although occasional patients with thalassemia intermedia or sideroblastic anemia with only slightly depressed hematocrit may give diagnostic difficulties.

FAMILY DETECTION FOR PREVENTION. Early treatment can remove increased iron stores that ultimately cause disease. Most importantly, treatment before the onset of cirrhosis most likely prevents the high frequency of hepatoma observed in hemochromatosis. All efforts should therefore be made to detect the disease as early as possible. Since the disease is an autosomal recessive trait, there is a 25 per cent chance that sibs of a patient will be similarly affected. Ideally all family members require a single determination of their HLA status to ascertain which sibs share all HLA determinants with the index case and therefore are homozygotes for the disease. Functional testing includes transferrin saturation, and serum ferritin. If full identity in HLA status and the characteristic iron metabolism abnormalities are found, a liver biopsy should be performed to assess the extent of iron storage. With iron overload, phlebotomies to remove iron should be initiated. Sib testing should be initiated at about puberty for males and after the age of 20 years for females. HLA-identical male sibs found to have a normal iron load should be restudied every two to three years, females somewhat less frequently. Frequent blood donations (three times a year) will prevent potentially toxic iron accumulation and are recommended for HLA-identical sibs. Parents and children of affected patients are obligate heterozygote carriers. Since the gene frequency of hemochromatosis appears to be high, matings of homozygotes with heterozygote carriers are not uncommon, and one half of the offspring of such couples will be homozygotes (pseudodominant vertical transmission). Thus, a parent or a child of a patient with hemochromatosis may also be a homozygote. Family detection therefore should include the entire family.

Occasionally, differentiation of heterozygotes from affected homozygotes may be difficult by serum ferritin and transferrin testing alone. HLA status may aid in such cases, since heterozygotes usually share only one half their HLA haplotypes with their homozygote sibs. Treatment to remove iron is rarely if ever required in heterozygotes.

TREATMENT. Excess iron can usually be removed by periodic venesections. The removal of one unit (approximately 500 ml) of blood depletes the body of 200 to 250 mg of iron. Weekly venesections are required for about two to three years to return iron stores to normal levels in patients with the full-blown disease and for lesser periods for those with early disease. Even though there is no scientific or medical contraindication to using blood from hemochromatic patients for blood transfusions, many blood banks do not use such blood.

Treatment should be monitored by frequent hematocrit determinations and plasma iron and ferritin levels six to ten times per year (Fig. 206–2). After an initial fall, hematocrit levels stabilize at approximately 90 per cent of pretreatment levels. Indicators of iron status do not change until significant depletion of iron stores has occurred. After iron stores have been normalized as shown by ferritin and transferrin levels,

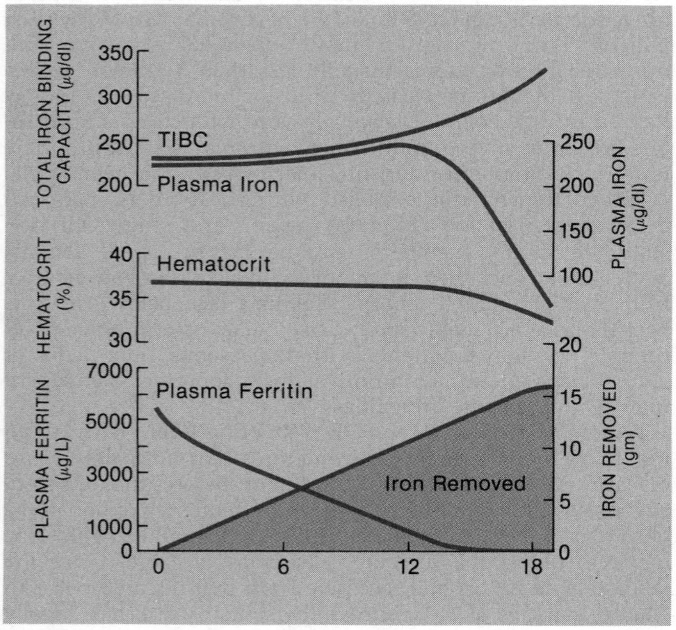

FIGURE 206–2. Serial changes in the hematocrit, plasma iron concentration, total iron-binding capacity, and plasma ferritin concentration in a subject with idiopathic hemochromatosis on repeated venesection therapy. (From Bothwell TH, Charlton RW, Cook JD, Finch CA: Idiopathic haemochromatosis. In Iron Metabolism in Man. Oxford, Blackwell Scientific Publications, 1979.)

venesections are required at two- to three-month intervals to prevent reaccumulation of iron. An iron-free diet is not necessary at any time during treatment. Treatment of hepatic, cardiac, endocrinologic, and metabolic complications is along conventional lines. Many manifestations of hemochromatosis *except* arthropathy, portal hypertension, and cirrhosis and hepatoma are dramatically improved by phlebotomy therapy.

PROGNOSIS. The five-year survival rate after diagnosis in untreated patients with the fully developed disease is 18 per cent and the ten-year survival rate 6 per cent. The principal cause of death in such patients relates to liver complications: hepatic failure and portal hypertension (30 per cent) and malignant hepatoma (30 per cent). An additional one third of patients die of cardiac failure.

Recently 163 treated patients whose disease was diagnosed between 1959 and 1983 were studied in West Germany. There were 53 deaths. Kaplan-Meier plots indicated cumulative survival of 92 per cent at 5 years, 76 per cent at 10 years, 59 per cent at 15 years, and 49 per cent at 20 years. Life expectancy was reduced significantly further in patients who had cirrhosis, diabetes, or required more than 18 months of venesection for iron depletion. Death was due to cirrhosis in 25 per cent and to hepatoma in 25 per cent. By contrast, in *treated patients without cirrhosis survival expectation was identical to that of the unaffected control population.* It is noteworthy that hepatoma has never been reported in any series among individuals with hemochromatosis who had not developed cirrhosis.

SECONDARY HEMOCHROMATOSIS. Classic hemochromatosis with iron deposits in parenchymal cells of the liver and other organs is observed in several anemias associated with erythroid marrow hyperplasia and ineffective erythropoiesis. Beta-thalassemia major and beta-thalassemia–hemoglobin E disease are the most common anemias of this type. Severe iron loading already occurs before transfusion therapy. Repeated blood transfusions produce further iron overload. In contrast to the HLA-linked hemochromatosis, iron overload in beta-thalassemia major occurs more rapidly and causes clinical symptoms early in life. Hepatic fibrosis is already common in children as is retarded growth and delayed puberty. Cardiac death usually occurs in adolescence or early adulthood unless iron removal is carried out.

Phlebotomies cannot be done since these patients are severely anemic. Chelation therapy with desferrioxamine together with frequent transfusions has improved the prognosis markedly. Death due to complications of iron storage can be prevented if iron removal can be initiated before clinical signs and symptoms of iron overload appear.

Patients with hypoplastic anemias do not absorb increased amounts of iron, but often require blood transfusions over prolonged periods. The transfused iron is largely stored in macrophages. No clinical signs or symptoms occur with storage of iron in macrophages. Redistribution to parenchymal cells with development of hepatic cirrhosis and/or other typical organ involvement occurs rarely.

Bothwell TH, Charlton RW, Motulsky AG: Idiopathic hemochromatosis. In Stanbury JB, Wyngaarden JB, Fredrickson DS, et al. (eds): The Metabolic Basis of Inherited Disease. 5th ed. New York, McGraw-Hill Book Company, 1983, pp 1269-1298. *A full discussion of all aspects of iron metabolism and genetics in HLA-linked and secondary hemochromatosis.*

Edwards CQ, Dadone MM, Skolnick MH, et al.: Hereditary haemochromatosis. Clin Haematol 11:411, 1982. *A comprehensive review of the disease based on the extensive Utah experience.*

Fairbanks VF, Baldus WP: Hemochromatosis: The neglected diagnosis. Mayo Clin Proc 61:296, 1986. *A succinct summary of this underdiagnosed disease and practical advice regarding laboratory tests.*

Halliday JW, Powell LW: Iron overload. Semin Hematol 19:42, 1982. *A balanced discussion of all aspects of idiopathic and secondary hemochromatosis.*

Milder MS, Cook JD, Stray S, et al.: Idiopathic hemochromatosis, an interim report. Medicine 59:34, 1980. *Clinical features and treatment of idiopathic hemochromatosis based on 34 cases.*

Niederau C, Fischer R, Sonnenberg A, et al.: Survival and causes of death in cirrhotic and in noncirrhotic patients with primary hemochromatosis. N Engl J Med 313:1256, 1985. *A detailed account of the natural history of treated hemochromatosis in 163 patients with 53 deaths.*

Simon M, Bourel M, Genetet B, et al.: Idiopathic hemochromatosis. Demonstration of recessive transmission and early detection by family HLA typing. N Engl J Med 297:1017, 1977. *Data to support HLA linkage and review of the inheritance of hemochromatosis with practical recommendations.*

Valberg LS, Ghent CN: Diagnosis and management of hereditary hemochromatosis. Annu Rev Med 36:27, 1985. *A useful review of the current status of diagnosis and management.*

207 PHOSPHORUS DEFICIENCY AND HYPOPHOSPHATEMIA

Lloyd H. Smith, Jr.

Phosphorus is necessary for the structural and functional integrity of all living things. In hydroxyapatite it is a key constituent of bone; as a part of phospholipids (lecithin, sphingomyelin) it is necessary for the structure of all cell membranes, both external and internal (endoplasmic reticulum, lysosomes, nuclear membranes). It furnishes the backbone of nucleic acids, captures and stores metabolic energy (~P), serves as a second messenger in endocrinology (cAMP, cGMP), regulates the release of O_2 by hemoglobin (2,3-diphosphoglycerate), and buffers urine. Even this partial list indicates that a severe deficiency of phosphorus would lead to widespread and serious consequences.

In an adult of average size there are approximately 700 to 800 grams (25 moles) of phosphorus, of which 80 to 85 per cent is in the skeleton and 10 per cent in muscle. Phosphate is the major anion of intracellular fluid (about 100 mM), where it is found mostly as phosphoproteins, phospholipids, or phosphosugars rather than as free orthophosphate. In extracellular fluid the normal concentration of phosphorus in adults is 2.7 to 4.5 mg per deciliter (0.9 to 1.5 mM), of which most is free; perhaps 10 per cent is protein bound. Serum phosphorus is normally higher in children (4.0 to 7.0 mg per deciliter). (It is conventional to express serum phosphate as the amount of elemental P, since pH influences the relative amounts of $H_2PO_4^-$ and $HPO_4^=$ present.) The average American diet contains about 1000 mg P, most of which is absorbed by active transport, increased by 1,25-dihydroxycholecalciferol. Approximately 90 per cent of that absorbed from the diet is excreted in the urine by a process involving filtration and partial renal tubular reabsorption. The tubular reabsorption of phosphate is diminished by parathyroid hormone (PTH), acting with cAMP as a second messenger. Through vitamin D, PTH, calcitonin, and the mineralization of osteoid, phosphate metabolism is closely linked with that of calcium. These interrelationships are discussed more completely in Ch. 244.

Hyperphosphatemia that is sustained occurs almost exclusively in three clinical conditions: (1) renal insufficiency (see Ch. 78), (2) hypoparathyroidism (including various types of pseudohypoparathyroidism) (see Ch. 247), and (3) acromegaly or gigantism (see Ch. 226). When severe, hyperphosphatemia may contribute to the acidosis of uremia, further reduce the extracellular fluid concentration of ionized calcium, or lead to metastatic calcification in extraosseous sites. Transient hyperphosphatemia may occur with acute tissue destruction, such as the tumor lysis syndrome or rhabdomyolysis.

CAUSES OF HYPOPHOSPHATEMIA. Hypophosphatemia (serum P <2.7 mg per deciliter) may be associated with a normal total body phosphate (representing a transient intracellular shift) or with phosphate deficiency. The two most common causes of transient hypophosphatemia are (1) ingestion of carbohydrates, which deplete phosphate in extracellular fluid in the process of their intracellular transport and metabolism, and (2) acute respiratory alkalosis, which leads to an intracellular shift of phosphate through mechanisms not fully explained.

TABLE 207–1. CAUSES OF HYPOPHOSPHATEMIA*

I. Moderate hypophosphatemia (P 1.0 to 2.5 mg per deciliter)
Hyperparathyroidism
Osteomalacia (usually with hyperparathyroidism), malabsorption, deficiency of vitamin D, familial hypophosphatemic rickets, vitamin D dependent rickets, oncogenic rickets
Carbohydrate administration or ingestion or enhanced metabolism—glucose, fructose, glycerol, lactate, insulin administration
Hypomagnesemia
ECF volume expansion
Acute alkalosis—bicarbonate infusion or moderate hyperventilation
Hemodialysis
II. Severe hypophosphatemia (P less than 1.0 mg per deciliter)
Chronic alcoholism and alcoholic withdrawal
Diabetic ketoacidosis, recovery phase
Enteric phosphate binding—excessive use of agents binding phosphate in the gut
Hyperalimentation
Nutritional recovery syndrome
Uptake by rapidly proliferating malignant tumors (rare)

*Modified from Knochel JP: Hypophosphatemia. West J Med 134:15, 1981.

It is convenient to summarize the causes of hypophosphatemia as those that usually result in only moderate reductions in serum P (1.0 to 2.5 mg per deciliter) and those that may result in severe hypophosphatemia (P <1.0 mg per deciliter) (Table 207–1). The latter may also be associated with lesser degrees of phosphate depletion as well.

Moderate hypophosphatemia may occur transiently during carbohydrate metabolism or alkalosis, as noted above, in the absence of phosphate depletion. Increased PTH, associated with either primary or secondary hyperparathyroidism, reduces the renal tubular reabsorption of phosphate and leads to renal phosphate wasting. In familial hypophosphatemic rickets there may be a primary defect in the renal tubular reabsorption of phosphate. The association of hypophosphatemia with hyperparathyroidism and the various types of osteomalacia or rickets is discussed more fully in Ch. 246 and 247. Hypomagnesemia and extracellular fluid volume expansion may result in reduced renal tubular reabsorption of phosphate and mild hypophosphatemia. Hemodialysis with equilibration against a dialysate deficient in phosphate may lead to overshoot hypophosphatemia. There are no well-defined acute metabolic consequences of moderate hypophosphatemia. Prolonged hypophosphatemia in this range may result in the defective mineralization of bone characteristic of osteomalacia or rickets.

Severe hypophosphatemia may cause serious metabolic consequences as described below. The most frequent cause of severe hypophosphatemia in clinical practice is *alcoholism*, especially during the withdrawal phase. The causes of phosphate depletion in alcoholics are complex and may include (1) poor dietary intake, (2) vomiting, (3) diarrhea, (4) the use of antacids which bind phosphate and reduce its absorption, (5) a possible phosphaturic effect of ethanol itself, (6) magnesium deficiency with phosphaturia, and (7) calcium deficiency with secondary hyperparathyroidism. The serum P level may be further reduced by the hyperventilation characteristic of alcohol withdrawal and by the therapeutic infusion of glucose. Patients with *uncontrolled diabetes mellitus* often become phosphate depleted through catabolism of intracellular organic phosphates and phosphaturia secondary to osmotic diuresis. Initial serum P levels are often normal or even high during diabetic ketoacidosis, but rapidly fall to hypophosphatemic levels during the first six to twelve hours of treatment with volume expansion, glucose, and insulin. Hyperventilation with *marked respiratory alkalosis* can cause profound hypophosphatemia within minutes; metabolic alkalosis of the same degree causes only moderate hypophosphatemia. Excessive ingestion of *phosphate binding antacids*, such as aluminum hydroxide, may inhibit phosphate absorption from the intestine sufficiently to cause chronic depletion, especially when combined with reduced dietary ingestion of phosphate. Excessive utilization of phosphate during tissue repletion may

TABLE 207–2. CONSEQUENCES OF SEVERE HYPOPHOSPHATEMIA

Acute—"metabolic"
- Hematologic
  - Red cell dysfunction and hemolysis
  - Leukocyte dysfunction
  - Platelet dysfunction
- Muscle
  - Weakness
  - Rhabdomyolysis
  - Myocardial dysfunction
- Central nervous system dysfunction
- Peripheral neuropathy
- Hepatic dysfunction

Chronic—"structural"
- Osteomalacia or rickets

occasionally result in severe hypophosphatemia during *hyperalimentation* (without adequate supplementary P) and during the *nutritional recovery syndrome* of refeeding patients with protein-calorie malnutrition or starvation. Whatever its cause, severe hypophosphatemia requires early attention because of its potential consequences.

CONSEQUENCES OF SEVERE HYPOPHOSPHATEMIA (Table 207–2). The long-term consequences of severe hypophosphatemia are largely structural, those of metabolic bone disease (see Ch. 246). The short-term consequences may be considered to be metabolic, although the distinction is an arbitrary one.

Red cell dysfunction in severe hypophosphatemia may result from two biochemical abnormalities, depletion of intracellular 2,3-diphosphoglycerate (2,3-DPG) and of ATP. Phosphate is a cofactor for glyceraldehyde-3-phosphate dehydrogenase, an enzyme in the pathway of the synthesis of 2,3-DPG. When intracellular erythrocytic phosphate decreases, a block in the glycolytic pathway results with accumulation of triose phosphates and depletion of 2,3-DPG. This molecule normally exercises a unique allosteric effect on the dissociation curve of oxyhemoglobin, shifting it "to the right" and thereby enhancing the tissue availability of oxygen (see Ch. 140). Reduction of erythrocytic 2,3-DPG, conversely, impairs effective oxygen delivery to the periphery. The same block in the glycolytic pathway reduces ATP synthesis. The degradation of AMP to inosine 5′-phosphate (IMP) by AMP deaminase is enhanced when the restraining influence of phosphate is reduced, further depleting the intracellular concentration of adenine nucleotides. As a result the concentration of erythrocytic ATP tends to fall in parallel with the reduction of serum phosphorus. At a critical level of ATP (usually with serum P <0.5 mg per deciliter), the energy metabolism of the erythrocyte may become inadequate to maintain the integrity of its membrane and *hemolysis* may occur.

Leukocyte dysfunction has been demonstrated during phosphate depletion in experimental animals, characterized by impaired chemotaxis, phagocytosis, and bactericidal function. These defects presumably result from inadequate ATP for normal cellular functions, possibly including the synthesis of phospholipids in membranes. Similarly *platelet dysfunction* occurs in experimental phosphate depletion, but no hemorrhagic diathesis has been attributed to phosphate deficiency in man.

Many patients with severe hypophosphatemia complain of *weakness*. This is often nonspecific and difficult to delineate from that caused by the associated disorder, but improved diaphragmatic contractility has been noted following the treatment of hypophosphatemia in patients with respiratory failure. *Rhabdomyolysis* is an occasional complication of severe hypophosphatemia, perhaps being somewhat analogous to hemolytic anemia in its pathogenesis, i.e., related to deficiency of ATP. The severity of rhabdomyolysis varies from that manifested solely by an elevated serum level of "muscle enzymes" (aldolase and creatine phosphokinase) to a full-fledged syndrome of muscle weakness, pain, tenderness, and stiffness associated with myoglobinuria. Interestingly, the release of phosphate from the necrosis of muscle may suffice to return the serum P level to normal. A few patients with severe phosphate depletion have exhibited congestive cardiomyopathy, which has seemed to respond to phosphate repletion. These clinical observations are strengthened by the demonstration of decreased myocardial contractility during experimental phosphate depletion in dogs.

Severe hypophosphatemia may result in *central nervous system dysfunction* with a constellation of symptoms and signs designated as metabolic brain disease or metabolic encephalopathy (see Ch. 457). These abnormalities may vary from irritability, weakness, and paresthesias to obtundation, seizures, and coma. It is presumed that this CNS dysfunction results from deranged energy metabolism of the brain secondary to ATP depletion. Observations have suggested that hepatic function is further impaired in alcoholics with severe hypophosphatemia, with early improvement during replacement therapy, but a clinical entity of *hypophosphatemic hepatic dysfunction* has not yet been well established.

TREATMENT OF HYPOPHOSPHATEMIA. The treatment of hypophosphatemia depends upon its cause, its acuteness, and its severity. Hypophosphatemia caused by acute respiratory alkalosis or the infusion of carbohydrates does not require replacement therapy. Chronic hypophosphatemia associated with aluminum hydroxide therapy, for example, may require reduction of the antacid and an oral source of supplemental phosphate such as milk (1 gram of P or 30 to 35 mmol per quart) or a balanced solution of phosphate salts (sodium or potassium salts as in Fleet enema solution or Neutra-Phos). It is rare that hypophosphatemia is so acute and severe as to require parenteral replacement therapy. When such treatment is undertaken it is well to remember that (1) it is unusual for hypophosphatemia to cause metabolic disturbances at concentrations greater than 1.0 mg per deciliter, so full parenteral replacement is neither necessary nor desirable; and (2) if hyperphosphatemia results, there is a danger of producing a decrease in ionized calcium (with tetany or convulsions) and/or metastatic calcification of soft tissues. It is usually safe and sufficient to administer intravenously 1 mmol of phosphate per kilogram of body weight evenly over a 24-hour period in the treatment of acute, severe hypophosphatemia associated with phosphate depletion. Since potassium depletion is so frequently associated with phosphate depletion both in alcoholics and in patients with diabetic ketoacidosis, it may be useful as a guideline to give half of parenterally administered potassium as its phosphate salt. Obviously parenteral phosphate should not be given in the face of hyperphosphatemia.

Agus ZS: Oncogenic hypophosphatemic osteomalacia. Kidney Int 24:113, 1983. *A description of the interesting syndrome of tumor-associated renal phosphate wasting.*

Janson D, Birnbaum G, Baker FJ: Hypophosphatemia. Ann Emerg Med 12:107, 1983. Knochel JP: Hypophosphatemia. West J Med 134:15, 1981. Yu GC, Lee DBN: Clinical disorders of phosphorus metabolism. West J Med (in press). *These three articles give excellent general reviews of the clinical and pathophysiologic aspects of phosphate deficiency syndromes in man and related disorders produced in experimental animals. They have useful bibliographies that allow the reader to pursue in depth the available information about each specific syndrome described above.*

Knochel JP: The clinical status of hypophosphatemia. N Engl J Med 313:447, 1985. *This useful editorial emphasizes the adverse effect of phosphate depletion on muscle function.*

208 DISORDERS OF MAGNESIUM METABOLISM

Lloyd H. Smith, Jr.

Magnesium is the fourth most common cation in the human body (after sodium, potassium, and calcium) and the cation in second highest concentration intracellularly. The average adult body contains about 25 grams (1000 mmol) of magnesium, of which 50 to 60 per cent is in bone. The normal serum magnesium concentration is 1.6 to 2.1 mEq per liter, approximately one fourth to one third being protein bound. The average American diet contains approximately 500 mg (20 mmol) of magnesium, much of this in chlorophyll. It has been estimated that about 0.15 mmol (3.5 to 4.5 mg) of dietary magnesium per kilogram per day is necessary to maintain a positive balance in adults. More is required in children. Magnesium is actively absorbed in the small intestine by a process that is enhanced by 1,25-dihydroxycholecalciferol, resulting in a net absorption of about 30 to 40 per cent of that ingested. This net absorption is balanced at equilibrium by renal excretion, which reflects filtration of the 65 to 75 per cent not protein bound followed by net renal tubular reabsorption of approximately 95 per cent. The kidney can control the excretion of magnesium over a wide range—from more than 250 mmol to less than 1 mmol per day. The factors that control the renal tubular reabsorption of magnesium are not completely understood, but include sodium excretion, calcium excretion, parathyroid hormone, and extracellular fluid volume. Excretion is also increased by ethanol and by many diuretic agents.

Magnesium has a structural role in bone crystal. It also serves as an activator of a large number of specific enzymes. Of particular importance it is a cofactor in all transphosphorylation reactions involving ATP, so that it is intimately involved in energy metabolism and the synthesis of macromolecules, for example. Perhaps even more basic in biology is its obligate role in the function of chlorophyll. By and large it has not been possible to correlate the signs or symptoms of magnesium deficiency or excess with any one of its specific biochemical functions.

HYPERMAGNESEMIA. Because of the ability of the normal kidney to excrete a magnesium load, significant hypermagnesemia is rarely seen in clinical practice. In the past magnesium ion was occasionally infused as a hypotensive agent in the treatment of acute hypertension with the secondary production of symptomatic hypermagnesemia. In patients with renal insufficiency the excessive use of magnesium, as in magnesium-containing antacids, may cause hypermagnesemia. The manifestations of hypermagnesemia are largely in the central nervous system and the cardiovascular system. Ionized magnesium is a sedative that depresses the function of the central nervous system and exerts a curare-like effect on the neuromuscular junction at high concentrations (>10 mEq per liter). The cardiovascular effects of hypermagnesemia are those of peripheral vasodilatation resulting in hypotension, generalized depression of the cardiac conduction system, bradyrhythmias, and asystole with cardiac arrest in diastole. The cardiac effects of Mg^{++} are usually manifested at serum concentration greater than 10 mEq per liter with asystole at levels greater than 25 mEq per liter, but a few patients have exhibited exceptional sensitivity with cardiotoxicity at levels of 4.5 to 5.5 mEq per liter. Factors that augment the cardiotoxicity of Mg^{++} include hypocalcemia, hyperkalemia, acidosis, digitalis therapy, and renal insufficiency (beyond its effect on the serum Mg^{++} level). Treatment of hypermagnesemia is usually limited to discontinuing its exogenous source. In severe hypermagnesemia, intravenous treatment with calcium may temporarily reverse many of the toxic effects because of the pharmacologic antagonism of ionized calcium and magnesium in the central nervous system.

HYPOMAGNESEMIA. Hypomagnesemia is a much more frequent metabolic derangement than hypermagnesemia, and usually occurs as one component of a complex deficiency state, affecting many minerals, vitamins, and nutrients.

Causes of Hypomagnesemia. Magnesium deficiency and hypomagnesemia result from decreased absorption or from increased excretion (Table 208–1). Very rarely it may result from "loss" into bone during excessive osteogenesis, the "hungry bone syndrome," during the repair of osteitis fibrosa generalisata following the removal of a parathyroid tumor (see Ch. 247). Serum levels may also fall, as do those of calcium, during acute pancreatitis. In general, decreased absorption of magnesium occurs in the same circumstances as does decreased calcium absorption, especially caused by dietary deficiency and malabsorption syndromes of whatever origin. Decreased absorption in uremia may result from deficiency of 1,25-dihydroxycholecalciferol. A few infants have been described with convulsions associated with hypocalcemia and hypomagnesemia in the absence of renal magnesium wasting. They have responded to continued high ingestion of magnesium, but not of calcium, and are thought to have a selective defect in gut absorption of magnesium. It is not clear whether ethanol diminishes magnesium absorption directly or only through diminished ingestion or vitamin D deficiency.

Increased loss of magnesium can occur from excessive vomiting, from diarrhea, or via the kidney. Rarely patients may exhibit what appears to be an inherited renal tubular defect in magnesium reabsorption. These patients have tended to have potassium wasting as well and to present with hypokalemia, hypomagnesemia, and hypocalcemia (secondary to hypomagnesemia). In general, magnesium clearance tends to parallel that of sodium and calcium and may be increased by diuretics (osmotic, thiazides, ethacrynic acid, furosemide), by ionized calcium, and possibly by ethanol. Renal magnesium wasting also occurs as a result of the renal tubular effect of certain drugs, especially aminoglycosides, amphotericin B, and cisplatin. The magnesium wasting of uncontrolled diabetes mellitus probably results from tissue catabolism and osmotic diuresis. Lactation hypomagnesemia is well described in cattle and has been documented in one woman whose serum Mg^{++} fell to 0.4 mEq per liter.

Consequences of Hypomagnesemia. Hypomagnesemia rarely occurs as a single deficiency so that it is not always possible to distinguish its signs and symptoms from those of associated deficiency states. Selective magnesium deficiency has been produced experimentally in man, however, and it is based on these observations, together with clinical correlations in patients, that the spectrum of manifestations listed in Table

TABLE 208–1. CAUSES OF HYPOMAGNESEMIA (SEEN MOST FREQUENTLY CLINICALLY IN ALCOHOLISM AND MALABSORPTION)

I. **Decreased absorption from dietary sources**
  - Diet poor in magnesium
  - Parenteral feeding without magnesium
  - Ethanol effect on absorption
  - Malabsorption syndromes
  - Uremia
  - Selective intestinal defect for magnesium absorption (rare)

II. **Increased loss of magnesium from the body**
  - Gastrointestinal tract—diarrhea, fistulas, suction
  - Kidney
    - Primary renal tubular defects
    - Secondary—diuretics, Ca^{++}, ethanol, expansion of ECF, diabetes mellitus, treatment with gentamicin, cisplatin, or amphotericin B
  - Breast—lactation hypomagnesemia (mostly in cattle, rarely in humans)

III. **Internal redistribution**
  - Acute pancreatitis
  - Increased loss into bone ("hungry bone syndrome")

TABLE 208–2. CONSEQUENCES OF MAGNESIUM DEFICIENCY

Neuromuscular	
	Lethargy, weakness, fatigue, decreased mentation, paresthesias
	Neuromuscular irritability, in part due to associated hypocalcemia
	Hyaline and vacuolar degeneration of myofibers with segmental necrosis
Gastrointestinal	
	Anorexia, nausea, vomiting
	Paralytic ileus
Cardiovascular	
	Increased sensitivity to digitalis glycosides
	Cardiac arrhythmias
Metabolic	
	Hypocalcemia—probably due to the combined result of decreased PTH secretion and decreased end-organ responsiveness to PTH
	Hypokalemia—tendency toward renal potassium wasting

208–2 has been described. Patients with magnesium deficiency are lethargic, weak, and irritable with decreased attention span. They may have tetany with positive Chvostek and Trousseau signs because of associated hypocalcemia (see below). In experimental magnesium deficiency, muscles are weak and may show hyaline and vacuolar degeneration of myofibers, sometimes followed by leukocytic infiltration, segmental necrosis, and early calcification. Patients with hypomagnesemia are generally anorectic and may have nausea, vomiting, and poor intestinal mobility. Hypomagnesemia may occur in congestive heart failure because of anorexia, malabsorption, and the excessive use of diuretic agents. Magnesium deficiency increases the sensitivity of the heart to digitalis glycosides so that digitalis toxicity occurs at a lower serum level and also tends to persist longer. Hypomagnesemia has also been associated with cardiac arrhythmias independent of digoxin–ventricular premature beats, ventricular tachycardia, and ventricular fibrillation. This association is often difficult to establish because other abnormalities generally coexist, especially hypokalemia.

Magnesium metabolism has a number of interesting interrelationships with that of calcium: (1) both are absorbed by the gut through mechanisms enhanced by vitamin D; (2) excess magnesium may inhibit calcium absorption, but not vice versa; (3) calcium and magnesium may compete for renal tubular reabsorption; (4) calcium and magnesium are physiologic antagonists in the central nervous system; and (5) magnesium is necessary for the normal secretion of parathyroid hormone (PTH) in response to hypocalcemia and also for the activity of PTH as a hormone at the site of its target organs. *Hypocalcemia* is one of the most consistent and important findings in magnesium deficiency with hypomagnesemia. Hypocalcemia responds promptly to magnesium replacement and is accompanied by a rise in plasma PTH. A burst of PTH secretion occurs within minutes after the infusion of magnesium intravenously into patients with combined hypocalcemia and hypomagnesemia. Many of these patients show evidence of resistance to exogenous PTH as well. Hypomagnesemia therefore results in a complex combination of hypoparathyroidism and acquired pseudohypoparathyroidism. This entity should be suspected especially in alcoholics or patients with malabsorption who present with hypocalcemia. *Hypokalemia* is frequently found with hypomagnesemia. Although some of the conditions that cause magnesium depletion also produce potassium depletion, there is evidence that magnesium deficiency itself enhances renal excretion of potassium. This associated hypokalemia is usually resistant to potassium replacement unless magnesium is replaced first.

Treatment of Hypomagnesemia. The treatment of hypomagnesemia is rarely an acute emergency. When rapid replacement therapy is judged to be vital (convulsions, tachyrhythmias), 2 grams of $MgSO_4$ (16.3 mEq) can be given intravenously over several minutes. This can be followed by a constant intravenous infusion of approximately 1 mEq of magnesium per kilogram per 24 hours, which usually suffices for initial replacement therapy. Ampules often contain 1 gram of $MgSO_4{\cdot}7H_2O$ which is 8.1 mEq Mg, so that initial replacement therapy usually requires 8 to 10 grams of $MgSO_4$ given either intravenously as above or intramuscularly as 2 grams every four hours for five doses. After the first day approximately 0.5 mEq of Mg per kilogram per 24 hours should be given intravenously or intramuscularly for two to five days, based on the return of the serum magnesium level to normal. Parenteral replacement therapy is often preferable to oral therapy because of the tendency of magnesium salts to cause diarrhea. When renal function is impaired, the aforementioned schedules for magnesium replacement must be followed with extra caution and with careful monitoring of serum levels. When there is chronic loss of magnesium (renal wasting, for example), oral therapy is preferred and can be carried out with various preparations as tolerated without diarrhea—magnesium hydroxide tablets, magnesium acetate solution, or liquid milk of magnesia.

Berkelhammer C, Bear RA: A clinical approach to common electrolyte problems. 4. Hypomagnesemia. Can Med Assoc J 132:360, 1985. *This succinct review is a very useful starting point from which to read more extensively about magnesium metabolism in man.*

Cronin RE, Knochel JP: Magnesium deficiency. Adv Intern Med 28:509, 1983. *An excellent general review of magnesium metabolism and the pathophysiology of magnesium deficiency (102 references).*

Dirko JH: The kidney and magnesium regulation. Kidney Int 23:771, 1983. *A succinct review of the role of the kidney in magnesium metabolism and of the causes of hypomagnesemia (36 references).*

Levine BS, Coburn JW: Magnesium, the mimac/antagonist of calcium. N Engl J Med 310:1253, 1984. *An editorial about the complex interactions of these important cations.*

Whang R: Magnesium deficiency: Pathogenesis, prevalence, and clinical implications. Am J Med 82(Suppl. 3A):24, 1987. *A succinct general review with a useful up-to-date list of 43 references.*

Other Hereditary Disorders

209 FAMILIAL MEDITERRANEAN FEVER

Daniel G. Wright

DEFINITION. Familial Mediterranean Fever (FMF) is an inherited, recurrent inflammatory disease of unknown cause. The disease is characterized by acute self-limited attacks of fever and peritonitis, sometimes accompanied by pleuritis, arthritis, and erythematous skin lesions. Among affected individuals in the Middle East and Europe, FMF is frequently complicated by amyloidosis and progressive renal failure. FMF has been given a number of other names: familial paroxysmal polyserositis, benign paroxysmal peritonitis, periodic peritonitis, and periodic disease. The first of these is descriptively accurate and an appropriate alternative name for the disease; the other terms, however, are misleading and should not be used. FMF is not a benign condition, given the potentially lethal complication of amyloidosis. Moreover, attacks of acute serositis in FMF affect sites other than the peritoneum, and they recur at irregular, unpredictable intervals that do not reflect true periodicity.

INCIDENCE, PREVALENCE, AND GENETICS. Although FMF has been recognized in many parts of the world, it is largely restricted to ethnic groups originating in the eastern

Mediterranean area. It is an uncommon disease, even in Israel where the largest number of cases are seen. Half the reported cases of FMF are in patients of Sephardic Jewish ancestry; approximately 20 per cent of patients are Armenian, and another 20 per cent are of Turkish or Arabic descent. Most of the remaining patients are of Italian, Greek, or Ashkenazic Jewish ancestry. However, the disease has also been recognized rarely in individuals with Anglo-Saxon or northern European origins. The disease is familial, and in well-studied, affected kindreds it appears to be inherited as an autosomal recessive trait. Nonetheless, nearly 50 per cent of patients do not give a positive family history for the disease. Among reported cases males predominate by a ratio of 3:2.

ETIOLOGY. Many pathogenetic explanations have been proposed for the acute inflammatory episodes of FMF. However, the etiology of this disease remains unknown. Extensive studies have failed to establish an infectious or allergic basis for the disease, and there is no good evidence to support suggestions that FMF represents a hormonal or psychosomatic disturbance. Recently, it has been suggested that FMF might be caused by a genetically determined defect in the normal regulation of acute inflammatory responses. Abnormalities of suppressor T lymphocytes, altered metabolism of lipoxygenase products of arachidonic acid, and absence of a normal inhibitor of the complement-derived anaphylatoxin C5a have been described in FMF. However, the etiologic significance (if any) of these observations remains to be clarified and confirmed.

PATHOLOGY. Pathologic findings in FMF are those of nonspecific, acute inflammation. Neutrophilic infiltration predominates in exudates recovered from peritoneal, pleural, or joint spaces at the time of acute attacks. Serosal thickening and secondary adhesions may occur, which in the abdomen can lead to mechanical bowel obstruction. Amyloidosis is the most serious histopathologic finding in FMF. In affected individuals, amyloid is deposited in the intima and media of arterioles and in the subendothelium of venules in all major organs. There is also parenchymal deposition of amyloid, particularly in the renal glomeruli, adrenals, spleen, and alveolar septa of the lung, while the liver and heart are characteristically spared.

CLINICAL MANIFESTATIONS. In most patients the signs and symptoms of FMF begin during the first two decades of life, usually between the ages of 5 and 15 years. Rarely, however, onset of the disease may occur in infancy or as late as the fifth or sixth decade. There is considerable variability in the duration and frequency of attacks even in the same patient. Acute attacks typically last for 24 to 48 hours and recur once or twice a month. However, attacks may recur as frequently as several times a week or as infrequently as once a year, and symptoms may persist for as long as a week during individual episodes. Some patients experience spontaneous remission that persists for years, followed by recurrence of frequent attacks. Pregnancy is often associated with remission of attacks, which then resume postpartum. Some patients relate the occurrence of attacks to cold weather and find that they experience attacks more frequently during winter than during summer. Recurrent attacks may also become less severe and/or less frequent as patients age or as they develop amyloidosis. Between attacks, patients typically feel entirely well.

Temperatures as high as 39° to 40°C occur with almost all attacks. Fevers may occur without concomitant evidence of serositis, but this is unusual. The rise in temperature is sometimes preceded by chills and typically peaks by 12 to 24 hours; diaphoresis frequently accompanies defervescence.

More than 95 per cent of patients experience abdominal pain and signs of peritonitis during acute attacks. Pain often begins in one quadrant and then becomes diffuse, sometimes with distension, rigidity, rebound tenderness, and ileus with nausea and vomiting. Pain may radiate to the back or to the shoulders, and upright abdominal roentgenograms may show small air-fluid levels and edema of the bowel. Although these signs and symptoms are self-limited, they can be indistinguishable from those of an acute abdominal emergency, and patients may undergo one or more exploratory laparotomies before the true nature of their disease is recognized. Potential uncertainties about the clinical management of acute abdominal episodes have led to the recommendation that elective appendectomy be carried out during a symptom-free period so that acute appendicitis will not confuse patients' subsequent care.

Pleuritic pain occurs during acute attacks in 75 per cent of patients. Symptoms of pleuritis may sometimes precede abdominal pain, and a few patients experience pleuritic attacks without abdominal symptoms. Chest pain is usually one sided and may be associated with diminished breath sounds, a friction rub, and transient pleural effusion.

Nonspecific, mild arthralgia is a common feature of febrile attacks, and acute, monoarticular or oligoarticular arthritis may occur. Although arthritis is unusual among patients in the United States, it is a frequently observed manifestation of FMF among Israeli patients. Arthritis usually affects large joints, the knee in particular, and effusions are common. While arthritic episodes are typically short lived, joint symptoms may also be protracted and follow a course that is distinct from the acute abdominal and/or pleuritic attacks. Roentgenographic findings are nonspecific.

As many as a third of patients experience transient, erysipelas-like skin lesions that appear typically on the lower leg, ankle, or dorsum of the foot. These lesions are well-circumscribed, painful, erythematous areas of swelling, 5 to 20 cm in diameter, that subside spontaneously within 24 to 48 hours.

Self-limited pericarditis, conjunctivitis, aseptic meningitis, and other forms of serositis have been reported as manifestations of this disease, but are very unusual. Migraine-like headaches and emotional lability have also been observed during acute attacks, but it is unclear whether there are primary or secondary manifestations.

The most serious complication of FMF is amyloidosis. The natural history of amyloidosis in this disease is one of relentless progression to renal failure and death, which may occur in adolescence or even earlier. While a high proportion of Turkish and Israeli patients develop amyloidosis, this complication has been very unusual among patients in the United States and in several well-studied Armenian kindreds. The genetic and/or environmental factors that explain these differences in the incidence of amyloidosis remain unclear. In Israel, 90 per cent of patients who develop amyloidosis (particularly common in Sephardic Jews) do so after first experiencing typical attacks of FMF (phenotype I); however, amyloidosis may also occur in asymptomatic siblings of FMF patients, or it may precede the onset of typical FMF attacks (phenotype II).

Laboratory findings in FMF are nonspecific. During acute attacks there is prominent leukocytosis (up to 30,000 per cu mm), and the erythrocyte sedimentation rate and acute phase reactants are increased. These values return to normal between attacks. With amyloidosis, laboratory abnormalities reflect the associated nephrotic syndrome and renal failure.

DIAGNOSIS. The diagnosis of FMF is based primarily upon clinical presentation and history, for there is as yet no clearly proven laboratory measurement or test that is specific for this disease. In individuals of appropriate ethnic background with typical recurrent, self-limited attacks, diagnosis should not be difficult; in such individuals, delay in recognizing the disease is usually because the diagnosis is not considered. Nonetheless, when a patient is first seen or when attacks are infrequent, a variety of other acute febrile conditions must be considered and excluded by appropriate diagnostic studies and follow-up, in particular appendicitis, pancreatitis, cholecystitis, and intestinal obstruction. Familial hyperlipidemia and porphyrias associated with abdominal symptoms must also be considered.

The diagnosis is usually most elusive when patients have a limited or atypical symptom complex. Isolated pleural attacks may closely mimic acute infections or pulmonary emboli. Arthritis, when it is a prominent manifestation, can at first be clinically indistinguishable from various infectious and noninfectious arthritides, and skin lesions on the lower legs may resemble cellulitis or superficial thrombophlebitis. Rare patients have febrile episodes without serositis, and these may require orderly evaluation to determine their origin. Recently it has been reported that infusion of metaraminol diluted in normal saline provokes acute signs and symptoms of FMF with a high degree of specificity for the disease. However, the appropriate role of such a test in establishing the diagnosis remains unclear. At present this procedure, which carries intrinsic risks from catecholamine effects and salt load, should be considered experimental and not for use in general practice.

Once FMF is diagnosed, a degree of diagnostic vigilance must be maintained, for patients are not immune to the more common acute illnesses that FMF mimics. Of note, these patients appear to be particularly prone to develop gallbladder disease.

TREATMENT. Colchicine treatment is effective in FMF. Several controlled clinical trials, together with extensive, uncontrolled clinical experience since the mid 1970's, have shown that prophylactic colchicine,* 0.6 mg orally two to three times a day, prevents or substantially reduces the acute attacks of FMF in 75 to 90 per cent of patients. Treatment failures are often associated with noncompliance and/or intolerance to the drug.

Some patients can abort attacks with intermittent courses of colchicine, beginning at the onset of attacks (0.6 mg orally every hour for 4 hours, then every 2 hours for 4 hours, then every 12 hours for 2 days). In general, patients who benefit from intermittent colchicine therapy are those who experience a recognizable, albeit vague, prodrome before developing fever and clear-cut acute symptoms. Colchicine does not alter fully developed attacks. Patients who experience gastrointestinal intolerance to colchicine may benefit from reduced doses. Although definite chronic complications from colchicine have not become apparent with its long-term use in FMF, it is still recommended that a trial of intermittent colchicine therapy be attempted, particularly in young patients, before long-term colchicine prophylaxis is used. Azoospermia and chromosomal nondisjunctions have been associated with use of this drug. This recommendation does not apply to individuals from ethnic groups and in geographic regions associated with a high risk of amyloidosis, for it is now evident that long-term colchicine therapy not only prevents the development of amyloidosis but may also arrest its progression in FMF.

Symptomatic and supportive treatment is indicated for patients who do not respond to colchicine. However, every effort should be made to avoid the use of narcotics. In the United States, addiction to narcotics has been the major long-term complication among FMF patients.

PROGNOSIS. The prognosis for normal longevity for patients in the United States with FMF is excellent, and since the recognition of colchicine's efficacy in this disease, most patients can be maintained almost entirely symptom-free. Except in very rare cases, this disease does not affect the physical growth and development of children. Long-term colchicine therapy has also clearly improved the prognosis of patients in the Middle East who are prone to develop amyloidosis, even those whose symptomatic attacks continue. However, among patients who are unable to tolerate colchicine or in whom amyloidosis has led to nephrotic syndrome or uremia, the likelihood of eventual death from renal failure remains great.

*This use of colchicine is not listed in the manufacturer's directive.

Sohar F, Gafni J, Pras M, et al.: Familial Mediterranean fever. A survey of 470 cases and review of the literature. Am J Med 43:227, 1967.

Schwabe AD, Peters RS: Familial Mediterranean fever in Armenians. Analysis of 100 cases. Medicine 53:453, 1974.

Meyerhoff J: Familial Mediterranean fever: Report of a large family, review of the literature, and discussion of the frequency of amyloidosis. Medicine 59:66, 1980. *These three articles provide extensive reviews of the clinical and pathologic manifestations of FMF. The last two discuss differences in the incidence of amyloidosis.*

Dinarello CA, Wolff SM, Goldfinger SE, et al.: Colchicine therapy for familial Mediterranean fever. A double-blind trial. N Engl J Med 291:934, 1974. *One of several controlled trials that clearly established the efficacy of prophylactic colchicine therapy in preventing FMF attacks.*

Wright DG, Wolff SM, Fauci AS, et al.: Efficacy of intermittent colchicine therapy in familial Mediterranean fever. Ann Intern Med 86:162, 1977. *A double-blind study that shows that intermittent courses of colchicine can successfully abort attacks in some patients with FMF.*

Zemer D, Pras M, Sohar E, et al.: Colchicine in the prevention and treatment of the amyloidosis of familial Mediterranean fever. N Engl J Med 314:1001, 1986. *A retrospective review of 1070 patients that provides convincing evidence that long-term colchicine therapy arrests the development of amyloidosis.*

210 THE AMYLOID DISEASES

Joel N. Buxbaum

DEFINITION. The amyloid diseases comprise a group of conditions of diverse causes characterized by the accumulation of ultrastructurally fibrillar material in various tissues such that vital organ function is compromised. The associated disease states may be inflammatory, hereditary, or neoplastic, and the deposition can be local or systemic. The clinical outcome may be benign or as malignant as the most aggressive of neoplasms. In many senses, amyloid deposition is a symptom of an underlying disorder, much as anemia is a symptom of a variety of pathologic states. The symptoms of the amyloidoses depend upon the amount and localization of deposition of amyloid.

In tissue sections with conventional staining techniques, all amyloid appears homogeneous and eosinophilic. All types bind Congo red and under polarized light emit an apple-green fluorescence when stained with this dye. Viewed with the electron microscope, all amyloid contains two discrete structures, a major fibrillar component with a characteristic periodicity and a minor rodlike component that, viewed on end, has the appearance of pentamer with a hollow core (the P-component). The P-component appears to be physically and chemically identical in all amyloids and normally circulates as a soluble serum protein. Its role in the process of tissue infiltration has not been established.

The deposited fibril, regardless of its chemical nature, when isolated and analyzed has the x-ray diffraction pattern characteristic of a beta-pleated sheet. It is insoluble at physiologic salt concentrations, but can be released from tissue deposits by extraction with distilled water. The latter observation, made in the early 1970's, allowed the chemical analysis of fibrils obtained from many preparations of amyloid from tissues of individuals with different diseases. These studies have, in turn, permitted a more precise, chemically based, classification of the various amyloid syndromes (Table 210–1).

The ability to analyze the deposited proteins has also allowed the identification of circulating precursors of the insoluble fibrils and given general insight into processes that may be common to all types of amyloid deposition. It appears that all amyloid fibrils have a soluble precursor. In those individuals with pathologic deposition, either the amount of precursor is increased or the precursor is processed in such a way as to render it insoluble under physiologic conditions. It is not clear when or how processing takes place vis-à-vis

TABLE 210–1. CHEMICAL CLASSIFICATION OF THE AMYLOIDOSES

Clinical Syndrome	Fibril Precursor	Fibril	Common	Chemical
Primary or Myeloma, with Amyloid	Ig L chain	L chain or fragment	AL	Aλ (1-n) or Aκ (1-n)
Secondary*	SAA	AA	AA	$AA_{prototype}$ $AA_{(trp)\ var}$
Hemodialysis-Associated	β2m	β2m monomer or dimer	β2m	$A_{\beta 2m}$
Senile				
Cardiac	TBPA or TT	TBPA or TT	AS_{c1}	A_{TBPA} (var) or A_{TT} (var)
Brain (Alzheimer's)	Unknown	β-protein	AS_{β}	$A_{\beta\text{-protein}}$
Pancreas	? Proin	? Proin	AS_{P}	—
Familial				
Neuropathic	TBPA (TT)	TBPA (TT)	AF†	A_{TBPA} (var)
Cardiomyopathic	TBPA (TT)	TBPA (TT)	AF_{Da}	A_{TBPA} (var)
Nephropathic	SAA	AA	AF†	AA
Vascular HCHWA (Iceland)	Cystatin‡ (gamma-trace)	Cystatin	AF_{HCHWA}	Cystatin (var)
Localized				
Endocrine			AE	
Medullary carcinoma, thyroid	(?) Procal	(?) Procal	AE_{t}	A_{procal}
Islet cell tumor	(?) Proins	(?) Proins	AE_{p}	A_{proins}
Skin	?	?	AD	?
Papular	?	?	AD_{p}	?
Macular	?	?	AD_{m}	?
Nodular	?	?	AD_{n}	?

*Inflammation associated.

†Familial amyloids have been designated by the geographic locale in which they have been found. The fibrils are identified by the notation AF with the country of origin indicated by a subscript, e.g., AF_{P} for the Portuguese.

‡Cystatin is a lysosomal proteinase inhibitor formerly known as gamma-trace.

β2m = beta-2-microglobulin, AF = amyloid fibril; Procal = procalcitonin; Proins = proinsulin; SAA = serum AA; TBPA = thyroxine-binding prealbumin; TT = transthyretin.

deposition. In some instances, it appears that structurally normal proteins, e.g., some intact Ig light chains, may be amyloidogenic even without extensive processing, and it is excessive production that leads to tissue deposition. In other conditions, synthesis of normal amounts of a structurally aberrant molecule leads to deposition with or without cleavage. It is also not certain what controls the site and rate of deposition. While some molecules undergo the entire process of synthesis, processing, and deposition in a confined locale, other equally amyloidogenic substances are deposited far from the site of synthesis.

Over the years, numerous attempts have been made to classify the amyloidoses. Histologic distribution, specific organ involvement, and the presence or absence of other overt disease have served as distinguishing parameters. Each of these classifications had some merit, but none of them was without overlap or inconsistencies. The currently utilized chemically based scheme is the result of the analysis of the structure of proteins making up the deposited fibrils (Table 210–1). What has become obvious is that the same protein may constitute the fibril in diseases of apparently different causes.

PATHOGENESIS. ***AA Amyloidosis.*** AA amyloid is most frequently found when deposition takes place in the course of chronic inflammatory disease. In the past, chronic infectious processes, such as tuberculosis and osteomyelitis, were the usual precipitating diseases. In recent years, the most commonly associated conditions have been the chronic noninfectious inflammatory diseases. Rheumatoid arthritis has a reported prevalence of up to 20 per cent in autopsy series with somewhat lower prevalence clinically (5 to 7 per cent). The prevalence in juvenile rheumatoid disease varies considerably in different countries (e.g., 0.14 per cent in the United States to 10 per cent in Poland). Other inflammatory joint diseases including the seronegative spondyloarthropathies, gout, and psoriasis as well as inflammatory bowel disease, even without arthritis, have been associated with amyloid deposition. Also at high risk for the development of AA disease are those individuals who inject foreign substances intracutaneously or subcutaneously. The chronic or recurrent skin inflammation found in these patients seems to be particularly effective in the induction of amyloidosis.

Renal deposition of the AA protein has been the ultimately fatal event in the course of some groups of patients with *familial Mediterranean fever* (FMF) (Ch. 209). In the past, approximately 90 per cent of North African patients with this disease succumbed to renal failure by the age of 40.

AA deposition is also seen with a variety of nonlymphoid tumors and some nonimmunoglobulin producing lymphomas. Renal and gastric carcinomas and Hodgkin's disease have been the tumors most frequently associated with AA amyloid.

Kidneys, liver, and spleen are the most important sites of AA deposition. The renal disease is characterized initially by proteinuria of the glomerular type. Early in the disease, the kidneys may be enlarged but with time they shrink and the ultimate course is one of progressive renal failure. A variety of tubular disorders have also been described, including renal tubular acidosis, because of impaired bicarbonate reabsorption, nephrogenic diabetes insipidus, glycosuria, and hyperkalemia caused by decreased potassium exchange. The liver disease is relatively nonspecific, usually resulting in only moderate hepatomegaly and liver function test abnormalities.

In the past, when chronic infections were the most frequent stimuli to amyloid deposition, a small number of cases were reported in which eradication of the infection resulted in arrest of progression or actual regression of the amyloidosis as documented by biopsy. In general, even without treatment the course of AA disease is more chronic than that of AL amyloid.

The deposited AA protein appears to be a discrete proteolytic product of the serum AA protein (SAA) that has a monomer molecular weight of 12,500, but circulates as a molecule of 220,000 to 235,000 molecular weight complexed to high-density lipoprotein. It has also been found complexed to albumin. It behaves as an acute phase protein, rising rapidly in the course of inflammation (infectious or noninfectious) and peaking and falling to normal levels with resolution of the inflammation. SAA levels are generally higher in the elderly, and high levels have also been noted in patients with myeloma. Its synthesis is stimulated by the monokine interleukin 1. It appears that the predisposition to develop AA deposition resides in the production of an amyloidogenic isotypical form of SAA, the inability to degrade SAA completely, or both occurring in the same individual.

AL Amyloidosis. AL (or light chain-related) deposition is the most common form of amyloidosis seen in current clinical practice. The proportion of the total number of cases that represents multiple myeloma or primary amyloid is difficult to judge, since marrow plasmacytosis may be significant in both and the diagnostic distinctions between the primary disease and myeloma blurred (Ch. 163). Functionally, both diseases are malignant. In the case of myeloma, the outcome is related primarily to the proliferative capacity of the neoplastic clone. When AL deposition is present, it contributes to the poor prognosis. In primary amyloid disease the growth of a dominant plasma cell clone appears to be limited, but the amyloidogenicity of its homogeneous product results in the ultimately fatal compromise of organ function, most commonly renal or cardiac.

AL deposition is more likely to occur in tongue, heart, lymph nodes, spleen, carpal ligaments, joints, peripheral nerves, and skin than in the AA type. Hence, cardiac failure, arrhythmias, carpal tunnel syndrome, peripheral neuropathy, and ecchymoses are more frequent in AL disease. A deficiency of clotting factor X has been reported with an attendant bleeding diathesis. There is evidence to suggest that some AL proteins may have affinity for the clotting factor with resultant lowering of the plasma levels. Removal of an amyloid-laden spleen has reversed the deficiency in some patients. Blood vessels tend to be fragile in AL patients, since the amyloid is deposited in vessel walls. When vessel walls become rigid, not only are they sensitive to trauma but they do not respond well in the reflex-mediated changes in body position. When this occurs, orthostatic hypotension may become a major clinical problem. Coronary artery amyloid deposition can result in clinical angina pectoris or myocardial infarction.

A large number of studies have now documented that the deposited fibrillar protein is related to the excess monoclonal light chain produced by the expanded plasma cell clone and found in the patient's serum, urine, or both. The actual tissue protein may represent the whole light chain or a fragment thereof, usually containing at least the variable region. Amino acid sequence analyses of tissue AL protein and the isolated light chain obtained from the same patient have demonstrated chemical identity.

Despite several detailed analyses, it is still not clear what makes a given light chain amyloidogenic. Of light chain types associated with either primary amyloid or myeloma-associated amyloid, it appears that lambda chains are more frequent than kappa, and that the $V\lambda_{VI}$ light chain subgroup is overly represented. It has been suggested that tissue affinity could be charge related or that the interaction between light chain and tissues could represent an autoantibody antigen interaction. Neither of these hypotheses has conclusive experimental support. Further, it has not been established whether amyloidogenesis involves only the processing of intact light chains to fragments or if some of the molecules are synthetic fragments that are predisposed to deposition. It is possible that both phenomena occur.

Most AL patients, even those with primary amyloid, have a detectable M-component, usually free light chains of a single class, found in the serum or urine. However, 5 to 15 per cent have not had such proteins detectable. Analyses of a small number of these patients indicate that in tissue culture their bone marrow cells synthesize an excess of free monoclonal light chains. Because of their low concentration in the serum and their presumed high affinity for tissues they cannot be detected by conventional immunochemical techniques. In no instance yet reported has an immunoglobulin heavy chain been found to make up the fibril isolated from human amyloid tissue.

Recently a number of patients have been reported in whom organ compromise has taken place because of infiltration with monoclonal light chains without discrete fibril formation. Some of these patients have had clinical multiple myeloma; others have not. It is likely that this condition is analogous to AL amyloid, but that the deposited proteins do not have the intrinsic properties necessary to form beta-pleated sheets of sufficient size and stability to make fibrils. While these proteins have been identified in tissue deposits by immunofluorescence, chemical studies of the circulatory and tissue forms have not yet been carried out; therefore, formal proof of their identity is lacking.

Senile Amyloidosis. The term *senile amyloid* has been used to describe Congo red–binding material found at autopsy in the tissues of elderly individuals. The material is most commonly found in the heart but has also been noted in the pancreas and brain. It is likely that it represents a variety of tissue-specific proteins.

The cerebral plaques identified in Alzheimer's disease are congophilic. It is not yet clear whether these are primary or secondary in the pathogenesis of the condition. Nonetheless, material isolated from the plaques and from amyloid-containing cerebral vessels of these patients, using techniques that allowed the characterization of other amyloids, has been found to consist of a polypeptide containing 28 amino acids that has no homology to any other sequenced protein. The material does not share antigenic determinants with the paired helical filaments that are also characteristic of Alzheimer's disease; hence the role of the sequenced "beta-protein" in the pathogenesis of the diseases is presently uncertain.

Amyloid material has also been noted in the brain lesions of Jakob-Creutzfeldt patients (Ch. 488.2) and animals suffering from scrapie. Immunohistochemical and nucleotide sequence analyses have indicated that the Alzheimer and Jakob-Creutzfeldt proteins are separate entities.

While many individuals in their eighth and ninth decades have scattered atrial deposits, clinically significant cardiac disease, characterized by either congestive heart failure or arrhythmia, appears to occur rarely. Once it does, the prognosis is poor. The presence of a chronic inflammatory disease (e.g., rheumatoid arthritis) or multiple myeloma does not increase the incidence of senile cardiac amyloid (SCA) deposition; this suggests an independent pathogenesis for all three diseases.

Recent studies have indicated that the fibril of SCA isolated from ventricular myocardium has an amino acid sequence homologous with serum thyroxine-binding prealbumin (transthyretin). Since prealbumin is not known to be synthesized by myocardial cells, SCA suggests that the precursor is produced at a remote site and localizes in its target organ by some unknown mechanism. Clinical studies have suggested that pulmonary involvement may also be associated with cardiac deposition, implying that deposition of the SCA protein may be more systemic than previously appreciated.

AL, AA, and SCA make up the bulk of the amyloid diseases encountered in clinical practice; however, there are additional, less common forms, the analysis of which has yielded insight into the genesis of these deposits. Localized forms have been noted in medullary carcinoma of the thyroid, in which the fibrillar protein is related to procalcitonin, and in insulinomas, in which the material appears to be antigenically related to insulin.

Congo red–binding structures are also seen in the pancreas of elderly patients with type II diabetes mellitus. Immunochemical analysis suggests that these may also be related to insulin.

Hemodialysis-Associated Amyloidosis. During the last decade a syndrome has been recognized in patients who have been maintained with long-term hemodialysis. It is characterized by carpal tunnel syndrome, i.e., compression of the median nerve by a thickened carpal ligament, and arthropathy, frequently severe enough to require joint replacement. Examination of the surgically removed ligaments and synovial and rectal biopsies from affected individuals have revealed amyloid. Chemical analysis of the fibrils shows that they consist of monomers and dimers of beta-2–microglobulin, the light chain of cell surface major histocompatibility antigens A, B, and C.

TABLE 210–2. FAMILIAL AMYLOID SYNDROMES*

Syndrome	Onset	Clinical	Fibril
Neuropathic			
Portuguese-Japanese (I)†	20–40	Lower limbs, autonomic	TPBA‡; Val 30→Met
Swiss-Indiana (II)	>40	Upper extremities, vitreous opacities	TBPA; Ile 84→Ser
Swedish	30–50	Upper and lower extremities, pupillary abnormalities, renal disease, autonomic and CNS dysfunction	TBPA; Val 30→Met
Iowa (III)	20–40	Upper and lower extremities, pupillary abnormalities, renal disease	Not known
Israel	20's	Upper and lower extremities, autonomic dysfunction, vitreous opacities	TBPA; Phe 33→Ile (?) Thr 49→Gly
Finland	40's	Facial, renal disease, lattice corneal dystrophy	Not known
Appalachian	40–60	Peripheral neuropathy, autonomic, cardiac	TBPA; Thr 60→Ala
Non-neuropathic			
Familial Mediterranean fever	10–30	Inflammatory serositis, nephropathy	AA
Derbyshire	10–30	Deafness, urticaria, fever, renal disease	Not known
Polish	40–60	Splenomegaly, hypertension, renal disease	Not known
Irish-American	40–60	Lung, renal	Not known
Iceland	20–40	Cerebral hemorrhage	Cystatin (var)
Denmark	30–70	Cardiac failure	TBPA (var)

*All appear to be autosomal dominants except for FMF, which is autosomal recessive.
†Roman numerals represent old clinical classification that applied when these were all called familial amyloidotic polyneuropathy.
‡Thyroxine-binding prealbumin or transthyretin (see Table 210–1).

Familial Amyloidosis. A series of genetically transmitted amyloid deposition diseases with characteristic clinical syndromes has been described; they are summarized in Table 210–2. The majority are primarily neuropathic with autosomal dominant inheritance. Other hereditary forms of primary nephropathic, cardiopathic, or cutaneous nature have also been described. The best studied of the renal forms, Familial Mediterranean Fever, is discussed in Ch. 209.

CLINICAL MANIFESTATIONS. Regardless of the type of protein, the clinical manifestations of amyloid deposition in a given organ are similar. The renal disease is primarily manifested by proteinuria, reflecting the glomerular localization of the deposition. Renal tubular defects have also been reported. Azotemia and renal failure usually occur late. The latter may be associated with vascular involvement. There is a 5 to 15 per cent incidence of renal vein thrombosis, particularly in patients with AA disease and the nephrotic syndrome. Amyloid renal disease may be associated with hypertension. The kidneys may be small, normal sized, or enlarged. Contraction of kidneys usually occurs late in the disease.

The most characteristic cardiac presentation is that of a restrictive cardiomyopathy with congestive heart failure. Supraventricular arrhythmias are common, as are varying degrees of A-V block. Echocardiographic studies usually show a thickened ventricular wall without a dilated ventricle and may reveal a characteristic sparkling of the myocardial echoes. Patients with myocardial amyloidosis tend to be sensitive to digitalis glycosides, and these drugs are generally not used. Pulmonary involvement tends to mirror cardiac involvement both in frequency and extent, but rarely it becomes a dominant clinical syndrome with impairment of both the mechanics of respiration and gas exchange. Localized upper and lower airway amyloid infiltration can present major mechanical problems requiring surgical intervention.

Gastrointestinal involvement is most frequently manifested by bleeding, although diarrhea and malabsorption due to either submucosal infiltration or autonomic neuropathy have been reported.

DIAGNOSIS. The diagnosis of amyloidosis is made by the demonstration of the characteristic tissue deposits. Over the years the choice of appropriate tissue for biopsy has become wider. In patients in whom the diagnosis is suspected on clinical grounds, recent data suggested that subcutaneous fat aspiration will yield Congo red-positive material in 90 to 95 per cent of cases of AL disease and two thirds of cases of AA deposition. Rectal biopsy in similar patients yields positive results in 75 to 85 per cent, if adequate mucosal and submucosal tissue is obtained. Gingival tissue will be positive in approximately one half of cases. Bone marrow biopsies have been positive in 40 to 50 per cent of patients with AL disease. These sites can be sampled with little chance of serious complications.

When there is evidence of involvement of a particular organ, diagnostic yields improve considerably. Operative specimens from carpal tunnel releases performed on patients with AL or hereditary neuropathic disease may show 95 per cent positivity. Renal biopsies in individuals with proteinuria have been reported to be positive in more than 90 per cent of patients. Liver biopsies also have a high yield; however, as with closed renal biopsies, significant, even fatal, bleeding has occurred. Hence these procedures are performed only after evaluation of bleeding tendencies and clotting factors. Liver biopsy is generally not carried out if a coagulopathy is present

In recent years it has become possible to distinguish the chemical types of amyloid in biopsy material. In the past a diagnosis of the AL type of disease could be inferred by the presence in the serum and urine of monoclonal Igs or light chains. With the use of potassium permanganate to bleach Congo red staining it is now possible to distinguish AA from AL in about two thirds of cases, AA staining being permanganate sensitive and the AL type resistant. More recently, antisera to the different light chain classes, AA proteins, beta-2-microglobulin, and prealbumin have been utilized either in the immunofluorescent or immunoperoxidase staining of biopsy samples. Since each of the deposited proteins arises from a different precursor, presumably in response to a different stimulus, it is reasonable to assume that these distinctions will eventually have therapeutic implications.

TREATMENT AND PROGNOSIS. AL deposition associated with multiple myeloma has been treated in the course of treating the neoplastic process. While 50 to 60 per cent of patients with myeloma will respond to treatment with alkylating agents and prednisone with extension of survival, the disease has not yet been cured nor has the amyloid deposition been reversed.

A number of patients with AL disease but without overt myeloma have been reported to show prolonged survival after therapy with myeloma-like protocols. However, these are anecdotal results at best and a single attempt at a randomized trial of alkylating agent therapy did not provide convincing evidence of prolonged survival. Nonetheless, it appears that some patients may respond to these regimens. There have also been occasional reports of improvement in AL disease during administration of the organic solvent dimethyl sulfoxide,* usually with concurrent alkylating agent therapy.

The most successful therapy of amyloid has been the prophylactic use of colchicine* in patients with North African Familial Mediterranean Fever (see Ch. 209). As a result of this experience and the observation that colchicine will also prevent experimental casein-induced murine AA deposition, several groups have instituted large-scale trials of colchicine in both AA and AL disease. Apart from the experience with Familial Mediterranean Fever, to date no regimen has been uniformly successful in the treatment of any form of amyloid deposition once it has become established.

Browning MJ, Banks RA, Tribe CR, et al.: Ten years' experience of an amyloid clinic. Q J Med 54:213, 1985. *The experience of a large British referral clinic, worth comparing with the Mayo experience in the last two references below.*

Glenner GG: The β-fibrilloses. N Engl J Med 302:1283; 1333, 1980. *A comprehensive review of the amyloidogenic proteins and the pathology of the disease in the context of newer information concerning the chemical structure of the fibrils.*

Glenner G, Osserman EF, Benditt EP, et al. (eds.): Amyloidosis. New York, Plenum Press, 1986. *The proceedings of the Fourth International Symposium, summarizing current work and thinking of most of the workers in the field, with the first formal interchange between individuals working primarily in Alzheimer's disease and those whose main interests lie in amyloid per se.*

Husby G, Sletten K: Chemical and clinical classification of amyloidosis 1985. Scand J Immunol 23:253, 1986. *An integrated review of the pathogenesis and molecular biology of the amyloidoses.*

Kyle RA: Amyloidosis: Review of 236 cases. Medicine 54:271, 1975. *The Mayo Clinic experience from 1960 to 1972 is described retrospectively. This is a very good review of the clinical features of the major syndromes seen in a large referred population.*

Kyle RA, Greipp PR: Amyloidosis (AL), clinical and laboratory features in 229 cases. Mayo Clin Proc 58:665, 1983. *This more recent reference extends the Mayo Clinic experience with an excellent description of the relevant features of this type of amyloidosis (117 references).*

*This use is not listed in the manufacturer's directive.

211 HEREDITARY SYNDROMES INVOLVING MULTIPLE ORGAN SYSTEMS

Arno G. Motulsky

The emergence of clinical genetics as a specialty has led to the definition of a large number of previously undifferentiated birth defects and syndromes. In some of these diseases the origin is monogenic, and multiple organ involvement is caused by the action of the mutant gene in various tissues. In other cases, a detectable chromosomal error or a known teratogen (such as Dilantin) causes multiorgan birth defects. Most frequently, neither a specific genetic nor environmental cause can be identified. Clinical genetics has grown rapidly, and most physicians are unable to keep abreast of the many newly described syndromes. While most of these conditions become manifest in infancy or childhood, adolescent and adult patients with such conditions often initially come to internists and primary care physicians, who should be aware of the various diagnostic, genetic, and management problems. A vague diagnosis of "multiple birth defects" or "genetic syndrome" usually is not sufficient. Appropriate genetic counseling ideally must be based on a definite diagnosis, optimal care often requires knowledge of the specific diagnosis and natural history of a given syndrome. The reader is referred to various textbooks and compendia for orientation and diagnostic approaches. Because of phenotypic variability in most syndromes, diagnosis may be difficult and new syndromes continue to be described. In this chapter a few selected syndromes are discussed briefly.

Cohen MM Jr: The Child with Multiple Birth Defects. New York, Random Press, 1982. *An excellent analytical introduction of approaches to syndromes and multiple birth defects.*

de Grouchy J, Turlean J: Clinical Atlas of Human Chromosomes. 2nd ed. New York, John Wiley & Sons, 1984. *A good general reference volume for standard syndromes associated with cytogenetic abnormalities.*

Emery AEH, Rimoin DL: Principles and Practice of Medical Genetics. 2 vol. New York, Churchill Livingstone, 1983. *The standard reference text in clinical genetics with full descriptions of disease entities and their genetics.*

Gorlin RJ, Pindborg JJ, Cohen MM Jr (eds.): Syndromes of the Head and Neck. 2nd ed. New York, McGraw-Hill Book Company, 1976. *Helpful for reference and differential diagnosis.*

McKusick V: Mendelian Inheritance in Man. 7th ed. Baltimore, Johns Hopkins University Press, 1986. *Standard reference book listing definite and possible monogenic disease, traits, and syndromes with short descriptions and literature citations.*

Schinzel A: Catalogue of Unbalanced Chromosome Aberrations in Man. New York, W. de Gruyter, 1984. *The definitive detailed reference for unbalanced chromosomal aberrations.*

Smith D: Recognizable Patterns of Human Malformation. 3rd ed. Philadelphia, W. B. Saunders Company, 1982. *The "bible" for description of malformation syndromes. Many photographs and short accounts of many different types of defects. Practically useful.*

WERNER'S SYNDROME

Werner's syndrome is a rare disorder with some clinical features that resemble early aging. Onset of clinical findings is usually in the second or third decade. Affected patients are short because of absence of the adolescent growth spurt and have slender limbs. There is premature graying and then loss of hair. Atrophy and hyperkeratosis of the skin with ulcerations around the feet are often seen. A characteristic squeaky voice and atrophy of muscle, fat, and bone of the extremities are the rule. Soft tissue calcifications usually develop. Atherosclerosis is premature with coronary heart disease and medial calcification of peripheral vessels. Juvenile cataracts and osteoporosis are typical. Hypogonadism occurs in both sexes, and mild diabetes is common. Malignant tumors occur in about 10 per cent of cases, with an unusually high occurrence of meningiomas and sarcomas. Mean age of death is in the early 40's. The phenotype of Werner's syndrome has been considered as a "caricature" of senescence rather than as a model of the normal aging process. The condition is inherited as an autosomal recessive trait. Altered glycosaminoglycan turnover in various tissues with increased excretion of hyaluronic acid in the urine has been frequently noted and suggests a fundamental abnormality affecting connective tissue. However, hyaluronic aciduria is not specific for Werner's syndrome. Fibroblasts from skin biopsies of patients with Werner's syndrome are difficult to culture. They grow more slowly, assume a senescent morphology more rapidly, and demonstrate a markedly reduced lifespan in vitro. DNA repair is normal. Karyotype preparations show a normal number of chromosomes, but variable stable chromosomal rearrangements such as translocations involving several chromosomes (variegated translocation mosaicism) are seen in over 90 per cent of cells (fibroblasts or lymphocytes). Werner's syndrome therefore can be classified among the group of chromosomal instability syndromes. No single enzymatic defect has been discovered yet to explain the multiple clinical, biochemical, and cytogenetic manifestations. Werner's syndrome is sometimes termed adult progeria, but it is entirely unrelated to the pediatric syndrome of progeria (Hutchinson-Gilford), in which death occurs in early adolescence from cardiac or cerebrovascular disease.

Epstein CJ, Martin GM, Schultz AL, et al.: The Werner's syndrome. Medicine 45:177, 1966. *A detailed summary of clinical and laboratory characteristics of 125 cases of Werner's syndrome.*

Salk W: Werner's syndrome. A review of recent research with an analysis of connective tissue metabolism, growth control of cultured cells, and chromosomal aberrations. Hum Genet 62:1, 1982. *A review of the current status of Werner's disease.*

SYNDROMES ASSOCIATED WITH HYPOGONADISM AND VARIOUS CONGENITAL ANOMALIES

LAURENCE-MOON-BARDET-BIEDL SYNDROME AND RELATED DISORDERS. The Laurence-Moon-Bardet-Biedl syndrome clinically exhibits the pentad of retinal dystrophy (usually pigmentary retinopathy), truncal obesity, mild to severe mental retardation, polydactyly, and hypogonadism. When not all of the five cardinal findings are seen, the diagnosis may be difficult. Electroretinography is useful for early diagnosis of the retinal dystrophy. Loss of central vision is gradual, and total blindness usually occurs after the age of 30 years. Although primary and secondary hypogonadism have been reported, hypogonadism is less frequently found in females. Interstitial nephritis may lead to renal failure.

Some investigators (the "splitters") distinguish between the Bardet-Biedl and the Laurence-Moon syndrome by the presence of spastic paraplegia and the absence of polydactyly and obesity in the latter condition. However, others (the "lumpers") believe that these distinctions relate to variable expression of a single disorder.

Alstrom's syndrome appears distinct and is also associated with retinal dystrophy and obesity. Affected patients are usually blind in early childhood and develop moderately severe deafness before age 10. Diabetes mellitus and slowly progressive chronic nephropathy in young adults are seen. Mental retardation and digital anomalies are not encountered.

Carpenter's syndrome (acrocephalopolysyndactyly) is a syndrome characterized by acrocephaly, syndactyly, and a characteristic facial appearance associated with polydactyly of the feet, obesity, mental retardation, and hypogonadism. The various characteristic skeletal findings should cause few diagnostic difficulties.

All these conditions (the syndromes of Laurence-Moon-Bardet-Biedl, Alstrom, Carpenter) are inherited as autosomal recessive traits.

PRADER-WILLI SYNDROME. In this not uncommon condition, infants are born with severe hypotonia and feeding difficulties; boys exhibit a small penis and cryptorchidism, and hypoplastic labia are seen in girls. Thin, turned-down upper lips and almond-shaped and up-slanting palpebral fissures are often seen. Skin and hair color tends to be fair. The feeding difficulties of infancy give way to compulsive hyperphagia with development of severe central obesity in later childhood. The limbs are relatively thin, and the hands and feet are characteristically small (acromicria). Young adults may present with pickwickian syndrome manifesting as cardiopulmonary compromise and somnolence. Severe obesity is the major cause of morbidity and mortality in this disorder. Affected patients are short, and there is hypogonadotrophic hypogonadism with sterility. Scoliosis and strabismus are common. Mild to severe mental retardation with behavioral and personality problems are the rule. Mild diabetes mellitus is often seen. Retinal abnormalities and polydactyly do not occur. In many cases a chromosome abnormality affecting band q11-12 of the long arm of chromosome 15 has been detected by high-resolution methods. The defect usually is a small deletion in the paternal chromosome 15, but more complex rearrangements affecting the relevant chromosomal segment have also been seen. Although the syndrome usually occurs as a sporadic event, rare familial cases have been reported. Parental chromosomes are usually normal. It is likely that an as yet undetectable chromosomal defect exists in those cases in which no visible chromosomal abnormality has been found. The relationship of the unique and specific chromosomal deletion to the pathogenesis of the syndrome remains unknown.

NOONAN'S PHENOTYPE. This phenotype is often diagnosed, but its boundaries are not sharply defined because of marked clinical variability. Its frequency has been estimated as 1 in 1000 to 1 in 2500. There are no chromosomal abnormalities, in contrast to the Turner syndrome (XO) that it somewhat resembles ("male" Turner syndrome). However, females can be affected as well. Previously suspected etiologic heterogeneity is contested by recent studies that suggest marked changes in the Noonan phenotype with age. Affected adolescents and adults are often but not always short and have a triangular micrognathic facial appearance with frequent hypertelorism, occasional ptosis, and posteriorly angulated low-set ears with a thick helix. A short webbed neck is common. The simultaneous presence of superior pectus carinatum and inferior pectus excavatum is helpful diagnostically. Pulmonary valve stenosis is seen frequently and can be accompanied by other types of congenital heart defects. Mild mental retardation is occasionally found. Lymphatic dysplasia causing lymphedema occurs sometimes.

Autosomal dominant inheritance can be frequently documented, but many cases are sporadic and presumably caused by new mutations. Careful examination of first-degree relatives often shows minor signs of the condition.

Allanson JE, Hall JG, Hughes HE, et al.: Noonan syndrome: The changing phenotype. Am J Med Genet 21:507, 1985. *Describes changes in Noonan phenotype from infancy to adulthood.*

Bray GA, Dahms WT, Swerdloff RS, et al.: The Prader-Willi syndrome. A study of 40 patients and a review of the literature. Medicine 62:59, 1983. *A comprehensive review of the syndrome.*

Cassidy SB: Prader-Willi syndrome. Curr Probl Pediatr 44:1, 1984. *An extensive review of the clinical, cytogenetic, behavioral, and management aspects, with many references.*

Goldstein J, Fialkow PJ: The Alstrom syndrome. Medicine 52:53, 1973. *Classic summary of the clinical, genetic, and pathophysiologic aspects of the syndrome.*

Klein D, Amman F: The syndrome of Laurence-Moon-Bardet-Biedl and allied disorders. J Neurol Sci 9:470, 1969. *Clinical description and differential diagnosis.*

Ledbetter DH, Mascarello JT, Riccardi VM, et al.: Chromosome 15 abnormalities and the Prader-Willi syndrome: A follow-up report of 40 cases. Am J Hum Genet 34:278, 1982. *Current status of the chromosomal defect affecting chromosome 15 q11-12.*

Mendez HMM, Opitz JM: Noonan syndrome: A review. Am J Med Genet 21:493, 1985. *Recent review of various manifestations with many references.*

INDEX

Page numbers in *Italics* refer to figures. Page numbers followed by a "t" refer to tables. For general terms such as "acute," "chronic," "idiopathic," look under the remaining portion of the term.